THE PHARMACOLOGICAL BASIS OF THERAPEUTICS

The Pharmacologica

EDITORS

Louis S. Goodman
M.A., M.D., D.Sc.(Hon.)

Distinguished Professor of Pharmacology,
University of Utah College of Medicine, Salt Lake City, Utah

Alfred Gilman
Ph.D.

Lecturer in Pharmacology,
Yale University School of Medicine, New Haven, Connecticut;
Professor of Pharmacology,
Albert Einstein College of Medicine of Yeshiva University, Bronx, New York

ASSOCIATE EDITORS

Alfred G. Gilman
M.D., Ph.D.

Associate Professor of Pharmacology,
University of Virginia School of Medicine, Charlottesville, Virginia

George B. Koelle
Ph.D., M.D., D.Sc.(Hon.), D.Med.(Hon.)

Elmer Holmes Bobst Professor and Chairman, Department of Pharmacology,
University of Pennsylvania School of Medicine, Philadelphia, Pennsylvania

Basis of Therapeutics

FIFTH EDITION

MACMILLAN PUBLISHING CO., INC.
New York

COLLIER MACMILLAN CANADA, LTD.
Toronto

BAILLIÈRE TINDALL
London

MACMILLAN PUBLISHING CO., INC.
866 Third Avenue · New York, N.Y. 10022

COLLIER MACMILLAN CANADA, LTD.

BAILLIÈRE TINDALL · London

Library of Congress catalog card number 75-15903
ISBN 0-02-344781-8
Baillière Tindall SBN 0 7020 0584 3

Printing: 3 4 5 6 7 8   Year: 6 7 8 9 0 1

The use of portions of the texts of the *United States Pharmacopeia,* Nineteenth Revision, official July 1, 1975, and of its first supplement is by permission received from the Board of Trustees of the United States Pharmacopeial Convention, Inc. The said Convention is not responsible for any inaccuracy of quotation, or for any false or misleading implication that may arise by reason of the separation of excerpts from the original context.

The use of portions of the texts of the *National Formulary,* Fourteenth Edition, official July 1, 1975, and of its first supplement is by permission received from the Board of Trustees of the United States Pharmacopeial Convention, Inc. Neither the U.S.P. Convention, Inc., nor the American Pharmaceutical Association, original publisher of the N.F., is responsible for any inaccuracy of quotation, or for any false or misleading implication that may arise by reason of the separation of excerpts from the original context.

In this textbook, reference to proprietary names of drugs is ordinarily made only in chapter sections dealing with preparations. Such names are given in SMALL-CAP TYPE, usually immediately following the official or nonproprietary titles. Proprietary names of drugs also appear in the Index.

PREFACE TO THE FIFTH EDITION

THE 35-year period since publication of the first edition of this textbook has witnessed an enormous change in the content, stature, and function of pharmacology; its role in the biomedical sciences; and its impact on the clinical sciences and rational therapeutics. Only the Preface to the First Edition is reprinted herein, because it clearly states the three primary objectives that have guided the writing of all subsequent editions.

The first edition was written when basic pharmacology had not yet attained its present importance and was not fully accepted by clinical colleagues as a meaningful or relevant discipline. The appearance of that book did much to change the picture. An eminent pharmacologist, commenting on the first edition many years after its appearance, stated that it provided a renaissance or perhaps more properly the *naissance* of the teaching and practice of pharmacology. The second edition, published in the mid-1950s, reflected the immense impact of the post–World War II burgeoning of biomedical research. The third and fourth editions were written as multiauthored works. Although the flood of new drugs had begun to ebb, fundamental advances highly pertinent to rational therapeutics were being made by the many flourishing subdisciplines of pharmacology. An authoritative textbook in such a diverse and active discipline could no longer be written by the two authors; however, as editors, they could devote their efforts to fulfill their original objectives.

It is possible in a preface to mention only a few examples of the major changes that appear in the present edition. Both the basic and applied aspects of pharmacokinetics have made impressive advances due to elegant analytical technics that can also be utilized clinically. The basic principles of pharmacokinetics are discussed separately as they relate to all drugs, and the practicing physician will find described valuable concepts now taught to the current generation of biomedical students. Applied principles are presented for individual drugs when altered biochemical disposition or impaired excretion requires changes in dosage regimens. In several cases the appropriate data are summarized in useful tabular form. Parallel advances have been made in the understanding of drug interactions. Again, the basic mechanisms of clinically relevant interactions are analyzed, and the applicable information is presented for individual drugs.

Studies on receptors for neurotransmitters, autacoids, hormones, and drugs have led to a better understanding of the mechanism of drug action and in certain instances to fruitful hypotheses or to more fundamental knowledge of the pathological physiology of disease states. An outstanding example is the inhibition of dopamine activation of adenylate cyclase by antipsychotic drugs in both the caudate nucleus and the limbic system. Indeed, discussion of the role of cyclic AMP as a "second messenger" and the effects of drugs thereon appears throughout the text. Prostaglandins are discussed both as primary drugs and as targets for the actions of drugs. In a similar manner the hypothalamic regulatory hormones are presented as primary therapeutic and diagnostic agents and in terms of mechanisms by which drugs can produce endocrinopathies. Needless to say, newly approved drugs are fully discussed as well as those that are still in the developmental stage but show considerable promise as future therapeutic agents. An outstanding example is the group of drugs that block the effects of histamine (and pentagastrin) on gastric secretion, the so-called H_2-receptor blocking drugs.

In order to prevent expansion of the present edition, less dynamic or outmoded areas have been condensed or eliminated, to allow adequate consideration of all important pharmacological and therapeutic advances. It is our estimate that well over one half of the text represents newly written or vigorously revised material.

Most of our contributors to the fourth edition were able and anxious to participate in the current undertaking, but it is with deep sadness that we record the untimely deaths of our friends and colleagues, Drs. Robert D. Dripps, Don W. Esplin, James E. P. Toman, and Louis G. Welt.

For the fifth edition, we have sought the assistance of two associate editors who are also contributors—Alfred G. Gilman, M.D., Ph.D., and George B. Koelle, Ph.D., M.D., D.Sc.(Hon.), D.Med.(Hon.). The former, a representative of the younger generation of pharmacologists, is broadly trained in general pharmacology and clinical science with major interests in biochemical pharmacology, molecular pharmacology, and cell biology; the latter, a contributor since the third edition, is a teacher of broad experience with a background of research in neuropharmacology and many important editorial responsibilities.

In addition to paying tribute to our collaborators, we gratefully acknowledge the advice and help received from scores of individuals, too numerous to mention by name. However, special thanks are due to George E. Downs, Pharm.D., Assistant Professor of Clinical Pharmacy, Philadelphia College of Pharmacy and Science, who gave us expert editorial help with regard to those sections of the text related to pharmaceutical preparations and dosages. We also wish to acknowledge the invaluable editorial assistance of Lou Ann Thomas, Carol Bennett, and Eloise Gabel Smyrl.

The editors and authors owe a great debt to Miss Joan Carolyn Zulch, Medical Editor, Macmillan Publishing Co., Inc. This being her fourth edition of this textbook, she qualifies as an expert, self-taught pharmacologist—knowledge that superbly complements her editorial excellence and the patience and sense of humor vital to her job. Just as Miss Zulch survived her work with us, so did the editors survive each other, and we again wish to pay tribute to our mutual friendship, which has grown ever firmer in the task of preparing this fifth edition.

LOUIS S. GOODMAN
ALFRED GILMAN

June, 1975

PREFACE TO THE FIRST EDITION

THREE objectives have guided the writing of this book—the correlation of pharmacology with related medical sciences, the reinterpretation of the actions and uses of drugs from the viewpoint of important advances in medicine, and the placing of emphasis on the applications of pharmacodynamics to therapeutics.

Although pharmacology is a basic medical science in its own right, it borrows freely from and contributes generously to the subject matter and technics of many medical disciplines, clinical as well as preclinical. Therefore, the correlation of strictly pharmacological information with medicine as a whole is essential for a proper presentation of pharmacology to students and physicians. Furthermore, the reinterpretation of the actions and uses of well-established therapeutic agents in the light of recent advances in the medical sciences is as important a function of a modern textbook of pharmacology as is the description of new drugs. In many instances these new interpretations necessitate radical departures from accepted but outworn concepts of the actions of drugs. Lastly, the emphasis throughout the book, as indicated in its title, has been clinical. This is mandatory because medical students must be taught pharmacology from the standpoint of the actions and uses of drugs in the prevention and treatment of disease. To the student, pharmacological data per se are valueless unless he is able to apply his information in the practice of medicine. This book has also been written for the practicing physician, to whom it offers an opportunity to keep abreast of recent advances in therapeutics and to acquire the basic principles necessary for the rational use of drugs in his daily practice.

The criteria for the selection of bibliographic references require comment. It is obviously unwise, if not impossible, to document every fact included in the text. Preference has therefore been given to articles of a review nature, to the literature on new drugs, and to original contributions in controversial fields. In most instances, only the more recent investigations have been cited. In order to encourage free use of the bibliography, references are chiefly to the available literature in the English language.

The authors are greatly indebted to their many colleagues at the Yale University School of Medicine for their generous help and criticism. In particular they are deeply grateful to Professor Henry Gray Barbour, whose constant encouragement and advice have been invaluable.

LOUIS S. GOODMAN
ALFRED GILMAN

New Haven, Connecticut
November 20, 1940

CONTRIBUTORS

Abildskov, J. A., M.D.   Professor of Medicine, University of Utah College of Medicine, Salt Lake City, Utah

Brazeau, Paul, Ph.D.   Professor of Pharmacology, Albert Einstein College of Medicine of Yeshiva University, Bronx, New York

Burns, J. J., Ph.D.   Vice President for Research, Hoffmann-La Roche, Inc., Nutley, New Jersey; Adjunct Professor of Pharmacology, Cornell University Medical College, New York, New York

Byck, Robert, M.D.   Associate Professor of Pharmacology and Psychiatry, Yale University School of Medicine; Associate Physician, Yale-New Haven Hospital, New Haven, Connecticut

Calabresi, Paul, M.D.   Professor and Chairman, Department of Medicine, Brown University; Physician-in-Chief, Roger Williams General Hospital, Providence, Rhode Island

Cohen, Peter J., M.D.   Professor and Chairman, Department of Anesthesiology, University of Colorado School of Medicine, Denver, Colorado

Cohn, Victor H., Ph.D.   Professor of Pharmacology, George Washington University School of Medicine, Washington, D.C.

Collier, Brian, Ph.D.   Associate Professor of Pharmacology and Therapeutics, McGill University Faculty of Medicine, Montreal, Quebec, Canada

Douglas, William W., Ch.B., M.D.   Professor of Pharmacology, Yale University School of Medicine, New Haven, Connecticut

Eder, Howard A., M.D.   Professor of Medicine, Albert Einstein College of Medicine of Yeshiva University; Attending Physician, Bronx Municipal Hospital Center, Bronx, New York

Farah, Alfred E., M.D.   Chairman, Sterling-Winthrop Research Institute, Rensselaer, New York

Fingl, Edward, Ph.D.   Professor of Pharmacology, University of Utah College of Medicine, Salt Lake City, Utah

Franz, Donald N., Ph.D.   Associate Professor of Pharmacology, University of Utah College of Medicine, Salt Lake City, Utah

Gilman, Alfred G., M.D., Ph.D.   Associate Professor of Pharmacology, University of Virginia School of Medicine, Charlottesville, Virginia

Greengard, Paul, Ph.D.   Professor of Pharmacology, Yale University School of Medicine, New Haven, Connecticut

Harvey, Stewart C., Ph.D.   Professor of Pharmacology, University of Utah College of Medicine, Salt Lake City, Utah

Haynes, Robert C., Jr., M.D., Ph.D.   Professor of Pharmacology, University of Virginia School of Medicine, Charlottesville, Virginia

Herbert, Victor, M.D., J.D.   Clinical Professor of Pathology and Clinical Professor of Medicine, Columbia University College of Physicians and Surgeons, New York, New York; Medical Investigator, U.S. Veterans Administration

Innes, Ian R., M.B., Ch.B., M.D.   Professor and Chairman, Department of Pharmacology and Therapeutics, University of Manitoba Faculty of Medicine, Winnipeg, Manitoba, Canada

Jaffe, Jerome H., M.D.   Professor of Psychiatry, Columbia University College of Physicians and Surgeons; Chief, Psychiatric Research, New York State Psychiatric Institute, New York, New York

Koelle, George B., Ph.D., M.D., D.Sc.(Hon.), D.Med.(Hon.).   Elmer Holmes Bobst Professor and Chairman, Department of Pharmacology, University of Pennsylvania School of Medicine, Philadelphia, Pennsylvania

Larner, Joseph, M.D., Ph.D.   Professor and Chairman, Department of Pharmacology, University of Virginia School of Medicine, Charlottesville, Virginia

Levine, Walter G., Ph.D. Associate Professor of Pharmacology, Albert Einstein College of Medicine of Yeshiva University, Bronx, New York

Mandel, H. George, Ph.D. Professor and Chairman, Department of Pharmacology, George Washington University School of Medicine, Washington, D.C.

Martin, William R., M.D. Chief, Addiction Research Center, National Institute of Mental Health, Lexington, Kentucky

Moe, Gordon K., Ph.D., M.D. Director of Research, Masonic Medical Research Laboratory, Utica, New York; Research Professor of Physiology, State University of New York, Upstate Medical Center, School of Medicine, Syracuse, New York

Mudge, Gilbert H., M.D. Professor of Medicine, Dartmouth Medical School, Hanover, New Hampshire

Murad, Ferid, M.D., Ph.D. Professor of Pharmacology, Professor of Medicine, and Director, Division of Clinical Pharmacology, University of Virginia School of Medicine, Charlottesville, Virginia

Nickerson, Mark, Ph.D., M.D. Professor of Pharmacology and Therapeutics, McGill University Faculty of Medicine, Montreal, Quebec, Canada

Parks, Robert E., Jr., M.D., Ph.D. Professor of Medical Science and Chairman, Section of Biochemical Pharmacology, Division of Biological and Medical Sciences, Brown University, Providence, Rhode Island

Peach, Michael J., Ph.D. Associate Professor of Pharmacology, University of Virginia School of Medicine, Charlottesville, Virginia

Price, Henry L., M.D. Professor and Chairman, Department of Anesthesiology, Hahnemann Medical College and Hospital, Philadelphia, Pennsylvania

Ritchie, J. Murdoch, Ph.D., D.Sc. Professor of Pharmacology, Yale University School of Medicine, New Haven, Connecticut

Rollo, Ian M., Ph.D. Professor of Pharmacology and Therapeutics, University of Manitoba Faculty of Medicine, Winnipeg, Manitoba, Canada

Ruedy, John, M.D. Professor of Pharmacology and Therapeutics, McGill University Faculty of Medicine, Montreal, Quebec, Canada

Smith, Theodore C., M.D. Professor of Anesthesia, University of Pennsylvania School of Medicine, Philadelphia, Pennsylvania

Straw, James A., Ph.D. Professor of Pharmacology, George Washington University School of Medicine, Washington, D.C.

Swinyard, Ewart A., M.S., Ph.D. Professor of Pharmacology and Dean, College of Pharmacy; Professor of Pharmacology, University of Utah College of Medicine, Salt Lake City, Utah

Volle, Robert L., Ph.D. Professor and Head, Department of Pharmacology, University of Connecticut School of Medicine, Farmington, Connecticut

Weinstein, Louis, Ph.D., M.D. Visiting Professor of Medicine, Harvard Medical School; Physician, Peter Bent Brigham Hospital, Boston, Massachusetts

Welt, Louis G., M.D. Late Professor and Chairman, Department of Medicine, Yale University School of Medicine, New Haven, Connecticut

Wollman, Harry, M.D. Robert Dunning Dripps Professor and Chairman, Department of Anesthesia, and Professor of Pharmacology, University of Pennsylvania School of Medicine, Philadelphia, Pennsylvania

Woodbury, Dixon M., Ph.D. Professor and Chairman, Department of Pharmacology, University of Utah College of Medicine, Salt Lake City, Utah

CONTENTS

SECTION

III

Local Anesthetics

SECTION

IV

Drugs Acting at Synaptic and Neuroeffector Junctional Sites

SECTION
XIV
Chemotherapy of Microbial Diseases

SECTION
XV
Chemotherapy of Neoplastic Diseases

SECTION
XVI
Drugs Acting on the Blood and the Blood-Forming Organs

THE PHARMACOLOGICAL
BASIS OF
THERAPEUTICS

SECTION

I

Introduction

CHAPTER

1 GENERAL PRINCIPLES

Edward Fingl and Dixon M. Woodbury

The basic pharmacological concepts summarized in this chapter apply to the characterization, evaluation, and comparison of all drugs. A clear understanding of these principles is essential for the subsequent study of the individual drugs. Many of these topics have been more extensively discussed in the textbooks by Melmon and Morrelli (1972), Levine (1973), and Goldstein and coworkers (1974).

In its entirety, *pharmacology* embraces the knowledge of the history, source, physical and chemical properties, compounding, biochemical and physiological effects, mechanisms of action, absorption, distribution, biotransformation and excretion, and therapeutic and other uses of drugs. Since a *drug* is broadly defined as any chemical agent that affects living processes, the subject of pharmacology is obviously quite extensive.

For the physician and the medical student, however, the scope of pharmacology is less expansive than indicated by the above definitions. The clinician is interested primarily in drugs that are useful in the prevention, diagnosis, and treatment of human disease, or in the prevention of pregnancy. His study of the pharmacology of these drugs can be reasonably limited to those aspects that provide the basis for their rational clinical use. Secondarily, the physician is also concerned with chemical agents that are not used in therapy but are commonly responsible for household and industrial poisoning as well as environmental pollution. His study of these substances is justifiably restricted to the general principles of prevention, recognition, and treatment of such toxicity or pollution. Finally, all physicians share in the responsibility to help resolve the continuing sociological problem of the abuse of drugs.

A brief consideration of its major subject areas will further clarify how the study of pharmacology is best approached from the standpoint of the specific requirements and interests of the medical student and practitioner. At one time, it was essential for the physician to have a broad botanical knowledge, since he had to select the proper plants from which to prepare his own crude medicinal preparations. However, fewer drugs are now obtained from natural sources, and, more importantly, most of these are highly purified or standardized and differ little from synthetic chemicals. Hence, the interests of the modern clinician in *pharmacognosy* are correspondingly limited. Nevertheless, scientific curiosity should stimulate the physician to learn something of the *sources* of drugs, and this knowledge often proves practically useful as well as interesting. He will find the *history* of drugs of similar value.

The preparing, compounding, and dispensing of medicines at one time lay within the province of the physician, but this work is now delegated almost completely to the pharmacist. However, to write intelligent prescription orders, the physician must have some knowledge of the *physical and chemical properties* of drugs and their available *dosage forms,* and he must have a basic familiarity with the *practice of pharmacy.* When the physician shirks his responsibility in this regard, he invariably fails to translate his knowledge of pharmacology and medicine into prescription orders and medication best suited for the individual patient. The few details essential to the writing of correct prescription orders are summarized in the Appendix.

Pharmacokinetics deals with the *absorption, distribution, biotransformation,* and *excretion* of drugs. These factors, coupled with dosage, determine the concentration of a drug at its sites of action and,

1

hence, the intensity of its effects as a function of time. Many basic principles of biochemistry and enzymology and the physical and chemical principles that govern the active and passive transfer and the distribution of substances across biological membranes are readily applied to the understanding of this important aspect of pharmacology.

The study of the biochemical and physiological *effects* of drugs and their *mechanisms of action* is termed *pharmacodynamics*. It is an experimental medical science that dates back only to the latter half of the nineteenth century. As a border science, pharmacodynamics borrows freely from both the subject matter and the experimental technics of physiology, biochemistry, microbiology, immunology, genetics, and pathology. It is unique mainly in that attention is focused on the characteristics of drugs. As the name implies, the subject is a dynamic one. The student who attempts merely to memorize the pharmacodynamic properties of drugs is foregoing one of the best opportunities for correlating the entire field of preclinical medicine. For example, the actions and effects of the saluretic agents can be fully understood only in terms of the basic principles of renal physiology and of the pathogenesis of edema. Conversely, no greater insight into normal and abnormal renal physiology can be gained than by the study of the pharmacodynamics of the saluretic agents.

Another ramification of pharmacodynamics is the correlation of the actions and effects of drugs with their chemical structures. Such *structure-activity relationships* are an integral link in the analysis of drug action, and exploitation of these relationships among established therapeutic agents has often led to the development of better drugs. However, the correlation of biological activity with chemical structure is usually of interest to the physician only when it provides the basis for summarizing other pharmacological information.

The physician is understandably interested mainly in the effects of drugs in man. This emphasis on *clinical pharmacology* is justified, since the effects of drugs are often characterized by significant interspecies variation, and since they may be further modified by disease. In addition, some drug effects, such as those on mood and behavior, can be adequately studied only in man. However, the pharmacological evaluation of drugs in man may be limited for technical, legal, and ethical reasons, and the choice of drugs must be based in part on their pharmacological evaluation in animals. Consequently, some knowledge of *animal pharmacology* and *comparative pharmacology* is helpful in deciding the extent to which claims for a drug based upon studies in animals can be reasonably extrapolated to man.

Pharmacotherapeutics deals with the use of drugs in the prevention and treatment of disease. Many drugs stimulate or depress biochemical or physiological function in man in a sufficiently reproducible manner to provide relief of symptoms or, ideally, to alter favorably the course of disease. Conversely, chemotherapeutic agents are useful in therapy because they have only minimal effects on man but can destroy or eliminate parasites. Whether a drug is useful for therapy is crucially dependent upon its ability to produce its desired effects with only tolerable undesired effects. Thus, from the standpoint of the physician interested in the therapeutic uses of a drug, the *selectivity* of its effects is one of its most important characteristics. Drug therapy is rationally based upon the correlation of the actions and effects of drugs with the physiological, biochemical, microbiological, immunological, and behavioral aspects of disease. Pharmacodynamics provides one of the best opportunities for this correlation during the study of both the preclinical and the clinical medical sciences.

Toxicology is that aspect of pharmacology that deals with the adverse effects of drugs. It is concerned not only with drugs used in therapy but also with the many other chemicals that may be responsible for household, environmental, or industrial intoxication. The adverse effects of the pharmacological agents employed in therapy are properly considered an integral part of their total pharmacology. The toxic effects of other chemicals is such an extensive subject that the physician must usually confine his attention to the general principles applicable to the prevention, recognition, and treatment of drug poisonings of any cause.

I. Pharmacokinetics

To produce its characteristic effects, a drug must be present in appropriate concentrations at its sites of action. Although obviously a function of the amount of drug administered, the concentrations attained also depend upon the extent and rate of its absorption, distribution, binding or localization in tissues, biotransformation, and excretion. These factors are depicted in Figure 1–1.

PHYSICOCHEMICAL FACTORS IN TRANSFER OF DRUGS ACROSS MEMBRANES

The absorption, distribution, biotransformation, and excretion of a drug all involve its passage across cell membranes. It is essential, therefore, to consider the mechanisms by which drugs cross membranes and the physicochemical properties of molecules and membranes that influence this transfer. Important characteristics of a drug are its molecular size and shape, degree of ionization, and relative lipid solubility of its ionized and nonionized forms.

When a drug permeates a cell, it must obviously traverse the cellular plasma membrane. Other barriers to drug movement may be a single layer of cells (intestinal epithe-

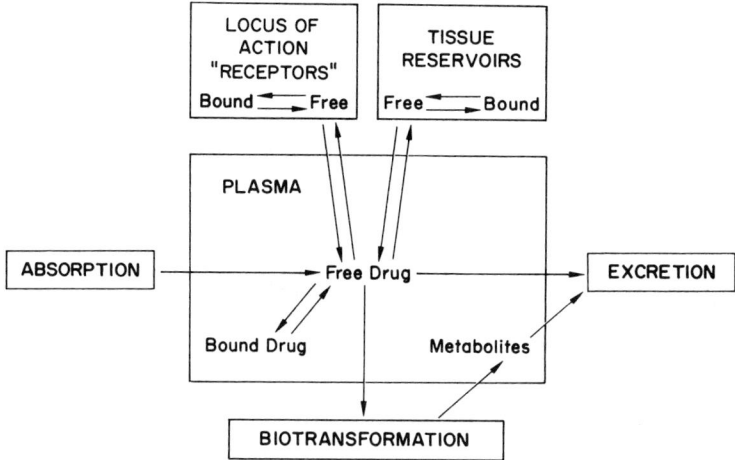

Figure 1-1. *Schematic representation of the interrelationship of the absorption, distribution, binding, biotransformation, and excretion of a drug and its concentration at its locus of action.*

Possible distribution and binding of metabolites are not depicted.

lium) or several layers of cells (skin). Despite these structural differences, the diffusion and transport of drugs across these various boundaries have many common characteristics, since drugs in general pass through cells rather than between them. The cellular plasma membrane thus represents the common barrier.

Cell Membranes. The classical observations by Overton and by Collander and Bärlund led to the theory that the cell (plasma) membrane was a thin layer of lipoid material interspersed with minute water-filled channels. Subsequent studies suggested that the plasma membrane consisted of a bimolecular lipoid sheet bound on both sides by protein, but this hypothesis has been broadened to a more dynamic model in which lipids and intrinsic and extrinsic proteins are viewed as being organized in a mosaic structure (Symposium, 1972). The intrinsic (integral) proteins are embedded or intercalated, in ordered or disordered arrangement, into a discontinuous lipid bilayer that forms the matrix of the mosaic. The intrinsic proteins are globular and bimodal, with their ionic and highly polar groups located largely on the membrane surfaces in contact with the extracellular and intracellular aqueous media, and with their nonpolar residues sequestered from contact with water in the membrane interior. Extrinsic proteins are bound to the exposed surfaces of the intrinsic proteins by electrostatic or hydrophobic interactions, but they are not involved in lipid-protein interactions that are critical to the membrane structure and its functions. Channels appear to be present in the central axes of the globular intrinsic proteins. Cell membranes are approximately 80 Å thick.

Passive Processes. Drugs cross membranes by either passive processes or by mechanisms involving the participation of components of the membrane. In the former, the drug molecules penetrate either by passage through aqueous channels in the membrane or by dissolving in the membrane. Both nonpolar lipid-soluble compounds and polar water-soluble substances that retain sufficient lipid solubility can cross the lipid portion of the membrane by *passive diffusion.* Such transfer is directly proportional to the concentration gradient across the membrane and the lipid:water partition coefficient of the drug. The greater the partition coefficient, the higher is the concentration of drug in the membrane and the faster is its diffusion. However, after a steady state is attained, the concentration of the free drug is the same on both sides of the membrane, if the drug is a nonelectrolyte. For ionic compounds, the steady-state concentrations will be dependent on the transmembrane potential and may be influenced by the state of ionization of the molecule on each side of the membrane. Passage through channels is called *filtration,* since it involves bulk flow of water as a result of a hydrostatic or osmotic difference across the membrane. The bulk flow of water carries with it any water-soluble molecule that is small enough to pass through the channels. Filtration is a common mechanism for transfer of many small, water-soluble, polar and nonpolar substances. The size of the membrane channels differs in the various body membranes. Capillary endothelial cells have large channels (40 Å), and molecules as large as albumin may pass to a limited extent from the plasma to the extracellular fluid. In contrast, the channels in the red-cell membrane, the intestinal epithelium, and most cell membranes are about 4 Å in diameter and permit passage only of water, urea, and other small, water-soluble molecules. Such substances generally do not pass through channels in cell membranes if their molecular weights are greater than 100 to 200.

Most inorganic ions are sufficiently small to penetrate the channels in membranes, but their concentration gradient across the cell membrane is generally determined by the transmembrane potential (*e.g.,* chloride ion) or by active transport (*e.g.,* sodium and potassium ions).

Weak Electrolytes and Influence of pH. Most drugs are weak acids or bases and are present in solution as both the nonionized and ionized species. The nonionized portion is usually lipid soluble and can readily diffuse across the cell membrane. In contrast, the ionized fraction is often unable to penetrate the lipoid membrane because of its low lipid solubility, or to traverse the membrane channels because of its size. If the ionized portion of a weak electrolyte can pass through the channels, or through the membrane, it will distribute according to the transmembrane potential in the same manner as an inorganic ion. For example, chloride, bicarbonate, bromide, and the ionized form of drugs, such as 5,5-dimethyl-2,4-oxazolidinedione, are distributed unequally across the red-blood-cell membrane.

The distribution of a weak electrolyte is usually determined by its pK_a and the pH gradient across the membrane. To illustrate the effect of pH on distribution of drugs, the partitioning of a weak acid ($pK_a = 4.4$) between plasma (pH = 7.4) and gastric juice (pH = 1.4) is depicted in Figure 1–2. It is assumed that the gastric mucosal membrane behaves as a simple lipoid barrier that is permeable only to the lipid-soluble, nonionized form of the acid. The ratio of nonionized to ionized drug at each pH can be calculated from the Henderson-Hasselbalch equation. Thus, in plasma, the ratio of nonionized to ionized drug is 1:1000; in gastric juice, the ratio is 1:0.001. The total concentration ratio between the plasma and the gastric juice would therefore be 1000:1 if such a system came to a steady state. For a weak base with a pK_a of 4.4 (BH$^+$ $\rightleftharpoons$ B + H$^+$), the ratio would be reversed. These considerations have obvious implications for the absorption and excretion of drugs, as will be discussed more specifically below. The establishment of concentration gradients of weak electrolytes across membranes with a pH gradient is a purely physical process and does not require an active transport system. All that is necessary is a membrane preferentially permeable to one form of the weak electrolyte and a pH gradient across the membrane. The establishment of the pH gradient is, however, an active process.

Carrier-Mediated Membrane Transport. *Active Transport.* Passive processes do not explain the passage of all drugs across cell membranes. Active transport is responsible for the rapid transfer of many organic acids and bases across the renal tubule, choroid plexus, and hepatic cells. *Active transport* differs from a passive process in that it exhibits selectivity, saturability, and a requirement for energy. The transported substance is transferred against an electrochemical gradient (uphill transport). Active transport is thought to be mediated by

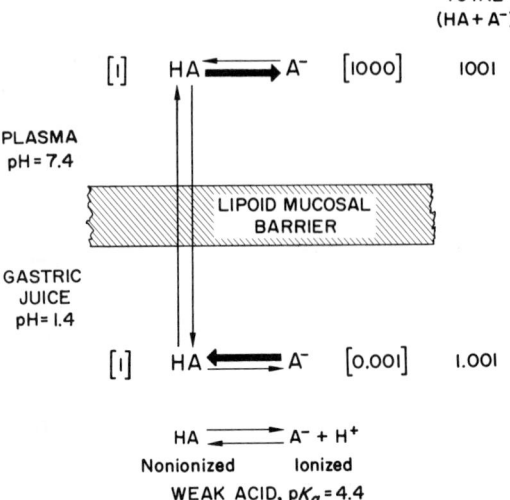

Figure 1–2. *Influence of pH on the distribution of a weak acid between plasma and gastric juice, separated by a lipoid barrier.*

Only the nonionized moiety can readily penetrate the membrane; hence, at equilibrium its concentration is the same in both compartments. The degree of dissociation of the acid on each side depends on the pH of the plasma and gastric juice. The total concentration difference between the two sides is a direct function of the pH gradient across the membrane.

The values in brackets represent relative concentrations of the ionized and nonionized forms on each side of the membrane. The thick horizontal arrows point in the direction of the predominant form of the weak acid at the indicated pH.

carriers—membrane components that form a complex with the substance to be transported. These processes are dependent in part upon the Na$^+$ gradient across the membrane and are influenced by drugs that modify Na-K transport.

Transcellular fluids are formed by the active transport of Na$^+$ across epithelial cells. So-called tight intercellular junctions between these cells prevent diffusion of fluids and solutes in both directions. Proteins and other macromolecules slowly cross epithelial cells by *pinocytosis,* a form of vesicular transport.

Facilitated Diffusion. Carrier-mediated transport that exhibits selectivity and saturability but in which the substance does not move against a concentration gradient is called *facilitated diffusion.* This is not an energy-dependent process. Glucose, for example, is transported into most cells by this process. Transport is facilitated by attachment to a carrier and is more rapid than simple diffusion. The transport of glucose across the gastrointestinal mucosa and by the kidney, however, is active and can proceed against a concentration gradient.

ABSORPTION OF DRUGS

It is of practical importance to know the manner in which drugs are absorbed. The rate of absorption influences the time course of drug effect, and it is an important factor in determining drug dosage. In addition, choice of the route by which a drug is administered is often influenced by considerations of drug absorption.

Factors That Modify Absorption. Many variables, in addition to the physicochemical factors discussed above, influence the absorption of drugs. Absorption from all sites of administration is dependent upon drug *solubility*. Drugs given in aqueous solution are more rapidly absorbed than those given in oily solution, suspension, or solid form. For those given in solid form, the rate of *dissolution* may be the limiting factor in their absorption. Local conditions at the site of absorption alter solubility. Thus, at the low pH of the gastric juice, many acidic drugs are absorbed slowly because they precipitate in the fluids of the stomach, and dissolution occurs very slowly. Highly insoluble substances may not be absorbed from the alimentary tract at all. The *concentration* of a drug influences its rate of absorption. Drugs ingested or injected in solutions of high concentration are absorbed more rapidly than are drugs in solutions of low concentration. The *circulation to the site of absorption* also affects drug absorption. Increased blood flow, brought about by massage or local application of heat, enhances absorption of a drug; decreased blood flow, produced by vasoconstrictors, shock, or other factors, slows absorption. The area of the *absorbing surface* to which a drug is exposed is one of the more important determinants of the rate of drug absorption. Drugs are absorbed very rapidly from large surface areas such as the pulmonary alveolar epithelium. The absorbing surface is determined largely by the *route of administration*.

Enteral (Oral) vs. Parenteral Administration. Often there is a choice of the route by which a therapeutic agent may be given, and a knowledge of the advantages and disadvantages of the different routes of administration is then of primary importance. Some characteristics of the major routes employed for systemic drug effect are compared in Table 1-1.

Oral ingestion is the most ancient method of drug administration. It is also the safest, most convenient, and most economical. Disadvantages to the oral route include emesis as a result of irritation to the gastrointestinal

Table 1-1. SOME CHARACTERISTICS OF COMMON ROUTES OF DRUG ADMINISTRATION *

ROUTE	ABSORPTION PATTERN	SPECIAL UTILITY	LIMITATIONS AND PRECAUTIONS
Intravenous	Absorption circumvented Potentially immediate effects	Valuable for emergency use Permits titration of dosage Suitable for large volumes and for irritating substances, if diluted	Increased risk of adverse effects Must inject solutions *slowly*, as a rule Not suitable for oily solutions or insoluble substances
Subcutaneous	Prompt, from aqueous solution Slow and sustained, from repository preparations	Suitable for some insoluble suspensions and for implantation of solid pellets	Not suitable for large volumes Possible slough from irritating substances
Intramuscular	Prompt, from aqueous solution Slow and sustained, from repository preparations	Suitable for moderate volumes, oily vehicles, and some irritating substances	Precluded during anticoagulant medication May interfere with interpretation of certain diagnostic tests (*e.g.,* creatine phosphokinase)
Oral ingestion	Variable; depends upon many factors (*see* text)	Most convenient, safe, and economical	Requires patient cooperation Absorption potentially erratic and incomplete for drugs that are poorly soluble and absorbed slowly

* *See* text for more complete discussion and for other routes.

mucosa, destruction of some drugs by digestive enzymes or low gastric pH, formation with food of complexes that cannot be absorbed, and necessity for cooperation on the part of the patient. In addition, drugs absorbed from the gastrointestinal tract may be extensively metabolized by the liver before they gain access to the general circulation.

The parenteral injection of medicinals has certain distinct advantages over oral administration. In some instances, parenteral administration is essential for the drug to be absorbed in active form. Absorption is usually more rapid and more predictable than when a drug is given by mouth. The effective dose can therefore be more accurately selected. In emergency therapy, parenteral administration is particularly serviceable. If a patient is unconscious, uncooperative, or unable to retain anything given by mouth, parenteral therapy may become a necessity. The injection of drugs also has its disadvantages. Strict asepsis must be maintained to avoid infection, an intravascular injection may occur when it is not intended, pain may accompany the injection, and it is often difficult for a patient to perform the injection himself if self-medication is a necessary procedure. Parenteral therapy is also more expensive and less safe than oral medication.

Oral Ingestion. Absorption of drugs from the gastrointestinal tract is for the most part understandable in terms of simple diffusion across the gastrointestinal epithelium. The rate of such diffusion is generally proportional to the lipid solubility of the compound in question. If the drug is a weak acid or base, its nonionized form is more lipid soluble, and the pH within the gastrointestinal tract becomes a major determinant. Alcohol, a lipid-soluble nonelectrolyte, is rapidly absorbed into the blood stream by diffusion across the gastric and intestinal mucosae. Quaternary ammonium compounds and other completely ionized, lipid-insoluble drugs are very slowly absorbed. Other drugs are poorly absorbed because even their nonionic forms are lipid insoluble.

Weak bases, such as quinidine and ephedrine, which are predominantly ionized at the pH of the gastric juice, are poorly absorbed through the gastric mucosa and are absorbed mainly through the intestinal mucosa. Weak acids, such as salicylates and barbiturates, which are predominantly nonionized in the acid gastric contents, are more readily absorbed from the stomach (see Figure 1–2). If the gastric contents are made alkaline, acidic compounds become more ionized and may be more slowly absorbed. Conversely, basic drugs become less ionized and may be more rapidly absorbed. However, *gastric pH* also influences *solubility* of the drug and *dissolution* of solid dosage forms. In addition, the net effect of change in gastric pH may be relatively minor, since absorption of most drugs occurs primarily from the intestine because of its greater *surface area*. For the same reason, the absorption of most drugs is delayed or reduced if *gastric emptying* is retarded.

Absorption from the alimentary tract may be decreased if the ingested drug is unstable in gastrointestinal fluid or if it is bound to food or other gastrointestinal contents. Simultaneous ingestion of food also delays absorption by delaying gastric emptying. Drugs that are destroyed by gastric juice or that cause gastric irritation are sometimes administered in dosage forms with a coating that prevents dissolution in the acid gastric contents. However, some *enteric-coated* preparations of a drug may also resist dissolution in the intestine, and very little of the drug may be absorbed.

Drugs related to the steroids, glucose, amino acids, and pyrimidines may be absorbed by active processes that are normally involved in the absorption of dietary and endogenous substances.

Timed-Release Preparations. The rate of absorption of a drug administered as a tablet or other solid oral-dosage form is dependent mainly upon its rate of dissolution in the gastrointestinal fluids. This factor is the basis for the so-called *timed-release, sustained-release,* or *prolonged-action* pharmaceutical preparations. Such preparations are designed to produce slow, uniform absorption of the drug and thereby provide a sustained effect for 8 hours or longer. Some are compounded to provide, in addition, rapid release of sufficient active ingredient to yield prompt onset of effect. Potential advantages of such preparations are reduction in the frequency of administration of the drug as compared with conventional dosage forms, possibly with improved compliance by the patient, maintenance of a therapeutic effect overnight, and decreased incidence of undesired effects by elimination of the peaks in drug concentration that often occur after administration of other dosage forms.

Some timed-release preparations fulfill these theoretical expectations. Unfortunately, not all marketed preparations are reliable. The dissolution rate of some preparations in gastrointestinal fluid may be quite irregular because of technical problems associated with their manufacture or because of variations in gastrointestinal pH, gastric emptying, intestinal motility, and other physiological factors that influence drug absorption. Moreover, slow absorption from the gastrointestinal tract is often incomplete and erratic. In addition, each drug must be evaluated separately for its suitability as a timed-release preparation. Drugs given for a brief therapeutic effect should not be in the timed-release form. Conversely, timed-release preparations are not needed for drugs with an inherent long duration of effect. Also, timed-release preparations of some drugs might not be safe. Since the total dose of drug ingested at one time may be several times the dose of the conventional form of the drug, faulty release of the entire amount at once could lead to toxicity. Finally, failure of adequate release may compromise the therapeutic effect. It is thus incumbent on the physician who uses preparations of this type to establish a need for a timed-release preparation and also to assure himself of its uniformity, reliability, and safety. This is especially necessary since the timed-release formulations of different manufacturers may vary considerably from each other.

Sublingual Administration. Absorption from the oral mucosa is rapid, and a higher concentration of the drug in the blood may be achieved by this route than by absorption lower in the alimentary tract. This can result because metabolism of drugs as a result of passage through the liver is minimized, and because the drug is not subjected to possible destruction by the gastrointestinal secretions or to formation of complexes with foods. However, substances that are distasteful or that are irritating should not be given by this route. The sublingual route of administration permits rapid absorption of nitroglycerin and other drugs. It is a convenient method when the drug is suitable for such administration.

Rectal Administration. The rectal route is often useful when oral ingestion is precluded by vomiting or when the patient is unconscious. In addition, the absorbed drug does not pass through the liver before entry into the systemic circulation. However, rectal absorption is often irregular and incomplete, and many drugs cause irritation of the rectal mucosa.

Parenteral Injection. The major routes of parenteral administration are intravenous, subcutaneous, and intramuscular. Absorption of lipid-soluble drugs from subcutaneous and intramuscular sites also occurs by simple diffusion through the capillary membranes into the blood and is directly proportional to the lipid:water partition coefficient of the drug. The rate of absorption is also influenced by the area of the absorbing capillary membranes and by the solubility of the substance in the interstitial fluid. Lipid-insoluble drugs are absorbed into the blood by penetration through the relatively large aqueous channels in the endothelial membrane; larger molecules, such as proteins, gain access to the circulation by way of lymphatic channels. Some large molecules and microcrystalline substances are absorbed from these sites by phagocytosis.

Intravenous. The factors concerned in absorption are circumvented by intravenous injection of drugs in aqueous solution, and the desired blood concentration of a drug is obtained with an accuracy and immediacy not possible by any other procedure. In some instances, as in the induction of surgical anesthesia by a barbiturate, the dose of a drug is not predetermined but is adjusted to the response of the patient. Also, certain irritating and hypertonic solutions can be given only in this manner, for the blood vessel walls are relatively insensitive and the drug, if injected slowly, is greatly diluted by the blood.

On the other hand, there are many dangers that attend intravenous injections. Unfavorable reactions are more prone to occur than when any other route is used. Once the drug is injected there is no retreat. Repeated intravenous injections are dependent upon the patency of veins. Drugs in an oily vehicle or those that precipitate blood constituents or hemolyze erythrocytes should not be given by this route. Unless specifically indicated, drugs should never be given directly into the blood stream. *Intravenous injection must usually be performed slowly.*

Subcutaneous. Injection at a subcutaneous site is often utilized for the administration of medicinals. It can be used only for drugs that are not irritating to tissue; otherwise, a slough may occur. The rate of absorption following subcutaneous injection of a drug is often sufficiently even and slow to provide a sustained effect. Moreover, it may be willfully varied by well-known technics. For example, the rate of absorption of a suspension of insoluble protamine insulin is slow compared with that of soluble insulin. The incorporation of a vasoconstrictor agent in a solution of a drug to be injected subcutaneously also retards absorption. This principle is utilized in the combination of epinephrine with local anesthetics. Absorption of drugs implanted under the skin in a solid pellet form occurs slowly over a period of weeks or months; several hormones are effectively administered in this manner.

Intramuscular. Drugs in aqueous solution are rapidly absorbed after intramuscular injection. Very slow, even absorption from the intramuscular site results if the drug is injected in solution in oil or suspended in various repository vehicles. Penicillin is often administered in this manner. Irritating substances that cannot be injected subcutaneously may often be given intramuscularly.

Intra-arterial. Occasionally a drug is injected directly into an artery to localize its effect in a particular tissue or organ. Antineoplastic agents are sometimes given in this manner for the treatment of localized tumors. Diagnostic agents are also sometimes injected by this route. Intra-arterial injection requires great care and should be reserved for experts.

Intrathecal. The blood-brain barrier and the blood-cerebrospinal fluid barrier often preclude or slow the entrance of drugs into the central nervous system (CNS). Therefore, when local and rapid effects of drugs on the meninges or cerebrospinal axis are desired, as in spinal anesthesia or acute CNS infections, drugs are sometimes injected directly into the spinal subarachnoid space.

Intraperitoneal. The peritoneal cavity offers a large absorbing surface from which drugs enter the circulation rapidly. Intraperitoneal injection is a common laboratory procedure, but it is seldom employed clinically. The dangers of infection and adhesions are too great to warrant the routine use of this route in man. However, peritoneal dialysis is sometimes a valuable procedure in the treatment of drug poisoning.

Pulmonary Absorption. Gaseous and volatile drugs may be inhaled and absorbed through the pulmonary epithelium and mucous membranes of the respiratory tract. Access to the circulation is rapid by this route, because the surface area is large. The principles governing absorption and excretion of the anesthetic gases and vapors are discussed in Chapter 5.

In addition, solutions of drugs can be atomized and the fine droplets in air (aerosol) inhaled. Advantages are the almost instantaneous absorption of a drug into the blood, if this is desired, and, in the case of pulmonary disease, local application of the drug at the desired site of action. For example, epinephrine can be given in this manner for the treatment of bronchial asthma. The main disadvantages are poor ability to regulate the dose, cumbersomeness of the methods of administration, and the fact that many gaseous and volatile drugs produce irritation of the pulmonary epithelium.

Topical Application. *Mucous Membranes.* Drugs are applied to the mucous membranes of the conjunctiva, nasopharynx, oropharynx, vagina, colon, urethra, and urinary bladder primarily for their local effects. Occasionally, as in the application of antidiuretic hormone to the nasal mucosa, systemic absorption is the goal. Absorption through mucous membranes occurs readily. In fact, local anesthetics applied for local effect may sometimes be absorbed so rapidly that they produce systemic toxicity.

Skin. Few drugs readily penetrate the intact skin. Absorption of those that do is proportional to their lipid solubility since the epidermis behaves as a lipoid barrier. The dermis, however, is freely permeable to many solutes; consequently, systemic absorption of drugs occurs much more readily through abraded or denuded skin. Toxic effects are sometimes produced by absorption through the skin of highly lipid-soluble substances (*e.g.,* a lipid-soluble insecticide in an organic solvent). Absorption through the skin can be enhanced by suspending the drug in an oily vehicle and rubbing the resulting preparation into the skin. This method of administration is known as *inunction.* Absorption through the skin is also increased by so-called occlusive dressings, which retain moisture and macerate the epidermis.

Bioavailability. Pharmaceutical formulations of a drug are termed *chemically equivalent* if they meet the chemical and physical standards established by governmental or other regulatory agencies. They are said to be *biologically equivalent* if they yield similar concentrations of drug in blood and tissues, and they are designated *therapeutically equivalent* if they provide equal therapeutic benefit in clinical trial. Pharmaceutical preparations that are chemically equivalent but not biologically or therapeutically equivalent are said to differ in their *bioavailability.* Dosage forms of a drug from different manufacturers and even different lots of preparations from a single manufacturer sometimes differ in their bioavailability. Such differences primarily involve oral dosage forms of poorly soluble, slowly absorbed drugs. They result from differences in crystal form, particle size, or other characteristics of the drug and from the many variables involved in the formulation and manufacture of the preparations. These factors affect the disintegration of the dosage form and dissolution of the drug and, hence, the rate and extent of drug absorption.

Biological nonequivalence of drug preparations is a particularly acute problem because bioavailability of a preparation in man has not always correlated with laboratory tests of tablet dissolution or with tests of bioavailability in animals. Biological non-equivalence of practical importance has been detected among the preparations of a number of important drugs, including the cardiac glycoside digoxin and several antibiotics. Responsible drug manufacturers, interested medical and pharmaceutical scientists, and governmental agencies are cooperating to speed resolution of the problem by establishing tests for bioavailability of pharmaceutical preparations in man and by devising *in-vitro* tests for drug dissolution that have satisfactory predictive value. The significance of possible nonequivalence of drug preparations is further discussed in connection with drug nomenclature and the choice of drug name in prescription order writing (*see* Appendix).

DISTRIBUTION OF DRUGS

After a drug is absorbed or injected into the blood stream, it may be distributed into the interstitial, cellular, and transcellular fluids. The rate, extent, and pattern of the initial distribution are determined by the physicochemical characteristics of the drug and by cardiac output and regional blood flow. Lipid-soluble drugs that readily cross membranes are distributed throughout all fluid compartments. They are distributed very promptly into heart, brain, liver, kidney, and other highly perfused tissues, less rapidly into muscle, and more slowly into fat. Drugs that do not readily cross membranes are restricted in their distribution and, hence, in their potential sites of action. Drugs may accumulate in tissues at higher concentration than in plasma as the result of pH gradients, binding, active transport, or dissolving in fat. Drug accumulated in tissues may serve as a reservoir that prolongs the effects of the drug.

Passage of Drugs into and across Cells. The capillary endothelium, except in the brain, does not restrict the distribution of drugs, and most drugs, whether ionized or nonionized, diffuse at least into the interstitial fluid. Distribution is limited, however, by plasma protein binding. Subsequent passage of drugs across other cell membranes involves the same factors discussed previously for membranes in general. Weak electrolytes penetrate cells by simple diffusion in the nonionized form in proportion to their lipid:water partition coefficient and are distributed between extracellular and intracellular fluids in proportion to the pH difference of the two fluids.

Since the pH difference between intracellular and extracellular fluids is small (7.0 versus 7.4), this factor can result in only a relatively small concentration gradient of drug across the plasma membrane. Weak bases are concentrated slightly inside of cells, while the concentration of weak acids is slightly lower in the cells than in extracellular fluids. Lowering the pH of extracellular fluid increases the intracellular concentration of weak acids and decreases that of weak bases, provided that the intracellular pH does not also change and that the pH change does not simultaneously affect the binding, biotransformation, or excretion of the drug. Elevating the pH produces the opposite effects.

Nonelectrolytes enter cells by diffusion and generally in proportion to their lipid solubility, but small molecules such as urea penetrate through aqueous channels in the membrane. Penetration of strong acids and bases that are completely ionized depends upon the permeability of the cell membrane; their distribution will also be influenced by the potential difference across the membrane. Subcellular membranes are also lipoid in nature, and penetration of drugs into mitochondria and certain other subcellular organelles follows the same principles as for cell membranes.

Central Nervous System and Cerebrospinal Fluid. The distribution of drugs in the CNS is unique mainly in that entry of drugs into the cerebral extracellular space and cerebrospinal fluid is restricted. Drugs that are ionized and/or lipid insoluble are largely excluded from the brain. Entry of the nonionized forms of weak acids and bases is somewhat restricted, but these substances enter in proportion to their lipid solubility. Because of the high cerebral blood flow, such drugs that are highly lipid soluble enter the brain quite rapidly.

Unlike other capillary endothelial cells, those of the brain not only restrict passage of drugs bound to plasma protein but also limit diffusion of drugs in general and particularly lipid-insoluble substances. Processes from glial cells (astrocytes) are in close approximation to the capillary endothelium and constitute another cellular barrier between the blood and the extracellular space. Entry of drugs into the brain by way of the cerebrospinal fluid is similarly limited by the cells of the choroid plexus.

In addition, organic ions are extruded from the cerebrospinal fluid into blood at the choroid plexus by transport processes similar to those in the renal tubule. Lipid-soluble substances leave the brain by diffusion through the capillaries and the blood–choroid plexus boundary. Drugs and endogenous metabolites, regardless of lipid solubility and molecular size, also exit with bulk flow of the cerebrospinal fluid through the arachnoid villi. (For a summary of the distribution of drugs in the CNS, *see* Rall, in La Du *et al.*, 1971; Davson, 1972.)

Drug Reservoirs. The body compartments in which a drug accumulates are potential reservoirs for the drug. If stored drug is in equilibrium with that in plasma and is released as the plasma concentration declines, a concentration of the drug in plasma and at its locus of action is sustained, and pharmacological effects of the drug are prolonged. However, the drug reservoir so alters the distribution of the drug that larger quantities of the drug are required initially to provide a therapeutically effective concentration.

Plasma Proteins and Other Extracellular Reservoirs. Many drugs are bound to plasma proteins, mostly to plasma albumin; binding to other plasma proteins generally occurs to a much smaller extent. The binding is usually reversible; occasionally, covalent binding occurs. The extent of the binding depends upon the particular drug. Some lipid-soluble organic acids, such as the penicillinase-resistant penicillins and the anticoagulant agent warfarin, are more than 90% bound. Lipid-soluble organic bases may also be highly bound to albumin, but to different sites. Fractional binding is a function of drug concentration but varies only slightly at drug concentrations less than 10 to 20 μg/ml. Drug bound to plasma protein may serve as a substantial drug reservoir. However, drugs that bind to plasma protein usually also bind to tissues, and the cellular reservoir may be even more significant.

Binding of a drug to plasma protein limits its concentration in tissues and at its locus of action, since only unbound drug is in equilibrium across membranes. Binding also limits glomerular filtration of the drug, but it does not generally limit renal tubular secretion or biotransformation, since drug-protein complexes usually dissociate rapidly. If a drug is avidly transported or metabolized

and its clearance, calculated on the basis of unbound drug, exceeds organ plasma flow, binding of the drug to plasma protein may be viewed as a transport mechanism that fosters drug elimination.

Since binding of drugs to plasma albumin is rather nonselective, many drugs with similar physicochemical characteristics compete with each other and with endogenous substances for these binding sites. Displacement of unconjugated bilirubin from binding to albumin by the sulfonamides and other organic anions is known to increase the risk of bilirubin encephalopathy in the newborn, and drug toxicity has sometimes been attributed to similar competition between drugs. Such interactions are often more complex than generally stated. Since drug displaced from plasma protein will redistribute into its full potential volume of distribution, the concentration of free drug in plasma and tissues after redistribution may be increased only slightly. The interaction may also involve altered elimination of the drug. Risk of adverse effect is greatest if the displaced drug has a limited volume of distribution, if the competition extends to the drug bound in tissues, if elimination of the drug is also reduced, or if the displacing drug is administered in high dosage by rapid intravenous injection. Competition of drugs for plasma protein binding sites may also cause misinterpretation of measured serum concentrations of drugs.

Some drugs are stored in connective tissue by binding to the strongly ionic groups of the mucopolysaccharides. The tetracycline antibiotics, heavy metals, and certain other drugs accumulate in bone, probably by adsorption of the substances to the bone-crystal surface or incorporation into the crystal lattice.

Cellular Reservoirs. Many drugs accumulate in muscle and other cells in higher concentrations than in the extracellular fluids. If the intracellular concentration is high and if the binding is reversible, the tissue involved may represent a sizable drug reservoir. During chronic administration of the antimalarial agent quinacrine, the concentration of the drug in liver may be several thousand times that in plasma. Accumulation in cells may be the result of active transport or, more commonly, binding. Tissue binding of drugs usually occurs with proteins, phospholipids, or nucleoproteins and is generally reversible.

Fat as a Reservoir. Many lipid-soluble drugs are stored by physical solution in the neutral fat. In obese persons, the fat content of the body may be as high as 50%, and even in starvation it constitutes 10% of body weight; hence, fat can serve as an important reservoir for lipid-soluble drugs. For example, as much as 70% of the highly lipid-soluble barbiturate thiopental may be present in body fat 3 hours after administration. However, fat is a rather sluggish reservoir because it has a relatively low blood flow.

Transcellular Reservoirs. Drugs also cross epithelial cells and may accumulate in the transcellular fluids. The major transcellular reservoir is the gastrointestinal tract. Weak bases are passively concentrated in the stomach from the blood, because of the large pH differential between the two fluids, and some drugs are secreted in the bile in an active form or as a conjugate that can be hydrolyzed in the intestine. In these cases and when an orally administered drug is slowly absorbed, the gastrointestinal tract serves as a drug reservoir.

Other transcellular fluids, including *cerebrospinal fluid, aqueous humor, endolymph,* and *joint fluids,* do not generally accumulate significant total amounts of drugs.

Redistribution. Termination of drug effect is usually by biotransformation and excretion, but it may also result from redistribution of the drug from its site of action into other tissues or sites. Redistribution is a factor in terminating drug effect primarily when a highly lipid-soluble drug that acts on the brain or cardiovascular system is administered rapidly by intravenous injection or by inhalation. Under these conditions, drug effect develops promptly as the drug quickly reaches its locus of action in the highly perfused tissue. However, drug effect also wanes rapidly, as the drug is redistributed from its locus of action to muscle and other less well perfused tissues. The drug may persist for an extended time but at a concentration below that necessary for effect. With repeated administration, drug redistribution will again occur rapidly, but the concentration now may not quickly fall below the critical level, and the duration of effect of successive doses thus increases. Termination of effect is now dependent upon drug elimination by biotransformation or excretion. The factors involved in redistribution of drugs have been

extensively studied for thiopental and are described in Chapter 9.

Placental Transfer of Drugs. A knowledge of the principles of transfer of drugs across the placenta is important, since drugs may cause congenital anomalies. Administered immediately prior to delivery, they may also have adverse effects upon the neonate. Drugs cross the placenta primarily by simple diffusion. Lipid-soluble, nonionized drugs readily enter the fetal blood from the maternal circulation. Penetration is least with drugs possessing a high degree of dissociation and/or low lipid solubility. The view that the placenta is a barrier to drugs is unrealistic. A more appropriate approximation is that the fetus is exposed to essentially all drugs taken by the mother.

BIOTRANSFORMATION OF DRUGS

Many drugs are lipid-soluble, weak organic acids or bases that are not readily eliminated from the body. For example, after filtration at the renal glomerulus they are readily reabsorbed by diffusion through the renal tubular cells. To be excreted more rapidly, they must be transformed into more polar compounds. These metabolites are usually less lipid soluble, more ionized at physiological pH, less bound to plasma and tissue proteins, less stored in fat, and less able to penetrate cell membranes. Thus, biotransformation not only fosters drug elimination but also often results in inactivation of the drug. If the metabolite is active, termination of action takes place by further biotransformation or by excretion of the active metabolite in the urine. (For excellent summaries of drug biotransformation, *see* Williams, 1959; La Du *et al.,* 1971; Goldstein *et al.,* 1974.)

Patterns of Biotransformation. The chemical reactions concerned in the biotransformation of drugs are classified as *nonsynthetic* and *synthetic.* The nonsynthetic reactions involve oxidation, reduction, or hydrolysis; they may result in activation, change in activity, or inactivation of the parent drug. The synthetic reactions, also called *conjugation reactions,* involve coupling between the drug or its metabolite and an endogenous substrate, usually a carbohydrate or an amino acid or a derivative of these, acetic acid, or inorganic sulfate. Synthetic reactions almost invariably result in inactivation of the parent drug.

Although many details of drug biotransformation are necessarily based upon observations in animals, the mechanisms in man are clearly similar. However, rates of the reactions in the various species are often quite different, and the patterns of biotransformation may be qualitatively different.

Various patterns of biotransformation, involving nonsynthetic and synthetic reactions and representing both activation and inactivation of drugs, are illustrated in Table 1–2. These reactions also emphasize that most drugs are converted concurrently or consecutively to multiple metabolites. The hepatic microsomal enzyme systems are responsible for the biotransformation of the majority of drugs. Other tissues, including plasma, kidney, and the gastrointestinal tract, also contribute to drug biotransformation.

The first reaction in Table 1–2, involving morphine, illustrates the common process of inactivation by glucuronide formation. The second series of reactions depicts the inactivation of the antiepileptic agent phenobarbital by oxidation. Subsequent conjugations of two types further facilitate excretion of the metabolite. The third reaction, oxidation of the antiepileptic agent trimethadione to the active metabolite dimethadione (DMO), demonstrates that oxidation need not inactivate a drug and that biotransformation does not always proceed to conjugation. DMO is not further metabolized but is slowly excreted in the urine. Oxidation may also result in conversion of an inactive drug to an active metabolite or the formation of a metabolite with qualitatively different activity than that of the parent drug. An example of the latter pattern is the biotransformation of the antipyretic-analgesic phenacetin to a metabolite that causes methemoglobin formation. The fourth reaction sequence illustrates that a drug may be converted concurrently to active and inactive metabolites. The sedative-hypnotic chloral hydrate is both oxidized to inactive trichloroacetic acid and reduced to trichloroethanol. The active metabolite is subsequently inactivated by conjugation. The time course of drug effect after administration of chloral hydrate thus depends upon the relative rates of the three reactions. The fifth series of reactions involves the third general type of nonsynthetic reaction, hydrolysis. The neuromuscular blocking agent succinylcholine is hydrolyzed to succinylmonocholine, and this metabolite with weak activity is then further hydrolyzed to inactive choline. The final reaction sequence illustrates that conjugation, in this case, of 6-mercaptopurine to its ribonucleotide, occasionally results in activation of a drug.

Table 1–2. REPRESENTATIVE PATTERNS OF DRUG BIOTRANSFORMATION

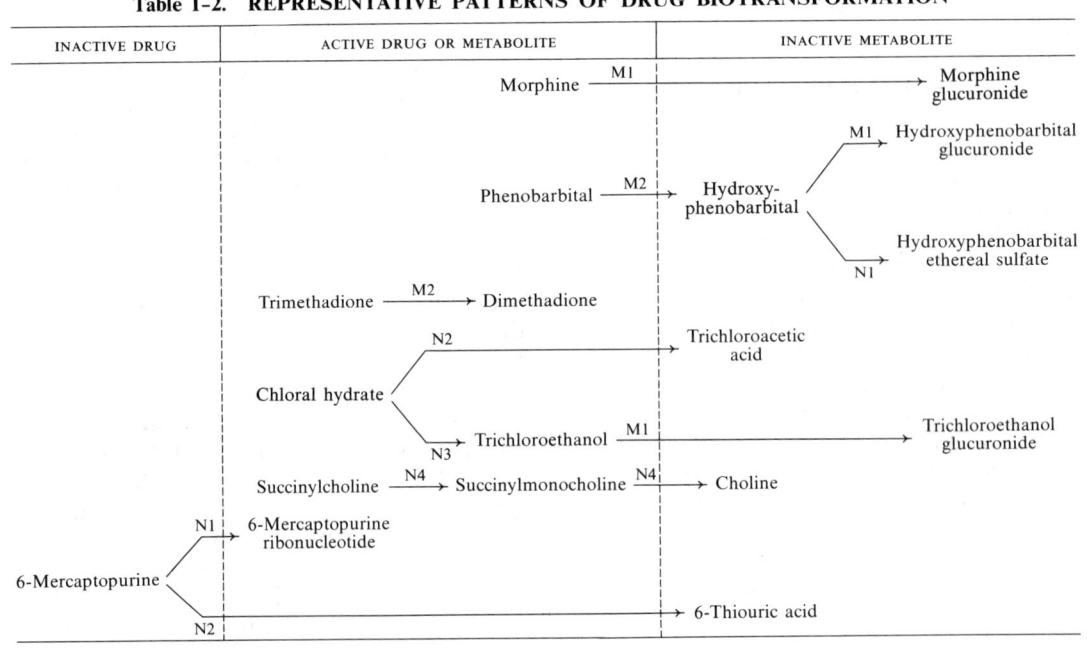

Site of reaction: M = microsomal
　　　　　　　　N = nonmicrosomal

Type of reaction: 1 = conjugation
　　　　　　　　　 2 = oxidation
　　　　　　　　　 3 = reduction
　　　　　　　　　 4 = hydrolysis

Hepatic Microsomal Drug-Metabolizing Systems.

The enzyme systems concerned in the biotransformation of many drugs are located in the hepatic endoplasmic reticulum. Fragments of this network are isolated by centrifugation of liver homogenates in the fraction generally called *microsomes.*

The endoplasmic reticulum resembles a canal system within the cell and may function also in the intracellular transport of various substances. It is continuous with the cell membrane and with the nuclear membrane but differs functionally from both. As identified by electron microscopy, the reticulum consists mainly of a membrane that often bears small ribonucleoprotein particles, called *ribosomes,* which cause the reticulum to have a rough surface. The rough-surfaced reticulum is concerned with protein synthesis, including the synthesis of the smooth-surfaced reticulum that contains the enzymes that metabolize drugs.

The microsomal enzymes catalyze glucuronide conjugations and most of the oxidations of drugs. Reduction and hydrolysis of drugs are catalyzed by both microsomal and nonmicrosomal enzymes. Lipid solubility is an important, but not the only, requirement for a drug to be metabolized by the hepatic microsomes since this property favors the penetration of a drug into the endoplasmic reticulum and its binding with cytochrome P-450, a primary component of the oxidative enzyme system. Most endogenous metabolic intermediates are polar compounds and are not substrates. However, the microsomal enzymes do contribute to the biotransformation of fatty acids and steroid hormones and also conjugate bilirubin.

The hepatic microsomal enzyme systems are notable; not only do they participate in the biotransformation of many drugs but also activity of these enzymes can be induced by many drugs and by chemicals encountered in the environment. Both normal interindividual differences in microsomal enzyme activity and susceptibility to induction are genetically determined. Rates of biotransformation of drugs among individuals may vary sixfold or more.

The evolutionary development of the drug-metabolizing system in hepatic endoplasmic reticulum is a fascinating story in comparative pharmacology but is beyond the scope of this chapter. An interesting summary has been presented by Brodie and Maickel in a symposium (1962).

Oxidation. The hepatic endoplasmic reticulum contains an important group of oxidative enzymes called *mixed-function oxidases* or *monooxygenases* that require both reduced nicotinamide adenine dinucleotide phosphate (NADPH) and molecular oxygen. These enzymes are involved in the biotransformation of many drugs. Epoxide intermediates in these reactions are capable of covalent binding with macromolecules and may be responsible for tissue necrosis, carcinogenicity, and other toxic effects of drugs.

The reactions catalyzed by the microsomal mixed-function oxidases include N- and O-dealkylation, aromatic ring and side chain hydroxylation, sulfoxide formation, N-oxidation, N-hydroxylation, deamination of primary and secondary amines, and the replacement of a sulfur by an oxygen atom (desulfuration). These reactions are depicted in Table 1–3.

The mixed-function oxidase system has not yet been fully characterized, since its components have not been purified in functional form. However, the electron-transport scheme is illustrated in Figure 1–3. The terminal oxidase is a hemoprotein (or group of proteins) designated cytochrome P-450, so named since it absorbs light at 450 nm when exposed to carbon monoxide. This property is also the basis for its analytical determination. Furthermore, carbon monoxide blocks the metabolism of many drugs by the system. The primary electron donor is NADPH; the electron transfer involves a flavoprotein, NADPH–cytochrome c reductase. A phospholipid is essential for activity of the reconstituted system

A drug substrate binds with oxidized cytochrome P-450 ($[Fe^{3+}]$ in Figure 1–3). The resulting drug-cytochrome complex is reduced by the reductase, and the reduced complex then combines with molecular oxygen. A second electron and two hydrogen ions are acquired from the donor system, and the subsequent products are oxidized metabolite and water, with regeneration of the oxidized cytochrome P-450.

Interactions of substrates and inhibitors with oxidized cytochrome P-450 produce characteristic changes in the absorbance spectrum of the microsomes. These provide the basis for designating drugs as type I or II and are indicative of two types of drug binding sites or at least two types of cytochrome P-450 molecules. Clarification of the relationships between these spectral changes and the binding of drugs to the components of cytochrome P-450 and the interaction of binding sites is an area of active research.

The rate of drug biotransformation by the mixed-function oxidase system is determined by the concentration of cytochrome P-450, the proportions of the various forms of cytochrome P-450 and their affinities for the substrate, the concentration of cyto-

Table 1-3. DRUG BIOTRANSFORMATION REACTIONS

I. *Oxidative Reactions* (Microsomal)

  (1) N- and O-Dealkylation

$$RNHCH_2CH_3 \xrightarrow{[O]} RNH_2 + CH_3CHO$$

$$ROCH_3 \xrightarrow{[O]} ROH + CH_2O$$

  (2) Side Chain (Aliphatic) and Aromatic Hydroxylation

$$RCH_2CH_3 \xrightarrow{[O]} R\overset{\displaystyle OH}{\overset{\displaystyle |}{C}}HCH_3$$

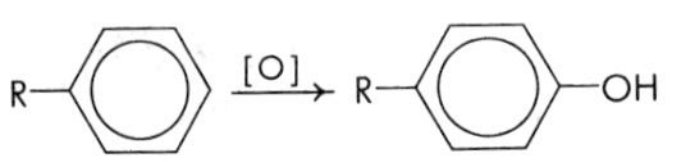

  (3) N-Oxidation and N-Hydroxylation

$$(R)_3N \xrightarrow{[O]} R_3N{=}O$$

$$RNHR' \xrightarrow{[O]} R\overset{\displaystyle OH}{\overset{\displaystyle |}{N}}R'$$

  (4) Sulfoxide Formation

$$RSR' \xrightarrow{[O]} R\overset{\displaystyle O}{\overset{\displaystyle \|}{S}}R'$$

  (5) Deamination of Amines

$$RCH_2NH_2 \xrightarrow{[O]} RCHO + NH_3$$

  (6) Desulfuration

$$RSH \xrightarrow{[O]} ROH$$

II. *Glucuronide Synthesis* (Microsomal)

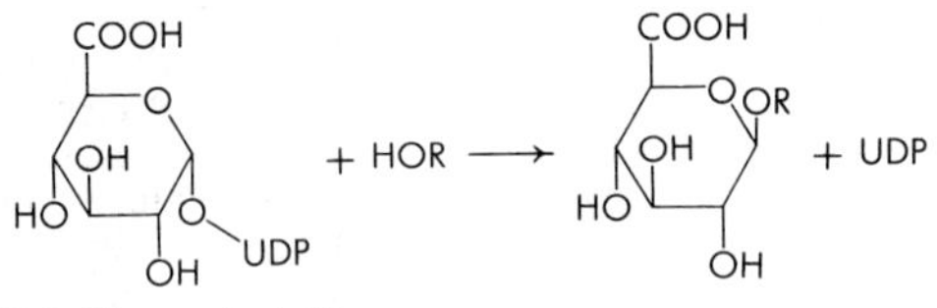

UDP–Glucuronic Acid

chrome c reductase, and the rate of reduction of the drug–cytochrome P-450 complex. Rate of biotransformation may also be influenced by competing endogenous and exogenous substrates. These many factors are responsible for the sometimes marked species, strain, and individual variations in drug metabolism by the microsomal system.

Glucuronide Synthesis. Glucuronides constitute the major proportion of metabolites of many phenols, alcohols, and carboxylic acids. Glucuronides are generally inactive and are rapidly secreted into the urine and bile by the transport mechanisms for anions. However, glucuronides eliminated in the bile may be subsequently hydrolyzed by

intestinal or bacterial β-glucuronidase, and the liberated drug may be reabsorbed. This enterohepatic cycling may prolong the action of the drug.

Glucuronide formation is catalyzed by various microsomal glucuronyltransferases, with uridine diphosphate–glucuronic acid (UDPGA) as the donor of glucuronic acid (Table 1–3). UDPGA is generated from glucose by enzymes in the cytosol. Glucuronide conjugation also occurs in the kidney and other tissues to a lesser extent.

Inhibition of Microsomal Drug Metabolism. Competitive inhibition between the many substrates for the microsomal enzymes

Table 1-3. DRUG BIOTRANSFORMATION REACTIONS (Continued)

III. *Other Conjugation Reactions*

(1) Acetylation

$$RNH_2 + CH_3\overset{O}{\overset{\|}{C}}SCoA \longrightarrow RNH\overset{O}{\overset{\|}{C}}CH_3 + CoA\text{---}SH$$
Acetyl CoA

(2) Conjugation with Glycine

$$RCOOH \longrightarrow R\overset{O}{\overset{\|}{C}}SCoA + NH_2CH_2COOH \longrightarrow R\overset{O}{\overset{\|}{C}}NHCH_2COOH + CoA\text{---}SH$$

(3) Conjugation with Sulfate

$$ROH + 3'\text{-phosphoadenosine } 5'\text{-phosphosulfate} \longrightarrow RO\overset{O}{\underset{O}{\overset{\|}{\underset{\|}{S}}}}OH + 3'\text{-phosphoadenosine } 5'\text{-phosphate}$$

(4) O-, S-, and N-Methylation

$$R\text{---}XH + S\text{-adenosylmethionine} \longrightarrow R\text{---}X\text{---}CH_3 + S\text{-adenosylhomocysteine}$$
$$(X = O, S, N)$$

IV. *Hydrolysis of Esters and Amides*

$$R\overset{O}{\overset{\|}{C}}OR' \longrightarrow RCOOH + R'OH$$

$$R\overset{O}{\overset{\|}{C}}NR' \longrightarrow RCOOH + R'NH_2$$

V. *Reduction*

(1) Azo Reduction

$$RN{=}NR' \longrightarrow RNH_2 + R'NH_2$$

(2) Nitro Reduction

$$RNO_2 \longrightarrow RNH_2$$

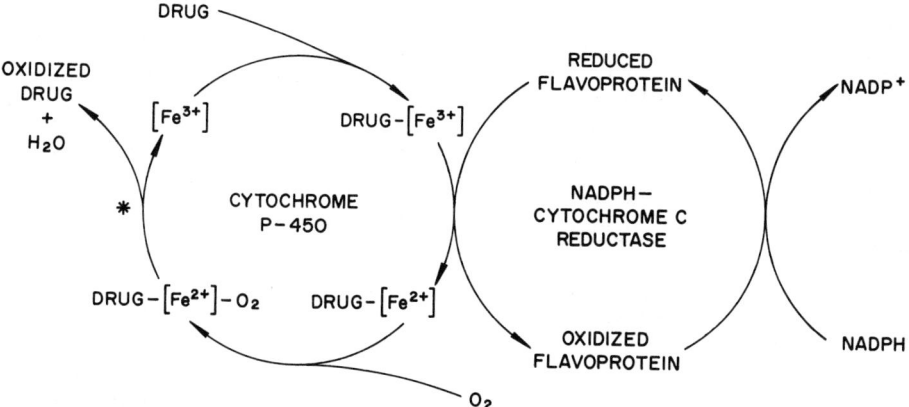

* Denotes contribution of a second electron and two hydrogen ions from NADH–flavoprotein–cytochrome b_5 or from NADPH–flavoprotein.

Figure 1-3. *Major components of the hepatic microsomal drug-metabolizing enzyme system.*

is readily demonstrated *in vitro*. Such inter-actions also occur *in vivo* but are not usually of practical significance. This is not unex-pected, since the inactivation of most drugs *in vivo* exhibits exponential (first-order) rather than linear (zero-order) kinetics. First-order kinetics usually applies, because drug concentrations are commonly well below those necessary to saturate metaboliz-ing enzymes, and competition between sub-strates is minimized under these conditions. An important corollary, however, is that sig-nificant mutual inhibition of drug metabo-lism is to be expected for drugs that normally exhibit zero-order inactivation kinetics. The best-established examples of inhibition of the metabolism of one drug by another during drug therapy do, in fact, involve phenytoin, dicumarol, and other drugs that exhibit zero-order elimination in the absence of other drugs.

The metabolism of a drug that is rapidly cleared by the liver is susceptible to changes in hepatic blood flow. An illustrative exam-ple is the inhibition of the hepatic metabo-lism of lidocaine by propranolol. Microsomal drug metabolism requires oxygen and is in-hibited by carbon monoxide and by hepato-toxic agents that destroy cytochrome P-450 or interfere with hepatic metabolism.

In animals, a number of agents are rather impres-sive inhibitors of microsomal drug metabolism. Pre-treatment with these compounds prolongs the effects of many other drugs by inhibition of their inacti-vation, or reduces the effects of those that are con-verted to active metabolites. The most extensively studied inhibitor is SKF 525A (β-diethylamino-ethyl-2,2-diphenylpentanoate; proadifen). Inhibition of drug metabolism by SKF 525A and related agents may be simply competitive but often involves multi-ple mechanisms, including both competitive and noncompetitive interference with the binding of substrates to cytochrome P-450 and with the reduc-tion of cytochrome P-450. These inhibitors may bind irreversibly with the enzyme, their metabolites may also be effective inhibitors, and most also cause induction of the microsomal system. In addition, such inhibitors may produce other pharmacological effects that contribute to drug interaction. Although not useful as therapeutic agents, they are valuable pharmacological tools for analysis of drug biotrans-formation and for characterization of the micro-somal enzyme systems.

Induction of Microsomal Enzyme Activity. The activity of the microsomal enzymes can be increased by administration of certain

drugs and by exposure to various chemicals in the environment. Not only is metabolism of the administered drug increased but also that of other drugs and endogenous sub-strates. The pharmacological effects of drugs that are inactivated by the microsomal en-zymes are correspondingly reduced; the effects of drugs that are converted to active metabolites may or may not be increased, depending upon the fate of the active me-tabolites. That a drug can increase its own metabolism and that of other substrates has wide implications for chronic toxicity tests, crossover drug studies in animals and man, chronic drug therapy with single or multiple drugs, and the development of tolerance to drugs. (For excellent reviews, *see* Conney, 1967; La Du *et al.,* 1971; Symposium, 1971.)

In animals, the several hundred compounds known to stimulate the microsomal enzyme systems are loosely classified into two types, namely, those that resemble phenobarbital and those that are simi-lar to the carcinogenic polycyclic hydrocarbons. Stimulation of the microsomal system by phenobar-bital results in altered biotransformation of a wide variety of substrates. The increase in enzyme activity is attributed to induced synthesis of cytochrome P-450, NADPH–cytochrome c reductase, and other enzymes involved in drug metabolism, since the increase has typical latency, cannot be produced *in vitro,* is associated with proliferation of the endo-plasmic reticulum, and can be prevented by inhibi-tors of nucleic acid and protein synthesis. Increased RNA polymerase activity and decreased microsomal ribonuclease activity have also been observed. Pheno-barbital, but not all other inducers, also increases liver weight, hepatic blood flow, bile flow, and other hepatic proteins, including those thought to be im-portant in the uptake of organic anions into the hepatocyte. Stimulation of the microsomal enzyme system by the polycyclic hydrocarbons is also attrib-uted to induced protein synthesis, but the increase in drug metabolism is limited to relatively few sub-strates, does not result in an increase in cytochrome c reductase, and is associated with the appearance of a qualitatively different terminal oxidase.

Enzyme induction also occurs to a limited extent in kidney, gastrointestinal tract, adrenal, lung, pla-centa, skin, and pancreas.

In man, susceptibility to induction is ge-netically determined and is greatest for indi-viduals with slowest drug metabolism prior to induction. Drug-metabolizing activity may increase as much as fourfold, but less than a twofold change is more common in pa-tients. The effect may be minimal if there has been prior induction. Induction develops and, upon removal of the inducing agent, wanes over a period of days or weeks, depending in part upon the time course for accumulation or elimination of the inducing agent.

Chronic administration of a drug may stimulate its own metabolism and that of other drugs. Concurrent administration of phenobarbital and warfarin results in lower plasma concentrations of warfarin and less anticoagulant effect than when the anticoagulant is administered alone. The desired therapeutic effect can be attained if dosage of the anticoagulant is increased. However, if the phenobarbital medication is stopped after the dosage of the anticoagulant has been adjusted, the plasma concentration and effect of warfarin increase, and severe bleeding may occur. Thus, during multiple-drug therapy involving an agent that stimulates drug metabolism, the effects of the other drugs must be carefully monitored, both when medication with the inducing agent is initiated and when it is discontinued.

Drug interactions frequently involve multiple mechanisms and are often variable. Administration of phenobarbital to patients previously maintained on phenytoin alone may result in a decrease, increase, or no change in the plasma concentration of phenytoin. These variable results are probably the net effect of both induction of the microsomal system and inhibition of phenytoin biotransformation.

Induction of the microsomal system also enhances the biotransformation of endogenous substrates such as bilirubin (*see* below) and the steroid hormones. This may be of practical importance when the glucocorticoids are administered as pharmacological agents. Normal endocrine balance will be altered only if the homeostatic mechanisms that regulate hormonal activity are inadequate.

Environmental Factors. Cigarette smoking and exposure to insecticides and other environmental chemicals also induce the hepatic microsomal drug-metabolizing enzymes in animals and man. *Cigarette smoking,* for example, enhances the metabolism of nicotine in man, and this may explain the tolerance to nicotine that occurs in smokers. To what extent smoking also stimulates the metabolism of commonly used drugs in man is an important but still largely unstudied problem. Individuals having intense, prolonged exposure to DDT and other *insecticides* also metabolize some drugs more rapidly than normal. The magnitude of the effect suggests that the less severe exposure sustained by the general population may not be of serious consequence, but this important problem deserves further study. *Ethanol* has two opposing effects on drug metabolism by the microsomal enzyme system. After acute ingestion of ethanol, microsomal metabolism may be inhibited; during chronic ingestion of ethanol, modest induction of the microsomal system may develop. Induction of the microsomal system is of limited practical significance for metabolism of ethanol, since ethanol is metabolized mainly by nonmicrosomal enzymes. However, microsomal induction by ethanol could influence the metabolism of other drugs; the opposing inhibitory effect of acute ethanol ingestion perhaps explains why the net effect is variable.

Drug Metabolism in the Neonate. Activity of the hepatic microsomal enzyme systems is low in the neonate, particularly premature babies. Reduced conjugating activity contributes to the hyperbilirubinemia of the neonate and the risk of bilirubin encephalopathy. It is also the basis of the increased toxicity in the neonate of drugs such as chloramphenicol that are inactivated by glucuronide formation. Activity of nonmicrosomal enzymes involved in drug biotransformation may also be reduced. Although many months are required for drug-metabolizing activity of the infant to approach (or exceed) that of the adult, significant increase occurs during the initial months of life.

Phenobarbital and other microsomal inducers have been employed in the treatment of hyperbilirubinemia in infants. The concentration of unconjugated bilirubin and the jaundice may be reduced. However, the effect may be of small magnitude and develops too slowly for acute management of hyperbilirubinemia. In addition, possible adverse effects of the drugs and of microsomal induction have not yet been adequately assessed.

Nonmicrosomal Drug Biotransformation. Although nonmicrosomal enzymes are involved in the biotransformation of fewer drugs than are the microsomal enzymes, nonmicrosomal drug metabolism is important. All conjugations other than glucuronide formation and some oxidation, reduction, and hydrolysis of drugs are catalyzed by nonmicrosomal enzymes. Such reactions contribute to the biotransformation of a number of common drugs, including aspirin and the sulfonamides. In addition, drugs that are only slowly metabolized may compete effectively with endogenous substrates. In certain such cases, as illustrated by the inhibition of xanthine oxidase by allopurinol, drug action and biotransformation are intimately related.

Nonmicrosomal biotransformation of drugs occurs primarily in the liver but also in plasma and other tissues. Although drug metabolism by the gastrointestinal tract and intestinal flora is usually minor relative to total drug elimination, biotransformation in the gastrointestinal tract sometimes contributes to what is superficially interpreted as poor oral absorption of a drug. In addition, minor metabolites from the intestinal metabolism of a drug may contribute to drug toxicity, and intestinal hydrolysis of glucuronides secreted in the bile is an integral link in the enterohepatic cycling of drugs.

Interindividual variation in rates of drug biotransformation is about the same for the nonmicrosomal enzymes as for the microsomal enzymes, namely, sixfold or greater. None of the nonmicrosomal enzymes involved in drug biotransformation is known to be inducible. Several, including pseudocholinesterase and the acetylating enzymes, exhibit genetic polymorphism. (*See* La Du *et al.,* 1971, for an excellent discussion of genetic modification of drug biotransformation.)

Conjugations. Inactivation of aromatic primary amines and hydrazines by conjugation with *acetic acid,* with acetyl coenzyme A as the acetyl donor, involves at least several N-acetyl transferases. Consequently, genetic polymorphism (slow or fast acetylation by different individuals) is exhibited only to some substrates, including isoniazid, hydralazine, and many sulfonamides.

Aromatic carboxylic acids, such as salicylic acid, are often inactivated by conjugation with *glycine.* A different enzyme is involved in the glycine conjugation of the bile acids. Drugs inactivated by glycine conjugation, such as salicylic acid, may exhibit dose-dependent elimination kinetics, that is, zero order at high concentrations and first order as the concentration is lowered.

Conjugation with *glutathione,* with subsequent formation of a mercapturate derivative, is not a quantitatively important route of biotransformation, but it contributes to inactivation of toxic epoxide intermediates produced by hydroxylation reactions.

Still other nonmicrosomal conjugations include *sulfate* conjugation of phenolic compounds, including steroids; *O-, S-,* and *N-methylation* of amines and phenols, including epinephrine and norepinephrine; and *ribonucleoside* and *ribonucleotide* formation, usually of analogs of the purines and pyrimidines to form active antimetabolites.

Hydrolysis. Esters, such as procaine, are hydrolyzed by a variety of nonspecific esterases in liver, plasma, gastrointestinal tract, and other tissues. Hydrolysis of amides, such as lidocaine, occurs primarily in the liver. Peptidases in plasma, erythrocytes, and many other tissues are involved in the biotransformation of the biologically active polypeptides.

Oxidation. Some drugs are oxidized by a variety of flavoprotein enzymes in mitochondria and cytosol of the liver and other tissues. Examples include the oxidation of alcohols and aldehydes by *alcohol and aldehyde dehydrogenases,* the purine antimetabolite 6-mercaptopurine by *xanthine oxidase,* and drugs related to the catecholamines by *tyrosine hydroxylase* and *monoamine oxidase.*

Reduction. Microsomal and nonmicrosomal enzymes in the liver and other tissues can catalyze the reduction of nitro groups and the cleavage and reduction of the azo linkage. Examples include the nitro reduction of chloramphenicol and the azo reduction of PRONTOSIL. However, reduction of nitro and azo compounds *in vivo* is probably catalyzed mainly by the intestinal flora in the anaerobic environment of the gut (Scheline, 1973).

EXCRETION OF DRUGS

Drugs are eliminated from the body either unchanged or as metabolites. Generally, the more polar compounds are excreted unchanged. The less polar, lipid-soluble drugs, however, are not readily eliminated until they are metabolized to more polar, less lipid-soluble compounds.

The kidney is the most important organ for elimination of drugs and their metabolites. Substances excreted in the feces are mainly unabsorbed orally ingested drugs or metabolites excreted in the bile and not reabsorbed from the intestinal tract. Excretion of drugs in milk is important not because of the amounts eliminated but because the excreted drugs are potential sources of unwanted pharmacological effects in the nursing infant. Pulmonary excretion is of importance mainly for the elimination of anesthetic gases and vapors (*see* Chapter 5); occasionally, small quantities of other drugs or metabolites are excreted by this route.

Renal Excretion. Excretion of drugs and metabolites in the urine involves three processes: glomerular filtration, active tubular secretion, and passive tubular reabsorption.

The amount of drug entering the tubular lumen by *filtration* is dependent on its fractional plasma protein binding and glomerular filtration rate. In the proximal renal tubule, certain organic anions and cations are added to the glomerular filtrate by active, carrier-mediated tubular *secretion.* Many organic acids, such as penicillin, and metabolites, such as glucuronides, are transported by the system that secretes naturally occurring substances such as uric acid; many organic bases, such as tetraethylammonium, are transported by another system that secretes choline, histamine, and other endogenous bases.

Both carrier systems are relatively nonselective, and organic ions of similar charge compete for transport. Both transport systems can also be bidirectional, and at least some drugs are both secreted and actively reabsorbed. However, transport of most exogenous ions is predominantly secretory. The outstanding example of the bidirectional tubular transport of an endogenous organic acid is uric acid. The characteristics of tubular transport systems are described in detail in Chapter 41.

In the proximal and distal tubules, the nonionized forms of weak acids and bases undergo net passive *reabsorption*. The concentration gradient for back diffusion is created by the reabsorption of water with sodium and other inorganic ions. Since the tubular cells are less permeable to the ionized forms of weak electrolytes, passive reabsorption of these substances is pH dependent. When the tubular urine is made more alkaline, weak acids are excreted more rapidly, primarily because they are more ionized and passive reabsorption is decreased. When the tubular urine is made more acid, the excretion of weak acids is reduced. Alkalinization and acidification of the urine have the opposite effects on the excretion of weak bases. In poisoning, the excretion of some drugs can be hastened by appropriate alkalinization or acidification of the urine. Whether alteration of urine pH results in significant change in drug elimination depends upon the extent and persistence of the pH change and the contribution of pH-dependent passive reabsorption to total drug elimination.

Biliary and Fecal Excretion. Many metabolites of drugs formed in the liver are excreted into the intestinal tract in the *bile*. These metabolites may be excreted in the feces; more commonly, they are reabsorbed into the blood and ultimately excreted in the urine. Both organic anions, including glucuronides, and organic cations are actively transported into bile by carrier systems similar to those that transport these substances across the renal tubule. Both transport systems are nonselective, and ions of like charge may compete for transport. Steroids and related substances are transported into bile by a third carrier system.

Excretion by Other Routes. Excretion of drugs into *sweat* and *saliva* is quantitatively unimportant.

Excretion by both routes is dependent mainly upon diffusion of the nonionized, lipid-soluble form of drugs through the epithelial cells of the glands and is pH dependent. Reabsorption of the nonionized drug from the primary secretion probably also occurs in the ducts of the glands, and active secretion of drugs across the ducts of the gland may also occur. Drugs excreted in the saliva enter the mouth, where they are usually swallowed. Their fate thereafter is the same as that of drugs taken orally.

The same principles apply to excretion of drugs in *milk*. Since milk is more acidic than plasma, basic compounds may be slightly concentrated in this fluid, and the concentration of acidic compounds in milk is lower than in plasma. Nonelectrolytes, such as ethanol and urea, readily enter milk and reach the same concentration as in plasma, independent of the pH of the milk. (*See* summary by Plaa, in La Du *et al.*, 1971.)

TIME COURSE OF DRUG EFFECT: PHARMACOKINETIC PRINCIPLES

Pharmacokinetic principles relate specifically to the variation with time of drug *concentration*, particularly in the blood, serum, or plasma. By extrapolation, they may be interpreted in terms of drug *effect*. Applied to therapy, pharmacokinetic principles aid in the selection and adjustment of drug dosage schedules and facilitate interpretation of measured serum concentrations of drugs. They are *not* a substitute for, but rather a supplement to, clinical monitoring and judgment.

Discussion in this section is limited to a summary of those fundamental pharmacokinetic principles that are conveniently applied to therapy.

Basic Concepts. Pharmacokinetic principles have wide utility as a guide to therapy. These principles are reliable, however, only if they are applied with appreciation of the assumptions upon which they are based. For example, the fundamental principles assume that the factors controlling drug elimination in the individual patient remain constant with time. Yet, drug elimination may change because of interaction with other drugs or following alterations in cardiovascular, renal, or hepatic function. Similarly, pharmacokinetic principles are most readily applied in terms of drug effect when effect is closely linked in time with drug concentration. However, the concentration-effect relationships for some drugs exhibit significant latency. These and other deviations from simple kinetic patterns must be recognized, and modifications of the fundamental principles must be adopted for specific drugs and for the individual patient.

The fundamental pharmacokinetic principles are based upon the most elementary kinetic *model.* The body is considered a *single compartment. Distribution* of the drug within the compartment is assumed to be relatively *uniform, or of no practical consequence if not uniform,* and to occur *rapidly* relative to absorption and elimination. For this model, *volume of distribution* of a drug is that in which it would *appear* to be distributed during the steady state, if it existed throughout that volume at the same concentration as in plasma. If a drug is highly concentrated in tissues, its *apparent volume of distribution* (V_d) may be many times total body water. Thus:

$$V_d = \frac{\text{Total amount of drug in body}}{\text{Concentration of drug in plasma}}$$

Absorption and elimination of the drug are assumed to follow *exponential (first-order)* kinetics; that is, a constant *fraction* of drug present is eliminated per unit of time. Elimination of most drugs is exponential, since drug concentrations usually do not approach those required for saturation of the elimination process. In certain exceptional cases, the drug elimination processes may become saturated, and zero-order kinetics will result; that is, a constant *amount* of the drug present is eliminated per unit of time.

The rate of an *exponential process* may be expressed by its *rate constant, k,* which expresses the *fractional change* per unit of time, or by its *half-time,* $t_{1/2}$, the time required for 50% completion of the process. The units of these two constants are time^{-1} and time, respectively. Both are independent of drug concentration (and dosage)—the hallmark of a first-order reaction. Simple calculations will reveal that the process is 93.75% complete after four half-times. A first-order rate constant and the half-time of the reaction are simply related ($kt_{1/2} = 0.693$) and may be interchanged accordingly. Total *body clearance* is the product of volume of distribution and elimination rate constant ($V_d k_e$) and expresses the volume of the V_d cleared per unit of time.

Single Doses. The time course of the plasma concentration of a hypothetical drug administered *intravenously* in a single dose is shown in Figure 1–4, *A.* As distribution of the drug occurs, the concentration falls rapidly. *Following* this initial distribution phase, the kinetics of drug elimination is apparent. Since first-order elimination kinetics dictates constant *fractional* drug loss per unit of time, a plot of the log of drug concentration versus time is linear during this phase (absorption is complete). The half-time for drug elimination can be accurately determined from such a graph. Furthermore, extrapolation of the first-order elimination line to the drug-concentration axis (time = 0) yields an estimate of the drug concentration that would have obtained if distribution were instantaneous. Since the total amount of drug is known at this "zero-time" (the dose administered), the apparent volume of distribution can be calculated from the dose and the concentration obtained by extrapolation.

An *effect* of a single dose of a drug may be characterized by its *latency, time of peak effect, magnitude of peak effect,* and *duration.* The influence of dosage and rates of absorption and elimination on these parameters is also illustrated in Figure 1–4.

Differences in rate of absorption (Figure 1–4, *B*), particularly the large differences that result from administration of a drug by different routes or in different dosage forms, have a significant influence on all characteristics of the time course of drug concentration (and effect). When absorption is rapid relative to elimination, differences in rate of absorption are of less consequence, peak effect approaches that achieved after intravenous administration, and latency and time of peak effect are determined primarily by the rate of absorption.

As *dosage* is increased (Figure 1–4, *C*), latency is reduced and the peak effect is increased without change in the time of peak effect. Duration of effect is increased proportionately less than peak effect. Reduced *elimination* (Figure 1–4, *D*) results in the expected prolongation of drug effect. If the drug is rapidly absorbed, differences in rate of elimination have relatively minor influence on peak effect. To minimize the consequences of interpatient differences in rates of absorption and elimination, when a choice

Figure 1–4. *Fundamental pharmacokinetic relationships for single doses of drugs.*

A. A drug (500 mg) is administered *intravenously* to a 65-kg man, and plasma samples are obtained for determination of drug concentration. The concentration falls rapidly initially, as distribution occurs. First-order elimination kinetics follows. Extrapolation of this line indicates a hypothetical plasma concentration of 12 μg/ml at zero-time. The V_d is thus 500/0.012, or 41.7 l. This is indicative of distribution in total body water or drug sequestration at some nonplasma site. The half-time of drug elimination is estimated to be 3 hours.

B. *Varied Absorption.* Patterns to illustrate the influence of absorption (*a*) 100 times as rapid as, (*b*) ten times as rapid as, and (*c*) equal to elimination.

C. *Varied Dosage.* Patterns to illustrate the influence of a twofold difference in dosage (absorption ten times as rapid as elimination).

D. *Varied Elimination.* Patterns to illustrate the influence of a twofold difference in rate of elimination (lower curve, absorption:elimination = 10:1; upper curve, absorption:elimination = 10:0.5).

Graphs B, C, and D are based upon the elementary one-compartment model:

$$C_t = \frac{fD}{V_d}\left(\frac{k_a}{k_a - k_e}\right)[\exp(-k_e t) - \exp(-k_a t)]$$

where C_t = concentration of drug in plasma (mg/l) at time t, D = dose (mg), f = fractional absorption, V_d = volume of distribution (l), k_a = absorption rate constant (time^{-1}), and k_e = elimination rate constant (time^{-1}).

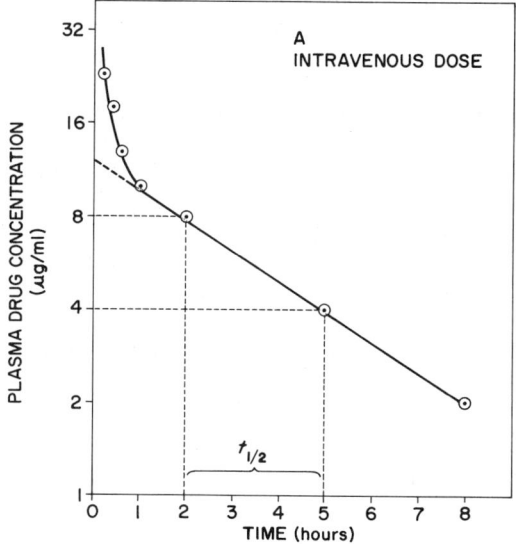

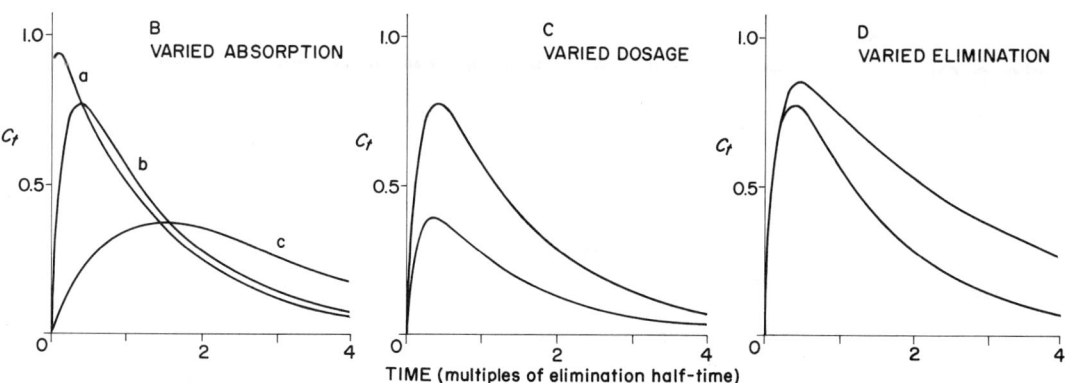

TIME (multiples of elimination half-time)

is possible, drug dosage forms and routes of administration that provide for rapid absorption should generally be preferred.

Repeated Doses. Since more than four half-times are required for complete exponential elimination, repeated administration of any drug at intervals shorter than this *must result in drug accumulation.* Drug accumulation will continue until the amount of drug eliminated per dose interval equals the amount administered per dose. When first-order elimination kinetics is followed, elimination of drug will increase as drug accumulation occurs, since a constant *fraction* of drug is eliminated per unit of time. Repeated administration of a drug is characterized by the *time course* of accumulation, the *extent* of accumulation, and the *fluctuations* between doses. The elimination half-time of a drug is an important determinant of all three characteristics. Administration of a drug at intervals equal to its elimination half-time is a convenient base for comparison of other dosage schedules.

If a drug is administered intermittently at constant intervals (that are short enough so that complete elimination is not achieved) or by constant intravenous infusion, it accumulates exponentially to a plateau, with a half-time equal to its elimination half-time (Figure 1-5). One thus attains 94% of the theoretical plateau value after four half-times. The *time* to attain the plateau is dependent *only* on the half-time for elimination, and this dependence of time course of drug accumulation on its elimination half-time is termed the *plateau principle*. It applies

not only to the initial accumulation of a drug but also to any increase or decrease from one plateau state to another, whether produced by a change in dosage or a change in elimination half-time.

The drug concentrations maintained during the plateau state are directly proportional to the total amount of drug given per unit of time (expressed as dose/dosage interval) and to the elimination half-time for the drug. These determinants may also be conceptualized as the amount of the individual dose and the number of such dosages given per half-time. (*See* legend for Figure 1-5.) When a drug is administered at intervals *equal to its elimination half-time,* the *average concentration* during the plateau state is about 1.5 times (actually 1.44 times) the peak concen-

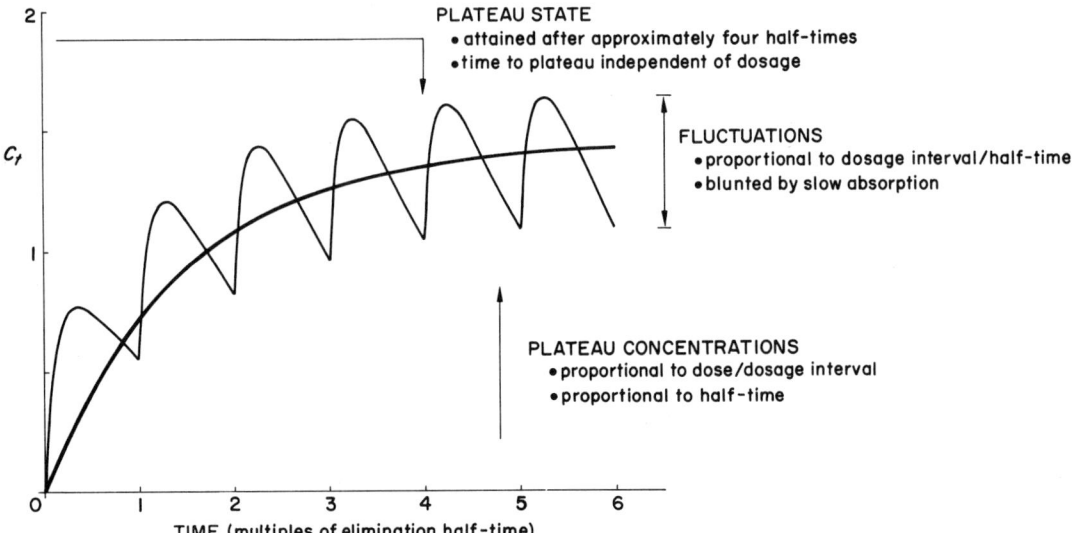

Figure 1-5. *Fundamental pharmacokinetic relationships for repeated administration of drugs.*

Light line is the pattern of drug accumulation during repeated administration of a drug at intervals equal to its elimination half-time, when drug absorption is ten times as rapid as elimination. As the relative rate of absorption increases, the concentration maxima approach 2 and the minima approach 1 during the plateau state. Heavy line depicts the pattern during administration of equivalent dosage by continuous intravenous infusion. Curves are based upon the elementary one-compartment model.

Average concentration ($\bar{C}_p$) when the *plateau state* is attained during intermittent drug administration:

$$\bar{C}_p = \frac{fD}{V_d k_e T} = \frac{1.44\, t_{1/2} fD}{V_d T}$$

where $t_{1/2}$ = elimination half-time (time), T = dosage interval (time), and other symbols are as indicated in Figure 1-4. By substitution of infusion rate for D/T, the formula also provides the concentration maintained during the plateau state during continuous intravenous infusion. Note that both $t_{1/2}$ and dosage interval must be expressed in identical units of time.

tration after the initial dose of the drug. If a drug has a half-time of 9 days and is administered once daily, it will therefore accumulate to an average concentration of 1.44 × 9, or 13 times that present after the first dose, and over 1 month will be required to achieve this result. These principles should be appreciated if the physician is to make rational decisions about dosage regimens.

For any given dosage, the average drug concentration during the plateau state is directly proportional to elimination half-time. Thus, if rates of elimination of a particular drug in a group of patients are known to vary by a factor of, say, sixfold, average drug concentrations during the plateau state in patients receiving the same dosage will differ by this same factor. Conversely, drug dosage will vary by this factor, if dosage is adjusted to provide the same average plateau concentration in all patients.

The fluctuations between doses during the plateau state are proportional to the ratio of the dosage interval and elimination half-time and are damped by slow absorption. When a rapidly absorbed drug is administered at intervals equal to its elimination half-time, the ratio of peak to minimum concentrations between doses approaches twofold. Half-doses at half-intervals will maintain the same average concentration with smaller fluctuations, an important achievement if the margin of safety of the drug is small.

Average drug concentration maintained during the plateau state is a function of maintenance dosage (dose/dosage interval), volume of distribution, and elimination half-time (Figure 1–5). If volume of distribution and elimination half-time are known, the appropriate maintenance dosage to sustain the desired concentration is readily calculated. Volume of distribution and elimination half-time are sometimes combined into a single factor identified as total body clearance or, simply, as the factor that relates plateau drug concentration and maintenance dosage.

Choice of Dosage Interval. Dosage interval should be selected primarily by consideration of the fluctuations in drug concentration that can be tolerated without excessive toxicity or loss of efficacy. On this basis, a dosage interval equal to or less than the elimination half-time is recommended

for most drugs. However, longer intervals may be satisfactory if larger fluctuations can be tolerated, or if the drug is slowly absorbed. In addition, choice of dosage interval must sometimes be tempered by consideration of patient convenience and compliance. For example, the penicillins in aqueous solution are often administered at intervals much greater than their half-times because a satisfactory effect can be achieved without toxicity despite the large fluctuations, and because the schedule is convenient for the patient.

Initial Loading Dose. When a drug is administered on a dosage schedule that is ultimately satisfactory for maintenance therapy, partial effect may occur promptly, but the full therapeutic and toxic effects of medication are necessarily delayed for the inevitable four elimination half-times. This may be a long time, indeed. If the therapeutic situation is not critical, such a dosage schedule may be preferred, since it minimizes the risk of excessive initial effect and permits adequate adjustment of dosage for the individual patient during the period of drug accumulation. If the desired full effect must be achieved more promptly, an initial so-called loading dose larger than the subsequent maintenance dose must be employed. It should be obvious, however, that if a dose larger than that required for maintenance is continued, accumulation will result and toxicity is the rule. If the dose given is only moderately greater than that required and if the elimination half-time is long, this toxicity may not become evident for an extended period of time. An estimated loading dose should be administered in divided fractions to permit at least some monitoring for efficacy and safety. Plateau concentrations during subsequent maintenance dosage are independent of the loading dose after the usual four half-times. Initial *total* loading dose (D^*), maintenance dosage (D/T; e.g., 100 mg/8 hr or 300 mg/24 hr), and elimination half-time ($t_{1/2}$, in the same units of time) are related as follows: $D^* = 1.4\, t_{1/2}\, D/T$. Arguments for and against an initial loading dose are further discussed in connection with various therapeutic agents, especially the cardiac glycosides, the antiarrhythmic drugs, and the oral anticoagulant agents (*see* Index).

Dose-Dependent Drug Elimination. Aspirin and phenytoin are examples of drugs that exhibit so-called dose-dependent elimination in the therapeutic range. As drug concentration (dosage) increases, elimination half-time and the time required to attain the plateau state also increase. In addition, plasma drug concentrations (and drug effects) during the plateau state increase disproportionately with increase in dosage. This pattern of deviation from simple kinetics is expected if the concentration of the drug approaches that required for saturation of the elimination process. Further increases in dosage result in no further increase in the rate of elimination (zero-order kinetics). Similar deviation can occur if a metabolite of the drug inhibits its elimination. Saturation of carrier-mediated uptake of the drug by the liver and changes in fractional oral absorption or fractional plasma protein binding are the basis of other patterns of dose-dependent deviation from simple first-order kinetics.

Adjustment of Dosage Schedules for Impaired Elimination.

To prevent excessive accumulation of a drug when its elimination is reduced in a patient with impaired renal, hepatic, or cardiovascular function, maintenance dosage (dose/dosage interval) must be reduced in proportion to the increase in elimination half-time. Whether the adjustment is accomplished by reducing the dose, increasing the dosage interval, or both depends upon the usual considerations of fluctuations and convenience. Since the therapeutic concentration desired has nothing to do with the rate of elimination, the initial loading dose need *not* be reduced for altered elimination *if the drug is rapidly absorbed,* but loading dose must be adjusted for altered volume of distribution. Plasma protein concentration and binding, factors in volume of distribution, may be reduced in both renal and hepatic disease. Volume of distribution may also be altered in patients with congestive heart disease. In patients with reduced renal function, consideration must be given not only to drugs excreted unchanged in the urine but also to renal elimination of metabolites of drugs.

Adjustment of dosage schedules on the basis of pharmacokinetic principles, whether estimated by rule of thumb or by computer, is necessarily only an approximation; final adjustment must be made on the basis of the usual patient monitoring, including measurement of serum drug concentrations, if feasible.

Adjustment of dosage schedules for patients with *impaired renal function* is reasonably satisfactory.

Drug elimination by the kidney is correlated with endogenous creatinine clearance, serum creatinine concentration, and blood urea nitrogen concentration. These indices of renal function (listed in order of decreasing preference) provide an estimate of the necessary adjustment. Formulas, graphs, nomographs, and computer programs have been devised for adjustment of dosage schedules for individual drugs, including the cardiac glycosides and aminoglycoside antibiotics. The following simple formula, proposed by Giusti and Hayton (1973), appears to provide a suitable approximation of the adjustment for all drugs:

$$G = 1 - f\left(1 - \frac{C_{Cr}^r}{C_{Cr}}\right)$$

where G is the fraction of the usual maintenance dose that may be administered at usual dosage intervals, f is the fraction of the drug excreted unchanged in the urine in patients with normal renal function, C_{Cr} is normal endogenous creatinine clearance, and C_{Cr}^r is endogenous creatinine clearance measured in the patient or estimated from serum creatinine concentration. Alternatively, $1/G$ is the factor by which the dosage interval should be increased, if the choice is to administer usual doses of the drug at longer intervals. The formula does *not* include adjustment for possible changes in plasma protein binding or volume of distribution.

Adjustment of dosage schedules for patients with *impaired hepatic function* is difficult, since hepatic drug elimination is not consistently correlated with any of the routine hepatic function tests. In addition, CNS depressants and other drugs can precipitate encephalopathy in the cirrhotic patient for reasons other than excessive accumulation of the drug secondary to reduced drug elimination. The possibility of developing a simple test for hepatic drug-metabolizing activity that has predictive value for a variety of drugs is under active investigation. Monitoring of drug concentrations in serum is a more direct approach to adjusting dosage schedules for patients with liver disease, when such tests are available. When necessary, one must in essence determine the half-time of elimination for the patient in question and then apply the fundamental principles already discussed.

Monitoring of Drug Concentrations in Serum.

Monitoring of drug concentrations in serum is particularly helpful in the use of drugs such as the antiepileptic agents, which are not readily monitored by direct clinical observation or other laboratory tests, and especially when these drugs are characterized by marked interpatient pharmacokinetic variation. This procedure is also a useful supplement to other monitoring in patients with impaired renal or hepatic function and whenever medication is unexpectedly ineffective or toxic. In addition, the patient's compliance may be improved merely by his knowing that drug concentrations are to be measured.

Serum drug concentrations are a reliable guide to therapy, however, only if the observations are interpreted in concert with other clinical information and with appropriate precautions. Serial measurements at selected intervals are always more useful than isolated determinations. Interpretation must include regard for the kinetic pattern for the particular drug, the interval between time of sampling and the last drug administration, and the plateau principle. Additional factors that must be considered include reliability of the analytical procedure, individual variation in serum concentrations associated with desired and undesired effects, possible active metabolites of the drug, factors that modify its concentration-effect relationship, concurrent medication, and possible drug tolerance. Finally, it must be recognized that the measured drug concentrations in serum, unless stated otherwise, represent both protein-bound and free drug. Potentially important differences in fractional binding of the drug are not detected by the usual measurements.

Studies with many drugs have shown that certain apparent variations in drug potency among different species and different individuals are due primarily to variations in the rate of drug disposition. When dosage is adjusted so that equivalent serum concentrations are maintained, quantitative differences in response tend to disappear. This is obviously important for the establishment of optimal dosage for the individual patient (*see* Brodie and Reid, 1967).

II. Pharmacodynamics

THE DOSE-EFFECT RELATIONSHIP

Ideally, the relationship between dose and effect is based upon the effects attained under equilibrium conditions. However, in practice, the dose-effect relationship is commonly derived from the peak effects after single doses of the drug. There is no single characteristic relationship between intensity of drug effect and drug dosage. A dose-effect curve may be linear, concave upward, concave downward, or sigmoid. Moreover, if the observed effect is the composite of several effects of the drug, such as the change in

blood pressure produced by a combination of cardiac, vascular, and reflex effects, the dose-effect curve need not be monotonic. However, a composite dose-effect curve can usually be resolved into simple curves for each of its components; and simple dose-effect curves, whatever their precise shape, can be viewed as having four characterizing parameters: potency, slope, maximal efficacy, and variability. These are illustrated in Figure 1-6 for the common sigmoid log

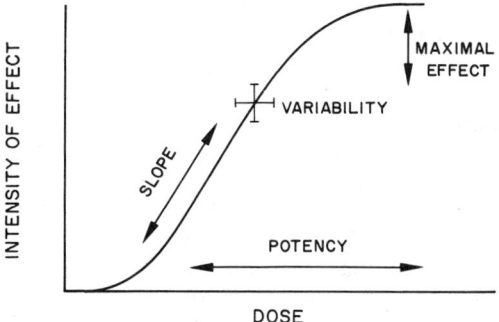

Figure 1-6. *The log dose-effect relationship.*

Representative log dose-effect curve, illustrating its four characterizing parameters (*see* text for explanation).

dose-effect curve. The logarithmic transformation of dosage is often employed for the dose-effect relationship, because it permits display of a wide range of doses on a single graph and because it has certain mathematical advantages when dose-effect curves are compared.

Potency. The location of its dose-effect curve along the *dose axis* is an expression of the potency of a drug. Potency is influenced by the absorption, distribution, biotransformation, and excretion of a drug, as well as being determined by its inherent ability to combine with its receptors. Potency is a relatively unimportant characteristic of a drug, since it makes little difference whether the effective dose of a drug is 1 μg or 100 mg, as long as the drug can be administered in appropriate dosage. Potency is not necessarily correlated with any other characteristic of a drug, and there is no justification for the view that the more potent of two drugs is clinically superior. Low potency is a disadvantage only if the effective dose is so large that it is awkward to administer. Extremely potent drugs, particularly if they are volatile or are absorbed through the skin, may be hazardous and may require special handling.

For therapeutic applications, the potency of a drug is necessarily stated in *absolute* dosage units (25 µg, 10 mg/kg, etc.); for comparison of drugs, *relative potency*, the ratio of equieffective doses (1/10 ×, 5 ×, etc.) is a more convenient expression.

Slope. While the slope of the more-or-less linear, central portion of the dose-effect curve is usually of more theoretical than practical importance, it can have therapeutic significance. For example, a steep dose-effect curve for a CNS depressant implies that there is a small ratio between the dose that produces coma and that which causes mild sedation, and that excessive or inadequate effect may occur if the dose of the drug is not carefully adjusted. Nevertheless, many factors influence the margin of safety of a drug and the variability of its effects, and these characteristics of a drug are properly expressed by methods that summarize the contributions of all factors (*see* below). It should be noted that doubling the dose of a drug does not necessarily produce twice the effect, and the quantitative relationships between dose and effect should not be confused in this manner.

The significance of the slope and shape of the dose-effect curve in analysis of drug action is beyond the scope of the present discussion. However, it deserves passing mention that mere parallelism of their log dose-effect curves is not a reliable basis for concluding that different drugs produce their effects by the same mechanism.

Maximal Efficacy. The maximal effect produced by a drug is referred to as its *maximal efficacy* or, simply, *efficacy*. Maximal efficacy of a drug may be determined by its inherent properties and be reflected as a plateau in the dose-effect curve, but it may also be imposed by other factors. If the undesired effects of a drug limit its dosage, its efficacy will be correspondingly limited, even though it is inherently capable of producing a greater effect. Maximal efficacy of a drug is clearly one of its major characteristics. One of many important differences between morphine and aspirin is the difference in their efficacy. The opioid provides relief of pain of nearly all intensities, whereas the salicylate is effective only against mild-to-moderate pain.

Efficacy and potency of a drug are not necessarily correlated, and these two characteristics of a drug should not be confused.

Biological Variation. The more important factors that modify drug effect are summarized later in this chapter. However, even when all known sources of variation are controlled or taken into account, drug effects are never identical in all patients, or even in a given patient on different occasions. A dose-effect curve applies only to a single individual at one time or to the average individual. The intersecting brackets in Figure 1–6 indicate that biological variation of the dose-effect relationship can be visualized in either of two ways. The vertical bracket expresses the fact that a range of effects will be produced if a given dose of a drug is administered to a group of individuals; alternatively, the horizontal bracket expresses the fact that a range of doses is required to produce a specified intensity of effect in all individuals.

Dose-Percent Curve. The dose of a drug required to produce a specified effect in an individual is termed the *individual effective dose*. This is a *quantal* rather than a graded response, since the specified effect is either present or absent. Individual effective doses of most drugs are lognormally distributed, which means that the familiar *normal curve* of variation is obtained if the logarithms of the individual effective doses for a group of patients are expressed as a frequency distribution (Figure 1–7, *A*). A cumulative frequency distribution of individual effective doses, that is, the percentage of individuals that exhibit the effect plotted as a function of logarithm of dose, is known as a dose-percent curve or a quantal dose-effect curve. This is the integrated form of the normal frequency distribution. Although also a sigmoid curve, the dose-percent curve is an expression of individual variability for a single effect and has a slightly different meaning from the graded dose-effect curve discussed above. However, the graded dose-effect curve can be viewed similarly as representing the integral (summation) of a large number of quantal (molecular) responses.

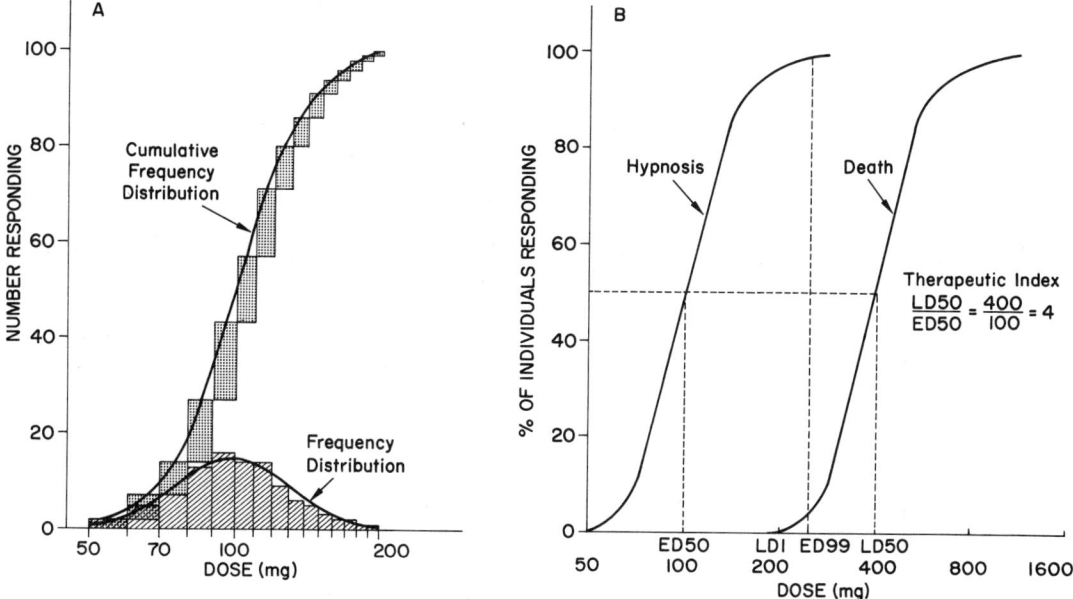

Figure 1-7. *Frequency distribution curves and quantal dose-effect curves.*

A. An experiment was performed on 100 subjects and the effective dose to produce a quantal response was determined for each individual. The number of subjects who required each dose is plotted, giving a lognormal frequency distribution (bars with diagonal lines). The stippled bars demonstrate that the normal frequency distribution, when summated, yields the cumulative frequency distribution—a sigmoidal curve that is a quantal dose-effect curve.

B. Quantal Dose-Effect Curves. Animals were injected with varying doses of a sedative-hypnotic, and the responses determined and plotted (*see* text for additional explanation).

The dose of a drug required to produce a specified intensity of effect in 50% of individuals is known as the *median effective dose* and is abbreviated ED50 (*not* ED_{50}) (Figure 1-7, *B*). If death is the end point, the median effective dose is termed the *median lethal dose* (LD50). The doses required to produce the stated effect in other percentages of the population are similarly expressed (ED20, LD90, etc.). Similar notations are also often used to refer to the dose of a drug required to produce a stated fraction of the maximal effect or a stated intensity of effect. These conflicting uses of the same abbreviations should not be confused.

Population variation requires consideration of the significance of ED99 and LD1. If variation is marked, these doses may overlap even though the ED50 and LD50 differ by a wide margin (*see* below).

Terminology. Specific terms are used to refer to individuals who are unusually sensitive or unusually resistant to a drug, and to describe those in whom a drug produces an unusual effect.

If a drug produces its usual effect at unexpectedly low dosage, the individual is said to be *hyperreactive.* Increased sensitivity to the usual effects of a drug should not be described as *hypersensitivity,* since this term is usually used to refer to the pattern of effects associated with drug allergy. Hyperreactivity to a drug should be termed *supersensitivity* only if the increased sensitivity is the result of denervation. If a drug produces its usual effect only at unusually large dosage, the individual is said to be *hyporeactive.* Decreased sensitivity is also described as *tolerance,* but this term has the connotation of hyporeactivity acquired as the result of prior exposure to the drug. Tolerance that develops rapidly after administration of only a few doses of a drug is termed *tachyphylaxis.* Reduced sensitivity should be described as *immunity* only if the acquired tolerance is the result of antibody formation.

An *unusual effect* of a drug, of whatever intensity and irrespective of dosage, that occurs in only a small percentage of individuals is often termed *idiosyncrasy*. However, this term is frequently considered a synonym for drug allergy and has so many other connotations that it probably should be abandoned. Unusual effects of drugs have also been called *meta reactions,* but this term has not gained wide acceptance. Perhaps unusual effects of drugs are best described as such or by terms that refer to the underlying mechanism; they are often types of drug allergy or a consequence of genetic differences.

Selectivity. A drug is usually described by its most prominent effect or by the action thought to be the basis of that effect. However, such descriptions should not obscure the fact that *no drug produces only a single effect.* Morphine is correctly described as an analgesic, but it also suppresses cough and causes sedation, respiratory depression, constipation, bronchiolar constriction, release of histamine, antidiuresis, and a variety of other effects. A drug is adequately characterized only in terms of its full *spectrum of effects.* The relationship between the doses of a drug required to produce undesired and desired effects is termed its *therapeutic index, margin of safety,* or *selectivity.* Rarely is a drug sufficiently selective to be described as being *specific.* For therapeutic applications, selectivity of a drug is clearly one of its more important characteristics.

In clinical studies, drug selectivity is often expressed indirectly by summarizing the pattern and incidence of adverse effects produced by therapeutic doses of the drug and by indicating the proportion of patients who were forced to decrease drug dosage or discontinue medication because of adverse effects. These indirect procedures are often adequate, but comparison of dose-effect curves for desired and undesired effects is more consistently meaningful and is preferred whenever feasible (Figure 1–7, *B*).

In laboratory studies, therapeutic index is usually defined as the ratio between the median toxic dose and the median effective dose (TD50/ED50) or the median lethal dose and median effective dose (LD50/ED50). Because the ideal drug produces its desired effect in all patients without causing toxic effects in any, and because dose-percent curves need

not be parallel, it can be logically argued that therapeutic index should be defined as the ratio between the minimum toxic dose and the maximum effective dose. However, minimum and maximum toxic and effective doses cannot be estimated with precision, particularly in the variable human population with which medical practice is concerned.

A drug does not have a single therapeutic index, but many. The margin of safety of aspirin for relief of headache is greater than its margin of safety for relief of arthritic pain, since the latter use requires larger dosage. Similarly, several therapeutic indices can be calculated for each desired effect. A synthetic opioid may cause less constipation than morphine and yet afford no advantage over the parent compound with regard to respiratory depression or sedation. Moreover, a drug may be selective within one context yet still be nonselective within another. The antihistamines are correctly described as selective antagonists of histamine, yet none of these drugs produces this selective peripheral effect without also causing significant central sedation. Finally, a drug may be correctly described as having an adequate margin of safety in most patients, but this description is meaningless for the patient who exhibits an unusual response to the drug. Penicillin is essentially nontoxic in the great majority of patients, yet it can cause death in those who have become allergic to it.

Biological Assay. Alkaloids and other highly purified drugs obtained from plants and animals can usually be standardized by their chemical or physical properties. However, drugs that are only partially purified, such as certain digitalis preparations and various hormones, vitamins, antibiotics, and vaccines, must be standardized by their biological properties. The estimation of the relative potencies of such preparations by comparison of their biochemical, pharmacological, or toxic effects is termed *biological assay* or, simply, *bioassay.* A dose-effect curve is determined for the preparation under study and is compared with that of a *reference standard.* The reference standard is usually a highly purified, often crystalline, preparation of the substance being assayed. The potency of a preparation standardized by biological assay is usually expressed in units, or weight equivalent, of the reference standard. Official drugs have legally required methods of assay, and both the assay procedure and the reference standard are rigidly defined. These are often the same as those specified by an appropriate international committee. Nonofficial preparations that are assayed by different methods or against different reference standards may vary considerably in relative potency.

MECHANISMS OF DRUG ACTION

The most fundamental aspect of pharmacodynamics is that which deals with the mechanisms of drug action. Before summarizing some general concepts pertaining to this fascinating subject, it is essential to emphasize the distinction between drug action and drug effect. It is also helpful clearly to define the objectives of analysis of drug action.

Although often considered as synonyms, the terms *action* and *effect* have useful pharmacological connotations that should be preserved. Most drugs produce their effects by combining with enzymes, cell membranes, or other specialized functional components of cells. Drug-cell interaction alters the function of the cell component and thereby initiates the series of biochemical and physiological changes that are characteristic of the drug. Only the initial consequence of drug-cell combination is correctly termed the *action* of the drug; the remaining events are properly called drug *effects*.

The objectives of analysis of drug action are identification of the primary action, delineation of the details of the chemical reaction between drug and cell, and characterization of the full action-effects sequence. Only the complete analysis provides a truly satisfactory basis for the therapeutic use of the drug.

Structure-Activity Relationship.

The actions of a drug are intimately related to its chemical structure. The relationship is frequently quite stringent, and relatively minor modifications in the drug molecule may result in major changes in pharmacological properties. Exploitation of structure-activity relationship has at times led to the synthesis of valuable therapeutic agents. Since changes in molecular configuration need not alter all actions and effects of a drug equally, it is sometimes possible to develop a *congener* with a more favorable therapeutic index or more acceptable secondary characteristics than those of the parent drug. In addition, effective therapeutic agents have been fashioned by developing structurally related competitive antagonists of other drugs or of endogenous substances known to be important in biochemical or physiological function.

Sometimes the structure-activity relationship appears quite broad. For example, many chemically dissimilar drugs exhibit local anesthetic activity, and compounds of totally different chemical structure produce similar CNS depressant effects. These examples do not negate the significance of the structure-activity relationship. They do, however, emphasize that much remains to be learned of the basic mechanisms of action of most drugs and that overtly similar effects may be produced by more than a single mechanism.

Drug Receptors.

The cell component directly involved in the initial action of a drug is usually termed its *receptive substance* or, simply, its *receptor*. The chemical groups that participate in drug-receptor combination and the adjacent portions of the receptor that favor or hinder access of the drug to these active groups are known as *receptor groups* or *receptor sites*. Drug-cell interactions that do not initiate drug action, such as the binding of drugs to plasma and cell proteins and to enzymes concerned with biotransformation and transport of drugs, are said to involve *secondary receptors, silent receptors,* or *storage sites*.

Receptors and Theories of Drug Action. As early as 1878, even before he coined the term *receptive substance,* Langley suggested that drug-cell combinations, and hence the actions and effects of drugs, were probably governed by the law of mass action. This view was extensively developed by A. J. Clark in the 1920s, and it remains the keystone of most theories of drug action. Thus, drug-receptor kinetic theory borrows freely from that developed for enzyme action, and the two obviously coalesce when drug effect results from a direct interaction with an enzyme.

For certain applications of receptor theory, it is necessary to assume some relationship between drug-receptor interaction and intensity of drug effect. In the classical receptor theory developed by Clark, it was assumed that drug effect is proportional to the fraction of receptors occupied by drug, and that maximal effect results when all receptors are occupied. While these assumptions are probably true in some cases, exceptions may be the rule. Subsequent modifications of *occupation theory* have assumed other relationships between receptor occupation and drug effect and have permitted the possibility that maximal effect may be achieved when only a critical portion of receptors is occupied. The latter concept is described as that of *spare receptors* or *receptor reserve*.

Still other modifications of receptor theory consider the possibilities that certain receptors may have multiple active sites or other drug binding (allosteric) sites. These sites may not act independently, and drug attachment at one point may alter the affinity for binding or reaction characteristics of agonists or antagonists at other locations. An interesting *rate theory* has also been proposed in which it is suggested that drug effect is a function not of receptor occupation but of the rate of drug-receptor combination. It should be pointed out that different kinetic descriptions (or receptor theories) may be required when there are fundamental differences in the mechanism of drug action. Thus, these theories are not mutually exclusive, and each may be true for individual situations.

Although receptors for most drugs have yet to be identified, there is little doubt that drug-cell combinations that obey mass-law kinetics are involved in drug actions. The many discrete relationships between chemical structure and biological activity and the competitive interaction of chemically similar drugs are difficult to explain except in these terms. Receptor groups, like the active centers of enzymes, are thought to be carboxyl, amino, sulfhydryl, phosphate, and similar reactive groups spatially oriented in a pattern complementary to that of the drugs with which they react. The binding of drugs to receptors, in various cases, involves all known types of bonds—ionic, hydrogen, van der Waals, and covalent. In most interactions it is likely that combinations of forces are involved.

Quantitative Descriptions of Drug Action. A drug that combines with a receptor, has an action, and initiates a sequence of effects is termed an *agonist*. If one assumes that such a drug interacts reversibly with its receptor and that the resultant effect is proportional to the number of receptors occupied, the following reaction equation can be written.

$$\text{Drug } (D) + \text{Receptor } (R) \underset{k_2}{\overset{k_1}{\rightleftharpoons}} DR \longrightarrow \text{Effect}$$

This reaction sequence is analogous to the interaction of substrate with enzyme, and the magnitude of effect can be analyzed in a manner similar to that for enzymatic product formation.

The applicable equation is identical in form with the Michaelis-Menten equation:

$$\text{Effect} = \frac{\text{Maximal Effect } (D)}{K_D + (D)}$$

where (D) = free drug concentration and K_D is the dissociation constant for the drug-receptor complex. This equation describes a simple rectangular hyperbola. There is no effect at $(D) = 0$; the effect is half-maximal when $(D) = K_D$, that is, when half of the receptors are occupied; the maximal effect is approached asymptotically as (D) increases above K_D. If the effect is plotted against log (D), the familiar sigmoidal dose-effect curve results (Figure 1–6).

Since straight lines greatly facilitate analysis of data, simple means have been devised to write a linear form of this equation. A linear relationship is obtained by taking the reciprocal of both sides of the expression and constructing the equivalent of a Lineweaver-Burk plot for enzyme kinetics:

$$\frac{1}{\text{Effect}} = \frac{K_D}{\text{Max. Effect } (D)} + \frac{1}{\text{Max. Effect}}$$

A plot of 1/Effect versus $1/(D)$ yields a straight line that intersects the Y-axis at 1/(Max. Effect) and that has a slope equal to K_D/(Max. Effect). Extrapolation of this line to the X-axis yields the value of the intercept, easily shown to be $-1/K_D$ (Figure 1–8, *A*). Thus, values for K_D and for the maximal effect can be readily calculated from such a plot. This representation is particularly useful for the analysis of drug antagonism.

Certain drugs interact with the receptor or with other components of the effector mechanism to inhibit the action of an agonist, while initiating no effect themselves. Such drugs are termed *antagonists*.

If the inhibition can be overcome by increasing the concentration of the agonist, ultimately achieving the same maximal effect, the antagonist is said to be *surmountable* or *competitive*. While this type of inhibition is commonly observed with antagonists that act reversibly at the receptor site, it will also result from reversible or irreversible interaction of the antagonist at other sites so that the affinity of the receptor for the agonist is altered. A conformational alteration of the receptor, with a reduction in affinity, could result from an action of an antagonist at a remote site. Since the maximal effect can still be achieved if sufficient agonist is used, the double reciprocal plots of agonist alone versus agonist plus competitive antagonist *must* meet at the 1/Effect axis, where the concentration of agonist is infinite. The lines diverge at lower agonist concentrations; the apparent affinity of agonist for receptor is lowered (Figure 1–8, *B*). In the presence of a competitive antagonist, the log dose-effect curve for the agonist is shifted to the right (Figure 1–8, *C*). The maximal efficacy is unaltered, but the agonist appears to be less potent.

A noncompetitive antagonist *prevents* the agonist from producing any effect at a given receptor site. This could result from irreversible interaction of the antagonist at any site to prevent binding of agonist. It would also follow reversible or irreversible interaction with any component of the system so as to prevent the successful initiation of effect following the binding of agonist. These results may be conceptualized as *removal* of receptor or response potential from the system. The maximal effect possible is reduced, but agonist can act normally at receptor-effector units not so influenced. The affinity of the agonist for the receptor and its potency are thus unaltered. The double reciprocal plot shows intersection of agonist and antagonist plus agonist lines on the $1/(D)$ axis at $-1/K_D$ (the affinity is unaltered). The maximal effect is different (Figure 1–8, *B*). Similarly, the log dose-effect curves show unaltered potency and reduced efficacy (Figure 1–8, *C*).

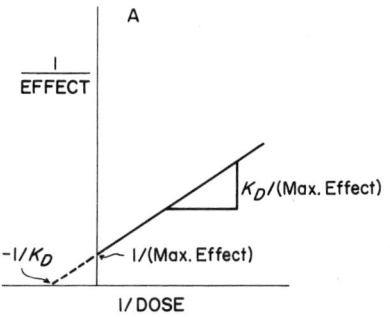

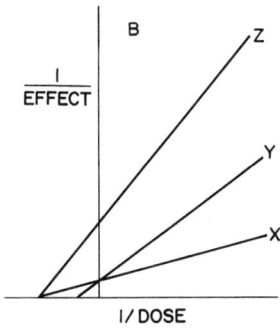

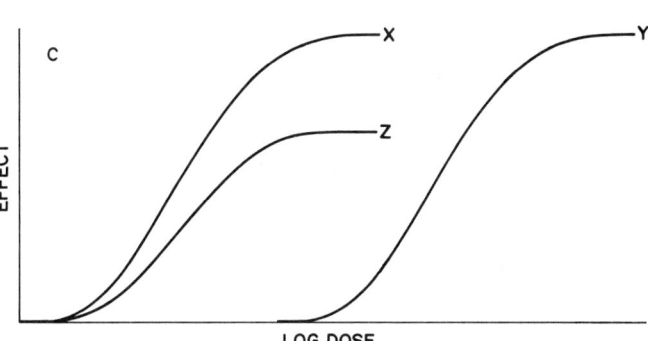

Figure 1–8. *Different representations of dose-effect curves, illustrating typical relationships between agonists and antagonists.*

A. A double-reciprocal plot of the concentration dependence of drug effect (*see* text for explanation).

B and C. Representative double-reciprocal plots (*B*) and log dose-effect curves (*C*).

Curves X and Y. Two agonists with similar efficacy but differing in potency (X more potent than Y) *or* an agonist in the absence (X) and presence (Y) of a competitive antagonist.

Curves X and Z. Two agonists with similar potency but differing in efficacy (full agonist, X, and partial agonist, Z) *or* an agonist in the absence (X) and presence (Z) of a noncompetitive antagonist.

Antagonists may thus be classified as acting reversibly or irreversibly. If the antagonist binds at the active site for the agonist, reversible antagonists will be competitive and irreversible antagonists will be noncompetitive. If binding is elsewhere, however, these simple rules do not hold, and any combination is possible.

When two drugs bind at the same site, why can one be an agonist and the other produce no effect—acting as an antagonist because of its presence? This question cannot be answered with precision, but it is assumed that fundamental differences in the physicochemical nature of the interaction must be operative. For example, fruitful interaction of receptor and agonist may produce a conformational change in the receptor (the drug action) necessary for the initiation of a sequence of effects. A corresponding change presumably does not result with the antagonist, even though binding occurs. Is this a quantal difference, or should not some compounds exhibit partial agonistic activity? This possibility is true in at least some cases; a *partial agonist* thus acts on the same receptor as does the agonist, but produces less than a maximal effect (Figure 1–8, *C*). If a partial agonist occupies a functionally significant fraction of the receptors, it will antagonize the actions of an agonist, while potentially producing little effect itself.

It is obvious that something less than a simple receptor-occupancy theory is involved, in that antagonists and partial agonists occupy receptors and do not produce maximal effects. It is thus necessary to extend the concept of *efficacy* to connote the *intrinsic activity* of drugs acting at the same receptor site. This concept can be quantified by the insertion

of a drug-dependent rate constant, k_3, in the fundamental equation:

$$D + R \underset{k_2}{\overset{k_1}{\rightleftharpoons}} DR \xrightarrow{k_3} \text{Effect}$$

For an antagonist, $k_3 = 0$.

The use of the word *efficacy* can, at times, be confusing. While an antagonist has no efficacy in this sense as an initiator of an action-effects sequence, it may have great therapeutic efficacy when used as an antagonist.

Even if the *action* of an agonist at a receptor site is proportional to its efficacy and to the number of receptor sites occupied, additional complications frequently make difficult the quantitative interpretation of the dose dependence of effect. This is particularly true when the drug-receptor interaction is but one event in a complex sequence of reactions ultimately resulting in an observable effect. For example, while occupancy of a certain number of receptors by agonist may initially lead to response, a later step in the pathway may become rate limiting at this stimulated level of function. Further receptor occupancy can then produce no additional effect. This is the concept of *spare receptors,* mentioned above. Conversely, if a drug is acting to inhibit a step in a reaction sequence, by interaction with its receptor, receptor occupancy will result in inhibition of the *ultimate effect* only when the step inhibited is or becomes the rate-limiting step. It may be necessary to occupy the majority of the receptors before any change in function is observed. In both of the situations described, it should be apparent that the concentration of drug producing a half-maximal effect bears no relationship to the dissociation constant for the drug-receptor complex. In the first example, the concentration of drug required for a half-maximal effect is less than K_D, whereas in the second case it is greater. Other examples of deviation from the fundamental receptor theory can be described; these form the basis for the other kinetic formulations of drug action mentioned above.

Classification of Receptors and Drug Effects. Drug receptors are classified and identified primarily on the basis of the effect, or lack of effect, of selective antagonists and by the relative potencies of representative agonists. For example, the effects of acetylcholine that mimic those of the alkaloid muscarine and that are selectively antagonized by atropine are termed *muscarinic effects.* Other effects of acetylcholine that mimic those of nicotine and that are not readily antagonized by atropine but are selectively blocked by other agents are described as *nicotinic effects.* By *extension,* these two types of cholinergic effects are said to be mediated by muscarinic or nicotinic receptors. Such classification of receptors results in an internally consistent scheme that gives support to the view that two receptor types are involved, but it contributes little to delineation of mechanism of drug action. It does provide a convenient basis for summarizing drug effects. If the effects and receptors in the various tissues have been classified, a statement that a drug activates a specified type of receptor is a succinct summary of its spectrum of effects and of the agents that will antagonize it. Similarly, a statement that a drug blocks a certain type of receptor specifies the agents that it will antagonize and at what sites.

Sites of Action. The receptor for a drug can be any functional macromolecular component that exists in the organism. This is a sweeping, but true, statement that has certain corollaries. One is that a drug is potentially capable of altering the rate at which any bodily function proceeds; a second is that, by virtue of interaction with such receptors, drugs do not create actions but simply modulate rates of ongoing function.

The two general, major determinants of the site of drug action will thus be the localization of receptors and the concentration of drug to which the receptor is exposed. Localization of drug action is not necessarily dependent upon selective distribution of the drug. However, even if drug *action* is localized, the effects of the drug may be widespread and disseminated by a variety of secondary forces, chemical and physical.

If a drug acts by interaction with a relatively nonspecialized receptor, that is, a receptor that serves functions common to most cells, its effects will be widespread. If this is a vital function, the drug will be particularly dangerous. Nevertheless, such a drug may be useful. Digitalis glycosides are potent inhibitors of a fundamental and vital ion transport process, common to most cells. As such, they can cause widespread toxicity, and their therapeutic index is dangerously low. Although their great utility is not to be denied, it would also be a boon to have a drug that accomplished the same therapeutic goal in a more selective way. Many similar examples could be cited, particularly in the area of cancer chemotherapy.

If a drug interacts with specialized receptors unique to specific types of differentiated cells, its effects are more specific. The hypothetical ideal drug would cause its therapeutic effect by virtue of such types of action. Side effects would be minimized, but toxicity might not be. If the differentiated function is a vital one, this type of drug could also be very dangerous. Some of the most lethal chemical agents known (*e.g.,* botulinus toxin) show such specificity and toxicity.

It must also be mentioned that several drugs do not act by virtue of combination with functional cellular components or receptors. Certain drugs may interact specifically with small molecules or ions that are normally or abnormally found in the body. The chelating agents, capable of forming strong bonds with a variety of metallic cations, are an excellent example. Certain drugs that are structural analogs of normal biological constituents may be incorporated into cellular components and thereby alter their function. This has been termed a "counterfeit incorporation mechanism" (*see* Goldstein *et al.,* 1974). Additionally, there is a group of agents that act by more physical mechanisms, some of which are poorly understood. A hint of this type of mechanism is provided by a lack of requirement for highly specific chemical structure. Stereo-isomers of such drugs would not be expected to differ in their potency or efficacy. For example, certain relatively benign compounds can be administered in large quantities, sufficient to increase the osmolarity of various body fluids. Appropriate changes in the distribution of water result. The volatile general anesthetic agents interact with membranes to depress excitability. Their diversity of structure suggests a biophysical mechanism of action, and their individual potencies correlate well with the physical property of their oil:water partition coefficients.

Not infrequently, analysis of drug action is limited by available physiological and biochemical knowledge. Elucidation of basic cellular function and further exploration of drug action then often proceed in parallel, with the drug frequently serving as an indispensable tool.

FACTORS THAT MODIFY DRUG EFFECTS AND DRUG DOSAGE

Many factors modify the effects of drugs. Some of these, such as the development of drug allergy, result in *qualitative* differences in the effects of a drug and may preclude its safe use. Others produce only *quantitative* changes in the usual effects of the drug and can be offset by appropriate adjustment of dosage. These variables must be taken into account before a drug is prescribed, and a stated *therapeutic dose* of a drug must be viewed only as the anticipated dose for the average patient or that from which to estimate the dose for an individual patient. Indeed, the optimal dosage for many drugs is determined for each patient only by careful monitoring of drug effect or drug concentration in serum. It is for this reason that it is appropriate to state that *the dose of a drug is "enough."*

The physician's legal responsibility if he deviates from dosages or uses approved by the U.S. Food and Drug Administration (FDA) for inclusion in the manufacturer's package insert and advertising has been summarized in a Council Conference (1969) and by the FDA (1972).

The following are the more important factors that modify drug effects and influence

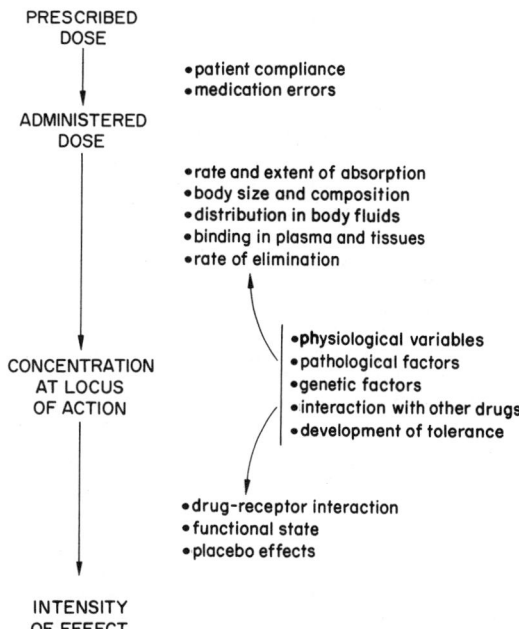

Figure 1-9. *Factors that determine the relationship between prescribed drug dosage and drug effect.* (Modified from Koch-Weser, 1972.)

the therapeutic dose of a drug. These factors are summarized schematically in Figure 1-9.

Medication Errors and Patient Compliance. A patient sometimes receives the wrong medication in the hospital, or his prescription order may not be written or filled correctly. These *medication errors* can be traced to inadequate checks in the medication system or to faulty communication between the physician and the nurse or pharmacist. More frequently, however, the patient himself is responsible for not taking medication as intended.

Only a minority of patients take medication exactly as intended; a significant fraction default completely, and some take drugs in excess of the amounts prescribed. A patient may comply well at one time but poorly at another. Many variables related to the therapeutic regimen, the patient, his illness, and the physician influence patient compliance. Directly or indirectly, however, the most important determinant of *patient compliance* is the quality of the physician-patient relationship. The nurse and pharmacist can aid in improving patient compliance by helping him understand his medication and the therapeutic directions. However, major responsibility for assuring patient compliance remains with the physician. He must not assume that a patient will follow his instructions and must work actively to promote patient compliance.

The important problems of medication errors and patient compliance are further discussed in the Appendix.

Placebo Effects. The net effect of drug therapy is the sum of the pharmacological effects of the drug and the nonspecific placebo effects associated with the therapeutic effort. Although identified specifically with administration of an inert substance in the guise of medication, *placebo effects are associated with the taking of any drug, active as well as inert.*

Placebo effects result from the physician-patient relationship, the significance of the therapeutic effort to the patient, and the mental "set" imparted by the therapeutic setting and by the physician. They vary significantly in different individuals and in any one patient at different times. Placebo effects are commonly manifest as alterations of mood, other subjective effects, and objective effects that are under autonomic or voluntary control. They may be favorable or unfavorable relative to the therapeutic objectives. Exploited to advantage, placebo effects can significantly supplement pharmacological effects and can represent the difference between success and failure of therapy. (*See* reviews by Wolf, 1959; Bourne, 1971.)

A placebo (in this context, better termed *dummy medication*) is an indispensable element of the controlled clinical trial. In contrast, a placebo has only a limited role in the routine practice of medicine. Although the inert medication may be an effective vehicle for a placebo effect, the physician-patient relationship is generally preferable. Relief or lack of relief of symptoms upon administration of a placebo is *not* a reliable basis for determining whether the symptoms have a "psychogenic" or "somatic" origin.

A *pure placebo* is a capsule of lactose, an injection of saline solution, or similar medication that is essentially inert. The term *impure placebo* refers to a substance with established pharmacological properties employed in subeffective dosage or in a setting in which its effects would not be expected to contribute to a favorable therapeutic outcome. In those limited circumstances in which a placebo is indicated in routine medical practice, the physician often prefers an impure placebo, because of the reduced risk of discovery by the patient. However, he risks deluding himself by erroneously attributing the resulting placebo effect to the pharmacological effects of the drug.

Body Weight and Volume of Distribution. Drug dosage should be suitably adjusted for abnormally lean or obese individuals and for those who are markedly dehydrated or edematous, with appropriate regard for whether the drug is distributed in fat or is restricted to the extracellular fluid compartment or lean body mass.

Age. Children are often more sensitive than adults to drug-induced changes in water and electrolyte or acid-base metabolism. Special precaution must also be taken in the use of hormones or other drugs that might influence growth and development.

Although drug dosage for older children may be calculated as a fraction of the adult dose on the basis of body weight or estimated body surface area, that for younger children, and especially for infants, should be learned as such and not calculated by

formula. Unfortunately, optimal doses for children have been established for relatively few drugs.

Adjustment of drug dosage for very young infants, particularly premature babies, is required because of differences in relative volumes of the body fluid compartments, reduced binding of drugs to plasma protein, immaturity of renal function or of the enzymatic mechanisms for drug inactivation, or incomplete development of the blood-brain barrier. The effects of drugs on the immature brain may also be somewhat unusual. Although many months are required for complete maturation, renal function increases significantly during the initial 2 to 3 postnatal weeks and hepatic function matures rapidly during the initial months of life.

Elderly individuals may respond to drugs in a somewhat abnormal manner, often because of impaired ability to inactivate or excrete drugs, or because of other concurrent pathology.

Sex. Women are thought to be more susceptible than men to the effects of certain drugs, in part because of smaller size. In some instances, this difference is considered sufficient to necessitate reduction in dosage.

During *pregnancy*, caution is necessary in the administration of drugs that might affect the uterus or fetus. A wise precaution is to avoid the use of all drugs except those essential to maintain pregnancy or the health of the mother (*e.g.,* iron salts, folic acid).

Route of Administration. Inasmuch as rate and extent of absorption and sometimes pattern of biotransformation differ with the route of administration, dosage must be adjusted to take this factor into account.

Time of Administration. The time at which a drug is administered sometimes influences dosage. This is especially true for oral therapy in relation to meals. Drug absorption proceeds more rapidly if the stomach and upper portion of the intestinal tract are free of food, and an amount of drug that is active before a meal may be ineffective if given after eating. On the other hand, irritating drugs are better tolerated if food is in the stomach.

Sedation and other minor adverse effects of a drug that is administered only once daily may be less annoying to the patient if the drug is taken upon retiring. Conversely, drugs that might interfere with sleep should not be administered near bedtime.

Diurnal and seasonal variations in the effects of drugs are well recognized in animals and may also be important in man.

Rate of Elimination. Adjustment of dosage schedules for patients with impaired renal or hepatic drug elimination has been discussed previously in connection with pharmacokinetic principles.

Tolerance. Tolerance may be acquired to the effects of many drugs, especially the opioids, barbiturates and other CNS depressants, nitrites, xanthines, and certain CNS stimulants. When this occurs, *cross-tolerance* may develop to the effects of pharmacologically related drugs, particularly those acting at the same receptor site, and drug dosage must be increased to maintain a given therapeutic effect. Since tolerance does not usually develop equally to all effects of a drug, the therapeutic index may decrease. However, there are also examples of the development of tolerance to the undesired effects of a drug and a resultant increase in its therapeutic index.

After tolerance develops, normal sensitivity may be regained only by suspending drug administration. For most drugs, the development of tolerance can be minimized by initiating therapy with the lowest effective dose and by avoiding continual administration of the drug at regular intervals. In contrast, the emergence of resistant microorganisms during chemotherapy is favored when only minimally effective dosage or intermittent medication is employed.

The mechanisms involved in the development of tolerance are only partially understood. In animals, tolerance often occurs as the result of induced synthesis of the hepatic microsomal enzymes concerned in drug biotransformation; the possible significance of this *drug-disposition* or *pharmacokinetic tolerance* during chronic medication in man is an area of continuing investigation. The most important factor in the development of tolerance to the opioids, barbiturates, and ethanol is some type of neuronal adaptation vaguely referred to as *cellular* or *pharmacodynamic tolerance*. Tachyphylaxis, such as that to histamine-releasing agents and to the sympathomimetic amines that act indirectly by releasing norepinephrine, has been attributed to depletion of available mediator, but other mechanisms may also contribute.

Physiological Variables. Water and electrolyte balance, acid-base status, body temperature, and other physiological variables also influence the effects of drugs. Unfortunately, no simple summary of the effect of these variables is possible. They must be considered for each drug individually.

The effects of drugs, just as those of disease, may be manifest as encroachment upon *physiological reserve* rather than as an overt effect, and this factor must also be considered when drugs are prescribed. Ganglionic blocking agents and other drugs that impair compensatory sympathetic reflexes may have minimal effects upon the blood pressure of a recumbent individual, yet cause orthostatic collapse when he assumes an upright posture. This principle is important in establishing proper dosage of drugs in the therapy of hypertension and in selecting drugs for preanesthetic medication. Similarly, respiratory depression may be manifest primarily as respiratory acidosis with only minimal reduction of rate or depth of breathing or of alveolar ventilation. Failure to appreciate this fact is often responsible for underestimation of the depressant effects of drugs on respiration.

Pathological Factors. The effects of drugs may also be modified by pathological factors. Patients with chronic pulmonary disease or increased intracranial pressure are often unusually sensitive to morphine and other respiratory depressants. Conversely, the hyperthyroid individual can tolerate larger doses of morphine than can the normal person, but he may be unusually responsive to a dose of epinephrine. *Nutritional* deficiencies may also modify the effects of drugs.

Genetic Factors. Genetic factors contribute to the normal variability of drug effects and are responsible for a number of striking quantitative and qualitative modifications of pharmacological activity. Many of these differences, such as the prolonged apnea in some patients after administration of usual doses of the neuromuscular blocking agent succinylcholine, have been traced to genetic influences on the enzymes involved in *drug biotransformation*. Other variations in drug effect, such as the greater incidence of drug-induced hemolytic anemia in non-Caucasians than in Caucasians, have been found to be related to genetic differences that modify the actions of drugs.

The objectives of *pharmacogenetics* include not only identification of differences in drug effects that have a genetic basis but also development of simple methods by which susceptible individuals can be recognized *before* the drug is administered.

Drug Interactions. The effects of a drug may be modified by prior or concurrent administration of another drug, and improved therapy is sometimes possible by judicious use of concurrent medication. However, since a patient usually receives many drugs during the course of an illness, the possibility of unplanned combination of drug effects must also be considered. Drug interactions may arise either from alteration of the absorption, distribution, biotransformation, or excretion of one drug by the other, or from combination of their actions or effects.

Multiple-Drug Therapy. Multiple-drug therapy is justified if it provides greater efficacy than can be achieved with full doses of single drugs, greater margin of safety, or more satisfactory onset or duration of effect. Sometimes a drug is administered in combination with another to prevent or antagonize an untoward effect. However, it is usually more desirable to reduce the dose of the toxic drug or to change medication, rather than to resort to combined medication. Whatever the rationale for multiple-drug therapy, the efficacy and safety of the combined medication must be evaluated in the same manner as for single drugs.

Drug Mixtures. A distinction must be made between the concurrent, but separate, administration of drugs and their administration together as a fixed-dose mixture. Most mixtures of drugs have distinct disadvantages, and their use may involve frank risk. Careful adjustment of dosage of each drug is almost always required to attain the maximum benefits from combined medication with a minimum of untoward effects. In some cases, proper timing of drug administration may also be important. The flexibility of dosage and timing essential for the success of combined medication is sacrificed if fixed-dose mixtures are used. In addition, the use of mixtures often complicates therapy, since if toxic effects occur it may be impossible to identify the component responsible, and all medication must then be discontinued. The use of mixtures also fosters multiple-drug therapy without first establishing the need for more than one drug. When this occurs, needless expense is imposed upon the patient, and he is unnecessarily exposed to the risk of toxicity from the superfluous components. Additionally, the indiscriminate use of drug mixtures encourages careless diagnosis and inappropriate therapy.

In a few instances, it has been established that in the great majority of patients a mixture of two or more drugs in a fixed ratio affords more satisfactory results than any single component. Fixed-dose mixtures may also be justified occasionally as a means to improve patient compliance. However, use of a drug mixture for the latter purpose is valid only if direct trial in the patient has established that multiple-drug therapy is superior to single-drug medication, and if an available fixed-dose mixture does, in fact, meet the dosage requirements for that patient.

Terminology. Descriptions of the combined effects of drugs are often ambiguous, because the terms *addition, summation, synergism, potentiation,* and *antagonism* are not employed consistently and some have imprecise quantitative connotations. The usage outlined here is largely that of Loewe (1953).

Two drugs are said to be *heterergic* for a particular effect if the effect is manifested by one of the drugs but is absent from the spectrum of the other. If the combined effect of heterergic drugs is greater than that of the active component alone, they are said to exhibit *synergism* or *potentiation;* if the combined effect is less than that of the active component alone, the interaction is termed *antagonism.*

Heterergic synergism and antagonism usually result from alterations in the absorption, distribution, biotransformation, or excretion of the active component. Such interactions are sometimes sought in therapy to achieve a more favorable duration of drug effect. They generally do not result in improvement of therapeutic index.

If two drugs produce the same overt effect, they are termed *homergic.* Descriptions of the combined effects of such drugs are intended to indicate whether they are equal to, or greater or less than, those expected by simple addition. However, two types of additive behavior can be distinguished. If the drugs are close congeners that act on the same receptors (*e.g.,* epinephrine and norepinephrine), *doses* of one drug should substitute for those of the other, in proportion to their relative potency, and, when combined, effects should be additive in the linear range of the dose-effect curve. Only drugs that exhibit this *dose addition* are properly described as *additive.* Deviations from dose addition are best termed *supra-additive* or *infra-additive.* Such descriptions imply that the drugs act by different mechanisms. Concurrent use of drugs that act by the same mechanism is rarely, if ever, superior to the use of appropriate dosage of one of the agents alone.

Descriptions of the combined effects of drugs are more appropriately directed at indicating whether the combination does or does not provide efficacy and/or safety that cannot be duplicated by single-drug therapy.

Prevention of Unplanned Drug Interactions. An interaction between drugs, if not recognized and corrected, can result in diminished drug efficacy or serious toxicity. It can be the immediate cause for hospitalization or prolong the stay of the inpatient. Drug interactions for particular agents are discussed throughout the text. Unfortunately, well-intended but uncritical tabulations of drug interactions have failed to maintain proper perspective. Advice to the physician for dealing with this important problem has suffered correspondingly.

The more extensive tabulations of drug interactions have included studies in animals that cannot be extrapolated to man, interactions that occur in man but are not of practical importance, isolated case reports of questionable significance, and frank speculation. Moreover, simple tabulation of interactions could not adequately stress that most interactions occur inconsistently or vary significantly.

Critical summaries of potential drug interactions have been prepared by Hansten (1973), the American Pharmaceutical Association (1973), and the Medical Letter (1975). An extensive tabulation of drug-induced modifications of clinical laboratory tests has been provided by Constantino and Kabat (1973).

Interactions of established clinical significance are properly considered an integral aspect of the basic pharmacology of the individual drugs or drug groups. They are sufficiently numerous to warrant that they be summarized by pharmacological class. However, individual agents in a class may deviate from such generalizations. For example, meperidine and morphine exhibit similar interactions with many CNS depressants but different interactions with the monoamine oxidase inhibitors. For this reason, identification of the mechanism of interaction is always informative. Classification of interactions by mechanism is also helpful for assessing the potential risk when it is not known whether a drug is or is not subject to a particular interaction.

Physicochemical interactions are those that occur in solution prior to administration. Such incompatibilities are discussed in the Appendix. Pharmacists are prepared to advise the physician on the possible incompatibility of drugs in solution.

Pharmacokinetic interactions are those that result in altered absorption, distribution, or elimination of a drug. Many mechanisms are involved, including changes in gastric pH or gastrointestinal motility, competition for plasma or tissue binding, inhibition of biotransformation, induction of the microsomal enzyme systems, competition for renal tubular secretion, and changes in urine pH. Important features of these mechanisms of interaction have been summarized in previous sections. Reduced absorption of drugs may also result from interaction in the gastrointestinal tract prior to absorption. Examples include the interactions between the tetracycline antibiotics and multivalent cations and the adsorption of drugs by the ion-exchange resin cholestyramine or the adsorbent kaolin. These interactions can usually be avoided by altering the timing of medications.

Pharmacodynamic interactions are those that involve the actions or effects of drugs. They include the obvious, yet sometimes overlooked, enhanced toxicity of drugs with similar adverse effects, such as that of ethanol and a barbiturate or two drugs with similar ototoxicity. They also include many interactions involving drug action that are not immediately obvious from the major effects of the agents. An example is the inhibition by the tricyclic antidepressants of the uptake of the antihypertensive agent guanethidine to its locus of action in the adrenergic neuron. Pharmacodynamic interactions also include drug-induced changes in electrolyte metabolism or other physiological variables that modify the action of another drug. An important example is the enhanced toxicity of the cardiac glycosides associated with hypokalemia produced by the saluretic agents. Pharmacodynamic interactions must obviously be considered individually for each pharmacological class.

The physician must be familiar with the drug interactions of established clinical significance. Interactions may involve not only the drugs that he prescribes but also those prescribed for the patient by other physicians, those taken without prescription, and certain foods. Obviously, the risk of interactions is reduced if medications are kept to a minimum. Appropriate monitoring is mandatory when drugs known to interact are employed concurrently. Depending upon the sequence of drug administration and subsequent dosage adjustments, many interactions may occur when medication is discontinued as well as initiated. Thus, increased vigilance is necessary whenever therapy is changed. Contributing factors include timing of medication, genetic differences, and concurrent pathology. For these many reasons, the physician must anticipate variability in the occurrence and magnitude of interactions and avoid complacency.

DRUG TOXICITY

No drug is free of toxic effects. The adverse effects of a drug during therapy are sometimes trivial, but they can be serious and may be fatal. Some appear promptly, but others may develop only after prolonged medication. Still others occur only in certain patients or only in combination with other drugs. Some toxic effects of drugs, such as orthostatic hypotension during antihypertensive medication, are an extension of the desired effects and can be reduced or controlled by proper adjustment of dosage. On the other hand, the desired and undesired effects of a drug may be different manifestations of the same primary action and thus be inseparable. In many instances, an effect of a drug that is sought in one patient becomes an undesired effect in another when the drug is employed for a different purpose.

Clinicians have long been aware of the drug-induced diseases. However, with the introduction into therapeutic practice of drugs of greater and broader efficacy, the problem of drug toxicity has increased. Although the incidence of adverse effects of drugs varies greatly, depending upon the drug and its manner of use, drug toxicity is a critical aspect of modern therapeutics. There is an urgent need for the development of methods in animals that more accurately predict the potential harmful effects of drugs in man. There is also need for more complete identification of the factors that increase the risk of toxicity and for better procedures for prompt collection, assessment, and dissemination of reports of clinical toxicity. However, adverse effects do not arise solely because of the inherent toxicity of drugs and the limitations of the methods for early detection of this toxicity. Most drug toxicity is predictable and attributable to excessive dosage of common drugs. Many of the adverse effects could be avoided if drugs were used more carefully and more wisely. The physician should avoid a toxic drug if a less toxic one will suffice; and he should, if possible, minimize the use of concurrent medication, since one drug may increase the toxicity of another. Moreover, he must be aware of the potential hazards of the drugs that he uses, and he must monitor adequately for occurrence of these adverse effects and be prepared to act promptly if toxicity occurs. He must be especially alert for the unexpected.

A brief consideration of several of the serious drug-induced diseases will introduce the reader to this important aspect of pharmacology.

Drug Allergy (Hypersensitivity). Although the incidence of allergic reactions to most drugs is low, drug allergy represents a major problem in the use of some drugs. There is an urgent need for reliable, safe methods for detecting susceptible individuals before drug administration. The development of such tests is complicated by the fact that metabolites of a drug, perhaps even minor metabolites that are not detected in usual biotransformation studies, as well as the drug itself and even trace impurities may serve as haptens. Also needed is more complete information on the risks of cross-sensitivity reactions between drugs in the same chemical and pharmacological classes.

Drug allergy may take many forms, including the full spectrum of immediate and delayed types of allergic reactions produced by foreign macromolecules. Skin reactions extend from mild rash to severe exfoliative dermatitis. Those of blood vessels range from acute urticaria and angioedema to severe arteritis with localized medial degeneration. Drug fever is an allergic phenomenon that very closely resembles serum sickness; it is manifested by fever, leukocytosis, arthralgia, and dermatitis. Rhinitis, asthma, and even anaphylactic shock are other familiar allergic responses that can be precipitated by drugs.

Various other adverse effects of drugs are thought to be allergic reactions because of their characteristics. Direct toxic effects of drugs can usually be produced in animals and occur in all patients if the dose is increased sufficiently. Toxic effects of drugs that cannot be produced in animals and develop only in some patients are often assumed to have an allergic basis, particularly if they occur in association with the more familiar manifestations of allergy and if the time course is typical of such reactions. Such assumptions can, however, be erroneous.

Blood Dyscrasias. Leukopenia, granulocytopenia, aplastic anemia, hemolytic anemia, thrombocytopenia, and, in some cases, defects in the clotting factors are serious, sometimes fatal, complications of drug therapy. Although drug allergy is responsible for many of the cytopenias, certain of the blood dyscrasias are believed to result from a direct toxic effect of drugs on bone marrow. The most common basis for drug-induced hemolytic anemia is a genetically determined deficiency in red-cell glucose-6-phosphate dehydrogenase activity.

Hepatotoxicity and Nephrotoxicity. Because drugs are concentrated in the liver and kidney, damage to these organs by a direct toxic effect of drugs is not uncommon. Hepatotoxicity and nephrotoxicity may also occur as forms of drug allergy.

Well-recognized adverse effects on the liver include hepatocellular toxicity, the potentially fatal viral hepatitis–like syndrome produced by the halogenated hydrocarbons and other drugs, and intrahepatic cholestasis, a type of hepatotoxicity that resembles obstructive jaundice and is produced by the phenothiazines, certain steroids, and other agents. Drugs may also interfere with bilirubin metabolism and with the many metabolic functions of the liver. In addition, a variety of drugs precipitate hepatic coma in patients with liver disease.

Glomerulopathy and a nephrotic syndrome clinically similar to poststreptococcal glomerulonephritis, interstitial nephritis, and tubular necrosis are important toxic effects of a number of drugs. Intrarenal precipitation of the less soluble sulfonamides is a major cause of the nephrotoxicity of these agents. Adverse effects of drugs on the kidney may also develop indirectly, secondary to hemolysis or hypotension.

Teratogenic Effects. Although the thalidomide tragedy dramatically emphasized that drugs may adversely influence fetal development, reliable clinical information about the possible teratogenic hazard of most drugs is still limited. For this reason, all unnecessary medication should be avoided during pregnancy. Moreover, since pregnancy is often not diagnosed at the time of greatest vulnerability of the fetus, all drugs not known to be reasonably safe on the basis of long usage should be avoided by women of childbearing age.

Behavioral Toxicity. This term refers to suppression of normal anxiety, reduction in motivation, impairment of memory and learning, distortion of judgment, nonpurposive or inappropriate behavior, and other adverse effects of drugs on mood, behavior, and psychological and psychometric functioning. Motor incoordination and impairment of ability to operate machinery or to drive a motor vehicle may also be considered a form of behavioral toxicity. The term has gained widest use in connection with psychopharmacological agents, but it applies to other drugs as well.

Drug Dependence and Drug Addiction. Any drug that alters mood or perception is likely to be abused and is potentially capable of producing *drug dependence* upon repeated administration. The drugs that are commonly abused include the opioids; the barbiturates, other sedative-hypnotics, and ethanol; the amphetamines, cocaine, and other CNS stimulants; LSD and other hallucinogens; and marihuana. The characteristics of drug dependence vary with the agent involved. However, one characteristic common to all types of drug dependence is *psychic dependence,* a drive or craving that requires periodic or chronic administration of the drug for pleasure or for relief of discomfort. Another feature of some types of drug dependence is *physical dependence,* a state characterized by the appearance of physical symptoms when administration of the drug is suspended. These symptoms are termed the *withdrawal* or *abstinence syndrome. Tolerance* is a characteristic of only certain types of drug dependence.

The term *drug dependence* was coined specifically to permit consideration of the pharmacological and medical aspects of *drug abuse* in isolation from the broader socioeconomic, moral, and legal aspects of the problem that are embraced by the term *drug addiction.* Unfortunately, the two terms continue to be used interchangeably. Abuse of drugs that markedly influence mood and behavior is a problem of continuing medical

and social importance. The subject is considered in detail in Chapter 16.

Drug Poisoning. Accidental poisoning is a health problem of major significance. Several thousand deaths from chemical poisoning occur annually in the United States, and it is estimated that the number of nonfatal poisonings exceeds 1 million per year. More than one tenth of these fatalities and over one half of all poisonings occur in children under 5 years of age. The tragedy of this high incidence of poisonings in childhood is that most could be avoided.

The physician should assume an active role in *prevention* of poisoning, particularly by fostering a more careful attitude toward drugs and chemicals in the home. Parents cannot be too strongly urged to keep drugs out of reach of children, preferably in a "locked" cabinet, and to teach them that medicinals are not candy. All drugs should be kept in "child-resistant" containers. The many common household articles that are poisonous should be made unavailable to children, and poisonous pesticides and herbicides should not be placed in the home. Indoctrination against accidental poisoning must also be directed to adults. They should be urged to read and heed labels on medicines, and they should be encouraged to discard residual prescription drugs that are no longer needed. Accidental poisoning among adults is not uncommon and usually results either from misguided attempts at self-medication or from mistaking one drug for another.

The number and variety of drugs and chemicals that might be encountered in poisonings are enormous. However, the physician should become familiar with the details of treatment for the more commonly encountered household poisons. He should also be prepared to treat intoxication caused by agents frequently used for suicidal purposes, such as the barbiturates, other CNS depressants, and carbon monoxide, and to detect and treat those types of industrial intoxications that might occur in his community. Additionally, he should take advantage of the services and information available to him through his regional Poison Control Center.

Diagnosis of Drug Poisoning. The diagnosis of poisoning may be difficult, since there is scarcely a syndrome produced by a toxic agent that cannot simulate disease. However, there are a number of clues that assist in the detection of acute poisoning, particularly if this possibility is included in the differential diagnosis. In this connection, contaminated foods are often the etiological agent. The onset of symptoms is usually sudden and follows the taking of food, drink, or medicine by an individual who has been previously well. In some cases, several individuals may suffer from similar symptoms after partaking of the same food. In addition, many drugs leave a telltale odor, produce irritation of the mucous membranes of the mouth and throat, or cause typical pharmacological effects. As a final check, simple chemical tests can sometimes confirm the diagnosis.

The diagnosis of chronic poisoning is often more difficult. At times, the symptoms and signs are not sufficiently characteristic to point to the toxic agent, and laboratory procedures may be essential. In many cases, only painstaking probing of the patient's history, habits, daily activities, and working conditions leads to the diagnosis. The more uncommon types of industrial poisoning may go undiagnosed until irreparable injury has been suffered by the patient.

Treatment of Drug Poisoning. Most emergency therapy of drug poisoning is symptomatic, since success often depends upon speed, and valuable time cannot be wasted in attempts at a positive identification of the specific cause of the patient's illness. However, therapy is facilitated if the responsible agent(s) and the degree of exposure or the amount ingested can be determined. The usual steps taken are (1) supportive or symptomatic therapy, (2) termination of exposure and removal of the poison from the body, and (3) administration of antidotes.

Adequate *supportive therapy,* identical to that in other medical emergencies, is the most important aspect of the treatment of drug poisoning. Serial measurement and charting of the vital signs and important reflexes are helpful procedures by which to judge the progress of the intoxication, the response to therapy, and the need for additional treatment. The patient should be kept in bed, under competent surveillance. Particular attention should be paid to the *respiration, circulation, hepatic and renal function, body temperature,* and *acid-base and fluid-and-electrolyte balance.* This usually necessitates hospitalization.

Poisons that have been applied externally are best removed by copious *washing* with water. Soap should be used on the skin, especially if the poison is not water soluble. Contaminated clothing should be discarded. Oral administration of *activated charcoal, induced vomiting,* and *gastric lavage* may be employed to reduce further absorption of an ingested poison. If gastric emptying has been delayed, such procedures may be of benefit even 8 hours after ingestion of the poison. Vomiting and gastric lavage are contraindicated in the treatment of poisoning by corrosive agents, strychnine, other convulsants, kerosene, or other hydrocarbon solvents.

Activated charcoal, administered orally as a fine powder suspended in water, adsorbs a wide variety of chemicals, but not cyanide, alcohols, mineral acids, or caustic alkalis. It is an effective procedure for retarding absorption of ingested poisons; many toxicologists rank it second in value only to support-

ive therapy. The so-called universal antidote, a mixture of activated charcoal, magnesium oxide, and tannic acid, has been abandoned, since it is less effective than activated charcoal alone. Household articles that are somewhat useful for dilution or adsorption of poisons are milk, beaten egg white, flour, and starch. Burnt toast is ineffective.

Much emphasis has been placed on the use of *emetics,* since vomiting may be as productive as gastric lavage and can be instituted more promptly. However, such drugs are contraindicated in the unconscious patient, and they may not be effective if the patient has ingested a CNS depressant. *Ipecac syrup* is orally effective, but vomiting may not occur for 20 to 30 minutes. It is not dependable if the patient has previously received activated charcoal. *Apomorphine* acts more promptly and certainly, but it must be administered parenterally. It may also cause protracted emesis and CNS depression. These adverse effects are antagonized by naloxone. Powdered mustard, administered orally as a suspension in warm water, is a household article that can be administered in an emergency. Mechanical stimulation of the oropharynx is unreliable and relatively ineffective.

Gastric lavage, when performed by a trained person, is an effective method for evacuation of the stomach. However, the procedure is time consuming and may not be reliable if the poison is insoluble. Care must be taken to prevent aspiration of gastric contents or lavage fluid into the lungs. After the stomach has been thoroughly emptied, a saline cathartic is sometimes administered through the stomach tube to diminish further intestinal absorption of the poison.

In some instances, the renal *excretion* of a drug can be increased by administration of an osmotic diuretic and by appropriate acidification or alkalinization of the urine. In cases of severe drug intoxication, elimination of the drug by *peritoneal dialysis,* often with a solution containing albumin, or by use of the *artificial kidney* is a highly effective procedure.

Antidotes serve only a limited role in the treatment of drug poisoning, even when the poison has been identified, because there are safe, effective, selective antagonists for relatively few drugs. Those that are available for individual poisons and drugs are discussed throughout the text. Outstanding examples are the use of chelating agents in metal poisoning, nitrites and thiosulfate in cyanide intoxication, methylene blue in methemoglobinemia, atropine and reactivators of acetylcholinesterase in poisoning by those insecticides and other drugs that inhibit the enzyme, and naloxone in opioid intoxication.

III. Development and Use of Drugs

DEVELOPMENT, EVALUATION, AND CONTROL OF DRUGS

The average practitioner is not usually directly concerned in the evaluation of drugs.

Nevertheless, he must know something about the development and evaluation of therapeutic agents, since this knowledge has an important bearing on his attitude toward new drugs and their use. The physician must also be familiar with the laws that regulate the use of medicinals.

Sources and Discovery of New Drugs. The earliest medicinals were crude powders, juices, or extracts from animal, plant, and mineral sources, and these continued to be the only drugs until early in the nineteenth century. However, once advances in chemistry permitted the isolation, purification, and identification of the active constituents, and as soon as advances in physiology, biochemistry, and pharmacology provided a rational basis for their evaluation and comparison, the stage was set for the preparation of chemically related drugs, the synthesis of new agents, and the beginning of the modern age of pharmacotherapy.

New therapeutic agents are discovered by screening, by structural modification of established drugs or endogenous substances, or by accident. Screening refers to the testing of large numbers of compounds, chosen in part at random, for selected types of pharmacological activity. The testing of thousands of soil samples for microorganisms capable of producing antibiotic activity is an example of this time-consuming, somewhat unsophisticated, relatively inefficient approach. However, it has the important advantage that it can uncover valuable new chemical classes of drugs.

Structural modifications of an established drug often yield congeners that differ only insignificantly from the parent and are aptly termed "me-too" drugs, the marketing of which is hard to justify. However, as discussed previously in the section on structure-activity relationship, such alterations at times yield a congener with pharmacological properties significantly different from those of the parent compound. For example, the first three sulfonamides introduced as chemotherapeutic agents, a milestone in the history of drug therapy, are now obsolete.

Another particularly fruitful approach has been the structural modification of endogenous molecules involved in cellular metabolism and function. This has led to the discovery, for example, of useful antimetabolites. Rapid advances in the elucidation of basic cellular mechanisms make it likely that more and more drugs of this type will be developed in the future.

Many significant advances in therapy in the past have resulted from fortuitous discovery of new drugs or new uses of established therapeutic agents by alert observation in the laboratory or clinic. Well-known examples of this approach are the discovery of penicillin by Fleming and the recognition of the saluretic activity of organic mercurials employed in the treatment of syphilis. Undesired effects of older agents have also been exploited in the development of new drugs, as illustrated by the evolution from the antibacterial sulfonamides of the carbonic anhydrase inhibitors, the antihypertensive thiazides, and the oral hypoglycemic agents.

Development and Evaluation of New Drugs. The development and evaluation of new drugs in the United States are rigidly controlled by federal regulations administered by the Food and Drug Administration (*see* below). A new drug may not be marketed for general clinical use until it has been subjected to thorough clinical pharmacological studies, and until "substantial evidence" of its efficacy and safety has been obtained from adequate, well-controlled clinical trials conducted by qualified investigators.

Before initial studies in man are permitted, the full pharmacological spectrum of a new drug and its pharmacokinetic characteristics must be thoroughly and extensively explored in *animals,* and both acute and chronic toxicity tests must be conducted on several species. Because of species variations, such studies are considered useful merely as evidence that the drug has promise and is sufficiently safe to warrant testing in man. Even the most extensive studies in animals cannot substitute for successful clinical trials as evidence of therapeutic efficacy.

The *initial clinical trials* of a new drug are necessarily cautious experiments, on volunteer normal subjects as well as patients, aimed primarily at establishing that the drug merits further study and providing pharmacokinetic information. If the initial trials in patients provide promise of clinical efficacy and adequate safety, the drug is subjected to thorough *clinical pharmacological studies,* and documentation of its efficacy and safety is sought in *controlled clinical trials.* Only under exceptional circumstances may a new drug be administered to an individual without his informed consent. All clinical studies of new drugs must comply with ethical principles and must be approved by peer-group review committees.

What constitutes an adequately controlled clinical trial necessarily varies, depending upon the drug effect being evaluated. The more important general requirements for all trials are an *appropriate and sensitive method* of evaluation, an *adequate number of subjects, lack of bias, concurrent comparison* of the new drug with a *reference drug* over a *range of doses,* and appropriate *statistical validation.* Many clinical trials must be conducted under so-called *blind* conditions. In a blind experiment, the nature of the medication is concealed from the patient (single-blind) or from both the patient and all persons associated with conduct and evaluation of the trial (double-blind). Blind conditions are essential for trials in which subjective effects of medication are being studied; they may also be necessary in evaluation of objective drug effects, if these are under voluntary control or otherwise easily biased. In addition to being compared with a reference drug, a new compound is often compared with inert *dummy* medication, to serve as a control for placebo effects and coincident effects, such as spontaneous remission of symptoms.

Because the capacity of existing facilities for conducting controlled clinical trials is limited, and for other practical reasons, controlled trials cannot possibly be conducted on all types of patients or under all varieties of clinical conditions. Consequently, evaluation of the efficacy of a drug may continue well into the period of its *general clinical use.* More important, since drug toxicity may occur only in a limited portion of the population, only after long chronic use, or only in combination with other variables, accurate assessment of the toxic potential of a new drug may not be possible until it has been in general use for several years.

Drug Regulations. There are a number of regulations and compendia concerned with the testing, labeling, purity, and quality of foods, drugs, and cosmetics. Such regulations are designed for the protection of the public health. The following regulations apply to the United States; other countries have similar codes.

The initial law was passed by Congress in 1906, as a result of the excessive adulteration and misbrandings of foods and drugs existing at that time. The subsequent modifications—in 1938 and 1962—were, unfortunately, a result of tragedies brought about by inadequate testing of new drugs or vehicles for drugs. Enforcement of the law and its amendments is entrusted to the Food and Drug Administration (FDA) of the Department of Health, Education, and Welfare.

The 1938 amendments assure the safety, quality, and purity of drugs, by requiring accurate labeling of all medicinals. Regulations resulting from the Drug Amendments Act of 1962 are concerned with establishing the efficacy as well as the safety of new drugs. In addition, they place responsibility with the FDA for continuing evaluation of drugs already in general use. Drugs found to be too dangerous in proportion to their therapeutic worth can be removed from the market. Other provisions of the Drug Amendments Act required retrospective evaluation of the efficacy of all drugs introduced from 1938 to 1962. The important and difficult review of prescription drugs was undertaken for the FDA by panels of experts organized by the Drug Research Board of the National Academy of Sciences–National Research Council. Their conclusions were reported in the *Federal Register* as Drug Efficacy Study Implementation (DESI) ratings. Review of so-called OTC drugs, those available "over the counter" without prescription, was initiated by the FDA in 1972.

Decisions as to whether drugs may be sold "over the counter" or dispensed only on prescription and the refilling of prescriptions are regulated by the FDA under the provisions incorporated in the Durham-Humphrey Amendment of 1952 (*see* Appendix). The FDA establishes special standards for vaccines and other biological preparations, insulin, antibiotics, and germicides and is responsible for certification of their safety and efficacy. Foods, food additives, and cosmetics are also under the jurisdiction of the FDA. Veterinary preparations are controlled as rigidly as are human medicinals. The FDA also administers the Poison Prevention Packaging Act of 1970, which requires that hazardous substances be dispensed in "child-resistant" containers.

The United States Pharmacopeia (U.S.P.) and The National Formulary (N.F.). The Federal Pure Food and Drugs Act of 1906 recognized the U.S.P. and the N.F. as "official compendia," thereby giving official status to the drugs and the standards set forth in these volumes. The approved therapeutic agents used in medical practice are described and defined with respect to source, chemistry, physical properties, tests for identity and purity, assay, storage, therapeutic dosage range, and class of use.

Although initially prepared as guides to the physician in his choice of drugs, these compendia serve primarily as official standards for the quality and purity of drugs and are now of more use to the pharmaceutical industry and the FDA than to physicians. Nevertheless, the prescribing of *official* drugs listed in either the U.S.P. or N.F. provides assurance to the physician that the patient will receive exactly what has been prescribed with respect to quality and chemical uniformity. However, no tests of biological equivalence of official drugs are required, but they are under serious consideration. Other nations have similar compendia; there is also a *Pharmacopoea Internationalis* (sponsored by WHO), as well as a *European Pharmacopoeia.*

U.S.P. The first *Pharmacopeia* in the United States was published in 1820; the current edition, U.S.P. XIX, became official in 1975. The U.S.P. is revised at 5-year intervals, with interim supplements, by a special Pharmacopeial Committee, the members of which donate their services in the interest of the important function they serve. The committee consists of outstanding pharmacologists, pharmacists, and physicians.

Most preparations in the U.S.P. are single drugs; instructions are provided for the preparation of those that must be compounded. The U.S.P. organization also provides reference standards for the assaying and testing of many of the U.S.P. drugs.

N.F. This compendium was first published in 1888 under the name *National Formulary of Unofficial Preparations.* After its designation as an official drug standard in 1906, the name was changed to the present title. Unlike the U.S.P., the N.F. also contains descriptions of many drug mixtures. The N.F. formerly contained drugs on the basis of demand as well as therapeutic value; beginning with N.F. XII the sole criterion for admission of drugs has been merit.

The current edition, N.F. XIV, became official in 1975. This is to be the last edition, inasmuch as the U.S.P. organization has assumed ownership of the laboratory control and publication activities of the N.F. Prior to 1975 the N.F. was revised at 5-year intervals, with interim supplements, by the American Pharmaceutical Association. It was prepared by a committee and advisory panels consisting mainly of outstanding pharmaceutical scientists and physicians.

Other Regulations. The Comprehensive Drug Abuse Prevention and Control Act of 1970, or more simply the Controlled Substances Act, regulates the distribution and dispensing of all CNS drugs with significant abuse potential. Morphine and other opioids, barbiturates and other sedative-hypnotic-tranquilizers, amphetamines and other stimulants, cocaine, marihuana, and LSD and other psychotomimetic agents are controlled under this law. It is enforced by the Drug Enforcement Administration, U.S. Department of Justice. Drugs liable to serious abuse are also regulated by state and city laws (*see* Appendix).

GUIDE TO THE "THERAPEUTIC JUNGLE"

The flood of new drugs in recent years has provided many dramatic improvements in therapy, but it has also created a number of problems of equal magnitude. Not the least of these is the "therapeutic jungle," the term used to refer to the combination of the overwhelming number of drugs, the confusion over nomenclature, and the associated uncertainty of the status of many of these drugs. A reduction in the marketing of close congeners and drug mixtures and an improvement in the quality of advertising are important ingredients in the remedy for the "therapeutic jungle." However, the physician can also contribute to the remedy by employing nonproprietary rather than proprietary names whenever appropriate, by using prototypes both as an instructional device and in clinical practice, by adopting a properly critical attitude toward new drugs, and by knowing and making use of reliable sources of pharmacological information. Most important, he should develop a "way of thinking about drugs" based upon pharmacological principles.

Drug Nomenclature. The existence of many names for each drug, even when reduced to a minimum, has led to a lamentable and confusing situation in drug nomenclature. In addition to its formal *chemical* name, a new drug is usually assigned a *code* name by the pharmaceutical manufacturer. If the drug appears promising, and the manufacturer wishes to place it on the market, a *United States Adopted Name* (USAN) is selected by the USAN Council, which is jointly sponsored by the American Medical Association, the American Pharmaceutical Association, and the United States Pharmacopeial Convention, Inc. This *nonproprietary* name is often referred to as the *generic* name. This term has become entrenched, but by definition it should be more properly reserved to designate a chemical or pharmacological class of drugs, such as sulfonamides or sympathomimetics. If the drug is eventually admitted to the U.S.P. or N.F., the

USAN becomes the *official* name. However, the nonproprietary name and the official name of an older drug may differ. Subsequently, the drug will also be assigned a *proprietary* name or *trademark* by the manufacturer. If the drug is marketed by more than one company, it may have several proprietary names. If mixtures of the drug with other agents are marketed, each such mixture may also have a separate proprietary name.

There is increasing worldwide adoption of the same name for each therapeutic substance. For newer drugs, the USAN is usually adopted for the nonproprietary name in other countries, but this is not true for older drugs. International agreement on drug names is mediated through the World Health Organization and the pertinent health agencies of the cooperating countries.

The nonproprietary or official name of a drug should be used whenever possible, and such a practice has been adopted in this textbook. The use of the nonproprietary name is clearly less confusing when the drug is available under multiple proprietary names, and when the nonproprietary name more readily identifies the drug with its pharmacological class. The best argument for the proprietary name is that it is frequently more easily pronounced and remembered as a result of advertising. For purposes of identification, proprietary names, designated by SMALL-CAP TYPE, appear throughout the text in chapter sections dealing with preparations as well as in the Index. This does not imply a complete listing of proprietary names, since the number for a single drug may be large and since proprietary names differ from country to country.

The question arises, however, whether the nonproprietary name or a proprietary name should be employed by the physician when he prescribes drugs. Use of the nonproprietary name, unless the source is designated, permits the pharmacist to dispense the preparation of any manufacturer, and this sometimes results in less expense for the patient. On the other hand, prescribing by nonproprietary name could result in the patient receiving a preparation of inferior quality or uncertain bioavailability. In many respects, the argument is academic, since many drugs are available from only a single manufacturer, especially during the years of their patent protection, and since the biological equivalence of most pharmaceutical preparations has not been evaluated. The FDA is attempting to establish standards for bioavailability. Thus, the immediate answer to the question for most drugs (and the ultimate answer for all drugs) is straightforward. The physician should prescribe by nonproprietary name. Until biological equivalence of preparations of all drugs is a certainty, the physician is well advised to identify those drugs for which nonequivalence of preparations is a potential problem (*e.g.,* many drugs employed for chronic use), and he should prescribe them in a manner that assures that his patient receives reliable medication. He can do this by prescribing by nonproprietary name, with addition of the name of the manufacturer desired. Occasionally, a particular dosage form or special pharmaceutical formulation of a drug can be identified only by proprietary name.

Use of Prototypes. For teaching purposes, as illustrated in this textbook, the confusion created by the welter of similar drugs is reduced by restricting major attention to prototypes in each pharmacological class. Focusing on the representative drugs results in better characterization of a class as a whole, and thereby permits sharper recognition of the occasional member that possesses unique properties. A teaching prototype is often the agent of choice for clinical use, but this is not always true. A particular drug may be retained as the prototype, even though a new congener is clinically superior, either because more is known about the older drug or because it is more illustrative for the entire class of agents.

The clinician will also find the prototype device helpful in his struggle with the surfeit of congeneric drugs, since his needs for therapeutic agents can usually be adequately satisfied by one or two drugs in each class. Which of a number of more-or-less equivalent drugs the physician actually chooses as his prototypes may be determined by differences in their duration of action or other secondary characteristics. The important consideration is that he restrict his attention to a limited number of drugs in each class and that he become thoroughly familiar with

their individual characteristics. If he does, he will inevitably use these agents more effectively than he would if he were to change repeatedly among a larger number of drugs. Moreover, the greater experience with a few drugs will provide a better base line of personal experience by which he may judge the claims for newer medicinals.

Attitude toward New Drugs. A reasonable attitude toward new drugs is summarized by the adage that advises the physician to be "neither the first to use a new drug nor the last to discard the old." This advice is intended as a reminder that only a minor fraction of the new drugs released each year represents significant therapeutic advance, and that the efficacy and safety of a new drug, particularly relative to older agents, may not be fully assessed until sometime after it has been in general clinical use. At the same time, it also stresses the physician's obligation to keep abreast of significant advances in pharmacotherapy. However, appropriate, timely change from the old drug to the new is possible only if the physician has access to prompt, unbiased, critical information about new drugs.

Information about Drugs. *Pharmacology textbooks* usually provide basic pharmacological principles, critical appraisal of the therapeutically useful classes of drugs, and detailed descriptions of the prototypes that serve as standards of reference for assessing new drugs. In addition, pharmacodynamics and pathological physiology are correlated. However, for obvious reasons, these textbooks cannot include information on the most recently introduced drugs, nor can they provide detailed descriptions of many of the older drugs.

Somewhat more current but not basic information about drugs is provided by *AMA Drug Evaluations (AMA-DE)*, a publication of the Department of Drugs of the American Medical Association. *AMA-DE* is a useful reference book that evaluates information on both old and new single-entity drugs and mixtures, arranged according to therapeutic category.

Information about drug products and dosage forms may be found in the *American Hospital Formulary Service, pharmIndex,* and the American Pharmaceutical Association's *Handbook of Non-Prescription Drugs.* The *Physicians' Desk Reference (PDR)* provides information about available products, dosage forms, contraindications, adverse effects, and allowable therapeutic claims, but it is *not* useful as a critical guide to therapy or for comparison of drugs. Legally, all information on a drug described in *PDR* must conform to the descriptive material in the package insert for that drug and must have the approval of the FDA.

A very useful source of information on new drugs and therapeutics is the biweekly publication, *The Medical Letter.* Its distinguished board of editors provides a distinct service to medicine and to physicians by furnishing prompt, unbiased, pointed assessment of new drugs. A British publication, the *Drug and Therapeutics Bulletin,* is also published fortnightly with the same high standards. *Rational Drug Therapy,* formerly titled *Pharmacology for Physicians,* is a monthly publication in which experts discuss the clinical pharmacology of drugs used for the therapy of particular diseases. Other current and critical sources of information on drugs, drug therapy, and drug toxicity include the editorials and short reviews in *Clinical Pharmacology and Therapeutics,* the *New England Journal of Medicine,* and similar periodicals. *Pharmacological Reviews* and *Annual Review of Pharmacology* are excellent sources of basic pharmacological information.

Additionally, the physician should not overlook the pharmacist as a valuable source of information about drugs. Many pharmacists are now being trained not merely in the traditional role as dispensers of drugs but as clinical pharmacists to provide information about drugs and other general assistance on problems related to drug use and drug toxicity.

The Application of Pharmacological Principles. Drug therapy is often less than optimal. Many factors contribute to these therapeutic failures, and the physician is not solely responsible. Nevertheless, suboptimal therapy and unnecessary adverse effects can frequently be traced to his prescribing a drug without valid indication or for only marginal reasons, improper choice of medication, inappropriate use of the proper agent, failure to employ appropriate ancillary therapy, or inadequate monitoring of therapy. Much of this improper use of drugs by the physician is simply a failure to apply pharmacological principles.

To ensure the rational use of drugs, the physician is advised to examine each therapeutic effort in a systematic manner, by questions similar to the following: Is there valid indication for this drug? Is it the agent of choice? Are its effects modified by the patient's illness or concurrent medication? Is the dosage schedule appropriate? Is ancillary medication indicated? What is the therapeutic objective and what evidence of efficacy and potential adverse effects should be monitored? Is the patient adequately informed and instructed about the medication and can his compliance be expected?

The above scheme provides a framework both for effective application of pharmacological principles and for developing a properly critical attitude toward drugs and their use. For the student, it will also serve as a study guide for the individual drugs and drug groups.

General References

Goldstein, A.; Aronow, L.; and Kalman, S. M. *Principles of Drug Action: The Basis of Pharmacology,* 2nd ed. John Wiley & Sons, Inc., New York, **1974.**
Levine, R. R. *Pharmacology: Drug Actions and Reactions.* Little, Brown & Co., Boston, **1973.**
Melmon, K. L., and Morrelli, H. F. (eds.). *Clinical Pharmacology: Basic Principles in Therapeutics.* Macmillan Publishing Co., Inc., New York, **1972.**

Historical Background

Holmstedt, B., and Liljestrand, G. (eds.). *Readings in Pharmacology.* Pergamon Press, Ltd., Oxford, **1963.**
Shuster, L. (ed.). *Readings in Pharmacology.* Little, Brown & Co., Boston, **1962.**

Absorption, Distribution, Biotransformation, and Excretion

Albert, A. Ionization, pH and biological activity. *Pharmac. Rev.,* **1952,** *4,* 136–167.
Brodie, B. B., and Hogben, C. A. M. Some physiochemical factors in drug action. *J. Pharm. Pharmac.,* **1957,** *9,* 345–380.
Conney, A. H. Pharmacological implications of microsomal enzyme induction. *Pharmac. Rev.,* **1967,** *19,* 317–366. (379 references.)
Davson, H. The blood-brain barrier. In, *The Structure and Function of Nervous Tissue,* Vol. 4. (Bourne, G. H., ed.) Academic Press, Inc., New York, **1972,** pp. 321–445.
Hartiala, K. Metabolism of hormones, drugs, and other substances by the gut. *Physiol. Rev.,* **1973,** *53,* 496–534.
La Du, B. N.; Mandel, H. G.; and Way, E. L. (eds.). *Fundamentals of Drug Metabolism and Drug Disposition.* The Williams & Wilkins Co., Baltimore, **1971.**

Reidenberg, M. M. *Renal Function and Drug Action.* W. B. Saunders Co., Philadelphia, **1971.**

Scheline, R. R. Metabolism of foreign compounds by gastrointestinal microorganisms. *Pharmac. Rev.,* **1973,** *25,* 451–523.

Symposium. (Various authors.) *Proceedings of the First International Pharmacological Meeting.* Vol. 6, *Metabolic Factors Controlling Duration of Drug Action.* (Brodie, B. B., and Erdos, E. G., eds.) Pergamon Press, Ltd., Oxford, **1962.**

Symposium. (Various authors.) Drug metabolism in man. (Vesell, E. S., ed.) *Ann. N.Y. Acad. Sci.,* **1971,** *179,* 1–773.

Symposium. (Various authors.) Membrane structure and its biological applications. (Green, D. E., ed.) *Ann. N.Y. Acad. Sci.,* **1972,** *195,* 1–519.

Symposium. (Various authors.) Drug-protein binding. (Anton, A. H., and Solomon, H. M., eds.) *Ann. N.Y. Acad. Sci.,* **1973,** *226,* 1–362.

Williams, R. T. *Detoxication Mechanisms: The Mechanism and Detoxication of Drugs, Toxic Substances and Other Organic Compounds,* 2nd ed. John Wiley & Sons, Inc., New York, **1959.**

Pharmacokinetic Principles

Brodie, B. B., and Reid, W. D. Some pharmacological consequences of species variation in rates of metabolism. *Fedn Proc. Fedn Am. Socs exp. Biol.,* **1967,** *26,* 1062–1070.

Giusti, D. L., and Hayton, W. L. Dosage regimen adjustments in renal impairment. *Drug Intell. clin. Pharm.,* **1973,** *7,* 382–387.

Teorell, T. Kinetics of distribution of substances administered to the body. I. The extravascular modes of administration. II. The intravascular modes of administration. *Archs int. Pharmacodyn. Thér.,* **1937,** *57,* 205–225, 226–240.

Wagner, J. G. *Biopharmaceutics and Relevant Pharmacokinetics.* Drug Intelligence, Hamilton, Ill., **1971.**

Biological Assay and Mathematics

Finney, D. J. *Statistical Method in Biological Assay,* 2nd ed. Hafner Publishing Co., New York; Charles Griffin & Co., Ltd., London, **1964.**

Gaddum, J. H. Bioassays and mathematics. *Pharmac. Rev.,* **1953,** *5,* 87–134. (208 references.)

Riggs, D. S. *The Mathematical Approach to Physiological Problems: A Critical Primer.* The Williams & Wilkins Co., Baltimore, **1963;** The M.I.T. Press, Cambridge, **1970.**

Mechanisms of Drug Action and Structure-Activity Relationship

Dikstein, S. (ed.). *Fundamentals of Cell Pharmacology.* Charles C Thomas, Pub., Springfield, Ill., **1973.**

Featherstone, R. M. (ed.). *A Guide to Molecular Pharmacology-Toxicology,* Parts I–II. Marcel Dekker, Inc., New York, **1973.**

Symposium. (Various authors.) *Advances in Chemistry Series.* Vol. 45, *Molecular Modification in Drug Design.* (Gould, R. F., ed.) American Chemical Soc., Washington, D. C., **1964.**

Drug Receptors

Clark, A. J. *The Mode of Action of Drugs on Cells.* E. Arnold & Co., London, **1933.**

Paton, W. D. M. A theory of drug action based on the rate of drug-receptor combination. *Proc. R. Soc., B,* **1961,** *154,* 21–69.

Porter, R., and O'Connor, M. (eds.). *Molecular Properties of Drug Receptors* (a Ciba Foundation symposium). J. & A. Churchill, Ltd., London, **1970.**

Rang, H. P. Receptor mechanisms: Fourth Gaddum Memorial Lecture, School of Pharmacy, University of London, January 1973. *Br. J. Pharmac.,* **1973,** *48,* 475–495.

Factors That Modify Drug Effects and Drug Dosage

Blackwell, B. Patient compliance. *New Engl. J. Med.,* **1973,** *289,* 249–252.

Bourne, H. R. The placebo—a poorly understood and neglected therapeutic agent. *Ration. Drug Ther.,* **1971,** *5,* No. 11, 1–6.

Council Conference. Notes on the package insert. *J. Am. med. Ass.,* **1969,** *207,* 1335–1338.

FDA. Use of drugs for unapproved indications: your legal responsibility. *FDA Drug Bull.,* Oct. **1972.**

Koch-Weser, J. Serum drug concentrations as therapeutic guides. *New Engl. J. Med.,* **1972,** *287,* 227–231.

Loewe, S. The problem of synergism and antagonism of combined drugs. *Arzneimittel-Forsch.,* **1953,** *3,* 285–290.

Symposium. (Various authors.) Symposium on pediatric pharmacology. (Yaffe, S. J., ed.) *Pediat. Clins N. Am.,* **1972,** *19,* 1–259.

Wolf, S. The pharmacology of placebos. *Pharmac. Rev.,* **1959,** *11,* 689–704.

Drug Interactions

American Pharmaceutical Association. *Evaluations of Drug Interactions—1973.* The Association, Washington, D. C., **1973.**

Constantino, N. V., and Kabat, H. F. Drug-induced modifications of laboratory test values—revised 1973. *Am. J. hosp. Pharm.,* **1973,** *30,* 24–71.

Hansten, P. D. *Drug Interactions: Clinical Significance of Drug-Drug Interactions and Drug Effects on Clinical Laboratory Results,* 2nd ed. Lea & Febiger, Philadelphia, **1973.**

Medical Letter. Adverse interactions of drugs. **1975,** *17,* 17–24.

Drug Toxicity

D'Arcy, P. F., and Griffin, J. P. *Iatrogenic Diseases.* Oxford University Press, London, **1972.**

Gardner, P., and Cluff, L. E. The epidemiology of adverse drug reactions: a review and perspective. *Johns Hopkins med. J.,* **1970,** *126,* 77–87.

Gleason, M. N.; Gosselin, R. E.; Hodge, H. C.; and Smith, R. P. *Clinical Toxicology of Commercial Products: Acute Poisoning,* 3rd ed. The Williams & Wilkins Co., Baltimore, **1969.**

Symposium. (Various authors.) Symposium on poisoning in children. (Coleman, A. B., and Alpert, J. J., eds.) *Pediat. Clins N. Am.,* **1970,** *17,* 471–758.

Development and Evaluation of Drugs

Ladimer, I., and Newman, R. W. (eds.). *Clinical Investigation in Medicine: Legal, Ethical, and Moral Aspects.* Boston University Law-Medicine Research Inst., Boston, **1962.**

Laurence, D. R. (ed.). *Quantitative Methods in Human Pharmacology and Therapeutics.* Pergamon Press, Ltd., Oxford, **1959.**

Talalay, P. (ed.). *Drugs in Our Society.* The Johns Hopkins Press, Baltimore, **1964.**

Wolstenholme, G., and Porter, R. (eds.). *Drug Responses in Man* (a Ciba Foundation volume). Little, Brown & Co., Boston, **1967.**

Official Drug Compendia

The National Formulary, 14th ed. (American Pharmaceutical Association.) Mack Printing Co., Easton, Pa., published **1974,** became official **1975.**

The Pharmacopeia of the United States of America, 19th rev. (The United States Pharmacopeial Convention, Inc.) Mack Printing Co., Easton, Pa., published **1974,** became official **1975.**

SECTION

II

Drugs Acting on the Central Nervous System

INTRODUCTION

Donald N. Franz

Drugs that exert their primary effects on the central nervous system (CNS) comprise the most widely employed group of pharmacologically active agents. In addition to their valid use in therapy, the consumption of drugs in the form of alcoholic and caffeinated beverages is socially accepted and widely practiced throughout the world. The burgeoning traffic in illicit drugs is confined exclusively to agents sought for their pronounced effects on the CNS. Drugs capable of influencing the mind have been available throughout recorded history, and their widespread abuse has become a significant social problem for which no satisfactory solutions are in sight.

Centrally acting drugs exert a broad spectrum of effects that are indispensable to therapeutics. Many modern surgical procedures obviously require the availability of general anesthetics. Highly selective effects on common symptoms such as pain and fever are very familiar, and debilitating neurological syndromes as diverse in etiology as epilepsy and parkinsonism can be effectively controlled by drug therapy. The introduction of potent psychotherapeutic agents in the past 2 decades has had a dramatic impact on the basic concepts and treatment of mental illness. In addition, pharmacological induction of psychic derangements resembling clinical psychoses continues to kindle speculation and investigation concerning the nature of psychiatric disorders.

Drugs other than those designated as centrally acting may exert profound effects on the CNS as part of their pharmacological actions. Many drugs administered for their peripheral action also produce side effects or toxic reactions that are referable to the CNS. The developing nervous system is especially vulnerable to permanent damage as a result of deviations from optimal levels of hormones, vitamins, and nutrients. Hormonal imbalance or vitamin deficiency may precipitate abnormal neurophysiological and psychic states that can be corrected by appropriate therapy.

Current knowledge of the CNS is quite incomplete. Nevertheless, it is possible to delineate guidelines and to outline principles that form the framework of current concepts of CNS pharmacology. Such principles depend upon physiological and biochemical schemes that are constantly undergoing revision.

Anatomical and Neurophysiological Considerations. No other biological system matches the human brain for complexity of organization. Full understanding of the integration and operation of approximately ten billion neurons and a greater number of glial cells that account for the enormously varied and complicated functions of the CNS represents the ultimate scientific challenge. Nevertheless, much has been learned about the basic properties of individual neurons, their modes of communication, and many aspects of their organization.

Anatomically, neurons are organized within various gross structures such as the cerebrum, cerebellum, brain stem, and spinal cord. Each gross division can be further subdivided into anatomically distinct collections of neuronal cell bodies (nuclei) or bundles of their axons (tracts). On a *functional* basis, the areas of the CNS concerned with one type of activity are linked together. Thus, it is possible to identify systems concerned with sensory functions, motor activity, regulation of autonomic functions, control of respiration, and memory and association. These systems do not operate independently; rather, they interact with one another to a considerable degree. Furthermore, certain anatomical regions of the CNS may participate in several of the functions mentioned. From the *evolutionary* standpoint some systems, such as those controlling respiration and the fundamental motor reflexes, are primitive and basic, whereas systems concerned with the fine control of movement and with association and memory are phylogenetically "newer."

Drug action is seldom, if ever, restricted to the neurons that comprise an anatomical or functional division of the CNS. Many drugs owe their usefulness in therapeutics to the fact that they selectively affect one system over another. Nevertheless, it should not be thought that they exert their actions solely on the neurons that participate in that function.

It is well established that communication between neurons in the CNS occurs primarily by chemical synaptic transmission. Electrical transmission as such is exceptional in the mammalian CNS, but synchronization among populations of functionally related neurons through ionic changes in their extracellular environment may be important at some sites. As in the periphery, synaptic connections in the CNS are characterized anatomically by presynaptic terminals containing synaptic vesicles and by areas of close apposition between presynaptic and postsynaptic membranes. Synapses are described as axodendritic, axosomatic, axoaxonic, or dendrodendritic to denote connections between the three different parts of neurons. Individual neurons differ enormously in the range and the complexity of their synaptic connections. A single neuron may receive thousands of synaptic connections, which in most cases probably represent a mixture of excitatory and inhibitory fibers (*see* Chapter 21).

Excitation in the CNS is similar in basic mechanism to that at synapses in the peripheral nervous system. The action potential in the excitatory presynaptic fiber causes release of a transmitter, which traverses the synaptic cleft and produces depolarization of the postsynaptic membrane. This depolarization, the excitatory postsynaptic potential (EPSP), is graded in amplitude according to the quantity of excitatory transmitter released. When the EPSP reaches a critical level, an action potential arises in the postjunctional neuron.

Inhibition may be exerted by several mechanisms. Two types of inhibition in the mammalian CNS currently are known. *Postsynaptic inhibition* is accomplished by the action of inhibitory transmitters on the postsynaptic membrane. The inhibitory transmitters stabilize the postsynaptic membrane by altering its ionic permeability or by modifying the activity of metabolically driven ion pumps. Thus, by direct action on the postsynaptic membrane, the inhibitory transmitters counteract the effect of the excitatory transmitter. In *presynaptic inhibition* the inhibitory fibers make connections with the presynaptic terminals of the excitatory fibers rather than with the postsynaptic membrane and, by depolarization of the presynaptic terminals, reduce the amount of excitatory transmitter released by the excitatory nerve impulse.

Throughout the CNS there are neuronal systems that produce either excitatory or inhibitory effects upon other areas. For example, certain portions of the reticular formation exert excitatory influences on many parts of the CNS; other portions of the reticular formation produce primarily inhibitory effects. Contained within the spinal cord are neuronal systems that are inhibitory to certain motoneurons and excitatory to others. Many of these systems are tonically active. Such excitatory and inhibitory systems are of extreme importance in regulating the level of activity of specific functional systems. They also serve to maintain the discreteness of reflex acts. Although the actions of drugs on these general excitatory and inhibitory systems are incompletely understood, it is known that in many cases they are of great importance in determining drug effect.

Neurochemical Considerations. The important discovery that synaptic transmission in the periphery is mediated by specific neurohumoral substances, primarily acetylcholine and norepinephrine, had a profound and enduring impact upon basic understanding of drug action in the nervous system (*see* Chapter 21). Likewise, synaptic excitation and inhibition in the CNS are accomplished by specific chemical transmitters; each neuron is thought to release the same transmitter from all of its synaptic terminals to produce either excitation or inhibition of the postsynaptic neurons that it innervates. It would be of great practical importance for elucidating central drug action to identify the transmitters at specific synapses in the CNS. However, the task of fulfilling the criteria for proof that a specific substance operates as a transmitter in the CNS presents a number of formidable obstacles that are not encountered in the far simpler organization of peripheral synapses. Nevertheless, progress toward identifying central transmitters is proceeding rapidly by a variety of sophisticated electrophysiological, pharmacological, biochemical, and histochemical approaches. Significant clues have also emerged from neuropathological studies. The list of putative central neuro-humoral transmitters, which can be substantiated to varying degrees, includes acetylcholine, norepinephrine, dopamine, 5-hydroxytryptamine, and several amino acids: glutamic, aspartic, and gamma-aminobutyric acids and glycine (*see* Chapter 21).

Although the identity of central transmitters offers considerable promise toward explaining mechanisms of drug action, full understanding must await comprehensive information on their metabolism and on their functional roles in the myriad of central pathways. Further-more, many centrally acting drugs owe their selectivity to mechanisms that are not confined to isolated effects on specific chemical synapses or transmitters (*see* below).

Classification of CNS Drugs. Some form of classification of CNS drugs is desirable. The most durable method would obviously be according to their mechanisms of action, but information at present is too scanty to permit classification on this basis. Therefore, the CNS drugs are classified according to their most prominent effect or the effect that establishes their therapeutic usefulness.

General (Nonselective) CNS Depressants. This category includes the anesthetic gases and vapors, the aliphatic alcohols, and the barbiturates and related sedative-hypnotic drugs. These agents, in contrast to selective depressants (*see* below), share the ability to depress excitable tissue at all levels of the CNS. In general, this action is accomplished by stabilization of neuronal membranes, including depression of presynaptic structures, with a consequent de-crease in amount of transmitter released by the nerve impulse, as well as depression of postsynaptic receptors.

General (Nonselective) CNS Stimulants. The drugs in this category are strychnine, picro-toxin, pentylenetetrazol, and related agents capable of powerful CNS excitation, and the xanthines, which have a much weaker action. General CNS stimulants exert their action throughout the CNS. Stimulation is accomplished by one of two general mechanisms: block-ade of inhibition (exemplified by strychnine) or direct neuronal excitation (exemplified by pentylenetetrazol). Direct excitation may include one or more of the following mechanisms: neuronal depolarization, increase in release of transmitter, more prolonged transmitter action, labilization of the neuronal membrane, or decrease in synaptic recovery time.

Drugs that Selectively Modify CNS Function. The agents in this group may exhibit either depressant or excitatory effects. In some instances, a drug may produce both effects simulta-neously on different systems. On the other hand, some agents in this category have little effect upon the level of excitability in doses used therapeutically. The principal classes of drugs are the following: anticonvulsants, antiparkinsonism drugs, narcotic-analgesics, and analgesic-antipyretics. Also included in this category is the heterogeneous group of agents employed as psychopharmacological drugs.

It must be pointed out that selectivity or nonselectivity of drug action in the CNS should be regarded as only relative and refers to more restricted versus more generalized effects on total brain function. For example, the use of general depressants would be very limited if central control of the respiratory and cardiovascular systems were not selectively spared to some degree. On the other hand, the very selective antagonism of one type of postsynaptic inhibition by the general stimulant strychnine occurs at many levels of the CNS.

Pharmacological effects of drugs from the "selective" category can be demonstrated experimentally on nervous pathways that are obviously not relevant to their therapeutic actions but, nevertheless, may provide clues to those actions. Although selectivity of drug effect may in some instances be remarkable, a drug usually affects a variety of functions of the CNS in varying degree. When only one constellation of effects is wanted in a therapeutic situation, the remaining effects produced by the drug are regarded as limitations in its selectivity or as "side effects." The imprecise boundary between wanted effects and side effects is illustrated by the aphorism: "One man's side effect is another man's remedy."

There is a tendency to exaggerate the selectivity of drugs. This is partly due to the fact that the drug is identified with the effect that is implied by the class name. Thus, the necessary process of classification usually creates overemphasis of drug selectivity. However, since all centrally acting drugs are more or less selective, it will be profitable to consider some of the probable bases for their selectivity; such considerations are inseparable from the mechanisms of their action.

Bases for Drug Selectivity; Mechanisms of Action.   The several processes that may contribute to the selective, in contrast to the general, effects of drugs on the CNS are as follows:

Differential Effects upon Neurohumoral Mechanisms.   Drugs may affect some step in the production or action of neurohumoral transmitters. At present the transmitter substances in the CNS are largely unproven; however, there is considerable evidence that actions upon transmitter mechanisms constitute one of the major bases for drug selectivity. Many concepts of drug effects on chemical transmission in the CNS are derived from knowledge of drug actions in the peripheral nervous system (*see* Chapter 21). Some potential mechanisms by which nervous system functions may be modified through actions on transmitter processes are as follows: mimicking the transmitter, prolonging the sojourn of the transmitter in the synaptic region, blocking the postsynaptic action of the transmitter, releasing the transmitter from presynaptic stores, depleting presynaptic stores of the transmitter, preventing the synthesis of the transmitter, enhancing the synthesis of the transmitter, preventing the release of the transmitter by the nerve impulse, and replacing the natural with a "false" transmitter.

Selective Neuronal Localization of the Drug.   Certain drugs are selectively concentrated by the neurons upon which they act. The terminal membranes of many neurons possess active uptake mechanisms that are selective for their particular transmitter or its precursors. However, the uptake mechanisms will often transport other substrates that are chemically related to the normal transmitter. Alteration of transmitter metabolism by foreign substrates is an established mechanism of selective drug action on neurohumoral mechanisms.

Selective Anatomical Localization of the Drug.   Differences in regional blood flow or in brain composition can account for some selective distribution of drugs to certain gross anatomical regions. Selective localization by such mechanisms may or may not be relevant to a particular drug effect.

Differential Actions on Different Cell or Synaptic Types.   Anatomically different types of cells may differ in their sensitivity to drugs. Factors such as cell size, and types and density of synaptic connections may be important in determining sensitivity to drugs. For example, synapses with a low safety factor for transmission are more readily blocked by general depressants than are those with a high safety factor.

Differential Effects Dependent upon Neuronal Organization.   Drugs that act equally on all cells of a given type may manifest a greater effect upon one type of neuronal organization than another. A clear example of this is the greater sensitivity of polysynaptic chains to depressant drugs as compared to pathways containing a single synapse.

Differential Effects Dependent upon the Functional State of Neurons.   An example of this mechanism is provided by agents that selectively affect synaptic recovery. The effect of such drugs is manifest primarily upon repetitively active systems. Another example is provided by antipyretic drugs, which lower temperature in a febrile but not in a normal individual.

On a less tangible level, it is clear that the effects of some psychopharmacological agents depend upon the psychic state of the individual.

Differential Effects upon Neuronal Metabolism. Drugs may affect transport or utilization of nutrients and metabolites, through actions on glial cells or by other means. By such mechanisms, drugs may differentially affect the level of metabolism of neurons, the degree of accumulation of metabolic products, or the rate of active ion pumping.

Differential Effects Resulting from Differences in Neuronal Biochemistry. The chemical receptor upon which a drug acts may be present in some neurons and absent from others. Drug receptors may be extracellular, within the neuronal membrane, or at intracellular structures. A drug would not affect neurons lacking its particular receptor.

Factors That Affect Intensity and Duration of CNS Drug Effect. Apart from the exceptional instances in which drugs are introduced directly into the CNS, the concentration of the agent in the blood after oral or parenteral administration has great bearing on the concentration in the CNS. However, this relationship is not so simple as for peripheral structures. The blood-brain barrier (Chapter 1) limits the passage of certain drugs into and out of the cerebrospinal fluid. In general, nonionized molecules pass this structure more readily than do ionized molecules. However, active transport of certain agents may occur across the barrier in either direction. In addition to this barrier, drugs in the cerebrospinal fluid may gain access to appropriate sites in the CNS at different rates.

Other factors may also influence the duration of drug effect. Where the action of a drug is to cause depletion of a transmitter substance, the effect of the drug may be delayed in appearance. Such depletion may lead to a prolonged effect that persists after the presence of the drug is no longer detectable. An example of this is provided by the drug reserpine, which depletes the stores of catecholamines in the central and peripheral nervous systems. The full effect of this drug appears many hours after it reaches a maximum concentration in the brain, and the consequences of depletion are apparent for a considerable time after all detectable reserpine has been eliminated from the body. Fixed binding of a drug to a receptor can also produce a prolonged effect. Certain cholinesterase inhibitors, such as di-*iso*propyl phosphorofluoridate, are bound by covalent linkage to the active receptor sites on the enzyme. Molecules of the inhibitor that are not so bound are eliminated from the body. Inhibition of the enzyme by the bound drug, however, persists until new enzyme molecules have been synthesized.

Repeated administration of certain drugs results in the development of *tolerance*. This represents still another mechanism by which drug effect and drug concentration are sometimes dissociated. Remarkable degrees of tolerance can develop to some CNS drugs that are chronically abused, particularly the opioids.

General Characteristics of CNS Drugs. The various levels of CNS excitability represent a continuum between the extremes of coma and convulsions. Decreases in excitability from normal are graded through sedation, hypnosis, general anesthesia, and coma. Increases in excitability from normal are graded through mild hyperexcitability, extreme hyperexcitability, and mild-to-severe convulsions. The agents included in the categories of *general CNS depressants* and *general CNS stimulants* are capable of modifying CNS excitability on this continuum. *Selective CNS drugs* are generally considered to be more restricted in their actions, but most of them can produce changes in excitability of some systems similar to those seen with nonselective agents. Combinations of centrally acting drugs are frequently administered for therapeutic advantage, but certain combinations of drugs may be detrimental because of interactions between their central effects. Some of the more common interactions are presented in relation to the following general characteristics of centrally acting drugs.

1. Individual drugs may differ from one another in both *potency* and *maximal effect* or *efficacy*. Although relative potency is seldom an important therapeutic consideration, the maximal effect that a drug can produce may be crucial. For example, differences in potency among narcotic analgesics have little bearing on the choice of drug, but the greater analgesic

efficacy of morphine than that of aspirin dictates the choice between them. Two agents with low efficacy may sometimes be combined to achieve a greater effect; on the other hand, lower doses of two agents with high efficacy may be combined to minimize toxicity.

2. Drug effect is additive with the physiological state and with the effect of other depressant and stimulant drugs. For example, a given amount of anesthetic agent will produce less anesthesia in a hyperexcitable than in a normal patient. The converse is true with respect to the effect of stimulant drugs. In general, depressant effects of drugs from all categories are additive. This summation is a major cause of drug interactions among general depressants and major and minor tranquilizers. Stimulant effects of drugs are also additive. Therefore, respiration adversely affected by morphine is further impaired by depressant drugs, whereas stimulant drugs can augment the excitatory effects of morphine to produce vomiting and convulsions.

3. Antagonism between depressants and stimulants is variable. Very few instances of true *pharmacological antagonism* among CNS drugs are known; for example, narcotic antagonists are very selective for the opioids, and trimethadione (an anticonvulsant) completely blocks the convulsions produced by pentylenetetrazol over a wide dosage range. Usually the antagonism exhibited is *physiological antagonism,* in which the antagonists do not act on precisely the same systems by opposite mechanisms. Thus, an individual who has received one drug cannot be returned entirely to normal by another. However, remarkable antagonism between depressants and stimulants may be noted with respect to certain functions.

4. An *excitatory effect* on some functions is commonly observed with low concentrations of some depressant drugs, due either to depression of inhibitory systems or to a transient increase in the release of excitatory transmitters. Examples are the "stage of excitement" during induction of general anesthesia by the anesthetic gases and vapors and the "stimulant" effects of alcohol. The excitatory phase occurs only with low concentrations of the depressant; uniform depression ensues with increasing drug concentration. The excitatory effects can be minimized by pretreatment with a depressant drug that is devoid of such effects.

5. Acute, excessive stimulation of the cerebrospinal axis is normally followed by depression, which is the consequence of neuronal fatigue and of exhaustion of metabolites and transmitter stores. This *postictal* depression is additive with the effects of depressant drugs.

6. Acute, drug-induced depression is not, as a rule, followed by stimulation. However, *chronic* drug sedation or depression is followed by prolonged hyperexcitability upon abrupt withdrawal of medication. This type of hyperexcitability can be effectively controlled by the same or another depressant drug. The reader is referred to the discussion of drug addiction (Chapter 16) for consideration of this phenomenon.

7. The selective effects of drugs on specific neurotransmitter systems may be additive or competitive. This potential for drug interactions must be considered whenever such drugs are administered concurrently. The prolonged duration of action of some, such as the monoamine oxidase inhibitors, necessitates a drug-free period before starting certain other drugs, to avoid interactions.

8. If two drugs with different mechanisms of action are both effective in the treatment of a given condition, a greater therapeutic effect may sometimes be achieved with their combined use than with either drug alone. This approach is frequently used to advantage in the therapy of epilepsy.

Perspectives.   The complexity of the CNS, as compared to other organs and systems of the body, humbles all who study it. Despite remarkable advances in neuropharmacology, the dearth of definitive information on the mechanisms by which specific drugs affect neuronal functions necessitates a considerable degree of empiricism in the therapeutic approach to both organic and functional diseases of the nervous system. Schemes purporting to show precisely how a drug acts to restore neuronal dysfunction must be regarded with considerable skepticism.

The actions of chemical substances of novel structure and congeners of old structures are constantly being investigated. Similarly, reinvestigation of old drugs reveals new properties and new central actions. Physiological advances continually indicate new points of drug attack, and pharmacological observations provide new clues to physiological mechanisms. Both areas of study often indicate new therapeutic approaches.

The problem of understanding the anatomical and functional complexities of the human nervous system poses the ultimate challenge for the mind of man. Progress in discovering and creating chemicals to ameliorate the undesirable consequences of functional and organic disturbances of the nervous system is steady but also marked by frequent reverses. While no limit should be placed upon our ultimate expectations, the problems of inadequate drug efficacy, drug toxicity, multiple actions and interactions of drugs, and side effects of drugs will plague therapeutics for a considerable time to come.

CHAPTER

2   HISTORY AND THEORIES OF GENERAL ANESTHESIA

Peter J. Cohen

HISTORY OF SURGICAL ANESTHESIA

Anesthetic agents have been employed since ancient times, their earliest use being lost in antiquity. The Egyptians, who practiced surgery widely, probably used narcotics of various sorts. The Chinese employed hashish (cannabis indica) for its analgesic properties. Pliny, Dioscorides, and Apuleius recommended mandragora (belladonna alkaloids) for use before operations. In addition to drugs, many bizarre and cruel physical methods were devised to render patients temporarily unconscious. For example, the Assyrians asphyxiated children by strangulation before circumcision, a practice used in Italy as late as the seventeenth century. Cerebral concussion, produced by striking a wooden bowl placed on the head, was also employed. The earliest written reference to anesthesia is believed to be in the treatise, *De Trinitate*, by St. Hilary of Poitiers *ca.* A.D. 350, who wrote, "The soul can be lulled to sleep by drugs, which overcome the pain and produce in the mind a deathlike forgetfulness of its power and sense" (cited by Montagu, 1946). Opium, belladonna, hemp, and alcoholic beverages were for many centuries the main drugs used to ease the pain of surgery.

The use of anesthetics for complete and safe abolition of pain in surgical operations is an accomplishment of an epoch-making 5-year period between 1842 and 1847. Before this, operations were horrible ordeals and the surgeon attempted to shorten the agony by working with great haste. Amputations, for example, were completed in a few seconds and surgeons boasted of their speed. Obviously, careful dissection and delicate treatment of tissues were impossible.

The first inhalational anesthetic to be discovered was nitrous oxide, by Priestley in 1776. Priestley accurately described the sensations occurring during inhalation of this agent as "analogous to gentle pressure on all the muscles, attended by an highly pleasurable thrilling, particularly in the chest and the extremities. . . . The sense of muscular power became greater, and at last an irresistible propensity to action was indulged in. . . . Whenever its operation was carried to the highest extent, the pleasurable thrilling . . . gradually diminished, the sense of pressure on the muscles was lost; impressions ceased to be perceived; vivid ideas passed rapidly through the mind, and voluntary power was altogether destroyed, so that the mouthpiece generally dropt from my unclosed lips." In 1799, Humphry Davy announced that nitrous oxide had the ability to destroy pain and suggested its use during surgical operations. For 43 years this suggestion lay unheeded. Pearson in 1795 recorded the use of ether inhalations to control the pain of colic, and Beddoes in the next year published a case report of deep sleep induced by ether. In 1818, Faraday reported on the analgesic effects of ether. Operations on animals depressed by carbon dioxide and hypoxia were performed by Hickman in 1824, in which year his famous pamphlet on suspended animation was published.

Despite these early stirrings, the discovery of surgical anesthesia was an American contribution. In the early 1840s, a peripatetic chemist-lecturer by the name of Colton traveled through New England giving public demonstrations of nitrous oxide, or "laughing gas," inhalation for an admission charge of 25 cents. On December 10, 1844, he arrived in Hartford, Connecticut and circulated the following advertisement:

A Grand Exhibition of the effects produced by inhaling Nitrous Oxid, Exhilarating or Laughing Gas! will be given at Union Hall this (Tuesday) Evening, Dec. 10th, 1844.

Forty gallons of Gas will be prepared and administered to all in the audience who desire to inhale it.

Twelve Young Men have volunteered to inhale the Gas, to commence the entertainment.

Eight Strong Men are engaged to occupy the front seats to protect those under the influence of the Gas from injuring themselves or others. This course is adopted that no apprehension of danger may be entertained. Probably no one will attempt to fight.

The effect of the Gas is to make those who inhale it either Laugh, Sing, Dance, Speak or Fight, and so forth, according to the leading trait of their character. They seem to retain consciousness enough not to say or do that which they would have occasion to regret.

N. B.—The Gas will be administered only to gentlemen of the first respectability. The object is to make the entertainment in every respect a genteel affair.

Horace Wells, a dentist in Hartford, attended the lecture. A drug clerk named Cooley volunteered to inhale the gas, and during the inhalation became dazed and belligerent. He jumped from the stage to fight with one of the "strong men" in the front row, but the latter fled. After him went Cooley, who during the chase jumped over a chair, tripped, and fell to the ground. The fall brought him to his senses and he returned to his seat sobered and apologetic. Suddenly he noticed that his leg was gashed and bleeding where he had struck the chair during the chase. He was astonished by the presence of the wound for he had experienced no pain. Wells carefully questioned him regarding this, but he insisted that there had been no pain with the injury. The very next day, Wells had one of his teeth extracted painlessly under nitrous oxide, Colton administering the gas. After the effect of the anesthetic had subsided, he exclaimed, "A new era in tooth-pulling!" He then used nitrous oxide in his dental practice in Hartford and gave the matter unrestricted publicity.

In January, 1845, Wells went to the Massachusetts General Hospital in Boston to exhibit his gas. The demonstration unfortunately failed, the patient awakening too soon and screaming in pain. Wells met with unjust ridicule because it was not then appreciated that the gas is hard to administer. The wonder is that without special apparatus Wells was successful at all.

The introduction of ether in the following year placed Wells and nitrous oxide in the background. Greatly embittered, Wells became insane and finally committed suicide. Wells must be given credit for appreciating the importance of nitrous oxide anesthesia and attempting to apply it in dental surgery. In the early 1860s, Colton, the traveling lecturer who 20 years before had by his demonstration initiated the work of Wells, revived the use of nitrous oxide and in a few years the gas was extensively employed in dentistry.

In March, 1842, over three centuries after the chemical discovery of ether by Valerius Cordus in 1540 (named "Aether" by August Siegmund Frobenius in 1730), Crawford W. Long of Jefferson, Georgia, had a friend inhale ether while he removed a small tumor from the neck. The subject felt no pain. American physicians were familiar with the effects of ether due chiefly to Faraday, who had written about the stupefying effects of the compound as early as 1818, as follows: "When the vapor of ether mixed with common air is inhaled, it produces effects similar to those occasioned by nitrous oxide." Nevertheless, in conservative medical circles, ether was considered to be dangerous in amounts causing loss of consciousness. Medical students and others had experimented with Faraday's observation by holding ether parties, or "jags" as they were called. Dr. Long often attended such ether frolics, having first witnessed them in Philadelphia several years before, and he became greatly interested in the possibilities of ether as an anesthetic. Finally, he used it for anesthesia on several occasions in his surgical practice. Unfortunately, Long failed to publish his experiences, and his findings remained unknown until ether anesthesia was rediscovered and properly developed by Morton and others as an accepted procedure in surgery.

William T. G. Morton of Boston, a former dental associate of Wells, was much interested in nitrous oxide anesthesia. He was also acquainted with the stupefying effects of ether. Morton entered the Harvard Medical School as a student and continued his practice of dentistry in order to defray his expenses. He consulted Prof. Charles T. Jackson, his chemistry teacher, concerning the problem of anesthesia. Morton apparently learned from Jackson that ether, to be useful, should be pure sulfuric ether, the kind that Burnell sold. Morton then practiced on himself, the family dog, cats, hens, and rats, and finally successfully extracted a tooth under ether on September 30, 1846. Soon he asked Dr. J. C. Warren, professor of surgery at Harvard Medical School, for permission to make a test trial of ether in a surgical operation. The request was allowed and the day set for the demonstration was October 16, 1846.

The story of this classical demonstration has been retold countless times. The operating room ("ether dome") at the Massachusetts General Hospital remains as a memorial to the first public demonstration of surgical anesthesia. In the gallery of this room skeptical spectators gathered, for the news had spread that a second-year medical student had developed a method for abolishing surgical pain. The patient, Gilbert Abbott, was brought in and Dr. Warren, the surgeon, waited in formal morning clothes, for gowns, masks, gloves, surgical asepsis, and the bacterial origin of infection were entirely unknown in that day. Everyone was ready and waiting, even the strong men to hold down the struggling patient, but Morton did not appear. Fifteen minutes passed, and the surgeon, becoming impatient, took his scalpel and turning to the gallery said, "As Dr. Morton has not arrived, I presume he is otherwise engaged." While the audience smiled and the patient cringed, the surgeon turned to make his incision. Just then Morton entered, his tardiness being due to the necessity for completing an apparatus with which to administer the ether. It is told that Dr. Warren stepped back, and pointing to the man strapped to the operating table said, "Well, sir, your patient is ready." Surrounded by a silent and unsympathetic audience, Morton went quietly to work. After a few minutes of ether inhalation, the patient was unconscious, whereupon Morton looked up and said, "Dr. Warren, *your* patient is ready." The operation was begun. The patient gave no sign of pain, yet he was alive and breathing. The strong men were not needed. When the operation was completed, Dr. Warren turned to the astonished audience and said, "Gentlemen, this is no humbug." Dr. Henry J. Bigelow, an eminent surgeon attending the demonstration, remarked, "I have seen something today that will go around the world."

The complete success of this demonstration resulted, after a short initial period of disbelief, doubt, and delay, in the rapid introduction of general anesthesia for surgical operations. Dr. Warren wrote, "A new era has opened on the operating surgeon. Who could have imagined that drawing a knife over the delicate skin of the face might produce a sensation of unmixed delight? That the contorting of an ankylosed joint should coexist with a celestial vision? If Ambrose Paré, and Louis, and Desault, and Chesselden and Hunter, and Cooper, could see what our eyes daily witness, how would they long to come among us and perform their exploits once more. And with what fresh vigor does the living surgeon, who is ready to resign the scalpel, grasp it, and wish again to go through his career under the new auspices." Dr. Oliver Wendell Holmes, in addressing his medical class at Harvard in the fall of 1847, said, "The knife is searching for disease—the pulleys are dragging back dislocated limbs—Nature herself is working out the primal curse which doomed the tenderest of her creatures to the sharpest of her trials, but the fierce extremity of suffering has been steeped in the waters of forgetfulness, and the deepest furrow in the knotted brow of agony has been smoothed forever."

The sequel to the story is an unhappy one. Acting on advice that subsequently proved to be poor, Morton obtained a government patent in 1846. This act and the allegedly unethical methods he used to obtain his patent raised a storm of protest, into which Jackson, Long, and Wells entered as parties in the contest for priority. Wells became insane and committed suicide; Jackson became insane; and Morton, embittered, impoverished, and unhappy, died of apoplexy. A monument erected by the citizens of Boston over the grave of Dr. Morton in Mt. Auburn Cemetery near Boston bears the following inscription written by Dr. Jacob Bigelow:

WILLIAM T. G. MORTON
Inventor and Revealer of Anaesthetic Inhalation.
Before Whom, in All Time, Surgery Was Agony.
By Whom Pain in Surgery Was Averted and Annulled.
Since Whom Science Has Control of Pain.

The search for other anesthetics was soon under way. Chloroform had been discovered in 1831, independently and simultaneously in the United States, France, and Germany, and 16 years later it was tried on animals by Flourens. In the same year (1847), a surgeon in Edinburgh by the name of James Young Simpson successfully tried chloroform anesthesia in humans. The suggestion to do so was made to Simpson by Waldie. It is said that during the first demonstration the attendant dropped and broke the bottle containing the chloroform. Inasmuch as there was no more immediately available, the operation was undertaken without anesthesia and the patient died almost with the first stroke of the knife. If this death had occurred while the chloroform was being used, it might have postponed the introduction of anesthesia in England for many years. Soon Simpson was employing chloroform routinely in his practice of obstetrics.

Strong opposition sprang up against the use of anesthesia in surgery and particularly its employment during childbirth. This opposition came especially from church circles. Simpson effectively met the not-unexpected attack by pointing out that God, the first surgeon, had used anesthesia by causing a deep sleep to fall upon Adam while He removed the rib from which Eve was made. It should be noted that this Biblical event (Gen. 2:21) occurred *before* the fall of Adam and Eve, while it was *after* the fall that God said, "In sorrow thou shalt bring forth children" (Gen. 3:16). Simpson was knighted for his contribution by Queen Victoria, to whom chloroform was administered during labor.

During the early years of the use of anesthesia, surgeons and nurses did not use the word *anesthesia;* the experience was a new one and there was no universally accepted expression to describe it. Such synonyms as narcotism, stupefaction, sopor, etherization, anodyne process, letheonization, hebetization, and apathisation were used. It is noteworthy that Bailey's *English Dictionary,* published in 1724, had already defined anesthesia as "a Defect of Sensation" (Beecher, 1968). It was Oliver Wendell Holmes who introduced the words *anesthesia, anesthetic,* and *anesthetist* into medicine. The following letter was written by Holmes to Morton:

Boston, November 21, 1846.
My Dear Sir: Everybody wants to have a hand in the great discovery. All I will do is to give you a hint or two as to names, or the name, to be applied to the state produced, and to the agent.
The state should, I think, be called "anaesthesia." This signifies insensibility, more particularly (as used by Linnaeus and Cullen) to objects of touch. The adjective will be "anaesthetic." Thus we might say the "state of anaesthesia," or the "anaesthetic state". . . .
I would have a name pretty soon, and consult some accomplished scholar, such as President Everett, or Dr. Bigelow, Sr., before fixing upon the term, *which will be repeated by the tongues of every civilized race of mankind.* . . . You could mention these words which I suggest for their consideration; but there may be others more appropriate and agreeable.

Yours respectfully,
O. W. Holmes

It was also Holmes who, when asked to decide whether Morton or another was the discoverer of ether so that the name might be carved on a monument to be dedicated for the purpose, evaded the ticklish question by saying, "Gentlemen, I propose that this monument be dedicated to ether." His true opinion, however, is revealed in the following statement from a letter written years later, on April 2, 1893, to Edward Snell: "Both these gentlemen [Jackson and Wells] deserve 'honorable mention' in connection with the discovery, but I have never a moment hesitated in awarding the essential credit of the great achievement to Dr. Morton." (*See* Morton, 1905; Keys, 1945.)

Regardless of the relative merits of the various contestants in the "ether controversy" for priority of discovery, the significance of the "death of pain" resulting from the introduction of surgical anesthesia has been beautifully described by the poet-physician Weir Mitchell, at the semicentennial anniversary of the discovery of ether anesthesia:

Whatever triumphs still shall hold the mind,
Whatever gift shall yet enrich mankind,
Ah! here no hour shall strike through all the years,
No hour as sweet, as when hope, doubt, and fears,
'Mid deepening stillness, watched one eager brain,
With Godlike will, decree the Death of Pain.

The subsequent history of anesthesia is a relatively recent chapter and is concerned with more than the introduction and development of new agents and technics. Anesthesiology has been added to medical school curricula. Anesthesiologists have assumed increasing responsibilities for patient care outside of the operating room, for example, in cases of barbiturate poisoning, tetanus, asphyxia neonatorum, pulmonary emphysema and fibrosis, extreme pain, circulatory collapse, and cardiac arrhythmias, to mention a few. The scientific aspects of the field have expanded in an explosive fashion. Research laboratories devoted to fundamental studies of narcosis and the pharmacological actions of drugs used by the anesthesiologist have increased in quality and quantity. As all of medicine has grown, so has anesthesiology.

THEORIES CONCERNING THE MECHANISMS OF ACTION OF ANESTHETICS

Despite the many advances in the field of central and peripheral nervous system physiology and much investigative work on the mechanism of action of anesthetic drugs, it is not possible, at the present time, to present a unified theory of narcosis. There are several difficulties immediately apparent. Although there is considerable information available dealing with neural transmission, the normal state of *consciousness* is still but poorly understood. In the absence of this knowledge it may, indeed, prove impossible to develop a fundamental theory that attempts to explain the *lack* of consciousness. In addition, although all anesthetics have the same general effect, that is, central nervous system (CNS) depression, it is equally true that their physical and chemical properties as well as their physiological effects are varied. Thus, their modes of action may very well differ and make necessary the formulation of a "theory of narcosis" for each agent or class of agents. Finally, many proposals are only *descriptive*. They describe the *effects* of anesthesia, for example, decreased synaptic transmission, decreased oxygen consumption, and changes in central electrical activity, rather than a mechanism by which these effects are produced (*see* Wall, 1967).

Colloid Theory. This theory, initially proposed by Claude Bernard (1875) and elaborated by Bancroft

and Richter (1931), was the first attempt to explain the state of anesthesia. They proposed that a reversible aggregation of cell colloids causes or accompanies anesthesia. Seifritz (1950), studying the slime mold, observed reversible cessation of protoplasmic streaming upon addition of chloroform, cyclopropane, and ethyl chloride, which he called *thixotropic setting*. Subsequently, Bruce and Christiansen (1965) demonstrated that diethyl ether and halothane inhibit movement and protoplasmic streaming in the ameba. Allison and Nunn (1968) ascribed production of narcosis to depolymerization of microtubules, structures that normally give rigidity to cytoplasm. However, Saubermann and Gallagher (1973) could find no changes in microtubular structure in the optic nerves of anesthetized mice.

Lipid Theory. The lipid theory was advanced initially by Meyer (1899, 1901) and Overton (1901). In its simplest terms, it proposes a direct parallelism between affinity of an anesthetic for lipid and its depressant action. Inasmuch as nerve cells and their membranes contain lipids, the anesthetic is thought to gain access to nerve tissue by virtue of its lipid solubility. Although there is an excellent correlation between anesthetic potency of a wide variety of inhalational anesthetics and their oil:gas partition coefficients (Eger *et al.*, 1965, 1969; Saidman *et al.*, 1967), these solubilities were examined *in vitro* with vegetable oils and water rather than with brain lipids and body fluids. In addition, alkaloids and inorganic ions do not comply with the theory, and many fat-soluble substances have no depressant action on the CNS or actually produce convulsions (Krantz *et al.*, 1958). It is now known that anesthetics may interact with proteins (Schoenborn and Nobbs, 1966; Schoenborn, 1967). Finally, this approach examines the site of localization or accumulation of agents, but not their mechanism of action.

Surface Tension or Adsorption Theory. Traube (1904) and Lillie (1909) related the potency of anesthetics to their ability to lower surface tension. Warburg (1921, 1930) proposed that the accumulation of narcotic agents at the cell surface could result in alteration of metabolic processes and neural transmission and thus cause anesthesia. Clements and Wilson (1962) have reformulated this theory and have demonstrated that nitrous oxide, cyclopropane, halothane, and chloroform lower the surface tension at a fat-water interface. They state that the adsorption of anesthetic agents may change the effective dielectric constant and permeability and may also alter critical structural relationships between those enzymes supporting oxidative phosphorylation and electron transport.

Cell Permeability Theory. Höber (1907), Lillie (1909), Loewe (1913), and Winterstein (1926) proposed that anesthetics cause a change in permeability of the cells of the CNS. Shanes (1958) reported that certain agents may physically stabilize the cell membrane by preventing the increase in ion permeability that normally accompanies depolarization. Yamaguchi and Okumura (1963) have shown that ether, chloroform, and urethan partially prevent the decrease in membrane resistance that normally occurs during excitation. Similarly, diethyl ether depresses the selective permeability of the cell to sodium ions (Shapovalor, 1963). Many other inhalational agents have been shown to influence sodium transport across the toad bladder and frog skin (*see* Andersen and Amaranath, 1973). Finally, the increase in red-cell permeability to glucose normally produced by carbon dioxide is inhibited by human anesthetic concentrations of halothane, methoxyflurane, and diethyl ether (Greene and Cervenko, 1967).

These observations of alterations in surface tension or cell membrane permeability are valuable descriptions of events that accompany or are associated with anesthetics. However, whether these changes *cause* anesthesia and, indeed, how these changes are produced remain questions to be answered.

Biochemical Theories. Various investigators have sought to explain anesthesia in terms of biochemical phenomena. Quastel (1952, 1963) has demonstrated the *in-vitro* inhibition of oxygen uptake by the brain after exposure to barbiturates, chloral hydrate, or urethan. He proposed that barbiturates interfere with the reoxidation of nicotinamide adenine dinucleotide (NADH). Barbiturates can also interfere with the synthesis of high-energy compounds by uncoupling oxidation from phosphorylation (*see* Bain, 1952; Brody and Bain, 1954). Both these phenomena occur at barbiturate concentrations considerably greater than those observed during clinical anesthesia. Recent investigations have demonstrated that clinically used concentrations of inhalational anesthetics markedly and reversibly depress the oxidation of glutamate and NADH (but *not* succinate) by rat liver mitochondria (Miller and Hunter, 1970; Cohen, 1973; Nahrwold and Cohen, 1973). Barbiturates and inhalational anesthetics inhibit the oxygen consumption of both monolayer cell cultures (Fink and Kenny, 1968; Fink *et al.*, 1969) and potassium-stimulated brain slices (Hoech *et al.*, 1966; Matteo *et al.*, 1969). Decreased cerebral oxygen consumption is observed in man anesthetized with a wide variety of inhalational and intravenous agents (Smith and Wollman, 1972). Calcium uptake by brain mitochondria is inhibited by halothane *in vitro* (Rosenberg and Haugaard, 1973). Since calcium plays a significant role in neuronal excitability, this finding may be of importance.

Again, however, these phenomena may only *accompany* anesthesia rather than *cause* it. In other words, the decreased CNS activity that occurs during anesthesia may, in turn, result in diminished need for oxygen. Since cellular energy stores remain normal during anesthesia (Nilsson and Siesjo, 1970), this is likely to be the case. Agents known to be uncouplers of oxidative phosphorylation, such as dinitrophenol, do not cause anesthesia. A convulsant barbiturate, 1,3-dimethyl-butyl-ethyl-barbiturate, also results in uncoupling of oxidative phosphorylation *in vitro*. Finally, the means by which anesthetics affect metabolism are incompletely understood at present.

Neurophysiological Theories. *In-vivo* and *in-vitro* studies in cats have shown decreased synaptic transmission in the superior cervical ganglion caused by chloroform, ether, ethanol, or pentobarbital; at the same time, axonal conduction remains unimpaired (*see* Larrabee and Holaday, 1952; Larrabee and Posternak, 1952). It is well known that changes in the EEG occur during anesthesia (*see* Chapter 3). It has been postulated that anesthetics inhibit the ascending reticular formation (Brazier, 1961; Magoun, 1961), which is apparently important for the maintenance of wakefulness. However, recent data suggest that, when subanesthetic concentrations of cyclopropane are administered to man, there is a profound effect upon diffuse projection systems in the brain while the subject remains *totally aware* of external stimuli (Clark *et al.*, 1969) (*see* page 64). Furthermore, there is no uniformity of neurophysiological effects of the anesthetics, and significant differences occur among them (Clark and Rosner, 1973; Rosner and Clark, 1973). Thus, this approach, although giving important information as to neuronal effects of anesthetics, does not propose a basic fundamental mechanism by which the agents produce these effects.

Physical Theories. Various workers have attempted to relate anesthetic potency to the thermodynamic activity or the molecular size of the agent. Increased anesthetic potency has been correlated with an increased magnitude of the van der Waals correlation factors that relate to molecular volume and attraction between molecules (Brink and Posternak, 1948; Wulf and Featherstone, 1957). Mullins (1954) has suggested that narcosis by chemically inert molecules appears to take place when a constant fraction of the total volume of some nonaqueous phase in the cell is occupied by narcotic molecules. He proposed that the occlusion of this critical portion of a free space in a membrane interferes with permeability to ions or molecules necessary to cell function. In these terms, the lipid theory could be restated as indicating a measurement of the van der Waals attraction between gas and lipid, while the adsorption theory deals with the attraction of a molecule between the surface and the interface. These approaches have been well reviewed by Featherstone and Muehlbaecher (1963).

Pauling (1961, 1964) and Miller (1961) independently proposed that anesthetic agents within the CNS are able to orient water molecules around them in an ordered manner. This interaction with water (rather than with lipid) results in the formation of hydrated microcrystals or clathrates, which can interfere with neuronal excitability. While it is true that hydrated crystal formation can take place at low temperatures, there is no experimental evidence that this occurs during anesthesia. In addition, careful standardized measurements of anesthetic potency disclose far better correlation of this parameter with lipid solubility than with hydrate dissociation pressure (Miller *et al.*, 1967, 1972). Finally, it is not possible to prepare hydrates of all the anesthetics *in vitro* (Eger *et al.*, 1969; Eger and Shargel, 1969). Thus, this approach must remain an attractive, but unproven, hypothesis.

Physicochemical Theories. A number of investigators (Miller et al., 1972, 1973; Seeman and Roth, 1972) have reevaluated the membrane as the primary site of anesthetic action. They postulate that general anesthetics can expand the lipid phase of the membrane, thus increasing fluidity or disorder or, perhaps, altering the shape of pores within the membrane. Narcosis may arise either as a direct result of these changes or be produced by changes in enzyme activity. High hydrostatic pressure (in the order of 100 atmospheres) can reverse anesthetic-induced expansion of the membrane; it also antagonizes anesthesia in the newt and mouse (Miller et al., 1973). Further support for this hypothesis comes from measurements of changes in electron-spin resonance produced in artificial phospholipid membranes by anesthetics and antagonized by pressure (Trudell et al., 1973a, 1973b, 1973c). This approach, which combines elements of a number of theories already presented, will be an important one for future investigation.

Summary. Theories of narcosis either have related the phenomenon of anesthesia to similarities in the physical or chemical properties of anesthetic agents or have described biochemical or physiological phenomena occurring during anesthesia. Through these observations, a vast amount of valuable information has been gathered. However, at the present time, a fundamental, predictive, and experimentally proven theory that can explain both the narcotic state and cellular changes produced by anesthesia is still lacking.

Allison, Z. C., and Nunn, J. F. Effects of general anaesthetics on microtubules. *Lancet*, **1968**, *2*, 1326–1329.

Andersen, N. B., and Amaranath, L. Anesthetic effects on transport across cell membranes. *Anesthesiology*, **1973**, *39*, 126–152.

Bain, J. A. Enzymatic aspects of barbiturate action. *Fedn Proc. Fedn Am. Socs exp. Biol.*, **1952**, *11*, 653–658.

Bancroft, W. S., and Richter, G. H. The chemistry of anesthesia. *J. phys. Chem.*, **1931**, *35*, 215–268.

Beecher, H. K. Oliver Wendell Holmes and anesthesia. *Anesthesiology*, **1968**, *29*, 1068.

Bernard, C. *Leçons sur les anésthesiques et sur l'asphyxie.* Baillière et fils, Paris, **1875**.

Brazier, M. A. B. Some effects of anaesthesia on the brain. *Br. J. Anaesth.*, **1961**, *33*, 194–204.

Brink, F., and Posternak, J. M. Thermodynamic analysis of relative effectiveness of narcotics. *J. cell. comp. Physiol.*, **1948**, *32*, 211–234.

Brody, T. M., and Bain, J. A. Barbiturates and oxidative phosphorylation. *J. Pharmac. exp. Ther.*, **1954**, *110*, 148–156.

Bruce, D., and Christiansen, R. Morphologic changes in the giant amoeba *Chaos chaos* induced by halothane and ether. *Expl Cell Res.*, **1965**, *40*, 544–553.

Clark, D. L.; Butler, R. A.; and Rosner, B. S. Dissociation of sensation and evoked responses by a general anesthetic in man. *J. comp. physiol. Psychol.*, **1969**, *68*, 315–319.

Clark, D. L., and Rosner, B. S. Neurophysiologic effects of general anesthetics. I. The electroencephalogram and sensory evoked responses in man. *Anesthesiology*, **1973**, *38*, 564–582.

Clements, J. A., and Wilson, K. M. The affinity of narcotic agents for interfacial films. *Proc. natn. Acad. Sci. U.S.A.*, **1962**, *48*, 1008–1014.

Cohen, P. J. Effect of anesthetics on mitochondrial function. *Anesthesiology*, **1973**, *39*, 153–164.

Davy, H. *Researches, Chemical and Philosophical; Chiefly Concerning Nitrous Oxide, or Dephlogisticated Nitrous Air, and Its Respiration.* J. Johnson, London, **1800**.

Eger, E. I., II; Brandstater, B.; Saidman, L. J.; Regan, M. J.; Severinghaus, J. W.; and Munson, E. S. Equipotent alveolar concentrations of methoxyflurane, halothane, diethyl ether, fluroxene, cyclopropane, xenon, and nitrous oxide in the dog. *Anesthesiology*, **1965**, *26*, 771–777.

Eger, E. I., II; Lundgren, C.; Miller, S. L.; and Stevens, W. C. Anesthetic potencies of sulfur hexafluoride, carbon tetrafluoride, chloroform and ethrane in dogs: correlation with the hydrate and lipid theories of anesthetic action. *Anesthesiology*, **1969**, *30*, 129–135.

Eger, E. I., II, and Shargel, R. O. The lack of hydrate formation at a temperature of 0° C of methoxyflurane, halothane, diethyl ether and fluroxene. *Anesthesiology*, **1969**, *30*, 136–137.

Faraday, M. Effects of inhaling the vapors of sulfuric ether. *Q. Jl Sci. Arts*, Miscellanea (art. xvi), **1818**, *4*, 158–159.

Featherstone, R. M., and Muehlbaecher, C. A. The current role of inert gases in the search for anesthesia mechanisms. *Pharmac. Rev.*, **1963**, *15*, 97–121.

Fink, B. R., and Kenny, G. E. Metabolic effects of volatile anesthetics in cell culture. *Anesthesiology*, **1968**, *29*, 505–516.

Fink, B. R.; Kenny, G. E.; and Simpson, W. E., III. Depression of oxygen uptake in cell culture by volatile, barbiturate and local anesthetics. *Anesthesiology*, **1969**, *30*, 150–155.

Greene, N. M., and Cervenko, F. W. Inhalational anesthetics, carbon dioxide, and glucose transport across red cell membranes. *Acta anaesth. scand.*, **1967**, *28*, Suppl., 1–18.

Hickman, H. H. *A Letter on Suspended Animation Containing Experiments Showing That It May Be Safely Employed on Animals, with the View of Ascertaining Its Probable Utility in Surgical Operations on the Human Subject.* W. Smith, Ironbridge, England, **1824**.

Höber, R. Beiträge zur physikalischen Chemie der Erregung und der Narkose. *Arch. ges. Physiol.*, **1907**, *120*, 492–516.

Hoech, G. P., Jr.; Matteo, R. F.; and Fink, B. R. Effect of halothane on oxygen consumption of rat brain, liver, and heart, and anaerobic glycolysis of rat brain. *Anesthesiology*, **1966**, *27*, 770–777.

Keys, T. E. *The History of Surgical Anesthesia.* Schuman's, New York, **1945**. (Profusely illustrated and excellent bibliography.)

Krantz, J. C., Jr.; Esquibel, A.; Truitt, E. B., Jr.; Ling, A. S. C.; and Kurland, A. A. Hexafluorodiethyl ether (INDOKLON)—an inhalant convulsant: its use in psychiatric treatment. *J. Am. med. Ass.*, **1958**, *166*, 1555–1562.

Larrabee, M. G., and Holaday, D. A. Depression of transmission through sympathetic ganglia during general anesthesia. *J. Pharmac. exp. Ther.*, **1952**, *105*, 400–408.

Larrabee, M. G., and Posternak, J. M. Selective action of anesthetics on synapses and axons in mammalian sympathetic ganglia. *J. Neurophysiol.*, **1952**, *15*, 91–114.

Lillie, R. S. On the connection between changes of permeability and stimulation on the significance of changes in permeability to carbon dioxide. *Am. J. Physiol.*, **1909**, *24*, 14–44.

Loewe, S. Membran und Narkose. *Biochem. Z.*, **1913**, *57*, 161–260.

Magoun, H. W. Brain mechanisms for wakefulness. *Br. J. Anaesth.*, **1961**, *33*, 183–193.

Matteo, R. S.; Hoech, G. P., Jr.; and Hoskin, F. C. G. The effects of cyclopropane and diethyl ether on tissue oxygen consumption and anaerobic glycolysis of brain in vitro. *Anesthesiology*, **1969**, *30*, 156–163.

Meyer, H. H. Zur Theorie de Alkoholnarkose. I. Mitt. Welche Eigenschaft der Anästhetika bedingt ihre narkotische Wirkung? *Arch. exp. Path. Pharmak.*, **1899**, *42*, 109.

——. Zur Theorie der Alkoholnarkose. III. Mitt. Der Einfluss wechselnder Temperatur auf Wirkungsstärke und Teilungskoeffizient der Narkotika. *Ibid.*, **1901**, *46*, 338.

Miller, K. W.; Paton, W. D. M.; and Smith, E. B. The anaesthetic pressures of certain fluorine-containing gases. *Br. J. Anaesth.*, **1967**, *39*, 910–918.

Miller, K. W.; Paton, W. D. M.; Smith, E. B.; and Smith, R. A. Physicochemical approaches to the mode of action of general anesthetics. *Anesthesiology*, **1972**, *36*, 339–351.

Miller, K. W.; Paton, W. D. M.; Smith, R. A.; and Smith, E. B. The pressure reversal of general anesthesia and the critical volume hypothesis. *Molec. Pharmac.*, **1973**, *9*, 131–143.

Miller, R. N., and Hunter, F. E., Jr. The effect of halothane on electron transport, oxidative phosphorylation, and swelling in rat liver mitochondria. *Molec. Pharmac.*, **1970**, *6*, 67–77.

Miller, S. L. A theory of gaseous anesthetics. *Proc. natn. Acad. Sci. U.S.A.*, **1961**, *47*, 1515–1524.

Montagu, M. F. A. A fourth century A.D. reference to anesthesia. *Bull. Hist. Med.*, **1946**, *19*, 113–114.

Morton, W. J. Memoranda relating to the discovery of surgical anesthesia, and Dr. William T. G. Morton's relation to this event. *Post-Graduate N.Y. post-grad. med. Sch.*, **1905**, *20*, 333–353.

Mullins, L. J. Some physical mechanisms in narcosis. *Chem. Rev.*, **1954**, *54*, 289–323.

Nahrwold, M. L., and Cohen, P. J. The effects of FORANE and fluroxene on mitochondrial respiration: correlation with lipid solubility and *in vivo* potency. *Anesthesiology*, **1973**, *38*, 437–444.

Nilsson, L., and Siesjo, B. K. The effect of anesthetics upon labile phosphates and upon extra- and intracellular lactate, pyruvate and bicarbonate concentrations in the rat brain. *Acta physiol. scand.*, **1970**, *80*, 235–248.

Overton, E. *Studien über die Narkose zugleich ein Beitrag zur allgemeinen Pharmakologie.* G. Fischer, Jena, **1901**.

Pauling, L. A molecular theory of general anesthesia. *Science, Wash.*, **1961**, *134*, 15–21.

——. The hydrate microcrystal theory of general anesthesia. *Anesth. Analg. curr. Res.*, **1964**, *43*, 1–10.

Quastel, J. H. Biochemical aspects of narcosis. *Curr. Res. Anesth. Analg.*, **1952**, *31*, 151–163.

——. Metabolic activity of neurons. *Ann. N.Y. Acad. Sci.*, **1963**, *109*, 436–450.

Rosenberg, H., and Haugaard, N. The effects of halothane on metabolism and calcium uptake in mitochondria of the rat liver and brain. *Anesthesiology*, **1973**, *39*, 44–53.

Rosner, B. S., and Clark, D. L. Neurophysiologic effects of general anesthetics. II. Sequential regional actions in the brain. *Anesthesiology*, **1973**, *39*, 59–81.

Saidman, L. J.; Eger, E. I., II; Munson, E. S.; Babad, A. A.; and Muallem, M. Minimum alveolar concentrations of methoxyflurane, halothane, and ether and cyclopropane in man: correlation with theories of anesthesia. *Anesthesiology*, **1967**, *28*, 994–1002.

Saubermann, A. J., and Gallagher, M. L. Mechanisms of general anesthesia: failure of pentobarbital and halothane to depolymerize microtubules in mouse optic nerve. *Anesthesiology*, **1973**, *38*, 25–29.

Schoenborn, B. P. Binding of cyclopropane to sperm whale myoglobin. *Nature, Lond.*, **1967**, *214*, 1120–1122.

Schoenborn, B. P., and Nobbs, C. L. The binding of xenon to sperm whale deoxymyoglobin. *Molec. Pharmac.*, **1966**, *2*, 491–498.

Seeman, P., and Roth, S. General anesthetics expand cell membranes at surgical concentrations. *Biochim. biophys. Acta*, **1972**, *255*, 171–177.

Seifritz, W. The effects of various anesthetic agents on protoplasm. *Anesthesiology*, **1950**, *11*, 24–32.

Shanes, A. M. Electrochemical aspects of physiological and pharmacological action in excitable cells. *Pharmac. Rev.*, **1958**, *10*, 59–164.

Shapovalov, A. I. [Intracellular microelectrode investigation of effect of anesthetics on transmission of excitation in the spinal cord.] *Farmak. Toks.*, **1963**, *26*, 150–153.

Smith, A. L., and Wollman, H. Cerebral blood flow and metabolism: effects of anesthetic drugs and techniques. *Anesthesiology*, **1972**, *36*, 378–400.

Traube, J. Theorie der Osmose und Narkose. *Arch. ges. Physiol.*, **1904**, *105*, 541–559.

Trudell, J. R.; Hubbell, W. L.; and Cohen, E. N. The effect of two inhalation anesthetics on the order of spin-labeled phospholipid vesicles. *Biochim. biophys. Acta*, **1973a**, *291*, 321–327.

——. Pressure reversal of inhalation anesthetic-induced disorder in spin-labeled phospholipid vesicles. *Ibid.*, **1973b**, *291*, 328–334.

Trudell, J. R.; Hubbell, W. L.; Cohen, E. N.; and Kendig, J. J. Pressure reversal of anesthesia: the extent of small-molecule exclusion from spin-labeled phospholipid model membranes. *Anesthesiology*, **1973c**, *39*, 207–211.

Wall, P. D. The mechanisms of general anesthesia. *Anesthesiology*, **1967**, *28*, 46–52.

Warburg, O. Physikalische Chemie der Zellatmung. *Biochem. Z.*, **1921**, *119*, 134–136.

——. The enzyme problem and biological oxidations. *Bull. Johns Hopkins Hosp.*, **1930**, *46*, 341–358.

Winterstein, H. *Die Narkose*, 2nd ed. Springer, Berlin, **1926**.

Wulf, R. J., and Featherstone, R. M. Correlation of van der Waals' constants with anesthetic potency. *Anesthesiology*, **1957**, *18*, 97–105.

Yamaguchi, T., and Okumura, H. Effects of anaesthetics on the electrical properties of the cell membrane of the frog muscle fibre. *Annotnes. zool. jap.*, **1963**, *36*, 109–117.

CHAPTER

3 SIGNS AND STAGES OF ANESTHESIA

Peter J. Cohen

Between 1847 and 1858, John Snow described certain signs that helped him determine the depth of anesthesia in patients receiving chloroform or ether. These included the onset of rhythmic, automatic breathing and the loss of winking in response to touching the conjunctiva as surgical anesthesia was reached, and the gradual disappearance of intercostal muscle activity and cessation of eyeball movement as anesthesia was deepened. In 1920 Guedel, using these and other signs, outlined four stages of general anesthesia, dividing the third stage, that of surgical anesthesia, into four planes. Guedel's observations related primarily to ether, a substance with such great solubility in blood that the onset and progressive deepening of anesthesia were predictably slow. Opportunity is thus afforded the anesthesiologist to watch the unfolding of a series of changes involving respiration, muscle tone, and reflex activity. The somewhat arbitrary division is as follows: I—stage of analgesia; II—stage of delirium; III—stage of surgical anesthesia; IV—stage of respiratory paralysis.

I. *Stage of Analgesia.* The first stage begins with the administration of the anesthetic and lasts until consciousness is lost. The patient himself can supply indices of depth, for example, by indicating if pain is present and by his ability to obey commands. Artusio (1954, 1955) has demonstrated that certain major operations requiring minimal muscular relaxation can be completed during the analgesia characterizing the lower half of this stage. The patient's trachea is intubated so that speech is denied him, but he can nod his head in response to questions, and open his eyes to indicate that he is not feeling pain.

An important aspect of the first stage is that analgesia is sufficiently profound for operation only if a greater depth of ether anesthesia has been initially reached and one then *ascends* toward the analgesic level. Most workers believe it difficult, if not impossible, to achieve adequate analgesia unless this procedure is followed. The pharmacological "history" of the patient is thus of importance, in that the response is determined to a considerable extent by what has transpired.

II. *Stage of Delirium.* This stage extends from the loss of consciousness to the beginning of surgical anesthesia. Excitement and involuntary activity may be minimal or marked. Under the latter circumstance, the patient may laugh, shout, sing, and thrash about. The jaw becomes set, skeletal muscular tone increases, and breathing is irregular. Incontinence of urine and feces may occur, as may retching or vomiting. The pupils may dilate. Hypertension and tachycardia may be marked. Because of the considerable exertion that may be involved, the duration and the intensity of this stage should be reduced to the minimum for patients in substandard health.

III. *Stage of Surgical Anesthesia.* The third stage extends from the end of the second stage until cessation of spontaneous respiration occurs. The transition to stage III can be recognized by the following signs. (1) The respiratory irregularity of stage II disappears. Respiration is entirely on an automatic basis, and regular breathing is present because psychic influences are absent and voluntary pathways are interrupted. (2) The eyelid and conjunctival reflexes are now absent; when the upper lid is gently lifted, it does not close when released. The eyelids no longer blink when the lashes are touched. (3) If the arm is elevated and released, it will now fall flaillike. The head can readily be moved from side to side without resistance. (4) If the anesthesiologist suddenly increases the concentration of anesthetic vapor, reflex respiratory arrest and swallowing no longer occur, whereas both of these reflex responses can be elicited during the second stage. (5) Roving movements of the eyeballs are characteristic of early stage III.

Planes of Anesthesia. The *physical signs* during surgical anesthesia depend on the particular plane of anesthesia. The third stage is divided into four planes, numbered from 1 to 4, in order of increasing depth of anesthesia. The major differences in physical signs in the various planes relate to the character of the *respiration,* the character of the *eyeball movements,* the presence or absence of certain *reflexes,* and the size of the *pupils* (Gillespie, 1943).

The usefulness of the above-mentioned physical signs in judging the planes of anesthesia may be illustrated by a few examples. (1) Full, regular, and automatic respirations that are equally abdominal and thoracic in character, associated with roving eyeballs, suggest plane 1. (2) When regular but less excursive respirations coincide with fixed eyeballs, the anesthesiologist knows that the depth of anesthesia has reached plane 2. (3) The beginning of plane 3 is indicated by increased abdominal respirations and delayed thoracic inspiratory effort, the latter reflecting the beginning paralysis of the intercostal muscles. (4) The transition from plane 3 to plane 4 is marked by complete intercostal paralysis. (5) Cessation of all respiratory effort marks the passage from plane 4 to stage IV. (6) The pupils start dilating in lower plane 2. The dilatation progresses as plane 3 advances, and is almost complete in plane 4, at which time the light reflex is lost.

IV. *Stage of Respiratory Paralysis.* This stage starts as soon as the weakened respiration of plane 4 ceases, and it ends with failure of the circulation. Stage IV is characterized in the Guedel system primarily by respiratory arrest, although vasomotor collapse will follow if the administration of ether is continued by means of artificial respiration. An attempt has been made to place many of these signs on a neuroanatomical basis (Dornette, 1964).

Since ether permits adequate alveolar ventilation throughout a wide range of inspired concentrations, and because considerable depth of anesthesia can be achieved without hypotension, it was natural for Guedel to emphasize the respiratory responses to increasing amounts of ether and to minimize the reactions of the circulation. However, these signs are not applicable during administration of many other general anesthetics. Cyclopropane, for example, causes apnea in a far lighter plane of anesthesia than does ether. Halothane causes hypotension more readily than does ether. Nitrous oxide is incapable of producing muscular relaxation; thus, neuromuscular blocking agents play an important role during anesthesia with nitrous oxide. The accompanying paralysis of respiration associated with neuromuscular blockade deprives the anesthesiologist of much information. Indeed, it is possible for the patient to be apneic and at the same time conscious and, perhaps, perceptive of pain. The skilled practitioner will therefore be alert to sweating, lacrimation, and changes in arterial blood pressure and pulse rate. Eye signs may be obscured by the intense pupillary constriction that accompanies administration of narcotic analgesics. Finally, while ether is a profound analgesic (*i.e.,* it is capable of abolishing pain without producing unconsciousness), certain other agents have no effect on the pain threshold of conscious man (Dundee *et al.,* 1962; Dundee, 1965). One may then ask by what means the modern practitioner is able to determine the depth of anesthesia.

Different goals of general anesthesia can be identified, for example, narcosis, muscular relaxation, and analgesia (Gray and Rees, 1952), or sensory block, mental quiet, motor block, and reduction of adverse reflex responses (Woodbridge, 1957, 1963). Such a diversity of purposes suggests that depth of anesthesia might be assessed according to each purpose. Thus, a given level of general anesthesia might be adequate for sedation but insufficient from the standpoint of analgesia or blocking of reflexes.

Clinicians often resort to this type of estimate of depth of anesthesia, chiefly because anesthesia today is rarely administered with a single agent. With the exception of cyclopropane and ether, most general anesthesia involves the use of a number of substances. Induction with thiopental is common, providing a rapid, smooth onset of unconsciousness, a situation highly acceptable to patients. Maintenance of anesthesia then frequently involves nitrous oxide in combination with various drugs, for example, halothane, methoxyflurane, enflurane, narcotics, or muscle relaxants.

The situation is further complicated when carbon dioxide tension is altered either deliberately or inadvertently. Hyperventilation is deliberately produced by many anesthesiologists because it can in turn produce muscular relaxation and depression of neural activity with need for a lesser amount of general anesthetic. Possible explanations of this include stimulation of inhibito-inspiratory Hering-Breuer reflexes by the intermittent increase in airway pressure necessary to raise alveolar ventilation above normal. Discharge over nerves to the muscles of respiration is dampened, and a quieter and more controllable operating field is thereby provided. Furthermore, hypocarbia appears to affect nerve cell activity in some parts of the central nervous system (CNS). In part, this may result directly from the change in carbon dioxide tension or pH. In addition, however, the reduction in cerebral blood flow produced by extreme hypocarbia (arterial carbon dioxide tension less than 20 torr, or mm Hg) is associated with chemical and EEG evidence of cerebral hypoxia (Cohen *et al.,* 1966; Alexander *et al.,* 1968; Granholm *et al.,* 1968; Plum *et al.,* 1968).

Additional difficulties in estimating depth of anesthesia occur when muscle relaxants are used. Complete muscular paralysis is readily achieved by such substances, thus eliminating all the skeletal muscular indices of depth, such as eyeball movement, changes in respiration, tightness of the jaw, and ability to phonate, swallow, move, or close the glottis.

A final problem is posed by the intensity of the stimulus applied to the anesthetized patient. Incision of the skin in a conscious individual evokes bright, burning, sharp pain. This remains a powerful stimulus during general anesthesia. Other intense stimuli involve manipulation of periosteum, cornea, urethral mucosa, or peritoneum, particularly if the latter is inflamed. There are also stimuli that evoke relatively little response, for example, cutting and sewing of the intestine or cutting of the brain substance. Stimuli of intermediate intensity are illustrated by those arising from manipulation of fascia, muscle, and fat. Thus, one may rightfully regard a given depth of anesthesia as "too light" for an intense stimulus but quite adequate for a stimulus of lesser strength.

Anesthetic Concentration. Depth of anesthesia depends, in part, upon the tension of the drug in the CNS. Eger and associates (1965) and Saidman and coworkers (1967) have developed the useful concept of minimum alveolar concentration (MAC). This value refers to the alveolar concentration (held constant for at least 15 minutes and, therefore, near equilibrium with that in the CNS) at which 50% of patients will not respond to the stimulus of skin incision. Values of MAC for commonly used general anesthetics (expressed in percent at 1 atmosphere pressure) are: methoxyflurane, 0.16; halothane, 0.77; enflurane, 1.68 (Gion and Saidman, 1971); ether, 1.92; fluroxene, 3.4; cyclopropane, 9.2; and nitrous oxide, 101.0. In using these figures, it must be remembered that the tensions of anesthetic gases are often quite different in brain, arterial blood, inspired gas, and the gas delivered to the breathing system. Furthermore, surgical requirements dictate that *all* patients not respond to skin incision. Finally, individual variation, acute tolerance, differing operative stimuli, and the presence of systemic disease often have a major influence on the response of the patient. For these reasons, the values on the flowmeters must not be permitted to be the sole consideration in governing administration of anesthesia.

The Electroencephalogram as an Index of Depth of General Anesthesia. In 1937 Gibbs and associates suggested that the EEG be used as a measure of the depth of anesthesia during surgical operations. Since that time a number of workers have classified the EEG changes produced by the inhalational agents and barbiturates (*see* Faulconer and Bickford, 1960; Clark and Rosner, 1973; Rosner and Clark, 1973).

Use of the EEG as the sole index of anesthetic depth may be unreliable, since many factors influence the activity of the CNS. Hypoxia, hypoglycemia, hypothermia, and inadequate cerebral circulation can markedly alter the EEG at a time when anesthetic concentration remains constant (Marshall *et al.,* 1965). Furthermore, although EEG changes produced by a given agent may correlate with brain concentration, they also vary widely when different anesthetics are compared.

An illustration of the EEG during cyclopropane anesthesia is shown in Figure 3-1. There is spontaneous electrical activity in the brain of conscious man, called alpha rhythm and best recorded with the subject's eyes closed. Its particular frequency and amplitude are said to be as characteristic of a person as his fingerprints. With the onset of general anesthesia, obvious EEG changes are observed. As anesthesia is deepened, the EEG waves become larger, slower, and more regular (Clark *et al.,* 1970). Decreased frequency and increased amplitude are also seen with increasing depth when anesthesia is produced by ether (Clark *et al.,* 1971). On the other hand, administration of enflurane is accompanied initially by *increased* frequency. As CNS concentration is increased, the EEG progresses to "spike-dome" complexes alternating with isoelectric periods (Clark *et al.,* 1971). These changes are not observed when isoflurane, an isomer of enflurane, is inhaled (Clark *et al.,* 1973).

Significant changes in arterial carbon dioxide tension (Pa_{CO_2}) often accompany general anesthesia and may exert profound effects on the EEG. During cyclopropane anesthesia, an increase in Pa_{CO_2} is associated with EEG changes indicative of greater

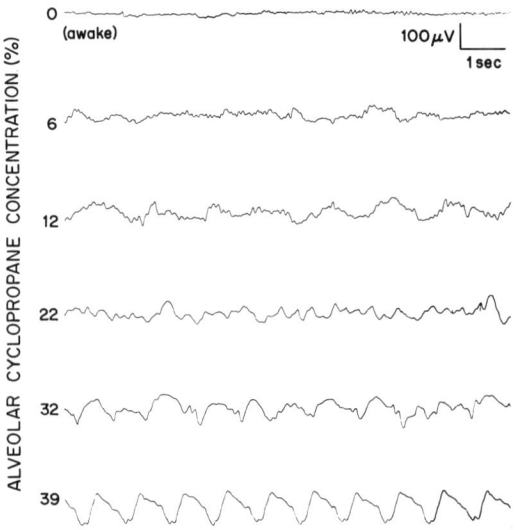

Figure 3-1. *EEG of normal man exposed to increasing concentrations of cyclopropane.*

Anesthetic tension in arterial and jugular venous blood is equal to that in the inspired gas. Therefore, the concentrations shown are directly related to the concentration of cyclopropane in the CNS. EEG recordings are monopolar (C_3).

depth of anesthesia (Clark *et al.*, 1970). Conversely, during anesthesia produced by enflurane, EEG alterations suggestive of increasing depth are observed when Pa_{CO_2} is decreased (Clark *et al.*, 1971). Decreasing Pa_{CO_2} during administration of enflurane results in EEG signs of cerebral excitability, a phenomenon not observed during isoflurane anesthesia (Neigh *et al.*, 1971; Clark *et al.*, 1973). The occurrence of these differing phenomena suggests different modes of action related to chemical structure of the anesthetic agent (Clark *et al.*, 1971). (For a detailed examination of this subject, the reader should consult Clark and Rosner, 1973; Rosner and Clark, 1973.)

Muscular Relaxation. In the absence of neuromuscular blocking drugs, suppression of spinal reflex activity is the major mechanism by which general anesthetics produce muscle relaxation (Ngai *et al.*, 1965). Thus, in both animals (de Jong and Robles, 1968; de Jong *et al.*, 1968) and man (de Jong *et al.*, 1967) there is an excellent correlation between anesthetic concentration, suppression of spinal reflex activity, and muscular relaxation. Observation of muscle tone can thus serve as an index of anesthetic depth. It should be stressed that the concentration required to produce muscle relaxation in the aged, debilitated patient is far less than that necessary in the robust young man.

Summary of Practical Considerations. The following approach is used for almost any general anesthetic. If the eyelids blink when the eyelashes are stroked, if the patient is swallowing, if respiration is irregular in rate and depth, and if one knows that not a great deal of anesthetic is in the body, surgical anesthesia is *not* present.

Loss of the eyelash reflex and the development of rhythmic respiration indicate the beginning of surgical anesthesia. If the skin incision is made at once, indications of "light" anesthesia may include an increase in respiratory rate or a rise in arterial blood pressure. Jaw muscles may become tight, and even if the mouth can be opened an oral airway may not be tolerated; an attempt to insert it may produce gagging, coughing, vomiting, or laryngospasm.

As anesthesia deepens, these responses are reduced in degree or abolished altogether. With most of the general anesthetics, an increase in depth brings progressive reduction in respiratory tidal volume. Tracheal tug may become evident as accessory muscles of respiration come into play. Diaphragmatic activity becomes jerky or snapping in character, and the lower chest is pulled in as the diaphragm descends. With some anesthetics,

such as ether and cyclopropane, pupillary dilatation increases progressively as deeper levels of anesthesia are reached. With others, for example, halothane and methoxyflurane, pupillary dilatation is not a useful sign, but arterial blood pressure tends to vary directly with anesthetic depth and hypotension can be used as an index of dosage. Suggestions that anesthesia is becoming "lighter" are the formation of tears, apnea following peritoneal stimulation, increasing resistance to inflation of the lungs, and the return of those indices of light anesthesia listed above.

Severe respiratory depression or cessation of breathing (excluding breath-holding seen during early phases of anesthesia) and marked hypotension or asystole must be regarded as evidence of deep anesthesia unless other causes, for example, the effect of muscle relaxants, blood loss, and hypoxia, or the influence of vagal reflexes, can explain these findings.

The concentration of anesthetic in gas and blood can be analyzed manometrically and by gas chromatography. The EEG sometimes furnishes useful information. Most important is the continuous observation of the individual response to the amount of drug administered. This takes the form of a titration of the patient's reaction to the dosage used. Allowance is made for the vigor of the patient, since with decreasing muscle tone there will be a less vigorous muscular reaction to stimuli. Recognition is made of the fact that the activity of protective reflexes diminishes with age. In general, the longer and more traumatic the operative procedure, the less anesthetic is needed. One attempts to determine whether surgical stimuli are harmful at any given time. For example, is the patient's skin clammy, and does the fullness of pulse, the cardiac rate, and the level of arterial blood pressure suggest undesirable circulatory depression from noxious surgical stimuli? If this is believed so, an increase in depth of anesthesia may be attempted. Reversal of untoward reactions indicates that the decision was correct. Worsening of the situation suggests other causes for the patient's problems.

Thus, common sense and experience, combined with constant attention to the patient and recording of his responses, permit the majority of individuals to be successfully anesthetized, although one often may not know precisely what depth of anesthesia is present at a particular time. If there were no surgical operation, that is, no added stimuli, and if a single anesthetic agent were added in gradually increasing amounts, it would be relatively easy to estimate depth of anesthesia. When one is forced to account for the influence not only of the anesthetic, or anesthetics, but also of the patient's physical condition, the state of alveolar ventilation, and the type and intensity of the surgical stimuli, the problem becomes more difficult. It is surprising and gratifying how often this can be satisfactorily solved.

The Neuropharmacological Basis for the Signs and Stages of Anesthesia. The neuropharmacological basis for the anesthetic stages should ultimately explain the patient's response to both the anesthetic drugs and the surgical stimuli. Although many facets are still imperfectly understood, much has been learned during the past 2 decades. A detailed analysis of the pathways of pain and the points at which anesthetics can act has been given by Wall (1967). It has long been considered that sensory impulses have two pathways by which they may reach the cortex. One is the classical lemniscal pathway, specific to the modality of the stimulus applied and also to its exact location; for example, in the lemniscal pathway the particular neuron involved in the transmission of tactile impulses from a particular point on one finger will be stimulated only by touch stimuli applied to that one spot. Such impulses reach the primary perception areas of the cortex. There are also extralemniscal pathways for sensory impulses. These are nonspecific as to both modality and location of stimuli. They travel up the spinoreticular, spinotectal, and spinothalamic tracts by way of the midbrain reticular substance and are projected in a nonspecific or diffuse manner onto the cortex.

The reticular core of the brain stem contains neurons and pathways involved in the maintenance of consciousness, the so-called reticular activating system (Moruzzi and Magoun, 1949). It also contains an inhibitory system that discharges upward, thereby reducing the level of excitability of the cortex. Both activation and inhibition of the cortex by the ascending reticular systems are active processes, and both can be blocked by anesthetics. It is the ascending *activating* influence of the brain stem core that may be primarily suppressed by most general anesthetics. (*See* French *et al.*, 1953; Davis *et al.*, 1957, 1958; Clutton-Brock, 1961; Abrahamian *et al.*, 1963.)

The ascending *inhibitory* system from the reticular formation to the cortex apparently can be selectively blocked by the barbiturates, thus facilitating the transmission of pain at very low dosage levels. This may account for the antialgesic properties of these drugs (Dundee, 1965). Accordingly, the relation between pain threshold and anesthetic depth is diphasic, the perception of pain increasing at first but

then diminishing below normal as the entire reticular system (both activating and inhibitory) becomes depressed by barbiturates.

In addition to blockade of reticular formation systems, there are sites of action of anesthetics higher in the CNS. Thus, ether in anesthetic doses blocks responses in the diencephalon, particularly in the centromedian nucleus and intralaminar cell groups of the thalamus, while barbiturates, chloralose, and tribromoethanol do not block. With very deep planes of anesthesia, almost regardless of the agent, depression of activity can be seen in the specific relay nuclei of the thalamus (Brazier, 1961). The effect of general anesthetics on the limbic system to alter "affect" rather than sensation or perception remains to be clarified.

To ascribe the state of general anesthesia to blockade of the reticular formation alone probably provides an oversimplified picture. Studies of the somatosensory evoked response (SER) in man have permitted evaluation of function of both the lemniscal and extralemniscal pathways. As in the case of EEG changes (*see* above) marked differences in drug effect were observed when various agents were compared. The data of Clark and associates (1969) suggest that an *awake* man breathing subanesthetic concentrations of cyclopropane shows marked depression of diffuse projection systems at a time when pain is consciously perceived. In essence, although there appears to be interference with pathways that are supposed to maintain wakefulness, the subject remains awake and in communication with his environment. In the presence of surgical anesthesia produced by cyclopropane, both specific and diffuse systems are depressed while peripheral nerves remain capable of conducting impulses (Clark *et al.*, 1970). When anesthesia is produced by inhaling 80% nitrous oxide and 2% ether, function of the reticular activating system is depressed while direct lemniscal transmission remains intact. When the concentration of ether is increased to 4%, both components of the SER are obliterated. Anesthesia produced by enflurane is accompanied by a SER with large increases in amplitude and latency (Clark *et al.*, 1971). On the other hand, its isomer, isoflurane, abolishes specific transmission during surgical anesthesia (Clark *et al.*, 1973). Different effects upon the SER are also observed when subanesthetic concentrations of these agents are administered (Hosick *et al.*, 1971). One should therefore be cautious in proposing a simplistic unitary approach to the neurophysiological effects of anesthesia (*see* Clark and Rosner, 1973; Rosner and Clark, 1973).

One can thus ask, "What is general anesthesia?" Is it a failure of the brain to receive impulses initiated by sensory stimuli, a failure of arriving sensory impulses to pass on into storage, or a failure of arriving sensory impulses to evoke "affect"? It seems likely that there are levels of anesthesia at which all three of these failures occur. There may be others at which only one is significant. For some anesthetics, data suggest that their effect is essentially an impairment of storage or memory, not of sensation. Are the sites of blockade on the route to perception or to storage?

A start has been made toward the identification of sites of action of anesthetics and the mechanisms by which narcosis is produced. The coming years promise excitement for workers involved in the study of the neurophysiology of the anesthetic state.

Abrahamian, H. A.; Allison, T.; Goff, W. R.; and Rosner, B. S. Effects of thiopental on human cerebral evoked responses. *Anesthesiology*, 1963, *24*, 650–657.

Alexander, S. C.; Smith, T. C.; Strobel, G.; Stephen, G. W.; and Wollman, H. Cerebral carbohydrate metabolism of man during respiratory and metabolic alkalosis. *J. appl. Physiol.*, 1968, *24*, 66–72.

Artusio, J. J., Jr. Di-ethyl ether analgesia: detailed description of the first stage of ether anesthesia in man. *J. Pharmac. exp. Ther.*, 1954, *111*, 343–398.

———. Ether analgesia during major surgery. *J. Am. med. Ass.*, 1955, *157*, 33–36.

Brazier, M. A. B. Some effects of anaesthesia on the brain. *Br. J. Anaesth.*, 1961, *33*, 194–204.

Clark, D. L.; Butler, R. A.; and Rosner, B. S. Dissociation of sensation and evoked responses by a general anesthetic in man. *J. comp. physiol. Psychol.*, 1969, *68*, 315–319.

Clark, D. L.; Hosick, E. C.; Adam, N.; Castro, A. D.; Rosner, B. S.; and Neigh, J. L. Neural effects of isoflurane (FORANE) in man. *Anesthesiology*, 1973, *39*, 261–270.

Clark, D. L.; Hosick, E. C.; and Rosner, B. S. Neurophysiological effects of different anesthetics in unconscious man. *J. appl. Physiol.*, 1971, *31*, 884–891.

Clark, D. L.; Rosner, B. S.; and Beck, C. Cerebral electrical activity during cyclopropane anesthesia in man. *J. appl. Physiol.*, 1970, *28*, 802–807.

Clutton-Brock, J. The importance of the central nervous effects of anaesthetic agents. *Br. J. Anaesth.*, 1961, *33*, 214–218.

Cohen, P. J.; Reivich, M.; and Greenbaum, L. J. Electroencephalographic changes induced by 100% oxygen breathing at 3 ata in awake man. In, *Proceedings of the Third International Conference on Hyperbaric Medicine.* (Brown, I. W., Jr., and Cox, B. G., eds.) National Academy of Sciences, Washington, D. C., 1966.

Davis, H. S.; Collins, W. F.; Randt, C. T.; and Dillon, W. H. Effect of anesthetic agents on evoked central nervous system responses: gaseous agents. *Anesthesiology*, 1957, *18*, 634–642.

Davis, H. S.; Dillon, W. H.; Collins, W. F.; and Randt, C. T. The effect of anesthetic agents on evoked central nervous system responses: muscle relaxants and volatile agents. *Anesthesiology*, 1958, *19*, 441–449.

de Jong, R. H.; Freund, F. G.; Robles, R.; and Morikawa, K. I. Anesthetic potency determined by depression of synaptic transmission. *Anesthesiology*, 1968, *29*, 1139–1144.

de Jong, R. H.; Hershey, W. N.; and Wagman, I. H. Measurement of a spinal reflex (H-reflex) during general anesthesia in man: association between reflex depression and muscular relaxation. *Anesthesiology*, 1967, *28*, 382–389.

de Jong, R. H., and Robles, R. Monosynaptic transmission in the cat's spinal cord: a quantitative measure of anesthetic dose. *Anesthesiology*, 1968, *29*, 887–891.

Dornette, W. H. L. The anatomic basis of the signs of anesthesia. *Anesth. Analg. curr. Res.*, 1964, *43*, 71–81.

Dundee, J. W. The anesthetist and analgesia. In, *Science and Practice in Anesthesia.* (Eckenhoff, J. E., ed.) J. B. Lippincott Co., Philadelphia, 1965.

Dundee, J. W.; Nicholl, R. M.; and Black, G. W. Alterations in response to somatic pain associated with anaesthesia. X. Further studies with inhalation agents. *Br. J. Anaesth.*, 1962, *34*, 158–160.

Eger, E. I., II; Saidman, L. J.; and Brandstater, B. Minimum alveolar anesthetic concentration: a standard of anesthetic potency. *Anesthesiology*, 1965, *26*, 756–763.

French, J. D.; Verzeano, M.; and Magoun, H. W. A neural basis of the anesthetic state. *A.M.A. Archs Neurol. Psychiatry*, 1953, *69*, 519–529.

Gibbs, F. A.; Gibbs, E. L.; and Lennox, W. G. Effect on the electroencephalogram of certain drugs which influence nervous activity. *Archs intern. Med.*, 1937, *60*, 154–166.

Gillespie, N. A. The signs of anaesthesia. *Curr. Res. Anesth. Analg.*, 1943, *22*, 275–282.

Gion, H., and Saidman, L. J. The minimum alveolar concentration of enflurane in man. *Anesthesiology*, 1971, *35*, 361–364.

Granholm, L.; Lukjanova, L.; and Siesjo, B. K. Evidence of cerebral hypoxia in pronounced hyperventilation. *Scand. J. clin. Lab. Invest.*, 1968, Suppl. 102, IV:C.

Gray, T. C., and Rees, G. J. The role of apnoea in anaesthesia for major surgery. *Br. med. J.*, 1952, *2*, 891–895.

Hosick, E. C.; Clark, D. L.; Adam, N.; and Rosner, B. S. Neurophysiological effects of different anesthetics in conscious man. *J. appl. Physiol.*, 1971, *31*, 892–898.

Marshall, M.; Longley, B. P.; and Stanton, W. H. Electroencephalography in anaesthetic practice. *Br. J. Anaesth.*, 1965, *37*, 845–857.

Moruzzi, G., and Magoun, W. H. Brain stem reticular formation and activation of the E.E.G. *Electroenceph. clin. Neurophysiol.*, 1949, *1*, 455–473.

Neigh, J. L.; Garman, J. K.; and Harp, J. R. The electroencephalographic pattern during anesthesia with ETHRANE: effects of depth of anesthesia, Pa_{CO_2}, and nitrous oxide. *Anesthesiology*, 1971, *35*, 482–487.

Ngai, S. H.; Hanks, E. C.; and Farhie, S. E. Effects of anesthetics on neuromuscular transmission and somatic reflexes. *Anesthesiology*, 1965, *26*, 162–167.

Plum, F.; Posner, J. B.; and Smith, W. W. Effect of hyperbaric-hyperoxic hyperventilation on blood, brain and CSF lactate. *Am. J. Physiol.*, 1968, *215*, 1240–1244.

Saidman, L. J.; Eger, E. I., II; Munson, E. S.; Babad, A. A.; and Muallem, M. Minimum alveolar concentrations of methoxyflurane, halothane, ether and cyclopropane in man: correlation with theories of anesthesia. *Anesthesiology*, 1967, *28*, 994–1002.

Wall, P. D. The mechanisms of general anesthesia. *Anesthesiology*, 1967, *28*, 46–52.

Woodbridge, P. D. Changing concepts concerning depth of anesthesia. *Anesthesiology*, 1957, *18*, 536–550.

———. The components of general anesthesia: a plea for the blocking of sensory pathways. *J. Am. med. Ass.*, 1963, *186*, 641–645.

Monographs and Reviews

Clark, D. L., and Rosner, B. S. Neurophysiologic effects of general anesthetics. I. The electroencephalogram and sensory evoked responses in man. *Anesthesiology*, 1973, *38*, 564–582.

Faulconer, A., Jr., and Bickford, R. G. *Electroencephalography in Anesthesiology.* Charles C Thomas, Pub., Springfield, Ill., 1960.

Guedel, A. E. *Inhalation Anesthesia: A Fundamental Guide*, 2nd ed. The Macmillan Co., New York, 1951.

Rosner, B. S., and Clark, D. L. Neurophysiologic effects of general anesthetics. II. Sequential regional actions in the brain. *Anesthesiology*, 1973, *39*, 59–81.

Snow, J. *The Inhalation of the Vapour of Ether in Surgical Operations.* John Churchill, London, 1847.

CHAPTER

4 PREANESTHETIC MEDICATION

Theodore C. Smith and Harry Wollman

Preanesthetic medication refers to the use of drugs prior to the administration of an anesthetic, with several purposes in mind. Preanesthetic medication should decrease anxiety without producing excessive drowsiness, facilitate a smooth, rapid induction without prolonging emergence, provide amnesia for the perioperative period while maintaining cooperation prior to loss of consciousness, and relieve preoperative and postoperative pain if it is present (Shearer, 1960, 1961). The drugs chosen for preanesthetic medication may in addition minimize some of the undesirable side effects of anesthetic agents, such as salivation, bradycardia, and postanesthetic vomiting. The accomplishment of these multiple purposes usually requires the concomitant use of two or three drugs. The most commonly employed classes include hypnotics, tranquilizers, opioids, antiemetics, and anticholinergics.

The wide variety of preanesthetic regimens in current use testifies to the lack of agreement on optimal combinations. Comparisons are difficult for a number of reasons. Many of the drugs produce similar or nearly indistinguishable effects (Elliot *et al.,* 1969). Premedication may produce differing results depending on the operative procedure; the choice of anesthetic drugs and technic; and the patient's disease, age, sex, physical status, and current drug therapy. The more ill, the more elderly, the less robust and active the patient, the greater are the effects exerted by sedatives, tranquilizers, and analgesics.

In addition, one must recognize that tranquility can result simply from an anesthesiologist's preoperative visit. Among patients who did not have a preoperative visit by an anesthesiologist, 58% in whom sedatives were omitted and 61% receiving pentobarbital claimed to be nervous on interview just prior to induction of anesthesia. On the other hand, nervousness existed in only 40% of those who received no drug but did have a preoperative visit from an anesthesiologist during which discussion concerned the patient's condition, the time of operation, the nature of the anesthetic, and the events of the next day (Egbert *et al.,* 1963). Factors other than drugs, therefore, favorably affect preoperative psychological preparation. Instruction, suggestion, and encouragement are useful nonpharmacological antidotes to anxiety and tension. A similar approach to the relief or avoidance of postoperative pain resulted in a 50% reduction of postoperative narcotic requirements (Egbert *et al.,* 1964).

The difficulties in evaluating preanesthetic regimens have fostered a move toward greater objectivity, and the number of double-blind studies has increased. Although much of the desired result is subjective, systems for grading responses have been developed (Morrison *et al.,* 1968; Norris, 1969). No single drug or combination has been proven superior to all others, and the choice of premedication remains largely an individual matter.

HYPNOTICS

While drowsiness does not imply loss of all anxiety, most drugs in use for preanesthetic medication have some of both effects. The important classes of hypnotics include barbiturates and nonbarbiturate sedatives and antihistamines.

Barbiturates. *Pentobarbital* and *secobarbital* are the barbituric acid derivatives used most frequently to provide sedation and relieve apprehension before operation. They may be administered orally or intramuscularly to adults in doses of 100 to 200 mg, and to infants and children in doses of 3 to 5 mg/kg of body weight. These drugs have minimal depressant action on respiration and circulation and rarely produce nausea or vomiting (*see* Andersen and Gravenstein, 1966). Patients receiving barbiturates for preanesthetic medication usually awaken more promptly from a general anesthetic than if a narcotic analgesic had been given, but the incidence of emergence excitement tends to be higher, presumably because of greater awareness of pain. Tolerance to the usually administered doses of barbiturates is observed in patients who have been taking many kinds of drugs, including other barbiturates, alcohol, and even aspirin and some anticoagulants.

Nonbarbiturate Sedatives. When it is desirable to avoid barbiturates for reasons of allergy or idiosyncrasy, the possibility of excitement, or physical incompatibility with other drugs, a number of alternate sedatives have found favor. *Paraldehyde, chloral hydrate,* and *glutethimide* have been used, but recent practice favors other compounds (*see* below).

Antihistamines. Sedation is a variable side effect of this group of drugs. *Hydroxyzine,* 50 to 150 mg intramuscularly, has found wide usage. It exhibits many minor benefits, such as bronchodilatory, antisialogogic, antiemetic, antiarrhythmic, and ataractic effects. It produces minimal circulatory and respiratory depression (Andersen and Gravenstein, 1966; Lauria *et al.,* 1968) and does not prolong anesthesia (Kim and Dobkin, 1973).

TRANQUILIZERS (ANTIANXIETY AGENTS)

Just as sedatives have some ataractic action, so do tranquilizers produce some sedation. The major groups include phenothiazines, butyrophenones, and benzodiazepines.

Phenothiazines. Many different phenothiazine derivatives and other tranquilizers have been recommended for preanesthetic medication. These substances were suggested because of sedative, antiarrhythmic, antihistaminic, and antiemetic properties. They are sometimes combined in reduced dosage with a barbiturate or an opioid for greater sedation. Prolongation of postanesthetic sleep and greater respiratory depression are probable, and decrease in blood pressure is possible (*see* Dobkin *et al.,* 1962a; Hoffman and Smith, 1970). *Chlorpromazine* has essentially been abandoned for preanesthetic purposes

because of an unacceptable incidence of arterial hypotension. Tachycardia is an occasional sequela, particularly of promazine. The value of phenothiazines in premedication must be carefully weighed against their side effects. Phenothiazines commonly used in premedication include *promazine, promethazine,* and *propiomazine,* all in intramuscular dosage of 20 to 50 mg. (For a comparative study of 16 different phenothiazines and a useful bibliography, *see* Dundee *et al.,* 1965a.)

Butyrophenones. This class of major tranquilizers exhibits some similarities to the phenothiazines. Butyrophenones, especially *droperidol,* have found their major use in anesthesia combined with synthetic opioids in "neurolept analgesia" technics (*see* Chapter 8). The combination of *fentanyl* with *droperidol* in a ratio of 1:50 (INNOVAR) does not produce respiratory depression to a clinically important extent (Kallos and Smith, 1969). The usual dose for premedication is 2.5 to 5 mg of droperidol, which provides 6 to 12 hours of ataraxia (*see* Downes *et al.,* 1967; Edmonds-Seal and Prys-Roberts, 1970). Some antiemetic activity can be expected, and there is reasonable cardiovascular stability despite slight α-adrenergic blocking activity. Both restlessness and extrapyramidal dyskinesia can occur, especially in children. These side effects can be successfully treated with atropine or benztropine mesylate.

Benzodiazepines. This class of drugs appears to allay apprehension with little soporific action and to provide amnesia, especially when combined with scopolamine (Clarke *et al.,* 1970; Dundee and Haslett, 1970). *Benzodiazepines* can raise the threshold for central nervous system toxicity of local anesthetics (de Jong and Heavner, 1973). *Diazepam* in doses of 5 to 10 mg has been most widely used. It is active orally but more predictable after intramuscular injection. It has little effect on respiration and does not potentiate opioid depression.

OPIOIDS

Surgical pain is often severe, and even minor preoperative pain is deleterious to smooth and pleasant induction of anesthesia. Therefore, when analgesics are used in premedication, only strong opioids have proven adequate. The major difference among opioids that governs the choice for premedication is duration of activity.

Morphine. Morphine in the usual doses of 8 to 10 mg intramuscularly is frequently used prior to operation. If pain is present before operation, it is one of the drugs of choice. If weak general anesthetic agents such as nitrous oxide or nonanalgesic drugs such as halothane or thiopental are selected, preoperative use of narcotics provides a smoother maintenance of anesthesia. It is the pain-relieving property that in all probability minimizes the incidence of restlessness or excitation during emergence from general anesthesia. The drug is useful also for depressing the cough reflex. Preanesthetic medication with a narcotic has been shown to reduce the amount of general anesthetic required by 10 to 20% (Saidman and Eger, 1964; Munson et al., 1965).

Unfortunately, morphine may have undesirable side effects. It often prolongs the awakening from general anesthesia since its clinical effects persist for 4 to 6 hours. Its stimulant effect on smooth muscle may cause spasm of the bile duct or of the ureters; colicky pain, often relieved by atropine but nearly always abolished by a narcotic antagonist, may result from this smooth muscle effect. Bronchiolar narrowing may develop in patients with asthma. Constipation and urinary retention may be annoying. Nausea and vomiting are not uncommon. A vagotonic effect may be evidenced by bradycardia (Marta et al., 1973). Hypotension can occur after the use of morphine or other narcotic analgesics. When given before cyclopropane, morphine tends to prevent or reverse the rise in cardiac output often seen with this agent in the absence of a preanesthetic narcotic. Its respiratory depressant action may increase intracranial pressure through retention of carbon dioxide and subsequent cerebral vasodilatation. While this can be undesirable in patients in whom intracranial pressure is already elevated, the effect can be abolished through adequate pulmonary ventilation. The respiratory and circulatory effects of narcotics have been reviewed by Eckenhoff

and Oech (1960), and differences among opioids have been considered by Loan and coworkers (1969) and Morrison and associates (1969).

Meperidine. This drug in 50- to 100-mg doses intramuscularly is used for preanesthetic medication, but it shares all the disadvantages of morphine. Like morphine it can depress blood pressure, cardiac output, and respiration, and it is a stimulant of smooth muscle. Tachycardia occasionally occurs, posing a problem in differential diagnosis. Respiratory depression lasts 2 to 3 hours (Downes et al., 1967).

Fentanyl. This synthetic opioid is useful in some cases because of its short duration of action, 1 to 2 hours (see Downes et al., 1967). The usual dose is 0.05 to 0.10 mg intramuscularly.

Pentazocine. This opioid possesses a very limited addiction liability but is not always effective against severe pain in the usual dose of 20 to 30 mg intramuscularly. It shares the same side effects as the other drugs of its class.

ANTIEMETICS

The newer halogenated ether and hydrocarbon anesthetics are less liable to cause nausea than are ether and cyclopropane. Often the sequelae of prophylactic antiemetics (notably hypotension) are as disturbing and frequent as emetic episodes. However, if a drug is otherwise useful in a given instance, its antiemetic effect is an additional welcome benefit. The ability of *phenothiazines* to reduce postanesthetic nausea and vomiting is real (Dundee et al., 1965b); however, many clinicians prefer to treat nausea and vomiting actively should it be necessary to do so after operation. *Droperidol* and *hydroxyzine* are sometimes used for their antiemetic effects. *Benzquinamide* is a mild tranquilizer with some respiratory stimulant activity, probably via peripheral chemoreceptors. It is also a mild vasopressor and hence does not share some of the drawbacks of other antiemetics (Klein et al., 1970). It is presently being studied in 25- to 50-mg doses for efficacy in anesthetic-induced vomiting.

Other drugs that have been shown to provide an antiemetic effect following intramuscular administration include scopolamine, 0.4 to 0.6 mg; cyclizine, 50 mg; and trimethobenzamide, 200 mg. None has gained wide usage.

ANTICHOLINERGIC DRUGS

In the early years of general anesthesia, the excessive respiratory tract secretions seen during open-drop administration of ether suggested the use of an anticholinergic drug prior to anesthetization. With the advent of less irritating anesthetic agents, secretions have become less of a problem. The emphasis has now shifted from the need for an antisialogogue to the requirement for a drug to counteract the vagal effects that occur frequently during anesthesia. Thus, atropine or a similar substance continues to be given by most anesthesiologists (Eger, 1962).

Atropine. Atropine produces oral dryness and blurred vision within 10 to 15 minutes after intramuscular injection of the standard 0.4- to 0.6-mg dose. The vagal blocking action of such an amount is small and of brief duration. It may not be sufficient to prevent parasympathetically induced cardiovascular effects such as hypotension and bradycardia that result from increase in ocular pressure, visceral traction, manipulation of the carotid sinus, or injection of multiple doses of succinylcholine. However, the intravenous injection of an additional dose of atropine often promptly restores the cardiac rate and the arterial pressure toward normal. Small doses may have a direct cardiac-slowing effect (Dauchot and Gravenstein, 1971).

Atropine administered systemically is not contraindicated in patients with glaucoma. Increased intraocular pressure does not result from the doses recommended (*see* Schwartz *et al.,* 1957). Some have advised that anticholinergic premedication be omitted in patients with asthma, for fear of inspissation of respiratory tract secretions. However, this has not proven to be a problem when the drugs are used in asthmatics. Their use in febrile patients may be unwise, since they depress the mechanism of heat loss by sweating.

Scopolamine. Scopolamine is superior to atropine as an antisialogogue but is less effective in preventing reflex bradycardia during general anesthesia, particularly in children (Freeman and Bachman, 1959). This may be the result of scopolamine's greater direct action to slow the cardiac pacemaker (*see* Gravenstein and Thornby, 1969). The sedative effect of scopolamine is more marked than that of atropine (*see* Domino and Corssen, 1967); occasionally, however, patients become restless or disoriented after scopolamine, and the incidence of emergence excitement appears greater after its administration (Eckenhoff *et al.,* 1961). The combination of scopolamine with a barbiturate is subjectively more unpleasant than scopolamine plus a narcotic analgesic, or atropine with a barbiturate or a narcotic analgesic (*see* Stephen *et al.,* 1969).

The effects of scopolamine or atropine alone on minute ventilation are minimal, although both increase respiratory dead space by dilating bronchi (Smith and DuBois, 1969). When scopolamine and secobarbital are combined, a moderate degree of respiratory depression occurs; but the combination of scopolamine and a narcotic analgesic produces less respiratory depression than does the narcotic alone (*see* Stephen *et al.,* 1969). Scopolamine is usually given intramuscularly, in a dose of 0.4 to 0.6 mg.

Other Drugs. Many other drugs have been used prior to anesthesia for their belladonna-like effects. These include synthetic anticholinergics such as methantheline and oxyphenonium, antihistamines such as hydroxyzine and diphenhydramine, and antiemetics such as cyclizine and promethazine (Dobkin *et al.,* 1962b). They do not possess any advantage over atropine or scopolamine, except perhaps in their longer duration of action.

Andersen, T. W., and Gravenstein, J. S. Cardiovascular effects of sedative doses of pentobarbital and hydroxyzine. *Anesthesiology,* **1966,** *27,* 272–278.

Clarke, P. R. F.; Eccersley, P. S.; Frisby, J. P.; and Thornton, J. A. The amnesic effect of diazepam (VALIUM). *Br. J. Anaesth.,* **1970,** *42,* 690–697.

Dauchot, P., and Gravenstein, J. S. Effects of atropine on the electrocardiogram in different age groups. *Clin. Pharmac. Ther.,* **1971,** *12,* 274–280.

de Jong, R. H., and Heavner, J. E. Diazepam and lidocaine-induced cardiovascular changes. *Anesthesiology,* **1973,** *39,* 633–638.

Dobkin, A. B.; Israel, J. S.; and Criswick, V. G. Prolongation of thiopental anaesthesia with hydroxyzine, SA 97, thiethylperazine, and thioridazine. *Can. Anaesth. Soc. J.,* **1962a,** *9,* 342–346.

Dobkin, A. B.; Woodworth, H.; and Israel, J. S. The antisialogogue effect of hydroxyzine, thiethylperazine, and N′-p-chloro-benzylhydryl-N′-methyl homopiperazine (SA 97). *Can. Anaesth. Soc. J.,* **1962b,** *9,* 234–238.

Domino, E. F., and Corssen, G. Central and peripheral effects of muscarinic cholinergic blocking agents in man. *Anesthesiology,* **1967,** *28,* 568–574.

Downes, J. J.; Kemp, R. V. F.; and Lambertsen, C. J. The magnitude and duration of respiratory depression due to fentanyl and meperidine in man. *J. Pharmac. exp. Ther.,* **1967,** *158,* 416–423.

Dundee, J. W., and Haslett, W. H. K. The benzodiazepines. *Br. J. Anaesth.,* **1970,** *42,* 217–234.

Dundee, J. W.; Moore, J.; Love, W. J.; Nicholl, R. M.; and Clarke, R. S. J. Studies of drugs given before anesthesia. VI. The phenothiazine derivatives. *Br. J. Anaesth.,* **1965a,** *37,* 332–353.

Dundee, J. W.; Nicholl, R. M.; Clarke, R. S. J.; Moore, J.; and Love, W. J. Studies of drugs given before anaesthesia. VII. Pethidine-phenothiazine combinations. *Br. J. Anaesth.,* **1965b,** *37,* 601–613.

Eckenhoff, J. E.; Kneale, D. H.; and Dripps, R. D. The incidence and etiology of postanesthetic excitement. *Anesthesiology,* **1961,** *22,* 667–673.

Edmonds-Seal, J., and Prys-Roberts, C. Pharmacology of drugs used in neuroleptanalgesia. *Br. J. Anaesth.,* **1970,** *42,* 207–216.

Egbert, L. D.; Battit, G. E.; Turndorf, H.; and Beecher, H. K. The value of the preoperative visit by an anesthetist. *J. Am. med. Ass.,* **1963,** *185,* 553–555.

Egbert, L. D.; Battit, G. E.; Welch, C. E.; and Bartlett, M. K. Reducing postoperative pain by encouragement and instruction of patients. *New Engl. J. Med.,* **1964,** *270,* 825–827.

Elliot, H. W.; Fisher, C. W.; de Lappe, A.; Davis, K.; and Botnik, E. Propiomazine, pentobarbital, hydroxyzine, and placebo: double-blind comparison of sedative effects. *Anesthesiology,* **1969,** *31,* 233–236.

Freeman, A., and Bachman, L. Pediatric anesthesia: an evaluation of preoperative medication. *Anesth. Analg. curr. Res.,* **1959,** *38,* 429–432.

Gravenstein, J. S., and Thornby, J. I. Scopolamine on heart rates in man. *Clin. Pharmac. Ther.,* **1969,** *10,* 395–400.

Hoffman, J. C., and Smith, T. C. The respiratory effects of meperidine and propiomazine in man. *Anesthesiology,* **1970,** *32,* 325–331.

Kallos, T., and Smith, T. C. The respiratory effects of INNOVAR given for premedication. *Br. J. Anaesth.,* **1969,** *41,* 303–306.

Kim, D., and Dobkin, A. B. Effect of premedication on duration of anaesthesia with halogenated vapours: chloroform, trichloroethylene, halothane, methoxyflurane, enflurane (ETHRANE) and isoflurane (FORANE). *Can. Anaesth. Soc. J.,* **1973,** *20,* 479–493.

Klein, R. L.; Graves, C. L.; Kim, Y.; and Blatnick, R. Inhibition of apomorphine-induced vomiting by benzquinamide. *Clin. Pharmac. Ther.,* **1970,** *11,* 530–537.

Lauria, J. I.; Markello, R.; and King, B. D. Circulatory and respiratory effects of hydroxyzine in volunteers and geriatric patients. *Anesth. Analg. curr. Res.,* **1968,** *47,* 378–382.

Loan, W. B.; Morrison, J. D.; Dundee, J. W.; Clarke, R. S. J.; Hamilton, R. C.; and Brown, S. S. Studies of drugs given before anaesthesia. XVII. The natural and semi-synthetic opiates. *Br. J. Anaesth.,* **1969,** *41,* 57–63.

Marta, J. A.; Davis, H. S.; and Eisele, J. H. Vagomimetic effects of morphine and INNOVAR in man. *Anesth. Analg. curr. Res.,* **1973,** *52,* 817–821.

Morrison, J. D.; Hill, G. B.; and Dundee, J. W. Studies of drugs given before anaesthesia. XV. Evaluation of the method of study after 10,000 observations. *Br. J. Anaesth.,* **1968,** *40,* 890–900.

Morrison, J. D.; Loan, W. B.; Dundee, J. W.; McDowell, S. A.; and Brown, S. S. Studies of drugs given before anaesthesia. XVIII. The synthetic opiates. *Br. J. Anaesth.,* **1969,** *41,* 987–993.

Munson, E. S.; Saidman, L. J.; and Eger, E. I., II. Effect of nitrous oxide and morphine on the minimum alveolar concentration of fluroxene. *Anesthesiology,* **1965,** *26,* 134–139.

Norris, W. The quantitative assessment of premedication. *Br. J. Anaesth.,* **1969,** *41,* 778–784.

Saidman, L. J., and Eger, E. I., II. Effect of nitrous oxide and of narcotic premedication on the alveolar concentration of halothane required for anesthesia. *Anesthesiology,* **1964,** *25,* 302–306.

Schwartz, H.; deRoetth, A., Jr.; and Papper, E. M. Preanesthetic use of atropine and scopolamine in patients with glaucoma. *J. Am. med. Ass.,* **1957,** *165,* 144–146.

Smith, T. C., and DuBois, A. B. The effects of scopolamine on the airways of man. *Anesthesiology,* **1969,** *30,* 12–18.

Stephen, G. W.; Banner, M. P.; Wollman, H.; and Smith, T. C. Respiratory pharmacology of mixtures of scopolamine with secobarbital and with fentanyl. *Anesthesiology,* **1969,** *31,* 237–242.

Monographs and Reviews

Eckenhoff, J. E., and Oech, S. R. The effects of narcotics and antagonists upon respiration and circulation in man. *Clin. Pharmac. Ther.,* **1960,** *1,* 483–524. (262 references.)

Eger, E. I., II. Atropine, scopolamine, and related compounds. *Anesthesiology,* **1962,** *23,* 365–383.

Shearer, W. M. The evolution of premedication. *Br. J. Anaesth.,* **1960,** *32,* 554–562; **1961,** *33,* 219–225.

5 UPTAKE, DISTRIBUTION, ELIMINATION, AND ADMINISTRATION OF INHALATIONAL ANESTHETICS

Harry Wollman and Theodore C. Smith

PRINCIPLES OF UPTAKE AND DISTRIBUTION

During general anesthesia produced with an inhalational agent, the depth of general anesthesia varies directly with the partial pressure (tension) of anesthetic agent in the brain, and the rates of induction and recovery depend upon the rate of change of tension in this tissue. The partial pressure of anesthetic agent in the brain changes at a rate determined by a number of factors, and is always approaching the tension in arterial blood. The factors that determine the tension of anesthetic gas in the arterial blood and in the brain must therefore be examined. These can be considered under four headings: (1) partial pressure of the anesthetic agent in inspired gas, (2) pulmonary ventilation delivering the anesthetic to the lungs, (3) transfer of the gas from the alveoli to the blood flowing through the lungs, and (4) loss of the agent from the arterial blood to all the tissues of the body. (*See* Kety, 1950, 1951.)

PARTIAL PRESSURE OF THE ANESTHETIC AGENT IN INSPIRED GAS

When an inhalational anesthetic agent is part of a gas mixture, its fractional concentration in that mixture is equal to its partial pressure divided by the total pressure. Thus, concentration is proportional to partial pressure (or tension) in gas mixtures, and one often refers to them interchangeably when speaking of the inspired gases.

When a constant tension is inhaled, the arterial blood tension approaches the tension of the agent in the inspired mixture, in the manner shown in Figure 5–1 for several different anesthetics. (The tension of the inspired vapor or gas is commonly called the "inspired tension.") For drugs such as cyclopropane and nitrous oxide, the arterial tension reaches 90% of the inspired tension in about 20 minutes. When ether is administered, 90% of the inspired tension is reached in arterial blood only after 20 hours.

In practice the inspired tension is rarely constant. An anesthetizing concentration of some agents may irritate the airway of an awake or lightly anesthetized patient, so that the inspired concentration must be increased slowly. In other cases, where the vapor is not irritating, the speed of induction may be increased by giving the inhalational anesthetics in concentrations greater than those ultimately desired. Anesthetic tensions are thus produced in blood and tissues sooner than would be possible if maintenance concentrations were used for induction. As anesthesia proceeds, the inspired concentration of anesthetic is reduced to a level suitable for the maintenance of anesthesia.

PULMONARY VENTILATION

Each inspiration delivers some anesthetic gas to the lung. If the respiratory minute ventilation is great, the anesthetic tension in alveoli increases quickly, as does its tension in arterial blood. Thus, the partial pressure of anesthetic gas in blood can be increased by control of respiration during induction in such a way as to ensure overventilation. Conversely, decreased ventilation (resulting, for instance, from respiratory depression by premedication or an anesthetic agent) can lead to a slower rate of change of arterial gas tension.

The effects of respiration are transient in the case of insoluble gases such as nitrous

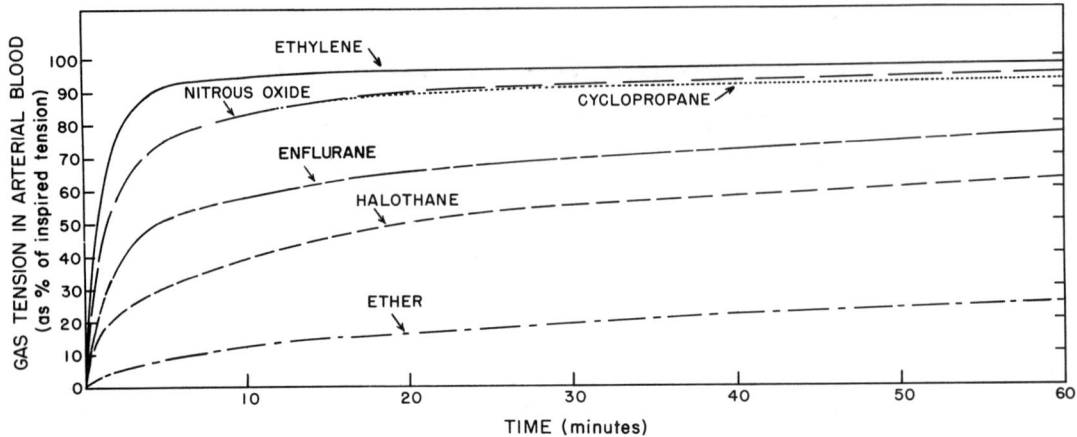

Figure 5-1. *The tensions of anesthetic gases in arterial blood.*

The curves demonstrate how arterial blood tension of the anesthetics increases toward the inspired tension. The increase in partial pressure is rapid for the relatively insoluble gases, and slower for those that are more soluble in blood. For the first comprehensive theoretical analysis of the shape of uptake curves, *see* Kety (1950, 1951). For an early experimental approach to the uptake of anesthetic gases, *see* Haggard (1924).

The course of events is illustrated here for an idealized situation, where the inhaled concentration remains constant, and pulmonary ventilation and cardiac output and its regional distribution remain constant at normal values. In fact, as anesthesia deepens, alveolar ventilation and cardiac output fall, and distribution of regional circulation and agent solubility are variably altered. These and other factors can result in up to 11% difference between predicted and actual concentration (Cowles *et al.,* 1972). Alinear analyses have been proposed that take these factors into consideration (Smith *et al.,* 1972; Munson *et al.,* 1973). (Modified from Mapleson, in the text by Papper and Kitz, 1963; also modified from Torri, Damia, Fabiani, and Frova, 1972.)

oxide, cyclopropane, and ethylene where left atrial blood concentration rapidly approaches the alveolar. However, the volume of respiration exerts a more significant and prolonged effect on the rate of uptake of more soluble and slowly equilibrating drugs such as halothane and ether. (For the reasons underlying these phenomena, *see* Eger, 1964.)

TRANSFER OF ANESTHETIC GASES FROM ALVEOLI TO BLOOD

The alveolar membrane allows rapid diffusion of anesthetic gases in both directions and poses no barrier to their transfer. Although the diffusion of anesthetic gases may be normal, certain situations can occur during clinical anesthesia that impede the efficient transfer of gases into blood flowing through the lung. One of these is underventilation of some of the alveoli, such as may occur in pulmonary emphysema. There is then a lower tension of anesthetic gas in the abnormal alveoli, and thus a lower anesthetic tension in the blood draining them. The con-

tribution of this blood to the arterial pool results in slowing of the rate of change of tension of the anesthetic in arterial blood. In fact, ventilation and perfusion of the alveoli are not always well matched during general anesthesia, and airway closure and atelectasis occasionally occur. The resulting mismatch of ventilation and perfusion in the lung produces a difference between alveolar and arterial tensions of anesthetic gases. This abnormal situation results in slowing of the rate of induction of, or recovery from, anesthesia (*see* Eger and Severinghaus, 1964).

In the absence of ventilation-perfusion disturbances, three factors determine how rapidly anesthetics pass from the inspired gases to blood. These are (1) the solubility of the agent in blood, (2) the rate of blood flow through the lung, and (3) the partial pressures of the agent in arterial and mixed venous blood.

Solubility of the Agent in Blood. This is usually expressed as the blood:gas partition coefficient, or λ, which represents the ratio of anesthetic concentration in blood to anesthetic concentration in a gas phase when the two are in equilibrium (*i.e.,* when the partial pressure is equal in both phases). The blood:gas partition coefficient is as high as 12 for very soluble agents such as ether and as low as 0.15 for relatively insoluble anesthetics such as ethylene. The more soluble an anesthetic is in blood, the more of it must be dissolved in blood to raise its partial pressure there appreciably. Therefore, the blood *tension* of *soluble* agents rises slowly. The potential reservoir for relatively insoluble gases is small and can be filled more quickly. Therefore, their tension in blood can increase more rapidly.

In column 1 of Table 5-1 are given the blood:gas partition coefficients for some of the anesthetic agents. The feature of the curves in Figure 5-1 that is largely determined by the blood solubility of the agents is the height and sharpness of the bend, or "knee," in the uptake curve. The more soluble the agent (*i.e.,* the higher the λ), the lower and less sharp is the "knee" of the curve, and the slower is the approach of blood tension to that of the inhaled gases.

Rate of Pulmonary Blood Flow. The pulmonary blood flow (*i.e.,* the cardiac output) affects the rate at which anesthetics pass from the alveolar gases into the arterial blood. An increase in pulmonary blood flow slows the initial portion of the arterial tension curve; but the latter part of the curve tends to catch up, with the overall result that there is little change in the total time required for complete equilibration. (For the reasons why this should be so, *see* Kety, 1950, 1951; Mapleson, 1963; Mapleson, in the text by Papper and Kitz, 1963; Eger, 1964.)

Partial Pressures in Arterial and Mixed Venous Blood. After taking up anesthetic gas in the lung, the blood circulates to the tissues, and anesthetic gas is transferred from the blood to all tissues of the body. Blood cannot approach equilibrium with inhaled gas tension until this process, which tends to decrease the blood tension, is nearly complete. The mixed venous blood returning to the lungs has more anesthetic gas in it with each passage through the body. After a few minutes of anesthesia the difference between arterial (or alveolar) and mixed venous gas tension decreases continuously. Since the rate of diffusion across the pulmonary membrane is proportional to the difference between alveolar and mixed venous gas tensions, the volume of gas transferred to arterial blood during each minute decreases as time passes. Thus, arterial tension rises more slowly in the final portion of the curves in Figure 5-1.

Table 5-1. PARTITION COEFFICIENTS AT BODY TEMPERATURE *

ANESTHETIC	Blood:Gas (1)	Tissue:Blood Brain Gray (2)	Brain White (3)	Heart (4)	Kidney (5)	Liver (6)	Muscle (7)	Fat (8)
Ethylene	0.15	—	—	1.0	—	—	—	6
Nitrous oxide	0.47	1.1	1.1	1.1	0.9	0.9	0.9	2.3
Cyclopropane	0.55	1.5	3.6	1.8	0.7	1.1	0.7	15
Fluroxene	1.4	1.1	1.7	—	0.9	1.4	1.4	23
Isoflurane	1.4	—	—	—	—	—	—	48
Enflurane	1.9	—	—	—	—	—	—	37
Halothane	2.4	2.1	3.3	2.9	1.5	2.5	2.5	65
Methoxyflurane	11	1.8	2.7	—	1.8	2.3	1.8	61
Ether	12	1.0	1.1	1.0	0.8	0.9	0.9	4.2

* These data have been calculated from the review of Steward and associates (1973). (*See also* Cowles *et al.,* 1971, for discussion of the problem involved in specifying precise coefficients for nonhomogeneous media.)

† There is considerable variation in blood:gas coefficients (column 1), which is reflected clinically in differing speeds of induction and of emergence after short administrations. The tissue:blood coefficients (columns 2 to 8) are close to unity for most agents, except in the case of fat:blood coefficients. These are considerably greater but vary widely and affect the tail of the uptake curve and the rate of emergence after long administrations.

THE CONCENTRATION EFFECT
AND THE SECOND-GAS EFFECT

The *concentration effect* may be defined as follows: when higher concentrations of an anesthetic gas are inhaled, arterial tension increases at a slightly greater rate than it would have if a lesser concentration of the anesthetic had been inhaled (*see* Eger, 1963). Consider a patient who is inhaling 75% nitrous oxide and 25% oxygen. Although nitrous oxide is relatively insoluble, when the inhaled concentration is high, the rate of uptake of the gas by blood and tissues may be as great as 1 liter per minute during the early minutes of anesthesia. As this volume of gas disappears from the lung, fresh gases are literally sucked into the lung from the breathing circuit to replace the volume taken up. The rate at which the inspired gas mixture is delivered to the lung is then 1 liter per minute greater than the minute ventilation would have provided without this effect. Therefore, the rate of rise of the arterial tension curve for nitrous oxide is increased during induction of anesthesia. However, if only 10% nitrous oxide is inhaled, the body's uptake of approximately 150 ml per minute results in no significant change in the rate of gas delivery to the lung, and there is little or no acceleration of the arterial tension.

The simultaneous presence of two anesthetic gases in the lung can introduce a closely related phenomenon known as the *second-gas effect*. An illustration may be taken in which 75% nitrous oxide and 1% halothane are administered together with 24% oxygen. The same disappearance of 1 liter per minute of nitrous oxide from the lung into the body takes place, and the rate at which 1% halothane is delivered to the alveoli becomes 1 liter per minute greater than the minute ventilation would otherwise have provided. As a result, the arterial tension of halothane rises a little more rapidly in the presence of nitrous oxide. (*See* Epstein *et al.*, 1964; for a discussion of the relation of the concentration and second-gas effects, *see* Stoelting and Eger, 1969a.)

LOSS OF ANESTHETIC GASES FROM
ARTERIAL BLOOD TO TISSUES

When the inhalational agents are delivered by arterial blood to the tissues, the tension rises in tissues to approach that in arterial blood. The rate at which a gas passes into tissues depends on (1) the solubility of the gas in the tissues, (2) the rate at which the gas is delivered to the tissues (*i.e.,* the blood flow to the various areas of the body), and (3) the partial pressures of the gas in arterial blood and tissues. Note that these three factors affecting transfer of the gas from blood to tissue are similar to the three that affect transfer of the anesthetic from lung to blood (*see* above).

Solubility of Gas in Tissues. This is expressed as a tissue : blood partition coefficient, a concept analogous to the blood : gas partition coefficient previously discussed. With most anesthetic agents, the tissue : blood partition is near unity for many of the body's lean tissues, as shown in columns 2 to 7 of Table 5–1; that is, these agents are equally soluble in lean tissue and blood. An anesthetic concentration in blood or tissue is the product of partial pressure and solubility. Thus, the concentration of most anesthetics in lean tissues, such as the gray matter of brain, approaches that in blood as tissue tension builds up toward arterial blood tension. On the other hand, the tissue : blood coefficient for all anesthetics is large for fatty tissues (column 8 of Table 5–1). Their concentration in the fatty tissue is much greater than that in blood at the time of equilibrium (when tissue tension equals blood tension).

Tissue solubility is of importance in determining the slope of the final portion, or "tail," of the gas tension curves (Figure 5–1). High tissue solubility, especially high fat solubility, tends to depress the rate of rise of the "tail" of the curve. This phenomenon is best seen by comparing the curves for nitrous oxide and the more fat-soluble gas cyclopropane. The cyclopropane curve coincides with that for nitrous oxide in the early minutes (they are about equally soluble in blood); but cyclopropane begins to lag behind nitrous oxide in the latter portion of the curve, where slope is affected by tissue solubility.

Tissue Blood Flow. The higher the blood flow to a tissue, the faster the delivery of the anesthetic agent, and the more rapidly will its tension and concentration rise in that area. This is illustrated in Figure 5–2, where the brain concentration of an inert gas approaches the arterial concentration more rapidly when cerebral blood flow is high, and more slowly when cerebral blood flow decreases. It has been suggested that anesthetic induction and emergence can be speeded by allowing the patient to inhale some carbon dioxide. This agent, by increasing ventilation, accelerates the rise in the arterial tension curve (*see* above). In addition, by dilating cerebral vessels, carbon dioxide increases cerebral blood flow and thus hastens the rate at which brain tension of the anesthetic

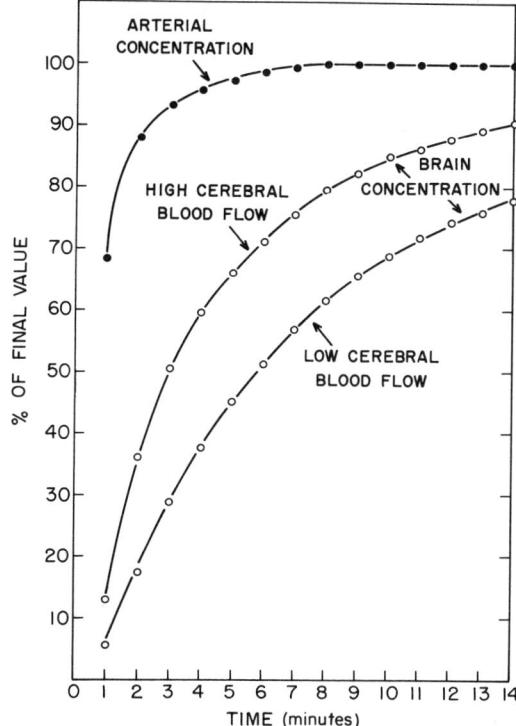

Figure 5-2. *Krypton-85 concentration in arterial blood and in brain.*

Mean values from six experiments are shown. The curves illustrate the increase in concentrations of ^{85}Kr, an inert gas, in arterial blood and in brain, when a constant concentration is inhaled. The arterial concentration increases rapidly toward its final value, as the gas is insoluble in blood. The brain concentration lags behind the arterial concentration in its approach toward its equilibrium (final) value. Brain concentration can be seen to increase more rapidly when cerebral blood flow is high, in this case due to carbon dioxide inhalation. (After Alexander, Wollman, Cohen, Melman, Chase, and Behar, 1964. Courtesy of *Anesthesiology.*)

tain a significant amount of anesthetic agent only after a considerable time has elapsed.

Partial Pressures in Arterial Blood and Tissues. As the tissues take up anesthetic agent, the partial pressure of the gas in tissues increases toward that of the arterial. Since the rate at which gas diffuses from arterial blood to tissues varies with the partial-pressure difference between them, tissue concentration changes rapidly in the early minutes of anesthesia; however, as the tissue tension comes closer to the arterial tension, the tissue uptake of gas slows (*see* Figure 5-2).

In *summary,* during the administration of an anesthetic, its tension in blood rises toward that in the inspired gas, at first rapidly, then more slowly. Tissue tensions increase concomitantly, approaching the arterial tension. The partial pressure increases most rapidly in tissues with high rates of blood flow, and lags considerably in areas where blood flow is slower.

INTERTISSUE DIFFUSION

Several other but less important factors influence the rate at which blood and tissues equilibrate with the inhaled tension of a gas. One is the diffusion of the gas between contiguous tissues. During the approach to equilibrium, the gas being inhaled may be present at different partial pressures in adjacent tissues, the partial pressure being higher in the areas with greater flow and in those where the gas is less soluble. The anesthetic will diffuse into the areas where its tension is lower. The rates of diffusion are such that tissue tensions are not much affected in areas with high blood flow and areas where the gas is relatively insoluble. However, tissue concentrations can be significantly changed by diffusion in areas where flow rates are low and gas solubility is high, as in adipose tissue (*see* Eger, 1973).

ELIMINATION OF INHALATIONAL ANESTHETICS

The major factors that affect rate of elimination of the anesthetics are the same as those that are important in the uptake phase: pulmonary ventilation, blood flow, and solubility in blood and tissue. However, the administration of anesthesia is usually completed before arterial tension has reached inspired tension, and long before tissues of low blood flow or high gas solubility have reached inspired tension. As ventilation with

changes. Since brain tension of the anesthetic is the important factor for anesthesia, this procedure results in more rapid induction or emergence but *not* in more profound anesthesia.

Only tissues with high rates of blood flow will exhibit rapid rises in concentration of anesthetic, and only high-flow areas take up significant amounts of the agent during the early stages of anesthesia. Since blood flow to adipose tissue is very slow, anesthetic gases will be delivered to, and taken up by, fatty tissues so slowly that these tissues con-

anesthetic-free gas washes out the lungs, the arterial blood tension declines first, followed by that in the tissues. An example of tissue concentrations during 60 minutes of nitrous oxide inhalation and 45 minutes of washout is shown in Figure 5-3 (*see* Cowles *et al.,* 1968). Notice that soon after elimination begins, the tension in lung and blood has fallen to very low (nonanesthetic) levels. Because of the high blood flow to brain, its tension of anesthetic gas decreases rapidly, accounting for the rapid awakening from anesthesia noted with relatively insoluble agents such as nitrous oxide. The agent persists for a longer time in tissues with lower blood flow such as muscle, and for yet longer times in fat where blood flow is very low, and from which the agent is therefore very slowly released.

DIFFUSION HYPOXIA

The reverse of the concentration effect (*see* above) can occur after the anesthetic has been discontinued, and will be illustrated for nitrous oxide. The elimination of nitrous oxide from blood to lung may proceed at a rate as great as the uptake. The additional gas added to the alveoli dilutes the available oxygen, and reduces alveolar oxygen concentration. The phenomenon is known as *diffusion hypoxia* (*see* Fink, 1955). It is seen in the early minutes following the end of a nitrous oxide administration, if the patient is breathing air. The hypoxia is usually mild, and is rarely a clinical threat. It can be prevented by oxygen inhalation for a few minutes at the end of the anesthetic administration.

Although *diffusion hypoxia* can theoretically occur after the withdrawal of any anesthetic agent, its magnitude is insignificant unless high concentrations of nitrous oxide have been inhaled for some time. Under these circumstances a considerable volume of inert gas has been dissolved in the body (up to 30 liters), and much of it is eliminated through the lungs in the first few minutes after its administration is discontinued. When lower concentrations of an agent (*e.g.,* 20% cyclopropane) are inhaled, even after a long time only a few liters will have been taken up in the body. When administration is discontinued, the elimination of about 300 ml per minute or less of cyclopropane is not sufficient to dilute the alveolar oxygen to hypoxic levels. When more soluble agents, such as ether, are inhaled for a long time, many liters of the gas are dissolved in blood and body tissues; but, following termination of the anesthetic, the slow rate of elimination of the gas results in little dilution of alveolar oxygen.

OTHER ROUTES OF ANESTHETIC ELIMINATION

The anesthetic gases are metabolized in the body to a small extent. This has been known for some time for trichloroethylene, but it is now clear that most other anesthetics are metabolized as well. Less than 3% of absorbed ether is oxidized, to carbon dioxide and water. Up to 4% of chloroform, 10% of fluroxene, 13% of halothane, and 20% of methoxyflurane are metabolized to various intermediate compounds, and in some cases to ionized halogens (Cohen, 1971). There is no direct evidence at present that nitrous oxide is metabolized.

Metabolism of anesthetic agents is generally accomplished by hepatic microsomal enzyme systems, which can be induced by a number of drugs, including preservatives added to liquid anesthetics, as well

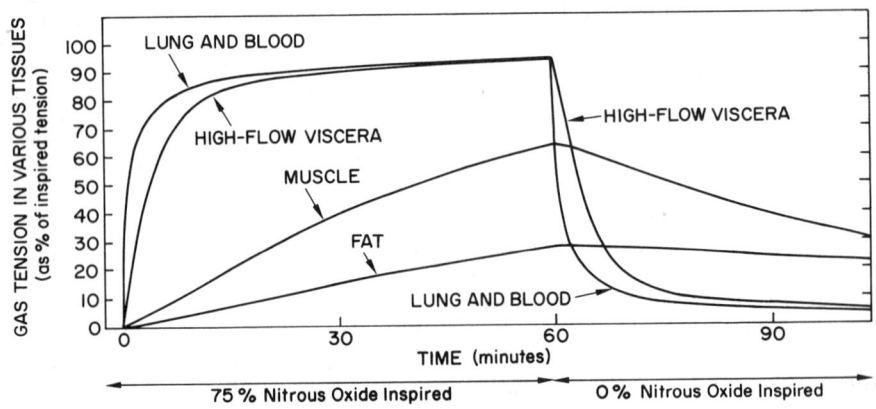

Figure 5-3. *Tissue tensions of an anesthetic gas during uptake and elimination.*

The curves demonstrate how tissue tensions of nitrous oxide approach the inspired tension during a 60-minute anesthetic uptake phase and a subsequent 45-minute elimination phase. The high-blood-flow viscera include brain, heart, and kidney. Liver and intestine have lower blood flows, and their tensions would lie between those of the high-blood-flow viscera and muscle. (Modified from Cowles, Borgstedt, and Gillies, 1968.)

as by the anesthetics themselves. For example, anesthesiologists who inhale anesthetic gases in the course of their practice have greater microsomal enzyme activity than do pharmacists. However, high concentrations of anesthetics inhibit their own metabolism. The bulk of metabolism of anesthetics occurs after clinical anesthesia has been discontinued, and is greatest for the more fat-soluble drugs (Berman *et al.*, 1973). The importance of the metabolism of anesthetic agents is not in the termination of their action; rather, it is hypothesized that metabolites of anesthetics may be responsible for certain of their toxic effects or aftereffects.

Additional small losses of anesthetic gases from the body occur by diffusion across skin and mucous membranes, and by means of urinary excretion of the agent or its breakdown products (Stoelting and Eger, 1969b; Cohen, 1971).

ADMINISTRATION OF INHALATIONAL ANESTHETICS

In the early years of anesthesia, anesthetics were administered by the open-drop technic. In a few instances this method of administration is used today. A liquid anesthetic is dripped onto a gauze-covered wire mask. The patient obtains oxygen from the room air, and the exhaled carbon dioxide and water vapor escape into the room. However, the anesthesiologist has little knowledge of the concentration of anesthetic vapor being breathed, and respiratory assistance is not possible with this technic while the anesthetic is being administered. Therefore, a breathing bag, a mask, and a source of oxygen should be at hand in case of respiratory emergencies. Anesthetic machines and modern breathing circuits are preferred.

ANESTHETIC MACHINES

With these devices, the anesthesiologist is able to deliver measured quantities of anesthetic gases and oxygen through accurate flowmeters, and with the use of special vaporizers it is possible to add the vapor of volatile anesthetic liquids to the gas stream. Tanks of oxygen and anesthetic gases are attached to the machine by fittings that are pin-indexed, so that a tank cannot be mounted in the wrong slot (*see* Epstein and Hunter, 1968).

Vaporizers. Liquid anesthetic agents can be vaporized in several ways (*see* Hill, 1968). They may be slowly dripped into the gas mixture, not unlike an open-drop technic. They may be vaporized by a gas stream that passes over the surface of the liquid, or past a wick saturated with the liquid. Some vaporizers with graduated dials can deliver a precisely known concentration of anesthetic vapor. Bimetalic valves incorporated in these vaporizers keep the output concentration constant over a range of room temperature, by altering the ratio of through flow to by-pass flow of gases. A gas may also be passed through the liquid, as in the modern, precise, "saturation-type" vaporizers such as the copper kettle. In these devices, gas bubbles pass through a liquid anesthetic in such a way that saturation of

the gas bubbles with the liquid agent is complete. Equilibration occurs within the vaporizer, the amount of liquid volatilized by the gas depending only upon the vapor pressure, which, in turn, is determined by the particular liquid and its temperature. Since vaporization of liquids tends to cool them, some vaporizers are made of materials that conduct heat well, and are thermally connected to the anesthesia machine, which provides a large heat reservoir. As a result, the temperature inside a copper kettle tends to remain constant, even when liquids are vaporized rapidly. The decrease in vapor pressure that occurs when temperature declines is thus minimized (Morris and Feldman, 1958).

As the vapor pressures of many liquid anesthetics are several hundred millimeters Hg at room temperature, saturation vaporizers can deliver far more than is necessary or desirable. Therefore, the outflow of gases from the vaporizer is diluted with additional flows of oxygen or nitrous oxide to attain the desired anesthetic concentrations. In Table 5–2 are shown the vapor pressures of some of the anesthetics, the concentrations that are delivered from saturation-type vaporizers, and the useful anesthetic concentrations that are attained by diluting the outflow of these vaporizers.

BREATHING CIRCUITS

The gases and vapors are delivered into a system of wide-bore tubes with valves, a distensible bag that provides a reservoir for the gases, and usually an absorber for expired carbon dioxide. Gases are administered to the patient by means of a face mask or endotracheal tube. Two types of gas delivery systems are illustrated in Figure 5–4. Generally, the components are made of electrically conductive materials, so that electrical potential differences and sparking are unlikely to occur, and explosive agents may be used more safely (*see* National Fire Prevention Association, 1971).

Valves. These may be one-way valves, which can act as non-rebreathing valves or can ensure that the gases are unidirectionally circulated in a *circle system.* They may be demand valves, which ensure that fresh gas can flow into the system only during inspiration and only in amounts required by the patient; or they may be pop-off valves, which permit the escape of excess gases from the circuit but do not allow entry of room air (*see* Foregger, 1959).

The Reservoir Bag. In the absence of a demand valve, there must be a reservoir of gas from which the patient can inhale. This is usually provided by a distensible bag that partially empties during inhalation and refills during exhalation. In non-rebreathing systems, the bag refills with fresh gases from the flowmeters. In rebreathing systems, it refills not only with fresh gas, but also with exhaled gases after they have passed through a carbon dioxide absorber. The bag also provides a means for the assistance or control of respiration by the anesthesiologist, who can compress the bag and thus force gas into the patient's lungs. When pressure on the bag is released, the lungs empty and the bag refills.

Table 5-2. CONSIDERATIONS AFFECTING THE USE OF VOLATILE ANESTHETICS IN SATURATION VAPORIZERS *

ANESTHETIC	(1) BOILING POINT (°C)	(2) VAPOR PRESSURE AT 20° C (MM HG)	(3) CONCENTRATION OF VAPOR DELIVERED BY A SATURATION VAPORIZER AT 20° C	(4) (5) USEFUL RANGES OF CONCENTRATION (INSPIRED GAS)	
				For Induction	*For Maintenance*
Ether	35	443	58%	10–40%	3–12%
Fluroxene	43	286	38%	4–12%	3–8%
Isoflurane	48	252	33%	2–6%	1–3%
Halothane	50	243	32%	1–4%	½–2%
Enflurane	57	180	24%	3–7%	1½–4%
Methoxyflurane	105	24	3%	Up to 3%	¼–1%

* Illustrations are given for six liquids that can be administered with saturation-type vaporizers. It will be noted that, as the boiling point (column 1) increases, the vapor pressure at room temperature (column 2) decreases. In column 3 are given the concentrations of these agents that could be delivered at room temperature by a saturation vaporizer, such as the copper kettle. It is clear that these concentrations are well above the useful anesthetic concentrations, roughly estimated in columns 4 and 5. Thus, in practice, the outflow of these vaporizers is diluted with additional flows of oxygen and/or nitrous oxide to attain more reasonable concentrations of the vaporized liquid. Only during induction of anesthesia with methoxyflurane can the kettle outflow be safely delivered directly to the patient without dilution.

The estimates of useful concentrations in columns 4 and 5 assume that the agent is being administered alone. If nitrous oxide is added to the mixture, lower concentrations of the volatile anesthetics can be used.

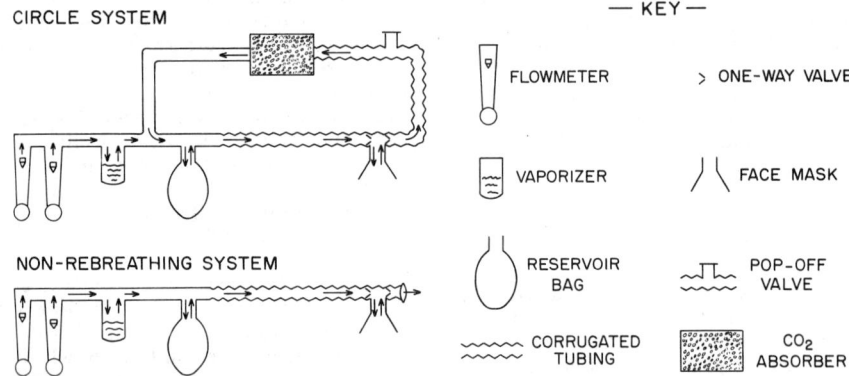

Figure 5-4. *Systems used for delivering inhalational anesthetics.*

Two breathing circuits are shown. It is easy to see that they are made up of similar components arranged in slightly different ways.

Circle System. Gases are delivered through flowmeters and past the vaporizer, and then circulate in one direction around the circle. If large amounts of fresh gas are added, the excess is eliminated through the one-way, pop-off valve. If, on the other hand, rebreathing of the exhaled gases takes place, only small amounts of fresh gases are added from the machine to replace the oxygen used by the patient in metabolism and the anesthetic gases taken up by the patient. In this case, no gas flows out through the pop-off valve, and the exhaled carbon dioxide is absorbed chemically. (For a discussion of optimal placement of the various components of circle systems, *see* Eger and Ethans, 1968.)

Non-rebreathing System. Gases are delivered through flowmeters and past the vaporizer, as in the circle system. They then pass to the reservoir bag and the patient. All exhaled gases escape through the one-way exhalation valve, and carbon dioxide absorption is unnecessary. Fresh gases must be delivered at a rate sufficient to supply the patient's minute ventilation.

If the one-way valve between the bag and the face mask is eliminated, this system becomes the popular Magill circuit, and the amount of rebreathing that takes place then depends on the flow rate of the gases (*see* Mapleson, 1954).

Carbon Dioxide Absorption or Elimination. In systems where rebreathing is permitted, one must provide for elimination of the exhaled carbon dioxide (*see* Gates and Adriani, 1962; Brown *et al.,* 1964). For this purpose, a canister of carbon dioxide–absorbing material can be included in the breathing circuit. This material is a basic substance, such as soda lime, that reacts with carbonic acid formed by carbon dioxide and water. As a result of the reaction, a carbonate and water are produced and heat is generated (*see* Bracken and Cox, 1968).

Another way in which carbon dioxide can be eliminated from an anesthetic system is by washout with high flows of fresh gases, the carbon dioxide being carried out in the overflow of other gases. The higher the flow rate, the greater is the overflow and the more complete the elimination of carbon dioxide (*see* Mapleson, 1954; Adriani, 1960; Brown *et al.,* 1964). In *non-rebreathing systems,* all the exhaled carbon dioxide is eliminated from the system by means of the non-rebreathing valve.

Nomenclature. Breathing systems are often described by the terms *closed, semiclosed, semiopen,* and *open.* However, variations in definition have resulted in disagreement among anesthesiologists over the name that should be attached to the particular system.

Since disagreements over nomenclature are so general, it seems most sensible to specify a system for the administration of anesthesia by simply describing the equipment of which it is composed, and the flow rates that are used (*see* Hamilton, 1964).

CHOICE OF AN ANESTHETIC SYSTEM

After the anesthesiologist has chosen the anesthetic agents, he selects a technic for their administration, considering such factors as the following. If, for instance, it is desired to confine an explosive agent such as cyclopropane within the breathing circuit, a low-flow technic with chemical absorption of carbon dioxide is indicated. Such systems also have the advantage of lower cost when expensive agents are used.

In some circumstances, either high-flow or non-rebreathing systems are useful, for example, when chemical absorption of carbon dioxide cannot be used (as when trichloroethylene is being administered). High-flow systems have the advantage that the anesthesiologist has a better idea of the concentrations of gases being inhaled. In addition, rapid changes in the inhaled concentrations are more readily achieved in these systems.

In still other circumstances it may be necessary or desirable to resort to the simplicity of open-drop administration, for instance, where minimal equipment is available far from a hospital.

GAS, HEAT, AND WATER EXCHANGE IN ANESTHETIC SYSTEMS

The rate of flow of fresh gases into the system and the presence or absence of valves determine several important factors; these include the rate of nitrogen elimination, the accumulation or loss of heat and water, and the reliability of information on the exact concentrations of gases being delivered.

Nitrogen Elimination. When an anesthetic diluted in oxygen is inhaled and the anesthetic mixture contains no nitrogen, the partial pressure of nitrogen in the alveoli of the lungs is rapidly reduced. Consequently, nitrogen is eliminated, first from the alveoli and subsequently from the blood and tissues. Three liters of nitrogen may be eliminated through the lungs during the first hour of anesthesia. In a low-flow system this will dilute the anesthetic mixture considerably. However, more anesthetic gas may be added to the mixture as necessary, and the oxygen concentration in closed systems can be maintained above 20% if enough additional oxygen is added. In a high-flow as well as in a non-rebreathing system, nitrogen elimination proceeds, as does carbon dioxide elimination, by a spillover of nitrogen with the excess gases through the expiratory valve (*see* Miles *et al.,* 1956).

Heat and Water Transfer. In normal conscious man, relatively dry gases are inhaled, and evaporation of water from the respiratory tract results in the exhalation of gases laden with water vapor. Heat and water are lost from the body when this evaporation takes place. Heat loss by this means is usually about 5 kcal per hour, or less than 10% of the basal metabolic rate. Water loss amounts to only about 10 ml per hour (*see* Burch, 1945). The same phenomenon occurs during anesthesia with non-rebreathing systems or high-flow systems where little rebreathing occurs. In systems with low flows of gas, water vapor accumulates, and the moist inhaled gases have less water vapor added to them in the respiratory tree. Thus, heat is lost through respiration at a slower rate than normal, as low as a fraction of 1 kcal per hour, and water loss can become as low as 3 ml per hour (*see* Clark *et al.,* 1954; Chase *et al.,* 1961).

The heat produced when carbon dioxide reacts with soda lime is usually not transferred to the patient, as there is most often a sufficient length of rubber tubing between the absorber and the patient to ensure that heat is dissipated before the gases reach him. Only in a to-and-fro closed system is the carbon dioxide absorber close enough to the patient to allow transfer of heat by way of the inhaled gases. In actual practice, heat loss or gain due to the anesthetic system is usually not large enough to represent a danger to the patient (*see* Wollman and Cannard, 1960).

Information on Exact Concentrations. The concentrations of anesthetics and oxygen being inhaled by the patient are identical to those being delivered by the machine only in non-rebreathing circuits. In these circuits, if the anesthesiologist has accurate flowmeters for gases and a dependable vaporizer for liquids, he can determine what concentrations of anesthetics and oxygen are being delivered to the patient. However, in systems where rebreathing occurs, the situation is considerably different. Denitrogenation of the patient dilutes the gases in the system; humidification of the gases in the system lowers their concentrations somewhat; oxygen is lost from the system as the patient utilizes it for metabolic requirements; and anesthetic gases are taken up by the patient at a changing rate. At the same time, small amounts of oxygen and anesthetic are added to the circuit. It is apparent that in a low-flow system, the inhaled gases are a mixture with a composition that is difficult to estimate. As the flow rates increase, the characteristics of the system become less like the low-flow and more like the non-rebreathing system, and the inhaled gas concentrations approach the concentrations being delivered from the flowmeters and the vaporizer. Nitrous oxide is most frequently delivered in high-flow systems; the anesthesiologist is then assured of at least 20% inhaled oxygen and very nearly 80% inhaled concentration of this rather impotent anesthetic gas (*see* Smith 1966).

Adriani, J. Disposal of carbon dioxide from devices used for inhalational anesthesia. *Anesthesiology,* **1960,** *21,* 742–748.

Alexander, S. C.; Wollman, H.; Cohen, P. J.; Melman, E.; Chase, P. E.; and Behar, M. G. Krypton[85] and nitrous oxide uptake of the human brain during anesthesia. *Anesthesiology,* **1964,** *25,* 37–42.

Berman, M. L.; Lowe, H. J.; Bochantin, J.; and Hagler, K. Uptake and elimination of methoxyflurane as influenced by enzyme induction in the rat. *Anesthesiology,* **1973,** *38,* 352–357.

Bracken, A., and Cox, L. A. Apparatus for carbon dioxide absorption. *Br. J. Anaesth.,* **1968,** *40,* 660–665.

Brown, E. S.; Seniff, A. M.; and Elam, J. O. Carbon dioxide elimination in semi-closed systems. *Anesthesiology,* **1964,** *25,* 31–36.

Burch, G. E. Rate of water and heat loss from the respiratory tract of normal subjects in a subtropical climate. *Archs intern. Med.,* **1945,** *76,* 315–327.

Chase, H. F.; Kilmore, M. A.; and Trotta, R. Respiratory water loss via anesthesia systems: mask breathing. *Anesthesiology,* **1961,** *22,* 205–209.

Clark, R. E.; Orkin, L. R.; and Rovenstine, E. A. Body temperature studies in anesthetized man: effect of environmental temperature, humidity, and anesthesia system. *J. Am. med. Ass.,* **1954,** *154,* 311–319.

Cowles, A. L.; Borgstedt, H. H.; and Gillies, A. J. Uptake and distribution of inhalation anesthetic agents in clinical practice. *Anesth. Analg. curr. Res.,* **1968,** *47,* 404–414.

———. Solubilities of ethylene, cyclopropane, halothane and diethyl ether in human and dog blood at low concentrations. *Anesthesiology,* **1971,** *35,* 203–211.

———. The uptake and distribution of four inhalation anesthetics in dogs. *Ibid.,* **1972,** *36,* 558–570.

Eger, E. I., II. Effect of inspired anesthetic concentration on the rate of rise of alveolar concentration. *Anesthesiology,* **1963,** *24,* 153–157.

———. Respiratory and circulatory factors in uptake and distribution of volatile anaesthetic agents. *Br. J. Anaesth.,* **1964,** *36,* 155–171.

———. Intertissue diffusion of anesthetics. *Anesthesiology,* **1973,** *38,* 201.

Eger, E. I., II, and Ethans, C. T. The effects of inflow, overflow, and valve placement on economy of the circle system. *Anesthesiology,* **1968,** *29,* 93–100.

Eger, E. I., II, and Severinghaus, J. W. Effect of uneven pulmonary distribution of blood and gas on induction with inhalation anesthetics. *Anesthesiology,* **1964,** *25,* 620–626.

Epstein, H. G., and Hunter, A. R. Anaesthetic apparatus: a pictorial review of the development of the modern anaesthetic machine. *Br. J. Anaesth.,* **1968,** *40,* 636–647.

Epstein, R. M.; Rackow, H.; Salanitre, E.; and Wolf, G. Influence of the concentration effect on the uptake of anesthetic mixtures: the second gas effect. *Anesthesiology,* **1964,** *25,* 364–371.

Fink, B. R. Diffusion anoxia. *Anesthesiology,* **1955,** *16,* 511–519.

Foregger, R. The classification and performance of respiratory valves. *Anesthesiology,* **1959,** *20,* 296–308.

Gates, G., and Adriani, J. Disposal of carbon dioxide from apparatus used for inhalational anesthesia. *Anesthesiology,* **1962,** *23,* 148–149.

Haggard, H. W. Absorption, distribution, and elimination of ethyl ether. *J. biol. Chem.,* **1924,** *59,* 737–802.

Hamilton, W. K. Nomenclature of inhalation anesthetic systems. *Anesthesiology,* **1964,** *25,* 3–5.

Hill, D. W. The design and calibration of vaporizers for volatile anaesthetic agents. *Br. J. Anaesth.,* **1968,** *40,* 648–659.

Kety, S. S. The physiological and physical factors governing the uptake of anesthetic gases by the body. *Anesthesiology,* **1950,** *11,* 517–526.

Mapleson, W. W. The elimination of rebreathing in various semi-closed anaesthesia systems. *Br. J. Anaesth.,* **1954,** *26,* 323–332.

———. An electric analogue for uptake and exchange of inert gases and other agents. *J. appl. Physiol.,* **1963,** *18,* 197–204.

Miles, G. G.; Martin, N. T.; and Adriani, J. Factors influencing the elimination of nitrogen using semiclosed inhalers. *Anesthesiology,* **1956,** *17,* 213–221.

Morris, L. E., and Feldman, S. A. Considerations in design and function of anesthetic vaporizers. *Anesthesiology,* **1958,** *19,* 642–649.

Munson, E. S.; Eger, E. I., II; and Bowers, D. L. Effects of anesthetic-depressed ventilation and cardiac output on anesthetic uptake: a computer nonlinear simulation. *Anesthesiology,* **1973,** *38,* 251–259.

Smith, N. T.; Zwart, A.; and Beneken, J. E. W. Interaction between the circulatory effects and the uptake and distribution of halothane: use of a multiple model. *Anesthesiology,* **1972,** *37,* 47–58.

Smith, T. C. Nitrous oxide and low inflow circle systems. *Anesthesiology,* **1966,** *27,* 266–271.

Stoelting, R. K., and Eger, E. I., II. An additional explanation for the second gas effect: a concentrating effect. *Anesthesiology,* **1969a,** *30,* 273–277.

———. Percutaneous loss of nitrous oxide, cyclopropane, ether and halothane in man. *Ibid.,* **1969b,** *30,* 278–289.

Torri, G.; Damia, G.; Fabiani, M. L.; and Frova, G. Uptake and elimination of enflurane in man: a comparative study between enflurane and halothane. *Br. J. Anaesth.,* **1972,** *44,* 789–794.

Wollman, H., and Cannard, T. H. Skeletal muscle, esophageal, and rectal temperatures in man during general anesthesia and operation. *Anesthesiology,* **1960,** *21,* 476–481.

Monographs and Reviews

Cohen, E. N. Metabolism of the volatile anesthetics. *Anesthesiology,* **1971,** *35,* 193–202.

Kety, S. S. The theory and applications of the exchange of inert gas at the lungs and tissues. *Pharmac. Rev.,* **1951,** *3,* 1–41. (133 references.)

National Fire Prevention Association. *Standard for the Use of Inhalational Anesthetics.* Bull. No. 56A, The Association, Boston (60 Batterymarch Street), **1971.**

Papper, E. M., and Kitz, R. J. (eds.). *Uptake and Distribution of Anesthetic Agents.* McGraw-Hill Book Co., New York, **1963.**

Steward, A.; Allott, P. R.; Cowles, A. L.; and Mapleson, W. W. Solubility coefficients for inhaled anaesthetics for water, oil, and biological media. *Br. J. Anaesth.,* **1973,** *45,* 282–293.

CHAPTER

6   GENERAL ANESTHETICS

Gaseous Anesthetics: Nitrous Oxide, Ethylene, and Cyclopropane

Henry L. Price

A decade ago, the three agents discussed in this chapter were used extensively as general anesthetics in the United States and elsewhere. With the development of some of the newer agents presented in the two chapters that follow, there has been a marked decline in the use of ethylene and cyclopropane; nitrous oxide, on the other hand, still retains an important place in the anesthesiologist's armamentarium (*see* Chenoweth, 1972). Emphasis will be given here to the important general principles that the drugs in this class illustrate.

NITROUS OXIDE

History. The early history of nitrous oxide anesthesia is presented in Chapter 2. Modern concepts began to emerge in 1868, when Andrews introduced oxygen administration with nitrous oxide, the manner of its present-day use. In 1879, Bert described the use of nitrous oxide–oxygen mixtures at pressures greater than 1 atmosphere. As a result of Bert's classical investigations, the first accurate knowledge of the action of nitrous oxide became available.

Chemistry, Preparations, and Properties. *Nitrous Oxide*, U.S.P. (dinitrogen monoxide; N_2O), is a colorless gas without appreciable odor or taste. It is marketed in steel cylinders as a colorless liquid under pressure. The vapor pressure at room temperature is approximately 50 atmospheres. As it is released from the cylinder, nitrous oxide returns to the gaseous state. The heat required for its vaporization is obtained from the walls of the cylinder and surrounding air, with the result that the tank becomes cold to the touch and may accumulate a deposit of frost. Nitrous oxide is heavier than air. It is the only inorganic gas that is practical for clinical anesthesia.

Nitrous oxide has relatively low solubility in blood, the blood:gas partition ratio at 37° C being 0.47. Nitrous oxide does not combine with hemoglobin and is carried in the blood in physical solution only. It is excreted unchanged through the lungs, but a small fraction, owing to the rapid diffusion of the gas, escapes through the skin.

The oxygen in the nitrous oxide molecule is un-available for tissue respiration because nitrous oxide does not decompose appreciably in the body. Seeds cannot germinate and plants cannot grow in nitrous oxide. A glowing ember, however, bursts into flame if thrust into the gas, just as if thrust into oxygen. Although nitrous oxide is not flammable, it supports combustion as actively as does oxygen when it is present in proper concentration with a flammable anesthetic. Fatal explosions have occurred with ether–nitrous oxide mixtures.

General Anesthetic Actions. The principal characteristics of the use of nitrous oxide result from its lack of potency. In 1879, Bert wrote that, "In order to achieve anesthesia at normal [atmospheric] pressure, it [is] necessary to inhale pure nitrous oxide; thus one [can] employ this gas only for very short operations since asphyxia threaten[s] the patient at the very moment when consciousness [is] lost." He was able to show in man that safe anesthesia with adequate oxygenation could be provided by the inhalation of 15% oxygen and 85% nitrous oxide, provided that the total atmospheric pressure could be increased (by using a pressure chamber) to 1.2 atmospheres. Obviously, it is not convenient to perform surgery routinely in a pressure chamber, and the use of nitrous oxide today is, except for very brief procedures, that of an adjunct to other more potent agents. Moreover, the discovery that the A-a (alveolar-arterial) difference for oxygen tension is considerably elevated during anesthesia has placed another limit on the concentration of nitrous oxide that can be inspired for prolonged periods without producing hypoxia. This limit is currently set at 65% nitrous oxide at sea level when the balance of the mixture is oxygen. During brief exposures or during the induction of anesthesia it is safe to give higher concentrations (85:15), because the uptake of nitrous oxide from the inspired air is initially so much more rapid than that of oxygen that the alveolar concentration of oxygen is higher than the inspired concentration.

When a 65:35 mixture of nitrous oxide and oxygen is inspired, most patients without premedication do not enter the second stage of anesthesia; in some, delirium is produced, and in only a few can surgical anesthesia be attained. For these reasons anesthesia is most frequently induced by means of an intravenous "sleep dose" of a rapidly acting barbiturate, followed by the inhalation of nitrous oxide in oxygen. As the effects of the initial dose of barbiturate wear off, surgical anesthesia can be continued by adding a small amount of a volatile anesthetic (*e.g.,* enflurane, halothane, or methoxyflurane) to the inspired mixture, by giving additional amounts of barbiturate, or by administering a narcotic analgesic (usually intravenously).

Analgesia. Nitrous oxide in subanesthetic concentrations is analgesic in man. As little as 10 volumes % can produce a substantial effect; inhalation of 20% of the gas in oxygen has been claimed as effective as 15 mg of morphine sulfate (Chapman *et al.,* 1943). The optimal concentration of nitrous oxide to produce a maximal degree of analgesia and yet maintain the cooperation of the subject approximates 35%.

Nitrous oxide analgesia has great value in the second stage of labor. The administration of 100% oxygen between contractions and the brief use of 100% nitrous oxide during contractions can produce analgesia without decreasing either uterine contraction or maternal oxygen saturation.

Other Actions. Although it is commonly believed that nitrous oxide has, in itself, no side actions, there are a number of effects worthy of mention.

Circulation. Eighty percent nitrous oxide in oxygen slightly depresses myocardial contractility by means of a direct action on the heart (Price and Helrich, 1955), and slightly increases the response of vascular smooth muscle to the sympathetic mediator norepinephrine. During anesthesia produced with halothane in oxygen, the addition of nitrous oxide increases peripheral vascular resistance, mean arterial blood pressure, and right atrial pressure; cardiac output is reduced (Smith *et al.,* 1968). Sympathetic nervous activity also increases.

Respiration. Fifty percent nitrous oxide in oxygen slightly elevates the resting respiratory minute volume without affecting the response to carbon dioxide (Eckenhoff and Helrich, 1958), but this concentration does not produce anesthesia. The respiratory effects of nitrous oxide anesthesia have not been measured. Following the induction of anesthesia with thiopental, the inhalation of nitrous oxide causes a reduction in the response to carbon dioxide.

Gastrointestinal Tract. The incidence of nausea and vomiting after minor operations performed under nitrous oxide is low, but not negligible; it averages about 15% and increases with the duration of anesthesia. Studies on the influence of the gas on the motility of the gastrointestinal tract in man are not available; in animals there is no marked effect in the absence of hypoxia (Miller, 1926).

Neuromuscular System. In the absence of other drugs or hypoxia, muscular relaxation during the inhalation of nitrous oxide cannot be produced in most subjects. Studies of neuromuscular function in man indicate little effect of nitrous oxide, even in combination with thiopental and meperidine (Brown, 1955).

Liver and Kidney. Effects of nitrous oxide on these organs are usually assumed to be negligible, but data are lacking.

Hematopoiesis. Exposure to nitrous oxide can depress the bone marrow, and death has been reported after prolonged exposure to the anesthetic (Lassen *et al.,* 1956; Wilson *et al.,* 1956). However, there is no evidence that this toxicity of nitrous oxide is important during exposures of 24 hours or less.

Diffusion of Nitrous Oxide. During the induction of anesthesia with nitrous oxide, the alveolar concentration of oxygen is increased because nitrous oxide enters the pulmonary capillaries more rapidly than does oxygen. At the termination of anesthesia the opposite process occurs, and the outward diffusion of nitrous oxide lowers the alveolar partial pressure of oxygen by about 10% during the first few minutes after nitrous oxide–oxygen anesthesia is concluded and the patient is breathing room air (Fink, 1955). It is, of course, possible and desirable to prevent hypoxia from occurring during this period by supplying additional oxygen.

In a similar fashion, the increased alveolar partial pressure of nitrous oxide that occurs when the gas is breathed will cause it to diffuse into the hollow structures of the body until it approaches equilibrium with the tension in the inspired gas mixture. This phenomenon can lead to distention of the gastrointestinal tract, provided both ends are closed. A pneumothorax will also increase in volume, as will any other closed air pockets, for example, cysts of the lung or kidney, air injected for pneumoencephalography, or air behind the eardrum.

Recovery. After administration of nitrous oxide–oxygen mixtures up to 65:35, the recovery from anesthesia is ordinarily rapid and devoid of unpleasant sequelae. Prolonged administration of nitrous oxide, however, may increase the incidence of postanesthetic nausea and vomiting and may delay awakening. The occurrence of hypoxia during the period of anesthesia further aggravates these problems. Other events occurring prior to the withdrawal of the anesthetic can influence recovery. The use of neuromuscular blocking agents in conjunction with nitrous oxide necessitates controlled or assisted respiration, with the possible consequence of hyperventilation and respiratory alkalosis. Hyperventilation and respiratory alkalosis may summate to depress function at a variety of central nervous sites, including the cerebral cortex. Increased pulmonary shunting and the ventilation perfusion abnormalities induced by the production of general anesthesia persist into the recovery period and will cause hypoxia if the inspired atmosphere is not enriched with oxygen. These changes typically revert to normal within 1 hour after anesthesia is discontinued.

Evaluation. The highest concentration of nitrous oxide that can safely be given for maintenance of anesthesia is 70%. Above this hypoxia will develop. This concentration of nitrous oxide is not sufficiently potent for most patients, and various supplementary drugs are used to complete the anesthesia. Preanesthetic medication with narcotics is helpful to increase the degree of analgesia. Thiopental can be added to provide further hypnosis. Common adjuvants are the volatile liquid anesthetics, such as halothane, methoxyflurane, enflurane, or ether. Narcotics and narcotic-tranquilizer mixtures such as fentanyl plus droperidol are also popular (*see* Chapter 8). The primary anesthetic is nitrous oxide, but the potency of the regimen is increased to whatever extent is demanded by the patient and the operation through the addition of the volatile liquid or narcotic. If muscular relaxation is required, a neuromuscular blocking drug is injected. Thus, one builds the total anesthetic regimen around nitrous oxide, for it cannot by itself provide sufficient hypnosis, analgesia, and muscular relaxation. It is difficult to decide whether

supplementation of nitrous oxide in this fashion is preferable to the use of a single potent anesthetic such as cyclopropane or enflurane; clinical impressions suggest a smoother postoperative course for the former technic, but convincing data are not yet available.

In *summary,* the principal limitation of nitrous oxide is its low anesthetic potency. This fact explains several of its dangers and drawbacks, namely, the potential hazards of hypoxia and unintentional overdosage with adjuvants such as narcotics, barbiturates, and neuromuscular blocking drugs. On the other hand, its nonflammability, lack of irritant actions, pleasant smell, and marked analgesic properties contribute to its value as a benign basal anesthetic upon which the actions of a variety of more potent, volatile anesthetic agents and muscle relaxants can be superimposed.

ETHYLENE

History. The anesthetic action of ethylene was noted as early as 1865, but little attention was paid to this observation until 1908, when it was observed that ethylene in high dilution was toxic to plants. In that year, certain carnation growers suffered heavy financial loss because the flowers shipped to Chicago greenhouses failed to open. Crocker and Knight of the Hull Botanical Laboratory studied the illuminating gas used in the greenhouses and found ethylene, which comprised 4% of the gas, to be the agent responsible. A dilution of 1:2,000,000 of ethylene in air is sufficient to affect carnations. The anesthetic action of ethylene on animals was rediscovered independently by Luckhardt and Lewis (1923) and Brown (1924). Luckhardt and Lewis were active in the successful development of ethylene as a surgical anesthetic. Operations on patients receiving ethylene were first performed in 1923.

Chemistry. *Ethylene,* $H_2C=CH_2$, is a colorless gas with an unpleasant, slightly sweet odor and taste. It has a boiling point of $-103.9°$ C. For use as an anesthetic, ethylene is purified and stored as a gas in steel cylinders. Ethylene is explosive and flammable when present in oxygen in concentrations of 2.9 to 80%. Ethylene is somewhat lighter than air, whereas ether, nitrous oxide, and cyclopropane are heavier; this property of ethylene is a further disadvantage since the explosive mixture tends to either rise or stratify, whereas operating rooms are designed for the safe use only of those flammable agents that sink to the floor because they are heavier than air.

Induction. In consequence of its very low partition ratio (blood:air = 0.14 at 37° C), the speed of induction is rapid, exceeding that of nitrous oxide. After the patient has taken six or more deep inhalations, mental clouding supervenes and unconsciousness soon follows. Induction is not disagreeable, although an occasional patient, surgeon, or anesthesiologist may complain of the odor of the gas. Ethylene in anesthetic concentrations does not irritate the respiratory mucosa. In order to speed induction, hypoxic mixtures of ethylene and oxygen (e.g., 85:15) are sometimes administered for a few minutes at the beginning of anesthesia.

Surgical Anesthesia. When an anesthetic mixture of ethylene and oxygen is inhaled, surgical anesthesia usually occurs in 2 to 5 minutes. After adequate preanesthetic medication, ethylene can carry anesthesia to the lower border of plane 1 in most cases, but some individuals cannot be anesthetized with a mixture containing an adequate proportion of oxygen. On the other hand, seriously ill patients can often be anesthetized with ethylene-oxygen mixtures alone. Subanesthetic concentrations of ethylene are analgesic, and the inhalation of 25 to 35 volumes % of the gas produces maximal analgesia without loss of consciousness or cooperativeness. On this basis, ethylene is only one tenth as potent as cyclopropane, which requires only 2 volumes % for analgesia without loss of awareness, and slightly more potent than nitrous oxide, which requires 35 to 40 volumes %.

Ethylene anesthesia will usually be adequate only for superficial operations. Muscular relaxation is essentially absent. Even with satisfactory preliminary medication, ethylene must be supplemented with other anesthetic agents or with a neuromuscular blocking agent when operations require muscular relaxation.

Respiration during surgical anesthesia under ethylene is not depressed; it may even be slightly stimulated through the chemoreceptor mechanism if the oxygen tension is lowered incident to the use of ethylene in concentrations over 80 volumes % (during induction). The *blood pressure* may rise moderately during the induction and early phase of surgical anesthesia, but it soon returns to normal and remains there throughout anesthesia. Cardiac arrhythmias occur infrequently when ethylene is used, and the cardiovascular effects of the gas are relatively benign. Pulmonary irritation does not occur, and the secretion of bronchial mucus is not stimulated. Salivation is negligible or absent. Renal and hepatic functions are relatively unimpaired by the gas. Neither metabolic nor respiratory acidosis occurs as often with ethylene as with ether. The respiratory mechanism of the fetus and the activity of the uterus are not depressed when ethylene is used in obstetrics, provided precautions are taken to avoid hypoxia.

Recovery. Recovery from ethylene anesthesia is rapid. As a rule, the patient is awake with a clear mind and able to talk within 2 or 3 minutes after administration of the gas is stopped. Ethylene is excreted almost quantitatively in the exhaled air and undergoes little chemical change in the body. Postanesthetic nausea and vomiting are less frequent and less severe than after ether.

Advantages. Ethylene has some advantages as an anesthetic agent. It permits a rapid induction of anesthesia. Excitement and struggle are minimal, and recovery from anesthesia is rapid. The myocardium is not "sensitized" to catecholamines by ethylene. Respiratory and vasomotor depression and metabolic disturbances are not conspicuous. Adverse pulmonary and renal effects are absent, and salivary and bronchial secretions are not stimulated.

Disadvantages. The chief disadvantage of ethylene is that it is explosive. Accidents with fatalities have occurred, especially in the early days of the use of the gas. The explosive range of ethylene-oxygen mixtures is broad, the most easily ignited range being 5 to 25% ethylene diluted with air or oxygen; the most critical time, therefore, is at the end of anesthesia when the gas is discontinued. This fact makes ethylene particularly unsuitable when it must be used intermittently, for example, during labor.

Status. The small increase in potency gained by using ethylene instead of nitrous oxide does not often outweigh the associated disadvantages, and the use of ethylene has declined markedly in recent years, particularly since the introduction of neuromuscular blocking drugs.

CYCLOPROPANE

History. Cyclopropane was first prepared in 1882 by von Freund, but its anesthetic properties were not appreciated. Years later, propylene ($CH_3 \cdot CH : CH_2$), an isomer of cyclopropane, was studied extensively for its usefulness as a general anesthetic but was found too depressant to the heart. In searching for the cause of this depression, Lucas and Henderson (1929) tested cyclopropane as a possible impurity. Cyclopropane not only was exonerated but also was found in itself to be a safe and potent anesthetic agent. After a 3-year period of study at the University of Wisconsin General Hospital, Waters and Schmidt (1934) published the first clinical report on the use of cyclopropane as a general anesthetic. An interesting account of the development of cyclopropane anesthesia has been given by a member of the group that discovered cyclopropane (Lucas, 1961).

Chemistry and Preparations. *Cyclopropane,* U.S.P. (*trimethylene*), is the simplest possible cyclic hydrocarbon, with the following structural formula:

$$H_2C - CH_2 \quad \overset{H_2}{\underset{}{C}}$$

Cyclopropane

It is a colorless gas with a not unpleasant, characteristic odor, resembling that of petroleum ether. It is stored in metal cylinders as a liquid under pressure, and remains stable indefinitely. Its blood:gas partition ratio at 37° C is 0.46. Cyclopropane is heavier than air, and it is flammable and explosive. The explosive range of cyclopropane in air is 2.4 to 10.3%; in oxygen, 2.5 to 60%.

PHARMACOLOGICAL PROPERTIES

General Anesthetic Actions. Cyclopropane is a relatively insoluble and extremely potent anesthetic gas. Unlike nitrous oxide, it can produce any desired level of anesthesia, and the deeper planes are accompanied by sufficient muscular relaxation to obviate the need for neuromuscular blocking agents, although these are frequently employed as supplements to permit use of a lessened amount of cyclopropane. The induction of surgical anesthesia with cyclopropane-oxygen requires only 2 to 3 minutes and is not unpleasant. Cyclopropane is minimally irritating to the respiratory tract, and, therefore, respiratory alterations such as breath-holding, tachypnea, and coughing are less frequent than with some anesthetics such as ether. Salivation is not prominent, provided a belladonna drug has been given; otherwise it can be troublesome. Laryngospasm may develop during induction or during very light anesthesia, but it is uncommon if anesthesia is conducted smoothly. Delirium during induction is not uncommon. Both problems are usually avoided by administering a sleep-inducing dose of thiopental intravenously before cyclopropane inhalation is begun.

Physical Signs. The signs of anesthesia are similar to those with other general anesthetic agents, with certain differences. The initial stimulation of respiration characteristic of the administration of ether is absent, and the tidal volume is progressively diminished as anesthetic depth increases. Pupillary size tends to increase both during profound anesthesia and during the emergence from anesthesia, although little dilatation may occur if morphine has been used as preanesthetic medication. Lacrimation may occur during very light anesthesia, but it is an unreliable sign of depth. Eyeball movements usually occur in plane 1; the eyes may remain eccentric even at deep planes of anesthesia. At profound levels proptosis is common. Arterial pressure is well maintained at all levels of anesthesia. Cardiac rate is typically normal, although it may slow gradually with the induction of anesthesia, particularly following premedication with morphine. Cardiac irregularities, usually ventricular in origin, can be caused either by excessive anesthetic depth or by hypercarbia. A sudden decrease in the palpable pulse usually indicates the development of bigeminal rhythm, only the normal beat giving rise to a perceptible pulse.

Cyclopropane causes *analgesia* without unconsciousness if continuously inhaled in concentrations as low as 1 volume %. Consciousness is lost when the alveolar concentration of cyclopropane reaches 7 to 10 volumes %. Because it is both flammable and expensive, cyclopropane is usually administered by closed circuit (*see* Chapter 5).

Respiration. In common with other general anesthetic agents, cyclopropane depresses the ventilatory response to carbon dioxide. However, the degree of depression is less than with halothane, methoxyflurane, or fluroxene, and spontaneous ventilation can be adequate at levels of anesthesia that suffice for surgical operations (Munson *et al.,* 1966). On the other hand, the nonirritant quality of the gas makes it easy to assume control of ventilation by means of intermittent, positive airway pressure. If spontaneous breathing is permitted, the rate of respiration accelerates as anesthesia is deepened, total volume decreases, and respiration is increasingly accomplished by means of diaphragmatic contractions.

Cardiovascular System. *Arterial Blood Pressure.* Arterial blood pressure is usually little affected by concentrations of cyclopropane causing surgical anesthesia, although severe reductions may occur when hemorrhage, myocardial disease, or sepsis is present. The modest elevation commonly observed is caused by an increase in total peripheral resistance. The increase in resistance stems both from an increased level of sympathetic nervous activity and from direct effects of the anesthetic upon vascular smooth muscle. Cardiac output is well maintained (Jones *et al.,* 1960). Central venous pressure is increased, as reflected by an increase in right ventricular work.

Cardiac Contractility. Cardiac contractility is also well maintained during cyclopropane anesthesia as the result of increased activity in sympathetic nerves supplying the myocardium; this, in turn, partially antagonizes the direct depressant effects of cyclopropane upon the heart (Price *et al.,* 1962).

Cardiac Rate. Cardiac rate tends to be either normal or somewhat slow during surgical anesthesia with cyclopropane, usually 60 to 70 beats per minute; bradycardia is especially evident if morphine is used for preanesthetic medication.

Cardiac Rhythm. A variety of arrhythmias may occur during the administration of cyclopropane, including sinus bradycardia, atrial extrasystoles, atrial fibrillation, A-V nodal rhythms, ventricular extrasystoles, and bigeminal rhythm. The intravenous administration of atropine can precipitate ventricular extrasystoles, as can various "pressor" drugs, the catecholamines in particular. Large doses of the latter agents can cause ventricular fibrillation.

Peripheral Circulation. Blood flow in the skin is greatly increased by cyclopropane, and can be increased in skeletal muscle as well. There is a tendency for increased bleeding of the wound during surgical operations performed during anesthesia with this agent. Cerebral and coronary blood flows are typically increased (Alexander *et al.,* 1968). In contrast, there is marked renal and splanchnic vasoconstriction with corresponding reductions in blood flow (Habif *et al.,* 1951; Price *et al.,* 1964); these changes are mediated through enhanced sympathetic nervous actions and can be reversed by ganglionic blocking drugs. Pulmonary arteriolar resistance is also increased.

Liver. The hepatic extraction of indocyanine green and other dyes is markedly reduced by cyclopropane inhalation in normal man, but splanchnic oxygen consumption is unaltered and there is no evidence that any functional changes result from ischemia despite the greatly reduced level of hepatic blood flow that occurs during anesthesia with this agent. The changes in parenchymal function represent direct anesthetic effects and are rapidly reversed when cyclopropane is discontinued. There is no evidence that cyclopropane is hepatotoxic, and unexplained hepatic necrosis has not been a problem with this agent, in contrast to certain halogenated anesthetics (*see* Chapter 7).

Miscellaneous Effects. As has been mentioned previously, cyclopropane increases sympathetic nervous activity (Price *et al.,* 1969). Metabolic derangements are mild or absent during cyclopropane anesthesia. The mild respiratory acidosis that occurs in the absence of respiratory assistance, either at deep levels of anesthesia or when opioids or muscle relaxants have been administered, can itself lead to metabolic acidosis (Holaday *et al.,* 1957). Bleeding time, clotting time, prothrombin time, thrombin time, platelet count, plasma fibrinogen concentration, and capillary fragility are not affected by cyclopropane (Vanderveen *et al.,* 1962). The hematocrit is usually increased as the result of a decrease in plasma volume. Experimental data indicate that the gas possesses parasympathomimetic properties, but these are usually of little clinical consequence when belladonna alkaloids are used for preanesthetic medication. Cyclopropane tends to enhance intestinal tone, due both to its parasympathomimetic effect and to a direct action on the intestinal smooth muscle. Smooth muscle of blood vessels, as well as that of the bronchi and bronchioles, tends to constrict when exposed to cyclopropane. For this reason, patients with a history of bronchial asthma may be poor choices for cyclopropane anesthesia. The gas exerts a positive inotropic action on skeletal muscle, resulting in an increase in the tension developed by both direct and indirect stimulation. It does not block the neuromuscular junction, and has no consistent effect upon transmission through autonomic ganglia. Occasionally priapism may develop under cyclopropane anesthesia.

Recovery. Recovery from cyclopropane anesthesia occurs within a few minutes after cessation of anesthetic administration. Nausea and vomiting are frequent but less severe than after ether. Emergence delirium is not infrequent, particularly in muscular males. It can often be avoided by administering a small dose of a narcotic analgesic prior to the termination of anesthesia. A marked decrease in blood pressure postoperatively may sometimes occur without tachycardia, pallor, or other signs of shock. Its most frequent cause is the reversal of a respiratory acidosis present during the period of cyclopropane administration (Dripps, 1947; Buckley *et al.*, 1953). Headache occurs more commonly than after most other general anesthetics.

Absorption, Metabolism, and Excretion. Cyclopropane is rapidly absorbed and almost entirely eliminated by way of the lungs; a small amount diffuses through the skin and an additional small amount (roughly 0.5%) is metabolized in the body and excreted as carbon dioxide and water (Van Dyke *et al.*, 1964). By the time of return of consciousness after cyclopropane anesthesia, the concentration of the agent in the expired gases has fallen to approximately 1%, and only traces are found at the end of 3 hours.

Disadvantages. Cyclopropane is explosive and flammable within the entire range of its anesthetic mixtures. Anesthesia with cyclopropane requires a closed or semiclosed circuit with a carbon dioxide absorption system, for both safety and economy. Some surgeons claim that cyclopropane produces capillary oozing, although others deny this. Postanesthetic hypotension, delirium, and headache are more frequent than after the use of other agents. Nausea and vomiting are common. Cyclopropane can cause disorders of cardiac rhythm, and various precautions must be observed to diminish their incidence.

Advantages, Indications, and Special Uses. Cyclopropane can be administered with a higher partial pressure of oxygen than can nitrous oxide or ethylene. It is nonirritating and usually does not cause respiratory irregularities in stage II. Concentrations producing light anesthesia do not depress the heart or circulation. Salivation is not prominent if a belladonna drug has been given as preanesthetic medication. Except for respiratory acidosis during spontaneous ventilation, deleterious metabolic effects are singularly absent. Injury to the liver or kidney as a direct result of cyclopropane apparently does not occur. Uterine tone is relatively well maintained. Postanesthetic recovery is rapid and smooth. Cyclopropane produces greater skeletal muscular relaxation than do the other anesthetic gases. There is a wide margin of safety between anesthetic and lethal concentrations, perhaps wider than that for any other anesthetic agent now in use.

Status. Cyclopropane continues to be a useful anesthetic agent, its outstanding merits being safety, controllability, and versatility. However, the fact that it is explosive has markedly limited its use and will do so further as increasingly satisfactory nonflammable agents become available.

Alexander, S. C.; James, F. M.; Colton, E. T.; Gleaton, H. R.; and Wollman, H. Effects of cyclopropane anesthesia on cerebral blood flow and carbohydrate metabolism in man. *Anesthesiology,* **1968,** *29,* 170–171.

Brown, R. C. The effect of anaesthetics on the response to stimulation of the ulnar nerve in man. *Br. J. Anaesth.,* **1955,** *27,* 471–476.

Brown, W. E. Ethylene as a general anesthetic. *Am. J. Surg., Anesth. Suppl.,* **1924,** *38,* 4–7.

Buckley, J. J.; Van Berger, F. H.; Dobkin, A. B.; Brown, E. B., Jr.; Miller, A. F.; and Varco, R. L. Postanesthetic hypotension following cyclopropane anesthesia: its relationship to hypercapnia. *Anesthesiology,* **1953,** *14,* 226–237.

Chapman, W. P.; Arrowood, J. G.; and Beecher, H. K. The analgetic effects of low concentrations of nitrous oxide compared in man with morphine sulphate. *J. clin. Invest.,* **1943,** *22,* 871–875.

Chenoweth, M. B. Foreword and commentary. In, *Modern Inhalation Anesthetics.* (Chenoweth, M. B., ed.) *Handb. exp. Pharmak.,* Springer-Verlag, Berlin, **1972,** *30,* 1–3.

Dripps, R. D. The immediate decrease in blood pressure seen at the conclusion of cyclopropane anesthesia: "cyclopropane shock." *Anesthesiology,* **1947,** *8,* 15–35.

Eckenhoff, J. E., and Helrich, M. The effect of narcotics, thiopental and nitrous oxide upon respiration and respiratory response to hypercapnia. *Anesthesiology,* **1958,** *19,* 240–253.

Fink, B. R. Diffusion anoxia. *Anesthesiology,* **1955,** *16,* 511–519.

Habif, D. V.; Papper, E. M.; Fitzpatrick, H. F.; Lowrance, P.; Smythe, C. McC.; and Bradley, S. E. The renal and hepatic blood flow, glomerular filtration rate, and urinary output of electrolytes during cyclopropane, ether, and thiopental anesthesia, operation, and the immediate postoperative period. *Surgery, St. Louis,* **1951,** *30,* 241–255.

Holaday, D. A.; Ma, D.; and Papper, E. M. The immediate effects of respiratory depression on acid-base balance in anesthetized man. *J. clin. Invest.,* **1957,** *36,* 1121–1129.

Jones, R. E.; Guldmann, N.; Linde, H. W.; Dripps, R. D.; and Price, H. L. Cyclopropane anesthesia. III. Effects of cyclopropane on respiration and circulation in normal man. *Anesthesiology,* **1960,** *21,* 380–393.

Keys, T. E. *The History of Surgical Anesthesia.* Schuman's, New York, **1945.**

Lassen, H. C. A.; Henriksen, E.; Neukirch, F.; and Kristensen, H. S. Treatment of tetanus: severe bone marrow depression after prolonged nitrous oxide anaesthesia. *Lancet,* **1956,** *1,* 527–530.

Lucas, G. H. W. The discovery of cyclopropane. *Anesth. Analg. curr. Res.,* **1961,** *40,* 15–27.

Lucas, G. H. W., and Henderson, V. E. New anesthetic gas: cyclopropane, preliminary report. *Can. med. Ass. J.,* **1929,** *21,* 173–175.

Luckhardt, A. B., and Lewis, D. Clinical experiences with ethylene-oxygen anesthesia. *J. Am. med. Ass.,* **1923,** *81,* 1851–1857.

Miller, G. H. Effects of general anesthesia on muscular activity of the gastrointestinal tract: a study of ether, chloroform, ethylene and nitrous oxide. *Curr. Res. Anesth. Analg.,* **1926,** *5,* 225–234.

Munson, E. S.; Larson, C. P., Jr.; Babad, A. A.; Regan, M. J.; Buechel, D. R.; and Eger, E. I., II. The effects of halothane, fluroxene and cyclopropane on ventilation: a comparative study in man. *Anesthesiology,* **1966,** *27,* 716–728.

Price, H. L.; Deutsch, S.; Cooperman, L. H.; Clement, A. J.; and Epstein, R. M. Effects of cyclopropane on splanchnic blood flow and metabolism in normal man. *J. clin. Invest.,* **1964,** *43,* 1244.

Price, H. L., and Helrich, M. The effect of cyclopropane, diethyl ether, nitrous oxide, thiopental, and hydrogen ion concentration on the myocardial function of the dog heart-lung preparation. *J. Pharmac. exp. Ther.,* **1955,** *115,* 206–216.

Price, H. L.; Jones, R. E.; Deutsch, S.; and Linde, H. W. Ventricular function and autonomic nervous activity during cyclopropane anesthesia in man. *J. clin. Invest.,* **1962,** *41,* 604–610.

Price, H. L.; Warden, J. C.; Cooperman, L. H.; and Millar, R. A. Central sympathetic excitation caused by cyclopropane. *Anesthesiology,* **1969,** *30,* 426–438.

Smith, T. N.; Eger, E. I., II; Whitcher, C. E.; Stoelting, R. K.; and Whayne, T. F. The circulatory effects of the addition of nitrous oxide to halothane anesthesia in man. *Anesthesiology,* **1968,** *29,* 212–213.

Vanderveen, J. L.; McGovern, J. J.; Bunker, J. P.; and Goldstein, R. Effects of anesthesia on hemostatic mechanisms in man. *Anesthesiology,* **1962,** *23,* 92–100.

Van Dyke, R. A.; Chenoweth, M. B.; and Van Poznak, A. Metabolism of volatile anesthetics. I. Conversion *in vivo* of several anesthetics to $^{14}CO_2$ and chloride. *Biochem. Pharmac.,* **1964,** *13,* 1239–1247.

Waters, R. M., and Schmidt, E. R. Cyclopropane anesthesia. *J. Am. med. Ass.,* **1934,** *103,* 975–983.

Wilson, P. E.; Martin, F. I. R.; and Last, P. M. Bone marrow depression in tetanus: report of a fatal case. *Lancet,* **1956,** *2,* 442–443.

7 GENERAL ANESTHETICS

[*Continued*]

Volatile Anesthetics: Ether, Halothane, Methoxyflurane, Enflurane, and Other Halogenated Volatile Anesthetics

Henry L. Price

Volatile anesthetics share three basic similarities: they are liquids at room temperature; they are potent in low concentrations; and they are more soluble in blood, cell water, and fat than are the anesthetic gases. Their solubility in blood and tissues retards equilibration and hence slows induction, and makes it inevitable that the ratio of the tensions of these agents in the alveoli and in the inspired anesthetic mixture will increase progressively as anesthesia continues. Consequently, the depth of anesthesia will increase with time unless the tension of the anesthetic in the inspired mixture is progressively reduced. Therefore, a concentration well above that required for maintenance may be administered initially, and progressively reduced to a lower level, thereby hastening the induction of anesthesia. During recovery, the relatively great solubility of the volatile agents in blood and tissue slows excretion via the lungs and retards the return of consciousness.

In current practice, these difficulties are reduced or obviated in many cases by using nitrous oxide as the basic anesthetic agent, supplemented by reduced amounts of a volatile agent. Muscular relaxation, when needed, is frequently secured by using a neuromuscular blocking agent.

ETHER

Despite the marked decline in its use, ether will be the first volatile anesthetic to be discussed in view of its long history and its safety as an anesthetic.

History. Ether was the first anesthetic to be employed successfully for a surgical operation (*see* Chapter 2). Prior to this the performance of any operation had necessitated the use of large, strong men who could restrain the involuntary thrashing of patients subjected to the excruciating pain that accompanied every surgical procedure.

Chemistry and Preparations. Diethyl ether $[(C_2H_5)_2{=}O]$ was discovered in 1540 by Valerius Cordis, but its anesthetic properties were not then recognized. It is a clear liquid with a boiling point of $36.5°$ C. It is official as *Ether,* U.S.P., in accordance with the specifications of which it must be packaged in containers not holding more than 3 kg, and used not longer than 24 hours after opening. Ether is supplied mixed with 3% ethanol to retard oxidation. There is some evidence that peroxides formed during exposure to air can enhance the danger of explosion. At $20°$ C, ether has a vapor pressure of 450 mm Hg. Its pungent odor precludes inhalation at concentrations exceeding a few percent unless anesthesia is first induced with another anesthetic agent. The minimal anesthetic concentration in man is 1.9%. It is explosive in concentrations above 1.8% in air, and above 2.1% in oxygen. The blood:gas partition ratio of ether in man is 15; the oil:water ratio is 3.2.

PHARMACOLOGICAL PROPERTIES

Central Nervous System. It is still not known how ether causes anesthesia in man (*see* Chapter 2). In low concentrations it suppresses medullary and mesencephalic reticular activity, as do many other agents, but at high concentrations ether causes generalized EEG seizure patterns not accompanied by overt signs of CNS activity.

Neuromuscular Blockade. Ether can produce profound muscular relaxation by means of both central (corticospinal) and peripheral (neuromuscular junction) blocking actions. Although the blockade by ether is unlike that caused by *d*-tubocurarine (only the latter can be effectively antagonized by neostigmine), the effects of *d*-tubocurarine are increased in the presence of ether. Ether also enhances the neuromuscular blocking effect of aminoglycoside and certain other antibiotics (*see* Chapter 28).

Respiration. Both the rate and the minute volume of ventilation tend to be elevated during the inhalation of ether and the arterial carbon dioxide tension (Pa_{CO_2}) remains within the normal range or is reduced during light anesthesia. Since the sensitivity of the respiratory response to elevated Pa_{CO_2} is reduced (Larson *et al.*, 1969), this observation suggests that respiration is driven reflexly by sensory receptors in the airway that are directly stimulated by ether.

Heart and Circulation. Ether produces relative circulatory stability, in part because its direct depressant action on the myocardium is antagonized by increased sympathetic nervous activity (Bhatia and Burn, 1933; Brewster *et al.*, 1953; Price, 1957). In the cat, the increase in sympathetic activity is accompanied by diminution of the barostatic reflexes (Skovsted and Price, 1970). Cardiac output is usually unaltered, although cardiac rate increases. Total peripheral resistance decreases. Ether does not sensitize the heart to the arrhythmogenic actions of catecholamines.

Other Actions. Nausea and vomiting are relatively common after administration of ether, probably as the result of central nervous actions. Ether causes renal vasoconstriction, decreases glomerular filtration, and decreases urinary output, probably as the result of liberation of antidiuretic hormone (ADH). Uterine relaxation can be secured with this agent, but it is safe for use during delivery since it does not directly depress the myometrium at the concentrations needed. Ether is not hepatotoxic, although it does depress hepatic function during its administration. Clotting time, bleeding time, prothrombin time, platelet count, and capillary fragility are unchanged during ether anesthesia.

Excretion and Metabolism. More than 90% of absorbed ether can be recovered unchanged in the expired air; metabolism in the body is not extensive (Van Dyke *et al.*, 1964), and the metabolites are not hepato-

toxic. Small amounts of unchanged ether are excreted in urine, milk, sweat, and other body fluids, and a tiny amount escapes through the intact skin.

Status. Ether is a versatile anesthetic of unexcelled safety, but it is flammable and irritating to breathe. Although countless medical students, interns, and anesthesia residents have learned through its use to appreciate "the signs of anesthesia," it is employed infrequently today except in teaching institutions or under conditions where proper equipment is lacking.

HALOTHANE

History. Halothane was introduced as an anesthetic under the aegis of the Committee on Nonexplosive Anesthetics, formed by the British Medical Research Council to consider what steps could be taken to find new nonexplosive anesthetics. Between 1951 and 1956, Suckling synthesized the compound, Raventos reported its use and actions in experimental animals, and Johnstone published his clinical experience with the drug. Within the next few years the use of halothane for surgical anesthesia became extremely popular.

Chemistry and Preparations. *Halothane*, U.S.P. (FLUOTHANE), is 2-bromo-2-chloro-1,1,1-trifluoroethane. It is supplied for anesthesia in amber-colored bottles, and its stability is further enhanced by the addition of 0.01% thymol. Soda lime does not accelerate the decomposition of halothane. Mixtures of halothane with air or oxygen are not explosive. The blood:gas partition ratio is 2.3 at 37° C.

All metals tested (silver, brass, copper, stainless steel, magnesium, aluminum, bronze, and tin) except nickel and titanium are tarnished or corroded by halothane. The compound interacts with rubber and some plastics, but not with polyethylene. The extreme solubility of halothane in rubber (Ostwald partition coefficient = 121) can theoretically slow the induction of anesthesia and retard emergence, in consequence of the uptake and release of the anesthetic by the walls of the rubber elements in the anesthetic equipment if low-flow technics are used.

PHARMACOLOGICAL PROPERTIES

General Anesthetic Actions. The signs of the depth of anesthesia are subtle. At usual levels of anesthesia the pupils are small, the eyes are closed, respirations are shallow but rapid, and the muscles of the hypopharynx are more relaxed than are those of the abdomen. The classical signs of ether anesthesia, first described by Guedel, are lacking. Frequently, the level of arterial blood pressure is most informative of depth of anesthesia. Any depth of anesthesia can be secured in the absence of hypoxia. (The minimal anesthetic concentration is 0.74 volume %.) As with the other volatile anesthetics, the alveolar tension of halothane increases progressively with time when it is inspired in a constant concentration.

The tendency of halothane to cause arterial hypotension at deeper levels of anesthesia, together with its lack of analgesic potency, has discouraged its use as a primary anesthetic agent. It is most frequently used as an adjuvant to nitrous oxide, and muscular relaxation, when desired, is usually produced by the injection of a neuromuscular blocking drug.

Respiration. Respiration is depressed by all anesthetic concentrations of halothane. At minimal anesthetic concentrations, there is less ventilation at any given level of Pa_{CO_2} than during the conscious state; however, ventilation will still increase to a satisfactory level as CO_2 builds up and Pa_{CO_2} is further increased. As anesthesia is deepened, the response to hypercarbia is progressively lost and ventilation becomes inadequate, irrespective of the level of Pa_{CO_2}. Paradoxically, the latter fact makes it safe to administer a high inspired tension of halothane provided that spontaneous ventilation is permitted and that the vehicle for halothane is pure oxygen. If ventilation is assisted, overdose may rapidly occur. If artificial respiration is to be employed, the inspired concentration of halothane must be kept within safe limits. Because the assumption of respiratory control by the anesthesiologist involves the loss of important information from the patient, inadvertent overdosage is particularly apt to occur under these conditions. Halothane obtunds laryngeal and pharyngeal reflexes to a marked degree, relaxes the masseter muscles, and inhibits salivation; this combination of effects renders tracheal intubation relatively simple. Laryngospasm, bronchospasm, and coughing are all inhibited by halothane. Although halothane has been thought on clinical grounds and from animal studies to produce bronchiolar dilatation by means of a direct action on smooth muscle, no such effect could be shown in man (Patterson *et al.*, 1968).

Circulation. Halothane directly depresses both the myocardium and the vascular smooth muscle. It also decreases efferent sympathetic nervous activity and interferes with the ability of the sympathetic mediator norepinephrine to antagonize peripheral vascular depression. Systemic arterial blood pressure, cardiac contractile force, cardiac output, and total peripheral resistance are all reduced by halothane in anesthetic concentrations (Deutsch *et al.*, 1962). These effects become more pronounced as the level of anesthesia is increased. Cardiac rate is less consistently affected. Constant attention to both the blood pressure and the pulse volume is essential to the safe conduct of anesthesia when halothane is used. There is some evidence that tolerance develops to the circulatory actions of halothane during continued exposure.

Halothane increases cerebral blood flow, largely by means of a direct vasodilator action on vascular smooth muscle (Wollman *et al.*, 1964). It also produces vasodilatation in skeletal muscle (Black and McArdle, 1962). In the splanchnic and renal circulations there is usually no pronounced change in resistance, and flow rate declines as systemic pressure is diminished (Epstein *et al.*, 1966).

Cardiac Rhythm. Halothane causes direct depression of the S-A node (Flacke and Alper, 1962); this fact apparently explains the observation that A-V nodal rhythm occurring during the administration of halothane may not respond to atropine. Ventricular arrhythmias are rare during the administration of halothane if respiratory acidosis, hypoxia, or other causes of sympathetic stimulation are avoided. Like chloroform, halothane "sensitizes" the ventricular conducting tissues to the actions of catecholamines, and serious arrhythmias may result if these substances are injected indiscriminately during the inhalation of halothane. The local injection of epinephrine to secure hemostasis may be permitted if (1) adequate ventilation of the patient is assured, (2) epinephrine in a concentration not greater than $1:100,000$ is used, and (3) the dose in adults does not exceed 10 ml (100 μg) in any 10-minute period or 30 ml (300 μg) per hour. The details of this topic are presented by Katz and associates (1962).

Liver. Halothane does not increase BSP retention any more than does cyclopropane or ether. However, hepatic damage has been reported to occur following the use of halothane, although the incidence is extremely low. Characteristically, there is a delay between exposure to halothane and the appearance of hepatic symptoms, ranging from 3 days to nearly 3 weeks. Women are affected more frequently than men. Repeated exposure to halothane apparently increases the likelihood of hepatic damage, and there is evidence that the reaction can be allergic in character (Klatskin, 1968). Indeed, there have been rare instances in which individuals chronically exposed to halothane vapor have developed this type of allergic hypersensitivity. The onset of the hepatic-injury syndrome is heralded by fever, anorexia, nausea, and vomiting. Occasionally a rash is present. Leukocytosis and increased levels of serum glutamic-oxaloacetic transaminase are almost invariably found. Death occurs rapidly in about half the cases; those who recover apparently do so completely. The outstanding pathological feature in all reported cases is extensive hepatocellular necrosis, predominantly centrilobular in location.

Halothane is metabolized to an important extent even after a brief exposure, and some of the products have been shown to be hepatotoxic (Rosenberg and Wahlstrom, 1971). Moreover, hepatic damage after halothane is increased in animals pretreated with phenobarbital, which causes microsomal enzyme induction and increased metabolism of halothane (Stenger and Johnson, 1972). Halothane can, under conditions of long exposure to low concentrations, be shown to behave as a true hepatotoxin in experimental animals.

The entire question of the possible role of halothane in the causation of hepatic disease is complicated by the possibility that many reported cases represent either infectious or serum hepatitis, which would have occurred even if halothane had not been given. The postanesthetic incidence of hepatitis is almost vanishingly small, and a cause-and-effect relationship is correspondingly difficult to establish (*see* Summary of the National Halothane Study, 1966; Ngai, 1972).

Gastrointestinal Tract. Halothane, in concentrations capable of producing anesthesia, depresses motility of the stomach, jejunum, and colon in dogs.

Activity returns promptly after the agent is discontinued. Halothane also antagonizes the contractions produced by neostigmine and morphine (Marshall, 1961).

Uterus. Halothane strongly inhibits myometrial tone, reduces the responses to ergot alkaloids and oxytocin, and should be employed with caution during delivery. However, its uterine actions make it useful in the maneuver of version and extraction.

Metabolism and Excretion. Rats given ^{36}Cl halothane exhale only 60% of the administered radioactivity in 30 hours; inorganic ^{36}Cl appears in the urine for more than 2 weeks (Van Dyke et al., 1964). This indicates substantial retention in the body and dechlorination of the parent molecule. In man trifluoroacetic acid, trifluoroethanol, and bromide have been found as metabolites in the urine; as much as 20% of the halothane taken up by the body may be broken down prior to its excretion (Rehder et al., 1967). These findings raise the question whether one is dealing with detoxification or an increased toxicity when halothane is transformed within the tissues (*see* above).

Disadvantages and Limitations. Halothane has a moderately high blood:gas solubility coefficient; consequently, the induction of anesthesia may be delayed and recovery is necessarily prolonged. Halothane is a relatively poor analgesic; it must often be supplemented with nitrous oxide, opiates, or muscle relaxants in order to provide satisfactory conditions for surgery. The cardiovascular actions of halothane lead to moderate or marked arterial hypotension. In addition, it sensitizes the conducting tissues of the heart to the arrhythmogenic actions of the catecholamines. During recovery, shivering is prominent, presumably as the result of heat loss to the environment during anesthesia. Cutaneous vasoconstriction during this phase can give the erroneous impression that the patient is in a state of shock or hypoxemia. Actually, vasoconstriction is purely superficial, and the differential diagnosis can be resolved by stroking or scratching the skin; the resulting hyperemia will demonstrate the adequacy of the oxygenation of the blood. A role of halothane in the causation of liver disease is likely, at least in some individuals. Finally, halothane is expensive.

Advantages and Uses. Halothane is non-flammable and nonirritating to the respiratory passages. It can produce profound anesthesia without restricting the supply of oxygen in the inspired mixture. It causes vasodilatation even in the presence of shock, and thereby permits an assessment of the status of blood loss and replacement on the basis of blood pressure alone. It also is useful in providing a "bloodless" field for plastic operations, when employed as an agent capable of inducing deliberate hypotension. Finally, it can be of value in the maneuver of version and extraction, by virtue of its relaxant actions on the myometrium.

Status. Halothane has become very popular in the relatively few years since its introduction. It is usually used in conjunction with nitrous oxide and muscle relaxants to provide general anesthesia for operations of every description, but it can also be given alone. Halothane appears likely to retain its popularity until it is displaced by a better agent or proved to be a cause of liver damage.

METHOXYFLURANE

History. First synthesized by Larsen in 1958, methoxyflurane was used clinically by Artusio in the following year and has since attracted a number of adherents. The drug is now used extensively in the United States, although it has yet to be fully evaluated.

Chemistry and Preparations. *Methoxyflurane,* N.F. (PENTHRANE), is 2,2-dichloro-1,1-difluoroethyl methyl ether. It is a clear, colorless liquid with a characteristic sweet, fruity odor. It is supplied for anesthesia in opaque bottles containing 0.01% butylated hydroxytoluene to retard decomposition. It is stable in the presence of soda lime, and nonflammable and nonexplosive in air or oxygen in anesthetic concentrations. The vapor tension at room temperature is relatively low (25 mm Hg at 20° C) and not far above that needed to induce anesthesia. Consequently, some have claimed that it is unnecessary to use a precisely calibrated vaporizer to administer methoxyflurane. The blood:gas partition ratio is 13 at 37° C.

PHARMACOLOGICAL PROPERTIES

General Anesthetic Actions. Methoxyflurane, the most potent of the inhalational anesthetic drugs (minimal anesthetic concentration, 0.16 volume %), can produce any desired depth of anesthesia in the absence of hypoxia, but its side effects (*see* below) are so prominent that it is often best employed together with nitrous oxide, barbiturates, and muscle relaxants. The induction of anesthesia is characteristically slow; as much as 20 minutes may occasionally be required. Delirium during induction is not uncommon. For these reasons, anesthesia is usually induced with a "sleep dose" of thiopental given intravenously.

The signs of anesthesia resemble those of halothane, except that respiratory depression and muscular relaxation are more prominent. For maintenance of anesthesia, concentrations of the anesthetic in the inspired mixture vary from 0.2 to 0.8 volume %. The blood:gas partition ratio is higher than that of halothane, and this accounts both for the relatively long induction time and for an emergence that is outstandingly slow. As with the other volatile anesthetics, the depth of anesthesia will increase with time unless the concentration of inspired methoxyflurane is progressively reduced following induction. Most patients awake quietly; some exhibit considerable analgesia even after fully regaining consciousness.

Respiration. The major difference between the respiratory actions of halothane and those of methoxyflurane is that the latter are more intense. It is frequently necessary to assist or control respiration. The use of an accurate ventilation meter is valuable, since it permits early detection of a diminished respiratory exchange. Because maintenance of a patent airway is vital and the need for respiratory assistance frequent, methoxyflurane is commonly administered by means of an endotracheal tube. Many anesthesiologists elect to preserve the patient's spontaneous ventilation. Although some degree of hypercarbia will develop, the character of respiration serves as a valuable sign of the depth of anesthesia while central respiratory depression automatically limits anesthetic dosage to a safe level.

Like halothane, methoxyflurane is nonirritating, does not stimulate tracheobronchial secretions, does not constrict bronchioles, and does not cause laryngospasm. Asthmatics tolerate the drug well.

Circulation. The circulatory actions of methoxyflurane are similar to, but less intense than, those of chloroform and halothane. Mild-to-moderate arterial hypotension, with or without bradycardia, is typical of light planes of anesthesia. Attempts to increase depth intensify these effects and may necessitate a reduction in the concentration of inspired vapor. Arterial hypotension is accompanied by reduced cardiac contractile force and cardiac output. Marked pallor of the skin is sometimes noted, and the surgical field exhibits relatively little oozing.

Cardiac Rhythm. The most frequent change in cardiac rhythm caused by methoxyflurane is sinus bradycardia, which responds well to atropine. A-V nodal rhythm develops occasionally, particularly during deep anesthesia. Ventricular arrhythmias are rare if sympathetic nervous stimulation is avoided. The most frequent causes of such stimulation include respiratory acidosis, tracheal intubation, and surgical stimulation during an inadequate depth of anesthesia. Like enflurane and halothane, methoxyflurane sensitizes the ventricles to catecholamines, and ominous ventricular rhythms are likely to occur if these drugs are administered indiscriminately during its use; however, the degree of sensitization is less than with the other two anesthetics.

Other Actions. In man, methoxyflurane increases BSP retention no more than does ether or cyclopropane. However, the unfortunate history of the halogenated anesthetics with respect to hepatic damage makes all of them suspect until proven safe. In dogs, renal damage could not be produced by methoxyflurane. However, in man a syndrome consisting of persistent diuresis with obvious dehydration has been described postoperatively in certain patients given methoxyflurane (Crandell *et al.,* 1966). More recently, Mazze and coworkers (1971) showed in a prospective randomized study that methoxyflurane in moderately high concentrations for prolonged periods of time caused high-output renal failure in the majority of patients studied. The diuresis was refractory to ADH and resembled that caused by fluoride intoxication. It is significant in this connection that methoxyflurane is, because of its high blood:gas and oil:water partition ratios, retained in the body for long periods and is extensively metabolized. In one study (Halsey *et al.,* 1971), roughly 50% was degraded. Uterine contractility is said to be relatively unaffected, and methoxyflurane has been recommended for use in obstetrical anesthesia. Nausea and vomiting are less frequent than after chloroform, ether, or cyclopropane.

Evaluation. Methoxyflurane has a number of interesting properties that may give it a unique place in anesthetic practice. At relatively light planes of anesthesia it provides substantial analgesia and muscular relaxation, and analgesia may persist after consciousness has returned. It is nonflammable, and does not sensitize the heart to catecholamines to the same degree as do the other halogenated agents in common use today. However, while any desired degree of muscular relaxation can be achieved by increasing anesthetic depth, the accompanying circulatory depression may be profound. For this reason methoxyflurane is most commonly used as an adjuvant to nitrous oxide, and profound relaxation is usually attained by neuromuscular blocking drugs. The slow onset of anesthesia and the slow recovery limit the usefulness of the drug, particularly in short operations. Finally, the status of the drug with respect to renal function appears dubious, and its use has been discontinued in several hospitals for this reason.

ENFLURANE

History. Enflurane was synthesized by Terrell in 1963, tested in animals and given clinical trial by Virtue and associates in 1966, and introduced for general human use in 1973.

Chemistry and Preparations. Chemically, *enflurane* (ETHRANE) is 2-chloro-1,1,2-trifluoroethyl difluoromethyl ether. It is a clear, colorless, nonflammable liquid with a mild, sweet odor. It is extremely stable chemically and does not contain a preservative. It does not attack aluminum, tin, brass, iron, or copper. The blood:gas partition ratio is 1.9. Its vapor pressure at 25° C is 218 mm Hg.

Enflurane is highly soluble in rubber (partition coefficient = 74), and the same considerations already described for halothane consequently apply to the use of this agent. The oil:water partition ratio is 120.

PHARMACOLOGICAL PROPERTIES

Central Nervous System. The earliest clinical report (Virtue *et al.,* 1966) indicated that enflurane could produce tonic-clonic seizures and involuntary motor activity. In cats with chronically implanted electrodes in selected nuclei of the limbic, sensory, and diffuse projection systems, enflurane induced bursts of high-voltage spikes separated by prolonged intervals of electrical silence (Julien and Kavan, 1972). Residual behavioral and EEG abnormalities persisted for 10 or more days. It was suggested that enflurane could be used to study mechanisms regulating cortical hyperexcitability, since anesthetic concentrations of the drug augmented evoked responses to peripheral stimulation by up to five times the control level.

On the other hand, recent clinical observations

suggest that seizure patterns are rare, except with hyperventilation during profound anesthesia, and such patterns are seldom associated with obvious movements (Clark *et al.,* 1971). Clinical anesthesia with enflurane resembles that produced by halothane or methoxyflurane, except that muscular relaxation is more pronounced and tachypnea is uncommon.

Any depth of anesthesia can be produced in the absence of hypoxia, but the occurrence of arterial hypotension limits the safe maintenance concentration to 3% or less. The minimal alveolar anesthetic tension is 1.7% in oxygen and 0.6% when given with 70% nitrous oxide. Although mask induction of anesthesia is not unpleasant, enflurane is usually given for maintenance following induction of anesthesia with a rapidly acting intravenous barbiturate.

Respiration. Enflurane causes the same degree of central respiratory depression as does halothane at concentrations that produce an equal depth of anesthesia. However, enflurane, unlike halothane, does not usually cause tachypnea when spontaneous ventilation is permitted, and it is thus superior under these conditions, particularly during abdominal surgery.

Circulation. Some degree of arterial hypotension is not uncommon, particularly prior to the beginning of surgery. Heart rate is not greatly affected and cardiac rhythm is usually normal. However, enflurane, like halothane, sensitizes the myocardium to catecholamines, and ventricular extrasystoles can be expected if these substances are given during anesthesia with this agent.

Cardiac output is slightly diminished, reflecting a similar reduction in the rate of whole-body oxygen consumption; however, the heart responds well to changes in venous return, cardiac output increasing substantially during mild hypercarbia and decreasing slightly during hypocarbia (Marshall *et al.,* 1972). Enflurane depresses contractility in isolated heart muscle to roughly the same extent as does halothane (Shimosato *et al.,* 1969; Brown and Crout, 1971).

The effects of enflurane on barostatic reflexes and preganglionic sympathetic nervous activity resemble those of halothane (Skovsted and Price, 1972).

Liver and Kidney. Although temporary depression of function is to be expected, there is to date no evidence for lasting adverse effects.

Gastrointestinal Tract. The actions of enflurane have not been fully evaluated, but they appear to resemble those of halothane.

Neuromuscular Junction. Muscular relaxation is adequate for intra-abdominal procedures at ordinary levels of anesthesia. Non-depolarizing muscle relaxants are markedly potentiated by enflurane. However, neostigmine does not reverse the direct neuromuscular blocking action of enflurane.

Metabolism and Excretion. Enflurane is metabolized in man to only a limited extent (2.5 to 10%), the principal products being inorganic fluoride and unidentified organic compounds. It is not presently known whether the amount of fluoride liberated is sufficient to affect renal function or whether the organic products are hepatotoxic. Roughly 85% of inhaled enflurane is recovered unchanged in the expired air.

Disadvantages and Limitations. Like halothane, enflurane markedly depresses myocardial contractile force, and it sensitizes the cardiac conducting system to the arrhythmogenic actions of catecholamines. Arterial hypotension may be bothersome in some patients. The seizure-like EEG patterns and involuntary movement sometimes encountered remain to be evaluated.

Advantages and Uses. Enflurane has all of the advantages of halothane. In addition, it is metabolized to a far lesser extent and has not as yet been implicated in cases of postoperative hepatic failure. Unlike halothane, it produces moderate muscular relaxation, probably by means of a direct effect on the neuromuscular junction. Finally, it does not cause tachypnea, and thus permits abdominal operations to be done during spontaneous respiration.

Status. Enflurane, although a relatively new drug, has many desirable properties as an anesthetic agent and has already achieved widespread popularity. Provided that no new hazardous side actions are uncovered, it appears likely to replace halothane in the near future. It is not yet an official drug.

OTHER HALOGENATED VOLATILE ANESTHETICS

FLUROXENE

Fluroxene, N.F. (FLUOROMAR), a halogenated ether (2,2,2-trifluoroethyl vinyl ether), possesses several properties similar to those of ether and cyclopropane. It is flammable but not explosive in ordinary concentrations, that is, 4 to 6% in oxygen. Fluroxene produces cardiovascular stability, in part because it excites sympathetic nervous activity, and it does not sensitize the heart to the arrhythmogenic actions of catecholamines. It has yet to be seriously implicated in the causation of hepatic necrosis or renal dysfunction in man, although it can decompose *in vitro* into trifluoroethanol, a known hepatotoxin, and acetaldehyde, as well as undergo polymerization. In order to retard these conversions, fluroxene is stored in dark bottles and is supplied with a stabilizer (0.01% N-phenyl-α-naphthylamine).

Its physical properties resemble those of halothane: vapor pressure at 20° C = 286 mm Hg; blood:gas partition ratio, 1.37 at 37° C; and oil:water partition ratio = 57. However, it is less potent than halothane; the minimal anesthetic alveolar concentration of fluroxene in man is 3.4% in oxygen and roughly 1% when it is used with 70% nitrous oxide.

The cardiovascular actions of fluroxene have caused the agent to be used in some clinics as a substitute for cyclopropane, that is, as a first choice in the presence of central or peripheral circulatory failure, including hemorrhagic shock. However, there is as yet no compelling evidence to substantiate claims of increased safety of fluroxene compared with other agents.

ISOFLURANE

Isoflurane (1-chloro-2,2,2-trifluoroethyl difluoromethyl ether; FORANE) is a new, nonflammable anesthetic likely to be released for general clinical use in the near future. Preliminary investigation indicates that isoflurane does not appear to be metabolized and that it may be free of hepatic and renal toxicity. Direct myocardial depression and sensitization of the heart to catecholamines are not obvious. Respiratory depression, however, and potentiation of neuromuscular blockade produced by *d*-tubocurarine are marked. Uptake and excretion of this agent are rapid when compared to halothane and methoxyflurane, since its blood:gas and oil:gas partition coefficients are lower (1.4 and 99, respectively, at 37° C). (*See* Vitcha, 1971.)

OBSOLETE ANESTHETICS

Certain volatile anesthetics, previously used for induction or maintenance of general anesthesia, are no longer of importance. They have been supplanted by nonflammable agents with more desirable properties. The discontinued compounds include *chloroform, vinyl ether, ethyl chloride, halopropane,* and *trichloroethylene.* The only advantage offered by any of them was that they were safe enough to be administered without accurate control or knowledge of respired tension.

Bhatia, B. B., and Burn, J. H. The action of ether on the sympathetic system. *J. Physiol., Lond.,* 1933, *78,* 257–270.

Black, G. W., and McArdle, L. The effects of halothane on the peripheral blood vessels. *Anaesthesia,* 1962, *17,* 82–89.

Brewster, W. R., Jr.; Isaacs, J. P.; and Wainø-Andersen, T. Depressant effect of ether on myocardium of the dog and its modification by reflex release of epinephrine and norepinephrine. *Am. J. Physiol.,* 1953, *175,* 399–414.

Brown, B. R., Jr., and Crout, J. R. A comparative study of the effects of five general anesthetics on myocardial contractility. *Anesthesiology,* 1971, *34,* 236.

Clark, D. L.; Hosick, E. D.; and Rosner, B. S. Neurophysiological effects of different anesthetics in unconscious man. *J. appl. Physiol.,* 1971, *31,* 884–891.

Crandell, W. B.; Pappas, S. G.; and MacDonald, A. Nephrotoxicity associated with methoxyflurane anesthesia. *Anesthesiology,* 1966, *27,* 591–607.

Deutsch, S.; Linde, H. W.; Dripps, R. D.; and Price, H. L. Circulatory and respiratory actions of halothane in normal man. *Anesthesiology,* 1962, *23,* 631–638.

Epstein, R. M.; Deutsch, S.; Cooperman, L. H.; Clement, A. J.; and Price, H. L. Splanchnic circulation during halothane anesthesia and hypercapnia in normal man. *Anesthesiology,* 1966, *27,* 654–661.

Flacke, W., and Alper, M. H. Actions of halothane and norepinephrine in the isolated mammalian heart. *Anesthesiology,* 1962, *23,* 793–801.

Halsey, M. J.; Sawyer, D. V. M.; Eger, E. I., II; Bahlman, S. H.; and Impelman, D. M. K. Hepatic metabolism of halothane, methoxyflurane, cyclopropane, ETHRANE,

and FORANE in miniature swine. *Anesthesiology,* 1971, *35,* 43–47.

Julien, R. M., and Kavan, E. M. Electrographic studies of a new volatile anesthetic agent: enflurane (ETHRANE). *J. Pharmac. exp. Ther.,* 1972, *183,* 393–403.

Katz, R. L.; Matteo, R. S.; and Papper, E. M. The injection of epinephrine during general anesthesia: halothane. *Anesthesiology,* 1962, *23,* 597–600.

Klatskin, G. Mechanism of toxic and drug induced hepatic injury. In, *Toxic Effects of Anesthetics.* (Fink, B. R., ed.) The Williams & Wilkins Co., Baltimore, 1968.

Larson, C. P.; Eger, E. I., II; Muallem, M.; Buechel, D. R.; Munson, E. S.; and Eisele, J. H. The effects of diethyl ether and methoxyflurane on ventilation. *Anesthesiology,* 1969, *30,* 174–185.

Marshall, B. E.; Cohen, P. J.; Klingenmaier, C. H.; Neigh, J. L.; and Pender, J. W. Some pulmonary and cardiovascular effects of enflurane (ETHRANE) anaesthesia with varying Pa_{CO_2} in man. *Br. J. Anaesth.,* 1972, *43,* 996–1002.

Marshall, F. N. Effects of halothane on gastrointestinal motility. *Anesthesiology,* 1961, *22,* 353–366.

Mazze, R. I.; Shue, G. L.; and Jackson, S. H. Renal dysfunction associated with methoxyflurane anesthesia. *J. Am. med. Ass.,* 1971, *216,* 278–288.

Ngai, S. H. Halothane. In, *Modern Inhalation Anesthetics.* (Chenoweth, M. B., ed.) *Handb. exp. Pharmak.,* Springer-Verlag, Berlin, 1972, *30,* 33–76.

Patterson, R. W.; Sullivan, S. F.; Malm, J. R.; Bowman, F. O., Jr.; and Papper, E. M. The effect of halothane on human airway mechanics. *Anesthesiology,* 1968, *29,* 900–907.

Price, H. L. Circulating adrenaline and noradrenaline during diethyl ether anesthesia in man. *Clin. Sci.,* 1957, *16,* 377–387.

Rehder, K.; Forbes, J.; Alter, H.; Hessler, O.; and Stier, A. Halothane biotransformation in man: a quantitative study. *Anesthesiology,* 1967, *28,* 711–715.

Rosenberg, P. H., and Wahlstrom, T. Hepatotoxicity of halothane metabolites *in vivo* and inhibition of fibroblast growth *in vitro. Acta pharmac. tox.,* 1971, *29,* 9–19.

Shimosato, S.; Sugai, N.; Iwatsuki, N.; and Etsten, B. E. The effect of ETHRANE on cardiac muscle mechanics. *Anesthesiology,* 1969, *30,* 513–518.

Skovsted, P., and Price, H. L. Central sympathetic activation caused by diethyl ether. *Anesthesiology,* 1970, *32,* 202–209.

———. The effects of ETHRANE on arterial pressure, preganglionic sympathetic activity and barostatic reflexes. *Ibid.,* 1972, *36,* 257–262.

Stenger, J. J., and Johnson, E. A. Effects of phenobarbital pretreatment on the response of rat liver to halothane administration. *Proc. Soc. exp. Biol. Med.,* 1972, *140,* 1319–1324.

Summary of the National Halothane Study. Possible association between halothane anesthesia and postoperative hepatic necrosis. *J. Am. med. Ass.,* 1966, *197,* 775–788.

Van Dyke, R. A.; Chenoweth, M. B.; and Van Poznak, A. Metabolism of volatile anesthetics. I. Conversion *in vivo* of several anesthetics to $^{14}CO_2$ and chloride. *Biochem. Pharmac.,* 1964, *13,* 1239–1247.

Virtue, R. W.; Lund, L. O.; Phelps, M., Jr.; Vogel, J. H. K.; Beckwitt, H.; and Heron, M. Difluoromethyl 1,1,2-trifluoro-2-chloroethyl ether as an anaesthetic agent: results with dogs, and a preliminary note on observations with man. *Can. Anaesth. Soc. J.,* 1966, *13,* 233–241.

Vitcha, J. F. A history of FORANE. *Anesthesiology,* 1971, *35,* 4–7.

Wollman, H.; Alexander, S. C.; Cohen, P. J.; Chase, P. E.; Melman, E.; and Behar, M. G. Cerebral circulation of man during halothane anesthesia. *Anesthesiology,* 1964, *25,* 180–191.

CHAPTER
8 GENERAL ANESTHETICS
[Continued]
Intravenous Anesthetics

Henry L. Price

BARBITURATES

History. The first genuine attempt at intravenous anesthesia was made in 1665, when Sigismund Elsholtz injected an opiate to produce insensibility. The first monograph on the subject appeared in 1875, when Oré published the results of his experiences with chloral hydrate. Oré was an enthusiastic votary of intravenous anesthesia, and believed it superior to ether and chloroform. But chloral hydrate was not well suited to anesthetic purposes, and the use of intravenous anesthesia did not become popular until the introduction of the ultrashort-acting barbiturates in the 1930s. The early barbiturates were slow in both onset and recovery and correspondingly difficult to employ clinically. The first practical intravenous anesthetic was hexobarbital, a barbiturate with a rapid hypnotic action. Its use was soon displaced by that of thiopental, introduced by Lundy in 1935. Since its introduction, thiopental has been widely used, and newer barbiturates with more desirable actions (with the possible exception of methohexital, *see* below) have not yet appeared.

Chemistry and Preparations. Thiopental as such is practically insoluble in water. (Its structure is given in Table 9–1, page 103.) It is supplied for clinical use as the sodium salt (*Thiopental Sodium for Injection,* U.S.P.), which is highly soluble in water but pharmacologically inactive. Included with each gram of thiopental sodium is 60 mg of sodium carbonate; hence solutions of the preparation are strongly alkaline (pH 11). Upon injection, the sodium carbonate is neutralized in the blood stream, and the thiopental is converted in large part to its acidic, or active, form. It does not form a precipitate in the blood, both because it is rapidly diluted and because it is strongly adsorbed on plasma proteins, albumin in particular. When thiopental sodium is dissolved in *Sterile Water for Injection,* U.S.P., a 2.8% solution is isotonic; concentrations less than 2.0% may cause hemolysis.

Methohexital is supplied for use as *Methohexital Sodium for Injection,* U.S.P. The pH of its aqueous solutions is 11. (Its structure is given in Table 9–1, page 103.)

Hexobarbital, N.F., is nearly insoluble in water; thus, it is also supplied as the sodium salt. The pH of aqueous solutions is 11. (Its structure is given in Table 9–1, page 103.)

PHARMACOLOGICAL PROPERTIES

The actions of barbiturates as a class are discussed in detail in Chapter 9. Only those properties particularly pertinent to intravenous anesthesia will be dealt with here. Since the actions of thiopental are typical of this class of agents, as well as being the most thoroughly documented, these will be emphasized. The effects of other intravenous agents will be mentioned only where they differ substantially.

Temporal Course of Effects. Intravenous anesthetics differ from inhalational agents in that, once injected, there is practically nothing that can be done to facilitate the removal of the drug. The temporal course of effects from induction and rapidly deepening anesthesia to gradual emergence depends almost entirely upon progressive redistribution of these drugs within the body (*see* Chapter 9). Metabolic degradation or excretion during the period of the ordinary anesthetic administration is negligible, except in the case of methohexital.

The most important property of the ultra-short-acting barbiturates is their ability to penetrate all tissues of the body without delay. For this reason their uptake by a given tissue depends only upon the local blood flow and the concentration of the drug in arterial blood. Because they are relatively well perfused, the viscera, including the brain, initially receive the bulk of a given dose of a rapidly acting barbiturate. The brain alone receives about one tenth of the dose within the first 40 seconds following an intravenous injection (Price *et al.,* 1960). As time passes, the relatively poorly perfused areas of the body (muscle, skin, connective tissue, fat, and

97

skeleton) gradually come to equilibrium with the blood concentration of barbiturate, with the result that concentrations in the blood and various viscera decline progressively. For the brain, the barbiturate level diminishes to about one half of its peak in 5 minutes, and to only one tenth by ½ hour following the injection. Recovery of consciousness usually occurs within this period following the administration of an ordinary induction dose. If the dose is unduly large, recovery is delayed for several reasons. First, the peak brain content will be excessive; second, the rate of removal may be reduced in consequence of circulatory depression; finally, the amount of drug in circulation will be relatively high even after saturation of the extracerebral tissues.

Anesthetic Actions. Like the inhalational anesthetics, the barbiturates produce unconsciousness primarily by blocking the central brain stem core ("reticular activating system"), which subserves wakefulness (Moruzzi and Magoun, 1949). However, the reticular core also contains an inhibitory component (Machne *et al.,* 1955; Magoun, 1958), and this is depressed by small doses of barbiturates. In terms of cortical responsiveness, the course of deepening barbiturate anesthesia follows a diphasic curve. At the lightest levels there is a release from inhibition in the extralemniscal systems, but on increasing depth the excitatory process also becomes depressed and cortical responsiveness declines. Curves of similar shape have been obtained when measurements of pain threshold are plotted against anesthetic depth, namely, that after low doses of thiopental there is an antianalgesic effect that is converted into an analgesic action as the dose is increased (Clutton-Brock, 1960, 1961; Dundee, 1960). However, the analgesia produced by barbiturates is not profound. This may be related to the fact that the classical (lemniscal) pain pathways are relatively unaffected by this class of anesthetic agents (Abrahamian *et al.,* 1963). In practice, nitrous oxide or some other inhalational anesthetic is usually administered following the induction of anesthesia with a barbiturate, in order to provide sufficient analgesia.

Respiration. The respiratory effects of the ultrashort-acting barbiturates are the result of direct depression of the medullary and pontine respiratory centers. Actions on the pulmonary stretch receptors, afferent and efferent nerves, and neuromuscular junction are negligible. Immediately following an injection of an ultrashort-acting barbiturate, respiratory depression may be pronounced. Central respiratory responses to carbon dioxide are depressed at all levels of anesthesia and are ultimately abolished as anesthesia is deepened. Responses to chemoreceptor excitation persist longer, but they are also extinguished at profound depths of anesthesia. At ordinary levels of anesthesia, tidal volume is diminished and respiratory rate is increased. Diaphragmatic activity persists after contractions of the intercostal muscles have become ineffective.

Cardiovascular System. Circulatory responses to the ultrashort-acting barbiturates are the complex result of a number of diverse and different primary actions. Myocardial contractility is depressed while vascular tone is increased by direct actions of these anesthetics. The medullary vasomotor center is depressed, but to a lesser extent than are hypothalamic centers regulating the force of cardiac contraction. Whole-body oxygen demand is reduced. Baroreceptor activation and conduction in afferent and efferent autonomic nerves are relatively unaffected; transmission in sympathetic ganglia is somewhat depressed. The end result is that cardiac output is reduced while total peripheral resistance increases. Consequently, the systemic arterial blood pressure is ordinarily little affected, although it may be reduced transiently immediately following the induction of anesthesia, when visceral concentrations of the barbiturate are high.

Vascular resistance in various areas of the body changes in characteristic fashion; that in the skin decreases as a consequence of diminished temperature regulation, and that in skeletal muscle, myocardium, liver, and kidney shows a modest increase. Vascular resistance in the central nervous system (CNS) increases by virtue of a reduction in metabolic demand, with a consequent reduction in the rate of carbon dioxide production (Pierce *et al.,* 1962).

The ultrashort-acting intravenous anesthetics do not sensitize the automatic tissues of the heart to catecholamines to any important degree.

Metabolism and Excretion. This subject is fully discussed in Chapter 9.

Uses in Anesthesia. The ultrashort-acting barbiturates have a number of uses, including their employment for general anesthesia and hypnosis.

General Anesthesia. The ultrashort-acting barbiturates are most commonly injected intravenously to induce or sustain surgical anesthesia. Since they are poor analgesics, they are seldom used alone, but are ordinarily supplemented with an inhalational anesthetic, usually nitrous oxide in oxygen.

Although the sodium salts of hexobarbital, kemithal, thiamylal, and methohexital are utilized as intravenous anesthetics, *thiopental sodium* is the most frequently employed. The use of thiopental increased steadily from its introduction in 1935, and in the succeeding 20 years attained a popularity probably unmatched by any other single anesthetic. The general principles that apply to the intravenous administration of barbiturates are the same as those that govern the use of other general anesthetic agents, and can be illustrated by thiopental as the prototype of its class.

With regard to *technic,* thiopental sodium can be administered intravenously by either intermittent injection or continuous infusion. For intermittent injection, a 2.5% aqueous solution is ordinarily used in preference to stronger solutions, which are more irritating. Care must be exercised to prevent intra-arterial injection or extravasation, which may result in tissue necrosis. One way of avoiding this complication is to inject only into a freely running intravenous infusion or to use dilute solutions (2.5% or less). Higher concentrations injected intra-arterially cause ischemia by producing vascular occlusion. The injury apparently results from the action of thiopental itself and not from its alkalinity. Sympathectomy or the administration of heparin diminishes the degree of necrosis, but intra-arterial injections of vasodilator drugs are ineffective (Kinmonth and Shepherd, 1959). No completely reliable therapy is known, perhaps because irreversible damage to the vessels occurs on first contact with the drug. Induction of anesthesia is usually performed slowly, by injecting 150 to 250 mg over a 15- to 30-second period; an inhalational anesthetic is then begun. Supplemental doses can be given as needed to maintain anesthesia. The total dose employed during the course of an ordinary operation rarely exceeds 1.0 g. It is impossible to estimate in advance how much barbiturate will be needed by a particular patient for an optimal level of anesthesia. Therefore, no categorical statements can be made about dosage and each case presents individual requirements.

When rapidly acting barbiturates are given intravenously for the production of anesthesia, the stages described in detail for the inhalational anesthetics are not easily delineated. During the course of a fairly rapid injection, the patient appears to fall asleep quite suddenly, sleep often interrupting his conversation in the middle of a sentence. When an injection is performed sufficiently slowly, the induction period resembles, in a general way, that noted with the inhalational anesthetics. The *stage of surgical anesthesia* is characterized by diminution or disappearance of eyelash and tendon reflexes; constricted or normal pupils and fixed eyeballs; relaxation of the pharyngeal structures, with a falling backward of the tongue; and shallow respiration and a decline in arterial blood pressure, especially marked in patients with essential hypertension. The safest indication of the depth of anesthesia is the degree of respiratory depression. Abdominal relaxation may be inadequate even in deep anesthesia. The signs vary with the amount of barbiturate administered and with the individual patient. When an overdose of the drug is given, muscular flaccidity is marked, respirations are seriously depressed or absent, and the blood pressure falls rapidly to alarmingly low levels.

Recovery is sometimes characterized by an initial period of restlessness, during which the patient may be irrational and hyperactive. This behavior is usually caused by pain, and may be related to the fact that thiopental and other rapidly acting barbiturates may have an antianalgesic effect at low concentrations. Shivering may occur, particularly following prolonged operations performed in chilly operating rooms. This phenomenon is associated with a decreased body temperature. In addition to shivering, a cold, clammy, and cyanotic skin may occasionally be present. The cyanosis is caused by peripheral vasoconstriction. After anesthesia of long duration and after large total doses of barbiturate, some patients may exhibit delayed awakening. This complication can best be avoided by limiting the total dose of barbiturate and by relying upon an inhalational anesthetic to provide analgesia. No specific barbiturate antagonist exists.

Hexobarbital causes a high incidence of muscle movements and hypotension, and is less satisfactory than thiopental or methohexital for this reason (Dundee, 1963). *Methohexital* also produces muscle movements in a large proportion of subjects. Its anesthetic effects last for a shorter period than those of thiopental or hexobarbital (Egbert *et al.,* 1959).

Among the *advantages* of intravenous barbiturate anesthesia are rapid and pleasant induction, reduction in the postanesthetic incidence of excitement and vomiting, quiet respiration, absence of salivation, nonexplosiveness, and speedy recovery after small doses.

Complications and undesirable features associated with the use of intravenous barbiturate anesthesia are extravenous injection (previously mentioned) and certain adverse respiratory actions, including apnea, coughing, laryngospasm, and bronchospasm. The last-mentioned effect may represent a true pharmacological response, particularly in individuals who are subject to allergic conditions such as bronchial asthma, but the other effects most frequently result from respiratory tract irritation caused, for example, by the aspiration of secretions or a premature attempt to insert an airway.

An important complication occurs in patients who have *acute intermittent porphyria*. This disease is exacerbated by the administration of barbiturates, and a rapidly fatal course thereafter is not uncommon. The cause of death is extensive demyelination of peripheral nerves (autonomic, sensory, and motor), including the cranial nerves. Lesions also occur within the CNS. Symptoms and signs include abdominal pain, motor weakness or paralysis, and the presence of porphobilinogen in the urine. Knowledge that a patient has acute intermittent porphyria constitutes an absolute contraindication to the use of intravenous barbiturate anesthesia (Dundee *et al.*, 1962).

The *principal limitation* affecting the use of barbiturates as general anesthetics is that they are poor analgesics. For this reason intravenous barbiturates are usually combined with inhalational anesthetics of limited potency, such as nitrous oxide or, very rarely, ethylene. Moreover, there is no practical way to control the amount of drug in the body, except to limit the dose to an amount that is usually safe.

Hypnosis. A slow intravenous infusion of a dilute solution of any of the ultrashort-acting barbiturates can be employed to induce a sleeplike state in which the recipient remains in partial contact with his surroundings. Under these conditions rapport can be established between a patient and his physician, as, for example, in psychotherapy, which permits the use of verbal suggestion, the acquisition of information that the fully conscious individual does not recognize, and the induction of "true," or drugless, hypnosis. This technic is particularly useful in states of increased anxiety, such as hysteria, and in cases of catatonia.

OTHER (NONBARBITURATE) AGENTS

NEUROLEPTIC-NARCOTIC COMBINATIONS

Neuroleptic compounds, such as *Droperidol*, N.F. ([1-{1[3-(*p*-fluorobenzoyl)propyl]-1,2,3,6-tetrahydro-4-pyridyl}-2-benzimidazolinone]; INAPSINE), have been combined with potent narcotic drugs to produce a state called "neurolept analgesia." Neuroleptics cause general quiescence and a state of psychic indifference to environmental stimuli, but do not produce sleep (*see* Chapter 12). Intravenous administration of a neuroleptic-narcotic mixture provides sufficient CNS action to permit certain procedures (*e.g.*, bronchoscopy, x-ray studies, burn dressings, or cystoscopy) to be performed without additional medication. If the combined actions of these drugs are supplemented by the inhalation of nitrous oxide, surgical operations are made possible.

The most popular fixed-dose mixture of this type, INNOVAR, consists (per milliliter) of 0.05 mg of the narcotic analgesic *Fentanyl Citrate*, U.S.P. ([N-{1-phenethyl-4-piperidyl} propionanilide citrate]; SUBLIMAZE CITRATE), and 2.5 mg of *droperidol*. The induction dose approximates 0.1 ml/kg of body weight and is injected intravenously over a period of 5 to 10 minutes. The onset of anesthesia is invariably slow, and 3 to 5 minutes must elapse between an injection of the mixture and the occurrence of a peak effect. Premature attempts to induce anesthesia with nitrous oxide frequently precipitate induction delirium, and positive pressure may cause laryngospasm (as in any patient too lightly anesthetized). Too rapid an injection may cause chest-wall spasm. For all these reasons, induction can be somewhat prolonged.

Beside the production of neurolepsis, the fentanyl-droperidol mixture may cause mild-to-moderate arterial hypotension and bradycardia, particularly during induction. Standard premedicating doses of atropine will prevent cardiac slowing in most cases. Respiratory depression is almost invariable, requiring assisted ventilation and, usually, tracheal intubation (Dunbar *et al.*, 1967). ECG abnormalities are rare, and epinephrine can be injected subcutaneously to secure hemostasis without fear of precipitating a cardiac arrhythmia. Tracheal secretions are minimal. Muscular rigidity may occur after rapid injections of the mixture. It can be antagonized with neuromuscular blocking agents.

Emergence from anesthesia is typically rapid, occurring within minutes after nitrous oxide inhalation is stopped, although postoperative respiratory depression is evident in about 40% of cases. This is due to the action of fentanyl and, consequently, can be counteracted with a narcotic antagonist (*see* Chapter 15). Nausea, retching, or vomiting occurs in approximately 10%, grogginess may persist for 24 hours or more in roughly 5%, and extrapyramidal movements (usually delayed for 6 to 12 hours) occur in about 1% of individuals given the mixture. The extrapyramidal movements, caused by droperidol, can ordinarily be controlled by antiparkinsonism drugs. Droperidol and other butyrophenones are contraindicated in patients with parkinsonism (*see* Wiklund and Ngai, 1971). Hazards associated with anesthesia produced by the fixed-ratio combination of drugs present in INNOVAR have been stressed (Medical Letter, 1974).

Status. Although the technic has a number of advocates, it has not as yet proven widely popular. The main drawbacks are the slow onset of anesthesia and the degree of respiratory depression it produces. Also, the two components of the mixture have widely different durations of action, that of droperidol markedly exceeding that of fentanyl. An important advantage is that analgesia frequently persists into the postoperative period. It has minimal toxic effects on the heart, liver, or kidneys, and may give protection against ventricular arrhythmias caused by the subcutaneous injection of epinephrine. It is valuable in procedures (such as "awake" intubation of the trachea) that are uncomfortable but are greatly facilitated by patient cooperation.

ARYLCYCLOALKYLAMINES

Several other chemically related nonbarbiturate drugs that produce what is called "dissociative anesthesia" have been used as anesthetics. The first of these, *phencyclidine*, caused unfortunate psychological effects, including hallucinations, and others had similar disadvantages. More recently a related drug, *Ketamine Hydrochloride*, N.F. (2-[*o*-chlorophenyl]-2-[methylamino] cyclohexanone hydrochloride; KETAJECT, KETALAR), has been synthesized and used clinically. This substance can be administered either intravenously or intramuscularly, in doses of 1 to 2 mg/kg and 4 to 6 mg/kg, respectively. When so used, it causes what has been described as dissociative anesthesia because, during induction, the recipient feels dissociated from his environment. Analgesia and amnesia are conspicuous, but muscular relaxation is poor. Respiration and respiratory resistance are little affected, and the ventilatory response to carbon dioxide is nearly normal. Arterial blood pressure, cardiac output, and heart rate are elevated. This compound is believed to act upon the cerebral cortex, particularly the limbic system, sparing medullary structures to a large extent. Awakening is prolonged, lasting several hours, and disagreeable dreams and hallucinations occasionally occur. In some patients the hallucinations recur unpredictably days or weeks after recovery from anesthesia. The drug may offer advantages in operations about the head and neck where the surgeon requires unhampered access to the operative field, and in emergency situations where hemorrhage is severe and rapid action without circulatory depression is needed (Virtue *et al.,* 1967). Ketamine is not indicated in intracranial operations because it increases cerebrospinal fluid pressure. It is often useful for diagnostic procedures in children and rarely produces hallucinations. Despite the relatively unobstructed airway which typifies anesthesia with ketamine, the cough reflex is depressed and aspiration has occurred.

Abrahamian, H. A.; Allison, T.; Goff, W. R., and Rosner, B. S. Effects of thiopental on human cerebral evoked responses. *Anesthesiology,* **1963,** *24,* 650–657.

Clutton-Brock, J. C. Some pain threshold studies with particular reference to thiopentone. *Anaesthesia,* **1960,** *15,* 71–79.

———. Pain and the barbiturates. *Ibid.,* **1961,** *16,* 80–88.

Dunbar, B. S.; Ovassapian, A.; Dripps, R. D.; and Smith, T. C. The respiratory response to carbon dioxide during INNOVAR nitrous oxide anaesthesia in man. *Br. J. Anaesth.,* **1967,** *39,* 861–866.

Dundee, J. W. Alterations in response to somatic pain associated with anaesthesia. II. The effect of thiopentone and pentobarbital. *Br. J. Anaesth.,* **1960,** *32,* 407–414.

———. Clinical studies of induction agents. VII. A comparison of eight intravenous anaesthetics as main agents for a standard operation. *Ibid.,* **1963,** *35,* 784–794.

Dundee, J. W.; McCleery, W. N. C.; and McLoughlin, G. The hazard of thiopental anesthesia in porphyria. *Anesth. Analg. curr. Res.,* **1962,** *41,* 567–574.

Egbert, L. D.; Oech, S. R.; and Eckenhoff, J. E. Comparison of the recovery from methohexital and thiopental anesthesia in man. *Surgery Gynec. Obstet.,* **1959,** *109,* 427–430.

Kinmonth, J. B., and Shepherd, R. C. Accidental injection of thiopentone into arteries: studies of pathology and treatment. *Br. med. J.,* **1959,** *2,* 914–918.

Lundy, J. S. Intravenous anesthesia: preliminary report of the use of two new thiobarbiturates. *Proc. Staff Meet. Mayo Clin.,* **1935,** *10,* 536–543.

Machne, X.; Calma, I.; and Magoun, H. W. Unit activity of central cephalic brainstem in E.E.G. arousal. *J. Neurophysiol.,* **1955,** *18,* 547–558.

Magoun, H. W. *The Waking Brain.* Charles C Thomas, Pub., Springfield, Ill., **1958.**

Medical Letter. Dangers of INNOVAR. **1974,** *16,* 42–43.

Moruzzi, G., and Magoun, H. W. Brainstem reticular formation and activation of the E.E.G. *Electroenceph. clin. Neurophysiol.,* **1949,** *1,* 455–473.

Pierce, E. C., Jr.; Lambertsen, C. J.; Deutsch, S.; Chase, P. E.; Linde, H. W.; Dripps, R. D.; and Price, H. L. Cerebral circulation and metabolism during thiopental anesthesia and hyperventilation in man. *J. clin. Invest.,* **1962,** *41,* 1664–1671.

Price, H. L.; Kovnak, P. H.; Safer, J. N.; Conner, E. H.; and Price, M. L. The uptake of thiopental by body tissues and its relation to the duration of narcosis. *Clin. Pharmac. Ther.,* **1960,** *1,* 16–22.

Virtue, R. W.; Alanis, J. M.; Mori, M.; Lafargue, R. T.; Vogel, J. H. K.; and Metcalf, D. R. An anesthetic agent: 2-orthochlorophenyl, 2-methylamino cyclohexanone HCl (CI-581). *Anesthesiology,* **1967,** *28,* 823–833.

Wiklund, R. A., and Ngai, S. H. Rigidity and pulmonary edema after INNOVAR in a patient on levodopa therapy: report of a case. *Anesthesiology,* **1971,** *35,* 545–547.

CHAPTER

9 HYPNOTICS AND SEDATIVES

The Barbiturates

Stewart C. Harvey

The principal use of sedative-hypnotic drugs is to produce drowsiness. The application of the term *sedative* to this group is somewhat misleading. It dates from the era when the sedative-hypnotic compounds were the only drugs (apart from alcohol, opiates, and belladonna) that could be used to calm anxious and disturbed patients. With the proliferation of "tranquilizing" agents, the drugs traditionally described as "sedative-hypnotics" have come to play a lesser, although still an important, role in daytime sedation. This role will be discussed briefly; a more detailed discussion of the pharmacotherapy of anxiety is presented in Chapter 12. In this and the following chapter, only drugs used specifically to treat sleep disorders are described.

Most of the modern sedative-hypnotic agents are *general depressants*. They depress a wide range of cellular functions in many vital organ systems. A rational approach to the therapeutic use of hypnotic compounds, and to the treatment of patients poisoned by such compounds, requires a thorough knowledge of the relative susceptibility of various organ systems to the depressant action of these drugs. The hypnotic agents tend to resemble one another with respect to their differential effects on various functions, and much of what is said of the barbiturates will be true of other hypnotic drugs. Hence, the properties of barbiturates will be set forth in some detail.

History. Barbituric acid (malonylurea) results from the condensation of malonic acid and urea. It was prepared in 1864 by Adolph von Baeyer, then a 29-year-old research assistant to Kekulé in Ghent. There are several stories about the origin of the term *barbituric acid*. For example, it is said that Baeyer celebrated the occasion of the synthesis of the new compound by visiting a nearby tavern frequented by artillery officers. It happened that it was the Day of St. Barbara, the patron saint of artillery officers,

and in the ensuing festivities *Barbara* was amalgamated with *urea* to give the new compound its name. Barbituric acid is not itself a central depressant. *Barbiturates* are derivatives of barbituric acid that have two substituents at position 5. The first hypnotic barbiturate, *diethylbarbituric acid* or *barbital,* was introduced into medicine by Fischer and von Mering in 1903, under the trade name of VERONAL. Barbital survived many years of clinical usage, and, although it has largely been supplanted by compounds with shorter durations of action, it is still considered an excellent hypnotic. The second oldest barbiturate is *phenobarbital;* it was introduced into therapeutics simultaneously and independently in 1912 by Loewe, Juliusburger, and Impens, and marketed under the trade name of LUMINAL. It is still a valuable central nervous system (CNS) depressant. In the following years, more than 2500 barbiturates were synthesized, many were carefully studied pharmacologically, and approximately 50 were marketed for clinical use. Today, a dozen or so barbiturates are widely used; of these, five or six would probably be sufficient to meet most therapeutic needs.

Chemical Structure. The ureides, formed from the combination of urea and various organic acids, include a large number of centrally acting agents. Ureides comprise two groups, monoureides and diureides. *Monoureides* (monoacyl ureas) are compounds in which only one amino group of urea is condensed with a carboxyl group, and include several weak hypnotics (*e.g., carbromal*). The five-membered ring structure, *hydantoin,* from which is derived a number of important antiepileptic agents as well as some rather toxic sedatives (*e.g.,* NIRVANOL), may be regarded as the condensation product of glycolic acid and urea. Acids such as malonic acid, with two carboxyl groups, may react with urea to form cyclic *diureides,* of which barbituric acid is an example. The reaction is depicted below.

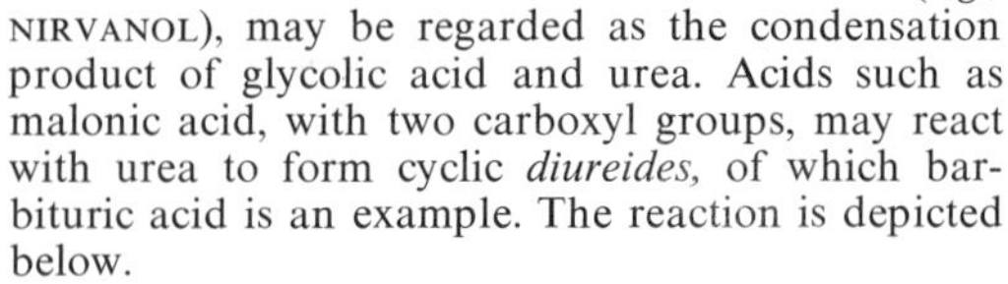

Urea   + Malonic Acid   Barbituric Acid

To obtain barbiturates with hypnotic action, both hydrogens on the carbon atom in position 5 must be replaced with alkyl or aryl groups. The substituents of the barbiturates marketed in the United States are shown in Table 9-1.

In the United States the names of all barbiturates end in *-al;* this suffix is an early misnomer that alludes to the carbonyl groups. In the British Commonwealth the ending *-one* is used. The carbonyl group at position 2 takes on acidic character because of lactam ("keto")–lactim ("enol") tautomerization favored by its location between the two electronegative amido nitrogens. The lactim form is favored in alkaline solution

$$\overset{O}{\underset{}{\|}}\overset{}{-C-NH-} \underset{H^+}{\overset{OH^-}{\rightleftharpoons}} \overset{O^-}{\underset{}{|}}\overset{}{-C=N-}$$

and salts result. The sodium salt of barbital may be considered to have the following structural formula:

Barbital Sodium

The barbituric acid derivatives do not dissolve readily in water, although they are quite soluble in nonpolar solvents (chloroform, oil, etc.), a feature that they share with many other organic compounds that depress the CNS. The sodium salts of barbiturates dissolve in water, forming alkaline and often unstable solutions.

Barbiturates in which the oxygen at C2 is replaced by sulfur are called *thiobarbiturates.* Although only those compounds having a barbituric acid ring (oxygen at C2) are properly called *barbiturates,* it has become common practice to refer to both groups of compounds as barbiturates and to distinguish between them, when necessary, by using the terms *thiobarbiturates* and *oxybarbiturates.*

Relation of Structure to Activity. The structure-activity relationship of the barbiturates has been widely studied, and certain regularities have been observed. In general, structural changes that increase lipid solubility decrease duration of action, decrease latency to onset of activity, accelerate metabolic degradation, and often increase hypnotic potency. Introduction of polar groups, such as ether, keto, hydroxyl, amino, or carboxyl groups, into alkyl side chains abolishes hypnotic activity. The correlation with hypnotic activity holds when the substituents are no longer than seven carbon atoms, but it is not known whether this limitation applies only to the racemic mixtures or to the S(−) antipodes as well. Lipid solubility also favors interaction with hydrophobic regions in proteins. It correlates roughly with binding to plasma protein and cytochrome P-450 and closely with binding to NADH–cytochrome c oxidoreductase.

Alkyl groups can also be substituted on one of the nitrogens in the barbituric acid ring to yield N-alkyl barbiturates. The only N-alkyl barbiturates employed clinically (mephobarbital, metharbital, hexobarbital, and methohexital [Table 9-1]) contain a methyl group on a nitrogen. Methylation of one of the nitrogens increases affinity for lipids, tending to decrease duration of action. Thus, methohexital has a shorter duration of action than do other currently available barbiturates. However, some N-methyl barbiturates are converted in the body to active,

Table 9-1. **BARBITURATES AVAILABLE CURRENTLY IN THE UNITED STATES: NAMES AND STRUCTURES**

GENERAL FORMULA:

BARBITURATE *	TRADE NAME	R_1	R_2	R_3	X
Amobarbital	AMYTAL	ethyl	isopentyl	H	O
Aprobarbital	ALURATE	allyl	isopropyl	H	O
Barbital	NEURONIDIA	ethyl	ethyl	H	O
Butabarbital	BUTISOL	ethyl	*sec*-butyl	H	O
Hexobarbital	SOMBULEX	methyl	1-cyclohexen-1-yl	CH_3	O
Mephobarbital	MEBARAL	ethyl	phenyl	CH_3	O
Metharbital	GEMONIL	ethyl	ethyl	CH_3	O
Methohexital	BREVITAL	allyl	1-methyl-2-pentynyl	CH_3	O
Pentobarbital	NEMBUTAL	ethyl	1-methylbutyl	H	O
Phenobarbital	LUMINAL	ethyl	phenyl	H	O
Probarbital	IPRAL	ethyl	isopropyl	H	O
Secobarbital	SECONAL	allyl	1-methylbutyl	H	O
Talbutal	LOTUSATE	allyl	*sec*-butyl	H	O
Thiamylal	SURITAL	allyl	1-methylbutyl	H	S
Thiopental	PENTOTHAL	ethyl	1-methylbutyl	H	S

* *See* Table 9-3 for currently official barbiturates.

demethylated, long-acting compounds; mephobarbital and metharbital are converted largely to phenobarbital and barbital, respectively.

A phenyl group at C5 or N confers selective anticonvulsant activity on a barbiturate. Thus, anticonvulsant activity and hypnotic potency are, to some extent, independently variable. Phenobarbital is much more potent as an anticonvulsant than as a sedative, and is often capable of being used as an antiepileptic in nonsedative doses. This is not true of other commonly employed barbiturates.

Slight changes in structure may convert barbituric acid derivatives into convulsants. Thus, if the alkyl side chains at C5 are too long, hypnotic activity diminishes and convulsant properties may appear. Alkyl groups attached to both of the N atoms also tend to yield convulsant compounds. The conversion of a depressant compound into a central stimulant by slight changes in structure is not uncommon in drugs affecting the CNS (e.g., local anesthetics, ethers); indeed, in some cases, the same drug may possess both stimulant and depressant properties depending on circumstances and dose. The R(+) optical isomers are also convulsants. Since all clinically used, asymmetrically substituted barbiturates are racemic mixtures, obviously the depressant S(−) antipode predominates over the R(+). Spirobarbiturates are also convulsants.

Thiobarbiturates are more lipid soluble than oxybarbiturates because the electronegativity of sulfur is nearly that of carbon; therefore, the $>$C$=$S group is nearly nonpolar. The thiobarbiturates have a very rapid onset and a short duration of CNS action and are more potent than the corresponding oxybarbiturates. The pharmacodynamic properties of thiobarbiturates differ slightly from those of oxybarbiturates; for example, thiobarbiturates tend to be somewhat more toxic. Numerous thiobarbiturates have been synthesized, but only those with a relatively high molecular weight have a satisfactory margin of safety for clinical use. The thiobarbiturates are employed almost solely as anesthetics for intravenous or rectal administration. Thiopental, the thio analog of pentobarbital, is taken as the prototype of the thiobarbiturates in this chapter.

MECHANISMS AND SITES OF ACTION

The barbiturates reversibly depress the activity of all excitable tissues. Not all tissues are affected at the same dose or concentration; the CNS is exquisitely sensitive, so that when barbiturates are given in sedative or hypnotic doses, very little effect on skeletal, cardiac, or smooth muscle occurs. Even in anesthetic concentrations, direct effects on peripheral excitable tissues are mild and do not create difficulties if the duration of anesthesia is not prolonged. Only if depression is extended, as in acute barbiturate intoxication, do serious deficits in cardiovascular and other peripheral functions occur. Conse-

quently, it is possible that the actions on the various excitable tissues do not derive from a common mechanism involving identical receptors. Nevertheless, it is probable that excitability in each tissue is depressed by an action on or in a membrane and that the ultimate mechanisms of depression among the excitable tissues are quite similar. Oxygen consumption in the various tissues, respiration in mitochondria, and the activities of several enzymes can be depressed by barbiturates in sundry concentrations, and it remains to be determined how some of these effects relate to the depression of excitability. In the sections that follow, attention will first be devoted to the actions of the drugs at a cellular level; subsequently, their effects on the CNS and other organ systems will be considered.

Local Anesthetic Action. Applied directly to peripheral nerves, barbiturates decrease the rate of rise and amplitude of the action potential and slow conduction; there is little or no effect on the resting membrane potential or transmembrane resistance. Blaustein (1968) found that in lobster axons barbiturates diminish the maximal transmembrane conductances of both sodium and potassium and the rate of increase of sodium conductance consequent to small depolarizing potentials. Unlike the amine local anesthetics, barbiturates do not affect the uptake of calcium (Krupp *et al.*, 1969). There is disagreement as to whether barbiturates act on axons in the ionized or nonionized form. Narahashi and coworkers (1971) have reported the most definitive findings, which strongly suggest that pentobarbital acts in the nonionized form. They employed the perfused giant axon of squid, in which not only could the pH of the intracellular and extracellular fluids be controlled independently but also the drug could be applied to either compartment. Pentobarbital was more effective when applied intracellularly, and it was more potent at pH 7 than pH 8. However, manipulation of pH affects the ionization of putative ionic receptor groups and the sequestration of calcium within membranes in addition to the ionization of barbiturates, so that activity in the ionized form cannot definitely be excluded.

On the desheathed frog sciatic nerve, pentobarbital is effective in a concentration of 5 mM, which is nearly two magnitudes higher than anesthetic concentrations in mammals. Consequently, it is not possible to state whether the central depressant effects of barbiturates are the result of local anesthetic actions on central neuronal structures. By analogy with the local anesthetics, unmyelinated, small-diameter structures like telodendria might be expected to be much more sensitive than axons. Thus, reservations based only on the high concentrations required for local anesthesia may not be justified. The discussion immediately following is relevant to this.

Chemical Transmission across Synaptic Junctions. It is generally believed that the synapse is the site of action of hypnotic compounds; indeed, chemical transmission across neuronal and neuroeffector junctions is far more susceptible to interference by the barbiturates than is conduction along nerve or muscle fibers.

Central Synapses. Barbiturates appear to affect different synapses in different ways. Synapses in several monosynaptic pathways in the spinal cord have been studied a number of times with intracellular or close extracellular microelectrodes (for references, *see* Weakly, 1969). The excitatory postsynaptic potential (EPSP) is depressed by barbiturates. Early workers attributed the effect to a stabilization of the postsynaptic membrane, because the threshold to electrical stimulation was found to be elevated; however, the doses of barbiturates were higher than anesthetic doses. In anesthetic doses, neither the postsynaptic membrane resistance nor excitability to electrical stimulation is affected, yet conduction into the presynaptic terminal also seems to be unimpaired. Weakly (1969) analyzed the quantum content from the EPSP in motoneurons of the *triceps surae* in cats and concluded that pentobarbital in anesthetic doses acts presynaptically to decrease the amount of transmitter released. Pentobarbital also appears to have a similar presynaptic action to decrease the EPSP elicited by stimulation of the lateral olfactory tract in isolated guinea pig cortex (Richards, 1972). In this preparation, barbiturates increase frequency potentiation, in contrast to certain monosynaptic pathways in the spinal cord, in which the response to repetitive stimulation is suppressed (Esplin, 1963). Posttetanic potentiation is unaffected in any preparation. In various inhibitory pathways, direct inhibition is enhanced, antagonized, or not affected (for references, *see* Richards, 1972). Certain other synapses also seem to be unaffected. In the cat cerebral cortex, barbiturates in anesthetic doses selectively abolish excitation but not inhibition elicited by norepinephrine applied directly to various synapses, but the effects of acetylcholine (ACh), 5-hydroxytryptamine, isoproterenol, or electrical stimulation are not influenced (Johnson *et al.,* 1969). The relevance of this antiadrenergic effect is unknown, but it is of interest that Chu and Bloom (1973) found that adrenergic neurons in the *locus ceruleus* of the cat were active during wakefulness and rapid-eye-movement (REM) sleep. In view of the presynaptic effects noted above, the fact that ACh is antagonized at the neuromuscular junction and in certain invertebrate ganglia, and the observation that adrenergic inhibition is not affected, the antiadrenergic effect noted by Johnson and coworkers (1969) should not be construed as evidence for a special affinity of barbiturates for adrenergic receptors; further analysis is required to establish whether the action is at the transmitter receptor or elsewhere in the response system.

Multineuronal Networks. The tendency of barbiturates to act selectively on synapses suggests that activity transmitted through polysynaptic pathways should be especially susceptible to barbiturate depression. Although it is probably true that polysynaptic pathways are somewhat more susceptible than monosynaptic reflexes to barbiturates, the degree of selectivity is not great (Wikler, 1945). Indeed, the effect of barbiturates to suppress evoked potentials in the reticular formation and yet not to suppress evoked callosal potentials (Golovchinsky and Plehotkina, 1971) reveals that factors other than morphological complexity predominate in determining the susceptibility of a neuronal pathway to barbiturates. Certainly, a selective action on polysynaptic pathways *per se* does not account for the hypnotic effects of the barbiturates, since many other drugs (*e.g.,* mephenesin) show a much higher degree of selectivity in depressing polysynaptic spinal reflexes and yet have comparatively little hypnotic effect.

There is reason to believe that both wakefulness and the development and spread of epileptiform activity in the CNS depend on repetitive activity in multineuronal networks, with the gradual recruitment of quiescent elements into an active pool until a critical size is attained for regenerative action and self-sustained discharge. The barbiturates exert marked effects on repetitive activity in a number of CNS pathways. In small doses, these drugs often have little effect on the response elicited by the initial stimulus in a train, sometimes even enhancing it; but the responses elicited by subsequent stimuli may be greatly depressed. Selective effects on repetitive activity have been observed in the spinal cord, retina, midbrain reticular system, thalamus, and cortex. The capacity of CNS pathways to respond to repetitive activity is dependent on the balance between inhibitory and excitatory influences following the wake of a volley of nerve impulses (*e.g.,* "long-circuited" facilitatory and inhibitory discharges, posttetanic potentiation, presynaptic inhibition, etc.). Drugs affect these delayed modulating influences differently. Depressant drugs may have differential effects on inhibitory and excitatory processes as well. Doubtless, the relative importance of the factors modulating transmission through multineuronal pathways differs from one part of the CNS to another. It is not yet possible to determine which of the various actions that the barbiturates have been shown to have at the cellular or synaptic level is responsible for their CNS depressant effects, and it is probable that such effects are the result of combined actions.

Autonomic Ganglia. Barbiturates selectively depress transmission in *sympathetic ganglia* in concentrations that are without detectable effect on nerve conduction, neuroeffector junctions, or cardiovascular or other smooth muscle (Exley, 1954). The effect is somewhat similar to that produced by tetraethylammonium inasmuch as the response of the ganglion cells to both preganglionic stimulation and choline esters is diminished. The ganglion cells are not depolarized, and they remain responsive to potassium chloride. Transmission is severely impaired by doses that do not prevent the release of ACh from preganglionic endings, although high doses of barbiturates may also reduce the efflux of ACh from the stimulated fibers. The ganglionic depressant action is sufficiently pronounced to be of clinical interest; it is observed with anesthetic concentrations and may account, at least in part, for the fall in blood pressure produced by intravenous oxybarbiturates and by severe barbiturate intoxication.

Neuroeffector Junctions. At *skeletal neuromuscular junctions,* barbiturates reduce the sensitivity of the postsynaptic membrane to the depolarizing effect of ACh (Thesleff, 1956), and the contractures elicited in chronically denervated muscle by intra-arterial ACh or decamethonium are reduced in amplitude. The neuromuscular blocking effects of both *d*-tubocurarine and decamethonium are enhanced by barbiturates. The curariform effect of barbiturates is not as pronounced as that of ether; however, it is demonstrable in animals receiving anesthetic doses.

In spite of the depressant action on transmission, the twitch response to a single electrical shock applied to the motor nerve may be augmented by subanesthetic concentrations of barbiturates. The relative capacities of the various barbiturates to augment twitch tension is highly correlated with their potency as CNS depressants. In a simple muscle twitch there is normally insufficient time, before relaxation sets in, for the full tension of the muscle to develop. It has been claimed that the augmentation of twitch by barbiturates is due to a slowing of conduction time and also that it is due to a selective depression of the biochemical process responsible for relaxation. In either case, there would be more time for the full muscle tension to develop.

Transmission in *autonomic neuroeffector junctions* is also affected by barbiturates. Amobarbital, for example, inhibits the response of the submaxillary gland to both ACh and stimulation of the chorda tympani. The response of intestinal smooth muscle to the excitatory effects of ACh is blocked by barbiturates; but the response to a variety of spasmogenic agents is also depressed, and it is therefore not certain that the barbiturates have a specific anticholinergic action. In the guinea pig vas deferens, the response to ACh is increased; however, the effect is nonspecific, since responses to histamine and catecholamines are also increased.

The effect of barbiturates on transmission at *adrenergic junctions* has been studied less extensively. Thiopental but not hexobarbital apparently releases norepinephrine from stores in or near vascular smooth muscle in perfused vessels of the rabbit ear (Burn and Hobbs, 1959); the resulting vasoconstriction is potentiated by cocaine and prevented by pretreatment with reserpine or tolazoline. Increases in the plasma level of catecholamines, probably of adrenal origin, have occasionally been observed in dogs after the intravenous injection of thiopental. Since all thiobarbiturates are alike in their ability to cause vasoconstriction in the rabbit ear and to decrease limb volume in dogs, they all probably release catecholamines locally.

Biochemical Effects. During anesthesia induced by barbiturates and other CNS depressants, there is a decrease in oxygen assimilation and an increase in high-energy phosphate and glycogen contents in the brain. It has not been established whether the depression of neuronal activity is the cause or the result of the decreased metabolic activity or whether the two effects are independent phenomena, perhaps linked to the same physicochemical properties of the

barbiturates. In this connection, interruption of the reticular activating system of experimental animals does not alter the effects of barbiturates on cerebral respiration (Cucchiara and Michenfelder, 1973); septal lesions increase both the anesthetic and metabolic effects (Roth and Harvey, 1968). It is also of interest that sodium succinate but not sodium pyruvate injected intracerebroventricularly in equimolar concentrations in the rat has been reported to shorten the duration of anesthesia caused by amobarbital (Reading and Wallwork, 1969), but it is not clear whether the mechanism is metabolic or osmolar. In rat brain cortex *in vitro,* Shankaran and Quastel (1972) reported that barbiturates suppress only that sodium uptake caused by agents that increase mitochondrial respiration; they suggest that the effect is mediated by calcium ions released from mitochondria. There has been a flurry of interest in barbiturate-induced inhibition of adenine nucleotide–dependent enzymes, but the effective concentrations are 100 to 1000 times higher than sedative concentrations. Barbiturates decrease the turnover of 5-hydroxytryptamine and catecholamines in the brains of experimental animals, but whether this is the cause or the effect of anesthesia is conjectural.

ACTIONS ON ORGAN SYSTEMS

Central Nervous System. The barbiturates produce all degrees of depression of the CNS, ranging from mild sedation to coma. The degree of depression obtained depends not only on the particular barbiturate, the dose, and the route of administration but also on the degree of excitability of the CNS at the time of administration and the extent to which previous experience with drugs has induced tolerance. As with ethanol, it should be kept in mind that sedative doses that exert no effects obvious to the untrained observer or the patient can cause impairment in learning, judgment, short-term memory, driving performance, and so forth, which is detectable by refined observation.

Sleep. The oxybarbiturates are used more for the production of sleep than for any other purpose. In most respects, barbiturate-induced sleep resembles physiological sleep. However, barbiturates reduce the amount of time spent in the REM phase of sleep, and, in this respect at least, barbiturate-induced sleep differs from physiological sleep (*see* Kay *et al.,* 1972). It has been claimed by some investigators that deprivation of this phase of sleep may have deleterious effects.

Subjects deprived of REM sleep for several nights exhibit a rebound increase in the proportion of time spent in REM sleep following the period of deprivation. During regular administration of barbiturates, the amount of REM sleep per night is reduced at first and then gradually returns to normal, as tolerance to the REM-suppressing effect of the drug develops. When the drug is withdrawn, there is a rebound increase in nightly REM sleep, and irregularities in REM sleep cycles may continue for many nights, associated with nightmares and a feeling of having slept badly (Oswald and Priest, 1965). Prolonged use of barbiturates increases restlessness during the late stages of sleep, causes anxiety, and increases plasma concentrations of growth hormone but decreases those of adrenocorticosteroids (*see* Ogunremi *et al.*, 1973).

In some individuals and in some circumstances, small doses of barbiturates produce overt excitement instead of sedation. In this respect, the action of barbiturates is not unlike that of alcohol; as in the case of alcohol, the effect is quite variable, depending on both personality and environment. With the racemic barbiturates, however, it is possible that the R(+) isomer makes an important contribution to the excitement phase.

Aftereffects. Drowsiness may last for only a few hours after a hypnotic dose of barbiturates, but subtle distortions of mood and impairment of judgment and fine motor skills may persist for many hours. Thus, 200-mg doses of secobarbital at bedtime have been shown to produce performance decrement 10 to 22 hours later in multidimensional tests designed to measure pilot proficiency in simulated air missions (McKenzie and Elliott, 1965).

The aftereffects of barbiturates may be manifested as overt excitement. Thus, an individual with a slowly waning concentration of barbiturate in his tissues may awaken slightly intoxicated and feel euphoric and energetic; later, as the demands of his daytime environment challenge his possibly impaired faculties, he may display irritability and temper.

It is not certain whether all aftereffects are due to residual concentrations of the active barbiturate or to certain isomers or metabolites. Aftereffects might also be *withdrawal symptoms,* which have been shown to occur after short periods of barbiturate or alcohol intoxication (*see* Chapter 16). Additionally, aftereffects may be caused by deprivation of some restorative process that occurs in natural sleep but not in barbiturate-induced sleep or by the retardation or interruption of certain diurnal cycles, with their possible desynchronization.

Occasionally, in experimental animals, very long-lasting aftereffects have been observed following 1 or 2 anesthetic doses of a barbiturate (Aston and Hibbeln, 1967).

The impairment of memory for events that occur during barbiturate sedation is not properly an aftereffect but, rather, an acute effect that interferes with the inscription of the memory trace.

Hyperalgesia. The barbiturates, unlike the gaseous and volatile anesthetics, lack significant ability to obtund the sense of pain without definite impairment of consciousness. By most experimental criteria, they are not classified as analgesics. Indeed, in small doses, the barbiturates may increase the reaction to painful stimuli (Dundee, 1960; Clutton-Brock, 1961). Taken by themselves, the barbiturates cannot be relied upon to relieve pain, or even to produce sedation or sleep in the presence of severe pain. On the basis of studies in mice, Neal (1965) has concluded that the hyperalgesic effect of barbiturates is not shared by most nonbarbiturate hypnotics. An adequate comparative study of the hyperalgesic properties of hypnotic compounds in man has not been made. Although barbiturates have been claimed to enhance analgesia from other drugs, a sound clinical assessment of their contribution to the efficacy of various analgesic drug combinations remains to be made. In experimental animals, barbiturates antagonize analgesics.

Anesthesia. The commonly used thiobarbiturates and certain ultrashort-acting oxybarbiturates may be administered intravenously to induce surgical anesthesia. This use is discussed in Chapter 8.

EEG Effects. When administered intravenously in small doses, or after oral ingestion, the barbiturates produce an increase in the energy of the high-frequency part of the EEG spectrum—initially at 25 to 35 Hz, then soon shifting to 15 to 25 Hz. This fast activity ("barbiturate activation") from the frontal cortex spreads to the parietal and occipital cortex and recedes in the reverse order as the effect of the drug wears off. It is accompanied by clouding of consciousness and, occasionally, euphoria. As the dose is increased, large-amplitude, random slow waves (5 to 12 Hz) similar to those occurring during sleep appear superimposed on the high-frequency waves and consciousness is lost, although the patient may continue to respond to strong painful stimuli. The 5- to 12-Hz waves usually appear in spindle-shaped bursts called spindles. The pacemaker for the spindles resides in the thalamus. Increasing the dose still further causes a decrease in the frequency of the waves to 1 to 3 Hz. At this point mild-to-moderate noxious stimuli fail to evoke responses. With still higher doses the amplitudes of the wave forms diminish, and there are occasional brief periods of electrical silence—the "burst-suppression" pattern. Major surgical procedures can be undertaken at this time. Although normal sleep interrupts

EEG coherence among certain limbic structures, even during "burst suppression" caused by thiopental this coherence is not affected (Brazier, 1967). The periods of electrical silence become longer as depression becomes more severe, and eventually all electrical activity disappears. The EEG patterns produced by barbiturates are grossly similar to those produced by gaseous and volatile anesthetic agents (Chapter 3); however, there are minor differences, particularly in the induction stage. The effects of barbiturates on the resting EEG and evoked responses have been reviewed by Clark and Rosner (1973) and Rosner and Clark (1973).

The Reticular Activating System. Although attempts have been made to localize the action of barbiturates to certain gross regions of the brain stem, such as the midbrain tegmentum or hypothalamus, drugs of this class apparently act at all levels of the neuraxis. Nevertheless, the reticular activating system is exquisitely sensitive to the depressant effects of the barbiturates and other sedative-hypnotic and anesthetic agents. Whatever may be the effects of barbiturates elsewhere in the CNS, it is the effect on the reticular system that seems to be responsible for the inability to maintain wakefulness under the influence of a barbiturate. The present view of the importance of effects on the reticular system in drug-induced sleep is based upon an enormous body of evidence accumulated by many investigators (*see* reviews by Killam, 1962; Rosner and Clark, 1973).

The early high-frequency response of the EEG to barbiturates resembles that from electrical arousal of the reticular formation, and the threshold for EEG arousal may be transiently lowered; however, the hippocampal component of the arousal response is missing, and true arousal does not occur. Ultimately, the threshold of the reticular system to direct electrical stimulation and the potentials evoked in the system by a variety of sensory stimuli are depressed; this effect occurs with doses that only slightly affect transmission in primary sensory pathways. The work of Magni and coworkers (1961) has shed some light on the phasic nature of the early EEG response. Evidence that depression of medullary structures is responsible for the high-frequency activity was obtained; in spinal cats with the basilar artery clamped, intracarotid injections of thiopental perfused the midbrain and produced the characteristic irregular, slow waves of sleep in the EEG, whereas intravertebral injections had the opposite effect, depressing the medullary structures and producing EEG activation.

Certain cerebellar effects of barbiturates once thought to result from an action on the mossy fiber system may be an indirect effect of an action on the reticulospinal tract and an alteration of modulation of spino-olivo-cerebellar transmission (Gordon *et al.*, 1972).

Anticonvulsant Action. In anesthetic doses, all the clinically employed barbiturates are capable of inhibiting convulsions, such as occur in strychnine poisoning, teta-nus, and status epilepticus. However, *phenobarbital* has a selective anticonvulsant effect, useful especially in the symptomatic therapy of grand mal epilepsy. This antiepileptic property is not shared by other barbiturates except *mephobarbital* and *metharbital*. It is unrelated to sedation, since nonsedative doses are often effective and because amphetamine counteracts the sedation without abolishing the anticonvulsant effect.

Studies of the effects of phenobarbital and other barbiturates on the epileptiform afterdischarges elicited by repetitive electrical stimulation of various brain structures have been reviewed by Domino (1962). In most structures the threshold for initiation of an afterdischarge is elevated and the duration of the afterdischarge shortened by the barbiturates, although exceptions have been noted. Phenobarbital increases the threshold for electrical stimulation of the motor cortex in doses that minimally affect the threshold of the reticular system (Aston and Domino, 1961). In this respect, phenobarbital more closely resembles phenytoin than it does barbiturates; however, it is improbable that the two drugs have the same mechanism of action, since, unlike phenobarbital, phenytoin does not suppress the convulsive activity that characterizes the barbiturate withdrawal syndrome (Essig and Carter, 1962). Additional details of the anticonvulsant properties of phenobarbital are given in Chapter 13.

Respiration. Barbiturates are respiratory depressants, affecting both the drive to respiration and the mechanism responsible for the rhythmic character of respiratory movements.

Respiratory Drive. Respiration is normally maintained by three physiological influences, or "drives," differentially affected by barbiturates and other depressant drugs: (1) a "neurogenic drive," possibly originating in the reticular activating system; (2) a chemical drive, dependent on the carbon dioxide tension (P_{CO_2}) and pH of arterial blood and cerebrospinal fluid; and (3) a hypoxic drive. The effects of hypoxia are mediated by the chemoreceptors of the carotid and aortic bodies, whereas the effects of changes in pH and P_{CO_2} are due principally to a direct action on medullary structures. The neurogenic drive is most sensitive to depression by hypnotics. (*See* Symposium, 1963a.)

In the waking state, normal ventilation is largely controlled by the neurogenic drive.

This drive is reduced by drug-induced sleep, and the control of respiration is then dominated by the direct action of CO_2 and hydrogen ions on medullary respiratory centers. The effects of an oral hypnotic dose of a barbiturate closely resemble those of natural sleep. During sleep there is a decrease in alveolar ventilation, an increase in alveolar CO_2 tension (3 to 5 mm Hg), and a slight decrease in the O_2 saturation of arterial blood. However, with low doses of barbiturates, the response to CO_2 is occasionally slightly enhanced (Brown et al., 1973).

As a dose of barbiturate is increased, the hypoxic and chemical drives to respiration are diminished roughly in proportion to dose. According to Harris and Slawson (1965), the hypoxic drive is measurably affected by hypnotic drugs at about three times the conventional dose. With this dose, the sensitivity of the medullary centers to CO_2 is affected little more than it is during natural sleep. However, the hypoxic drive persists at levels of intoxication causing complete insensitivity of the respiratory centers to CO_2. Thus, as intoxication becomes more severe, there is a shift in the control of respiration from the CO_2-sensitive areas of the medulla to the more primitive receptors of the carotid and aortic bodies. Eventually, if the concentration is increased still further, the powerful hypoxic drive also fails. However, the margin between the lighter planes of surgical anesthesia and dangerous respiratory depression is sufficient to permit the ultrashort-acting barbiturates to be used (with suitable precautions) as intravenous anesthetic agents.

Respiratory Reflexes and Rhythmicity. The barbiturates only slightly depress protective reflexes until the degree of intoxication is sufficient to produce severe respiratory depression. In animals the cough reflex is depressed only by doses that seriously embarrass respiration, and in this respect the barbiturates differ from opioids and other antitussives that may exert a selective effect on cough reflexes. Coughing, sneezing, hiccoughing, and laryngospasm occur not infrequently when barbiturates are employed as intravenous anesthetic agents. Indeed, laryngospasm is one of the chief respiratory complications of barbiturate anesthesia.

Cardiovascular System. In oral sedative or hypnotic doses, the barbiturates do not produce significant cardiovascular effects, except for a slight decrease in blood pressure and heart rate such as occurs in normal sleep. During thiopental anesthesia, there is usually either no change or a fall in mean arterial pressure, the latter being more pronounced in hypertensive patients. Hypotension is caused, in part, by the release of histamine. In some subjects, however, thiopental produces an increase in blood pressure. The medullary vasomotor center is depressed, but in normal subjects there is enough reserve in the compensatory reflexes to override partly the depressant effect. However, in congestive heart failure or hypovolemic shock, in which the reflexes are already quite active and the reflex reserve has been drawn upon, barbiturates can be expected to cause an exaggerated fall in blood pressure. Because barbiturates impair cardiovascular adjustments to inflation of the lung, positive-pressure respiration should be used cautiously, only when necessary for adequate pulmonary ventilation, in patients anesthetized with thiopental.

Apart from changes in blood pressure, the following cardiovascular changes have often been noted when thiopental and other intravenous thiobarbiturates are administered after conventional preanesthetic medication: a decrease in cardiac output; an increase in total calculated peripheral resistance, which develops only over a period of time and is probably partly compensatory to decreased cardiac output and partly central in origin; an increase or no change in heart rate; a decrease in intrathoracic blood volume; an increase in blood flow and volume in the extremities; a decrease or no change in the central, right atrial, and peripheral venous pressures; and a decrease in cerebral blood flow, with a marked fall in cerebrospinal fluid pressure. Although thiobarbiturates regularly cause cardiac arrhythmias in experimental animals, they rarely do so in man. Thiopental does not sensitize the automatic tissue of the heart to catecholamines. In general, the effects of thiopental anesthesia on the cardiovascular system are benign in comparison with the effects of other (volatile) anesthetic agents, and do not constitute a hazard in normal clinical practice. (For a detailed comparison of the effects of various anesthetic agents on hemodynamics, *see* the review by Price, 1960.)

Experimentally, high concentrations of barbiturates decrease myocardial contractility. There is no evidence that direct myocardial depression occurs in man or experimental animals with regular anesthetic doses, and a decrease in cardiac output can be explained by other mechanisms. In various *in-vitro* and *in-vivo* experimental preparations, the myocardial depressant concentration of pentobarbital ranges from about 125 to 250 mg per liter or kilogram, which is several times that required to cause anesthesia; heart failure in dogs occurs with doses that are approximately three times those necessary to cause respiratory failure. However, studies have not been made of the myocardial effects of smaller doses acting over a long period of time; it is possible that a direct action contributes to the myocardial depression that accompanies acute barbiturate poisoning. The intracellular distribution of calcium in the myocardium is altered by barbiturates (*see* Nayler and Szeto, 1972), and it is probable that such changes relate to the negative inotropic effects. Both cardiac glycosides and β-adrenergic agonists antagonize the myocardial depressant action.

In high concentrations, the barbiturates depress vascular smooth muscle, but this action is probably not significant in clinical doses, although it probably contributes to the cardiovascular depression that occurs in acute barbiturate intoxication. Intra-arterial oxybarbiturates cause vasodilatation, but thiobarbiturates result in vasoconstriction and intense pain followed by thrombosis of the artery.

Gastrointestinal Tract. The oxybarbiturates tend to decrease the tonus of the gastrointestinal musculature and the amplitude of rhythmic contractions. The locus of action is partly peripheral (*see* above) and partly central, depending on the dose. Hypnotic doses of amobarbital reduce the motility of the sigmoid colon in fasted human subjects; a similar effect occurs during physiological sleep. On emergence from barbiturate-induced sleep, there may be a period of intestinal and colonic hypermotility. A hypnotic dose does not significantly delay gastric emptying in man. Gastric secretions may be somewhat depressed by barbiturates. The relief of various gastrointestinal symptoms by sedative doses is probably largely due to the central depressant action.

Ureter, Urinary Bladder, and Uterus. In high concentrations not attained therapeutically except possibly during intravenous anesthesia, barbiturates depress the smooth muscle of the ureter and urinary bladder. Hypnotic doses do not significantly impair uterine activity during labor. Full anesthetic doses, on the other hand, decrease the force and frequency of uterine contractions. More important in the use of barbiturates during labor is their possible respiratory depressant effect on the infant, since the placenta offers no significant barrier to the passage of barbiturates to the fetus.

Kidney. In the concentrations required to produce deep anesthesia, the barbiturates exert direct effects on renal tubular transport mechanisms. In dogs anesthetized with pentobarbital, the Tm of *p*-aminohippurate may be depressed by as much as 15 to 25%; barbiturates in concentrations comparable to those in the plasma during anesthesia also depress the active uptake of *p*-aminohippurate by rat and rabbit renal cortex slices *in vitro*. When indirect, neurogenic, or hormonal effects are excluded, pentobarbital appears to depress the sodium and glucose reabsorptive processes by a direct action on tubular cells (Blake, 1957). However, the direct effects may be overshadowed, at least in part, by changes in renal hemodynamics that are largely the result of systemic hypotension, and by the tendency of barbiturates and certain other anesthetic agents to stimulate the secretion of antidiuretic hormone. The net effect is a decrease in urine flow. The effect on electrolyte excretion varies, depending on the previous state of the subject. In hydropenic dogs subjected to solute diuresis, urine osmolarity is not altered by pentobarbital anesthesia, whereas the drug may increase urine osmolarity in hydrated animals (West and Keller, 1955). The administration of a hypnotic dose of secobarbital to subjects undergoing maximal water diuresis is usually followed by a slight reduction in urine flow; this is attributable to a hemodynamic action rather than the release of antidiuretic hormone, since there is no corresponding increase in the osmolarity of the urine (Papper *et al.,* 1960). Severe oliguria or anuria may occur in acute barbiturate poisoning, largely as a result of the marked hypotension.

Liver. In the therapeutic dose range, barbiturates do not impair normal hepatic function. In patients hypersensitive to barbiturates, however, severe hepatic damage can occur from ordinary doses, usually associated with dermatitis and involvement of other parenchymatous organs.

Barbiturates exert remarkable actions on certain hepatic functions. Probably best known are those on the microsomal drug-metabolizing system (*see* Chapter 1), and there is now an enormous literature on the subject.

The barbiturates combine with cytochrome P-450 and thus competitively interfere with the biotransformations of a number of substrates of this enzyme, which include other drugs as well as endogenous substrates, such as steroids. Thus, adverse drug interactions and potential endocrine imbalance can result from such inhibition. The other substrates reciprocally inhibit barbiturate biotransformations. The nature of the inhibition is not simple, however, because barbiturates do not inhibit the biotransformations of all drugs that are substrates of the microsomal enzyme system. The barbiturates do not necessarily themselves need to be oxidized by the enzyme system during the time that they inhibit the biotransformations of other drugs. Various barbiturates differ in their affinity for cytochrome P-450. *In vitro,* allyl barbiturates actually destroy cytochrome P-450, but whether this effect occurs *in vivo* is unknown. Barbiturates also inhibit NADH cytochrome–c oxidoreductase, but it is not clear to what extent this effect contributes to the overall inhibition of the system. The biotransformations of barbiturates by the system are discussed on page 115.

The barbiturates cause a nonspecific increase in the activity of the hepatic microsomal enzyme system, which is the result of an increase in the enzyme content rather than a change in the properties of the enzymes. Not only is the rate of metabolism of a number of drugs increased but also that of steroids and certain other endogenous substrates. Glucuronyl transferase activity is increased. Parke (1971) lists (abridged) 49 biotransformations known to be accelerated. Not all biotransformations are affected equally, but a convenient rule of thumb is that at maximal induction in man the rate is approximately doubled. The inducing effect is not limited to the microsomal enzymes; for example, there is an increase in δ-aminolevulinic acid (ALA) synthetase, a mitochondrial enzyme, in aldehyde dehydrogenase, a cytoplasmic enzyme, and in the conjugation of sulfobromophthalein with glutathione. The effect on ALA synthetase results in an increase in porphyrin synthesis, which provides heme for the induced cytochrome P-450. Barbiturates increase the rate of synthesis of certain proteins, such as the Y and Z proteins, which are believed to regulate the entry of anionic compounds into hepatic cells; however, the synthesis of albumin and blood clotting factors is not affected. In addition to porphyrins and proteins, the synthesis and turnover of bile salts and cholesterol are increased. The induction of the microsomal enzymes gives rise to adverse drug interactions. For example, barbiturates can shorten the prothrombin time in patients receiving prothrombinopenic anticoagulants by causing a biotransformation-related decrease in the plasma concentrations of the drugs; the potency of digitoxin may be decreased by accelerated conversion to digoxin. The capacity of barbiturates to increase the synthesis of porphyrins is responsible for one of the more bizarre and dangerous side effects. In patients suffering from acute intermittent porphyria, the drugs may precipitate a severe attack, possibly culminating in paralysis and death. These patients already have a defect in the allosteric regulation of ALA synthetase, and barbiturates exacerbate an ongoing pathology. Hepatic enzyme induction also lends itself to certain clinical uses (page 119).

The inducing effect of the barbiturates is accompanied by a considerable hypertrophy of the endoplasmic reticulum and a moderate increase in weight of the liver. There are no apparent detrimental alterations in hepatic function. The principal mechanism of induction seems to be an intranuclear stabilization of preribosomal RNA, which is destined to be incorporated into membrane-bound polyribosomes. The effect requires several days of treatment to become maximal. There is, however, a short-term effect to increase the synthesis of cytoplasmic RNAs and to decrease the activity of both nuclear and cytoplasmic ribonucleases.

The effect of the biotransformable barbiturates to increase the rate of their own metabolism accounts for part of the tolerance to the drugs. Many sedative-hypnotics and various anesthetics and ethanol also induce the microsomal enzymes, and cross-tolerance is also thus partly accounted for. A number of other drugs, organochlorine insecticides, and certain food additives also can induce the microsomal enzymes and affect the elimination of barbiturates. The nutritional, pathological, and chemical factors that affect microsomal induction and related drug interactions are discussed in reviews by Conney (1967), Cooksley and Powell (1971), and Parke (1971), and in a symposium (1973).

Choleresis results from treatment with phenobarbital but not other barbiturates. In rats, increased bile flow appears to be independent of bile salt excretion; however, in man, both bile salt-dependent flow and bile salt–independent flow are increased (see Sharp and Mirkin, 1972; Stiehl et al., 1973). The biliary excretion of phospholipids, sulfobromophthalein, indocyanine green, rose bengal, and various drugs is also increased. The increase in bile salt secretion probably affects the absorption of various drugs and foodstuffs.

Tolerance. Both types of tolerance defined in Chapter 16 develop when barbiturates are taken repeatedly at short intervals. *Drug-disposition tolerance* to barbiturates results from the activation of drug-metabolizing enzyme systems in the liver, and is manifested by the more rapid detoxication of barbiturates, a decrease in sleeping time, and an increase in the average dose required to maintain a given tissue concentration. This type of tolerance can be demonstrated in animals after one or two administrations of the drugs, and is most marked for those agents with durations of action determined by the rate of metabolic degradation. *Pharmacodynamic tolerance* involves adaptation of nervous tissue to the presence of the drug. Barbiturate addicts often are resistant to the hypnotic effects of barbiturates and other general depressants, including ethanol and gaseous and volatile anesthetics. However, tolerance to the hypnotic effects of barbiturates evidently does not significantly increase the lethal dose.

Acute Tolerance. A number of investigators (see Maynert and Klingman, 1960) have reported that the plasma concentration at the time of awakening from barbiturate intoxication depends on the dose administered; the larger the dose, the higher is the plasma concentration at the time of return of consciousness. This suggests that the CNS may become resistant to the effects of the drugs even during a single administration, and the phenomenon is accordingly known as "acute tolerance." The mechanism of acute tolerance is unknown.

Dependence. The barbiturates have acquired a popular reputation as "addicting" drugs, especially likely to produce psychic and physical dependence. However, the barbiturates do not differ from other sedative-hypnotic drugs in this respect. The problem of addiction and a physiological basis for the development of physical dependence are discussed in Chapter 16. But it is important to emphasize here that, clinically, the most important preventive measures in patients without a history of previous abuse of drugs is to prescribe no more than the official or approved daily dose and to encourage the patient to do without the drug at the earliest possible time (*see* Clift, 1972).

The severity of the abstinence syndrome varies, depending on the depth, duration, and continuity of intoxication prior to withdrawal, and on the rate at which the drug is removed from the tissues by metabolic degradation and excretion. Persons dependent upon various barbiturates may be withdrawn more smoothly if the long-acting phenobarbital is substituted for a shorter-acting barbiturate prior to withdrawal (*see* Gay *et al.,* 1972). In epileptics, the discontinuation of barbiturate medication may result in status epilepticus, even when the patient has been taking a long-acting drug (*e.g.,* phenobarbital) in relatively small daily doses. Neither phenytoin nor chlorpromazine will prevent barbiturate abstinence convulsions.

Absorption and Routes of Administration. *Oral.* On principle, one would expect the short-acting, lipid-soluble barbiturates to be absorbed more rapidly than the long-acting barbiturates, and this is true for the extreme examples of lipid solubility. Thus, in man, oral thiopental may be completely absorbed from the stomach within 30 minutes, while the plasma concentration of phenobarbital or pentobarbital may still be increasing after 1½ hours or longer. However, the rate-limiting step in absorption is usually not passage through the gastrointestinal mucosa but the dissolution and dispersal of the drug in the gastrointestinal contents. Thus, Sjögren and associates (1965) found little difference in the rates of absorption of various short- and intermediate-acting compounds, when they were encapsulated in the form of free acids.

On the other hand, the sodium salts are more rapidly absorbed than the free acids (although they are extremely alkaline and may cause epigastric distress); the drugs are more rapidly absorbed when they are taken in dilute solution than in other forms; food in the stomach decreases the rate of absorption but not the amount absorbed.

Rectal. Barbiturates are absorbed from the colon, and rectal administration is occasionally used, as in infants or in prolonged convulsive states such as tetanus. The drug may be given in suspension or as a suppository; the soluble sodium salt may be incorporated in a retention enema.

Intramuscular. If necessary, the sodium salts of barbiturates can be injected intramuscularly in 10% solution. Subcutaneous injection may result in necrosis and sloughing, owing to the extreme alkalinity of the solution. Thiobarbiturates are not injected by these routes.

Intravenous. Intravenous administration should not be attempted except in an emergency or when adequate provisions are made for supporting respiration and circulation. In the emergency therapy of convulsive states, a 5% aqueous solution of a sodium salt of a barbiturate is employed. The injection must be made slowly, with due regard for the time required for the drug to penetrate the blood-brain barrier. In the case of long-acting agents such as phenobarbital, maximal central depression may not occur until 15 minutes or more after intravenous injection. The ultrashort-acting thiobarbiturates (administered in a 2.5% solution) and methohexital (1.0% solution) attain maximal concentrations in the brain in less than 30 seconds after intravenous injection. An alarming fall in blood pressure to shock levels is sometimes observed, especially after rapid injection. The intravenous injection of barbiturates often produces apnea, and occasionally laryngospasm, coughing, and other respiratory difficulties. Fatal accidents have resulted from the intravenous administration of barbiturates by inexperienced persons.

Distribution. There exists no impenetrable barrier to the diffusion of barbiturates in the body; consequently, if the sojourn of the drug in the plasma is sufficiently long, it will be distributed to all tissues and fluids. Small amounts of the barbiturates may appear in the milk after the ingestion of large doses. Barbiturates readily cross the placental barrier, and, within a few minutes after the injection of a short- or ultrashort-acting barbiturate, the concentration in the fetal blood approaches that in the maternal venous blood.

Physicochemical Factors. Barbiturates are preferentially concentrated in certain tissues, depending on the specific compound and the time after administration. The important physicochemical factors that determine the passage of drugs across cytostructural barriers and the manner in which they influence drug distribution and excretion have been presented in Chapter 1. In the case of barbiturates, the careful study of a large number of congeners has made these data particularly complete, and they are summarized in Table 9–2.

The three most important factors affecting the distribution and fate of the barbiturates are *lipid solubility* (partition coefficient), *protein binding,* and *extent of ionization.* In their undissociated form, the barbiturates have a rather high affinity for nonpolar solvents; however, there are enormous differences between the various compounds. When the drugs are ordered with respect to their affinity for a nonpolar solvent (Table 9–2), there is a correlation with pharmacological properties. Thus the more highly lipid-soluble compounds are short-acting agents with a rapid onset of action. They tend to be more rapidly degraded metabolically and are almost completely reabsorbed by the renal tubule.

Organ Tissues and Fluids. A fraction of the barbiturate in blood is reversibly bound to plasma protein, chiefly albumin. Protein binding appears to depend on the same structural feature that determines affinity for nonpolar solvents, since those drugs with the highest methylene chloride:water partition coefficients tend to be bound to the greatest extent (Table 9–2). Approximately 80% of the thiopental in blood is bound to plasma protein, whereas only a small fraction (perhaps 5%) of barbital is similarly bound. The intensity of CNS depression can be increased by acidic drugs such as aspirin or sulfonamides, which displace barbiturates from the plasma proteins.

The cerebrospinal fluid is virtually protein free. Accordingly, the maximal concentration of barbiturates attained in cerebrospinal fluid is less than the plasma concentration, being in most cases slightly less than the concentration in an ultrafiltrate of plasma. The concentration in ocular fluid is similar to that in cerebrospinal fluid.

In tissues, the barbiturate concentration is generally as high as or slightly higher than in plasma. With the exception of body fat, the capacity of tissues to concentrate barbiturates depends largely on protein binding, and the various barbiturates show the same relative affinities to tissue protein as to plasma protein. Somewhat higher concentrations are found in liver and kidney than in other tissues. Although fat depots have a potential greatly to concentrate the ultrashort-acting barbiturates, the binding to plasma protein, the slow rate of blood flow in fat, and the low surface:volume ratio of adipocytes make uptake slow in comparison to elimination, so that ultrahigh concentrations can be achieved only by repetitive dosage.

Distribution and Rate of Entry in Brain. Highly lipid-soluble drugs, such as thiopental, attain maximal concentrations in the brain within two or three passages of the blood. Barbital and phenobarbital, on the other hand, with low partition coefficients, penetrate the blood-brain barrier slowly, and 15 minutes or more may be required for the induction of sleep after their intravenous administration. If sufficient time is allowed after administration, both the short- and long-acting barbiturates tend to be uniformly distributed throughout the brain. During the first few minutes after injection, however, thiopental is found in the highest concentrations in those brain structures that have the greatest blood flow (cortex, geniculate bodies, and colliculi). Regional differences in blood flow have little effect on the distribution of the slowly penetrating agents. Certain pathological conditions (*e.g.,* meningitis) and certain drugs (*e.g.,* anticholinesterases) may increase the rate of entry of long-acting barbiturates into the brain.

Effect of Ionization. Partition as determined by pH favors a higher plasma than cytosol concentration of barbiturates. The intracerebral concentration is increased by lowering and decreased by elevating plasma pH, but only if intracellular pH is not affected proportionally (*see* Chapter 1). Thus, metabolic acid-base alterations have a greater effect on distribution of a barbiturate and depth of CNS depression than do respiratory acid-base disorders.

Table 9–2. BARBITURATES: RELATION BETWEEN PHYSICOCHEMICAL FACTORS, DISTRIBUTION, AND FATE

BARBITURATE	PARTITION COEFFICIENT *	PLASMA PROTEIN BINDING †	BRAIN PROTEIN BINDING ‡	DELAY IN ONSET OF ACTIVITY §	EXCRETED BY KIDNEY ¶	DEGRADATION BY LIVER SLICES #	pK_a **
Barbital	1	0.05	0.06	22	65–90	—	7.8
Phenobarbital	3	0.20	0.19	12	27–50	—	7.3
Pentobarbital	39	0.35	0.29	0.1	—	0.21	8.0
Secobarbital	52	0.44	0.39	0.1	—	0.28	7.9
Thiopental	580	0.65	0.50	—	—	0.38	7.4

* (Concentration in methylene chloride):(concentration in aqueous phase) of the nonionized form at approximately 25° C (Bush, 1963).

† Binding of 0.001 M barbituric acids by 1% bovine serum albumin in M/15 phosphate buffer at pH 7.4; fraction bound (Goldbaum and Smith, 1954).

‡ Fraction of barbiturate bound by rabbit brain homogenates (Goldbaum and Smith, 1954).

§ Minutes until anesthesia after intravenous injection in mice (Butler, 1942).

¶ Approximate percentage of total dose excreted unchanged in urine of man.

Fraction degraded *in vitro* by liver slices in 3 hours (Dorfman and Goldbaum, 1947).

** Ionization exponent at 25° C (Bush, 1963). The values have not been corrected thermodynamically.

Nevertheless, ventilation does affect the depth of anesthesia. Alterations in plasma pH affect urine pH, thus influencing tubular reabsorption and excretion of the barbiturates, as described below.

Termination of Activity. Three processes are responsible for the termination of the central depressant actions of the barbiturates: *physical redistribution, metabolic degradation,* and *renal excretion.* All reduce the plasma concentration of the barbiturate and result in the withdrawal of the drug from its site of action in the CNS. The fate of a specific barbiturate depends on its lipid solubility. Barbital, having low lipid solubility, is largely excreted unchanged by the kidney. Physical redistribution plays an especially important role in the case of the ultrashort-acting, highly lipid-soluble agents. Except for barbital, all barbiturates are primarily transformed, chiefly by the liver, and the metabolic products are excreted in the urine and, less commonly, in the feces.

Redistribution. The role of redistribution of the drug from brain to other tissues has been studied most thoroughly in the case of thiopental (*see* Symposium, 1963b). The rate of metabolism is much too slow (10 to 15% per hour) to account for the short duration of action of this compound. The rapid emergence from sleep after the administration of a single intravenous dose of thiopental depends on a shift of the drug from the brain to other tissue compartments. The rate at which the various tissue compartments take up the drug from the blood is related to their blood flow. Because of their high perfusion rates, the brain and certain visceral organs (liver, kidney, heart, etc.), which together receive 70% of the total cardiac output, exhibit maximal concentrations of thiopental within 30 seconds after its intravenous administration. On the other hand, about 15 to 30 minutes is required for muscle and skin to equilibrate with plasma, and more than an hour is required to redistribute to fat. As the muscle and fat take up thiopental, the plasma concentration falls, and the drug diffuses out of the brain along its concentration gradient. By 30 minutes, the brain and viscera may have given up as much as 90% of their initial peak concentrations to the nonvisceral lean tissues and fat depots. It is

for this reason that a patient may awaken within 15 to 30 minutes after a single intravenous injection of thiopental, even though the amount metabolized in this time is very small. Thus, small, single intravenous doses of an ultrashort-acting barbiturate have a transient action not because of rapid elimination or destruction of the drug but because the drug is redistributed from the brain to other tissues. In the first 15 to 20 minutes, the decline in brain concentration is due largely to the uptake of the drug by muscle. After that, uptake by fat and metabolic destruction account for the declining plasma concentration. The fact that thiopental remains in the body after it ceases to be active accounts for the cumulative effects of repeated doses of this agent, the persistent effect of large doses, and the characteristic "hangover" that may last for many hours after the emergence from thiopental-induced anesthesia.

The same principles apply to other ultrashort-acting, highly lipid-soluble compounds, including thiamylal, methitural, hexobarbital, methohexital, and thiohexital. However, metabolic degradation occurs more rapidly with some of these compounds than with thiopental, especially thiohexital, which has an average plasma half-time of 2.8 hours, which is shorter than that of any other barbiturate (Mark *et al.,* 1968).

Renal Excretion. Barbiturates not destroyed in the body are excreted unchanged in the urine. Only barbital is dependent mainly on renal excretion for the termination of its pharmacological action; 65 to 90% of the total dose appears in the urine unaltered. As much as 50% of a hypnotic dose of phenobarbital or aprobarbital may be excreted unchanged by the kidney. The other compounds rarely appear in the urine in unchanged form except in small or negligible quantities. Renal elimination occurs slowly. In normal adults, only 8% of an oral hypnotic dose of barbital is eliminated in the urine in the first 12 hours, 20% in 24 hours, and 35 to 65% in 48 hours. Traces of barbital may be detected in the urine as long as 8 to 12 days after the administration of a single hypnotic dose. Phenobarbital and aprobarbital are also eliminated slowly, over a period of several days.

The *renal clearance rate* of the barbiturates depends on a number of factors. Glomerular filtration of the drug is reduced by *binding to plasma proteins,* and is therefore less for phenobarbital than for barbital. The barbiturates in the glomerular filtrate are reabsorbed by *passive back diffusion* in a manner similar to that of urea. Since the tubular epithelium presents a lipid diffusion barrier to the barbiturates, only the relatively polar compounds (barbital, phenobarbital, etc.) escape tubular reabsorption to a significant degree. Back diffusion is proportional to the amount of water reabsorbed. In dogs, as much as 50 to 60% of the filtered barbital may be excreted during a marked osmotic diuresis, as compared with about 10% during water diuresis (Giotti and Maynert, 1951). At any given rate of urine flow, the clearance of phenobarbital is much greater in alkaline than in acid urine, because of the principle of partitioning according to pH. On the basis of experimental work on dogs, Waddell and Butler (1957) have estimated that it should be possible to triple the rate of elimination of phenobarbital by administration of sodium bicarbonate. These facts provide the rationale for the use of alkalis and diuresis in conjunction with diuretic agents in the treatment of intoxication with long-acting barbiturates.

When renal function is impaired, barbiturates that depend on the kidney for elimination may cause severe CNS depression and thereby may further reduce renal function. Furthermore, uremia may increase sensitivity to barbiturates and intensify the depression. Bilateral nephrectomy makes animals more susceptible to thiopental; this susceptibility does not occur immediately after the operation but gradually develops concomitantly with the increase in nonprotein nitrogen in the blood, and thus it cannot be attributed to any capacity of the kidney to degrade or sequester thiopental (Richards *et al.,* 1953). There is a decrease in the extent of protein binding of thiopental after nephrectomy, associated with a fall in the albumin fraction of plasma proteins. Thus, the unbound, freely diffusible thiopental in plasma may be abnormally high when this drug is administered to a patient with renal disease. Thiopental is more extensively bound to plasma protein than is hexobarbital, and the increase in barbiturate-induced depression following nephrectomy in animals is greater for thiopental than for hexobarbital (Taylor *et al.,* 1954).

Biliary Excretion. In rats, the metabolites of phenobarbital and pentobarbital are excreted into the bile in high concentration along with low concentrations of the unchanged drugs. The clinical implications of these facts require elucidation.

Site of Metabolic Degradation. Most barbiturates are transformed in the body to inactive metabolites. The principal site of biotransformation is the liver. The oxybarbiturates are transformed only by the liver; the thiobarbiturates may be transformed to a small extent in other tissues,

especially kidney and brain (Dorfman and Goldbaum, 1947; Gould and Shideman, 1952; Cooper and Brodie, 1955, 1957).

It has been reported that patients with impaired hepatic function require less thiopental to maintain surgical anesthesia than do those with normal hepatic function, and that the action of barbiturates may be prolonged in the presence of hepatic disease. However, the effects of barbiturates on patients with hepatic injury have rarely been studied quantitatively, and it appears that the specific dangers ascribed to barbiturates in patients with hepatic disease may have been overemphasized. Sessions and coworkers (1954) administered pentobarbital in hypnotic doses to patients with severe hepatic disease without observing ill effects; there was neither additional impairment of hepatic function nor increased CNS depression. The drug did not disappear less rapidly from the blood than in normal individuals. The hepatic enzymes responsible for metabolizing drugs may be able to function adequately in the presence of severe hepatic disease (Brodie *et al.,* 1959). However, cirrhotic patients may show increased sensitivity to hypnotics, even when adequate biochemical mechanisms for degrading the drug exist. Certainly, barbiturates should be administered with caution, and initially in reduced doses, to patients with hepatic damage. Barbiturates and other hypnotics should not be administered to patients showing the premonitory signs of hepatic coma.

The rates of biotransformation of certain drugs seem to have fixed ratios to one another, and it may be possible to predict the elimination rate and appropriate dose schedule of a barbiturate from the rate of elimination of an index drug, such as sulfinpyrazone (Kadar *et al.,* 1973). Since R(+) and S(−) enantiomorphs are metabolized differently, most of the half-life data on racemic barbiturates are not strictly valid.

Metabolic Products. The liver is the primary organ in terminating the central depressant action of oxybarbiturates. It transforms lipid-soluble agents into more polar derivatives that can then be excreted by the kidney. In mammals, by far the largest proportion of the products of barbiturate metabolism is excreted in the urine; however, a small fraction may appear in the feces by way of the bile.

In being converted into a form that can be excreted, most (but not all) barbiturates lose their pharmacological activity. A great deal of effort has been devoted to the identification of barbiturate metabolites, but in no single case have all the metabolites been accounted for. Barbiturates are transformed by four routes:

1. Oxidation of Radicals at C5. This is by far the most important pathway of metabolism for the barbiturates. The drugs are oxidized at the larger of the two 5-substituent groups, and the products are relatively polar alcohols, ketones, phenols, or carboxylic acids, which may appear in the urine both as free compounds and as glucuronic acid conjugates. As a rule, they do not possess hypnotic activity.

2. N-Dealkylation. In the dog, metharbital and mephobarbital are converted almost entirely into barbital and phenobarbital, respectively, as a result of N-demethylation. N-Demethylation occurs slowly, but barbital and phenobarbital themselves are eliminated even more slowly, so that they may accumulate during the administration of the N-methyl compounds. For example, in patients receiving mephobarbital regularly, the plasma concentration of phenobarbital may be three times that of mephobarbital. The ultrashort-acting agents, hexobarbital and methohexital, undergo N-demethylation to a very slight extent, but the rate of oxidation of the substituents at C5 is so much faster that the active N-demethylation products constitute only a minute fraction of the metabolites and do not contribute to the anesthetic action of the drugs.

3. Desulfuration of Thiobarbiturates. The sulfur of thiobarbiturates may be replaced by oxygen to yield the corresponding oxybarbiturates. The extent to which this process occurs in man is uncertain, but it is doubtful that this route accounts for more than a small fraction of the administered dose.

4. Destruction of the Barbituric Acid Ring. The barbituric acid ring is relatively stable *in vivo*, and hydrolytic cleavage of the ring, although it occurs, is of minor importance. The biotransformations of the barbiturates have been reviewed by Parke (1971).

Inhibition and stimulation of the microsomal enzyme system are discussed above (page 110). Details of the various functions of this system can be found in the various contributions to a symposium (1973).

Preparations and Dosage. Barbiturates are marketed in a bewildering array of preparations, often in mixtures with other drugs, including, for example, other barbiturates, bromides, tranquilizers, analgesics, belladonna alkaloids, sympathomimetic agents, xanthines, antihistamines, spasmolytics, vitamins, antibiotics, digestive enzymes, gastric antacids, and adsorbents. In the United States, phenobarbital is an ingredient in at least 80 different proprietary remedies, each with its own attractive trade name. The barbiturates, alone or in mixtures, may be obtained as powders, elixirs, syrups, drops, capsules, and tablets; in sustained-release forms; and as delayed-release, coated tablets. With few exceptions, proprietary mixtures should

be ignored. They offer little advantage, and whatever convenience they may appear to have is far outweighed by their cost. The physician can easily prescribe drugs for concurrent use, if necessary, and adjust the doses to the specific needs of his patients. Special slow-release forms of the drug would seem to be of little benefit in view of the duration of action of the longer-acting compounds, and their ingestion may greatly confuse the clinical picture should poisoning occur.

Oxybarbiturates are odorless, white crystalline powders that are slightly bitter to the taste, poorly soluble in cold water, but soluble in alcohol and hot water. Aqueous solutions are acid. The sodium salts are freely soluble in water, and their solutions are quite alkaline. Thiobarbiturates are yellow powders.

Only the preparations and doses for some of the more commonly used compounds are given here. The sedative dose is usually about one third to one fourth of the hypnotic dose, and may be repeated three or four times daily.

Amobarbital Sodium, U.S.P. (AMYTAL SODIUM). The hypnotic dose is 100 to 200 mg, ½ to 1 hour before bedtime. The drug is supplied as capsules containing 65 and 200 mg and as a sterile powder in ampuls containing 60, 125, 250, 500, or 1000 mg for injection. For sedation, *Amobarbital,* N.F., is used in a dose of 20 to 30 mg two or three times a day. It is supplied in tablets containing 15, 30, 50, or 100 mg and as elixirs (N.F.) containing 4.4 or 8.8 mg/ml.

Methohexital Sodium, U.S.P. (BREVITAL SODIUM). For induction of intravenous anesthesia, 75 mg is given at the rate of 2 mg per second; for maintenance, 20 to 40 mg is given, as needed.

Pentobarbital Sodium, U.S.P. (NEMBUTAL SODIUM). The sedative dose is 30 to 60 mg, two or three times daily; the hypnotic dose is 100 mg. It is available as a powder, as an elixir containing 4 mg/ml, and as capsules containing 30, 50, and 100 mg. The drug is also available in 100-mg tablets, and in suppositories containing 30 mg (for infants), 60 mg (for children up to 3 years), and 120 and 200 mg (for adults). For parenteral use, sterile solutions of pentobarbital sodium are available in ampuls (50 mg/ml) and in multiple-dose vials (50 mg/ml). Given intramuscularly to adults, the dose should not ordinarily exceed 200 mg, and the injection should be made in a large muscle mass to avoid irritation.

Phenobarbital, U.S.P. (LUMINAL). The sedative dose is 15 to 30 mg, repeated two to four times daily. The average hypnotic dose for adults is 100 mg. The daily intake should not exceed 600 mg. The drug is supplied as a powder, as an elixir containing 4 mg/ml, and as tablets containing 15, 30, 60, and 100 mg. *Phenobarbital Sodium,* U.S.P., is available for parenteral use in ampuls containing 60, 125, 200, and 300 mg of sterile powder, and in ampuls or vials containing solutions of 25, 50, 60, 125, or 150 mg/ml.

Secobarbital, U.S.P. (SECONAL). The average

adult hypnotic dose is 100 mg. Secobarbital is available as the powder, and as an elixir containing 4.4 mg/ml. *Secobarbital Sodium,* U.S.P., is available as a powder, and in capsules containing 30, 50, and 100 mg. The drug is also supplied in suppositories containing 30, 60, 120, and 200 mg. For parenteral administration, it is supplied as a sterile powder in ampuls containing 250 mg and as an injectable solution containing 50 mg/ml.

Thiopental Sodium, U.S.P. (PENTOTHAL SODIUM). For induction of intravenous anesthesia, 150 to 300 mg is given; for maintenance, 12.5 to 50 mg is administered as needed. Given rectally, the dose is 30 to 50 mg/kg, up to a total of 3 g; a 5 to 10% solution or 20% suspension in oil is employed.

Untoward Effects. Untoward effects of the barbiturates are sometimes in the form of "hangover," excitement, or pain. *Hangover* from relatively small hypnotic doses occurs especially in neurotic patients, particularly when the longer-acting barbiturates are employed. After the initial and characteristic period of depression has passed, lassitude, vertigo, nausea, vomiting, and diarrhea may be noted, and emotional disturbances and phobias may be accentuated. In some persons, barbiturates repeatedly produce *excitement* rather than depression, and the patient may appear to be inebriated. This type of idiosyncrasy is most frequent with phenobarbital and N-methylbarbiturates. Like other nonanalgesic hypnotic drugs, the barbiturates, when given in the presence of pain, may cause restlessness, excitement, and even delirium. Rarely, the use of barbiturates results in localized or diffuse myalgic, neuralgic, or arthritic *pain,* especially in psychoneurotic patients with insomnia. The pain may appear in paroxysms, is most intense in the early morning hours, and is most frequently located in the region of the neck, shoulder girdle, and upper limbs. Symptoms may last for days after the use of the drug is discontinued.

A personal or familial history of *acute intermittent porphyria* represents one of the few absolute contraindications to the use of barbiturates.

Acquired hypersensitivity to the barbiturates consists chiefly in allergic reactions that occur especially in persons who tend to have asthma, urticaria, angioedema, and similar conditions. Hypersensitivity reactions in this category include localized swellings, particularly of the eyelids, cheeks, or lips, and erythematous dermatitis. Rarely, exfoliative dermatitis may be caused by phenobarbital and can prove fatal; the skin eruption may be associated with fever, delirium, and marked degenerative changes in the liver and other parenchymatous organs. In a few cases, megaloblastic anemia has been associated with the chronic use of phenobarbital (Chapter 64).

Drug dependence, acute intoxication, and drug interactions are discussed elsewhere in this chapter.

THERAPEUTIC USES

The choice of a barbiturate for a particular therapeutic application is frequently determined by the duration of action that is required. The duration of action of the barbiturates ranges from 10 to 15 minutes for intravenously administered methohexital to a day or more for orally administered barbital. This range confers extraordinary versatility on the barbiturates as a class. They may be employed for almost any condition in which a relatively nonspecific depression of the CNS is desirable.

In Table 9–3, some official barbiturates are classified in the traditional way, with respect to duration of action. The "ultrashort-acting" agents listed in Table 9–3 are used principally as intravenous anesthetic agents, usually in conjunction with nitrous oxide or other inhalational agents (*see* Chapter 8). The "short- to intermediate-acting" compounds are used principally as sedative-hypnotic agents. The long-acting barbiturate phenobarbital has the broadest spectrum of therapeutic uses, being employed as a sedative-hypnotic as well as an antiepileptic agent. The other "long-acting" drugs are used principally in the treatment of epilepsy (*see* Chapter 13).

The distinction with respect to duration of action shown in Table 9–3 is often interpreted in a simplistic fashion, and such interpretations have been justly criticized (*see* Mark, 1969). The differences between the various categories are relative rather than absolute, and any attempt to ascribe to the drugs specific durations of action in hours would be quite misleading. Nevertheless, there are grounds for distinguishing the *relative* durations of actions in terms of their plasma and brain half-lives. However, the half-lives do not justify a distinction between short- and intermediate-acting barbiturates. Of

Table 9–3. OFFICIAL BARBITURATES: CLASSIFICATION AND PLASMA HALF-LIVES *

DRUG		HALF-LIFE
Long-Acting		
Phenobarbital †	U.S.P.	24–96 hr
Mephobarbital	N.F.	▲
Metharbital	N.F.	▲
Short- to Intermediate-Acting		
Amobarbital †	N.F.	14–42 hr
Butabarbital Sodium	N.F.	▲
Pentobarbital Sodium	U.S.P.	21–42 hr
Secobarbital	U.S.P.	20–28 hr
Talbutal	N.F.	▲
Ultrashort-Acting		
Hexobarbital	N.F.	5 hr
Methohexital Sodium	U.S.P.	3.5–6 hr ‡
Thiamylal Sodium	N.F.	▲
Thiopental Sodium	U.S.P.	3–8 hr ‡

* In man.

† Also official as the sodium salt.

▲ Half-life data for man unavailable.

‡ Half-life of the elimination phase after a single intravenous dose. The half-time for brain concentration is undoubtedly less than 30 min.

course, plasma half-life is only one of the factors affecting duration of action, and it varies among persons and in the same person from time to time.

Hypnosis. The recommended adult dose of the short- to intermediate-acting barbiturates for the purpose of inducing sleep is 0.1 to 0.2 g. Larger doses may be required for psychotic or disturbed patients, and smaller doses may be effective when the barbiturates are employed with other CNS depressants, for example, certain analgesics or tranquilizers. Under favorable conditions, in individuals who have not had much experience with depressant drugs, including alcohol, the recommended hypnotic doses will induce sleep that lasts for 6 or 7 hours without interruption. This does not mean that the soporific action of the drug continues unabated for 6 or 7 hours, or that the duration of soporific action is the same for all drugs. Environmental influences, diurnal rhythms, and "habits" of awakening at a certain hour may play a more important role in determining the time of awakening than do drug concentrations in the CNS. The rate of absorption, as determined by product formulation, also plays a role.

Within limits, a longer period of effective hypnotic action can be achieved by increasing the dose; however, it should be recalled that tolerance does not develop to the toxic effects of the drugs as readily as to their therapeutic effects, and the therapeutic ratio is not great. Needless to say, the dose is not left to the discretion of the patient. Although the physician should try to adjust the dose to the needs of the case, the patient emphatically should not. Persons suffering from chronic insomnia are frequently depressed, and depressed patients are often suicidal. *A physician who prescribes a large quantity of a hypnotic drug for his own convenience is therefore risking the life of his patient.* Setter and associates (1966) recommend that the physician limit the total quantity of the short-acting barbiturates prescribed at one time to less than 3 g (less than 30 100-mg capsules of secobarbital or pentobarbital) and the total quantity of phenobarbital to less than 5 g (less than 155 32-mg or 75 65-mg tablets). When the drug is being used as an hypnotic, it is difficult to see why more than ten full hypnotic doses should be needed, unless the patient is habituated to the drug or abusing it. Since patients requiring hypnotic agents usually have other drugs, including alcohol, available to them and since they may hoard drugs, limiting the total supply prescribed at any one time will not ensure absolute safety, but it is a reasonable precaution.

In view of the paucity of knowledge regarding aftereffects of hypnotic drugs, and the possible role of these aftereffects in establishing a vicious cycle in which the patient becomes habituated to the drug, it must be obvious that such drugs should be employed with reluctance. They are not substitutes for good sleep habits. Several nights of enforced regularity with respect to hours of retiring and arising, combined with scrupulous avoidance of caffeine, alcohol, and large snacks before bedtime until regular sleep habits are established, would probably obviate the need for hypnotic drugs in many cases. In this connection, a placebo may be beneficial in establishing a regular sleep routine. Numerous clinical studies have shown that it is difficult in cases of simple insomnia to distinguish the sleep-inducing properties of a placebo from those of a drug that is known on other grounds to be an effective hypnotic.

Although hypnotic drugs are often dispensed when advice and admonitions with regard to sleep habits would be more appropriate, the opposite sometimes occurs. In cases of severe insomnia when drug-induced sleep would provide most welcome relief, the well-meaning physician may refuse to prescribe hypnotic drugs because of his fear of addiction and physical dependence. There is a great deal of alarmist thinking about this facet of the problem. The danger of *severe* physical dependence is overemphasized. More pertinent is the fact that regular use of hypnotics may increase anxiety and exacerbate the insomnia, thus establishing a vicious cycle in which the patient becomes "habituated" to the drug. No general rule can be given. The possible consequences of persistent insomnia must be weighed against the possible dangers of the regular and habitual use of soporific drugs, the personality and environment of the patient being taken into account. Unfortunately, there is very little reliable information about the deleterious effects of either persistent insomnia or the regular use of hypnotic drugs in moderate doses.

Sedation. The sedative dose is from one third to one fourth the hypnotic dose, and may be given several times daily. The era when barbiturates, particularly phenobarbital, were virtually the only drugs recommended for daytime sedation has passed. They have been replaced largely by benzodiazepines and other compounds. Nevertheless, barbiturates are still employed as sedatives, especially to alter or augment the activity of other compounds; thus, barbiturates may diminish the excitement produced by dextroamphetamine and at the same time potentiate its mood-elevating and euphoric effects. The use of drugs for relieving anxiety and treating emotional disorders is discussed in Chapter 12.

Anticonvulsant Uses. Rapid onset of action is required when hypnotic drugs are used for *emergency treatment of convulsions,* such as occur in tetanus, eclampsia, status epilepticus, cerebral hemorrhage, and poisoning by convulsant agents. The barbiturates are still widely employed for this purpose. Some representative dose ranges for intravenous administration are as follows: phenobarbital sodium, 0.15 to 0.3 g; pentobarbital sodium, 0.3 to 0.5 g; amobarbital sodium, 0.4 to 0.8 g; thiopental sodium, 0.1 to 0.2 g. The injection should be made slowly, with the usual precautions necessary for intravenous administration. Phenobarbital sodium is of particular value because of its anticonvulsant efficacy. However, even when administered intravenously, 15 minutes or more may be required for it to attain peak concentrations in the brain. Thus, the practice of continuing to inject phenobarbital sodium until the convulsions stop has the consequence that the brain concentration will continue to rise and may eventually exceed that required to control the seizures. It is therefore important to use the minimal amount required, since the barbiturate-induced depression may summate with the postictal depression once the seizures are controlled, and to wait for the anticonvulsant effect to develop before deciding whether a second dose is necessary. In contrast to phenobarbital, the ultrashort- to intermediate-acting barbiturates have the disadvantage of being short lived, and of having a low ratio of anticonvulsant to hypnotic action. For the emergency treatment of certain convulsive disorders, and particularly for status epilepticus, *diazepam* is also a most useful drug.

The use of phenobarbital, mephobarbital, and metharbital in the symptomatic therapy of epilepsy is discussed in Chapter 13.

Miscellaneous Applications. The barbiturates may be used for preanesthetic medication and to produce basal anesthesia. The ultrashort-acting agents are employed principally as intravenous anesthetics. Short- and ultrashort-acting agents are occasionally used as adjuncts in the production of obstetrical analgesia. Although several studies have failed to show gross depression of infant respiration at birth, the drugs readily penetrate the placental barrier and are distributed to the fetal tissues. Evaluation of the effects of general depressants on the fetus and neonate is difficult, and the place that barbiturates should occupy in obstetrics is still controversial.

The barbiturates are employed as diagnostic and therapeutic aids in psychiatry, in *narcoanalysis* and *narcotherapy.* They are used to activate latent abnormalities in the EEG. In low concentrations, amobarbital has been administered directly into the carotid artery as a means of identifying the dominant cerebral hemisphere for speech prior to neurosurgery.

Because liver glucuronyl transferase and the bilirubin-binding Y protein are increased by the barbiturates, phenobarbital has been successfully used to treat *hyperbilirubinemia* and *kernicterus* in the neonate (*see* Crigler and Gold, 1969; Stern *et al.,* 1970); complete failure of this treatment (Cunningham *et al.,* 1969) can probably be attributed to discontinuing the drug prematurely. The nondepressant barbiturate phetharbital (N-phenylbarbital) works equally well (Hunter *et al.,* 1971). The effect of phenobarbital on bile salt metabolism and excretion has been employed in the treatment of selected cases of *cholestasis* (*see* Sharp and Mirkin, 1972; Linarelli *et al.,* 1973; Stiehl *et al.,* 1973).

BARBITURATE POISONING

Owing partly to the ready availability and promiscuous use of barbiturates, barbiturate poisoning has become a major therapeutic problem in large urban medical centers, and has increasingly engaged the attention of public health authorities. Death occurs in 0.5 to 12% of cases, depending upon local factors and the expertise of the treatment team.

Most of the cases are the result of deliberate attempts at suicide, but some are from accidental poisonings in children or drug abusers. A widely held concept is that poisoning often is the result of "drug automatism." It relates to the patient who fails to fall asleep after the first or second dose, becomes confused, and unwittingly ingests an overdose; on recovery, there is no memory of having taken the additional doses. The extent of poisoning from confusion during self-administration is perhaps overemphasized. Aitken and Proudfoot (1969) could attribute no more than two cases out of 994 to automatism; they believe the failure to recall suicidal intent is the result of psychogenic defense mechanisms. Nevertheless, Jansson (1961), after investigating 488 cases of intoxication, considered that it could be shown that approximately one fourth of these cases were classifiable as drug automatism; the automatism cases showed a noticeably higher proportion of cerebral lesions than did the patients with suicidal intent, and were thus probably more disposed to confusional states during mild intoxication.

The *lethal dose* of barbiturate varies with many factors and cannot be stated with certainty. One may assume that severe poisoning is likely to occur when more than ten times the full hypnotic dose has been ingested at once. The short-acting barbiturates are more potent and, of course, more toxic than the long-acting compounds. Lethal blood levels determined at autopsy may be as low as 6 mg/100 ml for long-acting and 1 mg/100 ml for intermediate- and short-acting barbiturates; if other depressant drugs or alcohol are also present, the lethal concentrations may be even lower. The finding of a high blood level in necropsy material does not in itself constitute *prima-facie* evidence of death from barbiturate poisoning. Patients with much higher blood levels than the above have recovered satisfactorily. Berman and coworkers (1956) reported a case of a 37.7-kg epileptic woman who consumed 25 g of phenobarbital with suicidal intent, and exhibited a peak blood level of 29 mg/100 ml, one of the highest ever recorded; she recovered after hemodialysis. Patients who ingest fatal amounts of the long-acting agents more frequently die in the hospital, whereas those who are poisoned by the short-acting agents are more frequently found dead. This would suggest that poisoning with the short-acting agents is somewhat more dangerous, since the therapeutic measures that are now available for the treatment of acute barbiturate intoxication are highly effective if they are instituted before serious respiratory and cardiovascular complications have developed.

Diagnosis of barbiturate poisoning may be difficult. Unstable individuals disposed toward self-destruction are likely to have a bountiful supply of CNS depressants on hand. The suicide attempt may follow the consumption of large quantities of alcohol, and the odor of the latter on the patient's breath may further confuse the picture. Physical examination alone is rarely sufficient to differentiate poisoning by the various agents and, particularly, by mixtures of CNS depressants. Circumstantial evidence, empty medicine bottles, characteristic color of capsules or tablets in the mouth or gastric contents, and other clues may be helpful. Ultimately, the differential diagnosis depends on the chemical identification of the compounds in body fluids.

The *signs and symptoms* of barbiturate poisoning are referable especially to the CNS and the cardiovascular system. Moderate intoxication resembles alcoholic inebriation. In severe intoxication, the patient is comatose, the level of reflex activity conforming in a general way to the intensity of the central depression. The deep reflexes may persist for some time despite coexistent coma. The Babinski sign is often positive. The EEG may be of the "burst-suppression" type with brief periods of electrical silence. The pupils may be constricted and react to light, but late in the course of barbiturate poisoning they may show hypoxic paralytic dilatation. Respiration is affected early. Breathing may be either slow, or rapid and shallow; Cheyne-Stokes rhythm may be present. Respiratory minute volume is diminished, and hypoxia and respiratory acidosis may develop. The blood pressure falls, owing partly to depression of medullary vasomotor centers; partly to a direct action of the drug on the myocardium, sympathetic ganglia, and vascular smooth muscle; and partly to hypoxia. The patient thus develops a typical shock syndrome, with a weak and rapid pulse, cold and sweaty skin, and a rise in the hematocrit. Respiratory complications (atelectasis, pulmonary edema, and bronchopneumonia) and renal failure are much dreaded and not infrequent concomitants of severe barbiturate poisoning. There is usually hypothermia, sometimes with temperatures as low as 32° C.

Not uncommonly, patients suffering from acute barbiturate intoxication develop sweat gland necrosis and bullous cutaneous lesions, evidently not due to hypersensitivity or hypothermia (*see* Beveridge, 1970). These lesions heal slowly, up to 2 months being required in some cases.

The optimal *treatment* of acute barbiturate intoxication has evolved from the "Scandinavian method," developed in the Poison Center of the Bispebjerg Hospital in Copenhagen (*see* Clemmesen and Nilsson, 1961), where the accumulated experience in the treatment of potentially lethal intoxication by sedative-hypnotics is in the tens of thousands of cases. Throughout the world, where the principles of the method are carefully adhered to, the collective mortality rate is less than 2% when the treatment is by experienced personnel and 5% when by the less experienced. At one time mortality ranged up to 40%. The method is applicable in most respects to the therapy of poisoning by CNS depressants as a class. It requires a highly organized intensive care unit, prepared for around-the-clock effort.

The depth of coma and adequacy of ventilation are first evaluated, and the initial step in management may be determined by the result. If the patient is still conscious, emesis can be considered. If more than 4 hours has elapsed since ingestion, often very little barbiturate can be recovered from the stomach (Matthew *et al.*, 1966); induction of emesis must be carried out quite soon after ingestion, if it is to be of value. Time is especially critical with the short- and intermediate-acting barbiturates, and some authorities recommend that emesis be induced before the patient is moved to the hospital. Although emesis is not without hazard, Mann and Sandberg (1970) recommend apomorphine (followed by levallorphan or nalorphine 1 minute after emesis has begun), especially in children. Evacuation of the stomach by emesis from *syrup of ipecac* is not as complete as with apomorphine. Emesis is more effective than lavage. The oral administration of activated charcoal may also be considered. Mann and Sandberg (1970) claim that 1 g of activated charcoal adsorbs as much as 300 to 350 mg of most barbiturates (700 mg of barbital), although it is not clear whether this efficiency applies *in vivo*. Although it is often too late for gastric lavage to be beneficial in comatose patients, if the bowel is quite hypotonic a significant fraction of the original dose may be recovered, even though lavage itself may wash some drug into the intestine. Mann and Sandberg suggest lavage with a 1:1 saline–castor oil emulsion to extract short-acting barbiturates. There is danger that some of the lavage fluid may be aspirated, thus contributing to the hazard of pulmonary complications.

Close and constant attention must be given to the maintenance of a patent airway. If the patient's reflexes permit, some form of oropharyngeal airway or endotracheal tube is passed; if the period of intubation is expected to exceed 4 days, tracheotomy should be undertaken. Oxygen, preferably not 100%, should be administered by a nasal catheter, or by catheter through the pharyngeal airway. When possible, blood P_{CO_2} and pH should be monitored; if inadequate respiratory exchange is suspected, mechanical ventilation is initiated. Chest x-rays are taken daily, and the patient is turned from one side to the other at least every 4 hours. Atelectasis, should it develop, is treated by tracheobronchial toilet and, if necessary, by bronchoscopy. A rise in temperature or evidence of pneumonia calls for appropriate therapy.

Measures should be taken to prevent further loss of body heat, but it is not universally agreed that it is necessary to restore the body temperature to normal.

In severe acute barbiturate intoxication, circulatory collapse is a major threat and at one time was the chief cause of death. Often the patient is admitted to hospital with severe hypotension, heralding the onset of shock. Robinson and coworkers (1971) recommend that slow intravenous infusion of 0.85% sodium chloride solution be started in *all* patients, to provide a ready vehicle for any intravenous medication as needed. Blood or other parenteral fluids are administered, according to the hematocrit, hemoglobin content, and plasma electrolyte concentrations. Once dehydration and hypovolemia have been corrected, further parenteral fluid treatment is determined by the assessment of renal function. Metaraminol or levarterenol may be used as a vasopressor agent, levarterenol being preferred for its cardiostimulatory actions; dopamine may possibly prove to be a superior choice. Acidosis can prevent an adequate pressor response. Shubin and Weil (1971) advocate the use of digitalis when central venous pressure is elevated by intravenous fluids and diuresis does not occur.

One of the most dangerous sequelae of shock and hypoxia is renal failure, accounting for one sixth of the deaths in the Copenhagen series. Furthermore, some long-acting barbiturates depend on the kidney for inactivation. Creatinine clearance is determined once a day during the first 4 days if any doubt exists regarding renal function, and, of course, urinary output is carefully followed. Anuria and uremia may be encountered late, even after the patient has recovered consciousness. Should renal failure occur, hemodialysis is required.

The most effective method of disposing of the poison is hemodialysis. According to Jørgensen and Wieth (1963), elimination of the drug is achieved 10 to 45 times faster by this procedure than by spontaneous means. Hemodialysis is more effective in removing long-acting than short-acting compounds because protein binding is less. More effective extraction of the lipid-soluble, short-acting barbiturates can be achieved by using a lipid-containing dialysate (Shinaberg *et al.*, 1965). Also, hemoperfusion through AMBERLITE AXD-2 anion-exchange resin or activated charcoal has been successfully used (*see* Rosenbaum *et al.*, 1971; Yatzidis, 1971). Peritoneal dialysis is only 25% as fast as hemodialysis in removing barbiturates from the body. If renal function is satisfactory, forced diuresis and alkalinization of the urine will significantly hasten the excretion of some but not all barbiturates. It is desirable to achieve a diuresis of 8 to 14 liters per day. Because antidiuretic hormone output is often increased in barbiturate intoxication, hypotonic solutions are less effective than osmotic or tubule-active diuretics. When diuresis of this magnitude is achieved, it is absolutely necessary to maintain water and electrolyte balance. Three factors militate against success with most short- and intermediate-acting barbiturates: low rate of glomerular filtration because of strong protein binding, rapid tubular reabsorption because of high lipid solubility, and high pK_a. Pentobarbital is only 33% ionized at urine pH 7.7, whereas phenobarbital is 71% ionized. Even though forced diuresis and alkalinization can increase the renal clearance of pentobarbital by as much as 15 times, the total rate of detoxication is increased by only 15 to 20%, because the principal mechanism of termination of activity is biotransformation (*see* Bloomer and Maddock, 1971). In contrast, the rates of detoxication of barbital, phenobarbital, apobarbital, and allobarbital, barbiturates for which renal excretion is a significant fraction of total elimination, are increased 30 to 180%; this effects a significant shortening of the duration of coma.

At one time, analeptics were widely used in the treatment of acute barbiturate intoxication. During the 1950s, numerous studies showed that mortality was much lower when analeptics were not used. Analepsis has no advocates today among the prominent workers in the treatment of barbiturate poisoning.

Various aspects of acute barbiturate intoxication and its management are discussed in reviews by Mann and Sandberg (1970), Matthew (1971), and Robinson and coworkers (1971).

Aitken, R. C. B., and Proudfoot, A. T. Barbiturate automatism—myth or malady? *Postgrad. med. J.,* **1969,** *45,* 612–616.

Aston, R., and Domino, E. F. Differential effects of phenobarbital, pentobarbital and diphenylhydantoin on motor cortical and reticular thresholds in the rhesus monkey. *Psychopharmacologia,* **1961,** *2,* 304–317.

Aston, R., and Hibbeln, P. Induced hypersensitivity to barbital in the female rat. *Science, Wash.,* **1967,** *157,* 1463–1464.

Berman, L. B.; Jeghers, H. J.; Schreiner, G. E.; and Pallota, A. Hemodialysis, an effective therapy for acute barbiturate poisoning. *J. Am. med. Ass.,* **1956,** *161,* 820–827.

Beveridge, G. W. Sweat gland necrosis in barbiturate poisoning. *Archs Derm.,* **1970,** *101,* 369.

Blake, W. Some effects of pentobarbital anesthesia on renal hemodynamics, water and electrolyte excretion in the dog. *Am. J. Physiol.,* **1957,** *191,* 393–398.

Blaustein, M. P. Barbiturates block sodium and potassium conductance increases in voltage-clamped lobster axons. *J. gen. Physiol.,* **1968,** *51,* 293–307.

Brazier, M. A. B. Thiopental: effects on subcortical mechanisms in temporal lobe epilepsy. *Anesthesiology,* **1967,** *28,* 192–200.

Brodie, B. B.; Burns, J. J.; and Weiner, M. Metabolism of drugs in subjects with Laennec's cirrhosis. *Medna exp.,* **1959,** *1,* 290–292.

Brown, C. R.; Forrest, W. H., Jr.; and Hayden, J. H. The respiratory effects of pentobarbital and secobarbital in clinical doses. *J. clin. Pharmac.,* **1973,** *13,* 28–35.

Burn, J. H., and Hobbs, R. Mechanism of arterial spasm following intra-arterial injection of thiopentone. *Lancet,* **1959,** *1,* 1112–1115.

Butler, T. C. The delay in onset of action of intravenously injected anesthetics. *J. Pharmac. exp. Ther.,* **1942,** *74,* 118–128.

Chu, N.-S., and Bloom, F. Norepinephrine-containing neurons: changes in spontaneous discharge patterns during sleep and waking. *Science, Wash.,* **1973,** *179,* 908–910.

Clift, A. D. Factors leading to dependence on hypnotic drugs. *Br. med. J.,* **1972,** *3,* 614–617.

Clutton-Brock, J. Pain and the barbiturates. *Anaesthesia,* **1961,** *16,* 80–88.

Cooper, J. C., and Brodie, B. B. The enzymatic metabolism of hexobarbital (EVIPAL). *J. Pharmac. exp. Ther.,* **1955,** *114,* 409–417.

———. Enzymatic oxidation of pentobarbital and thiopental. *Ibid.,* **1957,** *120,* 75–83.

Crigler, J. F., Jr., and Gold, N. I. Effect of sodium phenobarbital on bilirubin metabolism in an infant with congenital, nonhemolytic, unconjugated hyperbilirubinemia, and kernicterus. *J. clin. Invest.,* **1969,** *48,* 42–55.

Cucchiara, R. F., and Michenfelder, J. D. The effect of interruption of the reticular activating system on metabolism in canine cerebral hemispheres before and after thiopental. *Anesthesiology,* **1973,** *39,* 3–12.

Cunningham, M. D.; Mace, J. W.; and Peters, E. R. Clinical experience with phenobarbitone in icterus neonatorum. *Lancet,* **1969,** *1,* 550–551.

Dorfman, A., and Goldbaum, L. R. Detoxification of barbiturates. *J. Pharmac. exp. Ther.,* **1947,** *90,* 330–337.

Dundee, J. W. Alterations in response to somatic pain associated with anaesthesia. II. The effect of thiopentone and pentobarbitone. *Br. J. Anaesth.,* **1960,** *32,* 407–414.

Esplin, D. W. Criteria for assessing effects of depressant drugs on spinal cord synaptic transmission, with examples of drug selectivity. *Archs int. Pharmacodyn. Thér.,* **1963,** *143,* 479–497.

Essig, C. F., and Carter, W. W. Failure of diphenylhydantoin in preventing barbiturate withdrawal convulsions in the dog. *Neurology, Minneap.,* **1962,** *12,* 481–484.

Exley, K. A. Depression of autonomic ganglia by barbiturates. *Br. J. Pharmac. Chemother.,* **1954,** *9,* 170–181.

Gay, G. R.; Smith, D. E.; Wesson, D. R.; and Sheppard, C. W. Outpatient barbiturate withdrawal using phenobarbital. *Int. J. Addict.,* **1972,** *7,* 17–26.

Giotti, A., and Maynert, E. W. The renal clearance of barbital and the mechanism of its reabsorption. *J. Pharmac. exp. Ther.,* **1951,** *101,* 296–309.

Goldbaum, L. R., and Smith, P. K. The interaction of barbiturates with serum albumin and its possible relation to their disposition and pharmacological actions. *J. Pharmac. exp. Ther.,* **1954,** *111,* 197–209.

Golovchinsky, V. B., and Plehotkina, S. I. Difference in the sensitivity of the cerebral cortex and midbrain reticular formation to the action of diethylether and thialbarbital. *Brain Res.,* **1971,** *30,* 37–47.

Gordon, M.; Rubia, F. J.; and Strata, P. The effect of barbiturate anesthesia on the transmission to the cerebellar cortex. *Brain Res.,* **1972,** *43,* 677–680.

Gould, T., and Shideman, F. E. The *in vitro* metabolism of thiopental by a fortified, cell-free tissue preparation of the rat. *J. Pharmac. exp. Ther.,* **1952,** *104,* 427–439.

Harris, E., and Slawson, K. The respiratory effects of therapeutic doses of cyclobarbitone, TRICLOFOS, and

ethchlorvynol. *Br. J. Pharmac. Chemother.,* **1965,** *24,* 214–222.

Hunter, J.; Thompson, R. P. H.; Rake, M. O.; and Williams, R. Controlled trial of phetharbital, a non-hypnotic barbiturate, in unconjugated hyperbilirubinaemia. *Br. med. J.,* **1971,** *2,* 497–499.

Jansson, B. Drug automatism as a cause of pseudosuicide. *Postgrad. Med.,* **1961,** *30,* A34–A40.

Johnson, E. S.; Roberts, M. H. T.; and Straughn, D. W. The responses of cortical neurones to monoamines under different anesthetic conditions. *J. Physiol., Lond.,* **1969,** *203,* 261–280.

Jørgensen, H. E., and Wieth, J. O. Dialysable poisons: haemodialysis in the treatment of acute poisoning. *Lancet,* **1963,** *1,* 81–84.

Kadar, D.; Inaba, T.; Endrenyi, L.; Johnson, G. E.; and Kalow, W. Comparative drug elimination capacity in man—glutethimide, amobarbital, antipyrine, and sulfinpyrazone. *Clin. Pharmac. Ther.,* **1973,** *14,* 552–560.

Kay, D. C.; Jasinski, D. R.; and Eisenstein, R. B. Quantified human sleep after pentobarbital. *Clin. Pharmac. Ther.,* **1972,** *13,* 221–231.

Krupp, P.; Bianchi, C. P.; and Suarez-Kurtz, G. On the local anesthetic effect of barbiturates. *J. Pharm. Pharmac.,* **1969,** *21,* 763–768.

Linarelli, L. G.; Hengstenberg, F. H.; and Drash, A. L. Effect of phenobarbital on hyperlipemia in patients with intrahepatic and extrahepatic cholestasis. *J. Pediat.,* **1973,** *82,* 291–298.

McKenzie, R. E., and Elliott, L. L. Effects of secobarbital and *d*-amphetamine on performance during a simulated air mission. *Aerospace Med.,* **1965,** *36,* 774–779.

Magni, F.; Moruzzi, G.; Rossi, G. F.; and Zanchetti, A. EEG arousal following inactivation of the lower brain stem by selective injection of barbiturate into the vertebral circulation. *Archs ital. Biol.,* **1961,** *99,* 33–71.

Mark, L. C. Archaic classification of barbiturates. *Clin. Pharmac. Ther.,* **1969,** *10,* 287–291.

Mark, L. C.; Perel, J. M.; Brand, L.; and Dayton, P. G. Studies with thiohexital, an anesthetic barbiturate metabolized with unusual rapidity in man. *Anesthesiology,* **1968,** *29,* 1159–1166.

Matthew, H.; Mackintosh, T. F.; Thomsett, S. L.; and Cameron, J. C. Gastric aspiration and lavage in acute poisoning. *Br. med. J.,* **1966,** *1,* 1333–1337.

Maynert, E. W., and Klingman, G. I. Acute tolerance to intravenous anesthetics in dogs. *J. Pharmac. exp. Ther.,* **1960,** *128,* 192–200.

Narahashi, T.; Frazier, D. T.; Deguchi, T.; Cleaves, C. A.; and Ernau, M. C. The active form of pentobarbital in squid giant axons. *J. Pharmac. exp. Ther.,* **1971,** *177,* 25–33.

Nayler, W. G., and Szeto, J. Effect of sodium pentobarbital on calcium in mammalian heart muscle. *Am. J. Physiol.,* **1972,** *222,* 339–344.

Neal, J. The hyperalgesic action of barbiturates in mice. *Br. J. Pharmac. Chemother.,* **1965,** *24,* 170–177.

Ogunremi, O. O.; Adamson, L.; Březenová, V.; Hunter, W.; Maclean, A. W.; Oswald, I.; and Percy-Robb, I. W. Two antianxiety drugs: a psychoneuroendocrine study. *Br. med. J.,* **1973,** *2,* 202–205.

Oswald, I., and Priest, R. G. Five weeks to escape the sleeping-pill habit. *Br. med. J.,* **1965,** *2,* 1093–1099.

Papper, S.; Belsky, J. L.; Bleifer, K. H.; Saxon, L.; and Smith, W. P. Effect of meperidine and secobarbital upon renal excretion of water and solute in man. *J. Lab. clin. Med.,* **1960,** *56,* 727–733.

Reading, H. W., and Wallwork, J. Oxidation of succinate and pyruvate in rat brain and its effects on barbiturate anesthesia. *Biochem. Pharmac.,* **1969,** *18,* 2211–2214.

Richards, C. D. On the mechanism of barbiturate anesthesia. *J. Physiol., Lond.,* **1972,** *227,* 749–767.

Richards, R. K.; Taylor, J. D.; and Kueter, K. E. Effect of nephrectomy on the duration of sleep following administration of thiopental and hexobarbital. *J. Pharmac. exp. Ther.,* **1953,** *108,* 461–473.

Rosenbaum, J. L.; Kramer, M. S.; Raja, R.; and Boreyko, C. Resin hemoperfusion: a new treatment for acute drug intoxication. *New Engl. J. Med.,* **1971,** *284,* 874–877.

Roth, B. F., and Harvey, J. A. Altered response of cerebral respiration to thiopental and potassium ions *in vitro* after septal lesions. *J. Pharmac. exp. Ther.,* **1968,** *161,* 155–162.

Sessions, J. T., Jr.; Minkel, H. P.; Bullard, J. C.; and Inglefinger, F. J. The effect of barbiturates in patients with liver disease. *J. clin. Invest.,* **1954,** *33,* 1116–1127.

Setter, J. G.; Maher, J. F.; and Schreiner, G. E. Barbiturate intoxication. *Archs intern. Med.,* **1966,** *117,* 224–236.

Shankaran, R., and Quastel, J. H. Effects of anesthetics on sodium uptake into rat brain cortex *in vitro. Biochem. Pharmac.,* **1972,** *21,* 1763–1773.

Sharp, H. L., and Mirkin, B. L. Effect of phenobarbital on hyperbilirubinemia, bile acid metabolism, and microsomal enzyme activity in chronic intrahepatic cholestasis of childhood. *J. Pediat.,* **1972,** *81,* 116–126.

Shinaberg, J. H.; Shear, L.; Clayton, L. F.; Barry, K. G.; Knowlton, M.; and Goldbaum, L. R. Dialysis for intoxication with lipid soluble drugs: enhancement of glutethimide extraction with lipid dialysate. *Trans. Am. Soc. artif. internal Organs,* **1965,** *11,* 173–177.

Shubin, H., and Weil, M. H. Shock associated with barbiturate intoxication. *J. Am. med. Ass.,* **1971,** *215,* 263–268.

Sjögren, J.; Sölvell, L.; and Karlsson, I. Studies on the absorption rate of barbiturates in man. *Acta med. scand.,* **1965,** *178,* 553–559.

Stern, L.; Khanna, N. N.; Levy, G.; and Yaffe, S. J. Effect of phenobarbital on hyperbilirubinemia and glucuronide formation in newborns. *Am. J. Dis. Child.,* **1970,** *120,* 26–31.

Stiehl, A.; Thaler, M.; and Amirand, W. H. Effects of phenobarbital on bile salt metabolism in cholestasis due to intrahepatic bile duct hypoplasia. *Pediatrics, Springfield,* **1973,** *51,* 992–997.

Taylor, J. D.; Richards, R. K.; Davin, J. C.; and Asher, J. Plasma binding of thiopental in the nephrectomized rabbit. *J. Pharmac. exp. Ther.,* **1963,** *112,* 40–48.

Thesleff, S. The effect of anesthetic agents on skeletal muscle membrane. *Acta physiol. scand.,* **1956,** *37,* 335–349.

Waddell, W. J., and Butler, T. C. The distribution and excretion of phenobarbital. *J. clin. Invest.,* **1957,** *36,* 1217–1226.

Weakly, J. N. Effect of barbiturates on "quantal" synaptic transmission in spinal motorneurones. *J. Physiol., Lond.,* **1969,** *204,* 63–77.

West, C. D., and Keller, R. M. Effect of pentobarbital and chloralose anesthesia on renal function during solute diuresis in the dog. *Am. J. Physiol.,* **1955,** *180,* 167–172.

Wikler, A. Effects of morphine, NEMBUTAL, ether and eserine on two-neuron and multi-neuron reflexes in the cat. *Proc. Soc. exp. Biol. Med.,* **1945,** *58,* 193–196.

Yatzidis, H. The use of ion exchange resins and charcoal in acute barbiturate poisoning. Chapter 14 in, *Acute Barbiturate Poisoning.* (Matthew, H., ed.) Excerpta Medica, Amsterdam, **1971.**

Monographs and Reviews

Bloomer, H. A., and Maddock, R. K., Jr. An assessment of diuresis and dialysis for treating acute barbiturate poisoning. Chapter 15 in, *Acute Barbiturate Poisoning.* (Matthew, H., ed.) Excerpta Medica, Amsterdam, **1971.**

Bush, M. T. Sedatives and hypnotics. 1. Absorption, fate, and excretion. In, *Physiological Pharmacology.* Vol. 1, *The Nervous System—Part A: Central Nervous System Drugs.* (Root, W. S., and Hofmann, F. G., eds.) Academic Press, Inc., New York, **1963,** pp. 185–218.

Clark, D. L., and Rosner, B. S. Neurophysiologic effects of general anesthetics. I. The electroencephalogram and sensory evoked responses in man. *Anesthesiology,* **1973,** *38,* 564–582. (114 references.)

Clemmesen, C., and Nilsson, E. Therapeutic trends in the treatment of barbiturate poisoning. *Clin. Pharmac. Ther.,* **1961,** *2,* 220–229.

Conney, A. H. Pharmacological implications of microsomal enzyme induction. *Pharmac. Rev.,* **1967,** *19,* 317–366.

Cooksley, W. G. E., and Powell, L. W. Drug metabolism and interaction with particular reference to the liver. *Drugs,* **1971,** *2,* 177–189. (98 references.)

Domino, E. F. Sites of action of some central nervous depressants. *A. Rev. Pharmac.,* **1962,** *2,* 215–250.

Killam, E. K. Drug action on the brain-stem reticular formation. *Pharmac. Rev.,* **1962,** *14,* 175–224.

Mann, J. B., and Sandberg, D. H. Therapy of sedative overdosage. *Pediat. Clins N. Am.,* **1970,** *17,* 617–628.

Matthew, H. (ed.). *Acute Barbiturate Poisoning.* Excerpta Medica, Amsterdam, **1971.**

Parke, D. V. Biochemistry of the barbiturates. Chapter 2 in, *Acute Barbiturate Poisoning.* (Matthew, H., ed.) Excerpta Medica, Amsterdam, **1971.**

Price, H. L. General anesthesia and circulatory homeostasis. *Physiol. Rev.,* **1960,** *40,* 187–218.

Robinson, R. R.; Gunnells, J. C., Jr.; and Clapp, J. R. Treatment of acute barbiturate intoxication. *Mod. Treatm.,* **1971,** *8,* 561–579.

Rosner, B. S., and Clark, D. L. Neurophysiologic effects of general anesthetics. II. Sequential regional actions in the brain. *Anesthesiology,* **1973,** *39,* 59–81. (181 references.)

Symposium. (Various authors.) Regulation of respiration. (Nahas, G. G., ed.) *Ann. N.Y. Acad. Sci.,* **1963a,** *109,* 411–948.

Symposium. (Various authors.) *Uptake and Distribution of Anesthetic Agents.* (Papper, E. M., and Kitz, R. J., eds.) McGraw-Hill Book Co., New York, **1963b.**

Symposium. (Various authors.) Microsomes and drug oxidations. (Estabrook, R. W.; Gillette, J. R.; and Liebman, K. C.; eds.) *Drug Metab. Disposition,* **1973,** *1,* 1–486.

CHAPTER

10 HYPNOTICS AND SEDATIVES

[*Continued*]

Miscellaneous Agents

Stewart C. Harvey

Thousands of compounds with otherwise diverse chemical and pharmacological properties have in common the ability to produce a nonspecific, reversible depression of the central nervous system (CNS), and more are marketed for hypnotic use than are needed. Some were developed for other purposes, and their hypnotic use is not the culmination of a search for new hypnotic drugs. These drugs are mostly described elsewhere in this text (*see* especially Chapter 12).

It should be pointed out that nonbarbiturate hypnotic agents share most of the disadvantages of the barbiturates and usually have, in addition, the drawback that much less is known about their pharmacology and toxicology. This is true even of the older agents, chloral hydrate and paraldehyde. It scarcely needs to be said that the most frequent contraindication to the use of a sedative or hypnotic is ignorance on the part of the physician of its potential hazards. When patients complain that their insomnia or anxiety has not been relieved by their medication, it is probably more reasonable to attempt to adjust the dose of a familiar agent to the individual requirements of the patient than to try new drugs haphazardly.

In the management of insomnia, the following guidelines are offered. (1) Improve the sleep environment (*see* Wang and Wiener, 1973). (2) Eliminate organic causes of sleeplessness. (3) Select a short- or long-acting drug according to whether the insomniac has difficulty falling asleep or staying asleep. (4) Consider the possible drug interactions; unfortunately, not enough is known about most of the nonbarbiturate hypnotics. (5) Consider addiction liability. Although reliable comparative data are largely lacking, it is possible that there are

no great inherent differences among the hypnotic drugs in this regard. Continuous use of medication should be avoided and, after a good night's sleep is achieved, the drug should be discontinued for 2 to 3 days. The importance of avoiding dependence should be stressed to the patient (*see* Clift, 1972). Proceed cautiously with a patient who has a previous history of drug abuse. (6) It is probably best to choose the drug that least interferes with rapid-eye-movement (REM) sleep. The significance of the suppression of stage-4 sleep or of various alterations in the EEG is not known. (7) The importance of rapidity of onset of action is overly stressed. Differences in sleep latency after the various drugs is not great, and the time of administration can always be adjusted. The average sleep latency among insomniacs is usually less than an hour and, at best, drugs shorten this time by only 20 to 30 minutes. The total sleep time is actually not much increased by most hypnotic drugs.

The various drugs or drug classes are presented in alphabetical order.

BENZODIAZEPINES

The benzodiazepines differ among themselves, and it is difficult to characterize them as a class. Some of them appear to be more selective than the barbiturates in the suppression of anxiety, although the medical practice setting may determine which class of drugs is more efficacious (Rickels *et al.*, 1970). Benzodiazepines used especially in the treatment of anxiety, including chlordiazepoxide and diazepam, are discussed in Chapter 12.

All benzodiazepines have hypnotic actions, but the duration of action and side effects preclude the hypnotic use of some. They are considered to have a number of advantages over other sedative-hypnotics. The therapeutic index (lethal dose:hypnotic dose) appears to be quite high. For example, in 27 cases of overdose of nitrazepam (up to 40 times the hypnotic dose), there was no loss of consciousness and no respiratory depression (Matthew *et al.,* 1969). However, hypnotic doses of nitrazepam can cause carbon dioxide narcosis in patients with bronchopulmonary disease (Clark *et al.,* 1971). Diazepam in doses employed prior to endoscopy can cause respiratory depression (Rao *et al.,* 1973), and several benzodiazepines can cause more respiratory depression in animals than does thiopental; when diazepam is used in labor, there is a definite detrimental effect on the respiration and motor activity of the neonate. Benzodiazepines have a reputation for a low incidence of "hangover"; however, when measured objectively, the hangover from nitrazepam equals that from butabarbital (Walters and Lader, 1971) and amobarbital (Davies and Levine, 1967). The effects of benzodiazepines on the hepatic microsomal enzyme system appear to be slight; although they stimulate the system in rats, there is no effect on the elimination of warfarin or tricyclic antidepressants in man, and neither nitrazepam nor diazepam accelerates 6β-hydroxycortisol excretion, although chlordiazepoxide does. However, stimulators of the microsomal system do affect the metabolism of the benzodiazepines. Diazepam suppresses the nocturnal secretion of gastric acid in man by about half (Birnbaum *et al.,* 1971); this represents a distinct advantage for its hypnotic use in patients with peptic ulcer. Details of the actions and uses of the benzodiazepines can be found in the monograph edited by Garattini and associates (1973).

FLURAZEPAM HYDROCHLORIDE

Flurazepam is a somewhat more complex molecule than diazepam. Its structure is as follows:

Flurazepam Hydrochloride

The effects of flurazepam on the EEG differ from those of the barbiturates in that the fast activity seems to be increased only in the frontal lobe and does not spread to the occipital lobe (Frost *et al.,* 1973). In doses up to 30 mg it neither affects REM sleep nor causes a rebound after withdrawal, but doses of 60 mg suppress REM sleep without rebound. Flurazepam decreases sleep latency, the time in stage 4, and wake time, and increases total sleep time for as long as 22 nights of use. The efficacy of the drug beyond 22 consecutive nights of use is not known. (For the effects on sleep, *see* Dement *et al.,* 1973; Kales and Scharf, 1973.) In one study, patients rated flurazepam more highly than secobarbital (Boston Collaborative Drug Surveillance Program, 1972).

Flurazepam given orally is rapidly absorbed and distributed rather evenly throughout the body. It is metabolized in the liver. The diethylamine group is desethylated, then deaminated, eventually to yield the alcohol, the major metabolite in man. The alcohol is conjugated to form the glucuronide. The phenyl ring is also hydroxylated at the ortho position, then conjugated. The heterocyclic ring is also hydroxylated (*see* Schwartz, 1973). Flurazepam should be used cautiously when hepatic or renal function is impaired.

Although fewer persons discontinue the use of flurazepam than barbiturates, flurazepam causes an impressive number of side effects. The incidence appears to be about 7%. Excessive drowsiness occurs in about 2% of cases; in elderly or debilitated patients, this is more common, and there may also be vertigo, ataxia, and falling. Rare instances of faintness, slurred speech, lethargy, disorientation, and also coma can occur even in younger patients. "Hangover" appears to be infrequent. Idiosyncratic nervousness, talkativeness, irritability, apprehension, euphoria, excitement, and hallucinations have occurred. A large number of other minor side effects have also been reported; many of these effects (including rash) are observed after placebos, and they are normally common in the target population; it is thus not clear which of the effects are truly drug related (*see* review by Wolf, 1959). Elevated serum levels of the transaminases, alkaline phosphatase, and bilirubin have been reported on occasion; it would seem prudent to avoid the drug in patients with intermittent porphyria.

Prolonged use of supratherapeutic doses can result in psychic and physical dependence, and the same care to avoid abuse should be exercised as with other sedative-hypnotic drugs.

The hypnotic dose of *Flurazepam Hydrochloride,* N.F. (DALMANE), is 15 to 30 mg. It is available in capsules containing 15 or 30 mg.

NITRAZEPAM

Nitrazepam (MOGADON) has been used extensively in Europe and the British Commonwealth, and its release in the United States is probable. Some pertinent facts about this drug are noted above. Like the barbiturates, it increases EEG activity in the 15- to 35-Hz range, but it decreases alpha and theta activity, which barbiturates increase (Montagu, 1971). As a hypnotic in man, it is equiefficacious with short- and intermediate-acting barbiturates (Davies and Levine, 1967; Haider, 1968; Matthew *et al.,* 1969). After oral ingestion, about 78% is absorbed. Redistribution takes place over a period of 8 to 12 hours; after this time, the plasma concentration declines with a half-life of 21 to 25 hours (Rieder and Wendt, 1973), which may be the reason why the "hangover" is about the same as that following amobarbital.

BROMIDES

Bromides were introduced into medicine in 1857 and at one time were prescribed in enormous quantities. They were used as anticonvulsants and sedatives but not as hypnotics. The facts that therapeutic effects usually cannot be achieved without excessive drowsiness, that effective blood levels are quite close to those that cause intoxication (neurological and emotional disturbances, acneform and morbilliform rashes or Stevens-Johnson syndrome, and gastrointestinal disturbances), and that many days of medication are required before sedation occurs led to the virtual abandonment of these obsolete substances. They are still marketed in nonprescription products, fortunately in low-dosage units; in order to achieve a sedative effect, more must be taken than is stated on the label. The effective daily dose is 3 to 5 g. Bromides have anticonvulsant properties, for which they are no longer prescribed, except in very rare instances (see Chapter 13). The incidence of intoxication is now quite low. Nevertheless, it must be considered when a patient develops unexplained CNS depression, positive Babinski sign, tremors, dizziness, irritability, emotional disturbances, delirium, delusions, hallucinations, mania, lethargy, coma, or dermatological signs, especially in elderly patients, who may be clinging to a remedy from an earlier era. A plasma bromide level above 9 mEq per liter is suspect. The therapeutic and toxic effects all derive from the replacement of chloride by bromide in body fluids. Bromide ion is proportionately reabsorbed to a slightly greater extent than chloride by the renal tubules, so that it has a half-life of about 12 days. Treatment consists in increasing bromide excretion by the administration of sodium or ammonium chloride and a chloruretic diuretic; hemodialysis is also effective. A more detailed description of the actions and toxicity of bromide ion can be found in the *fourth edition* of this textbook.

CARBAMATES

The carbamates of the monohydric alcohols (urethanes), such as ethinamate, are relatively nonselective CNS depressants, similar to most barbiturates. The dicarbamates of the dihydric alcohols, such as meprobamate and mebutamate, often have a selective depressant action on polysynaptic reflexes, are muscle relaxants, and may have other activity as well.

ETHINAMATE

Ethinamate is more potent and less toxic than are the simple urethanes. Its chemical structure is as follows:

Ethinamate

It has a rapid onset and short duration of action. Consequently, it may be useful to the insomniac who has difficulty falling asleep but not to the one who has long periods of wakefulness during the night. Its effect on REM sleep is unknown.

Ethinamate is inactivated at least partly by the liver, by hydroxylation of the cyclohexyl ring; the product is conjugated and excreted as the glucuronide (Murata, 1961).

Side effects of ethinamate include nausea, occasional vomiting, and infrequently rash. Idiosyncratic excitement may occur, especially in children. Fever and thrombocytopenia occur rarely. The lethal dose is unknown; death has resulted from the ingestion of 15 g, but there has been recovery after 28 g. Chronic use of larger-than-recommended doses may lead to psychic and physical dependence. The abstinence syndrome is similar to that of the barbiturates (Ellinwood et al., 1962).

The hypnotic dose of *Ethinamate*, N.F. (VALMID), is 500 mg to 1 g. Although Gruber and coworkers (1954) found 500 mg to be equivalent to 100 mg of secobarbital, Rickels and Bass (1963) found this dose to be little better than a placebo and definitely inferior to the usual doses of other common hypnotics. It is marketed in 500-mg tablets.

MEPROBAMATE

The pharmacology of meprobamate is discussed in Chapter 12 because of the popular belief that it selectively relieves anxiety. However, of ten studies in which meprobamate was compared to barbiturates, only one showed meprobamate to be superior, one showed a barbiturate to be superior, and eight showed them to be equieffective (see Greenblatt and Shader, 1971). Thus, it is probable that meprobamate should be classified as a sedative-hypnotic drug. As such, meprobamate has no advantages over the barbiturates and certainly not over flurazepam. The hypnotic dose is 800 mg.

CHLORAL DERIVATIVES

The pharmacology and uses of the clinically employed chloral derivatives are the same, except for differences in the local actions. This is because they are all converted in the body to the same active intermediate. Therefore, whatever is said below about *chloral hydrate* applies equally well to *chloral betaine* and *triclofos sodium,* unless otherwise indicated.

History. Chloral hydrate, first made by Liebig in 1832, is the oldest member of the hypnotic group. In 1869, Liebreich, aware that chloral reacted with an alkali to form chloroform, anticipated that the compound would have hypnotic properties due to the slow release of chloroform *in vivo*. Although chloral hydrate is not converted into chloroform in the body, nevertheless, it proved to be an excellent hypnotic. The popularity of chloral hydrate waned when the barbiturates were introduced, but interest in the drug was renewed in the 1950s, and now in some hospitals as many as one third of patients receive the drug.

Chemistry. *Chloral* is the 2,2,2-trichloro derivative of acetaldehyde. Halogenation increases lipid solubility and usually enhances activity on the CNS. Thus, chloral is more of a central depressant than is acetaldehyde. Because chloral is an unstable, disagreeable oil that does not lend itself well to pharmaceutical formulations, it was introduced into medicine in the form of its hydrate, formed by adding one molecule of water to the carbonyl group. The formula of chloral hydrate is $CCl_3CH(OH)_2$.

Instead of water, various alcohols can be added to chloral to form hemiacetals of the general formula $CCl_3CH(OH)(OR)$; *chloral alcoholate* and *chloral betaine* are simple adducts, and the laboratory anesthetic α-*chloralose* is a complex adduct. The hemiacetals generate chloral hydrate *in vivo*. In the body, chloral hydrate is readily reduced to 2,2,2-trichloroethanol, CCl_3CH_2OH. Although this substance is an excellent hypnotic, it is not conveniently used as such, owing to its liquid and irritant properties; instead, it is used as the monosodium salt of the phosphate ester, *triclofos sodium,* $CCl_3CH_2OPO_3H^- \cdot Na^+$.

Local Actions. Chloral hydrate is quite irritating to the skin and mucous membranes, which accounts for its gastrointestinal side effects. These are particularly likely to occur if the drug is insufficiently diluted or if it is taken on an empty stomach. Chloral betaine and triclofos have low lipid solubility and little irritancy *per se,* but in the stomach the generation of some chloral causes some gastrointestinal irritation. They lack the disagreeable taste of chloral hydrate.

Systemic Actions. Like the barbiturates, chloral hydrate has little analgesic activity, and excitement or delirium may occur in the presence of pain. It is effective against experimentally induced convulsions produced by strychnine, pentylenetetrazol, and electroshock, and it has been used in the treatment of eclampsia and tetanus; however, the ratio of anticonvulsant to sedative effects is not great, and diazepam or barbiturates are preferable in the treatment of acute convulsive disorders. The margin of safety is too narrow to permit the drug to be used as a general anesthetic agent.

The effect of chloral hydrate on REM sleep is uncertain. Kales and associates (1970b) reported that neither 500 mg nor 1 g affected REM sleep, but Evans and Ogunremi (1970) found suppression by 800 mg. Even 1 g is only slightly effective as a hyp-

notic, and it is possible that in more effective doses a suppressant action on REM sleep may occur.

In therapeutic doses, respiration and blood pressure are affected by chloral hydrate little more than by ordinary sleep. Toxic doses produce severe respiratory depression and hypotension. Since chloral hydrate is a halogenated hydrocarbon, considerable attention has been devoted to its effects on the heart. In large doses, it depresses the contractility of the myocardium and shortens the refractory period, as do many hydrocarbon anesthetics. Untoward cardiac effects may occur when toxic doses are administered, especially to patients with heart disease; however, there is no evidence of deleterious effects on the heart from the continued use of the compound in therapeutic doses.

The pharmacological properties of *trichloroethanol* closely resemble those of chloral hydrate. Clinically, trichloroethanol is at least as effective as chloral hydrate (Owens *et al.,* 1955; Imboden and Lasagna, 1956). In the body, chloral hydrate is very rapidly reduced to trichloroethanol, and significant amounts of chloral hydrate have not been detected in the blood after its oral administration; therefore, it is generally believed that the central depressant effects are caused by the trichloroethanol. Grüner and coworkers (1973) have shown unequivocally that chloral hydrate itself possesses central depressant activity and that it is about equipotent with trichloroethanol. The equipotency means, however, that the usual small amounts of chloral hydrate present in the body after oral administration cannot make a significant contribution to the central depressant effects.

Distribution and Fate. Chloral hydrate and trichloroethanol readily penetrate membranes and enter cells throughout the body. Even though chloral hydrate is essentially undetectable in blood, it has been detected in cerebrospinal fluid, milk, and fetal blood (*see* Bernstine *et al.,* 1957). The more water-soluble derivatives, chloral betaine and triclofos, must first be hydrolyzed to chloral hydrate and trichloroethanol, respectively, before they can be comparably distributed. They are both rapidly and quantitatively converted to their respective parent compounds, and trichloroethanol is the final common metabolite.

Chloral hydrate is reduced by NADH to yield trichloroethanol, apparently by alcohol dehydrogenase in the liver; reduction can occur also in other locations, including erythrocytes. Ethanol accelerates the reduction, because its own dehydrogenation provides NADH to drive the reduction of chloral hydrate. A small but variable amount of chloral hydrate is oxidized to trichloroacetic acid by an NAD-dependent enzyme, mainly in the liver and kidney. The acid continues to accumulate for 1 or 2 days after the administration of chloral hydrate, which implies a chloral-trichloroethanol oxidoreductase system with an affinity, V_{max}, and equilibrium constant quite different from those of the system that effects the initial reduction of chloral hydrate. Trichloroethanol is mainly conjugated with glucuronic acid, and the glucuronide (*urochloralic acid*) is excreted mostly into the urine but also somewhat into the bile. The plasma half-life of trichloroethanol is about 8 hours. A rather thorough bibliography of the literature on the metabolism of chloral hydrate and trichloroethanol can be found in the article by Sellers and coworkers (1972b).

Untoward Effects. The irritant actions of chloral hydrate give rise to an unpleasant taste, epigastric distress, nausea, vomiting, and flatulence. Undesirable CNS effects include light-headedness, malaise, ataxia, and nightmares. "Hangover" may also occur, although it is less common than with barbiturates.

Rarely patients exhibit *idiosyncratic reactions* to chloral hydrate (Christianson and Perry, 1956). Occasionally, a patient becomes somnambulistic after receiving the drug, and he may be disoriented and incoherent and show paranoid behavior. *Allergic reactions* commonly include erythema, scarlatiniform exanthems, urticaria, and eczematoid dermatitis. The eruption usually begins on the face or back and spreads to the neck, chest, and arms; it may be followed by desquamation or exfoliation. The dermatitis may appear within several hours or as long as 10 days after ingestion of the drug. Eosinophilia and leukopenia may also occur. Chloral hydrate is contraindicated in patients with marked hepatic or renal impairment, and it should perhaps be avoided in patients with severe cardiac disease. If gastritis is present, the drug should not be given orally but may be administered in olive oil as a retention enema.

Although chloral hydrate and trichloroethanol are not themselves metabolized by the hepatic microsomal system, chloral hydrate in man appears to accelerate the rate of metabolic disposition of some drugs, for example, dicumarol and warfarin (Cucinell

et al., 1966), with a potentially fatal outcome. Possibly the metabolism of a large number of drugs is affected. The final effect on the action of other drugs may be complicated by the fact that trichloroacetic acid formed by the metabolism of chloral hydrate displaces acidic drugs from plasma proteins, thus temporarily increasing their blood levels in spite of shortening the half-life. Since many drugs are acidic and are protein bound, there may be a considerable potential for adverse interactions. At present, chloral derivatives probably should be used with care in intermittent porphyria. The subject of microsomal enzyme induction and displacement of protein-bound drugs by chloral derivatives has been reviewed by Greenblatt and Shader (1972).

Acute Intoxication. The toxic oral dose of chloral hydrate for adults is approximately 10 g, although death has been reported from as little as 4 g and individuals have survived after ingesting as much as 30 g. Poisoning by chloral hydrate resembles acute barbiturate intoxication, and the same supportive treatment is indicated. Gastric irritation may result in initial vomiting and even gastric necrosis (Vellar *et al.*, 1972). Pinpoint pupils may be seen, as in morphine poisoning. If the patient survives, icterus due to hepatic damage and albuminuria from renal irritation may appear.

The combination of chloral and ethanol (so-called knockout drops or "Mickey Finn") has long been thought to be especially toxic. Sellers and associates (1972a) studied the effects of chloral hydrate, 15 mg/kg, and ethanol, 500 mg/kg, after oral administration in man. Although motor performance and auditory vigilance were impaired more than when either substance was used alone, there was no obvious supra-addition or potentiation. Instead of a soporific effect, there was flushing, tachycardia (more than from ethanol alone), palpitation, and headache, reminiscent of the effects of acetaldehyde; the plasma acetaldehyde levels were actually lower than when ethanol was used alone, probably because trichloroethanol inhibits alcohol dehydrogenase. Unfortunately, the dose of chloral hydrate chosen for this study is only marginally hypnotic, and the dose of alcohol probably did not yield a blood level much above 0.03%, so that a pronounced soporific effect with higher doses cannot be ruled out. In rats, the combined effects of chloral hydrate and ethanol are somewhat supra-additive in certain combinations (Gessner and Cabana, 1970), but the combined effect is less than that anticipated from the popular lore of the "Mickey Finn." It has also been thought that the "knockout" effect is due to a distinct molecular species, namely, *chloral alcoholate,* generated in the victim's drink; however, chloral alcoholate is not sufficiently potent to account for the supposed effect; moreover, little alcoholate can form in a cold, dilute alcoholic beverage.

Chronic Intoxication. The habitual use of chloral hydrate may result in the development of tolerance, physical dependence, and addiction (Chapter 16). Chloral addicts may take enormous doses of the drug; for example, the poet-painter, Dante Gabriel Rossetti, is said to have taken as much as 12 g nightly. The chloral habit is similar to alcohol addiction, and sudden withdrawal may result in delirium. The chloral habitué may suddenly exhibit what was formerly termed a "break in tolerance," and death may occur, either as a result of an overdose or a failure of the detoxication mechanism due to hepatic damage. In patients suffering from chronic chloral intoxication, gastritis is common and skin eruptions may develop. Parenchymatous renal injury may also occur.

Dosage and Preparations. The usually recommended oral dose of chloral hydrate for the relief of insomnia in adults is 500 mg to 1 g; however, a number of well-controlled statistical studies in hospitalized patients have indicated that these doses are frequently too small. The time to onset of sleep may be somewhat shortened, but the time awake during the night is unaffected. In one study, for example, 1 g of chloral hydrate was only slightly better than a placebo, and was less effective than 300 mg of methyprylon, 800 mg of meprobamate, 500 mg of glutethimide, or 100 mg of secobarbital (Rickels and Bass, 1963). It would appear that many individuals may require 2 g of chloral hydrate. To minimize irritation, solutions of the drug should be taken well diluted with water or milk, but certainly not an alcoholic beverage. It is too irritating to be given hypodermically. *Chloral Hydrate,* U.S.P. (NOCTEC, SOMNOS), is supplied in syrups containing 50, 100, or 160 mg/ml; in capsules containing 250 or 500 mg, or 1.0 g; and unofficially in rectal suppositories (AQUACHLORAL) containing 300, 600, or 900 mg. *Chloral Betaine,* N.F. (BETA-CHLOR), is available in

870-mg tablets (equivalent to 500 mg of chloral hydrate); the dose is 870 mg to 1.74 g, which may be too small. It does not have the disagreeable taste of chloral hydrate.

The dose of *triclofos sodium* is 1.5 g, which will yield a blood level of trichloroethanol approximately equal to that from 900 mg of chloral hydrate. Brown and coworkers (1972) found 1.7 g to be equivalent to 100 mg of pentobarbital. Triclofos sodium (TRICLOS) is available in tablets containing 750 mg and in a liquid containing 100 mg/ml.

ETHCHLORVYNOL

Ethchlorvynol is a sedative-hypnotic drug with a rapid onset and short duration of action. It has the following structure:

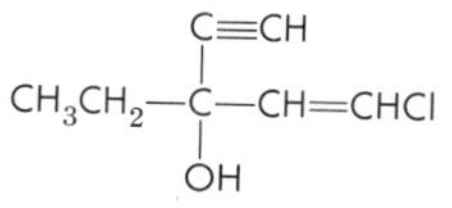

$$CH_3CH_2 - \overset{\overset{\displaystyle C \equiv CH}{|}}{\underset{\underset{\displaystyle OH}{|}}{C}} - CH = CHCl$$

Ethchlorvynol

CNS Effects. Ethchlorvynol has not only sedative-hypnotic activity but also anticonvulsant and muscle relaxant properties. Although the drug is said to produce less initial excitement than do the barbiturates, a valid clinical confirmation is needed. The EEG pattern following ethchlorvynol resembles that seen after barbiturates, with fast activity appearing first in the frontal lobes. The effect of the drug on REM sleep has not yet been investigated; however, with the usual dose, little effect would be expected because of the short duration of action. Because of the short half-life, it is better suited to the insomniac who has difficulty falling asleep than the one whose sleep is interrupted by long periods of wakefulness. If ethchlorvynol is taken along with ethanol, an exaggerated hypnotic effect may occur.

Absorption and Fate. After oral ingestion of 1 g of ethchlorvynol, symptoms of CNS depression occur within 15 to 30 minutes. The maximal blood level is attained in 1 to 1½ hours. The volume of distribution is greater than the volume of total body water. In acutely intoxicated patients, at least, the concentration in cerebrospinal fluid reaches 50% of that in plasma. After equilibrium following hypnotic doses, the blood level falls rapidly, with an average half-life of 5.6 hours (Cummins *et al.,* 1971). The drug is mainly destroyed in the liver, but approximately 10% of a usual dose is excreted into the urine. It is not known what hepatic enzymes are responsible for the metabolism of ethchlorvynol. Although the drug does not appear to stimulate the hepatic microsomal system in experimental animals, Johansson (1968) has reported that the drug suppresses the prothrombinopenic response to dicumarol.

Side Effects, Intoxication, and Abuse. The most common side effects caused by ethchlorvynol are aftertaste, dizziness, nausea, vomiting, hypotension, and facial numbness. In persons in whom absorption is especially rapid, giddiness and ataxia frequently occur; these effects can be controlled by giving the drug with food. Mild "hangover" is also relatively common, despite the short half-life of the drug. An occasional patient responds with exaggerated depression, which results in profound hypnosis, muscular weakness, and syncope unrelated to marked hypotension. Idiosyncratic responses range from mild stimulation to marked excitement and hysteria. Ethchlorvynol should not be used with antidepressants, because delirium may result. Hypersensitivity reactions include urticaria, rare but sometimes fatal thrombocytopenia (Jacobson, 1972), and occasionally cholestatic jaundice. Because of the possible effect to stimulate hepatic enzymes, the drug should be used cautiously in combination with drugs metabolized by the liver, and it is contraindicated in intermittent porphyria.

Acute intoxication is characterized by prolonged deep coma, severe respiratory depression, hypotension, relative bradycardia, and hypothermia. Although death has occurred with a blood level of 14 mg/100 ml, survival has been reported after a blood level of 16.6 mg/100 ml. The lethal dose usually ranges from 10 to 25 g, but death has followed a dose of 2.5 g (ethanol also present), and one patient has survived 50 g (with intensive care) after a coma lasting 7 days. Although present data are limited, it appears that the therapeutic index (lethal dose:hypnotic dose) of ethchlorvynol may not be much different than those of intermediate-acting barbiturates, if truly equivalent hypnotic doses are used in the comparison. Treatment is similar to that for acute barbiturate intoxication. Substantial amounts of ethchlorvynol have been recovered from the stomach by lavage as late as 5 hours after ingestion. Hemodialysis clears the blood at least three times faster than does forced diuresis or peritoneal dialysis (Teehan et al., 1970); oil dialysis is even more effective (Welch et al., 1972).

Chronic abuse of ethchlorvynol results in tolerance and physical dependence. Abusers may take up to 4 g of drug per day. Usually they show signs of intoxication, such as incoordination, tremors, ataxia, slurred speech, confusion, asthenia, hyperreflexia, nystagmus, diplopia, and sometimes toxic amblyopia, dyschromatopsia, scotoma, and peripheral neuritis. Withdrawal symptoms are similar to delirium tremens, sometimes suggestive of a schizophrenic reaction (see Flemenbaum and Gunby, 1971).

Preparations and Dosage. *Ethchlorvynol,* N.F. (PLACIDYL), is supplied in capsules containing 100, 200, 500, and 750 mg. The usual hypnotic dose is 500 mg, but this is somewhat small; Bellville and coworkers (1968) reported that 770 mg is equivalent to 100 mg of secobarbital. Up to 1 g may be required. If sleep is interrupted during the night, a supplemental dose of 100 to 200 mg may be given. Ethchlorvynol is not recommended for sedation because of the short duration of action.

METHAQUALONE

The 2,3-disubstituted quinazolinones possess hypnotic activity. Of these, only methaqualone is marketed. It has the structural formula as shown.

Methaqualone

Pharmacodynamics. Methaqualone has a wider spectrum of activity than do the barbiturates. In addition to sedative-hypnotic properties, it possesses anticonvulsant, antispasmodic, local anesthetic, and weak antihistaminic properties. It has an antitussive activity comparable to that of codeine (Boissier and Pagny, 1959); however, it lacks analgesic activity, although it enhances analgesia from codeine. Methaqualone also has been claimed to possess tranquilizing properties (Cromwell, 1968), but it is not clear that these are distinct from its sedative properties; evaluations from drug abusers suggest that they may be distinct (see below). In anesthetic doses, methaqualone exerts a myocardial depressant action that is the principal cause of hypotension.

The locus of the sedative-hypnotic action of methaqualone is not known. It has been claimed that in experimental animals the locus is cerebral cortical (see Brown and Goenechea, 1973); however, from what is known of the neurophysiology of sleep and the clinical toxicology, such a locus seems dubious. There is disagreement whether the REM phase of sleep is normal during methaqualone-induced sleep. Davison and coworkers (1970) reported that MANDRAX (a combination containing 250 mg of methaqualone and 25 mg of diphenhydramine) does not disturb the sleep pattern, whereas Kales and Kales (1970) state that 300 mg of methaqualone (as well as diphenhydramine) suppresses REM sleep; however, 150 mg does not. In high doses, the drug exerts a selective depressant action on polysynaptic pathways in the spinal cord. In rat brain and mitochondria, it appears to compete with Krebs cycle intermediates for NAD-dependent enzymes.

Absorption and Fate. In man, 99% of methaqualone is absorbed in 2 hours; the absorption of the hydrochloride is not dissolution limited and hence is faster. The drug is hydroxylated by the hepatic microsomal enzyme system, the N-tolyl group being the moiety affected. Nine hydroxyl metabolites result. These are conjugated and mainly excreted into the urine. In rats, methaqualone moderately increases the activity of the hepatic microsomal enzymes. In man, after 3 weeks of use in normal dosage, there is no significant change in the half-life of antipyrine or phenylbutazone or in the excretion of 6β-hydroxycortisol, but in hypnotic-dependent subjects the antipyrine half-life is moderately shortened, the effect being less than in barbiturate dependence (Stevenson et al., 1972). A substantial tolerance to methaqualone develops in abusers, but it is not necessarily metabolic in origin.

Uses, Dosage, and Preparations. For sedation, *Methaqualone,* N.F. (QUAALUDE, SOPOR), is used in a dose of 75 mg, three or four times a day; for hypnosis, the dose is 150 to 300 mg immediately before retiring. The drug is supplied in scored tablets containing 75, 150, or 300 mg. *Methaqualone Hydrochloride*, N.F. (OPTIMIL, PAREST), is used only for hypnosis. The dose is 200 to 400 mg (respectively equivalent to 175 or 350 mg of base). It is supplied in capsules containing 200 or 400 mg.

Side Effects, Intoxication, and Dependence. During sedation with methaqualone, fatigue and occasionally dizziness and torpor may occur. With hypnotic doses, there may be transient paresthesias preceding the onset of sleep. Persisting paresthesias and other signs of peripheral neuropathy that last for months to years have been reported, but the causal role of methaqualone is inconclusive (*see* Editorial, 1973). Occasionally, restlessness and anxiety occur instead of sedation and sleep. Although methaqualone has a shorter half-life than any barbiturate used for hypnosis, "hangover" is frequent. Other side effects include xerostomia, anorexia, nausea, vomiting, diarrhea, epigastric discomfort, sweating, bromidrosis, urticaria, and exanthems. Rarely, aplastic anemia has occurred, but the relationship to methaqualone has not been proven. Drug interactions involving methaqualone require more observations. At present, it must be considered to have the same potential for drug interactions as do the barbiturates, although it may not induce the synthesis of hepatic microsomal enzymes to the same extent. It has been used without difficulty in patients with intermittent porphyria.

Mild overdosage usually causes excessive central depression much like that from barbiturates, but restlessness and excitement sometimes result instead. With severe overdosage, delirium, pyramidal signs (such as hypertonicity, hyperreflexia, and myoclonus), and frank convulsions may occur. Myoclonic episodes and amnesia have occurred in one case with a dose as low as 400 mg (Waggoner *et al.*, 1973). During coma, cardiovascular and respiratory depression is less severe than with barbiturates. Coma has occurred after 2.4 g and death after 8 g. Suicidal intent has been indicated in a large proportion of cases. Most fatalities occur in persons who have also ingested ethanol. Treatment is primarily supportive. Hemodialysis is of questionable value, except, perhaps, with very high plasma levels of drug. Barbiturates must not be used to control convulsions; succinylcholine may be employed instead; the value of diazepam should be investigated.

Methaqualone is now regulated under the Comprehensive Drug Abuse Prevention and Control Act of 1970 (*see* Appendix). That it would come to be widely abused was quite predictable, despite the undeserved optimism of the pharmaceutical industry and many physicians. The unexpectedly explosive pace with which methaqualone became incorporated into the drug culture stems from a popular view among abusers that it has aphrodisiac activity and that it promotes unreserved interpersonal relations. Drug culturists contend also that it causes a dissociative "high" achieved without the drowsiness that barbiturates cause; in fact, many abusers liken the effects of methaqualone to those of heroin. Abusers employ doses of 75 mg to 2 g a day, with an average of about

725 mg. Severe grand mal convulsions may occur after withdrawal from high doses (Schwartzburg *et al.*, 1973). The subject of methaqualone abuse has been reviewed by Inaba and associates (1973), Pascarelli (1973), and Schwartzburg and colleagues (1973).

The biochemistry, experimental and clinical pharmacology, and toxicity of methaqualone have been reviewed by Brown and Goenechea (1973).

MONOUREIDES

The monoureides in general are short-acting sedative-hypnotics with a low therapeutic index. Consequently, they are very little used. *Capuride* (PACINOX) appears to have a more favorable therapeutic index, although it is not presently available in the United States. *Carbromal (bromodiethylacetylurea)* and *bromisovalum (α-bromoisovalerylurea)* are obsolete monoureides that are still available; they both release bromide ion and can thus give rise to bromide intoxication.

PARALDEHYDE

Chemistry. Paraldehyde was introduced into medicine by Cervello in 1882. Although it is a polymer of acetaldehyde, it is perhaps best regarded as a polyether of cyclic structure, as follows:

Paraldehyde

Paraldehyde is a colorless liquid with a strong aromatic odor and a burning, disagreeable taste. On exposure to light and air, it decomposes to acetaldehyde and is oxidized to acetic acid; it should therefore be stored in small, well-filled, tightly sealed, amber-colored containers. In at least eight cases of poisoning involving four fatalities, the use of deteriorated paraldehyde has been implicated. It is not uncommon to find the deteriorated drug. For example, a spot check in one large hospital revealed that only 11% of the samples collected from the wards met U.S.P. standards; one from the delivery floor was about 40% acetic acid by composition.

Pharmacological Actions. Despite the fact that paraldehyde has been in use for nearly a century, little is known about its pharmacology, metabolic fate, or toxicology. It is a rapidly acting hypnotic. When a dose of 4 to 8 ml is taken orally, sleep usually ensues in 10 to 15 minutes. The drug does not possess analgesic properties, and it may produce excitement or delirium in the presence of pain. It is effective against convulsions, and it has been used in the emergency therapy of tetanus, eclampsia, status epilepticus, and poisoning by convulsant drugs.

Paraldehyde has little effect on respiration and blood pressure in ordinary therapeutic doses. In large doses, it produces respiratory depression and hypotension.

Absorption, Fate, and Excretion. Oral paraldehyde is rapidly absorbed. About ½ hour is required for it to reach maximal concentrations in the brain after oral administration (Figot *et al.,* 1952). With hypnotic doses, 70 to 80% is metabolized in the liver, 11 to 28% is exhaled, and 0.1 to 2.5% is excreted in urine. In hepatic insufficiency, the rate of elimination is slowed, and the proportion excreted in the expired air is increased. Disulfiram increases the blood level of paraldehyde and acetaldehyde in animals (Keplinger and Wells, 1956), so that it is believed that paraldehyde is depolymerized to acetaldehyde in the liver, then oxidized by aldehyde dehydrogenase to acetic acid, which is ultimately metabolized to carbon dioxide and water.

The drug readily crosses the placental barrier and appears in the fetal circulation. Some delay in respiratory movements has been observed in neonates following its administration to the mother during labor.

Poisoning. Despite its low therapeutic index, paraldehyde was long regarded as an exceptionally safe hypnotic. It has not been widely used by ambulatory patients, owing to the unpleasant taste and disagreeable odor that it imparts to the breath. For the most part, the use of paraldehyde has been restricted to hospitalized patients or those under close medical supervision. In view of this, it is not surprising that paraldehyde poisoning is quite rare, although not so rare as is commonly believed. The lethal dose is difficult to ascertain; death has occurred from 25 g, but one person has survived 150 g. According to one estimate, the minimal lethal blood level is about 50 mg %.

The patient poisoned by paraldehyde commonly exhibits very rapid, labored respiratory movements, possibly due to the injurious effect of paraldehyde or its decomposition products on the lungs and possibly, in some cases, due to acidosis. Acidosis, bleeding gastritis, muscular irritability, azotemia, oliguria, albuminuria, leukocytosis, fatty changes in the liver and kidney with toxic hepatitis and nephrosis, pulmonary hemorrhages and edema, and dilatation of the right heart have all been observed in cases of severe acute or chronic paraldehyde poisoning.

Chronic paraldehyde intoxication results in *tolerance and dependence.* The paraldehyde addict may become acquainted with the drug when it is used in the treatment of alcoholism and then, surprisingly in view of its disagreeable taste and odor, prefer it to alcohol. Paraldehyde addiction resembles alcoholism, and withdrawal may result in delirium tremens and vivid hallucinations (Chapter 16).

Some paraldehyde habitués suffer from metabolic acidosis of unknown etiology (*see* Beier *et al.,* 1963). Normal persons are able to metabolize large amounts of acetic acid, so that a disturbance in intermediary metabolism or renal function may be involved; whether such disturbances are the direct effects of paraldehyde or indirectly the result of abnormal nutrition is speculative.

Preparations, Dosage, and Routes of Administration. *Paraldehyde,* U.S.P. (PARAL), is usually given orally in doses of 5 to 10 ml. When given rectally as a retention enema, the drug is usually added to 2 volumes of olive oil. Paraldehyde tends to produce local irritation of mucous membranes when it is administered frequently by mouth or rectum, especially if it is insufficiently diluted. The parenteral route should be avoided. The drug has been administered intramuscularly, the injections being made deep in the buttocks; however, severe and permanent sciatic nerve injury has occurred, as well as skin slough and sterile abscesses. Intravenous administration is extremely hazardous, although this route has been employed in the treatment of acute convulsive episodes. In no case should paraldehyde be taken from old, partially empty containers. It is best stored in 2- or 5-ml ampuls, which can be opened freshly and the unused contents discarded. Since paraldehyde reacts rapidly with certain plastics, it should be measured with glass syringes.

Therapeutic Uses. Paraldehyde has been used chiefly for the treatment of abstinence phenomena and other psychiatric states characterized by excitement; for the emergency treatment of convulsive episodes arising from tetanus, eclampsia, status epilepticus, and poisoning by convulsive drugs; and for basal and obstetrical anesthesia. However, in view of the disquieting increase in the frequency with which deaths have been attributed to paraldehyde intoxication, the tendency for the drug to become contaminated by corrosive decomposition products, and the serious and poorly understood manifestations of paraldehyde intoxication, it is doubtful whether its reputation as a safe (even if disagreeable) hypnotic is fully deserved. It may be that paraldehyde will be shown to have therapeutic virtues not possessed by other central depressants, but this has not yet been convincingly demonstrated. One rather specious argument in favor of its use in the treatment of patients showing abstinence phenomena is that it is less likely to be misused, owing to its unpleasant odor and taste.

PIPERIDINEDIONES

Glutethimide and *methyprylon* are both piperidinediones, but their respective pharmacological properties differ from each other more than the properties of methyprylon differ from those of the sedative-hypnotic barbiturates. The chemical structures are as follows:

Glutethimide   Methyprylon

GLUTETHIMIDE

Glutethimide was introduced in 1954, and within 1 year it became the sixth most prescribed hypnotic drug. Physicians naively believed that, because it was a nonbarbiturate, it had a high therapeutic index and was devoid of abuse potential. By 1964 it was quite clear that the addiction liability and severity of withdrawal symptoms were equal to those of the barbiturates and that certain features of acute intoxication made treatment more difficult. Today, glutethimide probably should not be regarded as just another sedative-hypnotic drug equivalent to a barbiturate; actually, it is inferior in several respects, and it is dubious whether it has enough virtue to recommend its continued use.

Pharmacological Actions. The pharmacology of glutethimide is like that of barbiturates in that it can induce hypnosis without selective analgesic, antitussive, or anticonvulsant action. It is also similar in its effects on the EEG pattern and in its suppression of REM sleep. It differs, however, in that doses that affect REM sleep do not alter the number of awakenings per night or the total sleep time (Kales *et al.,* 1970a). It also differs in that doses of 125 mg confer protection against motion sickness for 3 or 4 hours (Tyler, 1961). In acute intoxication, the ratio of cardiovascular to respiratory depression seems to be somewhat greater with glutethimide than with barbiturates. The drug exhibits pronounced anticholinergic activity, which is most prominent in the iris but which also is manifested by inhibition of salivary secretions and intestinal motility produced by cholinergic substances (Turrian and Gross, 1958).

Absorption and Fate. Glutethimide is quite erratically absorbed from the gastrointestinal tract. Blood levels vary over at least a twofold range and the equilibrium time over a sixfold range. This has been attributed to its very low aqueous solubility, but tablet disintegration time is also implicated because whole tablets have been recovered from the stomach of an acutely intoxicated patient 3 days after ingestion. The drug has a high lipid:water distribution coefficient, so that following intravenous injection it quickly penetrates the brain and then redistributes in the same manner as thiopental. About 50% of the drug is bound to plasma proteins. Less than 2% of a usual dose is excreted into the urine unchanged, most of the drug being metabolized in the liver. The average plasma half-life is 10 hours. Glutethimide is a racemate; both antipodes are hydroxylated, the *d* isomer on the piperidinedione ring and the *l* isomer on the phenyl substituent. Both hydroxylates are conjugated with glucuronic acid; the glucuronides pass into the enterohepatic circulation, and their excretion into the urine is quite slow. Approximately 2% of the *d* isomer is converted to α-phenyl-α-ethyl glutaconimide, which has hypnotic activity but which contributes insignificantly to the overall activity. The distribution and fate of glutethimide have been discussed by Keberle and associates (1962) and Curry and coworkers (1971).

Glutethimide stimulates the hepatic microsomal enzyme system. In one patient it was shown to diminish the half-life of antipyrine by about 80% and that of vitamin D_3 by about 50%, and to increase the excretion of 6β-hydroxycortisol by about eight times (Greenwood *et al.,* 1973). The excretion of D-glucaric acid and xylulose was also increased, and the plasma levels of 5-nucleotidase and γ-glutamyl transpeptidase were elevated. In animals, glutethimide increases δ-aminolevulinic acid (ALA) synthetase activity and the metabolism of barbiturates and other drugs, and it probably also does so in man. Glutethimide is contraindicated in intermittent porphyria.

Toxicity. With therapeutic doses, toxic side effects are rare and consist in "hangover," excitement, blurring of vision, gastric irritation, headache, and, infrequently, skin rashes, including exfoliative dermatitis. Thrombocytopenia, aplastic anemia, and leukopenia occur rarely.

Acute Intoxication. The symptoms of acute intoxication are similar to those of barbiturate poisoning. Respiratory depression is usually less severe than with barbiturate intoxication, but circulatory failure is at least equally severe. The antimuscarinic actions cause xerostomia, paralytic ileus, atony of the urinary bladder, and long-lasting mydriasis, which may persist for hours after the patient regains consciousness (Maher *et al.,* 1962). In some cases of glutethimide poisoning, occasional bouts of tonic muscular spasms, twitching, and even convulsions occur. The patient also tends to show cyclic variations in the level of intoxication, possibly owing to the delayed absorption of the drug (Schreiner *et al.,* 1958). A dose of 5 g is sufficient to produce severe intoxication. The lethal dose is between 10 and 20 g. In acute intoxication, the plasma half-life may be as long as 105 hours and averages about 40 hours; hemodialysis shortens the half-life to about 14 hours (Maher, 1970). The fall in plasma level may be followed by increased absorption from the intestinal tract, resulting in a rapid, secondary rise in blood level following the initial dialysis. Chazan and Garella (1971) have not found hemodialysis important to the successful management of intoxication.

Chronic Intoxication. Excessive use of glutethimide may lead to tolerance and psychic and physical dependence. The abstinence syndrome includes tremulousness, nausea, tachycardia, fever, tonic muscle spasms, and generalized convulsions. The same symptoms occasionally occur in patients who have been taking glutethimide regularly in moderate doses (0.5 to 3 g daily) even when there is no evidence of abstention (Zivin and Shalowitz, 1962), and also in patients being treated for acute intoxication who have no previous history of drug abuse. In the latter case, tonic muscular spasms and, infrequently, generalized convulsions are seen (*see* Maher *et al.,* 1962). Convulsive phenomena developing spontaneously during glutethimide administration, or during recovery from acute intoxication, are not understood. Possibly owing to the irregular absorption of the drug and its rapid metabolism, the blood level occasionally falls to a low value, resulting in the appearance of withdrawal phenomena. It is also possible that glutethimide, like other central depressants with a pronounced anticholinergic action, has mixed depressant and excitatory effects. Chronic use may also cause osteomalacia (Greenwood *et al.*, 1973).

Preparations and Dosage. *Glutethimide*, N.F. (DORIDEN), is supplied in capsules containing 500 mg and in 125-, 250-, and 500-mg tablets. The hypnotic dose is 500 mg, which may be repeated if necessary but not less than 4 hours before arising. The pre-anesthetic dose is 500 mg the night before surgery and 500 mg to 1 g an hour before anesthesia. The sedative dose is 125 to 250 mg, three times daily after meals.

METHYPRYLON

Methyprylon was introduced into medicine in 1955, but much still remains to be learned about its pharmacology and toxicology. In a dose of 300 mg, its hypnotic effect is indistinguishable from that of 200 mg of secobarbital (Rickels and Bass, 1963). This dose also suppresses REM sleep as much as does 100 mg of pentobarbital (Kales *et al.*, 1970c).

Little is known about the absorption and distribution of methyprylon. It is more water soluble than glutethimide, but it is not known whether gastrointestinal absorption is consequently less erratic. Approximately 97% of the drug appears to be metabolized, and only 3% is excreted in the urine unchanged. The metabolites are partly conjugated to glucuronides. Only 60% of the free metabolites and glucuronides is recoverable from urine. The plasma half-life is 4 hours, but it is longer in acute intoxication. Methyprylon stimulates the hepatic microsomal enzyme system and δ-ALA synthetase; it should probably be avoided in patients with intermittent porphyria.

Untoward effects of methyprylon are not frequent, but include "hangover," nausea, vomiting, epigastric distress, diarrhea, esophagitis, headache, and rash. Neutropenia and thrombocytopenia of unproven origin have occurred in persons taking methyprylon. An idiosyncratic excitement occasionally occurs.

Acute intoxication resembles that caused by barbiturates, and the general principles of management are the same. As with glutethimide, hypotension, shock, and pulmonary edema are more conspicuous features than is respiratory depression. Hemodialysis is an effective component of treatment. The lethal dose is unknown; death has occurred with 6 g, but recovery has occurred after 27 g. Coma may last for up to 5 days.

Habituation, tolerance, physical dependence, and addiction can occur. The abstinence syndrome is like that of the barbiturates and includes insomnia, confusion, hallucinations, and convulsions (Essig, 1964).

Preparations and Dosage. *Methyprylon,* N.F. (NOLUDAR), is supplied in 300-mg capsules and in 50- and 200-mg tablets. For adults, the oral hypnotic dose of methyprylon is 200 to 400 mg. The sedative dose is 50 to 100 mg, three or four times daily.

NONPRESCRIPTION SEDATIVE-HYPNOTIC DRUGS

Sedation and hypnosis occur as side effects with a number of drugs used for other purposes. Such effects occur with most antihistamines (Chapter 29), some antiparkinsonism anticholinergics (Chapter 14), and most phenothiazines (Chapters 4 and 12). Certain antihistamines (*e.g., methapyrilene, pyrilamine, diphenhydramine, promethazine,* and *hydroxyzine*) and anticholinergic drugs (*e.g., scopolamine, scopolamine-N-oxide,* and *benactyzine*) are promoted as sedative-hypnotics throughout the world. Among the nonprescription sedative-hypnotic drugs in the United States, methapyrilene (10 to 50 mg) is the most and scopolamine-N-oxide (0.15 to 0.25 mg) the second most used drug, and they are employed in combination in about half the products. Pyrilamine maleate and scopolamine are the only other organic sedative-hypnotic drugs available "over the counter," but inorganic bromides in small doses are also ingredients of nonprescription drug combinations. The doses of some nonprescription products are too low to be effective (*see* Rickels and Hesbacher, 1973).

Very little is known about the mode of CNS action of these nonprescription drugs. It has been suggested that a central antimuscarinic action is common to all (*see* White and Boyajy, 1960). Hypnotic doses of the anticholinergic compounds in animals cause the EEG and behavioral signs to become dissociated, and the EEG effects can be abolished by physostigmine. Diphenhydramine suppresses REM sleep, but it is not known whether all antihistamines do the same. Increasing doses of nonprescription hypnotic drugs generally do not deepen hypnosis, probably owing to a central stimulatory component of action that may cause excitatory effects, even convulsions. Tolerance to the sedative effects usually occurs during chronic use.

Beier, L. S.; Pitts, W. H.; and Gonick, H. C. Metabolic acidosis occurring during paraldehyde intoxication. *Ann. intern. Med.,* **1963,** *58,* 155–158.

Bellville, J. W.; Forrest, W. H.; Stevens, J.; and Beer, E. G. The hypnotic effects of ethchlorvynol and secobarbital in man. *Clin. Pharmac. Ther.,* **1968,** *9,* 625–630.

Bernstine, J. B.; Meyer, A. E.; and Bernstine, R. L. Maternal blood and cerebrospinal fluid estimation following the administration of chloral hydrate during the puerperium. *Am. J. Obstet. Gynec.,* **1957,** *73,* 801–804.

Birnbaum, D.; Karmeli, F.; and Tefera, M. The effect of diazepam on human gastric secretion. *Gut,* **1971,** *12,* 616–618.

Boissier, J.-R., and Pagny, J. Action antitussive d'un hypnotique non barbiturique, la métolquizolone. *Medna exp.,* **1959,** *1,* 368–372.

Boston Collaborative Drug Surveillance Program. A clinical evaluation of flurazepam. *J. clin. Pharmac.,* **1972,** *12,* 217–220.

Brown, C. R.; Shroff, P.; and Forrest, W. H. Relative potency of trichlorofos compared to pentobarbital as a hypnotic. *J. clin. Pharmac.,* **1972,** *12,* 306–312.

Chazan, J. A., and Garella, S. Glutethimide intoxication. A prospective study of 70 patients treated conservatively without hemodialysis. *Archs intern. Med.,* **1971,** *128,* 215–219.

Christianson, H. B., and Perry, H. O. Reactions to chloral hydrate. *A.M.A. Archs Derm.*, **1956**, *74*, 232–240.

Clark, T. J. H.; Collins, J. V.; and Tong, D. Respiratory depression caused by nitrazepam in patients with respiratory failure. *Lancet*, **1971**, *2*, 737–738.

Clift, A. D. Factors leading to dependence on hypnotic drugs. *Br. med. J.*, **1972**, *3*, 614–617.

Cromwell, H. A. Methaqualone—a sedative or mild tranquilizer for geriatric patients. *J. Am. Geriat. Soc.*, **1968**, *16*, 814–817.

Cucinell, S. A.; Oddesky, L.; Weiss, M.; and Dayton, P. G. The effect of chloral hydrate on bishydroxycoumarin metabolism. *J. Am. med. Ass.*, **1966**, *197*, 366–368.

Cummins, L. M.; Martin, Y. C.; and Scherfling, E. E. Serum and urine levels of ethchlorvynol in man. *J. pharm. Sci.*, **1971**, *60*, 261–263.

Curry, S. H.; Riddell, D.; Gordon, J. S.; Simpson, P.; Binns, T. B.; Rondel, R. K.; and McMartin, C. Disposition of glutethimide in man. *Clin. Pharmac. Ther.*, **1971**, *12*, 849–857.

Davies, C., and Levine, S. A controlled comparison of nitrazepam ("MOGADON") with sodium amylobarbitone as a sleep-inducing agent. *Br. J. Psychiat.*, **1967**, *113*, 1005–1008.

Davison, K.; Duffy, J. P.; and Osselton, J. W. A comparison of sleep patterns in natural and MANDRAX- and TUINAL-induced sleep. *Can. med. Ass. J.*, **1970**, *102*, 506–508.

Dement, W. C.; Zarcone, V. P.; Hoddes, E.; Smythe, H.; and Carskadon, M. Sleep laboratory and clinical studies with flurazepam. In, *The Benzodiazepines.* (Garattini, S.; Mussini, E.; and Randall, L. O.; eds.) Raven Press, New York, **1973**, pp. 599–611.

Editorial. Does methaqualone cause neuropathy? *Br. med. J.*, **1973**, *3*, 307.

Ellinwood, E. H., Jr.; Ewing, J. A.; and Hoaken, P. C. S. Habituation to ethinamate. *New Engl. J. Med.*, **1962**, *266*, 185–186.

Essig, C. F. Addiction to nonbarbiturate sedatives and tranquilizing drugs. *Clin. Pharmac. Ther.*, **1964**, *5*, 334–343.

Evans, J. I., and Ogunremi, O. Sleep and hypnotics. *Br. med. J.*, **1970**, *3*, 310–313.

Figot, P. P.; Hine, C. H.; and Way, E. L. The estimation and significance of paraldehyde levels in blood and brain. *Acta pharmac. tox.*, **1952**, *8*, 290–304.

Flemenbaum, A., and Gunby, B. Ethchlorvynol (PLACIDYL) abuse and withdrawal. (Review of clinical picture and report of 2 cases.) *Dis. nerv. Syst.*, **1971**, *32*, 188–192.

Frost, J. D., Jr.; Carrie, J. R. G.; Borda, R. P.; and Kellaway, P. The effects of DALMANE (flurazepam hydrochloride) on human EEG characteristics. *Electroenceph. clin. Neurophysiol.*, **1973**, *34*, 171–175.

Gessner, P. K., and Cabana, B. E. A study of the interaction of the hypnotic effects and of the toxic effects of chloral hydrate and ethanol. *J. Pharmac. exp. Ther.*, **1970**, *174*, 247–259.

Greenwood, R. H.; Prunty, F. T. G.; and Silver, J. Osteomalacia after prolonged glutethimide administration. *Br. med. J.*, **1973**, *1*, 643–645.

Gruber, C. M., Jr.; Kohlstaedt, K. G.; Moore, R. B.; and Peck, F. B., Jr. A study of the effects of "VALMID," a non-barbiturate central nervous system depressant, in humans. *J. Pharmac. exp. Ther.*, **1954**, *112*, 480–483.

Grüner, J.; Kriegelstein, J.; and Rieger, H. Comparison of the effects of chloral hydrate and trichloroethanol on the EEG of the isolated perfused rat brain. *Archs exp. Pharmac.*, **1973**, *277*, 333–348.

Haider, I. A double-blind controlled trial of a non-barbiturate hypnotic—nitrazepam. *Br. J. Psychiat.*, **1968**, *114*, 337–343.

Imboden, J., and Lasagna, L. An evaluation of hypnotic drugs in psychiatric patients. *Bull. Johns Hopkins Hosp.*, **1956**, *99*, 91–100.

Jacobson, E. S. Fatal immune thrombocytopenia induced by ethchlorvynol. *Ann. intern. Med.*, **1972**, *77*, 73–76.

Johansson, S.-A. Apparent resistance to oral anticoagulant therapy and influence of hypnotics on some coagulation factors. *Acta med. scand.*, **1968**, *184*, 297–300.

Kales, A.; Allen, C.; Scharf, M. B.; and Kales, J. Hypnotic drugs and their effectiveness. All night EEG studies of insomniac subjects. *Archs gen. Psychiat.*, **1970a**, *23*, 226–232.

Kales, A., and Kales, J. D. Sleep laboratory evaluation of psychoactive drugs. *Pharmac. Physns*, **1970**, *4*, No. 9, 1–6.

Kales, A.; Kales, J.; Scharf, M. B.; and Tjiauw-Ling, T. Hypnotics and altered sleep patterns. II. All-night EEG studies of chloral hydrate, flurazepam, and methaqualone. *Archs gen. Psychiat.*, **1970b**, *23*, 219–225.

Kales, A.; Preston, T. A.; Tjiauw-Ling, T.; and Allen, C. Hypnotics and altered sleepdream patterns. I. All-night EEG studies of glutethimide, methaprylon, and pentobarbital. *Archs gen. Psychiat.*, **1970c**, *23*, 211–218.

Kales, A., and Scharf, M. B. Sleep laboratory and clinical studies on the effects of benzodiazepines on sleep: flurazepam, diazepam, chlordiazepoxide, and RO 5-4200. In, *The Benzodiazepines.* (Garattini, S.; Mussini, E.; and Randall, L. O.; eds.) Raven Press, New York, **1973**, pp. 577–598.

Keberle, H.; Hoffmann, K.; and Bernhard, K. The metabolism of glutethimide (DORIDEN). *Experientia*, **1962**, *18*, 105–111.

Keplinger, M. L., and Wells, J. A. Effect of ANTABUSE on the action of paraldehyde in mice and dogs. *Fedn Proc. Fedn Am. Socs exp. Biol.*, **1956**, *15*, 445–446.

Maher, J. F. Determinants of serum half-life of glutethimide in intoxicated patients. *J. Pharmac. exp. Ther.*, **1970**, *174*, 450–455.

Maher, J. F.; Schreiner, G. E.; and Westervelt, F. B., Jr. Acute glutethimide poisoning. *Am. J. Med.*, **1962**, *33*, 70–82.

Matthew, H.; Proudfoot, A. T.; Aitkin, R. C. B.; Raeburn, J. A.; and Wright, N. Nitrazepam—a safe hypnotic. *Br. med. J.*, **1969**, *3*, 23–25.

Montagu, J. D. Effects of quinalbarbitone (secobarbital) and nitrazepam on the EEG in man: quantitative investigations. *Eur. J. Pharmac.*, **1971**, *14*, 238–249.

Murata, T. Metabolic fate of 1-ethynylcyclohexyl carbamate. II. Studies on the glucuronide excreted in the urine of humans receiving 1-ethynylcyclohexyl carbamate. *Chem. pharm. Bull., Tokyo*, **1961**, *9*, 146.

Owens, A. H., Jr.; Marshall, E. K., Jr.; Broun, G. O., Jr.; Zubrod, C. G.; and Lasagna, L. A comparative evaluation of the hypnotic potency of chloral hydrate and trichloroethanol. *Bull. Johns Hopkins Hosp.*, **1955**, *96*, 71–83.

Rao, S.; Sherbaniuk, R. W.; Prasad, K.; Lee, J. K.; and Sproule, B. J. Cardiopulmonary effects of diazepam. *Clin. Pharmac. Ther.*, **1973**, *14*, 182–189.

Rickels, K., and Bass, H. A comparative, controlled clinical trial of seven hypnotic agents in medical and psychiatric in-patients. *Am. J. med. Sci.*, **1963**, *245*, 142–152.

Rickels, K.; Clark, E. L.; Etezady, M. H.; Sachs, T.; Sapra, R. K.; and Yee, R. Butabarbital sodium and chlordiazepoxide in anxious neurotic patients: a collaborative controlled study. *Clin. Pharmac. Ther.*, **1970**, *11*, 538–550.

Rickels, K., and Hesbacher, P. T. Over-the-counter daytime sedatives. A controlled study. *J. Am. med. Ass.*, **1973**, *223*, 29–33.

Schreiner, G. E.; Berman, L. B.; Kovach, R.; and Bloomer, H. A. Acute glutethimide (DORIDEN) poisoning. *A.M.A. Archs intern. Med.*, **1958**, *101*, 899–911.

Schwartzburg, M.; Lieb, J.; and Schwartz, A. H. Methaqualone withdrawal. *Archs gen. Psychiat.*, **1973**, *29*, 46–47.

Sellers, E. M.; Carr, G.; Bernstein, J. G.; Sellers, S.; and Koch-Weser, J. Interaction of chloral hydrate and ethanol in man. II. Hemodynamics and performance. *Clin. Pharmac. Ther.*, **1972a**, *13*, 50–58.

Sellers, E. M.; Lang, M.; Koch-Weser, J.; LeBlanc, E.; and Kalant, H. Interaction of chloral hydrate and ethanol in man. I. Metabolism. *Clin. Pharmac. Ther.*, **1972b**, *13*, 37–49.

Stevenson, I. H.; Browning, M.; Crooks, J.; and O'Malley, K. Changes in human drug metabolism after long-term exposure to hypnotics. *Br. med. J.*, **1972**, *4*, 322–324.

Teehan, B. P.; Maher, J. D.; Carrey, J. J. H.; Flynn, P. D.; and Schreiner, G. S. Acute ethchlorvynol (PLACIDYL) intoxication. *Ann. intern. Med.*, **1970**, *72*, 875–882.

Turrian, H., and Gross, F. Anticholinergische Eigenschaften hypnotisch und antikonvulsiv wirkender Glutarsäureimide. *Helv. physiol. pharmac. Acta*, **1958**, *16*, 208–221.

Tyler, D. B. The use of α-ethyl-α-phenyl-glutarimide (DORIDEN), as a motion sickness preventive. *Curr. ther. Res.*, **1961**, *3*, 250–254.

Vellar, I. D. A.; Richardson, J. P.; Doyle, J. C.; and Keating, M. Gastric necrosis: a rare complication of chloral hydrate intoxication. *Br. J. Surg.*, **1972**, *59*, 317–319.

Waggoner, W. C.; Gagliardi, V. J.; and Lund, M. H. Excessive reaction to methaqualone HCl during bioavailability study. *Clin. Toxicol.*, **1973**, *6*, 317–323.

Walters, A. J., and Lader, M. H. Hangover effect of hypnotics in man. *Nature, Lond.*, **1971**, *229*, 637–638.

Welch, L. T.; Bower, J. D.; Ott, C. E.; and Hume, A. S. Oil dialysis for ethchlorvynol intoxication. *Clin. Pharmac. Ther.*, **1972**, *13*, 745–749.

White, R. P., and Boyajy, L. D. Neuropharmacological comparison of atropine, scopolamine, benactyzine, diphenhydramine and hydroxyzine. *Archs int. Pharmacodyn. Thér.*, **1960**, *128*, 260–273.

Zivin, I., and Shalowitz, M. Acute toxic reaction to prolonged glutethimide administration. *New Engl. J. Med.*, **1962**, *266*, 496–498.

Monographs and Reviews

Brown, S. S., and Goenechea, S. Methaqualone: metabolic, kinetic, and clinical pharmacologic observations. *Clin. Pharmac. Ther.*, **1973**, *14*, 314–324. (144 references.)

Garattini, S.; Mussini, E.; and Randall, L. O. (eds.). *The Benzodiazepines.* Raven Press, New York, **1973.**

Greenblatt, D. J., and Shader, R. I. Meprobamate: a study of irrational drug use. *Am. J. Psychiat.*, **1971**, *127*, 1297–1303. (72 references.)

——. The clinical choice of sedative-hypnotics. *Ann. intern. Med.*, **1972**, *77*, 91–100. (138 references.)

Inaba, D. S.; Gay, G. R.; Newmeyer, J. A.; and Whitehead, C. Methaqualone abuse. "Luding" out. *J. Am. med. Ass.*, **1973**, *224*, 1505–1509. (42 references.)

Pascarelli, E. F. Methaqualone abuse, the quiet epidemic. *J. Am. med. Ass.*, **1973**, *224*, 1512–1514. (35 references.)

Rieder, J., and Wendt, G. Pharmacokinetics and metabolism of the hypnotic nitrazepam. In, *The Benzodiazepines.* (Garattini, S.; Mussini, E.; and Randall, L. O.; eds.) Raven Press, New York, **1973**, pp. 99–127.

Schwartz, M. A. Pathways of metabolism of the benzodiazepines. In, *The Benzodiazepines.* (Garattini, S.; Mussini, E.; and Randall, L. O.; eds.) Raven Press, New York, **1973**, pp. 53–74.

Wang, R. I. H., and Wiener, M. Approach to the management of insomnia. *Drug Ther.*, **1973**, *3*, 77–83.

Wolf, S. The pharmacology of placebos. *Pharmac. Rev.*, **1959**, *11*, 689–704.

CHAPTER
11 THE ALIPHATIC ALCOHOLS

J. Murdoch Ritchie

ETHYL ALCOHOL

Alcoholic beverages have been used since the dawn of history, and the opinions and traditions of the past often cloud the discussion of this subject. The oldest alcoholic drinks were fermented beverages of relatively low alcohol content, that is, the beers and wines. When the Arabs introduced the then recent science of distilling into Europe in the Middle Ages, the alchemists believed that alcohol was the long-sought elixir of life. Alcohol was therefore held to be a remedy for practically all diseases, as indicated by the term *whisky* (Gaelic: *usquebaugh,* meaning "water of life"). It is now recognized that the therapeutic value of alcohol is much more limited than its social value.

PHARMACOLOGICAL ACTIONS

Local. Alcohol injures cells by precipitating and dehydrating protoplasm, and can therefore act as an astringent. It is also an irritant to denuded surfaces and to mucosae. The more concentrated the alcohol, the more pronounced are its effects.
Skin. Alcohol causes cooling of the skin by evaporation, and so alcohol sponges are commonly used in fever. Alcohol rubbed on the skin produces mild redness and burning, and it is therefore employed as a counterirritant and rubefacient. It is often used in bedridden patients to prevent bedsores and decubitus ulcers, for it hardens and cleans the skin and helps to prevent sweating.
Mucous Membranes. The irritant action of alcohol is particularly marked on mucosae. Strong concentrations may produce considerable inflammation of the gastric mucosa, for example. However, it is still unclear whether this, or malnutrition, is the cause of the chronic gastritis that is not uncommon in steady, heavy drinkers (*see* Lorber *et al.,* 1974).
Subcutaneous Tissues. Alcohol injected hypodermically causes considerable pain followed by anesthesia. If the injection is made close to nerves, neuritis and nerve degeneration may occur. Injections in or near nerves are deliberately used to cause anesthesia of protracted or even permanent character in the treatment of severe pain, for example, in *tic douloureux.*
Action on Bacteria. The bactericidal action of alcohol is discussed in Chapter 50.

Peripheral Nerves. Alcohol blocks conduction in peripheral nerve, by decreasing the maximal values of both the sodium and the potassium conductances (Armstrong and Binstock, 1964; Israel *et al.,* 1971). While it is tempting to ascribe the central effects of alcohol to its ability to block nervous conduction, the concentrations required, however, for peripheral blockade (about 5 to 10%) are greatly in excess of those needed to produce the central effects. It is interesting that ethyl alcohol produces a *de*polarization of peripheral nerve (Posternak and Arnold, 1954), cardiac muscle (Gimeno *et al.,* 1962), and skeletal muscle (Knutsson, 1961), whereas the higher aliphatic alcohols produce a *hyper*polarization of nerve (Posternak and Arnold, 1954).

Central Nervous System. The central nervous system (CNS) is more markedly affected by alcohol than is any other system of the body. The question whether alcohol is a "stimulant" has long been debated. Laymen in particular view alcoholic drinks as stimulating. However, there seems little doubt that alcohol is not a stimulant but, like other general anesthetics, is a primary and continuous depressant of the CNS. The apparent stimulation results from the unrestrained activity of various parts of the brain that have been freed from inhibition as a result of the depression of inhibitory control mechanisms.

Electrophysiological studies suggest that alcohol, like other general anesthetics (*see* Chapter 3), exerts its first depressant action upon those parts of the brain involved in the most highly integrated functions. The polysynaptic structures of the reticular activating system and certain cortical sites are particularly susceptible (Himwich and Callison, 1972). The cortex is thus released from its integrating control. As a result, the various processes related to thought occur in a jumbled, disorganized fashion and the smooth operation of motor processes becomes disrupted. The first mental processes to be affected are those that depend on training and previous experience and that usually make for sobriety and self-restraint. The finer grades of discrimination, memory, concentration, and insight are dulled and then lost. Confidence abounds, the personality becomes expansive and vivacious, and speech may become eloquent and occasionally brilliant. Mood swings are uncontrolled and emotional outbursts frequent. These psychic changes are accompanied by sensory and motor disturbances. For example, spinal reflexes are at first enhanced because they have been freed from central inhibitions; as intoxication becomes more advanced, however, this first phase of enhanced reflex activity is succeeded by a general impairment of nervous function and a condition of general anesthesia ultimately prevails.

Carefully performed experiments have shown that, in general, alcohol increases neither mental nor physical abilities. Although the individual often firmly believes that his performance is greatly improved, psychometric tests involving typewriting, target practice, and complicated mental problems indicate that efficiency is, in fact, decreased. Familiar and habitual tasks requiring less skill, thought, and attention are less markedly affected, especially if they are mechanical in nature (*see* Jellinek and McFarland, 1940). However, alcohol may cause some improvement in performance in *special* circumstances; for example, if a person's mental inhibitions prevent him from carrying out a task at which he is normally skilled, *moderate* amounts of alcohol, by relieving the inhibitions, may allow him to function more effectively.

In general, the effects of alcohol on the CNS are proportional to the concentration of alcohol in the blood. However, the effects are more marked when the concentration is rising than when it is falling. If the rate of absorption of alcohol from the gastrointestinal tract is rapid, a relatively high blood concentration may result from the ingestion of quite a small amount of alcohol. The same applies if the rate of distribution of alcohol to tissues, such as muscle, is low, perhaps because of a poor blood supply. Under both these circumstances, because the brain has an especially rich blood supply, the central effects may be rapidly obtained. However, redistribution of the alcohol soon occurs and the effects, as a result, are of relatively short duration.

Alcohol differs from the volatile general anesthetics in that over 90% of it is oxidized in the body and relatively little is excreted unchanged. The rate of oxidation is low, with the result that general anesthesia from alcohol lasts much longer than does that from conventional inhalational anesthetics. There is little margin between the full surgical anesthetic dose and that which is dangerous to respiration. For these reasons alcohol is not employed as a general anesthetic. It is still occasionally used as an analgesic and hypnotic, but much more so by the laity than by the medical profession. The ingestion of 60 ml of 95% alcohol raises the pain threshold approximately 35 to 40%, but it does not alter other sensory perceptions (Wikler *et al.,* 1945). Like morphine, alcohol also causes euphoria, and it changes the patient's reaction to pain from one of concern to one of relative detachment. The neurological and physiological effects of alcohol have been reviewed by Haggard and Jellinek (1942), Kalant (1961), Mardones (1963), Wallgren and Barry (1970), and Kissin and Begleiter (1971, 1972, 1974).

Respiration. Moderate amounts of alcohol in man may stimulate or depress respiration; the ventilatory response to carbon dioxide is, however, always depressed (Johnstone and Reier, 1973). Large amounts (sufficient to produce a blood concentration of 400 mg % or more) produce dangerous or lethal depression of respiration.

EEG. Alcohol produces a slowing of the alpha rhythm of the brain, and this effect becomes particularly prominent as intoxication develops. Chronic alcoholics, however, show no consistent, permanent pathological changes in rhythm (Begleiter and Platz, 1972).

Anticonvulsant Action. In laboratory animals, alcohol can effectively *suppress convulsions* induced by pentylenetetrazol and by electroshock (McQuarrie and Fingl, 1958; Workman *et al.,* 1958), but only in amounts that cause general depression of the CNS. The anticonvulsant action is followed by a period of hyperexcitability that lasts from 12 hours (after a single dose) to several days (after cessation of chronic administration). This is presumably one reason why alcohol may precipitate convulsions in man and why it is contraindicated in epilepsy. The subject is discussed more fully in Chapter 13.

Interaction with Other Drugs. The impairment of muscular coordination and of judgment that is associated with ingestion of a moderate amount of alcohol (sufficient to produce a blood concentration of up to 50 mg %) is very much enhanced in a person who has also taken sedatives, hypnotics, tranquilizers, or any of several analgesic agents. *Psychopharmacological agents are now so widely used that it is important for the physician to warn patients given such medication of the enhanced effects of alcohol and of the consequent increased danger of driving an automobile after drinking alcohol.*

Unusual side effects may occur when alcohol is taken in association with other drugs. For example, patients treated with oral hypoglycemic agents may experience unpleasant symptoms similar to those experienced by patients who take disulfiram after the ingestion of alcohol (*see* below). Furthermore, alcohol may interfere with the therapeutic actions of a wide variety of drugs, for example, the coumarin type of anticoagulant. The possible relationships between such interactions and the metabolism of alcohol by the hepatic microsomal oxidase system is discussed below (page 143). An excellent compendium of references to such interactions has been prepared by Polacsek and coworkers (1972). (*See also* Forney and Hughes, 1968; Kissin, 1974.)

Brain Metabolism. Many attempts have been made to find a metabolic basis for the effects of ethanol on the CNS, but these have not had much success. Thus, any effect of alcohol on tissue respiration in the whole animal or *in vitro* has been found to be slight or absent. Effects that are seen appear to be secondary to the functional changes in the neurons produced by alcohol (*see* Wallgren, 1971).

Cardiovascular System. The *immediate* effects of alcohol on the circulation are relatively minor. The blood pressure, cardiac output, and force of myocardial contraction do not change significantly after a moderate amount of alcohol. The pulse rate may increase, but this is usually due to muscular activity or reflex stimulation. The cardiovascular depression that is observed in acute severe alcoholic intoxication is due mainly to central vasomotor factors and to the respiratory depression. A direct depression of the heart by alcohol has been observed in rats (Haggard *et al.,* 1941b), but the concentration required (1250 mg %) is about 30% greater than that which produces respiratory arrest. However, recent studies make it clear that chronic excessive use of alcohol has a deleterious effect on the heart (*see* Myerson, 1971; Burch and Giles, 1974). Electron microscopic studies reveal characteristic intracellular lesions in the myocardium, associated with congestive heart failure; prognosis for return of muscle function is guarded. Other cardiovascular abnormalities occasionally observed in chronic heavy drinkers are largely the result of malnutrition and vitamin deficiency (*see* Hillman, 1974).

Alcohol in moderate doses causes vasodilatation, especially of the cutaneous vessels, and produces a warm and flushed skin. The vasodilatation is most likely the result of central vasomotor depression, because the direct action of alcohol on blood vessels is insignificant. The widespread belief that the coronary arteries are dilated and that the coronary blood flow is increased by moderate doses of alcohol is unsupported by acceptable laboratory or clinical evidence. Although alcohol compares favorably with nitroglycerin in its ability to prevent anginal pain in patients with coronary arteriosclerosis subjected to a standard exercise test, it does not prevent the characteristic changes in the RS-T segments and the T waves of the ECG (Russek *et al.,* 1950). This means that any salutary response to alcohol observed in angina pectoris must be due to its central depressant properties and not to any increase in coronary circulation. Alcohol administered to human subjects in doses sufficient to produce facial vasodilatation and mild inebriation causes no change in cerebral blood flow, cerebral metabolism, or cerebral vascular resistance. An amount that causes severe alcoholic intoxication (300 mg %) does indeed markedly increase mean cerebral blood flow and diminish cerebrovascular resistance. However, cerebral oxygen uptake is much reduced (*see* Wallgren, 1971). There is no rational basis, therefore, for the use of alcohol as a vasodilator in patients with cerebrovascular disease.

Skeletal Muscle. The total amount of work accomplished by an individual under the influence of small doses of alcohol may be increased. This is chiefly the result of the central action of the alcohol; for although alcohol is a readily available source of energy for muscular work and, in addition, may improve the circulation in muscle, the increased performance is largely due to a lessened appreciation of fatigue. Large doses of alcohol cause CNS depression and thereby decrease the amount of muscular work accomplished. Such doses also directly damage the muscle (Song and Rubin, 1972), causing an alcoholic skeletal myopathy similar in many respects to the alcoholic cardiomyopathy (*see* Myerson, 1971). There is a marked increase in the activity of serum creatine phosphokinase, indicative of muscle damage, and striking ultrastructural changes in the muscle.

Body Temperature. After ingestion of alcohol, there is a feeling of warmth because alcohol enhances cutaneous and gastric blood flow. Increased sweating may also occur. Heat is therefore lost more rapidly, and the internal temperature consequently falls. With large amounts of alcohol, the central temperature-regulating mechanism itself becomes depressed and the fall in body temperature may become pronounced. The action of alcohol in lowering body temperature is naturally greater when the environmental temperature is low, or when the mechanisms for dissipating heat are disturbed, as during fever. The taking of alcoholic beverages to "keep warm" in cold weather is obviously irrational, and may be dangerous if the conservation of body heat is essential. Those experienced in polar exploration are well acquainted with the dangers of this temptation.

Gastrointestinal Tract. The effects of various concentrations and types of alcoholic beverages on the gastrointestinal motor and secretory functions are influenced by a number of factors. Among these are the state of the digestive processes, the presence or absence of gastrointestinal disease, the amount and type of food present, the degree of tolerance for alcohol, accompanying psychological factors, and so forth.

Gastric secretions, like salivary secretions, are usually stimulated *psychically* by alcohol, especially if the individual likes it. The gastric juice produced in this way is rich in acid and normal in pepsin content. Alcohol may also *reflexly* stimulate the secretion of salivary and gastric juice by exciting sensory endings in the buccal and gastric mucosae. Finally, alcohol may evoke gastric secretion through a more *direct* action on the stomach, possibly involving the release of histamine; this could explain why alcohol-induced secretion is not inhibited by therapeutic doses of atropine. The involvement of histamine and gastrin has, however, been questioned (*see* Lorber *et al.,* 1974). Nevertheless, alcohol is a very effective stimulus for gastric acid secretion, and, clearly, the drinking of alcoholic beverages is inadvisable in patients with peptic ulcer. Alcohol is occasionally employed as a functional test for the ability of the gastric glands to secrete free hydrochloric acid.

The presence in the stomach of alcohol in concentrations of about 10% results in a gastric secretion rich in acid, but it is poor in pepsin unless psychic secretion is also elicited. However, although the pepsin content is decreased, there is no interference with peptic digestion, and gastric motility is not reduced. As the concentration of alcohol in ingested beverages is raised above about 20%, gastric secretion tends to be inhibited and peptic activity is depressed. Malt liquors and wine cause a similar inhibition even though the alcohol concentrations are relatively low, because they contain colloidal substances, tannins, and organic acids. Strong alcoholic drinks, of 40% concentration and over, are quite irritating to the mucosa and cause congestive hyperemia and inflammation. In such high concentrations alcohol produces an erosive gastritis (Leevy *et al.,* 1971) that is associated with a disruption of the barrier between the digestive juices and the gastric mucosa and a back diffusion of hydrogen ions from the lumen into the mucosa. This may explain why one out of three heavy drinkers suffers from chronic gastritis. The presence of food in the stomach tends to lessen irritation because it decreases the concentration of alcohol by dilution and the concentration of hydrogen ions by its buffering action. Further protection against excessive irritation is afforded by the stomach itself, which responds to the presence of alcohol by secreting mucus that both protects the mucosa and dilutes the alcohol. Aspirin, in the presence of hydrochloric acid, has been shown to produce severe gastric damage and brisk gastric bleeding in dogs (Davenport, 1969); this effect is much enhanced by alcohol.

The habitual use of immoderate amounts of alcohol may lead to constipation, due probably to an inadequate food intake and an insufficient bulk residue. On the other hand, diarrhea may occur, as a result of the irritant action of certain flavoring oils; in the chronic inebriate, however, it may signify vitamin deficiency. Alcohol taken in moderate amounts does not significantly influence the motor activity of the colon, but taken to the point of intoxication it results in virtual cessation of gastrointestinal secretory and motor functions. Absorption is delayed, and pylorospasm and vomiting may occur independently of any reflex due to local irritation.

Alcohol in moderate amounts apparently has little deleterious effect on intestinal functions. However, esophageal and duodenal abnormalities have been associated with chronic alcoholism. Alcohol is an etiological factor in acute and chronic pancreatitis (Pirola and Lieber, 1974). The latter may account for the deleterious effect of alcohol on the absorption of dietary fat and the fat-soluble vitamins (A, D, E, and K). Digestion in the small bowel is not likely to be impaired, perhaps because the alcohol reaching the intestine is considerably diluted by gastric secretions and mucus; and the secretion of pancreatic juice may actually be stimulated by small doses of alcohol.

Liver. Alcohol increases the rate at which isolated liver slices synthesize fat. This enhanced lipid anabolism seems to be caused by the increased NADH:NAD ratio that results from the oxidation of alcohol. This *direct* effect on the liver would therefore provide a plausible biochemical basis for the finding that alcohol promotes the hepatic accumulation of fat in animals. However, alcohol may also promote the accumulation of fat in the liver *indirectly,* for it causes the mobilization of fat from peripheral tissues. Even after the ingestion of relatively small amounts of alcohol, accumulation of fat in the liver of normal individuals can be demonstrated (*see* Feinman and Lieber, 1974). However, it is not quite clear how this condition of fatty liver is related to the alcoholic hepatitis or hepatic cirrhosis that is characteristic of many alcoholics (Galambos, 1972; Feinman and Lieber, 1974). Nor is it clear how much malnutrition and vitamin deficiency contribute to these conditions in man (Scheig, 1970; Galambos, 1972; Feinman and Lieber, 1974); in baboons, malnutrition does not seem to be involved in the development of alcoholic hepatitis (Rubin and Lieber, 1973). However, in spite of these effects, acute alcoholic intoxication in man is probably not associated with any great change in hepatic function, as indicated by a variety of simultaneously performed hepatic function tests (Beazell *et al.,* 1942).

It is not contended that the *continued* use of *large* amounts of alcohol has no serious effects on gastrointestinal and hepatic functions. The crucial problem centers about the occasional use of moderate amounts of alcoholic beverages. It seems that temperate amounts cannot be considered deleterious, and if one enjoys alcohol it may even affect digestion favorably if taken with meals. The influence of alcohol in the digestive tract has been extensively reviewed by Beazell and Ivy (1940) and by Wallgren and Barry (1970).

Kidney. That alcohol exerts a *diuretic effect* has been established by a number of investigators and by most consumers. Although the large amounts of fluid ordinarily ingested with alcoholic beverages undoubtedly contribute to the increased urine flow, alcohol in itself can be demonstrated to produce a marked diuretic response in man by virtue of a decrease in renal tubular reabsorption of water. Considerable evidence indicates that alcohol causes this diuresis by acting on the supraopticoneuro-hypophyseal system to inhibit the secretion of the posterior pituitary antidiuretic hormone. The diuretic effect is roughly proportional to the blood alcohol concentration and occurs when the concentration is rising but not when it is stationary or falling (*see* Haggard *et al.,* 1941a). Indeed, alcohol in repeated doses may have an antidiuretic effect (Beard and Knott, 1971).

Although the kidneys of habitual heavy drinkers may not be normal, this cannot necessarily be attributed to alcohol as such. With the possible exception of some individuals with arteriosclerotic nephritis, the ingestion of varying amounts of alcohol has no deleterious action on renal function either in normal subjects or in patients with acute or chronic nephritis. The effects of alcohol on the normal and pathological kidney have been reviewed by Bruger (1940).

Sexual Functions. Much of little worth has been written on the subject of the relation of alcohol to sexual activity. It is a popular notion that alcohol is an aphrodisiac; and, indeed, aggressive sexual behavior is often seen after alcohol, usually as a result of a loss of inhibition and restraint. Shakespeare, however, realized that inebriation interferes with coitus. In *Macbeth,* for example, the following conversation occurs (Act 2, scene 3):

MACDUFF: What three things does drink especially provoke?
PORTER: Marry, sir, nose-painting, sleep, and urine. Lechery, sir, it provokes, and unprovokes; it provokes the desire, but it takes away the performance. . . .

The experiments of Gantt (1952) on the effects of alcohol on the sexual reflexes of normal dogs support the observations of Shakespeare; in neurotic dogs, alcohol has some therapeutic value.

Endocrine Glands. Relatively large doses of alcohol stimulate the release of adrenocortical hormones by promoting the secretion of corticotropin (*see* Stokes, 1971).

Alcohol, even in moderate doses, produces a prompt increase in the urinary secretion of epinephrine, norepinephrine, and their metabolites. This is associated with an inhibition of the uptake of catecholamines into cells, leading to a decrease in the catecholamine content of the adrenal medulla and the CNS; 5-hydroxytryptamine is also released from the CNS (Feldstein, 1971). The increased concentration of circulating catecholamines might be partly responsible for the transient hyperglycemia, the pupillary dilatation, and the slight rise in blood pressure that often occur during the early stages of intoxication. It has been suggested that the altered CNS distribution of biogenic amines, particularly 5-hydroxytryptamine, mediates both the sleep and the tolerance associated with alcohol ingestion (see Truitt, 1973). Furthermore, the biogenic amines have been implicated in ethanol addiction: opium alkaloids are supposedly formed in the brain by a condensation between biogenic amines and acetaldehyde, a metabolite of ethanol (Davis and Walsh, 1970; however, see also Seevers, 1970, and Goldstein and Judson, 1971).

Blood. Alcohol produces a number of hematologic effects (see Lindenbaum, 1974). Some, such as sideroblastic and megaloblastic anemias, occur only if malnutrition coexists; alcohol also seemingly acts as a weak folate antagonist in man. Other effects, such as thrombocytopenia and vacuolization of the precursors of red and white cells, occur even when the diet is adequate and seem to result from a direct depressant action of alcohol on the bone marrow. There is also a depression of leukocyte migration into inflamed areas, which may partly account for the poor resistance of alcoholics to infection.

Absorption, Fate, and Excretion. *Absorption.* Alcohol is rapidly absorbed from the stomach, small intestine, and colon. Vaporized alcohol can be absorbed through the lungs, and fatal intoxication has occurred as a result of its inhalation. It can also be absorbed from subcutaneous sites; however, if the concentration is excessive the astringent action of alcohol prevails, with the result that the local blood supply is effectively shut off and, in consequence, absorption is limited. Absorption of alcohol through the human skin is negligible.

Many factors modify the absorption of alcohol from the *stomach*. At first absorption is rapid, but then it decreases to a very slow rate although the gastric concentration is still high. If the emptying of the stomach is delayed, for example, by pylorospasm due to high concentrations of alcohol, the subsequent absorption of alcohol from the intestine will also be delayed. The volume, character, and dilution of the alcoholic beverage, the presence of food, the period of time taken to ingest the drink, and individual peculiarities are major influences on the rate at which the stomach empties. Depending on these factors, complete absorption may require from 2 to 6 hours or more. With increasing concentration of ingested alcohol, absorption is facilitated until concentrations are reached that impede absorption. Most foods in the stomach tend to retard absorption, milk being especially efficacious. Beer exerts a retarding action, like that of food.

Absorption from the *small intestine* is extremely rapid and complete, and it is independent of both the concentration of alcohol and the presence of food in the stomach or intestine. The rapidity of absorption of alcohol from the small intestine is probably the reason why patients who have undergone massive gastrectomy may complain that they become intoxicated by amounts of alcohol that would have been innocuous prior to the operation (Muehlberger, 1958). Indeed, the time of gastric emptying and, consequently, of the onset of the phase of extremely rapid intestinal absorption may well be the prime factor that determines the wide variety of rates of absorption of ingested alcohol that are seen in different individuals and under different conditions.

Distribution in the Body. After absorption, alcohol is fairly uniformly distributed throughout all tissues and all fluids of the body. The plasma concentration is somewhat higher than that in erythrocytes. The placenta is permeable to alcohol; thus, alcohol gains free access to the fetal circulation, but it does not seem to harm the fetus. Inasmuch as alcohol affects primarily the CNS, much attention has been focused on the concentration in the brain, where, as a result of a large blood supply, the alcohol concentration quickly approaches that of the blood. The amount of alcohol in brains of persons dying of alcoholic intoxication was found to vary from 270 to 510 mg %. Alcohol is also present in cerebrospinal fluid, at a concentration lower than that in the blood when the blood concentration is rising and higher when the blood concentration is falling.

Metabolism. Ninety to 98% of the alcohol that enters the body is completely oxidized. The metabolism of alcohol differs from that of most substances in that the rate of oxidation is constant with time, and it is little increased by raising the concentration in the blood (zero-order kinetics). The amount of alcohol oxidized per unit of time is roughly proportional to body weight and probably to liver weight. In the adult, the *average* rate at which alcohol can be metabolized is about

10 ml per hour. Thus, the alcohol in about 120 ml (4 oz) of whisky or 1.2 liters (1.25 qt) of beer would require 5 to 6 hours to be oxidized by a person of average size. The relatively slow and constant rate of metabolism places a definite limit on the amount of alcohol that can be consumed over a given period of time without an individual becoming drunk due to an accumulation of alcohol. Direct determination in man indicates that the *maximal* daily metabolism of alcohol is about 450 ml (*see* Kalant, 1971). Various dietary, hormonal, and pharmacological factors have been reported to alter the metabolism of alcohol. For example, starvation lowers and insulin increases, whereas thyroid hormones leave unchanged the rate of oxidation of alcohol. However, any such effect is very slight and probably has little significance in the treatment of acute alcoholic intoxication (*see* Stokes, 1971).

The initial oxidation of alcohol occurs chiefly in the liver, and the rate of metabolism is considerably reduced in hepatectomized animals. The primary step is the oxidation of alcohol to acetaldehyde by *alcohol dehydrogenase,* which is a zinc-containing enzyme of molecular weight about 80,000 that utilizes NAD as the hydrogen acceptor (*see* Wartburg, 1971). The acetaldehyde is converted to acetyl coenzyme A, which is then oxidized through the citric acid cycle or utilized in the various anabolic reactions involved in the synthesis of cholesterol, fatty acids, and other tissue constituents. Many metabolic changes accompany or follow the metabolism of alcohol. Some changes, such as the increased production of lactate and fatty acid, the hyperuricemia, and, possibly, the decreases in the hepatic citric acid cycle activity and in fatty acid oxidation, seem to be a direct consequence of the increased NADH:NAD ratio produced by the oxidation of the alcohol (*see* Lieber *et al.,* 1971). The causes of a variety of other metabolic changes, including a decrease in urinary excretion of uric acid and an enhanced urinary loss of magnesium, calcium, and zinc, are obscure (Flink, 1971).

Alcohol has been shown also to be metabolized to acetaldehyde by another system of enzymes, namely, the microsomal mixed-function oxidases that occur in the smooth endoplasmic reticulum of the liver. The extent to which this system metabolizes ethanol in man is probably very small, but it provides a basis for the known interactions between ethanol and the host of other drugs also metabolized by this system (Lieber *et al.,* 1971). For example, ethanol first decreases and then increases the activity of the enzymes of the hepatic endoplasmic reticulum. Rubin and Lieber (1968) have suggested that this dual effect might explain why chronic alcoholics when inebriated are less resistant than normal individuals to barbiturates, but when sober are more resistant.

Excretion. Normally about 2% of ingested alcohol escapes oxidation; under special circumstances, such as when large doses of alcohol have been consumed, this value may be as high as 10%. Although small amounts of alcohol can be detected in sweat, tears, bile, gastric juice, saliva, and other secretions, most of the alcohol that escapes oxidation is excreted through the kidneys and lungs. Simple arithmetic explains why attempts to hasten significantly the emergence from intoxication by the use of diuretics or agents inducing hyperpnea are doomed to failure. At most, the concentration in the urine is slightly greater than, and the concentration in the alveolar air only 0.05%, that of the blood. A severely intoxicated individual with a blood alcohol concentration of 400 mg %, therefore, could lose at most about 4 g of alcohol per liter of urine and about 0.2 g per 100 liters of expired air.

Concentration of Alcohol in Body Fluids in Relation to Alcoholic Intoxication. Although the exact blood concentration of alcohol that indicates intoxication and drunkenness may be disputed, it is generally agreed that threshold effects (such as an increased reaction time, diminished fine motor control, and an impaired critical faculty) appear when the concentration of alcohol in the blood is 20 to 30 mg %; and more than 50% of persons are grossly intoxicated when the concentration is 150 mg %. The average concentration in fatal cases is about 400 mg % (Committee on Medicolegal Problems, 1968).

The determination of alcohol in body fluids is often important for medicolegal purposes to establish whether alcohol was ingested, or to aid in the diagnosis of drunkenness. Methods of determining the concentration of alcohol are given by the Committee on Medicolegal Problems (1968). For medicolegal tests the concentration of alcohol in the blood may be determined directly. Alternatively it can be estimated from the concentration either in expired air, which is about 0.05% that in the blood or, less frequently, in the urine, which is about 130% that in the blood.

Diagnosis of Intoxication. Much controversy exists concerning the definition and diagnosis of intoxication, and this divergence of opinion is particularly evident when the attempt is made to draft laws with regard to the driving of motor vehicles by persons who are drunk (*see* Turner *et al.,* 1958). All but a few states have passed laws embodying the recommendations of the National Safety Council and the American Medical Association. The recommendations in essence are as follows: if the defendant's blood has a concentration of alcohol of 100 mg % or over, he should be considered as being under the influence of intoxicating beverages; if 50 mg % or under, not under the influence; if between 50 and 100 mg %, this fact must be considered only with other competent positive evidence with regard to the guilt or innocence of the defendant. The fact that the average person with a blood alcohol concentration of 100 mg % or more is six to seven times more likely to have an accident than the driver with no alcohol in his blood emphasizes the importance of this legislation (*see* report by U.S. Department of Transportation, 1968).

The problem of the *intoxicated pedestrian* must also be recognized because negligence on the part of inebriated pedestrians may be an important factor in traffic accidents. For example, Gonzales and Gettler (1941) studied about 2500 pedestrians killed in highway accidents and found that about 30% were under the influence of alcohol and about 25% had a brain alcohol concentration of 100 to 250 mg % or more. Alcohol has also been found to be involved in 35% of general aviation crashes (*see* report by U.S. Department of Transportation, 1968). In addition, alcohol is a factor in a large number of *violent deaths* unassociated with traffic accidents. For example, studies in typical communities in the United States revealed that alcohol was a contributing or responsible factor in about 50% of violent deaths (*see* Tinklenberg, 1973).

From the medicolegal point of view the major factor in judging the degree of intoxication is the concentration of alcohol in the blood. The individual, on the other hand, is often concerned more with the *quantity* of alcohol he can safely drink. Unfortunately for him this is not a simple question because many factors, such as his weight and the rate of absorption from the gastrointestinal tract, determine the concentration of alcohol in the blood produced by the ingestion of a given amount of alcohol (*see* Haggard *et al.,* 1941c; Newman, 1941; Haggard and Jellinek, 1942). On the average, ingestion of 44 g of alcohol taken as whisky (4 oz) or martini cocktail (5.5 oz) on an empty stomach results in a maximal blood concentration of 67 to 92 mg %; after a mixed meal, 30 to 53 mg %. Ingestion of the same amount of alcohol taken as conventional-strength beer (1.2 liters, or 1.25 qt) on an empty stomach results in a maximal blood concentration of 41 to 49 mg %; after a mixed meal, 23 to 29 mg %. After gastrointestinal absorption is complete, the concentration in the blood at any time after ingestion can be estimated from the volume of distribution of the alcohol, which is 0.68 of the total body weight in man and 0.55 in

woman, and the metabolic rate of disappearance from the blood, which is about 18 mg % (range, 10 to 25 mg %) per hour (*see* Committee on Medicolegal Problems, 1968).

Tolerance and Addiction to Alcohol. The repeated use of alcohol results in the development of tolerance, so that larger doses must be taken in order to produce characteristic effects. However, the degree of tolerance is not as marked as for morphine and nicotine. Tolerance and addiction to alcohol are discussed in Chapter 16.

Alcohol as a Food. Alcohol is a ready, albeit expensive, source of energy that is utilized more rapidly than most foods because it is quickly absorbed from the gastrointestinal tract and requires no preliminary digestion. The energy released per gram of ethyl alcohol is approximately 7 kcal. Some alcoholic beverages also contain protein and carbohydrate; for example, beer contains about 500 kcal per liter, only half of which is provided by its alcohol content. In contrast, distilled spirits contain no such foodstuffs, and their calories are derived purely from alcohol. Moreover, they contain no vitamins.

Longevity and Heredity. Heavy drinkers have a shorter length of life on the average than do abstainers or moderate drinkers (*see* Schmidt and de Lint, 1973). However, there appears to be little or no difference in the life expectancy of abstainers as compared to *temperate* drinkers. Existing evidence does not support the claim that alcoholism injures human germ cells. The number of miscarriages tends to be higher in alcoholic women. This is mainly because they are prone to have a larger number of children, and the number of miscarriages increases as the number of conceptions increases. Likewise, infant mortality is higher in alcoholic families. This, in turn, is largely due to postnatal neglect and not to physically defective offspring.

Pathological Effects of Alcoholism and Relation to Disease and Infection. Abundant evidence indicates that certain diseases and syndromes, formerly attributed to the toxic effects of chronic ingestion of alcohol, are in reality a result of vitamin deficiencies incident to the poor food intake or the faulty gastrointestinal function of the alcoholic addict (*see* Hillman, 1974). This is true for neuropsychiatric syndromes such as polyneuritis, nicotinic acid deficiency encephalopathy, Wernicke's encephalopathy, and Korsakoff's psychosis (*see* Victor, 1958). Furthermore, the cirrhosis of the liver that occurs in 8% of chronic alcoholics in contrast to 1% of abstainers and temperate drinkers may be, at least in part, due to malnutrition (*see* Scheig, 1970; Lieber *et al.,* 1971). These diseases occur because the average heavy drinker may supply one half or more of his daily caloric requirements by drinking alcohol, and frequently continues doing so for many years. As a result, he may neglect to eat other foods that would balance his diet, and vitamin and other dietary deficiencies develop. These nutritional deficiencies account for the often poor physical state of the heavy drinker, which in turn often renders him more susceptible to infection.

Chemistry and Preparations. Alcohol is currently, and whisky, brandy, and sherry wine were formerly, official preparations. *Alcohol,* U.S.P. *(ethanol, ethyl alcohol)*, contains not less than 94.9% by volume of C_2H_5OH. *Diluted Alcohol,* U.S.P., contains about 49% C_2H_5OH by volume (about 41.5% by weight); it is thus nearly equivalent to 100-proof alcohol, which in the United States contains 50% C_2H_5OH by volume. (For an interesting account of the origin of the term *proof, see* Henderson, 1940.) *Whisky* (whiskey) and *brandy* are alcoholic liquids obtained by distillation of fermented mash and wholly or partly malted cereal grains, and the fermented juice of sound ripe grapes, respectively. They contain about 50% of C_2H_5OH by volume. *Sherry wine*, obtained by fermenting the juice of sound ripe grapes and fortifying it with brandy, contains approximately 20% of C_2H_5OH by volume. In addition, numerous other alcoholic beverages are commercially obtainable. *Rubbing Alcohol, N.F.*, contains about 70% (by volume) of ethanol, the remainder being acetone, methyl isobutyl ketone, coal tar colors, perfume oils, and water.

The relationship between chemical structure and pharmacological and toxicological action in a large number of aliphatic alcohols is reviewed in a monograph by Oettingen (1943), which also contains an extensive summary of the older literature on ethyl alcohol (*see also* Beer and Quastel, 1958; Rang, 1960; Grenell, 1971).

Therapeutic Uses of Alcohol.

Alcohol and alcoholic beverages are widely used by the laity for numerous ailments, and the proper delineation of their legitimate uses in medicine is sometimes difficult (*see* Leake and Silverman, 1966).

External. Alcohol is an excellent *solvent* for many drugs and is frequently employed for medicinal mixtures as a vehicle. Alcohol is a solvent for the *toxicodendrol* causing ivy poisoning; early and thorough washing of the affected parts with alcohol may abort or lessen the severity of the dermatitis. In *phenol skin burns* alcohol should be used immediately as a wash if castor oil is not available; it is not to be employed for gastric lavage, however, when phenol has been swallowed. Alcohol *cools* the skin when it is allowed to evaporate, and alcohol sponges are therefore used in fever. It is also *rubefacient* and is included in liniments. Alcohol (50 to 70% by volume) is employed as a rubbing agent on the skin of bedridden patients in order to prevent *decubitus ulcers*. It is also used to *decrease sweating,* and is an ingredient of many anhidrotic and astringent lotions. Ethyl alcohol still remains the most popular *skin disinfectant* (*see* Chapter 50).

Injection for Relief of Pain. Dehydrated alcohol may be injected in the close proximity of nerves or sympathetic ganglia for the relief of the long-lasting pain that occurs in *trigeminal neuralgia, inoperable carcinoma,* and other conditions. Epidural, subarachnoid, and lumbar paravertebral injections of alcohol have also been employed in appropriate circumstances. For example, lumbar paravertebral injections of alcohol may destroy sympathetic ganglia and thereby produce vasodilatation, relieve pain, and promote healing of lesions in patients with vascular disease of the lower extremities.

Alimentary Tract. Alcoholic beverages, if enjoyed by the patient, may be given before meals as a *stomachic* to improve appetite and digestion, especially in convalescent and debilitated or elderly patients. In cases of flatulence and colic, alcohol may give relief. The reflex stimulation arising from concentrated alcohol in the mouth, throat, and stomach is utilized to treat *fainting.*

Systemic Uses. Alcohol acts as a *hypnotic* and *antipyretic,* and is widely employed for these purposes by lay persons. Alcoholic beverages are sometimes valuable during convalescence as rapidly assimilable sources of energy or as remedies for insomnia. Although sometimes used for this purpose, alcohol is relatively ineffective in causing vasodilatation in persons with peripheral vascular disease or coronary artery disease; any benefits that may be noted from the ingestion of alcoholic beverages in such patients are probably due to a central depressant action rather than to an increase in peripheral or coronary blood flow.

For generations alcoholic beverages have been used to check impending *"head colds."* Perhaps the greatest therapeutic advantage of such therapy is to make the patient drowsy and sleepy so that he stays in bed, whereas otherwise he would be ambulant to the detriment of himself and his associates. Hamburger (1936) humorously advised the following therapy, culled from an old English book, to be instituted at the first inkling of a cold, namely, to hang one's hat on the bedpost, drink from a bottle of good whisky until two hats appear, and then get into bed and stay there.

Alcohol Inhalation in Acute Pulmonary Edema. Alcohol has been employed by inhalation as an *antifoaming agent* in the treatment of paroxysmal attacks of acute pulmonary edema secondary to left heart failure (*see* Luisada *et al.,* 1952). Alcohol, by its surface action, collapses the foam that obstructs the tracheobronchial airway. It can be inhaled from saturated gauze or administered as a vapor in oxygen by means of a face mask, nasal catheter, or respirator.

Contraindications.

In hepatic and severe renal disease, alcohol should probably not be used. Ulceration of the gastrointestinal tract and hyperacidity associated with digestive complaints are also contraindications. Alcohol should not be taken by epileptics because it may precipitate convulsions. In infections of the urinary tract, alcoholic beverages are to be avoided. Alcohol should be forbidden absolutely to patients who were once addicted to it (*see* Chapter 16). In general, the use of alcohol in the presence of any particular disease is a matter that the physician must decide in each individual case.

ACUTE ALCOHOLIC INTOXICATION

The characteristic signs and symptoms of alcoholic intoxication are well known. Nevertheless, the erroneous diagnosis of drunkenness is often made in patients who appear inebriated, but who have not ingested alcohol. Diabetic coma, for example, may be mistaken for severe alcoholic intoxication. Drug intoxications, cardiovascular accidents, schizophrenia, and fractured skulls, in the order named, seem to be the most common causes for the diagnostic errors (Jetter, 1938). The odor of the breath, which is *not* due to any alcohol vapor but, rather, to impurities in the alcoholic beverages or to other causes, is a notoriously unreliable guide and may often be seriously misleading. For medicolegal purposes, the concentration of alcohol in the blood, exhaled air, or urine should be determined.

In severe acute alcoholic intoxication the patient is stuporous or comatose. The skin is cold and clammy, the body temperature is low, respirations are slow and noisy, the pupils may be normal or dilated, and the heart rate is accelerated. If this condition persists for 8 or 10 hours, hypostatic pneumonia or increased intracranial pressure may ensue. Death is rare unless unconsciousness continues for many hours or trauma or infection complicates the case. Recovery is jeopardized if deep coma persists for over 12 hours.

Treatment. The patient should be kept warm. The stomach may be lavaged, but care must be taken to prevent pulmonary aspiration of the return flow. Analeptics such as pentylenetetrazol or caffeine have been employed to hasten emergence from acute alcoholic intoxication; such therapy may stimulate respiration and may help restore a comatose patient to consciousness without altering the blood concentration of alcohol. However, these agents are of questionable value, and great care must be taken not to precipitate convulsions. If significant respiratory depression is present, steps should be taken to protect the airway from aspiration and to provide ventilatory assistance if indicated. Increased intracranial pressure due to cerebral edema is treated by the usual medical measures, such as hypertonic mannitol solution intravenously, spinal fluid drainage, and so forth. Since ethanol is so freely miscible in water, it lends itself ideally to removal by hemodialysis (*see* Morgan and Cagan, 1974). In general, the therapy of the type of acute alcoholic intoxication where the patient is somnolent or comatose does not differ significantly from that of acute central depression caused by conventional general anesthetics or hypnotics. Reference should be made to the treatment of acute barbiturate intoxication for further measures (*see* Chapter 9).

Acute alcoholic intoxication is not always associated with coma. Usually therapy is not required, and it is sufficient for the patient to wait while his tissues metabolize the ingested alcohol at the characteristic constant rate until sobriety ensues. However, in some individuals the release of central inhibitory control of thought and action may lead to a condition that is characterized by nausea, vomiting, restlessness, hyperexcitability, and hyperactivity often of an extremely violent nature. Sedatives and hypnotics such as paraldehyde, chloral hydrate, and barbiturates have been extensively employed to quiet such a patient. Great care must be taken, however, when sedatives are used to treat a patient who has already treated himself to an excessive amount of a CNS depressant, namely, alcohol; and physical restraints may be safer. Phenothiazines are sometimes used to treat violent patients (Morgan and Cagan, 1974), and have been employed both to relieve the nausea and to produce relaxation and control of the patient's excessive motor activity without causing any dangerous increase in the degree of central depression. This topic is discussed in Chapter 16 in connection with chronic alcoholism. The subject of acute alcoholic intoxication has been extensively reviewed by various authors (*see* Newman, 1941; Block, 1956; Koppanyi *et al.,* 1961; Morgan and Cagan, 1974).

METHYL ALCOHOL

Methyl alcohol (CH_3OH), also called *methanol, wood alcohol,* and *Columbian spirit,* is the simplest of the alcohols. The pharmacology, biochemistry, and toxicology of methyl alcohol have been extensively reviewed by Oettingen (1943), Røe (1946), Cooper and Kini (1962), and Morgan and Cagan (1974). It is widely employed industrially as a solvent. It is also used as an adulterant to "denature," and thereby make unfit to drink, the ethyl alcohol that is used for cleaning purposes, paint removal, and a variety of other uses. Such alcohol, being tax free, is considerably less expensive than more conventional alcoholic beverages and, unless denatured, offers considerable temptation to the derelict. Methyl alcohol is purely of toxicological interest. Poisoning results from its ingestion as a substitute for, or as an adulterant of, ethyl alcohol. For example, 6% of all blindness in the United States Armed Forces during World War II was caused by methanol (Greear, 1950). The clinical, therapeutic, and laboratory aspects of an outbreak of methanol poisoning in Atlanta, Georgia in 1951, in which there were 41 deaths, were studied by Cooper and associates (1952); the ocular effects were analyzed by Benton and Calhoun (1952). Serious or fatal poisoning can also occur from industrial exposure.

Fate in the Body. After absorption, methyl alcohol is widely distributed in body tissues. It is found in the cerebrospinal fluid in a concentration higher than that in the blood and is secreted in the gastric juice. Although rats may exhale about 15%, and dogs about 50%, of an ingested dose, it is doubtful whether a significant amount is eliminated by this channel in man. A small percentage is excreted in the urine.

Methyl alcohol is largely oxidized in the body to formaldehyde and formic acid. Animals differ in their ability to oxidize methanol to formic acid and to oxidize formic acid itself. In the rabbit only 1% is excreted as formic acid in the urine, compared with 20% in the dog; an intermediate value is obtained in man. The concentrations of formic acid in blood and urine are directly related to the amount of methyl alcohol consumed and, therefore, serve as indices to the severity of poisoning (*see* Bastrup, 1947; Lund, 1948).

The oxidation of methanol, like that of ethanol, proceeds independently of the concentration in the blood. The rate, however, is only one seventh that of ethanol, so that complete oxidation and excretion of methyl alcohol usually require several days. Oxidation occurs mainly in the liver and kidney (Bartlett, 1950).

Relation of Methanol to Ethanol Oxidation. Although experiments with isolated rat-liver slices have emphasized the importance of liver catalase in oxidizing methanol (Smith, 1961; Makar and Mannering, 1968), it is still generally agreed that in the monkey and in man alcohol dehydrogenase is involved in the first step of oxidation (*see* Cooper and Kini, 1962). The fact that it is this same enzyme that is responsible for the oxidation of ethyl alcohol is presumably the explanation for the finding *in vitro* that ethanol very considerably depresses the rate of oxidation of methanol. The common biochemical pathway of oxidation of both alcohols also accounts for the clinical observations that simultaneous administration of ethanol may ameliorate the toxic sequelae of methanol poisoning (Røe, 1946; Smith, 1961). This is because the products of oxidation of methanol are toxic rather than methanol itself, and, therefore, the degree of poisoning is minimized if the rate of oxidation of methanol is reduced as much as possible.

Methyl Alcohol Poisoning. Poisoning due to methyl alcohol results from a combination of the following: (1) a minor factor of CNS depression, similar to that produced by ethyl alcohol; (2) a major factor of acidosis due to the production of formic and other organic acids; and (3) a specific toxicity of the oxidation products of methanol (probably formaldehyde) for the retinal cells.

Symptoms. Methanol is less inebriating than ethanol; indeed, inebriation is not a prominent symptom of methanol intoxication unless a very large amount is consumed or ethanol is also ingested. An asymptomatic latent period of 8 to 36 hours may precede the onset of symptoms; if ethanol is simultaneously imbibed in sufficient amount, methanol poisoning may be considerably delayed, or, on occasion, even averted. In such cases ethanol intoxication is prominent, and methanol ingestion may not be suspected.

Symptoms and *signs* of methanol poisoning consist in headache, vertigo, vomiting, severe upper abdominal pain, back pain, dyspnea, motor restlessness, cold clammy extremities, blurring of vision, hyperemia of the optic disc, and, occasionally, diarrhea. Blood pressure is usually unaffected. The pulse is slow in severely ill patients, and bradycardia constitutes a grave prognostic sign. The visual disturbance can proceed to blindness, and the pupils then do not react to light. Restlessness and delirium may be marked. Despite the severe acidosis, Kussmaul respiration is not common. Coma can develop with amazing rapidity in relatively asymptomatic subjects. In moribund patients the respiration is slow, shallow, gasping, and "fish mouth" in type. Death may be sudden, or it may occur only after many hours of coma. Death occurs in inspiratory apnea, with terminal opisthotonos and convulsions.

Laboratory findings include evidence of severe acidosis (low blood pH, low serum bicarbonate concentration), methanol and formic acid in blood and urine, moderate ketonemia, normal serum sodium and potassium concentrations, albuminuria, and slight or moderate acetonuria. The ketonemia and acetonuria are mild in comparison with the severity of the acidosis. Cerebral blood flow and cerebral oxygen consumption are both markedly reduced during methanol poisoning (Battey *et al.,* 1956). Serum amylase is elevated as a result of pancreatitis; indeed, the pancreatic injury probably accounts for the violent epigastric pain. Cerebrospinal fluid pressure is often elevated. The ECG usually exhibits minor abnormalities.

Death from methanol is nearly always preceded by blindness. As little as 15 ml of methanol has caused blindness, and ingestion of 70 to 100 ml is usually fatal. The formaldehyde is probably the cause of the selective injury to the retinal cells (Kini and Cooper, 1962; Kini *et al.,* 1962).

Treatment and Prognosis. The cardinal feature of methanol poisoning is the acidosis, and the correction of acidosis is the keystone of proper therapy if the patient is to survive. It is also believed that the prognosis with respect to salvage of vision is directly dependent on the rapidity and the completeness of the correction of the acidosis (Benton and Calhoun, 1952). However, the acidosis itself is not the cause of the ocular disturbances, because these phenomena are not observed in other types of acidosis. Indeed, retinal changes may occur in methanol poisoning despite seemingly adequate therapy with alkali (*see* Benton and Calhoun, 1952; Potts, 1955). Furthermore, it has been shown in experiments on rabbits in which various substances were injected intraocularly (Kini *et al.,* 1962) that, whereas formaldehyde causes distinct histological changes in the retina, methanol and sodium formate are without effect. All the available evidence is therefore consistent with the idea that blindness is induced by an intermediary product of methanol metabolism, possibly formaldehyde, the effect of which is *enhanced* by acidosis (Mardones, 1963). Because of the slow oxidation of methanol the risk of recurrence of acidosis after a period of successful treatment is great, and hence close observation and proper therapy should be continued for several days to prevent sudden relapse and death. The metabolic acidosis is treated with alkalis (*see* Chapter 36); hypokalemia from alkali therapy may require administration of potassium salts. In general, water and electrolyte balance and nutrition must be maintained. The use of hemodialysis or peritoneal dialysis will hasten the removal of methanol from the body (Wenzl *et al.,* 1968). The patient should be kept warm and his eyes protected from strong light.

The administration of ethanol is recommended on

the basis that it retards the oxidation of methanol, as explained above, and is a specific measure for the prevention of blindness that may otherwise follow. Ethanol administration may also be a lifesaving procedure if alkali therapy must be postponed for any reason. Neurological damage, giving rise to a permanent motor dysfunction, may follow methanol poisoning; the rigidity and hypokinesis may be relieved by levodopa (Guggenheim *et al.*, 1971). There are many reviews of the clinical, pathological, and therapeutic aspects of methanol poisoning (*see* Chew *et al.*, 1946; Røe, 1946; Cooper *et al.*, 1952; Morgan and Cagan, 1974).

DISULFIRAM

History. Williams (1937) noted that workers exposed to tetra*methyl*thiuram disulfide developed a hypersensitivity to ethanol. He even suggested that it be used as a cure for alcoholism, but his suggestion was not acted upon. The ethyl congener, *tetraethylthiuram disulfide (disulfiram)*, had been used in the rubber industry as an antioxidant. Workers exposed to disulfiram also developed a hypersensitivity to ethanol. No published report on this subject appeared until two Danish physicians, who had taken disulfiram in the course of an investigation of its potential anthelmintic usefulness, became ill at a cocktail party. Quick to realize that the disulfiram had altered their response to alcohol, they then initiated a series of pharmacological and clinical studies that provided the basis for the use of disulfiram as an adjunct in the treatment of chronic alcoholism (*see* Hald and Jacobsen, 1948; Hald *et al.*, 1948). Similar sensitization is produced by industrial exposure to cyanamide (Hald *et al.*, 1952), by eating the fungus *Coprinus atramentarius* (Fischer, 1945), or by the ingestion of *animal charcoal* (Clark and Hulpieu, 1958).

Chemistry and Preparation. The chemical structure of disulfiram is as follows:

Disulfiram

The drug is a white or light-gray, odorless, almost tasteless, crystalline powder that is almost insoluble in water. It forms chemical complexes with certain metals, especially iron and copper. The structure-activity relationship of disulfiram and its congeners has been reported by Hald and coworkers (1952). *Disulfiram*, N.F. (ANTABUSE), is available in the form of oral, scored tablets that contain 250 or 500 mg of the drug.

Absorption, Fate, and Excretion. Disulfiram is rapidly absorbed from the human gastrointestinal tract. However, a period of 12 hours is required for its full action, perhaps because its high fat solubility allows it to accumulate in the fat depots. Elimination is relatively slow, and about one fifth still remains in the body at the end of a week. The greater part of the absorbed drug is oxidized, probably chiefly in the liver, and excreted in the urine as the sulfate, partly free and partly esterified.

Mechanism of Action. Disulfiram, given by itself, is a relatively nontoxic substance, and few untoward effects are observed when it is administered alone in reasonable doses in animals or in man. However, disulfiram markedly alters the intermediary metabolism of alcohol. When ethanol is given to an animal or to an individual previously treated with disulfiram, the blood acetaldehyde concentration rises five to ten times higher than in an untreated animal or individual. This effect is accompanied by marked signs and symptoms, known as the *acetaldehyde syndrome*. Within about 5 to 10 minutes the face feels hot, and soon afterwards it is flushed and scarlet in appearance. As the vasodilatation spreads over the whole body, intense throbbing is felt in the head and neck, and a pulsating headache may develop. Respiratory difficulties, nausea, copious vomiting, sweating, thirst, chest pain, considerable hypotension, orthostatic syncope, marked uneasiness, weakness, vertigo, blurred vision, and confusion are observed. The facial flush is replaced by pallor, and the blood pressure may fall to shock level. As little as 7 ml of alcohol will cause mild symptoms in sensitive persons, and the effect, once elicited, lasts between 30 minutes (in mild cases) and several hours (in severe cases). After the symptoms wear off, the patient is exhausted and may sleep for several hours, after which he is well again.

Most of the signs and symptoms observed after the ingestion of disulfiram plus alcohol are attributable to the resulting increase in the concentration of acetaldehyde in the body. They can, in fact, be produced in normal humans by the intravenous injection of acetaldehyde (Asmussen *et al.*, 1948). Acetaldehyde is produced as a result of the initial oxidation of ethanol by the alcohol dehydrogenase of the liver. It does not accumulate in the tissues because it is further oxidized almost as soon as it is formed, most likely primarily by the enzyme aldehyde dehydrogenase. In the presence of disulfiram, however, the concentration of acetaldehyde rises because disulfiram seems to compete with NAD for the active centers of the enzyme aldehyde dehydrogenase and thereby reduces the rate of oxidation of the acetaldehyde. Disulfiram also markedly decreases the oxygen consumption and the xanthine oxidase, succinic dehydrogenase, and catalase activity of liver homogenates. Some aspects of the disulfiram-ethanol reaction, however, are still obscure. For example, *hypo*tension is characteristic of the disulfiram-ethanol reaction, whereas injection of acetaldehyde into animals usually causes *hyper*tension (*see* Perman, 1962). The hypotension could result from the known inhibition by disulfiram of dopamine-β-hydroxylase, with a consequent reduction of norepinephrine synthesis in sympathetic nerve terminals (*see* Morgan and Cagan, 1974).

Toxic Reactions and Contraindications. Disulfiram by itself is largely, but not completely, innocuous. It may cause acneform eruptions, allergic dermatitis, urticaria, lassitude, fatigue, tremor, restlessness, reduced sexual potency, headache, dizziness, a garlic-like or metallic taste, and mild gastrointestinal disturbances. In contrast to these relatively mild effects, however, alarming reactions may result from the ingestion of even small amounts of alcohol in persons treated with disulfiram. Marked respiratory depression, cardiovascular collapse, cardiac arrhythmias, myocardial infarction, acute congestive heart failure, unconsciousness, convulsions, and sudden and unexplained fatalities have occurred. Obviously the use of disulfiram as a therapeutic agent is not without danger, and should be attempted only under careful medical and nursing supervision. The patient must be warned that, as long as he is taking disulfiram, the ingestion of alcohol in any form will make him sick and may endanger his life. He must learn to avoid disguised forms of alcohol, such as sauces, fermented vinegar, cough syrups, and even aftershave lotions and backrubs.

Administration and Dosage. Disulfiram should be administered only by a physician, and therapy is usually commenced in the hospital. The maintenance dose is about 0.5 g per day, although sometimes it may have to be reduced to 0.25 g or less if unpleasant side effects appear. The daily dose should be taken in the morning, the time when the resolve not to drink may be strongest. Sensitization to alcohol lasts for 6 to 12 days after the ingestion of disulfiram because of its slow rate of elimination.

Therapeutic Use. The only therapeutic use of disulfiram is in the treatment of *chronic alcoholism.* Disulfiram is not a cure for alcoholism, but merely affords the volunteer a crutch by which the sincere desire to stop drinking can be fortified. The rationale for its use is that the patient knows that if he is to avoid the devastating experience of the "acetaldehyde syndrome" he cannot drink for at least 3 or 4 days after taking disulfiram. The subject is further discussed in Chapter 16, which deals with the therapy of chronic alcoholism.

DISULFIRAM-LIKE DRUGS

The severity of the disulfiram-ethanol reaction has prompted a search for other drugs with a disulfiram-like action that is sufficiently powerful to discourage drinking but does not endanger life. Ferguson (1956) has suggested *citrated calcium carbimide,* also called TEMPOSIL, as another drug in the treatment of alcoholism. Its effects and mode of action seem to be similar to those of disulfiram, but its onset and duration of action are briefer (Mitchell, 1958) and it seems to produce alarming circulatory changes less frequently than does disulfiram. The drug is no longer marketed.

The antiprotozoal drug *metronidazole* and the hypoglycemic *sulfonylureas* may produce a reaction similar to the disulfiram-ethanol reaction; the latter group of drugs cause the acetaldehyde concentration of the blood to rise (Truitt *et al.,* 1962). The mechanism of action remains to be elucidated.

Armstrong, C. M., and Binstock, L. The effects of several alcohols on the properties of the squid giant axon. *J. gen. Physiol.,* **1964,** *48,* 265–277.

Asmussen, E.; Hald, J.; and Larsen, V. The pharmacological action of acetaldehyde on the human organism. *Acta pharmac. tox.,* **1948,** *4,* 311–320.

Bartlett, G. R. Combustion of C[14] labeled methanol in intact rat and its isolated tissues. *Am. J. Physiol.,* **1950,** *163,* 614–618.

Bastrup, J. T. On the excretion of formic acid in experimental poisoning with methyl alcohol. *Acta pharmac. tox.,* **1947,** *3,* 312–322.

Battey, L. I.; Patterson, J. L.; and Heyman, A. Effects of methyl alcohol on cerebral blood flow and metabolism. *A.M.A. Archs Neurol. Psychiatry,* **1956,** *76,* 252–256.

Beazell, J. M.; Berman, A. L.; Hough, V. H.; and Ivy, A. C. The effect of acute alcoholic intoxication on hepatic function. *Am. J. dig. Dis.,* **1942,** *9,* 82–85.

Beer, C. T., and Quastel, J. H. The effects of aliphatic alcohols on the respiration of rat brain cortex slices and rat brain mitochondria. *Can. J. Biochem. Physiol.,* **1958,** *36,* 543–556.

Benton, C. D., Jr., and Calhoun, F. P., Jr. The ocular effects of methyl alcohol poisoning: report of a catastrophe involving three hundred and twenty persons. *Trans. Am. Acad. Ophthal. Oto-lar.,* **1952,** *56,* 875–883.

Block, M. A. Medical treatment of alcoholism. *J. Am. med. Ass.,* **1956,** *162,* 1610–1619.

Chew, W. B.; Berger, E. H.; Brines, O. A.; and Capron, M. J. Alkali treatment of methyl alcohol poisoning. *J. Am. med. Ass.,* **1946,** *130,* 61–64.

Clark, W. C., and Hulpieu, H. R. The disulfiram-like activity of animal charcoal. *J. Pharmac. exp. Ther.,* **1958,** *123,* 74–80.

Cooper, J. R., and Kini, M. M. Biochemical aspects of methanol poisoning. *Biochem. Pharmac.,* **1962,** *11,* 405–416.

Cooper, M. N.; Mitchell, G. L., Jr.; Bennett, I. L., Jr.; and Cary, F. H. Methyl alcohol poisoning: an account of the 1951 Atlanta epidemic. *J. med. Ass. Ga.,* **1952,** *41,* 48–51.

Davenport, H. W. Gastric mucosal hemorrhage in dogs. Effects of acid, aspirin, and alcohol. *Gastroenterology,* **1969,** *56,* 439–449.

Davis, V. E., and Walsh, J. J. Alcohol, amines, and alkaloids: a possible biochemical basis for alcohol addiction. *Science, Wash.,* **1970,** *167,* 1005–1006.

Ferguson, J. K. W. A new drug for alcoholism treatment. *Can. med. Ass. J.,* **1956,** *74,* 793–795.

Fischer, I. Säregen svampforgiftning. *Svenska Läkartidn.,* **1945,** *42,* 2513–2515.

Gantt, W. H. Effect of alcohol on the sexual reflexes of normal and neurotic male dogs. *Psychosom. Med.,* **1952,** *14,* 174–181.

Gimeno, A. L.; Gimeno, M. F.; and Webb, J. L. Effects of ethanol on cellular membrane potential and contraction of isolated rat atrium. *Am. J. Physiol.,* **1962,** *203,* 194–196.

Goldstein, A., and Judson, B. Alcohol dependence and opiate dependence: lack of a relationship in mice. *Science, Wash.,* **1971,** *172,* 290–292.

Gonzales, T. A., and Gettler, A. Alcohol and the pedestrian in traffic accidents. *J. Am. med. Ass.,* **1941,** *117,* 1523–1525.

Greear, J. N. The causes of blindness. In, *Blindness: Modern Approaches to the Unseen Environment.* (Zahl, P. A., ed.) Princeton University Press, Princeton, N.J., **1950.**

Guggenheim, M. A.; Couch, J. R.; and Weinberger, W. Motor dysfunction as a permanent complication of methanol ingestion. *Archs Neurol., Chicago,* **1971,** *24,* 550–554.

Haggard, H. W.; Greenberg, L. A.; and Carroll, R. P. Studies in the absorption, distribution and elimination of alcohol. VIII. The diuresis from alcohol and its influence on the elimination of alcohol in the urine. *J. Pharmac. exp. Ther.*, **1941a**, *71*, 348–357.

Haggard, H. W.; Greenberg, L. A.; Cohen, L. H.; and Rakieten, N. Studies on the absorption, distribution and elimination of alcohol. IX. The concentration of alcohol in the blood causing primary cardiac failure. *J. Pharmac. exp. Ther.*, **1941b**, *71*, 358–361.

Haggard, H. W.; Greenberg, L. A.; and Lolli, G. The absorption of alcohol with special reference to its influence on the concentration of alcohol appearing in the blood. *Q. Jl Stud. Alcohol*, **1941c**, *1*, 684–726.

Hald, J., and Jacobsen, E. A drug sensitising the organism to ethyl alcohol. *Lancet*, **1948**, *2*, 1001–1004.

Hald, J.; Jacobsen, E.; and Larsen, V. The sensitizing effect of tetraethylthiuramdisulphide (ANTABUSE) to ethyl alcohol. *Acta pharmac. tox.*, **1948**, *4*, 285–296.

———. The ANTABUSE effect of some compounds related to ANTABUSE and cyanamide. *Ibid.*, **1952**, *8*, 329–337.

Hamburger, L. P. Some minor ailments: their importance in the medical curriculum. *Yale J. Biol. Med.*, **1936**, *8*, 365–386.

Henderson, Y. The high proof of liquor as a factor in the production of alcoholism. *Q. Jl Stud. Alcohol*, **1940**, *1*, 1–12.

Jellinek, E. M., and McFarland, R. A. Analysis of psychological experiments on the effects of alcohol. *Q. Jl Stud. Alcohol*, **1940**, *1*, 272–371.

Jetter, W. W. Studies in alcohol. I. The diagnosis of acute alcoholic intoxication by a correlation of clinical and chemical findings. *Am. J. med. Sci.*, **1938**, *196*, 475–487.

Johnstone, R. E., and Reier, C. E. Acute respiratory effects of ethanol in man. *Clin. Pharmac. Ther.*, **1973**, *14*, 501–508.

Kini, M. M., and Cooper, J. R. Biochemistry of methanol poisoning: the effect of methanol and its metabolites on retinal metabolism. *Biochem. J.*, **1962**, *82*, 164–172.

Kini, M. M.; King, D. W., Jr.; and Cooper, J. R. Biochemistry of methanol poisoning. V. Histological and biochemical correlates of effects of methanol and its metabolites on the rabbit retina. *J. Neurochem.*, **1962**, *9*, 119–124.

Knutsson, E. Effects of ethanol on the membrane potential and membrane resistance of frog muscle fibres. *Acta physiol. scand.*, **1961**, *52*, 242–253.

Koppanyi, T.; Canary, J. J.; and Maengwyn-Davies, G. D. Problems in acute alcohol poisoning. *Q. Jl Stud. Alcohol*, **1961**, *22*, Suppl. 1, 24–36.

Lieber, C. S. Alcoholic fatty liver, hyperlipemia and hyperuricemia. In, *Biochemical Factors in Alcoholism.* (Maickel, R. P., ed.) Pergamon Press, Ltd., Oxford, **1967**, pp. 167–183.

Lieber, C. S., and DeCarli, L. M. Ethanol oxidation by hepatic microsomes: adaptive increase after ethanol feeding. *Science, Wash.*, **1968**, *162*, 917–918.

Luisada, A. A.; Goldman, M. A.; and Weyl, R. Alcohol vapor by inhalation in the treatment of acute pulmonary edema. *Circulation*, **1952**, *5*, 363–369.

Lund, A. Excretion of methanol and formic acid in man after methanol consumption. *Acta pharmac. tox.*, **1948**, *4*, 205–212.

McQuarrie, D. G., and Fingl, E. Effects of single doses and chronic administration of ethanol on experimental seizures in mice. *J. Pharmac. exp. Ther.*, **1958**, *124*, 264–271.

Makar, A. B., and Mannering, J. G. Role of the intracellular distribution of hepatic catalase in the peroxidative oxidation of methanol. *Molec. Pharmac.*, **1968**, *4*, 484–491.

Mitchell, E. H. Use of citrated calcium carbimide in alcoholism. *J. Am. med. Ass.*, **1958**, *168*, 2008–2009.

Muehlberger, C. W. The physiological action of alcohol. *J. Am. med. Ass.*, **1958**, *167*, 1842–1845.

Perman, E. S. Studies on the ANTABUSE-alcohol reaction in rabbits. *Acta physiol. scand.*, **1962**, *55*, Suppl. 190, 1–46.

Posternak, J., and Arnold, E. Action de l'anélectrotonus et d'une solution hypersodique sur la conduction dans un nerf narcotisé. *J. Physiol., Paris*, **1954**, *46*, 502–505.

Potts, A. M. The visual toxicity of methanol. VI. The clinical aspects of experimental methanol poisoning treated with base. *Am. J. Ophthal.*, **1955**, *39*, 86–92.

Rang, H. P. Unspecific drug action: the effects of a homologous series of primary alcohols. *Br. J. Pharmac. Chemother.*, **1960**, *15*, 185–200.

Røe, O. Methanol poisoning: its clinical course, pathogenesis and treatment. *Acta med. scand.*, **1946**, *126*, Suppl. 182, 1–253.

Rubin, E., and Lieber, C. S. Hepatic microsomal enzymes in man and rat: induction and inhibition by ethanol. *Science, Wash.*, **1968**, *162*, 690–691.

———. Experimental alcoholic hepatitis: a new primate model. *Ibid.*, **1973**, *182*, 712–713.

Russek, H. I.; Naegele, C. F.; and Ragan, F. D. Alcohol in the treatment of angina pectoris. *J. Am. med. Ass.*, **1950**, *143*, 355–357.

Scheig, R. Effects of ethanol on the liver. *Am. J. clin. Nutr.*, **1970**, *23*, 467–473.

Schmidt, W., and de Lint, J. Causes of death of alcoholics. *Q. Jl Stud. Alcohol*, **1973**, *33*, 171–185.

Seevers, M. H. Morphine and ethanol physical dependence: a critique of a hypothesis. *Science, Wash.*, **1970**, *170*, 1113–1114.

Smith, M. E. Interrelations in ethanol and methanol metabolism. *J. Pharmac. exp. Ther.*, **1961**, *134*, 233–237.

Song, S. K., and Rubin, E. Ethanol produces muscle damage in human volunteers. *Science, Wash.*, **1972**, *175*, 327–328.

Truitt, E. B.; Duritz, G.; Moran, A. M.; and Prouty, R. W. Disulfiram-like actions produced by hypoglycemic sulfonylurea compounds. *Q. Jl Stud. Alcohol*, **1962**, *23*, 197–207.

Turner, R. F.; Heise, H. A.; and Muehlberger, C. W. Interpretation of tests for intoxication. *J. Am. med. Ass.*, **1958**, *168*, 1359–1362.

Victor, M. Alcohol and nutritional diseases of the nervous system. *J. Am. med. Ass.*, **1958**, *167*, 65–71.

Wenzl, J. E.; Mills, S. D.; and McCall, J. T. Methanol poisoning in an infant. Successful treatment with peritoneal dialysis. *Am. J. Dis. Child.*, **1968**, *116*, 445–447.

Wikler, A.; Goodell, H.; and Wolff, H. G. Studies on pain: the effects of analgesic agents on sensations other than pain. *J. Pharmac. exp. Ther.*, **1945**, *83*, 294–299.

Williams, E. E. Effects of alcohol on workers with carbon disulfide. *J. Am. med. Ass.*, **1937**, *109*, 1472–1473.

Workman, R. L., Jr.; Swinyard, E. A.; Rigby, O. F.; and Swinyard, C. A. Correlation between anticonvulsant activity and plasma concentration of ethanol. *J. Am. pharm. Ass., Sci. Ed.*, **1958**, *47*, 769–772.

Monographs and Reviews

Beard, J. O., and Knott, D. H. The effect of alcohol on fluid and electrolyte metabolism. In, *The Biology of Alcoholism.* Vol. 1, *Biochemistry.* (Kissin, B., and Begleiter, H., eds.) Plenum Press, New York, **1971**, pp. 353–376.

Beazell, J. M., and Ivy, A. C. The influence of alcohol in the digestive tract. *Q. Jl Stud. Alcohol*, **1940**, *1*, 45–73.

Begleiter, H., and Platz, A. The effects of alcohol on the central nervous system in humans. In, *The Biology of Alcoholism.* Vol. 2, *Physiology and Behavior.* (Kissin, B., and Begleiter, H., eds.) Plenum Press, New York, **1972**, pp. 293–343.

Bruger, M. The effects of alcohol on the normal and pathologic kidney: a review. *Q. Jl Stud. Alcohol*, **1940**, *1*, 85–94.

Burch, G. E., and Giles, T. D. Alcoholic cardiomyopathy. In, *The Biology of Alcoholism.* Vol. 3, *Clinical Pathology.* (Kissin, B., and Begleiter, H., eds.) Plenum Press, New York, **1974**, pp. 435–460.

Committee on Medicolegal Problems. *Alcohol and the Impaired Driver: A Manual on the Medicolegal Aspects of Chemical Tests for Intoxication.* American Medical Association, Chicago, **1968.**

Feinman, L., and Lieber, C. S. Liver disease in alcoholism. In, *The Biology of Alcoholism.* Vol. 3, *Clinical Pathology.* (Kissin, B., and Begleiter, H., eds.) Plenum Press, New York, **1974,** pp. 303–338.

Feldstein, A. Effect of ethanol on neurohumoral amine metabolism. In, *The Biology of Alcoholism.* Vol. 1, *Biochemistry.* (Kissin, B., and Begleiter, H., eds.) Plenum Press, New York, **1971,** pp. 127–159.

Flink, E. B. Mineral metabolism in alcoholism. In, *The Biology of Alcoholism.* Vol. 1, *Biochemistry.* (Kissin, B., and Begleiter, H., eds.) Plenum Press, New York, **1971,** pp. 377–395.

Forney, R. B., and Hughes, F. W. *Combined Effects of Alcohol and Other Drugs.* Charles C Thomas, Pub., Springfield, Ill., **1968.**

Galambos, J. T. Alcoholic hepatitis: its therapy and prognosis. *Prog. liver Dis.,* **1972,** *4,* 567–588.

Grenell, R. Effects of alcohol on the neuron. In, *The Biology of Alcoholism.* Vol. 1, *Biochemistry.* (Kissin, B., and Begleiter, H., eds.) Plenum Press, New York, **1971,** pp. 1–19.

Haggard, H. W., and Jellinek, E. M. *Alcohol Explored.* Doubleday, Doran & Co., Inc., Garden City, N.Y., **1942.**

Hillman, R. W. Alcoholism and malnutrition. In, *The Biology of Alcoholism.* Vol. 3, *Clinical Pathology.* (Kissin, B., and Begleiter, H., eds.) Plenum Press, New York, **1974,** pp. 513–586.

Himwich, H. E., and Callison, D. A. The effects of alcohol on evoked potentials of various parts of the central nervous system of the cat. In, *The Biology of Alcoholism.* Vol. 2, *Physiology and Behavior.* (Kissin, B., and Begleiter, H., eds.) Plenum Press, New York, **1972,** pp. 67–84.

Israel, Y.; Rosenmann, E.; Hein, S.; Colombo, G.; and Canessa-Fischer, M. Effects of alcohol on the nerve cell. In, *Biological Basis of Alcoholism.* (Israel, Y., and Mardones, J., eds.) John Wiley & Sons, Inc., New York, **1971,** pp. 53–72.

Jacobsen, E. The metabolism of ethyl alcohol. *Pharmac. Rev.,* **1952,** *4,* 107–135.

Kalant, H. The pharmacology of alcohol intoxication. *Q. Jl Stud. Alcohol,* **1961,** *22,* Suppl. 1, 1–23.

———. Absorption, diffusion, distribution, and elimination of ethanol: effects on biological membranes. In, *The Biology of Alcoholism.* Vol. 1, *Biochemistry.* (Kissin, B., and Begleiter, H., eds.) Plenum Press, New York, **1971,** pp. 1–62.

Kissin, B. Interactions of ethyl alcohol and other drugs. In, *The Biology of Alcoholism.* Vol. 3, *Clinical Pathology.* (Kissin, B., and Begleiter, H., eds.) Plenum Press, New York, **1974,** pp. 109–161.

Kissin, B., and Begleiter, H. (eds.). *The Biology of Alcoholism.* Vol. 1, *Biochemistry.* Plenum Press, New York, **1971.**

———. *Ibid.* Vol. 2, *Physiology and Behavior.* Plenum Press, New York, **1972.**

———. *Ibid.* Vol. 3, *Clinical Pathology.* Plenum Press, New York, **1974.**

Leake, C. D., and Silverman, M. *Alcoholic Beverages in Clinical Medicine.* Year Book Medical Publishers, Inc., Chicago, **1966.**

Leevy, C. M.; Tanribilir, A. K.; and Smith, F. Biochemistry of gastrointestinal and liver disease in alcoholism. In, *The Biology of Alcoholism.* Vol. 1, *Biochemistry.* (Kissin, B., and Begleiter, H., eds.) Plenum Press, New York, **1971,** pp. 307–325.

Lieber, C. S.; Rubin, E.; and DeCarli, L. M. Effects of ethanol on lipid, uric acid, intermediary and drug metabolism, including the pathogenesis of the alcoholic fatty liver. In, *The Biology of Alcoholism.* Vol. 1, *Biochemistry.* (Kissin, B., and Begleiter, H., eds.) Plenum Press, New York, **1971,** pp. 263–305.

Lindenbaum, J. Hematologic effects of alcohol. In, *The Biology of Alcoholism.* Vol. 3, *Clinical Pathology.* (Kissin, B., and Begleiter, H., eds.) Plenum Press, New York, **1974,** pp. 461–480.

Lorber, S. H.; Dinoso, V. P., Jr.; and Chey, W. Y. Diseases of the gastrointestinal tract. In, *The Biology of Alcoholism.* Vol. 3, *Clinical Pathology.* (Kissin, B., and Begleiter, H., eds.) Plenum Press, New York, **1974,** pp. 339–357.

Mardones, J. The alcohols. In, *Physiological Pharmacology,* Vol. 1. (Root, W. S., and Hofmann, F. G., eds.) Academic Press, Inc., New York, **1963.**

Morgan, R., and Cagan, E. J. Acute alcohol intoxication, the disulfiram reaction, and methyl alcohol intoxication. In, *The Biology of Alcoholism.* Vol. 3, *Clinical Pathology.* (Kissin, B., and Begleiter, H., eds.) Plenum Press, New York, **1974,** pp. 163–189.

Myerson, R. M. Effects of alcohol on cardiac and muscular function. In, *Biological Basis of Alcoholism.* (Israel, Y., and Mardones, J., eds.) John Wiley & Sons, Inc., New York, **1971,** pp. 183–208.

Newman, H. W. *Acute Alcoholic Intoxication: A Critical Review.* Stanford University Press, Stanford, Calif., **1941.**

Oettingen, W. F. von. *The Aliphatic Alcohols: Their Toxicity and Potential Dangers in Relation to Their Chemical Constitution and Their Fate in Metabolism.* Public Health Bulletin No. 281, U.S. Government Printing Office, Washington, D. C., **1943.**

Pirola, R. C., and Lieber, C. S. Acute and chronic pancreatitis. In, *The Biology of Alcoholism.* Vol. 3, *Clinical Pathology.* (Kissin, B., and Begleiter, H., eds.) Plenum Press, New York, **1974,** pp. 359–402.

Polacsek, E.; Barnes, T.; Turner, N.; Hall, R.; and Weise, C. *Interaction of Alcohol and Other Drugs.* Addiction Research Foundation, Toronto, **1972.**

Stokes, P. E. Alcohol-endocrine relationships. In, *The Biology of Alcoholism.* Vol. 1, *Biochemistry.* (Kissin, B., and Begleiter, H., eds.) Plenum Press, New York, **1971,** pp. 397–436.

Tinklenberg, J. R. Alcohol and violence. In, *Alcoholism. Progress in Research and Treatment.* (Bourne, P. G., and Fox, R., eds.) Academic Press, Inc., New York, **1973,** pp. 195–210.

Truitt, E. B. A biogenic amine hypothesis for alcohol tolerance. *Ann. N.Y. Acad. Sci.,* **1973,** *215,* 177–182.

U.S. Department of Transportation. *Alcohol and Highway Safety.* (A Report to the Congress from the Secretary of Transportation.) The Department, Washington, D. C., **1968.**

Wallgren, H. Effect of ethanol on intracellular respiration and cerebral function. In, *The Biology of Alcoholism.* Vol. 1, *Biochemistry.* (Kissin, B., and Begleiter, H., eds.) Plenum Press, New York, **1971,** pp. 103–125.

Wallgren, H., and Barry, H., III. *Actions of Alcohol,* Vols. I and II. American Elsevier Publishing Co., Inc., New York, **1970.**

Wartburg, J. P. von. The metabolism of alcohol in normals and alcoholics: enzymes. In, *The Biology of Alcoholism.* Vol. 1, *Biochemistry.* (Kissin, B., and Begleiter, H., eds.) Plenum Press, New York, **1971,** pp. 63–102.

12 DRUGS AND THE TREATMENT OF PSYCHIATRIC DISORDERS

Robert Byck

Twenty percent of the prescriptions written in an average community in the United States are for medications intended to affect mental processes, namely, to stimulate, sedate, or otherwise change behavior. A large number of the drugs administered by physicians primarily for other purposes also modify thought, mood, and emotion. In this chapter two groups of agents will be discussed. The first are drugs used in the treatment of psychiatric disorders. The second group may so alter the function of the central nervous system (CNS), either as main or side effects, to warrant their being called psychotoxic drugs. The members of both groups are often described as *psychoactive* or *psychotropic* drugs. Over 1500 compounds classified primarily as psychotropic agents have been described (Usdin and Efron, 1972). Their use has become widespread since the early 1950s.

Psychotherapeutic drugs are intended to treat abnormalities of mental function. Because of a widespread desire to modify "normal" feelings, several such drugs have become important in the life pattern of a vast number of people in many countries. For this reason, the effects of psychotropic agents on normal subjects will also be described.

Many diverse discoveries have led to the development of "biological psychiatry," a discipline concerned with the chemical pathophysiology of psychiatric illnesses. An attempt will be made in this chapter to summarize what is known about the biological basis of mental illness in order to help elucidate the possible mechanisms of action of the psychotropic drugs.

In the presentation of each drug group, a prototype drug will be used to exemplify the characteristics of the class. Important differences from the prototype drug will be discussed when appropriate. Sections on the rational use of these drugs in the treatment of the major psychiatric disorders will comprise an important part of this chapter. An attempt will also be made to define the characteristics of treatable conditions, and to suggest a pattern in which drugs may be used in treatment.

There are considerable problems in the terminology of psychoactive drugs and in the nosology of psychiatric illnesses. The classification of psychotherapeutic agents in this chapter will be as follows: *antipsychotic* drugs, *mood-stabilizing* and *antidepressant* drugs, and *antianxiety-sedative* drugs.

Psychotoxic agents have a variety of actions; some can reproducibly cause psychotic states and are therefore termed *psychotogenic* agents. These include the drugs that induce *delirium* and the *psychedelic* drugs (*e.g.,* marihuana). Some agents improve mood and hence are called *euphoriants;* but in higher doses they may cause a paranoid psychosis and thus are both euphoriant and psychotogenic (*e.g.,* amphetamines). For this reason a simple nomenclature is not possible. Many of the psychotoxic drugs are euphoriant in low doses and are widely abused (*see* Chapter 16).

The use of drugs in the treatment of psychiatric disorders is complicated by many of the diagnostic uncertainties and inaccuracies that have plagued psychiatry. In most areas of therapeutics, physicians are reasonably certain about the diagnosis and nature of a disease before specific drug therapy is instituted. In psychiatry, despite the best efforts, blurring of diagnostic entities is a rule rather than an exception, and consequently the use of psychotropic drugs frequently lacks the elegance and precision possible in other areas of medicine. In this chapter diagnostic terms that imply discrete disease entities will be used whenever possible. There is often polar disagreement among psychiatrists as to what constitutes a treatable disease process, but the impreciseness of the diagnostic entities does not invalidate the many salutary drug effects on mental symptoms. The current diagnostic terminology often employed in the United States is described in the American Psychiatric Association's *Diagnostic and Statistical Manual of Mental Disorders: II* (1968).

History. Modification of behavior, mood, and emotion by drugs has always been a favorite indulgence of mankind. The use of psychoactive drugs evolved along two related paths. The first was in the use of drugs to modify normal behavior and to produce models of madness. The second was to alleviate or cure mental ailments. The two paths are conceptually related in that specific drug treatment implies a pathophysiological basis of mental symptoms. Until recent times, the search for such a basis was barren and frustrating.

A definitive older account of the history and characteristics of many psychoactive compounds is presented by Lewin (1924). A more modern review is that of Holmstedt (1967). In 1845, Moreau proposed that hashish intoxication provided a model psychosis useful in the study of insanity. Three decades later, Freud presented his study of cocaine and suggested its potential uses in pharmacotherapy (*see* Byck, 1974). Soon thereafter, Kraepelin founded the first laboratory of clinical psychopharmacology in Dorpat, where he evaluated psychological effects of drugs in man. In 1931, Sen and Bose published the first report of the use of *Rauwolfia serpentina* in the treatment of insanity. Insulin shock, pentylenetetrazol-induced convulsions, and electroconvulsive therapy followed in 1933, 1934, and 1937, respectively, and treatment of both depression and schizophrenia thus became available. Amphetamine was the first synthetic drug to provide a model psychosis. In 1943, Hofmann purposefully ingested a minute amount of lysergic acid diethylamide (LSD) to experience its psychic effects. His report of the high potency of LSD made the concept that a toxic metabolic product might be the cause of mental illness more acceptable, thereby renewing the search for a model psychosis. Accounts of this and other early experiments in psychopharmacology have been presented by the original participants (*see* Ayd and Blackwell, 1970). The historical background for the major psychoactive drugs is presented later in the chapter.

The first report on the treatment of mania with lithium was that of Cade (1949). This discovery was slow in gaining general acceptance by the psychiatric community. In 1950, *chlorpromazine* was synthesized in France. The recognition of the unique effects of chlorpromazine by Laborit and its use in psychiatric patients by Delay and Deniker (1952) marked the beginnings of modern psychopharmacology. Thus, agents with selective antipsychotic effects became available. In 1953 the term *tranquilizer* was introduced by Yonkman to characterize the psychic effect of reserpine. Despite its popularity this term will not be used in this chapter.

The report on *meprobamate* by Berger (1954) marked the beginning of investigations of antianxiety drugs. In 1958, Kuhn recognized the antidepressant effect of *imipramine;* an antituberculosis drug, *iproniazid,* introduced in the same year, was soon recognized as a monoamine oxidase inhibitor and antidepressant. *Chlordiazepoxide,* the first of the antianxiety benzodiazepines, was introduced in 1957. In the following year Janssen discovered the antipsychotic properties of *haloperidol,* a butyrophenone, and thus still another class of antipsychotic agents became available.

During the 1960s there was a rapid expansion of psychopharmacological research, and many new theories of psychoactive drug effects were introduced. The clinical efficacy of many of these agents was firmly established during this decade.

In recent years, emphasis has centered on biogenic amines in the CNS and their possible causal involvement in mental illness. In addition, much attention is being paid to the liabilities of treatment with psychotherapeutic drugs, and a balanced view of their advantages and disadvantages is beginning to emerge.

Nosology. The physician's use of psychotherapeutic drugs is frequently governed by the therapeutic value implied in the names of drug classes. It is therefore important to recognize the commonly accepted definitions of major diagnostic terms. "Patients are described as *psychotic* when their mental functioning is sufficiently impaired to interfere grossly with their capacity to meet the ordinary demands of life. The impairment may result from a serious distortion in their capacity to recognize reality. Hallucinations and delusions may, for example, distort their perceptions" (American Psychiatric Association, 1968). Klein and Davis (1969) have stated that "the hallmark of psychosis is the apparently inexplicable nature of the misevaluation or misperception which has the force of reality." Unfortunately, as Detre and Jarecki (1971) have commented, ". . . the borderline between 'neurosis' and 'psychosis' is fluid; cognitive disturbances are ubiquitous in psychiatric disorders and the severity of the incapacitation does not necessarily distinguish the two." Patients who have a schizophrenic psychosis in remission may be only slightly if at all impaired, whereas an obsessive-compulsive neurosis may be completely crippling.

In view of these complexities, emphasis will be placed on the effects of drugs on specific *symptoms* and *symptom complexes* that frequently characterize psychiatric illnesses. Some clear definitions for the diagnosis of many psychiatric illnesses are given by Feighner and colleagues (1972). Operational criteria for a cross-cultural diagnosis of schizophrenia have been derived from a study sponsored by the World Health Organization (Carpenter *et al.*, 1973). Specific nosological problems will be discussed as they are relevant to drug actions and uses.

Biological Theories of Mental Illness. *Schizophrenia.* This disease affects mood, behavior, emotion, and cognitive processes. The modification of a number of biological variables in the disorder suggests that a biochemical basis should be sought. The argument for a biochemical basis of schizophrenia comes from four types of evidence. Whether this evidence will also lead to an explanation for *vulnerability* to the disease remains moot. The masterful critique of Kety (1959) still holds today in evaluating research in this area. Reviews of this subject have been published by Wyatt and coworkers (1971), Kety and Matthysse (1972), and Snyder and associates (1974).

The four evidential areas are *physiological-biochemical, model pharmacological, pharmacological,* and *genetic.* There is, of course, considerable conceptual overlap in this research, and no unitary theory has as yet been accepted.

The *physiological-biochemical evidence* is based either on abnormal physiological responsiveness or on the presence of abnormal substances in the tissues, blood, or urine of schizophrenic patients. For example, there are differences both in blood histamine concentrations and in responsiveness to histamine between schizophrenics and normal subjects. Characterization of this difference has been difficult because both high and low blood histamine concentrations have been found, but schizophrenics do consistently respond less to histamine administered intradermally than do normal individuals. The evidence for excretion of abnormal substances by schizophrenics is typified by a substance causing a "pink spot" on test of urine. This is presumed to be an abnormally methylated dopamine metabolite, 3,4-dimethoxyphenethylamine (DMPEA). DMPEA does not cause a schizophrenic psychosis when administered to normal individuals. Small quantities of its acid metabolite are produced in the body, but the evidence is equivocal as to whether its presence in urine is unique to schizophrenics or whether it reflects dietary or other exogenous factors. The interest in the pink spot is based on the appealing but unproven transmethylation theory. Some methylated products of normally occurring biogenic amines are hallucinogenic. Thus, bufotenine, dimethyltryptamine, and mescaline are produced by methylation of indole, tryptamine, and dopamine, respectively. Methionine, as well as other methyl donors for certain transmethylation reactions, can cause an exacerbation of psychosis (*see* Snyder *et al.*, 1974). Whether amine-induced psychosis is closely related to schizophrenia is an open question.

Evidence for the significance of other presumed urine and blood abnormalities in schizophrenia is equally tenuous and lacks the pharmacological appeal of the transmethylation theory. There are obvious difficulties in deducing information about brain chemistry from analyses of urine and blood. Reported abnormalities in brain chemistry such as the alleged deficiency of dopamine β-hydroxylase in the brains of schizophrenic subjects are suspect because of many methodological difficulties, but this field of research may prove fruitful, particularly in view of the success in Parkinson's disease.

The *model-pharmacological theory* of schizophrenia is also concerned with dopamine and methylated amines. A model psychosis presumably related to schizophrenia can be produced by abnormal metabolism of amines or by exogenous substances that affect their storage or release. The paranoid psychosis produced by large doses of amphetamine and blocked by the phenothiazines is hypothesized to be the result of excess dopaminergic activity. A number of psychedelic drugs, such as indoleamines and methylated phenethylamines, can produce symptoms that are similar in certain respects to those observed in naturally occurring psychoses. It is known that dimethyltryptamine, a methylated indoleamine, can be produced in the body.

Pharmacological hypotheses of schizophrenia have been based on analyses of the actions common to the antipsychotic drugs. The most consistent finding is that all known antipsychotic drugs seem to block the effects of dopamine. Originally there appeared to be other similarities among antipsychotic drugs, such as the production of catalepsy in animals, parkinsonism in man, blocking of conditioned avoidance response, and "stabilization" of neuronal membranes; however, these shared actions were eliminated as essential for antipsychotic action when new drugs were found not to possess them (*see* Matthysse, 1973; Snyder *et al.*, 1974). In this area of research, two requirements for identification of the pathophysiological substrate of schizophrenia are that all antipsychotic drugs possess a common specific action and that this specific action can be related to an abnormal characteristic found in the CNS of schizophrenics. The concept of a dopamine-receptor abnormality in particular does not meet the second requirement. Since there are no animal models for schizophrenia, this research path will continue to be difficult. The possibility that any common action of antipsychotic drugs has neurophysiological effects two or three steps removed from the presumed defect in schizophrenia is another difficulty. For example, the drugs may correct imbalances between neural systems controlled or modulated by different neuro-transmitter substances.

The *genetic approach* seeks to establish a biological basis for schizophrenia by an examination of the heredity of persons afflicted with the disease. Kallmann (1953) found that the concordance rate for schizophrenia varied directly with the closeness of blood relationship. The incidence of schizophrenia in the immediate families of schizophrenics is consistently higher than that in the population at large. Neither of these facts rules out the effects of precipitating psychological factors in the rearing of children. However, if monozygotic twins are reared apart, the concordance rate is about the same as if they were reared together. When children with a schizophrenic heritage are reared by foster parents together with children without this heritage, the former group shows a higher incidence of the disorder. This same result has been found in five studies in three countries (*see* Kety and Matthysse, 1972). These genetic studies now provide strong but not conclusive evidence for a biological substrate of schizophrenia.

Affective Disorders. The biological basis of affective disorders (mania and depression) is on firmer ground than that for schizophrenia. As with schizophrenia, a major problem is with the definition of the disorders (*see* subsequent section on drug treatment of affective disorders, page 185), and the research pathways are the same as described above. The impetus for research in depression and mania comes both from the elucidation of the metabolic pathways of the biogenic amines (*see* Axelrod, 1971; Axelrod and Weinshilboum, 1972) and from the effects of antidepressant drugs on aminergic systems. The immense literature in these areas has been reviewed by Davis (1970) and Schildkraut (1973).

The *physiological-biochemical evidence* has centered on the presence of various amine metabolites in body fluids. Almost all the metabolites of norepinephrine, dopamine, and 5-hydroxytryptamine (5-HT), as well as substances such as cyclic adenosine 3′,5′-monophosphate (cyclic AMP), have been examined in the blood and urine of depressed and manic patients. The original source of these substances may or may not be the brain. Studies of the norepinephrine metabolite 3-methoxy,4-hydroxyphenethylene glycol in the urine of depressed patients have indicated that there may be a subgroup of these patients who consistently excrete low levels of this substance. Another and perhaps overlapping group of depressed patients shows low concentrations of the 5-HT metabolite 5-hydroxyindoleacetic acid in their spinal fluid. There is some hope that biochemically defined subgroups of depressed patients will respond specifically to selected drug therapy.

With regard to the *model-pharmacological area* of research, pharmacologically induced depression as a side effect of reserpine treatment was among the original clues in the formulation of the "catecholamine hypothesis" by Jacobsen (1964). This hypothesis, later elaborated by Bunney and Davis (1965), Schildkraut (1965), and Schildkraut and Kety (1967), postulates that depression is the result of a functional deficiency of brain catecholamines. Additional pharmacological support was provided by the antidepressant effects of monoamine oxidase inhibitors, which can produce a state resembling mania; these inhibitors increase available biogenic amines by preventing their enzymatic destruction.

Pharmacological hypotheses for a chemical pathogenesis of depression are based on the fact that all drugs currently used in affective disorders have actions on aminergic systems. In general, antidepressants act to increase the amount of amines at central synapses, either by blocking re-uptake or preventing the breakdown of amines. Even electroconvulsive therapy affects norepinephrine turnover and metabolism in the CNS. Further discussions of the actions of antidepressant drugs appear later in the chapter.

The view that mania had a *genetic basis* was first proposed by the French psychiatrist Esquirol in 1837. Kraepelin, in 1921, considered heredity to be paramount in the etiology of manic-depressive illness. Evidence that manic-depressive illness is an X chromosome–linked hereditary disease is presented in some detail in the monograph by Winokur and coworkers (1969). It is now commonly accepted that there is at least a genetic predisposition to "bipolar" manic-depressive illness. The evidence for a genetic basis for other forms of depression is less well established.

In *summary,* there is evidence that both schizophrenia and manic-depressive illness are diseases that have biological bases, even though the exact nature of these illnesses is not yet clear. The concept of deranged cerebral chemistry is well enough established to justify continued research on how drugs affect neuronal mechanisms in psychiatric patients. Nevertheless, physicians give drugs to *people,* and the effects of drugs are greatly modified by psychological phenomena. For this reason, interpersonal and social factors should never be minimized in the use of psychoactive drugs.

Animal Experiments and Psychopharmacology. Because the essential characteristics of human mental disease cannot be reproduced in animals, studies of etiology and treatment are greatly hampered. In man, psychiatric illness can manifest itself by disturbances in interpersonal relationships and communication. Internal conflict, anxiety, and depression are often revealed only through verbalization. Social structure and communication in subhuman animals are so rudimentary as to make the human achievements in this area unique. The intellectual superiority of man over even the highest other primates is so great as to make comparison of respective psychopathology exceedingly difficult.

Although the study of animal behavior has not yet yielded much information concerning the mode of action of drugs in abnormal human behavior, such studies have led to screening procedures for the selection of drugs in the treatment of mental illness. The usefulness of many compounds in the treatment of psychiatric disorders was discovered fortuitously in patients receiving them for other purposes. However, many psychiatrically useful phenothiazines and drugs such as haloperidol, chlordiazepoxide, and others were discovered by means of animal screening technics. Once a therapeutically useful drug has been found, its properties in animal tests can be ascertained and new compounds with similar actions can be synthesized. The chance of discovering a unique therapeutic agent with this method is small, but variations in efficacy and toxicity may be found.

Clinical Evaluation of Psychotropic Drugs. Although there are problems in the evaluation of the efficacy of any drug in a particular disease syndrome, the difficulties in evaluating psychoactive drugs frequently seem almost insurmountable. Despite this, the physician must be able to evaluate the literature of clinical psychopharmacology and have in mind standards by which a particular study can be judged. Assessment of change and improvement in psychiatric illness has never been an easy task. This was true before the advent of drug therapy and, although methods of evaluation have become more and more sophisticated, it is true today. Perhaps the most striking example of this problem is found in literature concerning the efficacy of psychotherapy. Although it is eminently clear that psychotherapy does have salutary effects in individual patients, nonetheless no study has demonstrated this in a scientifically acceptable way. The problem would appear to be simpler in the evaluation of pharmacotherapy, for here one presumes that the agent is uniform and administered to all patients in the same way. Unfortunately, the results are still frequently equivocal.

The problems that have to be faced cannot be outlined in detail, but the following criteria should be applied for the evaluation of studies in this field. (1) The pathological syndrome to be studied should be carefully defined and as homogeneous a group of patients as possible should be selected on this basis. (2) The treatment setting is of importance, especially as it relates to patient compliance. (3) The natural history of many psychiatric disorders is so unpredictable that double-blind, placebo-controlled studies are essential. (4) If two drugs are to be compared with respect to efficacy, they cannot be evaluated on the basis of an arbitrary fixed dose of each drug; dose-response studies are essential. (5) The number of patients studied should be sufficiently large to apply statistical analysis, and the rating scales employed for the evaluation of the drug should be of such a nature as to permit factor analysis. A critical review of the principles and problems in establishing the efficacy and safety of psychotropic drugs has been presented by Levine and associates (1971).

The discussions of psychotropic drugs in the following sections will place major emphasis on the results of carefully controlled studies whenever these are available. Unfortunately, in many areas controlled studies have never been done; here, the best available evidence will be used in evaluating drug efficacy. Since the literature is so vast, reference will often be made to review articles. As with all classes of drugs, the prudent physician will employ only a limited number of proven agents and become thoroughly familiar with their use.

I. Drugs Used in the Treatment of Psychoses

Several classes of drugs are effective in the symptomatic treatment of psychoses. They are most appropriately used in the therapy of schizophrenia, organic psychoses, and the manic phase of manic-depressive illness. Their occasional use may be indicated in depression or in severe anxiety. Structurally these classes comprise the phenothiazines and thioxanthenes, the butyrophenones, the dibenzodiazepines, and the rauwolfia alkaloids. Since these drugs share certain effects, information about side effects and therapeutic uses pertinent to all antipsychotic drugs is presented in a single section after the specific descriptions of chemical groups. The use of these drugs in practice is not limited to the treatment of psychoses, as evident from the fact that an estimated 250 million people had received drugs in these classes by the end of 1970. The liabilities of their widespread use have been emphasized (Crane, 1973).

PHENOTHIAZINES AND THIOXANTHENES

The phenothiazines as a class, and especially chlorpromazine, the prototype, are among the most widely used drugs in the practice of medicine today. Chlorpromazine and related phenothiazine derivatives are employed primarily in the treatment of psychiatric patients. They are also of importance for the control of nausea and vomiting. Other phenothiazines are of value for their antihistaminic effect. One phenothiazine, methotrimeprazine, is used as an analgesic. Uses other than antipsychotic or antiemetic are discussed elsewhere (*see* Index). Presently, there are more than 2-dozen phenothiazine drugs used in medicine, about half of them for psychiatric conditions. Since there are great similarities among these latter compounds, they will not be treated separately except where they are sufficiently different from chlorpromazine to warrant a discussion of the distinction.

History. Although phenothiazine itself was synthesized in 1883, it was not until 1934 that it was first used as an anthelmintic, urinary antiseptic, and insecticide. In the late 1930s a derivative of phenothiazine, promethazine, was found to have antihistaminic properties and, like many antihistaminic drugs, a strong sedative effect. Abortive attempts had been made to treat psychoses with antihistamines, and in 1950 promethazine was tried in the treatment of motor agitation in mental disease but without much success.

Meanwhile, the ability of promethazine to cause a marked prolongation of barbiturate sleeping time in mice was discovered, and in 1952 the French surgeon Laborit introduced the drug into clinical anesthesia as a potentiating agent (*see* Laborit *et al.,* 1952). This prompted a search for other phenothiazine derivatives with potentiating actions as well as greater central activities, and in that same year Charpentier synthesized chlorpromazine. Soon thereafter, Laborit and coworkers described the ability of this compound to potentiate anesthetics and produce "artificial hibernation." They noted that chlorpromazine by itself did not cause a loss of consciousness but produced only a tendency to sleep and a marked lack of interest in what was going on.

Courvoisier and her associates (1953) described an amazingly large number of actions manifested by chlorpromazine. These included gangliolytic, adrenolytic, antifibrillatory, antiedema, antipyretic, antishock, anticonvulsant, and antiemetic properties. In addition, chlorpromazine was found to enhance the activity of a number of analgesic and central depressant drugs.

The first report on the treatment of mental illness by chlorpromazine alone was made by Delay and Deniker (1952). They were convinced that chlorpromazine achieved more than symptomatic relief of agitation or anxiety and that it could have an ameliorative effect upon psychotic processes with quite diverse symptomatology. In 1954, Lehmann and Hanrahan reported, for the first time in the Western Hemisphere, the use of chlorpromazine in the treatment of psychomotor excitement and manic states. Subsequently, the drug was released for marketing in the United States. It was first employed clinically as an antiemetic, but it was also noted that it produced sedation, relaxation, and hypothermia. In addition, it was considered promising as a potentiating agent for a variety of other centrally acting drugs. Clinical studies soon revealed that the most important use of chlorpromazine was in the treatment of psychotic states, and it has since been used primarily for psychiatric purposes.

Chemistry and Structure-Activity Relationship. Phenothiazine has a three-ring structure in which two benzene rings are linked by a sulfur and a nitrogen atom (*see* Table 12–2, page 170). If the nitrogen at position 10 is replaced by a carbon atom with a double bond to the side chain, the compound becomes a thioxanthene. Usual substitutions are at positions 2 and 10. Substitution of a chlorine or methoxy group in position 2 increases the potency of phenothiazines for depressing motor activity and conditioned avoidance responses in animals and for altering psychotic behavior in humans. Acetyl or thiomethyl substitution at position 2 also provides useful antipsychotic compounds (acetophenazine and thioridazine, respectively). A CF_3 substitution in this position greatly increases antipsychotic and antiemetic potency as well as the tendency to produce extrapyramidal symptoms (*e.g.,* trifluopromazine, fluphenazine).

The nature of the substituent at position 10 also influences pharmacological activity. As can be seen in Table 12–2 (page 170), the phenothiazines can be divided into three groups on the basis of substitution at this site. The group with an aliphatic side chain includes chlorpromazine and trifluopromazine. Methotrimeprazine is a methoxy-substituted compound with antipsychotic effects, but it is used primarily as a parenteral analgesic. The second group, with approximately the same order of clinical potency, contains a piperidine moiety in the side chain; it includes thioridazine, as well as mepazine and mesoridazine (not shown in Table 12–2). There appears to be a lower incidence of extrapyramidal side effects with this substitution. Mepazine, however, is a less effective antipsychotic drug than chlorpromazine. The most potent phenothiazine antipsychotic compounds are those of the third group, which have a piperazine (or piperazinyl) group, such as perphenazine, fluphenazine, acetophenazine, prochlor-perazine, and trifluoperazine.

The thioxanthene analog of chlorpromazine is chlorprothixene. The piperazine-substituted thioxanthene, thiothixene, is a high-potency antipsychotic drug. This compound has markedly augmented antiemetic properties and a greater tendency to produce parkinsonism, but diminished sedative effects.

All the phenothiazines used in psychiatry have a three-carbon bridge between the nitrogen atom of the ring and that of the side chain. This is in contrast to anticholinergic phenothiazines used in the treatment of parkinsonism (*e.g.*, ethopropazine, diethazine) and to antihistaminic phenothiazines (*e.g.*, promethazine), which have only two carbons separating the nitrogens. Similarities between the structures of chlorpromazine and of dopamine, epinephrine, and norepinephrine have been noted on the basis of stereochemical models and crystallographic data (Horn and Snyder, 1971). These similarities are not apparent when the two-dimensional structural formulas are compared.

Pharmacological Properties

The phenothiazine derivatives have many pharmacological actions and therapeutic applications in common. Chlorpromazine may be taken as the prototype drug, since it has been given to many more patients and studied more extensively than any of its congeners.

General Psychophysiological and Behavioral Effects. Effects of chlorpromazine frequently differ between psychotic and normal subjects. The changes produced by the drug may represent a move toward normality on the part of the psychotic, but a dysphoria and a move away from "normal" in the nonanxious normal subject. Chlorpromazine produces a considerable degree of sedation when given initially. If a single oral dose of 100 mg of chlorpromazine is given to a normal subject, profound effects on both physiological and mental processes occur. These include a fall in blood pressure, tachycardia, a slight decrease in respiratory rate, decreased salivary secretion, miosis, and decreased motor activity. The subject will sit in silence and show an indifference to the events around him, responding minimally to external stimuli, even those that might arouse emotion during his normal state. His palms will be dry and, if in a cold room, his temperature will drop slightly. If questioned, he might show a general reduction in anxiety.

This pattern of response indicates a wide variety of central and peripheral actions of the drug. The psychological syndrome characterized by psychomotor slowing, emotional quieting, and affective indifference was called the *neuroleptic syndrome* by Delay and Deniker (1952).

The sedative effect may be useful in the treatment of anxious and agitated psychotic patients but must be differentiated from the antipsychotic effect, which may take several weeks to develop fully. Tolerance occurs rather rapidly to sedation but not to the ameliorative effect upon psychotic behavior. Furthermore, some congeners, particularly the position 10–substituted piperazine derivatives, possess effective antipsychotic activity but lack the sedative property. The sedative effect of chlorpromazine differs from that of the barbiturates in that the phenothiazine causes little ataxia and incoordination and the patient may be easily aroused.

Effects on Sleep. Chlorpromazine may either inhibit or enhance rapid-eye-movement (REM) sleep, depending on dosage. The effect of antipsychotic drugs on sleep patterns is not clear, but they tend to normalize the sleep disturbance characteristic of many psychoses. The ability to prolong and enhance the effect of narcotic and hypnotic drugs appears to parallel the marked sedative potency of the particular phenothiazine. The piperazine derivatives that do not cause drowsiness, such as prochlorperazine or fluphenazine, have little ability to affect hypnosis produced by other drugs.

Effects on Conditioned Responses. Courvoisier and her colleagues (1953) found that chlorpromazine impairs the ability of animals to make a conditioned avoidance response (to a learned auditory cue that signals the onset of punishing shock avoidable by climbing a pole). Under the influence of small doses of the drug, animals ignore the warning signal but are still able to escape by climbing the pole once the shock is applied. Barbiturates affect both avoidance (the conditioned response) and escape (the unconditioned response) to approximately the same extent. This test and its many variations has become the basis for commonly used screening procedures for psychotherapeutic drugs.

Cook and Weidley (1957) confirmed and extended these observations on chlorpromazine, and showed that barbiturates and meprobamate affect the conditioned as well as the unconditioned responses to about the same extent, and only in doses that produce ataxia or hypnosis.

Effects on Complex Behavior. Chlorpromazine impairs vigilance in human subjects performing a variety of tasks, such as continuous pursuit-rotor and tapping-speed tests. The drug produces relatively little impairment of digit-symbol substitution, a test of intellectual functioning. On the other hand, secobarbital causes greater impairment in performance in digit-symbol substitution than in continuous performance and other vigilance tests. In normal subjects chlorpromazine may inhibit the performance of complex intellectual tasks such as story writing, but such experiments are difficult to design and interpret.

Effects on Motor Activity. All the phenothiazines used in psychiatry can diminish spontaneous motor activity in every species of animal studied, including man. However, one of the more disturbing side effects of chlorpromazine, *akathisia,* is manifested by a marked increase in motor activity (page 169). Some phenothiazines produce cataleptic effects in animals so that the bodies and limbs can be molded into various postures and remain immobile for long periods of time. Catalepsy resembles but is not the same as the *catatonia* seen in some schizophrenics. In man, catatonic symptoms are relieved by phenothiazines.

Effects on Specific Areas of the Nervous System. The effects of chlorpromazine are apparent at all levels in the nervous system. Only those that are clinically relevant or pertinent to the presumed mechanism of action will be described.

Cortex. Since psychosis obviously involves a disorder of higher functions and thought processes, relevant cortical effects of antipsychotic drugs are of great interest. Chlorpromazine and other antipsychotic drugs inhibit the re-uptake of norepinephrine and 5-HT in rat cerebral cortex but do not affect the re-uptake of gamma-aminobutyric acid.

EEG. When chlorpromazine is administered to man, there is a slowing of the EEG pattern with an increase in the occurrence of theta waves, some increase in burst activity, and spiking. There is a decrease in the variability of frequencies and an increase in voltage. Haloperidol, the thioxanthenes, and thioridazine share this effect. The piperazine derivatives of phenothiazine cause slowing with increased alpha and theta waves. Promazine and prochlorperazine cause a slowing, a decrease in alpha activity, and seizure activity (Fink, 1969).

Seizure Threshold. Chlorpromazine can lower the convulsive threshold. Drug-induced seizures are more likely to be seen in patients who have either a history of a seizure disorder or a condition that predisposes toward seizures. Phenothiazines should be used with extreme caution, if at all, in untreated epileptic patients and in patients undergoing withdrawal from central depressant drugs such as alcohol and barbiturates. Phenothiazines may be used in epileptics if concomitant anticonvulsant drug therapy is maintained.

Basal Ganglia. Because the extrapyramidal effects of most antipsychotic drugs are prominent, a great deal of interest has centered on the specific actions of these compounds in this region. The pathophysiology of Parkinson's disease involves the destruction of a dopamine-containing pathway that connects the substantia nigra with the corpus striatum (*see* Chapter 14). With the exception of reserpine, all antipsychotic drugs, including the phenothiazines, block the dopamine receptors and increase the turnover rate of dopamine in the corpus striatum. The increased turnover rate is believed to be the result of a neuronal feedback mechanism. In an elegant series of experiments, Bunney and coworkers (1973) showed that several antipsychotic phenothiazines and haloperidol reverse the amphetamine-induced depression of firing rates of identified dopaminergic neurons in the substantia nigra and ventral tegmental areas. Spontaneous firing of these cells is also increased by antipsychotic phenothiazines. Promethazine, which has no antipsychotic activity, has no effect. A dopamine-sensitive adenylate cyclase has been demonstrated in the caudate nucleus of the rat brain. Greengard and associates showed that the antipsychotic drugs chlorpromazine and haloperidol were potent competitive inhibitors of the stimulatory effects of dopamine on the enzyme (*see* Kebabian *et al.*, 1972). The locus of action of the antipsychotic drugs, at least in the rat caudate nucleus, may be this presumed "dopamine receptor." Similar findings in the dopaminergic mesolimbic system, discussed below, support this concept. Furthermore, the administration of levodopa to rats results in a rapid increase in the concentration of cyclic AMP in the caudate nucleus, due to its conversion to dopamine and the activation of adenylate cyclase (Garelis and Neff, 1974).

One proposed screening method for antipsychotic drugs utilizes the peculiar turning behavior of rats given amphetamine after a unilateral lesion is produced in the nigroneostriatal pathway. Chlorpromazine blocks this turning presumably by an effect on dopamine-sensitive neurons (Christie and Crow, 1971). The effects of these agents on dopamine-stimulated adenylate cyclase activity should also prove a useful screen.

Hypothalamus. Chlorpromazine inhibits the release of growth hormone, perhaps by an action on the hypothalamus, and also may antagonize the secretion of prolactin release-inhibiting hormone (Martin, 1973). Dopamine can also inhibit prolactin release by a direct action on the pituitary, and the phenothiazines and butyrophenones are potent blockers of this effect (*see* Chapter 66). Prolactin release is thus enhanced by these drugs, and they can cause galactorrhea. Chlorpromazine also appears to cause a reduction in the secretion of corticotropin-regulatory hormone in response to certain stresses (Frohman, 1972). The interference with temperature regulation by chlorpromazine is presumed to be a hypothalamic action.

Limbic System. Histochemical technics have demonstrated that neurons in the mesolimbic system, particularly in the nucleus accumbens, contain dopamine. Moreover, dopamine turnover rate in the limbic system is increased by antipsychotic drugs. This increase in turnover rate, while blocked by the antiparkinsonism, anticholinergic agent trihexyphenidyl in the striatum, is not blocked in the limbic system (Anden, 1972). The obvious relationship of the emotional disturbances in schizophrenia to the functions of the limbic system has led to speculation that the site of antipsychotic drug activity rests in these areas.

There is an adenylate cyclase in the limbic system, as well as in the caudate nucleus, that is specifically activated by dopamine. Furthermore, Clement-Cormier and associates (1974) showed that the activation of the limbic enzyme is also blocked by the antipsychotic phenothiazines and other classes of antipsychotic drugs. They postulated that the relevant dopamine receptors in both the caudate nucleus and the limbic system may be linked to adenylate cyclase and proposed that the extrapyramidal symptoms (caudate) and the antipsychotic effects (limbic) could be explained by one basic mechanism of action. These investigators studied many compounds for their comparative efficacy in inhibiting the activation by dopamine of the adenylate cyclases from the two sites. For each of the drugs tested, the ratio of the K_i for the enzyme derived from either site was essentially unity. Moreover, the inhibitory activity of individual drugs corresponded to their therapeutic efficacy as antipsychotic agents but not to their proclivity to produce extrapyramidal symptoms.

These observations in no way weaken the concept that the mechanism of action of antipsychotic drugs with respect to therapeutic efficacy and side effects may relate to the inhibition of the dopamine activation of adenylate cyclase. Rather, it would appear that the marked differences between antipsychotic drugs in their therapeutic efficacy and their proclivity to produce extrapyramidal symptoms might best be explained by an additional action on the caudate nucleus of those drugs that exhibit the lowest incidence of extrapyramidal effects, that is, an anticholinergic action (*see* Snyder *et al.*, 1974).

Brain Stem. Chlorpromazine has effects upon the brain stem that are ultimately expressed as depression of function. Ordinarily clinical doses of the phenothiazines have little effect upon *respiration*. In human subjects, slight depression of respiratory minute and tidal volumes has been reported following a single intravenous or intramuscular injection (Dobkin *et al.*, 1954). *Vasomotor reflexes* mediated by either the hypothalamus or the brain stem are depressed by relatively low doses of chlorpromazine. This effect might occur at many points in the reflex pathway, and the net result is a centrally mediated fall in blood pressure.

The action of chlorpromazine upon the *brain stem reticular system* appears to be more complex than that of the barbiturates, which directly depress this system. Killam and Killam (1958) believe that chlorpromazine increases reticular activity, which, in turn, stimulates filtering mechanisms in the reticular formation that act to reduce the inflow of stimuli in a selective manner. Within this framework, the reactivity to direct stimulation of the reticular formation after chlorpromazine may be due to a decrease in spontaneous activity, the effect of which ordinarily tends to occlude the response to direct stimulation.

Chemoreceptor Trigger Zone (CTZ). Chlorpromazine has a marked protective action against the effects of apomorphine, a dopamine-receptor stimulant, on the CTZ of the medulla. Chlorpromazine inhibits not only apomorphine-induced emesis but also that produced by dihydrogenated ergot alkaloids. The antiemetic effect of chlorpromazine occurs with very low doses. By contrast, thioridazine inhibits apomorphine-induced emesis but has no clinical efficacy as an antiemetic in man. Drugs or other stimuli that cause emesis by an action on the nodose ganglion or locally on the gastrointestinal tract are not antagonized by chlorpromazine, nor is chlorpromazine effective against nausea due to vestibular stimulation.

Spinal Cord. Disagreement exists concerning the effects of chlorpromazine upon spinal reflexes; certain investigators claim that chlorpromazine has little or no effect upon such reflexes, while others claim depression of one or another.

Peripheral Nerves. Chlorpromazine is a potent local anesthetic, but the drug has never been used for this purpose.

Autonomic Nervous System. As one might expect, a drug with peripheral cholinergic blocking activity, α-adrenergic blocking actions, and adrenergic activity (secondary to the block of re-uptake of amines) has complex effects on the autonomic nervous system. The antihistaminic and antitryptamin-ergic effects further complicate the picture. Chlorpromazine either blocks or reverses the pressor effects of epinephrine. In contrast, the tricyclic antidepressants and monoamine oxidase inhibitors can markedly increase responses to pressor amines in man. The arrhythmogenic effects of epinephrine in rabbits and dogs are also blocked by chlorpromazine.

The cholinergic blocking effects of the drug are weak, but the blurring of vision commonly experienced with chlorpromazine may be due to an anticholinergic action on the ciliary muscle. Chlorpromazine regularly produces a miosis in man, which can be due to α-adrenergic blockade. Other phenothiazines, such as perphenazine and trifluoperazine, can cause mydriasis.

Constipation and decreased gastric secretion and motility are observed in patients given chlorpromazine. Doses of 1 to 3 mg/kg can block the effects of physostigmine on intestinal tone and peristalsis, presumably as a result of cholinergic blockade. Decreased sweating and salivation are other manifestations of the anticholinergic effects of the phenothiazines. Urinary retention is rare.

The phenothiazines inhibit ejaculation without interfering with erection. Thioridazine produces this effect with some regularity, and there are thus problems in its acceptance by male patients. The attribution of this effect to adrenergic blockade is logical but unsubstantiated inasmuch as thioridazine is less potent than chlorpromazine in its antiadrenergic effects.

Chlorpromazine exhibits a variety of other antagonistic actions at other receptor sites. The drug has only slight *antihistaminic* effects. Chlorpromazine blocks the actions of *5-HT* quite effectively, both *in vivo* and *in vitro;* however, it remains to be demonstrated whether this antagonism plays any role in the therapeutic efficacy of the phenothiazines. There is little, if any, ganglionic blocking effect.

For further discussion of the autonomic pharmacology of the phenothiazines, the exhaustive monograph by Gordon (1967) should be consulted. Reviews by Sigg (1968), Klein and Davis (1969), and Shader and DiMascio (1970) also describe the autonomic side effects of numerous psychotropic drugs.

Skeletal Muscle Tone and Movement. Chlorpromazine causes skeletal muscular relaxation in some types of spastic conditions. Since it has little effect at spinal levels, actions on motor activity must be mediated at a higher level, perhaps in the medulla or the basal ganglia. The drug does not produce blockade of the neuromuscular junction.

Phenothiazines and other antipsychotic drugs often produce parkinsonism and other extrapyramidal effects. Theories on mechanism have been discussed above. The clinical syndrome produced by all groups of antipsychotic drugs is described below (page 169).

Endocrine System. The effects of chlorpromazine on hypothalamic regulatory hormones result in profound changes in the endocrine system, as mentioned above. The release and/or action of the prolactin release–inhibiting hormone is impaired; the drug has also been shown to reduce urinary concentrations of gonadotropins, as well as estrogens and progestins. As a result of these derangements, galactorrhea and gynecomastia can occur. Amenorrhea is also seen with chlorpromazine, but this is relatively infrequent. In animals, the drug can block ovulation, suppress the estrous cycle, cause infertility and pseudopregnancy, and maintain an endometrial decidual reaction. Inhibition of gonadotropin secretion also can result in decreased testicular weight.

Nonreproductive functions are also affected. Chlorpromazine may cause a decrease in the secretion of adrenocorticosteroids as a result of diminished release of corticotropin. It interferes with growth by inhibiting the secretion of pituitary growth hormone, an effect utilized in the treatment of acromegaly (Kolodny et al., 1971). In addition, chlorpromazine can decrease the secretion of neurohypophyseal hormones. Weight gain and an increase in appetite occur with all phenothiazines but not with haloperidol. Peripheral edema occurs in 1 to 3% of patients and may be of endocrine origin.

Kidney. Chlorpromazine may have diuretic effects in animals and man, due either to a depressant action upon the secretion of antidiuretic hormone (ADH) or to inhibition of reabsorption of water and electrolytes by a direct action on the renal tubule, or both. It may prevent the fall in renal blood flow occurring in shock. The slight fall in blood pressure that occurs with chlorpromazine is not found to be associated with any significant change in glomerular filtration rate, and there is a tendency toward an increase in renal blood flow.

Cardiovascular System. The actions of chlorpromazine on the cardiovascular system are complex because the drug produces direct effects on the heart and blood vessels, and also indirect ones through actions on CNS and autonomic reflexes. In normal man, the intravenous administration of chlorpromazine causes *orthostatic hypotension,* due to a combination of central actions and peripheral α-adrenergic blockade, and reflex *tachycardia.* Oral therapy causes mild hypotension, systolic blood pressure being affected more than diastolic. Tolerance develops to the hypotensive effect, so that after several weeks of chronic administration the pressures return toward normal (Sakalis et al., 1972). However, some degree of orthostatic hypotension may persist indefinitely. The orthostatic hypotension occurs more frequently with chlorpromazine and thioridazine, and less so with piperazine derivatives such as perphenazine. Chlorpromazine also has a direct depressant action on the heart; cat papillary muscle shows a negative inotropic response to relatively low concentrations of chlorpromazine. The drug has a vasodilating action due to both its effects on the autonomic nervous system and a direct action on blood vessels. An increase in coronary blood flow may result from administration of the drug.

Chlorpromazine has an antiarrhythmic effect upon the heart, which may be due either to a quinidine-like action or to a local anesthetic effect. EEG changes include prolongation of the Q-T and P-R intervals, blunting of T waves, and S-T segment depression. Thioridazine, in particular, causes a high incidence of T wave changes. Cardiotoxicity of a more severe nature has been reported in young patients (Alexander and Nino, 1969).

Liver. Aside from the hypersensitivity reactions occasionally seen after administration of the phenothiazines, such as an obstructive form of jaundice (*see* below), these drugs have no characteristic hepatic effects. There is a suggestion that chlorpromazine may produce an increase in bile viscosity unaccompanied by clinical signs. The drugs may be used in patients with liver disease, but caution is advisable since their metabolism may be delayed or modified and they may compromise an already diseased liver.

Absorption, Fate, and Excretion. The absorption of orally administered chlorpromazine is dependent on the dosage form, the elixir giving the highest plasma concentration of drug. Peak plasma levels are reached at 2 to 3 hours. There is a wide intersubject variability (ten times or more) in the plasma concentrations achieved. They may be decreased significantly by food in the stomach and by the concomitant administration of anticholinergic antiparkinsonism drugs. Although a relatively short plasma half-life (6 hours or less) has been reported, metabolites of chlorpromazine are excreted in the urine for 2 to 6 weeks after cessation of medication. The concentration reached in brain may be four to five times that in plasma. More than 90% of the drug in the plasma is bound to proteins.

Chlorpromazine is metabolized in the liver and excreted in both urine and feces. A reciprocal relationship exists between the amounts excreted by each route. In man, after chronic dosage the highest concentration of unconjugated chlorpromazine metabolites is found in the lung and liver. The 7-hydroxy chlorpromazine that is found in body tissues appears to be an active metabolite. This may account for the fact that most investigators report that plasma concentrations of free chlorpromazine do not correlate with the therapeutic responses. Plasma concentrations of concurrently measured free, protein-bound, and 7-hydroxy chlorpromazine may, in the future, provide a guide for dosage. Since there is some evidence that chlorpromazine can cause hepatic microsomal enzyme induction, it may accelerate its own metabolism; this may account for progressively decreasing plasma concentrations of free drug during maintenance of a fixed dosage schedule.

One hundred sixty-eight possible metabolites of chlorpromazine have been postulated and many of them actually isolated from human urine (Williams and Parke, 1964). Hydroxylation in the 3 and 7 positions and subsequent conjugation with glucuronic acid represent the principal metabolic pathway. The formation of the sulfoxides is the next most common. Metabolic alterations in the side chain also occur. Approximately half of the metabolites of the commonly used phenothiazines are found in the urine and the rest in the feces. *The ultimate sojourn of the phenothiazine drugs in the body is exceedingly long.* Six months after discontinuation of these drugs, various metabolites are detectable in the urine.

The sulfoxides of the phenothiazines have been intensively studied and found to be significantly less potent than the parent compound. In man, urinary excretion of chlorpromazine plus its sulfoxides varies from 1 to 20% of the daily dose administered (Huang and Kurland, 1961). The average ratio of free chlorpromazine to the sulfoxide in the urine is about 1:16. There is much evidence that the sulfoxide undergoes additional metabolism, probably to the sulfone. The various phenothiazine congeners of chlorpromazine undergo similar metabolic degradation.

Demethylation is another method of detoxication by the liver. It is interesting that certain phenothiazines may be converted by demethylation to drugs with antidepressant properties resembling those of imipramine.

Tolerance and Physical Dependence. The phenothiazines do not appear to be addicting, as the term is defined in Chapter 16. However, some degree of physical dependence may occur. There are reports of muscular discomfort and difficulty in sleeping that develop several days after abrupt discontinuation. EEG changes upon sudden withdrawal have not been detected. Monkeys given 2 mg/kg, four times a day, for over a month showed no obvious withdrawal symptoms when the drug was discontinued.

Tolerance develops to the sedative effects of chlorpromazine and other phenothiazines. This takes place over a period of days or weeks, and has been demonstrated by a variety of objective tests.

Preparations and Dosage. The very large number of phenothiazines and antipsychotic drugs precludes a presentation of all available members of the group and their preparations and dosage forms. Table 12–2 (page 170) provides this information for selected drugs based upon extent of use and unique properties. Detailed information on dosage appears in the discussion of drug treatment of psychoses (page 173).

Toxic Reactions and Side Effects. The phenothiazines have a high therapeutic index and are remarkably safe agents. Furthermore, most phenothiazines have a relatively flat dose-response curve, so that they can be used over a wide range of dosages. Although occasional deaths from overdosage have been reported, this is a rare event. Side effects are often extensions of the many pharmacological actions of the drugs, which have already been discussed and will not be repeated or will only be mentioned here. The most important are those on the *CNS, cardiovascular system, autonomic nervous system,* and *endocrine functions.* The *extrapyramidal effects,* which are of great importance, are discussed in detail on page 169 for antipsychotic drugs in general (*see also* Shader and DiMascio, 1970). The most dangerous effects of the phenothiazines are those resulting from hypersensitivity reactions, particularly blood dyscrasias.

Therapeutic doses of phenothiazines, such as chlorpromazine, may cause faintness, palpitation, nasal stuffiness, dry mouth, and some slight constipation. The patient may complain of being cold, drowsy, or weak. The most troublesome side effect is *orthostatic hypotension,* which may result in syncope. A fall in blood pressure is most likely to occur from administration of the phenothiazines with aliphatic side chains. Congeners of the piperazine type produce less hypotension and may be used when this side effect is to be avoided. A mild elevation of temperature may be seen during the first few days, particularly if the drug is given parenterally. On the other hand, hypothermia can occur and may be due both to the action on the heat-regulating center and to direct peripheral vasodilatation. Sensitivity and adaptation to environmental temperature change are impaired so that fatal hyperthermia and heat stroke are possible complications.

Jaundice. Jaundice was observed in patients shortly after the introduction of chlorpromazine into psychiatric therapy and was the cause for some alarm. The incidence of this complication is relatively low, not more than 2 to 4%. Commonly oc-

curring during the second to fourth week of therapy, it is characterized by bile in the urine and abnormally high levels of alkaline phosphatase associated with high plasma bilirubin concentrations. There is usually a normal cephalin flocculation. The jaundice is generally mild, with the plasma bilirubin rarely rising higher than 15 mg/100 ml; the direct bilirubin is higher than the indirect. Fever, anorexia, and hepatic tenderness are usually not present but may be prodromal symptoms of an impending jaundice. Despite the presence of jaundice, patients rarely complain of pruritus.

The jaundice is of the obstructive type; this has been confirmed by liver biopsy and at autopsy. The biopsy specimens show centralobular cholestasis, with little or no parenchymatous damage and with mild inflammatory response. It is thought that the presence of inspissated bile in the hepatic canaliculi is caused by an increase in viscosity of the bile or by periductal edema. In one comparative study, forcing of fluids decreased the incidence of jaundice dramatically. This was attributed to dilution of the bile.

There is general agreement that the jaundice following phenothiazine administration is a hypersensitivity manifestation. Eosinophilic infiltration of the liver as well as eosinophilia are frequently present, there is prompt recurrence of jaundice when the patient is again given the same drug, and there is no correlation between the dose administered and the appearance of jaundice. Ayd (1962) has indicated that desensitization to chlorpromazine may occur with repeated administration in individuals exhibiting jaundice. If jaundice is not observed within the first month of treatment with a phenothiazine, the chance of its later occurrence decreases with time. Since there is always the possibility of shifting a patient from one drug to another without the recurrence of a hypersensitivity reaction, it is felt by some investigators that therapy should be carefully continued in cases of jaundice when the psychiatric disorder calls for uninterrupted drug therapy.

Blood Dyscrasias. Leukocytosis, leukopenia, and eosinophilia occur with phenothiazine medication. Leukopenia appears to be particularly frequent in patients whose white-blood-cell counts were low before the institution of drug therapy. It is difficult to determine whether a leukopenia occurring during the administration of a phenothiazine is a forewarning of impending agranulocytosis. This serious complication occurs in approximately 1 in 10,000 patients receiving chlorpromazine, usually during the first 6 weeks of treatment and more often in older women than in men. Since the onset of blood dyscrasia may be sudden, the appearance of an apparent upper respiratory infection in a patient being started on antipsychotic drugs should be followed immediately by a complete blood count.

Skin Reactions. Dermatological reactions to the phenothiazines are not uncommon. Urticaria or dermatitis occurs in about 5% of patients receiving chlorpromazine. Three types of skin disorders are associated with the use of phenothiazines. The first is a hypersensitivity reaction that may be urticarial, maculopapular, petechial, or edematous. It usually occurs between the first and fifth week of treatment.

The skin clears following discontinuation of the drug and may remain so even if drug therapy is reinstituted. Secondly, contact dermatitis may occur in personnel who handle chlorpromazine, and there may be a certain degree of cross-sensitivity to the other phenothiazines. Thirdly, photosensitivity occurs, the reaction resembling that seen with severe sunburn. This complication may be prevented simply by keeping the patient well covered. An effective sunscreen preparation containing para-aminobenzoic acid should be prescribed for outpatients during the summer.

Abnormal pigmentation induced by long-term administration of phenothiazines in high doses to chronic schizophrenics has been reported. Patients showing this effect have generally received any of a number of phenothiazines, but chlorpromazine is the drug most commonly implicated. The reaction manifests itself as a gray-blue pigmentation in regions exposed to the sun. The dermis contains deposits of melanin located throughout the depth of the corium. Ultraviolet light with wavelengths above 3200 Å seems to be primarily responsible for the effects.

Epithelial keratopathy is often observed in patients on long-term therapy with chlorpromazine, and opacities in the cornea and in the lens of the eye have also been noted. In very extreme cases the deposits in the lens may result in impairment of vision. Pigmentary retinopathy, which has been reported particularly following the use of thioridazine, may be a closely related toxic effect of the phenothiazines (Zelickson and Zeller, 1964; Prien *et al.,* 1970); thus far it has been reported only with doses of thioridazine in excess of 1000 mg per day.

Metabolic Effects. It has been observed that chlorpromazine raises plasma cholesterol levels consistently and significantly (Clark *et al.,* 1967).

Interaction with Other Drugs. The phenothiazines markedly affect the actions of a number of other drugs, and cognizance must be taken of this fact. Chlorpromazine and other antipsychotic drugs, in common with the tricyclic antidepressants, may block the antihypertensive effects of guanethidine. Patients being treated with phenothiazines should be advised that their susceptibility to alcohol may be increased. Chlorpromazine has been shown to increase the miotic and sedative effects of morphine. It markedly enhances the respiratory depression produced by meperidine. The enhancement of the effects of a variety of drugs, particularly CNS depressants, is not due to inhibition of hepatic microsomal enzymes. In fact, phenothiazines promote induction of these enzymes (*see* Conney, 1967). Chlorpromazine can also interfere with a number of laboratory tests (*see* Young *et al.,* 1972, for a complete listing and references). Abnormal glucose tolerance tests are commonly reported.

THERAPEUTIC USES

The use of the phenothiazine antipsychotics in various *psychiatric disorders* is discussed on page 172.

Alcoholism. The use of phenothiazines in the treatment of drug abuse is discussed in Chapter 16.

Table 12-1. PHENOTHIAZINES USED IN THE TREATMENT OF NAUSEA AND VOMITING

DRUG	ROUTE, DOSAGE FORM, AND DOSE		
	Oral T = tablet S = syrup	*Suppository*	*Intramuscular*
Chlorpromazine, U.S.P. (THORAZINE)		25–100 mg, 3–4 times/day	
Chlorpromazine Hydrochloride, U.S.P.	(T) (S) 10–25 mg, 4–6 times/day		25–50 mg, 6–8 times/day
Triflupromazine Hydrochloride, N.F. (VESPRIN)	(T) 10–20 mg (up to 20–30 mg/day)		5–15 mg, every 4 hr (up to 60 mg/day)
Prochlorperazine, U.S.P. (COMPAZINE)		25 mg, 2 times/day	
Prochlorperazine Edisylate, U.S.P.	(S) 5–10 mg, every 4–6 hr		5–10 mg, every 4–6 hr
Prochlorperazine Maleate, U.S.P.	(T) 5–10 mg, every 4–6 hr		
Promazine Hydrochloride, N.F. (SPARINE)	(T) 25–50 mg, every 4–6 hr (S) 5–10 mg, every 4–6 hr		25–50 mg, every 4–6 hr
Promethazine Hydrochloride, U.S.P. (PHENERGAN)	(T) (S) 25–50 mg, daily	25–50 mg, daily	12.5–25 mg, every 4–6 hr
Thiethylperazine Maleate, N.F. (TORECAN)	(T) 10–30 mg, daily	10–30 mg, daily	10–30 mg, daily

By and large, they do not seem to be particularly useful in withdrawal from narcotics, but they do help in alcoholic hallucinosis, a syndrome that should be differentiated from delirium tremens.

Nausea and Vomiting. Chlorpromazine, in relatively low, nonsedative doses, can prevent vomiting of certain origins. The potent and selective antiemetic action of the drug has found useful clinical application in a number of disorders characterized by vomiting, such as uremia, gastroenteritis, carcinomatosis, radiation sickness, and emesis caused by a number of drugs including estrogens, the tetracyclines, morphine, meperidine, agents used in the chemotherapy of malignancy, and disulfiram. Chlorpromazine has also been used in nausea and vomiting of pregnancy, but pregnant patients should not be given the drug for this purpose. The compound does not appear to control motion sickness. Although prochlorperazine is a very potent antiemetic agent, it produces a very high incidence of dystonias, especially when given intramuscularly, and hence should be used with caution. The same precautions should be observed in the use of phenothiazines for nausea and vomiting as with the use of potent analgesics in the treatment of pain, because they may mask diagnostic symptoms in acute surgical conditions or neurological syndromes. Not all the phenothiazines with antipsychotic activity are equally effective as antiemetics. The preparations and dosages of phenothiazines that are effective in the treatment of nausea and vomiting are listed in Table 12–1. Surprisingly, nausea is occasionally seen as a side effect of antipsychotic drugs.

Hiccough. An interesting use of chlorpromazine is in the control of *intractable hiccough*. The mechanism of action in this disorder is unknown, but the close proximity of the medullary areas for the integration of respiration and vomiting should be noted.

BUTYROPHENONES

Haloperidol, a butyrophenone, was synthesized by Janssen and introduced for the treatment of psychoses in Europe in 1958. It was first marketed in the United States in 1967 and has proven to be an effective alternative to the more familiar antipsychotic phenothiazine drugs. This agent grew out of efforts to increase the analgesic potency of a series of 4-phenylpiperidines related to meperidine. Haloperidol is the only butyrophenone used in psychiatry in the United States, but *droperidol,* a related compound, is used in anesthesia for its neuroleptic and antiemetic effects (*see* Chapter 8). The structural formula of haloperidol is given in Table 12–2 (page 171).

PHARMACOLOGICAL PROPERTIES

Although structurally different from the phenothiazines, the butyrophenones share many of their pharmacological properties. Haloperidol may be considered as the prototype drug.

In normal man, haloperidol resembles the piperazine phenothiazines in its actions. It is an extremely potent antipsychotic agent and has been shown to be effective both in the treatment of the manic phase of manic-depressive illness and in schizophrenia. In most respects, the pharmacology of haloperidol differs in degree but not in kind from the piperazine phenothiazines. Since it shares with phenothiazines the ability to block the effects of dopamine and to increase its turnover rate, the presumed mechanism of action is the same.

Central Nervous System. Haloperidol calms and induces sleep in excited patients. This sedative effect is less prominent than that of chlorpromazine. The effects on the EEG resemble those with chlorpromazine, that is, slowing with an increase in theta waves. Haloperidol may lower the convulsive threshold. Since many of the hypothalamic effects of chlorpromazine are the result of dopaminergic blockade, it is not surprising that haloperidol exhibits these same effects to about the same degree. It also blocks apomorphine-induced emesis.

Autonomic Nervous System. Haloperidol has less prominent autonomic effects than do the other antipsychotic drugs. It has little anticholinergic activity but can cause blurring of vision. It blocks the activation of α receptors by sympathomimetic amines but is much less potent than chlorpromazine in this action.

Cardiovascular and Respiratory System. Hypotension occurs with the use of haloperidol but is less severe and less common than that seen with phenothiazines. Although ECG changes attributable to the drug have not been reported, tachycardia does occur. A potentiation of respiratory depressant drugs can be expected with haloperidol as with the phenothiazines.

Endocrine Effects. Weight gain does not seem to be a side effect of haloperidol. Galactorrhea and the other endocrine responses common to the phenothiazines do occur.

Absorption, Fate, and Excretion. Haloperidol is readily absorbed from the gastrointestinal tract. Peak plasma levels occur 2 to 6 hours after ingestion and may plateau for as long as 72 hours, with persistence of detectable levels for weeks. The drug is concentrated in the liver, and about 15% of a given dose is excreted in the bile. Excretion also occurs by way of the kidney and proceeds slowly; about 40% is eliminated by this route during the first 5 days after a single dose.

Preparations and Dosage. These are described in Table 12–2 (page 171). Dosage is more thoroughly discussed in the section dealing with drug treatment of psychoses (page 172).

Side Effects and Toxicity. Haloperidol produces a high incidence of *extrapyramidal reactions* (page 169). These seem to be more prominent in younger patients. Haloperidol therapy should be initiated with caution. Reports of depression with use of the drug may represent a true side effect or a reversion from a manic state. Severe hematological effects are rare, but *leukopenia* has been reported frequently; agranulocytosis has also occurred. Although the drug has been reported to cause jaundice, the incidence is so low that a causal relationship is hard to establish. Other side effects of haloperidol are those to be expected from the pharmacological actions that are discussed above. It is prudent to avoid the use of haloperidol in pregnant women until it is certain that the drug has no teratogenic effect on the fetus (*see* Kopelman *et al.*, 1975).

Therapeutic Uses. The major use of haloperidol, namely, the *treatment of psychoses,* is described below (page 172).

The butyrophenone is reported to be an effective treatment for the syndrome of Gilles de la Tourette (Shapiro and Shapiro, 1968). This is a peculiar neurological disorder manifested by violent muscular jerks, grimacing, and explosive utterances of foul expletives (coprolalia).

DIBENZODIAZEPINES

Although no member of this class of drugs is available for clinical use at this time in the United States, the dibenzodiazepines are of considerable research and therapeutic interest. A group of these compounds was synthesized as potential sedative-antianxiety drugs. Since some members appeared to have an appreciable degree of antipsychotic activity as revealed by animal screening and clinical trials, a congener, *clozapine,* was further tested in man and found to have demonstrable antipsychotic action. The structure of clozapine is as follows:

Clozapine

Clozapine does not meet many of the usual laboratory criteria for an antipsychotic drug. It is relatively inactive in producing catalepsy. It does not appear to antagonize apomorphine- or amphetamine-induced stereotyped behavior as do other antipsychotics. Moreover, it has low potency in blocking conditioned avoidance responses in animals. Nonetheless, it is antipsychotic in man. It produces a marked increase in REM sleep (Blum and Girke, 1973). It is also unique in that few extrapyramidal side effects have been seen in patients treated with this drug (DeMaio, 1972). Snyder and associates (1974) have suggested that this may be due to its high level of central anticholinergic activity. The oral antipsychotic dose for adults in reported studies has been about 300 mg per day.

Clozapine has provided a tool for the examination of the properties of antipsychotic agents. It increases turnover rate of cerebral dopamine and perhaps norepinephrine. It shows a different spectrum of action on dopaminergic systems than does haloperidol, producing greater dopamine turnover changes in the limbic system than in the corpus striatum (Anden and Stock, 1973). However, it is as potent as chlorpromazine in its ability to inhibit the dopamine activation of the adenylate cyclase from both the caudate nucleus and limbic system (Clement-Cormier *et al.*, 1974). If its early clinical promise is confirmed, it will provide a useful addition to the available antipsychotic agents.

RAUWOLFIA ALKALOIDS

Reserpine, the principal alkaloid of *Rauwolfia serpentina,* is now mainly of historical interest in psychiatry. It is less effective as an antipsychotic than are other available drugs and is rarely used for this purpose. In some instances, it may be employed in patients who cannot tolerate other classes of antipsychotic agents. Goodwin and colleagues (1972) have reviewed the psychiatric effects of reserpine in man.

History. Descriptions of the use of extracts of plants resembling rauwolfia may be traced back to ancient Hindu ayurvedic writings. They were used in primitive Hindu medicine for a variety of diseases, including snakebite (because of the resemblance of the root to a snake), hypertension, insomnia, and insanity.

Rauwolfia serpentina (Benth) is a climbing shrub of the Apocynaceae family, indigenous to India and neighboring countries. A French botanist, Plumier, in 1703 named the plant *Rauwolfia serpentina* in honor of Dr. Leonhard Rauwolf of Augsburg, a sixteenth century botanist who never saw the plant or even knew of its existence. Therapeutic applications of the whole root for the treatment of psychoses and hypertension were described in an Indian medical journal in 1931 by Sen and Bose. Little attention was paid to this finding until 1955, when Vakil wrote the first report in a Western medical journal of its antihypertensive effects.

In 1954, Kline reported that rauwolfia or reserpine was helpful in the treatment of psychotic patients. Subsequent discovery of the ability of rauwolfia alkaloids and related compounds to release biogenic amines from storage sites in the body initiated a great number of investigations directed at elucidating the interactions between these amines and reserpine (*see* Chapter 26).

Chemistry. There are a number of rauwolfia alkaloids with complex structures. The structure of reserpine is as follows:

Reserpine

PHARMACOLOGICAL PROPERTIES

Central Nervous System. The central effects of the rauwolfia alkaloids resemble those of the phenothiazine derivatives, but they are by no means identical. It can only be presumed that the central effects of reserpine are due to depletion of stores of catecholamines and 5-HT in the brain (*see* Chapters 21 and 26). Reserpine produces a state of indifference to environmental stimuli, a tendency to sleep, ptosis, and easy arousability by strong stimuli, unaccompanied by ataxia or disequilibrium. Following prolonged administration of high doses, *extrapyramidal* effects are noted (*see* below).

While small doses of reserpine may stimulate *res-*

piration, larger doses decrease respiratory rate, depth, and minute volume, and death ultimately results from central respiratory depression. Reserpine lowers *body temperature,* but only in large doses.

Reserpine differs from the phenothiazines in that it has little or no antihistaminic, cholinergic blocking, or direct adrenergic blocking effect. The peripheral effects of reserpine are discussed in Chapter 26.

Absorption, Fate, and Excretion. The rauwolfia alkaloids are absorbed readily from the gastrointestinal tract and from parenteral sites of injection. Reserpine is a "hit-and-run" drug. Both behavioral effects and amine depletion are initiated slowly and persist long after the drug is gone from the body. Reserpine binds persistently to sites involved with storage of biogenic amines. Identified metabolic products are reserpic acid, syringic acid, and syringoyl methyl reserpate. Reserpine appears to be taken up rapidly by lipid-containing tissues, and the drug is distributed fairly uniformly in different parts of the brain.

Preparations and Dosage. Several alkaloids have been isolated from rauwolfia, including reserpine and rescinnamine, and the major pharmacological actions of rauwolfia are attributed to them. Since the effects of the alkaloids vary qualitatively as well as quantitatively, preparations of the whole root and partially purified mixtures of the alkaloids must be standardized by bioassay.

The rauwolfia fractions, alkaloids, and semisynthetic derivatives are available in a large variety of preparations; only the two that are official are described here. The whole root, *Rauwolfia Serpentina,* N.F. (RAUDIXIN), is supplied in 50- and 100-mg tablets; the average dose is 200 to 400 mg daily. *Reserpine,* U.S.P. (RAURINE, RAU-SED, RESERPOID, SANDRIL, SERPASIL, SERPATE, VIO-SERPINE), is available in 0.25- and 0.5-mg capsules; as an elixir, 0.05 mg/ml; in solution (for injection), 5 mg/2 ml and 25 or 50 mg/10 ml; and as tablets (0.1, 0.25, 0.5, 1, 2, and 5 mg). In psychoses, doses as high as 5 mg daily, taken orally, or 10 mg daily by intramuscular injection have been prescribed, but the drug is now rarely used for this purpose.

Toxicity. A variety of mildly unpleasant effects associated with the clinical administration of reserpine may be considered to be an extension of its pharmacological actions. They are due largely to a combination of depletion of norepinephrine from sympathetic fibers and depletion of 5-HT from the various stores. Among them are drowsiness, nightmares, and parasympathetic predominance, including bradycardia, excessive salivation, cutaneous vasodilatation, nausea, and diarrhea. Nasal congestion is quite common. Orthostatic hypotension may occur following parenteral doses. Excessive gastric secretion with activation of peptic ulcer has been reported repeatedly.

By far the most serious adverse effect produced by the rauwolfia alkaloids is *depression.* About 6%

of patients on reserpine have serious depressions requiring hospitalization or electroconvulsive therapy (Goodwin *et al.,* 1972).

Parkinsonism occurs following large doses of rauwolfia derivatives. Dystonic reactions and akathisia are much less frequent with the rauwolfia drugs than with phenothiazines. Nevertheless, choreoathetosis and cerebellar signs have been reported. Convulsive episodes have occurred following large doses of reserpine.

Allergic reactions to the rauwolfia alkaloids are relatively rare. Purpura associated with a fall in platelet count has been seen in a number of individuals. Patients with allergic disorders may suffer exacerbation of symptoms. Allergic rhinitis may be aggravated by the additional nasal congestion. Bronchiolar secretion and constriction may be enhanced by rauwolfia and dermatological disorders aggravated by cutaneous vasodilatation.

Weight gain occurs following administration of reserpine and related compounds. Edema is not uncommon, and frank heart failure has been reported.

Reserpine inhibits the ovarian cycle and menstruation and depresses fertility, apparently by blocking the secretion of hypothalamic regulatory hormones. Feminization has been reported in males as well as impairment of sexual function.

Additional aspects of the toxicity of reserpine are discussed in Chapter 26.

NEUROLOGICAL SYNDROMES: SIDE EFFECTS COMMON TO ALL CLASSES OF ANTIPSYCHOTIC DRUGS

A variety of neurological syndromes, involving particularly the extrapyramidal system, occur following the use of almost all antipsychotic drugs. These reactions are particularly prominent during treatment with the piperazine group of phenothiazine drugs and with haloperidol. There is less likelihood of acute extrapyramidal side effects with thioridazine and the dibenzodiazepines. Extrapyramidal symptoms may also be associated with the administration of tricyclic antidepressants; however, this is a rare side effect. A special review of neurological effects associated with antipsychotic drug use (American College of Neuropsychopharmacology Task Force, 1973) is helpful in the differential diagnosis of these syndromes.

There are four varieties of extrapyramidal syndromes associated with the use of antipsychotic drugs. Three of these usually appear concomitantly with the administration of the drug, and one is a late-appearing syndrome that occurs either after the drug is discontinued or during prolonged treatment.

A *parkinsonian syndrome* that may be indistinguishable from idiopathic parkinsonism may develop during administration of antipsychotic drugs. Its incidence varies with different agents (Table 12-2), and in some patients it may not be seen at all. Clinically, there is a generalized slowing of volitional movement (akinesia) with mask facies and a reduction in arm movements. The most noticeable signs are *rigidity* and *tremor at rest,* especially involving the upper extremities. "Pill-rolling" movements may be seen. Parkinsonian side effects may be mistaken for depression since the flat facial expression and retarded movements resemble signs of depression.

Another extrapyramidal effect seen during antipsychotic drug therapy is *akathisia.* This term refers to the compelling need of the patient to be in constant movement rather than to any specific movement pattern. The patient feels that he must get up and walk or continuously move about, and he may be unable to keep this under control. Akathisia can be mistaken for agitation in psychotic patients; the distinction is critical, since agitation might be appropriately treated with an increase in dosage. Parenteral administration of benztropine allows a differential diagnosis between the two conditions, inasmuch as psychotic agitation will not respond to this drug. Treatment of akathisia requires reduction of antipsychotic drug dosage.

Acute dystonic reactions are occasionally seen with the initiation of antipsychotic drug therapy. Facial grimacing and torticollis can occur and may be associated with oculogyric crisis. These syndromes may be mistaken for hysterical reaction or seizures, but like akathisia they respond dramatically to parenteral administration of anticholinergic antiparkinsonism drugs. Once again, the differential diagnosis is important.

Tardive dyskinesia is a late-appearing neurological syndrome associated with antipsychotic drug use. It occurs more frequently in older patients, and an incidence as high as 20% has been reported in chronically institutionalized patients. It may be more common in females and those with a history of prior brain damage. Its incidence with specific drug groups is not known. Tardive dyskinesia is characterized by stereotyped involuntary movements consisting in sucking and smacking of the lips, lateral jaw movements, and fly-catching dartings of the tongue. There may be choreiform and purposeless, quick movements of the extremities. All these movements disappear during sleep, as they do in parkinsonism. Unfortunately, the tardive dyskinesias may be masked by large doses of antipsychotic drugs, but under no circumstances should the dose of the offending drug be increased. Symptoms may persist indefinitely after discontinuation of the medication, although sometimes tardive dyskinesias in younger patients will disappear with time. There is no evidence that they respond to treatment with antiparkinsonism drugs, and no adequate therapy has as

Table 12-2. SELECTED ANTIPSYCHOTIC DRUGS: CHEMICAL STRUCTURES, DOSES, SIDE EFFECTS, AND DOSAGE FORMS

Phenothiazines — general structure with positions 1–9, S, N, R_1, R_2.

NONPROPRIETARY NAME / TRADE NAME	R_2	R_1	DOSE — Antipsychotic Dose Range—Daily Dosage (Usual, mg)	DOSE — Extreme* (mg)	Single Intramuscular Dose† (mg)	SIDE EFFECTS — Sedative Effects	SIDE EFFECTS — Extrapyramidal Effects	SIDE EFFECTS — Hypotensive Effects	DOSAGE FORMS — Oral (T = tablet mg; C = capsule mg; S = syrup; E = elixir; C = concentrate)	DOSAGE FORMS — Injection (A = ampul; V = vial; S = syringe)
Chlorpromazine Hydrochloride, U.S.P. THORAZINE	—Cl	—(CH$_2$)$_3$—N(CH$_3$)$_2$	200–800	25–2000	25–50	+++	++	I.M. +++ Oral ++	(T) 10, 25, 50, 100, 200 (C) sustained release; 30, 75, 150, 200, 300 (S) 10 mg/5 ml (C) 30 mg/ml, 100 mg/ml ‡	(A) 25 mg/ml, 50 mg/2 ml (V) 25 mg/ml in 10 ml
Triflupromazine Hydrochloride, N.F. VESPRIN	—CF$_3$	—(CH$_2$)$_3$—N(CH$_3$)$_2$	50–200	50–400	20–50	++	+++	++	(T) 10, 25, 50 (S) 50 mg/5 ml	(V) 10 mg/ml in 10 ml (S) 10 mg/ml
Thioridazine Hydrochloride, U.S.P. MELLARIL	—SCH$_3$	—(CH$_2$)$_2$—[N-methylpiperidine], —CH$_3$	100–600	50–800		+++	+	++	(T) 10, 25, 50, 100, 150, 200 (C) 30 mg/ml	
Perphenazine, N.F. TRILAFON	—Cl	—(CH$_2$)$_3$—N[piperazine]—N—(CH$_2$)$_2$—OH	8–32	4–64	5–10	++	+++	+	(T) 2, 4, 8, 16 (T) sustained release; 8 (S) 2 mg/5 ml (C) 16 mg/5 ml	(A) 5 mg/ml (V) 5 mg/ml
Prochlorperazine Edisylate, U.S.P. Prochlorperazine Maleate, U.S.P. COMPAZINE	—Cl	—(CH$_2$)$_3$—N[piperazine]—N—CH$_3$	75–100	15–150	5–10	++	+++	+	(T) 5, 10, 25 (C) sustained release; 10, 15, 30, 75 (S) 5 mg/5 ml (C) 10 mg/ml ‡	(A) 5 mg/ml

Fluphenazine Enanthate, U.S.P.
Fluphenazine decanoate

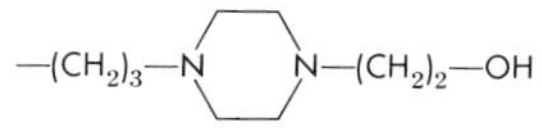

$-(CH_2)_3-N$⟨N⟩$N-(CH_2)_2-OH$

PERMITIL, PROLIXIN
(HYDROCHLORIDE, ENANTHATE,
AND DECANOATE)

10 ml, enanthate and decanoate
(S) 25 mg/ml
(V) 25 mg/ml in 5 ml
(E) 0.5 mg/ml	2.5, 5, 10 (T) sustained release; 1
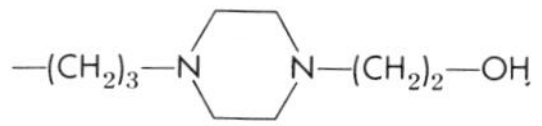 (decanoate or enanthate: 25–50 every 2 weeks)	40–80	20–150

Acetophenazine Maleate, N.F.

$-(CH_2)_3-N$⟨N⟩$N-(CH_2)_2-OH$ $-COCH_3$

TINDAL

| ++ | ++ | + | (T) 20 |

| 40–80 | 20–150 |

Trifluoperazine Hydrochloride, N.F.

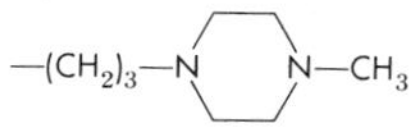

$-(CH_2)_3-N$⟨N⟩$N-CH_3$ $-CF_3$

STELAZINE

| + | +++ | + | (T) 1, 2, 5, 10 | (C) 10 mg/ml | (V) 2 mg/ml in 10 ml |

| 4–15 | 2–64 | 1–2 |

Thioxanthenes §

Chlorprothixene, N.F.

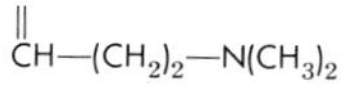

$CH-(CH_2)_2-N(CH_3)_2$ $-Cl$

TARACTAN

| +++ | ++ | ++ | (T) 10, 25, 50, 100 | (C) 100 mg/5 ml | (A) 25 mg/2 ml |

| 50–400 | 30–600 | 25–50 |

Thiothixene Hydrochloride, N.F.

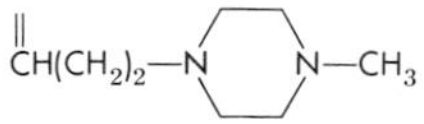

$CH(CH_2)_2-N$⟨N⟩$N-CH_3$ $-SO_2N(CH_3)_2$

NAVANE

| + to ++ | ++ | ++ | (C) 1, 2, 5, 10, 20 ‡ | (C) 5 mg/ml | (A) 4 mg/2 ml |

| 6–30 | 6–60 | 2–6 |

Butyrophenones

Haloperidol, U.S.P.

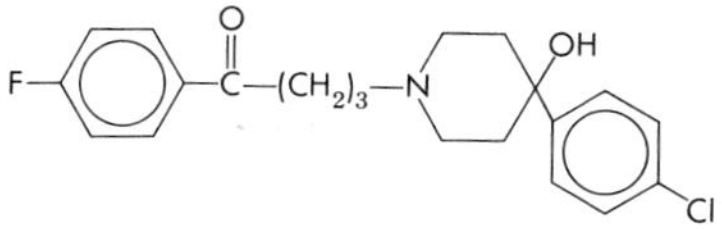

HALDOL

| + | +++ | + | (T) 0.5, 1, 2, 5 | (C) 2 mg/ml | (A) 5 mg/ml |

| 2–6 | 1–30 | 3–5 |

* Extreme dosage ranges should not be exceeded except when all other appropriate measures have failed.

† Except for the enanthate and decanoate forms of fluphenazine, dosage is given I.M. every 4 to 6 hours for agitated patients.

‡ Chlorpromazine, U.S.P., is available as the free base in rectal suppositories in 25- and 100-mg sizes; Prochlorperazine, U.S.P., suppositories contain 2.5, 5, or 15 mg of the free base; Thiothixene, N.F., is available as the free base in 1-, 2-, 5-, and 10-mg capsules.

§ C=replaces N at position 10 in the general formula of phenothiazines (*see* structure at top of first column).

171

yet been devised. Lesions in the substantia nigra have been seen at autopsy in patients with tardive dyskinesias (Christiansen *et al.,* 1970).

The *prevention* of neurological syndromes as complications of antipsychotic drug use is of major importance. Certain therapeutic rules should be followed: *Routine* administration of antiparkinsonism agents should be avoided with most antipsychotic drug regimens. In certain instances, with the use of drugs such as haloperidol or fluphenazine where a high incidence of extrapyramidal reactions occurs, antiparkinsonism medication should be held in readiness. If these drugs are used on an outpatient basis, some antiparkinsonism medication may be prescribed when absolutely needed. For most antipsychotic drugs this will not be necessary. Since it is known that there is a diminution in extrapyramidal symptoms after the first 6 months of antipsychotic drug treatment, all patients on antiparkinsonism medication should be withdrawn from this medication after this period to see whether there is a recrudescence of extrapyramidal symptoms. *Many authorities advise that the only appropriate treatment of extrapyramidal symptoms is reduction of antipsychotic drug dosage.* This may not be practical in some patients with uncontrollable psychotic symptomatology, but it is advisable in all other patients. Since all the antiparkinsonism drugs cause side effects of their own (*see* Chapter 14), and may increase patient discomfort as well as decrease the effectiveness of some antipsychotic drugs, they should not be used except when there is no other alternative (*i.e.,* reduction of the dose of antipsychotic drug or a change to a drug that is less likely to cause extrapyramidal symptoms). Since the extrapyramidal effects of the antipsychotic drugs may persist for some time, it may be necessary to initiate or continue antiparkinsonism medication after withdrawal of the antipsychotic drug. It should be recalled that levodopa does not antagonize the extrapyramidal effects of antipsychotic agents.

The use of minimal effective dosages of antipsychotic drugs for long-term therapy, as well as discontinuation of treatment as soon as it seems clinically indicated (*see* below), is the best preventive practice.

DRUG TREATMENT OF PSYCHOSES

The efficacy of the antipsychotic drugs in the treatment of *schizophrenia* has been demonstrated beyond question (*see* National Institute of Mental Health Study Group, 1964; Davis, 1965; May, 1968). Nonetheless, as May (1968) states, "Elegance in . . . drug therapy . . . calls for the [relatively rare] combination of expertise in drug effect, continuous understanding of the patient and of the process of his illness and sensitivity to the nuances of the patient therapist relationship."

The first requirement for successful treatment is *accuracy* in *diagnosis* and *evaluation.* In order to assess changes in the patient's condition, an accurate evaluation of his mental and physical status at the start of therapy is necessary. Treatment goals should then be defined. Although rating scales for symptom complexes are available (*see* Levine *et al.,* 1971), the physician can define treatable target symptoms on the basis of clinical interviews or simple scales. Phenothiazines and other antipsychotic drugs favorably modify the pathognomonic symptoms of schizophrenia, that is, thought disorder; blunted affect, withdrawal, and retardation; and autistic behavior and mannerisms. Favorable changes in belligerence, resistiveness, perceptual disturbances, and paranoid projection also occur with the use of antipsychotic drugs (for operational definitions, *see* Carpenter *et al.,* 1973). Other symptoms of psychosis may respond variably to different antipsychotic drug regimens, but there is no present evidence that any one drug has a selective effect on a particular symptom complex. Since compliance with medication schedules can be poor on both inpatient and outpatient services, it is important to make sure that the patient is receiving the drug.

If there is any doubt about compliance, the patient should be treated with weekly or biweekly injections of fluphenazine decanoate or enanthate, long-acting preparations. Since delusional paranoid patients frequently believe that the medicine is "poison," this group is particularly appropriate for the administration of long-acting injectable preparations.

Since the choice of a drug cannot be made on the basis of anticipated therapeutic effect, the *selection* of a particular medication for treatment often depends on side effects. If a patient has responded well to a drug in the past, it should again be used. If the patient's history does not indicate either a drug of choice or one to be avoided, the following guidelines might be used. (1) If the risk of unknown or unforeseen complications is an important consideration, the most thoroughly studied drug, chlorpromazine, should be used. (2) If there is a high probability of noncompliance with prescribed regimens, the oral dosage of fluphenazine should be established and then the patient can be switched to parenteral fluphenazine enanthate or decanoate on a biweekly injection schedule. (3) If the patient has a history of cardiovascular disease or stroke and the threat from hypotension is serious, a piperazine phenothiazine or haloperidol should be used. (4) If because of age, medical condition, or disease factors there is a marked risk of development of extrapyramidal symptoms, thioridazine should be the first choice. (5) If the patient would be seriously discomforted by interference with ejaculation, thioridazine should be avoided. (6) If sedative effects are considered undesirable, a piperazine phenothiazine or haloperidol is preferable. (7) If the patient has compromised hepatic function or if there is a potential threat of jaundice, haloperidol is probably the safest starting drug. Choice can also be conditioned by the physician's experience in the use of a particular drug, a factor that can outweigh all others. Skill in the use of these drugs also depends on selection of an adequate dosage level, knowledge of what to expect, and judgment as to when to stop therapy or change drugs.

Some patients do not respond to antipsychotic drug treatment and their disease may even get worse. In general, it can be anticipated that female patients with good premorbid adjustment who show acute paranoid symptomatology will respond most favorably to antipsychotic medication (*see* Judd *et al.,* 1973; Klein and Rosen, 1973). Since the individual nonresponder cannot be identified beforehand with certainty, the physician must accept the fact that there is a small subgroup of patients who do worse on medication than on no drug at all. If a patient does not show clinical improvement after a course of adequate treatment (*see* below) and if he fails to respond to another drug given in adequate dosage, therapy should be discontinued and the working diagnosis reevaluated.

The *time course of response* to antipsychotic drugs is such that 3 weeks or more is required to demonstrate positive effects in hospitalized schizophrenics (National Institute of Mental Health, 1964). Full effect may require 6 weeks to 6 months. In contrast, improvement of acute schizophrenic patients within 48 hours can be seen on global assessment after treatment with parenteral antipsychotic drugs (Shopsin *et al.,* 1969). On some scales, amobarbital is equally effective within this time span, so the possibility that sedative rather than selective antipsychotic effects are responsible for the improvement must be considered. A patient should show improvement within the first 3 weeks of treatment. If not, either the dose should be increased or a different antipsychotic drug administered.

After the initial response of the patient, drugs are frequently used in conjunction with psychotherapy. Although there is no clear statistical evidence that this greatly affects prognosis (Grinspoon *et al.,* 1968; May, 1968; Feinsilver and Gunderson, 1972), psychotherapy and other treatment will assist the patient in adjusting to his environment. Intensive work with the families of psychotic patients may improve the outcome of drug treatment. In the care of outpatients in particular, the acceptance of pharmacotherapy by the family may be critical in ensuring adequate treatment. A change in the unfavorable environment that frequently surrounds schizophrenic patients will help them to function better, even if symptoms are only reduced and not eliminated.

There is no convincing evidence that combinations of antipsychotic drugs offer any advantage. A combination of an antipsychotic drug and an antidepressant may be useful in some cases.

The *duration of treatment* has received a great deal of attention. Prien and Klett (1972), in a review of this subject, found that withdrawal of drugs from chronic schizophrenic patients resulted in a 40% or greater relapse rate within 6 months. Patients who have been maintained on low doses have a lower relapse rate when their medication is stopped. Often dosage in chronic cases can be lowered to 100 to 300 mg of chlorpromazine (or its equivalent) per day without any signs of relapse. Intermittent therapy can be useful, particularly in reducing the incidence of side effects. Effective maintenance with monthly injections of fluphenazine decanoate has been reported (Hirsch *et al.,* 1973).

Dosage of antipsychotic drugs is often difficult to determine because of the variable dose-response curve and the difficulties in defining an end point of therapeutic response. In the treatment of acute psychoses, one should start with a low dose and increase it quite rapidly, within 2 or 3 days, to achieve control of symptoms. The dose is then adjusted to a maintenance level during the next month, as the patient's condition warrants. In acutely agitated patients, parenteral medication is often indicated and the doses should be small (25 to 50 mg of intramuscular chlorpromazine) but given as often as every 40 minutes to obtain the desired response. However, the relatively slow onset of antipsychotic effect cannot be overemphasized. Some antipsychotic drugs, such as haloperidol and fluphenazine, have been given over a thousandfold dosage range without disaster. When doses higher than those usually recommended are given, plasma concentrations should be obtained if possible, to determine whether the drug is being absorbed. There is wide variability in plasma concentrations of antipsychotic drugs among individuals (Sakalis *et al.,* 1972). After an initial stabilization period, regimens based on a single daily dose have been shown to be efficacious.

Table 12–2 (page 170) gives "usual" and "extreme" ranges of dosage for selected antipsychotic agents. These ranges are only for the treatment of schizophrenia and are only approximate guidelines; higher and lower doses have been used but cannot be recommended. The idea that inpatients will require larger doses than outpatients is unsubstantiated. Careful observation of the patient's changing response in target symptoms is the best guide to appropriate dosage.

The treatment of *organic brain syndromes,* both chronic and acute, is another use of the antipsychotic drugs. Once again there is no drug of choice (*see* review by Prien, 1973). In acute brain syndromes without likelihood of seizures, frequent small (4-mg) doses of a drug such as perphenazine, which has less hypotensive effect than chlorpromazine, may effectively control agitation. The antipsychotic drugs are less liable to cause paradoxical excitement, such as that seen with barbiturates. Almost any antipsychotic drug can be used, but the doses should be low. Thioridazine is often preferred in older patients because of the lower incidence of extrapyramidal side effects.

The use of antipsychotic drugs in *mania* and *depression* has met with some success. Haloperidol and chlorpromazine are both effective in the treatment of mania and are often used concomitantly with the institution of lithium therapy (*see* below). Often high dosage must be used to control mania. The treatment of depression with phenothiazines is more controversial. Controlled studies have demonstrated the efficacy of certain phenothiazines in depressive syndromes (*see* Overall *et al.,* 1964). This subject is discussed subsequently in the section on drug treatment of affective disorders (page 187).

Anxiety is considered by some to be an indication for the use of antipsychotic drugs. In view of the wide range of disturbing and serious side effects, it would seem that the use of these drugs is inappropriate. However, if there is underlying psychosis manifested by thought disorder, phenothiazines may be more effective than conventional antianxiety agents (*see* Harrow *et al.,* 1972). In general, however, the use of antipsychotic drugs should be reserved for the more serious and disabling psychiatric disorders. If patients have crippling anxieties that do not respond to the sedative-antianxiety agents, a trial of antipsychotic drugs in low dosage may be warranted. Furthermore, there is a type of patient who tends to abuse the sedative-antianxiety drugs. Since the abuse potential of the phenothiazines is low or nonexistent, they might be appropriate in such a circumstance. Whenever nonpsychotic patients are treated with antipsychotic drugs, the physician should take cognizance of the lower tolerance of such patients to the dysphoric effects, especially those of phenothiazines.

The status of the drug treatment of *childhood psychosis* and behavior disorders of childhood is confused by diagnostic inconsistencies and an almost total absence of rigorously controlled studies. Some success has been achieved with phenothiazines in the treatment of psychotic children; however, many children do worse on antipsychotic medication than on no medication at all. Chlorpromazine and trifluoperazine have been reported effective in severely impaired autistic children, and the differential diagnosis of this group from the so-called *minimal-brain-damage* (*MBD*) *syndrome* in children is essential. MBD has been treated with antipsychotic drugs. However, CNS stimulants (amphetamine, methylphenidate) seem more effective, although they may cause depression of growth (Safer *et al.,* 1972). Unfortunately, the term *MBD* is clearly a misnomer since no brain damage, minimal or otherwise, has been detected in most of these children. (For reviews of the diagnosis and treatment of MBD, *see* De La Cruz *et al.,* 1973; Sroufe and Stewart, 1973.)

II. Drugs Used in the Treatment of Affective Disorders

Affective disorders—*mania* and *depression*—are characterized by changes in mood state as the primary symptoms. Either of these two extremes of mood may be accompanied by psychosis with disordered thought and delusional perceptions. Psychosis may have, as a secondary symptom, a change in mood, and it is this overlap that causes much confusion in diagnosis. Severe mood changes without psychosis frequently occur and are often accompanied by *anxiety* (*see* below). The decision to use an antidepressant drug rather than an antipsychotic agent, for example, may rest on such factors as predominant symptomatology, family history, and precise information on the onset and course of the current episode of the disease.

Mania, characterized by elation, hyperactivity, and uncontrollable thought and speech, is treated both with antipsychotic drugs and with lithium carbonate. Depression, characterized by feelings of intense sadness and self-deprecation and by physical and mental slowing, can be treated with the tricyclic antidepressant drugs, the monoamine oxidase inhibitors, some antipsychotic agents, lithium carbonate, and electroconvulsive shock. There is no obvious chemical similarity between the various therapeutic modalities, but there are striking similarities in their effects on brain amines. Problems of selection of treatment as well as the decision to treat affective disorders are discussed at the end of this section.

TRICYCLIC ANTIDEPRESSANTS

Imipramine (a dibenzazepine derivative), *amitriptyline* (a dibenzocycloheptadiene derivative), and other closely related compounds are the drugs currently most widely used for the treatment of depression. Because of their structure (*see* below), they are often referred to as the tricyclic antidepressants. Their efficacy in alleviating depression has been well established.

History. In 1889, Thiele and Holzinger synthesized iminodibenzyl and described its chemical characteristics in detail. The pharmacological properties were not investigated until 1948, when Häfliger synthesized a series of more than 40 derivatives of iminodibenzyl for possible uses as antihistamines, sedatives, analgesics, and antiparkinsonism drugs. One of these was *imipramine*, a dibenzazepine compound, which differs from the phenothiazines only by replacement of the sulfur with an ethylene linkage. Following screening in animals, a few compounds, including imipramine, were selected on the basis of sedative or hypnotic properties for therapeutic trial.

During clinical investigation of these phenothiazine analogs, Kuhn (1958) found quite fortuitously that, unlike the phenothiazines, imipramine was relatively ineffective in quieting agitated psychotic patients. Instead, it apparently bestowed remarkable benefit upon certain depressed patients. Subsequently, Kuhn administered imipramine to approximately 50 patients suffering from a variety of depressive syndromes and concluded that it was most useful in "endogenous" depressions characterized by regression and inactivity, whereas patients with hyperactive, agitated, and anxious depressions were made worse by the drug. Since then, further evidence for the effectiveness of this compound has accumulated.

The search for chemically related compounds has

Table 12-3. TRICYCLIC ANTIDEPRESSANTS

$CH_2CH_2CH_2N(CH_3)_2$
Imipramine

$CHCH_2CH_2N(CH_3)_2$
Amitriptyline

$CHCH_2CH_2N(CH_3)_2$
Doxepin

$CH_2CH_2CH_2NHCH_3$
Desipramine

$CHCH_2CH_2NHCH_3$
Nortriptyline

$CH_2CH_2CH_2NHCH_3$
Protriptyline

yielded to date *amitriptyline, desipramine, nortriptyline, protriptyline,* and *doxepin.* There is no convincing evidence that these substances are more effective than imipramine in clinical usage.

Chemistry. The structures of the tricyclic compounds are given in Table 12-3. Imipramine and promazine are identical except for the linkage between the two benzene rings. Structurally, in the phenothiazine ring system, the sulfur atom enables conjugation of the benzene rings to occur, whereas the $-CH_2-CH_2-$ group in imipramine prevents such conjugation. The physicochemical properties of promazine and imipramine are strikingly similar. The demethylated derivative of imipramine, desipramine (the secondary amine), is a metabolic product of imipramine and has been suggested as the active agent responsible for antidepressant effects.

Amitriptyline has a carbon substituted for the nitrogen in the central ring structure, and the side chain is attached to the ring by a double bond. This is analogous to the conversion of a phenothiazine to a thioxanthene. Nortriptyline, the desmethyl derivative of amitriptyline (also the secondary amine and a metabolic product of amitriptyline), is likewise available as an antidepressant agent. If an oxygen atom is substituted for one of the methylene groups in the center ring of amitriptyline, another antidepressant agent, doxepin, is formed.

PHARMACOLOGICAL PROPERTIES

Central Nervous System. One might expect an effective antidepressant drug to have a stimulating or mood-elevating effect when given to a normal subject. Although this may occur with the monoamine oxidase (MAO) inhibitors, it is not true of the tricyclic antidepressants.

If a dose of 100 mg of imipramine is given to a normal subject, he feels sleepy and tends to be quieter, his blood pressure falls slightly, and he feels light-headed. Often unpleasant anticholinergic effects (dry mouth and blurred vision) appear. There is little, if any, change in pupillary size. His gait may become unsteady, and he feels tired and clumsy. These drug effects are usually perceived as unpleasant, and cause a feeling of "unhappiness" and an *increase* in anxiety. There may be a deterioration in tests of performance (DiMascio *et al.,* 1964). The acute drug effects clearly resemble those seen with certain phenothiazines.

Repeated administration for several days leads to accentuation of these symptoms and, in addition, to difficulty in concentrating and thinking, comparable to that experienced during the course of similar treatment with chlorpromazine (Grunthal, 1958). Imipramine seems to produce greater impairment of cognitive and affective processes and lesser reduction in physical movement than does chlorpromazine.

In contrast, if the drug is given over a period of time to depressed patients, an elevation of mood occurs. *About 2 to 3 weeks must pass before the therapeutic effects of the drug are evident.* For this reason, the tricyclic antidepressants should never be prescribed on an "as-needed" basis. The explanation of the slow onset of effects may relate to changes in the metabolism of biogenic amines that occur (*see* below).

The manner in which imipramine relieves the signs and symptoms of depression is not clear. Its effect has been described as a dulling of depressive ideation rather than as the euphoric stimulation produced by the MAO inhibitors, but a definitively discriminative experiment is yet to be performed. However, reports of manic excitement as well as of euphoria and insomnia indicate that imipramine does have a stimulant action under certain circumstances. In a collaborative study a relatively high incidence of manic reactions was reported in patients treated with imipramine (Prien *et al.*, 1972). Hallucinations and excitement have been reported in a small percentage of patients receiving imipramine (Lehmann *et al.*, 1958). This may represent a delirium-like syndrome secondary to central anticholinergic effects (*see* below).

Effects on Sleep. The tricyclic antidepressants occasionally have been used as hypnotics because of their sedative property. Although this effect may be useful in the initial therapy of a depressed patient with sleep loss, their general use for hypnosis is not recommended. In adequate doses they cause hangover and are not as effective as a conventional hypnotic. The drugs do decrease the number of awakenings, increase stage-4 sleep, and markedly decrease REM time. There is no convincing evidence for any difference among the various tricyclic drugs in their hypnotic properties.

EEG Effects. EEG studies in man have shown that imipramine and amitriptyline decrease the percentage-time alpha and the total electrical activity, but increase theta activity. Some increase in delta, beta, and burst activity is seen (Fink, 1969).

Effects on Animal Behavior. Despite its clinical antidepressant effects, imipramine produces depression of spontaneous motor activity in laboratory animals. Like the phenothiazines, it also prolongs hexobarbital sleeping time and alcohol narcosis, decreases body temperature, and causes ataxia. It impairs both acquisition and performance of conditioned avoidance responses. In all these tests, it is far less potent than chlorpromazine.

Although imipramine decreases spontaneous motor activity in animals, it is also capable of stimulating a great variety of behavior patterns. Blockade of the reserpine-induced sedative or "depressive" patterns in animals is a characteristic of all the tricyclic antidepressants. The latter drugs must be given before the reserpine because an intact CNS store of amines must be present for this blocking effect to become evident. Since reserpine depletes the brain of both 5-HT and norepinephrine, it is not clear which amine, if not both, is important for this action. Although this blocking effect is used as an animal screening test for antidepressants, its meaning in relation to human depression is unclear.

Actions on Brain Amines. The action of the tricyclic antidepressants on the metabolism of catecholamines and indoleamines in the brain has contributed significantly to the "biogenic amine hypothesis" of depression.

The field is so complex that only a brief outline is presented here. The reviews of Davis (1970) and Schildkraut (1973) should be consulted for fuller expositions and references. The amines of primary interest are 5-HT and norepinephrine. Unlike the antipsychotic drugs, the tricyclic antidepressants do not have a significant effect on dopamine receptors. All tricyclic antidepressants block the re-uptake of norepinephrine by adrenergic nerve terminals. The demethylated analogs are more potent in this action, whereas the methylated drugs are more potent in the blockade of 5-HT re-uptake. Imipramine slows the turnover rate of 5-HT, an effect not shared by desipramine, while the turnover rate of norepinephrine is increased by the demethylated drugs nortriptyline and desipramine. The exact relationship of these effects to the actions of the tricyclic antidepressants in human depression is not known.

The aminergic pathophysiology of depression is presented here in an attempt to explicate the actions of the antidepressant drugs. A disorder of amine metabolism exists in a subgroup of depressed patients as yet not clearly defined. Presumably it is these patients who respond favorably to the antidepressant drugs. A disorder of amine metabolism may also afflict some patients with mania. Although other neurotransmitter substances may be involved, it is known that all drugs and treatments that modify depression or mania have significant effects on the metabolism of norepinephrine. No more explicit statement can be made at this time, but there is considerable hope that eventually a consistent explanation of depression and its treatment will evolve.

Autonomic Nervous System. In contrast to the weak anticholinergic effects of the phenothiazines, the anticholinergic responses to therapeutic doses of the tricyclic antidepressants are prominent. These are manifested in blurred vision, dry mouth, constipation, and urinary retention. Protriptyline seems to cause the highest incidence of these effects. Tachycardia is frequent and may in part be an adrenergic effect caused by the blockade of norepinephrine re-uptake in the heart. Since the autonomic changes that accompany depression may include some of these symptoms, the determination of what is a true autonomic side effect of a tricyclic antidepressant must rest on a careful physical examination and history obtained before the initiation of drug therapy.

Cardiovascular System. Tricyclic antidepressants have marked effects on the cardiovascular system even in therapeutic doses (*see* Raisfeld, 1972). Imipramine lowers the blood pressure in anesthetized dogs and obtunds various cardiovascular reflexes, including the carotid occlusion reflex, the Bezold-Jarisch reflex, and postural responses. There is an increased tendency for arrhythmias to develop in patients on tricyclic drugs, and there have been several reports of unexpected deaths (Williams and Sherter, 1971; Moir *et al.,* 1972). These adverse reactions may be related to the blockade of amine re-uptake by these drugs and the resultant high concentrations of norepinephrine in cardiac tissue. Orthostatic hypotension is commonly observed with therapeutic doses. Myocardial infarction and the precipitation of congestive heart failure during the course of treatment have been attributed to imipramine administration. Tachycardia is a common finding. The most prominent ECG change observed following the use of imipramine consists in inversion or flattening of the T waves.

Since the tricyclic antidepressants can cause orthostatic hypotension, produce arrhythmias, and interact in deleterious ways with other drugs (*see* below), great caution must be observed in their use in patients with significant cardiac disease. Unfortunately, since many depressed patients fall in an age group where cardiac problems are common and coexistence of depressive illness and cardiovascular disease is frequent, the physician is faced with a dilemma. This can be resolved by consideration of the usual self-limited time course of depressions, treatment of associated anxiety and sleep disorders with other appropriate medication (*see* below), and use of electroconvulsive therapy (ECT) in serious depressions. ECT exposes the patient to a very short period of high risk, during which time he can be under the supervision of trained personnel.

Respiration. In man, imipramine in clinical doses produces little effect on respiration. Respiratory depression has been observed following poisoning with imipramine and with amitriptyline (*see* below).

Preparations, Dosage, and Routes of Administration. These are presented in Table 12-4. A further consideration of dosage ap-

Table 12-4. ANTIDEPRESSANT DRUGS: PREPARATIONS, DOSAGE FORMS, AND DOSES

NONPROPRIETARY NAME	TRADE NAME	DOSAGE FORMS *	DAILY DOSE— FIRST WEEK (*mg*)	USUAL RANGE OF DAILY DOSE AFTER FIRST 2 WEEKS (*mg*)
Tricyclics				
Imipramine Hydrochloride, U.S.P.	PRESAMINE TOFRANIL	(T) 10, 25, 50 mg (A) 25 mg/2 ml	50–100	75–300
Desipramine Hydrochloride, N.F.	NORPRAMIN PERTOFRANE	(C) 25, 50 mg (T) 25, 50 mg	50–150	75–300
Amitriptyline Hydrochloride, U.S.P.	ELAVIL	(T) 10, 25, 50 mg (V) 10 mg/ml	50–100	75–300
Nortriptyline Hydrochloride, N.F.	AVENTYL	(C) 10, 25 mg (S) 10 mg/5 ml	25–50	50–100
Protriptyline Hydrochloride, N.F.	VIVACTYL	(T) 5, 10 mg	10–30	15–60
Doxepin Hydrochloride, N.F.	SINEQUAN	(C) 10, 25, 50 mg	50–100	75–150
Monoamine Oxidase Inhibitors				
Isocarboxazid, N.F.	MARPLAN	(T) 10 mg	10–30	10–50
Phenelzine Sulfate, N.F.	NARDIL	(T) 15 mg	30–45	15–75
Tranylcypromine Sulfate, N.F.	PARNATE	(T) 10 mg	20–30	10–40

* T = tablet; C = capsule; V = vial for I.M. injection; A = ampul for I.M. injection; S = oral solution.

pears in the discussion of drug treatment of affective disorders (page 186).

Absorption, Distribution, Fate, and Excretion. Imipramine is well absorbed from the gastrointestinal tract. In man, imipramine is rapidly distributed and metabolized by demethylation, oxidation, and aromatic hydroxylation. Demethylation converts the drug to an active metabolite, desipramine. Pharmacological activity is lost after 2-hydroxylation. The pharmacologically active metabolites of imipramine are highly but variably bound to plasma protein (Glassman and Perel, 1973).

There is a wide interpatient variation in the steady-state plasma concentrations of tricyclic antidepressants. This variation seems to be genetically determined; identical twins show virtually identical plasma concentrations and half-lives after oral administration of nortriptyline (Alexanderson and Sjöqvist, 1971). Plasma concentrations of the tricyclic antidepressants can be increased by concomitant administration of drugs that inhibit hepatic hydroxylating enzymes. Some investigators have found a correlation between steady-state plasma concentrations and therapeutic response (Åsberg *et al.,* 1971), whereas others have not. Glassman and coworkers (1974) have discussed these disparate results.

Excretion of the tricyclic antidepressants is rapid, in contrast to the long latency of onset of action of the drugs. Approximately 40% of a dose of radioactive imipramine appears in the urine in 24 hours and a total of 70% during the first 72 hours. The remainder appears in the feces. A small portion can be recovered as unchanged drug or as the active desmethyl derivative. The larger portion is excreted as the N-oxide or as the nonconjugated or conjugated 2-OH derivative.

With the exception of demethylation, desipramine would be expected to follow the same metabolic pathway as imipramine, since most of the excretory products of the parent compound are demethylated. The metabolic fate of amitriptyline is very similar to that of imipramine. It involves demethylation, hydroxylation of the central ring, and conjugation.

Tolerance and Physical Dependence. Tolerance to the anticholinergic effects, such as dry mouth, constipation, blurred vision, and tachycardia, tends to develop with continued use of imipramine. Orthostatic hypotension similar to that seen with the phenothiazines may occur initially, but tolerance to this effect is acquired. Occasional patients will show physical or psychic dependence on the tricyclic antidepressants (Shatan, 1966). A withdrawal syndrome consisting in malaise, chills, coryza, and muscle aching has been reported to follow abrupt discontinuation of high doses of imipramine.

Toxic Reactions and Side Effects. Since imipramine was the first of the tricyclic antidepressants to be introduced into therapy, most is known of its toxic potentialities. However, in all probability, the discussion that follows applies to all members of the group. The most frequent untoward reactions caused by imipramine and amitriptyline are those attributable to anticholinergic effects, including dry mouth, constipation, dizziness, tachycardia, palpitations, blurred vision, and urinary retention. Special precautions should be taken in patients with benign prostatic hypertrophy. Paradoxically, excessive sweating is a fairly common complaint; the mechanism of this response is not known. Weakness and fatigue are attributable to central effects of the drug and may resemble those seen with the phenothiazines. Headache is fairly common, as are muscle tremors and epigastric distress. There are marked individual differences in the type and the frequency of these side effects, and they may be related to plasma concentrations of active drug. Older patients tend to suffer more from dizziness, postural hypotension, constipation, delayed micturition, edema, and muscle tremors. Various types of cardiovascular difficulties have already been discussed in detail.

Another undesirable effect of imipramine is a transition from depression to hypomanic or manic excitement in certain patients. In others, hallucinations and delusions may occur. Psychotic manifestations can be managed by the administration of phenothiazines without interfering with the antidepressant effects of imipramine.

A persistent fine tremor occurs in about 10% of those receiving the drug. Severe, sudden tremors have been reported in elderly individuals when the daily dosage reaches 250 mg. A mild parkinsonian syndrome resembling that occurring with the phenothiazines may be seen in some patients, particularly older persons taking large doses. As with the phenothiazines, high doses of imipramine may produce grand mal seizures even in patients without a history of convulsions.

Imipramine may produce an allergic type of obstructive jaundice similar to that caused by the phenothiazines; it clears when the drug is discontinued. Agranulocytosis has been reported from imipramine, as from the phenothiazine derivatives; it represents a hypersensitivity reaction. Eosinophilia may also occur. Skin rashes appear on occasion, including photosensitization similar to that produced by the phenothiazines.

Toxicity due to *acute overdosage* is characterized by hyperpyrexia, hypertension, seizures, and coma (Noble and Matthew, 1969). In some cases of poisoning in children, the drug has caused cardiac conduction defects and arrhythmias including multifocal ectopic beats.

Treatment of poisoning by tricyclic antidepressants should follow the same principles as for poisoning with the phenothiazines. Gastric lavage is useful in acute overdosage. Vital signs and ECG should be monitored continuously, and all cases should be treated in an intensive care unit. Treatment will depend upon the particular signs exhibited. Convulsions may be controlled with diazepam administered intravenously. Hypertension may be treated with short-acting α-adrenergic blocking agents, but caution is desirable. Temperature can be reduced and respiration assisted with physical methods. Propranolol and lidocaine are useful in controlling the arrhythmias; however, the availability of resuscitative equipment is important. Patients should not be discharged in less than 3 days under any circumstances.

Several clinical reports indicate that *physostigmine,* an anticholinesterase capable of crossing the blood-brain barrier, can effectively reverse the anticholinergic CNS manifestations of severe poisoning by the tricyclic antidepressants, including coma, myoclonus, choreoathetosis, and delirium. Dramatic improvement has been recorded; indeed, its use may be lifesaving. Physostigmine salicylate is given intramuscularly or by slow intravenous injection in an initial dose of 2 mg for adults. This dose is repeated in 20 minutes if there is no response. In cases responding favorably, 1 to 4 mg may have to be given every 30 to 60 minutes over a period of many hours. The tachycardia and tachypnea may also be counteracted by such therapy. (*See* Slovis *et al.,* 1971; Burks *et al.,* 1974; Snyder *et al.,* 1974.)

Interaction with Other Drugs. Administration of tricyclic antidepressants concurrently with or shortly after treatment with MAO inhibitors has resulted in severe reactions, consisting in signs and symptoms resembling those of atropine toxicity. A dose as low as 25 mg of imipramine, taken 3 days after the discontinuation of therapeutic doses of tranylcypromine, has been reported capable of producing a severe reaction characterized by convulsions, coma, and hyperpyrexia. Their concurrent use is thus contraindicated. Ten days to 2 weeks should elapse between discontinuance of MAO inhibitors and initiation of tricyclic antidepressant therapy. If the situation is desperate, ECT may be employed during the interval.

Other interactions include the potentiation of central depressant drugs, blockade of the antihypertensive effects of guanethidine, and augmentation of the pressor effects of sympathomimetic amines. Interactions with thyroid preparations, methylphenidate, and phenothiazines, all of which may enhance the therapeutic effect of the tricyclic antidepressants, have been reported.

Therapeutic Uses. The use of the tricyclic drugs for the *treatment of depression* is presented below (page 186).

The tricyclic antidepressants have also been employed for a variety of other ailments, but because of their toxicity indiscriminate use should be avoided. Imipramine has been reported to be of value in the treatment of *enuresis in childhood.* It is not within the scope of this text to discuss the selection of patients, dosage, duration of treatment, and other judgmental decisions (*see* Medical Letter, 1974). Some success has been reported in the treatment of *severe obsessive-compulsive neurosis,* and when this condition is incapacitating a trial may be warranted (*see* Detre and Jarecki, 1971).

MONOAMINE OXIDASE (MAO) INHIBITORS

The MAO inhibitors comprise a rather heterogeneous group of drugs that have in common the ability to block oxidative deamination of naturally occurring monoamines. However, the relationship between MAO inhibition and some of the ancillary therapeutic actions of these drugs is not firmly established. These drugs have numerous other effects, many of which are still poorly understood. For example, they lower blood pressure and thus have some limited usefulness in the treatment of hypertension.

History. Pathways of biosynthesis and metabolic degradation of naturally occurring amines have been studied with great interest for the past 4 decades (*see* Axelrod, 1971). Only during the past 20 years, however, have drugs been utilized specifically to inhibit oxidative deamination of biogenic amines. In 1951, *isoniazid* and its isopropyl derivative, *iproniazid,* were developed for the treatment of tuberculosis. It was soon found that both compounds, but especially iproniazid, had mood-elevating effects in tuberculous patients. In 1952, Delay and collaborators investigated the action of isoniazid in the treatment of depressed states. Zeller and coworkers (1952) had found that iproniazid, in contrast to isoniazid, was capable of inhibiting the enzyme MAO. Because of its marked central stimulating effects, the use of iproniazid was discontinued in the treatment of tuberculosis. However, in 1957, following investigations by Kline and colleagues and by Crane, it was introduced into psychiatry for the treatment of depressed patients. Kline referred to the compound as a psychic energizer, but the term *psychomotor stimulant* is more appropriate. Success was soon reported in the treatment of both hospitalized patients with psychotic depressions and nonhospitalized patients suffering from neurotic depressions. Such reports led to the development and clinical trial of many new compounds that also had the capacity to inhibit MAO.

Because of toxicity, there has been a great deal of flux in the introduction and withdrawal of MAO inhibitors. Drugs no longer available include *iproniazid, pheniprazine,* and *etryptamine.* Tranylcypromine was withdrawn from the market for some months during 1964, but again became available for use in patients under close medical observation. At present, the MAO inhibitors marketed for use in psychiatric depression are *isocarboxazid, nialamide, phenelzine,* and *tranylcypromine.*

Chemistry and Structure-Activity Relationship. The first MAO inhibitors to be used in the treatment of depression were hydrazide derivatives of hydrazine, a highly hepatotoxic substance. Subsequently, compounds unrelated to hydrazine were found to be very potent MAO inhibitors. Several of these agents were structurally related to amphetamine and were synthesized in an attempt to enhance central stimulant properties.

Cyclization of the side chain of amphetamine resulted in the nonhydrazide MAO inhibitor *tranylcypromine.* Another nonhydrazide MAO inhibitor, *pargyline,* employed as an antihypertensive agent, resulted from modification of the phenylalkylamine side chain to include an acetylenic moiety. The structures of tranylcypromine and phenelzine, a hydrazide that is still employed as an antidepressant, are as follows:

Tranylcypromine

Phenelzine

PHARMACOLOGICAL PROPERTIES

Two prototype drugs, *phenelzine* and *tranylcypromine,* exemplify the MAO inhibitors. The effects of these inhibitors are seen mainly in organ systems that are influenced by sympathomimetic amines and 5-HT. MAO inhibitors inhibit not only the enzyme after which they are named but also many other enzymes as well. In addition, they have numerous effects that are probably unrelated to enzyme inhibition. Since many pharmacological actions have been ascribed to alterations in MAO activity, a brief description of the role of that enzyme, as it is currently understood, is warranted.

Distribution of MAO and Its Substrates. Both MAO and catechol-O-methyl transferase (COMT) are of major importance in the regulation of metabolic degradation of epinephrine, norepinephrine, and dopamine; in addition, MAO oxidatively deaminates 5-HT. MAO is localized mainly in the mitochondrial fraction within the cell. At present it is felt that MAO plays a major role in the degradation of intracellular biogenic amines while COMT is more important for the metabolism of circulating catecholamines. The details of their role in the inactivation of norepinephrine and related biogenic amines are presented in Chapter 21.

In contrast to the catecholamines, the metabolic disposition of 5-HT depends almost entirely on oxidation by MAO. The distribution and possible physiological functions of 5-HT are discussed in Chapter 29. An extensive discussion of MAO and its inhibitors can be found in the monograph edited by Costa and Sandler (1972).

Relationship of Enzyme Inhibition to Pharmacological Actions. Clinically available MAO inhibitors produce irreversible inactivation of MAO by forming stable complexes with the enzyme. Since the synthesis of biogenic amines is apparently not inhibited, and since MAO normally limits intracellular amine levels, amine concentrations within the cell increase.

After administration of a single large dose of inhibitor, one can measure an increase in endogenous norepinephrine, epinephrine, dopamine, and 5-HT in various tissues, including brain, heart, intestine, and blood. There is an initial *decrease* in the synthesis of amines for a period of hours concomitant with the early rise in amine levels (Glowinski *et al.*, 1972). MAO inhibitors also enhance the effects of exogenously administered amines, such as 5-HT and norepinephrine, as well as precursors, such as 3,4-hydroxyphenylalanine (dopa) and 5-hydroxytryptophan. These amino acids are capable of penetrating the blood-brain barrier and are decarboxylated in the brain to the corresponding amines. In contrast to the precursors, the amines penetrate the barrier with difficulty. There is evidence that some MAO inhibitors prevent the release of norepinephrine from nerve endings by nerve impulses. However, MAO inhibitors do not interfere with the release of biogenic amines by pharmacological agents such as tyramine and amphetamine, a property that relates to the clinical toxicity of this class of drugs (*see* below).

Specificity of Actions of MAO Inhibitors. There are several *amine oxidases,* of which MAO is but one. The clinically useful MAO inhibitors are not entirely specific for monoamines since they interfere with the metabolic degradation of many drugs. They are, however, not inhibitors of enzymes that oxidize a number of naturally occurring biogenic amines such as histamine (which is acted upon by diamine oxidase).

The degree to which MAO is inhibited in a particular organ of the body varies with the particular MAO inhibitor. Since MAO inhibition cannot be easily monitored in clinical situations (because of long latency and duration of action), the drugs are never administered parenterally. In their clinical use they probably have a major effect on the enzymes in the liver.

MAO activity has been assayed in human subjects by a number of indirect methods, including chromatography of urinary amines, fluorometric measurement of urinary tryptamine and tyramine, and the measurement of the conversion of 5-HT to 5-hydroxyindoleacetic acid (5-HIAA) after administration of a standard test dose. More direct measurements are achieved by the assay of MAO activity in tissue obtained by jejunal biopsy and in platelets.

Psychological Effects. The most useful effect of the various MAO inhibitors is to elevate the mood of depressed patients. Objective measurement of this effect presents a difficult problem. In some cases, treatment may result in hypomanic or manic reactions consisting in agitation and talkativeness. This may represent either drug influence upon the natural history of the disease or a toxic psychokinetic reaction. Further discussion of antidepressive effects appears below. It may take weeks to obtain a discernible response in depressed patients, but the amphetamine-like effects of tranylcypromine can become apparent within a much shorter time. Signs of central stimulation are commonly seen in patients receiving pargyline for the treatment of hypertension. This effect takes several weeks to become manifest.

Effects on Sleep. MAO inhibitors are among the most effective REM suppressors known. This effect has been used therapeutically in the treatment of narcolepsy (Wyatt *et al.*, 1971). Moreover, when they are effective in the treatment of depression, MAO inhibitors correct the accompanying disorder of sleep, whether it is an increase or decrease of sleep time.

EEG Effects. In man, the effects of the MAO inhibitors upon the EEG are slight. Tranylcypromine decreases the frequency variability of the EEG.

Animal Behavior. The administration of single doses of an MAO inhibitor produces either minor changes in the behavior of animals or none at all, even when biochemical studies reveal marked alteration in the activity of the enzymes in the brain and significant elevations of brain concentrations of dopamine, norepinephrine, and 5-HT. However, when these drugs are combined with other agents, marked effects upon behavior and CNS function may be seen. Thus, in animals pretreated with MAO inhibitors, reserpine and tetrabenazine produce excitement rather than sedation, hexobarbital sleeping time is prolonged, and the actions of many other CNS depressants and stimulants may be augmented.

Cardiovascular System. MAO inhibitors lower blood pressure and provide symptomatic relief in angina pectoris. Their cardiovascular effects are discussed in detail in Chapter 33.

Absorption, Fate, and Excretion. All the currently employed MAO inhibitors are readily absorbed when given by mouth. The rate at which these drugs produce inhibition of MAO is not known, but pargyline takes about a day to produce measurable MAO inhibition in jejunal tissue; it reaches a maximum by the second or third day of daily administration of the drug (*see* Levine and Sjoerdsma, 1963). These agents are probably present in the body for only a short time, but they produce long-lasting effects by irreversible inactivation of the enzyme. The termination of drug effect depends upon enzyme regeneration, a process taking weeks.

The hydrazide MAO inhibitors are thought to be cleaved, with resultant liberation of active products. On the other hand, the nonhydrazide MAO inhibitors apparently combine directly with the enzyme. The hydrazide MAO inhibitors are inactivated primarily by acetylation. About one half the population are slow acetylators of the hydrazide-type drugs, including phenelzine, and this may explain the exaggerated effects observed in some patients given conventional doses of phenelzine (Vesell, 1972).

Toxic Reactions and Side Effects. *Acute Toxicity.* Toxic reactions from overdosage may occur in a matter of hours despite the long delay in onset of a therapeutic response. Reported effects of overdosage include agitation, hallucinations, hyperreflexia, hyperpyrexia, and convulsions. Both hypotension and hypertension have been reported. Treatment of such intoxication presents a problem since various types of supra-additive effects from antidotal drugs may be expected. There is a strong temptation to give sympathomimetic amines to combat hypotension and barbiturates to reduce CNS hyperexcitability, but these agents should be used with extreme caution. Conservative treatment aimed at maintaining normal temperature, respiration, blood pressure, and proper fluid and electrolyte balance has proven successful in most of the reported cases. Since the inhibition of the enzyme is irreversible, late toxic effects may appear. Patients with known overdosage of MAO inhibitors should be observed in the hospital for at least a week after the poisoning.

Chronic Toxicity. The toxic effects of the MAO inhibitors are greater than those of any other group of psychotherapeutic agents. The most dangerous are those involving the liver, the brain, and the cardiovascular system. Hepatotoxicity does not seem to be related to dosage or duration of therapy. Hypersensitivity may be the responsible mechanism, although activation of a viral infection has also been suggested as an etiological factor. The incidence of hepatic toxicity with currently used MAO inhibitors is low.

Excessive central stimulation consisting in tremors, insomnia, and hyperhydrosis may occur and might be considered extensions of the pharmacological effects. Agitation and hypomanic behavior may also occur, and on rare occasions hallucinations and confusion are observed. It may be that these behavioral toxicities, like those seen with imipramine, develop only in certain susceptible individuals (*see* below). *Convulsions* have also been reported. Peripheral neuropathy following the use of hydrazides may possibly be related to a pyridoxine deficiency.

Orthostatic hypotension occurs with the use of all the MAO inhibitors currently employed. The immediate condition readily yields to recumbency, but the dose may have to be reduced or the medication withdrawn.

A variety of other less serious side effects have been reported, including dizziness and vertigo (perhaps related to orthostatic hypotension), headache, inhibition of ejaculation, difficulty in urination, weakness, fatigue, dry mouth, blurred vision, and skin rashes. Constipation is common, but the cause is not known.

Interaction with Other Drugs. The paucity of grossly observable signs following the administration of MAO inhibitors is deceptive, for major changes have occurred in the body's capacity to handle endogenous biogenic amines and to respond to a wide spectrum of pharmacological agents. When MAO is inhibited, biogenic amines are not deaminated but are able to leave the cell in an active form and produce behavioral and pharmacodynamic effects.

Because of their interference with various enzymes, the MAO inhibitors are able to prolong and intensify the effects of other drugs and to interfere with the metabolism of various naturally occurring substances. There is considerable evidence that administration of *precursors of biogenic amines* may cause marked effects when administered following MAO inhibitors. Thus, the administration of dopa and 5-hydroxytryptophan increases the brain levels of catecholamines and 5-HT, respectively, and produces signs of central excitation in animals.

The actions of *sympathomimetic amines* are potentiated following the use of MAO inhibitors. The effect is much greater with indirectly acting amines (*e.g.,* amphetamine and tyramine) than with directly acting amines, which are potentiated in man to a greater degree by the tricyclic antidepressants. Since administered catecholamines are largely destroyed by COMT, the MAO inhibitors will have relatively little effect in prolonging and intensifying their action. On the other hand, inasmuch as certain sympathomimetic amines such as amphetamine and tyramine act peripherally, primarily by releasing the stores of catecholamines in nerve endings, and since the level of amines is raised by MAO inhibitors, profound potentiation of effects such as pressor responses may be expected (*see* below).

MAO inhibitors also interfere with detoxication mechanisms for certain other drugs. They prolong and intensify the effects of central depressant agents, such as barbiturates, alcohol, and potent analgesics; of anticholinergic agents, particularly those used in the treatment of parkinsonism; and of antidepressant agents, especially imipramine and amitriptyline. A serious hyperpyrexic reaction occurs after the concomitant use of meperidine. This reaction seems to be mediated by the release of 5-HT and does not occur in experimental animals if they are pretreated with inhibitors of 5-HT synthesis.

Hypertensive crisis is the most serious toxic effect of MAO inhibitors related to drug interaction. A combination of chance and clinical acumen led a number of investigators to note that hypertensive crises could be associated with the ingestion of cheese in patients receiving MAO inhibitors, particularly tranylcypromine and phenelzine but also other agents in this class. Acting on the suggestion of an alert pharmacist, Blackwell suggested that certain cheeses might contain a pressor amine or substance capable of liberating stored catecholamines (*see* Ayd and Blackwell, 1970). *Tyramine* was soon implicated as the culpable substance. The average meal of natural or aged cheeses contains enough tyramine to provoke a marked rise in blood pressure and other cardiovascular changes. Presumably as a result of hepatic MAO inhibition, the tyramine escapes oxidative deamination that would normally occur in the liver, and releases norepinephrine that is present in supranormal amounts in nerve endings. Other foods implicated in this syndrome include beer, wine, pickled herring, chicken liver, yeast, coffee, broad-

bean pods, and canned figs (*see* Marley and Blackwell, 1970). Patients being treated with MAO inhibitors and their families should be given a list of foods to be avoided and a general warning about the use of *any* medication by the patient without permission. Care must even be exercised here, since certain depressed patients have used such a list as a compilation of potential suicidal agents.

In certain instances, intracranial bleeding has occurred, and death has sometimes followed. Headache is a common symptom, and fever frequently accompanies the hypertensive episode. There is a clinical similarity of the hypertensive syndrome to that seen in pheochromocytoma, particularly following the provocative use of histamine to release catecholamines from the tumor. Such episodes may also be encountered when MAO inhibitors are used with sympathomimetic amines, methyldopa, dopamine, and tryptophan. It should be noted that tranylcypromine can cause a reaction if administered when the effect of phenelzine is still present. Switching a patient from one MAO inhibitor to another or to a tricyclic antidepressant requires a rest period of 10 to 14 days.

Treatment of the hypertensive crisis is directed at lowering the blood pressure. For this purpose a short-acting α-adrenergic blocking agent (*e.g.,* phentolamine) is recommended. Fever may be reduced by external cooling.

The actual incidence of serious side effects is very difficult to determine. It has been estimated that by 1970 3.5 million patients had used tranylcypromine and, of these, 50 persons sustained cerebrovascular accidents and 15 died. Coincidental presence of nondrug-induced pathology probably plays an important role. There is no evidence that the relative incidence of hypertensive crises is any greater with tranylcypromine than with the other agents in this class, but the absolute number of patients treated with the latter drugs is considerably smaller.

Therapeutic Uses. The MAO inhibitors have been used primarily in the treatment of *depression* and certain *phobic-anxiety states.* Their possible use in *narcolepsy* is mentioned above; since the specific indication for their use is not yet clear and their toxicity relatively great, they have been reserved mainly for patients refractory to other treatments. They are also employed in the therapy of hypertension, although this is now uncommon (*see* Chapter 33). The use of

MAO inhibitors in psychiatry is discussed in detail below in connection with the drug treatment of affective disorders.

LITHIUM CARBONATE

The introduction of lithium into psychiatric treatment has been marked by both exorbitant claims and caviling denials about its efficacy in various conditions. It is not a catholicon for all forms of cyclical illness, but it is effective in the treatment of the manic phase of manic-depressive illness, as a mood-stabilizing drug when used chronically in manic-depressives, and as an antidepressant in an ill-defined group of patients.

The general pharmacology of lithium, including possible mechanisms of actions and effects upon a variety of organ systems, is discussed in Chapter 37. The following presentation will be limited to actions on the CNS; absorption, fate, and excretion as they relate to dosage regimens; toxic reactions and side effects; drug interactions that accompany therapeutic use; and the applications of lithium in the treatment of affective disorders.

History. Lithium was used as a treatment for gout by Garrod in 1859. The bromide salt was employed as a hypnotic in the 1920s, and in 1940 lithium chloride was used as a sodium substitute with disastrous consequences, including deaths. Cade in Australia, while looking for toxic nitrogenous substances in mental patients by injecting their urine into guinea pigs, administered lithium salts to his experimental animals in an attempt to increase the solubility of urates. Lithium carbonate made the guinea pigs lethargic. In an inductive leap, Cade gave lithium carbonate to manic patients. In 1949, he reported that lithium seemed to have a specific effect on mania. For a more detailed history, *see* Schou (1968) and Ayd and Blackwell (1970). The drug was then investigated in other countries with encouraging results and was introduced as an experimental drug in the United States in the 1960s.

Chemistry and Preparations. Lithium is a monovalent cation that is the lightest of the alkali metals. The ion is easily measured spectrophotometrically. It occurs in trace amounts in the body, and, like sodium and potassium, its salts are highly soluble in water. *Lithium Carbonate,* U.S.P., is available as official tablets or capsules, each containing 300 mg.

PHARMACOLOGICAL PROPERTIES

In normal man, lithium in therapeutic doses has almost no discernible psychotropic effect. It is not sedative like the phenothiazines, nor is it euphoriant. This lack of psychoactivity in normal subjects differentiates lithium from all other drugs used in psychiatry.

Central Nervous System. A great deal of interest has centered on the modifications of brain amine metabolism by lithium. It is by no means certain that these actions are responsible for the therapeutic effects of lithium in manic-depressive illness. Lithium inhibits the release of norepinephrine and 5-HT, increases re-uptake of norepinephrine, and possibly increases synthesis and the turnover rate of 5-HT. It apparently has little effect on dopaminergic systems. The ion inhibits the activation of adenylate cyclase within the CNS when given in high doses to experimental animals, and alters the concentrations of γ-aminobutyric acid and glutamate. Considerable modification of hormonal responses can result from the actions of lithium (*see* Chapter 37). Thus, lithium has many effects on the chemical transmitter systems believed to be involved in the pathophysiology of depression and mania.

Effects on Sleep. When given to manic patients who characteristically sleep little or not at all, lithium corrects the sleep disorder. It appears to be a REM suppressant when used therapeutically.

Absorption, Fate, and Excretion. Lithium ions are readily absorbed when given orally. A plasma lithium peak is reached 1 to 3 hours after ingestion of lithium carbonate. Decrease in plasma concentration occurs in two phases. There is a steep drop for 5 to 6 hours, and this is followed by a slower elimination over the next 24 hours or more. For this reason it is essential to measure lithium plasma levels 8 to 10 hours after the last dose and always at the same time for a particular patient. It is tempting to attribute this biphasic excretion to mobilization from extracellular and intracellular sites, respectively.

Lithium is not bound to plasma proteins. The concentration in cerebrospinal fluid is only about half of that in plasma. The main route of excretion is by the kidneys. Under normal conditions the renal lithium clearance is of the order of 15 to 30 ml per minute, with an excretion fraction of approximately 0.2. About half of a single dose of lithium is excreted in 24 hours. Plasma lithium concentrations may not represent the most accurate method of determining effective lithium concentration in tissue, and for this reason some investigators utilize lithium concentrations in erythrocytes, either independently or in relation to the plasma level.

When sodium intake is lowered, lithium excretion is slower and severe intoxication may ensue. Thus, lithium should not be given to patients on a salt-free diet. Conversely, administration of large amounts of sodium increases the excretion of lithium. Although this procedure for the mobilization of excess lithium is advocated by some investigators (Platman and Fieve, 1969), others have not found it so successful (Schou, 1968). The administration of potassium has also been suggested as a means of speeding the excretion of lithium following intoxication, and this has theoretical merit.

Plasma Lithium Concentrations and Therapeutic Response. Lithium dosage is routinely monitored by the measurement of plasma lithium. In acute mania daily doses of about 1800 mg, administered in 4 divided doses, produce plasma lithium concentrations of 0.9 to 1.4 mEq per liter; this seems to be an effective plasma level in this condition (Prien *et al.,* 1972). Although patients with mania are reported to retain lithium, this becomes apparent only when measurements of urinary excretion are made, possibly indicating a greater intracellular distribution. There seems to be no clinical advantage in attaining plasma concentrations higher than 1.5 mEq per liter, and the side effects increase greatly above this value. Lithium maintenance therapy is reported to be effective in prevention of both mania and depression, with a dose of about 1200 mg per day resulting in a median plasma concentration of 0.8 mEq per liter (Prien *et al.,* 1972).

Toxic Reactions and Side Effects. Patients on therapeutic doses of lithium may complain of fatigue and muscular weakness. Slurred speech, ataxia, and a fine tremor of the hands are commonly noticed. Nausea, vomiting, and diarrhea may occur. A neph-

rogenic diabetes insipidus accompanied by excessive thirst is frequently seen. Exophthalmos has been reported. Leukocytosis occurs in many patients. A few patients have developed diffuse nontoxic goiters. While most mild side effects disappear after a week or so of continued treatment, thirst, excessive urination, and tremor persist.

When plasma concentrations rise above 2 mEq per liter, more serious toxic effects occur. The CNS is primarily affected. Consciousness is impaired, and even coma may occur. Muscular rigidity, hyperactive deep reflexes, and marked tremor and muscle fasciculations are observed. Epileptic seizures occur in some patients. EEG abnormalities are common.

Interactions with Other Drugs. Lithium treatment should only be conducted in patients with normal sodium intake. Compensation should be made for abnormal sodium loss, such as that caused by increased sweating in the summer. Lithium decreases the pressor response to norepinephrine in man. Thiazide diuretics may correct the diabetes insipidus caused by lithium, but they increase retention of lithium, probably by altering sodium balance. Lithium is often used in conjunction with antipsychotic and antidepressant drugs. The antipsychotic drugs may block the nausea, which can be a sign of lithium toxicity. Urinary retention due to the anticholinergic effects of the tricyclic antidepressants can become particularly uncomfortable in the presence of a lithium-induced diuresis. There is, however, no absolute contraindication to the concurrent use of lithium and other psychotropic drugs.

Therapeutic Uses. The use of lithium in *manic-depressive illness* is discussed below.

DRUG TREATMENT OF AFFECTIVE DISORDERS

Mood changes are natural variations familiar to all people. When these changes, either an elevation or depression of mood, extend beyond the range of normal and become intolerable to an individual, they constitute incapacitating illnesses. Since mood varies over a continuum and a person's or society's tolerance to either depression or elation may vary, the decision when to treat either mania or depression may depend on external factors.

Mania. Mania, which in its milder form is called *hypomania*, is a mood state characterized by elation. The occurrence of manic or hypomanic states in a patient's history is fundamental to the diagnosis of *manic-depressive illness.* Definitions and diagnosis have been reviewed by Winokur and coworkers (1969). This affective disorder is primarily treated with lithium carbonate, both as maintenance therapy and as an adjunctive or primary treatment of acute episodes. (*See* above for dosage and details of therapy.) Manic-depressive illness may be either *bipolar,* characterized by episodes of *both* mania and depression, or *unipolar,* characterized by recurrent episodes of *either* mania or depression. Unipolar manic disorders are rare, and bipolar disorders do not necessarily involve an *alternation* of two mood states. A differential diagnosis from schizoaffective illness (a variation of schizophrenia with mood alternation) must be made since lithium is ineffective in this disease.

Acute mania is treated with lithium or antipsychotic drugs and frequently with both concomitantly. Since the patients are often destructive and unmanageable, vigorous therapy may be indicated. Studies in the treatment of acute mania show that, while intramuscular haloperidol or chlorpromazine is effective, often the episode can be treated successfully with lithium alone (Johnson *et al.*, 1971). In patients unresponsive to large doses of antipsychotic drugs, ECT may be used.

Maintenance therapy of patients with bipolar manic-depressive illness should be instituted with lithium carbonate if a clear diagnosis can be made. A collaborative study has also demonstrated the effectiveness of maintenance therapy with lithium carbonate in unipolar depressive disorders (Prien *et al.*, 1972); the same study showed that imipramine also has some advantage for this purpose.

Depression. The clinical use of the antidepressant drugs has been reviewed by Glassman and Perel (1973), American Psychiatric Association (1974), and Schildkraut (1974). Depending on the observer, the patient, and the situation, depression may be viewed as a symptom, a syndrome, or a disease entity, and the lack of uniformity in classifying the diverse clinical pictures subsumed under the rubric of depression constitutes a major obstacle to the assessment of any treatment modality. Most commonly, an attempt is made to differentiate among the various clinical pictures on the basis of severity, precipitating factors, or the presence of a hypothetical underlying biological disorder.

Most individuals have cyclic variations in mood, and some sad days are part of the human condition. Normal individuals will also exhibit marked sadness following the death of a loved one, a major illness, a failure in business, or a severe blow to self-esteem. This response may be so exaggerated or prolonged in a neurotic individual that it becomes incapacitating, but the precipitating factor can usually be identified and the sadness often seems understandable. Such *reactive* (neurotic) depressions may be quite severe and are sometimes prolonged. There are still other individuals who seem to have been depressed all of their lives; they seem to find little joy in any form of social interaction, and their self-esteem is chronically low. This picture is common among patients who exhibit alcoholism, narcotic addiction, or sociopathic behavior. Another major group consists of those patients whose symptoms have a definite onset, but the onset seems unrelated to significant external events. Such patients are usually older, and the depressions are often considered to be *endogenous.* When the depression occurs in later life, it is then termed *involutional.* In this group, the depressive picture is often characterized by marked retardation, feelings of guilt and worthlessness, and vegetative signs such as early-morning awakening, decreased appetite, constipation, and weight loss. Some patients, particularly those with bipolar manic-depressive illness, may show an *increase* in sleep and general anergy and retardation. Still others in this older group may exhibit only a loss of energy and interest associated with a persistent preoccupation with bodily complaints. Many psychiatrists use the term *endogenous depression* interchangeably with *psychotic depression.* In the severe cases, especially where there is delusion of guilt, unreasonable hopelessness, suicidal preoccupation, or agitation, the term *psychotic depression* seems quite appropriate. Severe depression may also occur in the context of a schizophrenic psychotic episode. A discussion of various classification systems has been given by Robins and Guze (1972).

The treatment of depression can involve a number of therapeutic measures. Psychotherapy, family therapy, hospitalization, ECT, tricyclic antidepressants, MAO inhibitors, antipsychotic drugs, lithium carbonate, antianxiety drugs, and other measures may be required in various combinations.

First one must decide *whether* to treat depression. This usually involves a differential diagnosis with a consideration of other medical illnesses such as cancer and congestive heart failure, which can present with depressive symptomatology. The "depression" may clear only when the medical illness has been successfully treated. Since many depressions resolve spontaneously, the physician should consider the length of the illness, the age of the patient, and his previous history. If there are vegetative signs present and the mood state is disabling, a decision to treat should be made.

The next question is the treatment setting. Suicidal patients should be hospitalized. Hospitalization for others depends on the severity of the symptoms and the ability of the patient to function in the outside world.

A tricyclic antidepressant, such as amitriptyline, should be instituted with a single 50-mg dose at bedtime and increasing to a total dose of about 150 mg per day by the end of the first week. Most of the daily dose can be given at bedtime. If the patient shows no response in the first 2 weeks, the dose can be increased to a maximum of 300 mg per day. If the patient does not respond to amitriptyline, imipramine can be tried (*see* Schildkraut, 1974). If the patient is unresponsive or unmanageable, ECT may be necessary. ECT is also indicated in the presence of a persistent refusal to take drugs, or a previous history of failure to respond to an adequate trial of antidepressant drugs. Hostility, rather than anxiety, as a prominent symptom of depression can be considered a relative contraindication to the use of either imipramine or diazepam (*see* American Psychiatric Association, 1974). In such patients the phenothiazines are more effective than the tricyclic antidepressants.

Kuhn (1958) had originally observed that imipramine seemed more effective in *endogenous* depressions. A more extensive survey by Kiloh and Garside (1963) indicated that both ECT and the various drug therapies for depression were most effective in the endogenous varieties whereas, regardless of severity or the presence of a definable precipitating cause, psychotherapy was more beneficial in reactive or neurotic depression. Although it is generally agreed that ECT is still the most effective treatment in endogenous depression, with perhaps 70 to 90% of patients showing a satisfactory remission, controlled studies indicate that in adequate doses the response to tricyclic compounds may approach (but not exceed) that obtained with ECT. The percentage of patients showing improvement with tricyclic drugs varies widely (32 to 80%), depending on criteria for diagnosis and improvement and on dosage schedules. However, most psychiatrists report improvement in approximately 60 to 70% of depressed patients (*see* American Psychiatric Association, 1974). ECT and a tricyclic antidepressant may be given concurrently, but it is not clear if this reduces the amount of ECT required. The idea that drugs are relatively ineffective in neurotic depressions has not found universal support; a few controlled studies indicate that, even in younger patients with clear-cut precipitating factors, imipramine is superior to a placebo (*see* Wittenborn *et al.,* 1962; Rickels *et al.,* 1970; American Psychiatric Association, 1974).

MAO inhibitors should be used if (1) there is a previous history of good response to these agents, (2) the patient is reliable enough to be trusted with a potentially highly toxic drug, (3) there has been a failure of tricyclic drug therapy and ECT is contraindicated, and/or (4) the patient has a syndrome known to be responsive to these agents.

There have been few well-controlled comparative studies of the different MAO inhibitors. The general opinion is that tranylcypromine is the most effective of the group, but phenelzine is also useful. When MAO inhibitors are used, the concomitant use of pressor amines, meperidine, tricyclic antidepressants, and other substances listed previously is absolutely contraindicated.

For the present, considerations of both efficacy and potential toxicity indicate that the use of tricyclic compounds should be the initial pharmacological approach to depression. It is usually possible to predict the eventual outcome of treatment from the response obtained in the first 2 to 3 weeks. If the response is not satisfactory, the physician must then weigh the relative toxicities of ECT and MAO inhibitors against the probabilities that they will produce improvement. He must also weigh the fact that

perhaps 80% or more of depressed patients will eventually recover without treatment.

The concurrent administration of antidepressant drugs and sedative agents, such as diazepam, is thought to be helpful in depressions when anxiety is a prominent feature. Alternatively, a combination of a phenothiazine and a tricyclic antidepressant can be used. Amphetamine and related substances capable of producing mood elevation in relatively normal individuals have not been proven effective in depressions.

For the sadness and grief that are an inevitable part of living and for those individuals for whom depression has become a way of life, antidepressant medication is of little value; the drugs are potentially toxic and should not be used unless the risk is balanced by the expectation of some benefit.

Phobic Anxiety States. A number of investigators have described a syndrome consisting in the sudden onset of episodic panic attacks that result in marked phobic constriction of travel and activities. The patients often complain of depression, apathy, and somatic difficulties, but between panic attacks they are lively and friendly although somewhat manipulative and demanding. In many such patients, the onset of symptoms occurs upon threatened or actual separation from a valued person; in a number of others, onset is associated with a period of endocrine fluctuation (*e.g.,* ante-partum, post-partum, or post-oophorectomy periods). The syndrome does not respond readily to psychotherapy, sedatives, phenothiazines, or ECT. It does show a remarkable change after the administration of tricyclic antidepressants or MAO inhibitors, and these two therapies seem equally effective. The phobic attitudes may continue, but the episodic panic attacks cease, only to recur when the medication is discontinued. This response to antidepressant drugs has caused some psychiatrists to view such syndromes as one type of "atypical" or "masked" depression; however, the term *phobic-anxiety state* seems preferable. (*See* Roth, 1960.)

III. Drugs Used in the Treatment of Anxiety

Sedative-antianxiety drugs, or more simply and less accurately, *antianxiety drugs,* are prescribed more frequently than any other group of therapeutic agents. The chemical diversity of these compounds defies coherent description. The two most widely used classes are the propanediol carbamates (meprobamate and congeners) and the benzodiazepines (diazepam and congeners). The antihistaminic sedatives are discussed briefly here and elsewhere, and the barbiturate members of the group are described in Chapter 9. No consistent mode of action has been hypothesized for these drugs, and their diverse pharmacological actions do not fit into simple patterns. These drugs are frequently prescribed without adequate indication, as discussed below.

PROPANEDIOL CARBAMATES

Meprobamate may be taken as the prototype drug in this class since it is the most widely used. Meprobamate is clearly different from either the rauwolfia alkaloids or the phenothiazines since, unlike these drugs, it is of little value in the treatment of psychoses, does not produce extrapyramidal effects or selectively suppress conditioned avoidance responses, and has anticonvulsant properties.

History. Developed by Berger (1954) as a longer-acting successor to mephenesin, meprobamate was originally synthesized as a potential muscle relaxant in 1951. Mephenesin had been tried in different types of psychiatric disorders, but its usefulness was limited because of its short duration of action and unreliable absorption. Over 1200 compounds were investigated before meprobamate was selected and its pharmacological properties were described, including the ability to allay anxiety. Meprobamate quickly grew in popularity, and within 2 years after its introduction it was very widely prescribed.

Chemistry and Structure-Activity Relationship. *Meprobamate* is a simple aliphatic compound with the following structural formula:

$$H_2N-\overset{\overset{O}{\|}}{C}-OCH_2-\overset{\overset{C_3H_7}{|}}{\underset{\underset{CH_3}{|}}{C}}-CH_2O-\overset{\overset{O}{\|}}{C}-NH_2$$

Meprobamate

The substitution of a butyl group in place of a hydrogen on one of the carbamyl nitrogen atoms produces *tybamate,* a shorter-acting antianxiety agent. Isopropyl substitution at the same position results in *carisoprodol,* a muscle relaxant (*see* Chapter 14). The structure-activity relationship and pharmacological properties of this group have been reviewed by Ludwig and Potterfield (1971).

Pharmacological Properties

The pharmacological effects of meprobamate are very similar to those of the barbiturates. Indeed, in clinical usage it is difficult, if not impossible, to differentiate between the drugs. Only by careful pharmacological analysis can certain distinctions be discerned.

Central Nervous System. The locus and mode of action of meprobamate on the CNS are not known. A variety of neurophysiological effects have been reported (*see* Ludwig and Potterfield, 1971). *Anticonvulsant* properties are ascribed to meprobamate, but it is of no clinical use for this purpose and may aggravate grand mal epilepsy. Convulsions are seen on withdrawal from large doses of meprobamate. Meprobamate has no specific depressant effects on the reticular activating system. If the effect of a sufficiently large dose of meprobamate is examined with a highly sensitive test, psychological impairment will be found. With the usual single clinical dose of 400 mg, the effect of the drug is not reflected in performance of psychological tests. With 800 mg some impairment of learning may be detected, and with 1600 mg there is definite impairment of learning, motor coordination, and reaction time (Kornetsky, 1958). McNair (1973) critically reviewed all studies of the effects of antianxiety agents on human performance. Lack of adequate dose-response data and inconsistent measurement technics led him to the conclusion that no real conclusion could be drawn.

In animals, meprobamate resembles the barbiturates more closely than the phenothiazines and rauwolfia alkaloids in its effects upon conditioned avoidance responses. Effects upon conditioned responses are obtained with meprobamate, but only when doses are employed that also obtund unconditioned responses.

EEG Effects. Meprobamate produces increased fast activity with increased amplitude of the EEG. Beta waves (13 to 33 Hz) are particularly prominent. This EEG pattern is shared with barbiturates and benzodiazepines (Fink, 1969). After low doses of the drug the changes in the EEG cannot be distinguished from those caused by a placebo.

Effects on Sleep. Meprobamate suppresses REM sleep, as do the barbiturates. REM rebound after withdrawal of the drug has been reported. This agent offers no apparent advantages as a hypnotic over other commonly used drugs.

Autonomic Nervous System. No autonomic effects of meprobamate are seen after clinically used doses.

Muscle. Although skeletal muscle relaxation can presumably be measured objectively, quantitative data comparing the effect of meprobamate and other agents upon muscle spasm are difficult to obtain. There is evidence that sedation from meprobamate plays an important role in muscle relaxation (Domino, 1962). Some congeners of meprobamate are said to produce muscle relaxation with lesser sedative effects (*see* Chapter 14).

Cardiovascular and Respiratory Systems. In toxic doses meprobamate causes respiratory depression. Hypotension occurs occasionally with therapeutic doses.

Absorption, Fate, and Excretion. Meprobamate is well absorbed from the gastrointestinal tract, reaches a peak plasma concentration and systemic effect at about 2 to 3 hours, and has a half-life of 10 hours. Meprobamate can induce microsomal enzyme systems in the liver, and accelerated drug disposition, pharmacodynamic tolerance, and interactions with other drugs thus occur. In contrast, tybamate, which has a half-life of 3 hours, does not cause tolerance of either kind. The brief action of tybamate is an advantage in some situations. Meprobamate is quite uniformly distributed in the body, and about 10% of the drug is excreted in an unchanged form in the urine. The rest is excreted as hydroxymeprobamate and as a glucuronide.

Toxic Reactions and Side Effects. The major side effects of meprobamate are sleepiness and ataxia. Hypotension may occur. Allergic reactions have been reported in from 0.2 to 3.4% of different series of patients and appear most frequently in those with a history of dermatological or allergic conditions. Urticaria or an erythematous rash is the most common manifestation. Acute nonthrombocytopenic purpura has also been reported, and angioedema and bronchospasm have occasionally occurred. Meprobamate has been found to be associated with the development of aplastic anemia, thrombocytopenia, leukopenia, agranulocytosis, and erythroid hypoplasia; the number of reported cases has been very small.

Exacerbation of acute intermittent porphyria similar to that seen with barbiturates may be caused by meprobamate. *Suicide attempts* with meprobamate are not uncommon. Although a single dose of 12 g has been fatal, the usual lethal dose is considered to be 40 g or more. Coma, low blood pressure, shock, pulmonary edema, and respiratory depression characterize massive overdosage. Management of suicide attempts should follow the principles set forth for barbiturate overdose.

Tolerance and *physical dependence* occur with meprobamate but not with tybamate. A characteristic CNS depressant withdrawal syndrome consisting of delirium and convulsions is seen frequently in patients who have been given doses of 2 g or more a day. The withdrawal syndrome appears in 36 to 48 hours (*see* Bulla *et al.,* 1959).

Preparations and Dosage. These are presented in Table 12–5 (page 192).

BENZODIAZEPINE COMPOUNDS

Six benzodiazepine derivatives are presently available. *Chlordiazepoxide, diazepam, oxazepam,* and *clorazepate,* which are used mainly for treating anxiety, although there are other therapeutic indications for their use, are discussed here. *Flurazepam* and *nitrazepam* are considered to be hypnotics and are discussed in Chapter 10.

History. Compounds of this type were initially synthesized in 1933. Animal tests indicated that chlordiazepoxide had interesting muscle relaxant, antistrychnine, and spinal reflex–blocking properties. Randall and coworkers (1960) reported that it produced "taming" of a number of species of animals in doses much lower than those producing ataxia or measurable hypnosis. The difficult problem of defining "taming" in animals and of relating this effect to human therapeutic needs has been discussed by Cook and Kelleher (1963), but this "taming" effect in monkeys led to the clinical trial of the drug in man for the determination of antianxiety effects (Randall and Kappell, 1973).

Chemistry and Structure-Activity Relationship. Over 2000 benzodiazepines have been synthesized. The structure-activity relationship of this group has been reviewed by Sternbach (1973). Chlordiazepoxide was the first compound introduced for clinical use, but several useful congeners have been developed. Oxazepam is a N-demethylated 3-hydroxylated metabolic product of diazepam. Clorazepate is probably converted to N-dimethyl diazepam, which is then oxidized to oxazepam. The structures of the four available antianxiety benzodiazepines are shown on the following page.

Chlordiazepoxide   Diazepam

Oxazepam   Clorazepate

PHARMACOLOGICAL PROPERTIES

Chlordiazepoxide and diazepam can be considered prototype drugs for their class. They have achieved wide use as antianxiety agents but have other therapeutic applications as well.

Central Nervous System. *Behavioral and Neurophysiological Effects.* The effects of the benzodiazepines in the relief of anxiety can readily be demonstrated in experimental animals. In conflict punishment procedures, benzodiazepines greatly reduce the suppressive effects of punishment. Positive effects in this experimental model are not seen with antidepressants and antipsychotics (*see* Cook and Davidson, 1973). However, anxiety in rats and man can hardly be equated.

Earlier in this chapter, the difficulties in evaluating the therapeutic efficacy of psychotropic drugs in man were outlined. These difficulties are particularly great in the evaluation of antianxiety drugs. Therefore, it is readily understandable why disparate results have been obtained, since very few investigations meet the criteria that are necessary for definitive conclusions.

Many studies have shown that chlordiazepoxide is more effective than a placebo in the treatment of varied groups of anxious neurotic patients (*see* Klein and Davis, 1969; Wheatley, 1973). However, negative results have also been reported (*see* Gottschalk *et al.*, 1973). Since the neurophysiological or biochemical basis of anxiety is unknown, assessment of efficacy must be based on the general acceptance of benzodiazepine compounds by the medical profession. The clinical popularity of these drugs apparently is the result of a mechanism of action that is as yet undefinable.

In common with barbiturates, chlordiazepoxide blocks EEG arousal from stimulation of the brain stem reticular formation. The effects of this compound upon the brain are not yet well known. Przybyla and Wang (1968) found that the major locus of central depressant action of diazepam on spinal reflexes is the brain stem reticular system. Like meprobamate and the barbiturates, chlordiazepoxide depresses the duration of electrical afterdischarge in the limbic system, including the septal region, the amygdala, and the hippocampus.

Effects on Sleep. Benzodiazepines can be used effectively as hypnotics in conjunction with their use as antianxiety drugs. They do not suppress REM sleep in usual doses but do markedly diminish or eliminate stage-4 sleep. The significance of this is not known, but diazepam has been used in the treatment of "night terrors" that arise out of stage-4 sleep. Diazepam seems to be more effective than chlordiazepoxide in its hypnotic action (Kales and Scharf, 1973).

EEG Effects. The benzodiazepines cause an increase in fast beta activity with an increase in amplitude of the EEG. This is a pattern similar to that of meprobamate. All the benzodiazepines increase *seizure threshold* and are anticonvulsant. Diazepam is used clinically for this purpose, especially in status epilepticus (*see* Chapter 13).

Cardiovascular and Respiratory Systems. Considerable attention must be paid to the cardiovascular effects of the benzodiazepines since they are used so widely in cardiac patients. Diazepam, in an intravenous dose of about 60 mg, causes a slight decrease in respiration, blood pressure, and left ventricular stroke work. Increase in heart rate and decrease in cardiac output can also occur (Rao *et al.*, 1973). The effects are minimal, and it is unlikely that there is significant depression of cardiovascular function when the benzodiazepines are given in usual therapeutic doses by the oral route.

Skeletal Muscle. Diazepam is widely used as a muscle relaxant although controlled studies rarely show any advantage of any benzodiazepine over either placebo or aspirin (*see* Medical Letter, 1973). Some muscle relaxation occurs after administration of any of the CNS depressants, and there seems to be no particular advantage to any one of them when given by the oral route. The combined sedative and relaxing properties of parenteral diazepam have been used to advantage prior to such procedures as electrical conversion of cardiac arrhythmias. (*See* Chapter 14 for a discussion of centrally acting muscle relaxants.)

Absorption, Fate, and Excretion. Chlordiazepoxide is slowly absorbed and may take several hours to reach a peak plasma concentration. The half-life of the drug in the circulation is 1 to 2 days, and with continued administration several days are thus required for the plasma concentrations to reach a plateau. Two active metabolites, a lactam and a demethylated derivative, are formed. Small amounts of free and conjugated chlordiazepoxide are excreted in the urine. Diazepam, in contrast, is rapidly absorbed, reaching peak plasma concentrations in 1 hour. Drug elimination follows a biphasic pattern, with a rapid phase ($t_{1/2} = 2$ to 3 hours) followed by a slow decay with a half-time of 2 to 8 days. After steady-state concentrations are achieved (in about a week), a half-life of 3 days is found (Berlin *et al.,* 1972). Diazepam is metabolized to active products, including oxazepam. One third is excreted as oxazepam, and 70% of the metabolites appears in the urine. Oxazepam reaches a peak plasma concentration in 4 hours and is excreted in the urine as the glucuronide conjugate.

Tolerance and Physical Dependence. These occur with the benzodiazepines as with all drugs of this class. High doses must be given before marked withdrawal symptoms, including seizures, appear. Habituation to the benzodiazepines is common; however, because of the long half-lives and conversion to active metabolites, withdrawal symptoms after chronic use may not appear for a week after discontinuation of the drug. In most instances after usual doses, the withdrawal syndrome is benign.

Toxic Reactions and Side Effects. The expected side effects of drowsiness and ataxia are extensions of the pharmacological actions of these drugs. An increase in hostility has been reported as a possible pharmacological action of all the benzodiazepines, except oxazepam (*see* DiMascio, 1973). As with the more familiar alcohol-released aggression, the possibility of such a paradoxical effect should be kept in mind. Equally paradoxical is an *increase* in anxiety, but such a response can occur in patients whose need for mastery of their situation is dulled by the sedative effects of antianxiety agents. Both psychoses and sudden suicidal impulses have been reported in patients receiving high doses of benzodiazepines.

In general, the clinical toxicity of the benzodiazepines is low. Weight gain, which may be the result of renewed appetite, occurs in some patients. Many of the side effects reported for these drugs so overlap with symptoms of anxiety that unless a careful history is taken one is hard put to ascribe these effects to the drug. Among the other toxic reactions seen with chlordiazepoxide are skin rash, nausea, headache, impairment of sexual function, vertigo, and light-headedness. Agranulocytosis has also been reported. Menstrual irregularities have been noted, and women may fail to ovulate while taking benzodiazepines.

Overdosage with the benzodiazepines is frequent, but serious sequelae are rare. A few deaths have been reported at doses greater than 700 mg (Detre and Jarecki, 1971). The striking advantage of this group of drugs is the remarkable margin of safety. Treatment for overdosage is purely supportive of respiratory and cardiovascular function.

Drug Interactions. These are infrequent with the benzodiazepines. Except for an additive effect with other CNS depressants, they are not significant. Cigarette smoking may decrease the effectiveness of usual doses of these drugs. The relative lack of either side effects or drug interactions frequently makes these drugs the agents of choice in the treatment of anxiety states.

Preparations and Dosage. These are presented in Table 12–5.

Table 12-5. ANTIANXIETY DRUGS: PREPARATIONS, DOSAGE FORMS, AND DOSES

NONPROPRIETARY NAME	TRADE NAME	DOSAGE FORMS *	INITIAL SINGLE ADULT DOSE (mg)	USUAL RANGE DAILY DOSAGE (mg)
Benzodiazepines				
Chlordiazepoxide Hydrochloride, U.S.P.	LIBRIUM	(C) 5, 10, 25 mg (A) 100 mg	10	20–60
Chlordiazepoxide, N.F.	LIBRITABS	(T) 5, 10, 25 mg		
Clorazepate Dipotassium	TRANXENE	(C) 3.75, 7.5, 15 mg		
Diazepam, U.S.P.	VALIUM	(T) 2, 5, 10 mg (A) 10 mg/2 ml (V) 50 mg/10 ml	5	5–20
Oxazepam, N.F.	SERAX	(T) 15 mg (C) 10, 15, 30 mg	10	30–90
Propanediol Carbamates				
Meprobamate, U.S.P.	EQUANIL MILTOWN (others)	(T) 200, 400 mg	600	400–1200
Tybamate	SOLACEN TYBATRAN	(C) 125, 250, 350 mg	500	500–1500
Antihistamines				
Hydroxyzine Hydrochloride, N.F.	ATARAX	(T) 10, 25, 50, 100 mg	25	25–150
Hydroxyzine Pamoate, N.F.	VISTARIL	(C) 25, 50, 100 mg (SU) 25 mg/5 ml (S) 10 mg/5 ml (V) 50 mg/ml (2 and 5 ml)		

* C = capsule; S = syrup; SU = suspension; T = tablet; A = ampul; V = vial.

Therapeutic Uses. The benzodiazepines are used in the treatment of *anxiety* (*see* below). In addition, chlordiazepoxide has been widely employed in the treatment of *alcohol withdrawal syndromes* (*see* Chapter 16). The substitution of an antianxiety agent for alcohol in chronic alcoholism is a common practice, but this does not appear significantly to reduce alcohol intake or in any way to be an effective treatment of alcoholism. Other uses are as premedication in *anesthesia,* and in *obstetrics* during labor. When used for the latter purpose, the need for meperidine is greatly reduced. Diazepam administered to the mother can cause both hypothermia and hypotonia in the infant (Forfar and Nelson, 1973). An increase in fetal heart rate is also noted after diazepam is given to the mother. All effects are of short duration.

Diazepam has also been employed as a skeletal muscle relaxant. It has been used successfully in the treatment of *tetanus* in the intravenous dose of 2 to 20 mg at intervals of 2 to 8 hours. In conventional doses it has been claimed to relieve the muscular spasticity of *upper motoneuron* disorders; however, as is the case with most centrally acting muscle relaxants, superiority to a placebo response is difficult to prove. On the other hand, there is evidence from controlled studies that diazepam is effective in relieving spasticity and athetosis in patients with *cerebral palsy.* (For a representative publication, *see* Engle, 1966.) The use of diazepam in *cardioversion* is well documented, and for this purpose it is given intravenously in doses of from 5 to 30 mg. The uses of diazepam in *convulsive disorders* are discussed in Chapter 13.

SEDATIVE ANTIHISTAMINES AND OTHER COMPOUNDS

A wide variety of drugs with sedative action have been used for their antianxiety effects. These include such diverse agents as hydroxyzine and other antihistaminic sedatives, and scopolamine. Since their spectrum of action differs from the other groups, they offer an alternative, albeit one without a notable record of proven efficacy in the treatment of anxiety (*see* Chapter 10).

DRUG TREATMENT OF ANXIETY

Anxiety, a cardinal symptom of many psychiatric disorders, is a universal human experience widely treated with drugs. It is a symptom, a manifestation of another process, and rarely a disease in itself. Anxiety may permeate a person's existence or be an intermittent and transient phenomenon. The internal and external stimuli that can produce anxiety encompass most of the events of man's life. A wide range of drugs that can relieve anxiety is available. There is an obvious lack of similarity in chemical structure and spectrum of action. Some drugs will decrease anxiety in one person and paradoxically increase it in another. There are certain prerequisites for the medical treatment of anxiety that must be met before drugs are used. The first of these is *diagnosis*.

Anxiety is defined as an emotional state, unpleasant in nature, associated with an uneasiness or disquietude and resembling fear in its psychophysiological concomitants. When one is considering drug use, the distinctions about the nuances of this emotional state and its differentiation from fear become academic. Since anxiety is a *response* to stimuli, it frequently is terminated by the removal of these stimuli, be they internal or external. Anxiety is a regular part of the symptom pattern in most medical and psychiatric illnesses. The potential value of reducing this symptomatic component of an illness or of reducing a possibly crippling emotion in response to appropriate fear-producing situations should not be deprecated. Unfortunately, since anxiety about other symptoms is the universal driving force that brings patients to doctors, almost all patients will be anxious. If a broader diagnosis such as depression, psychosis, or systemic disease can be made, the initial therapeutic effort should be directed toward specific therapy. Past that point, and when anxiety worsens the intercurrent illness, the treatment of the symptom is warranted. The expected time course of the anxiety should be estimated and the course of treatment planned accordingly. Long-term prescription orders for antianxiety medication are unwise.

The *selection* of an antianxiety drug is less of a problem than the initial decision to use one. Frequently, in older patients or in those not tolerant to its effects, an alcoholic beverage may be the drug of choice. Phenobarbital and amobarbital should not be ignored in the selection process; they are inexpensive and well tolerated. Patient preference can be important if a course of therapy is to be followed, and here the evidence seems to indicate general acceptability for the benzodiazepines. There is little to guide one in the selection of a specific member of this class. When interactions with other drugs may be a problem, the benzodiazepines are also the drugs of choice. The brief duration of action of tybamate may offer an advantage in some situations. The dosage regimen used should be guided by the characteristics of the associated symptoms and causes. If loss of sleep is a complicating factor, there is usually no need to use a hypnotic drug. Since most of these drugs have half-lives of a day or longer, arranging dosage so that two thirds of the daily dose is taken at bedtime and the other third in two divided doses during the day provides hypnotic and continuous antianxiety effect. Long courses of treatment are rarely needed or useful since tolerance develops to CNS depressants and anxiety is usually self-limited.

Prolonged therapy can lead to habituation and little therapeutic effect other than the warding off of withdrawal symptomatology.

The antianxiety agents have found some usefulness in the treatment of mild depressions and may provide considerable relief in these self-limited diseases. Since suicide is often a possibility during a depressed state, the low toxicity of the benzodiazepines gives them a marked safety advantage. If habituation is a distinct possibility, an antihistamine sedative or a low dose of one of the antipsychotic drugs should be considered.

Many times antianxiety drugs are given indiscriminately to medical and surgical patients. Long-term or renewable prescription orders for patients who see doctors infrequently are not advisable. Short courses of therapy or intermittent use is always desirable with sedative-antianxiety agents. The effective drugs in this category are class-IV prescription items in the United States (*see* Appendix). A lucid account of trials of antianxiety agents in general practice, placebo responses, and straightforward scales for evaluation can be found in the publication of Wheatley (1973).

IV. Psychotoxic Drugs

The drugs discussed in this section can be divided into two categories. Many of them, although used for established therapeutic purposes, can produce pathological states that resemble the psychoses and other disorders of mental function. Presumably, they can provide some insight into the mechanism of mental disorders. Others are used or abused primarily for their psychotoxic effects. Terminology in this area is extremely difficult. The terms that will be used describe specific psychiatric syndromes that can be adequately characterized. The drugs, in general, may be divided into those that produce *psychosis*—the psychotogenic agents; those that produce a *mood change*—either depression or mania; and, finally, a heterogeneous group of compounds that may, in some individuals, produce *anxiety*. In each instance, the psychological syndrome produced by a prototype drug will be described as well as what is known of its mechanism of action. Treatment will also be considered. Further reference to some of the drugs in this class is made in Chapter 16.

PSYCHOTOGENIC DRUGS

All these drugs may, in low doses, produce euphoria, but in higher doses they inevitably produce psychological syndromes that can be characterized as psychoses. Such psychoses are distinguishable by their overt psychological characteristics and by their autonomic concomitants. The dose-effect curves vary considerably. Certain compounds, for example, marihuana, usually cause only mood changes, but in high doses they produce a psychosis. The response to others, such as LSD, rapidly changes from euphoria to psychosis as the dose is slightly increased. A few agents must be given in extremely high doses in order to produce a psychosis; deoxyethyltryptamine (DOET) is an example.

DRUGS THAT INDUCE DELIRIUM

This group of drugs is well known, and many are among the oldest therapeutic agents. Some drugs produce delirium while they are being administered and others only as a result of cessation of medication. Alcohol is the most familiar member of the latter group, but the occurrence of such delirium on withdrawal is characteristic of most CNS depressant drugs.

A prototype of the delirium-inducing drugs is *atropine*. The psychological effects of atropine and other anticholinergic agents have been described by Ketchum and co-workers (1973). Any drug with atropine-like effects, including the tricyclic antidepressants and the phenothiazines, can induce this syndrome. As the dose is increased above that necessary to elicit the expected peripheral autonomic effects, central disturbances such as euphoria, somnolence, restlessness, ataxia and incoordination, hyperreflexia, and hyperthermia supervene, followed by distorted awareness, loss of attentiveness, and inability to speak coherently or interpret stimuli realistically. As the psychosis develops, prominent symptoms are impairment in memory, particularly for recent events; disorientation as to time, place, and person; and disturbance in perception of time, as is characteristic of delirium. Visual hallucinations, enhanced by the paralysis of accommodation, frequently occur. *Treatment* of atropine-induced delirium with physostigmine is discussed in Chapter 25. Treatment of this syndrome with phenothiazine drugs is contraindicated.

DRUGS THAT INDUCE PARANOID PSYCHOSES

Although cocaine was the first drug reported to produce a paranoid psychosis (*see* Byck, 1974), the modern and most widely studied example is *amphetamine*. The psychosis produced by amphetamine and similar central stimulants has been shown to be dose related and reproducible (Angrist and Gershon, 1972; Snyder, 1972). Amphetamine has effects on both noradrenergic and dopaminergic systems and increases the turnover rates of norepinephrine and dopamine, as described more fully in Chapter 24. Conventional doses of dextroamphetamine produce CNS excitation and mild euphoria. However, as the acute oral dose is increased to about 100 mg, a psychosis characterized by extreme suspicion and fear of the environment ensues. Visual hallucinations and misperceptions may occur, but the subject is, for the most part, aware of his surroundings and able to respond to them, and he is usually oriented in time and space. This syndrome has been mistaken for paranoid schizophrenia. The differential diagnosis may be difficult, but it is aided by signs of peripheral sympathomimetic activity and particularly by a confirmed history or evidence of the use of drugs of the stimulant type. *Treatment* of psychoses such as that induced by amphetamine is effectively accomplished with antipsychotic drugs such as chlorpromazine and haloperidol.

DRUGS THAT INDUCE PSYCHEDELIC STATES

These drugs, among which *LSD* may be considered the prototype, have been widely used, abused, and reviewed. They are considered by some to provide a drug model of psychosis. They produce a different syndrome than the two described above, which has certain of the characteristics of the acute schizophrenic episode (*see* Bowers and Freedman, 1966). The alterations in consciousness, mood, and perception caused by LSD have been described as follows: "Psychotomimetic drugs such as [LSD] reliably and consistently produce periods of altered perception and experience without [a] clouded consciousness or marked physiological changes; mental processes that are usually dormant and transient during wakefulness become 'locked' into a persistent state. The usual boundaries which structure thought and perception become fluid; awareness becomes vivid while control over input is markedly diminished; customary inputs and modes of thought . . .

become novel, illusory and portentous; and with the loss of customary controlling anchors, dependence on the surroundings, on prior expectations [and fears], or on a mystique for structure and support is enhanced. Psychiatrists recognize these primary changes as a background state out of which a number of secondary psychological states can ensue, depending on motive, capacity and circumstance" (*see* Giarman and Freedman, 1965).

Hofmann's description of the LSD experience was as follows: ". . . my field of vision swayed before me, and objects appeared distorted like images in curved mirrors. I had the impression of being unable to move from the spot, although my assistant told me afterwards that we had cycled at a good pace. . . . As far as I remember, the following were the most outstanding symptoms: vertigo, visual disturbances; the faces of those around me appeared as grotesque, colored masks; . . . [I had] clear recognition of my condition, in which state I sometimes observed, in the manner of an independent, neutral observer, that I shouted half insanely or babbled incoherent words. Occasionally I felt as if I were out of my body. . . . When I closed my eyes, an unending series of colorful, very realistic and fantastic images surged in upon me. A remarkable feature was the manner in which all acoustic perceptions (*e.g.,* the noise of a passing car) were transformed into optical effects, every sound evoking a corresponding colored hallucination constantly changing in shape and color like pictures in a kaleidoscope. . . . I fell asleep and awoke next morning feeling perfectly well" (Hofmann, 1970).

The other pharmacological effects of LSD are largely sympathomimetic, such as mydriasis, increase in blood pressure, tachycardia, hyperreflexia, tremor, piloerection, muscular weakness, increased body temperature, and an elevation of free fatty acids in the blood. Somatic symptoms such as drowsiness, dizziness, nausea, and paresthesias also occur occasionally. LSD causes an antidiuretic effect and decreases the urinary clearance of creatinine.

Mechanism of Action of LSD. How LSD produces its effects is not fully known. There are two major views, which are not mutually exclusive. One, couched in physiological terms and first put forth by Bradley and Elkes (1953), holds that LSD increases the responsivity of the brain stem reticular formation to input from sensory collaterals, although it does not lower the threshold for direct stimulation. The other, framed in more pharmacological terms, holds that LSD exerts its effects through modifying the actions of 5-HT in the brain.

LSD is a potent antagonist of certain of the peripheral actions of 5-HT *in vitro,* and the concept that its psychological effects are due to blockade of 5-HT within the CNS was one of the earliest theories of its mechanism of action. (The possible role of 5-HT in CNS function is considered in Chapter 29.) It is now clear that no simple blockade theory will account for the effects of LSD and related drugs. The following observations support a role for 5-HT in the action of LSD and related drugs. Drugs in this class produce activation of the EEG and behavioral alerting only when connections between midbrain and medulla are intact. 5-HT in the brain is contained primarily within neurons whose cell bodies are located in the brain stem raphe nuclei. The effects of LSD at the brain stem level appear to be confined to these neurons, and when the drug is given parenterally it produces a *decrease* in the rate of firing of neurons in raphe nuclei. The work of Aghajanian and coworkers demonstrated that the 5-HT–containing neurons in the raphe nuclei are selectively and exquisitely sensitive to small parenteral doses of LSD. Although certain studies suggest that LSD may act on this neuronal system by blockade of 5-HT, the prevailing view is that, at doses that produce psychological effects, LSD mimics 5-HT at central synapses and that the decrease in the firing rate of raphe nuclei neurons and the decreased turnover rate of 5-HT seen after parenteral LSD are a result of a negative feedback within the affected neuronal system (*see* Aghajanian and Haigler, 1974; Haigler and Aghajanian, 1974). Studies showing that the neurons in the raphe are excited by iontophoretically applied 5-HT, an effect blocked by LSD, and that low doses of LSD administered chronically to rats produce an increase in 5-HT turnover rate, indicate that our understanding of this drug is far from adequate.

Absorption, Fate, and Excretion of LSD. After oral administration, LSD is rapidly absorbed and distributed throughout the body. Although the highest concentrations are found in lung, liver, kidney, and brain, actually only a small percentage of an administered dose reaches the brain. The drug is metabolized to 2-oxy-LSD by enzymes in hepatic microsomes. LSD is excreted largely in the feces. The half-life is 7 minutes in the mouse, 100 minutes in the monkey, and approximately 175 minutes in man, following an intravenous dose.

Miscellaneous Psychedelic Drugs. *Mescaline* is another drug that produces a psychedelic state. It shares this property with a large number of other substances, including many *substituted phenethylamines.* The relationship of these drugs to the development of the concept of the biochemical basis of mental illness has been discussed previously. This subject has been reviewed by Efron (1970), Brawley and Duffield (1972), and Snyder and associates (1974).

The effects of *marihuana* are described elsewhere (*see* Chapter 16). Although the full syndrome of marihuana intoxication resembles that of the psychedelics, it is often classified separately because of its usage pattern. The mode of action of Δ^9-tetrahydrocannabinol (Δ^9-THC), one of the major active psychedelic ingredients in marihuana, is not known. Byck and Ritchie (1973) have suggested that its action may be on nerve fiber tracts, rather than on synaptic transmission as may be the case with other psychedelic drugs. Although Δ^9-THC is a β-adrenergic agonist and its peripheral effects are blocked by propranolol, the psychic effects are not. In man, increase in pulse rate and conjunctival injection are regular effects of Δ^9-THC. Effects on pupil size, blood pressure, and respiratory rate are variable. α-Methyl-p-tyrosine, an inhibitor of tyrosine hydroxylase, also does not modify the psychological effect of Δ^9-THC in man.

Studies with radioactive Δ^9-THC given intravenously (Lemberger et al., 1971) have demonstrated that the drug is rapidly metabolized, partially to the psychoactive 11-OH-Δ^9-tetrahydrocannabinol, and that its disappearance from blood is biphasic. There is a rapid disappearance in the first hour and then a prolonged (3 days or more) excretion of the rest of the drug and its metabolites.

Other drugs known to produce psychedelic states, but with less constancy, are cyclazocine, pentazocine, ethosuximide, phenytoin, and a wide variety of natural substances of which psilocybin is the prototype. (For more extensive discussion, see Lewin, 1931; Holmstedt, 1967; Efron, 1970.) Psychoses produced by anticonvulsants may be either true drug effects or an unmasking of a suppressed psychotic process.

Treatment of Psychedelic Drug Intoxication. When a diagnosis can be made, treatment of the psychedelic drug intoxication should be conservative. The presence of familiar persons and "talking down" the patient are appropriate for these time-limited reactions. Sedative barbiturates and diazepam given parenterally are reported to be helpful. Continued observation and periodic reevaluation of the diagnosis are important. Intramuscular doses of antipsychotic drugs are rarely needed and are of questionable value. However, if psychosis persists beyond the expected duration of drug action, antipsychotic medication is indicated.

DRUGS THAT INDUCE AFFECTIVE DISORDERS

Both depression and mania can be induced by drugs, but these effects are not as constant as the psychotogenic effects discussed above. Although reserpine has always been the prototype of a depression-producing drug, the effect is inconstant. There is some evidence that reserpine-induced depressions occur with greater frequency in patients with a previous history of affective disorder (Goodwin et al., 1972). Levodopa, propranolol, methyldopa, and various steroids have been associated with depressive syndromes in some patients (Medical Letter, 1972). The possible depression-inducing properties of digitalis are reviewed by Greenblatt and Shader (1972). The depression produced by the above-mentioned drugs is indistinguishable from the naturally occurring disease, but it can usually be diagnosed by a history of drug ingestion. Depression that occurs after the use of the antipsychotic agents (fluphenazine and haloperidol are frequently cited) is probably either an unmasking process or part of the natural resolution of the psychosis. Treatment with tricyclic antidepressants is usually effective despite continuation of the antipsychotic drug.

The treatment of drug-induced depression simply involves removal of the offending substance if circumstances permit. Recovery may, nonetheless, take weeks to occur. As indicated above, tricyclic antidepressant therapy is occasionally required.

Mania and hypomanic responses have been reported after the use of levodopa and various corticosteroids. The steroids are of particular interest because they can produce almost any form of psychiatric disorder. However, a hypomanic state extending to true mania is a common and predictable dose-related effect of the steroids. One of the most compelling descriptions of mania induced by a corticosteroid was presented by Roueché (1957). The patient described it thusly: "I hadn't felt so good in years. I don't mean just physically. It was more than that. I felt bright as a button—capable of anything. It was really extraordinary. It was almost as though I'd never been fully awake before. . . . My mind was like some wonderful precision instrument. Everything I did was right, and absolutely effortless." The patient's wife saw his behavior as follows: "Everything he said was a joke. He was absolutely bursting with high spirits. . . . exaltation had become his natural state. Every impulse seemed to quicken it. . . . Only he talked so fast he was almost incoherent." The mania disappeared after cessation of the steroid therapy.

DRUGS THAT INDUCE ANXIETY REACTIONS

Drug-induced anxiety reactions are both common and difficult to document. The attribution of increased anxiety to the effect of a drug depends on a strict time congruence of drug administration and onset of anxiety, paralleled by relief of the anxiety when the drug is discontinued. Almost all of the sympathomimetic amines can produce an autonomic state that is perceived as anxiety. This effect can feed back on itself and cause panic reactions.

Drugs that restrict either consciousness or movement may in themselves cause increased anxiety. This may occur with the sedative-antianxiety agents, the antipsychotic drugs, and the antidepressants. Antihistamines occasionally produce nervousness or anxiety that appears to be an idiosyncratic drug response. The major characteristic of drug-induced anxiety reactions is their apparent inexplicable nature. The patient does not perceive anything that would make him nervous, but nonetheless the symptoms persist. Acute anxiety reactions in normal persons who feel that the anxiety state is unjustified should always cause the physician to suspect drug-induced anxiety. Treatment—drug withdrawal—is, as mentioned, crucial to the diagnosis.

Alexander, C. S., and Nino, A. Cardiovascular complications in young patients taking psychotropic drugs. Am. Heart J., **1969**, 78, 757–769.

Alexanderson, B., and Sjöqvist, F. Individual differences in the pharmacokinetics of monomethylated tricyclic antidepressants: role of genetic and environmental factors and clinical importance. Ann. N.Y. Acad. Sci., **1971**, 179, 739–751.

American College of Neuropsychopharmacology Task Force. Drug therapy: neurological syndromes associated with antipsychotic-drug use. *New Engl. J. Med.,* **1973,** *289,* 20–23.

Anden, N.-E. Dopamine turnover in the corpus striatum and the limbic system after treatment with neuroleptic and antiacetylcholine drugs. *J. Pharm. Pharmac.,* **1972,** *24,* 905–906.

Anden, N.-E., and Stock, G. Effect of clozapine on the turnover of dopamine in the corpus striatum and in the limbic system. *J. Pharm. Pharmac.,* **1973,** *25,* 346–348.

Åsberg, M.; Crönholm, B.; Sjöqvist, F.; and Tuck, D. Relationship between plasma level and therapeutic effect of nortriptyline. *Br. med. J.,* **1971,** *3,* 331–334.

Ayd, F. J., Jr. A critical appraisal of chlordiazepoxide. *J. Neuropsychiat.,* **1962,** *3,* 177–180.

Berger, F. M. The pharmacological properties of 2-methyl-2-*n*-propyl-1,3-propanediol dicarbamate (MIL-TOWN), a new interneuronal blocking agent. *J. Pharmac. exp. Ther.,* **1954,** *112,* 413–423.

Berlin, A.; Siwers, B.; Agurell, S.; Hiort, A.; Sjöqvist, F.; and Strom, S. Determination of bioavailability of diazepam in various formulations from steady state plasma concentration data. *Clin. Pharmac. Ther.,* **1972,** *13,* 733–744.

Blum, A., and Girke, W. Marked increase in REM sleep produced by a new antipsychotic compound. *Clin. Electroenceph.,* **1973,** *4,* 80–84.

Bowers, M. B., Jr., and Freedman, D. X. "Psychedelic" experiences in acute psychoses. *Archs gen. Psychiat.,* **1966,** *15,* 240–248.

Bradley, P. B., and Elkes, J. The effect of amphetamine and *d*-lysergic acid diethylamide (LSD-25) on the electrical activity of the brain of the conscious cat. *J. Physiol., Lond.,* **1953,** *120,* 13–15.

Bulla, J. D.; Ewing, J. A.; and Buffaloe, W. J. Further controlled studies of meprobamate. *Am. Practnr Dig. Treat.,* **1959,** *10,* 1961–1964.

Bunney, B. S.; Walters, J. R.; Roth, R. H.; and Aghajanian, G. K. Dopaminergic neurons: effect of antipsychotic drugs and amphetamine on single cell activity. *J. Pharmac. exp. Ther.,* **1973,** *185,* 560–571.

Bunney, W. E., Jr., and Davis, J. M. Norepinephrine in depressive reactions. *Archs gen. Psychiat.,* **1965,** *13,* 483–494.

Burks, J. S.; Walker, J. E.; Rumack, B. H.; and Ott, J. E. Tricyclic antidepressant poisoning. Reversal of coma, choreoathetosis, and myoclonus by physostigmine. *J. Am. med. Ass.,* **1974,** *230,* 1405–1407.

Byck, R., and Ritchie, J. M. Δ⁹ Tetrahydrocannabinol effects on mammalian nonmyelinated nerve fibers. *Science, Wash.,* **1973,** *180,* 84–85.

Cade, J. F. J. Lithium salts in the treatment of psychotic excitement. *Med. J. Aust.,* **1949,** *2,* 349–352.

Carpenter, W. T., Jr.; Strauss, J. S.; and Bartko, J. J. Flexible system for the diagnosis of schizophrenia: report from the WHO international pilot study of schizophrenia. *Science, Wash.,* **1973,** *182,* 1275–1277.

Christiansen, E.; Møller, J. E.; and Eaurbye, A. Neuropathological investigation of 28 brains from patients with dyskinesia. *Acta psychiat. neurol. scand.,* **1970,** *46,* 14–23.

Christie, J. E., and Crow, T. J. Turning behaviour as an index of the action of amphetamines and ephedrines on central dopamine-containing neurones. *Br. J. Pharmac.,* **1971,** *43,* 658–667.

Clark, M. L.; Ray, T. S.; Paredes, A.; Ragland, R. E.; Costilee, J. P.; Smith, C. W.; and Wolf, S. Chlorpromazine in women with chronic schizophrenia: the effect on cholesterol levels and cholesterol-behavior relationships. *Psychosom. Med.,* **1967,** *29,* 634–642.

Clement-Cormier, Y. C.; Kebabian, J. W.; Petzold, G. L.; and Greengard, P. Dopamine-sensitive adenylate cyclase in mammalian brain: a possible site of action of antipsychotic drugs. *Proc. natn. Acad. Sci. U.S.A.,* **1974,** *71,* 1113–1117.

Cook, L., and Davidson, A. B. Effects of behaviorally active drugs in a conflict-punishment procedure in rats. In, *The Benzodiazepines.* (Garattini, S.; Mussini, E.; and Randall, L. O.; eds.) Raven Press, New York, **1973,** pp. 327–346.

Cook, L., and Weidley, E. Behavioral effects of some psychopharmacological agents. *Ann. N.Y. Acad. Sci.,* **1957,** *66,* 740–752.

Courvoisier, S.; Fournel, J.; Ducrot, R.; Kolsky, M.; and Koetschet, P. Propiérties pharmacodynamiques du chlorhydrate de chloro-3(dimethylamino-3′propyl)-10 phenothiazine (4560 RP). *Archs int. Pharmacodyn. Thér.,* **1953,** *92,* 305–361.

Delay, J., and Deniker, P. Trente-huit cas de psychoses traitées par la cure prolongée et continue de 4560 RP. Le Congrès des Al. et Neurol. de Langue Fr. In, *Compte rendu du Congrès.* Masson et Cie, Paris, **1952.**

DeMaio, D. Clozapine, a novel major tranquilizer. *Arzneimittel-Forsch.,* **1972,** *22,* 919–923.

DiMascio, A.; Heninger, G.; and Klerman, G. L. Psychopharmacology of imipramine and desipramine: a comparative study of their effects in normal males. *Psychopharmacologia,* **1964,** *5,* 361–371.

Dobkin, A. B.; Gilbert, R. G. B.; and Lamoureu, L. Physiological effects of chlorpromazine. *Anaesthesia,* **1954,** *9,* 157–174.

Domino, E. F. Human pharmacology of tranquilizing drugs. *Clin. Pharmac. Ther.,* **1962,** *3,* 599–664.

Engle, H. A. The effect of diazepam (VALIUM) in children with cerebral palsy; a double blind study. *Devl Med. Child Neurol.,* **1966,** *8,* 661–667.

Forfar, J. O., and Nelson, M. M. Epidemiology of drugs taken by pregnant women: drugs that may affect the fetus adversely. *Clin. Pharmac. Ther.,* **1973,** *14,* Part 2, 632–642.

Garelis, E., and Neff, N. H. Cyclic adenosine monophosphate; selective increase in caudate nucleus after administration of L-dopa. *Science, Wash.,* **1974,** *183,* 532–533.

Glassman, A.; Hurwic, M. J.; Kanzler, M.; Shostak, M.; and Perel, J. M. Imipramine steady-state studies and plasma binding. In, *Proceedings of the Third International Symposium on Phenothiazines and Structurally Related Compounds.* Raven Press, New York, **1974,** pp. 457–463.

Glowinski, J.; Hamon, M.; Javoy, F.; and Morot Gaudry, Y. Rapid effects of monoamine oxidase inhibitors on synthesis and release of central monoamines. In, *Monoamine Oxidases—New Vistas. Advances in Biochemical Psychopharmacology,* Vol. 5. (Costa, E., and Sandler, M., eds.) Raven Press, New York, **1972,** pp. 423–440.

Gottschalk, L. A.; Noble, E. P.; Stolzoff, G. E.; Bates, D. E.; Cable, C. G.; Uliana, R. L.; Birch, H.; and Fleming, E. W. Relationships of chlordiazepoxide blood levels to psychological and biochemical responses. In, *The Benzodiazepines.* (Garattini, S.; Mussini, E.; and Randall, L. O.; eds.) Raven Press, New York, **1973,** pp. 257–280.

Grinspoon, L.; Ewalt, J. R.; and Shader, R. Psychotherapy and pharmacotherapy in chronic schizophrenia. *Am. J. Psychiat.,* **1968,** *124,* 1645–1652.

Grunthal, E. Untersuchungen über die besondere psychologische Wirkung des Thymolepticums TOFRANIL. *Psychiat.-neurol. Wschr.,* **1958,** *136,* 402–408.

Haigler, H. J., and Aghajanian, G. K. Lysergic acid diethylamide and serotonin: a comparison of effects on serotonergic neurons and neurons receiving a serotonergic input. *J. Pharmac. exp. Ther.,* **1974,** *88,* 688–699.

Harrow, M.; Himmelhoch, J.; Tucker, G.; Hersh, J.; and Quinlan, D. Over-inclusive thinking in acute schizophrenic patients. *J. abnorm. soc. Psychol.,* **1972,** *79,* 161–168.

Himmelhoch, J. M.; Detre, T.; Kupfer, D. J.; Swartzburg, M.; and Byck, R. Treatment of previously intractable depressions with tranylcypromine and lithium. *J. nerv. ment. Dis.,* **1972,** *155,* 216–220.

Hirsch, S. R.; Gaind, R.; Rohde, P. D.; Stevens, B. C.; and Wing, J. K. Outpatient maintenance of chronic schizophrenic patients with long-acting fluphenazine: double-blind placebo trial. *Br. med. J.*, **1973**, *1*, 633–637.

Hofmann, A. The discovery of LSD and subsequent investigations on naturally occurring hallucinogens. In, *Discoveries in Biological Psychiatry.* (Ayd, F. J., Jr., and Blackwell, B., eds.) J. B. Lippincott Co., Philadelphia, **1970**, pp. 93–94.

Horn, A. S., and Snyder, S. H. Chlorpromazine and dopamine: conformational similarities that correlate with the antischizophrenic activity of phenothiazine drugs. *Proc. natn. Acad. Sci. U.S.A.*, **1971**, *68*, 2325–2328.

Huang, C. L., and Kurland, A. A. A quantitative study of chlorpromazine and its sulfoxides in the urine of psychotic patients. *Am. J. Psychiat.*, **1961**, *118*, 428–437.

Jacobsen, E. The theoretical basis of the chemotherapy of depression. In, *Depression: Proceedings of the Symposium Held at Cambridge, 22–26 Sept. 1959.* (Davies, E. B., ed.) Cambridge University Press, London, **1964**, pp. 208–213.

Johnson, G.; Gershon, S.; Burdock, E. I.; Floyd, A.; and Hekimian, L. Comparative effects of lithium and chlorpromazine in the treatment of acute manic states. *Br. J. Psychiat.*, **1971**, *119*, 267–276.

Judd, L. L.; Goldstein, M. J.; Rodnick, E. H.; and Jackson, N. L. P. Phenothiazine effects in good premorbid schizophrenics divided into paranoid-nonparanoid status. *Archs gen. Psychiat.*, **1973**, *29*, 207–211.

Kales, A., and Scharf, M. B. Sleep laboratory and clinical studies of the effects of benzodiazepines on sleep. In, *The Benzodiazepines.* (Garattini, S.; Mussini, E.; and Randall, L. O.; eds.) Raven Press, New York, **1973**, pp. 577–598.

Kebabian, J. W.; Petzold, G. L.; and Greengard, P. Dopamine-sensitive adenylate cyclase in caudate nucleus of rat brain, and its similarity to the "dopamine receptor." *Proc. natn. Acad. Sci. U.S.A.*, **1972**, *69*, 2145–2149.

Ketchum, J. S.; Sidell, F. R.; Crowell, E. B., Jr.; Aghajanian, G. K.; and Hayes, A. H., Jr. Atropine, scopolamine, and ditran: comparative pharmacology and antagonists in man. *Psychopharmacologia*, **1973**, *28*, 121–145.

Kiloh, L. G., and Garside, R. F. The independence of neurotic depression and endogenous depression. *Br. J. Psychiat.*, **1963**, *109*, 451–463.

Klein, D. F. Importance of psychiatric diagnosis in prediction of clinical drug effects. *Archs gen. Psychiat.*, **1967**, *16*, 118–126.

Klein, D. F., and Rosen, B. Premorbid asocial adjustment and response to phenothiazine treatment among schizophrenic inpatients. *Archs gen. Psychiat.*, **1973**, *29*, 480–485.

Kolodny, H. D.; Sherman, L.; Singh, A.; Kim, S.; and Benjamin, F. Acromegaly treated with chlorpromazine. *New Engl. J. Med.*, **1971**, *284*, 819–822.

Kopelman, A. E.; McCullar, F. W.; and Heggeness, L. Limb malformations following maternal use of haloperidol. *J. Am. med. Ass.*, **1975**, *231*, 62–64.

Kornetsky, C. Effects of meprobamate, phenobarbital and dextroamphetamine on reaction time and learning in man. *J. Pharmac. exp. Ther.*, **1958**, *123*, 216–219.

Kuhn, R. The treatment of depressive states with G22355 (imipramine hydrochloride). *Am. J. Psychiat.*, **1958**, *115*, 459–464.

Laborit, H.; Huguenard, P.; and Alluaume, R. Un nouveau stabilisateur vegetatif, le 4560 RP. *Presse méd.*, **1952**, *60*, 206–208.

Lehmann, H. E.; Cahn, C. H.; and de Vertouil, R. L. The treatment of depressive conditions with imipramine (G22355). *Can. psychiat. Ass. J.*, **1958**, *3*, 155–164.

Lehmann, H. E., and Hanrahan, G. E. Chlorpromazine, a new inhibiting agent for psychomotor excitement and manic states. *A.M.A. Archs Neurol. Psychiatry*, **1954**, *71*, 227–257.

Lemberger, L.; Axelrod, J.; and Kopin, I. J. Metabolism and disposition of Δ^9-tetrahydrocannabinol in man. *Pharmac. Rev.*, **1971**, *23*, 371–380.

Levine, R. J., and Sjoerdsma, A. Estimation of monoamine oxidase activity in man: techniques and applications. *Ann. N.Y. Acad. Sci.*, **1963**, *107*, 966–974.

Medical Letter. Drugs that cause depression. **1972**, *14*, 35–36.

———. Diazepam as a muscle relaxant. **1973**, *15*, 57–58.

———. Imipramine for enuresis. **1974**, *16*, 22–24.

Moir, D. C.; Cornwell, W. B.; Dingwall-Fordyce, I.; Crooks, J.; O'Malley, K.; Turnbull, M. J.; and Weir, R. D. Cardiotoxicity of amitriptyline. *Lancet*, **1972**, *2*, 561–564.

Overall, J. E., and Henry, B. W. Decisions about drug therapy. III. Selection of treatment for psychiatric inpatients. *Archs gen. Psychiat.*, **1973**, *28*, 81–89.

Overall, J. E.; Hollister, L. E.; Meyer, F.; Kimball, I.; and Shelton, J. Imipramine and thioridazine in depressed and schizophrenic patients. *J. Am. med. Ass.*, **1964**, *189*, 93–96.

Platman, S. F., and Fieve, R. R. Lithium retention and excretion. *Archs gen. Psychiat.*, **1969**, *20*, 285–289.

Prien, R. F.; Caffey, E. M.; and Klett, C. J. Relationship between serum lithium level and clinical response in acute mania treated with lithium. *Br. J. Psychiat.*, **1972**, *120*, 409–414.

Prien, R. F.; DeLong, S. L.; Cole, J. O.; and Levine, J. Ocular changes occurring with prolonged high dose chlorpromazine therapy. *Archs gen. Psychiat.*, **1970**, *23*, 464–468.

Prien, R. F., and Klett, C. J. An appraisal of the long-term use of tranquilizing medication with hospitalized schizophrenics: a review of the literature. *Schizophrenia Bull.*, **1972**, *5*, 64–73.

Prien, R. F.; Klett, C. J.; and Caffey, E. M. Lithium carbonate and imipramine in prevention of affective episodes. *Archs gen. Psychiat.*, **1972**, *29*, 420–425.

Przybyla, A. C., and Wang, S. C. Locus of central depressant action of diazepam. *J. Pharmac. exp. Ther.*, **1968**, *163*, 439–447.

Raisfeld, I. H. Cardiovascular complications of antidepressant therapy. *Am. Heart J.*, **1972**, *83*, 129–133.

Randall, L. O.; Schallek, W.; Heise, G. A.; Keith, E. F.; and Bagdon, R. E. The psychosedative properties of methaminodiazepoxide. *J. Pharmac. exp. Ther.*, **1960**, *129*, 163–171.

Rao, S.; Sherbaniuk, R. W.; Prasad, K.; Lee, S. J. K.; and Sproule, B. J. Cardiopulmonary effects of diazepam. *Clin. Pharmac. Ther.*, **1973**, *14*, 182–189.

Rickels, K.; Gordon, P.; Weise, C. C.; Bazilian, S. E.; Feldman, H. S.; and Wilson, D. A. Amitriptyline and trimipramine in neurotic depressed outpatients: a collaborative study. *Am. J. Psychiat.*, **1970**, *127*, 208–218.

Rivera-Calimlim, L.; Castaneda, L.; and Lasagna, L. Effects of mode of management on plasma chlorpromazine in psychiatric patients. *Clin. Pharmac. Ther.*, **1973**, *14*, 978–986.

Roueché, B. Ten feet tall. In, *The Incurable Wound.* Little, Brown & Co., Boston, **1957**; Berkley Publishing Corp., New York, **1958**, pp. 121 *et seq.*

Safer, D.; Allen, R.; and Barr, E. Depression of growth in hyperactive children on stimulant drugs. *New Engl. J. Med.*, **1972**, *287*, 217–220.

Sakalis, G.; Curry, S. H.; Mould, G. P.; and Lader, M. H. Physiologic and clinical effects of chlorpromazine and their relationship to plasma level. *Clin. Pharmac. Ther.*, **1972**, *13*, 931–946.

Sen, G., and Bose, K. C. *Rauwolfia serpentina*, a new Indian drug for insanity and high blood pressure. *Indian med. Wld*, **1931**, *2*, 194–201.

Shapiro, A. K., and Shapiro, E. Treatment of Gilles de la Tourette's syndrome with haloperidol. *Br. J. Psychiat.*, **1968**, *114*, 345–350.

Shatan, C. Withdrawal symptoms after abrupt termination of imipramine. *Can. psychiat. Ass. J.*, **1966**, *2*, 150–157.

Shopsin, B.; Hekimian, L. J.; Gershon, S.; and Floyd, A. A controlled evaluation of haloperidol, chlorpromazine, and sodium amobarbital: intramuscular short-term use in acute psychotic patients. *Curr. ther. Res.,* **1969,** *11,* 561–573.

Slovis, T. L.; Ott, J. E.; Teitelbaum, D. T.; and Lipscomb, W. Physostigmine therapy in acute tricyclic antidepressant poisoning. *Clin. Toxicol.,* **1971,** *4,* 451–459.

Snyder, B. D.; Blonde, L.; and McWhirter, W. R. Reversal of amitriptyline intoxication by physostigmine. *J. Am. med. Ass.,* **1974,** *230,* 1433–1434.

Snyder, S. H. Catecholamines in brain as mediators of amphetamine psychosis. *Archs gen. Psychiat.,* **1972,** *27,* 169–179.

Wittenborn, J. R.; Plante, M.; Burgess, F.; and Maurer, H. A comparison of imipramine, electroconvulsive therapy and placebo in the treatment of depressions. *J. nerv. ment. Dis.,* **1962,** *135,* 131–137.

Wyatt, R. J.; Fram, D. H.; Buchbinder, R.; and Snyder, F. Treatment of intractable narcolepsy with a monoamine oxidase inhibitor. *New Engl. J. Med.,* **1971,** *285,* 987–991.

Zelickson, A. S., and Zeller, H. C. A new and unusual reaction to chlorpromazine. *J. Am. med. Ass.,* **1964,** *188,* 394–396.

Zeller, E. A.; Barsky, J.; Fouts, J. R.; Kirchheimer, W. F.; and Van Orden, L. S. Influence of isonicotinic acid hydrazide (INH) and 1-isonicotinyl-2-isopropyl hydrazide (IIH) on bacterial and mammalian enzymes. *Experientia,* **1952,** *8,* 349–350.

Monographs and Reviews

Aghajanian, G. K., and Haigler, H. J. Mode of action of LSD on serotonergic neurons. In, *Serotonin—New Vistas. Advances in Biochemical Psychopharmacology,* Vol. 10. (Costa, E.; Gessa, G. L.; and Sandler, M.; eds.) Raven Press, New York, **1974,** pp. 167–177.

American Psychiatric Association. *Diagnostic and Statistical Manual of Mental Disorders: II.* The Association, Washington, D. C., **1968.**

———. Special section: drug treatment of affective disorders. *Am. J. Psychiat.,* **1974,** *131,* 181–205.

Angrist, B. M., and Gershon, S. Psychiatric sequelae of amphetamine use. In, *Psychiatric Complications of Medical Drugs.* (Shader, R. I., ed.) Raven Press, New York, **1972,** pp. 175–199.

Axelrod, J. Noradrenaline: fate and control of its biosynthesis. *Science, Wash.,* **1971,** *173,* 598–606.

Axelrod, J., and Weinshilboum, R. Catecholamines. *New Engl. J. Med.,* **1972,** *287,* 237–242.

Ayd, F. J., Jr., and Blackwell, B. (eds.). *Discoveries in Biological Psychiatry.* J. B. Lippincott Co., Philadelphia, **1970.**

Bleuler, E. *Dementia Praecox or the Group of Schizophrenias.* (Zinkin, J., trans.) International Universities Press, New York, **1950.**

Brawley, P., and Duffield, J. C. The pharmacology of hallucinogens. *Pharmac. Rev.,* **1972,** *24,* 31–66.

Byck, R. (ed.). *Cocaine Papers: Sigmund Freud.* Stonehill Publishing Co., New York, **1974.**

Clark, W. G., and del Guidice, J. (eds.). *Principles of Psychopharmacology.* Academic Press, Inc., New York, **1970.**

Cole, J. O.; Freedman, A. M.; and Friedhoff, A. J. (eds.). *Psychopathology and Psychopharmacology.* Johns Hopkins University Press, Baltimore, **1973.**

Conney, A. H. Pharmacological implications of microsomal enzyme induction. *Pharmac. Rev.,* **1967,** *19,* 317–366.

Cook, L., and Kelleher, R. T. Effects of drugs on behavior. *A. Rev. Pharmac.,* **1963,** *3,* 205–222.

Costa, E., and Sandler, M. (eds.). *Monoamine Oxidases—New Vistas. Advances in Biochemical Psychopharmacology,* Vol. 5. Raven Press, New York, **1972.**

Crane, G. E. Clinical psychopharmacology in its 20th year. *Science, Wash.,* **1973,** *181,* 124–128.

Davis, J. M. The efficacy of the tranquilizing and antidepressant drugs. *Archs gen. Psychiat.,* **1965,** *13,* 552–572.

———. Theories of biological etiology of affective disorders. *Int. Rev. Neurobiol.,* **1970,** *12,* 145–175.

Davis, J. M., and Fann, W. E. Lithium. *A. Rev. Pharmac.,* **1971,** *11,* 285–302.

De La Cruz, F. F.; Fox, B. H.; and Roberts, R. H. (eds.). Minimal brain dysfunction. *Ann. N.Y. Acad. Sci.,* **1973,** *205,* 1–396.

Detre, T. P., and Jarecki, H. G. *Modern Psychiatric Treatment.* J. B. Lippincott Co., Philadelphia, **1971.**

DiMascio, A. The effects of benzodiazepines on aggression: reduced or increased? In, *The Benzodiazepines.* (Garattini, S.; Mussini, E.; and Randall, L. O.; eds.) Raven Press, New York, **1973,** pp. 433–440.

Efron, D. H. *Psychotomimetic Drugs.* Raven Press, New York, **1970.**

Feighner, J. P.; Robins, E.; Guze, S. B.; Woodruff, R. A., Jr.; Winokur, G.; and Munoz, R. Diagnostic criteria for use in psychiatric research. *Archs gen. Psychiat.,* **1972,** *26,* 57–63.

Feinsilver, D., and Gunderson, J. Psychotherapy for schizophrenics—is it indicated? A review of the relevant literature. *Schizophrenia Bull.,* **1972,** *6,* 11–23.

Fink, M. EEG and human psychopharmacology. *A. Rev. Pharmac.,* **1969,** *9,* 241–258.

Forrest, I. S.; Carr, C. J.; and Usdin, E. (eds.). *Phenothiazines and Structurally Related Drugs. Advances in Biochemical Psychopharmacology,* Vol. 9. Raven Press, New York, **1974.**

Frohman, L. A. Clinical neuropharmacology of hypothalamic releasing factors. *New Engl. J. Med.,* **1972,** *286,* 1391–1398.

Galbrecht, C. R., and Klett, C. J. Predicting response to phenothiazines: the right drug for the right patient. *J. nerv. ment. Dis.,* **1968,** *147,* 173–183.

Garattini, S.; Mussini, E.; and Randall, L. O. (eds.). *The Benzodiazepines.* Raven Press, New York, **1973.**

Giarman, N. J., and Freedman, D. X. Biochemical aspects of the actions of psychotomimetic drugs. *Pharmac. Rev.,* **1965,** *17,* 1–25.

Glassman, A. H., and Perel, J. M. The clinical pharmacology of imipramine. *Archs gen. Psychiat.,* **1973,** *28,* 649–653.

Glowinski, J., and Axelrod, J. Effects of drugs on the disposition of H^3-norepinephrine in the rat brain. *Pharmac. Rev.,* **1966,** *18,* 775–785.

Goodwin, F. K.; Ebert, M. H.; and Bunney, W. E., Jr. Mental effects of reserpine in man: a review. In, *Psychiatric Complications of Medical Drugs.* (Shader, R. I., ed.) Raven Press, New York, **1972,** pp. 73–101.

Gordon, M. (ed.). *Psychopharmacological Agents,* Vol. II. Academic Press, Inc., New York, **1967.**

Greenblatt, D. J., and Shader, R. I. Digitalis toxicity. In, *Psychiatric Complications of Medical Drugs.* (Shader, R. I., ed.) Raven Press, New York, **1972,** 25–47.

———. *Benzodiazepines in Clinical Practice.* Raven Press, New York, **1974.**

Hingtgen, J. N., and Bryson, C. Q. Recent developments in the study of early childhood psychoses: infantile autism, childhood schizophrenia, and related disorders. *Schizophrenia Bull.,* **1972,** *5,* 8–53.

Hollister, L. E.; Caffey, E. M., Jr.; and Klett, C. J. Abnormal symptoms, signs and laboratory tests during treatment with phenothiazine derivatives. *Clin. Pharmac. Ther.,* **1960,** *1,* 284–293.

Holmstedt, B. Historical survey. In, *Ethnopharmacologic Search for Psychoactive Drugs.* (Efron, D. H.; Holmstedt, B.; and Kline, N. S.; eds.) Public Health Service Publication No. 1645, U.S. Government Printing Office, Washington, D. C., **1967,** pp. 3–32.

Kaim, S. C. Benzodiazepines in the treatment of alcohol withdrawal states. In, *The Benzodiazepines.* (Garattini, S.; Mussini, E.; and Randall, L. O.; eds.) Raven Press, New York, **1973,** pp. 571–575.

Kallmann, F. J. *Heredity in Health and Mental Disorder: Principles of Psychiatric Genetics in the Light of Compar-*

ative Twin Studies. W. W. Norton & Co., Inc., New York, **1953.**

Kety, S. S. Biochemical theories of schizophrenia. *Science, Wash.,* **1959,** *29,* 1528–1532, 1590–1596.

——. Toward hypotheses for a biochemical component in the vulnerability to schizophrenia. *Semin. Psychiat.,* **1972,** *4,* 233–238.

Kety, S. S., and Matthysse, S. (eds.). Prospects for research on schizophrenia: a report based on an NRP work session. *Neurosci. Res. Prog. Bull.,* **1972,** *10,* 370–507.

Killam, K. F., and Killam, E. K. Drug action on pathways involving the reticular formation. In, *Reticular Formation of the Brain.* (Jasper, H. H.; Proctor, L. D.; Knighton, S. S.; Noshay, W. C.; and Costell, R. T.; eds.) Little, Brown & Co., Boston, **1958,** pp. 111–222.

Klein, D. F., and Davis, J. M. *Diagnosis and Drug Treatment of Psychiatric Disorders.* The Williams & Wilkins Co., Baltimore, **1969.**

Klerman, G. L., and Cole, J. O. Clinical pharmacology of imipramine and related antidepressant compounds. *Pharmac. Rev.,* **1965,** *17,* 101–141.

Levine, J.; Schiele, B. C.; and Bouthilet, L. (eds.). *Principles and Problems in Establishing the Efficacy of Psychotropic Agents.* Public Health Service Publication No. 2138, U.S. Government Printing Office, Washington, D. C., **1971.**

Lewin, L. *Phantastica, Narcotic and Stimulating Drugs; Their Use and Abuse.* Berlin, **1924;** English translation, London, **1931;** E. P. Dutton & Co., New York, **1931.**

Ludwig, B. J., and Potterfield, J. R. The pharmacology of propanediol carbamates. *Adv. Pharmac. Chemother.,* **1971,** *9,* 173–240.

McNair, D. M. Antianxiety drugs and human performance. *Archs gen. Psychiat.,* **1973,** *29,* 611–617.

Marley, E., and Blackwell, B. Interactions of monoamine oxidase inhibitors, amines, and foodstuffs. *Adv. Pharmac. Chemother.,* **1970,** *8,* 185–239.

Martin, J. B. Neural regulation of growth hormone secretion. *New Engl. J. Med.,* **1973,** *288,* 1384–1393.

Matthysse, S. Antipsychotic drug actions: a clue to the neuropathology of schizophrenia? *Fedn Proc. Fedn Am. Socs exp. Biol.,* **1973,** *32,* 200–205.

May, P. R. A. *Treatment of Schizophrenia: A Comparative Study of Five Treatment Methods.* Science House, Inc., New York, **1968.**

Mendels, J., and Frazer, A. Intracellular lithium concentration and clinical response: towards a membrane theory of depression. *J. psychiat. Res.,* **1973,** *10,* 9–18.

National Institute of Mental Health, Psychopharmacology Service Center Collaborative Study Group. Phenothiazine treatment in acute schizophrenia. *Archs gen. Psychiat.,* **1964,** *10,* 246–261.

Noble, J., and Matthew, H. Acute poisoning by tricyclic antidepressants: clinical features and management of 100 patients. *Clin. Toxicol.,* **1969,** *2,* 403–421.

Prien, R. F. Chemotherapy in chronic organic brain syndrome—a review of the literature. *Psychopharmac. Bull.,* **1973,** *9,* 5–20.

Randall, L. O., and Kappell, B. Pharmacological activity of some benzodiazepines and their metabolites. In, *The Benzodiazepines.* (Garattini, S.; Mussini, E.; and Randall, L. O.; eds.) Raven Press, New York, **1973,** pp. 27–51.

Rickels, K. *Non-specific Factors in Drug Therapy.* Charles C Thomas, Pub., Springfield, Ill., **1968.**

——. Drug use in outpatient treatment. *Am. J. Psychiat.,* **1968,** *124,* 20–31.

Robins, E., and Guze, S. B. Classification of affective disorders: the primary, secondary, the endogenous-reactive, and the neurotic psychotic concepts. In, *Recent Advances in the Psychobiology of the Depressive Illnesses.* (Williams, T. A.; Katz, M. M.; and Shield, J. A.; eds.) DHEW Publication No. (HSM) 70-9053, U.S. Government Printing Office, Washington, D. C., **1972,** pp. 283–293.

Roth, M. The phobic anxiety-depersonalization syndrome

and some general aetiological problems in psychiatry. *J. Neuropsychiat.,* **1960,** *1,* 293–306.

Schildkraut, J. J. The catecholamine hypothesis of affective disorders: a review of supporting evidence. *Am. J. Psychiat.,* **1965,** *122,* 509–522.

——. Neuropharmacology of the affective disorders. *A. Rev. Pharmac.,* **1973,** *13,* 427–454.

——. The current status of biological criteria for classifying the depressive disorders and predicting responses to treatment. *Psychopharmac. Bull.,* **1974,** *10,* 5–25.

Schildkraut, J. J., and Kety, S. S. Biogenic amines and emotion. *Science, Wash.,* **1967,** *156,* 21–30.

Schou, M. Lithium in psychiatry—a review. In, *Psychopharmacology: A Review of Progress, 1957–1967.* (Efron, D. H.; Cole, J. O.; Levine, J.; and Wittenborn, J. R.; eds.) Public Health Service Publication No. 1836, U.S. Government Printing Office, Washington, D. C., **1968,** pp. 701–718.

Shader, R. I., and DiMascio, A. *Psychotropic Drug Side Effects: Clinical and Theoretical Perspectives.* The Williams & Wilkins Co., Baltimore, **1970.**

Sigg, E. B. Autonomic side-effects induced by psychotherapeutic agents. In, *Psychopharmacology: A Review of Progress, 1957–1967.* (Efron, D. H.; Cole, J. O.; Levine, J.; and Wittenborn, J. R.; eds.) Public Health Service Publication No. 1836, U.S. Government Printing Office, Washington, D. C., **1968,** pp. 581–588.

Singer, I., and Rotenberg, D. Mechanisms of lithium action. *New Engl. J. Med.,* **1973,** *289,* 254–260.

Snyder, S. H.; Banerjee, S. P.; Yamamura, H. I.; and Greenberg, D. Drugs, neurotransmitters, and schizophrenia. *Science, Wash.,* **1974,** *184,* 1243–1253.

Sroufe, L. A., and Stewart, M. A. Treating problem children with stimulant drugs. *New Engl. J. Med.,* **1973,** *289,* 407–413.

Steinberg, H. (ed.). *Animal Behavior and Drug Action.* J. & A. Churchill, Ltd., London, **1964.**

Sternbach, L. H. Chemistry of 1,5-benzodiazepines and some aspects of the structure-activity relationship. In, *The Benzodiazepines.* (Garattini, S.; Mussini, E.; and Randall, L. O.; eds.) Raven Press, New York, **1973,** pp. 1–26.

Stevens, J. R. An anatomy of schizophrenia? *Archs gen. Psychiat.,* **1973,** *29,* 177–189.

Taylor, M. A. Schneiderian first-rank symptoms and clinical prognostic features in schizophrenia. *Archs gen. Psychiat.,* **1972,** *26,* 64–67.

Usdin, E., and Efron, D. H. *Psychotropic Drugs and Related Compounds,* 2nd ed. DHEW Publication No. (HSM) 72-9074, U.S. Government Printing Office, Washington, D. C., **1972.**

Vesell, E. S. Pharmacogenetics. *New Engl. J. Med.,* **1972,** *287,* 904–909.

Wheatley, D. *Psychopharmacology in Family Practice.* William Heinemann Medical Books, Ltd., London, **1973.**

Wikler, A. Clinical and social aspects of marihuana intoxication. *Archs gen. Psychiat.,* **1970,** *23,* 320–325.

Williams, R. B., and Sherter, C. Cardiac complications of tricyclic antidepressant therapy. *Ann. intern. Med.,* **1971,** *74,* 395–398.

Williams, R. T., and Parke, D. V. The metabolic fate of drugs. *A. Rev. Pharmac.,* **1964,** *4,* 85–114.

Winokur, G.; Clayton, P. J.; and Reich, T. *Manic Depressive Illness.* C. V. Mosby Co., St. Louis, **1969.**

Wyatt, R. J.; Termini, B. A.; and Davis, J. I. Biochemical and sleep studies of schizophrenia: a review of the literature—1960–1970. I. Biochemical studies. II. Sleep studies. *Schizophrenia Bull.,* **1971,** *4,* 10–66.

Young, D. S.; Thomas, D. W.; Friedman, R. B.; and Pestaner, L. C. Bibliography: drug interferences with clinical laboratory tests. *Clin. Chem.,* **1972,** *18,* 1041–1304. (Over 1000 references.)

Zbinden, G., and Randall, L. O. Pharmacology of benzodiazepines: laboratory and clinical correlations. *Adv. Pharmac.,* **1967,** *5,* 213–291.

13 DRUGS EFFECTIVE IN THE THERAPY OF THE EPILEPSIES

Dixon M. Woodbury and Edward Fingl

GENERAL CONSIDERATIONS

Classification of Epileptic Seizures. The term *epilepsies* is a collective designation for a group of chronic central nervous system (CNS) disorders having in common the spontaneous occurrence of brief episodes (seizures) associated with loss or disturbance of consciousness, usually but not always with characteristic body movements (convulsions) and sometimes autonomic hyperactivity, and always correlated with abnormal and excessive EEG discharges.

Epileptic seizures in an individual patient are classified on the basis of the clinical manifestations of the attacks and the EEG pattern. Accurate diagnosis is essential since pharmacotherapy is selective for a particular type of epilepsy. A simplified form of the International Classification of Epileptic Seizures (Gastaut, 1970), useful for purposes of antiepileptic therapy, is presented in Table 13–1. A more complete description of the various types of seizures has been provided by Aird and Woodbury (1974).

For study of the antiepileptic agents, the classification may be further condensed. *Absence* (petit mal) seizures respond well to one group of drugs, and *generalized tonic-clonic* (grand mal) and *cortical focal* convulsions are usually adequately controlled by another. *Temporal lobe* (psychomotor) seizures tend to be refractory to therapy and respond only to some of the agents in the second group. *Infantile* myoclonus and the types of epilepsy that occur in *young children* represent a group for which therapy is generally unsatisfactory. Multiple-drug therapy is often required, since two or more seizure types may occur in the same patient. Generalized tonic-clonic seizures are common in patients with other minor types of attack, since the grand mal convulsion is essentially the invasion of the entire brain by convulsive activity restrained to limited foci and pathways in all other lesser seizure types. For purposes of drug treatment it appears to make little difference whether the convulsive disorder is considered to be *idiopathic* (cause unknown) or *symptomatic* (cerebral organic pathology presumed).

Nature and Mechanisms of Seizures. Almost a century ago John Hughlings Jackson, the father of modern concepts of epilepsy, proposed that seizures were caused by "occasional, sudden, excessive, rapid and local discharges of gray matter," and that a generalized convulsion resulted when normal brain tissue was invaded by the seizure activity initiated in the abnormal focus. In the intervening years little has been added to Jackson's concepts except for the electrical proof of their correctness. The EEG amply demonstrates that seizures are in fact electrical explosions of the brain and serves as the basic method of modern differential diagnosis of the epilepsies (Gibbs and Gibbs, 1954, 1964).

Application of alumina cream to the motor cortex of the monkey creates an epileptogenic focus that causes chronically recurring, spontaneous clinical seizures of focal onset—the fundamental characteristics of human epilepsy. This experimental model is easily manipulated and has been used by many investigators to explore the nature and mechanisms of seizures (*see* Ward, in Symposium, 1969, 1972b). In such models and also in man, anatomical and neurophysiological studies suggest that "epileptic" neurons are responsible for initiating seizure discharges.

An abnormal feature of the neuron engaged in seizure activity is the "paroxysmal depolarizing shift" (PDS), often associated with high-frequency action-potential bursts, loss of inhibitory postsynaptic potentials, and synchronous discharge of other cells of the same columnar group; the PDS correlates well with the familiar, bizarre seizure wave of the gross-surface EEG. Neurons in a chronic-seizure focus exhibit a kind of denervation sensitivity with regard to excitatory stimuli, and may also be rela-

Table 13-1. CLASSIFICATION OF THE EPILEPSIES *

SEIZURE TYPE †		CHARACTERISTICS
I. *Partial Seizures* (Focal Seizures)	A. Partial seizures with elementary symptomatology (*cortical focal*)	Various manifestations, generally without impairment of consciousness, including convulsions confined to a single limb or muscle group (*Jacksonian motor epilepsy*), specific and localized sensory disturbances (*Jacksonian sensory epilepsy*), and other limited signs and symptoms depending upon the particular cortical area producing the abnormal discharge
	B. Partial seizures with complex symptomatology (*temporal lobe, psychomotor*)	Attacks of confused behavior, generally with impairment of consciousness, with a wide variety of clinical manifestations, associated with bizarre generalized EEG activity during the seizure but with evidence of anterior temporal lobe focal abnormalities even in the interseizure period in many cases
	C. Partial seizures secondarily generalized	
II. *Generalized Seizures* (Bilateral, Symmetrical Seizures)	A. Absences (*petit mal*)	Brief and abrupt loss of consciousness associated with high-voltage, bilaterally synchronous, 3-per-second spike-and-wave pattern in the EEG, usually with some symmetrical clonic motor activity varying from eyelid blinking to jerking of the entire body, sometimes with no motor activity
	B. Bilateral massive epileptic myoclonus	Isolated clonic jerks associated with brief bursts of multiple spikes in the EEG
	C. Infantile spasms	Progressive disorder in infants with motor spasms or other convulsive signs, bizarre diffuse changes in the interseizure EEG (hypsarhythmia), and progressive mental deterioration
	D. Clonic seizures	In young children, rhythmic clonic contractions of all muscles, loss of consciousness, and marked autonomic manifestations
	E. Tonic seizures	In young children, opisthotonus, loss of consciousness, and marked autonomic manifestations
	F. Tonic-clonic seizures (*grand mal*)	Major convulsions, usually a sequence of maximal tonic spasm of all body musculature followed by synchronous clonic jerking and a prolonged depression of all central functions
	G. Atonic seizures	Loss of postural tone, with sagging of the head or falling
	H. Akinetic seizures	Impairment of consciousness and complete relaxation of all musculature, secondary to excessive inhibitory discharge

* Modified from the International Classification of Epileptic Seizures (Gastaut, 1970).

† Some classifications include unilateral seizures as a distinct category. Additional seizure types are presently unclassified due to incomplete data.

tively lacking in inhibitory input. The pharmacological properties of these damaged hyperactive cells may differ from the properties of more normal neighboring neurons.

There is as yet no definitive explanation of the cause of high-frequency firing in the seizure focus of a typical epileptic patient. Local biochemical changes, ischemia, and loss of vulnerable small-cell inhibitory systems are among the possible mechanisms. The pathological origins of such foci include congenital defects, head trauma and hypoxia at birth, inflammatory vascular changes subsequent to infectious illnesses of childhood, concussion or depressed skull fracture, abscess, neoplasm, and vascular occlusion of whatever etiology. Although these different lesions have somewhat different predilections for various brain areas, the type of chronic stable focus appears to be similar, and the type of seizure pattern shown by the patient seems more related to the anatomical connections of the focus than to the original etiology.

The seizure focus may remain quiescent over long periods of time, discharging only intermittently as revealed by EEG analysis, and may cause no signs or symptoms. The spread of convulsive activity to neighboring normal cells is presumably restrained by normally present inhibitory mechanisms. However, physiological changes that cannot in themselves cause seizures may trigger the focus or facilitate seizure spread to normal tissue. Among such factors are blood sugar concentration, blood gas tensions, plasma pH, total osmotic pressure and electrolyte composition of extracellular fluid, endocrine changes, fatigue, emotional stress, and nutritional deficiencies. A seizure focus, particularly in the hippocampus, which normally has a low threshold for discharge, might also be triggered by an increase in potassium ion concentration in brain interstitial space. Accumulation of the cation could occur during excessive neuronal activity in the presence of defective transport of the cation from the cerebrospinal fluid (CSF) or impairment of the normal glial function to buffer increases in potassium ion concentration (Pollen and Tractenberg, 1970; Glaser, in Symposium, 1972b).

Thus, many contributory factors interplay to precipitate seizures in a brain predisposed by injury or inherited defect, and the physician should not be perplexed when patients with seemingly identical seizure patterns often respond quite differently to drug therapy.

Given a seizure focus and suitable precipitating circumstances, the abnormal activity may spread to normal brain tissue. If the spread is sufficiently extensive, the entire brain is activated and a tonic-clonic convulsion with unconsciousness ensues. If the spread is localized, the seizure produces signs and symptoms characteristic of the anatomical focus. More distant areas and centers may be driven indirectly without themselves participating in the production of high-frequency seizure discharges, but with disruption of their normal function. For example, a driving focus is suggested by the characteristic cortical EEG dysrhythmia (3-per-second spike and wave) and the associated unconsciousness of absence seizures, which disappear as abruptly as they began with no evidence of cortical postseizure fatigue.

Once initiated, a seizure is undoubtedly maintained by reentry of excitatory impulses in a closed feedback pathway that need not include the original seizure focus. Contributing toward self-maintenance and spread is the phenomenon of posttetanic potentiation (PTP), a progressive enhancement of synaptic transmission during rapid, repetitive stimulation; PTP is of particular interest because it can be abolished by the anticonvulsant phenytoin (diphenylhydantoin) (Esplin, 1957). Contributing to the self-limitation and eventual abrupt collapse of the seizure are the elevated threshold and prolonged refractoriness that result from hyperactivity, and also inhibition from pathways external to the seizure loop. Metabolic factors, such as accumulation of carbon dioxide and depletion of oxygen and high-energy phosphate intermediates, undoubtedly also contribute to self-limitation of seizure discharge.

Mechanisms of Anticonvulsant Effects. The mechanisms of seizures suggest several general ways in which drugs might abolish or attenuate them (Toman and Goodman, 1948): (1) effects on nonneural lesions, such as normalization of the ischemic blood supply of typical cortical seizure foci; (2) effects confined to the pathologically altered neurons of the seizure focus to prevent their excessive discharge; (3) effects on normal neurons to prevent their detonation by the seizure focus.

Most, if not all, presently available antiepileptic agents act at least in part by the third mechanism, since all modify the ability of the brain to respond to various seizure-evoking stimuli. Specific neurophysiological effects include reduction of PTP, elevation of excitatory synaptic threshold, potentiation of presynaptic or postsynaptic inhibition, and prolongation of refractory period. All these effects generally embarrass normal functions of the brain and lead to undesired central side effects. Furthermore, a particular drug might have more than one effect.

The more plausible mechanisms of anticonvulsant effect will be discussed during subsequent consideration of the individual agents. The question "Which drug works best?" can receive but an empirical and provisional answer. Pursuit of the question "Why does it work at all?" contributes to the rational use of a drug and opens the door to the discovery of new and better therapy.

Chemical Structure and Antiepileptic Selectivity. Most clinically useful antiepileptic agents are closely related in structure to phenobarbital, the oldest drug of the group, and contain the following structural common denominator:

$$R_1 \diagdown \underset{R_2 \diagup}{\overset{X}{C_5}} \cdots \overset{\displaystyle C=O}{\underset{\displaystyle O=C \text{---} N \text{---} R_3}{\underset{3}{\vert}}}$$

The substituent at X varies with the chemical class:

Barbiturates	—CO—NH—
Deoxybarbiturates	—CH$_2$—NH—
Hydantoins	—NH—
Oxazolidinediones	—O—
Succinimides	—CH$_2$—
Acetylureas	—NH$_2$

The clinical selectivity of the drugs in these classes is summarized in Table 13–2 (page 220). Except for agents selectively active against absence seizures, a phenyl or similar aromatic group at R_1 or R_2 appears essential for antiepileptic activity. For those interested in the structure-activity relationship, a wealth of results from laboratory anticonvulsant tests on thousands of organic compounds is summarized and catalogued in an excellent monograph by Close and Spielman (1961).

As illustrated by the sulfonamide carbonic anhydrase inhibitors, drugs may have anticonvulsant properties even though they lack the structural common denominator of the major antiepileptic agents. Since such drugs often have a novel mechanism of action, they provide incentive for the continuing search for new agents unrelated to the primary clinical antiepileptics. An example of current interest is *dipropylacetic acid* (DÉPAKINE, ERGENYL); its anticonvulsant effects are thought to be associated with an increase in brain gamma-aminobutyric acid (GABA), a putative inhibitory transmitter. Even if such agents prove unsatisfactory for antiepileptic therapy, their study in the laboratory and clinic provides basic information about mechanisms of seizures and drug action that ultimately should lead to significant advance.

Therapeutic Aspects. The prime objective of therapy of epilepsy is complete suppression of all seizures without impairment of CNS functions. It is commonly accepted that, with patience and persistence, 70 to 80% of all epileptic patients are significantly benefited by currently available pharmacotherapy. Unfortunately, there have been relatively few adequately controlled clinical trials of these agents, and this estimate of efficacy is based largely on clinical impression (Coatsworth and Penry, in Symposium, 1972a). Nevertheless, even if the true percentage of patients benefited is less, drug therapy is the mainstay for control of the

epilepsies. Surgery, obviously indicated in epilepsy secondary to cerebral neoplasm, may be of permanent benefit to a very small minority of patients with discrete focal cortical lesions amenable to resection. Moreover, even these neurosurgical cases sometimes require continuing pharmacotherapy because of secondary foci. Adjuvant measures, such as fluid and dietary restrictions and psychotherapy, may be helpful; however, with the possible exception of the ketogenic diet in the management of absence seizures, they are rarely adequate substitutes for modern pharmacotherapy.

The general principles of the drug therapy of the epilepsies are summarized below, following discussion of the individual agents. Details of diagnosis and therapy can be found in the monographs and reviews listed at the end of the chapter.

Plasma Concentrations of Antiepileptic Drugs. Measurement of plasma drug concentrations greatly facilitates antiepileptic medication, especially multiple-drug therapy (Symposium, 1972a; Aird and Woodbury, 1974). Plasma drug concentrations recommended for maintenance antiepileptic therapy, as well as other pharmacokinetic characteristics essential for interpretation of measured plasma drug concentrations and for devising drug dosage schedules, are summarized for the individual agents in Table 13–2. The value of monitoring plasma concentrations of the antiepileptic agents is discussed further at the end of the chapter.

HYDANTOINS

PHENYTOIN (DIPHENYLHYDANTOIN)

Phenytoin (diphenylhydantoin) is a primary drug for all types of epilepsy except absence seizures. It has been more thoroughly studied in the laboratory and clinic than any other antiepileptic agent.

History. Phenytoin was introduced for the symptomatic treatment of epilepsy by Merritt and Putnam in 1938. In contrast to the earlier chance discovery of the anticonvulsant properties of bromide and phenobarbital, phenytoin was the product of a planned search for new chemicals capable of suppressing electroshock convulsions in laboratory animals. The discovery of phenytoin was a signal advance. Since it is not a sedative in ordinary doses, it established that antiepileptics need not impair consciousness; and since, unlike phenobarbital, it is effective in some cases of temporal lobe epilepsy, it encouraged the search for basic differences between the various convulsive disorders and for drugs with selective anticonvulsant action. In addition, it demonstrated the value of laboratory anticonvulsant testing, opened a new era in the study of structure-activity relationship, and provided a valuable laboratory tool for the study of the neurophysiological and neurochemical basis of seizures.

Structure-Activity Relationship. Phenytoin has the following structural formula:

Phenytoin

It contains the structural common denominator characteristic of many of the antiepileptic agents. As noted previously, a 5-phenyl or other aromatic substituent appears essential for activity against clinical generalized tonic-clonic seizures and for abolition of the maximal electroshock seizure pattern in laboratory animals. Alkyl substituents in position 5 contribute to sedation, a property absent in phenytoin. The 5 carbon permits asymmetry, as in mephenytoin, but there appears to be little difference in activity between isomers. Methylation of N3 changes the spectrum somewhat, but the methyl group is removed in the liver. (*See* Toman and Goodman, 1948; Close and Spielman, 1961.)

Pharmacological Effects. *Central Nervous System.* Phenytoin exerts antiepileptic activity without causing general depression of the CNS. In toxic doses it may produce excitatory signs and at lethal levels a type of decerebrate rigidity. The most easily demonstrated properties of phenytoin are its ability to limit the development of maximal seizure activity and to reduce the spread of the seizure process from an active focus. Both features are undoubtedly related to its clinical usefulness.

The anticonvulsant properties of phenytoin have been reviewed by Toman and Goodman (1948) and Woodbury (Symposium, 1969). Unlike phenobarbital, phenytoin does not elevate the threshold for seizures induced by injection of such convulsant drugs as strychnine, picrotoxin, or pentylenetetrazol. It also has only limited ability to elevate threshold for electroshock seizures. Phenytoin does, however, restore abnormally increased excitability toward normal.

Probably the most significant effect of phenytoin is its ability to modify the pattern of maximal electroshock seizures. The characteristic tonic phase can be abolished completely, but the residual clonic seizure may be exaggerated and prolonged. The EEG during such modified seizures shows a reduction both in voltage and frequency of convulsive discharges (Bárány and Stein-Jensen, 1946; Toman *et al.,* 1946). The drug produces similar alterations in the convulsions of psychiatric patients undergoing electroconvulsive therapy (Toman *et al.,* 1947) and in maximal seizures induced in animals by picrotoxin and pentylenetetrazol. This seizure-modifying action is observed also with other typical antiepileptics effective against generalized tonic-clonic seizures. Phenytoin does not abolish the tonic seizure induced by strychnine, which acts by blockade of postsynaptic inhibition. This and other evidence suggest that most of the effects of the drug are related to presynaptic rather than postsynaptic actions.

The mechanism of anticonvulsant effect of phenytoin has been extensively explored by detailed neurophysiological studies (Delgado and Mihailović, 1956; Gangloff and Monnier, 1957; Strobos and Spudis, 1960; Vastola and Rosen, 1960; Aston and Domino, 1961; Schallek and Kuehn, 1963; Rosati *et al.,* 1967; and others). In various species, as revealed by a variety of stimulation-recording technics, the ability of phenytoin to reduce the duration of afterdischarge and to limit the spread of seizure activity is more prominent than its effect on threshold for stimulation. Moreover, elevation of threshold is relatively selective for the cerebral cortex and hippocampus. Morrell and coworkers (1959) noted that phenytoin was superior to phenobarbital in blocking cortical spread of focal seizure activity but inferior to the barbiturate in suppressing focal activity. They considered these differences significant to their clinical efficacy. Phenytoin therapy can induce complete remission of generalized tonic-clonic and certain other partial seizures but does not completely eliminate the sensory aura or other prodromal signs.

An *excitatory* effect on the cerebellum, to activate inhibitory pathways that extend to the cerebral cortex, may also contribute to the anticonvulsant effect of phenytoin. Halpern and Julien (1972) and Julien and Halpern (1972) noted that reduction of seizure activity in a cortical epileptogenic focus by the drug was associated with increased cerebellar Purkinje cell discharge. After cerebellectomy, cortical focal seizure activity increased and phenytoin was less effective. The effects of the drug in developing animals are also of interest. In the early postnatal period, phenytoin has predominantly excitatory effects on the CNS (Vernadakis and Woodbury, 1969, and in Symposium, 1969). These excitatory effects become less prominent and the anticonvulsant effects more consistent as the animal develops, in parallel with maturation of postsynaptic inhibitory systems.

A *stabilizing* effect of phenytoin is apparent on all neuronal membranes, including peripheral nerve, and probably on all nonexcitable as well as excitable membranes (Korey, 1951; Toman, 1952; Morrell *et al.,* 1958; Brumlik and Moretti, 1966; Fromm and Killian, 1967; Rosenberg and Bartels, 1967; Toman and Sabelli, 1969). Except in toxic doses, it does not interfere with normal cell function. This stabilizing effect on membranes may underlie the relief of pain by phenytoin in trigeminal and glossopharyngeal neuralgias (Iannone et al., 1958) and may be the basis of its reduction of ventricular ectopic activity in digitalis-induced arrhythmias (see Chapter 32). The effects of phenytoin on cardiac, skeletal, and smooth muscle have been reviewed by Woodbury (Symposium, 1969).

An important mechanism in the development of high-frequency trains of impulses in cerebral excitatory feedback circuits and in the spread of seizure activity is PTP, the enhancement of synaptic transmission following rapid, repetitive presynaptic stimulation. Phenytoin reduces PTP of synaptic transmission in the spinal cord and in the stellate ganglion of the cat (Esplin, 1957). Since it has no other notable effect on synaptic transmission, phenytoin probably alters seizure manifestations only insofar as they involve PTP (see Woodbury and Esplin, 1959; Woodbury and Kemp, 1971).

Mechanism of Action. Considerable evidence indicates that the PTP-preventing and membrane-stabilizing effects of phenytoin result directly or indirectly from effects on the movement of ions across cell membranes.

Based upon its effects on calculated intracellular cation concentrations and other indirect evidence, Woodbury (1955) suggested that phenytoin might stimulate active Na^+ transport in the brain and at other sites. Although the anticonvulsant may inhibit Na^+, K^+-activated adenosine triphosphatase (Na^+, K^+-ATPase) activity when the $Na^+:K^+$ ratio is low, it does appear to increase enzyme activity when the $Na^+:K^+$ ratio is high. Phenytoin enhances active Na^+ and K^+ transport in synaptosomes isolated from primary epileptogenic foci (Escueta and Reilly, 1971), and it increases both enzyme activity and Na^+ and K^+ transport in the intestinal mucosa. Of particular interest are the observations that phenytoin increases active K^+ influx into lobster axons but does not affect passive K^+ efflux (Fertziger et al., 1971). In choroid plexus and other nonexcitable epithelial cells, Na^+ flux is enhanced in part indirectly by an increase in Na^+ permeability of the mucosal surface (Williams et al., 1971; Woodbury and Kemp, 1971; Watson and Woodbury, 1972). Stimulation of ion transport by phenytoin would increase K^+ uptake and Na^+ extrusion by neurons and/or glia and enhance the removal of K^+ from the CSF and cerebral interstitial fluid at the choroid plexus. Such effects would oppose the alterations in these cations that occur during seizure activity (Fertziger and Ranck, 1970) and could explain the characteristic anticonvulsant effects of phenytoin.

However, the observations on Na^+, K^+-ATPase activity have been conflicting (Festoff and Appel, 1968; Rawson and Pincus, 1968; Formby, 1970; Peter, 1970; Lewin and Bleck, 1971a, 1971b; Siegel and Goodwin, 1971), and phenytoin has still other effects on cell membranes. It decreases permeability of neuronal cell membranes to Na^+ (Pincus and Rawson, 1969; Pincus et al., 1970; Swanson and Crane, 1970) and acts similarly to tetrodotoxin on the voltage-clamped squid giant axon to block sodium channels (Lipicky et al., 1972). Decreased Na^+ permeability or conductance could also explain inhibition of PTP and other effects of phenytoin. In addition, it has been suggested that a fundamental effect of the anticonvulsant is reduction of Ca^{2+} permeability of the membrane, and part of its anticonvulsant effects could also result from direct or indirect effects on neurotransmitters (see Woodbury, in Symposium, 1969).

Whether a single basic action will ultimately explain these varied effects of phenytoin remains to be determined.

Absorption, Distribution, Biotransformation, and Excretion. The pharmacokinetic characteristics of phenytoin are markedly influenced by its limited aqueous solubility and its dose-dependent elimination. Its inactivation by the hepatic microsomal enzyme system is susceptible to inhibition by other drugs.

Phenytoin is a weak acid with a pK_a of about 8.3; its aqueous solubility is limited, even in the intestine. Upon intramuscular injection, the drug precipitates at the injection site and is slowly absorbed, as if it had been administered in a repository preparation.

Absorption of phenytoin after oral ingestion is slow, sometimes variable, and occasionally incomplete. Significant differences in bioavailability of oral pharmaceutical preparations have been detected (Glazko, 1972). Peak plasma concentration after a single dose may occur as early as 3 hours or as late as 12 hours. Slow absorption during chronic medication blunts the fluctuations of drug concentration between doses.

Phenytoin is 70 to 95% bound to plasma proteins, mainly albumin. A greater fraction remains unbound in the neonate, in patients with hypoalbuminemia, and in uremic patients (Rane et al., 1971; Reidenberg et al., 1971). The drug is widely distributed in all tissues. Fractional binding in tissues, including brain, is about the same as in plasma. Thus, its apparent volume of distribution is about 70% of body weight, but would be about seven times larger if calculated on the basis of unbound drug. Concentration in the CSF is equal to the unbound fraction in plasma.

Less than 5% of phenytoin is excreted unchanged in the urine. The remainder is metabolized primarily by the hepatic microsomal enzymes. The major metabolite, the parahydroxyphenyl derivative, is inactive. It accounts for 60 to 70% of a single dose of the drug and a somewhat smaller fraction during chronic medication. It is excreted initially in the bile and subsequently in the urine, in large part as the glucuronide. Other apparently inactive metabolites include the dihydroxy catechol and its 3-methoxy derivative, and the dihydrodiol. At plasma concentrations below 10 μg/ml, elimination is exponential (first order); plasma half-time averages about 24 hours but varies at least fourfold. At higher concentrations, dose-dependent elimination is apparent; plasma half-time increases with concentration (dose), perhaps because the hydroxylation reaction approaches saturation or is inhibited by the metabolites. A genetically determined limitation in ability to metabolize phenytoin has been detected (Kutt et al., 1964). (See Dill et al., 1956; Arnold and Gerber, 1970; Chang et al., 1970, 1972; Symposium, 1972a; Glazko, 1973.)

Toxicity. The toxic effects of phenytoin depend upon the route and duration of exposure as well as dosage. When it is administered intravenously at an excessive rate in the emergency treatment of cardiac arrhythmias or status epilepticus, the most notable toxic signs are *cardiovascular collapse* and/or *CNS depression*. Acute overdosage by the oral route features primarily signs referable to the cerebellum and vestibular system. Toxic effects associated with chronic medication are also primarily dose-related *cerebellar-vestibular effects* but include other CNS effects, *behavioral changes, increased frequency of seizures, gastrointestinal symptoms, gingival hyperplasia, osteomalacia,* and *megaloblastic anemia. Hirsutism* is an annoying untoward effect in young females. These adverse effects can usually be made bearable by proper adjustment of dosage and do not usually interfere with therapy. Serious adverse effects, including those on the skin, bone marrow, and liver, are probably manifestations of *drug allergy.* Although rare, they necessitate withdrawal of the drug.

The toxicity of phenytoin has been extensively reviewed in a symposium (1972a).

Central nervous system toxicity is the most consistent effect of phenytoin overdosage. *Nystagmus, ataxia, diplopia,* and *vertigo* and other cerebellar-vestibular effects are common. *Blurred vision, mydriasis,* and *hyperactive tendon reflexes* also occur. *Behavioral* effects include *hyperactivity, silliness, confusion, dullness, drowsiness,* and *hallucinations. Peripheral neuropathy,* sometimes with absent tendon reflexes, has been reported in 7 to 30% of patients, particularly the elderly, who have received the drug in high dosage for many years. The relationship to cyanocobalamin metabolism remains uncertain (see Symposium, 1972a). Cerebellar Purkinje cells exhibit damage following high doses of phenytoin only in the presence of concurrent hypoxia (Dam, 1972; Symposium, 1972a).

Gingival hyperplasia occurs in about 20% of all patients during chronic therapy and is probably the most common manifestation of phenytoin toxicity in children and young adolescents. The hyperplasia appears to involve altered collagen metabolism (Symposium, 1972a). Toothless portions of the gums are not affected. The condition does not require

withdrawal of medication. It can be minimized by good oral hygiene.

Gastrointestinal disturbances, including *nausea, vomiting, epigastric pain,* and *anorexia,* can be minimized by taking the drug with meals or in more frequent divided doses.

A variety of *endocrine* effects have been reported. Inhibition of release of *antidiuretic hormone* (ADH) has been observed in patients with inappropriate ADH secretion. *Hyperglycemia* and *glycosuria* appear to be due to inhibition of insulin secretion (Kiser et al., 1970; Levin et al., 1970). *Osteomalacia,* with hypocalcemia and elevated alkaline phosphatase activity, has been attributed to both altered vitamin D metabolism and inhibition of intestinal calcium absorption (Symposium, 1972a). This condition is relatively resistant to vitamin D administration.

Hypersensitivity reactions include *morbilliform rash* in 2 to 5% of patients and occasionally more serious skin reactions, including *Stevens-Johnson syndrome. Systemic lupus erythematosus* and potentially fatal *hepatic necrosis* have been reported rarely. *Hematological* reactions include *neutropenia, leukopenia, thrombocytopenia, agranulocytosis,* and *aplastic anemia. Megaloblastic anemia* has been attributed to altered folate absorption but probably also involves altered folate metabolism (Symposium, 1972a). It is rare and responds to administration of folic acid. Similar effects have been reported during medication with phenobarbital, primidone, and mephenytoin. *Lymphadenopathy,* resembling Hodgkin's disease and malignant lymphoma, is associated with reduced immunoglobulin A (IgA) production (Sorrell et al., 1971). *Hypoprothrombinemia* and *hemorrhage* have occurred in the newborn of mothers who received phenytoin during pregnancy; vitamin K is effective treatment or prophylaxis.

Preparations and Dosage. *Phenytoin Sodium,* U.S.P. *(diphenylhydantoin sodium;* DILANTIN), is available as 30- and 100-mg capsules for oral use, and as a sterile solution of 50 mg/ml, with a special solvent, for parenteral use. Official preparations of *Phenytoin,* U.S.P., include 50-mg tablets and an oral suspension containing 125 mg/5 ml.

Choice and adjustment of phenytoin dosage and interpretation of measured plasma drug concentrations must be dominated by recognition of the dose-dependent elimination of the drug. As dosage is increased, plasma half-life and the time required to attain the plateau state increase. Plasma drug concentration increases disproportionately as dosage is increased.

Initial daily dosage for adults is 3 to 4 mg/kg (100 mg, twice daily). Dosage is subsequently increased, preferably with monitoring of plasma concentration, as needed for control of seizures or as limited by toxicity. Increments in dosage may be made at 1-week intervals at low dosage but at 2-week intervals when dosage exceeds 300 mg daily. Doses greater than 500 mg daily are rarely tolerated if taken regularly. Because of its relatively long half-life and slow absorption, a single daily dose is often satisfactory for adults, but gastric intolerance may dictate divided dosage. Divided dosage is recommended for children. If loading dosage is deemed necessary, 600 to 1000 mg, in divided portions over 8 to 12 hours, will provide effective plasma concentrations within 24 hours in most patients.

Intravenous administration of phenytoin should not exceed 50 mg per minute. A slower rate is preferred, especially in elderly patients. Intramuscular administration is not recommended.

Plasma Drug Concentrations. During chronic medication, plasma drug concentration is not linearly related to daily dose. However, in the therapeutic range, it averages about 3 to 4 $\mu g/ml$ per mg/kg daily dose. The plateau state is attained in 5 to 7 days at low doses and 10 to 14 days at high doses. Plasma concentrations of 10 to 20 $\mu g/ml$ are optimal. Concentrations as low as 8 $\mu g/ml$ may be adequate for seizure control in some patients. Nystagmus is usually evident at 20 $\mu g/ml$, ataxia is apparent at 30 $\mu g/ml$, and lethargy occurs at 40 $\mu g/ml$ or higher. Association between plasma concentration and other adverse effects has not been established. The possibility that the blood:plasma or erythrocyte:plasma phenytoin ratio might provide a reliable estimate of the concentration of drug not bound to plasma protein is being explored. (*See* Buchthal *et al.,* 1960; Symposium, 1972a.)

Drug Interactions. Interaction between phenytoin and *phenobarbital* is variable. Phenobarbital may increase the biotransformation of phenytoin, by induction of the hepatic microsomal enzyme system, but may also decrease its inactivation, apparently by competitive inhibition. In addition, phenobarbital may reduce the oral absorption of phenytoin. Conversely, the phenobarbital concentration is sometimes increased by phenytoin. *Ethanol* has similar opposing effects on the inactivation of phenytoin.

Well-documented *increase* in phenytoin plasma concentration, by inhibition of its inactivation, has occurred during concurrent administration of *chloramphenicol, dicumarol, disulfiram, isoniazid,* or *sulthiame.* Less well documented or variable increase has been reported for a variety of other drugs. Inhibition of phenytoin inactivation should be suspected for other agents that are also hydroxylated by the microsomal enzyme system. Well-documented *decrease* in phenytoin concentration has been reported for *carbamazepine.* Conversely, the carbamazepine concentration may be reduced by phenytoin.

Interactions involving displacement of bound phenytoin by other drugs are possible and have been much studied *in vitro* but not documented *in vivo.* Phenytoin is only a weak inducer of the hepatic microsomal enzyme system in man.

Therapeutic Uses. *Epilepsy.* Many experienced clinical investigators consider phenytoin the drug of first choice in all forms of epilepsy except in absence seizures (*see* Gibbs and Stamps, 1958; Lennox and Lennox, 1960). Others favor phenobarbital, especially in children. The two drugs are often employed concurrently.

The use of phenytoin and other agents in the therapy of the epilepsies is discussed further at the end of the chapter.

Other Uses. Phenytoin has been used for the treatment of *disturbed nonepileptic psychotic patients* with variable results. A favorable response is more likely when there is initially an abnormal EEG, especially when the abnormality is of a paroxysmal type that suggests that an underlying seizure mechanism is disrupting normal behavior. Some cases of *trigeminal and related neuralgias* respond well to phenytoin, but carbamazepine is the preferred agent. The use of phenytoin in the treatment of *cardiac arrhythmias* is discussed in Chapter 32.

OTHER HYDANTOINS

Mephenytoin. *Mephenytoin,* N.F. (MESANTOIN), 3-methyl-5,5-phenylethylhydantoin, is N-demethylated to NIRVANOL (Butler, 1953). This metabolite was employed clinically in the 1920s but was abandoned because of a high incidence of serious toxicity. The metabolite probably accounts, at least in part, for the therapeutic benefit and toxicity of chronic mephenytoin medication.

Pharmacological Effects. Mephenytoin is active in most anticonvulsant tests in animals (Toman *et al.,* 1947; Goodman *et al.,* 1948; Brown *et al.,* 1953). Like phenytoin, it inhibits PTP. Unlike phenytoin, it antagonizes pentylenetetrazol, elevates seizure threshold, and is a sedative. Also unlike phenytoin, mephenytoin is rapidly absorbed after oral administration. Its N-demethylation and the subsequent inactivation of the metabolite by hydroxylation are catalyzed by the hepatic microsomal enzymes.

Therapeutic Uses and Toxicity. Mephenytoin was introduced in 1945 for the treatment of epilepsy (*see* Loscalzo, 1952). Its antiepileptic spectrum is the same as that of phenytoin, and it may exacerbate absence seizures. Very limited pharmacokinetic information is available (Plaa and Hine, 1960). Although sometimes dramatically superior to phenytoin therapeutically (Lennox and Lennox, 1960), this advantage is offset by its toxicity. Mephenytoin causes significantly less ataxia, gingival hyperplasia, gastric distress, and hirsutism than does phenytoin and less sedation than does phenobarbital. However, serious toxicity is common. These adverse effects include morbilliform rash (in 10% of patients), fever, lymphadenopathy, leukopenia, pancytopenia, agranulocytosis, hepatotoxicity, periarteritis nodosa, and lupus erythematosus. Death attributed to aplastic anemia has occurred. Acute overdosage results in coma.

When mephenytoin is used, it is generally concurrently with other agents, in the lowest dose possible, and only in patients who fail to respond to or do not tolerate safer agents. Because of its sedative effects, mephenytoin is more rationally employed concurrently with phenytoin than with phenobarbital or primidone.

Preparations and Dosage. Typical daily dosage is 300 to 600 mg in adults and 100 to 400 mg in children. The drug is available in 100-mg tablets.

Ethotoin. *Ethotoin* (PEGANONE) is 3-ethyl-5-phenylhydantoin. Introduced by Schwade and co-workers (1956), it appeared to be of some value in the treatment of temporal lobe as well as generalized tonic-clonic seizures and to be relatively free of the typical adverse effects of phenytoin. However, because of its low efficacy, it is employed only occasionally, mostly as an adjunct to other agents, in the therapy of generalized tonic-clonic seizures. The usual daily dose for adults is 2.0 to 3.0 g. Ethotoin is available in 250- and 500-mg tablets.

Skin rash, gastrointestinal distress, and drowsiness are the common adverse effects of ethotoin. Lymphadenopathy has also been reported. Metabolites, produced by the hepatic microsomal enzymes, include the N-dealkyl and parahydroxyphenyl derivatives.

ANTICONVULSANT BARBITURATES

The pharmacology of the barbiturates as a class is considered in Chapter 9; discussion in this chapter is limited to the three barbiturates employed for therapy of the epilepsies.

PHENOBARBITAL

Phenobarbital was the first effective organic antiepileptic agent (Hauptmann, 1912). It is the least toxic, the least expensive, and still one of the most effective and widely used.

Structure-Activity Relationship. The structural formula of phenobarbital is shown in Table 9–1 (page 103). As noted previously, most other antiepileptic agents were developed as structural variations of phenobarbital.

Anticonvulsant Properties. Phenobarbital is active in most anticonvulsant tests in animals but is relatively nonselective. It limits the spread of seizure activity and also elevates seizure threshold. Many of its characteristics were noted during the previous discussion of phenytoin.

Absorption, Distribution, Biotransformation, and Excretion. Oral absorption of phenobarbital is complete but somewhat slow; peak plasma concentration occurs several hours after a single dose. It is 40 to 60% bound to plasma proteins and bound to a similar extent in tissues, including brain. Ten to 25% of phenobarbital is eliminated by pH-dependent renal excretion; the remainder is inactivated by the hepatic microsomal enzymes. The major metabolite, the para-hydroxyphenyl derivative, is inactive and is excreted in the urine partly as the sulfate conjugate (Butler, 1956). The plasma half-life of phenobarbital is 2 to 6 days in adults and somewhat shorter and more variable in children.

Toxicity. The adverse effects of phenobarbital have been reviewed by Browning and Maynert (Symposium, 1972a). *Sedation,* the most frequent undesired effect of phenobarbital, is apparent to some extent in all patients upon initiation of therapy, but tolerance develops during chronic medication. *Nystagmus* and *ataxia* occur at excessive dosage. Phenobarbital sometimes produces *irritability* and *hyperactivity* in children and *confusion* in the elderly.

Scarlatiniform or *morbilliform rash,* possibly with other manifestations of drug allergy, occurs in 1 to 2% of patients. Fatal *exfoliative dermatitis* is rare. *Hypoprothrombinemia* with hemorrhage has been observed in the newborn of mothers who have received phenobarbital during pregnancy; vitamin K is effective for treatment or prophylaxis. *Megaloblastic anemia* that responds to folate and *osteomalacia* that responds to high doses of vitamin D occur during chronic phenobarbital therapy of epilepsy, as they do during phenytoin medication. Other adverse effects of phenobarbital are discussed in Chapter 9.

Preparations and Dosage. *Phenobarbital,* U.S.P., and *Phenobarbital Sodium,* U.S.P., are available in a variety of dosage forms for oral and parenteral use. The usual daily dose for *adults* is 1 to 3 mg/kg (60 to 200 mg). Since plasma half-time averages 4 days, several weeks are required to attain the plateau state. Double dosage for the initial 4 days provides an effective plasma drug concentration more promptly, but sedation will be prominent. The usual initial daily dose for *children* is 2 to 3 mg/kg, in two divided portions. Dosage is subsequently increased or adjusted, as required for control of seizures or as limited by toxicity.

Plasma Drug Concentrations. During chronic medication in adults, plasma concentration of phenobarbital averages 10 μg/ml per mg/kg daily dose; in children, the value is 5 to 7 μg/ml per mg/kg. Although higher concentrations are frequently maintained, particularly in institutionalized patients with refractory seizures, plasma concentrations of 10 to 30 μg/ml are usually recommended for control of epilepsy; 15 μg/ml is the minimum for prophylaxis against febrile convulsions. Whether tolerance develops to the antiepileptic effects of phenobarbital is uncertain.

The relationship between plasma concentration of phenobarbital and adverse effects varies with the development of tolerance. Sedation, nystagmus, and ataxia are usually absent at concentrations below 30 μg/ml during chronic medication, but adverse effects may be apparent for several days at lower concentrations when therapy is initiated or whenever dosage is increased. Concentrations greater than 60 μg/ml may be associated with marked intoxication in the nontolerant individual.

Since significant behavioral toxicity may be present despite the absence of overt signs of toxicity, the tendency to maintain patients, particularly children, on excessively high doses of phenobarbital should be resisted. Plasma phenobarbital concentration should be increased above 30 to 40 μg/ml only if the increment is adequately tolerated and only if it contributes significantly to seizure control. (*See* Svensmark and Buchthal, 1963; Buchthal *et al.*, 1968; Buchthal and Svensmark, 1971; Symposium, 1972a.)

Drug Interactions. Interactions between phenobarbital and other drugs usually involve induction of the hepatic microsomal enzyme system by phenobarbital (*see* Chapters 1 and 9). The variable interaction with phenytoin has been discussed previously (page 208).

Therapeutic Uses. Phenobarbital is an effective agent for *generalized tonic-clonic (grand mal)* and *cortical focal seizures.* Its efficacy, low toxicity, and low cost make it the agent of choice for these types of epilepsy, particularly in children. It is also useful for interruption of *status epilepticus* and for prophylaxis or treatment of *febrile convulsions* in young children (Melchior *et al.*, 1971; Symposium, 1972a). Phenobarbital is of limited value in *temporal lobe epilepsy* and may exacerbate absence seizures. Phenobarbital medication must always be withdrawn gradually; abrupt withdrawal may increase seizure frequency or precipitate status epilepticus.

The use of phenobarbital in the therapy of the epilepsies is discussed further at the end of the chapter.

OTHER BARBITURATES

Mephobarbital. *Mephobarbital,* N.F. (MEBARAL), is N-methylphenobarbital. It is N-demethylated by the hepatic microsomal enzymes, and most of its activity during chronic medication can be attributed to the accumulation of phenobarbital produced by this conversion. Consequently, the pharmacological properties, toxicity, and clinical uses of mephobarbital are the same as those for phenobarbital. However, oral absorption of mephobarbital is usually incomplete, and its dose is approximately twice that

of phenobarbital. The plasma concentration of phenobarbital provides a guide to adjustment of mephobarbital dosage.

Metharbital. *Metharbital,* N.F. (GEMONIL), is N-methylbarbital. It is N-demethylated by the hepatic microsomal enzymes to barbital, which is excreted unchanged in the urine. Most of the activity of metharbital during chronic medication is probably attributable to the metabolite. Metharbital has greater sedative and less antiepileptic activity than does phenobarbital. It has been reported to be effective for infantile myoclonic spasms (Perlstein, 1950, 1957). The initial dosage for infants and small children is 50 mg, one to three times daily; for adults, 100 mg, two to three times daily.

DEOXYBARBITURATES

PRIMIDONE

Primidone is an effective agent for treatment of all types of epilepsy except absence seizures.

Chemistry. Primidone may be viewed as a congener of phenobarbital in which the carbonyl oxygen of the urea moiety is replaced by two hydrogen atoms:

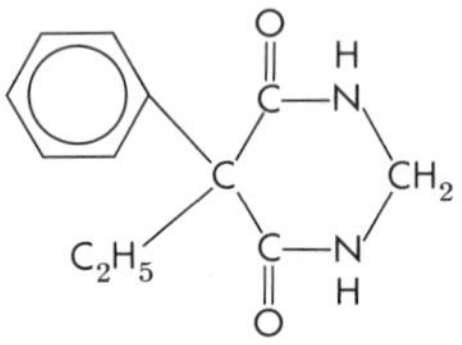

Primidone

Anticonvulsant Effects. Primidone resembles phenobarbital in many laboratory anticonvulsant effects, but it is rather more selective in modifying electroshock seizure pattern in animals and man (Bogue and Carrington, 1953; Goodman *et al.*, 1953). The anticonvulsant effects of administered primidone in animals are attributed to both the parent drug and its active metabolites (Symposium, 1972a).

Absorption, Distribution, Biotransformation, and Excretion. Primidone is converted to two active metabolites, phenobarbital and phenylethylmalonamide (PEMA). The plasma half-time of PEMA is 24 to 48 hours; both it and phenobarbital (plasma half-time: 48 to 120 hours) accumulate during chronic medication. The appearance of phenobarbital in plasma may be delayed several days upon initiation of therapy. The plasma half-time of primidone varies from 3 to 24 hours. In animals, both primidone and PEMA are excreted unchanged in the urine. Renal excretion in man has not been studied. Neither primidone nor PEMA is bound significantly to plasma proteins. Peak plasma concentration after a single dose of primidone occurs between ½ and 9 hours. (*See* Gallagher and Baumel, in Symposium, 1972a.)

Toxicity. The toxicity of primidone has been reviewed by Booker (Symposium, 1972a). The more common complaints are *sedation, vertigo, dizziness, nausea, vomiting, ataxia, diplopia,* and *nystagmus.* The relationship of adverse effects to dosage is complex, since they result from both the parent drug and its two active metabolites and since tolerance develops during chronic medication. Side effects are occasionally quite severe when therapy is initiated.

Serious adverse effects are relatively uncommon, but *maculopapular* and *morbilliform rash, leukopenia, thrombocytopenia, systemic lupus erythematosus,* as well as *lymphadenopathy* have been reported. Acute *psychotic reactions,* usually in patients with temporal lobe epilepsy, have also occurred. *Hemorrhagic disease* in the neonate, *megaloblastic anemia,* and *osteomalacia* similar to those discussed previously in connection with phenytoin and phenobarbital have also been described.

Preparations and Dosage. *Primidone,* U.S.P. (MYSOLINE), is available as 50- and 250-mg tablets and as an oral suspension (250 mg/5 ml). The usual daily dose for adults is 500 to 1500 mg; for children, 5 to 20 mg/kg. Therapy should be initiated at lower dosage and increased gradually. Lower dosage may be possible or necessary when the drug is used concurrently with phenytoin.

Plasma Drug Concentrations. During chronic medication, the plasma concentration of phenobarbital generated by biotransformation of primidone averages 2 μg/ml per mg/kg daily dose of primidone. The plasma concentration of primidone fluctuates significantly between doses but averages about 1 μg/ml per mg/kg daily dose of primidone. The plasma concentration of the active metabolite PEMA is usually intermediate between those of primidone and phenobarbital. Dosage of primidone may be adjusted primarily with reference to the concentration of phenobarbital, as outlined previously for administered phenobarbital, and secondarily with reference to the concentration of the parent drug. Concentrations of primidone greater than 10 μg/ml are usually associated with significant ataxia and lethargy. A disproportionately high primidone:phenobarbital concentration ratio during chronic medication usually implies that medication has not been taken regularly. The relationship of plasma concentration of PEMA to efficacy and toxicity has not been established. (*See* Booker and Gallagher and Baumel, in Symposium, 1972a.)

Drug Interactions. Interactions between primidone and other drugs have not been reported but are presumably similar to those for phenobarbital.

Therapeutic Uses. Clinical antiepileptic efficacy of primidone was first reported by Handley and Stewart (1952). It is useful against *generalized tonic-clonic, cortical focal,* and *temporal lobe epilepsy.* It may be effective alone in patients refractory to other medications but is more effective when used concurrently with phenytoin. Its use in combination with phenobarbital is illogical. Primidone is ineffective against absence seizures but sometimes useful against myoclonic seizures in young children.

The therapeutic use of primidone and other antiepileptic agents is discussed further at the end of the chapter.

IMINOSTILBENES

CARBAMAZEPINE

Carbamazepine, U.S.P. (TEGRETOL), is chemically and pharmacologically related to the tricyclic antidepressants (Chapter 12). While it is a promising agent for therapy of temporal lobe epilepsy, its status will remain uncertain until its potential for serious toxicity has been more clearly defined. It is the primary agent for treatment of trigeminal and related neuralgias. The drug has also been reported to be effective in terminating attacks of intractable hiccough.

Pharmacological Properties. The anticonvulsant effects of carbamazepine in animals resemble those of phenytoin. It blocks PTP, abolishes the tonic extensor component of the maximal electroshock seizure, has limited ability to elevate seizure threshold, and does not antagonize pentylenetetrazol.

Pharmacokinetic information on carbamazepine is incomplete and variable. Oral absorption is adequate. Its plasma half-time is said to be 15 to 30 hours but may sometimes be significantly longer. It is highly bound to plasma proteins and tissues. Unchanged drug and at least seven unidentified metabolites are excreted in the urine.

Toxicity. Carbamazepine has caused deaths from *aplastic anemia* and from its *cardiovascular effects;* nevertheless, it is a potentially valuable drug (Livingston *et al.,* 1974). Serious adverse effects, in addition to bone-marrow depression, include *leukopenia, thrombocytopenic purpura, hepatocellular* and *cholestatic jaundice, acute oliguria* with *hypertension, thrombophlebitis, left ventricular failure,* and *cardiovascular collapse. Skin rash,* often with other manifestations of drug allergy, is said to occur in 3% of patients. *Stevens-Johnson syndrome, exfoliative dermatitis, photosensitivity, altered skin pigmentation,* and *systemic lupus erythematosus* have been reported.

The more frequent untoward effects of carbamazepine include *diplopia, blurred vision, drowsiness, dizziness, nausea, vomiting,* and *ataxia.* A wide variety of other CNS, gastrointestinal, cardiovascular, and dermatological effects have also been reported. Other adverse effects and precautions are similar to those for the tricyclic antidepressants. Some tolerance develops to the untoward effects of carbamazepine, and they can be minimized by gradual increase in dosage and adjustment of maintenance dosage.

Therapeutic Uses. *Epilepsy.* Carbamazepine is said to control or benefit at least two thirds of patients with *temporal lobe epilepsy,* occurring alone or combined with *generalized tonic-clonic seizures,* and to be somewhat less effective against generalized convulsions alone. However, until its efficacy has been established in adequately controlled clinical trials, and particularly until its potential for serious toxicity is more clearly defined, carbamazepine should be employed only for treatment of susceptible seizures that are refractory to the established agents. When it is employed, requisite precautions and careful monitoring of renal, hepatic, and bone-marrow function are mandatory. Its alleged psychotropic effect in patients with temporal lobe epilepsy also remains to be established. It is not effective for absence seizures or infantile myoclonus. A brief but informative summary of the status of carbamazepine has been provided by Cereghino and coworkers (1974).

The usual daily dose for adults has been 600 to 1200 mg, attained gradually from an initial dose of 100 mg, twice daily. Plasma drug concentrations associated with efficacy and toxicity have not been established. Plasma concentrations of 1 to 10 μg/ml are usually attained during chronic medication but are variable and may be lower in patients also receiving phenobarbital or phenytoin (Christiansen and Dam, 1973). Carbamazepine may decrease phenytoin concentration.

Neuralgia. Carbamazepine was introduced by Blom in the early 1960s and is now the primary agent for treatment of *trigeminal* and *glossopharyngeal neuralgias (see* Crill, 1973). It is also effective for *lightning tabetic pain.* Carbamazepine is *not* an analgesic and should *not* be employed for relief of other types of pain.

Most patients with neuralgia are benefited initially, but only 70% obtain continuing relief. Adverse effects have required discontinuation of medication in 5 to 20% of patients. Concurrent medication with phenytoin may be useful when carbamazepine alone is not satisfactory. The usual adult maintenance dose is 400 to 800 mg daily, attained by gradual increase from an initial dose of 100 mg, twice daily.

SUCCINIMIDES

ETHOSUXIMIDE

The succinimides evolved from a systematic search for effective agents less toxic than the oxazolidinediones for the treatment of absence seizures. Ethosuximide is the agent of choice for this type of epilepsy.

Structure-Activity Relationship. Ethosuximide has the following structural formula:

Ethosuximide

The structure-activity relationship of the succinimides is in accord with that for other anticonvulsant classes (Chen *et al.,* 1963). Methsuximide and phensuximide have phenyl substituents and are more active against maximal electroshock seizures. Ethosuximide, with alkyl substituents, is the most active against pentylenetetrazol seizures and is the most selective for clinical absence seizures.

Anticonvulsant Properties. The anticonvulsant spectrum of ethosuximide in animals resembles that of trimethadione. The most prominent characteristic of both drugs is protection against pentylenetetrazol seizures. Ethosuximide also elevates threshold for electroshock seizures, but it abolishes the tonic extensor component of maximal electroshock seizures only in anesthetic doses. Neurophysiological analysis of ethosuximide is incomplete. However, it does block spiking activity in both the primary and secondary foci and the associated clonic seizure activity produced by the local application of cobalt to the frontal cortex of the rat.

Absorption, Distribution, Biotransformation, and Excretion. Ethosuximide is essentially completely absorbed from the gastrointestinal tract. Peak plasma concentration after a single oral dose occurs in 1 to 7 hours. Ethosuximide is not significantly bound to plasma proteins; during chronic medication, the concentration in the CSF is similar to that in plasma. In animals, it is relatively evenly distributed in all tissues and does not accumulate in fat.

In man, 10 to 20% of the drug is excreted unchanged in the urine. The remainder is metabolized by hepatic microsomal enzymes. The major metabolite, the hydroxyethyl derivative, accounts for about 40% of administered drug, is inactive, and is excreted as such and as the glucuronide in the urine. Other metabolites include the corresponding ketone derivative and an open-ring succinamic acid compound. The plasma half-time of ethosuximide averages about 30 hours in children and 60 hours in adults (*see* Symposium, 1972a).

Toxicity. The toxicity of ethosuximide has been reviewed by Buchanan (Symposium, 1972a). The most common dose-related side effects are *gastrointestinal* complaints (*nausea, vomiting*, and *anorexia*) and *CNS* effects (*drowsiness, lethargy, euphoria, dizziness, headache*, and *hiccough*). Some tolerance to these effects develops. *Parkinson-like symptoms* and *photophobia* have also been reported. *Restlessness, agitation, anxiety, aggressiveness, inability to concentrate*, and other behavioral effects have occurred primarily in patients with a prior history of psychiatric disturbance.

Urticaria and other skin reactions, including *Stevens-Johnson syndrome, systemic lupus erythematosus, eosinophilia, leukopenia, thrombocytopenia, pancytopenia*, and *aplastic anemia*, have also been attributed to the drug. The leukopenia may be transient, despite continuation of the drug, but several deaths have resulted from bone-marrow depression. Renal or hepatic toxicity has not been reported.

Preparations and Dosage. *Ethosuximide*, U.S.P. (ZARONTIN), is available for oral administration as 250-mg capsules and as a syrup (250 mg/5 ml). An initial daily dose of 250 mg in children and 500 mg in adults is increased by 250-mg increments at weekly intervals until seizures are adequately controlled or toxicity intervenes. Usual maintenance dosage is 20 to 40 mg/kg. Increased caution is required if daily dosage exceeds 1500 mg in adults or 750 to 1000 mg in children.

Plasma Drug Concentrations. During chronic medication in children, the plasma concentration of ethosuximide averages 2 to 4 μg/ml per mg/kg daily dose. The plateau state is attained in 4 to 6 days. A plasma concentration of 40 to 100 μg/ml is required for satisfactory control of absence seizures in most patients. However, some patients may be completely controlled at lower concentrations, and others are incompletely controlled at higher concentrations. A relationship between plasma concentration and adverse effects has not been established. Concentrations as high as 160 μg/ml have been tolerated without excessive toxicity. (*See* Symposium, 1972a.)

Drug Interactions. Interactions between ethosuximide and other drugs have not been reported. Increased toxicity should be anticipated with other drugs having similar dose-related adverse effects.

Therapeutic Uses. Ethosuximide is more effective than trimethadione against *absence seizures* (Vossen, 1958; Zimmerman and Burgemeister, 1958; Symposium, 1972a) and has a lower risk of serious adverse effects; it is the agent of choice for this type of epilepsy. Concurrent medication with phenytoin or primidone against associated or unmasked generalized tonic-clonic seizures is required in the majority of patients. Ethosuximide is ineffective for control of other types of epilepsy.

The use of ethosuximide and the other antiepileptic agents is discussed further at the end of the chapter.

OTHER SUCCINIMIDES

Methsuximide. Methsuximide, N,2-dimethyl-2-phenylsuccinimide, was introduced by Zimmerman (1956) for the therapy of absence seizures. Ethosuximide subsequently proved more effective. Methsuximide, particularly when given concurrently with other drugs, may also be useful in the treatment of temporal lobe epilepsy. Adverse gastrointestinal and central effects are similar in pattern to those of ethosuximide. Severe depression, skin rash, fever, periorbital edema, leukopenia, aplastic anemia, nephropathy, and hepatotoxicity have also been reported.

Methsuximide, N.F. (CELONTIN), is available as 150- and 300-mg capsules. Medication is initiated with 300 mg, given daily. The usual daily dose for adults is 600 to 1200 mg. Patients receiving higher doses, especially in multiple-drug therapy, should be carefully monitored.

Methsuximide is rapidly absorbed and metabolized (Symposium, 1972a). It is not bound significantly to plasma proteins, and less than 1% is excreted unchanged in the urine. Metabolism by the hepatic microsomal enzymes in the dog yields N-demethyl and parahydroxyphenyl derivatives and their glucuronides (Dudley *et al.*, 1974). The N-demethyl metabolite has been implicated in the production of delayed coma after acute overdosage of methsuximide (Karch, 1973) and has been detected in much higher concentration than the parent drug in the plasma of patients during chronic methsuximide therapy (Strong *et al.*, 1974). Inadequate study of this active metabolite limits the value of the meager pharmacokinetic information on methsuximide.

Phensuximide. The first succinimide introduced for the therapy of absence seizures (Zimmerman, 1951) was phensuximide, N-methyl-2-phenylsuccinimide. Low efficacy has relegated it to secondary status. Adverse gastrointestinal and central effects are similar to those for ethosuximide. A dreamlike state, skin rash, fever, granulocytopenia, leukopenia, and reversible nephropathy have also been reported.

Phensuximide, N.F. (MILONTIN), is available as 250- and 500-mg capsules and as a suspension containing 300 mg/5 ml. The usual daily dose for adults is 2.0 to 4.0 g.

Pharmacokinetic information on phensuximide is meager (Symposium, 1972a), and its value is limited by inadequate study of the possible contribution of the N-demethyl metabolite to its efficacy and toxicity. The parent drug is absorbed promptly and is not bound to plasma proteins. Renal excretion of unchanged drug is negligible. Phensuximide is rapidly metabolized by the hepatic microsomal and other enzymes, in part to the parahydroxyphenyl derivative. Other metabolites identified in the dog include the N-demethyl compound and an open-ring succinamic acid derivative (Dudley *et al.*, 1972).

OXAZOLIDINEDIONES

TRIMETHADIONE

Although no longer the clinical agent of choice, trimethadione has been extensively studied in the laboratory and clinic, and, in this regard, it may still be considered the prototype for agents useful against absence (petit mal) seizures.

History. The demonstration by Perlstein and the confirmation by many others of the selectivity of trimethadione in the treatment of absence seizures was an important advance in the therapy of the epilepsies (Lennox, 1945; Goodman *et al.*, 1946; Perlstein and Andelman, 1946; Richards and Perlstein, 1946). It provided the first clear indication that drugs could be selective for the various types of epilepsy and spurred research on the basic physiological mechanism of the absence seizures, which previously had been refractory to therapy. Moreover, it provided a new pharmacological tool for such investigations. In addition, it reemphasized the value of a systematic search for new anticonvulsants by means of laboratory tests (Everett and Richards, 1944; Goodman *et al.*, 1946).

Structure-Activity Relationship. Trimethadione has the structural formula as shown.

Trimethadione

The oxazolidinediones contain the structural common denominator typical of many other classes of antiepileptic agents. The alkyl substituents on the carbon in position 5 appear important for the selectivity of the oxazolidinediones both as antagonists of pentylenetetrazol in animals and as clinically useful agents in the therapy of absence seizures. The same is true for the succinimides. The structure-activity relationship for these compounds has been reviewed by Toman and Goodman (1948), Close and Spielman (1961), and Chen and coworkers (1963).

Pharmacological Effects. The outstanding anticonvulsant property of trimethadione in laboratory animals is its protective effect against pentylenetetrazol seizures, in which property it differs markedly from phenytoin (Everett and Richards, 1944; Toman and Goodman, 1948). Conversely, it is far inferior to phenytoin in its ability to modify the maximal electroshock seizure pattern.

Dimethadione, the N-demethyl metabolite of trimethadione, is active and resembles the parent drug in most respects. In general, compared with the parent drug, the metabolite is more potent (Withrow *et al.*, 1968).

In laboratory animals, in nondepressant doses trimethadione prevents completely all evidence of central excitation from pentylenetetrazol, including EEG signs. Conversely, central depression by large doses of trimethadione is completely antagonized by pentylenetetrazol. Thus, the two drugs are mutual antagonists. Trimethadione, like the barbiturates, is protective to a variable extent against other chemical convulsants and elevates the threshold for electroshock seizures. In higher dosage, it can abolish the tonic component of maximal seizures (Toman *et al.*, 1946; Brown *et al.*, 1953; and others). Unlike typical antiepileptic barbiturates and hydantoins, it fails to modify the maximal seizure pattern in psychiatric patients undergoing electroconvulsive therapy, even in doses well above the accepted level for suppression of clinical absence seizures (Toman *et al.*, 1947).

Neurophysiological studies have also identified significant differences between the effects of trimethadione and phenytoin. Schallek and Kuehn (1963) observed that trimethadione considerably elevates the threshold for seizure discharge by repetitive stimulation of the central lateral nucleus of the thalamus of the cat, in doses lower than required for other areas and in contrast to the lack of effect of phenytoin on the thalamus. Morrell and associates (1959) noted that trimethadione depressed the projection of seizure activity from cortical foci to thalamus while leaving cortical spread relatively unaffected. Phenytoin produces the opposite effect. Although trimethadione also elevates the cortical seizure threshold (Delgado and Mihailović, 1956), some thalamic nuclei are particularly sensitive to the drug. Since the thalamocortical system appears particularly important in the genesis of absence seizures, the relatively selective effect of trimethadione on thalamic nuclei could account for its clinical efficacy against this type of epilepsy.

The effects of trimethadione on spinal cord synaptic transmission are also of interest (Esplin and Curto, 1957; Woodbury and Esplin, 1959). Trimethadione can selectively depress polysynaptic transmission in acute spinal cats without affecting monosynaptic transmission. Carbon dioxide and acetazolamide produce the opposite pattern. Trimethadione also markedly decreases spinal cord transmission during repetitive stimulation without modifying transmission of single impulses, and it antagonizes the effects of pentylenetetrazol on the spinal cord. Transmission in the stellate ganglion during repetitive stimulation is also blocked. Unlike phenytoin, trimethadione has no effect on PTP in the spinal cord or stellate ganglia. It does, however, modify convulsions produced by spinal cord stimulation, by markedly diminishing the duration of poststimulation discharge without blocking the initiation of the discharge (Esplin and Freston, 1960).

It is unlikely that trimethadione alters presynaptic or postsynaptic inhibition, since it does not antagonize strychnine. In addition, it does not raise the resting threshold for synaptic excitation. It does, however, intensify posttransmission depression and is competitive with pentylenetetrazol, which is thought to stimulate excitatory synapses. Its main effect is to block transmission of repetitive impulses without impairing transmission of single impulses. This effect could decrease the tendency for self-sustained discharge and probably underlies the ability of trimethadione to elevate seizure threshold.

The molecular basis for the anticonvulsant effect of trimethadione has not been elucidated, but the underlying mechanism may be a reduction of potassium permeability of neurons. Gross and Woodbury (1972) noted that pentylenetetrazol increases the short-circuit current across the epithelial cells of the toad bladder, by increasing the outward K^+ flux across the serosal surface. This effect was inhibited by trimethadione in concentrations comparable to those that antagonize pentylenetetrazol convulsions in mice. For reasons noted above, a similar reduction of K^+ permeability of neurons by trimethadione could explain its anticonvulsant effects.

Absorption, Distribution, Biotransformation, and Excretion. Trimethadione is rapidly absorbed from the gastrointestinal tract; the peak plasma concentration after a single dose occurs in ½ to 2 hours (Frey and Schulz, 1970). It is not bound significantly to plasma proteins and is uniformly distributed in tissues, including brain. Its apparent volume of distribution is 60% of body weight. Trimethadione is largely demethylated by the hepatic microsomal enzymes to the active metabolite dimethadione (Butler et al., 1965). Dimethadione is not further metabolized but is excreted unchanged in the urine with a half-time of 6 to 13 days. During chronic medication, the metabolite accumulates and is responsible for the major activity of the medication. (See Symposium, 1972a.)

Toxicity. The most common undesired effects of trimethadione are *sedation* and *hemeralopia* (blurring of vision in bright light or glare effect). The latter appears to be an effect upon the neural layers of the retina rather than on the photochemical process (Sloan and Gilger, 1947). Hemeralopia does not usually require discontinuation of medication and can be overcome by the use of tinted glasses. Children are not as susceptible as adults. Drowsiness tends to diminish with continued medication. Trimethadione may also precipitate generalized *tonic-clonic seizures* in some patients with absence seizures associated with grand mal.

Less common but more serious untoward effects include *exfoliative dermatitis* and other *skin rashes, blood dyscrasias, hepatitis,* and *nephrosis.* Fatalities have been reported. Moderate *neutropenia* is not uncommon (incidence as high as 20%); fulminating *pancytopenia* and *aplastic anemia* have occurred. *Lupus erythematosus* and *lymphadenopathy* have been observed. A *myasthenic syndrome* has also been reported (Booker et al., 1968). (See Gallagher, in Symposium, 1972a.)

Preparations and Dosage. *Trimethadione,* U.S.P. (TRIDIONE), is available for oral use as 300-mg capsules, 150-mg sweetened tablets, and a flavored solution (40 mg/ml). The usual daily dose is 900 to 2100 mg for adults and 20 to 60 mg/kg (300 to 900 mg) for children. However, larger doses are sometimes necessary, and dosage is individualized for each patient to provide maximal efficacy with minimal side effects. Although commonly administered in divided doses, once-daily medication may be satisfactory.

Plasma Drug Concentrations. During chronic medication, plasma concentration of trimethadione averages 0.6 µg/ml per mg/kg daily dose, with moderate fluctuations between doses. Plasma concentration of the active metabolite dimethadione averages 20 times higher (12 μg/ml per mg/kg) and provides the guide for adjustment of dosage. Several weeks are required to attain the plateau state when therapy is initiated and when dosage is changed. A disproportionately high trimethadione:dimethadione concentration ratio usually implies that the patient has not been taking medication regularly. The plasma concentration of dimethadione must usually be maintained above 700 μg/ml for control of seizures. The relationship between plasma concentration and adverse effects has not been established. (*See* Jensen, 1962; Chamberlin *et al.*, 1965; Symposium, 1972a.)

Drug Interactions. Interactions between trimethadione and other drugs have not been reported. It is prudent to avoid concurrent administration of drugs that produce similar dose-related adverse effects.

Therapeutic Uses. Trimethadione is employed only in the treatment of *absence seizures,* and usually only in patients who are inadequately controlled by or do not tolerate ethosuximide. Because of its potential for serious toxicity, treatment with trimethadione necessitates close medical supervision of the patient, especially during the initial year of therapy. However, its side effects should not prevent full employment of trimethadione when it is indicated and if medication can be adequately supervised.

The therapeutic use of trimethadione and other agents in the treatment of absence seizures is discussed further at the end of the chapter.

PARAMETHADIONE

Paramethadione was first reported to be clinically useful for *absence seizures* by Davis and Lennox (1947). It differs from trimethadione only in the replacement of one of the methyl groups on the carbon in the 5 position by an ethyl substituent. Its pharmacological properties, therapeutic uses, dosage, and toxicity are similar to those of trimethadione.

Paramethadione, U.S.P. (PARADIONE), is available as 150- and 300-mg capsules and in a flavored solution (300 mg/ml).

Although the undesired effects of paramethadione and trimethadione are similar, the reported incidence of serious adverse effects may be less for paramethadione (Lennox and Lennox, 1960). More importantly perhaps, individuals who do not tolerate one of the oxazolidinediones may tolerate the other.

Paramethadione is N-demethylated by the hepatic microsomal enzymes to an active metabolite that is slowly excreted in the urine (Butler and Waddell, 1955). The metabolite accumulates during chronic medication and is probably responsible for most of the anticonvulsant activity of the parent drug, as dimethadione is for trimethadione.

BENZODIAZEPINES

The benzodiazepines are employed clinically primarily as sedative-antianxiety drugs; their pharmacology is presented in detail in Chapters 10 and 12. Discussion in this chapter is limited to consideration of their possible usefulness in the therapy of the epilepsies; in this context, diazepam may be considered the prototype.

DIAZEPAM

Chemistry. The structural formula of diazepam is shown on page 190. Although superficially unrelated chemically, the benzodiazepines and the other antiepileptic agents have a similar steric configuration (Camerman and Camerman, 1970).

Anticonvulsant Properties. In animals, prevention of pentylenetetrazol seizures by the benzodiazepines is more prominent than their modification of the maximal electroshock seizure pattern (Swinyard and Castellion, 1966; Millichap, 1969). In experimental models of epilepsy, they suppress the spread of seizure activity produced by epileptogenic foci in the cortex, thalamus, and limbic structures but do not abolish the abnormal discharge of the focus (*see* Browne and Penry, 1973; Symposium, 1973). In low dosage, the benzodiazepines suppress polysynaptic activity in the spinal cord and decrease neuronal activity in the mesencephalic reticular system. It has been suggested that the anticonvulsant properties (as well as other CNS effects) of the benzodiazepines may result from their mimicking the effects of the putative inhibitory neurotransmitter glycine at strychnine-sensitive synapses (Young *et al.*, 1974).

Absorption, Distribution, Biotransformation, and Excretion. After *intravenous* administration, diazepam exhibits the redistribution kinetics typical of highly lipid-soluble agents. Central effects develop promptly but wane rapidly as the drug is redistributed to other tissues.

Oral absorption of diazepam is adequate, and the peak plasma concentration occurs within 1 to 3 hours after a single dose. Diazepam is highly bound to plasma proteins and tissues. The major metabolite, the N-demethyl derivative, is active; other active metabolites, also produced by the hepatic microsomal enzymes, include the ring-hydroxylated derivative and oxazepam, the product of both reactions. Most of the drug is eliminated in the urine as glucuronides and other inactive metabolites. Both the active parent drug and the active demethyl metabolite have a plasma half-time of 1 to 2 days or longer and accumulate during chronic medication. Their pharmacokinetics have not been adequately characterized. (*See* Symposium, 1973.)

Toxicity. *Cardiovascular* and *respiratory depression* may occur after *intravenous* administration of diazepam, particularly if other anticonvulsants or central depressants have been administered previously. The toxicity of intravenous diazepam has been reviewed by Greenblatt and Koch-Weser (1973).

Sedation is the most prominent side effect of diazepam during *chronic oral* medication; *ataxia* and *incoordination* are also common. Although partial tolerance develops to these effects, they persist to a significant extent. Other undesired effects include *dysarthria, dizziness, inattention,* and *hypotonia. Excitement* occurs occasionally. Effects on behavior are varied but have included *acute psychotic episodes.* Either *increased appetite,* with weight gain, or *anorexia,* with weight loss, may occur. *Increased salivary* and *bronchial secretions* may be troublesome in children. *Seizures* are sometimes exacerbated (*see* below).

Other aspects of the toxicity of the benzodiazepines are discussed in Chapter 12.

Preparations. *Diazepam,* U.S.P. (VALIUM), is available as 2-, 5-, and 10-mg tablets and in solution (5 mg/ml) for injection. The solvent for the commercial parenteral preparation is a propylene glycol-ethanol–water mixture and should not be diluted with aqueous solutions.

Plasma Drug Concentrations. Plasma concentrations of diazepam and its active N-demethyl metabolite associated with clinical efficacy and toxicity have not been established. During chronic oral medication, the concentration of each compound has commonly been between 0.1 and 1 μg/ml. Immediately after intravenous injection, at the time that recurrent seizures are interrupted, the plasma concentration of the parent drug is probably greater than 0.5 μg/ml.

Drug Interactions. Interactions between the benzodiazepines and other drugs are not well documented. Diazepam may increase the plasma concentration of concurrently administered phenytoin and phenobarbital; inducers of the hepatic microsomal enzymes are said to increase the biotransformation of the benzodiazepines.

Therapeutic Uses. The antiepileptic effects of the benzodiazepines have been reviewed by Browne and Penry (1973). Diazepam, administered intravenously, is the agent of choice for interruption of *status epilepticus.* The role of diazepam and the other benzodiazepines for chronic oral therapy of the epilepsies is not well defined but is clearly limited. The use of the benzodiazepines in the treatment of *alcohol* and *sedative-hypnotic withdrawal syndromes* is discussed in Chapter 16.

Status Epilepticus. Administered slowly intravenously, diazepam interrupts recurrent seizures in 80 to 90% of cases, for the most part independently of seizure type or etiology. The usual dose for adults and older children is 5 to 10 mg, as required; as much as 30 mg has been employed. Equipment for maintenance of an airway and for mechanical support of ventilation must be immediately available. Since the effects of intravenous diazepam are terminated by redistribution of the drug, seizures may recur within 30 to 60 minutes and may require additional doses. Appropriate maintenance therapy with other agents should be instituted promptly.

Chronic Oral Therapy. The status of diazepam and the other benzodiazepines for chronic oral therapy of the epilepsies remains uncertain. Most clinical trials have not been adequately controlled, the benzodiazepines have usually been added to other medication, and the various congeners have not been compared with each other or with the established antiepileptic agents. Clinical experience is actually greater with new investigational agents than with those already available for clinical use.

Clinical trials of the benzodiazepines for generalized tonic-clonic, cortical focal, and temporal lobe epilepsy have not been encouraging, and generalized tonic-clonic seizures may be exacerbated. The benzodiazepines may also precipitate status epilepticus in patients with the Lennox-Gastaut syndrome (petit mal variant).

Promising results with the benzodiazepines have been reported for therapy of *infantile myoclonus,* other types of *myoclonic* and *akinetic epilepsy,* and *absence seizures.* Unfortunately, tolerance frequently develops to the antiepileptic effects of the benzodiazepines in these patients. Although efficacy may be regained by increase in dosage, sedation and other undesired effects may become prominent. The recommended daily dose of diazepam, as an adjunct to other therapy in infantile myoclonus and other seizures in young children, is 0.1 to 1 mg/kg (Millichap, 1971). Medication is initiated at low dosage and gradually increased, to minimize the sedative effects.

OTHER BENZODIAZEPINES

Benzodiazepines in addition to diazepam that have had clinical trial as antiepileptic agents include *chlordiazepoxide* (LIBRIUM), *oxazepam* (SERAX), *chlorazepate* (TRANXENE), *nitrazepam* (MOGADON), and *clonazepam* (CLONOPIN). As noted above in the discussion of diazepam, clinical trial of these agents for chronic oral therapy of the epilepsies has been somewhat encouraging but inconclusive. Their status will remain uncertain until they are compared with each other and with the established antiepileptic agents in adequately controlled trials and, most importantly, until the tolerance to their antiepileptic effects is more thoroughly studied and assessed. Similarly, much additional clinical experience is required for evaluation of the role of the more lipid-soluble congeners as intravenous agents for control of status epilepticus.

OTHER ANTIEPILEPTIC AGENTS

ACETYLUREAS

Phenacemide. Phenacemide (phenylacetylurea) is the straight-chain analog of 5-phenylhydantoin. It was introduced by Gibbs and coworkers (1949). Even if its efficacy remained unchallenged, its clinical value and use would be severely limited by its potential for serious toxicity. It has been termed a "drug of last resort" (Coatsworth and Penry, in Symposium, 1972a). Phenacemide should be used only in the therapy of temporal lobe epilepsy refractory to other agents, in association with other drugs, and only if adequate supervision and monitoring are possible. Periodic assessment of hepatic, renal, and bone-marrow function is mandatory. The patient and his family must be alerted to the possible hazards of the drug.

Phenacemide, N.F. (PHENURONE), is available as 500-mg tablets. Usual daily dosage in adults has varied from 1.5 to 5.0 g. Phenacemide is almost completely absorbed from the gastrointestinal tract. Biotransformation by hepatic microsomal enzymes includes inactivation by parahydroxylation of the phenyl substituent; ring closure to form a hydantoin does not occur. Unchanged drug is not excreted in the urine (Everett and Richards, 1952). Plasma concentrations associated with efficacy and safety have not been established.

Serious *adverse effects* of phenacemide severely limit its use and often necessitate withdrawal of the drug. As summarized by Tyler and King (1951), behavioral effects may occur in 17% of patients and include personality changes, aggressive behavior, paranoid and depressive reactions, and acute psychosis. Other adverse effects include gastrointestinal symptoms (8%), skin rash (5%), drowsiness (4%), aplastic anemia (2%), hepatitis (2%), and occasional nephritis. Deaths from aplastic anemia have occurred.

Phenacemide has a broad spectrum of anticonvulsant activity in experimental animals. In nontoxic doses, it abolishes the tonic extensor phase of maximal electroshock seizures, elevates the threshold for electroshock convulsions in normal and hyponatremic animals, and prevents or modifies pentylenetetrazol seizures (Swinyard and Toman, 1950; Brown *et al.,* 1953). High doses of phenacemide in animals cause CNS depression.

Pheneturide. Pheneturide (phenylethylacetylurea, ethylphenacemide; BENURIDE) is not available for clinical use in the United States. It resembles phenacemide in most respects, including the potential for serious adverse effects (Wright, 1965; Vas and Parsonage, 1967). It may increase the plasma concentration of concurrently administered phenobarbital or phenytoin (Huismin *et al.,* 1970). Pheneturide should be employed only in combination with other agents in the therapy of refractory temporal lobe epilepsy. Typical daily dosage for adults is 300 to 1000 mg.

SULFONAMIDES: CARBONIC ANHYDRASE INHIBITORS

Acetazolamide. Acetazolamide, the prototype for the carbonic anhydrase inhibitors, is discussed with the saluretic agents in Chapter 39. It has anticonvulsant properties in animals and is sometimes an effective antiepileptic agent, particularly against absence seizures. However, its usefulness is limited by the rapid development of tolerance. (*See* Lombroso and Forsythe, 1960; Millichap, 1971.) *Acetazolamide,* U.S.P. (DIAMOX), is available as 125- and 250-mg tablets, 500-mg sustained-release capsules, and as a solution (500 mg per vial) for parenteral use.

Acetazolamide is rapidly absorbed from the gastrointestinal tract, is highly bound to plasma proteins, and is eliminated unchanged in the urine. Some pharmacokinetic characteristics are provided in Table 13-2; its effects on acid-base metabolism and its toxicity are discussed in detail in Chapter 39. Adverse effects are minimal when it is employed in moderate dosage for limited periods. Drowsiness and paresthesias may occur at high doses and during prolonged medication. Skin rash and other allergic reactions are not common.

The anticonvulsant properties of the carbonic anhydrase inhibitors resemble those of carbon dioxide. In animals, they abolish the tonic extensor component of maximal electroshock convulsions, elevate seizure threshold, and protect against audiogenic seizures and those produced by withdrawal from high concentrations of carbon dioxide. In the spinal cord, monosynaptic pathways are selectively depressed without effect on synaptic recovery or posttetanic potentiation. Threshold for stimulation of the diencephalon is also increased. These effects may result from inhibition of glial cell carbonic anhydrase, with subsequent accumulation of carbon dioxide and reduced flux of sodium into neurons. (*See* Woodbury and Kemp, 1970.)

Sulthiame. Sulthiame (OSPOLOT, TROLONE) is another carbonic anhydrase inhibitor. It is not available in the United States but has been employed for several years in Europe as an antiepileptic agent, usually in combination with other drugs. Its status is uncertain. Its anticonvulsant properties resemble those of acetazolamide. However, unlike acetazolamide, it is partially inactivated by hydroxylation by hepatic microsomal enzymes. When employed clinically, it may significantly increase the plasma concentration of concurrently administered phenytoin, apparently by inhibition of its inactivation. Such interaction has undoubtedly contributed to its total antiepileptic activity and has caused phenytoin toxicity (Hansen *et al.*, 1968; Houghton and Richens, 1974).

BROMIDE

Bromide, the oldest of the antiepileptic agents, is discussed with the sedative-hypnotics in Chapter 10. It is effective only against generalized tonic-clonic seizures. It has been made obsolete, at least in the United States, by the organic antiepileptic agents.

GENERAL PRINCIPLES AND CHOICE OF DRUGS FOR THE THERAPY OF THE EPILEPSIES

The initial choice of the best possible drug or combination is made on the basis of seizure type, as established by history and EEG. *Medication is selected to "fit the fit."* The physician should become skilled in the *use of the primary agents* (Table 13–2) rather than dabble in sporadic trials of a variety of drugs of limited or uncertain value.

Essential to optimal management of epilepsy is the *filling-out of a seizure chart* by the patient or a relative; *frequent visits to the physician or seizure clinic,* particularly in the early period of treatment, since hematological and other possible somatic side effects require consideration of change in medication; and *long-term follow-up,* including repetition of EEG and neurological examination. Most crucial for successful management is *regularity of medication.*

Even when it is anticipated that multiple-drug therapy will be required, *medication is initiated with a single drug. Initial dosage* is usually that expected to provide a plasma drug concentration during the plateau state at least in the lower portion of the range associated with clinical efficacy. However, to minimize dose-related adverse effects, therapy with some drugs is initiated at reduced dosage, and the clinically effective amount is attained gradually. Loading dosage is employed only if the urgency for control of

seizures exceeds the risk of adverse effects during the initial therapy.

The results of the initial medication should be assessed with appropriate regard for the time required to attain the plateau state, the usual variability of incidence of seizures, and the anticipation that some tolerance usually develops to the sedative and other minor adverse effects of these drugs. Dosage is increased at appropriate intervals, as required for control of seizures or as limited by toxicity, and such adjustment is preferably assisted by monitoring of plasma drug concentration.

If a single drug fails to provide adequate control of seizures in maximal tolerated dosage, *another drug should be substituted or a second drug may be added.* The choice between these alternatives is usually determined by consideration of the adverse effects of the drug in the individual patient. Unless serious adverse effects of the drug dictate otherwise, *drug dosage should always be reduced gradually* when a drug is being discontinued, to minimize the risk of precipitating status epilepticus. No drug should be discarded as useless unless obvious toxicity or monitoring of plasma drug concentration indicates that the patient has actually been taking the medication as prescribed.

Common *causes of failure* of antiepileptic medication are improper diagnosis of the type of seizure, incorrect choice of drug, inadequate or excessive dosage, too frequent changes in medication without regard for the time required for transition between plateau states, failure to utilize fully the advantages of multiple-drug medication, inattention to ancillary aspects of therapy, and poor compliance by the patient. Poor compliance may take the form of erratic medication, with only partial control of seizures; consistent failure to take medication, with failure ever to attain adequate drug concentration; or excessive medication, with needless toxicity. Poor compliance sometimes persists despite the best efforts of the physician, but it can usually be corrected. Similarly, failure of therapy because of inattention to recommendations about diet, rest, avoidance of alcohol, and similar ancillary factors can usually be prevented.

Measurement of *plasma drug concentration* at appropriate intervals greatly facilitates the

Table 13-2. TYPICAL THERAPEUTIC USES, USUAL DOSAGE, AND SOME PHARMACOKINETIC CHARACTERISTICS OF ANTIEPILEPTIC AGENTS

DRUG	TYPICAL THERAPEUTIC USES *	USUAL ORAL MAINTENANCE DOSE † Adults (mg/day)	Children (mg/kg/day)	PLASMA PROTEIN BINDING (%)	PLASMA HALF-TIME ‡ Adults	PLASMA CONCENTRATION FOR EFFICACY §,¶ (µg/ml)
Primary Agents						
Phenobarbital	GTC, CF, F	60–300	2–5	40–60	2–6 days[a]	10–30[b]
Primidone	GTC, CF, TL	500–1500	5–20	0	Primidone: 3–12+ hr PEMA: 1–2 days Phenobarbital: 2–6 days	Judged by phenobarbital metabolite: as above[c]
Phenytoin	GTC, CF, TL	200–400	4–8	70–95	Low concentration: 7–42 hr[d] High concentration: dose dependent	10–20[e]
Ethosuximide	A	750–2000	20–60	0	2–3 days[f]	40–100
Other Barbiturates						
Mephobarbital	GTC, CF	120–600	4–10		Mephobarbital: shorter than phenobarbital Phenobarbital: 2–6 days	Judged by phenobarbital metabolite: as above
Other Hydantoins						
Mephenytoin	GTC, CF, TL	300–600	3–10		Mephenytoin: shorter than metabolite Metabolite: NIRVANOL; half-time not reported	—[g]
Ethotoin	GTC	2000–3000				
Other Succinimides						
Methsuximide	A, TL	300–1200	20–60	0	Methsuximide: 2–4 hr Metabolite: longer than methsuximide Phensuximide: about 4 hr	—[g]

Drug	Seizure types				Half-time (t½)	Plasma concentration (µg/ml)
...imethadione				0	...imethadione: 12–24 hr	
Paramethadione	A	900–2100	20–60	0	Dimethadione: 6–13 days Paramethadione: shorter than metabolite Metabolite: similar to dimethadione	Judged by dimethadione metabolite: 700 —g
Other Agents						
Carbamazepine	GTC, CF, TL	600–1200		80	Carbamazepine: 12–30+ hr	—g,h
Diazepam	M		0.1–1	80–90	Diazepam: 1–2+ days Metabolite: 1–2+ days	
Acetazolamide	A, GTC, CF	500–1000	10–30	90	4–10 hr	—h
Phenacemide	TL	1500–5000			12 days	—i
Bromide	GTC	not recommended		0		

* GTC Generalized tonic-clonic (grand mal) seizures
CF Cortical focal seizures
TL Temporal lobe (psychomotor) seizures
A Absence (petit mal) seizures
M Myoclonic spasms
F Febrile convulsions
† See text for parenteral doses for status epilepticus.
‡ Compounds listed include active metabolites.
§ Range that provides at least partial control and possibly complete control in the majority of patients.
¶ For most drugs, plasma concentration associated with toxicity varies with the development of tolerance (see text).

a Phenobarbital half-time for children: 36 to 72 hr.
b For prophylaxis against febrile convulsions, phenobarbital concentration must be maintained above 15 µg/ml.
c Significant ataxia and lethargy occur in most patients if primidone concentration exceeds 10 µg/ml.
d Phenytoin half-time for children: shorter than for adults and also dose dependent.
e Efficacy may be attained at phenytoin concentration as low as 8 µg/ml; nystagmus may be present at concentrations as low as 15 µg/ml.
f Ethosuximide half-time for children: 1 to 2 days.
g Active metabolite contributes significantly to efficacy and must be considered in interpretation of plasma drug concentrations.
h Tolerance develops to antiepileptic effect.
i Bromide intoxication should be suspected if the plasma concentration exceeds 9 mEq per liter.

initial adjustment of dosage for individual differences in drug elimination and the *subsequent adjustment* of dosage to minimize dose-related adverse effects without sacrifice of seizure control. If seizure control is less than complete, monitoring can assist in the choice between adjusting dosage of the existing medication, substituting an alternative drug, or adding a second drug. Periodic monitoring during *maintenance therapy* can detect failure of the patient to take the medication as prescribed; for the patient with infrequent seizures and apparent control, periodic monitoring can provide assurance that seizure control is, in fact, being maintained. Knowledge of plasma drug concentration can be especially helpful during *multiple-drug therapy.* If toxicity occurs, monitoring helps to identify the particular drug responsible, and, if pharmacokinetic drug interaction occurs, it can guide readjustment of dosage. In general, monitoring of plasma drug concentrations during antiepileptic therapy is likely to be an aid whenever therapy is less than satisfactory or whenever it is associated with toxicity or an unexpected or atypical clinical response.

The following paragraphs present a brief summary of the choice of drugs for specific types of epilepsy.

Generalized Tonic-Clonic (Grand Mal) and Cortical Focal Seizures. Phenytoin may abolish generalized tonic-clonic seizures completely in 60 to 65% of patients and reduce their frequency and severity in another 20%. Phenobarbital is somewhat less effective but is usually the agent of choice since it is less toxic and less expensive. Concurrent administration of the two drugs is often advantageous. The differing side effects of these two drugs permit full dosage of each and, therefore, a relatively greater common anticonvulsant effect. The combined use is also of value because the full effect of phenytoin alone may leave a residuum of focal seizures, aura or prodromata, or a subclinical focal EEG dysrhythmia. This residuum can be prevented by concurrent use of phenobarbital. Conversely, the combined use of the two drugs is advantageous in mixed generalized tonic-clonic and temporal lobe seizures because phenobarbital alone is usually ineffective against the latter component.

Primidone alone may be effective in patients refractory to phenytoin and phenobarbital. However, it is more commonly employed concurrently with phenytoin. Since it is metabolized in part to phenobarbital, primidone is logically a substitute for, not a supplement to, phenobarbital. Mephenytoin is sometimes dramatically superior to phenytoin, but

the advantage is offset by the greater risk of serious toxicity.

Cortical focal seizures of most types, motor or sensory, respond almost as well to appropriate medication as do generalized tonic-clonic seizures.

Absence (Petit Mal) Seizures. Trimethadione was the first agent of selective benefit against absence seizures in children (Lennox, 1945; Richards and Perlstein, 1946). As a result, its reputation has somewhat exceeded its true worth. Ethosuximide is more effective and has a lower risk of serious toxicity; it is now considered the agent of choice. Complete control of absence seizures can be attained in about 50% of patients and significant reduction in seizure frequency is achieved in another 25%. Trimethadione or the other agents effective against absence seizures are employed in patients refractory to ethosuximide.

Phenytoin, phenobarbital, and primidone are ineffective against absence seizures and may increase their frequency, but medication with one of these agents is required in the majority of patients as additional therapy against the emergence of generalized tonic-clonic seizures (Livingston *et al.,* 1965).

Partial Seizures with Complex Symptomatology (Temporal Lobe, Psychomotor Seizures). Temporal lobe seizures are often more refractory to medication than are other cortical focal types. Phenobarbital is rarely effective; phenytoin and primidone are the agents of choice. Although either agent alone may be effective, combined use of the two is more frequently satisfactory. If necessary, mephenytoin may be substituted for phenytoin, or methsuximide may be added. The ultimate position of carbamazepine in this sequence will depend upon clarification of its toxic potential. Phenacemide, in combination with other agents, may be employed if safer medications fail.

Seizures in Infants and Young Children. *Infantile myoclonic spasms* with *hypsarhythmia* are refractory to the usual antiepileptic agents; corticotropin or the adrenocorticosteroids are the agents of choice. The earlier the diagnosis is established and treatment initiated, the more successful is therapy. Diazepam or another benzodiazepine may be a useful adjunct, but tolerance is usually prominent.

Primidone, possibly with a benzodiazepine as an adjunct, may be effective against *myoclonic, akinetic,* and *atonic* seizures in young children. Phenobarbital provides effective prophylaxis against *febrile* convulsions; it may also be employed, with appropriate antipyretic therapy, for treatment of febrile convulsions.

Phenytoin is relatively ineffective and may produce restlessness and hyperactivity when employed in young children (Laurance, 1970). Phenobarbital is the drug of choice for generalized tonic-clonic seizures in children under 5 years of age.

Status Epilepticus and Other Convulsive Emergencies. Diazepam, administered intravenously, is the agent of choice for control of *status epilepticus.* It is effective in 80 to 90% of cases, largely independent of seizure type or etiology. Phenobarbital or phenytoin may also be employed intravenously. The latter agent must be administered at a rate less than 50 mg per minute, and even more slowly in elderly patients, to minimize the risk of central and cardiovascular toxicity. Whatever agent is employed, equipment for maintenance of an airway and for mechanical support of ventilation must be immediately available.

As discussed in Chapter 9, convulsive emergencies associated with *drug poisoning* and *drug-induced seizures* in previously nonepileptic patients during medication with agents such as the local anesthetics may also be controlled by diazepam or phenobarbital or another barbiturate. The control of *drug-withdrawal seizures* associated with abuse of alcohol, barbiturates, or related sedative-hypnotics is discussed in Chapter 16.

Antiepileptic Therapy and Pregnancy. Children of epileptic mothers who received anticonvulsant medication during the early months of pregnancy have a twofold to threefold increase in incidence of a variety of birth defects. Evidence is greatest for therapy with phenobarbital or phenytoin, and there is suggestive evidence for a similar relationship for other antiepileptic agents. None can yet be absolved.

Most (> 90%) epileptic mothers treated with antiepileptic drugs bear normal children. In addition, epilepsy itself probably carries a risk of fetal defects, and abrupt discontinuation of medication incurs a definite risk of status epilepticus and its hazards for the fetus and mother. For these reasons, antiepileptic medication should *not* be discontinued in pregnant epileptic women for whom the medication is necessary for the prevention of major seizures. However, depending upon the frequency and severity of seizures in the *individual patient,* cautious reduction of dosage to a minimum may be feasible and advisable, particularly in the first trimester. Folic acid deficiency, if present, should be corrected. (*See* Fedrick, 1973; Lowe, 1973; Monson *et al.,* 1973.)

The newborn of mothers who received phenobarbital, primidone, or phenytoin during pregnancy may also develop a deficiency of vitamin K–dependent clotting factors, and serious hemorrhage may occur during the first 24 hours of life. Bleeding can be prevented by administration of vitamin K.

Arnold, K., and Gerber, N. The rate of decline of diphenylhydantoin in human plasma. *Clin. Pharmac. Ther.,* **1970,** *11,* 121–134.

Aston, R., and Domino, E. F. Differential effects of phenobarbital, pentobarbital and diphenylhydantoin on motor cortical and reticular thresholds in the rhesus monkey. *Psychopharmacologia,* **1961,** *2,* 304–317.

Bárány, E. H., and Stein-Jensen, E. The mode of action of anticonvulsant drugs on electrically induced convulsions in the rabbit. *Archs int. Pharmacodyn. Thér.,* **1946,** *73,* 1–47.

Blom, S. Tic douloureux treated with new anticonvulsant. *Archs Neurol., Chicago,* **1963,** *9,* 285–290.

Bogue, J. Y., and Carrington, H. C. The evaluation of "MYSOLINE"—a new anticonvulsant drug. *Br. J. Pharmac. Chemother.,* **1953,** *8,* 230–236.

Booker, H. E.; Chun, R. W. M.; and Sanguino, M. Myasthenic syndrome associated with trimethadione. *Neurology, Minneap.,* **1968,** *18,* 274.

Brown, W. C.; Schiffman, D. O.; Swinyard, E. A.; and Goodman, L. S. Comparative assay of antiepileptic drugs by "psychomotor" seizure test and minimal electroshock threshold test. *J. Pharmac. exp. Ther.,* **1953,** *107,* 273–283.

Browne, T. R., and Penry, J. K. Benzodiazepines in the treatment of epilepsy: a review. *Epilepsia,* **1973,** *14,* 277–310.

Brumlik, J., and Moretti, L. The effect of diphenylhydantoin on nerve conduction velocity. *Neurology, Minneap.,* **1966,** *16,* 1217–1218.

Buchthal, F., and Svensmark, O. Serum concentrations of diphenylhydantoin (phenytoin) and phenobarbital and their relation to therapeutic and toxic effects. *Psychiat. Neurol. Neurochir.,* **1971,** *74,* 117–136.

Buchthal, F.; Svensmark, O.; and Schiller, P. J. Clinical and electroencephalographic correlation with serum levels of diphenylhydantoin. *Archs Neurol., Chicago,* **1960,** *2,* 624–630.

Buchthal, F.; Svensmark, O.; and Simonsen, H. Relation of EEG and seizures to phenobarbital in serum. *Archs Neurol., Chicago,* **1968,** *19,* 567–572.

Butler, T. C. Quantitative studies of the physiological disposition of 3-methyl-5-ethyl-5-phenyl hydantoin (MESANTOIN) and 5-ethyl-5-phenyl hydantoin (NIRVANOL). *J. Pharmac. exp. Ther.,* **1953,** *109,* 340–345.

——. The metabolic hydroxylation of phenobarbital. *Ibid.,* **1956,** *116,* 326–336.

Butler, T. C., and Waddell, W. J. A pharmacological comparison of the optical isomers of 5-ethyl-5-methyl-2,4-oxazolidinedione and of 3,4-dimethyl-5-ethyl-2,4-oxazolidinedione (paramethadione, PARADIONE). *J. Pharmac. exp. Ther.,* **1955,** *113,* 238–240.

Butler, T. C.; Waddell, W. J.; and Poole, D. T. Demethylation of trimethadione and metharbital by rat liver microsomal enzymes: substrate concentration-yield relationships and competition between substrates. *Biochem. Pharmac.,* **1965,** *14,* 937–942.

Camerman, A., and Camerman, M. Diphenylhydantoin and diazepam. Molecular structure similarities and steric basis of anticonvulsant activity. *Science, Wash.,* **1970,** *168,* 1457–1458.

Cereghino, J. J.; Brock, J. T.; Van Meter, J. C.; Penry, J. K.; Smith, L. D.; and White, B. G. Carbamazepine for epilepsy. A controlled prospective evaluation. *Neurology, Minneap.,* **1974,** *24,* 401–410.

Chamberlin, H. R.; Waddell, W. J.; and Butler, T. C. A study of the product of demethylation of trimethadione in the control of petit mal epilepsy. *Neurology, Minneap.,* **1965,** *15,* 449–454.

Chang, T.; Okerholm, R. A.; and Glazko, A. J. Identification of 5-(3,4-dihydroxyphenyl)-5-phenylhydantoin: a metabolite of 5,5-diphenylhydantoin (DILANTIN) in rat urine. *Anal. Letters,* **1972,** *5,* 195–202.

Chang, T.; Savory, A.; and Glazko, A. J. A new metabolite of 5,5-diphenylhydantoin (DILANTIN). *Biochem. biophys. Res. Commun.,* **1970,** *38,* 444–449.

Chen, G.; Weston, J. K.; and Bratton, A. C., Jr. Anticonvulsant activity and toxicity of phensuximide, methsuximide and ethosuximide. *Epilepsia,* **1963,** *4,* 66–76.

Christiansen, J., and Dam, M. Influence of phenobarbital and diphenylhydantoin on plasma carbamazepine levels in patients with epilepsy. *Acta neurol. scand.,* **1973,** *49,* 543–546.

Crill, W. E. Carbamazepine. *Ann. intern. Med.,* **1973,** *79,* 844–847.

Dam, M. The density and ultrastructure of the Purkinje cells following diphenylhydantoin treatment in animals and man. *Acta neurol. scand.,* **1972,** *48,* Suppl. 49, 1–65.

Davis, J. P., and Lennox, W. G. The effect of trimethyloxazolidine dione and dimethyl ethyloxazolidine dione on seizures and on the blood. *Proc. Ass. Res. nerv. ment. Dis.,* **1947,** *36,* 423–436.

Delgado, J. M. R., and Mihailović, L. Use of intracerebral electrodes to evaluate drugs that act on the central nervous system. *Ann. N.Y. Acad. Sci.,* **1956,** *64,* 644–666.

Dill, W. A.; Kazenko, A.; Wolf, L. M.; and Glazko, A. J. Studies on 5,5-diphenylhydantoin (DILANTIN) in animals and man. *J. Pharmac. exp. Ther.,* **1956,** *118,* 270–279.

Dudley, K. H.; Bius, D. L.; and Grace, M. E. Metabolic fates of N-methyl-α-phenylsuccinimide (phensuximide, MILONTIN) and of α-phenylsuccinimide in the dog. *J. Pharmac. exp. Ther.,* **1972,** *180,* 167–179.

Dudley, K. H.; Bius, D. L.; and Waldrop, C. D. Urinary metabolites of N-methyl-α-methyl-α-phenylsuccinimide (methsuximide) in the dog. *Drug Metab. Disposition,* **1974,** *2,* 113–122.

Escueta, A. V., and Reilly, E. L. The effects of diphenylhydantoin on potassium transport within synaptic terminals of the epileptogenic foci. *Neurology, Minneap.,* **1971,** *21,* 418.

Esplin, D. W. Effects of diphenylhydantoin on synaptic transmission in cat spinal cord and stellate ganglion. *J. Pharmac. exp. Ther.,* **1957,** *120,* 301–323.

Esplin, D. W., and Curto, E. M. Effects of trimethadione on synaptic transmission in the spinal cord; antagonism of trimethadione and pentylenetetrazol. *J. Pharmac. exp. Ther.,* **1957,** *121,* 457–467.

Esplin, D. W., and Freston, J. W. Physiological and pharmacological analysis of spinal cord convulsions. *J. Pharmac. exp. Ther.,* **1960,** *130,* 68–80.

Everett, G. M., and Richards, R. K. Comparative anticonvulsant action of 3,5,5-trimethyloxazolidine-2,4-dione (TRIDIONE), DILANTIN and phenobarbital. *J. Pharmac. exp. Ther.,* **1944,** *81,* 402–407.

———. Pharmacological studies of phenacetylurea (PHENURONE), an anticonvulsant drug. *Ibid.,* **1952,** *106,* 303–313.

Fedrick, J. Epilepsy and pregnancy: a report from the Oxford Record Linkage Study. *Br. med. J.,* **1973,** *2,* 442–448.

Fertziger, A. P.; Liuzzi, S. E.; and Dunham, P. B. Diphenylhydantoin (DILANTIN): stimulation of potassium influx in lobster axons. *Brain Res.,* **1971,** *33,* 592–596.

Fertziger, A. P., and Ranck, J. B., Jr. Potassium accumulation in interstitial space during epileptiform seizures. *Expl Neurol.,* **1970,** *26,* 571–585.

Festoff, B. W., and Appel, S. H. Effect of diphenylhydantoin on synaptosome sodium-potassium-ATPase. *J. clin. Invest.,* **1968,** *47,* 2752–2758.

Formby, B. The *in vivo* and *in vitro* effect of diphenylhydantoin and phenobarbitone on K⁺-activated phosphohydrolase and (Na⁺,K⁺)-activated ATPase in particulate membrane fractions from rat brain. *J. Pharm. Pharmac.,* **1970,** *22,* 81–85.

Frey, H. H., and Schulz, R. Time course of the demethylation of trimethadione. *Acta pharmac. tox.,* **1970,** *28,* 477–483.

Fromm, G. H., and Killian, J. M. Effect of some anticonvulsant drugs on the spinal trigeminal nucleus. *Neurology, Minneap.,* **1967,** *17,* 275–280.

Gangloff, H., and Monnier, M. The action of anticonvul-

sant drugs tested by electrical stimulation of the rabbit cortex, diencephalon and rhinencephalon in the unanesthetized rabbit. *Electroenceph. clin. Neurophysiol.,* **1957,** *9,* 43–58.

Gastaut, H. Clinical and electroencephalographical classification of epileptic seizures. *Epilepsia,* **1970,** *11,* 102–113.

Gibbs, F. A.; Everett, G. M.; and Richards, R. K. PHENURONE in epilepsy. *Dis. nerv. Syst.,* **1949,** *10,* 47–49.

Glazko, A. J. Diphenylhydantoin. *Pharmacology,* **1972,** *8,* 163–177.

———. Diphenylhydantoin metabolism: a prospective review. *Drug Metab. Disposition,* **1973,** *1,* 711–714.

Goodman, L. S.; Swinyard, E. A.; Brown, W. C.; Schiffman, D. O.; Grewal, M. S.; and Bliss, E. L. Anticonvulsant properties of 5-phenyl-5-ethyl-hexahydropyrimidine-4,6-dione (MYSOLINE), a new antiepileptic. *J. Pharmac. exp. Ther.,* **1953,** *108,* 428–436.

Goodman, L. S.; Toman, J. E. P.; and Swinyard, E. A. The anticonvulsant properties of TRIDIONE: laboratory and clinical investigations. *Am. J. Med.,* **1946,** *1,* 213–228.

———. Anticonvulsant properties of 5,5-phenyl thienyl hydantoin in comparison with DILANTIN and MESANTOIN. *Proc. Soc. exp. Biol. Med.,* **1948,** *68,* 584–587.

Greenblatt, D. J., and Koch-Weser, J. Adverse reactions to intravenous diazepam: a report from the Boston Collaborative Drug Surveillance Program. *Am. J. med. Sci.,* **1973,** *266,* 261–266.

Gross, G. J., and Woodbury, D. M. Effects of pentylenetetrazol on ion transport in the isolated toad bladder. *J. Pharmac. exp. Ther.,* **1972,** *181,* 257–272.

Halpern, L. M., and Julien, R. M. Augmentation of cerebellar Purkinje cell discharge rate after diphenylhydantoin. *Epilepsia,* **1972,** *13,* 377–385.

Handley, R., and Stewart, A. S. R. MYSOLINE: a new drug in the treatment of epilepsy. *Lancet,* **1952,** *1,* 742–744.

Hansen, J. M.; Kristensen, M.; and Skovsted, L. Sulthiame (OSPOLOT) as inhibitor of diphenylhydantoin metabolism. *Epilepsia,* **1968,** *9,* 17–22.

Hauptmann, A. LUMINAL bei Epilepsie. *Münch. med. Wschr.,* **1912,** *59,* 1907–1909.

Houghton, G. W., and Richens, A. Inhibition of phenytoin metabolism by sulthiame in epileptic patients. *Br. J. clin. Pharmac.,* **1974,** *1,* 59–66.

Huisman, J. W.; Van Heycop Ten Ham, M. W.; and Van Zije, C. H. Influence of ethylphenacemide on serum levels of other anti-epileptic drugs. *Epilepsia,* **1970,** *11,* 207–215.

Iannone, A.; Baker, A. B.; and Morrell, F. DILANTIN in the treatment of neuralgia. *Neurology, Minneap.,* **1958,** *8,* 126–128.

Jensen, B. N. Trimethadione in serum of patients with petit mal epilepsy. *Dan. med. Bull.,* **1962,** *9,* 74–79.

Julien, R. M., and Halpern, L. M. Effects of diphenylhydantoin and other antiepileptic drugs on epileptiform activity and Purkinje cell discharge rates. *Epilepsia,* **1972,** *13,* 387–400.

Karch, S. B. Methsuximide overdose: delayed onset of profound coma. *J. Am. med. Ass.,* **1973,** *223,* 1463–1465.

Kiser, J. S.; Vargas-Cordon, M.; Brendel, K.; and Bressler, R. The *in vitro* inhibition of insulin secretion by diphenylhydantoin. *J. clin. Invest.,* **1970,** *49,* 1942–1948.

Korey, S. R. Effects of DILANTIN and MESANTOIN on the giant axon of the squid. *Proc. Soc. exp. Biol. Med.,* **1951,** *76,* 297–299.

Kutt, H.; Wolk, M.; Scherman, R.; and McDowell, F. Insufficient parahydroxylation as a cause of diphenylhydantoin toxicity. *Neurology, Minneap.,* **1964,** *14,* 542–548.

Laurance, B. M. Idiopathic epilepsy. *Practitioner,* **1970,** *205,* 331–332.

Lennox, W. G. The petit mal epilepsies: their treatment with TRIDIONE. *J. Am. med. Ass.,* **1945,** *129,* 1069–1073.

Levin, S. R.; Booker, J., Jr.; Smith, D. F.; and Grodsky, G. M. Inhibition of insulin secretion by diphenylhydantoin in the isolated perfused pancreas. *J. clin. Endocr. Metab.*, **1970**, *30*, 400–401.

Lewin, E., and Bleck, V. The effect of diphenylhydantoin administration on cortex potassium-activated phosphatase. *Neurology, Minneap.*, **1971a**, *21*, 417–418.

——. The effect of diphenylhydantoin administration on sodium-potassium-activated ATPase in cortex. *Ibid.*, **1971b**, *21*, 647–651.

Lipicky, R. J.; Gilbert, D. L.; and Stillman, I. M. Diphenylhydantoin inhibition of sodium conductance in the squid giant axon. *Proc. natn. Acad. Sci. U.S.A.*, **1972**, *69*, 1758–1760.

Livingston, S.; Pauli, L. L.; and German, W. Carbamazepine (TEGRETOL) in epilepsy. Nine year follow-up study with special emphasis on untoward reactions. *Dis. nerv. Syst.*, **1974**, *35*, 103–107.

Livingston, S.; Torres, I.; Pauli, L. L.; and Rider, R. V. Petit mal epilepsy: results of a prolonged follow-up study of 117 patients. *J. Am. med. Ass.*, **1965**, *194*, 227–232.

Lombroso, C. T., and Forsythe, I. A long term follow-up of acetazolamide (DIAMOX) in the treatment of epilepsy. *Epilepsia*, **1960**, *1*, 493–500.

Loscalzo, A. E. MESANTOIN in the control of epilepsy. *Neurology, Minneap.*, **1952**, *2*, 403–411.

Lowe, C. R. Congenital malformations among infants born to epileptic women. *Lancet*, **1973**, *1*, 9–10.

Melchior, J. C.; Buchthal, F.; and Lennox-Buchthal, M. The ineffectiveness of diphenylhydantoin in preventing febrile convulsions in the age of greatest risk, under three years. *Epilepsia*, **1971**, *12*, 55–62.

Merritt, H. H., and Putnam, T. J. A new series of anticonvulsant drugs tested by experiments on animals. *Archs Neurol. Psychiat., Chicago*, **1938a**, *39*, 1003–1015.

——. Sodium diphenyl hydantoinate in treatment of convulsive disorders. *J. Am. med. Ass.*, **1938b**, *111*, 1068–1073.

Millichap, J. G. Relation of laboratory evaluation to clinical effectiveness of antiepileptic drugs. *Epilepsia*, **1969**, *10*, 315–328.

——. Drug therapy and management of the child with epilepsy. *Drug Ther.*, **1971**, *1*, No. 10, 15–29.

Monson, R. R.; Rosenberg, L.; Hartz, S. C.; Shapiro, S.; Heinonen, O. P.; and Slone, D. Diphenylhydantoin and selected congenital malformations. *New Engl. J. Med.*, **1973**, *289*, 1049–1052.

Morrell, F.; Bradley, W.; and Ptashne, M. Effect of diphenylhydantoin on peripheral nerve. *Neurology, Minneap.*, **1958**, *8*, 140–144.

——. Effects of drugs on discharge characteristics of chronic epileptogenic lesions. *Ibid.*, **1959**, *9*, 492–498.

Perlstein, M. A. GEMONAL (5,5-diethyl 1-methyl barbituric acid): a new drug for convulsive and related disorders. *Pediatrics, Springfield*, **1950**, *5*, 448–451.

——. Metharbital (GEMONIL) in myoclonic spasms of infancy and related disorders. *A.M.A. J. Dis. Child.*, **1957**, *93*, 425–429.

Perlstein, M. A., and Andelman, M. B. TRIDIONE: its use in convulsive and related disorders. *J. Pediat.*, **1946**, *29*, 20–40.

Peter, J. B. A (Na$^+$K$^+$)-ATPase of sarcolemma from skeletal muscle. *Biochem. biophys. Res. Commun.*, **1970**, *40*, 1362–1367.

Pincus, J. H.; Grove, I.; Marino, B. B.; and Glaser, G. E. Studies on the mechanisms of action of diphenylhydantoin. *Archs Neurol., Chicago*, **1970**, *22*, 566–577.

Pincus, J. H., and Rawson, M. D. Diphenylhydantoin and intracellular sodium concentration. *Neurology, Minneap.*, **1969**, *19*, 419–422.

Plaa, G. L., and Hine, C. H. Hydantoin and barbiturate blood levels observed in epileptics. *Archs int. Pharmacodyn. Thér.*, **1960**, *78*, 375–382.

Pollen, D. A., and Tractenberg, M. C. Neuroglia: gliosis and focal epilepsy. *Science, Wash.*, **1970**, *167*, 1252–1253.

Rane, A.; Lunde, P. K. M.; Jalling, B.; Yaffee, S. J.; and

Sjöqvist, F. Plasma protein binding of diphenylhydantoin in normal and hyperbilirubinemic infants. *Pediat. Pharmac. Ther.*, **1971**, *78*, 877–882.

Rawson, M. D., and Pincus, J. H. The effect of diphenylhydantoin on sodium, potassium, magnesium-activated adenosine triphosphatase in microsomal fractions of rat and guinea pig brain and on whole homogenates of human brain. *Biochem. Pharmac.*, **1968**, *17*, 573–579.

Reidenberg, M. M.; Odar-Cedarlöf, I.; von Bahr, C.; Borgå, O.; and Sjöqvist, F. Protein binding of diphenylhydantoin and desmethylimipramine in plasma from patients with poor renal function. *New Engl. J. Med.*, **1971**, *285*, 264–267.

Richards, R. K., and Perlstein, M. A. TRIDIONE, a new drug for the treatment of convulsive and related disorders. *Archs Neurol. Psychiat., Chicago*, **1946**, *55*, 164–165.

Rosati, R. A.; Alexander, J. A.; Schaals, S. F.; and Wallace, A. G. Influence of diphenylhydantoin on electrophysiological properties of the canine heart. *Circulation Res.*, **1967**, *21*, 757–765.

Rosenberg, P., and Bartels, E. Drug effects on the spontaneous electrical activity of the squid giant axon. *J. Pharmac. exp. Ther.*, **1967**, *155*, 532–544.

Schallek, W., and Kuehn, A. Effects of trimethadione, diphenylhydantoin, and chlordiazepoxide on afterdischarges in brain of cat. *Proc. Soc. exp. Biol. Med.*, **1963**, *112*, 813–817.

Schwade, E. D.; Richards, R. K.; and Everett, G. M. PEGANONE, a new antiepileptic drug. *Dis. nerv. Syst.*, **1956**, *17*, 155–158.

Siegel, G. J., and Goodwin, B. B. Effects of 5,5-diphenylhydantoin (DPH) and 5-p-hydroxyphenyl-5-phenylhydantoin (HPPH) on brain Na$^+$-K$^+$-ATPase. *Neurology, Minneap.*, **1971**, *21*, 417.

Sloan, L. L., and Gilger, A. P. Visual effects of TRIDIONE. *Am. J. Ophthal.*, **1947**, *30*, 1387–1405.

Sorrell, T. C.; Forbes, I. J.; Burness, F. R.; and Rischbieth, R. H. C. Depression of immunological function in patients treated with phenytoin sodium (sodium diphenylhydantoin). *Lancet*, **1971**, *2*, 1233–1235.

Strobos, R. R. J., and Spudis, E. V. Effect of anticonvulsant drugs on cortical and subcortical seizure discharges in cats. *Archs Neurol., Chicago*, **1960**, *2*, 399–406.

Strong, J. M.; Abe, T.; Gibbs, E. L.; and Atkinson, A. J., Jr. Plasma levels of methsuximide and N-desmethylmethsuximide during methsuximide therapy. *Neurology, Minneap.*, **1974**, *24*, 250–255.

Svensmark, O., and Buchthal, F. Accumulation of phenobarbital in man. *Epilepsia*, **1963**, *4*, 199–206.

Swanson, P. D., and Crane, P. Diphenylhydantoin and the cations and phosphates of electrically stimulated brain slices. *Neurology, Minneap.*, **1970**, *20*, 1119–1123.

Swinyard, E. A., and Castellion, A. W. Anticonvulsant properties of some benzodiazepines. *J. Pharmac. exp. Ther.*, **1966**, *151*, 369–375.

Swinyard, E. A., and Toman, J. E. P. A comparison of the anticonvulsant actions of some phenylhydantoins and their corresponding phenylacetylureas. *J. Pharmac. exp. Ther.*, **1950**, *100*, 151–157.

Toman, J. E. P.; Loewe, S.; and Goodman, L. S. Physiology and therapy of convulsive disorders. I. Effect of anticonvulsant drugs on electroshock seizures in man. *Archs Neurol. Psychiat., Chicago*, **1947**, *58*, 312–324.

Toman, J. E. P., and Sabelli, H. C. Comparative neuronal mechanisms. *Epilepsia*, **1969**, *10*, 179–192.

Toman, J. E. P.; Swinyard, E. A.; and Goodman, L. S. Properties of maximal seizures, and their alteration by anticonvulsant drugs and other agents. *J. Neurophysiol.*, **1946**, *9*, 231–240.

Tyler, M. W., and King, E. Q. Phenacemide in treatment of epilepsy. *J. Am. med. Ass.*, **1951**, *147*, 17–21.

Vas, C. J., and Parsonage, M. J. Treatment of intractable temporal lobe epilepsy with pheneturide. *Acta psychiat. neurol. scand.*, **1967**, *43*, 580–586.

Vastola, E. F., and Rosen, A. Suppression by anticonvulsants of focal electrical seizures in the neocortex. *Electroenceph. clin. Neurophysiol.,* **1960,** *12,* 327–332.

Vernadakis, A., and Woodbury, D. M. The developing animal as a model. *Epilepsia,* **1969,** *10,* 163–178.

Vossen, R. On the anticonvulsant effect of succinimides. *Dt. med. Wschr.,* **1958,** *83,* 1227–1230.

Watson, E., and Woodbury, D. M. Effects of diphenylhydantoin on active sodium transport in frog skin. *J. Pharmac. exp. Ther.,* **1972,** *180,* 767–776.

Williams, J. A.; Withrow, C. D.; and Woodbury, D. M. Effects of ouabain and diphenylhydantoin on transmembrane potentials, intracellular electrolytes and cell pH of rat muscle and liver *in vivo. J. Physiol., Lond.,* **1971,** *212,* 101–115.

Withrow, C. D.; Stout, R. J.; Barton, L. J.; Beacham, W. S.; and Woodbury, D. M. Anticonvulsant effects of 5,5-dimethyl-2,4-oxazolidinedione (DMO). *J. Pharmac. exp. Ther.,* **1968,** *161,* 335–341.

Woodbury, D. M. Effects of diphenylhydantoin on electrolytes and radiosodium turnover in brain and other tissues of normal, hyponatremic and postictal rats. *J. Pharmac. exp. Ther.,* **1955,** *115,* 74–95.

Wright, J. A. TRINURIDE in the treatment of major epilepsy. *Epilepsia,* **1965,** *6,* 67–74.

Young, A. B.; Zukin, S. R.; and Snyder, S. H. Interaction of benzodiazepines with central nervous glycine receptors: possible mechanism of action. *Proc. natn. Acad. Sci. U.S.A.,* **1974,** *71,* 2246–2250.

Zimmerman, F. T. Use of methylphenylsuccinimide in treatment of petit mal epilepsy. *A.M.A. Archs Neurol. Psychiatry,* **1951,** *66,* 156–162.

———. Evaluation of N-α,α-methylphenyl succinimide in the treatment of petit mal epilepsy. *N. Y. St. J. Med.,* **1956,** *56,* 1460–1465.

Zimmerman, F. T., and Burgemeister, B. B. A new drug for petit mal epilepsy. *Neurology, Minneap.,* **1958,** *8,* 769–775.

Monographs and Reviews

Aird, R. B., and Woodbury, D. M. *Management of Epilepsy.* Charles C Thomas, Pub., Springfield, Ill., **1974.**

Close, W. J., and Spielman, M. A. Anticonvulsant drugs. In, *Medicinal Chemistry,* Vol. 5. (Hartung, W. H., ed.) John Wiley & Sons, Inc., New York, **1961.**

Gibbs, F. A., and Gibbs, E. L. *Atlas of Electroencephalography,* Vols. 2 and 3. Addison-Wesley Press, Reading, Mass., **1954** and **1964.**

Gibbs, F. A., and Stamps, F. W. *Epilepsy Handbook.* Charles C Thomas, Pub., Springfield, Ill., **1958.**

Jackson, J. H. On epilepsy and epileptiform convulsions. In, *Selected Writings of John Hughlings Jackson,* Vol. 1. (Taylor, J., ed.) Hodder & Stoughton, London, **1931.**

Lennox, W. G., and Lennox, M. A. *Epilepsy and Related Disorders.* Little, Brown & Co., Boston, **1960.** (Two volumes, 1128 references.)

Livingston, S. *Comprehensive Management of Epilepsy in Infancy, Childhood and Adolescence.* Charles C Thomas, Pub., Springfield, Ill., **1972.**

Mercier, J. (ed.). *Anticonvulsant Drugs,* Vols. 1 and 2. *International Encyclopedia of Pharmacology and Therapeutics,* Sect. 19. Pergamon Press, Ltd., Oxford, **1973.**

Penfield, W., and Jasper, H. H. *Epilepsy and the Functional Anatomy of the Human Brain.* Little, Brown & Co., Boston, **1954.**

Symposium. (Various authors.) *Basic Mechanisms of the Epilepsies.* (Jasper, H. H.; Ward, A. A., Jr.; and Pope, A.; eds.) Little, Brown & Co., Boston, **1969.**

Symposium. (Various authors.) *Antiepileptic Drugs.* (Woodbury, D. M.; Penry, J. K.; and Schmidt, R. P.; eds.) Raven Press, New York, **1972a.**

Symposium. (Various authors.) *Experimental Models of Epilepsy: A Manual for the Laboratory Worker.* (Purpura, D. P.; Penry, J. K.; Tower, D.; Woodbury, D. M.; and Walter, R.; eds.) Raven Press, New York, **1972b.**

Symposium. (Various authors.) *The Benzodiazepines.* (Garattini, S.; Mussini, E.; and Randall, L. O.; eds.) Raven Press, New York, **1973.**

Temkin, O. *The Falling Sickness: A History of Epilepsy from the Greeks to the Beginning of Modern Neurology.* The Johns Hopkins Press, Baltimore, **1945.**

Toman, J. E. P. Neuropharmacology of peripheral nerve. *Pharmac. Rev.,* **1952,** *4,* 168–218. (298 references.)

Toman, J. E. P., and Goodman, L. S. Anticonvulsants. *Physiol. Rev.,* **1948,** *28,* 409–432. (216 references.)

Woodbury, D. M., and Esplin, D. W. Neuropharmacology and neurochemistry of anticonvulsant drugs. *Proc. Ass. Res. nerv. ment. Dis.,* **1959,** *37,* 24–56.

Woodbury, D. M., and Kemp, J. W. Some possible mechanisms of action of antiepileptic drugs. *Pharmakopsychiat. Neuro-Psychopharmak.,* **1970,** *3,* 201–226.

———. Pharmacology and mechanisms of action of diphenylhydantoin. *Psychiat. Neurol. Neurochir.,* **1971,** *74,* 91–115.

CHAPTER

14 DRUGS FOR PARKINSON'S DISEASE; CENTRALLY ACTING MUSCLE RELAXANTS

Donald N. Franz

Drugs described in this chapter have in common the ability to diminish skeletal muscle tone by actions on the central nervous system (CNS). The agents fall into two distinct categories on the basis of pharmacological properties and therapeutic uses. One group includes agents useful in treating Parkinson's disease and related syndromes. The introduction of levodopa (L-dihydroxy-phenylalanine) for the therapy of parkinsonism constitutes a major advance and represents a clinical return from the investment of 2 decades of research into the nature of synaptic transmitters in the CNS. The synthetic anticholinergic agents, formerly the only ameliorating drugs, are still useful for parkinsonism, but they are in general much less effective than levodopa. The other group of drugs, the centrally acting muscle relaxants, depress with varying degrees of selectivity certain neuronal systems controlling muscle tone and are used for treating acute muscle spasm, tetanus, and some orthopedic conditions. They are not employed in parkinsonism.

I. Drugs for Parkinson's Disease

Parkinson's disease (paralysis agitans), first described by James Parkinson in 1817, is one of the more prevalent serious neurological diseases, afflicting more than one million persons in the United States. The vast majority of cases are idiopathic, but a diminishing number are attributable to latent neurological manifestations of von Economo's encephalitis lethargica, pandemic from 1918 to 1926. A parkinsonism-like syndrome may also arise from cerebral hypoxia, resulting from atherosclerosis or carbon monoxide poisoning or from chronic exposure to man-

ganese. In addition, the extrapyramidal side effects from phenothiazines and related antipsychotic drugs resemble parkinsonism, especially in older patients (*see* Chapter 12).

Regardless of the etiology, Parkinson's syndrome is characterized by chronic, progressive motor dysfunction as a result of *tremor, rigidity,* and *akinesia.* A persistent tremor is superimposed on hypertonicity of agonist and antagonist muscle groups, initiation of movements becomes increasingly difficult and slow, and associated automatic and auxiliary movements are progressively reduced. In advanced stages, patients become virtually "frozen" and are unable to care for themselves. Loss of motor function accounts for a host of signs and symptoms of parkinsonism, such as masklike facies, impairment of postural reflexes, reduced blinking, impaired ocular convergence, microphonia, and micrographia. Autonomic symptoms of sialorrhea, seborrhea, and hyperhidrosis are also common. Oculogyric crises occur in some cases of postencephalitic but not in idiopathic parkinsonism.

For 100 years drug therapy of parkinsonism depended primarily on the limited efficacy of belladonna alkaloids and, subsequently, related synthetic agents. Therapy was often supplemented with antihistamines, amphetamine, or related drugs. Although optimal combinations of these drugs produce limited objective improvement, this can mean the difference between ambulation and incapacitation. However, side effects of these agents are troublesome, and characteristic progression of the disease continues unabated.

A new era in pharmacotherapy was opened by the discovery that large doses of levodopa produce dramatic improvement in the symptoms of parkinsonism in a large majority of patients. Numerous clinical trials in thousands of patients have established that levodopa is the most effective treatment currently available and that it is considerably more effective than previous therapy. The introduction of levodopa is also significant because it is an outstanding example of the successful therapeutic application of biochemically derived information to a chronic, degenerative neurological disorder. The expectation that similar neurochemical approaches will ultimately lead to advances in therapy for other debilitating nervous system diseases has kindled enthusiasm for the future of research in this field.

LEVODOPA (L-DOPA)

The initial report describing dramatic symptomatic improvement in a small number of parkinsonian patients placed on large, oral doses of racemic dopa (Cotzias *et al.*, 1967) was soon followed by more extensive clinical trials that confirmed the efficacy and safety of the levo isomer. Since its approval for general use in the United States in 1970, many thousands of patients have benefited from its unique therapeutic effects. The effectiveness of levodopa requires penetration of the drug into the CNS and its subsequent enzymatic conversion to dopamine, a central neurotransmitter. Progressive degeneration of the predominant dopaminergic pathway between the substantia nigra and the corpus striatum is considered largely responsible for the symptoms of Parkinson's disease. Dopamine is inhibitory to neurons in the caudate nucleus, whereas acetylcholine appears to be an excitatory transmitter in a second pathway to the same neurons. Consequently, progressive loss of the dopaminergic nigrostriatal fibers is considered to permit excitatory predominance by the intact cholinergic pathways, and may also render the neurons of the caudate nucleus supersensitive to dopamine (*see* Papeschi, 1972; Sourkes, 1972). The implication that levodopa supplies an increased amount of the missing transmitter, dopamine, and thereby restores functional capacity to the system is the most attractive of several hypotheses for its mechanism of action (*see* below). Several symposia (*see* Symposium, 1970, 1971, 1972) and extensive reviews (Barbeau and McDowell, 1970; Brogden *et al.*, 1971; Barbeau, 1974) on the use of levodopa in parkinsonism have been published.

History. Events leading up to the discovery of L-dopa as a therapeutic agent actually began in the early 1950s with the important clinical observation that *reserpine* could induce a parkinsonian syndrome as a dose-dependent side effect. Reserpine was soon shown to release and deplete brain stores of 5-hydroxytryptamine (5-HT) and catecholamines, and Carlsson and coworkers (1957) found that the akinesia and sedation produced by reserpine in mice could be reversed by dopa but not by 5-hydroxytryptophan, the precursor of 5-HT. The presence of dopamine in the brain, first reported by Montagu (1957), was confirmed by Carlsson's group, who also showed its depletion by reserpine and replenishment by dopa and suggested that it may serve an independent role in brain function (Carlsson *et al.*, 1958).

Measurements of regional dopamine concentrations in human brains provided the basic link between laboratory studies and clinical application. Bertler and Rosengren (1959) and Carlsson (1959) found that about 80% of human brain dopamine is concentrated in the basal ganglia, mostly in the caudate nucleus and putamen (corpus striatum), and they suggested its possible importance in extrapyramidal function or malfunction. The fundamental discovery by Hornykiewicz and coworkers (Ehringer and Hornykiewicz, 1960; Hornykiewicz, 1966) that striatal dopamine concentrations are markedly deficient (one tenth or less of normal) in the brains of patients with parkinsonism furnished the crucial evidence linking dopamine with the disease state. The degree of dopamine deficiency correlated with the loss of melanin-containing neurons in the pars compacta of the substantia nigra, the most consistent pathological finding in parkinsonism. Since it was known that dopa but not dopamine could cross the blood-brain barrier and raise central dopamine levels, the former was the logical drug for therapeutic trial. The results of early clinical trials with intravenously administered dopa were equivocal (*see* review by Barbeau, 1969). Cotzias and associates then tested the effects of high oral doses of D,L-dopa in 16 patients with Parkinson's disease. Complete or appreciable, sustained improvement occurred in 8 of the 16 patients (Cotzias *et al.*, 1967). These results were quickly confirmed and extended in a number of trials with the active isomer, L-dopa, which proved less toxic and more effective than the D,L mixture.

Chemistry. Levodopa (L-dopa) is formed in mammals from L-tyrosine as an intermediary metabolite in the enzymatic synthesis of catecholamines. Dopamine is formed directly from levodopa by the cytoplasmic enzyme, aromatic L-amino acid decarboxylase. The structures of levodopa and dopamine are shown in Figure 14–1 (page 231). Dopamine is structurally related to apomorphine, with which it shares certain pharmacological properties. Both agents produce nausea and vomiting by actions on the medullary chemoreceptor trigger zone (CTZ), and both are effective in controlling the symptoms of parkinsonism (*see* Cotzias *et al.*, 1970). Nonemetic congeners of apomorphine might profitably be explored for potential use in parkinsonism.

Pharmacological Properties

The main effects of levodopa are produced by the product of its decarboxylation, dopamine; levodopa, as such, is practically inert pharmacologically. Since about 95% of orally administered levodopa is rapidly decarboxylated in the periphery to dopamine, which does not penetrate the blood-brain barrier, large doses must be taken to allow sufficient penetration of levodopa into the brain to raise central dopamine concentrations. Tolerance to the necessarily large dosage is achieved only by gradual upward titration over a period of weeks or months until a maximal clinical response is obtained or until the emergence of limiting side effects.

Central Nervous System. The pharmacological effects of levodopa on muscle tone and movement are not seen in normal individuals or in patients with neurological disorders other than parkinsonism. Akinesia and rigidity usually respond more quickly and consistently than does tremor, but a significant reduction in tremor is often obtained with continued therapy. Amelioration of neurological symptoms is accompanied by similar improvements in functional ability and alleviation of secondary symptoms. The secondary motor manifestations such as disturbances in posture, gait, associated movements, facial expression, speech, handwriting, swallowing, and respiration are proportionately improved.

Psychic Effects. In most patients, levodopa at least partially relieves the changes in mood characteristic of Parkinson's disease. Early in therapy, feelings of apathy and depression are generally replaced by increased vigor and a sense of well-being. It is described as a general alerting response, characterized by apparent improvement in mental function, and an increased interest in self, surroundings, and family. A stormy attempt to regain an active role in family affairs after a long period of dependency may be misdiagnosed as being a drug-induced psychosis. The importance of positive family support for successful levodopa therapy has been emphasized by many experts. However, a significant number of patients do develop serious behavioral side effects, as discussed below.

Cardiovascular System. Peripheral decarboxylation of levodopa leads to marked increases in blood concentrations of dopamine. *Dopamine* is a pharmacologically active catecholamine with prominent effects on α- and β-adrenergic receptors, although its potency is much less than that of epinephrine, norepinephrine, or isoproterenol. The reluctance of early investigators to test the effects of high doses of levodopa for parkinsonism rested largely on the expectation of potentially toxic cardiovascular effects, particularly hypertension. Contrary to such expectation, therapeutic doses of levodopa cause significant *orthostatic hypotension* in both parkinsonian patients and normal subjects; however, usually it is asymptomatic and tolerance develops within a few months.

The mechanism by which oral levodopa produces hypotension is not fully understood. Peripheral dopamine does not appear to be involved, since both in man (Watanabe *et al.,* 1970) and in animals (Henning and Rubenson, 1970) the hypotension is not prevented by the use of a peripheral decarboxylase inhibitor. This suggests a central mechanism. Franz and collaborators found a depressant effect of levodopa on sympathetic preganglionic neurons in the spinal cord and proposed that this might account for the hypotension (Hare *et al.,* 1972; Neumayr *et al.,* 1974).

Therapeutic doses of levodopa produce *cardiac stimulation* by an action of dopamine on β-adrenergic receptors. Transient tachycardia occurs in some patients, and myocardial contractility may be increased for several hours after a large dose, especially early in therapy. Tolerance to the cardiac effects also develops after several months. Since dopamine increases the incidence of arrhythmias in susceptible patients, this constitutes a potentially serious side effect of levodopa (Goldberg and Whitsett, 1971). The cardiac effects of levodopa mediated by dopamine are usually prevented by β-adrenergic antagonists such as propranolol and by peripherally acting decarboxylase inhibitors (*see* below).

Gastrointestinal System. Nausea, vomiting, and anorexia are common but unpredictable effects of oral levodopa therapy and may limit the amount of drug that can be given. Most patients become tolerant to these effects, especially if the dosage of levodopa is increased slowly. In fact, these symptoms generally determine the rate at which the dosage can be increased during initial therapy. They can usually be ameliorated by taking levodopa with food, thereby slowing its absorption.

Levodopa produces nausea and vomiting through the action of dopamine on the CTZ in the area postrema of the medulla. The CTZ appears to lie outside the blood-brain barrier since prevention of the peripheral decarboxylation of levodopa minimizes its emetic effect.

Metabolic and Endocrine Effects. The decreased rate of glucose utilization associated with deficient insulin secretion reported in some patients with Parkinson's disease is not altered by levodopa therapy; virtually no change in mean fasting blood sugar concentration occurs (Langrall and Joseph, 1972). On the other hand, Sirtori and associates (1972) found significantly elevated plasma concentrations of *growth hormone* 2 to 3 hours after administration of a therapeutic dose of levodopa, both early and late in the course of treatment; some impairment of glucose utilization associated with delayed hypersecretion of insulin was also noted. These metabolic changes may reflect the enhanced secretion of growth hormone after each dose. The plasma free fatty acid concentration was transiently increased after each dose, and serum cholesterol was increased by 10% after 1 year. Augmented secretion of growth hormone by levodopa has also been reported by others (*see* Eddy *et al.,* 1971), and administration of levodopa is used as a probative test for the ability to secrete growth hormone. The consequences of long-term stimulation of growth hormone secretion by levodopa are unknown. In contrast, levodopa can inhibit the secretion of prolactin (*see* Chapter 66).

Mechanism of Action. Since its introduction into therapy for parkinsonism, levodopa has been assumed to act by replenishing deficient stores of dopamine in the corpus striatum. The severe depletion of dopamine in the caudate nucleus and putamen leaves little doubt that the parkinsonian syndrome is neurochemically a "striatal dopamine-deficiency syndrome." The severity of symptoms is positively correlated with the degree of deficiency, which in turn is related to the loss of nigrostriatal neurons; furthermore, the brains of parkinsonian patients who had been on high doses of levodopa until death contain dopamine concentrations in the striatum that not only are five to eight times higher than found in untreated patients but also are directly correlated with their clinical response to the drug. These findings indicate that dopamine storage capacity of the terminals of the nigrostriatal fibers is not completely lost in parkinsonism. The striatal concentration of aromatic L-amino acid decarboxylase, the enzyme that converts levodopa to dopamine, is markedly reduced in parkinsonism, but sufficient enzymatic activity remains to account for the replenishment of dopamine by levodopa therapy. (*See* Bernheimer *et al.,* 1973; Hornykiewicz, 1973a, 1973b.)

If levodopa improves neurological function by replenishing or enhancing dopamine stores in residual terminals of a degenerating nigrostriatal system, there should be a good correlation between the clinical response and the severity of the disease. However, although some correlation exists, the large number of exceptions has prompted other explanations as to how levodopa exerts its benefit. For example, it has been suggested that dopamine may be formed at nondopaminergic sites. Ng and coworkers (1972) marshaled experimental support for their proposal that levodopa may be taken up by nondopaminergic neurons containing the decarboxylase enzyme, converted to dopamine, and released as a "false transmitter" to stimulate nearby dopamine receptors. The criteria necessary for such a role are met by a large group of 5-HT–containing neurons that remain functionally intact in Parkinson's disease

and terminate in the same striatal areas that are also normally innervated by dopaminergic neurons. This concept of transmitter exchange in central neurons raises interesting theoretical questions regarding neuronal plasticity in the CNS. Enzymatic or non-enzymatic decarboxylation of levodopa in other areas or elements of the brain provides additional possible mechanisms for the generation of dopamine (Sandler, 1971).

The ability of dopamine to activate adenylate cyclase and to increase the concentration of cyclic adenosine 3',5'-monophosphate in the caudate nucleus suggests that a dopamine-sensitive adenylate cyclase may be a receptor for dopamine in the mammalian brain (*see* page 160).

Among other explanations for the mechanism of action of levodopa are proposals that metabolites of the drug other than dopamine may have antiparkinsonism activity (Sourkes, 1971; Sandler *et al.,* 1973).

Absorption, Distribution, Fate, and Excretion. Levodopa is rapidly absorbed from the gastrointestinal tract, and peak plasma concentrations occur within 1 to 3 hours after its ingestion when the stomach is empty. Since gastric absorption is limited whereas intestinal absorption is quite rapid, the rate and time of absorption depend on gastric emptying. In addition, a significant amount of levodopa is metabolized in the lumen of the stomach and intestine. Administration of antacid has been shown to facilitate gastric emptying and levodopa absorption in patients with low basal gastric pH (Rivera-Calimlim *et al.,* 1971).

More than 95% of levodopa is decarboxylated in the periphery by the widely distributed extracerebral aromatic L-amino acid decarboxylase. Absorbed levodopa is extensively decarboxylated in its first passage through the liver, which is rich in decarboxylase, so that relatively little unchanged drug reaches the cerebral circulation and probably less than 1% penetrates into the CNS. Inhibition of peripheral decarboxylase markedly increases the proportion of levodopa that crosses the blood-brain barrier (*see* below).

The principal metabolic pathways for levodopa are depicted in Figure 14–1. A small amount is methylated to 3-O-methyldopa, which accumulates in the CNS due to its long half-life. Most is converted to dopamine, small amounts of which in turn are metabolized to norepinephrine and epinephrine. Biotransformation of dopamine proceeds rapidly to the principal excretion products, 3,4-dihydroxyphenylacetic acid

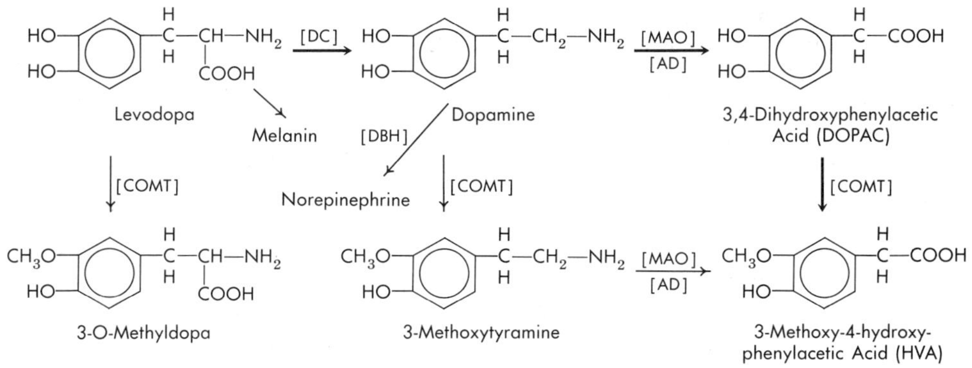

Figure 14-1. *Important catabolic pathways of levodopa* (L-*dopa*).

Major pathways are shown by heavy arrows; minor pathways, by light arrows. *AD*, aldehyde dehydrogenase; *COMT*, catechol-O-methyltransferase; *DBH*, dopamine-β-hydroxylase; *DC*, aromatic L-amino acid decarboxylase; *MAO*, monoamine oxidase. (For biosynthetic pathway, see Figure 21–4, page 423.)

(DOPAC) and 3-methoxy-4-hydroxyphenylacetic acid (homovanillic acid, HVA). Some biochemical evidence indicates that an acceleration of levodopa metabolism occurs during prolonged therapy, possibly due to enzyme induction.

Dopamine metabolites are rapidly excreted in the urine, about 80% of a radioactively labeled dose being recovered within 24 hours. The principal metabolites, DOPAC and HVA, account for up to 50% of the administered dose. These metabolites, as well as small amounts of levodopa and dopamine, also appear in the cerebrospinal fluid. Negligible amounts are found in the feces. After prolonged therapy with levodopa, the ratio of DOPAC to HVA excreted may increase, probably reflecting a depletion of labile methyl groups available for methylation; it is estimated that about three fourths of dietary methionine is utilized for the metabolism of large therapeutic doses of levodopa.

Preparations and Dosage. *Levodopa*, U.S.P. (BENDOPA, DOPAR, LARODOPA), is available for *oral* use as tablets or capsules containing 100, 250, or 500 mg.

The optimal maintenance dosage of levodopa is determined by careful titration in each patient. The usual initial dose is 0.5 to 1.0 g daily, divided into two or three equal portions. The total daily dosage is then gradually increased by increments of 100 mg to 750 mg, every 2 to 3 days. The rate of increase in dosage is determined primarily by the patient's tolerance to nausea and vomiting or to orthostatic hypotension. Significant objective improvement may appear during the second or third week as the daily dosage reaches 2.5 to 3.0 g. Further benefit accrues gradually with increasing dosage and even after the dose is stabilized at an apparently optimal level. Good therapeutic responses are not reached in some patients for 3 or 4 months; therefore, levodopa should not be considered ineffective until full doses have been administered for such periods. In general, younger patients with less severe symptoms derive greater benefit than do severely debilitated, elderly patients in whom maximal tolerated doses are often limited by side effects. However, it is impossible to predict accurately the efficacy of levodopa in individual cases. The usual daily maintenance dose ranges from 3 to 6 g, taken in at least three equally divided and spaced amounts with food. More frequent administration of smaller doses may reduce side effects and yield better results. Total daily dosage should not exceed 8 g. With the concurrent administration of a dopa decarboxylase inhibitor, the dosage range of levodopa is reduced by approximately 75% (*see* below).

Side Effects and Toxicity. The majority of parkinsonian patients treated with levodopa experience side effects. Their intensity and type vary greatly and appear and disappear at different stages of therapy. Although many are relatively innocuous, others are troublesome and necessitate reduction in dosage or complete withdrawal of the drug. Side effects are generally dose dependent and reversible, but elderly patients and those with postencephalitic parkinsonism tend to be intolerant of large doses.

The most common side effects *early* in therapy with levodopa are nausea, vomiting, and orthostatic hypotension; the last-named effect is usually asymptomatic. Cardiac arrhythmias occur in some patients, especially those with preexisting disturbances in cardiac conduction. The majority of patients on *long-term* therapy develop abnormal involuntary movements, which vary considerably in pattern and severity and often limit the tolerated dosage of levodopa. Numerous psychiatric disturbances are produced by levodopa in a significant proportion of patients and frequently are dose limiting. All the side effects are reversible and can generally be controlled by a reduction in dosage. Although levodopa appears to be relatively free of serious toxicity, it should be noted that its long-term safety has not yet been established.

Gastrointestinal. About 80% of patients experience anorexia, nausea, or vomiting early in therapy with levodopa. The mechanism has been discussed above. Nausea is most likely to occur if dosage is increased too rapidly, if individual doses are too large, or if the drug is taken without food. Anorexia may result in transient weight loss in some patients. Gastrointestinal side effects tend to disappear with continuing therapy as tolerance develops. Bleeding and perforation of peptic ulcers have been reported in a few patients (Keenan, 1970; Langrall and Joseph, 1972). Infrequent complaints include diarrhea or constipation, epigastric distress, abdominal pain, and flatulence.

Hypotension. Parkinsonian patients have a lower mean blood pressure than is normal for their age group. Blood pressure, especially in the erect position, is further reduced during levodopa therapy. About 30% of patients develop significant orthostatic hypotension early in therapy. It is usually asymptomatic, but some patients experience dizziness and, rarely, syncope, which can result in serious injury from falling. Careful regulation of dosage is necessary in such individuals, and the usual measures for controlling orthostatic hypotension should be employed. As tolerance develops to the hypotension, blood pressure tends to return to predrug levels, but some patients experience recurrent episodes of hypotension for months. In individuals with essential hypertension, levodopa therapy may lower the blood pressure toward normal.

Cardiac Irregularities. Cardiac arrhythmias are not uncommon in the older-age group of patients with Parkinson's disease, and consequently a direct association between the development of arrhythmias and levodopa therapy is difficult to establish. However, the β-adrenergic action of dopamine on the heart presents a potentially serious side effect of levodopa. Fortunately, the incidence of arrhythmia is low. Sinus tachycardia, atrial and ventricular extrasystoles, atrial flutter and fibrillation, and ventricular tachycardia have all been reported. The more serious disturbances occur in patients with preexisting irregularities, and levodopa treatment of such patients should be initiated in a hospital situation (Goldberg and Whitsett, 1971; Hunter *et al.*, 1971). The increased myocardial contractility produced by levodopa may be detrimental in patients with coronary artery insufficiency. The concurrent use of a β-adrenergic blocking agent may be indicated in some cases.

Abnormal Involuntary Movements. These occur in most parkinsonian patients treated with optimal doses of levodopa and are the most common dose-limiting side effects of the drug. They appear with increasing frequency during continuing drug administration and are directly related to the dose of the drug and to the degree of clinical improvement. About 80% of patients on full therapeutic doses for a year or longer will develop some abnormal movements; they have been described as adventitious, choreoathetoid, or dyskinetic, and range in intensity and duration from minor and fleeting to severe, continuous, and disabling. Initially and most common is the faciolingual type, consisting of grotesque facial grimacing, exaggerated chewing, twisting and protrusion of the tongue, and rhythmic opening and closing of the mouth. Bobbing or waving movements of the head and neck or gross head turning may occur. There may be limb or trunk involvement with rhythmic or jerking movements of the hands and arms, which can progress to ballismus; the lower extremities may also be affected. Rocking movements of the trunk may occur. Opisthotonus, myoclonic contractions, and painful dystonias are among the more severe symptoms. Rarely, exaggerated respiratory movements can produce an irregular gasping pattern or hyperventilation. (*See* Barbeau *et al.*, 1970.)

Abnormal involuntary movements are obviously distressing to the patient and his family and frequently become intolerable. Tolerance does not develop to this side effect; in fact, the symptoms tend to increase in severity if the dosage is not reduced. They are completely reversible by reduction in dosage of levodopa, sometimes by only a small amount, but this is more difficult to achieve in patients on long-term therapy. Unfortunately, some return or increase in parkinsonian symptoms invariably accompanies dosage reduction. The onset of involuntary movements usually occurs at the dosage level providing maximal therapeutic benefit, and a compromise must be sought between relief of the disorder and the occurrence of abnormal movements. No satisfactory means, pharmacological or otherwise, has yet been found selectively to antagonize this side effect.

The dyskinesias caused by levodopa do not occur in normal subjects or in patients with other neurological diseases not involving the extrapyramidal system. In patients with hemiparkinsonism, abnormal movements are confined to the affected side. Therefore, it appears that extrapyramidal neuronal damage is a necessary condition for the levodopa-induced dyskinesias. Patients not benefited by the drug seldom develop abnormal movements (Markham, 1971). This suggests a close biochemical linkage between successful therapy and involuntary movements, both involving activation of neostriatal dopamine receptors. Carlsson (1970) has proposed that levodopa therapy cannot simulate the normal physiological control of dopamine release at its receptor sites and that, in parkinsonian states, levodopa-induced dyskinesias may result from stimulation of supersensitive denervated receptors by dopamine.

An occasional patient experiences sudden attacks of akinesia with *hypotonia* rather than rigidity, termed "akinesia paradoxica." The mechanism is unknown but may involve effects of the drug on the cerebellum or central effects of levodopa metabolites.

Psychiatric and Behavioral Disturbances. The *mild* reactions in this category are generally not serious and seldom necessitate dosage reduction or withdrawal. Episodes of nervousness, anxiety, or agitation early in therapy are not uncommon. Some patients experience insomnia, vivid dreams, and nightmares, whereas others sleep better or, rarely, suffer attacks of daytime somnolence. These side effects usually subside with time.

Serious psychiatric disturbances occur in about 15% of patients on levodopa and usually require dosage reduction or, for some patients, complete withdrawal of the drug. Many factors contribute to their occurrence, especially mental status before therapy, and they vary greatly in character and time of onset after levodopa therapy is initiated. One of the more common disturbances resembles an organic brain syndrome and is characterized by *confusion,* sometimes progressing to frank *delirium.* Although the mental depression of many patients is often improved by levodopa, some appear to develop a more severe *depression,* which in a few cases has led to suicidal gestures. Tricyclic antidepressant drug therapy has been helpful in some cases. Fully developed *psychotic reactions* with paranoid delusions or hallucinations are most likely to occur in patients with a history of mental disorder, organic brain syndrome including dementia, or postencephalitic parkinsonism (Celesia and Barr, 1970; Sacks *et al.,* 1972). A few patients develop classical symptoms of *hypomania,* one manifestation of which may be inappropriate or excessive sexual behavior. Barbeau (1971) has described more subtle mental changes in patients who had been taking levodopa for more than 2 years; these include a gradual decrease in attention span, loss of memory for recent events, and insouciance. (*See* Goodwin, 1971; Goodwin *et al.,* 1971; Malitz, 1972; Markham, 1972.)

Laboratory Abnormalities. Careful laboratory monitoring of numerous biochemical indices in several thousand patients has revealed only mild and transient abnormalities; these have not been associated with any evidence of organ toxicity and almost always return to normal without interruption of levodopa therapy (*see* Brogden *et al.,* 1971; McDowell, 1971; Langrall and Joseph, 1972). Urinary metabolites of levodopa cause false-positive tests for ketoacidosis by the dip-stick test and color the urine red, then black, on exposure to air or alkali.

Miscellaneous Side Effects. Many minor side effects, some probably not directly related to levodopa, have been reported. Among the more common are changes in taste sensation, sweating, excessive nasal discharge, and widening of the palpebral fissures. Less frequent side effects are burning sensation in the tongue, urinary frequency or retention,

and increased pain related to preexisting chronic pain syndromes. Drug rash and other hypersensitivity reactions are quite rare. Both mydriasis and miosis have been observed. Severely ill patients with postencephalitic parkinsonism may develop oculogyric crises.

Contraindications and Precautions. Levodopa is contraindicated in patients with narrow-angle glaucoma, acute psychosis, or severe psychoneurosis. It should not be administered to patients with *uncompensated* endocrine, renal, hepatic, cardiovascular, or pulmonary disease. The additive effects of levodopa and other adrenergic agents dictate extreme caution in patients with asthma or emphysema who may require sympathomimetic drugs. Patients with cardiac arrhythmias or a history of myocardial infarction should undergo initial therapy with levodopa only in a facility equipped for intensive coronary care. Since control of diabetic patients may be adversely affected by levodopa, they should be carefully monitored for any necessity to modify their regimen. Caution is also necessary in patients with a history of peptic ulcer, convulsions, or psychiatric disorder. Patients with chronic wide-angle glaucoma may be given levodopa provided intraocular pressure is monitored and remains well controlled. Discontinuation of levodopa therapy for 6 to 24 hours prior to general anesthesia is recommended although no untoward reactions have been reported. The safety of levodopa during pregnancy has not been established; however, infants should not be nursed by mothers receiving the drug since it may appear in the milk. Furthermore, the drug may inhibit lactation. Since levodopa therapy has been associated with increased growth of *melanoma,* patients with known melanomas or pigmented lesions should be carefully monitored for changes in such lesions and the drug should be withdrawn if changes occur (Lieberman and Shupack, 1974).

Interactions with Other Drugs. *Pyridoxine* rapidly reverses the therapeutic effects of levodopa in parkinsonism; even small doses of pyridoxine such as found in "over-the-counter" multivitamin preparations can decrease its efficacy. The enzymatic conversion of levodopa to dopamine by aromatic L-amino acid decarboxylase requires pyridoxyl-5-phosphate as a coenzyme; administration of supplemental pyridoxine increases decarboxylase activity so that more levodopa is converted to dopamine in the periphery and less is available for penetration into the CNS. This effect of pyridoxine is readily prevented by selective inhibition of peripheral decarboxylase.

Monoamine oxidase inhibitors are definitely contraindicated in patients taking levodopa because hypertension may result. Such medication should be withdrawn at least 14 days, preferably a month, prior to levodopa administration. The cardiovascular system may also be adversely affected by *sympathomimetic drugs* in the presence of levodopa. Epinephrine–local anesthetic combinations represent a potential hazard in this regard. The hypotensive effect of levodopa may necessitate reduction in the dose of antihypertensive drugs.

The *antipsychotic drugs* (reserpine, phenothiazines, and butyrophenones) can produce parkinsonian syndromes, reserpine by depleting central dopamine stores and the others by blocking dopamine receptors. Since these drugs antagonize the therapeutic effects of levodopa, they are contraindicated. Although patients taking levodopa have been treated with tricyclic antidepressant drugs without adverse effects, these agents tend to produce extrapyramidal side effects that may diminish the benefit from levodopa.

Parkinsonian symptoms are exacerbated in untreated but not in levodopa-treated patients by intravenous injection of small doses of physostigmine, presumably by enhancement of cholinergic transmission in the extrapyramidal system (Weintraub and Van Woert, 1971; *see also* review by Bianchine and Sunyapridakul, 1973).

Decarboxylase Inhibitors. Concurrent administration of decarboxylase inhibitors that do not enter the brain decreases the decarboxylation of levodopa in the periphery. Extensive laboratory investigations and clinical trials have been conducted with two such inhibitors, *carbidopa* (MK-486) and *benserazide hydrochloride* (Ro 4-4602). They have the following structural formulas:

Carbidopa

Benserazide Hydrochloride

Clinical studies to date have clearly demonstrated distinct advantages of therapy with the use of one of these drugs concurrently with levodopa: (1) The optimally effective dose of levodopa can be reduced by about 75%, inasmuch as a much larger proportion of levodopa enters the brain. (2) Nausea and vomiting from stimulation of dopamine receptors in the medullary CTZ are largely eliminated. Likewise, the cardiac side effects are diminished or prevented. (3) Effective dose levels of levodopa during initial therapy can be achieved much more quickly since the necessity to develop tolerance to the peripheral effects of dopamine is minimized. (4) Antagonism of the therapeutic efficacy of levodopa by pyridoxine is avoided. (5) The frequency and intensity of diurnal variations in control of symptoms by levodopa are reduced, presumably by avoidance of large fluctuations in central dopamine concentration. The number of divided doses per day may often be reduced without loss of control. (6) The percentage of patients improved and the degree of improvement appear to be somewhat greater.

However, some of the problems of levodopa therapy are not resolved by the concomitant use of peripheral decarboxylase inhibitors. The incidence of orthostatic hypotension is essentially unchanged, evidence that it is mediated primarily by an action of dopamine in the CNS. Abnormal involuntary movements not only occur with the same frequency but also tend to develop earlier in therapy and may be more severe, and they often persist for a longer period after the dosage of levodopa is reduced. Adverse mental effects also occur with about the same frequency but appear earlier in the course of therapy. In recommended doses the currently employed peripheral decarboxylase inhibitors are essentially devoid of pharmacological activity, and toxic effects have not been observed. (*See* Chase and Watanabe, 1972; Papavasiliou *et al.*, 1972; Rinne *et al.*, 1972; Mars, 1973; *see also* monograph edited by Yahr, 1973.)

Preparations and Dosage. Although *carbidopa* and *benserazide hydrochloride* can be prescribed in several countries abroad, neither drug is yet available for general use in the United States; it is anticipated that carbidopa may become available for prescription use in the United States in the near future. In contrast to the general reservations concerning the prescribing of fixed-dose combinations of two or more active drugs, treatment with *carbidopa* and levodopa is accomplished most satisfactorily when the drugs are given together in a ratio of 1:10 by weight (available as SINEMET); with *benserazide* and levodopa, in a ratio of 1:4 (MADOPAR). The present dosage form of carbidopa consists of tablets containing 10 mg of carbidopa plus 100 mg of levodopa (SINEMET-100), or 25 mg of carbidopa plus 250 mg of levodopa (SINEMET-250). In such a combination, therapy is generally initiated with 600 mg of levodopa daily, in divided doses, and increased as required to a maximal daily dose of 2 g of levodopa. For patients treated previously with levodopa alone, therapy should be withheld for at least 8 hours after the last dose of levodopa; combined carbidopa-levodopa medication is then initiated, but the total daily dose of levodopa is reduced to one fourth of that taken previously.

THERAPEUTIC USES

Many aspects of the therapeutic use of levodopa have been described in the preceding pages, particularly in the discussion of the CNS effects of the drug. Levodopa is the agent of choice for treating *Parkinson's disease.* In general, cases of idiopathic parkinsonism respond somewhat better than do those with a postencephalitic or atherosclerotic etiology, but many of these patients are also markedly benefited.

Between two thirds and three fourths of patients experience substantial improvement, and some become almost or completely asymptomatic. Some patients derive only mild-to-moderate benefit, and about 10% experience little or no improvement. Patients with previous stereotaxic surgery often obtain a good-to-excellent response from levodopa therapy. A few patients cannot tolerate the side effects of the drug. The results of large collaborative studies are summarized by Keenan (1970) and Langrall and Joseph (1972).

Levodopa affords only symptomatic relief of parkinsonism. If the drug is stopped, all the preexisting symptoms gradually return within a week or two; upon resumption of levodopa therapy after a period of withdrawal, the previous therapeutic response is reestablished after a week or more. Although some experienced observers have reported an apparent arrest or slowing in the natural progression of the disease, an extensive 3-year study by Hunter and associates (1973) indicates that parkinsonian disabilities continue to progress after 2 years of levodopa therapy (*see also* Birdsong and McKinney, 1974). The ultimate status of the influence of levodopa treatment on the progressive nature of the disease process can be determined only by further careful, long-term assessment.

Parkinsonian symptoms resulting from *chronic manganese poisoning* are often dramatically reduced by levodopa therapy (Mena *et al.,* 1970). Extrapyramidal symptoms but not dementia in patients with *parkinsonism-dementia of Guam* also respond favorably to the drug (Schnur *et al.,* 1971). Levodopa has produced marked and sustained improvement in parkinsonian symptoms resulting from *carbon monoxide poisoning* in at least one patient in whom it has been tested (Ringel and Klawans, 1972). *The drug is not useful in controlling or reversing the extrapyramidal side effects induced by antipsychotic drugs*

such as the phenothiazines and butyrophenones, since these drugs presumably block the activation of dopamine receptors.

The efficacy of levodopa for parkinsonism has prompted clinical trials of the drug for a number of other neurological conditions characterized by disordered extrapyramidal function. Some improvement in motor symptoms has been reported in some patients with *torsion dystonias* (*see* Eldridge, 1970), *athetoid cerebral palsy* (Rosenthal *et al.,* 1972), and *progressive supranuclear palsy* (Klawans and Ringel, 1971), but the results have not been impressive. Levodopa therapy may improve the mental and circulatory status of patients in *hepatic failure* (Parkes *et al.,* 1970a; Fischer and Baldessarini, 1971; Abramsky and Goldschmidt, 1974). Levodopa has not been found useful in the treatment of any psychiatric disorder; in fact, the drug tends to exacerbate latent or active psychotic states, both organic and functional (*see* Malitz, 1972).

AMANTADINE

The antiparkinsonism activity of the antiviral agent amantadine (Chapter 61) was discovered fortuitously by Schwab and coworkers (1969), who noted symptomatic improvement in a parkinsonian patient receiving the drug to prevent A_2 influenza. A number of subsequent clinical trials have established that amantadine is more effective in relieving the symptoms of parkinsonism than are the anticholinergic drugs. Although the majority of patients are benefited by amantadine, the degree of objective improvement is clearly less than that achieved with levodopa, and the efficacy of amantadine in most patients tends to diminish with time. An additive effect of amantadine with levodopa has been demonstrated repeatedly, especially in patients unable to tolerate full therapeutic doses of levodopa. However, patients receiving near-maximal benefit from levodopa generally gain little additional improvement from amantadine. The drug is effective in all types of parkinsonism, and the degree of improvement does not appear to be related to age, sex, duration or severity of the disease, or previous thalamotomy. The rapid onset of optimal benefit from amantadine, within 2 weeks, affords an advantage over levodopa. Amantadine also produces fewer side effects than either levodopa or the anticholinergic agents. The value of concomitant use of anticholinergic drugs and amantadine is not established; in fact, amantadine appears to enhance the side effects of the anticholinergic agents. (*See* Parkes *et al.,* 1970b; Forssman *et al.,* 1972; Mawdsley *et al.,* 1972; Schwab *et al.,* 1972.)

The *usual dosage* of amantadine for parkinsonism is 200 mg daily, in two equal doses. Some patients may derive additional benefit from a third 100-mg dose, but the incidence of side effects is thereby increased. Amantadine is readily absorbed from the gastrointestinal tract and has a relatively long duration of action. It is excreted unchanged in the urine and may accumulate in the body when renal function is inadequate.

Table 14-1. MISCELLANEOUS DRUGS FOR PARKINSONISM

Anticholinergic Agents

CLASS AND NONPROPRIETARY NAME	CHEMICAL STRUCTURE	TRADE NAME	PREPARATION	SINGLE ORAL DOSE (INITIAL)
Benztropine Mesylate, U.S.P.		COGENTIN	Tablets, 0.5, 1, and 2 mg; Injection, 2 mg/2 ml	0.5–1 mg
Trihexyphenidyl Hydrochloride, U.S.P.		ARTANE, PIPANOL, TREMIN	Tablets, 2 and 5 mg; Sustained-release capsules, 5 mg; Elixir, 2 mg/5 ml	1–2 mg
Biperiden Hydrochloride, N.F.		AKINETON	Tablets, 2 mg; Injection, 5 mg of biperiden lactate per ml	1–2 mg
Cycrimine Hydrochloride, N.F.		PAGITANE	Tablets, 1.25 and 2.5 mg	1.25–5 mg

Hydrochloride, N.F.	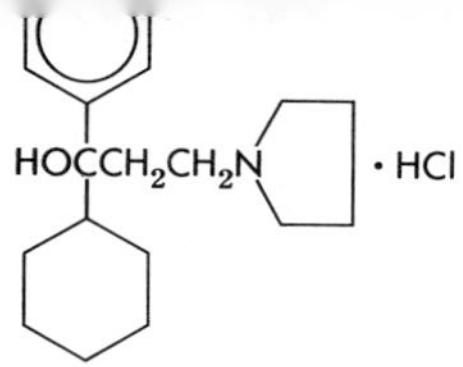HOCCH2CH2N · HCl			
Antihistamines				
Chlorphenoxamine Hydrochloride, N.F.	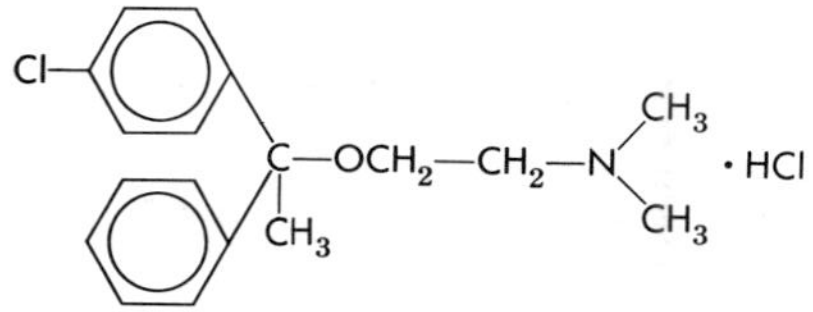Cl C—OCH2—CH2—N CH3 CH3 CH3 · HCl	PHENOXENE	Tablets, 50 mg	50 mg
Orphenadrine Hydrochloride	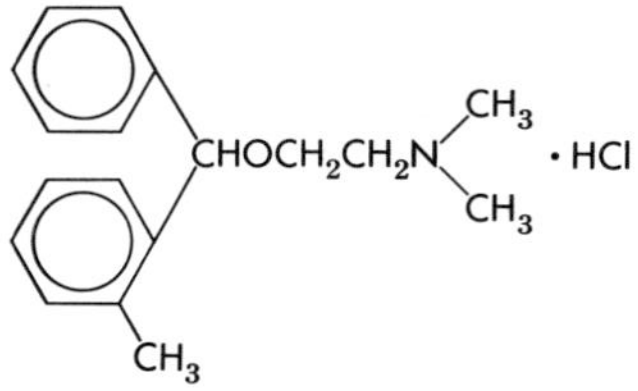CHOCH2CH2N CH3 CH3 · HCl CH3	DISIPAL	Tablets, 50 mg	50 mg
Phenothiazines *				
Ethopropazine Hydrochloride, U.S.P.	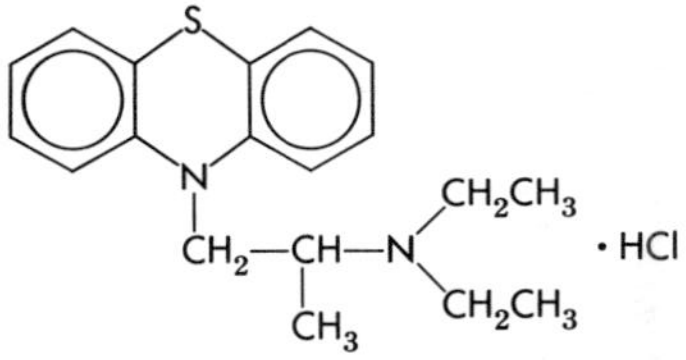S N CH2—CH—N CH3 CH2CH3 CH2CH3 · HCl	PARSIDOL	Tablets, 10, 50, and 100 mg	50 mg

* Promethazine Hydrochloride, U.S.P., is also used for parkinsonism (*see* Index).

Mechanism of Action. Amantadine releases dopamine from peripheral neuronal storage sites in animals primed with dopamine (Grelak *et al.,* 1970); this peripheral effect suggested that amantadine may exert a similar action on the residual, intact dopaminergic terminals in the striatum of parkinsonian patients. Farnebo and coworkers (1971), Von Voigtlander and Moore (1971), and others have demonstrated experimentally that amantadine causes release of dopamine from central neurons and facilitates its release by nerve impulses. Such a mechanism would account for the clinical observation that the efficacy of amantadine is usually enhanced by the addition of relatively small doses of levodopa. Release of dopamine by amantadine could also occur from central sites other than nigrostriatal neurons.

Side Effects. Compared to levodopa or anticholinergic agents, amantadine is relatively free of side effects. They are generally mild, often transient, and always reversible. Their incidence and severity increase markedly when the daily dosage exceeds 200 mg. A common untoward effect, *livedo reticularis* in the extremities and associated ankle edema, may be due to the vasoconstrictor effects of catecholamines released by amantadine (*see* Pearce *et al.,* 1974). Insomnia, dizziness, lethargy, drowsiness, and slurred speech have been reported. Nausea, vomiting, anorexia, and constipation occur infrequently. More serious adverse reactions include congestive heart failure, orthostatic hypotension, urinary retention, and, rarely, convulsions. Amantadine may cause severe mental symptoms in patients with a history of psychiatric disorders and may be contraindicated in such individuals. Hallucinations, confusion, and nightmares are more common when the drug is coadministered with anticholinergic agents.

Preparations. *Amantadine Hydrochloride,* N.F. (SYMMETREL), is available as 100-mg capsules and as a syrup containing 50 mg/5 ml.

Status. The use of amantadine in parkinsonian states is relatively new. A more complete assessment of its value and toxicity, alone and with other agents, must await the results of additional experience.

MISCELLANEOUS DRUGS FOR PARKINSONISM

For more than a century, *anticholinergic agents* were the drugs of choice for treating parkinsonism. Initially, the naturally occurring belladonna alkaloids were used, but synthetic anticholinergic agents with more selective central effects have been favored since their introduction in the 1940s (*see* Cunningham *et al.,* 1949). Some antihistamines were also considered useful as ancillary drugs. However, the introduction of levodopa has relegated these agents to a secondary status for the treatment of parkinsonism. At best, combinations of the older drugs can produce only limited improvement in symptoms in about 75% of patients and are obviously much less effective than levodopa. Optimal dosage is limited by numerous side effects, and the natural course of the disease is not abated. Nevertheless, the anticholinergic drugs are still very useful for patients with minimal symptoms, for those unable to tolerate levodopa because of side effects or contraindications, for those who are not benefited by levodopa or amantadine, and as an adjunct to levodopa therapy. The majority of patients receiving levodopa also require an anticholinergic agent for optimal improvement. Furthermore, the anticholinergic drugs effectively counteract *drug-induced parkinsonism and dystonias,* although they should not be used routinely to mask these side effects of neuroleptic agents (*see* Chapter 12). The anticholinergic and antihistaminic drugs used for parkinsonism are listed in Table 14–1. Although phenothiazines that are effective as neuroleptics are contraindicated in parkinsonism, a few with prominent anticholinergic properties have been found useful in some patients and are also included in the table.

Pharmacological Properties. The anticholinergic drugs, typified by *trihexyphenidyl,* are effective in all forms of parkinsonism and favorably influence akinesia, rigidity, and tremor as well as secondary symptoms such as depressed mood, sialorrhea, and hyperhidrosis. Although the peripheral side effects (dry mouth, cycloplegia, constipation, and urinary retention) of the synthetic agents are less prominent than those of the natural alkaloids, they usually limit dosage. Large doses produce typical central symptoms of atropine intoxication, including mental confusion, delirium, ataxia, hallucinations, somnolence, and, rarely, coma. Although there is essentially no difference pharmacologically among the anticholinergic agents, some patients may tolerate one better than another.

The *antihistamines* listed in Table 14–1 are structurally related to diphenhydramine, which is also used for parkinsonism. They possess some central anticholinergic properties and are well tolerated, especially by the elderly, who are likely to be less tolerant to the anticholinergics. The antihistamines produce fewer peripheral side effects, but they do not benefit the tremor and sialorrhea as much as do the anticholinergic drugs. Their sedative effect may be helpful in some patients, and they tend to improve mood and muscular strength.

Benztropine combines the chemical features of atropine and diphenhydramine and exhibits the pharmacological properties of both. It has a long duration of action and is a useful alternative when tolerance develops to the other anticholinergic drugs. The *phenothiazines* listed have prominent anticholinergic and slight antihistaminic or neuroleptic properties and may be especially helpful for controlling tremor.

Mechanism of Action. At least part of the symptoms of parkinsonism are thought to result from the effects of excitatory cholinergic pathways that terminate in the basal ganglia; they predominate when the inhibitory control from the nigrostriatal dopaminergic pathways is gradually lost. Partial blockade of the striatal cholinergic receptors by centrally acting anticholinergic agents tends to return the balance of excitation and inhibition toward normal. The observation that the anticholinergic drugs can also block the re-uptake of dopamine by nerve terminals in the striatum and thereby make more of the transmitter available to the receptors suggests a second possibility for their mechanism of action (Coyle and Snyder, 1969). However, the tricyclic antidepressants are more selective blockers of such dopamine reuptake, but they are not particularly effective in controlling the symptoms of parkinsonism.

Dosage. Patients should be started on the single oral doses listed in Table 14–1, given two or three times daily. Dosage should then be gradually increased until there is maximal improvement or, more likely, until the onset of intolerable side effects. Many patients are eventually able to tolerate daily doses that are two to four times the starting dose. It is especially important to tailor the medication in order to achieve the optimal balance between control of the disabling symptoms and the adverse reactions to the drugs. The optimal dose of a given drug for a particular individual cannot be stated. In general, elderly patients are less able to tolerate large doses of the drugs than are young patients. Changes in medication from one agent to another are frequently required. When such a change is made, the first drug is gradually withdrawn as the dosage of the second drug is increased by daily increments. The drugs with prominent peripheral anticholinergic effects must be used with great caution in individuals suffering from glaucoma or urinary retention secondary to disorders of the prostate. Patients obtaining benefit from levodopa frequently obtain further benefit from one of these secondary agents.

Drug-Induced Parkinsonism. Parkinsonism and acute dyskinesias and dystonias induced by the phenothiazines and other antipsychotic agents usually respond readily to low doses of anticholinergic drugs. *Such therapy is valid only for their rapid control and not to prevent their possible occurrence or to mask their actual occurrence.* The development of a permanent extrapyramidal syndrome, *tardive dyskinesia,* is sometimes a disastrous result of antipsychotic medication. Hence extrapyramidal symptoms must be recognized early, and this is not possible if the patient is also receiving anticholinergic drugs. (*See* Chapter 12.)

II. Centrally Acting Muscle Relaxants

Studies in France in 1910 disclosed that *phenoxypropanediol* (ANTODYNE) caused reversible flaccid paralysis in animals. In 1943, Goodman reported similar effects of benzimidazole, a distinctly different chemical compound. Interest in the relaxant property of the glycerol ethers related to phenoxypropanediol was renewed as a result of the studies of Berger and Bradley (1946), who reported on the properties of mephenesin. The early studies concerning muscle relaxants are reviewed by Berger (1949).

A sedative effect is exhibited to some degree by all muscle relaxants. Both laboratory and clinical testing indicate that for some drugs sedative effects appear to predominate over selective muscle relaxant activity. This has created some confusion concerning proper classification; improper classification, in turn, has blurred the distinction between the two pharmacologically separable effects, and certain agents have been promoted for both uses. Among the agents that combine a prominent sedative action with muscle relaxant properties are some of the antianxiety agents—meprobamate, tybamate, chlormezanone, and diazepam; their use in the treatment of emotional disturbances is discussed in Chapter 12. Drugs used primarily for their centrally acting muscle relaxant properties are listed in Table 14–2.

Although *mephenesin* is little used clinically at the present time, it is the oldest and probably the most extensively studied of the drugs in this class. The pharmacological actions of the newer agents are, in general, qualitatively similar to those of mephenesin. It may appropriately be taken as the prototype for the drugs that produce relaxation of skeletal muscle by a central action and that cause relatively little sedation. Smith (1965) has reviewed in depth the chemical properties and pharmacological actions of drugs possessing muscle relaxant activity.

PHARMACOLOGICAL ACTIONS

Muscle relaxants cause skeletal muscular relaxation, without loss of consciousness, as a result of a selective action upon the CNS. Administration of mephenesin or its surrogates to *normal animals* reduces spontaneous activity and decreases skeletal muscle tone. Sufficiently large doses cause a transient, flaccid paralysis. Death from respiratory depression occurs after very large doses. All types of *experimental hypertonia and hyperreflexia,* such as produced by decerebration or by spinal or supraspinal lesions, are diminished by nonparalyzing doses of muscle relaxants. They also afford protection against certain convulsive agents, particularly strychnine, and against electroshock seizures (Roszkowski, 1960).

In *man,* slow intravenous administration of 30 mg/kg of mephenesin has little effect on voluntary motor power or sensation; it causes coarse nystagmus, disturbance of convergence, only slight mental obtundation, and insignificant changes in the EEG. A feeling of warmth and relaxation may

Table 14–2. **CENTRALLY ACTING MUSCLE RELAXANTS CURRENTLY AVAILABLE**

NONPROPRIETARY NAME	CHEMICAL STRUCTURE	TRADE NAME	PREPARATION	SINGLE DOSE
Methocarbamol, N.F.		ROBAXIN	Tablets, 500 and 750 mg	1–2 g, oral
			Injection, 1 g/10 ml	1–3 g, i.v., slowly
Orphenadrine Citrate, N.F.		NORFLEX	Tablets, 100 mg	100 mg, oral
			Injection, 60 mg/2 ml	60 mg, i.m. or i.v.
Carisoprodal		RELA, SOMA	Tablets, 350 mg Capsules, 250 mg	250–350 mg
Chlorphenesin Carbamate		MAOLATE	Tablets, 400 mg	800 mg
Chlorzoxazone		PARAFLEX	Tablets, 250 mg	250–750 mg
Mephenesin		———	Tablets, 500 mg	1–2 g
Metaxalone		SKELAXIN	Tablets, 400 mg	800 mg

be noted, particularly if the drug is administered rapidly.

The *mechanism of action* of muscle relaxants is quite different from that of curare. Neuronal conduction, neuromuscular transmission, and muscle excitability are not depressed except after nearly lethal doses. A prominent effect of muscle relaxants is to depress spinal polysynaptic reflexes preferentially over monosynaptic reflexes. This effect of mephenesin was recognized early and is exhibited by the other muscle relaxants; it has led to their characterization as *interneuronal blocking agents*. However, this characterization is imprecise because depression is not restricted to interneurons. Furthermore, certain agents that do not produce muscular relaxation also show some preferential depression of polysynaptic reflexes; therefore, this effect is not an identifying characteristic of the class.

The actions of mephenesin on the CNS have been investigated more than those of other muscle relaxants. Mephenesin has been shown to depress transmission through a number of spinal and supraspinal polysynaptic pathways. Significantly, both facilitation and inhibition of muscle stretch reflexes resulting from stimulation of appropriate areas in the reticular formation are depressed by mephenesin. On the other hand, the central polysynaptic pathways concerned with arousal elicited by stimulation of the midbrain reticular formation are little affected by the drug. In the intact animal, actions of mephenesin at both spinal and supraspinal sites apparently contribute to the muscular relaxation. Mephenesin has been shown to prolong synaptic recovery time and to reduce repetitive interneuron discharges. Such effects may underlie the selectivity of the drug for certain tonically active systems controlling muscle tone. Diazepam appears to have a more selective action on reticular neuronal mechanisms that control muscle tone than on spinal interneuronal activity, whereas mephenesin-like drugs exhibit no such selectivity (Tseng and Wang, 1971). The mechanisms of action of muscle relaxants remain to be elucidated. (*See* Henneman *et al.,* 1949; Kaada, 1950; Longo, 1961; Esplin, 1963; and reviews by Domino, 1956, and Smith, 1965.)

Side Effects. Centrally acting muscle relaxants commonly produce drowsiness, dizziness, headache, blurred vision, weakness, lethargy, ataxia, and nystagmus. Nausea, vomiting, heartburn, and abdominal distress are also observed, especially after large oral doses. Hypersensitivity reactions include skin rash and pruritus and, rarely, anaphylactoid reactions and leukopenia. Chlorzoxazone has been reported to cause jaundice. Intravenous injection or oral ingestion of large doses may produce hypotension, tachycardia, flaccid paralysis, and respiratory depression.

THERAPEUTIC STATUS

Muscle relaxants administered intravenously have established value in treating acute muscle spasms associated with trauma and inflammation. They are also beneficial in producing muscle relaxation for certain orthopedic manipulations. These drugs may temporarily abate some of the symptoms of cerebral palsy, but they have a minor role in the overall management of this disease (*see* Denhoff and Robinault, 1960). Muscle relaxants are of little value in Parkinson's disease or in other motor dysfunctions resulting from diseases of the brain or spinal cord (*see* Schwab, 1964). Mephenesin and methocarbamol have been employed in the treatment of tetanus, but diazepam is superior for this purpose. However, none of the centrally acting drugs surpasses neuromuscular blocking agents in the control of tetanic spasms, but the use of the latter agents necessitates mechanical respiratory assistance.

All centrally acting muscle relaxants produce some sedation, at least at the highest doses employed clinically. Conversely, a number of agents with major clinical uses based upon sedative and antianxiety effects possess some of the pharmacological properties of muscle relaxants; meprobamate, chemically related to carisoprodol, is an example of such a drug.

Orally administered muscle relaxants do not produce the flaccidity obtainable in animals and man after intravenous administration of these agents. Studies in experimental animals (*see* Smith, 1965) indicate that the oral doses of mephenesin or methocarbamol necessary to produce demonstrable muscular relaxation are some five to ten times greater than effective intravenous doses. In other words, muscular relaxation following oral administration of the agents mentioned could not be expected with the doses commonly used clinically.

Many agents with muscle relaxant properties produce notable sedation in ordinary oral doses. Such agents enjoy particularly wide use in the treatment of muscle tension and pains associated with anxiety states and psychosomatic disorders. Favorable reports of the effects of such drugs for the conditions mentioned are numerous; however, the benefits attributable to the sedative effect of the drug or to a placebo effect have not been determined. In many instances, particularly with numerous proprietary drug mixtures, the dose of the purported muscle relaxant is so small that a discernible effect on the central pathways controlling muscle tone would be surprising. In the absence of definitive studies it appears reasonable to ascribe the beneficial effects of such agents to their sedative properties.

DANTROLENE

Dantrolene represents a new class of skeletal muscle relaxants (Snyder *et al.,* 1967). It exerts its effects by a direct action on skeletal muscle. Dantrolene has the following chemical structure:

$$O_2N\text{—}\underset{}{\bigcirc}\text{—}\underset{O}{\bigcirc}\text{—}CH=N\text{—}N\underset{O}{\overset{O}{\bigcirc}}NH$$

Dantrolene

Pharmacological Properties. Dantrolene produces relaxation and reduces contraction of skeletal muscle by a direct action on excitation-contraction coupling, perhaps by decreasing the amount of calcium released from the sarcoplasmic reticulum. It does not affect the membrane potential or electrical excitability of skeletal muscle, nor does it alter neuromuscular transmission (*see* Ellis and Carpenter, 1972, 1974; Putney and Bianchi, 1974). Although the drug produces some CNS depressant effects, it does not depress polysynaptic reflexes preferentially as do the centrally acting muscle relaxants. Dantrolene diminishes the force of electrically induced twitches in man without altering muscle action potentials, and it reduces reflex more than voluntary contraction (Herman *et al.,* 1972). In patients with upper motoneuron lesions, spasticity is generally diminished by dantrolene therapy and functional capacity is often improved. However, the drug also tends to induce a generalized muscle weakness that can be detrimental to functional improvement.

Absorption of dantrolene from the gastrointestinal tract is slow and incomplete but sufficiently consistent to provide dose-related plasma concentrations. The mean half-life of the drug in adults is about 9 hours after a 100-mg dose. It is slowly metabolized by the liver, and the 5-hydroxy and acetamido metabolites are excreted with unchanged drug in the urine.

Preparations and Dosage. *Dantrolene sodium* (DANTRIUM) is available for oral use in capsules containing 25 or 100 mg. The starting dose of 25 mg twice a day is gradually increased weekly by increments of 50 to 100 mg per day to a maximal dose of 400 mg daily, given in four divided doses. For children, the recommended starting dose of 1 mg/kg twice a day is gradually increased to a maximum of 3 mg/kg four times a day, but not to exceed 400 mg daily.

Side Effects and Precautions. The major side effect of dantrolene is weakness, probably an extension of its effect on skeletal muscle. Although weakness may be transient or mild, its persistence in some ambulatory patients may compromise therapeutic benefit. Euphoria, light-headedness, dizziness, drowsiness, and fatigue often occur early in treatment, but these side effects are generally transient; nevertheless, patients should be cautioned against driving or participating in hazardous occupations. Although the diarrhea that occurs in some patients can usually be controlled by a more gradual increase in dosage, it may necessitate withdrawal of the drug. In older patients on the drug for more than 60 days, hepatotoxicity and death may rarely occur.

Dantrolene should be used with caution in patients with impaired pulmonary function or severe myocardial disease. The central effects of dantrolene may be enhanced by sedative-antianxiety drugs. As with any new drug, the long-term safety of dantrolene has not been established.

Therapeutic Uses. Dantrolene provides significant and sustained reduction of spasticity and improves functional capacity for the majority of *paraplegic* and *hemiplegic* patients; clonus, mass-reflex movements, and abnormal resistance to passive stretch are reduced. About one half of patients with *athetoid cerebral palsy* or *multiple sclerosis* are also sufficiently improved to warrant continued treatment. Dantrolene represents a significant advance in the medical management of these above-indicated diseases. In general, patients whose functional rehabilitation is retarded by spasticity appear to gain most from the drug. Tolerance to its therapeutic effect does not appear to develop. (*See* Chyatte and Basmajian, 1973; Chyatte *et al.*, 1973; Gelenberg and Poskanzer, 1973; Mayer *et al.*, 1973; Symposium, 1974.)

The status of dantrolene in the treatment of other conditions characterized by overactivity of skeletal muscle has not been established. The drug is *not indicated* for muscle spasm associated with rheumatoid disorders.

BULBOCAPNINE

Bulbocapnine is not a central relaxant; it is described here because it acts centrally to modify skeletal muscle tone. The drug is derived from tubers of several species of *Corydalis* or *cava* plant, commonly known as "Dutchman's breeches." Chemically, the alkaloid bears a striking resemblance to apomorphine. The slight difference in chemical structure of bulbocapnine divests it of the emetic action so characteristic of apomorphine. Apomorphine exhibits antiparkinsonism activity similar to that of levodopa, and both antagonize bulbocapnine-induced catalepsy, presumably by direct activation of central dopamine receptors. As long ago as the sixteenth century, bulbocapnine was recommended for diseases of the head and nerves and for trembling of the hands, and it has been used sporadically for

tremor. The history and actions of the drug have been reviewed by de Jong (1945).

The administration of bulbocapnine to animals results in a peculiar state of catalepsy. When an adequate dose is injected subcutaneously into a cat, there occurs in about 10 minutes a "fixed posture" that is maintained for several hours. Voluntary motion is absent, and a peculiar plastic rigidity ensues that allows the animal to be bent like a lead pipe and placed in many bizarre positions. Some degree of sedation and lethargy is also noted, especially in rabbits and guinea pigs. Recovery with no aftereffects is complete within 18 hours. When larger doses are given, tonic and clonic convulsions appear and death may follow.

The effects of bulbocapnine are prevented by pretreatment with trihexyphenidyl, diphenhydramine, amantadine, and imipramine (Loizzo *et al.*, 1971). Transient catalepsy is produced by bilateral injection of small amounts of bulbocapnine into the striatum, which appears to be its primary site of action (Tseng *et al.*, 1973). The pharmacological actions and interactions of bulbocapnine support the proposal by Ernst (1969) that it blocks central dopamine receptors. Further studies of this interesting drug may contribute to greater understanding of the central control of skeletal muscle tone and movement. It is not currently used in therapy. (*See* Papeschi, 1972.)

Abramsky, O., and Goldschmidt, Z. Treatment and prevention of acute hepatic encephalopathy by intravenous levodopa. *Surgery, St. Louis,* **1974,** *75,* 188–193.

Barbeau, A. Long-term side-effects of levodopa. *Lancet,* **1971,** *1,* 395.

Barbeau, A.; Mars, H.; Gillo-Joffroy, L.; and Arsenault, A. A proposed classification of dopa-induced dyskinesias. In, *L-Dopa and Parkinsonism.* (Barbeau, A., and McDowell, F. H., eds.) F. A. Davis Co., Philadelphia, **1970,** pp. 118–121.

Berger, F. M., and Bradley, W. The pharmacological properties of α:β-dihydroxy-γ-(2-methylphenoxy)-propane (MYANESIN). *Br. J. Pharmac. Chemother.,* **1946,** *1,* 265–272.

Bertler, Å., and Rosengren, E. Occurrence and distribution of dopamine in brain and other tissues. *Experientia,* **1959,** *15,* 10–11.

Birdsong, J. H., and McKinney, A. S. Long-range motor performance changes in levodopa-treated patients with Parkinson's disease. *Neurology, Minneap.,* **1974,** *24,* 107–115.

Carlsson, A. The occurrence, distribution, and physiological role of catecholamines in the nervous system. *Pharmac. Rev.,* **1959,** *11,* 490–493.

————. Biochemical implications of dopa-induced actions on the central nervous system, with particular reference to abnormal movements. In, *L-Dopa and Parkinsonism.* (Barbeau, A., and McDowell, F. H., eds.) F. A. Davis Co., Philadelphia, **1970,** pp. 205–213.

Carlsson, A.; Lindqvist, M.; and Magnusson, T. 3,4-Dihydroxyphenylalanine and 5-hydroxytryptophan as reserpine antagonists. *Nature, Lond.,* **1957,** *180,* 1200.

Carlsson, A.; Lindqvist, M.; Magnusson, T.; and Waldeck, B. On the presence of 3-hydroxytyramine in brain. *Science, Wash.,* **1958,** *127,* 471.

Celesia, G. G., and Barr, A. N. Psychosis and other manifestations of levodopa therapy. *Archs Neurol., Chicago,* **1970,** *23,* 193–200.

Chase, T. N., and Watanabe, A. M. Methyldopahydrazine as an adjunct to L-dopa therapy in parkinsonism. *Neurology, Minneap.,* **1972,** *22,* 384–392.

Chyatte, S. B., and Basmajian, J. V. Dantrolene sodium: long-term effects in severe spasticity. *Archs phys. Med. Rehabil.,* **1973,** *54,* 311–315.

Chyatte, S. B.; Birdsong, J. H.; and Roberson, D. L. Dantrolene sodium in athetoid cerebral palsy. *Archs phys. Med. Rehabil.,* **1973,** *54,* 365–368.

Cotzias, G. C.; Papavasiliou, P. S.; Fehling, C.; Kaufman, B.; and Mena, I. Similarities between neurologic effects of L-dopa and of apomorphine. *New Engl. J. Med.,* **1970,** *282,* 31–33.

Cotzias, G. C.; Van Woert, M. H.; and Schiffer, L. M. Aromatic amino acids and modification of parkinsonism. *New Engl. J. Med.,* **1967,** *276,* 374–379.

Coyle, J. T., and Snyder, S. H. Antiparkinsonian drugs: inhibition of dopamine uptake in the corpus striatum as a possible mechanism of action. *Science, Wash.,* **1969,** *166,* 899–901.

Cunningham, R. W.; Harned, B. K.; Clark, M. C.; Cosgrove, R. R.; Daugherty, N. S.; Hine, C. H.; Vessey, R. E.; and Yuda, N. N. The pharmacology of 3-(N-piperidyl)-1-phenyl-1-cyclohexyl-1-propanol HCl (ARTANE) and related compounds: new antispasmodic agents. *J. Pharmac. exp. Ther.,* **1949,** *96,* 151–165.

Eddy, R. L.; Jones, A. L.; Chakmakjian, Z. H.; and Silverthorne, M. C. Effect of levodopa (L-dopa) on human hypophyseal trophic hormone release. *J. clin. Endocr. Metab.,* **1971,** *33,* 709–712.

Ehringer, H., and Hornykiewicz, O. Verteilung von Noradrenalin und Dopamin (3-hydroxytyramin) im Gehirn des Menschen und ihr Verhalten bei Erkrankungen des extrapyramidalen Systems. *Klin. Wschr.,* **1960,** *38,* 1236–1239.

Ellis, K. O., and Carpenter, J. F. Studies on the mechanism of action of dantrolene sodium, a skeletal muscle relaxant. *Naunyn-Schmiedebergs Archs Pharmac.,* **1972,** *275,* 83–94.

————. Mechanism of control of skeletal-muscle contraction by dantrolene sodium. *Archs phys. Med. Rehabil.,* **1974,** *55,* 362–369.

Ernst, A. M. The role of biogenic amines in the extrapyramidal system. *Acta physiol. pharmac. néerl.,* **1969,** *15,* 141–154.

Esplin, D. W. Criteria for assessing effects of depressant drugs on spinal cord synaptic transmission, with examples of drug selectivity. *Archs int. Pharmacodyn. Thér.,* **1963,** *143,* 479–497.

Farnebo, L.-O.; Fuxe, K.; Goldstein, M.; Hamberger, B.; and Ungerstedt, U. Dopamine and noradrenaline releasing action of amantadine in the central and peripheral nervous system: a possible mode of action in Parkinson's disease. *Eur. J. Pharmac.,* **1971,** *16,* 27–38.

Fischer, J. E., and Baldessarini, R. J. False neurotransmitters and hepatic failure. *Lancet,* **1971,** *2,* 75–80.

Forssman, B.; Kihlstrand, S.; and Larsson, L.-E. Amantadine therapy in parkinsonism. *Acta neurol. scand.,* **1972,** *48,* 1–18.

Gelenberg, A. J., and Poskanzer, D. C. The effect of dantrolene sodium on spasticity in multiple sclerosis. *Neurology, Minneap.,* **1973,** *23,* 1313–1315.

Goldberg, L. I., and Whitsett, T. L. Cardiovascular effects of levodopa. *Clin. Pharmac. Ther.,* **1971,** *12,* 376–382.

Goodman, L. The pharmacodynamic actions of benzimidazole: a preliminary report. *Bull. New Engl. med. Cent.,* **1943,** *5,* 97–100.

Goodwin, F. K. Psychiatric side effects of levodopa in man. *J. Am. med. Ass.,* **1971,** *218,* 1915–1920.

Goodwin, F. K.; Murphy, D. L.; Brodie, H. K. H.; and Bunney, W. E. Levodopa: alterations in behavior. *Clin. Pharmac. Ther.,* **1971,** *12,* 383–396.

Grelak, R. P.; Clark, R.; Stump, J. M.; and Vernier, V. G. Amantadine-dopamine interaction: possible mode of action in parkinsonism. *Science, Wash.,* **1970,** *169,* 203–204.

Hare, B. D.; Neumayr, R. J.; and Franz, D. N. Opposite effects of L-dopa and 5-HTP on spinal sympathetic reflexes. *Nature, Lond.,* **1972,** *239,* 336–337.

Henneman, E.; Kaplan, A.; and Unna, K. A neuropharmacological study on the effect of MYANESIN (TOLSEROL) on motor systems. *J. Pharmac. exp. Ther.,* **1949,** *97,* 331–341.

Henning, M., and Rubenson, A. Central hypotensive effect of L-3,4-dihydroxyphenylalanine in the rat. *J. Pharm. Pharmac.,* **1970,** *22,* 553–560.

Herman, R.; Mayer, N.; and Mecomber, S. A. Clinical pharmaco-physiology of dantrolene sodium. *Am. J. phys. Med.,* **1972,** *51,* 296–311.

Hunter, K. R.; Hollman, A.; Laurence, D. R.; and Stern, G. M. Levodopa in parkinsonian patients with heart-disease. *Lancet,* **1971,** *1,* 932–934.

Hunter, K. R.; Laurence, D. R.; Shaw, K. M.; and Stern, G. M. Sustained levodopa therapy in parkinsonism. *Lancet,* **1973,** *2,* 929–931.

Kaada, B. R. Site of action of MYANESIN (mephenesin, TOLSEROL) in the central nervous system. *J. Neurophysiol.,* **1950,** *13,* 89–104.

Keenan, R. E. The Eaton Collaborative Study of levodopa therapy in parkinsonism: a summary. *Neurology, Minneap.,* **1970,** *20* (No. 12, Part 2), 46–59.

Klawans, H., and Ringel, P. Observations on the efficacy of L-dopa in progressive supranuclear palsy. *Eur. Neurol.,* **1971,** *5,* 115–129.

Langrall, H. M., and Joseph, C. Evaluation of safety and efficacy of levodopa in Parkinson's disease and syndrome; results of a collaborative study. *Neurology, Minneap.,* **1972,** *22* (No. 5, Part 2), 3–16.

Lieberman, A. N., and Shupack, J. L. Levodopa and melanoma. *Neurology, Minneap.,* **1974,** *24,* 340–343.

Loizzo, A.; Scotti de Carolis, A.; and Longo, V. G. Studies on the central effects of bulbocapnine. *Psychopharmacologia,* **1971,** *22,* 234–249.

Longo, V. G. Effects of mephenesin on the repetitive discharge of spinal cord interneurones. *Archs int. Pharmacodyn. Thér.,* **1961,** *132,* 222–236.

McDowell, F. Clinical laboratory abnormalities. *Clin. Pharmac. Ther.,* **1971,** *12,* 335–339.

Markham, C. H. The choreoathetoid movement disorder induced by levodopa. *Clin. Pharmac. Ther.,* **1971,** *12,* 340–343.

————. Thirty months' trial of levodopa in Parkinson's disease. *Neurology, Minneap.,* **1972,** *22,* Suppl., 17–21.

Mars, H. Modification of levodopa effect by systemic decarboxylase inhibition. *Archs Neurol., Chicago,* **1973,** *28,* 91–95.

Mawdsley, C.; Williams, I. R.; Pullar, I. A.; Davidson, D. L.; and Kinloch, N. E. Treatment of parkinsonism by amantadine and levodopa. *Clin. Pharmac. Ther.,* **1972,** *13,* 575–583.

Mayer, N.; Mecomber, S. A.; and Herman, R. Treatment of spasticity with dantrolene sodium. *Am. J. phys. Med.,* **1973,** *52,* 18–29.

Mena, I.; Court, J.; Fuenzalida, S.; Papavasiliou, P. S.; and Cotzias, G. C. Modification of chronic manganese poisoning; treatment with L-dopa or 5-OH tryptophane. *New Engl. J. Med.,* **1970,** *282,* 5–10.

Montagu, K. A. Catechol compounds in rat tissues and in brains of different animals. *Nature, Lond.,* **1957,** *180,* 244–245.

Neumayr, R. J.; Hare, B. D.; and Franz, D. N. Evidence for bulbospinal control of sympathetic preganglionic neurons by monoaminergic pathways. *Life Sci.,* **1974,** *14,* 793–806.

Ng, L. K. Y.; Chase, T. N.; Colburn, R. W.; and Kopin, I. J. L-Dopa in parkinsonism. A possible mechanism of action. *Neurology, Minneap.,* **1972,** *22,* 688–696.

Papavasiliou, P. S.; Cotzias, G. C.; Düby, S. E.; Steck, A. J.;

Fehling, C.; and Bell, M. A. Levodopa in parkinsonism: potentiation of central effects with a peripheral inhibitor. *New Engl. J. Med.,* **1972,** *285,* 8–14.

Parkes, J. D.; Sharpstone, P.; and Williams, R. Levodopa in hepatic coma. *Lancet,* **1970a,** *2,* 1341–1343.

Parkes, J. D.; Zilkha, K. J.; Calver, D. M.; and Knill-Jones, R. P. Controlled trial of amantadine hydrochloride in Parkinson's disease. *Lancet,* **1970b,** *1,* 259–262.

Pearce, L. A.; Waterbury, L. D.; and Green, H. D. Amantadine hydrochloride: alteration in peripheral circulation. *Neurology, Minneap.,* **1974,** *24,* 46–48.

Putney, J. W., Jr., and Bianchi, C. P. Site of action of dantrolene in frog sartorius muscle. *J. Pharmac. exp. Ther.,* **1974,** *189,* 202–212.

Ringel, S. P., and Klawans, H. L., Jr. Carbon monoxide-induced parkinsonism. *J. neurol. Sci.,* **1972,** *16,* 245–251.

Rinne, U. K.; Sonninen, V.; and Siirtola, T. Treatment of Parkinson's disease with L-dopa and decarboxylase inhibitor. *Z. Neurol.,* **1972,** *202,* 1–20.

Rivera-Calimlim, L.; Dujovne, C. A.; Morgan, J. P.; Lasagna, L.; and Bianchine, J. R. Absorption and metabolism of L-dopa by the human stomach. *Eur. J. clin. Invest.,* **1971,** *1,* 313–320.

Rosenthal, R. K.; McDowell, F. H.; and Cooper, W. Levodopa therapy in athetoid cerebral palsy. *Neurology, Minneap.,* **1972,** *22,* 1–11.

Roszkowski, A. P. A pharmacological comparison of therapeutically useful centrally acting skeletal muscle relaxants. *J. Pharmac. exp. Ther.,* **1960,** *129,* 75–81.

Sacks, O. W.; Kohl, M. S.; Messeloff, C. R.; and Schwartz, W. F. Effects of levodopa in parkinsonian patients with dementia. *Neurology, Minneap.,* **1972,** *22,* 516–519.

Sandler, M. How does L-dopa work in parkinsonism? *Lancet,* **1971,** *1,* 784–785.

Sandler, M.; Carter, S. B.; Hunter, K. R.; and Stern, G. M. Tetrahydroisoquinoline alkaloids: *in vivo* metabolites of L-dopa in man. *Nature, Lond.,* **1973,** *241,* 439–443.

Schnur, J. A.; Chase, T. N.; and Brody, J. A. Parkinsonism-dementia of Guam: treatment with L-dopa. *Neurology, Minneap.,* **1971,** *21,* 1236–1242.

Schwab, R. S. Muscle relaxants. *Practitioner,* **1964,** *192,* 104–108.

Schwab, R. S.; England, A. C., Jr.; Poskanzer, D. C.; and Young, R. R. Amantadine in the treatment of Parkinson's disease. *J. Am. med. Ass.,* **1969,** *208,* 1168–1170.

Schwab, R. S.; Poskanzer, D. C.; England, A. C.; and Young, R. R. Amantadine in Parkinson's disease. Review of more than two years' experience. *J. Am. med. Ass.,* **1972,** *222,* 792–795.

Sirtori, C. R.; Bolme, P.; and Azarnoff, D. L. Metabolic responses to acute and chronic L-dopa administration in patients with parkinsonism. *New Engl. J. Med.,* **1972,** *287,* 729–733.

Snyder, H. R., Jr.; Davis, C. S.; Bickerton, R. K.; and Halliday, R. P. 1-[(5-Arylfurfurylidene)amino]hydantoins. A new class of muscle relaxants. *J. mednl pharm. Chem.,* **1967,** *10,* 807–810.

Sourkes, T. L. Possible new metabolites mediating actions of L-dopa. *Nature, Lond.,* **1971,** *229,* 413–414.

Tseng, L. F.; Wei, E.; and Loh, H. H. Brain areas associated with bulbocapnine catalepsy. *Eur. J. Pharmac.,* **1973,** *22,* 363–366.

Tseng, T. -C., and Wang, S. C. Locus of action of centrally acting muscle relaxants, diazepam and tybamate. *J. Pharmac. exp. Ther.,* **1971,** *178,* 350–360.

Von Voigtlander, P. F., and Moore, K. E. Dopamine: release from the brain *in vivo* by amantadine. *Science, Wash.,* **1971,** *174,* 408–410.

Watanabe, A. M.; Chase, T. N.; and Cardon, P. V. Effect of L-dopa alone and in combination with an extracerebral decarboxylase inhibitor on blood pressure and some cardiovascular reflexes. *Clin. Pharmac. Ther.,* **1970,** *11,* 740–746.

Weintraub, M. I., and Van Woert, M. H. Reversal by levodopa of cholinergic hypersensitivity in Parkinson's disease. *New Engl. J. Med.,* **1971,** *284,* 412–415.

Monographs and Reviews

Barbeau, A. L-Dopa therapy in Parkinson's disease: a critical review of nine years' experience. *Can. med. Ass. J.,* **1969,** *101,* 791–800.

———. Drugs affecting movement disorders. *A. Rev. Pharmac.,* **1974,** *14,* 91–113.

Barbeau, A., and McDowell, F. H. (eds.). *L-Dopa and Parkinsonism.* F. A. Davis Co., Philadelphia, **1970.**

Berger, F. M. Spinal cord depressant drugs. *Pharmac. Rev.,* **1949,** *1,* 243–278. (136 references.)

Bernheimer, H.; Birkmayer, W.; Hornykiewicz, O.; Jellinger, K.; and Seitelberger, F. Brain dopamine and the syndromes of Parkinson and Huntington. *J. neurol. Sci.,* **1973,** *20,* 415–455. (115 references.)

Bianchine, J. R., and Sunyapridakul, L. Interactions between levodopa and other drugs: significance in the treatment of Parkinson's disease. *Drugs,* **1973,** *6,* 364–388. (118 references.)

Brogden, R. N.; Speight, T. M.; and Avery, G. S. Levodopa: a review of its pharmacological properties and therapeutic uses with particular reference to parkinsonism. *Drugs,* **1971,** *2,* 262–408. (337 references.)

de Jong, H. H. *Experimental Catatonia.* The Williams & Wilkins Co., Baltimore, **1945.**

Denhoff, E., and Robinault, I. *Cerebral Palsy and Related Disorders: A Developmental Approach to Dysfunction.* McGraw-Hill Book Co., New York, **1960.**

Domino, E. F. The correlation between animal testing procedures and clinical effectiveness of centrally acting muscle relaxants of the mephenesin type. *Ann. N.Y. Acad. Sci.,* **1956,** *64,* 705–729. (177 references.)

Eldridge, R. (ed.). Conference on the torsion dystonias (dystonia musculorum deformans). *Neurology, Minneap.,* **1970,** *20* (No. 11, Part 2), 1–154.

Hornykiewicz, O. Dopamine (3-hydroxytyramine) and brain function. *Pharmac. Rev.,* **1966,** *18* (Part 2), 925–964.

———. Parkinson's disease: from brain homogenate to treatment. *Fedn Proc. Fedn Am. Socs exp. Biol.,* **1973a,** *32,* 183–190.

———. Dopamine in the basal ganglia. *Br. med. Bull.,* **1973b,** *29,* 172–178.

Malitz, S. (ed.). *L-Dopa and Behavior.* Raven Press, New York, **1972.**

Papeschi, R. Dopamine, extrapyramidal system, and psychomotor function. *Psychiat. Neurol. Neurochir.,* **1972,** *75,* 13–48.

Smith, C. M. Relaxants of skeletal muscle. In, *Physiological Pharmacology.* Vol. 2, *The Nervous System—Part B: Central Nervous System Drugs.* (Root, W. S., and Hofmann, F. G., eds.) Academic Press, Inc., New York, **1965,** pp. 2–96. (459 references.)

Sourkes, T. L. Central actions of dopa and dopamine. *Revue can. Biol.,* **1972,** *31,* 153–168.

Symposium. (Various authors.) Pharmacologic and clinical experiences with levodopa. *Neurology, Minneap.,* **1970,** *20* (No. 12, Part 2), 1–66.

Symposium. (Various authors.) Symposium on levodopa in Parkinson's disease. Clinical and pharmacological aspects. *Clin. Pharmac. Ther.,* **1971,** *12,* 317–416.

Symposium. (Various authors.) Symposium on levodopa in Parkinson's disease. *Neurology, Minneap.,* **1972,** *22* (No. 5, Part 2), 1–102.

Symposium. (Various authors.) Spasticity—its etiology, physiology and the pharmacology of a new agent. *Archs phys. Med. Rehabil.,* **1974,** *55,* 331–392.

Yahr, M. D. (ed.). *Advances in Neurology.* Vol. 2, *Treatment of Parkinsonism—The Role of Dopa Decarboxylase Inhibitors.* Raven Press, New York, **1973.**

CHAPTER

15 NARCOTIC ANALGESICS AND ANTAGONISTS

Jerome H. Jaffe and William R. Martin

This chapter presents the pharmacological properties and therapeutic uses of the *opioids, opioid antagonists,* and *related analgesics.* The term *opioid* refers to any natural or synthetic drug that has morphine-like pharmacological actions; it is used interchangeably with the term *narcotic analgesic.* The opioids are employed primarily for the relief of pain, but their use entails the risk of producing physical and sometimes psychological dependence. There are as yet no agents effective against severe pain that are entirely free of this risk.

MORPHINE AND OTHER OPIUM ALKALOIDS

In 1680, Sydenham wrote, "Among the remedies which it has pleased Almighty God to give to man to relieve his sufferings, none is so universal and so efficacious as opium." Morphine, the alkaloid that gives opium its analgesic actions, remains the standard against which new analgesics are measured. Although newer analgesics possess special properties, none is clinically superior in relieving pain.

History. The psychological effects of opium may have been known to the ancient Sumerians (*ca.* 4000 B.C.) whose ideograph for the poppy was *hul* ("joy") plus *gil* ("plants"), but the first undisputed reference to poppy juice is found in the writings of Theophrastus in the third century B.C. The word *opium* itself is derived from the Greek name for juice, the drug being obtained from the juice of the poppy capsules. Arabian physicians were well versed in the uses of opium; Arabian traders introduced the drug to the Orient, where it was employed mainly for the control of dysenteries. By the middle of the sixteenth century, the uses of opium that are still valid were fairly well understood in Europe. Paracelsus (1493–1541) is credited with the compounding of "laudanum," which remains in use today.

In the eighteenth century opium smoking became popular in the Orient. At that time the use of opiates for their subjective effects was considerably more acceptable than it is at present. In Europe, the ready availability of opium led to some degree of overuse, but the problem of opium eating (actually the drinking of laudanum) never became as prevalent or as socially destructive as the abuse of alcohol.

In 1803, a young German pharmacist, Sertürner, isolated and described an opium alkaloid that he named morphine, after Morpheus, the Greek god of dreams. The discovery of other alkaloids in opium quickly followed that of morphine (codeine by Robiquet in 1832, papaverine by Merck in 1848), and by the middle of the nineteenth century the use of pure alkaloids rather than crude opium preparations began to spread throughout the medical world.

The invention of the hypodermic needle and the parenteral use of morphine tended to produce a more severe variety of compulsive drug use. In the United States, the extent of the opiate-use problem was accentuated by the influx of opium-smoking Chinese laborers, the widespread use of morphine among wounded Civil War soldiers, and the unrestricted availability of opium that prevailed until the early years of this century. The recognition of this serious liability of morphine stimulated a search for potent analgesics that would not lead to compulsive drug use, a search not yet ended.

The reader interested in the history of opium and its alkaloids and the problem of addiction is referred to the accounts of Terry and Pellens (1928), Lewin (1931), and Musto (1973).

Source and Composition of Opium. Opium is obtained from the milky exudate of the incised unripe seed capsules of the poppy plant, *Papaver somniferum,* indigenous to Asia Minor. The milky juice is dried in the air and forms a brownish, gummy mass. This is further dried and powdered to make the official powdered opium, containing well over a score of alkaloids. Only a few—morphine, codeine, and papaverine—have clinical usefulness. The alkaloids constitute about 25% by weight of opium. They can be divided into two distinct chemical classes, *phenanthrenes* and *benzylisoquinolines,* which contrast sharply in their pharmacological properties. Those of medical interest and their approximate percentages are shown in Table 15–1.

Table 15–1. ALKALOIDS OF OPIUM

CLASS	NATURAL ALKALOID	PERCENTAGE IN OPIUM
Phenanthrene	Morphine	10.0
	Codeine	0.5
	Thebaine	0.2
Benzylisoquinoline	Papaverine	1.0
	Noscapine	6.0

The major opium alkaloid of the benzylisoquinoline group is *papaverine*. It lacks morphine-like effects and is discussed as a smooth muscle relaxant in Chapter 34.

Chemistry of the Opium Alkaloids. Morphine and codeine are by far the most important phenanthrene alkaloids of opium. The structure of morphine originally proposed by Gulland and Robinson in 1925, and ultimately proven to be correct, is as follows:

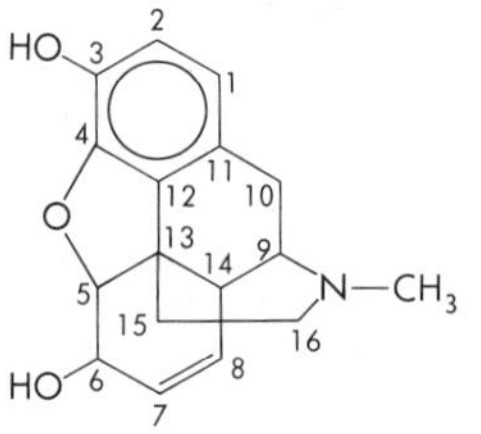

Morphine

Although morphine can be synthesized in the laboratory with great difficulty, many semisynthetic derivatives are made by relatively simple modifications of the morphine or thebaine molecule. *Codeine* is methylmorphine, the methyl substitution being on the phenolic OH. *Thebaine* differs from morphine only in that both OH groups are methylated and that there are two double bonds in the ring ($\Delta^{6,7}$, $\Delta^{8,14}$), but it is practically devoid of analgesic action and produces seizures at a relatively low dosage. Certain derivatives of thebaine are more than 1000 times as potent as morphine (*e.g.*, etorphine). *Diacetylmorphine*, or *heroin*, is made from morphine by the acetylation of both the phenolic and the alcoholic OH groups. *Apomorphine* is structurally similar to

morphine and can be prepared from it. It is a potent emetic and dopaminergic substance that has been tried experimentally in the treatment of Parkinson's disease. *Hydromorphone, oxymorphone, hydrocodone, and oxycodone* are also made by modifying the morphine molecule. The structural relationship between morphine and some of its surrogates and antagonists is shown in Table 15–2.

Structure-Activity Relationship of the Opioids. In addition to morphine, codeine, and the semisynthetic derivatives of the natural opium alkaloids (often referred to as *opiates* because of their derivation from opium), there are a number of other structurally distinct chemical classes of drugs with pharmacological actions remarkably similar to those of morphine. These diverse groups share the capacity to produce analgesia, respiratory depression, gastrointestinal spasm, and morphine-like physical dependence. Toxic doses commonly produce convulsions, and the analgesic, gastrointestinal, depressant, and convulsant effects can be antagonized by naloxone and related antagonists. Clinically useful compounds include the morphinans, benzomorphans, methadones, phenylpiperidines, and propionanilides. In addition, *thiambutene* and *benzimidazole* derivatives possess narcotic activity (for references, *see* Braenden *et al.*, 1955). Although the flat two-dimensional representations of these chemically diverse compounds appear to be quite different, an examination of molecular models suggests that all of them include or can simulate a piperidine ring. The probable structure of the opioid receptor and the structure-activity relationship among the diverse compounds with analgesic actions are discussed by Hardy and Howell (1965), May and Sargent (1965), Lewis and associates (1971), and Lowney and co-workers (1974). Examples of chemical modifications

Table 15–2. STRUCTURES OF OPIOIDS AND NARCOTIC ANTAGONISTS CHEMICALLY RELATED TO MORPHINE

NONPROPRIETARY NAME	CHEMICAL RADICALS AND POSITIONS			OTHER CHANGES †
	3 *	6 *	17 *	
Morphine	—OH	—OH	—CH$_3$	—
Heroin	—OCOCH$_3$	—OCOCH$_3$	—CH$_3$	—
Hydromorphone	—OH	=O	—CH$_3$	(1)
Metopon	—OH	=O	—CH$_3$	(1),(2)
Oxymorphone	—OH	=O	—CH$_3$	(1),(3)
Levorphanol	—OH	—H	—CH$_3$	(1),(4)
Codeine	—OCH$_3$	—OH	—CH$_3$	—
Hydrocodone	—OCH$_3$	=O	—CH$_3$	(1)
Oxycodone	—OCH$_3$	=O	—CH$_3$	(1),(3)
Nalorphine	—OH	—OH	—CH$_2$CH=CH$_2$	—
Naloxone	—OH	=O	—CH$_2$CH=CH$_2$	(1)
Naltrexone	—OH	=O	$-\mathrm{CH_2CH}\overset{\textstyle CH_2}{\overbrace{}}\mathrm{CH_2}$	(1)

* The numbers 3, 6, and 16 refer to positions in the morphine molecule, as shown above.
† Other changes in the morphine molecule are as follows:
   (1) Single instead of double bond between C7 and C8.
   (2) CH$_3$ added at C5.
   (3) OH added to C14.
   (4) No oxygen between C4 and C5.

that produce clinically significant alterations are presented in connection with the individual drugs.

PHARMACOLOGICAL PROPERTIES

Morphine and its surrogates produce their major effects on the central nervous system (CNS) and the bowel. The older literature on the opium alkaloids has been reviewed by Reynolds and Randall (1957). Additional reviews are those of Winter (1965), Lim (1966), Martin (1967), Domino (1968), and Lewis and associates (1971). Opioid actions and uses have also been the subject of a number of symposia (see Soulairac et al., 1968; Wikler, 1968; Clouet, 1971; Kosterlitz et al., 1973; Braude et al., 1974).

Mechanism of Action. At present, the mechanisms by which the opioids exert their effects remain uncertain. Stereospecific saturable receptors for opioids and opioid antagonists have been studied in vertebrate neural tissues by several investigators (Goldstein et al., 1971; Pert and Snyder, 1973, 1974; Simon et al., 1973; Lowney et al., 1974). The distribution of these receptors in the nervous system does not correlate precisely with the distribution of any one putative neurotransmitter or any recognized neural subsystem, although the limbic system and periaqueductal gray matter, areas that may play a role in opioid analgesia, are particularly enriched (Hiller et al., 1973; Kuhar et al., 1973). It is likely that the receptors thus far studied will prove to be heterogeneous (see also page 272).

There is ample evidence that opioids interact with more than one neurotransmitter, either directly or indirectly. Opioids decrease the release of acetylcholine (ACh) from some peripheral and central cholinergic neurons, elevate brain ACh levels (see Harris and Dewey, 1973; Lees et al., 1973), and antagonize the ACh-depleting effects of hemicholinium (Domino and Wilson, 1973). Opioids seem to inhibit the release of catecholamines from certain peripheral neurons, but increase the release, synthesis, and turnover of catecholamines in the CNS (see Way and Shen, 1971; Lees et al., 1973; Smith and Sheldon, 1973). In some preparations morphine blocks the effects of 5-hydroxytryptamine (5-HT), but it can also stimulate its release from the gut. Chronic administration increases the turnover of 5-HT in the brain without altering the steady-state concentrations in the brain (see Way and Shen, 1971).

Since the opioids have multiple effects on the CNS, it is quite possible that a given neurotransmitter may play a more critical role in one effect (e.g., analgesia) than it does in another (e.g., stimulation of locomotor activity, increased bowel tone, or emesis). Nevertheless, attempts to understand the role of various transmitters in any one specific opioid action, such as analgesia, have not yielded clear-cut results. For example, in man, opioid-induced euphoria and analgesia are enhanced by the simultaneous administration of amphetamines, suggesting at least an additive role for norepinephrine or dopamine. Animal studies in which precursors, blockers, and depletors of catecholamines have been used to manipulate central adrenergic processes in order to determine their role in opioid analgesia have yielded conflicting results (see Way and Shen, 1971; Buxbaum et al., 1973; Calcutt et al., 1973; Cicero et al., 1974). Nevertheless, the preponderance of evidence suggests that central noradrenergic mechanisms may produce analgesia and euphoria that may add to the effects of opioids. Attempts to elucidate the role of 5-HT in opioid analgesia are plagued by similar apparent inconsistencies in the data, although there is a trend suggesting that 5-HT is synergistic with opioids in producing analgesia (see Chapter 29). The equally complex role of neurotransmitters in the development of opioid tolerance and physical dependence is discussed in Chapter 16.

Central Nervous System. In man, morphine produces *analgesia, drowsiness, changes in mood,* and *mental clouding.* A significant feature of the analgesia is that it occurs without loss of consciousness. When small-to-moderate amounts of morphine (5 to 10 mg) are given to patients with pain, discomfort, worry, tension, or other complaints, any or all of these effects occur. Patients with pain report that it is entirely gone, or less intense, or that they are less distressed by it. Drowsiness occurs commonly both in volunteers and in patients with clinical pain. The extremities feel heavy and the body warm, the face and especially the nose may itch, and the mouth becomes dry. In addition to relief of distress, some patients experience euphoria. If the external situation is favorable, sleep may ensue.

When morphine in the same dose is given to a presumably normal, pain-free individual, the experience is not always pleasant; sometimes *dysphoria* rather than euphoria results, consisting in mild anxiety or fear; frequently there is nausea and occasionally vomiting. Morphine also produces *mental clouding* characterized by drowsiness and inability to concentrate, difficulty in mentation, apathy, lessened physical activity, reduced visual acuity, and lethargy. In post-addict volunteers, mental clouding is less prominent than in normal subjects, and the euphoria is more pronounced.

As the dose is increased, subjective effects become more pronounced; there is increased drowsiness that leads to sleep; in individuals who experience euphoria, the euphoric effect is accentuated; patients with severe pain that is not adequately relieved by smaller doses of morphine are usually relieved by larger doses (15 to 20 mg). The incidence of nausea and vomiting is also increased, and respiratory depression, the major toxic effect of morphine-like drugs, may become pronounced; but even large doses are not anticonvulsant and do not cause slurred speech or significant motor incoordination.

Analgesia. The relief of pain by morphine and its surrogates is relatively selective, in that other sensory modalities (touch, vibration, vision, hearing, etc.) are not obtunded. Indeed, with therapeutic doses of morphine the painful stimulus itself may be recognized but it may not be perceived as painful. Thus, patients frequently report that the pain is still present but that they feel more comfortable (*see* below).

Continuous dull pain is relieved more effectively than sharp intermittent pain, but with sufficient amounts of morphine it is possible to relieve even the severe pain associated with renal or biliary colic. Although there are some types of pain that are not adequately relieved by safe doses of morphine, it is much more significant that most types of pain respond to about the same degree.

The selectivity of opioid-induced analgesia is greater than that of other drugs acting on the CNS. Thus, the inhalation of nitrous oxide (20 to 40 volumes %), while producing analgesia that is approximately equivalent to 15 mg of morphine, also produces an overall impairment of consciousness, marked drowsiness, alterations in judgment, impairment of immediate and delayed memory, and nausea. Similarly, low concentrations of ether, high doses of barbiturates, or gross intoxication with alcohol produce significant analgesia, but only in association with sedation and impairment of motor coordination, intellectual acuity, emotional control, and judgment (*see* Parbrook, 1967). For a given degree of analgesia, the mental clouding produced by therapeutic doses of morphine is considerably less pronounced and of a qualitatively different character; morphine and related drugs rarely produce the garrulous, silly, and emotionally labile behavior frequently seen in alcohol and barbiturate intoxication. The characteristics of the subjective effects produced by narcotic analgesics have been extensively studied in patients and nonaddict volunteers by Beecher, Keats, Lasagna, and their coworkers (*see* Beecher, 1959; Smith *et al.*, 1962), while the comparative effects of morphine, barbiturates, and other drugs in postaddicts have been studied at the Addiction Research Center, Lexington, Kentucky (*see* Wikler, 1958; Hill *et al.*, 1963; Haertzen, 1966).

Any meaningful discussion of the action of analgesic agents must include some distinction between *pain as a specific sensation,* subserved by distinct neurophysiological structures, and *pain as suffering* (the original sensation plus the reactions evoked by the sensation). There is general agreement that all types of painful experiences, whether produced with experimental technics or occurring clinically as a result of pathology, include both the *original sensation* and the *reaction to that sensation.* However, clinical and laboratory situations differ considerably in the degree to which the *reactive component* plays a role. Thus, a cooperative subject can reliably report when a thermal stimulus to the forehead first becomes painful (the pain threshold), but this situation is considerably different from that of pathological pain that cannot be terminated at will and where the meaning of the sensation and the distress it engenders are markedly affected by the individual's previous experiences and current expectations.

The effects of analgesics on both experimentally produced and pathological pain have been carefully studied in man. The experimental measurements of the effects of morphine on *pain threshold* have not always been consistent; some workers find that analgesics reliably elevate the threshold, while many others do not obtain consistent changes. By contrast, moderate doses of morphine are quite effective in relieving clinical pain and increasing the capacity to *tolerate* experimentally induced pain (*see* Wolff *et al.*, 1966, 1969; Smith *et al.*, 1968). One possible interpretation is that at usual therapeutic doses the opioids act primarily on those systems responsible for the affective responses to noxious stimuli. This effect is best assessed by asking patients with clinical pain about the degree of relief produced by the drug administered. When pain does not evoke its usual responses (anxiety, fear, panic, and suffering), *a patient's ability to tolerate the pain may be markedly increased even when the capacity to perceive the sensation is relatively unaltered (see* Beecher, 1959).

It would, however, be an oversimplification to ascribe all of narcotic-induced analgesia to alterations in the reactive component, even though such a view may be reasonably accurate when one is dealing with most types of clinical pain and the usual therapeutic doses of morphine. It would also be an oversimplification to consider the reactive component of pain as being identical or equivalent to anxiety, in the sense that this term is used in other contexts (fear and apprehension without an obvious external stimulus). Noxious stimulation elicits distinct defensive response patterns even at the spinal level (*see* below), and it is quite conceivable that other specific nociceptive defensive reactions not identical to those evoked by fear and anxiety-producing situations are evoked at higher levels. Drugs such as the barbiturates and benzodiazepines that are quite effective antianxiety agents in doses not producing gross intoxication are not particularly effective as analgesics.

Sites of Morphine-Induced Analgesia. The analgesic effects of morphine are due to its actions on the CNS. The opioids neither alter the threshold or responsivity of *nerve endings* to noxious stimulation nor impair the conduction of the nerve impulse along peripheral nerves. The neurophysiological effects of the opioids have been subjected to extensive investigation (*see* reviews by Wikler, 1958; Martin, 1963; Lim, 1966; Domino, 1968; Soulairac *et al.,* 1968). It is difficult to state precisely what sites within the nervous system are responsible for the analgesic and sedative effects of morphine, or for its euphoric and behavioral effects.

At the level of the *spinal cord,* nociceptive reflexes (*e.g.,* the ipsilateral flexor, crossed extensor, and C-fiber reflexes) are depressed by morphine and related drugs in doses that have relatively little effect on the patellar reflex. The effect of morphine on multineuronal pathways may be due to a depressant action on the mechanisms involved in the temporal summation characteristic of responses mediated by such pathways. Nociceptive responses characterized by afterdischarge are probably a consequence of persisting repetitive firing of interneurons, and are selectively depressed by opioids. Conventional tests of analgesic drugs (*e.g.,* the tail flick in rats or the skin twitch in dogs in response to thermal stimuli) are, in part at least, a measurement of effects on spinal multineuronal reflexes. In humans with complete spinal cord transection, morphine depresses nociceptive flexor withdrawal reflexes. The drug may also affect the balance of supraspinal inhibitory and facilitatory influences on the cord and thus exert an indirect suppression of spinal reflexes. (*See* Wikler, 1958; Martin, 1963; Melzack and Wall, 1965; Mayer *et al.,* 1971.)

The effects of morphine at higher levels in the CNS are quite complex. There are probably multiple sites in the brain involved in the perception of pain and the modulation of nociceptive reflexes. In the rat, electrical stimulation in the region of the midbrain central gray matter produces analgesia sufficient for laparotomy without loss of general motor responsiveness (Reynolds, 1969). Furthermore, stimulation at mesencephalic and diencephalic sites abolishes the response to intense pain while leaving other sensory modalities mainly unaffected. In this situation, the field of analgesia can be restricted to one limb, so that painful stimulation to another limb elicits a normal reaction (Mayer *et al.,* 1971). Minute amounts of opioids injected into the cerebral ventricles or into various sites within the brain also produce analgesia, and microinjections of narcotic antagonists into the midbrain tegmentum can antagonize the analgesic effects of systemically administered opioids (*see* Martin, 1967; Herz *et al.,* 1970; Jacquet and Lajtha, 1973).

Animals pressing a lever to avoid an electrical stimulus to the Gasserian ganglion or other brain sites that seem to produce aversive effects reduce their lever-pressing activity after the administration of morphine in doses that do not cause gross sedation. However, the pressing activity again increases if the stimulus intensity is increased. In such situations, it appears that the effect of morphine is to increase the threshold stimulus required to produce pain. The effects of morphine on self-stimulation at "reward" or "pleasure centers" is inconsistent; both lowered and raised thresholds have been reported.

The effect of morphine on the *limbic system* suggests that it is qualitatively quite distinct from that of agents commonly used in the treatment of anxiety (barbiturates, meprobamate, and chlordiazepoxide). Such agents share the capacity to raise the threshold and shorten the duration of afterdischarges in the hippocampus. The cortical potentials evoked by direct stimulation of limbic structures are not altered by morphine (Monnier *et al.,* 1962; McKenzie, 1964). However, the alterations in electrical activity in the amygdala and hippocampus produced by peripheral stimulation are depressed by analgesic doses of opioids. For example, strong electrical shocks that cause vocalization also produce high-voltage waves in the hippocampus, which outlast the stimulus; opioids shorten the duration of this response or prevent it entirely.

Opioid-induced alteration of the limbic system responses to painful stimuli without significant alteration of transmission through classical sensory pathways is consistent with the clinical observation that, in usual doses, the opioids reduce the affective response to nociceptive stimulation and increase pain tolerance without altering the threshold for perception of the stimulus (*see* above).

While it is not yet certain that the stereospecific opioid receptors identified in mammalian brain (*see* above) are those responsible for opioid analgesia, it is noteworthy that these receptors are found in high concentrations in the limbic system and closely related areas of the brain.

Hypothalamic and Centrally Induced Endocrinological Effects. Morphine decreases the response of the hypothalamus to afferent stimulation, but does not significantly alter its response to direct electrical stimulation. In many species it alters the equilibrium point of the hypothalamic heat-regulatory mechanisms so that an animal will maintain a lower body temperature. Thus, in the dog, morphine initiates a period of panting that gradually subsides as the temperature decreases; the panting reappears if attempts are made to raise body temperature to the pre-morphine level. In man, body temperature falls slightly after single therapeutic doses of morphine, although it appears to be increased by chronic high dosage. In the cat and other animals in which morphine causes excitement and mania, body temperature is increased.

Morphine and most narcotics cause a release of antidiuretic hormone (ADH) and thereby a decrease in urinary output. This effect is mediated by the hypothalamus and can be produced by the injection of minute amounts of morphine into the supraoptic nucleus. However, in some animals the oliguria seen after morphine may also involve other mechanisms, such as decreased glomerular filtration due to hypotension. Morphine also decreases the effect of diuretics in patients with congestive heart failure.

The acute effects of opioids on corticotropin (ACTH) release and adrenocortical activity are inconsistent and depend upon the species and circumstances of administration. Morphine may, however, inhibit the adrenocortical response to stress and the diurnal pattern of release. In man, chronically administered morphine depresses adrenocortical function, probably through an action on the anterior pituitary gland, and thereby decreases plasma and urinary 17-hydroxycorticosteroid and 17-ketosteroid concentrations (*see* George, 1971; Sloan, 1971).

Morphine-like drugs may also suppress the release of follicle-stimulating hormone (FSH), luteinizing hormone (LH), and thyrotropin (TSH). Growth hormone concentrations are not markedly altered (*see* Dole, 1970; Martin *et al.*, 1973a).

Consistent with these findings on adenohypophyseal hormones is a dose-related reduction of plasma testosterone concentrations. However, there may be some tolerance to a number of the endocrinological effects, since many patients maintained on methadone have testosterone and luteinizing hormone values within the normal range (*see* Chapter 16).

In man, a modest elevation of blood sugar may occur with doses of morphine in the therapeutic range. This hyperglycemia is quite prominent in other species and seems to be due to the effects of morphine on discrete receptor sites that are distinct from the central sites involved in epinephrine-induced hyperglycemia (Borison *et al.*, 1962; Feldberg and Shaligram, 1972). The hyperglycemia ultimately involves the secretion of epinephrine from the adrenal medulla and requires an intact pathway from the CNS to that organ.

EEG. In man, single therapeutic doses of opioids produce a shift toward increased voltage and lower frequencies in the EEG, such as occurs in natural sleep or after very low doses of barbiturates. In postaddicts, single doses of morphine suppress the rapid-eye-movement (REM) or "paradoxical sleep" phase of the EEG; slow-wave sleep is also reduced, while light sleep and waking time are increased. With repeated administration, some tolerance develops to these effects; whether these effects are also seen with other opioids such as methadone is not clear (Kay *et al.*, 1969).

Pupil. Morphine and many of its surrogates cause constriction of the pupil in man. The exact mechanism remains uncertain, but it is primarily due to a central effect by way of an action on the Edinger-Westphal nucleus of the oculomotor nerve, rather than an effect on the pupillary sphincter itself. Whereas morphine greatly enhances the pupillary responses to light, miosis occurs even in total darkness. Atropine and related drugs counteract morphine-induced miosis. Following toxic doses of opioids, *the miosis is marked and pinpoint pupils are pathognomonic;* however, marked mydriasis occurs when asphyxia intervenes. Tolerance to the miotic effect of morphine is not prominent, and the morphine or heroin addict continues to have constricted pupils.

The pupillary effects of morphine vary with the species. Cats (excited by morphine) and monkeys (sedated by morphine) show mydriasis. Therapeutic doses of morphine increase accommodative power and lower intraocular tension in both normal and glaucomatous eyes.

Excitatory Effects. Extremely high doses of morphine and its surrogates produce convulsions. Supraspinal structures are more sensitive to the convulsant effect than is the spinal cord since convulsant doses produce seizures above the level of a cord transection but not below it. The cortex seems to be directly affected since morphine applied topically or administered systemically produces a prolongation of induced afterdischarge in isolated cortex, and seizure-like activity can be seen unilaterally in the electrocorticograms of dogs given large systemic doses of morphine or methadone (Wikler and Altschul, 1950). With most opioids, convulsant effects are seen only at dose levels far in excess of those required to produce profound analgesia, often 100 times as high; however, with some agents convulsant effects may occur at doses only moderately higher than those required for analgesia. In some instances, metabolites may have more convulsant activity than the parent drug, as is the case with meperidine. Excitatory effects may be responsible for the muscular rigidity seen when very high doses of meperidine or fentanyl are used for anesthesia.

In some species, relatively low doses of morphine produce gross excitation and hyperthermia.. In the cat, for example, suitable doses produce not only analgesia but also a state in which the animal is continually restless, seems frightened, and cowers and scrambles to avoid being handled. Larger doses lead to seizures and death. These effects can be antagonized by naloxone and prevented by phenytoin, and do not occur after lesions in the caudal hypothalamus. Following high doses of opioids, mice show increased locomotor activity. Differences between animals that appear excited rather than sedated by opioids do not seem to be related to differences in metabolism (*see* Way, 1968). Animals stimulated rather than sedated by morphine include pigs, cows, sheep, goats, lions, tigers, bears, and horses.

Respiration. Morphine is a primary and continuous depressant of respiration, at least in part by virtue of a direct effect on the brain stem respiratory centers. The respiratory depression is discernible even with doses too small to produce sleep or disturb consciousness, and increases progressively as the dose is increased. In man, death from morphine poisoning is nearly always due to respiratory arrest. Therapeutic doses of morphine in man depress all phases of respiratory activity (rate, minute volume, and tidal exchange). The diminished respiratory volume is due primarily to a slower rate of breathing, and with toxic amounts the rate may fall to 3 or 4 per minute. Morphine and related narcotics may also produce irregular and periodic breathing; in man this is often seen even after therapeutic doses.

Maximal respiratory depression occurs within approximately 7 minutes after intravenous administration of morphine, but may not be seen for as long as 30 minutes after intramuscular administration or as long as 90 minutes following subcutaneous administration. The sensitivity of the respiratory center begins to return toward normal within 2 to 3 hours; however, respiratory minute volume is still considerably below normal for as long as 4 to 5 hours following therapeutic doses.

The *mechanism* of respiratory depression by morphine and related narcotic analgesics involves a reduction in the responsiveness of the brain stem respiratory centers to increases in carbon dioxide tension (P_{CO_2}). They also depress the pontine and medullary centers involved in regulating respiratory rhythmicity and the responsiveness of medullary respiratory centers to electrical stimulation (*see* Pentiah *et al.*, 1966; Flórez *et al.*, 1968).

The influence of various afferent stimuli on the respiratory center is not affected to the same degree. Hypoxic stimulation of the chemoreceptors may still be effective when the respiratory center shows decreased responsiveness to CO_2. When the main stimulus to respiration is hypoxia, the inhalation of high tensions of O_2 may produce apnea. In addition to a marked depression of the automatic regulation of respiration, voluntary control of respiration may also be altered. After large doses of morphine or synthetic narcotics, patients will breathe if instructed to do so, but without such instruction they may remain relatively apneic. This indifference to respiration may account, in part, for the usefulness of these agents in pulmonary edema and other situations in which the patient's struggle to breathe aggravates the basic pathology.

Within minutes after an intravenous therapeutic dose of morphine, there is a decrease in minute volume, followed by an increase in CO_2 in the blood and alveolar air. The accumulation of CO_2 may then result in an increase in the activity of the respiratory center and an increase in minute volume, tidal volume, and rate toward predrug values. In this way, respiratory function may appear to be relatively unaffected at a time when the sensitivity of the respiratory center to CO_2 has been considerably diminished. Thus, respiratory rate and sometimes even minute volume can be unreliable indicators of the degree of respiratory depression. Natural sleep also produces a decrease in the sensitivity of the medullary center to CO_2, and the effects of morphine and sleep are additive. (*See* reviews by Eckenhoff and Oech, 1960; Martin, 1963.)

Effects of Other Opioids. In equianalgesic doses, respiration in man is depressed by parenteral codeine and morphine to about the same degree (120 mg of codeine, 10 mg of morphine), but death as a result of codeine overdosage is rare. Numerous studies have compared morphine with other opioids with respect to their ratios of analgesic to respiratory depressant activities. It is clear that all the opioids are capable of producing respiratory depression, and most studies have found that, when equianalgesic doses are used, the degree of respiratory depression observed is not significantly different from that seen with morphine (*see* Eckenhoff and Oech, 1960).

Morphine and related narcotic analgesics also depress the *cough reflex*, at least in part by a direct effect on a cough center in the medulla (Chakravarty *et al.*, 1956). There is, however, no obligatory relationship between depression of respiration and depression of coughing, and effective antitussive agents are available that do not depress respiration (*see* below).

Nauseant and Emetic Effects. Nausea and vomiting produced by morphine and its derivatives are unpleasant side effects caused by direct stimulation of the chemoreceptor trigger zone (CTZ) for emesis, in the area postrema of the medulla. Apomorphine, a drug with dopaminomimetic activity, also causes vomiting by stimulation of the CTZ. The emetic effect of morphine is counteracted by narcotic antagonists and by some phenothiazine derivatives, particularly those with potent dopamine-blocking action (*see* Chapter 12). Certain individuals never vomit after morphine, whereas others do so each time the drug is administered.

Nausea and vomiting are relatively uncommon in recumbent patients given therapeutic doses of morphine, but nausea occurs in approximately 40% and vomiting in 15% of ambulatory patients given 15 mg of the drug subcutaneously. This suggests that a vestibular component is also operative. Indeed, it has been shown that the nauseant and emetic effects of morphine in man are markedly enhanced by vestibular stimulation, and that morphine and synthetic narcotic analgesics produce an increase in vestibular sensitivity (Gutner *et al.*, 1952). Drugs that are useful in motion sickness are sometimes helpful in reducing opioid-induced nausea in ambulatory patients.

In addition to stimulating the CTZ, *morphine depresses the vomiting center.* After a therapeutic dose of morphine, subsequent doses are unlikely to produce vomiting; other emetics are also ineffective after morphine. All clinically useful narcotic analgesics produce some degree of nausea and vomiting. Careful, controlled clinical studies usually demonstrate that in equianalgesic dosage the incidence of such side effects is not significantly lower than that seen with morphine. For example, when the dose of codeine is increased to the point where it is equianalgesic with 10 mg of morphine, the incidence of side effects, including nausea and vomiting, is comparable to that seen with morphine.

Cardiovascular System. In the supine patient, therapeutic doses of morphine or synthetic narcotics have no major effect on blood pressure or heart rate and rhythm. Changes that occur are usually secondary to sleep or lessened physical activity. The vasomotor center in man is but little affected by doses of morphine that cause obvious respiratory depression. Even after toxic doses, the blood pressure is usually maintained until relatively late in the course of intoxication, and falls largely as a result of hypoxia. This is evident from the fact that artificial respiration or administration of oxygen may cause the blood pressure to rise despite the persisting medullary depression. Morphine and most narcotics decrease the capacity of the cardiovascular system to respond to gravitational shifts and, therefore, when supine patients assume the head-up position, ortho-

static hypotension and fainting may occur, due primarily to peripheral vasodilatation.

Peripheral vasodilatation due to morphine and other narcotics does not seem to be the result of a centrally mediated effect. Morphine and most other natural and synthetic narcotics release *histamine,* and such release plays a large role in the narcotic-induced hypotension. However, this is not the sole mechanism involved since less histamine is detectable after morphine-induced hypotension than is found during hypotension caused by other histamine liberators, and the hypotension is only partially blocked by antihistamines (*see* Eckenhoff and Oech, 1960). Direct depression of the vasomotor center is not a prominent effect of narcotics, although it could conceivably be present but masked by the stimulant action of accumulated CO_2.

Effects on the myocardium are not significant in normal man; the heart rate is either unaffected or slightly increased, and there is no consistent effect on cardiac output. The ECG is not altered. In patients with coronary artery disease but no acute medical problems, 8 mg of morphine intravenously produces a decrease in oxygen consumption, cardiac index, left ventricular end-diastolic pressure, and cardiac work (Alderman *et al.,* 1972). In patients with acute myocardial infarction, the cardiovascular response to morphine may be more variable than in normal subjects, and the magnitude of changes (*e.g.,* the decrease in blood pressure) may be more pronounced (Thomas *et al.,* 1965).

Morphine and other narcotics should be used with caution in patients who have a decreased blood volume since they are prone to develop hypotension. Morphine should be used with great caution in patients with cor pulmonale, since deaths following ordinary therapeutic doses have been reported. The concurrent use of certain phenothiazines may increase the risk of morphine-induced hypotension.

Cerebral circulation is not directly affected by therapeutic doses of morphine. However, respiratory depression and CO_2 retention result in cerebral vasodilatation and an increase in cerebrospinal fluid pressure; the pressure increase does not occur when P_{CO_2} is maintained at normal levels by artificial ventilation.

Gastrointestinal Tract. The use of opium for relief of diarrhea and dysentery preceded by many centuries its employment for analgesia. The observed effects of morphine and related drugs on the bowel may vary widely, depending on the species, the dose, and the experimental technics. Therefore, the present discussion will concentrate on the effects observed in man.

Stomach. Morphine and related drugs cause some decrease in the secretion of hydrochloric acid; this can be overcome by chemical or psychic stimulation. A more pronounced effect is the decrease in motility associated with an increase in the tone of the antral portion of the stomach. There is also an increase in the tone of the first part of the duodenum, which often makes therapeutic intubation exceedingly difficult and delays the passage of the gastric contents through the duodenum for as much as 12 hours. This delay accounts for about one half of the total gastrointestinal delay, which is the basis of morphine constipation.

Small Intestine. Both biliary and pancreatic secretions are diminished by morphine, and digestion of food in the small intestine is delayed. There is an increase in resting tone, and periodic spasms are observed. The amplitude of the nonpropulsive type of rhythmic contractions is usually enhanced, but *propulsive contractions are markedly decreased.* The upper part of the small intestine, particularly the duodenum, is affected more than the ileum. A period of relative atony may follow the hypertonicity. Water is more completely absorbed from the chyme because of the delayed passage of the bowel contents, and the viscosity of the chyme is thereby increased. The tone of the ileocecal valve is enhanced. Large doses of atropine may counteract, in part, the gastrointestinal responses to morphine, but resection of the extrinsic nerves and ganglionic blocking agents do not do so. The actions of morphine on the small intestine are thought to cause about one fourth of the total constipating effect of the alkaloid. (*See* Chapman *et al.,* 1950; Vaughan Williams and Streeten, 1950; Daniel *et al.,* 1959.)

Large Intestine. Propulsive peristaltic waves in the colon are diminished or abolished after morphine, and tone is increased to the point of spasm. The resulting delay in the passage of the contents causes considerable desiccation of the feces, which, in turn, retards its advance through the colon. The amplitude of the nonpropulsive type of rhythmic contractions of the colon is usually enhanced. The tone of the anal sphincter is greatly augmented, and this, combined with inattention to the normal sensory stimuli for the defecation reflex due to the central actions of the drug, further contributes to morphine-induced constipation. The actions of morphine on the large intestine combine to contribute about one fourth of the entire constipating effect.

Atropine partially antagonizes the spasmogenic action on the human colon, but it has little effect on the decreased propulsive activity produced by morphine.

Whereas the intestinal responses to opium and morphine are unpleasant side effects when the drugs are given for analgesia, they can be desirable therapeutic objectives in themselves, especially in patients with exhausting diarrhea or dysentery. In patients with chronic ulcerative colitis, opioids may stimulate colonic motility, and the use of opioids during acute episodes of the disease sometimes leads to a toxic dilatation of the colon (Garrett *et al.,* 1967). Codeine and all the morphine surrogates produce qualitatively similar effects on the motility of the bowel. There are, however, quantitative differences, and not all narcotic analgesics are useful in the treatment of diarrheas.

Mechanism of Action on the Bowel. Neither the administration of ganglionic blocking agents nor the removal of the extrinsic innervation of the bowel prevents the characteristic actions of morphine and its surrogates in the unanesthetized animal. At present, it appears that the effects of morphine are exerted on nerve plexuses within the bowel wall (*see* Weinstock, 1971). The spasmogenic action of opioids may involve the local release of 5-HT (Burks, 1973).

Biliary Tract. Therapeutic doses of morphine, codeine, and other morphine surrogates can cause a marked increase in biliary tract pressure. For example, after 10 mg of subcutaneous morphine sulfate the pressure in the common bile duct rises from the normal of less than 20 mm of water to a level of 200 to 300 mm. The response begins within 5 minutes after injection, reaches its peak in 15 minutes, and persists for 2 hours or more. Symptoms often accompany the increased pressure and vary from epigastric distress to typical biliary colic.

Some patients with biliary colic may experience exacerbation and not relief of pain when given these drugs. Furthermore, an occasional individual complains of pain in the epigastrium or right hypo-chondrium after morphine, probably due to duo-denal or biliary tract spasm. Biliary tract spasm produced by morphine is evident roentgenographi-cally as well as manometrically, and a sharp con-striction becomes apparent at the lower end of the common bile duct (sphincter of Oddi). This spasm prevents emptying and thus causes the intraductal pressure to rise, and is probably responsible for the elevations of plasma amylase and lipase that are sometimes found after patients have been given morphine. Such elevations may persist for 24 hours after therapeutic doses and may confuse the diagno-sis of intra-abdominal pathology, especially when acute pancreatitis is one of the diseases under con-sideration (*see* Bogoch *et al.,* 1954). Biliary spasm is not, however, a consistent effect of therapeutic doses of morphine, and some patients show no changes in bile duct size or pressure. Atropine only partially prevents morphine-induced biliary spasm, but nalorphine prevents or relieves it. Nitroglycerin (0.6 mg) administered sublingually also decreases the elevated intrabiliary pressure, but the relaxation is less marked, although more prolonged, than that afforded by inhalation of amyl nitrite. Some anal-gesics such as meperidine, phenoperidine, and penta-zocine seem to produce less pronounced increases in biliary pressure (Hopton and Torrance, 1967; Economou and Ward-McQuaid, 1971).

Other Smooth Muscle. *Ureter and Urinary Blad-der.* Therapeutic doses of morphine increase the tone and amplitude of contractions of the *ureter,* especially of the lower third. The response of the ureters in man to narcotic agents is quite variable. When the antidiuretic effects of the drugs are promi-nent and urine flow decreases, the ureter may be-come quiescent.

The tone of the detrusor muscle of the *urinary bladder* is augmented by morphine; this sometimes causes urinary urgency. The tone of the vesical sphincter is also enhanced by morphine; this effect may make urination difficult, and catheterization is sometimes required following therapeutic doses of morphine. The central effects of these drugs may make the patient inattentive to the stimuli arising in the bladder and may play a role in morphine-induced urinary retention.

Uterus. The administration of large doses of morphine and most of its surrogates in animals sig-nificantly prolongs labor, increases the amount of contamination in the fetal respiratory passages, and increases neonatal mortality. Studies of the effects of therapeutic doses of morphine in women also suggest that labor may be somewhat prolonged (*see* Campbell *et al.,* 1961). The mechanism involved is not clear, for the normally contracting human uterus at term does not appear to be significantly affected by analgesic doses of morphine. However, it has been noted that, if the uterus is made hyperactive by oxytocics, morphine tends to restore tone, fre-quency, and amplitude of contractions to normal. In addition, the central effects of morphine may affect the degree to which the parturient is able to cooper-ate in the delivery.

Bronchial Musculature. Although large doses of morphine and meperidine produce constriction of the bronchi, this effect is rarely seen after therapeutic doses in man. The possible role of morphine-induced bronchoconstriction in the aggravation of asthma is discussed below.

Skin. In man, therapeutic doses of morphine cause cutaneous blood vessels to dilate. The skin of the face, neck, and upper thorax frequently becomes flushed and warm. These changes in cuta-neous circulation may, in part, be due to the release of histamine and may be responsible for the *pruritus* and the *sweating* that commonly follow the adminis-tration of morphine. Histamine release probably accounts for the urticaria commonly seen at the site of injection.

Tolerance, Physical Dependence, and Abuse Liability. The development of toler-ance and physical dependence with repeated use is a characteristic feature of all the opioid drugs, and the possibility of developing psy-chological dependence on the effects of these drugs is one of the major limitations of their clinical use. It is important to emphasize that the overall abuse liability of an agent is not established by any one single factor; rather, it is a composite based on a number of fac-tors. These include: (1) the capacity of the drug to produce the kind of physical de-pendence in which drug withdrawal causes sufficient distress to bring about drug-seeking behavior; (2) its ability to suppress with-drawal symptoms caused by withdrawal of other agents; (3) the degree to which it in-duces euphoria similar to that produced by morphine and other opioids; (4) the patterns of toxicity that occur when the dose is in-creased beyond the usual therapeutic range; and (5) physical characteristics of the drug, such as water solubility, that may determine whether it is likely to be abused by the par-enteral route. There is evidence to suggest that the overall abuse liability of some of the analgesics related to the opioid antagonists is lower than that of morphine. The implica-tions of the differences in abuse potential for the choice of agents in therapy are discussed below, and the subject of compulsive drug use is elaborated in detail in Chapter 16.

Absorption, Distribution, Fate, and Excre-tion. *Absorption.* The opioids are readily absorbed from the gastrointestinal tract; they are also absorbed from the nasal mucosa and the lung (as when heroin is used as snuff or opium is smoked), and after subcutaneous or intramuscular injection. With most opioids, including morphine, the effect of a given dose is considerably less after oral than after parenteral administration. However, the shape of the time-effect curve also varies with the route of administration, so that the duration of action is often somewhat longer with the oral route. Such differences in time-effect curves are illustrated in Figure 15–1.

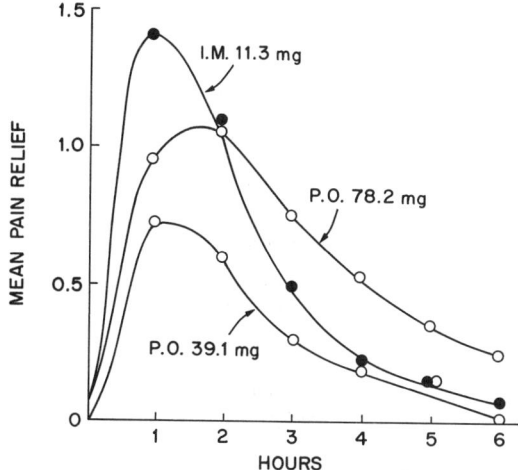

Figure 15–1. *Time-effect curves for oral* (P.O.) *and intramuscular* (I.M.) *morphine.*

Changes in pain relief in cancer patients are plotted on an arbitrary scale against time after drug administration. The oral doses represent the logarithmic means of the upper and lower oral doses from a series of sequential experiments. The intramuscular dose represents the mean of an 8- and 16-mg standard used in the same experiments. All drugs were administered in a random order to 25 patients with pain due to cancer. Differences in the configuration of the time-effect curves indicate that the orally administered drug cannot be considered as being merely less active than the parenterally administered drug, and that estimates of relative potency will vary depending on which criterion one uses: peak effect, duration of effect, or total effect. (After Houde, Wallenstein, and Beaver, 1965. Courtesy of Academic Press, Inc.)

When morphine and most of its congeners are given intravenously, they act promptly. However, the more lipid-soluble surrogates have a somewhat more rapid onset of action after subcutaneous administration due to differences in the rate of absorption. The durations of action show relatively little variation (*see* Table 15–3).

Distribution and Fate. The metabolism and excretion of morphine have been studied extensively. Like most basic amines, free morphine rapidly leaves the blood and is concentrated in parenchymatous tissues, such as the kidney, lung, liver, and spleen. Skeletal muscle has a somewhat lower level of morphine, but because of its mass it accounts for the major fraction of the drug in the body. Morphine does not accumulate in tissues, and 24 hours after the last dose tissue concentrations are quite low. However, very sensitive methods can detect morphine or its metabolites in urine for several days after the last dose.

Although the primary site of action of morphine is in the CNS, in the adult animal only small quantities pass the blood-brain barrier. Compared to other opioids such as codeine, heroin, and methadone, morphine crosses the blood-brain barrier in considerably smaller amounts (*see* Oldendorf *et al.,* 1972). Transport of opioids by the choroid plexus has been noted, but its significance remains uncertain (*see* Hug, 1971).

The major pathway for the detoxication of morphine is conjugation with glucuronic acid, and after the intravenous administration of morphine the tissue concentrations of free morphine decline progressively while those of conjugated morphine (morphine-3-monoglucuronide) increase and then decline more slowly. For many narcotics, N-demethylation occurs in several mammalian species including man, but in the case of morphine it does not appear to be a major pathway in man.

Excretion. Small amounts of free morphine and larger amounts of conjugated morphine are found in the urine, and these account for most of the administered drug. Although traces of morphine are detectable in the urine for well over 48 hours, 90% of the total excretion takes place in the first 24 hours. The major route of elimination is by glomerular filtration. Active secretion of dihydromorphine by the proximal portion of the renal tubules in dogs has been observed, but its significance remains uncertain. A measurable amount of conjugated morphine can be found in the bile. About 7 to 10% of administered morphine eventually appears in the feces, and this comes almost exclusively from the bile.

**Table 15-3. A COMPARISON OF NARCOTIC ANALGESICS WITH
RESPECT TO DOSAGE, DURATION OF ACTION, WITHDRAWAL SYMPTOMS,
AND DISTINGUISHING FEATURES**

NONPROPRIETARY NAME	TRADE NAME	DOSE * (mg)	DURATION OF ACTION * (hours)	WITHDRAWAL SYMPTOMS	DISTIN- GUISHING FEATURES ▲
Morphine		10	4–5	*see* text	*see* text
Heroin (diacetyl-morphine)		3 (2–8)	3–4	like morphine	2
Hydromorphone (dihydromorphinone)	DILAUDID	1.5	4–5	like morphine	
Oxymorphone (dihydro-hydroxymorphinone)	NUMORPHAN	1.0–1.5	4–5	like morphine	
Metopon (methyldihydro-morphinone)	METOPON	3.5	4–5	like morphine	3
Codeine		120 (10–30)	(4–6)	*see* text	*see* text
Hydrocodone (dihydro-codeinone)	HYCODAN †	(5–10)	(4–8)	between morphine and codeine	4
Dihydrocodeine	PARACODIN	60	4–5	between morphine and codeine	3
Oxycodone (dihydro-hydroxycodeinone)	PERCODAN †.	10–15 (3–5)	4–5 (4–5)	close to morphine	
Pholcodine (β-morph-olinylethylmorphine)	ETHNINE, PHOLDINE	(10–15)	(4–5)	much less than codeine	3, 4, 5
Levorphanol	LEVO-DROMORAN	2–3	4–5	like morphine	7
Phenazocine	PRINADOL	3	4–5	between metha-done and morphine	6, 10
Methadone	DOLOPHINE, etc.	7.5–10	3–5	*see* text	6, 8
Dextromoramide	PALFIUM	5–7.5	4–5	like methadone	3, 6, 8
Dipipanone	PIPADONE	20–25	4–5	like methadone	3, 6, 8, 9
Phenadoxone	HEPTALGIN, etc.	10–20	1–3	less than mor-phine	3, 9
Meperidine	DEMEROL, etc.	80–100	2–4	*see* text	1, 7
Alphaprodine	NISENTIL	40–60	1–2	like meperidine	1, 7
Anileridine	LERITINE	25–30	2–4	like meperidine	1, 7
Piminodine	ALVODINE	7.5–10	2–4	like meperidine	1, 7

* *Dose* shown is the amount given *subcutaneously* that produces approximately the same analgesic effects as 10 mg of morphine administered subcutaneously. The figures in *parentheses* are the *doses* and the *duration* of action for *oral, antitussive* doses; they are not necessarily equieffective doses. *Duration of action* shown is for *subcutaneous* administration; after *intravenous* administration, peak effects are somewhat more pronounced but overall effects are of shorter duration.

▲ 1 = causes little or no constipation; 2 = manufacture or importation into the United States illegal; 3 = not available in the United States; 4 = by tradition used mainly as an antitussive; 5 = little or no analgesic or euphorigenic activity; 6 = may exhibit cumulative effects on repeated dosage; 7 = retains fair degree of efficacy when given orally; 8 = retains most of its analgesic efficacy when given orally; 9 = marked irritation at injection sites; 10 = *see* previous edition of this textbook for description.

† The products marketed in the United States with these trade names contain additional ingredients.

The doses and durations shown in this table are based on papers reviewed by Eddy and coworkers, 1957; Reynolds and Randall, 1957; Murphree, 1962; and Lasagna, 1964.

Codeine, in contrast to morphine, is approximately two thirds as effective orally as parenterally, both as an analgesic and as a respiratory depressant. Very few opioids have so high an oral-parenteral potency ratio; also in this group is oxycodone. Their greater oral efficacy may be due to better absorption. However, the action of morphine is terminated largely by glucuronide conjugation at the 3 position; the methoxy group at the 3 position in codeine and oxycodone may serve to protect these drugs from rapid biotransformation by the liver. Once absorbed, codeine is metabolized by the liver and excreted chiefly in the urine, largely in inactive forms. A small fraction (approximately 10%) of administered codeine is demethylated to form morphine, and both free and conjugated morphine can be found in the urine after therapeutic doses of codeine. There is indirect evidence that in some species the conversion to morphine contributes significantly to the effect of codeine (*see* Way, 1968). To what extent this is true in man is still not clear. However, codeine has an exceptionally low binding constant for the hypothetical opioid receptor.

Heroin (diacetylmorphine) is rapidly hydrolyzed to monoacetylmorphine (MAM), which, in turn, is hydrolyzed to morphine. In the adult, the blood-brain barrier tends to impede entry of morphine into the brain; the barrier is considerably less effective against heroin and MAM since both are more lipid soluble than morphine. Most of the current evidence suggests that morphine is responsible for the pharmacological actions of heroin. Heroin is mainly excreted in the urine largely as free and conjugated morphine.

The absorption, fate, and distribution of morphine-like drugs have been critically analyzed in the reviews by Way and Adler (1960, 1962), Way (1968), Mulé (1971), and Scrafani and Clouet (1971).

Idiosyncrasy, Variations in Response, and Precautions. Opiates and related narcotics produce a wide spectrum of unwanted effects, such as nausea, vomiting, dizziness, mental clouding, dysphoria, constipation, and increased pressure in the biliary tract. These occur so commonly that they cannot be considered idiosyncratic, even though there are many patients who do not experience such effects. Rarely, a patient may develop a delirium, and an occasional patient may experience insomnia rather than sedation. *Increased sensitivity* to pain after the analgesia has worn off sometimes occurs.

Allergic phenomena occur with opioid analgesics, but they are not common. They are usually manifested as urticaria and other types of skin rashes; contact dermatitis in nurses and pharmaceutical workers has been reported. Wheals at the site of injection of morphine, codeine, and related drugs are probably related to histamine release, and also occur with many synthetic narcotics that are also histamine releasers. Anaphylactoid reactions have been reported after intravenous codeine and morphine, but such reactions are quite rare; however, it has been suggested that they are responsible for some of the sudden deaths, episodes of pulmonary edema, and other complications that occur among addicts who use heroin intravenously (*see* Sapira, 1968; Challenor *et al.,* 1973).

A number of factors may alter the sensitivity to opiate analgesics, including the integrity of the blood-brain barrier. For example, when morphine is administered to the mother prior to delivery, the newborn infant may exhibit respiratory depression even though the drug produced no significant depression in the mother. This increased sensitivity of the newborn is due to an immature blood-brain barrier, which permits a larger amount of administered morphine to gain access to the CNS (*see* Way *et al.,* 1965). Since the blood-brain barrier does not play as prominent a role in limiting the access of all opioids to the CNS, some such as meperi-

dine will be found to produce no more respiratory depression in the newborn than in the adult. After the neonatal period, there is little change in analgesic response to opioids until late in life. In patients over 60 years old there seems to be both a decrease in sensitivity to pain and an increased analgesic response to opioids (Bellville *et al.,* 1971).

Pain seems to be the physiological antidote to the depressant effects of narcotics, and the patient with severe pain may tolerate larger doses of morphine (3 to 4 therapeutic doses over a period of a few hours) but may exhibit subjective and respiratory depression should the pain suddenly subside. *Illnesses* of various types may increase or decrease the sensitivity to morphine and related drugs. Patients with *myxedema* are allegedly more sensitive to the depressant effects, whereas *hyperthyroid* patients seem more tolerant; controlled studies, however, are lacking. Chronic nephritis is not a major contraindication to the use of morphine, since the fate of the drug is primarily dependent upon biotransformation in the liver. When there is evidence of hepatic insufficiency from whatever cause, one may expect the duration of action to be prolonged and cumulative effects should be anticipated. However, patients with *cirrhosis without hepatic insufficiency* seem to tolerate morphine reasonably well, and even *patients with cirrhosis who have had hepatic coma* do not have serious reactions after single therapeutic doses of morphine. Since all the narcotic analgesics are metabolized by the liver, the same precautions should also apply; however, since the metabolic pathways for some synthetic opioids are different from those for morphine, it is possible that some narcotics might be safer than others (*see* Way and Adler, 1962).

Patients with *reduced blood volume* are considerably more susceptible to the hypotensive effects of morphine and related drugs, and these agents must be employed with caution in patients with any type of hemorrhage. The respiratory depressant effects of morphine and the related capacity to elevate intracranial pressure may be markedly exaggerated in the presence of head injury or of an already elevated cerebrospinal fluid pressure produced by trauma. Therefore, while *head injury per se* does not constitute an absolute contraindication to the use of narcotics, the possibility of exaggerated depression of respiration must be considered. Furthermore, the likelihood that narcotics will produce mental clouding and side effects such as miosis and vomiting, which are important signs in following the clinical course of patients with head injuries, must be carefully weighed before such agents are used. In patients with *prostatic hypertrophy,* morphine may precipitate acute urinary retention, requiring repeated catheterization.

Morphine and related narcotics must be used with great caution in any situation in which there is decreased respiratory reserve, such as *emphysema, kyphoscoliosis,* or even severe *obesity.* In patients with chronic *cor pulmonale,* death has occurred following therapeutic doses of morphine. Although many patients with such conditions seem to be functioning within normal limits, they are already utilizing compensatory mechanisms, such as increased respiratory rate. Many have chronically elevated levels of plasma CO_2, and may be less sensitive to the stimulating actions of CO_2. The further imposition of the depressant effects of narcotics can be disastrous.

Narcotics have been reported to precipitate attacks of *asthma* in anesthetized patients, but the risk does not seem to be high. There is general agreement, however, that during an asthmatic attack morphine and related drugs should be avoided. All narcotic analgesics depress the respiratory center, release histamine, depress the cough reflex, and tend to dry secretions. Giving such agents to asthmatic patients, in whom the airway resistance may be many times greater than normal, invites disaster by producing a decrease in respiratory drive without a corresponding decrease in airway resistance. It is worth noting, however, that some clinicians (and some patients) have found narcotics beneficial in spite of these risks. Many addicts state that their asthmatic attacks respond to narcotics better than to conventional medications, and Weinberg and Sensiba (1956) reported the successful use of 5 mg of methadone or 50 mg of meperidine along with scopolamine intravenously as emergency treatment for status asthmaticus.

Interactions with Other Drugs. The depressant effects of some opioids may be exaggerated and prolonged by phenothiazines, monoamine oxidase inhibitors, and tricyclic antidepressants; the mechanism of this supra-additive effect is not fully understood, but may involve alterations in the rate of metabolic transformation of the opioid or alterations in neurotransmitters involved in opioid actions. Some, but not all, phenothiazines reduce the amount of narcotic required to produce a given level of analgesia. However, the respiratory depressant effects seem also to be enhanced, the degree of sedation is increased, and the hypotensive effects of phenothiazines become an additional complication. *Some phenothiazine derivatives enhance the sedative effects, but at the same time seem to be antianalgesic* and increase the amount of narcotic required to produce satisfactory relief from pain (Moore and Dundee, 1961).

Preparations, Dosage, and Routes of Administration of Opium and Its Alkaloids. *Powdered Opium,* U.S.P., is a light-brown powder, supplied for clinical use in capsule, tablet, or pill form. The official morphine content of opium is 10.0 to 10.5% by weight. Thus, a dose of 60 mg taken orally is equivalent to 6 mg of morphine. PANTOPON is the proprietary name of a commonly used preparation of purified opium alkaloids. *Opium tincture (laudanum, deodorized opium tincture)* is a hydroalcoholic solution containing 10% of opium (1.0% of morphine). The average adult dose is 0.6 to 1.5 ml (equivalent to 6 to 15 mg of morphine), taken orally. *Opium (gum opium)* is still official in the U.S.P.; the dose is the same as for the powder. These preparations are infrequently employed. *Paregoric,* U.S.P. (*camphorated opium tincture*), is a hydroalcoholic preparation in which there is also benzoic acid, camphor, and anise oil. The usual adult dose is 5 to 10 ml, which corresponds to 20 to 40 mg of opium or 2 to 4 mg of morphine. Paregoric represents a needlessly complex therapeutic survival of a former day.

Morphine. Morphine is available as the alkaloidal base, but it is prescribed only in the form of its water-soluble salts. The two most common salts are *Morphine Sulfate,* U.S.P., and *morphine hydrochloride.* The salts are bitter, white powders that are quite soluble in water and exhibit characteristic alkaloidal incompatibilities. Solutions of morphine salts are not irritating on injection. *Morphine Sulfate Injection,* U.S.P., is a sterile aqueous solution for parenteral use, and usually contains 8, 10, 15, or 30 mg in 1 ml.

Hypodermically, 10 mg/70 kg of body weight is generally considered to be an optimal initial dose of morphine. It is optimal in that it provides satisfactory analgesia in approximately 70% of patients with moderate-to-severe pain (*e.g.,* postoperative pain) with only a moderate incidence of side effects. Subsequent doses may be higher or lower, depending on the analgesic response and the side effects produced. The average *oral* adult dose of morphine is often stated as 8 to 20 mg. However, controlled studies have shown that oral administration is only about one sixth to one fifteenth as effective as parenteral administration (depending on whether *peak* or *total analgesia* is measured) (*see* Figure 15–1).

Occasionally morphine sulfate is given *intravenously,* and it has been employed by this route for the control of severe postoperative pain and restlessness, for preoperative medication in emergencies, for minor surgical procedures when general anesthesia is not indicated, for severe cardiac pain, for severe renal colic, and for pulmonary edema. The usual dose is 4 to 10 mg. The analgesic effect starts immediately and reaches its peak in 20 minutes; the maximal respiratory depression is manifest within 10 minutes.

The dose of opiates for *infants and children* is best learned as such and modified to suit the particular case. In general, however, the dose may be calculated on the basis of body weight.

Codeine. Codeine is available as the free alkaloidal base (*Codeine,* N.F.) and in the form of its water-soluble salts. The most common salts of codeine are *Codeine Sulfate,* N.F., and *Codeine Phosphate,* U.S.P. Both are available as official tablets containing 15, 30, or 60 mg of the drug. *Codeine Phosphate Injection,* U.S.P., contains 15, 30, or 60 mg/ml of the salt. Codeine phosphate has the advantage of being much more soluble in water than is the sulfate. Also available is *Terpin Hydrate and Codeine Elixir,* N.F., used mainly for cough and containing 10 mg in a 5-ml dose.

Although a dose of 120 mg of codeine, administered hypodermically, produces analgesia equivalent to that resulting from 10 mg of morphine, the former drug has few advantages over morphine when used parenterally. However, codeine has a high oral-parenteral potency ratio, and in this respect it has definite advantages over morphine. Orally, a dose of 32 mg of codeine is approximately equianalgesic with 325 to 600 mg of aspirin; when these two drugs are combined, the analgesic effect equals or sometimes exceeds that of 65 mg of codeine (Houde *et al.,* 1965). The variability of the analgesic response at this dosage level is considerable (*see* Beaver, 1966; Miller *et al.,* 1970). The effects of 15 mg of codeine orally can be demonstrated by objective technics to reduce the frequency of pathological cough, and progressively greater cough suppression is seen as the dose is increased up to 60 mg (Sevelius *et al.,* 1971). The abuse liability of codeine is much lower than that of morphine, as discussed more fully in Chapter 16.

Apomorphine. Apomorphine is obtained by treating the morphine molecule with strong mineral acids. Its analgesic properties are diminished, but it retains the capacity to stimulate the medullary CTZ and to produce a combination of CNS excitation and depression. Its primary therapeutic use is in the production of emesis, particularly in cases of poisoning by orally ingested substances (*see* Done, 1969). The usual dose is 0.1 mg/kg, given subcutaneously; vomiting ordinarily occurs within a few minutes and is preceded by nausea and salivation. If the first dose does not produce emesis, subsequent doses are even less likely to do so. Since the drug can also produce respiratory depression, it must be used with caution when there is CNS depression from whatever cause. *Apomorphine Hydrochloride,* N.F., and *Apomorphine Hydrochloride Tablets,* N.F., are the available preparations. The emetic effect of apomorphine can be counteracted by opioid antagonists.

Etorphine hydrochloride (M-99; IMMOBILON) is an analog of thebaine used exclusively for immobilizing large animals (*see* Harthoorn, 1967). In man, it is 400 times as potent as morphine in producing subjective effects and suppressing opioid withdrawal. Its duration of action is relatively short. Poisoning with etorphine should be treated in the same way as morphine poisoning.

Other Semisynthetic Morphine and Codeine Derivatives. There are many drugs that can substitute for morphine and codeine. Their names, doses, and special characteristics are shown in Table 15-3.

Hydromorphone Hydrochloride, N.F. (DILAUDID), is available in 1-, 2-, 3-, and 4-mg tablets; in ampuls containing 2, 3, and 4 mg; and as 3-mg rectal suppositories. *Hydromorphone Sulfate Injection,* N.F., is available in multiple-dose vials containing 2 mg/ml.

Hydrocodone Bitartrate, N.F., is used in combination with other ingredients in a variety of proprietary antitussive and analgesic-antipyretic mixtures (*e.g.,* HYCODAN). Similarly, *oxycodone* is available only as an ingredient in analgesic and antitussive mixtures (*e.g.,* PERCODAN). *Oxymorphone Hydrochloride,* N.F., is listed as an official preparation but is not commercially available at present.

ACUTE OPIOID POISONING

Acute opioid poisoning may result from clinical overdosage, accidental overdosage in addicts, or attempts at suicide. Occasionally, a delayed type of poisoning may occur from the injection of an opioid into chilled skin areas or in patients with low blood pressure and shock. The drug is not fully absorbed, and, therefore, a subsequent dose may be given. When normal circulation is established, an excessive amount may suddenly be absorbed. Because tolerance to the opioids develops so rapidly, and because there is great individual variation in sensitivity, it is difficult to state the exact amount of any opioid that is toxic or lethal to man. Recent experiences with methadone indicate that in nontolerant individuals serious toxicity may follow the oral ingestion of 40 to 60 mg. Older literature suggests that, in the case of morphine, a normal, pain-free adult is not likely to die after oral doses of less than 120 mg, or to have serious toxicity with less than 30 mg parenterally.

Symptoms and Diagnosis. By the time he is seen by the physician, the patient who has taken an overdose of an opioid is usually asleep or stuporous. If a large overdose has been taken, he cannot be aroused and may be in a *profound coma.* The *respiratory rate* is quite low (sometimes only 2 to 4 per minute), and *cyanosis* may be present. As the respiratory exchange becomes poorer, *blood pressure,* at first maintained near normal, falls progressively. If adequate oxygenation is restored early, the blood pressure will improve; if hypoxia persists untreated, however, there may be capillary damage, and measures to combat *shock* may then be required. The *pupils* are symmetrical and pinpoint in size; however, if hypoxia is severe, they may be dilated. *Urine formation* is depressed, not only by the antidiuretic effect of the drug but also as a result of low blood pressure. *Body temperature* falls, and the skin becomes cold and clammy. The *skeletal muscles* are flaccid, the jaw is relaxed, and the tongue may fall back and block the airway. Frank convulsions may occasionally be noted in infants and children. When death occurs, it is nearly always due to respiratory failure. Sometimes, even if respiration is restored, death may still occur as a result of complications, such as pneumonia or shock, that develop during the period of coma. Pulmonary edema is commonly seen with opioid poisoning. It is probably not due to contaminants or to anaphylactoid reactions, and has been observed following toxic doses of morphine, methadone, propoxyphene, and uncontaminated heroin (*see* Levine and Grimes, 1973; Tennant, 1973).

The triad of *coma, pinpoint pupils,* and *depressed respiration* strongly suggests opioid poisoning. Since deliberate or accidental overdosage is common among addicts, the finding of needle marks suggestive of addiction further supports the diagnosis. Mixed poisonings, however, are not uncommon. In such cases, other agents such as barbiturate or alcohol may also be contributing to the clinical picture. Chemical examination of the urine and gastric contents for morphine and other CNS depressants may help to clarify the diagnosis, but the results usually become available too late to influence treatment.

Treatment. The first step is to establish a patent airway and ventilate the patient. Narcotic antagonists such as naloxone can produce dramatic reversal of severe narcotic-induced respiratory depression (*see* below), and the use of naloxone is now the treatment of choice. If naloxone is unavailable, older narcotic antagonists, such as nalorphine or levallorphan, are still of great value, but some additional caution is indicated (*see* below). The safest approach is the administration of small intravenous doses (*e.g.,* 0.4 to 0.8 mg of naloxone), judiciously repeated over the course of 20 to 30 minutes. The response to such treatment is so predictable that, if no effect is seen after 10 mg of naloxone has been administered, one can reasonably question the accuracy of the diagnosis. Pulmonary edema sometimes associated with opioid overdosage may be countered by positive-pressure respiration. Grand mal seizures, occasionally seen as part of the toxic syndrome with meperidine and propoxyphene, are ameliorated by treatment with naloxone.

Narcotic antagonists, such as nalorphine and levallorphan, that also have agonistic actions should be used with care since they may further embarrass respiration that has been depressed by alcohol, barbiturates, or related CNS depressants. Since naloxone has no direct respiratory depressant action, it is the drug of choice when there is any question about the cause of the respiratory depression. The presence of alcohol or a barbiturate does not prevent the salutary effect of an antagonist, and in cases of mixed intoxications the situation will be improved insofar as the respiratory depression is due to the narcotic. Although narcotic antagonists also counteract the sedative effects of morphine, one need not attempt to restore the patient to full consciousness. The duration of action of antagonists is usually much shorter than that of the corresponding narcotics; hence, the patient must be carefully watched, lest he slip back into coma. This is particularly important when the overdosage is due to methadone or *l*-acetylmethadol. The depressant effects of these drugs may persist for 24 to 72 hours, and fatalities have occurred as a result of premature discontinuation of treatment with an antagonist drug.

The use of a narcotic antagonist to treat acute poisoning in an addict should be undertaken with care, since the antagonist may precipitate a severe withdrawal syndrome that cannot be readily suppressed during the period of action of the antagonist. In some situations, this withdrawal syndrome can be more life threatening than the respiratory depression itself. It is usually possible, however, to administer a small dose of naloxone that will antagonize respiratory depression without producing severe withdrawal symptoms.

These principles are appropriate in treating acute poisoning with codeine, all of the semisynthetic narcotics, and almost all the synthetic narcotics. Toxicity due to overdose of pentazocine and cyclazocine-like drugs can be partially alleviated by high doses of naloxone, which, unlike nalorphine, antagonizes the agonistic effects of these agents. The pharmacological actions of narcotic antagonists are discussed in more detail below.

THERAPEUTIC USES

Sir William Osler referred to morphine as "God's own medicine." The years since Osler have seen the introduction of scores of synthetic and semisynthetic agents that are equal to morphine in their ability to produce analgesia; undoubtedly the search for better analgesics will continue. For the present, however, the opioids retain their very special place in the treatment of pain.

General Principles. It bears reemphasis that, when narcotic analgesics are administered for the relief of pain, cough, or diarrhea, only symptomatic treatment is being provided and the underlying pathology remains. The physician must constantly weigh the benefits of this relief against its costs and risks to the patient. Such costs and risks are frequently quite different, depending upon whether the symptom is a manifestation of an acute or a chronic disease.

In acute problems, narcotics may obscure the symptoms or the progress of the disease. In many situations, *pain is a chief diagnostic symptom,* and its total abolition may seriously handicap the discovery of the nature of the patient's illness. While the old rule that *opioids should not be given until the diagnosis is made* remains generally valid, the skillful use of a narcotic analgesic may sometimes aid in the diagnosis of acute abdominal conditions.

The problems that arise in the *treatment of chronic conditions* involve more complex considerations. With repeated daily administration tolerance will eventually develop to the therapeutic effects of the drug, as will some degree of physical dependence. The degree will depend on the particular drug, the frequency of administration, and the quantity administered. The risk of developing emotional dependency is always present. Thus, a decision to relieve any chronic symptom, especially pain, by the parenteral administration of a narcotic may be short-sighted and can be a disservice to the patient. Furthermore, the patient who must cope with a chronic illness is more likely to develop an emotional overdependence on narcotics. Measures other than drugs should be employed to relieve chronic pain when they are effective and available. To cite but one example, cutaneous stimulation or stimulation of the dorsal columns may be of some value in alleviating chronic pain (*see* Shealy *et al.,* 1970). The general principles to be observed in order to minimize the incidence of medical addiction are discussed in Chapter 16.

In the usual doses, narcotic analgesics relieve suffering primarily by altering the emotional component of the painful experience; the physician who views his patient as a whole person responding to a physically and emotionally stressful illness, who realizes the importance of his own relationship to the patient, and who utilizes this relationship to provide psychological support and a realistic perspective will need to prescribe considerably less narcotic than a physician who cannot offer this kind of psychological support and attempts to use a drug in its place. In addition to emotional support, the physician should also take into account the substantial variability in both the capacity to tolerate pain and the response to narcotic analgesics. Some patients may require considerably more than the average dose of a drug to experience any pain relief at all; others, perhaps because of more rapid metabolic disposition, may require a drug at shorter intervals. Some clinicians, out of an exaggerated concern for the possibility of inducing addiction, tend to prescribe initial doses of narcotics that are too low or too infrequent to alleviate pain, and then respond to the patient's continued complaints with an even more exaggerated concern about dependence, despite the high probability that the request for more drug is only the expected consequence of the inadequate dosage prescribed (*see* Marks and Sachar, 1973).

Pain. In many instances even relatively severe pain can be considerably relieved by parenteral doses of morphine (10 mg) that cause little stupefaction or respiratory depression.

The Selection of a Drug. The differences between morphine and its semisynthetic and synthetic surrogates have been considerably overestimated (*see* Table 15-3). In equianalgesic doses, most of these drugs produce approximately the same incidence and degree of unwanted side effects. Nevertheless, there are some patients who may have side effects with one agent and not with another. Some drugs have shorter durations of action, others are particularly efficacious when given by mouth, and a few are considered to have a lower risk for producing opioid dependence. The availability of a wide range of surrogates provides for therapeutic flexibility. When pain is not too severe, codeine, oxycodone, or hydrocodone orally will often provide very satisfactory relief, especially when given with a non-narcotic analgesic such as aspirin. When the pain is associated with biliary spasm, meperidine may produce less increase in the spasm than will an equianalgesic dose of morphine. When the pain is likely to be of short duration (*e.g.,* diagnostic procedures, cystoscopy, orthopedic manipulation, etc.), a drug with a shorter duration of action, such as meperidine or alphaprodine, might be preferable to morphine or methadone.

The Pain of Terminal Illness. Although they are not requisite or even desirable in all cases of terminal cancer, the euphoria, tranquility, and relief of pain afforded by the wise use of narcotics are a blessing to the patient and his family. Some degree of physical dependence and tolerance develops whenever a narcotic is given in therapeutic dosage several times a day over a prolonged period. In patients with painful terminal illnesses such considerations should not in any way prevent the physician from fulfilling his primary obligation to ease the patient's discomfort. The physician should not wait until the pain becomes agonizing; *no patient should ever wish for death because of his physician's reluctance to use adequate amounts of effective narcotics.* Such patients, while they may be physically dependent, are not considered "addicts" even though they may need large doses on a regular basis; in states that require the reporting of addicts, patients with terminal illnesses are not reportable. The use of narcotics should be reserved until nonnarcotic drugs or other measures no longer give adequate relief. Thus, oral codeine, propoxyphene, or pentazocine should be employed together with nonnarcotic sedatives and analgesics and the doses increased until pain can no longer be controlled without the more effective narcotic analgesics. Since one wishes to be able to provide relief for the longest period possible and to reserve a margin of susceptibility in order to cope with the terminal stages when the pain may become more severe, the doses should not be increased faster than is necessary to keep the patient comfortable. When opiates and other analgesics are no longer satisfactory, nerve block by injections of alcohol, chordotomy, or other types of neurosurgical intervention such as neurostimulation may be required if the nature of the lesion permits.

Postoperative Pain. Narcotic analgesics are commonly employed to control pain and discomfort in the immediate postoperative period, but they should be considered two-edged swords. If used indiscriminately, they may obscure the outcome of surgery and the course of recovery, and prevent the early recognition of complications. They may also decrease the effectiveness of coughing, decrease respiratory ventilation, predispose to pneumonitis, reduce bowel motility, and cause urinary retention. On the other hand, the reduction of pain associated with movements of the chest can increase the patient's ability to breathe deeply and to cough voluntarily, and can also facilitate early ambulation. When pain is not too severe, oral codeine with aspirin often provides adequate analgesia without the side effects associated with the use of usual doses of morphine.

Headache. Headache is often a recurrent problem, sometimes reflecting emotional disturbances, and narcotic analgesics, with the possible exception of codeine, should not be employed unless all other measures have failed. Even then, considerable care should be employed to minimize psychological dependence and addiction.

Obstetrical Analgesia. The use of morphine and its synthetic surrogates in obstetrical analgesia is a highly specialized field requiring experience and sound judgment to ensure safety. For any given agent, three factors must be considered: efficacy in relieving pain, effect on the progress of labor, and effect on the fetus. All the available, fully effective narcotics are powerful respiratory depressants, and the fetus seems more susceptible to their respiratory depressant effects than does the mother. In equianalgesic doses, morphine and methadone appear somewhat more depressant to the fetus than are meperidine and closely related drugs (*see* Eddy *et al.,* 1957; Campbell *et al.,* 1961). The pharmacological basis for this difference has been presented above. The differences are sufficient to justify the selection of other drugs in preference to morphine and the available semisynthetics for obstetrical use. Regardless of the specific opioid analgesic that is selected, opioid-induced respiratory depression in

the newborn can be immediately reversed by a small dose of naloxone injected into the umbilical vein.

Sedation and Sleep. Whenever possible, drugs other than narcotics should be prescribed for sedation, tranquility, or sleep. However, nonnarcotic sedatives such as the barbiturates and chloral hydrate produce little analgesia. When sleeplessness is due to *pain* or *cough,* opiates are often necessary, and when properly used they foster rest and thus conserve the patient's strength. Long years of use have demonstrated the value of narcotic analgesics for preanesthetic medication. However, extensive controlled clinical studies (Eckenhoff and Helrich, 1958; Beecher, 1959) suggest that nonnarcotic preanesthetic medication, such as with pentobarbital, is just as effective in reducing preoperative apprehension and does not cause vomiting. While narcotics will continue to be valuable for the preoperative sedation of patients in pain, their routine use in pain-free patients is difficult to justify on the basis of available evidence.

Cough. The opiates remain among the most effective agents available for suppressing cough. This antitussive effect can be demonstrated experimentally against the coughing induced by electrical stimulation of the medulla or by chemical or mechanical irritation of the respiratory tract. The dose of any given narcotic required to suppress cough induced by these technics seems to be lower than that required for analgesia. A 15-mg oral dose of codeine, although analgesically ineffective, produces a demonstrable antitussive effect, and higher doses of codeine produce even more suppression of chronic cough. Interestingly, the degree of relief reported by patients does not necessarily correlate with actual reduction in the frequency of coughing (Sevelius *et al.,* 1971), and it has been suggested that the usual doses of opioids produce their major effect on the patient's subjective reactions to the cough, rather than on the frequency and intensity of coughing (*see* Beecher, 1959).

Considerable progress has been made in separating analgesic actions from antitussive activity, and there are now a number of effective nonnarcotic, nonaddictive antitussives available for clinical use (*see* below).

Dyspnea. Certain forms of dyspnea may be markedly relieved by morphine. This is especially true of the dyspnea of *acute left ventricular failure* and *pulmonary edema,* in which the response to intravenous morphine may be dramatic. The mechanism underlying this relief is still not clear. It may involve an alteration of the patient's reaction to impaired respiratory function and an indirect reduction of the work of the heart due to reduced fear and apprehension. However, it is more probable that the major benefit is due to cardiovascular effects such as decreased peripheral resistance and an increased capacity of the peripheral vascular compartment (*see* Vasko *et al.,* 1966). Opioids are contraindicated in pulmonary edema due to respiratory irritants unless severe pain is also present; their use in asthma has already been discussed.

Constipating Effects. The opioids remain the most effective agents for causing constipation or treating diarrhea. Mild constipation and a drier stool are often desirable after ileostomy or colostomy, whereas the constipating action is especially valuable in treating exhausting diarrhea and dysenteries due to a number of causes. When diarrhea is caused by food or drug poisoning, the toxic agent should be evacuated before instituting therapy, and the treatment of chronic diarrheas with narcotics should be undertaken only with a full appreciation of the risk of psychological and physical dependence. As in the case for cough, it requires considerably less morphine to affect the gut than to produce analgesia. Traditionally, opium preparations (opium tincture, 0.5 to 1.0 ml; paregoric, 4 ml) rather than the pure alkaloids are used; the morphine content of these doses cannot provide significant analgesia (especially by the oral route), but such dosage is, nevertheless, effective treatment for diarrhea. Synthetic opioids also produce a decrease in bowel motility; one of these, *diphenoxylate,* is used exclusively for this purpose (*see* below).

Special Anesthesia. High doses of morphine or other opioids have been used as the primary anesthetic agents in certain surgical procedures. Although respiration is so depressed that physical assistance is required, the patient retains consciousness (*see* Arens *et al.,* 1972).

LEVORPHANOL AND CONGENERS

Levorphanol is the only commercially available analgesic congener of the morphinan series. It more closely resembles morphine than does any other synthetic narcotic. The *d* isomer (*dextrorphan*) is relatively devoid of analgesic action and makes little contribution to the activity of the racemate (*racemorphan*). The structure of levorphanol is indicated in Table 15–2.

The *pharmacological effects* of levorphanol in all species including man closely parallel those of morphine (for references, *see* Reynolds and Randall, 1957). It is more potent than morphine as an analgesic, but depression of respiration, stimulation of smooth muscle, and addiction liability are also proportionately increased. However, clinical reports suggest that it produces less nausea and vomiting. The nonanalgesic isomer *dextrorphan* possesses considerable antitussive activity (*see* below). Levorphanol is promptly absorbed from subcutaneous sites. Although it is less effective when given orally, its oral-parenteral potency ratio is considerably better than that of morphine. The average dose, 2 to 3 mg subcutaneously, is approximately equianalgesic with 10 mg of morphine. Maximal analgesia occurs 60 to 90 minutes after subcutaneous injection. Clinical studies of levorphanol have been reviewed by Eddy and coworkers (1957) and by Lasagna (1964); its absorption, fate, and excretion have been reviewed by Way and Adler (1962). The drug is available as *Levorphanol Tartrate,* N.F. (LEVO-DROMORAN), as *Levorphanol Tartrate Tablets,* N.F., containing 2 mg, and as *Levorphanol Tartrate Injection,* N.F., containing 2 mg/ml.

MEPERIDINE AND CONGENERS

History. Meperidine is a synthetic, analgesic drug introduced by Eisleb and Schaumann in 1939. Originally studied as an atropine-like agent, it was soon discovered to have considerable analgesic activity. It is chemically quite dissimilar to morphine, and for a long time was thought to be free of many of its undesirable properties. Many years of clinical experience were required to correct some of the original misconceptions about the pharmacological actions of this drug, which, after morphine and codeine, is probably the most widely used, effective narcotic analgesic.

Chemistry. Meperidine and its congeneric phenylpiperidine derivatives have the following structural formulas:

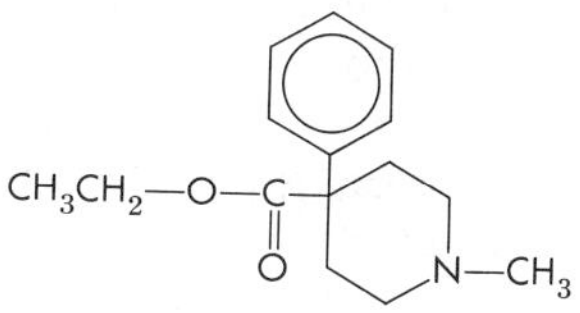

Meperidine

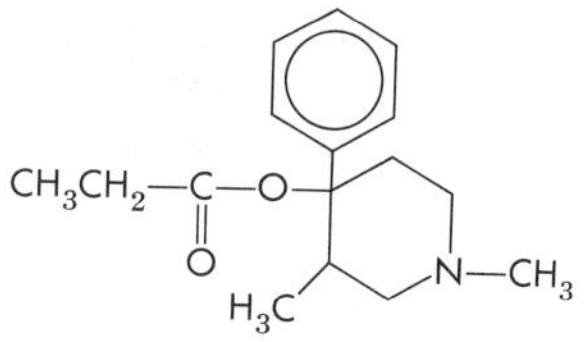

Alphaprodine

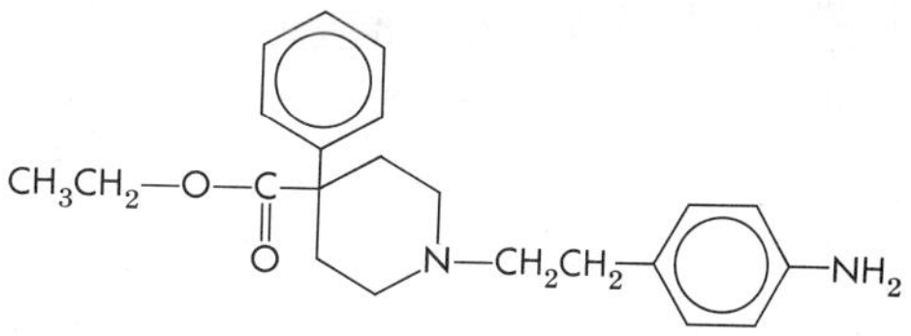

Anileridine

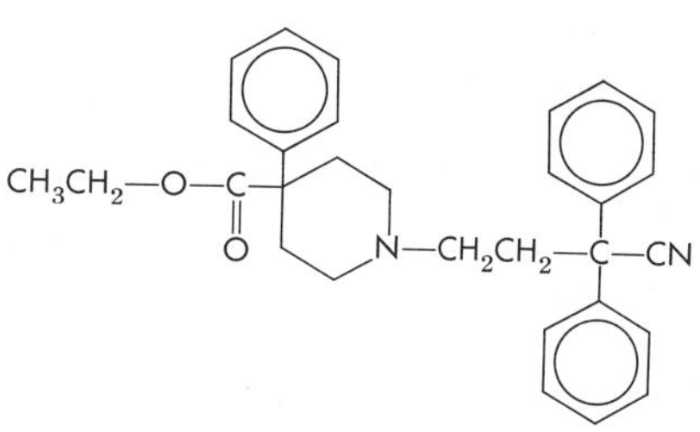

Diphenoxylate

With the exception of diphenoxylate, all form acid salts that are readily soluble in water. Meperidine is only one of a series of congeners with very similar pharmacological properties. Other structurally related substances are briefly described below. Although the two-dimensional representation of the structure of meperidine does not resemble that of morphine, the molecule does conform to the steric configuration of the opioid receptor.

PHARMACOLOGICAL PROPERTIES

Meperidine, like most narcotic analgesics, exerts its chief pharmacological actions on the CNS.

Central Nervous System.   Therapeutic doses of meperidine produce analgesia, sedation, euphoria, respiratory depression, and other diverse CNS effects comparable to those described for morphine.

Analgesia.   In patients or experimental subjects, the analgesic effects of meperidine are detectable about 15 minutes after oral administration, reach a peak in about an hour, and subside gradually over several hours. The onset of analgesic effect is somewhat more prompt (within 10 minutes) after subcutaneous or intramuscular administration, but the duration of action is shorter than that of morphine, being approximately 2 to 4 hours. This necessitates a shorter interval between injections for the relief of continuing pain.

In general, 80 to 100 mg of meperidine by the parenteral route is approximately equivalent to 10 mg of morphine. Since neither morphine nor meperidine in these doses produces satisfactory analgesia in all patients in all situations, there are times when larger doses are appropriate; when larger doses are used, due consideration should be given to the increased toxicity and side effects that occur. In terms of total analgesic effect, meperidine is less than one half as effective when given by mouth as when given parenterally (*see* review by Lasagna, 1964).

Sedation, Euphoria, and Excitation.   In equianalgesic doses, meperidine produces as much sedation as does morphine (Eckenhoff and Helrich, 1958) and as much euphoria (10 to 20% of patients). A few patients may experience dysphoria. Meperidine differs from morphine in that toxic doses sometimes cause CNS excitation, characterized by tremors, muscle twitches, and seizures (*see* below).

Respiration.   In equianalgesic doses, meperidine depresses respiration to the same degree as does morphine. Peak respiratory depression is observed within 1 hour after intramuscular administration, and after usual therapeutic doses there is a return toward normal starting at about 2 hours, although minute volume is usually measurably depressed for as long as 4 hours (Lambertsen *et al.*, 1961). The respiratory depression produced by meperidine can be antagonized by naloxone, nalorphine, and related narcotic antagonists.

Miscellaneous Nervous System Effects.   After systemic administration, meperidine may obtund or abolish the corneal reflex. Like other opioids, meperidine causes pupillary constriction. It has considerable local anesthetic activity but is somewhat irritating when applied locally. Meperidine appears to increase the sensitivity of the labyrinthine apparatus in human subjects (Gutner *et al.*, 1952), a fact that may partially explain the higher incidence of dizziness, nausea, and vomiting encountered when the drug is given to ambulatory patients; it lacks anticonvulsant activity. Meperidine causes the release of ADH, and stimulates the CTZ, thereby causing nausea and vomiting. The drug may also inhibit the release of ACTH and gonadotropic hormones, thereby affecting the respective target organs; it produces a rise in blood sugar by a mechanism similar to that described for morphine.

EEG.   Single doses of meperidine have no significant effect on cortical electrical activity in man. However, upon continued administration of large doses at short intervals, slow waves appear in the EEG after a few days, and then become progressively slower and of greater amplitude. The slow waves persist even after tolerance has developed to the drug. The EEG changes differ from those observed after morphine in that abnormal slow-wave activity occurs only when morphine is administered more rapidly than tolerance develops. The meperidine-induced alterations persist for about 48 hours after withdrawal of the drug, after which time the EEG record slowly returns to its original character. Large doses of meperidine regularly produce EEG evidence of convulsive activity in animals.

Cardiovascular System.   In therapeutic doses, meperidine has no significant untoward effects on the cardiovascular system, particularly in recumbent patients; myocardial contractility is not depressed and the ECG is unaltered. Ambulatory patients given meperidine may experience syncope associated with a fall in blood pressure, but symptoms rapidly clear if the recumbent position is assumed. After the intravenous administration of meperidine, there is an increase in peripheral blood flow and a decrease in peripheral arterial and venous resistance, effects that are not blocked by prior oral administration of antihistamines (Nadasdi and Zsotér, 1969). The mechanisms involved may be similar to those described above for morphine. Intramuscular administration of meperidine does not significantly affect heart rate, but intravenous administration frequently produces an increased rate that is sometimes alarming. As with morphine, respiratory depression is responsible for an accumulation of CO_2, which, in turn, produces cerebrovascular dilatation, increase in cerebral blood flow, and elevation of cerebrospinal fluid pressure (see Eckenhoff and Oech, 1960).

Smooth Muscle. Meperidine has a spasmogenic effect on certain smooth muscles, similar to that observed with morphine, methadone, and other synthetic narcotic analgesics.

Gastrointestinal Tract. Experiments on the intact gastrointestinal tract in animals and man usually demonstrate a moderate spasmogenic effect of meperidine on the stomach and small intestine, with a decrease in propulsive activity; these effects are qualitatively similar to those of morphine. Both propulsive and nonpropulsive contractions are diminished, but intermittent spasms and sudden elevations of tone appear. However, clinical observations indicate that it does not cause as much constipation when given over prolonged periods of time; this may be related to its shorter duration of action, which permits periods of normal function, or to a more favorable ratio of analgesic to gastrointestinal effects. In contrast to the opiates, meperidine is not of value in the treatment of diarrhea. After equianalgesic doses, the spasm in the biliary tract, as well as the rise in pressure in the common bile duct, induced by meperidine is less than that caused by morphine but greater than that by codeine.

Bronchial Musculature. Although meperidine is capable of opposing bronchospasm induced by agents such as histamine and methacholine, it has little effect on the normal bronchial musculature when given in therapeutic doses. When given in large doses meperidine is capable of producing bronchoconstriction (see Eckenhoff and Oech, 1960).

Ureter. After therapeutic doses of meperidine, peristaltic activity in the intact human ureter decreases. This seems to be related to a diminution in the secretion of urine, related to both antidiuretic activity and decreased glomerular filtration.

Uterus. The intact uterus of nonpregnant women is usually mildly stimulated by meperidine. Late in pregnancy, the drug does not significantly alter the activity of the normally contracting uterus, but appears to increase the tone and the frequency and intensity of contraction in the uterus made hyperactive by oxytocics. Administered prior to an oxytocic, meperidine does not exert any antioxytocic effect. Therapeutic doses given during labor appear neither to delay the birth process nor to alter the rhythmic uterine contractions (see Eddy et al., 1957). The drug does not interfere with normal postpartum contraction or involution of the uterus, and it does not increase the incidence of post-partum hemorrhage.

Absorption, Fate, and Excretion. Meperidine is absorbed by all routes of administration. After oral ingestion of single doses, peak plasma concentrations are obtained between the first and second hours. After intravenous administration, plasma values decline rapidly for the first 1 or 2 hours, and more slowly thereafter. Approximately 40% of meperidine is bound to plasma proteins. The drug is metabolized chiefly in the liver.

In man, meperidine is hydrolyzed to merperidinic acid, which, in turn, is partially conjugated. Meperidine is also N-demethylated to normeperidine, which may then be hydrolyzed to normeperidinic acid and subsequently conjugated. About one third of administered meperidine can be accounted for in the urine as N-demethylated derivatives; the clinical significance of the formation of normeperidine is discussed further under toxicity. Very little meperidine is excreted unchanged (see Way and Adler, 1962; Way, 1968).

Preparations, Routes of Administration, and Dosage. Trade names for meperidine include DEMEROL, DOLANTIN, DOLANTAL, DOLOSAL, and PETHOID. The international nonproprietary name is *pethidine. Meperidine Hydrochloride,* U.S.P., *Meperidine Hydrochloride Injection,* U.S.P., *Merperidine Hydrochloride Tablets,* U.S.P., and *Meperidine Hydrochloride Syrup,* N.F., are the official preparations. The drug is available for oral use in 50- and 100-mg tablets, and as an elixir containing 50 mg/5 ml; for parenteral use it is available in 0.5-, 1.0-, 1.5-, and 2.0-ml ampuls, and in 10- and 30-ml vials containing 50 mg/ml. It is also available in 1-ml ampuls and 20-ml vials containing 100 mg/ml and in 1- or 2-ml disposable syringes containing 50, 75, or 100 mg/ml. It is usually given orally or intramuscularly. Intravenous use increases the incidence and severity of untoward effects and subcutaneous administration causes local irritation and tissue induration. The dose varies with the clinical situation. Most patients with moderate-to-severe pain are relieved by 100 mg parenterally. The effectiveness of the drug by the oral route is not reduced to the same degree as is that of morphine. Doses for infants and children may be calculated on a weight basis. The drug is subject to the same narcotic regulations as apply to the opium alkaloids (see Appendix).

Of the several available meperidine congeners, only those that are official are described here. *Alphaprodine Hydrochloride,* N.F. (NISENTIL), is available in 1-ml ampuls containing 40 or 60 mg/ml, and in 10-ml multiple-dose vials containing 60 mg/ml. *Anileridine Hydrochloride,* N.F. (LERITINE), is available as 25-mg tablets. *Anileridine Injection,* N.F., is marketed for parenteral administration in ampuls and multiple-dose vials containing 25 mg/ml of anileridine phosphate. *Piminodine Esylate,* N.F. (ALVODINE), is available as an official injection containing 20 mg/ml, and as official tablets containing 50 mg. Doses, durations of action, and distinguishing pharmacological features of alphaprodine, anileridine, and piminodine are shown in Table 15-3.

Diphenoxylate. Diphenoxylate is a meperidine congener that has a definite constipating effect in man. While it has been proposed as a maintenance drug in the treatment of opioid dependence, its only recognized use is in the treatment of diarrhea. Although single doses in the therapeutic range (*see* below) produce no morphine-like subjective effects, at high doses (40 to 60 mg) the drug shows typical opioid activity, including euphoria, suppression of morphine abstinence, and a morphine-like physical dependence after chronic administration. Diphenoxylate is unusual in that even its salts are virtually insoluble in aqueous solution, thus obviating the possibility of abuse by the parenteral route (Fraser and Isbell, 1961). *Diphenoxylate Hydrochloride,* U.S.P., *Diphenoxylate Hydrochloride and Atropine Sulfate Solution,* U.S.P., and *Diphenoxylate Hydrochloride and Atropine Sulfate Tablets,* U.S.P., are the official preparations. In the combination (LOMOTIL), each tablet or 5 ml contains 2.5 mg of diphenoxylate and 25 μg of atropine sulfate. The recommended daily dosage for treatment of *diarrhea* in adults is 20 mg, in divided doses. It is a schedule-V narcotic (*see* Appendix). *Difenoxin* (diphenoxylic acid) is one of the metabolites of diphenoxylate; it has morphine-like actions similar to those of the parent compound, and is likely to become available for clinical use in the near future.

Ethoheptazine. Ethoheptazine (1-methyl-4-carbethoxy-4-phenylhexamethyleneimine) is structurally related to meperidine. It produces analgesic effects by an action on the CNS. The abuse potential is extremely low, but its efficacy as an analgesic is not impressive. *Ethoheptazine citrate* (ZACTANE) is available as tablets containing 75 mg, and as tablets containing 75 mg in combination with 325 mg of aspirin (ZACTIRIN).

Untoward Effects, Precautions, and Contraindications. The untoward effects that may occur after therapeutic doses of meperidine are similar to those seen with morphine and include dizziness, sweating, euphoria, dry mouth, nausea, vomiting, weakness, visual disturbances, palpitation, dysphoria, syncope, and sedation. The incidence and severity of these responses are greater in ambulatory patients than in those confined to bed. The overall incidence of the individual side effects is quite similar to that observed after equianalgesic doses of morphine, except that constipation and urinary retention do not occur as frequently after meperidine.

Tolerance to some of the untoward effects of meperidine, such as nausea, vomiting, and sedation, usually develops during the course of chronic administration. Patients who experience nausea and vomiting with morphine may not do so with meperidine; the converse may also be true. As far as is known, the use of meperidine is not contraindicated in any particular disease or syndrome, but it should be employed with caution in situations where the use of morphine entails a risk (*see* above).

Interaction with Other Drugs. Therapeutic doses of *atropine* or *scopolamine* do not seem to interfere with the intensity of the analgesia produced by meperidine, but concomitant administration of *amphetamine* has been reported to enhance the analgesic effects of meperidine and its congeners. Severe reactions may occur when meperidine is administered to patients being treated with *monoamine oxidase inhibitors;* these are characterized by excitation, delirium, hyperpyrexia, and convulsions, or by severe respiratory depression and cyanosis without hypotension. Similar reactions do not appear to occur with morphine (*see* Shee, 1960). The mechanism is still uncertain.

When therapeutic doses of meperidine are injected concurrently with *phenothiazines,* there may be exaggeration of the respiratory depressant effects; maximal respiratory depression does not occur until 1½ hours and persists close to maximum for 3½ hours. This is in contrast to maximal depression at 1 hour with approximately 50% recovery at the end of 3½ hours when meperidine is given alone (Lambertsen *et al.,* 1961). Meperidine-induced respiratory depression may also be enhanced by tricyclic antidepressants; it is not enhanced by intramuscular administration of 100 mg of chlordiazepoxide or 10 mg of diazepam. These effects may be due to reduction in the rate of meperidine metabolism. Some phenothiazines may antagonize the analgesic effects of meperidine (*see* above).

Toxicity. In nontolerant man, toxic parenteral doses of meperidine commonly produce respiratory depression that can be antagonized by naloxone or nalorphine. In addicts tolerant to the depressant effects of meperidine, large doses repeated at short intervals produce tremors, muscle twitches, dilated pupils, hyperactive reflexes, and convulsions.

Normeperidine, a metabolite of meperidine, differs from meperidine in having greater excitant and less depressant effect. When toxic doses of meperidine are given parenterally, the rate of absorption exceeds the rate of normeperidine formation, and the picture is primarily one of CNS depression. When toxic doses of meperidine are given orally, the rate of absorption does not exceed the capacity of the liver to convert meperidine to normeperidine. Hence the ratio of normeperidine to meperidine increases, producing a picture of mixed stupor and convulsions (Deneau and Nakai, 1961).

When nalorphine is given to a patient who has received an extremely large dose of meperidine, the respiratory depression is antagonized but convulsions may ensue, necessitating the use of a barbiturate. Development of tolerance also alters the toxicity of meperidine.

Tolerance, Physical Dependence, and Abuse Liability. The duration of action of meperidine is considerably shorter than that of morphine, and continuous depression of the CNS is attained only when the drug is used at less than 4-hour intervals. This may account for the slower development of tolerance to meperidine. Tolerance to the excitatory effects of meperidine does not seem to develop even after prolonged use of high doses. When patients who have become tolerant to the respiratory depressant effects of meperidine are given high doses at frequent intervals, twitches, tremors, jitteriness, and hypersensitivity to external stimuli may occur, as well as hallucinations and seizures (*see* Chapter 16).

The pattern of withdrawal symptoms after abrupt discontinuation of meperidine differs somewhat from that after morphine in that there is less in the way of autonomic effects and the symptoms develop more rapidly and are of shorter duration. It should be emphasized that the degree of physical dependence that a drug induces is only one factor in determining its abuse liability (*see* above). Actually, the need to use a drug repeatedly at short intervals can be viewed as a factor favoring the reinforcement of drug-seeking behavior. Some congeners of meperidine can produce a marked degree of physical dependence, and withdrawal symptoms following abrupt discontinuation result in a severe morphine-like withdrawal syndrome. The abuse potential of the clinically available meperidine congeners is similar to that of meperidine.

THERAPEUTIC USES

The major use of meperidine is for analgesia. Unlike morphine and its congeners, meperidine is not useful for the treatment of cough and diarrhea.

Analgesia. Meperidine can be used in any situation where a narcotic analgesic is required. However, there are a number of clinical conditions in which its relatively shorter duration of action or its lesser spasmogenic effects make meperidine preferable to morphine. For example, in equianalgesic doses meperidine has less spasmogenic effect on the biliary tract than does morphine. On the other hand, in bronchoscopy the relative lack of antitussive activity of meperidine makes it less valuable. Because of concern about drug dependence, many clinicians prescribe doses of meperidine that are too low or too infrequent, thereby causing unnecessary suffering. This is discussed above, in the section on therapeutic uses of morphine.

Meperidine crosses the placental barrier and even in reasonable analgesic doses causes a significant increase in the percentage of babies who show delayed respiration, decreased respiratory minute volume, or decreased oxygen saturation, or who require resuscitation (*see* review by Eddy *et al.*, 1957). However, meperidine produces less respiratory depression in the newborn than does an equianalgesic dose of morphine or methadone. It is also possible that, due to the shorter duration of action of meperidine compared to morphine, the baby is less liable to be delivered at the peak of respiratory depressant effects. Several studies have shown that after equianalgesic doses pentazocine crosses the placenta to a significantly lesser degree than does meperidine. Whether this is associated with a significantly decreased frequency of fetal depression is not clear. Concurrent use of meperidine and certain phenothiazines reduces the amount of narcotic required to produce a given degree of obstetrical analgesia, possibly by slowing the metabolism of meperidine. The claims that there are advantages to such therapy require evaluation in controlled studies.

Other Uses. Meperidine cannot be considered an innocuous drug for use in patients with bronchial asthma, since it depresses respiratory drive without decreasing respiratory resistance. Judiciously used, narcotic analgesics such as meperidine can be of great value in allaying apprehension and sometimes in aborting the progression of an asthmatic attack to status asthmaticus. On the other hand, deaths have occurred in patients given meperidine during an asthmatic episode. Deaths in asthmatic patients who received narcotics are usually not a result of bronchoconstriction. At post-mortem examination, thick, viscid secretions are found occluding the bronchial tree, suggesting that death was related to a combination of depression of respiratory drive, decrease in cough reflex, and drying of secretions.

FENTANYL

Fentanyl is a synthetic opioid related to the phenylpiperidines. It has the following structural formula:

Fentanyl

As an analgesic it is estimated to be 80 times as potent as morphine. Its respiratory depressant effect is of shorter duration than that of meperidine (Downes *et al.,* 1967); its analgesic and euphoric effects are antagonized by opioid antagonists, but are not significantly prolonged or intensified by *droperidol,* a "neuroleptic" agent with which it is usually combined for use as an intravenous anesthetic (*see* Chapter 8). The subjective effects of the combination depend on the relative proportions of the two agents (Gorodetsky and Martin, 1965). High doses of fentanyl produce marked muscular rigidity, probably through actions on the CNS (*see* Sokoll *et al.,* 1972); this effect can be antagonized by naloxone. Fentanyl is used exclusively for anesthesia. It is available as *Fentanyl Citrate,* U.S.P., and *Fentanyl Citrate Injection,* U.S.P. (SUBLIMAZE), containing 50 µg of fentanyl citrate per milliliter in 2- and 5-ml ampuls.

TILIDINE

Tilidine (VALORON) is a representative of a distinct pharmacological class that structurally resembles the phenylpiperidines. Subcutaneously, it is approximately one tenth to one twentieth as potent as morphine in producing analgesia and morphine-like subjective effects and suppressing signs of morphine abstinence. Administered orally, tilidine is approximately twice as potent as orally administered codeine in producing morphine-like effects and is probably more potent than codeine as an analgesic. The drug appears to be more potent orally than parenterally; this suggests that a metabolite is the active form of the drug. Very large doses produce anxiety, tremor, and hyperactive tendon reflexes. Tilidine is not available as yet for clinical use.

METHADONE AND CONGENERS

Methadone was synthesized by German chemists and came into clinical use at the end of World War II. The pharmacological properties of methadone are qualitatively similar to those of morphine.

Chemistry. Methadone has the following structural formula:

Methadone

In spite of the fact that the two-dimensional structure of methadone does not remotely resemble that of morphine, steric factors force the molecule to simulate the pseudopiperidine ring configuration that appears to be essential for opioid activity (*see* Goldstein *et al.,* 1974). The analgesic activity of the racemate is almost entirely the result of its content of *l*-methadone, which is 8 to 50 times more potent than the *d* isomer (depending upon the species and analgesic test employed). *d*-Methadone also lacks significant respiratory depressant action and addiction liability, but it does possess antitussive activity.

A larger number of structural isomers and congeners of methadone have been synthesized and compared pharmacologically with methadone and morphine (*see* Braenden *et al.,* 1955). As analgesics, these drugs have no demonstrable superiority over the parent compound. The dose, durations of action, and other effects of the congeners are compared to those of other narcotic analgesics in Table 15–3.

Pharmacological Actions. The pharmacological actions of single doses of methadone are qualitatively identical to those of morphine. The outstanding properties of methadone are its effective analgesic activity, its efficacy by the oral route, its extended duration of action in suppressing withdrawal symptoms in physically dependent individuals, and its tendency to show persistent effects with repeated administration. The drug also causes sedation and respiratory depression, and exhibits effects upon smooth muscle and the cardiovascular system similar to those of morphine.

Central Nervous System. After parenteral administration in man, a single dose of methadone is an effective analgesic, equal in potency and duration of action to morphine. Single doses of methadone may be slightly less hypnotic than comparable doses of morphine; however, upon repeated administration, marked sedative effects are seen in some patients (Isbell *et al.,* 1948; Martin *et al.,* 1973a). Methadone, like morphine, produces respiratory depression, miosis, antitussive effects, hyperglycemia, hypothermia, release of ADH, and suppression of release of gonadotropic hormones by the anterior pituitary gland. In equianalgesic doses, its actions on these systems are equivalent to those of morphine.

Smooth Muscle. In the intact, unanesthetized animal, methadone, like morphine, increases intestinal tone, diminishes the amplitude of contractions, and produces a marked decrease in propulsive activity. In man, methadone is constipating and causes biliary tract spasm. After therapeutic doses, the ureters become quiescent, perhaps because of the antidiuretic effect. The uterus at term is not significantly affected.

Cardiovascular System. The effects of methadone upon the cardiovascular system, especially in the recumbent individual, are not prominent; peripheral vasodilatation may contribute to orthostatic hypotension. The ECG remains unchanged except for the occasional appearance of sinus bradycardia. Methadone does not interfere with cardiovascular reflexes.

Absorption, Fate, and Excretion. Appreciable concentrations of methadone can be found in the plasma within 10 minutes after its subcutaneous injection. It is also well absorbed from the gastrointestinal tract and can be detected in plasma within 30 minutes after oral ingestion; it reaches peak concentrations at about 4 hours. After therapeutic doses, about 85% of methadone is bound to plasma proteins (Olsen, 1973). Like most of the other narcotic analgesics, the drug rapidly leaves the blood and becomes localized in tissues such as lung, liver, kidney, and spleen; only a small fraction enters the brain. Peak concentrations occur in the brain within 1 or 2 hours after subcutaneous or intramuscular administration, and this correlates well with the intensity and duration of analgesia. Methadone appears to be firmly bound to protein in various tissues, including brain. Some of its effects after repeated administration are due to its gradual accumulation in tissues. When administration is discontinued, low plasma concentrations are maintained by slow release from extravascular binding sites (Misra and Mulé, 1972; Dole and Kreek, 1973).

Methadone undergoes extensive biotransformation in the liver. The major metabolites, the results of N-demethylation and cyclization to form pyrrolidines, are excreted in the urine and the bile along with small amounts of unchanged drug. The amount of methadone excreted in the urine is increased when the urine is acidified. In nontolerant subjects, the mean apparent half-life of methadone after a single dose is approximately 15 hours (Inturrisi and Verebely, 1972a, 1972b).

The use of methadone in the treatment of compulsive heroin users has revived interest in other methadone congeners, such as α-*dl*- and *l*-acetylmethadol (methadyl acetate). In subjects physically dependent on α-*dl*-acetylmethadol, opioid withdrawal symptoms are not perceived for 72 to 96 hours after the last oral dose, and subjects are entirely comfortable when given a single dose of the drug as infrequently as every 72 hours (Fraser and Isbell, 1952; Jaffe *et al.*, 1972). The relatively slow onset and protracted duration of action of this drug, which is probably inactive, are thought to be due in part to its conversion to active metabolites (noracetylmethadol and normethadol) that are slowly further metabolized or excreted (*see* reviews by Way and Adler, 1962; Way, 1968).

Preparations, Routes of Administration, and Dosage. *Methadone Hydrochloride,* U.S.P., is a bitter white powder, soluble in water and ethanol. Trade names of methadone include AMIDONE, BUTALGIN, DOLOPHINE, METHADON, MIADONE, PHYSEPTONE, and POLAMIDON. All conventional routes of administration may be used, but subcutaneous administration may cause local irritation. *Methadone Hydrochloride Tablets,* U.S.P., are available for oral use in 5- and 10-mg amounts. *Methadone Hydrochloride Injection,* U.S.P., is available in single ampuls and multiple-dose vials containing 10 mg/ml. *Methadone hydrochloride syrup* contains 5 mg/15 ml. The *oral analgesic dose* for adults is 5 to 15 mg, depending on the severity of the pain and the response of the patient; the initial parenteral dose is usually 5 to 10 mg.

In the United States, special controls on methadone have been enacted in an effort to prevent its unregulated large-scale use in the treatment of narcotics addiction. Under these controls, even for use in treatment of pain, methadone is available only through specially licensed addiction treatment programs and special pharmacies, primarily those associated with hospitals. Nevertheless, the indications for the use of methadone remain unchanged. Specialized dosage forms used in narcotics addiction are discussed in Chapter 16.

Side Effects, Toxicity, and Precautions. Side effects caused by methadone are similar to those caused by morphine. As with morphine and meperidine, certain of these side effects occur more frequently in ambulatory than in bed patients. Delirium, transient hallucinations, and hemorrhagic urticaria have been reported, but are quite rare. The principal danger of overdosage is diminished pulmonary ventilation. The conditions that alter sensitivity to methadone are similar to those outlined for morphine, and the therapy of acute methadone intoxication is the same as for morphine.

Tolerance, Physical Dependence, and Abuse Liability. The abuse liability of methadone and its congeners in man has been thoroughly assessed. Volunteer postaddicts who received subcutaneous or oral methadone daily developed partial *tolerance* to the nauseant, anorectic, miotic, sedative, respiratory depressant, and cardiovascular effects of methadone. Tolerance develops more slowly to methadone than to morphine in some patients, especially with respect to the depressant effects. However, this may be related in part to cumulative effects of the drug or its metabolites. Sedation with concomitant slowing of the EEG occurs during experimental addiction (Martin *et al.*, 1973a). Tolerance to the constipating effect of methadone does not develop as fully as does tolerance to other effects. The behavior of the addicts who use methadone parenterally is strikingly similar to that of the morphine addict, but many former heroin users treated with oral methadone show virtually no overt behavioral effects (*see* Chapter 16).

Development of physical dependence during the chronic administration of methadone can be demonstrated by drug withdrawal or by administration of a narcotic antagonist (*see* Chapter 16). Subcutaneous administration of 10 to 20 mg of methadone in former narcotics addicts produces definite euphoria, equal in duration to that caused by morphine. On the basis of definitive studies, the overall abuse potential of methadone is rated comparable to that of morphine (Isbell *et al.*, 1948; Martin *et al.*, 1973a).

Therapeutic Uses. The primary uses of methadone are relief of pain, treatment of narcotic abstinence syndromes, and treatment of heroin users. It is not widely used as an antiperistaltic agent, but it is an effective antitussive. It should be used with extreme caution, if at all, in labor.

Analgesia. Methadone provides relief from all types of pain, comparable to that obtained with morphine (*see* review by Lasagna, 1964). The dose is in the same range as that of morphine. The onset of analgesia occurs 10 to 20 minutes following parenteral administration and 30 to 60 minutes after oral medication. The duration of action of single doses is essentially the same as that of morphine. With repeated usage, some cumulative effects are seen, so that either lower dosage or longer intervals between doses become possible. *In contrast to morphine, methadone and many of its congeners retain a considerable degree of their effectiveness when given orally.* In terms of total analgesic effects, methadone given orally is about 50% as effective as the same dose administered intramuscularly; however, the oral-parenteral potency ratio is considerably lower when peak analgesic effect is considered (Beaver *et al.*, 1967). In equianalgesic doses, the pattern and incidence of untoward effects caused by methadone and morphine are similar.

PROPOXYPHENE

Of the four stereoisomers, only the alpha racemate, known as *propoxyphene*, has analgesic activity. Its analgesic effect resides in the dextrorotatory isomer, *d*-propoxyphene (dextropropoxyphene). However, levopropoxyphene seems to have some antitussive activity. As can be seen from the following formula, it is related structurally to methadone.

Propoxyphene

Pharmacological Actions. Propoxyphene produces analgesia by acting on the CNS. It also produces other CNS effects that are qualitatively similar to those seen with codeine and other opioids. It has no significant antipyretic or anti-inflammatory effects. It is likely that at equianalgesic doses the incidence of side effects such as nausea, anorexia, constipation, abdominal pain, and drowsiness would be similar to those of codeine.

There is some question about the minimal dosage required to relieve pain in clinical situations. Some studies have reported that 32 mg of propoxyphene is no better than a placebo; other studies indicate this dosage to be demonstrably effective. Higher doses produce analgesia somewhat more reliably. Beaver (1966) estimated that it requires 90 to 120 mg of propoxyphene orally to equal the analgesic effects of 60 mg of codeine, a dose that produces about as much analgesia as 600 mg of aspirin. The statement that, at the usual clinical dosage, propoxyphene or codeine is no more effective than aspirin is probably true, but it can be misleading. The analgesic effectiveness of aspirin in relieving moderate pain has been repeatedly demonstrated; it is about one fifth to one tenth as potent as codeine. Higher doses of either propoxyphene or codeine would probably yield more analgesia, that is, have greater efficacy, albeit with an increased incidence of side effects. Furthermore, combinations of propoxyphene and aspirin (like combinations of codeine and aspirin) afford a higher level of analgesia than does either agent given alone (*see* Lasagna, 1964; Beaver, 1966; Merck, 1970; Miller *et al.*, 1970).

Absorption, Fate, and Excretion. Propoxyphene is absorbed after oral or parenteral administration. After oral administration the water-soluble hydrochloride appears to be absorbed somewhat more rapidly than the relatively water-insoluble napsylate. However, differences in peak plasma concentrations between the two preparations are small. Despite the differences in solubility, their administration with a high-fat meal does not appreciably alter their absorption rates. Plasma concentrations are detectable within an hour, reach their highest values at about 2 hours, then slowly decrease. The mean half-life of propoxyphene following oral administration is approximately 3½ hours, which is twice the value obtained after intravenous injection. With repeated oral administration every 6 hours, plasma concentrations increase, reaching a steady state after about 2 days. There is great variability between subjects in terms of the plasma concentration achieved (Wolen *et al.,* 1971a, 1971b). In man, the major route of metabolism is N-demethylation to yield norpropoxyphene, which is then excreted in the urine (McMahon *et al.,* 1971).

Toxicity. In the usual therapeutic doses propoxyphene produces no significant effects on the cardiovascular system. Given orally, it is approximately one third as potent as orally administered codeine in depressing respiration (Bellville and Seed, 1968). Moderately toxic doses usually produce CNS and respiratory depression, but with still larger doses the clinical picture may be complicated by convulsions in addition to respiratory depression. Delusions, hallucinations, and confusion have also been noted following the ingestion of toxic doses, and deaths due to propoxyphene overdosage are often accompanied by pulmonary edema (Tennant, 1973). Naloxone reverses the toxic effects of propoxyphene, but the effects of other antagonists such as nalorphine seem to be more variable.

Abuse Liability. The abuse liability of propoxyphene is somewhat lower than that of codeine. Very large doses (800 mg of the hydrochloride per day) reduce the intensity of the morphine withdrawal syndrome somewhat less effectively than do 1500-mg doses of codeine. For most would-be abusers, use of higher doses of propoxyphene is prevented by untoward side effects and the occurrence of toxic psychoses. When very large doses are used in morphine-tolerant addicts, some respiratory depression is seen, suggesting that there is not a high degree of cross-tolerance between propoxyphene and morphine. Abrupt discontinuation of chronically administered propoxyphene hydrochloride (up to 800 mg per day, given for almost 2 months) results in mild abstinence phenomena, and large oral doses (300 to 600 mg) produce subjective effects that are considered pleasurable by postaddicts but are not necessarily identified as morphine-like. Administered intravenously, it is recognized as a narcotic; however, the drug is quite irritating when administered either intravenously or subcutaneously, so that abuse by these routes results in severe damage to veins and soft tissues, which limits the time the drug can be used parenterally (Fraser and Isbell, 1960; Tennant, 1973).

Since its introduction almost 2 decades ago the drug has not been subjected to strict narcotic controls, and while there have been a number of cases of dependence reported (*see* Miller *et al.,* 1970) they have been quite uncommon when measured against the widespread clinical use of the drug. A brief outbreak of serious dependence, including intravenous use, was reported, and it subsided only when more stringent accounting and prescribing regulations were introduced (Tennant, 1973). At present, the drug is still not subject to special controls in the United States.

Preparations, Dosage, and Therapeutic Uses. Although it has been used experimentally for the suppression of withdrawal symptoms in cases of opioid addiction, the only recognized use of propoxyphene is for the treatment of mild-to-moderate pain that is not adequately relieved by aspirin. When appropriate doses are selected, combinations of aspirin and propoxyphene can be as effective as the combination of codeine and aspirin. However, the latter combination is considerably less costly; inasmuch as the situations calling for analgesics of this type are commonly chronic conditions, the factor of cost cannot be discounted. The current wide popularity of propoxyphene in clinical situations in which codeine was once used seems to be largely a result of unrealistic overconcern about the addictive potential of codeine.

The drug is available as *Propoxyphene Hydrochloride,* U.S.P. (DARVON, DOLENE, SK-65); *Propoxyphene Hydrochloride Capsules,* U.S.P., which contain 32 or 65 mg of the hydrochloride; and *propoxyphene hydrochloride and aspirin capsules* (DARVON WITH A.S.A.), containing 65 mg of the hydrochloride and 325 mg of aspirin. It is also available as *Propoxyphene Napsylate,* N.F. (DARVON-N). Because of differences in molecular weight of the salts, a dose of 100 mg of propoxyphene napsylate is required to supply an amount of propoxyphene equivalent to that present in 65 mg of propoxyphene hydrochloride. *Propoxyphene Napsylate Tablets,* N.F., are supplied in 50- and 100-mg sizes; *Propoxyphene Napsylate Oral Suspension,* N.F. (50 mg/5 ml), and *propoxyphene napsylate* in combination with aspirin (DARVON-N WITH A.S.A.) are also available.

NARCOTIC ANTAGONISTS AND PARTIAL AGONISTS

History. In 1915, Pohl observed that N-allylnorcodeine prevented or abolished morphine- and heroin-induced respiratory depression. More than 25 years elapsed before Unna as well as Hart and McCawley independently described the more pronounced morphine-antagonizing properties of nalorphine. The clinical significance of this antagonistic effect was not explored until 1951, when Eckenhoff and coworkers reported the use of nalorphine as an antidote for morphine poisoning in man. Then, in 1953, Wikler and associates demonstrated that nalorphine would precipitate acute abstinence syndromes in postaddicts who had received morphine, methadone, or heroin for brief periods, and that in the majority of nonaddicted subjects large doses of nalorphine produced dysphoria and anxiety rather than euphoria. Shortly thereafter, Lasagna and Beecher noted that, although nalorphine antagonized the analgesic effects of morphine, it was, nevertheless, an effective analgesic when given to patients with postoperative pain. The dysphoric side effects produced by nalorphine make it unsuitable for clinical use as an analgesic; however, since the low abuse potential of nalorphine had already been observed, the report of its analgesic effects raised the hope that other narcotic antagonists might be free of these dysphoric effects and still have analgesic activity. The search for compounds useful as narcotic antagonists led to the discovery of new drugs, such as *naloxone, penta-*

zocine, and *propiram,* that enlarged the physician's therapeutic armamentarium, changed the views as to how these drugs act, and even changed the terminology used to describe them.

Chemistry. With the discovery of drugs that have both morphine-antagonistic effects and morphine-like subjective effects, the study of the structure-activity relationship among opioids and opioid antagonists became more complex and more exciting. Whereas the substitution of an allyl group for the N-methyl group in codeine, morphine, levorphanol, oxymorphone, and phenazocine produces drugs with antagonistic actions, it is now clear that such simple substitutions do not necessarily guarantee an analog that is antagonistic. Furthermore, some substitutions produce congeners that are relatively pure antagonists, whereas others produce drugs that have marked agonistic actions along with their antagonistic effects. The chemistry and structure-activity relationship of opioid antagonists have been reviewed by Lewis and associates (1971), Archer and coworkers (1973), and Harris (1974). The structural formulas of *naloxone* (N-allyl-noroxymorphone), *naltrexone* (N-cyclopropylmethyl-noroxymorphone), and *nalorphine* (N-allyl-normorphine) are shown in Table 15–2. Cyclazocine has the following structural formula:

Cyclazocine

Pharmacological Properties

The drugs now considered as opioid antagonists or partial agonists have widely differing actions that necessitate some changes in terminology. The use of the term *opioid antagonist* for drugs such as naloxone presents no difficulty, since naloxone is almost a *pure antagonist.* However, drugs such as nalorphine, levallorphan, and cyclazocine, in addition to their powerful antagonistic actions, also produce autonomic, endocrine, analgesic, and respiratory depressant effects similar to those of morphine. Accordingly, they can be thought of as *agonist-antagonists* or *partial agonists of the nalorphine type.* There are drugs such as profadol and propiram that are almost entirely morphine-like in their actions, except that they can precipitate withdrawal symptoms in subjects maintained on high doses of morphine, while actually suppressing withdrawal in subjects

maintained on low doses. These drugs are referred to here as *partial agonists of the morphine type.* Lastly, there are a number of drugs such as pentazocine that, although exerting weak antagonistic activity, also produce agonistic effects that are not as clearly nalorphine-like and are, at present, difficult to classify. The literature on opioid antagonists has been reviewed by Martin (1967) and in several symposia (*see* Kosterlitz *et al.,* 1973; Braude *et al.,* 1974). In this section, *naloxone* will be described as the prototype of a *relatively pure opioid antagonist; nalorphine* will be presented as an example of an antagonist that is also a *partial agonist of the nalorphine type;* and *propiram* will be discussed as an example of a *partial agonist of the morphine type.* Because *pentazocine* is used clinically and is not easily classified, it is presented separately in greater detail. In each of these groups, the pharmacological effects of the drug depend upon whether morphine or some other opioid has been previously administered.

Mechanism of Action. There is ample evidence that opioid antagonists compete with morphine-like drugs for stereospecific opioid receptor sites and apparently occupy these sites without initiating any response. Goldstein and associates have extracted and partially purified a membrane-bound proteolipid of mouse brain that exhibited highly selective, stereospecific binding of the opioid agonist levorphanol; the binding was inhibited competitively by naloxone. From these and related observations it was proposed that the proteolipid, which has an estimated mass of approximately 60,000 daltons, is probably a major opioid receptor. The authors hypothesized that combination of the receptor with the agonist, but not with the antagonist, produces a conformational change that initiates certain pharmacological responses. They acknowledged the possible existence of additional opioid receptors where agonists or partial agonists might act to produce other pharmacological effects. (*See* Goldstein, 1973, 1974; Lowney *et al.,* 1974.)

A concept of simple competitive antagonism at a single receptor site does not account readily for a number of interactions between opioids and drugs with opioid antagonist actions. Among these are the following: (1) some antagonists (*e.g.,* nalorphine, cyclazocine) produce psychotomimetic and other subjective effects that are qualitatively distinct from those produced by morphine; (2) antagonists of the nalorphine type produce a variety of physical dependence that results in a withdrawal syndrome qualitatively distinct from that seen after withdrawal of morphine; (3) antagonists of the nalorphine type are quite effective against severe but not mild opioid-induced respiratory depression; (4) it requires progressively less of an antagonist to precipitate withdrawal symptoms or to antagonize morphine effects as physical dependence develops; (5) partial agonists of the nalorphine type precipitate the withdrawal syndrome in subjects who are dependent on high levels of morphine, but substitute for morphine at lower levels of such physical dependence. To account for these observations, Martin (1967) has proposed that, in addition to the major opioid receptor, there is a similar but distinct receptor (the nalorphine receptor) at which antagonists such as nalorphine and cyclazocine produce their agonistic effects. Within the framework of a dual- or multiple-receptor hypothesis, a drug could have varying degrees of agonistic activity at the morphine receptor, the nalorphine receptor, or both. For example, naloxone is viewed as having affinity for both receptors, but no activity at either. Nalorphine and cyclazocine are seen as exerting agonist activity at the nalorphine receptor, and acting as competitive antagonists at the morphine receptor, where they are presumed to have high affinity but no activity.

Also related to these interactions at the receptor level are the changes that accompany the development of physical dependence. When prolonged action at the opioid receptors causes physical dependence, the physiological systems involved develop what has been described as latent hyperexcitability. In this situation, apparently very little displacement of the opioid by an antagonist is needed to increase the activity in the system. Substantial displacement (and replacement with an antagonist or partial agonist) will result in marked hyperexcitability. The net effect that is seen when an opioid is competitively displaced can be viewed as the sum of the agonistic activity of antagonist or partial agonist at both the morphine and the nalorphine receptors, the proportions of the receptors of each variety that were occupied, and the degree of physical dependence that developed prior to the administration of the antagonist or partial agonist.

Pert and Snyder (1974) have proposed a related hypothesis on the nature of the receptor to account for their observations on the binding of opioid agonists and antagonists to a putative receptor in brain homogenates. Binding of antagonists is enhanced by sodium ion, while that of agonists is inhibited; partial agonists assume an intermediate position. These data are consistent with a model in which the receptor can exist in two conformations, one to which agonists bind most readily and the other to which antagonists are preferentially bound. Partial agonists hypothetically have affinity for both forms of the receptor, and sodium is thought to alter the position of the equilibrium between the two forms by an action at an allosteric site. This system could serve as an *in-vitro* test for relative agonist and antagonist activities of new compounds.

Effects in the Absence of Opioid Drugs.

Naloxone is almost devoid of agonistic effects. In man, subcutaneous doses up to 12 mg produce no discernible subjective effects, and 24 mg causes only slight drowsiness. Oral doses of more than 1 g have been administered without producing any major subjective or physiological effects (Zaks *et al.*, 1971). *Naltrexone* also appears to be a relatively pure antagonist, but with higher oral efficacy and a somewhat longer duration of action (Martin *et al.*, 1973b).

Small doses (5 to 15 mg) of *nalorphine* in man produce certain autonomic effects resembling those produced by morphine. There is lowering of body temperature, slight decrease in heart rate, and constriction of the pupils. Respiratory minute volume and the sensitivity of the respiratory center to CO_2 are reduced to the same degree as that seen after low doses of morphine. Some antagonists of the nalorphine type also induce diuresis by inhibiting the release of ADH.

The subjective effects of nalorphine in man depend largely upon the dose, the subject, and the situation. In patients with postoperative pain, a dose of 10 to 15 mg of nalorphine is about as effective as 10 mg of morphine in producing analgesia. While most patients show relaxation and drowsiness, a significant percentage experience unpleasant reactions that range from anxiety, "crazy feelings," and vivid, disturbing, "unreal" daydreams to frank hallucinatory phenomena, usually visual. Other side effects include difficulty in focusing the eyes, sweating, nausea, and the feeling of being groggy or drunk and of being sleepy but unable to sleep. These dysphoric and psychotomimetic effects appear more frequently as the dose is increased, but there is not a consistent increase in analgesia. Postaddicts report that the effects of low doses of nalorphine are more like those of short-acting barbiturates or alcohol than those of morphine. The dysphoric effects can be antagonized by large doses of naloxone.

In contrast to morphine, the respiratory depression produced by nalorphine does not increase as the dose is raised. For example, a dose of 75 mg does not produce significantly greater respiratory depression than is seen with 10 to 20 mg (Keats *et al.*, 1960). Deaths from nalorphine in man have not been reported. Antagonists of the nalorphine type might thus be considered to have only very limited actions at the opioid receptor but significant agonistic actions at the nalorphine receptor. It requires a considerably higher dose of naloxone to antagonize the effects of nalorphine than those of morphine.

In man, *profadol* and *propiram* produce subjective and physiological effects that are quite similar to those of morphine (*i.e.,* euphoria, analgesia, miosis, respiratory depression). Even at high doses, nalorphine-like subjective effects are usually not seen, and the agonist effects can be antagonized by either nalorphine or naloxone. Thus, in terms of the dual-receptor hypothesis profadol and propiram would appear to have actions only at the morphine receptor.

Antagonistic Actions. Small doses (0.4 to 0.8 mg) of *naloxone* given intramuscularly or intravenously in man prevent or promptly reverse the effects of opioid drugs. In patients with respiratory depression, there is an increase in respiratory rate within 1 or 2 minutes. Sedative effects are reversed and blood pressure, if depressed, returns to normal. One milligram of naloxone intravenously completely blocks the effects of 25 mg of heroin (Zaks *et al.,* 1971). Antagonistic effects last from 1 to 4 hours, depending on the dose of naloxone. It can also reverse the psychotomimetic and dysphoric effects of nalorphine and cyclazocine, but higher doses (10 to 15 mg) are required. Thus, naloxone might be viewed as having greater affinity for the morphine receptor than for the nalorphine receptor (*see* Jasinski *et al.,* 1970). Antagonism of opioid effects by naloxone is often accompanied by "overshoot" phenomena; for example, respiratory rate depressed by opioids transiently becomes higher than that prior to the period of depression. This "overshoot" is probably related to the "unmasking" of acute physical dependence (*see* below).

Nalorphine also prevents or abolishes opioid-induced CNS and gastrointestinal effects, with certain minor exceptions. Antagonism of morphine-induced antidiuretic, hypothermic, and antitussive effects may be masked by the capacity of nalorphine to produce these same actions. In patients with severe respiratory depression the antagonism of opioid effects is seen within 1 or 2 minutes after the intravenous injection of 5 to 10 mg of nalorphine and lasts 1 to 4 hours. Patients may not show complete reversal of sedative effects.

Opioid antagonists do not alter the respiratory depressant effects of barbiturates, alcohol, or other nonopioid CNS depressants. Instead, the respiratory depressant actions of the nalorphine-type antagonists may add to existing respiratory depression produced by CNS depressants. Pure opioid antagonists such as naloxone, which produce no respiratory depression themselves, have significant advantages in situations where the etiology of the respiratory depression is not clear.

The degree of antagonism produced depends not only on the dose of the antagonist but also on the dose of the opioid that has been given and the degree to which opioid physical dependence has developed. Thus, 10 mg of nalorphine does not antagonize the relatively mild respiratory depression produced by 10 mg of morphine, probably because its antagonistic effects are masked by its agonistic effects. However, smaller doses of nalorphine antagonize the severe depression produced by 70 mg of morphine. In patients who are physically dependent, very small doses (2 to 5 mg) of nalorphine may be sufficient not only to antagonize respiratory depression but also to precipitate withdrawal phenomena. In such individuals, large doses of nalorphine or other opioid antagonists can produce severe withdrawal symptoms that cannot be readily reversed even by large doses of morphine during the period of action of the antagonist. Nalorphine does not antagonize the agonistic effects of cyclazocine and other partial agonists of the nalorphine type.

Effects in Physical Dependence. In opioid-dependent subjects, small subcutaneous doses of naloxone (0.5 mg) precipitate a moderate-to-severe withdrawal syndrome that is very similar to that seen after abrupt withdrawal of opioids, except that the syndrome appears within minutes after administration and subsides in about 2 hours. The severity and duration of the syndrome are related to the dose of the antagonist and the degree of dependence.

Nalorphine is about one seventh as potent as naloxone in precipitating withdrawal symptoms in morphine-dependent subjects. With nalorphine it is possible to demonstrate mild abstinence phenomena in man after as little as 15 mg of morphine given four times a day for 2 to 3 days. If given within 12 to 24 hours after a large dose of morphine, nalorphine produces mydriasis or no effect, rather than its characteristic miosis. However, the agonistic effects of nalorphine tend to obscure the rather remarkable rapidity with which opioid physical dependence develops in both man and animals. Naloxone produces "overshoot" phenomena suggestive of early acute physical dependence 24 hours after a single large dose of morphine, and it precipitates withdrawal symptoms 5 days after a single 40-mg dose of methadone (Nutt and Jasinski, 1974).

Antagonists of the nalorphine-type do not precipitate withdrawal symptoms after chronic use of pentazocine, but do precipitate a morphine type of withdrawal syndrome following use of propiram and profadol. Naloxone precipitates a withdrawal syndrome after chronic doses of pentazocine, but the doses required are larger than those needed to precipitate the morphine withdrawal syndrome. High doses of profadol and propiram precipitate withdrawal symptoms in subjects dependent on high doses of morphine, but suppress such symptoms in subjects dependent on low doses.

Tolerance, Physical Dependence, and Abuse Potential. Tolerance develops to the agonistic but not to the antagonistic effects of opioid antagonists and partial agonists. Tolerance to the subjective effects, including the dysphoric and the psychotomimetic responses to both nalorphine and cyclazocine, has been demonstrated in man; cross-tolerance between these agents has also been shown (*see* Martin, 1967). However, even in subjects highly tolerant to the dysphoric, sedative, and motor effects of cyclazocine, a small (4-mg) dose continues to prevent the euphoric, miotic, respiratory depressant, and physical dependence-producing properties of morphine and heroin.

Even after prolonged administration of high doses, discontinuation of naloxone is not followed by any recognizable withdrawal syndrome, and the withdrawal of *naltrexone,* another relatively pure antagonist, produces very few signs and symptoms. However, after chronic administration of high dosage, abrupt discontinuation of either *nalorphine* or *cyclazocine* causes a characteristic withdrawal syndrome that is similar for both drugs. One early sign is repeated brief episodes of a sensation that is described by some subjects as "electric shocks to the head" and by others as light-headedness or fainting spells. It does not appear to be a convulsive phenomenon, and consciousness is not lost. Later signs and symptoms include lacrimation, rhinorrhea, yawning, chills, diarrhea, fever, and loss of appetite and body weight. Although the intensity of these withdrawal signs and symptoms in the nalorphine withdrawal syndrome is generally less than comparable manifestations of the morphine withdrawal syndrome, a more striking contrast is the absence of "craving" or drug-seeking behavior. Drug-seeking behavior is present in the pentazocine withdrawal syndrome, which has characteristics of both the nalorphine- and the morphine-type withdrawal syndrome; such behavior is prominent following withdrawal of profadol or propiram, where the pattern of signs and symptoms is similar to that seen with morphine withdrawal.

Since nalorphine, cyclazocine, and naloxone (1) do not support physical dependence of the morphine type, (2) are viewed by postaddicts as either neutral or unpleasant drugs in terms of their subjective effects, and (3) do not produce a variety of physical dependence that leads to drug-seeking behavior, they are considered to have little or no abuse potential. Because propiram and profadol are similar to morphine except for their capacity to precipitate abstinence at high levels of morphine physical dependence, they are judged to have an abuse potential approaching that of morphine and related opioids (for references, *see* Martin, 1967; Jasinski *et al.,* 1971; Jasinski, 1973). The abuse potential of pentazocine is discussed below.

Absorption, Fate, and Excretion. The effects of *naloxone* are seen almost immediately after its intravenous administration. The drug is metabolized in the liver primarily by conjugation with glucuronic acid; other metabolites are produced in small amounts (Weinstein *et al.,* 1974). Following parenteral administration, the duration of action of naloxone is about 1 to 4 hours. The drug is absorbed after oral administration, but it is metabolized so rapidly in its first passage through the liver that it is only one fiftieth as potent as when given parenterally (*see* Nutt and Jasinski, 1974). Oral doses of more than 1 g are almost completely metabolized in less than 24 hours.

Like naloxone, *nalorphine* is much more effective after parenteral than oral administration, probably because of rapid biotransformation in the liver (mainly conjugation with glucuronic acid). Following parenteral administration of nalorphine, concentrations in the brain are three to four times higher than after comparable doses of morphine. Brain concentrations fall rapidly and only trace amounts are found after 4 hours. The onset and duration of action of *levallorphan* are similar to those of nalorphine.

Unlike nalorphine, *cyclazocine* and *naltrexone,* both of which have cyclopropylmethyl substitutions on the nitrogen, retain much of their efficacy by the oral route, and their durations of action are longer, approaching 24 hours after moderate oral doses (*see* Martin *et al.,* 1973b).

Preparations. *Naloxone Hydrochloride Injection,* U.S.P. (NARCAN), is available in 1-ml ampuls and 10-ml multiple-dose vials in a concentration of 0.4 mg/ml. It is the drug of choice in most situations where an opioid antagonistic effect is required. *Nalorphine Hydrochloride Injection,* N.F. (NALLINE), is available for pediatric use in 1-ml ampuls containing 0.2 mg. It is also available in 1-, 2-, and 10-ml ampuls containing 5 mg/ml. The narcotic status of nalorphine is described in the Appendix to this book. The dose is highly dependent on the clinical situation. *Levallorphan Tartrate,* N.F., and *Levallorphan Tartrate Injection,* N.F. (LORFAN), are also available, the latter in a concentration of 1 mg/ml. It is approximately ten times as potent as nalorphine, and its therapeutic indications are virtually identical.

Therapeutic Uses. Narcotic antagonists are used in the treatment of narcotic-induced respiratory depression. They are also used in the diagnosis of physical dependence on narcotic drugs and as therapeutic agents in the treatment of compulsive narcotics users, as discussed in Chapter 16. Partial agonists are also used as analgesics (*see* Table 15–3).

Treatment of Narcotic Overdosage. The dramatic effects of opioid antagonists in reversing narcotic-induced respiratory depression in the adult have already been discussed. Narcotic antagonists have also been effectively employed to decrease neonatal respiratory depression secondary to the administration of narcotics to the mother. When employed for this purpose, the antagonist may be given either to the mother shortly before delivery (preferable) or to the infant by way of the umbilical vein following delivery. The usual dose of naloxone is 0.4 or 0.8 mg for the mother; a therapeutic dose has not been established for the newborn, but 5 μg/kg has been given without adverse effects. Narcotic antagonists cannot be expected to decrease apnea of the newborn caused by trauma of delivery or other factors; they are not effective antagonists against drugs other than opioid narcotics. There is an overwhelming body of evidence showing that all known narcotics, even in reasonable therapeutic doses (*e.g.,* 10 mg of morphine, 100 mg of meperidine), produce a significant increase in the incidence of neonatal depression compared to deliveries in which no general anesthetic or narcotic is used. This increased depression is not great; however, even if the use of narcotic antagonists results in only a slight decrease in the incidence of such respiratory depression, their routine use would still appear justified whenever narcotics are administered during labor (*see* review by Eddy *et al.,* 1957). Antagonists with agonistic actions, such as nalorphine or levallorphan, should be used only when naloxone is unavailable.

Analgesia. Pure opioid antagonists are of no value as analgesics and, because of their unpleasant side effects, agonists of the nalorphine type have not been widely used. Partial agonists of the morphine type, such as propiram, may be used in the near future. Pentazocine is discussed separately, below.

It should be emphasized that the risk of dependence is not a major limiting factor in the use of opioid analgesics for the relief of pain in acute situations. Thus, the major advantage of analgesics with low abuse liability is limited to conditions where analgesics must be given chronically or to persons whose personalities suggest a predisposition to develop psychological dependence.

PENTAZOCINE

Pentazocine is one of the many compounds synthesized as part of a deliberate effort to develop an effective analgesic with little or no abuse potential. A benzomorphan derivative, pentazocine has both agonistic actions and weak opioid antagonistic activity. It is too weak an antagonist to be classed with nalorphine, and it is also inappropriate to group it with morphine and the other opioids. The pharma-

cology of pentazocine has been reviewed by Brogden and associates (1973).

Chemistry. Pentazocine, a white powder soluble in acidic aqueous solutions, has the following structural formula:

Pentazocine

The analgesic and respiratory depressant activity of the racemate is due mainly to the *l* isomer.

Pharmacological Actions. Like most opioids, pentazocine exerts its major effects on the CNS and smooth muscle. The pattern of *CNS effects* is generally similar to that of the opioids, including analgesia, sedation, and respiratory depression. A dose of approximately 20 mg of the racemate or 13 mg of the *l* isomer produces the same degree of respiratory depression as does a 10-mg dose of morphine (*see* Bellville and Forrest, 1968). Increasing the dose of pentazocine beyond 30 mg does not ordinarily produce proportionate increases in respiratory depression (Engineer and Jennett, 1972). However, at doses of 60 to 90 mg, nalorphine-like dysphoric and psychotomimetic effects may occur that can be antagonized by naloxone but not by nalorphine.

The effects of pentazocine on the *gastrointestinal tract* are qualitatively similar to those of the opioids. Relatively small intramuscular doses (15 mg) significantly decrease gastric emptying time; higher doses (30 to 45 mg) increase the transit time through the intestinal tract (Danhof, 1967), but produce less elevation of biliary pressure than equianalgesic doses of morphine (Economou and Ward-McQuaid, 1971).

The *cardiovascular responses* to pentazocine differ somewhat from those seen with the opioids, in that high doses cause an increase in blood pressure and heart rate. In normal subjects, pentazocine causes a decrease in effective renal plasma flow but no decrease in glomerular filtration rate (Sigman and Elwood, 1967). In patients with coronary artery disease, pentazocine (intravenously) elevates mean aortic pressure, left ventricular end-diastolic pressure, and mean pulmonary artery pressure, and causes an increase in cardiac work (Alderman *et al.,* 1972). Pentazocine produces a rise in plasma epinephrine and norepinephrine, and this may account for its effects on blood pressure (Tammisto *et al.,* 1971).

The effects of pentazocine on *uterine contractility* do not appear to differ from those of meperidine.

Pentazocine also has weak narcotic antagonistic activity (approximately one fiftieth as potent as nalorphine). It does not antagonize the respiratory depression produced by morphine; however, when given to patients who have been receiving opioids on a regular basis, it may precipitate opioid withdrawal symptoms (Beaver *et al.*, 1966). In patients tolerant to opioids, pentazocine reduces the analgesia produced by morphine, even when clear-cut withdrawal symptoms are not produced.

Absorption, Fate, and Excretion. Pentazocine is well absorbed from the gastrointestinal tract and from subcutaneous and intramuscular sites. Plasma levels coincide closely with the onset, duration, and intensity of analgesia; peak concentrations occur 15 minutes to 1 hour after intramuscular administration and 1 to 3 hours after oral administration. Plasma half-life after intramuscular administration is about 2 hours; plasma levels are still elevated at 5 hours after oral administration (Berkowitz *et al.*, 1969).

Although some free pentazocine is excreted in the urine, the action of the drug is terminated largely by biotransformation in the liver; the metabolites, products of the oxidation of the terminal methyl groups and glucuronide conjugates, are excreted by the kidney, and approximately 60% of the total dose is eliminated within the first 24 hours. There is considerable variability between individuals in terms of rate of pentazocine metabolism, and this may account for the variability of analgesic response (*see* Brogden *et al.*, 1973). Pentazocine passes the placental barrier but to a lesser extent than does meperidine (Beckett and Taylor, 1967).

Preparations, Routes of Administration, and Dosage. *Pentazocine Lactate Injection*, N.F. (FORTRAL, TALWIN), is available in 1-, 1.5-, and 2-ml ampuls and 10-ml multiple-dose vials, each milliliter containing an amount equivalent to 30 mg of the base. *Pentazocine Hydrochloride Tablets*, N.F., for oral use contain 50 mg of the base. Pentazocine is somewhat irritating when administered subcutaneously or intramuscularly. In terms of analgesic effect, a 30- to 50-mg dose given parenterally is approximately equivalent to 10 mg of morphine. A dose of about 50 mg of oral pentazocine results in analgesia equivalent to that produced by 60 mg of codeine. In terms of peak effect, pentazocine is approximately one fourth as potent orally as parenterally; in terms of total analgesic effect, one third as potent. (*See* Beaver *et al.*, 1966, 1968; Kantor *et al.*, 1966; Morrison *et al.*, 1971.)

Side Effects, Toxicity, and Precautions. Side effects from pentazocine differ somewhat from those of opioids. The most commonly reported effect is sedation, followed by sweating, and dizziness or light-headedness; nausea also occurs, but vomiting is less common than with morphine. Nalorphine-like psychotomimetic effects such as anxiety, nightmares, weird thoughts, and hallucinations have been reported. These are not common with doses in the therapeutic range (*see* Paddock *et al.*, 1969) but are seen with increasing frequency with doses above 60 mg. The clinical picture of overdosage has not been well defined. High doses produce marked respiratory depression associated with increased blood pressure and tachycardia. The respiratory depression is antagonized by naloxone but not by nalorphine.

Patients who have been receiving opioids on a regular basis may experience withdrawal symptoms when given pentazocine. After an opioid-free interval of 1 to 2 days, it is usually possible to administer pentazocine without producing such withdrawal effects.

Tolerance, Physical Dependence, and Abuse Potential. With frequent and repeated use, some tolerance develops to the analgesic and subjective effects of pentazocine; however, it is not clear if the rate of development of this tolerance is comparable to that seen with narcotic analgesics or is the same for all effects of the drug. When given intravenously or subcutaneously to postaddicts, pentazocine (40 mg) produces essentially morphine-like effects; when the dose is increased to 60 mg, the effects begin to resemble the nervousness and loss of energy produced by nalorphine. In contrast to morphine and other opioids, pentazocine does not prevent or ameliorate the morphine withdrawal syndrome when substituted in subjects physically dependent on morphine. Instead, when high doses of pentazocine are given to such subjects, its antagonistic actions, although weak, precipitate withdrawal symptoms.

Postaddicts given high doses spaced closely enough to produce continuous action on the nervous system (*e.g.*, 60 to 90 mg every 4 hours) consistently develop physical dependence that can be demonstrated by abrupt withdrawal or precipitated by naloxone but not by nalorphine. The withdrawal syndrome after chronic doses of more than 500 mg per day is similar in some respects to that seen after withdrawal of nalorphine, but it also has some of the characteristics of opioid withdrawal and, although milder, may be associated with drug-seeking behavior; that is, subjects request additional medicine to alleviate the withdrawal syndrome (Jasinski *et al.*, 1970).

In the original evaluation of the abuse potential of pentazocine, most postaddicts who were offered the opportunity to continue taking the drug elected not to do so, and few subjects in the chronic administration studies reached sufficiently high dosage to exhibit withdrawal phenomena upon abrupt discontinuation (Fraser and Rosenberg, 1964). Pentazocine was not considered to have a significant abuse potential, and it was released for general use subject to neither narcotic laws nor dangerous drug laws. Many physicians believed that the drug had no abuse potential at all and, therefore, were less than cautious in prescribing it, in permitting unlimited refilling of prescriptions, and in allowing its self-administration by ambulatory patients. Subsequently, cases of compulsive self-administration primarily of *parenteral* pentazocine were reported. Many, but not all, of these individuals previously had been dependent on opioids; most would have preferred opioids if the latter had been legal and equally available. The withdrawal symptoms seen in many of these cases included abdominal cramps, anxiety, chills, elevated temperature, vomiting, sweating, lacrimation, and drug-seeking behavior.

As the abuse potential of parenteral pentazocine became more widely appreciated, more supervision was exercised by physicians and pharmacists. The availability of the oral preparation reduced the tendency to prescribe the parenteral form when the oral form was more appropriate, and the oral preparation seemed to pose less risk for abuse.

In spite of its easy availability, the drug has not been widely abused by heroin addicts. Since it does not substitute for opioids in sustaining opioid physical dependence, and since in most subjects increases in dose do not produce a progressively intense euphoria, pentazocine is considered to have an abuse potential that is probably lower than that of codeine or propoxyphene. In spite of the reported cases of pentazocine abuse, experience over the last few years still supports this general assessment; but clearly pentazocine should be used with prudence (*see* Lewis, 1973). When it is necessary to relieve pentazocine withdrawal symptoms, the predominant opinion is that this should be done with gradual reduction of pentazocine itself, rather than by substitution of low doses of methadone.

Therapeutic Uses. Pentazocine is used primarily as an analgesic. Because it may be employed in situations where there is chronic severe pain or where the risk of drug dependence is higher than average (*e.g.,* individuals with past histories of alcoholism or excessive self-administration of drugs), it is likely that cases of dependence will continue to develop. Because abuse patterns appear to be less likely to develop with oral administration, this route should be used whenever possible. The problem will remain one in which the physician must choose among a number of unattractive alternatives—inadequate relief of pain, risk of dependence on pentazocine, or risk of dependence on an opioid of higher abuse potential. Pentazocine may have advantages when it is important to minimize the risk of compulsive drug use.

NONNARCOTIC ANTITUSSIVES

Cough is a useful physiological mechanism serving to clear the respiratory passages of foreign material and excess secretions. It should not be suppressed indiscriminately. There are, however, many situations in which cough does not serve any useful purpose but may, instead, only annoy the patient or prevent rest and sleep. In such situations the physician should use a drug that will reduce the frequency or intensity of the coughing. The cough reflex is complex, involving the central and peripheral nervous systems as well as the smooth muscle of the bronchial tree. It has been suggested that irritation of the bronchial mucosa does not lead directly to stimulation of cough receptors (which probably represent a specialized type of stretch receptor), but first causes bronchoconstriction, which, in turn, stimulates cough receptors located in tracheobronchial pas-

sages (*see* Salem and Aviado, 1970). The afferent supply of these receptors is by way of the vagus nerve, and central components of the reflex probably involve several mechanisms or centers that are distinct from the mechanisms involved in the regulation of respiration.

The drugs that can affect this complex mechanism directly or indirectly are quite diverse. For example, drugs that cause bronchodilation could alter the initiation of coughing without having any significant central effects; other drugs might act primarily on the central or the peripheral nervous system components of the cough reflex. The literature on antitussives has been exhaustively reviewed by Salem and Aviado (1970). This section describes a few of the many drugs that have been in clinical use and that are believed to act on the nervous system in modifying cough.

A number of drugs are known to reduce cough as a result of their central actions, although the exact mechanisms are still not entirely clear. Included among them are the opioid analgesics discussed above as well as a number of nonnarcotic agents. In selecting a specific agent for a particular patient, *the advantages of a low abuse potential per se should not be overvalued.* It is true that narcotics addicts who cannot obtain their drug of choice, and occasionally adolescents seeking new experiences, often turn to cough preparations containing opioids or to paregoric; however, despite the extensive use and ready availability of such preparations, the number of persons dependent on them is exceedingly small. Nonnarcotic antitussives having no significant abuse liability would seem to be most advantageous in treating *chronic cough* or in treating individuals who seem *psychologically predisposed* to drug dependence; nevertheless, in the overwhelming majority of situations requiring a cough suppressant, abuse liability need not be a major consideration.

Much more significant considerations are the *antitussive efficacy against pathological cough* and the *incidence of side effects.* Most of the nonnarcotic agents now offered as antitussives are effective against cough induced by a variety of experimental technics. Some of these technics are able to distinguish 30 mg of codeine from a placebo, but their validity for predicting clinical efficacy is still open to question. With the exception of dextromethorphan, described below, well-controlled clinical studies demonstrating the effectiveness of many of the marketed non-narcotic antitussives against pathological cough are few in number. Admittedly, clinical assessments are difficult since the subjective ratings of relief by patients do not correlate with objective measures (tape recordings) of the frequency of cough (Woolf and Rosenberg, 1964; Sevelius *et al.*, 1971).

Dextromethorphan. *Dextromethorphan* (*d*-3-methoxy-N-methylmorphinan) is the *d* isomer of the codeine analog of levorphanol; however, unlike the *l* isomer, it has no analgesic or addictive properties. The drug acts centrally to elevate the threshold for coughing. Its effectiveness in patients with pathological cough has been demonstrated in controlled studies, where it was found to be about the equal of codeine. Unlike codeine, it rarely produces drowsiness or gastrointestinal disturbances. In therapeutic dosage the drug does not inhibit ciliary activity. Its toxicity is quite low, but extremely high doses may produce CNS depression.

Dextromethorphan Hydrobromide, N.F., is available as a syrup containing 15 mg/5 ml. The average adult dose is 15 to 30 mg, three to four times daily; however, as is the case with codeine, higher doses are often required. *Terpin Hydrate and Dextromethorphan Hydrobromide Elixir*, N.F., containing 10 mg/5 ml, is also available. The drug is generally marketed for "over-the-counter" sale in syrups and lozenges, or in combinations with an antihistamine for prescription orders under multiple brand names in many countries throughout the world.

Levopropoxyphene Napsylate, N.F. (NOVRAD), in doses of 50 to 100 mg orally appears to suppress cough to about the same degree as does 30 mg of dextromethorphan. Unlike dextropropoxyphene, levopropoxyphene has little or no analgesic activity.

Noscapine is a naturally occurring opium alkaloid of the benzylisoquinoline group; except for its antitussive effect, it has no significant actions on the CNS in doses within the therapeutic range. In dogs, the drug is a potent releaser of histamine, and large doses cause bronchoconstriction and transient hypotension. Toxic doses produce convulsions in animals. The average adult dose is 15 to 30 mg, three or four times daily, but single doses of 60 mg have been used. It is the primary ingredient in several proprietary mixtures.

Other drugs that have been used as centrally acting antitussives include *pipazethate, carbetapentane, caramiphen,* and *oxolamine*. Each is a member of a distinct pharmacological class unrelated to the opioids; in general their toxicity is low, but controlled clinical studies are still insufficient to determine whether they merit consideration as alternatives to more thoroughly studied agents.

Benzonatate, N.F. (TESSALON), is a long-chain polyglycol derivative chemically related to procaine and believed to exert its antitussive action on stretch or cough receptors in the lung (*see* Bucher, 1958). It has been administered by all routes; the oral dose is about 100 mg, but higher doses have been used.

Alderman, E. L.; Barry, W. H.; Graham, A. F.; and Harrison, D. C. Hemodynamic effects of morphine and pentazocine differ in cardiac patients. *New Engl. J. Med.*, **1972**, *287*, 623–627.

Arens, J. F.; Benbow, B. P.; Ochsner, J. L.; and Theard, R. Morphine anesthesia for aortocoronary bypass procedures. *Anesth. Analg. curr. Res.*, **1972**, *51*, 901–913.

Beaver, W. T.; Wallenstein, S. L.; Houde, R. W.; and Rogers, A. A comparison of the analgesic effects of pentazocine and morphine in patients with cancer. *Clin. Pharmac. Ther.*, **1966**, *7*, 740–751.

————. A clinical comparison of the analgesic effects of methadone and morphine administered intramuscularly, and of orally and parenterally administered methadone. *Ibid.*, **1967**, *8*, 415–426.

————. A clinical comparison of the effects of oral and intramuscular administration of analgesics: pentazocine and phenazocine. *Ibid.*, **1968**, *9*, 582–597.

Beckett, A. H., and Taylor, J. F. Blood concentrations of pethidine and pentazocine in mother and infant at time of birth. *J. Pharm. Pharmac.*, **1967**, *19*, Suppl., 50s–52s.

Bellville, J. W., and Forrest, W. H., Jr. Respiratory and subjective effects of *d*- and *l*-pentazocine. *Clin. Pharmac. Ther.*, **1968**, *9*, 142–151.

Bellville, J. W.; Forrest, W. H., Jr.; Miller, E.; and Brown, B. W. Influence of age on pain relief from analgesics. *J. Am. med. Ass.*, **1971**, *217*, 1835–1841.

Bellville, J. W., and Seed, J. C. A comparison of the respiratory depressant effects of dextropropoxyphene and codeine in man. *Clin. Pharmac. Ther.*, **1968**, *9*, 428–434.

Berkowitz, B. A.; Asling, J. H.; Shnider, S. M.; and Way, E. L. Relationship of pentazocine plasma levels to pharmacological activity in man. *Clin. Pharmac. Ther.*, **1969**, *10*, 320–328.

Bogoch, A.; Roth, J. L. A.; and Bockus, H. L. The effects of morphine on serum amylase and lipase. *Gastroenterology*, **1954**, *26*, 697–708.

Borison, H. L.; Fishburn, B. R.; Bhide, N. K.; and McCarthy, L. E. Morphine-induced hyperglycemia in the cat. *J. Pharmac. exp. Ther.*, **1962**, *138*, 229–235.

Burks, T. F. Mediation by 5-hydroxytryptamine of morphine stimulant actions in dog intestine. *J. Pharmac. exp. Ther.*, **1973**, *185*, 530–539.

Buxbaum, D. M.; Yarbrough, G. G.; and Carter, M. E. Biogenic amines and narcotic effects. I. Modification of morphine-induced analgesia and motor activity after alteration of cerebral amine levels. *J. Pharmac. exp. Ther.*, **1973**, *185*, 317–327.

Calcutt, C. R.; Handley, S. L.; Sparkes, C. G.; and Spencer, P. S. J. Roles of noradrenaline and 5-hydroxytryptamine in the antinociceptive effects of morphine. In, *Agonist and Antagonist Actions of Narcotic Analgesic Drugs.* (Kosterlitz, H. W.; Collier, H. O. J.; and Villarreal, J. E.; eds.) University Park Press, Baltimore, **1973**, pp. 176–191.

Campbell, C.; Phillips, O. C.; and Frazier, T. M. Analgesia during labor: a comparison of pentobarbital, meperidine, and morphine. *Obstet. Gynec., N.Y.,* **1961**, *17*, 714–718.

Chakravarty, N. K.; Matallana, A.; Jensen, R.; and Borison, H. L. Central effects of antitussive drugs on cough and respiration. *J. Pharmac. exp. Ther.*, **1956**, *117*, 127–135.

Challenor, Y. B.; Richter, R. W.; Brunn, B.; and Pearson, J. Nontraumatic plexitis and heroin addiction. *J. Am. med. Ass.,* **1973,** *225,* 958–961.

Chapman, W. P.; Rowlands, E. N.; and Jones, C. M. Multiple-balloon kymographic recording of the comparative action of DEMEROL, morphine and placebos on the motility of the upper small intestine in man. *New Engl. J. Med.,* **1950,** *243,* 171–177.

Cicero, T. J.; Meyer, E. R.; and Smithloff, B. R. Alpha adrenergic blocking agents: antinociceptive activity and enhancement of morphine-induced analgesia. *J. Pharmac. exp. Ther.,* **1974,** *189,* 72–82.

Danhof, I. E. Pentazocine effects on gastrointestinal motor functions in man. *Am. J. Gastroent., N.Y.,* **1967,** *48,* 295–310.

Daniel, E. E.; Sutherland, W. H.; Bogoch, A.; (and Kent, J. T. [tech. asst.]). Effects of morphine and other drugs on the motility of the terminal ileum. *Gastroenterology,* **1959,** *36,* 510–523.

Deneau, G. A., and Nakai, K. The toxicity of meperidine in the monkey as influenced by its rate of absorption. In, *Minutes of 23rd Meeting of Committee on Drug Addiction and Narcotics,* Appen. 6. NAS–NRC, Washington, D. C., **1961.**

Dole, V. P., and Kreek, M. J. Methadone plasma level: sustained by a reservoir of drug in tissue. *Proc. natn. Acad. Sci. U.S.A.,* **1973,** *70,* 10.

Domino, E. F., and Wilson, A. Effects of narcotic analgesic agonists and antagonists on rat brain acetylcholine. *J. Pharmac. exp. Ther.,* **1973,** *184,* 18–32.

Done, A. K. Pharmacologic principles in the treatment of poisoning. *Pharmac. Physcns,* **1969,** *3,* 1–10.

Downes, J. J.; Kemp, R. A.; and Lambertsen, C. J. The magnitude and duration of respiratory depression due to fentanyl and meperidine in man. *J. Pharmac. exp. Ther.,* **1967,** *158,* 416–420.

Eckenhoff, J. E., and Helrich, M. Study of narcotics and sedatives for use in preanesthetic medication. *J. Am. med. Ass.,* **1958,** *167,* 415–422.

Economou, G., and Ward-McQuaid, J. N. A cross-over comparison of the effect of morphine, pethidine, pentazocine, and phenazocine on biliary pressure. *Gut,* **1971,** *12,* 218–221.

Engineer, S., and Jennett, S. Respiratory depression following single and repeated doses of pentazocine and pethidine. *Br. J. Anaesth.,* **1972,** *44,* 795–801.

Feldberg, W., and Shaligram, S. V. The hyperglycemic effect of morphine. *Br. J. Pharmac.,* **1972,** *46,* 602–618.

Flórez, J.; McCarthy, L. E.; and Borison, H. L. A comparative study in the cat of the respiratory effects of morphine injected intravenously and into the cerebrospinal fluid. *J. Pharmac. exp. Ther.,* **1968,** *163,* 448–455.

Fraser, H. F., and Isbell, H. Actions and addiction liabilities of alpha-acetylmethadols in man. *J. Pharmac. exp. Ther.,* **1952,** *105,* 458–465.

——. Human pharmacology and addiction liability of *dl*- and *d*-propoxyphene. *Bull. Narcot.,* **1960,** *12,* 9–14.

——. Human pharmacology and addictiveness of ethyl 1-(3-cyano-3,3-phenylpropyl)-4-phenyl-4-piperidine carboxylate hydrochloride (R-1132, diphenoxylate). *Ibid.,* **1961,** *13,* 29–43.

Fraser, H. F., and Rosenberg, D. E. Studies on the human addiction liability of 2′-hydroxy-5,9-dimethyl-2-(3,3-dimethyl-allyl)6,7-benzomorphan (WIN 20, 228): a weak narcotic antagonist. *J. Pharmac. exp. Ther.,* **1964,** *143,* 149–156.

Garrett, J. M.; Sauer, W. G.; and Moertel, C. G. Colonic motility in ulcerative colitis after opiate administration. *Gastroenterology,* **1967,** *53,* 93–100.

Goldstein, A. The search for the opiate receptor. In, *Pharmacology and the Future of Man: Proceedings of the Fifth International Congress on Pharmacology,* Vol. I. (Acheson, G. H., and Cochin, J., eds.) S. Karger, Basel, **1973,** pp. 140–150.

——. Interactions of narcotic antagonists with receptor sites. In, *Narcotic Antagonists.* (Braude, M. C.; Harris, L. S.; May, E. L.; Smith, J. P.; and Villarreal, J. E.; eds.) Raven Press, New York, **1974,** pp. 471–481.

Goldstein, A.; Lowney, L. I.; and Pal, B. K. Stereospecific and non-specific interactions of the morphine congener levorphanol in subcellular fractions of mouse brain. *Proc. natn. Acad. Sci. U.S.A.,* **1971,** *68,* 1742–1747.

Gorodetsky, C. W., and Martin, W. R. A comparison of fentanyl, droperidol and morphine. *Clin. Pharmac. Ther.,* **1965,** *6,* 731–739.

Gutner, L. B.; Gould, W. J.; and Batterman, R. C. The effects of potent analgesics upon vestibular function. *J. clin. Invest.,* **1952,** *31,* 259–266.

Haertzen, C. A. Development of scales based on patterns of drug effects, using the Addiction Research Center Inventory (ARCI). *Psychol. Rep.,* **1966,** *18,* 163–194.

Herz, A.; Albus, K.; Metyš, J.; Schubert, P.; and Teschenmacher, H. J. On the central sites for the antinociceptive action of morphine and fentanyl. *Neuropharmacology,* **1970,** *9,* 539–551.

Hill, H. E.; Haertzen, C. A.; Wolbach, A. B., Jr.; and Miner, E. J. The Addiction Research Center Inventory: standardization of scales which evaluate subjective effects of morphine, amphetamine, pentobarbital, alcohol, LSD-25, pyrahexyl and chlorpromazine. *Psychopharmacologia,* **1963,** *4,* 167–205.

Hiller, J. M.; Pearson, J.; and Simon, E. J. Distribution of stereospecific binding of the potent narcotic analgesic etorphine in the human brain: predominance in the limbic system. *Res. Commun. chem. Path. Pharmac.,* **1973,** *6,* 1052–1062.

Hopton, D. S., and Torrance, H. B. Action of various new analgesic drugs on the human common bile duct. *Gut,* **1967,** *8,* 296–300.

Houde, R. W.; Wallenstein, S. L.; and Beaver, W. T. Clinical measurement of pain. In, *Analgetics.* (deStevens, G., ed.) Academic Press, Inc., New York, **1965,** pp. 75–122.

Inturrisi, C. E., and Verebely, K. The levels of methadone in the plasma in methadone maintenance. *Clin. Pharmac. Ther.,* **1972a,** *13,* 633–637.

——. Disposition of methadone in man after single oral dose. *Ibid.,* **1972b,** *13,* 923–930.

Isbell, H.; Wikler, A.; Eisenman, A. J.; Daingerfield, M.; and Frank, K. Liability of addiction to 6-dimethylamino-4-4-diphenyl-3-heptanone (METHADON, "AMIDONE," or "10820") in man. *Archs intern. Med.,* **1948,** *82,* 362–392.

Jacquet, Y. F., and Lajtha, A. Morphine action at central nervous system sites in the rat; analgesia or hyperalgesia depending on site and dose. *Science, Wash.,* **1973,** *182,* 490–492.

Jaffe, J. H.; Senay, E. C.; Schuster, C. R.; Renault, P. R.; Smith, B.; and DiMenza, S. Methadyl acetate vs methadone. A double-blind study in heroin users. *J. Am. med. Ass.,* **1972,** *222,* 437–442.

Jasinski, D. R. Effects in man of partial morphine agonists. In, *Agonist and Antagonist Actions of Narcotic Analgesic Drugs.* (Kosterlitz, H. W.; Collier, H. O. J.; and Villarreal, J. E.; eds.) University Park Press, Baltimore, **1973,** pp. 94–103.

Jasinski, D. R.; Martin, W. R.; and Hoeldtke, R. D. Effects of short- and long-term administration of pentazocine in man. *Clin. Pharmac. Ther.,* **1970,** *11,* 385–403.

——. Studies of the dependence-producing properties of GPA-1657, profadol, and propiram in man. *Ibid.,* **1971,** *12,* 613–649.

Kantor, T. G.; Sunshine, A.; Laska, E.; Meisner, M.; and Hopper, M. Oral analgesic studies: pentazocine hydrochloride, codeine, aspirin, and placebo and their influence on response to placebo. *Clin. Pharmac. Ther.,* **1966,** *7,* 447–454.

Kay, D. C.; Eisenstein, R. B.; and Jasinski, D. R. Morphine effects on human REM state, waking state, and NREM sleep. *Psychopharmacologia,* **1969,** *14,* 404–416.

Keats, A. S.; Telford, J.; Kurosu, Y.; and Papadopoulos, C. N. Morphine antagonists as analgesics in man. In, *Minutes of 21st Meeting of Committee on Drug Addiction and Narcotics,* Appen. 2. NAS–NRC, Washington, D. C., **1960.**

Kuhar, M. J.; Pert, C. B.; and Snyder, S. H. Regional distribution of opiate receptor binding in human and monkey brain. *Nature, Lond.,* **1973,** *245,* 447–450.

Lambertsen, C. J.; Wendel, H.; and Longenhagen, J. B. The separate and combined respiratory effects of chlorpromazine and meperidine in normal men controlled at 46 mm Hg alveolar pCO_2. *J. Pharmac. exp. Ther.,* **1961,** *131,* 381–393.

Levine, S. B., and Grimes, E. T. Pulmonary edema and heroin overdose in Vietnam. *Archs Path.,* **1973,** *95,* 330–332.

Lewis, J. R. Use and misuse of pentazocine. *J. Am. med. Ass.,* **1973,** *225,* 1530–1531.

Lowney, L. I.; Schulz, K.; Lowery, P. J.; and Goldstein, A. Partial purification of an opiate receptor from mouse brain. *Science, Wash.,* **1974,** *183,* 749–753.

McKenzie, J. S. The influence of morphine and pethidine on somatic evoked responses in the hippocampal formation of the cat. *Electroenceph. clin. Neurophysiol.,* **1964,** *17,* 428–431.

McMahon, R. E.; Ridolfo, A. S.; Culp, H. W.; Wolen, R. L.; and Marshall, F. J. The fate of radiocarbon-labeled propoxyphene in rat, dog, and human. *Toxic. appl. Pharmac.,* **1971,** *19,* 427–444.

Marks, R. M., and Sachar, E. J. Undertreatment of medical inpatients with narcotic analgesics. *Ann. intern. Med.,* **1973,** *78,* 173–181.

Martin, W. R.; Jasinski, D. R.; Haertzen, C. A.; Kay, D. C.; Jones, B. E.; Mansky, P. A.; and Carpenter, R. W. Methadone—a reevaluation. *Archs gen. Psychiat.,* **1973a,** *28,* 286–295.

Martin, W. R.; Jasinski, D. R.; and Mansky, P. A. Naltrexone, an antagonist for the treatment of heroin dependence. *Archs gen. Psychiat.,* **1973b,** *28,* 784–791.

Mayer, D. J.; Wolfle, T. L.; Akil, H.; Carder, B.; and Liebeskind, J. C. Analgesia from electrical stimulation in the brainstem of the rat. *Science, Wash.,* **1971,** *174,* 1351–1354.

Melzack, R., and Wall, P. D. Pain mechanisms: a new theory. *Science, Wash.,* **1965,** *150,* 971–979.

Misra, A. L., and Mulé, S. J. Persistence of methadone-^{3}H and metabolite in rat brain after a single injection and its implications on pharmacological tolerance. *Nature, Lond.,* **1972,** *238,* 155–156.

Monnier, M.; Nosal, G.; and Radouco-Thomas, C. Central mechanisms of pain analysed by the action of analgesics. In, *The Assessment of Pain in Man and Animals.* (Keele, C. A., and Smith, R., eds.) Universities Federation for Animal Welfare, London, **1962.**

Moore, J., and Dundee, J. W. Alterations in response to somatic pain associated with anaesthesia. VII. The effect of nine phenothiazine derivatives. *Br. J. Anaesth.,* **1961,** *33,* 422–431.

Morrison, J. D.; Loan, W. B.; and Dundee, J. W. Controlled comparison of the efficacy of fourteen preparations for the relief of postoperative pain. *Br. med. J.,* **1971,** *3,* 287–290.

Nadasdi, M., and Zsotér, T. T. The effect of meperidine on the peripheral circulation. *Clin. Pharmac. Ther.,* **1969,** *10,* 239–243.

Nutt, J. G., and Jasinski, D. R. Methadone-naloxone mixtures for use in methadone maintenance programs. I. An evaluation in man of their pharmacological feasibility. II. Demonstration of acute physical dependence. *Clin. Pharmac. Ther.,* **1974,** *15,* 156–166.

Oldendorf, W. H.; Hyman, S.; Braun, L.; and Oldendorf, S. Z. Blood-brain barrier penetration of morphine, co-

deine, heroin, and methadone after carotid injection. *Science, Wash.,* **1972,** *178,* 984–986.

Olsen, G. D. Methadone binding to human plasma proteins. *Clin. Pharmac. Ther.,* **1973,** *14,* 338–343.

Paddock, R.; Beer, E. G.; Bellville, J. W.; Ciliberti, B. J.; Forrest, W. H., Jr.; and Miller, E. V. Analgesic and side effects of pentazocine and morphine in a large population of postoperative patients. *Clin. Pharmac. Ther.,* **1969,** *10,* 355–365.

Parbrook, G. D. Techniques of inhalational analgesia in the postoperative period. *Br. J. Anaesth.,* **1967,** *39,* 730–735.

Pentiah, P.; Reilly, F.; and Borison, H. L. Interactions of morphine sulfate and sodium salicylate on respiration in cats. *J. Pharmac. exp. Ther.,* **1966,** *154,* 110–118.

Pert, C. B., and Snyder, S. H. Opiate receptor: its demonstration in nervous tissue. *Science, Wash.,* **1973,** *179,* 1011–1014.

———. Opiate receptor binding of agonists and antagonists affected differentially by sodium. *Molec. Pharmac.,* **1974,** *10,* 868–879.

Reynolds, D. V. Surgery in the rat during electrical analgesia induced by focal brain stimulation. *Science, Wash.,* **1969,** *164,* 444–445.

Sevelius, H.; McCoy, J. F.; and Colmore, J. P. Dose response to codeine in patients with chronic cough. *Clin. Pharmac. Ther.,* **1971,** *12,* 449–455.

Shealy, C. N.; Mortimer, J. T.; and Hagfors, N. R. Dorsal column electroanalgesia. *J. Neurosurg.,* **1970,** *32,* 560–564.

Shee, J. C. Dangerous potentiation of pethidine by iproniazid and its treatment. *Br. med. J.,* **1960,** *2,* 507–509.

Sigman, E. M., and Elwood, C. M. Effect of intramuscular pentazocine on renal hemodynamics in normal human subjects. *Anesth. Analg. curr. Res.,* **1967,** *46,* 57–60.

Simon, E. J.; Hiller, J. M.; and Edelman, I. Stereospecific binding of the potent narcotic analgesic ^{3}H etorphine to rat-brain homogenate. *Proc. natn. Acad. Sci. U.S.A.,* **1973,** *70,* 1947–1949.

Smith, C. B., and Sheldon, M. I. Effects of narcotic analgesic drugs on brain noradrenergic mechanisms. In, *Agonist and Antagonist Actions of Narcotic Analgesic Drugs.* (Kosterlitz, H. W.; Collier, H. O. J.; and Villarreal, J. E.; eds.) University Park Press, Baltimore, **1973,** pp. 164–175.

Smith, G. M.; Lowenstein, E.; Hubbard, J. H.; and Beecher, H. K. Experimental pain produced by the submaximum effort tourniquet technique: further evidence of validity. *J. Pharmac. exp. Ther.,* **1968,** *163,* 468–474.

Smith, G. M.; Semke, C. W.; and Beecher, H. K. Objective evidence of mental effects of heroin, morphine and placebo in normal subjects. *J. Pharmac. exp. Ther.,* **1962,** *136,* 53–58.

Sokoll, M. D.; Hoyt, J. L.; and Gergis, S. D. Studies in muscle rigidity, nitrous oxide, and narcotic analgesic agents. *Anesth. Analg. curr. Res.,* **1972,** *51,* 16–20.

Tammisto, T.; Jaattela, A.; Nikki, P.; and Takki, S. Effect of pentazocine and pethidine on plasma catecholamine levels. *Ann. clin. Res.,* **1971,** *3,* 22–29.

Tennant, F. S., Jr. Complications of propoxyphene abuse. *Archs intern. Med.,* **1973,** *132,* 191–194.

Thomas, M.; Malmcrona, R.; Fillmore, S.; and Shillingford, J. Haemodynamic effects of morphine in patients with acute myocardial infarction. *Br. Heart J.,* **1965,** *27,* 863–875.

Vasko, J. S.; Henney, R. P.; Oldham, H. N.; Brawley, R. K.; and Morrow, A. G. Mechanisms of action of morphine in the treatment of experimental pulmonary edema. *Am. J. Cardiol.,* **1966,** *18,* 876–883.

Vaughan Williams, E. M., and Streeten, D. H. P. The action of morphine, pethidine, and AMIDONE upon the intestinal motility of conscious dogs. *Br. J. Pharmac. Chemother.,* **1950,** *5,* 584–603.

Way, W. L.; Costley, E. C.; and Way, E. L. Respiratory

sensitivity of the newborn infant to meperidine and morphine. *Clin. Pharmac. Ther.,* **1965,** *6,* 454–461.

Weinberg, S. J., and Sensiba, S. W. Scopolamine-METHADON-DEMEROL treatment of emergency status asthmaticus. *Dis. Chest,* **1956,** *30,* 580–582.

Weinstein, S. H.; Pfeffer, M.; and Schor, J. Metabolism and pharmacokinetics of naloxone. In, *Narcotic Antagonists.* (Braude, M. C.; Harris, L. S.; May, E. L.; Smith, J. P.; and Villarreal, J. E.; eds.) Raven Press, New York, **1974,** pp. 525–535.

Wikler, A., and Altschul, S. Effects of methadone and morphine on the electroencephalogram of the dog. *J. Pharmac. exp. Ther.,* **1950,** *98,* 437–446.

Wolen, R. L.; Gruber, C. M., Jr.; Kiplinger, G. F.; and Scholz, N. E. Concentration of propoxyphene in human plasma following oral, intramuscular, and intravenous administration. *Toxic. appl. Pharmac.,* **1971a,** *19,* 480–492.

———. Concentration of propoxyphene in human plasma following repeated oral doses. *Ibid.,* **1971b,** *19,* 493–497.

Wolff, B. B.; Kantor, T. G.; Jarvik, M. E.; and Laska, E. Response of experimental pain to analgesic drugs. I. Morphine, aspirin and placebo. *Clin. Pharmac. Ther.,* **1966,** *7,* 224–238.

———. Response of experimental pain to analgesic drugs. III. Codeine, aspirin, secobarbital, and placebo. *Ibid.,* **1969,** *10,* 217–228.

Woolf, C. R., and Rosenberg, A. Objective assessment of cough suppressants under clinical conditions using a tape recorder system. *Thorax,* **1964,** *19,* 125–130.

Zaks, A.; Jones, T.; Fink, M.; and Freedman, A. Treatment of opiate dependence with high dose oral naloxone. *J. Am. med. Ass.,* **1971,** *215,* 2108–2110.

Monographs and Reviews

Archer, S.; Albertson, N. F.; and Pierson, A. K. Structure-activity relationships in the opioid antagonists. In, *Agonist and Antagonist Actions of Narcotic Analgesic Drugs.* (Kosterlitz, H. W.; Collier, H. O. J.; and Villarreal, J. E.; eds.) University Park Press, Baltimore, **1973,** pp. 25–29.

Beaver, W. T. Mild analgesics, a review of their clinical pharmacology (Part II). *Am. J. med. Sci.,* **1966,** *251,* 576–599.

Beecher, H. K. *The Measurement of Subjective Responses: Quantitative Effects of Drugs.* Oxford University Press, New York, **1959.**

Braenden, O. J.; Eddy, N. B.; and Halbach, H. Synthetic substances with morphine-like effect. Relationship between chemical structure and analgesic action. *Bull. Wld Hlth Org.,* **1955,** *13,* 937–998.

Braude, M. C.; Harris, L. S.; May, E. L.; Smith, J. P.; and Villarreal, J. E. (eds.). *Narcotic Antagonists.* Raven Press, New York, **1974.**

Brogden, R. N.; Speight, T. M.; and Avery, G. S. Pentazocine: a review of its pharmacological properties, therapeutic efficacy and dependence liability. *Drugs,* **1973,** *5,* 6–91. (181 references.)

Bucher, K. Pathophysiology and pharmacology of cough. *Pharmac. Rev.,* **1958,** *10,* 43–58.

Clouet, D. H. (ed.). *Narcotic Drugs: Biochemical Pharmacology.* Plenum Press, New York, **1971.**

Dole, V. P. Biochemistry of addiction. *A. Rev. Biochem.,* **1970,** *39,* 821–840.

Domino, E. F. Effects of narcotic analgesics on sensory input, activating system and motor output. *Proc. Ass. Res. nerv. ment. Dis.,* **1968,** *46,* 117–149.

Eckenhoff, J. E., and Oech, S. R. The effects of narcotics and antagonists upon respiration and circulation in man. *Clin. Pharmac. Ther.,* **1960,** *1,* 483–524. (262 references.)

Eddy, N. B.; Halbach, H.; and Braenden, O. J. Synthetic substances with morphine-like effect. Clinical experience: potency, side-effects, addiction liability. *Bull. Wld Hlth Org.,* **1957,** *17,* 569–863.

George, R. Hypothalamus: anterior pituitary gland. In, *Narcotic Drugs: Biochemical Pharmacology.* (Clouet, D. H., ed.) Plenum Press, New York, **1971,** pp. 283–299. (98 references.)

Goldstein, A.; Aronow, L.; and Kalman, S. M. *Principles of Drug Action: The Basis of Pharmacology,* 2nd ed. John Wiley & Sons, Inc., New York, **1974.**

Hardy, R. A., Jr., and Howell, M. G. Synthetic analgesics with morphine-like actions. In, *Analgetics.* Vol. 5, *Medicinal Chemistry.* (deStevens, G., ed.) Academic Press, Inc., New York, **1965,** pp. 179–279. (385 references.)

Harris, L. S. Narcotic antagonists: structure-activity relationships. In, *Narcotic Antagonists.* (Braude, M. C.; Harris, L. S.; May, E. L.; Smith, J. P.; and Villarreal, J. E.; eds.) Raven Press, New York, **1974,** pp. 13–20. (51 references.)

Harris, L. S., and Dewey, W. L. Role of cholinergic systems in the central action of narcotic agonists and antagonists. In, *Agonist and Antagonist Actions of Narcotic Analgesic Drugs.* (Kosterlitz, H. W.; Collier, H. O. J.; and Villarreal, J. E.; eds.) University Park Press, Baltimore, **1973,** pp. 198–206.

Harthoorn, A. M. Comparative pharmacological reactions of certain wild and domestic mammals to thebaine derivatives in the M-series of compounds. *Fedn Proc. Fedn Am. Socs exp. Biol.,* **1967,** *26,* 1251–1261.

Hug, C. C., Jr. The metabolic disposition of narcotic analgesic drugs: transport in the central nervous system. In, *Narcotic Drugs: Biochemical Pharmacology.* (Clouet, D. H., ed.) Plenum Press, New York, **1971,** pp. 122–136. (116 references.)

Kosterlitz, H. W.; Collier, H. O. J.; and Villarreal, J. E. (eds.). *Agonist and Antagonist Actions of Narcotic Analgesic Drugs.* University Park Press, Baltimore, **1973.**

Lasagna, L. The clinical evaluation of morphine and its substitutes as analgesics. *Pharmac. Rev.,* **1964,** *16,* 47–83. (160 references.)

Lees, G. M.; Kosterlitz, H. W.; and Waterfield, A. A. Characteristics of morphine-sensitive release of neurotransmitter substances. In, *Agonist and Antagonist Actions of Narcotic Analgesic Drugs.* (Kosterlitz, H. W.; Collier, H. O. J.; and Villarreal, J. E.; eds.) University Park Press, Baltimore, **1973,** pp. 142–152.

Lewin, L. *Phantastica, Narcotic and Stimulating Drugs; Their Use and Abuse.* Berlin, **1924;** English translation, London, **1931;** E. P. Dutton & Co., Inc., New York, **1931.**

Lewis, J. W.; Bentley, K. W.; and Cowan, A. Narcotic analgesics and antagonists. *A. Rev. Pharmac.,* **1971,** *11,* 241–270. (305 references.)

Lim, R. K. S. A revised concept of the mechanism of analgesia and pain. In, *Pain.* (Knighton, R. S., and Cumke, P. R., eds.) Little, Brown & Co., Boston, **1966.** (197 references.)

Martin, W. R. Analgesic and antipyretic drugs: strong analgesics. In, *Physiological Pharmacology.* Vol. 1, *The Nervous System—Part A: Central Nervous System Drugs.* (Root, W. S., and Hofmann, F. G., eds.) Academic Press, Inc., New York, **1963,** pp. 275–312.

———. Opioid antagonists. *Pharmac. Rev.,* **1967,** *19,* 463–521. (373 references.)

May, E. L., and Sargent, L. J. Morphine and its modifications. In, *Analgetics.* Vol. 5, *Medicinal Chemistry.* (deStevens, G., ed.) Academic Press, Inc., New York, **1965,** pp. 123–177.

Merck Sharp & Dohme Research Laboratories. *Codeine and Certain Other Analgesic and Antitussive Agents: A Review.* Merck & Co., Inc., Rahway, N. J., **1970.**

Miller, R. R.; Feingold, A.; and Paxinos, J. Propoxyphene hydrochloride: a critical review. *J. Am. med. Ass.,* **1970,** *213,* 996–1006.

Mulé, S. J. Physiological disposition of narcotic agonists and antagonists. In, *Narcotic Drugs: Biochemical Pharmacology.* (Clouet, D. H., ed.) Plenum Press, New York, **1971,** pp. 99–121. (116 references.)

Murphree, H. B. Clinical pharmacology of potent analgesics. *Clin. Pharmac. Ther.,* **1962,** *3,* 473–504.

Musto, D. F. *The American Disease.* Yale University Press, New Haven, **1973.**

Reynolds, A. K., and Randall, L. O. *Morphine and Allied Drugs.* University of Toronto Press, Toronto, **1957.** (More than 1600 references.)

Salem, H., and Aviado, D. M. (eds.). *Antitussive Agents,* Vols. 1, 2, and 3. *International Encyclopedia of Pharmacology and Therapeutics,* Sect. 27. Pergamon Press, Ltd., Oxford, **1970.**

Sapira, J. D. The narcotic addict as a medical patient. *Am. J. Med.,* **1968,** *45,* 555–588.

Scrafani, J. T., and Clouet, D. H. The metabolic disposition of narcotic analgesic drugs: biotransformations. In, *Narcotic Drugs: Biochemical Pharmacology.* (Clouet, D. H., ed.) Plenum Press, New York, **1971,** pp. 137–158. (138 references.)

Sloan, J. W. The effects of narcotic analgesic drugs on specific systems: corticosteroid hormones. In, *Narcotic Drugs: Biochemical Pharmacology.* (Clouet, D. H., ed.) Plenum Press, New York, **1971,** pp. 262–282. (139 references.)

Soulairac, A.; Cahn, J.; and Charpentier, J. (eds.). *Pain.* Academic Press, Inc., New York, **1968.**

Terry, C. E., and Pellens, M. *The Opium Problem.* Bureau of Social Hygiene, Inc., New York, **1928.**

Way, E. L. Distribution and metabolism of morphine and its surrogates. *Proc. Ass. Res. nerv. ment. Dis.,* **1968,** *46,* 13–31.

Way, E. L., and Adler, T. K. The pharmacologic implications of the fate of morphine and its surrogates. *Pharmac. Rev.,* **1960,** *12,* 383–446.

———. *The Biological Disposition of Morphine and Its Surrogates.* World Health Organization, Geneva, **1962.**

Way, E. L., and Shen, F. H. Effects of narcotic analgesic drugs on specific systems: catecholamines and 5-hydroxy-tryptamine. In, *Narcotic Drugs: Biochemical Pharmacology.* (Clouet, D. H., ed.) Plenum Press, New York, **1971,** pp. 229–253. (134 references.)

Weinstock, M. Sites of action of narcotic analgesic drugs: in peripheral tissues. In, *Narcotic Drugs: Biochemical Pharmacology.* (Clouet, D. H., ed.) Plenum Press, New York, **1971,** pp. 394–407.

Wikler, A. *Mechanisms of Action of Opiates and Opiate Antagonists: A Review of Their Mechanisms of Action in Relation to Clinical Problems.* Public Health Monograph No. 52, U.S. Government Printing Office, Washington, D. C., **1958.** (195 references.)

Wikler, A. (ed.). *The Addictive States.* The Williams & Wilkins Co., Baltimore, **1968.**

Winter, C. A. The physiology and pharmacology of pain and its relief. In, *Analgetics.* Vol. 5, *Medicinal Chemistry.* (deStevens, G., ed.) Academic Press, Inc., New York, **1965,** pp. 10–74. (283 references.)

16 DRUG ADDICTION AND DRUG ABUSE

Jerome H. Jaffe

As far back as recorded history, every society has used drugs producing profound effects on mood, thought, and feeling. Moreover, there were always a few individuals who digressed from custom with respect to the time, the amount, and the situation in which these drugs were to be used. Thus, both the nonmedical use of drugs and the problem of drug abuse are as old as civilization itself.

Problems of Terminology. *Drug abuse* refers to the use, usually by self-administration, of any drug in a manner that deviates from the approved medical or social patterns within a given culture. The term conveys the notion of social disapproval, and it is not necessarily descriptive of any particular pattern of drug use or its potential adverse consequences.

Since this definition is largely a social one, it is not surprising that for any particular drug there is a great variation in what is considered abuse, not only from culture to culture but also from time to time and from one situation to another within the same culture. For example, in Western society, chronic intoxication with alcohol is usually considered drug abuse, yet on certain occasions gross intoxication with alcohol is not. The use of medically prescribed barbiturates to induce sleep is permissible, but the self-administration of the same amount of barbiturates to induce euphoria in a social situation would be abuse. The use of medically prescribed opioid analgesics for the relief of pain or the treatment of gastrointestinal disorders is quite proper; however, the self-administration of the same drugs, in the same dosages, for relief of depression or tension is considered flagrant abuse. Temporal variations are common. For example, little more than a decade ago the use of psychedelic (hallucinogenic, psychotomimetic, psychotogenic) compounds was a practice limited to a few college students and research workers in the United States. It was not illegal, and there was no social condemnation of the users. By the mid-1960s, experimentation with psychedelic drugs was widespread among both college and high school students; the use of these drugs had become equivalent to abuse; and the possession, manufacture, or sale of such drugs had been made a criminal offense under federal law.

Nonmedical drug use is a less pejorative term but is so general that it encompasses behaviors ranging from the occasional use of alcohol to compulsive use of opioids, and includes behaviors that may or may not be associated with any adverse effects. Nonmedical drug use may consist in *experimental use* of a drug on one or a few occasions, because of curiosity about its effects, or in order to conform to the expectations of peer groups. It may involve the *casual* or *"recreational" use* of modest amounts of a drug for its pleasurable effects, or *circumstantial use*, in which certain drug effects are sought because they are helpful in particular circumstances, as when students or truck drivers take amphetamines to alleviate fatigue. These various forms of nonmedical use may then lead to more *intensive patterns* of use in terms of frequency or amount and, in some cases, to patterns of *compulsive drug use*.

Compulsive Drug Use. One of the hazards in the use of drugs to alter mood and feeling is that some individuals eventually behave as if *the effects produced by a drug, or the conditions associated with its use, are necessary to maintain an optimal state of well-being.* Such individuals are said to have a *psychological dependence* on the drug (*habituation*). The intensity of this dependence may vary from a mild desire to a "craving" or "compulsion" to use the drug. This need or psychological dependence may then give rise to behavior (*compulsive drug use*) characterized by a preoccupation with the use and procurement of the drug. In extreme forms, the behavior exhibits the characteristics of a chronic relapsing disease. Since *intense reliance* on the effects of self-administered drugs *per se* is generally a deviation from approved and expected patterns of use, the terms *compulsive drug use* and *compulsive abuse* are often interchangeable.

However, there are often striking inconsistencies in the way the terms *drug use* and *drug abuse* are employed.

Currently, in Western society, the attitude toward the use of tobacco is still so permissive that even chronic, heavy, compulsive use damaging to the user's health, and over which he may have little control, was, until very recently, rarely thought of as compulsive abuse. There are now some signs that this overly permissive attitude toward tobacco is changing, and that compulsive smoking is beginning to emerge as a form of behavior that is appropriately grouped with other drug dependencies (*see* Russell, 1971; World Health Organization, 1973).

Compulsive drug use is usually detrimental both to the user and to the society of which he is a part. However, detrimental effects can be determined only after an evaluation of the pattern of use by a given individual and a consideration of the available alternatives. For example, if the only alternative to the use of opioids is the compulsive use of alcohol, there are many who would take the view that opioid dependence is far less destructive to the individual and society, and that some provision should be made to permit that particular individual to use opioid drugs.

Compulsive drug use is commonly, but not necessarily, associated with the development of tolerance and physical dependence. *Tolerance* has developed when, after repeated administration, a given dose of a drug produces a decreased effect or, conversely, when increasingly larger doses must be administered to obtain the effects observed with the original dose. *Physical dependence* refers to an altered physiological state produced by the repeated administration of a drug, which necessitates the continued administration of the drug to prevent the appearance of a stereotyped syndrome, *the withdrawal or abstinence syndrome,* characteristic for the particular drug. The theoretical bases for the phenomena of tolerance and physical dependence are discussed below.

Addiction. It is possible to describe all known patterns of drug use without employing the terms *addict* or *addiction.* In many respects this would be advantageous, for the term *addiction,* like the term *abuse,* has been used in so many ways that it can no longer be employed without further qualification or elaboration. However, since it is not likely that the term will be dropped from the language, it is appropriate to make an effort to delimit its meaning. The definition used here is somewhat arbitrary, and it is not necessarily identical with other definitions of addiction or drug dependence (*see* Eddy *et al.,* 1965; National Commission, 1973; World Health Organization, 1973). In this chapter, the term *addiction* will be used to mean *a behavioral pattern of compulsive drug use, characterized by overwhelming involvement with the use of a drug, the securing of its supply, and a high tendency to relapse after withdrawal.* Addiction is thus viewed as an extreme on a continuum of involvement with drug use and refers in a *quantitative* rather than a *qualitative* sense to the degree to which drug use pervades the total life activity of the user. In most instances it will not be possible to state with precision at what point compulsive use should be considered addiction. Anyone who is addicted would be considered drug dependent within the WHO definitions, but *within the set of definitions used here the term* addiction *cannot be used interchangeably with* physical dependence. *It is possible to be physically dependent on drugs without being addicted and to be addicted without being physically dependent* (*see* below).

Risks of Nonmedical Drug Use. The risk of compulsive drug use is only one of a number of hazards related to the nonmedical use of drugs. The particular hazards vary considerably and depend on the drug, the dose, the route of administration, the setting in which it is used, and the psychological state and drug-related experiences of the user. Certain risks are not limited to more intensive drug-use patterns, but may be associated with experimental, recreational, or circumstantial use as well. For example, if the dose is excessive, even the first experiment with a drug may produce serious toxicity, and even occasional parenteral drug use can cause infections if hygienic precautions are inadequate. Other risks may be entirely unrelated to the pharmacological actions of the drugs used. In many societies certain forms of nonmedical drug use may lead to social ostracism or criminal prosecution. However, in this chapter the emphasis will be on the pharmacological and biochemical aspects of nonmedical drug use.

GENESIS OF DRUG USE AND DEPENDENCE

Whether the use of a drug is socially acceptable or subject to extreme disapproval, multiple factors determine who will experiment with the drug and experience its effects; other factors determine who will continue to use it casually or recreationally; and still other factors decide who will progress from casual to intensive or compulsive use.

Experimentation is largely a matter of availability, curiosity, the attitude and drug-using behavior of one's friends, the social acceptability of a given form of drug use, the risks believed to be associated with experimental use, and the tendency of the individual to respect social norms. Sometimes, drug experimentation may involve the use of substances that produce unpleasant effects. The host of materials ingested over the centuries for supposed aphrodisiac effects bears witness to this. However, from the thousands of substances that have been self-administered over the years, only a few have become staples in mankind's pharmacopoeia of drugs for nonmedical use; of these, still fewer give rise to serious problems of dependence. A full exploration of the interactions between man, environment, and drugs is beyond the scope of this chapter. (*See* Brecher, 1972; Government of Canada, 1973; National Commission, 1973; World Health Organization, 1973, 1974.)

The emphasis here will be on the interactions of man and drug, and on those aspects of the interaction that are relevant to clinical situations and to the development of compulsive drug use.

Drugs as Reinforcers.   Man's tendency to take drugs is shared with other mammals. Laboratory animals quickly learn to self-administer most of the drugs commonly used for nonmedical purposes, including opioids, barbiturates, alcohol, volatile solvents, central nervous system (CNS) stimulants, nicotine, and caffeine. Whether an animal will self-administer a drug depends on a number of factors, including the properties of the drug itself, the route of administration, the size of the individual dose, the amount of work required to obtain a dose (schedule of reinforcement), the presence of other drugs, and the kinds of drugs the animal has been given previously (*see* Schuster and Thompson, 1969). When given continuous access, animals show patterns of self-administration that are strikingly similar to those exhibited by human users of the same drug. Such observations suggest that preexisting psychopathology is not a requisite for initial or even continued drug taking, and that drugs themselves are powerful reinforcers, even in the absence of physical dependence.

Some drugs (*e.g.,* chlorpromazine) are never self-administered; they appear instead to have aversive properties, and animals learn to avoid maneuvers that result in small injections of such drugs. On the other hand, animals will press a lever more than four thousand times to get a single injection of cocaine, and when given free access, they immediately begin self-administering high daily doses that may produce severe toxic effects and induce self-mutilating behavior. With stimulants such as amphetamine and cocaine, periods of self-imposed abstinence alternate

with periods of drug administration; generally the animals die of toxic effects and inanition after a period of several weeks of continuous use. If saline solution is substituted for cocaine or amphetamine, there is a burst of rapid lever pressing for several hours, then abruptly all responding ceases and is not resumed. In contrast, animals self-administering morphine gradually raise the daily dose over a period of weeks, then self-administer the drug at a steady rate that avoids both gross toxicity and withdrawal symptoms. When saline solution is substituted for morphine, however, the animal continues to press the lever (except during the peak of withdrawal) and does so at a slow but steady rate over a period of weeks (*see* Thompson and Pickens, 1970).

Tolerance and Physical Dependence.   In addition to the primary reinforcing effects, when drugs are used chronically other factors come into play that profoundly affect the pattern of use and the likelihood that the drug use will be continued. Among these are the capacities of some substances, but not others, to produce *tolerance* and/or *physical dependence.* These phenomena, as previously defined, are often assumed to be inextricably linked to each other and to the problem of compulsive drug use. Neither of these assumptions is valid. Tolerance and physical dependence develop not only with narcotics, alcohol, and hypnotics but also after chronic administration of a wide variety of drugs that are not self-administered by animals or used compulsively by man. Such drugs include anticholinergics, chlorpromazine, imipramine, and cyclazocine, a synthetic narcotic antagonist (*see* Chapter 15). Nor does physical dependence invariably occur in every situation where tolerance develops. Tolerance is a very general phenomenon observed with a host of substances and involves many independent mechanisms. In any given case, more than one of these mechanisms may be operative (*see* Kalant *et al.,* 1971; Hug, 1972). Here are considered only those aspects of tolerance that are relevant to problems of nonmedical drug use.

Tolerance to Opioids.   Tolerance does not develop uniformly to all the actions of a narcotic drug. There may be complete tolerance to some actions concurrent with undiminished responses to others. Opioid tolerance is characterized by a shortened duration and decreased intensity of the analgesic, euphorigenic, sedative, and other CNS depressant effects as well as by a marked elevation in the average lethal dose. While animals that are tolerant to opioids may metabolize them somewhat more rapidly, changes in the rate of drug disposition cannot fully account for all the phenomena of opioid tolerance, including the observation that tolerant animals are less depressed with brain concentrations of morphine or methadone that produce severe depression in nontolerant animals. Most of the tolerance seen with opioids must be attributed to some form of adaptation of cells in the nervous system to the drug's action ("pharmacodynamic," "tissue," or "cellular" tolerance).

Although tolerance itself does not necessarily affect the likelihood of continued use, it can affect patterns of use by increasing the amount of drug that must be taken to produce a given effect (*e.g.,* euphoria). The use of increased amounts may in turn enhance the risk of toxic effects or produce other problems if the drug is expensive or obtained illicitly.

The essential mechanisms underlying tolerance to opioids are not known. The mechanisms that are finally elucidated will have to account for: (1) the interference with the development of tolerance by drugs that inhibit synthesis of proteins or the synthesis of certain neurotransmitters; (2) the acceleration of the development of tolerance by precursors of 5-hydroxytryptamine (5-HT); (3) the rapidity with which some forms of tolerance develop; and (4) under certain conditions, its remarkable persistence. In the dog, considerable recovery from behavioral depression occurs during the course of a continuous 8-hour infusion of morphine (acute tolerance). In man, a dosage of 500 mg of morphine per day can be reached within 10 days (Fraser *et al.,* 1957). Some residual tolerance is seen in the rat many months after a single dose of morphine.

Many lines of investigation are under study. Martin (1968) has proposed that homeostatic mechanisms can account for some of the phenomena of acute tolerance, whereas the more chronic form may be due to redundant pathways in the CNS that take over function when other pathways are blocked by opioids. Other investigators have suggested that tolerance to morphine may involve an increased synthesis of catecholamines or of 5-HT (*see* Way, 1973), or the development of some form of immune reaction (*see* Cochin, 1973). Several theories (extracellular and intracellular receptors that induce opposing responses, enzyme expansion, disuse supersensitivity, and increase in receptors) postulate a single mechanism to account for both tolerance and physical dependence. These are considered below in the discussion of physical dependence.

Tolerance to Alcohol, Barbiturates, and Related Hypnotics. Some form of pharmacodynamic tolerance to alcohol and barbiturates must be assumed, inasmuch as animals tolerant to barbiturates or alcohol show significantly less sedation and ataxia than do nontolerant animals at the same blood concentrations. However, as the blood concentrations are increased, there is progressively less difference between tolerant and nontolerant animals in the degree of CNS depression and, in contrast to the tolerance seen with opioids, animals tolerant to alcohol or barbiturates show no dramatic elevation of the lethal blood concentration.

In the case of short-acting barbiturates (*e.g.,* hexobarbital, pentobarbital), alcohol, and a number of nonbarbiturate hypnotics (glutethimide, meprobamate, etc.), a more rapid enzymatic degradation of the drug can also be demonstrated in tolerant animals. Thus, in the same animal two independent mechanisms, *pharmacodynamic* tolerance and *drug-disposition* tolerance, contribute to the decreased duration and intensity of the response to a given dose. Both modes of adaptation are relevant to clinical problems. Drug-disposition tolerance, however, does not seem closely related to the phenomena of physical dependence and pharmacodynamic tolerance; changes in the rate of enzymatic degradation of barbiturates can be induced by pretreatment with substances that do not in themselves produce CNS depression or pharmacodynamic tolerance.

With this group of drugs, as with the opioids, tolerance does not directly increase the probability of continued or compulsive use. However, tolerance to toxic effects may not develop in parallel with tolerance to CNS depression and, in the case of alcohol particularly, the consumption of more drug in order to obtain CNS effects may increase the likelihood of direct drug-induced organ damage (*see* Lieber, 1972). Furthermore, the shortened duration of action may increase the frequency of drug taking, thereby increasing the number of times that drug-taking behavior will be reinforced.

Some aspects of tolerance to general CNS depressants develop with surprising rapidity. Thus, in man, when the blood concentration is falling after administration of a large dose of alcohol, the signs and symptoms of intoxication disappear at a concentration that was associated with gross intoxication when the blood level was rising. This apparently rapid or *acute* CNS tolerance has also been observed in dogs with pentobarbital, thiopental, paraldehyde, and trichloroethanol, and the degree of tolerance that develops (as measured by the blood concentration of the drug when signs of ataxia disappear) seems directly related to the depth of the CNS depression that was produced by the drug (Maynert and Klingman, 1960). It is not clear whether the mechanisms underlying acute tolerance are related to those involved in the tolerance that develops over longer periods. The subject of tolerance to alcohol and related general CNS depressants has been reviewed by Kalant and associates (1971) and Hug (1972). Tolerance to CNS sympathomimetics, nicotine, cannabinoids, and psychedelics is discussed under clinical characteristics of their abuse.

Physical Dependence. Physical dependence has been studied after chronic administration of opioids, general depressants of the CNS (alcohol, barbiturates, and related hypnotics), amphetamines, nicotine, and opioid antagonists. Several research workers have pointed out that the withdrawal symptoms associated with many of these classes of agents are characterized by rebound effects in those same physiological systems that were modified initially by the drug (*rebound hyperexcitability*). For example, general depressants elevate the seizure threshold, but spontaneous seizures are seen during withdrawal; morphine depresses the flexor and crossed extensor spinal reflexes, but these same polysynaptic reflexes are hyperexcitable during morphine withdrawal. Amphetamines alleviate fatigue, suppress appetite, and elevate mood; amphetamine withdrawal is characterized by lack of energy, hyperphagia, and depression. Nicotine tends to suppress anger; irritability is a common complaint following abrupt cessation in heavy smokers. It is not certain whether all the complex patterns of symptoms seen during withdrawal from opioids or general depressants should be considered rebound effects, nor whether such a generalization is applicable to the stereotyped, distinct syndromes observed after abrupt withdrawal of drugs such as chlorpromazine, imipramine, and cyclazocine.

Time Required. The time required to produce physical dependence on any drug depends on a number of factors, but the most important seem to be the degree to which function in the CNS is altered by the drug and the continuity of this alteration. However, whether a withdrawal syndrome is clinically observable depends on (1) the criteria for withdrawal symptoms, (2) the sensitivity of technics used to detect withdrawal phenomena, and (3) the rate at which the drug is removed from its site of action.

Patients who have received therapeutic doses of morphine several times a day for 1 to 2 weeks will have only mild symptoms that may not be recognized as withdrawal symptomatology when the drug is stopped; symptoms are even less pronounced when the opioid is one that is slowly eliminated. However, if the drug is not simply discontinued but an opioid antagonist (naloxone) is used to induce withdrawal, it is possible to demonstrate withdrawal symptoms in man after therapeutic doses of morphine, methadone, or heroin given four times per day for as short a period as 2 to 3 days (Wikler *et al.,* 1953). In former heroin addicts naloxone precipitates mild withdrawal symptoms 1 week after a single 40-mg dose of methadone, indicating the presence of an otherwise subclinical level of physical dependence. In short, the phenomenon of opioid physical dependence is initiated by the first dose, and this rapid development has important clinical implications (*see* below).

The time required to produce physical dependence with general CNS depressants is likewise short; when rapidly metabolized drugs are used, the earliest signs of rebound excitability can be detected after surprisingly brief periods of CNS depression. Using the threshold for seizures in mice as a measure, McQuarrie and Fingl (1958) were able to demonstrate that a single large dose of alcohol produces an elevation of the seizure threshold that is followed by a period of subnormal threshold. After 3 days of chronic exposure to ethanol, mice develop marked physical dependence, with spontaneous seizures upon abrupt withdrawal (Goldstein, 1973). With short-acting barbiturates it may require weeks of *mild intoxication* to produce clinically significant physical dependence, but 10% of patients who were kept *deeply intoxicated* (semicomatose) for 16 to 20 hours per day, for 10 to 12 days, became so physically dependent that they developed seizures and delirium on abrupt withdrawal (Alexander, 1951). In cats, evidence of withdrawal hyperexcitability can be demonstrated after as little as 26 hours of deep pentobarbital intoxication.

In contrast to the short-acting drugs,

abrupt discontinuation of long-acting drugs, such as methadone or acetylmethadol, produces withdrawal symptoms that are slow in onset and generally less severe. This is true also of long-acting hypnotics and sedatives such as phenobarbital and chlordiazepoxide when contrasted with pentobarbital or meprobamate. Conversely, when methadone is displaced from the receptors by an antagonist, a severe withdrawal syndrome ensues. It is as if a great deal of latent hyperexcitability is explosively released rather than gradually dissipated over a period of time. Thus, it is necessary to distinguish between the degree of *latent* hyperexcitability and the amount manifested when the drug is stopped. Continuous action at the receptor theoretically produces a greater degree of physical dependence. However, such factors as tissue binding or slow metabolism may result in a very slow reversal of the process, a slower onset of withdrawal phenomena, and a generally less severe clinical syndrome.

These observations suggest that the adaptational processes that eventually produce grossly observable withdrawal symptoms, at least with opioids and general CNS depressants, actually begin with the first dose. This has obvious implications not only for the problem of deciding just when physical dependence is present but also for the problem of determining the causes of compulsive abuse. It is quite conceivable that individuals who use short-acting drugs to induce euphoria or reduce tensions can perceive an exacerbation of these same tensions (rebound effects) as the drug effects wane. Such increases in tension might then contribute to the motivation to repeat the use of the drug, and the alleviation of withdrawal phenomena might increase the effectiveness of the drug as a reinforcer of drug-using behavior. Whether similar subtle post-drug-use effects are seen with amphetamines or nicotine is not clear.

The relationship between compulsive drug use and physical dependence is more variable and far more complex than was previously realized. For example, some degree of physical dependence develops in medical patients who receive opioids regularly for more than a few days. The overwhelming majority of such patients do not exhibit drug-seeking behavior, do not become compulsive users, and discontinue the drug when the medical condition is relieved. Furthermore, drug-seeking behavior has not been observed in patients with affective disorders treated with opioids or in chronic schizophrenic patients made physically dependent on morphine. A large proportion of the young men who served in the United States Army in Vietnam used heroin, and about half of this group became physically dependent. Nevertheless, a substantial percentage simply stopped their heroin use before their return to the United States, and many did so without benefit of any special treatment (*see* Robins, 1974).

It is probable that at least some degree of physical dependence on CNS depressants (including alcohol) develops after relatively brief periods of continuous use, yet the majority of individuals are able to tolerate minor withdrawal phenomena and do not become compulsive drug users.

Thus, although some compulsive users attribute their drug problems entirely to "getting hooked" (either iatrogenically or out of ignorance in the course of using drugs illicitly), physical dependence is currently viewed not so much as a direct cause of compulsive use but as one of several factors that contribute to its development and to the tendency to relapse after withdrawal (*see* below).

Degree of Physical Dependence and Locus of Changes. At the present time, the degree of physical dependence can be measured only by the severity of the withdrawal syndrome produced either by abrupt withdrawal or by use of drug antagonists. With opioid drugs, there appears to be an upper limit to the degree of physical dependence. This upper limit seems to be an exponential function of total daily dose, so that increasing the daily dose in man beyond the equivalent of 500 mg of morphine does not significantly increase the severity of the withdrawal syndrome. As mentioned above, such dosage levels can be reached within 2 weeks. Since the abrupt withdrawal of hypnotics or alcohol after high dosage produces seizures and delirium that can be fatal in man and animals, it is difficult to establish an upper limit of physical dependence on these agents.

Physical dependence and withdrawal symptoms are due to drug-induced alterations within the nervous system, with the most prominent changes occurring in the CNS. Abundant evidence indicates that, in the case of opioids, these changes are not limited to any one part of the CNS but occur throughout the entire neuraxis. Withdrawal phenomena can be demonstrated in decorticate and decerebrate animals and in the spinal cord of man and animals after cord transection (*see* Wikler, 1958). Similarly, decorticate dogs still develop seizures during barbiturate withdrawal (*see* Essig, 1967). It is probable that the entire neuraxis is also involved in physical dependence on hypnotics and alcohol. However, in the case of opioids, some areas of the CNS, such as the medial thalamus and medial areas of the diencephalic-mesencephalic structures, may be more involved than others (*see* Wei *et al.,* 1973).

Cross-Dependence. The ability of one drug to suppress the manifestations of physical dependence produced by another and to maintain the physically dependent state is referred to as *cross-dependence.* Cross-dependence may be partial or complete, and the degree is more closely related to pharmacological effects than to chemical similarities.

In general, any potent opioid will show cross-dependence with other opioids. Partial cross-dependence is also seen between alcohol and barbiturates, whereby in man alcohol can very substantially but not completely suppress the symptoms of barbiturate withdrawal (Fraser *et al.,* 1957). Animal studies show a high degree of cross-dependence among general CNS depressants; most sedative-hypnotics (*e.g.,* paraldehyde, chloral hydrate, meprobamate, chlordiazepoxide, etc.) will show a reasonable degree of cross-dependence with each other and with alcohol and barbiturates. There is also some cross-dependence between barbiturates and volatile anesthetics. Clinical reports are consistent with these findings, although there are few well-controlled studies.

If a long-acting drug such as methadone is substituted over several days for morphine, abrupt discontinuation produces a withdrawal syndrome characteristic of the long-acting drug rather than that of morphine. This aspect of cross-dependence has important clinical implications, since the withdrawal symptoms that occur with drugs with longer half-lives (methadone, phenobarbital, chlordiazepoxide) are generally less severe but more protracted (*see* Isbell *et al.,* 1948; Wulff, 1959; Hollister *et al.,* 1961). This phenomenon is the basis for the substitution treatment of physical dependence for both opioids and CNS depressants.

Theories of Physical Dependence. Despite considerable research effort, the basic mechanisms responsible for physical dependence on opioids and general CNS depressants are still unclear. Most theories postulate some form of CNS counteradaptation to the agonistic actions of the drugs. Counteradaptation results in the development of a "latent hyperexcitability" that becomes manifest in the form of withdrawal phenomena when the drugs are stopped or, in the case of opioids, when they are displaced from the receptor by an antagonist. The theories differ largely in the level of explanation or in the mechanisms proposed to account for the counteradaptive changes; most involve models that account for the observation that physical dependence is generally accompanied by tolerance and that the two phenomena develop and decay at about the same rate.

Martin (1968) has proposed a homeostatic and redundancy model in which tolerance is due to the opening of redundant pathways within the CNS when the primary pathway is blocked by the action of the drug. With drug withdrawal, activity in the primary pathway is restored, which in combination with continuing activity in the redundant pathway results in a rebound hyperexcitability of the pathways once depressed by the drug. While developed largely to account for opioid physical dependence, this theory is applicable to other drugs as well. Others have speculated that decreased neural activity in any functional system results in a "disuse supersensitivity" analogous to the denervation supersensitivity that develops in peripheral autonomic structures. The supersensitivity is thought to begin as soon as input is reduced and to account for decreased drug effect (tolerance); abrupt withdrawal of the drug or its displacement by an antagonist restores input to supersensitive elements, producing a "rebound" hyperactivity in the very systems that were depressed by the drug (*see* Jaffe and Sharpless, 1968). This model does not require that the drug be present on the ultimate neuronal receptor itself. A related theory postulates that alterations in neural input cause an increase in the number of receptors, which in turn may be "active" or "silent." An increase in receptors for neurotransmitters would account for tolerance, and the rebound effects occur when drug withdrawal restores normal neurotransmitter activity to a system with excess receptors (*see* Collier, 1966). With the assay of saturable stereospecific opioid binding sites in brain, this hypothesis has become a subject of intense interest.

Enzyme expansion theories postulate that drugs that cause dependence inhibit an enzyme that synthesizes a product important for cell activity (*e.g.,* a neurotransmitter), and that the level of the enzyme itself is regulated by its product, the neurotransmitter. The initial drug effect is a result of the decrease in transmitter concentration, but this decrease also leads to increased synthesis of the enzyme and a new steady-state level that restores transmitter concentration, resulting in tolerance; when the drug is withdrawn there is excess enzyme, which then causes excess synthesis of transmitter, and this produces rebound effects until the enzyme activity falls to a new steady state (*see* Goldstein and Goldstein, 1968; Shuster, 1971). These theories are applicable to both opioid and CNS-depressant types of physical dependence.

Apart from general theories, there has been much research on biochemical changes in the CNS during the development of physical dependence on opioids, as well as on barbiturates, alcohol, and CNS stimulants. Almost every substance with postulated neurotransmitter function has been explored. While the data are not entirely consistent, many studies tend to show that in opioid physical dependence there is an increased rate of synthesis of 5-HT in the brain, and that the degree of tolerance and physical dependence is reduced by agents that interfere with the synthesis of protein or of 5-HT. Other studies have emphasized the role of increased synthesis of catecholamines in opioid dependence. Similar efforts to explore the role of putative neurotransmitters in barbiturate and alcohol dependence indicate that, while depletion of catecholamines aggravates the alcohol withdrawal syndrome, only drugs that induce cross-dependence or that raise brain concentrations of gamma-aminobutyric acid (GABA) have an ameliorative effect (see Goldstein, 1973); this is consistent with the observed fall in brain GABA concentration during ethanol withdrawal (Patel and Lal, 1973).

At present no single model is able to account for all the complex phenomena that are seen with the many classes of drugs producing tolerance and physical dependence. It is likely that multiple mechanisms are involved, and that each model may reflect a facet of truth. For the present, the more heuristic models are the more challenging. Opioid tolerance and physical dependence have been reviewed by Dole (1970), Shuster (1971), Wikler (1972), and Way (1973), and nonopioid tolerance and physical dependence by Kalant and associates (1971); tolerance to a variety of CNS agents has been reviewed by Hug (1972).

Learning, Conditioning, and Relapse. Within the framework of learning theory, drug use, whether casual or compulsive, can be viewed as behavior that is maintained by its consequences; consequences that strengthen a behavior pattern are reinforcers. Drugs may reinforce the antecedent drug-taking behavior by inducing pleasurable effects (positive reinforcement) or by terminating some aversive or unpleasant situation (negative reinforcement), as when a drug alleviates pain or anxiety. Secondary or social reinforcement entirely independent of pharmacological effects may also play a role, as is the case when drug use results in special status, membership in a desired group, or the approval of friends. Sometimes social reinforcement maintains experimental behavior until the individual comes to appreciate the primary drug effect or becomes tolerant to some initial aversive effects of the particular drug. This seems to be the case with many young people who do not like the initial effects of tobacco or who perceive nothing pleasurable about the initial effects of smoking marihuana. Although it is not as widely appreciated, some individuals find the effects of an initial dose of heroin, with its associated nausea and vomiting, somewhat unpleasant; however, social reinforcers may maintain the behavior until tolerance develops to these effects.

The development of physical dependence gives rise to the possibility of another variety of reinforcement; each time drug use alleviates withdrawal distress the antecedent drug-using behavior is further reinforced. Even when tolerance attenuates the initial reinforcing effects, drugs that induce physical dependence create a regularly recurring sense of distress that is immediately eliminated by another dose of the drug. During the withdrawal state, drug use can simultaneously alleviate distress and produce euphoria, a particularly powerful reinforcement.

Recent studies have described a protracted opioid abstinence syndrome characterized by physiological and psychological abnormalities that persist for many weeks after withdrawal. Since the subjective sense of not being quite normal is immediately relieved by very small doses of opioid drugs, the protracted abstinence syndrome may predispose to relapse by creating a prolonged period of increased vulnerability during which the effects of opioids are especially reinforcing (see Dole, 1972; Cushman and Dole, 1973; Martin et al., 1973).

Animal work has also demonstrated that acute drug effects, withdrawal phenomena, and relief of withdrawal symptoms by drugs can be conditioned to environmental stimuli (see Roffman et al., 1973; Wikler, 1973). Such conditioning helps to explain how the rituals and circumstances surrounding drug use can act as secondary reinforcers, and how the mere taking of an inert pill or the use of a needle and syringe containing no drug can evoke the feelings (including relief of withdrawal symptoms) previously produced when the pill or syringe contained an active substance. The observation that withdrawal distress can become conditioned to the environment in which it occurs may underlie reports that former narcotics addicts may experience sensations very similar to withdrawal symptoms, including an intensified craving for drugs, when they return to an environment where drugs are available. Alcoholics may have similar experiences, particularly when they are exposed to the sight and smell of alcohol (Ludwig et al., 1974). Conditioned abstinence is thought to play a significant role in relapse to opioid use; it is possible that similar mechanisms are operative in relapse to tobacco, barbiturates, and alcohol.

Vulnerability. In man, drugs may produce effects experienced as pleasurable, novel, or tension reducing, but these effects are not such powerful reinforcers that repetitive drug use is inevitable. Much research has centered on why some individuals stop after experimentation, others continue drug use but do not become dependent, and still others become compulsive drug users.

Individuals who later become regular users of socially disapproved drugs tend to be more impulsive, more rebellious with respect to social norms, and less tolerant of frustration, but they do not fall into any single diagnostic category. To date, no clearly recognized addictive personality or constellation of traits has been identified that is equally applicable to all varieties of compulsive drug users. Indeed, given the different pharmacological effects of various drugs, it would be surprising if all compulsive drug users were similar.

There are many factors that could contribute to increased vulnerability to continued or compulsive drug use. Some individuals may experience a more intense response to the initial reinforcing properties of the drugs, such as a more intense euphoria or a more profound reduction of unpleasant feelings of anger, depression, or anxiety. Such intense reactions, in turn, could be due to differences in sensitivity to drug effects or to initially higher levels of distress. Thus, for some, drug use may be viewed as self-treatment for internal distress. Although the agent selected or the pattern of use may sometimes run counter to social norms, for some individuals the alternative may be a state of tension that may be felt to be intolerable. On the other hand, the contributory factors may be entirely social, as in the case of young people who continue to smoke cigarettes (despite some initial unpleasant reactions) more to conform to the pressures from friends than because of an especially intense need for the pharmacological effects of nicotine. Still other possibilities include differences in the intensity of withdrawal phenomena as experienced by different users (*see* above).

Efforts to delineate the factors that contribute to vulnerability have included studies of the personalities and family structures of different types of drug users, and the role of peer groups, social factors, and economic conditions in generating tension and frustration. In some cases, constitutional and genetic factors have been identified that might be responsible either for abnormal states of tension or for unusually positive or negative responses to drug use or drug withdrawal (*see* Goodwin *et al.*, 1973). But it would appear that for any given pattern of continued drug use the outcome is the result of an interaction between social, biological, and environmental factors.

Sociological Factors. It would be difficult to overestimate the effects of social organization on the incidence, prevalence, and consequences of nonmedical drug use. Social factors have a major influence on which individuals have access to various drugs, and social attitudes determine which drugs are acceptable for casual or "recreational" use, which may be used for relief of tension, and which are prohibited. In addition, the nature of a society often determines the kinds of tensions induced in its members, as well as the kinds of behaviors that are viewed as socially acceptable. Thus, until recently in Western cultures the pressures to perform sexually and aggressively were greater for males than for females, while the pressures against use of opioids or alcohol were greater for females than for males. In general, when the use of a drug is widely accepted, the number of users tends to be large and their personal characteristics are quite diverse, including the characteristics of the small proportion who become compulsive users. When a particular form of drug use meets with severe disapproval, those who use it despite such sanctions tend to be very different from the average person in society in terms of attitudes and emotional adjustment even before use. Consequently, a high proportion may become intensive or compulsive users, sometimes leading to the erroneous conclusion that the particular drug is "more addicting" than those drugs used by larger and more diverse populations.

The acceptability of a drug may increase or decrease with time in a fadlike fashion. Sometimes the use of a drug may become identified with acceptance of the values of particular groups within a society, and individuals may participate in drug-using behavior as a way of symbolizing their group affiliation. Membership, even in highly deviant groups, may in turn represent an attempted solution to problems of personal identity, since some groups have elaborate sets of behavioral norms.

Chronic drug use may establish a complex equilibrium among family members, and abstinence on the part of the user, with its attendant changes in behavior and role, can also induce tension in other members of the family. Relapse to drugs or alcohol sometimes restores the previous pathological equilibrium. Cultural attitudes toward addicts and alcoholics and the legal or medical complications of drug use further increase the drug user's difficulties in obtaining realistic gratifications (alternative reinforcers) and simultaneously foster his return to an environment (the local bar or group of heroin addicts) where he is accepted, where the drug is available, and where its use is acceptable and has been repeatedly reinforced.

CLINICAL CHARACTERISTICS

Most of the pharmacological agents commonly used for subjective purposes (excluding caffeine) can be placed into six major classes, as follows: (1) opioid analgesics, (2) general CNS depressants, (3) CNS sympathomimetics, (4) nicotine, (5) cannabinoids, and (6) psychedelics (hallucinogens, psychotomimetics, psychotogens). Although within each class the agents have many actions in common, there are also differences, and the classification is offered merely for its didactic convenience.

OPIOIDS

Incidence and Patterns of Use. In the late 1960s the use of heroin increased considerably, both in the United States and in Great Britain. The reasons for the increase are still not entirely clear, but some of the factors include changes in social attitudes toward drug use and toward established social norms in general, increased availability of drugs, and the substantial increase in the adolescent population (a result of the sharp increase in births following World War II), with its associated social changes.

In the United States, heroin use is still mainly centered in large urban areas, such as New York and Chicago, and members of racial and ethnic groups from lower socioeconomic strata continue to be overrepresented. However, heroin use is now observed with greater frequency among more affluent members of society. There are no reliable estimates of the number of people who are addicted to narcotics in the United States, and the estimates that do exist are confounded by the tendency to equate experimental and "recreational" use with compulsive use or addiction. It is likely that over the 10-year period ending in 1974, well over a million people had experimented with heroin (see National Commission, 1973), and that during the period of peak prevalence (probably 1970–1972) there were more than 250,000 heroin addicts.

In the United States there are two basic patterns of opioid use and dependence. One involves individuals whose drug use begins in the context of medical treatment and who obtain their initial supplies through medical channels. This group constitutes a very small percentage of the addicted population. The other pattern begins with experimental or "recreational" drug use, progresses to more intensive use, and involves primarily adolescents and young adults, with males far outnumbering females.

Most users are introduced to the drug by other users. This is true both of the initial contact and of those subsequent contacts leading to relapse after periods of withdrawal. The way in which drug use spreads from one friend to another in epidemic fashion has been well documented (de Alarcon,

1969; Hughes *et al.*, 1972). In general, the professional "peddler" or "pusher" does not play a major role in enticing nonusers to try either narcotics or marihuana. This is not a matter of the pusher's scruples; it simply reflects the fact that the risks are high. The professional "pusher" feels safe only when selling to a known addict.

A user's first experience with opioids is often quite unpleasant, with nausea and vomiting as the outstanding features. Some may not try again for days or weeks; others, however, discover a new world of inner satisfaction with the first dose and make a conscious decision to continue to use the drug as frequently as their finances will permit. Some may struggle with the impulse to use it again and may do so only intermittently for many months or years before becoming regular users; some may never become compulsive users. Although there are no statistics to support the notion, the most common pattern may be to try the drug once or twice and then, with awareness of the dangers, to avoid it thereafter (see Robins and Murphy, 1967; National Commission, 1973). Despite the medical and legal risks, where group values support opioid use and relatively pure drugs are easily available, a very high percentage of users may become physically dependent. In 1971, about 42% of United States Army enlisted men in Vietnam used opioids at least once, and about half of these users reported that at some time during their year in Vietnam they were physically dependent (Robins, 1974).

The incidence of opioid addiction among physicians, nurses, and those in the related health professions is many times higher than in any group with comparable educational background. Most physician-addicts state that they first took the drug to overcome fatigue or to alleviate some bodily ailment, and few indicate that they were seeking thrills; the original motive, however, has little effect on the pattern and the consequences of the addiction that later develops. These are often related more to chance factors, such as whether they are prosecuted by enforcement agencies for their drug use. Considering the frequency with which opioid analgesics are used in clinical medicine, addiction as a complication of medical treatment is quite uncommon. When it does occur, the pattern it follows depends on both the emotional adjustment of the patient prior to involvement with opioids and the source of the drug. Those individuals who continue to obtain it from physicians usually avoid the problems associated with illicit drugs. Those who must obtain drugs from illicit traffic encounter the same problems that are faced by heroin users. The personality characteristics of physician-addicts, and probably those of "medical" addicts in general, are distinct from those of the urban heroin addict.

Rapid intravenous injection of an opioid produces a warm flushing of the skin and sensations in the lower abdomen described by addicts as similar in intensity and quality to sexual orgasm, and known as a "rush," "kick," or "thrill." Although heroin is the most commonly used illicit opioid, it has few special pharmacological properties that account for its popularity. Given subcutaneously, even experienced users cannot reliably distinguish heroin from morphine. This is understandable, since heroin is rapidly converted into morphine in the body. When these two drugs are given intravenously, addicts are better able to distinguish between them. Because of the greater lipid solubility of heroin in comparison to morphine, a larger fraction crosses the blood-brain barrier, thus producing a rapid onset of opioid effects. In the brain, heroin is rapidly deacetylated to 6-monoacetyl morphine and to morphine. In this sense, heroin carries morphine rapidly into the brain. On a weight basis, heroin is about two and one-half times as potent as morphine, but it does not produce more euphoria, greater physical dependence, or fewer side effects (Martin and Fraser, 1961). Its popularity in illicit trade may be related in part to its ease of manufacture and its relatively smaller bulk.

Symptoms and Effects of Compulsive Opioid Use. Many previously held views about the behavior and physical state of opioid users and addicts are now being revised in the light of careful clinical observation of a wide diversity of drug users and addicts under very different conditions. The major finding is that behavior, social adjustment, and medical problems are surprisingly varied. Experience with thousands of patients maintained on high daily doses of methadone for periods of more than 8 years has shown no direct injurious effects (Kreek, 1973; Wilmarth and Goldstein, 1974). Good health and productive work are thus not incompatible with regular use of opioids. However, it is now clear that the behavior of the individual prior to opioid use and the purposes and patterns of use determine the social and physiological consequences.

Even in England, where chronic narcotics users may still obtain pure heroin from legitimate medical sources at no cost, the patterns of social adjustment are extremely varied. The majority of narcotics users in Britain are young people who were introduced to drug use by friends, began out of curiosity, and continue because of the euphoric effects. The preferred route of administration is intravenous. The patterns of adjustment among the patients receiving treatment at London clinics are similar to those observed in the United States. Four major patterns have been noted: (1) "stables"—patients who are legitimately employed, do not engage in criminal activity, do not associate with other addicts, and do not buy extra heroin illicitly; (2) "junkies"—patients who are the opposite of the stable patients in these respects; (3) "loners"—patients who are on welfare rather than engaging in crime, do not associate with other addicts, but do use a wide variety of drugs not prescribed by the clinic; and (4) "two-worlders"—patients who are employed but associate with other addicts, buy extra drugs, and engage in criminal activities. The disorganized behavior and criminality of the "junkies" and the organized behavior of the "stables" antedated the addiction (Stimson, 1973). Despite the legal source of drugs, those receiving heroin at London clinics have a high incidence of infections (due to neglect of hygienic procedures or to shared needles) and a surprisingly high mortality rate, ranging from 2 to 6% per year (Stimson, 1973). Similar variations in patterns of behavior, social adjustment, and impaired health have been noted among heroin addicts in the United States despite the exclusively illegal sources of their drugs.

Undoubtedly, the high cost and impurities of illicit drugs in the United States exact their toll. Many females earn their drug money through prostitution, and there is a high incidence of venereal disease among female heroin addicts. The average annual death rate among young-adult heroin addicts is several times higher than that for nonaddicts of similar age and ethnic backgrounds. In the younger group, much of this increase is due to fatal narcotic overdosage that is usually an accidental outcome of the dangerous fluctuations in the purity of illicit heroin. Another frequent cause of sudden death has been termed an "anaphylactoid reaction," which probably results from the intravenous injection of a drug containing certain impurities. The suicide rate among adult addicts is likewise considerably higher than that of the general population, and a surprisingly high percentage die violent deaths at the hands of others. The medical complications common among drug users include infections (*e.g.*, septicemia, endocarditis, hepatitis, tetanus, and pulmonary, cerebral, and subcutaneous abscesses) due to shared needles and unhygienic procedures, foreign body emboli, granulomata due to injection of contaminants, and a variety of neurological, musculoskeletal, and other lesions that may be due to hypersensitivity reactions. The medical problems associated with opioid use have been reviewed by Sapira (1968) and Thornton and Thornton (1974).

The health and social adjustment of patients maintained on oral methadone are equally varied. Many hold jobs, raise children, commit no crimes, and use no socially disapproved drugs. Yet other patients continue to commit crimes, do not obtain employment, and use other drugs or excessive amounts of alcohol. The mortality rate among patients in maintenance programs is higher than that among others of comparable age and socioeconomic status, but the general consensus is that the high rate is not related to the effects of oral methadone *per se,* but directly or indirectly to problems that antedated methadone use.

Opioids reduce pain, aggression, and sexual drives, and their use, therefore, is unlikely to induce crime. However, many individuals committed crimes prior to opioid use, and they do not necessarily stop when opioid use begins. In addition, many individuals who did not engage in crime previously may begin to do so in order to obtain money to buy opioids, since the cost is generally beyond the amount they can obtain legitimately. The complex relationship between opioid use and crime has been discussed in detail by several special commissions (*see* Task Force, 1967; Government of Canada, 1973; National Commission, 1973).

Tolerance, Physical Dependence, and Withdrawal Symptoms. A remarkable degree of tolerance develops to the respiratory depressant, analgesic, sedative, emetic, and euphorigenic effects of opioids; however, the rate at which this tolerance develops, in either the addict or the medical patient, depends on the pattern of use. With intermittent use, it is possible to obtain desired analgesic and sedative effects from doses in the therapeutic range for an indefinite period. It is only when there is a more or less continuous drug action that significant tolerance develops. Thus, if the drug is used frequently, the addict who is primarily seeking to get a "kick" or to maintain a state of dreamy indifference (a "high") must constantly increase the dose. In this way, some addicts can build up to phenomenally large doses. In one verified case a dose of 5 g of morphine was used each day. With the development of tolerance, the lethal dose is greatly altered. A case is recorded in which an addict was injected intravenously with 2 g of morphine over a period of 2½ hours without significant change in blood pressure, pulse rate, or respiration; the usual dose for this individual was 0.25 g. However, tolerance is not absolute. With all opioid analgesics a dose always exists that is capable of producing death from respiratory depression, even in tolerant individuals.

Tolerance does not develop equally or at the same rate to all the effects of opioids, and even users highly tolerant to respiratory depressant effects continue to exhibit miosis and to complain of constipation. Although in the dog considerable tolerance to morphine develops during the course of an 8-hour intravenous infusion, such acute tolerance does not appear to develop in man (Elliot *et al.*, 1971). Subjects maintained on daily oral doses of 100 mg of methadone for more than 8 weeks still seemed sedated and apathetic, and had constricted pupils and decreased respiratory rates (Martin *et al.*, 1973). However, experience with thousands of patients maintained on methadone for periods of several years suggests that, while constipation is a continuing problem, substantial sedation and apathy are easily managed by modest reductions in dosage. Indeed, without laboratory technics even skilled clinicians cannot distinguish between patients maintained on methadone and patients who are drug free. Some patients are eager to be withdrawn from methadone, which again underscores the distinction between physical dependence and addiction.

Meperidine addicts may use large daily doses (3 to 4 g per day), but significant tolerance does not develop to the drug's excitant and atropine-like actions. When very high doses of meperidine are used, even the tolerant addict may show dilated pupils, increased muscular activity, twitching, tremors, mental confusion, and, occasionally, grand mal seizures (Isbell and White, 1953).

A high degree of cross-tolerance between drugs with similar pharmacological actions is a constant finding, and *an individual tolerant to one opioid analgesic will be tolerant to another even if the two are chemically quite dissimilar.* Tolerance to opioids largely disappears when withdrawal has been completed, and many addicts have taken fatal overdoses by returning to their previous dosage immediately after undergoing withdrawal.

The character and the severity of the withdrawal symptoms that appear when an opioid is discontinued depend upon many factors, including the particular drug, the total daily dose used, the interval between doses, the duration of use, and the health and personality of the addict. The details of the time and the dosage required to induce physical dependence have been discussed above.

It is helpful to view the total clinical picture of the abstinence syndrome as made up of *purposive behavior,* which is goal oriented, highly dependent on the observer and the environment, and directed at getting more drug, and *nonpurposive behavior,* which is not goal oriented and relatively independent of the observer and the environment. The purposive phenomena, including complaints, pleas, demands, manipulations, and simulations, are as varied as the imagination of the drug-using population. In the hospital setting, they are considerably less pronounced when the patient is certain that his behavior does not affect the decision to give him a drug.

In the case of morphine or heroin, the first withdrawal signs are usually noted shortly before the time of the next scheduled dose. At this time, purposive behavior is prominent; it increases in intensity, reaching a peak at 36 to 72 hours after the last dose, and then gradually subsides. Nonpurposive symptoms, such as lacrimation, rhinorrhea, yawning, and sweating, appear about 8 to 12 hours after the last dose. About 12 to 14 hours after the last dose, the addict may fall into a tossing, restless sleep known as the "yen," which may last several hours but from which he awakens more restless and more miserable than before. As the syndrome progresses, additional signs and symptoms appear, consisting in dilated pupils, anorexia, gooseflesh, restlessness, irritability, and tremor. With morphine and heroin, nonpurposive symptoms reach their peak at 48 to 72 hours. As the syndrome approaches peak intensity, the patient exhibits increasing irritability, insomnia, marked anorexia, violent yawning, severe sneezing, lacrimation, and coryza. Weakness and depression are pronounced. Nausea and vomiting are common, as are intestinal spasm and diarrhea. Heart rate and blood pressure are elevated. Marked chilliness, alternating with flushing and excessive sweating, is characteristic. Pilomotor activity resulting in waves of gooseflesh is prominent, and the skin resembles that of a plucked turkey. This feature is the basis of the expression "cold turkey" to signify abrupt withdrawal without treatment. Abdominal cramps and pains in the bones and muscles of the back and extremities are also characteristic, as are the muscle spasms and kicking movements that may be the basis for the expression "kicking the habit." Other signs of CNS hyperexcitability

include ejaculation in men and orgasm in women. The respiratory response to CO_2, which is decreased during opioid administration, is exaggerated during withdrawal. Rebound phenomena are also observed in the endocrine system. During addiction, urinary 17-ketosteroid levels are decreased; during withdrawal, they increase markedly (Eisenman *et al.,* 1958). Leukocytosis is common, and white-cell counts above 14,000/cu mm are often seen.

The failure to take food and fluids, combined with vomiting, sweating, and diarrhea, results in marked weight loss, dehydration, ketosis, and disturbance in acid-base balance. Occasionally there is cardiovascular collapse. At any point in the course of withdrawal, the administration of a suitable opioid will completely and dramatically suppress the symptoms of withdrawal. Obviously, administration of a drug cannot immediately restore body fluids or acid-base balance, and in this sense the syndrome is not completely reversible. Without treatment, the syndrome runs its course and most of the grossly observable symptoms disappear in 7 to 10 days, but it is not certain how long it takes to restore physiological equilibrium completely.

It is now clear that the recovery process is complex and protracted, and that the early opioid abstinence syndrome characterized by the signs and symptoms described above is followed by a *protracted abstinence syndrome* during which a number of physiological variables attain subnormal values. For example, a period of hyposensitivity to the respiratory stimulant effects of CO_2 persists for many weeks after the exaggerated sensitivity of the early abstinence period subsides. In addition, there seem to be subtle behavioral manifestations of protracted abstinence that include an incapacity to tolerate stress, a poor self-image, and overconcern about discomfort. It is not unreasonable to postulate that these altered states contribute to the tendency of compulsive opioid users to relapse after withdrawal (*see* Dole, 1972; Martin *et al.,* 1973).

The *abrupt withdrawal of methadone* produces a syndrome that is qualitatively similar to that of morphine, but it develops more slowly and is more prolonged, although usually less intense. The addict has few or no symptoms until 24 to 48 hours after the last dose, and then complains of weakness, anxiety, anorexia, insomnia, abdominal discomfort, headache, sweating, pain in muscles and bones, and hot and cold flashes. As with morphine withdrawal, there is nausea, vomiting, and an increase in body temperature, blood pressure, pulse, respiratory rate, and pupillary size. In general, after abrupt withdrawal, the primary or early abstinence syndrome reaches its maximal intensity by about the third day, may not begin to decrease until the third week, and apparent recovery may not occur until the sixth or seventh week. The early abstinence syndrome is followed by a secondary or protracted abstinence syndrome in which a number of previously elevated physiological parameters attain and remain at subnormal values through the twenty-fourth postwithdrawal week, and there are concomitant psychological disturbances such as tiredness, weakness, hypochondriasis, and feelings of lessened efficiency (Isbell *et al.*, 1948; Martin *et al.*, 1973). Even with very slow reduction in dosage, patients who have been maintained on high doses of methadone experience qualitatively similar withdrawal symptoms during and following the period of dosage reduction (Cushman and Dole, 1973).

The *meperidine abstinence syndrome* usually develops within 3 hours after the last dose, reaches its peak within 8 to 12 hours, and then declines, so that few symptoms are apparent after 4 to 5 days. Craving may be intense, but the nonpurposive autonomic signs, while present, are not as prominent; the pupils may not be widely dilated, and there is usually little nausea, vomiting, or diarrhea. However, at peak intensity the muscle twitching, restlessness, and nervousness may be worse than during morphine withdrawal (Isbell and White, 1953).

Although *codeine* can partially suppress morphine withdrawal, withdrawal symptoms after codeine (1200 to 1800 mg per day), while qualitatively similar to those of morphine, are considerably less intense.

Withdrawal symptoms after semisynthetic and synthetic opioids are qualitatively similar to those after morphine, and they seem to follow the general rule that drugs with shorter durations of action tend to produce shorter, more intense abstinence syndromes while those drugs that are slowly eliminated produce withdrawal syndromes that are prolonged but mild. Some differences between the opioid withdrawal syndrome and those seen with agonist-antagonists are described in Chapter 15.

Withdrawal in the Newborn. Babies born to mothers who have been taking opioids regularly prior to delivery will be physically dependent. The withdrawal signs include irritability and excessive crying, tremors, hyperactive reflexes, increased respiratory rate, increased stools, sneezing, yawning, vomiting, and fever. With heroin or methadone, signs most commonly appear within the first few days of life. The intensity of the syndrome does not always correlate with the duration of maternal opioid use or dose. There is no consensus on the best method of managing withdrawal. Some clinicians use paregoric; others use phenobarbital or chlorpromazine (*see* Kahn *et al.*, 1969; Reddy *et al.*, 1971; Lipsitz and Blatman, 1974). Some investigators have expressed the view that babies born to mothers taking low doses of heroin fare better than those of mothers maintained on methadone, but the evidence for this is unconvincing (*see* Wilmarth and Goldstein, 1974).

Narcotic Antagonists. The abstinence syndromes described above are those seen when the drugs are abruptly withdrawn. If, however, the drug is not withdrawn but simply displaced from its site of action by an antagonist such as naloxone, a withdrawal syndrome develops within a few minutes after hypodermic administration and reaches its peak intensity within ½ hour. Until the antagonist is eliminated, even large doses of the previously used opioid cannot suppress the syndrome; partial suppression is possible, but only by using extremely large doses of opioid, which may then produce respiratory depression when the action of the antagonist is over. The intensity of naloxone-precipitated withdrawal is usually more severe than that seen after abrupt withdrawal of the drug. Methadone withdrawal produced in this way is especially severe.

With improvements in chemical methods for drug detection, narcotic antagonists are no longer used to detect drug use. Some clinicians have advocated their use in screening out nonphysically dependent opioid users seeking treatment in opioid maintenance programs. However, since antagonists may induce acute withdrawal phenomena after only a few days of opioid use (*see* Chapter 15), this procedure requires considerable experience.

GENERAL CNS DEPRESSANTS: BARBITURATES AND RELATED SEDATIVE-HYPNOTIC DRUGS

The subjective effects of barbiturates and related sedatives and antianxiety agents are detailed elsewhere. In general, they are similar to those of alcohol, and the effects vary considerably with the dose, the situation, and the personality of the user.

Prevalence, Agents Employed, and Patterns of Use. The incidence and prevalence of nonmedical and compulsive use of barbiturates and related drugs cannot be stated with accuracy, but it is believed to exceed greatly that of the opioids (*see* National

Commission, 1973). Illegal traffic in these drugs is common; in the jargon of the drug-using subculture, barbiturates are known as "goofballs" or "downs." Opioid users frequently take barbiturates or glutethimide to augment the effects of weak heroin, and many heroin users are physically dependent on both heroin and hypnotics. Some alcoholics use these agents to relieve the alcohol withdrawal syndrome or to produce a state of intoxication devoid of the odor of alcohol (Devenyi and Wilson, 1971; Freed, 1973). The short-acting barbiturates such as pentobarbital ("yellow jackets") or secobarbital ("red devils") are preferred to long-acting agents such as phenobarbital. Since the user is more interested in the pharmacological effects than in chemical classifications, it is not surprising that nonbarbiturates such as meprobamate, glutethimide, methyprylon, methaqualone, and some of the benzodiazepines are also abused. Paraldehyde and chloral hydrate, subject to considerable abuse in the past, have now been largely replaced by the other agents mentioned. Meprobamate seems less acceptable as a barbiturate substitute; and chlordiazepoxide, with its minimal euphoriant actions and slow onset of effects, is quite uncommon as a drug of abuse. Most users take the drugs orally, but there are a few individuals who inject barbiturates intravenously or intramuscularly. Such users can be recognized by the large abscesses that cover the accessible areas of their bodies.

The patterns of nonmedical use are as varied as those for alcohol and range from infrequent sprees of gross intoxication, lasting a few days, to the prolonged, compulsive, daily use of huge quantities and a preoccupation with securing and maintaining adequate supplies. The original contact with the drug may have been through a physician's prescription or through illicit drug trade. In the medical patient, the development of the problem may be a gradual one, beginning with prolonged use for insomnia and progressing through increased dosage at night to a few capsules for sedation in the morning. Eventually, the drug is a major part of the user's life. In such situations, what at one point could be considered a habituation at another is clearly an addiction; there is no sharp line that can be drawn between appro-

priate use, abuse, habituation, and addiction.

It has been observed that the combination of amphetamines and barbiturates produces more elevation of mood than either drug alone. The mechanisms of this supra-additive effect are not yet clear (Legge and Steinberg, 1962), but competition for the same microsomal enzyme system and hence production of higher blood concentrations of the drugs could be involved. Whether this phenomenon is responsible for the very common practice of simultaneous abuse of amphetamine and barbiturate is not certain.

The amount of hypnotic that may be taken varies considerably, but an average daily dose of 1.5 g of short-acting barbiturate is not uncommon, and some individuals have consumed as much as 2.5 g daily over many months. Similar multiples of the usual daily therapeutic doses are taken by the compulsive users of meprobamate, glutethimide, methyprylon, methaqualone, and diazepam. The abuse of sedative agents has been reviewed by Essig (1964, 1968).

Signs and Symptoms. Both the acute and the chronic effects of mild intoxication with barbiturates and related drugs resemble those of intoxication with alcohol. The intoxicated individual shows a general sluggishness, difficulty in thinking, slowness of speech and comprehension, poor memory, faulty judgment, narrowed range of attention, emotional lability, and exaggeration of basic personality traits. Irritability, quarrelsomeness, and moroseness are common. There may be laughing or crying without provocation, untidiness in personal habits, hostile and paranoid ideas, and suicidal tendencies (Isbell et al., 1950; Fraser et al., 1954).

The psychic and psychomotor effects of chronic barbiturate intoxication were studied in detail by Kornetsky (1951) and Hill and Belleville (1953). Chronic intoxication with pharmacologically similar agents has not been studied in as controlled a manner, but the clinical descriptions of isolated cases of abuse of high doses of meprobamate, chlordiazepoxide, and glutethimide are quite similar to the picture of chronic barbiturate intoxication. Neurological effects described here are those for barbiturates. These effects include thick, slurred speech, nystagmus, diplopia, strabismus, difficulty in accommodation, vertigo, ataxic gait, positive Romberg's sign, hypotonia, dysmetria, and decreased superficial reflexes; deep reflexes, pupillary responses, and sensation are usually unaltered. Occasionally transient ankle clonus and Babinski's signs are elicitable. Nutrition is usually unimpaired. Skin rashes may develop; they may be erythematous, urticarial, purpuric, or scarlatiniform. The urine may contain albumin and casts.

Tolerance, Physical Dependence, and Withdrawal Symptoms. Chronic intoxication with short-acting barbiturates and related hypnotics results in both drug-disposition and pharmacodynamic tolerance. The overall tolerance has an upper limit that gives chronic intoxication with hypnotics a very characteristic picture. For example, an individual tolerant to 1.2 g of pentobarbital per day may show little evidence of intoxication on that dose; however, if the dose is raised by as little as 0.1 g per day, prolonged and perhaps cumulative intoxication may occur (Isbell and White, 1953). It is also characteristic of adaptation to this class of agents that, while there may be considerable tolerance to the sedative and intoxicating effects, the lethal dose is not much greater in addicts than in normal individuals. Consequently, acute barbiturate or meprobamate poisoning may be accidentally or willfully superimposed on chronic intoxication at any time.

There are marked similarities between the withdrawal syndromes seen with barbiturates and those seen with meprobamate, glutethimide, methaqualone, and related drugs. It seems justified, therefore, to use the term *general depressant withdrawal syndrome* to refer to the manifestations of withdrawal from any of these agents. In its mildest form, the general depressant withdrawal syndrome may consist in only paroxysmal EEG abnormalities. Somewhat greater degrees of physical dependence result in tremulousness, anxiety, weakness, and insomnia. When the syndrome is severe, there may be, in addition, grand mal seizures and delirium.

The amount of barbiturate required to produce physical dependence in man has been carefully studied (Fraser *et al.,* 1958). It has been found that 0.2 g of pentobarbital per day can be ingested over many months without the development of any toler-

ance or physical dependence. After a daily dose of 0.4 g for 3 months, abrupt withdrawal produces paroxysmal EEG changes without other significant symptoms in about 30% of subjects. After 0.6 g per day for 1 to 2 months, 50% of subjects show minor withdrawal symptoms such as insomnia, anorexia, tremor, and EEG changes, and 10% may have a single seizure. When subjects are continuously intoxicated (0.9 to 2.2 g per day) for several months, 75% may have seizures and 66% delirium, and all experience insomnia, tremor, and anorexia on abrupt withdrawal. Haizlip and Ewing (1958) observed significant symptoms, similar to those described for barbiturates, after withdrawal of meprobamate that had been given at doses of 3.2 and 6.4 g for 40 days. Other hypnotics have not been as carefully studied (*see* Essig, 1964). Nonmedical use of methaqualone has been described by Inaba and associates (1973).

The typical course of withdrawal from large amounts of short-acting barbiturates is as follows: over the first 12 to 16 hours, as the blood concentration declines and the intoxication clears, the patient seems to improve but then becomes increasingly restless, anxious, tremulous, and weak. There may be complaints of abdominal cramps, nausea, and vomiting. Orthostatic hypotension is characteristic and may produce fainting if the patient stands up quickly. Within the first 24 hours, he may become too weak to get out of bed; coarse tremors of the hands are prominent, deep reflexes may be hyperactive, and the blink reflex is increased. During this period, *purposive behavior* is prominent and the patient may plead for his drug. With the short-acting barbiturates and meprobamate, the symptoms usually reach their peak during the second and third days of abstinence; convulsions, when they occur, are usually seen within this period. The number of seizures varies from a single one to *status epilepticus.*

With the longer-acting barbiturates and chlordiazepoxide, symptoms reach their peak more slowly, and seizures may not occur at all or may occur as late as the seventh to eighth day (Wulff, 1959; Hollister *et al.,* 1961). In Wulff's (1959) series, when the rate of elimination of the barbiturate was slower than 20% per day, EEG changes and withdrawal symptoms were not seen. Some patients who have seizures may begin to show improvement after the third day, but more than half go on to develop delirium. Anxiety mounts with time, and frightening dreams may be succeeded by a refractory insomnia. Visual hallucinations, usually of a persecutory nature, may occur, generally at the same time that sensorial clouding begins. Disorientation for time and place completes the picture of a full-blown delirium. Once the delirium develops, even the administration of large doses of barbiturate may not suppress it immediately. This is also true of the delirium that develops during the withdrawal of alcohol. The reason for this relative irreversibility is not clear.

During the delirium, which usually occurs between the fourth and seventh day, agitation and hyperthermia can lead to exhaustion and cardiovascular collapse. A number of deaths due to withdrawal of general depressants have been reported. The withdrawal syndrome, even if untreated, usually clears by about the eighth day, and clearing is generally preceded by a period of prolonged sleep. When hallucinations persist for several months, the situation would seem analogous to chronic alcoholic hallucinosis, which is felt by many investigators to be a manifestation of an underlying psychosis.

The spontaneous EEG during the second and third days of short-acting barbiturate withdrawal is characterized by dysrhythmias in the form of diffuse slowing, random slow waves, recurrent spikes, and high-voltage paroxysmal discharges of various sorts. Wulff (1959) has shown that photic stimulation will produce paroxysmal EEG changes in many patients who show no abnormalities in the resting EEG. Such changes were seen in over 90% of patients who exhibited abstinence phenomena and, therefore, may be of diagnostic significance.

Chronic use of multiple doses of hypnotics produces a decrease in rapid-eye-movement (REM) sleep and a marked decrease in stages 3 and 4. During drug withdrawal there is a large increase in REM sleep associated with an increase in frequency of dreaming. Sleep stages 3 and 4 return to normal without rebound (Kales *et al.,* 1974).

Babies born to mothers physically dependent on general CNS depressants will manifest withdrawal syndromes of varying severity (Desmond *et al.,* 1972). The signs are similar to those seen in the opioid withdrawal syndrome of the newborn.

ALCOHOL

Prevalence and Patterns of Use. In Western society, alcohol has the unique distinction of being the only potent pharmacological agent with which obvious self-induced intoxication is socially acceptable. In the United States, two thirds of all adults use alcohol occasionally, and at least 12% of the users can be considered "heavy" drinkers. If cigarette smoking is excluded, alcoholism is by far the most serious drug problem in the United States and most other countries. Measured in terms of accidents, lost productivity, crime, death, or damaged health, the combined social costs of problem drinking in the United States have been estimated to exceed 15 billion dollars annually. The cost in broken homes, wasted lives, loss to society, and human misery is beyond calculation.

There are different patterns of alcoholism in which there are varying degrees of psychological and nutritional complications, physical dependence (inability to abstain), "loss of control," and episodic use. In addition, problem drinkers may also abuse other drugs such as sedatives and amphetamines. Sometimes these are used in combination with alcohol; at other times, such drugs are taken in preference to alcohol, and alcohol is used only when the drug of choice is not available (*see* Freed, 1973).

The wide spectrum of alcohol use associated with adverse consequences makes it difficult to formulate any simple definition of alcoholism. The problem of definition has been addressed by the National Council on Alcoholism (1972), which has developed a set of comprehensive diagnostic criteria. Different people use alcohol for different reasons. For some it produces euphoria and releases emotions; for others it relieves depression or anxiety. However, other modes of reinforcement must come into play with chronic use since, after the first few days of drinking, alcoholics in laboratory settings often become more anxious and more depressed as drinking continues.

Tolerance, Physical Dependence, and Special Complications. Chronic use of alcohol results in an increased capacity to metabolize alcohol, which declines after several weeks of abstinence, so that abstinent alcoholics and normal individuals metabolize alcohol at about the same rate. Chronic use of alcohol also produces pharmacodynamic tolerance, so that a higher blood concentration is necessary to produce intoxication in tolerant than in normal individuals. Some alcoholics can perform well on difficult tasks when their blood alcohol concentrations are above 200 mg %, twice the value that in most states is legally defined as significant intoxication. However, as is the case with barbiturates, there is no marked elevation of the lethal dose, and severe acute intoxication with respiratory depression may be superimposed on chronic alcoholic intoxication at any time.

Cross-tolerance between alcohol and other drugs may be due to pharmacodynamic tolerance in the CNS or to more rapid metabolism, since alcohol use increases hepatic microsomal enzyme activity. Individuals tolerant to alcohol usually show cross-tolerance to general anesthetics; this cross-tolerance is probably a result of pharmacodynamic tolerance. There is also cross-tolerance to a variety of other sedative-hypnotics, which results from both pharmacodynamic (CNS) tolerance and from more rapid metabolism. However, cross-tolerance is seen only in the relatively sober alcoholic. When blood concentrations of alcohol are high, the effects of other drugs are additive to those of alcohol. In addition, there is some mutual inhibition of metabolism as a result of competition for shared enzymatic systems (*see* Kalant *et al.,* 1971; Hawkins and Kalant, 1972; Hug, 1972; Lieber, 1972; Sellers *et al.,* 1972). There is no cross-tolerance between alcohol and opioid drugs.

Maintenance of chronic high blood concentrations of alcohol produces a state of physical dependence. The signs and symptoms of the alcohol withdrawal syndrome are quite similar to those described for barbiturate withdrawal (*see* above). The intensity of the alcohol withdrawal syndrome correlates only partially with the amount of alcohol consumed and the duration of use. The poor correlation is probably due to the way in which alcohol is metabolized. The body is able to metabolize the alcoholic content of about 30 ml (1 oz) of whisky in an hour, so that if the intake is sufficiently spread out over the day the alcohol may be metabolized without any substantial increase in blood concentration. On the other hand, the ingestion of only modestly larger amounts, but spaced so that the body's metabolic capacity is exceeded (*e.g.,* 120 ml [4 oz] of whisky every 3 hours), can produce much higher blood concentrations, which can induce clinically significant physical dependence in a matter of a few days (*see* above). Withdrawal phenomena most commonly appear within 12 to 72 hours after total cessation of drinking. However, even a relative decline in blood concentration (*e.g.,* from 300 to 100 mg%) may precipitate the syndrome, and such declines may occur with changes in the pattern of drinking, as well as with decreases in the total daily intake.

The clinical picture of alcohol withdrawal described by Victor and Adams (1953) is still the basis for the delineation of three somewhat distinct withdrawal states—the tremulous syndrome, alcohol-related seizure disorders, and delirium tremens. However, there is much *overlapping,* as the following description indicates.

Tremulousness, which appears within a few hours after the last drink, is often accompanied by nausea, weakness, anxiety, and sweating. Purposive behavior directed toward obtaining alcohol or a suitable substitute is prominent. There may be cramps and vomiting. Hyperreflexia is prominent. Tremors may be mild or so marked that the patient may be unable to lift a glass. The subject may begin to "see things," at first only when the eyes are closed but later even while the eyes are open. Insight is at first retained, and the subject remains oriented. The syndrome at this point is often referred to as *acute alcoholic hallucinosis.* However, some experts feel that hallucinosis is not necessarily an index of the severity of the withdrawal syndrome; it is sometimes seen while alcoholics are severely intoxicated. Grand mal seizures can occur, but they are less common in alcohol withdrawal than in barbiturate withdrawal. The spontaneous EEG shows mild but definite dysrhythmias, in contrast to the major alterations seen during withdrawal of short-acting barbiturates (Wikler *et al.,* 1956). As in the case of barbiturates, however, photic stimulation often reveals paroxysmal abnormalities even when the spontaneous record appears normal. The REM phase of sleep that is depressed by alcohol shows a rebound increase during alcohol withdrawal.

The tremulous state reaches peak intensity within 24 to 48 hours, and seizures are most likely to occur within the first 24 hours after cessation of drinking. If the syndrome progresses further, insight is lost; the subject becomes weaker, more confused, disoriented, and agitated. He may be terrified by his persecutory hallucinations. They are often so vivid that the subject, even after recovery, sometimes doubts their unreality. At this stage, which appears around the third day of withdrawal, the picture is that of the *tremulous delirium,* which was first described by Thomas Sutton in 1813. Hyperthermia is common, and exhaustion and cardiovascular collapse may occur.

The alcohol abstinence syndrome is self-limited. If the patient does not die, recovery usually occurs within 5 to 7 days, without treatment. Those patients in whom the sensorium is clear but hallucinations persist well beyond the usual period of recovery are frequently found to be paranoid schizophrenics.

Babies born to mothers who drink heavily during pregnancy not only experience alcohol withdrawal after delivery but also, in some cases, are believed to suffer permanent mental retardation (Jones *et al.,* 1974).

A number of special problems are seen in chronic alcoholism that are not seen with other types of drug abuse. Most of these special problems are now thought to be related to multiple nutritional deficiencies that are, in turn, the result of the capacity of alcohol to supply calories and depress appetite without supplying essential vitamins and amino acids. They include peripheral polyneuropathies, pellagra, nutritional amblyopia, Wernicke's encephalopathy, and Korsakoff's psychosis. However, other disorders, such as fatty liver, cirrhosis of the liver, and damage to cardiac and skeletal muscle, once thought to be related to nutritional aberrations, may be due to direct toxic effects of alcohol itself (*see* Lieber, 1972; Chapter 11).

CNS Sympathomimetics:
Amphetamine and Related Drugs

The subjective effects of CNS sympathomimetics, like those of all centrally active drugs, are dependent on the user, the environment, the dose of the drug, and the route of administration. For example, moderate doses of amphetamine given orally to normal subjects commonly produce an elevation of mood, a sense of increased energy and alertness, and decreased appetite; task performance that has been impaired by fatigue or boredom is improved. Some individuals may become anxious, irritable, or loquacious. A few may experience transient drowsiness (Tecce and Cole, 1974), but insomnia is more common. As the dose is increased toward toxic levels, the effects of individual experiences and of environment become less significant. The general pharmacology of these agents is described in Chapter 24. When equated for differences in potency, a number of other CNS sympathomimetics and related agents can produce subjective effects that resemble those of amphetamine. These drugs include dextroamphetamine, methamphetamine, phenmetrazine, methylphenidate, and diethylpropion (*see* Martin *et al.,* 1971).

Cocaine addicts describe the euphoric effects of cocaine in terms that are almost indistinguishable from those used by amphetamine addicts. Cocaine also produces increased feelings of well-being in depressed patients (Post *et al.,* 1974), and the toxic syndrome seen with cocaine seems clinically indistinguishable from that produced by amphetamines. In addition, animals exhibit similar patterns of cocaine and amphetamine self-administration. The chewing of coca leaves is still common among the Peruvian Indians of the Andes. However, in the latter setting neither the intense preoccupation with drug use nor drug toxicity seems to occur (*see* Murphy *et al.,* 1969). In short, while it is commonly assumed that the subjective effects of cocaine are more intense and its abuse potential more significant than those of the amphetamines, reliable evidence for this assumption is difficult to obtain, and in this discussion cocaine will be considered as equivalent to a CNS sympathomimetic.

Considering these drugs as a class does not imply that they have identical mechanisms of action or that drug abusers cannot distinguish among them. For example, after intravenous administration of cocaine the effects are brief, lasting only a matter of minutes, whereas those of methamphetamine may last for hours. However, they cause very similar subjective effects, produce similar toxic syndromes, and, when one drug is unavailable for nonmedical use, others within the group may be substituted.

In summarizing the effects and nonmedical-use patterns of this group, *amphetamine will be taken as a prototype,* with significant differences pointed out where they occur.

Elevation of mood is the typical, rather than the atypical, response to CNS sympathomimetics. Perhaps it is the capacity of so many normal individuals to experience the drug-induced mood elevation without becoming compulsive users that made it difficult fully to appreciate the abuse potential of the amphetamine-like drugs. However, this attitude has been revised as a result of both the waves of amphetamine abuse that have occurred throughout the United States and a number of Western European countries, and the belated appreciation of the significance of the epidemic of intravenous methamphetamine addiction that occurred in Japan immediately after World War II (*see* Kalant, 1966). Amphetamines and several related drugs are now covered by the same federal regulations applicable to the opioids, and illicit transactions are subject to the same penalties.

Incidence and Patterns of Use. It is difficult to estimate the prevalence of use of sympathomimetic CNS stimulants in the general population. Nonmedical use of these drugs fluctuates widely over time in response to cycles of popularity. During the early 1970s there was a surprisingly high rate of nonmedical use among both civilian and military populations (*see* National Commission, 1973; Robins, 1974). Presently, in the United States there seems to be a substantial increase in the use of cocaine, but the use of intravenous amphetamines has decreased sharply compared to the period of the late 1960s. Increases in prevalence among young people often occur first among populations of delinquents or the emotionally disturbed.

There are a number of different patterns of amphetamine abuse. One involves those who first obtain the drug from a physician in the course of treatment for obesity or depression and then pass through a phase of habituation as described for barbiturates. Truck drivers and students who use the drug to stay awake may also follow this pattern. More often, the individual obtains the drug specifically for its euphoric effects. "Bennies" (BENZEDRINE), "dexies" (dextroamphetamine), and "ups" are terms commonly used to refer to oral preparations. Those who inject the drugs intravenously may dissolve oral tablets or use crystalline methamphetamine ("crystal") manufactured in illegal laboratories. Used intravenously, amphetamine and methamphetamine are known as "speed."

During the early phases of intravenous use, three or four doses of 20 to 40 mg of amphetamine are usually considered sufficient. In addition to the marked euphoria, the user experiences a sense of markedly enhanced physical strength and mental capacity, and feels little need for either sleep or food. Difficult to substantiate by objective means is the claim made by many users that orgasm in both male and female is delayed, permitting extended periods of sexual activity finally culminating in orgasms reported to be more intense and pleasurable (*see* Kramer *et al.,* 1967). The sensation of "flash" or "rush" that immediately follows intravenous administration, while qualitatively distinct from the opioid "rush," is nevertheless described as being intensely pleasurable and somewhat akin to sexual orgasm.

With time, tolerance develops; higher and more frequent doses are used, and toxic symptoms and signs then appear. These include bruxism, touching and picking of the face and extremities, suspiciousness, and a feeling of being watched. In addition, the user seems fascinated or preoccupied with his own thinking processes and with philosophical concerns about "meanings" and "essences." Stereotyped, repetitive behavior is common. Many patients who later show a full-blown toxic psychosis exhibit a compulsion to take apart mechanical objects. They also have a compulsion to put them together, but are usually too disorganized to do so. Both cocaine and amphetamine users commonly attempt to antagonize these effects with other drugs. The mixture of an opioid (the preferred antagonist) and either cocaine or an amphetamine is known as a "speedball." Many amphetamine users simultaneously consume large amounts of barbiturates or alcohol. Interestingly, subjects taking high doses of amphetamine in experimental settings generally exhibit depression and irritability rather than euphoria (Griffith *et al.,* 1972). Nevertheless, the amphetamine user continues his drug in spite of the toxic effects. The drug may be injected every 2 to 3 hours around the clock for periods of several days, during which time he may eat little and remain awake continuously. Such an episode or "run" commonly ends when the user is out of drug or too disorganized or paranoid to continue. Stopping is followed within a few hours by a deep sleep, which usually lasts 12 to 18 hours but which may last longer if the "run" has been an unusually long one. Upon awakening, users are extremely hungry and lethargic. Some are depressed. Much of the paranoid ideation is gone. The lethargy may persist for many days; reinitiation of drug use eliminates the lethargy and also starts a new cycle. During a "run" some addicts are reported to use as much as 1 g of methamphetamine intravenously every few hours.

Stereotyped behavior is also seen in animals given large doses of amphetamines. It is thought to involve dopaminergic structures in the corpus striatum and is blocked by selective lesions or dopamine antagonists (*see* Randrup and Munkvad, 1972). Animals self-administering cocaine or amphetamines often show a cyclic pattern of use with periods of spontaneous abstinence interposed between periods of use. With round-the-clock access to the drugs there is weight loss, self-mutilation, and death within about 2 weeks (*see* Yokel and Pickens, 1973).

Excessive doses of amphetamine may cause severe chest pain and unconsciousness. Excessive doses of cocaine may cause seizures and death from respiratory failure.

Unlike the user of morphine, whose drives are usually decreased, the user of CNS sympathomimetics is hyperactive and during a toxic episode may act in response to his persecutory delusions, carrying weapons and using them on the alleged persecutors. The stereotype of the "depraved dope fiend," once so inappropriately used to describe the opioid user, is not entirely unjustified when applied to the user of CNS sympathomimetics who develops toxic symptoms (*see* Ellinwood, 1971). Some individuals seem able to use the drug for months or years without developing a toxic paranoid syndrome, yet such symptoms can develop in the course of a single "run." (*See* Chapter 12.)

A small percentage of amphetamine addicts seem able to restrict drug intake and function productively (stabilized addicts). Others show progressive social and occupational deterioration, punctuated by periods of hospitalization for toxic psychosis. In terms of the compulsion to continue use, the degree to which a drug pervades the life of the user, and the tendency to relapse following withdrawal, the compulsive user of amphetamine or cocaine is an addict. It is not clear whether the amphetamine syndrome is as persistent as that produced by opioids. In the United States the waves of amphetamine use did not leave large numbers of chronic users in their wake. However, many intravenous users eventually became heroin users. Most observers have noted considerable psychopathology in compulsive amphetamine users and their families, which appeared to have antedated the drug use (*see* Connell, 1958; Kramer *et al.*, 1967; Angrist and Gershon, 1969; Ellinwood, 1969).

Tolerance, Toxicity, Physical Dependence, and Withdrawal Symptoms. Tolerance develops to the central effects of amphetamines, and the chronic user often increases the dose to continue to obtain the desired effect. Some users are able to take several hundred milligrams per day over prolonged periods. By suppressing appetite, high doses of amphetamine may foster ketosis; and, since amphetamine is excreted much more rapidly in acidic urine, some of the apparent tolerance may be due to more rapid elimination of the drug.

There is some question whether tolerance develops to cocaine. Cocaine addicts have been reported to use up to 10 g in a single day. However, it has been observed that after a period of abstinence an individual may be able to tolerate the same large individual doses that had been reached gradually during the period of chronic use. Given this observation and the known capacity of the liver to detoxicate cocaine rapidly, even the huge doses used by addicts do not necessarily demonstrate tolerance to cocaine. Animals self-administering cocaine reach high but stable dosage levels within a few days.

Cross-tolerance between the amphetamine-like sympathomimetics has been observed clinically, but cross-tolerance between cocaine and the amphetamine-like agents has not been reported. Tolerance to certain of the toxic effects on the CNS does not develop, and a toxic psychosis may occur after periods of weeks to months of continued use. Tolerance to amphetamines has been reviewed by Kalant and associates (1971) and Hug (1972).

The fully developed toxic syndrome from amphetamine is characterized by vivid visual, auditory, and sometimes tactile hallucinations; picking and excoriation of the skin and delusions of parasitosis are not uncommon. There is also paranoid ideation, loosening of associations, and changes in affect occurring in association with a *clear sensorium*. In chronic users, there may be a striking paucity of sympathomimetic effects, and the blood pressure is not unduly elevated. It is often extremely difficult to differentiate this syndrome from a schizophrenic reaction (Connell, 1958; Angrist and Gershon, 1969; Ellinwood, 1969). Although the psychotic symptoms are slower to appear than after the use of cocaine, the syndrome may be seen as soon as 36 to 48 hours after the ingestion of a single large dose of amphetamine. In apparently sensitive individuals, psychosis may be produced by single large doses, for example, 55 to 75 mg of dextroamphetamine. Probably, with high enough doses, psychosis can be induced in anyone (Griffith *et al.*, 1972). Although there are obvious differences in sensitivity to the toxic effects, in general those who become psychotic are users of larger doses. After single large doses, amphetamine is slowly excreted over 5 to 7 days (Connell, 1958), suggesting the possibility that cumulative effects might occur with repeated adminis- tration. Unless the individual continues to use the drug, the psychosis usually clears within a week, the hallucinations being the first symptoms to disappear. Acidic urine is associated with a shorter plasma half-life of amphetamine and a more rapid clearing of the psychosis. Some work suggests that metabolites may play a role in amphetamine psychosis (Ånggård et al., 1973).

For a long time it was believed that, except for drug craving, prolonged sleep, general fatigue, lassitude, and depression, there were no withdrawal symptoms from ampheta- mine-like drugs and, therefore, no physical dependence. However, this view has been under reconsideration for some time. It is still considered true that abrupt discontinuation of sympathomimetic amines does not cause major, grossly observable, physiological dis- ruptions that would necessitate the gradual withdrawal of the drug. But the prolonged sleep, lassitude, fatigue, and hyperphagia, as well as the occasionally reported profound depression, that follow discontinuation of these drugs are difficult to attribute merely to the preceding loss of sleep and weight. In addition, amphetamines suppress the REM phase of sleep, and after abrupt withdrawal of large doses the EEG pattern shows a re- bound increase in this phase of sleep (Oswald and Thacore, 1963). Similar REM suppression followed by rebound is seen after chronic administration of cocaine (Post et al., 1974). Most observers now recognize the existence of a withdrawal syndrome fol- lowing discontinuation of amphetamine-like drugs. Its role in perpetuating drug use or relapse is not clear.

NICOTINE (TOBACCO)

The use of tobacco is so common that it is super- fluous to describe the varied patterns of use or the overt behavior of the users. Indeed, smoking is so widespread that it is rarely viewed as a form of drug "abuse" or as an addiction even though it fits all of the accepted criteria for drug dependence (see Russell, 1971; Brecher, 1972). The pharmacological effects of nicotine and some of the adverse conse- quences of smoking tobacco are considered in Chapter 27.

Tobacco use is unique, in that all its potential adverse effects are associated with chronic rather than experimental or occasional use. Public aware- ness of the serious health consequences of smoking has not had any dramatic effect on tobacco use for the population as a whole, and in the United States the incidence and prevalence of cigarette smoking are now increasing among young people.

There is considerable evidence that nico- tine is the reinforcing constituent that gives tobacco its universal popularity (see Domino, 1973; Jarvik, 1973). While animals will self- administer nicotine, it is not a particularly powerful reinforcer as compared to other drugs. Why it creates so enduring a pattern of self-administration is still uncertain. It does seem clear that smokers may continue to smoke for very different reasons; some smoke for enjoyment or social reinforcement, some to alleviate primary distress such as anger, fear, or shame, and some to avoid the distress experienced when deprived of to- bacco.

It seems clear that pharmacological factors interact with environmental stimuli and so- cial reinforcers so that after thousands of repetitions a puff on a cigarette has consid- erably more reinforcing effect than it did originally. (For references, see Russell, 1971; Dunn, 1973.)

Tolerance, Physical Dependence, and Re- lapse. Tolerance develops to some, but not all, of the effects of nicotine. The question of nicotine physical dependence is somewhat controversial. While some heavy smokers state that they feel few effects even when they stop smoking abruptly, others report a syndrome of irritability, aggressiveness, hostility, depression, and difficulty in con- centrating that lasts for several days after discontinuation. These symptoms are ac- companied by changes in the EEG and autonomic function. Many of these phe- nomena can be considered rebound effects from the actions of nicotine (see Russell, 1971; Dunn, 1973). Whether some smokers also have a protracted abstinence syndrome or whether abstinence phenomena become conditioned to environmental stimuli is still unclear. However, it is clear that the rate of relapse among compulsive smokers who seek treatment is discouragingly high, with only 25% still not smoking 2 years after cessation, regardless of the specific treatment used (see Brecher, 1972). A Bibliography on Smoking *and Health* published annually is available from the U.S. Government Printing Office.

CANNABINOIDS (MARIHUANA)

History and Source. *Cannabis,* obtained from the flowering tops of *hemp* plants, is a very ancient drug. Other names for cannabis or its products include *hashish, charas, bhang, ganja, dagga,* and *marihuana.* The common hemp is an herbaceous annual, of which *Cannabis sativa* is the sole species and *Cannabis sativa* var. *indica* and var. *americana* are two varieties. While all parts of both the male and the female plant contain psychoactive substances (cannabinoids), the highest cannabinoid concentrations are found in the flowering tops. In the Middle East and North Africa the dried resinous exudate of the tops is called *hashish;* in the Far East it is called *charas.* The dried leaves and flowering shoots of the plant, containing smaller amounts of the active substance, are called *bhang,* and the resinous mass from the small leaves and brackets of inflorescence is called *ganja.* In the United States, the term *marihuana* is used to refer to any part of the plant or extract therefrom that induces somatic and psychic changes in man. Most commonly, the plant is cut, dried, chopped, and incorporated into cigarettes.

Chemistry. Among the cannabinoids synthesized by the hemp plant are cannabinol, cannabidiol, cannabinolic acid, cannabigerol, cannabicyclol, and several isomers of tetrahydrocannabinol. The isomer believed responsible for most of the characteristic psychological effects of marihuana is *l*-Δ^9-tetrahydrocannabinol (Δ^9-THC), also referred to as *l*-Δ^1-THC. The effects of *l*-Δ^8-THC, which occurs in minute amounts in marihuana, are similar to those of *l*-Δ^9-THC. Both isomers are viscous, noncrystalline, water-insoluble compounds.

Δ^9-THC has the following structure:

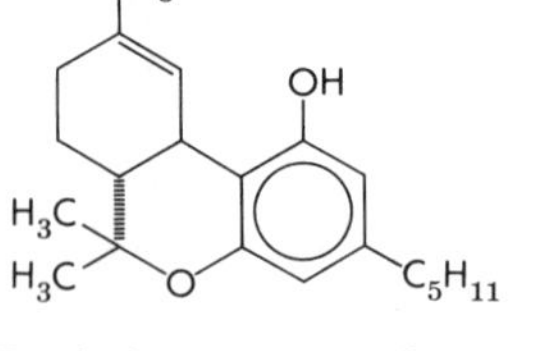

Tetrahydrocannabinol (Δ^9-THC)

Many derivatives of tetrahydrocannabinol have been synthesized and studied, and some of these are more potent than the natural plant products.

Pharmacological Effects in Animals. In rats and mice, Δ^9-THC or extracts of cannabis produce a decrease in spontaneous behavior associated with an altered responsivity to stimuli. There is a dose-dependent hypothermia. In monkeys, both Δ^9-THC and Δ^8-THC produce sedation, decrease in aggressive behavior, loss of ability or motivation to perform complex tasks, and apparent hallucinations. Δ^9-THC and several of its synthetic congeners have a number of actions not unlike those of the barbiturates. They prolong hexobarbital sleeping time, exhibit anti-convulsant activity, raise the threshold for EEG and behavioral arousal, and depress polysynaptic reflexes. Yet they may also prolong the stimulant action of amphetamine.

Pharmacological Effects in Man. Δ^9-THC exerts its most prominent effects on the CNS and cardiovascular system. Because of differences due to dose, route of administration, setting, and the experience and expectations of subjects, condensed descriptions of the behavioral responses to Δ^9-THC are difficult and sometimes misleading.

In the United States, an average marihuana cigarette delivers the equivalent of 2.5 to 5 mg of Δ^9-THC. Doses in this range or slightly higher produce effects on mood, memory, motor coordination, cognitive ability, sensorium, time sense, and self-perception. Most commonly there is an increased sense of well-being or euphoria, accompanied by feelings of relaxation and sleepiness when subjects are alone; where users can interact, sleepiness is less pronounced and there is often spontaneous laughter (Hollister, 1971; Jones, 1971; Secretary, 1972). The sleepiness contrasts with the effects of LSD and related hallucinogens, which induce a state of arousal. With oral doses of Δ^9-THC that are equivalent to several cigarettes, short-term memory is impaired and there is a deterioration in capacity to carry out tasks requiring multiple mental steps to reach a specific goal. This effect on memory-dependent, goal-directed behavior has been called "temporal disintegration," and is correlated with a tendency to confuse past, present, and future, and with depersonalization—a sense of strangeness and unreality about the self (Melges *et al.,* 1970). Balance and stability of stance are affected even at low doses (Evans *et al.,* 1973), effects that are more apparent when the eyes are closed. Decreases in muscle strength and hand steadiness can be demonstrated. Although performance of relatively simple motor tasks and simple reaction times are relatively unimpaired until higher doses are reached, more complex tasks, such as those involved in driving, may be affected by doses equivalent to two cigarettes (*see* Rafaelsen *et al.,* 1973). Research subjects routinely report that they feel unable to drive while "high" on oral doses of Δ^9-THC.

Marihuana smokers frequently report increased hunger, dry mouth and throat, more vivid visual imagery, and a keener sense of hearing. Subtle visual and auditory stimuli previously ignored may take on a novel quality, and the nondominant senses of touch, taste, and smell seem to be enhanced. Altered time perception is a consistent effect of cannabinoids. Time seems to pass more slowly—minutes may seem like hours (*see* Hollister, 1971; Secretary, 1972). The effects on the EEG are not prominent, resembling those seen in the drowsy state. In a single case, electrodes in deep brain structures recorded high-voltage, slow-wave activity in septal leads, corresponding to the subjective elevation of mood (Heath, 1972).

Higher doses of Δ^9-THC can induce frank hallucinations, delusions, and paranoid feelings. Thinking becomes confused and disorganized; depersonalization and altered time sense are accentuated. Anxiety reaching panic proportions may replace euphoria, often as a result of the feeling that the drug-induced state will never end. With high enough doses, the clinical picture is that of a toxic psychosis with hallucinations, depersonalization, and loss of insight (*see* Nahas, 1973; Chopra and Smith, 1974). Because of the rapid onset of effects when marihuana is smoked and the low Δ^9-THC content of marihuana grown in the United States, most users are able to regulate their intake in order to avoid the excessive dosage that produces these unpleasant effects; psychiatric emergencies as a result of smoking marihuana are quite uncommon.

The most consistent effects on the cardiovascular system are an increase in heart rate and a marked reddening of the conjunctivae. Propranolol, a β-adrenergic blocking agent, prevents the tachycardia produced by Δ^9-THC, but it does not interfere with the subjective and behavioral effects (*see* Drew *et al.*, 1972). The increase in heart rate is dose related, and its onset and duration correlate well with blood concentrations of Δ^9-THC. Increases of 20 to 50 beats per minute are usual, but a tachycardia of 140 beats per minute is not uncommon. Urinary excretion of free epinephrine is increased, but the amount of free norepinephrine is unchanged (Weiss *et al.*, 1972). There are no consistent changes in respiratory rate or deep-tendon reflexes. There is a very slight tendency toward lowered oral temperature. Pupillary size is not significantly altered, although intraocular pressure may be decreased.

While there are similarities between the subjective effects of Δ^9-THC at high doses and those of LSD, there are also substantial differences, and cannabinoids should therefore be considered as a separate and distinct pharmacological class. The mechanism of action of Δ^9-THC is unknown. The psychological effects are not prevented by pretreatment with alpha-methylparatyrosine (Hollister, 1974), which reduces brain concentrations of dopamine and norepinephrine, although such pretreatment does eliminate the euphoria produced by amphetamine and partially eliminates the euphoria produced by ethanol. Patients maintained on lithium or methadone continue to experience the effects of marihuana without apparent alteration. Applied directly to a vagus nerve preparation, Δ^9-THC reduces the size of the compound action potential recorded from nonmyelinated fibers (Byck and·Ritchie, 1973). In animals, high doses of Δ^9-THC alter brain concentrations of 5-HT, but substantial behavioral effects of Δ^9-THC are seen with lower doses that have no effects on brain 5-HT.

Chronic smoking of marihuana and hashish has long been associated with bronchitis and asthma. While suppression of immune responses (Nahas *et al.*, 1974) and decreased plasma testosterone (Kolodny *et al.*, 1974) in man have been reported, studies of predominantly lower-income chronic users in several parts of the world did not reveal any striking impairment of physical health or psychological functioning (*see* Secretary, 1972; Beaubrun and Knight, 1973). However, some United States Army enlisted men using high doses of hashish on a chronic basis exhibited apathy, dullness, and impairment of judgment, concentration, and memory, associated with a loss of interest in personal appearance, hygiene, and diet. After discontinuation, memory, alertness, concentration, and calculating ability returned to normal within 2 to 4 weeks, but several men seemed to exhibit continued intermittent residual symptoms (memory loss, confusion, inability to calculate and concentrate) similar to those seen with organic brain disease (Tennant and Groesbeck, 1972). Such *chronic high-dosage* use is not common in the United States, but some clinicians have described subtle changes in personality and decreased interest in achievement and pursuit of conventional goals (the amotivational syndrome) in young marihuana users who regularly smoke a few cigarettes a day. At present, there is no evidence to suggest that any such personality changes are due to organic brain damage. Differences between chronic users and nonusers may be due to factors that antedate drug use, but the possibility of an adverse effect of frequent or chronic low levels of intoxication on developing personality cannot be dismissed.

Absorption, Fate, and Excretion. Low-grade marihuana may contain less than 0.5% Δ^9-THC, while some Asian varieties may contain more than 3%. It is estimated that, even when smoked with maximal efficiency, no more than 50% of Δ^9-THC in a marihuana cigarette is actually absorbed. Thus, a 500-mg cigarette containing 1% Δ^9-THC would deliver at most 2.5 mg of Δ^9-THC to the lungs. Pharmacological effects occur within minutes after smoking begins and plasma concentrations reach their peak at 10 to 30 minutes. Unless more is smoked, the effects of a cigarette seldom last longer than 2 or 3 hours. After oral administration, the onset of effects usually occurs at about ½ to 1 hour; peak effects may not occur until the second or third hour and correlate well with plasma concentrations. Effects may persist for 3 to 5 hours. Although gastrointestinal absorption is largely complete, Δ^9-THC is approximately three times more potent when smoked than when taken by mouth (*see* Hollister, 1971; Secretary, 1972).

Δ^9-THC is rapidly converted into an active metabolite, 11-hydroxy-Δ^9-THC, which produces effects identical to those of the parent compound. 11-Hydroxy-Δ^9-THC is, in turn, converted into a more polar, inactive metabolite (8,11-dihydroxy-THC), which is then excreted in the urine and feces. Metabolites excreted in the bile may be reabsorbed. Very little unmetabolized Δ^9-THC is found in the urine. After reaching their peaks, plasma concentrations of Δ^9-THC and 11-hydroxy-Δ^9-THC fall rapidly at first (half-time of minutes), reflecting the redistribution of these lipophilic compounds to lipid-rich tissues, including the CNS. This first phase of rapid decline is followed by a much slower phase (half-time of days), reflecting the gradual metabolism and elimination of the drug from the body. Traces of Δ^9-THC and its metabolites persist in the plasma of man for several days and can be detected in the fat and brain of animals for days after a single administration. Metabolites can be found in the urine for days or weeks (*see* Hollister, 1971; Lemberger *et al.*, 1972; Perez-Reyes *et al.*, 1972; Secretary, 1972). Δ^9-THC crosses the placental barrier. Consumption of repeated oral doses of Δ^9-THC by man for several days or its daily smoking for several weeks does not seem to produce clinically detectable evidence of accumulation, but this does not preclude the possibility that such would not occur over a more prolonged period or with higher doses. Chronic marihuana smokers metabolize Δ^9-THC more rapidly than do nonsmokers (Lemberger *et al.*, 1971).

Tolerance and Physical Dependence. In animals, tolerance develops to the lethal, hypothermic, and some of the behavioral effects of cannabinoids. While in certain species the degree of tolerance is remarkable, it may not develop to all the effects of the drug. Its duration after the drug is discontinued is dependent on the dose, frequency of administration, and the particular species. It is not clear how much of the tolerance is due to a more rapid metabolic disposition of the drug and how much is due to functional or pharmacodynamic adaptations in the CNS (*see* Harris, 1971; Secretary, 1972; Nahas, 1973).

Reports from many countries throughout the world indicate that a number of regular users of hashish consume amounts of Δ^9-THC that would produce toxic effects in most Western users. Some American soldiers in Europe smoked amounts of hashish that were equivalent to 5000 to 6000 marihuana cigarettes per month (Tennant and Groesbeck, 1972). Volunteers in chronic experiments tend to increase the number of marihuana cigarettes or oral intake of synthetic cannabinoid as the experiment progresses and to show decreased drug effects (Williams *et al.*, 1946; Mendelson and Meyer, 1972). However, if the total dosage used is low, subjects continue to experience a "high" after the first cigarette of the day (Mendelson and Meyer, 1972). Daily use of low doses may not be sufficient to induce any remarkable degree of tolerance. Experienced users may actually report more subjective effects from smoking marihuana than naive subjects. However, they generally show less impairment of perceptual and motor functions, as well as smaller increases in heart rate. At the same time, experienced users may be less able to discriminate between cigarettes that contain Δ^9-THC and cigarettes that do not. Either they tend to get "high" on placebos, or there are conditioned aspects to the subjective effects for which the act of smoking marihuana not containing Δ^9-THC is an adequate stimulus (*see* Jones, 1971; Secretary, 1972).

Some degree of cross-tolerance between alcohol and Δ^9-THC has been observed in rats. However, there is no cross-tolerance between cannabinoids and the psychedelics (hallucinogens).

While there are reports that abrupt discontinuation of cannabinoids after chronic use of high dosage is followed by irritability, restlessness, nervousness, and insomnia, there is no generally recognized or sharply defined cannabinoid withdrawal syndrome. However, some heavy chronic users may have considerable difficulty in giving up the use of marihuana (*see* Jones, 1971; Nahas, 1973).

Therapeutic Uses. Although cannabis was once used for a wide variety of clinical disorders and has even been demonstrated to have antibacterial activity, there are at present no substantiated indications for its use. Despite its capacity to elevate mood, Δ^9-THC does not seem to have clinically useful antidepressant actions (Kotin *et al.*, 1973).

Patterns of Use and Related Social Issues. Over the past decade the smoking of marihuana (also known as grass, pot, tea, reefer, weed, and Mary Jane) has increased greatly in the United States and in other English-speaking and European countries. The concern about the increased use and the illegal status of marihuana was a major factor in the creation of a special commission to study drug-use problems in several countries (*e.g.,* the United States, Canada, New Zealand, Great Britain). In the United States, by 1972, 16% of the adult and 14% of the juvenile population had used marihuana at least once, and 8 and 7%, respectively, continued to use it at least occasionally. However, only a small percentage of those who continue to use marihuana do so on a daily basis (National Commission, 1972, 1973). While use still occurs primarily among adolescents and young adults, by 1972 older adults were beginning to experiment with marihuana, including substantial numbers of younger physicians, medical students, nurses, lawyers, and teachers.

The National Commission (1973) concluded that the risks associated with current patterns of use in the United States did not warrant *criminal* penalties for possession of small amounts for personal use, and recommended that such penalties should be eliminated, that use should be discouraged, and that only sale should be subject to criminal sanctions. The Canadian Commission made similar recommendations with respect to marihuana (*see* Government of Canada, 1973). It is likely that "recreational" use by large numbers of people will eventually be associated with chronic heavy use by a few. It remains to be seen just what the long-term medical and public health consequences of such heavy use will be.

PSYCHEDELICS (HALLUCINOGENS, PSYCHOTOMIMETICS, PSYCHOTOGENS)

There is no sharp line that divides the psychedelics from other classes of centrally active drugs. Under certain conditions, or at toxic dosage, several classes of drugs (anticholinergics, bromides, antimalarials, opioid antagonists, cocaine, amphetamines, and corticosteroids) can induce illusions, hallucinations, delusions, paranoid ideations, and other alterations of mood and thinking that are observed in spontaneously occurring psychotic states. However, despite the legal terminology that defines lysergic acid diethylamide (LSD) and related drugs as hallucinogens, the production of hallucinations is not the most useful way to describe the very interesting pharmacological effects of this group of drugs.

The psychedelic drugs to be discussed here can, indeed, produce such pathological effects as the terms *hallucinogenic, psychotomimetic,* and *psychotogenic* imply, but the feature that distinguishes the psychedelic agents from other classes of drugs is their capacity reliably to induce or compel states of altered perception, thought, and feeling that are not (or cannot be) experienced otherwise except in dreams or at times of religious exaltation.

Most descriptions of the "psychedelic state" include several major effects. There is heightened awareness of sensory input, often accompanied by an enhanced sense of clarity, but a diminished control over what is

experienced. Frequently there is a feeling that one part of the self seems to be a passive observer (a "spectator ego") rather than an active organizing and directing force, while another part of the self participates and receives the vivid and unusual sensory experiences. The environment may be perceived as novel, often beautiful, and harmonious. The attention of the user is turned inward, preempted by the seeming clarity and portentous quality of his own thinking processes. In this state the slightest sensation may take on profound meaning. Indeed, "meaningfulness" seems more important than what is meant, and the "sense of truth" more significant than what is true. Commonly, there is a diminished capacity to differentiate the boundaries of one object from another and of the self from the environment. Associated with the loss of boundaries there may be a sense of union with "mankind" or the "cosmos." To the extent that these drugs reveal this innate capacity of the mind to see more than it can tell and to experience and believe more than it can explain, the term *mind expanding* is not entirely inappropriate (Freedman, 1968).

As with any scheme of classification, the choice of agents to include or exclude is somewhat arbitrary. Most of the drugs that are generally included among the psychedelics are related either to the indolealkylamines, such as LSD, psilocybin, psilocin, dimethyltryptamine (DMT), and diethyltryptamine (DET), or to the phenylethylamines (mescaline) or phenylisopropylamines, such as 2,5-dimethoxy-4-methylamphetamine (DOM, "STP"), 2,5-dimethoxy-4-ethylamphetamine (DOE), and 3-methoxy-4,5-methylenedioxyamphetamine (MMDA). While the cannabinoids produce a number of psychological effects that are quite similar to those of drugs that are classified here as psychedelics, they also exhibit sufficient differences to justify a separate classification. The descriptions of the subjective effects of nitrous oxide and ethyl ether (not included here as psychedelics) are in some ways similar to those of the agents considered here (*see* Nagle, 1968), illustrating the arbitrary nature of classification schemes.

LSD and Related Compounds. The history, chemistry, research uses, and mechanisms of action of LSD and related drugs are presented in Chapter 12. Attention is here directed to their effects in man and to the patterns and consequences of their self-administration.

Pharmacological Effects. In man, oral

doses of LSD as low as 20 to 25 μg produce CNS effects in susceptible individuals. At such doses there are few detectable effects on other organ systems.

Some of the features that distinguish the psychedelic state from other effects produced by drugs have already been described. In addition, LSD produces somatic effects largely sympathomimetic in nature, such as pupillary dilatation, increase in blood pressure, tachycardia, hyperreflexia, tremor, nausea, piloerection, muscular weakness, and increased body temperature.

Following oral doses of 0.5 to 2.0 μg/kg the somatic symptoms are usually perceived within a few minutes. These include dizziness, weakness, drowsiness, nausea, and paresthesias. They may be followed by a feeling of inner tension relieved by laughing or crying. Several feelings may seem to coexist at the same time. In the second or third hour, visual illusions, wavelike recurrences of perceptual changes (*e.g.,* micropsia, macropsia), and affective symptoms may occur. There may be difficulty in locating the source of a sound; the user may be hypervigilant or withdrawn, or may alternate between these states. With many subjects there is a fear of fragmentation or disintegration of the self. Afterimages are prolonged, and the overlapping of present and preceding perceptions occurs. Some subjects recognize these confluences, whereas others elaborate them into hallucinations. In contrast to naturally occurring psychoses, auditory hallucinations are rare. Synesthesias, the overflow from one sensory modality to another, may occur. Colors are heard and sounds may be seen. Subjective time is also seriously altered, so that clock time seems to pass extremely slowly. The loss of boundaries and the fear of fragmentation create a need for a structuring or supporting environment; and, in the sense that they create a need for experienced companions and an explanatory system, these drugs are "cultogenic." During the "trip," thoughts and memories can vividly emerge under self-guidance or unexpectedly, to the user's distress. There may be a crossover of the affect of what is recalled with the content of what is presently perceived. Mood may be labile, shifting from depression to gaiety, from elation to fear. Tension and anxiety may mount and reach panic proportions. After about 4 to 5 hours, if a major panic episode does not occur, there may be a sense of detachment and the conviction that one is magically in control.

Between the dose ranges of 1 to 16 μg/kg, the severity of the psychophysiological effects of LSD is proportional to the dose. The entire syndrome, including the pupillary dilatation, begins to clear after about 12 hours, although the half-life of the drug in man is approximately 3 hours. (For references and more detailed description, *see* Cohen, 1967; Freedman, 1969.)

Miscellaneous effects include decreased free-water clearance due to an antidiuretic action, decreased urinary clearance of creatinine and phosphorus, and an elevation of plasma free fatty acids, effects that are also seen with mescaline.

While the user may be greatly impressed with the drug experience and feel a greater sensitivity for art, music, human feelings, and the harmony of the universe, there is little evidence for long-term changes in personality, beliefs, values, or behavior (McGlothlin and Arnold, 1971).

Although the patterns of psychological and biochemical effects seen with other agents are quite similar to those with LSD, there are significant differences in potency, absorption, metabolism, duration of action, and the slope of the dose-response curves. DMT, for example, is inactive by mouth and must be injected, sniffed, or smoked to produce effects. LSD is longer acting and more than 100 times as potent as psilocybin and psilocin, the active alkaloids in the Mexican "magic mushroom"; it is 4000 times as potent as mescaline in producing altered states of consciousness. There may also be some differences in the frequency of somatic effects, such as more vomiting with mescaline. The effects of an oral dose of mescaline (about 5 mg/kg) persist for about 12 hours. DOM and DOE are particularly interesting in that at low doses they produce mild euphoria and enhanced self-awareness without perceptual distortion or hallucinogenic effects. At higher doses DOM has typical psychedelic activity, but with DOE there appears to be a rather wide dose range over which euphoria and self-awareness are produced without perceptual distortions (Snyder *et al.,* 1971).

Incidence and Patterns of Use. In the United States, the use of LSD ("acid") and related psychedelics reached a peak of popularity in the late 1960s and thereafter gradually declined. While they are now controlled by federal and state laws prescribing severe penalties for their possession or distribution, psychedelic drugs are manufactured illegally and are still available through illicit channels. The decline in popularity appears to be related to a fuller realization of the real and potential hazards of these drugs (*see* below), and to a decrease in their fascination for the mass media, whose repeated and seductive descriptions of the psychedelic subculture and its prophets contributed greatly to the epidemic and to a saturation of the "population at risk." As noted already, these drugs in general do not give rise to patterns of repetitive use over prolonged periods.

Used more by college students, the affluent, and the artistic than by the poor or the sociopathic, the most common psychedelic-use pattern is the occasional "trip," separated by intervals of weeks or months during which marihuana is used with variable frequency. The "acid head," or chronic user, is quite uncommon, and even among this group "trips" are rarely more frequent than biweekly. Chronic users may complain of memory difficulties and seem to exhibit extreme passivity. They tend to avoid competitive situations, equating these with anger and aggression. The relationship of such characteristics to the repeated drug experience is not clear (*see* Blacker *et al.*, 1968). For purposes of "trip" taking, other psychedelics (*e.g.*, mescaline, psilocybin, DMT, DOM) are generally viewed as interchangeable with LSD, although users are generally cognizant of the differences in potency, somatic side effects, and durations of action. At the peak of concern over the possible effects of LSD on chromosomes, most users of psychedelics made an effort to purchase mescaline. However, almost all the "mescaline" that was being sold on the illicit market was actually LSD. For most users the "psychedelic scene" tends to become less interesting with time. Even though the smoking of marihuana may continue, the use of the potent psychedelics is generally discontinued (*see* McGlothlin and Arnold, 1971).

Tolerance, Toxicity, and Physical Dependence. A high degree of tolerance to the behavioral effects of LSD develops after three or four daily doses; sensitivity returns after a comparable drug-free interval. There is considerable cross-tolerance between LSD, mescaline, and psilocybin, but none between LSD and the amphetamines. Withdrawal phenomena are not seen after abrupt discontinuation.

The "therapeutic ratio" of LSD is exceedingly high if the dose required to produce psychological effects is compared with the lethal dose. In man, deaths attributable to direct drug effects are unknown, although fatal accidents and suicides during states of LSD intoxication have been reported. Death due to overdosage in animals results from respiratory failure, but in rabbits there is a marked hyperthermia as well. In spite of the concern about chromosomal aberrations and teratogenic effects induced by LSD, the evidence is contradictory and of uncertain significance. First, the chromosomal damage from LSD may be no greater than that produced by many common drugs. In addition, heavy drug users, regardless of the type of drug used, may differ from nondrug users in terms of nutrition and frequency of viral infections, so that even clear-cut differences may not be drug related. Lastly, the medical significance of chromosomal breakage is unknown (*see* Kato and Jarvik, 1969; Gilmour *et al.*, 1971). Improvements in cytogenetic technics should clarify this problem. Similarly, whereas LSD given to animals during pregnancy can produce abortions, stillbirths, and deformities, it is not clear that these effects occur with the doses used by man. Among women who received pure LSD in medical settings months or years prior to conception, there was a slightly higher risk of spontaneous abortion, but no significant increase in birth defects. However, the effects of LSD during pregnancy are still uncertain (*see* Jacobson and Berlin, 1972). Among American Indian tribes that have used mescaline for several generations there appears to be no striking increase in genetic abnormalities or congenital malformations.

The evidence for significant psychological hazards in the use of psychedelic agents is unambiguous. The most common adverse effect is a temporary (24-hour) episode of panic—a "bad trip." This can be treated by reassurance in a supportive environment, antianxiety agents, phenothiazines, or induction of sleep with barbiturates. Such "bad trips" cannot be reliably prevented and have been experienced even by users who had previous "good trips." Recurrences of drug effects without the drug, "flashbacks," are a puzzling but treatable phenomenon. In some individuals the use of psychedelics can precipitate serious depressions, paranoid behavior, or prolonged psychotic episodes. Whether such episodes would have occurred without the drug is not clear (*see* Cohen, 1967; Freedman, 1969). Prolonged psychotic episodes following repeated use of LSD tend to resemble the schizophreniform psychotic state and may require large doses of a phenothiazine for their control (Bowers, 1972). There is the possibility that repeated use of LSD can induce subtle deficits in the capacity for abstract thinking (McGlothlin *et al.*, 1969; Tucker *et al.*, 1972), although recent reviews examining the same clinical findings have tended to minimize this risk (*see* McWilliams and Tuttle, 1973).

Therapeutic Uses. LSD is not an approved drug, and its uses can only be considered to be experimental. Over the past 30 years, it has been proposed as an aid in psychotherapy, as an adjunct to the treatment of alcoholism and opioid addiction, and as a device to induce tranquility and reduce the need for opioid analgesics in cases of terminal cancer. In each situation, the use has largely been abandoned either because controlled studies have failed to demonstrate the value of LSD or because the elaborate precautions required to minimize adverse psychological reactions dampened enthusiasm and rendered its therapeutic use impractical.

MISCELLANEOUS SUBSTANCES USED FOR SUBJECTIVE EFFECTS

The catalog of agents that have been used to produce subjective changes is impressive, and each generation not only adds a few new substances but seems impelled to reevaluate the old.

Hydrocarbons and Anesthetics. The intoxicating and euphorigenic effects of both nitrous oxide and ethyl ether were recognized before their potential as anesthetics was appreciated. In the nineteenth century, efforts to reduce alcoholism in Ireland by means of ether were markedly successful, but the use of ether became so widespread that it was necessary to take steps to reeducate the public to the use of alcohol. When access to alcohol or other intoxicants is restricted by finances, laws, or incarceration, substances with marked toxicity such as antifreeze, paint thinner, and other industrial solvents may be used. Since adolescents are usually prohibited from using alcoholic beverages, "glue sniffing" falls into this category. However, prohibition of alcohol cannot fully explain such behavior. Young adults who can afford and obtain alcohol have also engaged in the inhalation of glue, solvents, and even propellants used in aerosols, sometimes with fatal consequences. The causes of the fatalities are not clear; inhaling from a plastic bag (a common practice) may result in hypoxia as well as an extremely high vapor concentration. Studies in dogs have shown that aerosol propellants containing fluorinated hydrocarbons produce cardiac arrhythmias (Flowers and Horan, 1972). Because of the great variability among these solvents, no general statement can be made with respect to direct toxicity. Certainly the halogenated hydrocarbons have the theoretical potential for producing serious organ damage. The subject has been reviewed by Kupperstein and Sussman (1968).

Other Agents. In large amounts, the common household spice *nutmeg* produces marked subjective changes. It is commonly used for this purpose by the inmates of prisons. The oral ingestion of the equivalent of two grated nutmegs produces, after a latency of several hours, leaden feelings in the extremities and a mental state that may include feelings of depersonalization and unreality. Agitation and apprehension are also common. Dry mouth, thirst, rapid heart rate, and red, flushed face are common and may mimic atropine poisoning (*see* Weil, 1967).

The medically inappropriate, excessive use of *nonnarcotic analgesic mixtures* (containing aspirin, phenacetin, caffeine, etc.) has been reported. Such use, however, is not characterized by extreme psychological dependence. Conceivably, excessive use of such drugs may be related to the mood-elevating effects of the *caffeine*, or to certain misconceptions about the capacity of such mixtures to relieve tension and increase the user's ability to concentrate on tedious tasks. Most investigators feel that tolerance and a limited degree of psychological dependence develop with caffeine. Dreisbach and Pfeiffer (1943) have demonstrated that withdrawal of caffeine in tolerant subjects produces a throbbing headache.

For untold generations, *peyote, ololiuqui* (from the seeds of the morning glory, *Rivea corymbosa*), and "*magic mushrooms*" have been used to produce altered states of consciousness by the Indians of the North American continent. Throughout the world, many other substances are used for similar mind- and mood-changing effects. These include the use of *kava* in the South Pacific, *indole-containing snuff* among the Amazonian Indians in Brazil, and *fly agaric* among the Uralic-speaking tribes of Siberia. A discussion of the pharmacology and the use patterns of these substances is beyond the scope of this chapter. The interested reader should consult Lewin (1931), Efron and associates (1967), and Farnsworth (1968).

TREATMENT

The indications for treatment vary with the drugs being used as well as with the social and cultural factors determining the particular pattern of drug use. Some patterns of drug use, such as the "recreational" use of marihuana, do not require treatment any more than does the occasional smoking of tobacco or the social use of alcohol. Such casual use is not without hazard, but this does not imply a treatable disorder. It is likely that changing views about drug use will continue to create gray areas where the indications for treatment are unclear. However, there is general agreement that treatment is appropriate for the adverse consequences of drug use and for the compulsive drug user who voluntarily seeks help.

WITHDRAWAL TECHNICS

Over the past decade, many entrenched views about withdrawal of drugs have been modified. No longer do all clinicians adhere to the view that drug withdrawal must be the first step in treatment or that it requires a carefully controlled drug-free environment. Under appropriate circumstances successful withdrawal from opioids, alcohol, barbiturates, and amphetamines has been accomplished on an ambulatory basis. However, such ambulatory withdrawal requires the establishment of a positive therapeutic relationship and considerable clinical experience. Withdrawal from tobacco is an exception and is typically an outpatient procedure. For the other drugs, withdrawal is usually better managed in an inpatient or residential setting where access to drugs can be controlled, the withdrawal syndrome observed, and appropriate treatment provided. When many addicted patients are being treated in the same hospital unit, drug smuggling can cause problems. However, when only an occasional patient is involved, it merely delays or prevents the completion of withdrawal; it should not unduly discourage attempts at treatment.

Certain general principles apply irrespective of the particular drug or drugs the patient has been using. (1) The *degree of physical dependence,* if any, that may have developed to each drug the patient has been using should be estimated. (2) A *medical history* should be taken and a physical examination carried out, to determine if there are any indications that the usual withdrawal technics should be modified. For example, a more gradual reduction of opioids would be appropriate in patients with angina pectoris, ulcerative colitis, pulmonary insufficiency, or other debilitating illness. Needless to say, patients who are experiencing severe pain from obvious causes are not appropriate candidates for withdrawal of opioid analgesics until some alternative method of managing the pain is available. (3) The patient should be given sufficient quantities of whichever *drugs* are necessary *to suppress severe withdrawal symptoms,* and the dose of these drugs is then gradually reduced.

Estimating the degree of physical dependence to opioids or to general CNS depressants from the history alone is difficult, since addicted patients often distort their history of drug use. However, their motives vary widely, and so does the manner in which the history is distorted. For example, heroin users are usually unaware of the purity of the drugs they have been using. They tend to exaggerate their usage considerably and may also claim to be using large quantities of barbiturates or other sedatives in the hope that the doctor will then provide them with more generous amounts of opioids or hypnotics. Conversely, some individuals who use illicit drugs may completely deny the intake of barbiturates, even when they have been using a sufficient quantity to produce a dangerous degree of physical dependence. Others, who have used paregoric or cough medicines in an alcoholic vehicle, are often unaware of the large amounts of alcohol they consume. The possibility of physical dependence on general CNS depressants should always be considered when a patient who has had sufficient opioids to suppress withdrawal symptoms remains sleepless and jittery. In striking contrast are those addicts, such as physicians and nurses, who do not obtain their drugs through illicit traffic and who may attempt to minimize the extent of their use. The difficulty in getting an accurate history means that the physician must place great reliance on observation of the patient and on his familiarity with the symptoms of withdrawal from both opioids and general depressants.

The Withdrawal of Opioids. Even with very gradual reduction in dosage, most patients will perceive some withdrawal symptoms. Patients should be told from the outset to expect some discomfort, particularly if the degree of physical dependence has been significant and if the goal is to complete the process within a matter of days. It may be possible, of course, to continue to give the patient the drug he was using (heroin, morphine, meperidine, etc.) and simply reduce the dose over a period of several days. However, for reasons already discussed, methadone is quite suitable for suppressing withdrawal symptoms and can be substituted for any of the natural or synthetic opioid analgesics currently in use. With *methadone substitution,* now considered the most satisfactory technic, the opioid withdrawal symptoms are rarely worse than those of a moderate "influenza-like" syndrome. The dose of methadone will vary with the degree of physical dependence and the medical condition of the patient.

In otherwise-healthy individuals, even abrupt withdrawal of opioids is rarely fatal. However, unless the degree of physical dependence is quite low, abrupt withdrawal is seldom justifiable. The patient is observed and, if significant withdrawal symptoms appear, an initial dose of methadone that rarely needs to exceed 15 to 20 mg is given orally. Additional methadone can be given if the symptoms are not suppressed or each time withdrawal symptoms reappear. After the patient has been observed for 24 to 36 hours and given methadone as described, it becomes a relatively simple matter to calculate a stabilization dose. Usually 1 mg of methadone can substitute for 4 mg of morphine, 2 mg of heroin, or 20 mg of meperidine. Reduction can be started immediately. Empirically it has been found that a reduction each day of 20% of the total daily dose is well tolerated and causes little discomfort. If the patient is not vomiting, methadone should be given by mouth and need not be given more frequently than twice a day. The majority of patients can be completely withdrawn from opioids in less than 10 days, although very mild abstinence symptoms may persist for a number of days after the last dose of methadone. The protracted abstinence syndrome has been described above.

A number of clinicians have found that after a period of social stabilization (usually 6 to 18 months) many former heroin addicts maintained on methadone can be gradually withdrawn from methadone entirely on an ambulatory basis. Even though the dosage is reduced very slowly (*e.g.,* 3 mg per week), when the daily dosage of methadone is reduced to about 10 to 30 mg, many of these patients experience opioid withdrawal symptoms. Some patients are able to tolerate the discomfort and the psychological difficulties, complete the withdrawal process, and do not relapse to opioid use. Others complete the withdrawal process but later relapse to heroin use, and still others elect to discontinue withdrawal and remain on maintenance doses of methadone. Among the symptoms experienced over a period lasting up to several months after withdrawal are insomnia, irritability, restlessness, malaise, pain, fatigue, premature ejaculation, and gastrointestinal hyperactivity (Cushman and Dole, 1973).

Many nonopioids have been used for the opioid withdrawal syndrome; few have proven to have significant value. Certain drugs such as reserpine have a demonstrably aggravating effect on the course of withdrawal. The phenothiazines have not been demonstrated to be of significant help, although pilot studies suggest that haloperidol has possibilities (*see* Karkalas and Lal, 1973). Nighttime sedation with the barbiturates or related sedative-hypnotics is helpful, but complete suppression of opioid withdrawal symptoms with such agents alone cannot be achieved short of anesthetic doses.

The Withdrawal of General CNS Depressants (Barbiturates and Related Drugs). Abrupt withdrawal of general CNS depressants that have been used in high doses over prolonged periods can be fatal. Nevertheless, some European clinicians with considerable experience feel that abrupt withdrawal has its advantages; they administer sedatives only if a delirium develops or if the patient has more than one seizure (Wulff, 1959). In the United States, where there is considerably more abuse of short-acting barbiturates, abrupt withdrawal is not considered a safe technic, and the administration of a suitable general CNS depressant is usually started before major withdrawal symptoms develop. Pentobarbital (orally) can be substituted for any barbiturate the patient has been using. Clinical observations suggest that it is also a suitable substitute for glutethi-

mide, paraldehyde, chloral hydrate, and meprobamate and for the suppression of the alcohol withdrawal syndrome. Sufficient pentobarbital should be given to produce mild intoxication, that is, slight ataxia, nystagmus, and slurred speech. Most patients require from 0.2 to 0.4 g every 6 hours, but some may need up to 2.5 g over a 24-hour period. The daily dose can be estimated from the response to a 200-mg pentobarbital test dose (Wikler, 1968). Once a level of mild intoxication has been achieved, the dosage of pentobarbital should be maintained for at least 24 to 36 hours. At this level, the patient should be free of tremulousness, irritability, and insomnia. The amount of barbiturate required for this initial period becomes the *stabilization level.*

Once the above-described stabilization level has been reliably established and the patient observed for 1 to 2 days, gradual withdrawal can be started. Clinical experience has shown that most patients can tolerate reductions of 0.1 g of pentobarbital per day without significant discomfort. However, the patient should be observed daily; if insomnia, tremulousness, or orthostatic hypotension occurs, further withdrawal should be suspended for 1 to 2 days. If such symptoms are severe, a single extra dose of 0.2 g will usually suppress them. However, once a withdrawal delirium develops, increasing the amount of pentobarbital will not immediately restore equilibrium; the delirium and disorientation may persist for several days. With the use of the pentobarbital-substitution technic, withdrawal may take from 10 days to 3 weeks. It cannot safely be hurried. Patients who are taking large amounts of lesser-known sedatives or longer-acting benzodiazepines should probably be gradually withdrawn from the original drug of abuse without substitution therapy (*see* Wikler, 1968).

Some clinicians feel that the longer duration of action of phenobarbital has advantages for managing withdrawal of general CNS depressants, and use 30 mg of phenobarbital for each hypnotic dose of the drug of dependence (*e.g.,* for each 100 mg of pentobarbital), divided and given four times each day. Phenobarbital is then reduced by 30 mg per day (Smith and Wesson, 1971).

The Withdrawal of Alcohol. There are certain distinctions between the overall effects of chronic abuse of alcohol and those of other general CNS depressants, which necessitate differences in the therapeutic approach. Chronic ingestion of large amounts of alcohol is very frequently associated with various degrees of malnutrition and avitaminosis, especially vitamin B deficiencies. Whereas the well-nourished alcoholic may sometimes be overhydrated during withdrawal (Beard and Knott, 1968), others may be severely dehydrated because of vomiting caused by alcoholic gastritis or withdrawal and also, perhaps, because of the diuretic effects of alcohol. Pneumonitis is also a frequent complication. Thus, injections of vitamins, attention to fluid balance, and administration of antibiotics are often a necessary part of treatment, but *these are obviously not substitutes for measures that suppress the general-depressant withdrawal syndrome.*

As is the case with mild degrees of physical dependence of any type, in the milder forms of alcohol withdrawal a wide variety of drugs (phenothiazines, sedatives, antianxiety agents) will provide some symptomatic relief (*see* Victor, 1966). When there is a significant degree of physical dependence, drugs that show cross-dependence with alcohol are demonstrably superior in reducing mortality and morbidity to those that do not show such cross-dependence. Unfortunately, the tremulousness, which in some patients may be the most severe manifestation of physical dependence, may in others be the prodrome of the more severe epileptiform and delirious states. It is not possible to know in advance which patients are only mildly physically dependent and which patients will develop delirium tremens. Since delirium tremens always carries with it a certain risk of a fatal outcome, it seems appropriate to treat all but the mildest cases of alcoholic withdrawal with agents that show cross-dependence with alcohol. Theoretically, alcohol itself should be quite effective in the suppression of the alcohol withdrawal syndrome. However, its short duration of action and narrow range of safety make it a poor therapeutic agent. In practice, alcohol is always abruptly stopped and more effective agents are substituted. If given in adequate quantities, pentobarbital, phenobarbital, chloral hydrate, paraldehyde, chlordiazepoxide, and diazepam have all been shown to be effective in preventing the development of withdrawal symptoms or suppressing the syndrome once it develops. The general technic is similar to that used in the management of physical dependence on barbiturates, in that the patient is brought to a stabilization level of mild intoxication and the drug is then gradually withdrawn. Chlordiazepoxide is now the most widely used drug for withdrawal, even though in some well-controlled studies it has not seemed as effective as a paraldehyde–chloral hydrate combination (Golbert *et al.,* 1967). Yet in some ways the long duration of action and slow elimination of chlordiazepoxide make its use in the treatment of physical dependence on alcohol analogous to the use of methadone in the treatment of physical dependence on opioids. The rate at which chlordiazepoxide dosage should subsequently be reduced has not been carefully studied; the clinician's adjustment of doses should be guided by the degree of intoxication and the appearance of tremulousness and insomnia. The suppression of alcoholic withdrawal symptoms often requires 0.6 to 1.2 g of pentobarbital, 40 to 80 ml of paraldehyde, or 300 to 500 mg of chlordiazepoxide per day.

Although the phenothiazines appear to have little or no cross-dependence with alcohol, some clinicians continue to use them or to use related drugs such as haloperidol. When compared to the time required for gradual withdrawal of general CNS depressants, the use of such drugs may shorten the period of hospitalization. However, several carefully controlled studies have shown that, when the physical dependence is at all severe, the use of phenothiazines (*e.g.,* promazine and chlorpromazine) does not prevent the development of delirium tremens and that the mortality rate is significantly higher than in patients treated with paraldehyde or chlordiazepoxide (*see* Thomas and Freedman, 1964; Golbert *et al.,* 1967; Kaim *et al.,* 1969).

Withdrawal Technics in Mixed Patterns of Abuse. It is not uncommon to encounter individuals who abuse several classes of drugs at the same time. The abrupt withdrawal of CNS sympathomimetics, psychedelics, or tobacco does not produce any major physiological disturbances. At present, standard medical practice does not involve attempts to ameliorate the withdrawal of CNS sympathomimetics or tobacco. Depending on the quantities involved, individuals may be physically dependent on both opioids and general CNS depressants. The therapeutic regimen in such situations combines the procedures described above. General CNS depressants are given in sufficient quantity to produce mild intoxication, and a stabilization dose is determined. This is followed by gradual reduction. At the same time the patient is observed for the autonomic signs of opioid withdrawal, and sufficient methadone or another suitable opioid is given to suppress such symptoms. After stabilization, the opioid is reduced as previously described. Since insomnia, weakness, and restlessness form a part of both withdrawal syndromes, the evaluation is simplified by not attempting to reduce the opioid dose until the withdrawal of the general CNS depressant is well controlled. Simultaneous withdrawal of both classes of drugs at appropriate rates is not contraindicated, but this procedure requires considerable experience.

APPROACHES TO BEHAVIORAL MODIFICATION

A number of very different approaches to modifying patterns of compulsive drug abuse are currently in use. They differ not only in the way the problem is conceptualized but also in the goals given priority, the methods used, and the patterns of change induced. No longer do all approaches use total abstinence as the sole criterion of successful treatment. Instead, there is a growing emphasis on achieving productive and socially acceptable behavior and on improving physical health and interpersonal relationships. Sometimes marked changes occur in these areas even when the pattern of drug use has only been modified rather than eliminated.

Some treatments place emphasis on emotional problems that are believed to increase vulnerability to compulsive drug use; others aim at providing alternative gratifications or modifying life styles; still others use various forms of external pressure and threats of adverse consequences to change drug-use patterns; some employ pharmacological agents to modify the response to the drugs themselves. In practice, several of these methods are combined in any one treatment program (Glasscote et al., 1972; Meyer, 1972). Although similar themes appear in programs designed to modify compulsive use of different drugs, the great differences in pharmacological effects and social attitudes make it convenient to discuss treatment approaches to each drug separately. The nonpharmacological methods can be only briefly summarized here.

In assessing the value of any form of treatment it is essential to recognize that the recovery rate with little or no intervention is sometimes surprisingly high. Several workers have described a process wherein many opioid users voluntarily and spontaneously stop using the drugs in the fourth or fifth decade of life (Robins and Murphy, 1967; Ball and Snarr, 1969; Vaillant, 1973). The onset of opioid abuse in adolescence has been related to the intensification of conflicts about identity and the expression of aggression and sexuality during this period; the "maturing-out" process may be associated with a decline in the intensity of these same conflicts. For some young people major changes in associates and environment lead to rapid abandonment of drug

use (Robins, 1974). Cessation of opioid use does not necessarily mean total abstinence; on follow-up, former users may be consuming a variety of other drugs (see O'Donnell, 1968).

Hospitalization and Psychotherapy. For many years, it was felt that for the first few months following drug withdrawal rehabilitation should be carried out in a drug-free environment (closed institution). Measured by the percentage of patients who remained abstinent, the results of such prolonged institutional rehabilitation were quite disappointing, not only for opioid users but also for patients addicted to alcohol, barbiturates, or amphetamines. The use of prolonged hospitalization (more than 3 weeks) is now on the decline. It may seem logical that for most patients hospitalization should last for at least a few weeks longer than the acute withdrawal period, but the case for prolonged hospitalization per se as a therapeutic measure has not been demonstrated.

There is little evidence to show that traditional individual psychotherapy is of any value in the treatment of the compulsive drug user. Over the past decade specialized forms of group psychotherapy have been developed, but there is no way of predicting the type of drug user who will be helped by one or another of the many technics now in use. There is general agreement that compulsive drug users cannot regain the ability to employ the drug of abuse in moderation, but even on this point there are dissenting opinions.

Voluntary Groups and Self-Regulatory Communities. Alcoholics Anonymous, Narcotics Anonymous, Synanon, Daytop Village, and similar groups have been helpful in the rehabilitation of certain types of compulsive drug users. Their efficacy may be due to a number of factors, including a reduction in the sense of isolation and a gratification of the need to belong. Equally important is the absence of a hard line between "patient" and "staff." The organizations are usually operated by former drug users, and the new member is immediately confronted by individuals who at once convey understanding and concern, and provide role models for responsible behavior. Also important is the participation itself, which keeps the individual away from the environment in which drug use occurred and in the company of people who share his concerns about drug use in a way that amounts to a ritualization of sobriety. Only a small percentage of compulsive drug users seem motivated to seek admission to such groups; fewer still actually enter after learning what is expected of members, and many leave within weeks after joining. Those who remain in residential programs do well while they are members and many continue to do well after they leave, but there are no satisfactory follow-up studies of individuals who have returned to the outside community with the approval of the group (Glasscote et al., 1972).

Supervisory-Deterrent Approaches. Some approaches emphasize the maintenance of abstinence and involve a period in a hospital, prison, or special facility followed by careful supervision of the individual in the community. If the chemical analysis of urine specimens shows return to drug use, the supervisee, who has usually been paroled or civilly committed to the program, is reinstitutionalized. Although certain forms of psychological treatment are sometimes available within the institution, the critical element of the system is thought to be the deterrent effect of reinstitutionalization. In theory, this approach can be used with all types of compulsive drug abuse. While it is believed that this system was highly effective in Japan in controlling serious epidemics of amphetamine and heroin addiction, the experience in the United States has been far less impressive. Very few individuals under such supervision were able to remain totally abstinent, and by the end of the first year after discharge more than two thirds had been reinstitutionalized. Inasmuch as individuals so supervised may spend less than half of the period of supervision in good standing outside of institutions (Kramer and Bass, 1969), the economic and social cost of such an approach has led to a major decline in its use for compulsive drug users. However, there is now increasing use of external pressure (*e.g.,* threat of job loss) to motivate the working problem drinker to remain in treatment.

The Role of Pharmacological Agents.

With every form of drug dependence, other drugs have been tried as therapeutic agents on a variety of theoretical grounds. Sometimes the therapeutic agents are directed at some postulated underlying psychological difficulty (*e.g.,* anxiety or depression) that is felt to contribute to the motivation to use the drug of dependence. Sometimes the therapeutic agent is intended to substitute, in whole or in part, for the effects of the drug being used, or at least to suppress any subclinical withdrawal phenomena (*e.g.,* lobeline for nicotine, methadone for heroin). Still other agents are intended to interfere in a variety of ways with the reinforcing or satisfying properties of the dependence-producing drug (*e.g.,* opioid antagonists), or to create situations where their use becomes unpleasant (*e.g.,* disulfiram).

Opioid Maintenance. Methadone maintenance was originally based on the hypothesis that, as a result of repeated use of opioids, the addict has sustained a metabolic alteration such that opioids produce a euphoria not experienced by nonaddicts, and that for months or years after withdrawal the addict experiences a feeling of abnormality (opioid hunger) relieved only by opioids (Dole *et al.,* 1966). Since the original pilot studies of Dole and Nyswander, the use of this approach has been greatly expanded and the procedures and dosages have been substantially modified. Most commonly the procedure consists in the daily administration of 40 to 100 mg of methadone, orally in a flavored vehicle, combined with efforts at social rehabilitation. At the stabilization level (achieved by gradually increasing the dose over a period of several weeks), there is a high degree of cross-tolerance to all opioids so that the euphoric effects of even high doses of intravenous opioid are generally not experienced. Dole and coworkers (1966) have referred to this state as "narcotic blockade." While many patients report little or no craving for illicit opioids, in most treatment programs and under experimental conditions there are usually some patients who continue to seek out and use intravenous opioids despite the attenuated effects. This treatment explicitly emphasizes law-abiding and productive behavior rather than abstinence *per se,* and its relative efficacy in reaching its goals is well documented (Dole *et al.,* 1968; Wilmarth and Goldstein, 1974). The acceptability of this approach to both the medical profession and the opioid users themselves combined with its relative effectiveness has had an impact of revolutionary proportions on the treatment of opioid addiction in the United States. However, the expansion of programs to provide treatment to all addicts who want it has generated considerable controversy, and there are a number of questions still unresolved (*see* Goldstein, 1972; Jaffe, 1972). Methadone maintenance is no longer considered experimental, but it is subject to special regulations and is restricted to special clinics.

The use of methadone should not be confused with the British practice of prescribing heroin for self-administration. With methadone the route is exclusively oral, thus eliminating both the sharp ups and downs that characterize the effects of repeated doses of intravenous heroin and the complications that occur when addicts inject themselves without benefit of hygienic technic. Equally important, the duration of action of methadone is such that it need be given only once a day. Although the plasma concentrations of methadone do change over the course of 24 hours (*see* Chapter 15), the decline is not great enough to produce withdrawal phenomena. Therefore, the ingestion of all medication can be supervised by scheduled visits to the clinic, thus obviating the possibility of illicit redistribution by patients.

Controlling illicit redistribution from treatment programs is an important and controversial issue. The sharp increase in young heroin users that occurred in Great Britain during the 1960s is generally attributed to a few physicians who, by prescribing heroin for a few patients in excess of their needs, made it possible for these patients to initiate new users by giving away or selling the excess. On the basis of this experience the British approach to heroin addiction was modified so that the prescribing of heroin for addicts is now restricted to clinics staffed by specialists. However, the existence of these clinics has not prevented the development of an illicit traffic in heroin that serves those who do not use the clinics and those who feel the clinics are not generous enough in their prescribing habits (*see* Bewley, 1973; Stimson, 1973). In practice, most methadone treatment programs permit patients to take some drug home, and there has been some illicit diversion. Concern about this has led to efforts to develop longer-acting opioids for clinical use. One such drug is *acetylmethadol*, which suppresses opioid withdrawal for up to 72 hours after a single dose and, theoretically, all doses can be ingested under direct supervision when patients come to the clinics three times per week. In clinical trials it appears to be similar to methadone in its overall effects (*see* Jaffe *et al.*, 1972). It is still an investigational drug.

Narcotic Antagonists. These drugs have also been used in the treatment of compulsive opioid users. When the opioid receptors in the CNS are continuously occupied by antagonists, the effects of ordinary doses of opioids are attenuated or entirely blocked. Under these conditions even the repeated administration of opioids for several weeks does not induce a significant degree of physical dependence since, presumably, the opioids do not produce their actions at the relevant receptor sites.

Theoretically, the use of opioid antagonists might be helpful in several ways. If compulsive opioid use is a result of the reinforcement of drug-seeking behavior due to drug effects, then the repeated use of opioids without effect (as would be the case if the patient were taking adequate amounts of an antagonist) would tend to produce extinction. Furthermore, if the development of physical dependence could be prevented, then conditioned abstinence phenomena should also be extinguished and the protracted abstinence syndrome should eventually subside. It is important to point out that, independent of the reinforcement model, prevention of the development of physical dependence in ambulatory patients may be of considerable value in that it may stop occasional illicit use from progressing quickly into regular and compulsive use. A number of specific opioid antagonists (cyclazocine, naloxone, and naltrexone) have been subjected to clinical trial. Patients must first be withdrawn from opioids, since antagonists precipitate abstinence symptoms in physically dependent individuals.

Cyclazocine is relatively long acting, and significant blockade of intravenous opioids persists for approximately 24 hours after a 4- to 6-mg oral dose. The side effects, tolerance, and characteristic variety of physical dependence produced by cyclazocine are described in Chapter 15. *Naloxone* is relatively free of the side effects that commonly occur with cyclazocine; however, it has a short duration of action, and its oral efficacy is so low that it has not proven to be a practical drug for treatment. There is currently some optimism about *naltrexone*, since it is orally effective, seems relatively free of side effects, and, depending on the dose, can produce blockade for more than 24 hours (Martin *et al.*, 1973). A depot naltrexone preparation has also been developed but has not yet been tested adequately. The results obtained with opioid antagonists in terms of the percentage of patients becoming socially productive and remaining abstinent are less impressive than those reported for the methadone-maintenance approach (*see* Fink *et al.*, 1973).

Other Pharmacological Procedures. Maintenance approaches for compulsive users of general CNS depressants and amphetamine-like drugs have not been well studied. With the exception of patients dependent on very small doses of such drugs, most practitioners strive for total withdrawal. Drugs that interfere with the synthesis or effects of catecholamines can attenuate or antagonize the effects of amphetamines (Jönsson *et al.*, 1971), but the clinical significance of this observation is uncertain. Except for the very heavy smoker, drugs such as lobeline or even nicotine itself do not contribute to the likelihood of successful abstinence from smoking.

Disulfiram and related agents have been used in the treatment of alcoholism for a number of years. When an individual who has been taking disulfiram ingests alcohol, a syndrome characterized by nausea, vomiting, flushing and hypotension, anxiety, and palpitations develops within minutes. The details of the administration and the potential hazards of disulfiram and related agents are discussed in Chapter 11. Disulfiram can be administered only with the patient's cooperation and, therefore, is useful only for selected patients. Other factors being equal, patients who take disulfiram relapse less rapidly than those who do not. Depot forms of disulfiram have also been employed. The use of disulfiram has been reviewed by Lundwall and Baekeland (1971).

Conditioned aversion technics have been tried in alcoholism, smoking, and other forms of drug abuse. This usually involves the administration of an emetic agent (apomorphine or ipecac), followed shortly thereafter by a dose of the drug (*e.g.*, a small amount of whisky or other agent) so that nausea and vomiting occur soon after the drug is ingested. In this way, the taking of alcohol or the drug of abuse becomes a conditioned stimulus that produces a sensation of nausea. Succinylcholine has been used to induce an anxiety-producing paralysis that is then linked with drinking or drug use. Enthusiasm for the aversion technics has declined as their limitations have become clearer. Sedatives, antianxiety agents, and antidepressants have also been explored in the search for drugs that would reduce the relapse rate in alcoholism. None has been demonstrated to be more than partially useful (*see* Kissin and Gross, 1968).

THE ROLE OF THE MEDICAL PROFESSION IN PREVENTION

Given the relationship between availability of certain drugs and the prevalence of their self-administration, consideration must be given to regulation of the manufacture, prescription, and dispensing of those drugs considered to have an "abuse liability." Developing reasonable regulations requires efforts in several areas, including (1) methods for assessing the likelihood that a particular drug will be self-administered, (2) guidelines for classifying drugs in order to provide for different degrees of control at the levels of manufacturing, prescribing, and dispensing, and (3) general guidelines for medical practitioners who must prescribe these drugs for patients. The use of drugs with an abuse potential in the treatment of compulsive drug users creates special problems because of the belief that such individuals are particularly likely to sell or give some of their prescribed medication to others. While special concern about prescribing drugs for this group is often based on moral and political issues, there is a core of legitimate concern linked to the effort to control availability of drugs used illicitly.

Addicting and Nonaddicting Drugs: Assessing Abuse Potential. In most cases it is not possible to predict from the chemical structure the likelihood that a given drug will produce effects that might lead to its abuse. At present such evaluations are best accomplished by determining how many properties a new drug shares with prototypal drugs known to be abused. The technics used with opioid-like agents are well established. Thus, a drug is considered to be nonopioid with respect to abuse liability (1) if it does not suppress the opioid withdrawal syndrome when tested in subjects physically dependent on morphine, (2) if it does not produce morphine-like physical dependence when given chronically, and (3) if postaddicts neither consistently identify it as "dope" (morphine-like) nor repeatedly request it when offered the opportunity to do so. On the other hand, if a compound is found to share these key characteristics with morphine, it is considered to have a high abuse liability and is recommended for appropriate controls. Some drugs share a few characteristics but not others. For example, cyclazocine produces a variety of physical dependence in which the withdrawal symptoms are not associated with drug-seeking behavior; other drugs may be somewhat morphine-like with respect to one or two characteristics, but because of differences in solubility or toxicity they are considered to present a lower order of risk. Such agents may be recommended for less stringent controls than those applied to the opioids. The difficulties in assessing abuse liability of agonist-antagonists are described in Chapter 15.

It is possible to estimate the cross-dependence of a drug with barbiturates in both man and animals. The assessment of the abuse potential of other classes of drugs is less well established. Until recently, procedures for estimating abuse potential were employed routinely prior to release only for the opioids. New drugs that have pharmacological actions similar to those of amphetamines or general CNS depressants are now required to be evaluated for abuse potential prior to marketing for general use. The general procedures for assessing abuse potential have been reviewed by Fraser (1972) and Yanagita (1973).

Treating the Compulsive Drug User. In the United States, the effort to control drug availability previously included severe restrictions on the use of opioids and certain other controlled drugs in the treatment of compulsive drug users. Musto (1973) has documented the history of the interactions between the medical profession and regulatory authorities. This situation has changed substantially since 1970, and opioids are now used both for easing withdrawal and for maintenance. However, it is likely that further changes will be made in laws and rules as practitioners and regulators strive for a balance between flexibility for treatment and control of illicit diversion. At present, continued administration of opioids to patients with chronic, incurable, and painful conditions is not considered "maintenance of an addiction" and, although the practice varies from state to state, such individuals are not generally reported to health authorities as narcotics addicts.

The treatment of compulsive narcotics users who do not have an obvious medical problem is more complicated. Methadone and similar drugs for both the ambulatory withdrawal and maintenance treatment of heroin addiction are now used in the treatment of more than 70,000 individuals at several hundred separate centers throughout the United States. While such a treatment system has many advantages, already discussed, it also creates certain problems and public health risks. Patients participating in programs can be sources of illicit diversion of the drug prescribed (especially if they are permitted to take home substantial quantities), thus creating the potential of primary addiction to methadone in others. In addition, some intermittent heroin users may become severely physically dependent if inappropriately admitted to maintenance programs. In an attempt to reduce such problems, the federal government promulgated regulations that legitimized the use of methadone, but at the same time attempted to minimize the amount of take-home medication permitted in such programs and to reduce the likelihood that patients would obtain methadone from more than one source. As part of these regulations, the distribution of methadone has been restricted to certain pharmacies. It is still medically appropriate to administer an opioid to relieve acute withdrawal symptoms. However, it is expected that, where there are nearby specialized detoxication or maintenance programs, the patient will be referred to these specialized facilities. The use of opioid maintenance is restricted to specially licensed centers and to clinicians affiliated with them. Since there are also state regulations, interested clinicians should contact the appropriate state agencies.

Thus far there are no specific regulations or constraints at the federal level that would prohibit the use of CNS stimulants or general CNS depressants in the treatment of compulsive users of nonopioid drugs. However, there is a prevalent view that with few exceptions chronic maintenance programs for these drugs are of little benefit to the patient.

In practice, the physician must often administer potent analgesics or sedatives even to persons who seem predisposed to develop psychological dependence on such drugs. There are a few general rules applicable to opioids that, if followed in all cases, will minimize the probability of such a complication. The patient should not be given an opioid when another drug of lower abuse potential will suffice. The patient should not be permitted to self-administer such drugs parenterally. Only a few days' supply should be dispensed at any given time, and a return to nonopioids should be undertaken as soon as the situation permits. If the drug has been administered repeatedly for more than a few weeks, a change to a long-acting drug a few days prior to discontinuation will minimize withdrawal symptomatology. On the other hand, the tendency to avoid the use of opioid analgesics should not be carried to unwarranted extremes; the patient who needs a potent analgesic should not be left in pain because of the physician's fear of causing addiction.

Most physicians now exercise great care in prescribing potent opioids. They are beginning to exercise similar prudence in the prescription of sedatives, antianxiety agents, and CNS sympathomimetics. New regulations limiting the number of times a prescription order for controlled drugs can be renewed should result in more careful periodic reassessment of the need for such drugs.

Drugs given for the relief of fluctuating levels of pain, anxiety, or feelings of depression can be taken in several ways. They can be requested or taken by the patient each time the distress becomes too intense to tolerate, that is, for *relief* of distress; or they can be taken in anticipation of the recurrence of distress, that is, to *avoid* distress. With respect to inducing drug dependence, both ways carry risks. When used for *relief,* minimal amounts of drug will be used, since the time of drug action will correspond to the time when its action is required. However, each time relief is promptly obtained, the act of self-administration of the drug will be reinforced. Drugs with slower onset and longer duration of action may minimize this reinforcement process. Self-administration to *avoid* distress may be less reinforcing of each drug-taking act, but the patient never waits long enough to find out whether the drug is needed at all. Even the idea of discontinuing may cause anticipation of the return of distress. From a pharmacological viewpoint, the avoidance schedule leads to the regular and frequent use of unnecessary amounts of drug, maximizing the development of physical dependence (where this phenomenon is relevant). Although there are no easy solutions to this therapeutic dilemma, the physician should be aware of the factors that may be operative and suggest to the patient the approach best suited to the individual situation. It would also be helpful if, when appropriate, the physician took advantage of his own relationship with the patient to reinforce efforts other than the use of drugs to cope with psychic and physical distress. Furthermore, physicians cannot escape their responsibilities as role models. Doctors who smoke, drink too much, or use any drug to excess obviously do not present the proper model to their patients.

A final caveat is in order. Undoubtedly, whether drugs are used for producing pleasure or for the avoidance or relief of distress, it is the *self-administration* of drugs and the *self-induced* changes in mood that are the critical factors in the development of com-

pulsive abuse. The physician would do well to remember this, not only in his treatment of patients but also when he considers treating himself.

IMPACT OF LEGISLATION AND SOCIAL ATTITUDES ON THE PATTERNS AND TREATMENT OF DRUG ABUSE

Every measure taken to regulate drug use has its social costs as well as its potential benefits. For example, harsh penalties for the mere possession of certain drugs (*e.g.,* heroin, cocaine, marihuana) undoubtedly retard their acceptance as substances for social and "recreational" purposes, in the sense that alcohol and tobacco are so used. Whatever the advantages of such a retardation may be, costs must be measured in money, in the criminal stigmatization of many otherwise law-abiding citizens, and in the development of systems of illicit drug distribution. The eventual impact of restrictive laws and criminal sanctions is usually difficult to predict. To the extent that they may foster the development of socially stigmatized drug-using subcultures where there is social reinforcement of both drug use and deviant behavior, the problems of treating compulsive drug users are made more difficult. Yet, to the extent that overall drug use and adverse drug effects are reduced, there may be corresponding benefits. Experience seems to show, however, that within a culture that accepts the use of some psychoactive agents total prohibition of selected classes of drugs tends to produce a shift toward the use of other agents, at least among individuals who have already developed patterns of compulsive drug use. Thus, some opioid users shift to alcohol and barbiturates in preference to no drug at all, but they often return to opioids whenever the availability increases. Based on pharmacological considerations, such shifts are of dubious benefit to society or to the individual concerned. Furthermore, prohibitions against specific classes of drugs and the social attitudes associated with such prohibitions create selective processes that determine the characteristics of users of prohibited drugs. For example, if the penalties and attitudes are such that a particular drug (*e.g.,* heroin) is available only by interacting with a deviant and antisocial subculture, then only those willing to engage in such interaction are likely to persist in the use of that particular drug. The effects of subculture membership, the drug-using experience, and the initial selective process interact to produce many of the characteristics sometimes thought to be due to the drug experience alone. Whether control of availability reduces the overall prevalence of compulsive drug use is an unsettled question. But it seems reasonable to assume that many people will develop drug-related problems when exposed to certain drugs who would not do so if such drugs were not readily available. The complex relationship between social responses and drug-use patterns has been extensively reviewed (*see* Brecher, 1972; Government of Canada, 1973; National Commission, 1973; World Health Organization, 1973, 1974).

Alexander, E. J. Withdrawal effects of SODIUM AMYTAL. *Dis. nerv. Syst.,* **1951,** *12,* 77–82.

Änggård, E.; Jönsson, L.-E.; Hogmark, A.-L.; and Gunne, L.-M. Amphetamine metabolism in amphetamine psychosis. *Clin. Pharmac. Ther.,* **1973,** *14,* 870–880.

Angrist, B. M., and Gershon, S. Amphetamine abuse in New York City—1966–1968. *Semin. Psychiat.,* **1969,** *1,* 195–207.

Ball, J. C., and Snarr, R. W. A test of the maturation hypothesis with respect to opiate addiction. *Bull. Narcot.,* **1969,** *21,* 9–13.

Beard, J. D., and Knott, D. H. Fluid and electrolyte balance during acute withdrawal in chronic alcoholic patients. *J. Am. med. Ass.,* **1968,** *204,* 133–138.

Beaubrun, M. H., and Knight, F. Psychiatric assessment of 30 chronic users of cannabis and 30 matched controls. *Am. J. Psychiat.,* **1973,** *130,* 309–311.

Bewley, T. H. Treatment of opiate addiction in Great Britain. In, *Opiate Addiction: Origins and Treatment.* (Fisher, S., and Freedman, A. M., eds.) V. H. Winston & Sons, Inc., Washington, D. C., **1973,** pp. 141–161.

Blacker, K. H.; Reese, T. J.; Stone, G. C.; and Pfefferbaum, D. Chronic users of LSD: the "acidheads." *Am. J. Psychiat.,* **1968,** *125,* 341–351.

Bowers, M. B., Jr. Acute psychosis induced by psychotomimetic drug abuse. I. Clinical findings. II. Neurochemical findings. *Archs gen. Psychiat.,* **1972,** *27,* 437–442.

Byck, R., and Ritchie, J. M. Δ⁹-Tetrahydrocannabinol: effects on mammalian nonmyelinated nerve fibers. *Science, Wash.,* **1973,** *180,* 84–85.

Chopra, G. S., and Smith, J. W. Psychotic reactions following cannabis use in East Indians. *Archs gen. Psychiat.,* **1974,** *30,* 24–27.

Cochin, J. Factors influencing tolerance to and dependence on narcotic analgesics. In, *Opiate Addiction: Origins and Treatment.* (Fisher, S., and Freedman, A. M., eds.) V. H. Winston & Sons, Inc., Washington, D. C., **1973,** pp. 23–42.

Collier, H. O. J. Tolerance, physical dependence and receptors: a theory of the genesis of tolerance and physical dependence through drug-induced changes in the number of receptors. *Adv. Drug Res.,* **1966,** *3,* 171–188.

Cushman, P., and Dole, V. P. Detoxification of rehabilitated methadone-maintained patients. *J. Am. med. Ass.,* **1973,** *226,* 747–752.

de Alarcon, R. The spread of heroin abuse in a community. *Bull. Narcot.,* **1969,** *21,* 17–22.

Desmond, M. M.; Schwaneke, R. P.; Wilson, G. S.; Yasunaga, S.; and Burgdorff, I. Maternal barbiturate utilization and neonatal withdrawal symptomatology. *J. Pediat.,* **1972,** *80,* 190–197.

Devenyi, P., and Wilson, M. Abuse of barbiturates in an alcoholic population. *Can. med. Ass. J.,* **1971,** *104,* 219–221.

Dole, V. P. Narcotic addiction, physical dependence and relapse. *New Engl. J. Med.,* **1972,** *286,* 988–992.

Dole, V. P.; Nyswander, M. E.; and Kreek, M. J. Narcotic blockade. *Archs intern. Med.,* **1966,** *118,* 304–309.

Dole, V. P.; Nyswander, M. E.; and Warner, A. Successful treatment of 750 criminal addicts. *J. Am. med. Ass.,* **1968,** *206,* 2708–2711.

Dreisbach, R. H., and Pfeiffer, C. Caffeine-withdrawal headache. *J. Lab. clin. Med.,* **1943,** *28,* 1212–1218.

Drew, W. G.; Kiplinger, G. F.; Miller, L. L.; and Marx, M. Effects of propranolol on marihuana-induced cognitive dysfunctioning. *Clin. Pharmac. Ther.,* **1972,** *13,* 526–533.

Eddy, N. B.; Halbach, H.; Isbell, H.; and Seevers, M. Drug dependence: its significance and characteristics. *Bull. Wld Hlth Org.,* **1965,** *32,* 721–733.

Eisenman, A. J.; Fraser, H. F.; Sloan, J.; and Isbell, H. Urinary 17-ketosteroid excretion during a cycle of addiction to morphine. *J. Pharmac. exp. Ther.,* **1958,** *124,* 305–311.

Ellinwood, E. H., Jr. Amphetamine psychosis: a multidimensional process. *Semin. Psychiat.,* **1969,** *1,* 208–226.

————. Assault and homicide associated with amphetamine abuse. *Am. J. Psychiat.,* **1971,** *127,* 90–95.

Elliot, H. W.; Parker, K. D.; Crim, M.; Wright, J. A.; and Nomof, N. Actions and metabolism of heroin administered by continuous intravenous infusion to man. *Clin. Pharmac. Ther.,* **1971,** *12,* 806–814.

Essig, C. F. Clinical and experimental aspects of barbiturate withdrawal convulsions. *Epilepsia,* **1967,** *8,* 21–30.

Evans, M. A.; Martz, R.; Brown, D. J.; Rodda, B. E.; Kiplinger, G. F.; Lemberger, L.; and Forney, R. B. Impairment of performance with low doses of marihuana. *Clin. Pharmac. Ther.,* **1973,** *14,* 936–940.

Fink, M.; Freedman, A. M.; Resnick, R.; and Zaks, A. Clinical status of the narcotic antagonists in opiate dependence. In, *Agonist and Antagonist Actions of Narcotic Analgesic Drugs.* (Kosterlitz, H. W.; Collier, H. O. J.; and Villarreal, J. E.; eds.) University Park Press, Baltimore, **1973,** pp. 266–276.

Flowers, N. C., and Horan, L. G. Nonanoxic aerosol arrhythmias. *J. Am. med. Ass.,* **1972,** *219,* 33–37.

Fraser, H. F. Criteria for evaluating physical dependence and overall abuse potential of drugs in man. In, *Chemical and Biological Aspects of Drug Dependence.* (Mulé, S. J., and Brill, H., eds.) CRC Press, Cleveland, **1972,** pp. 85–95.

Fraser, H. F.; Isbell, H.; Eisenman, A. J.; Wikler, A.; and Pescor, F. T. Chronic barbiturate intoxication: further studies. *A.M.A. Archs intern. Med.,* **1954,** *94,* 34–41.

Fraser, H. F.; Wikler, A.; Essig, C. F.; and Isbell, H. Degree of physical dependence induced by secobarbital or phenobarbital. *J. Am. med. Ass.,* **1958,** *166,* 126–129.

Fraser, H. F.; Wikler, A.; Isbell, H.; and Johnson, N. K. Partial equivalence of chronic alcohol and barbiturate intoxications. *Q. Jl Stud. Alcohol,* **1957,** *18,* 541–551.

Freedman, D. X. The use and abuse of LSD. *Archs gen. Psychiat.,* **1968,** *18,* 300–347.

Gilmour, D. G.; Bloom, A. D.; Lele, K. P.; Robbins, E. S.; and Maximilian, C. Chromosomal aberrations in users of psychoactive drugs. *Archs gen. Psychiat.,* **1971,** *24,* 268–272.

Golbert, T. M.; Sanz, C. J.; Rose, H. D.; and Leitschuh, T. H. Comparative evaluation of treatments of alcohol withdrawal syndromes. *J. Am. med. Ass.,* **1967,** *201,* 99–102.

Goldstein, A., and Goldstein, D. B. Enzyme expansion theory of drug tolerance and physical dependence. *Proc. Ass. Res. nerv. ment. Dis.,* **1968,** *46,* 265–267.

Goldstein, D. B. Alcohol withdrawal reaction in mice: effects of drugs that modify neurotransmission. *J. Pharmac. exp. Ther.,* **1973,** *186,* 1–9.

Goodwin, D. W.; Schulsinger, F.; Hermansen, L.; Guze, S. B.; and Winokur, G. Alcohol problems in adoptees raised apart from alcoholic biological parents. *Archs gen. Psychiat.,* **1973,** *28,* 238–243.

Griffith, J. D.; Cavanaugh, J.; Held, J.; and Oates, J. A. Dextroamphetamine. *Archs gen. Psychiat.,* **1972,** *26,* 97–100.

Haizlip, T. M., and Ewing, J. A. Meprobamate habituation: a controlled clinical study. *New Engl. J. Med.,* **1958,** *258,* 1181–1186.

Heath, R. G. Marihuana. *Archs gen. Psychiat.,* **1972,** *26,* 577–584.

Hill, H. E., and Belleville, R. E. Effects of chronic barbiturate intoxication on motivation and muscular coordination. *A.M.A. Archs Neurol. Psychiatry,* **1953,** *70,* 180–188.

Hollister, L. E. Interactions in man of delta-9-tetrahydrocannabinol. I. Alphamethylparatyrosine. *Clin. Pharmac. Ther.,* **1974,** *15,* 18–21.

Hollister, L. E.; Motzenbecker, F. P.; and Degan, R. O. Withdrawal reactions from chlordiazepoxide (LIBRIUM). *Psychopharmacologia,* **1961,** *2,* 63–68.

Hughes, P.; Barker, N.; Crawford, G.; and Jaffe, J. H. The natural history of a heroin epidemic. *Am. J. publ. Hlth*, **1972,** *62,* 995–1001.

Inaba, D. S.; Gay, G. R.; Newmeyer, J. A.; and White-head, C. Methaqualone abuse—"luding out." *J. Am. med. Ass.,* **1973,** *224,* 1505–1509.

Isbell, H.; Altschul, S.; Kornetsky, C. H.; Eisenman, A. J.; Flanary, H. G.; and Fraser, H. F. Chronic barbiturate intoxication: an experimental study. *Archs Neurol. Psychiat., Chicago,* **1950,** *64.* 1–28.

Isbell, H., and White, W. M. Clinical characteristics of addictions. *Am. J. Med.,* **1953,** *14,* 558–565.

Isbell, H.; Wikler, A.; Eisenman, A. J.; Daingerfield, M.; and Frank, K. Liability of addiction to 6-dimethylamino-4-4-diphenyl-3-heptanone (METHADON, "AMIDONE" or "10820") in man. *Archs intern. Med.,* **1948,** *82,* 362–392.

Jacobson, C. B., and Berlin, C. M. Possible reproductive detriment in LSD users. *J. Am. med. Ass.,* **1972,** *222,* 1367–1373.

Jaffe, J. H. The maintenance approach to the management of opioid dependence. In, *Drug Abuse: Proceedings of the International Conference.* (Zarafonetis, C. J. D., ed.) Lea & Febiger, Philadelphia, **1972,** pp. 161–169.

Jaffe, J. H.; Senay, E. C.; Schuster, C. R.; Renault, P. R.; Smith, B.; and DiMenza, S. Methadyl acetate vs methadone. A double-blind study in heroin users. *J. Am. med. Ass.,* **1972,** *222,* 437–442.

Jaffe, J. H., and Sharpless, S. K. Pharmacological denervation supersensitivity in the central nervous system: a theory of physical dependence. *Proc. Ass. Res. nerv. ment. Dis.,* **1968,** *46,* 226–246.

Jarvik, M. E. Further observations on nicotine as the reinforcing agent in smoking. In, *Smoking Behavior: Motives and Incentives.* (Dunn, W. L., Jr., ed.) V. H. Winston & Sons, Inc., Washington, D. C., **1973,** pp. 33–49.

Jones, K. L.; Smith, D. W.; Streissguth, A.; and Myrianthopoulos, N. C. Outcome in offspring of chronic alcoholic women. *Lancet,* **1974,** *1,* 1076–1077.

Jones, R. T. Marihuana-induced "high": influence of expectation, setting and previous drug experience. *Pharmac. Rev.,* **1971,** *23,* 359–369.

Jönsson, L.-E.; Änggård, E.; and Gunne, L.-M. Blockade of intravenous amphetamine euphoria in man. *Clin. Pharmac. Ther.,* **1971,** *12,* 889–896.

Kahn, E. J.; Neumann, L. L.; and Polk, G. A. The course of the heroin withdrawal syndrome in newborn infants treated with phenobarbital or chlorpromazine. *J. Pediat.,* **1969,** *77,* 495–500.

Kaim, S. C.; Klett, C. J.; and Rothfield, B. Treatment of acute alcohol withdrawal state. *Am. J. Psychiat.,* **1969,** *25,* 1640–1646.

Kales, A.; Bixler, E. O.; Tan, T. L.; Scharf, M. B.; and Kales, J. D. Chronic hypnotic use: ineffectiveness, drug withdrawal insomnia and hypnotic drug dependence. *J. Am. med. Ass.,* **1974,** *227,* 513–517.

Karkalas, J., and Lal, H. A comparison of haloperidol with methadone in blocking heroin-withdrawal symptoms. *Int. Pharmacopsychiat.,* **1973,** *8,* 248–251.

Kato, T., and Jarvik, L. LSD-25 and genetic damage. *Dis. nerv. Syst.,* **1969,** *30,* 42–46.

Kissin, B., and Gross, M. M. Drug therapy in alcoholism. *Am. J. Psychiat.,* **1968,** *125,* 31–41.

Kolodny, R. C.; Masters, W. H.; Kolodner, R. M.; and Toro, G. Depression of plasma testosterone levels after chronic intensive marihuana use. *New Engl. J. Med.,* **1974,** *290,* 872–874.

Kornetsky, C. H. Psychological effects of chronic barbiturate intoxication. *A.M.A. Archs Neurol. Psychiatry,* **1951,** *65,* 557–567.

Kotin, J.; Post, R. M.; and Goodwin, F. K. Δ^9-Tetrahydrocannabinol in depressed patients. *Archs gen. Psychiat.,* **1973,** *28,* 345–348.

Kramer, J. C., and Bass, R. A. Institutionalization patterns among civilly committed addicts. *J. Am. med. Ass.,* **1969,** *208,* 2297–2301.

Kramer, J. C.; Fischman, V. S.; and Littlefield, D. C. Amphetamine abuse. *J. Am. med. Ass.,* **1967,** *201,* 305–309.

Kreek, M. J. Medical safety and side effects of methadone in tolerant individuals. *J. Am. med. Ass.,* **1973,** *223,* 665–668.

Legge, D., and Steinberg, H. Actions of a mixture of amphetamine and a barbiturate in man. *Br. J. Pharmac. Chemother.,* **1962,** *18,* 490–500.

Lemberger, L.; Crabtree, R. E.; and Rowe, H. M. 11-Hydroxy-Δ^9-tetrahydrocannabinol: pharmacology, disposition, and metabolism of a major metabolite of marihuana in man. *Science, Wash.,* **1972,** *177,* 62–64.

Lemberger, L.; Tamarkin, N. R.; Axelrod, J.; and Kopin, I. J. Delta-9-tetrahydrocannabinol: metabolism and disposition in long-term marihuana smokers. *Science, Wash.,* **1971,** *173,* 72–73.

Lipsitz, P. J., and Blatman, S. Newborn infants of mothers on methadone maintenance. *N.Y. St. J. Med.,* **1974,** *74,* 994–999.

Ludwig, A. M.; Wikler, A.; and Stark, L. H. The first drink: psychological aspects of craving. *Archs gen. Psychiat.,* **1974,** *30,* 539–547.

McGlothlin, W. H., and Arnold, D. O. LSD revisited. *Archs gen. Psychiat.,* **1971,** *24,* 35–49.

McGlothlin, W. H.; Arnold, D. O.; and Freedman, D. X. Organicity measures following repeated LSD ingestion. *Archs gen. Psychiat.,* **1969,** *21,* 704–709.

McQuarrie, D. G., and Fingl, E. Effects of single doses and chronic administration of ethanol on experimental seizures in mice. *J. Pharmac. exp. Ther.,* **1958,** *124,* 264–271.

Martin, W. R. A homeostatic and redundancy theory of tolerance to and dependence on narcotic analgesics. *Proc. Ass. Res. nerv. ment. Dis.,* **1968,** *46,* 206–225.

Martin, W. R., and Fraser, H. F. A comparative study of physiological and subjective effects of heroin and morphine administered intravenously in postaddicts. *J. Pharmac. exp. Ther.,* **1961,** *133,* 388–399.

Martin, W. R.; Jasinski, D. R.; Haertzen, C. A.; Kay, D. C.; Jones, B. E.; Mansky, P. A.; and Carpenter, R. W. Methadone—a reevaluation. *Archs gen. Psychiat.,* **1973,** *28,* 286–295.

Martin, W. R.; Jasinski, D. R.; and Mansky, P. A. Naltrexone, an antagonist for the treatment of heroin dependence. *Archs gen. Psychiat.,* **1973,** *28,* 784–791.

Martin, W. R.; Sloan, J. W.; Sapira, J. D.; and Jasinski, D. R. Physiologic, subjective, and behavioral effects of amphetamine, methamphetamine, ephedrine, phenmetrazine, and methylphenidate in man. *Clin. Pharmac. Ther.,* **1971,** *12,* 245–258.

Maynert, E. W., and Klingman, C. I. Acute tolerance to intravenous anesthetics in dogs. *J. Pharmac. exp. Ther.,* **1960,** *128,* 192–200.

Melges, F. T.; Tinklenberg, J. R.; Hollister, L. E.; and Gillespie, H. K. Temporal disintegration and depersonalization during marihuana intoxication. *Archs gen. Psychiat.,* **1970,** *23,* 204–210.

Mendelson, J. H., and Meyer, R. E. Behavioral and biological concomitants of chronic marihuana smoking by heavy and casual users. In, *Technical Papers of the First Report of the National Commission on Marihuana and Drug Abuse.* Appendix, Vol. I. U.S. Government Printing Office, Washington, D. C., **1972,** pp. 68–98.

Murphy, H. B. M.; Rios, O.; and Negrete, J. C. The effects of abstinence and of re-training on the chewer of cocaleaf. *Bull. Narcot.,* **1969,** *21,* 41–47.

Nahas, G. G.; Suciu-Foca, N.; Armand, J.-P.; and Morishima, A. Inhibition of cellular mediated immunity in marihuana smokers. *Science, Wash.,* **1974,** *183,* 419–420.

National Council on Alcoholism. Criteria for the diagnosis of alcoholism. *Am. J. Psychiat.*, **1972**, *129*, 214–216.

O'Donnell, J. A. Social factors and follow-up studies in opioid addiction. *Proc. Ass. Res. nerv. ment. Dis.*, **1968**, *46*, 333–346.

Oswald, I., and Thacore, V. R. Amphetamine and phenmetrazine addiction: physiological abnormalities in the abstinence syndrome. *Br. med. J.*, **1963**, *2*, 427–431.

Patel, G. J., and Lal, H. Reduction in brain γ-aminobutyric acid and in barbital narcosis during ethanol withdrawal. *J. Pharmac. exp. Ther.*, **1973**, *186*, 625–629.

Perez-Reyes, M.; Timmons, M. C.; Lipton, M. A.; Davis, K. H.; and Wall, M. E. Intravenous injection in man of Δ⁹-tetrahydrocannabinol and 11-OH-Δ⁹-tetrahydrocannabinol. *Science, Wash.*, **1972**, *177*, 633–634.

Post, R. M.; Kotin, J.; and Goodwin, F. K. The effects of cocaine on depressed patients. *Am. J. Psychiat.*, **1974**, *131*, 511–517.

Rafaelsen, O. J.; Bech, P.; Christiansen, J.; Christrup, H.; Nyboe, J.; and Rafaelsen, L. Cannabis and alcohol: effects on simulated car driving. *Science, Wash.*, **1973**, *179*, 920–923.

Randrup, A., and Munkvad, I. Correlation between specific effects of amphetamines on the brain and on behavior. In, *Current Concepts on Amphetamine Abuse.* (Ellinwood, E. H., and Cohen, S., eds.) U.S. Government Printing Office, Washington, D. C., **1972**, pp. 17–25.

Reddy, A. M.; Harper, R. G.; and Stern, G. Observations on heroin and methadone withdrawal in the newborn. *Pediatrics, Springfield*, **1971**, *48*, 353–358.

Robins, L. *The Vietnam Drug User Returns: Final Report, Sept. 1973.* Special Action Office Monograph, Ser. A, No. 2, U.S. Government Printing Office, Washington, D. C., **1974**.

Robins, L. N., and Murphy, G. E. Drug use in a normal population of young Negro men. *Am. J. publ. Hlth*, **1967**, *57*, 1580–1596.

Roffman, M.; Reddy, C.; and Lal, H. Control of morphine-withdrawal hypothermia by conditional stimuli. *Psychopharmacologia*, **1973**, *29*, 197–201.

Russell, M. A. H. Cigarette smoking: a natural history of a dependence disorder. *Br. J. med. Psychol.*, **1971**, *44*, 1–16.

Sellers, E. M.; Lang, M.; Koch-Weser, J.; LeBlanc, E.; and Kalant, H. Interaction of chloral hydrate and ethanol in man. I. Metabolism. *Clin. Pharmac. Ther.*, **1972**, *13*, 37–49.

Smith, D. E., and Wesson, D. R. Phenobarbital technique for treatment of barbiturate dependence. *Archs gen. Psychiat.*, **1971**, *24*, 56–60.

Snyder, S. H.; Weingartner, H.; and Faillace, L. A. DOET (2,5-dimethoxy-4-ethylamphetamine), a new psychotropic drug. Effects of varying doses in man. *Archs gen. Psychiat.*, **1971**, *24*, 50–55.

Tecce, J. J., and Cole, J. O. Amphetamine effects in man: paradoxical drowsiness and lowered electrical brain activity (CNV). *Science, Wash.*, **1974**, *185*, 451–453.

Tennant, F. S., Jr., and Groesbeck, C. J. Psychiatric effects of hashish. *Archs gen. Psychiat.*, **1972**, *27*, 133–136.

Thomas, D. W., and Freedman, D. X. Treatment of the alcohol withdrawal syndrome: comparison of promazine and paraldehyde. *J. Am. med. Ass.*, **1964**, *188*, 316–318.

Thompson, T., and Pickens, R. Stimulant self-administration by animals: some comparisons with opiate self-administration. *Fedn Proc. Fedn Am. Socs exp. Biol.*, **1970**, *29*, 6–12.

Tucker, G. J.; Quinlan, D.; and Harrow, M. Chronic hallucinogenic drug use and thought disturbance. *Archs gen. Psychiat.*, **1972**, *27*, 443–447.

Vaillant, G. E. 20-year follow-up of New York narcotic addicts. *Archs gen. Psychiat.*, **1973**, *29*, 237–241.

Victor, M. Treatment of alcoholic intoxication and the withdrawal syndrome. *Psychosom. Med.*, **1966**, *28*, 636–650.

Victor, M., and Adams, R. D. The effect of alcohol on the nervous system. *Res. Publs Ass. Res. nerv. ment. Dis.*, **1953**, *32*, 526–573.

Wei, E.; Loh, H. H.; and Way, E. L. Brain sites of precipitated abstinence in morphine-dependent rats. *J. Pharmac. exp. Ther.*, **1973**, *185*, 108–115.

Weil, A. T. Nutmeg as a psychoactive drug. In, *Ethnopharmacologic Search for Psychoactive Drugs.* (Efron, D. H.; Holmstedt, B.; and Kline, N. S.; eds.) Public Health Service Publication No. 1645, U.S. Government Printing Office, Washington, D. C., **1967**, pp. 188–201.

Weiss, J. L.; Watanabe, A. M.; Lemberger, L.; Tamarkin, N. R.; and Cardon, P. V. Cardiovascular effects of delta-9-tetrahydrocannabinol in man. *Clin. Pharmac. Ther.*, **1972**, *13*, 671–684.

Wikler, A. Diagnosis and treatment of drug dependence of the barbiturate type. *Am. J. Psychiat.*, **1968**, *125*, 758–765.

———. Dynamics of drug dependence. Implications of a conditioning theory for research and treatment. *Archs gen. Psychiat.*, **1973**, *28*, 611–616.

Wikler, A.; Fraser, H. F.; and Isbell, H. N-Allylnormorphine: effects of single doses and precipitation of "abstinence syndromes" during addiction to morphine, methadone or heroin in man (post-addicts). *J. Pharmac. exp. Ther.*, **1953**, *109*, 8–20.

Wikler, A.; Pescor, F. T.; Fraser, H. F.; and Isbell, H. Electroencephalographic changes associated with chronic alcoholic intoxication and the alcohol abstinence syndrome. *Am. J. Psychiat.*, **1956**, *113*, 106–114.

Williams, E. G.; Himmelsbach, C. K.; Wikler, A.; Ruble, D. C.; and Lloyd, B. L., Jr. Studies of marihuana and pyrahexyl compound. *Publ. Hlth Rep., Wash.*, **1946**, *61*, 1059–1083.

Yanagita, T. An experimental framework for evaluation of dependence liability of various types of drugs in monkeys. *Bull. Narcot.*, **1973**, *25*, 57–64.

Yokel, R. A., and Pickens, R. Self-administration of optical isomers of amphetamine and methylamphetamine by rats. *J. Pharmac. exp. Ther.*, **1973**, *187*, 27–33.

Monographs and Reviews

Brecher, E. M. *Licit and Illicit Drugs.* Consumers Union of United States, Inc., Mt. Vernon, N.Y., **1972**.

Cohen, S. Psychotomimetic agents. *A. Rev. Pharmac.*, **1967**, *7*, 301–316.

Connell, P. H. *Amphetamine Psychosis: Maudsley Monographs, No. 5, Institute of Psychiatry.* Chapman & Hall, Ltd., London, **1958**.

Dole, V. P. Biochemistry of addiction. *A. Rev. Biochem.*, **1970**, *39*, 821–840. (194 references.)

Domino, E. F. Neuropsychopharmacology of nicotine and tobacco smoking. In, *Smoking Behavior: Motives and Incentives.* (Dunn, W. L., Jr., ed.) V. H. Winston & Sons, Inc., Washington, D. C., **1973**, pp. 5–31.

Dunn, W. L., Jr. (ed.). *Smoking Behavior: Motives and Incentives.* V. H. Winston & Sons, Inc., Washington, D. C., **1973**.

Efron, D. H.; Holmstedt, B.; and Kline, N. S. (eds.). *Ethnopharmacologic Search for Psychoactive Drugs.* Public Health Service Publication No. 1645, U.S. Government Printing Office, Washington, D. C., **1967**.

Essig, C. F. Addiction to non-barbiturate sedatives and tranquilizing drugs. *Clin. Pharmac. Ther.*, **1964**, *5*, 334–343.

———. Addiction to barbiturate and nonbarbiturate sedative drugs. *Proc. Ass. Res. nerv. ment. Dis.*, **1968**, *46*, 188–198.

Farnsworth, N. R. Hallucinogenic plants. *Science, Wash.*, **1968**, *162*, 1086–1092.

Freed, E. X. Drug abuse by alcoholics: a review. *Int. J. Addict.*, **1973**, *8*, 451–473. (150 references.)

Freedman, D. X. The psychopharmacology of hallucinogenic agents. *A. Rev. Med.*, **1969**, *20*, 409–418.

Glasscote, R.; Sussex, J. N.; Jaffe, J. H.; Ball, J.; and Brill, L. *The Treatment of Drug Abuse: Programs, Problems, Prospects.* Joint Information Service, Washington, D. C., **1972.**

Goldstein, A. Heroin addiction and the role of methadone in its treatment. *Archs gen. Psychiat.,* **1972,** *26,* 291–297.

Government of Canada. *Final Report of the Commission of Inquiry into the Non-medical Use of Drugs.* Queen's Printer, Ottawa, Ontario, **1973.**

Harris, L. S. General and behavioral pharmacology. *Pharmac. Rev.,* **1971,** *23,* 285–294.

Hawkins, R. D., and Kalant, H. The metabolism of ethanol and its metabolic effects. *Pharmac. Rev.,* **1972,** *24,* 67–157. (641 references.)

Hollister, L. E. Marihuana in man: three years later. *Science, Wash.,* **1971,** *172,* 21–29.

Hug, C. C., Jr. Characteristics and theories related to acute and chronic tolerance development. In, *Chemical and Biological Aspects of Drug Dependence.* (Mulé, S. J., and Brill, H., eds.) CRC Press, Cleveland, **1972,** pp. 307–358.

Kalant, H.; LeBlanc, A. E.; and Gibbins, R. J. Tolerance to and dependence on some non-opiate psychotropic drugs. *Pharmac. Rev.,* **1971,** *23,* 135–191. (402 references.)

Kalant, O. J. *The Amphetamines: Toxicity and Addiction.* Charles C Thomas, Pub., Springfield, Ill., **1966.**

Kupperstein, L. R., and Sussman, R. M. A bibliography on the inhalation of glue fumes and other toxic vapors—a substance abuse practice among adolescents. *Int. J. Addict.,* **1968,** *3,* 177–198.

Lewin, L. *Phantastica, Narcotic and Stimulating Drugs; Their Use and Abuse.* Berlin, **1924.** English translation, London, **1931;** E. P. Dutton & Co., Inc., New York, **1931.**

Lieber, C. S. Chemical characteristics of drugs inducing physical and/or psychic dependence to alcohol. In, *Chemical and Biological Aspects of Drug Dependence.* (Mulé, S. J., and Brill, H., eds.) CRC Press, Cleveland, **1972,** pp. 135–161. (206 references.)

Lundwall, L., and Baekeland, F. Disulfiram treatment of alcoholism. *J. nerv. ment. Dis.,* **1971,** *153,* 381–394.

McWilliams, S. A., and Tuttle, R. J. Long-term psychological effects of LSD. *Psychol. Bull.,* **1973,** *79,* 341–351.

Meyer, R. E. *Guide to Drug Rehabilitation: A Public Health Approach.* Beacon Press, Boston, **1972.**

Musto, D. F. *The American Disease.* Yale University Press, New Haven, **1973.**

Nagle, D. R. Anesthetic addiction and drunkenness: a contemporary and historical survey. *Int. J. Addict.,* **1968,** *3,* 25–40.

Nahas, G. G. *Marihuana: Deceptive Weed.* Raven Press, New York, **1973.**

National Commission on Marihuana and Drug Abuse.

First Report. *Marihuana: A Signal of Misunderstanding.* U.S. Government Printing Office, Washington, D. C., **1972.**

———. Second Report. *Drug Use in America: Problem in Perspective.* U.S. Government Printing Office, Washington, D. C., **1973.**

Sapira, J. D. The narcotic addict as a medical patient. *Am. J. Med.,* **1968,** *45,* 555–588.

Schuster, C. R., and Thompson, T. Self administration of and behavioral dependence on drugs. *A. Rev. Pharmac.,* **1969,** *9,* 483–502.

Secretary of Health, Education, and Welfare. *Marihuana and Health: Second Annual Report to Congress.* U.S. Government Printing Office, Washington, D. C., **1972.**

Shuster, L. Tolerance and physical dependence. In, *Narcotic Drugs: Biochemical Pharmacology.* (Clouet, D. H., ed.) Plenum Press, New York, **1971,** pp. 408–423.

Stimson, G. V. *Heroin and Behavior: Diversity among Addicts Attending London Clinics.* John Wiley & Sons, Inc., New York, **1973.**

Task Force on Narcotics and Drug Abuse: The President's Commission on Law Enforcement and Administration of Justice. *Task Force Report: Narcotics and Drug Abuse.* U.S. Government Printing Office, Washington, D. C., **1967.**

Thornton, W. E., and Thornton, B. P. Narcotic poisoning: a review of the literature. *Am. J. Psychiat.,* **1974,** *131,* 867–869.

Way, E. L. Some biochemical aspects of morphine tolerance and physical dependence. In, *Opiate Addiction: Origins and Treatment.* (Fisher, S., and Freedman, A. M., eds.) V. H. Winston & Sons, Inc., Washington, D. C., **1973,** pp. 99–120.

Wikler, A. *Mechanisms of Action of Opiates and Opiate Antagonists: A Review of Their Mechanisms and Action in Relation to Clinical Problems.* Public Health Monograph No. 52, U.S. Government Printing Office, Washington, D. C., **1958.** (195 references.)

———. Theories related to physical dependence. In, *Chemical and Biological Aspects of Drug Dependence.* (Mulé, S. J., and Brill, H., eds.) CRC Press, Cleveland, **1972,** pp. 359–377. (111 references.)

Wilmarth, S. S., and Goldstein, A. *Therapeutic Effectiveness of Methadone Maintenance Programs in the U.S.A.* Offset Publication No. 3, World Health Organization, Geneva, **1974.**

World Health Organization. *Youth and Drugs.* Technical Report No. 516, WHO, Geneva, **1973.**

———. *Expert Committee on Drug Dependence: Twentieth Report.* Technical Report No. 551, WHO, Geneva, **1974.**

Wulff, M. H. The barbiturate withdrawal syndrome: a clinical and electroencephalographic study. *Electroenceph. clin. Neurophysiol.,* **1959,** Suppl. 14, 1–173.

17 ANALGESIC-ANTIPYRETICS, ANTI-INFLAMMATORY AGENTS, AND DRUGS EMPLOYED IN THE THERAPY OF GOUT

Dixon M. Woodbury and Edward Fingl

This chapter deals primarily with the *salicylates* and agents with similar analgesic, antipyretic, and anti-inflammatory properties. Also included are *colchicine* and *allopurinol,* unrelated drugs employed in the treatment of gout and hyperuricemia.

The salicylates and related agents differ significantly in their toxicity and, hence, in their therapeutic uses. Only a few are sufficiently safe to share usefulness with aspirin as general-purpose analgesic-antipyretics. In this context, these drugs are described as *antipyretic, nonnarcotic, anti-inflammatory,* or *mild analgesics,* to distinguish them from the opioid or narcotic analgesics. The opioids, administered parenterally, provide relief of most types and degrees of pain, solely by a central mechanism; their use is associated with significant tolerance, physical dependence, and abuse liability. In contrast, aspirin and the salicylate-like agents, administered orally, provide relief of only mild-to-moderate pain, in major part by a peripheral anti-inflammatory effect; they are not characterized by significant tolerance or physical dependence liability.

Most of the salicylate-like agents are too toxic to be employed as general analgesic-antipyretics, and toxicity also limits their value as anti-inflammatory agents. They do, however, have some therapeutic usefulness as supplements to aspirin in the therapy of rheumatoid arthritis and related inflammatory disorders. Considered in this context, these drugs are referred to as *salicylate-like* or *nonsteroidal anti-inflammatory* agents. The ideal anti-inflammatory and antirheumatic agent has yet to be discovered, and aspirin remains the agent of choice for such therapy. Gold salts, antimalarial agents, and other drugs employed in the therapy of rheumatoid arthritis are described in other chapters (*see* Index).

Gout and rheumatoid arthritis provide an informative contrast in pharmacotherapy. The etiology of rheumatoid arthritis remains elusive, and therapy is necessarily based primarily on the salicylates and related nonselective anti-inflammatory agents. Such therapy is of distinct benefit but is by no means entirely satisfactory and is often limited by drug toxicity; in addition, although development of crippling deformities is reduced, the basic course of the disease is not altered. In contrast, since the therapy of gouty arthritis can be rationally and selectively directed toward control of the underlying hyperuricemia, it is more uniformly effective and satisfactory. More effective therapy of rheumatoid arthritis should be possible when its etiology is established and the specific characteristics of the inflammatory process are unraveled.

Historical Background. The scarcity and the consequent high price of quinine during the last third of the nineteenth century motivated the search for synthetic antipyretics. As a result, a large number of compounds were introduced into medicine and, although they differ considerably from quinine both chemically and in their lack of antimalarial efficacy, they share with cinchona the ability to produce antipyretic, analgesic, and anti-inflammatory effects. The salicylates and several others have survived and proven their usefulness, not so much as antipyretics but as analgesics and anti-inflammatory agents.

Other salicylate-like anti-inflammatory agents are of more recent origin and are the product of the continuing search for agents with anti-inflammatory effects superior to those of aspirin or, more importantly, effective anti-inflammatory agents with a greater margin of safety. Curiously, major impetus to research in this area was provided by recognition of the value and the limitations of the adrenocorticosteroids for the chronic therapy of inflammatory disorders. The early history of the antirheumatic drugs has been summarized by Rodnan and Benedek (1970).

THE SALICYLATES

Aspirin, acetylsalicylic acid, is the most extensively employed analgesic-antipyretic and anti-inflammatory agent. It is the prototype for both the salicylates and other drugs with similar effects and is the standard of reference for comparison and evaluation of these agents.

As a therapeutic agent, aspirin presents something of a paradox. The layman relies upon it as the "common household analgesic"; yet, because the drug is so generally available, he often underrates its analgesic efficacy. Likewise, the pharmacologist and clinician praise the efficacy and safety of aspirin as an analgesic and antirheumatic agent; yet they find it necessary to warn constantly of its role as the most common cause of drug poisoning in young children and its potential for serious toxicity, if it is used improperly.

History and Source. *Willow bark* (*Salix alba*), the antipyretic property of which was known to the ancients, yields a bitter glycoside called *salicin,* first discovered by Leroux in 1827. On hydrolysis, salicin liberates glucose and *salicylic alcohol* (saligenin). Piria, in 1838, made *salicylic acid* from salicin. Six years later, salicylic acid was prepared from *oil of gaultheria* (oil of wintergreen) by Cahours. The synthetic manufacture of this acid from phenol was accomplished in 1860 by Kolbe and Lautemann. *Sodium salicylate* was first used as an antipyretic and for rheumatic fever by Buss in 1875, and in the following year its value in *rheumatic fever* was discovered independently by Stricker and MacLagan. In 1879, Sée observed that salicylates increased the urinary excretion of uric acid, and this property was utilized in the treatment of gout by Campbell in 1879. *Phenyl salicylate* was introduced into medicine in 1886 by Nencki, and *aspirin* (acetylsalicylic acid) in 1899 by Dreser. The synthetic salicylates soon completely displaced the more expensive compounds obtained from natural sources.

The older literature on salicylates has been summarized by Hanzlik (1927); subsequent developments have been reviewed extensively. (*See* Gross and Greenberg, 1948; Randall, 1963; Symposium, 1963, 1966; Smith and Smith, 1966.)

Chemistry. Salicylic acid (orthohydroxybenzoic acid) is so irritating that it can only be used externally and, therefore, various derivatives of this acid have been synthesized for systemic use. These com-

prise two large classes, namely, *esters of salicylic acid* obtained by substitution in the carboxyl group, and *salicylate esters of organic acids* in which the carboxyl group of salicylic acid is retained and substitution is made in the OH group. For example, aspirin is an ester of acetic acid. In addition, there are salts of salicylic acid. The chemical relationships can be seen clearly from the structural formulas shown in Table 17–1.

Table 17–1. STRUCTURAL FORMULAS OF THE SALICYLATES

All the above compounds are referred to collectively as the "salicylates" or the "salicyl" drugs, the salicyl radical being $C_6H_4(OH) \cdot CO \cdot O^-$. The salicylates will be discussed as a class, and significant differences between them will be noted as the occasion arises.

Structure-Activity Relationship. Salicylates generally act by virtue of their salicylic acid content, although some of the effects of aspirin are due to its ability to acetylate proteins (*see* below). Substitutions on the carboxyl or hydroxyl groups serve only to change the potency or toxicity of the compound. The ortho position of the OH is an important feature for the action of salicylate. Benzoic acid, C_6H_5COOH, shares many of the actions of salicylic acid but is much weaker. The effects of substitutions on the benzene ring have been extensively studied by use of a variety of model systems, but no drug superior to those shown in Table 17–1 has as yet resulted from such investigations.

PHARMACOLOGICAL PROPERTIES

Analgesia. The types of pain amenable to relief by salicylates are those of low intensity, whether circumscribed or widespread in origin; particularly amenable are headache, myalgia, arthralgia, and other pains arising from integumental structures rather than from viscera. The salicylates have lower maximal effects than do the narcotic analgesics and hence are used only for pain of slight-to-moderate intensity. The salicylates are more widely used for pain relief than is any other class of drugs. They have the advantage that chronic use does not lead to tolerance or addiction and that toxicity is lower than that of more potent analgesics.

The salicylates alleviate pain by virtue of both a peripheral and a central nervous system (CNS) effect. A peripheral effect of salicylates has been well documented and emphasized by Lim (1966). Relief of pain results from modification of the cause of pain at the site of origin, which is often the locus of inflammation. Salicylates, by inhibiting the synthesis of prostaglandins that occurs in inflamed tissues, prevent the sensitization of the pain receptors to mechanical stimulation or to chemicals, such as bradykinin, that appear to mediate the pain response (*see* Chapter 30; *see also* Ferreira and Vane, 1974).

Direct effects of salicylates on the CNS have been described and suggest a hypothalamic site for the analgesic as well as the antipyretic effects. This is supported by the fact that analgesic doses do not cause mental disturbances, hypnosis, or changes in modalities of sensation other than pain. Neither do salicylates appear to affect the reticular pathways involved in arousal and in domination of attention caused by pain. Both the peripheral and CNS factors contribute significantly to the pain relief afforded by this class of drugs (*see* Winder, 1959; Paalzow, 1969; Dubas and Parker, 1971).

Because of the relatively weak analgesic effectiveness of the salicylates, experimental evaluation of this effect has presented many problems (*e.g., see* Smith and Beecher, 1969; Bloomfield and Hurwitz, 1970). However, careful analysis has confirmed that salicylates do possess definite and useful analgesic properties. Pathological pain appears to be more susceptible to relief by salicylates than is experimentally induced pain (*see* review by Beecher, 1957). Suitably controlled experiments have repeatedly shown aspirin to be superior to placebo in pathological pain of a wide variety of causes. Aspirin has approximately one tenth the milligram potency of codeine. For example, in one study of chronic pathological pain, 325 mg of aspirin was found to be equivalent to 32 mg of codeine. However, reported values have varied from one twentieth to one fifth (for summary, *see* Beaver, 1965, 1966). The efficacy of aspirin in combination with other drugs is discussed later in this chapter.

Antipyresis. Salicylates lower body temperature. The antipyretic effect is usually rapid and effective in febrile patients, but it is rarely demonstrable when the temperature is normal. Regulation of body temperature requires a delicate balance between heat production and heat loss. The CNS, especially the hypothalamic nuclei, plays an indispensable role in regulating the peripheral mechanisms concerned with the production and loss of body heat. The hypothalamus regulates the set point at which body temperature is maintained. In fever, the balance between heat production and heat loss still persists except that the set point is at a higher level. The salicylates act to reset the "thermostat" for normal temperature. Heat production is not inhibited, but heat dissipation is augmented by increased peripheral blood flow and sweating.

There is evidence that fevers of varied etiology, such as those produced by bacterial endotoxins or viruses, are caused by endogenous pyrogen derived from polymorphonuclear leukocytes. Endogenous pyrogen acts directly on the thermoregulatory center in the hypothalamus to increase the set-point temperature. The ratio between sodium and calcium ions appears to determine the discharge rate of the thermoregulatory neurons in the hypothalamus, and leukocytic pyrogen removes the inhibitory influence of calcium ions on the permeability of these neurons to sodium (Feldberg and Saxena, 1970; Myers and Tytell, 1972).

The temperature-elevating effect of leukocytic pyrogen is inhibited by salicylates in various species including man and by acetaminophen in cats (Adler *et al.,* 1969; Clark and Moyer, 1972). The site of antipyretic action of these agents is predominantly central. Both antagonize the pyretic effect of intracerebrally injected leukocytic or bacterial pyrogens, given either intravenously or intracerebrally, probably by competing with the pyrogens for receptor sites in the thermoregulatory centers of the hypothalamus (Wit and Wang, 1968; Cranston *et al.,* 1970; Clark and Coldwell, 1972; Clark and Moyer, 1972).

The antipyretic effects of salicylates are not, however, due to a direct effect on hypothalamic neurons since they neither lower normal body temperature nor prevent the fever induced by local cooling of the hypothalamus (Cranston *et al.,* 1970). Rather, the antipyretic effect, like the analgesic effect, appears to involve inhibition of the synthesis of prostaglandins. Prostaglandin E_1 is a powerful pyrogen when injected into the anterior hypothalamus or cerebral ventricles, the same region where pyrogens act, and this effect is *not* blocked by antipyretic agents. Pyrogens cause generation of prostaglandin E-like substance in the brain; this effect is inhibited by salicylates.

Whereas salicylates in moderate doses lower an elevated body temperature, they also increase oxygen consumption and metabolic rate, and, in toxic doses, produce a pyretic effect that results in sweating, thus enhancing the dehydration that occurs in salicylate intoxication (*see* below).

Miscellaneous Neurological Effects. In high doses, salicylates have toxic effects on the CNS, consisting in stimulation (including convulsions) followed by depression. Confusion, dizziness, tinnitus, high-tone deafness, delirium, psychosis, stupor, and coma may occur. The *tinnitus* and *hearing loss* caused by salicylate poisoning are similar to those seen in Ménière's disease and are due to increased labyrinthine pressure (Waltner, 1955) and/or an effect on the hair cells of the cochlea. There is a close relation between the hearing loss in decibels and the plasma salicylate concentration. The loss is completely reversible within 2 or 3 days after withdrawal of the drug (Myers et al., 1965).

Nausea and *vomiting* are induced by salicylates and result from stimulation of receptors that are accessible from the cerebrospinal fluid, probably in the medullary chemoreceptor trigger zone (CTZ). Simultaneous afferent input to the vomiting center from central and peripheral receptors is necessary to evoke a normal-threshold emetic response to intravenously administered salicylates (Bhargava et al., 1963; Clark et al., 1972). Either supradiaphragmatic vagotomy or ablation of the CTZ greatly elevates the emetic threshold; spinal cord pathways also are involved in mediating salicylate-induced emesis. Thus, mucosal receptors stimulated by gastric irritation, the CTZ, and some as-yet-unknown central receptors are involved in the nausea and vomiting induced by salicylates. In man, centrally induced nausea and vomiting generally appear at plasma salicylate concentrations of about 270 μg/ml, but these same effects may occur at much lower plasma values as a result of local gastric irritation.

Respiration. The effects of salicylate on respiration are of paramount importance because they contribute to the serious acid-base balance disturbances that characterize poisoning by this class of compounds. Salicylates stimulate respiration directly and indirectly. Full therapeutic doses of salicylates increase oxygen consumption and CO_2 production in experimental animals and man. This effect of salicylate occurs primarily in skeletal muscle and is a result of salicylate-induced uncoupling of oxidative phosphorylation (*see* below). The increased production of CO_2 stimulates respiration. The increased alveolar ventilation balances the increased CO_2 production, and thus plasma CO_2 tension (P_{CO_2}) does not change. The *initial* increase in alveolar ventilation is characterized mainly by an increase in depth of respiration and only a slight increase in rate, a pattern similar to that produced by inhalation of CO_2 and by exercise. If a barbiturate or morphine is administered to depress the respiratory response to CO_2, plasma P_{CO_2} increases markedly and a respiratory acidosis develops.

As salicylate gains access to the medulla, it directly stimulates the respiratory center. This results in marked hyperventilation characterized by an increase in depth and a pronounced increase in rate. During the initial phase of salicylate toxicity in dogs, alve-

olar ventilation and respiratory rate may double; during the later phase of direct central stimulation, respiratory minute volume is increased as much as tenfold, alveolar and plasma P_{CO_2} fall, the latter to as low as 16 mm Hg, and *respiratory alkalosis* ensues. Similarly, dramatic changes occur in patients with salicylate poisoning. Plasma salicylate concentrations of 350 μg/ml are nearly always associated with hyperventilation in man, and marked hyperpnea occurs when the level approaches 500 μg/ml.

The mechanism by which salicylate causes *hyperventilation* has not been fully elucidated. In dogs and cats, functional denervation of the carotid bodies and section of the vagi do not abolish the increase in alveolar ventilation following intravenous salicylate (Tenney and Miller, 1955; Cochran and Ramsay, 1956). Moreover, direct application of a low concentration of salicylate to the medulla or into the cerebral ventricles is followed by a prompt and dramatic increase in ventilation, a fall in alveolar P_{CO_2}, a rise in arterial pH, and no change or an increase in cerebrospinal fluid (CSF) pH. Hence, there is no evidence that its central stimulant effect on respiration is due to a primary CSF acidosis. As a result of this direct central effect of salicylate, the sensitivity of the respiratory centers to CO_2 is markedly increased, as demonstrated in both experimental animals and man (Tenney and Miller, 1955; Samet et al., 1960). Further localization of the salicylate effect has been provided by Rosenstein and Borison (1963), who observed that in decerebrate or pentobarbital-anesthetized cats salicylate differs from CO_2 in its CNS actions. CO_2 acts at the supramedullary level, whereas salicylate exerts both direct stimulant and depressant effects on the medulla. CO_2 stimulates depth more than rate of respiration, whereas salicylate stimulates rate more than depth. They suggested that the central stimulating effect of salicylate predominates over that of CO_2 since the consequent reduction in plasma P_{CO_2} did not counteract the effect of salicylate. Indeed, it was not possible to produce apnea in salicylate-treated animals by forced mechanical hyperventilation. The major central respiratory effect of salicylate thus appears to be directly on the medulla to drive that portion of the respiratory center concerned with control of respiratory rate. However, morphine blocks salicylate-induced stimulation of rate but not that of depth, and this has been interpreted to indicate an influence of salicylate on the pontine modulator of respiration in addition to its effect on the medullary pacemaker (Pentiah et al., 1966).

The *depressant* effect of salicylate on the medulla appears after high doses or after prolonged exposure. Toxic doses of salicylates cause central respiratory paralysis as well as circulatory collapse secondary to vasomotor depression. Since enhanced CO_2 production continues, respiratory acidosis ensues (*see* below). High doses of salicylate also induce pulmonary edema, probably central in origin; the edema tends to limit gas exchange in the alveoli and thereby enhances the respiratory acidosis. In persons hypersensitive to salicylate, an asthmatic attack may embarrass respiration.

Acid-Base Balance and Electrolyte Pattern. Therapeutic doses of salicylate produce definite changes in the acid-base balance and electrolyte pattern. The initial event, as discussed above, is an extracellular and intracellular *respiratory alkalosis. Compensation* for the respiratory alkalosis promptly ensues. Renal excretion of bicarbonate accompanied by sodium and potassium is increased, plasma bicarbonate is thus lowered, and blood pH returns toward normal. This is the stage of *compensated respiratory alkalosis.*

This phase of the acid-base sequence is most often seen in adults given intensive salicylate therapy and seldom proceeds further. The severity of the respiratory alkalosis is proportional to the dose of salicylate and the duration of medication. In ten healthy adults given 12 g of aspirin over a period of 9 hours, Farber and coworkers (1949) observed the following changes: an average increase of 4 liters per minute in respiratory volume, and a respiratory alkalosis with an increase in plasma pH of 0.06 unit, a decrease in plasma P_{CO_2} of 10.5 mm Hg, and a decrease in plasma bicarbonate of 3.0 mEq per liter. The maximal acid-base change occurred 2 to 4 hours after the peak plasma salicylate concentration (390 µg/ml) was reached; significant alterations were still discernible 20 hours after the last dose of drug. Salicylism occurred in eight of the ten subjects.

Subsequent changes in acid-base status generally occur only when toxic doses of salicylates are ingested by infants and children and occasionally (2%) after large doses in adults. In infants and children, the phase of respiratory alkalosis may not be observed by the physician, since the child with salicylate intoxication is rarely seen early enough. The stage generally present is characterized by a decrease in blood pH, a low plasma bicarbonate concentration, and a normal or nearly normal plasma P_{CO_2}, changes consistent, except for P_{CO_2}, with the picture of metabolic acidosis. However, in reality there is a *combination of respiratory acidosis and metabolic acidosis* produced as follows. The respiratory depression from toxic doses of salicylate permits the enhanced production of CO_2 to outstrip its alveolar excretion; consequently, plasma P_{CO_2} increases and blood pH decreases. Since

plasma bicarbonate level is already low due to increased renal bicarbonate excretion, the acid-base status at this stage is essentially an uncompensated respiratory acidosis. Superimposed, however, is a true metabolic acidosis caused by accumulation of acids as a result of three processes. First, salicylic acid derivatives dissociate at plasma pH, and in toxic doses displace about 2 to 3 mEq per liter of plasma bicarbonate. Second, vasomotor depression caused by toxic doses of salicylate impairs renal function with consequent accumulation of strong acids of metabolic origin, namely, sulfuric and phosphoric acids. Third, organic acids accumulate secondary to salicylate-induced derangement of carbohydrate metabolism, especially pyruvic, lactic, and acetoacetic acids. Hence, metabolic acidosis is further enhanced. (For summaries of the acid-base effects of salicylate, *see* Tenney and Miller, 1955; Winters *et al.,* 1959; Symposium, 1963.)

The series of events that produce acid-base disturbances in salicylate intoxication also cause alterations of *water and electrolyte balance.* The low plasma P_{CO_2} leads to decreased renal tubular reabsorption of bicarbonate and increased renal excretion of sodium, potassium, and water (*see* introduction to Section VIII). In addition, water is lost by salicylate-induced sweating and by insensible water loss through the lungs during hyperventilation, and dehydration rapidly occurs. Since more water than electrolyte is lost by way of the sweat and lungs, the dehydration is associated with hypernatremia.

Prolonged exposure to high doses of salicylate also causes *potassium depletion* due to both renal and extrarenal factors. Respiratory alkalosis is known to produce hypokalemia (Chapter 36). In addition, salicylate promotes increased urinary excretion of potassium by a direct effect on the renal tubules (Robin *et al.,* 1959). Also, like other agents that uncouple oxidative phosphorylation, salicylates inhibit the active system for Na-K transport in cells; as a result, sodium and water accumulate in cells, potassium is lost, and intracellular volume increases. If renal function is compromised in salicylate intoxication, the potassium lost from cells accumulates in the extracellular fluid and potassium intoxication may occur. Salicylate can also cause cellular loss of potassium by increasing its rate of passive efflux. The drug has been shown to increase the permeability of cellular and subcellular membranes to potassium, a process that *in vivo* is probably secondary to the respiratory alkalosis; it also decreases permeability to chloride ion. (*See* Hicklin, 1959; Charnock *et al.,* 1961; Symposium, 1963; Schorderet and Straub, 1971; Levitan and Barker, 1972.)

Cardiovascular Effects. Ordinary therapeutic doses of salicylates have no important direct cardiovascular actions. The peripheral vessels tend to dilate after large doses, due to a direct effect on their smooth muscle. Toxic amounts depress the circulation directly and by central vasomotor paralysis.

In experimental animals and man, salicylates increase cardiac output and right ventricular and systemic pressures by increasing the contractile force of the heart (Tenney and Miller, 1955; Walton and Darby, 1958; Alexander and Smith, 1962). As a consequence, left ventricular work is increased. Aspirin and indomethacin, which inhibit prostaglandin synthesis, enhance the coronary dilatation induced by increased cardiac activity; it has been suggested that they might be useful in preventing coronary insufficiency in conditions of cardiac stress (*see* Talesnik and Sunahara, 1973).

In patients given large doses of sodium salicylate or aspirin, such as are used in acute rheumatic fever, the circulating plasma volume increases (about 20%), the hematocrit falls, and cardiac output and work are increased. Consequently, in patients with clear evidence of carditis, such alterations can cause congestive failure and pulmonary edema, and high doses are best avoided in such individuals (Alexander and Smith, 1962).

Gastrointestinal Effects. The ingestion of salicylate may result in epigastric distress, nausea, and vomiting. The mechanism of the emetic effect is discussed above. Salicylate may also cause gastric ulceration and even hemorrhage in experimental animals and in man. Exacerbation of peptic ulcer symptoms (heartburn, dyspepsia), gastrointestinal hemorrhage, and erosive gastritis have all been reported in patients on high-dose therapy, but may rarely occur with low doses as a hypersensitivity response. The salicylate-induced gastric bleeding is painless and frequently leads to blood loss in the stool and occasionally to an iron-deficiency anemia. In most cases, however, blood loss is not significant.

The occurrence of these effects in *man* has been demonstrated by many investigators (for reviews, *see* Symposium, 1963; Smith and Smith, 1966; Cooke, 1973; Paulus and Whitehouse, 1973). For example, ingestion of 4 or 5 g of aspirin per day for 26 days, a dose that produces plasma salicylate concentrations in the usual range for anti-inflammatory therapy (120 to 350 μg/ml), results in an average fecal blood loss of about 3 to 8 ml per day as compared with approximately 0.6 ml per day in untreated subjects (Leonards and Levy, 1973). Gastroscopic or direct examination in salicylate-treated subjects reveals discrete ulcerative and hemorrhagic lesions of the gastric mucosa; in many cases, multiple hemorrhagic lesions with sharply demarcated areas

of focal necrosis are observed. The bleeding is associated with exfoliation of gastric mucosal cells. Salicylates have been incriminated as a cause of peptic ulcer, and ulceration and bleeding are enhanced by these drugs in patients with peptic ulcer. In a massive survey of hospital admissions (Levy, 1974), a history of heavy aspirin use, for 4 or more days a week, was more common in patients with gastrointestinal bleeding but without evidence of duodenal ulcer and in those with newly diagnosed benign gastric ulcer, than in control subjects who were admitted for conditions in other categories.

The mechanism by which high local concentrations of salicylates injure gastric mucosal cells is unknown. However, gastric acidity plays an important role, and other factors are also involved. Salicylates break down the normal gastric mucosal barrier against back diffusion of hydrogen ions and leakage of other ions, which then may injure the submucosal capillaries with subsequent necrosis and bleeding. Other salicylate-induced factors include inhibition of secretion of the protective gastric mucus, increased bleeding as a result of inhibition of platelet aggregation, and reduced synthesis of prostaglandin, which inhibits gastric acid secretion. The incidence of bleeding is highest with insoluble salicylates that tend to deposit in the gastric mucosal folds. Occult blood loss can be reduced or prevented by administering aspirin in solution or in a dosage form that provides reliable disintegration and dissolution. Ethanol ingestion may increase the occult blood loss induced by aspirin.

All anti-inflammatory agents of diverse structure, of which the adrenocorticosteroids provide the most striking example, share the ulcerogenic property of the salicylates. Therefore, the explanation of the etiology of such gastric lesions may be intimately related to the mechanism of anti-inflammatory action.

Hepatic and Renal Effects. Salicylate, even in large dosage, does not appear to damage the hepatic parenchyma, as indicated by the results of ordinary clinical tests for hepatic function. Whether the changes in plasma prothrombin and fibrinogen content are due to some subtle action of salicylate on the liver is unknown (*see* below). The salicylates cause an increase in the volume output of bile, but they decrease the total cholate excretion; this *choleretic effect* is apparently due to a direct action on liver cells. In severe salicylate intoxication, fatty infiltration of the liver and kidney may occur.

Urinary changes are infrequent, even after high therapeutic doses and prolonged use of salicylate, and normal renal function is unaltered. However, after large toxic doses, salicylate increases the clearance of water, sodium, chloride, potassium, urate, and phosphate, all partly independent of the respiratory alkalosis it produces; glucose reabsorption is also reduced, as is renal concentrating capacity. If the alkalosis and saluresis are severe and prolonged, dehydration and oliguria may develop; renal failure often occurs in the late stages of salicylate intoxication. High doses of salicylate initially increase the number of erythrocytes and tubular epithelial cells in the urine; with continued drug administration this effect subsides within a few days, but persists to some extent during prolonged drug administration (*see* Prescott, 1965). The significance of this phenomenon in relation to analgesic nephrotoxicity is discussed below.

Effects on the Blood. Salicylate medication does not ordinarily alter the *leukocyte* or *erythrocyte* count, the hematocrit, or the hemoglobin content, nor does it produce methemoglobinemia. The mechanism of the salicylate reduction in leukocytosis and in the elevated *erythrocyte sedimentation rate* in acute rheumatic fever is not understood. The *plasma iron concentration* is markedly decreased and *erythrocyte survival time* shortened by doses of 3 to 4 g per day. Aspirin is included among the drugs that can cause a mild degree of hemolysis in individuals with a glucose-6-phosphate dehydrogenase deficiency.

Effects on Platelets. Ingestion of aspirin by normal individuals causes a definite prolongation of the bleeding time; this is not due to hypoprothrombinemia (*see* below) and can occur with a dose as small as 0.3 g. For example, a single dose of 0.65 g of aspirin approximately doubles the mean bleeding time of normal persons for a period of 4 to 7 days.

Hemostasis in injured blood vessels begins with adherence of platelets to exposed connective tissue, followed by release of adenosine diphosphate (ADP) from storage organelles of the adherent platelets. The released ADP makes other platelets "sticky" and causes them to aggregate and release their ADP and to form an occlusive plug subsequently stabilized by fibrin formation. Aspirin blocks the adhesion of platelets to connective tissue or collagen fibers, possibly through inhibition of collagen glucosyltransferase present in membranes of platelets. Aspirin also inhibits ADP release from platelets and the resultant aggregation induced by connective tissue or collagen. The release of platelet-bound 5-hydroxytryptamine is also suppressed by aspirin, as is the synthesis of prostaglandins in platelets. The latter effect is perhaps relevant since prostaglandin E_1 also prevents platelet aggregation by ADP, but it appears to have no specific effect on the release reaction. The similar effects of acetic anhydride and the substantially greater potency of aspirin than sodium salicylate suggest that platelet acetylation by aspirin is responsible for the blocking effect on aggregation, but this point is disputed. The effect of aspirin may be irreversible and thus account for the inhibition of platelet aggregation and the prolongation of bleeding time for several days after a single dose (*see* Chapter 65 and summaries by Mustard and Pack-ham, 1970; O'Reilly, 1971; Davis, 1973; and many others).

Aspirin should be avoided in patients with severe hepatic damage, hypoprothrombinemia, vitamin K deficiency, or hemophilia, because the inhibition of platelet hemostasis can result in hemorrhage. Also, aspirin therapy should be stopped at least 1 week prior to surgery. Additionally, care should be exercised in the use of aspirin during long-term treatment with oral anticoagulant agents, because of the possible danger of blood loss from the gastric mucosa. However, the intentional use of aspirin and other drugs inhibiting platelet aggregation, in conjunction with oral anticoagulants, is being actively explored for the prophylaxis of coronary and cerebral arterial thrombosis.

Prothrombinopenic Effect. Salicylate in large doses (over 6 g per day) reduces the plasma prothrombin level. Link and associates (1943) first demonstrated in the rat that salicylic acid induces a hypoprothrombinemia that is preventable by vitamin K, and nearly all subsequent workers have confirmed that salicylates slightly prolong prothrombin time; this effect is too small to be of much clinical significance. It has been suggested that salicylate interferes with the role of vitamin K in prothrombin synthesis (*see* Chapter 65; *see also* Quick and Clesceri, 1960).

Uricosuric Effects. Appropriate doses of salicylate increase the urinary excretion of urates, and the drug was once used in acute and chronic gout. The uricosuric action is markedly dependent on the dose (Yü and Gutman, 1959). Low doses (1 or 2 g per day) may actually decrease urate excretion and elevate plasma urate concentrations; intermediate doses (2 or 3 g per day) usually do not alter urate excretion; large doses (over 5 g per day) induce uricosuria and lower plasma urate levels. Such large doses are poorly tolerated. Even small doses of salicylate should not be given concomitantly with probenecid and other uricosuric agents that decrease tubular reabsorption of uric acid, because it annuls their effect. More effective uricosuric agents are available (*see* Index).

Effects on Rheumatic, Inflammatory, and Immunological Processes, and on Connective Tissue Metabolism. For almost 100 years the salicylates have retained their preeminent position in the treatment of the rheumatic diseases. Although they suppress the clinical signs and even improve the histological picture in acute rheumatic fever, subsequent tissue damage such as cardiac lesions and other visceral involvement is unaffected.

The basic mechanism of action of salicylates in rheumatic diseases appears to be concerned with effects on inflammatory and immunological processes in mesenchymal and connective tissue. The results of considerable investigation still do not provide an explanation for the antirheumatic effects, but certain trends are emerging.

A variety of experimentally induced inflammatory and "arthritis-like" syndromes in animals are suppressed by salicylates; however, the relevance to rheumatic diseases in man is not clear, except that drugs that block these syndromes are also effective in the rheumatic diseases of man.

Inflammation in patients with rheumatoid arthritis involves the combination of an antigen (gamma globulin) with an antibody (rheumatoid factor) and complement, causing the local release of chemotactic factors that attract leukocytes. The leukocytes phagocytize the antigen-antibody-complement complexes and also release the many enzymes contained in their lysosomes. These lysosomal enzymes then cause injury to cartilage and other tissues and enhance the inflammation. Cell-mediated immunity may also be involved. Prostaglandins are also formed by leukocytes during phagocytosis, secondary to release of phospholipases from lysosomes and the subsequent hydrolysis of phospholipids to yield fatty acids such as arachidonic acid, which are precursors of prostaglandins. Local injection of either prostaglandin E_1 or E_2 causes marked vasodilatation and hyperemia; increases permeability, swelling, and pain; and induces leukocyte migration into the area. If injected into the synovial cavity, these prostaglandins cause arthritic manifestations. Although prostaglandins E_1 and E_2 evoke only some of the local and systemic manifestations of inflammation produced by histamine, bradykinin, and 5-hydroxytryptamine, known chemical mediators of inflammation, they intensify the effects of these mediators in doses that have little effect by themselves. Therapeutic doses of salicylates, indomethacin, and other anti-inflammatory drugs block an early step in the synthesis of prostaglandins from precursor fatty acids, by inhibition of prostaglandin synthetase. The evidence that the anti-inflammatory and many other effects of salicylates and related drugs are due to inhibition of prostaglandin synthesis has been summarized by Ferreira and Vane (1974) and is discussed further in Chapter 30. Other processes that might underly their anti-inflammatory effect, such as uncoupling of oxidative phosphorylation, inhibition of leukocyte phagocytosis, and stabilization of lysosomal membranes, generally require drug concentrations higher than those achieved with therapeutic doses. The provocative theory that anti-inflammatory drugs act by displacing endogenous anti-inflammatory peptides from their binding sites on plasma proteins requires confirmation (see McArthur et al., 1971).

Because of the known relationship between rheumatic fever and immunological processes, attention has been directed to the effects of salicylates on antigen-antibody reactions. These agents suppress a variety of such reactions. Several different mechanisms are involved, including suppression of antibody production, interference with antigen-antibody aggregation, inhibition in vitro of antigen-induced release of histamine, and nonspecific stabilization of changes in capillary permeability in the presence of immunological insults. The relation of the suppressive effects of salicylates on immunological processes to their antirheumatic efficacy in man is yet to be elucidated.

Drugs useful as antirheumatic and anti-inflammatory agents influence the metabolism of connective tissue, and these effects may be involved in their anti-inflammatory action. For example, salicylates can affect the composition, biosynthesis, or metabolism of connective tissue mucopolysaccharides concerned with the ground substance that provides barriers to spread of infection and inflammation. (See Whitehouse, 1965; Smith and Smith, 1966; Paulus and Whitehouse, 1973; Ferreira and Vane, 1974.)

Metabolic Effects. The salicylates have a multiplicity of effects on metabolic processes, some of which have already been discussed. Only a few pertinent aspects will be presented here. (See Symposium, 1963; Whitehouse, 1965; Smith and Smith, 1966; Smith and Dawkins, 1971; Paulus and Whitehouse, 1973; Ferreira and Vane, 1974.)

Oxidative Phosphorylation. The uncoupling of oxidative phosphorylation by salicylate is similar to that induced by 2,4-dinitrophenol, in that intact mitochondrial membranes are not essential (Miyahara and Karler, 1965); the terminal phosphorylation step concerned with the oxidation of cytochrome c appears to be especially sensitive to both agents, and both stimulate mitochondrial adenosine triphosphatase activity in vitro. The effect occurs in man with doses of salicylate used in the treatment of rheumatoid arthritis.

As a result of the uncoupling action of salicylates, a number of adenosine triphosphate (ATP)–dependent reactions are inhibited. The salicylate-induced increase in oxygen uptake and carbon dioxide production, described above, is due to the uncoupling action of the drug and the enhanced oxidation compensatory to the relative inefficiency of the phosphorylating mechanisms. The salicylate-induced depletion of hepatic glycogen can also be explained by this mechanism. The pyretic effect of toxic doses of salicylate can be similarly explained since the oxidatively derived energy normally used for the conversion of inorganic phosphate to ATP is dissipated principally as heat. Salicylate in toxic doses may decrease aerobic metabolism as a result of inhibition of various dehydrogenases, by competing with the pyridine nucleotide coenzymes, and inhibition of some oxidases that require nucleotides as coenzymes, such as xanthine oxidase.

Carbohydrate Metabolism. The effects of salicylate on carbohydrate metabolism are complex. Multiple factors appear to be involved, some tending to lower and others to raise the blood sugar level. In both animals and man, large doses of salicylates may cause hyperglycemia and glycosuria and deplete liver and muscle glycogen; these effects are partly explained by the release of epinephrine, through activation of central sympathetic centers. Such large doses also reduce aerobic metabolism of glucose and increase glucose-6-phosphatase activity, effects tending to increase the blood sugar level. In addition, by an increase in adrenocortical activity, prolonged hyperglycemia occurs in salicylate intoxication.

In certain diabetic patients and in experimental animals with endocrine imbalances, salicylate can lower the blood sugar and reduce the glycosuria. Indeed, salicylates were among the earliest agents used to lower the blood sugar of diabetics. The hypoglycemia is not a result of insulin release, and sensitivity to insulin is not modified by salicylate; it is accompanied by protein catabolism and loss of intracellular potassium, effects opposite to those of insulin. The conclusion from considerable experimental evidence is that salicylate-induced hypoglycemia is due to increased utilization of glucose by peripheral tissues; decreased synthesis of carbohydrate, however, is involved since key regulatory enzymes for gluconeogenesis are inhibited by salicylates.

Nitrogen Metabolism. Salicylate in toxic doses causes a significant negative nitrogen balance, characterized by an aminoaciduria. Adrenocortical activation may contribute to the negative nitrogen balance by enhancing protein catabolism. The mechanism of the aminoaciduria produced by salicylates is not known; it is probably the result of a combination of decreased protein synthesis due to preferential inhibition of aminoacyl-tRNA synthetases, accelerated breakdown of proteins, and inhibition of the active renal tubular reabsorption of amino acids—all processes that involve ATP—as well as inhibition of aminotransferases involved in amino acid interconversions.

Fat Metabolism. Salicylates reduce lipogenesis by partially blocking incorporation of acetate into fatty acids; they also inhibit epinephrine-stimulated lipolysis in fat cells and displace long-chain fatty acids from binding sites on human plasma proteins. The combination of these effects leads to increased entry and enhanced oxidation of fatty acids in muscle, liver, and other tissues, and to the lowering of concentrations of plasma free fatty acids, phospholipid, and cholesterol; the oxidation of ketone bodies is also increased.

Endocrine Effects.

Salicylate directly or indirectly influences the function of a number of endocrine systems; such effects are in part responsible for some of the metabolic and pharmacological responses to the drug.

Adrenal Medulla. As mentioned above, high doses of salicylate activate central sympathetic centers and thereby cause release of epinephrine from the adrenal medulla. The released epinephrine is partly responsible for the hyperglycemia and the depletion of liver glycogen observed after large amounts of the drug.

Adrenal Cortex. Very large doses of salicylate stimulate steroid secretion by the adrenal cortex through an effect on the hypothalamus and increase transiently the plasma concentrations of free adreno-

corticosteroids by displacement from plasma proteins. However, there is abundant evidence that the anti-inflammatory effects of salicylate are independent of these effects on adrenocorticosteroids (*see* Domenjoz, 1966; Smith and Smith, 1966; Paulus and Whitehouse, 1973).

Thyroid Gland. Chronic administration of salicylate decreases the plasma protein-bound iodine and thyroidal uptake and clearance of iodine, but increases oxygen consumption and rate of disappearance of thyroxine and triiodothyronine from the circulation. These effects are probably due to the competitive displacement by salicylate of thyroxine and triiodothyronine from prealbumin and the thyroxine-binding globulin in plasma; consequently, the plasma concentrations of free thyroxine and triiodothyronine are increased. This causes inhibition of thyrotropin secretion, which results in decreases in thyroid activity, iodine uptake, and hormonal release. These events lead to a new equilibrium at a lower concentration of protein-bound iodine, but with slightly elevated concentrations of free circulating thyroxine and triiodothyronine for at least 8 to 10 days. Most of the calorigenic effect of salicylate is directly on peripheral tissues, but an immediate and transient calorigenic effect may be mediated in part through release of thyroxine and triiodothyronine from binding sites. (*See* Smith and Smith, 1966; Larsen, 1972.)

Salicylates and Pregnancy. After doses close to lethal for the embryo and highly toxic to the mother, *teratogenic effects* occur in experimental animals during the early stages of development. However, there is no evidence that therapeutic doses of salicylates cause fetal damage in human beings, and their use in moderation during pregnancy does not appear to be contraindicated. Nevertheless, chronic high-dose salicylate therapy of pregnant women for rheumatoid arthritis increases the length of gestation and the frequency of postmaturity, and prolongs spontaneous labor, presumably due to inhibition of prostaglandin synthesis (Lewis and Schulman, 1973).

Local Irritant Effects. Salicylic acid is quite irritating to skin and mucosa and destroys epithelial cells. The keratolytic action of the free acid is employed for the local treatment of warts, corns, fungal infections, and certain types of eczematous dermatitis. The tissue cells swell, soften, and desquamate. The salts of salicylic acid are innocuous to the unbroken skin; however, if the free acid is released in the stomach, the gastric mucosa may be irritated. Methyl salicylate (oil of wintergreen) is irritating to both skin and gastric mucosa and is only used externally, in liniments as a counterirritant.

Absorption, Distribution, Biotransformation, and Excretion. These important aspects of the salicylates have been reviewed by Davison (1971).

Absorption. Orally ingested salicylates are absorbed rapidly, partly from the stomach but mostly from the upper small intestine.

Appreciable plasma concentrations are found in less than 30 minutes; after a single dose, a peak value is reached in about 2 hours and then gradually declines. Rate of absorption is determined by many factors, particularly the disintegration and dissolution rates if tablets are given, the pH at the mucosal surfaces, and gastric emptying time.

Salicylate absorption occurs by passive diffusion primarily of the nondissociated lipid-soluble molecules (salicylic acid and acetylsalicylic acid) across gastrointestinal membranes and hence is influenced by gastric pH. If the pH is increased, salicylate is more ionized and this tends to decrease rate of absorption; however, a rise in pH also increases solubility of salicylate, which has the opposite effect on absorption. Actually, there is little meaningful difference between the rates of absorption of sodium salicylate, aspirin, and the numerous buffered preparations of salicylates. For example, in man the absorption half-time for unbuffered aspirin is about 30 minutes, for buffered aspirin about 20 minutes, and for an aspirin solution only slightly less. The presence of food delays absorption of salicylates.

Rectal absorption of salicylate is usually slower, incomplete, and unreliable; rectal administration is therefore not advisable when high plasma concentrations of the drug are required. Salicylic acid is rapidly absorbed from the intact *skin,* especially when applied in oily liniments or ointments, and systemic poisoning has occurred from its application to large areas of skin. Methyl salicylate is likewise speedily absorbed when applied cutaneously; its gastrointestinal absorption may be delayed many hours and, therefore, gastric lavage should be performed even in cases of poisoning that are seen late.

When the nonionized salicylate molecules in the gastric lumen enter the mucosal cells, they dissociate predominantly to the ionized form at the intracellular pH of 7.0 and accumulate there in large amounts; for example, the concentration of salicylate anion in mucosal cells may be 15 to 20 times that in the gastric lumen. As a result, gastric mucosal damage may occur.

Distribution. After absorption, salicylate is rapidly distributed throughout all body tissues and most transcellular fluids, primarily by pH-dependent passive processes. For example, it can be detected in synovial, spinal, and peritoneal fluid, and in saliva and milk. Salicylate is actively transported by a low-capacity, saturable system out of the CSF across the choroid plexus (Spector and Lorenzo, 1973). The drug readily crosses the placental barrier. It is not secreted in gastric juice. Only traces of salicylate are present in sweat, bile, and feces.

The volumes of distribution of aspirin and sodium salicylate in normal subjects average about 150 ml/kg of body weight, a value equivalent to that of the extracellular space; since salicylate is present within cells in various tissues, this suggests a markedly uneven distribution of salicylate in the body. The concentration of salicylate in intracellular fluid is lower than in plasma, in part because of the lower pH of the former. The movement of salicylate across some cell membranes is pH dependent and appears also to be insulin dependent. Salicylate does not accumulate in pathological fluids, such as joint effusions in acute rheumatic fever; hence, a selective distribution is not the basis for its therapeutic effects.

Ingested aspirin is mainly absorbed as such, but some enters the systemic circulation as salicylic acid, consequent to hydrolysis by esterases in the gastrointestinal mucosa and the liver. Aspirin can be detected in the plasma only for a short time; for example, 30 minutes after a dose of 0.65 g, only 27% of the total plasma salicylate is in the acetylated form. The absorbed ester is rapidly hydrolyzed to salicylic acid in plasma, liver, and erythrocytes, and more slowly in synovial fluid. As a result of the rapid hydrolysis, plasma concentrations of aspirin are always low and rarely exceed 20 µg/ml at ordinary therapeutic doses. Aspirin *per se* is pharmacologically active and does not require hydrolysis to salicylic acid for its effects. Methyl salicylate is also rapidly hydrolyzed to salicylic acid, mainly in the liver.

At concentrations encountered clinically, from 50 to 90% of the salicylate is bound to plasma proteins, especially albumin. Hypoalbuminemia, as may occur in rheumatoid arthritis, is associated with a proportionately higher level of free salicylate in the plasma. Salicylate competes with thyroxine, triiodothyronine, penicillin, thiopental, phenytoin, sulfinpyrazone, bilirubin, tryptophan, certain peptides, possibly steroids, uric acid, and naproxen for plasma protein binding sites. Aspirin as such is bound to only a very limited extent; however, it acetylates human plasma albumin *in vivo* by reaction with the ∊-amino group of lysine. This may result in alteration of the antigenicity of albumin and be related to the syndrome of aspirin hypersensitivity (Hawkins *et al.,* 1969). Hormones, DNA, platelets, and hemoglobin and other proteins are also acetylated. The binding of phenylbutazone and flufenamic acid to albumin is modified as a result of acetylation of this protein by aspirin. The acetylation of human serum albumin by aspirin is inhibited by salicylate anion.

Biotransformation and Excretion. The *biotransformation* of salicylate takes place in many tissues, but particularly in the microsomal system and mitochondria of liver. The three chief metabolic products are salicyluric acid (the glycine conjugate), the ether or phenolic glucuronide, and the ester or acyl glucuronide. In addition, a small fraction is oxidized to gentisic acid (2,5-dihydroxybenzoic acid) and to 2,3-dihydroxybenzoic and 2,3,5-trihydroxybenzoic acids. These metabolites are found in the urine; the conjugates and gentisic acid have also been identified in plasma, liver, and some other tissues. The concentration of the metabolites in plasma is generally only about 1% of the total plasma salicylate.

Salicylates are *excreted* mainly by the kidney, and in much smaller amounts through other channels. Practically all of a given dose can be recovered in the urine as free, unaltered salicylate and as the metabolites described above, the nature and the relative amounts of which vary in health and disease, with the dosage, and with the pH of the urine. Studies in man indicate that salicylate is excreted in the urine as free salicylic acid (10%), salicyluric acid (75%), salicylic phenolic (10%) and acyl (5%) glucuronides, and gentisic acid (<1%). However, excretion of free salicylate is extremely variable. In alkaline urine up to 85% of the ingested drug is eliminated as free salicylate, whereas in acidic urine this may be as low as 5%.

The plasma half-life for aspirin is approximately 20 minutes; that for salicylate is 3 to 6 hours in low doses and 15 to 30 hours at high doses. This dose-dependent elimination is the result of the limited ability of the liver to form salicyluric acid and the phenolic glucuronide (Levy *et al.*, 1972).

The plasma concentration of salicylate is increased by conditions that decrease glomerular filtration rate or reduce the secretory Tm of the proximal tubules, such as renal disease or the presence of inhibitors that compete for the transport system (*e.g.*, probenecid). Changes in urinary pH in the acid range have negligible effects on salicylate clearance; however, the mean clearance is about four times as great at pH 8.0 as at pH 6.0. The clearance is well above the glomerular filtration rate at pH 8.0 but considerably below it when the urine is acidic. This is due to the fact that salicylate and salicylurate are highly ionized at pH 8.0, and little diffuses back from the renal tubular lumen. At a urinary pH of 6.0, large amounts of salicylate and salicylurate are nonionized and readily back-diffuse. High rates of urine flow decrease tubular back diffusion, whereas the opposite is true in oliguria. The conjugates of salicylic acid with glycine and glucuronic acid are water-soluble organic acids that do not readily back-diffuse across the renal tubular cells. Their excretion, therefore, is both by glomerular filtration and proximal tubular secretion and is not pH dependent. (*See* Smith and Smith, 1966; Morgan and Polak, 1971.)

Preparations, Dosage, and Routes of Administration. The two most commonly used preparations of salicylate for systemic effects are *sodium salicylate* and *aspirin* (*acetylsalicylic acid*).

Sodium Salicylate, N.F., is a white, water-soluble powder with a sweet, saline taste. It is available as official tablets that contain 300 or 600 mg of drug.

Aspirin, U.S.P., is a white powder, poorly soluble in water (1:300). It is available as official tablets ranging from 65 to 650 mg, capsules (300 mg), and suppositories ranging from 65 to 1300 mg.

Methyl Salicylate, U.S.P. (*sweet birch oil, wintergreen oil, gaultheria oil, betula oil*), is a colorless, yellowish, or reddish liquid having the characteristic odor and taste of wintergreen. It is employed only for cutaneous counterirritation in the form of salves and liniments.

Salicylic Acid, U.S.P., is a white powder poorly soluble in water (1:460) but quite soluble in alcohol (1:3). Its use is reserved for local application as a keratolytic agent, in official plasters and collodion, and as a component of *Benzoic Acid and Salicylic Acid Ointment,* U.S.P., and *Zinc Oxide Paste with Salicylic Acid,* N.F.

The *dose* of salicylate depends on the condition being treated. The usual single dose of sodium salicylate or aspirin in adults is 300 mg to 1.0 g. This may be repeated every 4 hours. In acute rheumatic fever and rheumatoid arthritis more intensive medication is employed (*see* below).

The *route of administration* is practically always oral. There is rarely any necessity for parenteral administration. The *rectal* administration of aspirin suppositories or sodium salicylate (2%) in thin starch or acacia solution may be necessary in infants or when oral medication is not retained. Salicylates are conveniently taken in tablets or capsules with a full glass of water to minimize gastric irritation. Aspirin is poorly soluble, has many chemical incompatibilities, and should be dispensed only in solid dry form.

Timed-release preparations are of limited value, since the half-time for elimination of salicylate is so long. Absorption from *enteric-coated* tablets is sometimes incomplete.

SALICYLATE INTOXICATION

Salicylates are widely used in medicine and are indiscriminately employed by the laity for every conceivable ailment. When one considers their abuse and their availability, the high incidence of toxic reactions to salicylate is not surprising. Fortunately, most of these cases are mild and inconsequential. However, salicylate poisoning can result in death, and the drug should not be viewed as a harmless household remedy. The toxicity of the salicylates is underestimated by both the laity and physicians. Hypersensitivity is also a cause of untoward responses to salicylate. Furthermore, renal or hepatic insufficiency or hypoprothrombinemia or other bleeding disorder enhances the possibility of salicylate toxicity. Children with fever and dehydration are particularly prone to intoxication from relatively small doses of salicylate.

Acute Salicylate Poisoning. The *fatal dose* varies with the preparation of salicylate. From 10 to 30 g of sodium salicylate or aspirin has caused death in adults, but much larger amounts (130 g of aspirin, in one case) have been ingested without fatal outcome. The lethal dose of methyl salicylate is considerably less than that of sodium salicylate. As little as 4 ml (4.7 g) of methyl salicylate may be fatal in children.

Symptoms and Signs. Mild chronic salicylate intoxication is termed *salicylism.* This condition usually occurs only after repeated administration of large doses. When fully developed, the syndrome consists chiefly in headache, dizziness, ringing in the ears, difficulty in hearing, dimness of vision, mental confusion, lassitude, drowsiness, sweating, thirst, hyperventilation, nausea, vomiting, and occasionally diarrhea. Care should be exercised in prescribing salicylate to patients with aural disease. A more severe degree of salicylate intoxication is characterized by CNS disturbances (including EEG abnormalities), skin eruptions, and marked alterations in acid-base balance. The above-mentioned CNS effects are more pronounced; in addition, restlessness, garrulity, incoherent speech, apprehension, vertigo, tremor, diplopia, maniacal delirium, hallucinations, generalized convulsions, and coma may occur. The mental disturbances, sometimes referred to as "salicylate jag," simulate alcoholic inebriation; euphoria and elation are absent, however, and the experience is rather a melancholy affair.

A pustular acneform *skin eruption* simulating that of bromism may develop, but it is usually not observed unless salicylate medication has been continued for longer than 1 week. Other salicylate-induced cutaneous lesions are erythematous, scarlatiniform, pruritic, eczematoid, or desquamative in character. Rarely, the eruptions may be bullous or purpuric, and hemorrhages may occur from mucous membranes. Fever is usually prominent, especially in children. Dehydration often occurs as a result of hyperpyrexia, sweating, vomiting, and the loss of water vapor during hyperventilation.

Gastrointestinal symptoms are often conspicuous and include epigastric distress, nausea, vomiting, anorexia, and occasionally abdominal pain. Approximately 50% of all individuals with plasma salicylate concentrations of more than 300 µg/ml experience nausea.

A most prominent feature of salicylate intoxication is the *disturbance in acid-base balance and electrolyte composition of the plasma,* the characteristics of which have already been presented. The most severe metabolic disturbances occur in infants and very young children who become intoxicated as the result of therapeutic overdosage for some febrile illness, usually a minor respiratory infection; most of the acidotic patients seen with salicylate intoxication are in this group. Higher doses of the drug and a longer duration of intoxication intensify the metabolic effects and the acidosis. In older patients the intoxication is generally due to accidental or suicidal ingestion of a large single dose.

Hemorrhagic phenomena are occasionally seen during salicylate poisoning, the mechanism and significance of which have been discussed. Petechial hemorrhages are a prominent post-mortem feature. Thrombocytopenic purpura is a rare complication. *Hypoglycemia* may be a serious consequence of salicylate toxicity in young children. It should be seriously considered in any young child with coma, convulsions, or cardiovascular collapse.

Severe toxic *encephalopathy* may be a prominent feature of salicylate poisoning and may be difficult to differentiate from chorea or rheumatic encephalopathy. As poisoning progresses, central stimulation is replaced by increasing depression, stupor, and coma. Cardiovascular collapse and respiratory insufficiency ensue, and terminal asphyxial convulsions and pulmonary edema sometimes appear. Death usually results from respiratory failure after a period of unconsciousness.

Symptoms of poisoning by *methyl salicylate* differ little from those just described. Poisoning occurs most frequently in children who mistake this aromatic oil for candy. Central excitation, intense hyperpnea, and hyperpyrexia are prominent features. The odor of the drug can easily be detected on the breath and in the urine and vomitus. *Methyl salicylate should always be kept where children cannot gain access to it.* Poisoning by *salicylic acid* differs only in the increased prominence of gastrointestinal symptoms due to the marked local irritation. *Phenyl salicylate* intoxication is unique in that the most conspicuous symptoms are due to the phenol that is liberated by hydrolysis, probably in the tissues.

Treatment. Salicylate poisoning represents an acute medical emergency. The treatment is largely symptomatic and not entirely satisfactory. Death may result despite all recommended procedures. Salicylate medication is withdrawn as soon as intoxication is suspected. The patient should be hospitalized and a most guarded prognosis given. *Hospitalization is particularly advisable in the case of methyl salicylate poisoning because children have been known to succumb within a few hours after the parents had been informed that recovery seemed assured or that the intoxication was inconsequential.* Blood should be obtained for plasma salicylate determinations and acid-base and electrolyte studies. Done (1960) has demonstrated that the salicylate concentration is reasonably well correlated with clinical severity, when corrected for the duration of the intoxication, and is of value in assessing the type of therapy to be instituted. Absorption of salicylate from the gastrointestinal tract can be reduced by emesis, gastric lavage, administration of activated charcoal, or a combination of these. Emesis is usually induced with syrup of ipecac (*see* Index).

Hyperthermia and dehydration are the immediate threats to life, and the initial therapy must be directed to their correction and to the maintenance of adequate renal function. External sponging with tepid water should be provided quickly to any child who has a rectal temperature over 104° F. Adequate amounts of intravenous fluids must be given promptly. The type and amount of repair solutions to be employed depend upon the interpretation of the laboratory data on acid-base balance. If the patient presents with an acidosis, correction of the low blood pH is essential, especially since acidosis results in a shift of salicylate from plasma into brain and other tissues; alkalosis reverses this process and also increases salicylate excretion (Hill, 1971). Death may result from the high concentrations of salicylate in brain tissue during the acidotic phase; hence, avoidance or correction of acidosis should be a primary therapeutic goal (Hill, 1973). Bicarbonate solution should be infused intravenously to combat the acidosis and, if possible, to maintain alkaline diuresis. Excessively rapid infusion of bicarbonate can cause pulmonary edema or other unwanted effects. Frequent monitoring of blood pH, plasma P_{CO_2}, and plasma glucose concentration are necessary. Correction of ketosis and hypoglycemia by administration of glucose is also essential for complete control of the metabolic acidosis; however, the ketosis clears only slowly. If potassium deficiency occurs during salicylate intoxication, it should be treated by adding the cation to the intravenous fluids once it has been determined that urine formation is adequate. Plasma transfusion may be beneficial, especially if the shock syndrome intervenes. Any attempt to obtund the salicylate-induced hyperventilation by giving a barbiturate or a narcotic is dangerous and may rapidly lead to respiratory acidosis and coma. Hemorrhagic phenomena may necessitate whole-blood transfusion and vitamin K_1 or its oxide.

Measures to rid the body rapidly of salicylate should be immediately undertaken. Sodium bicarbonate administration is effective and rapid, if an alkaline urine can be produced. Forced diuresis with alkalinizing solution appears to be better than alkali alone; acetazolamide can be added to this combination if a more rapid effect is necessary and only if systemic acidosis is avoided (Hill, 1973; Reimold et al., 1973). Potassium should be administered with the bicarbonate to prevent further depletion of intracellular potassium.

In severe intoxication, extrarenal measures such as exchange transfusion, peritoneal dialysis, hemodialysis, and hemoperfusion are the most effective measures available for the removal of salicylate. Hemodialysis in adults and older children and exchange transfusion or peritoneal dialysis in infants should be considered seriously in all salicylate-intoxicated patients whose clinical condition is deteriorating despite appropriate therapy and in those who have associated serious disease. (See Smith and Smith, 1966; Symposium, 1968; Done and Temple, 1971; Hill, 1973.)

Hypersensitivity. Hypersensitivity to salicylate usually manifests itself in the form of skin rashes and anaphylactic phenomena. These can occur after a small dose of salicylate. The previous ingestion of salicylate without ill effects is no guarantee against the subsequent occurrence of allergic reactions to the drug. Aspirin is the compound most often involved; sensitivity to sodium salicylate and salicylic acid is rare, and cross-sensitivity between these agents and aspirin is uncommon. However, many aspirin-hypersensitive patients are also hypersensitive to indomethacin, another anti-inflammatory agent (see below). Allergic responses also take the form of

angioedema and asthma. If laryngeal swelling occurs, alarming asphyxial symptoms may develop. Edema of the eyelids, tongue, lips, face, and intestinal tract is not uncommon; an erysipelatous swelling of the entire face may occur. Many patients who react badly to aspirin have a history of allergic disease, especially asthma, and nasal polyps are also frequently present. Asthma constitutes the chief allergic manifestation in most individuals sensitive to aspirin; death may result. One should therefore observe care in prescribing aspirin for patients with asthma.

Individuals with hypersensitivity to aspirin should be warned against taking proprietary mixtures, which often contain this drug. Aspirin hypersensitivity cannot be predicted by skin tests; hence, a clinical history is the only satisfactory method for its diagnosis. Aspirin hypersensitivity probably involves acetylation of protein to produce an antigenic substance; an impurity in aspirin, acetylsalicylsalicylic acid, is another possible immunogenic compound involved in allergic reactions to this drug.

The overall incidence of hypersensitivity to aspirin is probably of the order of 0.2 to 0.9%. Treatment of allergic responses to salicylates does not differ from that ordinarily employed in acute anaphylactic reactions. Epinephrine is the drug of choice and usually controls angioedema and urticaria without difficulty, but asthma induced by aspirin may at times prove refractory to therapy. (See Samter and Beers, 1968; Giraldo et al., 1969; Chafee and Settipane, 1974; Settipane et al., 1974.)

THERAPEUTIC USES

There are many *systemic* and a few *local* uses of the salicylates. Several are based on tradition and empirical results rather than on a clear understanding of the mechanism of therapeutic benefit. The laity often attributes properties to the salicylates that have no existence in fact.

Systemic Uses. *Antipyresis.* Antipyretic therapy is reserved for cases in which fever in itself may be deleterious, and for patients who experience considerable relief when a fever is lowered. Little is known concerning the relationship between fever and the acceleration of immune processes; it may at times be a protective physiological mechanism. The course of the patient's illness may be obscured by the relief of symptoms and the reduction of fever from the use of antipyretic drugs; otherwise the effect of salicylate is nonspecific and does not influence the course of the underlying disease (see Done, 1973). The antipyretic dose of salicylate for adults is 325 mg to 1.0 g, orally every 3 or 4 hours; for children, 10 to 20 mg/kg every 6 hours, not to exceed a total daily dose of 3.6 g.

Analgesia. Salicylate is valuable for the nonspecific relief of certain types of pain, for example, *headache, arthritis, dysmenorrhea, neuralgia,* and *myalgia.* For this purpose, it is prescribed in the same doses and manner as for antipyresis. The use of salicylate in combination with other analgesics, sedatives, and so forth is discussed later in the chapter.

"Colds" and Other Minor Respiratory Infections. Salicylate does not influence the course of the common cold or upper respiratory infections. It may make the patient more comfortable by reducing fever and relieving headache and muscle aching. If the symptomatic improvement tempts the individual to be ambulatory and active during his infection, the drug may do more harm than good. The use of gargles containing aspirin has no value.

Gout. Salicylates are no longer used for the treatment of gout. Allopurinol, probenecid, and sulfinpyrazone are preferred for the chronic therapy of gout, and colchicine is of particular value in the treatment of acute attacks (*see* Index).

Acute Rheumatic Fever. In this disease, the salicylates suppress the acute exudative inflammatory process of the disease but do not affect the progression of the disease or the later phases of granulomatous inflammation or scar formation. Within 24 to 48 hours after adequate doses of salicylate, there is usually considerable or complete relief of pain, swelling, immobility, local heat, and redness of the involved joints; fever and pulse rate are lowered and the patient feels much improved. Further joint involvement usually does not occur while appropriate salicylate medication is being given. Other aspects of the management of acute rheumatic fever are not altered as a result of salicylate medication. Salicylate-induced improvement should not be mistaken for control of the disease. The drug is effective only in relieving certain features of the exudative process (joint, pericardial, and pleural effusions, etc.) and does not in any way alter the proliferative reactions. Thus, cardiac complications, chorea, encephalopathy, subcutaneous nodules, and other features are not prevented or benefited, and the duration of the disease is not shortened. However, if a patient has severe carditis and heart failure, the nonspecific anti-inflammatory effect of salicylates and particularly of adrenocorticosteroids may be invaluable in reducing the burden upon the heart; occasionally this salutary effect may tilt the balance in favor of survival in a critically ill patient.

Dosage. For maximal suppression of rheumatic inflammation, doses that provide a plasma salicylate concentration of 250 to 350 μg/ml should be maintained, but polyarthritis and fever usually respond to smaller amounts. For adults, a total daily dosage of 5 to 8 g, given at intervals in 1-g amounts, usually suffices. Children are given 100 to 125 mg/kg per day, in divided portions every 4 to 6 hours, for up to 1 week; the dose is then reduced in stepwise fashion at weekly intervals to 60 mg/kg per day (10 mg/kg every 4 hours, or 15 mg/kg every 6 hours) and maintained as long as necessary. Anorexia, tinnitus, nausea, and vomiting are common during the first 3 or 4 days of therapy, but tend to subside despite continuation of medication. There is no fixed dose or schedule that will give optimal results in all patients, and such treatment by rote may be harmful. Large doses should be employed only if smaller amounts fail to give relief; indeed, relatively small doses (5 g per day) may occasionally cause very high plasma salicylate levels. Ordinarily, full doses are continued until at least 2 weeks after the patient is asymptomatic and all evidence of active infection (elevated leukocyte count and erythrocyte sedimentation rate, fever, ECG abnormalities, etc.) has disappeared. The drug is then gradually discontinued over a period of 7 to 10 days. If symptoms and signs of the disease reappear, salicylate therapy is reinstituted. Aspirin is recommended and sodium salicylate should be avoided, because restricted sodium intake is advisable. Therapy with adrenocorticosteroids does not yield overall results superior to those obtained with the salicylates. Salicylate and adrenocorticosteroid are additive in their effects; an advantage of their concurrent use is the reduction of dosage of the steroid and thereby its side effects. The effect of adrenocorticosteroids on the rheumatic process is discussed elsewhere. If carditis is not evident, salicylates and not steroids should be used. However, if acute severe carditis is present, most investigators believe adrenocorticosteroids should be given instead of salicylates, at least initially. (*See* McEwen, 1959; Combined Rheumatic Fever Study Group, 1960, 1965; United Kingdom and United States Joint Report, 1960.)

Rheumatoid Arthritis. Despite the development of several newer agents, salicylates are still the cornerstone of therapy and the drugs of first choice for the treatment of rheumatoid arthritis. In addition to the analgesia that allows more effective therapeutic exercises, there is improvement in appetite and a feeling of well-being. Salicylates also reduce the inflammation in joint tissues and surrounding structures. Damage to joints is the most difficult aspect of rheumatoid arthritis to manage, and any agent that reduces the inflammation is important in lessening or delaying the development of crippling. Salicylates can be shown to produce objectively measurable anti-inflammatory changes when given in large doses for long periods to patients with active rheumatoid disease (*see* Boardman and Hart, 1967a; Deodhar *et al.,* 1973). If necessary, other drugs that favorably affect the course of the arthritis can be used concurrently to good advantage. Fairly large doses of salicylate slightly below those that produce tinnitus (5 to 6 g daily) are advised, but some patients respond well to 3.6 g daily (Multz *et al.,* 1974). In addition to drug therapy and other measures, meticulous attention should be paid to therapeutic exercises to maintain as full range of normal joint motion as possible and to improve muscle strength.

The majority of patients with rheumatoid arthritis can be controlled with salicylates alone. Only a few require more aggressive therapy with the more toxic drugs available. When salicylate therapy is not appropriate, other anti-inflammatory agents, gold salts (Chapter 46), antimalarials (Chapter 52), adrenocorticosteroids (Chapter 70), and immunosuppressive agents (Chapter 62) can be used. These more toxic drugs often ameliorate the disease in selected patients and, in the case of gold salts and immunosuppressive agents, may reduce bony erosions.

Other Uses. The inhibitory effect of low doses of aspirin on platelet aggregation has led to several potential therapeutic uses of this drug. These uses require further evaluation, but all are sufficiently important to mention. Thus, the prophylactic administration of aspirin has been shown to exert a protective effect equivalent to that of oral anticoagulant agents against *venous thrombosis* and *pulmonary embolism* in patients undergoing certain orthopedic operations. Aspirin also has been used to abolish both the increased platelet aggregability and the *transient ischemic episodes* in patients with multiple episodes of transient *monocular blindness* (amaurosis fugax) secondary to retinal emboli. In addition, aspirin is undergoing study in the prophylaxis of *coronary thrombosis.* There is some evidence that aspirin may prevent the *cartilage degeneration* that occurs secondary to patellar dislocations and other joint injuries, when given immediately after injury.

Relation of Plasma Salicylate Concentration to Therapeutic Effect and Toxicity. For optimal anti-inflammatory effect for patients with rheumatic diseases, plasma salicylate concentrations of 150 to 300 μg/ml are required. Because salicylate elimination is dose dependent in this range, large individual variations occur in the concentrations obtained with the same total daily dose. Hence, optimal intensive salicylate therapy can be achieved only by individualizing the total dose of aspirin. This is especially important since the range of plasma salicylate concentrations needed for optimal anti-inflammatory effects may overlap that at which tinnitus is noted. In a study of patients with rheumatoid arthritis by Mongan and coworkers (1973), the range of plasma salicylate concentrations at which tinnitus occurred varied from 196 to 458 μg/ml. Daily dosage varied from 3.6 to 10.8 g. Tinnitus was a reliable index of therapeutic plasma concentration in those patients with normal hearing, but not in those with a pre-existing hearing loss. In the latter patients, plasma salicylate concentrations may be a useful guideline. Hyperventilation generally occurs at concentrations greater than 350 μg/ml and other signs of intoxication, such as acidosis, at concentrations greater than 460 μg/ml. Single analgesic-antipyretic doses of salicylate usually yield plasma concentrations below 60 μg/ml; in this range first-order kinetics applies.

The plasma concentration of salicylate is generally little affected by other drugs, but concurrent administration of aspirin lowers the concentrations of indomethacin, naproxen, and fenoprofen, at least in part by displacement from plasma proteins. Other interactions of aspirin include the antagonism of spironolactone-induced natriuresis and the blockade of the active transport of aminosalicylic acid and penicillin from CSF to blood.

Local Uses. *Salicylic acid* is applied topically as a *keratolytic agent.* In combination with benzoic acid, it is often prescribed for *epidermophytosis.* Salicylic acid is also employed as a *wart* and *corn* remover (10 to 20% in collodion). It is sometimes prescribed in talc (2 to 4%) for *hyperhidrosis.*

Methyl salicylate is reserved for external use as a *counterirritant.* It is employed for painful muscles or joints, in an ointment or liniment. Absorption of methyl salicylate can occur through the skin, and death has resulted from systemic poisoning from the local misapplication of the drug. It is a common *pediatric poison,* and its use should be strongly discouraged. It is also used as a *flavoring agent.*

SALICYLATE-LIKE ANTI-INFLAMMATORY AGENTS

PHENYLBUTAZONE

Phenylbutazone, a congener of antipyrine and aminopyrine (*see* below), was employed originally as a solubilizing agent for aminopyrine. It was introduced in 1949 for the treatment of rheumatoid arthritis and allied disorders. Phenylbutazone is an effective anti-inflammatory agent, but toxicity precludes its use in long-term therapy.

Chemistry. Phenylbutazone is 3,5-dioxo-1,2-diphenyl-4-*n*-butylpyrazolidine, a pyrazolon derivative. The structural formula is as follows:

Phenylbutazone

The pharmacological properties of phenylbutazone are profoundly affected by slight changes in its chemical structure, probably because metabolites contribute significantly to its pharmacological effects. (*See* Burns *et al.,* 1960; Gutman et al., 1960.)

Pharmacological Properties. The anti-inflammatory effects of phenylbutazone are similar to those of salicylate, but the toxic effects of the two drugs differ significantly. Like aminopyrine, phenylbutazone can cause agranulocytosis. The pharmacology and toxicology of phenylbutazone and its metabolites and congeners have been reviewed by Randall (1963).

Anti-inflammatory Effects. Phenylbutazone has prominent anti-inflammatory effects in animals, and comparable effects are demonstrable in patients with rheumatoid arthritis and related disorders. The mechanism of the anti-inflammatory effects of phenylbutazone is not known. Like salicylates, phenylbutazone inhibits the biosynthesis of prostaglandins, uncouples oxidative phosphorylation, and inhibits the ATP-dependent biosynthesis of mucopolysaccharide sulfates in cartilage. (*See* Domenjoz, 1960, 1966; Randall, 1963; Whitehouse, 1965; Ferreira and Vane, 1974.)

Antipyretic and Analgesic Effects. The *antipyretic* effect of phenylbutazone has been little studied in man. For pain of nonrheumatic origin, its *analgesic* efficacy is inferior to that of salicylates. Because of its toxicity, phenylbutazone should not be used as a general-purpose analgesic or antipyretic.

Uricosuric Effect. Phenylbutazone has a mild uricosuric effect in experimental animals and man, probably attributable to one of its metabolites. The uricosuric effect results from diminished tubular reabsorption of uric acid. Low concentrations of the drug inhibit tubular secretion of uric acid and cause urate retention. A congener, *sulfinpyrazone,* is much more effective than phenylbutazone as a uricosuric agent and is useful for the treatment of chronic gout (*see* Chapter 41).

Water and Electrolyte Effects. Phenylbutazone causes significant retention of sodium and chloride, accompanied by a reduction in urine volume; edema may result in some cases. The excretion of potassium is not changed. Plasma volume frequently increases as much as 50%; as a result, cardiac decompensation and acute pulmonary edema have occurred in patients given the drug. The expansion of plasma volume accounts, in part, for the anemia observed during medication. The retention of sodium and chloride represents a direct effect of the drug on the renal tubules. The mechanism has not been elucidated. On cessation of medication, the excess of sodium and chloride is excreted and a compensatory diuresis results.

Other Effects. Phenylbutazone reduces the uptake of iodine by the thyroid gland, apparently by a direct effect on the thyroid to inhibit synthesis of organic iodine compounds. Goiter and myxedema may occasionally result from this effect. Phenylbutazone also inhibits enzymes of the Krebs cycle; the resulting diminished energy production may contribute to its toxicity.

Absorption, Distribution, Biotransformation, and Excretion. Phenylbutazone is rapidly and completely absorbed from the gastrointestinal tract, and peak plasma concentration is reached in 2 hours. After therapeutic doses, phenylbutazone is 98% bound to plasma proteins; at higher plasma concentrations of phenylbutazone, the bound fraction may be only 90%.

The plasma half-time of phenylbutazone is 50 to 100 hours. Biotransformation by the hepatic microsomal system yields two metabolites, *oxyphenbutazone* (phenolic group in para position of benzene ring) and γ-hydroxyphenylbutazone (a compound with an alcoholic OH in the 3 position of the butyl side chain). Oxyphenbutazone has antirheumatic and sodium-retaining activities similar to those of phenylbutazone. Also like the parent drug, oxyphenbutazone is extensively bound to plasma proteins and has a plasma half-time of several days. It accumulates significantly during chronic phenylbutazone administration and contributes to the pharmacological and toxic effects of the parent drug. In animals, oxyphenbutazone inhibits the biotransformation of phenylbutazone. The other metabolite of phenylbutazone has marked uricosuric effect but little antirheumatic or sodium-retaining effect. It is extensively bound to plasma proteins. Its plasma half-time is about 12 hours.

Phenylbutazone and oxyphenbutazone are only slowly excreted in the urine, since binding to plasma protein limits their glomerular filtration, and since both have a relatively high pK_a, which favors passive reabsorption in the distal tubule. Only a trace of unchanged phenylbutazone is excreted in the urine; about 4% appears as oxyphenbutazone and about 15% as the uricosuric metabolite. (*See* Burns *et al.,* 1953, 1955; Gutman *et al.,* 1960.)

Drug Interactions. Other *anti-inflammatory* agents, *oral anticoagulant* agents, *oral hypoglycemics, sulfonamides,* and other drugs may be displaced from binding to plasma proteins by phenylbutazone. The net result may be increased pharmacological or toxic effects of the displaced drug, depending upon the drug and its disposition after being displaced (*see* Chapter 1). The well-documented increased risk of bleeding associated with concurrent phenylbutazone-warfarin medication involves such displacement, but phenylbutazone also modifies the action of the oral anticoagulant agent and influences platelet function. The gastrointestinal effects of phenylbutazone also contribute to the hazard. Displacement of plasma protein–bound thyroid hormone complicates the interpretation of *thyroid function tests.*

Phenylbutazone may cause induction of hepatic microsomal enzymes, and it may also inhibit inactivation of other drugs that are hydroxylated by the microsomal system. It has been said to increase the effect of *insulin.* Oral absorption of phenylbutazone is reduced by concurrently administered *cholestyramine.* The anabolic steroid *methandrostenolone* increases plasma concentrations of administered oxyphenbutazone, but features of the interaction have been inconsistent.

Toxic Effects. Phenylbutazone is poorly tolerated by many patients. Some type of side effect is noted in 10 to 45% of patients, and medication may have to be discontinued in 10 to 15%. Nausea, vomiting, epigastric discomfort, and skin rashes are the most frequently reported untoward effects. Diarrhea, vertigo, insomnia, euphoria, nervousness, hematuria (enhanced by concomitant anticoagulant administration), and blurred vision have also been observed. In addition, water and electrolyte retention and edema formation occur.

More serious forms of adverse effects include peptic ulcer (or its reactivation) with hemorrhage or perforation, hypersensitivity reactions of the serum-sickness type, ulcerative stomatitis, hepatitis, nephritis, aplastic anemia, leukopenia, agranulocytosis, and thrombocytopenia. A number of deaths have occurred, especially from aplastic anemia and agranulocytosis.

If phenylbutazone is employed, close medical supervision of the patient, periodic blood examinations, and dietary electrolyte restriction are mandatory. Its use should be limited to short-term therapy of not more than 1 week during any one treatment period. Even then, the incidence of disturbing side effects is about 10%. The patient must be told to discontinue the drug and promptly report to the physician if he develops fever, sore throat or other oral lesions, skin rash, pruritus, jaundice, weight increase, or tarry stools. The drug is contraindicated in patients with hypertension; cardiac, renal, or hepatic dysfunction; or a history of peptic ulcer or hypersensitivity to the drug. The toxic effects of the drug are more severe in elderly persons, and its use in this group is inadvisable. (*See* Mauer, 1955; Clinicopathologic Conference, 1961; and many others.)

Preparations and Dosage. *Phenylbutazone,* U.S.P. (BUTAZOLIDIN), is available in 100-mg coated tablets for oral administration. Daily maintenance doses of 400 to 600 mg for brief periods provide maximal therapeutic effects; higher doses only increase toxicity. The drug should be taken with meals to lessen gastric irritation.

Therapeutic Uses. Phenylbutazone is used for the therapy of *acute gout* and for the treatment of *rheumatoid arthritis and allied disorders.* Acute exacerbations of these conditions respond particularly well to the drug, and its use should be reserved for such episodes.

Phenylbutazone should be employed only after other drugs have failed and then only after careful consideration of the risks involved as compared with the advantage to the patient. If doses of 400 to 600 mg of phenylbutazone per day for 7 days do not produce improvement, the drug should be discontinued. Indiscriminate use of phenylbutazone in the therapy of trivial acute or chronic *musculoskeletal disorders* can only be condemned. It should not be employed as a general analgesic or antipyretic. (*See* Brodie *et al.,* 1954; Graham, 1958; Steinbrocker and Argyros, 1960.)

Phenylbutazone is an effective alternative to colchicine in *acute gout.* Excellent relief can be attained with a brief course of medication, and about 85 to 95% of acute attacks are controlled within 24 to 36 hours. Phenylbutazone causes fewer gastrointestinal side effects than does colchicine and is more reliable when initiation of medication has been delayed. Dosage recommendations have varied: 800 mg daily for 2 days; 800 mg the first day, followed by 300 mg daily for 3 days; or an initial dose of 400 mg, followed by 100 mg every 4 hours until articular inflammation subsides. The relative merits and dangers of phenylbutazone, compared with colchicine, have been discussed by Goldfinger (1971) and Yü (1974). Prophylactic use of phenylbutazone is not advised, and the drug should not be used as a uricosuric agent.

Phenylbutazone has a *limited* role in the therapy of *rheumatoid arthritis,* primarily for relief of acute exacerbations of the disorder that are not relieved by other measures (Gifford, 1973). Synovitis is often reduced by a brief regimen (600 mg on the first day, followed by 400 mg daily for 3 days). Because of the high incidence of adverse effects, long-term therapy is not recommended. Brief courses of the drug, *if justified,* may be of similar benefit for acute exacerbations of *ankylosing spondylitis* and *osteoarthritis.*

OXYPHENBUTAZONE

Oxyphenbutazone is a hydroxy analog of phenylbutazone and one of the major active metabolites of the parent drug. Various aspects of its pharmacology and metabolism are discussed above, in comparison with phenylbutazone. Oxyphenbutazone has the same spectrum of activity, therapeutic uses, interactions, and toxicity as the parent compound, and

it shares the same indications, dangers, and contraindications for clinical use. Oxyphenbutazone is said to cause somewhat less gastric irritation.

Oxyphenbutazone, N.F. (TANDEARIL), is marketed in 100-mg tablets. It should be taken in three or four divided portions after meals to lessen gastric irritation. Dosage of oxyphenbutazone is the same as that of phenylbutazone.

INDOMETHACIN

Indomethacin was the product of a laboratory search for drugs with anti-inflammatory properties. It was introduced in 1963 for the treatment of rheumatoid arthritis and related disorders. Although it is an effective anti-inflammatory agent, toxicity often limits its use.

Chemistry. Indomethacin is 1-(*p*-chlorobenzoyl)-5-methoxy-2-methylindole-3-acetic acid. Its structural formula is as follows:

Indomethacin

Pharmacological Properties. Indomethacin has prominent anti-inflammatory and antipyretic properties in experimental animals similar to those of the salicylates (Winter *et al.,* 1963). Comparable effects have been demonstrated in man.

The *anti-inflammatory* effects of indomethacin are evident in patients with rheumatoid and other types of arthritis and in acute gout. Although indomethacin is more potent than aspirin, the anti-inflammatory effects of tolerated doses of indomethacin in rheumatoid arthritis are not superior to those of salicylate.

Whether indomethacin has *analgesic* properties distinct from its anti-inflammatory effects remains uncertain. However, in patients with acute postoperative and posttraumatic pain of mild-to-moderate intensity, single 50-mg doses of indomethacin provide relief approximately equivalent to that of 600 mg of aspirin. The *antipyretic* effect of indomethacin has also been readily demonstrated in patients with fever. Single doses of indomethacin are usually adequately tolerated; however, because of its potential toxicity, indomethacin is not recommended as a general analgesic-antipyretic.

Like the salicylates and related anti-inflammatory agents, indomethacin inhibits the biosynthesis of prostaglandins; this action may be the basis of its anti-inflammatory and antipyretic properties and certain of its other effects (Ferreira and Vane, 1974). Like colchicine, it inhibits motility of polymorphonuclear leukocytes; like salicylate, it uncouples oxidative phosphorylation in cartilaginous and hepatic mitochondria.

Absorption, Distribution, Biotransformation, and Excretion. Indomethacin is rapidly and almost completely absorbed from the gastrointestinal tract following oral ingestion. Peak plasma concentration is attained within 3 hours in the fasting subject but may be somewhat delayed when the drug is taken after meals. Indomethacin is 90% bound to plasma proteins and also extensively bound in tissues. The concentration of the drug in the CSF is low.

Contrary to initial impression, indomethacin is largely converted to inactive metabolites (Duggan *et al.,* 1972). About half of a single oral dose is O-demethylated and about 10% is conjugated with glucuronic acid by the hepatic microsomal enzymes. A portion is also N-deacylated by a nonmicrosomal system. Some of these metabolites are detectable in plasma, and free and conjugated metabolites are eliminated in the urine, bile, and feces. Enterohepatic cycling of the conjugates occurs. Ten to 20% of the drug is excreted unchanged in the urine, in part by tubular secretion. The plasma half-time of the unchanged drug is about 2 hours.

Drug Interactions. The reported antagonism between indomethacin and *aspirin* in some laboratory tests for anti-inflammatory activity has provoked speculation that similar antagonism might occur during therapy. In man, the slight reduction in the plasma concentration of indomethacin by aspirin does not appear to be of practical significance (Champion *et al.,* 1972). Whether it reflects displacement of bound indomethacin from plasma protein has not been determined. The crucial question, whether favorable or unfavorable combined effects result when the two drugs are administered concurrently for the therapy of rheumatoid arthritis, remains unanswered.

The total plasma concentration of indomethacin plus its inactive metabolites is increased by concurrent administration of *probenecid.* However, it has not been determined whether the concentration of unchanged indomethacin not bound to plasma protein is altered, or whether the dosage of indomethacin must be adjusted when the two drugs are employed together. Indomethacin does not interfere with the uricosuric effect of probenecid. Indomethacin is said not to modify the effect of the *oral anticoagulant* agents. However, concurrent administration could be hazardous because of the increased risk of gastrointestinal bleeding.

Toxic Effects and Precautions. Approximately 35 to 50% of patients receiving usual therapeutic doses of indomethacin experience untoward symptoms, and about 20% must discontinue its use. Most adverse effects are dose related (Boardman and Hart, 1967b).

Gastrointestinal complaints and complications consist in anorexia, nausea, abdominal pain, and peptic ulcers, often with bleeding and perforation. Acute pancreatitis has also been reported. Diarrhea

may occur and is sometimes associated with ulcerative lesions of the bowel. Hepatic involvement has been rare.

The most frequent *CNS* effect is severe frontal headache, occurring in 25 to 50% of patients who take the drug chronically. Dizziness, vertigo, lightheadedness, and mental confusion are frequent. Severe depression, psychosis, hallucinations, and suicide have been reported. Corneal opacities, visual-field changes, and pallor of the optic disc have also occurred.

Hematopoietic reactions consist in neutropenia, thrombocytopenia, and, rarely, aplastic anemia. Deaths in children have occurred from what was probably overwhelming sepsis due to activation of latent infections. *Hypersensitivity* reactions are manifested as rashes, itching, urticaria, and, more seriously, acute attacks of asthma. Patients allergic to *aspirin* may exhibit cross-reaction to indomethacin.

Indomethacin should not be used in pregnant women, children, persons operating machinery, or patients with psychiatric disorders, epilepsy, or parkinsonism. It is also contraindicated in individuals with renal disease or ulcerative lesions of the stomach or intestines.

Preparations and Dosage. *Indomethacin,* N.F. (INDOCIN), is available for oral use. Official capsules contain 25 or 50 mg of the drug.

The initial dose is 25 mg, twice daily, and this can be increased by 25-mg increments at weekly intervals until the total daily dose is 100 to 150 mg. Few patients tolerate more than 100 mg per day without severe side effects. The drug should be taken in divided portions with food or immediately after meals, to lessen gastric distress. A dose of indomethacin taken with milk at bedtime is said to reduce the incidence of morning headache.

Suppositories of indomethacin have been used but have not provided consistent therapeutic effect. Compressed tablets have been discontinued since they harden on storage and are absorbed erratically.

Therapeutic Uses. Because of the high incidence and severity of side effects associated with chronic administration, the use of indomethacin as a general analgesic or antipyretic is not recommended. However, it has proven useful as an antipyretic in *Hodgkin's disease* when the fever has been refractory to other therapy.

Clinical trials of indomethacin as an anti-inflammatory agent have been reviewed by O'Brien (1968). Its role in the therapy of *rheumatoid arthritis* has been succinctly summarized by Gifford (1973). Indomethacin relieves pain, reduces swelling and tenderness of the joints, and increases grip strength. However, since it is not superior to aspirin, and since aspirin is also better tolerated, the salicylate remains the primary agent of choice. Nevertheless, since about 25% of patients show good or excellent improvement with indomethacin, the drug is worthy of trial if aspirin is ineffective or not tolerated. Because of possible drug interaction (*see* below), aspirin should be discontinued during the trial. If indomethacin (75 to 100 mg, daily) fails to provide benefit in 2 to 3 weeks, alternative therapy must be considered.

Indomethacin has been claimed to be useful in *ankylosing spondylitis, osteoarthrosis,* and *psoriatic arthritis.* However, clinical trials of the drug have not been adequate to establish its status in these disorders, and aspirin or other therapy remains the treatment of choice. Acute attacks of *gout* also respond to indomethacin, but colchicine or phenylbutazone is generally preferred.

OTHER SALICYLATE-LIKE
ANTI-INFLAMMATORY AGENTS

In recent years, literally thousands of compounds have been screened in the laboratory for anti-inflammatory activity, and perhaps a score have had at least cursory clinical trial. The yield in new therapeutic agents has been minimal. All closely resemble the salicylates but differ somewhat in their spectra of toxicity. None has been shown to possess clinical anti-inflammatory efficacy superior to that of aspirin. Their role is mainly as alternative therapy when aspirin is ineffective or not tolerated. Research in this area has, however, provided steady progress in unraveling the complexities of the inflammatory processes and their modifications by drugs, the necessary prelude to the development of superior therapeutic agents.

A brief summary of the anthranilic acid derivatives and the arylalkanoic acids will illustrate the results of the continuing search for new anti-inflammatory agents. Both groups of compounds are organic acids that bind extensively to plasma protein and compete with other organic acids, including the oral anticoagulant agents. Their antipyretic, analgesic, and anti-inflammatory effects are similar to those of the salicylates; they are ulcerogenic, influence platelet function, and inhibit the biosynthesis of prostaglandins.

Mefenamic Acid and Related Agents. Mefenamic acid is a derivative of anthranilic acid, the amine analog of salicylic acid. It is the only fenamate available for clinical use in the United States, but it was released in 1967 only for restricted use as an analgesic. Although other anthranilic acid derivatives may have somewhat better anti-inflammatory activity, the toxicity of mefenamic acid tends to discourage interest in the group.

Mefenamic acid (PONSTEL), in recommended doses of 250 or 500 mg, provides analgesia in man similar to that produced by aspirin. However, diarrhea is common and often severe, and gastrointestinal ulceration and bleeding have been reported. Exacerbation of asthma, autoimmune hemolytic anemia, albuminuria, and slight elevation of blood urea nitrogen may occur. Agranulocytosis, thrombocytopenic purpura, megaloblastic anemia, and pancytopenia have been reported. Other undesired effects include drowsiness, nausea, dizziness, nervousness, and headache. The effects of oral anticoagulant agents are enhanced.

Since it is not superior to established analgesics and can cause serious toxicity, the use of mefenamic acid is *not recommended.* If it is used, administration should not be extended beyond 7 days. If diarrhea occurs, the drug must be discontinued and not used again. It should not be used in children or in women of childbearing age.

Ibuprofen and Other Arylalkanoic Acids. Several arylalkanoic acids are available for clinical use in other countries, but most are not yet marketed in the United States. The arylalkanoic acids offer promise of anti-inflammatory activity with less gastrointestinal distress; additional clinical experience is required for their assessment.

Ibuprofen (MOTRIN), a phenylpropionic acid derivative, has been used clinically in some countries since the late 1960s. It is now also marketed in the United States. In recommended dosage, its anti-inflammatory effects in rheumatoid arthritis are inferior to those of full doses of aspirin. In low dosage, ibuprofen may provide relief of pain without objective anti-inflammatory effect. Compared with aspirin, ibuprofen causes less occult bleeding and fewer complaints of gastrointestinal distress. However, exacerbation of peptic ulcer has been reported, and its efficacy and safety for long-term therapy are still incompletely established. Headache and other central effects occur in some patients, and alterations in hepatic function tests have been noted. Decreased visual acuity and visual-field defects have also occurred. The recommended dose for the symptomatic treatment of rheumatoid arthritis is 900 to 1600 mg per day. The drug is expensive.

Investigational arylalkanoic acids, such as *naproxen* (NAPROSYN) and *ketoprofen* (ORUDIS), have had only limited clinical trial. However, they appear to be more effective than ibuprofen as anti-inflammatory agents in man. Although they cause fewer complaints of gastrointestinal distress than does aspirin, the use of naproxen has been associated with a significant incidence of serious gastrointestinal bleeding. Much additional clinical experience is required to assess the status of the arylalkanoic acids.

SALICYLATE-LIKE ANALGESIC-ANTIPYRETICS

PARA-AMINOPHENOL DERIVATIVES:
ACETAMINOPHEN AND PHENACETIN

Acetaminophen and phenacetin are effective alternatives to aspirin for its analgesic and antipyretic uses. Acetaminophen has somewhat less overall toxicity and is preferred over phenacetin. Because acetaminophen is well tolerated and lacks many of the undesired effects of aspirin, it has been gaining favor as the "common household analgesic." However, its suitability for this purpose is questionable; in acute overdosage, acetaminophen can cause fatal hepatic necrosis.

History. Although not a para-aminophenol derivative, *acetanilid* is considered the parent member of this group of drugs. It was introduced into medicine in 1886 under the name of *antifebrin* by Cahn and Hepp, who had accidentally discovered its antipyretic action. However, acetanilid proved to be excessively toxic and is now only of historical interest.

The early reports of poisoning from acetanilid prompted the search for less toxic compounds. *Para-aminophenol* itself was tried in the belief that the body oxidized acetanilid to this compound. Toxicity was not lessened, however, and a number of chemical derivatives of para-aminophenol were then tested. One of the more satisfactory of these was *phenacetin (acetophenetidin)*. It was introduced into therapy in 1887 and is still extensively employed, although largely in analgesic mixtures.

Acetaminophen (paracetamol; N-acetyl-para-aminophenol) was first used in medicine by von Mering in 1893. However, it has gained popularity only since 1949, after it was recognized as the major active metabolite of both acetanilid and phenacetin.

Chemistry and Structure-Activity Relationship. The relationship between the drugs under discussion and their metabolites is depicted in Table 17-2. The antipyretic activity of the compounds resides in the aminobenzene structure, but aniline itself is too toxic for clinical use. Introduction of other radicals into the OH of para-aminophenol and into the free amino group of aniline reduces toxicity without loss of antipyretic action. Best results are obtained when an alkyl group is substituted in the OH (ethyl in phenacetin) and/or an acid group is introduced in

the NH_2 of aniline (acetyl in phenacetin and acetaminophen).

Pharmacological Effects. Acetaminophen and phenacetin have analgesic and antipyretic effects similar to those of aspirin. However, they have only weak anti-inflammatory effects and do not share the antirheumatic uses of the salicylates. The pharmacological effects of administered phenacetin are a combination of its inherent effects (Conney *et al.*, 1966) and those of acetaminophen, its major metabolite. Minor metabolites contribute significantly to the toxic effects of both drugs. The pharmacological properties of acetaminophen and phenacetin have been reviewed by Smith (1958), Randall (1963), and Beaver (1965, 1966).

Analgesia and Antipyresis. Like the salicylates, acetaminophen and phenacetin relieve pain of moderate intensity, such as usually occurs in headache and dysmenorrhea, and in many muscle, joint, and peripheral nerve disorders. Intense pain or that arising from smooth muscle spasm in hollow viscera is not alleviated. Also like the salicylates, acetaminophen and phenacetin reduce fever by a direct effect on the heat-regulating centers to increase dissipation of body heat.

Acetaminophen reduces fever not by interfering with the release of endogenous pyrogen from leukocytes but by inhibiting the action of endogenous pyrogen on the hypothalamic heat-regulating centers (Clark and Moyer, 1972). The locus of the analgesic effect is uncertain. Laboratory tests have been interpreted to indicate that it is solely a central effect, solely a peripheral effect, or a combination of both. The mechanism of the antipyretic and analgesic effects is also uncertain. Acetaminophen is more active than aspirin as an inhibitor of prostaglandin synthetase of brain, but it is only a very weak inhibitor of prostaglandin synthesis by a preparation from spleen (Ferreira and Vane, 1974).

Although adequately controlled clinical trials are limited (*see* Beaver, 1965, 1966), acetaminophen and phenacetin are generally considered approximately equipotent with aspirin both as analgesics and as antipyretics. The time course of these effects is also similar to that of aspirin. The ceiling effect for analgesia has not been determined.

Subjective Effects and Abuse Liability. Phenacetin has been said to cause relaxation, drowsiness, euphoria, stimulation, and increased efficiency; such effects have been thought to contribute to its abuse liability. In patients, minor subjective effects may well occur secondary to relief of pain or fever. In healthy subjects, with double-blind assessment by

Table 17-2. STRUCTURAL FORMULAS OF MAJOR PARA-AMINOPHENOL DERIVATIVES, AND THEIR INTERRELATIONS

questionnaire (Eade and Lasagna, 1967), the subjective effects of a single 2-g dose of acetaminophen or aspirin could not be distinguished from those of dummy medication. In the same dose, phenacetin produced a sedative effect characterized as less prominent but more unpleasant than that of pentobarbital, 150 mg. Similar subjective effects of phenacetin, often with light-headedness, dizziness, and a sense of unreality and detachment, have also been noted during pharmacokinetic studies. Restlessness and excitement may occur for 3 or 4 days when chronic abuse of phenacetin is discontinued.

Other Effects.   Single or repeated therapeutic doses of phenacetin or acetaminophen are benign to the cardiovascular and respiratory systems. Acid-base changes do not occur. Neither drug produces the gastric irritation, erosion, or bleeding that may occur after salicylates, nor do they have an effect upon platelets or uric acid excretion. Acetaminophen, like vasopressin, enhances transport of water across toad urinary bladder, and has been used in patients with diabetes insipidus with some success (Nusynowitz and Forsham, 1966).

Absorption, Distribution, Biotransformation, and Excretion.   Acetaminophen and phenacetin are metabolized primarily by the hepatic microsomal enzymes. The major pathways of biotransformation are depicted in Table 17–2 (*see* Brodie and Axelrod, 1949; Prescott, 1969; Abel, 1971).

Acetaminophen is rapidly and practically completely absorbed from the gastrointestinal tract. Plasma concentration reaches a peak in ½ to 1 hour; the plasma half-time is 1 to 3 hours. Acetaminophen is relatively uniformly distributed throughout most body fluids. Binding of the drug to plasma proteins is variable; 20 to 50% may be bound at the concentrations encountered during acute intoxication.

About 3% of acetaminophen is excreted unchanged in the urine, and about 80% is excreted in the urine after conjugation in the liver, predominantly with glucuronic acid and to a small extent with sulfuric acid. The glucuronide accumulates in plasma before excretion. A conjugate with cysteine and metabolites produced by hydroxylation and deacetylation have also been detected. The hydroxylated metabolites are responsible for methemoglobin formation and hepatotoxicity.

In the normal individual, 75 to 80% of administered phenacetin is rapidly metabolized to acetaminophen. Peak plasma concentration of unchanged phenacetin usually occurs in about 1 hour, and that of derived acetaminophen in 1 to 2 hours. However, oral absorption of phenacetin is markedly influenced by the particle size of the administered drug, and the plasma concentrations of phenacetin and acetaminophen are correspondingly variable.

The fate of derived acetaminophen is the same as that of administered acetaminophen. Phenacetin is converted to at least a dozen other metabolites, by N-deacetylation to para-phenetidin and by hydroxylation and further metabolism of phenacetin and para-phenetidin. The hydroxylated metabolites are responsible for methemoglobin formation and hemolysis of red blood cells. A contaminant in some commercial preparations of phenacetin, 4-chloroacetanilid, also contributes to these toxic effects. Metabolites of phenacetin in voided urine may darken upon standing to a red-brown or brown-black pigment. Less than 1% of phenacetin is excreted unchanged in the urine.

Individuals with a genetically determined limitation in ability to metabolize phenacetin to acetaminophen convert a greater fraction of administered phenacetin to the toxic metabolites, possibly with propensity for serious methemoglobin formation and hemolysis. Administration of acetaminophen or phenacetin to patients with impaired renal function results in increased accumulation of conjugated acetaminophen in plasma but only minor changes in the plasma concentrations of phenacetin and free acetaminophen.

Drug Interactions.   Acetaminophen and phenacetin can induce synthesis of the hepatic microsomal enzymes, but the effect is not seen with usual doses. Similarly, the prothrombinopenic effect of the *oral anticoagulant* agents may be increased by chronic administration of full doses of acetaminophen, but intermittent doses of the drug have only little such effect.

Toxicity.   In recommended therapeutic dosage, acetaminophen and phenacetin are usually well tolerated. *Skin rash* and other allergic reactions occur occasionally. The rash is usually erythematous or urticarial but sometimes more serious and may be accompanied by *drug fever* and mucosal lesions. Patients allergic to the salicylates do not exhibit cross-sensitivity to the para-aminophenols. In a few cases, the use of acetaminophen has been associated with the occurrence of *neutropenia, pancytopenia,* and *leukopenia;* further information on this association is required.

The most serious adverse effect of acute overdosage of acetaminophen and phenacetin is dose-dependent, potentially fatal *hepatic necrosis.* Renal tubular necrosis and hypoglycemic coma may also occur. Phenacetin may cause *methemoglobinemia* and *hemolytic anemia* as a form of acute toxicity but more commonly as a consequence of chronic overdosage. Acetaminophen causes less methemoglobin formation and has not been incriminated in the hemolytic reactions, but it has caused *thrombocytopenia.* The *nephrotoxicity* associated with chronic abuse of acetaminophen, phenacetin, and other analgesics is discussed later (page 349).

Hepatotoxicity.   In adults, hepatotoxicity may occur after ingestion of a single dose of 10 to 15 g

(200 to 250 mg/kg) of acetaminophen; a dose of 25 g or more is potentially fatal. Symptoms during the first 2 days of acute poisoning by acetaminophen do not reflect the potential seriousness of the intoxication. Nausea, vomiting, anorexia, and abdominal pain occur during the initial 24 hours and may persist for a week or more. Liver injury may become manifest the second day, initially by elevation of serum transaminase and lactic dehydrogenase activity, increased serum bilirubin concentration, and prolongation of prothrombin time. Alkaline phosphatase activity and serum albumin concentration may remain normal. The hepatotoxicity may progress to encephalopathy, coma, and death. Transient azotemia is apparent in most patients and acute renal failure occurs in some. Hypoglycemia may occur, but glycosuria and impaired glucose tolerance have also been reported. Both metabolic acidosis and metabolic alkalosis have been noted; cerebral edema and nonspecific myocardial depression have also occurred. Biopsy reveals centralobular necrosis with sparing of the periportal area. In nonfatal cases, the hepatic lesions are reversible over a period of weeks or months. (*See* Proudfoot and Wright, 1970; Prescott *et al.*, 1971; Clark *et al.*, 1973.)

Measurement of the plasma half-time of acetaminophen during the first day of acute poisoning provides an early indication of the severity of the liver injury. Hepatic necrosis should be anticipated if the half-time exceeds 4 hours, and hepatic coma is likely if the half-time is greater than 12 hours. A single determination of serum acetaminophen concentration is a less reliable predictor of hepatic injury. However, only minimal liver damage has developed when the serum concentration was below 120 μg/ml at 4 hours or less than 50 μg/ml at 12 hours after ingestion of the drug. Encephalopathy should also be anticipated if serum bilirubin concentration exceeds 4 mg/100 ml during the first 5 days.

Toxic doses of acetaminophen in animals produce liver injury with histological features similar to those in man. The hepatotoxicity is dose dependent and has been attributed to a covalently bound metabolite, possibly the N-hydroxyl derivative (Mitchell *et al.*, 1973a, 1973b). Since the severity of the liver injury can be varied by *pretreatments* that modify the rate of biotransformation of acetaminophen or that alter the hepatic stores of glutathione, it has been suggested that hepatotoxicity occurs when production of the toxic metabolite exceeds the capacity of available glutathione for its inactivation. The extent to which these factors influence acetaminophen-induced hepatotoxicity in man remains to be determined. Whether administration of sulfhydryl compounds *after* exposure to acetaminophen can minimize the hepatic insult is being explored.

Treatment of acute acetaminophen overdosage is purely symptomatic; vigorous supportive therapy is essential in severe intoxication. Since the hepatic injury is dose dependent and occurs early in the course of intoxication, procedures to limit continuing absorption of the drug must be initiated promptly. Induction of vomiting or gastric lavage should be performed in all cases, and such treatment should be followed by oral administration of activated charcoal. Although there is as yet no evidence that

reduction of plasma drug concentration alters the severity or the course of the hepatic injury, hemodialysis, if it can be initiated within the first 12 hours, has been advocated for all patients with a plasma acetaminophen concentration greater than 120 μg/ml 4 hours after drug ingestion (Farid *et al.*, 1972). Peritoneal dialysis without albumin in the dialysate has not been useful, but dialysis with albumin merits trial. Forced diuresis has also been advocated but has not been shown to increase drug elimination significantly and could be hazardous if renal function is impaired. There are no known antidotes for acetaminophen. Adrenocorticosteroids and antihistamines have been employed but have not been of obvious benefit. Antihistamines increase acetaminophen toxicity in animals.

Hemolytic Anemia. Phenacetin-induced hemolytic anemia has been most frequently associated with *chronic* ingestion of the drug. Hemolysis is apparently caused by metabolites that oxidize glutathione and components of the red-blood-cell membrane and shorten erythrocyte survival. The anemia is usually mild, with slight reticulocytosis, but may be progressive and severe in the presence of uremia or other exacerbating factors. Splenomegaly has been reported. Methemoglobinemia, sulfhemoglobin formation, and Heinz bodies are not consistently present; the blood film may contain characteristic irregularly contracted and fragmented erythrocytes. (*See* Duggan, 1970; Davidson, 1971.)

Hemolytic anemia may also occur following *acute* administration of phenacetin. Although such a reaction is not common, the anemia is usually severe and may be accompanied by intravascular hemolysis, hemoglobinuria, and acute anuria. These reactions occur in patients with red-blood-cell glucose-6-phosphate dehydrogenase deficiency (*see* Chapter 52) or as an immunological reaction of the "innocent bystander" type (Wintrobe, 1969). Although the antibodies are directed to the drug or metabolite, adsorption of the antigen-antibody complexes on the red-blood-cell surface leads to activation of complement and damage to the membrane.

Methemoglobinemia. Marked methemoglobinemia, sulfhemoglobin formation, cyanosis, and functional anemia were prominent characteristics of poisoning by acetanilid, the parent member of the aminophenol group. Phenacetin causes much less methemoglobinemia and sulfhemoglobin formation, and acetaminophen even less. Since a single 2-g dose of phenacetin in adults converts only 1 to 3% of the total hemoglobin to methemoglobin, the methemoglobinemia produced by therapeutic doses of acetaminophen or phenacetin is not usually of clinical significance. However, in acute overdosage or during chronic abuse, methemoglobinemia may contribute to the total toxicity. Methemoglobinemia may be prominent in individuals who convert a greater fraction of phenacetin to the hydroxylated metabolites, and commercial preparations of phenacetin contaminated with 4-chloroacetanilid cause a greater degree of methemoglobinemia.

Preparations and Dosage. *Acetaminophen,* U.S.P. (*paracetamol;* N-acetyl-para-aminophenol), is marketed under many trade names (*e.g.,* TEMPRA, TYLE-

NOL). Official preparations include tablets (120 and 325 mg) and an elixir and syrup (120 mg/5 ml); a solution (60 mg/0.6 ml) is also available.

The conventional oral dosage is 325 to 650 mg every 4 hours for adults and older children. The total daily dose should not exceed 2.6 g. For young children, the single dose is 60 to 120 mg, depending upon age and weight; total daily dosage should not exceed 1.2 g. Acetaminophen should not be administered for more than 10 days or to young children except upon advice of a physician.

Phenacetin (acetophenetidin) is no longer an official drug. It is too insoluble to be prescribed in aqueous solution, and is usually administered orally in powder, capsule, or tablet form. In recent years it has been employed primarily in analgesic mixtures. The average single dose for adults is 300 mg; the total daily dose should not exceed 2.4 g.

Therapeutic Uses. Acetaminophen or phenacetin is a suitable substitute for aspirin for its analgesic or antipyretic uses in patients who are allergic to aspirin or when aspirin is contraindicated, as in patients with gout or peptic ulcer. Acetaminophen has somewhat less overall toxicity and is preferred over phenacetin. Neither drug is an effective antirheumatic agent. An additional minor convenience of acetaminophen is its availability in a liquid dosage form for oral ingestion.

Analgesia. For headache, dysmenorrhea, arthralgia, myalgia, and similar disorders, a therapeutic dose of acetaminophen or phenacetin may be given every 3 or 4 hours. Self-medication over a period of days is not advised. If ordinary doses are ineffective, larger amounts as a rule do not give relief. Acetaminophen is definitely less effective than aspirin in patients with active rheumatoid arthritis, and any relief obtained is due to the analgesic effect. Analgesic combinations containing acetaminophen and phenacetin are discussed below.

Antipyresis. The use of acetaminophen or phenacetin to reduce fever is similar to that of aspirin. The indications and the rationale for reducing body temperature are discussed in connection with the salicylates.

PYRAZOLON DERIVATIVES:
ANTIPYRINE AND AMINOPYRINE

Antipyrine (phenazone) and *aminopyrine (amidopyrine)* were introduced into medicine in the late nineteenth century as antipyretics and subsequently were also widely used as analgesics and anti-inflammatory agents. However, clinical use of aminopyrine was sharply curtailed after its potentially fatal bone-marrow toxicity was recognized, and antipyrine has also lost favor. Both drugs have virtually disappeared from the therapeutic scene in the United States, but antipyrine is still employed in some countries, usually in analgesic mixtures. A variety of related pyrazolon derivatives have enjoyed sporadic popularity. The congeneric phenylbutazone has limited usefulness as an anti-inflammatory agent (*see above*).

Chemistry and Pharmacological Properties. Antipyrine and aminopyrine are closely related phenylpyrazolon derivatives. Their structural formulas are as follows:

Antipyrine

Aminopyrine

The pharmacology and toxicology of antipyrine and aminopyrine have been reviewed by Greenberg (1950), Randall (1963), and Beaver (1965, 1966). In both animals and man, the pyrazolon derivatives exhibit *analgesic, antipyretic,* and *anti-inflammatory* properties similar to those of the salicylates. Neither antipyrine nor aminopyrine has been subjected to adequately controlled clinical trial by current standards. However, aminopyrine was considered the superior anti-inflammatory agent and equivalent to aspirin for therapy of acute rheumatic fever. Unlike salicylate, the pyrazolon derivatives are not organic acids, are only slightly bound to plasma protein, and do not have uricosuric properties. They do not cause gastric irritation or produce the acid-base or metabolic effects of salicylate.

Aminopyrine Agranulocytosis. Aminopyrine and its close congener *dipyrone* cause a high incidence of agranulocytosis. This allergic reaction is characterized by the presence in the plasma of antibodies to granulocytes (*see* Wintrobe, 1969). In rare individuals, instead of frank agranulocytosis, each administration of aminopyrine produces a sharp fall in total leukocyte count associated with a severe chill, spiking fever, headache, and pain in muscles and joints; the attack is over within a few hours. The incidence of aminopyrine-induced agranulocytosis has been variously estimated between 0.01 and 0.86%. The mortality rate has been 20 to 50% (*see* Huguley, 1964).

Antipyrine. Reports of agranulocytosis attributed to antipyrine have been rare. Nevertheless, because it is closely related to aminopyrine and because it is not superior to safer drugs, the use of antipyrine as an analgesic and antipyretic is not recommended. Whether antipyrine has clinically useful antirheumatic properties has never been adequately determined. It is no longer an official drug.

Antipyrine is employed as a *pharmacological tool* for measurement of total body water and for assessment of hepatic microsomal mixed-function oxidase activity. It is rapidly and essentially completely absorbed from the gastrointestinal tract. Peak plasma concentration is usually attained in 1 to 2 hours. It is less than 10% bound to plasma proteins and is distributed in various tissues in proportion to their water content. About 30 to 40% of the drug is converted to 4-hydroxyantipyrine. This metabolite is rapidly and almost completely conjugated with glucuronic, and perhaps sulfuric, acid and excreted in the urine. Only about 5% of unaltered antipyrine is eliminated in the urine. Hydroxylation of the side chain also occurs, but the fate of a significant fraction of the drug remains uncertain. The plasma half-time for the unchanged drug is 7 to 20 hours (*see* Brodie and Axelrod, 1950).

Antipyrine causes induction of the hepatic microsomal enzyme system and modifies the biotransformation of other drugs, including the oral anticoagulant agents.

Aminopyrine and Dipyrone. "Over-the-counter" sale of *aminopyrine* in the United States has been prohibited since 1938, and federal regulations require that preparations of aminopyrine and dipyrone bear a warning on the labels stating that *the drug may cause fatal agranulocytosis.*

Although it is an excellent antipyretic, analgesic, and anti-inflammatory agent, and despite its advantages over salicylate, *aminopyrine* ordinarily should not be employed because of the danger of agranulocytosis. In some cases of prolonged intractable fever, as in Hodgkin's disease and periarteritis nodosa, aminopyrine is capable of controlling the disability and may be justified. *Dipyrone,* the methanesulfonate derivative of aminopyrine, has similar pharmacological and toxicological properties, including the potential to cause fatal agranulocytosis. It differs only in being more soluble and available for parenteral administration.

If used at all in the treatment of intractable fever, aminopyrine or dipyrone should be employed only after safer drugs and other measures have proven ineffective, and only with proper supervision and monitoring. Administration of dipyrone with chlorpromazine can result in serious hypothermia, and such use is contraindicated. Dipyrone can aggravate a bleeding tendency or prothrombin deficiency.

SALICYLAMIDE

Salicylamide, the amide of salicylic acid, is no longer an official drug. Its effects in man are not reliable, and its use is not recommended. The small doses included in "over-the-counter" analgesic and sedative mixtures are probably ineffective.

Although not metabolized to salicylate in the body, salicylamide has antipyretic, analgesic, and anti-inflammatory effects similar to those of salicylate. It also has sedative and hypotensive effects. However, the drug is very rapidly inactivated during

absorption and the initial circulation through the liver. Concentrations of active drug in the systemic circulation are markedly influenced by the dosage form, and they are disproportionately low after low doses. Salicylamide may inhibit the metabolism of other drugs by the liver.

ANALGESIC COMBINATIONS AND MIXTURES

Aspirin, acetaminophen, and phenacetin are frequently administered with each other and a variety of other drugs, including caffeine, sedatives, and the opioid analgesics. Concurrent administration of an opioid and an analgesic-antipyretic, such as codeine and aspirin, has a valid role in analgesic medication. However, none of the mixtures of analgesic-antipyretics, including the traditional aspirin-phenacetin-caffeine combination, has been shown to provide significant advantage over medication with aspirin alone.

Irrational analgesic mixtures, such as those with a hazardous component or presumed active ingredients that are in fact inert, can be expected to disappear from the therapeutic scene when the assessment of "over-the-counter" medications currently being conducted by the FDA is completed and the recommendations of its panel are implemented.

Combined Opioid and Analgesic-Antipyretic Medication. In most controlled clinical trials, codeine, 65 mg, has been found to add significantly to the analgesic effect of aspirin, 650 mg. The combined codeine-aspirin effect can be duplicated by larger doses of codeine alone, but considerations of toxicity and abuse favor restricting the dosage of the opioid. Thus, combined codeine-aspirin analgesia is justified if aspirin alone in full dosage is ineffective. Gastrointestinal and central side effects typical of the opioids are the price for the increased analgesia provided by this multiple-drug therapy. Parenteral opioids are still required for relief of severe pain.

In adequate dosage, other orally effective opioids add similarly to the analgesic effect of aspirin. In general, a dose of an opioid that given alone provides uncertain analgesia adds only equivocally to the analgesic effect of aspirin. Although it is likely that an effective dose of an opioid adds to the analgesic effect of acetaminophen as it does to that of aspirin, clinical documentation is required. The usual arguments for and against the use of fixed-dose mixtures versus concurrent but separate administration of the components apply to combined opioid and analgesic-antipyretic medication (*see* Chapter 1).

Mixtures of Analgesic-Antipyretics. The many mixtures of aspirin with acetaminophen or phenacetin, and often with caffeine and other drugs, are promoted with claims that they provide greater analgesia and/or cause fewer adverse effects than does aspirin alone. Neither claim withstands critical scrutiny. In most controlled clinical trials, relief of pain by an analgesic mixture has not been superior to that of aspirin alone. In the occasional trial in which a mixture has provided somewhat greater pain relief, the difference has been of doubtful practical significance, or aspirin would probably have been as effective if it had been employed in comparable dosage.

All analgesic-antipyretics, alone or in combination, are adequately tolerated in recommended dosage. Differences in the incidence of gastrointestinal distress and other minor adverse effects are generally inconsistent and of doubtful practical significance. On the other hand, the contraindications to aspirin, such as allergy to the drug, are not satisfied by the reduction in dosage of aspirin afforded by a mixture, but only by total avoidance of salicylate. An important criticism of an analgesic mixture is that its aspirin content is sometimes not recognized, and toxicity results when the mixture is inadvertently taken by a patient for whom such medication is contraindicated.

Mixtures with Caffeine. Caffeine is included in many analgesic mixtures, presumably in the belief that it increases the analgesic effect in general, has unique value for relief of headache, or exerts a favorable influence on mood. In patients with cancer, the analgesia provided by aspirin, 650 mg, is not increased by concurrent administration of caffeine, 65 mg (Moertel *et al.*, 1974). In controlled trials, analgesic mixtures containing caffeine have not been found superior to aspirin for relief of headache, nor has caffeine been shown to contribute other favorable effects. It is pertinent that the dose of caffeine employed with the ergot alkaloids for relief of migraine headache is 100 mg, and that a cup of coffee contains 100 to 150 mg of caffeine; yet the caffeine content of the usual two tablets of an analgesic mixture is only 16 to 65 mg.

Analgesic-Sedative Mixtures. A sedative is administered concurrently with an analgesic either to provide both sedation and analgesia or in the belief that sedation increases the analgesic effect. In low but sufficient dosage to produce detectable sedative effect, neither pentobarbital, 32 mg, nor promazine, 25 mg, increases the analgesic effect of aspirin, 650 mg (Moertel *et al.*, 1974). Increased sedation without enhanced analgesia is also the usual result when a sedative is administered concurrently with an opioid analgesic.

The sedative component of most analgesic-sedative mixtures usually has a weak central depressant effect of questionable reliability. Whether such mixtures do, in fact, provide sedation as well as analgesia has not been established for most of these mixtures. When sedation as well as analgesia is desired, it is best achieved by separate administration of a reliable agent in appropriate dosage.

Analgesic Nephropathy. Since the early 1950s increasing efforts have been devoted to analysis of the association between nephropathy and chronic abuse of analgesic mixtures. Despite numerous clinical observations and experimental studies in animals and man, crucial details of the problem remain uncertain. Critical analyses of analgesic nephropathy have been provided by Schreiner (1962), Gilman (1964), Shelley (1967), Gault and coworkers (1968), and Abel (1971).

Although phenacetin has been implicated by some as the nephrotoxic component of analgesic mixtures, it is premature to single out any particular ingredient as the causative factor. It is also impossible to absolve any one component. A more balanced view is that chronic abuse of any of the analgesic-antipyretics or analgesic mixtures may, in the susceptible individual, or in concert with other variables, cause renal injury.

As for other forms of drug abuse, prevention and correction require education. Patients must be convinced that *daily consumption of analgesics or analgesic mixtures in large amounts or for long periods must be avoided.*

Certain individuals consume analgesic mixtures in prodigious amounts over periods of years without medical supervision. Chronic toxicity from these mixtures is usually characterized by a high incidence of gastrointestinal disturbances (including peptic ulcer), anemia, methemoglobinemia, splenomegaly, and renal injury. Females are involved more frequently than males, and there is often a history of frequent urinary tract infection. Emotional disturbances are common, and other drugs may be abused concurrently.

The primary renal lesion appears to be *papillary necrosis,* with secondary *chronic interstitial nephritis.* The injury is often insidious in onset, is usually manifest initially as reduced tubular function and concentrating ability, and may progress to renal insufficiency if misuse of analgesics continues.

Attempts to identify the nephrotoxic component of the analgesic mixtures have not been conclusive, but some progress has been made. In the 1950s phenacetin was implicated by some because it was a drug common to all analgesic mixtures. However, also common to all mixtures are potent anti-inflammatory agents such as salicylate or antipyrine. Prescott (1965) demonstrated in volunteer subjects that aspirin alone (3.6 g, daily) causes a marked increase in renal tubular cells in the urine. Similar but less prominent and less consistent effects are produced by phenacetin, caffeine, and acetaminophen. Although a relationship between these short-term experimental observations and the injury that occurs after chronic analgesic abuse is uncertain, such studies emphasize that analgesics other than phenacetin, as well as caffeine, may be involved. Experimental studies in animals have also been inconclusive, particularly because large doses of drug are required to produce renal lesions. Nevertheless, they, too, indicate that salicylates, other analgesic-antipyretics, and caffeine can be nephrotoxic.

The phenacetin component in many analgesic mixtures has been replaced by other analgesic-antipyretics; the use of phenacetin by itself has been restricted to prescription in some countries. In the United States, warning labels are required on all analgesic drug mixtures containing phenacetin, to the effect that damage to the kidney may occur when such a mixture is used in large amount or for long periods. Such warning is appropriate for all analgesics and analgesic mixtures.

Only a minority of patients who consume analgesic mixtures in excess develop renal injury, and there are striking geographical differences in the incidence of analgesic nephropathy. For these and other reasons, it has been suggested that genetically determined differences in drug metabolism or in susceptibility to drug injury may be an important determinant of the toxicity. Other possible variables include a contaminant in some commercial preparations of phenacetin and differences in interaction between the components of the various mixtures or with other drugs consumed concurrently. It has also been proposed that analgesics may increase the susceptibility to urinary tract infection, or that infection may predispose to drug toxicity. Thoughtful reviewers of the problem of analgesic nephropathy have consistently called for prospective epidemiological studies to clarify the role of the individual drugs, and to identify the major risk factors. They warn, however, that even extensive studies on the general population may be inconclusive because analgesics other than aspirin are not widely taken alone, individuals often consume a variety of analgesic mixtures, and their personal estimates of analgesic consumption are frequently unreliable. Careful analysis of subpopulations in which these variables can be eliminated or controlled will probably provide more reliable conclusions.

DRUGS EMPLOYED IN THE THERAPY OF GOUT

Discussion in this section of the drugs used in the therapy of gout is limited to *colchicine* and *allopurinol*. The pharmacology of the uricosuric agents is presented in Chapter 41. Progress in the treatment of gout during the past 25 years has been authoritatively reviewed by Gutman (1973) and Yü (1974).

COLCHICINE

Colchicine is a unique anti-inflammatory agent in that it is effective essentially only against gouty arthritis. It provides dramatic relief of acute attacks of gout and is an effective prophylactic agent against such attacks.

History. Colchicine is an alkaloid of *Colchicum autumnale* (autumn crocus, meadow saffron), a plant so named because it grew in Colchis in Asia Minor. Although the poisonous action of colchicum was known to Dioscorides, preparations of the plant were not recommended for pain of articular origin until the sixth century A.D. Colchicum was introduced for the therapy of acute gout by von Störck in 1763, and its specificity for this syndrome soon resulted in its incorporation in a number of "gout mixtures" popularized by charlatans. Benjamin Franklin, himself a sufferer from gout, is reputed to have introduced colchicum therapy in the United States. The alkaloid *colchicine* was isolated from colchicum in 1820 by Pelletier and Caventou.

Chemistry. The structural formula of colchicine is as follows:

Colchicine

The structure-activity relationship of colchicine and related agents has been discussed by Wallace (1961).

Pharmacological Properties. The anti-inflammatory effect of colchicine in acute gouty arthritis is selective for this disorder. Colchicine is only occasionally effective in other types of arthritis; it is not an analgesic and does not provide relief of other types of pain.

Colchicine is also an antimitotic agent and has been widely employed as an experimental tool in the study of normal and abnormal cell division and cell function.

Effect in Gout. Analysis of the processes involved in precipitation of an acute attack of gouty arthritis has helped to elucidate the mechanism of the anti-inflammatory effect of colchicine (*see* Seegmiller *et al.,* 1963; Malawista, 1968). The drug does not influence the renal excretion of uric acid, its concentration in blood, or the miscible pool of uric acid. An acute attack of gout apparently occurs as a result of an inflammatory reaction to crystals of monosodium urate that are deposited in the joint tissue from hyperuric body fluids. The inflammatory response involves local infiltration of granulocytes that phagocytize the urate crystals. In synovial tissues and in leukocytes associated with the inflammatory process, lactic acid production is high and this favors a local decrease in pH that fosters further uric acid deposition. Colchicine inhibits migration of granulocytes to the inflammatory area and reduces the increased lactic acid production associated with phagocytosis. By these and possibly other effects on leukocytes, colchicine interrupts the cycle of urate crystal deposition and inflammatory response that sustains the acute attack.

Effect on Cell Division. Colchicine can arrest plant and animal cell division *in vitro* and *in vivo*. Pernice in 1889 was the first to note that colchicum influenced mitosis, but the details were first elucidated by Lits (1934) and Amoroso (1935). Mitosis is arrested in the metaphase, due to failure of spindle formation. Bizarre and abnormal nuclear configurations ensue, and the cells often die. Cells with the highest rates of division are affected earliest. High concentrations may completely prevent cells from entering mitosis. Both normal and cancer cells are similarly affected. The effect is not specific for colchicine and is exhibited by the vinca alkaloids (vincristine and vinblastine), podophyllotoxin, griseofulvin, and other agents. The extensive studies of the effects of colchicine on cell division and its use as a pharmacological tool have been summarized by Dustin (1963).

Mechanism of Action. The antimitotic and anti-inflammatory effects of colchicine may have a common denominator (*see* Malawista, 1968). By virtue of its ability to bind to microtubular protein, colchicine interferes with the function of the mitotic spindles and causes depolymerization and disappearance of the fibrillar microtubules in granulocytes and other motile cells. This latter effect could explain the interference with the mobilization of leukocytes during inflammation and the other effects on leukocytes. Vinblastine and griseofulvin, both metaphase-arresting agents, also exhibit anti-inflammatory properties and colchicine-like effects on leukocytes and their microtubules. Colchicine also inhibits the release of histamine granules from mast cells, the secretion of insulin from islet beta cells, and the movement of melanin granules in melanophores, processes that may involve the translocation of granules by the microtubule system. Details of the effects of colchicine and related agents on microtubules have been reviewed in a symposium (1974).

Other Effects. Colchicine exhibits a variety of other pharmacological effects. It lowers body temperature, increases the sensitivity to central depressants, depresses the respiratory center, enhances the response to sympathomimetic agents, constricts blood vessels and induces hypertension by central vasomotor stimulation, enhances gastrointestinal activity by neurogenic stimulation but depresses it by a direct effect, and alters neuromuscular function (*see* Ferguson, 1952).

Absorption, Distribution, Biotransformation, and Excretion. Colchicine is rapidly absorbed after oral administration, but large amounts of drug and metabolites enter the intestinal tract in the bile and intestinal secretions. This fact, plus the rapid turnover of intestinal epithelium, probably explains the prominence of intestinal manifestations in colchicine

poisoning. Administered intravenously, colchicine rapidly leaves the blood and distributes in a space larger than that of the body water. The kidney, liver, spleen, and intestinal tract contain high concentrations of colchicine, but it is apparently absent from heart, skeletal muscle, and brain. The drug can be detected in leukocytes for at least 9 days after a single intravenous dose.

Colchicine is partially deacetylated in the liver, and most of the drug and its metabolites are eliminated in the feces. In normal individuals, 10 to 20% of the drug, in part unchanged, is excreted in the urine. In patients with liver disease, hepatic uptake and elimination are reduced and a greater fraction of the drug is excreted in the urine (*see* Wallace *et al.*, 1970).

Drug Interactions. Interactions between colchicine and allopurinol, the uricosuric agents, and other drugs have not been reported.

Toxicity. *Nausea, vomiting, diarrhea,* and *abdominal pain* are the most common and earliest untoward effects of colchicine overdosage. To avoid more serious toxicity, administration of the drug is discontinued as soon as these symptoms occur. A latent period of several hours or more occurs between the administration of the drug and the onset of symptoms. This interval is not altered by dosage or route of administration. For this reason, and because of individual variation, adverse effects may be unavoidable during an initial course of colchicine medication. However, the patient often remains relatively consistent in his response to the drug, and therefore toxicity can be minimized or avoided during subsequent courses of therapy.

In *acute poisoning,* the diarrhea soon becomes profuse, watery, and bloody due to a *hemorrhagic gastroenteritis.* Considerable fluid, electrolyte, and plasma are lost through the bowel. Altered function of the ileal mucosa results in reversible malabsorption of cyanocobalamin and the actively transported sugars. Even when given by injection, colchicine causes gastrointestinal irritation. Burning of the throat and skin are also prominent symptoms. Because of the extensive vascular damage, shock occurs. The *kidney* is also injured, and hematuria and oliguria ensue. *Muscular depression* is pronounced, an ascending *paralysis* of the CNS develops, and death results from respiratory arrest usually within 1 to 2 days.

The *fatal dose* varies considerably. As little as 7 mg of colchicine has proved fatal, but much larger doses have been survived. *Treatment* of acute colchicine poisoning should be directed very early against shock. The remaining measures are purely symptomatic and supportive. Atropine and morphine aid in relieving abdominal pain.

Colchicine produces a temporary leukopenia that is soon replaced by a leukocytosis, sometimes due to a striking increase in the number of basophilic granulocytes. The site of action is apparently directly on the bone marrow. *Chronic administration* of colchicine entails some risk of *agranulocytosis, aplastic anemia, myopathy,* and *alopecia.*

Preparations. *Colchicine,* U.S.P., is available as official tablets (0.5 or 0.6 mg); they should be stored in tight, light-resistant containers. Sterile solution (0.5 mg/ml) is also available for injection.

Therapeutic Uses. Colchicine provides dramatic relief of *acute attacks* of gout. The effect is sufficiently selective that the drug has been used for diagnostic purposes, but the test is not infallible. Colchicine also has an established role to *prevent* and to *abort* acute attacks of gout. (*See* Seegmiller and Grayzel, 1960; Yü and Gutman, 1961; Gutman, 1973; Yü, 1974.)

Acute Attacks. When colchicine is given promptly within the first few hours of an attack, less than 5% of patients fail to obtain relief. A patient who is in helpless agony with a tumefied, red, hot joint is sufficiently relieved so that he can walk about in a few hours. Pain, swelling, and redness abate within 12 hours and are completely gone in 48 to 72 hours.

The former practice of administering colchicine at hourly intervals is no longer recommended (Yü, 1974). An initial dose of 1 mg is followed by 0.5 mg every 2 to 3 hours; drug administration is stopped as soon as the pain disappears or gastrointestinal symptoms develop. The total dose usually required to alleviate an attack is 4 to 10 mg, and the latter amount should not be exceeded. Opioids or other drugs may be required for the diarrhea. In subsequent attacks, the patient may be able to stop medication short of the amount causing toxic reactions. To avoid cumulative toxicity, the course of colchicine should not be repeated within 3 days. If necessary, colchicine may be administered intravenously. A single dose of 2 mg, diluted in 10 to 20 ml of 0.9% sodium chloride solution, is usually adequate. Extravasation must be avoided.

Great care should be exercised in prescribing colchicine for aged or feeble patients, and for those with cardiac, renal, or gastrointestinal disease. In these patients and in those who do not tolerate or respond to colchicine, a short course of phenylbutazone (*see* above), followed by prophylactic doses of colchicine, may be employed.

When corticotropin or corticosteroid therapy is employed for acute attacks, prophylactic doses of colchicine should be given concurrently and continued after withdrawal of the hormone or steroid, to prevent the precipitation of an acute attack of gout that may follow such withdrawal.

Prophylactic Uses. For patients with chronic gout, colchicine has established value as a prophylactic agent during the asymptomatic intercritical period. It has a preeminent place in the prevention of acute gout when there is frequent recurrence of attacks. The regular ingestion of colchicine effectively minimizes the frequency and the intensity of acute episodes; by reducing stiffness and aching, it often permits relatively normal activity in a person who otherwise would be incapacitated. Prophylactic medication is also indicated upon initiation of chronic medication with allopurinol or the uricosuric agents, since acute attacks often increase in frequency during the early months of such therapy.

The usual *prophylactic dose* of colchicine is 0.5 to 2.0 mg or more every night or every other night, as required by the individual patient. Tolerance does not develop to the alkaloid.

Colchicine should be taken in larger abortive doses immediately upon the first twinge of articular pain or the appearance of any prodrome of an acute attack. Thus, the patient should always have the drug with him. The judicious ingestion of colchicine during the premonitory, incipient, and inflorescent stages of acute gouty arthritis will abort paroxysms and prevent chronic gouty arthritis.

Prior to and following surgery in patients with gout, colchicine should be given for a few days (0.5 mg, three times a day); this greatly reduces the very high incidence of acute attacks of gouty arthritis precipitated by operative procedures.

Encouraging results have been obtained with the daily use of colchicine for the prevention of attacks of *familial Mediterranean fever* (familial paroxysmal polyserositis).

ALLOPURINOL

Allopurinol is an effective drug for the therapy of both the primary hyperuricemia of gout and that secondary to hematological disorders or antineoplastic therapy. In contrast with the uricosuric agents that increase the renal excretion of urate, allopurinol inhibits the terminal steps in uric acid biosynthesis. Since overproduction of uric acid is a contributing factor in most patients with gout and a characteristic of most types of secondary hyperuricemia, allopurinol represents a rational approach to therapy.

History. The introduction of allopurinol by Hitchings, Elion, and associates provides an elegant example of the development of a drug on a rational biochemical basis. Originally synthesized as a candidate antineoplastic agent, allopurinol was found to lack antimetabolite activity but, by *in-vitro* test, it proved to be a substrate for and an inhibitor of xanthine oxidase. Inhibition of xanthine oxidase *in vivo* was initially established in leukemic patients receiving treatment with the antimetabolite 6-mercaptopurine. Allopurinol delayed inactivation of 6-mercaptopurine by xanthine oxidase and also reduced the plasma concentration and renal excretion of uric acid. Subsequent clinical trial for treatment of gout by Rundles and coworkers was successful and quickly confirmed. (*See* Elion *et al.,* 1963; Rundles *et al.,* 1963.)

Chemistry and Pharmacological Effects. Allopurinol (4-hydroxypyrazolo[3,4-*d*]pyrimidine) is a structural analog of hypoxanthine (*see* Table 17–3). Both allopurinol and its primary metabolite alloxanthine (oxypurinol) are inhibitors of xanthine oxidase. Inhibition of this enzyme accounts for the major pharmacological effects of allopurinol. (*See* Rundles *et al.,* 1963, 1966; Yü and Gutman, 1964.)

Uric acid in man is formed primarily by the xanthine oxidase–catalyzed oxidation of hypoxanthine and xanthine (*see* Table 17–3). At low concentrations, allopurinol is a substrate for and competitive inhibitor of the enzyme; at high concentrations, it is a noncompetitive inhibitor. Alloxanthine, the metabolite formed by the action of xanthine oxidase, is a noncompetitive inhibitor of the enzyme. Inhibition of the penultimate and ultimate steps in uric acid biosynthesis reduces the plasma concentration and urinary excretion of uric acid and increases the plasma concentrations and renal excretion of the more soluble oxypurine precursors.

Before allopurinol treatment of hyperuricemia, the urinary purine content is almost solely uric acid. During such treatment, the urinary purine load is divided among hypoxanthine, xanthine, and uric acid. Since each has its independent solubility, plasma uric acid concentration is reduced without exposing the urinary tract to an excessive load of uric acid and the likelihood of calculus formation.

The alterations in purine metabolism produced by allopurinol explain its salutary effects in gout. By lowering the uric acid concentration in plasma below its limit of solubility, the dissolution of tophi is facilitated and the development or progression of chronic gouty arthritis is prevented. The formation of uric acid stones virtually disappears with therapy, and this prevents the development of nephropathy. The incidence of acute attacks of arthritis may increase during the early months of therapy but is subsequently reduced.

Tissue deposition of xanthine and hypoxanthine does not usually occur during allopurinol therapy because the renal clearance of the oxypurines is rapid; their plasma concentrations are only slightly increased and do not exceed their solubility. Although xanthine constitutes about 50% of total oxypurine excreted in the urine and is relatively insoluble, xanthine stone formation during allopurinol therapy has occurred only in an occasional patient with very high uric acid production prior to treatment. The risk can be minimized by alkalinization of the urine and by increasing the daily fluid intake during allopurinol administration. In some patients, the allopurinol-induced increase in excretion of oxypurines is less than the reduction in uric acid excretion; this disparity is primarily a result of reutilization of oxypurines and feedback inhibition of *de-novo* purine biosynthesis. Increased oxypurine excretion matches the reduction in uric acid excretion in patients with phosphoribosyltransferase deficiency; such individuals are unable to reutilize oxypurines.

Absorption, Distribution, Biotransformation and Excretion. Allopurinol is relatively rapidly absorbed after oral ingestion, and peak plasma concentration is reached in from 2 to 6 hours. About

Table 17–3. STEPS IN ALLOPURINOL INHIBITION OF URIC ACID FORMATION

20% is excreted in the feces in 48 to 72 hours, presumably as unabsorbed drug. Allopurinol is rapidly cleared from plasma with a half-time of 2 to 3 hours, primarily by conversion to alloxanthine. Less than 10% of a single dose or about 30% of the drug ingested during chronic medication is excreted unchanged in the urine. Self-inhibition of the metabolism of allopurinol to alloxanthine explains this dose-dependent elimination. Alloxanthine is slowly excreted in the urine by the net balance of glomerular filtration and probenecid-sensitive tubular reabsorption. The plasma half-time of alloxanthine is 18 to 30 hours in patients with normal renal function and increases in proportion to the reduction of glomerular filtration in patients with renal impairment. Although alloxanthine is a less potent inhibitor of xanthine oxidase than is the parent drug, the metabolite accumulates in the body during chronic administration of allopurinol and contributes significantly to the therapeutic effects of the medication. Patients with a genetic deficiency of xanthine oxidase (xanthinuria) do not convert allopurinol to alloxanthine. (*See* Elion *et al.*, 1966, 1968.)

Allopurinol and its metabolite alloxanthine are distributed in total tissue water, with the exception of brain, in which their concentration is about half that in other tissues. Neither compound is bound to plasma proteins.

Drug Interactions. Interactions between allopurinol and *probenecid* and other *uricosuric* agents and those between allopurinol and *6-mercaptopurine, azathioprine,* and other *antineoplastic* agents have already been discussed (*see* above). Allopurinol may also interfere with the hepatic inactivation of other drugs, including the *oral anticoagulant* agents (Vesell *et al.,* 1970; Rawlins and Smith, 1973). Although the effect is variable and of clinical significance only in some patients, increased monitoring of prothrombin activity is recommended in patients receiving both medications.

Whether the increased incidence of skin rash in patients receiving concurrent allopurinol-*ampicillin* medication, compared with that of these agents administered individually, should be ascribed to allopurinol or to hyperuricemia remains to be established (Boston Collaborative Drug Surveillance Program, 1972).

The reported interference by allopurinol with mobilization of hepatic *iron* has not been confirmed (Grace *et al.,* 1970), and the proposed role of xanthine oxidase in iron metabolism remains unestablished. Nevertheless, concurrent administration of iron during allopurinol medication is not recommended.

Toxicity. Allopurinol is adequately tolerated by most patients. The most common adverse effects are *hypersensitivity* reactions involving the skin and blood. They may occur even after months or years of chronic medication. These usually subside within a few days after medication is discontinued.

Serious reactions preclude further use of the drug.

Attacks of acute gout may occur more frequently during the initial months of allopurinol medication and may require concurrent prophylactic colchicine therapy (*see* above).

The cutaneous reaction is predominantly a pruritic, erythematous, or maculopapular eruption, but occasionally the lesion is exfoliative, urticarial, or purpuric. Fever, malaise, and muscle aching may also occur. Such effects are noted in about 3% of patients with normal renal function but more frequently in those with renal impairment.

Transient leukopenia or leukocytosis and eosinophilia are rare reactions but may require cessation of therapy. A few cases of hepatomegaly and elevated levels of serum glutamic oxalacetic acid transaminase have been recorded, and there have been isolated reports of peripheral neuritis, bone-marrow depression, and cataract. Eosinophilia with epidermal necrolysis has resulted in renal failure.

Undesirable side effects such as headache, drowsiness, nausea, vomiting, vertigo, diarrhea, and gastric irritation occur occasionally but do not usually require that therapy be stopped.

Inhibition of xanthine oxidase by allopurinol is not known to cause significant adverse effects. However, the drug does have effects on purine and pyrimidine metabolism. These effects are still incompletely explored, and their significance, especially during long-term therapy, remains to be determined.

Preparations and Dosage. *Allopurinol,* U.S.P. (ZYLOPRIM), is available as 100- and 300-mg scored tablets for oral use.

For control of hyperuricemia in gout, the aim of therapy is to reduce plasma uric acid concentration below 6 mg %. Medication must not be initiated during an acute attack of arthritis, and it is started at low doses to minimize the risk of precipitating such attacks. Concurrent prophylactic colchicine therapy is also recommended during and sometimes beyond the initial months of therapy. Fluid intake should be sufficient to maintain daily urinary volume above 2 liters; slightly alkaline urine is preferred. An initial daily dose of 100 mg is increased by 100-mg increments at weekly intervals. The usual daily maintenance dose for adults is 300 mg; a single daily dose is satisfactory. Dosage must be reduced in patients with renal impairment in proportion to the reduction in glomerular filtration; 100 mg daily or 300 mg twice weekly is often satisfactory.

In the treatment of secondary hyperuricemias, as for the prevention of uric acid nephropathy during vigorous therapy of certain neoplastic diseases, a dose of 200 to 800 mg daily for 2 to 3 days or longer is advisable, together with a high fluid intake. In children with secondary hyperuricemias associated with malignancies, the usual daily dose is 150 to 300 mg, depending upon age.

Therapeutic Uses. Allopurinol provides effective therapy for both the primary *hyperuricemia* of gout and that secondary to polycythemia vera, myeloid metaplasia, or other blood dyscrasias. (*See* Rundles *et al.,* 1963, 1966; Yü and Gutman, 1964; Klinenberg *et al.,* 1965; Krakoff, 1967; Muggia *et al.,* 1967; Gutman, 1973; Yü, 1974.) Allopurinol is contraindicated in patients who have exhibited serious adverse effects from the medication, nursing mothers, and children, except those with malignancy.

In *gout,* allopurinol is generally used in the severe chronic forms characterized by one or more of the following conditions: gouty nephropathy, tophaceous deposits, renal urate stones, impaired renal function, or hyperuricemia not readily controlled by the uricosuric drugs. In the absence of these indications, the uricosuric agents should be favored (Goldfinger, 1971; Rastegar and Thier, 1974).

When given in effective doses and over prolonged periods, allopurinol fosters resorption of tophi and improvement of joint function in patients with tophaceous gout; this occurs *pari passu* with the reduction in plasma uric acid concentration. By decreasing the amount of uric acid excreted and thereby preventing the development of nephrolithiasis, allopurinol eliminates the major cause of renal injury in patients with gout. It also appears likely that gouty nephropathy can be reversed by the drug if therapy is begun at a reasonably early stage, before renal function is severely compromised; however, there is little evidence of improvement in advanced renal disease.

Since attacks of acute gout occur in patients on allopurinol, particularly during the initial stage of treatment, colchicine is used prophylactically when therapy is begun and continued if necessary to prevent such attacks. Concurrent allopurinol and uricosuric therapy is also employed occasionally, especially in patients with large tophaceous deposits in whom it is desirable both to reduce uric acid production and to increase urate elimination. Such combined medication is valid, but interaction between these drugs is sometimes complex. The uricosuric agents increase the renal excretion of alloxanthine and thus cause a reduction in allopurinol effect. Conversely, allopurinol may delay elimination of probenecid and increase its plasma concentration (Tjandramaga *et al.,* 1972).

Allopurinol is also administered prophylactically to reduce the hyperuricemia and to prevent urate deposition or renal calculi in patients with leukemias, lymphomas, or other malignancies, particularly when *antineoplastic* or *radiation* therapy is initiated. Allopurinol inhibits the enzymatic inactivation of 6-mercaptopurine by xanthine oxidase. Thus, when allopurinol is used concomitantly with 6-mercaptopurine or azathioprine, dosage of the antineoplastic agent must be reduced to one fourth to one third of the usual dose. The risk of bone-marrow suppression is also increased when allopurinol is administered with cytotoxic agents that are not metabolized by xanthine oxidase, particularly cyclophosphamide (Boston Collaborative Drug Surveillance Program, 1974).

The *iatrogenic hyperuricemia* sometimes induced by the thiazides and other drugs can be prevented or reversed by concurrent allopurinol medication. Allopurinol is also useful in lowering the high plasma concentrations of uric acid in patients with the *Lesch-Nyhan syndrome* and thereby prevents the complications resulting from hyperuricemia; there is no evidence that it alters the progressive neurological and behavioral abnormalities characteristic of the disease.

Abel, J. A. Analgesic nephropathy—a review of the literature, 1967–1970. *Clin. Pharmac. Ther.,* **1971,** *12,* 583–598.

Adler, R. D.; Rawlins, M.; Rosendorff, C.; and Cranston, W. I. The effect of salicylate on pyrogen-induced fever in man. *Clin. Sci.,* **1969,** *37,* 91–97.

Alexander, W. D., and Smith, G. Disadvantageous circulatory effects of salicylate in rheumatic fever. *Lancet,* **1962,** *1,* 768–771.

Amoroso, E. C. Colchicine and tumour growth. *Nature, Lond.,* **1935,** *135,* 266–267.

Bhargava, K. P.; Chandra, O. M.; and Verma, D. R. The mechanism of the emetic action of sodium salicylate. *Br. J. Pharmac. Chemother.,* **1963,** *21,* 45–50.

Bloomfield, S. S., and Hurwitz, H. N. Tourniquet and episiotomy pain as test models for aspirin-like analgesics. *J. clin. Pharmac.,* **1970,** *10,* 361–369.

Boardman, P. L., and Hart, E. D. Clinical measurement of the anti-inflammatory effects of salicylates in rheumatoid arthritis. *Br. med. J.,* **1967a,** *4,* 264–268.

———. Side-effects of indomethacin. *Ann. rheum. Dis.,* **1967b,** *26,* 127–132.

Boston Collaborative Drug Surveillance Program. Excess of ampicillin rashes associated with allopurinol or hyperuricemia. *New Engl. J. Med.,* **1972,** *286,* 505–507.

———. Allopurinol and cytotoxic drugs: interaction in relation to bone marrow depression. *J. Am. med. Ass.,* **1974,** *227,* 1036–1040.

Brodie, B. B., and Axelrod, J. The fate of acetophenetidin (phenacetin) in man and methods for the estimation of acetophenetidin and its metabolites in biological material. *J. Pharmac. exp. Ther.,* **1949,** *97,* 58–67.

———. The fate of antipyrine in man. *Ibid.,* **1950,** *98,* 97–104.

Brodie, B. B.; Lowman, E. W.; Burns, J. J.; Lee, P. R.; Chenkin, T.; Goldman, A.; Weiner, M.; and Steele, J. M. Observations on the antirheumatic and physiologic effects of phenylbutazone (BUTAZOLIDIN) and some comparisons with cortisone. *Am. J. Med.,* **1954,** *16,* 181–190.

Burns, J. J.; Rose, R. K.; Chenkin, T.; Goldman, A.; Schulert, A.; and Brodie, B. B. The physiological disposition of phenylbutazone (BUTAZOLIDIN) in man and a method for its estimation in biological material. *J. Pharmac. exp. Ther.,* **1953,** *109,* 346–357.

Burns, J. J.; Rose, R. K.; Goodwin, S.; Reichenthal, J.; Horning, E. C.; and Brodie, B. B. The metabolic fate of phenylbutazone (BUTAZOLIDIN) in man. *J. Pharmac. exp. Ther.,* **1955,** *113,* 481–489.

Burns, J. J.; Yü, T.-F.; Dayton, P. G.; Gutman, A. B.; and Brodie, B. B. Biochemical and pharmacological considerations of phenylbutazone and its analogues. *Ann. N.Y. Acad. Sci.,* **1960,** *86,* 253–262.

Chafee, F. H., and Settipane, G. A. Aspirin intolerance. I. Frequency in an allergic population. *J. Allergy clin. Immun.,* **1974,** *53,* 193–199.

Champion, G. D.; Paulus, H. E.; Mongan, E.; Okun, R.; Pearson, C. M.; and Sarkissian, E. The effect of aspirin on serum indomethacin. *Clin. Pharmac. Ther.,* **1972,** *13,* 239–244.

Charnock, J. S.; Opit, L. J.; and Hetzel, B. S. Electrolyte distribution in rats following salicylate. *Metabolism,* **1961,** *10,* 874–882.

Clark, R.; Thompson, R. P. H.; Borirakchanyavat, V.; Widdop, B.; Davidson, A. R.; Goulding, R.; and Williams, R. Hepatic damage and death from overdose of paracetamol. *Lancet,* **1973,** *1,* 66–69.

Clark, W. G., and Coldwell, B. A. Competitive antagonism of leukocytic pyrogen by sodium salicylate and acetaminophen. *Proc. Soc. exp. Biol. Med.,* **1972,** *141,* 669–672.

Clark, W. G.; Montoya, S. F., Jr.; and Pomarantz, S. D. Sites of emetic action of sodium salicylate in the cat. *Toxic. appl. Pharmac.,* **1972,** *23,* 191–196.

Clark, W. G., and Moyer, S. G. The effects of acetaminophen and sodium salicylate on the release and activity of leukocytic pyrogen in the cat. *J. Pharmac. exp. Ther.,* **1972,** *181,* 183–191.

Clinicopathologic Conference. Agranulocytosis and anuria during phenylbutazone therapy of rheumatoid arthritis. *Am. J. Med.,* **1961,** *30,* 268–280.

Cochran, J. B., and Ramsay, A. G. The hyperpnoea produced by intravenous administration of salicylates. *Br. J. Pharmac. Chemother.,* **1956,** *11,* 364–366.

Combined Rheumatic Fever Study Group. A comparison of the effect of prednisone and acetylsalicylic acid on the incidence of residual rheumatic heart disease. *New Engl. J. Med.,* **1960,** *262,* 895–902.

———. A comparison of short-term, intensive prednisone and acetylsalicylic acid therapy in the treatment of acute rheumatic fever. *Ibid.,* **1965,** *272,* 63–70.

Conney, A. H.; Sansur, M.; Soroko, F.; Koster, R.; and Burns, J. J. Enzyme induction and inhibition in studies on the pharmacological actions of acetophenetidin. *J. Pharmac. exp. Ther.,* **1966,** *151,* 133–138.

Cooke, A. R. The role of acid in the pathogenesis of aspirin-induced gastrointestinal erosions and hemorrhage. *Am. J. dig. Dis.,* **1973,** *18,* 225–237.

Cranston, W. I.; Hellon, R. F.; Luff, R. H.; Rawlins, M. D.; and Rosendorff, C. Observations on the mechanism of salicylate-induced antipyresis. *J. Physiol., Lond.,* **1970,** *210,* 593–600.

Davidson, R. J. L. Phenacetin-induced haemolytic anaemia. *J. clin. Path.,* **1971,** *24,* 537–541.

Davis, J. W. The potential danger of aspirin to patients with intracranial bleeding. *J. Med., Basel,* **1973,** *4,* 371–376.

Deodhar, S. D.; Dick, W. C.; Hodgkinson, R.; and Buchanan, W. W. Measurement of clinical response to anti-inflammatory drug therapy in rheumatoid arthritis. *Q. Jl Med.,* **1973,** *42,* 387–401.

Domenjoz, R. The pharmacology of phenylbutazone analogues. *Ann. N.Y. Acad. Sci.,* **1960,** *86,* 263–291.

Done, A. K. Salicylate intoxication: significance of measurements of salicylate in blood in cases of acute ingestion. *Pediatrics, Springfield,* **1960,** *26,* 800–807.

———. Antipyretics. *Pediat. Clins N. Am.,* **1973,** *19,* 167–177.

Done, A. K., and Temple, A. R. Treatment of salicylate poisoning. *Mod. Treatm.,* **1971,** *8,* 528–551.

Dubas, T. S., and Parker, J. M. A central component in the analgesic action of sodium salicylate. *Archs int. Pharmacodyn. Thér.,* **1971,** *194,* 117–122.

Duggan, D. E.; Hogans, A. F.; Kwan, K. C.; and McMahon, F. G. The metabolism of indomethacin in man. *J. Pharmac. exp. Ther.,* **1972,** *181,* 563–575.

Duggan, J. M. Splenomegaly in analgesic takers. *Med. J. Aust.,* **1970,** *2,* 580–583.

Eade, N. R., and Lasagna, L. A comparison of acetophenetidin and acetaminophen. II. Subjective effects in

healthy volunteers. *J. Pharmac. exp. Ther.,* **1967,** *155,* 301–308.

Elion, G. B.; Callahan, S.; Rundles, R. W.; and Hitchings, G. H. Relationship between metabolic fates and antitumor activities of thiopurines. *Cancer Res.,* **1963,** *23,* 1207–1217.

Elion, G. B.; Kovensky, A.; Hitchings, G. H.; Metz, E.; and Rundles, R. W. Metabolic studies of allopurinol, an inhibitor of xanthine oxidase. *Biochem. Pharmac.,* **1966,** *15,* 863–880.

Elion, G. B.; Yü, T.-F.; Gutman, A. B.; and Hitchings, G. H. Renal clearance of oxipurinol, the chief metabolite of allopurinol. *Am. J. Med.,* **1968,** *45,* 69–77.

Farber, H. R.; Yiengst, M. J.; and Shock, N. W. The effect of therapeutic doses of aspirin on the acid-base balance of the blood in normal adults. *Am. J. med. Sci.,* **1949,** *217,* 256–262.

Farid, N. R.; Glynn, J. P.; and Kerr, D. N. S. Hemodialysis in paracetamol self-poisoning. *Lancet,* **1972,** *2,* 396–398.

Feldberg, W., and Saxena, P. N. Mechanism of action of pyrogen. *J. Physiol., Lond.,* **1970,** *211,* 245–261.

Ferguson, F. C., Jr. Colchicine. I. General pharmacology. *J. Pharmac. exp. Ther.,* **1952,** *106,* 261–270.

Gault, M. H.; Rudwal, T. C.; Engles, W. D.; and Dossetor, J. B. Syndrome associated with abuse of analgesics. *Ann. intern. Med.,* **1968,** *68,* 906–925.

Gifford, R. H. Chemotherapy for rheumatoid arthritis. *Ration. Drug Ther.,* **1973,** *7,* No. 12, 1–7.

Gilman, A. Analgesic nephrotoxicity: a pharmacological analysis. *Am. J. Med.,* **1964,** *36,* 167–173.

Giraldo, B.; Blumenthal, M. N.; and Spink, W. W. Aspirin intolerance and asthma. A clinical and immunological study. *Ann. intern. Med.,* **1969,** *71,* 479–496.

Goldfinger, S. E. Treatment of gout. *New Engl. J. Med.,* **1971,** *285,* 1303–1306.

Grace, N. D.; Greenwald, M. A.; and Greenberg, M. S. Effect of allopurinol on iron mobilization. *Gastroenterology,* **1970,** *59,* 103–108.

Graham, W. The status of phenylbutazone (BUTAZOLIDIN) in the treatment of rheumatic disorders. *Can. med. Ass. J.,* **1958,** *79,* 634–638.

Gutman, A. B. The past four decades of progress in the knowledge of gout, with an assessment of the present status. *Arthritis Rheum.,* **1973,** *16,* 431–445.

Gutman, A. B.; Dayton, P. G.; Yü, T.-F.; Berger, L.; Chen, W.; Sicam, L. E.; and Burns, J. J. A study of the inverse relationship between pK_a and rate of renal excretion of phenylbutazone analogs in man and dog. *Am. J. Med.,* **1960,** *29,* 1017–1033.

Hawkins, D.; Pinckard, R. N.; Crawford, I. P.; and Farr, R. S. Structural changes in human serum albumin induced by ingestion of acetylsalicylic acid. *J. clin. Invest.,* **1969,** *48,* 536–542.

Hicklin, J. A. Salicylate and potassium fluxes of rat diaphragm. *Nature, Lond.,* **1959,** *184,* 2029–2030.

Hill, J. B. Experimental salicylate poisoning: observations on the effects of altering blood pH on tissue and plasma salicylate concentrations. *Pediatrics, Springfield,* **1971,** *47,* 658–665.

———. Salicylate intoxication. *New Engl. J. Med.,* **1973,** *288,* 1110–1113.

Huguley, C. M., Jr. Agranulocytosis induced by dipyrone, a hazardous antipyretic and analgesic. *J. Am. med. Ass.,* **1964,** *189,* 938–941.

Klinenberg, J. R.; Goldfinger, S. E.; and Seegmiller, J. E. The effectiveness of the xanthine oxidase inhibitor allopurinol in the treatment of gout. *Ann. intern. Med.,* **1965,** *62,* 639–647.

Krakoff, I. H. Clinical pharmacology of drugs which influence uric acid production and excretion. *Clin. Pharmac. Ther.,* **1967,** *8,* 124–138.

Larsen, P. R. Salicylate-induced increases in free triiodothyronine in human serum. Evidence of inhibition of triiodothyronine binding to thyroxine-binding globulin and thyroxine-binding prealbumin. *J. clin. Invest.,* **1972,** *51,* 1125–1134.

Leonards, J. R., and Levy, G.   Gastrointestinal blood loss during prolonged aspirin administration. *New Engl. J. Med.,* **1973,** *289,* 1020–1022.

Levitan, H., and Barker, J. L.   Salicylate: a structure-activity study of its effects on membrane permeability. *Science, Wash.,* **1972,** *176,* 1423–1425.

Levy, G.; Tsuchiya, T.; and Amsol, L. P.   Limited capacity for salicyl phenolic glucuronide formation and its effect on the kinetics of salicylate elimination in man. *Clin. Pharmac. Ther.,* **1972,** *13,* 258–268.

Levy, M.   Aspirin use in patients with major upper gastro-intestinal bleeding and peptic-ulcer disease. A report from the Boston Collaborative Drug Surveillance Program, Boston University Medical Center. *New Engl. J. Med.,* **1974,** *290,* 1158–1162.

Lewis, R. B., and Schulman, J. D.   Influence of acetyl-salicylic acid, an inhibitor of prostaglandin synthesis on the duration of human gestation and labour. *Lancet,* **1973,** *2,* 1159–1161.

Lim, R. K. S.   Salicylate analgesia. In, *The Salicylates: A Critical Bibliographic Review.* (Smith, M. J. H., and Smith, P. K., eds.) John Wiley & Sons, Inc., New York, **1966.**

Link, K. P.; Overman, R. S.; Sullivan, W. R.; Huebner, C. F.; and Scheel, L. D.   Studies on the hemorrhagic sweet clover disease. XI. Hypoprothrombinemia in the rat induced by salicylic acid. *J. biol. Chem.,* **1943,** *147,* 463–474.

Lits, F. J.   Contribution à l'étude des réactions cellulaires provoquées par la colchicine. *C. r. Séanc. Soc. Biol.,* **1934,** *115,* 1421–1423.

McArthur, J. N.; Dawkins, P. D.; Smith, M. J. H.; and Hamilton, E. B. D.   Mode of action of antirheumatic drugs. *Br. med. J.,* **1971,** *2,* 677–679.

McEwen, C.   Current status of therapy in rheumatic fever. *J. Am. med. Ass.,* **1959,** *170,* 1056–1062.

Malawista, S. E.   Colchicine: a common mechanism for its anti-inflammatory and anti-mitotic effects. *Arthritis Rheum.,* **1968,** *11,* 191–197.

Mauer, E. F.   The toxic effects of phenylbutazone (BUTA-ZOLIDIN): review of literature and report of the twenty-third death following its use. *New Engl. J. Med.,* **1955,** *253,* 404–410.

Mitchell, J. R.; Jollow, D. J.; Gillette, J. R.; and Brodie, B. B.   Drug metabolism as a cause of drug toxicity. *Drug Metab. Disposition,* **1973a,** *1,* 418–423.

Mitchell, J. R.; Jollow, D. J.; Potter, W. Z.; Gillette, J. R.; and Brodie, B. B.   Acetaminophen-induced hepatic necrosis. IV. Protective role of glutathione. *J. Pharmac. exp. Ther.,* **1973b,** *187,* 211–217.

Miyahara, J. T., and Karler, R.   Effect of salicylate on oxidative phosphorylation and respiration of mitochon-drial fragments. *Biochem. J.,* **1965,** *97,* 194–198.

Moertel, C. G.; Ahmann, D. L.; Taylor, W. F.; and Schwartau, N.   Relief of pain by oral medications: a controlled evaluation of analgesic combinations. *J. Am. med. Ass.,* **1974,** *229,* 55–59.

Mongan, E.; Kelly, P.; Nies, K.; Porter, W. W.; and Paulus, H. E.   Tinnitus as an indication of therapeutic serum salicylate levels. *J. Am. med. Ass.,* **1973,** *226,* 142–145.

Morgan, A. G., and Polak, A.   The excretion of salicylate in salicylate poisoning. *Clin. Sci.,* **1971,** *41,* 475–484.

Muggia, F.; Ball, T. J., Jr.; and Ultmann, J. E.   Allopurinol in the treatment of neoplastic disease complicated by hyperuricemia. *Archs intern. Med.,* **1967,** *120,* 12–18.

Multz, C. V.; Bernhard, G. C.; Blechman, W. C.; Zane, S.; Restifo, R. A.; and Varady, J. C.   A comparison of intermediate-dose aspirin and placebo in rheumatoid arthritis. *Clin. Pharmac. Ther.,* **1974,** *15,* 310–315.

Mustard, J. F., and Packham, M. A.   Factors influencing platelet function: adhesion, release and aggregation. *Pharmac. Rev.,* **1970,** *22,* 97–187.

Myers, E. N.; Bernstein, J. M.; and Fostiropolous, G.   Salicylate ototoxicity: a clinical study. *New Engl. J. Med.,* **1965,** *273,* 587–590.

Myers, R. D., and Tytell, M.   Fever: reciprocal shift in brain sodium to calcium ratio as the set-point temperature rises. *Science, Wash.,* **1972,** *178,* 765–767.

Nusynowitz, M. L., and Forsham, P. H.   The antidiuretic action of acetaminophen. *Am. J. med. Sci.,* **1966,** *252,* 429–435.

O'Brien, W. M.   Indomethacin: a survey of clinical trials. *Clin. Pharmac. Ther.,* **1968,** *9,* 94–107.

O'Reilly, R. A.   Impact of aspirin and chlorthalidone on the pharmacodynamics of oral anticoagulant drugs in man. *Ann. N.Y. Acad. Sci.,* **1971,** *179,* 173–186.

Paalzow, L.   An electrical method for estimation of analgesic activity in mice. *Acta pharm. suec.,* **1969,** *6,* 207–226.

Pentiah, P.; Reilly, F.; and Borison, H. L.   Interactions of morphine sulfate and sodium salicylate on respiration in cats. *J. Pharmac. exp. Ther.,* **1966,** *154,* 110–118.

Prescott, L. F.   Effects of acetylsalicylic acid, phenacetin, paracetamol, and caffeine on renal tubular epithelium. *Lancet,* **1965,** *2,* 91–96.

———.   The metabolism of phenacetin in patients with renal disease. *Clin. Pharmac. Ther.,* **1969,** *10,* 383–394.

Prescott, L. F.; Wright, N.; Roscoe, P.; and Brown, S. S.   Plasma-paracetamol half-life and hepatic necrosis in patients with paracetamol overdosage. *Lancet,* **1971,** *1,* 519–522.

Proudfoot, A. T., and Wright, N.   Acute paracetamol poisoning. *Br. med. J.,* **1970,** *3,* 557–558.

Quick, A. J., and Clesceri, L.   Influence of acetylsalicylic acid and salicylamide on the coagulation of blood. *J. Pharmac. exp. Ther.,* **1960,** *128,* 95–98.

Rastegar, A., and Thier, S. O.   The treatment of hyperuricemia in gout. *Ration. Drug Ther.,* **1974,** *8,* No. 3, 1–4.

Rawlins, M. D., and Smith, S. E.   Influence of allopurinol on drug metabolism in man. *Br. J. Pharmac.,* **1973,** *48,* 693–698.

Reimold, E.; Worthen, H. G.; and Reilly, T. P., Jr.   Salicylate poisoning: comparison of acetazolamide administration and alkaline diuresis in the treatment of experimental salicylate intoxication in puppies. *Am. J. Dis. Child.,* **1973,** *125,* 668–674.

Robin, E. D.; Davis, R. P.; and Rees, S. B.   Salicylate intoxication with special reference to the development of hypokalemia. *Am. J. Med.,* **1959,** *26,* 869–882.

Rodnan, G. P., and Benedek, T. G.   The early history of antirheumatic drugs. *Arthritis Rheum.,* **1970,** *13,* 145–165.

Rosenstein, R., and Borison, H. L.   Actions of carbon dioxide and sodium salicylate on central control of respiration in cats. *J. Pharmac. exp. Ther.,* **1963,** *139,* 361–367.

Rundles, R. W.; Metz, E. N.; and Silberman, H. R.   Allopurinol in the treatment of gout. *Ann. intern. Med.,* **1966,** *64,* 229–258.

Rundles, R. W.; Wyngaarden, J. B.; Hitchings, G. H.; Elion, G. B.; and Silberman, H. R.   Effects of a xanthine oxidase inhibitor on thiopurine metabolism, hyperuricemia and gout. *Trans. Ass. Am. Physns,* **1963,** *76,* 126–140.

Samet, P.; Fierer, E. M.; and Bernstein, W. H.   Effect of salicylates on ventilatory response to inhaled carbon dioxide in normal subjects. *J. appl. Physiol.,* **1960,** *15,* 826–828.

Samter, M., and Beers, R. F., Jr.   Intolerance to aspirin: clinical studies and consideration of its pathogenesis. *Ann. intern. Med.,* **1968,** *68,* 975–983.

Schordberet, M., and Straub, R. W.   Effects of non-narcotic analgesics and nonsteroid anti-inflammatory agents upon inorganic phosphates, intracellular potassium and impulse conduction in mammalian nerve fibers. *Biochem. Pharmac.,* **1971,** *20,* 1355–1361.

Schreiner, G. E. The nephrotoxicity of analgesic abuse. *Ann. intern. Med.,* **1962,** *57,* 1047–1052.

Seegmiller, J. E., and Grayzel, A. I. Use of the newer uricosuric agents in the management of gout. *J. Am. Med. Ass.,* **1960,** *173,* 1076–1080.

Settipane, G. A.; Chafee, F. H.; and Klein, D. E. Aspirin intolerance. II. A prospective study in an atopic and normal population. *J. Allergy clin. Immun.,* **1974,** *53,* 200–204.

Shelley, J. H. Phenacetin, through the looking glass. *Clin. Pharmac. Ther.,* **1967,** *8,* 427–471.

Smith, G. M., and Beecher, H. K. Experimental production of pain in man: sensitivity of a new method to 600 mg of aspirin. *Clin. Pharmac. Ther.,* **1969,** *10,* 213–216.

Spector, R., and Lorenzo, A. V. The transport and metabolism of salicylate in the central nervous system: *in vivo* studies. *J. Pharmac. exp. Ther.,* **1973,** *185,* 276–286.

Steinbrocker, O., and Argyros, T. G. Phenylbutazone as a therapeutic agent in rheumatic disease: its present status. *Arthritis Rheum.,* **1960,** *3,* 368–375.

Talesnik, J., and Sunahara, F. A. Enhancement of metabolic coronary dilatation by aspirin-like substances by suppression of prostaglandin feed-back control? *Nature, Lond.,* **1973,** *244,* 351–353.

Tenney, S. M., and Miller, R. M. The respiratory and circulatory actions of salicylate. *Am. J. Med.,* **1955,** *19,* 498–508.

Tjandramaga, T. B.; Cucinell, S. A.; Israili, Z. H.; Perel, J. M.; Dayton, P. G.; Yü, T.-F.; and Gutman, A. B. Observations on the disposition of probenecid in patients receiving allopurinol. *Pharmacology,* **1972,** *8,* 259–272.

United Kingdom and United States Joint Report. The evaluation of rheumatic heart disease in children: five-year report of a cooperative clinical trial of ACTH, cortisone and aspirin. *Circulation,* **1960,** *22,* 503–515.

Vesell, E. S.; Passananti, G. T.; and Greene, F. E. Impairment of drug metabolism in man by allopurinol and nortriptyline. *New Engl. J. Med.,* **1970,** *283,* 1484–1488.

Wallace, S. L. Colchicine: clinical pharmacology in acute gouty arthritis. *Am. J. Med.,* **1961,** *30,* 439–448.

Wallace, S. L.; Omokoku, B.; and Ertel, N. H. Colchicine plasma levels: implications as to pharmacology and mechanism of action. *Am. J. Med.,* **1970,** *48,* 443–448.

Waltner, J. G. The effect of salicylates on the inner ear. *Ann. Otol. Rhinol. Lar.,* **1955,** *64,* 617–622.

Walton, R. P., and Darby, T. D. Circulatory effects of salicylates. *Circulation Res.,* **1958,** *6,* 155–158.

Winder, C. V. Aspirin and algesimetry. *Nature, Lond.,* **1959,** *184,* 494–497.

Winter, C. A.; Risley, E. A.; and Nuss, G. W. Anti-inflammatory and antipyretic activities of indomethacin, 1-(*p*-chlorobenzoyl)-5-methoxy-2-methylindole-3-acetic acid. *J. Pharmac. exp. Ther.,* **1963,** *141,* 369–376.

Winters, R. W.; White, J. S.; Hughes, M. C.; and Ordway, N. K. Disturbances of acid-base equilibrium in salicylate intoxication. *Pediatrics, Springfield,* **1959,** *23,* 260–285.

Wintrobe, M. M. The therapeutic millennium and its price: a view from the haematopoietic system, the Lilly Lecture, 1968. *Jl R. Coll. Physns Lond.,* **1969,** *3,* 99–119.

Wit, A., and Wang, S. C. Temperature-sensitive neurons in preoptic/anterior hypothalamic region: actions of pyrogen and acetylsalicylate. *Am. J. Physiol.,* **1968,** *215,* 1160–1169.

Yü, T.-F. Milestones in the treatment of gout. *Am. J. Med.,* **1974,** *56,* 676–685.

Yü, T.-F., and Gutman, A. B. Study of the paradoxical effects of salicylate in low, intermediate and high dosage on the renal mechanisms for excretion of urate in man. *J. clin. Invest.,* **1959,** *38,* 1298–1315.

———. Efficacy of colchicine prophylaxis in gout: prevention of recurrent gouty arthritis over a mean period of five years in 208 gouty subjects. *Ann. intern. Med.,* **1961,** *55,* 179–192.

———. Effect of allopurinol (4-hydroxypyrazolo-[3,4-*d*] pyrimidine) on serum and urinary uric acid in primary and secondary gout. *Am. J. Med.,* **1964,** *37,* 885–898.

Monographs and Reviews

Beaver, W. T. Mild analgesics: a review of their clinical pharmacology. *Am. J. med. Sci.,* **1965,** *250,* 577–604; **1966,** *251,* 576–599. (392 references.)

Beecher, H. K. The measurement of pain. Prototype for the quantitative study of subjective responses. *Pharmac. Rev.,* **1957,** *9,* 59–209. (687 references.)

Davison, C. Salicylate metabolism in man. *Ann. N.Y. Acad. Sci.,* **1971,** *179,* 249–268.

Domenjoz, R. Synthetic anti-inflammatory drugs: concepts of their mode of action. *Adv. Pharmac.,* **1966,** *4,* 143–217. (520 references.)

Dustin, P., Jr. New aspects of the pharmacology of antimitotic agents. *Pharmac. Rev.,* **1963,** *15,* 449–480.

Ferreira, S. H., and Vane, J. R. New aspects of the mode of action of nonsteroid anti-inflammatory drugs. *A. Rev. Pharmac.,* **1974,** *14,* 57–73.

Greenberg, L. A. *Antipyrine: A Critical Bibliographic Review.* Hillhouse Press, New Haven, Conn., **1950.** (1735 references.)

Gross, M., and Greenberg, L. A. *The Salicylates: A Critical Bibliographic Review.* Hillhouse Press, New Haven, Conn., **1948.** (4093 references.)

Hanzlik, P. J. *Actions and Uses of the Salicylates and Cinchophen in Medicine.* The Williams & Wilkins Co., Baltimore, **1927.**

Paulus, H. E., and Whitehouse, M. W. Nonsteroid anti-inflammatory agents. *A. Rev. Pharmac.,* **1973,** *13,* 107–125.

Randall, L. O. 2. Non-narcotic analgesics. In, *Physiological Pharmacology.* Vol. 1, *The Nervous System—Part A: Central Nervous System Drugs.* (Root, W. S., and Hofmann, F. G., eds.) Academic Press, Inc., New York, **1963,** pp. 313–416. (231 references.)

Salter, R. H. Aspirin and gastrointestinal bleeding. *Am. J. dig. Dis.,* **1968,** *13,* 38–58.

Seegmiller, J. E.; Lester, L.; and Howell, R. R. Medical progress: biochemistry of uric acid and its relation to gout. *New Engl. J. Med.,* **1963,** *268,* 712–716, 764–773, 821–827.

Smith, M. J. H., and Dawkins, P. O. Salicylate and enzymes. *J. Pharm. Pharmac.,* **1971,** *23,* 729–744.

Smith, M. J. H., and Smith, P. K. (eds.) *The Salicylates: A Critical Bibliographic Review.* John Wiley & Sons, Inc., New York, **1966.**

Smith, P. K. *Acetophenetidin: A Critical Bibliographic Review.* Interscience Publishers, Inc., New York, **1958.** (529 references.)

Symposium. (Various authors.) *Salicylates: An International Symposium.* (Dixon, A. St. J.; Martin, B. K.; Smith, M. J. H.; and Wood, P. H. N.; eds.) J. & A. Churchill, Ltd., London, **1963.**

Symposium. (Various authors.) *Proceedings of the Conference on Effects of Chronic Salicylate Administration.* (Lamont-Honers, R. W., and Wagner, B. M., eds.) National Institutes of Health, NIAMD, Bethesda, **1966.**

Symposium. (Various authors.) Aspirin and salicylates. *Clin. Toxicol.,* **1968,** *1,* 379–473.

Symposium. (Various authors.) Pharmacological and biochemical properties of microtubule proteins. *Fedn Proc. Fedn Am. Socs exp. Biol.,* **1974,** *33,* 151–174.

Whitehouse, M. W. Some biochemical and pharmacological properties of anti-inflammatory drugs. *Prog. Drug Res.,* **1965,** *8,* 301–429. (404 references.)

CHAPTER

18 CENTRAL NERVOUS SYSTEM STIMULANTS

Strychnine, Picrotoxin, Pentylenetetrazol, and Miscellaneous Agents (Doxapram, Ethamivan, Nikethamide, Flurothyl, Methylphenidate)

Donald N. Franz

Stimulation of the central nervous system (CNS) can be produced in man and animals by a large number of natural and synthetic substances. Only a few have been used therapeutically. Some drugs exhibit prominent central stimulation at toxic levels, and others produce mild stimulation as a side effect. This chapter includes those drugs that produce central stimulation as their most prominent action and are generally classified as *analeptics* or *convulsants*.

Although some analeptics were formerly used in attempts to counteract severe intoxication by general depressants, this practice has been overwhelmingly discredited by the far greater success achieved with more conservative measures that stress intensive supportive care. Several analeptics have limited uses for combating depressed respiration in pulmonary disease or for hastening recovery from general anesthesia. A few have very specialized applications. All are capable of producing generalized convulsions in sufficient doses. Unfortunately, the margin of safety of doses for stimulation of central respiratory centers is generally very narrow and unpredictable. No totally safe, selective respiratory stimulant is currently available.

The excitability of the CNS reflects a balance between excitatory and inhibitory influences that is normally maintained within relatively narrow limits. Drugs can increase excitability either by blocking inhibition or by enhancing excitation. Strychnine and picrotoxin selectively block inhibition in the CNS; these drugs are important research tools employed to study inhibitory transmitters and receptor types. The other analeptics described in this chapter do not affect inhibitory processes and, therefore, presumably act by enhancing excitation. The pharmacology of analeptics has been reviewed by Hahn (1960) and by Esplin and Zablocka-Esplin (1969).

STRYCHNINE

Strychnine has no demonstrated therapeutic value, despite a long history of unwarranted popularity. However, strychnine holds a singular position as the only centrally acting drug for which the detailed mechanism of action is thoroughly understood in terms of central synaptic transmission.

Source and Chemistry. Strychnine is the principal alkaloid present in *nux vomica,* the seeds of a tree native to India, *Strychnos nux-vomica.* The term *nux vomica* has been erroneously translated as "emetic nut." Actually, strychnine is not an emetic, and the word *vomica* means depression or cavity, a feature of the strychnos seed attributed by legend to the digital imprint of the Creator.

Nux vomica was introduced into Germany in the sixteenth century as a poison for rats and other animal pests. Its use as a rat poison persists to this day and is a source of accidental strychnine poisoning of children. Strychnine was first employed in medicine in 1540, but it did not gain wide usage until 200 years later.

In addition to strychnine, the closely related alkaloid *brucine* is found in nux vomica. Brucine is much less potent than strychnine. The structural formula of strychnine is as follows:

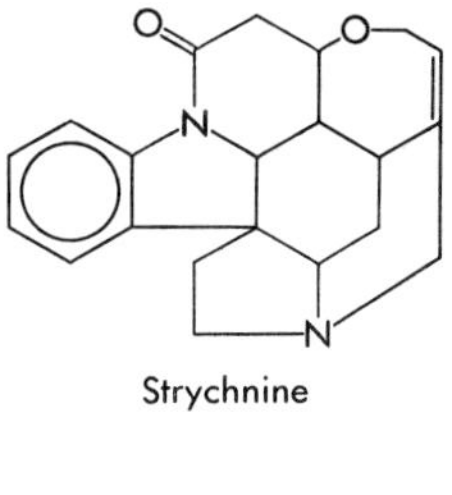

Strychnine

Pharmacological Actions. *Central Nervous System.* Strychnine produces excitation of all portions of the CNS. This effect, however, does not result from direct synaptic excitation. Strychnine increases the level of neuronal excitability by selectively

359

blocking inhibition. Nerve impulses are normally confined to appropriate pathways by inhibitory influences. When inhibition is blocked by strychnine, ongoing neuronal activity is enhanced and sensory stimuli produce exaggerated reflex effects.

Strychnine is a powerful convulsant, and the convulsion has a characteristic motor pattern. Inasmuch as strychnine reduces inhibition, including the reciprocal inhibition existing between antagonistic muscles, the pattern of convulsion is determined by the most powerful muscles acting at a given joint. In most laboratory animals, this convulsion is characterized by tonic extension of the body and of all limbs. Tonic extension is preceded and followed during the phase of postictal depression by phasic *symmetrical* extensor thrusts that may be initiated by any modality of sensory stimulus. The sloth presents an interesting exception. In this animal, the powerful antigravity muscles are flexors, and the strychnine convulsion is characterized by tonic flexion of all limbs (Esplin and Woodbury, 1961). The pattern of the strychnine convulsion therefore contrasts sharply with that produced by drugs that directly excite central neurons.

Typical strychnine convulsions also occur in spinal animals. For this reason the effects of strychnine are often ascribed to a spinal locus of action, and the convulsion is frequently termed a *spinal convulsion*. In fact, other portions of the CNS are fully excited by doses that produce the characteristic motor manifestations in a spinal animal. The tonic extensor convulsion reflects the action of strychnine to reduce inhibition, rather than the characteristic response of the spinal cord to a convulsant drug. Convulsions in spinal animals produced by drugs that directly excite neurons are asymmetrical and incoordinated, in contrast to the pattern observed with strychnine. The medulla, likewise, is affected by strychnine at dosages that produce hyperexcitability throughout the CNS. However, strychnine does not selectively stimulate the medulla, and the drug is not therapeutically useful as a respiratory analeptic.

Cardiovascular System. Strychnine has no direct effects on the heart or blood vessels. Complex changes in blood pressure that occur during strychnine convulsions are related to the effects of the drug on vasomotor centers, including those in the spinal cord.

Gastrointestinal Tract. Strychnine was at one time employed for atonic constipation on the basis of a presumed stimulatory effect of the drug on the gastrointestinal tract. Experiments in both animals and man have failed to demonstrate such stimulation with concentrations of the agent that can be obtained clinically. The bitter taste of strychnine, which is detectable in very dilute solutions, has led to the use of the drug as a stomachic and bitter. Bitters supposedly stimulate the taste buds, increase the appetite, and reflexly stimulate gastric secretion.

Skeletal Muscle. Convulsive doses of strychnine have no detectable effect on skeletal muscle. Increased muscle tone is the result purely of the central actions of the drug. In supraconvulsive doses, a curariform action on the neuromuscular junction is observed.

Mechanism of Action. Strychnine has been the object of many experimental investigations. The convulsant action of the drug has often been attributed to interference with central inhibitory processes. Blockade of spinal inhibition by subconvulsive doses of strychnine was first demonstrated by Eccles and coworkers (Bradley *et al.,* 1953). Strychnine interferes only with *postsynaptic* inhibition. Postsynaptic inhibition is mediated by many known pathways in the brain and spinal cord, and, when allowances are made for differences in functional organization, the pathways appear to be about equally sensitive to blockade by strychnine. Well-known examples of postsynaptic inhibition are the inhibitory influences existing between the motoneurons of antagonistic muscle groups and recurrent spinal inhibition mediated by the Renshaw cell. Renshaw cells are excited by intraspinal collaterals of motoneuron axons that liberate acetylcholine. Strychnine blocks recurrent inhibition at the Renshaw cell–motoneuron synapse.

Compelling evidence has accumulated to implicate *glycine* as the predominant postsynaptic inhibitory transmitter to motoneurons and interneurons in the spinal cord. An important part of this evidence rests on the ability of strychnine to block selectively both synaptically evoked postsynaptic inhibition and the identical inhibitory effects of glycine on spinal neurons. Strychnine acts as a competitive antagonist of the inhibitory transmitter at postsynaptic inhibitory sites in the same manner as curare blocks acetylcholine at the neuromuscular junction (Kuno and Weakly, 1972). Tetanus toxin also blocks postsynaptic inhibition, but it acts by preventing release of glycine from inhibitory interneurons. Strychnine-sensitive postsynaptic inhibition in higher centers of the CNS may also be mediated by glycine. The pharmacology of postsynaptic inhibition has been reviewed by Curtis (1969). An interesting parallelism between the effects of drugs on postsynaptic inhibition and on peripheral cholinergic synapses is discussed by Esplin and Zablocka-Esplin (1969).

Absorption, Fate, and Excretion. Strychnine is readily absorbed from the gastrointestinal tract and parenteral sites of injection. It is carried in the blood by both plasma and erythrocytes and rapidly leaves the circulation for the tissues. The CNS does not contain a higher concentration of the drug than do other organs. Strychnine is readily metabolized, mainly by the enzymes of hepatic microsomes (Adamson and Fouts, 1959). Approximately 20% of the alkaloid escapes into the urine. The rate of destruction of strychnine is such that approximately two lethal doses can be given over a period of 24 hours without noticeable toxic symptoms or cumulative effects.

Toxicology. Despite the fact that strychnine preparations are less available than formerly, poisoning by strychnine still occurs from rodenticides and sugar-coated proprietary cathartic and tonic tablets. The majority of cases of accidental poisoning are in children, who may succumb to as little as 15 mg. The fatal adult oral dose is about 50 to 100 mg, but 30 mg has been lethal (Gleason *et al.,* 1969; Polson and Tattersall, 1969).

Symptoms of Strychnine Poisoning. The effects of strychnine in man closely resemble those described above for laboratory animals. The first effect that is noticed is stiffness of the face and neck muscles. Heightened reflex excitability soon becomes evident. Any sensory stimulus may produce a violent motor response. In the early stages this is a coordinated extensor thrust, and in the later stages it may be a full tetanic convulsion. In this convulsion, the body is arched in hyperextension (opisthotonos) so that only the crown of the head and the heels of the patient may be touching the ground. All voluntary muscles, including those of the face, are in full contraction. Respiration ceases due to the contraction of the diaphragm and the thoracic and abdominal muscles. Convulsive episodes may recur repeatedly with intermittent periods of depression; the frequency and severity of the convulsions are increased by sensory stimulation. Death results from medullary paralysis, which is due primarily to the hypoxia resulting from the periods of impaired respiration. In the early stages the patient not only is conscious but also is acutely perceptive to all stimuli. The muscle contractions are quite painful, and the patient is extremely apprehensive and fearful of impending death as he awaits the next tetanic spasm. If untreated, death from strychnine often occurs after the second to fifth full convulsion, but the first may be fatal if sustained.

Treatment of Strychnine Poisoning. The most urgent objectives in the treatment of strychnine poisoning are the prevention of convulsions and the support of respiration. CNS depressants antagonize the effect of strychnine so that effective respiration is possible even if heightened reflex activity is still present.

Although short-acting barbiturates have long been the mainstay for combating strychnine convulsions, limited clinical experience indicates that *diazepam* is superior to the barbiturates and should be considered the drug of choice. Prompt and continuous control of convulsions by diazepam with little accompanying sedation affords distinct advantages over the more depressant barbiturates (Hardin and Griggs, 1971; Jackson *et al.,* 1971; Maron *et al.,* 1971; Herishanu and Landau, 1972). Nearly anesthetic levels of barbiturates may be required for adequate control of convulsions, thereby augmenting existing respiratory depression due to postictal depression or medullary hypoxia. However, CNS depression from effective doses of diazepam is minimal. Antagonism of strychnine convulsions by diazepam probably resides largely in its selective anticonvulsant and centrally acting muscle relaxant properties.

In adults, convulsions may be terminated by 10 mg of diazepam, intravenously, which should be repeated as subsequent prodromal symptoms arise. Children may require smaller doses. All forms of sensory stimulation should be minimized. If adequate respiratory ventilation is not restored by the termination of convulsions, intubation and mechanical assistance are essential.

Gastric lavage may be performed if there is a possibility that some strychnine has remained in the stomach, but only after convulsions are controlled. Potassium permanganate is an effective chemical antidote and may be used for gastric lavage in a 1:5000 concentration. Iodine tincture diluted with water (1:250), tannic acid solution (2.0%, or in the form of strong tea), or activated charcoal may also be employed.

Therapeutic Uses. Strychnine has an undeserved reputation as a useful therapeutic agent. To the drug have been ascribed properties that it does not possess or that it exhibits only when administered in toxic doses. Nevertheless, strychnine has a background of long usage and it continues to enjoy unwarranted popularity. Strychnine is sometimes employed as a *tonic.* This "tonic" effect is supposedly comprised of three aspects of strychnine action: the bitter taste, stimulation of the gastrointestinal tract, and an increase in tone of voluntary muscle. As a bitter, strychnine is in no way unique. The remaining two actions are not manifested by therapeutic doses. There is no rational basis for the use of strychnine in therapy and, consequently, no justification for the presence of strychnine in any proprietary medication. There are no official strychnine preparations.

PICROTOXIN

Picrotoxin is obtained from *Anamirta cocculus,* a climbing shrub indigenous to Malabar and the East Indies. The drug is present in the seeds of the plant, commonly known as fishberries, a name derived from the practice of throwing the bruised berries upon the water as a means of catching fish. The fish, after devouring the berries, are incapacitated and rise to the surface.

Chemistry. Picrotoxin is a nonnitrogenous neutral principle, having the empirical formula $C_{30}H_{34}O_{13}$. It can be broken down into two dilactones: *picrotoxinin* ($C_{15}H_{16}O_6$) and *picrotin* ($C_{15}H_{18}O_7$). Picrotin is inactive. Picrotoxinin, the active component, has the following structural formula:

Picrotoxinin

Pharmacological Actions. Picrotoxin is a powerful stimulant and affects all portions of the CNS. Larger doses of picrotoxin are required to produce convulsions in a spinal animal than in an intact animal; in this respect picrotoxin differs strikingly from strychnine.

No appreciable effect of picrotoxin is seen until convulsive doses are given. The resultant convulsion is clonic and incoordinated, and the pattern resembles that produced by pentylenetetrazol (*see* below). With large doses of picrotoxin a tonic-clonic seizure may occur in which tonic flexion precedes tonic extension. Accompanying the convulsive movements are salivation, elevation of blood pressure due to vasomotor stimulation, and frequently emesis. Respiratory stimulation with picrotoxin is quite evident, but only in doses approaching convulsant levels.

Mechanism of Action. In mammals it has been shown that picrotoxin blocks *presynaptic* inhibition and strychnine-resistant *postsynaptic* inhibition in the CNS. Picrotoxin has been known for some time to antagonize the inhibitory transmitter gamma-aminobutyric acid (GABA) in invertebrates. Subsequently such antagonism has been convincingly demonstrated at many sites in the mammalian CNS. The nearly identical effects of GABA and natural inhibition and the selective antagonism of both by picrotoxin have made GABA a leading candidate as a central inhibitory transmitter, especially in higher centers. Another convulsant and selective GABA antagonist, *bicuculline,* has also contributed to this possibility. The relative importance of blockade of presynaptic or postsynaptic inhibition for the convulsant activity of picrotoxin is unknown. (*See* review by Obata, 1972; and Chapter 21.)

Absorption, Fate, and Excretion. Although picrotoxin is absorbed by all routes, the full effect on the CNS is not seen for several minutes even when the drug is administered intravenously. Its distribution in the body is unknown. Picrotoxin is probably destroyed quite readily, and this accounts for its relatively brief duration of action.

Toxicology. Picrotoxin is a highly toxic substance, and a dose of 20 mg may produce symptoms of severe poisoning. The fatal dose for man is unknown. A barbiturate is an effective antidote for poisoning by picrotoxin, and the procedure outlined for the treatment of strychnine poisoning, except for the use of chemical antidotes, applies also to picrotoxin. The use of diazepam has not been reported.

Preparations. *Picrotoxin* is a microcrystalline, odorless powder, stable in air but affected by light. It is also available in a sterile isotonic saline solution. The concentration of marketed preparations is 3 mg/ml.

Therapeutic Uses. Formerly employed in the treatment of poisoning by CNS depressants, picrotoxin is no longer regarded as a useful therapeutic agent. However, it remains an important laboratory tool for studying inhibition in the CNS.

PENTYLENETETRAZOL

Pentylenetetrazol (pentamethylenetetrazol) is a synthetic compound with the following structural formula:

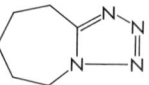

Pentylenetetrazol

Pharmacological Actions. Pentylenetetrazol has been widely studied in man and experimental animals. The actions of the drug are exerted primarily on the CNS. All levels of the cerebrospinal axis are stimulated by the drug; however, the dose required to produce convulsive movements in an animal with the spinal cord transected is several times that needed in the intact animal.

Pentylenetetrazol is a useful laboratory tool for screening anticonvulsant drugs. In experimental animals, threshold convulsive doses of the drug produce motor activity characterized by forelimb and jaw clonus. This convulsion resembles that produced by electrical stimulation of the brain with current of just threshold intensity. With slightly larger doses of pentylenetetrazol, generalized, asynchronized clonic movements are observed. This phase is usually superseded by a tonic convulsion; such a convulsion resembles that produced by supramaximal brain stimulation in that the movements of the limbs consist of flexion followed by extension. Thus, the pentylenetetrazol convulsion contrasts markedly with that produced by strychnine (*see* above), which is characterized by extension only.

Mechanism of Action. Pentylenetetrazol does not block either presynaptic or postsynaptic inhibition. Studies of the drug on single spinal motoneurons and interneurons have thus far failed to reveal the mechanism of its stimulant action (*see* Esplin and Zablocka-Esplin, 1969). There is evidence that the excitatory effect of pentylenetetrazol may be due to a decrease in neuronal recovery time. Eyzaguirre and Lilienthal (1949) observed that the relative refractory period of nerve tested *in vivo* was shortened by large doses of pentylenetetrazol and that a single stimulus produced repetitive discharge. Lewin and Esplin (1961) demonstrated that pentylenetetrazol decreased the time for recovery in the monosynaptic pathway of the spinal cord. It is of interest in this regard that pentylenetetrazol and trimethadione exhibit markedly antagonistic actions, both in the whole animal and in simple neuronal systems; the prominent action of trimethadione on spinal synaptic systems is prolongation of the time required for synaptic recovery (Esplin and Curto, 1957).

In a novel approach toward elucidating its mechanism of action, Gross and Woodbury (1972) found that pentylenetetrazol increased the permeability of toad bladder to potassium ions; this effect was antagonized by trimethadione in the same dose ratio that protects against pentylenetetrazol-induced convulsions in animals. The relative potencies of a series of related structural analogs on toad bladder bore a strong correlation to their convulsant potencies. Similar permeability changes in the CNS could raise extraneuronal potassium, which would partially depolarize neuronal membranes and thereby increase their excitability. Such a mechanism may account for the convulsive activity of pentylenetetrazol.

Absorption, Fate, and Excretion. Pentylenetetrazol is readily absorbed from all sites of administration. Following absorption, the drug is rapidly and equally distributed throughout the tissues. Pentylenetetrazol is largely and quite rapidly inactivated in the body, and the liver appears to be the primary or sole organ responsible. Studies with radioactive pentylenetetrazol (Esplin and Woodbury, 1956; Rowles *et al.,* 1971) have shown that 75% of the injected radioactive material is excreted in the urine. The excretory products have not been identified, but they are presumed to be inactive inasmuch as nephrectomy does not prolong the biological activity of pentylenetetrazol.

Preparations. *Pentylenetetrazol* (METRAZOL, NIORIC) occurs as white crystals that are freely soluble in water. Available marketed preparations include oral tablets (0.1 g), a sterile 10% solution in 1-ml ampuls and 30-ml vials, and an elixir (100 mg/5 ml).

Therapeutic Uses. As a diagnostic aid in *epilepsy,* pentylenetetrazol finds a valid use as an EEG activator. For this purpose, the drug is injected intravenously while EEG records are being taken. Subconvulsive doses of the drug, alone or together with flashing light, will often activate latent epileptogenic foci. In addition, the pentylenetetrazol-induced convulsions are of value in characterizing the underlying cerebral disorders in patients with proven epilepsy (Ajmone-Marsan and Ralston, 1957).

At one time pentylenetetrazol was employed as a convulsant drug in the so-called *shock treatment* of certain mental diseases. Flurothyl is probably superior for this purpose (*see* below). This method of treating mental disorders, aside from electroconvulsive therapy (ECT) when indicated, has declined in popularity with the increasing number of psychopharmacological agents available (*see* Chapter 12).

Pentylenetetrazol has received trial in the management of regressed geriatric patients. Despite 2 decades of use and many clinical trials, opinion on its beneficial effects in such patients is still divided (*see* Stotsky *et al.,* 1972).

Pentylenetetrazol is no longer used as a respiratory stimulant.

Bemegride. *Bemegride* (MEGIMIDE), a glutarimide derivative, resembles pentylenetetrazol in many of its actions. It has also been used for EEG activation but does not appear to have advantages over pentylenetetrazol. It is available in ampuls that contain 5 mg/ml.

DOXAPRAM, ETHAMIVAN, AND NIKETHAMIDE

These agents are nonspecific analeptics capable of producing widespread stimulation of the CNS. Their use as stimulants for depressed respiration is predicated on a dubious ability to stimulate central respiratory centers selectively without affecting other motor centers in the CNS. While this is admittedly a worthwhile therapeutic goal in several clinical situations, no agent with such selectivity is currently available; indeed, the complexity of central integration may exclude specific stimulation of discrete functional areas by drugs. Nevertheless, laboratory and clinical demonstrations of limited selective effects on respiration by doxapram, ethamivan, and nikethamide have led to their use as respiratory stimulants. Their chemical structures are as follows:

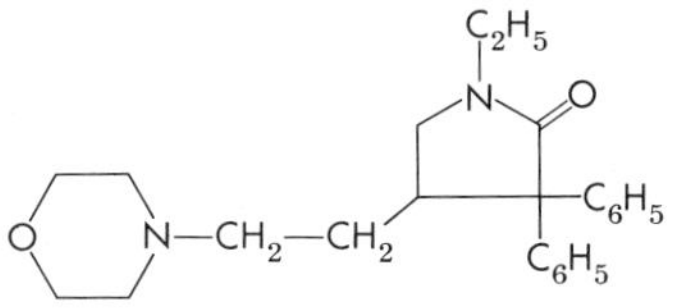

Doxapram

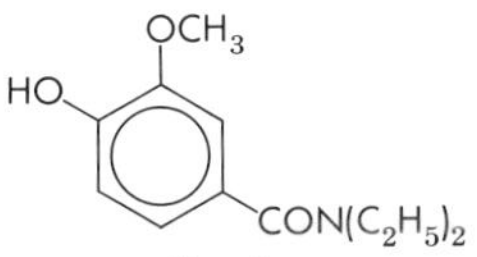

Ethamivan

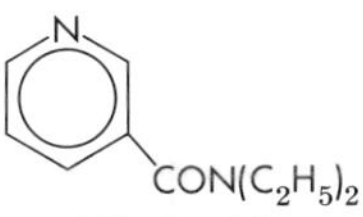

Nikethamide

Pharmacological Actions. Doxapram, ethamivan, and nikethamide stimulate all levels of the cerebrospinal axis. Adequate doses produce tonic-clonic convulsions similar in pattern to those produced by pentylenetetrazol. They presumably act by enhancing excitation rather than by blocking central inhibition.

Respiration can be stimulated by each of the three agents in doses that produce little generalized excitation. Direct medullary stimulation is largely responsible for this effect, but indirect stimulation by activation of peripheral chemoreceptors may also contribute. The duration of stimulation is transient after a single intravenous dose and seldom lasts for more than 5 or 10 minutes. Since it is doubtful that the drugs are metabolized so rapidly, the brief duration of action may reflect a "bolus effect" on respiratory centers with subsequent redistribution to other areas. This may in part account for more widespread stimulation after repeated doses, since the convulsant dose is generally not much larger than the respiratory stimulant dose. Limited clinical experience indicates that the margin of safety is greater for doxapram than for ethamivan and nikethamide (Wolfson et al., 1965; Edwards and Leszczynski, 1967). However, side effects indicative of subconvulsive CNS stimulation are common with all three: hypertension, tachycardia, arrhythmias, coughing, sneezing, vomiting, itching, tremors, muscle rigidity, sweating, flushing, and hyperpyrexia. Where needed most, in deeply comatose patients, analeptics are virtually ineffective in doses below those producing convulsions; postictal depression following convulsions further intensifies the coma (see Mark, 1967).

Preparations and Dosage. *Doxapram Hydrochloride,* N.F. (DOPRAM), is supplied for injection in 20-ml vials containing 20 mg/ml. Single or divided intravenous doses in the range of 0.5 to 1.5 mg/kg are employed to produce the desired effect. The drug may also be given by intravenous infusion at an initial rate of 5 mg per minute, later reduced 50% or more.

Ethamivan, N.F. (EMIVAN), is available for intravenous injection (*Ethamivan Injection,* N.F.) in 2- and 10-ml ampuls containing 50 mg/ml. The intravenous dose is 0.5 to 2.0 mg/kg, given slowly as a single injection. Intravenous infusion at a rate of 0.05 to 0.15 mg/kg per minute is also employed.

Nikethamide (CORAMINE, NIKORIN) is available in 25% aqueous solution, marketed in bulk for oral use and in 1.5-ml sterile ampuls for parenteral administration. Intravenous or intramuscular doses range from 1 to 15 ml of the 25% parenteral solution.

Therapeutic Uses and Status. Successful treatment of *acute sedative-hypnotic intoxication* emphasizes an orderly regimen of supportive therapy *without* the use of respiratory stimulants (Clemmesen and Nilsson, 1961; see Chapter 9). Systematic improvements in physiological support during 3 decades have reduced mortality rates from 25% during the height of analeptic therapy to a present rate of less than 1%. Mechanical assistance to depressed respiration is established as being far safer, more reliable, and more effective than erratic stimulation by drugs. Present opinion is unanimous in the condemnation

of analeptics for the management of poisoning from any sedative-hypnotic drug (Mark, 1967; Lawson and Proudfoot, 1971; Picchioni, 1971).

Doxapram, ethamivan, and nikethamide have been used as temporary measures to correct acute respiratory insufficiency in patients with *chronic obstructive pulmonary disease.* Intermittent or continuous infusion is necessary for sustained respiratory stimulation and reduction in carbon dioxide tension; however, potential improvement in oxygen tension is offset by a disproportionate increase in oxygen consumption. Typical side effects are common. Consequently, the value of analeptics in the therapy of pulmonary disease is very limited (Bader and Bader, 1965; Bickerman and Chusid, 1970). They may be of some short-term value to alleviate respiratory depression induced by oxygen therapy in these patients (Woolf, 1970; Moser et al., 1973). Recommended oral doses of analeptics are ineffective.

Analeptics have been advocated to hasten *recovery from anesthesia* by stimulating respiration and contributing to the postoperative "stir-up" regimen. However, there is no evidence to indicate a reduction in postanesthetic complications by routine use of central stimulants. The brief respiratory stimulation obtained after intravenous injection is usually not accompanied by improved oxygenation. Many clinicians prefer manual or mechanical methods of ventilatory assistance when necessary. Furthermore, potential nonspecific side effects of central stimulation may complicate recovery (Wolfson et al., 1965; Mark, 1967). An analeptic may assist in determining whether postanesthetic apnea is the result of respiratory depression or residual muscular paralysis; however, this can be more safely assessed by the use of a peripheral nerve stimulator. If an analeptic is elected, doxapram probably has some advantage in margin of safety. Untoward cardiovascular effects of doxapram may be accentuated in patients receiving sympathomimetic drugs or monoamine oxidase inhibitors.

FLUROTHYL

Flurothyl (hexafluorodiethyl ether) is *bis*(2,2,2-trifluoroethyl) ether. Krantz and coworkers (1957) showed that this volatile agent produced clonic and tonic convulsions in laboratory animals when the vapor was inhaled or when the liquid was administered systemically. Flurothyl is rapidly eliminated by the lungs, and the convulsions produced by a single exposure to the drug are brief.

Preparations and Dosage. *Flurothyl,* N.F. (INDOKLON), is supplied in ampuls containing 2 ml of the pure liquid. It is administered by inhalation from a vaporizer. The smallest amount needed to induce a convulsion, usually 0.5 to 1 ml, is employed. Convulsions usually occur within 40 seconds.

Therapeutic Uses and Status. Flurothyl is employed as a convulsive agent for the therapy of mental disorders. Trials of the drug for this use have not indicated serious untoward reactions provided premedication and other precautions appropriate to convulsive therapy are observed. No consistent pathological lesions were noted in dogs or rats subjected to repeated convulsions with flurothyl. Comparisons of flurothyl convulsions with ECT indicate that the two procedures are similar in safety, efficacy, and side effects (*see* Report of the Council, 1966; Laurell, 1970). However, ECT is still employed much more frequently.

METHYLPHENIDATE

Methylphenidate is a piperidine derivative that is structurally related to amphetamine and has the following formula:

Methylphenidate

Pharmacological Actions. In contrast to the other drugs discussed in this chapter, methylphenidate is a mild CNS stimulant with more prominent effects on mental than on motor activities. However, large doses produce signs of generalized CNS stimulation that may lead to convulsions in man and animals. Its pharmacological properties are essentially the same as those of the amphetamines. Methylphenidate also shares the abuse potential of the amphetamines.

Preparations and Dosage. *Methylphenidate Hydrochloride,* U.S.P. (RITALIN), is available as official tablets that contain 5, 10, or 20 mg of drug. The usual adult dose is 10 mg, given two or three times daily. The dosage recommended for hyperkinetic children is initially 0.25 mg/kg daily (Millichap, 1968). This dose is doubled each week, if untoward effects are not observed, until the optimal daily dosage of 2 mg/kg is reached. The drug is given in equal portions before breakfast and lunch.

Therapeutic Uses and Status. Methylphenidate has received extensive trial in various types of depression, in the treatment of overdosage from depressant drugs, and in relieving lassitude from various causes. Its effectiveness for these uses is not well established.

Methylphenidate is an important adjunct in the therapy of *hyperkinetic syndromes* in children characterized as having *minimal brain dysfunction* (MBD). Millichap (1968, 1973) has concluded that methylphenidate is superior to amphetamine and is the drug of choice in such children. Double-blind studies with placebo control (*see* Knights and

Hinton, 1969) have clearly demonstrated that methylphenidate can improve both behavior and learning ability in 50 to 75% of these children. However, indiscriminate use of stimulant drugs for "problem" children and sole dependence on drug therapy for MBD should be discouraged (*see* Erenberg, 1972; Sroufe and Stewart, 1973). Reports of growth suppression (Safer *et al.,* 1972) and increases in heart rate (Knights and Hinton, 1969) by methylphenidate, especially at high dose levels, further emphasize the advisability of judicious therapy. Acute episodes of hallucinosis early in therapy with methylphenidate may represent idiosyncratic reactions (Lucas and Weiss, 1971). It is generally assumed but unproved that the basic mechanism of action of methylphenidate in patients with MBD is the same as that of amphetamine.

Methylphenidate is effective in the treatment of *narcolepsy,* either alone or in combination with a tricyclic antidepressant (Zarcone, 1973).

Adamson, R. H., and Fouts, J. R. Enzymatic metabolism of strychnine. *J. Pharmac. exp. Ther.,* **1959,** *127,* 87–91.

Bader, M. E., and Bader, R. A. Respiratory stimulants in obstructive lung disease. *Am. J. Med.,* **1965,** *38,* 165–171.

Bickerman, H. A., and Chusid, E. L. The case against the use of respiratory stimulants. *Chest,* **1970,** *58,* 53–56.

Bradley, K.; Easton, D. M.; and Eccles, J. C. An investigation of primary or direct inhibition. *J. Physiol., Lond.,* **1953,** *122,* 474–488.

Clemmesen, C., and Nilsson, E. Therapeutic trends in the treatment of barbiturate poisoning—the Scandinavian method. *Clin. Pharmac. Ther.,* **1961,** *2,* 220–229.

Edwards, G., and Leszczynski, S. O. A double-blind trial of five respiratory stimulants in patients in acute ventilatory failure. *Lancet,* **1967,** *2,* 226–229.

Erenberg, G. Drug therapy in minimal brain dysfunction: a commentary. *J. Pediat.,* **1972,** *81,* 359–365.

Esplin, D. W., and Curto, E. M. Effects of trimethadione on synaptic transmission in the spinal cord; antagonism of trimethadione and pentylenetetrazol. *J. Pharmac. exp. Ther.,* **1957,** *121,* 457–467.

Esplin, D. W., and Woodbury, D. M. The fate and excretion of C^{14}-labeled pentylenetetrazol in the rat, with comments on analytical methods for pentylenetetrazol. *J. Pharmac. exp. Ther.,* **1956,** *118,* 129–138.

———. Spinal reflexes and seizure patterns in the two-toed sloth. *Science, Wash.,* **1961,** *133,* 1426–1427.

Eyzaguirre, C., and Lilienthal, J. L., Jr. Veratrinic effects of pentamethylenetetrazol (METRAZOL) and 2,2-bis(*p*-chlorophenyl) 1,1,1 trichloroethane (DDT) on mammalian neuromuscular function. *Proc. Soc. exp. Biol. Med.,* **1949,** *70,* 272–275.

Gleason, M. N.; Gosselin, R. E.; Hodge, H. C.; and Smith, R. P. *Clinical Toxicology of Commercial Products,* 3rd ed., Sect. III. The Williams & Wilkins Co., Baltimore, **1969,** pp. 214–217.

Gross, G. J., and Woodbury, D. M. Effects of pentylenetetrazol on ion transport in the isolated toad bladder. *J. Pharmac. exp. Ther.,* **1972,** *181,* 257–272.

Hardin, J. A., and Griggs, R. C. Diazepam treatment in a case of strychnine poisoning. *Lancet,* **1971,** *2,* 372–373.

Herishanu, Y., and Landau, H. Diazepam in the treatment of strychnine poisoning. *Br. J. Anaesth.,* **1972,** *44,* 747–748.

Jackson, G.; Ng, S. H.; Diggle, G. E.; and Bourke, I. G. Strychnine poisoning treated successfully with diazepam. *Br. med. J.,* **1971,** *3,* 519–520.

Knights, R. M., and Hinton, G. S. The effects of methylphenidate (RITALIN) on the motor skills and behaviour of children with learning problems. *J. nerv. ment. Dis.,* **1969,** *148,* 643–653.

Krantz, J. C., Jr.; Truitt, E. B., Jr.; Ling, A. S. C.; and Speers, L. Anesthesia. IV. The pharmacological response to hexafluorodiethyl ether. *J. Pharmac. exp. Ther.,* **1957,** *121,* 362–368.

Kuno, M., and Weakly, J. N. Quantal components of the inhibitory synaptic potential in spinal motoneurones of the cat. *J. Physiol., Lond.,* **1972,** *224,* 287–303.

Lawson, A. A. H., and Proudfoot, A. T. Medical management of acute barbiturate poisoning. In, *Acute Barbiturate Poisoning.* (Matthew, H., ed.) Excerpta Medica, Amsterdam, **1971,** pp. 175–193.

Lewin, J., and Esplin, D. W. Analysis of the spinal excitatory action of pentylenetetrazol. *J. Pharmac. exp. Ther.,* **1961,** *132,* 245–250.

Lucas, A. R., and Weiss, M. Methylphenidate hallucinosis. *J. Am. med. Ass.,* **1971,** *217,* 1079–1081.

Mark, L. C. Analeptics: changing concepts, declining status. *Am. J. med. Sci.,* **1967,** *254,* 296–302.

Maron, B. J.; Krupp, J. R.; and Tune, B. Strychnine poisoning successfully treated with diazepam. *J. Pediat.,* **1971,** *78,* 697–699.

Millichap, J. G. Drugs in management of hyperkinetic and perceptually handicapped children. *J. Am. med. Ass.,* **1968,** *206,* 1527–1530.

———. Drugs in management of minimal brain dysfunction. *Ann. N.Y. Acad. Sci.,* **1973,** *205,* 321–334.

Moser, K. M.; Luchsinger, P. C.; Adamson, J. S.; McMahon, S. L.; Schlueter, D. P.; Spivack, M.; and Weg, J. G. Respiratory stimulation with intravenous doxapram in respiratory failure. *New Engl. J. Med.,* **1973,** *288,* 427–431.

Picchioni, A. L. Clinical status and toxicology of analeptic drugs. *Am. J. hosp. Pharm.,* **1971,** *28,* 201–203.

Polson, C. J., and Tattersall, R. N. *Clinical Toxicology.* J. B. Lippincott Co., Philadelphia, **1969,** pp. 558–568.

Report of the Council. A convulsant agent for psychiatric use: flurothyl (INDOKLON). *J. Am. med. Ass.,* **1966,** *196,* 29–30.

Rowles, S. G.; Born, G. S.; Russell, H. T.; Kessler, W. V.; and Christian, J. E. Biological disposition of pentylenetetrazol-10-^{14}C in rats and humans. *J. pharm. Sci.,* **1971,** *60,* 725–727.

Safer, D.; Allen, R.; and Barr, E. Depression of growth in hyperactive children on stimulant drugs. *New Engl. J. Med.,* **1972,** *287,* 217–220.

Sroufe, L. A., and Stewart, M. A. Treating problem children with stimulant drugs. *New Engl. J. Med.,* **1973,** *289,* 407–413.

Stotsky, B. A.; Cole, J. O.; Lu, L.-M.; and Sniffin, C. M. A controlled study of the efficacy of pentylenetetrazol (METRAZOL) with hard-core hospitalized psychogeriatric patients. *Am. J. Psychiat.,* **1972,** *129,* 387–391.

Wolfson, B.; Siker, E. S.; and Ciccarelli, H. E. A double blind comparison of doxapram, ethamivan and methylphenidate. *Am. J. med. Sci.,* **1965,** *249,* 391–398.

Woolf, C. R. The use of "respiratory stimulant" drugs. *Chest,* **1970,** *58,* 49–53.

Zarcone, V. Narcolepsy. *New Engl. J. Med.,* **1973,** *288,* 1156–1166.

Monographs and Reviews

Ajmone-Marsan, C., and Ralston, B. L. *The Epileptic Seizure: Its Functional Morphology and Diagnostic Significance.* Charles C Thomas, Pub., Springfield, Ill., **1957.**

Curtis, D. R. The pharmacology of postsynaptic inhibition. *Prog. Brain Res.,* **1969,** *31,* 171–189.

Esplin, D. W., and Zablocka-Esplin, B. Mechanisms of action of convulsants. In, *Basic Mechanisms of the Epilepsies.* (Jasper, H. H.; Ward, A. A., Jr.; and Pope, A.; eds.) Little, Brown & Co., Boston, **1969,** pp. 167–183. (67 references.)

Hahn, F. Analeptics. *Pharmac. Rev.,* **1960,** *12,* 447–530. (724 references.)

Laurell, B. Flurothyl convulsive therapy. *Acta psychiat. neurol. scand.,* **1970,** Suppl. 213, 1–79.

Obata, K. The inhibitory action of γ-aminobutyric acid, a probable synaptic transmitter. *Int. Rev. Neurobiol.,* **1972,** *15,* 167–187.

19 CENTRAL NERVOUS SYSTEM STIMULANTS

[*Continued*]

The Xanthines

J. Murdoch Ritchie

CAFFEINE, THEOPHYLLINE, AND THEOBROMINE

Source and History. Caffeine, theophylline, and theobromine are three closely related alkaloids that occur in plants widely distributed throughout the world. From earliest times, man has made beverages from aqueous extracts of these plants. *Coffee,* the seeds of *Coffea arabica* and related species, contains caffeine. *Tea,* the leaves of *Thea sinensis,* contains caffeine and theophylline. *Cocoa,* obtained from the seeds of *Theobroma cacao,* contains caffeine and theobromine. *Maté,* the national drink of many South American countries, contains caffeine. Even some so-called soft drinks, particularly the cola-flavored drinks popular in the United States, contain caffeine because they are made from the nuts of the tree, *Cola acuminata.* These kola nuts, the guru nuts chewed by the natives of the Sudan, contain about 2% caffeine.

The earliest history of these drinks is lost in considerable obscurity, the absence of fact being compensated by a profusion of conjectural statements and mythical stories. For example, legend credits the discovery of coffee to a prior of an Arabian convent. Shepherds reported that goats that had eaten the berries of the coffee plant gamboled and frisked about all through the night instead of sleeping. The prior, mindful of the long nights of prayer that he had to endure, instructed the shepherds to pick the berries so that he might make a beverage from them. The success of his experiment is obvious from the fierce opposition stirred up by the more orthodox section of the priests against the use of this devotional antisoporific, and from the popularity of coffee today. More than a billion kilograms are consumed annually in the United States alone.

Modern pharmacological studies of caffeine have amply confirmed the ancient belief that caffeine has a stimulant action, which is the basis for the popularity of all the caffeine-containing beverages. Caffeine and related compounds, however, possess other important pharmacological properties and are valuable therapeutic agents.

Chemistry. Caffeine, theophylline, and theobromine are methylated xanthines. They are often spoken of as *xanthine derivatives, methylxanthines,* or merely *xanthines.* Xanthine itself is dioxypurine and is structurally related to uric acid. Caffeine is

1,3,7-trimethylxanthine; theophylline, 1,3-dimethylxanthine; and theobromine, 3,7-dimethylxanthine. The structural formulas of purine, uric acid, xanthine, and the three pharmacologically important xanthine derivatives are as follows:

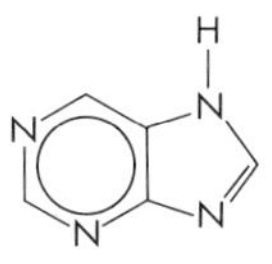

Purine 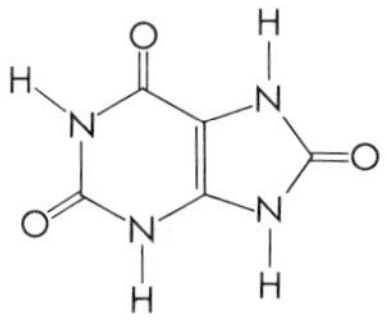   Uric Acid

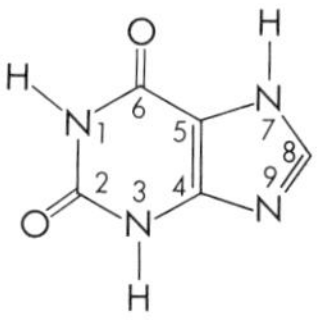

Xanthine 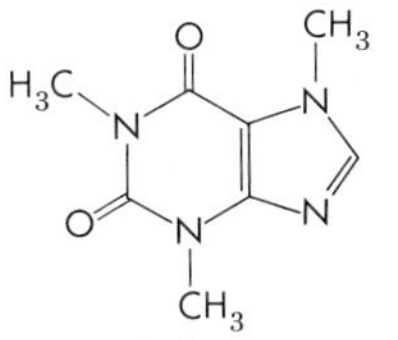   Caffeine

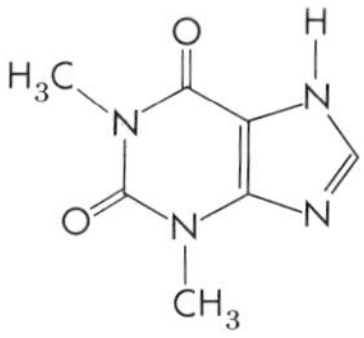

Theophylline 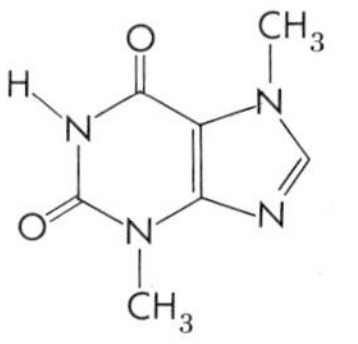   Theobromine

Studies of the actions of congeners of the methylxanthines have revealed structure-activity relationships of a complex nature (Scott *et al.,* 1946; Quimby *et al.,* 1958; Armitage *et al.,* 1961). Inhibition of cyclic nucleotide phosphodiesterase, a well-known action of the methylxanthines, is associated with small nonpolar substitutions at positions 1 and 3. 1-Methyl,3-isobutyl xanthine is particularly potent in this regard (Beavo *et al.,* 1970). Although these investigations are of theoretical interest and experimental value, the synthetic compounds have not yet been shown to offer any therapeutic advantage over naturally occurring xanthines.

The solubility of the methylxanthines is low and is much enhanced by the formation of complexes (usually 1:1) with a wide variety of compounds (Higuchi and Zuck, 1953). These include, in addition to those discussed below, barbiturates, local anesthetics, salicylates, and sulfonamides (Higuchi and Lach, 1954).

PHARMACOLOGICAL PROPERTIES

Caffeine, theophylline, and theobromine share in common several pharmacological actions of therapeutic interest. They stimulate the central nervous system (CNS), act on the kidney to produce diuresis, stimulate cardiac muscle, and relax smooth muscle, notably bronchial muscle. Because the various xanthines differ markedly in the intensity of their actions on various structures, one particular xanthine is usually more suitable than another for any specific therapeutic effect and has fewer side actions. Table 19–1 depicts the relative potencies of the xanthines in producing various effects.

Central Nervous System. Caffeine is a powerful CNS stimulant; theophylline is less so; and theobromine is virtually inactive in this respect. Thus, caffeine is the xanthine usually employed clinically for its central action, although theophylline also has specific uses as a respiratory stimulant. Caffeine excites the CNS at all levels. The cortex is first affected and then the medulla, while the cord is stimulated only by very large amounts.

Cortex. Caffeine stimulates all portions of the cortex. Its main action is to produce a more rapid and clearer flow of thought, and to allay drowsiness and fatigue. After taking caffeine one is capable of a greater sustained intellectual effort and a more perfect association of ideas. There is also a keener appreciation of sensory stimuli, and reaction time is appreciably diminished. This accounts for the hyperesthesia, sometimes unpleasant, which some persons experience after drinking too much coffee. In addition, motor activity is increased; typists, for example, work faster and with fewer errors. However, re-

cently acquired motor skill in a task involving delicate muscular coordination and accurate timing may not be improved (Goldstein *et al.*, 1965) or may even be adversely affected. These effects may be brought on by the administration of 150 to 250 mg of caffeine, the amount contained in 1 or 2 cups of coffee or tea.

Medulla. Caffeine also stimulates the medullary respiratory, vasomotor, and vagal centers. This stimulant action may be of some therapeutic value when the medulla is depressed by barbiturates and other drugs. High blood concentrations of caffeine are required. For example, a dose of caffeine of 150 to 250 mg taken orally produces little change in respiration; however, the same amount administered parenterally definitely stimulates the respiratory center by sensitizing it to CO_2 (Richmond, 1949) or by lowering its threshold to CO_2 (Dowell, 1965). Parenterally administered theophylline also increases the rate and the depth of respiration, even in normal individuals. The stimulation of the vasomotor and vagal centers by xanthines can best be demonstrated in medullary perfusion experiments, because after systemic administration the peripheral effects of the drug on the circulation tend to mask the central actions (*see* below).

Cord. After the administration of large amounts of caffeine or theophylline, the entire CNS, including the spinal cord, is stimulated. Reflex excitability is increased, and lower motor centers may be directly excited. In experimental animals this may lead to clonic convulsions and death. However, in man the toxic dose of caffeine is so large (over 10 g) that human fatality is unlikely.

There is no doubt that the excitation of the CNS produced by large amounts of caffeine is followed by depression. There has been considerable controversy, however, as to whether this is also true after the mild

Table 19–1. RELATIVE PHARMACOLOGICAL ACTIVITY OF THE XANTHINES

XANTHINE	CNS AND RESPIRATORY STIMULATION	CARDIAC STIMULATION	CORONARY DILATATION	SMOOTH MUSCLE RELAXATION	SKELETAL MUSCLE STIMULATION	DIURESIS
Caffeine	1 *	3	3	3	1	3
Theophylline	2	1	1	1	2	1
Theobromine	3	2	2	2	3	2

* 1 = most active.

physiological stimulation produced by the small amounts contained in the average cup of tea or coffee.

Cardiovascular System. The xanthines, especially theophylline, have important, clinically useful actions on the circulatory system. Even caffeine, which is the least active in this respect, has a powerful effect on the circulation, but its side effects on the CNS preclude its clinical use for cardiovascular effects.

All parts of the circulatory system are affected in some way by the xanthines. In several instances these various actions are antagonistic. Therefore, the observation of a single function, for example, the blood pressure, is deceiving because the drugs may act on a variety of circulatory factors in such a way that the blood pressure may remain essentially unchanged.

Heart. The xanthines stimulate the myocardium directly. When they are added to the perfusion fluid of an isolated mammalian heart, the force of contraction, the rate, and the cardiac output increase; in experimental animals, this inotropic effect is accompanied by an increase in duration of the action potential of atrial muscle (Gubareff and Sleator, 1965).

In papillary muscle, both the rate of development of tension and the time to attain peak tension are increased (Marcus *et al.,* 1972); in contrast, the catecholamines decrease the time required to reach peak tension. When the xanthines are given to an intact animal, however, some of these effects may be masked because these agents, especially caffeine, stimulate the medullary vagal nuclei and thus tend to produce a decrease in heart rate. Consequently, as a result of these two opposing actions, there may be a slight bradycardia, a tachycardia, or no change at all in heart rate. After large doses of caffeine in both man and experimental animals, the direct stimulation of the myocardium predominates and a definite tachycardia ensues. Eventually this stimulation may become so great that it causes cardiac irregularities. Occasionally, arrhythmias are encountered in persons who use caffeine beverages to excess.

The direct myocardial action of the xanthines, particularly theophylline, causes an increase in cardiac output, which may occur even in the absence of tachycardia. There is an accompanying decrease in the venous filling pressure, which is caused at least partly by the more complete emptying of the heart. In normal individuals the lowering of filling pressure may outlast the stimulation of the myocardium, so that the rise in cardiac output is brief and may be followed by a fall below the initial level. In heart failure, however, the venous pressure is initially rather high; consequently the cardiac stimulation, together with the lowering of venous pressure produced by theophylline, leads to a marked increase in cardiac output that occurs almost immediately and persists for 30 minutes or more after intravenous administration (Howarth *et al.,* 1947; Fowell *et al.,* 1949). Thus, theophylline is a valuable drug in the emergency treatment of congestive heart failure.

The xanthines can markedly potentiate the cardiac inotropic responses to β-adrenergic agonists (Rall and West, 1963) and to glucagon (Marcus *et al.,* 1971). This supraadditive interaction is presumably explained by the effects of these drugs on the metabolism of cyclic adenosine $3',5'$-monophosphate (cyclic AMP) (*see* below).

The methylxanthines can also stimulate release of catecholamines from the adrenal medulla (Peach, 1972; Poisner, 1973), and large increases in the urinary excretion of epinephrine occur following the intravenous infusion of a therapeutic dose of aminophylline in man (Atuk *et al.,* 1967). Similar release of norepinephrine apparently occurs from the adrenergic nerve endings of the isolated heart and contributes to the inotropic effects of the xanthines *in vitro* (Westfall and Fleming, 1968).

Blood Vessels. Caffeine dilates the coronary, pulmonary, and general systemic blood vessels by a direct action on the vascular musculature. Caffeine also tends to constrict blood vessels by stimulating the medullary vasomotor center. After therapeutic doses, the peripheral vasodilator action predominates. Oncometric studies in animals show that there is a definite increase in organ volume following the administration of xanthines. Vasodilatation, coupled with an augmented cardiac output, results in an increased blood flow. However, in man the increase in peripheral blood flow is short lived (Stewart and Jack, 1940) and is not of sufficient magnitude and duration to be of value in the treatment of peripheral vascular disease.

Cerebral Circulation. In contrast to their direct dilating effect upon the systemic blood vessels, the xanthines cause a marked increase in cerebral vascular resistance with an accompanying decrease in cerebral blood flow and in the oxygen tension of the brain (Wechsler *et al.,* 1950; Moyer *et al.,* 1952a, 1952b). The xanthines probably act directly on the musculature of the cerebral arterioles. It is this vasoconstriction, rather than the decrease in cerebrospinal fluid pressure that may also occur, that is believed to be responsible for the striking relief of hypertensive headache by the xanthines.

Coronary Circulation. Experimentally, it can be demonstrated that the xanthines dilate coronary arteries and increase coronary blood flow. This has led to their use in the treatment of coronary artery disease. However, opinion as to their value is divided and the evidence in this field is controversial. There seems to be general agreement in the studies on man that under certain conditions the xanthines increase coronary blood flow. There is also abundant evidence that the drugs increase the work of the heart. The outstanding question is whether the blood supply to the myocardium increases to a greater extent than does the oxygen demand. Regardless of controversial claims and disappointing clinical results, the xanthines continue to be employed by some physicians in the treatment of coronary insufficiency. (*See* Charlier, 1961; Modell, 1972.)

Blood Pressure. From the previous discussion it is obvious that the effect of xanthines on the systemic blood pressure is unpredictable. Both the central vasomotor and the direct myocardial stimulation favor an increase in blood pressure. Conversely, the central vagal stimulation and the peripheral vasodilatation favor a decrease. The end result of the opposing actions on blood pressure is not striking; usually there is a slight rise, seldom amounting to more than 10 mm Hg. The combination of vasodilatation and enhanced cardiac output raises the pulse pressure, produces a more rapid blood flow, and leads to a more efficient circulation. In

man the pulmonary arterial pressure is usually reduced (Parker *et al.,* 1966; Ježek *et al.,* 1970).

Smooth Muscle. The xanthines also act on smooth muscles other than those of blood vessels. Their most important action in this respect is their ability to relax the smooth muscles of the *bronchi,* especially if the bronchi have been constricted either experimentally by histamine or clinically in asthma. Theophylline is the most effective and produces a definite increase in vital capacity. It is, therefore, of value in the treatment of bronchial asthma.

The xanthines may also overcome spasm of the biliary tract produced in man by the injection of morphine or other opioids. Theophylline-containing compounds, in particular, have therefore been employed in the treatment of biliary colic.

The action of the xanthines on the motor activity of the *gastrointestinal tract* is unimportant therapeutically. Dilute solutions increase, and high concentrations depress, the tone and strength of contraction of isolated intestinal strips. The intravenous injection of aminophylline in man causes a transient suppression of motility in the large and small bowel.

Skeletal Muscle. Xanthines strengthen the contraction of isolated skeletal muscle elicited by either direct or indirect electrical stimulation and render the muscle less susceptible to fatigue (Huidobro, 1945; Goffart and Ritchie, 1952). The facilitation of neuromuscular transmission may be due to increased release of acetylcholine (Wilson, 1973); additional mechanisms are discussed below.

The xanthines, particularly caffeine, increase capacity for muscular work; theobromine is the least effective. Because the increase in work performance is produced only by doses of caffeine that also cause subjective symptoms of central stimulation (Foltz *et al.,* 1942), it has been argued that the central effects of the xanthines account for the increased capacity for muscular work. Until evidence is produced to the contrary, however, the peripheral effects cannot be discounted.

Diuretic Actions. Xanthines increase the production of urine. Theophylline is the most powerful xanthine diuretic, but its action is of short duration. Theobromine is less active, but its effect is more sustained. Caffeine is the least powerful. A more detailed analysis of the diuretic action is given in Chapter 39.

Gastric Secretion. In man, moderate doses of caffeine result in a prolonged augmentation of gastric secretion (Roth and Ivy, 1944a). The combined action of caffeine and histamine is greater than the sum of their individual actions with respect to the secretion of both acid and pepsin (Grossman et al., 1945). Moreover, a number of investigators have shown that the administration of caffeine to animals in large single doses, in smaller repeated daily doses, or by intramuscular injection in beeswax results in pathological changes in the gastrointestinal tract and ulcer formation (see Merendino et al., 1945). The significance of experimental peptic ulcers produced in this way has been questioned because of the high doses used. However, in view of the responsiveness of the human gastric mucosa to caffeine, cognizance must be taken of the ubiquitous use of coffee and cola beverages in the pathogenesis of peptic ulcer and in the management of the ulcer patient (Roth et al., 1944; Roth and Ivy, 1944b).

The secretory response evoked by caffeine shows characteristic patterns in normal individuals, and in patients with gastric or duodenal ulcers. Moreover, the distinction is greater than that obtainable with an alcohol test meal. There is also evidence that individuals with a predisposition toward peptic ulcers, or patients with peptic ulcers who are in remission, exhibit an abnormal response. These considerations led Roth and coworkers to suggest that the use of a caffeine test meal may be of diagnostic and prognostic value (see Littman et al., 1955).

Blood Clotting. It has been known since 1920 that, following the administration of aminophylline to man, the coagulation time of the blood is shortened. The methylxanthines can also antagonize the effects of the hypoprothrombinemia caused by coumarin derivatives and can prevent the clotting defect associated with hepatic injury. The main action seems to result from an increase in the concentration of factor V (Ac-globulin) in the plasma (see Chapter 65), which, in turn, may be caused by an increase in the plasma concentration of free fatty acids produced by the xanthines (Bellet et al., 1968); this action indirectly causes any circulating prothrombin to be more effective; there are also increases in the concentrations of circulating prothrombin and fibrinogen. Clinical studies in man, however, have failed to show that *therapeutic* doses of xanthines have a measurable effect on the coagulation time of the blood.

Metabolism. The xanthines, especially caffeine, cause a slight increase in the basal metabolic rate, which can be observed in habitual coffee drinkers. Numerous investigators have reported that the ingestion of 0.5 g of caffeine may increase the basal metabolic rate by an average of 10% and occasionally 25%. The maximal change occurs from 1 to 3 hours after the administration of the drug. During the early phase, the medullary stimulation increases the respiratory minute volume and results in an excessive elimination of carbon dioxide. This produces a rise in respiratory quotient that is later followed by a compensatory fall (Haldi et al., 1941).

Caffeine has certain actions on processes of intermediary metabolism. For example, it depresses the formation of urea from ammonium salts both in liver slices *in vitro* and in experimental animals. It also promotes creatinuria in man. In sufficient concentration, the xanthines can mimic the metabolic effects of the catecholamines. These include stimulation of lipolysis, glycogenolysis, and gluconeogenesis.

Tolerance. Some degree of tolerance may develop to certain effects of the xanthines, especially the diuretic and the salivary-stimulating actions and the disturbance of sleep (Colton et al., 1968). Cross-tolerance between the members of the group also occurs. Little or no tolerance develops to the central stimulation. Habituation is discussed under caffeine beverages.

Cellular Basis for the Action of the Xanthines. Two types of effects of the methylxanthines have received major attention in studies of their mechanism of action: those mediated by cyclic nucleotides and those associated with intracellular translocations of calcium. Of interest at present is the question of whether both types of effect have a common basis. Sutherland and associates have revealed a biochemical mechanism that may underlie certain of the metabolic and physiological effects of methylxanthines. Having first established the critical role of cyclic AMP in promoting glycogenolysis in certain tissues (*see* Chapter 21), they showed that the methylxanthines, particularly theophylline, are competitive inhibitors of at least certain forms of cyclic nucleotide phosphodiesterase, the enzymes that catalyze the conversion of cyclic AMP to 5′-AMP (Butcher and Sutherland, 1962). Cyclic AMP concentrations are thus elevated in some tissues following exposure to methylxanthines. The catecholamines (and several other hormones and neurohumors) also increase the concentration of cyclic AMP in many tissues, but by the different mechanism of stimulation of cyclic AMP synthesis (*see* Chapter 24). Thus, both the methylxanthines and the catecholamines would be expected to have those particular pharmacological properties that are thought to depend on their common ability to increase the cyclic AMP concentration in the tissues. By virtue of their differing sites of action, these effects of methylxanthines could be expected to result in a potentiation of, rather than simple addition with, those effects of catecholamines that are due to production of increased concentrations of cyclic AMP. For example, this may account for the fact that the xanthines markedly potentiate the cardiac inotropic responses to the catecholamines. It should be noted that the effects of xanthines alone on cyclic AMP concentrations may be minimal in the absence of a stimulation of cyclic AMP synthesis, since the basal rate of cyclic AMP formation may be low.

The methylxanthines have other rather opposite effects on cyclic AMP metabolism in special situations. Adenosine appears to act as a hormone-like stimulator of cyclic AMP synthesis at certain sites, particularly in the brain (Sattin and Rall, 1970). Theophylline and other xanthines *inhibit* this stimulatory effect of adenosine and may act as competitive antagonists at a specialized adenosine receptor. It is unknown if xanthine-induced increases or decreases of cyclic AMP concentration offer any explanation for the effects of these compounds on the CNS.

The current literature is replete with studies on the interactions between numerous hormones that stimulate cyclic AMP synthesis and methylxanthines, with interpretations of the data centering primarily around the possible involvement of the cyclic nucle-

otide (*see* Robison *et al.*, 1971). While the methylxanthines have been of considerable value in the study of cyclic AMP action, other effects of these compounds have been demonstrated and must be borne in mind.

Complementary studies, particularly on skeletal muscle, have emphasized the involvement of *calcium* in the pharmacological action of caffeine. When isolated frog sartorius muscle is exposed to increasing concentrations of caffeine in the bathing fluid, a series of successive electrical and mechanical effects is recorded that can be related to changes in the distribution of calcium at various intracellular sites. At 0.5 to 1 mM caffeine, the twitch response to stimulation of the motor nerve is increased in rapidity of onset, height, and duration; the predominant site of action probably involves the coupling step between the spread of the muscle action potential and the release of Ca^{2+} to the myoplasm thereby induced. Contraction is initiated by combination of free myoplasmic Ca^{2+} with the troponin protein of the thin filaments; this inactivates an inhibitory influence and allows combination of the actin of the thin filaments with the myosin of the thick filaments, which in turn initiates contraction. Caffeine at this concentration probably sensitizes the Ca^{2+} release mechanism of the terminal cisternae of the sarcoplasmic reticulum. At intermediate concentrations (1 to 5 mM) caffeine also produces reversible contracture, which at concentrations above 5 mM becomes irreversible (*i.e.*, rigor). These effects are probably due to an increase in Ca^{2+} permeability of the membranes of the sarcoplasmic reticulum, which normally terminates the contractile process by active uptake and sequestration of Ca^{2+}, as well as the membranes of the mitochondrial Ca^{2+} storage sites and the muscle fiber. The net result is the persistence of the myoplasmic free-Ca^{2+} level above 0.1 μM, the threshold for contraction. (See reviews by Bianchi, 1968, 1975.) The effects of methylxanthines on contraction and Ca^{2+} distribution in cardiac muscle resemble in general those obtained with skeletal muscle (Blinks *et al.*, 1972).

Of particular interest is the demonstration that the clinical condition of *malignant hyperthermia*, which is induced in certain genetically determined patients by various general anesthetics, can be mimicked *in vitro* by exposure of caffeine-treated frog muscle to halothane. Both conditions are characterized by contracture, which is probably due to impairment of the uptake of Ca^{2+} by the sarcoplasmic reticulum. Contracture in the model system is reversed effectively by procainamide but not by lidocaine (Strobel and Bianchi, 1971).

The precise relationship between the xanthines, calcium, and cyclic AMP is thus complex, particularly since both calcium and cyclic AMP are rather ubiquitous regulators of cellular functions and often interact to share a role in the modulation of certain functions (*see* Rasmussen, 1970). Further complexities are in sight, since calcium and xanthines can both influence the metabolism of another cyclic nucleotide, cyclic guanosine 3′,5′-monophosphate (cyclic GMP). Certain of the actions of cyclic GMP may be opposite in direction to those of cyclic AMP. It is thus difficult to assign the pharmacological effects of the xanthines to one mechanistic class or another. The ability to potentiate effects of catecholamines and other hormones is perhaps more readily interpreted in terms of cyclic AMP, as may be the effects on smooth muscle. Effects on skeletal muscle and neuromuscular transmission and stimulation of catecholamine secretion from the adrenal medulla may relate more to calcium mobilization. The effects on the heart are particularly difficult, and multiple actions of the xanthines are apparent. Potentiation of catecholamines by inhibition of cyclic AMP catabolism, direct effects of calcium on the contractile apparatus, and release of catecholamines may all be involved.

Toxicology. A fatal dose of caffeine given to an animal produces convulsions because of the central stimulating effect. Early in the poisoning, these are epileptiform in nature; as the action of the drug on the spinal cord becomes manifest, strychnine-like convulsions may appear. Death results from respiratory failure.

In man the fatal oral dose of caffeine is estimated to be about 10 g, but death from overdosage is highly unlikely. Untoward reactions, however, may be observed following the ingestion of 1 g or more of caffeine. These are mainly referable to the central nervous and circulatory systems. Insomnia, restlessness, and excitement are the early symptoms, which may progress to mild delirium. Sensory disturbances such as ringing in the ears and flashes of light are common. The muscles become tense and tremulous. Tachycardia and extrasystoles are frequent, and respiration is quickened. The diuretic action may be prominent. The central symptoms of caffeine poisoning can be readily controlled by the administration of depressants of the CNS; the short-acting barbiturates are effective and convenient for this purpose.

Theophylline, on the other hand, can be quite toxic and has occasionally proved fatal. Aminophylline (theophylline ethylenediamine) must be injected slowly when given by the intravenous route; otherwise, headache, palpitation, dizziness, nausea, fall in blood pressure, and even precordial pain may occur. The wisdom of injecting xanthines intravenously in patients with severe myocardial damage has been questioned. However, the incidence of untoward responses appears to be very low provided adequate care is taken. The intramuscular injection of aminophylline is accompanied by local pain that may persist for many hours.

Toxic effects may occur whatever the route of administration. For example, studies on children have shown that the same set of symptoms occurs during severe intoxication with aminophylline, whether the drug is given by the oral, rectal, or intravenous route. It is characterized by frequent vomiting, unusual thirst, and maniacal agitation leading in the severest cases to convulsions, shock, and death (Bacal *et al.,* 1959).

Mutagenic Effects. Caffeine induces chromosomal breakage in the fruit fly, higher plants, and a variety of microorganisms. It has similar effects in man (Ostertag *et al.,* 1965). However, these effects are obtained only with concentrations of caffeine much in excess of those used therapeutically or resulting from drinking tea or coffee (Thayer *et al.,* 1971; Thayer and Kensler, 1973). The latter observations, in fact, indicate that caffeine does not increase the mutation rate much above the small natural rate, and so does not seem to present any significant toxic hazard in man.

Relation to Myocardial Infarction. The lack of convincing evidence for a beneficial effect of the methylxanthines in the treatment of coronary insufficiency has already been discussed. Much interest has recently developed concerning a possible deleterious effect of these agents, particularly caffeine, in the etiology of acute myocardial infarction. Jick and coworkers (1973) reported that individuals drinking more than 5 to 6 cups of coffee per day are about twice as liable to suffer myocardial infarction. However, in an equally careful study Klatsky and associates (1973) found no independent association between coffee drinking and a subsequent first myocardial infarction; they suggest that the discrepancy in the findings of the two groups may be related to factors such as cigarette smoking or the selection of control subjects.

Absorption, Fate, and Excretion. The xanthines are readily absorbed after oral, rectal, or parenteral administration. The rate at which they are absorbed depends on the xanthine preparation used and on the route of administration (*see* Lillehei, 1968). The oral route is the most convenient, but absorption of the simple alkaloids from the gastrointestinal tract may be erratic, perhaps because of their poor aqueous solubility (about 2% for caffeine, 1% for theophylline, and less than 0.1% for theobromine). Furthermore, oral administration may give rise to gastric irritation, nausea, and vomiting. These considerations have led to the xanthines, especially theophylline, being given by rectal suppository or retention enema (*see* Ridolfo and Kohlstaedt, 1959); absorption, however, may still be slow and erratic. Another approach has been to use xanthine compounds that are both more soluble and less irritating. True salts (*e.g.,* choline theophyllinate) or one of the double salts that the xanthines form with a number of compounds (*e.g.,* caffeine and sodium benzoate) are employed. The most widely used theophylline compound is aminophylline, which is a combination of theophylline with ethylenediamine. The ethylenediamine seems to be therapeutically inert, but its presence is important because it increases the amount of theophylline in solution about 20-fold.

The effect of the xanthines is greatest and most rapid when these complex salts are administered intravenously. Great care, however, must be exercised when they are administered by this route, especially in patients with severe myocardial damage, for high local concentrations may result in the precipitation of free alkaloids when salts are exposed to the pH of the blood. This may be responsible for the sharp, usually transient, fall in blood pressure that often occurs when injection is too rapid.

In the body the xanthines are only partially demethylated and oxidized. They are largely excreted as methyluric acids or as methylxanthines. Cornish and Christman (1957) found that in man theophylline is converted mainly to 1,3-dimethyluric acid, theobromine is excreted largely as both 3- and 7-methylxanthines, and caffeine is excreted as 1-methyluric acid and 1-methylxanthine in relatively equal amounts. About 10% of the alkaloids is excreted unchanged. Because none of the xanthines is completely demethylated, there is no increase in the excretion of uric acid. Therefore, the xanthines are not contraindicated in gout.

The enzymes responsible for the metabolic degradation of the methylated xanthines are not known, but xanthine oxidase is not involved. The half-time for disappearance of theophylline from plasma is approximately 4 hours following intravenous administration (Mitenko and Ogilvie, 1973a).

Preparations. The xanthines are weakly basic alkaloids. They are usually dispensed in the form of soluble double salts that they form with a number of compounds. For oral administration either the free base or one of the double salts may be used; for parenteral administration, however, it is necessary to employ one of the salts.

Caffeine, U.S.P., is a white crystalline, glistening substance soluble in water to the extent of 1:50.

Caffeine and Sodium Benzoate Injection, U.S.P., and *citrated caffeine* are white, rather bitter, water-soluble compounds. The former is the preparation of choice for hypodermic administration and is available in ampuls containing 500 mg/2 ml of solution for intramuscular injection. Citrated caffeine is available as tablets in 60-mg size for oral use.

Theophylline, U.S.P., is a white crystalline, bitter powder that is only slightly soluble in water (1%). *Theophylline Tablets,* N.F., are available for oral use. ELIXOPHYLLIN is a preparation containing free theophylline dissolved in 20% ethanol. Oral doses are claimed to be rapidly absorbed and to produce little gastric irritation. Theophylline is also available as the loose complexes and double salts described below, the percentage of anhydrous theophylline by weight being indicated in parentheses after each heading.

Aminophylline, U.S.P. (*theophylline ethylenediamine*) (85%), is the most widely used of the soluble theophylline salts. It occurs as white or slightly yellowish granules or powder with a slightly ammoniacal odor and a bitter taste; 1 g dissolves in about 5 ml of water. The following official (U.S.P.) preparations of aminophylline are available: solutions in ampuls that contain 250 mg/10 ml and 500 mg/20 ml, for intravenous administration; tablets in 100- and 200-mg sizes, for oral administration; rectal suppositories in 125-, 250-, and 500-mg sizes.

Theophylline Sodium Glycinate, N.F. (51%), a white crystalline powder freely soluble in water, is claimed to produce little gastric irritation. Tablets, ampuls, suppositories, and elixirs are available.

Oxtriphylline, N.F. (64%), also called *choline theophyllinate* and CHOLEDYL, differs from the preparations described above in that it is a true salt of theophylline in which the hydrogen atom at position 7 has been replaced by the choline cation. It is freely soluble in water to yield a solution of pH 9.7. Compared to aminophylline, it is more soluble, more stable, better absorbed from the gastrointestinal tract, and less irritating to the gastric mucosa. Tablets in 100- and 200-mg sizes and an elixir (100 mg/5 ml) are available.

Dyphylline, also called NEOTHYLLINE and LUFYLLIN, is 7-(2,3-dihydroxypropyl)theophylline. This neutral derivative of theophylline is stable in gastric juice. It produces less gastric irritation than most theophylline compounds. Tablets (200 mg), an elixir (100 mg/15 ml), and ampuls (500 mg/2 ml) are available.

Theobromine is available as the free alkaloid; the drug is also available as a variety of complexes containing roughly equimolecular proportions of theobromine and some other compound. These preparations are given only by the oral route. The approximate percentage by weight of theobromine is indicated after each heading below.

Theobromine calcium salicylate (48%) (THEOCAL-CIN) is a white odorless powder only slightly soluble in water, available as tablets (500 mg).

Theobromine sodium salicylate (56%), a freely soluble white powder, is available in 500-mg tablets.

THERAPEUTIC USES

The diverse pharmacological actions of the xanthines find many therapeutic applications. The drugs are of particular value for their effects on the *myocardium, smooth muscle, CNS,* and *kidney.* The preparations of caffeine are usually utilized only as central stimulants. Theophylline preparations, usually aminophylline, are used to relax bronchial smooth muscle and to stimulate the myocardium.

Cardiac Uses. The direct myocardial stimulation produced by the xanthines is of considerable value in treating acute episodes of congestive heart failure. Their chief usefulness is for the relief of paroxysmal dyspnea associated with left heart failure. In this condition the immediate effects on cardiac output, venous pressure, and the bronchial muscle combine to afford rapid relief of pulmonary edema and dyspnea. Sole reliance is not placed upon the xanthines, and their use is combined with other conventional procedures, such as phlebotomy or the application of tourniquets to reduce venous return, morphine therapy to relieve dyspnea, and administration of oxygen to relieve hypoxia. The preparation of choice is aminophylline, which is given in the dose of 0.5 g by slow intravenous or by intramuscular injection. If indicated, this may be followed by intravenous digitalization. The action of the aminophylline is rapid in onset and lasts until that of the cardiac glycoside begins.

The xanthines have been employed to reduce the frequency and severity of attacks of *angina pectoris.* However, the literature, as mentioned above, is highly controversial, and there is no proof of efficacy.

Bronchial Asthma. Theophylline compounds, particularly aminophylline, play an important role in the management of the asthmatic patient. They are useful as prophylactic drugs and are valuable adjuncts in the treatment of prolonged attacks and in the management of status asthmaticus.

Although adrenocorticosteroids may be necessary for the treatment of prolonged attacks of asthma, bronchodilator drugs occupy a dominant place in therapy. The successful treatment of status asthmaticus calls for a variety of measures, including the use of oxygen or oxygen-helium mixtures, sympathomimetic drugs, expectorants, sedatives, and bronchial aspiration (*see* Safar, 1969). One of the most effective bronchodilating agents is aminophylline. For treatment of intractable bronchial asthma, aminophylline is first given by slow intravenous injection in a dose of 0.5 g. A high percentage of patients experience almost immediate relief for a period of time. It is necessary, however, to continue therapy in order to prevent recurrence. For this purpose, aminophylline can be given rectally either as a suppository containing 0.5 g, or more effectively as a retention enema containing 0.5 to 0.7 g in 20 ml of tap water. Rectal instillations are given morning and night for at least a week. When this therapy is combined with appropriate ancillary measures, prolonged periods of remission can sometimes be achieved.

Studies on asthmatic subjects reveal that plasma concentrations of theophylline of 5 to 20 μg/ml are associated with therapeutic effects. Toxicity is particularly apparent at concentrations greater than 20 μg/ml. A loading dose of aminophylline of 5.6 mg/kg intravenously followed by 0.9 mg/kg per hour results in plasma concentrations of approximately 10 μg/ml (Mitenko and Ogilvie, 1973b; Nicholson and Chick, 1973).

Aminophylline or some other theophylline compound may be given over prolonged periods by mouth to reduce the number and severity of asthmatic attacks. The drug may be combined with ephedrine, which acts additively; a barbiturate may also be incorporated to counteract the combined central stimulant actions of the xanthine and the sympathomimetic. A single dose of 0.25 g of the theophylline compound is repeated three or four times daily.

The bronchodilating, respiratory-stimulating, and hemodynamic actions of aminophylline, or theophylline, are used in the treatment of a variety of other respiratory disorders, such as Cheyne-Stokes respiration, bronchitis, obstructive pulmonary disease, and emphysema (Dowell, 1965; Parker *et al.,* 1966; Ježek *et al.,* 1970; McIntosh, 1971).

Central Nervous System. The central action of the xanthines, particularly caffeine, is occasionally used in treating cases of poisoning by central depressants. The drug is given by intramuscular injection, usually as caffeine and sodium benzoate (0.5 to 1.0 g).

Kidney. The use of xanthines as diuretics is discussed in Chapter 39.

Miscellaneous Uses. The intravenous injection of aminophylline has been shown to be effective in relieving the pain of acute biliary colic. The dose is 0.25 to 0.5 g, given slowly by the intravenous route.

The xanthines are widely employed in the treatment of *headache.* When effective, they probably act as the result of a direct vasoconstrictor effect on cerebral blood vessels. Caffeine, the preparation most commonly used, is seldom employed alone;

rather, it is used in combination with an analgesic, such as a salicylate, in the treatment of ordinary types of headache, and in combination with an ergot alkaloid in the treatment of migraine. It is of interest that the withdrawal of caffeine from individuals habituated to it may also result in headaches. This "caffeine-withdrawal" headache can be relieved by the administration of caffeine. It is not unlikely that the incidence of this type of headache is high and provides a further explanation for the benefit obtained from the use of caffeine in analgesic mixtures.

XANTHINE BEVERAGES

The most popular xanthine beverages are coffee, tea, cocoa, and cola-flavored drinks. Coffee and tea contain caffeine, whereas cocoa contains theobromine. The caffeine content of tea leaves (about 2.0%) is higher than that of coffee beans (0.7 to 2.0%), but the beverages as finally prepared contain about equal amounts of the alkaloid. A 360-ml (12-oz) bottle of a cola drink contains 35 to 55 mg of caffeine. The average cup of coffee contains between 100 and 150 mg of caffeine, approximately a therapeutic dose. Naturally, the daily ingestion of even this amount of a potent alkaloid is bound to exert some pharmacological action. In addition to alkaloids, coffee contains certain oils, and there is an appreciable amount of tannin in tea.

There is little doubt that the popularity of the xanthine beverages depends on their stimulant action, although most people are unaware of any stimulation. The degree to which an individual is stimulated by a given amount of caffeine varies. For example, some persons boast of their ability to drink several cups of coffee in the evening and yet "sleep like a log." On the other hand, there are rare persons who are so sensitive to caffeine that even a single cup of coffee will cause a response bordering on the toxic. Decaffeinated coffee, containing only 1 to 6 mg caffeine per cup, may be an acceptable substitute.

The xanthine beverages present a medical problem in that they are a dietary source of a stimulant of the CNS. Often the physician is faced with the question whether to deny caffeine-containing beverages to patients. Children are more susceptible than adults to excitation by xanthines. For this reason, tea and coffee should be excluded from their diet. Even cocoa is of doubtful value. It has a high tannin content, and the theobromine content may be more than 200 mg per cup.

A patient with an active peptic ulcer should restrict his intake of caffeine-containing beverages. Even decaffeinated coffee stimulates gastric secretion to a limited extent because of other constituents of the bean. Individuals with peptic ulcer should consume their coffee (if at all) during meals, well diluted with cream because the buffering capacity of coffee is negligible.

Xanthine beverages are often denied to individuals with hypertension because of the action on the cardiovascular and nervous systems. Obviously, in a disease in which sedation may be an important factor, stimulation by a xanthine would not be desired. However, most authorities take the attitude that the complete denial of coffee to an individual who enjoys it is apt to be more disturbing than any stimulation he may receive from the beverage.

Overindulgence in xanthine beverages may lead to a condition that might be considered one of chronic poisoning. Central nervous stimulation results in restlessness and disturbed sleep; myocardial stimulation is reflected in premature systoles and tachycardia. The essential oils of coffee may cause some gastrointestinal irritation, and diarrhea is a common symptom. The high tannin content of tea, on the other hand, is apt to cause constipation.

There is no doubt that a certain degree of tolerance (Colton *et al.,* 1968) and of psychic dependence (*i.e.,* habituation) develops to the xanthine beverages. This is probably true even in those individuals who do not partake to excess. However, the morning cup of coffee is so much a part of American and European dietary habit that one seldom looks upon its consumption as a drug habit, and there is no evidence that the practice is in any way harmful. The feeling of well-being and the increased performance it affords, although possibly obtained at the expense of decreased efficiency later in the day, are experiences that few individuals would care to give up.

Armitage, A. K.; Boswood, J.; and Large, B. J. Structure/activity relations in a series of 6-thioxanthines with bronchodilator and coronary dilator properties. *Br. J. Pharmac. Chemother.,* **1961,** *17,* 196–207.

Atuk, N. O.; Blaydes, M. C.; Westervelt, F. B.; and Wood, J. E. Effect of aminophylline on urinary excretion of epinephrine and norepinephrine in man. *Circulation,* **1967,** *35,* 745–753.

Bacal, H. L.; Linegar, K.; Denton, R. L.; and Gourdeau, R. Aminophylline poisoning in children. *Can. med. Ass. J.,* **1959,** *80,* 6–9.

Beavo, J. A.; Rogers, N. L.; Crofford, O. B.; Hardman, J. G.; Sutherland, E. W.; and Newman, E. V. Effects of xanthine derivatives on lipolysis and on adenosine 3′,5′-monophosphate phosphodiesterase activity. *Molec. Pharmac.,* **1970,** *6,* 597–603.

Bellet, S.; Feinberg, L. J.; Sandberg, H.; and Hirabayashi, M. The effects of caffeine on free fatty acids and blood coagulation parameters of dogs. *J. Pharmac. exp. Ther.,* **1968,** *159,* 250–254.

Bianchi, C. P. Pharmacological actions on excitation-contraction coupling in striated muscle. *Fedn Proc. Fedn Am. Socs exp. Biol.,* **1968,** *27,* 126–131.

——. Cellular pharmacology of contraction of skeletal muscle. In, *Cellular Pharmacology of Excitable Tissues.* (Narahashi, T., ed.) Charles C Thomas, Pub., Springfield, Ill., **1975.**

Blinks, J. R.; Olson, C. B.; Jewell, B. R.; and Braveny, P. Influence of caffeine and other methylxanthines on mechanical properties of isolated mammalian heart muscle. Evidence for a dual mechanism of action. *Circulation Res.,* **1972,** *30,* 367–392.

Butcher, R. W., and Sutherland, E. W. Adenosine 3′,5′-phosphate in biological materials. *J. biol. Chem.,* **1962,** *237,* 1244–1250.

Charlier, R. *Coronary Vasodilators.* Pergamon Press, Ltd., Oxford, **1961.**

Colton, T.; Gosselin, R. E.; and Smith, R. P. The tolerance of coffee drinkers to caffeine. *Clin. Pharmac. Ther.,* **1968,** *9,* 31–39.

Cornish, H. H., and Christman, A. A. A study of the metabolism of theobromine, theophylline, and caffeine in man. *J. biol. Chem.,* **1957,** *228,* 315–323.

Dowell, A. R. Effect of aminophylline on respiratory center sensitivity in Cheyne-Stokes respiration and in pulmonary emphysema. *New Engl. J. Med.,* **1965,** *273,* 1447–1453.

Foltz, E.; Ivy, A. C.; and Barborka, C. J. The use of double work periods in the study of fatigue and the influence of caffeine on recovery. *Am. J. Physiol.,* **1942,** *136,* 79–86.

Fowell, D. M.; Winslow, J. A.; Sydenstricker, V. P.; and Wheeler, N. C. Circulatory and diuretic effects of theophylline isopropanolamine. *Archs intern. Med.,* **1949,** *83,* 150–157.

Goffart, M., and Ritchie, J. M. The effect of adrenaline on the contraction of mammalian skeletal muscle. *J. Physiol., Lond.,* **1952,** *116,* 357–371.

Goldstein, A.; Kaizer, S.; and Warren, R. Psychotropic effects of caffeine in man. II. Alertness, psychomotor coordination, and mood. *J. Pharmac. exp. Ther.,* **1965,** *150,* 146–151.

Grossman, M. I.; Roth, J. A.; and Ivy, A. C. Pepsin secretion in response to caffeine. *Gastroenterology,* **1945,** *4,* 251–256.

Gubareff, T. de, and Sleator, W., Jr. Effects of caffeine on mammalian atrial muscle, and its interaction with calcium. *J. Pharmac. exp. Ther.,* **1965,** *148,* 202–214.

Haldi, J.; Bachman, G.; Ensor, C.; and Wynn, W. The effect of various amounts of caffeine on the gaseous exchange and the respiratory quotient in man. *J. Nutr.,* **1941,** *21,* 307–320.

Higuchi, T., and Lach, J. L. Investigation of some complexes formed in solution by caffeine. IV. Interactions between caffeine, sulfathiazole, sulfadiazine, *p*-aminobenzoic acid, benzocaine, phenobarbital, and barbital. *J. Am. pharm. Ass., Sci. Ed.,* **1954,** *43,* 349–354.

Higuchi, T., and Zuck, D. A. Investigation of some complexes formed in solution by caffeine. II. Benzoic acid and benzoate ion. *J. Am. pharm. Ass., Sci. Ed.,* **1953,** *42,* 132–145.

Howarth, S.; McMichael, J.; and Sharpey-Schafer, E. P. The circulatory action of theophylline ethylene diamine. *Clin. Sci.,* **1947,** *6,* 125–135.

Huidobro, F. A comparative study of the effectiveness of 1,3,7 trimethylxanthine and certain dimethylxanthines (1,3 dimethylxanthine and 3,7 dimethylxanthine) against fatigue. *J. Pharmac. exp. Ther.,* **1945,** *84,* 380–386.

Ježek, V.; Ouředník, A.; Stěpánek, J.; and Boudík, F. The effect of aminophylline on the respiration and pulmonary circulation. *Clin. Sci.,* **1970,** *38,* 549–554.

Jick, J.; Miettinen, O. S.; Neff, R. K.; Shapiro, S.; Heinonen, O. P.; and Slone, D. Coffee and myocardial infarction. *New Engl. J. Med.,* **1973,** *289,* 63–67.

Klatsky, A. L.; Friedman, G. D.; and Siegelaub, A. B. Coffee drinking prior to acute myocardial infarction. Results from the Kaiser-Permanente epidemiologic study of myocardial infarction. *J. Am. med. Ass.,* **1973,** *226,* 540–543.

Lillehei, J. P. Aminophylline. Oral vs. rectal administration. *J. Am. med. Ass.,* **1968,** *205,* 530–533.

Littman, A.; Fox, B. W.; Kammerling, E. M.; and Fox, N. I. A single aspiration gastric analysis in duodenal ulcer and control patients. *Gastroenterology,* **1955,** *28,* 953–963.

McIntosh, D. A. Comparative assessment of choline theophyllinate and sustained-release theophylline in patients attending a chest clinic. *Br. J. clin. Pract.,* **1971,** *25,* 233–235.

Marcus, M. L.; Skelton, C. L.; Grauer, L. E.; and Epstein, S. E. Effects of theophylline on myocardial mechanics. *Am. J. Physiol.,* **1972,** *222,* 1361–1365.

Marcus, M. L.; Skelton, C. L.; Prindle, K. H., Jr.; and Epstein, S. E. Potentiation of the inotropic effects of glucagon by theophylline. *J. Pharmac. exp. Ther.,* **1971,** *179,* 331–337.

Merendino, K. A.; Judd, E. S.; Baronofsky, I.; Litow, S. S.;

Lannin, B. G.; and Wangensteen, O. H. Influence of caffeine on ulcer genesis. *Surgery, St. Louis,* **1945,** *17,* 650–666.

Mitenko, P. A., and Ogilvie, R. I. Pharmacokinetics of intravenous theophylline. *Clin. Pharmac. Ther.,* **1973a,** *14,* 509–513.

———. Rational intravenous doses of theophylline. *New Engl. J. Med.,* **1973b,** *289,* 600–603.

Modell, W. (ed.). *Drugs of Choice.* C. V. Mosby Co., St. Louis, **1972.**

Moyer, J. H.; Miller, S. I.; Tashnek, A. B.; and Bowman, R. The effect of theophylline with ethylenediamine (aminophylline) on cerebral hemodynamics in the presence of cardiac failure with and without Cheyne-Stokes respiration. *J. clin. Invest.,* **1952a,** *31,* 267–272.

Moyer, J. H.; Tashnek, A. B.; Miller, S. I.; Snyder, H.; and Bowman, R. O. The effect of theophylline with ethylenediamine (aminophylline) and caffeine on cerebral hemodynamics and cerebrospinal fluid pressure in patients with hypertension headaches. *Am. J. med. Sci.,* **1952b,** *224,* 377–385.

Nicholson, D. P., and Chick, T. W. A re-evaluation of parenteral aminophylline. *Am. Rev. resp. Dis.,* **1973,** *108,* 241–247.

Ostertag, W.; Duisberg, E.; and Stürmann, M. The mutagenic activity of caffeine in man. *Mutat. Res.,* **1965,** *2,* 293–296.

Parker, J. O.; Kelkar, K.; and West, O. R. Hemodynamic effects of aminophylline in cor pulmonale. *Circulation,* **1966,** *33,* 17–25.

Peach, M. J. Stimulation of release of adrenal catecholamine by adenosine 3′,5′-cyclic monophosphate and theophylline in the absence of extracellular Ca^{2+}. *Proc. natn. Acad. Sci. U.S.A.,* **1972,** *69,* 834–836.

Poisner, A. M. Direct stimulant effect of aminophylline on catecholamine release from the adrenal medulla. *Biochem. Pharmac.,* **1973,** *22,* 469–476.

Quimby, C. W.; Aviado, D. M.; and Schmidt, C. F. The effects of aminophylline and other xanthines on the pulmonary circulation. *J. Pharmac. exp. Ther.,* **1958,** *122,* 396–405.

Rall, T. W., and West, T. C. The potentiation of cardiac inotropic responses to norepinephrine by theophylline. *J. Pharmac. exp. Ther.,* **1963,** *139,* 269–274.

Rasmussen, H. Cell communication, calcium ion, and cyclic adenosine monophosphate. *Science, Wash.,* **1970,** *170,* 404–412.

Richmond, G. H. Action of caffeine and aminophylline as respiratory stimulants in man. *J. appl. Physiol.,* **1949,** *2,* 16–23.

Ridolfo, A. S., and Kohlstaedt, K. G. A simplified method for the rectal instillation of theophylline. *Am. J. med. Sci.,* **1959,** *237,* 585–589.

Robison, G. A.; Butcher, R. W.; and Sutherland, E. W. *Cyclic AMP.* Academic Press, Inc., New York, **1971.**

Roth, J. A., and Ivy, A. C. The effect of caffeine upon gastric secretion in the dog, cat and man. *Am. J. Physiol.,* **1944a,** *141,* 454–461.

———. The synergistic effect of caffeine upon histamine in relation to gastric secretion. *Ibid.,* **1944b,** *142,* 107–113.

Roth, J. A.; Ivy, A. C.; and Atkinson, A. J. Caffeine and "peptic" ulcer. *J. Am. med. Ass.,* **1944,** *126,* 814–820.

Safar, P. Recognition and management of airway obstruction. *J. Am. med. Ass.,* **1969,** *208,* 1008–1011.

Sattin, A., and Rall, T. W. The effect of adenosine and adenine nucleotides on the adenosine 3′,5′-phosphate content of guinea pig cerebral cortex slices. *Molec. Pharmac.,* **1970,** *6,* 13–23.

Scott, C. C.; Anderson, R. C.; and Chen, K. K. Further study of some 1-substituted theobromine compounds. *J. Pharmac. exp. Ther.,* **1946,** *86,* 113–119.

Stewart, H. J., and Jack, N. B. The effect of aminophyllin on peripheral blood flow. *Am. Heart J.,* **1940,** *20,* 205–222.

Strobel, G. E., and Bianchi, C. P. An *in vitro* model of anesthetic hypertonic hyperpyrexia, halothane-caffeine-induced muscle contractures: prevention of contracture by procainamide. *Anesthesiology,* **1971,** *35,* 465–473.

Thayer, P. S.; Himmelfarb, P.; Liss, R. H.; and Carlson, B. L. Continuous exposure of HeLa cells to caffeine. *Mutat. Res.,* **1971,** *12,* 197–203.

Thayer, P. S., and Kensler, C. J. Genetic tests in mice of caffeine alone and in combination with mutagens. *Toxic. appl. Pharmac.,* **1973,** *25,* 157–168.

Wechsler, R. L.; Kleiss, L. M.; and Kety, S. S. The effects of intravenously administered aminophylline on cerebral circulation and metabolism in man. *J. clin. Invest.,* **1950,** *29,* 28–30.

Westfall, D. P., and Fleming, W. W. Sensitivity changes in the dog heart to norepinephrine, calcium and aminophylline resulting from pretreatment with reserpine. *J. Pharmac. exp. Ther.,* **1968,** *159,* 98–106.

Wilson, D. F. Effects of caffeine on neuromuscular transmission in the rat. *Am. J. Physiol.,* **1973,** *225,* 862–865.

Local Anesthetics

20 COCAINE; PROCAINE AND OTHER SYNTHETIC LOCAL ANESTHETICS

J. Murdoch Ritchie and Peter J. Cohen

THE GENERAL PHARMACOLOGY OF THE LOCAL ANESTHETICS

Local anesthetics are drugs that block nerve conduction when applied locally to nerve tissue in appropriate concentrations. They act on any part of the nervous system and on every type of nerve fiber. For example, when they are applied to the motor cortex impulse transmission from that area stops, and when they are injected into the skin they prevent the initiation and the transmission of sensory impulses. A local anesthetic in contact with a nerve trunk can cause both sensory and motor paralysis in the area innervated. Many kinds of compounds interfere with conduction, but they often permanently damage the nerve cells. The great practical advantage of the local anesthetics is that their action is reversible; their use is followed by complete recovery in nerve function with no evidence of structural damage to nerve fibers or cells.

Since ionic mechanisms of excitability are similar in nerve and muscle, it is not surprising that these agents also can have prominent actions on all types of muscular tissue.

History. The first local anesthetic to be discovered was cocaine, an alkaloid contained in large amounts (0.6 to 1.8%) in the leaves of *Erythroxylon coca,* a shrub growing in the Andes Mountains 3000 to 9000 ft above sea level. Nearly 9 million kilograms of these leaves are consumed annually by about 2 million inhabitants of the highlands of Peru, who chew or suck the leaves for the sake of the cocaine; little or no coca is consumed at lower altitudes. For many centuries it has played an important role in the social and political life of these people because of the sense of well-being it produces.

The pure alkaloid was first isolated by Niemann, a pupil of Wöhler, who noted that it had a bitter taste and produced a peculiar effect on the tongue, making it numb and almost devoid of sensation. Von Anrep in 1880 studied its pharmacological actions and observed that the skin became insensitive to the prick of a pin when cocaine was infiltrated subcutaneously. He recommended that the alkaloid be used clinically as a local anesthetic. His suggestion, however, was not acted upon, and credit for the introduction of cocaine into clinical use as a local anesthetic is usually given to two young Viennese physicians, Sigmund Freud and Karl Koller. In 1884, Freud made a general study of the physiological effects of cocaine. He was particularly impressed by the central actions of the drug and used it to wean one of his colleagues from morphine. He was successful in this attempt, but at the cost of producing one of the first-known cocaine addicts of modern times. Koller quickly appreciated that the anesthetizing properties of cocaine had great practical importance and soon introduced cocaine into ophthalmology as a local anesthetic.

The acceptance of cocaine as a local anesthetic was immediate, and in this way the history of local anesthesia differs sharply from that of general anesthesia. Other investigators rapidly extended Koller's initial observation. Within a short time, Hall in 1884 introduced local anesthesia into dentistry, and the next year Halsted, by demonstrating that cocaine could stop transmission in nerve trunks, laid the foundation for nerve block anesthesia in surgery. Corning in 1885 produced spinal anesthesia in dogs, but several years passed before his technic was employed in clinical surgery.

A chemical search for synthetic substitutes for

cocaine started in 1892 with the work of Einhorn and his colleagues. This resulted in 1905 in the synthesis of procaine, which today is still widely employed. Chemical investigation still continues, however, because no available local anesthetic is free of undesirable properties. As a result, an unnecessarily large number of compounds are marketed for clinical use. Most of these differ little in therapeutic efficacy, and only a few have distinctive features to recommend their preferential use.

Properties Desirable in Local Anesthetics. A good local anesthetic should combine several properties. It should not be irritating to the tissue to which it is applied, nor should it cause any permanent damage to nerve structure; most local anesthetics in common use fulfill these requirements. Its systemic toxicity should be low because it is eventually absorbed from its site of application. Therefore, the therapeutic index is an important factor in evaluating the efficacy and safety of local anesthetic agents. Since this can vary greatly among local anesthetics, there is a constant search for new, more effective, and safer agents. The ideal local anesthetic must be effective regardless of whether it is injected into the tissue or whether it is applied locally to mucous membranes. It is usually important that the time required for the onset of anesthesia should be as short as possible. Furthermore, the action must last long enough to allow time for the contemplated surgery, yet not so long as to entail an extended period of recovery. There are many agents that satisfy this latter requirement. Occasionally, a local anesthetic action lasting for days or even weeks or months is desirable, for example, in the control of chronic pain. Unfortunately, the available compounds employed for anesthesia of such long duration have high local toxicity. Neurolysis with slough and necrosis of surrounding tissues occurs, and partial or complete transverse injury of the cord with permanent paralysis may result if such a reaction occurs in the vicinity of the spinal cord.

GENERAL PROPERTIES OF LOCAL ANESTHETIC DRUGS

The local anesthetics have many actions in common, and before discussing the pharmacology of the individual members these general properties will be considered.

Chemistry and Structure-Activity Relationship. Table 20–1 shows that all the useful local anesthetics consist of three parts. There is a hydrophilic amino group that is connected by an intermediate group to a lipophilic aromatic residue. The amino group is either a tertiary amine (*e.g.,* procaine) or a secondary amine (*e.g.,* hexylcaine). The link between the intermediate group and the aromatic residue is either an amide bond, as in lidocaine and dibucaine, or an ester linkage. The ester link is important because it is this bond that is hydrolyzed during metabolic degradation and inactivation in the body. Procaine is typical of local anesthetics with the esteratic link. The structure of procaine is shown at the top of Table 20–1. It is evident that the procaine molecule can be divided into three main portions: the aromatic acid (para-aminobenzoic), the alcohol (ethanol), and the tertiary amino group (diethylamino). Changes in any part of the molecule alter the anesthetic potency and the toxicity of the compound, a fact that provides the basis for the vast number of available local anesthetics. Increasing the length of the alcohol group leads to a greater anesthetic potency. It also leads to an increase in toxicity so that compounds with an ethyl ester, such as procaine, exhibit the least toxicity. The length of the two terminal groups on the tertiary amino nitrogen is similarly important. The structure-activity relationship and the physicochemical properties of local anesthetics have been reviewed by Büchi and Perlia (1971).

Mechanism of Action. Local anesthetics prevent both the generation and the conduction of the nerve impulse. Their main site of action is the cell membrane, and there is seemingly little direct action of physiological importance on the axoplasm. Those axoplasmic effects that do occur may be secondary to the membrane action. The work of Hodgkin, Huxley, and their colleagues has led to a better understanding of the nature of the nerve impulse, and it is now relatively easy to explain, at least partially, the action of local anesthetics within the framework of the ionic theory of nervous activity.

Local anesthetics and other classes of agents (*e.g.,* alcohols and barbiturates) block conduction by interfering with the process fundamental to the generation of the nerve action potential, namely, the large *transient* increase in the permeability of the membrane to sodium ions that is produced by a slight depolarization of the membrane (Taylor, 1959). As the anesthetic action progressively develops in a nerve, the threshold for electrical excitability gradually increases and the safety factor for conduction decreases; when this action is sufficiently well developed, block of conduction is produced.

Local anesthetics block conduction in nerve perhaps by competing with calcium at some site that controls the permeability of the membrane (Blaustein and Goldman, 1966; Strichartz, 1973). Calcium is also involved in the action of local anesthetics on smooth muscle (Feinstein, 1966) and on the adrenal medulla (*see* Jaanus *et al.,* 1967).

The local anesthetics also reduce the permeability of *resting* nerve to potassium as well as to sodium ions. This accounts for the

AROMATIC RESIDUE	INTERMEDI- ATE CHAIN	AMINO GROUP	AROMATIC RESIDUE	INTERMEDI- ATE CHAIN	AMINO GROUP
Procaine — H_2N—(ring)	$COOCH_2CH_2$—N	C_2H_5, C_2H_5	Lidocaine — (ring with CH_3, CH_3)	$NHCOCH_2$—N	C_2H_5, C_2H_5
Bupivacaine — (ring with CH_3, CH_3)	$NHCO$—	N C_4H_9 (piperidine)	Mepivacaine — (ring with CH_3, CH_3)	$NHCO$—	N CH_3 (piperidine)
Chloroprocaine — H_2N—(ring, Cl)	$COOCH_2CH_2$—N	C_2H_5, C_2H_5	Phenacaine — H_5C_2O—(ring)	$N{=}C(CH_3)$—N	H, (ring OC_2H_5)
Cocaine — (ring)	$COOCHCH_2CH$—N, CH_2CH_2—CH, $CH(COOCH_3)$	CH_3	Piperocaine — (ring)	$COOCH_2CH_2CH_2$—N	CH_3 (piperidine)
Cyclomethycaine — (cyclohexyloxy ring)	$COOCH_2CH_2CH_2$—N	CH_3 (piperidine)	Pramoxine — H_9C_4O—(ring)	$OCH_2CH_2CH_2$—N	(morpholine, O)
Dibucaine — (quinoline, OC_4H_9)	$CONHCH_2CH_2$—N	C_2H_5, C_2H_5	Prilocaine — (ring with CH_3)	$NHCOCH(CH_3)$—N	H, C_3H_7
Dimethisoquin — (isoquinoline, H_9C_4, N)	OCH_2CH_2—N	CH_3, CH_3	Proparacaine — H_2N—(ring), H_7C_3O—	$COOCH_2CH_2$—N	C_2H_5, C_2H_5
Dyclonine — H_9C_4O—(ring)	$COCH_2CH_2$—N	(piperidine)	Tetracaine — H_9C_4—N (H)—(ring)	$COOCH_2CH_2$—N	CH_3, CH_3
Hexylcaine — (ring)	$COOCH(CH_3)CH_2$—N	H, (cyclohexyl)			

381

observation that the block in conduction is not accompanied by any large or consistent change in the resting potential.

A small fall in potential or no change has been described. Straub (1956) has shown that it is the initial physiological state of the nerve fiber that determines whether a local anesthetic produces a rise, a fall, or no change in potential. For example, procaine produces a slight rise in potential in a normal nerve, a slight fall in a nerve in the catelectrotonic state, and no change in a nerve in the anelectrotonic state. This may be explained by the supposition that local anesthetics generally reduce the permeability of the resting nerve membrane to sodium, potassium, and other ions. A similar reduction in permeability also occurs in the membrane of skeletal muscle, both in the resting state (Shanes, 1950) and during the generation of an action potential (Inoue and Frank, 1962).

Quaternary analogs of local anesthetics block conduction when applied internally to perfused giant axons of squid, but they are relatively ineffective when applied externally. These observations, together with others on the effects of varying pH on the potency of related tertiary amines, led Narahashi and colleagues to conclude that the site at which local anesthetics act, at least in their charged form, is accessible only from the inner surface of the membrane (Narahashi and Frazier, 1971). Local anesthetics applied externally must therefore first cross the membrane, in the uncharged form, before they can exert a blocking action. Furthermore, Strichartz (1973) has shown that the binding of the charged form of the local anesthetic to the receptor is voltage dependent, in a way that suggests that the receptor is about halfway down the sodium channel.

The exact mechanism whereby a local anesthetic influences the permeability of the membrane is at present unknown, but it is interesting that the relative anesthetic potency of a series of compounds exactly parallels their effectiveness in increasing the surface pressure of monomolecular films of lipids (see Skou, 1961). On the basis of this work, Shanes (1958, 1963) suggested that local anesthetics achieve block by increasing the surface pressure of the lipid layer that constitutes the nerve membrane, thereby closing the pores through which ions move. This would cause a general decrease in the resting permeability and would also limit the increase in sodium permeability, the fundamental change necessary for the generation of the action potential. More recently, however, Metcalfe and Burgen (1968) have suggested that local anesthetics affect permeability by increasing the degree of disorder of the membrane (see Ritchie, 1971).

Differential Sensitivity of Nerve Fibers to Local Anesthetics. As a general rule, small nerve fibers are more susceptible to the action of local anesthetics than are large fibers. This was clearly established for the myelinated A fibers by Gasser and Erlanger

(1929), who showed that when cocaine is applied to a cutaneous nerve the gamma waves (from small cutaneous afferent fibers) are the first and the alpha waves (from large fibers) the last to disappear. The smallest mammalian nerve fibers are nonmyelinated and, on the whole, are blocked more readily than the myelinated fibers. However, the spectrum of sensitivity of the nonmyelinated fibers overlaps that of the myelinated fibers to some extent. Thus, Nathan and Sears (1961) have shown that some myelinated A delta fibers are blocked earlier, and with lower concentrations of anesthetic, than are most of the C fibers. The sensitivity to local anesthetics is not determined by fiber size alone, therefore, but also by the anatomical fiber type. This is not surprising in view of the great difference between the physiological mode of conduction in the myelinated fibers, in which conduction is saltatory, and that of the nonmyelinated fibers, in which it is continuous. Still other factors as yet unknown may determine the susceptibility of a fiber to a local anesthetic. For example, it is not known whether myelinated autonomic B fibers and myelinated A fibers of the same diameter differ in sensitivity. Although there is general agreement on the differential *rate* of blockade produced by local anesthetics in fibers of different sizes, there is some question whether a similar differential effect obtains after sufficient time has been allowed for full equilibration of the local anesthetic with the tissue. Indeed, Franz and Perry (1974) found that *absolute* differential blockade occurred only when the length of nerve exposed to the anesthetic was limited to a few millimeters.

The sensitivity of a fiber to local anesthetics does not seem to depend on whether it is sensory or motor, in spite of a widespread belief to the contrary. The misconception seems to have arisen in the following way. When a local anesthetic is applied to a muscle-nerve trunk, which contains both sensory and motor fibers, the contractions elicited reflexly, by jerking a tendon, for example, are blocked before those elicited by electrical stimulation of the nerve. This led to the belief that an appropriate concentration of anesthetic could block completely the sensory fibers without abolishing the conduction of impulses in motor fibers. In 1957, however, Matthews and Rushworth made the first direct comparison of the relative sensitivity of muscle proprioceptive afferent and muscle efferent fibers, both of which are of the same large diameter. These investigators found that the two types of fibers were *equally* sensitive. However, the smaller gamma *motor* fibers supplying the muscle spindles were much more rapidly blocked by the local anesthetic, and it is this preferential blockade of the smaller motor fibers, rather than the sensory fibers, that leads to the preferential loss of the muscle reflexes. Franz and Perry (1974) suggest that differential block cannot result from differences in minimal concentrations necessary to block axons of different diameters. Rather, it results from differences in the critical lengths of axons that must be exposed to the anesthetic, smaller axons having shorter critical lengths because of their smaller internodal distances. In the early stages of development of anesthetic action, small discrete lengths of the most accessible portions of the nerve trunk are the first to be exposed to the anesthetic as it diffuses inward along various intrafascicular routes. Smaller fibers with their shorter critical lengths are thus blocked more quickly by anesthetic solutions than are larger fibers; the same reasoning accounts for their slower recovery when the process is reversed.

The differential sensitivity exhibited by fibers of varying sizes to block is of great practical importance and may explain why there is a definite order in which the sensory functions of a nerve are affected by local anesthetics. Fortunately for the patient, the sensation of pain is usually the first modality to disappear, and it is followed in turn by the sensations of cold, warmth, touch, and deep pressure, although there is a great individual variation. Gasser and Erlanger (1929) were impressed by the fact that, when pressure was applied to a nerve, the resulting anesthesia appeared in a sequence roughly *opposite* to that observed after block by anesthetic drugs; that is, pain was the last sensation to disappear and touch the first. They suggested that touch is mediated by the largest sensory fibers in a nerve, pain by the smallest sensory fibers, and temperature by fibers of intermediate diameters. Although open to certain criticisms (Douglas and Ritchie, 1962), this suggestion has been extremely useful in the analysis of sensory function.

Effect of pH. The local anesthetics in the form of the unprotonated amine tend to be only slightly soluble and unstable in solution. Therefore, they are generally marketed in the form of their water-soluble salts, usually the hydrochlorides. Inasmuch as the local anesthetics are weak bases, these salt solutions are quite acid, a condition that fortunately increases the stability of the local anesthetic and any accompanying vasoconstrictor substance. There is abundant evidence to show that the acid salt must be neutralized in the tissues and the free amine liberated before the drug can penetrate the tissues and produce an anesthetic action.

Numerous investigations have shown that the addition of base to local anesthetic solutions enhances activity. This is especially true when anesthetics are applied to isolated nerve trunks or to the cornea, where the buffering capacity of the tissue fluids is limited. It has been predicted, therefore, that previous alkalinization of an anesthetic solution, or the use of a salt of a weak acid such as the borate salt of the local anesthetic, will increase its clinical efficacy. However, objective tests have failed to substantiate this point, and more alkaline preparations have the disadvantage of being relatively unstable. The explanation probably is that, under conditions usually encountered in clinical use, the pH of the local anesthetic is rapidly brought to that of the extracellular fluids, regardless of the pH of the solution in which it is injected.

All the commonly used local anesthetics contain a tertiary (or secondary) nitrogen atom and, therefore, can exist either as the uncharged tertiary (or secondary) amine or as the positively charged substituted ammonium cation, depending on the dissociation constant (pK_a) of the compound and the pH of the solution. The ionization of a typical local anesthetic may be depicted as follows:

$$\begin{array}{c} R_1 \\ R_2-\overset{+}{N}H \\ R_3 \end{array} \rightleftharpoons \begin{array}{c} R_1 \\ R_2-N \\ R_3 \end{array} + H^+$$

The pK_a of any typical local anesthetic in common use lies between 8.0 and 9.0, so that only 5 to 20% will be in the form of the unprotonated amine at the pH of the tissues. This fraction, although small, is important because the drug usually has to diffuse through connective tissue and other cellular membranes to get to its site of action, and it is generally agreed that it can do so only in the form of the uncharged amine. There has been a difference of opinion as to which form is active once the anesthetic has reached the nerve. Krahl and coworkers (1940) made a careful study of the action of local anesthetics in inhibiting cell division in sea urchin eggs and concluded that the intracellular presence of the cationic form was responsible for the inhibition. Largely on the basis of these experiments, it was suggested that the form of the molecule active in nerve fibers is the cation. This conclusion has been supported by the results of experiments on anesthetized mammalian nonmyelinated fibers (Ritchie and Greengard, 1966) in which conduction could be blocked or unblocked merely by setting the pH of the bathing medium at pH 7.2 or pH 9.6, respectively, without altering the amount of anesthetic present. When the pH is low, and conduction is blocked, most of the anesthetic must be in its cationic form. This seems to indicate that the cation is the molecular form that combines with some receptor in the membrane to prevent the generation of an action potential (*see also* Ariëns and Simonis, 1963). While it is now clear that both molecular forms possess anesthetic activity (Ritchie and Ritchie, 1968), the *major* role of the cation is clearly demonstrated by Narahashi and colleagues using quaternary analogs of the amine local anesthetics (Narahashi and Frazier, 1968).

Prolongation of Action by Vasoconstrictors. The duration of action of a local anesthetic is proportional to the time during which it is in actual contact with nervous tissues. Consequently, procedures that maintain the localization of the drug at the nerve greatly prolong the period of anesthesia. Cocaine itself constricts blood vessels and, therefore, prevents its own absorption. For this reason, the duration of cocaine anesthesia is greater than that of most local anesthetics that do not cause vasoconstriction. Braun in 1903 demonstrated that the addition of epinephrine to local anesthetic solutions greatly prolongs and intensifies their action. In clinical practice, therefore, the solution of a local anesthetic usually also contains epinephrine (1 part in 50,000 to 1 part in 500,000), norepinephrine (1 part in 100,000), or a suitable synthetic congener, for example, phenylephrine. In general, the concentration of such constrictor agents should be kept at the minimal effective level. The epinephrine performs a dual service. By decreasing the rate of absorption, epinephrine not only localizes the anesthetic at the desired site but also allows the rate at which it is destroyed in the body to keep pace with the rate at which it is absorbed into the circulation. This reduces its systemic toxicity.

Some of the vasoconstrictor agent may be absorbed systemically, perhaps to an excessive extent, and may occasionally lead to untoward reactions such as restlessness, an increase in heart rate, palpitation, and chest pain. This could be avoided by the use of pure α-adrenergic agonists. There may also be a delay in wound healing, tissue edema, or necrosis after local anesthesia; these effects seem to occur because sympathomimetic amines produce an increase in the oxygen consumption of the tissue, and this, together with the vasoconstriction, leads to hypoxia and local tissue damage. Because of these considerations, vasopressin has been tried as the constrictor substance (Klingenström and Westermark, 1963; Hansson, 1971). Pure synthetic vasopressin causes vasoconstriction without increasing the metabolism of the tissue and seems to cause less local tissue damage. The local anesthetics themselves may inhibit cell motility and delay wound healing.

Pharmacological Actions. In addition to blocking conduction in nerve axons in the peripheral nervous system, local anesthetics interfere with the function of all organs in which conduction or transmission of impulses occurs. Thus, they have important effects on the central nervous system (CNS), the autonomic ganglia, the neuromuscular junction, and all forms of muscle fiber.

Central Nervous System. Following absorption, all nitrogenous local anesthetics may cause stimulation of the CNS, producing restlessness and tremor that may proceed to clonic convulsions. In general, the more potent the anesthetic the more readily convulsions may be produced. Alterations of CNS activity are thus predictable from the local anesthetic agent in question and the blood concentration achieved. Central stimulation is followed by depression, and death is usually due to respiratory failure. It is possible to protect animals from several lethal doses of a local anesthetic by the use of artificial respiration.

Frank and Sanders (1963) have suggested that the apparent stimulation and the subsequent depression produced by applying local anesthetics to the CNS are both, in fact, due solely to *depression* of neuronal activity. The apparent stimulation is due perhaps to a selective depression of inhibitory neurons. The evidence for this theory is that, when procaine is applied to the cortical neurons in isolated slabs of cerebral cortex, only depression of the directly evoked electrical responses is obtained. Depression of activity is also the only effect that procaine produces in monosynaptic and polysynaptic spinal reflexes (Taverner, 1960). This depressant action also accounts for the findings in laboratory animals that local anesthetics can produce a condition indistinguishable from general anesthesia when given after subanesthetic doses of a general anesthetic. It would also account for the suppressive effects of local anesthetics against convulsions produced by electric shock and by pentylenetetrazol (Tanaka, 1955) and is the rationale for their use as antiepileptic agents (Bernhard and Bohm, 1965).

The support of respiration is the essential feature of treatment in the late stage of intoxication. While the barbiturates are capable of arresting convulsions resulting from toxic doses of local anesthetics, a near-anesthetic dose of barbiturate is required to prevent such seizures. The usual clinical dose merely provides psychic sedation and affords little protection (*see* page 392).

All the local anesthetics stimulate the CNS, but cocaine is unique in having a powerful action on the cortex. This property of cocaine and its ability to produce addiction are discussed in Chapter 16. The synthetic local anesthetics, in contrast, are less stimulating to the higher cerebral centers and do not cause addiction.

Neuromuscular Junction and Ganglionic Synapse. The local anesthetics also affect transmission at the neuromuscular junction. Harvey (1939) observed that the close intra-arterial injection of as little as 0.2 mg of procaine into the cat's tibialis anterior muscle reduced twitches and tetanic responses evoked by maximal motor-nerve volleys, and the response of the muscle to injected acetylcholine. The muscle, however, responded normally to direct electrical stimulation. Other work (Hirst and Wood, 1971) suggests that procaine also diminishes the release of acetylcholine by the motor-nerve endings. The effects of procaine and physostigmine are antagonistic, and those of procaine and curare additive. The postsynaptic action of procaine, however, differs from that of curare in that the end-plate current is much prolonged by procaine (Deguchi and Narahashi, 1971; Hirst and Wood, 1971).

Similarly, when procaine is added to the fluid perfusing a ganglion, preganglionic stimulation fails to elicit postganglionic discharges and the ganglion cells become insensitive to stimulation by acetylcholine. Furthermore, the production of acetylcholine in response to preganglionic stimulation is diminished, showing that, unlike curare, procaine has a marked effect on the synaptic endings of the preganglionic fibers as well as on the ganglion cells.

Cardiovascular System. Following systemic absorption, local anesthetics act on the cardiovascular system. The primary site of action is the myocardium, where decreases in electrical excitability, conduction rate, and force of contraction occur. In addition, most local anesthetics cause arteriolar dilatation. The cardiovascular effects are usually seen only after high systemic concentrations are attained. However, on rare occasion small amounts of anesthetic employed for simple infiltration anesthesia will cause cardiovascular collapse and death. The exact mechanism is unknown, but it probably results from cardiac arrest due to either an action on the pacemaker or the sudden onset of ventricular fibrillation. Such a reaction may follow inadvertent intravascular administration of the agent. Both the ionized and the nonionized forms of the local anesthetic may be important for these effects. It has been suggested that the effects on threshold and conduction time depend on the presence of the procaine cations in the extracellular medium; on the other hand, the effect on the strength of the myocardial contractions depends exclusively on the presence of the nonionized form of procaine, presumably indicating that this is an intracellular action (Baird and Hardman, 1961).

Studies on isolated atrial and ventricular muscle reveal that procaine resembles quinidine in its cardiac action in that it increases the effective refractory period, raises the threshold for stimulation, and prolongs conduction time. These cardiac actions of procaine, and the accompanying characteristic changes in the ECG, would be of therapeutic interest were it not for the rapid metabolic destruction of the compound and the propensity of procaine and other local anesthetics to cause central stimulation. Therefore, studies of procaine congeners were undertaken to find a compound that possessed the quinidine-like action on the heart but not the other undesirable properties. The result was the introduction of procainamide. Procaine and other local anesthetics share completely the cardiac actions of procainamide, as more fully discussed in Chapter 32.

Smooth Muscle. The local anesthetics depress contractions in strips of isolated intestine and in the intact bowel (*see* Zipf and Dittmann, 1971). On the isolated intestine, there is little correlation between anesthetic potency and antispasmodic efficacy, and this spasmolytic action, which can antagonize the spasm produced by a variety of chemical agents, seems to be caused by a direct depression of smooth muscle.

Spinal and epidural anesthesia, as well as instillation of local anesthetics into the peritoneal cavity, cause sympathetic nervous system paralysis that can result in increased tone of gastrointestinal musculature. Some local anesthetics may increase the tone of human uterine muscle (*see* de Jong, 1970).

Hypersensitivity to Local Anesthetics.

Rare individuals exhibit a hypersensitivity to local anesthetics. This may manifest itself as an allergic dermatitis, a typical asthmatic attack, or a fatal anaphylactic reaction (*see* Adriani, 1960). Hypersensitivity seems to occur most prominently in response to local anesthetics of the *ester type* and frequently extends to chemically related compounds. Agents of the amide type are essentially free of this problem, and substitution of such a compound to avoid group specificity is usually possible. Certain antihistamines are occasionally used as local anesthetics for individuals who have become hypersensitive to all the conventional agents. These antihistamines presumably have the general structural features necessary for local anesthetic activity without sharing the specific antigenic determinants of the conventional drugs.

Fate of Local Anesthetics.

The metabolic fate of local anesthetics is of great practical importance because their toxicity depends largely on the balance between their rate of absorption and their rate of destruction. As noted above, the rate of absorption of anesthetic agents can be reduced considerably by the incorporation of a vasoconstrictor agent in the anesthetic solution. However, the rate at which they are destroyed varies greatly, and this is a major factor in determining the safety of a particular anesthetic agent. Furthermore, binding of the anesthetic to tissues reduces the amount that appears in the systemic circulation and, consequently, reduces toxicity. Many of the common local anesthetics are esters, and their toxicity is usually lost as the result of hydrolysis, which in most animals occurs in both the liver and the plasma. Animals with experimentally produced hepatic damage are much more susceptible to the toxic actions of local anesthetics, so that the extensive use of a local anesthetic in patients with severe hepatic damage should perhaps be avoided. However, the ester type of local anesthetic is degraded not only by liver esterase but also by a plasma esterase, probably plasma cho-

linesterase. Metabolic degradation by the plasma esterase is particularly important in man, whose plasma can hydrolyze local anesthetics of the ester type 4 to 20 times faster than can the plasma of any other animal (Foldes *et al.*, 1956). Indeed, Brodie and coworkers (1948) have shown that in man the hydrolysis of procaine occurs mainly in the plasma and only to a small extent in the liver. Since spinal fluid contains little or no esterase, anesthesia produced by the intrathecal injection of an anesthetic agent will persist until the local anesthetic agent has been absorbed into the blood.

The metabolism of the amide-linked local anesthetics is more complex (*see* Hansson, 1971). Lidocaine is degraded by hepatic microsomes, the initial reactions involving N-dealkylation and subsequent hydrolysis. The general features of the metabolism of mepivacaine and prilocaine are probably similar.

Those anesthetic agents that are slowly destroyed by the liver are in small part eliminated in the urine.

COCAINE

Source. Cocaine is obtained from the leaves of *Erythroxylon coca* and other species of *Erythroxylon*, trees indigenous to Peru and Bolivia, where its leaves have been used for centuries by the natives to increase endurance (central stimulation).

Chemistry. Cocaine is benzoylmethylecgonine. Ecgonine is an amino alcohol base closely related to tropine, the amino alcohol in atropine. Cocaine is thus an ester of benzoic acid and a nitrogen-containing base. It has the fundamental structure previously described for the synthetic local anesthetics. The structural formula of cocaine is as follows:

$$H_2C-CH-CH \cdot COOCH_3$$
$$N \cdot CH_3 \quad CH \cdot OOC$$
$$H_2C-CH-CH_2$$

Cocaine

Pharmacological Actions. The most important action of cocaine clinically is its ability to block nerve conduction following local application. Its most striking systemic effect is stimulation of the CNS. In addition, cocaine has numerous important side actions.

Central Nervous System. Cocaine stimulates the CNS from above downward. The first recognizable action is on the cortex. In man, this is manifested in garrulousness, restlessness, and excitement. Mental powers may be increased. There may also be an increased capacity for muscular work, probably due to a lessened sense of fatigue. Sir Arthur Conan Doyle's famous Sherlock Holmes took advantage of the central effects of cocaine, much to the perturbation of Dr. Watson. Other actions on the cerebral cortex are discussed under *cocaine addiction* (*see* Chapter 16). In laboratory animals, the cortical action is manifested mainly by increased motor activity. After small amounts of cocaine motor activity is well coordinated, but as the dose is increased the lower centers also are affected. Stimulation of lower motor centers causes tremors and convulsive movements. Cord reflexes are increased and eventually clonic-tonic convulsions appear. As has been mentioned earlier, these "stimulating" effects may actually be the result of depression of inhibitory neurons.

The action of cocaine on the medulla results in an increase in the respiratory rate. At first the depth of respiration is unaffected, but soon it is diminished so that breathing is rapid and shallow. The vasomotor and vomiting centers may also share in the stimulation, and emesis is not uncommon.

Central stimulation is soon followed by depression. The higher centers are the first to be depressed, and this may occur when the lower portions of the cerebrospinal axis are still in the stage of excitation. Eventually the vital medullary centers are depressed, and death results from respiratory failure.

Cardiovascular System. Small doses of cocaine given systemically may slow the heart as a result of central vagal stimulation, but after moderate doses the heart rate is increased. The increased cardiac rate probably results from increased central sympathetic stimulation as well as from the peripheral effects of cocaine on the sympathetic nervous system, as discussed below. Although the blood pressure may finally fall, there is at first a prominent rise in blood pressure due to centrally mediated tachycardia and vasoconstriction. A large intravenous dose of cocaine may cause immediate death from cardiac failure due to a direct toxic action on the heart muscle.

Skeletal Muscle. There is no evidence that cocaine increases the intrinsic strength of muscular contraction. The relief of fatigue by cocaine seems to result from central stimulation, which masks the sensation of fatigue.

Body Temperature. Cocaine is markedly pyrogenic. The increased muscular activity attending stimulation by cocaine augments heat production. Vasoconstriction due to central vasomotor stimulation decreases heat loss. Also, there is reason to believe that cocaine has a direct action on the heat-regulating centers, for the onset of cocaine fever is often heralded by a chill, which indicates that the body is adjusting its temperature to a higher level. Cocaine pyrexia is often a striking feature of cocaine poisoning and can easily be elicited in animals by sublethal doses.

Sympathetic Nervous System. Cocaine potentiates both the excitatory and the inhibitory responses of sympathetically innervated organs to epinephrine, norepinephrine, and sympathetic nerve stimulation. Cocaine potentiation was first observed by Frölich and Loewi in 1910, and many explanations have been offered to account for the phenomenon. It now seems well established that cocaine does this by blocking the uptake of catecholamines at adrenergic nerve endings, the process of which is primarily responsible for terminating the actions of both adrenergic impulses and circulating catecholamines (*see* Chapter 21; and Figure 21-5, page 425).

Cocaine is the only local anesthetic that is known to interfere with the uptake of norepinephrine by the adrenergic nerve terminals and, therefore, is the only local anesthetic to produce sensitization to catecholamines. This provides a plausible explanation of why cocaine, unlike other local anesthetics, produces vasoconstriction and mydriasis. The peripheral component of the cardioacceleration produced by cocaine is probably of similar origin.

Local Anesthetic Actions. The most important local action of cocaine is its ability to block nerve conduction when brought into direct contact with nerve tissue. Cocaine blocks terminal sensory nerve fibers in a concentration as low as 0.02%. Higher concentrations are required to block conduction in nerve trunks or to produce anesthesia by direct contact with mucous membranes.

Eye. The local actions of cocaine on the eye are of historical importance because cocaine was at one time used extensively in ophthalmological procedures. The cornea can be anesthetized with solutions of 0.25 to 0.5%. There is an accompanying constriction of the conjunctival vessels, and the sclera is blanched. Anesthesia may extend to the iris. Mydriasis also occurs (*see* above). The pupil of the cocainized eye responds to light, and pilocarpine and physostigmine still produce miosis. Further mydriasis by atropine can be superimposed on that of cocaine and *vice versa*. Cocaine in high concentration causes cycloplegia, and varying effects on intraocular pressure. In most instances it causes a reduction of intraocular pressure through vasoconstriction; however, it has precipitated attacks of acute glaucoma. In concentrations that were once employed for anesthesia, cocaine has a deleterious effect on the cornea; it may become clouded and pitted, and ulceration may follow. This toxic action of cocaine is enhanced because the normal protective eyelid reflexes are abolished by the corneal anesthesia.

It is obvious that there are many properties of cocaine that detract from its value as a local anesthetic in ophthalmology. Consequently, cocaine has been replaced in this field by the agents discussed later in this chapter.

Absorption, Fate, and Excretion. While the local vasoconstriction caused by cocaine limits the rate of its absorption, this may easily exceed the rate of detoxication and excretion. Thus, cocaine can be highly toxic. Cocaine is absorbed from all sites of application, including mucous membranes. Absorption occurs even from the urinary bladder if inflammation is present. When given orally, cocaine is largely hydrolyzed in the gastrointestinal tract and rendered ineffective.

After absorption, cocaine is metabolized by the liver although some may be excreted unchanged in the urine. It has been estimated that the liver can detoxicate one minimal lethal dose of cocaine an hour. Cocaine is not destroyed as fast as many of the synthetic local anesthetics. Therefore, it is more toxic after subcutaneous administration than are many of its substitutes.

Tolerance and Addiction. Cocaine is a powerful cortical stimulant and is often abused for this effect. Both addiction and tolerance can result from the continued use of cocaine. These phenomena and the treatment of the cocaine addict are dealt with in Chapter 16.

Acute Cocaine Poisoning. The fatal dose of cocaine in man has been stated to be 1.2 g, obviously only an approximate figure. Severe toxic effects have been reported from doses as low as 20 mg.

The symptoms of cocaine poisoning are mainly referable to the CNS. The patient quickly becomes excited, restless, garrulous, anxious, and confused. Reflexes are enhanced. Additional signs and symptoms may include headache, tachycardia, irregular respiration, chill, fever, mydriasis, exophthalmos, and formication. Nausea, vomiting, and abdominal pain are frequent. Delirium, Cheyne-Stokes respiration, convulsions, and unconsciousness occur terminally. Death results from respiratory arrest. Acute poisoning by cocaine can result in almost immediate death, the patient often collapsing and dying before the physician realizes what has occurred. This type of response probably results from an anaphylactoid reaction to impurities present in "street" preparations or from rapid absorption or intravascular administration.

Treatment. The specific treatment of CNS excitation in acute cocaine poisoning is the intravenous administration of diazepam or a barbiturate. The intravenous route is necessary because symptoms progress with such great rapidity. The same principles of dosage apply as for the therapy of strychnine poisoning. Artificial respiration is necessary. It is important to limit absorption of the drug. The circulation from the site of cocaine absorption should be stopped by a tourniquet or in any other way possible. If the entrance of the drug into the circulation can be checked and respiratory exchange maintained, the prognosis is favorable because cocaine is destroyed fairly rapidly. The prophylaxis and treatment of untoward responses to cocaine are discussed under the clinical uses of local anesthetics.

Preparations and Dosage. *Cocaine,* N.F., and *Cocaine Hydrochloride,* U.S.P., are the official preparations of the alkaloid. Both are white crystalline powders. The alkaloidal base is freely soluble in organic solvents; the hydrochloride salt, in water. Cocaine is not used internally or injected. Solutions employed clinically for surface anesthesia vary from 1.0 to 4.0% (cornea) and 5 to 10% (nose and throat), depending on the mucosa being anesthetized. Epinephrine is usually incorporated in these solutions. Occasionally, dry cocaine powder is moistened with epinephrine solution to form so-called cocaine mud for use on the nasal mucosa. In view of the dangerous potentiative interaction between cocaine and catecholamines, this practice is to be condemned.

Cocaine, because of its addicting potency, is included among the drugs controlled by the federal drug-abuse regulations (*see* Appendix).

PROCAINE

Procaine was synthesized by Einhorn in 1905 and introduced under the trade name NOVOCAIN. It is still a useful local anesthetic. The chemical structure of procaine has already been discussed.

Pharmacological Actions. The pharmacological actions that procaine shares with other local anesthetic drugs have been presented. However, one property unique to procaine and some related drugs deserves consideration.

Procaine-Sulfonamide Antagonism. Procaine and many other local anesthetics are hydrolyzed in the body to produce para-aminobenzoic acid, which inhibits the action of the sulfonamides. This fact is of practical importance. For example, despite adequate sulfonamide therapy local infections have occurred in areas infiltrated with procaine prior to diagnostic punctures in meningitis and drainage procedures in empyema. Therefore, procaine and other local anesthetic derivatives of para-aminobenzoic acid should not be used in any condition in which therapy with a sulfonamide drug is being employed. Procaine and its congeners also interfere with the chemical determination of sulfonamide concentration in biological fluids. Local anesthetics other than derivatives of para-aminobenzoic acid do not affect sulfonamide activity and, therefore, can be used under all these circumstances.

Absorption, Fate, and Excretion. Procaine is readily absorbed following parenteral administration and thus does not long remain at the site of injection. In order to retard absorption, vasoconstrictor drugs may be added to procaine solutions. Following absorption, procaine is rapidly hydrolyzed, mostly in the circulation, by an esterase, presumably plasma cholinesterase. The products of the enzymatic hydrolysis of procaine are para-aminobenzoic acid and diethylaminoethanol. The former is excreted in the urine to the extent of about 80%, either unchanged or in conjugated form. Only 30% of the diethylaminoethanol can be recovered in the urine; the remainder undergoes metabolic degradation (Brodie *et al.,* 1948).

Toxicity. The usual spectrum of CNS and cardiovascular toxicity may be seen with procaine. Toxicity is greatly decreased if absorption is slowed by vasoconstrictors. There is a high incidence of allergic reactions to procaine, and sensitive individuals usually also react to structurally similar compounds (*e.g.,* tetracaine).

Preparations. *Procaine Hydrochloride,* U.S.P. (NOVOCAIN), occurs as a white crystalline powder that is freely soluble in water. It is available as an official injection. Market preparations include the following: ampuls or vials of a 0.5, 1, 2, or 10% solution without epinephrine, or 1 or 2% solution with epinephrine in a concentration of 1:50,000 to 1:100,000, for infiltration and nerve block; 5 to 20% solution in ampuls, for spinal anesthesia; ampuls of sterile procaine hydrochloride crystals (50 to 500 mg), for spinal anesthesia; 0.1 or 0.2% procaine hydrochloride in isotonic sodium chloride solution, for intravenous infusion.

Dosage. Procaine solutions are used for infiltration anesthesia (0.25 to 0.5%), nerve block (1.0 or 2.0%), and spinal anesthesia (dose varies with the technic employed). For continuous caudal analgesia, the usual initial dose is 30 ml of a 1.5% solution. Procaine is not an efficient local anesthetic for topical application to mucous membranes and is seldom employed as such, a concentration of 10 to 20% being necessary for adequate anesthesia.

Clinical Uses. The various clinical uses of procaine as a local anesthetic are discussed later in this chapter.
Procaine Salts of Other Drugs. Procaine can form poorly soluble salts or conjugate with other drugs and prolong their action. This property is unrelated to the ability of procaine to produce local anesthesia. For example, after the intramuscular injection of procaine penicillin G, the antibiotic is absorbed very slowly so that detectable concentrations of penicillin exist in the blood and urine for prolonged periods, as discussed in more detail in Chapter 57. The possibility of allergy to procaine must be considered when hypersensitivity to such preparations occurs.

LIDOCAINE

Lidocaine, introduced in 1948, is one of the most widely used local anesthetics.

Pharmacological Actions. The pharmacological actions that lidocaine shares with other local anesthetic drugs have been presented. Lidocaine produces more prompt, more intense, longer-lasting, and more extensive anesthesia than does an equal concentration of procaine. Unlike procaine it is an aminoethylamide. It is an agent of choice, therefore, in individuals sensitive to procaine and other ester-type local anesthetics.

Absorption, Fate, and Excretion. Lidocaine is relatively quickly absorbed after parenteral administration and from the gastrointestinal tract (*see* Boyes *et al.*, 1971; Hansson, 1971; Keenaghan and Boyes, 1972). Although it is effective when used without any vasoconstrictor, in the presence of epinephrine the rate of absorption and the toxicity are thereby decreased and the duration of action is prolonged. Lidocaine is metabolized in the liver by the microsomal mixed-function oxidases by dealkylation to monoethylglycine and xylidide. The latter compound retains significant local anesthetic and toxic activity. In man about 75% of xylidide is excreted in the urine as the further metabolite, 4-hydroxy-2,6-dimethylaniline (Keenaghan and Boyes, 1972).

Toxicity. Lidocaine has approximately the same toxicity as procaine when administered subcutaneously in a 0.5% solution. When stronger solutions (2%) are injected, lidocaine is more toxic than procaine. It is nonirritating and highly stable. Because it is metabolized in the liver, lidocaine seems to be more toxic in individuals with diminished hepatic function (Selden and Sasahara, 1967). In experimental animals overdosage of lidocaine produces death from ventricular fibrillation or cardiac arrest; procaine, on the other hand, tends to depress respiration rather than the circulation (de Jong, 1970). A notable side effect of lidocaine is sleepiness. There is also a high incidence of dizziness, which may be caused by a metabolite rather than by lidocaine itself (Boyes *et al.*, 1971).

Preparations. *Lidocaine Hydrochloride,* U.S.P. (*lignocaine;* XYLOCAINE), is an odorless, white crystalline powder that is very soluble in water and alcohol. The official preparations are an *injection* and a *jelly.* Market preparations (0.5 to 4.0%), available in ampuls, vials, or prefilled syringes with and without epinephrine (1:100,000 to 1:200,000), are suitable for infiltration (0.5%), block (1 to 2%), and topical mucosal anesthesia (1 to 2%). *Lidocaine Ointment,* U.S.P. (2.5 to 5%), *Lidocaine Hydrochloride Jelly,* U.S.P. (2%), and *Lidocaine Aerosol,* N.F. (100 mg/1 g), are also available.

Clinical Uses. Lidocaine has a variety of clinical uses as a local anesthetic, as discussed below. In addition, lidocaine is used intravenously as an antiarrhythmic agent, as described in Chapter 32.

OTHER SYNTHETIC LOCAL ANESTHETICS

The number of synthetic local anesthetics is so large that it is impractical to consider all of them. Therefore, a discussion of the individual members of this series will be limited mainly to those that are official in the U.S.P. or N.F.

Some local anesthetic agents are too toxic to be given by injection. Their use is restricted to topical application to the eye, the mucous membranes, or the skin. Many local anesthetics are suitable, however, for infiltration or injection to produce nerve block; some of them are also useful for topical application. The main categories of local anesthetics are given below; the agents are listed in alphabetical order.

LOCAL ANESTHETICS SUITABLE FOR INJECTION

Bupivacaine hydrochloride (MARCAINE) is a relatively new local anesthetic of the amide type, structurally related to mepivacaine. It is a potent agent capable of producing prolonged analgesia. Its mean duration of action is greater than that of tetracaine, while the toxicity of the two compounds is similar. The onset of analgesia with bupivacaine is similar to that of lidocaine, mepivacaine, and tetracaine. Bupivacaine hydrochloride is available in solutions for injection (0.25, 0.5, and 0.75%) with or without epinephrine (1:200,000).

Chloroprocaine Hydrochloride, N.F. (NESACAINE), is a halogenated derivative of procaine, the pharmacological properties of which it shares almost completely. Its anesthetic potency is at least twice as great as that of procaine, and its toxicity is lower. Chloroprocaine hydrochloride is available in solution for injection (1.0 and 2.0%).

Dibucaine Hydrochloride, N.F. (*cinchocaine;* NUPERCAINE), is a quinoline derivative. It is one of the most potent, most toxic, and longest acting of the commonly employed local anesthetics. It is about 15 times as potent and as toxic as procaine, and its anesthetic action lasts about three times as long. Dibucaine hydrochloride is infrequently used either topically or by injection.

Hexylcaine Hydrochloride, N.F. (CYCLAINE), was previously used for infiltration, spinal, topical, and nerve block anesthesia. It is about twice as potent as procaine. Hexylcaine hydrochloride is available for topical application as a 5% solution and for injection as a 1% solution.

Mepivacaine Hydrochloride, U.S.P. (CARBOCAINE), is a local anesthetic of the amide type. Its pharmacological properties are somewhat similar to those of lidocaine, which it resembles chemically. Its action is more rapid in onset and somewhat more prolonged than that of lidocaine. It has been employed for all types of infiltration and regional nerve block anesthesia as well as for spinal anesthesia. Mepivacaine hydrochloride is marketed in solutions for injection (1.0, 1.5, 2.0, and 3.0% without, and 2% with, levonordefrin).

Piperocaine hydrochloride (METYCAINE) is an ester of benzoic acid and an ethanolamine whose nitrogen atom is contained in a methylpiperidine ring. It is about three times as toxic as procaine upon intravenous injection, but after subcutaneous administration its toxicity is approximately the same as that of procaine. It is about as potent an anesthetic as procaine. Piperocaine is now infrequently used topically or by injection.

Prilocaine Hydrochloride, N.F. (CITANEST), is a local anesthetic of the amide type. Its pharmacological properties resemble those of lidocaine. Its onset and duration of action are longer than those of lidocaine. Like lidocaine, it may produce sleepiness. A unique toxic aftereffect is methemoglobinemia, and its use is declining for this reason. It has been employed for all types of infiltration and regional nerve block anesthesia as well as for spinal anesthesia. Prilocaine hydrochloride is marketed in solutions for injection (1.0, 2.0, 3.0, and 4.0%).

Tetracaine Hydrochloride, U.S.P. (AMETHOCAINE, PONTOCAINE), is a derivative of para-aminobenzoic acid in which a butyl group has been substituted for one of the hydrogens of the para-amino group. It is about ten times more toxic and more active than procaine after intravenous injection. For topical anesthesia of the eye, a 0.5% solution is used; for the mucous membranes of the nose and throat, a 2.0% solution. For spinal anesthesia, a total dose of 10 to 20 mg is adequate. Tetracaine has been rather extensively employed for continuous caudal anesthesia, but its onset of action at this site is very slow. The initial dose usually consists of 30 ml of a 0.25% solution. The effects are longer lasting than those of procaine. Tetracaine hydrochloride is available in

solutions and in ampuls containing the dry salt. An official ophthalmic solution of tetracaine and an official ophthalmic ointment of 0.5% tetracaine base in white petrolatum are also marketed.

LOCAL ANESTHETICS LARGELY RESTRICTED TO OPHTHALMOLOGICAL USE

While certain of the agents described above can be used in the eye, the following local anesthetic agents are largely restricted to the production of corneal anesthesia. Their main advantage over the prototype, cocaine, is that they produce little or no mydriasis or corneal injury.

Benoxinate Hydrochloride, N.F. (DORSACAINE), is a benzoic acid ester related to procaine. It is an effective surface anesthetic agent that is useful in ophthalmology. A single instillation of 0.08 ml of a 0.4% solution produces within 60 seconds a sufficient degree of anesthesia to permit tonometry. It is marketed as a 0.4% solution.

Naepaine hydrochloride (AMYLSINE) is a derivative of para-aminobenzoic acid and is distinctive in that it is a secondary rather than a tertiary amino ester. It is used exclusively for producing corneal anesthesia and is available as a 4% solution.

Phenacaine Hydrochloride, N.F. (HOLOCAINE, TANICAINE), was one of the earliest local anesthetics to be introduced. It is not an ester and differs greatly in chemical structure from the majority of local anesthetics. Upon intravenous injection it is as toxic as cocaine. It is used solely to produce topical anesthesia, especially of the eye. Both an ophthalmic solution (1%) and an ophthalmic ointment (1%) are marketed preparations. Phenacaine hydrochloride is slightly irritating, and anesthesia is preceded by smarting.

Proparacaine Hydrochloride, U.S.P. (OPHTHAINE, OPHTHETIC), is a benzoic ester, but it is chemically distinct from procaine, benoxinate, and tetracaine. This difference in chemical structure may explain the lack of cross-sensitization between proparacaine and other local anesthetic agents. It is about as potent as tetracaine. Unlike some topical anesthetics, proparacaine hydrochloride produces little or no initial irritation. It is available in a 0.5% official ophthalmic solution for topical application.

LOCAL ANESTHETICS USED MAINLY TO ANESTHETIZE THE LESS DELICATE MUCOUS MEMBRANES AND THE SKIN

Some anesthetics are either too irritating or too ineffective to be applied to the eye. However, they are useful as topical anesthetic agents on the skin and the less delicate mucous membranes. These preparations are effective in the symptomatic relief of anal and genital pruritus, ivy poisoning, and numerous other acute and chronic dermatoses.

Cyclomethycaine Sulfate, N.F. (SURFACAINE), acts on damaged or diseased skin and on the mucosa of the rectum and genitourinary system, but it is relatively ineffective on the mucous membranes of the mouth, nose, bronchi, and eye. The compound is marketed as a cream (0.5%), an ointment (1.0%), a jelly for urethral application (0.75%), and suppositories containing 10 mg, all of which are official in the N.F.

Dimethisoquin Hydrochloride, N.F. (QUOTANE), is an active surface anesthetic that is not of the benzoate ester type. The high anesthetic potency of dimethisoquin makes it of unique value as an antipruritic for the relief of itching and pain associated with various dermatological lesions. The compound appears to be less sensitizing when applied topically than antipruritic ointments containing antihistaminic drugs, but isolated cases of contact dermatitis have been reported. Dimethisoquin is marketed as a skin lotion (0.5%) and as an ointment for rectal application (0.5%). Both are official preparations.

Dyclonine Hydrochloride, N.F. (DYCLONE), has a rapid onset of action and a duration of effect comparable to that of procaine. It is absorbed through the skin and mucous membranes. The compound is used as a 0.5 to 1.0% solution for topical anesthesia in otolaryngology.

Pramoxine Hydrochloride, N.F. (TRONOTHANE), is a surface anesthetic agent that is not of the benzoate ester type. Its distinct chemical structure is likely to minimize the danger of cross-sensitivity reactions in patients allergic to other local anesthetics. Pramoxine produces satisfactory surface anesthesia and is reasonably well tolerated on the skin and less delicate mucous membranes. It is too irritating to be used on the eye or in the nose. Official preparations are available for topical application as a 1% cream or jelly.

ANESTHETICS OF LOW SOLUBILITY

Some local anesthetics are poorly soluble in water and, consequently, too slowly absorbed to be toxic. They can be applied directly to wounds and ulcerated surfaces where they remain localized for long periods of time, which accounts for their sustained anesthetic action. Chemically, they are esters of para-aminobenzoic acid that lack the terminal tertiary or secondary amino group possessed by the previously described local anesthetics. The most important members of the series are *Benzocaine,* N.F. (*ethyl aminobenzoate;* ANESTHESIN), *Butyl Aminobenzoate,* N.F., and *orthoform.* All are white crystalline, insoluble powders whose structural formulas are shown below:

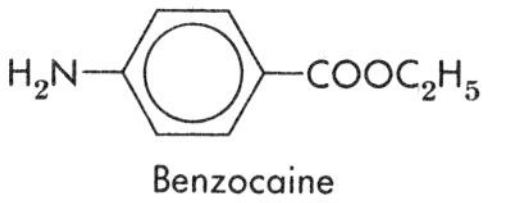

Benzocaine

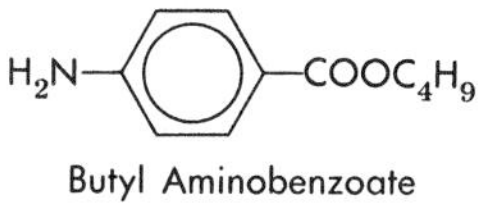

Butyl Aminobenzoate

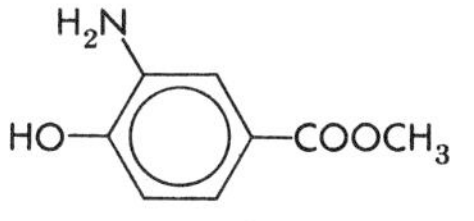

Orthoform

They may be applied as dusting powders, undiluted or diluted with sterile talc. They are soluble in oil and may be incorporated in oily solutions, ointments, and suppositories.

Some salts of the tertiary amino group of local anesthetics are of extremely low solubility. The hydroiodide salt of tetracaine, for example, is very insoluble and may produce anesthesia of 45-hours'

duration when sprinkled in a surgical wound (Cherney, 1963).

TETRODOTOXIN AND SAXITOXIN

These toxins are two of the most potent poisons known, the minimal lethal dose of each in the mouse being about 8 μg/kg. Both toxins are responsible for outbreaks of fatal poisoning in man. Tetrodotoxin is found in the gonads and other tissues of some fish of the suborder Gymnodontes (to which the Japanese *fugu,* or puffer fish, belongs); it also occurs in the skin of some newts of the family Salamandridae. Saxitoxin, elaborated by the dinoflagellate *Gonyaulax catenella,* is retained in the tissues of clams and other shellfish that eat these organisms. Given the right conditions of temperature and light the *Gonyaulax* may multiply so rapidly as to discolor the ocean—hence the term "red tide." Shellfish feeding on *Gonyaulax* at this time become extremely toxic to man and are responsible for the periodic outbreaks of *paralytic shellfish poisoning* (*see* Kao, 1966, 1972).

Although the toxins are chemically different from each other, their *mechanism of action* seems identical (*see* Narahashi, 1972). Both toxins, in nanomolar concentrations, specifically block the sodium channels in the membranes of excitable cells. As a result, the sodium currents are inhibited and the action potential is blocked. Blockade of vasomotor nerves, together with a relaxation of vascular smooth muscle, seems to be responsible for the hypotension that is characteristic of tetrodotoxin poisoning (Kao, 1972). Both toxins cause death by paralysis of the respiratory muscles. The *treatment* of severe cases of poisoning therefore requires artificial ventilation. Early gastric lavage and therapy to support the blood pressure are also indicated. If the patient survives paralytic shellfish poisoning for 24 hours, the prognosis is good (*see* Ogura, 1971; Schantz, 1971).

Apart from toxicological considerations, there are two other reasons for current interest in these toxins. First, since the toxins are much more specific and potent than the local anesthetics described above, they might serve as prototypes for new chemical classes of local anesthetics. For a variety of reasons neither toxin itself seems suitable; it is unfortunate, therefore, that all modifications of the toxin molecule examined so far have led to a more-or-less total loss of activity. Second, they are important in the analysis of the molecular basis of the action potential. Indeed, experiments with radioactively labeled toxins have already been used to determine the density of sodium channels in a variety of nerves (Henderson *et al.,* 1974).

CLINICAL USES OF LOCAL ANESTHETICS

The following discussion will indicate the fields of usefulness of the local anesthetic agents, together with the principles and precautions to be observed during their administration.

PREVENTION AND TREATMENT OF
TOXIC REACTIONS

The major cause of systemic reactions to local anesthetics is a high blood concentration of the drug. Absorption from the pharynx, trachea, and pulmonary alveoli results in blood levels that may approach those achieved with a rapid intravenous injection (Adriani and Campbell, 1956). Instillation of the drug into the pyriform fossa, for example, will give a peak concentration in 4 to 6 minutes that is 33 to 50% of that achieved with an intravenous injection. Figure 20–1 indicates that the peak level reached when a drug is applied to the pharynx is lower and flatter than that obtained with intravascular injection; however, it is higher and attained more rapidly than that after subcutaneous or perineural infiltration. Following paracervical block for relief of pain of labor, the rapid absorption of local anesthetic (with a peak concentration at 10 to 20 minutes) followed by transplacental passage has been associated with fetal bradycardia (Gordon, 1968) and, on rare occasion, with convulsions and death of the newborn (Rosefsky and Petersiel, 1968). Absorption does not take place from the stomach, esophagus, or bladder if the mucosa is intact (Campbell and Adriani, 1958).

Because of the threat of high blood concentrations whenever local anesthetics are used, it is important to administer the smallest amount that will be effective. Fractional doses administered over a period of time, especially when applied topically, result in a far lower blood level than when the entire dose is given at once. Since there is a latent period of varying duration before the onset of anesthesia, regardless of the site of administration, one must allow this time to pass before giving additional drug. The addition of epinephrine will delay systemic absorption except when the drug has been applied topically. Epinephrine may result in tachycardia, palpitations, restlessness, and anxiety. These may be confused with a toxic reaction to the anesthetic agent.

Hypnotics and anticonvulsants have been used to attempt to prevent CNS toxicity from local anesthetics. A sedative dose of barbiturate (*e.g.*, 100 to 200 mg of secobarbital or pentobarbital) will not protect against convulsions caused by local anesthetics. Even intravenous thiopental in doses sufficient to cause sleep (2 to 4 mg/kg) will not prevent a convulsion; rather, it will only increase the dose of local anesthetic required to produce a convulsion (Usubiaga *et al.,* 1966). On the other hand, while the intravenous administration of diazepam (0.25 mg/kg) produces little change in behavior in the unanesthetized cat, it doubles the dose of lidocaine required to produce seizures (de Jong and Heavner, 1971). Clinical experience also suggests that diazepam is useful to prevent convulsions from local anesthetics.

Treatment of Systemic Reactions. Convulsions and cardiovascular and respiratory collapse are the

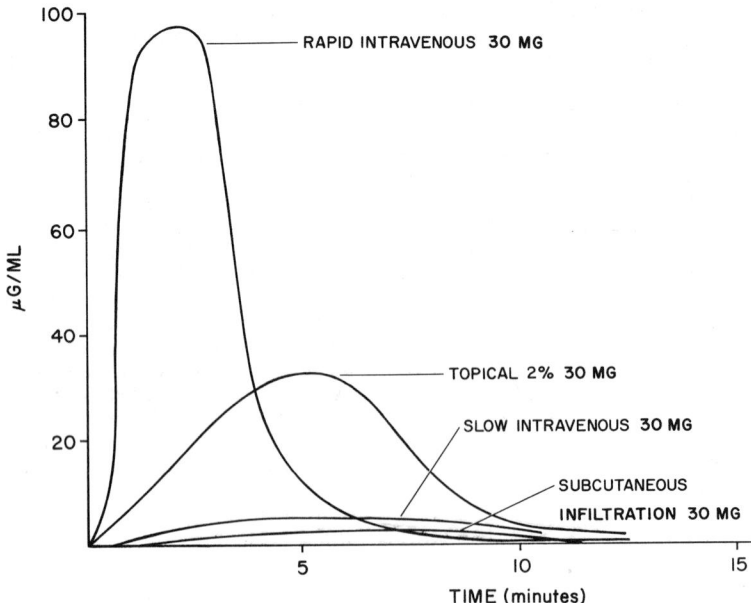

Figure 20–1. *Blood concentrations of local anesthetics.*

Comparison of blood concentrations obtained after injecting 30 mg of tetracaine in dogs intravenously and rapidly over a 30- to 60-second interval, after application topically to the pharyngeal mucous membranes, after subcutaneous infiltration, and after slow intravenous infusion. (After Adriani and Campbell, 1956. Courtesy of the *Journal of the American Medical Association.*)

complications most to be feared. Immediate therapy must have as its goal reversal of these events. Convulsions may result in bodily injury, aspiration of vomitus, or respiratory arrest followed by hypoxic brain damage and cardiac arrest. Thus, prevention of hypoxia is of paramount importance. Although convulsions increase cerebral metabolism, both brain oxygenation and subsequent cerebral function remain normal provided that pulmonary ventilation is restored and arterial blood pressure does not decrease (Plum et al., 1968). Thus, Moore and Bridenbaugh (1960) administer only succinylcholine, which suppresses skeletal muscle activity and facilitates the institution of artificial ventilation with oxygen. However, convulsions are most often treated with a rapidly acting barbiturate given intravenously. Such drug reactions are obviously dangerous; *large* doses of local anesthetics should be administered only where proper facilities, drugs, and personnel are available. Since intravenous diazepam (0.1 mg/kg) rapidly terminates convulsions produced by local anesthetics in the monkey (Munson and Wagman, 1972), it is likely that this agent when administered in dosages that have minimal effects on ventilation and circulation will prove effective in the therapy of local anesthetic–induced seizures.

If respiration is inadequate, oxygenation must be restored immediately by artificial ventilation. Arterial hypotension should be treated with intravenously administered fluids and pressor drugs until normal pressure has been restored. If effective cardiac action has ceased, immediate therapy must be undertaken; closed-chest cardiac massage with artificial ventilation is the treatment of choice until an ECG diagnosis can be made (Dripps et al., 1972). If cardiovascular collapse is due to ventricular fibrillation, electrical defibrillation should be attempted. If the myocardium was previously normal and immediate treatment has been instituted, restoration of spontaneous cardiac activity and of normal cerebral function can be expected. Thus, with what was once thought to be heroic treatment, excellent results may now be anticipated. Measures that fall short of this will usually prove inadequate.

CHOICE OF ANESTHETIC

There is a wide variety of local anesthetic agents available (Tables 20–1, 20–2). The experienced anesthesiologist may use a number of drugs and would be remiss if he failed

Table 20–2. SUGGESTED USES, CONCENTRATIONS, AND MAXIMAL DOSAGES OF SELECTED LOCAL ANESTHETICS *

DRUGS	TOPICAL †	DOSE (mg)	INJECTION	DOSE (mg)
Bupivacaine hydrochloride	No data		Infiltration and peripheral nerves 0.25–0.75%	500
Chloroprocaine hydrochloride	Ineffective		Infiltration 0.5% (200 ml) Peripheral nerves 2% (50 ml)	1000
Cocaine hydrochloride	Respiratory tract 5–10% (4–2 ml)	200	Not employed	
Lidocaine hydrochloride	Respiratory tract 2–4% (10–5 ml)	200	Infiltration 0.5% (100 ml) Peripheral nerves 1–2% (50–25 ml)	500
Mepivacaine hydrochloride	Ineffective		Infiltration 0.5–1.0% (100–50 ml) Peripheral nerves 1–2%	500
Piperocaine hydrochloride	Infrequently used Urethra 2% (30 ml)	600	Infiltration 0.5% (200 ml) Peripheral nerves 1.0–1.5% (100–65 ml)	1000
Prilocaine hydrochloride	Poorly effective		Infiltration 0.5% (120 ml)	600
Procaine hydrochloride	Ineffective		Infiltration 0.5% (200 ml) Peripheral nerves 1–2% (100–50 ml)	1000
Tetracaine hydrochloride	Respiratory tract 1–2% (8–4 ml)	80	Infrequently used for infiltration and nerve injection 0.1 to 0.25%	100

* Modified from Dripps, Eckenhoff, and Vandam, 1972.
† *See* text for specific recommendations regarding use on cornea, other mucous membranes, intact or abraded skin, etc.

to afford new preparations a therapeutic trial. However, the less experienced practitioner need gain experience with only a few agents. In this way he can become familiar with their effective concentrations, limitations, and toxicity. A working knowledge of one surface anesthetic and one for injection should suffice. Lidocaine is an excellent agent of choice. It is stable, and can be stored indefinitely and autoclaved repeatedly. The onset of action is rapid, and, once injected, the agent diffuses rapidly through tissue and into the nerve. It is an excellent surface analgesic. The duration of action after infiltration is 90 to 120 minutes. Bupivacaine is attaining rapid clinical acceptance since its duration of action is significantly longer than that of other agents in current use.

TECHNICS FOR LOCAL ANESTHESIA

Surface Anesthesia. The aqueous solutions of salts of local anesthetics do not penetrate significantly the intact epidermis. Preparations of the anesthetic bases in ointments accomplish this to a limited extent. For application to wounds, ulcers, and burns for the relief of pain, the insoluble compounds already described are the preparations of choice. They are relatively safe and, if properly used, do not interfere with tissue healing. A 2% solution of lidocaine in carboxymethylcellulose (viscous lidocaine) has been used for the relief of pain in the mucous membranes of the mouth, pharynx, and esophagus. It provides relief after tooth extraction and tonsillectomy, and may prevent gagging when a gastric tube is passed. Repeated use may, however, cause significant absorption, cumulation, and toxicity.

Anesthesia of the mucous membranes of the nose, throat, tracheobronchial tree, and genitourinary tract may be produced by the application of any of the agents that penetrate these membranes. As has already been pointed out, topical application in these areas involves the risk of rapid systemic absorption. Most difficulties arise when more than one fourth to one third of the limit recommended for infiltration has been exceeded topically. The important principles of topical anesthesia have been summarized by Adriani and associates (1964). There is a maximal effective concentration for each topical anesthetic; increasing the concentration above this does not result in greater analgesia or increased duration. Procaine and mepivacaine are not practical as topical anesthetics because of the high concentrations required. The addition of vasoconstrictors to a topical anesthetic does not alter the duration of action of the drug or the time course of systemic absorption. The use of hyaluronidase, cations such as calcium, potassium, sodium, magnesium, or ammonium, or surface-wetting agents has no effect on the duration or intensity of analgesia. If the mucous membrane is alkalinized with 5.0% sodium bicarbonate solution, the latent period and the duration of action will be

shorter while the intensity of analgesia will be increased; this is true only of basic nitrogen-containing agents. Detectable drug levels in the blood are present after application to abraded skin and the raw surface of a third-degree burn; there is no significant absorption from first- or second-degree burns. The agents that are most effective clinically are the least injurious locally but, unfortunately, have the greatest systemic toxicity.

The cornea is easily anesthetized by topical application of solutions of local anesthetics. The advantages of several synthetic compounds over cocaine for corneal anesthesia have already been described. Anesthetic agents may also be applied to the eye and mucous membranes in the form of ointments. However, chronic ophthalmic use of local anesthesia can permanently damage the corneal epithelium.

Infiltration Anesthesia. The purpose of this technic is to anesthetize nerve endings by their direct exposure to the drug. The solution may be injected into the papillary layer of the skin (intradermal). The onset of cutaneous anesthesia is almost immediate, and only small amounts of the anesthetic need be employed. Subcutaneous injection carries the anesthesia to a deeper level but allows for greater absorption. A short interval is required before the onset of anesthesia. After the skin is anesthetized, the deeper structures may be infiltrated if such is required by the surgical procedure. A type of infiltration commonly employed is known as *ring block*. In this procedure the anesthetic is infiltrated subcutaneously in a circular manner around the field of operation, effectively blocking sensory nerves supplying the skin over the operative field. When ring block is employed to anesthetize the digits or penis, epinephrine should be avoided because of the possibility of producing ischemic necrosis.

Block Anesthesia. A variety of technics exist for interrupting conduction in the autonomic and somatic nervous system by local anesthetic drugs. These range from block of a single nerve (*e.g.,* occipital nerve) through various plexus blocks (brachial or celiac plexus) to epidural and spinal anesthesia. These technics can be used for surgical procedures as well as for diagnosis and therapy. Detailed discussion of the uses and technics of nerve block may be found in specialized textbooks (*see* Moore, 1965). A comprehensive discussion of the physiological events involved in nerve block has been presented by de Jong (1970).

Hyaluronidase and Carbonation in Surface, Infiltration, and Block Anesthesia. The enzyme hyaluronidase has been incorporated in local anesthetic solutions to facilitate distribution of the anesthetic agent. There is, however, a higher rate of systemic reactions to the anesthetic drugs when hyaluronidase is used. When it is employed in nerve blocks in which the anesthetic is confined within a fascial plane, the success rate is not increased. Use of hyaluronidase is no substitute for anatomical knowledge, skill, or experience. In addition, in certain blocks, spread of the anesthetic drug is undesirable;

for example, when hyaluronidase is used in blocking the stellate ganglion, there is an increased incidence of recurrent laryngeal nerve block. Because of the disadvantages of the agent as well as its cost, hyaluronidase is little used at present.

Equilibration of a local anesthetic amine with carbon dioxide produces the carbonic acid salt. Bromage (1967a) has reported that use of these carbonated solutions results in a shorter latent period, a decreased dose requirement, as well as an increased intensity and a slight prolongation of analgesia when compared with the conventional hydrochloride. Use of carbonated local anesthetics has not been widespread in the United States because of difficulties in obtaining the drugs commercially.

SPINAL ANESTHESIA

Sequence of Anesthesia and Site of Action. Following the intrathecal injection of a local anesthetic, there is a definite sequence in which nerve block is established. Sympathetic and parasympathetic nerves are affected first, followed by involvement of nerves mediating the sensations of cold, warmth, pain, touch, and deep pressure. Finally, somatic motor function, vibratory sense, and proprioception are blocked. As the anesthesia wears off, function is regained in the reverse order, motor activity being the first to be restored.

The site of action of a local anesthetic introduced into the spinal subarachnoid space is a matter of interest. Howarth (1949) and Cohen (1968) have demonstrated that radioactive local anesthetics are concentrated within spinal nerve roots as well as the posterior and lateral columns of the spinal cord. The observation that the border of analgesia may differ from the dorsolaterally slanting pattern that would result were the site of action at the nerve root alone provides further evidence that local anesthetics may act on structures inside the spinal cord (Urban, 1973). The site of action of minimally effective concentrations of procaine, which block sensory but not motor impulses, is the dorsal root ganglia (Frumin *et al.*, 1953). Thus, the onset of analgesia following the intrathecal administration of a local anesthetic drug depends upon passage of the drug from the spinal fluid into spinal nerve roots, ganglia, and possibly the spinal cord itself.

Duration of Anesthesia and Fate of Anesthetic Agents. The rate of enzymatic hydrolysis of local anesthetic agents by spinal fluid is slow. Studies with radioactive dibromoprocaine in animals indicate that the greatest portion leaves the subarachnoid space by way of the venous drainage and a much smaller portion by way of lymphatics (Howarth, 1949). The duration of anesthesia depends upon the rate at which the drug is removed from the cerebrospinal fluid and from the nerve roots where it exerts its action.

The average duration of anesthesia with commonly used drugs is 60 minutes with procaine, 120 minutes with tetracaine, and even longer with bupivacaine, but the range is considerable and unpredictable. Duration of anesthesia can be lengthened somewhat by increasing the concentration of anes-

thetic agent in the injected solution, further extended by the addition of a vasoconstrictor drug to the anesthetic solution, and maintained essentially indefinitely by the use of continuous spinal anesthesia (*see* below).

The effect of a vasoconstrictor drug in the subarachnoid space is to retard the rate of removal of the local anesthetic. Analysis of the cerebrospinal fluid for local anesthetic drugs shows a higher concentration following the use of epinephrine. This results in a greater amount of the drug being initially available for entrance into neural tissue and offers at least some explanation for the prolongation of anesthesia. Epinephrine (0.2 to 0.5 mg) and phenylephrine (3 to 10 mg) are effective. Systemic actions are not apparent after the intrathecal administration of a sympathomimetic vasoconstrictor, nor is there any evidence that neural tissue is adversely affected.

Level of Anesthesia. Local anesthetics are usually injected into the subarachnoid space between the conus medullaris and the terminal portion of the subarachnoid space, in order to avoid injury to the spinal cord. In the adult, therefore, the injection is ordinarily made through one of the vertebral interspaces between the second and fifth lumbar levels. Obviously upward diffusion of the anesthetic agent must take place in order to obtain extensive sensory blockade, and the topography of the anesthetized area depends upon the extent of this diffusion. The upward passage of an anesthetic agent in the subarachnoid space depends upon many factors, among them being the position of the patient, the specific gravity of the injected solution, the natural curvature of the spine, movements or coughing by the patient, and the size of the subarachnoid space. The last-named factor appears to be increased by anything that raises intra-abdominal pressure, such as pregnancy at term, obesity, ascites, or a large ovarian cyst.

Specific Gravity. The specific gravity of solutions of local anesthetics can be varied by changing their composition. The specific gravity of normal cerebrospinal fluid is approximately 1.007. An anesthetic solution with a specific gravity higher than that of spinal fluid is known as a *hyperbaric* solution. This is often achieved by the addition of glucose. Conversely, by dissolving local anesthetics in hypotonic solutions of sodium chloride or in distilled water, it is possible to obtain a *hypobaric* solution.

Position of the Patient. Many anesthesiologists partially regulate the level of spinal anesthesia by relating the position of the patient (or given portions of his vertebral column) to the specific gravity of the anesthetic solution. Flexing the legs on the hips minimizes the normal lumbar lordosis. If this maneuver is carried out for 2 to 3 minutes after the injection of the local anesthetic, there is less cephalad spread of the drug (Smith, 1968). Finally, if a low level of anesthesia is sought, the patient should sit up during the injection of a hyperbaric solution and for 5 minutes thereafter, or the patient should be in the recumbent head-down position during the injection of a hypobaric solution.

Other Factors. The role of the volume of solution injected, the concentration of the local anesthetic drug, and the rate of injection in determining the level and duration of block is difficult to determine. Most statements relating these factors are based mainly on impressions.

Respiration. With sensory blockade as high as T_2, arterial oxygen and carbon dioxide tensions remain unaltered (Askrog et al., 1964; de Jong, 1965; Ward et al., 1965). Similarly, spinal anesthesia with a thoracic sensory level does not impair gas exchange in either the obese or the emphysematous patient (Paskin et al., 1969). Due to the sparing of upper intercostal and diaphragmatic muscular activity, tidal volume and respiratory rate are not significantly affected. However, functions that depend upon the ability to inspire fully or to move air rapidly are affected. Vital capacity, maximal breathing capacity, expiratory reserve volume, forced expiratory flow rates, and the ability to cough are decreased during spinal anesthesia (Freund et al., 1967; Paskin et al., 1969). The position of the patient (e.g., as in lateral decubitus position with flexion) and the placement of packs within the abdominal cavity during operation may reduce pulmonary exchange during spinal anesthesia.

Extreme hypotension during spinal anesthesia may result in inadequate medullary blood flow; this, in turn, can produce respiratory arrest. Such arrest is not caused by direct action of the local anesthetic on the medulla, since an injection of 1 ml of 5% or 0.5 ml of 10% procaine solution into the fourth ventricle of dogs has no effect upon respiration. Often, respiratory arrest is caused by motor-nerve paralysis. The anesthesiologist must therefore be constantly on the alert to ascertain how high motor paralysis has extended. It may even be as long as 50 minutes before the anesthetic has become "fixed" and the level constant. Signs of impending respiratory paralysis are diminution of thoracic respiration with increasing diaphragmatic excursions, whispering followed by loss of spoken voice, dilatation of the alae nasi, and use of the accessory muscles of respiration. A failing respiration during spinal anesthesia calls for immediate use of artificial ventilation.

The incidence of postoperative pneumonia and atelectasis has been found to be the same following either spinal or general anesthesia. The major determinant of this complication is the type of operative procedure undertaken and not the method of anesthesia.

Cardiovascular System. Following the intrathecal injection of a local anesthetic in a concentration sufficient to produce nerve block, profound circulatory changes occur. Arterial blood pressure, cardiac output and index, stroke volume, arterial pressure, pulmonary arterial pressure, total peripheral resistance, and left ventricular work decrease (Ward et al., 1965). These changes are variable and unpredictable, although in general they are roughly proportional to the area of anesthesia. Cardiac rate may decrease.

Spinal anesthesia results in arteriolar dilatation in those vascular beds to which sympathetic efferent fibers have been blocked. A blockade of tonic constrictor impulses to veins can cause decreased venous tone, postarteriolar pooling of blood, and diminished venous return to the heart. These effects will contribute to a decrease in systolic pressure by reducing stroke volume and cardiac output. Compensatory reflexes effect vasoconstriction in unanesthetized areas. The position of the patient (head-up tilt, prone-jackknife) or the presence of packs and retractors in the abdominal cavity or weight of the gravid uterus on the great veins may also compromise venous return and produce arterial hypotension. These changes may not be as great in the young individual whose vessels may have considerable autonomy and who may have increased ability to compensate for regional sympathetic blockade. Hypotension may occur when a spinal anesthetic is given in the presence of hypovolemia. The final circulatory status will depend, then, upon the relative contributions of each of the above variables. The subject of circulatory changes during spinal anesthesia has been reviewed by Greene (1970).

Prophylaxis and Treatment of Arterial Hypotension. A rational approach to the prevention or therapy of the hypotension caused by spinal anesthesia may be derived from a consideration of the mechanisms already discussed. Decreased venous return may be restored toward normal by elevation of the legs; one may wrap the legs in elastic bandages prior to the administration of a spinal anesthetic in order to prevent pooling in this area. The rapid infusion of intravenous fluids will fill a dilated vascular bed and result in a more adequate venous return.

Sympathomimetic amines may be given intramuscularly 5 minutes before the local anesthetic is injected into the subarachnoid space to minimize hypotension, or intravenously once hypotension has developed. A variety of drugs has been used, and each has its proponents. Ephedrine, phenylephrine, hydroxyamphetamine, and methoxamine have proven of value. In treating the hypotension that may accompany spinal anesthesia, the clinician must consider the effects of drugs on regional circulation. For example, methoxamine, metaraminol, and ephedrine will all return arterial pressure to normal in the pregnant female at term when spinal anesthesia has produced hypotension. However, ephedrine will have the most beneficial effect in restoring uterine blood flow to normal and assuring a favorable acid-base status in the fetus (Shnider et al., 1968, 1970).

Regional Circulation. *Brain.* The cerebral circulation has a high degree of autonomy. Sympathetic innervation plays little or no role in its control, and cerebral blood flow tends to remain constant over a wide range of arterial blood pressure. However, marked hypotension during spinal anesthesia may result in insufficient blood being delivered through the cerebral circulation, particularly in patients with hypertension or atherosclerosis. If symptoms of cerebral hypoxia (nausea, vomiting, syncope) occur as a result of arterial hypotension, they should be promptly treated.

Heart. Hypotension produced by spinal anesthesia in man and experimental animals causes a parallel reduction in both coronary blood flow and myocardial work. Thus, there tends to be little or no change in coronary sinus oxygen saturation (Hackel et al., 1956).

Kidney. During spinal anesthesia, as in an unanesthetized man, if arterial blood pressure is lowered sufficiently, renal blood flow and urinary output will be diminished; sufficient blood will still perfuse the kidney to support its metabolism, and, therefore, the effects are transient in nature. Renal function will be restored to normal when blood pressure rises as the effects of the spinal anesthetic cease. If blood pressure is markedly lowered, insufficient renal perfusion may result in postoperative renal shutdown. (*See* Papper et al., 1950; Greene et al., 1954.)

Liver. The hepatic effects of spinal anesthesia in man not undergoing operation or receiving vasopressor drugs are of interest. Estimated hepatic blood flow was reduced by 25% if the sensory level was below T_4 and by 33% if the level was above T_4. At the same time, changes in splanchnic vascular resistance were not seen and it was concluded that the lowered hepatic blood flow was secondary to arterial hypotension. Despite the lowered hepatic blood flow, changes in hepatic oxygen consumption were not observed (Mueller et al., 1952). Increased retention of BSP in the postoperative period following a spinal anesthetic has been noted by many workers. Greene and coworkers (1954) could find no correlation between excretion of BSP and the degree of hypotension produced by the spinal anesthetic. A variety of tests of hepatic function on the first, third, and fifth postoperative days showed significant abnormalities in BSP retention (first postoperative day) and urine urobilinogen (fifth postoperative day). These results do not differ appreciably from those found in patients with similar operations conducted under cyclopropane, ether, or nitrous oxide–ether anesthesia (French et al., 1952). It may therefore be concluded that these abnormalities, unrelated to the duration of anesthesia, are a manifestation of the "stress" of operation rather than a result of the anesthetic agent used.

Effects on Other Organs. *Adrenal.* The effect of spinal anesthesia and the surgical procedure upon adrenocortical function as judged by plasma 17-hydroxycorticosteroid levels has been studied. An increase was not seen either following the administration of the anesthetic (Oyama and Matsuki, 1970) or during the operation (Vandam and Moore, 1960). In the postoperative period, however, plasma corticosteroids rose to values found after operations conducted under general anesthesia. Normally, the increase in plasma corticosteroids seen after operations is due to afferent nerve impulses arising from the site of operation that enter the CNS. Complete isolation of the operative site from the CNS by spinal anesthesia may be responsible for the failure of plasma corticosteroids to increase during operation.

Gastrointestinal Tract. The sympathetic denervation produced by spinal anesthesia causes contraction of the bowel due to unopposed parasympathetic action. Although perforation of a weakened area of bowel could theoretically result, such an event must be very rare. The nausea and vomiting that sometimes occur during spinal anesthesia may be due to increased gastric motility; if such symptoms occur, one must be certain that this, rather than cerebral hypoxia (*see* above), is the cause.

Neurological Complications. Neurological complications may follow lumbar puncture, injection of a local anesthetic agent into the subarachnoid space, or such unrelated factors as improper positioning of the patient during the operative procedure. *Trauma* occurring during a lumbar puncture can involve the ligaments, periosteum, annulus fibrosis, perivertebral plexus of veins, meninges, nerve roots, or spinal cord. *Leakage of cerebrospinal fluid* can result in headache or visual and auditory symptoms (syndrome of decreased intracranial pressure). The *cauda equina syndrome* may follow a spinal anesthetic. Inasmuch as the nerves involved are those exposed to the highest concentration of local anesthetic, the lesion may be attributed to a direct toxic action of the drug on nerve tissue. The signs and symptoms of the cauda equina syndrome consist in a loss of control of the sphincters of the bladder and bowel and varying degrees of sensory and motor disturbance in the lower extremities. Recovery may occur slowly or not at all. Another grave complication is *chronic progressive adhesive arachnoiditis* in which there is progressive proliferation of the pia-arachnoid. Eventually, the subarachnoid space may be completely obliterated and circulation to the spinal cord seriously compromised. This entity often begins with involvement of the lumbosacral cord and progresses to thoracic, phrenic, and bulbar dysfunction, resulting in death. Bacterial contamination may result in septic meningitis.

An extensive prospective study of 10,098 spinal anesthetics administered between 1948 and 1951 to 8460 patients who were then carefully followed for at least 6 months (some for over 5 years) has been made; major neurological sequelae did not occur in this group of patients. In the many patients similarly anesthetized during the subsequent 13 years at the Hospital of the University of Pennsylvania, this finding still remained true. The study also analyzed in detail the incidence of minor neurological untoward effects and technics for their prevention. (*See* Dripps and Vandam, 1951, 1954; Vandam and Dripps, 1960.)

Advantages of Spinal Anesthesia. Every patient who is to undergo operation presents individual physiological and psychological characteristics that must be analyzed before a method of anesthesia is selected. In some circumstances, spinal anesthesia offers advantages. Analgesia and complete muscular relaxation can be produced, and the patient need not lose consciousness. For some individuals who fear "going to sleep" this last-named feature removes a source of apprehension.

Spinal anesthesia is useful in operations on the lower extremities, in rectal and perineal surgery, and in procedures such as transurethral resection of the prostate. The deliberate production of hypotension may be of value in aiding hemostasis.

Disadvantages of Spinal Anesthesia. Certain disadvantages (hypotension, neurological sequelae) have been discussed. Additional problems will now be considered. Nausea and vomiting may accompany spinal anesthesia and are apt to be caused by hypotension or by traction on viscera. Feelings of pain, nausea, vomiting, or an indescribable sensation of discomfort may occur with traction on or manipulation of intra-abdominal structures; these are very likely mediated by vagal afferents that are not blocked by the anesthetic. This discomfort may be minimized by the use of a narcotic analgesic as preanesthetic medication, but will not be completely eliminated. For this reason, it is usually best to supplement a spinal anesthetic with general anesthesia for surgery that involves intra-abdominal procedures.

Discomfort is caused by the presence of a tourniquet on the leg in the presence of skin analgesia up to the midabdomen. Loss of proprioception, inability to localize one's legs in space, and development of a "phantom" limb sensation have been described. The deafferentation produced by a high sensory level may be quite disagreeable to some patients. A difficulty inherent in both spinal and epidural anesthesia arises in the patient receiving anticoagulant therapy; in such an individual an epidural hematoma may follow injury to even a small vessel in the epidural space.

The principal disadvantage of the technic lies in its unpredictability. The level of spinal anesthesia is not controllable, and its duration of action is variable. Indeed, there are a certain number of cases in which analgesia fails to develop at all, probably because the drug is not deposited in the subarachnoid space.

Continuous Spinal Anesthesia. The objective of continuous spinal anesthesia is to overcome some of the disadvantages of single-dose spinal anesthesia, namely, the failure of the single-dose method to produce the level, degree, and duration of anesthesia desired. This is accomplished by leaving a needle or catheter within the spinal subarachnoid space. In this manner, both the extent and the duration of spinal anesthesia become more controllable through the ability to inject fractional repeated doses of the anesthesic agent. A local anesthetic of short duration, such as procaine, can be used to increase controllability further. There are a number of disadvantages of this technic. Tachyphylaxis is seen sometimes, and may result from acidification of cerebrospinal fluid by the local anesthetic (*see* Cohen *et al.,* 1968). The effect of prolonged contact of anesthetic solutions with nervous tissue might be expected to increase the incidence of nerve injury. This has not proven to be the case. The danger of infection, irritation, or direct injury from the continuous presence of the spinal needle or catheter is a challenge to careful technic. Finally, the most significant disadvantage of continuous spinal anesthesia is the necessity for a large-gauge needle through which the catheter must be placed. This results in an increased incidence of symptoms related to reduced cerebrospinal fluid pressure.

Epidural Anesthesia. Epidural anesthesia is an extensive block anesthesia produced by injecting a local anesthetic into the epidural space. With this technic, sensory anesthesia extending as high as the chin can be produced. A single dose of the local anesthetic may be administered or a continuous technic may be used.

Technic. Segmental epidural anesthesia may be performed by introducing the needle through any interspace. In carrying out lumbar epidural anesthesia, the usual procedure is to enter the space below the level of L_2. The entrance of the needle can be conveniently detected by a number of methods inasmuch as a negative pressure exists in the epidural space. After a "test dose" of 2 to 3 ml to determine if inadvertent subarachnoid puncture has been made, the anesthetic solution is slowly administered.

Epinephrine, when used to prolong duration of anesthesia, has no effect on the spread of analgesia but does increase both its duration and intensity (Bromage *et al.,* 1964). Sympathetic block may be produced with 0.5 to 1.0% lidocaine solution, while 1.0 to 1.5% lidocaine solution will cause sensory loss. Motor blockade will result from the injection of 2% lidocaine solution.

Action of Local Anesthetics in the Epidural Space. Epidural anesthesia derives its name from the site of injection rather than from the site of nerve block. Within the epidural space the spinal nerves are covered with a thick layer of dura, and it is not until the nerves leave the intervertebral foramina that this protection is lost. It is likely that after epidural injection the local anesthetic solution diffuses along the perineural lymphatics to leave the epidural space at the intervertebral foramina and to block the spinal nerves outside of the spinal canal. Thus, epidural anesthesia may be an extensive paravertebral block. However, it has been shown that, following the introduction of procaine into the epidural space in the usual anesthetic dose, a significant concentration is achieved in the spinal fluid (Frumin *et al.,* 1953). Since a local anesthetic can pass from the epidural to the subarachnoid space, perhaps through the arachnoid villi, this also must be considered a mechanism of epidural anesthesia. It has been possible to demonstrate the presence of radioactive lidocaine and mepivacaine in the thoracic and lumbosacral spinal cord after epidural injection. Lesser amounts have been seen within the cervical cord and the medulla (Bromage, 1967b). Furthermore, it has been demonstrated that the concentration of chloroprocaine in the spinal fluid is three times higher at the end of anesthesia than at its onset (Foldes *et al.,* 1956). An excellent review relating the anatomy of the epidural space to the site of action of epidural anesthesia is that of Shantha and Evans (1972).

In *summary,* the site of action of local anesthetic agents placed in the epidural space is not completely known but may include: (1) mixed nerves in paravertebral spaces, (2) dura-covered nerve roots within the epidural space, (3) subarachnoid nerve roots after drug diffusion across the dura, and (4) the neuraxis itself.

The diffusion of a local anesthetic along the spinal epidural space and its egress through the many intervertebral foramina or through the dura into the subarachnoid space are relatively slow processes, and for this reason there is an appreciable latent period between the injection and the onset of anesthesia. Complete surgical anesthesia may require 15 to 30 minutes to develop.

Evaluation of Epidural Anesthesia. Epidural anesthesia possesses most of the advantages of spinal anesthesia with many of its disadvantages. Its main advantage lies in the fact that the subarachnoid space is not entered. Thus, headache and other neurological sequelae of spinal anesthesia are avoided. Segmental anesthesia is more predictable with epidural anesthesia. Difficulty in technic and a latent period considerably longer than that observed with spinal anesthesia constitute disadvantages of epidural anesthesia. Another major disadvantage is the large amount of drug that must be employed; therefore, systemic absorption of the agent may be significant. The somnolence often seen when lidocaine is used may be due to this absorption. The effects on respiration are similar to those produced by spinal anesthesia (Ward *et al.,* 1965). There is also inability to block discomfort from visceral manipulation.

Circulatory effects of epidural anesthesia are complex and may differ somewhat from alterations following subarachnoid block. These reflect the effects not only of sympathetic blockade but also of reflex responses, as well as possibly direct peripheral effects of the local anesthetic and of epinephrine if it is present in the injection solution. Bonica and associates (1970) found that, when lidocaine alone produced epidural anesthesia to T_4 or below, mean arterial blood pressure (MABP), cardiac output (CO), and total peripheral resistance (TPR) did not change. When the same agent produced blockage to a level of T_{2-3}, MABP and CO increased by 5 and 23%, respectively, while TPR decreased by 15%. Blockade to the T_1 dermatome or higher produced a decrease of 16% in MABP and 19% in TPR, while CO was slightly greater than normal. In contrast, when anesthesia to the T_5 dermatome was produced by lidocaine with epinephrine (1:200,000), there was a 10% decrease in MABP, a 49% increase in CO, and a 37% decrease in TPR. These changes reflect β-adrenergic stimulation produced by the epinephrine. In the presence of hemorrhage, the sympathetic block produced by epidural anesthesia becomes extremely significant and may result in rapid and deleterious circulatory changes (Bonica *et al.,* 1972).

Caudal Anesthesia. Caudal anesthesia is a type of epidural anesthesia in which the anesthetic solution is introduced into the sacral canal through the sacral hiatus. The technic of injecting anesthetic solutions into the sacral canal is described by Moore (1965) and will not be considered here. The two outstanding dangers are (1) introducing the needle into the venous plexus lining the sacral canal, with the resultant intravascular injection of drug, and (2) penetrating the dura, with the development of a high level of spinal anesthesia. Usually a maximum of 30 ml of 1.0 to 1.5% lidocaine or mepivacaine in isotonic sodium chloride solution will suffice. Epi-

nephrine solution (1:100,000) is often added to the local anesthetic to delay systemic absorption.

Continuous Epidural Analgesia. Continuous epidural analgesia may be used for any procedure in which epidural analgesia is indicated and prolonged duration is sought. It may be administered by the lumbar or caudal route. It is of value in obstetrics in that sensory block of the uterus and relaxation of the perineum can be attained, often without significant disturbance to the rhythmic activity of the uterus or the tone of the abdominal muscles.

The visceral afferent fibers from the uterus are supplied by the eleventh and twelfth thoracic nerves; sensory fibers from the cervix and upper vagina travel in the sacral parasympathetic nerves; both the sensory and motor fibers of the lower vagina, perineum, and pelvic floor travel in the perineal and pudendal nerves, which arise from the lower somatic sacral nerves. Thus, an anesthetic solution in the sacral canal will block pain impulses from the birth canal and at the same time cause muscular relaxation in that area. If the anesthetic solution rises in the epidural space to the level of T_{11} and T_{12}, impulses arising from uterine contractions are blocked. On the other hand, autonomic efferent motor nerves to the body of the uterus arise for the most part from the fifth to tenth thoracic segments. Thus, it is possible for an anesthetic agent to block all sensory impulses from the uterus without interfering seriously with motor activity, provided the agent does not ascend in the epidural space above the level of T_{11}.

Evaluation. When properly performed, continuous epidural analgesia can obliterate the pain of labor. Moreover, it does not cause fetal depression if hypotension is avoided, a point of special importance in premature births. During the course of labor, patients are alert and cooperative, and do not tend to become exhausted. Manipulative procedures are facilitated by the relaxation produced; manual or forceps rotation is easily accomplished and delivery achieved as a rule with a minimum of trauma to mother and child. The method is useful for patients who have recently eaten.

The outstanding disadvantage of continuous epidural analgesia is the fact that the incidence of operative deliveries is greatly increased, because the analgesia removes the patient's incentive to "bear down." Furthermore, motor block of the abdominal and pelvic muscles interferes with internal rotation. Thus, there is an increased incidence of posterior positions and transverse arrests. This may be prevented by the use of a more dilute solution of the local anesthetic, which produces sensory but not motor blockade. Hypotension due to sympathetic block may occur; if this is not treated rapidly, fetal hypoxia may result. Although local anesthetics are rapidly absorbed from the epidural space and transmitted across the placenta to the fetus, umbilical venous concentration at birth is only one half that found in maternal arterial blood. Occasionally, however, a high fetal concentration of the drug is associated with mild depression of the newborn infant (*see* Shnider and Way, 1968). An extremely rare event is the accidental injection of the local anesthetic directly into the fetus; this results in apnea, bradycardia, and convulsions in the first minutes of life (Sinclair *et al.,* 1965).

OTHER TECHNICS FOR LOCAL ANESTHESIA

Intravenous Regional Anesthesia. The technic of producing surgical anesthesia by the intravenous injection of a local anesthetic into a limb whose circulation has been interrupted by a tourniquet was developed over 6 decades ago and still enjoys considerable popularity (Atkinson *et al.,* 1965). The site of action of the local anesthetic may be the nerve trunk (Raj *et al.,* 1972). A dose of 40 ml of 0.5% lidocaine or mepivacaine or 0.25% bupivacaine (*without epinephrine*) will suffice to produce intense analgesia in the adult arm. The low incidence of cardiovascular and CNS effects accompanying this technic is undoubtedly due to rapid tissue uptake of the drug from blood (Knapp, 1967). With intravenous regional anesthesia the concentration in the plasma is actually less than with conventional axillary block or lumbar epidural anesthesia. Furthermore, blood levels following release of the tourniquet are lower than those associated with CNS toxicity.

Therapeutic Nerve Block. A number of clinical conditions respond to nerve block. Appropriate sympathetic blocks are of use in the treatment of such entities as causalgia, the shoulder-hand syndrome, acute pancreatitis, acute arterial occlusion, and thrombophlebitis. Blocks of somatic afferent paths are used primarily to relieve pain. Symptomatic relief frequently outlasts the duration of action of the local anesthetic agent used. The explanation for this is unknown. Epidural or intercostal block may be used to provide analgesia in the postoperative period. This provides rapid restoration of normal pulmonary function (since coughing and deep breathing may be prevented by pain) and may have advantages over narcotic analgesics (Hollmen and Saukkonen, 1972; Holmdahl *et al.,* 1972; Bridenbaugh *et al.,* 1973).

Neurolytic drugs have been placed in the subarachnoid space primarily for relief of pain and spasticity. Such procedures demand extreme care for they are potentially hazardous. *Absolute alcohol* (0.4 to 0.5 ml) has a specific gravity of 0.806 and its site of action can be somewhat controlled by tilting the patient, the substance acting like a bubble in a carpenter's level. Injection is usually made in the lumbar region. Pain relief when obtained lasts for 6 weeks to 6 months.

Phenol (1.0 to 1.5 ml of 5 to 15% solution in glycerin or iophendylate) is also injected intrathecally. As usually given, it is hyperbaric (specific gravity, 1.250) and the patient is positioned accordingly. If 5% phenol is used, only pain sensation will be affected; touch, proprioception, and motor function will remain intact. More concentrated solutions can cause motor block. In the case of spasticity, motor block may indeed be of great use and is often sought intentionally (Maher, 1957).

ADDITIONAL USES OF LOCAL ANESTHETICS

Treatment of Cardiac Arrhythmias. The use of *lidocaine* in the treatment of ventricular arrhythmias is discussed in Chapter 32.

Supplementation of General Anesthesia. Lidocaine, in doses smaller than those that produce marked respiratory depression, suppresses coughing in response to an endotracheal tube. In contrast, thiopental and meperidine produce respiratory depression or apnea before coughing is stopped (Steinhaus and Gaskin, 1963). De Clive-Lowe and associates (1958) have combined lidocaine with a thiopental–nitrous oxide–succinylcholine anesthesia, claiming the following advantages: (1) less succinylcholine required to produce muscular relaxation and (2) decreased requirement for postoperative sedation and narcotic analgesics.

Use as an Intravenous Analgesic. Intravenous procaine has been used with success by some workers as an analgesic. However, the side effects of tachycardia, dyspnea, anxiety, and disorientation are considered by some to preclude its use. Keats and associates (1951) have concluded that, unless intravenous procaine can be demonstrated to produce significant beneficial effects on specific disease processes, it has no place in the treatment of pain. Yet, Gilbert and coworkers (1951) have had some success in treating the pain of malignancy by the use of 0.5% lidocaine solution given as an intravenous drip; in some patients pain relief persisted for 1 to 10 hours after cessation of drug administration.

Adriani, J., and Campbell, B. Fatalities following topical application of local anesthetics to mucous membranes. *J. Am. med. Ass.,* **1956**, *162,* 1527–1530.

Adriani, J.; Zepernick, R.; Arens, J.; and Authement, E. The comparative potency and effectiveness of topical anesthetics in man. *Clin. Pharmac. Ther.,* **1964**, *5,* 49–62.

Ariëns, E. J., and Simonis, A. M. pH and drug action. *Archs int. Pharmacodyn. Thér.,* **1963**, *141,* 309–330.

Askrog, V. F.; Smith, T. C.; and Eckenhoff, J. E. Changes in pulmonary ventilation during spinal anesthesia. *Surgery Gynec. Obstet.,* **1964**, *119,* 563–567.

Atkinson, D. I.; Modell, J.; and Moya, F. Intravenous regional anesthesia. *Anesth. Analg. curr. Res.,* **1965**, *44,* 313–317.

Baird, W. M., and Hardman, H. F. An analysis of the effect of pH, procaine cation, nonionized procaine and procaine ethylchloride cation upon cardiac conduction time, stimulation threshold, amplitude of contraction and the relationship of these parameters to antiarrhythmic activity. *J. Pharmac. exp. Ther.,* **1961**, *132,* 382–391.

Blaustein, M. P., and Goldman, D. E. Competitive action of calcium and procaine on lobster axon. *J. gen. Physiol.,* **1966**, *49,* 1043–1063.

Bonica, J. J.; Berges, P. U.; and Morikawa, K. I. Circulatory effects of peridural block. I. Effects of level of analgesia and dose of lidocaine. *Anesthesiology,* **1970**, *33,* 619–626.

Bonica, J. J.; Kennedy, W. F., Jr.; Akamatsu, T. J.; and Gerbershagen, H. U. Circulatory effects of peridural block. III. Effects of acute blood loss. *Anesthesiology,* **1972**, *36,* 219–227.

Boyes, R. N.; Scott, D. B.; Jebson, P. J.; Godman, M. J.; and Julian, D. G. Pharmacokinetics of lidocaine in man. *Clin. Pharmac. Ther.,* **1971**, *12,* 105–116.

Bridenbaugh, P. O.; DuPen, S. L.; Moore, D. C.; Bridenbaugh, L. D.; and Thompson, G. E. Postoperative intercostal nerve block analgesia versus narcotic analgesia. *Anesth. Analg. curr. Res.,* **1973,** *52,* 81–85.

Brodie, B. B.; Lief, P. A.; and Poet, R. The fate of procaine in man following its intravenous administration and methods for the estimation of procaine and diethylaminoethanol. *J. Pharmac. exp. Ther.,* **1948,** *94,* 359–366.

Bromage, P. R. Improved conduction blockage in surgery and obstetrics: carbonated local anesthetics. *Can. med. Ass. J.,* **1967a,** *97,* 1377–1384.

Bromage, P. R.; Burfoot, M. F.; Crowell, D. E.; and Pettigrew, R. T. Quantity of epidural blockage. I. Influence of physical factors. *Br. J. Anaesth.,* **1964,** *36,* 342–352.

Campbell, D., and Adriani, J. Absorption of local anesthetics. *J. Am. med. Ass.,* **1958,** *168,* 873–877.

Cherney, L. S. Tetracaine hydroiodide: a long-lasting local anesthetic agent for the relief of pain. *Anesth. Analg. curr. Res.,* **1963,** *42,* 477–481.

Cohen, E. N. Distribution of local anesthetic agents in the neuraxis of the dog. *Anesthesiology,* **1968,** *29,* 1002–1005.

Cohen, E. N.; Levine, D. A.; Colliss, J. E.; and Gunther, R. E. The role of pH in the development of tachyphylaxis to local anesthetic agents. *Anesthesiology,* **1968,** *29,* 994–1001.

De Clive-Lowe, S. G.; Desmond, J.; and North, J. Intravenous lignocaine anesthesia. *Anesthesiology,* **1958,** *13,* 138–146.

Deguchi, T., and Narahashi, T. Effects of procaine on ionic conductances of end-plate membranes. *J. Pharmac. exp. Ther.,* **1971,** *176,* 424–433.

de Jong, R. H. Arterial carbon dioxide and oxygen tensions during spinal block. *J. Am. med. Ass.,* **1965,** *191,* 698–702.

de Jong, R. H., and Heavner, J. E. Diazepam prevents local anesthetic seizures. *Anesthesiology,* **1971,** *34,* 523–531.

Douglas, W. W., and Ritchie, J. M. Mammalian nonmyelinated nerve fibers. *Physiol. Rev.,* **1962,** *42,* 297–334.

Dripps, R. D., and Vandam, L. D. Hazards of lumbar puncture. *J. Am. med. Ass.,* **1951,** *147,* 1118–1121.

———. Long-term follow-up of patients who received 10,098 spinal anesthetics: failure to discover major neurological sequelae. *Ibid.,* **1954,** *156,* 1486–1491.

Feinstein, M. B. Inhibition of contraction and calcium exchangeability in rat uterus by local anesthetics. *J. Pharmac. exp. Ther.,* **1966,** *152,* 516–524.

Foldes, F. F.; Colavincenzo, J. W.; and Birch, J. H. Epidural anesthesia: a reappraisal. *Curr. Res. Anesth. Analg.,* **1956,** *35,* 33–47.

Frank, G. B., and Sanders, H. D. A proposed common mechanism of action for general and local anesthetics in the central nervous system. *Br. J. Pharmac. Chemother.,* **1963,** *21,* 1–9.

Franz, D. N., and Perry, R. S. Mechanisms for differential block among single myelinated and non-myelinated axons by procaine. *J. Physiol., Lond.,* **1974,** *236,* 193–210.

French, A. B.; Barss, T. P.; Fairlie, C. S.; Bengle, A. L., Jr.; Jones, C. M.; Linton, R. R.; and Beecher, H. K. Metabolic effects of anesthesia in man. V. A comparison of the effects of ether and cyclopropane anesthesia on the abnormal liver. *Ann. Surg.,* **1952,** *135,* 145–163.

Freund, F. G.; Bonica, J. J.; Ward, R. J.; Akamatsu, T. J.; and Kennedy, W. F., Jr. Ventilatory reserve and level of motor block during high spinal and epidural anesthesia. *Anesthesiology,* **1967,** *28,* 834–837.

Frumin, M. J.; Schwartz, H.; Burns, J. J.; Brodie, B. B.; and Papper, E. M. The appearance of procaine in the spinal fluid during peridural block in man. *J. Pharmac. exp. Ther.,* **1953,** *109,* 102–105.

Gasser, H. S., and Erlanger, J. The role of fiber size in the establishment of a nerve block by pressure or cocaine. *Am. J. Physiol.,* **1929,** *88,* 581–591.

Gilbert, C. R. A.; Hanson, I. R.; Brown, A. B.; and Hingson, R. A. Intravenous uses of XYLOCAINE. *Curr. Res. Anesth. Analg.,* **1951,** *30,* 301–313.

Gordon, H. R. Fetal bradycardia after paracervical block: correlation with fetal and maternal blood levels of local anesthetic (mepivacaine). *New Engl. J. Med.,* **1968,** *279,* 910–914.

Greene, N. M.; Bunker, J. P.; Kerr, W. S.; Felsinger, J. M. von; Keller, J. W.; and Beecher, H. K. Hypotensive spinal anesthesia: respiratory, metabolic, hepatic, renal, and cerebral effects. *Ann. Surg.,* **1954,** *140,* 641–651.

Hackel, D. B.; Sancetta, S. M.; and Kleinerman, J. Effect of hypotension due to spinal anesthesia on coronary blood flow and myocardial metabolism in man. *Circulation,* **1956,** *13,* 92–97.

Harvey, A. M. The actions of procaine on neuromuscular transmission. *Bull. Johns Hopkins Hosp.,* **1939,** *65,* 223–238.

Henderson, R.; Ritchie, J. M.; and Strichartz, G. R. The binding of labelled saxitoxin to the sodium channels in nerve membranes. *J. Physiol., Lond.,* **1974,** *235,* 789–804.

Hirst, G. D. S., and Wood, D. R. On the neuromuscular paralysis produced by procaine. *Br. J. Pharmac.,* **1971,** *41,* 94–104.

Hollmen, A., and Saukkonen, J. The effects of postoperative epidural analgesia versus centrally acting opiate on physiological shunt after upper abdominal operation. *Acta anaesth. scand.,* **1972,** *16,* 147–154.

Holmdahl, M. H.; Sjorgren, S.; Strom, G.; and Wright, B. Clinical aspects of continuous epidural blockade for postoperative pain relief. *Upsala J. med. Sci.,* **1972,** *77,* 47–56.

Howarth, F. Studies with a radioactive spinal anesthetic. *Br. J. Pharmac. Chemother.,* **1949,** *4,* 333–347.

Inoue, F., and Frank, G. B. Action of procaine on frog skeletal muscle. *J. Pharmac. exp. Ther.,* **1962,** *136,* 190–196.

Jaanus, S. D.; Miele, E.; and Rubin, R. P. The analysis of the inhibitory effect of local anesthetics and propranolol on adrenomedullary secretion evoked by calcium or acetylcholine. *Br. J. Pharmac. Chemother.,* **1967,** *31,* 319–330.

Keats, A. S.; D'Alessandro, G. L.; and Beecher, H. K. A controlled study of pain relief by intravenous procaine. *J. Am. med. Ass.,* **1951,** *147,* 1761–1763.

Keenaghan, J. B., and Boyes, R. N. The tissue distribution, metabolism and excretion of lidocaine in rats, guinea pigs, dogs and man. *J. Pharmac. exp. Ther.,* **1972,** *180,* 454–463.

Klingenström, P., and Westermark, L. Local effects of adrenaline and phenylalanyl-lysyl-vasopressin in local anaesthesia. *Acta anaesth. scand.,* **1963,** *7,* 131–137.

Knapp, R. B. Drug distribution following intravenous regional anesthesia. *J. Am. med. Ass.,* **1967,** *199,* 760–762.

Krahl, M. E.; Keltch, A. K.; and Clowes, G. H. A. The role of changes in extracellular and intracellular hydrogen ion concentration in the action of local anesthetic bases. *J. Pharmac. exp. Ther.,* **1940,** *68,* 330–350.

Maher, R. M. Neurone selection in relief of pain: further experiences with intrathecal injections. *Lancet,* **1957,** *1,* 16–19.

Matthews, P. B. C., and Rushworth, G. The relative sensitivity of muscle nerve fibres to procaine. *J. Physiol., Lond.,* **1957,** *135,* 263–269.

Metcalfe, J. C., and Burgen, A. S. V. Relaxation of anaesthetics in the presence of cyto-membranes. *Nature, Lond.,* **1968,** *220,* 587–588.

Moore, D. C., and Bridenbaugh, L. D. Oxygen: the antidote for systemic toxic reactions from local anesthetic drugs. *J. Am. med. Ass.,* **1960,** *174,* 842–847.

Mueller, R. P.; Lynn, R. B.; and Sancetta, S. M. Studies of hemodynamic changes in humans following induction of low and high spinal anesthesia. II. Changes in splanchnic blood flow, oxygen extraction and consumption and splanchnic vascular resistance in humans not undergoing surgery. *Circulation*, **1952**, *6*, 894–901.

Munson, E. S., and Wagman, I. H. Diazepam treatment of local anesthetic-induced seizures. *Anesthesiology*, **1972**, *37*, 523–528.

Narahashi, T., and Frazier, D. T. Site of action and active form of local anesthetics in nerve fibers. *Fedn Proc. Fedn Am. Socs exp. Biol.*, **1968**, *27*, 408.

Nathan, P. W., and Sears, T. A. Some factors concerned in differential nerve block by local anaesthetics. *J. Physiol., Lond.*, **1961**, *157*, 565–580.

Oyama, T., and Matsuki, A. Plasma levels of corticol in man during spinal anaesthesia and surgery. *Can. Anaesth. Soc. J.*, **1970**, *17*, 234–241.

Papper, E. M.; Habif, D. V.; and Bradley, S. E. Studies of renal and hepatic function in normal man during thiopental, cyclopropane, and high spinal anesthesia. *J. clin. Invest.*, **1950**, *29*, 838.

Paskin, S.; Rodman, T.; and Smith, T. C. The effect of spinal anesthesia on the pulmonary function of patients with chronic obstructive pulmonary disease. *Ann. Surg.*, **1969**, *169*, 35–41.

Plum, F.; Posner, J. B.; and Troy, B. Cerebral metabolic and circulatory responses to induced convulsions in animals. *Archs Neurol., Chicago*, **1968**, *18*, 1–13.

Raj, P. P.; Garcia, C. E.; Burleson, J. W.; and Jenkins, M. T. The site of action of intravenous regional anesthesia. *Anesth. Analg. curr. Res.*, **1972**, *51*, 776–786.

Ritchie, J. M., and Ritchie, B. R. Local anesthetics: effect of pH on activity. *Science, Wash.*, **1968**, *162*, 1394–1395.

Rosefsky, J. B., and Petersiel, M. E. Perinatal deaths associated with mepivacaine paracervical block anesthesia in labor. *New Engl. J. Med.*, **1968**, *278*, 530–533.

Selden, R., and Sasahara, A. A. Central nervous system toxicity induced by lidocaine: report of a case in a patient with liver disease. *J. Am. med. Ass.*, **1967**, *202*, 908–910.

Shanes, A. M. Drug and ion effects in frog muscle. *J. gen. Physiol.*, **1950**, *33*, 729–744.

———. Drugs and nerve conduction. *A. Rev. Pharmac.*, **1963**, *3*, 185–204.

Shantha, T. R., and Evans, J. A. The relationship of epidural anesthesia to neural membranes and arachnoid villi. *Anesthesiology*, **1972**, *37*, 543–557.

Shnider, S. M.; DeLorimer, A. A.; Holl, J. W.; Chapler, F. K.; and Morishima, H. O. Vasopressors in obstetrics. I. Correction of fetal acidosis with ephedrine during spinal hypotension. *Am. J. Obstet. Gynec.*, **1968**, *102*, 911–919.

Shnider, S. M.; DeLorimer, A. A.; and Steffenson, J. L. Vasopressors in obstetrics. III. Fetal effects of metaraminol infusion during obstetric spinal hypotension. *Am. J. Obstet. Gynec.*, **1970**, *108*, 1017–1022.

Shnider, S. M., and Way, E. L. Plasma levels of lidocaine (XYLOCAINE) in mother and newborn following obstetrical conduction anesthesia: clinical applications. *Anesthesiology*, **1968**, *29*, 951–958.

Sinclair, J. C.; Fox, H. A.; Lentz, J. F.; Fuld, G. L.; and Murphy, J. Intoxication of the fetus by a local anesthetic: a newly recognized complication of maternal caudal anesthesia. *New Engl. J. Med.*, **1965**, *273*, 1173–1177.

Skou, J. C. The effect of drugs on cell membranes with special reference to local anaesthetics. *J. Pharm. Pharmac.*, **1961**, *13*, 204–217.

Smith, T. C. The lumbar spine and subarachnoid block. *Anesthesiology*, **1968**, *29*, 60–64.

Steinhaus, J. E., and Gaskin, L. A study of intravenous lidocaine as a suppressant of cough reflex. *Anesthesiology*, **1963**, *24*, 285–290.

Straub, R. Effects of local anesthetics on resting potential of myelinated nerve fibres. *Experientia*, **1956**, *12*, 182–187.

Strichartz, G. R. The inhibition of sodium currents in myelinated nerve by quaternary derivatives of lidocaine. *J. gen. Physiol.*, **1973**, *62*, 37–57.

Tanaka, K. Anticonvulsant properties of procaine, cocaine, adiphenine and related structures. *Proc. Soc. exp. Biol. Med.*, **1955**, *90*, 192–195.

Taverner, D. The action of local anaesthetics on the spinal cord of the cat. *Br. J. Pharmac. Chemother.*, **1960**, *15*, 201–206.

Taylor, R. E. Effect of procaine on electrical properties of squid axon membrane. *Am. J. Physiol.*, **1959**, *196*, 1071–1078.

Urban, B. J. Clinical observations suggesting a changing site of action during induction and recession of spinal and epidural anesthesia. *Anesthesiology*, **1973**, *39*, 496–503.

Usubiaga, J. E.; Wikinski, J.; Ferrero, R.; Usubiaga, L. E.; and Wikinski, R. Local anesthetic-induced convulsions in man: an electroencephalographic study. *Anesth. Analg. curr. Res.*, **1966**, *45*, 611–620.

Vandam, L. D., and Dripps, R. D. Long-term follow-up of patients who received 10,098 spinal anesthetics. IV. Neurological disease incident to traumatic lumbar puncture during spinal anesthesia. *J. Am. med. Ass.*, **1960**, *172*, 1483–1487.

Vandam, L. D., and Moore, F. D. Adrenocortical mechanisms related to anesthesia. *Anesthesiology*, **1960**, *21*, 531–552.

Ward, R. J.; Bonica, J. J.; Freund, F. G.; Akamatsu, T.; Danziger, F.; and Englesson, S. Epidural and subarachnoid anesthesia: cardiovascular and respiratory effects. *J. Am. med. Ass.*, **1965**, *191*, 275–278.

Monographs and Reviews

Adriani, J. The clinical pharmacology of local anesthetics. *Clin. Pharmac. Ther.*, **1960**, *1*, 645–673.

Bernard, C. G., and Bohm, E. *Local Anesthetics as Anticonvulsants: A Study on Experimental and Clinical Epilepsy.* Almqvist & Wiksell, Stockholm, **1965**.

Bromage, P. R. Physiology and pharmacology of epidural analgesia. *Anesthesiology*, **1967b**, *28*, 592–622.

Büchi, J., and Perlia, X. Structure-activity relations and physicochemical properties of local anesthetics. In, *Local Anesthetics*, Vol. 1. *International Encyclopedia of Pharmacology and Therapeutics*, Sect. 8. (Lechat, P., ed.) Pergamon Press, Ltd., Oxford, **1971**, pp. 39–130.

de Jong, R. H. *Physiology and Pharmacology of Local Anesthesia.* Charles C Thomas, Pub., Springfield, Ill., **1970**.

Dripps, R. D.; Eckenhoff, J. E.; and Vandam, L. D. *Introduction to Anesthesia: The Principles of Safe Practice*, 4th ed. W. B. Saunders Co., Philadelphia, **1972**.

Geddes, I. C. A review of local anaesthetics. *Br. J. Anaesth.*, **1954**, *26*, 208–224.

Greene, N. N. *Physiology of Spinal Anesthesia*, 2nd ed. The Williams & Wilkins Co., Baltimore, **1970**.

Hansson, E. Absorption, distribution, metabolism and excretion of local anesthetics. In, *Local Anesthetics*, Vol. 1. *International Encyclopedia of Pharmacology and Therapeutics*, Sect. 8. (Lechat, P., ed.) Pergamon Press, Ltd., Oxford, **1971**, pp. 239–260.

Kao, C. Y. Tetrodotoxin, saxitoxin and their significance in the study of excitation phenomena. *Pharmac. Rev.*, **1966**, *18*, 997–1049.

———. Pharmacology of tetrodotoxin and saxitoxin. *Fedn Proc. Fedn Am. Socs exp. Biol.*, **1972**, *31*, 1117–1123.

Macintosh, R. R. *Lumbar Puncture and Spinal Analgesia.* The Williams & Wilkins Co., Baltimore, **1951**.

Moore, D. C. *Regional Block*, 4th ed. Charles C Thomas, Pub., Springfield, Ill., **1965**.

Mullins, L. J. Workshop on effects of anesthesia on metabolism and cellular functions. (Bunker, J. P., and Vandam, L. D., cochairmen.) *Pharmac. Rev.*, **1965**, *17*, 214–217.

Narahashi, T. Mechanism of action of tetrodotoxin and

saxitoxin on excitable membranes. *Fedn Proc. Fedn Am. Socs exp. Biol.,* **1972,** *31,* 1124–1132.

Narahashi, T., and Frazier, D. T. Site of action and active form of local anesthetics. *Neurosci. Res.,* **1971,** *4,* 65–99.

Ogura, Y. Fugu (puffer-fish) poisoning and the pharmacology of crystalline tetrodotoxin poisoning. In, *Neuropoisons: Their Pathophysiological Actions.* Vol. 1, *Poisons of Animal Origin.* (Simpson, L. L., ed.) Plenum Press, New York, **1971,** pp. 139–156.

Ritchie, J. M. The mechanism of action of local anesthetic agents. In, *Local Anesthetics,* Vol. 1. *International Encyclopedia of Pharmacology and Therapeutics,* Sect. 8. (Lechat, P., ed.) Pergamon Press, Ltd., Oxford, **1971,** pp. 131–166.

Ritchie, J. M., and Greengard, P. On the mode of action of local anesthetics. *A. Rev. Pharmac.,* **1966,** *6,* 405–430.

Schantz, E. J. Paralytic shellfish poisoning and saxitoxin. In, *Neuropoisons: Their Pathophysiological Actions.* Vol. 1, *Poisons of Animal Origin.* (Simpson, L. L., ed.) Plenum Press, New York, **1971,** pp. 159–168.

Shanes, A. M. Electrochemical aspects of physiological and pharmacological action in excitable cells. *Pharmac. Rev.,* **1958,** *10,* 59–273.

Zipf, H. F., and Dittmann, E. C. General pharmacological effects of local anesthetics. In, *Local Anesthetics,* Vol. 1. *International Encyclopedia of Pharmacology and Therapeutics,* Sect. 8. (Lechat, P., ed.) Pergamon Press, Ltd., Oxford, **1971,** pp. 191–238.

SECTION

IV

Drugs Acting at Synaptic and Neuroeffector Junctional Sites

CHAPTER

21 NEUROHUMORAL TRANSMISSION AND THE AUTONOMIC NERVOUS SYSTEM

George B. Koelle

The theory of *neurohumoral transmission* received direct experimental validation over half a century ago, and extensive investigation during the ensuing years has led to its general acceptance. The theory states that nerves transmit their impulses across most synapses and neuroeffector junctions by means of specific chemical agents known as *neurohumoral transmitters.* The actions of most drugs affecting smooth muscle and gland cells, the so-called autonomic drugs, can be interpreted in terms of their mimicking or modifying the actions of the neurohumoral transmitters released by the autonomic fibers at either the ganglia or the effector cells.

Most of the general principles concerning the *physiology* and *pharmacology* of the peripheral autonomic nervous system and its effector organs apply with certain modifications to the neuromuscular junctions of skeletal muscle also, and in a more limited sense to the central nervous system (CNS).

A clear understanding of the anatomy and physiology of the autonomic nervous system is essential to a study of the pharmacology of the *autonomic drugs.* One can often predict the actions of an autonomic agent on various organs of the body if the responses to nerve impulses are known.

ANATOMY AND GENERAL FUNCTIONS OF THE AUTONOMIC NERVOUS SYSTEM

The autonomic nervous system is also called the visceral, vegetative, or involuntary nervous system. Its peripheral representation consists of nerves, ganglia, and plexuses that provide the innervation to the heart, blood vessels, glands, viscera, and smooth muscles. It is therefore widely distributed throughout the body and controls the so-called automatic, or vegetative, functions.

Differences between Autonomic and Somatic Nerves. A major difference between autonomic and somatic nerves is that of the structures innervated. The motor nerves of the involuntary system supply all structures of the body except skeletal muscle, which is innervated by somatic nerves. The most distal synaptic junctions in the autonomic reflex arc occur in ganglia that are entirely outside of the cerebrospinal axis, whereas the synapses of somatic nerves are entirely within the CNS. Autonomic nerves form extensive peripheral plexuses, whereas such networks are absent from the somatic system. The motor nerves to skeletal muscles are myelinated, whereas the postganglionic autonomic nerves are generally nonmyelinated. When the cerebrospinal nerves are interrupted, the skeletal muscles that they innervate are completely paralyzed and undergo atrophy, whereas smooth muscles and glands generally show some level of automatic activity independent of intact innervation. There are, however, certain similarities between these two nervous systems, as will be described later.

Visceral Afferent Fibers. The *afferent* fibers from visceral structures are the first link in the *reflex arcs of the autonomic system.* With certain exceptions, such as axon reflexes, most visceral reflexes are mediated through the CNS. The afferents are, for the most part, nonmyelinated fibers and are carried into the cerebrospinal axis by the vagus, pelvic, splanchnic, and other autonomic nerves. For example, about four fifths of the vagal nerve fibers are sensory. Other autonomic afferents from blood vessels in skeletal muscles and from certain integumental structures are carried in the somatic nerves. The cell bodies of visceral afferent fibers lie in the dorsal root ganglia of the spinal nerves and in the corresponding sensory ganglia of certain cranial nerves, such as the nodose ganglion of the vagus. The *efferent* link of the autonomic reflex arc is discussed in the sections that follow.

The autonomic afferent fibers are concerned with the mediation of visceral sensation (including pain and referred pain); with vasomotor, respiratory, and viscerosomatic reflexes; and with the regulation of interrelated visceral activities. A special example of an autonomic afferent system is that arising from the pressoreceptive endings in the carotid sinus and the aortic arch, and from the chemoreceptor cells in the carotid and aortic bodies; this system is important in the reflex control of blood pressure, heart rate, and respiration, and its afferent fibers pass in the glossopharyngeal and vagus nerves to the medulla.

There are no important physiological differences between visceral and somatic afferent fibers, and their responses to drugs do not differ significantly. The clinical importance of such fibers arises especially in connection with the relief of visceral pain by surgery or by local anesthetic block.

Central Autonomic Connections. There are probably no purely autonomic or somatic centers of integration, and extensive overlap occurs. Somatic responses are always accompanied by visceral responses and *vice versa.* Autonomic reflexes can be elicited at the level of the *spinal cord.* They are clearly demonstrable in the spinal animal, including man, and are manifested in sweating, blood pressure alterations, vasomotor responses to temperature changes, and reflex emptying of the urinary bladder, rectum, and seminal vesicles. Extensive central ramifications of the autonomic nervous system exist above the level of the spinal cord. The integration of the control of blood pressure and respiration in the *medulla oblongata* is well known, but there are even higher levels of integration of autonomic func-

tions, especially in the hypothalamus and cortex. The *hypothalamus* is the principal locus of integration of the entire autonomic system and is concerned in the regulation of body temperature, water balance, carbohydrate and fat metabolism, blood pressure, emotions, sleep, and sexual reflexes. Much information concerning central integration of autonomic functions has come not only from physiological experimentation but also from clinical investigation of such syndromes as diabetes insipidus, dystrophia adiposogenitalis, narcolepsy, hypothermia, hyperthermia, and diencephalic autonomic epilepsy. The hypothalamic nuclei that lie posteriorly and laterally are sympathetic in their main connections, and their stimulation results in massive discharge of the sympathoadrenal system. Parasympathetic functions are evidently integrated by the midline nuclei in the region of the tuber cinereum and by nuclei lying anteriorly. The supraoptic nuclei are involved in water metabolism through their connections with the posterior lobe of the hypophysis. This hypothalamiconeurohypophyseal system represents a centrally located autonomic mechanism that exerts its peripheral effects on the kidney by means of the antidiuretic hormone (ADH). *Thalamic* and *striatal* levels of autonomic representation have not been sufficiently investigated; however, the neostriatum is probably concerned in the regulation of certain vegetative functions, as indicated clinically by the autonomic disturbances accompanying lesions in this region. The *cortex* provides another suprasegmental level of integration for sympathetic and parasympathetic functions. It is also a locus for correlation between somatic and vegetative functions, both sensory and motor. The activities of the cardiovascular, gastrointestinal, and many other systems are partially regulated at this highest level. Of considerable theoretical and potentially therapeutic interest are attempts to control blood pressure and other autonomic functions through conditioning initiated at a level of conscious effort (Miller *et al.,* 1970). Attention has also been focused on the importance of the *limbic* system, which includes the olfactory lobe, hippocampal formation, and the pyriform lobe, in the integration of emotional state with motor and visceral activities (*see* review by MacLean, 1970).

The actions of autonomic drugs on central nuclei, although poorly understood, are often prominent and may at times overshadow the peripheral effects (*e.g.,* scopolamine, dextroamphetamine, di*iso*propyl phosphorofluoridate, etc.). Likewise, nonautonomic drugs, the primary actions of which are to stimulate or depress the CNS, may exert important visceral effects (*e.g.,* phenothiazines, barbiturates, morphine, pentylenetetrazol, etc.). The central control of the peripheral vegetative system has been reviewed by Chase and Clemente (1968).

Divisions of the Peripheral Autonomic System. On the efferent or motor side, the autonomic nervous system consists of two large divisions: (1) the *sympathetic* or *thorocolumbar* outflow and (2) the *parasympathetic* or *craniosacral* outflow. Only the briefest outline of those anatomical features necessary for an understanding of the actions of autonomic drugs will be given here.

The arrangement of the principal parts of the peripheral autonomic nervous system is presented schematically in Figure 21-1. As will be discussed subsequently, the neurohumoral transmitter of all preganglionic autonomic fibers, all postganglionic parasympathetic fibers, and a few postganglionic sympathetic fibers is *acetylcholine* (ACh); these so-called *cholinergic fibers* are depicted in *blue.* The *adrenergic fibers,* shown in *red,* comprise the majority of the postganglionic sympathetic fibers; here the transmitter is *norepinephrine (noradrenaline, levarterenol).* The transmitter of the *primary afferent fibers,* shown in *green,* has not been identified conclusively. The terms *cholinergic* and *adrenergic* were proposed originally by Dale to describe neurons that liberate ACh and norepinephrine (at that time, "sympathin"), respectively. Subsequently, Dale (1954) suggested the terms *cholinoceptive* and *adrenoceptive* to denote postjunctional sites that are acted upon by the respective transmitters.

Sympathetic Nervous System. The cells that give rise to the *preganglionic fibers* of this divison lie mainly in the intermediolateral columns of the spinal cord and extend from the eighth cervical to the second or third lumbar segment. The axons from these cells are carried in the anterior nerve roots and synapse with neurons lying in sympathetic ganglia outside the cerebrospinal axis. The sympathetic ganglia comprise three groups—vertebral, prevertebral, and terminal.

The *vertebral sympathetic ganglia* consist of 22 pairs that lie on either side of the vertebral column to form the lateral chains. The ganglia are connected to each other by nerve trunks and to the spinal nerves by rami communicantes. The *white rami* are restricted to the segments of the thoracolumbar outflow; they carry the preganglionic myelinated fibers that issue from the spinal cord by way of the anterior spinal roots. The *gray rami* arise from the ganglia and carry postganglionic fibers back to the spinal nerves for distribution to sweat glands and pilomotor muscles, and to blood vessels of skeletal muscle and skin. The *prevertebral ganglia* lie in the abdomen and the pelvis near the ventral surface of the bony vertebral column, and consist mainly of the celiac (solar), superior mesenteric, aorticorenal, and inferior mesenteric ganglia. The *terminal ganglia* are few in number, lie near the organs that they innervate, and consist especially of those connected with the urinary bladder and rectum. In addition to the above ganglionic system, there are small *intermediate ganglia,* especially in the thoracolumbar region, that lie outside the conventional vertebral chain. They are variable in number and location, but are usually in close proximity to the communicating rami and the anterior spinal nerve roots. Since they are not readily accessible to surgical resection, their continued presence after conventional types of sympathectomy may explain some of the poor results after surgery and the apparent return of autonomic functions.

Postganglionic fibers issuing from sympathetic ganglia reach all the visceral structures of the thorax, abdomen, head, and neck. The trunk and the limbs are supplied by means of sympathetic fibers in spinal nerves, as previously described. The prevertebral ganglia contain cell bodies the axons of which innervate the glands and the smooth muscles of the abdominal and the pelvic viscera. Many of the upper thoracic sympathetic fibers from the vertebral ganglia form *terminal plexuses,* such as the cardiac, esophageal, and pulmonary. The sympathetic distribution to the head and the neck (vasomotor, pupillodilator, secretory, and pilomotor) is by way of the cervical sympathetic chain and its three ganglia. All postganglionic fibers in this chain arise from cell bodies located in these three ganglia; all preganglionic fibers arise from the upper thoracic segments of the spinal cord, there being no sympathetic fibers that leave the CNS above the first thoracic level. However, immunohistofluorescence studies have suggested the possibility that neurons situated along the fourth ventricle in the medulla and pons may be equivalent in origin and function to sympathetic ganglion cells and may innervate the cerebral vasculature (Hartman and Udenfriend, 1972).

Preganglionic fibers issuing from the spinal cord may synapse with the neurons of more than one sympathetic ganglion by means of collaterals issued en route. Their principal ganglia of termination need not correspond to the original level of issuance of the preganglionic fiber from the spinal cord. Many of the preganglionic fibers from the fifth to the last thoracic segment pass through the vertebral ganglia and form the *splanchnic nerves.* Most of the splanchnic nerve fibers do not synapse until they reach the celiac ganglion.

The *adrenal medulla* is embryologically, anatomically, and functionally homologous to the sympathetic ganglia, although the former differs in that the principal catecholamine it releases is *epinephrine (adrenaline).* The secretory chromaffin cells originate from the same region of the neural crest as do the sympathetic ganglion cells. Furthermore, the chromaffin cells are innervated by typical preganglionic fibers.

Parasympathetic Nervous System. This system consists of three outflows of preganglionic fibers from the CNS and their postganglionic connections. The regions of central origin are the midbrain, the medulla oblongata, and the sacral part of the spinal cord. The *midbrain* or tectal outflow consists of fibers arising from the Edinger-Westphal nucleus of the *third* cranial nerve and going to the ciliary ganglion in the orbit. The *medullary* outflow comprises the parasympathetic components of the seventh, ninth, and tenth cranial nerves. The fibers in the *facial* nerve form the chorda tympani, which innervates the ganglia lying on the submaxillary and sublingual glands. They also form the greater superficial petro-

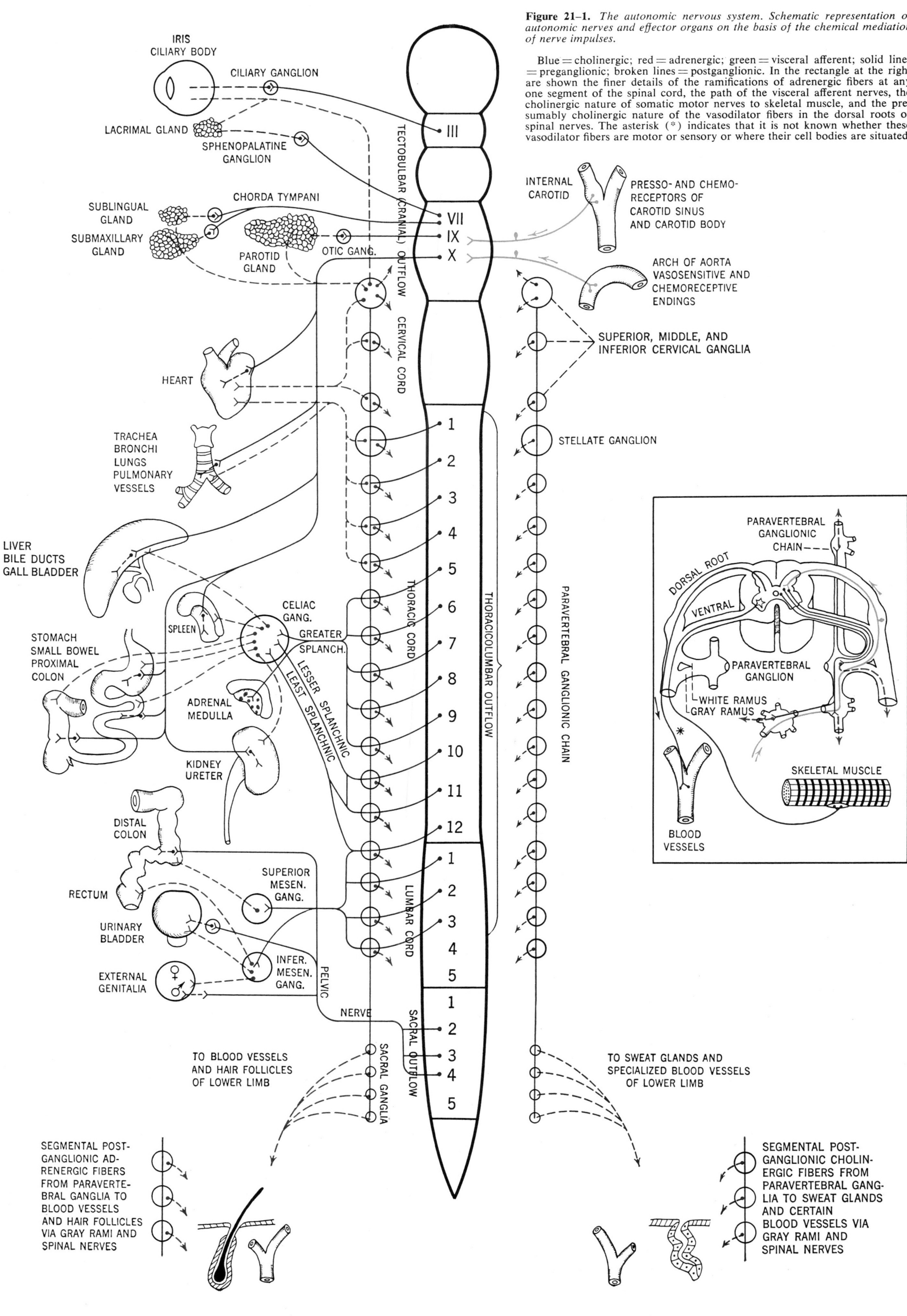

Figure 21–1. *The autonomic nervous system. Schematic representation of autonomic nerves and effector organs on the basis of the chemical mediation of nerve impulses.*

Blue = cholinergic; red = adrenergic; green = visceral afferent; solid lines = preganglionic; broken lines = postganglionic. In the rectangle at the right are shown the finer details of the ramifications of adrenergic fibers at any one segment of the spinal cord, the path of the visceral afferent nerves, the cholinergic nature of somatic motor nerves to skeletal muscle, and the presumably cholinergic nature of the vasodilator fibers in the dorsal roots of spinal nerves. The asterisk (*) indicates that it is not known whether these vasodilator fibers are motor or sensory or where their cell bodies are situated.

sal nerve, which contributes to the Vidian nerve innervating the sphenopalatine ganglion. The *glossopharyngeal* autonomic components innervate the otic ganglion. From the aforementioned peripheral ganglia, postganglionic parasympathetic fibers originate that supply the sphincter of the iris, the ciliary muscle, the salivary and lacrimal glands, and the mucous glands of the nose, mouth, and pharynx. These fibers also include vasodilator nerves to the organs mentioned. The *vagus* nerves arise in the medulla and contain preganglionic fibers, most of which do not synapse until they reach the many small ganglia lying directly on or in the viscera of the thorax and abdomen. In the intestinal wall, the vagal fibers terminate around ganglion cells in the plexuses of Auerbach and Meissner. The preganglionic fibers are thus very long and the postganglionic fibers quite short. The vagus nerve in addition carries a far greater number of afferent fibers (but apparently not pain fibers) from the viscera into the medulla; the cell bodies of these fibers lie mainly in the nodose ganglion. The *sacral* outflow consists of axons that arise from cells in the second, third, and fourth segments of the sacral cord and proceed as preganglionic fibers to form the pelvic nerves (nervi erigentes). They synapse in terminal ganglia lying near or within the bladder, rectum, and sexual organs. The vagal and sacral outflows provide motor, secretory, and vasodilator fibers to thoracic, abdominal, and pelvic organs, as indicated in Figure 21-1. The functions of these nerves are subsequently described.

Differences between Sympathetic and Parasympathetic Nerves. The *sympathetic system* is distributed to effectors throughout the body whereas the parasympathetic distribution is much more limited. Furthermore, the *sympathetic fibers* ramify to a much greater extent. A preganglionic sympathetic fiber may traverse a considerable distance of the sympathetic chain and pass through several ganglia before it finally synapses with a postganglionic neuron; also, its terminals make contact with a large number of postganglionic neurons. In some ganglia, the ratio of preganglionic axons to ganglion cells may be 1:20 or more. In this manner, a diffuse discharge of the sympathetic system is possible. In addition, there is an overlapping of synaptic innervation so that one ganglion cell is supplied by several preganglionic fibers.

The *parasympathetic system,* on the other hand, has its terminal ganglia very near to the organs innervated and thus is more discrete and limited in its discharge of impulses. In some organs, there appears to be a 1:1 relationship between the number of preganglionic and postganglionic fibers. On the other hand, the ratio of preganglionic vagal fibers to ganglion cells in Auerbach's plexus has been estimated as 1:8000. Hence, this distinction between the two systems does not apply to all sites.

Details of Innervation of Neurons and Effector Organs. Electron microscopic studies have added greatly to our knowledge of the detailed structure of synaptic and neuroeffector junctions. Of importance to the present topic is the correlation that can now be drawn, or postulated, between certain details of junctional ultrastructure and mechanisms of drug action.

Within the *CNS*, which has been most extensively studied to date, there are enormous variations in the types and numbers of presynaptic terminals, or boutons, that may impinge on the soma, dendrites, or axon hillock of a given neuron. It has been estimated for a *motoneuron* of the spinal cord that approximately four fifths of its surface is covered by several thousand presynaptic terminals. This has provided a dramatic demonstration of Sherrington's designation of such cells as the *final common pathway* of a vast complexity of excitatory and inhibitory impulses. Between the presynaptic and postsynaptic membranes is a space approximately 200 Å in width, the synaptic cleft, which is probably continuous with the limited volume of extracellular fluid and contains no interposed glial elements. Both membranes show at intervals apposed regions of increased opacity; at such regions the presynaptic axoplasm contains varying numbers of vesicular structures that are concentrated near the membrane. These "synaptic vesicles" are believed to contain the neurohumoral transmitter (*see* De Robertis, 1964; Gray, 1971).

The axon of each somatic *motoneuron* divides into many branches, each of which innervates a single muscle fiber, so that more than 100 muscle fibers may be supplied by one motoneuron to form a *motor unit.* At each neuromuscular junction, or *motor endplate,* the axonal terminal loses its myelin sheath and forms a terminal arborization that lies in an invagination of the sarcoplasmic membrane. Within the axonal terminal is a high density of mitochondria and a collection of synaptic vesicles concentrated near the membrane.

As was evident from earlier studies, the terminations of the *postganglionic autonomic fibers* at smooth muscle and gland cells show certain distinct differences from the foregoing pattern. In most autonomic effector organs, the innervation forms a rich plexus or terminal reticulum. The earlier literature has been reviewed critically by Hillarp (1959), according to whose interpretation, supported by subsequent histochemical and electron microscopic observations, the terminal reticulum is a triad. This consists of the final ramifications of the postganglionic sympathetic (adrenergic), parasympathetic (cholinergic), and visceral afferent fibers, all of which are enclosed within a frequently interrupted sheath of satellite or Schwann cells. At such interruptions, the efferent nerve fibers show varicosities that are packed with synaptic vesicles (Thaemert, 1963). Such junctions between a given axon and effector cell may occur at repeated intervals when the two course in close

Table 21-1. RESPONSES OF EFFECTOR ORGANS TO AUTONOMIC NERVE IMPULSES

EFFECTOR ORGANS	ADRENERGIC IMPULSES[1] Receptor Type	ADRENERGIC IMPULSES[1] Responses[2]	CHOLINERGIC IMPULSES[1] Responses[2]
Eye			
Radial muscle, iris	α	Contraction (mydriasis) + +	———
Sphincter muscle, iris		———	Contraction (miosis) + + +
Ciliary muscle	β	Relaxation for far vision (slight effect)	Contraction for near vision + + +
Heart			
S-A node	β[3]	Increase in heart rate + +	Decrease in heart rate; vagal arrest + + +
Atria	β[3]	Increase in contractility and conduction velocity + +	Decrease in contractility, and (usually) increase in conduction velocity + +
A-V node	β[3]	Increase in automaticity and conduction velocity + +	Decrease in conduction velocity; A-V block + + +
His-Purkinje system	β[3]	Increase in automaticity and conduction velocity + + +	Little effect
Ventricles	β[3]	Increase in contractility, conduction velocity, automaticity, and rate of idioventricular pacemakers + + +	Slight decrease in contractility claimed by some
Arterioles			
Coronary	α,β	Constriction +; dilatation[4] + +	Dilatation $\pm$
Skin and mucosa	α	Constriction + + +	Dilatation[5]
Skeletal muscle	α,β	Constriction + +; dilatation[6] + +	Dilatation[7] +
Cerebral	α	Constriction (slight)	Dilatation[5]
Pulmonary	α,β	Constriction +; dilatation[4]	Dilatation[5]
Abdominal viscera; renal	α,β	Constriction + + +; dilatation[6] +	———
Salivary glands	α	Constriction + + +	Dilatation + +
Veins (Systemic)	α	Constriction + +	———
Lung			
Bronchial muscle	β	Relaxation +	Contraction + +
Bronchial glands		Inhibition (?)	Stimulation + + +
Stomach			
Motility and tone	β	Decrease (usually)[8] +	Increase + + +
Sphincters	α	Contraction (usually) +	Relaxation (usually) +
Secretion		Inhibition (?)	Stimulation + + +
Intestine			
Motility and tone	α,β	Decrease[8] +	Increase + +
Sphincters	α	Contraction (usually) +	Relaxation (usually) +
Secretion		Inhibition (?)	Stimulation + +
Gallbladder and Ducts		Relaxation +	Contraction +
Urinary Bladder			
Detrusor	β	Relaxation (usually) +	Contraction + + +
Trigone and sphincter	α	Contraction + +	Relaxation + +
Ureter			
Motility and tone		Increase (usually)	Increase (?)
Uterus	α,β	Pregnant: contraction (α); nonpregnant: relaxation (β)	Variable[9]
Sex Organs, Male		Ejaculation + + +	Erection + + +
Skin			
Pilomotor muscles	α	Contraction + +	———
Sweat glands	α	Localized secretion[10] +	Generalized secretion + + +
Spleen Capsule	α,β	Contraction + + +; relaxation +	———
Adrenal Medulla		———	Secretion of epinephrine and norepinephrine

Table 21-1. RESPONSES OF EFFECTOR ORGANS TO AUTONOMIC NERVE IMPULSES (Continued)

EFFECTOR ORGANS	ADRENERGIC IMPULSES[1]		CHOLINERGIC IMPULSES[1]
	Receptor Type	*Responses*[2]	*Responses*[2]
Liver	β	Glycogenolysis, gluconeogenesis, etc. $+++$	Glycogen synthesis $+$
Pancreas			
Acini	α	Decreased secretion $+$	Secretion $++$
Islets (β cells)	α	Decreased secretion $+++$	————
	β	Increased secretion $+$	————
Fat Cells	β	Lipolysis $+++$	————
Salivary Glands	α	Potassium and water secretion[11] $+$	Potassium and water secretion $+++$
	β	Amylase secretion $+$	
Lacrimal Glands		————	Secretion $+++$
Nasopharyngeal Glands		————	Secretion $++$
Pineal Gland	β	Melatonin synthesis	————

[1] The anatomical classes of adrenergic and cholinergic nerve fibers are described on page 405 and depicted in Figure 21-1 in red and blue, respectively.

[2] Responses are designated 1+ to 3+ to provide an approximate indication of the importance of adrenergic and cholinergic nerve activity in the control of the various organs and functions listed.

[3] β Receptors of the heart, activation of which produces excitatory responses, have been classified as β_1, and most of the remainder, where inhibition is produced, as β_2.

[4] Dilatation predominates *in situ* due to autoregulatory phenomena.

[5] Cholinergic vasodilatation at these sites is of questionable physiological significance.

[6] Over the usual concentration range of physiologically released, circulating epinephrine, β-receptor response (vasodilatation) predominates in blood vessels of skeletal muscle and liver; α-receptor response (vasoconstriction), in blood vessels of other abdominal viscera. The renal and mesenteric vessels also contain specific dopaminergic receptors, activation of which causes dilatation, but their physiological significance has not been established (*see* review by Goldberg, 1972).

[7] Sympathetic cholinergic system causes vasodilatation in skeletal muscle, but this is not involved in most physiological responses.

[8] It has been proposed that adrenergic fibers terminate at inhibitory β receptors on smooth muscle fibers, and at inhibitory α receptors on parasympathetic cholinergic (excitatory) ganglion cells of Auerbach's plexus.

[9] Depends on stage of menstrual cycle, amount of circulating estrogen and progesterone, and other factors.

[10] Palms of hands and some other sites ("adrenergic sweating").

[11] Parotid glands lack adrenergic innervation.

apposition for a considerable length, but it is not certain whether every effector cell receives its own autonomic innervation in most organs. There is apparently wide variation in the distance between the nerve varicosities and the smooth muscle fibers, ranging from 200 Å in the vas deferens to 10,000 Å in certain blood vessels. In some instances, nerve fibers appear actually to penetrate smooth muscle fibers (*see* review by Burnstock and Iwayama, 1971).

Between the smooth muscle fibers themselves, "protoplasmic bridges" have been described, which are believed to permit the conduction of impulses from cell to cell without the intervention of nervous elements. By such a mechanism, the direct actions of neurohumoral transmitters or drugs on a limited portion of the total cell population could be extended indirectly to large numbers of effector cells.

A structure long favored by physiologists as a relatively simple model for the study of synaptic transmission, the superior cervical *sympathetic ganglion* of the cat, has been shown to be extremely complex, both anatomically (Elfvin, 1963a, 1963b) and pharmacologically (Chapter 27). The preganglionic fibers lose their myelin sheaths, and divide repeatedly into a vast number of end fibers with diameters ranging from 0.1 to 0.3 μm; except at points of synaptic contact, they retain their satellite-cell sheaths. The vast majority of synapses are axo-dendritic. Apparently, a given axonal terminal may synapse with one or more dendritic processes at several points, as in the case of the innervation of smooth muscle described above. It is of interest that there are points of apparently intimate contact between neighboring ganglion cells that are dendro-dendritic and dendrosomatic; the physiological significance of such contacts is not known. Additional elements of yet-unknown function that are present in varying numbers in sympathetic ganglia are small, catecholamine-containing chromaffin cells, some of which appear to make synaptic contact with ganglion cells. Others are clustered predominantly around blood vessels (*see* Elfvin, 1971; Eränkö and Eränkö, 1971).

The Responses of Effector Organs to Autonomic Nerve Impulses. A clear understanding of the response of the various effector organs to autonomic nerve impulses makes it possible to anticipate the actions of drugs that mimic or inhibit the actions of these nerves. In general, the sympathetic and parasympathetic systems are viewed as physiological antagonists. If one system inhibits a certain function, the other usually augments that function. Most viscera are innervated by both divisions of the autonomic nervous system, and the level of activity at any one moment is the algebraic sum of the two component influences. The action of one system is brought into relief by surgical removal or drug-induced paralysis of the opposing system. However, despite the conventional concept of antagonism between the two portions of the autonomic nervous system, their activities as manifested in certain structures may be either different and independent or correlated synergistically. Data appropriate to the problem will be presented in this and subsequent chapters, as the occasion arises. The effects of stimulating the sympathetic (adrenergic) and parasympathetic (cholinergic) nerves to various organs, visceral structures, and effector cells are summarized in Table 21-1.

General Functions of the Autonomic Nervous System. The integrating action of the autonomic nervous system is of vital importance for the well-being of the organism. In general, the autonomic nervous system regulates the activities of structures that are not under voluntary control and that, as a rule function below the level of consciousness. Thus, respiration, circulation, digestion, body temperature, metabolism, sweating, and the secretions of certain endocrine glands are regulated, in part or entirely, by the autonomic nervous system and its central connections. As Claude Bernard (1878–1879) and Cannon (1929, 1932) have emphasized, the constancy of the internal environment of the organism is to a large extent controlled by the vegetative, or autonomic, nervous system.

The sympathetic and parasympathetic systems have contrasting functions in regulating the internal environment. The *sympathetic system* and its associated adrenal medulla are not essential to life, and animals completely deprived of the sympathoadrenal system can continue a fairly normal existence within the sheltered confines of the laboratory. Under circumstances of stress, however, the lack of the sympathoadrenal functions becomes evident. In cats, for example, body temperature cannot be regulated when environmental temperature varies; the blood sugar level does not rise in response to urgent need; compensatory vascular responses to hemor-

rhage, oxygen want, excitement, and work are lacking; resistance to fatigue is lessened; sympathetic components of instinctive reactions to fright and danger are lost; pilomotor responses are absent; and other serious deficiencies in the protective forces of the body are discernible.

The *sympathetic system* is normally active at all times, the degree of activity varying from moment to moment and from organ to organ; in this manner, the finer adjustments to a constantly changing environment are accomplished. The *sympathoadrenal system* can also discharge as a unit. This occurs especially during rage and fright, under which circumstances sympathetically innervated structures over the entire body are affected simultaneously. The heart rate is accelerated; the blood pressure rises; red blood cells are poured into the circulation from the spleen (in certain species); the blood is shifted from the skin and splanchnic bed to the skeletal muscles; the concentration of blood sugar rises; the bronchioles and pupils dilate; and, on the whole, the organism is better prepared for "fight or flight." Many of these effects result primarily from, or are reinforced by, the actions of epinephrine, secreted by the adrenal medulla (*see* below).

The *parasympathetic system* is organized mainly for discrete and localized discharge and not for mass responses. It is concerned primarily with the functions of conservation and restoration of energy rather than with the expenditure of energy. It slows the heart rate, lowers the blood pressure, stimulates the gastrointestinal movements and secretions, aids absorption of nutrients, protects the retina from excessive light, and empties the urinary bladder and rectum. No useful purpose would be served in the body if the parasympathetic nerves all discharged at once.

NEUROHUMORAL TRANSMISSION

The concept of *neurohumoral transmission* holds that nerve impulses elicit responses in smooth, cardiac, and skeletal muscles, exocrine glands, and postsynaptic neurons through liberation of specific chemical substances. The steps involved and the evidence for them will be outlined in some detail because the concept of chemical mediation of nerve impulses profoundly affects our knowledge of the mechanism of action of drugs at these sites.

HISTORICAL ASPECTS

The earliest concrete proposal of a neurohumoral mechanism was made shortly after the turn of the present century. Lewandowsky (1898) and Langley (1901) noted independently the similarity between the effects of injection of extracts of the adrenal gland and stimulation of sympathetic nerves. A few years later, in 1905, T. R. Elliott, while a student at Cambridge, England, extended these observations and postulated that sympathetic nerve impulses release minute amounts of an epinephrine-like substance in immediate contact with effector cells. He considered this substance to be the chemical step in the process of transmission. He also noted that long after sympathetic nerves had degenerated the effector organs still responded characteristically to the hormone of the adrenal medulla. In 1905, Langley suggested that effector cells have excitatory and inhibitory "receptive substances," and that the response to epinephrine depended on which type of substance was present. In 1907, Dixon was so impressed by the correspondence between the effects of the alkaloid muscarine and the responses to vagal stimulation that he advanced the important idea that the vagus nerve liberated a muscarine-like substance that acted as a chemical transmitter of its impulses. In the same year, Reid Hunt announced his studies of acetylcholine (ACh) and other choline esters. In 1914, Dale thoroughly reinvestigated the pharmacological properties of ACh. He was so intrigued with the remarkable fidelity with which this drug reproduced the responses to stimulation of parasympathetic nerves that he introduced the term *parasympathomimetic* to characterize its effects. Dale also noted the brief duration of the action of this chemical and proposed that an esterase in the tissues rapidly splits ACh to acetic acid and choline, the latter being a much less potent compound.

The brilliant researches of Otto Loewi, begun in the winter of 1921, established the first real proof of the chemical mediation of nerve impulses by the peripheral release of specific chemical agents. Loewi's studies deserve description because the technic employed is basic to investigations in this field. He stimulated the vagus nerve of a perfused (donor) frog heart and allowed the perfusion fluid to come in contact with a second (recipient) frog heart used as a test object. A substance was liberated from the first organ that slowed the rate of the second. Loewi referred to this chemical substance as *Vagusstoff* ("vagus-substance"; parasympathin); subsequently, Loewi and Navratil (1926) presented evidence for its identification as *ACh*. Loewi also discovered that an accelerator substance similar to epinephrine was liberated into the perfusion fluid in summer, when the action of the sympathetic fibers in the frog's vagus, a mixed nerve, predominated over that of the inhibitory fibers. Loewi's discoveries were eventually confirmed and are now universally accepted. The essential features of the experiments are shown in Figure 21–2, which illustrates Bain's (1932) modification of Loewi's technic.

Feldberg and Krayer (1933) extended the field by providing strong evidence that the cardiac vagus-substance is also ACh in mammals. Many other investigations established quite conclusively that a chemical mediator, ACh, is instrumental in the transmission of parasympathetic impulses in mammals to other structures, including the iris, salivary glands, stomach, and small intestine.

In addition to its role as the neurohumoral transmitter of all postganglionic parasympathetic fibers and of a few postganglionic sympathetic fibers, such as those to the sweat glands (Dale and Feldberg, 1934) and the sympathetic vasodilator fibers (Uvnäs, 1954), ACh has been shown to have this transmitter function in three additional classes of nerves: (1) preganglionic fibers of both the sympathetic (Feldberg and Gaddum, 1934) and the parasympathetic (Perry and Talesnik, 1953) systems, (2) motor nerves to skeletal muscle (Dale *et al.,* 1936), and (3) certain neurons within the CNS (*see* Feldberg, 1945, for early references). Subsequent evidence for this is discussed below.

Figure 21–2. *Bain's modification of Loewi's technic for demonstrating the release of the vagus-substance upon stimulation of the cardiac nerve to the frog's heart.*

The donor heart (*D*) with nerves intact is perfused at constant pressure with a balanced salt solution. The perfusion fluid then passes to the isolated recipient heart (*R*). Cardiac contractions are recorded by means of writing levers; time (*T*), in 5-second intervals. The vagus fibers to the donor heart are stimulated (*S*) for 40 seconds, and the donor heart is quickly arrested. Slowing of the recipient heart is apparent within 15 seconds after arrest of the donor heart, and asystole occurs shortly thereafter. (After Bain, 1932. Courtesy of the *Quarterly Journal of Experimental Physiology and Cognate Medical Sciences* and Sir Edward Sharpey-Schafer's trustees.)

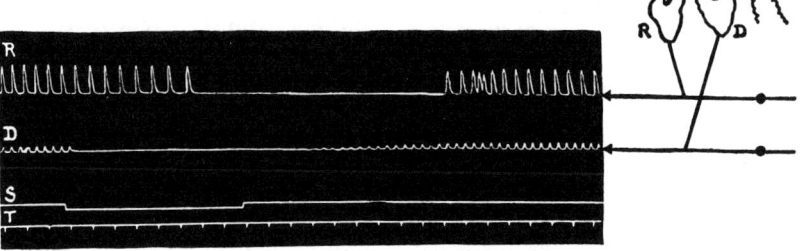

Mention has already been made of Loewi's discovery of an accelerator substance released from frog hearts under certain conditions. In the same year, Cannon and Uridil (1921) reported that the liver, upon stimulation of the sympathetic hepatic nerves, released an epinephrine-like substance that increased the blood pressure and the heart rate but did not dilate the pupil. Subsequent experiments, mainly by Cannon and coworkers, firmly established that this substance is the chemical mediator liberated by sympathetic nerve impulses at neuroeffector junctions. The mediator was originally called "sympathin" by Cannon in order to avoid premature implications regarding its chemical structure.

Just as there are biological indicators for the presence of ACh, there are specific tests for detecting "sympathin," such as acceleration of the rate of the denervated heart, elevation of blood pressure, and retraction of the denervated nictitating membrane of the cat. With such tests it has been repeatedly demonstrated that, when postganglionic sympathetic nerves are stimulated, there is released at the neuroeffector junctions a chemical substance that has sympathomimetic properties. The numerous important experiments by various investigators and the progressive steps by which Cannon and associates developed the concept of "sympathin" can be found in the monograph by Cannon and Rosenblueth (1937).

In many of its pharmacological and chemical properties, Cannon's "sympathin" closely resembled epinephrine, but the two substances differed in certain important respects. When epinephrine is injected into the body, it elicits both excitatory and inhibitory effects. Thus, it accelerates the rate of the heart but simultaneously dilates certain vascular beds while constricting others. In contrast, the excitatory effects of "sympathin" could be elicited separately. As early as 1910, Barger and Dale noted that the effects of sympathetic nerve stimulation were more closely reproduced by the injection of sympathomimetic primary amines than by that of epinephrine or other secondary amines. The possibility that demethylated epinephrine (*norepinephrine, levarterenol, noradrenaline*) might be "sympathin" had been repeatedly advanced by Z. M. Bacq and others, but definitive evidence for its role as the sympathetic nerve mediator was not obtained until specific chemical and biological assay methods were developed for the *quantitative* determination of small amounts of sympathomimetic amines in extracts of tissues and body fluids. Euler in 1946 found that the sympathomimetic substance in highly purified extracts of sympathetic nerves and effector organs bore a strong resemblance to norepinephrine by all criteria used. He proposed that the sympathetic transmitter is norepinephrine and that sympathetic nerve stimulation on some occasions may, in addition, liberate small quantities of epinephrine itself. Numerous workers have confirmed and extended these observations, and all available evidence indicates that *norepinephrine* is the predominant sympathomimetic substance in postganglionic sympathetic nerves and is the adrenergic mediator liberated by their stimulation. (*See* review by Euler, 1972a.)

It now seems clear that norepinephrine is also the neurohumoral transmitter in certain tracts in the CNS. The evidence for this is based both on pharmacological findings and on quantitative and direct histofluorescence demonstrations of the selective occurrence of norepinephrine and other monoamines in various central pathways (*see* reviews by Rothballer, 1959; Hillarp *et al.*, 1966; Salmoiraghi, 1966; Marley and Stephenson, 1972). In addition, its immediate precursor, *dopamine*, probably serves as the major adrenergic transmitter in the mammalian extrapyramidal system and limbic system as well as throughout the nervous system of certain invertebrates (*see* reviews by Carlsson, 1959; Hornykiewicz, 1966). Of particular significance is the demonstration that in Parkinson's disease the major biochemical lesion is the depletion of dopamine from the nigrostriatal tract. A practical consequence of this has been the introduction of levodopa (L-dihydroxyphenylalanine), the immediate precursor of dopamine, for the treatment of parkinsonism (*see* Chapter 14). The question of the occurrence of epinephrine in the hypothalamus and olfactory bulb and tubercle of the mammalian brain is still controversial (*see* review by Wurtman *et al.*, 1972).

STEPS INVOLVED IN NEUROHUMORAL TRANSMISSION

The sequence of events involved in neurohumoral transmission is of particular importance pharmacologically, since the actions of a great number of drugs, particularly those affecting the autonomic nervous system, can be related directly to the individual steps. In conformity with the usual convention, the term *conduction* will be reserved for the passage of an impulse along an axon or muscle fiber; *transmission* refers to the passage of an impulse across a synaptic or neuroeffector junction. With the exception of the local anesthetics, which are infiltrated in high concentrations in the immediate vicinity of nerve trunks, very few drugs modify axonal conduction in the doses employed therapeutically. Hence, this process will be described only briefly in order to introduce its role in triggering the first step in transmission.

Axonal Conduction. The most acceptable present hypothesis of conduction stems largely from the investigative work of Hodgkin and Huxley (1952).

At rest, the interior of the typical mammalian axon is approximately 70 mV negative to the exterior. The *resting potential* is essentially a *diffusion potential*, based chiefly on the 30- to 50-fold higher concentration of potassium ion in the axoplasm as compared with the extracellular fluid, and the relatively high permeability of the resting axonal membrane to potassium ions. Sodium and chloride ions are present in higher concentrations in the extracellular fluid than in the axoplasm, but their concentration gradients across the membrane are somewhat lower than that of potassium, and the axonal membrane at rest is considerably less permeable to these ions; hence their contribution to the resting potential is relatively minor. These ionic gradients are maintained by an energy-dependent active-transport or pump mechanism, involving an adenosine triphosphatase (ATPase) activated by sodium at the inner and by potassium at the outer surface of the membrane (*see* Chapter 31 and reviews by Albers, 1967; Thomas, 1972). At some sites, an electrogenic sodium pump may also contribute to the net resting potential (Casteels *et al.,* 1971).

In response to a stimulus above the threshold level, a nerve *action potential* (AP) or nerve impulse is initiated at a local region of the membrane. This is detectable first by a rapid deflection of the internal resting potential from its negative value toward zero, and continuing uninterruptedly to a positive overshoot. This local reversal of the membrane potential is due to a sudden, selective increase in the permeability of the membrane to *sodium* ions, which flow rapidly inward, in the direction of their concentration gradient. Repolarization of the membrane follows immediately and results from the rapid replacement of this change by one of increased permeability to *potassium*. The transmembrane ionic currents produce local circuit currents around the axon. By such currents, adjacent inactive regions of the axon are activated, and excitation of the next excitable portion of the axonal membrane occurs. This brings about the propagation of the AP. The AP is therefore conducted without decrement along the axon. The region that has just been active remains momentarily in a refractory state. In myelinated fibers, permeability changes occur only at the nodes of Ranvier, thus causing a rapidly progressing type of jumping, or saltatory, conduction. The puffer fish poison, *tetrodotoxin,* is one of the few compounds that selectively block axonal conduction; it does so by preventing the increase in permeability to sodium ion associated with the rising phase of the AP (Kao, 1966). In contrast, *batrachotoxin,* an extremely potent steroidal alkaloid secreted by a South American frog, produces paralysis through a selective increase in sodium permeability, which induces a persistent depolarization (Albuquerque *et al.,* 1973). The physiological and pharmacological aspects of axonal conduction have been reviewed in detail by Shanes (1958a, 1958b), Katz (1966), and Cole (1968).

Junctional Transmission. The arrival of the AP at the axonal terminals initiates a series of events that effect the neurohumoral transmission of an excitatory or inhibitory impulse across the synapse or neuroeffector junction (*see* reviews by Eccles, 1964, 1973; Katz, 1966; McLennan, 1970; Krnjević, 1974). These events, diagramed in Figure 21–3, are as follows:

1. *Release of the Transmitter.* The neurohumoral transmitters are probably synthesized in the region of the axonal terminals and stored there within the synaptic vesicles (*see* below), either in highly concentrated ionic form, as in the case of ACh, or as a readily dissociable complex or salt, as that of norepinephrine with adenosine triphosphate (ATP) and a specific protein. During the resting state, there is a continual, slow release of isolated quanta of the transmitter, ordinarily insufficient to cause initiation of a propagated impulse at the postjunctional site. The AP causes the synchronous release of several hundred quanta. The depolarization of the axonal terminal triggers this process; however, the intermediate steps are uncertain. One step is the mobilization of calcium ion, which enters the intra-axonal medium and is believed to promote fusion of the vesicular and axoplasmic membranes. The contents of the vesicles are then discharged to the exterior by a process termed *exocytosis.*

2. *Combination of the Transmitter with Postjunctional Receptors and Production of the Postjunctional Potential.* The transmitter diffuses across the synaptic or junctional cleft, a distance of 100 to 500 Å, and combines with specialized macromolecular receptors on the postjunctional membrane; this results generally in a localized, nonpropagated increase in the ionic permeability, or conductance, of the membrane. With certain exceptions, noted below, either of two types of permeability change can occur: (1) a generalized increase in permeability to all types of ions, resulting in a localized depolarization of the membrane, that is, an *excitatory postsynaptic potential* (EPSP); or (2) a selective increase in permeability to only the smaller ions (*e.g.,* potassium, chloride), resulting in stabilization or actual hyperpolarization of the membrane, which constitutes an *inhibitory postsynaptic potential* (IPSP).

It should be emphasized that the potential changes associated with the EPSP and IPSP at most sites are the results of passive flows of extracellular and/or intracellular ions down their concentration gradients. As a result of the action of the transmitter, membrane resistance at the immediate vicinity of the receptors is reduced to values lower than those of the surrounding membrane; the postsynaptic potential that results is due to the rapid, brief increase in permeability. Takeuchi and Takeuchi (1960), using

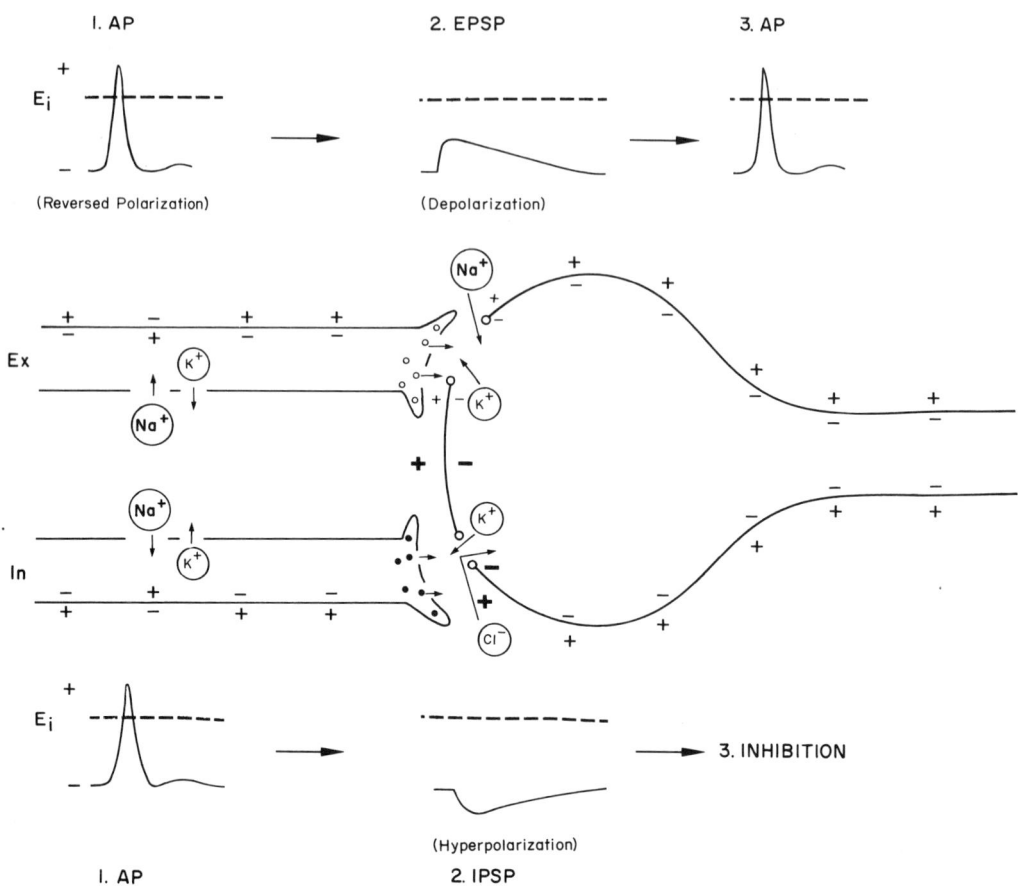

Figure 21-3. *Steps involved in excitatory* (Ex) *and inhibitory* (In) *neurohumoral transmission.*

1. The nerve action potential (AP), consisting in a self-propagated *reversal* of negativity (the internal potential, E_i, goes from a negative value, through zero potential, indicated by the broken line, to a positive value) of the axonal membrane, arrives at the presynaptic terminal and causes release of the excitatory (o) or inhibitory (●) transmitter.

2. Combination of the excitatory transmitter with postsynaptic receptors produces a localized depolarization, the excitatory postsynaptic potential (EPSP), through an increase in permeability to all ions (Na^+ and K^+ chiefly involved). The inhibitory transmitter causes a selective increase in permeability to the smaller ions (K^+ and Cl^- chiefly involved), resulting in a localized hyperpolarization, the inhibitory postsynaptic potential (IPSP).

3. The EPSP initiates a conducted AP in the postsynaptic neuron; this can, however, be prevented by the hyperpolarization induced by a concurrent IPSP.

The transmitter is dissipated by enzymatic destruction, by re-uptake into the presynaptic terminal or adjacent glial cells, or by diffusion. (After Eccles, 1964, 1973; Katz, 1966; and others.)

the voltage clamp technic, have indicated that at the motor end-plate of skeletal muscle the end-plate potential (EPP) produced by ACh is due to an increase in permeability to Na^+ and K^+ but not to Cl^-.

At most excitatory synapses of the CNS, the EPSP presumably also results from an increase in permeability to Na^+ and K^+, whereas IPSPs are believed to result from a permeability increase to Cl^-, K^+, or both. The net potential change attained is determined by the degree to which each participating ion approaches its *equilibrium potential*, that is, that which would result from the difference in ex-

tracellular and intracellular concentrations in the absence of any permeability barrier. At some invertebrate postsynaptic sites, a metabolically dependent, electrogenic sodium pump may contribute to the potential change induced by the transmitter (Kerkut *et al.*, 1969).

While most receptors have not been isolated and purified and their properties are thus still largely conjectural, the evidence for their existence now seems irrefutable (*see* Michelson and Zeimal, 1973; symposium edited by Rang, 1973). The evidence stems particularly from pharmacological investigations described in the chapters that follow. Present information concerning the nature of the cholinergic receptor at the motor end-plate of skeletal muscle, which has been studied most thoroughly, is summarized in Chapter 28.

3. *Initiation of Postjunctional Activity.* If an EPSP exceeds a certain threshold value, it initiates a propagated AP in a neuron or a muscle AP in most skeletal muscles and in cardiac muscle. In certain types of tonic skeletal muscle and in smooth muscle, in which propagated impulses do not occur, an EPSP initiates a localized contractile response; in gland cells, it initiates secretion. An IPSP will tend to oppose excitatory potentials initiated by other neuronal sources at the same time and site; whether a propagated impulse or other response ensues will depend on the algebraic sum of all these effects. In the CNS, and possibly at other sites, inhibition can also result from a relatively prolonged depolarizing action of a transmitter on presynaptic terminals, which in turn brings about a reduction in the amount of transmitter released by the terminals in response to nerve impulses (Eccles, 1964). This phenomenon of *presynaptic inhibition* has provided a tentative explanation of the mechanism of action of some centrally acting drugs (*see* Chapter 18).

4. *Destruction or Dissipation of the Transmitter.* When impulses can be transmitted across junctions at frequencies ranging from a few up to several hundred per second, it is obvious that there must be some efficient means of disposing of the transmitter following each impulse. At most cholinergic junctions, a highly specialized enzyme, *acetylcholinesterase* (AChE), is available for this function. It has been calculated that diffusion may account for termination of the action of ACh at some synapses. It is unlikely that any particular enzyme is directly involved in terminating the action of the adrenergic transmitter at the immediate receptor site in most organs; this is probably effected by a combination of re-uptake of most of the released norepinephrine by the axonal terminals, and simple diffusion (*see* Iversen, 1967).

EVIDENCE FOR NEUROHUMORAL
TRANSMISSION

The concept of neurohumoral transmission was first developed primarily to explain observations

relating to the transmission of impulses from postganglionic autonomic fibers to effector cells. The general lines of evidence in its support have included: (1) demonstration of the presence of a physiologically active compound, and of the enzymes necessary for its synthesis and breakdown, at appropriate sites; (2) recovery of the compound from the perfusate of an innervated structure during periods of nerve stimulation, but not (or in greatly reduced amounts) in the absence of stimulation; (3) demonstration that the compound, when administered appropriately, is capable of producing responses identical with those to nerve stimulation; and (4) demonstration that the responses to nerve stimulation and to the administered compound are modified in the same manner by various drugs. With the fulfillment of the foregoing criteria to varying degrees at several autonomic effector organs, the concept soon gained practically unanimous acceptance for these sites.

General acceptance of neurohumoral, rather than electrogenic, transmission at autonomic ganglia and the neuromuscular junction of skeletal muscle was withheld for a considerable period, chiefly for two reasons: (1) the extremely rapid time factors involved, in contrast to those at autonomic effector sites; and (2) discrepancies between the amount of the putative transmitter, ACh, recovered during nerve stimulation and that required to produce characteristic responses. Both objections have, for the most part, been answered satisfactorily through the development of modern technics of intracellular recording and microiontophoretic application of drugs, as will be described. The anatomical complexities and cellular barriers of the CNS are such that it is exceedingly difficult to stimulate isolated fiber tracts to, and recover uncontaminated perfusates from, selected groups of neurons. However, studies of individual neurons of the spinal cord and brain, particularly in the brilliant investigations of Eccles and his colleagues, have provided evidence of central neurohumoral transmission that has become increasingly convincing (*see* monographs by Eccles, 1964, 1973).

One important feature of junctional transmission that supports the concept of a neurohumoral mechanism is *the irreducible latent period between the arrival of an impulse at the axonal terminal and the appearance of the postjunctional potential.* Physiologists had long recognized a synaptic delay, sometimes as brief as a fraction of a millisecond, that could not be accounted for in terms of known conduction velocities in the presynaptic or postsynaptic neurons. However, there remained the possible explanation that conduction might be considerably slowed in the fine preterminal axonal branches. This limitation was overcome in an investigation of the giant synapse of the squid. Bullock and Hagiwara (1957) inserted fine-recording micropipettes into the presynaptic and postsynaptic fibers and simultaneously recorded from both following presynaptic stimulation. There was invariably a delay of 0.5 to 2.0 milliseconds, depending upon the temperature, between the arrival of the impulse at the presynaptic electrode and the recording of postsynaptic activity; furthermore, depolarization or hyperpolarization of either the presynaptic or the postsynaptic element induced no detectable change in the potential of the other (Hagiwara and Tasaki, 1958). These findings are consistent only with the chemical mediation of synaptic transmission and not with the direct spread of electrical current across the synapse.

In further support of neurohumoral transmission as a general phenomenon is the considerable indirect evidence indicating that most postsynaptic and postjunctional membranes are electrically inexcitable. The interested reader is referred to the reviews by Grundfest (1957a) and Eccles (1964) for documentation and critical analysis.

There are isolated instances of synapses where transmission undoubtedly does occur by the direct spread of current across the junction. The only such sites known in mammals are in the CNS (Horcholle-Bossavit and Tyc-Dumont, 1971; Sotelo and Llinás, 1972). These cases seem to be exceptional and are associated with unusual anatomical arrangements.

CHOLINERGIC TRANSMISSION

Mention has been made of Loewi and Navratil's (1926) tentative identification of the *Vagusstoff* as *acetylcholine (ACh)* and of the subsequent extension of this work to the implication that ACh is the neurohumoral transmitter at a wide variety of neuroeffector junctions and synaptic sites. In close association with the transmitter are the two enzymes *choline acetyltransferase* and *acetylcholinesterase (AChE)*, which are involved in its synthesis and hydrolysis, respectively.

Acetylcholine. Originally, pharmacological tests or bioassays were required to demonstrate this ester in extracts and perfusates of biological origin. Although several chemical and physical tests for ACh are also known, many do not have the requisite sensitivity or specificity (*see* Whittaker, 1963). In recent years, however, several excellent methods have been devised that involve various combinations of the technics of electrophoresis, fluorimetry, radioisotopic labeling, gas chromatography, and mass spectroscopy (*see* Hanin, 1974). Since some of these require elaborate equipment and methodology, they have by no means eliminated the use of the more sensitive of the bioassays. The latter also illustrate several important general pharmacological principles.

Inasmuch as none of the pharmacological tests is specific, certain other criteria must be met in order to establish the identity of the material in tissue extracts as ACh. Chang and Gaddum in 1933 de-

scribed the following indices, various combinations of which have been employed in most subsequent studies of the distribution or release of ACh. (1) Inhibition of cholinesterase in the test object (leech muscle, frog heart, denervated skeletal muscle, etc.) usually increases the response obtained. (2) The presence of blood or tissue extract decreases or destroys the activity of ACh, and this destruction is prevented by cholinesterase inhibitors. (3) ACh is quickly destroyed by hydrolysis in an alkaline medium. (4) Boiling for several minutes in weakly acidic solution does not destroy ACh. (5) Atropine, curare, and nicotine individually block certain specific pharmacological actions of ACh, but they do not interfere significantly with the release of ACh at nerve terminals. (6) The responses of various biological indicators to ACh bear a definite quantitative relation to each other, and the chemical mediator being studied must give these same relative values before it can be tentatively accepted as ACh. The cholinergic mediator at most sites fulfills all the requirements mentioned. Still other reasons for identifying it as ACh are that both are dialyzable, soluble in alcohol but not in ether, and restored to activity by acetylation after inactivation by cholinesterases.

Chang and Gaddum's pharmacological tests for ACh have subsequently been considerably modified and expanded. Procedures have been developed for concentrating and purifying extracts so that the active substance can be applied to single neurons by microiontophoresis, in the case of ionized compounds such as ACh, or by electro-osmosis for nonionized compounds (Krnjević and Whittaker, 1965). Remarkable sensitivity has been achieved. By means of its iontophoretic application to the denervated motor end-plate of frog muscle, it is possible to detect as little as 5×10^{-15} mole of ACh (Nastuk and Levine, 1961). The same level of sensitivity has been obtained by a much more simple procedure with a clam heart as the test object (Cottrell *et al.,* 1970).

Several additional choline esters of biological origin have been discovered, and most of these act qualitatively similarly to ACh or as ACh antagonists. The list includes *murexine (urocanylcholine; β-imidazolyl,-4[5]-acrylylcholine,* from the hypobranchial glands of a marine snail), *propionylcholine* (from ox spleen), *α-aminobutyrylcholine* (in mammalian brain), and *acrylylcholine* and its derivatives *senecioylcholine* and *sinapylcholine* (in various marine snails). However, it is questionable whether any of these compounds plays a role in neurohumoral transmission in mammals (*see* Whittaker, 1963).

Choline Acetyltransferase (Choline Acetylase). This enzyme, a basic protein with a molecular weight of approximately 65,000, was first studied in cell-free extracts of the electric organ of the Amazonian electric eel, *Electrophorus electricus*. It has been partially purified from this and other sources by Nachmansohn and associates, who have played the major role in elucidating its properties (*see* Nachmansohn, 1959). Choline acetyltransferase catalyzes the final step in the synthesis of ACh—the acetylation of choline with acetyl coenzyme A (CoA).

The acetyl CoA for this reaction is derived from pyruvate via the multistep pyruvate dehydrogenase reaction or by the "acetate-activating reaction." This latter process, catalyzed by acetate thiokinase, first involves reaction of acetate with ATP to form an enzyme-bound acyladenylate (acetyl-AMP). In the presence of CoA, transacetylation and acetyl CoA synthesis proceed.

Tremendous variations in choline acetyltransferase activity occur in mammalian nerve tissue. In general, high concentrations have been reported for peripheral cholinergic nerves (*e.g.*, ventral spinal roots, superior cervical ganglion) and thousandfold lower values are detected in afferent nerves (*e.g.*, dorsal spinal roots, optic nerve). Similar differences have been found by ultramicro determination of the concentrations of choline acetyltransferase in single cholinergic and noncholinergic neurons of autonomic ganglia (Buckley *et al.*, 1967). Various regions of the CNS also differ markedly in their ability to synthesize ACh (*see* Nachmansohn, 1959; Hebb, 1963). It is of interest that the human placenta, which is devoid of nervous tissue, also contains a high concentration of the enzyme (Kato, 1960).

Choline acetyltransferase, like other protein constituents of the neuron, is synthesized within the perikaryon and is then transported by unknown mechanisms along the length of the axon to its terminal. The synaptic vesicles may be formed at the terminal, rather than in the perikaryon. In addition to the vesicles, the axonal terminals contain a large number of mitochondria, where acetyl CoA is synthesized as described. Choline is taken up from the extracellular fluid into the axoplasm by active transport. The final step in the synthesis probably occurs within the cytoplasm, following which most of the ACh is sequestered within the synaptic vesicles (*see* Potter, 1972). Moderately potent, selective inhibitors of choline acetyltransferase have become available (Cavallito *et al.*, 1969). The storage and release of ACh are discussed below.

Acetylcholinesterase. For ACh to serve as the neurohumoral agent in peripheral junctional transmission, the ester must be removed or inactivated within the time limits imposed by the response characteristics of visceral neuroeffector junctions, motor endplates, and various types of neurons. These limits range from over a second to less than a millisecond. At the latter extreme, the mediator must be destroyed almost immediately—with "flashlike suddenness," as Dale has expressed it. Body fluids and tissues contain enzymes, first called *choline esterase,* that

are capable of rapidly hydrolyzing ACh to choline and acetic acid. The choline produced is pharmacologically weak in comparison with its acetylated precursor; for example, it possesses only 10^{-5} the vasodepressor potency of ACh. The general characteristics and distribution of acetylcholinesterase are discussed below; a more complete account of its molecular structure and its reactions with ACh and various inhibitors is presented in Chapter 22.

Acetylcholinesterase (AChE; also known as specific or true ChE) occurs in neurons, at the neuromuscular junction, and in certain other tissues (*see* below); it is responsible for the hydrolysis of ACh released in the process of cholinergic transmission. *Butyrocholinesterase* (BuChE; also known as cholinesterase, ChE, nonspecific ChE, or pseudo-ChE) is present in various types of glial or satellite cells but only to a limited extent in neuronal elements of the central and peripheral nervous systems, and in the plasma, liver, and other organs; its physiological function is unknown. Although both types of enzyme can hydrolyze ACh and certain other aliphatic and aromatic esters and as a group are inhibited selectively by physostigmine, they can be distinguished by several criteria.

The main reason for distinguishing between AChE and BuChE is that practically all the pharmacological effects of the anti-ChE agents (Chapter 22 *et seq.*) are due to the inhibition of the AChE, with the consequent accumulation of endogenous ACh; inhibition of BuChE at most sites produces no apparent functional derangement (*see* monograph by Goedde *et al.*, 1967).

AChE hydrolyzes ACh at a greater velocity than any other choline ester; it hydrolyzes acetyl-β-methylcholine (methacholine), but not benzoylcholine; and it is inhibited selectively by low concentrations of several *bis*-quaternary ammonium bases and by other agents. BuChE, on the other hand, exhibits a maximal velocity of hydrolysis with butyrylcholine as substrate; it hydrolyzes benzoylcholine, but not methacholine; and it is more sensitive to inhibition by several organophosphorus agents, such as di*iso*propyl phosphorofluoridate (DFP) and mipafox, and certain quaternary ammonium compounds than is AChE. (For complete descriptions of the properties and methods for determination of these enzymes, *see* Holmstedt, 1959; Augustinsson, 1963.)

Knowledge of the *cytological distribution* of AChE has been considerably expanded in recent years, chiefly by the use of two approaches: microgasometric analysis by the Cartesian-diver (Giacobini, 1959) and the magnetic-diver (Brzin *et al.*, 1966) technics, and microscopic histochemistry (Schwarzacher, 1961; Koelle, 1963). The former technic permits the quantitation of AChE activity in individual neurons, and even in their constituent parts (*e.g.*, axonal segment, nucleolus). With methods of the latter type it is possible to visualize, by light and more recently by electron microscopy, the sites of enzyme activity in relation to the various structural components of tissues and cells. The major findings from such studies will be summarized briefly. The reader is referred to the references quoted above for details of this subject.

Neurons that give rise to the three categories of peripheral cholinergic fibers (postganglionic parasympathetic, preganglionic autonomic, somatic motor) contain relatively high concentrations of AChE throughout their entire length (dendrites, perikarya, axons). The concentrations in noncholinergic peripheral neurons (adrenergic, primary afferent) are, in general, considerably lower, but there are marked species variations. A small percentage of sympathetic ganglion cells in most species contains concentrations of AChE equivalent to those of their respective parasympathetic ganglion cells; evidence has been obtained that in the cat the former give rise to the cholinergic sympathetic fibers that innervate the sweat glands (Sjöqvist, 1963). The presence of AChE in presumably noncholinergic neurons has led to some speculation concerning its function at such sites (*see* below).

Within the CNS, marked variations in AChE activity occur. With certain exceptions, notably the cerebellum, there are good correlations between the concentrations of AChE, ACh, and choline acetyltransferase (Silver, 1967). In neurons of some regions, such as the caudate nucleus and the putamen, the concentration of AChE is extremely high; the neurons of other areas can be classified as showing intermediate, low, or little or no activity on the basis of their specific staining reactions. The polarity of AChE-staining tracts in the CNS can be determined following chronic transection, which results in the accumulation of AChE on the proximal side, and its loss from the side distal to the cell bodies. By such an approach, it has been shown that in the rat two major AChE-staining pathways arise from the reticular and tegmental nuclei of the brain stem and project diffusely throughout the subcortical and cortical regions (Lewis and Shute, 1967; Shute and Lewis, 1967; Ramon-Moliner, 1972). These probably represent, at least in part, the mesodiencephalic activating system, which pharmacological studies have shown to contain an important cholinergic component (*see* below).

At the motor end-plates of skeletal muscle, most of the AChE is localized at the surface and infoldings of the postjunctional membrane, or subneural apparatus (Davis and Koelle, 1967; Couteaux, 1972). Accordingly, it is situated strategically for the rapid hydrolysis of ACh following the production of the EPP. The distribution of AChE is more complex in autonomic ganglia. Here both histochemical and pharmacological findings suggest that the neuronal AChE consists of two fractions: a functional portion, with its active sites directed externally to the surface of the cell membrane and directly concerned in the hydrolysis of ACh; and an internal or reserve portion, representing enzyme more recently synthesized within the endoplasmic reticulum and serving as a source of replacement for the former in the course of the cell's cycle of protein turnover (Koelle and Koelle, 1959; McIsaac and Koelle, 1959). Although

essentially all the functional AChE disappears from sympathetic ganglia of the cat following preganglionic denervation, this is perhaps due in part to the loss of a trophic factor, since more recent electron microscopic studies have shown that the enzyme is present normally at both the presynaptic and postsynaptic membranes (Koelle *et al.*, 1975).

In skeletal muscle, there are several additional sites of AChE activity, such as the musculotendinous junction, for which no definite functional role can be assigned. The same is true regarding the occurrence of the enzyme at several other locations, including the erythrocytes, thrombocytes, and placenta.

Storage and Release of Acetylcholine. In 1950, Fatt and Katz (1952) recorded at the motor end-plate of skeletal muscle and observed the random occurrence of small (approximately 0.1 to 3.0 mV) spontaneous depolarizations at a frequency of approximately one per second. The magnitude of these miniature end-plate potentials (m.e.p.p.s) is considerably below the threshold required to fire a muscle AP; that they are due to the release of ACh is indicated by their enhancement by neostigmine and their blockade by *d*-tubocurarine. This was the first evidence that ACh is stored in and released from motor-nerve endings in constant amounts or *quanta*. The morphological counterpart of this phenomenon was discovered shortly thereafter, in the form of synaptic vesicles noted in electron micrographs of nerve terminals by De Robertis and Bennett (1955). The storage and release of ACh have been investigated most extensively at motor end-plates; nevertheless, most of the principles discovered at this locus probably apply to other sites of cholinergic transmission as well, and in many respects to noncholinergic transmission (*see* reviews by McLennan, 1970; Phillis, 1970; Kuno, 1971; Potter, 1972; Hubbard, 1973; Krnjević, 1974).

While there is general agreement regarding certain steps involved in the storage and release of ACh, many of the details are still moot or unknown, as reference to the reviews listed above will disclose. Estimates of the ACh content of the synaptic vesicles range from 1000 to over 50,000 molecules per vesicle, and it has been calculated that a single motor-nerve terminal contains 300,000 or more vesicles. In addition, an uncertain but significant amount of ACh is present in the extravesicular cytoplasm. Mathematical treatment of the data obtained from postsynaptic recording at the motor end-plate during the continuous application of ACh to resting muscle has permitted estimation of the potential change induced by a single molecule of ACh (3×10^{-7} V); from such calculations, it is evident that even the lower estimate of the ACh content per vesicle (1000 molecules) is sufficient to account for the magnitude of the m.e.p.p.s (Katz and Miledi, 1972).

In the superior cervical ganglion of the cat, approximately 85% of the total ACh content is stored in a releasable "depot" form, which is subdivided into more readily and less readily releasable reservoirs. The remaining 15% of the extractable ACh is in a "stationary" form and is perhaps located centrally to the axonal terminals. An additional "surplus" portion that may exceed the total depot ACh accumulates in the presence of an anti-ChE agent. The ganglion is able to support a remarkably high rate of ACh synthesis and release; when it is perfused with plasma and stimulated supramaximally at a frequency of 20 cycles per second, the ACh output during 1 hour is approximately six times the original content (Birks and MacIntosh, 1961).

When an AP arrives at the motor-nerve terminal, there is an explosive release of 100 or more quanta (or vesicles) of ACh, following a latent period of approximately 0.75 millisecond (Katz and Miledi, 1965). The intermediate steps appear to be as follows: the depolarization of the terminal permits the inflow of calcium ions, which hypothetically then bind to negative charges or other sites on the internal surface of the terminal axoplasmic membrane. This could facilitate fusion of axonal and vesicular membranes, resulting in the extrusion of the contents of the vesicles. The presence of calcium ions in the extracellular fluid is essential for the release of ACh elicited by the nerve impulse, and this effect is in turn antagonized by magnesium ions. An extensive analysis of the factors involved in transmitter release has been published by Cooke and associates (1973).

Characteristics of Cholinergic Transmission at Various Sites. From the comparisons noted above, it is obvious that there are marked differences between various sites of cholinergic transmission with respect to general-architectural and fine-structural arrangements, the distributions of AChE, and the temporal factors involved in normal functioning. For example, in skeletal muscle the junctional sites occupy a small, discrete portion of the surface of the individual fibers and are relatively isolated from those of adjacent fibers; in the superior cervical ganglion, in contrast, approximately 100,000 ganglion cells are packed within a volume of a few cubic millimeters, and both the presynaptic and postsynaptic neuronal processes form complicated patterns of intertwining ramifications. It is therefore to be expected that the specific features of cholinergic transmission will vary markedly at different sites.

1. *Skeletal Muscle.* In early studies it was shown that stimulation of a motor nerve resulted in the output of ACh from the corresponding perfused muscle, and that the close intra-arterial injection of ACh produced muscular contraction similar to that elicited by stimulation of the motor nerve. However, the strength of this evidence for cholinergic transmision at the neuromuscular junction was weakened by the large quantitative difference between the amount of ACh required to produce contraction over the amount recovered following nerve stimulation. The discrepancy was eventually resolved by the demonstration that the amount of ACh (10^{-17} mole) required to elicit an EPP following its microiontophoretic application to the motor end-plate of a rat diaphragm muscle fiber is equivalent to that recovered from each fiber following stimulation of the phrenic nerve (Krnjević and Miledi, 1958; Krnjević and Mitchell, 1961).

The combination of ACh with the receptors at the external surface of the postjunctional membrane induces an immediate, marked increase in permeability to Na^+ and K^+; it has been estimated that for each molecule of ACh that combines there is a flow of 50,000 cations across the postjunctional membrane (Katz and Miledi, 1972). This is the basis for the localized depolarizing EPP, which triggers the conducted muscle AP, and the latter in turn leads to contraction. Further details concerning these events and their modification by neuromuscular blocking agents are presented in Chapter 28.

Following section and degeneration of the motor nerve to skeletal muscle or of the postganglionic fibers to autonomic effectors, there is a marked reduction in the threshold doses of the transmitters and of certain other drugs required to elicit a response, that is, *denervation supersensitivity* (*see* monograph by Cannon and Rosenblueth, 1949). It has been shown that in skeletal muscle this change is accompanied by a spread of the cholinoceptive sites from the end-plate region to the adjacent portions of the sarcoplasmic membrane, which eventually involves practically its entirety (Axelsson and Thesleff, 1959). Some have suggested that this and other changes in the muscle fibers are due primarily to the loss of an unidentified *neurotrophic factor* that is normally secreted by the axonal terminals, rather than to deprivation of the transmitter, ACh (Albuquerque et al., 1972).

It has been mentioned that the *electric organs* of certain fish are rich sources of AChE and choline acetyltransferase. These structures represent evolutionary modifications of skeletal muscle; in some genera (*e.g., Electrophorus*), the individual electroplaques are homologous to the entire muscle fiber, and the electrical impulse generated in response to a nerve impulse or to the application of ACh is comprised of a localized postjunctional potential and a propagated AP. In other genera (*e.g., Torpedo, Raia*), only a postjunctional potential is produced, so that here the structure represents only the homolog of the motor end-plate. By the simultaneous discharge of hundreds of individual electroplaques arranged in series and in parallel, impulses of several hundred volts, with currents ranging up to 1 A, can be produced. The unique features of these remarkable structures are of particular value for physiological investigation, and much of our knowledge of neurohumoral transmission has been derived from their study (*see* reviews by Grundfest, 1957b; Chagas and Paes-de-Carvalho, 1961). The electric organ of *Electrophorus* has also been employed in attempts to identify and characterize the cholinergic receptor (*see* Chapter 28).

2. *Autonomic Effectors.* In contrast to other cholinergically innervated cells (*i.e.,* skeletal muscle and neurons), smooth muscle and the cardiac conduction system (S-A node, atrium, A-V node, and the His-Purkinje system) normally exhibit intrinsic activity, both electrical and mechanical, that is modified but not initiated by nerve impulses. In the basal condition, smooth muscle and the cardiac conduction system exhibit spikes, or waves of reversed membrane polarization, that are propagated from cell to cell at rates considerably slower than the AP of axons or skeletal muscle. The spikes are apparently initiated by rhythmic fluctuations in the membrane resting potential; in intestinal smooth muscle, the site of the pacemaker activity continually shifts, whereas in the heart it normally arises from the S-A node but can under certain circumstances arise from any part of the conduction system (*see* Chapter 32). As in skeletal muscle, the spike initiates a contraction.

The addition of ACh (10^{-7} to 10^{-6} M) to isolated intestinal muscle causes a fall in the resting potential and an increase in the frequency of spike production, followed by a rise in tension. The primary action of ACh in initiating these effects is probably the partial depolarization of the cell membrane, brought about by an increase in sodium conductance; while there are changes in the conductances of potassium and chloride also, their significance is uncertain (*see* review by Bolton, 1973). It is of interest, however, that ACh can also produce contraction of smooth muscle when the membrane has been completely depolarized by immersion in potassium-Ringer solution, provided calcium is present. Although the physiological significance of this observation is uncertain, there is increasing evidence that calcium ion fluxes are in some way affected by ACh, and that calcium ion is released by ACh and is directly involved in regulating the permeability of the membrane to sodium and in coupling membrane depolarization with contraction (*see* review by Bennett, 1972).

In the cardiac conduction system, particularly from the S-A to the A-V node, stimulation of the cholinergic innervation (represented preganglionically by the vagal trunk) or the direct application of ACh causes inhibition, associated with hyperpolarization of the fiber membrane and a marked decrease in the rate of depolarization. These effects are due to a selective increase in permeability to potassium (Burgen and Terroux, 1953; Trautwein *et al.,* 1956). At the same time, the presence of a basal level of ACh may be essential for the maintenance of the transmembrane potential above a critical value of 60 mV, below which the rate of sodium entry is too slow to produce depolarization and impulses can no longer be conducted.

Although direct evidence is lacking, it is likely that, in those smooth muscle fibers where cholinergic impulses are inhibitory, ACh produces inhibition by the same mechanism as described above.

3. *Autonomic Ganglia.* The evidence for cholinergic transmission in autonomic ganglia is similar to that obtained at the neuromuscular junction of skeletal muscle. When the perfusate from the isolated cat superior cervical ganglion is tested, ACh appears in the perfusion fluid after preganglionic but not after antidromic stimulation; it is not liberated spontaneously in significant amounts. The ganglion cells can be discharged by injecting very small amounts of ACh into the perfusion fluid or into the blood supply to the normally circulated ganglion (Feldberg and Gaddum, 1934; Emmelin and MacIntosh, 1956).

The ability of preganglionic impulses to discharge ganglion cells goes hand in hand with the ability of such impulses to release ACh into the perfusates. For example, when Locke's solution *without glucose* is perfused through a sympathetic ganglion, continued stimulation of the preganglionic nerve rapidly exhausts the mechanism of synaptic transmission, and the output of ACh from the ganglion simultaneously fails; both are restored at the same time when choline and glucose, lactate, or pyruvate are added to the perfusion fluid. When the Locke's solution lacks *calcium,* synaptic transmission and release of ACh by preganglionic nerve impulses fail at the same time; both are promptly and simultaneously restored by addition of calcium to the perfusion fluid. These effects of calcium are antagonized by *magnesium,* just as at the motor end-plate. After *preganglionic nerve section,* synaptic transmission and release of ACh by preganglionic impulses disappear together, at a time when conduction is still unimpaired in the severed fiber.

Subsequent studies have disclosed that ganglionic transmission is a highly complex process, combining many of the features of transmission at the neuromuscular junctions of both skeletal and smooth muscle. Interneurons and additional transmitters may also be involved. An account of these events and their modification by drugs is presented in Chapter 27.

4. *Central Nervous System.* Numerous investigations have been concerned with elucidating the role of ACh in central synaptic transmission. In general, the same lines of experimentation have been employed as for ganglionic and neuromuscular transmission. The extreme difficulties involved in obtaining data bearing on the neurohumoral function of ACh and other agents in the CNS, as compared with various peripheral sites, have already been discussed. This applies in particular to the problem of recovering perfusates from homogeneous

groups of axonal terminations and identifying therein a putative transmitter following selective stimulation of the corresponding nerve fibers; to date, this has not been accomplished. However, the weight of other kinds of evidence now makes it seem undeniable that cholinergic transmission occurs at some sites in the CNS. It is equally evident that ACh is not a universal central transmitter. While the evidence for a transmitter role is not as great for any other agent as it is for ACh, several possible candidates are discussed in the sections that follow. The early studies relating to the central neurohumoral transmitter role of ACh have been examined critically by Feldberg (1945), and subsequent general reviews have considered more recent aspects of this topic (Curtis and Crawford, 1969; McLennan, 1970; Phillis, 1970; Krnjević, 1974).

As noted above, there is a reasonably close parallelism between the concentrations of ACh, choline acetyltransferase, and AChE in most parts of the CNS, varying from high in some regions to very low in others. This suggests that there are both cholinergic and noncholinergic neuronal systems. While ACh has not been recovered from localized perfusates, it has been collected from the pia-arachnoid surface of the cerebral cortex (Mitchell, 1963). The rate of release is markedly increased by pharmacological or electrical stimulation of the brain or groups of peripheral nerves and is diminished by undercutting of cortical slabs in chronic experiments. This procedure does not compromise the cortical circulation, but it causes a marked decrease in the concentrations of choline acetyltransferase and AChE.

The *injection of ACh* (0.1 to 1.0 μg) into the internal carotid artery of the rabbit produces a diffuse *EEG arousal response,* along with a generalized motor response; small intravenous doses of atropine (1 to 3 mg/kg) antagonize the arousal response to ACh and to external stimuli (Longo, 1955). This evidence that cholinergic fibers are involved in the mesodiencephalic activating system is supported by the localization of AChE in corresponding tracts, described above, and by the increased release of ACh from the cerebral cortex that follows stimulation of the reticular formation (Phillis, 1968).

A major difficulty in studying the effects of ACh and other drugs on the CNS is the *blood-brain barrier,* which markedly limits the penetration of charged compounds or ions. Another severe handicap is the impossibility of confining the distribution of a drug to a limited or homogeneous group of synaptic sites, following its intravascular injection. These factors probably account largely for the inconsistency of early results. Attempts to circumvent some of these problems have led to the use of other routes of drug administration, such as local application to the surface of the brain and spinal cord and injection into the cerebral ventricles. ACh and anti-ChE agents given by such routes produce in some instances marked effects upon the CNS, but the effects do not clearly point to transmitter functions of ACh at specific sites.

Rapid iontophoretic application of minute amounts of ACh and other agents through micropipettes close to the surface of individual neurons,

with simultaneous intracellular recording of their responses, has overcome many of these obstacles. Individual neurons at a variety of sites in the CNS have been shown to respond with some degree of selectivity to ACh; the implication that ACh is the neurohumoral transmitter at such sites is strengthened when the effects of both applied ACh and stimulation of immediately afferent fibers are blocked by antagonists of either the nicotinic (*e.g.,* *d*-tubocurarine, dihydro-β-erythroidine) or the muscarinic (atropine) type (*see* page 435 for explanation of *nicotinic* and *muscarinic* receptors).

Investigation of recurrent inhibition of spinal motoneurons has provided the most convincing evidence of a central cholinergic pathway obtained to date. The findings and conclusions of Eccles and colleagues are, briefly, as follows. The axons of spinal motoneurons give off collaterals in the ventromedial portion of the cord to closely adjacent interneurons known as Renshaw cells; the latter, in turn, are primarily inhibitory to the motoneurons of the same segmental level. All the pharmacological data indicate that transmission from the motoneuron collaterals to the Renshaw cells is cholinergic, and that the receptors are predominantly *nicotinic.* Thus, activation of the latter by orthodromic or antidromic impulses over the ventral roots or by iontophoretically applied ACh is prolonged and intensified by anti-ChE agents, such as physostigmine, and nearly completely blocked by dihydro-β-erythroidine. These findings are consistent with Dale's (1934) principle that a given neuron liberates the same transmitter at all synaptic terminals, since the axon from which the collaterals arise innervates skeletal muscle fibers. The fibers from the Renshaw cells, which apparently end on the motoneuron, release an unidentified inhibitory transmitter that causes hyperpolarization of the postsynaptic membrane. Strychnine (*see* Chapter 18) and tetanus toxin cause exaggeration of spinal reflexes through interaction with the transmitter of the Renshaw cells and of other inhibitory fibers, either by competing with it at the postjunctional site or by interfering with its release. (*See* reviews by Eccles, 1964, 1973; Willis, 1971.)

In contrast to the Renshaw cells, most of the neurons at higher levels of the CNS that are activated by the microiontophoretic application of ACh have predominantly *muscarinic* receptors. Firing comes on slowly and persists several seconds after the application of ACh; the depolarization is blocked by atropine, and is due probably to a decrease in potassium conductance (Krnjević *et al.,* 1971). Neurons with these characteristics are distributed widely throughout the brain, and, in addition, many neurons throughout the CNS are inhibited by the action of ACh on muscarinic receptors.

Actions of Acetylcholine at Prejunctional Sites: Hypothetical Implications. Considerable attention has been focused on the possible involvement of *prejunctional cholinoceptive sites* in both cholinergic and noncholinergic transmission and in the actions of various drugs. The intra-arterial injection of ACh or an anti-ChE agent (physostigmine or neostigmine) produces both fasciculations (synchronous contractions of the skeletal muscle fibers of *entire motor units*) and antidromic APs that are conducted from the terminals of the motor nerves to the ventral spinal roots. Both effects are blocked by curare. These and related observations suggest that the compounds act at the prejunctional axonal terminals as well as at the postjunctional cholinoceptive sites. Several investigators, particularly Riker and associates (1957, 1969), have amplified and extended these observations. The theoretical and practical implications of their findings are discussed in Chapter 28.

In order to relate a number of pharmacological findings on the cat superior cervical ganglion to the histochemical localization of AChE in the same structure, a hypothesis was proposed that involves a *positive-feedback* step in ganglionic transmission (Koelle, 1962). In terms of the hypothesis, the ACh released initially by the nerve impulse acts at the presynaptic terminals to prolong briefly the depolarized state and thus amplify the amount of ACh available to act postsynaptically; the process was assumed to be terminated by a combination of desensitization of the presynaptic receptors and enzymatic hydrolysis by AChE. Subsequent work has demonstrated the presence of ganglionic presynaptic cholinoreceptors, but enhancement of ACh release following their activation has been recorded only occasionally (Nishi, 1970). The present status of the hypothesis has been reviewed by Hubbard (1970) and Koelle (1971).

Participation of Acetylcholine in Transmission by Noncholinergic Neurons. Burn and Rand in 1959 introduced the concept of a *cholinergic link* in *adrenergic transmission.* According to this hypothesis, stimulation of *sympathetic fibers* results first in the release of ACh, which, in turn, causes the release of norepinephrine to act on the effector organs. The evidence to support this proposal includes the finding at several sites that, following a dose of atropine sufficient to block the direct effects of ACh on autonomic effector cells, injection of ACh produces sympathomimetic effects; if the animal is pretreated with reserpine to deplete adrenergic fibers of their norepinephrine content, the sympathomimetic response can no longer be obtained; but, when the sympathetic nerves of reserpine-treated animals are stimulated, ACh-like effects are produced; and finally, anti-ChE agents and other drugs modify the responses to stimulation of sympathetic nerves at certain sites in a manner consistent with the proposal. The concept is by no means generally accepted at present, and some observations are apparently at variance with it (*see* reviews by Burn and Rand, 1965; Ferry, 1966). However, no other explanation has been forthcoming for all the supporting observations, particularly on eccrine sweat glands (Lloyd, 1965).

There is both histochemical and pharmacological evidence for a similar role of ACh in releasing the neurosecretory products of the *hypothalamiconeurohypophyseal* tract (oxytocin and vasopressin), and the unidentified neurohumoral transmitters at a variety of central sites, including the terminations of the *vagal afferent* fibers, the *olivocochlear bundle,* the

amacrine cells of the retina, and the *Renshaw cells* of the spinal cord (Koelle, 1971). It should be emphasized that these schemes are to be regarded only as working hypotheses to relate a group of findings not readily explainable otherwise.

Proposed Functions of Acetylcholine at Nonjunctional Sites. The presence of various concentrations of ACh, choline acetyltransferase, and AChE at numerous nonjunctional sites, and indeed in some cells that are devoid of innervation, has led naturally to speculation and experimentation to elucidate the physiological function of ACh in such locations. Most attention has been directed toward establishing a role of ACh in axonal conduction, as a local hormone, and in the regulation of membrane permeability and transport. However, there has been little recent work in this area (*see* Koelle, 1963).

In the description of the Hodgkin-Huxley hypothesis of the mechanism of propagation of the nerve AP (page 413), it was pointed out that local ionic currents produced at an active region of the membrane bring about the changes in permeability at an adjacent, inactive site that lead to the development there of the spike. Nachmansohn (1959, 1973) has proposed that ACh is the missing factor linking electrical events to the permeability changes. According to his hypothesis, the local currents trigger the release of ACh, at successive intervals along the axon, which combines with axonal receptors to effect the permeability changes; its action is then terminated by its rapid hydrolysis by AChE. When the impulse reaches the axonal terminal, transmission across the synapse is visualized as being effected by the same mechanism: the release of ACh at the postsynaptic site by the current flowing across the synaptic cleft. Accordingly, axonal conduction and synaptic transmission are presented as identical processes. Among the findings that are still inconsistent with the hypothesis are (1) the extreme variations in the concentrations of ACh, choline acetyltransferase, and AChE in various types of axons; (2) differences of one or two orders of magnitude between the concentrations of anti-ChE agents required to block axonal conduction over those that produce inactivation of all detectable AChE; and (3) the irreducible latent period of junctional transmission, discussed earlier. The interested reader is referred to the reviews cited above for full documentation and interpretation of the evidence.

ADRENERGIC TRANSMISSION

Under this general heading are included *norepinephrine,* the transmitter of most sympathetic postganglionic fibers and probably of certain tracts in the CNS, and *dopamine,* the predominant transmitter of the mammalian extrapyramidal system, as well as *epinephrine,* the major hormone of the adrenal medulla.

A tremendous amount of information has accumulated concerning catecholamines and related compounds during recent years. Two major reasons for this have been the application of new technics, especially radioisotopic labeling and histofluorescence localization of catecholamines, and indications of the importance of interactions between the endogenous catecholamines and many of the drugs now used in the treatment of hypertension, mental disorders, and a variety of other conditions. The details of these interactions and of the pharmacology of the sympathomimetic amines themselves will be found in subsequent chapters. (*See also* symposia edited by Acheson, 1966; Blaschko and Muscholl, 1972; Cotten, 1972; Usdin and Snyder, 1973.) The basic physiological, biochemical, and pharmacological features are presented briefly here.

Synthesis, Storage, and Release of Catecholamines. The *synthesis* of epinephrine from phenylalanine, by the steps shown in Figure 21-4, was proposed by Blaschko in 1939. The overall conversion was not actually demonstrated until several years later when Gurin and Delluva (1947) gave radioactively

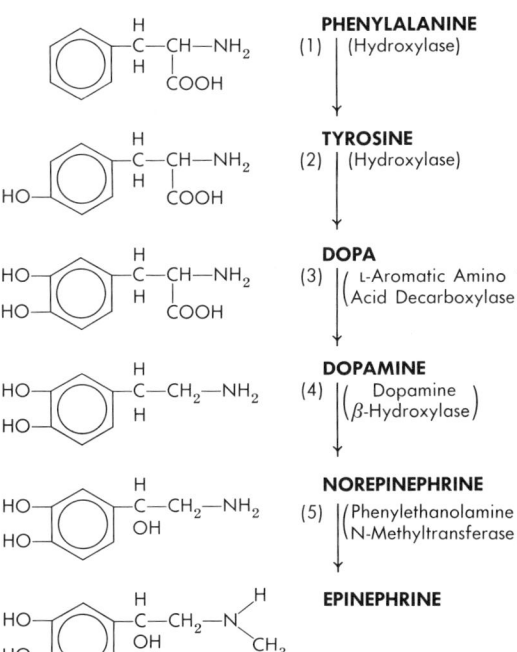

Figure 21-4. *Steps in enzymatic synthesis of norepinephrine and epinephrine.* (After Blaschko, 1939; Gurin and Delluva, 1947; Levin *et al.*, 1960; and others.)

labeled phenylalanine to rats and recovered radioactive epinephrine from the adrenal gland. This sequence has now been confirmed, and the enzymes involved have been identified and characterized. It is important to note that none of these enzymes is highly specific; consequently, many other endogenous substances as well as certain drugs are similarly acted upon at the various steps. For example, 5-hydroxytryptamine (5-HT, serotonin), tyramine, and histamine can be produced by L-aromatic amino acid decarboxylase, or dopa decarboxylase (step 3), from their corresponding amino acids. Tyramine, in turn, can be oxidized (step 4) to octopamine, the phenol analog of norepinephrine; while octopamine is present only in small amounts in mammals (Molinoff and Axelrod, 1969), it is probably the major adrenergic transmitter in certain invertebrates (Barker *et al.*, 1972b). Dopa decarboxylase can also convert the drug α-methyldopa to α-methyldopamine (Hess *et al.*, 1961), which, in turn, is converted by dopamine β-hydroxylase to the "false transmitter," α-methylnorepinephrine.

Another aspect of prime pharmacological significance is that of the relative velocities of each of these enzymatic steps in the body. One approach to the treatment of hypertension has consisted in attempts to block the synthesis of norepinephrine by compounds that inhibit the various enzymes involved. However, this mode of attack can be expected to be fruitful only if the reaction involved is the *rate-limiting* one, tyrosine hydroxylase (step 2) (Levitt *et al.*, 1965).

Current knowledge concerning the *cellular sites and mechanisms of synthesis, storage, and release* of catecholamines has been derived from studies of both adrenergically innervated organs and adrenal medullary tissue. Nearly all the *norepinephrine* content of the former is confined to the postganglionic sympathetic fibers; it disappears within a few days after section of the nerves. The small amount of residual catecholamine is largely *epinephrine,* which is presumably localized in chromaffin cells.

Formaldehyde-vapor histofluorescence studies have revealed the presence of a dense network of catecholamine-containing nerve fibers in smooth and cardiac muscle, blood vessels, and certain exocrine glands, which represents the postganglionic adrenergic component of the terminal reticular apparatus. Most of the catecholamine is present in frequently occurring vesicular swellings that are in close apposition to the muscle and gland cells (Carlsson et al., 1962). By modifications of the same technic, certain tracts in the CNS have been characterized as containing norepinephrine, dopamine, or 5-HT (Hillarp et al., 1966). The latter findings have greatly strengthened both earlier proposals and current indications, based largely on pharmacological evidence, of the central neurohumoral roles of these monoamines (see reviews by Brodie et al., 1959; Rothballer, 1959; McLennan, 1970; Kety, 1972).

More recently, the purification of most of the enzymes that participate in the synthesis of norepinephrine has permitted the preparation of highly specific antisera against them. When the antisera, in turn, are purified and coupled with fluorescein isothiocyanate, they can then be applied to tissue sections for the cytological localization of the enzymes by appropriate *immunohistofluorescence* technics. Similar principles have been employed for the development of extremely sensitive *radioimmunoassays* for the quantification of norepinephrine, epinephrine, and their precursors and metabolites in serum and tissues (see Goldstein et al., 1972; Hartman and Udenfriend, 1972).

Another approach that promises to be of considerable value for investigating the functions of adrenergic innervation has been the development of means of producing *immunosympathectomy* and *chemosympathectomy*. The former arose from observations that a protein, *nerve-growth factor,* present in various sources including salivary glands, produces a marked hypertrophy of sympathetic ganglia, both in tissue culture and in newborn animals. When an *antiserum* to the nerve-growth factor is injected into newborn animals under proper conditions, it suppresses the development of the peripheral sympathetic system (Levi-Montalcini and Angeletti, 1968). The same result can be obtained more simply in both newborn and adult animals by the administration of the chemosympathectomizing agent 6-hydroxydopamine. This compound is taken up selectively by adrenergic fibers and results in their destruction (Thoenen, 1972).

The main features of the mechanisms of synthesis, storage, and release of catecholamines and their modifications by drugs are summarized in Figure 21–5. Osmophilic granules, 0.05 to 0.2 μm in diameter, have been isolated from the adrenal medulla, splenic nerves, and various regions of the CNS; they correspond to similar structures noted in electron micrographs of tissue sections (Bloom, 1973). The granules contain extremely high concentrations of catecholamines (approximately 21% dry weight) and ATP, in a molecular ratio of 4:1, as well as a specific protein, *chromogranin,* and the enzyme dopamine β-hydroxylase. While the intragranular catecholamine-nucleotide-protein complex constitutes the *reserve pool,* which is the major storage depot of epinephrine in the adrenal medulla, it is uncertain whether a corresponding complex with norepinephrine is the major storage form of the transmitter in the terminals of adrenergic fibers (DePotter, 1971). Nevertheless, some reserve pool undoubtedly exists in active equilibrium with considerably smaller *mobile pools* within the *granules* (II) and the *cytoplasm* (I). In the course of synthesis (Figure 21–4), the hydroxylation of tyrosine to dopa and the decarboxylation of dopa to dopamine (steps 2 and 3) take place in the cytoplasm. Dopamine then enters the granules, where it is converted to norepinephrine (step 4). In the adrenal medulla, most of the norepinephrine leaves the granules, is methylated in the cytoplasm to epinephrine (step 5), and then reenters a different group of intracellular granules, where it is stored until released. Thus, in the human adult, epinephrine accounts for approximately 80% of the catecholamines of the adrenal medulla, with norepinephrine making up most of the remainder. (See reviews by Axelrod, 1963; Euler, 1972a; Stjärne, 1972.)

In addition to its synthesis *de novo,* outlined above, there is a second major source of the norepinephrine of the terminal portions of the adrenergic fibers, namely, recapture by active transport of norepinephrine previously released to the extracellular fluid. This process, in fact, is probably the major one responsible for the termination of the effects of adrenergic impulses in most organs; the blood vessels apparently constitute an exception, where the immediate disposition of released norepinephrine is accomplished largely by a combination of enzymatic breakdown and diffusion (Spector et al., 1972). In order to effect the re-uptake of norepinephrine and to maintain the concentration gradients of synthesized norepinephrine within the aforementioned pools, at least two active transport systems are probably involved: one, across the axoplasmic membrane from the extracellular fluid to the *cytoplasmic mobile pool* (*I*); and the other, from I to the *intragranular mobile pool* (*II*). Evidence for the former transport system is largely indirect and is based on the selective actions of various drugs, as discussed below.

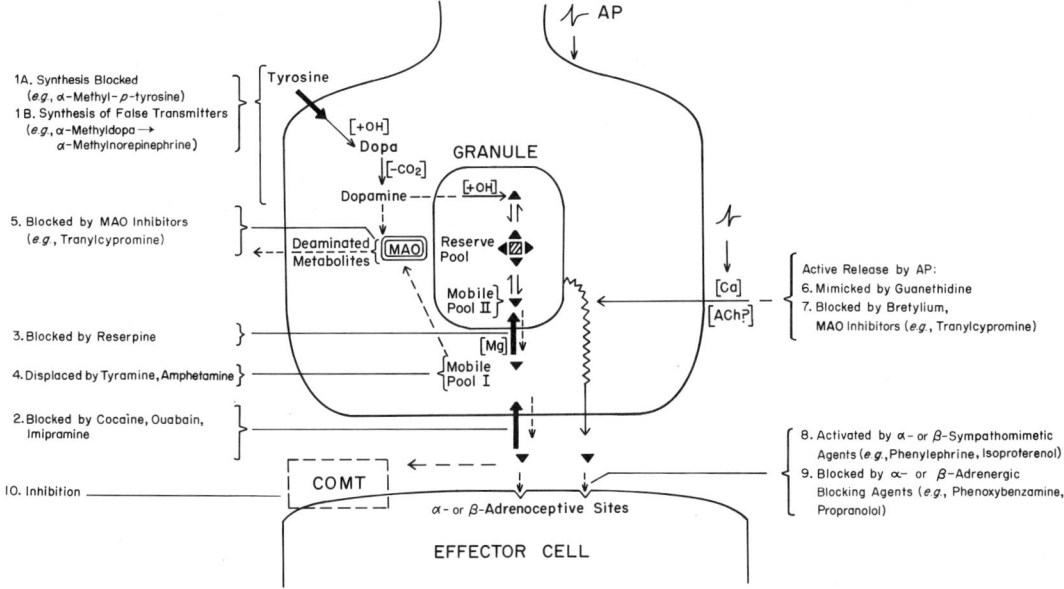

Figure 21-5. *Proposed sites of action of drugs that modify synthesis, uptake, release, and actions of norepinephrine at adrenergic nerve terminals.*

Norepinephrine (▼) within the nerve terminal is partitioned into a cytoplasmic mobile pool (*I*) and intragranular pools through equilibria between active transport (heavy arrows), passive diffusion (dash arrows), enzymatic synthesis (light arrows), and destruction (mitochondrial monoamine oxidase, MAO). Intragranular reserve pool consists of catecholamine-ATP (▨) salt (combined in a ratio of 4:1, along with a specific protein) in equilibrium with an intragranular mobile pool (*II*). As shown at right, norepinephrine is discharged rapidly to the exterior by the nerve action potential (AP) through the mobilization of calcium ion, with possible involvement of acetylcholine (Burn and Rand hypothesis). On the basis of pharmacological data, the norepinephrine released by the AP is shown to come from the intragranular pools. The contents of the granule are presumably released by exocytosis (*see* page 426). Following release of norepinephrine and its action at adrenoceptive sites of effector cells, excess is removed from extracellular region largely by return to axonal terminal through active transport and to some extent by diffusion and subsequent enzymatic inactivation by extraneuronal catechol-O-methyl-transferase (COMT).

Drugs may exert their effects by modifying these processes as follows:

1. Interference with synthesis of transmitter: (*A*) inhibition of rate-limiting enzyme (tyrosine hydroxylase), leading to depletion of norepinephrine (*e.g.*, α-methyl-*p*-tyrosine); (*B*) enzymatic transformation by same pathway as normal precursor, leading to synthesis of "false transmitter" (*e.g.*, α-methyldopa → α-methylnorepinephrine).

2. Blockade of active transport from extracellular fluid to cytoplasmic mobile pool (*I*), causing augmentation of norepinephrine action at adrenoceptive sites (*e.g.*, cocaine, imipramine, chlorpromazine).

3. Blockade of active transport from cytoplasmic (*I*) to intragranular (*II*) pools, leading to depletion of latter, and enzymatic deamination within cytoplasm by mitochondrial MAO (*e.g.*, reserpine).

4. Displacement of norepinephrine from cytoplasmic mobile pool (*I*), leading to sympatho-mimetic effects (*e.g.*, tyramine, amphetamine). Similar displacement could also occur from granular storage sites.

5. Inhibition of MAO, leading to accumulation of norepinephrine at central and possibly other sites (*e.g.*, tranylcypromine). See also 7.

6. Active release from intragranular mobile pool (*II*), leading to transient sympathomimetic effects followed by depletion of reserve pool (*e.g.*, guanethidine).

7. Interference with release by AP, causing block of adrenergic nerve activity (*e.g.*, bretylium, certain MAO inhibitors).

8. Activation of effector cells by sympathomimetic agents at α- or β-adrenoceptive sites (*e.g.*, phenylephrine, isoproterenol).

9. Blockade by adrenergic blocking agents at α- or β-adrenoceptive sites (*e.g.*, phenoxy-benzamine, propranolol).

10. Inhibition of COMT (no important present examples).

(*See* text for references.)

Due to the relative ease of isolating pure preparations of granules, especially from the adrenal medulla, the second transport system has been characterized more fully. It can concentrate catecholamines against a 200-fold gradient across the granular membrane to the *intragranular mobile pool (II)*, which then is in equilibrium with the catecholamine-ATP-protein complex that constitutes the *reserve pool.* The system is activated by ATP and the magnesium ion, and is blocked by very low concentrations (4×10^{-8} M) of reserpine (Kirshner, 1962; Carlsson *et al.,* 1963). The transport system across the axoplasmic membrane is blocked selectively by a number of other drugs, including *cocaine, imipramine,* and *ouabain.* Certain sympathomimetic drugs (*e.g., ephedrine, tyramine*) produce most of their effects indirectly, chiefly by displacing norepinephrine from the cytoplasmic mobile pool (I) to the extracellular fluid, where the released endogenous transmitter then acts at the receptor sites of the effector cells. The relationship between these activities and the important effects of such drugs is discussed below.

Adrenergic fibers can sustain the output of norepinephrine during prolonged periods of stimulation without exhausting their reserve supply, provided the mechanisms of synthesis and uptake of the transmitter are unimpaired.

Many years ago it was noted that the urinary output of *norepinephrine* in man is greater following periods of activity than after rest, suggesting that the synthesis of norepinephrine is enhanced by increased activity of the sympathetic nervous system (Euler, 1954). This relationship has been considerably amplified and confirmed through a variety of experimental procedures, and with the use of modern methods for the estimation of norephinephrine, its precursors, and metabolites. It appears that at least two mechanisms are responsible, both of which involve primarily the rate-limiting enzyme in the synthesis of norepinephrine, tyrosine hydroxylase (step 2). First, as a negative-feedback system, tyrosine hydroxylase is inhibited by the ultimate end product, norepinephrine. This inhibitory action of norepinephrine is apparently exerted by binding to the normal site for the enzyme's cofactor, tetrahydropteridine. Thus, with a decrease in the concentration of norepinephrine in the cytoplasmic mobile pool (I), as would follow brief periods of rapid firing and the uptake of norepinephrine by depleted granules, the activity of the enzyme is relatively enhanced. Conversely, when the level of cytoplasmic norepinephrine is raised by a monoamine oxidase inhibitor (*see* below), tyrosine hydroxylase is in turn inhibited, and the rate of norepinephrine synthesis falls. The second mechanism is based on changes in the concentration of the enzyme itself. Sustained periods of high frequency of preganglionic firing, as would result from heightened reflex activity due to denervation of the baroreceptors or the chronic administration of a hypotensive drug, induce an increase in the level of tyrosine hydroxylase (and of dopamine β-hydroxylase) in the postsynaptic adrenergic neurons, which can enhance the amount of norepinephrine formed and released at adrenergic terminals (*see* reviews by Axelrod, 1972; Kopin, 1972; Weiner *et al.,* 1972).

A major factor that controls the rate of synthesis of *epinephrine,* and hence the size of the store available for release from the adrenal medulla, is the level of glucocorticoids secreted by the adrenal cortex. The latter hormones are carried in high concentration, by the intra-adrenal portal vascular system, directly to the adrenal medullary chromaffin cells, where they induce the synthesis of phenylethanolamine-N-methyltransferase (step 5), the enzyme that methylates norepinephrine to epinephrine. Thus, any stress that persists sufficiently to invoke an enhanced secretion of corticotropin (*see* Chapter 70) will mobilize the appropriate hormones of both the adrenal cortex (predominantly cortisol) and medulla (epinephrine) (*see* review by Wurtman *et al.,* 1972).

This remarkable relationship is present only in certain mammals, including man, where the adrenal chromaffin cells are enveloped entirely by steroid-secreting cortical cells. In the dogfish, for example, where the chromaffin cells and steroid-secreting cells are located in independent, noncontiguous glands, no epinephrine is formed (*see* review by Coupland, 1972).

It is likely that the enzymes discussed above, which participate in the synthesis of norepinephrine, are synthesized in the perikaryonal cell bodies of the adrenergic neurons and are then transported along the axons to their terminals. This can occur either slowly (1 to 3 mm per day) by bulk flow through axoplasm, as appears to be the case for tyrosine hydroxylase, or much more rapidly (1 to 10 mm per hour), as with dopamine β-hydroxylase. The microtubular system may participate in such rapid axonal transport and also in the formation of the granules and in their extrusion following nerve impulses (*see* review by Kopin and Silberstein, 1972).

The full sequence of steps by which the *nerve impulse* effects the *release of norepinephrine* from adrenergic fibers is not known. In the adrenal medulla, the triggering event is the liberation of ACh by the preganglionic fibers and its combination with receptors on the chromaffin cells to produce a localized depolarization; a succeeding step is the entrance of calcium ions into these cells, which results in the extrusion by exocytosis of the granular contents (epinephrine, ATP, chromogranin, dopamine β-hydroxylase) to the extracellular fluid and hence into the circulation (Douglas, 1968). Calcium likewise appears to play an essential role in coupling the nerve impulse with the release of norepinephrine at adrenergic nerve terminals (Burn and Gibbons, 1965), as has been demonstrated also at cholinergic terminals. In terms of the above-discussed Burn and Rand hypothesis, ACh release is postulated to be an essential or facilitatory step in the liberation of norepinephrine, but this is still controversial. Evidence that exocytosis is the primary event in the release of norepinephrine from granules in adrenergic nerve terminals is not yet as firmly established as is that for the adrenal medulla for technical reasons. However, enhanced activity of the sympathetic nervous system is accompanied by an increased concentration of both dopamine β-hydroxylase and chromogranin in the circulation. This should result only if the entire contents of the granule were released. As discussed below, drugs can act at these steps either by promoting actively the release of norepinephrine, in much the same manner as the nerve impulse (*e.g., guanethidine*), or by blocking this process (*e.g., bretylium*, certain inhibitors of monoamine oxidase [MAO]).

Metabolic Disposition. The two enzymes of major importance in the initial steps of metabolic transformation of catecholamines in the mammal are MAO and catechol-O-methyltransferase (COMT) (*see* reviews by Blaschko, 1952; Axelrod, 1963, 1966; Costa and Sandler, 1972; Kopin, 1972). Yet it is unlikely, at sites other than blood vessels, that either of these enzymes is of importance in the termination of the effects of adrenergic impulses, in relation to other processes such as re-uptake by the axonal terminals, diffusion, temporary adsorption to plasma proteins, and reflex adjustments. As Blaschko (1952) has pointed out, the narrow spatial and temporal limitations of the action of the transmitter that are essential for efficient functioning at most sites of cholinergic transmission probably do not apply to adrenergic transmission at peripheral autonomic effectors.

Both MAO and COMT are widely distributed throughout the body, including the brain; the highest concentrations of each are in the liver and the kidney. However, there are distinct differences in their cytological locations; whereas MAO is associated chiefly with mitochondria, including those within the terminals of adrenergic fibers, COMT is confined largely to the soluble cytoplasmic fraction and apparently has no selective association with adrenergic nerves. These factors are of importance both in determining the primary metabolic pathways followed by catecholamines in various circumstances and in explaining the effects of certain drugs.

From a variety of studies in which isotopically labeled catecholamines were used, it appears that most of the epinephrine and norepinephrine that enters the circulation, from the adrenal medulla or from exogenous administration, or that is released rapidly from adrenergic fibers is first methylated by COMT to metanephrine or normetanephrine, respectively (Figure 21-6). Norepinephrine that is released slowly, either by drugs such as reserpine or by nerve impulses of low frequency, is probably initially deaminated by the MAO of intra-axonal mitochondria to the corresponding aldehyde (not shown in Figure 21-6) and then converted rapidly at extraneuronal sites to 3,4-dihydroxymandelic acid. In either case, most of the metabolite resulting from attack by the initial enzyme is then converted by the other to the common product, 3-methoxy-4-hydroxy-mandelic acid, generally but incorrectly called "vanillylmandelic acid (VMA)," which constitutes the major metabolite of catecholamines excreted in the urine. The corresponding product of the metabolic degradation of dopamine, which contains no hydroxyl group in the side chain, is homovanillic acid (HVA). In the human brain, and throughout the body of the rat and certain other species, the aldehyde oxidation products of MAO are reduced rather than oxidized, resulting in the ultimate formation of 3-methoxy-4-hydroxyphenylglycol (Figure 21-6, dashed arrows). Variable amounts of all these metabolites are conjugated to the corresponding sulfates or glucuronides prior to urinary excretion.

The quantitative relationship between the foregoing pathways is illustrated by the results of an investigation in which isotopically labeled epinephrine was administered intravenously to human subjects in amounts equivalent to those secreted normally by the adrenal medulla (LaBrosse *et al.*, 1961). Approximately 40% of the dose given was recovered from the urine as 3-methoxy-4-hydroxymandelic acid, 40% as metanephrine (free and conjugated), 7% as 3-methoxy-4-hydroxyphenylglycol sulfate, and small amounts as 3,4-dihydroxymandelic acid and unchanged epinephrine. Normally the 24-hour urinary excretion includes 2 to 4 mg of 3-methoxy-4-hydroxymandelic acid (representing chiefly norepinephrine produced by adrenergic fibers and deaminated within them by MAO prior to release), 100 to 300 μg of normetanephrine (representing physiologically active norepinephrine released by adrenergic fibers), 100 to 200 μg of metanephrine (representing part of the epinephrine released by the adrenal medulla), 25 to 50 μg of norepinephrine, and 2 to 5 μg of epinephrine.

Inhibitors of MAO (*e.g., pargyline, nialamide*) can cause an increase in the level of norepinephrine in the brain and other tissues accompanied by a variety of pharmacological effects; however, some of the

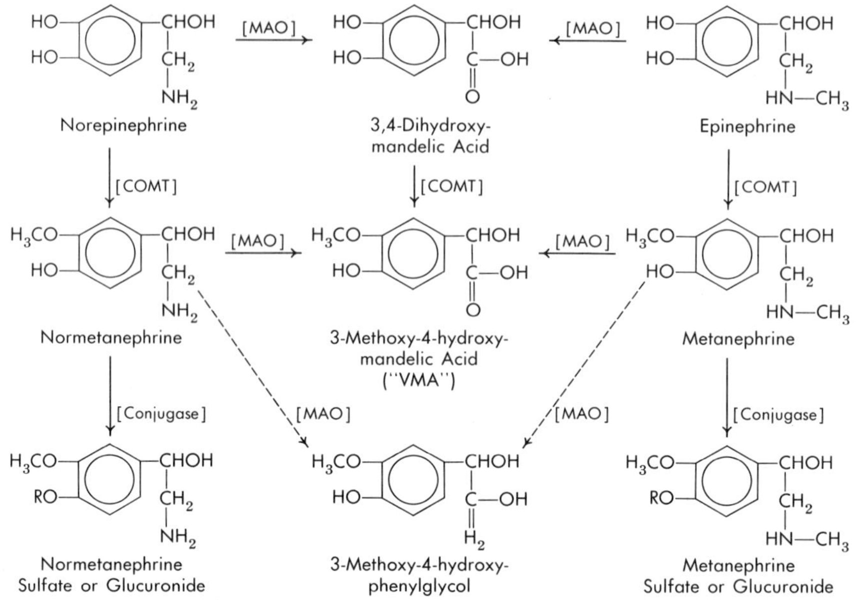

Figure 21-6. *Steps in the metabolic disposition of catecholamines.*

Both norepinephrine and epinephrine can initially be oxidatively deaminated by monoamine oxidase (MAO) to the corresponding aldehyde (not shown) and thence oxidized to 3,4-dihydroxy-mandelic acid; alternatively, they can first be methylated by catechol-O-methyltransferase (COMT) to normetanephrine and metanephrine, respectively. Most of the products of either type of reaction are then metabolized by the other enzyme to form the major excretory product, 3-methoxy-4-hydroxymandelic acid (frequently misnamed vanillylmandelic acid ["VMA"], a convention that unfortunately has become generally established). Small amounts of normeta-nephrine and metanephrine are conjugated to the corresponding sulfates or glucuronides, and small portions of their initial aldehyde oxidation products are reduced to 3-methoxy-4-hydroxy-phenylglycol (dashed arrows); the latter step occurs to a greater extent in the CNS. (After Axelrod, 1963, and others.)

effects may be due to additional, unrelated actions of these compounds, as discussed below. No striking pharmacological action can be attributed to the inhibition of COMT.

General Actions of Adrenergic Transmitters. The effects of norepinephrine released by adrenergic nerve impulses at various effector organs are listed in Table 21-1, and the actions of the catecholamines and other sympathomimetic agents are presented in detail in Chapter 24. Hence, it is necessary here to mention only the general principles relating to the role of the catecholamines as neurohumoral transmitters. Norepinephrine, epinephrine, and other catecholamines can cause either excitation or inhibition of *smooth muscle,* depending on the site, the dose, and the catecholamine chosen. Norepinephrine is the most potent excitatory catecholamine and has correspondingly low ac-

tivity as an inhibitor; *isoproterenol* exhibits the reverse pattern of activity. Epinephrine is relatively potent both as an excitor and as an inhibitor of smooth muscle. On the basis of such observations, Ahlquist (1948) proposed the terms α and β *receptors* for adrenoceptive sites on smooth muscles where catecholamines produce excitation and inhibition, respectively. The gut is generally relaxed by catecholamines, but here the inhibitory response is mediated by both α and β receptors. The cardiac nodes and muscle respond to catecholamines and adrenergic impulses with an increase in rate and force of contraction (positive chronotropic and inotropic effects), but these have essentially the pharmacological properties of β-adrenergic responses. Isoproterenol is thus the most potent agent in producing these effects. This classification of receptors has been corroborated by the findings that certain drugs (*e.g., phenoxybenzamine*) produce selective blockade of the effects of adrenergic nerve impulses and sympathomimetic agents at α-receptor sites, whereas others (*e.g., propranolol*) produce selective β-adrenergic blockade.

It has also been shown that the β receptors can be subdivided into β_1 receptors (chiefly at cardiac sites) and β_2 receptors (elsewhere) on the basis of the relative selectivity of effects of both excitatory agents and antagonists (Lands *et al.*, 1967). The future development of highly selective drugs in these categories would offer distinct therapeutic advantages.

In the smooth muscle of the guinea pig *vas deferens*, where adrenergic nerve impulses cause contraction by activation of α receptors, Burnstock and Holman (1961) have shown that effects at the muscle fiber membrane are quite similar to those produced by ACh on smooth muscles where the ester has an excitatory effect. Each adrenergic nerve impulse causes localized, partial depolarization; when the summation of successive responses attains a critical level of depolarization, a spike potential is induced; this is conducted over the adjacent muscle fibers and is followed by contraction. These effects are due primarily to an increase in Na^+ conductance (Magaribuchi *et al.*, 1971).

In contrast, in the guinea pig *taenia coli*, where the spontaneous rhythmic activity is inhibited by adrenergic nerve impulses through activation of both α and β receptors, the opposite effects are produced: suppression of spike discharges, abolition of conducted responses to electrical stimulation, and hyperpolarization. The basis for these effects is considerably more complex. The inhibitory response mediated by the α receptors is due to an increase in K^+ conductance. The β-receptor inhibitory component is apparently not associated with any significant change in ionic conductance; it may be due to an increase in the binding of calcium to the cell membrane, which results in a stabilizing effect, and is probably based in turn on an increase in intracellular cyclic adenosine 3',5'-monophosphate (cyclic AMP), as discussed below (*see* review by Bülbring, 1973). An additional complication is introduced by the possibility that the α-inhibitory effects of catecholamines on the gastrointestinal tract are brought about primarily at the level of the cholinergic parasympathetic neurons in Auerbach's plexus (Reddy and Moran, 1968).

In addition to the foregoing pharmacodynamic effects, epinephrine and its congeners produce an important group of *metabolic effects,* the manifestations of which include hyperglycemia, hyperlactacidemia, hyperlipemia, increased oxygen consumption, and hyperkalemia (*see* reviews by Haugaard and Hess, 1965; Ellis, 1967; Himms-Hagen, 1967, 1972). The key compound that is involved in the mediation of these effects, as well as those of a great number of other hormones, is *cyclic AMP,* as has been demonstrated in a brilliant series of investigations initiated by Sutherland, Rall, and their associates (*see* Robison *et al.,* 1971; Rall, 1972; Introduction to Section XVII, this text). Epinephrine enhances the accumulation of intracellular cyclic AMP by activating (via a β receptor) a membrane-bound enzyme, adenylate cyclase, which catalyzes the conversion of ATP to cyclic AMP. Cyclic AMP then initiates a series of intracellular alterations, resulting in the characteristic metabolic effects of the catecholamines and probably in many of their pharmacodynamic effects as well.

The β receptors are presumably located in the cell membranes with their catecholamine-binding sites oriented externally; the mechanism of interaction of the receptor with adenylate cyclase is unknown. It may be relatively direct or by means of yet-unidentified chemical messengers. Numerous difficulties have been encountered in attempts to study binding of catecholamines to the β-adrenergic receptor (*see* Maguire *et al.,* 1974). New technics appear promising, however, and progress in the isolation and characterization of the receptor may soon be forthcoming (Aurbach *et al.,* 1974).

Hyperglycemia induced by catecholamines and by glucagon is attributable in part to activation, via cyclic AMP, of hepatic *glycogen phosphorylase.* This enzyme converts glycogen to glucose-1-phosphate—the rate-limiting step in *glycogenolysis.* In addition, the action of cyclic AMP results in the inactivation of *glycogen synthase,* the enzyme that catalyzes the transfer of glucosyl units from UDP-glucose to glycogen. These two effects of cyclic AMP thus summate to increase the output of glucose from the liver.

The mechanism of action of cyclic AMP to produce these enzymatic changes is complex and is the result of the initiation of cascading series of protein phosphorylation reactions (Figure 21–7). Cyclic AMP interacts with its intracellular receptor, a *cyclic AMP–dependent protein kinase,* and causes the dissociation of this enzyme into an activated catalytic subunit and a regulatory subunit (the cyclic AMP-binding component). The activated protein kinase can phosphorylate a variety of proteins, ATP being used as a substrate. Thus, protein kinase phosphorylates glycogen synthase, and the result is *inactivation* of the enzyme by its conversion from a form that is independent (I) of a cofactor (glucose-6-phosphate) for activity to a form that is dependent (D) on the cofactor. Concurrently, the activated protein kinase phosphorylates and *activates* the enzyme *phosphorylase kinase.* Phosphorylase kinase is in fact another protein kinase, and it catalyzes the phosphorylation and *activation* of phosphorylase. In

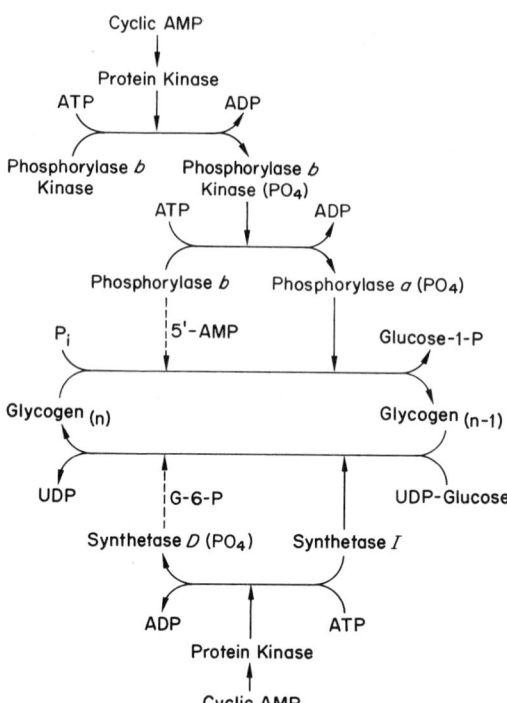

Figure 21-7. *Regulation of glycogen metabolism in muscle by cyclic AMP.*

The details are described in the text. Various protein phosphatases that catalyze the removal of phosphate from the phosphorylated proteins have been omitted for simplification. Dashed arrows indicate activation of phosphorylase *b* and synthase *D* by 5'-AMP and glucose-6-phosphate (G-6-P), respectively. The reactions in liver are analogous, except that the two forms of phosphorylase are referred to as *inactive* and *active*, and there is little effect of 5'-AMP. (After Rall and Gilman, 1970. Courtesy of *Neurosciences Research Program Bulletin.*)

muscle, the phosphorylation of phosphorylase results in its conversion from the *b* form (dependent on 5'-AMP for activity) to the *a* (independent) form. In liver, a similar activation occurs, although *inactive* hepatic phosphorylase is only little affected by 5'-AMP.

Since muscle does not contain glucose-6-phosphatase, an end product of glycogenolysis in muscle is lactate, and *hyperlactacidemia* results.

Hyperglycemia is also promoted by other catecholamine-induced mechanisms:

1. *Gluconeogenesis* from lactate and amino acids is stimulated, via cyclic AMP, by catecholamines and glucagon. The mechanism of this action is less precisely understood. The critical reactions occur in mitochondria and involve the metabolic transformation of pyruvate to oxaloacetate to phosphoenolpyruvate. The latter is then converted to glucose by the action of several cytoplasmic en-

zymes. This is also an important action of glucocorticoids (*see* Chapter 70), by mechanisms not directly involving cyclic AMP. Catecholamines also act on adipose tissue, through cyclic AMP, to enhance *lipolysis,* with a resultant outpouring of free fatty acids and glycerol into the bloodstream. The metabolism of fatty acids by various tissues can spare their utilization of glucose.

2. Catecholamines have both an inhibitory effect on the secretion of insulin by the β cells of the pancreatic islets, via α receptors, and a cyclic AMP–mediated stimulatory effect, by means of β receptors. The inhibitory effect predominates strongly *in vivo.* Since insulin can antagonize many of the metabolic effects of catecholamines and glucagon, this inhibitory effect on the secretion of insulin reinforces the actions described above.

The catecholamine-induced efflux of potassium from the liver, following a transient influx, is probably mediated by cyclic AMP, as is the briefer outflow of calcium. In the heart, catecholamines and glucagon increase the uptake of calcium.

The important question of a causal relationship between the accumulation of cyclic AMP induced by catecholamines and the pharmacodynamic actions of these agents at autonomic effector and synaptic sites is currently a subject of extensive investigation. Most if not all the actions of catecholamines at *β-receptor* sites appear to be brought about by activation of adenylate cyclase and the consequent increase in the intracellular concentrations of cyclic AMP. This applies to inhibitory effects on smooth muscle, excitatory effects on the myocardium, secretory responses of exocrine glands, and quite possibly the action of norepinephrine as an inhibitory neurohumoral transmitter in the CNS. No such relationship has been demonstrated for α-receptor activation; indeed, this has been shown in some tissues to inhibit adenylate cyclase activity, but the physiological significance of this inhibition is unknown.

The positive inotropic effect of epinephrine on the *myocardium,* which is brought about predominantly by activation of β receptors, has been investigated extensively in an effort to determine whether it is related causally to the concurrent increase in cyclic AMP. There is a large amount of indirect and direct evidence to suggest that this is the case. However, the positive inotropic effect does not result from stimulated cardiac glycogenolysis, as was earlier suspected. Subsequently, emphasis has been placed on phosphorylation of proteins important in the regulation of contraction (*e.g.,* troponin) or on possible cyclic AMP–mediated alterations of Ca^{2+} transport by the sarcoplasmic reticulum. Yet, as pointed out in a critical review by Sobel and Mayer (1973), one should not exclude the possibility that catecholamines have other actions on the myocardium, independent of cyclic AMP, that may also be involved in the inotropic response.

Of particular interest is the role of cyclic AMP in the CNS (*see* reviews by Rall and Gilman, 1970; Rall, 1972). High concentrations of adenylate cyclase are present in the CNS, where catecholamines and other putative transmitters can produce marked increases in the concentrations of cyclic AMP. However, some of these receptors may be located in glial cells, the functions of which are largely unknown (Gilman and Nirenberg, 1971).

Bloom and associates have investigated the mechanism of the inhibitory effect of a tract of norepinephrine-containing fibers that arise in the locus ceruleus of the pons and terminate on the dendrites of the Purkinje cells of the *cerebellar cortex* of the rat (*see* Hoffer *et al.*, 1973). Stimulation of the locus ceruleus, or microiontophoretic application of norepinephrine or cyclic AMP to the Purkinje cells, produces inhibition of the latter, characterized in each case by (1) decreased rate of spontaneous discharge, (2) hyperpolarization with decrease in membrane conductance (in contrast to the increased conductance that generally accompanies the IPSP), (3) delayed onset and decline of the inhibitory response, (4) enhancement of such by inhibitors of cyclic AMP degradation, and (5) antagonism by β-adrenergic blocking agents of the foregoing effects following electrical stimulation of the nerve tracts or application of norepinephrine, but not following application of cyclic AMP. Thus, these findings appear not only to fulfill most of the standard criteria for identifying norepinephrine as the inhibitory transmitter at the site studied but also to provide strong evidence that its inhibitory action is mediated by cyclic AMP.

OTHER NEUROHUMORAL TRANSMITTERS

From the foregoing account, it is evident that ACh has been established as the neurohumoral transmitter agent at most efferent sites in the peripheral nervous system; the major exception is the terminals of most postganglionic sympathetic fibers, where norepinephrine has this function. In addition, ACh, norepinephrine, and dopamine probably serve as transmitters at certain sites within the CNS. Accordingly, there remain to be defined the transmitting agents of the primary afferent fibers, of certain exceptional postganglionic autonomic fibers (discussed below), and of the presumed majority of various excitatory and inhibitory fibers of the CNS that are neither cholinergic nor adrenergic. Although many naturally occurring compounds have been proposed for these roles, none has as yet been definitely established as a transmitter substance. The most likely candidates are discussed briefly below.

Amino Acids. By means of microiontophoretic application of compounds to neurons in various regions of the CNS, exhaustive searches for agents that might simulate the effects of impinging excitatory and inhibitory nerve impulses were conducted by Curtis and Watkins (1960), Krnjević and

Phillis (1963), and others. A major outcome of these collective efforts was the focusing of attention on a group of amino acids, which appear to fulfill to a considerable degree the criteria established for the identification of neurohumoral transmitters. Parallel investigations of synaptic and neuromuscular transmission in crustaceans have provided even stronger evidence that two amino acids, gamma-aminobutyric acid (GABA) and L-glutamic acid, function there as inhibitory and excitatory transmitters, respectively. At present, the two most promising candidates of this class for roles as inhibitory transmitters in the mammalian CNS are the monocarboxylic amino acids, *GABA* and *glycine*. Two dicarboxylic amino acids, L-*glutamic acid* and L-*aspartic acid*, qualify most closely as excitatory transmitters. (For documentation, *see* reviews by Curtis and Crawford, 1969; McLennan, 1970; Phillis, 1970; Curtis and Johnston, 1974; Krnjević, 1974.)

GABA was first proposed as an inhibitory transmitter or modulator of the mammalian CNS by Hayashi (1954) on the basis of its known presence in the brain and its anticonvulsant activity. In the same year, Florey (1954) extracted a synaptic inhibitory substance from various parts of the CNS, which was later identified as GABA (Bazemore *et al.*, 1957). Subsequently GABA was shown to produce inhibition accompanied by hyperpolarization, through an increase in chloride conductance, at cortical neurons and at cerebellar neurons of Deiter's nucleus; the latter effect was identical with that obtained by stimulation of inhibitory axons arising from Purkinje cells in the cerebellar cortex. By means of a remarkably sensitive enzymatic cycling method that permits determination of the GABA content of single mammalian neurons, Otsuka and Miyata (1972) have obtained evidence that the inhibitory terminations of the Purkinje cell axons on the Deiter's neurons contain extremely high concentrations of GABA. GABA may also produce presynaptic inhibition by depolarization of afferent terminals in the spinal cord (Davidoff, 1972).

The identification of GABA as an inhibitory transmitter has been strengthened further by the more or less selective blocking action obtained with *picrotoxin*, the alkaloid *bicuculline*, and more recently *penicillin* against both GABA and inhibitory nerve impulses at various sites. At the same time, these observations have provided an explanation for the mechanism of the convulsant action of these drugs. Semicarbazide and other pyridoxal-complexing hydrazides may produce convulsions through inhibition of the enzyme that synthesizes GABA, glutamate decarboxylase, resulting in a lowering of the level of GABA in the brain.

In *summary*, GABA has been established as an

inhibitory transmitter beyond reasonable doubt at the crustacean neuromuscular junction and with high probability in the mammalian CNS. (*See also* reviews by Roberts, 1968; Iversen, 1972; Otsuka, 1972.)

Glycine likewise meets many of the criteria for an inhibitory transmitter in the mammalian CNS; in contrast to GABA, its actions and distribution suggest that it functions in this capacity predominantly in the spinal cord and brain stem. Like GABA, it produces hyperpolarization of the postsynaptic membrane through an increase in chloride conductance, and its action may be terminated by active uptake into both neuronal and glial elements.

Strychnine, which produces convulsions by blocking spinal inhibitory pathways, was shown to block the inhibitory action of glycine at spinal motoneurons, an observation that supports the proposal that glycine is the transmitter of spinal inhibitory interneurons. However, this action is not specific, since strychnine also antagonizes the inhibitory effects of a variety of endogenous compounds on cerebral cortical neurons and can prevent the release of ACh from cholinergic fibers.

L-*Glutamate* produces excitation of practically all cells tested in the mammalian CNS; its depolarizing action on neuronal membranes is associated with an increase in both Na^+ and K^+ conductance, which may result in turn from displacement of Ca^{2+} from critical sites at the neuronal membrane where cation permeability is controlled (Curtis *et al.,* 1972; Zieglgänsberger and Puil, 1973). While glutamate is found in greater amounts than any other amino acid in the brain, its concentration is particularly high at certain sites, including the forebrain, cerebellum, and dorsal roots and dorsal gray matter of the spinal cord. On the basis of its actions and distribution, glutamate has been proposed as the transmitter of the primary afferent fibers, and as an excitatory transmitter at various other sites in the CNS. Like the inhibitory amino acids, its action is probably terminated by rapid uptake into both neuronal and glial cells. To date, no compounds have been shown convincingly to produce selective blockade of the actions of glutamate, although several have been proposed (Halderman and McLennan, 1972). *Aspartate* is similar to glutamate in its actions, and is found in moderate concentrations in various parts of the CNS. The relative potencies of the two compounds vary according to the sites tested.

A considerable body of evidence now indicates that glutamate is the excitatory transmitter at the neuromuscular junctions of crustaceans and other arthropods (Kravitz *et al.,* 1970); recent findings suggest that in the same phylum ACh may function as the neurotransmitter of primary afferent fibers (Barker *et al.,* 1972a). Thus, it would appear that in the course of evolution the arthropods and vertebrates may have adopted the same two compounds as neurotransmitters between the CNS and the periphery; however, in the divergence of the two phyla from a common primordial stock, the efferent and afferent roles of ACh and glutamate were reversed.

Adenosine Triphosphate. ATP was once proposed as the possible neurohumoral transmitter of primary afferent fibers (Holton, 1959), but confirmatory evidence is lacking. More recently, a stronger case has been presented by Burnstock (1972) and associates that ATP may function as an inhibitory transmitter in the gastrointestinal tract, where it is presumed to be released by certain postganglionic fibers arising from Auerbach's plexus, and as an excitatory transmitter in the urinary bladder. Such hypothetical fibers have been designated as "purinergic." While this proposal is still tentative, it would explain certain long-puzzling pharmacological anomalies. For example, responses of the bladder to nerve impulses are notably resistant to both adrenergic and cholinergic antagonists.

Adenosine and certain adenine nucleotides are prominent stimulators of cyclic AMP synthesis in the CNS (Sattin and Rall, 1970). Since adenosine is released from brain cells by depolarization and adenine nucleotides are released with catecholamines from the adrenal medulla, it seems possible that adenosine and/or adenine nucleotides may be transmitters or modulators of synaptic transmission in the CNS.

Other Compounds. Several other possible transmitters at various central sites are discussed elsewhere. These include *5-hydroxytryptamine* and *histamine* (Chapter 29) and various *peptides* and *prostaglandins* (Chapter 30).

The Relationship between the Nervous and the Endocrine Systems

The concept that "humors" are secreted at certain sites to act elsewhere in the body can be traced back to Aristotle. In modern terms, the theory of neurohumoral transmission by its very designation implies at least a superficial resemblance between the nervous and the endocrine systems. Yet it should now be clear that the similarities extend considerably deeper, particularly with respect to the autonomic nervous system. In the regulation of homeostasis, the autonomic nervous system is responsible for rapid adjustments to changes in the total environment, which it effects at both its ganglionic relays and postganglionic terminals by the liberation of chemical agents that act transiently at their immediate sites of release. The endocrine system, in contrast, regulates slower, more generalized adaptations by releasing its hormonal agents into the systemic circulation to act at distant, widespread sites over periods of hours or days. Both systems have their major central representations in the hypothalamus, where they are integrated with each other and with subcortical, cortical, and spinal influences. Furthermore, there are structures that defy strict classification as belonging to the nervous system or to the endocrine system. One example is the *adrenal medulla*. Another is the *hypothalamico-neurohypophyseal tract*, which is analogous to the neurosecretory cells in certain invertebrates and fish (*see* reviews by Welsh, 1955; Scharrer, 1972). In fish, such cells exhibit both synaptic excitability and impulse conduction, as they presumably do in their mammalian counterpart. The neurohumoral theory may thus be said to provide a unitary concept of the evolution and functioning of the nervous and the endocrine systems, in which the differences are essentially only quantitative.

PHARMACOLOGICAL CONSIDERATIONS

In the foregoing sections, there are numerous references to the actions of drugs considered primarily as tools for the dissection and elucidation of physiological mechanisms. Here will be presented a classification of drugs that act upon the nervous system and its effector organs at some stage of neurohumoral transmission. In the immediately succeeding chapters, as well as elsewhere in the text, the systematic pharmacology of the important members of each of these classes is described.

Before proceeding with any classification of drugs, it is essential to emphasize an important general principle. The "first adage" of pharmacology is: "No drug has a single effect." Thus, a drug may be classified as an "anti-ChE agent," but this does not preclude its having direct effects at postsynaptic cholinoceptive sites or elsewhere. Likewise, as has already been mentioned, iproniazid and other chemically related MAO inhibitors have also been shown to block the release of norepinephrine from adrenergic fibers; their therapeutic effect in the treatment of essential hypertension may be due to this blockade of release. While drugs are placed in a given class on the basis of what appears to be their primary or predominant action, the decision must often be an arbitrary one. Their additional effects or side effects constitute the major limitation to the usefulness of drugs as tools in the analysis of physiological and pharmacological mechanisms. In addition to such pharmacological side effects,

there are what might be called "clinical side effects"; these may compromise the value of certain drugs when they are employed therapeutically. For example, when ganglionic blocking agents were employed in the treatment of essential hypertension to lower blood pressure by blocking sympathetic vasoconstrictor impulses, they also produced blurring of vision, constipation, and urinary retention; such undesirable effects are due not to extraganglionic actions but to the blockade of parasympathetic ganglia. For these reasons both the pharmacologist and the clinician are constantly seeking drugs that have more selective effects, with respect to both mechanism and site.

Each step involved in neurohumoral transmission (Figure 21-3) represents a potential point of drug attack. This is illustrated in the more detailed diagram of the adrenergic terminal and its postjunctional site, in Figure 21-5. It is now profitable to consider the prototype drugs that affect processes concerned in each step of transmission at both cholinergic and adrenergic junctions. Table 21-2 includes representative agents that act by the mechanisms listed below.

Interference with the Synthesis or Release of the Transmitter. *Cholinergic.* *Hemicholinium* (HC-3), a synthetic compound, blocks the transport system by which choline accumulates in the terminals of cholinergic fibers and thus it limits the synthesis of the ACh store available for release (Birks and MacIntosh, 1957). *Botulinus toxin,* the causative agent in certain cases of severe food poisoning, has been shown to prevent the release of ACh by all types of cholinergic fibers studied; fatality results from peripheral respiratory paralysis. Apparently, the toxin blocks conduction at the preterminal portion of the axon, but why this effect is confined to cholinergic fibers is not known.

Adrenergic. Several drugs in this category are discussed above as well as elsewhere (*see* Index). α-*Methyl-p-tyrosine* blocks the synthesis of norepinephrine by inhibiting tyrosine hydroxylase, the enzyme representing the rate-limiting step. On the other hand, α-*methyldopa*, like dopa itself, is successively decarboxylated and hydroxylated in its side chain to form the "false neurotransmitter," α-*methylnorepinephrine*. The significance of

Table 21-2. TYPES OF ACTION OF REPRESENTATIVE DRUGS AT PERIPHERAL CHOLINERGIC AND ADRENERGIC SYNAPSES AND NEUROEFFECTOR JUNCTIONS *

MECHANISM OF ACTION	SYSTEM	DRUGS	EFFECT
1. Interference with synthesis of transmitter	Cholinergic	Hemicholinium	Depletion of ACh
	Adrenergic	α-Methyl-p-tyrosine	Depletion of norepinephrine
2. Metabolic transformation by same pathway as precursor of transmitter	Adrenergic	α-Methyldopa	Displacement of norepinephrine by false transmitter (α-methylnorepinephrine)
3. Blockade of transport system of membrane of nerve terminal	Adrenergic	Imipramine, amitriptyline	Accumulation of norepinephrine at extracellular sites
4. Blockade of transport system of storage granule membrane	Adrenergic	Reserpine	Destruction of norepinephrine by mitochondrial MAO, and depletion from adrenergic terminals
5. Displacement of transmitter from axonal terminal	Cholinergic	Carbachol	Cholinomimetic
	Adrenergic (rapid, brief)	Amphetamine, tyramine	Sympathomimetic
	Adrenergic (slow, prolonged)	Guanethidine	Depletion of norepinephrine from adrenergic terminal
6. Prevention of release of transmitter	Cholinergic	Botulinus toxin	Anticholinergic
	Adrenergic	Bretylium	Antiadrenergic
7. Mimicry of transmitter at postsynaptic receptor	Cholinergic Muscarinic Nicotinic	Methacholine Nicotine	Cholinomimetic Cholinomimetic
	Adrenergic Alpha Beta Beta$_2$	Phenylephrine Isoproterenol Salbutamol	Sympathomimetic Sympathomimetic Selective sympathomimetic (inhibition of smooth muscle)
8. Blockade of endogenous transmitter at postsynaptic receptor	Cholinergic Muscarinic Nicotinic	Atropine d-Tubocurarine, hexamethonium	Cholinergic blockade Cholinergic blockade
	Adrenergic Alpha Beta Beta$_1$	Phenoxybenzamine Propranolol Practolol	α-Adrenergic blockade β-Adrenergic blockade Selective adrenergic blockade (cardiac)
9. Inhibition of enzymatic breakdown of transmitter	Cholinergic	Anti-ChE agents (physostigmine, diisopropyl phosphorofluoridate [DFP])	Cholinomimetic
	Adrenergic	MAO inhibitors (pargyline, nialamide, tranylcypromine)	Accumulation of norepinephrine at certain sites; potentiation of tyramine

* Modified from Koelle, 1968.

434

these metabolic transformations of the drug is discussed in Chapter 33 (*see* review by Muscholl, 1972). *Bretylium* and *iproniazid* act by preventing the release of norepinephrine by the nerve impulse. Blockade of the synthesis of 5-HT, with its consequent depletion from the brain, is produced selectively by p-*chlorophenylalanine,* a selective inhibitor of tryptophan hydroxylase (*see* review by Bloom and Giarman, 1968).

Promotion of the Release of the Transmitter. *Cholinergic. Carbachol* (carbamylcholine) has been proposed to act by release of ACh at certain vascular smooth muscle neuroeffector junctions and in sympathetic ganglia (Renshaw *et al.,* 1938; Volle and Koelle, 1961). In addition, it probably acts directly at all postjunctional cholinergic receptors, as it does at the motor end-plate of skeletal muscle. *Tetraethylammonium* (TEA), which is classified as a ganglionic blocking agent, also promotes the release of ACh from certain cholinergic terminals (Koketsu, 1958).

Adrenergic. Several drugs that promote the release of the adrenergic mediator have already been discussed. On the basis of the *rate* and the *duration* of the drug-induced release of norepinephrine from adrenergic terminals, one of two opposite effects can predominate. Thus, *tyramine, ephedrine, amphetamine,* and related drugs cause a relatively rapid, brief liberation of the transmitter and hence produce a sympathomimetic effect. On the other hand, *reserpine* and *guanethidine* bring about a slow, prolonged depletion of the transmitter, which is largely metabolized by MAO prior to its release; consequently, their sympathomimetic effects are slight, and their major effects are equivalent to adrenergic blockade. As mentioned earlier, reserpine and guanethidine also cause the release of 5-HT and possibly other, unidentified amines from central and peripheral sites, and many of their major effects may be based on this action.

Combination with Postjunctional Receptor Sites. *Cholinergic.* With the development of the theory of cholinergic transmission, the focus of attention was transferred from the nerve terminal to the postjunctional site as the probable locus of action of a large number of peripherally acting stimulating and blocking drugs. This viewpoint has been of great value in the clarification and the classification of the effects of the majority of currently employed drugs in this category, and its application has led to the development of several new, more selectively acting compounds. Since ACh is the neurohumoral transmitter at various peripheral junctions, it can be assumed that the postjunctional cholinergic receptors all share certain common features. However, it has long been known that individual drugs vary with respect to their potency relative to that of ACh at different cholinoceptive sites. The various receptors must therefore have certain distinctive features, in addition to their common ones, based on specific chemical groupings or steric factors in their immediate vicinity. This constitutes the major basis of selectivity of drug action (*see* Figure 21-8). When a drug combines with a cholinergic receptor, it may produce one of two effects: the same effect as that of ACh (*i.e., cholinomimetic*); or no apparent direct effect but, by occupation of the receptor site, prevention of the action of endogenous ACh (*i.e., cholinergic blockade*). Many drugs produce the two effects in sequence; nicotine is an outstanding example of such an agent.

The effects of the alkaloids *muscarine* and *nicotine* on cholinergic junctions provided the basis for Dale's classical differentiation of receptor types, which is still accurate for both the peripheral and central nervous systems. The parasympathomimetic effects of muscarine were well known at the turn of the century and, in fact, prompted the early speculations by Dixon and Loewi concerning the possibility of neurohumoral transmission in the autonomic nervous system. By convention, the cholinomimetic effects of drugs at *autonomic effector cells,* including those of ACh itself, are referred to as *muscarinic effects,* since the alkaloid activates these receptors. From the early work of Langley it is known that nicotine in low doses stimulates, and in higher doses paralyzes, autonomic ganglia; the same sequence was later shown to occur at the motor end-plates of certain types of skeletal muscle. The stimulation and then blockade of *autonomic ganglia* and the *end-plates of skeletal muscle,* as exhibited by ACh and various other drugs, are

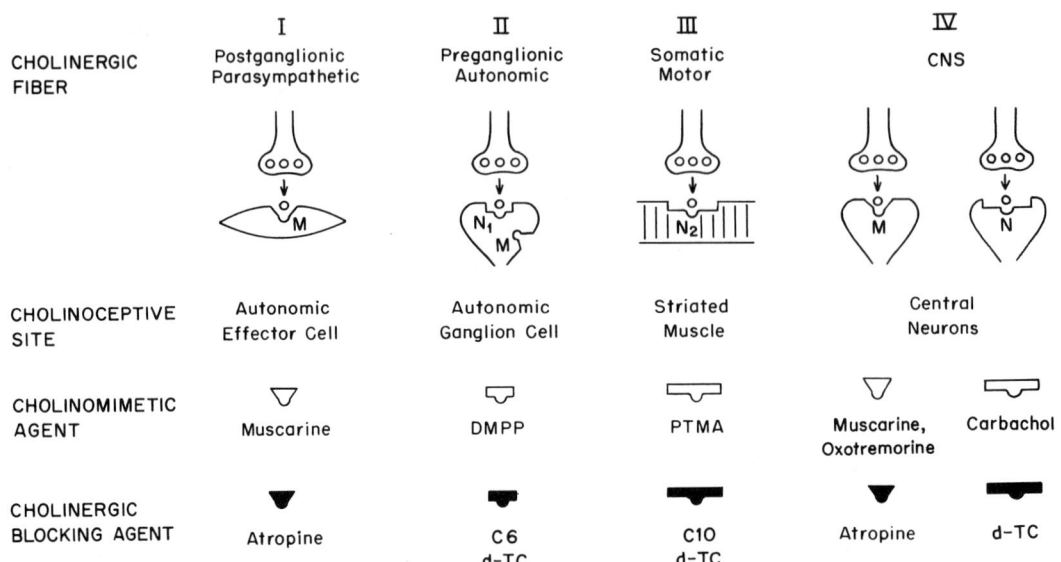

Figure 21-8. *Relative specificity of action of cholinomimetic and cholinergic blocking agents.*

Acetylcholine (ACh; depicted above as o), released by the nerve action potential from the four classes of cholinergic fibers (*I–IV*) or introduced from an exogenous source, can combine with the cholinoceptive sites of the corresponding postjunctional cells (*I–IV*) to produce its characteristic transmitter effects. Individual chemical configurations on the postjunctional membranes immediately adjacent to the ACh receptors are assumed to confer relative specificity by limiting the approach of various ACh-like drugs, according to their "shape" or "fit" with the total receptor complex. The receptors of autonomic effector cells (*I*) are classified as *muscarinic* (*M*), and those of autonomic ganglion cells (*II*) and striated muscle (*III*) are classified as *nicotinic* (*N*). Although certain drugs act at nicotinic receptors on both *II* and *III* (e.g., *d*-tubocurarine, *d*-TC), others are relatively selective for *II* (e.g., hexamethonium, C6) or *III* (e.g., decamethonium, C10); hence, their designation here as N_1 and N_2, respectively. Autonomic ganglion cells (*II*) also contain muscarinic receptors, although these may not participate in normal ganglionic transmission. Cholinoceptive neurons of the CNS have predominantly either nicotinic (spinal cord) or muscarinic (thalamus, cerebral cortex) receptors.

Examples of drugs that act selectively to produce cholinomimetic effects at the foregoing cholinoceptive sites are muscarine (*I*), dimethylphenylpiperazinium (DMPP) (*II*), phenyltrimethylammonium (PTMA) (*III*), muscarine or oxotremorine (*IV-M*), and carbachol (*IV-N*). Cholinergic blocking agents also combine relatively selectively at such sites but have no important effects directly; their effects are due to blockade of the approach of endogenous ACh or exogenous cholinomimetic agents. Examples of drugs acting in this manner are atropine (*I*), hexamethonium (C6) (*II*), decamethonium (C10) (*III*), atropine (*IV-M*), and *d*-tubocurarine (*IV-N*).

Nicotine acts at nicotinic sites to produce stimulation in low doses, blockade in high doses.

thus termed *nicotinic effects*. It must be emphasized that these effects by no means describe the full pharmacological spectra of muscarine and nicotine, which also have marked effects on the CNS and elsewhere.

The nicotinic and muscarinic actions of ACh can be strikingly demonstrated in the intestinal tract of a primitive fish, the tench. This fish has an intestine composed of two muscular coats, the outer one being striated muscle and the inner one smooth muscle; both types of muscle, however, are supplied by the vagus nerve and, therefore, receive cholinergic innervation. The outer muscle coat responds to stimulation with a rapid contraction characteristic of skele-

tal muscle, as schematically presented in Figure 21-9. When the vagus is stimulated, the released ACh excites both sets of muscle to contract, the recorded result appearing as diagramed in the figure. After *curare*, vagal stimulation elicits only the smooth muscle or muscarinic component of contraction because the striated muscle is paralyzed. If *atropine* is applied and the vagus then stimulated, only the striated muscle or nicotinic component of contraction is evoked because atropine blocks the response of smooth muscle to ACh. When *both curare and atropine* are given and the vagus is stimulated, no contraction occurs because both the nicotinic and the muscarinic actions of ACh are blocked. An additional observation from the field of comparative pharmacology serves to illustrate some of the foregoing drug actions. The iris sphincter of birds is composed of striated rather than smooth muscle. Consequently, the miotic response to stimulation of its cholinergic postganglionic nerves is blocked by tubocurarine but not by atropine.

The "nicotinic" receptors of autonomic ganglia and skeletal muscle are not completely identical since they respond differently to certain stimulating and blocking agents, as can be seen in Figure 21–8. *Dimethylphenylpiperazinium* (DMPP) and *phenyltrimethylammonium* (PTMA) are highly selective stimulants of autonomic ganglion cells and end-plates of skeletal muscle, respectively. *Tetraethylammonium* and *hexamethonium* are likewise selective ganglionic blocking agents. d-*Tubocurarine,* on the other hand, effectively blocks transmission at both motor end-plates and autonomic ganglia, although its action at the former site predominates, whereas *decamethonium,* a depolarizing agent, produces selective neuromuscular blockade. Some evidence suggests that the muscarinic receptors of smooth muscle may also be separable into more than one type (Burgen and Spero, 1968). The situation at autonomic ganglia is complicated further by the fact that the ganglion cells also have a secondary component of muscarinic receptors; these may not participate normally in ganglionic transmission, but they are selectively activated by anti-ChE agents and muscarinic drugs and blocked by atropine (*see* Chapters 22 and 27).

It now seems clear that cholinergic receptors on various neurons of the CNS are also either nicotinic or muscarinic; the former predominate on the Renshaw cells of the spinal cord, whereas most of those at cortical and subcortical sites are muscarinic.

Atropine selectively blocks all the muscarinic responses to injected ACh and related cholinomimetic drugs, whether they are excitatory, as in the intestine, or inhibitory, as in the heart. However, it is less effective in blocking responses to stimulation of certain postganglionic parasympathetic fibers. For example, although small doses of atropine prevent cardiac slowing or salivary secretion after nerve stimulation, even large doses will not abolish fully the responses of the smooth muscle of the intestine and urinary bladder to nerve impulses. A possible explanation is that such impulses are mediated in fact by purinergic, or ATP-releasing, fibers. Other belladonna alkaloids related to atropine and many synthetic compounds have similar blocking actions at cholinergic neuroeffector junctions.

With regard to the possible molecular basis for the difference between muscarinic and nicotinic receptors, it has been pointed out that ACh as well as numerous nicotinic and muscarinic activating and blocking drugs possess two features in common: a quaternary ammonium group or its equivalent; and an atom capable of forming a hydrogen bond, through an unshared pair of electrons, at an appropriate distance from the former. With the muscarinic agents, the distance between the two atoms is 4.3 to

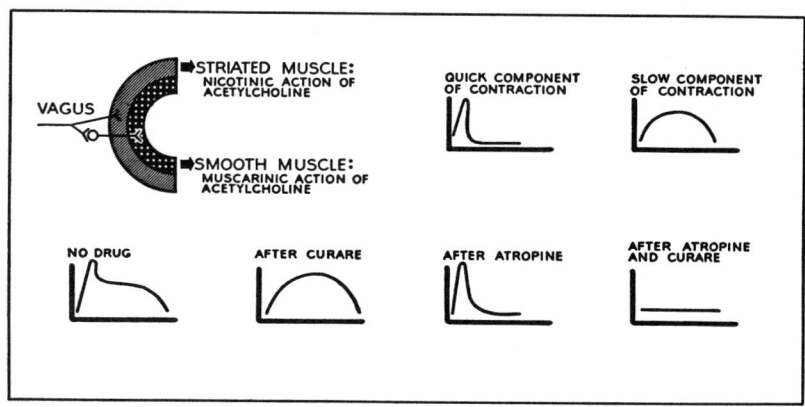

Figure 21–9. *Schematic representation of the nicotinic and muscarinic actions of acetylcholine* (*ACh*).

The two muscle coats of the intestinal wall of the tench are shown in the upper left diagram. The types of response elicited by vagal stimulation before and after administration of autonomic blocking agents are illustrated. The details are described in the text.

4.4 Å, corresponding to that between the N^+ and the ester-O atom of ACh. For the nicotinic agents, the corresponding distance is 5.9 Å, which is equivalent to that between the N^+ and carbonyl-O of ACh. The presence of hydrophobic groups (*e.g.,* the methyl groups on the N^+ of ACh) is proposed to be involved both in the attraction of the drugs to the receptor and in the transition from activating to blocking activity (Beers and Reich, 1970). A somewhat different interpretation of similar data has also been proposed, namely, that opposite sides of ACh react at muscarinic and nicotinic receptors (Chothia, 1970). Thus, a picture of the receptors emerges that includes an anionic group, a nucleophilic group, and adjacent hydrophobic areas, not unlike that for the active centers of AChE, as discussed in Chapter 22.

Adrenergic. A vast number of synthetic compounds that bear structural resemblance to the naturally occurring catecholamines can combine at α- or β-adrenoceptive sites, or both, and produce sympathomimetic effects (*see* Chapter 24). *Phenylephrine* acts relatively selectively at α-receptor sites, whereas *isoproterenol* exhibits an even greater degree of selective action at β adrenoreceptors. More recently, drugs have been sought for selective activation of β_1 or β_2 receptors. As an example of the latter type, *salbutamol* has been shown to produce effective bronchodilatation with minimal effects on the heart (Brittain, 1971). The main features of adrenergic blockade, including the selectivity of various blocking agents for α and β receptors, have been discussed. Here too, dissociation of effects at β_1 and β_2 adrenoreceptors has been achieved, as exemplified by the β_1-blocking agent, *practolol*, which blocks the cardiac actions of catecholamines without causing an equivalent degree of antagonism at bronchioles (Dunlop and Shanks, 1968). It should be recalled that several important drugs promoting or preventing the release of norepinephrine produce effects that resemble those of either direct activators or blockers of the postjunctional adrenoceptive sites, according to the rate and the duration of their action and other factors. To date, there are relatively few examples of cholinomimetic drugs that have been demonstrated to act by comparable presynaptic mechanisms.

Interference with the Destruction or Dissipation of the Transmitter. *Cholinergic.* The *anti-ChE agents* (Chapter 22) constitute a large group of compounds, the primary action of which is the brief or prolonged inhibition of AChE, with the consequent accumulation and action of endogenous ACh at sites of cholinergic transmission. Many drugs in this class probably have, in addition, direct actions at cholinoceptive sites and elsewhere, the importance of which varies with the individual compounds, the dose, the site of action, and other factors.

Adrenergic. As mentioned previously, there appears to be no parallelism between the role of either COMT or MAO in terminating the action of the adrenergic transmitter and that of AChE in terminating the action of the cholinergic transmitter. The re-uptake of norepinephrine by the adrenergic nerve terminals is probably the major mechanism for terminating its transmitter action. Interference with this process has been proposed as the basis of the potentiating effect of *cocaine* on responses to adrenergic impulses and injected catecholamines; the antidepressant effect of *imipramine* and related drugs is perhaps due to a similar action at putative adrenergic synapses in the CNS. Inhibitors of COMT, such as pyrogallol and tropolone, produce only slight enhancement of the actions of catecholamines, whereas MAO inhibitors, such as *tranylcypromine,* potentiate the effects of tyramine but not of catecholamines. There is an interesting consequence of the latter action that is of considerable importance clinically. Patients who are being treated with MAO inhibitors may develop severe hypertensive episodes following the ingestion of foods rich in tyramine, such as Roquefort cheese, pickled herring, and certain wines. This is because tyramine, which is normally metabolized by the MAO of the gut and the liver following absorption, now gains access to the systemic circulation and releases large amounts of norepinephrine from adrenergic nerve terminals.

Actions Unrelated to Neurohumoral Transmitters. The mechanisms of action of the great majority of currently employed drugs that affect primarily the peripheral nervous system and its effector organs can be classified within the four categories discussed above. This cannot be said of most centrally acting agents, at least at present. However, there is a growing number of examples of drugs, such as *strychnine, atropine,* the *anti-ChE agents,* the *antidepressant drugs, antiparkinsonism agents,* and the *antipsychotic phenothiazines* and *butyrophenones,* where reasonable evidence exists that their major effects are due to modification of neurohumoral transmission in the CNS. However, there are virtually no indications of this mechanism for such large and important classes of therapeutic agents as the *general anesthetics, anticonvulsant agents,* and *sedatives.* It now appears likely that such compounds act by modifying the stability of neuronal membranes through mechanisms that are still poorly understood.

From many lines of current investigation, including the study of individual central neurons during application of drugs to them by microiontophoresis, data on the pharmacological properties of central receptors are rapidly accumulating. As is evident, such studies have led to the development of compounds with sufficient selectivity of action at such central sites to provide new and unique therapeutic agents. Stated more precisely, the study of the mechanism of action of many of these drugs, after their therapeutic efficacy has been recognized by empirical observations, has led to a more complete understanding of central synaptic transmission and the putative neurohumors that are involved.

Ahlquist, R. P. A study of the adrenotropic receptors. *Am. J. Physiol.,* **1948,** *153,* 586–600.

Albuquerque, E. X.; Seyama, I.; and Narahashi, T. Characterization of batrachotoxin-induced depolarization of the squid giant axons. *J. Pharmac. exp. Ther.,* **1973,** *184,* 308–314.

Albuquerque, E. X.; Warnick, J. E.; Tasse, J. R.; and Sansone, F. M. Effects of vinblastine and colchicine on neural regulation of the fast and slow skeletal muscles of the rat. *Expl Neurol.,* **1972,** *37,* 607–634.

Aurbach, G. D.; Fedak, S. A.; Woodward, C. J.; Palmer, J. S.; Hauser, D.; and Troxler, F. β-Adrenergic receptor: stereospecific interaction of iodinated β-blocking agent with high affinity site. *Science, Wash.,* **1974,** *186,* 1223–1224.

Axelsson, J., and Thesleff, S. A study of supersensitivity in denervated mammalian skeletal muscle. *J. Physiol., Lond.,* **1959,** *147,* 178–193.

Bain, W. A. Method of demonstrating humor transmission of effects of cardiac vagus stimulation in frog. *Q. Jl exp. Physiol.,* **1932,** *22,* 269–274.

Barger, G., and Dale, H. H. Chemical structure and sympathomimetic action of amines. *J. Physiol., Lond.,* **1910,** *41,* 19–59.

Barker, D. L.; Herbert, E.; Hildebrand, J. G.; and Kravitz, E. A. Acetylcholine and lobster sensory neurones. *J. Physiol., Lond.,* **1972a,** *226,* 205–229.

Barker, D. L.; Molinoff, P. B.; and Kravitz, E. A. Octo-

pamine in the lobster nervous system. *Nature, New Biol.,* **1972b,** *236,* 61–63.

Bazemore, A. W.; Elliott, K. A. C.; and Florey, E. Isolation of factor I. *J. Neurochem.,* **1957,** *1,* 334–339.

Beers, W. H., and Reich, E. Structure and activity of acetylcholine. *Nature, Lond.,* **1970,** *228,* 917–922.

Birks, R. I., and MacIntosh, F. C. Acetylcholine metabolism of a sympathetic ganglion. *Can. J. Biochem. Physiol.,* **1961,** *39,* 787–827.

Blaschko, H. The specific action of L-dopa decarboxylase. *J. Physiol., Lond.,* **1939,** *96,* 50P–51P.

Brittain, R. T. A comparison of the pharmacology of salbutamol with that of isoprenaline, orciprenaline and trimetoquinol. *Postgrad. med. J.,* **1971,** *47,* Suppl., 11–16.

Brzin, M.; Tennyson, V. M.; and Duffy, P. E. Acetylcholinesterase in frog sympathetic and dorsal root ganglia: a study by electron microscope cytochemistry and microgasometric analysis with the magnetic diver. *J. cell Biol.,* **1966,** *31,* 215–242.

Buckley, G.; Consolo, S.; Giacobini, E.; and Sjöqvist, F. Cholinacetylase in innervated and denervated sympathetic ganglia and ganglion cells of the cat. *Acta physiol. scand.,* **1967,** *71,* 348–356.

Bullock, T. H., and Hagiwara, S. Intracellular recording from the giant synapse of the squid. *J. gen. Physiol.,* **1957,** *40,* 565–577.

Burgen, A. S. V., and Spero, L. The action of acetylcholine and other drugs on the efflux of potassium and rubidium from smooth muscle of the guinea-pig intestine. *Br. J. Pharmac.,* **1968,** *34,* 99–115.

Burgen, A. S. V., and Terroux, K. G. On the negative inotropic effects in the cat's auricle. *J. Physiol., Lond.,* **1953,** *120,* 449–464.

Burn, J. H., and Gibbons, W. R. The release of noradrenaline from sympathetic fibres in relation to calcium concentrations. *J. Physiol., Lond.,* **1965,** *181,* 214–223.

Burn, J. H., and Rand, M. J. Sympathetic postganglionic mechanism. *Nature, Lond.,* **1959,** *184,* 163–165.

Burnstock, G., and Holman, M. E. The transmission of excitation from autonomic nerve to smooth muscle. *J. Physiol., Lond.,* **1961,** *155,* 115–133.

Cannon, W. B., and Uridil, J. E. Studies on the conditions of activity in endocrine glands. VIII. Some effects on the denervated heart of stimulating the nerves of the liver. *Am. J. Physiol.,* **1921,** *58,* 353–354.

Carlsson, A.; Falck, B.; and Hillarp, N.-Å. Cellular localization of brain monoamines. *Acta physiol. scand.,* **1962,** *56,* Suppl. 196, 1–27.

Carlsson, A.; Hillarp, N.-Å.; and Waldeck, B. Analysis of the Mg^{++}-ATP dependent storage mechanism in the amine granules of the adrenal medulla. *Acta physiol. scand.,* **1963,** *59,* Suppl. 215, 1–38.

Casteels, R.; Droogmans, G.; and Hendrickx, H. Electrogenic sodium pump in smooth muscle cells of the guinea-pig's taenia coli. *J. Physiol., Lond.,* **1971,** *217,* 297–313.

Cavallito, C. J.; Yun, H. S.; Smith, J. C.; and Foldes, F. F. Choline acetyltransferase inhibitors. Configurational and electronic features of styrylpyridine analogs. *J. mednl Chem.,* **1969,** *12,* 134–138.

Chang, H. C., and Gaddum, J. H. Choline esters in tissue extracts. *J. Physiol., Lond.,* **1933,** *79,* 255–285.

Chothia, C. Interaction of acetylcholine with different cholinergic nerve receptors. *Nature, Lond.,* **1970,** *225,* 36–38.

Cooke, J. D.; Okamoto, K.; and Quastel, D. M. J. The role of calcium in depolarization-secretion coupling at the motor nerve terminal. *J. Physiol., Lond.,* **1973,** *228,* 459–497. (*See also* immediately preceding papers by same group on pages 377, 407, and 435.)

Cottrell, G. A.; Powell, B.; and Stanton, M. A simple method for measuring a picogram of acetylcholine using the clam (*Mya arenaria*) heart. *Br. J. Pharmac.,* **1970,** *40,* 866–870.

Curtis, D. R.; Game, C. J. A.; Johnston, G. A. R.; McCulloch, R. M.; and MacLachlan, R. M. Convulsive action of penicillin. *Brain Res.*, **1972**, *43*, 242–245.

Curtis, D. R., and Watkins, J. C. The excitation and depression of spinal neurones by structurally related amino acids. *J. Neurochem.*, **1960**, *6*, 117–141.

Dale, H. H. The action of certain esters and ethers of choline, and their relation to muscarine. *J. Pharmac. exp. Ther.*, **1914**, *6*, 147–190.

Dale, H. H., and Feldberg, W. Chemical transmission of secretory impulses to sweat glands of cat. *J. Physiol., Lond.*, **1934**, *82*, 121–128.

Dale, H. H.; Feldberg, W.; and Vogt, M. Release of acetylcholine at voluntary motor nerve endings. *J. Physiol., Lond.*, **1936**, *86*, 353–380.

Davidoff, R. A. Gamma-aminobutyric acid antagonism and presynaptic inhibition in the frog spinal cord. *Science, Wash.*, **1972**, *175*, 331–333.

Davis, R., and Koelle, G. B. Electron microscopic localization of acetylcholinesterase and nonspecific cholinesterase at the neuromuscular junction by the gold-thiocholine and gold-thiolacetic acid methods. *J. cell Biol.*, **1967**, *34*, 157–171.

DePotter, W. P. Noradrenaline storage particles in the splenic nerve. *Phil. Trans. R. Soc., Lond., B*, **1971**, *261*, 313–317.

De Robertis, E., and Bennett, H. S. Some features of the submicroscopic morphology of synapses in frog and earthworm. *J. biophys. biochem. Cytol.*, **1955**, *1*, 47–58.

Dixon, W. E. On the mode of action of drugs. *Med. Mag., Lond.*, **1907**, *16*, 454–457.

Dunlop, D., and Shanks, R. G. Selective blockade of adrenoceptive beta receptors in the heart. *Br. J. Pharmac.*, **1968**, *32*, 201–218.

Elfvin, L.-G. The ultrastructure of the superior cervical sympathetic ganglion of the cat. I. The structure of the ganglion cell processes as studied by serial sections. *J. ultrastruct. Res.*, **1963a**, *8*, 403–440. II. The structure of the preganglionic end fibers and the synapses as studied by serial sections. *Ibid.*, **1963b**, *8*, 441–476.

———. Ultrastructural studies on the synaptology of the inferior mesenteric ganglion of the cat. *Ibid.*, **1971**, *37*, 411–425.

Elliott, T. R. The action of adrenalin. *J. Physiol., Lond.*, **1905**, *32*, 401–467.

Emmelin, N., and MacIntosh, F. C. The release of acetylcholine from perfused sympathetic ganglia and skeletal muscles. *J. Physiol., Lond.*, **1956**, *131*, 447–496.

Euler, U. S. von. Adrenaline and noradrenaline. Distribution and action. *Pharmac. Rev.*, **1954**, *6*, 15–22.

Fatt, P., and Katz, B. Spontaneous subthreshold activity at motor nerve endings. *J. Physiol., Lond.*, **1952**, *117*, 109–128.

Feldberg, W., and Gaddum, J. H. The chemical transmitter at synapses in a sympathetic ganglion. *J. Physiol., Lond.*, **1934**, *81*, 305–319.

Feldberg, W., and Krayer, O. Das Auftreten eines azetylcholinartigen Stoffes im Herzvenenblut von Warmblütern bei Beizung der Nervi vagi. *Naunyn-Schmiedebergs Arch. exp. Path. Pharmak.*, **1933**, *172*, 170–193.

Florey, E. An inhibitory and excitatory factor of mammalian central nervous system, and their action on a single sensory neuron. *Archs int. Physiol.*, **1954**, *62*, 33–53.

Giacobini, E. The distribution and localization of cholinesterases in nerve cells. *Acta physiol. scand.*, **1959**, *45*, Suppl. 156, 1–45.

Gilman, A. G., and Nirenberg, M. Effect of catecholamines on the adenosine 3′:5′-cyclic monophosphate concentrations of clonal satellite cells of neurons. *Proc. natn. Acad. Sci. U.S.A.*, **1971**, *68*, 2165–2168.

Goldstein, M.; Fuxe, K.; and Hökfelt, T. Characterization and tissue localization of catecholamine synthesizing enzymes. *Pharmac. Rev.*, **1972**, *24*, 293–309.

Gurin, S., and Delluva, A. The biological synthesis of radioactive adrenalin from phenylalanine. *J. biol. Chem.*, **1947**, *170*, 545–550.

Hagiwara, S., and Tasaki, I. A study of the mechanism of impulse transmission across the giant synapse of the squid. *J. Physiol., Lond.*, **1958**, *143*, 114–137.

Halderman, S., and McLennan, H. The antagonistic action of glutamic acid diethylester towards amino acid–induced and synaptic excitations of central neurones. *Brain Res.*, **1972**, *45*, 393–400.

Hartman, B. K., and Udenfriend, S. The application of immunological techniques to the study of enzymes regulating catecholamine synthesis and degradation. *Pharmac. Rev.*, **1972**, *24*, 311–330.

Hayashi, T. Effects of sodium glutamate on the nervous system. *Keio J. Med.*, **1954**, *3*, 183–192.

Hess, S. M.; Connamacher, R. H.; Ozaki, M.; and Udenfriend, S. The effects of α-methyl-dopa and α-methyl-meta-tyrosine on the metabolism of norepinephrine and serotonin *in vivo*. *J. Pharmac. exp. Ther.*, **1961**, *134*, 129–138.

Hillarp, N.-Å.; Fuxe, K.; and Dahlström, A. Demonstration and mapping of central neurons containing dopamine, noradrenaline, and 5-hydroxytryptamine and their reactions to psychopharmaca. *Pharmac. Rev.*, **1966**, *18*, 727–741.

Hodgkin, A. L., and Huxley, A. F. A quantitative description of membrane current and its application to conduction and excitation in nerve. *J. Physiol., Lond.*, **1952**, *117*, 500–544.

Hoffer, B. J.; Siggins, G. R.; Oliver, A. P.; and Bloom, F. E. Activation of the pathway from locus coeruleus to rat cerebellar Purkinje neurons: pharmacological evidence of noradrenergic central inhibition. *J. Pharmac. exp. Ther.*, **1973**, *184*, 553–569.

Holton, P. The liberation of adenosine triphosphate on antidromic stimulation of sensory nerves. *J. Physiol., Lond.*, **1959**, *145*, 494–504.

Horcholle-Bossavit, G., and Tyc-Dumont, S. Evidence for a rapid transmission in the cat vestibular-ocular pathway. *Expl Brain Res.*, **1971**, *13*, 327–338.

Kato, J. Choline acetylase of human placenta. *J. Biochem., Tokyo*, **1960**, *48*, 768–772.

Katz, B., and Miledi, R. The measurement of synaptic delay, and the time course of acetylcholine release at the neuromuscular junction. *Proc. R. Soc., B*, **1965**, *161*, 483–495.

———. The statistical nature of the acetylcholine potential and its molecular components. *J. Physiol., Lond.*, **1972**, *224*, 665–699.

Kerkut, G. A.; Brown, L. C.; and Walker, R. J. Postsynaptic stimulation of the electrogenic sodium pump. *Life Sci.*, **1969**, *8*, 297–300.

Kirshner, N. Uptake of catecholamines by a particulate fraction of the adrenal medulla. *J. biol. Chem.*, **1962**, *237*, 2311–2317.

Koelle, G. B.; Davis, R.; Koelle, W. A.; Smyrl, E. G.; and Fine, A. V. The electron microscopic localization of acetylcholinesterase and pseudocholinesterase in autonomic ganglia. In, *Cholinergic Mechanisms.* (Waser, P. G., ed.) Raven Press, New York, **1975**, pp. 251–255.

Koelle, W. A., and Koelle, G. B. The localization of external or functional acetylcholinesterase at the synapses of autonomic ganglia. *J. Pharmac. exp. Ther.*, **1959**, *126*, 1–8.

Koketsu, K. Action of tetraethylammonium chloride on neuromuscular transmission in frogs. *Am. J. Physiol.*, **1958**, *193*, 213–218.

Kravitz, E. A.; Slater, C. R.; Takahashi, K.; Bownds, M. D.; and Grossfeld, R. M. Excitatory transmission in vertebrates—glutamate as a potential neuromuscular transmitter compound. In, *Excitatory Synaptic Mechanisms.* (Andersen, P., and Jansen, J. K. S., eds.) Universitetsforlaget, Oslo, **1970**, pp. 85–93.

Krnjević, K., and Miledi, R. Acetylcholine in mammalian

neuromuscular transmission. *Nature, Lond.,* **1958,** *182,* 805–806.

Krnjević, K., and Mitchell, J. F.   The release of acetylcholine in the isolated rat diaphragm. *J. Physiol., Lond.,* **1961,** *155,* 246–262.

Krnjević, K., and Phillis, J. W.   Iontophoretic studies of neurones in the mammalian cerebral cortex. *J. Physiol., Lond.,* **1963,** *165,* 274–304.

Krnjević, K.; Pumain, R.; and Renaud, L.   The mechanism of excitation by acetylcholine in the cerebral cortex. *J. Physiol., Lond.,* **1971,** *215,* 247–268.

Krnjević, K., and Whittaker, V. P.   Excitation and depression of cortical neurones by brain fractions released from micropipettes. *J. Physiol., Lond.,* **1965,** *179,* 298–322.

LaBrosse, E. H.; Axelrod, J.; Kopin, I. J.; and Kety, S. S.   Metabolism of 7-H³-epinephrine-*d*-bitartrate in normal young men. *J. clin. Invest.,* **1961,** *40,* 253–260.

Lands, A. M.; Arnold, A.; McAuliff, J. P.; Luduena, F. P.; and Brown, R. G., Jr.   Differentiation of receptor systems activated by sympathomimetic amines. *Nature, Lond.,* **1967,** *214,* 597–598.

Langley, J. N.   Observations on the physiological action of extracts of the supra-renal bodies. *J. Physiol., Lond.,* **1901,** *27,* 237–256.

Levin, E. Y.; Levenberg, B.; and Kaufman, S.   The enzymatic conversion of 3,4-dihydroxyphenylethylamine to norepinephrine. *J. biol. Chem.,* **1960,** *235,* 2080–2086.

Levitt, M.; Spector, S.; Sjoerdsma, A.; and Udenfriend, S.   Elucidation of the rate-limiting step in norepinephrine biosynthesis in the perfused guinea pig heart. *J. Pharmac. exp. Ther.,* **1965,** *148,* 1–8.

Lewandowsky, M.   Ueber eine Wirkung des Nebennierenextractes auf das Auge. *ZentBl. Physiol.,* **1898,** *12,* 599–600.

Lewis, P. R., and Shute, C. C. D.   The cholinergic limbic system: projection to hippocampal formation, medial cortex, nuclei of the ascending cholinergic reticular system, and the subfornical organ and supra-optic crest. *Brain,* **1967,** *90,* 521–540.

Loewi, O.   Über humorale Übertragbarkeit der Herznervenwirkung. *Pflügers Arch. ges. Physiol.,* **1921,** *189,* 239–242.

Loewi, O., and Navratil, E.   Über humorale Übertragbarkeit der Herznervenwirkung. X. Mitteilung. Über das Schicksal des Vagusstoff. *Pflügers Arch. ges. Physiol.,* **1926,** *214,* 678–688.

Longo, V. G.   Acetylcholine, cholinergic drugs, and cortical electrical activity. *Experientia,* **1955,** *11,* 76–78.

McIsaac, R. J., and Koelle, G. B.   Comparison of the effects of inhibition of external, internal and total acetylcholinesterase upon ganglionic transmission. *J. Pharmac. exp. Ther.,* **1959,** *126,* 9–20.

Magaribuchi, T.; Ito, Y.; and Kuriyama, H.   Effects of catecholamines on the guinea-pig vas deferens in various ionic environments. *Jap. J. Physiol.,* **1971,** *21,* 691–708.

Maguire, M. E.; Goldmann, P. H.; and Gilman, A. G.   The reaction of [³H] norepinephrine with particulate fractions of cells responsive to catecholamines. *Molec. Pharmac.,* **1974,** *10,* 563–581.

Miller, N. E.; DiCara, L. V.; Solomon, H.; Weiss, J. M.; and Dworkin, B.   Learned modifications of autonomic functions: a review and some new data. *Circulation Res.,* **1970,** *26–27,* Suppl. 1, 3–11.

Mitchell, J. F.   The spontaneous and evoked release of acetylcholine from the cerebral cortex. *J. Physiol., Lond.,* **1963,** *165,* 98–116.

Molinoff, P., and Axelrod, J.   Octopamine: normal occurrence in sympathetic nerves of rats. *Science, Wash.,* **1969,** *164,* 428–429.

Nastuk, W. L., and Levine, L.   A microbioassay for acetylcholine. *Proc. Soc. exp. Biol. Med.,* **1961,** *106,* 502–505.

Otsuka, M., and Miyata, Y.   Application of enzymatic cycling to the measurement of gamma-aminobutyric acid in single neurons of the mammalian central nervous system. In, *Studies of Neurotransmitters at the Synaptic Level. Advances in Biochemical Psychopharmacology,* Vol. 6. (Costa, E.; Iversen, L. L.; and Paoletti, R.; eds.) Raven Press, New York, **1972,** pp. 61–74.

Perry, W. L. M., and Talesnik, J.   The role of acetylcholine in synaptic transmission at parasympathetic ganglia. *J. Physiol., Lond.,* **1953,** *119,* 455–469.

Phillis, J. W.   Acetylcholine release from the cerebral cortex: its role in cortical arousal. *Brain Res.,* **1968,** *7,* 378–389.

Ramon-Moliner, E.   Acetylthiocholinesterase distribution in the brain stem of the cat. *Ergebn. Anat. EntwGesch.,* **1972,** *46,* 3–53.

Reddy, V., and Moran, N. C.   An evaluation of the adrenergic receptor types in isolated segments of the small intestine of the rabbit. *Archs int. Pharmacodyn. Thér.,* **1968,** *176,* 326–336.

Renshaw, R. R.; Green, D.; and Ziff, M.   A basis for the acetylcholine action of choline derivatives. *J. Pharmac. exp. Ther.,* **1938,** *62,* 430–448.

Riker, W. F.; Roberts, J.; Standaert, F. G.; and Fujimoru, H.   The motor nerve terminal as the primary focus for drug-induced facilitation of neuromuscular transmission. *J. Pharmac. exp. Ther.,* **1957,** *121,* 286–312.

Sattin, A., and Rall, T. W.   The effect of adenosine and adenine nucleotides on the adenosine 3′,5′-phosphate content of guinea pig cerebral cortex slices. *Molec. Pharmac.,* **1970,** *6,* 13–23.

Shute, C. C. D., and Lewis, P. R.   The ascending cholinergic reticular system: neocortical, olfactory and subcortical projections. *Brain,* **1967,** *90,* 497–520.

Sjöqvist, F.   Pharmacological analysis of acetylcholinesterase-rich ganglion cells in the lumbo-sacral sympathetic system of the cat. *Acta physiol. scand.,* **1963,** *157,* 352–362.

Sotelo, C., and Llinás, R.   Specialized membrane junctions between neurons in the vertebrate cerebellar cortex. *J. cell Biol.,* **1972,** *53,* 271–289.

Spector, S.; Tarver, J.; and Berkowitz, B.   Effects of drugs and physiological factors in the disposition of catecholamines in blood vessels. *Pharmac. Rev.,* **1972,** *24,* 191–202.

Takeuchi, A., and Takeuchi, N.   On the permeability of end-plate membrane during the action of transmitter. *J. Physiol., Lond.,* **1960,** *154,* 52–67.

Thaemert, J. C.   The ultrastructure and disposition of vesiculated nerve processes in smooth muscle. *J. cell Biol.,* **1963,** *16,* 361–377.

Trautwein, W.; Kuffler, S. W.; and Edwards, C.   Changes in membrane characteristics of heart muscle during inhibition. *J. gen. Physiol.,* **1956,** *40,* 135–145.

Volle, R. L., and Koelle, G. B.   The physiological role of acetylcholinesterase (AChE) in sympathetic ganglia. *J. Pharmac. exp. Ther.,* **1961,** *133,* 223–240.

Zieglgänsberger, W., and Puil, E. A.   Actions of glutamic acid on spinal neurons. *Expl Brain Res.,* **1973,** *17,* 35–49.

Monographs and Reviews

Acheson, G. H. (ed.).   Second symposium on catecholamines. *Pharmac. Rev.,* **1966,** *18,* Part 1, 1–803.

Albers, R. W.   Biochemical aspects of active transport. *A. Rev. Biochem.,* **1967,** *36,* 727–756.

Augustinsson, K.-B.   Classification and comparative enzymology of the cholinesterases and methods for their determination. In, *Cholinesterases and Anticholinesterase Agents.* (Koelle, G. B., ed.) *Handb. exp. Pharmak.,* Vol. 15. Springer-Verlag, Berlin, **1963,** pp. 89–128.

Axelrod, J.   The formation, metabolism, uptake and release of noradrenaline and adrenaline. In, *The Clinical Chemistry of Monoamines.* (Varley, H., and Gowenlock, A. H., eds.) Elsevier Publishing Co., Amsterdam, **1963,** pp. 5–18.

———.   Methylation reactions in the formation and metabolism of catecholamines and other biogenic amines: the enzymatic conversion of norepinephrine (NE) to epinephrine (E). *Pharmac. Rev.,* **1966,** *18,* 95–113.

———.   Dopamine-β-hydroxylase: regulation of its synthesis and release from nerve terminals. *Ibid.*, 1972, *24*, 233–243.

Bennett, M. R. *Autonomic Neuromuscular Transmission.* Cambridge University Press, London, 1972.

Bernard, C. *Leçons sur les phénomènes de la vie communs aux animaux et aux végétaux.* Baillière, Paris, 1878–1879. (Two volumes.)

Birks, R. I., and MacIntosh, F. C. Acetylcholine metabolism at nerve-endings. *Br. med. Bull.*, 1957, *13*, 157–161.

Blaschko, H. Amine oxidase and amine metabolism. *Pharmac. Rev.*, 1952, *4*, 415–458.

Blaschko, H., and Muscholl, E. (eds.). *Catecholamines. Handb. exp. Pharmak.*, Vol. 33. Springer-Verlag, Berlin, 1972.

Bloom, F. E. Ultrastructural identification of catecholamine-containing central synaptic terminals. *J. Histochem. Cytochem.*, 1973, *21*, 333–348.

Bloom, F. E., and Giarman, N. J. Physiologic and pharmacologic considerations of biogenic amines in the nervous system. *A. Rev. Pharmac.*, 1968, *8*, 229–258.

Bolton, T. B. The permeability change produced by acetylcholine in smooth muscle. In, *Drug Receptors.* (Rang, H. P., ed.) University Park Press, Baltimore, 1973, pp. 87–104.

Brodie, B. B.; Spector, S.; and Shore, P. A. Interactions of drugs with norepinephrine in the brain. *Pharmac. Rev.*, 1959, *11*, 548–564.

Bülbring, E. Actions of catecholamines on smooth muscle cell membrane. In, *Drug Receptors.* (Rang, H. P., ed.) University Park Press, Baltimore, 1973, pp. 1–13.

Burn, J. H., and Rand, M. J. Acetylcholine in adrenergic transmission. *A. Rev. Pharmac.*, 1965, *5*, 163–182.

Burnstock, G. Purinergic nerves. *Pharmac. Rev.*, 1972, *24*, 509–581.

Burnstock, G., and Iwayama, T. Fine-structural identification of autonomic nerves and their relation to smooth muscle. In, *Histochemistry of Nervous Transmission.* (Eränkö, O., ed.) Elsevier Publishing Co., Amsterdam, 1971, pp. 389–404.

Cannon, W. B. Organization for physiological homeostasis. *Physiol. Rev.*, 1929, *9*, 399–431.

————. *The Wisdom of the Body.* W. W. Norton & Co., Inc., New York, 1932.

Cannon, W. B., and Rosenblueth, A. *Autonomic Neuroeffector Systems.* The Macmillan Co., New York, 1937.

————. *The Supersensitivity of Denervated Structures: A Law of Denervation.* The Macmillan Co., New York, 1949.

Carlsson, A. The occurrence, distribution and physiological role of catecholamines in the nervous system. *Pharmac. Rev.*, 1959, *11*, 233–566.

Chagas, C., and Paes-de-Carvalho, A. (eds.). *Bioelectrogenesis: A Comparative Survey of Its Mechanisms, with Particular Emphasis on Electric Fishes.* Elsevier Publishing Co., Amsterdam, 1961.

Chase, M. H., and Clemente, C. D. Central neural components of the autonomic nervous system. *Anesthesiology*, 1968, *29*, 625–633.

Cole, K. S. *Membranes, Ions and Impulses: A Chapter of Classical Biophysics.* University of California Press, Berkeley, 1968.

Costa, E., and Sandler, M. (eds.). *Monoamine Oxidases—New Vistas. Advances in Biochemical Psychopharmacology*, Vol. 5. Raven Press, New York, 1972.

Cotten, M. deV. (ed.). Regulation of catecholamine metabolism in the sympathetic nervous system (N.Y. Heart Association Symposium). *Pharmac. Rev.*, 1972, *24*, 161–434.

Coupland, R. E. The chromaffin system. In, *Catecholamines.* (Blaschko, H., and Muscholl, E., eds.) *Handb. exp. Pharmak.*, Vol. 33. Springer-Verlag, Berlin, 1972, pp. 16–45.

Couteaux, R. Structure and cytochemical characteristics of the neuromuscular junction. In, *Neuromuscular Blocking and Stimulating Agents*, Vol. 1. *International Encyclopedia of Pharmacology and Therapeutics*, Sect. 14. (Cheymol, J., ed.) Pergamon Press, Ltd., Oxford, 1972, pp. 7–56.

Curtis, D. R., and Crawford, J. M. Central synaptic transmission—microelectrophoretic studies. *A. Rev. Pharmac.*, 1969, *9*, 209–240.

Curtis, D. R., and Johnston, G. A. R. Amino acid transmitters in the mammalian central nervous system. *Ergebn. Physiol.*, 1974, *69*, 97–188.

Dale, H. H. Chemical transmission of the effects of nerve impulses. *Br. med. J.*, 1934, *1*, 835–841.

————. The beginnings and the prospects of neurohumoral transmission. *Pharmac. Rev.*, 1954, *6*, 7–13.

De Robertis, E. *Histophysiology of Synapses and Neurosecretion.* Pergamon Press, Ltd., Oxford, 1964.

Douglas, W. W. Stimulus-secretion coupling: the concept and clues from chromaffin and other cells (the First Gaddum Memorial Lecture, Cambridge, September 1967). *Br. J. Pharmac.*, 1968, *34*, 451–474.

Eccles, J. C. *The Physiology of Synapses.* Springer-Verlag, Berlin; Academic Press, Inc., New York, 1964.

————. *The Understanding of the Brain.* McGraw-Hill Book Co., New York, 1973.

Ellis, S. The effects of sympathomimetic amines and adrenergic blocking agents on metabolism. In, *Physiological Pharmacology.* Vol. 4, *The Nervous System—Part D: Autonomic Nervous System Drugs.* (Root, W. S., and Hofmann, F. G., eds.) Academic Press, Inc., New York, 1967, pp. 179–241.

Eränkö, O., and Eränkö, L. Small, intensely fluorescent granule-containing cells in the sympathetic ganglion of the rat. In, *Histochemistry of Nervous Transmission.* (Eränkö, O., ed.) Elsevier Publishing Co., Amsterdam, 1971, pp. 39–51.

Euler, U. S. von. Synthesis, uptake and storage of catecholamines in adrenergic nerves. The effects of drugs. In, *Catecholamines.* (Blaschko, H., and Muscholl, E., eds.) *Handb. exp. Pharmak.*, Vol. 33. Springer-Verlag, Berlin, 1972a, pp. 186–230.

————. Regulation of catecholamine metabolism in the sympathetic nervous system. *Pharmac. Rev.*, 1972b, *24*, 365–369.

Feldberg, W. Present views on the mode of action of acetylcholine in the central nervous system. *Physiol. Rev.*, 1945, *25*, 596–642.

Ferry, C. B. Cholinergic link hypothesis in adrenergic neuroeffector transmission. *Physiol. Rev.*, 1966, *46*, 420–456.

Goedde, H. W.; Doenicke, A.; and Altland, K. *Pseudocholinesterasen.* Springer-Verlag, Berlin, 1967.

Goldberg, L. I. Cardiovascular and renal actions of dopamine: potential clinical applications. *Pharmac. Rev.*, 1972, *24*, 1–29.

Gray, E. G. The fine structural characterization of different types of synapse. In, *Histochemistry of Nervous Transmission.* (Eränkö, O., ed.) Elsevier Publishing Co., Amsterdam, 1971, pp. 149–160.

Grundfest, H. Electrical inexcitability of synapses and some consequences in the central nervous system. *Physiol. Rev.*, 1957a, *37*, 337–361.

————. The mechanisms of discharge of the electric organs in relation to general and comparative electrophysiology. *Prog. Biophys. biophys. Chem.*, 1957b, *7*, 3–71.

Hanin, I. (ed.). *Choline and Acetylcholine: Handbook of Chemical Assay Methods.* Raven Press, New York, 1974.

Haugaard, N., and Hess, M. E. Actions of autonomic drugs on phosphorylase activity and function. *Pharmac. Rev.*, 1965, *17*, 27–69.

Hebb, C. O. Formation, storage, and liberation of acetylcholine. In, *Cholinesterases and Anticholinesterase Agents.* (Koelle, G. B., ed.) *Handb. exp. Pharmak.*, Vol. 15. Springer-Verlag, Berlin, 1963, pp. 56–88.

Hillarp, N.-Å. The construction and functional organization of the autonomic innervation apparatus. *Acta physiol. scand.,* **1959,** *46,* Suppl. 157, 1–39.

Himms-Hagen, J. Sympathetic regulation of metabolism. *Pharmac. Rev.,* **1967,** *19,* 367–461.

———. Effects of catecholamines on metabolism. In, *Catecholamines.* (Blaschko, H., and Muscholl, E., eds.) *Handb. exp. Pharmak.,* Vol. 33. Springer-Verlag, Berlin, **1972,** pp. 363–462.

Holmstedt, B. Pharmacology of organophosphorus cholinesterase inhibitors. *Pharmac. Rev.,* **1959,** *11,* 567–688.

Hornykiewicz, O. Dopamine (3-hydroxytyramine) and brain function. *Pharmac. Rev.,* **1966,** *18,* 925–964.

Hubbard, J. I. Mechanism of transmitter release. In, *Progress in Biophysics and Molecular Biology,* Vol. 21. (Butler, J. A. V., and Noble, D., eds.) Pergamon Press, Ltd., Oxford, **1970,** pp. 33–124.

———. Microphysiology of vertebrate neuromuscular transmission. *Physiol. Rev.,* **1973,** *53,* 674–723.

Iversen, L. L. *The Uptake and Storage of Noradrenaline in Sympathetic Nerves.* Cambridge University Press, London, **1967.**

———. The uptake, storage, release and metabolism of GABA in inhibitory nerves. In, *Perspectives in Neuropharmacology.* (Snyder, S. H., ed.) Oxford University Press, New York, **1972,** pp. 75–111.

Kao, C. Y. Tetrodotoxin, saxitoxin and their significance in the study of excitation phenomena. *Pharmac. Rev.,* **1966,** *18,* 997–1049.

Katz, B. *Nerve, Muscle, and Synapse.* McGraw-Hill Book Co., New York, **1966.**

Kety, S. S. Norepinephrine in the central nervous system and its correlations with behavior. In, *Brain and Human Behavior.* (Karczmar, A. G., and Eccles, J. C., eds.) Springer-Verlag, Berlin, **1972,** pp. 115–129.

Koelle, G. B. A new general concept of the neurohumoral function of acetylcholine and acetylcholinesterase. *J. Pharm. Pharmac.,* **1962,** *14,* 65–90.

———. Cytological distributions and physiological functions of cholinesterases. In, *Cholinesterases and Anticholinesterase Agents.* (Koelle, G. B., ed.) *Handb. exp. Pharmak.,* Vol. 15. Springer-Verlag, Berlin, **1963,** pp. 187–298.

———. Functional anatomy of synaptic transmission. *Anesthesiology,* **1968,** *29,* 643–653.

———. Current concepts of synaptic structure and function. *Ann. N.Y. Acad. Sci.,* **1971,** *183,* 5–20.

Kopin, I. J. Metabolic degradation of catecholamines. The relative importance of different pathways under physiological conditions and after administration of drugs. In, *Catecholamines.* (Blaschko, H., and Muscholl, E., eds.) *Handb. exp. Pharmak.,* Vol. 33. Springer-Verlag, Berlin, **1972,** pp. 271–282.

Kopin, I. J., and Silberstein, S. D. Axons of sympathetic neurons: transport of enzymes *in vivo* and properties of axonal sprouts *in vitro. Pharmac. Rev.,* **1972,** *24,* 245–254.

Krnjević, K. Chemical nature of synaptic transmission in vertebrates. *Physiol. Rev.,* **1974,** *54,* 418–540.

Kuno, M. Quantum aspects of central and ganglionic synaptic transmission in vertebrates. *Physiol. Rev.,* **1971,** *51,* 647–678.

Levi-Montalcini, R., and Angeletti, P. U. Nerve growth factor. *Physiol. Rev.,* **1968,** *48,* 534–569.

Lloyd, D. P. C. Cholinergy and adrenergy in the neural control of sweat glands. In, *Studies in Physiology.* (Curtis, D. R., and McIntyre, A. K., eds.) Springer-Verlag, New York, **1965,** pp. 169–178.

MacLean, P. D. The limbic brain in relation to the psychoses. In, *Physiological Correlates of Emotion.* (Black, P., ed.) Academic Press, Inc., New York, **1970,** pp. 130–146.

McLennan, H. *Synaptic Transmission,* 2nd ed. W. B. Saunders Co., Philadelphia, **1970.**

Marley, E., and Stephenson, J. D. Central actions of catecholamines. In, *Catecholamines.* (Blaschko, H., and

Muscholl, E., eds.) *Handb. exp. Pharmak.,* Vol. 33. Springer-Verlag, Berlin, **1972,** pp. 186–230.

Michelson, M. J., and Zeimal, E. V. *Acetylcholine: An Approach to the Molecular Mechanism of Action.* Pergamon Press, Ltd., Oxford, **1973.**

Muscholl, E. Adrenergic false transmitters. In, *Catecholamines.* (Blaschko, H., and Muscholl, E., eds.) *Handb. exp. Pharmak.,* Vol. 33. Springer-Verlag, Berlin, **1972,** pp. 618–660.

Nachmansohn, D. *Chemical and Molecular Basis of Nerve Activity.* Academic Press, Inc., New York, **1959.**

———. The neuromuscular junction—the role of acetylcholine in excitable membranes. In, *The Structure and Function of Muscle,* 2nd ed., Vol. 3. (Bourne, G. H., ed.) Academic Press, Inc., New York, **1973,** pp. 31–116.

Nishi, S. Cholinergic and adrenergic receptors at sympathetic preganglionic nerve terminals. *Fedn Proc. Fedn Am. Socs exp. Biol.,* **1970,** *29,* 1957–1965.

Otsuka, M. α-Aminobutyric acid in the nervous system. In, *The Structure and Function of Nervous Tissue,* Vol. 4. (Bourne, G. H., ed.) Academic Press, Inc., New York, **1972,** pp. 249–289.

Phillis, J. W. *The Pharmacology of Synapses.* Pergamon Press, Ltd., Oxford, **1970.**

Potter, L. T. Synthesis, storage, and release of acetylcholine from nerve terminals. In, *The Structure and Function of Nervous Tissue,* Vol. 4. (Bourne, G. H., ed.) Academic Press, Inc., New York, **1972,** pp. 105–128.

Rall, T. W. Role of adenosine 3′,5′-monophosphate (cyclic AMP) in actions of catecholamines. *Pharmac. Rev.,* **1972,** *24,* 399–410.

Rall, T. W., and Gilman, A. G. (eds.). The role of cyclic AMP in the nervous system. *Neurosci. Res. Prog. Bull.,* **1970,** *8,* 221–323.

Rang, H. P. (ed.). *Drug Receptors.* University Park Press, Baltimore, **1973.**

Riker, W. F., Jr., and Okamoto, M. Pharmacology of motor nerve terminals. *A. Rev. Pharmac.,* **1969,** *9,* 173–208.

Roberts, E. Some biochemical-physiological correlations in studies in γ-aminobutyric acid. In, *Structure and Function of Inhibitory Neuronal Mechanisms.* (Euler, C. von; Skoglund, S.; and Soderberg, U.; eds.) Pergamon Press, Ltd., Oxford, **1968,** pp. 401–418.

Robison, G. A.; Butcher, R. W.; and Sutherland, E. W. *Cyclic AMP.* Academic Press, Inc., New York, **1971.**

Rothballer, A. B. The effects of catecholamines on the central nervous system. *Pharmac. Rev.,* **1959,** *11,* 494–547.

Salmoiraghi, G. C. Central adrenergic synapses. *Pharmac. Rev.,* **1966,** *18,* 717–726.

Scharrer, B. Comparative aspects of neuroendocrine communication. *Gen. comp. Endocr.,* **1972,** Suppl. 3, 515–517.

Schwarzacher, H. G. (ed.). *Histochemistry of Cholinesterase. Biblphie anat.,* **1961,** *2,* 1–255.

Shanes, A. M. Electrochemical aspects of physiological and pharmacological action in excitable cells. I. The resting cell and its alteration by extrinsic factors. *Pharmac. Rev.,* **1958a,** *10,* 59–164. II. The action potential and excitation. *Ibid.,* **1958b,** *10,* 165–273.

Silver, A. Cholinesterases of the central nervous system with special reference to the cerebellum. *Int. Rev. Neurobiol.,* **1967,** *10,* 57–109.

Sobel, B. E., and Mayer, S. E. Cyclic adenosine monophosphate and cardiac contractility. *Circulation Res.,* **1973,** *32,* 407–414.

Stjärne, L. The synthesis, uptake and storage of catecholamines in the adrenal medulla. The effects of drugs. In, *Catecholamines.* (Blaschko, H., and Muscholl, E., eds.) *Handb. exp. Pharmak.,* Vol. 33. Springer-Verlag, Berlin, **1972,** pp. 231–269.

Thoenen, H. Surgical, immunological, and chemical sympathectomy. In, *Catecholamines.* (Blaschko, H., and Muscholl, E., eds.) *Handb. exp. Pharmak.,* Vol. 33. Springer-Verlag, Berlin, **1972,** pp. 813–844.

Thomas, R. C. Electrogenic sodium pump in nerve and muscle cells. *Physiol. Rev.,* **1972,** *52,* 563–594.

Usdin, E., and Snyder, S. (eds.). *Frontiers in Catecholamine Research.* Pergamon Press, Ltd., Oxford, **1973.**

Uvnäs, B. Sympathetic dilator outflow. *Physiol. Rev.,* **1954,** *34,* 608–618.

Weiner, N.; Cloutier, G.; Bjur, R.; and Pfeffer, R. I. Modification of norepinephrine synthesis in intact tissue by drugs and during short-term adrenergic nerve stimulation. *Pharmac. Rev.,* **1972,** *24,* 203–232.

Welsh, J. H. Neurohormones. *Hormones, Lond.,* **1955,** *3,* 97–151.

Whittaker, V. P. Identification of acetylcholine and related esters of biological origin. In, *Cholinesterases and Anticholinesterase Agents.* (Koelle, G. B., ed.) *Handb. exp. Pharmak.,* Vol. 15. Springer-Verlag, Berlin, **1963,** pp. 1–39.

Willis, W. D. The case for the Renshaw cell. *Brain Behav. Evol.,* **1971,** *4,* 5–52.

Wurtman, R. J.; Pohorecky, L. A.; and Baliga, B. S. Adrenocortical control of the biosynthesis of epinephrine and proteins in the adrenal medulla. *Pharmac. Rev.,* **1972,** *24,* 411–426.

CHAPTER

22 ANTICHOLINESTERASE AGENTS

George B. Koelle

The role of acetylcholinesterase (AChE) in terminating the transmitter action of acetylcholine (ACh) at the junctions of the various cholinergic nerve endings with their effector organs or postsynaptic sites is presented in Chapter 21. Drugs that inhibit or inactivate AChE are called *anticholinesterase* (anti-ChE) agents. They cause ACh to accumulate at cholinoceptive sites and thus are potentially capable of producing effects equivalent to continuous stimulation of cholinergic fibers throughout the central and peripheral nervous systems. In view of the widespread distribution of cholinergic neurons, it is not surprising that the anti-ChE agents as a group have assumed more extensive practical application as toxic agents, in the form of agricultural insecticides and potential chemical-warfare "nerve gases," than as drugs. Nevertheless, there are certain representatives that are clinically useful.

Prior to World War II, only the "reversible" anti-ChE agents were generally known, of which *physostigmine (eserine)* is the outstanding example. Shortly before and during World War II, a comparatively new class of highly toxic chemicals, the *organophosphates,* was developed chiefly by Schrader, of I.G. Farbenindustrie, first as agricultural insecticides and later as potential chemical-warfare agents. The extreme toxicity of these compounds was found to be due to their "irreversible" inactivation of AChE, thereby exerting their effects for considerably longer periods than do the classical inhibitors. Since the pharmacological actions of both classes of anti-ChE agents are qualitatively similar, they will be discussed as a group, and the important special features of the individual classes or compounds noted. Certain effects of anti-ChE agents and their interactions with other drugs at autonomic ganglia and the neuromuscular junctions of skeletal muscle are described in Chapters 27 and 28.

History. *Physostigmine,* also called *eserine,* is an alkaloid obtained from the Calabar or ordeal bean, the dried ripe seed of *Physostigma venenosum* Balfour, a perennial woody climber growing on the banks of streams in tropical West Africa. The Calabar bean, also called Esére nut, chop nut, or bean of Etu Esére, was once used by native tribes of West Africa as an "ordeal poison" in trials for witchcraft.

The Calabar bean was brought to England in 1840 by Daniell, a British medical officer stationed in Calabar, and early investigations of its pharmacological properties were conducted by Christioson (1855), Fraser (1863), and Argyll-Robertson (1863). A pure alkaloid was isolated by Jobst and Hesse in 1864 and named *physostigmine;* the following year, Vee and Leven obtained the same alkaloid, which they named *eserine*. The first therapeutic use of the drug was in 1877 by Laqueur, in the treatment of glaucoma, one of its few clinical uses today. M. and M. Polonovski (1923) and Stedman and Barger (1925) elucidated the chemical structure of physostigmine, and its synthesis was accomplished by Julian and Pikl in 1935. Interesting accounts of the history of physostigmine have been presented by Rodin (1947), Karczmar (1970), and Holmstedt (1972).

As a result of the basic research of Stedman (1929a, 1929b) and associates in elucidating the chemical basis of the activity of physostigmine, Aeschlimann and Reinert (1931) systematically investigated a series of substituted phenyl esters of alkyl carbamic acids. *Neostigmine,* a most promising member of this series, was introduced into therapeutics in 1931 for its stimulant action on the intestinal tract. It was reported independently by Remen (1932) and Walker (1935) to be effective in the symptomatic therapy of myasthenia gravis. Additional anti-ChE agents that bear a general structural resemblance to neostigmine were introduced subsequently for the treatment of myasthenia gravis; chief among these are *pyridostigmine* and *ambenonium. Edrophonium,* a drug of simpler structure and with an extremely brief duration of action, is used in the diagnosis and evaluation of therapy of the same disease, as well as for the treatment of overdosage with curariform drugs.

It is remarkable that the first account of the synthesis of a highly potent compound of the *organophosphorus anti-ChE* series, *tetraethylpyrophosphate* (TEPP), was published by Clermont in 1854, 10 years prior to the isolation of physostigmine. More remarkable still, as Holmstedt (1963) has pointed out, is the fact that the investigator survived to report on the compound's taste; a few drops of the pure compound placed on the tongue would be expected to prove rapidly fatal. Modern investigations of the organophosphorus compounds, and the first hint of their toxicity, date from the 1932 publication of

Lange and Krueger on the synthesis of dimethyl and diethyl phosphorofluoridates. The authors' statement that inhalation of the vapors of these compounds caused a persistent choking sensation and blurred vision apparently was instrumental in leading Schrader to explore this class for insecticidal activity.

During the synthesis and investigation of approximately 2000 compounds, Schrader (1952) defined the structural requirements for insecticidal (and, as learned subsequently, for anti-ChE) activity (*see* below). One compound in this early series, *parathion,* later became the most widely employed insecticide of this class. During World War II, the efforts of Schrader's group were directed toward the development of chemical-warfare agents. The synthesis of several compounds of much greater toxicity than parathion, such as *sarin, soman,* and *tabun,* resulted. It is estimated that over 10,000 tons of the last-mentioned agent was manufactured at one German plant for this purpose. Investigators in the Allied countries also followed Lange and Krueger's lead in the search for potentially toxic compounds; di*iso*propyl phosphorofluoridate (DFP), synthesized by McCombie and Saunders (1946), was the organophosphorus compound studied most extensively by British and American scientists. It has been estimated that over 50,000 organophosphorus compounds have by now been synthesized and screened for insecticidal potency, of which over 3 dozen have been produced commercially (Chadwick, 1963).

In the 1950s, a series of heterocyclic, aromatic, and naphthyl *carbamates* was synthesized and found to have a high degree of selective toxicity against insects and to be potent anti-ChE agents (Gysin, 1954). Among those currently employed as insecticides are 1-naphthyl N-methylcarbamate (CARBARYL, SEVIN) and 2-isopropoxyphenyl N-methylcarbamate (BAYGON) (*see* Fukuto, 1972).

Mechanism of Action. The anti-ChE agents are among the relatively few drugs for which the mechanism of action can presently be described in precise molecular terms. This can be related directly to their overall pharmacological effects and has led to the development of useful compounds capable of reversing the actions of anti-ChE agents. The interactions between most of the anti-ChE agents and the enzyme AChE differ primarily in quantitative respects from the reaction between AChE and its normal substrate, ACh.

The general characteristics of AChE (acetylcholine hydrolase), its distinction from butyrocholinesterase (BuChE, nonspecific ChE, or pseudo-ChE), and its distribution are presented in Chapter 21.

Earlier work on the purification and characterization of AChE from the electric organ of the eel, *Electrophorus electricus,* led to its crystallization (Leuzinger *et al.,* 1968). The unit structure of AChE from both electric organs and mammalian sources is a protein with a molecular weight of 80,000; the units are grouped as tetramers, which are obtained in extracts along with aggregates of two and three tetramers (Dudai *et al.,* 1973; Hollinger and Niklasson, 1973; Rieger *et al.,* 1973). In skeletal muscle, the largest aggregate appears to be associated specifically with the postjunctional membrane, while only the smaller complexes are found in extracts of the noninnervated portions of muscle and of the motor nerve (Hall, 1973).

From studies initiated by Wilson and Bergmann (1950) and extended by Wilson and others, it has been established that the active surface of the enzyme unit consists of two sites, an anionic and an esteratic site. At the anionic site (a negative charge, probably of the free carboxyl group of a dicarboxylic amino acid), the positively charged quaternary N atom of ACh is attracted by electrostatic forces; bonding is enhanced by hydrophobic forces exerted on the N-methyl groups and by London–van der Waals dispersion forces. The esteratic site consists of essentially two components, located 2.5 and 5 Å, respectively, from the anionic site: a potentially acidic function (the hydroxyl group of serine) and a basic nucleophilic group (an imidazole group of histidine). The imidazole group, by hydrogen bonding, enhances the nucleophilic activity of the serine hydroxyl group, thus enabling it to interact with the electrophilic carbonyl C atom of ACh. A covalent bond is formed, with the production of an acetylated enzyme intermediate and the release of choline (Figure 22-1, *I*). The electrophilic C atom of the acetyl group then undergoes nucleophilic attack by the electronegative oxygen atom of a water molecule. The acetyl-enzyme complex is thus hydrolyzed, and the products are the regenerated enzyme and acetic acid. The rate constants in this reaction sequence are extremely high; thus, the time required for the complete hydrolysis of one ACh molecule (the turnover time) is only 80 microseconds (Wilson *et al.,* 1960). (*See also* Froede and Wilson, 1971; Kitz, 1973; and references therein.)

The mechanisms of action of compounds that typify the three classes of anti-ChE agents are also shown in Figure 21-1 (*II, III, IV*).

Simple quaternary compounds, such as *tetraethylammonium* ion, inhibit the enzyme reversibly by combining with it only at the anionic site and thus blocking attachment of the substrate. Much more potent reversible inhibitors, such as *edrophonium,* combine in addition with the imidazole nitrogen atom of the esteratic site by hydrogen bonding (Figure 22-1, *II*). In all such cases, inhibition is rapidly reversible, and such drugs have a very brief duration of action following systemic administration.

It was at one time generally assumed that *physostigmine, neostigmine,* and related potent inhibitors that possess a carbamyl ester linkage or urethan structure, in addition to a tertiary amino or quaternary ammonium group, inhibit the enzyme in the same reversible fashion. However, careful kinetic studies have since shown that only a negligible amount of an inhibitor of this type is released reversibly from the enzyme; actually, physostigmine and neostigmine are hydrolyzed extremely slowly by cholinesterase (Goldstein and Hamlisch, 1952; Myers, 1952, 1956; Wilson *et al.*, 1960). It is likely that inhibitors of this class form complexes in which the inhibitor is attached to the enzyme at both the anionic and esteratic sites, following which their hydrolysis proceeds in a manner analogous to that of ACh (Figure 22–1, *III*); the alcoholic moiety is split off, leaving a carbamylated enzyme that reacts with water to release a substituted carbamic acid and the regenerated enzyme. The main difference between the hydrolysis of the natural substrate, ACh, and of the inhibitor, neostigmine, is the velocity of the final step; the half-life of dimethylcarbamyl-AChE, formed by the reaction with neostigmine, is more than 40 million times that of the acetylated enzyme (30 minutes and 42 microseconds, respectively) (Wilson and Harrison, 1961). Thus, these drugs and the newer carbamate insecticides are called "competitive substrates" or "acid-transferring inhibitors" and can be distinguished from the simply reversible inhibitors described above.

The reaction between AChE and most *organophosphorus inhibitors,* such as DFP, occurs only at the esteratic site but proceeds in a comparable fashion (Figure 22–1, *IV*). Here, the resultant phosphorylated enzyme is extremely stable: if the attached alkyl groups are methyl or ethyl, significant regeneration of the enzyme by hydrolytic cleavage requires several hours; with *iso*propyl groups, as in the example given, virtually no hydrolysis occurs, and the return of AChE activity is dependent upon synthesis of new enzyme, a process requiring days to months. Certain quaternary organophosphorus compounds (*e.g.,* echothiophate) combine at both the esteratic and anionic sites, which probably contributes to their extreme potency and specificity. (*See* Burgen and Hobbiger, 1951; Cohen and Oosterbaan, 1963; Holmstedt, 1963.)

An additional group of acid-transferring inhibitors is composed of the methanesulfonates; these compounds react with the enzyme in a similar manner to produce methylsulfonyl-AChE, which, like phosphorylated AChE, is extremely resistant to hydrolytic reactivation (Kitz and Wilson, 1963). Essentially irreversible alkylation of the *anionic site* of AChE is obtained with certain other compounds, including N,N-dimethyl-2-chloro-2-phenethylamine (Belleau and Tani, 1966) and *p*-(trimethylammonium)benzene-diazonium fluoborate (Wofsy and Michaeli, 1967). Neither these agents nor the methanesulfonates have been employed clinically to date.

From the foregoing account, it is apparent that the terms "reversible" and "irreversible," as applied to the carbamyl ester and organophosphorus anti-ChE agents, respec-

tively, reflect only quantitative differences, and that both classes of drugs react with the enzyme in essentially the same manner as does ACh.

The competitive interactions between the two types of inhibitor and the substrate at the active site of the enzyme are illustrated by the observation that the presence of a sufficient concentration of ACh, physostigmine, or neostigmine prevents alkylphosphorylation of AChE by DFP. Occupation of the active sites of the enzyme by the shorter-acting drug prevents their more prolonged alkylphosphorylation by the organophosphorus compound, as has been shown *in vitro* (Koelle, 1946) and *in vivo* (Leopold and McDonald, 1948).

Action at Effector Organs. The characteristic pharmacological effects of the anti-ChE agents are due primarily to the inhibition or inactivation of AChE at sites of cholinergic transmission, with the consequent accumulation and actions of endogenous ACh liberated both by cholinergic nerve impulses and, in much smaller amounts, by continual leakage during the resting stage. With some of the organophosphorus agents, such as DFP, virtually all the acute effects of moderate doses are attributable to this action. Thus, the characteristic miotic effect following local application of DFP to the eye is not observed in the chronically postganglionically denervated eye, where there is no effective source of endogenous ACh.

Among the classical anti-ChE agents, physostigmine, a tertiary amine, exerts a minimum of effects not related to ACh inhibition. At sufficiently high dosage, however, it has a direct blocking action at autonomic ganglia (Paton and Perry, 1953). The quaternary ammonium anti-ChE compounds all have additional direct actions at some cholinoceptive sites, either cholinomimetic or cholinergic blockade. This is not surprising, since both the tetrameric grouping and the charge characteristics of the AChE subunit are quite similar to those of the nicotinic cholinergic receptor (*see* Chapter 28). The importance of the "direct" actions varies with the individual drug, the dose, the species, the site, and other factors. For example, the effects of *neostigmine* on the spinal cord and neuromuscular junction are based on a combination of its anti-ChE and direct cholinomimetic actions; on the other hand, like DFP

I

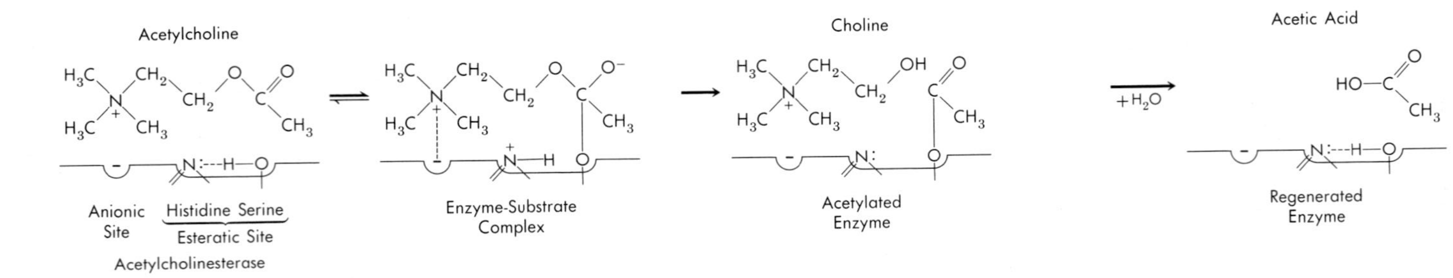
Acetylcholine
Anionic Site
Histidine Serine
Esteratic Site
Acetylcholinesterase
Enzyme-Substrate Complex
Choline
Acetylated Enzyme
+H2O
Acetic Acid
Regenerated Enzyme

II

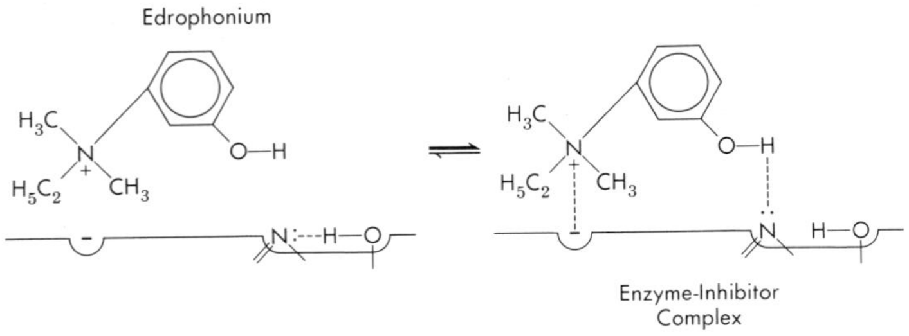
Edrophonium
Enzyme-Inhibitor Complex

III

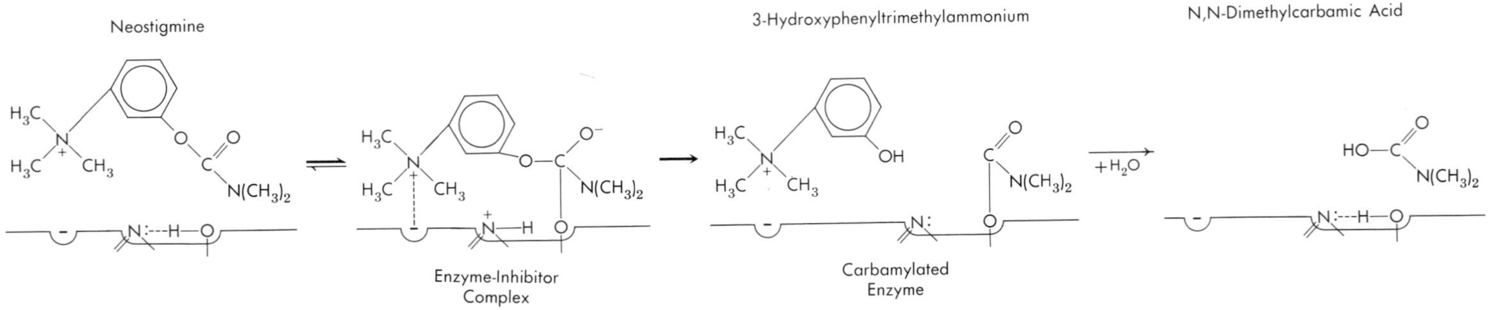
Neostigmine
Enzyme-Inhibitor Complex
3-Hydroxyphenyltrimethylammonium
Carbamylated Enzyme
+H2O
N,N-Dimethylcarbamic Acid

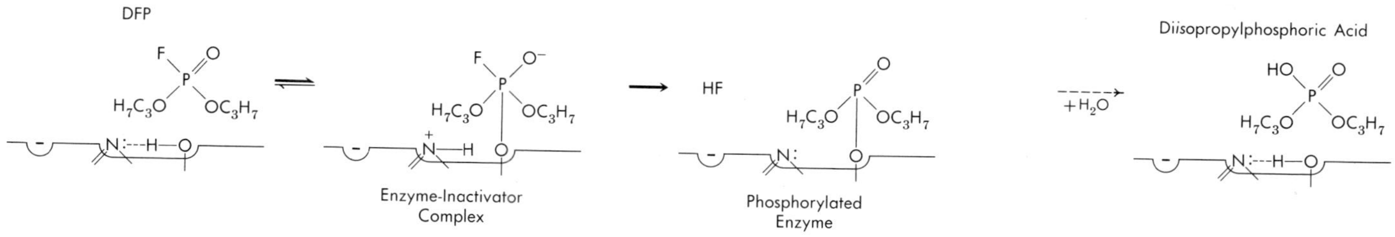

Figure 22-1. *Steps involved in the hydrolysis of acetylcholine (ACh) by acetylcholinesterase (AChE) (I), and in the inhibition of AChE by reversible (II), carbamyl ester (III), and organophosphorus (IV) agents.*

I. The substrate, ACh, combines with an active unit of the enzyme to form a complex, by electrostatic attraction between the quaternary N^+ atom of the choline moiety and the *anionic site* of the enzyme, and by interaction between the electrophilic C atom of the carbonyl group and the serine hydroxyl group of the esteratic site (the nucleophilicity of which is enhanced by the histidine imidazole group). Choline is then split off, leaving the acetylated enzyme. The latter reacts rapidly with water to produce acetic acid and the regenerated active enzyme.

II. Edrophonium combines electrostatically at the anionic site and by H bonding to the imidazole N atom of histidine at the esteratic site to form an enzyme-inhibitor complex.

III. Neostigmine and related ammonium- or amino-carbamate esters react with the enzyme in the same manner as does the substrate; however, the carbamylated enzyme reacts with water at less than a millionth the rate of the corresponding acetylated form to regenerate the active enzyme.

IV. DFP and similar organophosphorus inhibitors react only at the esteratic site to form a phosphorylated enzyme; in the case of diisopropylphosphoryl-AChE, essentially no spontaneous hydrolytic reactivation occurs.

Heavy, light, and dash arrows represent extremely rapid, intermediate, and extremely slow or insignificant reaction velocities, respectively. *See* text for more complete account.

(After Nachmansohn and Wilson, 1951; Wilson, 1954, 1967; Froede and Wilson, 1971; Kitz, 1973; H. A. Friedman, personal communication; and others.)

and physostigmine, it has no detectable miotic action when applied to the chronically denervated iris.

Chemistry and Structure-Activity Relationship. A large number of drugs have been demonstrated to have anti-ChE activity *in vitro.* However, AChE is present in most tissues in a quantity in excess of that required for normal function. To exert a significant effect *in vivo,* therefore, an anti-ChE agent must generally inhibit from 50 to 90% of the functional AChE at a given site (*see* Chapter 21). This can readily be achieved, since most of the compounds to be discussed produce 50% inhibition of the enzyme at concentrations of 10^{-7} M or lower. These facts must be considered in evaluating attempts to relate the pharmacological properties of certain drugs to a degree of AChE inhibition of dubious significance.

The structure-activity relationship of anti-ChE drugs has been reviewed extensively for the "reversible" inhibitors (Augustinsson, 1948; Long, 1963), the organophosphorus agents (Holmstedt, 1959, 1963), and both classes of compounds (Koelle and Gilman, 1949; Karczmar, 1967a; Usdin, 1970). Only those agents that are of general therapeutic or toxicological interest will be considered here.

"Reversible" Carbamate Inhibitors. Drugs of this class that are of therapeutic interest are shown in Table 22–1. After the structure of physostigmine was established, Stedman (1929a, 1929b) and associates undertook a systematic investigation of a number of related synthetic compounds. They concluded that

the essential moiety of the physostigmine molecule was the methyl carbamate of a basically substituted simple phenol (left of the dash line in Table 22–1). The quaternary ammonium derivative, *neostigmine,* is a compound of greater stability and equal or greater potency. The simple analogs of neostigmine that lack the carbamyl group, such as *edrophonium,* are less potent and much shorter-acting anti-ChE agents, since they produce a truly reversible inhibition as described above.

Retention of the dimethylcarbamate side chain in the *meta* position, but incorporation of the quaternary N atom within the ring, to form a pyridyl nucleus, results in compounds with anti-ChE and pharmacological properties similar to those of neostigmine. *Pyridostigmine* is a drug of this class employed in the treatment of myasthenia gravis.

A marked increase in anti-ChE potency and duration of action can result from the linking of two quaternary ammonium nuclei by a chain of appropriate structure and length. One such example is the miotic agent *demecarium,* which consists of two neostigmine molecules connected at their carbamate nitrogen atoms by a series of ten methylene groups. It is likely that this compound combines with the anionic and esteratic sites of two adjacent AChE units within the same tetramer, just as the *bis*-quaternary neuromuscular blocking agent *decamethonium* is presumed to act at two adjacent cholinoreceptors (Chapter 28). Another class of *bis*-quaternary compounds is represented by the dioxamide *ambenonium,* used in the treatment of myasthenia gravis. In addition to its potent anti-ChE activity, this drug has a variety of actions at both

Table 22-1.   REPRESENTATIVE "REVERSIBLE" ANTICHOLINESTERASE AGENTS EMPLOYED CLINICALLY

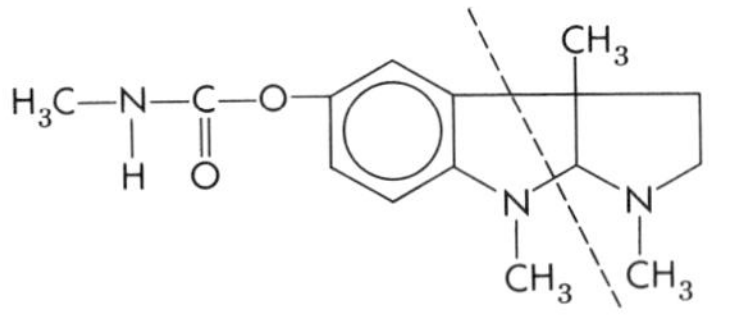

Physostigmine

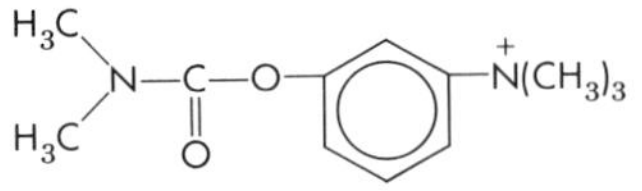

Neostigmine

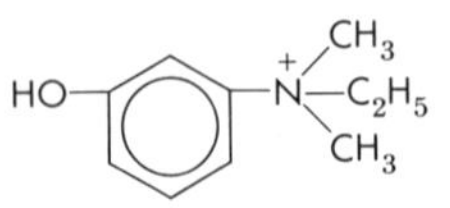

Edrophonium

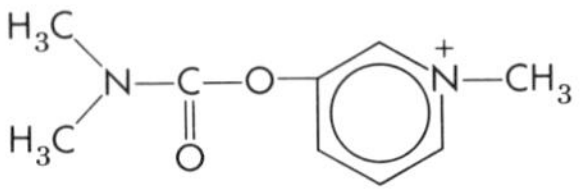

Pyridostigmine

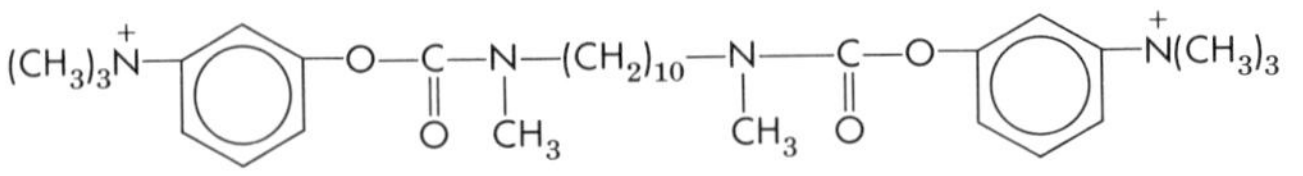

Demecarium

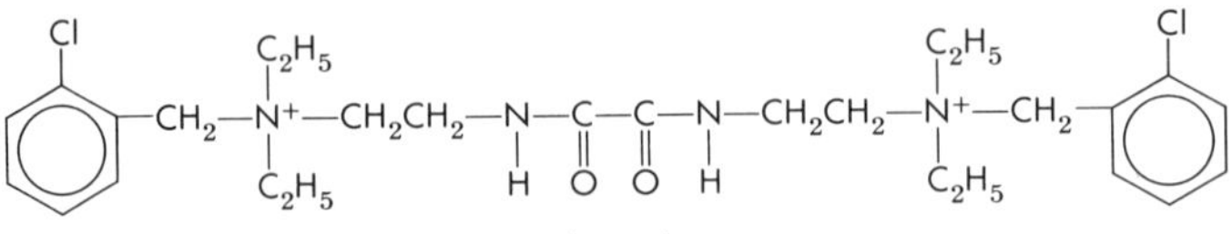

Ambenonium

Table 22-2. CHEMICAL CLASSIFICATION OF REPRESENTATIVE ORGANOPHOSPHORUS COMPOUNDS OF PARTICULAR PHARMACOLOGICAL OR TOXICOLOGICAL INTEREST *

General formula (Schrader, 1952):

$$R_1 \diagdown \underset{R_2 \diagup}{P} \diagup \overset{O}{\diagdown} X$$

Group A, X = halogen, cyanide, or thiocyanate; group B, X = alkyl, alkoxy, or aryloxy; group C, thiol- or thionophosphorus compounds; group D, pyrophosphates and similar compounds; group E, quaternary ammonium compounds

GROUP	STRUCTURAL FORMULA	COMMON, CHEMICAL, AND OTHER NAMES	COMMENTS
A	$i\text{-}C_3H_7O$, $i\text{-}C_3H_7O$, O, F on P	DFP Diisopropyl phosphorofluoridate	Potent, irreversible inactivator
	$i\text{-}C_3H_7NH$, $i\text{-}C_3H_7NH$, O, F on P	Mipafox, Isopestox N,N'-Diisopropyl-phosphorodiamidic fluoride	Early insectide; selective inhibitor of nonspecific ChE (BuChE)
	$(CH_3)_2N$, C_2H_5O, O, CN on P	Tabun Ethyl N-dimethylphosphoramido-cyanidate	Extremely toxic "nerve gas"
	$i\text{-}C_3H_7O$, CH_3, O, F on P	Sarin (GB) Isopropyl methylphosphono-fluoridate	Extremely toxic "nerve gas"
	$(CH_3)_3CCHO$ (CH$_3$), CH_3, O, F on P	Soman Pinacolyl methylphosphono-fluoridate	Extremely toxic "nerve gas"
B	C_2H_5O, C_2H_5O, O, O-phenyl-NO_2 on P	Paraoxon, Mintacol, E 600 Diethyl 4-nitrophenyl phosphate	Active metabolite of parathion
C	C_2H_5O, C_2H_5O, S, O-phenyl-NO_2 on P	Parathion, Thiophos, E 605 (see list of trade names in text) Diethyl O-(4-nitrophenyl) phosphorothioate	Widely employed agricultural insecticide, resulting in numerous cases of accidental poisoning
	C_2H_5O, phenyl, S, O-phenyl-NO_2 on P	EPN O-Ethyl O-(4-nitrophenyl) phenylphosphonothioate	Widely employed agricultural insecticide
	CH_3O, CH_3O, S, S—CHCOOC$_2$H$_5$ / CH$_2$COOC$_2$H$_5$ on P	Malathion O,O-Dimethyl S-(1,2-dicarbe-thoxyethyl) phosphorodi-thioate	Widely employed insecticide of greater safety than parathion or EPN because of rapid metabolism by higher organisms
D	C_2H_5O, C_2H_5O, O, P—O—P, OC$_2$H$_5$, OC$_2$H$_5$	TEPP Tetraethyl pyrophosphate	Early insecticide
	$(CH_3)_2N$, $(CH_3)_2N$, O, P—O—P, N(CH$_3$)$_2$, N(CH$_3$)$_2$	OMPA, Schradan Octamethyl pyrophosphoramide	Insecticide; inactive in vitro, but metabolized by animals and plants to potent anti-ChE agent
E	C_2H_5O, C_2H_5O, O, $SCH_2CH_2\overset{+}{N}(CH_3)_3$ on P, I$^-$	Echothiophate, Phospholine, 217MI Diethoxyphosphinylthiocholine iodide	Extremely potent choline deriva-tive; employed in treatment of glaucoma; relatively stable in aqueous solution

* After Holmstedt, 1959, 1963; see also Usdin, 1970.

the prejunctional and postjunctional membranes of the skeletal muscle motor end-plate (Karczmar, 1967b).

Organophosphorus Inhibitors. The general formula for this class of cholinesterase inhibitors is presented in Table 22–2. A great variety of substituents is possible: R_1 and R_2 may be alkyl, alkoxy, aryloxy, amido, mercaptan, or other groups, and X may represent a halide, cyanide, thiocyanate, phenoxy, thiophenoxy, phosphate, or carboxylate group. It is obviously impossible to list here more than a few representative compounds of the more than 50,000 that have been prepared. A useful chemical classification of the compounds in this class that are of particular pharmacological or toxicological interest has been developed by Holmstedt (1959, 1963), upon which the listing in Table 22–2 is based.

Diisopropyl phosphorofluoridate (DFP) is perhaps the best known and most extensively studied compound of this general class, as the result both of its early development and toxicological evaluation during World War II and of certain of its properties that render it particularly valuable as an investigative tool. The latter include the virtually irreversible inactivation that it produces by alkylphosphorylation of AChE and certain other esterases; its high lipid solubility, resulting in penetration into the central nervous system (CNS); and its specificity. Its diamide analog, *mipafox*, was formerly employed as an insecticide; in low concentrations, it inhibits BuChE selectively.

The "nerve gases," *tabun, sarin,* and *soman,* are among the most potent synthetic toxic agents known; they are lethal to laboratory animals in minute doses.

Parathion has been used extensively throughout the world as an agricultural insecticide. In original form, its anti-ChE activity is extremely low; however, it is metabolized to the much more active agent, *paraoxon,* to which most of its pharmacological and toxicological effects are due; the same sequence occurs with other phosphorothioate agents, such as EPN. Parathion has probably been responsible for more cases of accidental poisoning and death than any other organophosphorus compound. The trade names under which it is marketed and the code names that have been employed to designate the compound include THIOPHOS, NIRAN, APHAMITE, GENITHION, MACKOTHION, ALKRON, COROTHION, PENPHOS, PHOS-KIL, VAPOPHOS, PLANTTHION, E-605, COMPOUND 3422, DNTP, AAT, and DPP. (*See* Report to the Council, 1953, and Gleason *et al.,* 1968, for listings of many pesticides and their trade names and synonyms.)

Organophosphorus compounds with selective toxicity to insects have been sought. *Malathion* is metabolized to inactive products much more rapidly in higher animals than in insects; consequently, it is less dangerous to man, other mammals, and birds at insecticidal concentrations. However, its use is not without risk when protective measures are inadequate. *TEPP* has been used as an insecticide. A tetramide derivative of the same structural class, *OMPA,* is practically devoid of anti-ChE activity; but, like parathion, it is metabolized to an extremely active product, probably the N oxide or the isomeric hydroxymethyl compound. Apparently a similar transformation takes place in plants.

Among the quaternary ammonium organophosphorus compounds (group E, Table 22–2), only *echothiophate* has useful clinical application at present. It is relatively resistant to spontaneous hydrolysis and can thus be stored for several weeks in aqueous solution.

PHARMACOLOGICAL PROPERTIES

It should be possible to predict the pharmacological properties of anti-ChE agents merely by knowing those loci where ACh is physiologically released by nerve impulses and the responses of the corresponding effector organs to the chemical mediator (*see* Table 21–1, page 408). While this is true in the main, several factors prevent the rigid application of such an assumption. Potentially, the anti-ChE agents can produce all the following effects: (1) cholinomimetic actions of the muscarinic type at autonomic effector organs; (2) stimulation, followed by depression or paralysis, of all autonomic ganglia and skeletal muscle (nicotinic actions); and (3) stimulation, with subsequent depression, of cholinoceptive sites in the CNS. Following toxic or lethal doses of anti-ChE agents, most of these effects can actually be noted (*see* below). However, with smaller doses, particularly those employed therapeutically, several modifying factors are present. As stated previously, the final response of autonomic structures to an anti-ChE agent depends on the balance between the ganglionic and peripheral components of its action. The response of effectors also depends on whether they receive cholinergic nerve impulses continuously or phasically. Moreover, little is known concerning the relative degree to which the drugs inactivate AChE in various tissues *in vivo.* In general, compounds containing a quaternary ammonium group do not penetrate cell membranes readily; hence, anti-ChE agents in this category are absorbed poorly from the gastrointestinal tract and are excluded by the blood-brain barrier from exerting significant action on the CNS after moderate doses. On the other hand, such compounds act relatively selectively at the neuromuscular junctions of skeletal muscle, through both their anti-ChE and direct cholinomimetic mechanisms, and have comparatively less effect at autonomic effector sites; their ganglionic actions are generally intermediate. In contrast, the more lipid-soluble agents, such as tertiary amines and most organophosphorus compounds, are well absorbed after oral administration and have ubiquitous effects at both peripheral and central cholinoceptive sites.

The actions of anti-ChE agents on autonomic effector cells and on cortical and subcortical sites in the CNS, where the receptors are largely of the muscarinic type, are blocked by *atropine.* Likewise, atropine blocks most of the excitatory actions of anti-ChE agents on autonomic ganglia, since such agents activate predominantly or exclusively muscarinic receptors of the ganglion cells, rather than the nicotinic receptors normally involved in ganglionic synaptic transmission (*see* Chapter 27).

The main actions of anti-ChE agents that are of therapeutic importance are concerned with the *eye,* the *intestine,* and the *skeletal neuromuscular junction;* most of the other actions are of toxicological interest.

Eye. When applied locally to the conjunctiva, anti-ChE agents cause conjunctival hyperemia and constriction of the iris sphincter (miosis) and ciliary muscle (spasm of accommodation). Miosis is apparent in a few minutes and becomes maximal in ½ hour. Although the pupil may be "pinpoint" in size, it generally contracts further when exposed to light. The pupil gradually returns to its normal size in a few hours to several days, depending upon the drug and its concentration. The spasm of accommodation is more transient and generally disappears considerably before termination of the miosis. Intraocular pressure usually falls concomitantly, as the result of facilitation of resorption of the aqueous humor; the reduction in tension is likely to be particularly marked in eyes in which the pressure is elevated. However, in some cases anti-ChE agents may cause an initial increase in intraocular pressure due to dilatation of the finer blood vessels and to increased permeability of the blood–aqueous humor barrier; this is generally followed by a fall below initial pressure. (A more complete account of these processes is given below in the discussion of glaucoma.)

Gastrointestinal Tract. While the actions of various anti-ChE agents on the gastrointestinal tract are nearly identical, *neostigmine* has been studied most extensively in

this regard. In man, neostigmine enhances *gastric* contractions and increases the secretion of acid gastric juice. The drug tends to counteract the inhibition of gastric tone and motility induced by atropine, and enhances the stimulatory effect of morphine. After bilateral vagotomy, the gastric motor effects of neostigmine are greatly reduced and, therefore, the drug is not very helpful in relieving atony of the stomach that may result from this operation. The lower portion of the *esophagus* is stimulated by neostigmine; in patients with marked achalasia and dilatation of the esophagus, the drug has been shown to cause a salutary increase in tone and peristalsis.

Neostigmine augments the motor activity of the *small and large bowel;* the colon is particularly stimulated. Atony is overcome or prevented, propulsive waves are increased in amplitude and frequency, and transport is thus promoted. These features make neostigmine a drug of choice for facilitating transport and expulsion of intestinal contents in patients with nonobstructive paralytic ileus, particularly because side effects are minimal. Atropine inhibits but does not completely abolish the intestinal effects of neostigmine.

The total effect of anti-ChE agents on intestinal motility probably represents a combination of actions at the ganglion cells of Auerbach's plexus and at the muscle fibers, as a result of the preservation of ACh released by the cholinergic preganglionic and postganglionic fibers, respectively.

Skeletal Neuromuscular Junction. The physiology of cholinergic transmission at the neuromuscular junction is considered in Chapters 21 and 28. Most of the known effects of neostigmine and other potent anti-ChE drugs on muscle fibers can be adequately explained on the basis of their inhibition of AChE at neuromuscular junctions (*see* review by Werner and Kuperman, 1963). However, there is good evidence for an accessory component of *direct action* of neostigmine and other quaternary ammonium anti-ChE agents on skeletal muscle. For example, the intra-arterial injection of neostigmine into chronically denervated muscle, or into normally innervated muscle in which essentially all the AChE has been inactivated by a prior dose of DFP, evokes an immediate contraction, whereas physostigmine does not

(Riker and Wescoe, 1946). When precise measurements of the end-plate current are made by intracellular recording with the voltage-clamp technic, even such "pure" anti-ChE agents as DFP can be shown to have additional, direct effects at the cholinergic receptor site (Kuba *et al.*, 1973).

Normally, a single nerve impulse in a terminal motor-axon branch liberates enough ACh to produce a localized depolarization, the end-plate potential, of sufficient magnitude to initiate a propagated muscle action potential. The liberated ACh is so rapidly hydrolyzed by AChE that its concentration falls below the threshold concentration during the refractory period of the muscle. Therefore, each motor-nerve impulse initiates only one muscle contraction. After partial inhibition of AChE, however, the ACh liberated by a single nerve impulse may persist long enough to set up repetitive muscle action potentials, with a resultant increase in strength of contraction. Furthermore, sufficient ACh may diffuse to neighboring muscle fibers to excite them as well, resulting in asynchronous contractions or *fibrillation*. In addition, the persistent action of ACh on the axonal terminal can initiate its antidromic firing with the resultant activation of the motoneuron, leading in turn to the synchronous contraction of an entire motor unit, or *fasciculation*. Finally, after a sufficiently high dose of an anti-ChE agent, the local concentration of ACh may reach the level required to produce a depolarizing *blockade* of the neuromuscular junction (*see* Chapter 28). Thus, a small dose of physostigmine or neostigmine may increase the skeletal muscle contraction produced by a single maximal nerve stimulus, but larger doses or repetitive nerve stimulation at a rapid rate may result in depression or block.

The various actions of anti-ChE agents on skeletal muscle are augmented by epinephrine or ephedrine, decreased only slightly by very large doses of atropine, and blocked by *d*-tubocurarine. Conversely, the anti-ChE agents act as "decurarizing" drugs (*see* Chapter 28). Neostigmine is not effective against the skeletal muscle paralysis caused by decamethonium, succinylcholine, or benzoquinonium, since these agents also produce neuromuscular blockade by sustained depolarization or desensitization of the motor end-plate.

Actions at Other Sites. *Secretory glands* that are innervated by postganglionic cholin-

ergic fibers include the bronchial, lacrimal, sweat, salivary, gastric, intestinal, and acinar pancreatic glands; low doses of anti-ChE agents cause, in general, an augmentation of their secretory responses to nerve stimulation, and higher doses produce an increase in the resting rate of secretion.

Smooth muscle fibers of the bronchioles and ureters are contracted by these drugs, and the ureters may show increased peristaltic activity.

The *cardiovascular actions* of anti-ChE agents are extremely complex, since they reflect at any given moment the algebraic sum of the excitatory and inhibitory actions of accumulated endogenous ACh at several levels of the innervation of the heart and blood vessels. The predominant effect on the *heart* from the peripheral action of accumulated ACh is bradycardia, resulting in a fall in cardiac output and hypotension.

The effective refractory period of cardiac muscle fibers is shortened, and the refractory period and conduction time of the conducting tissue are increased. The *blood vessels* are in general dilated, although the coronary and pulmonary circulation may show the opposite response. The sum of the foregoing effects should result in hypotension, but at the ganglionic level ACh has first an excitatory and at higher concentrations an inhibitory action. Hence, the excitatory action on the parasympathetic ganglion cells would tend to reinforce the above effects, whereas the opposite sequence would result from the action of ACh on sympathetic ganglion cells. Excitation followed by inhibition is also produced by ACh at the medullary vasomotor and cardiac centers. All these effects are complicated further by the hypoxia resulting from the bronchoconstrictor and other actions of accumulated ACh on the respiratory system; this would reinforce both sympathetic tone and ACh-induced discharge of epinephrine from the adrenal medulla. Hence, it is not surprising that a wide variety of hemodynamic effects has been reported following anti-ChE agents, depending on the drug, dose, route of administration, species, and other factors.

At *autonomic ganglia*, as indicated above, low concentrations of ACh or of anti-ChE agents cause spontaneous firing of the ganglion cells in response to submaximal preganglionic stimulation. This effect results from the activation of *muscarinic* receptors. The ganglionic blockade from higher concentrations of anti-ChE drugs apparently results from persistent depolarization of the cell membrane induced at the *nicotinic* receptors, which masks the preceding excitatory effect (Dolivo and Koelle, 1970; *see also* Chapter 27).

The effects of anti-ChE drugs on the CNS are likewise characterized by stimulation or facilitation at various sites, succeeded by inhibition or paralysis at higher concentrations. In the EEG, for example, the initial characteristic change noted is desynchronization, or the appearance of waves of low voltage and high frequency, probably reflecting a stimulant action on the ascending reticular activating system. The respiratory and other subcortical centers likewise show stimulation after low doses and depression with higher or toxic doses. The stimulant effects are antagonized by atropine, although not as completely as are the muscarinic effects at autonomic effector sites.

Absorption, Fate, and Excretion. *Physostigmine* is readily absorbed from the gastrointestinal tract, subcutaneous tissues, and mucous membranes. The conjunctival instillation of solutions of the drug may result in systemic effects if measures (*e.g.*, pressure on inner canthus) are not taken to prevent absorption from the nasal mucosa. The alkaloid is largely destroyed in the body, mainly by hydrolytic cleavage at the ester linkage by cholinesterases; renal excretion plays only a minor role in its disposal. In man, a 1-mg dose of physostigmine injected subcutaneously is largely destroyed in 2 hours.

Neostigmine and related quaternary ammonium drugs are absorbed poorly after oral administration, such that much larger doses are needed than by the parenteral route. Whereas the effective parenteral dose of neostigmine in man is 0.5 to 2.0 mg, the equivalent oral dose may be 30 mg or more. Large oral doses may prove toxic if intestinal absorption is enhanced for any reason. The exact fate of neostigmine is unknown; it is probably both destroyed by cholinesterases and excreted in the urine. In rats, the ester bond can apparently be cleaved by hepatic microsomal enzymes (Roberts *et al.*, 1968). Pyridostigmine and its analogous metabolite are primarily found in the urine after treatment of man with this drug (Somani *et al.*, 1972).

The commonly encountered *organophosphorus anti-ChE agents* are, with certain exceptions (*e.g.*, echothiophate), highly lipid-soluble liquids; many have high vapor

pressures at ordinary temperatures. The less volatile agents that are commonly employed as agricultural insecticides (*e.g.*, parathion, malathion) are generally dispersed as aerosols or as dusts consisting of the organophosphorus compound adsorbed to an inert, finely particulate material. Consequently, the compounds are rapidly and effectively *absorbed* by practically all routes, including the gastrointestinal tract, as well as through the skin and mucous membranes following contact with the liquid form, and by the lungs after inhalation of the vapors or finely dispersed dusts or aerosols.

Following their absorption, most organophosphorus compounds are *excreted* almost entirely as metabolic breakdown products in the urine. Between the time of absorption and excretion, there are varying periods during which the original compound or its metabolites remain bound to proteins in the blood and tissues. Both *hydrolytic* and *oxidative enzymes* are involved in the metabolism of the organophosphorus compounds.

The organophosphorus anti-ChE agents are hydrolyzed in the body by a group of enzymes known as "phosphorylphosphatases." These are widely distributed throughout the various tissues and can hydrolyze a large number of organophosphorus compounds (*e.g.*, DFP, tabun, sarin, paraoxon, TEPP) by splitting the anhydride-like P—F (or P—CN) bond. They also hydrolyze several aliphatic (*e.g.*, ethyl acetate) and aromatic (*e.g.*, phenyl acetate) esters. The enzymes are not inhibited by organophosphorus compounds, presumably because the phosphorylated active site reacts rapidly with water to regenerate the free form, in contrast to its high stability in the case of the cholinesterases. It has been suggested that acquired resistance of insects to certain insecticides of this class results from the adaptive development of such enzymes (*see* reviews by Holmstedt, 1959; Mounter, 1963).

Another point of hydrolytic cleavage of malathion (Table 22–2) and certain related compounds is at the two carboxylic ester linkages of the succinate side chain. The presence in mammalian liver of enzymes that can effect this type of reaction and their relative paucity in insects account for the selective insecticidal action of such agents. On the other hand, certain acyl ester organophosphorus compounds are rendered more toxic in mammals and insects by enzymatic cleavage of the equivalent linkage.

Because of the above reactions, the effects of exposure to two organophosphorus insecticides may be supra-additive. For example, it has been found that, when malathion is administered to animals in combination with EPN, the resulting toxicity is as much as 50 times what would be expected from the sum of their individual toxicities. This is apparently due primarily to the inhibition by EPN of the enzyme systems that normally metabolize malathion to inactive products. Other combinations of organophosphorus insecticides have also shown supra-addition of toxic effects. The chief interest in the *oxidative* reactions that organophosphorus compounds may undergo in the body lies in the resultant conversion of inactive to highly active anti-ChE agents, as discussed above. (*See* reviews by Chadwick, 1963; Mounter, 1963; Usdin, 1970.)

TOXICOLOGY

The toxicological aspects of the anti-ChE agents are of practical importance to the physician. In addition to numerous cases of accidental intoxication from the use and manufacture of organophosphorus compounds as agricultural insecticides, these agents have been employed frequently for homicidal and suicidal purposes, largely on the basis of their ready accessibility. In addition, several organophosphorus compounds and triarylphosphates can produce a peculiar syndrome of neuronal degeneration, associated with demyelination, following chronic exposure; these effects are apparently not due to inhibition of AChE or other cholinesterases. Severe outbreaks of this form of intoxication have resulted from the repeated ingestion of such compounds as contaminants or adulterants of beverages and cooking oils.

Acute Intoxication. The effects of acute intoxication by anti-ChE agents are manifested by muscarinic and nicotinic signs and symptoms and, except for compounds of extremely low lipid solubility, by signs referable to the CNS. Effects may be *localized* or *generalized.* Local effects are due to the action of vapors or aerosols at their site of contact with the eyes or respiratory tract, or to the local absorption after liquid contamination of the skin or mucous membranes, including those of the gastrointestinal tract. General effects rapidly follow systemic absorption by any route; they appear most rapidly after inhalation of vapors or aerosols, and severe effects may then be present within a few minutes. In contrast, after gastrointestinal and percutaneous absorption, the onset of symptoms is delayed. The *duration* of effects is determined largely by the nature of the compound; it may vary from a matter of minutes, as after an overdose of edrophonium, to several days or even weeks following irreversible alkylphosphorylation of AChE by DFP or sarin.

After *local exposure* to vapors or aerosols or after their *inhalation,* ocular and respiratory effects generally appear first. Ocular effects include marked miosis, conjunctival congestion, ciliary spasm, and brow ache, along with watery nasal discharge; respiratory effects consist in "tightness" in the chest and wheezing respiration, due to the combination of bronchoconstriction and increased bronchial secretion. Gastrointestinal symptoms occur earliest after *ingestion,* and include anorexia, nausea and vomiting, abdominal cramps, and diarrhea. With *percutaneous absorption* of liquid, localized sweating and muscular fasciculation in the immediate vicinity are generally the earliest manifestations.

Additional *muscarinic* effects include those discussed above, under pharmacological properties; severe intoxication is manifested by extreme salivation, involuntary defecation and urination, sweating, lacrimation, bradycardia, and hypotension.

Nicotinic actions at the *neuromuscular junctions* of skeletal muscle usually consist in fatigability and generalized weakness, involuntary twitchings, scattered fasciculations, and eventually severe weakness and paralysis; undoubtedly a central component of action contributes to some of these effects. The most serious consequence of the neuromuscular actions is paralysis of the respiratory muscles.

The broad spectrum of effects on the CNS include confusion, ataxia, slurred speech, loss of reflexes, Cheyne-Stokes respiration, generalized convulsions, coma, and central respiratory paralysis. Actions on the vasomotor and other cardiovascular centers further complicate the hemodynamic pattern.

The *time of death* after a single acute exposure may range from less than 5 minutes to nearly 24 hours, depending upon the dose, route, agent, and other factors. Effective therapy must obviously be instituted with the least possible delay.

The *cause of death* is primarily *respiratory failure,* usually accompanied by a secondary *cardiovascular* component. Muscarinic, nicotinic, and central actions all contribute to respiratory embarrassment; they include laryngospasm, bronchoconstriction, increased tracheobronchial and salivary secretion, and peripheral and central respiratory paralysis. Although the blood pressure may fall to alarmingly low levels and cardiac irregularities intervene, these effects probably result as much from hypoxia as from the specific actions mentioned, since they are often reversed by the establishment of adequate pulmonary ventilation.

Diagnosis and Treatment. The *diagnosis* of severe, acute anti-ChE intoxication is readily made from the history of exposure and the characteristic signs and symptoms. In suspected cases of milder acute or chronic intoxication, determination of the plasma and erythrocyte ChE activities will generally establish the diagnosis. Although these values show considerable variation in the normal population, they will usually be depressed well below the normal range before any symptoms due to systemic anti-ChE intoxication are evident. Such figures do not reflect with any accuracy the activities of the corresponding enzymes in the tissues, the depression of which is the basis of the toxic effects.

Treatment is both specific and highly effective. *Atropine* in sufficient dosage (*see* below) effectively antagonizes the actions at muscarinic receptor sites, including the increased tracheobronchial and salivary secretion, the bronchoconstriction, the autonomic ganglionic stimulation, and to a moderate extent the central actions. It is virtually without effect against the peripheral neuromuscular activation and subsequent paralysis. The last-mentioned action of the anti-ChE agents as well as all other peripheral effects can be reversed by *pralidoxime*, a cholinesterase reactivator that is discussed in detail below.

In moderate or severe anti-ChE intoxication, the recommended adult dose of pralidoxime is 1 g, injected intravenously within not less than 2 minutes. If weakness is not relieved or if it recurs after 20 minutes, the dose may be repeated. Early treatment is very important to assure that the oxime reaches the phosphorylated AChE while the latter can still be reactivated.

In addition, certain general measures may be necessary. These include (1) termination of exposure, by removal of the patient or application of a gas mask if the atmosphere is contaminated, copious washing of contaminated skin or mucous membranes with water, or gastric lavage; (2) maintenance of a patent airway; (3) artificial respiration, if required; (4) oxygen administration; (5) alleviation of persistent convulsions by trimethadione (1 g, intravenously every 15 minutes, to a maximum of 5 g) or sodium thiopental (2.5% solution, intravenously); and (6) treatment of shock (*see* Grob, 1963a; Wills, 1963, 1970). Diazepam deserves clinical trial for the control of seizures occurring in patients poisoned by anti-ChE agents.

Atropine should be given in heroic doses. Following an initial injection of 2 to 4 mg, given intravenously if possible, otherwise intramuscularly, the 2-mg dose should be repeated every 3 to 10 minutes until muscarinic symptoms disappear, and also if they reappear. As much as 50 mg may be required the first day. A mild degree of atropinization should then be maintained, by the oral administration of 1 or 2 mg at intervals of several hours, as long as symptoms are in evidence. Whereas the AChE *reactivators* represent a major advance in the therapy of anti-ChE intoxication (*see* below), their use should still be supplemented by the administration of atropine as described.

Pralidoxime has been proposed for *prophylactic use* in agricultural workers and others who are

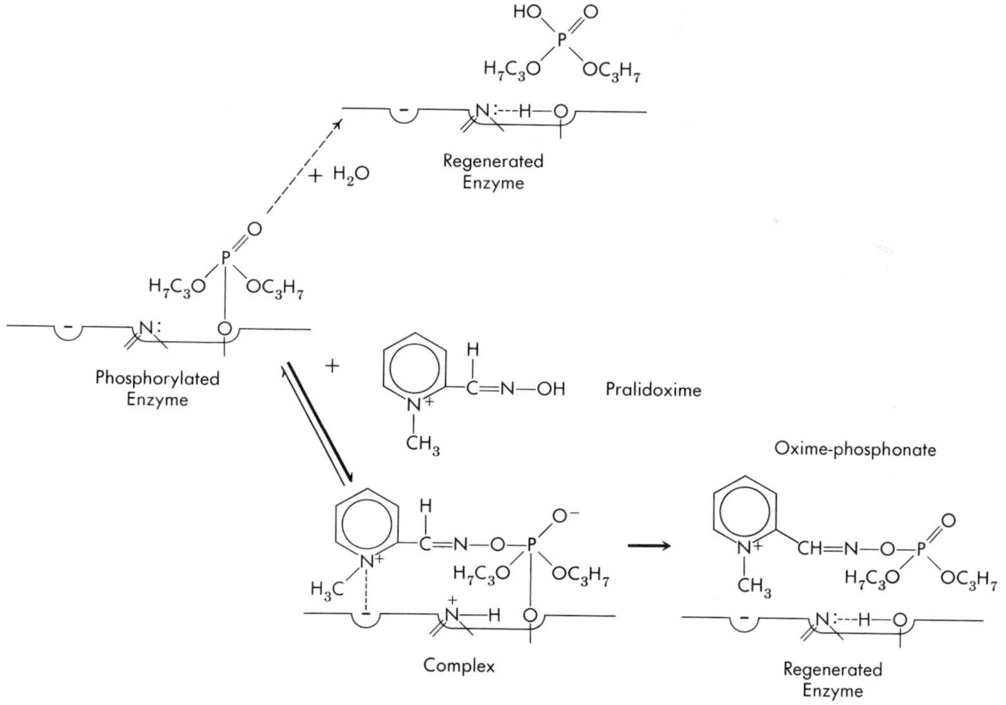

Figure 22-2. *Reactivation of alkylphosphorylated acetylcholinesterase (AChE).*

Following alkylphosphorylation of AChE by DFP (at left), spontaneous hydrolytic reactivation occurs at an insignificant rate (upper reaction), as indicated by dash arrow.

Pralidoxime (in lower reaction) combines with the anionic site by electrostatic attraction of its quaternary N^+ atom, which orients the nucleophilic oxime group to react with the electrophilic P atom; the oxime-phosphonate is split off, leaving the regenerated enzyme. (After Wilson, 1959; Froede and Wilson, 1971; and others.)

Table 22–3. CHOLINESTERASE REACTIVATORS

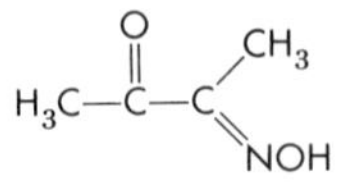

Diacetyl Monoxime (DAM)

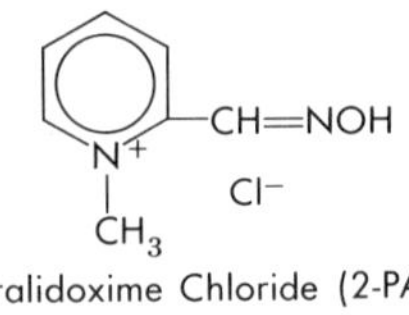

Pralidoxime Chloride (2-PAM)

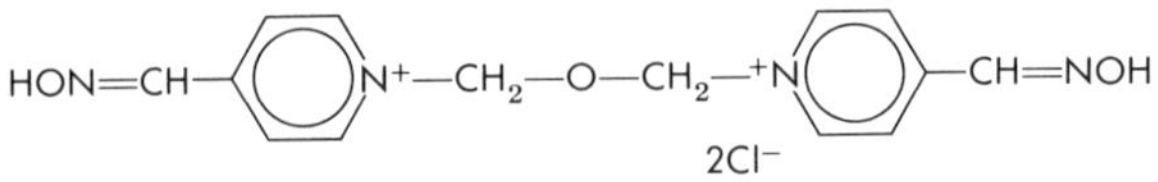

Obidoxime Chloride

known to be exposed to organophosphorus agents; however, there is not as yet sufficient information on the effect of prolonged therapy to recommend its use for this purpose.

Cholinesterase Reactivators. While the phosphorylated esteratic site of AChE undergoes hydrolytic regeneration at a slow or negligible rate (Figure 22–2, upper reaction), Wilson (1951) found that the nucleophilic agent hydroxylamine (H_2NOH) can reactivate the enzyme much more rapidly. In the search for more effective reactivators that followed, a large number of hydroxamic acids (RCONHOH) and oximes (RCH=NOH) were shown to have this property, for example, diacetyl monoxime (DAM; Table 22–3). From the data that accrued, it was predicted that highly effective reactivation should be produced by a molecule containing both a quaternary N atom and an oxime group, spaced at an appropriate distance. This goal was achieved to a remarkable degree by Wilson and Ginsburg (1955) with pyridine-2-aldoxime methyl chloride (2-PAM, 2-formyl-1-methylpyridinium chloride oxime, *pralidoxime;* Table 22–3); reactivation with this compound occurs at a million times the rate of that with hydroxylamine (Heilbronn-Wikström, 1965). Certain *bis*-quaternary oximes were subsequently shown to be even more potent as reactivators; an example is *obidoxime chloride* (1,1′-[oxydimethylene]*bis*[4-formylpyridinium] dichloride dioxime; *see* Table 22–3) (Hobbiger and Vojvodić, 1966).

Mechanism of Action. When the quaternary ammonium group of pralidoxime is attracted electrostatically to the anionic site of the enzyme, the oxime group of the former is oriented optimally to exert nucleophilic attack on the electrophilic phosphorus atom of the phosphorylated esteratic site; the oxime-phosphonate is then split off, leaving the regenerated enzyme (Figure 22–2, lower reaction) (Wilson, 1959).

The velocity of reactivation of phosphorylated AChE by pralidoxime varies with the nature of the phosphoryl group, and in general follows the same sequence as the order for spontaneous hydrolytic reactivation, that is, dimethylphosphoryl-AChE > diethylphosphoryl-AChE > di*iso*propyl-AChE, and so forth. The unidentified phosphorylated AChE formed by the active metabolite of OMPA is not reactivated by the oximes and hydroxamic acids. Moreover, all types of phosphorylated AChE undergo a fairly rapid process of "aging," so that within the course of minutes or hours they become completely resistant to the reactivators. The "aging" is probably due to the splitting-off of one alkyl or alkoxy group, leaving a much more stable monoalkyl- or monoalkoxy-phosphoryl-AChE (Berends *et al.,* 1959; Fleisher and Harris, 1965). It is debatable whether pralidoxime and related agents can effectively antagonize the effects of intoxication by neostigmine and other carbamyl ester inhibitors. (*See* Hobbiger, 1963; Usdin, 1970.)

Pharmacology, Toxicology, and Disposition. The reactivating action of oximes and hydroxamic acids *in vivo* is most marked at the skeletal neuromuscular junction. Following a dose of an organophosphorus compound that produces total blockade of transmission, the intravenous injection of an oxime can restore the response to stimulation of the motor nerve within a few minutes. Antidotal effects are less striking at autonomic effector sites and insignificant in the CNS (except with the nonquaternary compounds, such as DAM).

High doses of pralidoxime and related compounds can in themselves cause neuromuscular blockade and other effects, including inhibition of AChE; such actions are minimal at the doses recommended for clinical use. If pralidoxime is injected intravenously more rapidly than the recommended rate of 500 mg per minute, it can cause mild weakness, blurred vision, diplopia, dizziness, headache, nausea, and tachycardia.

The oximes as a group are largely metabolized by the liver, and the breakdown products are excreted by the· kidney.

Chronic Neurotoxicity of Organophosphorus Compounds.

Certain fluorine-containing alkylorganophosphorus anti-ChE agents (*e.g.,* DFP, mipafox) have in common with a number of triarylphosphates, of which triorthocresylphosphate (TOCP) is the classical example, the property of inducing a peculiar type of delayed neurotoxicity. This syndrome first received widespread attention following the demonstration that TOCP, an adulterant of Jamaica ginger, was responsible for an outbreak of thousands of cases of paralysis that occurred in the southern United States during prohibition. Several similar outbreaks attributable to the ingestion of triarylphosphate compounds have been recorded since then; the one occurring in 1959 in Meknes, North Africa, involving approximately 10,000 people, resulted from the use of olive oil mixed with a lubricating oil containing triorthocresylphosphate. The development of a similar syndrome in a subject following prolonged exposure to mipafox led to the intensive experimental investigation of the organophosphorus anti-ChE agents for this potential hazard.

The *clinical picture* is that of a severe polyneuritis that begins several days after exposure to a sufficient single or cumulative amount of the toxic compound. It is manifested initially by weakness and ready fatigability of the legs, and to a lesser extent of the arms, accompanied by reduced tendon reflexes and the presence of muscle twitching, fasciculation, and tenderness to palpation. In severe cases, the weakness may progress eventually to complete flaccid paralysis that, over the course of weeks or months, is often succeeded by a spastic paralysis with a concomitant exaggeration of reflexes. During these phases, the muscles show marked wasting. Recovery may require 2 or more years.

Only certain triarylphosphates and only fluorine-containing alkylphosphates have been found to produce the characteristic neurotoxic pattern, clinically and experimentally. Accordingly, it does not seem to be dependent upon inhibition of AChE or other cholinesterases. The *pathological lesion,* studied most thoroughly in the chicken, is characterized by *axonal* swelling, segmentation, and eventual breakdown into granular debris; the marked *demyelination* is probably secondary to the aforementioned axonal changes. Only the motoneurons of the lumbar cord have been found to show chromatolysis. The pathways involved include the sciatic nerve; the spinocerebellar tract, posterior columns, and anterior tracts in the spinal cord; and the lateral tracts of the medulla. Neither the biochemical basis nor any specific therapy for the neurotoxic syndrome is known (*see* Bidstrup *et al.,* 1953; Davies, 1963; Usdin, 1970).

Preparations. The compounds described here are those commonly used as anti-ChE drugs and cholinesterase reactivators in the United States. *Conventional dosages* and *routes of administration* are given in the discussion of therapeutic applications of these agents (*see* below).

Physostigmine, U.S.P. (*eserine*), *Physostigmine Salicylate,* U.S.P., and *Physostigmine Sulfate,* U.S.P., are available as crystalline powders for compounding oral and parenteral preparations in suitable dosage forms. Physostigmine salicylate (ANTILIRIUM) injection contains 2-mg amounts in 2-ml ampuls. The U.S.P. also describes official ophthalmic ointments, containing either the salicylate or sulfate salt, and an ophthalmic solution of the salicylate salt.

Neostigmine Bromide, U.S.P. (PROSTIGMIN), is available for *oral* use in 15-mg tablets. *Neostigmine Methylsulfate,* U.S.P. (PROSTIGMIN METHYLSULFATE), is marketed for *parenteral* injection in sterile solution in ampuls and vials containing 0.25, 0.5, or 1.0 mg/ml.

Ambenonium Chloride, N.F. (MYTELASE), is available for *oral* use in 10- and 25-mg tablets.

Pyridostigmine Bromide, U.S.P. (MESTINON), is available for *oral* use in 60-mg tablets, in 180-mg sustained-release tablets, and in a syrup that contains 12 mg/ml.

Edrophonium Chloride, U.S.P. (TENSILON), is marketed for *parenteral* injection in ampuls and vials containing 10 mg/ml.

Demecarium Bromide Ophthalmic Solution, N.F. (HUMORSOL), is available in concentrations of 0.125 and 0.25%.

Echothiophate Iodide for Ophthalmic Solution, U.S.P. (PHOSPHOLINE), is marketed as a powder in 3.0-, 6.25-, 12.5-, and 25-mg amounts. Solutions of appropriate strength must be freshly prepared by the pharmacist, in a diluent supplied by the manufacturer. Once prepared, the solution is stable for about a year if kept refrigerated. The powder must not be applied to the eye.

Isoflurophate Ophthalmic Solution, U.S.P., is a sterile solution of 0.1% isoflurophate (*diisopropyl phosphorofluoridate,* DFP; FLOROPRYL) in a suitable vegetable oil. *Isoflurophate Ophthalmic Ointment,* U.S.P., contains 0.025% isoflurophate in a suitable anhydrous base.

Pralidoxime Chloride, U.S.P. (PROTOPAM), is the only AChE reactivator currently available for general use in the United States. It is dispensed in ampuls in sterile, 1-g amounts for extemporaneous solution in 20 ml of sterile distilled water. It is also marketed in official 500-mg tablets.

Other reactivators of AChE not currently available in the United States include *obidoxime chloride* (TOXOGONIN), its analog *trimedoxime,* and *diacetyl monoxime* (DAM). *Obidoxime* is more potent than pralidoxime; the recommended dose is 3 to 6 mg/kg, injected intravenously over 5 to 10 minutes. The dose of *diacetyl monoxime* is 1 to 2 g, injected intravenously at a rate of 200 mg per minute; unlike pralidoxime or obidoxime, it penetrates the blood-brain barrier and reactivates AChE in the CNS. Both drugs can also be repeated in the same doses after 20 minutes.

THERAPEUTIC USES

Although anti-ChE agents have been recommended for the treatment of a wide variety of conditions, their superiority to other drugs and widespread acceptability have been established mainly in three areas: *atony of the smooth muscle of the intestinal tract and urinary bladder, glaucoma,* and *myasthenia gravis.* In these conditions, certain anti-ChE agents can be recommended as the drugs of choice, either generally or in specific stages or categories of the disease; other classes of drugs may sometimes be indicated as adjuncts or in preference to the anti-ChE agents. *Physostigmine* is also of benefit in the treatment of *atropine intoxication* (*see* below) and of *tricyclic antidepressant poisoning* (page 179). *Edrophonium* can be used for terminating attacks of *paroxysmal supraventricular tachycardia.*

Paralytic Ileus and Atony of the Urinary Bladder. In the treatment of both these conditions, *neostigmine* is generally the most satisfactory of the anti-ChE agents. The direct parasympathomimetic agents, discussed in Chapter 23, are employed for the same purposes.

Neostigmine is used for the relief of *abdominal distention* from a variety of medical and surgical causes. The usual subcutaneous dose of neostigmine methylsulfate for postoperative paralytic ileus is 0.5 to 1.0 mg. Peristaltic activity commences in 10 to 30 minutes after parenteral administration, whereas 2 to 4 hours is required after oral administration of neostigmine bromide (15 mg). A rectal tube should be inserted to facilitate expulsion of gas, and it may be necessary to assist evacuation with a small low enema. The drug is not to be employed when there is mechanical obstruction of the intestine or urinary bladder, when peritonitis is present, or when the viability of the bowel is doubtful. Other medical measures are not to be neglected, including intubation and suction as well as appropriate fluid and electrolyte therapy. Indeed, neostigmine and other drugs are to be viewed mainly as adjuvant agents in the treatment of distention.

When neostigmine is employed for the treatment of atony of the detrusor muscle of the *urinary bladder,* postoperative dysuria is relieved and the time interval between operation and spontaneous urination is shortened. The drug is used in the same dose and manner as in the management of paralytic ileus.

Glaucoma. Glaucoma is a disease complex characterized chiefly by an increase in intraocular pres-

sure that, if sufficiently high and persistent, leads to irreversible blindness. Of the three types—primary, secondary, and congenital—anti-ChE agents are of great value in the management of the primary as well as of certain categories of the secondary type (*e.g.,* aphakic glaucoma, following cataract extraction); the congenital type rarely responds to other than surgical treatment. Primary glaucoma is subdivided into narrow-angle (acute congestive) and wide-angle (chronic simple) types, based on the configuration of the angle of the anterior chamber where reabsorption of the aqueous humor occurs. Anti-ChE agents produce a fall in intraocular pressure in both types of primary glaucoma, chiefly by lowering the resistance to outflow of the aqueous humor. Effects on the volumes of the various intraocular vascular beds (*e.g.,* those of the iris, ciliary body, etc.) and on the rate of secretion of the aqueous humor into the posterior chamber may contribute secondarily to the lowering of pressure, or conversely may produce a rise in pressure preceding the fall. In narrow-angle glaucoma, the aqueous outflow is facilitated by the freeing of the entrance to the trabecular space at the canal of Schlemm from blockade by the iris, as the result of the drug-induced contraction of the iris sphincter. The mechanism of the improvement in aqueous outflow in the wide-angle type is not clear, since no such block by the iris exists. Here, contraction of the iris sphincter, and perhaps more importantly of the ciliary muscle, may realign the trabecular meshwork so as to improve reabsorption, or the effect on outflow may result primarily from vasomotor effects at the canal of Schlemm or intrascleral plexus (*see* reviews by Leopold and Krishna, 1963; Watson, 1972).

The foregoing distinctions are of great importance for therapy, since the roles of miotic drugs, including the anti-ChE agents, are quite different in the management of the two types of primary glaucoma. Acute congestive (narrow-angle) glaucoma is nearly always a medical emergency in which the drugs are essential in controlling the acute attack, but the long-range management is usually based predominantly on surgery (*e.g.,* peripheral or complete iridectomy). Chronic simple, or wide-angle, glaucoma, on the other hand, has a gradual, insidious onset and is not generally amenable to surgical improvement; in this type, control of intraocular pressure is usually dependent upon drug therapy on a permanent basis.

Acute congestive glaucoma may be precipitated by the injudicious use of a mydriatic agent in patients over 40, or by a variety of factors that can cause pupillary dilatation or engorgement of intraocular vessels. The cardinal signs and symptoms include marked ocular inflammation, a semidilated pupil, severe pain, and nausea. Every effort must be made to reduce the intraocular pressure to the normal level and maintain it there for the duration of the attack. In general, an anti-ChE agent is instilled in the conjunctival sac in combination with a parasympathomimetic agent for greatest effectiveness. One such combination that is frequently employed is a solution of *physostigmine salicylate,* 1%, plus *pilocarpine nitrate,* 4%. This combination should be instilled six times at 10-minute intervals, then three times at 30-minute intervals, and thereafter as required. *Ad-*

junctive therapy should include the intravenous administration of a carbonic anhydrase inhibitor, such as *acetazolamide*, to reduce the secretion of aqueous humor, or of an osmotic agent, such as *urea*, to induce intraocular dehydration.

Chronic simple glaucoma and *secondary glaucoma* require careful consideration of the needs of the individual patient in selecting the drug or combination of drugs to be employed. The choices available include (1) parasympathomimetic agents (*e.g., pilocarpine nitrate,* 0.5 to 4%; *see* Chapter 23); (2) anti-ChE agents that are short acting (*e.g., physostigmine salicylate,* 0.02 to 1%) and long acting (*demecarium bromide,* 0.1 to 0.5%; *echothiophate,* 0.03 to 0.25%; *isoflurophate,* 0.005 to 0.2%); and, paradoxically, (3) sympathomimetic agents (*e.g., epinephrine,* 1 to 2%; *phenylephrine,* 10%; *see* Chapter 24). Drugs of the last-mentioned class reduce intraocular pressure both by increasing outflow and by decreasing the rate of secretion of aqueous humor.

A new approach to the treatment of chronic glaucoma is the production of chemosympathectomy of the anterior segment by means of *6-hydroxydopamine* (Holland and Mims, 1971; *see also* Chapter 21).

Formerly the long-acting anti-ChE agents were generally preferred, since they offered the dual advantage of convenience with respect to frequency of instillation and more satisfactory control of pressure overnight. However, their use entails the risk of development of lenticular opacities, discussed below. Of the organophosphorus agents, *DFP* has the longest duration of action and is extremely potent when applied locally; solutions in peanut or sesame oil require instillation from once daily to once weekly, and may control intraocular pressure in severe cases that are resistant to other drugs. The oily vehicle is unpleasant to most patients. Consequently, DFP has largely been replaced by echothiophate.

Untoward Effects. It has now been established that treatment of glaucoma with potent, long-acting anti-ChE agents (including demecarium, echothiophate, and isoflurophate) for 6 months or longer carries a high risk of the development of a specific type of *cataract,* described as anterior subcapsular vacuoles (Axelsson and Holmberg, 1966; de Roetth, 1966; Shaffer and Hetherington, 1966). The incidence of lenticular opacities under such circumstances has been found to be as high as 50%; the hazard is apparently increased in proportion to the strength of the solution, frequency of instillation, duration of therapy, and age of the patient. The underlying mechanism remains elusive (*see* Laties, 1969). In contrast, treatment with *pilocarpine* (4%), alone or in combination with *physostigmine* (0.2%), one to five times daily, was found to entail no higher incidence of the development of lenticular opacities than appeared spontaneously in untreated patients in comparable age groups (Axelsson, 1969). At present, it seems clear that pilocarpine and other shorter-acting miotic drugs should be employed as long as they provide adequate control of intraocular tension. If they fail to do so, the hazards of cataract development must be balanced against those of increased intraocular pressure before resorting to the use of the potent, long-acting anti-ChE agents. When

such drugs are used, patients should be examined for the appearance of lenticular opacities at intervals of 6 months or less.

Miscellaneous ocular side effects that may occur following local instillation of anti-ChE agents are headache, brow pain, blurred vision, phacodinesis, pericorneal injection, congestive iritis, various allergic reactions, and, rarely, retinal detachment. The temporary rise in intraocular pressure that may precede the fall has already been mentioned. When anti-ChE drugs are instilled intraconjunctivally at frequent intervals, sufficient absorption may occur to produce various systemic effects, including potentiation of the neuromuscular blocking agent succinylcholine (*see* Chapter 28); this possibility can be minimized by applying pressure just below the inner angle of the eye during and for a short period following instillation of the drug.

Anti-ChE agents have been employed locally in the treatment of a variety of other ophthalmological conditions, including accommodative esotropia and myasthenia gravis confined to the extraocular and eyelid muscles, and, in alternation with a mydriatic drug such as atropine, for the breaking of adhesions between the iris and the lens or cornea. (For a complete account of the use of anti-ChE agents in ocular therapy, *see* Leopold and Krishna, 1963.)

Myasthenia Gravis. The major characteristic features of myasthenia gravis are weakness and rapid fatigability of skeletal muscle (*see* Grob, 1963b; Whipple, 1966; Fields, 1971; Osserman *et al.,* 1972). Exacerbations and remissions often occur unpredictably. Another feature of the disease is the high incidence of thymoma. In 1895, Jolly noted the resemblance between the signs of myasthenia gravis and those of curare poisoning in animals and, accordingly, suggested that physostigmine, known to antagonize curare, might be of therapeutic value. Following an unsuccessful attempt in 1895 by A. Murri, nearly 40 years elapsed before this suggestion was again acted upon by Walker (1934). Remen (1932) and Walker (1935) independently reported superior results with *neostigmine.* Since that time, numerous investigations have established neostigmine as the standard drug for the therapy of myasthenia gravis, against which newer agents are compared.

The site of the physiological defect in myasthenia gravis, as in curare poisoning, is the neuromuscular junction. When a motor nerve of a normal subject is stimulated at a frequency of 25 per second, both the electrical and the mechanical responses are well sustained. In the affected muscles of a myasthenic patient, the initial responses may be normal, but they rapidly decrease and may shortly fail altogether ("Jolly's reaction"); this finding explains why the patient is unable to maintain voluntary muscular contractions for more than brief periods. If the patient is then given an appropriate dose of neostigmine, the response to tetanic stimulation improves concomitantly with a symptomatic improvement in strength, so that both may approach the normal level; there is no accompanying fasciculation or repetitive response to single stimuli. Contrariwise, the same dose of neostigmine in a *normal* subject causes a *reduction* in the original and subsequent responses to tetanic stimulation of the motor nerve, localized weakness or paralysis of voluntary contraction, fascicular twitching, and repetitive muscle action potentials in response to a single stimulus (Harvey *et al.*, 1941; Grob, 1963b). From these and related physiological findings, it is generally agreed that in myasthenia gravis the essential defect, reversible by anti-ChE agents, is the failure of an appropriate amount of ACh to reach the cholinoceptive sites of the postjunctional membrane following rapidly repetitive nerve impulses. The main basis of this defect may be a marked decrease in the ACh content of the individual quanta, or synaptic vesicles, of the motor-nerve terminals. This was suggested by the close resemblance between the defect in neuromuscular transmission produced in cats by hemicholinium (HC-3), which causes depletion of the store of ACh (*see* Chapter 21), and that recorded in myasthenic patients (Desmedt, 1966). Direct corroborative evidence was obtained by Elmqvist (1965), Thesleff (1966), and their associates by *in-vitro* studies of isolated intercostal nerve–muscle fiber preparations obtained by biopsy from patients with myasthenia gravis. Miniature end-plate potentials were recorded at the same frequency as those in similar preparations from normal subjects, but they averaged only one fifth the amplitude of the latter; there appeared to be no reduction in sensitivity of the postjunctional membrane. However, studies by Acheson and coworkers (1948), Churchill-Davidson and Richardson (1953), Grob and associates (1966), and Grob (1971) have indicated that the latter factor may also be involved. Thus, the relative importance of a prejunctional and postjunctional defect in myasthenia gravis is still uncertain. The etiology of the disease also remains obscure, although hypotheses involving autoimmune phenomena and the thymus have been proposed.

Treatment. Neostigmine, pyridostigmine, and *ambenonium* are the standard anti-ChE drugs used in the symptomatic treatment of myasthenia gravis. All can increase the response of myasthenic muscle to repetitive nerve impulses, probably primarily by the preservation of endogenous ACh and secondarily by their direct cholinomimetic action.

When the diagnosis of myasthenia gravis has been established (*see* below), treatment can be instituted with any of these drugs, then changed if optimal improvement in strength is not achieved, initially or at any time subsequently. The optimal single oral dose can be determined by either of two empirical methods involving oral or intravenous titration.

In the oral test, baseline recordings are made of grip strength, vital capacity, and a number of signs and symptoms that reflect the strength of various muscle groups. The patient is then given an oral dose of neostigmine (7.5 mg), pyridostigmine (30 mg), or ambenonium (2.5 mg). The improvement in muscle strength and changes in other signs and symptoms are noted at frequent intervals until there is a return to the basal state. After an hour or longer in the basal state, the drug is given again with the dose increased to one and one-half times the initial amount, and the same observations are repeated. This sequence is continued, with increasing increments of one half

the initial dose, until the optimal response is obtained; the result can be confirmed by the *edrophonium test* (*see* below). The optimal single oral dose may range from the initial doses given above to more than ten times these amounts.

Alternatively, the optimal dose can be determined by an intravenous titration test, as described in detail by Osserman (1958) and Osserman and associates (1972). This involves recording of the same parameters as above, before and following the intravenous injection of successive, small increments of neostigmine (0.125 mg) or pyridostigmine (0.5 mg), at intervals of a few minutes. Prior to injection of the anti-ChE agent, the patient is given an intravenous injection of 0.4 to 0.6 mg of atropine to prevent muscarinic side effects. When the optimal total intravenous dose has been established, and confirmed by the edrophonium test, the optimal single oral dose is estimated as approximately 30 times that amount.

The duration of action of these drugs is such that the interval between oral doses required to maintain a reasonably even level of strength is usually 2 to 4 hours for neostigmine and 3 to 6 hours for pyridostigmine or ambenonium. However, the amount required may vary from day to day, and physical or emotional stress, intercurrent infections, and menstruation usually necessitate an increase in the frequency or size of the dose. In addition, unpredictable exacerbations and remissions of the myasthenic state may require adjustment of the dosage upward or downward. Although all patients with myasthenia gravis should be seen by a physician at regular intervals, most can be taught to modify their dosage regimens according to their changing requirements. *Pyridostigmine* is available as time-span tablets containing a total of 180 mg, of which 60 mg is released immediately and 120 mg over several hours; this preparation is of particular value in maintaining patients overnight. Muscarinic cardiovascular and gastrointestinal side effects of anti-ChE agents can generally be controlled by atropine or other anticholinergic drugs (Chapter 25); in most patients, tolerance is developed eventually to the muscarinic effects, so that anticholinergic medication can be suspended. Intestinal or urinary obstruction and bronchial asthma present particular hazards with respect to the muscarinic actions. A number of drugs, including curariform agents and certain antibiotics and general anesthetics, interfere with neuromuscular transmission; their administration to patients with myasthenia gravis is hazardous without proper adjustment of anti-ChE dosage and other appropriate precautions.

Parenteral administration of the standard anti-ChE agents is sometimes required in desperately ill myasthenic patients who do not respond adequately to oral medication; the subcutaneous, intramuscular, or intravenous route may be used. Ambulatory patients who have difficulty in eating may be benefited by a small subcutaneous dose injected ½ hour prior to mealtime.

Edrophonium, the reversible, short-acting anti-ChE agent discussed above, is of value in establishing the diagnosis of myasthenia gravis, and in determining the adequacy of anti-ChE medication initially and in certain emergency situations.

Although the diagnosis can usually be made from the history, signs, and symptoms, its differentiation from certain neurasthenic, infectious, endocrine, neoplastic, and degenerative neuromuscular diseases may sometimes be difficult. However, myasthenia gravis is the only condition in which the aforementioned deficiencies can be improved dramatically by anti-ChE medication. The *edrophonium test* is performed by injecting intravenously 2 mg of edrophonium chloride, followed 45 seconds later by an additional 8 mg if the first dose causes no reaction; a positive response consists in brief improvement in strength, unaccompanied by lingual fasciculation (which generally occurs in nonmyasthenic patients). *Atropine sulfate,* 0.6 mg or more intravenously, should be given immediately if a severe reaction ensues (for complete details, *see* Osserman and Genkins, 1966; Osserman *et al.,* 1972).

When the optimal single oral dose of anti-ChE drug is first determined, the edrophonium test can be employed to confirm its adequacy. In this situation, a total dose of only 2 mg of edrophonium is given. If the dose of the standard anti-ChE agent is insufficient, further improvement of strength will result. If the dose is adequate or excessive, edrophonium will cause no change or a reduction in strength. The same principle is the basis for the use of the edrophonium test in making the differential diagnosis between *cholinergic crisis* and *myasthenic weakness.* The former condition results from overdosage with anti-ChE drugs; it is characterized by weakness resulting from excessive depolarization of the motor end-plate and the other possible factors discussed earlier. It may closely resemble myasthenic weakness, which is due to insufficient anti-ChE medication. The distinction is of obvious practical importance, since the former is treated by withholding, and the latter by administering, the anti-ChE agent. When the edrophonium test is performed cautiously, limiting the dose to 1 or 2 mg, and with facilities for respiratory resuscitation immediately available, a further decrease in strength indicates cholinergic crisis, while improvement signifies myasthenic weakness.

If the patient suspected of having myasthenia gravis exhibits minimal symptoms at the time of examination, a provocative test can be performed by injecting intravenously 0.1 to 0.5 mg of *d*-tubocurarine chloride. A positive response consists in the rapid precipitation of the characteristic weakness and associated symptoms; it should be reversed by the immediate intravenous injection of 2.0 mg of neostigmine methylsulfate. The *d*-tubocurarine test is a potentially hazardous procedure; it should be performed only by a physician who has been especially trained in its use and with facilities for respiratory and cardiovascular resuscitation immediately at hand.

Adjuvant drugs of established value in myasthenia gravis include ephedrine, potassium, and, in special circumstances (*see* below), adrenocorticotropic hormone (ACTH). *Ephedrine sulfate,* 25 or 50 mg orally, one to three times daily, provides further improvement in strength in some patients, probably by enhancing ACh release at the motor end-plate, either directly or via interaction with endogenous catecholamine (*see* Chapter 21); in addition, it opposes some of the muscarinic side effects of anti-ChE therapy. *Potassium chloride,* 1 to 2 g orally, taken as a liquid preparation with each dose of anti-ChE agent, is frequently beneficial; it may also enhance ACh release, as well as replace intracellular potassium lost during prolonged depolarization of the motor end-plates.

Anti-ChE insensitivity and generalized deterioration may develop in advanced cases and present a serious emergency. Therapy is directed toward supporting respiration by means of a mechanical respirator and, if necessary, tracheostomy; correcting any electrolyte or endocrine imbalance; combating intercurrent infections; and, specifically, instituting a course of ACTH therapy. This should be conducted under constant careful supervision. It consists in a daily dose of 100 U.S.P. units of ACTH, given by intravenous infusion over 8 hours or by a single intramuscular injection of a gel preparation, for 10 days. After a rest period of a few to 10 days, the course may be repeated. Thereafter, the patient may be given single intramuscular injections of 100 units at intervals of 1 to 3 weeks. During the course of therapy, the dose of anti-ChE drug is reduced to approximately one half the previous amount and adjusted subsequently in accordance with the patient's needs. Most patients exhibit a marked further *decrease* in strength during the course of ACTH therapy, but generally develop a remarkable degree of remission thereafter, which may persist for several months. The underlying mechanisms of the response have not been explained (Namba *et al.,* 1971).

Thymectomy should be considered in every case of myasthenia gravis, and the risks weighed against the potential benefits. In certain categories of patients, the likelihood of an improved prognosis is high, whereas in others there is little chance of modifying advantageously the course of the disease (*see* Papatestas *et al.,* 1971; Perlo *et al.,* 1971).

Atropine Intoxication. Many of the serious peripheral and central effects of poisoning by atropine and related anticholinergic drugs (Chapter 25) can be reversed by the intravenous injection of *physostigmine salicylate.* The recommended initial dose is 0.5 to 2 mg for adults and half these amounts for children. The lower dose should be injected cautiously first, and additional increments can then be given as indicated. Neostigmine and related quaternary ammonium anti-ChE agents do not effectively penetrate the brain to relieve CNS symptoms.

Acheson, G. H.; Langohr, J. L.; and Stanbury, J. B. Sensitivity of skeletal muscle to intra-arterial acetylcholine in normal and myasthenic man. *J. clin. Invest.,* **1948,** *27,* 439–445.

Aeschlimann, J. A., and Reinert, M. Pharmacological action of some analogues of physostigmine. *J. Pharmac. exp. Ther.,* **1931,** *43,* 413–444.

Argyll-Robertson, D. The Calabar bean as a new agent in ophthalmic practice. *Edinb. med. J.,* **1863,** *8,* 815–820.

Axelsson, U. Glaucoma miotic therapy and cataract. *Acta ophthal.,* **1969,** Suppl. 102, 1–37.

Axelsson, U., and Holmberg, A. The frequency of cataract after miotic therapy. *Acta ophthal.,* **1966,** *44,* 421–429.

Belleau, B., and Tani, H. A novel irreversible inhibitor of acetylcholinesterase specifically directed at the anionic binding site: structure-activity relationships. *Molec. Pharmac.*, **1966**, *2*, 411–422.

Berends, F.; Posthumus, C. H.; Sluys, I. v.d.; and Deierkauf, F. A. The chemical basis of the "ageing process" of DFP-inhibited pseudocholinesterase. *Biochim. biophys. Acta*, **1959**, *34*, 576–579.

Bidstrup, P. L.; Bonnell, J. A.; and Beckett, A. G. Paralysis following poisoning by a new organic phosphorus insecticide (mipafox). *Br. med. J.*, **1953**, *1*, 1068–1072.

Burgen, A. S. V., and Hobbiger, F. The inhibition of cholinesterases by alkylphosphates and alkylphenolphosphates. *Br. J. Pharmac. Chemother.*, **1951**, *6*, 593–605.

Christioson, R. On the properties of the ordeal bean of Old Calabar. *Mon. J. Med., Lond.*, **1855**, *20*, 193–204.

Churchill-Davidson, H. C., and Richardson, A. T. Neuromuscular transmission in myasthenia gravis. *J. Physiol., Lond.*, **1953**, *122*, 252–263.

Clermont, P. de. Chimie organique—note sur la préparation de quelques éthers. *C. r. hebd. Séanc. Acad. Sci., Paris*, **1854**, *39*, 338–341.

de Roetth, A., Jr. Lenticular opacities in glaucoma patients receiving echothiophate iodide therapy. *J. Am. med. Ass.*, **1966**, *195*, 664–666.

Desmedt, J. E. Presynaptic mechanisms in myasthenia gravis. *Ann. N.Y. Acad. Sci.*, **1966**, *135*, 209–246.

Dolivo, M., and Koelle, G. B. Properties of nicotinic and muscarinic receptors in isolated rat ganglia. *Experientia*, **1970**, *26*, 679.

Dudai, Y.; Herzberg, M.; and Silman, I. Molecular structures of acetylcholinesterase from electric organ tissue of the electric eel. *Proc. natn. Acad. Sci. U.S.A.*, **1973**, *70*, 2473–2476.

Elmqvist, D. Neuromuscular transmission with special reference to myasthenia gravis. *Acta physiol. scand.*, **1965**, *64*, Suppl. 249, 1–34.

Fleisher, J. H., and Harris, L. W. Dealkylation as a mechanism for aging of cholinesterase after poisoning with pinacolyl methylphosphonofluoridate. *Biochem. Pharmac.*, **1965**, *14*, 641–650.

Fraser, T. R. On the characters, actions and therapeutical uses of the ordeal bean of Calabar (*Physostigma venenosum*, Balfour). *Edinb. med. J.*, **1863**, *9*, 36–56, 123–132, 235–248.

Goldstein, A., and Hamlisch, R. E. Properties and behavior of purified human plasma cholinesterase. IV. Enzymatic destruction of the inhibitors prostigmine and physostigmine. *Archs Biochem. Biophys.*, **1952**, *35*, 12–22.

Grob, D. Spontaneous end-plate activity in normal subjects and in patients with myasthenia gravis. *Ann. N.Y. Acad. Sci.*, **1971**, *183*, 248–269.

Grob, D.; Namba, T.; and Feldman, D. S. Alterations in reactivity to acetylcholine in myasthenia gravis and carcinomatous myopathy. *Ann. N.Y. Acad. Sci.*, **1966**, *135*, 247–275.

Gysin, H. Über einige neue Insektizide. *Chimia*, **1954**, *8*, 205–210, 221–228.

Hall, Z. W. Multiple forms of acetylcholinesterase and their distribution in endplate and non-endplate regions of rat diaphragm muscle. *J. Neurobiol.*, **1973**, *4*, 343–361.

Harvey, A. M.; Lilienthal, J. L., Jr.; and Talbot, S. A. Observations on the nature of myasthenia gravis: the phenomena of facilitation and depression of neuromuscular transmission. *Bull. Johns Hopkins Hosp.*, **1941**, *69*, 547–565.

Heilbronn-Wikström, E. Phosphorylated cholinesterases, their formation, reactions and induced hydrolysis. *Svensk kem. Tidskr.*, **1965**, *77*, 11–43.

Hobbiger, F., and Vojvodić, V. The reactivating and antidotal actions of N,N′-trimethylenebis(pyridinium-4-aldoxime)(TMB-4) and N,N′-oxydimethylenebis(pyridinium-4-aldoxime) (toxogenin) with particular reference to

their effect on phosphorylated acetylcholinesterase in brain. *Biochem. Pharmac.*, **1966**, *15*, 1677–1690.

Holland, M. G., and Mims, J. L. Anterior segment chemical sympathectomy by 6-hydroxy-dopamine. *Invest. Ophthal.*, **1971**, *10*, 120–143.

Hollinger, E. G., and Niklasson, B. H. The release and molecular state of mammalian brain acetylcholinesterase. *J. Neurochem.*, **1973**, *20*, 821–836.

Jolly, F. Pseudoparalysis myasthenica. *Neurol. Zbl.*, **1895**, *14*, 34.

Julian, P. L., and Pikl, J. Studies in indole series. V. Complete synthesis of physostigmine (eserine). *J. Am. chem. Soc.*, **1935**, *57*, 755–757.

Kitz, R., and Wilson, I. B. Acceleration of the rate of reaction and methanesulfonyl fluoride and acetylcholinesterase by substituted ammonium ions. *J. biol. Chem.*, **1963**, *238*, 745–748.

Koelle, G. B. Protection of cholinesterase against irreversible inactivation by di-isopropyl fluorophosphate *in vitro*. *J. Pharmac. exp. Ther.*, **1946**, *88*, 232–237.

Kuba, K.; Albuquerque, E. X.; and Barnard, E. A. Di-isopropylfluorophosphate: suppression of ionic conductance of the cholinergic receptor. *Science, Wash.*, **1973**, *181*, 853–856.

Lange, W., and Krueger, G. von. Über Ester der Monofluorphosphorsäure. *Ber. dt. chem. Ges.*, **1932**, *65*, 1598–1601.

Laqueur, L. Ueber Atropin und Physostigmin in ihre Wirkung auf den intraocularen Druck: Ein Beitrag zur Therapie des Glaucoms. *Albrecht v. Graefes Arch. Ophthal.*, **1877**, *23*, 149–176.

Laties, A. M. Localization in cornea and lens of topically-applied irreversible cholinesterase inhibitors. *Am. J. Ophthal.*, **1969**, *68*, 848–857.

Leopold, I. H., and McDonald, P. R. Di-isopropyl fluorophosphate (DFP) in treatment of glaucoma: further observations. *Archs Ophthal., N.Y.*, **1948**, *40*, 176–186.

Leuzinger, W.; Baker, A. L.; and Cauvin, E. Acetylcholinesterase. II. Crystallization, absorption spectra, isoionic point. *Proc. natn. Acad. Sci. U.S.A.*, **1968**, *59*, 620–623.

McCombie, H., and Saunders, B. C. Alkyl fluorophosphonates: preparation and physiological properties. *Nature, Lond.*, **1946**, *157*, 287–289.

Myers, D. K. Studies on cholinesterase. 8. Determination of reaction velocity constants with a reversible inhibitor of pseudo-cholinesterase. *Biochem. J.*, **1952**, *52*, 46–53.

———. Studies on cholinesterase. 10. Return of cholinesterase activity in the rat after inhibition by carbamoyl fluorides. *Ibid.*, **1956**, *62*, 556–563.

Namba, T.; Brunner, N. G.; Shapiro, M. S.; and Grob, D. Corticotropin therapy in myasthenia gravis: effects, indications, and limitations. *Neurology, Minneap.*, **1971**, *21*, 1008–1018.

Osserman, K. E., and Genkins, G. Critical reappraisal of the use of edrophonium (TENSILON) chloride tests in myasthenia gravis and significance of clinical classification. *Ann. N.Y. Acad. Sci.*, **1966**, *135*, 312–326.

Papatestas, A. E.; Alpert, L. I.; Osserman, K. E.; Osserman, R. S.; and Kark, A. E. Studies in myasthenia gravis: effects of thymectomy. *Am. J. Med.*, **1971**, *50*, 465–476.

Paton, W. D. M., and Perry, W. L. M. The relationship between depolarization and block in the cat's superior cervical ganglion. *J. Physiol., Lond.*, **1953**, *119*, 43–57.

Perlo, V. P.; Arnason, B.; Poskanzer, D.; Castleman, B.; Schwab, R. S.; Osserman, K. E.; Papatestis, A.; Alpert, L.; and Kark, A. The role of thymectomy in the treatment of myasthenia gravis. *Ann. N.Y. Acad. Sci.*, **1971**, *183*, 308–315.

Polonovski, M., and Polonovski, M. Etúde sur les alcaloïdes de la fève de Calabar (XI). Quelques hypothèses sur la constitution de l'ésérine. *Bull. Soc. chim. Fr.*, **1923**, *33*, 1117–1131.

Remen, L. Zur Pathogenese und Therapie der Myasthenia

gravis pseudoparalytic. *Dt. Z. NervHeilk.*, **1932**, *128*, 66–78.

Report to the Council. Use and abuse of generic (coined common) names for pesticides. *J. Am. med. Ass.*, **1953**, *152*, 818–821.

Rieger, F.; Bon, S.; Massoulié, J.; and Cartaud, J. Observation par microscopie électronique des formes allongées et globulaires de l'acétylcholinestérase de gymnote (*Electrophorus electricus*). *Eur. J. Biochem.*, **1973**, *34*, 539–547.

Riker, W. F., Jr., and Wescoe, W. C. The direct action of prostigmine on skeletal muscle: its relationship to the choline esters. *J. Pharmac. exp. Ther.*, **1946**, *88*, 58–66.

Roberts, J. B.; Thomas, B. H.; and Wilson, A. Metabolism of neostigmine *in vitro. Biochem. Pharmac.*, **1968**, *17*, 9–12.

Rodin, F. H. Eserine: its history in the practice of ophthalmology (physostigmine): *Physostigma venenosum* (Balfour): (Calabar bean). *Am. J. Ophthal.*, **1947**, *30*, 19–28.

Shaffer, R. N., and Hetherington, J., Jr. Anticholinesterase drugs and cataracts. *Am. J. Ophthal.*, **1966**, *62*, 613–618.

Somani, S. M.; Roberts, J. B.; and Wilson, A. Pyridostigmine metabolism in man. *Clin. Pharmac. Ther.*, **1972**, *13*, 393–399.

Stedman, E. III. Studies on the relationship between chemical constitution and physiological action. Part II. The miotic activity of urethanes derived from the isomeric hydroxybenzyldimethylamines. *Biochem. J.*, **1929a**, *23*, 17–24.

———. Chemical constitution and miotic action. *Am. J. Physiol.*, **1929b**, *90*, 528–529.

Stedman, E., and Barger, G. Physostigmine (eserine). Part III. *J. chem. Soc.*, **1925**, *127*, 247–258.

Thesleff, S. Acetylcholine utilization in myasthenia gravis. *Ann. N.Y. Acad. Sci.*, **1966**, *135*, 195–206.

Walker, M. B. Treatment of myasthenia gravis with physostigmine. *Lancet*, **1934**, *1*, 1200–1201.

———. Case showing effect of prostigmine on myasthenia gravis. *Proc. R. Soc. Med.*, **1935**, *28*, 759–761.

Wilson, I. B. Acetylcholinesterase. XI. Reversibility of tetraethyl pyrophosphate inhibition. *J. biol. Chem.*, **1951**, *190*, 111–117.

———. Conformation changes in acetylcholinesterase. *Ann. N.Y. Acad. Sci.*, **1967**, *144*, 664–674.

Wilson, I. B., and Bergmann, F. Acetylcholinesterase. VIII. Dissociation constants of the active groups. *J. biol. Chem.*, **1950**, *186*, 683–692.

Wilson, I. B., and Ginsburg, S. A powerful reactivator of alkyl phosphate–inhibited acetylcholinesterase. *Biochim. biophys. Acta*, **1955**, *18*, 168–170.

Wilson, I. B., and Harrison, M. A. Turnover number of acetylcholinesterase. *J. biol. Chem.*, **1961**, *236*, 2292–2295.

Wilson, I. B.; Hatch, M. A.; and Ginsburg, S. Carbamylation of acetylcholinesterase. *J. biol. Chem.*, **1960**, *235*, 2312–2315.

Wofsy, L., and Michaeli, D. Affinity labeling of the anionic site of acetylcholinesterase. *Proc. natn. Acad. Sci. U.S.A.*, **1967**, *58*, 2296–2298.

Monographs and Reviews

Augustinsson, K.-B. A study in comparative enzymology. *Acta physiol. scand.*, **1948**, *15*, Suppl. 52, 1–182.

Chadwick, L. E. Actions on insects and other invertebrates. In, *Cholinesterases and Anticholinesterase Agents.* (Koelle, G. B., ed.) *Handb. exp. Pharmak.*, Vol. 15. Springer-Verlag, Berlin, **1963**, pp. 741–798.

Cohen, J. A., and Oosterbaan, R. A. The active site of acetylcholinesterase and related esterases and its reactivity towards substrates and inhibitors. In, *Cholinesterases and Anticholinesterase Agents.* (Koelle, G. B., ed.) *Handb. exp. Pharmak.*, Vol. 15. Springer-Verlag, Berlin, **1963**, pp. 299–373.

Davies, D. R. Neurotoxicity of organophosphorus compounds. In, *Cholinesterases and Anticholinesterase Agents.*

(Koelle, G. B., ed.) *Handb. exp. Pharmak.*, Vol. 15. Springer-Verlag, Berlin, **1963**, pp. 860–882.

Ehrenpreis, S. (ed.). Cholinergic mechanisms. *Ann. N.Y. Acad. Sci.*, **1967**, *144*, 383–935.

Fields, W. S. (ed.). Myasthenia gravis. *Ann. N.Y. Acad. Sci.*, **1971**, *183*, 1–386.

Froede, H. C., and Wilson, I. B. Acetylcholinesterase. In, *The Enzymes*, Vol. 5. (Boyer, P. D., ed.) Academic Press, Inc., New York, **1971**, pp. 87–114.

Fukuto, T. R. Metabolism of carbamate insecticides. *Drug Metab. Rev.*, **1972**, *1*, 117–151.

Gleason, M. R.; Gosselin, R. E.; and Hodge, H. C. *Clinical Toxicology of Commercial Products*, 3rd ed. The Williams & Wilkins Co., Baltimore, **1968**.

Grob, D. Anticholinesterase intoxication in man and its treatment. In, *Cholinesterases and Anticholinesterase Agents.* (Koelle, G. B., ed.) *Handb. exp. Pharmak.*, Vol. 15. Springer-Verlag, Berlin, **1963a**, pp. 989–1027.

———. Therapy of myasthenia gravis. *Ibid.*, **1963b**, pp. 1028–1050.

Hobbiger, F. Reactivation of phosphorylated acetylcholinesterase. In, *Cholinesterases and Anticholinesterase Agents.* (Koelle, G. B., ed.) *Handb. exp. Pharmak.*, Vol. 15. Springer-Verlag, Berlin, **1963**, pp. 921–988.

Holmstedt, B. Pharmacology of organophosphorus cholinesterase inhibitors. *Pharmac. Rev.*, **1959**, *11*, 567–688. (764 references.)

———. Structure-activity relationships of the organophosphorus anticholinesterase agents. In, *Cholinesterases and Anticholinesterase Agents.* (Koelle, G. B., ed.) *Handb. exp. Pharmak.*, Vol. 15. Springer-Verlag, Berlin, **1963**, pp. 428–485.

———. The ordeal bean of Old Calabar: the pageant of *Physostigma venenosum* in medicine. In, *Plants in the Development of Modern Medicine.* (Swain, T., ed.) Harvard University Press, Cambridge, **1972**, pp. 303–360.

Karczmar, A. G. Pharmacologic, toxicologic, and therapeutic properties of anticholinesterase agents. In, *Physiological Pharmacology.* Vol. 3, *The Nervous System—Part C: Autonomic Nervous System Drugs.* (Root, W. S., and Hofmann, F. G., eds.) Academic Press, Inc., New York, **1967a**, pp. 163–322.

———. Multiple mechanisms of action of drugs at the neuromyal junction as studied in the light of the phenomenon of "reversal." *Laval méd.*, **1967b**, *38*, 465–480.

———. History of the research with anticholinesterase agents. In, *Anticholinesterase Agents*, Vol. 1. *International Encyclopedia of Pharmacology and Therapeutics*, Sect. 13. (Karczmar, A. G., ed.) Pergamon Press, Ltd., Oxford, **1970**, pp. 1–44.

Kitz, R. J. Molecular pharmacology of acetylcholinesterase. In, *Modern Pharmacology.* Part 1, *A Guide to Molecular Pharmacology-Toxicology.* (Featherstone. R. M., ed.) Marcel Dekker, Inc., New York, **1973**, pp. 333–374.

Koelle, G. B., and Gilman, A. Anticholinesterase drugs. *Pharmac. Rev.*, **1949**, *1*, 166–216. (322 references.)

Leopold, I. H., and Krishna, N. Local use of anticholinesterase agents in ocular therapy. In, *Cholinesterases and Anticholinesterase Agents.* (Koelle, G. B., ed.) *Handb. exp. Pharmak.*, Vol. 15. Springer-Verlag, Berlin, **1963**, pp. 1051–1080.

Long, J. P. Structure-activity relationships of the reversible anticholinesterase agents. In, *Cholinesterases and Anticholinesterase Agents.* (Koelle, G. B., ed.) *Handb. exp. Pharmak.*, Vol. 15. Springer-Verlag, Berlin, **1963**, pp. 374–427.

Mounter, L. A. Metabolism of organophosphorus anticholinesterase agents. In, *Cholinesterases and Anticholinesterase Agents.* (Koelle, G. B., ed.) *Handb. exp. Pharmak.*, Vol. 15. Springer-Verlag, Berlin, **1963**, pp. 486–504.

Nachmansohn, D., and Wilson, I. B. The enzymic hydrolysis and synthesis of acetylcholine. *Adv. Enzymol.,* **1951,** *12,* 259–339.

Osserman, K. E. *Myasthenia Gravis.* Grune & Stratton, Inc., New York, **1958.**

Osserman, K. E.; Foldes, F. F.; and Genkins, G. Myasthenia gravis. In, *Neuromuscular Blocking and Stimulating Agents,* Vol. 11. *International Encyclopedia of Pharmacology and Therapeutics,* Sect. 14. (Cheymol, J., ed.) Pergamon Press, Ltd., Oxford, **1972,** pp. 561–618.

Schrader, G. *Die Entwicklung neuer Insektizide auf Grundlage von Organischen Fluor- und Phosphorverbindungen.* Monographie No. 62, Verlag Chemie, Weinheim, **1952.**

Usdin, E. Reactions of cholinesterases with substrates inhibitors and reactivators. In, *Anticholinesterase Agents,* Vol. 1. *International Encyclopedia of Pharmacology and Therapeutics,* Sect. 13. (Karczmar, A. G., ed.) Pergamon Press, Ltd., Oxford, **1970,** pp. 47–354.

Watson, P. G. (ed.). Glaucoma. *Br. J. Ophthal.,* **1972,** *56,* 145–318.

Werner, G., and Kuperman, A. S. Actions at the neuromuscular junction. In, *Cholinesterases and Anticholines-terase Agents.* (Koelle, G. B., ed.) *Handb. exp. Pharmak.,* Vol. 15. Springer-Verlag, Berlin, **1963,** pp. 570–678.

Whipple, K. S. (ed.). Myasthenia gravis. *Ann. N.Y. Acad. Sci.,* **1966,** *135,* 1–680.

Wills, J. H. Pharmacological antagonists of the anticholinesterase agents. In, *Cholinesterases and Anticholinesterase Agents.* (Koelle, G. B., ed.) *Handb. exp. Pharmak.,* Vol. 15. Springer-Verlag, Berlin, **1963,** pp. 883–920.

————. Toxicity of anticholinesterases and treatment of poisoning. In, *Anticholinesterase Agents,* Vol. 1. *International Encyclopedia of Pharmacology and Therapeutics,* Sect. 13. (Karczmar, A. G., ed.) Pergamon Press, Ltd., Oxford, **1970,** pp. 355–471.

Wilson, I. B. The mechanism of enzyme hydrolysis studied with acetylcholinesterase. In, *Symposium on the Mechanism of Enzyme Action.* (McElroy, W. D., and Glass, B., eds.) The Johns Hopkins Press, Baltimore, **1954,** pp. 642–657.

————. Molecular complementarity and antidotes for alkyl phosphate poisoning. *Fedn Proc. Fedn Am. Socs exp. Biol.,* **1959,** *18,* 752–758.

CHAPTER

23 PARASYMPATHOMIMETIC AGENTS

George B. Koelle

Parasympathomimetic agents have as their primary action the excitation or inhibition of autonomic effector cells that are innervated by postganglionic parasympathetic, or cholinergic, nerve impulses. Additional actions are exerted on cells that are not so innervated but nevertheless possess cholinergic receptors. These drugs may be divided into two groups: (1) acetylcholine (ACh) and several synthetic choline esters and related derivatives; and (2) the naturally occurring cholinomimetic alkaloids (particularly pilocarpine, muscarine, and arecoline) and certain chemically related synthetic compounds. In addition, the anticholinesterase (anti-ChE) agents (Chapter 22) and ganglionic stimulants (Chapter 27) have parasympathomimetic actions, but these are accompanied by prominent effects at other sites of cholinergic transmission.

CHOLINE ESTERS

Acetylcholine (ACh) has had virtually no therapeutic applications because of its diffuseness of action and its rapid hydrolysis by both acetylcholinesterase (AChE) and nonspecific cholinesterase. Consequently, numerous derivatives have been synthesized in attempts to obtain drugs with more selective and prolonged actions.

History. ACh was first synthesized by Baeyer in 1867. Investigations culminating in its identification as a neurohumoral transmitter are described in Chapter 21.

Of several hundred synthetic choline derivatives investigated, only methacholine, carbachol, and bethanechol have had clinical application. The structures of these compounds are shown in Table 23–1. Although *methacholine,* the β-methyl analog of ACh, was studied by Hunt and Taveau as early as 1911, it was not until the systematic investigations of this compound by Simonart (1932) and Starr and associates (1933) that the drug received adequate therapeutic trial. *Carbachol,* the carbamyl ester of choline, and *bethanechol,* its β-methyl analog, were synthesized in the early 1930s; their pharmacological

actions were investigated by Molitor (1936) and others.

Mechanism of Action. The mechanisms of action of endogenous ACh at the postjunctional membranes of the effector cells and neurons that correspond to the four classes of cholinergic nerves are treated in detail in Chapter 21. By way of recapitulation, these are (1) postganglionic parasympathetic fibers to autonomic effector cells, (2) preganglionic autonomic fibers to sympathetic and parasympathetic ganglion cells and to the adrenal medulla, (3) somatic motor nerves to skeletal muscle, and (4) certain fiber tracts within the central nervous system (CNS). When ACh is administered systemically, it has the potential to produce the same effects, although as a quaternary ammonium compound its penetration to sites within the CNS is limited. Since muscarine was characterized originally as acting relatively selectively at *autonomic effector cells* to produce qualitatively the same effects as ACh, actions of ACh and related drugs at these sites are referred to as *muscarinic.* Accordingly, the *muscarinic,* or *parasympathomimetic,* actions of the drugs considered in this chapter are practically equivalent to the effects of postganglionic parasympathetic nerve impulses listed in Table 21–1 (page 408); the differences between the actions of the individual drugs are largely quantitative and a matter of relative selectivity for one organ system or another. It is now known that varying proportions of *muscarinic* receptors are also present on autonomic ganglion cells and on certain cortical and subcortical neurons, and hence the drugs of this class may have secondary effects at these sites. All the actions of ACh and other parasympathomimetic drugs at muscarinic receptors can be blocked by *atropine (see* Chapter 25). The *nicotinic* actions of such drugs refer to their initial stimulation, and in high doses to subsequent blockade, of autonomic ganglion

467

Table 23-1. STRUCTURAL FORMULAS OF CHOLINE, ACETYLCHOLINE, AND CLINICALLY EMPLOYED CHOLINE ESTERS

Choline chloride	$(CH_3)_3N^+CH_2CH_2OH$	Cl^-
Acetylcholine chloride	$(CH_3)_3N^+CH_2CH_2O\overset{\displaystyle O}{\overset{\|}{C}}CH_3$	Cl^-
Methacholine chloride	$(CH_3)_3N^+CH_2\underset{CH_3}{CH}O\overset{\displaystyle O}{\overset{\|}{C}}CH_3$	Cl^-
Carbachol chloride	$(CH_3)_3N^+CH_2CH_2O\overset{\displaystyle O}{\overset{\|}{C}}NH_2$	Cl^-
Bethanechol chloride	$(CH_3)_3N^+CH_2\underset{CH_3}{CH}O\overset{\displaystyle O}{\overset{\|}{C}}NH_2$	Cl^-

cells and the neuromuscular junction, actions comparable to those of nicotine.

Structure-Activity Relationship. The structure-activity relationship of parasympathomimetic agents has been described in detail (Simonart, 1932; Brücke, 1956; Waser, 1961; Bebbington and Brimblecombe, 1965; Kosterlitz, 1967; Rand and Stafford, 1967). Attention is confined here only to those drugs that are of therapeutic interest.

Acetyl-β-methylcholine (methacholine) differs from ACh chiefly in its greater duration and selectivity of action. Its action is more prolonged because it is hydrolyzed by AChE at a considerably slower rate than ACh and is almost totally resistant to hydrolysis by nonspecific cholinesterase or pseudocholinesterase. Its selectivity is manifested by a lack of significant nicotinic and a predominance of muscarinic actions, the latter being most marked on the cardiovascular system (Table 23-2).

Carbachol and *bethanechol* are virtually totally resistant to hydrolysis by either AChE or nonspecific cholinesterase; bethanechol has mainly muscarinic actions, but both drugs act relatively selectively on the smooth muscle of the gastrointestinal tract and urinary bladder. Carbachol retains a high level of nicotinic activity, particularly on autonomic ganglia. It is likely that both its peripheral and its ganglionic actions are due, at least in part, to the release of endogenous ACh from the terminals of cholinergic fibers (*see* Chapter 21). Carbachol probably shares this mechanism of action with numerous other parasympathomimetic choline esters and alkyltrimethylammonium compounds (Takagi *et al.*, 1968).

PHARMACOLOGICAL PROPERTIES

Cardiovascular System. ACh has three primary effects upon the cardiovascular system: *vasodilatation,* a decrease in the rate of the heart beat (the *negative chronotropic* effect), and a decrease in the force of cardiac contraction (the *negative inotropic* effect). The latter is particularly true of atrial muscle. However, certain of these effects can be partially or totally obscured by a number of factors, especially including the release by ACh of catecholamines from both cardiac and extracardiac tissues and the dampening of the direct effects of ACh by baroreceptor and other reflexes.

Although ACh is rarely given systemically as a drug, its cardiac actions are of importance because of the involvement of cholinergic vagal impulses in the actions of the cardiac glycosides, antiarrhythmic agents, and many other drugs. The intravenous injection of a small (1 to 5 μg/kg) dose of ACh in an anesthetized animal produces an evanescent fall in blood pressure due to generalized vasodilatation, accompanied usually

Table 23-2. SOME PHARMACOLOGICAL PROPERTIES OF CHOLINE ESTERS

CHOLINE ESTER	SUSCEPTIBILITY TO CHOLINESTERASES	Muscarinic				Antagonism by Atropine	*Nicotinic*
		Cardiovascular	Gastrointestinal	Urinary Bladder	Eye (topical)		
Acetylcholine	+++	++	++	++	+	+++	++
Methacholine	+	+++	++	++	+	+++	+
Carbachol	−	+	+++	+++	++	+	+++
Bethanechol	−	±	+++	+++	++	+++	−

by reflex tachycardia. A considerably larger dose is required to elicit bradycardia from the direct action of ACh on the heart. In *man,* intravenous infusions of ACh (20 to 60 mg per minute) produce little change other than vasodilatation and a slight fall in blood pressure, because of the rapid enzymatic hydrolysis of ACh and the efficient compensatory cardiovascular reflexes mediated through the caroticoaortic baroreceptors. In addition, sympathoadrenal discharge produced by the nicotinic action of ACh tends to prevent any marked alterations in heart rate and blood pressure. When large doses (90 to 140 mg per minute) are administered intravenously, the complete pattern of bradycardia, hypotension, and the expected responses of other autonomic effectors is obtained.

ACh, whether released by cholinergic fibers or injected, produces *dilatation* of essentially *all vascular beds,* including the pulmonary (Aviado, 1965) and coronary (Levy and Zieske, 1969). However, it is unlikely that either parasympathetic vasodilator or sympathetic vasoconstrictor tone plays a major role in the regulation of coronary blood flow, in comparison with the effects of local oxygen tension and autoregulatory metabolic factors such as adenosine (Berne, 1964). The effect of choline esters to dilate vascular beds is due to the presence of muscarinic receptors at these sites, despite the lack of apparent cholinergic innervation of many vascular beds.

ACh has important actions on all types of specialized cardiac cells; the same is qualitatively true of vagal impulses, since it has been demonstrated that cholinergic parasympathetic fibers are distributed extensively to the S-A and A-V nodes and the atrial muscle. The innervation of the ventricular and papillary muscle is more limited (Kamijo and Koelle, 1955; Gerebtzoff, 1959; Jacobowitz *et al.,* 1967).

In the *S-A node,* each normal cardiac impulse is initiated by the spontaneous depolarization of the pacemaker fibers, due to a progressive fall in potassium conductance. At a critical level, the threshold potential, this depolarization initiates an action potential (AP). The AP is conducted over the course of the atrial fibers to the A-V node and thence through the Purkinje system to the

ventricular muscles. ACh slows the heart rate by decreasing the rate of diastolic depolarization at the S-A node, thereby delaying the attainment of the threshold potential and the succeeding events in the cardiac cycle.

In *atrial muscle,* ACh decreases the strength of contraction. It also slows the rate of conduction of the AP and shortens the durations of the AP and the effective refractory period. The combination of these factors is the basis for the perpetuation or exacerbation by vagal impulses of atrial flutter or fibrillation arising at an ectopic focus. In contrast, primarily in the *A-V node* and to a much lesser extent in the *Purkinje conducting system,* ACh slows conduction but increases the refractory period. With an increase in vagal tone, such as is produced by the digitalis glycosides, these effects can contribute to the reduction in the frequency with which aberrant atrial impulses are transmitted to the ventricle, and thus decrease the ventricular rate during atrial flutter or fibrillation. ACh normally decreases the strength of contraction of the ventricle; at excessive concentrations, it exhibits a positive inotropic effect, mainly through the local release of catecholamine (Buccino *et al.,* 1966). (*See also* Rand and Stafford, 1967; Higgins *et al.,* 1973.)

The effects produced in man by constant *intravenous* infusion of *methacholine* are identical with those obtained with ACh, but the effective dose is only about $\frac{1}{200}$ as large. After a *subcutaneous* dose of 20 mg, a transient fall in blood pressure and a compensatory tachycardia occur. When methacholine is administered *orally,* doses 50 to 100 times as large as the effective subcutaneous dose have to be employed before significant effects are observed; these are gradual in onset and mild in character. For example, after an oral dose of 1 g the blood pressure falls only moderately, the pulse rate slows, the typical flush appears, and the skin temperature of the extremities rises, indicative of vasodilatation. Methacholine administered parenterally, either alone or concomitantly with neostigmine, can cause *cardiac arrhythmias,* such as various degrees of heart block including complete A-V dissociation. Cardiac arrhythmias caused by methacholine are particularly prone to occur in patients with hyperthyroidism, especially transient atrial fibrillation; alterations in the ventricular complex, displacements of the S-T segment, and inversion of the T wave also occur.

In contrast to ACh and methacholine, the cardiovascular effects of *carbachol* and *bethanechol* ordinarily are inconspicuous following usual subcutaneous or oral doses, and generally consist only in a slight, transient fall in diastolic pressure accompanied by a mild reflex tachycardia.

Gastrointestinal System. All the compounds of this class are capable of producing increases in tone, amplitude of contractions, and peristaltic activity of the stomach and intestines, as well as enhanced secretory activity of the gastrointestinal tract. The motor effects may be accompanied by nausea, belching, vomiting, intestinal cramps, and defecation. *Carbachol* and *bethanechol* produce the foregoing responses with a minimum of cardiovascular effects after appropriate oral or subcutaneous doses; by contrast, *ACh* and *methacholine* elicit enteric responses only after doses that also induce relatively prominent cardiovascular effects.

Urinary Tract. *Carbachol* and *bethanechol,* in contrast to ACh and methacholine, stimulate selectively the urinary tract as well as the gastrointestinal tract. The choline esters contract the detrusor muscle of the urinary bladder and decrease bladder capacity. In animals with experimental lesions of the spinal cord or sacral roots, they bring about satisfactory evacuation of the neurogenic bladder. The frequency of ureteral peristaltic waves is enhanced.

Miscellaneous Effects. ACh and its analogs activate secretion by all *glands* that receive parasympathetic innervation, including the lacrimal, tracheobronchial, salivary, digestive, and exocrine sweat glands. The effects on the *respiratory system,* in addition to increased tracheobronchial secretion, include bronchoconstriction and stimulation of the chemoreceptors of the carotid and aortic bodies. When instilled intraconjunctivally, they produce *miosis;* however, the resultant fall in intraocular tension may be preceded by a temporary elevation due to an increase in the permeability of the blood–aqueous humor barrier.

The effects of ACh at the neuromuscular junction of skeletal muscle and on autonomic ganglia are described in Chapter 21; while its derivatives considered here have been shown to produce similar

effects in the laboratory, these are not significant with the doses employed clinically, with the possible exception of carbachol. Likewise, these drugs exhibit cholinomimetic effects on the *CNS* when administered by special technics, but their failure to penetrate the blood-brain barrier following ordinary doses precludes such effects under ordinary circumstances.

Synergisms and Antagonisms. ACh and methacholine are hydrolyzed by AChE, and their effects are markedly enhanced by the prior administration of anti-ChE agents. The latter drugs produce only additive effects with the stable analogs, carbachol and bethanechol.

The *muscarinic* actions of all the drugs of this class are blocked selectively by atropine, through competitive occupation of cholinoceptive sites on the autonomic effector cells and on the secondary muscarinic receptors of autonomic ganglion cells. Epinephrine and other sympathomimetic amines likewise antagonize most of their muscarinic effects at sites where adrenergic and cholinergic impulses produce opposing effects (Table 21–1, page 408).

The *nicotinic* actions of ACh and its derivatives at autonomic ganglia are blocked by hexamethonium and related drugs; their actions at the neuromuscular junction of skeletal muscle are antagonized by *d*-tubocurarine and other competitive blocking agents, and are augmented by depolarizing neuromuscular blocking agents.

Preparations, Routes of Administration, and Dosage. *Acetylcholine chloride* is used practically exclusively for compounding *acetylcholine chloride for ophthalmic solution* (MIOCHOL). The latter is available in vials for the extemporaneous preparation of a 1% solution in 5% mannitol.

While several preparations of *methacholine* (*acetyl-β-methacholine*) are official (*Methacholine Bromide,* N.F.; *Methacholine Bromide Tablets,* N.F.; *Methacholine Chloride,* N.F.; *Methacholine Chloride, Sterile,* N.F.), the drug is now rarely used clinically.

Bethanechol Chloride, N.F. (*carbamylmethylcholine chloride;* MYOTONACHOL, URECHOLINE), is available as official 5-, 10-, and 25-mg scored tablets and as an official injection (5 mg/ml). It is used to stimulate contraction of the gastrointestinal tract and the urinary bladder. The *oral* dose for adults varies from 5 to 30 mg; the *subcutaneous* dose is 2.5 to 5.0 mg. The single dose may be given three to four times daily. *The drug should not be administered by the intramuscular or intravenous route.*

Carbachol, U.S.P. (*carbamylcholine chloride*), is available in bulk form but is used solely as *Car-*

bachol Ophthalmic Solution, U.S.P., in concentrations of 0.75, 1.5, 2.25, and 3.0%.

Precautions, Toxicity, and Contraindications. The drugs of this class should be administered only by the *oral* or *subcutaneous* route for systemic effects, or by *intraconjunctival instillation.* If they are given intravenously or intramuscularly, their relative selectivity of action no longer holds, and the incidence and severity of toxic side effects are greatly increased. In order to *counteract* any serious toxic reactions to these drugs, *atropine sulfate* (0.5 to 1.0 mg) should be given intramuscularly or intravenously, and should be readily available. *Epinephrine* (0.1 to 1.0 mg, subcutaneously) is also of value in overcoming severe cardiovascular or bronchoconstrictor responses.

Among the major *contraindications* to the use of the choline esters are *asthma, hyperthyroidism, coronary insufficiency,* and *peptic ulcer.* As noted previously, their bronchoconstrictor action is liable to precipitate an asthmatic attack, and hyperthyroid patients may develop atrial fibrillation, particularly after methacholine. Hypotension induced by these agents can severely reduce coronary flow, especially if it is already compromised. The gastric acid secretion produced by the choline esters will aggravate the symptoms of peptic ulcer.

A number of *untoward clinical reactions* can follow the administration of *methacholine,* including nausea and vomiting, substernal pain or pressure, dyspnea, fainting, and transient complete heart block. Patients with hypertension may react to the drug with a precipitous fall in blood pressure. Overdosage may result in an alarming but transient syncopal reaction, with cardiac arrest and loss of consciousness.

While the same reactions observed after methacholine administration are possible after *bethanechol,* untoward effects related to the cardiovascular system are less liable to occur. Undesirable effects may include flushing, sweating, epigastric distress, abdominal cramps, belching, a sensation of tightness in the urinary bladder, difficulty in visual accommodation, headache, and salivation.

THERAPEUTIC USES

The choline esters have to a large extent been replaced by other drugs. This applies particularly to *methacholine* as a vasodilator and cardiac vagomimetic agent. *Bethanechol* is still used as a stimulant of the smooth muscle of the gastrointestinal tract and uri-

nary bladder; *carbachol* is obsolete for these purposes because of its relatively higher component of nicotinic action at autonomic ganglia. All these drugs, as well as *ACh,* can be employed as miotics in certain situations.

Paroxysmal Supraventricular Tachycardia. In some patients reflex vagal stimulation (through pressure on the carotid sinus or eye, induction of emesis, postural and breathing maneuvers, etc.) will arrest attacks of paroxysmal S-A nodal or atrial tachycardia. In the past, methacholine was sometimes given to accomplish reversion to normal sinus rhythm, but this use has been abandoned because of the numerous side effects. A more satisfactory drug that acts indirectly in the same manner is the short-acting anti-ChE agent edrophonium. Other drugs that may be used for this purpose include the digitalis glycosides, sympathomimetic (pressor) amines that have a minimum of β-receptor stimulatory activity (such as phenylephrine, methoxamine, or hydroxyamphetamine), or a suitable antiarrhythmic agent (Chapter 32); in refractory cases, electrical cardioversion may be necessary.

Gastrointestinal Disorders. Bethanechol is of value in certain cases of *postoperative abdominal distention.* The oral route is preferred; the usual dose is 10 to 20 mg, three or four times daily. It may be necessary to insert a rectal tube to facilitate passage of flatus. The drug has likewise been used to advantage in certain cases of adynamic ileus secondary to toxic states. *Gastric atony and retention following bilateral vagotomy* for peptic ulcer are often satisfactorily relieved by bethanechol; in this condition, neostigmine is ineffective. Bethanechol is given by mouth with each main meal in cases without complete retention; when gastric retention is complete and nothing passes into the duodenum, the subcutaneous route is necessary because the drug is not adequately absorbed from the stomach. Bethanechol increases the volume and the acidity of secretion of the vagotomized stomach and hence should be given only with meals. The drug may also be employed for postoperative gastric atony other than that associated with vagotomy. Bethanechol is of value in selected cases of *congenital megacolon.*

Urinary Bladder Disorders. Bethanechol may be useful in combating *urinary retention* when organic obstruction is absent, as in postoperative and postpartum retention and in certain cases of neurogenic bladder. Catheterization, with its attendant risk of urinary tract infection, can thus be avoided. For *acute retention,* the drug is injected subcutaneously in the usual dose of 5 mg, which can be repeated after 15 to 30 minutes if necessary. A bedpan or urinal should be available to the patient. The stomach should be empty at the time the drug is injected. In *chronic cases,* 10 mg of the drug may be given orally, three times daily, until voluntary or automatic voiding begins and then its administration is slowly withdrawn.

Ophthalmological Uses. *Acetylcholine,* 1%, is used in cataract extractions and certain other surgical procedures on the anterior segment when it is desired to produce rapid, brief miosis (Rizzuti, 1967). *Methacholine,* in concentrations up to 20%, in combination with neostigmine bromide, 5%, instilled intraconjunctivally at frequent intervals, has been recommended for the emergency treatment of acute attacks of *congestive glaucoma.* For the chronic therapy of noncongestive, wide-angle glaucoma, *carbachol* (0.25 to 1.5%) and *bethanechol* (1.0%) have been employed; however, both these drugs penetrate the cornea poorly, and for this reason are generally compounded with a wetting agent. Other drugs used in this condition include pilocarpine and aceclidine, as well as the anti-ChE agents.

Diagnostic Uses. If a patient is suspected of having poisoning due to atropine or other belladonna alkaloids, 10 to 30 mg of *methacholine* may be injected subcutaneously. The failure of appearance of the characteristic flush, sweating, lacrimation, rhinorrhea, salivation, and enhanced peristalsis is pathognomonic of *belladonna intoxication.* The specific antidote for this condition is *physostigmine.*

Methacholine and *bethanechol* have also been employed diagnostically in place of secretin as a test for *pancreatic enzymatic function;* by simultaneously stimulating secretion and constricting the ampullary mechanism, the drugs should normally cause an increase in the serum amylase level.

CHOLINOMIMETIC NATURAL ALKALOIDS AND SYNTHETIC ANALOGS

The three major natural alkaloids in this group—*pilocarpine, muscarine,* and *arecoline* —have as their principal action the stimulation of the same autonomic effector cells as those acted upon by cholinergic postganglionic nerve impulses. In this respect they resemble the choline esters discussed above. Muscarine acts almost exclusively at *muscarinic* receptor sites—their classification as such being derived from this fact. Arecoline acts in addition at *nicotinic* receptors. On the basis of this information, most of their pharmacological actions can be predicted. However, there are certain inconsistencies in their actions, particularly those of pilocarpine on the sweat glands and the cardiovascular system, that have not been adequately explained.

Although these naturally occurring alkaloids are of great value as pharmacological tools and have enjoyed a certain degree of popularity as therapeutic agents in the past, their present clinical use is largely restricted

to the employment of pilocarpine as a miotic agent.

History and Sources. *Pilocarpine* is the chief alkaloid obtained from the leaflets of South American shrubs of the genus *Pilocarpus.* Although it was long known by the natives that the chewing of leaves of *Pilocarpus* plants caused salivation, the first experiments were apparently performed in 1874 by a Brazilian physician named Coutinhou. The alkaloid was isolated in 1875, and shortly thereafter the actions of pilocarpine on the pupil as well as on the sweat and salivary glands were described by Weber.

The poisonous effects of certain species of mushrooms have been known since ancient times, but it was not until Schmiedeberg isolated the alkaloid *muscarine* from *Amanita muscaria* that the properties of the drug could be systematically investigated. Schmiedeberg and Koppe published the first careful pharmacological study of muscarine in 1869. The role played by muscarine in the development of the neurohumoral theory has been recounted in Chapter 21.

Arecoline is the chief alkaloid of areca or betel nuts, the seeds of *Areca catechu.* The *betel nut* has been consumed as a euphoretic by the natives of the East Indies from early times in a masticatory mixture known as *betel* and composed of the nut, shell lime, and leaves of *Piper betle,* a climbing species of pepper. The mixture stains the teeth black. The use of betel nut as a vermifuge was known to the Chinese as early as the sixth century, and the nut is still employed for this purpose in China.

Structure-Activity Relationship. The parasympathomimetic alkaloids show marked differences as well as interesting relationships in structure (Table 23-3). *Arecoline* and *pilocarpine* are tertiary amines, but the former has been shown to be pharmacologically active chiefly in the protonated form (Burgen, 1965); arecoline bears a certain structural resemblance to nicotine, as does pilocarpine to histamine.

A synthetic compound that resembles arecoline, 3-acetoxyquinuclidine (*aceclidine,* Table 23-3), was shown by Mashkovsky and Zaitseva (1968) to act as a typical parasympathomimetic agent. Its quaternary methiodide derivative is considerably less potent, but can be regarded as a conformationally rigid analog of methacholine. Resolution of its enantiomorphs and examination of their pharmacological properties by Belleau and associates has provided information regarding the stereospecific properties of both the muscarinic receptor and acetylcholinesterase (Robinson *et al.,* 1969).

Muscarine, a quaternary ammonium compound containing a tetrahydrofuran ring, has three asymmetrical carbon atoms; all four pairs of its possible enantiomorphs have been synthesized (Eugster *et al.,* 1958), including the naturally occurring L(+) form. A synthetic compound that has proven extremely valuable as an investigative tool in the search for antiparkinsonism drugs and in other studies of the pharmacology of the CNS is *oxotremorine* (Table 23-3). In the periphery, it acts as a potent muscarinic agent. Its parkinsonism-like central effects include

Table 23-3. STRUCTURAL FORMULAS OF CHOLINOMIMETIC NATURAL ALKALOIDS AND SYNTHETIC ANALOGS

Arecoline   Pilocarpine   Muscarine

Aceclidine   Oxotremorine

tremor, ataxia, and spasticity, which result apparently from activation of muscarinic receptors in the basal ganglia and elsewhere (Cho *et al.,* 1962). Although oxotremorine bears superficially little resemblance to muscarine, the distances between the presumed active centers of the two compounds are remarkably close (Bebbington and Brimblecombe, 1965).

The chemistry and pharmacology of many natural and synthetic muscarinic compounds have been reviewed by Waser (1961), Bebbington and Brimblecombe (1965), Kosterlitz (1967), and Miller and Lewis (1969).

Mechanism of Action. While these compounds act primarily at muscarinic receptors of autonomic effector cells, ganglionic effects can also be observed. This is particularly true of pilocarpine, although its ganglionic action also involves stimulation of muscarinic receptors, and hence is blocked by relatively low doses of atropine (*see* Chapter 27). Ganglionic actions of *muscarine* defy strict categorization. Although muscarine stimulates the superior cervical ganglion of the cat, the dose required is considerably higher than that which acts peripherally; the ganglionic action is blocked by moderate doses of either atropine or hexamethonium (Ambache *et al.,* 1956). The ganglionic stimulant action of *arecoline* is due predominantly to activation of nicotinic receptors, in that it is blocked by nicotine and is relatively resistant to atropine (Euler and Domeij, 1945).

PHARMACOLOGICAL PROPERTIES

Smooth Muscle. Pilocarpine, when applied locally to the *eye,* causes pupillary constriction, spasm of accommodation, and a transitory rise in intraocular pressure, followed by a more persistent fall. Miosis lasts from several hours to a day, but fixation of the lens for near vision disappears in about 2 hours. The *smooth muscles of other organs* respond in general to both pilocarpine and muscarine as would be predicted on the basis of their responses to cholinergic nerve stimulation. Thus, these drugs stimulate the smooth muscles of the *intestinal tract,* thereby increasing tone and motility; large doses cause marked spasm and tenesmus. The

bronchial musculature is also stimulated; asthmatic patients uniformly respond to pilocarpine with a reduction in vital capacity, and a typical asthmatic attack may be precipitated. The tone and motility of the *ureters, urinary bladder, gallbladder,* and *biliary ducts* are also enhanced by pilocarpine and muscarine. The *spleen* contracts after pilocarpine due to stimulation of its capsular musculature; this is probably the basis for the observed *leukocytosis* and *increased erythrocyte count.* When muscarine is applied to various isolated organs *in vitro,* the response of the smooth muscle is generally more delayed and considerably more prolonged than that following equipotent doses of ACh.

Sweat Glands. Pilocarpine (10 to 15 mg, subcutaneously) causes marked diaphoresis in man; 2 to 3 liters of sweat may be secreted. Accompanying side effects may include hiccough, salivation, nausea, vomiting, weakness, and occasionally collapse. Muscarine and arecoline are also potent diaphoretic agents.

The intradermal injection of a solution of pilocarpine or ACh in normally innervated skin causes local sweating and vasodilatation, the responses to ACh being enhanced by physostigmine; atropine injected into the same area causes prompt cessation of both sweating and vasodilatation. Preganglionic sympathectomy of cutaneous areas in man does not prevent secretion of sweat in response to parenteral pilocarpine. In contrast, postganglionically denervated sweat glands do not respond even to the intracutaneous injection of pilocarpine or ACh despite their responsiveness to intense local heat and to catecholamines. The reason for this anomaly is not clear. One would expect that denervated effector cells would respond excessively to neurochemical transmitters and closely allied drugs (*see* Lloyd, 1965).

Other Glands. The salivary, lacrimal, gastric, pancreatic, and intestinal glands, and the mucous cells of the respiratory tract are also stimulated by these alkaloids. Normal saliva is one of the few hypotonic fluids that the body elaborates and is also unique in containing a larger amount of potassium than does the extracellular fluid from which it is derived; after pilocarpine, the composition of the saliva tends to approach that of an ultrafiltrate of the plasma (Dreisbach, 1961, 1963).

The *gastric glands* are stimulated to secrete a juice rich in acid but especially abundant in pepsin and mucin, resembling that resulting from vagal stimulation. Few choline esters exceed pilocarpine in the ability to stimulate the secretion of pepsin (Hollander, 1944). The effects of the alkaloids on *pancreatic, intestinal,* and *hepatic biliary* secretions are not prominent. Large doses can produce sufficient *bronchiolar secretion* to cause pulmonary edema.

Cardiovascular System. The most prominent cardiovascular effects following the intravenous injection of extremely small doses (0.01 to 0.03 μg/kg) of *muscarine* in various species are a marked fall in the blood pressure and a slowing or temporary cessation of the heart beat.

The actions of *pilocarpine* on the cardiovascular system are complex and defy satisfactory explanation. An intravenous injection of 0.1 mg/kg of pilocarpine produces a brief fall in blood pressure. However, if this is preceded by an appropriate dose of a nicotinic blocking agent, pilocarpine produces a marked rise in pressure. Both the vasodepressor and pressor responses are prevented by atropine; the latter effect is also abolished by α-adrenergic blocking agents (Koppanyi, 1939; Levy and Ahlquist, 1962). A possible explanation is that pilocarpine acts at nicotinic receptors at the terminals of cholinergic fibers to release ACh and causes initial vasodepression, and at excitatory muscarinic receptors on sympathetic ganglion cells and adrenomedullary chromaffin cells to cause hypertension.

Central Nervous System. Many years ago it was shown that the injection of *pilocarpine* into the cerebral ventricles of man or the rabbit produced a variety of autonomic and somatic motor effects that suggested the activation of paraventricular hypothalamic nuclei (Cushing, 1932; Light *et al.,* 1933). Subsequently, pilocarpine, muscarine, and arecoline have been found to evoke a characteristic cortical arousal or activation response in cats following the intravenous injection of relatively small doses, similar to that produced by the injection of ACh or anti-ChE agents, or by electrical stimulation of the brain stem reticular formation. The arousal response to all these drugs is reduced or blocked by atropine and related agents (Rinaldi and Himwich, 1955a, 1955b). Pilocarpine has also been shown to produce a variety of stimulant and depressant effects on the CNS, the analysis of which indicates that it acts at cholinoceptive sites and also elicits strychnine-like effects (Zablocka and Esplin, 1964). There is likewise evidence that pilocarpine acts presynaptically to cause release and then depletion of the postsynaptic inhibitory neurotransmitter (Turkanis and Esplin, 1968). The spectrum of the known central actions of this group of drugs, ranging from those at individual neurons to the modification of complex behavioral processes, has been reviewed by Votava (1967), Curtis and Crawford (1969), and Krnjević (1974).

The hallucinogenic effects that follow the consumption of various species of *Amanita,* and that were presumably the basis of the wild fury of the Scandinavian Berserkers (Fabing, 1956), are probably not due to muscarine but to the related compound, ibotinic acid (*see* Farnsworth, 1968).

Toxicology. Poisoning from pilocarpine, muscarine, or arecoline is characterized chiefly by exaggeration of their various parasympathomimetic effects, and resembles that produced by consumption of mushrooms of the genus *Inocybe* (*see* below). *Treatment* consists in the parenteral administration of atropine, and in adequate measures to support the respiration and the circulation and to counteract pulmonary edema.

Preparations and Dosage. *Pilocarpine Hydrochloride* and *Pilocarpine Nitrate* are official in the U.S.P., both as the salts and as *ophthalmic solutions.* The average oral or hypodermic dose of pilocarpine, now rarely used, is 5 to 10 mg.

A device for achieving the sustained release of pilocarpine into the cul-de-sac of the eye is also available (OCUSERT). This is an elliptically shaped unit consisting of a pilocarpine-containing reservoir surrounded by a permeable membrane. Following placement by the patient, different forms of the unit are designed to release pilocarpine at a rate of either 20 or 40 μg per hour for 1 week. Intraocular pressure is reduced continuously, conveniently, and with considerably less total drug than by other methods.

Arecoline is used in veterinary medicine as a vermifuge.

Fate and Excretion. Little definitive information is available on the fate and elimination of pilocarpine. It is partly destroyed in the body, but the larger fraction is excreted in the urine in combined form.

THERAPEUTIC USES

Pilocarpine is used in the treatment of *glaucoma* (*see* page 460), where it has generally been administered as a 0.5 to 4.0% aqueous solution. It can also be given in an ointment or as lamellae. Experience with the sustained-release device described above is limited, but it may offer several advantages. The miotic action of pilocarpine is useful in overcoming the mydriasis produced by atropine; alternated with mydriatics, pilocarpine is employed to break adhesions between the iris and the lens.

Aceclidine (GLAUCOSTAT), in concentrations of 0.5 to 2.0%, has been shown to be approximately as effective as pilocarpine in reducing intraocular pressure in glaucoma, and it is a useful alternative for patients in whom the latter drug is unsatisfactory (Lieberman and Leopold, 1967; Romano, 1970). The drug is employed extensively in Europe but is not currently available in the United States.

Muscarine and *arecoline* are not employed clinically in man.

MUSHROOM POISONING (MYCETISMUS)

Mushroom poisoning has been known for centuries. The Greek poet Euripides (fifth century B.C.)

is said to have lost his wife and three children from this cause. Mushrooms were employed by professional poisoners in ancient times.

Although *Amanita muscaria* is the source from which *muscarine* has generally been isolated, its content of the alkaloid is so low (approximately 0.003%) that it is considered unlikely that muscarine could be responsible for the major toxic effects. Much higher concentrations of muscarine are present in various species of *Inocybe*. The symptoms of intoxication attributable to muscarine develop within ½ to 2 hours following ingestion of species of *Inocybe*; they include salivation, lacrimation, nausea, vomiting, headache, visual disturbances, abdominal colic, diarrhea, dyspnea, bradycardia, profound hypotension, and shock. Treatment with atropine (2 mg, parenterally) should effectively block all these effects. Intoxication produced by *A. muscaria* may present a combination of some of the foregoing symptoms along with a variety of central effects, including irritability, restlessness, ataxia, anxiety, mania, hallucinations, delirium, and even convulsions. Substances responsible for the central effects may include the muscarine-like compound *ibotinic acid,* or any of a series of indole derivatives that have been only partially identified. Treatment is dependent largely on the use of sedatives (Waser, 1961).

The most serious form of mycetismus is produced by *A. phalloides* and related species, which are fairly common in both North America and Europe. Prodromal gastrointestinal symptoms are followed in a day or longer by signs of severe impairment of hepatic and renal function caused by two groups of cyclic peptides: the *phallotoxins,* a group of cyclic heptapeptides that appear to inhibit protein synthesis; and the *amatoxins,* cyclic octapeptides that interfere with ribonucleic acid synthesis (Wieland, 1968). A member of the latter group, α-amanitin, has been shown to be an extremely potent and selective inhibitor of RNA polymerase B (Kedinger *et al.,* 1970). The prognosis is grave; death usually occurs in 5 to 8 days after ingestion of the mushrooms. Treatment is purely symptomatic and supportive, and includes prolonged rest in bed, opioids for pain, and therapy for shock when indicated. The value of antitoxic sera in cases of poisoning by *A. phalloides* is unproved.

Ambache, N.; Perry, W. L. M.; and Robertson, P. A. The effect of muscarine on perfused superior cervical ganglia of cats. *Br. J. Pharmac. Chemother.,* **1956,** *11,* 442–448.

Baeyer, A. Ueber das Neurin. *Justus Liebigs Annln Chem.,* **1867,** *142,* 322–326.

Buccino, R. A.; Sonnenblick, E. H.; Cooper, T.; and Braunwald, E. Direct positive inotropic effect of acetylcholine on myocardium. Evidence for multiple cholinergic receptors in the heart. *Circulation Res.,* **1966,** *11,* 1097–1108.

Burgen, A. S. V. The role of ionic interaction at the muscarinic receptor. *Br. J. Pharmac. Chemother.,* **1965,** *25,* 4–17.

Cho, A. K.; Haslett, W. L.; and Jenden, D. J. The peripheral actions of oxotremorine, a metabolite of tremorine. *J. Pharmac. exp. Ther.,* **1962,** *138,* 249–257.

Dreisbach, R. H. Effect of pilocarpine on transfer of Ca⁴⁵ and K⁴² to rat submaxillary gland and kidney. *J. Pharmac. exp. Ther.,* **1961,** *131,* 257–260.

———. Effect of parasympathetic stimulants on Ca⁴⁵ transfer in rat parotid glands *in vitro. Am. J. Physiol.,* **1963,** *204,* 497–500.

Eugster, C. H.; Häfliger, F.; Denss, R.; and Girod, E. Die Spaltung von d,l-Muscarin in die optischen Antipoden. *Helv. chim. Acta.,* **1958,** *41,* 886–888.

Euler, U. S. von, and Domeij, B. Nicotine-like action of arecoline. *Acta pharmac. tox.,* **1945,** *1,* 263–269.

Fabing, H. D. On going berserk: a neurochemical inquiry. *Scient. Mon., N.Y.,* **1956,** *82,* 232–237.

Hollander, F. The secretion of gastric mucus and hydrochloric acid in response to pilocarpine: a review of the literature. *Gastroenterology,* **1944,** *2,* 201–211.

Hunt, R., and Taveau, R. DeM. The effects of a number of derivatives of choline and analogous compounds on the blood pressure. *U.S. Hyg. Lab. Bull.,* No. 73, Washington, D. C., **1911.**

Jacobowitz, D.; Cooper, T.; and Barner, H. B. Histochemical and chemical studies of the localization of adrenergic and cholinergic nerves in normal and denervated cat hearts. *Circulation Res.,* **1967,** *20,* 289–298.

Kamijo, K., and Koelle, G. B. The histochemical localization of specific cholinesterase in the conduction system of beef heart. *J. Pharmac. exp. Ther.,* **1955,** *113,* 30.

Kedinger, C.; Gniazdowski, M.; Mandel, J. L., Jr.; Gissinger, F.; and Chambon, P. α-Amanitin: a specific inhibitor of one of two DNA-dependent RNA polymerase activities from calf thymus. *Biochem. biophys. Res. Commun.,* **1970,** *38,* 165–171.

Koppanyi, T. The hemodynamic effect of pilocarpine. *J. Pharmac. exp. Ther.,* **1939,** *66,* 19–20.

Levy, B., and Ahlquist, R. P. A study of sympathetic ganglionic stimulants. *J. Pharmac. exp. Ther.,* **1962,** *137,* 219–228.

Levy, M. N., and Zieske, H. Comparison of the cardiac effects of vagus nerve stimulation and acetylcholine infusions. *Am. J. Physiol.,* **1969,** *216,* 890–897.

Lieberman, T. W., and Leopold, I. H. The use of aceclydine in the treatment of glaucoma. *Am. J. Ophthal.,* **1967,** *64,* 405–415.

Light, R. U.; Bishop, C. C.; and Kendall, L. G. The response of the rabbit to pilocarpine administered into the cerebrospinal fluid. *J. Pharmac. exp. Ther.,* **1933,** *47,* 37–45.

Mashkovsky, M. D., and Zaitseva, C. A. The cholinomimetic activity of 3-acetoxyquinuclidine (aceclidine). *Arzneimittel-Forsch.,* **1968,** *18,* 320–322.

Molitor, H. A comparative study of the effects of five choline compounds used in therapeutics: acetylcholine chloride, acetyl-beta-methylcholine chloride, carbaminoyl choline, ethyl ether beta-methylcholine chloride, carbaminoyl beta-methylcholine chloride. *J. Pharmac. exp. Ther.,* **1936,** *58,* 337–360.

Rinaldi, F., and Himwich, H. E. Alerting responses and actions of atropine and cholinergic drugs. *A.M.A. Archs Neurol. Psychiatry,* **1955a,** *73,* 387–395.

———. Cholinergic mechanism involved in function of mesodiencephalic activating system. *Ibid.,* **1955b,** *73,* 396–402.

Rizzuti, A. B. Acetylcholine in surgery of the lens, iris and cornea. *Am. J. Ophthal.,* **1967,** *63,* 484–487.

Robinson, J. B.; Belleau, B.; and Cox, B. 3-Acetoxyquinuclidine methiodide. Resolution, absolute configuration, and stereospecificity of interaction with the acetylcholine binding sites. *J. mednl Chem.,* **1969,** *12,* 848–854.

Romano, J. H. Double-blind cross-over comparison of aceclidine and pilocarpine in open-angle glaucoma. *Br. J. Ophthal.,* **1970,** *54,* 510–521.

Simonart, A. On the action of certain derivatives of choline. *J. Pharmac. exp. Ther.,* **1932,** *46,* 157–193.

Starr, I., Jr.; Elsom, K. A.; Reisinger, J. A.; and Richards, A. N. Acetyl-β-methylcholin: action on normal persons with note on action of ethyl ether of β-methylcholin. *Am. J. med. Sci.,* **1933,** *186,* 313–323.

Takagi, K.; Takayanagi, I.; and Maezima, Y. An analysis of the sites of action of some partial agonists. *Eur. J. Pharmac.*, **1968**, *3*, 52–57.

Turkanis, S. A., and Esplin, D. W. Evidence for the release and depletion of the postsynaptic inhibitory transmitter by pilocarpine. *Archs int. Pharmacodyn. Thér.*, **1968**, *173*, 195–200.

Zablocka, B., and Esplin, D. W. Central excitatory and neuromuscular paralyzant effects of pilocarpine in cats. *Archs int. Pharmacodyn. Thér.*, **1964**, *147*, 490–496.

Monographs and Reviews

Aviado, D. M. Acetylcholine and other parasympathomimetics. In, *The Lung Circulation*. Vol. 1, *Physiology and Pharmacology*. Pergamon Press, Ltd., Oxford, **1965**, pp. 329–341.

Bebbington, A., and Brimblecombe, R. W. Muscarinic receptors in the peripheral and central nervous systems. *Adv. Drug Res.*, **1965**, *2*, 143–172.

Berne, R. M. Regulation of coronary blood flow. *Physiol. Rev.*, **1964**, *44*, 1–29.

Brücke, F. von. Dicholinesters of α,ω-dicarboxylic acids and related substances. *Pharmac. Rev.*, **1956**, *8*, 265–335. (376 references.)

Curtis, D. R., and Crawford, J. M. Central synaptic transmission—micro-electrophoretic studies. *A. Rev. Pharmac.*, **1969**, *9*, 209–240.

Cushing, H. *Papers Relating to the Pituitary Body, Hypothalamus and Parasympathetic Nervous System.* Charles C Thomas, Pub., Springfield, Ill., **1932**.

Farnsworth, N. R. Hallucinogenic plants. *Science, Wash.*, **1968**, *162*, 1086–1092.

Gerebtzoff, M. A. *Cholinesterases: A Histochemical Contribution to the Solution of Some Functional Problems.* Pergamon Press, Ltd., Oxford, **1959**.

Higgins, C. B.; Vatner, S. F.; and Braunwald, E. Parasympathetic control of the heart. *Pharmac. Rev.*, **1973**, *25*, 119–155.

Kosterlitz, H. W. Effects of choline esters on smooth muscle and secretions. In, *Physiological Pharmacology*. Vol. 3, *The Nervous System—Part C: Autonomic Nervous System Drugs*. (Root, W. S., and Hofmann, F. G., eds.) Academic Press, Inc., New York, **1967**, pp. 97–161.

Krnjević, K. Chemical nature of synaptic transmission in vertebrates. *Physiol. Rev.*, **1974**, *54*, 418–540.

Lloyd, D. P. C. Cholinergy and adrenergy in the neural control of sweat glands. In, *Studies in Physiology*. (Curtis, D. R., and McIntyre, A. K., eds.) Springer-Verlag, New York, **1965**, pp. 169–178.

Miller, J. W., and Lewis, J. E. Drugs affecting smooth muscle. *A. Rev. Pharmac.*, **1969**, *9*, 147–172.

Rand, M. J., and Stafford, A. Cardiovascular effects of choline esters. In, *Physiological Pharmacology*. Vol. 3, *The Nervous System—Part C: Autonomic Nervous System Drugs*. (Root, W. S., and Hofmann, F. G., eds.) Academic Press, Inc., New York, **1967**, pp. 1–95.

Schmiedeberg, O., and Koppe, R. *Das Muscarin, das giftige Alkaloid des Fliegenpilzes.* F. C. W. Vogel, Leipzig, **1869**.

Votava, Z. Pharmacology of the central cholinergic synapses. *A. Rev. Pharmac.*, **1967**, *7*, 223–240.

Waser, P. G. Chemistry and pharmacology of muscarine, muscarone, and some related compounds. *Pharmac. Rev.*, **1961**, *13*, 465–515. (104 references.)

Wieland, T. Poisonous principles of mushrooms of the genus Amanita. *Science, Wash.*, **1968**, *159*, 946–952.

24 NOREPINEPHRINE, EPINEPHRINE, AND THE SYMPATHOMIMETIC AMINES

Ian R. Innes and Mark Nickerson

The sympathomimetic drugs make up one of the most extensively studied groups of pharmacological agents and, consequently, many are known and widely used. In general, their effects resemble the responses to stimulation of adrenergic nerves, but there are often differences in the details and the intensity of action of the drugs. Several have additional properties, such as profound effects on the central nervous system (CNS), that are of value in specific clinical conditions. Sympathomimetic agents are used for a variety of purposes in therapeutics, and the physician must therefore understand the general pharmacology of the group and the differences between the effects of individual members.

Most of the actions of sympathomimetic agents can be classified into five broad types: (1) a *peripheral excitatory action* on certain types of smooth muscle, such as those in blood vessels supplying skin and mucous membranes, and also on salivary and certain sweat glands; (2) a *peripheral inhibitory action* on certain other types of smooth muscle, such as those in the wall of the gut, in the bronchial tree, and in blood vessels supplying skeletal muscle; (3) a *cardiac excitatory action,* responsible for an increase in heart rate and force of contraction; (4) *metabolic actions,* such as an increase in rate of glycogenolysis in liver and muscle, and liberation of free fatty acids from adipose tissue; and (5) *CNS excitatory actions,* such as respiratory stimulation and, with some of the drugs, an increase in wakefulness and a reduction in appetite. All sympathomimetic drugs do not show each of the above types of action to the same degree. Thus, doses of epinephrine and norepinephrine that cause an equal rise in arterial blood pressure have quite different effects on bronchial musculature, heart rate, and glycogen stores. However, many differences in the effects of the

sympathomimetic amines are only quantitative, and a description of the effects of each individual compound would be unnecessarily repetitive. Therefore, the pharmacological properties of these drugs as a class are described in detail for the prototype agent, *epinephrine.* Indeed, most of the fundamental studies on the many properties of this class of drugs have been made with epinephrine as the model agent. Differences in the effects of the various congeners are particularly pronounced in the cardiovascular responses they evoke. These variations are largely due to differences in the intensity and the duration of their effects at the many possible sites where their sympathomimetic actions can occur, and also to differences in the reflex responses of homeostatic mechanisms. Such factors are discussed below.

History. The pressor effect of suprarenal extracts was first shown by Oliver and Schäfer in 1895. The active principle was named epinephrine by Abel in 1899 and synthesized independently by Stolz and Dakin. The history of its isolation and identification has been reviewed by Hartung (1931). The development of our knowledge of epinephrine and norepinephrine as neurohumoral transmitters is outlined in Chapter 21. Barger and Dale (1910) studied the pharmacological activity of a large series of synthetic amines related to epinephrine and termed their action *sympathomimetic.* This important study determined the basic structural requirements for activity and indicated that the sympathomimetic amines had qualitatively similar effects but that there were considerable quantitative differences. When it was found that cocaine or chronic denervation of effector organs reduced their responses to ephedrine and tyramine but enhanced the effects of epinephrine (Tainter and Chang, 1927; Burn and Tainter, 1931), it became clear that the differences between sympathomimetic amines were not simply quantitative. It was then suggested that epinephrine acted directly on the effector cell while ephedrine and tyramine had an indirect effect by acting on the nerve endings. The discovery that reserpine depletes tissues of norepinephrine, first made by Bertler and coworkers (1956), was followed by evidence that tyramine does not act on reserpinized tissues

(Carlsson *et al.*, 1957). Burn and Rand (1958), confirming these observations, concluded that some sympathomimetic amines act by releasing endogenous norepinephrine. Many subsequent investigations have been directed toward clarifying this mechanism.

Sites and Mechanism of Action. α *and* β *Receptors or Adrenoceptors.* One of the more important factors in determining the effects of a sympathomimetic drug is that there are two major types of receptors with which it can react to elicit a response in sympathetic effector cells. Ahlquist (1948) classified these receptor sites as α and β, on the basis of their responses to a series of sympathomimetic amines. The concept of α- and β-receptor sites simplifies the classification of both sympathomimetic drugs and adrenergic blocking agents. The adrenergic blocking action of many compounds, such as imidazolines and haloalkylamines, is selective for α receptors, whereas others, such as propranolol, block only β receptors (*see* Chapter 26).

In general, the effect on α receptors in smooth muscle is excitatory and that on β receptors at such sites is inhibitory, although this is not an absolute rule and no such scheme is applicable elsewhere (*see* Table 21-1, page 408). Thus, activation of β-adrenergic receptors results in stimulation of various secretions (*e.g.*, that of insulin). Furthermore, the stimulatory effects of catecholamines on the heart are mediated by β receptors. While both α- and β-receptor activation results in inhibition of intestinal smooth muscle, the effect of α receptors may be largely indirect, through inhibition of excitatory parasympathetic ganglion cells of Auerbach's plexus; nevertheless, the presence of both an α- and a β-blocking agent is required to prevent completely the inhibitory effect of epinephrine on the intestine (Ahlquist and Levy, 1959).

Sympathetic effector cells may have α or β receptors or both. For example, the smooth muscle of blood vessels supplying skeletal muscles has both β receptors, the activation of which by low concentrations of epinephrine causes vasodilatation, and α receptors that allow epinephrine to constrict these vessels. Thus, it appears that in this tissue the threshold concentration of epinephrine for activation of β receptors is lower, but when both types of receptor are activated the re-

sponse to α receptors predominates. The predominant type of adrenergic receptor in tissues where it has been determined is given in Table 21-1 (page 408). In some cases, the receptors have as yet been studied only in animal tissues; however, where the receptors have been classified in man, no striking species differences have appeared.

The responses to sympathomimetic drugs can often be clearly predicted on the basis of a knowledge of their selectivity in reacting with α or β receptors. Thus, isoproterenol, which acts on β receptors and has little or no action on α receptors, increases the heart rate and force of contraction, dilates skeletal muscle vascular beds to lower mean blood pressure, and relaxes bronchial muscle. On the other hand, phenylephrine, which acts on α receptors but has little action on β receptors, has little direct cardiac effect and does not relax bronchial muscle, but it raises the blood pressure by contracting peripheral vascular beds.

Differences in the sensitivity of β receptors of different organs to β-receptor stimulants and β-blocking agents of varied chemical structure are sufficient to differentiate two distinct types: β_1 in heart and small intestine, and β_2 in bronchi, vascular beds, and uterus (Lands *et al.*, 1967). Thus, there are β-blocking agents that are sufficiently selective to block either β_1 or β_2 receptors without affecting markedly the other type (Levy and Wilkenfeld, 1969). Similarly, salbutamol (albuterol), which is used to treat bronchial asthma, selectively activates β_2 receptors and thereby relaxes bronchial smooth muscle with little accompanying undesirable cardiac stimulation (Choo-Kang *et al.*, 1970).

The above-described classification of adrenergic receptors is most applicable to relatively simple actions of catecholamines that have been studied in isolation. Receptors for their metabolic and CNS actions are sometimes not so readily classified into α and β types. For example, the relative potencies of norepinephrine, epinephrine, and isoproterenol in causing hyperglycemia in man follow the α-receptor pattern, and the effects of α- and β-adrenergic antagonists are complex (*see* Chapter 26). Since the concentration of plasma glucose is the *composite* of multiple factors, many of which are influenced by catecholamines, this is not surprising. When examined in isolation, many of the metabolic effects of catecholamines appear to be mediated by β receptors; there are, however, anomalies and confusing variation from species to species and from tissue to tissue.

Release of Stored Norepinephrine. Many sympathomimetic drugs, such as *amphetamine* and *ephedrine,* act indirectly by releasing norepinephrine from storage sites in the sympathetic nerves to the effector organ. The responses they elicit are therefore similar to those of norepinephrine but are slower in onset and generally longer lasting than those of a single equipressor dose of norepinephrine. They also exhibit tachyphylaxis; that is, repeated injections or continuous infusions of these indirectly acting drugs become less effective as the norepinephrine stores are diminished by continued release. Many sympathomimetic drugs owe only part of their effect to norepinephrine release and also act directly on adrenergic receptors.

Much of the present knowledge of norepinephrine-releasing sympathomimetic amines is based on experimental work with *tyramine.* Intravenous injection of tyramine increases the amount of norepinephrine in the venous outflow of several organs *in vivo* and in the effluent of isolated perfused organs, and infusion of large amounts of tyramine reduces the organ content of norepinephrine. The effects of tyramine, ephedrine, and many other noncatecholamines are strikingly reduced in organs where norepinephrine stores have been depleted either by removal of the adrenergic nerve supply or by treatment of the animal with reserpine. Release of catecholamine from the adrenal medulla plays little part in the action of tyramine. In animals depleted of norepinephrine by reserpine, an intravenous infusion of norepinephrine briefly restores responses to tyramine. The indirect action of tyramine involves only a small part of the norepinephrine store, since replacement of as little as 1% restores much of the response to tyramine. On the basis of this and other evidence, it is likely that tyramine displaces norepinephrine from a relatively small mobile pool that is bound loosely to some unidentified component of the nerve cytoplasm or storage granules. (*See* Trendelenburg, 1972; Smith, 1973; Chapters 21 and 26.)

Such indirectly acting sympathomimetic amines must be transported into the adrenergic nerve terminals before they are able to displace norepinephrine. Various drugs, such as *imipramine* and *cocaine,* can interfere with the uptake process, and these agents will thus antagonize the actions of indirectly acting sympathomimetic amines. Inhibition of the same transport mechanism by these drugs potentiates the effects of norepinephrine, since this blocks an important means of removal of catecholamines from the area of the receptors.

Reflex Effects. Compensatory reflexes play a large part in determining cardiovascular responses to sympathomimetic drugs. One of the most striking effects of many sympathomimetic amines is a rise in arterial blood pressure due to stimulation of α receptors in vascular beds. This elicits compensatory reflexes through the caroticoaortic baroreceptor system, resulting in a diminution of overall sympathetic tone that tends to lessen the effect of the sympathomimetic drugs and is accompanied by an increase in vagal tone that slows the heart. This compensatory mechanism is of special importance for drugs having little β-receptor activity and, therefore, little direct cardioaccelerator action. To cite a clinical application, methoxamine, a drug with negligible β-receptor activity, is used to treat paroxysmal atrial or nodal tachycardia because it raises blood pressure and thereby reflexly lessens sympathetic cardioaccelerator tone and increases parasympathetic cardiodecelerator tone, the combined effects of which may be enough to end the episode of tachycardia.

Reflex effects also enter into the cardiac responses to norepinephrine. Epinephrine and norepinephrine have different effects on the heart rate. Both increase reflex vagal tone by raising the blood pressure, but the vagal activity after epinephrine is less than that after norepinephrine, since the β-receptor vasodilator activity of epinephrine on blood vessels of skeletal muscle keeps the diastolic pressure comparatively low (*see* Figure 24-1, page 484). Thus, epinephrine is opposed by less vagal tone, so that its usual overall effect on the heart rate is tachycardia; after norepinephrine, the predominant effect is bradycardia.

Reflex inhibition of sympathetic tone is of value during spinal anesthesia. Beside blocking the sensory and motor nerve supply to the lower part of the body, spinal anesthesia may block the sympathetic nerve supply to the vasculature of the lower extremities and the abdomen, and thus cause vasodilatation and a consequent fall in blood pressure. The homeostatic mechanisms respond to produce intense vasoconstriction in the upper part of the body. This may be relieved by the injection of an α-receptor stimulant that constricts vessels throughout the body. The resulting vasoconstriction in the lower part of the body raises the blood pressure and permits relaxation of the compensatory sympathetic tone in the upper part. Vasoconstriction is thus redistributed more equitably in the various vascular beds.

Reflex effects also modify responses to drugs acting on β receptors. Such drugs dilate blood vessels supplying skeletal muscle, thus lowering mean arterial blood pressure; the compensatory reflex increase in sympathetic tone constricts other vascular beds and, along with reduced vagal tone, augments the rate and force of cardiac contraction. These effects, in turn, tend to return the blood pressure toward its original level. The cardiac response to these drugs is especially pronounced since the reflex effects and the direct β-receptor cardiac stimulant action are in the same direction.

Mechanism of Direct Action on Sympathetic Effectors. Catecholamines act directly on sympathetic effector cells following interaction with receptors located particularly in cellular plasma membranes. Sympathomimetic drugs influence biochemical reactions as well as functional responses in virtually all tissues they affect, and the relation between these effects has been extensively studied. Production of cyclic adenosine 3',5'-monophosphate (cyclic AMP) by stimulation of adenylate cyclase has had particular attention as a possible step linking β-receptor activation to both functional and metabolic changes. This subject is discussed in Chapter 21.

The relationship of electrical phenomena, ion fluxes, and changes of tension in smooth muscle has been extensively studied without the establishment of a general pattern. The ionic movements differ between α- and β-receptor activation, and probably between smooth muscles. Visceral smooth muscle contractions are generally associated with slow waves of partial depolarization, in some muscles with superimposed action potentials that travel for some distance along adjacent cells. Contractions due to α-receptor stimulation are accompanied in some muscles by graded depolarization only; in others, there is a concomitant appearance or increased frequency of superimposed action potentials. The ionic mechanisms associated with these changes are also discussed in Chapter 21. In muscles inhibited by β-receptor stimulation the membrane becomes hyperpolarized and action potentials disappear or are less frequent. These changes are not consistently accompanied by potassium movement. The relationship of hyperpolarization to sodium movement is in dispute, and entry of calcium has been proposed

as a component of the complex ionic mechanism. (*See* Somlyo and Somlyo, 1968; Daniel *et al.,* 1970; Marshall, 1973.) Although the effects of epinephrine appear to be related to changes in *transmembrane potentials,* neither its excitatory nor inhibitory actions can depend entirely on the electrical changes. Isolated smooth muscle preparations, depolarized by being bathed in a solution with a high potassium content, can still be stimulated or inhibited by epinephrine; the muscle contraction due to epinephrine is reduced to about half by such depolarization. Both α- and β-adrenergic blocking agents have their usual effects on epinephrine-induced actions on depolarized muscles. These observations do not necessarily exclude a mechanism of action involving ionic movements; in depolarized preparations epinephrine increases the permeability of the cell membrane to ions, and does not cause contraction in the absence of calcium. Observations on the rabbit stomach, where hyperpolarization instead of depolarization accompanies contraction due to epinephrine, also indicate that broad generalizations should not be made about the nature and importance of electrical changes (*see* Furchgott, 1960; Schild, 1960).

Chemistry and Structure-Activity Relationship of Sympathomimetic Amines. β-Phenylethylamine (Table 24–1) can be viewed as the parent compound of the sympathomimetic amines, consisting of an aromatic nucleus (a benzene ring) and an aliphatic portion, ethylamine. The structure permits substitutions to be made on the aromatic ring, the α- and β-carbon atoms, and the terminal amino group, to yield a great variety of compounds with sympathomimetic activity. Norepinephrine, epinephrine, and isoproterenol have OH groups substituted in the 3 and 4 positions of the benzene ring. Since *o*-dihydroxybenzene is also known as *catechol,* sympathomimetic amines with these OH substitutions in the aromatic ring are termed *catecholamines.*

The structure-activity relationship (SAR) of sympathomimetic drugs has been studied extensively since the classical investigations of Barger and Dale (1910). The pressor effects have been investigated more than other properties of the drugs. However, the pressor responses are the resultant of many effects on a complex system and involve many interacting factors that preclude their exact interpretation. The current classification of the actions of sympathomimetic drugs into those on α and β receptors, norepinephrine stores, and nonadrenergic receptors, along with the complication of diverse reflex effects, makes many of the early investigations meaningless. This is obvious when it is appreciated that most sympathomimetic drugs influence both α and β receptors, but that the ratio of the α and β activity varies tremendously between drugs, in a continuous spectrum from an almost pure α activity (phenylephrine) to an almost pure β activity (isoproterenol). Since α activity on vascular beds raises the blood pressure and β activity on vascular beds lowers the blood pressure, it is virtually impossible to determine SAR from measurements of blood pressure alone unless one class of receptors has been blocked by a selective adrenergic blocking agent.

Table 24-1. CHEMICAL STRUCTURES AND MAIN CLINICAL USES OF IMPORTANT SYMPATHOMIMETIC DRUGS †

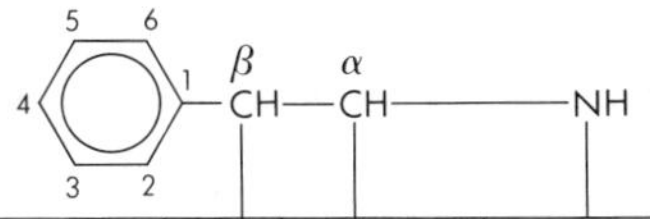

Prototype formula (ring positions 5, 6 top; 4, 3, 2 around ring; position 1 attachment):

$$4\text{-}[ring]\text{-}1\text{—}\overset{\beta}{C}H\text{—}\overset{\alpha}{C}H\text{—NH}$$

Drug	Ring substituents	β	α	N	α Receptor A N P V	β Receptor B C M	CNS,0
Phenylethylamine		H	H	H			
Epinephrine	3-OH,4-OH	OH	H	CH$_3$	A, P,V	B,C	
Norepinephrine	3-OH,4-OH	OH	H	H	P		
Dopamine	3-OH,4-OH	H	H	H	P		
Nordefrin	3-OH,4-OH	OH	CH$_3$	H	V		
Isoproterenol	3-OH,4-OH	OH	H	CH(CH$_3$)$_2$		B,C	
Isoetharine	3-OH,4-OH	OH	CH$_2$CH$_3$	CH(CH$_3$)$_2$		B	
Metaproterenol	3-OH,5-OH	OH	H	CH(CH$_3$)$_2$		B	
Terbutaline	3-OH,5-OH	OH	H	C(CH$_3$)$_3$		B	
Fenoterol	3-OH,5-OH	OH	H	1 *		B	
Metaraminol	3-OH	OH	CH$_3$	H	P		
Phenylephrine	3-OH	OH	H	CH$_3$	N,P		
Tyramine	4-OH	H	H	H			
Hydroxyamphetamine	4-OH	H	CH$_3$	H	N,P	C	
Nylidrin	4-OH	OH	CH$_3$	2 *		M	
Isoxsuprine	4 OH	OH	CH$_3$	3 *		M	
Ritodrine	4-OH	OH	CH$_3$	4 *		B	
Methoxyphenamine	2-OCH$_3$	H	CH$_3$	CH$_3$		B	
Methoxamine	2-OCH$_3$,5-OCH$_3$	OH	CH$_3$	H	P		
Salbutamol	3-CH$_2$OH,4-OH	OH	H	C(CH$_3$)$_3$		B	
Soterenol	3-NHSO$_2$CH$_3$,4-OH	OH	H	CH(CH$_3$)$_2$		B	
Amphetamine		H	CH$_3$	H			CNS,0
Methamphetamine		H	CH$_3$	CH$_3$	P		CNS,0
Benzphetamine		H	CH$_3$	5 *			0
Ephedrine		OH	CH$_3$	CH$_3$	N,P	B,C	
Phenylpropanolamine		OH	CH$_3$	H	N		
Mephentermine		H	6 *	CH$_3$	N,P		
Phentermine		H	6 *	H			0
Chlorphentermine	4-Cl	H	6 *	H			0
Fenfluramine	3-CF$_3$	H	CH$_3$	C$_2$H$_5$			0
Quinterenol	7 *	OH	H	CH(CH$_3$)$_2$		B	
Tuaminoheptane	CH$_3$(CH$_2$)$_3$	H	CH$_3$	H	N		
Cyclopentamine	8 *	H	CH$_3$	CH$_3$	N		
Propylhexedrine	9 *	H	CH$_3$	CH$_3$	N		
Diethylpropion	10 *						0
Phenmetrazine	11 *						0
Phendimetrazine	12 *						0

Substituent/replacement structures (numbered):

1. —CH—CH$_3$; CH$_2$—[ring]—OH
2. —CH—CH$_3$; CH$_2$—CH$_2$—[ring]
3. CH$_3$; —CH—CH$_2$—O—[ring]
4. —CH$_2$; CH$_2$—[ring]—OH
5. CH$_3$; —N ; CH$_2$—[ring]
6. CH$_3$; —C— ; CH$_3$
7. [8-hydroxyquinoline ring]
8. [cyclopentane ring]
9. [cyclohexane ring]
10. —C—CH—N—C$_2$H$_5$; O CH$_3$ C$_2$H$_5$
11. O—CH$_2$; —CH   CH$_2$; CH—NH ; CH$_3$
12. O—CH$_2$; —CH   CH$_2$; CH—N ; CH$_3$ CH$_3$

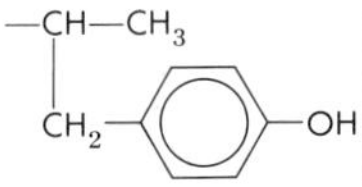

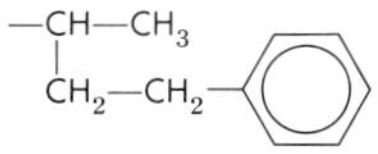

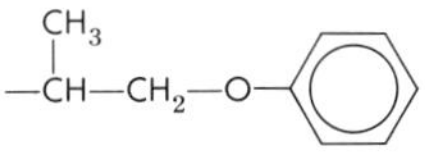

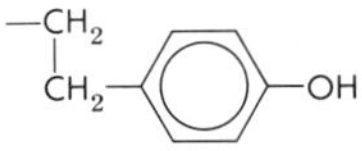

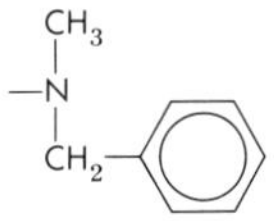

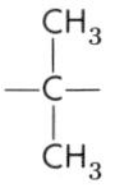

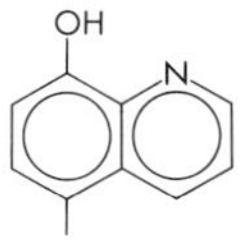

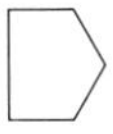

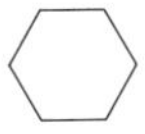

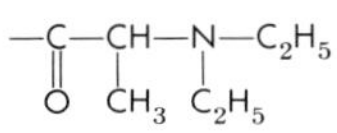

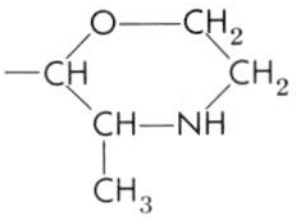

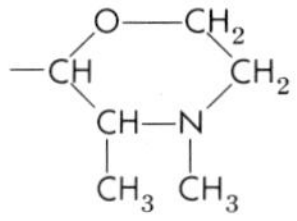

α Activity
A = Allergic reactions
N = Nasal decongestion
P = Pressor (may include β action)
V = Other local vasoconstriction (*e.g.*, in local anesthesia)

β Activity
B = Bronchodilator
C = Cardiac
M = Muscle vessel dilatation

CNS = Central nervous system
0 = Anorectic

* Numbers bearing an asterisk refer to the substituents numbered in the bottom rows of the table; substituents 7, 8, and 9 replace the phenyl ring, and 10, 11, and 12 are attached directly to the phenyl ring, replacing the ethylamine side chain.
† The α and β in the prototype formula refer to positions of the C atoms in the ethylamine side chain.

There is a similarly wide spectrum in the ratio between direct action on adrenergic receptors and indirect effects through the release of norepinephrine. SAR has been studied in simplified systems where norepinephrine stores have been depleted by denervation or by drugs such as reserpine, or where release of stored norepinephrine is inhibited by drugs. However, each of these procedures presents additional complications, the main problem being the fact that one cannot assume that the drugs used to simplify the preparations have no effects other than depletion or inhibition of release of norepinephrine stores; for example, they often cause an unequal augmentation of the effects of the various directly acting agents. Among the sympathomimetic amines, only the catecholamines do not release norepinephrine stores to any significant degree. Despite the multiplicity of the sites of action of sympathomimetic amines, several generalizations can be made, as presented below.

Separation of Aromatic Ring and Amino Group. By far the greatest sympathomimetic activity occurs when two carbon atoms separate the ring from the amino group. This rule applies with few exceptions to all types of action.

Substitution on the Amino Group. The effects of amino substitution are most readily seen in the actions of catecholamines on α and β receptors. Increase in the size of the alkyl substituent increases β-receptor activity. Norepinephrine has, in general, rather feeble β_2 activity; this is greatly increased in epinephrine with the addition of a methyl group, and both β_1 and β_2 activity are maximal in isoproterenol with an isopropyl substituent. Selective β_2-receptor stimulants require a large amino substituent, but depend on other substitutions for their selectivity for β_2 rather than for β_1 receptors. α-Receptor activity is also modified by alkyl substitution on the amino group. In general, the less the substitution on the amino group the greater is the selectivity for α activity, although N-methylation increases the potency of primary amines. Thus, α activity is maximal in epinephrine, less in norepinephrine, and almost absent in isoproterenol. Norepinephrine activity, however, is predominantly on α receptors.

Substitution on the Aromatic Nucleus. Maximal α and β activity depends on the presence of OH groups in the 3 and 4 positions. When one or both of these groups are absent, without other aromatic substitution, the overall potency is reduced and there is especially a reduction in β activity. Phenylphrine is therefore less potent than epinephrine on both α and β receptors, with β activity almost completely lacking; phenylephrine raises blood pressure without appreciably stimulating the heart. Hydroxy groups in the 3 and 5 positions confer β_2-receptor selectivity on compounds with large amino substituents. Thus, metaproterenol, terbutaline, and fenoterol relax the bronchial musculature in asthma without causing significant tachycardia. The ratio of α and β activity varies among noncatecholamines, which owe part of their action to released norepinephrine. The low β_2 activity of norepinephrine probably partly accounts for the relatively low potency of many noncatecholamines on β_2 receptors.

Noncatecholamines that lack both OH groups on the ring can produce greater CNS stimulation than epinephrine in doses that can be safely given. Thus, ephedrine, amphetamine, and methamphetamine are powerful central stimulants. However, this difference may be regarded primarily as a relatively greater loss of peripheral α and β activity rather than as an increase in central stimulation, although qualitatively different central effects also occur. A dose of 50 mg of ephedrine elicits central effects without inordinate cardiovascular effects; effects on the respiratory center can be seen with epinephrine in doses of 20 μg or less. An amount of epinephrine large enough to produce central effects comparable to those of ephedrine cannot safely be given because of intense peripheral α and β actions.

Catecholamines have only a brief duration of action and are ineffective after oral administration because they are rapidly inactivated in the gut wall and in the liver before reaching the systemic circulation (*see* Chapter 21). Absence of one or both OH substituents, particularly the 3-OH group, increases the oral effectiveness and the duration of action.

Groups other than OH have been substituted on the aromatic ring. In general, potency on α receptors is reduced and β-receptor activity is minimal; the compounds may even block β receptors. For example, methoxamine, with methoxy substituents on positions 2 and 5, has highly selective α-stimulating activity and in large doses blocks β receptors. Salbutamol (albuterol), a selective β_2-receptor stimulant useful in the treatment of asthmatic attacks, has a CH_2OH substituent on position 3 and is an important exception to the general rule of low β activity.

Substitution on the α-Carbon Atom. This substitution blocks oxidation by monoamine oxidase (MAO), thus greatly prolonging the duration of action of noncatecholamines, the detoxication of which depends largely on breakdown by MAO since they are unaffected by catechol-O-methyltransferase (COMT). The duration of action of nordefrine (α-methylnorepinephrine) is not prolonged, whereas the duration of action of noncatecholamines with an α-methyl group, such as ephedrine or amphetamine, is measured in hours rather than in minutes.

Substitution on the β-Carbon Atom. Substitution of an OH group on the β carbon generally decreases central stimulant action and increases both α and β activity. Thus, ephedrine is less potent than methamphetamine as a central stimulant, but it is more powerful in dilating bronchioles and increasing blood pressure and heart rate. Similarly epinine is less potent than epinephrine on both α and β receptors.

Absence of the Benzene Ring. CNS stimulant activity is reduced without a corresponding decrease in α and β activity when the benzene ring is replaced by an appropriate aliphatic chain (*e.g.,* tuaminoheptane, methylhexaneamine), by a saturated ring (*e.g.,* cyclopentamine, propylhexedrine), or by a different unsaturated ring (*e.g.,* naphazoline; Table 24–2). Naphazoline, in fact, is a powerful α-receptor stimulant, but it differs from other sympathomimetic amines in that it depresses instead of stimulates the CNS. The proportion of α to β activity varies with the compound; however, in general these amines

Table 24-2. CHEMICAL STRUCTURES OF IMIDAZOLINE DERIVATIVES

| Naphazoline | Tetrahydrozoline | Oxymetazoline | Xylometazoline |

have rather more marked α than β activity, fitting them for use as nasal decongestants by virtue of their vasoconstrictor properties.

Optical Isomerism. Substitution on either α or β carbon yields optical isomers. Levorotatory substitution on the β carbon confers the greater peripheral activity, so that the naturally occurring *l*-epinephrine and *l*-norepinephrine are ten or more times as potent as their unnatural *d* isomers. Dextrorotatory substitution on the α carbon generally provides a more potent compound than the *l* isomer in peripheral and central stimulant activity. *d*-Amphetamine is more potent than *l*-amphetamine in central but not peripheral activity.

I. Catecholamines

EPINEPHRINE

PHARMACOLOGICAL PROPERTIES

In general, the responses to epinephrine resemble the effects of stimulation of adrenergic nerves. However, they are not identical due to differences between epinephrine and the adrenergic mediator, norepinephrine, in the proportion of their α- to β-receptor activity. Most of the responses listed in Table 21–1 (page 408) are seen after injection of epinephrine in man, but sweating, piloerection, and mydriasis occur only under special circumstances. Particularly prominent are the actions on the heart and the vascular and other smooth muscle. So enormous is the literature on almost every aspect of the many changes in bodily function caused by epinephrine that this discussion is limited largely to the actions of the drug in man and refers to the more abundant results in animals when studies in man are limited.

Blood Pressure. Epinephrine is one of the most potent vasopressor drugs known. Given rapidly *intravenously* it evokes a characteristic effect on blood pressure, which rises rapidly to a peak that is proportional to the dose. The increase in systolic pressure is greater than in diastolic pressure, so that the pulse pressure increases. The pressure then falls below normal before returning to the control level. Repeated doses of epinephrine continue to have the same pressor effect, in sharp contrast to amines that owe a major part of their effect to release of norepinephrine.

The mechanism of the rise in blood pressure due to epinephrine is threefold: a direct myocardial stimulation that increases the strength of ventricular contraction, an increased heart rate, and, most important, vasoconstriction in many vascular beds, especially in the precapillary resistance vessels of skin, mucosa, and kidney, along with marked constriction of the veins. The pulse rate, at first accelerated, may be slowed markedly at the height of the rise by compensatory vagal discharge. This bradycardia is absent if the effects of vagal discharge are blocked by atropine. Minute doses of epinephrine (0.1 μg/kg) may cause the blood pressure to fall. The depressor effect of small doses and the diphasic response to larger doses are due to greater sensitivity to epinephrine of vasodilator β_2 receptors than of constrictor α receptors.

The effects are somewhat different when the drug is given by slow *intravenous infusion* or by *subcutaneous injection*. Absorption of epinephrine after subcutaneous injection is slow due to the drug's local vasoconstrictor action; the effects of doses as large as 0.5 to 1.5 mg can be duplicated by intravenous infusion at a rate of 10 to 30 μg per minute. There is a moderate increase in systolic pressure, but the *diastolic pressure* usually *falls* (Figure 24–1). Pulse pressure is increased, but the mean blood pressure is seldom greatly elevated. Peripheral resistance decreases, due to action on β_2 receptors of vessels in skeletal muscle, where blood flow is

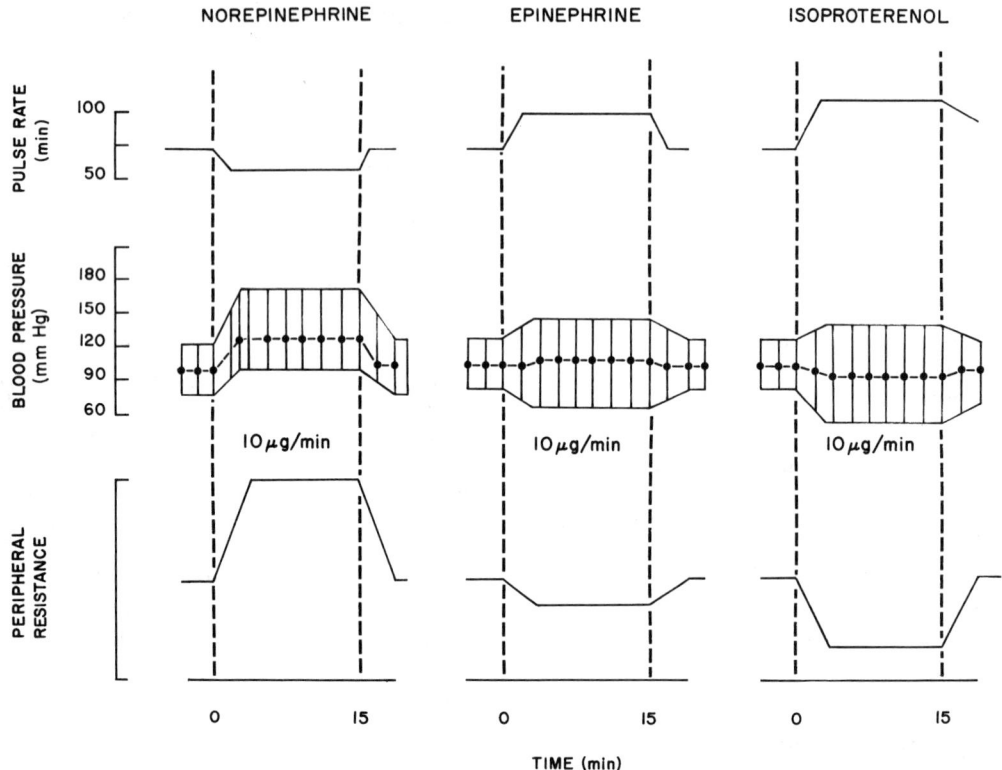

Figure 24-1. *The effects of intravenous infusion of norepinephrine, epinephrine, and isoproterenol in man.* (After Allwood, Cobbold, and Ginsburg, 1963. Courtesy of the *British Medical Bulletin.*)

enhanced, often doubled after a subcutaneous dose of 0.5 to 1.0 mg. Since the blood pressure is not, as a rule, greatly elevated, compensatory reflexes do not antagonize appreciably the direct cardiac actions. Heart rate, cardiac output, stroke volume, and left ventricular work per beat are increased due to direct cardiac stimulation and to increased venous return to the heart, which is reflected by an increase in right atrial pressure. The details of the effects of intravenous infusion of epinephrine, norepinephrine, and isoproterenol in man are compared in Table 24–3 and Figure 24–1. Ordinarily the vasodilator effect of epinephrine dominates the circulatory pattern, and the rise in systolic pressure is largely due to an increase in cardiac output. Occasionally there is no change or even a slight rise in peripheral resistance and diastolic pressure, clearly dependent upon the ratio of α to β response in the various vascular beds.

Vascular Effects. The chief vascular action of epinephrine is exerted on the smaller arterioles and precapillary sphincters, although veins and large arteries also respond to the drug. Various vascular beds react differently (*see* Table 21–1, page 408). The blood vessels to *skin, mucosa,* and *kidney* are constricted by the action on their α receptors. The vessels to *skeletal muscles* are dilated after low doses by the action on their β_2 receptors, which are sensitive to much lower concentrations of epinephrine than are the α receptors; larger doses activate α receptors in addition, and the overall effect of full activation of both α and β receptors is an increase in peripheral resistance and, consequently, a rise in blood pressure. When enough epinephrine has been eliminated to end its effect on the less sensitive but predominant α receptors, the effect on β receptors persists for a time, thus accounting for the secondary hypotension of the diphasic response. The α and β components of the vascular action of epinephrine can be separated by selective α- and β-blocking agents.

Injected epinephrine markedly reduces *cutaneous blood flow,* constricting precapillary vessels and subpapillary venules. However, skin pallor due to cutaneous vasoconstriction during "flight-or-fight" reactions is mainly due to increased sympathetic discharge rather than to released epinephrine. Release of endogenous epinephrine from the adrenal glands plays little part in cardiovascular reactions except in extremely stressful circumstances such as asphyxia. Cutaneous vasoconstriction accounts for a marked decrease in blood flow in the hands and feet. The "aftercongestion" of mucosae following the vasoconstriction from locally applied epinephrine is probably due to changes in vascular reactivity as a result of tissue hypoxia rather than to β-receptor activity of the drug on mucosal vessels.

Blood flow to *skeletal muscles* is increased by therapeutic doses in man. Epinephrine infused intravenously in man at the rate of 30 μg per minute causes a very large but transient increase in blood flow, followed by a fall to about double the resting flow. This is due to a powerful β_2-receptor vasodilator action followed by a partially counterbalancing vasoconstrictor action on the α receptors that are also present in this vascular bed. After α-blocking agents, the pronounced vasodilatation in muscle due to epinephrine is sustained; after β-blocking agents, only vasoconstriction occurs. These vascular effects are independent of cardiac or central reflex effects and occur also in sympathectomized limbs.

The effect of epinephrine on *cerebral circulation* is related to systemic blood pressure. The drug has no significant constrictor action on cerebral arterioles; moreover, autoregulatory mechanisms tend to limit the increase in cerebral blood flow due to increased blood pressure. In man, intravenous infusion of pressor doses (20 to 70 μg per minute) increases both cerebral blood flow and oxygen uptake without altering cerebrovascular resistance (King *et al.*, 1952). Intravenous infusion of 0.1 μg/kg per minute in man markedly increases *hepatic blood flow* and decreases *splanchnic vascular resistance,* concomitantly with a large increase in hepatic glucose output and in the consumption of oxygen as measured in the splanchnic vascular bed (*see* Bearn *et al.*, 1951; Greenway and Stark, 1971).

The effects of epinephrine on *renal function* are variable, but the *renal vascular*

changes in man are clear (Smythe *et al.*, 1952; Gombos *et al.*, 1962). Doses of epinephrine (3 to 23 μg per minute, intravenously) that have little effect on mean arterial pressure consistently increase renal vascular resistance and reduce renal blood flow by as much as 40%. All segments of the renal vascular bed contribute to the increased resistance. Renin secretion is increased. Since the glomerular filtration rate is only slightly and variably altered, the filtration fraction is consistently increased. Excretion of sodium, potassium, and chloride is decreased; urine volume may be increased, decreased, or unchanged. Maximal tubular reabsorptive (glucose Tm) and excretory (iodopyracet Tm) capacities are unchanged.

Arterial and venous *pulmonary pressures* are raised. Although direct pulmonary vasoconstriction can be shown under suitable conditions, the increase in pulmonary pressure in man is predominantly, if not entirely,

Table 24–3. COMPARISON OF THE EFFECTS OF INTRAVENOUS INFUSION OF EPINEPHRINE AND LEVARTERENOL IN MAN *

	EPINEPH-RINE	LEVARTER-ENOL
Cardiac		
Heart rate	+	− †
Stroke volume	+ +	+ +
Cardiac output	+ + +	0, −
Arrhythmias	+ + + +	+ + + +
Coronary blood flow	+ +	+ +
Blood Pressure		
Systolic arterial	+ + +	+ + +
Mean arterial	+	+ +
Diastolic arterial	+,0,−	+ +
Mean pulmonary	+ +	+ +
Peripheral Circulation		
Total peripheral resistance	−	+ +
Cerebral blood flow	+	0, −
Muscle blood flow	+ + +	0, −
Cutaneous blood flow	− −	− −
Renal blood flow	−	−
Splanchnic blood flow	+ + +	0, +
Metabolic Effects		
Oxygen consumption	+ +	0, +
Blood sugar	+ + +	0, +
Blood lactic acid	+ + +	0, +
Eosinopenic response	+	0
Central Nervous System		
Respiration	+	+
Subjective sensations	+	+

* 0.1 to 0.4 μg/kg/min
+ = increase; 0 = no change; − = decrease; † = after atropine, +
(After Goldenberg, Aranow, Smith, and Faber, 1950. Courtesy of *Archives of Internal Medicine.*)

secondary to an increase in left atrial pressure. Redistribution of blood from the systemic to the pulmonary circulation, due to constriction of the more powerful musculature in the systemic great veins, doubtless plays an important part in the increase in pulmonary pressure. Overdosage of epinephrine may cause death by pulmonary edema precipitated by elevated pulmonary capillary filtration pressure.

Coronary blood flow is enhanced by epinephrine or by cardiac sympathetic stimulation in man as well as in animals. The increased flow occurs even with doses that do not increase the aortic blood pressure and is the algebraic resultant of three factors. The first factor is the increase in mechanical compression of the coronary vessels due to more forcible contraction of the surrounding myocardium, tending to reduce coronary flow; however, an opposite effect results from the increased duration of diastole (*see* below). The second factor is the direct action of the drug on coronary vessels, which have both α and β receptors; in man this is predominantly constrictor via α receptors (Anderson *et al.,* 1972). The effect of direct action is of little importance compared to the overriding influence of the third factor, a metabolic dilator effect consequent upon the increased strength of contraction, and due to locally produced metabolites (such as adenosine) resulting from a relative myocardial hypoxia. If aortic blood pressure is enhanced and diastolic time per minute is increased, the above-mentioned effects tend to contribute to an increase rather than a decrease in coronary blood flow. (*See* Gregg and Fisher, 1963; Dempsey and Cooper, 1972.)

Cardiac Effects. Epinephrine is a powerful cardiac stimulant. It acts directly on β_1 receptors of the myocardium and of the cells of the pacemaker and conducting tissues. This stimulation is independent of alterations in cardiac function secondary to increased venous return and other peripheral vascular effects. The heart rate increases and the rhythm is often altered. Cardiac systole is shorter and more powerful, cardiac output is enhanced, and the work of the heart and its oxygen consumption are markedly increased. Cardiac efficiency (work done relative to oxygen consumption) is lessened. The

direct actions of epinephrine uncomplicated by secondary effects can be most readily observed in isolated preparations from animals. Examples are responses of the isolated papillary muscle of the cat, where the actions include increases in contractile force, rate of rise of tension in isometric contractions, excitability, and oxygen consumption and acceleration of the rate of spontaneously beating muscles, as well as induction of automaticity in quiescent muscles.

In accelerating the heart within the physiological range, epinephrine shortens systole more than diastole so that the duration of diastole per minute is increased. Epinephrine speeds the heart by accelerating the slow depolarization of S-A cells that takes place during diastole, that is, during phase 4 of microelectrode recordings. Thus, the transmembrane potential of the pacemaker cells falls more rapidly to the threshold level at which sodium conductance suddenly increases and precipitates the action potential. The amplitude of the action potential and the maximal rate of depolarization are also increased. A shift in the location of the pacemaker in the S-A node often occurs, indicating the activation of latent pacemaker cells. In Purkinje fibers, epinephrine accelerates diastolic depolarization and further facilitates activation of latent pacemaker cells. These changes do not occur in atrial and ventricular muscle fibers, where epinephrine has little effect on the stable, phase-4 resting potential after repolarization. Some effects of epinephrine on cardiac tissues are largely secondary to the increase in heart rate, and are small or inconsistent in preparations where the heart rate is kept constant. For example, the effect of epinephrine on repolarization of atrium, Purkinje fibers, or ventricle is small if the heart rate is unchanged; the duration of the action potential may be shortened or prolonged, with differences between species. When the heart rate is increased, the action-potential duration is consistently shortened, and the refractory period is correspondingly decreased. Similarly, acceleration of the heart rate plays an important part in increasing the conduction velocity in the bundle of His, Purkinje fibers, and ventricle. Thus, the drug shortens the refractory period of atrial and ventricular muscle and speeds A-V conduction. It also decreases the grade of A-V block occurring as a result of disease, drugs, or vagal stimulation.

Conduction through the Purkinje system depends on the level of membrane potential at the time of excitation. Excessive reduction of this potential results in conduction disturbances, ranging from slowed conduction to complete inexcitability. Epinephrine increases the membrane potential and improves conduction in canine Purkinje fibers that have been excessively depolarized. Since circumstances favoring such excessive depolarization are common in diseased hearts, a similar mechanism has been proposed to account for the salutary effects of epinephrine in various human arrhythmias—as, for example, in patients with complete heart block until more definitive measures can be taken (Singer *et al.,* 1967). If large doses of epinephrine are given, premature ventricular systoles occur and may herald more serious ventricular arrhythmias. This is rarely seen with conventional doses in man, but ventricular extrasystoles, tachycardia, or even fibrillation may be precipitated by release of endogenous epinephrine when the heart has been sensitized to this action of epinephrine by certain anesthetics or in cases of myocardial infarction. The mechanism of induction of these cardiac arrhythmias is not clear. During anesthesia, some of the arrhythmias, such as ventricular tachycardia, may not be due to the emergence of ventricular pacemakers but to the effect of epinephrine in modifying impulse conduction through areas of cardiac tissue in which conduction has been depressed by the anesthetic agent, thus permitting irregular reentry of delayed impulses to unaffected areas of the conduction system and contractile tissue (*see* Dresel *et al.,* 1960). The dangers and prevention of this complication of anesthesia are presented elsewhere (*see* Index).

The refractory period of the human A-V node is normally shortened by epinephrine, but may be prolonged by doses that slow the heart through reflex vagal discharge, an effect reversed by atropine. Supraventricular arrhythmias are apt to occur from the combination of epinephrine and cholinergic stimulation. Depression of sinus rate and A-V conduction by vagal discharge probably plays a part in epinephrine-induced ventricular arrhythmias, since various drugs that block the vagal effect confer some protection. The cardiac arrest occasionally caused by vagal discharge due to pressure on the eyeball or carotid sinus can be abolished by epinephrine, which induces or accelerates impulse formation in the ventricles. The action of epinephrine in inducing cardiac automaticity and its action in causing arrhythmias are effectively antagonized by β-blocking agents, which inhibit its chronotropic and inotropic effects. However, α-blocking agents such as phenoxybenzamine protect against epinephrine-induced cardiac irregularities during anesthesia; protection is due in part to prevention of the rise in blood pressure (which sensitizes the myocardium to epinephrine-induced ectopic rhythms) and in part to a direct effect of phenoxybenzamine on the myocardium (*see* Nickerson and Nomaguchi, 1949). This leaves in doubt whether the arrhythmic action is entirely on β receptors or partly on α receptors in addition. There are α receptors in at least some regions of the heart, since the α-receptor stimulant phenylephrine and, during β-receptor block, epinephrine prolong the refractory period and strengthen contractions of isolated atria; these effects are antagonized by α-blocking agents (Benfey and Varma, 1967).

Cardiac arrhythmias have been recorded in man after accidental intravenous administration of conventional subcutaneous doses of epinephrine. Systolic and diastolic pressures rise alarmingly, sometimes as high as 400/300 mm Hg for a short time; cerebro-vascular hemorrhage has occurred from this error. Venous pressure rises, hyperventilation occurs (occasionally preceded by a brief period of apnea), pallor and palpitation are prominent, and heart rate is accelerated after a transient bradycardia. Ventricular premature systoles usually appear within the first minute after injection, frequently followed by multifocal ventricular tachycardia (prefibrillation rhythm). As the effects on the ventricle subside 1 or 2 minutes after their appearance, a marked atrial tachycardia ensues, occasionally associated with A-V block.

In the human *ECG,* epinephrine decreases the T wave amplitude in all leads in normal persons. In animals given relatively larger doses, additional effects are seen on the T wave and S-T segment. After being decreased in amplitude, the T wave may become diphasic and the S-T segment deviates either above or below the isoelectric line before abnormal ventricular deflections appear. Such S-T segment changes are similar to the downward deviation found in patients with *angina pectoris* during spontaneous or epinephrine-induced attacks of pain. These electrical changes have therefore been attributed to myocardial hypoxia due to inability of the coronary blood flow to keep pace with the increased oxygen requirement of the heart stimulated by epinephrine.

Effects on Smooth Muscles. The effects of epinephrine on the smooth muscles of different organs and systems depend upon the type of adrenergic receptor in the muscle and are qualitatively similar to the effects of adrenergic nerve impulses, as shown in Table 21–1 (page 408). The effects on smooth muscle of blood vessels have already been described; the effects on bronchial smooth muscle are discussed below under respiratory effects. Gastrointestinal smooth muscle is, in general, relaxed by epinephrine. Intestinal tone and the frequency and amplitude of spontaneous contractions are reduced. The stomach is usually relaxed and the pyloric and ileocecal sphincters are contracted, but these effects depend upon the preexisting state of activity of the muscle. If tone is already high, epinephrine causes relaxation; if low, contraction. Epinephrine contracts the *splenic capsule* and reduces the size of the spleen; in some species, but not in man, this partly accounts for the increase in red blood cells in the peripheral circulation after epinephrine, thus providing a physiological mechanism for increasing the amount of circulating hemoglobin during acute hypoxia, hemorrhage, and other stresses that evoke the secretion of epinephrine.

The responses of *uterine muscle* to epinephrine vary with species, phase of the sexual cycle, state of gestation, and the dose given. The response of the human uterus is important because the drug may be given during pregnancy or labor. Epinephrine contracts strips of pregnant or nonpregnant human uterus *in vitro* in any effective concentration. The effects of epinephrine on the human uterus *in situ*, however, differ. During the last month of pregnancy and at parturition, epinephrine inhibits uterine tone and contractions; this effect is of no clinical value because it is brief and accompanied by cardiovascular effects. However, other more selective β_2-receptor stimulants, such as salbutamol (albuterol) or ritodrine, have been used successfully to delay premature labor. (*See* Bieniarz *et al.,* 1972; Liggins and Vaughan, 1973.)

Respiratory Effects. Epinephrine stimulates respiration, but this effect is brief and has no clinical value. Given intravenously to animals or man, epinephrine may cause a brief period of apnea ("epinephrine apnea") before stimulation is seen. The apnea is probably due in part to a transient reflex inhibition of the respiratory center through the baroreceptor mechanism and in part to direct inhibition of the center.

Epinephrine can also affect respiration by its peripheral actions, particularly by relaxing bronchial muscle. It has a powerful bronchodilator action, most evident when bronchial muscle is contracted due to disease, as in bronchial asthma, or to drugs and autacoids such as histamine, choline esters, pilocarpine, bradykinin, slow-reacting substance, or prostaglandin $F_{2\alpha}$. In such situations, epinephrine has a striking therapeutic effect as a physiological antagonist to the constrictor influences since it is not limited to specific competitive antagonism such as occurs with antihistaminic drugs against hista-

mine-induced bronchoconstriction. Epinephrine also alters respiration by its α-receptor action in both normal and asthmatic persons; it increases vital capacity by relieving congestion of the bronchial mucosa and, when its action is limited as much as possible to the pulmonary vascular bed by administration as an aerosol, by constricting pulmonary vessels. Its effect in asthma may be due in part to an additional action shown by Assem and Schild (1969), namely, inhibition of antigen-induced release of histamine; this action is shared by selective β_2-receptor stimulants.

Epinephrine increases respiratory rate and tidal volume, and thereby reduces alveolar carbon dioxide content in normal subjects. As already discussed, lethal doses in man may cause death by interference with gaseous exchange due to development of pulmonary edema. Administration of a rapidly acting α-blocking agent or intermittent positive-pressure respiration (to increase intraalveolar pressure) may be lifesaving.

Effects on Central Nervous System. Epinephrine in conventional therapeutic doses is not a powerful CNS stimulant and, therefore, is not useful as an analeptic, as are certain of its noncatechol congeners. Nevertheless, the drug may cause restlessness, apprehension, headache, and tremor in many persons. In animals, small intravenous doses cause arousal from natural sleep and large doses cause stupor, emesis, exaggerated knee jerks, spasticity, and even convulsions. In patients with Parkinson's disease, epinephrine increases the rigidity and tremor, but the locus and mechanism of action are unclear.

Reports of the effects of epinephrine on the *EEG* in man differ and have included insignificant changes, a shift to faster frequencies, an intensification of alpha rhythm, and the appearance of slow waves. Clinical doses probably have no specific EEG effect.

Metabolic Effects. Epinephrine has a number of important influences on metabolic processes. These are probably the only effects of endogenous epinephrine that are of major importance under physiological conditions. Epinephrine elevates *blood glucose* and *lactate* concentrations by the series of enzyme activations described in Chapter 21. In addition, *insulin secretion* is predominantly inhibited via α receptors. Epinephrine also decreases the uptake of glucose by peripheral tissues. Glycosuria rarely occurs. The effect of epinephrine to stimulate glycogenolysis in most tissues and in most species involves β receptors, while the receptor type responsible for hepatic gluconeogenesis is less clear (Tolbert *et al.,* 1973).

Epinephrine raises the blood concentration of *free fatty acids* by activation of triglyceride lipase, which accelerates the breakdown of triglycerides to form free fatty acids and glycerol. Fat is deposited in muscle and liver, probably due to the increased amount of free fatty acid in the blood. This lipolytic action also appears to be mediated by cyclic AMP via β-adrenergic receptors. The effects on other lipids are less clear, but infusions of epinephrine generally increase plasma cholesterol, phospholipid, and low-density lipoproteins. The *calorigenic action* of epinephrine (increase in metabolism) is reflected in man by an increase of 20 to 30% in oxygen consumption after conventional doses. Animal studies have shown that this effect, although composite, is mainly through enhanced breakdown of triglycerides in brown adipose tissue, providing an increase in oxidizable material. (*See* Himms-Hagen, 1967, 1972; Porte and Robertson, 1973; Chapter 21.)

Epinephrine produces a transient rise in *plasma potassium* concentration, mainly due to release of potassium from the liver. This hyperkalemia is followed by a more prolonged fall in plasma potassium. During these changes liver potassium rapidly enters the blood and is taken up by muscle; subsequently the muscle potassium falls during the period of hypokalemia and is transferred to the liver. *Inorganic phosphate* concentration in plasma is decreased by epinephrine.

Miscellaneous Effects. Epinephrine reduces circulating *plasma volume* by loss of protein-free fluid to the extracellular space, thereby increasing *erythrocyte* and *plasma protein concentrations.* However, conventional doses of epinephrine in man do not significantly alter plasma volume or packed red-cell volume under normal conditions, although such doses are reported to have variable effects in shock, hemorrhage, hypotension, and anesthesia. Epinephrine increases *total leukocyte count* but causes *eosinopenia.* Epinephrine has long been known to accelerate blood coagulation in animals and man, an effect probably due to increased activity of factor V (Forwell and Ingram, 1957).

The effects of epinephrine on *secretory glands* are not marked; in most glands secretion is usually inhibited, partly due to reduced blood flow caused by vasoconstriction. Epinephrine stimulates *lacrimation* and a scanty mucous secretion from salivary glands. *Sweating* and *pilomotor activity* are not seen after systemic administration of epinephrine, but occur after intradermal injection of very dilute solutions of either epinephrine or norepinephrine. Such effects are inhibited by α-blocking agents. Epinephrine-induced sweating is part of the indirect evidence for an adrenergic sweating mechanism in man.

Mydriasis is not readily produced in animals or man by epinephrine instilled into the conjunctival sac of normal eyes. However, epinephrine thus applied causes mydriasis after postganglionic sympathetic denervation of the pupil and also in patients with diabetic coma, chronic renal hypertension, hyperthyroidism, and acute pancreatitis, and in certain cases of glaucoma. Epinephrine usually lowers *intraocular pressure* from normal levels and in open-angle glaucoma; the mechanism is not clear, but both reduced production of aqueous humor due to vasoconstriction and enhanced outflow probably occur (*see* Grant, 1969).

Although epinephrine does not directly excite *skeletal muscle,* it facilitates neuromuscular transmission by a prejunctional α-receptor action that appears to increase the amount of acetylcholine (ACh) liberated from the nerve with each impulse. It also acts directly on the muscle cell, a β-receptor action that prolongs the active state of white, fast-contracting fibers and shortens the active state of red, slow-contracting fibers. Epinephrine temporarily abolishes fatigue due to prolonged rapid stimulation of the motor nerve; its effect may equal that of an hour or more of complete rest. The prejunctional α receptors are largely responsible for this effect, but the direct action on fast-contracting fibers also plays a part. (*See* Bowman and Nott, 1969.) Given intra-arterially in patients with myasthenia gravis, epinephrine causes a very real increase in motor power of the injected limb for 30 minutes or more. Given orally, ephedrine and amphetamine have this same effect; although these two drugs have been used clinically in this condition, the improvement in muscle strength does not approach that seen after neostigmine. Skeletal muscles of hypocalcemic patients are hypersensitive to epinephrine, which causes immediate local tetany upon intra-arterial injection; the mechanism of this action is not known.

Large or repeated doses of epinephrine or other sympathomimetic amines given to experimental animals lead to *damage to arterial walls and myocardium,* so severe as to cause the appearance of necrotic areas, indistinguishable in the heart from myocardial infarcts. The mechanism of this injury is not yet clear, but verapamil (which inhibits entry of calcium into the myocardial cell), propranolol, dipyridamole, indomethacin, or aspirin gives substantial protection against the damage. Similar lesions occur in many patients with pheochromocytoma or after prolonged infusions of norepinephrine (*see* Vliet *et al.,* 1966).

Absorption, Fate, and Excretion. *Absorption.* Epinephrine does not reach pharmacologically active concentrations in the body after oral administration because it is destroyed in the gastrointestinal tract and rapidly conjugated and oxidized in the liver. Absorption occurs from subcutaneous tissues and can be hastened by massage of the injection site. Absorption is more rapid after intramuscular than after subcutaneous injection. When strong solutions (1%) are nebulized and inhaled, the actions of the drug are largely restricted to the respiratory tract; although systemic reactions may occur from such inhalation, they are usually mild unless large amounts are used.

Fate and Excretion. Epinephrine is rapidly inactivated in the body despite its stability in the blood. The liver, which is rich in both of the enzymes responsible for destruction of circulating epinephrine, is an important, although not essential, tissue in the degradation process. While only small amounts appear in the urine of normal persons, the urine of patients with pheochromocytoma contains large amounts of epinephrine and norepinephrine.

The greater part of a dose of epinephrine injected into man is accounted for by excretion of metabolites in the urine. Most of the injected drug is first metabolized by COMT and MAO, as already described (*see* page 427 and Figure 21–6, page 428), and excreted as the inactivated compounds. When either MAO or COMT is inhibited, destruction of epinephrine by the remaining enzyme occurs. Congeners of epinephrine are metabolized by the same enzyme systems; amines lacking the 3-OH group are unaffected by COMT, and their disposal depends upon MAO. Destruction of these amines is generally slower than that of epinephrine, and inhibition of MAO by a variety of drugs may prolong their action in the body. (*See* Sharman, 1973.)

Preparations, Dosage, and Routes of Administration. Many preparations of epinephrine are available. Epinephrine is the official U.S.P. term; Adrenaline, the B.P. term. The use of trade names (*e.g.,* ADRENALIN, SUPRARENIN), common in medical parlance, leads to confusion and is not advised.

Epinephrine, U.S.P., is the *l* form of β-(3,4-dihydroxyphenyl)-α-methylaminoethanol (*see* Table 24–1). It is only very slightly soluble in water but forms water-soluble salts with acids. It is unstable in alkaline solution and on exposure to air or light, turning pink from oxidation to adrenochrome and then brown from formation of melanin. Epinephrine may be given by injection, usually subcutaneously, inhaled as an aerosol, or applied locally to mucous membranes or abraded surfaces, as an aqueous solution, ointment, or suppository.

Epinephrine Injection, U.S.P., is a 1:1000 sterile solution of epinephrine hydrochloride in distilled water for parenteral injection, and is available in 1-ml ampuls and 30-ml vials. The solution is nearly colorless and slightly acid; it withstands a short period of boiling and keeps fairly well when undiluted and sterile, but deteriorates in a few hours when diluted. Colored solutions should be rejected. The usual adult dose given *subcutaneously* ranges from 0.1 to 0.5 ml (0.1 to 0.5 mg). The *intravenous* route is rarely used. If the solution is given by vein, it must be adequately diluted and injected *very slowly.* The dose is seldom as much as 0.25 mg. *Intracardiac* injection is occasionally used for resuscitation in extreme emergencies. The *intramuscular* route is generally used only when a prolonged action is desired; for this purpose, *Sterile Epinephrine Oil Suspension,* U.S.P., a suspension of epinephrine in vegetable oil (2 mg/ml) is available in 1-ml ampuls. The dose for adults is 0.2 to 1.0 ml (0.4 to 2.0 mg) every 8 to 16 hours, but the initial dose should not exceed 0.5 ml and doses over 1.0 ml may be dangerous. Although the duration of action is prolonged by delaying complete absorption of the drug, the onset of action is usually as rapid as with subcutaneously administered *epinephrine injection.* Subcutaneous injection should be avoided, since the oil may cause irritation and local reactions. Intramuscular injections are occasionally painful, even when made slowly, and some patients are allergic to the oil. An unofficial aqueous 1:200 suspension of crystalline epinephrine (SUS-PHRINE) depends for prolonged action on its insolubility. Injected subcutaneously the initial adult dose is 0.1 ml, and the maximum is 0.3 ml, repeated no sooner than after 4 hours. *Epinephrine suspensions must never be injected intravenously.*

Epinephrine Inhalation, U.S.P., is a nonsterile 1% aqueous solution of epinephrine hydrochloride for oral (not nasal) inhalation, either from a nebulizer or from an intermittent positive-pressure breathing apparatus. It is used to relieve bronchial constriction and is available in 5-ml vials. *Every precaution must be taken not to confuse this 1:100 solution with the 1:1000 solution designed for parenteral administration.* Injection of the 1:100 solution has caused death.

Epinephrine Nasal Solution, U.S.P., is a 1:1000 preparation of epinephrine hydrochloride identical with *epinephrine injection* except that it is not sterile. It is generally used in preparing more dilute solutions (1:50,000 to 1:2000) for sprays to constrict vessels of mucosa or abraded skin. *Epinephrine Bitartrate,* U.S.P., is available as an official *ophthalmic* solution in concentrations of 0.25, 0.5, 0.55, 1.0, and

1.1% of epinephrine base, and as an unofficial pressurized *aerosol* (MEDIHALER-EPI) delivering measured doses of 0.3 mg (0.16 mg of epinephrine base) for oral inhalation.

Toxicity, Side Effects, and Contraindications. Epinephrine may cause disturbing reactions, such as *fear, anxiety, tenseness, restlessness, throbbing headache, tremor, weakness, dizziness, pallor, respiratory difficulty,* and *palpitation.* The effects rapidly subside with rest, quiet, recumbency, and reassurance, but the patient is often alarmed and should perhaps be forewarned. Hyperthyroid and hypertensive individuals are particularly susceptible to the untoward and pressor responses to epinephrine. In psychoneurotic individuals, existing symptoms are often markedly aggravated by the administration of epinephrine.

More serious accidents consist in *cerebral hemorrhage* and *cardiac arrhythmias.* The use of large doses or the accidental *intravenous* injection of epinephrine may result in cerebral hemorrhage from the sharp rise in blood pressure. Subarachnoid hemorrhage and hemiplegia have occurred even after a subcutaneous dose of 0.5 ml of the 1 : 1000 U.S.P. injection. In contrast, doses as large as 5 to 20 mg injected by mistake have caused no permanent ill effects. Rapidly acting vasodilators such as the nitrites can counteract the marked pressor effects of large doses of epinephrine. The rapidly acting α-blocking agents may also be of use.

Ventricular arrhythmias may follow the administration of epinephrine. If ventricular fibrillation develops, it is usually fatal unless immediate remedial measures are employed; it is particularly prone to occur if the drug is used unwisely during anesthesia, especially with cyclopropane or halogenated hydrocarbon anesthetics, or in individuals with organic heart disease. Patients with longstanding bronchial asthma and a significant degree of emphysema, who have reached the age in which degenerative heart disease is prevalent, must be given epinephrine only with considerable caution. In patients suffering from shock, the drug may accentuate the underlying disorder. Anginal pain is readily induced by epinephrine in patients with angina pectoris, probably due to the great increase in cardiac work, which accentuates the insufficiency of the coronary circulation.

Therapeutic Uses. Epinephrine has a wide variety of clinical uses in medicine and surgery. In general, these are based on the actions of the drug on blood vessels, heart, and bronchial muscle. The most common uses of epinephrine are to relieve respiratory distress due to *bronchospasm,* to provide rapid relief of *hypersensitivity reactions* to drugs and other allergens, and to *prolong the action of infiltration anesthetics.* Its cardiac effects may be of use in restoring cardiac rhythm in *cardiac arrest* due to various causes, but it is not used in cardiac failure or in hemorrhagic, traumatic, or cardiogenic shock. It is also used as a *topical hemostatic* on bleeding surfaces. The therapeutic uses of epinephrine are further discussed later in this chapter, together with those of other sympathomimetic drugs.

LEVARTERENOL (NOREPINEPHRINE)

Levarterenol (*l*-arterenol, *l*-norepinephrine, *l*-noradrenaline, *l*-β-[3,4-dihydroxyphenyl]-α-aminoethanol) is the chemical mediator liberated by postganglionic adrenergic nerves. It differs from epinephrine only by lacking the methyl substitution in the amino group (*see* Table 24–1). As with epinephrine, the *d* isomer has pharmacological properties similar to those of the *l* form, but it is much less active. Levarterenol constitutes 10 to 20% of the catecholamine content of human adrenal medulla and as much as 97% in some pheochromocytomas. The history of its discovery and its role as a neurohumoral mediator are discussed in Chapter 21; the structure-activity relationship of levarterenol to other sympathomimetic amines has been described above.

Pharmacological Actions. The pharmacological actions of levarterenol and epinephrine have been extensively compared *in vivo* and *in vitro* (*see* Table 24–3). Both drugs act directly on effector cells, and their actions differ mainly in the ratio of their effectiveness in stimulating α and β receptors. Levarterenol acts predominantly on α receptors and has little action on β receptors, except in the heart. Even on α receptors, levarterenol is somewhat less potent than epinephrine on most test objects, requiring larger doses to produce equal effects. Its β_2 receptor actions are much feebler than those of epinephrine. There are some differences in the effects of adrenergic blocking agents on the net cardiovascular responses to the two amines, due to the relative lack of β_2-receptor activity of levarterenol.

Cardiovascular Effects. The cardiovascular effects of intravenous infusion of 10 μg of levarterenol per minute in man are shown in Figure 24–1. Systolic and diastolic pressures and usually pulse pressure are increased. Cardiac output is unchanged or decreased, and the total peripheral resistance is raised. Compensatory vagal reflex activity slows the heart, overcoming the direct cardioaccelerator action, and the stroke volume is thus increased. The peripheral vascular resistance increases in most vascular beds, and the blood flow is reduced through kidney, brain, liver, and usually skeletal muscle. A marked venoconstriction contributes to the increased resistance. Glomerular filtration rate is maintained unless the decrease in renal blood flow is quite marked. With the reduction in cerebral blood flow there is an accompanying fall in cerebral oxygen consumption. Levarterenol constricts mesenteric vessels and reduces splanchnic and hepatic blood flow in man. Coronary flow is substantially increased, probably due to both indirectly induced coronary dilatation, as with epinephrine, and elevated blood pressure. Unlike epinephrine, small doses of levarterenol do not cause vasodilatation or lower blood pressure, since the blood vessels of skeletal muscle are constricted instead of dilated; α-blocking agents therefore abolish the pressor effects but do not cause significant reversal. The circulating blood volume is reduced by loss of protein-free fluid to the extracellular space, probably due to postcapillary vasoconstriction. The usual ECG change is sinus bradycardia due to a reflex increase in vagal tone, with or without prolongation of the P-R interval. Nodal rhythm, A-V dissociation, bigeminal rhythm, ventricular tachycardia, and fibrillation have also been observed.

Other Effects. Other responses to levarterenol are not prominent in man. The drug causes hyperglycemia and other metabolic effects similar to those produced by epinephrine, but these are observed only when larger doses are given. Respiratory minute volume is slightly increased. Other effects on the CNS are somewhat less prominent than those of epinephrine. Intradermal injection of suitable doses in man causes sweating that is not blocked by atropine. Increased frequency of contraction of the pregnant human uterus has been observed, but the effects on the other smooth muscles are slight.

Absorption, Fate, and Excretion. Levarterenol, like epinephrine, is ineffective when given orally and is absorbed poorly from sites of subcutaneous injection. It is rapidly inactivated in the body by the same enzymatic processes that methylate and oxidize epinephrine (*see* above). Only 4 to 16% of an administered dose is excreted unchanged in the urine. Negligible amounts are normally found in the urine, but as much as 15 mg per day may be excreted by persons with pheochromocytoma.

Preparations, Dosage, and Administration. *Levarterenol Bitartrate,* U.S.P. (LEVOPHED BITARTRATE), is the water-soluble, crystalline monohydrate salt. Like epinephrine, it is readily oxidized. *Levarterenol Bitartrate Injection,* U.S.P., is a 0.2% sterile solution of the bitartrate, equivalent to 0.1% of levarterenol base. It is usually given by *intravenous infusion,* as a solution containing 4 μg/ml of levarterenol base, obtained by diluting 4 ml of the official injection in 1000 ml of 5% dextrose injection, which may also contain a variable amount of sodium chloride. After the cardiovascular response to a test dose of 0.1 to 0.2 μg/kg of body weight is observed, the infusion is adjusted to obtain the desired pressor response. Normally the infusion of 2 to 4 μg of base per minute (0.5 to 1.0 ml per minute) is adequate. The pressor response to the drug can be readily controlled since it disappears within 1 or 2 minutes after the infusion is stopped. In patients in whom intravenous infusion of large volumes of fluid is undesirable, less dilute solutions may be used cautiously. Oral administration is ineffective.

Toxicity, Side Effects, and Precautions. The untoward effects of levarterenol are similar to those of epinephrine, but they are usually minimal and less frequent. Anxiety, respiratory difficulty, awareness of the slow, forceful heart beat, and transient headache are the most common effects. Overdoses or conventional doses in hypersensitive persons (*e.g.,* hyperthyroid patients) cause severe hypertension with violent headache, photophobia, stabbing retrosternal and pharyngeal pain, pallor, intense sweating, and vomiting. The risk of cardiac arrhythmias contraindicates the use of the drug during anesthesia with agents that sensitize the automatic tissue of the heart. Transitory swelling and engorgement of the thyroid has occurred in a few cases; the cause is unknown.

Care must be taken that *necrosis* and

sloughing do not occur at the site of intravenous injection, due to extravasation of the drug. The infusion should be made high in the limb, preferably through a long plastic cannula extending centrally, and the site of infusion should be changed at least every 12 hours. Impaired circulation at injection sites, with or without extravasation of levarterenol, may be relieved by hot packs and infiltration of the area with phentolamine or a local anesthetic. Levarterenol infusions should never be left unattended. Blood pressure must be determined at least every 15 minutes during the infusion and more frequently during initial adjustment of the rate. Blood pressure should not be raised to more than normotensive levels. Reduced blood flow to vital areas is a constant danger in the use of levarterenol. The drug should not be used in pregnant women because of its contractile action on the pregnant uterus.

Therapeutic Uses and Status. Although levarterenol is vital in maintaining homeostasis, it has only a limited and somewhat doubtful therapeutic value. The therapeutic use of levarterenol and of other sympathomimetic amines in hypotension due to shock is discussed later in this chapter.

ISOPROTERENOL

Isoproterenol (isopropylarterenol, isopropylnorepinephrine, isoprenaline, isopropylnoradrenaline, *dl*-β-[3,4-dihydroxyphenyl]-α-isopropylaminoethanol) (Table 24–1) is the most active of the sympathomimetic amines that act almost exclusively on β receptors by virtue of their N-alkyl substitution. First studied by Konzett (1940), it has since been the subject of extensive animal and clinical research.

Pharmacological Actions. Isoproterenol has a powerful action on all β receptors and almost no action on α receptors. Its main actions, therefore, are on the heart, the smooth muscle of bronchi, skeletal muscle vasculature, and the alimentary tract. The major cardiovascular effects of isoproterenol, epinephrine, and levarterenol in man are compared in Figure 24–1. The *l* isomer is 50 times as powerful as the *d* isomer in circulatory activity in man.

Cardiovascular System. Intravenous infusion of isoproterenol in man lowers peripheral vascular resistance, mainly in skeletal muscle but also in renal and mesenteric vascular beds, and diastolic pressure falls (*see* Figure 24–1). Cardiac output is raised by an increase in the venous return to the heart, combined with the positive inotropic and chronotropic actions of the drug. With usual doses of isoproterenol in man, the increase in cardiac output is generally enough to maintain or raise the systolic pressure, although the mean pressure is reduced. Renal blood flow is decreased in normotensive subjects but is markedly increased in patients in cardiogenic or septicemic shock. Pulmonary arterial pressure is unchanged. Larger doses (*e.g.*, 1 μg/kg) cause a striking fall in mean blood pressure.

Smooth Muscle. Isoproterenol relaxes almost all varieties of smooth muscle when the tone is high, but this action is most pronounced on bronchial and gastrointestinal smooth muscle. It prevents or relieves bronchoconstriction due to drugs in animals and to drugs and bronchial asthma in man, but tolerance to this effect develops with overuse of the drug. Its effect in asthma may be due in part to an additional action to inhibit antigen-induced release of histamine (Assem and Schild, 1969); this action is shared by selective β₂-receptor stimulants. The drug decreases the tone and motility of intestinal musculature and inhibits uterine motility even when epinephrine causes contraction. An additional α-receptor action occurs in some muscles with high doses, especially after β-receptor block, and blanching of the skin occurs when the compound is injected intradermally in man.

Metabolic and Central Nervous System Actions. In man, isoproterenol causes less hyperglycemia than does epinephrine, but it is as effective as epinephrine in releasing *free fatty acid*. Insulin secretion is stimulated both by glucose and by direct β-adrenergic activation of pancreatic islet cells. The *calorigenic* actions of isoproterenol and epinephrine are similar. Like epinephrine, it can cause central excitation, but this is not significant with clinically used doses.

Absorption, Fate, and Excretion. Isoproterenol is readily absorbed when given parenterally or as an aerosol. Absorption of sublingual or oral doses is unreliable. It is metabolized and eliminated by the same routes as epinephrine, and its effects are of approximately the same duration.

Preparations. *Isoproterenol Hydrochloride,* U.S.P. (ISUPREL), is a white, water-soluble powder; it is oxidized on exposure to air or alkali. *Isoproterenol Hydrochloride Inhalation,* U.S.P., is available as a 0.25% aerosol (ISUPREL MISTOMETER, NORISODRINE AEROTROL) and as solutions (0.5 and 1%). A usual dose to relieve bronchoconstriction in asthma is 0.5 ml of the 0.5% solution. The drug is also available as *Isoproterenol Hydrochloride Injection,* U.S.P., containing 10, 20, or 200 μg/ml. Sublingual tablets (10 and 15 mg) are marketed, but their absorption is variable and unreliable and pronounced systemic effects are more frequent than with inhalation. Unofficial sustained-action tablets for oral use are also marketed, but they are less reliable than ephedrine, a long-acting sympathomimetic drug used in the same clinical conditions and readily absorbed after oral administration. *Isoproterenol Sulfate,* N.F. (NORISODRINE), is supplied as a powder inhalant (10 or 25% with lactose). An unofficial aerosol of 0.2% (MEDIHALER-ISO) is available, delivering a dose of 75 μg for each oral inhalation.

Toxicity and Side Effects. The acute toxicity of isoproterenol in animals is much less than that of epinephrine. However, cardiac arrhythmias can occur readily, and large or repeated doses in animals may lead to myocardial necrosis as with epinephrine, or to cardiac arrest when the heart is subjected to an increased work load (Lockett, 1965). *Palpitation, tachycardia, headache,* and *flushing* of the skin are common; serious *arrhythmias, anginal pain, nausea, tremor, dizziness, weakness,* and *sweating* occasionally occur. Serious *cardiac reactions* are rare, but death may follow an overdose. The toxicity associated with the use of pressurized aerosols containing isoproterenol is discussed below (page 509).

Therapeutic Uses. Isoproterenol is employed clinically only as a *bronchodilator* in respiratory disorders and as a *cardiac stimulant* in heart block, cardiogenic shock after myocardial infarction, and septicemic shock. Its use in these conditions and its value in relation to other sympathomimetic agents are discussed later in this chapter.

DOPAMINE

Dopamine (3,4-dihydroxyphenylethylamine) (Table 24–1) is the immediate precursor in the synthesis of norepinephrine in the body (*see* Chapter 21). In *animals,* higher doses than have usually been used in man increase peripheral resistance and cardiac output and raise arterial blood pressure. In normal *man,* infusion of the drug decreases peripheral resistance and causes mesenteric and renal vasodilatation. Renal blood flow, glomerular filtration rate, urine flow, and sodium excretion are enhanced. Dopamine also has a direct inotropic effect on the heart; cardiac output is increased, but there is usually little change in arterial blood pressure or heart rate. The drug is less prone to cause tachycardia and arrhythmias than are other catecholamines. The major cardiovascular effects are the result of actions of the drug on α- and β-adrenergic receptors and on specific dopamine receptors in the mesenteric and renal vascular beds; the renal and mesenteric vasodilatation is not blocked by α- or β-blocking agents. In patients in shock the blood pressure is elevated by dopamine therapy, particularly the systolic pressure, and the increase in urine flow is prominent. Many aspects of the pharmacology of dopamine have been reviewed by Goldberg (1972).

Although there are specific dopamine receptors in the CNS, injected dopamine has no central effects because it does not cross the blood-brain barrier (*see* Chapters 14 and 21).

Preparations, Dosage, and Routes of Administration. *Dopamine hydrochloride* (INTROPIN) is a water-soluble, light-sensitive, white crystalline powder, marketed in solution in 5-ml ampuls containing 40 mg/ml of the drug. It is used only by the intravenous route. The contents of the ampul must be diluted in 250 or 500 ml of an appropriate, non-alkaline, sterile solution (0.9% sodium chloride or 5% dextrose), to yield a final concentration of 800 or 400 μg/ml. It is given for the treatment of shock by metered, drip infusion at an initial rate of 2.5 μg/kg per minute, and the dose is gradually increased to 10 to 20 μg/kg or more per minute, if necessary. Frequent monitoring of the rate of urine flow is essential, because this is the best index of a satisfactory response. The duration of action of dopamine is quite brief and hence the rate of administration can be used effectively to control the intensity of effect.

Precautions, Adverse Reactions, and Contraindications. Before dopamine is administered to patients in shock, hypovolemia should be corrected by transfusion of whole blood, plasma, or appropriate fluids. The blood pressure, heart rate, and urine flow rate should be continuously monitored and the dosage adjusted accordingly. Untoward effects include nausea, vomiting, tachycardia, ectopic beats, precordial pain, dyspnea, headache, and vasoconstriction as indicated by a disproportionate rise in diastolic pressure. Occasionally hypertension and azotemia may develop. Since dopamine is metabolized by MAO, the dose must be greatly reduced in patients who have recently received drugs that inhibit this enzyme. Dopamine should not be used in individuals with tachyarrhythmias or known to have pheochromocytoma. Experience with dopamine therapy in children is as yet limited.

Therapeutic Uses. Dopamine has been employed in the treatment of *shock syndromes* from various causes, including trauma, myocardial infarction, and endotoxic septicemia. The prognosis is more favorable when therapy is instituted early and especially before the rate of urine flow is seriously decreased (below 0.3 ml per minute). Dopamine is a relatively new drug, and the full spectrum of its therapeutic value, limitations, and adverse effects is still to be assessed. The management of shock is more fully discussed later in this chapter. Dopamine may also be of value in the treatment of *chronic refractory congestive heart failure* (*see* Goldberg, 1974).

II. Noncatecholamines

A great many sympathomimetic drugs lacking the catechol nucleus have been studied, and several are used clinically. As already discussed, their effects depend in part upon release of norepinephrine from stores in adrenergic nerve terminals and in part upon a direct action on effector cells.

The ratio of direct to indirect action varies widely among these compounds (Trendelenburg *et al.,* 1962; Schmidt and Fleming, 1963). Even for an individual compound this ratio varies from species to species and from tissue to tissue within the same species. The methods presently available for determining this ratio are complex and imprecise. Nevertheless, an indication of the importance of some structural groups can be obtained. Catecholamines do not owe any significant part of their action to a release of norepinephrine. The position of the OH in the benzene ring appears to be of great importance in determining direct action. Compounds with only the 3-OH have a very high ratio of direct to indirect action. For example, phenylephrine, lacking only the 4-OH of epinephrine, very largely depends for its effects on its direct action. In contrast, compounds with only a 4-OH owe the larger part of their effects to indirect action; indeed, tyramine, with this OH

group, is the prototype with which most of the fundamental investigations of this indirect action have been made.

Since the actions of norepinephrine are more marked on α than on β receptors, many noncatecholamines that release norepinephrine have predominantly α-receptor effects. However, many noncatecholamines show powerful β-receptor action and are widely used in clinical conditions that require sympathomimetic drugs with β activity. Thus, ephedrine, although dependent upon norepinephrine release for some of its effect, relieves bronchospasm by its β-receptor action on bronchial muscle, an effect virtually absent with norepinephrine. In contrast, some noncatecholamines may lack actions typical of norepinephrine. For example, phenylephrine mainly acts directly on effector cells and exhibits little of the cardiac excitatory effect that is so pronounced with norepinephrine. It is therefore impossible to predict the characteristic effects of noncatecholamines simply on the basis that they all release at least some norepinephrine.

With few exceptions the actions and effects of noncatecholamines, except those on the CNS, fit within the framework of α- and β-receptor activity as listed in Table 21–1 (page 408) and, therefore, only the main differences in their properties will be presented. The additional CNS effects, most prominent with sympathomimetic amines lacking substituents on the benzene ring, have been most extensively studied with amphetamine and, consequently, are discussed in detail in relation to the properties and clinical uses of this drug.

Absorption, Distribution, and Fate of Noncatecholamines. In contrast to the catecholamines, most of the clinically used noncatecholamines are effective when given orally and many act for long periods. These properties are due in part to resistance to the inactivating enzymes of liver and other tissues and in part to the fact that relatively large amounts are given. The amount of inactivation by the liver after oral administration of various sympathomimetics has not been adequately studied. Phenylisopropylamines, the most commonly used noncatecholamines, become localized in tissues soon after their administration; and, in contrast to catecholamines, which cross the blood-brain barrier with difficulty, they are found in high concentration in brain and cerebrospinal fluid. This accounts in part for their relatively powerful CNS activity. Although several pathways, including *p*-hydroxylation, N-demethylation, deamination, and conjugation in the liver, take part in their disposal, a substantial part of these drugs is excreted in the urine. Urinary excretion of amphetamine and many other noncatecholamines is greatly influenced by urinary pH. Since the pK_a of amphetamine is 9.93, the percentage of nonionized drug increases in alkaline urine, and the drug is readily reabsorbed by the renal tubules; at pH 8.0 only 2 to 3% is excreted. If the urine is acidic, urinary excretion may be as much as 80% (Beckett and Rowland, 1965). The effects of amphetamine are greatly prolonged in patients with alkaline urine, and acidification of the urine by the administration of ammonium chloride is a logical procedure in the treatment of amphetamine poisoning. A large number of noncatecholamines have pK_a values between 9.0 and 10.3 (Vree *et al.*, 1969), and similar striking effects of urinary pH can be expected.

Both amphetamine and ephedrine are resistant to the action of MAO and, indeed, inhibit its action on other substrates. This property has led to the highly speculative suggestion, for which there is no direct evidence, that inhibition of MAO in the brain is the cause of their central effects.

Patients treated with MAO inhibitors, now used clinically only occasionally, should not take noncatecholamines or ingest certain cheeses, wines, and yeast products containing sympathomimetic agents, such as tyramine, that are normally inactivated by MAO (page 183).

AMPHETAMINE

Amphetamine, racemic β-phenylisopropylamine (Table 24-1), has powerful CNS stimulant actions in addition to the peripheral α and β actions common to sympathomimetic drugs. Unlike epinephrine, it is effective after oral administration and its effects last for several hours.

History. The pressor effects of amphetamine were first described by Piness and associates (1930). Alles (1933) observed its bronchodilator, respiratory stimulant, and analeptic actions and, comparing it with epinephrine, found its cardiovascular effects to be of much longer duration but its potency to be only about 0.5 to 1.0%. The central stimulant effects of amphetamine were first used clinically by Prinzmetal and Bloomberg (1935) to treat narcolepsy and have since been employed in a variety of conditions, including obesity, fatigue, parkinsonism, and poisoning by CNS depressants.

PHARMACOLOGICAL PROPERTIES

Cardiovascular Responses. In man and animals, amphetamine given orally raises both systolic and diastolic blood pressures. The pulse pressure is usually increased, since amphetamine has β- as well as α-receptor activity. Heart rate is often reflexly slowed; with large doses, cardiac arrhythmias may occur. Cardiac output is not enhanced by therapeutic doses, and cerebral blood flow is little changed. The *l* isomer is slightly more potent than the *d* isomer in its cardiovascular actions.

Other Smooth Muscles. In general, smooth muscles respond to amphetamine as they do to other sympathomimetics. Bronchial muscle is relaxed, but the effect is not sufficiently marked to be of therapeutic value. The contractile effect on the urinary bladder sphincter is particularly marked, and has been used in treating enuresis and incontinence. Pain and difficulty in micturition occasionally occur. The gastrointestinal effects of amphetamine are unpredictable. If enteric activity is pronounced, amphetamine may cause relaxation and delay the movement of intestinal contents; if the gut is already relaxed, the opposite effect may be seen. The response of the human uterus varies, but usually there is an increase in tone.

Central Nervous System. Amphetamine is one of the most potent sympathomimetic amines with respect to stimulation of the CNS. It is an effective agent for stimulating the medullary respiratory center, lessening the degree of central depression caused by various drugs, and stimulating the normal cerebrospinal axis. Animals given sufficient doses of amphetamine show tremor, restlessness, increased motor activity, agitation, and sleeplessness; these effects are thought to be due to cortical stimulation and possibly to stimulation of the reticular activating system. In contrast, the drug can obtund the maximal electroshock seizure discharge and prolong the ensuing period of depression; these properties may be related to the usefulness of amphetamine in certain cases of epilepsy. In elicitation of CNS excitatory effects, the *d* isomer (dextroamphetamine) is three to four times as potent as the *l* isomer.

In man, the marked *analeptic* action is exemplified by the fact that anesthesia produced by 0.5 g of amobarbital sodium given intravenously can be greatly lessened by 10 to 30 mg of amphetamine injected intravenously. The *psychic* effects depend on the dose and the mental state and personality of the individual. The main results of an oral dose of 10 to 30 mg are as follows: wakefulness, alertness, and a decreased sense of fatigue; elevation of mood, with increased initiative, confidence, and ability to concentrate; often elation and euphoria; increase in motor and speech activity. Performance of only simple mental tasks is improved; and, although more work may be accomplished, the number of errors is not necessarily decreased. Physical performance, for example, in athletes, is improved. These effects are not invariable, and may be reversed by overdosage or repeated usage. Prolonged use or large doses are nearly always followed by mental depression and fatigue. Many individuals given amphetamine experience headache, palpitation, dizziness, vasomotor disturbances, agitation, confusion, dysphoria, apprehension, delirium, or fatigue. (*See* review by Weiss and Laties, 1962.)

Fatigue and Sleep. Prevention and reversal of fatigue by amphetamine have been studied extensively in the laboratory, in military field studies, and in athletics. In general, the duration of adequate performance is prolonged before fatigue appears and the effects of fatigue are at least partly reversed. The most striking improvement due to amphetamine appears to occur when performance has been reduced by fatigue and lack of sleep. Such improvement may be partly due to alteration of unfavorable attitudes toward the task. However, amphetamine reduces the occurrence of microsleeps, the brief losses of vigilance that impair performance after

prolonged sleep deprivation, and thus improves execution of tasks requiring sustained attention. The drug is effective in postponing sleep and promoting wakefulness. Rapid-eye-movement (REM) sleep is reduced to about 10%, less than half the normal proportion of total sleeping time. The need for sleep may be postponed, but it obviously cannot be indefinitely avoided. When the drug is discontinued after long use, total sleep increases, and REM sleep appears more rapidly than usual and is unduly prolonged. The pattern of sleep may take as long as 2 months to return to normal. Because the beneficial effects of the drug have to be repaid in the coin of fatigue and often depression, and because of the variable reactions in patients, amphetamine should not be used indiscriminately. (*See* reviews by Weiss and Laties, 1962; Oswald, 1968.)

Analgesia. Although amphetamine and some other sympathomimetic amines have a small analgesic effect in man and experimental animals, no therapeutic advantage in the use of amphetamine for analgesia, either alone or given with other drugs, has been established.

EEG. In general, amphetamine accelerates and desynchronizes the EEG. It causes a shift of the resting EEG toward the higher frequencies in man, but to a smaller degree than that occurring during attention. It reduces the amplitude and the duration of the large delta waves that are present during sleep after prolonged insomnia and in narcolepsy. The postconvulsive confusion and slow-wave EEG observed after electroshock seizures in monkeys are counteracted by amphetamine. In some children with petit mal and typical 3-per-second spike-and-dome dysrhythmia, amphetamine may abolish both the seizures and the abnormal EEG discharges; this may be due, in part, to an effect on alertness and activity. In children with behavioral disorders and abnormal EEG (6-cycle-per-second rhythm), amphetamine may improve behavior with or without altering the EEG. The EEG cannot be fully relied on as a criterion for the effects of amphetamine, since the drug can cause behavioral arousal even when desynchronization of the EEG is prevented by atropine (Bradley, 1958). (*See* review by Toman and Davis, 1949.)

Spinal Cord, Reticular Formation, and Respiratory Center. Amphetamine facilitates monosynaptic and polysynaptic transmission in the spinal cord. In common with ephedrine, it enhances excitatory activity, promotes righting movements and postural activity, and speeds the recovery of responses in spinal, decerebrate, and decorticate animals. Amphetamine can reverse the depressant effect of barbiturates on the reticular formation, and it lowers the threshold for arousal by electrical stimulation of this region (Bradley and Key, 1958).

The *respiratory center* is stimulated by

amphetamine in animals, and the rate and depth of respiration are increased. In normal man, usual doses of the drug do not appreciably increase respiratory rate or minute volume. Nevertheless, when respiration is depressed by centrally acting drugs, amphetamine may stimulate respiration.

Depression of Appetite. Amphetamine and similar drugs have been widely used in the treatment of obesity, although the wisdom of this use is at best questionable. Weight loss in obese humans treated with amphetamine is almost entirely due to reduced food intake and only in small measure to increased metabolism. The site of action is central and is probably in the lateral hypothalamic feeding center; injection of amphetamine into this area, but not into the ventromedial satiety center, suppresses food intake (*see* Blundell and Leshem, 1973). In man, some drug-induced loss of acuity of smell and taste has been described, and increased physical activity may also contribute to the loss of weight. In dogs, the effect is powerful and may lead to complete starvation if amphetamine is given each day 1 hour before the daily meal; food is refused even if offered for 45 minutes. The effect is much less in man, and tolerance to acceptable doses develops rapidly. The effect is insufficient to reduce weight continuously in obese individuals without dietary restriction. Amphetamine has little effect in reducing food intake in those persons whose overeating is impelled by psychological factors.

Mechanisms of the CNS Effects. Although these mechanisms are not fully clear, the alerting action appears to depend on local release of norepinephrine in the brain. Activation of reticular-arousal-system neurons by locally applied amphetamine mimics the effect of norepinephrine; this is prevented by reserpine, which causes depletion of catecholamines and 5-hydroxytryptamine(5-HT), by α-methyl-*p*-tyrosine, which causes depletion of catecholamines but not of 5-HT, and by agents that deplete the brain of norepinephrine but not dopamine (Boakes *et al.,* 1972). Similarly, catecholamines have been implicated in the anorectic effect of amphetamine, but its congener fenfluramine may act by releasing 5-HT. Antagonists of 5-HT block the effect of fenfluramine but not that of amphetamine, while chlorphentermine, which inhibits re-uptake of 5-HT, antagonizes fenfluramine but potentiates amphetamine (Jespersen and Scheel-Krüger, 1973). For other CNS effects of amphetamine, a direct action on adrenergic receptors has not yet been excluded.

Metabolic Effects. Although large doses of amphetamine markedly increase oxygen consumption in animals, conventional therapeutic doses cause either no change, a small fall, or a modest rise (10 to 15%) in the metabolic rate in man. When an increase does occur, it is neither as constant nor as significant as that caused by epinephrine, but it is more sustained. Some patients show a slight increase in body temperature. The apparent calorigenic action may be due to restlessness caused by the drug. Amphetamine increases the plasma concentration of free fatty acids but, in contrast to epinephrine, does not modify carbohydrate utilization or increase the concentration of blood glucose or lactate, and the respiratory quotient is unaltered.

Preparations, Administration, and Dosage. *Amphetamine sulfate* (BENZEDRINE) is a white, water-soluble powder, available in 5- and 10-mg tablets and 15-mg slow-release capsules. The *d* isomer is available as *Dextroamphetamine Phosphate,* N.F., in 5-mg tablets; and as *Dextroamphetamine Sulfate,* U.S.P. (DEXEDRINE), in official 5- and 10-mg tablets, in an official elixir (1 mg/ml), as an injection (20 mg/ml), and in 5-, 10-, and 15-mg slow-release capsules. *Amphetamine base* is a volatile liquid that changes to the carbonate when exposed to air; it was formerly used in inhalers to treat nasal congestion. For this purpose it has been replaced by various sympathomimetic amines that have considerably less central stimulant action.

With the usual oral dose of 2.5 to 5.0 mg of dextroamphetamine, the effects appear within ½ to 1 hour. The patient's sensitivity should first be tested with a dose of 2.5 mg. For chronic medication the usual dosage is 5 mg, two or three times daily. The last dose is generally given not later than 4 P.M., to avoid insomnia. Parenterally, intramuscular injection is preferable to the intravenous route. Vascular effects appear within 5 minutes. For treatment of poisoning by central depressants, 10 to 20 mg of dextroamphetamine may be given initially, and repeated at ½-hour intervals depending on the patient's response. A 1% aqueous solution of amphetamine sulfate may be applied locally as a mydriatic or nasal decongestant.

The amphetamines are schedule-II drugs under federal regulations (*see* Appendix).

Toxicity and Side Effects. The *acute toxic effects* of amphetamine are usually extensions of its therapeutic actions and, as a rule, result from overdosage. The *central effects* commonly include restlessness, dizziness, tremor, hyperactive reflexes, talkativeness, tenseness, irritability, weakness, insomnia, fever, and sometimes euphoria. Confusion, assaultiveness, increased libido, anxiety, delirium, hallucinations, panic states, and suicidal or homicidal tendencies occur, especially in mentally ill patients. Fatigue and depression usually follow the central stimulation. *Cardiovascular effects* are common and include headache, chilliness, pallor or flushing, palpitation, cardiac arrhythmias, anginal pain, hypertension or hypotension, and circulatory collapse. Excessive sweating occurs. Symptoms referable to the *gastrointestinal system* include dry mouth, metallic taste, anorexia, nausea, vomiting, diarrhea, and abdominal cramps. Fatal poisoning usually terminates in convulsions and coma, and cerebral hemorrhages are the main pathological finding.

The *toxic dose* of amphetamine varies widely. Toxic manifestations occasionally occur as an idiosyncrasy after as little as 2 mg, but are rare with doses of less than 15 mg. Severe reactions have occurred with 30 mg, yet doses of 400 to 500 mg have been survived. Death has followed rapid injection of 120 mg. Larger doses can be tolerated after chronic use of the drug.

Treatment of acute amphetamine intoxication should include acidification of the urine by administration of ammonium chloride. Excretion of amphetamine is negligible in alkaline urine, and is vastly increased in acidic urine. Chlorpromazine is effective treatment for the CNS symptoms, and additionally its α-receptor blocking action reduces the elevated blood pressure; a nitrite or a rapidly acting α-receptor blocking agent may also be required if hypertension is marked.

Chronic amphetamine intoxication causes symptoms similar to those of acute overdosage, but abnormal mental conditions are more common. Weight loss may be marked, and occasionally dermatitis occurs. A psychotic reaction with vivid hallucinations and paranoid delusions, often mistaken for schizophrenia, is the most common serious effect. Recovery is usually rapid after withdrawal of the drug, but occasionally the condition becomes chronic. In these persons amphetamine may act as a precipitating factor hastening the onset of an incipient schizophrenia. (*See* Angrist and Gershon, 1972; Chapter 12.)

Precautions and Contraindications. The abuse of amphetamine by the laity as a means of overcoming sleepiness and of increasing energy and alertness should be discouraged. The drug should be used only under medical supervision. The additional *contraindications* and *precautions* in the use of amphetamine are generally similar to those described above for epinephrine. Its use is inadvisable in patients with anorexia, insomnia, asthenia, psychopathic personality, or a history of homicidal or suicidal tendencies.

Addiction and Tolerance. *Addiction* often occurs to amphetamine and dextroamphetamine, as discussed in Chapter 16. *Tolerance* almost invariably develops to the anorexigenic effect of amphetamines, and is often seen also in the need for increasing doses to maintain improvement of mood in psychiatric patients. A period without the drug usually restores the patient's sensitivity. Tolerance is striking in addicts, and a daily intake of 1700 mg without apparent ill effects has been reported. Development of tolerance is not invariable, and cases of narcolepsy have been treated for years without requiring an increase in the initially effective dose.

Therapeutic Uses. Amphetamine and dextroamphetamine are used chiefly for their CNS effects. They have been largely supplanted by other sympathomimetic agents for their peripheral effects. Dextroamphetamine, with greater CNS action and less peripheral action, is generally preferred to amphetamine; it is used in obesity, narcolepsy, parkinsonism, behavior disorders, and absence seizures. These uses are discussed later in this chapter.

METHAMPHETAMINE

Methamphetamine is closely related chemically to amphetamine and ephedrine (Table 24–1). Its *pharmacological actions* are similar to those of amphetamine, but it exhibits a different ratio between central and peripheral actions. Small doses have prominent central stimulant effects without significant peripheral actions; somewhat larger doses produce a sustained rise in systolic and diastolic blood pressure, due in man mainly to cardiac stimulation. Cardiac output is increased, although the heart rate may be reflexly slowed. The drug has considerable β-receptor stimulant activity and increases blood flow in skeletal muscle. Peripheral venous pressure is increased and venous constriction occurs. These factors tend to increase the venous return and, therefore, the cardiac output. Pulmonary arterial pressure is raised, probably secondary to increased cardiac output. Renal blood flow is also enhanced. Although moderate doses stimulate cardiac contraction, excessive doses depress the myocardium. (*See* Aviado, 1959, 1970; Eckstein and Abboud, 1962.)

Preparations and Dosage. *Methamphetamine hydrochloride* (DESOXYN, FETAMIN) is the *d* isomer. It is available in tablets containing 2.5 or 5 mg; in sustained-release tablets containing 5, 10, or 15 mg; and as an injection containing 20 mg/ml. The usual oral dose for central effects varies from 2.5 mg daily to 5 mg three times daily. For the pressor effect, a dose of 10 to 30 mg is given intramuscularly.

Methamphetamine is a schedule-II drug under federal regulations (*see* Appendix).

Therapeutic Uses. Methamphetamine is principally used for its *central effects,* which are more pronounced than those of amphetamine and are accompanied by less prominent peripheral actions. It has also been used to maintain blood pressure in certain *hypotensive states* (*e.g.,* in spinal anesthesia). These uses are discussed below in the therapeutic section of this chapter.

EPHEDRINE

Ephedrine occurs naturally in various plants. It was used in China for over 5000 years before being introduced into Western medicine in 1924 (*see* Chen and Schmidt, 1930). Prepared synthetically in 1927, it has since been used extensively for clinical conditions in which either peripheral or CNS actions of sympathomimetic drugs are desired. Its central actions are less pronounced than those of the amphetamines, which have therefore superseded ephedrine for all except peripheral effects. Ephedrine stimulates both α and β receptors and has clinical uses related to both types of action. The drug owes part of its peripheral action to release of norepinephrine, but it also has direct effects on receptors and exhibits substantial effects in reserpine-treated animals and man (Krogsgaard, 1956). Tachyphylaxis develops to its peripheral actions, and rapidly repeated doses become less effective, probably as a result of the depletion of norepinephrine stores.

Since ephedrine contains two asymmetrical carbon atoms, four compounds are possible. Only *l*-ephedrine and racemic ephedrine are commonly used clinically; their pharmacological properties and uses are essentially similar. The structure of ephedrine is depicted in Table 24–1.

Pharmacological Actions. Ephedrine differs from epinephrine mainly in its efficacy after oral administration, its much longer duration of action, its more pronounced central actions, and its much lower potency. *Cardiovascular effects* of ephedrine are in many ways similar to those of epinephrine, but they persist seven to ten times as long. The drug elevates the systolic and usually also the diastolic pressure in man, and pulse pressure increases. Pressor responses are due partly to vasoconstriction but mainly to cardiac stimulation, provided venous return is adequate. The heart rate may not be altered, but it increases if vagal reflexes are blocked. The force of myocardial contraction and cardiac output are augmented by the drug; the renal and splanchnic blood flows are decreased whereas the coronary, cerebral, and muscle blood flows are increased. The pressor responses to ephedrine are blocked by α-blocking agents, but reversal, if it occurs, is slight.

Bronchial muscle relaxation is less prominent but more sustained with ephedrine than with epinephrine. Consequently, ephedrine is of value only in milder cases of acute asthma and in chronic cases that need continued medication. *Mydriasis* occurs after local application of the drug to the eye. Reflexes to light are not abolished, accommodation is unaffected, and intraocular pressure is unchanged. Ephedrine and other sympathomimetics are of little use as mydriatics in the presence of inflammation. The drug is less effective in individuals who have heavily pigmented irides than in those in whom the iris is light colored, a difference attributed by Angenent and Koelle (1953) to a greater content of *o*-diphenol oxidase in heavily pigmented irides. Other smooth muscles are generally affected by ephedrine in the same manner as by epinephrine. However, the activity of the human *uterus* is usually reduced by ephedrine, regardless of the effect of epinephrine, and thus this agent has been used to relieve the pain of dysmenorrhea. Ephedrine is less effective than epinephrine in elevating the concentration of *blood sugar.* The *CNS effects* of ephedrine are similar to those of amphetamine but are considerably less marked.

Preparations, Administration, and Dosage. *Ephedrine Sulfate,* U.S.P., is the *l* isomer. It is available in 25- and 50-mg tablets and capsules and in a 4-mg/ml syrup; the oral dose varies from 15 to 50 mg. For continued medication small doses are given at 3- to 4-hour intervals. Sterile solutions (20, 25, and 50 mg/ml) are available; in hypotensive states, 15 to 50 mg may be given subcutaneously or, if a rapid response is necessary, 20 mg can be injected intravenously. Solutions of 1 and 3% in water and 1% in jelly are available for nasal mucosal decongestion, and aqueous solutions of 3 to 5% are applied to the eye to produce mydriasis.

Toxic Reactions. These are similar to the untoward reactions observed after epinephrine, with additional reactions referable to the CNS effects of ephedrine. Insomnia is common with continued medication, but it is readily counteracted by barbiturates. *Precautions* in the use of ephedrine are similar to those outlined for epinephrine and the amphetamines.

Therapeutic Uses. The main clinical applications of ephedrine are in *bronchospasm,* in *Stokes-Adams syndrome,* as a *nasal decongestant,* as a *mydriatic,* and in certain *allergic disorders.* The drug has also been employed as a *pressor* agent, particularly during spinal anesthesia, and for its central stimulant action in *narcolepsy.* These uses are discussed below in the therapeutic section of this chapter.

MEPHENTERMINE

Mephentermine is N-methyl-ω-phenyl-*tertiary*-butylamine (Table 24–1). It is one of several pressor agents currently used in various hypotensive conditions. Its duration of action is prolonged, pressor effects lasting 30 to 60 minutes after subcutaneous and up to 4 hours after intramuscular doses. Its peripheral actions and effects appear to be similar to those of methamphetamine, but its central actions are relatively feeble and of no clinical use. Mephentermine acts both directly and by release of endogenous norepinephrine. Cardiac contraction is enhanced, and cardiac output and systolic and diastolic pressures are usually increased. The change in heart rate is variable, depending

on the degree of vagal tone; large doses can depress the heart. The pressor response involves both increased cardiac output and peripheral vasoconstriction. In some cases the net vascular effect may be vasodilatation, which appears not to involve β receptors (Caldwell and Goldberg, 1970). Coronary blood flow is increased, forearm blood flow is reduced, and venous tone is increased. Marked mucosal vasoconstriction can be produced by local application of the drug. CNS effects may occur with large doses of mephentermine. These include drowsiness, weeping, incoherence, and convulsions, and rapidly disappear on withdrawal of the drug. (For references, *see* Aviado, 1959, 1970; Eckstein and Abboud, 1962; Zaimis, 1968.)

Preparations and Dosage. *Mephentermine Sulfate,* N.F. (WYAMINE), is available in sterile solution (15 and 30 mg/ml) for parenteral injection. Given *subcutaneously* or *intramuscularly* the dose is usually 10 to 30 mg. Slow *intravenous infusions* are also given, the rate being varied to produce the desired pressor effect. Oral tablets containing 12.5 or 25 mg and a nasal inhaler are also marketed.

Therapeutic Uses. Mephentermine is mainly used as a pressor agent in various *hypotensive states,* as discussed below in the therapeutic section of this chapter.

HYDROXYAMPHETAMINE

Hydroxyamphetamine, synthesized in Germany in 1913, came into clinical use only after reinvestigation 2 decades later (Alles, 1933; Alles and Prinzmetal, 1933). Its chemical structure differs from that of amphetamine only by the addition of a 4-OH group (*see* Table 24–1).

Pharmacological Actions. In many respects the actions of hydroxyamphetamine resemble those of ephedrine, with the exception that the drug almost entirely lacks CNS stimulant activity. The duration of action after oral or subcutaneous administration is from 90 to 120 minutes; after intravenous injection, 20 to 30 minutes.

Cardiovascular Actions. In man, as in other species, the drug elevates systolic and diastolic pressures; the increase is apparently due more to cardiac stimulation than to enhanced peripheral resistance, although the latter does occur. Heart rate is often reflexly slowed at the height of the pressor response, and cardiac irregularities, probably due to reflex vagal activity, have been reported. The cardiac stimulant action of the drug has been used to maintain an adequate ventricular rate in Stokes-Adams syndrome. Reflex vagal activity does not, of course, alter the effects of hydroxyamphetamine or other sympathomimetic drugs on the ventricle when complete heart block is present. In dogs, cardiac output and coronary blood flow increase, while cutaneous, splanchnic, and renal blood flows decrease. Pulmonary vessels are not constricted by the drug. The effects of hydroxyamphetamine on various vascular beds in man have not been established. Responses of cutaneous blood vessels in man are anomalous in that they are not effectively constricted by the drug, and systemic doses do not lower skin temperature. Hydroxyamphetamine constricts the vessels of the nasal mucosa, and this property has been used clinically. Venous constriction may play a role in causing the pressor response. (*See* Aviado, 1959, 1970.)

Smooth Muscle. Hydroxyamphetamine exerts both α and β activity on smooth muscle. Actions on α receptors are put to effective clinical use for mydriasis, by instillation of the drug in the eye, and for nasal decongestion, by application of nasal drops or a spray. The β-receptor activity of the compound is reflected in relaxation of bronchial muscle, but this is too feeble to be of value.

Preparations and Dosage. *Hydroxyamphetamine Hydrobromide,* N.F. (PAREDRINE), is available in 20-mg tablets and as a 1% ophthalmic solution. The oral dose in Stokes-Adams syndrome and orthostatic hypotension varies from 20 to 60 mg, three to five times daily.

Therapeutic Uses. The clinical applications, mainly in *hypotensive states,* in *Stokes-Adams syndrome,* as a *mydriatic,* and as a *nasal decongestant,* are discussed below in the therapeutic section of this chapter.

METARAMINOL

Metaraminol, 3-hydroxyphenylisopropanolamine (Table 24-1), is used almost exclusively for the treatment of hypotensive states. It has both direct and indirect actions and its overall effects are similar to those of norepinephrine, but it is much less potent

and has a more prolonged action. It lacks CNS stimulant effects. Metaraminol is absorbed after oral administration; however, for equal effects, oral doses must be five or six times greater than doses given intramuscularly or intravenously. The pressor effect of an intramuscular dose of 5 mg lasts for about 1½ hours.

Cardiovascular Actions. The cardiovascular actions in man are reflected in a sustained rise in systolic and diastolic pressures, almost entirely due to vasoconstriction and usually accompanied by a marked reflex bradycardia. Occasionally sinus arrhythmia also occurs. In normotensive subjects, cardiac output is unchanged or may decrease slightly, but the force of myocardial contraction is enhanced. Cardiac output increases strikingly when slowing of the heart is prevented by atropine. Increased cardiac output may play a larger role in patients with hypotension and shock, in which conditions the drug increases cardiac output as well as peripheral resistance. Metaraminol increases venous tone and decreases renal and cerebral blood flows, the latter even when blood pressure is raised as much as 40%. In dogs, limb and splanchnic blood flows are also decreased and coronary blood flow is increased, but these effects have not yet been confirmed in man. Pulmonary vasoconstriction occurs in man, and the pulmonary blood pressure is elevated by the drug even when cardiac output is reduced. (*See* Aviado, 1959, 1970; Eckstein and Abboud, 1962; Zaimis, 1968.)

Preparations and Dosage. *Metaraminol Bitartrate,* U.S.P. (ARAMINE), is available in 1-ml ampuls and 10-ml vials as a sterile solution (10 mg/ml) for intramuscular injection, usually in a dose of 5 to 10 mg, or, after suitable dilution, for intravenous infusion. The rate of administration is regulated according to the individual's response to the drug. Subcutaneous injections should be avoided since tissue sloughing may occur.

Therapeutic Uses. The principal use of metaraminol is as a pressor agent in certain *hypotensive states,* the treatment of which is discussed below in the therapeutic section of this chapter.

PHENYLEPHRINE

Phenylephrine differs chemically from epinephrine only in lacking an OH in the 4 position on the benzene ring (Table 24-1).

It was first studied by Barger and Dale (1910), but was not used clinically until years later when it was found to have greater potency than other monohydroxyl derivatives. Phenylephrine is a powerful α-receptor stimulant with little effect on the β receptors of the heart. A direct action on receptors accounts for the greater part of its effects, only a small part being due to its ability to release norepinephrine. Central stimulant action is minimal.

Cardiovascular Actions. The predominant actions of phenylephrine are on the *cardiovascular system.* Intravenous, subcutaneous, or oral administration causes a rise in systolic and diastolic pressures in man and other species. Responses are more sustained than those to epinephrine, lasting 20 minutes after intravenous and as long as 50 minutes after subcutaneous injection. Accompanying the pressor response to phenylephrine is a marked reflex bradycardia that can be blocked by atropine; after atropine, large doses of the drug increase the heart rate only slightly. In man, cardiac output is slightly decreased and peripheral resistance is considerably increased. Circulation time is slightly prolonged, and venous pressure is slightly increased; venous constriction is not marked. Most vascular beds are constricted, and renal, splanchnic, cutaneous, and limb blood flows are reduced but coronary blood flow is increased. Pulmonary vessels are constricted, and pulmonary arterial pressure is raised. The drug is a powerful vasoconstrictor, with properties very similar to those of norepinephrine but almost completely lacking the chronotropic and inotropic actions on the heart. Cardiac irregularities are seen only very rarely even with large doses, and the reflex slowing is sufficient to permit use of the drug to end attacks of paroxysmal atrial tachycardia. (*See* Aviado, 1959, 1970; Eckstein and Abboud, 1962.)

Preparations, Administration, and Dosage. *Phenylephrine Hydrochloride,* U.S.P. (ISOPHRIN, NEO-SYNEPHRINE), is the *l* isomer. It is available as a sterile solution (10 mg/ml) for parenteral use, an elixir (1 mg/ml), various nasal (0.125, 0.25, 0.5, and 1.0%) and ophthalmic (2.5 and 10%) solutions, and a viscous ophthalmic solution (10%). For children, the weaker solutions should be used because of the possibility of toxic effects. Roughly equipressor doses are 0.8 mg intravenously, 5 mg subcutaneously or intramuscularly, and 250 mg orally. However, absorption after oral administration is unreliable. For treatment of hypotension during spinal anesthesia, the usual dose is 5 to 10 mg, administered intramuscularly. The rate of intravenous infusion in hypotensive states should be regulated according to the patient's response.

Therapeutic Uses. Phenylephrine is used mainly as a *nasal decongestant,* a pressor agent in *hypotensive states,* a *mydriatic,* a local vasoconstrictor (0.005%) in solutions of local anesthetics, and in the relief of *paroxysmal atrial tachycardia.* These uses are discussed below in the therapeutic section of this chapter.

METHOXAMINE

Methoxamine is β-hydroxy-β-(2,5-dimethoxyphenyl) isopropylamine (Table 24–1). Its pharmacological properties are almost exclusively those characteristic of α-receptor stimulation. The outstanding effect is an increase in blood pressure due entirely to vasoconstriction. The drug has virtually no stimulant action on the heart and lacks β-receptor action on smooth muscle. It causes little or no CNS stimulation.

Cardiovascular Actions. Methoxamine, given intravenously or intramuscularly in man, causes a rise in systolic and diastolic blood pressures that persists for 60 to 90 minutes. The pressor effect is due almost exclusively to an increase in peripheral resistance. Cardiac output is decreased or unchanged. Renal blood flow is reduced in man to a greater extent than after equipressor doses of norepinephrine or metaraminol. Cerebral, splanchnic, and limb blood flows are reduced in dogs, and coronary blood flow is unchanged; whether the effects are similar in man is not known. In man, the venous pressure increases, but the constrictor action on forearm veins is feeble. Methoxamine has no significant stimulant action on the heart, and does not increase the ventricular rate in patients with heart block. Reflex bradycardia is prominent, and, therefore, the drug is used clinically to relieve attacks of paroxysmal atrial tachycardia. When the vagal effects are blocked by atropine, methoxamine often slows the heart slightly. This is probably due to a direct action on α receptors. Injection of the drug into the artery leading to the sinus node slows the heart, an effect blocked by phentolamine (James *et al.,* 1968). Methoxamine does not appear to precipitate cardiac arrhythmias. In contrast to epinephrine, methoxamine prolongs ventricular muscle action potentials and refractory period and slows A-V conduction (Gilbert *et al.,* 1958). Tachyphylaxis to the drug occurs in experimental animals, but has not been reported in man. (*See* Aviado, 1959, 1970; Eckstein and Abboud, 1962; Zaimis, 1968.)

In man, pressor doses of methoxamine cause pilomotor stimulation and often a desire to micturate. Occasionally tingling of the extremities and a feeling of coldness follow intravenous injection of the drug.

Preparations, Administration, and Dosage. *Methoxamine Hydrochloride,* U.S.P. (VASOXYL), is available as a solution (10 or 20 mg/ml) for intramuscular injection. The dose varies from 10 to 20 mg. Intravenous injections of 5 to 10 mg may also be given with the precautions properly accorded to intravenous injections of sympathomimetic amines.

Therapeutic Uses. Methoxamine is almost solely used as a pressor agent in *hypotensive states* and to end attacks of *paroxysmal atrial tachycardia.* These conditions are discussed below in the therapeutic section of this chapter.

METHOXYPHENAMINE

Methoxyphenamine, β-(*o*-methoxyphenyl) isopropylmethylamine, differs from methamphetamine only in having a methoxy substituent in the 2 position on the benzene ring (Table 24–1), but its pharmacological properties differ greatly. Its main sympathomimetic action is on β receptors of smooth muscle. By this action, the drug causes *bronchodilatation,* its usual clinical use. Its bronchodilator effect is greater than that of ephedrine, and the accompanying cardiovascular effects are considerably less. The α-receptor and central stimulant actions of the drug are minimal. Methoxyphenamine also exhibits weak antihistaminic properties.

Preparations and Dosage. *Methoxyphenamine hydrochloride* (ORTHOXINE) is marketed in 100-mg tablets and in a syrup (10 mg/ml). The usual oral dose is 50 to 100 mg, repeated every 3 or 4 hours if necessary.

Therapeutic Uses. Methoxyphenamine is used mainly in mild cases of *asthma* and other *allergic conditions,* as discussed below.

SELECTIVE β_2-RECEPTOR STIMULANTS

Various drugs that act selectively on β_2 receptors have been developed, primarily for the treatment of *bronchial asthma.* These include *metaproterenol (orciprenaline;* ALUPENT, METAPREL), *salbutamol (albuterol;* VENTOLIN), *terbutaline* (BRICANYL), *fenoterol* (BEROTEC), *ritodrine* (PREMAR), *isoetharine* (DILABRON), *quinterenol (quinprenaline),* and *soterenol.* Their chemical structures are shown in Table 24–1. Through their specificity for β_2 receptors they relax smooth muscle of the bronchi, uterus, and vascular supply to skeletal muscle, but have much less stimulant action on the heart than does isoproterenol. Thus, in asthmatic patients salbutamol and isoproterenol are approximately equipotent as bronchodilators when given by aerosol, whereas ten times the dose of salbutamol is required to cause equal cardioacceleration. Metaproterenol is somewhat less selective than salbutamol for β_2 receptors, but cardiac stimulation is sufficiently limited to give the drug a considerable therapeutic advantage over isoproterenol. The drugs cause little change in blood pressure. Side effects include nervousness, weakness, and drowsiness; tremor is common, particularly after oral administration. Inhaled as aerosols they act as promptly and efficiently as does isoproterenol, and remain effective for about 4 hours. With the exception of isoetharine (a catecholamine) they are resistant to COMT; the details of their disposal are not fully known, but some form inactive conjugates. For example, both free and conjugated salbutamol are excreted in the urine. The proportion of the excreted conjugate is much greater after administration orally or as a metered aerosol than after administration intravenously or by bronchoscope, indicating both that metabolism takes place in the gastrointestinal tract and that much of an aerosol is swallowed (Evans *et al.,* 1973). (*See* Lewis, 1971.)

Metaproterenol, ritodrine, and salbutamol have been used successfully by continuous intravenous infusion to *delay delivery in premature labor.* Side effects are more prominent with the large doses required and include nervousness, tremor, headache, nausea and vomiting, hypotension, and maternal and fetal tachycardia (*see* Liggins and Vaughan, 1973).

Metaproterenol is available in the United States as 20-mg oral tablets and as a metered aerosol (0.65 mg per dose). In other countries, the metered aerosol is available as 0.75 mg per dose; other marketed preparations of the drug include a syrup (2 mg/ml), a 5% inhalant solution, and a sterile solution (0.5 mg/ml) for parenteral use. Usual doses are 20 mg orally, four times daily; or 0.5 mg intramuscularly, repeated after 30 minutes if necessary. *Salbutamol* is widely used in Europe and Canada as a metered aerosol (0.1 mg per dose), and is under clinical investigation in the United States. Several other selective β_2-receptor stimulants are also available in Europe either as aerosols or oral tablets, including a slow-release tablet of isoetharine. None appears to present significant advantages over salbutamol.

NYLIDRIN AND ISOXSUPRINE

The chemical structures of these agents are shown in Table 24-1. Both are well absorbed when given orally, and have a long duration of action. Their main effects are dilatation of blood vessels in skeletal muscle and cardiac stimulation. The actions thus follow the pattern of β-receptor stimulation but the vasodilatation is resistant to doses of propranolol that block vasodilatation due to isoproterenol. Blood flow in muscle increases and peripheral resistance falls. Heart rate and cardiac output increase. Systolic pressure usually rises slightly and diastolic pressure falls; mean arterial pressure changes little. Cerebral blood flow may increase slightly. *Disturbing side effects* occasionally occur, including nervousness, trembling, weakness, dizziness, palpitation, nausea, and vomiting. For its uterine relaxant action, isoxsuprine has been used to treat *dysmenorrhea* and *premature labor,* but its usefulness in these conditions has not been established. Both drugs have been proposed for the treatment of peripheral vascular disorders. These uses are discussed later in this chapter.

Preparations, Administration, and Dosage. *Nylidrin Hydrochloride,* N.F. (ARLIDIN), is available in 6- and 12-mg oral tablets. *Isoxsuprine Hydrochloride,* N.F. (VASODILAN), is marketed as 10- and 20-mg oral tablets. The usual doses are 3 to 12 mg, three or four times daily, for nylidrin; and 10 to 20 mg, three or four times daily, for isoxsuprine. Isoxsuprine is available in a sterile solution (5 mg/ml) for intramuscular injection; the dose is 5 to 10 mg.

MISCELLANEOUS SYMPATHO-MIMETIC DRUGS

Several sympathomimetic drugs are used primarily as vasoconstrictors for local application to the nasal mucous membrane or the eye. Their structures are depicted in Tables 24-1 and 24-2. They vary from simple aliphatic amines to complex imidazoline derivatives. Their nonproprietary and trade names as well as available preparations are as follows: *Propylhexedrine,* N.F. (BENZEDREX), nasal inhaler (250 mg); *Tuaminoheptane Sulfate,* N.F. (TUAMINE), 1% nasal solution and a nasal inhaler (325 mg); *Naphazoline Hydrochloride,* U.S.P. (PRIVINE), 0.05% nebulizer or nasal solution and 0.1% ophthalmic solution; *Tetrahydrozoline Hydrochloride,* U.S.P., 0.05 and 0.1% nasal solutions (TYZINE) and 0.05% ophthalmic solution (VISINE); *Oxymetazoline Hydrochloride,* U.S.P. (AFRIN), 0.05% nasal solution; *Xylometazoline Hydrochloride,* N.F. (OTRIVIN), 0.05 and 0.1% nasal solutions.

Cyclopentamine Hydrochloride, N.F. (CLOPANE), is available as a 0.5 or 1.0% nasal solution. It also has been used as a pressor agent and causes little central excitation. The intramuscular dose is 25 mg.

Phenylpropanolamine Hydrochloride, N.F. (PROPADRINE), shares the pharmacological properties of ephedrine and is approximately equal in potency except that it causes less CNS stimulation. The drug is available in 25- and 50-mg capsules and in an elixir (4 mg/ml). It is also the ingredient of numerous proprietary mixtures that are marketed for the oral treatment of nasal and sinus congestion, usually in combination with an antihistaminic drug.

THERAPEUTIC USES OF SYM-PATHOMIMETIC DRUGS

As a result of the ubiquitous distribution of sympathetic nerves and adrenergic receptor systems in the body and their involvement in a variety of clinical disorders, and because sympathomimetic agents not only exhibit α- and β-receptor activity but also exert, in several instances, prominent CNS excitatory effects, it is not surprising that drugs in this class have a large number of important therapeutic uses. These clinical applications are considered in the following pages.

Use of Vascular Effects. *Control of Hemorrhage.* The vasoconstrictor action of epinephrine may control superficial hemorrhage from skin and mucous membranes when the drug is applied topically as a spray or on cotton or gauze pledgets. It is effective only against bleeding from arterioles and capillaries and does not control venous oozing or hemorrhage from larger vessels.

Decongestion of Mucous Membranes. Sympathomimetic amines with α-receptor action cause marked vasoconstriction and blanching when applied to nasal and pharyngeal mucosal surfaces. They are therefore useful in the treatment of mucosal congestion accompanying *hay fever, allergic rhinitis, acute coryza, sinusitis,* and other respiratory conditions. The short duration of action of many of the amines, such as epinephrine, limits their value in shrinking the nasal mucosa, and longer-acting congeners are more commonly used in these conditions. Some of the sympathomimetic amines more widely used for nasal decongestion are indicated as *N* in Table 24–1. All have the disadvantage that their use may be followed by "aftercongestion" and that prolonged use often results in chronic rhinitis. Some (*e.g.,* naphazoline) also irritate the nasal mucosa, causing a brief but sharp stinging sensation when first applied. Sufficient absorption of any of the imidazoline derivatives (Table 24–2) may cause CNS depression, leading to coma and marked reduction in body temperature, especially in infants. These drugs should not be used in young children. Some nasal decongestants and their usual concentrations as nasal drops or spray are as follow: amphetamine, 1%; ephedrine, 1%; hydroxyamphetamine, 1%; mephentermine, 0.5%; methoxamine, 0.5%; and phenylephrine, 0.125, 0.25, and 0.5%. Others are described above, under miscellaneous sympathomimetic drugs.

Epinephrine is used in many surgical procedures on the nose, throat, and larynx, to shrink the mucosa and improve visualization by limiting hemorrhage. Since epinephrine is relatively nonirritating, it is especially suitable for use in treatment of congestion of the conjunctiva.

The efficacy of locally applied sympathomimetic vasoconstrictors in shrinking the nasal mucosa has led to the use of amines that may have this effect when given orally. Since the vessels of the nasal mucosa have not been shown to be more sensitive than most other vessels to sympathomimetic drugs, doses of orally administered sympathomimetics large enough to afford relief from nasal congestion will be expected to constrict other vascular beds and to raise the blood pressure. Ephedrine and pseudoephedrine have been given orally as nasal decongestants; their effects on nasal congestion due to colds are not of much consequence, but *allergic rhinitis* often responds well. While they do not raise blood pressure to any marked extent in doses that have this decongestant effect, they redistribute blood flow and cause cardiac stimulation. Several oral preparations promoted for the relief of colds and other upper respiratory conditions contain a sympathomimetic amine in combination with a variety of other agents (*e.g.,* antihistamines, antimuscarinic drugs, antipyretic-analgesics, caffeine, antitussives). Benefit from these blunderbuss preparations depends largely on the effects of the other drugs. In addition, the placebo effect in improving the patient's feeling of well-being should not be underestimated. No convincing evidence of benefit from oral use of sympathomimetics to relieve nasal congestion in colds has yet been presented.

Use with Local Anesthetics. Epinephrine is widely used in concentrations of 1:100,000 to 1:20,000 in solutions of local anesthetics. It slows absorption of the local anesthetic by local vasoconstriction and thus prolongs the duration of anesthesia, decreases the amount of anesthetic needed, and lessens the danger of systemic toxicity. Furthermore, hemorrhage from surgical procedures in the area of infiltration is decreased. However, careful surgical hemostasis is more necessary than ever because small vessels that have been cut but are constricted by epinephrine may escape detection. Stronger concentrations may cause tissue damage from ischemia. The total amount of epinephrine injected with a local anesthetic solution should not exceed 1 mg. Small amounts of epinephrine can also be added to the local anesthetic solution injected intrathecally for spinal anesthesia. Here also it delays absorption of the local anesthetic and intensifies and prolongs anesthesia. Since epinephrine is the most potent α-receptor stimulant, lower concentrations of epinephrine than of any other sympathomimetic amine are effective. Nordefrine, methoxamine, and phenylephrine are the usual alternatives to epinephrine. The combined use of epinephrine and local anesthetics is further discussed in Chapter 20.

Hypotension. The use of sympathomimetic amines to relieve hypotension occurring during spinal anesthesia or from overdosage of antihypertensive agents has a rational basis in temporarily constricting resistance vessels relaxed by release from adrenergic vasoconstrictor tone. Agents with predominantly α-receptor action are clearly the most suitable for this purpose, but levarterenol is not frequently used because its intravenous administration demands attention that is not necessary with longer-acting sympathomimetics that can be given intramuscularly.

Given before *spinal anesthesia,* intramuscular injections of ephedrine, hydroxyamphetamine, mephentermine, metaraminol, methamphetamine, methoxamine, or phenylephrine are often effective in preventing a substantial fall in blood pressure (*see* Aviado, 1959). This is not recommended as a routine procedure, but only in those cases where a significant fall in blood pressure is predictable. Where hypotension is marked in spite of the initial prophylactic injection, a second intramuscular dose may be required to restore blood pressure. However, if the operative conditions permit, the blood pressure may usually be restored to an acceptable level without drugs by tilting the operating table to elevate the legs and thereby improve the venous return to the heart. Persistent hypotension during operation usually indicates hypovolemia and should be treated by replacement of the circulating blood volume with blood or plasma volume expanders. Treatment with sympathomimetics is unwise in cases of hypotension occurring in patients under *general anesthesia* with cyclopropane, halothane, and other drugs that sensitize the heart to the arrhythmic action. Even the feeble cardiac-stimulant action of phenylephrine may then be enough to precipitate ventricular arrhythmias. If administration of a pressor drug appears to be imperative, the choice of a sympathomimetic should be limited to one with minimal cardiac excitatory actions, such as phenylephrine or methoxamine. Methoxamine has been reported to inhibit the development of cardiac arrhythmias, perhaps by a β-blocking action.

Administration of sympathomimetic agents for their pressor effect may be a useful *emergency measure* until other therapy can be instituted in certain hypotensive states (*e.g.,* in acute hemorrhage). Sympathomimetics may be used to raise the blood pressure and sustain the coronary and cerebral circulation until measures can be taken to restore an adequate circulating blood volume. However, this therapy must be regarded as only a temporary expedient that can obscure the extent of blood volume replacement required and can in itself cause loss of fluid from the vascular compartment. Vasopressor therapy can thus increase the risk of further circulatory deterioration.

The release of large amounts of catecholamines during operation on patients with *pheochromocytoma* can lead to a considerable decrease in the circulating blood volume, and the blood pressure may drop precipitously as soon as the tumor has been removed. Levarterenol infusion has been used to sustain the blood pressure postoperatively, but adequate fluid-volume replacement appears to be more rational therapy. Alternatively, the loss of circulating volume can be largely prevented and the postoperative fall in pressure much reduced or eliminated by inhibiting the vasoconstriction due to released catecholamines with an α-adrenergic blocking agent (*see* Chapter 26).

The blood pressure of patients with *orthostatic hypotension* due to various factors, including neurological diseases such as syringomyelia and tabes dorsalis, may be supported by treatment orally with ephedrine, amphetamine, or other long-acting pressor sympathomimetic agents. However, responses are highly variable and control of the blood pressure in these conditions remains a very difficult problem.

Shock. Intravenous infusions of levarterenol or of other sympathomimetics have been widely used in the treatment of shock associated with trauma, hemorrhage, septicemia, or myocardial infarction. This treatment is directed toward raising the blood pressure on the assumption that this will improve nutrition of vital organs. The rationale, however, is questionable. Shock of other than cardiogenic etiology is usually characterized by a relative deficiency in circulating blood volume, and compensatory mechanisms will have already initiated intense peripheral vasoconstriction. Renal and splanchnic blood flows are already much reduced, and further vasoconstriction in these regions by the action of a sympathomimetic drug can seriously impair the blood supply to the kidney, liver, and other vital organs. In addition, it is probably of importance that sympathomimetic vasoconstriction can itself reduce circulating blood volume. Continuous infusion of levarterenol in animals can cause lethal shock, and the injudicious use of this drug or other sympathomimetic agents in man can produce the same effect (Spoerel *et al.*, 1964). The first consideration in the treatment of most types of shock should be adequate replacement of blood volume; this tends to reduce sympathetic tone and restore adequate circulation to vital areas.

Isoproterenol, which activates β_1 and β_2 receptors, has the advantage of improving circulation by increasing cardiac output while producing dilatation in essentially all arteriolar beds; when infused at a rate of approximately 5 μg per minute, the net effect in patients with shock is frequently an increase in arterial pressure accompanied by a fall in central venous pressure. However, patients must be monitored constantly, and the infusion terminated if the heart rate rises to a dangerous level or if any sign of arrhythmia develops. Infusion of dopamine may improve circulation in the compromised mesenteric and renal vascular beds by dilatation of these vessels. Administration of an α-adrenergic blocking agent may supplement fluid therapy in some cases by further reducing adrenergic vasoconstriction. This aspect of shock therapy is discussed in Chapter 26. Successful results in treating shock with levarterenol or other vasopressor agents are the subject of many reports; however, assessment of such results is notoriously difficult, and it is seldom clear whether survival was due to or in spite of this treatment (*see* Nickerson, 1962; Hardaway, 1968; Aviado, 1970).

Shock following *myocardial infarction* differs in that reduced cardiac output is probably primary and not, as in other types of shock, secondary to inadequate venous return. A suitable vasopressor agent can raise the blood pressure in most cases of myocardial shock and may somewhat improve survival, although the mortality rate remains high. The elevated blood pressure increases coronary flow and presumably the nutrition of uninvolved myocardium and areas of marginal viability. However, it also increases the myocardial work required for any given level of cardiac output, and the effect of sympathomimetic vasopressor agents on the balance between these two opposing factors doubtless varies with patients. Sympathomimetic agents that stimulate the heart are generally agreed to be the most appropriate therapeutic agents, but myocardial infarction predisposes to the arrhythmic action of these drugs. Isoproterenol, which stimulates the heart but lacks vasoconstrictor action, is less effective in increasing coronary perfusion than are levarterenol and metaraminol, which have both actions. Although isoproterenol may increase cardiac output, myocardial lactate production increases, an indication of greater cardiac hypoxia. With levarterenol, lactate production decreases. Dopamine has also been used, but it has not presented substantial advantages in the treatment of shock caused by myocardial infarction. In contrast, dopamine has given encouraging results in cardiogenic shock following cardiac surgery; with dopamine therapy several patients unresponsive to other sympathomimetic amines have recovered, although prolonged infusion was often needed, in one patient for 14 days (Rosenblum and Frieden, 1972). Metabolic acidosis due to poor tissue perfusion after myocardial infarction should be corrected since it adds to the cardiac depression and inhibits the response to sympathomimetic vasoconstrictor drugs. For patients with inadequate venous return, a plasma volume expander may also be used, with due care to avoid circulatory overload leading to acute heart failure. Despite all measures, therapy of myocardial shock has only limited success and the mortality rate remains very high. (*See* Kuhn, 1970.)

Peripheral Vascular Disease. Nylidrin and isoxsuprine, which are long-acting, orally effective sympathomimetic amines with predominant β-receptor action, have been used in the treatment of intermittent claudication due to peripheral vascular disease. Although both drugs increase the resting blood flow of skeletal muscle in normal persons, clinical results have been disappointing, probably due to the fact that control of the blood flow in skeletal muscle normally depends largely on dilatation of the blood vessels by locally produced metabolites. Such metabolites maximally dilate the blood vessels before symptoms of claudication appear. There is no evidence that blood vessels maximally dilated by local factors can be further dilated by sympathomimetics. In addition, only those vessels least affected by the pathological changes in diseases such as arteriosclerosis obliterans can be expected to dilate, and benefit can be obtained only when there is an element of arteriolar spasm. Thus, in a study by Caliva and associates (1959), doses of nylidrin that normally increased blood flow in the calf by 33% had no effect on the blood flow in eight patients with arteriosclerosis obliterans; in patients with venous disease and segmental atherosclerosis, the flow at rest was increased but there was no improvement in tolerance to walking. There is no rational basis for the use of these drugs in conditions where the blood supply to the skin is reduced, since their effects on cutaneous blood flow are negligible.

The use of nylidrin has been proposed to increase cerebral blood flow in cerebrovascular disease. However, it is not likely that severely sclerotic cerebral vessels are capable of dilatation. In addition, the degree of dilatation of cerebral vessels depends largely on local factors that will already have induced the greatest dilatation of which these vessels are capable. No evidence of improvement due to nylidrin has been found in patients with longstanding hemiplegia or in recent cerebral infarction.

Use of Reflex Cardiac Effects of Pressor Drugs. Attacks of *paroxysmal atrial* or *nodal tachycardia* may be ended by reflex vagal discharge caused by pressor responses to phenylephrine or methoxamine, drugs without significant cardiac excitatory action. The dose, given slowly intravenously, should not raise the blood pressure above 160 mm Hg; for phenylephrine, the dose may be 0.15 to 0.8 mg; for methoxamine, 3 to 5 mg. A short-acting anticholinesterase agent such as edrophonium may be safer for this purpose (*see* Chapter 22).

Use of Cardiac Effects. *Cardiac Arrest and Heart Block with Syncopal Seizures.* Syncope in *Stokes-Adams syndrome,* generally occurring at the transition from partial to complete A-V block, may be due to ventricular standstill or to prefibrillatory rhythm leading to ventricular fibrillation. Epinephrine and isoproterenol are of value in prophylaxis and symptomatic treatment of the attacks, but physical measures should be applied first in the acute attack. Circulation may sometimes be restored by a precordial blow followed by external cardiac compression or, if readily at hand, by an electrical pacemaker or defibrillator. Next, cardiac puncture with or without intracardiac injection of epinephrine may be effective and, as a last resort, thoracotomy and manual cardiac massage may rarely be required. External cardiac massage by compression of the chest can maintain circulation for considerable periods. To restore the intrinsic cardiac rhythm once some circulation has been established, intravenous infusion of epinephrine or isoproterenol may be necessary. These catecholamines are likely to precipitate ventricular fibrillation if injudiciously used in patients

with prefibrillatory rhythm and, therefore, extreme care should be taken in their *intravenous* administration. When the indications are less urgent, repeated subcutaneous injections of epinephrine, intramuscular injections of epinephrine in oil, or sublingual doses of isoproterenol may give the desired results. Epinephrine has been used to maintain an adequate ventricular rate (30 to 40 beats or more per minute) for as long as a week, but other sympathomimetic amines are more suitable for prolonged and prophylactic treatment. Isoproterenol can be given sublingually or in sustained-action oral tablets, but absorption, especially after its oral administration, is unreliable. Ephedrine and hydroxyamphetamine are both orally effective and longer acting. Either can prevent recurrence of syncopal attacks. *However, drug therapy is now regarded as a temporary measure only to be used until an electrical pacemaker can be fitted to supply optimal and reliable ventricular regulation.*

The problem of reviving patients apparently dead from *drowning, electrocution,* or *anesthetic accidents* is not substantially different from that of the syncope in Stokes-Adams syndrome, and the same principles apply. In all cases of cardiac arrest, hypoxia is an important additional factor necessitating adequate artificial ventilation. Anesthetic cardiac accidents may be due either to asystole or to ventricular fibrillation. Since the heart is sensitized to the arrhythmic action of epinephrine by many anesthetics, the drug may convert asystole to ventricular fibrillation. Physical measures, especially the use of an electrical pacemaker, which should be available in the operating room, are obviously more appropriate. Electrical countershock followed by mechanical compression of the heart is indicated in ventricular fibrillation. Although the use of epinephrine in anesthetic accidents is theoretically inadvisable in cardiac arrest or after defibrillation, many patients have recovered when the drug has been administered. It is impossible to decide whether recovery is due to the drug, to mechanical stimulation of the myocardium by the needle prick, or to other procedures simultaneously applied. In patients who do not respond to other measures, it is not unreasonable to resort to the cardiac excitatory action of epinephrine. (*See* Bellet, 1960; Zoll and Linenthal, 1963; and many others.)

Acute Cardiac Failure. The treatment of acute cardiac failure does not include the use of epinephrine or other sympathomimetic drugs. The drug treatment of the acute attack of left-heart failure characterized by *"cardiac asthma"* or *pulmonary edema* is primarily with morphine, aminophylline, highly potent diuretics, digoxin, and oxygen. Emergency treatment with epinephrine to stimulate the heart should be avoided, since this procedure increases the demand of the heart for oxygen. A more effective and rational emergency measure is the application of venous tourniquets to the limbs, thereby reducing venous return and decreasing the load on the heart. A mistaken diagnosis of dyspnea due to bronchial asthma has sometimes led to treatment of cardiac asthma (dyspnea due to left ventricular failure) with epinephrine, in some cases with benefit. This can be expected only when there is a degree of bronchospasm superimposed on the basic pulmonary vascular congestion due to the cardiac failure and cannot be relied on as a basis for routine treatment of acute cardiac failure with epinephrine.

Uses in Allergic Disorders. *Bronchial Asthma.* Epinephrine, isoproterenol, and the newer selective β_2-receptor stimulants are the mainstay of the symptomatic treatment of respiratory distress due to bronchospasm. Relief is due to the β_2-receptor action that relaxes smooth muscle; with epinephrine, a contributory factor may be an α-receptor action that constricts bronchial mucosal vessels, thereby reducing congestion and edema. Acute asthmatic attacks are usually relieved within 3 to 5 minutes after subcutaneous injection of 0.2 to 0.5 mg of epinephrine or after oral inhalation of a 1% solution of epinephrine, a 0.5 or 1% solution of isoproterenol, or a 5% solution of metaproterenol from a nebulizer. The decrease in vital capacity and the increase in residual air characteristic of these attacks are rapidly corrected, and maximal breathing capacity and velocity of expiration increase. Although airway obstruction is relieved, the lowered Pa_{O_2} is often not increased and may even fall further, indicating that the ventilation-perfusion disturbance is not remedied. Pressurized aerosols of these drugs and the more selective β_2 stimulants such as salbutamol or terbutaline are also rapidly effective. The latter drugs have the advantage that they are powerful long-acting bronchodilators with little action on the heart and are therefore less likely to cause the palpitations that are troublesome with the use of epinephrine and isoproterenol. In addition, they do not lower Pa_{O_2}.

Whatever the drug or route of administration, the smallest dose affording relief should be used. Inhalations of isoproterenol or epinephrine may have to be repeated at intervals of 2 or 3 minutes, and subcutaneous injections of epinephrine at 15- to 20-minute intervals until relief occurs. If symptoms recur, massage of the site of injection may give relief by enhancing absorption of the drug. With the longer-acting β_2-receptor stimulants, 1 or 2 inhalations are often sufficient and repetition is unnecessary for 4 hours. *Very slow intravenous infusion* of epinephrine has been used in patients who failed to respond to subcutaneous injection, but *this procedure is hazardous* and presents no advantage. Tolerance to injected epinephrine may occur after repeated use, and larger doses are then needed. In these patients inhalation of epinephrine or another β-receptor stimulant may prove effective.

Complete refractoriness to epinephrine and isoproterenol is not uncommon after protracted therapy in severe cases and in status asthmaticus, especially when bronchospasm is associated with the presence of viscid mucus plugs in the bronchi. Epinephrine reduces bronchial secretion and may make these plugs more viscid and difficult to dislodge. Measures to facilitate removal of mucus plugs are important in these cases and include expectorants and increased hydration of the patient to liquefy the plugs, and mechanical removal of retained secretion by bronchoscopic suction. Suitable chemotherapy is used to combat respiratory infection when this common precipitating cause is present.

Pressurized aerosols containing isoproterenol or epinephrine became readily available about 1960 and are widely accepted as effective and convenient therapy. Some experts believe that the delivery of the dose is so rapid that the drug is distributed throughout only a part of the inspired air and some regions of the lungs are not reached; this objection would apply less to the slower delivery by manually propelled inhalant solutions. In many countries, but not in North America, the mortality from asthma increased through the 1960s, an increase coinciding with the growing use of pressurized aerosols. Since attention was drawn to this association the mortality rate has dropped, probably because warnings have been given against undisciplined use of such aerosols. Stolley (1972) pointed out that in countries that escaped the increased mortality the aerosol solution was much weaker than the aerosol available in the affected countries. The cause of death is not clear. It is possible that rapidly repeated use of the aerosol after refractoriness has developed leads to vasodilatation, fall in the ventilation-perfusion ratio, and a fatal lowering of Pa_{O_2} and increase in Pa_{CO_2}. A more likely alternative is the toxicity of the chlorofluorinated hydrocarbons used as propellants; these compounds can produce bronchoconstriction, cardiac arrhythmias, and sensitization of the myocardium to the arrhythmogenic action of epinephrine and isoproterenol (*see* Taylor and Harris, 1970; Reinhardt *et al.,* 1971; Chapter 44). At present, the use of pressurized aerosols of this type should be discouraged.

In cases of *refractory asthma,* intravenous administration of aminophylline is sometimes useful, but intravenous injection of adrenocorticosteroids is often required to break into the severe asthmatic cycle. Because of the serious side effects of prolonged use of such steroids (*see* Chapter 70), their administration should be discontinued as early as practicable; fortunately, such discontinuation is possible in virtually all cases. Withdrawal from steroids may become exceptionally difficult if delayed. Susceptibility to small doses of epinephrine and other sympathomimetic amines is usually restored once repeated and progressive bronchial relaxation has been achieved. For prolonged relief from bronchospasm, usually in chronic asthma, *epinephrine in oil* is sometimes used, and a dose of 1 ml may permit a night's sleep free from attacks. The longer-acting oral sympathomimetics with prominent β-receptor action are more commonly used to prevent attacks. Ephedrine, 20 to 50 mg given at 4-hour intervals, is an effective prophylactic. Methoxyphenamine and metaproterenol are effective substitutes without significant CNS activity. The CNS stimulant action of ephedrine tends to cause wakefulness and irritability, and a barbiturate is commonly given in addition. Many drug mixtures have been proposed for the treatment of asthma; they have the obvious disadvantage of all mixtures in that the dose of each ingredient cannot be individually regulated to the patient's specific and changing requirements.

Miscellaneous Allergic Disorders. Epinephrine is the drug of first choice to relieve the symptoms of acute hypersensitivity reactions to drugs (*e.g.,* penicillin) and of other acute reactions to sera and other allergens. A subcutaneous injection of epinephrine rapidly relieves itching, urticaria, and swelling of lips, eyelids, and tongue, and the drug may be life-saving when edema of the glottis threatens suffocation. Only epinephrine is administered to relieve these acute reactions since it acts particularly rapidly; however, ephedrine, having a more prolonged action, can be used for the continued treatment of allergic disorders, such as hay fever. Epinephrine may also give symptomatic relief in certain forms of eczematoid dermatitis. When skin tests are performed for hypersensitivity to various foods, drugs, pollens, or other allergens, epinephrine should always be at hand to control acute untoward reactions. If chronic medication with ephedrine is being used for allergic conditions, the drug should not be given for at least 12 hours before sensitivity tests are made; otherwise, positive reactions may be prevented. When conjunctival tests for serum or drug hypersensitivity are made, epinephrine solution instilled into the eye readily controls the local discomfort of positive reactions.

Ophthalmic Uses. Local application of various sympathomimetic amines to the conjunctiva is used to dilate the pupil, mainly to permit adequate examination of the fundus. The mydriatic effect of these drugs, notably ephedrine (3 to 5%), amphetamine (1%), hydroxyamphetamine (1 to 3%), and phenylephrine (1 to 2%), lasts for only a few hours. The sympathomimetics have the additional advantage that they do not cause cycloplegia and usually do not increase intraocular pressure. Sympathomimetic mydriatics are also used to reduce the incidence of posterior synechiae in uveitis, and epinephrine (1 to 2%) or phenylephrine (10%) is used to treat open-angle glaucoma, reducing the intraocular pressure by their local vasoconstrictor action, which decreases production of aqueous humor.

Use of Central Effects. Apart from a series of drugs used only as anorectics (*see* below), the main sympathomimetics used for central effects are ephedrine, amphetamine, dextroamphetamine, methamphetamine, and mephentermine. Of these, dextroamphetamine and methamphetamine are most widely employed. The peripheral actions of ephedrine, mephentermine, and, to a lesser extent, amphetamine are disproportionately great, and central effects cannot be obtained without side effects from the peripheral actions.

Narcolepsy. Ephedrine, amphetamine, methamphetamine, and dextroamphetamine have been used to treat narcoleptic patients. The amphetamines largely prevent attacks of sleep in nearly all patients, and cataplexy is often much improved. The usual dose of dextroamphetamine varies from 30 to 50 mg daily, in divided portions, the last dose being taken not later than 4 P.M. so that the nocturnal sleep is not prevented. Tolerance does not appear to develop to these agents in the treatment of narcolepsy.

Parkinsonism. Dextroamphetamine partially alleviates various symptoms of parkinsonism, but it has been superseded by levodopa and other antiparkinsonism drugs. It may, however, be of value if levodopa cannot be tolerated, when it can be given as an adjuvant to the other drugs. It has little effect on tremor, but decreases rigidity in many patients and frequently relieves oculogyric crises. The drug brings about a better sleep cycle, a subjective improvement in muscle strength and rigidity, and elevates the mood, a most important objective in the treatment of the patients. The total daily dose varies from 10 to 50 mg or more. In certain other diseases of the extrapyramidal system, such as *spasmodic torticollis* and spasmodic movements of a limb, dextroamphetamine may relieve symptoms.

Obesity and Weight Reduction. Whatever the etiology of obesity, a factor common to all cases is necessarily an intake of amounts of food that supply more energy than the body uses. Of the two possible measures to correct this imbalance, attempts to reduce food intake have been more popular in Western civilization. Persistent dietary restraint has proven both essential and difficult to achieve, and various sympathomimetic and related drugs that depress appetite have been used to make a low-calorie diet more tolerable. These appetite depressants are of no value without an accompanying stringent dietary regimen, and it has been regularly demonstrated that, without consistent supervision, no prescribed regimen of drug or diet is predictably successful. Several factors have a part in determining this unsatisfactory situation. In many patients the etiology of obesity is psychological, and compulsive overeating is difficult to eradicate even with psychiatric help. The central stimulant and anorectic effects of most of these drugs have proven inseparable. This prevents their use in the latter part of the day; given after 4 P.M., they interfere with sleep at night. Since much of the overeating takes place in the evening, their value is obviously limited. The anorectic agents are often given with a barbiturate to overcome this difficulty, but without conspicuous success. In addition, tolerance develops within a few weeks and increased dosage is limited both by the peripheral actions that these drugs exert and by such symptoms of central stimulation as nervousness and irritability. Even during the early period of administration, peripheral effects, although seldom pronounced, are rarely completely absent. However, the use of an anorectic by obese individuals who are well motivated to reduce their food intake may ease the discomfort of adherence to a restricted diet, and may be of help in the earlier part of a regimen while new dietary patterns are being established.

None of the drugs used in obesity has proved superior to dextroamphetamine or methamphetamine, either in effectiveness or in lack of peripheral side effects. However, certain other agents have not so far presented a significant problem of drug abuse and, therefore, are preferable. In contrast to other amphetamine derivatives, fenfluramine (Table 24–1) causes drowsiness and does not interfere with REM sleep. Although this agent may be more acceptable for evening administration, it has been no more effective than other drugs (*see* Modell, 1960). The preparations are as follows: *benzphetamine hydrochloride* (DIDREX), 25- and 50-mg tablets; *chlorphentermine hydrochloride* (PRE-SATE), 65-mg slow-release tablets; *Diethylpropion Hydrochloride*, N.F. (TENUATE, TEPANIL), 25-mg tablets and 75-mg slow-release tablets; *fenfluramine hydrochloride* (PONDIMIN),

20-mg tablets; *phendimetrazine tartrate* (PLEGINE), 35-mg tablets; *Phenmetrazine Hydrochloride, N.F.* (PRELUDIN), 25-mg tablets and 50- and 75-mg slow-release tablets; *phentermine hydrochloride* (IONAMIN, WILPO), 8-, 15-, and 30-mg slow-release capsules. The usual dose is one tablet three times a day, but the effect of a single dose should be first be tested; a single slow-release dose should be taken at least 12 hours before bedtime.

Depressant Drug Poisoning. The central stimulant sympathomimetics can lessen the degree of depression caused by moderate doses of anesthetics and hypnotics, but it is questionable whether they have any significant effect in persons poisoned with large doses of depressants. There is little need for their use in patients with adequate respiration and active reflexes. In patients in whom central depression is greater, maintenance of adequate ventilation and general measures to support the circulation should be the primary objective (*see* Chapter 9). There is little evidence that this objective is better attained when a sympathomimetic or other analeptic is added to supportive measures.

Psychogenic Disorders. Amphetamines have been used in mild mental disorders such as mood disturbances, chronic nervous exhaustion, and psychoneuroses. In most conditions they have been superseded by other psychoactive drugs. Their indiscriminate use in patients with mental disorders should be avoided (*see* Chapter 12).

Hyperkinetic Syndrome. The amphetamines have a dramatic effect in calming a high proportion of abnormally hyperactive children. Restlessness, distractibility, and impulsive behavior are reduced, attention span is lengthened, and behavior becomes more tolerable to parents and teachers. Concomitant psychotherapy and parent counseling are necessary. Long term drug therapy is essential; withdrawal leads to deterioration of performance. However, since the demands of school aggravate the condition, the drug can often be stopped during vacations. The usual dose of dextroamphetamine is 5 to 10 mg three times daily. Tolerance to this effect does not appear to develop. Side effects include insomnia, headache, irritability, depression, periods of excessive crying, and gastrointestinal cramps, but these do not often require discontinuation of the drug. Continued use of dextroamphetamine depresses growth in these children; a rebound weight gain occurs when the drug is stopped. Methylphenidate, which is equally effective, may cause less inhibition of growth. It is not yet known if the long-term use of these stimulant drugs leads to subsequent abuse of the drug. It is alarming that the number of hyperkinetic children is estimated at 5%. A careful assessment of the condition must be made before therapy is begun. (*See* Sroufe and Stewart, 1973; Chapters 12 and 18.)

The mechanism of action of amphetamine in children with the hyperkinetic syndrome is probably related to the effect of the drug on CNS neurotransmitters (*see* Snyder, 1973). It is not difficult to correlate the alerting and attention-span effects of the drug with its central actions, but the calming effect seems paradoxical.

Epilepsy. In *grand mal*, dextroamphetamine may be a valuable adjunct to phenobarbital, counter-acting the ataxia and drowsiness produced by the barbiturate and thus allowing effective amounts to be given. It is also useful in *absence seizures* (petit mal) to counteract the sedative effect of trimethadione if this is troublesome. In some cases of petit mal, dextroamphetamine, either alone or in conjunction with an oxazolidinedione or succinimide, may prevent the attacks and restore the EEG to normal.

Fatigue. The effects and limitations of amphetamines in preventing and alleviating fatigue and sleepiness have already been discussed. The drugs should be used for such purposes only sparingly and with medical advice.

Miscellaneous Uses. Ephedrine and amphetamine have been reported to prevent *syncopal reactions* of the vagal or vasodepressor type due to abnormal sensitivity of the carotid sinuses. Ephedrine, amphetamine, and other sympathomimetics have been used with variable success to treat *urinary incontinence* and *nocturnal enuresis*. The benefit may be due partly to central effects of the drugs and partly to contraction of the vesical sphincter. Dextroamphetamine may be helpful in relieving *premenstrual tension*. Ephedrine and amphetamine, although quite unreliable as uterine relaxants and often excitatory, have been reported to relieve the pain of *dysmenorrhea*. Epinephrine has been replaced by *glucagon* for the emergency treatment of severe hypoglycemia due to *hyperinsulinism*, prior to the infusion of glucose. The use of salbutamol and other selective β_2 agonists to delay delivery in *premature labor* has been mentioned.

Ahlquist, R. P. A study of adrenotropic receptors. *Am. J. Physiol.,* **1948,** *153,* 586–600.

Ahlquist, R. P., and Levy, B. Adrenergic receptive mechanism of canine ileum. *J. Pharmac. exp. Ther.,* **1959,** *127,* 146–149.

Alles, G. A. The comparative physiological actions of *dl-β*-phenylisopropylamines. I. Pressor effect and toxicity. *J. Pharmac. exp. Ther.,* **1933,** *47,* 339–354.

Alles, G. A., and Prinzmetal, M. The comparative physiological actions of *dl-β*-phenylisopropylamines. II. Bronchial effect. *J. Pharmac. exp. Ther.,* **1933,** *48,* 161–174.

Anderson, R.; Holmberg, S.; Svedmyr, N.; and Åberg, G. Adrenergic α- and β-receptors in coronary vessels in man: an *in vitro* study. *Acta med. scand.,* **1972,** *191,* 241–244.

Angenent, W. J., and Koelle, G. B. A possible enzymatic basis for the differential action of mydriatics on light and dark irides. *J. Physiol., Lond.,* **1953,** *119,* 102–117.

Assem, E. S. K., and Schild, H. O. Inhibition by sympathomimetic amines of histamine release induced by antigen in passively sensitized human lung. *Nature, Lond.,* **1969,** *224,* 1028–1029.

Barger, G., and Dale, H. H. Chemical structure and sympathomimetic action of amines. *J. Physiol., Lond.,* **1910,** *41,* 19–59.

Bearn, A. G.; Billing, B.; and Sherlock, S. The effect of adrenaline and noradrenaline on hepatic blood flow and splanchnic carbohydrate metabolism in man. *J. Physiol., Lond.,* **1951,** *115,* 430–441.

Beckett, A. H., and Rowland, M. Urinary excretion kinetics of amphetamine in man. *J. Pharm. Pharmac.,* **1965,** *17,* 628–639.

Benfey, B. G., and Varma, D. R. Interactions of sympathomimetic drugs, propranolol and phentolamine, on atrial refractory period and contractility. *Br. J. Pharmac. Chemother.,* **1967,** *30,* 603–611.

Bertler, A.; Carlsson, A.; and Rosengren, E. Release by reserpine of catecholamines from rabbit hearts. *Naturwissenschaften*, **1956**, *43*, 521.

Bieniarz, J.; Motew, M.; and Scommegna, A. Uterine and cardiovascular effects of ritodrine in premature labor. *Obstet. Gynec., Hagerstown*, **1972**, *40*, 65–73.

Blundell, J. E., and Leshem, M. B. Dissociation of the anorexic effects of fenfluramine and amphetamine following intrahypothalamic injection. *Br. J. Pharmac.*, **1973**, *47*, 183–185.

Boakes, R. J.; Bradley, P. B.; and Candy, J. M. A neuronal basis for the alerting action of (+)-amphetamine. *Br. J. Pharmac.*, **1972**, *45*, 391–403.

Bradley, P. B. The central action of certain drugs in relation to the reticular formation. In, *Reticular Formation of the Brain.* (Jasper, H. H.; Proctor, L. D.; Knighton, R. S.; Noshay, W. C.; and Costello, R. T.; eds.) Little, Brown & Co., Boston, **1958**, pp. 123–149.

Bradley, P. B., and Key, B. J. The effect of drugs on arousal responses produced by electrical stimulation of the reticular formation of the brain. *Electroenceph. clin. Neurophysiol.*, **1958**, *10*, 97–110.

Burn, J. H., and Rand, M. J. The action of sympathomimetic amines in animals treated with reserpine. *J. Physiol., Lond.*, **1958**, *144*, 314–336.

Burn, J. H., and Tainter, M. L. An analysis of the effect of cocaine on the actions of adrenaline and tyramine. *J. Physiol., Lond.*, **1931**, *71*, 169–193.

Caldwell, R. W., and Goldberg, L. I. An evaluation of the vasodilation produced by mephentermine and certain other sympathomimetic amines. *J. Pharmac. exp. Ther.*, **1970**, *172*, 297–309.

Caliva, F. S.; Eich, R.; Taylor, H. L.; and Lyons, R. H. Some cardiovascular effects of phenyl-2-butyl-norsupifren hydrochloride (ARLIDIN). *Am. J. med. Sci.*, **1959**, *238*, 174–179.

Carlsson, A.; Rosengren, E.; Bertler, A.; and Nilsson, J. Effect of reserpine on the metabolism of catecholamines. In, *Psychotropic Drugs.* (Garattini, S., and Ghetti, V., eds.) Elsevier Publishing Co., Amsterdam, **1957**.

Choo-Kang, Y. F. J.; Parker, S. S.; and Grant, I. W. B. Response of asthmatics to isoprenaline and salbutamol aerosols administered by intermittent positive-pressure ventilation. *Br. med. J.*, **1970**, *4*, 465–468.

Dresel, P. E.; MacCannell, K. L.; and Nickerson, M. Cardiac arrhythmias induced by minimal doses of epinephrine in cyclopropane-anesthetized dogs. *Circulation Res.*, **1960**, *8*, 948–955.

Evans, M. E.; Walker, S. R.; Brittain, R. T.; and Paterson, J. W. The metabolism of salbutamol. *Xenobiotica*, **1973**, *3*, 113–120.

Forwell, G. D., and Ingram, G. I. C. The effect of adrenaline infusion on human blood coagulation. *J. Physiol., Lond.*, **1957**, *135*, 371–383.

Furchgott, R. F. Receptors for sympathomimetic amines. In, *Adrenergic Mechanisms* (a Ciba Foundation symposium). (Vane, J. R.; Wolstenholme, G. E. W.; and O'Connor, M.; eds.) Little, Brown & Co., Boston; J. & A. Churchill, Ltd., London, **1960**, pp. 246–252.

Gilbert, J. L.; Lange, G.; Polevoy, I.; and Brooks, C. McC. Effects of vasoconstrictor agents on cardiac irritability. *J. Pharmac. exp. Ther.*, **1958**, *123*, 9–15.

Goldberg, L. I. Dopamine—clinical uses of an endogenous catecholamine. *New Engl. J. Med.*, **1974**, *291*, 707–710.

Goldenberg, M.; Aranow, H., Jr.; Smith, A. A.; and Faber, M. Pheochromocytoma and essential hypertensive vascular disease. *Archs intern. Med.*, **1950**, *86*, 823–836.

Gombos, E. A.; Hulet, W. H.; Bopp, P.; Goldring, W.; Baldwin, D. S.; and Chasis, H. Reactivity of renal and systemic circulations to vasoconstrictor agents in normotensive and hypertensive subjects. *J. clin. Invest.*, **1962**, *41*, 203–217.

Hartung, W. H. Epinephrine and related compounds: influence of structure on physiologic activity. *Chem. Rev.*, **1931**, *9*, 389–465.

James, T. N.; Bear, E. S.; Lang, K. F.; and Green, E. W. Evidence for adrenergic alpha receptor depressant activity in the heart. *Am. J. Physiol.*, **1968**, *215*, 1366–1375.

Jespersen, S., and Scheel-Krüger, J. Evidence for a difference in mechanism of action between fenfluramine- and amphetamine-induced anorexia. *J. Pharm. Pharmac.*, **1973**, *25*, 49–54.

King, B. D.; Sokoloff, L.; and Wechsler, R. L. The effects of *l*-epinephrine and *l*-norepinephrine upon cerebral circulation and metabolism in man. *J. clin. Invest.*, **1952**, *31*, 273–279.

Konzett, H. Neue broncholytisch hochwirksame Körper der Adrenalinreihe. *Naunyn-Schmiedebergs Arch. exp. Path. Pharmak.*, **1940**, *197*, 27–40.

Krogsgaard, A. R. The effect of intravenously injected reserpine on blood pressure, renal function and sodium excretion. *Acta med. scand.*, **1956**, *154*, 41–51.

Lands, A. M.; Arnold, A.; McAuliff, J. P.; Luduena, F. P.; and Brown, T. G., Jr. Differentiation of receptor systems activated by sympathomimetic amines. *Nature, Lond.*, **1967**, *214*, 597–598.

Levy, B., and Wilkenfeld, B. E. An analysis of selective beta receptor blockade. *Eur. J. Pharmac.*, **1969**, *5*, 227–234.

Liggins, G. C., and Vaughan, G. S. Intravenous infusion of salbutamol in the management of premature labour. *J. Obstet. Gynaec. Br. Commonw.*, **1973**, *80*, 29–33.

Lockett, M. Dangerous effects of isoprenaline in myocardial failure. *Lancet*, **1965**, *2*, 104–106.

Nickerson, M., and Nomaguchi, G. M. Mechanism of DIBENAMINE protection against cyclopropane-epinephrine cardiac arrhythmias. *J. Pharmac. exp. Ther.*, **1949**, *95*, 1–11.

Oliver, G., and Schäfer, E. A. The physiological effects of extracts from the suprarenal capsules. *J. Physiol., Lond.*, **1895**, *18*, 230–276.

Piness, G.; Miller, H.; and Alles, G. A. Clinical observations on phenylaminoethanol sulphate. *J. Am. med. Ass.*, **1930**, *94*, 790–791.

Prinzmetal, M., and Bloomberg, W. The use of BENZEDRINE for the treatment of narcolepsy. *J. Am. med. Ass.*, **1935**, *105*, 2051–2054.

Reinhardt, C. F.; Azar, A.; Maxfield, M. E.; Smith, P. E.; and Mullin, L. S. Cardiac arrhythmias and aerosol "sniffing." *Archs envir. Hlth*, **1971**, *22*, 265–279.

Rosenblum, R., and Frieden, J. Intravenous dopamine in the treatment of myocardial dysfunction after open-heart surgery. *Am. Heart J.*, **1972**, *83*, 743–748.

Schild, H. O. Effect of adrenaline on depolarized smooth muscle. In, *Adrenergic Mechanisms* (a Ciba Foundation symposium). (Vane, J. R.; Wolstenholme, G. E. W.; and O'Connor, M.; eds.) Little, Brown & Co., Boston; J. & A. Churchill, Ltd., London, **1960**, pp. 288–292.

Schmidt, J. L., and Fleming, W. W. The structure of sympathomimetics as related to reserpine induced sensitivity changes in the rabbit ileum. *J. Pharmac. exp. Ther.*, **1963**, *139*, 230–237.

Singer, D. H.; Lazzara, R.; and Hoffman, B. F. Interrelationships between automaticity and conduction in Purkinje fibers. *Circulation Res.*, **1967**, *21*, 537–558.

Smythe, C. McC.; Nickel, J. F.; and Bradley, S. E. The effect of epinephrine (USP), *l*-epinephrine and *l*-norepinephrine on glomerular filtration rate, renal plasma flow and the urinary excretion of sodium, potassium and water in normal man. *J. clin. Invest.*, **1952**, *31*, 499–506.

Snyder, S. H. How amphetamine acts in minimal brain dysfunction. *Ann. N.Y. Acad. Sci.*, **1973**, *205*, 310–320.

Spoerel, W. E.; Seleny, F. L.; and Williamson, R. D. Shock caused by continuous infusion of metaraminol bitartrate (ARAMINE). *Can. med. Ass. J.*, **1964**, *90*, 349–353.

Stolley, P. D. Asthma mortality—why the United States was spared an epidemic of deaths due to asthma. *Am. Rev. resp. Dis.,* **1972,** *105,* 883–890.

Tainter, M. L., and Chang, D. K. The antagonism of the pressor action of tyramine by cocaine. *J. Pharmac. exp. Ther.,* **1927,** *30,* 193–207.

Taylor, G. V., ɪv, and Harris, W. S. Cardiac toxicity of aerosol propellants. *J. Am. med. Ass.,* **1970,** *214,* 81–85.

Tolbert, M. E. M.; Butcher, F. R.; and Fain, J. N. Lack of correlation between catecholamine effects of cyclic adenosine 3′:5′-monophosphate and gluconeogenesis in isolated rat liver cells. *J. biol. Chem.,* **1973,** *248,* 5686–5692.

Trendelenburg, U.; Muskus, A.; Fleming, W. W.; and de la Sierra, B. G. A. Modification by reserpine of the action of sympathomimetic amines in spinal cats: a classification of sympathomimetic amines. *J. Pharmac. exp. Ther.,* **1962,** *138,* 170–180.

Vliet, P. D. V.; Burchell, H. B.; and Titus, J. L. Focal myocarditis associated with pheochromocytoma. *New Engl. J. Med.,* **1966,** *274,* 1102–1108.

Vree, T. B.; Muskens, A. T. J. M.; and van Rossum, J. M. Some physicochemical properties of amphetamine and related drugs. *J. Pharm. Pharmac.,* **1969,** *21,* 774–775.

Monographs and Reviews

Allwood, M. J.; Cobbold, A. F.; and Ginsburg, J. Peripheral vascular effects of noradrenaline, isopropylnoradrenaline and dopamine. *Br. med. Bull.,* **1963,** *19,* 132–136.

Angrist, B. M., and Gershon, S. Psychiatric sequelae of amphetamine use. In, *Psychiatric Complications of Medical Drugs.* (Shader, R. I., ed.) Raven Press, New York, **1972,** pp. 175–199.

Aviado, D. M., Jr. Cardiovascular effects of some commonly used pressor amines. *Anesthesiology,* **1959,** *20,* 71–97. (228 references.)

———. *Sympathomimetic Drugs.* Charles C Thomas, Pub., Springfield, Ill., **1970.**

Bellet, S. Mechanism and treatment of A-V heart block and Adams-Stokes syndrome. *Prog. cardiovasc. Dis.,* **1960,** *2,* 691–705.

Bowman, W. C., and Nott, M. W. Actions of sympathomimetic amines and their antagonists on skeletal muscle. *Pharmac. Rev.,* **1969,** *21,* 27–72.

Chen, K. K., and Schmidt, C. F. Ephedrine and related substances. *Medicine, Baltimore,* **1930,** *9,* 1–117.

Daniel, E. E.; Paton, D. M.; Taylor, G. S.; and Hodgson, B. J. Adrenergic receptors for catecholamine effects on tissue electrolytes. *Fedn Proc. Fedn Am. Socs exp. Biol.,* **1970,** *29,* 1410–1425.

Dempsey, P. J., and Cooper, T. Pharmacology of the coronary circulation. *A. Rev. Pharmac.,* **1972,** *12,* 99–110.

Eckstein, J. W., and Abboud, F. M. Circulatory effects of sympathomimetic amines. *Am. Heart J.,* **1962,** *63,* 119–135.

Goldberg, L. I. Cardiovascular and renal actions of dopamine: potential clinical applications. *Pharmac. Rev.,* **1972,** *24,* 1–29.

Grant, W. M. Action of drugs on movement of ocular fluids. *A. Rev. Pharmac.,* **1969,** *9,* 85–94.

Greenway, C. V., and Stark, R. D. Hepatic vascular bed. *Physiol. Rev.,* **1971,** *51,* 23–65.

Gregg, D. E., and Fisher, L. C. Blood supply to the heart. In, *Circulation,* Vol. II. *Handbook of Physiology,* Sect. II. (Hamilton, W. F., ed.) American Physiological Society, Washington, D. C., **1963,** pp. 1517–1584.

Hardaway, R. M., ɪɪɪ. *Clinical Management of Shock: Surgical and Medical.* Charles C Thomas, Pub., Springfield, Ill., **1968.**

Himms-Hagen, J. Sympathetic regulation of metabolism. *Pharmac. Rev.,* **1967,** *19,* 367–461.

———. Effects of catecholamines on metabolism. In, *Catecholamines.* (Blaschko, H., and Muscholl, E., eds.) *Handb. exp. Pharmak.,* Vol. 33. Springer-Verlag, Berlin, **1972,** pp. 363–462.

Kuhn, L. A. Shock in myocardial infarction—medical treatment. *Am. J. Cardiol.,* **1970,** *26,* 578–587.

Lewis, A. A. G. (ed.). Salbutamol. Proceedings of an international symposium. *Postgrad. med. J.,* **1971,** *47,* Suppl., 1–133.

Marshall, J. M. Effects of catecholamines on the smooth muscle of the female reproductive tract. *A. Rev. Pharmac.,* **1973,** *13,* 19–32.

Modell, W. Status and prospect of drugs for overeating. *J. Am. med. Ass.,* **1960,** *173,* 1131–1136.

Nickerson, M. Drug therapy of shock. In, *Shock: Pathogenesis and Therapy* (a Ciba Foundation symposium). (Bock, K. D., ed.) Springer-Verlag, Berlin, **1962,** pp. 356–370.

Oswald, I. Drugs and sleep. *Pharmac. Rev.,* **1968,** *20,* 273–303. (134 references.)

Porte, D., Jr., and Robertson, R. P. Control of insulin secretion by catecholamines, stress, and the sympathetic nervous system. *Fedn Proc. Fedn Am. Socs exp. Biol.,* **1973,** *32,* 1792–1796.

Sharman, D. F. The catabolism of catecholamines: recent studies. *Br. med. Bull.,* **1973,** *29,* 110–115.

Smith, A. D. Mechanisms involved in the release of noradrenaline from sympathetic nerves. *Br. med. Bull.,* **1973,** *29,* 123–129.

Somlyo, A. P., and Somlyo, A. V. Vascular smooth muscles. I. Normal structure, pathology, biochemistry and biophysics. *Pharmac. Rev.,* **1968,** *20,* 197–272.

Sroufe, L. A., and Stewart, M. A. Treating problem children with stimulant drugs. *New Engl. J. Med.,* **1973,** *289,* 407–413.

Toman, J. E. P., and Davis, J. P. The effects of drugs upon the electrical activity of the brain. *Pharmac. Rev.,* **1949,** *1,* 425–492.

Trendelenburg, U. Factors influencing the concentration of catecholamines at the receptors. In, *Catecholamines.* (Blaschko, H., and Muscholl, E., eds.) *Handb. exp. Pharmak.,* Vol. 33. Springer-Verlag, Berlin, **1972,** pp. 726–761.

Weiss, B., and Laties, V. G. Enhancement of human performance by caffeine and the amphetamines. *Pharmac. Rev.,* **1962,** *14,* 1–36. (118 references.)

Zaimis, E. Vasopressor drugs and catecholamines. *Anesthesiology,* **1968,** *29,* 732–762. (162 references.)

Zoll, P. M., and Linenthal, A. J. A program for Stokes-Adams disease and cardiac arrest. *Circulation,* **1963,** *27,* 1–4.

25 ATROPINE, SCOPOLAMINE, AND RELATED ANTIMUSCARINIC DRUGS

Ian R. Innes and Mark Nickerson

The drugs described in this chapter inhibit the actions of acetylcholine (ACh) on autonomic effectors innervated by postganglionic cholinergic nerves as well as on smooth muscles that lack cholinergic innervation; that is, they antagonize the muscarinic actions of ACh. They are therefore known as *antimuscarinic* agents. Because the main actions of all members of this class of drugs are qualitatively similar to those of the best-known member, atropine, the terms *atropinic* and *atropine-like* are also appropriately used. Such drugs have also been variously termed *antiparasympathetic, anticholinergic, cholinolytic, parasympatholytic, antispasmodic,* or *spasmolytic*. Most of these terms are misleading or insufficiently descriptive.

In general, antimuscarinic agents have little effect on the actions of ACh at nicotinic receptor sites. Thus, at autonomic ganglia, where transmission normally involves predominantly nicotinic receptors, atropine produces partial block only at relatively high doses. At the neuromuscular junction, where the receptors are probably exclusively nicotinic, extremely high doses of atropine or related drugs are required to demonstrate any degree of blockade; in such circumstances, it is equally possible that blockade is due to actions unrelated to specific antagonism at ACh-receptor sites. However, quaternary ammonium analogs of atropine and related drugs generally exhibit varying degrees of nicotinic blocking activity and, consequently, are more likely to interfere with ganglionic or neuromuscular transmission in doses of the same magnitude as those that produce muscarinic block. In the central nervous system (CNS), cholinergic transmission appears to be predominantly nicotinic in the spinal cord and predominantly muscarinic at both subcortical and cortical levels in the brain. Accordingly, many or most of the CNS effects of atropine-like drugs at ordinary doses are probably attributable to their anticholinergic central actions. At high or toxic doses, the central effects of atropine and related drugs consist, in general, of stimulation followed by depression; these are probably due to a combination of antimuscarinic and unrelated actions. Since quaternary compounds penetrate the blood-brain barrier poorly, antimuscarinic drugs of this type show little in the way of central effects. (*See* Chapter 21.)

All parasympathetic neuroeffector junctions are not equally sensitive to the antimuscarinic agents. However, the order of sensitivity of various parasympathetically innervated organs to block by atropinic agents varies little between drugs. Small doses depress salivary, bronchial, and sweat secretion. With larger doses, the pupil dilates, accommodation of the eye is inhibited, and vagal effects on the heart are blocked so that the heart rate is increased. Larger doses inhibit the parasympathetic control of the urinary bladder and gastrointestinal tract, thus inhibiting micturition and decreasing the tone and motility of the gut. Still larger doses are required to inhibit gastric secretion. Since only the primary phase of gastric secretion is controlled by the vagus, the remaining hormonally controlled secretion remains unaffected. Thus, doses of any antimuscarinic drug that reduce the tone and motility of the stomach and the duodenum and depress gastric secretion also invariably affect salivary secretion and ocular accommodation and often slow micturition. The drugs therefore produce the functional equivalent of resection or paralysis of postganglionic cholinergic nerves. The end result often simulates overactivity of the sympathetic system, since the balance between sympathetic and parasympathetic tone, with opposing effects in so many organs, is upset and the responses to sympathetic impulses become dominant.

The actions and effects of the anti-muscarinic agents usually differ only quantitatively from those of atropine, which is considered in detail as the prototype of the group. The properties of other antimuscarinic drugs are discussed in terms of their differences from those of atropine.

History. The naturally occurring antimuscarinic drugs are the alkaloids of the belladonna plants. The most important of these are *atropine* and *scopolamine*. Preparations of belladonna were known to the ancient Hindus and have been used by physicians for many centuries. Poisoners of the Middle Ages frequently used the deadly nightshade plant to cause obscure and often prolonged poisoning. This prompted Linné to name the shrub *Atropa belladonna*, after Atropos, the oldest of the Three Fates, who cuts the thread of life.

Accurate study of the actions of belladonna dates from the isolation of atropine in pure form by Mein in 1831. In 1867, Bezold and Bloebaum showed that atropine blocks the cardiac effects of vagal stimulation, and 5 years later Heidenhain found that it prevents salivary secretion due to stimulation of the chorda tympani. These fundamental observations were quickly followed by many others, and today there is an extensive and secure body of experimental and clinical information on the pharmacological actions of the belladonna alkaloids. Many semisynthetic congeners of the belladonna alkaloids, usually quaternary ammonium derivatives, and a large number of synthetic antimuscarinic compounds with structures often quite unrelated to those of the natural alkaloids have been prepared, primarily with the objective of depressing gastric secretion without undesired antimuscarinic effects on

other organs. These drugs have few advantages over the naturally occurring alkaloids and their derivatives.

ATROPINE, SCOPOLAMINE, AND RELATED BELLADONNA ALKALOIDS

Sources and Members. The belladonna drugs are widely distributed in nature, especially in the Solanaceae plants. *Atropa belladonna,* the deadly nightshade, yields mainly the alkaloid *atropine (dl-hyoscyamine).* The same alkaloid is found in *Datura stramonium,* known as Jamestown or Jimson weed, stinkweed, thorn-apple, and devil's apple. The alkaloid *scopolamine (hyoscine)* is found chiefly in the shrub *Hyoscyamus niger* (henbane) and *Scopolia carniolica.* The official tincture of belladonna acts chiefly by virtue of its atropine content.

Chemistry. These alkaloids are organic esters formed by combination of an aromatic acid, *tropic acid,* and complex organic bases, either *tropine* (tropanol) or *scopine.* Scopine differs from tropine only in having an oxygen bridge between the carbon atoms designated as 6 and 7 in the structural formulas in Table 25-1. This oxygen bridge is the sole chemical difference between atropine and scopolamine. Homatropine is a semisynthetic compound produced by combining the base tropine with mandelic acid. *Atropine methylnitrate, methscopolamine bromide,* and *homatropine methylbromide* are the corresponding quaternary ammonium derivatives (Table 25-1).

Structure-Activity Relationship. The basis of the selective antimuscarinic action of atropine resides

Table 25-1.   BELLADONNA ALKALOIDS AND CLOSELY ALLIED SYNTHETIC SUBSTANCES

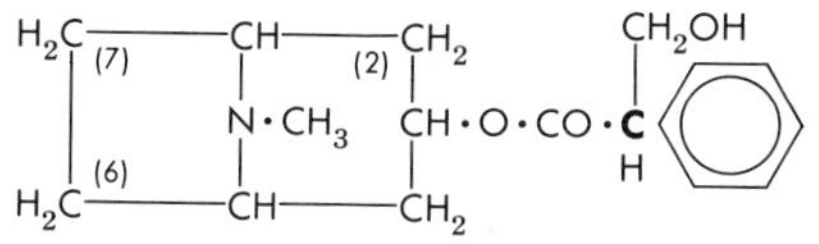

Atropine

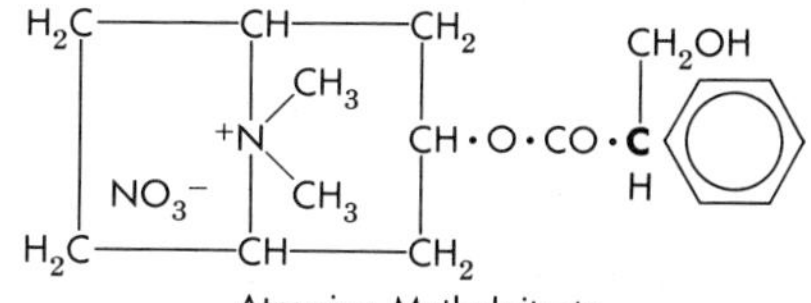

Scopolamine

Homatropine

Atropine Methylnitrate

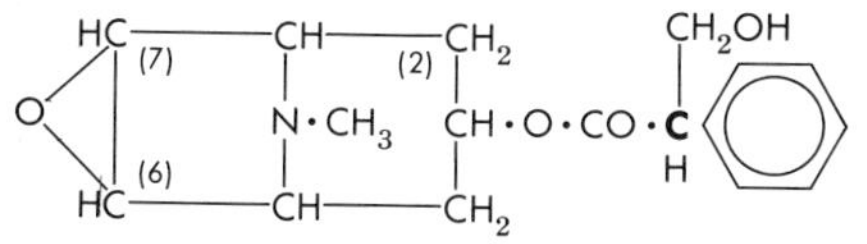

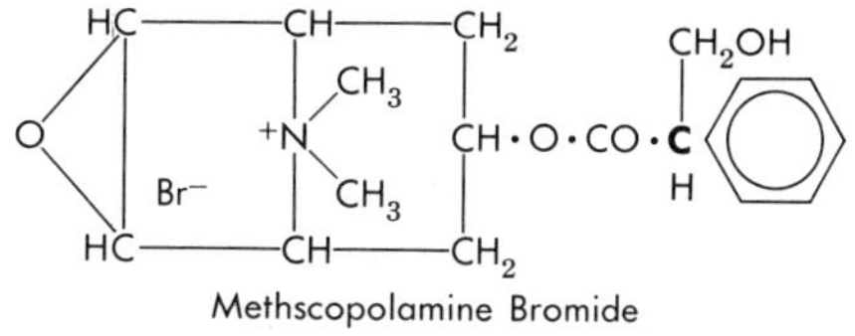

Methscopolamine Bromide

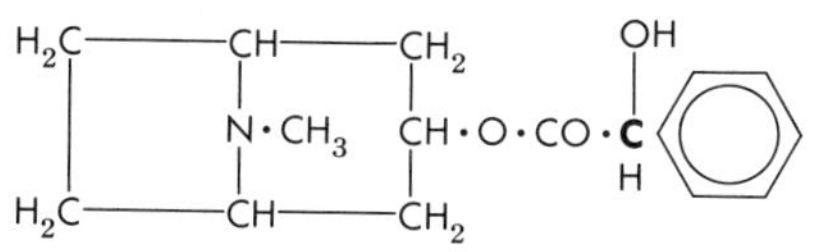

Homatropine Methylbromide

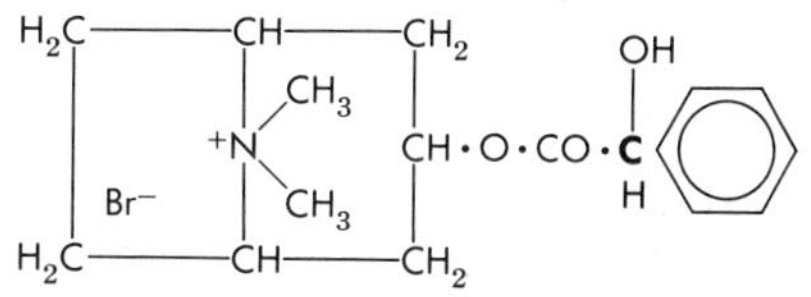

not in the tropine base, which is relatively inactive, but in an ester of tropic acid and a tertiary amino alcohol. The presence of a free OH group in the acid portion of the ester is also important. Substitution of other aromatic acids for tropic acid modifies but does not necessarily abolish the antimuscarinic activity. When given parenterally, quaternary ammonium derivatives of atropine and scopolamine are, in general, more potent than their parent compounds in both antimuscarinic and ganglionic blocking activity, and lack CNS activity because of poor penetration into the brain. Given orally, they are poorly and unreliably absorbed, as are other quaternary ammonium compounds.

The presence of an asymmetrical carbon atom in tropic and mandelic acids (boldface **C** in the formulas in Table 25–1) allows for optical activity and stereoisomerism. Scopolamine is *l*-hyoscine and is much more active than *d*-hyoscine. Atropine is racemized during extraction and consists of a mixture of equal parts of *d*- and *l*-hyoscyamine, but the antimuscarinic activity is almost wholly due to the naturally occurring *l* form. *l*-Hyoscyamine is thus twice as potent as atropine in its antimuscarinic activity. In central activity, *l*-hyoscyamine is 8 to 50 times as potent as the *d* isomer.

Antimuscarinic agents vary in chemical structure probably more than do the members of any other single class of pharmacologically active drugs. They include various isomers or congeners of muscarine, which range from partial agonists to purely competitive antagonists (Rossum, 1960); drugs such as dibutoline, a congener of carbachol; belladonna alkaloids and their quaternary derivatives (*see* Ing, 1946; Stoll, 1948; Lands, 1951; and others); many other tropanes; and a wide variety of drugs with chemical structures apparently not resembling those of the classical antimuscarinic alkaloids (*see* Pierce, 1960; Bebbington and Brimblecombe, 1965).

Mechanism of Action. The major action of the antimuscarinic agents is a *competitive* or *surmountable* antagonism to ACh and other muscarinic agents. The antagonism can therefore be overcome by increasing sufficiently the concentration of ACh at receptor sites of the effector organ, for example, by anticholinesterase (anti-ChE) agents. The receptors affected are those peripheral structures that are either stimulated or inhibited by muscarine, that is, exocrine glands and smooth and cardiac muscle. The drugs can block all muscarinic actions of ACh and other choline esters. Responses to postganglionic cholinergic nerve stimulation may also be inhibited, but less readily than are responses to injected choline esters. The difference may be due to release of ACh by cholinergic nerve terminals so close to receptors that diffusion limits the concentration of antagonist that can be attained in the very narrow synaptic cleft. A comparable rela-

tionship exists for α-adrenergic blocking agents (*see* Chapter 26).

Atropine-induced parasympathetic block may be preceded by a transient phase of mild stimulation. Thus, small doses of atropine usually slow the heart rate by several beats per minute. This is probably due largely to central vagal stimulation by doses of atropine too small to block the peripheral muscarinic receptors. However, an additional direct action on the heart is also likely, since a small dose of atropine methylbromide, which does not cross the blood-brain barrier, also slows the heart (Kottmeier and Gravenstein, 1968). Low concentrations of atropine may also stimulate isolated tissues directly (*see* Averill and Lamb, 1959; Ashford *et al.*, 1962). Thus, some antimuscarinic agents may have a dual action, as agonists in low doses and as antagonists in higher doses (partial agonists). However, the peripheral stimulant action of atropine is of little significance except on the heart.

Selectivity of Antagonism. Atropine is a highly selective antagonist of muscarinic agents at the corresponding receptors of smooth and cardiac muscle and exocrine gland cells. This antagonism is so selective that atropine blockade of the actions of a noncholinomimetic drug has been taken as evidence that the drug acts indirectly through ACh release or some other cholinergic mechanism. For example, the stimulant action of 5-hydroxytryptamine (5-HT) on guinea pig ileum has been attributed to activation of intramural cholinergic neurons because it is blocked by atropine. However, atropine and other antimuscarinic agents are no exceptions to the rule that selectivity of antagonism is rarely absolute and is usually lost when high doses are used. Conclusions based on selectivity of antagonism by atropine are therefore acceptable only when they are supported by more direct evidence. Under appropriate experimental conditions and usually in higher doses than are needed to antagonize ACh, atropine may block or reduce responses to histamine, 5-HT, and norepinephrine. Atropine is moderately active in relieving histamine-induced bronchoconstriction in man and experimental animals. It also antagonizes the action of 5-HT on rat uterus, the respiratory tract smooth muscle of guinea pig and cat, guinea pig atria, and the aneural smooth muscle of chick amnion, where 5-HT may be presumed to act directly. Atropine in large doses (1.4 to 4.0 mg/kg) depresses contraction of the cat nictitating membrane induced by norepinephrine. In all cases, the antagonism of other types of agonists is less complete than that of ACh.

PHARMACOLOGICAL PROPERTIES

The discussion in this section is centered chiefly on atropine, but differences in the pharmacological properties of the other alkaloids will be mentioned when necessary. Atropine and scopolamine differ quantitatively in antimuscarinic actions. Scopolamine has a stronger action on the iris, ciliary body, and certain secretory (salivary, bronchial, and sweat) glands, but atropine is the more potent on heart, intestine, and bronchial muscle, and has a more prolonged action. Atropine does not depress the CNS in clinical doses and, therefore, is used in preference to scopolamine for most purposes. Where some central depressant effect is no disadvantage or is desired, as in preanesthetic medication, scopolamine is frequently used. Reference to Table 21–1 (page 408) and Figure 21–1 (facing page 406) will indicate the effector cells and responses that are inhibited.

Central Nervous System. *Atropine* stimulates the medulla and higher cerebral centers. In clinical doses (0.5 to 1.0 mg), this effect is usually confined to mild vagal excitation. The rate and occasionally the depth of breathing are increased, but this effect is probably the result of bronchiolar dilatation and the subsequent increase in physiological "dead space." When respiration is seriously depressed, atropinic drugs cannot be relied on as stimulants. Instead, large or repeated doses may depress respiration even further. With toxic doses of atropine, central excitation becomes more prominent, leading to restlessness, irritability, disorientation, hallucinations, or delirium (*see* the discussion of atropine poisoning). With still larger doses, stimulation is followed by depression, coma ensues, and medullary paralysis causes death. Even moderate doses of atropine may depress certain central motor mechanisms controlling muscle tone and movement, as seen in the salutary effect on the tremor and rigidity of parkinsonism (*see* Chapter 14).

Scopolamine in therapeutic doses normally causes drowsiness, euphoria, amnesia, fatigue, and dreamless sleep with a reduction in rapid-eye-movement (REM) sleep. However, the same doses occasionally cause excitement, restlessness, hallucinations, or delirium, especially in the presence of severe pain. They resemble the central effects of toxic doses of atropine, and occur regularly after large doses of scopolamine. The use of scopolamine with morphine for obstetrical analgesia, *twilight sleep,* depends upon its action in causing amnesia, which does not occur if atropine is used instead.

Central Anticholinergic Action. Antagonism by atropine of many of the central effects of ACh, physostigmine, and di*iso*propyl phosphorofluoridate (DFP) is part of the indirect evidence that ACh acts as a chemical mediator in the brain (*see* Chapter 21). However, it is not known whether the observed effects on the CNS are due to direct actions on neurons or to antagonism of a central synaptic transmitter. Doses of atropine required to inhibit peripheral responses to choline esters or anti-ChE agents have themselves almost no detectable central effects. Large doses are required for central effects. This may reflect nonspecific antagonistic or depressant actions, or difficulty of penetration of the drug into the CNS. Reversal by physostigmine of atropine-induced depression of the hypothalamus and reticular activating system in animals and of the central effects of atropine poisoning in man points to a specific antagonism. Also in animals atropine antagonizes the action of ACh applied locally to cerebral cortex and spinal cord. However, atropine also depresses the effects of noncholinergic stimuli, indicating that the drug has central actions other than blocking cholinergic synapses. (*See* Krnjević, 1969, 1974.)

EEG. Atropine promptly restores to normal the increased EEG activity due to DFP. Given alone, it reduces the voltage and frequency of the *alpha* rhythm and consistently shifts the EEG rhythm to slow activity, a pattern typical of the EEG in drowsiness. Both atropine and scopolamine also depress the EEG arousal response to photostimulation (Ostfeld and Arguete, 1962). In experimental animals, atropine and particularly scopolamine antagonize EEG activation by hypothalamic or reticular formation stimulation and by several drugs, including sympathomimetics. In therapeutic doses, atropine reduced abnormal EEG waves in about one half of a group of patients with *grand mal* (Grob et al., 1947). It has also been reported to reduce spike-and-dome paroxysms in certain cases of *petit mal* and to prevent exacerbations of these attacks by cholinomimetic drugs. Atropine or scopolamine disrupts several behaviorial responses in experimental animals at the same time as the EEG is altered. Although in many cases physostigmine promptly and simultaneously restores both to normal, the correlation between EEG and behavioral changes has not been established. (*See* reviews by Toman and Davis, 1949; Longo, 1966.)

Antitremor Activity. The belladonna alkaloids have long been used in parkinsonism. A central anticholinergic mechanism is likely since physostigmine reverses the beneficial effects of antimuscarinic drugs and aggravates the symptoms in untreated patients (Duvoisin, 1967). In animals, effectiveness against parkinsonism-like tremor induced by surgical lesions or by the experimental cholinomimetic drug oxotremorine is difficult to correlate with peripheral antimuscarinic potency; scopolamine is more potent than atropine, and both are more potent than the synthetic antiparkinsonism agents trihexyphenidyl and caramiphen (Vernier and Unna,

1956; Farquharson and Johnston, 1959). The salutary effect of levodopa in parkinsonism has led to considerable insight into the relations between cholinergic and dopaminergic mechanisms in this disease (*see* Chapter 14).

Vestibular Function. Scopolamine is effective in preventing motion sickness. This action is probably either on the cortex or more peripherally on the maculae of the utricle and saccule.

Eye. The atropinic drugs block the responses of the sphincter muscle of the iris and the ciliary muscle of the lens to cholinergic stimulation (Table 25–4, page 528). Thus, they dilate the pupil (*mydriasis*) and paralyze accommodation (*cycloplegia*). The wide pupillary dilatation results in photophobia; the lens is fixed for far vision, near objects are blurred, and sometimes micropsia occurs. The full drug effect is to abolish the normal pupillary reflex constriction to light or upon convergence of the eyes. These effects can occur after either local or systemic administration of the alkaloids, but conventional doses of atropine (0.6 mg) have little ocular effect, in contrast to equal doses of scopolamine, which cause definite mydriasis and loss of accommodation. After subcutaneous injection of atropinic drugs, the ocular effects develop more slowly and last longer than do the effects on salivary secretion and heart rate. Locally applied atropine or scopolamine produces ocular effects of considerable duration; accommodation and pupillary reflexes may not fully recover for 7 to 12 days. The atropinic mydriatics differ from the sympathomimetic agents in that the latter cause pupillary dilatation without loss of accommodation. As the mydriatic and cycloplegic effects of the belladonna alkaloids depend on competitive antagonism, pilocarpine, choline esters, physostigmine, and DFP in sufficient concentrations can surmount the antagonism and constrict the pupil by increasing the local concentration of agonist.

Atropinic drugs when administered systemically have little effect on *intraocular pressure* except in patients with narrow-angle glaucoma, where the pressure may occasionally rise dangerously. This effect is due to the iris, crowded back into the angle of the anterior chamber of the eye, interfering with drainage of aqueous humor. The drugs may precipitate a first attack in unrecognized cases of this rare condition. In wide-angle glaucoma a significant rise in pressure is unusual and the drugs can generally be used safely (*see* Medical Letter, 1974).

Respiratory Tract. The belladonna alkaloids inhibit secretions of the nose, mouth, pharynx, and bronchi, and thus dry the mucous membranes of the respiratory tract. This action is especially marked if there is excessive secretion, and is the basis for the use of atropine and scopolamine in preanesthetic medication. The smooth muscles of bronchi and bronchioles are relaxed, with a resulting slight widening of the airway, which decreases airway resistance but increases the volume of residual air. The increase in "dead space" due to bronchiolar dilatation may be the basis of the respiratory stimulation produced by atropine. Atropine is more potent than scopolamine as a bronchodilator. It is particularly effective against bronchoconstriction produced by parasympathomimetic drugs such as methacholine and anticholinesterase agents, but it is also moderately active in histamine-induced experimental asthma in both animals and man. However, atropine is generally considered to be less potent than epinephrine or isoproterenol as a bronchial relaxant, even against bronchoconstriction from electrical stimulation of the vagus. The role of cholinergic factors in the causation of bronchial asthmatic attacks remains to be elucidated.

Atropine and scopolamine reduce the occurrence of laryngospasm during general anesthesia. This appears to be due to depression of respiratory tract secretions that can precipitate reflex laryngospasm, caused by contraction of the laryngeal skeletal muscle, which is not blocked by atropine.

Cardiovascular System. *Heart.* The main effect of atropine on the heart is to alter *rate*. With average clinical doses (0.4 to 0.6 mg), the rate often decreases, as discussed above. The slowing is rarely marked, about 4 to 8 beats per minute, and is usually absent after rapid intravenous injection. There are no accompanying changes in blood pressure or cardiac output. Larger doses cause progressively increasing tachycardia by blocking vagal effects on the S-A pacemaker. The resting heart rate is increased by about 35 to 40 beats per minute in young men given 2 mg intramuscularly; the maximal heart rate (*e.g.*, in response to exercise) is not altered by atropine. The influence of atropine is most noticeable in healthy young adults, in whom vagal tone is at its height. In infancy and old age, even large doses of atropine may fail to accelerate the heart. With low doses of scopolamine (0.1 or 0.2 mg) the cardiac slowing is greater than with atropine. With higher doses the cardioacceleration is at first equal, but it is short lived and is followed within 30 minutes by a return to the normal rate or by bradycardia. Thus, after a short initial period, doses of scopolamine that produce ocular effects do not speed the heart; with atropine, ocular effects are accompanied by tachycardia. Atropine often causes cardiac arrhythmias, but without significant cardiovascular symptoms. Atrial arrhythmias and atrioventricular dissociation occur, the former most commonly in children given small doses that slow the heart, the latter usually in adults after small or large doses (Dauchot and Gravenstein, 1971; Hayes et al., 1971).

Adequate doses of atropine can abolish many types of reflex vagal cardiac slowing or asystole, for example, from inhalation of irritant vapors, stimulation of the carotid sinus, pressure on the eyeballs, peritoneal stimulation, central stimulation of vagal nuclei, or the normal afferent impulses causing respiratory arrhythmia. It also prevents or abruptly abolishes bradycardia or asystole from injection of choline esters, anti-ChE agents, or other parasympathomimetic drugs, as well as cardiac arrest from electrical stimulation of the vagus.

The removal of vagal influence on the heart by atropine may also cause changes in *conduction*. A-V conduction time is decreased, even when heart rate is kept constant by atrial pacing, and the P-R interval is shortened. In certain cases of partial heart block, in which vagal activity is an etiological factor, atropine may lessen the degree of block. In some patients with complete heart block, the idioventricular rate may be accelerated by atropine; in others it is stabilized. Atropine may improve the clinical condition of patients with early myocardial infarction by relieving severe sinus or nodal bradycardia or A-V block (see Adgey et al., 1968; and below). In contrast, toxic doses and, occasionally, a large therapeutic dose of atropine may cause A-V block and nodal rhythm. The main change produced by atropine (1.2 mg, subcutaneously) in the human ECG is a significant lowering of the T waves, usually in all three limb leads.

Circulation. Atropine, in clinical doses, completely counteracts the peripheral vasodilatation and sharp fall in blood pressure caused by choline esters. Yet, when given alone, its effect on blood vessels and blood pressure is neither striking nor constant. This is not unexpected, because most vascular beds probably lack significant cholinergic innervation and the cholinergic sympathetic vasodilator fibers to vessels supplying skeletal muscle do not appear to be involved to any important extent in the normal regulation of tone. Intra-arterial injections of atropine do not normally alter blood flow in the human forearm (Gaskell, 1956). However, inhibition of vasodilatation in this area by atropine is part of the evidence that there are some cholinergic vasodilators in the region (see Shepherd, 1963). Atropine reduces forearm vasodilatation due to emotional stress, only temporarily decreases the vasodilator response to body heating, and has no effect on cold vasodilatation.

Systemic doses of 2 to 5 mg of atropine slightly raise systolic and lower diastolic pressures (Cullumbine et al., 1955). Doses of 2 mg slightly increase cardiac output and decrease central venous pressure (Berry et al., 1959); right atrial and pulmonary artery pressures and pulmonary blood volume decrease (Daly et al., 1963). The cause of these effects is not clear. Late in the course of atropine poisoning, the blood pressure may fall markedly, but this is probably due to central vasomotor depression. Toxic amounts of atropine usually, and therapeutic doses occasionally, dilate cutaneous blood vessels, especially those in the blush area (*atropine flush*). The mechanism of this anomalous vascular response is unknown. It may be a compensatory reaction permitting the radiation of heat to offset the atropine-induced rise in temperature. On the other hand, it may represent a direct vasodilator action unrelated to cholinergic blockade. The scarlet appearance of the flushed skin, coupled with fever, has caused atropine intoxication to be mistakenly diagnosed as scarlet fever.

Atropine has been reported to increase coronary blood flow in normal man, but this is probably directly related to metabolic changes due to an increase in heart rate. This effect is unlikely to be useful in the myocardium where metabolites have already accumulated after infarction. (See review by Eger, 1962.)

Gastrointestinal Tract. Many gaps still exist in our knowledge of the effects of belladonna alkaloids on the secretory and motor activity of the gastrointestinal tract. Experiments, particularly on man, involve many complicating factors so that the results of different investigators are often at variance. Among these factors are the particular alkaloid used, the dose and route of administration, the time at which the effects are observed, the technic of measurement of secretory or motor activity, psychic factors, the presence or absence of disease (especially peptic ulcer), the level of functional activity of the gastrointestinal tract at the time of drug administration, and the type of gastric secretory stimulus used (various test meals, alcohol, histamine, hypoglycemia, caffeine, etc.). Interest in the actions of antimuscarinic drugs on the stomach and intestine stems from their wide use in the treatment of peptic ulcer and as antispasmodic agents for gastrointestinal disorders. Although atropine can completely abolish the effects of ACh (and other parasympathomimetic drugs) on the gastrointestinal tract, it inhibits only incompletely the effects of vagal impulses. This difference is particularly striking in the effects of atropine on motility of the gut. The cause is not known; it may be due to the involvement of neurohumoral transmitters other than ACh and norepinephrine (*see* Chapter 21).

Secretion. Salivary secretion is particularly sensitive to inhibition by antimuscarinic agents, which can completely abolish the copious, watery, parasympathetically induced secretion. The mouth becomes dry, and swallowing and talking become difficult. Although salivary secretion is abolished, the accompanying vasodilatation in the glands due to release of bradykinin is unaffected.

Gastric secretion is reduced in volume and total acid content. This reduction is notable only when relatively large doses are given to experimental animals. In the *dog*, the results are fairly clear-cut, largely because technics are available for quantitative collection of pure gastric juice. Atropine in full doses depresses normal interdigestive secretion and all phases of the gastric secretory response to food. The response to histamine is partly inhibited; although the total acid output is decreased, the concentration of acid may rise somewhat because of a decreased secretion of buffering substances.

In *man,* the effect of atropine on gastric secretion depends on the many factors listed above. On the whole, gastric secretion is not greatly altered by conventional doses of the belladonna drugs; to be effective, doses must usually be given (1 mg or more) that invariably cause dry mouth, increase in heart rate, ocular disturbances, and other side effects. Secretion during both psychic and gastric phases is reduced but not abolished. Volume is usually reduced, but the concentration of acid is not necessarily lowered. The intestinal phase of gastric secretion may be somewhat inhibited. Full doses of atropine diminish and may completely abolish the interdigestive (fasting) secretion of acid; this action is less prominent in peptic ulcer patients. The duration of the effect of atropine on gastric secretion is brief when compared with that on salivary glands. Secretion induced by histamine, alcohol, or caffeine is reduced but not abolished by the doses of atropine tested in man.

The gastric cells that secrete mucin and enzymes are more directly under vagal influence than are the acid-secreting cells, and full doses of atropine may decrease the concentration of these organic constituents. Atropine completely blocks the copious secretion of gastric juice, rich in both acid and proteolytic

enzyme, elicited by injection of choline esters (methacholine and carbachol) or pilocarpine. (*See* the classical review by Code, 1951.)

Atropine has little effect on the secretion of *pancreatic juice, bile,* or *succus entericus,* processes largely under hormonal rather than vagal control.

Motility. The belladonna alkaloids have marked effects on motility of the gastrointestinal tract, since the parasympathetic nerves almost exclusively supply the extrinsic nervous motor control of the gut; sympathetic nerve impulses play a relatively small part in the physiological regulation of tone and motility. The parasympathetic nerves enhance both tone and motility, and relax sphincters, thereby favoring the passage of chyme through the gut. However, the gut has a complex system of intramural nerve plexuses that are mainly responsible for motility, and impulses from the CNS only modify the effects of the intrinsic reflexes. The terminal neurons of the intramural plexuses are cholinergic, and the effects of their activity can be blocked by atropine. However, atropine-resistant tone and movements of the gut are also observed; early recovery of spontaneous gastrointestinal movements may follow their inhibition by atropine, and further doses may have little additional effect.

Both in normal subjects and in patients with gastrointestinal disease, full therapeutic doses of atropine produce definite and prolonged inhibitory effects on the motor activity of the stomach, duodenum, jejunum, ileum, and colon, characterized by a decrease in tone and in amplitude and frequency of peristaltic contractions. These effects have been shown with many technics (fluoroscopy; intubation; gastric, ileal, or colonic fistulas; etc.); because they are more readily accessible, the stomach and the colon have been studied more thoroughly than has the small intestine. It should be noted that the doses needed to produce inhibition are more than enough to depress salivary secretion and usually produce ocular and cardiac effects. Excessive motility and hypertonus (as produced by morphine, insulin hypoglycemia, parasympathomimetic drugs, and certain emotional stimuli) are readily inhibited by appropriate doses of atropine, and more normal motor activity is usually restored. Atropine (0.8 mg, subcutaneously) inhibits, and at times completely abolishes, the tone and propulsive motility of the human colon. It also antagonizes in large measure the stimulant effects of morphine on the large intestine.

Atropine abolishes or prevents the excess motor activity of the gastrointestinal tract induced by parasympathomimetic drugs and anti-ChE agents. In moderate doses, the alkaloids do not block responses to other directly acting stimulants, such as histamine and vasopressin, that do not act on ACh receptors. However, responses to drugs acting through the intramural plexuses, such as nicotine and 5-HT, are inhibited.

Other Smooth Muscle. *Urinary Tract.* Intravenous urographic studies in man indicate that atropine (1.2 mg, intravenously) dilates the pelves, calyces, ureters, and bladder, and increases the visibility of the kidneys. Atropine decreases the normal tone and amplitude of contractions of the *ureter* and often eliminates drug-induced enhancement of ureteral tone. Contraction of the urinary bladder due to parasympathetic nerve stimulation is only partly inhibited; the residual contraction may be due to release by noncholinergic fibers of a chemical transmitter resistant to atropine.

Biliary Tract. Atropine exerts a mild antispasmodic action on the gallbladder and bile ducts in man. However, this is not sufficient to overcome or prevent the marked spasm and increase in biliary duct pressure induced by morphine, meperidine, or methadone. Both nitrites and theophylline are more effective than atropine in this respect. Atropine has no consistent effect on the choledochal sphincter mechanism in man. At times it causes relaxation; at other times, increased resistance. Emptying of the human gallbladder in response to a fat meal is delayed by prior administration of atropine. There is little basis for the use of atropine alone as a biliary antispasmodic.

Uterus. Atropine has negligible effects on the human uterus and, therefore, is useless in treating dysmenorrhea. Given to women in labor to cause amnesia, scopolamine does not alter or interfere with uterine contractions or increase the duration of labor; although the drug crosses the placental barrier, the fetus is not adversely affected, and the respiration of the newborn is not depressed.

Secretory Glands. The effects of belladonna alkaloids on respiratory and alimentary tract secretions have been discussed. Even small doses of atropine or scopolamine inhibit the activity of *sweat glands,* despite the vasodilatation the drugs may cause in some skin areas. The skin becomes hot and dry; sweating may be depressed enough to raise the body temperature, but only notably so after toxic doses. Atropine more readily blocks sweating induced by injected muscarinic agents than it does thermoregulatory sweating. The anhidrotic action of atropine and stimulation of sweating by muscarinic agents appeared for many years to be a pharmacological anomaly, as the sweat glands are supplied only by nerves that are anatomically sympathetic. However, these fibers are, in fact, mainly cholinergic. The alkaloids also inhibit, although not strikingly, the *lacrimal glands. Milk secretion* is not significantly affected.

Body Temperature. The rise in body temperature due to the belladonna alkaloids is usually significant only after large doses. Nevertheless, in infants and small children moderate doses induce "atropine fever." In atropine poisoning in infants, the temperature may reach 43° C or higher. Suppression of sweating is doubtless a considerable factor in the production of the fever, especially when the environmental temperature is high, but other mechanisms may be important when large doses are taken. It has been suggested that atropine may exert a central effect on temperature regulation; however, animals that do not sweat, such as the dog, do not exhibit fever after atropine.

Miscellaneous Effects. In man, atropine in usual doses has little effect on the *basal metabolic rate* or *respiratory quotient,* but large doses may increase metabolic rate. Alveolar ventilation may be increased and alveolar carbon dioxide tension (P_{CO_2}) lowered. Leukocytosis may occur in children given atropine. As already indicated, extremely high doses of atropine are required to block nicotinic receptors. Hence, in doses employed clinically the drug has little or no effect on ganglionic or neuromuscular transmission. Very large doses produce antidiuresis by increasing renal tubular reabsorption of water; this effect is probably mediated by the release of antidiuretic hormone (ADH) from the neurohypophysis. The drug inhibits postcoital ovulation in rabbits; it reduces release of various adenohypophyseal hormones, suggesting a possible cholinergic link in the release mechanism (*see* de Wied and de Jong, 1974).

Tolerance. Tolerance to the belladonna drugs occurs in man to a limited extent. Habituation and addiction do not occur, although vomiting, malaise, sweating, and salivation have been recorded in patients with parkinsonism upon sudden withdrawal of the large doses required for therapeutic benefit.

Absorption, Fate, and Excretion. The belladonna alkaloids are absorbed rapidly from the gastrointestinal tract. They also enter the circulation when applied locally to the mucosal surfaces of the body. Only limited absorption occurs from the eye and the intact skin. The total absorption of quaternary ammonium derivatives of the alkaloids after an oral dose is only about 25% (Levine, 1959); nevertheless, some of these compounds, applied locally to the eye, can cause mydriasis and cycloplegia. Atropine disappears rapidly from the blood and is distributed throughout the entire body. Most is excreted in the urine within the first 12 hours, in part unchanged, varying from 13 to 50%, and the remainder as a metabolite that has not yet been definitely identified (*see* Kalser, 1971). Only about 1% of an oral dose of scopolamine is eliminated in the urine. Traces of atropine are found in various secretions, including milk.

Some species of animals, especially certain rodents and marsupials, tolerate large doses of belladonna alkaloids. This is commonly seen in some varieties of rabbit, which show no toxic effects when fed on a diet of belladonna leaves. The resistance of these rabbits is genetically determined and depends on the presence of an enzyme, *atropine esterase,* found in the blood and liver, that destroys the alkaloid. The enzyme is not present in man. (*See* Sawin and Glick, 1943.)

Poisoning by Belladonna Alkaloids.

Atropine and scopolamine are the most important drugs of the belladonna group from the standpoint of poisoning. Infants and young children are especially susceptible to the alkaloids (*see* Unna *et al.,* 1950). Indeed, many cases of intoxication in children have resulted from conjunctival instillation of atropinic drugs, systemic absorption occurring from the nasal mucosa after the drug has traversed the nasolacrimal duct or from the intestinal tract if it is swallowed. Delirium or toxic psychoses, without undue peripheral manifestations, have been reported in adults after instillation of atropine eyedrops. Serious poisoning has followed the error of substituting scopolamine or atropine for the weaker homatropine. Atropine in medicinal mixtures given to children for enuresis has caused poisoning. Patients using belladonna in ascending doses should be warned of the early signs of intoxication. Poisoning occurs from overdose of the many "over-the-counter" sleeping medicines containing scopolamine, and from purposeful ingestion, for hallucinatory effects, of nonprescription asthma remedies containing stramonium and belladonna. Serious intoxication may occur in children who ingest berries or seeds containing belladonna alkaloids. Reports of stramonium poisoning due to tea made from Jimson weed seeds date as far back as 1676 in the United States and are described in early editions of this textbook.

Fatalities from atropine and scopolamine are rare, but sometimes occur in children. Of all the potent alkaloids, atropine has one of the widest margins of safety. The *fatal dose* of atropine is not known; 200-mg doses have often been used therapeutically for mental illness, and doses of as much as 1000 mg have been survived. In children, 10 mg or less may be lethal. Scopolamine is usually stated to be more toxic than atropine, but the evidence for this is inconclusive; doses of 500 mg have been survived. Idiosyncrasy is more common with scopolamine than with atropine, and ordinary therapeutic doses sometimes cause alarming reactions. Homatropine methylbromide is well tolerated in doses much larger than the therapeutic and is only about $\frac{1}{50}$ as toxic as atropine. Table 25–2 shows the doses of atropine giving undesirable responses or symptoms of overdosage.

Table 25–2. EFFECTS OF ATROPINE IN RELATION TO DOSAGE

DOSE	EFFECTS
0.5 mg	Slight cardiac slowing; some dryness of mouth; inhibition of sweating
1.0 mg	Definite dryness of mouth; thirst; acceleration of heart, sometimes preceded by slowing; mild dilatation of pupil
2.0 mg	Rapid heart rate; palpitation; marked dryness of mouth; dilated pupils; some blurring of near vision
5.0 mg	All the above symptoms marked; speech disturbed; difficulty in swallowing; restlessness and fatigue; headache; dry, hot skin; difficulty in micturition; reduced intestinal peristalsis
10.0 mg and more	Above symptoms more marked; pulse rapid and weak; iris practically obliterated; vision very blurred; skin flushed, hot, dry, and scarlet; ataxia, restlessness, and excitement; hallucinations and delirium; coma

Symptoms and Signs. These develop promptly after ingestion of the drug. The mouth becomes dry and burns; swallowing and talking are difficult or impossible, and there is marked thirst. The vision is blurred, and photophobia is prominent. The skin is hot, dry, and flushed. A rash may appear, especially over the face, neck, and upper part of the trunk; desquamation may follow. An atropine rash is more likely to occur in children. The body temperature rises, especially in infants. The pulse is weak and very rapid, but in infants and old people tachycardia may not be pronounced. Palpitation is prominent, and the blood pressure may be elevated. Urinary urgency and difficulty in micturition are sometimes noted. Abdominal distention may develop, especially in infants.

The patient is restless, excited, and confused, and exhibits weakness, giddiness, and muscular incoordination. Gait and speech are disturbed. Nausea and vomiting sometimes occur. The behavior and mental symptoms may suggest an acute organic psychosis. Memory is disturbed, orientation is faulty, hallucinations (especially visual) are common, the sensorium is clouded, and mania and delirium are not unusual (*see* Ketchum *et al.,* 1973). The diagnosis of an acute schizophrenic episode or alcoholic delirium has been mistakenly made, and some patients have been committed to psychiatric institutions for observation and diagnosis. The syndrome often lasts 48 hours or longer and may be punctuated by convulsions. Depression and circulatory collapse occur only in cases of severe intoxication; the blood pressure declines, respiration becomes inadequate, and death due to respiratory failure follows after a period of paralysis and coma (*see* Shader and Greenblatt, 1972).

Diagnosis. Careful analysis of the symptoms readily indicates widespread paralysis of organs innervated by parasympathetic nerves. This should immediately arouse suspicion of belladonna poisoning. Particularly significant are the dry mucous membranes, widely dilated and unresponsive pupils, tachycardia, cutaneous flush, and fever. However, the mental symptoms may distract attention from the obvious peripheral autonomic signs. *Any patient with an acute onset of bizarre mental and neurological symptoms should be suspected of poisoning by drugs, including atropinic drugs.* A history of prior belladonna medication may help to confirm the diagnosis. If belladonna poisoning is still doubtful, subcutaneous injection of 1 mg of the anti-ChE agent physostigmine may be diagnostic. If the typical salivation, sweating, and intestinal hyperactivity do not occur, belladonna intoxication is almost certain, because the alkaloids antagonize the muscarinic effects of physostigmine.

Treatment. When the poison has been taken orally, gastric lavage and other measures to limit intestinal absorption should be initiated without delay. *Physostigmine,* long overlooked as a possible antidote to atropine poisoning, is the rational therapy. For example, the slow intravenous injection of 1 to 4 mg of physostigmine (0.5 to 1.0 mg in children) rapidly abolishes the delirium and coma caused by large doses of atropine. Since physostigmine is rapidly destroyed, the patient may again lapse into coma within 1 to 2 hours, and repeated doses may be needed (*see* Forrer and Miller, 1958; Ketchum *et al.,* 1973; Rumack, 1973). If marked excitement is present and more specific treatment is not available, diazepam is most suitable for sedation and for control of convulsions. Large doses should be avoided because the central depressant action may coincide with the depression occurring late in belladonna poisoning. Phenothiazines should not be used because their antimuscarinic action is likely to intensify toxicity and may plunge the patient into coma. Artificial respiration with oxygen may be necessary. Ice bags and alcohol sponges help to reduce fever, especially in children.

Preparations, Dosage, and Routes of Administration. *Belladonna Tincture,* U.S.P., is a widely used preparation that consists of an aqueous-alcoholic extract of belladonna leaves. The adult dose is 0.6 to 1.0 ml, which contains approximately 0.2 to 0.3 mg, respectively, of the alkaloids of the leaf (mainly atropine). *Belladonna Extract,* N.F., may be given in pills or capsules; the dose is 15 mg, equivalent to approximately 0.2 mg of atropine. *Belladonna Leaf,* U.S.P., is used for the preparation of the tincture and extract. *Atropine,* N.F., is the main alkaloid of belladonna as the free base. The readily soluble salt, *Atropine Sulfate,* U.S.P., is official as a powder, in tablet form, as an injectable solution, and as an ophthalmic solution. The average adult dose of atropine sulfate is 0.5 mg. It is usually given orally, but may be injected subcutaneously or intravenously. *Scopolamine (l-*hyoscine) is marketed as the readily soluble salt, *Scopolamine Hydrobromide,* U.S.P. (*hyoscine hydrobromide*). The adult oral or parenteral dose is 0.6 mg. Preparations of stramonium and hyoscyamus are no longer official; they are now rarely used except in "over-the-counter" preparations and are not recommended because of their uncertain actions.

SYNTHETIC AND SEMISYNTHETIC SUBSTITUTES FOR BELLADONNA ALKALOIDS

The lack of selectivity of the belladonna alkaloids for those parasympathetic functions that might profitably be blocked in various diseases has led to intensive efforts to discover antimuscarinic drugs with more selective effects. Success has been limited, and the continuing appearance on the market of new antimuscarinic drugs that are promoted for the treatment of peptic ulcer and other gastrointestinal disorders makes it clear that the agents now available leave something to be desired. Although there are minor variations, the sequence of block in various organ systems is very similar for all antimuscarinics now used clinically. An important comparison of the effects of several drugs was made by Herxheimer (1958). In general, it can be stated that all antimuscarinic drugs fail to block gastrointestinal function in doses that do not have the usual atropinic effects on other structures, as outlined above.

The main differences in pharmacological properties are seen with those compounds having a quaternary ammonium structure. These drugs are poorly and unreliably absorbed after oral administration, and valid comparisons of their potencies with those of the belladonna alkaloids can be made only after parenteral administration. Penetration of the conjunctiva is also poor, so that most quaternary ammonium compounds are of little value in ophthalmology. Central effects are generally lacking, because these agents do not readily pass the blood-brain barrier. The quaternary ammonium compounds usually have a somewhat more prolonged action; little is known of the fate and excretion of most of these agents. The ratio of ganglionic blocking to antimuscarinic activity is greater for compounds with the quaternary ammonium structure because of their greater potency at nicotinic receptors; some of the side effects seen after high doses are due to ganglionic blockade. Thus, impotence and postural hypotension occur and urinary retention is not uncommon in patients with prostatic hypertrophy who are given these drugs. Poisoning with quaternary ammonium compounds may also cause a curariform neuromuscular block, leading to respiratory paralysis. Toxic doses of these agents produce, therefore, the usual manifestations of antimuscarinic poisoning with additional effects of ganglionic and, rarely, neuromuscular block, but usually without significant CNS involvement.

There is a clinical impression that the quaternary ammonium compounds have a relatively greater effect on gastrointestinal activity and that the doses necessary to treat gastrointestinal disorders are, consequently, somewhat more readily tolerated; this has been attributed to the additional element of ganglionic block. However, no drug of this class has yet been shown to produce adequate control of gastric secretion or gastrointestinal motility at doses that are devoid of significant side effects due to muscarinic blockade at other sites.

The pharmacological properties of the drugs discussed below differ little from those of other agents in the same general category and range between those of atropine and those of oxyphenonium and methantheline, the quaternary ammonium compounds with the greatest ratio of ganglionic blocking to antimuscarinic activity. The names, chemical structures, dosage forms, and usual clinical doses of these and other drugs of the same class are given in Table 25–3.

Homatropine. This drug (Table 25–1) has about one tenth the potency of atropine. It is used solely as a topical *mydriatic* and *cycloplegic* in the form of 2 to 5% *Homatropine Hydrobromide Ophthalmic Solution*, U.S.P., or of the unofficial hydrochloride, for which purposes it is preferable to atropine in many cases because of its rapid onset and short duration of action (Table 25–4). Accommodation is usually normal within 24 hours, but a briefer cycloplegia can be obtained by a 1% solution, often used in combination with a sympathomimetic drug (*e.g.,* ephedrine). Homatropine does not usually cause complete cycloplegia in children. Some conjunctival vasodilatation occurs after instillation of the drug.

QUATERNARY AMMONIUM DERIVATIVES OF
BELLADONNA ALKALOIDS

Atropine Methylnitrate. When given parenterally, *atropine methylnitrate* (EKOMINE, METROPINE) (Table 25–1) has more potent antimuscarinic properties than has atropine. It also has strong ganglionic blocking activity, being more potent in this respect than tetraethylammonium.

Methscopolamine Bromide. *Methscopolamine Bromide,* N.F. (PAMINE) (Table 25–1), lacks the central actions of scopolamine. It is less potent than

atropine and is less well absorbed, but its action is more prolonged, the usual oral dose (2.5 mg) acting for 8 hours. Its limited use has been chiefly in gastrointestinal diseases.

Homatropine Methylbromide. Used mainly in gastrointestinal disorders and sometimes for preanesthetic medication, *Homatropine Methylbromide,* N.F. (Table 25–1), is less potent than atropine in antimuscarinic activity (oral dose, 2.5 to 5.0 mg), but it is four times more potent as a ganglionic blocking agent. Homatropine methylbromide may have a more favorable therapeutic ratio than atropine, requiring relatively larger doses to produce minimal toxic effects, but this point has not been fully established.

SYNTHETIC QUATERNARY AMMONIUM
COMPOUNDS

Methantheline. *Methantheline Bromide,* N.F. (BANTHINE), is a widely used and extensively studied synthetic quaternary ammonium compound (Table 25–3) that differs from atropine in having a particularly high ratio of ganglionic blocking to antimuscarinic activity. High doses may cause impotence, an effect rarely produced by purely antimuscarinic drugs and indicative of ganglionic block. Toxic doses may paralyze respiration by neuromuscular block. CNS manifestations of restlessness, euphoria, fatigue, or, very rarely, acute psychotic episodes may appear in occasional patients. Gastrointestinal effects of methantheline appear to be relatively greater than those of atropine, and many clinicians have the impression that the doses of methantheline used in the treatment of gastrointestinal disorders cause fewer antimuscarinic side effects than does atropine. The action is somewhat more prolonged than that of atropine, the effects of a therapeutic dose lasting 6 hours. An additional toxic manifestation unrelated to the blocking actions is the occasional appearance of skin rashes, including exfoliative dermatitis.

Propantheline. Closely related chemically to methantheline, *Propantheline Bromide,* U.S.P. (PROBANTHINE) (Table 25–3), has similar properties but is two to five times more potent in antimuscarinic activity and about one and one-half times more potent as a ganglionic blocking agent. Very high doses block the skeletal neuromuscular junction. The usual clinical dose (15 mg) acts for about 6 hours.

Oxyphenonium. *Oxyphenonium bromide* (ANTRENYL) (Table 25–3) is somewhat more potent than methantheline and also has a particularly high ratio of ganglionic blocking to antimuscarinic activity. Nevertheless, usual doses exert their main effects because of the antimuscarinic action. Large doses block ganglionic transmission, and toxic doses may block neuromuscular transmission. CNS activity is lacking.

OTHER SYNTHETIC ANTIMUSCARINIC
COMPOUNDS

The synthetic drugs in this group do not have the quaternary ammonium structure. Most are well ab-

Table 25–3. REPRESENTATIVE SYNTHETIC ANTIMUSCARINIC DRUGS

DRUG, DOSAGE FORM, AND USUAL SINGLE DOSE	CHEMICAL STRUCTURE
Quaternary Ammonium Compounds Anisotropine methylbromide VALPIN Tablets: 10 mg Elixir: 2 mg/ml 10 mg	
Diphemanil Methylsulfate, N.F. PRANTAL *† Tablets: 100 mg 50 to 100 mg	
Glycopyrrolate, N.F. ROBINUL * Tablets: 1 and 2 mg 1 to 2 mg	
Hexocyclium Methylsulfate, N.F. TRAL † Tablets: 25 mg 25 mg	
Isopropamide Iodide, N.F. DARBID Tablets: 5 mg 5 mg	
Mepenzolate Bromide, N.F. CANTIL Tablets: 25 mg Liquid: 5 mg/ml 25 to 50 mg	
Methantheline Bromide, N.F. BANTHINE * Tablets: 50 mg 25 to 50 mg	
Oxyphenonium bromide ANTRENYL Tablets: 5 mg 10 mg	

Most of the drugs are given four times daily, before meals and at bedtime.
* Also available in a solution or as a powder for dissolution for injection.
† Also available as a sustained-release tablet.
‡ Not available in the United States under this trade name.

525

Table 25–3. REPRESENTATIVE SYNTHETIC ANTIMUSCARINIC DRUGS (Continued)

DRUG, DOSAGE FORM, AND USUAL SINGLE DOSE	CHEMICAL STRUCTURE
Quaternary Ammonium Compounds (*Cont.*) Poldine Methylsulfate, N.F. NACTON Tablets: 4 mg 4 mg	
Propantheline Bromide, U.S.P. PRO-BANTHINE * Tablets: 7.5 and 15 mg 15 mg	
Tridihexethyl Chloride, N.F. PATHILON *† Tablets: 25 mg 25 mg	
Other Synthetic Antimuscarinic Compounds Cyclopentolate Hydrochloride, U.S.P. CYCLOGYL Ophthalmic solution: 0.5, 1.0, and 2.0%	
Eucatropine Hydrochloride, U.S.P. EUPHTHALMINE ‡ Ophthalmic solution: 2 to 5%	
Oxyphencyclimine Hydrochloride, N.F. DARICON Tablets: 10 mg 10 mg	
Piperidolate Hydrochloride, N.F. DACTIL Tablets: 50 mg 50 mg	
Thiphenamil hydrochloride TROCINATE Tablets: 100 and 400 mg 400 mg	

Table 25-3.   REPRESENTATIVE SYNTHETIC ANTIMUSCARINIC DRUGS (Continued)

DRUG, DOSAGE FORM, AND USUAL SINGLE DOSE	CHEMICAL STRUCTURE
Other Synthetic Antimuscarinic Compounds (Cont.) Tropicamide, U.S.P. MYDRIACYL Ophthalmic solution: 0.5 and 1%	
Antispasmodics with Little Antimuscarinic Activity Adiphenine hydrochloride TRASENTINE Tablets: 75 mg 75 to 150 mg	
Dicyclomine Hydrochloride, U.S.P. BENTYL * Capsules: 10 mg Tablets: 20 mg Syrup: 2 mg/ml 10 to 20 mg	

Most of the drugs are given four times daily, before meals and at bedtime.
* Also available in a solution or as a powder for dissolution for injection.
† Also available as a sustained-release tablet.
‡ Not available in the United States under this trade name.

sorbed after oral administration, and some (*e.g.,* cyclopentolate and tropicamide) are useful in ophthalmology. Their pharmacological properties are very similar to those of atropine and, therefore, do not require separate discussion.

OTHER AGENTS PROPERLY CLASSIFIED AS
NONSPECIFIC SMOOTH MUSCLE RELAXANTS

Two drugs, often classified with antimuscarinic agents as "antispasmodics," do not properly belong to the group of antimuscarinic agents. These drugs—*adiphenine hydrochloride* (TRASENTINE) and *Dicyclomine Hydrochloride,* U.S.P. (BENTYL) (Table 25–3)—decrease spasm of the gastrointestinal tract, biliary tract, ureter, and uterus without producing characteristic atropinic effects on the salivary, sweat, or gastrointestinal glands, the eye, or the cardiovascular system, except in large doses. Their major action appears to be a nonspecific direct relaxant action on smooth muscle rather than a competitive antagonism of ACh. Neither of the drugs bears a chemical resemblance to the belladonna alkaloids, but adiphenine is chemically related to the local anesthetics and has local anesthetic activity. Anesthesia of the oral mucosa results when tablets of the drug are chewed. It has been suggested that the orally ingested drug may relax intestinal smooth muscle by a local anesthetic action that interrupts local reflexes regulating tone and motility. Secretory activity is unaffected. Clinical use of these drugs has been disappointing.

THERAPEUTIC USES OF ANTIMUSCARINIC DRUGS

The belladonna alkaloids have been employed in a wide variety of clinical conditions, predominantly to inhibit effects of parasympathetic nervous system activity. However, the lack of selectivity of the antimuscarinic agents makes it difficult to obtain desired therapeutic responses without concomitant side effects. The latter usually are not serious but are sufficiently disturbing to the patient to limit sharply the dosage tolerated and therefore the usefulness of these agents, particularly for chronic administration. Certain of the synthetic belladonna substitutes are used much more extensively than are the natural alkaloids in a number of clinical conditions. However, there are few situations in which this preference is supported by acceptable evidence. Where a particular agent or group of agents has been proved superior to others for a specific clinical use on the basis of selectivity, duration of action, or other properties, this advantage is pointed out in the following sections.

Central Nervous System. For many years the belladonna alkaloids and subsequently the tertiary-amine synthetic substitutes were the only agents helpful in the treatment of *parkinsonism.* Levodopa is now the treatment of choice, but concurrent therapy with the synthetic agents may be required (*see* Chapter 14). The synthetic agents are also useful in the treatment of parkinsonism-like symptoms induced by phenothiazines or butyrophenones (*see* Chapter 12).

The belladonna alkaloids were among the first drugs to be used in the prevention of *motion sickness.* Scopolamine is the most effective prophylactic agent for short (4- to 6-hour) exposures to severe motion, and probably for periods up to several days. Oral doses of 0.1 mg protect 75% of susceptible persons, and do not affect vision and rarely cause dryness of the mouth. Intramuscular injection of 0.2 mg controls symptoms of most seasick individuals; sedation is the major disadvantage. (*See* Brand and Whittingham, 1970.) The superiority of scopolamine is more apparent the more susceptible the subjects and the more severe the stress. The drug is not recommended for nausea and vomiting due to most other causes. All agents used to combat motion sickness should be given *prophylactically;* they are much less effective after severe nausea or vomiting has developed. (For further discussion of motion sickness, *see* Chapter 29.) Scopolamine has also been successfully used for prophylaxis in the premonitory phase in Ménière's disease.

The sedation, tranquilization, and amnesia produced by scopolamine are useful in several circumstances, including *labor, delirium tremens, toxic psychoses,* and *maniacal states.* In these conditions, it is almost always combined with agents producing analgesia or sedation. Given alone in the presence of pain or severe anxiety, scopolamine may induce outbursts of uncontrolled behavior.

Uses in Anesthesia. The belladonna alkaloids are well established as a component of *preanesthetic medication,* mainly to inhibit excessive salivation and respiratory tract secretion due to irritant anesthetics;

their concomitant bronchodilator action is also of value. The increasing use of relatively nonirritating anesthetics lessens the importance of antimuscarinic agents for this purpose. Scopolamine may contribute to tranquilization and amnesia. Atropine is commonly given with neostigmine to counteract its parasympathomimetic effects when the latter agent is used to end curarization after surgery. Serious cardiac arrhythmias have occasionally occurred, perhaps due to the combination of initial central vagal stimulation by atropine and the cholinomimetic effect of neostigmine. (For details, *see* Chapters 4 and 28.)

Uses in Ophthalmology. Effects limited to the eye are obtained by local administration of an antimuscarinic drug to produce mydriasis and cycloplegia. Cycloplegia is not attainable without mydriasis and requires higher concentrations or more prolonged application of a given agent. Mydriasis is often necessary for thorough examination of the retina and optic disc and in the therapy of *acute iritis, iridocyclitis,* and *keratitis.* The belladonna mydriatics may be alternated with miotics for breaking or preventing the development of adhesions between the iris and the lens. Complete cycloplegia may be necessary in the treatment of *iridocyclitis* and *choroiditis* and for accurate *measurement of refractive errors.* Details of the drugs commonly used and the duration of action of the usual solutions are given in Table 25–4. One or 2 drops of an aqueous solution, often containing a surface-active agent to facilitate penetration, is instilled into the conjunctival sac and repeated as necessary to produce the desired intensity and duration of effect. The values given vary with the frequency and duration of contact with the solution and with individual susceptibility. Although the effect of a single drop of a solution of atropine on healthy eyes is very prolonged, in acute inflammation two or three instillations a day may be required to maintain a full effect. Atropine occasionally causes local irritation of the eye, and in susceptible persons it may produce swelling of the eyelids and conjunctivitis. With continued use, the

Table 25–4. MYDRIATIC AND CYCLOPLEGIC PROPERTIES OF ANTIMUSCARINIC AGENTS

DRUG	STRENGTH OF SOLUTION * (*percent*)	MYDRIASIS		PARALYSIS OF ACCOMMODATION	
		Maximal (*minutes*)	*Recovery* † (*days*)	*Maximal* (*hours*)	*Recovery* ‡ (*days*)
Atropine sulfate	1.0	30–40	7–10	1–3	7–12
Scopolamine hydrobromide	0.5	20–30	3–7	½–1	5–7
Homatropine hydrobromide	1.0 §	40–60	1–3	½–1	1–3
Eucatropine hydrochloride	2.0–5.0	30	¼	None	—
Cyclopentolate hydrochloride	0.5–1.0	30–60	1	½–1	1
Tropicamide	0.5–1.0 ‖	20–40	¼	½	<¼

* One instillation of 1 drop of solution.

† To within 1 mm of original pupillary diameter.

‡ To within 2 diopters of original accommodative power; ability to read fine print is possible by the third day after atropine or scopolamine and by 6 hours after homatropine instillation.

§ Full mydriasis and accommodation loss require instillation of a 5% solution.

‖ Adequate accommodation loss lasting about 30 minutes requires instillation of a 1% solution.

conjunctivitis may become chronic. Therapy with antihistaminic agents may control the atropine conjunctivitis, or therapy may be continued with another agent (*e.g.,* scopolamine).

Shorter-acting substitutes for atropine or scopolamine are used when prolonged mydriasis and cycloplegia are not required or may pose a hazard to the patient. The standard agents for this purpose are homatropine, cyclopentolate, eucatropine, and tropicamide. Of these homatropine has the longest action but may not provide adequate cycloplegia even with 5% solutions. Where mydriasis alone is desired, the weaker solutions of cyclopentolate, eucatropine, or tropicamide may be used, if necessary in combination with a sympathomimetic drug such as phenylephrine. Psychotic reactions, behavioral disturbances, and convulsions have appeared after ophthalmic use of cyclopentolate; these adverse effects have not yet been reported with eucatropine or tropicamide.

It is of great importance to recognize patients who are predisposed to narrow-angle glaucoma. The ophthalmic use of any of the antimuscarinic drugs may increase intraocular pressure in eyes with a narrow angle between iris and cornea, precipitating an attack of *acute glaucoma* with the potential hazard of ensuing blindness, particularly if mydriasis is prolonged. Atropine and scopolamine are therefore particularly dangerous. Systemic use of the antimuscarinic agents can also precipitate glaucoma in such predisposed patients. In wide-angle glaucoma the drugs do not cause dangerous elevation of intraocular pressure. Although narrow-angle glaucoma is a very rare condition, the use of drugs with antimuscarinic properties is not; careful ophthalmological evaluation, including examination with tonometer and gonioscope, should be undertaken to detect the possible presence of a narrow-angle anterior chamber before starting therapy with these agents, particularly if therapy is to be intensive or prolonged. Mydriasis due to the shorter-acting agents may be counteracted by local application of pilocarpine (1 to 4%); mydriasis from atropine and scopolamine is usually only partly counteracted, even by physostigmine (0.25%) or isoflurophate (0.1%).

The photophobia associated with mydriasis may require that the patient wear dark glasses. Although absorption into the blood stream from the conjunctival sac is minimal, systemic toxicity can occur from an antimuscarinic agent that reaches more absorptive mucosal surfaces by way of the nasolacrimal duct, and this danger should be minimized by pressure on the inner canthus of the eye for a few minutes after each instillation. This precaution is particularly important in small children, who are highly susceptible to the toxic effects of belladonna alkaloids.

Respiratory Tract. Atropine and other belladonna alkaloids and substitutes reduce secretion in both the upper and the lower respiratory tract, and they are common constituents of proprietary "cold" tablets. This effect in the nasopharynx may provide some symptomatic relief of *acute rhinitis* associated with *coryza* or *hay fever,* but such therapy does not affect the natural course of the condition. It is probable that the contribution of antihistamines employed in "cold" mixtures is also primarily due to their antimuscarinic properties, except in conditions with an allergic basis. The belladonna alkaloids can induce bronchial dilatation and were formerly in common use as a remedy for bronchial asthma.

All antimuscarinic agents reduce the volume of bronchial secretion, which may result in decreased fluidity and subsequent inspissation of the residual secretion. This viscid material is difficult to remove from the respiratory tree, and its presence can dangerously obstruct airflow and predispose to infection. Because of the effect on bronchial secretion, repeated administration of any antimuscarinic drug to a patient with chronic lung disease is considered by some authorities to be potentially hazardous.

Cardiovascular System. Aside from inhibition of certain reflexes during anesthesia and surgery, the cardiovascular effects of the belladonna alkaloids have limited clinical application, and the synthetic substitutes are little used in this field. Atropine is a specific antidote for the cardiovascular collapse that may result from the injudicious administration of a choline ester.

Atropine may be of value in the initial treatment of carefully selected cases of *acute myocardial infarction* in which excessive vagal tone causes sinus or nodal bradycardia accompanied by a falling blood pressure and a low cardiac output, or a high-grade A-V block resulting in ectopic ventricular tachyarrhythmia (*see* Thomas and Woodgate, 1966; Adgey *et al.,* 1968). Intravenously administered atropine may restore a normal heart rate and increase the blood pressure to an adequate level within a few minutes. It has been suggested that some of the deaths occurring in the first few hours after myocardial infarction are related to excessive vagal tone and may be avoided by the use of atropine. In such patients who develop the above-indicated cardiovascular evidence of excessive vagal activity, there may also be other signs of such activity, including nausea, vomiting, and gastrointestinal hypermotility. The administration of small doses of atropine (0.2 to 0.4 mg) intravenously seems justified. A major concern is obviously the status of the coronary circulation. Hypotension may contribute to extension of the myocardial infarction; if hypotension is due to bradycardia, atropine may prevent such extension. However, if the heart rate is accelerated by atropine without improvement of coronary perfusion pressure, further ischemia will result. Tachycardia, ventricular arrhythmias, and fibrillation may also occur (*see* Richman, 1974). Controlled studies of the effects of atropine in properly selected patients seen soon after myocardial infarction (especially in mobile coronary-care facilities) are needed to settle the question of the precise indications for atropine and the benefits to be derived from its use.

Atropine is occasionally useful in reducing the severe bradycardia and syncope associated with a *hyperactive carotid sinus reflex.* It has little effect on most ventricular rhythms. In some cases atropine may eliminate ventricular premature contractions associated with a very slow atrial rate. It may also reduce the degree of A-V block when increased vagal tone is a major factor in the conduction defect. Atropine is occasionally useful in the diagnosis of *anomalous A-V conduction* (Wolff-Parkinson-White syndrome) by restoring the QRS complex to normal duration.

Gastrointestinal Tract. Antimuscarinic agents have been used extensively as adjuncts to dietary and antacid treatment of *peptic ulcer,* but their value in this condition is extremely difficult to assess. The rationale of therapy is theoretically sound; the drugs reduce gastric secretion, provided the dose is increased to the limits of tolerance of side effects. Inhibition of motility in the ulcerated region should also contribute to the relief of pain. An additional theoretical factor is delayed gastric emptying, which would prolong the neutralizing effect of antacids; this effect, however, might be counteracted by equally prolonged production of acid because of the continued presence of food in the stomach. High expectations on theoretical grounds have not materialized. Peptic ulcer is a chronic recurrent disease characterized by remissions and exacerbations, and radiological assessment of healing is notoriously difficult. Evidence of healing has therefore been based mainly on subjective symptoms. In controlled trials these symptoms have frequently improved equally well with placebo medication. The long-term effects of antimuscarinic therapy have been equally disappointing (*see* Sun, 1964; Trevino *et al.,* 1967).

The inadequacy of the belladonna alkaloids in peptic ulcer and the extensive potential market for more effective therapy have led to the development and promotion of many synthetic substitutes. Although many of the quaternary ammonium agents have additional ganglion blocking activity, none has proven distinctly superior to the natural alkaloids either in therapeutic effect or in reduction of atropinic side effects. If an antimuscarinic drug is to be used, the official belladonna tincture is the most economical and the most readily titrated to each patient's optimal dose. In order to obtain significant relief of pain, the dose must be increased to the limit the patient will tolerate, which generally entails acceptance of some unpleasant side effects. A relatively high dose is less troublesome if taken at bedtime, so that peak side effects as well as inhibition of gastric secretion occur during sleep.

It can be predicted that improvement in the therapy of peptic ulcer will be provided in the near future by the further development of effective and safe antihistaminic agents that block selectively H_2 receptors (*see* Chapter 29).

The belladonna alkaloids and their synthetic substitutes have been employed and recommended in a wide variety of conditions known or supposed to involve increased tone (*"spasticity"*) or motility of the gastrointestinal tract. These agents reduce tone and motility when administered in maximal tolerated doses, and can be expected to have a real although often incomplete effect if the condition in question is in fact due to excessive smooth muscle contraction, a point that is often in doubt. The antimuscarinic agents do not consistently correct disordered motor activity. In some patients with *irritable colon syndrome,* the drugs may give some initial relief of symptoms but do not cause consistent or continued improvement. The intestinal hypermotility and increased frequency of stools associated with administration of two antihypertensive agents, guanethidine and reserpine, are frequently well controlled. Similarly, diarrhea sometimes associated with irritative conditions of the lower bowel, such as mild *dysenteries* and *diverticulitis,* may respond to such therapy. In these conditions, both the frequency of bowel movements and the associated abdominal cramps may be reduced or fully controlled. However, more severe conditions such as *salmonella dysenteries, ulcerative colitis,* and *regional enteritis* respond poorly. Large single parenteral doses of an antimuscarinic agent occasionally assist the roentgenological differentiation of morphological defects and functional spasm of the gastrointestinal tract. *Constipation* associated with increased tone of the large bowel may be favorably affected. Such increased tone is an obvious component of morphine-induced obstipation and lead colic, and atropine may provide partial relief. Responses in the more common cases of *"spastic constipation"* associated with anxiety, travel, misuse of laxatives, and other causes are variable, and in most reports it is impossible to distinguish between pharmacodynamic and placebo benefit. The cardiac, pyloric, and ileocecal sphincters in man contract in response to cholinergic stimuli (Bennet and Whitney, 1966), and this may account for the favorable responses observed after antimuscarinic agents in such conditions as *pylorospasm* and *cardiospasm.*

The belladonna alkaloids and synthetic substitutes are very effective in reducing *excessive salivation,* such as that associated with heavy-metal poisoning or parkinsonism; indeed, the dosage must be adjusted carefully to avoid reducing secretion to the point where dry mouth is troublesome. Although these agents are rarely effective alone in relieving *biliary colic,* they are commonly administered with morphine or another narcotic; this would seem to be a rational combination, but the extent to which the antimuscarinic component contributes to the relief obtained is difficult to define. Antimuscarinic agents can reduce the volume and tryptic activity of pancreatic secretion, perhaps largely secondary to retarded entry of acid gastric contents into the duodenum and thus delayed release of secretin. Several agents, particularly methantheline and propantheline, have been tried in the treatment of *acute pancreatitis,* and have been reported to decrease pain and plasma amylase activity in some cases. However, the results have been highly variable and, in general, disappointing.

Genitourinary Tract. Almost all the antimuscarinic and antispasmodic drugs available for clinical use may relieve the pain of *dysmenorrhea* for one or a few menstrual periods when first administered, but none is consistently effective.

Atropine is commonly given with a narcotic in the treatment of *renal colic* in the hope that it will relax the ureteral smooth muscle; however, as in biliary colic, it probably does not make a major contribution to the relief of pain. The belladonna alkaloids and several synthetic substitutes can lower intravesicular pressure, increase capacity, and reduce the frequency of urinary bladder contractions by antagonizing the parasympathetic control of this organ. The block is less complete than in many other organs, but it has been taken as a basis for the use of such agents in *enuresis* in children, particularly when a progressive increase in bladder capacity is the objective, to reduce urinary frequency in spastic paraplegia, and to increase the capacity of the bladder in conditions in which irritation has led to hypertonicity. However, it has not been established that antimuscarinic drugs make a major contribution to the treatment of any of these conditions.

Anticholinesterase and Mushroom Poisoning. The use of atropine in large doses for the treatment of poisoning by anti-ChE organophosphorus insecticides is discussed in detail in Chapter 22. Atropine may also be used to antagonize the parasympathomimetic effects of neostigmine or other anti-ChE agents administered in the treatment of myasthenia gravis. It does not interfere with the salutary effects at the skeletal neuromuscular junction, and is particularly useful early in therapy, before tolerance to muscarinic side effects has developed.

Atropine is a specific antidote for the so-called *rapid type* of *mushroom poisoning* due to the cholinomimetic alkaloid muscarine, found in *Amanita muscaria* and a few other fungi. Atropine is of no value in the *delayed type* of mushroom poisoning due to the toxins of *A. phalloides* and certain other species of the same genus. (*See* Chapter 23.)

Adgey, A. A. J.; Geddes, J. S.; Mulholland, H. C.; Keegan, D. A. J.; and Pantridge, J. F. Incidence, significance, and management of early bradyarrhythmia complicating acute myocardial infarction. *Lancet,* **1968,** *2,* 1097–1101.

Ashford, A.; Penn, G. B.; and Ross, J. W. Cholinergic activity of atropine. *Nature, Lond.,* **1962,** *193,* 1082–1083.

Averill, K. H., and Lamb, L. E. Less commonly recognized actions of atropine on cardiac rhythm. *Am. J. med. Sci.,* **1959,** *237,* 304–318.

Bennet, A., and Whitney, W. A pharmacological study of the motility of the human gastrointestinal tract. *Gut,* **1966,** *7,* 307–316.

Berry, J. N.; Thompson, H. K., Jr.; and Miller, D. E. Changes in cardiac output, stroke volume, and central venous pressure induced by atropine in man. *Am. Heart J.,* **1959,** *58,* 204–213.

Brand, J. J., and Whittingham, P. Intramuscular hyoscine in control of motion sickness. *Lancet,* **1970,** *2,* 232–234.

Cullumbine, H.; McKee, W. H. E.; and Creasy, N. H. The effects of atropine sulphate upon healthy male subjects. *Q. Jl exp. Physiol.,* **1955,** *40,* 309–319.

Daly, W. J.; Ross, J. C.; and Behnke, R. H. The effect of changes in the pulmonary vascular bed produced by atropine, pulmonary engorgement, and positive-pressure breathing on diffusing and mechanical properties of the lung. *J. clin. Invest.,* **1963,** *42,* 1083–1094.

Dauchot, P., and Gravenstein, J. S. Effects of atropine on the electrocardiogram in different age groups. *Clin. Pharmac. Ther.,* **1971,** *12,* 274–280.

Duvoisin, R. C. Cholinergic-anticholinergic antagonism in parkinsonism. *Archs Neurol., Chicago,* **1967,** *17,* 124–136.

Farquharson, M. E., and Johnston, R. G. Antagonism of the effects of tremorine by tropine derivatives. *Br. J. Pharmac. Chemother.,* **1959,** *14,* 559–566.

Forrer, G. R., and Miller, J. J. Atropine coma: a somatic therapy in psychiatry. *Am. J. Psychiat.,* **1958,** *115,* 455–458.

Gaskell, P. The effect of intra-arterial atropine infusions on the blood flow through the human hand and forearm. *J. Physiol., Lond.,* **1956,** *131,* 639–646.

Grob, D.; Harvey, A. M.; Langworthy, O. R.; and Lilienthal, J. L., Jr. The administration of di-isopropylfluorophosphate (DFP) to man. III. Effect on the central nervous system with special reference to the electrical activity of the brain. *Bull. Johns Hopkins Hosp.,* **1947,** *81,* 257–266.

Hayes, A. H., Jr.; Copelan, H. W.; and Ketchum, J. S. Effects of large intramuscular doses of atropine on cardiac rhythm. *Clin. Pharmac. Ther.,* **1971,** *12,* 482–486.

Herxheimer, A. A comparison of some atropine-like drugs in man, with particular reference to their end-organ specificity. *Br. J. Pharmac. Chemother.,* **1958,** *13,* 184–192.

Ing, H. R. Synthetic substitutes for atropine. *Br. med. Bull.,* **1946,** *4,* 91–95.

Kalser, S. C. The fate of atropine in man. *Ann. N.Y. Acad. Sci.,* **1971,** *179,* 667–683.

Ketchum, J. S.; Sidell, F. R.; Crowell, E. B., Jr.; Aghajanian, G. K.; and Hayes, A. H., Jr. Atropine, scopolamine, and ditran: comparative pharmacology and antagonists in man. *Psychopharmacologia,* **1973,** *28,* 121–145.

Kottmeier, C. A., and Gravenstein, J. S. The parasympathomimetic activity of atropine and atropine methylbromide. *Anesthesiology,* **1968,** *29,* 1125–1133.

Lands, A. M. An investigation of the molecular configurations favorable for stimulation or blockade of the acetylcholine-sensitive receptors of visceral organs. *J. Pharmac. exp. Ther.,* **1951,** *102,* 219–236.

Levine, R. M. The intestinal absorption of the quaternary derivatives of atropine and scopolamine. *Archs int. Pharmacodyn. Thér.,* **1959,** *121,* 146–149.

Medical Letter. Effects of systemic drugs with anticholinergic properties on glaucoma. **1974,** *16,* 28.

Ostfeld, A. M., and Arguete, A. Central nervous system effects of hyoscine in man. *J. Pharmac. exp. Ther.,* **1962,** *137,* 133–139.

Richman, S. Adverse effect of atropine during myocardial infarction. Enhancement of ischemia following intravenously administered atropine. *J. Am. med. Ass.,* **1974,** *228,* 1414–1416.

Rossum, J. M. van. Atropine-like actions of muscarine isomers. *Science, Wash.,* **1960,** *132,* 954–956.

Rumack, B. H. Anticholinergic poisoning: treatment with physostigmine. *Pediatrics, Springfield,* **1973,** *52,* 449–451.

Sawin, P. B., and Glick, D. Atropinesterase, genetically determined enzymes in rabbit. *Proc. natn. Acad. Sci. U.S.A.,* **1943,** *29,* 55–59.

Stoll, H. C. Pharmacodynamic considerations of atropine and related compounds. *Am. J. med. Sci.,* **1948,** *215,* 577–592.

Sun, D. C. H. Long-term anticholinergic therapy for prevention of recurrences in duodenal ulcer. *Am. J. dig. Dis.,* **1964,** *9,* 706–716.

Thomas, M., and Woodgate, D. Effect of atropine on bradycardia and hypotension in acute myocardial infarction. *Br. Heart J.,* **1966,** *28,* 409–413.

Trevino, H.; Anderson, J.; Davey, P. G.; and Henley, K. S. The effect of glycopyrrolate on the course of symptomatic duodenal ulcer. *Am. J. dig. Dis.,* **1967,** *12,* 983–987.

Unna, K. R.; Glaser, K.; Lipton, E.; and Patterson, P. R. Dosage of drugs in infants and children. I. Atropine. *Pediatrics, Springfield,* **1950,** *6,* 197–207.

Vernier, V. G., and Unna, K. R. The experimental evaluation of antiparkinsonian compounds. *Ann. N.Y. Acad. Sci.,* **1956,** *64,* 690–704.

Monographs and Reviews

Ambache, N. The use and limitations of atropine for pharmacological studies on autonomic effectors. *Pharmac. Rev.,* **1955,** *7,* 467–494.

Bachrach, W. H. Anticholinergic drugs: survey of the literature and some experimental observations. *Am. J. dig. Dis.,* **1958,** *3,* 743–799.

Bebbington, A., and Brimblecombe, R. S. Muscarinic receptors in the peripheral and central nervous systems. *Adv. Drug Res.,* **1965,** *2,* 143–172.

Code, C. F. The inhibition of gastric secretion: a review. *Pharmac. Rev.,* **1951,** *3,* 59–106. (336 references.)

de Wied, D., and de Jong, W. Drug effects and hypothalamic–anterior pituitary function. *A. Rev. Pharmac.,* **1974,** *14,* 389–412.

Eger, E. I., ii. Atropine, scopolamine, and related compounds. *Anesthesiology,* **1962,** *23,* 365–383. (294 references.)

Krnjević, K. Central cholinergic pathways. *Fedn Proc. Fedn Am. Socs exp. Biol.,* **1969,** *28,* 113–120. (64 references.)

———. Chemical nature of synaptic transmission in vertebrates. *Physiol. Rev.,* **1974,** *54,* 418–540.

Longo, V. G. Behavioral and electroencephalographic effects of atropine and related compounds. *Pharmac. Rev.,* **1966,** *18,* 965–996. (184 references.)

Pierce, J. S. Antispasmodics and antiulcer drugs. In, *Medicinal Chemistry.* (Burger, A., ed.) Interscience Publishers, Inc., New York, **1960,** pp. 463–493. (128 references.)

Shader, R. I., and Greenblatt, D. J. Belladonna alkaloids and synthetic anticholinergics: uses and toxicity. In, *Psychiatric Complications of Medical Drugs.* (Shader, R. I., ed.) Raven Press, New York, **1972,** pp. 103–147.

Shepherd, J. T. *Physiology of the Circulation in Human Limbs in Health and Disease.* W. B. Saunders Co., Philadelphia, **1963.**

Toman, J. E. P., and Davis, J. P. The effects of drugs upon the electrical activity of the brain. *Pharmac. Rev.,* **1949,** *1,* 425–492. (349 references.)

26 DRUGS INHIBITING ADRENERGIC NERVES AND STRUCTURES INNERVATED BY THEM

Mark Nickerson and Brian Collier

History and Terminology. Since the classical paper in which Dale (1906) described the alteration of responses to sympathetic nerve stimulation and to sympathomimetic amines by certain ergot preparations, many natural and synthetic compounds have been found to block various of these responses. Adrenergic blocking drugs have contributed much to our understanding of sympathetic nervous system function, and several are now of considerable therapeutic importance.

The term *adrenergic blocking agent* designates a compound that selectively inhibits certain responses to adrenergic nerve activity and to epinephrine, norepinephrine, and other sympathomimetic amines. The locus of action is the effector cell, and this criterion distinguishes such agents from substances that prevent sympathoadrenal discharge by blocking nerve impulse transmission within the cerebrospinal axis, in autonomic ganglia, or along peripheral neurons, or that interfere with the release of adrenergic mediator (norepinephrine). The terms *adrenolytic* and *sympatholytic* are sometimes applied to agents that block responses to epinephrine and to adrenergic nerve activity, respectively, but these have been used to refer to a wide variety of pharmacological actions and their meaning is often unclear. All known adrenergic blocking agents can inhibit responses to both circulating sympathomimetic drugs and sympathetic nerve activity. While the former effect is practically always obtained at a lower dose, the relative effectiveness against these two types of stimuli varies considerably.

Before 1958, all known adrenergic blocking agents affected mainly α-adrenergic receptors and were unable to prevent responses such as myocardial stimulation, bronchial smooth muscle relaxation, and vasodilatation in skeletal muscle. Since that time, several compounds have been found to inhibit selec-

tively responses mediated by β-adrenergic receptors. (*See* Table 21-1, page 408, for distribution of α- and β-adrenergic receptors.) Sympathomimetic amines show a wide quantitative variation in their relative actions on α- and β-adrenergic receptors, but the antagonists are more selective for one or the other and are classified as α- and β-adrenergic blocking agents.

Many compounds are now known to prevent responses to adrenergic nerve activity by interfering with the normal release of norepinephrine at nerve terminals. Such compounds may be referred to as *adrenergic neuron blocking agents,* and they differ from adrenergic blocking agents in many important respects. The basis for many of these differences is that adrenergic neuron blocking agents inhibit responses to nerve activity irrespective of whether α or β receptors are involved.

Because the effects of both adrenergic and adrenergic neuron blocking agents are dependent on the type and degree of adrenergic control of various organs and systems, a rational approach to this subject requires knowledge of the general principles of autonomic physiology and pharmacology presented in Chapter 21, and summarized in Tables 21-1 (page 408) and 21-2 (page 434), as well as in Figures 21-1 (facing page 406) and 21-5 (page 425).

I. α-Adrenergic Blocking Agents

PHENOXYBENZAMINE AND RELATED HALOALKYLAMINES

The effects of members of this series will be discussed as representative of α-adrenergic blockade *per se*. Although these drugs effectively block other types of receptors, they produce few effects in intact laboratory animals or man that cannot be attributed to α-adrenergic blockade, and thus provide a clearer picture of the results of this action than do agents of most other chemical classes.

Practically all of the many active members of the haloalkylamine series possess similar adrenergic blocking properties. *Dibenamine* and *phenoxybenzamine* will be taken as examples of the group, the former because it was the first to be discovered (Nickerson and Goodman, 1947), and the latter because it is the compound most commonly used at the present time and the only member of the series that has been studied extensively in man. Their pharmacological properties are qualitatively the same, the major differences being that phenoxybenzamine is six to ten times as potent as dibenamine, is somewhat better absorbed after oral administration, and has a higher antihistaminic activity.

Chemistry. Dibenamine is N,N-dibenzyl-β-chloroethylamine, and phenoxybenzamine differs from it only in the replacement of one benzyl group by a phenoxyisopropyl moiety. Their structural formulas are as follows:

Dibenamine

Phenoxybenzamine

The haloalkylamine adrenergic blocking agents are closely related chemically to the nitrogen mustards; like the latter, the tertiary amine cyclizes to form a reactive ethylenimonium intermediate (Chapter 62). The molecular configuration directly responsible for blockade is probably a highly reactive carbonium ion formed when the three-membered ring breaks. The relatively slow onset of action, even after intravenous administration, is probably due to the time required for the formation of these reactive intermediates, which can then alkylate various biological materials. The exact nature of the groupings on or near α-adrenergic receptors with which the haloalkylamines react has not been determined.

All tertiary β-haloalkylamines probably react in a qualitatively similar manner by way of ethylenimonium intermediates, and α-adrenergic blocking activity is dependent on other substituents. The major structural requirements for production of the characteristic nonequilibrium blockade have been reviewed by Nickerson and Gump (1949) and Graham (1962).

Locus and Mechanism of Action. α-Adrenergic blockade is due to a direct action on α-adrenergic receptors and is independent of any effects on adrenergic nerves or on the basic response mechanisms of effector cells. β-Adrenergic receptors are not affected.

The presence of a catecholamine or an α-adrenergic blocking agent of the competitive type during the development of blockade by a haloalkylamine can decrease the degree of block attained (Nickerson and Gump, 1949; Furchgott, 1954). This appears to involve a competition for the same population of receptors, and indicates that the initial approximation of the haloalkylamine to its site of action is due to the same relatively weak forces (ionic, hydrogen bond, etc.) involved in the actions of most agonists and of adrenergic blocking agents of most other chemical classes (competitive antagonists). The fact that occupancy of a specific type of receptor by an agonist or competitive antagonist during the first stage of action of a haloalkylamine inhibits the blockade of this type but not of other types of receptors ("receptor protection") provides the basis for the most specific method now available to determine the type of receptor with which a given agent interacts (Furchgott, 1954; Nickerson, 1956; Innes, 1962). It was anticipated that a labeled haloalkylamine could be used in combination with agonist protection of specific receptors to identify and characterize the α-adrenergic receptors. However, the many attempts to date have been unsuccessful, probably because the receptors represent too small a percentage of the total binding sites to be clearly detected (*see* Yong and Nickerson, 1973). This explanation is in agreement with the very diffuse distribution of ³H-phenoxybenzamine found with radioautography.

After blockade by a haloalkylamine has fully developed, it is unaltered by exposure to another drug capable of interacting with the same receptors. This stage may be referred to as *nonequilibrium blockade* and is the result of stable covalent bond formation between the antagonist and the receptor (Nickerson, 1957). This mechanism also appears to be responsible for both the completeness and the persistence of the blockade produced by agents of this series (Nickerson, 1962b). The many reports of a "deblocking" effect of sympathomimetics, antihistamines, β-adrenergic blocking agents, and other drugs appear to arise from the measurement of complex responses under conditions of only partial blockade of the α-adrenergic receptors. Thus, blockade of opposing vascular β-adrenergic receptors or elimination of their significance by prior maximal vasodilatation can allow the activation of a few unblocked α receptors to be measured. However, a relatively specific deblock by trypsin has been reported, associated with release of labeled haloalkylamine, apparently bound to a small peptide (*see* Graham and Mottram, 1971).

In addition to producing α-adrenergic blockade, the haloalkylamines, and to varying degrees other classes of α-adrenergic blocking agents, exert important effects on catecholamine metabolism. Phenoxybenzamine increases the rate of peripheral norepinephrine turnover, which is associated with increased tyrosine hydroxylase activity. In intact animals, these effects are probably predominantly due to reflexly increased sympathetic nerve activity, but a facilitation of release has also been demonstrated. The latter has been differentiated from inhibition of re-uptake by parallel increases in norepinephrine and dopamine-β-hydroxylase output (Potter *et al.,* 1971).

Phenoxybenzamine and many congeners inhibit the uptake of catecholamines into both adrenergic nerve terminals (Uptake$_1$) and extraneuronal tissues (Uptake$_2$). The ratios of effectiveness against these two processes vary considerably among members of the series (Iversen *et al.,* 1972), but the block of Uptake$_2$ is probably the more important in causing potentiation of responses and augmentation of the outflow of norepinephrine during stimulation of sympathetic nerves to an organ. The output is increased much more than by cocaine, and the ratio of norepinephrine to metabolites is greatly increased (Su and Bevan, 1970). In smooth muscle preparations where the capacity of Uptake$_2$ without enzymatic backup is relatively limited, a haloalkylamine may appear to have an effect almost identical to that of inhibiting both monoamine oxidase (MAO) and catechol-O-methyltransferase (Kalsner and Nickerson, 1969b). A large part of the potentiation of responses to catecholamines by a haloalkylamine, as by cocaine, is due to a postjunctional mechanism completely unrelated to amine inactivation (Kalsner and Nickerson, 1969b). In contrast to cocaine, haloalkylamines can increase responses to tyramine, and they can inhibit norepinephrine release by nicotine and guanethidine. The haloalkylamines also block the renal tubular transport of organic bases (Ross *et al.,* 1968). Although the relative potencies of different haloalkylamines in producing these varied effects are not closely correlated with their α-adrenergic blocking activity, it is not surprising that drugs characterized by their ability to combine with a subcellular configuration involved in one action of sympathomimetics can affect other tissue constituents with which these agonists interact.

PHARMACOLOGICAL PROPERTIES

Phenoxybenzamine and dibenamine effectively prevent responses that are mediated by α-adrenergic receptors, predominantly excitatory responses of smooth muscle and exocrine glands (Table 21–1, page 408). The blocking agents may be considered to act by reducing the total population of α receptors;

consequently, the *actions* of various sympathomimetics are inhibited essentially to the same extent. However, the *net effects* of different sympathomimetics on a complex parameter such as blood pressure may be antagonized to very different degrees. For example, a dose of phenoxybenzamine that completely eliminates the pressor response to epinephrine or converts it to a depressor response may produce only a 50% inhibition of the pressor response to norepinephrine. Epinephrine produces both vasoconstriction and vasodilatation, and moderate inhibition of the former may allow the latter to predominate; norepinephrine, on the other hand, has very little vasodilator action, and all of the residual constriction is manifested in the pressor response. It should also be emphasized that the effects of any blocking agent are highly dependent on the state of activity of the system on which it acts. Thus, the vasodilatation induced by phenoxybenzamine may vary markedly in different vascular beds, depending on their degree of adrenergic vasomotor control, and may vary over a wide range in a single vascular bed, depending on its physiological state (*see* Nickerson and Hollenberg, 1967).

Blockade by most haloalkylamines develops relatively slowly, and the peak effect is usually not attained in less than an hour after intravenous administration. However, the maximum is approached asymptotically, and a considerable percentage of the blockade is established in a much shorter period. The blockade produced by a single dose of dibenamine or phenoxybenzamine disappears with a half-life of roughly 24 hours in intact laboratory animals and man, and can be detected for at least 3 or 4 days. Thus, the effects of daily administration are cumulative for nearly a week. With increasing doses of the blocking agent, the dose-response curve for an agonist is shifted progressively to the right as the number of available receptors is reduced. Because the antagonist is not in equilibrium with the receptors, the maximum may be proportionately reduced. However, some normal tissues contain receptors much in excess of the number required for a full response to most agonists (the "spare receptors"), and a considerable proportion can be inactivated before the tissue is incapable of a maximal response. Many aspects of the general pharmacology of the haloalkylamines are reviewed by Graham (1962) and Nickerson and Hollenberg (1967).

α-Adrenergic blocking agents have generally been observed to block responses to circulating sympathomimetics more readily than those to adrenergic nerve activity. For some agents such as piperoxan this differential is very large. However, it has been reported that the reverse is true for phenoxybenzamine. Unfortunately, these experiments were done in intact vascular beds and there is no clear evidence that the distribution of resistance in sequential segments is the same with nerve stimulation and injected norepinephrine. The results of other experiments with isolated preparations are difficult to interpret because maximal responses to the different stimuli were unequal. It may be that block of the two types of stimuli by phenoxybenzamine is essentially equal, but clearly definitive experiments have not yet been done. (*See* Wyse and Beck, 1972.)

In addition to the blockade of α-adrenergic receptors, the haloalkylamines can inhibit responses to 5-hydroxytryptamine (5-HT, serotonin), histamine, and acetylcholine (ACh). Blockade of these other types of agonists has the same general pharmacological characteristics as does the adrenergic blockade. Although nonequilibrium blockade of responses to histamine and 5-HT requires the same basic chemical configuration as does α-adrenergic blocking activity and the same intermediate transformations are probably involved, potency with respect to these properties varies considerably. For example, dibenamine has relatively low antihistaminic activity, whereas phenoxybenzamine and a number of phenoxyethyl and l-naphthylmethyl congeners are as potent in this regard as many of the antihistamines now employed clinically. Effective blockade of responses to ACh usually requires relatively high doses of haloalkylamine. The possible involvement of these various receptor types should always be determined when a haloalkylamine is used as a pharmacological tool. However, in the absence of a specific nonadrenergic stimulus, most of the effects observed in laboratory animals and man are due to α-adrenergic blockade.

Cardiovascular System. *Blood Pressure.* The usual blocking dose of phenoxybenzamine (1.0 mg/kg in man) or of dibenamine infused slowly intravenously into healthy, recumbent, normovolemic subjects causes little change in systemic blood pressure, although the diastolic pressure tends to fall somewhat. However, a sharp drop may occur in any situation involving compensatory sympathetic vasoconstriction, such as upright posture or hypovolemia. Thus, a prominent effect of the blockade is *postural hypotension*. In addition, impairment of compensatory vasoconstriction sensitizes to the hypotensive effects of a variety of agents and conditions that tend to produce vasodilatation, including hypercapnia and analgesics such as morphine and meperidine. Rapid injection of a haloalkylamine can cause a precipitous fall in blood pressure, which probably involves factors other than α-adrenergic blockade.

Blood Flows. Phenoxybenzamine produces a considerable, progressive increase in cardiac output and decrease in total peripheral resistance in normal recumbent subjects. However, the changes in blood flow and resistance induced in specific vascular beds vary widely with the conditions under which the blocking agent is administered. In general, the responses are predictable from a knowledge of the level of adrenergic vasomotor control. Cerebral and coronary resistances are not significantly altered by α-adrenergic blockade *per se*. Cerebral flow is little affected unless the blood pressure is greatly reduced, and coronary flow increases in parallel with reflex cardiac stimulation. Phenoxybenzamine increases resting muscle blood flow and, in a cool environment, enhances cutaneous blood flow. However, sympathetic vasoconstriction exerts little restraint on muscle blood flow during exercise or on cutaneous blood flow in a warm environment, and under these conditions α-adrenergic blockade produces little change. Splanchnic and renal blood flows are not altered remarkably in the normovolemic subject at rest; however, in the presence of the increased adrenergic vasoconstrictor tone induced by circumstances such as hypovolemia or norepinephrine infusion, phenoxybenzamine increases flow to a major degree in both these areas. In the kidney, perfusion of the outer cortex is most markedly affected. Pulmonary arteries and veins are also relaxed; however, because of a greater systemic vasodilatation, blood volume in the pulmonary circuit is usually decreased.

Only a few of the almost limitless variations in the effects of α-adrenergic blockade on resistance and flow under various physiological and pathological conditions can be presented here. However, the examples given above are representative of the general relation of level of adrenergic vasomotor tone and response to blockade. This relation is discussed in more detail by Nickerson and Hollenberg (1967). Other important effects of haloalkylamines, and of other agents that inhibit sympathetic vasoconstriction, are diversion of a higher percentage of the total blood flow through channels that exchange metabolites effectively with tissue cells ("nutrient channels"), and movement of fluid from the interstitial to the vascular compartment, the result of differential effects on precapillary and postcapillary resistance vessels (Nickerson and Hollenberg, 1967; Hollenberg and Nickerson, 1970).

Responses to Adrenergic Stimuli. Pressor responses to epinephrine and other sympathomimetic amines are blocked or reversed by phenoxybenzamine, dibenamine, and their active congeners (Figure 26–1). A reduction in the pressor response without reversal is usually seen when the capacity for adrenergic vasodilatation is limited by any factor, for example, the species (rabbits), the sympathomimetic used (norepinephrine or

phenylephrine), or the preparation (pithed animals). Because norepinephrine has little vasodilator action and endogenous circulating catecholamines play a very limited role in cardiovascular responses to electrical or reflex activation of the sympathetic system, these are usually not reversed. However, if the total response involves a vasodilating influence of any type, a change from constrictor to dilator or from pressor to depressor response may be induced by α-adrenergic blockade. Blockade of the effects of sympathetic nerve stimulation on muscle vascular beds is illustrative (Folkow *et al.,* 1948). The nerves involved contain both adrenergic constrictor and cholinergic dilator fibers. Before blockade, an apparently pure constrictor response is produced. Dibenamine easily converts this to vasodilatation of considerable magnitude, but subsequent administration of atropine can reveal a residual con-

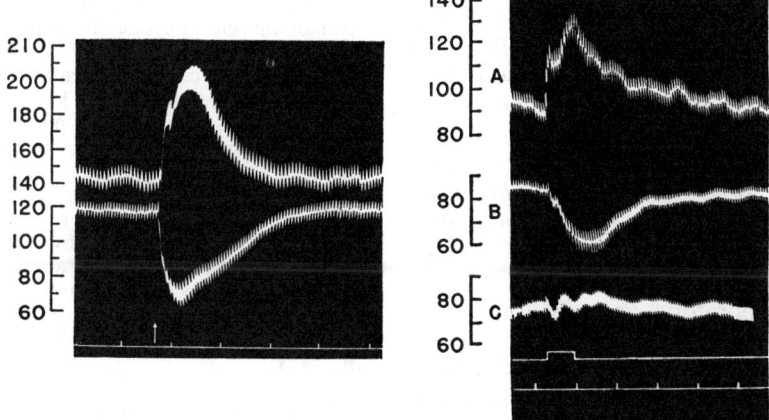

Figure 26–1. *Effect of dibenamine on blood pressure responses of anesthetized cat.*

Left. Responses to a small dose of epinephrine. Upper record before and lower record after intravenous administration of dibenamine (15 mg/kg). The arrow indicates intravenous injections of epinephrine (2.5 μg/kg). The pressor response is converted to depressor by selective blockade of the vasoconstrictor (α-receptor) action of epinephrine, which allows expression of the concurrent vasodilator (β-receptor) action. Ordinate, blood pressure in mm Hg; abscissa, time in minutes.

Right. Responses to splanchnic nerve stimulation. *A* before and *B* after dibenamine; *C* after dibenamine and removal of adrenal glands. Ordinate, blood pressure in mm Hg; abscissa, time in minutes. Period of stimulation is indicated by upward deflection of signal line. The initial sharp component of the pressor response in tracing *A* is due to the local effect of norepinephrine released from sympathetic nerve endings in splanchnic vessels. The subsequent slower component of the rise is predominantly due to catecholamines released from the adrenal medulla. In tracing *B* each of the two components of the original pressor response is reversed. The initial rapid fall is small. The second, slower component of the reversal represents the vasodilator response to circulating catecholamines, predominantly the effect of epinephrine. After removal of the adrenal glands, only the local (splanchnic) component of the response remains. (After Nickerson and Goodman, 1947. Courtesy of the *Journal of Pharmacology and Experimental Therapeutics.*)

strictor response. Thus, if only net changes in resistance are considered, atropine appears to antagonize the action of dibenamine or "deblock."

Many effects induced directly or indirectly by stimulation of α-adrenergic receptors of vascular smooth muscle are prevented by the haloalkylamines. These include the lethal effects of epinephrine and many other sympathomimetic amines, the changes in erythrocyte and leukocyte counts induced by fright or struggle, and the pulmonary lesions resulting from exposure to oxygen at high pressure. Similarly, a number of secondary pathological effects of infused epinephrine or norepinephrine, including pulmonary edema, reduction in plasma volume, accumulation of pericardial fluid, adrenocortical necrosis, and changes in hepatic cells, are effectively blocked.

Cardiac Effects. The chronotropic and inotropic effects of epinephrine, norepinephrine, and direct or reflex sympathetic nerve stimulation on the mammalian myocardium are not inhibited by the haloalkylamines or by other α-adrenergic blocking agents (Nickerson and Chan, 1961). Indeed, the tachycardia in intact animals is usually exaggerated because the pressor response is prevented. Phenoxybenzamine and dibenamine induce reflex tachycardia; this is a characteristic component of the response to peripheral vasodilatation, and may be accentuated by altered norepinephrine release and inactivation, as well as by "postjunctional" potentiation.

In both laboratory animals and man, haloalkylamines effectively inhibit cardiac arrhythmias that involve catecholamines in their genesis, with or without specific sensitization of the myocardium by drugs such as cyclopropane or chloroform. Both inhibition of the adrenergic pressor response and a direct blocking effect on the heart are involved, but it is not known if the latter is related to the same small component of α-adrenergic receptors demonstrable under other conditions. Arrhythmias following acute coronary artery occlusion or precipitated by hypothermia are not similarly inhibited.

Although the heart is predominantly under the control of β-adrenergic receptors, some α receptors are present, and these are effectively blocked by haloalkylamines (Benfey, 1973). Many years ago it was observed that dibenamine could block responses of "winter" but not those of "summer" frog hearts

to epinephrine (Nickerson and Nomaguchi, 1950), and it has now been demonstrated that the characteristics of both amphibian and mammalian myocardial adrenergic receptors can change from β to α at temperatures below 20° C (Kunos et al., 1973). This remarkable phenomenon has not yet been explained.

Metabolic Effects. The receptors involved in metabolic responses to catecholamines are predominantly β, but important α-adrenergic actions also participate. The effects of phenoxybenzamine *in vivo* appear particularly complex, primarily because many of the measured responses are composite. For example, agents such as epinephrine stimulate hepatic glycogenolysis (β) and inhibit insulin secretion (α). However, there is also a weaker β-adrenergic stimulatory effect on insulin secretion. In the presence of phenoxybenzamine, the inhibitory action of epinephrine on insulin secretion is blocked, and the response to β-receptor stimulation and the direct effect of glucose are revealed. The subsequent rise in insulin concentration may facilitate glucose uptake to the extent that hyperglycemia (from glycogenolysis) is obscured. The result is an *apparent* block of the glycogenolytic effect of epinephrine by phenoxybenzamine when, in fact, this is not the case. Phenoxybenzamine does not specifically antagonize the effects of catecholamines on glycogenolysis in liver or muscle, nor does it inhibit catecholamine-augmented lipolysis. In some circumstances α-adrenergic blockade can considerably increase norepinephrine-induced lipolysis in human adipose tissue. (*See* Himms-Hagen, 1967; Symposium, 1970.)

Dibenamine and phenoxybenzamine do not alter the normal blood potassium concentration, but they do promote the disappearance of infused potassium from the blood stream and prevent the rapid increase that can be induced by epinephrine. These effects are not dependent on altered glycogenolysis or circulatory effects. They may be related to block of a specific potassium-releasing action of catecholamines mediated by α-adrenergic receptors (Batzri et al., 1973).

Central Nervous System. Interest in possible physiological functions of catecholamines in the central nervous system (CNS) has led to many studies of the central effects of α-adrenergic blocking agents. The complications involved in conducting and interpreting such studies have been discussed in Chapter 21.

Excitation and inhibition of single neurons in the CNS have been produced by norepinephrine applied locally by microiontophoresis. Some inhibitory responses are blocked by β-adrenergic blocking drugs, and some excitatory responses are blocked by α-adrenergic antagonists. However, there are many exceptions, and some responses are not readily inhibited by blocking agents of either class. The effects on locomotor activity, learned behavior, body temperature, and blood pressure produced by catecholamines injected into the cerebral ventricles appear to be more frequently antagonized by α- than by β-adrenergic blocking drugs, but many of the results are difficult to interpret. Studies of the relative potencies of a series of amines and of the effectiveness of α- and β-adrenergic blocking agents may indicate quite different conclusions regarding the type of receptors involved in a response. The effects of catecholamines on the CNS and their inhibition by various drugs are extensively reviewed by Marley and Stephenson (1972).

Dibenamine, phenoxybenzamine, and congeners can stimulate the CNS to cause nausea, vomiting, hyperventilation, motor excitability, and even convulsions, particularly when a relatively large dose is rapidly injected intravenously. In man, a characteristic loss of time perception may occur. These effects develop and terminate much more rapidly than does the blockade, and hydrolysis products of the active agents, which do not block α receptors, are also effective CNS stimulants. Mild-to-moderate sedation commonly results from the slow intravenous infusion of the usual blocking dose of phenoxybenzamine in man, and tiredness and lethargy may accompany oral medication. This sedation is very similar to that produced by drugs that appear to activate central α-adrenergic receptors (*e.g.*, clonidine). There is little basis for assuming that the CNS effects of the haloalkylamines are a reflection of central α-adrenergic blockade.

Other Effects. Phenoxybenzamine and dibenamine effectively antagonize the wide variety of responses to endogenous and exogenous sympathomimetic amines that are mediated by α-adrenergic receptors. These include contractions of the nictitating membrane, retractor penis, arrector pili, and the uteri of several species. Motility of the nonpregnant human uterus *in situ* is reduced and stimulation by norepinephrine is prevented (Wansbrough *et al.*, 1968). Estrogen-induced tubal block of ovum transport is inhibited in rabbits, and it is of interest that the circular fibers of the human tubal isthmus have a particularly dense adrenergic innervation (Owman *et al.*, 1967). However, phenoxybenzamine and estrogen have very similar central effects in inhibiting luteinizing hormone (LH) release in ovariectomized monkeys (Bhattacharya *et al.*, 1972). Salivary secretion of water and electrolytes evoked by cervical sympathetic nerve stimulation or injected sympathomimetic drugs is blocked. The volume and enzyme content of pancreatic exocrine secretion are increased by α- and decreased by β-adrenergic blockade. The limited adrenergic sweating observed in man, particularly of the hands and axillae, is also blocked. Sweating responses in various animal species reflect a complex involvement of α- and β-adrenergic and cholinergic receptors, and generalizations are difficult (*see* Nickerson and Hollenberg, 1967). Stimulation of the radial fibers of the iris is readily blocked, and miosis is a prominent component of the response to phenoxybenzamine in man, but accommodation is not significantly affected.

Inasmuch as the predominantly inhibitory effects of sympathomimetics on the gastrointestinal tract are mediated by α as well as by β receptors, combined α- and β-adrenergic blockade is usually required to inhibit completely relaxation by epinephrine or norepinephrine. A very limited overall effect of α-adrenergic blockade on gastrointestinal sphincters is indicated by the fact that dibenamine and phenoxybenzamine do not appreciably alter the rate of passage of barium sulfate along the human gastrointestinal tract.

Absorption, Fate, and Excretion. Haloalkylamine adrenergic blocking agents are effective when administered by all routes, but injection should be only intravenously because of their irritant properties. Absorption from the gastrointestinal tract is incomplete and somewhat capricious; 20 to 30% of orally administered phenoxybenzamine appears to be absorbed in active form.

Phenoxybenzamine and dibenamine have a high lipid solubility at body pH, and accumulation in fat may occur after large doses. However, a stable bonding to tissue constituents rather than slow release from "fat depots" is responsible for the prolonged action (Nickerson, 1962b). The metabolic fate of these highly unstable agents is poorly understood. Over 50% of the radioactivity of intravenously administered phenoxybenzamine is excreted in 12 hours and over 80% in 24 hours, but small amounts remain in various tissues for at least a week.

Preparations, Routes of Administration, and Dosage. *Phenoxybenzamine Hydrochloride*, N.F. (DIBENZYLINE), is available for *oral* use in 10-mg capsules; ampuls for intravenous use (100 mg of the drug in 2 ml) are available for investigational purposes. The oral dose usually varies between 20 and 200 mg per day and must be attained by small increments. When administered *intravenously,* phenoxybenzamine must be well diluted and infused slowly. Most commonly a dose of 1.0 mg/kg is diluted in 250 to 500 ml of 5% glucose or 0.9% sodium chloride solution and infused over a period of at least 1 hour.

Toxicity, Side Effects, and Precautions. Untoward effects of phenoxybenzamine are largely due to the blockade of α-adrenergic receptors. Loss of vasomotor control can result in postural hypotension and reflex tachycardia in ambulatory patients, or a sharp fall in blood pressure in those who are hypovolemic. The postural hypotension and palpitation may disappear despite continued blockade, but can reappear under conditions that promote vasodilatation, such as exercise, eating a large meal, or consuming alcohol. Because of the danger of severe hypotension when the drug is administered in the presence of hypovolemia, intravenous administration must be slow, the patient must be kept under constant observation, and blood or an appropriate plasma-volume expander must be on hand to correct any deficit revealed by the hemodynamic response. Inhibition of compensatory vasoconstriction also exaggerates the depressor effects of narcotics and other agents that act directly to relax vascular smooth muscle. Other results of α-receptor blockade include miosis, nasal stuffiness, and inhibition of ejaculation. Effects not clearly related to blockade are local tissue irritation, sedation, and a generalized feeling of weakness and tiredness. Local irritation is probably involved in the nausea and occasional vomiting that may follow large oral doses, particularly if administered on an empty stomach. Specific liver, kidney, or bone-marrow damage has not been observed in either experimental animals or man. However, the clinical use of phenoxybenzamine has been too limited to allow definitive statements regarding its toxicity.

Therapeutic Uses. The clinical uses of haloalkylamines are discussed below, along with those of other α-adrenergic blocking agents.

ERGOT ALKALOIDS

The ergot alkaloids were the first adrenergic blocking agents to be discovered, and most aspects of their general pharmacology were disclosed by the classical studies of Dale (1906). Unfortunately, emphasis on their adrenergic blocking activity has frequently caused other important pharmacological properties, particularly direct stimulation of smooth muscle and complex excitation and depression of the CNS, to be overlooked, with consequent misinterpretation of experimental and clinical responses.

Chemistry. Details of the chemistry of the ergot alkaloids are presented elsewhere (Chapter 42). However, certain aspects are significant for the present discussion of α-adrenergic blockade. Compounds of the *ergonovine* type, which lack a polypeptide side chain, have no adrenergic blocking activity. Of the natural ergot preparations, "ergotoxine" has the greatest α-adrenergic blocking potency. It was studied for almost 40 years before it was shown to be a mixture of three alkaloids— *ergocornine, ergocristine,* and *ergocryptine;* fortunately, these have very similar pharmacological

properties. Dihydrogenation of the lysergic acid nucleus increases α-adrenergic blocking activity and decreases, but does not eliminate, the ability to stimulate smooth muscle.

PHARMACOLOGICAL PROPERTIES

Both the natural and the dihydrogenated peptide alkaloids produce *α-adrenergic blockade.* This is relatively persistent for a competitive antagonist, but it is of much shorter duration than that produced by a haloalkylamine. These drugs also are effective antagonists of 5-HT. Although the hydrogenated ergot alkaloids are among the most potent α-adrenergic blocking agents known, side effects prevent the administration of doses that could produce more than minimal blockade in man.

Although commonly classified as α-adrenergic blocking agents, the most important effects of all the ergot alkaloids are due to actions on the CNS and direct stimulation of smooth muscle. The latter occurs in many different organs (*see* Chapter 42), and even dihydroergotoxine has been observed to produce spastic contractions of the intestine in man. In some organs the stimulation has been shown to be due to an action on the same receptors involved in responses to catecholamines (Innes, 1962). Thus, the ergot alkaloids can be considered to be a series of partial agonists, with blocking activity increasing and intrinsic activity decreasing from ergotamine to dihydroergotoxine.

The peptide ergot alkaloids can reverse the pressor response to epinephrine to depressor (α-adrenergic blockade), but they can also convert the depressor response to isoproterenol to pressor. The latter effect appears to be due to an increase in cardiac output in the presence of a vascular bed already constricted by the alkaloid. All the *natural ergot alkaloids* cause a significant rise in blood pressure as a result of direct peripheral vasoconstriction, which is more pronounced in postcapillary than in precapillary vessels (Mellander and Nordenfelt, 1970). Although hydrogenation reduces this action, dihydroergotamine is still an effective vasoconstrictor, and a residual constrictor action of dihydroergotoxine is also demonstrable. Ergotamine, and probably all other ergot alkaloids, can produce coronary vasoconstriction, often with associated ischemic changes in the ECG and anginal pain in patients with coronary artery disease. *Dihydroergotoxine* produces only limited vasoconstriction, and its overall effects include peripheral vasodilatation and a fall in arterial pressure. These effects are predominantly due to central depression of vasomotor nerve activity (Barcroft *et al.*, 1951). The ergot alkaloids usually induce bradycardia even when the blood pressure is not increased. This is predominantly due to increased vagal activity, but a central reduction in sympathetic tone and direct myocardial depression may also be involved. The cardiovascular effects of central actions of ergot alkaloids are qualitatively similar to those of clonidine (*see* Chapter 33), and are more likely due to direct actions on the CNS than to central adrenergic blockade.

Actions of the ergot alkaloids on the CNS occur with doses lower than those required to produce significant α-adrenergic blockade in the periphery. Vasomotor activity is decreased, respiration is depressed, and the characteristic effects of carbon dioxide on both respiration and blood pressure are reduced. Cardiovascular responses to carotid baroreceptor and chemoreceptor stimuli are also inhibited, and temperature regulation is impaired. Several ergot alkaloids have been shown to block the secretion of anterior pituitary hormones (*see* Chapter 66). A *bromo derivative of ergocryptine* (*CB 154*) appears to block spontaneous and drug-induced prolactin secretion with fewer peripheral effects than other alkaloids, and has been used clinically to inhibit aberrant galactorrhea and puerperal lactation (*see* Besser *et al.*, 1972). All the peptide ergot alkaloids have potent *emetic* properties due to stimulation of the chemoreceptor trigger zone in the medulla oblongata.

The natural and hydrogenated ergot alkaloids all inhibit epinephrine-induced hepatic glycogenolysis and hyperglycemia more effectively than do other α-adrenergic blocking agents. This is not correlated with the blockade of cardiovascular or other smooth muscle responses, and appears not to be a specific α-receptor effect. Glycogenolysis in skeletal muscle and the consequent lactacidemia are not similarly inhibited.

Several aspects of the pharmacology of the ergot alkaloids are discussed in more detail by Rothlin (1947), Nickerson (1949), and Nickerson and Hollenberg (1967).

Toxicity and Side Effects. The dose of dihydroergotoxine in man is strictly limited by the production of nausea and vomiting. Prolonged or excessive administration of any of the natural peptide ergot alkaloids can cause vascular insufficiency and gangrene of the extremities. This is particularly prone to occur in the presence of preexisting vascular pathology or infection. In severe cases, prompt vasodilatation is essential. There have been no comparative studies on the treatment of this sporadic condition, but a direct-acting drug such as *nitroprusside* appears to be most effective (Carliner *et al.*, 1974). Toxic effects of the ergot alkaloids are described in more detail in Chapter 42.

Preparations, Routes of Administration, and Dosage. *Dihydroergotoxine mesylate* (HYDERGINE) is available for parenteral use in 1.0-ml ampuls containing 0.3 mg of drug. It also is available in 0.5-mg sublingual tablets. The usual intramuscular or intravenous dose is 0.3 to 1.0 mg. Absorption after sublingual or oral administration is very limited. Preparations used for their direct effects on smooth muscle are described in Chapter 42.

Therapeutic Uses. Use of dihydroergotoxine as a peripheral vasodilator and antihypertensive agent was never widespread in North America, and has now been largely abandoned. Dihydroergotoxine has recently been used to treat "mental and emotional complaints of the aged," presumed to be due to inadequacies of cerebral blood flow. Several reports of "double-blind" studies have claimed statistically significant improvement in one or more of a wide variety of criteria, such as tension, irritability, emotional lability, alertness, depressive moods, disorientation, confusion, forgetfulness, self-care, motor retardation, conceptual disorganization, hostility, and blunted affect. However, the parameters affected are not consistent, and it has not been shown that the drug can augment the vasodilatation due to accumulated carbon dioxide in low-flow areas of the brain (*see* McHenry *et al.*, 1971) or that significant amounts are absorbed after oral or sublingual administration. Reports over the past several years do not provide a basis for altering an earlier negative opinion of the efficacy of dihydroergotoxine in CNS problems of elderly patients (*see* Medical Letter, 1970). Other uses of the ergot alkaloids are described in Chapter 42.

TOLAZOLINE AND PHENTOLAMINE

Tolazoline (2-benzyl-2-imidazoline) was first reported in the pharmacological literature as a vasodepressor agent with effects similar to those of histamine. Its α-adrenergic blocking action was noted only during subsequent investigations. *Phentolamine* was introduced later, with particular attention to its α-adrenergic blocking activity.

Chemistry. The 2-substituted imidazolines have a wide range of pharmacological actions, including adrenergic blocking, sympathomimetic, antihypertensive, antihistaminic, histamine-like, and cholinomimetic; slight changes in structure may make one or another of these properties dominant. At the present time, members of the series are marketed for each of the first four properties listed. The structural formulas of *tolazoline* and *phentolamine* are as follows:

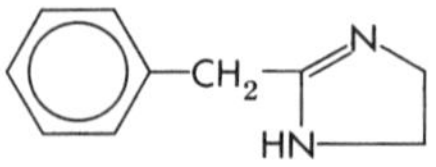

Tolazoline

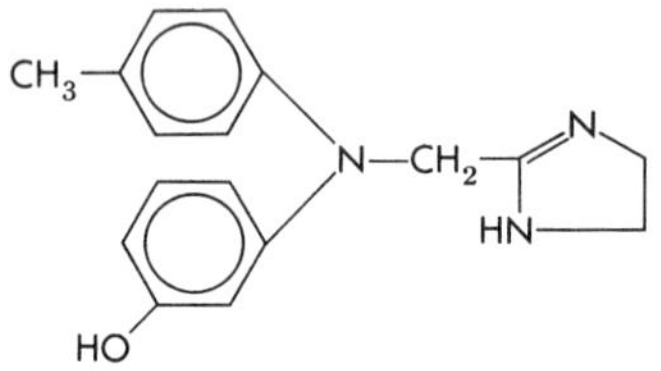

Phentolamine

PHARMACOLOGICAL PROPERTIES

Tolazoline and *phentolamine* produce a moderately effective competitive α-adrenergic blockade that is relatively transient. Responses to 5-HT are also inhibited. In addition, they have important actions on cardiac and smooth muscle that may be divided into three classes: (1) "sympathomimetic," including cardiac stimulation; (2) "parasympathomimetic," including gastrointestinal tract stimulation that is blocked by atropine; and (3) "histamine-like," including stimulation of gastric secretion and peripheral vasodilatation (*see* Nickerson, 1949). Phentolamine is a considerably more potent α-adrenergic blocking agent than is tolazoline, and its other effects are somewhat less prominent.

The usual clinical doses of tolazoline produce very little α-adrenergic blockade, and the block produced by tolerated doses of phentolamine in man is far from complete. Tolazoline or phentolamine given intravenously produces vasodilatation and cardiac stimulation; the blood pressure response varies with the relative contributions of the two effects. Phentolamine usually causes a fall in pressure, but the net effect of tolazoline commonly is pressor. Both agents can decrease peripheral resistance and increase venous capacity. The dilatation is predominantly due to a *direct action on vascular smooth muscle* in the dose range now usually employed in man (Taylor *et al.,* 1965). However, high doses of phentolamine can produce a hemodynamic picture characteristic of α-adrenergic blockade (Moyer and Caplovitz, 1953); at this dose level side effects are severe. Pulmonary arterial pressure and vascular resistance are usually reduced by tolazoline or phentolamine. The acute response is variable, but is of considerable magnitude in some patients with elevated pulmonary pressures; significant chronic reductions have not been achieved. A paradoxical increase in pulmonary resistance has been reported, and it has been suggested that these drugs may have a direct vasoconstrictor action that is usually masked (*see* Yoran and Glassman, 1973). Many imidazoline derivatives are α-adrenergic partial agonists.

Therapeutic doses of phentolamine and tolazoline cause cardiac stimulation that is more than just a reflex response to peripheral vasodilatation, and this can be associated with cardiac arrhythmias in both laboratory animals and man. The stimulation appears to involve endogenous norepinephrine (Das and Parratt, 1971), and both increased release of and interference with inactivation of mediator may be involved.

Tolazoline and phentolamine can block many responses that involve α-adrenergic receptors. However, the intrinsic eye muscles are relatively resistant, and in intact laboratory animals and man tolazoline may cause mydriasis rather than miosis. The imidazoline blocking agents stimulate salivary, lacrimal, respiratory tract, and pancreatic secretion, and tolazoline can cause profuse sweating in man. This is probably a direct effect because tolazoline has been reported to induce secretion by denervated salivary glands. Tolazoline and phentolamine produce hyperperistalsis and diarrhea in laboratory animals and man, effects that are blocked by atropine. Abdominal discomfort is a very common side effect of phentolamine administration. Phentolamine and tolazoline stimulate gastric secretion of both acid and pepsin.

Absorption, Fate, and Excretion. *Tolazoline* is well absorbed after both parenteral and oral administration. However, it is considerably less effective when given orally because rapid renal excretion prevents accumulation of adequate concentrations during the slow absorption from the gastrointestinal tract. It is largely excreted unchanged by the organic-base transport system of the renal tubules. Little is known about the fate of *phentolamine* in the body. It is not more than 20% as active after oral as after parenteral administration, and only 10% of an injected dose can be recovered in the urine in active form.

Toxicity, Side Effects, and Precautions. The most disturbing clinical side effects of tolazoline and phentolamine are attributable to cardiac and gastrointestinal stimulation. Both drugs can cause alarming tachycardia, cardiac arrhythmias, and anginal pain, most frequently after parenteral administration. Tolazoline has been implicated as a precipitating factor in myocardial infarction and occasionally may produce severe hypertension. Gastrointestinal stimulation may result in abdominal pain, nausea, vomiting, diarrhea, and exacerbation of peptic ulcer. Effective doses of tolazoline quite frequently produce piloerection, chilliness, and apprehension. The imidazoline blocking agents should be used with caution in patients with gastritis, peptic ulcer, or coronary artery disease.

Preparations, Routes of Administration, and Dosage. *Tolazoline Hydrochloride,* N.F. (PRISCOLINE), is marketed for oral use in official tablets containing 25 mg, and an official injection in 10-ml multiple-dose vials (25 mg/ml). The most commonly employed oral dosage is 25 or 50 mg three times a day, although considerably larger doses are required to produce significant α-adrenergic blockade. A full parenteral dose is 50 to 200 mg, given intravenously, intramuscularly, or subcutaneously. However, tolazoline is infrequently administered parenterally except for investigational purposes.
Phentolamine Mesylate, U.S.P. (REGITINE MESYLATE), is marketed for parenteral use in sterile ampuls containing 5 mg. The standard dose that has been employed in the diagnosis of pheochromocytoma in adults is 5 mg, given intravenously. *Phentolamine Hydrochloride,* N.F. (REGITINE), is available for oral use in tablets containing 50 mg.

Therapeutic Uses. Clinical applications of the adrenergic blocking and vasodilating actions of tolazoline and phentolamine are discussed with those of other α-adrenergic blocking agents later in this chapter (*see also* Chapter 34).

OTHER α-ADRENERGIC BLOCKING AGENTS

Natural and synthetic compounds of several other chemical classes have in the past attracted attention because of their α-adrenergic blocking activity. A number of these are discussed in the reviews of Bovet and Bovet-Nitti (1948) and Nickerson (1949). Many drugs, in addition to those studied primarily because of their α-adrenergic blocking activity, depress responses to adrenergic stimuli. In many cases the blocking effects are weak and of questionable selectivity. However, important exceptions are found among the *phenothiazines* and *butyrophenones,* which are of interest primarily for their effects on the CNS (*see* Chapter 12). *Chlorpromazine, haloperidol,* and several related drugs produce significant α-adrenergic blockade in both laboratory animals and man. At the same time, chlorpromazine can prolong and, under appropriate conditions, enhance the pressor response to norepinephrine, or the response to norepinephrine may be unaltered while that to epinephrine is dramatically reversed. Haloperidol also inhibits dopamine-induced renal vasodilatation, which is not affected by the common α- or β-adrenergic blocking agents. (*See* Webster, 1965; Yeh *et al.,* 1969; Goldberg, 1972.) α-Adrenergic blocking activity is not shared by all of the antipsychotic phenothiazines; while it has not been proven that any of their central effects are due to inhibition of responses to endogenous catecholamines, interest centers around their blocking actions at receptor sites for dopamine.

Benzodioxans. Many members of this series, which was first described over 40 years ago by Fourneau and Bovet, produce a relatively transient, competitive α-adrenergic blockade. Some compounds, such as *piperoxan,* inhibit responses to circulating catecholamines much more effectively than those to adrenergic nerve activity. *Dibozane* is a later addition to the series. The benzodioxans have many and varied actions in addition to adrenergic blockade (*see* reviews by Bovet and Bovet-Nitti, 1948; Nickerson, 1949).

Yohimbine. Yohimbine is an indolealkylamine alkaloid with a chemical similarity to reserpine. Yohimbine and a diastereoisomer, *corynanthine,* and a derivative, *ethyl yohimbine,* produce competitive α-adrenergic blockade of limited duration. Yohimbine also blocks peripheral 5-HT receptors. It has little direct effect on smooth muscle, but readily penetrates the CNS and produces a complex pattern of responses in doses lower than required to produce peripheral α-adrenergic blockade. These include antidiuresis, due to vasopressin release, and a general picture of central excitation, including elevations of blood pressure and heart rate, increased motor activity, irritability, and tremor in both unanesthetized laboratory animals and man. Sweating, nausea, and vomiting are also common after parenteral administration in man (Garfield *et al.,* 1967). Yohimbine, but not corynanthine, can modify 5-HT metabolism by inhibiting trytophan pyrrolase (Papeschi *et al.,* 1971). Yohimbine has been sporadically promoted as an aphrodisiac, but there is no convincing evidence for such an effect. It has no proven therapeutic uses.

EEDQ. EEDQ (N-ethoxycarbonyl-2-ethoxy-1,2-dihydroquinoline) produces a nonequilibrium block of α-adrenergic receptors that is superficially very similar to that produced by the haloalkylamines.

This type of compound has been utilized in peptide bond synthesis as a specific activator of carboxyl functions, and it has been postulated that α-adrenergic receptor inactivation involves such a group (Belleau *et al.,* 1969). Observations of its interactions with related drugs have been interpreted as indicating at least three distinct points of attachment for agonists and antagonists in the vicinity of α-adrenergic receptors (Kalsner, 1973).

EEDQ also blocks 5-HT receptors, and 5-HT inhibits this action. It has little effect on responses of smooth muscle to histamine, ACh, or potassium but may reduce sensitivity of the neuromuscular junction to ACh. EEDQ can produce a persistent α-adrenergic block in intact anesthetized animals and a reversal of pressor responses to epinephrine and protection against epinephrine-induced cardiac arrhythmias. In unanesthetized animals, EEDQ produces CNS depression and, in larger doses, catalepsy, but there is no evidence that these effects are due to α-adrenergic blockade.

Azapetine. Azapetine (6-allyl-6,7-dihydro-5H-dibenz[*c,e*]azepine) has blocking and direct vasodilating actions that are qualitatively and quantitatively very similar to those of tolazoline. Most smooth muscle responses mediated by α-adrenergic receptors are blocked about equally. Azapetine tends to lower the blood pressure more than does tolazoline, probably because it causes less cardiac stimulation. (*See* review by Nickerson and Hollenberg, 1967.)

THERAPEUTIC USES OF α-ADRENERGIC BLOCKING AGENTS

α-Adrenergic blockade has been employed or suggested as therapy in a wide variety of conditions, but it has few well-established uses. Quite possibly the clinical application of these drugs will always be severely limited by the fact that efferent sympathetic pathways operating through α-adrenergic receptors are critical to the cardiovascular reflexes that allow man to function as a biped, and it is often difficult to balance the therapeutic benefits of blockade against the disadvantages of disrupting this essential regulatory function.

Cardiovascular Uses. Because the control of peripheral vessels is more thoroughly understood than most other adrenergic functions, α-adrenergic blocking agents have received most attention in this area.

Hypertension. Although several drugs currently used in the treatment of essential hypertension act by inhibiting sympathetic vasoconstrictor tone, results with α-adrenergic blocking agents in this condition have been disappointing. An important factor is that β receptors are unaffected, and reflex tachy-cardia and palpitation are added to the other side effects associated with inhibition of sympathetic vasoconstriction. However, small doses of phenoxybenzamine have been found useful in patients who have developed resistance to adrenergic neuron blocking drugs on the basis of vascular supersensitivity to catecholamines (Sandler *et al.,* 1968). Phenoxybenzamine and phentolamine have also been used successfully to control acute hypertensive episodes due to sympathomimetics, and to certain foods and drugs in the presence of MAO inhibition. The general treatment of hypertension is discussed in Chapter 33.

Pheochromocytoma. Many pharmacological tests for the diagnosis of pheochromocytoma have been employed in the past, including provocative tests with histamine, methacholine, and glucagon, as well as blocking tests with piperoxan and phentolamine. Determination of the amounts of catecholamines and their metabolites, particularly metanephrine and normetanephrine, in the urine is now generally accepted as the most reliable method of diagnosis, and the pharmacological tests are now obsolete. (*See* review by Wolf *et al.,* 1970.)

Adrenergic blocking agents are useful in the *preoperative management* of cases of pheochromocytoma, for the *prolonged treatment* of cases not amenable to surgery, and to prevent paroxysmal hypertension during *operative manipulation* of the tumor. Oral phenoxybenzamine is the agent of choice in the first two of these situations. The stable, persistent blockade may allow improvement in the general cardiovascular status of the patient prior to operation, and it permits expansion of the blood volume, which may be severely reduced as a result of the excessive adrenergic vasoconstriction. Patients with inoperable tumors have been adequately controlled with phenoxybenzamine for many years (*see* Engelman and Sjoerdsma, 1964). In the operative management of pheochromocytoma, phenoxybenzamine (1.0 mg/kg) administered intravenously 36 hours and again approximately 12 hours prior to surgery provides essentially complete protection against both pressor episodes and cardiac arrhythmias, irrespective of the amount of catecholamine released. In addition, the otherwise-common complication of postoperative hypotension rarely occurs in patients operated on while under the effects of full phenoxybenzamine blockade. Oral phenoxybenzamine provides less complete block, and addition of a β-adrenergic blocking agent or special anesthetic procedures may be necessary to prevent arrhythmias (*see* Ross *et al.,* 1967; Crout and Brown, 1969).

Shock. Largely because of preoccupation with low blood pressure as a criterion of shock, vasopressor agents have been used extensively in its treatment. However, vasoconstriction is a prominent feature of shock *per se,* and there is little evidence that its accentuation by drugs is beneficial. Indeed, hyperactivity of the sympathetic nervous system or infusion of a vasoconstrictor such as norepinephrine can accentuate the development of shock initiated by hemorrhage, trauma, or infection, and can itself induce lethal shock in both laboratory animals and man.

Many agents that induce vasodilatation by inhibiting sympathetic vasoconstriction or by directly relaxing vascular smooth muscle improve the survival rate of experimental animals subjected to various shock-inducing procedures. However, the haloalkylamine adrenergic blocking agents have been most thoroughly investigated in this regard and, where direct comparison is possible, appear to be the most effective. Protection can be attributed to at least three distinct cardiovascular effects: (1) increased cardiac output and total blood flow, particularly in the abdominal viscera; (2) local redistribution of blood flow so that a larger percentage passes through channels that readily exchange metabolites with tissue cells, presumably true capillaries; and (3) reversal of the vasoconstriction-induced shift of fluid from the vascular to the interstitial compartment. Although the contribution of intravascular coagulation in the progression of shock is not fully defined, it may be significant that phenoxybenzamine effectively prevents the formation of microthrombi and the subsequent intravascular hemolysis induced by catecholamines (McKay et al., 1969). A similar mechanism is probably involved in inhibition of the generalized Shwartzman reaction induced by endotoxin.

Phenoxybenzamine is under investigation as a treatment for clinical shock resulting from *hemorrhage, trauma,* and *infection,* and the results have been very encouraging. In addition to its specific "antishock" effects, seen clearly in patients who have not responded to fully adequate replacement of intravascular fluid volume, two other effects of phenoxybenzamine can make important contributions to the practical clinical management of this condition: (1) The fall in blood pressure induced when it is administered in the presence of hypovolemia provides a quick and reliable indication of the adequacy of intravascular fluid–volume replacement, a point often difficult to determine even with careful monitoring of the central venous pressure. (2) The shift of blood from the pulmonary to the systemic vascular bed associated with blockade of sympathetic vasomotor tone allows administration of larger volumes of fluid more rapidly than would otherwise be possible, particularly in patients with some myocardial inadequacy. It should be emphasized that any drug therapy in shock is secondary to fully adequate replacement of intravascular fluid volume with blood or other appropriate fluids. *Phenoxybenzamine should not be given unless the central venous pressure has been elevated by fluid administration without an adequate circulatory response;* inhibition of vasoconstrictor reflexes makes the circulation highly vulnerable to hypovolemia. In addition, the blocking agent must be administered slowly and suitable fluids must be immediately available for use if a sharp drop in blood pressure indicates that replacement has in fact been inadequate. (*See* Nickerson, 1962a; Hardaway, 1968.)

The mortality from *cardiogenic shock,* usually following myocardial infarction, is approximately 80% and it has not been appreciably reduced by any type of therapy tried to date. Cardiogenic shock has many features in common with shock of other etiology: cardiac output is usually low and peripheral vascular resistance elevated; major deficits in plasma volume can develop; and survival is inversely related to the blood lactate concentration, which reflects inadequacies of systemic tissue perfusion. However, in contrast to shock precipitated by other events, perfusion of at least parts of the coronary vascular bed is a limiting factor. This perfusion is directly related to the aortic diastolic pressure and inversely related to the intraventricular diastolic pressure. As in other types of shock, α-adrenergic blockade with a drug such as phenoxybenzamine can decrease peripheral resistance, blood lactate, and intraventricular diastolic pressure, and can allow an increase in cardiac output without a comparable increase in myocardial work. However, it also tends to decrease aortic diastolic pressure, and blockade must be established very slowly, with constant monitoring. No overall improvement in survival rate has yet been demonstrated with this type of therapy, but some cases appear to respond dramatically (Freeman, 1969; Riordan and Walters, 1969). Further work may allow selection of a subgroup of patients in whom peripheral vasoconstriction is a major deleterious factor and in whom any fall in aortic diastolic pressure can be limited.

Several other applications of α-adrenergic blockade are based on considerations very similar to those involved in the treatment of shock. Preoperative administration of phenoxybenzamine has been shown to improve postoperative cardiovascular and renal function following extended periods of extracorporeal circulation associated with cardiac surgery (Burack et al., 1972). The drug has also been used to reduce renal vasospasm and to improve perfusion, particularly of the outer cortex, during short-term preservation of both animal and human kidneys for transplantation (Pryor et al., 1971; McCabe and Fitzpatrick, 1972). Phenoxybenzamine also may increase the viability of renal and hepatic cells subjected to periods of interrupted blood flow to these organs (Rangel et al., 1969), and the drug has been shown to improve the survival of experimental skin flaps (Palmer, 1972). Improvements in microvascular flow appear to be involved in the reported increased survival in experimental malaria, and in the rapid improvement in renal function induced by phenoxybenzamine in some cases of malaria-induced acute renal failure in man (Sitprija, 1971).

Peripheral Vascular Disease. Many α-adrenergic blocking drugs, direct-acting vasodilators (*see also* Chapter 34), and drugs with mixed actions are promoted for the treatment of inadequacies of blood flow, particularly to the skin and muscles of the extremities. Ischemia in these areas arises from a variety of pathological processes, but morphological changes that limit flow in relatively large vessels are commonly involved. In general, the results of drug therapy in this broad group of diseases have been disappointing, and vasoactive drugs should not be given precedence over conservative medical management or surgery, where the latter is indicated and possible.

Intravenous phenoxybenzamine can increase blood flow in the limbs only slightly less than does regional local anesthetic nerve block; tolazoline and dihydroergotoxine in the doses usually employed clinically induce smaller increases. The response in skin is relatively greater than that in muscle, probably because cutaneous vessels are predominantly controlled by adrenergic vasoconstrictor nerves. In occlusive arterial disease the increase in cutaneous blood flow tends to vary inversely with the severity of the ischemia (Thomas *et al.*, 1968). The less severe cases may represent those in which collateral vessels exist that are capable of dilatation, and some benefit could result from drug therapy; however, it is also possible for a vasodilator to divert blood from the most ischemic areas because their vessels are the least capable of dilatation.

Although no fully controlled studies of clinical efficacy are available, the very large component of sympathetic control of skin vessels lends credence to the reported beneficial effects of α-adrenergic blocking agents on some *cutaneous manifestations of atherosclerosis, phlebitis* and *phlebothrombosis, trauma,* and *frostbite sequelae.* It has been shown that α-adrenergic blockade can increase skin blood flow in cases of occlusive arterial disease in which muscle flow is unaltered (Myers *et al.*, 1968). In ambulatory patients, postural hypotension precludes the use of doses of phenoxybenzamine that produce extensive blockade. In acute peripheral vascular insufficiency in hospitalized patients, maximal inhibition of sympathetic vasoconstrictor tone with phenoxybenzamine may be desirable, but such therapy should not be substituted for or allowed to delay surgical intervention where this is possible. Several α-adrenergic blocking agents have been administered intra-arterially to patients with peripheral vascular disease, but the questionable benefits obtained do not justify the risks of this route of administration.

The above considerations do not apply to inadequacies of skeletal muscle blood flow, where the vessels are predominantly under the control of local metabolic factors. There are many reports of the efficacy of α-adrenergic blocking agents and of other vasodilatators in *intermittent claudication.* However, there is no convincing evidence that any agent or procedure can increase skeletal muscle blood flow beyond the level produced by exercise to the limit of tolerance. Such exercise is also generally accepted as the most effective mechanism for improving the collateral circulation to ischemic muscle.

Although cerebral vascular resistance is predominantly controlled by local carbon dioxide tension (P_{CO_2}), there may be an adrenergic component to responses of large intracranial vessels. Phenoxybenzamine has been shown experimentally to inhibit vascular spasm induced by application of free blood, and has been given by intracarotid injection to prevent vascular spasm following operations on intracranial aneurysms, with apparently good results (Cummins and Griffith, 1971).

The most favorable clinical responses to α-adrenergic blockade are in conditions with a large component of adrenergic vasoconstriction, such as *Raynaud's syndrome* and *acrocyanosis.* These are less common and threatening than occlusive arterial disease, but even here drug therapy is probably secondary to other measures. Phenoxybenzamine and tolazoline have been observed to relieve vasospasm and reduce sensitivity to cold in Raynaud's syndrome. Satisfactory results are obtained in most cases with oral doses that produce only a relatively low level of adrenergic blockade (Friend and Edwards, 1954; Gifford, 1971). Vasospasm induced by an exogenous sympathomimetic is readily antagonized, and local infiltration with 2.5 to 5.0 mg of phentolamine or addition of the drug to the intravenous solution effectively prevents the severe local vasoconstriction and skin necrosis that can be associated with infusion of a vasoconstrictor such as norepinephrine, particularly if there is some extravasation.

Other Cardiovascular Uses. High spinal cord transection commonly leads to autonomic hyperreflexia with paroxysmal elevations in blood pressure from both cutaneous and visceral stimuli, particularly those from the urinary bladder. It has been reported that these pressor episodes and the associated signs and symptoms can be well controlled by relatively small oral doses of phenoxybenzamine (Sizemore and Winternitz, 1970).

Any inadequacy of cardiac output, particularly of relatively acute onset, can cause an increase in sympathetic vasomotor tone, which increases peripheral resistance and decreases venous compliance. Because the constriction is greater in the systemic bed, blood is shifted to the pulmonary circuit, and increased pulmonary blood volume and pressure can cause *pulmonary congestion and edema.* It has been repeatedly shown that block of sympathetic vasoconstriction can rapidly reverse these processes and decrease myocardial work and pulmonary congestion. α-Adrenergic blockade has been shown to be beneficial in heart failure with pulmonary edema (*see* Majid *et al.*, 1971), and in acute myocardial infarction where pain can accentuate the vasoconstriction (Kelly *et al.*, 1973). Other vasodilator drugs such as nitroprusside (*see* Chapter 33) are also effective, but pathogenetic considerations suggest that α-adrenergic blockade with an agent such as phenoxybenzamine would be the most rational therapy.

Miscellaneous Uses. The obvious "sympathomimetic" nature of many of the signs and symptoms of hyperthyroidism has led to attempts at symptomatic control with adrenergic blocking agents. The results have been inconsistent, but α-adrenergic blockade appears to have less effect than β blockade. The more fundamental matter of altering endocrine function by blocking agents is just beginning to be explored on the basis of recent observations on adrenergic involvement in the control of hormone secretion. However, it has been reported that α-adrenergic blockade can restore the insulin response to glucose after stress and can decrease the blood glucose in *juvenile diabetes,* apparently by antagonizing adrenergic suppression of insulin release (Cegrell, 1972; Robertson *et al.*, 1972), and can decrease plasma growth hormone concentrations in *acromegaly* (Nakagawa and Mashimo, 1973).

Adrenergic stimuli are known to increase the motility of human ureters, but there has been little information on their involvement in the spasms of *ureteral colic.* It has been reported that relatively large intravenous doses of phentolamine (40 to 50 mg) relaxed the ureters and gave almost complete relief of pain in over half of the patients studied; propranolol was ineffective (Kubacz and Catchpole, 1972).

II. β-Adrenergic Blocking Agents

PROPRANOLOL AND RELATED DRUGS

The first drug shown to produce a selective blockade of β-adrenergic receptors was *dichloroisoproterenol (DCI)* (Powell and Slater, 1958). Studies with DCI made a substantial contribution to the understanding of adrenergic effects mediated by β receptors, but it was not used in man, largely because it has a prominent β-receptor stimulant action; that is, it is a partial agonist. *Pronethalol* has weaker agonist properties and was used therapeutically, but following reports that it produces tumors in animals it was replaced by propranolol, which has little or no agonist activity. *Propranolol* is currently the only β-adrenergic blocking agent on the market in the United States and Canada, although others are available elsewhere. Many β-adrenergic antagonists have been synthesized and tested (*see* Karow *et al.,* 1971). They differ in potency, β-receptor selectivity, agonist activity, and membrane-stabilizing actions (local anesthetic and quinidine-like properties). The β-adrenergic receptors of various tissues can be differentiated pharmacologically as β_1 (heart) and β_2 (most smooth muscle) (Levy and Wilkenfeld, 1970). For example, it is possible to inhibit cardiac responses selectively with a drug such as *practolol* or *sotalol,* but the differentiation is not absolute and larger doses can block all β-adrenergic receptors. None of the presently available β-adrenergic blocking agents is ideal, and the search for new drugs of this class continues; for example, preliminary reports indicate that *tolamol* (4-[(2-hydroxy-3-*o*-tolyloxypropylamino)ethoxy]benzamide) is a cardioselective β-adrenergic blocking agent equal in potency to propranolol and with no intrinsic activity.

Propranolol will be considered the prototype compound because it has been much more extensively studied than any other β-adrenergic blocking drug, and *practolol* will be considered as representative of cardioselective blocking agents.

Chemistry. Most of the more effective β-adrenergic blocking agents can be considered to be derivatives of the β-receptor agonist isoproterenol. The structural formulas of several of the most thoroughly studied drugs are as follows:

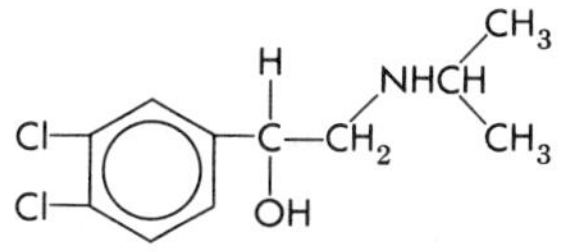

Dichloroisoproterenol (DCI)

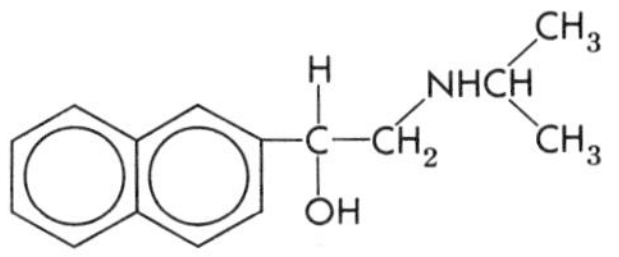

Pronethalol

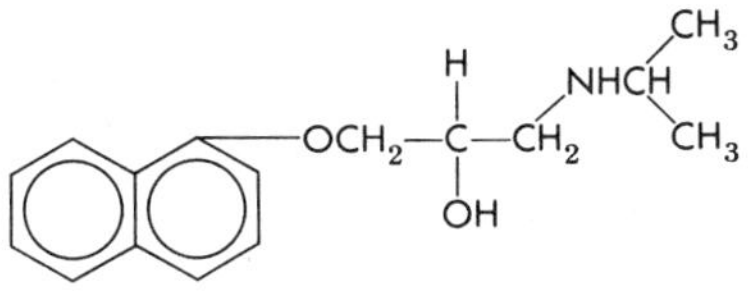

Propranolol

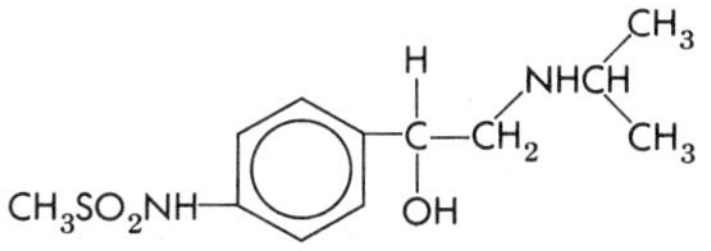

Sotalol

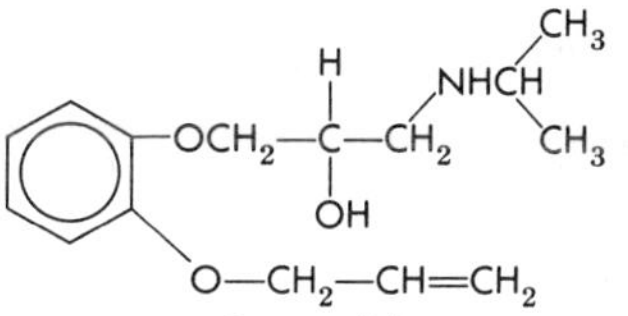

Oxprenolol

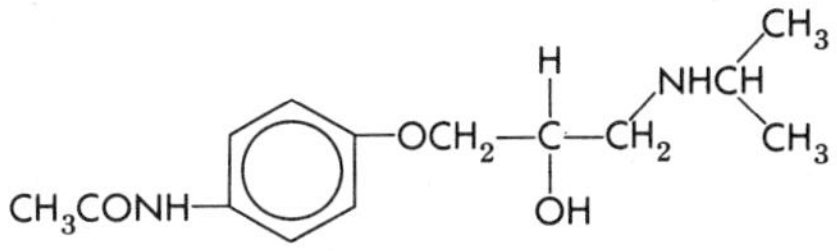

Practolol

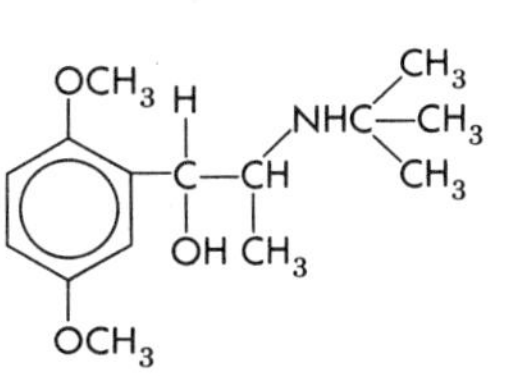

Butoxamine

The structural similarity between β-receptor agonists and antagonists is much closer than in the case of drugs acting at α receptors. The side chain with an isopropyl-substituted secondary amine appears to favor interaction with β receptors; the N-tertiary butyl substituent, as in butoxamine, confers the same type of selectivity but resists metabolic degradation (Burns *et al.,* 1967). The nature of substituents on the aromatic ring determines whether the effect will be predominantly activation or blockade. These substituents also affect cardioselectivity. The aliphatic hydroxyl appears to be essential for activity. It gives the molecule optical activity, and the (−) forms of both β-adrenergic agonists and antagonists are much more potent than the (+) forms. This difference is useful in distinguishing the effects of β-receptor blockade from those of other pharmacological actions of the molecule; for example, the (+) form of propranolol has less than 1% of the potency of the (−) form of propranolol in blocking β-adrenergic receptors, but the two isomers are equipotent as local anesthetics (Barrett and Cullum, 1968).

PHARMACOLOGICAL PROPERTIES

As in the case of the α-adrenergic blocking agents, much of the pharmacology of β-adrenergic blockade can be deduced from a knowledge of the functions subserved by the involved receptors (Table 21–1, page 408) and the physiological or pathological conditions under which they are activated. Thus, β-receptor blockade has little effect on the normal heart with the subject at complete rest, but may have profound effects when sympathetic control of the heart is high, as during exercise. The overall response to a β-adrenergic blocking agent may also be modified by other properties of the drug in question. β-Receptor stimulation ("intrinsic sympathomimetic activity") is an important component of the response to some β blockers. Some β-adrenergic antagonists also have important direct actions on cell membranes, which are commonly described as membrane stabilizing, local anesthetic, and quinidine-like. The local anesthetic potencies of pronethalol and propranolol are about equal to that of lidocaine; oxprenolol is about half as potent, and sotalol and practolol are almost devoid of this property. The membrane-stabilizing action of propranolol has contributed to reported cardiac effects in laboratory experiments, but it appears to be of little clinical importance with the usual therapeutic doses. Other results of this action include inhibition of osmotic lysis of erythrocytes (Langslet, 1970), inhibition of 5-HT uptake by blood platelets (Lemmer *et al.,* 1972), and inhibition of norepinephrine release from and uptake by adrenergic nerves (Mylecharane and Raper, 1973). Doses of propranolol well within the therapeutic range can reduce the oxygen affinity of hemoglobin in intact erythrocytes *in vivo* by a mechanism unrelated to β-adrenergic receptors (Oski *et al.,* 1972; Pendleton *et al.,* 1972).

Cardiovascular System. As in the case of α blockade, the most important effects of β-adrenergic blocking drugs are on the cardiovascular system, predominantly due to actions on the heart.

β-Adrenergic Receptor Blockade. β-Adrenergic antagonists without intrinsic sympathomimetic activity, such as propranolol, decrease heart rate and cardiac output, prolong and decrease the velocity of mechanical systole, and slightly decrease blood pressure in resting subjects (Robin *et al.,* 1967; Helfant *et al.,* 1971). Peripheral resistance is increased as a result of compensatory sympathetic reflexes, and blood flow to all tissues except the brain is reduced (Nies *et al.,* 1973). β-Adrenergic blocking agents have minimal direct effects on the peripheral vasculature, although propranolol causes a brief vasodilatation unrelated to β-receptor blockade when injected intra-arterially (Shanks, 1967). The major effects of propranolol on the heart are absent in animals whose norepinephrine stores have been depleted (Shanks, 1966). Reported differences in the responses of resting and anesthetized subjects probably reflect differences in residual sympathetic control of the heart due to either physiological or emotional factors. Chronic treatment of hypertensive patients with a β-adrenergic blocking agent results in a slowly developing reduction in blood pressure. The mechanism responsible for this antihypertensive effect is not clear, but one likely explanation is that there is a gradual loss of the reflex increase of peripheral resistance in response to the reduced cardiac output (Tarazi and Dustan, 1972).

The cardiac effects of β-adrenergic blockade are often reflected in changes in sodium excretion. The normal diurnal pattern is reversed, as in patients with moderate myocardial inadequacy, and there is a slow adjustment to a new steady state with increased total body sodium and extracellular fluid volume. These effects are most obvious in patients with some preexisting myocardial inadequacy. In some patients with severe heart disease, β-adrenergic blockade can cause progressive accumulation of sodium and water, edema, and frank congestive heart failure (Epstein and Braunwald, 1966). These effects on sodium excretion probably result from intrarenal hemodynamic changes that are part of the adjustment to the decreased cardiac output (Nies *et al.*, 1971). The magnitude of the effect appears to parallel the dependence of the heart on adrenergic stimulation to maintain adequate function. Occasionally a β-adrenergic blocking agent, particularly when given intravenously, can precipitate acute heart failure.

The effect of β-adrenergic blockade on the heart is more marked under conditions of increased demand and sympathetic tone. The cardiac response to fluid load is reduced, as is the tachycardia associated with exercise, nitrite hypotension, or the Valsalva maneuver (Black and Prichard, 1973). Ventricular dimensions and contractility are little affected in normal, supine, resting subjects, but the decreases in end-diastolic and end-systolic ventricular size and the increase in myocardial contractility associated with exercise are reduced. In patients with occlusive coronary artery disease, propranolol can cause significant increases in ventricular end-diastolic volumes and pressures, and in the tension-time index; it can also cause or increase ventricular asynergy (*see* Robin *et al.*, 1967; Helfant *et al.*, 1971). Maximal exercise tolerance is considerably decreased in normal individuals, but can be increased in patients with angina pectoris by both propranolol and practolol (Sowton *et al.*, 1971). During moderate exercise, adjusted to the cardiac status of the subject, the inadequate increase in cardiac output is compensated for by increased oxygen extraction, but during maximal exercise total oxygen consumption is decreased. Total coronary blood flow and myocardial oxygen consumption are also decreased (Wolfson and Gorlin, 1969). The reduction is predominantly in subepicardial blood flow, which leads to a relative redistribution of flow (Gross and Winbury, 1973). A similar internal shunting after β-adrenergic blockade allows blood flow to ischemic areas of the heart to be altered less than that to other regions (Pitt and Craven, 1970).

In appropriate doses, all β-adrenergic blocking drugs reduce the chronotropic and inotropic effects of cardiac sympathetic nerve activity and of circulating β-receptor agonists. Stimulation by other agents, including calcium, barium, methylxanthines, and digitalis, is little affected. The relative effectiveness of various β-adrenergic antagonists against circulating and locally released catecholamines is not entirely clear, but it appears that propranolol blocks the two types of stimuli about equally (Ledsome *et al.*, 1974). All currently available β-adrenergic blocking drugs are competitive antagonists, and the block can therefore be overcome by an increased concentration of agonist.

Propranolol and other nonselective β-adrenergic blocking drugs inhibit the vasodepressor and vasodilator effects of isoproterenol, and augment the pressor effect of epinephrine. Pressor responses to norepinephrine may be slightly decreased because its cardiac actions are blocked, but those to phenylephrine are unchanged. These effects are entirely predictable from a knowledge of the relative activities of different sympathomimetics on vascular α and β receptors. Vascular β receptors make only a limited contribution to the circulatory status under most physiological and pathological conditions; in intact laboratory animals and man, the effect of their blockade is obscured by the reflex response to myocardial blockade. Vasodilatation due to histamine, ACh, and nitroglycerin is unaffected. β-Adrenergic blockade does not inhibit renal vasodilatation induced by dopamine, although the limited response to isoproterenol in this vascular bed and to dopamine in the femoral vasculature are eliminated (McNay and Goldberg, 1966). A cardioselective (β_1) drug such as practolol blocks the cardiac effects of isoproterenol with only minimal reduction of the vasodilatation and hypotension produced. The pressor effect of epinephrine is reduced rather than enhanced, presumably because cardiac stimulation is inhibited. Isoproterenol-induced tachycardia is not completely prevented in unanesthetized animals unless atropine is also given to eliminate the vagal component of the reflex response to the decrease in blood pressure. Butoxamine, in contrast, blocks β_2 vasodilator and other smooth muscle inhibitory effects of isoproterenol, but relatively little antagonism of the cardiac effects is observed in anesthetized animals; in unanesthetized dogs, however, it blocks the chronotropic action (Levy, 1966; Burns *et al.*, 1967).

β-Adrenergic Receptor Stimulation. Some β-adrenergic blocking agents can cause β-receptor stimulation both *in vitro* and *in vivo* in the same doses that inhibit responses to β agonists. This agonist action is most prominent with DCI, slight with oxprenolol and practolol, and virtually absent with propranolol and sotalol. Agonist activity might be a disadvantage when drugs of this class are used in the treatment of angina pectoris.

Quinidine-like Effects. The β-adrenergic blocking drugs with local anesthetic activity also have a quinidine-like action on the heart, but the relative potencies with respect to these two properties are not always the same (*see* Singh and Vaughan Williams, 1971). In isolated atria, pronethalol, propranolol, and oxprenolol decrease spontaneous frequency, maximal driving frequency, and contractility, and increase electrical threshold. They also increase A-V conduction time in intact hearts. Resting membrane potential and repolarization are not greatly affected by propranolol, but the height and rate of rise of the action potential are reduced because the drug decreases the inward sodium current (Tarr *et al.,* 1973). These quinidine-like effects are associated with generalized depression of myocardial function, which can cause death with large doses. It has been suggested that β-adrenergic blocking agents without membrane-stabilizing activity are less likely than propranolol to precipitate heart failure. However, direct myocardial depression requires doses much higher than those necessary for β-adrenergic blockade, and it appears that block of sympathetic stimulation is by far the most important factor in the occasional precipitation of heart failure in a patient with an inadequate myocardium. The quinidine-like effects of β-adrenergic blocking drugs appear to contribute little to the treatment of cardiac arrhythmias; effective blood levels of propranolol are below those that cause much membrane stabilization, and β blockers without this property are also effective antiarrhythmic agents (*see* Black and Prichard, 1973).

Central Nervous System. Propranolol readily penetrates the brain, but it has few, if any, effects that can be clearly attributed to block of β-adrenergic receptors in the CNS. The usual therapeutic doses of propranolol produce no CNS effects in most patients. Large doses have usually been found to be depressant in laboratory animals. The negligible central effects of practolol and the fact that it is an effective antihypertensive drug appear to rule out the possibility that this effect of the β-adrenergic blocking agents is due to an action on the CNS. There are several reports that β-adrenergic antagonists reduce anxiety, but there is little evidence that this is due to any action on the CNS; the observations can be adequately explained by the relief of symptoms that the drug achieves. Propranolol antagonizes the effects of stimuli that inhibit growth hormone secretion, and this may represent blockade of some central action of dopamine (Collu *et al.,* 1972); most reports indicate that it has little effect on plasma growth hormone concentrations in normal individuals (*see* Blackard and Hubbell, 1970).

Metabolic Effects. β-Adrenergic blocking agents can considerably modify carbohydrate and fat metabolism, although many species and tissue variations as well as composite effects confuse this complex field (*see* reviews by Himms-Hagen, 1967, and several articles in Symposium, 1970). The effects of catecholamines on carbohydrate and fat metabolism are mediated by β receptors and changes in adenylate cyclase activity, with resultant production of cyclic adenosine 3',5'-monophosphate (cyclic AMP). Adrenergic blocking agents that inhibit metabolic responses act on this sequence of events. In man, propranolol inhibits the rise in plasma free fatty acids induced by sympathomimetic amines or by enhanced sympathetic nervous system activity. It also effectively and selectively inhibits the lipolytic action of catecholamines on isolated adipose tissue of several species, and practolol and butoxamine appear to have similar effects. The actions of adrenergic blocking agents on carbohydrate metabolism are more complicated. The hyperglycemic response to epinephrine is reduced by β-adrenergic blocking drugs in most species and by α blockers in only a few. The effects of the latter agents also involve actions on insulin secretion (*see* above). Glycogenolysis in heart and skeletal muscle is inhibited by β- and not by α-adrenergic blocking drugs. That in liver is inhibited by both types of antagonist in some species, but the effects of α blockers appear to be nonspecific (*see* Newton and Hornbrook, 1972). The release of insulin by isoproterenol is blocked by propranolol, but apparently not by practolol (Loubatieres *et al.,* 1971). Propranolol does not affect plasma glucose or insulin concentrations in normal individuals, or the rate or magnitude of the fall of plasma glucose after insulin, but it does slow the subsequent recovery of glucose concentration and prevents the usual rebound of plasma glycerol. These effects are presumably due to inhibition of the glycogenolytic and lipolytic actions of endogenous catecholamines released in response to hypoglycemia. Consequently, β-adrenergic blocking agents must be used with caution in patients prone to hypoglycemia and particularly in diabetics treated with insulin. Many aspects of the adrenergic control of insulin secretion have been reviewed by Porte and Robertson (1973).

Other Effects. Propranolol blocks the action of sympathomimetic amines on β-adrenergic receptors in many structures. However, when administered in the absence of a specific agonist, the most important response to β blockade outside of the cardiovascular system is that of the bronchi and bronchioles. Adrenergic bronchodilatation is mediated by β receptors, but the presence of significant intrinsic adrenergic bronchodilator activity was not demonstrated before the clinical availability of β-adrenergic blocking agents. Propranolol consistently increases airway resistance. This effect is small and of no clinical significance in normal individuals, but it can be marked and potentially dangerous in asthmatics. Because bronchodilatation is a $β_2$-adrenergic response, practolol is much less likely than propranolol to induce bronchoconstriction (MacDonald and McNeill, 1968), and it has been used in asthmatic patients with minimal effects on airway resistance (*see* Formgren, 1972). Practolol effectively inhibits the cardiac stimulation but not the bronchodilatation caused by isoproterenol inhaled or injected in the treatment of asthma (*see* Howard *et al.,* 1972). However, practolol has been reported to cause bronchial irritation in some asthmatics (*see* Waal-Manning and Simpson, 1971). Both propranolol and practolol have been reported to potentiate bronchospasm induced by ACh, methacholine, histamine, and 5-HT, and this potentiation is greater in asthmatic than in nonasthmatic subjects (*see* Nicolaescu *et al.,* 1972).

β-Adrenergic blocking agents antagonize relaxation of the uterus by catecholamines, but they have no effect under conditions in which the response is excitatory (Tothill, 1967). Propranolol increases the activity of the human uterus, more in the nonpregnant than in the pregnant state (Wansbrough *et al.,* 1968). β-Receptor blockade inhibits the action of epinephrine that prevents local edema formation in response to the injection of a variety of irritants in the rat paw (*see* Green, 1972), and both propranolol and practolol block the "antianaphylactic" effect of catecholamines on antigen-induced histamine release from sensitized lung (Assem and Schild, 1971). Circulating eosinophils increase in man during the administration of propranolol, and the reduction characteristically induced by epinephrine is blocked (Koch-Weser, 1968).

The effects of β-adrenergic blocking agents on skeletal neuromuscular transmission are variable, and appear to be unrelated to either β-adrenergic blockade or local anesthetic activity (Wislicki, 1969). Drugs that block β-adrenergic receptors antagonize epinephrine-induced tremor in man, and large doses of propranolol can reduce tremorine-induced tremor in laboratory animals. However, propranolol is not consistently effective in controlling essential tremor or the tremor of parkinsonism (Gilligan *et al.,* 1972). It is likely that the antitremor effect is peripheral, and it probably is observed only in cases where tremor is accentuated by emotional stress.

β-Adrenergic blocking drugs antagonize the release of renin from the juxtaglomerular apparatus of the kidney by sympathomimetic amines or sympathetic nerve activity (*see* Ganong, 1973). They also reduce, but do not completely block, the increase in plasma renin activity induced by sodium deprivation (Michelakis and McAllister, 1972). However, reduction of plasma renin activity is not necessary for the antihypertensive effect of β-adrenergic blocking drugs (Stokes *et al.,* 1974). (*See also* Chapters 30 and 33.)

Absorption, Fate, and Excretion. *Propranolol* is well absorbed after oral administration. It is concentrated in the lungs and

to a lesser extent in brain, liver, kidney, and heart, and is excreted in the urine after being almost completely metabolized (Hayes and Cooper, 1971). More than 90% of circulating propranolol is bound to plasma protein (Evans *et al.,* 1973a). The plasma half-life in man is approximately 3 hours (Shand *et al.,* 1970). Details of the metabolic fate of propranolol are still not clear; eight metabolites have been recovered from the urine of dogs or man (Walle and Gaffney, 1972). One important metabolite, 4-hydroxypropranolol, found only after oral or intraportal administration, has blocking activity similar to that of propranolol (Fitzgerald and O'Donnell, 1971). The metabolism of propranolol occurs mostly in the liver, which has a saturable, high-affinity binding mechanism for the drug; low concentrations can be removed completely during a single passage (Evans *et al.,* 1973b). *Practolol* is readily absorbed from the gastrointestinal tract, and is rapidly distributed throughout the body, except for the brain. More than 85% is excreted unchanged in the urine, but at least 18 metabolites have been identified. The plasma half-life of practolol is 6 to 8 hours after oral administration in man (*see* Schneck *et al.,* 1972).

Preparations, Routes of Administration, and Dosage. *Propranolol Hydrochloride,* U.S.P. (INDERAL), is available in tablets containing 10 and 40 mg for oral administration, and in 1-ml ampuls containing 1.0 mg for intravenous use. The most usual oral doses are 20 to 40 mg, three or four times a day, but much higher doses have been employed when necessary. The usual intravenous dose is 1 to 3 mg, which should be injected over several minutes or in increments of 0.5 mg with continuous monitoring of the ECG. Considerably larger doses are commonly infused to assure β-receptor blockade when the drug is used as a tool in clinical investigation.

None of the other β-adrenergic blocking drugs discussed in this section is currently available for general clinical use in the United States or Canada.

Toxicity, Side Effects, and Precautions.
The major dangers of therapy with propranolol or other β-adrenergic blocking drugs are related to the blockade *per se.* Serious cardiac depression is uncommon, but heart failure may develop suddenly or slowly, usually in patients whose hearts are severely compromised by disease or by other drugs (*e.g.,* anesthetics). Acute failure is rare with oral administration. Propranolol should

be given with caution to any patient with inadequate myocardial function, but it may be beneficial if a treatable arrhythmia or excessive sinus rate contributes significantly to the inadequacy. The inotropic action of digitalis is not prevented by propranolol, but both drugs depress A-V conduction. Propranolol can cause A-V dissociation and cardiac arrest in patients with preexisting partial heart block due to digitalis or other factors.

A second important danger from β-adrenergic blockade is an increase in airway resistance, which can be life threatening in asthmatics. Asthma is a contraindication to the use of propranolol. Agents such as practolol, which are much less liable to cause bronchoconstriction, will probably replace propranolol for use in asthmatics and other patients with a history of severe allergy. The effectiveness of epinephrine in the treatment of acute allergic reactions may be reduced in patients on chronic medication with this drug.

Propranolol augments the hypoglycemic action of insulin by reducing the compensatory effect of sympathoadrenal activation, and masks the tachycardia that is an important sign of developing hypoglycemia. Consequently, any patient susceptible to episodes of hypoglycemia must be watched carefully for untoward reactions.

Side effects of propranolol that are not extensions of the desired pharmacological action are usually not serious and frequently disappear during continued drug administration. Nausea, vomiting, mild diarrhea, and constipation have been reported. CNS effects are not common, but many have been observed, including hallucinations, nightmares, insomnia, lassitude, and depression (*see* Greenblatt and Shader, 1972). In double-blind studies, many of these CNS complaints occurred with equal frequency during placebo administration. Rash, fever, and purpura probably reflect an allergic response; they are infrequent but require discontinuation of the drug. Unwanted effects of propranolol have been reviewed by Greenblatt and Koch-Weser (1973).

Therapeutic Uses. The β-adrenergic receptors most important to the body economy are those of the heart, and this organ has received primary attention in the clinical application of β-adrenergic blocking agents. The clinical use of propranolol in the treatment of certain *cardiac arrhythmias* is discussed in Chapter 32. The other important cardiovascular uses of β-adrenergic blocking drugs are in the treatment of *angina pectoris* (*see* Chapter 34) and *hypertension* (*see* Chapter 33).

Propranolol is also used in *hypertrophic obstructive cardiomyopathies*. In these conditions forceful contraction of the myocardium along a ventricular outflow tract can greatly increase outflow resistance, particularly during exercise. β-Adrenergic blockade may have little effect when the patient is at rest, but it has been shown to improve hemodynamic parameters considerably during exercise, and relatively long-term treatment has been reported to be beneficial (*see* Shand *et al.*, 1971). Propranolol is sometimes useful in the management of tachycardia and arrhythmias in patients with *pheochromocytoma*. However, it is less important than α-adrenergic blockade in this condition and should not be given except in the presence of the latter. When used alone, β-adrenergic blocking drugs can cause a dangerous increase in blood pressure. Similarly, they can accentuate vasospasm in conditions such as Raynaud's syndrome.

β-Adrenergic blockade has been shown to have palliative value in a variety of conditions that involve adrenergic signs and symptoms. In *hyperthyroidism* propranolol has been reported to decrease heart rate, cardiac output, and tremor, and it has been used to control the signs and symptoms of the iatrogenic hyperthyroidism that may be associated with the use of dextrothyroxine in the treatment of hypercholesterolemia. β-Adrenergic blockade can produce rapid, dramatic improvement in thyroid crises (*see* Malcolm, 1972; Chapter 67). A central mechanism of action has been suggested to explain the beneficial effects of propranolol in various *anxiety states*, but peripheral block of symptoms such as palpitation and tremor, which tend to sustain the condition by a positive feedback, appears to be the most likely mechanism (*see* Bonn *et al.*, 1972).

III. Adrenergic Neuron Blocking Agents

Interference with chemical mediation at postganglionic adrenergic nerve endings can occur by several mechanisms, including depletion of the stores of mediator and direct prevention of its release. However, many drugs in this class appear to act by more than one mechanism, and the contribution of each to a given effect is often unclear. It is particularly difficult to assess the contribution of reduced norepinephrine content to adrenergic neuron blockade. In some cases block occurs only after extensive depletion, in others with only minor changes in total content. Any given observation can be explained by assumptions regarding "functional compartments" of mediator. However, such explanations are hazardous when different observations require very different and sometimes mutually exclusive assumptions.

GUANETHIDINE

Guanethidine may be considered representative of drugs that depress the function of postganglionic adrenergic nerves. Its mechanism of action initially appeared to be quite different from that of the first reported adrenergic neuron blocking agents, TM10 and bretylium (*see* below), but it now appears that these drugs have common actions and differ predominantly in the quantitative importance of each. Assessment of the structure-activity relationship among adrenergic neuron blocking drugs is complicated by the fact that many have a pattern of action intermediate between those of guanethidine and bretylium (*see* Boura and Green, 1965); all compounds within this spectrum have a strongly basic moiety such as the guanidine grouping or a quaternary nitrogen. The structural formulas of guanethidine and bretylium are as follows:

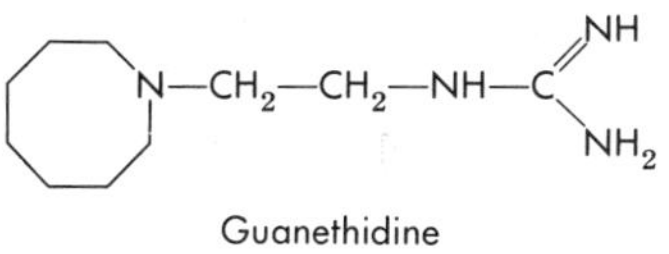

Guanethidine

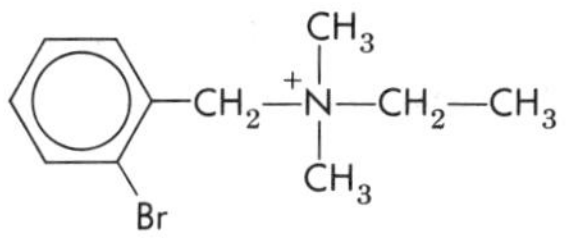

Bretylium

Locus and Mechanism of Action. The major effect of guanethidine is inhibition of responses to sympathetic adrenergic nerve activation and to indirect-acting sympathomimetic amines (*e.g.,* tyramine, amphetamine). Since guanethidine also sensitizes effector cells to catecholamines, effective block must mean that the amount of mediator released is drastically reduced. Gua-

nethidine has considerable local anesthetic activity, but concentrations that prevent responses to adrenergic nerve stimulation do not block conduction along adrenergic axons. Essentially complete inhibition of responses to adrenergic nerve activity can develop very rapidly prior to a detectable change in tissue catecholamine stores, which subsequently decline slowly. It is of interest that there have been no reports of important differences in the characteristics of the neuron block shortly after exposure to guanethidine and after prolonged administration. Chronic administration can greatly reduce tissue concentrations of norepinephrine, and the depletion persists for several days after the drug has been discontinued. It has been reported that depletion of mediator from short adrenergic neurons, such as those in the vas deferens, can last for many months (Evans *et al.,* 1973). Guanethidine has little effect on the catecholamine content of the adrenal medulla, and penetrates the CNS very poorly after systemic administration. In contrast to reserpine, it has little effect on the 5-HT content of most organs. Although it appears reasonable that depletion of norepinephrine stores should impair adrenergic nerve function, the blockade without depletion demonstrable during the early stage of guanethidine action could also explain all observed inhibition of responses to nerve activity and to indirect-acting sympathomimetics. In addition, depletion of tissue norepinephrine and inhibition of responses to adrenergic nerve stimulation are readily dissociable among congeners of guanethidine (Fielden and Green, 1967). Many of the actions and effects of guanethidine and related drugs have been reviewed by Boura and Green (1965).

Guanethidine is taken up by and stored in adrenergic nerves, and this accumulation is essential for its action. Uptake involves the same mechanism responsible for the nerve membrane transport of norepinephrine, and the uptake and subsequent action of guanethidine can be inhibited by sympathomimetics, phenoxybenzamine, cocaine, and tricyclic antidepressants. Guanethidine apparently accumulates in and displaces norepinephrine from intraneuronal storage granules, and is itself released by nerve stimulation. Thus, it fits the definition of a "false transmitter," but this mechanism appears not to be responsible for its effects. Guanethidine can also be released by reserpine, amphetamine, and tyramine; while release by the latter two drugs is associated with a decreased response, it is not clear whether the granule-bound or some other pool of guanethidine with which it is in equilibrium is primarily responsible for the nerve block. (*See* Mitchell and Oates, 1970; Kirpekar and Furchgott, 1972; Shand *et al.*, 1973.) There is little direct evidence to support the suggestion that guanethidine, bretylium, and related adrenergic neuron blocking drugs act by interfering with the alleged cholinergic link in adrenergic transmission.

A considerable part of the norepinephrine released from adrenergic nerve terminals by guanethidine is first deaminated by intraneuronal MAO. The percentage is less than that deaminated during release by reserpine, but more than with tyramine. However, sufficient amounts of unchanged norepinephrine are released initially to produce sympathomimetic effects, including hypertension, contraction of the nictitating membrane, piloerection, and cardiac stimulation. Guanethidine directly depresses the myocardium previously depleted of catecholamines. In addition to its indirect effects, guanethidine has been shown to produce vasodilatation in animals pretreated with reserpine; this is at least partly prevented by β-adrenergic blockade, which suggests a direct action on β-adrenergic receptors.

Chronic administration of guanethidine produces a supersensitivity of effector cells that is very similar to that due to sympathetic postganglionic denervation. It reaches a maximum in 10 to 14 days, is greater for norepinephrine than for epinephrine, and can be explained by chronic absence of released mediator (Emmelin and Engström, 1961). Guanethidine can also cause an acute increase in the sensitivity of tissues to catecholamines. This could involve a "presynaptic" component due to competition for the amine transport mechanism at the nerve membrane, but it is at least partly due to an action unrelated to adrenergic nerves (Maxwell, 1965).

PHARMACOLOGICAL PROPERTIES

The most important effects of guanethidine are attributable to reduction of responses to sympathetic nerve activation. In contrast to adrenergic blocking agents, responses mediated by α- and β-adrenergic receptors are suppressed about equally. Guanethidine usually causes a roughly parallel shift to the right of frequency-response curves for stimulation of adrenergic nerves, but with some preferential block of responses to low frequencies. This effect is similar to that of reserpine, but both drugs differ significantly from bretylium, which decreases the slope of the curve. *In-vivo* responses that involve the adrenal medulla (*e.g.*, to splanchnic nerve stimulation) may be unaffected or even augmented.

Overall responses after guanethidine administration are a resultant of decreased release of mediator from adrenergic nerve endings and increased sensitivity of effector cells to the mediator. Indeed, with appropriate doses and durations of guanethidine administration, and with appropriate frequencies of nerve stimulation, it is possible to obtain augmented responses. This combination of effects makes guanethidine a hazardous pharmacological tool, particularly in man where the dose is limited by side effects. (*See* reviews by Boura and Green, 1965; Furst, 1967.)

Cardiovascular System. Rapid intravenous injection of guanethidine produces a characteristic triphasic response. There is an initial rapid fall in blood pressure associated with increased cardiac output and decreased peripheral resistance; the latter is probably due to a transient direct action of the drug on resistance vessels. The fall in blood pressure is followed by hypertension, which may persist for several hours and is much accentuated by prior ganglionic blockade or spinal cord section. Infusion of the doses employed in man causes a definite, but relatively small and transient increase in blood pressure.

In both laboratory animals and man, the initial changes are followed by a progressive fall in both systemic and pulmonary arterial pressures that may last for several days. This period of hypotension is usually associated with bradycardia, decreased pulse pressure, and decreased cardiac output. Systolic pressure in the erect position is most markedly reduced, and changes in supine blood pressure are often small. Peripheral resistance is not usually decreased, but the absence of a consistently increased peripheral resistance in the presence of decreased transmural pressure indicates some relaxation of peripheral arterioles. At least under resting conditions the distribution of blood flow is not greatly affected, although the hepatosplanchnic and renal beds may receive a smaller percentage of the cardiac output after guanethidine.

During chronic administration the cardiac output may return toward or to normal, probably as a result of the sodium and water retention and increased blood volume induced by guanethidine. The heart rate is usually decreased for the duration of the antihypertensive response. The effect of guanethidine on plasma renin activity has received little attention, but it appears to cause a decrease, as do most other drugs and procedures that decrease β-adrenergic effects on the kidneys (Stokes *et al.*, 1970).

Guanethidine inhibits cardiovascular reflexes such as those elicited by bilateral carotid artery occlusion in laboratory animals or by the Valsalva maneuver or cold pressor test in man. Blockade may be incomplete with the doses usually employed in man. However, a significant antihypertensive effect is always associated with some impairment of cardiovascular adjustments, and postural and exercise hypotension are common. (*See* review by Sannerstedt and Conway, 1970.)

Other Effects. Guanethidine has been studied primarily for its cardiovascular effects. However, it has been shown to produce a generalized depression of responses to sympathetic nerve stimulation and augmentation of responses to catecholamines in both *in-vivo* and *in-vitro* experiments on a large number of tissues and organs.

Guanethidine and most other adrenergic neuron blocking drugs increase *gastrointestinal motility* and can cause diarrhea. This is commonly attributed to parasympathetic predominance after blockade of adrenergic fibers, but it is not well correlated with such blockade; for example, reserpine causes relatively more and bethanidine relatively less diarrhea than does guanethidine. The effect of guanethidine on gastrointestinal motility has been roughly correlated with release of intestinal 5-HT (Cass and Spriggs, 1961), but this mechanism is not fully established. It has also been suggested that altered histamine metabolism may be involved (LeBlanc *et al.*, 1972). The *salt and water retention* commonly seen in hypertensive patients treated with guanethidine can probably be accounted for by hemodynamic effects, but the drug has been shown to stimulate sodium transport in frog skin and a renal tubular effect in man has not been ruled out.

Absorption, Fate, and Excretion. Under the usual conditions of chronic oral administration, absorption of guanethidine can vary from 3 to about 30%; it appears to be relatively constant in a given patient. However, differences in absorption account for only part of the wide variation in dose required for a satisfactory antihypertensive effect. Guanethidine is rapidly cleared by the kidney, but small amounts may remain in the body for as long as 14 days; retention probably involves both specific (adrenergic nerves) and nonspecific tissue uptake. Almost all the guanethidine that enters the circulation in man is accounted for by renal excretion of the parent compound and of two more polar and much less active metabolites. Metabolism appears to be by hepatic microsomal enzymes, and the percentage metabolized is considerably higher after oral than after parenteral administration. (*See* McMartin and Simpson, 1971.)

Preparations, Routes of Administration, and Dosage. *Guanethidine Sulfate*, U.S.P. (ISMELIN), is available in 10- and 25-mg tablets for oral administration. The usual daily dose is 25 to 50 mg, but it varies widely; because of its long duration of action, a single daily dose is satisfactory. The starting dose for ambulatory patients is usually 10 mg, and this may be increased at intervals of about 1 week until the desired effects are obtained or unacceptable side effects supervene. Carefully supervised patients in the hospital may receive a somewhat higher initial dose, and it may be increased more rapidly.

Toxicity, Side Effects, and Precautions. The effects of guanethidine are cumulative over extended periods. Adverse effects can appear or progress for many days or even weeks after an increase in dosage, and may not subside for several days after complete cessation of therapy. The therapeutic effect of guanethidine can be antagonized by tricyclic antidepressants (Mitchell *et al.*, 1970), and a similar antagonism has been reported with chlorpromazine. Sensitization by guanethidine to some sympathomimetics found in "cold remedies" can result in hypertensive crises. The most important complication of guanethidine therapy is postural hypotension; it is most prominent shortly after arising from sleep and may be accentuated by hot weather, alcohol, or exercise. Hypotensive episodes may be associated with symptoms of cerebral and myocardial ischemia. It is important that both standing and supine blood pressures be considered in adjusting dosage. A generalized subjective "weakness" is common; it is partially but not entirely attributable to postural hypotension. Fluid retention occurs and can lead to edema and resistance to the antihypertensive effect if a diuretic is not given concurrently. Guanethidine can also decrease myocardial competence by decreasing adrenergic nerve effects, and this plus fluid accumulation can lead to frank heart failure in patients with limited cardiac reserve. Some tendency to diarrhea is associated with guanethidine therapy in a high percentage of cases, but this can often be controlled by relatively small doses of an anticholinergic agent, paregoric, or a kaolin-pectin preparation. In contrast to the ganglionic blocking agents, guanethidine *per se* does not produce impotence. However, inhibition of ejaculation is common, and impotence may be a psychogenic aftermath. Guanethidine can cause severe hypertensive reactions in patients with pheochromocytoma. In spite of extensive use, no hepatic or bone-marrow damage attributable to guanethidine has been reported.

Therapeutic Uses. The only major use of guanethidine is in the treatment of *hypertension,* as discussed in detail in Chapter 33. It also effectively controls the pressor episodes associated with the hyperreflexia of high spinal cord lesions. Local application of guanethidine has received limited trial in the treatment of *glaucoma,* sometimes in combination with epinephrine (Roth, 1973), and to produce a partial Horner's syndrome in cases of *abnormal eyelid retraction* (Gay *et al.,* 1967).

BRETYLIUM

Choline 2,6-xylyl ether (TM10) was the first of many strongly basic compounds shown to inhibit responses to adrenergic nerve stimulation without impairing responses to exogenous catecholamines or to stimulation of cholinergic nerves. Other properties, particularly a relatively strong cholinomimetic action, eliminated TM10 as a possible therapeutic agent. However, interest in this type of specific blockade of adrenergic nerves led to the study of many congeners, of which *bretylium* was the first to be used in man. Its pharmacology will be discussed in comparison with that of guanethidine. Its structural formula is given above.

Pharmacological Properties. Bretylium and guanethidine produce very similar early inhibition of responses to adrenergic nerve stimulation and to amphetamine and other indirect-acting sympathomimetics, although the action of bretylium is more readily antagonized by such drugs. Agents that block the amine transport mechanism at adrenergic nerve-terminal membranes, such as imipramine, inhibit the action of both guanethidine and bretylium, but they antagonize only the latter if administered after the neuron block has been established (Toda, 1972). In contrast to guanethidine, a single blocking dose of bretylium produces little reduction in tissue catecholamine levels, although a relatively early decrease in a "soluble fraction," or the mobile pools, of norepinephrine has been reported (Abbs and Robertson, 1970). Only large, repeated doses produce essentially total depletion. Bretylium can

cause an initial increase in tissue catecholamines, antagonize the depleting action of guanethidine, and delay the release of norepinephrine during nerve degeneration. The initial "sympathomimetic" effects of bretylium are less prominent and more transient than those of guanethidine, but seem to be produced via endogenous catecholamines. High concentrations of bretylium accumulate in adrenergic nerves. It is an effective local anesthetic, and the possibility that this action may be involved in the failure of mediator release is suggested, but not proved, by the observation that block of responses occurs at about the same time as failure of antidromic conduction (Haeusler *et al.,* 1969). However, failure of axonal conduction appears not to be responsible for the block, because responses to field stimulation are effectively inhibited. Like guanethidine, bretylium does not block release of catecholamines from the adrenal medulla, and responses of effector cells to circulating catecholamines may be much increased.

The major cardiovascular effects of bretylium are very similar to those of guanethidine. The reduction in blood pressure by either drug is predominantly postural and is augmented by exercise; the tachycardia of exertion is reduced or absent. The duration of action of bretylium is considerably shorter than that of guanethidine, from 6 to 24 hours depending on the dose. The pharmacology of bretylium has been discussed by Boura and Green (1965).

At one time bretylium was quite widely used in the treatment of hypertension. However, poor absorption after oral administration, side effects, and the development of tolerance made bretylium a less desirable antihypertensive agent than guanethidine. It is used occasionally in the treatment of cardiac arrhythmias (*see* Chapter 32).

INTERMEDIATE COMPOUNDS

A large number of compounds within the general guanethidine-bretylium spectrum of activity have been synthesized and tested. The most successful from a therapeutic standpoint have combined a very basic guanidine or amidine moiety, similar to that in guanethidine, with an aromatic ring constituent, as in bretylium. Two of these compounds, *bethanidine* (1-benzyl-2,3-dimethylguanidine) and *debrisoquin* (3,4-dihydro-2[1H]-isoquinolinecarboxamidine; DECLINAX), have proved to be useful antihypertensive drugs. Their hemodynamic effects are essentially the same as those of guanethidine or bretylium, and the reduction in blood pressure has a large postural component. In other respects their pharmacological properties appear to be similar to those of bretylium. Compared to guanethidine, their durations of action are much shorter, they produce lesser sympathomimetic effects when injected intravenously, and they cause considerably less depletion of norepinephrine stores. (*See* Moe *et al.,* 1964; Boura and Green, 1965.) In occasional patients the shorter duration of action of bethanidine and debrisoquin or the lesser tendency to produce diarrhea may be a significant advantage, but in general they have the same role as guanethidine in antihypertensive therapy. (*See* Chapter 33.)

RESERPINE

Rauwolfia serpentina (Benth) is a climbing shrub of the family Apocynaceae that is indigenous to India and neighboring countries, where crude preparations of the plant have been used for centuries to treat a great variety of diseases. There are over 100 *Rauwolfia* species, and *R. serpentina* itself contains at least 20 alkaloids. However, reserpine is by far the most extensively used and studied, and none of the currently available alkaloids or mixtures differs qualitatively from it in pharmacological or therapeutic properties. (*See* Bein, 1956, for a review of the pharmacology of a number of other rauwolfia alkaloids.) Much of the interest in reserpine has centered on its CNS effects, which are covered in Chapter 12. The present discussion will be limited to *cardiovascular* and other pharmacological effects pertinent to the treatment of hypertension.

Locus and Mechanism of Action. Reserpine depletes stores of catecholamines and 5-HT in many organs, including the brain and adrenal medulla, and most of its pharmacological effects have been attributed to this action. Depletion is slower and less complete in the adrenal medulla than in other tissues. The action of reserpine on the CNS appears not to play an important role in the reduction in sympathetic nerve effects; there is no reduction and may even be a reflex increase in sympathetic outflow (Iggo and Vogt, 1960; MacLeod, 1972).

Reduced concentrations of catecholamines can be measured within an hour after reserpine administration, and depletion is maximal by 24 hours. Most of the catecholamine is deaminated intraneuronally, and pharmacological effects of the released mediator are minimal unless MAO has been inhibited. The doses used in most laboratory experiments reduce tissue catecholamines to negligible levels. Major impairment of adrenergic nerve function usually begins at levels below 30% of normal, and is roughly related to the degree of depletion. Tissue catecholamines are restored slowly; consequently, repeated doses have a cumulative action when administered even at intervals of up to a week or longer. Chronic administration of reserpine in doses of less than 1.0 mg per day has been shown greatly to decrease the norepinephrine content of the human myocardium (Chidsey *et al.*, 1963).

Depletion of catecholamines by reserpine is at least partially dependent on nerve activity and can be reduced by spinal cord section or ganglionic blockade. However, in contrast to normal release by exocytosis, reserpine releases catecholamines without releasing dopamine-β-hydroxylase (Viveros *et al.*, 1969). Studies with labeled drug indicate that reserpine itself is not released by nerve activity even in the period up to 18 hours after administration when some of the drug is reversibly bound; all reserpine remaining in tissues after 24 to 30 hours is firmly bound and may persist for many days (Norn and Shore, 1971).

It is clear that reserpine interferes with intracellular storage of catecholamines, but the amounts of reserpine in tissues are much too small to assume a stoichiometric displacement. It competitively antagonizes the uptake of norepinephrine by isolated chromaffin granules, apparently by inhibiting the ATP-Mg^{2+}–dependent uptake mechanism of the granule membrane. This may be irreversible, because it appears that restoration of normal intraneuronal stores of norepinephrine is dependent on transport of new storage vesicles down the axon (Häggendal and Dahlström, 1972). A number of observations are explained by the hypothesis of competition between reserpine and catecholamine at the storage granule membrane. For example, inhibition of reserpine-induced catecholamine depletion by MAO inhibitors has been attributed to an increased intracellular concentration of free amine that competes with reserpine for granule membrane sites, and the decrease in norepinephrine synthesis induced by reserpine may be due to block of dopamine uptake into storage granules that contain the hydroxylating enzyme. A compensatory increased firing of adrenergic nerves after reserpine and other drugs that inhibit their effects causes an increase in tyrosine hydroxylase activity, and chronic reserpine administration is associated with an increased norepinephrine turnover rate. (*See* Weiner, 1970.)

Reserpine reduces the overall "uptake" of catecholamines by adrenergic neurons, and it has been assumed that this leaves more free agonist to react with tissue receptors and, thus, accounts for the *supersensitivity to catecholamines* produced by this drug. Altered nerve uptake can undoubtedly contribute to supersensitivity under some circumstances. However, it has been shown that the overall rate of termination of the action of norepinephrine in vascular tissue is not decreased by reserpine, and the sensitization produced in this tissue must be due to other actions (Kalsner and Nickerson, 1969a); it has been suggested that an increased availability of calcium in effector cells is involved (Carrier and Jurevics, 1973).

A number of observations suggest that reserpine has other actions. Reserpine administered intraarterially produces peripheral vasodilatation in both normal and sympathectomized human extremities. It directly depresses several parameters of myocardial function (Nayler, 1962), and chronic administration of small doses has been reported to produce morphological changes in the myocardium. Reserpine can also produce an acute block of norepinephrine release that is antagonized by increased extracellular sodium and is probably due to an action on the nerve membrane (Misu *et al.*, 1972). Release of gastrin via a central vagal mechanism appears to be involved in the increased gastric acid secretion induced by reserpine (Emås and Fyrö, 1965). The drug can produce a variety of endocrine changes in experimental animals (*see* Gaunt *et al.*, 1963), but similar effects have not been shown to result from administration of the usual antihypertensive doses in man.

Pharmacological Properties. Reserpine acts centrally to produce characteristic sedation and tranquilization (*see* Chapter 12). After a transient "sympathomimetic" effect, seen only after parenteral administration of relatively large doses, reserpine causes a slowly developing fall in blood pressure frequently associated with bradycardia. In recumbent subjects, the reduction in blood pressure may involve a decrease in peripheral resistance; this is most marked in the skin, and cutaneous blood flow may be increased. However, the antihypertensive effect of chronic administration of reserpine is usually associated with a reduced cardiac output (Cohen *et al.*, 1968). Pressor responses, such as those induced by carotid artery occlusion or stimulation of the central end of the cut vagus nerve, are effectively inhibited by the doses of reserpine commonly employed in experimental animals. Most observations in man indicate that cardiovascular reflexes are only partially inhibited, probably because of the small doses administered. However, reflex responses of veins can be comparably depressed by guanethidine and reserpine, and the two drugs appear to have a similar potential to decrease cardiac output and produce postural hypotension at equivalent levels of inhibition of efferent nerve function. Responses to indirect-acting sympathomimetic amines are potentiated during the initial phase of reserpine action, but later they are depressed. (*See* reviews by Alper *et al.*, 1963; Sannerstedt and Conway, 1970.)

Routes of Administration and Dosage. The oral antihypertensive dose of reserpine ranges from 0.1 to 1.0 mg daily, usually taken in two or three divided doses. Higher doses are now rarely employed because of increased side effects. It requires up to 3 weeks for the full antihypertensive effect to develop. (Details of the available rauwolfia preparations are given in Chapter 12.)

Toxicity, Side Effects, and Precautions. Untoward responses to reserpine are predominantly referable to the CNS and the gastrointestinal tract, and have resulted in a progressive reduction in the doses employed in the treatment of hypertension. The mild sedative effect of small doses may be desirable in some apprehensive patients. However, even doses as small as 0.25 mg per day can produce a considerable incidence of nightmares and psychic depression (Quetsch *et al.*, 1959), sometimes severe enough to require hospitalization or to end in suicide. *Reserpine should not be administered to patients with a history of depressive episodes,* and it should be discontinued if suggestive signs or symptoms develop. Extrapyramidal disturbances rarely occur with the usual antihypertensive dose. Reserpine commonly increases gastrointestinal tone and motility, with abdominal cramps and diarrhea. Single doses of 0.25 mg or more quite consistently increase gastric acid secretion. The secretory effects of chronic administration and their relation to reports of gastrointestinal ulceration and hemorrhage are less clear-cut, but reserpine probably should not be given to patients with a history of peptic ulcer and it should be discontinued if signs or symptoms of peptic ulceration appear. Reserpine quite commonly causes weight gain.

Hypotensive episodes are rare with doses of less than 1.0 mg of reserpine per day, but patients may be sensitized to this reaction following a cerebrovascular accident. Vascular side effects include flushing and nasal congestion; these are usually of minor importance, but the latter may occasionally cause serious respiratory problems in infants born of mothers receiving reserpine. Reserpine has been accused of producing cardiovascular lability during anesthesia, but careful studies have failed to substantiate this, and it does not appear necessary to discontinue the drug prior to anesthesia and surgery (Munson and Jenicek, 1962).

In a retrospective study in the United States, subsequently confirmed in the United Kingdom and Finland, it was found that the long-term administration of reserpine as an antihypertensive drug in women was associated with over a threefold increase in the incidence of *carcinoma of the breast* (*see* Boston Collaborative Drug Surveillance Program, 1974; Editorial, 1974). Whether chronic reserpine therapy is similarly associated with the occurrence of other types of malignancy in women or men is currently under investigation. The mechanism of this effect of reserpine is unknown, but compounds that deplete dopamine from the CNS or antagonize its action can enhance the secretion of prolactin and cause mammary tumors in experimental animals (*see* Chapter 66).

Therapeutic Uses. The only important application of the cardiovascular effects of reserpine is in the treatment of *hypertension,* as discussed in detail in Chapter 33. It is occasionally used in the management of *Raynaud's syndrome.*

SPECIFIC INHIBITORS OF CATECHOLAMINE SYNTHESIS

Much of the work on adrenergic neuron blocking drugs has assumed a cause-and-effect relationship between depletion of norepinephrine stores and failure of nerve function. Consequently, it appeared that inhibition of norepinephrine synthesis would represent the ultimate mechanism of adrenergic neuron blockade. Inhibitors of each step of the biosynthesis have been studied, but major depletion occurs only with drugs that act on the rate-limiting step, the hydroxylation of tyrosine. Of these inhibitors, α-methyl-*p*-tyrosine (α-MT) is the most thoroughly studied and one of the most effective. The pattern of effects produced by α-MT differs considerably from that of the classical adrenergic neuron blocking drugs. Almost complete depletion of norepinephrine stores in brain and peripheral tissues in laboratory animals by α-MT does not lower blood pressure, and only limited signs of sympathetic inadequacy have been reported; responses to both tyramine and norepinephrine are depressed (Spector *et al.,* 1965). Conversely, it has been reported that a single intravenous dose of α-MT can considerably inhibit the reduction in hindlimb perfusion induced by sympathetic nerve stimulation at a time when the norepinephrine content of arterial walls is unaltered (Redisch *et al.,* 1969). Norepinephrine synthesis has been decreased by about 70% in man by α-MT; this produces considerable improvement in patients with pheochromocytoma, but has little effect on the blood pressure of those with essential hypertension (Engelman *et al.,* 1968).

α-MT appears to be a useful tool in assessing norepinephrine turnover rates in laboratory animals where synthesis can be almost completely prevented by an excess of inhibitor. It has also been employed in a variety of studies on adrenergic mechanisms in the CNS. However, in very few of these has the time course of the effects been related to catecholamine stores, and in many studies no determinations of norepinephrine content are reported. (*See* review by Moore and Dominic, 1971.) Until the relationship between norepinephrine "pools" and nerve function can be more adequately established, effects of cate-cholamine-depleting drugs should be interpreted with caution in the assessment of adrenergic functions in the CNS.

DRUGS THAT DESTROY ADRENERGIC NERVE FIBERS

Interest in 6-hydroxydopamine (6-OHDA) was first aroused by the observation that it caused a prolonged decrease in the catecholamine content of the heart (Porter *et al.,* 1963). This effect was subsequently shown to be due to destruction of sympathetic nerve endings. Most peripheral sympathetic nerves are affected by adequate doses, but there are some quantitative differences in sensitivity that appear to be inversely related to the density of innervation. The adrenal medulla and peripheral cholinergic neurons are unaffected. Reductions in the norepinephrine and tyrosine hydroxylase contents of tissues are well correlated, and it appears that determination of the former provides a relatively accurate index of the extent of nerve-terminal destruction. 6-OHDA does not damage peripheral adrenergic nerve-cell bodies or proximal axons in adult animals, and regeneration of the terminals is usually complete. Regeneration is usually faster than after surgical sympathectomy, probably because a shorter segment of the terminal axon is involved, but may vary from a few days to over a month. In newborn animals the entire neuron may be destroyed and a permanent "sympathectomy" produced. This is usually more complete than that produced by antisera against the nerve-growth factor (immunosympathectomy) (*see* Levi-Montalcini and Angeletti, 1966).

The action of 6-OHDA on peripheral adrenergic nerves is dependent on its accumulation by the nerve-membrane amine pump and can be prevented by drugs such as desipramine that block this process. Although 6-OHDA is taken up by intraneuronal storage granules, this step appears not to be necessary for nerve damage because the drug is fully effective in animals pretreated with reserpine.

Morphological changes in adrenergic nerve endings have been detected as early as 1 hour after administration of 6-OHDA, and subsequent events are similar to those following nerve section. The first responses to 6-OHDA administration are "sympathomimetic," due to the release of endogenous norepinephrine. These early effects can be observed with doses too small to destroy nerve terminals and may last for many hours after larger doses. Later effects are very similar to those due to guanethidine or surgical sympathectomy and have an intermediate time course. Responses to nerve stimulation and to indirect-acting sympathomimetics are inhibited, and those to catecholamines are enhanced. The supersensitivity involves both prejunctional and postjunctional components.

6-OHDA does not penetrate the CNS from the blood stream, but it can act on central neurons after local or intraventricular administration; 6-hydroxydopa administered systemically with an MAO inhibitor can affect both central and peripheral neurons (Sachs and Jonsson, 1972). 6-OHDA has been shown by histological and analytical technics to damage central neurons containing either norepinephrine or dopamine; the former are usually considered to be the more susceptible. However, selectivity with respect to neurons in the CNS is not fully established, and there may be only a small differential in the amounts required to damage "monoaminergic" neurons and to affect all other cellular elements (Poirier et al., 1972). In contrast to peripheral neurons, many cell bodies in the CNS are damaged and little regeneration occurs. Although extensive destruction of norepinephrine- and dopamine-containing neurons, and perhaps other cellular elements of the brain, has been achieved, the only clear behavioral effect seems to be a persistent hyperirritability. Prior treatment with 6-OHDA has been reported to alter responses to a number of drugs acting on the CNS, including morphine, cocaine, and amphetamine, but the results do not yet provide a readily interpretable pattern.

The pharmacology of 6-OHDA has been reviewed by Thoenen and Tranzer (1973) and Kostrzewa and Jacobowitz (1974).

Abbs, E. T., and Robertson, M. I. Selective depletion of noradrenaline: a proposed mechanism of the adrenergic neurone-blocking action of bretylium. *Br. J. Pharmac.,* **1970,** *38,* 776–791.

Assem, E. S. K., and Schild, H. O. Antagonism by β-adrenoceptor blocking agents of the antianaphylactic effect of isoprenaline. *Br. J. Pharmac.,* **1971,** *42,* 620–630.

Barcroft, H.; Konzett, H.; and Swan, H. J. C. Observations on the action of the hydrogenated alkaloids of the ergotoxine group on the circulation in man. *J. Physiol., Lond.,* **1951,** *112,* 273–291.

Barrett, A. M., and Cullum, V. A. The biological properties of the optical isomers of propranolol and their effects on cardiac arrhythmias. *Br. J. Pharmac.,* **1968,** *34,* 43–55.

Batzri, S.; Selinger, Z.; Schramm, M.; and Rabinovitch, M. R. Potassium release mediated by the epinephrine α-receptor in rat parotid slices. *J. biol. Chem.,* **1973,** *248,* 361–368.

Belleau, B.; DiTullio, V.; and Godin, D. The mechanism of irreversible adrenergic blockade by N-carbethoxydihydroquinolines—model studies with typical serine hydrolases. *Biochem. Pharmac.,* **1969,** *18,* 1039–1044.

Benfey, B. G. Characterization of α-adrenoceptors in the myocardium. *Br. J. Pharmac.,* **1973,** *48,* 132–138.

Besser, G. M.; Parke, L.; Edwards, C. R. W.; Forsyth, I. A.; and McNeilly, A. S. Galactorrhoea: successful treatment with reduction of plasma prolactin levels by bromergocryptine. *Br. med. J.,* **1972,** *3,* 669–672.

Bhattacharya, A. N.; Dierschke, D. J.; Yamaji, T.; and Knobil, E. The pharmacologic blockade of the circhoral mode of LH secretion in the ovariectomized rhesus monkey. *Endocrinology,* **1972,** *90,* 778–786.

Blackard, W. G., and Hubbell, G. J. Stimulatory effect of exogenous catecholamines on plasma HGH concentrations in presence of beta adrenergic blockade. *Metabolism,* **1970,** *19,* 547–552.

Bonn, J. A.; Turner, P.; and Hicks, D. C. Beta-adrenergic receptor blockade with practolol in treatment of anxiety. *Lancet,* **1972,** *1,* 814–815.

Boston Collaborative Drug Surveillance Program. Reserpine and breast cancer. *Lancet,* **1974,** *2,* 669–671.

Burack, B.; Marcus, D.; Miyamoto, A.; Escher, D. J. W.; and Robinson, G. Response of class IV patients to alpha blockade prior to open-heart surgery. *Am. Heart J.,* **1972,** *84,* 456–462.

Burns, J. J.; Salvador, R. A.; and Lemberger, L. Metabolic blockade by methoxamine and its analogs. *Ann. N.Y. Acad. Sci.,* **1967,** *139,* 833–840.

Carliner, N. H.; Denune, D. P.; Finch, C. S., Jr.; and Goldberg, L. I. Sodium nitroprusside treatment of ergotamine-induced peripheral ischemia. *J. Am. med. Ass.,* **1974,** *227,* 308–309.

Carrier, O., Jr., and Jurevics, H. A. The role of calcium in "nonspecific" supersensitivity of vascular muscle. *J. Pharmac. exp. Ther.,* **1973,** *184,* 81–94.

Cass, R., and Spriggs, T. L. B. Tissue amine levels and sympathetic blockade after guanethidine and bretylium. *Br. J. Pharmac. Chemother.,* **1961,** *17,* 442–450.

Cegrell, L. Phentolamine and juvenile diabetes. *Lancet,* **1972,** *2,* 1421.

Chidsey, C. A.; Braunwald, E.; Morrow, A. G.; and Mason, D. T. Myocardial norepinephrine concentration in man. Effects of reserpine and of congestive heart failure. *New Engl. J. Med.,* **1963,** *269,* 653–658.

Cohen, S. I.; Young, M. W.; Lau, S. H.; Haft, J. I.; and Damato, A. N. Effects of reserpine therapy on cardiac output and atrioventricular conduction during rest and controlled heart rates in patients with essential hypertension. *Circulation,* **1968,** *37,* 738–746.

Collu, R.; Fraschini, F.; Visconti, P.; and Martini, L. Adrenergic and serotinergic control of growth hormone secretion in adult male rats. *Endocrinology,* **1972,** *90,* 1231–1237.

Crout, J. R., and Brown, B. R., Jr. Anesthetic management of pheochromocytoma: the value of phenoxybenzamine and methoxyflurane. *Anesthesiology,* **1969,** *30,* 29–36.

Cummins, B. H., and Griffith, H. B. Intracarotid phenoxybenzamine for cerebral arterial spasm. *Br. med. J.,* **1971,** *1,* 382–383.

Das, P. K., and Parratt, J. R. Myocardial and haemodynamic effects of phentolamine. *Br. J. Pharmac.,* **1971,** *41,* 437–444.

Editorial. Rauwolfia derivatives and cancer. *Lancet,* **1974,** *2,* 701–702.

Emås, S., and Fyrö, B. Vagal release of gastrin in cats following reserpine. *Acta physiol. scand.,* **1965,** *63,* 358–369.

Emmelin, N., and Engström, J. Supersensitivity of salivary glands following treatment with bretylium or guanethidine. *Br. J. Pharmac. Chemother.,* **1961,** *16,* 315–319.

Engelman, K.; Horwitz, D.; Jéquier, E.; and Sjoerdsma, A. Biochemical and pharmacologic effects of α-methyltyrosine in man. *J. clin. Invest.,* **1968,** *47,* 577–594.

Engelman, K., and Sjoerdsma, A. Chronic medical therapy for pheochromocytoma: a report of four cases. *Ann. intern. Med.,* **1964,** *61,* 229–241.

Epstein, S. E., and Braunwald, E. The effect of β-adrenergic blockade on patterns of urinary sodium excretion: studies in normal subjects and in patients with heart disease. *Ann. intern. Med.,* **1966,** *65,* 20–27.

Evans, B.; Iwayama, T.; and Burnstock, G. Long-lasting supersensitivity of the rat vas deferens to norepinephrine after chronic guanethidine administration. *J. Pharmac. exp. Ther.,* **1973,** *185,* 60–69.

Evans, G. H.; Nies, A. S.; and Shand, D. G. The disposition of propranolol. III. Decreased half-life and volume of distribution as a result of plasma binding in man, monkey, dog and rat. *J. Pharmac. exp. Ther.,* **1973a,** *186,* 114–122.

Evans, G. H.; Wilkinson, G. R.; and Shand, D. G. The disposition of propranolol. IV. A dominant role for tissue uptake in the dose-dependent extraction of propranolol by the perfused rat liver. *J. Pharmac. exp. Ther.,* **1973b,** *186,* 447–454.

Fielden, R., and Green, A. L. A comparative study of the noradrenaline-depleting and sympathetic-blocking actions of guanethidine and (−)-β-hydroxyphenethylguanidine. *Br. J. Pharmac. Chemother.,* **1967,** *30,* 155–165.

Fitzgerald, J. D., and O'Donnell, S. R. Pharmacology of 4-hydroxypropranolol, a metabolite of propranolol. *Br. J. Pharmac.,* **1971,** *43,* 222–235.

Folkow, B.; Haeger, K.; and Uvnäs, B. Cholinergic vasodilator nerves in the sympathetic outflow to the muscles of the hind limbs of the cat. *Acta physiol. scand.,* **1948,** *15,* 401–411.

Formgren, H. Practolol in the treatment of tachyarrhythmias in patients with bronchial asthma. *Am. Heart J.,* **1972,** *84,* 710–712.

Freeman, J. Phenoxybenzamine in the treatment of cardiogenic shock. *Med. J. Aust.,* **1969,** *2,* 1151–1154.

Friend, D. G., and Edwards, E. A. Use of DIBENZYLINE as a vasodilator in patients with severe digital ischemia. *A.M.A. Archs intern. Med.,* **1954,** *93,* 928–937.

Furchgott, R. F. Dibenamine blockade in strips of rabbit aorta and its use in differentiating receptors. *J. Pharmac. exp. Ther.,* **1954,** *111,* 265–284.

Garfield, S. L.; Gershon, S.; Sletten, I.; Sundland, D. M.; and Ballou, S. Chemically induced anxiety. *Int. J. Neuropsychiat.,* **1967,** *3,* 426–433.

Gay, A. J.; Salmon, M. L.; and Wolkstein, M. A. Topical sympatholytic therapy for pathologic lid retraction. *Archs Ophthal., N.Y.,* **1967,** *77,* 341–344.

Gifford, R. W., Jr. The arteriospastic diseases: clinical significance and management. *Cardiovasc. Clins,* **1971,** *3,* No. 1, 128–139.

Gilligan, B. S.; Veale, J. L.; and Wodak, J. Propranolol in the treatment of tremor. *Med. J. Aust.,* **1972,** *1,* 320–322.

Graham, J. D. P., and Mottram, D. R. Binding of N-(2-bromoethyl)-N-ethyl-N^1-naphthylmethylamine HBr (SY 28) to the proteins of guinea-pig vas deferens. *Br. J. Pharmac.,* **1971,** *42,* 428–436.

Green, K. L. The anti-inflammatory effect of catecholamines in the peritoneal cavity and hind paw of the mouse. *Br. J. Pharmac.,* **1972,** *45,* 322–332.

Gross, G. J., and Winbury, M. M. *Beta* adrenergic blockade on intramyocardial distribution of coronary blood flow. *J. Pharmac. exp. Ther.,* **1973,** *187,* 451–464.

Haeusler, G.; Haefly, W.; and Huerlimann, A. On the mechanism of the adrenergic nerve blocking action of bretylium. *Naunyn-Schmiedebergs Arch. Pharmak.,* **1969,** *265,* 260–277.

Häggendal, J., and Dahlström, A. The recovery of the capacity for uptake-retention of [^{3}H] noradrenaline in rat adrenergic nerves after reserpine. *J. Pharm. Pharmac.,* **1972,** *24,* 565–574.

Hayes, A., and Cooper, R. G. Studies on the absorption, distribution and excretion of propranolol in rat, dog and monkey. *J. Pharmac. exp. Ther.,* **1971,** *176,* 302–311.

Helfant, R. H.; Herman, M. V.; and Gorlin, R. Abnormalities of left ventricular contraction induced by beta adrenergic blockade. *Circulation,* **1971,** *43,* 641–647.

Hollenberg, N. K., and Nickerson, M. Changes in pre- and postcapillary resistance in pathogenesis of hemorrhagic shock. *Am. J. Physiol.,* **1970,** *219,* 1483–1489.

Howard, J. C.; Cochrane, P.; and Conway, M. Practolol and isoprenaline in status asthmaticus. *Lancet,* **1972,** *2,* 47–48.

Iggo, A., and Vogt, M. Preganglionic sympathetic activity in normal and in reserpine-treated cats. *J. Physiol., Lond.,* **1960,** *150,* 114–133.

Innes, I. R. Identification of the smooth muscle excitatory receptors for ergot alkaloids. *Br. J. Pharmac. Chemother.,* **1962,** *19,* 120–128.

Iversen, L. L.; Salt, P. J.; and Wilson, H. A. Inhibition of catecholamine uptake in the isolated rat heart by haloalkylamines related to phenoxybenzamine. *Br. J. Pharmac.,* **1972,** *46,* 647–657.

Kalsner, S. Mechanism of potentiation by amines of nonequilibrium blockade of the α-adrenoceptor. *Br. J. Pharmac.,* **1973,** *47,* 386–397.

Kalsner, S., and Nickerson, M. Effects of reserpine on the disposition of sympathomimetic amines in vascular tissue. *Br. J. Pharmac.,* **1969a,** *35,* 394–405.

———. Effects of a haloalkylamine on responses to and disposition of sympathomimetic amines. *Ibid.,* **1969b,** *35,* 440–445.

Kelly, D. T.; Delgado, C. E.; Taylor, D. R.; Pitt, B.; and Ross, R. S. Use of phentolamine in acute myocardial infarction associated with hypertension and left ventricular failure. *Circulation,* **1973,** *47,* 729–735.

Kirpekar, S. M., and Furchgott, R. F. Interaction of tyramine and guanethidine in the spleen of the cat. *J. Pharmac. exp. Ther.,* **1972,** *180,* 38–46.

Koch-Weser, J. Beta adrenergic blockade and circulating eosinophils. *Archs intern. Med.,* **1968,** *121,* 255–258.

Kubacz, G. J., and Catchpole, B. N. The role of adrenergic blockade in the treatment of ureteral colic. *J. Urol.,* **1972,** *107,* 949–951.

Kunos, G.; Yong, M. S.; and Nickerson, M. Transformation of adrenergic receptors in the myocardium. *Nature, New Biol.,* **1973,** *241,* 119–120.

Langslet, A. Membrane stabilization and cardiac effects of d,l-propranolol, d-propranolol and chlorpromazine. *Eur. J. Pharmac.,* **1970,** *13,* 6–14.

LeBlanc, J.; Côté, J.; Doré, F.; and Rousseau, S. Effects of guanethidine and related compounds on histamine excretion. *Can. J. Physiol. Pharmac.,* **1972,** *50,* 539–544.

Ledsome, J. R.; Kellett, R. P.; and Burkhart, S. M. The ability of propranolol to antagonize induced changes in heart rate. *J. Pharmac. exp. Ther.,* **1974,** *188,* 198–206.

Lemmer, B.; Wiethold, G.; Hellenbrecht, D.; Bak, I. J.; and Grobecker, H. Human blood platelets as cellular models for investigation of membrane active drugs: beta-adrenergic blocking agents. *Naunyn-Schmiedebergs Archs Pharmac.,* **1972,** *275,* 299–313.

Levy, B. The adrenergic blocking activity of N-*tert*-butylmethoxamine (butoxamine). *J. Pharmac. exp. Ther.,* **1966,** *151,* 413–422.

Loubatieres, A.; Mariani, M. M.; Sorel, G.; and Savi, L. The action of β-adrenergic blocking and stimulating agents on insulin secretion. Characterization of the type of β receptor. *Diabetologia,* **1971,** *7,* 127–132.

McCabe, R. E., Jr., and Fitzpatrick, H. F. The preservation of human cadaver kidneys for transplantation. *J. Am. med. Ass.,* **1972,** *219,* 1056–1059.

MacDonald, A. G., and McNeill, R. S. A comparison of the effect on airway resistance of a new beta blocking drug, ICI 50,172, and propranolol. *Br. J. Anaesth.,* **1968,** *40,* 508–510.

McHenry, L. C., Jr.; Jaffe, M. E.; Kawamura, J.; and Goldberg, H. I. HYDERGINE effect on cerebral circulation in cerebrovascular disease. *J. neurol. Sci.,* **1971,** *13,* 475–481.

McKay, D. G.; Whitaker, A. N.; and Cruse, V. Studies of catecholamine shock. II. An experimental model of microangiopathic hemolysis. *Am. J. Path.,* **1969,** *56,* 177–200.

MacLeod, V. H. The influence of some centrally acting drugs on sympathetic nerve activity. *Br. J. Pharmac.,* **1972,** *45,* 194P–195P.

McMartin, C., and Simpson, P. The absorption and metabolism of guanethidine in hypertensive patients requiring different doses of the drug. *Clin. Pharmac. Ther.,* **1971,** *12,* 73–77.

McNay, J. L., and Goldberg, L. I. Comparison of the effects of dopamine, isoproterenol, norepinephrine and bradykinin on canine renal and femoral blood flow. *J. Pharmac. exp. Ther.,* **1966,** *151,* 23–31.

Majid, P. A.; Sharma, B.; and Taylor, S. H. Phentolamine for vasodilator treatment of severe heart-failure. *Lancet,* **1971,** *2,* 719–724.

Maxwell, R. A. Concerning the mode of action of guanethidine and some derivatives in augmenting the vasomotor action of adrenergic amines in vascular tissues of the rabbit. *J. Pharmac. exp. Ther.,* **1965,** *148,* 320–328.

Medical Letter. Dihydrogenated ergot alkaloids (HYDERGINE) and cerebrovascular insufficiency. **1970,** *12,* 27–28.

Mellander, S., and Nordenfelt, I. Comparative effects of

dihydroergotamine and noradrenaline on resistance, exchange and capacitance functions in the peripheral circulation. *Clin. Sci.,* **1970,** *39,* 183–201.

Michelakis, A. M., and McAllister, R. G. The effect of chronic adrenergic receptor blockade in plasma renin activity in man. *J. clin. Endocr. Metab.,* **1972,** *34,* 386–394.

Misu, Y.; Kubo, T.; and Nishio, H. Acute partial sympathetic blockade by reserpine in the isolated rabbits' hearts. *Eur. J. Pharmac.,* **1972,** *19,* 267–275.

Mitchell, J. R.; Cavanaugh, J. H.; Arias, L.; and Oates, J. A. Guanethidine and related agents. III. Antagonism by drugs which inhibit the norepinephrine pump in man. *J. clin. Invest.,* **1970,** *49,* 1596–1604.

Mitchell, J. R., and Oates, J. A. Guanethidine and related agents. I. Mechanism of the selective blockade of adrenergic neurons and its antagonism by drugs. *J. Pharmac. exp. Ther.,* **1970,** *172,* 100–107.

Moe, R. A.; Bates, H. M.; Palkoski, Z. M.; and Banziger, R. Cardiovascular effects of 3,4-dihydro-2(1H) isoquinoline carboxamidine (DECLINAX). *Curr. ther. Res.,* **1964,** *6,* 299–318.

Moyer, J. H., and Caplovitz, C. The clinical results of oral and parenteral administration of 2-(N′-p-tolyl-N′-m-hydroxyphenylaminomethyl) imidazoline hydrochloride (REGITINE) in the treatment of hypertension and an evaluation of cerebral hemodynamics. *Am. Heart J.,* **1953,** *45,* 602–610.

Munson, W. M., and Jenicek, J. A. Effect of anesthetic agents on patients receiving reserpine therapy. *Anesthesiology,* **1962,** *23,* 741–746.

Myers, K. A.; Hobbs, J. T.; and Irvine, W. T. Haemodynamic action of thymoxamine (an alpha-adrenergic blocking agent) in occlusive peripheral arterial disease. *Cardiovasc. Res.,* **1968,** *4,* 360–366.

Mylecharane, E. J., and Raper, C. Further studies on the adrenergic neuron blocking activity of some β-adrenoceptor antagonists and guanethidine. *J. Pharm. Pharmac.,* **1973,** *25,* 213–220.

Nakagawa, K., and Mashimo, K. Suppressibility of plasma growth hormone levels in acromegaly with dexamethasone and phentolamine. *J. clin. Endocr. Metab.,* **1973,** *37,* 238–246.

Nayler, W. G. A direct effect of reserpine on ventricular contractility. *J. Pharmac. exp. Ther.,* **1962,** *139,* 222–229.

Newton, N. E., and Hornbrook, K. R. Effects of adrenergic agents on carbohydrate metabolism of rat liver: activities of adenyl cyclase and glycogen phosphorylase. *J. Pharmac. exp. Ther.,* **1972,** *181,* 479–488.

Nickerson, M. Receptor occupancy and tissue response. *Nature, Lond.,* **1956,** *178,* 697–698.

————. Mechanism of the prolonged adrenergic blockade produced by haloalkylamines. *Archs int. Pharmacodyn. Thér.,* **1962b,** *140,* 237–250.

Nickerson, M., and Chan, G. C.-M. Blockade of responses of isolated myocardium to epinephrine. *J. Pharmac. exp. Ther.,* **1961,** *133,* 186–191.

Nickerson, M., and Goodman, L. S. Pharmacological properties of a new adrenergic blocking agent: N,N-dibenzyl-β-chloroethylamine (dibenamine). *J. Pharmac. exp. Ther.,* **1947,** *89,* 167–185.

Nickerson, M., and Gump, W. S. The chemical basis for adrenergic blocking activity in compounds related to dibenamine. *J. Pharmac. exp. Ther.,* **1949,** *97,* 25–47.

Nickerson, M., and Nomaguchi, G. M. Blockade of epinephrine-induced cardioacceleration in the frog. *Am. J. Physiol.,* **1950,** *163,* 484–504.

Nicolaescu, V.; Manicatide, M.; and Stroescu, V. β-Adrenergic blockade with practolol in acetylcholine-sensitive asthma patients. *Respiration,* **1972,** *29,* 139–154.

Nies, A. S.; Evans, G. H.; and Shand, D. G. Regional hemodynamic effects of beta-adrenergic blockade with propranolol in the unanesthetized primate. *Am. Heart J.,* **1973,** *85,* 97–102.

Nies, A. S.; McNeil, J. S.; and Schrier, R. W. Mechanism of increased sodium reabsorption during propranolol administration. *Circulation,* **1971,** *44,* 596–604.

Norn, S., and Shore, P. A. Failure to affect tissue reserpine concentrations by alteration of adrenergic nerve activity. *Biochem. Pharmac.,* **1971,** *20,* 2133–2135.

Oski, F. A.; Miller, L. D.; Delivoria-Papadopoulos, M.; Manchester, J. H.; and Shelburn, J. C. Oxygen affinity in red cells: changes induced *in vivo* by propranolol. *Science, Wash.,* **1972,** *175,* 1372–1373.

Owman, C.; Rosengren, E.; and Sjöberg, N.-O. Adrenergic innervation of the human female reproductive organs: a histochemical and chemical investigation. *Obstet. Gynec., N.Y.,* **1967,** *30,* 763–773.

Palmer, B. The influence of stress on the survival of experimental skin flaps. *Scand. J. plast. reconstr. Surg.,* **1972,** *6,* 110–113.

Papeschi, R.; Sourkes, T. L.; and Youdim, M. B. H. The effect of yohimbine on brain serotonin metabolism, motor behavior and body temperature of the rat. *Eur. J. Pharmac.,* **1971,** *15,* 318–326.

Pendleton, R. G.; Newman, D. J.; Sherman, S. S.; Brann, E. G.; and Maya, W. E. Effect of propranolol upon the hemoglobin-oxygen dissociation curve. *J. Pharmac. exp. Ther.,* **1972,** *180,* 647–656.

Pitt, B., and Craven, P. Effect of propranolol on regional myocardial blood flow in acute ischaemia. *Cardiovasc. Res.,* **1970,** *4,* 176–179.

Poirier, L. J.; Langelier, P.; Roberge, A.; Boucher, R.; and Kitsikis, A. Non-specific histopathological changes induced by the intracerebral injection of 6-hydroxydopamine (6-OH-DA). *J. neurol. Sci.,* **1972,** *16,* 401–416.

Porter, C. C.; Totaro, J. A.; and Stone, C. A. Effect of 6-hydroxydopamine and some other compounds on the concentration of norepinephrine in the hearts of mice. *J. Pharmac. exp. Ther.,* **1963,** *140,* 308–316.

Potter, W. P. de; Chubb, I. W.; Put, A.; and Schaepdryver, A. F. de. Facilitation of the release of noradrenaline and dopamine-β-hydroxylase at low stimulation frequencies by α-blocking agents. *Archs int. Pharmacodyn. Thér.,* **1971,** *193,* 191–197.

Powell, C. E., and Slater, I. H. Blocking of inhibitory adrenergic receptors by a dichloro analog of isoproterenol. *J. Pharmac. exp. Ther.,* **1958,** *122,* 480–488.

Pryor, J. P.; Keaveny, T. V.; Reed, T. W.; and Belzer, F. O. Improved immediate function of experimental cadaver renal allografts by elimination of agonal vasospasm. *Br. J. Surg.,* **1971,** *58,* 184–187.

Quetsch, R. M.; Achor, R. W. P.; Litin, E. M.; and Faucett, R. L. Depressive reactions in hypertensive patients: a comparison of those treated with rauwolfia and those receiving no specific antihypertensive treatment. *Circulation,* **1959,** *19,* 366–375.

Rangel, D. M.; Bruckner, W. L.; Byfield, J. E.; Dinbar, A.; Yakeishi, Y.; Stevens, G. H.; and Fonkalsrud, E. W. Enzymatic evaluation of hepatic preservation using cell-stabilizing drugs. *Surgery Gynec. Obstet.,* **1969,** *129,* 963–972.

Redisch, W.; Terry, E. N.; Rouen, L. R.; and Clauss, R. H. Effects of alpha-methyl-tyrosine upon catecholamine levels in arterial tissue and plasma and upon peripheral blood flow measurements in the anesthetized dog. *J. cardiovasc. Surg.,* **1969,** *10,* 291–298.

Riordan, J. F., and Walters, G. Effects of phenoxybenzamine in shock due to myocardial infarction. *Br. med. J.,* **1969,** *1,* 155–158.

Robertson, R. P.; Brunzell, J. O.; Hazzard, W. R.; Lerner, R. L.; and Porte, D., Jr. Paradoxical hypoinsulinaemia: an alpha-adrenergic-mediated response to glucose. *Lancet,* **1972,** *2,* 787–789.

Robin, E.; Cowan, C.; Puri, P.; Ganguly, S.; DeBoyrie, E.; Martinez, M.; Stock, T.; and Bing, R. J. A comparative study of nitroglycerin and propranolol. *Circulation,* **1967,** *36,* 175–186.

Ross, C. R.; Pessah, N. I.; and Farah, A. Inhibitory effects of β-haloalkylamines on the renal transport of N-methyl-nicotinamide. *J. Pharmac. exp. Ther.,* **1968,** *160,* 375–380.

Ross, E. J.; Prichard, B. N. C.; Kaufman, L.; Robertson, A. I. G.; and Harries, B. J. Preoperative and operative management of patients with phaeochromocytoma. *Br. med. J.,* **1967,** *1,* 191–198.

Roth, J. A. Guanethidine and adrenaline used in combination in chronic simple glaucoma. *Br. J. Ophthal.,* **1973,** *57,* 507–510.

Sachs, C., and Jonsson, G. Degeneration of central and peripheral noradrenaline neurons produced by 6-hydroxy-dopa. *J. Neurochem.,* **1972,** *19,* 1561–1575.

Sandler, G.; Leishman, A. W. D.; and Humberstone, P. M. Guanethidine-resistant hypertension. *Circulation,* **1968,** *38,* 542–551.

Schneck, D. W.; Aoki, V. S.; Kroetz, F. W.; and Wilson, W. R. Correlation of beta-blockade with serum practolol levels after oral administration. *Clin. Pharmac. Ther.,* **1972,** *13,* 685–693.

Shand, D. G.; Morgan, D. H.; and Oates, J. A. The release of guanethidine and bethanidine by splenic nerve stimulation: a quantitative evaluation showing dissociation from adrenergic blockade. *J. Pharmac. exp. Ther.,* **1973,** *184,* 73–80.

Shand, D. G.; Nuckolls, E. M.; and Oates, J. A. Plasma propranolol levels in adults with observations in four children. *Clin. Pharmac. Ther.,* **1970,** *11,* 112–120.

Shand, D. G.; Sell, C. G.; and Oates, J. A. Hypertrophic obstructive cardiomyopathy in an infant—propranolol therapy for three years. *New Engl. J. Med.,* **1971,** *285,* 843–844.

Shanks, R. G. The pharmacology of beta sympathetic blockade. *Am. J. Cardiol.,* **1966,** *18,* 308–316.

————. The peripheral vascular effects of propranolol and related compounds. *Br. J. Pharmac. Chemother.,* **1967,** *29,* 204–217.

Singh, B. N., and Vaughan Williams, E. M. Effects on cardiac muscle of the β-adrenoceptor blocking drugs INPEA and LB 46 in relation to their local anaesthetic action on nerve. *Br. J. Pharmac.,* **1971,** *43,* 10–22.

Sitprija, V. Urinary excretion patterns in renal failure due to malaria: the effects of phenoxybenzamine in two cases. *Aust. N.Z. J. Med.,* **1971,** *1,* 44–48.

Sizemore, G. W., and Winternitz, W. W. Autonomic hyper-reflexia—suppression with alpha-adrenergic blocking agents. *New Engl. J. Med.,* **1970,** *282,* 795.

Sowton, E.; Smithen, C.; Leaver, D.; and Barr, I. Effect of practolol on exercise tolerance in patients with angina pectoris. *Am. J. Med.,* **1971,** *51,* 63–70.

Spector, S.; Sjoerdsma, A.; and Udenfriend, S. Blockade of endogenous norepinephrine synthesis by α-methyl-tyrosine, an inhibitor of tyrosine hydroxylase. *J. Pharmac. exp. Ther.,* **1965,** *147,* 86–95.

Stokes, G. S.; Goldsmith, R. F.; Starr, L. M.; Gentle, J. L.; Mani, M. K.; and Stewart, J. H. Plasma renin activity in human hypertension. *Circulation Res.,* **1970,** *27,* Suppl. 2, II-207–II-214.

Stokes, G. S.; Weber, M. A.; and Thornell, I. R. β-Blockers and plasma renin activity in hypertension. *Br. med. J.,* **1974,** *1,* 60–62.

Su, C., and Bevan, J. A. The release of H³-norepinephrine in arterial strips studied by the technique of superfusion and transmural stimulation. *J. Pharmac. exp. Ther.,* **1970,** *172,* 62–68.

Tarazi, R. C., and Dustan, H. P. Beta adrenergic blockade in hypertension. Practical and theoretical implications of long-term hemodynamic variations. *Am. J. Cardiol.,* **1972,** *29,* 633–640.

Tarr, M.; Luckstead, E. F.; Jurewicz, P. A.; and Haas, H. G. Effect of propranolol on the fast inward sodium current in frog atrial muscle. *J. Pharmac. exp. Ther.,* **1973,** *184,* 599–610.

Taylor, S. H.; Sutherland, G. R.; MacKenzie, G. J.; Staunton, H. P.; and Donald, K. W. The circulatory effects

of phentolamine in man with particular respect to changes in forearm blood flow. *Clin. Sci.,* **1965,** *28,* 265–284.

Thomas, M.; Campbell, H.; and Heard, G. The effect of vasodilator drugs on skin blood flow in peripheral vascular occlusion. A double-blind trial using tolazoline. *Br. J. Surg.,* **1968,** *55,* 588–590.

Toda, N. Interactions of bretylium and drugs that inhibit the neuronal membrane transport of norepinephrine in isolated rabbit atria and aortae. *J. Pharmac. exp. Ther.,* **1972,** *181,* 318–327.

Tothill, A. Investigation of adrenaline reversal in the rat uterus by the induction of resistance to isoprenaline. *Br. J. Pharmac. Chemother.,* **1967,** *29,* 291–301.

Viveros, O. H.; Arqueros, L.; Connett, R. J.; and Kirshner, N. Mechanism of secretion from the adrenal medulla. IV. The fate of the storage vesicles following insulin and reserpine administration. *Molec. Pharmac.,* **1969,** *5,* 69–82.

Waal-Manning, H. J., and Simpson, F. O. Practolol treatment in asthmatics. *Lancet,* **1971,** *2,* 1264–1265.

Walle, T., and Gaffney, T. E. Propranolol metabolism in man and dog: mass spectrometric identification of six new metabolites. *J. Pharmac. exp. Ther.,* **1972,** *182,* 83–92.

Wansbrough, H.; Nakanishi, H.; and Wood, C. The effect of adrenergic receptor blocking drugs on the human uterus. *J. Obstet. Gynaec. Br. Commonw.,* **1968,** *75,* 189–198.

Webster, R. A. The antiadrenaline activity of some phenothiazine derivatives. *Br. J. Pharmac. Chemother.,* **1965,** *25,* 566–576.

Wislicki, L. Excitatory and depressant effects of β-adrenoceptor blocking agents on skeletal muscle. *Archs int. Pharmacodyn. Thér.,* **1969,** *182,* 310–317.

Wolfson, S., and Gorlin, R. Cardiovascular pharmacology of propranolol in man. *Circulation,* **1969,** *40,* 501–511.

Wyse, D. G., and Beck, L. Phenoxybenzamine blockade of neural and exogenous noradrenaline. *J. Pharm. Pharmac.,* **1972,** *24,* 478–481.

Yeh, B. K.; McNay, J. L.; and Goldberg, L. I. Attenuation of dopamine renal and mesenteric vasodilatation by haloperidol: evidence for a specific dopamine receptor. *J. Pharmac. exp. Ther.,* **1969,** *168,* 303–309.

Yong, M. S., and Nickerson, M. Dissociation of *alpha* adrenergic receptor protection from inhibition of ³H-phenoxybenzamine binding in vascular tissue. *J. Pharmac. exp. Ther.,* **1973,** *186,* 100–108.

Yoran, C., and Glassman, E. The paradoxic effect of tolazoline hydrochloride on pulmonary hypertension of mitral stenosis. *Chest,* **1973,** *63,* 843–846.

Monographs and Reviews

Alper, M. H.; Flacke, W.; and Krayer, O. Pharmacology of reserpine and its implications for anesthesia. *Anesthesiology,* **1963,** *24,* 524–542.

Bein, H. J. The pharmacology of rauwolfia. *Pharmac. Rev.,* **1956,** *8,* 435–483.

Black, J. W., and Prichard, B. N. C. Activation and blockade of β adrenoceptors in common cardiac disorders. *Br. med. Bull.,* **1973,** *29,* 163–167.

Boura, A. L. A., and Green, A. F. Adrenergic neurone blocking agents. *A. Rev. Pharmac.,* **1965,** *5,* 183–212.

Bovet, D., and Bovet-Nitti, F. *Médicaments du Système Nerveaux Végétatif.* S. Karger, Basel, **1948.**

Dale, H. H. On some physiological actions of ergot. *J. Physiol., Lond.* **1906,** *34,* 163–206.

Furst, C. I. The biochemistry of guanethidine. *Adv. Drug Res.,* **1967,** *4,* 133–161.

Ganong, W. F. Biogenic amines, sympathetic nerves, and renin secretion. *Fedn Proc. Fedn Am. Socs exp. Biol.,* **1973,** *32,* 1782–1784.

Gaunt, R.; Chart, J. J.; and Renzi, A. A. Interactions of drugs with endocrines. *A. Rev. Pharmac.,* **1963,** *3,* 109–128.

Goldberg, L. I. Cardiovascular and renal actions of dopamine: potential clinical applications. *Pharmac. Rev.,* **1972,** *24,* 1–29.

Graham, J. D. P. 2-Halogenoalkylamines. *Prog. med. Chem.,* **1962,** *2,* 132–175.

Greenblatt, D. J., and Koch-Weser, J. Adverse reactions to propranolol in hospitalized medical patients: a report from the Boston Collaborative Drug Surveillance Program. *Am. Heart J.,* **1973,** *86,* 478–484.

Greenblatt, D. J., and Shader, R. I. On the psychopharmacology of beta adrenergic blockade. *Curr. ther. Res.,* **1972,** *14.* 615–625.

Hardaway, R. M., III. *Clinical Management of Shock.* Charles C Thomas, Pub., Springfield, Ill., **1968.**

Himms-Hagen, J. Sympathetic regulation of metabolism. *Pharmac. Rev.,* **1967,** *19,* 367–461.

Karow, A. M., Jr.; Riley, M. W.; and Ahlquist, R. P. Pharmacology of clinically useful beta-adrenergic blocking drugs. *Fortschr. ArzneimittForsch.,* **1971,** *15,* 103–122.

Kostrzewa, R. M., and Jacobowitz, D. M. Pharmacological actions of 6-hydroxydopamine. *Pharmac. Rev.,* **1974,** *26,* 199–288.

Levi-Montalcini, R., and Angeletti, P. U. Immunosympathectomy. *Pharmac. Rev.,* **1966,** *18,* 619–628.

Levy, B., and Wilkenfeld, B. E. Selective interactions with beta adrenergic receptors. *Fedn Proc. Fedn Am. Socs exp. Biol.,* **1970,** *29,* 1362–1364.

Malcolm, J. Adrenergic beta receptor inhibition and hyperthyroidism. *Acta cardiol.,* **1972,** Suppl. 15, 307–326.

Marley, E., and Stephenson, J. D. Central actions of catecholamines. In, *Catecholamines.* (Blaschko, H., and Muscholl, E., eds.) *Handb. exp. Pharmak.,* Vol. 33. Springer-Verlag, Berlin, **1972,** pp. 463–537.

Moore, K. E., and Dominic, J. A. Tyrosine hydroxylase inhibitors. *Fedn Proc. Fedn Am. Socs exp. Biol.,* **1971,** *30,* 859–870.

Nickerson, M. The pharmacology of adrenergic blockade. *Pharmac. Rev.,* **1949,** *1,* 27–101.

———. Nonequilibrium drug antagonism. *Pharmac. Rev.,* **1957,** *9,* 246–259.

———. Drug therapy of shock. In, *Shock: Pathogenesis and Therapy* (a Ciba Foundation symposium). (Bock, D. K., ed.) Springer-Verlag, Berlin, **1962a,** pp. 356–370.

Nickerson, M., and Hollenberg, N. K. Blockade of α-adrenergic receptors. In, *Physiological Pharmacology.* Vol. 4, *The Nervous System—Part D: Autonomic Nervous System Drugs.* (Root, W. S., and Hofmann, F. G., eds.) Academic Press, Inc., New York, **1967,** pp. 243–305.

Porte, D., Jr., and Robertson, R. P. Control of insulin secretion by catecholamines, stress, and the sympathetic nervous system. *Fedn Proc. Fedn Am. Socs exp. Biol.,* **1973,** *32,* 1792–1796.

Rothlin, E. The pharmacology of the natural and dihydrogenated alkaloids of ergot. *Bull. schweiz. Akad. med. Wiss.,* **1947,** *2,* 249–273.

Sannerstedt, R., and Conway, J. Hemodynamic and vascular responses to antihypertensive treatment with adrenergic blocking agents: a review. *Am. Heart J.,* **1970,** *79,* 122–127.

Symposium. (Various authors.) Adrenergic receptors mediating metabolic responses. *Fedn Proc. Fedn Am. Socs exp. Biol.,* **1970,** *29,* 1350–1429.

Thoenen, H., and Tranzer, J. P. The pharmacology of 6-hydroxydopamine. *A. Rev. Pharmac.,* **1973,** *13,* 169–180.

Weiner, N. Regulation of norepinephrine biosynthesis. *A. Rev. Pharmac.,* **1970,** *10,* 273–290.

Wolf, R. L.; Mendlowitz, M.; and Fruchter, A. Diagnosis and treatment of pheochromocytoma. *Mt. Sinai J. Med.,* **1970,** *37,* 549–567.

27 GANGLIONIC STIMULATING AND BLOCKING AGENTS

Robert L. Volle and George B. Koelle

The pharmacology of ganglionic transmission is based primarily on modifications of the acetylcholine (ACh)–acetylcholinesterase (AChE) system. Accordingly, the passage of impulses in autonomic ganglia can be impaired by drugs that (1) interfere with the storage and synthesis of the transmitter (*e.g.,* hemicholinium), (2) prevent the liberation of ACh from the preganglionic nerve endings (*e.g.,* botulinus toxin, local anesthetics), (3) inactivate ganglionic cholinesterases (*e.g.,* physostigmine, DFP), and (4) either mimic or prevent the interactions between ACh and its ganglionic cholinoceptive sites.

Transmission in autonomic ganglia is more complex than formerly believed. It is now clear that there are at least three forms of transmission in autonomic ganglia (Eccles and Libet, 1961; Nishi and Koketsu, 1968; Libet, 1970). In addition to the *primary* pathway involving the ACh depolarization of postsynaptic sites that are sensitive to specific non-depolarizing ganglionic blocking agents, *secondary* pathways for the transmission of excitatory and inhibitory impulses that are insensitive to blockade by such agents have also been described. In a variety of sympathetic ganglia, ACh released from the presynaptic nerve terminals causes a triphasic pattern of postsynaptic potentials consisting, in sequence, of an initial excitatory postsynaptic potential (EPSP with a latency of 1 millisecond), an inhibitory postsynaptic potential (IPSP with a latency of approximately 35 milliseconds), and a late EPSP (latency of several hundred milliseconds). Fundamental differences exist in the sensitivity of the several postsynaptic mechanisms to blockade by drugs and among the electrogenic mechanisms giving rise to the three postsynaptic potentials. (*See* Figure 27–1.)

The initial EPSP is suppressed by conventional non-depolarizing ganglionic blocking agents and represents the first step in the process of initiating the action potentials of the *primary* pathway for ganglionic transmission. Action-potential generation occurs in the postganglionic neuron when the initial EPSP attains a critical amplitude. It has been estimated that eight to ten synapses must be activated in mammalian sympathetic ganglia for transmission to be effective. By the judicious application of ACh, it is possible to match the amplitude and time course of the ACh-evoked depolarization with that of the initial EPSP. Both the initial EPSP and the ACh-evoked depolarization can be attributed to an increase in sodium and potassium conductances of the ganglion cell.

The late EPSP is enhanced or unaffected by conventional ganglionic blocking agents, but it is quite sensitive to blockade by atropine. There is evidence to show that the late EPSP may act to facilitate transmission of impulses through the primary pathway and may serve as an alternate pathway for transmission when the primary pathway is blocked. Under some circumstances, complete ganglionic blockade can be achieved only when a specific ganglionic blocking agent and an atropine-like drug are applied simultaneously. The application of ACh or acetyl-β-methylcholine (MCh) to sympathetic ganglion cells causes a delayed depolarization that is sensitive to blockade by atropine (Koketsu *et al.,* 1968; Libet, 1970). Some controversy exists about the electrogenic mechanism of the late EPSP or depolarization caused by muscarinic drugs. There is no change in membrane conductance during the late EPSP in mammalian sympathetic ganglion cells (Kobayashi and Libet, 1968); in contrast, there is an *increase* in membrane resistance in frog sympathetic ganglion cells that can be attributed to a decrease in potassium conductance (Weight and Votava, 1970).

Like the late EPSP, the IPSP is unaffected by the traditional ganglionic blocking agents but is sensitive to blockade by atropine. Several lines of evidence point toward the participation of a catecholamine in the generation of the IPSP. Dopamine and norepinephrine cause ganglionic hyperpolarization, and both the IPSP and the catecholamine-induced hyperpolarization are blocked by selected α-adrenergic blocking agents. A model (Figure 27–1) has been proposed that suggests that ACh released from the nerve terminals acts upon a catecholamine-containing cell or interneuron within the ganglion to cause the release of dopamine (or norepinephrine), which in turn acts upon the ganglion cell to cause hyperpolarization (IPSP) (Eccles and Libet, 1961; Libet, 1970). This model accounts for the susceptibility of the IPSP to blockade by both atropine and α-adrenergic antagonists. Moreover, morphological evidence has been obtained of catecholamine-containing cells, in addition to the ganglion cells themselves, in sympathetic ganglia; these include the dopamine-containing small, intensely fluorescent (SIF) cells and adrenergic nerve terminals. Although the participation of the SIF cells in ganglionic transmission has not been established, evidence has been obtained

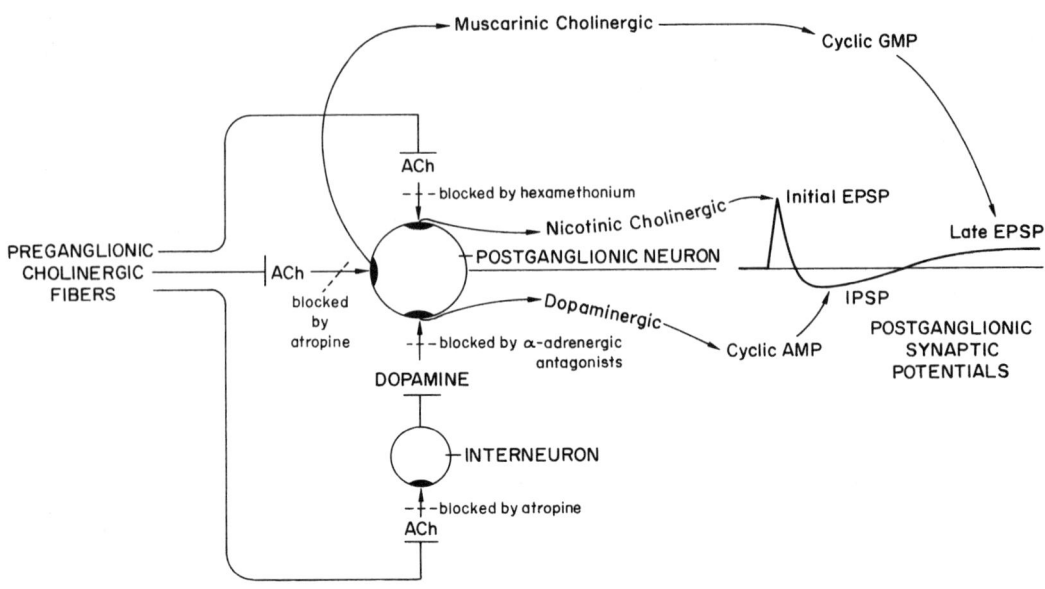

Figure 27-1. *Schematic representation of multiple cholinoceptive and adrenoceptive sites in mammalian superior cervical ganglion and the postulated role of cyclic nucleotides.*

The diagram shows the relationship between the various neuronal elements, the neurotransmitters released at the various synapses, the sensitivity of the synaptic receptors to different classes of specific antagonists, the electrical signs that accompany activation of the various postganglionic receptors following preganglionic stimulation, and the postulated involvement of cyclic nucleotides in the production of the electrophysiological responses. (After Greengard and Kebabian, 1974. Courtesy of *Federation Proceedings.*)

that adrenergic fibers inhibit transmission in parasympathetic ganglia of the bladder (de Groat and Saum, 1972). The electrogenic mechanism for the IPSP or hyperpolarization produced by catecholamines is not yet understood. Some studies indicate the involvement of an electrogenic pump (Nishi and Koketsu, 1968), whereas others implicate an increased potassium conductance (Kosterlitz *et al.,* 1968) or a decreased sodium conductance (Weight and Padjen, 1973).

Cyclic adenosine 3′,5′-monophosphate (cyclic AMP) may mediate the hyperpolarizing effect of catecholamines. Thus, dopamine stimulates cyclic AMP synthesis in the ganglion, and application of cyclic AMP to the ganglion reproduces the physiological effect of dopamine (Greengard and Kebabian, 1974). Related studies indicate that another cyclic nucleotide, cyclic guanosine 3′,5′-monophosphate (cyclic GMP), could be involved in the generation of the late EPSP (Figure 27-1).

Although the technics used in most studies have been adequate to demonstrate the three cholinergic synaptic events, the procedures used for the activation of the atropine-sensitive sites are somewhat complicated, and the question of a physiological role for the several sites is unanswered. For example, in the clinical use of conventional non-depolarizing ganglionic blocking agents, transmission at these sites is adequately depressed without the concomitant use of atropine. In addition, neither the depletion of ganglionic stores of catecholamines by re-

serpine nor the blockade of the inhibitory system by either atropine or α-adrenergic blocking agents causes any change in ganglionic transmission by the primary pathway. Nonetheless, it is quite clear that multiple, heterogeneous cholinoceptive sites do exist in sympathetic ganglia and play a role in the pharmacology and pathophysiology of ganglionic transmission. (*See* reviews by Volle, 1969; Haefely, 1972.)

Drugs that stimulate autonomic ganglia at cholinoceptive sites can be grouped into two major categories. The first group consists of drugs with nicotinic actions, including *nicotine* itself. Their excitatory effects on ganglia are rapid in onset, are blocked by non-depolarizing ganglionic blocking agents, and mimic *the initial EPSP.* The second group is composed of drugs such as *muscarine* and *methacholine,* and the *anticholinesterase* (anti-ChE) *agents.* Their excitatory effects on ganglia are delayed in onset, blocked by atropine-like drugs, and mimic *the late EPSP* (Figure 27-1).

Ganglionic blocking agents impair transmission by actions at the primary nicotinic receptor and also may be classified into two groups. The *first group* includes those drugs that initially stimulate the ganglia by an ACh-like action and then block because of a persistent depolarization (*e.g.*, nicotine); this results in desensitization of the cholinoceptive site and a prolonged blockade. (*See* reviews by Volle, 1969; Haefely, 1972.) There is also evidence that the nicotine-like drugs may cause a block of transmission by actions on the nerve endings. The blockade of autonomic ganglia produced by the *second group* of blocking drugs, of which *hexamethonium* can be regarded as a prototype, does not involve prior ganglionic stimulation or changes in the ganglionic potentials. Such agents impair transmission by competing with ACh for ganglionic cholinoceptive sites and, in a manner analogous to the blockade of transmission at the neuromuscular junction by curare, prevent the development of the postsynaptic depolarization (initial EPSP) (Figure 27–1). Compounds in this group have no effect on nerve conduction or on the release of transmitter substance from the nerve terminals. It is this class of conventional ganglionic blocking agents that is employed in therapy (*see* below).

GANGLIONIC STIMULATING DRUGS

Although the ganglionic stimulating drugs have no essential therapeutic uses, they are of considerable interest as experimental tools.

History. Two natural alkaloids, nicotine and lobeline, owe much of their pharmacological activity to their actions at autonomic ganglia. *Nicotine* was first isolated from leaves of tobacco, *Nicotiana tabacum*, by Posselt and Reiman in 1828. Orfila initiated the first pharmacological studies of the alkaloid in 1843, and Langley and Dickinson described the actions of the drug on autonomic ganglia in 1889. *Lobelia* (Indian tobacco) is obtained from the dried leaves and tops of an herb, *Lobelia inflata*. *Lobeline* is the chief constituent of lobelia and was first obtained in crystalline form by Wieland in 1915. Lobeline has many of the same actions in the body as nicotine but is less potent.

A number of synthetic compounds also have prominent actions at ganglionic receptor sites. The actions of the *onium compounds,* of which *tetramethylammonium* (TMA) is the simplest prototype, were explored in considerable detail in the last half of the nineteenth century and in the early decades of the twentieth century. The structure-activity relationship of the onium compounds has been reviewed by Ing (1936). In 1951, Chen and coworkers described the ganglionic stimulating properties of *1,1-dimethyl-4-phenylpiperazinium (DMPP) iodide.*

Chemistry. *Nicotine* is one of the few natural liquid alkaloids. It is colorless, volatile, and strongly alkaline in reaction; on exposure to air it turns brown and acquires the odor of tobacco. The alkaloid is readily soluble in water and forms water-soluble salts. Nicotine is a combination of a pyridine and a pyrrolidine ring, as follows:

Nicotine

Nicotine and the closely related alkaloid nornicotine (demethylated nicotine) possess asymmetrical carbon atoms. The *d* and *l* forms of nicotine appear to have the same potency. (*See* review by Jackson, 1941.)

Lobeline (α-lobeline, *l*-lobeline) is a substituted piperidine compound that is sparingly soluble in water but forms water-soluble salts. Its structural formula is as follows:

Lobeline

Tetramethylammonium is the simplest molecule of the tetra-alkylammonium series. Like the other onium compounds, its most striking chemical feature is the positively charged nitrogen atom.

NICOTINE

Nicotine has no therapeutic application. However, its high toxicity and presence in tobacco give nicotine a considerable measure of medical importance.

Pharmacological Actions. The complex and often unpredictable changes that occur in the body after administration of nicotine are due not only to its actions on a variety of neuroeffector junctions but also to the fact that the alkaloid has both stimulant and depressant phases of action. The ultimate response of any one structure or system represents the summation of the several different and opposing effects of nicotine. For example, the drug can increase the heart rate by excitation of sympathetic or paralysis of parasympathetic cardiac ganglia, and it can slow the heart rate by paralysis of sympathetic or stimulation of parasympathetic cardiac ganglia. In addition, the effects of the drug on the chemoreceptors of the carotid and aortic bodies and on medullary centers influence heart rate, as do also the cardiovascular compensatory reflexes resulting from changes in blood pressure caused by nicotine. Finally, nicotine causes a discharge of epinephrine from the adrenal medulla, and this hormone accelerates cardiac rate and raises blood pressure.

Peripheral Nervous System. The major action of

nicotine consists initially in transient stimulation and subsequently in a more persistent depression of all autonomic ganglia. Small doses of nicotine stimulate the ganglion cells directly and facilitate the transmission of impulses. When larger doses of the drug are applied, the initial stimulation is followed very quickly by a blockade of transmission. Whereas stimulation of the ganglion cells coincides with their depolarization, depression of transmission by adequate doses of nicotine occurs both during the depolarization and after it has subsided (Ginsborg and Guerrero, 1964). Nicotine also possesses a biphasic action on the adrenal medulla; small doses evoke the discharge of catecholamines, and larger doses prevent their release in response to splanchnic nerve stimulation.

Nicotine also causes the release of catecholamines in a number of isolated organs. This action results in a sympathomimetic response to nicotine that is blocked by drugs known to prevent the effects of catecholamines (see Burn et al., 1959; Ferry, 1963).

The effects of nicotine on the neuromuscular junction are similar to those on ganglia. However, with the exception of avian and denervated mammalian muscle, the stimulant phase is largely obscured by the rapidly developing paralysis. In the latter stage, nicotine produces neuromuscular blockade due to receptor desensitization that is largely the basis for the toxic effect of the alkaloid on respiration. In contrast to autonomic ganglia, where lobeline causes depolarization and acts like nicotine, the end-plate of skeletal muscle fibers is blocked but not depolarized by lobeline. However, the neuromuscular blockade caused by lobeline, like that of nicotine, does appear to be noncompetitive (Steinberg and Volle, 1972).

Nicotine, like ACh, is known to stimulate a number of sensory receptors. These include mechanoreceptors that respond to stretch or pressure of the skin, mesentery, tongue, lung, and stomach; chemoreceptors of the carotid body; thermal receptors of the skin and tongue; and pain receptors. Prior administration of hexamethonium prevents the stimulation of the sensory receptors by nicotine, but has little effect, if any, on the activation of the sensory receptors by physiological stimuli. The explanation of these observations is controversial (Douglas and Gray, 1953; Armette and Ritchie, 1961).

Central Nervous System. Nicotine markedly stimulates the central nervous system (CNS). Appropriate doses produce *tremors* in both man and laboratory animals; with somewhat larger doses, the tremor is followed by *convulsions*. These central actions can be blocked by a variety of agents, including antiparkinsonism drugs, curariform drugs, anticonvulsants, adrenergic blocking agents, and hypnotics. The *excitation of respiration* is a particularly prominent action of nicotine; although large doses act directly on the medulla oblongata, smaller doses augment respiration reflexly by excitation of the chemoreceptors of the carotid and aortic bodies, as first demonstrated by Heymans and coworkers (1931). Stimulation of the CNS is followed by depression, and death results from failure of respiration due to both central paralysis and peripheral blockade of muscles of respiration.

Nicotine and lobeline cause *vomiting* by a complex of central and peripheral actions. The central component of the vomiting response is due to stimulation of the emetic chemoreceptor trigger zone in the area postrema of the medulla oblongata (Laffan and Borison, 1957). In addition, nicotine activates a number of vagal and spinal afferent nerves that form the sensory input of the reflex pathways involved in the act of vomiting.

Nicotine exerts an *antidiuretic action* as the result of stimulation of the hypothalamiconeurohypophyseal system with the consequent release of antidiuretic hormone (ADH). The actions of nicotine on the CNS have been reviewed extensively by Silvette and associates (1962).

Cardiovascular System. In general, the cardiovascular responses to nicotine are due to stimulation of sympathetic ganglia and the adrenal medulla, together with the discharge of catecholamines from sympathetic nerve endings and chromaffin tissues of various organs (Gebber, 1969). Also contributing to the sympathomimetic response to nicotine is the activation of chemoreceptors of the aortic and carotid bodies, which reflexly results in *vasoconstriction, tachycardia,* and *elevated blood pressure.* In addition, there is evidence that nicotine increases *coronary blood flow* as a consequence of the increased cardiac work, elevated blood pressure, and increased cardiac output that it produces.

Gastrointestinal Tract. In contrast to the cardiovascular actions of nicotine, the effects of the drug on the gastrointestinal tract are due largely to parasympathetic stimulation. The combined activation of parasympathetic ganglia and cholinergic nerve endings results in increased tone and motor activity of the bowel and occasionally in diarrhea.

Exocrine Glands. Nicotine causes an initial stimulation of salivary and bronchial secretions that is followed by inhibition. Salivation caused by smoking is reflexly produced by the irritant smoke rather than by a systemic effect of nicotine.

Absorption, Fate, and Excretion. Nicotine is readily absorbed not only from the oral and gastrointestinal mucosa and from the respiratory tract but also from the skin. Indeed, severe poisoning has resulted from percutaneous absorption.

Approximately 80 to 90% of nicotine is altered in the body, mainly in the liver but also in the kidney and lung. The major detoxication products of nicotine are cotinine, γ-(3-pyridyl)-γ-oxobutyric acid, 3-pyridylacetic acid, and isomethylnicotinium ion. Nicotine, together with its detoxication products, is eliminated completely and rapidly by the kidney. The rate of urinary excretion of nicotine is dependent upon the pH of the urine; when the urine is alkaline, only one fourth as much nicotine is excreted as when the urine is acid.

Nicotine is also excreted in the *milk* of lactating women who smoke, the amount of the drug being directly related to the amount of tobacco used. The milk of heavy smokers may contain 0.5 mg per liter.

Acute Nicotine Poisoning. Nicotine is one of the most toxic of all drugs; it acts at a rate comparable to that of cyanide. Poisoning may occur from accidental ingestion of insecticide sprays in which nicotine is present as the effective agent or in children from ingestion of tobacco products. The acutely fatal dose of nicotine for an adult is probably about 60 mg; some cigarettes contain 20 to 30 mg. Apparently the gastric absorption of nicotine from tobacco taken by mouth is delayed, so that vomiting caused by the central effect of the initially absorbed fraction removes much of the tobacco remaining in the stomach.

The onset of symptoms of acute, severe nicotine poisoning is rapid; they include nausea, salivation, abdominal pain, vomiting, diarrhea, cold sweat, headache, dizziness, disturbed hearing and vision, mental confusion, and marked weakness. Faintness and prostration ensue; the blood pressure falls; breathing is difficult; the pulse is weak, rapid, and irregular; and collapse may be followed by terminal convulsions. Death may result within a few minutes from respiratory failure caused by paralysis of the muscles of respiration.

Therapy. Vomiting should be induced with syrup of ipecac, or gastric lavage should be performed in order to remove the nicotine. A sludge of activated charcoal is then passed through the tube and left in the stomach. Artificial respiration with oxygen should be instituted if needed and continued for as long as necessary. Other therapy, including treatment of shock, is purely symptomatic.

TOBACCO AND CHRONIC NICOTINE POISONING

Tobacco is the dried leaf of *Nicotiana tabacum,* a plant indigenous to America but now grown in many parts of the world. The use of tobacco for smoking, chewing, or snuffing is indulged in by many millions of people throughout the world. About 800 billion cigarettes are smoked annually in the United States alone.

Chemical Composition of Tobacco. The percentage of nicotine in tobacco varies considerably and may range from 0.5 to 8.0%. The smoke of the average cigarette may yield 6 to 8 mg, and that of a cigar may contain from 15 to more than 40 mg of nicotine. Approximately 90% of the nicotine in *inhaled* smoke is absorbed compared to only 25 to 50% of that in smoke that is drawn into the mouth and then expelled. Nearly 500 compounds have been isolated from the particulate and gaseous phases of tobacco smoke. In addition to nicotine, tobacco contains pyridine and other nitrogenous bases, a family of isoprenoid compounds, volatile acids, tarry and phenolic substances, and, especially, furfural and acrolein. These chemicals undoubtedly contribute to the irritation of the mucous membranes produced by tobacco and tobacco smoke. Substances such as polonium-210 and nickel have been identified in tobacco smoke and implicated as causative factors in the induction of lung cancer. Appreciable amounts of carbon monoxide may be present in tobacco smoke; 5 to 10% of the circulating hemoglobin may be converted to carboxyhemoglobin as a result of fairly continuous smoking of cigarettes.

Chronic Effects of Tobacco. While tolerance to many of the pharmacodynamic effects of nicotine

develops when the compound is taken repeatedly, the chronic use of tobacco by a large part of the population raises the problem of the *chronic toxicity* of nicotine and, of unquestionably greater importance, the other constituents of tobacco smoke. The relationship between the increased use of cigarettes and a variety of medical problems has received considerable attention and is described in *Smoking and Health* and *The Health Consequences of Smoking,* detailed and authoritative reports by the Surgeon General of the United States Public Health Service (*see* Report, 1964, 1967). It has been estimated that 360,000 persons die annually in the United States because of tobacco use. The devastating statistical calculation has been made that one's life is shortened 14 minutes for every cigarette smoked. Smoking is thus the greatest public health hazard in the United States and the nation's most preventable cause of death (*see* Ochsner, 1971).

In epidemiological studies, a positive correlation was observed between the incidence of *lung cancer* and cigarette smoking (*see* Report, 1964, 1967). These studies have shown that approximately 11 cigarette smokers die from cancer of the lung for each nonsmoker who dies from the same cause. Heavy use of tobacco in this century is apparently responsible for the fact that carcinoma of the lung is now the most common cancer among American men. Similar studies have shown a relation between the use of cigarettes and cancer of the oral cavity, larynx, and esophagus, as well as mucosal epitheliomas. A *smoker's respiratory syndrome* has been described, characterized by dyspnea, wheezing, pharyngeal constriction, pain in the chest, and frequent upper respiratory infections; often mistaken for asthma, the condition disappears when smoking is eliminated. Many of the symptoms may be due to depression of the ciliary defense mechanism of the respiratory tree by the constituents of tobacco smoke. There is evidence that smoking may impair ventilatory efficiency. The incidence of chronic obstructive pulmonary disease is also greater for chronic smokers than for nonsmokers. Objective and subjective evidence of pulmonary damage can even be observed in high school students with 1 to 5 years of smoking experience (Seely *et al.,* 1971).

Considerable attention has been focused on the effects of tobacco smoking on the cardiovascular system. Cigarette smokers have a higher death rate from coronary heart disease than do abstainers. There also appears to be a similar association between smoking and cerebrovascular disorders. The excessive use of tobacco may cause premature systoles, paroxysmal attacks of atrial tachycardia, or a decrease in amplitude or an inversion of the T wave. The observation that cigarette smoke may enhance thrombus formation suggests an additional contributory factor in coronary heart disease (Levine, 1973). The use of tobacco has long been suspected of being etiologically related to *Buerger's disease,* but the exact connection is far from clear. More than 90% of all patients with thromboangiitis obliterans are smokers. Smoking of tobacco under controlled conditions is known to produce *peripheral vasoconstriction,* especially in the skin.

Epidemiological evidence suggests that smoking is

also associated with an increased incidence of peptic ulcer and death therefrom. Psychological factors have often been invoked, since increased formation of gastric acid is not usually observed. However, the secretion of bicarbonate into the small intestine is depressed by nicotine, and this could be a provocative factor (Konturek *et al.*, 1971).

Cigarette smoking also appears to be responsible for a variety of reproductive disorders, including preeclampsia, fewer pregnancies, more abortions, and a higher incidence of neonatal mortality. The birth weights of infants born of mothers who smoke during pregnancy is reduced significantly (Butler *et al.*, 1972).

Tobacco amblyopia is a relatively rare sequela of the tobacco habit. It is usually characterized by a gradual but sometimes by a sudden decrease of visual acuity, most prominent in the central field, especially for colored objects. If untreated, the condition may progress to optic nerve atrophy and permanent injury to vision. Complete cessation of the use of tobacco is indicated.

OTHER GANGLIONIC STIMULANTS

It has been noted earlier that parasympathomimetic drugs (*e.g.*, muscarine, pilocarpine, and some synthetic choline esters) possess the ability to stimulate autonomic ganglia and the adrenal medulla. In contrast to the ganglionic stimulation produced by nicotine, TMA, and DMPP, the stimulation evoked by this group of cholinomimetic drugs is blocked by atropine. For most of these agents, however, the effects of ganglionic stimulation are usually overshadowed by more prominent actions on peripheral neuroeffector junctions.

In addition to the ganglionic stimulating agents related to the ACh-AChE system, *histamine, 5-hydroxytryptamine,* and *angiotensin II* stimulate the sympathetic ganglia and the adrenal medulla. Since the actions of these substances are not antagonized by either hexamethonium or atropine, noncholinergic ganglionic receptors are involved.

Catecholamines have mixed excitatory and inhibitory actions on sympathetic ganglia (*see* de Groat, 1967). *Isoproterenol* causes depolarization of the ganglion cells and facilitates transmission of impulses in both curare- and atropine-sensitive cholinergic pathways. The excitatory actions of isoproterenol are prevented by β-adrenergic blocking compounds. *Norepinephrine, epinephrine,* and *dopamine* usually cause a depression of transmission and hyperpolarization of the ganglion cells. When these inhibitory effects are prevented by α-adrenergic blocking compounds, norepinephrine and epinephrine display the excitatory actions of isoproterenol. Catecholamines also depress transmitter release, and this action may contribute to ganglionic blockade (Christ and Nishi, 1971).

GANGLIONIC BLOCKING DRUGS

In contrast to nicotine and related compounds, a number of drugs block transmission in autonomic ganglia without pro-

ducing any preceding or concomitant change in the membrane potentials of ganglion cells (Figure 27–1). In general, they do not modify the conduction of impulses in preganglionic or postganglionic fibers and do not prevent release of ACh by preganglionic impulses. They produce ganglionic blockade by occupying receptor sites and by stabilizing the postsynaptic membranes against the actions of ACh liberated from presynaptic nerve endings.

The chemical diversity of compounds sharing this action on autonomic ganglia is illustrated in Table 27–1. Although the finer mechanisms of ganglionic blockade have not been studied in detail for each drug, there is considerable presumptive evidence that they depress ganglionic transmission by the same general process. The structure-activity relationship of these compounds has been extensively analyzed and reviewed (Paton and Zaimis, 1952; Ing, 1956), and will not be considered here except as it relates to the differences in absorption, distribution, excretion, and side effects of the several drugs.

Table 27–1. NON-DEPOLARIZING GANGLIONIC BLOCKING AGENTS

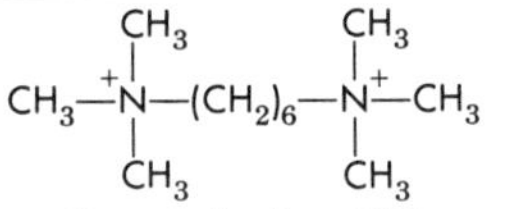

Hexamethonium (C6)

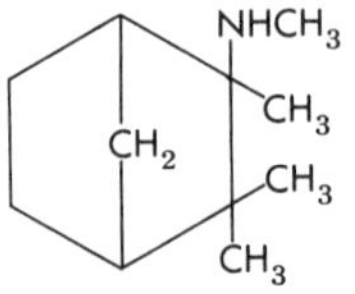

Mecamylamine

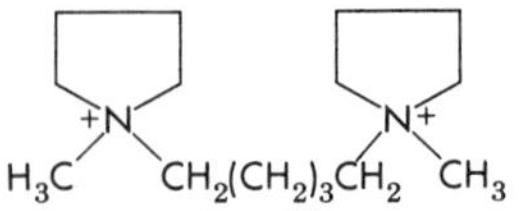

Pentolinium

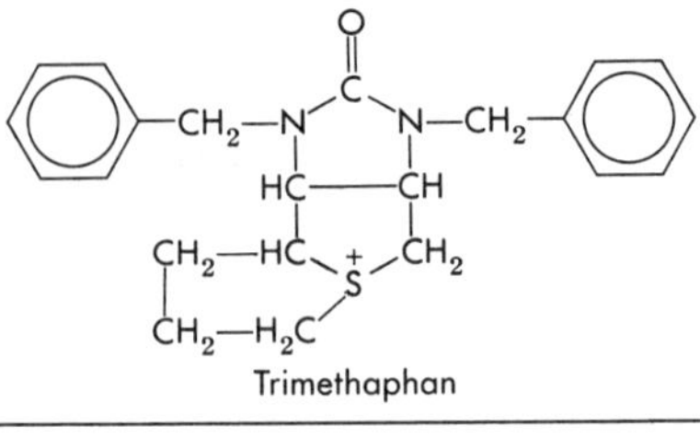

Trimethaphan

HEXAMETHONIUM AND RELATED DRUGS

History and Structure-Activity Relationship. Although Marshall (1913) and Burn and Dale (1915) first described the "nicotine paralyzing" action of *tetraethylammonium* (TEA) on ganglia, and other investigators had reported certain additional pharmacological properties, TEA was largely overlooked until Acheson and Moe (1946) and Acheson and Pereira (1946) published their definitive analyses of the effects of the ion on the cardiovascular system and autonomic ganglia. The *bis*-quaternary ammonium salts were developed and studied independently by Barlow and Ing (1948) and Paton and Zaimis (1949, 1952).

The prototype ganglionic blocking drug in this series, *hexamethonium* (C6), has a bridge of six methylene groups between the two quaternary nitrogen atoms (Table 27–1). Subsequently, several series of *bis*-quaternary ammonium compounds were investigated for ganglionic blocking activity, and some drugs so discovered have been employed clinically, including *chlorisondamine* and *trimethidinium*. Of these, the only one that is still official is *pentolinium* (Table 27–1). Triethylsulfonium salts, like the quaternary and *bis*-quaternary ammonium ions, possess ganglionic blocking actions. This knowledge led to the development of other sulfonium ganglionic blocking agents and culminated in the synthesis of *trimethaphan* (Randall *et al.,* 1949) (Table 27–1).

The synthesis of secondary amines with ganglionic blocking activity represented somewhat of a departure in the chemistry of these agents. The pharmacological properties of *mecamylamine* (Table 27–1) were first reported in the mid-1950s, and the drug was soon thereafter introduced into therapy (Stone *et al.,* 1956). *Pempidine,* a tertiary amine with similar properties, was introduced shortly thereafter.

Pharmacological Properties. Nearly all of the physiological alterations observed after the administration of hexamethonium and related drugs can be attributed to the blockade of transmission in autonomic ganglia by the mechanisms already considered. Since all members of this group of drugs exhibit essentially the same pharmacological activity, their actions in the body can be discussed together.

The alteration of physiological processes attending ganglionic blockade can be anticipated with reasonable accuracy by a careful inspection of Figure 21–1 (facing page 406) and by knowing which division of the autonomic nervous system exercises dominant control of various organs (Table 27–2). For example, blockade of sympathetic ganglia interrupts adrenergic control of arterioles and results in vasodilatation, improved peripheral blood flow of some vascular beds, and a fall in blood pressure.

In addition, generalized ganglionic blockade may result also in atony of the bladder and gastrointestinal tract, cycloplegia, xerostomia, diminished perspiration, and, by abolishing circulatory reflex pathways, postural hypotension. Many of these changes represent the generally undesirable features of ganglionic blockade, which limit the therapeutic efficacy of ganglionic blocking agents.

Cardiovascular System. The importance of existing sympathetic tone in determining the degree to which blood pressure is lowered by ganglionic blockade is illustrated by the fact that blood pressure may be decreased only minimally in recumbent normotensive subjects but may fall markedly in sitting or standing subjects. In the latter situation, *postural hypotension* occurs and may cause syncope. Postural hypotension persists longer than recumbent hypotension and is a major problem in ambulatory patients receiving ganglionic blocking drugs; it is relieved to some extent by muscular activity and completely by recumbency, and tends to become less prominent after continued medication. Sympathetically mediated vasomotor reflexes are inhibited or abolished, and the cold pressor response is reduced. The drugs induce a hypotensive response even in sympathectomized patients, probably because there are ganglionic vasoconstrictor pathways not removed by surgery.

Changes in *cardiac rate* following ganglionic blockade depend largely on existing vagal tone. In man, mild tachycardia usually accompanies the hypotension, a sign that indicates fairly complete ganglionic blockade. However, a decrease may occur if the heart rate is initially high.

Cardiac output is often reduced by ganglionic blocking drugs in patients with normal cardiac function, probably as a consequence of diminished venous return resulting from venous dilatation and peripheral pooling of the blood. In patients with cardiac failure, ganglionic blockade frequently results in increased cardiac output due to a reduction in peripheral resistance and to decreased right-heart pressure resulting from a decrease in venous return.

Table 27–2. USUAL PREDOMINANCE OF SYMPATHETIC (ADRENERGIC) OR PARASYMPATHETIC (CHOLINERGIC) TONE AT VARIOUS EFFECTOR SITES, WITH CONSEQUENT EFFECTS OF AUTONOMIC GANGLIONIC BLOCKADE

SITE	PREDOMINANT TONE	EFFECT OF GANGLIONIC BLOCKADE
Arterioles	Sympathetic (adrenergic)	Vasodilatation; increased peripheral flow; hypotension
Veins	Sympathetic (adrenergic)	Dilatation; pooling of blood; decreased venous return; decreased cardiac output
Heart	Parasympathetic (cholinergic)	Tachycardia
Iris	Parasympathetic (cholinergic)	Mydriasis
Ciliary muscle	Parasympathetic (cholinergic)	Cycloplegia
Gastrointestinal tract	Parasympathetic (cholinergic)	Reduced tone and motility; constipation
Urinary bladder	Parasympathetic (cholinergic)	Urinary retention
Salivary glands	Parasympathetic (cholinergic)	Xerostomia
Sweat glands	Sympathetic (cholinergic)	Anhidrosis

In hypertensive subjects, cardiac output, stroke volume, and left ventricular work are diminished.

Although *total systemic vascular resistance* is decreased in patients undergoing therapy with the ganglionic blocking agents, the changes in *blood flow* and *vascular resistance* of individual vascular beds are variable. The *skin temperature* is elevated mostly in the skin areas of the hands and feet. The retinal and choroidal vessels dilate. Full parenteral doses of hexamethonium cause essentially the same degree of increase in blood flow to the leg as does lumbar epidural or intrathecal block by a local anesthetic. On the other hand, *skeletal muscle blood flow* is unaltered and *splanchnic blood flow* decreases following ganglionic blockade. There is usually a reduction in *cerebral blood flow,* although the reduction is less than would be anticipated from the change in blood pressure. In hypertensive patients with retinopathy, hexamethonium has been shown to reduce equally *cerebrovascular resistance* and mean arterial pressure without producing a significant alteration in cerebral blood flow, changes that are favorable for cerebral hemodynamics in hypertension. Hexamethonium has variable effects on *coronary blood flow.* (*See* review by Aviado, 1960.)

The *renal effects* of ganglionic blockade in normotensive subjects include a decrease in glomerular filtration rate (GFR) and renal blood flow (RBF) and an increase in renal vascular resistance (RVR) (Moyer *et al.,* 1955). In some hypertensive subjects, ganglionic blocking agents produce the same renal changes as occur in normotensive individuals; in others, RBF is increased or unchanged, and RVR is reduced.

Gastrointestinal Tract. The volume and the acidity of *gastric secretions* are generally decreased by the ganglionic blocking agents. The secretory response to insulin-induced hypoglycemia is diminished, as is the increase in *pancreatic secretions* stimulated by the consumption of a test meal of milk. *Salivary secretion* is also diminished. The *tone* and *motility* of the gastrointestinal tract in man are reduced, and propulsive movements of the small intestine may be completely stopped.

Other Effects. Ganglionic blockade causes partial or total impairment of the voiding contractions of the *urinary bladder,* with a resultant increase in vesical capacity. This is due to blockade of parasympathetic ganglia along the efferent pathways of the spinal reflex concerned with micturition, so that bladder distention causes no urge to void. Moderate dosage in some subjects may result in incomplete emptying of the bladder and a large residual urine. Ganglionic blockade causes incomplete *mydriasis* and partial loss of *accommodation* as a result of impaired transmission in the ciliary ganglion. *Sweating* is reduced.

Untoward Responses and Severe Reactions.
Among the milder untoward responses observed are visual disturbances (such as mydriasis and difficulty in accommodation), dry mouth, conjunctival suffusion, urinary hesitancy, decreased potentia, subjective chilliness, moderate constipation, occasional diarrhea, abdominal discomfort, anorexia, heartburn, nausea, eructation and bitter taste, and the signs and symptoms of syncope caused by postural hypotension. These side effects tend to become less pronounced as administration of the drug is continued.

More severe reactions include *marked hypotension, constipation, paralytic ileus,* and *urinary retention.* Anginal pain may be precipitated in patients with angina pectoris if the hypotension is excessive. Syncope may occur without warning, and hypotension and collapse may be profound.

Unlike the quaternary ammonium ganglionic blocking agents, which do not readily reach the CNS, *mecamylamine* can produce *prominent central effects,* resulting in tremors, mental confusion, seizures, mania, or depression; these effects of the secondary- and tertiary-amine ganglionic blocking drugs have been related either to an anti-ACh action or, because of structural considerations, to direct central effects (*see* Freis, 1959).

Absorption, Fate, and Excretion. The absorption of quaternary ammonium compounds from the enteric tract is incomplete, erratic, and unpredictable. This is due both to the limited ability of quaternary ammonium ions to penetrate cell membranes and to the depression of propulsive movements of the stomach and small intestine. Gastric emptying time may be so delayed that two or three doses may be retained in the stomach; the gastric contents may then suddenly enter the duodenum, and the absorption of the accumulated toxic amounts of drug can cause severe hypotension and collapse. Although the absorption of mecamylamine is less erratic, the danger persists of reduced bowel activity leading to frank paralytic ileus.

After absorption, the quaternary ammonium blocking agents are confined primarily to the extracellular space. Penetration of the blood-brain barrier is limited. Most of a parenteral dose is excreted unchanged by the kidney. Mecamylamine is not confined to the extracellular space; high concentrations accumulate in the liver and kidney. In addition, the drug traverses the blood-brain barrier and the placental barrier. Mecamylamine is excreted slowly by the kidney in unchanged form. The rate of its renal elimination is influenced markedly by urinary pH; alkalinization of the urine reduces and acidification promotes renal excretion of the drug. (*See* review by Peters, 1960.)

Preparations, Administration, and Dosage. Of the numerous ganglionic blocking agents that have appeared on the therapeutic scene, only *mecamylamine, pentolinium,* and *trimethaphan* are currently official.

Mecamylamine Hydrochloride, N.F. (INVERSINE), is available for oral administration in scored and quarter-sectioned tablets containing 2.5 and 10 mg, respectively.

Pentolinium Tartrate, N.F. (ANSOLYSEN), is available as official tablets containing 20, 40, or 100 mg and as an injection in 10-ml vials containing 10 mg/ml. The injection should be administered only subcutaneously or intramuscularly; if given intravenously, the response is unpredictable.

Trimethaphan Camsylate, U.S.P. (ARFONAD), is available as an injection, in 10-ml ampuls containing 50 mg/ml.

THERAPEUTIC USES

Historically the major therapeutic use of the ganglionic blocking agents has been in the management of *hypertensive cardiovascular disease*. Their use for this purpose has diminished considerably with the advent of other therapeutic agents (*see* Chapter 33). The same is true with respect to most of their other uses.

The extremely short-acting ganglionic blocking agent *trimethaphan* can be given by intravenous infusion of a solution containing 1.0 mg/ml (0.1%) in 5% glucose solution to anesthetized patients in order to produce *controlled hypotension* for certain surgical procedures (plastic, neurological, ophthalmological) in which it is important to reduce hemorrhage in the operative field to a minimum. The operative region is elevated insofar as possible, and an initial rate of infusion of 1 to 4 mg of trimethaphan per minute is subsequently adjusted to maintain the desired level of blood pressure. The same method of administration is employed for the emergency treatment of *hypertensive crises*, particularly when complicated by acute cardiac failure and pulmonary edema. In this situation, the recommended initial rate of infusion is 0.1 to 1 mg per minute. Abrupt reduction of blood pressure, particularly to levels below the normal range, is dangerous in patients with coronary or cerebrovascular insufficiency. Infusion should be terminated gradually while the blood pressure is carefully monitored. Since trimethaphan causes histamine release, it should be avoided or used with extreme caution in patients who have a history of allergy (*see* Larson, 1964).

Acheson, G. H., and Moe, G. K. The action of tetraethylammonium ion on the mammalian circulation. *J. Pharmac. exp. Ther.*, **1946**, *87*, 220–236.

Acheson, G. H., and Pereira, S. A. The blocking effect of tetraethylammonium ion on the superior cervical ganglion of the cat. *J. Pharmac. exp. Ther.*, **1946**, *87*, 273–280.

Armette, C. J., and Ritchie, J. M. The action of acetylcholine and some related substances on conduction in mammalian non-myelinated nerve fibers. *J. Physiol., Lond.*, **1961**, *155*, 372–384.

Barlow, R. B., and Ing, H. R. Curare-like action of polymethylene bis-quaternary ammonium salts. *Br. J. Pharmac. Chemother.*, **1948**, *3*, 298–304.

Burn, J. H., and Dale, H. H. The action of certain quaternary ammonium bases. *J. Pharmac. exp. Ther.*, **1915**, *6*, 417–438.

Burn, J. H.; Leach, E. H.; Rand, M. J.; and Thompson, J. W. Peripheral effects of nicotine and acetylcholine resembling those of sympathetic stimulation. *J. Physiol., Lond.*, **1959**, *148*, 332–352.

Butler, N. R.; Goldstein, H.; and Ross, E. M. Cigarette smoking in pregnancy: its influence on birth weight and perinatal mortality. *Br. med J.*, **1972**, *2*, 127–130.

Chen, G.; Portman, R.; and Wickel, A. Pharmacology of 1,1-dimethyl-4-phenylpiperazinium iodide, a ganglionstimulating agent. *J. Pharmac. exp. Ther.*, **1951**, *103*, 330–336.

Christ, D. D., and Nishi, S. Site of adrenaline blockade in the superior cervical ganglion of the rabbit. *J. Physiol., Lond.*, **1971**, *213*, 107–117.

de Groat, W. C. Actions of the catecholamines in sympathetic ganglia. *Circulation Res.*, **1967**, *21*, Suppl. 3, 135–145.

de Groat, W. C., and Saum, W. R. Sympathetic inhibition of the urinary bladder and of pelvic ganglionic transmission in the cat. *J. Physiol., Lond*, **1972**, *220*, 297–314.

Douglas, W. W., and Gray, J. A. B. The excitant action of acetylcholine and other substances on cutaneous sensory pathways and its prevention by hexamethonium and *d*-tubocurarine. *J. Physiol., Lond*, **1953**, *119*, 118–128.

Eccles, R. M., and Libet, B. Origin and blockade of the synaptic responses of curarized sympathetic ganglia. *J. Physiol., Lond.*, **1961**, *157*, 484–503.

Ferry, C. B. The sympathomimetic effect of acetylcholine on the spleen of the cat. *J. Physiol., Lond.*, **1963**, *167*, 487–504.

Freis, E. D. Clinical uses of ganglionic blocking agents in the treatment of hypertension and a comparison of different blocking agents. In, *Hypertension.* (Moyer, J., ed.) W. B. Saunders Co., Philadelphia, **1959**, pp. 429–433.

Gebber, G. L. Neurogenic basis for the rise in blood pressure evoked by nicotine in the cat. *J. Pharmac. exp. Ther.*, **1969**, *166*, 255–269.

Ginsborg, B. L., and Guerrero, S. On the action of depolarizing drugs on sympathetic ganglion cells of the frog. *J. Physiol., Lond.*, **1964**, *172*, 189–206.

Greengard, P., and Kebabian, J. W. Role of cyclic AMP in synaptic transmission in the mammalian peripheral nervous system. *Fedn Proc. Fedn Am. Socs exp. Biol,* **1974**, *33*, 1059–1067.

Heymans, C.; Bouckaert, J. J.; and Dautrebande, I. Sinus carotidien et réflexes respiratoires. III. Sensibilité des sinus carotidiens aux substances chimiques. Action stimulante respiratoire réflexe du sulfure de sodium, du cyanure de potassium, de la nicotine et de la lobéline. *Archs int. Pharmacodyn. Thér.*, **1931**, *40*, 54–91.

Kobayashi, H., and Libet, B. Generation of slow postsynaptic potentials without increase in ionic conductance. *Proc. natn. Acad. Sci. U.S.A.,* **1968**, *60*, 1304–1311.

Koketsu, K.; Nishi, S.; and Soeda, H. Calcium and acetylcholine-potential of bullfrog sympathetic ganglion cell membrane. *Life Sci.*, **1968**, *7*, 955–963.

Konturek, S. J.; Solomon, T. E.; McCreight, W. G.; Johnson, L. R.; and Jacobson, E. D. Effects of nicotine on gastrointestinal secretions. *Gastroenterology*, **1971**, *60*, 1098–1105.

Kosterlitz, H. W.; Lees, G. M.; and Wallis, D. I. Resting and action potentials recorded by the sucrose-gap method in the superior cervical ganglia of the rabbit. *J. Physiol., Lond.*, **1968**, *195*, 39–53.

Laffan, R. J., and Borison, H. L. Emetic action of nicotine and lobeline. *J. Pharmac. exp. Ther.*, **1957**, *121*, 468–476.

Langley, J. N., and Dickinson, W. L. On the local paralysis of peripheral ganglia, and on the connexion of different classes of nerve fibers with them. *Proc. R. Soc., B,* **1889**, *46*, 423–431.

Levine, P. N. An acute effect of cigarette smoking on platelet function. A possible link between smoking and arterial thrombosis. *Circulation*, **1973**, *48*, 619–623.

Marshall, C. R. Studies on the pharmaceutical action of tetra-alkyl-ammonium compounds. *Trans. R. Soc. Edinb.*, **1913**, *1*, 17–40.

Moyer, J. H.; McConn, R.; and Morris, G. C. Effect of controlled hypotension with PENDIOMIDE (as used in surgery) on renal hemodynamics and water and electrolyte excretion—a comparison with hexamethonium and ARFONAD and the effect of norepinephrine on these responses. *Anesthesiology*, **1955**, *16*, 355–364.

Nishi, S., and Koketsu, K. Early and late after-discharges of amphibian sympathetic ganglion cells. *J. Neurophysiol.*, **1968**, *31*, 109–121.

Ochsner, A. The health menace of tobacco. *Am. Scient.,* **1971**, *59*, 246–252.

Paton, W. D. M., and Zaimis, E. J. The pharmacological actions of polymethylene bistrimethylammonium salts. *Br. J. Pharmac. Chemother.*, **1949**, *4*, 381–400.

Randall, L. O.; Peterson, W. G.; and Lehmann, G. The

ganglionic blocking action of thiophanium derivatives. *J. Pharmac. exp. Ther.,* **1949,** *97,* 48–57.

Seely, J. E.; Zuskin, E.; and Bouhuys, A. Cigarette smoking: objective evidence for lung damage in teen-agers. *Science, Wash.,* **1971,** *172,* 741–743.

Steinberg, M. I., and Volle, R. L. A comparison of lobeline and nicotine at the frog neuromuscular junction. *Naunyn-Schmiedebergs Archs Pharmac.,* **1972,** *272,* 16–31.

Stone, C. A.; Torchiana, M. L.; Navarro, A.; and Beyer, K. H. Ganglionic blocking properties of 3-methyl-amino-isocamphane hydrochloride (mecamylamine): a secondary amine. *J. Pharmac. exp. Ther.,* **1956,** *117,* 169–183.

Weight, F., and Padjen, A. Slow postsynaptic inhibition: evidence for synaptic inactivation of sodium conductance in sympathetic ganglion cells. *Brain Res.,* **1973,** *55,* 219–224.

Weight, F., and Votava, J. Slow synaptic excitation in sympathetic ganglion cells: evidence for synaptic inactivation of potassium conductance. *Science, Wash.,* **1970,** *170,* 755–758.

Monographs and Reviews

Aviado, D. M. Hemodynamic effects of ganglion blocking drugs. *Circulation Res.,* **1960,** *8,* 304–314.

Haefely, W. Electrophysiology of the adrenergic neuron. In, *Catecholamines.* (Blaschko, H., and Muscholl, E., eds.) *Handb. exp. Pharmak.,* Vol. 33. Springer-Verlag, Berlin, **1972,** pp. 661–725.

Ing, H. R. The curariform action of onium salts. *Physiol. Rev.,* **1936,** *16,* 527–544.

———. Structure-action relationships of hypotensive drugs. In, *Hypotensive Drugs.* (Harrington, M., ed.) Pergamon Press, Ltd., Oxford, **1956,** pp. 7–22.

Jackson, K. E. Alkaloids of tobacco. *Chem. Rev.,* **1941,** *29,* 123–197. (278 references.)

Larson, A. G. Deliberate hypotension. *Anesthesiology,* **1964,** *25,* 682–706.

Libet, B. Generation of slow inhibitory and excitatory postsynaptic potentials. *Fedn Proc. Fedn Am. Socs exp. Biol.,* **1970,** *29,* 1945–1956.

Paton, W. D. M., and Zaimis, E. J. The methonium compounds. *Pharmac. Rev.,* **1952,** *4,* 219–253. (187 references.)

Peters, L. Renal tubular excretion of organic bases. *Pharmac. Rev.,* **1960,** *12,* 1–35. (104 references.)

Report. *Smoking and Health: Report of the Advisory Committee to the Surgeon General of the Public Health Service.* Public Health Service Publication No. 1103, U.S. Government Printing Office, Washington, D.C., **1964.**

Report. *The Health Consequences of Smoking: A Public Health Service Review.* Public Health Service Publication No. 1696, U.S. Government Printing Office, Washington, D.C., **1967.**

Silvette, H.; Hoff, E. C.; Larson, P. S.; and Haag, H. B. The action of nicotine on central nervous system function. *Pharmac. Rev.,* **1962,** *14,* 137–173. (184 references.)

Trendelenburg, U. Some aspects of the pharmacology of autonomic ganglion cells. *Ergebn. Physiol.,* **1967,** *59,* 1–85.

Volle, R. L. Ganglionic transmission. *A. Rev. Pharmac.,* **1969,** *9,* 135–146.

Volle, R. L., and Hancock, J. C. Transmission in sympathetic ganglia. *Fedn Proc. Fedn Am. Socs exp. Biol.,* **1970,** *29,* 1913–1918.

CHAPTER

28 NEUROMUSCULAR BLOCKING AGENTS

George B. Koelle

Several drugs employed clinically have as their major action the interruption of transmission of the nerve impulse at the skeletal neuromuscular junction. On the basis of a characteristic feature associated with the production of this effect, they are classified either as *competitive* (*stabilizing*) agents, of which curare is the classical example, or as *depolarizing* agents, such as succinylcholine. The neuromuscular blocking agents also have other important sites of action, including autonomic ganglia.

History, Sources, and Chemistry. *Curare* is a generic term for various South American arrow poisons. The drug has a long and romantic history. It has been employed for centuries by the Indians along the Amazon and Orinoco Rivers and in other parts of the continent for killing wild animals used for food; death results from paralysis of skeletal muscles. The technic of preparation of curare by the South American Indians was long shrouded in mystery and was entrusted only to tribal witch doctors. Soon after the discovery of the American continent, Sir Walter Raleigh and other early explorers and botanists became interested in curare, and late in the sixteenth century samples of the native preparations were brought to Europe for examination and investigation. Following the pioneering work of the scientist-explorer von Humboldt, in 1805, the *botanical sources* of curare quite early became the object of much field search, and active investigation still continues. The curares from eastern Amazonia contain various species of *Strychnos* as their chief ingredient. It is noteworthy that most of the South American species of *Strychnos* examined contain chiefly quaternary, neuromuscular blocking alkaloids, whereas the Asiatic, African, and Australian species nearly all contain tertiary, strychnine-like alkaloids. Certain species of *Chondrodendron* also yield curare and are employed by natives in the western Amazon regions; *C. tomentosum* in particular is a source of *d*-tubocurarine. Research on curare was greatly accelerated by the work of Gill (1940), who, after prolonged and intimate study of the native methods of preparing curare, brought to the United States a sufficient amount of the authentic drug prepared from *C. tomentosum* to permit chemical and pharmacological investigations.

The modern clinical use of curare probably dates from 1932, when West employed highly purified fractions in patients with tetanus and spastic disorders. In 1940, Bennett introduced the drug as an adjuvant in the pentylenetetrazol shock treatment of psychiatric disorders. The first trial of curare for promoting muscular relaxation in general anesthesia was reported by Griffith and Johnson (1942); this application of the drug was soon greatly expanded and now represents its chief therapeutic use.

The fascinating history of curare, the reports of early travelers, and the complex problems of botanical source, nomenclature, and chemical identification have been presented in extensive monographic reviews (*see* McIntyre, 1947, 1972; Bovet *et al.,* 1959; and previous editions of this text).

Crude curare contains a number of closely related alkaloids that exert similar pharmacological actions, but attention was focused chiefly on *d-tubocurarine*, the essential structure of which was established by King (1935). Until recently it was assumed to be a *bis*-quaternary ammonium compound, but one of the N atoms constitutes a tertiary amine (Everett *et al.,* 1970; Table 28–1). A semisynthetic derivative of *d*-tubocurarine employed clinically is its dimethyl ether (*dimethyl tubocurarine*); this agent is about three times as potent as *d*-tubocurarine in man.

The most potent of all curare alkaloids are the *toxiferines* obtained from *S. toxifera* (*see* Waser, 1972). A semisynthetic derivative, *alcuronium chloride* (*diallylbisnortoxiferin*), is employed clinically in Europe (Table 28–1).

The seeds of the trees and shrubs of the genus *Erythrina*, widely distributed in the tropical and subtropical areas of the American continent and of Asia, Africa, and Australia, contain substances with curare-like activity. Of 105 known species, the seeds from more than 50 have been tested and all were found to contain alkaloids with curariform properties (Folkers and Unna, 1939). *Erythroidine*, a tertiary nitrogenous base obtained from *E. americana*, was the first crystalline alkaloid of the group to be isolated. It consists of at least two isomeric alkaloids, *alpha* and *beta* erythroidine (Table 28–1). A hydrogenated derivative, *dihydro-β-erythroidine*, has been studied most carefully and subjected to clinical trial.

Gallamine (Table 28–1) is one of a series of synthetic curare substitutes first reported on extensively by Bovet and coworkers in 1949 (*see* review by Bovet, 1972). Their work in this field started with the synthesis of structures related to, but less complicated than, *d*-tubocurarine. The same approach led to the development of the *polymethylene bis-trimethylammonium series* (referred to herein by the generic term *methonium compounds*) simultaneously and independently by Barlow and Ing (1948) and Paton and Zaimis (1949 *et seq.*). Because *d*-tubocurarine appeared to contain two quaternary nitrogen atoms and since "onium cations" possessed the general property of curare-like blockade of neuromuscular

Table 28-1. STRUCTURAL FORMULAS OF MAJOR NEUROMUSCULAR BLOCKING AGENTS

COMPETITIVE AGENTS

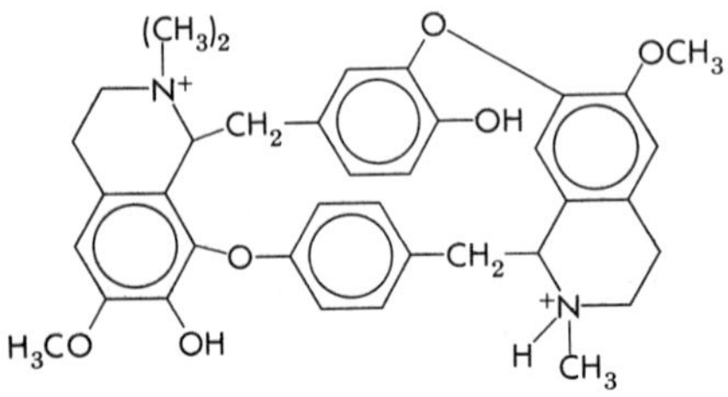

d-Tubocurarine

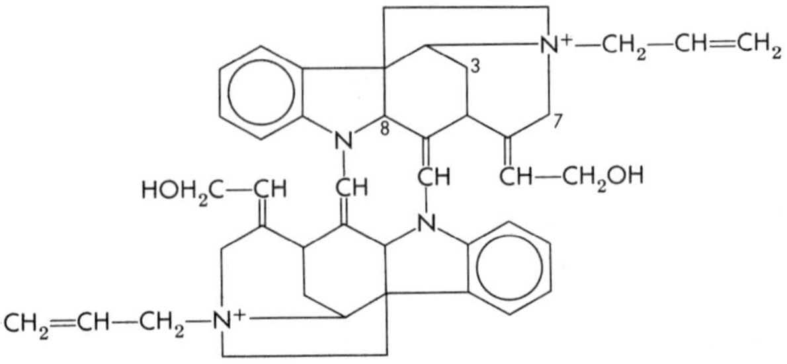

Alcuronium

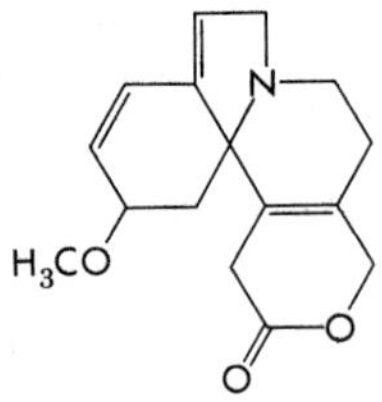

β-Erythroidine

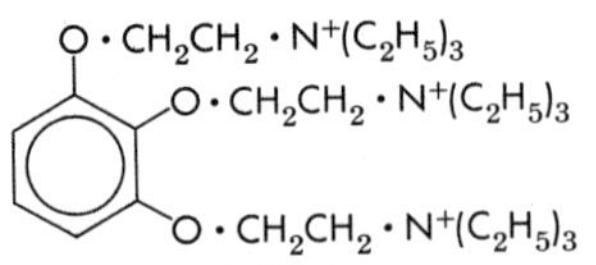

Gallamine

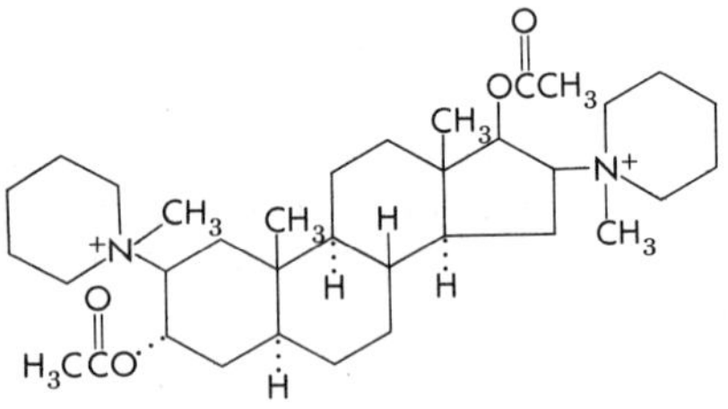

Pancuronium

DEPOLARIZING AGENTS

$(CH_3)_3\overset{+}{N}-(CH_2)_{10}-\overset{+}{N}(CH_3)_3$

Decamethonium

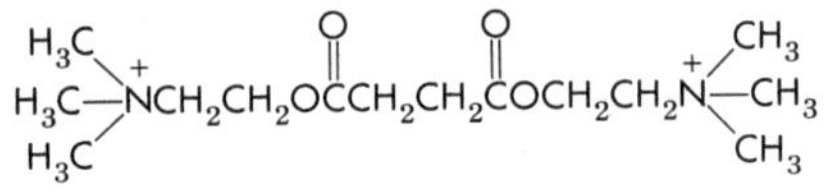

Succinylcholine

COMBINED ACTION

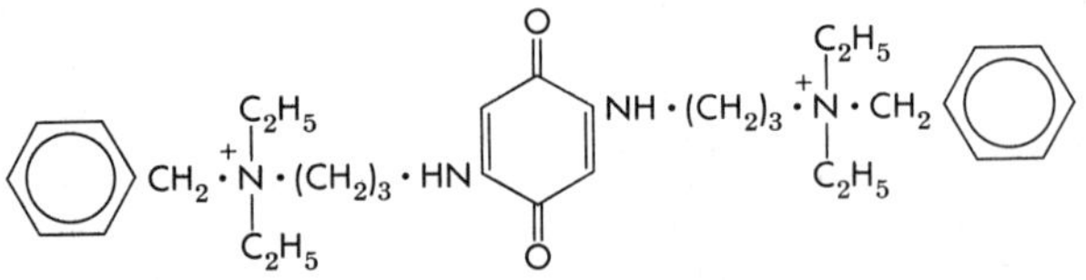

Benzoquinonium

---

transmission, both groups of investigators prepared and tested a number of simple *bis*-quaternary ammonium salts in which the nitrogen atoms were directly attached to the terminal carbons of polymethylene chains of different length; potency was greatest in the *bis*-trimethylammonium series, and unusually high activity was found when the chain contained ten carbon atoms (*decamethonium* [*C10*], Table 28-1). The member of the series containing six carbon atoms in the chain, *hexamethonium* (*C6*), was found to be particularly effective as a ganglionic blocking agent (*see* Chapter 27).

The use of curarized animals by Hunt and Taveau in 1906 in experiments on *succinylcholine* (Table 28-1) prevented them from observing the neuromuscular blocking activity of the drug, and this property went unrecognized for more than 40 years.

In 1949, the curariform action of the compound was described independently by workers in Italy, Great Britain, and the United States, and its clinical application soon followed.

Benzoquinonium is a synthetic neuromuscular blocking agent obtained by quaternization of a compound originally synthesized as a candidate antibacterial substance (Hoppe, 1950; Table 28-1). It combines certain features of both the competitive and depolarizing agents, and in addition has considerable anticholinesterase (anti-ChE) activity.

Pancuronium is a member of a series of *bis*-quaternary ammonium steroids that were synthesized in 1964. Extensive pharmacological and clinical studies have shown that it is approximately five times as potent as *d*-tubocurarine as a competitive neuromuscular blocking agent, with minimal cardiovascular and little or no histamine-releasing or hormonal actions (Buckett *et al.,* 1968; Speight and Avery, 1972).

Structure-Activity Relationship. The first attempts to analyze the structure-activity relationship (SAR) of drugs were made in the field of curarimimetic substances (*see* Crum Brown and Fraser, 1868, 1869), although neither the structure of the active ingredients of curare nor the role of acetylcholine (ACh) in neuromuscular transmission was then known. Recent work has served as much to complicate the picture as to simplify it. This is due in particular to the contrasting features, as well as the similarities, of the *competitive* (stabilizing) and *depolarizing* agents. Furthermore, an agent may depolarize in one species and stabilize in another, or it may act oppositely on different muscles in the same species; both types of action may be exerted simultaneously or consecutively on the same muscle. In addition, local anesthetic, anti-ChE, and ACh-releasing properties of certain drugs complicate SAR interpretation (*see* Karczmar *et al.,* 1972). The term *curarimimetic* will be used here as a general designation for neuromuscular blockade without regard to mechanism.

The functional relationship of curare to ACh focuses attention on the role of *quaternary ammonium groups* in curarimimetic agents. Only a few quaternary ammonium compounds, among them the simple esters of betaine, have been found to lack curarimimetic activity when properly tested, although many of them are quite weak. Many well-known drugs (atropine, quinine, strychnine, etc.) show a marked increase in curarimimetic potency when their nitrogen atom is quaternized. On the other hand, many nonquaternary ammonium compounds have a curare-like activity (quinine, nicotine, *erythroidine derivatives,* etc.). The curarimimetic activity of β-erythroidine and dihydro-β-erythroidine is actually abolished by quaternization of the nitrogen. Other atoms can substitute for cationic quaternary nitrogen; thus, curarimimetic activity has been reported for sulfonium, phosphonium, arsonium, stibonium, and iodinium compounds.

Some essential factors that determine the activity of neuromuscular blocking agents of either the *competitive* or *depolarizing* class have been summarized by Cavallito (1962, 1967) as *coulombic-bonding characteristics, steric influences,* and the *lipophilic-hydrophilic balance* of the molecule. (*See also* Bovet, 1972; Cheymol and Bourillet, 1972; Waser, 1972.)

The *bis*-quaternary ammonium structure of most of the compounds in Table 28–1 suggests that *electrostatic* or *coulombic bonding* occurs between the two *completely ionized cationic centers* of the drug and certain *anionic groups* of the receptor site; for example, replacement of one quaternary group of decamethonium by an incompletely ionized primary amine group results in a considerable weakening of potency (Barlow *et al.,* 1955). The *concentration of charge* on the nitrogen atom undoubtedly contributes also to potency; substitution of a *methyl* group by an *ethyl* or *aromatic* group dissipates the charge, particularly in the latter case, and results in a decrease in neuromuscular blocking potency; however,

with such substitutions it is difficult to distinguish between the relative importance of changes in charge density and of steric factors. Such substituents will also modify the polarity, or *hydrophilic-lipophilic balance,* of the molecule, a characteristic that has been correlated with either an increase or a decrease in competitive neuromuscular blockade.

Optical isomerism is an additional factor of considerable importance in determining potency; *d*-tubocurarine is 20 to 60 times more potent than the *l* isomer.

For both theoretical and practical reasons, the structural features that distinguish *competitive* from primarily *depolarizing* neuromuscular blocking agents have received particular attention. Although numerous exceptions can be cited to all proposals made to date in this regard, a few useful generalizations can be drawn. The *competitive* or *stabilizing* agents are for the most part relatively bulky, rigid molecules (*e.g., d*-tubocurarine, the toxiferines, β-erythroidine, gallamine, pancuronium), whereas the *depolarizing* agents (*e.g.,* decamethonium, succinylcholine) have generally a more slender, flexible structure (*see* Table 28–1).

With the elucidation of the structure of *d*-tubocurarine and the finding that the distance between the quaternary and the protonated-tertiary nitrogen atoms is approximately 12.5 Å, it has been assumed that this feature is critical for typical curariform action, although exceptions have been cited (Loewe and Harvey, 1952). With further increase in the length of the polymethylene chain of the *methonium compounds,* a second peak has been found for potency of depolarizing neuromuscular blockade at C14 to C18, representing a distance between the quaternary ammonium groups of approximately 20 Å (Barlow and Zoller, 1964). Similar peaks of neuromuscular blocking potency at 12 to 14 Å and at 20 Å between quaternary ammonium groups have been noted for various related series of blocking agents (*see* Khromov-Borisov and Michelson, 1966). These observations have led to the interesting deduction of a tetrameric arrangement of the cholinoreceptive sites.

The Cholinoceptive Site. The concept of nicotinic cholinergic receptors, with which ACh combines to initiate the end-plate potential (EPP), and where the neuromuscular blocking agents interfere with this process, is introduced in Chapter 21. Early attempts to characterize the receptors were based largely on indirect evidence from kinetic data and from studies of the SARs of agonists and antagonists. From such data, it has been deduced that the nicotinic receptor possesses an anionic group, to which the quaternary N atom of ACh and of blocking agents is attracted by coulombic forces, and a hydrogen-bonding site that reacts with the carbonyl O atoms of ACh or an equivalent atom of the blocking agents, along with an immediately adjacent nucleophilic group that can exert a dipole-dipole attraction at the carbonyl C atom of ACh. In addition, hydrophobic areas near the anionic group are presumed to attract alkyl or similar groups on the quaternary N atom by van der Waals forces (*see* Beers and Reich, 1970; Paton,

1970; Michelson and Zeimal, 1973; Goldstein *et al.,* 1974).

Direct determination of the molecular structure of receptors can now be approached by the use of affinity labeling reagents, that is, isotopically labeled compounds that combine specifically with the receptors and thus allow their identification during extraction and isolation (*see* Hammes *et al.,* 1973; Rang, 1973). An extremely useful tool of this type was provided by the discovery by C. Y. Lee and associates that an active principle of a cobra venom, α-*bungarotoxin* (a polypeptide with a molecular weight of approximately 8000), combines irreversibly and with high specificity with nicotinic receptors (Chang and Lee, 1963; Changeaux *et al.,* 1970). Reversibly bound ligands can be used with greater difficulty, but they offer the advantage of allowing the recovery of an underivatized receptor. With these technics, purification of nicotinic receptors present in high concentrations in electric organs of certain eels and rays has been achieved. The receptor molecule appears to be a lipoprotein with a subunit molecular weight of approximately 50,000. The putative receptor can be convincingly separated from acetylcholinesterase (AChE).

Radioautography, following exposure of tissue to labeled compounds, has been used to study the receptor at the skeletal muscle end-plate (MEP) (*see* Waser, 1970; Hammes *et al.,* 1973). These studies suggest that there are approximately 5×10^7 receptors per MEP, a density that could account for 20% of the membrane surface. A similar number of AChE molecules may be present.

The major question, of course, is how interaction between cholinergic agonists or antagonists and their receptor results ultimately in alterations of ionic permeability or the prevention of such. Current hypotheses envision an interaction between the receptors and *ionophores,* defined generally as macromolecular components (carriers, pores, channels) that serve to facilitate *specifically* the passive movements of ions. However, it is possible that the receptor alone possesses the molecular features necessary for the translocation of ions. Michaelson and Raftery (1974) have reconstituted a vesicular membrane system from the purified ACh receptor of *Torpedo californica* electroplax and lipids of the same organism. The reconstituted system responds to ACh and carbamylcholine with increased $^{22}Na^+$ conductance.

PHARMACOLOGICAL PROPERTIES

Skeletal Muscle. The peripheral locus of the paralytic action of curare was first adequately described by Bernard (1856, 1857). His classical experiments on the localization, as described below, are still instructively performed with the purified alkaloid, *d*-tubocurarine, by students in the pharmacological laboratory.

If the hindleg of a pithed frog is ligatured in a manner that deprives the limb of its circulation but

allows the sciatic nerve to remain free, the injection of curare into the ventral lymph sac produces typical effects in all parts of the frog except in the ligatured limb. In this unpoisoned leg, electrical stimulation of the sciatic nerve produces typical muscular contraction, whereas the opposite poisoned extremity is unresponsive to nerve stimulation. Furthermore, afferent stimulation of the sciatic nerve of the poisoned limb elicits crossed-reflex responses in the unpoisoned extremity. It is thus clear that curare, in producing the observed effects, does not act centrally (spinal cord) or on peripheral nerve, but must reach skeletal muscle in order to exert its effect. Further localization is accomplished by showing that the curarized muscle is electrically excitable when stimulated directly and that the sciatic nerve, when soaked in a solution of curare, is still capable of carrying impulses. This places the site of action at the neuromuscular junction.

Mechanism of Action. The cellular locus and mechanism of action of *d-tubocurarine* and other *competitive* neuromuscular blocking agents have been well defined by modern technics, including microiontophoretic application of drugs and intracellular recording. In brief, *d*-tubocurarine combines with the cholinoceptive sites at the postjunctional membrane and thereby blocks the transmitter action of ACh. When the drug is applied directly to the end-plate of a single isolated muscle fiber under microscopic control, the muscle cell becomes insensitive to motor-nerve impulses and to directly applied ACh; however, the end-plate region and the remainder of the muscle fiber membrane retain their normal sensitivity to the application of potassium ions, and the muscle fiber still responds to direct electrical stimulation.

The steps involved in the release of ACh by the nerve action potential (AP), and the sequential production of the postjunctional EPP, the muscle AP, and contraction have been described in Chapter 21 (page 413). During progressive curarization of a muscle, the EPP is gradually diminished in amplitude and shortened in duration, before the muscle AP is affected; when the amplitude of the EPP falls below approximately 70% of its normal value, it is insufficient to initiate the propagated muscle AP, and thus contraction does not occur in response to a single nerve impulse. *d*-Tubocurarine also partially prevents the increase and prolongation of the EPP by physostigmine and other anti-ChE agents (Eccles *et al.,* 1942; Kuffler, 1942; Fatt and Katz, 1951). Within certain concentration limits these effects provide the basis for the therapeutically useful antagonism between competitive blocking drugs and anti-ChE agents. However, large amounts of anti-ChE agents also block transmission at the end-plate, as discussed below. (Recent reviews of this field include those by Cheymol and Bourillet, 1972; Waser, 1972.)

The *depolarizing agents succinylcholine* and *decamethonium* act by a different mechanism. Their initial effect is to depolarize the membrane in the same manner as ACh but more persistently, which results in a brief period of firing manifested by transient muscular fasciculation. This phase is succeeded shortly by neuromuscular paralysis, the mechanism and even the primary site of which are still uncertain and controversial. The blockade exhibits several distinct differences from that produced by *d*-tubocurarine and related drugs; these are listed in Table 28-2.

The explanation of these distinctive features of neuromuscular blockade by the depolarizing agents appeared at one time to be provided by the discovery by Burns and Paton (1951) that, in contrast to the stabilizing action of *d*-tubocurarine on the motor end-plate, decamethonium produces an immediate and persistent depolarization of both the end-plate and the immediately adjacent area of the sarcoplasmic membrane in the gracilis muscle of the cat. Much the same result is obtained with high, paralyzing doses of ACh in the presence of an anti-ChE

agent. Thus, it was assumed that neuromuscular blockade was due to the inability of the depolarized area just beyond the end-plate to initiate propagated muscle APs in response to the continued depolarization of the end-plate itself. However, this proposal was inadequate to explain several subsequent observations, particularly the persistence of neuromuscular blockade considerably beyond the period of depolarization of the end-plate (*see* below).

Many of the characteristics of depolarizing blocking agents listed in Table 28-2 apply only to man and to the twitch ("white") muscles of the cat. In all muscles investigated in the monkey, dog, rabbit, and rat, and in the slowly contracting soleus muscle of the cat, decamethonium and succinylcholine produce a type of blockade that combines certain features of both the depolarizing and the competitive agents described above and that has some characteristics not associated with either; this type of action has been termed a "dual" mechanism by Zaimis (1953, 1959). In such cases, the depolarizing agents produce initially the characteristic fasciculations and potentiation of the maximal twitch; however, with the onset of blockade, there is a poorly sustained response to tetanic stimulation of the motor nerve, intensification of the block by *d*-tubocurarine, and antagonism by anti-ChE agents. As a unique feature in "dual" blockade, there is marked tachyphylaxis, that is, a reduction in the effect of subsequent doses of the same drug. Neither the purely depolarizing blockade observed in man nor the "dual" type obtained in certain other species has been demonstrated to change to the other type during the course

Table 28-2. COMPARISON OF COMPETITIVE (*d*-TUBOCURARINE) AND DEPOLARIZING (DECAMETHONIUM) BLOCKING AGENTS *

	d-TUBOCURARINE	DECAMETHONIUM (C10)
Effect of *d*-tubocurarine chloride administered previously	Additive	Antagonistic
Effect of decamethonium administered previously	No effect, or antagonistic	Some tachyphylaxis; usually no cumulative effect
Effect of anti-ChE agents on block	Decurarization	No antagonism
Effect on motor end-plate	Elevated threshold to ACh	Partial, persisting depolarization
Initial excitatory effect on striated muscle	None	Transient fasciculations
Character of muscle response to indirect tetanic stimulation during *partial* block	Poorly sustained contraction	Well-sustained contraction
Effect of KCl or of a tetanus on block	Transient decurarization	No antagonism
Effect of current applied to endplate region:		
—cathodal	Lessens paralysis	Intensifies paralysis
—anodal	Intensifies paralysis	Lessens paralysis
Effect of lowering muscle temperature on block	Antagonism and shortening of effect	Amplification and prolongation of effect
Effect on denervated mammalian muscle	Transient fibrillation	Contracture
Effect on avian muscle	Flaccid paralysis	Contracture, spastic paralysis
Mammalian species sensitivity	Rat $>$ Mouse $>$ Rabbit $>$ Cat	Cat $>$ Rabbit $>$ Monkey $>$ Mouse $>$ Rat
	$\dfrac{\text{Activity in cat}}{\text{Activity in rat}} \doteq 0.5$	$\dfrac{\text{Activity in cat}}{\text{Activity in rat}} \doteq 200$
Muscle selectivity (cat)	Paralyzes respiratory ("red") muscles more than limb ("white") muscles	Paralyzes respiratory muscles less than limb muscles

* Based on data in Paton and Zaimis, 1949, 1952.

of prolonged infusions *in vivo* (Zaimis, 1959), although this can be observed *in vitro*.

Most difficult to reconcile with the concept of depolarization blockade presented above are the findings of Thesleff (1955, 1958), Castillo and Katz (1957), and others on the relative durations of depolarization and of blockade recorded intracellularly following the microiontophoretic application of various agents at the motor end-plates of frog, rat, and cat muscles *in vitro*. The rapid application of ACh, decamethonium, or succinylcholine under such conditions produces a brief depolarization of the end-plate that resembles closely that obtained with stimulation of the motor nerve. When *d*-tubocurarine or gallamine is applied continuously by the same method, it causes no change in the EPP but prevents or reduces the depolarizing effect of ACh. However, with the continuous application of decamethonium, succinylcholine, or ACh for 5 to 10 seconds, the initial depolarization usually disappears almost completely, but the depolarizing effect of ACh remains blocked. Such findings have led to the concept that the *depolarization* produced by decamethonium and related drugs is succeeded under certain conditions by a *desensitization* of the receptors. However, this term illuminates little.

From a practical viewpoint it should be emphasized that, while there have been suggestions to the contrary, most of the evidence to date indicates that in *man* both decamethonium and succinylcholine produce and maintain a neuromuscular blockade that has all the characteristics of a *depolarizing* blockade, as listed in Table 28–2; this applies in particular to its *intensification* by edrophonium, neostigmine, and other anti-ChE agents that antagonize competitive block.

The observations by Masland and Wigton (1940) that the muscular fasciculation produced by the intra-arterial injection of ACh or neostigmine is accompanied by antidromic nerve impulses in the ventral roots and that both effects are blocked by curare were confirmed and amplified by Riker and associates (1957). Subsequent work by the latter investigators and others has led to the proposal that the *prejunctional motor-nerve terminal* is the primary site of action of the competitive and depolarizing neuromuscular blocking agents (*see* Riker and Okamoto, 1969). Evidence to the contrary has been presented by Karczmar (1967), Foldes (1971), and Karczmar and associates (1972). Inasmuch as fasciculation is dependent upon the synchronous contraction of an entire motor unit (*i.e.,* the 100 or so muscle fibers innervated by a single anterior horn cell), its production by axon reflexes initiated at one or more of the terminals of the same mononeurons does appear to be the most plausible explanation for this phase of the action of the depolarizing agents. However, the doses of *d*-tubocurarine that terminate this effect are far below those that are required to produce neuromuscular blockade (Standaert, 1964), and quantities of succinylcholine that induce maximal fasciculation and related excitatory effects produce only partial neuromuscular blockade (Standaert and Adams, 1965). Thus, the postjunctional membrane seems to be the primary site of blockade of transmission by drugs of both classes.

Further substantiation of this conclusion is provided by the work of Katz and Miledi (1965), Blaber (1970), and Auerbach and Betz (1971).

According to a *kinetic theory* of drug action proposed by Paton (1961), the excitatory action of a drug is determined not by the *number* of receptors occupied by it at a given moment but by the *rate* of association and dissociation of the drug with the receptors. While somewhat at variance with the concepts of Ariëns and associates (1964) and Stephenson (1956) that a drug's excitatory or inhibitory potency is determined by the proportion of receptors occupied and its *intrinsic activity,* the theory might apply to the distinction between competitive and depolarizing blocking agents. Thus, evidence has been assembled by Paton (1967) to indicate that the former have a low and the latter a high rate of dissociation from the receptors.

Many ions, drugs, and toxins block neuromuscular transmission by other mechanisms, such as interference with the synthesis or release of ACh (*see* Chapter 21); but these agents are not employed clinically for this purpose, and hence they are not considered in detail here. The sites of action and interrelationship of some of them are indicated in Figure 28–1.

Sequence and Characteristics of Paralysis. *Animals* poisoned by *d*-tubocurarine or other *competitive blocking agents* first exhibit motor weakness, and ultimately the muscles become totally flaccid and inexcitable through their motor innervation. Small, rapidly moving muscles such as those of the fingers, toes, eyes, and ears are involved before those of the limbs, neck, and trunk. Ultimately the intercostal muscles and finally the diaphragm are paralyzed, and respiration then ceases. Death is caused by hypoxia secondary to peripheral respiratory paralysis. Terminal asphyxial convulsions may appear, but these are mild owing to the almost complete muscular paralysis. Life can be saved by artificial respiration, particularly because the duration of action of *d*-tubocurarine is relatively brief. Recovery of muscles usually occurs in the reverse order to that of their paralysis, and thus the diaphragm is ordinarily the first to regain function. The action of *d*-tubocurarine is entirely reversible so that recovery is eventually complete.

When an appropriate dose of *d*-tubocurarine (10 to 15 mg) is injected *intravenously in man,* the onset of effects is very rapid. Slight dizziness and a sensation of warmth are first experienced. Difficulty in focusing and weakness in the jaw muscles are then observed, and difficulty in speech and in keeping the eyelids open soon follows. Ptosis, strabismus, diplopia, dysarthria, and dysphagia are indicative of the

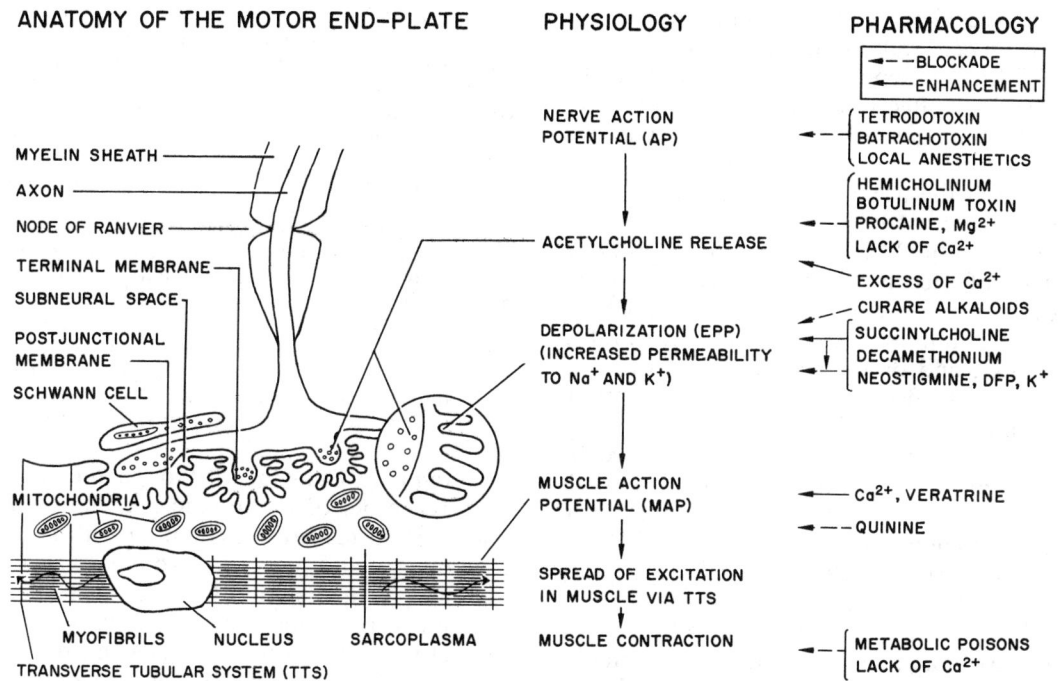

ANATOMY OF THE MOTOR END-PLATE PHYSIOLOGY PHARMACOLOGY

Figure 28-1. *Sites of action of agents at the neuromuscular junction and adjacent structures.*

The anatomy of the motor end-plate, shown at the left, and the sequence of events from liberation of acetylcholine (ACh) by the nerve action potential (AP) to contraction of the muscle fiber, indicated in the middle column, are described in some detail in Chapter 21. The modification of these processes by various agents is shown on the right; the dashed arrows indicate inhibition or block; the solid arrows, enhancement or activation. The circled insert is an enlargement of the indicated structures. (Modified from Waser, 1958.)

early involvement of the small muscles of the head and neck. Relaxation of the small muscles of the middle ear improves acuity of hearing for low tones. The limbs feel heavy and are difficult to move. Respiratory movements become more diaphragmatic as the intercostal muscles are involved. Despite adequate artificially controlled respiration, "shortness of breath" is experienced. The accumulation of unswallowed saliva in the pharynx may prove most annoying and causes the sensation of choking. Head movement soon becomes impossible, and ultimately the ability to move the limbs and trunk is lost. Throughout the stage of complete muscular paralysis, consciousness and sensorium remain entirely undisturbed (*see* below). The experience is definitely unpleasant. Facial and diaphragmatic muscles are the first to recover, followed in order by those of the legs, arms, shoulder girdle, trunk, larynx, hands, feet, and pharynx.

The *small motor-nerve system* in mammals innervates the intrafusal fibers of muscle spindles; when the intrafusal fibers shorten, afferent volleys are discharged from the activated spindles and initiate spinal reflexes that enhance skeletal muscle tone. *d*-Tubocurarine has been shown to block the responses of intrafusal fibers to small motor-nerve stimulation and to ACh, just as it blocks the parallel responses of ordinary skeletal muscle fibers; whether

there is selectivity of this action has not been established. (*See* Hunt and Kuffler, 1950; Smith, 1963.)

Prior to causing paralysis, the *depolarizing agents* decamethonium and succinylcholine evoke transient muscular fasciculation, observed especially over the chest and abdomen; however, these are uncommon in the anesthetized patient. As the paralytic effect progresses, the neck, arm, and leg muscles are involved at a time when there is only slight weakness of facial, masticatory, lingual, pharyngeal, and laryngeal muscles; at this stage, respiratory muscular weakness is not pronounced and vital capacity is reduced only 25%. On the basis of the foregoing pattern, it has been claimed that *decamethonium,* in contrast with *d*-tubocurarine, causes muscular relaxation in doses that spare the respiratory muscles. While this claim is supported by certain experimental studies, it still remains to be shown conclusively that the sparing of respiration alleged to occur in certain species of animals obtains in man (*see* Unna *et al.,* 1950; Foldes, 1966; Grob, 1967).

With the exception of succinylcholine, the foregoing effects of the neuromuscular blocking agents become apparent within a few minutes after the intravenous administration of the usual clinical dose and persist over the course of 20 to 40 minutes.

After a single intravenous dose of 10 to 30 mg of succinylcholine, muscular fasciculation ensues briefly; then relaxation occurs within 1 minute, becomes maximal within 2 minutes, and disappears as a rule within 5 minutes. Transient apnea usually occurs at the time of maximal effect. Muscular relaxation of longer duration can be achieved by repeated injections at appropriate intervals or by continuous intravenous infusion. Even after discontinuance of an infusion, the effects of the drug usually disappear rapidly because of its rapid hydrolysis by the pseudocholinesterase of the plasma and liver. The degree of muscular relaxation can usually be altered within 30 to 60 seconds by a change in the rate of infusion. Muscle soreness may follow the administration of succinylcholine. The duration of action of succinylcholine can be greatly enhanced and the initial muscular fasciculation practically abolished by the prior administration of *hexafluorenium bromide,* 0.4 mg/kg, intravenously, a drug that has the combined actions of inhibition of pseudocholinesterase and mild, competitive neuromuscular blockade (Torda *et al.,* 1967).

Central Nervous System. *d*-Tubocurarine and other quaternary neuromuscular blocking agents are virtually devoid of central effects following the intravenous administration of ordinary clinical doses because of their inability to penetrate effectively the blood-brain barrier. On the other hand, the tertiary-amine erythrina alkaloids cause central depression in clinical doses. However, ever since Brodie stated in 1812 that "woorara acts on the brain," the possibility of curare having central effects has been a subject of speculation and experimentation.

The most decisive experiment performed to settle the problem whether curare significantly affects central functions in the dose range employed clinically is that of Smith and associates (1947). Smith (an anesthesiologist) permitted himself to receive intravenously two and one-half times the amount of

d-tubocurarine necessary for paralysis of all skeletal muscles. Adequate respiratory exhange was maintained by artificial respiration with oxygen. Included among the various functions continuously or repeatedly examined were the EEG, sensorium, pain threshold, mentation and memory, vision, smell and hearing, neurological signs, ECG, pulse rate, respiration, and blood pressure. At no time was there any evidence of lapse of consciousness, impairment of memory, clouding of sensorium, analgesia, disturbance of special senses, or alteration in the resting EEG or its response to pattern vision. No evidence of central respiratory or vasomotor stimulation was observed. It was concluded that *d*-tubocurarine given intravenously even in large doses has no significant central stimulant, depressant, or analgesic effect in man, and that its sole action of value in anesthesia is the peripheral paralytic effect on skeletal muscle.

Autonomic Ganglia. Although the nicotinic receptors of autonomic ganglion cells have certain features in common with those at the motor end-plate, the two types are not identical, as discussed in Chapter 21. Hence, neuromuscular blocking agents vary with respect to their relative potencies in producing ganglionic blockade. Just as at the motor end-plate, ganglionic blockade by *d*-tubocurarine and other stabilizing drugs is antagonized effectively by anti-ChE agents, such as neostigmine; however, in ganglia, the antagonism is reinforced by the additional action of endogenous ACh at the muscarinic receptors of the ganglion cells, as described in Chapters 22 and 27.

At the doses of *d*-tubocurarine and dimethyl tubocurarine employed clinically, some degree of blockade is probably produced, both at autonomic ganglia and at the adrenal medulla, which results in a fall in blood pressure. Gallamine in clinically useful doses blocks selectively the cardiac vagus nerve, but whether this occurs at the ganglionic or at a more peripheral site is uncertain; this action results in sinus tachycardia and occasionally in other cardiac arrhythmias and hypertension. Pancuronium and alcuronium have minimal ganglionic effects at ordinary clinical doses.

Of the *depolarizing agents,* decamethonium rarely exhibits effects attributable to ganglionic blockade; although instances of bradycardia, tachycardia, and even cardiac arrest have been reported, it is generally difficult if not impossible to dissociate such occurrences from the actions of the anesthetic agent or other circumstances. Succinylcholine, on the other hand, more frequently exhibits cardiovascular effects that are probably due to the successive stimulation of vagal ganglia (manifest by bradycardia, which may be severe and cause hypotension) and of sympathetic ganglia (resulting in hypertension and tachycardia). With extremely high doses, ganglionic blockade may ensue (*see* Foldes, 1966; Dijl, 1972).

Histamine Release. Following the demonstration by Alam and coworkers (1939) that histamine is released from muscle by the intra-arterial injection of curare in dogs, Comroe and Dripps (1946) discovered that *d*-tubocurarine produces typical histamine-like wheals when injected intracutaneously or intra-arterially in man. They suggested that certain phenomena (bronchospasm, hypotension, excessive bronchial and salivary secretion) observed in the clinical use of *d*-tubocurarine might be caused by the release of histamine, and that antihistaminic drugs might be used to advantage to overcome such effects. Subsequently, many workers verified and extended these findings and conclusions. The decreased coagulability of the blood that has been noted after *d*-tubocurarine is probably due to the concomitant release of heparin from the mast cells. Dimethyl tubocurarine and succinylcholine likewise cause histamine release to a significant degree. Decamethonium and gallamine apparently release detectable amounts of histamine only when administered in very high doses. Pancuronium and alcuronium are practically devoid of histamine-releasing activity following ordinary doses.

Cardiovascular System. The rapid intravenous injection of large doses of *d*-tubocurarine in man may cause a fall in blood pressure, at times precipitous. The major cause of the hypotension is peripheral vasodilatation from curare-induced release of histamine, together with sympathetic ganglionic blockade, as discussed above. An additional factor in the production of cardiovascular collapse is diminished venous return due to loss of skeletal muscle tone, diminished respiratory excursion, and the use of intermittent positive pressure in the airway for the purpose of restoring respiratory adequacy. A further complication can arise through the release of epinephrine from the adrenal medulla by histamine.

The cardiovascular and certain other side effects of *benzoquinonium* are due primarily to its anti-ChE activity, which is approximately one fourth that of neostigmine. They include bradycardia, hypotension, and possible circulatory collapse, and require complete atropinization as a precautionary measure; ephedrine is useful in cases of syncope.

Miscellaneous Actions. Most of the additional side effects of the neuromuscular blocking agents are probably based on the ganglionic and histamine-releasing actions already considered. Ganglionic blockade is chiefly responsible for the decreased tone and motility of the gastrointestinal tract and for the blockade of the cardiac vagus produced by high doses of *d*-tubocurarine. Decamethonium and succinylcholine exhibit muscarinic actions, but only in extremely high doses; the latter drug may cause an increase in intraocular tension. The anti-ChE activity of *benzoquinonium* has been discussed. Both the competitive and the depolarizing agents have been reported to release potassium from intracellular sites; this may be a factor in the production of prolonged apnea that has been noted in patients· who receive these drugs while in electrolyte imbalance (Dripps, 1953). Such alterations in the distribution of potassium may be of particular importance in patients with congestive heart failure who are receiving digitalis or diuretics.

Synergisms and Antagonisms. The interactions between the competitive and depolarizing neuromuscular blocking agents have already been considered. From a clinical viewpoint, the most important pharmacological interactions of these drugs are with certain *general anesthetics,* certain *antibiotics,* and *anti-ChE compounds* used as "decurarizing agents."

Ether exerts a stabilizing effect on the postjunctional membrane and, therefore, acts synergistically with the *competitive blocking agents,* including benzoquinonium. Consequently, when such blocking drugs are employed for muscular relaxation as adjuncts to ether anesthesia, their doses should be reduced to a range of one third to one half the standard doses employed. *Halothane, cyclopropane, fluroxene, methoxyflurane,* and *enflurane* likewise act synergistically with the competitive blocking agents, but to a lesser extent (*see* Foldes, 1966).

Streptomycin in sufficiently high doses was shown by Brazil and Corrado (1957) to produce neuromuscular blockade in much the same manner as do magnesium ions, by inhibition of ACh release from the preganglionic terminal (through competition with calcium ions) and to a lesser extent by stabilization of the postjunctional membrane. The blockade is antagonized by calcium salts, but only inconsistently by anti-ChE agents. This action is shared to varying degrees by several additional *aminoglycoside antibiotics,* particularly *neomycin* and *kanamycin,* and to a lesser extent by gentamicin, viomycin, and paromomycin. The *tetracycline antibiotics* can also produce neuromuscular block, possibly by chelation of calcium ions. Additional antibiotics that have neuromuscular blocking action, through unidentified mechanisms, include the *polypeptides* (*polymyxins A* and *B, colistin*) and *lincomycin.* (*See* review by Pittinger and Adamson, 1972.) Accordingly, when neuromuscular blocking agents are to be administered to patients who are receiving any of these antibiotics, special consideration should be given to the dose and to the judicious use of a calcium salt as an antagonist if recovery of spontaneous respiration is delayed.

Since the anti-ChE agents neostigmine and edrophonium preserve endogenous ACh and also act directly on the neuromuscular junction, they can be employed as "decurarizing" agents in the treatment of overdosage with *d*-tubocurarine and related competitive blocking compounds. Because of its very potent anti-ChE activity, benzoquinonium is not antagonized satisfactorily by these agents, and its blocking action may even be intensified. Likewise, the anti-ChE agents generally show a synergism with the depolarizing blocking drugs and a consequent increase in paralysis. Claims that the depolarizing drugs exhibit a "dual" action in man, with eventual susceptibility to antagonism by edrophonium and neostigmine, require considerable substantiation before this procedure can be recommended. The use of *hexafluorenium*, a selective inhibitor of pseudocholinesterase, to prolong the blocking action of succinylcholine has been mentioned. Patients receiving other anti-ChE agents will similarly show greatly potentiated responses to succinylcholine.

Epinephrine and *norepinephrine* exert an anticurare effect, probably by increasing the amount of ACh released at the nerve terminal (*see* Bowman and Nott, 1969).

Miscellaneous drugs that may have significant interactions with either competitive or depolarizing neuromuscular blocking agents include *trimethaphan, hexamethonium, narcotic analgesics, procaine, lidocaine, quinidine, phenelzine, propranolol, magnesium salts, corticosteroids, digitalis glycosides,* and *diuretics* (*see* Dijl, 1972; Hansten, 1973).

Toxicology. Poisoning from the neuromuscular blocking agents is almost always the result of clinical overdosage or their injudicious use. The important untoward responses are *prolonged apnea, cardiovascular collapse,* and those resulting from *histamine release.*

Failure of respiration to become adequate in the postoperative period after use of these relaxants may represent cause-effect or coincidence. Coincidental possibilities for subnormal alveolar ventilation include the inhibitory effects of a foreign body in the respiratory tract (almost always the inflated cuff on an endotracheal tube), decreased arterial carbon dioxide tension secondary to hyperventilation during the operative procedure, or the neuromuscular depressant effect of excessive amounts of neostigmine used to reverse the action of the competitive blocking drugs. Directly related factors may also include alterations in body temperature (an increased temperature potentiating the "curare-like" drugs, and a decreased temperature exerting the same effect on the action of the depolarizing substances); electrolyte imbalance (*e.g.*, hypokalemia prolonging and intensifying the effect of the competitive

blockers); decreased plasma cholinesterase (*e.g.*, congenital deficiency or liver disease, resulting in reduction in the rate of destruction of succinylcholine); the presence of latent myasthenia gravis or of malignant disease such as oat-cell carcinoma of the lung; reduced blood flow to skeletal muscles causing delayed removal of the blocking drugs; decreased elimination of the relaxants secondary to reduced renal function; and interactions with any of the drugs noted above. Great care should be taken when administering muscle relaxants to dehydrated or desperately ill patients. Prolongation of drug effects has also been noted in patients with collagen diseases, familial periodic paralysis, porphyria, and thyroid disorders (Dijl, 1972).

A severe rapid rise in temperature, which may be accompanied by marked neuromuscular rigidity, has occurred occasionally in patients receiving *halothane* and *succinylcholine,* and more rarely with other combinations of general anesthetics and neuromuscular blocking agents. This condition, known as *malignant hyperthermia,* has a familial tendency. It should be treated by rapid cooling, 100% oxygen inhalation, and control of the acidosis that is generally present; intravenous procainamide has also been reported to be effective (Dijl, 1972; Gordon *et al.*, 1973).

Treatment of respiratory paralysis should be by positive-pressure artificial respiration with oxygen and maintenance of a patent airway until the complete recovery of normal respiration is assured. With the competitive blocking agents, this may be hastened by the administration of neostigmine methylsulfate (1 to 3 mg, intravenously, combined with 0.6 to 1.2 mg of atropine sulfate) or edrophonium (10 mg, intravenously, repeated as required). Other measures include direct treatment of the additional causative factors listed above.

Neostigmine antagonizes only the skeletal muscular blocking action of the competitive blocking agents, and it may aggravate such side effects as hypotension or bronchospasm. Sympathomimetic amines may be given to support the blood pressure. The position of the patient should be such as to favor the return of venous blood from the flaccid musculature. Antihistamines are of definite benefit in counteracting histamine-like reactions only if administered prior to the blocking agent.

Absorption, Fate, and Excretion. Quaternary ammonium neuromuscular blocking agents are very poorly and irregularly absorbed from the gastrointestinal tract. *d*-Tubocurarine and its derivatives are inactive after oral administration, unless huge doses are ingested; this fact was well known to the South American Indians, who ate with impunity the flesh of game killed with curare-poisoned arrows. Absorption is quite adequate from intramuscular sites, a fact made use of in infants in whom intravenous injection may be difficult to accomplish.

When a single moderate dose of *d*-tubocurarine is injected intravenously, the action begins to wear off in about 20 minutes, yet some residual effect is still discernible after 2 to 4 hours or more. However, when a second dose is given as late as 24 hours after a first, less drug is needed for an equivalent degree of paralysis. The brief duration of paralysis following the initial dose is probably due chiefly to redistribution of the drug; when repeated doses are administered, the tissues become saturated and factors of degradation and excretion then directly influence intensity and duration of action. In man, about one third of an administered dose of *d*-tubocurarine is excreted in the urine over a period of several hours, independent of dose and parenteral route of injection, and a variable amount is metabolized (Cohen *et al.*, 1967). In patients with renal insufficiency, cumulation may occur following multiple doses (Gibaldi *et al.*, 1972). For practical purposes, no significant amount of *d*-tubocurarine crosses the placenta late in pregnancy to reach the fetus.

The distribution and elimination of *dimethyl tubocurarine* are probably similar to those of *d*-tubocurarine, although the duration of action of the former drug is somewhat shorter. The metabolism of *alcuronium* is not yet elucidated. *Gallamine* and *decamethonium* are almost entirely excreted by the kidney, with no apparent metabolic degradation. Approximately 75% of an injected dose of *benzoquinonium* is excreted unchanged.

The extremely brief duration of action of *succinylcholine* is due largely to its rapid hydrolysis by the pseudocholinesterase of liver and plasma. The initial metabolite, *succinylmonocholine,* has a much weaker, predominantly competitive type of neuromuscular blocking action. It is, in turn, hydrolyzed more slowly to succinic acid and choline; approximately 10% of the original drug is excreted unchanged. Among the occasional patients who exhibit prolonged apnea following the administration of succinylcholine, a considerable number have been found to have an atypical plasma cholinesterase or a deficiency of the enzyme, due to a genetic factor, hepatic disease, or a nutritional disturbance; however, in some the level of the enzyme in the plasma has been normal (Kalow and Gunn, 1957; Kalow, 1965).

Preparations, Routes of Administration, and Dosage. Neuromuscular blocking agents are administered parenterally and nearly always *intravenously*. Detailed information on *dosage* can be found in anesthesiology textbooks (*see* Foldes, 1966; Siker *et al.*, 1969) and in the package inserts accompanying the marketed drugs. Only examples of dose schedules are given below. No categorical statements can be made about dosage, and each patient presents numerous individualized requirements that vary considerably with the many factors influencing the neuromuscular blockade produced by these agents. *The neuromuscular blocking agents are potentially hazardous drugs. Consequently, they should be administered to patients only by anesthesiologists and other clinicians who have had extensive training in their use and in a setting where facilities for respiratory and cardiovascular resuscitation are immediately at hand.*

Tubocurarine Chloride, U.S.P. (*d-tubocurarine chloride;* TUBARINE), is marketed as a sterile solution containing 3 or 15 mg/ml. The solution containing 15 mg/ml should always be diluted before injection. The use of *d*-tubocurarine to produce muscular relaxation for surgical purposes may be cited as an example of one dose schedule employed. In conjunction with usual preanesthetic medication and light surgical anesthesia other than with ether, 6 to 9 mg of the drug may be given as a single intravenous injection in adults. One half of this dose may be given after 3 to 5 minutes, if necessary, and small supplements employed later, as required. If *ether* is used, only one third the recommended dose should be given; with certain other general anesthetics, intermediate doses should be employed.

Dimethyl Tubocurarine Iodide, N.F. (METUBINE), is available as a solution containing 2 mg/ml. Since this drug is approximately three times as potent as *d*-tubocurarine in man, the doses employed are only one third those of the parent alkaloid.

Gallamine Triethiodide, U.S.P. (FLAXEDIL), is available as a sterile solution containing 20 or 100 mg/ml. For muscular relaxation in conjunction with surgical anesthesia, gallamine triethiodide is usually injected intravenously in a dose not exceeding 1.0 mg/kg of body weight, and an additional amount (0.5 to 1.0 mg/kg) may be given after 40 to 50 minutes, if necessary.

Succinylcholine Chloride, U.S.P. (ANECTINE, QUELICIN, SCOLINE, SUCOSTRIN, SUX-CERT), is marketed as a sterile powder (0.5 and 1.0 g) and as a sterile solution containing 20, 50, or 100 mg/ml. For brief surgical procedures in adults, the usual intravenous dose is 20 mg, but the optimal dose varies considerably (10 to 30 mg or more). The drug is given by intravenous drip infusion for more prolonged procedures, in order to obtain sustained muscular relaxation; the dose varies widely from patient to patient (0.5 to 5.0 mg or more per minute), and must be highly individualized. Moment-to-moment control of relaxation can be obtained by careful attention to the rate of infusion and the response of the patient.

Hexafluorenium Bromide, N.F. (MYLAXEN; hexamethylenebis [9-fluorenyldimethylammonium]), is a selective inhibitor of plasma cholinesterase with mild competitive neuromuscular blocking potency. It is given to prolong the blocking action of *succinylcholine* and to minimize the fasciculation that occurs prior to neuromuscular block with this agent. The drug is available in a solution in 10-ml vials (20 mg/ml). Following an intravenous dose of hexafluorenium of 0.4 mg/kg (not to exceed a total dose of 36 mg), the initial dose of succinylcholine is 0.2 mg/kg, intravenously (not to exceed a total dose of 18 mg), which causes muscular relaxation for 20 to 30 minutes.

Decamethonium Bromide, N.F. (SYNCURINE), is marketed as a sterile solution containing 1 mg/ml. The initial intravenous dose in adults varies from 0.5 to 3.0 mg, injected at the rate of 0.5 mg per minute. Supplements may be injected at 10- to 30-minute intervals, if required.

Pancuronium bromide (PAVULON) is available in ampuls containing 2 mg/ml. The usual intravenous dose is 0.04 to 0.08 mg/kg.

Alcuronium chloride (diallylbisnortoxiferin chloride, ALLOFERIN) is provided in ampuls containing 5 mg/ml; the recommended intravenous dose is 10 to 15 mg. The drug is not yet marketed in the United States.

THERAPEUTIC USES

The main clinical use of the neuromuscular blocking agents is as an *adjuvant in surgical anesthesia* to obtain relaxation of skeletal muscle, particularly of the abdominal wall, so that operative manipulations are facilitated. With muscular relaxation no longer dependent upon general anesthesia, a much lighter level of anesthesia suffices.

The drugs are also of value in various *orthopedic procedures,* such as the correction of dislocations and the alignment of fractures. They have also been used to advantage to facilitate *laryngoscopy, bronchoscopy,* and *esophagoscopy,* usually in combination with general anesthesia.

Use to Prevent Trauma in Shock Therapy. The chemoconvulsive or electroconvulsive therapy of psychiatric disorders is occasionally complicated by trauma to the patient; the grand mal seizures induced may cause dislocations or fractures. Inasmuch as the muscular component of the convulsion is not essential for benefit to be obtained from the procedure, various means have been tried to "soften" the overt motor manifestation of the seizure. Among these is the use of neuromuscular blocking agents and thiopental. The combination of the blocking drug, the anesthetic agent, and postictal depression usually results in respiratory depression or temporary apnea. An endotracheal tube and oxygen should always be available, and the previously described precautions must be rigidly observed. An oropharyngeal airway should be inserted as soon as the jaw muscles relax (after the seizure) and provision made to prevent aspiration of mucus and saliva. Since the introduction of curare for this purpose in 1940, practically all the neuromuscular blocking agents have been similarly employed. Succinylcholine is now most often used because of the brevity of its effect.

Miscellaneous Uses. *d*-Tubocurarine has been sporadically employed for its "lissive" action in the symptomatic therapy of a variety of *spastic disorders,* but the results have been disappointing. Curare has had sporadic clinical trial for the symptomatic control of muscular spasms in *acute convulsive states,* such as *tetanus, status epilepticus, convulsant drug intoxication,* and *other convulsions* (e.g., following the bite of the *black widow spider*); its major limitation in such conditions is the narrow margin between the dose that affords relief and that which produces respiratory paralysis.

Diagnostic Uses. Curare is of value for the *differentiation between muscle spasm and organic changes in joints* that exhibit limitation of passive motion. The drug can also be employed diagnostically for the *detection of pain due to nerve-root compression* masked by painful spasm of muscles involved in protective splinting. The use of *d*-tubocurarine to assist in the *diagnosis of myasthenia gravis* is presented in Chapter 22.

Alam, M.; Anrep, G. V.; Barsoum, G. S.; Talaat, M.; and Wieninger, E. Liberation of histamine from the skeletal muscle by curare. *J. Physiol., Lond.,* **1939**, *95,* 148–158.

Auerbach, A., and Betz, W. Does curare affect transmitter release? *J. Physiol., Lond.,* **1971**, *213,* 691–705.

Barlow, R. B.; Blaschko, H.; Himms, J. M.; and Trendelenburg, U. Observations on Ω-amino-polymethylene trimethylammonium compounds. *Br. J. Pharmac. Chemother.*, **1955**, *10,* 116–123.

Barlow, R. B., and Ing, H. R. Curare-like action of polymethylene *bis*-quaternary ammonium salts. *Br. J. Pharmac. Chemother.*, **1948**, *3,* 298–304.

Barlow, R. B., and Zoller, A. Some effects of long chain polymethylene bis-onium salts on junctional transmission in the peripheral nervous system. *Br. J. Pharmac. Chemother.*, **1964**, *23,* 131–150.

Beers, W. H., and Reich, E. Structure and activity of acetylcholine. *Nature, Lond.,* **1970**, *228,* 917–922.

Bennett, A. E. Preventing traumatic complications in convulsive shock therapy by curare. *J. Am. med. Ass.,* **1940**, *114,* 322–324.

Bernard, C. Analyse physiologique des propriétés des systèmes musculaire et nerveux au moyer du curare. *C.r. hebd. Séanc. Acad. Sci., Paris,* **1856**, *43,* 825–829.

Blaber, L. C. The effect of facilitatory concentrations of decamethonium on the storage and release of transmitter at the neuromuscular junction of the cat. *J. Pharmac. exp. Ther.,* **1970**, *175,* 664–672.

Brazil, O. V., and Corrado, A. P. The curariform action of streptomycin. *J. Pharmac. exp. Ther.,* **1957**, *120,* 452–459.

Buckett, W. R.; Marjoribanks, C. E. B.; Marwick, F. A.; and Morton, M. B. The pharmacology of pancuronium bromide (Org. NA97), a new potent steroidal neuromuscular blocking agent. *Br. J. Pharmac. Chemother.,* **1968**, *32,* 671–682.

Burns, B. D., and Paton, W. D. M. Depolarization of the motor end-plate by decamethonium and acetylcholine. *J. Physiol., Lond.,* **1951**, *115,* 41–73.

Castillo, J. del, and Katz, B. A comparison of acetylcholine and stable depolarizing agents. *Proc. R. Soc., B,* **1957**, *146,* 362–368.

Chang, C. C., and Lee, C. Y. Isolation of neurotoxins from the venom of *Bungarus multicinctus* and their modes of neuromuscular blocking action. *Archs int. Pharmacodyn. Thér.,* **1963**, *144,* 241–257.

Changeux, J.-P.; Kasai, M.; and Lee, C. Y. Use of a snake venom toxin to characterize the cholinergic receptor protein. *Proc. natn. Acad. Sci. U.S.A.,* **1970**, *67,* 1241–1247.

Cohen, E. N.; Brewer, H. W.; and Smith, D. The metabolism and excretion of *d*-tubocurarine-H³. *Anesthesiology,* **1967**, *28,* 309–317.

Comroe, J. H., Jr., and Dripps, R. D. The histamine-like action of curare and tubocurarine injected intracutaneously and intra-arterially in man. *Anesthesiology,* **1946**, *7,* 260–262.

Crum Brown, A., and Fraser, T. R. On the connection between chemical constitution and physiological action. Part I. On the physiological action of the salts of the ammonium bases, derived from strychnia, brucia, thebaia, codeia, morphia, and nicotia. *Trans. R. Soc. Edinb.,* **1868**, *25,* 151–203.

———. Part II. On the physiological action of the ammonium bases derived from atropia and conia. *Ibid.,* **1869**, *25,* 693–739.

Dripps, R. D. Abnormal respiratory responses to various "curare" drugs during surgical anesthesia: incidence, etiology and treatment. *Ann. Surg.,* **1953**, *137,* 145–155.

Eccles, J. C.; Katz, B.; and Kuffler, S. W. Effect of eserine on neuromuscular transmission. *J. Neurophysiol.,* **1942**, *5,* 211–230.

Everett, A. J.; Lowe, L. A.; and Wilkinson, S. Revision of the structure of (+)-tubocurarine chloride and (+)-chondrocurine. *Chem. Commun.,* **1970**, 1020–1021.

Fatt, P., and Katz, B. An analysis of the end-plate potential recorded with an intra-cellular electrode. *J. Physiol., Lond.,* **1951**, *115,* 320–369.

Folkers, K., and Unna, K. Erythrina alkaloids. V. Comparative curare-like potencies of species of the genus *Erythrina. J. Am. pharm. Ass., Sci. Ed.,* **1939**, *28,* 1019–1028.

Gibaldi, M.; Levy, G.; and Hayton, W. L. Tubocurarine and renal failure. *Br. J. Anaesth.,* **1972**, *44,* 163–165.

Griffith, H. R., and Johnson, G. E. The use of curare in general anesthesia. *Anesthesiology,* **1942**, *3,* 418–420.

Hoppe, J. O. A pharmacological investigation of 2,5-*bis*-(3-diethylaminopropylamino) benzoquinone-*bis*-benzylchloride (WIN 2747): a new curarimimetic drug. *J. Pharmac. exp. Ther.,* **1950**, *100,* 333–345.

Hunt, R., and Taveau, R. M. On the physiological action of certain choline derivatives and new methods for detecting choline. *Br. med. J.,* **1906**, *2,* 1788–1791.

Kalow, W., and Gunn, D. R. The relation between dose of succinylcholine and duration of apnea in man. *J. Pharmac. exp. Ther.,* **1957**, *120,* 203–214.

Katz, B., and Miledi, R. Propagation of electric activity in motor nerve terminals. *Proc. R. Soc., B,* **1965**, *161,* 453–482.

King, H. Curare alkaloids. I. Tubocurarine. *J. chem. Soc.,* **1935**, 1381–1389.

Kuffler, S. W. Further study on transmission in an isolated nerve-muscle fibre preparation. *J. Neurophysiol.,* **1942**, *5,* 309–322.

Loewe, S., and Harvey, S. C. Equidistance concept and structure-activity relationship of curarizing drugs. *Naunyn-Schmiedebergs Arch. exp. Path. Pharmak.,* **1952**, *214,* 214–226.

Masland, R. L., and Wigton, R. S. Nerve activity accompanying fasciculation produced by prostigmin. *J. Neurophysiol.,* **1940**, *3,* 269–275.

Michaelson, D. M., and Raftery, M. A. Purified acetylcholine receptor: its reconstitution to a chemically excitable membrane. *Proc. natn. Acad. Sci. U.S.A.,* **1974**, *71,* 4768–4772.

Paton, W. D. M., and Zaimis, E. J. The pharmacological actions of polymethylene bistrimethylammonium salts. *Br. J. Pharmac. Chemother.,* **1949**, *4,* 381–400.

Riker, W. F.; Roberts, J.; Standaert, F. G.; and Fujimoru, H. The motor nerve terminal as the primary focus for drug-induced facilitation of neuromuscular transmission. *J. Pharmac. exp. Ther.,* **1957**, *121,* 286–312.

Smith, S. M.; Brown, H. O.; Toman, J. E. P.; and Goodman, L. S. The lack of cerebral effects of *d*-tubocurarine. *Anesthesiology,* **1947**, *8,* 1–14.

Standaert, F. G. The action of *d*-tubocurarine on the motor nerve terminal. *J. Pharmac. exp. Ther.,* **1964**, *143,* 181–186.

Standaert, F. G., and Adams, J. E. The actions of succinylcholine on the mammalian motor nerve terminal. *J. Pharmac. exp. Ther.,* **1965**, *149,* 113–123.

Stephenson, R. P. A modification of receptor theory. *Br. J. Pharmac. Chemother.,* **1956**, *11,* 379–393.

Thesleff, S. The mode of neuromuscular block caused by acetylcholine, nicotine, decamethonium and succinylcholine. *Acta physiol. scand.,* **1955**, *34,* 218–231.

———. A study of the interaction between neuromuscular blocking agents and acetylcholine at the mammalian motor end-plate. *Acta anaesth. scand.,* **1958**, *2,* 69–79.

Torda, T. A. G.; Foldes, F. F.; Bailey, M. B.; Klonymus, D. H.; and Kuwabara, S. The interactions of neuromuscular blocking agents in man: the role of hexafluorenium. *Anesthesiology,* **1967**, *28,* 1010–1019.

Unna, K. R.; Pelikan, E. W.; Macfarlane, D. W.; Cazort, R. J.; Sadove, M. S.; Nelson, J. T.; and Drucker, A. P. Evaluation of curarizing drugs in man. I. Potency, duration of action, and effects on vital capacity of *d*-tubocurarine, dimethyl-*d*-tubocurarine, and decamethylene-*bis* (trimethylammonium bromide). *J. Pharmac. exp. Ther.,* **1950**, *98,* 318–329.

Waser, P. Pharmakologie der Muskelendplatten. *Schweizer Arch. Neurol. Psychiat.,* **1958**, *82,* 298–319.

West, R. Curare in man. *Proc. R. Soc. Med.,* **1932**, *25,* 1107–1116.

Zaimis, E. J. Motor end-plate differences as a determining factor in the mode of action of neuromuscular blocking substances. *J. Physiol., Lond.*, **1953**, *122*, 238–251.

Monographs and Reviews

Ariëns, E. J.; Simonis, A. M.; and van Rossum, J. M. Drug-receptor interaction: interaction of one or more drugs with one receptor system. In, *Molecular Pharmacology*. (Ariëns, E. J., ed.) Academic Press, Inc., New York, **1964**, pp. 119–286.

Bernard, C. *Leçons sur les effets des substances toxiques et médicamenteuses.* J.-B. Baillière et Fils, Paris, **1857**.

Bovet, D. Synthetic inhibitors of neuromuscular transmission, chemical structures and structure activity relationships. In, *Neuromuscular Blocking and Stimulating Agents*, Vol. 1. *International Encyclopedia of Pharmacology and Therapeutics*, Sect. 14. (Cheymol, J., ed.) Pergamon Press, Ltd., Oxford, **1972**, pp. 243–294.

Bovet, D.; Bovet-Nitti, F.; and Marini-Bettòlo, G. B. (eds.). *Curare and Curare-like Agents.* Elsevier Publishing Co., Amsterdam, **1959**.

Bowman, W. C., and Nott, M. W. Actions of sympathomimetic amines and their antagonists on skeletal muscle. *Pharmac. Rev.*, **1969**, *21*, 27–72. (385 references.)

Cavallito, C. J. Structure-action relations throwing light on the receptor. In, *Curare and Curare-like Agents* (a Ciba Foundation study group). (De Reuck, A. V. S., ed.) Little, Brown & Co., Boston, **1962**, pp. 55–70.

——. Bonding characteristics of acetylcholine simulants and antagonists and cholinergic receptors. *Ann. N.Y. Acad. Sci.*, **1967**, *144*, 900–912.

Cheymol, J., and Bourillet, F. Inhibitors of post-synaptic receptors. In, *Neuromuscular Blocking and Stimulating Agents*, Vol. 1. *International Encyclopedia of Pharmacology and Therapeutics*, Sect. 14. (Cheymol, J., ed.) Pergamon Press, Ltd., Oxford, **1972**, pp. 297–356.

Dijl, W., van. Neuromuscular blocking agents. In, *Side Effects of Drugs*, Vol. 7. (Meyler, L., and Herxheimer, A., eds.) Excerpta Medica, Amsterdam, **1972**, pp. 209–223.

Foldes, F. F. (ed.). *Muscle Relaxants.* F. A. Davis Co., Philadelphia, **1966**.

Foldes, F. F. Presynaptic aspects of neuromuscular transmission and block. *Anaesthetist*, **1971**, *20*, 6–19.

Gill, R. C. *White Waters and Black Magic.* Henry Holt & Co., New York, **1940**.

Goldstein, A.; Aronow, L.; and Kalman, S. M. *Principles of Drug Action: The Basis of Pharmacology*, 2nd ed. John Wiley & Sons, Inc., New York, **1974**.

Gordon, R. A.; Britt, B. A.; and Kalow, E. (eds.). *International Symposium on Malignant Hyperthermia.* Charles C Thomas, Pub., Springfield, Ill., **1973**.

Grob, D. Neuromuscular blocking drugs. In, *Physiological Pharmacology.* Vol. 3, *The Nervous System—Part C: Autonomic Nervous System Drugs.* (Root, W. S., and Hofmann, F. G., eds.) Academic Press, Inc., New York, **1967**, pp. 389–460.

Hammes, G. G.; Molinoff, P. B.; and Bloom, F. E. Receptor biophysics and biochemistry. *Neurosci. Res. Prog. Bull.*, **1973**, *11*, 156–294.

Hansten, P. D. *Drug Interactions*, 2nd ed. Lea & Febiger, Philadelphia, **1973**.

Hunt, C. C., and Kuffler, S. W. Pharmacology of the neuromuscular junction. *Pharmac. Rev.*, **1950**, *2*, 96–120.

Kalow, W. Genetic factors in relation to drugs. *A. Rev. Pharmac.*, **1965**, *5*, 9–26.

Karczmar, A. G. Neuromuscular pharmacology. *A. Rev. Pharmac.*, **1967**, *7*, 241–276.

Karczmar, A. G.; Nishi, S.; and Blaber, L. C. Synaptic modulations. In, *Brain and Human Behavior.* (Karczmar, A. G., and Eccles, J. C., eds.) Springer-Verlag, Berlin, **1972**, pp. 63–92.

Khromov-Borisov, N. V., and Michelson, M. J. The mutual disposition of cholinoreceptors of locomotor muscles, and the changes in their disposition in the course of evolution. *Pharmac. Rev.*, **1966**, *18*, 1051–1090.

McIntyre, A. R. *Curare: Its History, Nature, and Clinical Use.* University of Chicago Press, Chicago, **1947**.

——. History of curare. In, *Neuromuscular Blocking and Stimulating Agents*, Vol. 1. *International Encyclopedia of Pharmacology and Therapeutics*, Sect. 14. (Cheymol, J., ed.) Pergamon Press, Ltd., Oxford, **1972**, pp. 187–203.

Michelson, M. J., and Zeimal, E. V. *Acetylcholine: An Approach to the Molecular Mechanism of Action.* Pergamon Press, Ltd., Oxford, **1973**.

Paton, W. D. M. A theory of drug action based on the rate of drug-receptor combination. *Proc. R. Soc., B*, **1961**, *154*, 21–69.

——. Kinetic theories of drug action with special reference to the acetylcholine group of agonists and antagonists. *Ann. N.Y. Acad. Sci.*, **1967**, *144*, 869–881.

——. Receptors as defined by their pharmacological properties. In, *Molecular Properties of Drug Receptors* (a Ciba Foundation symposium). (Porter, R., and O'Connor, M., eds.) J. & A. Churchill, Ltd., London, **1970**, pp. 3–32.

Paton, W. D. M., and Zaimis, E. J. The methonium compounds. *Pharmac. Rev.*, **1952**, *4*, 219–253.

Pittinger, C., and Adamson, R. Antibiotic blockade of neuromuscular function. *A. Rev. Pharmac.*, **1972**, *12*, 169–184.

Rang, H. P. (ed.). *Drug Receptors.* University Park Press, Baltimore, **1973**.

Riker, W. F., and Okamoto, M. Pharmacology of motor nerve terminals. *A. Rev. Pharmac.*, **1969**, *9*, 173–208.

Siker, E. S.; Wolfson, B.; and Schaner, P. J. Muscle relaxants: advances in the last decade. *Clin. Anesth.*, **1969**, *3*, 416–457.

Smith, C. M. Neuromuscular pharmacology: drugs and muscle spindles. *A. Rev. Pharmac.*, **1963**, *3*, 223–242.

Speight, T. M., and Avery, G. S. Pancuronium bromide: a review of its pharmacological properties and clinical application. *Drugs*, **1972**, *4*, 163–226.

Waser, P. G. On receptors in the postsynaptic membrane of the motor endplate. In, *Molecular Properties of Drug Receptors* (a Ciba Foundation symposium). (Porter, R., and O'Connor, M., eds.) J. & A. Churchill, Ltd., London, **1970**, pp. 59–75.

——. Chemistry and pharmacology of natural curare compounds. In, *Neuromuscular Blocking and Stimulating Agents*, Vol. 1. *International Encyclopedia of Pharmacology and Therapeutics*, Sect. 14. (Cheymol, J., ed.) Pergamon Press, Ltd., Oxford, **1972**, pp. 205–239.

Zaimis, E. J. Mechanisms of neuromuscular blockade. In, *Curare and Curare-like Agents.* (Bovet, D.; Bovet-Nitti, F.; and Marini-Bettòlo, G. B.; eds.) Elsevier Publishing Co., Amsterdam, **1959**, pp. 191–203.

Autacoids

INTRODUCTION

William W. Douglas

Assembled for consideration in this section are a number of substances with widely differing structures and pharmacological activities; although disparate in these respects, they are grouped together here because they share in common a natural occurrence in the body. At the same time, the opportunity is taken to discuss drugs antagonizing their actions, wherever such drugs are available. The oldest and most familiar substances in the group, histamine and the antihistamines, are dealt with in Chapter 29. The same chapter is concerned with another endogenous amine, *5-hydroxytryptamine (5-HT, serotonin, enteramine)*, and its antagonists. Chapter 30 is devoted to the polypeptides—*angiotensin, bradykinin,* and *kalidin*—and to the lipids known as the *prostaglandins.* The section thus includes a motley of substances of intense pharmacological activity that are normally present in the body or may be formed there, and that cannot conveniently be classed with other members of this broad group, such as the neurohumors and hormones. These different substances have been variously described as *local hormones, autopharmacological agents,* and the like; but a generic term that is at once shorter, more accurate, and euphonious is *autacoid,* a word derived from the Greek *autos* ("self") and *akos* ("medicinal agent" or "remedy"). This term was devised by Sir Edward Schäfer (1916), later Sharpey-Schafer, as a substitute for Starling's word *hormone,* which, being derived from the Greek *hormaein* (meaning "to stir up"), is a misnomer for the inhibitory substances that also came to be embraced by this designation. However, Starling's term *hormone,* albeit unsatisfactory from the etymological standpoint, has won the day, and Schäfer's has passed into limbo. Such a good word deserves a better fate, and hence its revival here. All the substances described in this section can probably lay claim to the title without distortion of its sense.

What of the significance of this group of autacoids? What is their role in the body? What is their value as drugs and what is their place in therapeutics? Unfortunately, only rather imprecise answers can be given to these questions. The very fact that the substances have been classified under the noncommittal title of *autacoids* is, in a sense, a confession that the evidence does not at present permit a more precise functional classification such as, for example, hormone or neurohumor. This is not to say that such functions are foreign to the autacoids. On the contrary, as the evidence concerning their possible roles in the body is unfolded, it will be apparent to the reader that both such functions may be displayed by the substances under consideration. But the core of the matter is that, while the autacoids possess an astonishingly wide range of pharmacological activities and in vanishingly small amounts, there are comparatively few instances where a physiological role can be stated with assurance. After the example of Pirandello, who named one of his plays *Six Characters in Search of an Author,* the present section might well have been entitled "Various Autacoids in Search of a Function." The problem, as will become clear from what follows, is not so much with a dearth of hypotheses as with a surfeit of them. But while scientists dispute the rival claims of the different hypotheses, there is general agreement that each of the autacoids to be discussed is of importance in the body's economy. All are agents that the body employs in the execution of various functions in health and disease; they are clearly part and parcel of the physiological and pathological phenomena that provide the rationale for drug therapy; and their discovery has provided new possibilities for therapeutic intervention by the use of drugs that antagonize their action or interfere in one way or another with their metabolism. Together these facts thrust the autacoids squarely to the center of interest for those who are concerned with the pharmacological basis of therapeutics.

CHAPTER

29 HISTAMINE AND ANTIHISTAMINES; 5-HYDROXYTRYPTAMINE AND ANTAGONISTS

William W. Douglas

HISTAMINE

History. The history of β-imidazolylethylamine, or histamine, shows several close parallels with that of acetylcholine (ACh). Both compounds were synthesized as chemical curiosities before their biological significance was recognized; both were first detected as uterine stimulants in extracts of ergot, from which they were subsequently isolated; and both proved to be casual contaminants of ergot, resulting from bacterial action.

When Dale and Laidlaw (1910, 1911) subjected histamine to intensive pharmacological study, they discovered, *inter alia,* that it stimulated a host of smooth muscles and had an intense depressor action. With rare acumen they drew attention to the fact that the pharmacological activity of histamine resembled that of many tissue extracts and, further, that the immediate symptoms with which an animal responds to an injection of a normally inert protein, to which it has been sensitized, are to a large extent those of poisoning by β-imidazolylethylamine (histamine). Their prescient comments anticipated by many years the events that were to thrust histamine to the center of physiological interest, namely, the discovery of its occurrence in the body and its release upon cellular injury. Although histamine had been identified chemically in tissue extracts previously, it was suspected that it might have arisen from putrefaction. It was not until 1927 that Best, Dale, Dudley, and Thorpe isolated histamine from impeccably fresh samples of liver and lung, thereby establishing beyond doubt that this amine is a natural constituent of the body. Demonstrations of its presence in a variety of other tissues soon followed—hence the name *histamine* after the Greek word for tissue, *histos.*

Meanwhile, Lewis and his colleagues, in a series of brilliant experiments, had amassed evidence that a substance with the properties of histamine ("H-substance") was liberated from the cells of the skin by injurious stimuli, including the union of antigen and antibody (Lewis, 1927). Given the chemical evidence of histamine's presence in the body, there remained little impediment to supposing that Lewis' "H-substance" was histamine itself. This conception was advanced with telling force by Dale in his Croonian lectures of 1929 and stimulated the growth of interest in histamine to a rare luxuriance. Now, nearly half a century later, it is evident that histamine is involved in many other diverse physiological processes quite apart from reaction to injury. Moreover, painstaking studies, carried out over many years, indicate that histamine receptors in various tissues fall into two broad classes: H_1 (Ash and Schild, 1966) and H_2 (Black *et al.,* 1972). The recent introduction by Black and associates of drugs that effectively block H_2 receptors—an action not shared by former antihistamines—promises to generate new interest and understanding of histamine's functions.

Chemistry. Histamine is 5-(2-aminoethyl)-imidazole (or β-imidazolylethylamine). It may be formed by decarboxylation of the amino acid histidine, a reaction effected by the enzyme L-histidine decarboxylase (Figure 29–2, page 600).

There are many drugs with histamine-like properties, and most contain the following fragment:

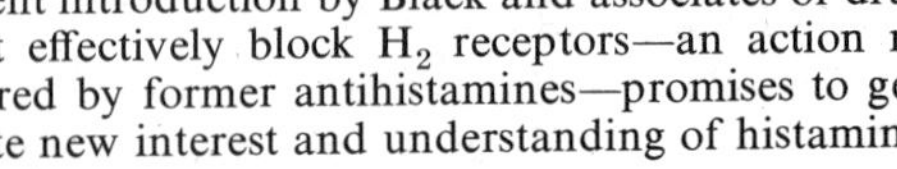

However, there are a number of exceptions, and one can say only that compounds with appreciable histamine-like activity consist of small, nitrogen-containing heterocyclic rings to which are attached 2-aminoethyl side chains. Among the histamine analogs there is a striking lack of correlation between their action on gastric secretion and their other histamine-like actions. Some, for example, are powerful gastric secretagogues but have feeble actions on smooth muscle and blood pressure, while others show the opposite pattern.

PHARMACOLOGICAL EFFECTS: H_1 AND H_2 RECEPTORS

Histamine contracts many smooth muscles, such as those of the bronchi and gut, but powerfully relaxes others, including those of fine blood vessels. It is also a very potent stimulus to gastric acid production and elicits various other exocrine secretions. Effects attributable to these actions dominate the overall response to the drug; however, there are several others, of which edema formation and stimulation of sensory nerve endings are perhaps the most familiar. Some of these effects, such as bronchoconstriction and contraction of the gut, are readily antagonized by the long-available antihistamines such as pyrilamine, and are considered to

involve H_1 receptors. Others, most notably gastric secretion, are completely refractory to such antagonists, involve activation of H_2 receptors, and are susceptible to inhibition by newly developed histamine antagonists (Black *et al.*, 1972). Still others, such as the hypotension resulting from vascular dilatation, are mediated by receptors of both H_1 and H_2 types, and are annulled only by a combination of H_1 and H_2 histamine antagonists. Various congeners of histamine can activate the different receptors with relative selectivity, as is illustrated in Figure 29-1, where the relative activity of various methyl derivatives of histamine on guinea pig ileum and atrium are shown. Although most of the derivatives are roughly equipotent in the two test systems, 2-methylhistamine is more active on ileum than atrium; the opposite is true of 4-methylhistamine, which has only negligible effects on the ileum. Moreover, the substances that are effective on the atrium are potent stimulants of gastric acid secretion whereas those with little effect on the atrium fail to stimulate gastric secretion. Thus, in cats 4-methylhistamine, N-methylhistamine,

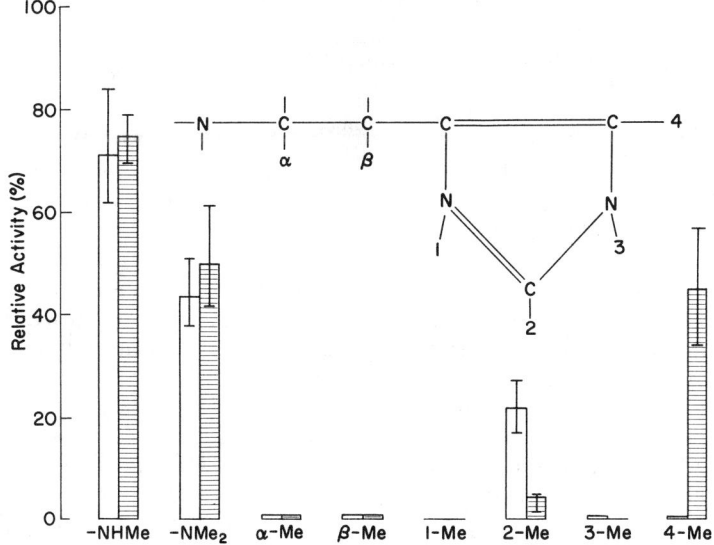

Figure 29-1. *Structure-activity relationship of histamine derivatives.*

Bar graph showing activity of methyl derivatives of histamine relative to histamine (equal to 100), estimated on both ileum (white columns) and atrium (hatched columns). Each bar gives mean relative activity (with 95% confidence limits). Nomenclature of the derivatives follows from the system, customary for histidine, in which (a) the ring nitrogen adjacent to the side chain is named position 1 and the second ring nitrogen becomes position 3, and (b) the carbon atom adjacent to the side chain nitrogen is called the alpha position. (After Black, Duncan, Durant, Ganellin, and Parsons, 1972. Courtesy of *Nature*.)

and N,N-dimethylhistamine are as potent as or more potent than histamine itself (Code *et al.,* 1971; Impicciatore and Grossman, 1973). These and other differential effects of histamine-like agonists, together with the differential effects of histamine antagonists (Black *et al.,* 1972), provide the experimental basis for the division of histamine receptors into H_1 and H_2 types. Note also (Figure 29-1) the great loss of potency resulting from methyl substitution on the α or β carbon atom of the side chain or the ring nitrogen atoms.

Cardiovascular System. Histamine was early recognized to be a powerful and consistent stimulant of smooth muscle in a variety of preparations, including isolated arteries and veins, and vasoconstriction had been demonstrated in perfused arterial beds from all the common laboratory species. In line with these findings, histamine was found to raise blood pressure in the rabbit. However, no such rise occurred in the cat and dog; on the contrary, histamine causes a sharp fall of blood pressure in these species. The explanation was provided by Dale and Laidlaw (1919), who showed that, in addition to its constrictor actions on larger blood vessels and arterioles (which vary with species and are comparatively feeble in carnivores), histamine has powerful dilator actions on the minute blood vessels, capillaries, and venules. They suggested that the effect of histamine on vascular resistance and blood pressure results from a balance between the two opposed actions.

"Capillary" Dilatation. This is the most characteristic action of histamine on the vascular tree and by far the most important in man. It results from some direct action of histamine on the vessels and is independent of innervation. All the "capillaries" in the body are involved, but the response following parenteral injection in man is most obvious in the skin of the face and upper part of the body, the so-called blushing area, which becomes hot and flushed.

Increased "Capillary" Permeability. This is the second of the classical effects of histamine on the fine vessels and results in outward passage of plasma protein and fluid into the extracellular spaces and formation of edema.

While it is traditional to ascribe these effects to an action of histamine on "capillaries," it should be understood that, when so used, the word is a generic term for the vessels of the microcirculation. Neither the fall in resistance nor the increase in permeability following histamine is attributable to the very finest vessels, only a few micrometers in diameter, that are capillaries in the most rigorous morphological sense and devoid of smooth muscle. Dilator responses are mainly attributable to inhibitory effects of histamine on the smooth muscle of somewhat larger vessels upstream (terminal arterioles); such dilatation as occurs in the postcapillary venules, which up to about 50 μm in diameter are devoid of smooth muscle, seems to be mainly passive, due, on the one hand, to the fall in resistance upstream (and increased blood flow) and, on the other, to a rise in pressure in larger veins that histamine tends to constrict (*see* below). By contrast, increased permeability results mainly from actions of histamine on postcapillary venules, mostly those of about 20 to 30 μm in diameter, where histamine causes the endothelial cells to separate at their boundaries and thus to expose the basement membrane, which is freely permeable to plasma protein and fluid. The gaps (or "stomata") between endothelial cells may also permit passage of particles such as platelets or injected colloidal drugs and dyes that become trapped between the cells and the basement membrane. Although the separation of the endothelial cells responsible for increased permeability is doubtless favored by the dilatation of the small venules just described, such dilatation, or "stretching," is not the primary cause. Rather, this seems to be a direct contractile response of the endothelial cells to histamine, resulting in "shrinkage." (*See* Rocha e Silva, 1966; Majno *et al.,* 1969.)

Triple Response. When histamine is injected intradermally, it produces a characteristic triad of phenomena known as the "triple response" (Lewis, 1927), comprising the following: (1) a localized red spot, extending for a few millimeters around the site of injection, coming on within a few seconds, reaching a maximum in about a minute, and soon acquiring a bluish tint; (2) a brighter red flush, or "flare," of irregular outline, extending for 1 cm or so beyond the original red spot and developing somewhat more slowly; and (3) localized edema fluid, forming a wheal that is discernible in about 1½ minutes and occupies the same area as the original small red spot at the injection site. The first component is due to local dilatation of the minute blood vessels (capillaries, venules, and terminal arterioles) in direct response to histamine; the surrounding flush results from widespread dilatation of neighboring arterioles through the medium of a local axon reflex mechanism (the nature of which is still poorly understood); wheal formation is separable from the vasodilator effect of histamine and is due to a direct action of the drug on the walls of the fine blood vessels to increase their permeability.

Arterioles. The response of arterioles to histamine changes as one ascends the zoological scale (Dale, 1929). The predominant effect in rodents is strong arteriolar constriction; in cats, slight arteriolar constriction; in the dog, monkey, and man, arteriolar dilatation.

Veins. Although histamine dilates the finer vessels on the venous side of the capillary bed, it constricts larger veins (Sharpey-Schafer and Ginsburg, 1962).

Cerebral Vessels. The cerebral vessels are sensitive to quite small doses of histamine and respond with brisk dilatation. An important consequence of this response in man is headache, which may be very severe.

Histamine Headache. Histamine headache is preceded by flushing of the face and a gradually developing sense of pulsating fullness in the head. Following intravenous injections of the drug, it appears in about a minute, reaches a peak shortly thereafter, and slowly diminishes in intensity to terminate in about 5 to 10 minutes. At first it has a throbbing character coincident with pulsations observable in the temporal artery; later it becomes more or less continuous and is felt as a dull ache deep in the head, often worst in the frontal and temporal regions. Before the headache begins, blood pressure falls sharply and cerebrospinal fluid pressure rises; but when headache is at its peak both these parameters have usually returned toward normal. At this time, however, measurement of cerebrospinal fluid pressure shows violent pulsations, and it is therefore supposed that the headache is due to stretching of sensory endings in and around the cranial arteries. The headache can be suppressed by various maneuvers that lower systemic blood pressure or raise the cerebrospinal fluid pressure. A somewhat similar headache is produced by other potent vasodilators, such as amyl nitrite.

Heart. In the intact animal given conventional doses of histamine, direct cardiac actions are not evident; but barosensory reflexes, evoked by the falling blood pressure, stimulate heart rate and tend to augment cardiac output. Venoconstriction and increased venous return contribute to the rise in cardiac output in the early phases of the response. In addition, depending on species and dose, direct chronotropic and inotropic

effects of histamine may also be involved. Cardiac output falls later as blood pools in the peripheral vascular bed. Coronary flow is usually increased. The ECG may show minor changes of little functional consequence.

In a variety of cardiac preparations, histamine can be shown to have positive inotropic and chronotropic effects. This is due, in part, to release of catecholamines (*see* under adrenal medulla, below). But the effects are not abolished when the heart is depleted of catecholamines by reserpine nor when β receptors are blocked with appropriate drugs; thus, there is clearly a direct component mediated through histamine receptors. High doses of histamine have negative inotropic effects, retard impulse propagation in the conducting system, and may induce extrasystoles and ventricular fibrillation. (*See* Euler, 1966; Flacke *et al.,* 1967; Black *et al.,* 1972; Hughes and Coret, 1972; Mannaioni, 1972.)

Blood Pressure. In man and many other species, the extreme dilatation of terminal arterioles in response to histamine causes an impressive fall in *systemic blood pressure,* which, however, recovers rapidly after moderate doses as compensatory reflexes are activated and the drug is inactivated.

Effects of histamine on the *pulmonary circulation* are variable. In the dog, intravenous injection of histamine is rapidly followed by increase in the pressure in the right atrium, pulmonary artery, and pulmonary vein; pulmonary vascular volume rises and flow increases. Pressure in the pulmonary circulation subsequently drops as systemic hypotension develops and cardiac output falls. The pattern of pressure changes appears to reflect mainly changes in pulmonary blood flow in response to variations in venous return and cardiac output. In various isolated preparations a constriction of both pulmonary arteries and veins has been observed. In man, however, a fall in pulmonary artery pressure and resistance has been reported following subcutaneous injection of histamine. (*See* Storstein *et al.,* 1959; Colebatch, 1970.)

Histamine Shock. Histamine in large doses causes a profound and progressive fall in blood pressure. Dale and Laidlaw (1919), who called the phenomenon "histamine shock," showed that as the minute blood vessels dilate, they trap large amounts of blood and, as their permeability increases, plasma escapes from the circulation. These effects diminish the effective blood volume, reduce venous return, and greatly lower cardiac output. The condition resembles surgical or traumatic shock. The heart continues to beat forcefully, although ineffectually, and the pulse is thready. Large vessels, arteries and veins, are collapsed and emptied of blood, while the fine vessels are engorged and mucous membranes are heavily injected and take on a dusky-red hue. Edema is apparent in delicate structures such as the pancreas. As blood volume falls, the hematocrit may rise to 150% of normal. In contrast, the blood is poor in leukocytes. Lymphatics are engorged, and lymph flow is increased.

Extravascular Smooth Muscle. Histamine stimulates, or more rarely relaxes, various smooth muscles. There are wide variations in the responses of different tissues, species, and even individuals. *Bronchial muscle* of guinea pigs is exquisitely sensitive, and bronchoconstriction leads to death. Minute doses of histamine will also evoke intense bronchoconstriction in human beings with bronchial asthma and certain other pulmonary diseases. In normal man and many animals, the effect is much less pronounced and exceptionally, as in the sheep bronchus or cat trachea, histamine causes relaxation (*see* Eyre, 1973). Likewise, the *uterus* of some species contracts to histamine while that of the rat relaxes; in the human uterus, gravid or not, the response is negligible. Responses of *intestinal muscle* also vary with species and region, but the classical effect is contraction; the contractile response of the terminal ileum of the guinea pig forms the basis for the common bioassay of histamine. *Bladder, iris,* and many other smooth muscle preparations are affected little or inconsistently by histamine.

A direct action on smooth muscle is generally responsible for most of these effects. However, an indirect component involving stimulation of neural elements has been detected in isolated intestinal preparations (Paton and Vane, 1963), and a reflex contribution to bronchoconstriction has been reported.

Plasma Potassium. Efflux of potassium from smooth muscle in response to histamine may raise the plasma potassium concentration significantly (Macmillan and Vane, 1956).

Exocrine Glands. *Gastric Glands.* Histamine is a remarkably powerful gastric secretagogue and evokes a copious secretion of gastric juice of high acidity in doses below those that influence the blood pressure. Its effect on the composition of gastric juice varies somewhat with species and dose (Ivy and Bachrach, 1966), but in man the output of pepsin is increased along with that of acid. The effect is well maintained during prolonged intravenous infusions of histamine. While these actions are believed to be exerted directly on the gland cells (both parietal and chief), the presence of an intact vagus permits a higher rate of secretion. After vagotomy in man the maximal secretory response to histamine may fall to about one third of the value found before the operation (Payne and Kay, 1962).

Other Exocrine Glands. The effects of histamine on glands outside the stomach are relatively unimportant. The drug has some stimulant actions on salivary, pancreatic, intestinal, bronchial, and lacrimal secretions, but these are generally inconstant, fleeting, and feeble. In salivary glands, where the action of histamine has been most closely studied, it is possible to show some stimulation after chronic denervation, which is thus direct; however, in normally innervated glands, much of the effect seems to be mediated through the nerves (*see* Emmelin, 1966).

Sensory Nerve Endings: Pain and Itch. The "flare" component of the triple response is but one example of histamine's capacity to stimulate nerve endings. It causes itching when introduced into the most superficial layers of the skin by a variety of technics, including pricking, injection, and iontophoresis; when administered more deeply in the skin, especially in higher doses, it evokes pain, sometimes accompanied by itching. Afferent discharges evoked by histamine have been recorded in cutaneous nerves (*see* Keele and Armstrong, 1964).

Stimulant effects on nerve endings, motor as well as sensory, contribute to the indirect effects of histamine on smooth muscle preparations and glands that are blocked, for example, by atropine or hexamethonium; an action on sympathetic nerve endings would explain the release of norepinephrine from the isolated heart provoked by histamine in high doses (*see* Paton and Vane, 1963; Rocha e Silva, 1966).

Adrenal Medulla and Ganglia. Many substances that excite nerve endings also stimulate ganglion cells and chromaffin cells in the adrenal medulla and elsewhere. This is true of histamine (Euler, 1966; Brezenoff and Gertner, 1972). However, these cells respond vigorously only when histamine is administered in large amounts or by close arterial injection, and not when conventional doses are given intravenously. Nevertheless, a secondary rise in blood pressure attributable to adrenal medullary stimulation is seen in experimental animals given large doses of histamine intravenously and in patients with pheochromocytoma given modest doses. In addition to its direct action on the chromaffin cells, demonstrable by intracellular recording (Douglas *et al.*, 1967), histamine also evokes medullary secretion indirectly by effects mediated through the splanchnic nerves (Staszewska-Barczak and Vane, 1965).

Mode of Action. H_1 and H_2 Receptors.

Due to the relatively brief experience with H_2 antagonists, there is insufficient evidence for a confident classification of all the many effects of histamine into those mediated by H_1 receptors, H_2 receptors, or both. Indeed, it may yet be shown that more than two histamine receptors exist. Nevertheless, the concept of two types, H_1 and H_2, merits adoption. The classical (pre-1972) "antihistamines" are all, it appears, capable of blocking effectively H_1 receptors only; and any response to histamine that is inhibited by such agents is *a priori* an H_1 effect (Ash and Schild, 1966). H_2 receptors, on the other hand, are refractory to block by such antihistamines but are inhibited preferentially by H_2-receptor antagonists such as metiamide (Black *et al.*, 1972, 1973). As noted earlier, H_2 receptors are entirely responsible for histamine's important effect on gastric secretion. They also play a major role in histamine's stimulant effect on the heart, in its relaxant effect on the rat uterus and sheep bronchus, and in biochemical responses of brain tissue (Shimizu *et al.*, 1970). Both H_1 and H_2 receptors seem to be involved in a synergistic manner in vasodilatation and in edema formation. Such combinations, however, apparently act in antagonistic fashion in some species and systems (Turker, 1973).

Mechanisms at the Cellular Level. Many responses to histamine are clearly attributable to an increase in membrane permeability that allows the common inorganic ions (mainly cations) to flow down electrochemical gradients and alter transmembrane potential. It doubtless explains the stimulant actions of histamine (and other autacoids to be discussed) on *nerve endings* or *ganglion cells* to effect depolarization and initiation of impulses. Moreover, an essentially similar action appears to account for *secretion*, at least as it occurs in the *chromaffin cells of the adrenal medulla.* Here histamine and each of several other autacoids of quite different structure, including 5-hydroxytryptamine (5-HT), angiotensin, and bradykinin, mimic the physiological secretagogue ACh in depolarizing the plasmalemma (Douglas *et al.*, 1967). It has been suggested that such membrane effects involving calcium influx or mobilization may provide a general mechanism of *"stimulus-secretion coupling"* common to a variety of secretagogues and cells (Douglas, 1968, 1974). An

action on the cell membrane to facilitate calcium entry probably also explains the stimulant effect of histamine and other autacoids on *smooth muscle contraction.* In several smooth muscles, the depolarizing and impulse-generating currents are carried by calcium ions, in contrast to skeletal muscles and nerves where sodium is the current-carrying cation, and this is clearly an important device for increasing intracellular calcium. It should, however, be emphasized that the essential event for the contractile response is the increase in the intracellular concentration of free calcium ions and not the changes in membrane potential. Thus, histamine and the other autacoids continue to evoke contraction in smooth muscles already completely depolarized by excess potassium. The contractile responses of cardiac tissue (and possibly endothelial cells) to histamine and some of the other autacoids may be explained similarly. (*See* Ebashi and Endo, 1968; Somlyo and Somlyo, 1970.)

The mode of action of histamine and other autacoids to produce *smooth muscle relaxation,* including *vasodilatation,* has not been defined. A reasonable assumption is that these agents somehow lower the intracellular concentration of free calcium ions either by inhibiting calcium influx (hyperpolarizing effects consistent with this concept have been observed) or by promoting sequestration or extrusion of calcium ions. Again, changes in membrane potential *per se* do not appear to be critical since inhibitory responses are also obtainable in depolarized smooth muscle (*see* reviews cited above, and Ash and Schild, 1966).

The involvement of cyclic adenosine 3′,5′-monophosphate (cyclic AMP) in so many diverse physiological processes has raised the question whether histamine's effects are mediated, at least in part, by this nucleotide. Histamine has been found to increase adenylate cyclase activity and the concentration of cyclic AMP in several tissues, including heart (Klein and Levey, 1971), gastric mucosa (Nakajima *et al.*, 1971; Domschke *et al.*, 1973), and brain (Kakiuchi and Rall, 1968). There is in this pattern an indication of preferential involvement of H_2 receptors, but the degree of correlation has yet to be established.

ENDOGENOUS HISTAMINE: DISTRIBUTION AND BIOSYNTHESIS

There are numerous reasons for supposing that histamine has important functions in the body's economy. Although some of the most familiar hypotheses on the function of histamine have been concerned with pathological physiology and, in particular, with anaphylaxis, allergy, injury, and shock, indications of a normal physiological function are accumulating apace with the development of highly refined methods of study. For example, there is now impressive evidence that endogenous histamine is the final common mediator of gastric secretory responses, and there are some grounds for supposing it to be involved in tissue growth and repair, in regulation of the microcirculation, and in the functioning of the central nervous system (CNS) (*see* Kahlson and Rosengren, 1971).

Distribution. Histamine is widely, if unevenly, distributed throughout the animal kingdom and is present in many venoms, noxious secretions, bacteria, and plants (Reite, 1972). Almost all mammalian tissues contain preformed histamine. The concentration is particularly high in the skin, intestinal mucosa, and lungs. Of no less importance than concentration, and often unrelated to it, is histamine-forming capacity. Some tissues synthesize and turn over histamine at a remarkably high rate.

Origin, Synthesis, and Storage. It appears unlikely that ingested histamine or that formed by bacteria in the gastrointestinal tract contributes significantly to the endogenous pool, despite evidence that injected histamine can be taken up by various tissues (*see* Symposium, 1967). Most absorbed histamine is catabolized by the liver, and the remainder is largely destroyed in the lungs and other tissues or eliminated in the urine. Every mammalian tissue that contains histamine, including white blood cells, appears capable of synthesizing the amine from histidine. The conversion of histidine to histamine can be catalyzed *in vitro*, and in exceptional instances *in vivo*, by nonspecific aromatic L-amino acid decarboxylase (dopa decarboxylase); however, the principal enzyme involved *in vivo* is a specific histidine decarboxylase, which is specific for the substrate L-histidine. In many tissues the chief site of histamine storage is the *mast cell* or, in the case of blood, the *basophil* (a circulating counterpart of the fixed-tissue mast cell). These cells synthesize histamine and store it as a complex with heparin in membrane-limited secretory granules. The turnover rate is slow. When tissues rich in mast cells are depleted of their histamine stores, it may take weeks before they are repleted. The histamine of mast cells and basophils, as will be described shortly, has an important role in the pathological physiology of anaphylaxis, allergy, and injury, and in the responses to certain drugs.

Mast cells are by no means the only tissue source of histamine. The amine is present in substantial amounts in the human epidermis, the CNS, and the gastrointestinal mucosa. Moreover, histamine in such sites, in contrast to that in mast cells, is commonly undergoing a brisk turnover and is released rather than stored. It contributes importantly to the daily excretion of histamine and its metabolites in the urine. Furthermore, since L-histidine decarboxylase is an inducible enzyme, the histamine-forming capacity of such nonmast-cell sites is subject to regulation by various physiological and other factors. It is around the physiological functions of the "induced" or "nascent" histamine formed in nonmast-cell sites that much current opinion and speculation revolve. (*See* Schayer, 1965; Rocha e Silva, 1966; Kahlson and Rosengren, 1971; Johnson *et al.*, 1973.)

ENDOGENOUS HISTAMINE:
FUNCTIONS

In the following discussion the now-classical involvement of histamine release from mast cells and basophils in various pathological processes will be considered before the later work implicating nonmast-cell histamine in various physiological processes. There is no significance to this order other than convenience and approximation to the historical sequence of development of the field.

Histamine Release in Anaphylaxis and Allergy. Although Dale and Laidlaw had drawn attention to the close correspondence between the effects of poisoning with histamine and anaphylactic shock as early as 1910, many years elapsed before the meaning of this correspondence became apparent. Three major clues were provided by (1) the work of Dale (1913), which showed convincingly that the hypersensitivity phenomenon involved a reaction of antigen with cell-fixed antibody; (2) the work of Lewis (1927), demonstrating that a histamine-like agent ("H-substance") was liberated in the skin during the local anaphylactic reaction; and (3) the work of Best and associates (1927), establishing beyond doubt that histamine is a natural constituent of the tissues of the body. The first two clues prompted Lewis (1927) to enunciate the hypothesis that the antigen-antibody reaction caused the cells to liberate a substance with the properties of histamine that was responsible for the characteristic physiological accompaniments of the phenomenon, that is, vasodilatation, itching, and edema formation. The third clue allowed Dale (1929) to argue forcibly that this "H-substance" was histamine itself. Within a few years, the release of histamine during the antigen-antibody reaction had been successfully demonstrated by Bartosch and coworkers (1932) and by Dragstedt and Gebauer-Fuelnegg (1932), and the histamine hypothesis of the mediation of hypersensitivity phenomena won wide acceptance. When, following World War II, the newly discovered histamine antagonists were found to reduce the intensity of various hypersensitivity reactions, the importance of histamine was established beyond all reasonable doubt.

Mechanism. The principal target cells of the hypersensitivity reactions of the immediate type are the mast cells and basophils. Within the secretory granules of these cells, the histamine is stored along with a heparin-protein complex to which it is loosely bound by ionic forces, probably involving carboxyl groups. Release is brought about by a series of reactions leading to expulsion of the contents of the secretory granules by the process of exocytosis. The chain of events is initiated by interaction of specific antigen and cell-bound reaginic (IgE) antibody, is calcium dependent, requires metabolic energy, and shows various features indicative of an enzymatic process (Mongar and Schild, 1962; Rocha e Silva, 1966; Symposium, 1967; McIntyre, 1973). Such an active secretory process is to be distinguished from gross cell damage (cytolysis) and resembles the secretory responses of various endocrine and exocrine cells to their appropriate secretagogues. The exocytotic response of mast cells involves the serial fusion of many granule membranes and is of the type termed "sequential" or "compound," such as occurs most commonly in certain exocrine cells (*see* Douglas, 1974). The essential point is that this mechanism allows for selective discharge of granule contents without cell disruption. The underlying hypothesis is that the effect of the antigen-antibody reaction on the structure of the cell membrane increases its permeability to calcium. Thus, it has been shown that the response to antigen proceeds in two stages: the first, "activation," does not require calcium; the second, which results in histamine release, does require calcium and occurs even when antigen has been removed. Moreover, during the course of exposure to antigen, histamine release can be arrested promptly by calcium chelators (Lichtenstein, 1971). Calcium ionophores, drugs known to promote transmembrane fluxes of calcium (Pressman, 1973), release histamine (Foreman and Mongar, 1973). Furthermore, mast cells pretreated with these drugs or subjected to other conditions probably facilitating calcium entry have been shown to extrude granules in characteristic exocytotic fashion when calcium is introduced (Cochrane and Douglas, 1974; Kagayama and Douglas, 1974). Finally, granule extrusion has been observed following microinjection of calcium ions into mast cells (Kanno *et al.,* 1973). This "calcium-influx-exocytosis" hypothesis does not exclude the operation of alternative mechanisms of hypersensitivity-induced histamine release for which there is also evidence (*see* Symposium, 1968a, 1968b; McIntyre, 1973).

Limitations of the Histamine Hypothesis of Hypersensitivity Reactions. *Involvement of Other Autacoids.* It is now evident that the classical histamine hypothesis does not provide a full explanation of all the effects accompanying immediate hypersensitivity (antigen–antibody) reactions. At least part of the explanation resides in the fact that during such reactions various other autacoids are liberated or produced along with histamine, the nature and relative importance of which vary with species and tissue. These additional autacoids are considered below and in the chapter that follows.

Direct Effects of Antigen. An additional explanation for the anaphylactic and allergic responses that are apparently independent of histamine or other known autacoids may lie in the observation that antigens can act directly on the membranes of sensitized muscle cells to cause depolarization and contraction (Alonso–De Florida *et al.,* 1968).

Histamine Release by Drugs, Macromolecules, and Venoms. Drugs or other substances to which an individual has become allergic will, of course, release histamine indirectly by the hypersensitivity reaction. In addition, many compounds, including numerous therapeutic agents, have the capacity to elicit histamine release directly and quite independently of development of allergy. Among them are amides, amidines, diamidines, quaternary ammonium compounds, piperidine derivatives, pyridinium compounds, alkaloids, antibiotic bases, and dyes. Not uncommonly, therapeutic administration of such substances, especially by the intravenous route, has

rather dramatic consequences attributable to histamine release. Drugs that exhibit this side effect are discussed throughout the text.

Histamine Liberators. There are certain other basic compounds with histamine-releasing power so far transcending their other pharmacological actions that they are commonly referred to as histamine liberators, although they might more properly be described as "mast-cell depletors," since they commonly cause these cells to void the entire contents of their secretory granules. The prototype and most thoroughly studied is compound 48/80, a mixture of condensation products formed from formaldehyde and p-methoxy-N-methylphenethylamine, consisting of dimers, trimers and higher polymers— of which the hexamer is probably most active (Goth, 1973). Such drugs elicit the syndrome of histamine release in its purest form. Within seconds of their intravenous injection, human subjects experience a burning, itching sensation, as if a bundle of nettles had been placed on the skin. This effect, most marked in the palms of the hand and in the face, scalp, and ears, is soon followed by a feeling of intense warmth. The skin reddens, and the color rapidly spreads over the trunk. Blood pressure falls, the heart rate accelerates, and the subject complains of headache, often intense. After a few minutes, blood pressure recovers, and edema and crops of giant hives appear in the skin, particularly over the thorax and abdomen. There is colic, nausea, hypersecretion of acid with acid vomitus, and moderate bronchospasm. This anaphylactoid reaction may occasionally be seen with therapeutic agents that are strong histamine releasers; sometimes it is referred to as a "nitritoid crisis." The effect becomes less intense with successive injections as mast-cell stores of histamine are depleted. The drug does not deplete tissues of nonmast-cell histamine.

Mechanism. The prototypic basic histamine liberator, compound 48/80, acts on rat mast cells to set in motion an active granule-extrusion process (compound exocytosis) resembling that induced by the hypersensitivity reaction in its dependence on energy and calcium. The mechanism of action is uncertain. These basic histamine liberators may act like antigen at the cell surface, as suggested by their affinity for acid mucopolysaccharides present in the membrane (Goth, 1973), or the essential component of their action may be a mobilization of cellular calcium (Douglas, 1974). Some other basic compounds with surfactant properties, such as decylamine, seem to have a nonspecific membrane-disrupting, detergent-like effect or may even displace histamine from intracellular granules without frank rupture. These nonspecific effects require neither calcium ions nor energy.

Basic polypeptides and *proteins* such as protamine, polylysine, histones, and lysosomal proteins release histamine. Some of these are themselves released by tissue damage and could be regarded as physiological stimuli participating in histamine release following injury. Among them are some vasoactive polypeptides, including bradykinin, kallidin, and substance P, which seem to initiate the specific exocytotic response. *Venoms* and *toxins* of many sorts also release histamine, because of their content of basic polypeptides and/or enzymes such as phospholipase A, which may initiate the specific degranulating response or lyse cells. (*See* Beraldo and Dias da Silva, 1966; Goth, 1973; Johnson and Erdös, 1973.)

Histamine Release by Physical or Chemical Insult. Any physical process involving mechanical, thermal, or radiant energies sufficiently intense to damage cells, particularly mast cells, will liberate histamine. The redness and urtication seen when the skin is scratched is a familiar example, as is "cold urticaria." Histamine release also occurs on overexposure to sunlight or intense ionizing radiation, although its relative contribution to the ensuing response is debatable. Indeed, histamine has some protective effect against ionizing radiation (Bacq, 1973). Chemicals causing gross cell damage, such as detergents, bile salts, and lysolecithin, will also release histamine as will osmotic shock.

Injury, Stress, "Induced Histamine," and Microcirculation. Schayer (1963) suggested that "induced histamine," which is not stored but immediately freed, has a role in *regulating the microcirculation* to satisfy locally increased requirements for blood resulting from injurious stimuli. Histamine was also proposed to account for the delayed phase of vasodilatation occurring in *inflammation.* This view is still controversial, and the factors regulating microcirculation remain a complex puzzle. (*See* Zweifach, 1973.)

Tissue Growth and Repair. Kahlson and colleagues have marshaled evidence that a conspicuously high histamine-forming capacity is present in many tissues undergoing rapid growth or repair, such as embryonic tissue, regenerating liver, bone marrow, wound and granulation tissue, and malignant growths in various species, principally the rat. The histamine formed, which they refer to as "nascent histamine," is not stored but free to diffuse (compare with Schayer's "induced histamine," above). They have shown that inhibition of L-histidine decarboxylase arrests fetal development in the rat and, conversely, that drugs elevating histamine-forming capacity accelerate wound healing. Their evidence has led them to suggest that "nascent histamine" has a role in anabolic processes (*see* Kahlson and Rosengren, 1971).

Gastric Secretion. In 1920, Popielski and also Keeton and associates reported that histamine stimulates gastric secretion, and the latter investigators proposed that endogenous histamine might be the final common mediator of acid secretion whether evoked by nervous, mechanical, or chemical means. In subsequent years this prescient scheme has found support in numerous observations resulting from improved methods of studying histamine metabolism and its relation to physiologically induced gastric secretion. In 1965, Code could restate, with increasingly convincing argument, that "stimulation of gastric secretion is a physiological function of histamine"; with still more evidence at their disposal,

Kahlson and Rosengren (1968) could write, "the role of accelerated histamine formation in the mucosa is not a mere hypothesis, but a fact." It must be recognized, however, that uncertainties remain, and the nature and extent of histamine's physiological role are still vigorously debated. One of the principal impediments to analysis in the past has been the absence of antagonists to the stimulant effect of histamine and its congeners on gastric secretion. Recently, this difficulty has been overcome with the discovery of the H_2-receptor blocking agents (*see* below), and new inroads into this old problem of histamine's function in gastric secretion can be expected. The demonstration that such H_2-blocking drugs reduce acid secretion in response not only to histamine but also to feeding and to pentagastrin (Black *et al.,* 1972, 1973) lends fresh support to the histamine hypothesis. Information on the identity of the histamine-containing or -producing cells and their relation to the acid-producing parietal cells is fragmentary (Håkanson *et al.,* 1971).

As described above, most of the histamine that is absorbed from the gastrointestinal tract is destroyed by passage through the liver, but traces survive and appear in the arterial blood. Usually the amounts are too low to stimulate gastric secretion, but this is not so when hepatic destruction is impaired. Thus, when blood is diverted past the liver by a portacaval shunt (Eck fistula), the output of acid in response to a meat meal is greatly increased. Such an effect could explain the high incidence of peptic ulceration in hepatic cirrhosis.

Nerves and Brain. *Afferent Nerves.* Histamine, liberated by one means or another, is frequently involved in initiation of sensory impulses evoking *pain and itch* (Keele and Armstrong, 1964).

Efferent Nerves. The possibility that reflex vasodilatation involves an active component in addition to inhibition of sympathetic vasoconstrictor activity and that this *"active reflex vasodilatation"* may be mediated by histamine liberated by efferent nervous function continues to be debated. There is, as yet, no convincing evidence of peripheral histaminergic nerves. Although histamine has been shown in peripheral nerve trunks, much seems to be present there in mast cells.

Brain. Within the CNS, except for restricted areas, mast cells are absent, and the histamine there must reside in some other component. The distribution of histamine in the brain is very uneven and is reminiscent of that of other biogenic amines; the concentration is highest in the hypothalamus, intermediate in the midbrain, and lowest in the cerebral cortex and white matter. Moreover, subcellular distribution indicates its presence in nerve endings. In addition, the brain has enzymes for both the formation and the inactivation of histamine: L-histidine decarboxylase on the one hand and N-methyltransferase and monoamine oxidase (MAO) on the other (Schayer and Reilly, 1973). Turnover of brain histamine is rapid and is augmented by stressful stimuli that also increase L-histidine decarboxylase activity; inhibitors of the latter enzyme, such as α-hydrazinohistidine, lower brain histamine concentrations.

Finally, histamine can be released from brain tissue by depolarizing stimuli, and this effect requires calcium (*see* Taylor *et al.,* 1972). These observations, in addition to evidence that histamine introduced directly into the brain elicits a spectrum of effects, that various centrally active drugs can modify brain histamine concentrations, and that various antihistamines have obvious central effects, combine to suggest that histamine has a function in the CNS, possibly as a neurotransmitter. (*See* Snyder and Taylor, 1972.)

Headache. Because injected histamine can cause intense headache, endogenous histamine has been implicated in the genesis of a variety of headaches, particularly the syndrome named *histaminic cephalalgia* by Horton (1941). The headache encountered in this syndrome is, however, quite different from that which occurs in response to histamine injections in the normal individual, and cannot be mimicked by liberation of endogenous histamine, which yields the same sort of headache as produced by exogenous histamine. These and other considerations have led to the view that histamine is unlikely to play any part in the genesis of "Horton's headache" (*see* Lecomte, 1957).

Growths of Mast Cells and Basophils. In *urticaria pigmentosa,* aggregates of mast cells form in the upper corium and give rise to pigmented cutaneous lesions in the form of macules, papules, or nodules that urticate when stroked. In *systemic mastocytosis,* similar aggregates are found in other organs. Patients with these syndromes excrete abnormally high amounts of histamine and its metabolites in the urine. They also suffer a constellation of signs and symptoms attributable to excessive histamine release, including, in addition to urticaria and dermographism, pruritus, headache, weakness, hypotension, flushing of the face, and a variety of gastrointestinal effects such as peptic ulceration. The signs and symptoms are precipitated or exacerbated by a variety of stimuli—the friction of toweling the skin or exposure to drugs that release histamine directly or to which patients are allergic. Excessive numbers of basophils are present in the blood in *myelogenous leukemia* and raise its histamine content to high levels. This histamine seems to be rather tightly bound and usually produces no pharmacological responses. Curiously, excessive amounts of histamine are not excreted in the urine of patients with the disease. How the histamine is disposed of is a mystery (Code *et al.,* 1964). *Gastric carcinoid* tumors secrete histamine, and this apparently contributes to the patchy "geographical" flush.

ADDITIONAL CONSIDERATIONS

Absorption, Fate, and Excretion. Histamine is readily absorbed after parenteral injection and acts rapidly when given by the subcutaneous or intramuscular route. Its action is evanescent, since it diffuses into tissues and is rapidly metabolized. Very large amounts of histamine can be given orally, however, without causing effects, since much is converted by intestinal bacteria to inactive N-acetylhistamine, and the free histamine absorbed is mostly inactivated as it traverses the intestinal wall or passes through the liver.

In man there are two major paths of histamine metabolism (*see* Figure 29–2). The more important one involves ring methylation and is catalyzed by the enzyme histamine-N-methyltransferase (imidazole-N-methyltransferase, INMT). Most of the product, methylhistamine, is converted by MAO to methyl imidazole acetic acid (methyl ImAA). In the other path, histamine undergoes oxidative deamination catalyzed mainly by diaminoxidase (DAO), also called "histaminase," which actually comprises nonspecific enzymes found in most tissues that deaminate various aromatic or aliphatic diamines. The products are imidazole acetic acid (ImAA) and, eventually, its riboside. The various metabolites, which have little or no pharmacological activity, are excreted in the urine. The relative roles of these enzymes in the metabolism of endogenous histamine have not yet been established. Some inhibitors of INMT and DAO are known, but their significance is mainly experimental and their contribution to clinical responses uncertain. Amodiaquine and some other antimalarials inhibit INMT (*see* Schayer and Reilly, 1973). DAO activity can be inhibited by aminoguanidine, by many MAO inhibitors, and by isoniazid and hydralazine.

The DAO activity of plasma rises sharply during the first trimester of pregnancy and remains high until term. Its origin is the maternal placenta, but its function is uncertain (Torok *et al.,* 1970). High plasma levels of DAO occur also in medullary carcinoma of the thyroid, a tumor that synthesizes large amounts of the enzyme (Baylin *et al.,* 1972).

Toxicity. Overdosage with histamine is rare, and symptoms are generally not dangerous. However, massive doses cause intense headache, flushing, profound fall of blood pressure, bronchospasm, dyspnea, a metallic taste, vomiting, and diarrhea. The prompt injection of histamine antagonists will suppress these reactions, especially if absorption of the histamine can be delayed by application of a tourniquet.

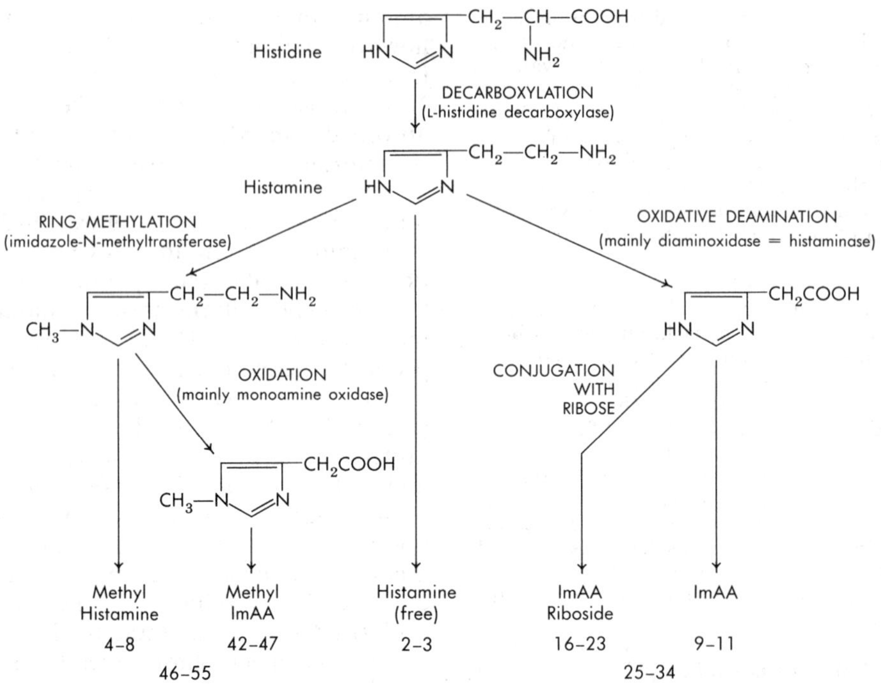

Histidine HN—N ... CH_2—CH—$COOH$ | NH_2

DECARBOXYLATION
(L-histidine decarboxylase)

Histamine HN—N ... CH_2—CH_2—NH_2

RING METHYLATION
(imidazole-N-methyltransferase)

OXIDATIVE DEAMINATION
(mainly diaminoxidase = histaminase)

CH_3—N—N ... CH_2—CH_2—NH_2

HN—N ... CH_2COOH

OXIDATION
(mainly monoamine oxidase)

CONJUGATION
WITH
RIBOSE

CH_3—N—N ... CH_2COOH

Methyl Histamine	Methyl ImAA	Histamine (free)	ImAA Riboside	ImAA
4–8	42–47	2–3	16–23	9–11
46–55			25–34	

Figure 29-2. *Synthesis and catabolism of histamine.*

Percent recovery of histamine and metabolites in the urine in 12 hours following intradermal ^{14}C-histamine in human males (values from Schayer and Cooper, 1956).

Preparations. *Histamine Phosphate,* U.S.P., and *histamine dihydrochloride* are water-soluble, colorless crystals. *Histamine Phosphate Injection, U.S.P.,* contains 1 mg of the salt (0.36 mg of histamine base) in 1 ml. Other available preparations contain 0.275 and 2.75 mg of histamine phosphate in 1 ml (0.1 and 1 mg of histamine base in 1 ml), and are packaged in 1- or 5-ml ampuls.

CLINICAL USES

The practical applications of histamine fall into two categories: first, its uses as a diagnostic agent, which for the most part are on a sound physiological basis; and, second, its more controversial uses in therapy, especially of diseases of allergy.

Diagnostic Uses. *Gastric Secretion.* Histamine is a valuable tool for assessing the ability of the stomach to secrete acid. The standard test for many years was to give histamine subcutaneously, in a dose (0.3 to 0.7 mg of histamine base) that represents a compromise between that maximally effective on acid secretion and that causing intolerable side effects. Kay (1953) made use of the fact that the stimulant effect of histamine on gastric secretion is unopposed by classical antihistamines (H_1-blocking drugs) to devise an *augmented histamine test.* Patients protected against the more distressing side effects of

histamine by such a drug are given histamine in a dose sufficient to produce a maximal secretory response. In this test, total acid production correlates well with parietal cell mass. The histamine analog betazole and the polypeptide pentagastrin (*see* below) offer alternative and in some respects advantageous methods of testing gastric secretory function.

Other Diagnostic Uses. Histamine has various other minor diagnostic uses. The fact that intradermal histamine causes a "flare" that is mediated by axon reflexes allows a test for the *integrity of sensory nerves,* of value in certain neurological conditions. The ability of intradermal histamine to cause wheal formation provides a test for *circulatory competency* in limb extremities of doubtful viability; there is no edema formation unless circulation is adequate. Finally, the stimulant effect of histamine on chromaffin cells has been applied in a provocative test for *pheochromocytoma.* Diagnosis may be made with much less risk by measurement of 24-hour urinary catecholamine excretion.

Therapeutic Uses. In various diseases in which histamine is suspected of being involved in the etiology, such as in allergies, Ménière's disease, and various vascular headaches, attempts have been made to desensitize the patient with courses of histamine injections. There is no experimental evidence that such regimens induce significant tolerance, however, and the procedure has not met with general acceptance.

BETAZOLE

Betazole is an isomer of histamine with preferential effects on gastric secretion (Rosière and Grossman, 1951).

Chemistry. Betazole has the following structural formula:

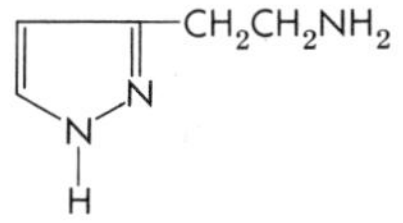

Betazole

Pharmacological Properties. Betazole possesses, in attenuated form, the characteristic actions of histamine on gastric acid secretion, smooth muscle, and blood pressure. However, in contrast to histamine, its stimulant effect on gastric acid is much more prominent than are its other histamine-like effects.

Clinical Use. Betazole is a convenient alternative to histamine in gastric function tests. It is no less effective than histamine in assessing the capacity of the stomach to secrete acid. Moreover, its side effects are probably no worse than those of histamine itself and compare favorably with those occurring with equieffective doses of histamine "covered" with an antihistamine, as in the augmented histamine test. The use of betazole avoids the need for an antihistamine that may have its own undesirable side effects (*see* Breuer and Kirsner, 1967).

Preparation. *Betazole Hydrochloride,* U.S.P. (HISTALOG), is a water-soluble powder, available in ampuls containing 50 mg in 1 ml. The usual adult dose is 100 mg.

GASTRIN; PENTAGASTRIN

For many years there was a widely prevalent view that gastrin, the antral hormone, was simply histamine. Largely due to the work of Gregory and Tracy (*see* their review of 1966), this view was finally proven erroneous, and the potent physiological gastric secretagogue released by vagal and gastric responses to feeding was shown to be a heptadecapeptide. Gastrin activity also occurs as larger peptides in the circulation. The hormone is produced by specialized endocrine cells (G-cells) in the pyloric mucosa in intimate contact with the lumen of the pyloric glands (*see* Grossman, 1970; Andersson, 1973).

The studies by Gregory and Tracy (1966) and Morley (1968) demonstrated that the full spectrum of gastrin-like activity is present in smaller fragments of the peptide, the smallest effective compound being the C-terminal tetrapeptide amide: Trp-Met-Asp-Phe-NH$_2$. This has about 10% of the potency of gastrin. A synthetic pentapeptide derivative, *pentagastrin,* proved still more active and has been adopted for gastric function tests as an alternative to histamine or betazole.

Chemistry. Pentagastrin is N-*t*-butyloxycarbonyl-β-alanyl-L-tryptophyl-L-methionyl-L-aspartyl-L-phenylalanine amide. It has the structural formula shown at the bottom of the page.

Pharmacological Effects. The most prominent action of pentagastrin is to stimulate the secretion of gastric acid, pepsin, and intrinsic factor of Castle; additionally, it stimulates pancreatic secretion, inhibits absorption of water and electrolytes from the ileum, contracts the smooth muscle of the lower esophageal sphincter and stomach (but delays gastric emptying time), relaxes the sphincter of Oddi, increases blood flow in the gastric mucosa, stimulates L-histidine decarboxylase activity in rat gastric mucosa, and, *in high doses,* stimulates a variety of smooth muscles in different species. It also mimics or blocks the effects of the polypeptides pancreozymin-cholecystokinin, secretin, and caerulin, a naturally occurring decapeptide that, along with pancreozymin-cholecystokinin, shares a common C-terminal heptapeptide residue with gastrin. The half-life of pentagastrin in the circulation appears to be about 10 minutes (Merchant *et al.,* 1972). Pentagastrin activates adenylate cyclase in gastric mucosa; it is of interest, in the light of the histamine hypothesis (*see* Kahlson and Rosengren, 1971), that this effect is not additive with histamine (Ruoff and Sewing, 1973).

Clinical Use. Pentagastrin has been used widely in Europe since 1966 to measure the maximal acid secretory capacity of the stomach. It elicits reproducible secretory responses comparable to those induced by histamine or betazole and offers several advantages. The pentagastrin test requires only a single subcutaneous or intramuscular injection; it is relatively short in duration, and side effects are minor and transient. These may include nausea, dizziness, faintness, flushing, and a sensation of warmth.

Preparation. *Pentagastrin* (PEPTAVLON) is marketed in vials containing 0.5 mg in 2 ml. The diagnostic dose is 6 μg/kg, administered by subcutaneous injection. The drug is not yet available in the United States.

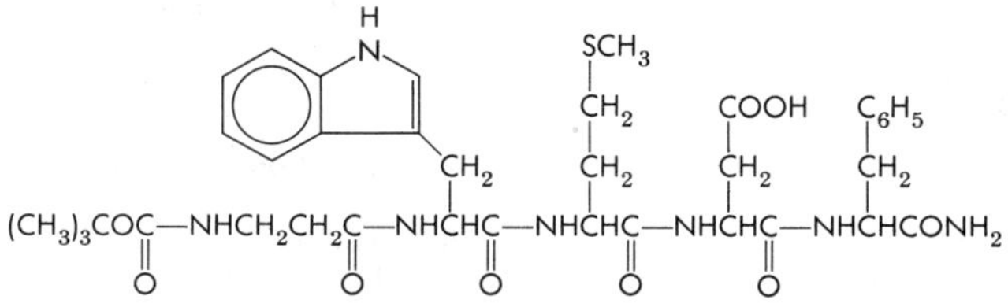

Pentagastrin

INHIBITION OF ALLERGIC RELEASE OF HISTAMINE AND OTHER AUTACOIDS

The above heading relates to a therapeutic objective rather than to an accomplishment. To be completely effective a therapeutic approach based solely on antagonism of the autacoids that are released or formed during the hypersensitivity response would require combined therapy with a battery of antagonists. However, available antagonists to autacoids other than histamine are of limited value, and there is no certainty that all the relevant autacoids have been identified. Furthermore, such a blunderbuss approach would almost certainly be less than optimally effective and would be cumbersome. One can also criticize the traditional use of "physiological" antagonists such as epinephrine to reverse the effects of histamine and other autacoids as nonspecific and purely symptomatic. Obviously it would be preferable to prevent release or formation of the various autacoids. A general suppression of the immune response is clearly an unsound approach, and it remains to be determined whether selective suppression of cytotropic reactions involved in the release of autacoids is feasible. There are indications that pharmacological suppression of release may be obtained in some clinical conditions including asthma. The drug that has focused attention on the therapeutic possibility of suppressing autacoid release is *cromolyn;* although the benefits of this drug are clearly limited, they have generated interest in the general therapeutic approach of suppressing autacoid release.

An alternative pharmacological approach could involve the cyclic AMP system. In contrast to most secretory systems where elevation of intracellular cyclic AMP concentration promotes release, stimulation of adenylate cyclase has an inhibitory effect on release of autacoids from mast cells and basophils. How much the clinical benefits from the use of agents that elevate cyclic AMP (catecholamines, methylxanthines) are related to this inhibitory effect on autacoid release is uncertain. The main point is that in such observations there is clearly an opening toward a new therapeutic approach to the problem. The various drugs acting through cyclic AMP seem to exert their effects at the first stage of the antigen-antibody reaction involving "activation" of the cell and not at the subsequent calcium-dependent step (*see* Koopman *et al.,* 1970; Bourne *et al.,* 1974).

CROMOLYN SODIUM

Cromolyn sodium, the disodium salt of 1,3-*bis*(2-carboxychromon-5-yloxy)-2-hydroxypropane, has the following structure:

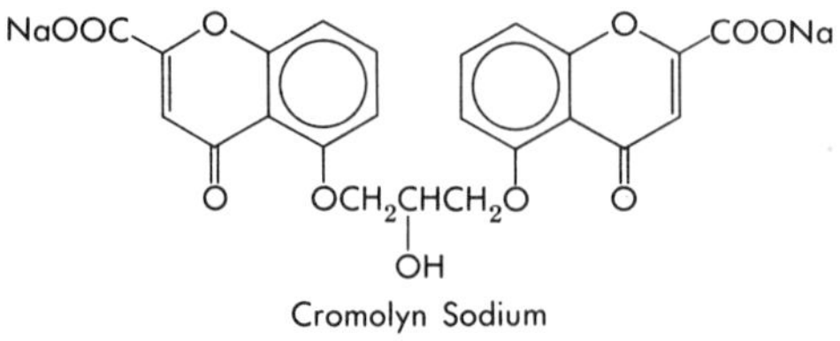

Cromolyn Sodium

History. This synthetic drug was found to inhibit experimental asthma induced by pollen inhalation, as a result of a systematic search for drugs capable of diminishing asthmatic attacks. The chemical approach was based on the long-known smooth muscle–relaxing effects of plant extracts containing khellin, to which it is chemically related. However, the antiasthmatic properties of cromolyn are not attributable to smooth muscle–relaxing effects, which the drug does not possess, but to another action seemingly involving suppression of autacoid release (*see* Cox *et al.,* 1970).

Pharmacological Effects. Cromolyn is not a bronchodilator nor does it relax various other smooth muscles. It does not inhibit significantly responses of smooth muscles to any agonist. It is devoid of significant anti-inflammatory activity. It does, however, inhibit release of histamine and slow-reacting substance in anaphylaxis (SRS-A) from human lung during allergic responses (reaginic, IgE mediated). Both these substances, especially SRS-A, are potent bronchial spasmogens. The action of cromolyn is apparently on the pulmonary mast cells, the primary target cells in the acute hypersensitivity reaction in this tissue. An inhibitory action on antigen-induced production of histamine and SRS-A can be demonstrated in peritoneal mast cells *in vivo* and *in vitro* (Garland and Mongar, 1974). Cromolyn does not inhibit fixation of antibodies, nor does it seem to interfere with the antigen-antibody reaction; rather, it suppresses the response to this reaction. Moreover, the action in suppressing histamine release is not a general one; histamine release from mast cells in response to releasing drugs such as compound 48/80 or bee venom is unaffected. Furthermore, it does not prevent mast-cell–mediated hypersensitivity reactions ("flare" and whealing) in human skin. There are clearly both tissue and species variations in the response to the drug (Assem and Mongar, 1970; Cox *et al.,* 1970; Orange and Austen, 1971).

Clinical Use. Since its introduction in 1968, cromolyn has been widely used in Europe in the prophylaxis of severe bronchial asthma, especially the type that is clearly attributable to inhalation of allergens. Beneficial effects have been corroborated in a study sponsored by the American Academy of Allergy (Bernstein *et al.,* 1972) in which cromolyn-treated patients showed symptomatic improvement and decreased requirement for bronchodilator drugs and steroids (*see also* Dykes, 1974). The benefits of the drug are exclusively prophylactic; cromolyn is without value after an asthmatic attack has begun. Asthma is an extremely complex syndrome that involves a constellation of factors (*see* Study Group, 1971), and it is still too early for full appraisal of the drug's prophylactic worth or even for a convincing explanation of its mode of action.

Preparation. Cromolyn sodium (AARANE, INTAL) is available in capsules containing 20 mg of powder administered by a special inhaler. One capsule is usually inhaled four times daily.

HISTAMINE ANTAGONISTS (ANTIHISTAMINES)

History. It was long obvious that drugs able to antagonize the actions of histamine would be of great interest both as investigative tools and as therapeutic agents. Histamine-blocking activity was first detected by Bovet and Staub (1937) in one of a series of amines with a phenolic ether function synthesized by Fourneau. This substance, 2-isopropyl-5-methyl-phenoxyethyldiethylamine, protected guinea pigs against several lethal doses of histamine, antagonized histamine-induced spasms of various smooth muscles, and, most significantly, lessened the symptoms of anaphylactic shock (Staub and Bovet, 1937). Although the drug was too weak and too toxic for clinical use, this was a most exciting beginning. A more effective drug was uncovered in diethylamino-ethyl-N-ethylaniline. This, too, was rather toxic, but a dimethylamine derivative prepared by Mosnier and investigated by Halpern (1942) proved acceptable for clinical use. This substance, ANTERGAN, was the first antihistaminic drug, or antihistamine, to be employed in therapy. NEO-ANTERGAN, introduced shortly thereafter (Bovet *et al.,* 1944), the official name of which is *pyrilamine maleate,* is still one of the most effective antihistamines. While these developments were taking place in wartime France, the leads offered by the original Fourneau compounds were also being followed in the United States and resulted in the discovery of the highly effective histamine antagonists *diphenhydramine* (Loew *et al.,* 1946) and *tripelennamine* (Yonkman *et al.,* 1946).

By the late 1940s, it was obvious that numerous compounds possessed significant antihistaminic properties. This circumstance, coupled with the unrestrained enthusiasm of some early clinical reports, encouraged a frenzy of syntheses. Most of the efforts were successful, and the physician was shortly confronted with scores of antihistamines to choose from, mostly offering little or no advantage over the original compounds.

All these traditional antihistamines, while effectively antagonizing many important responses to histamine, uniformly failed to inhibit others, most conspicuously gastric acid secretion. The discovery by Black and colleagues in 1972 of agents preferentially blocking gastric secretion and other histamine-induced effects refractory to the traditional antihistamines thus signaled a breakthrough in the field. The discovery at once offered important new tools for probing the significance of histamine in physiological and pathophysiological processes and held out promise of a new and potentially important class of therapeutic agents, the H_2 antagonists.

Antagonism of Histamine H_1 and H_2 Receptors: Terminology. The traditional antihistamines, such as those listed in Tables 29-1 and 29-2 (pages 604 and 609), are effective against many responses to histamine on smooth muscle or other systems that are apparently mediated by a pharmacologically distinct class of histamine receptors, the H_1 receptors of Ash and Schild (1966). The new class of histamine antagonists blocks actions of histamine on receptors of a different type, termed histamine H_2 receptors, and have been referred to as H_2-receptor antagonists (Black *et al.,* 1972). By analogy one might thus refer to the classical antihistamines as histamine H_1-receptor antagonists. However, such terminology is somewhat cumbersome and it might be permissible, by analogy with the field of catecholamines with its α-blocking drugs and β-blocking drugs, to refer simply to H_1-blocking drugs and H_2-blocking drugs (or even H_1 and H_2 blockers) provided the context is clear.

Mechanism of Action. Drugs used to block histamine receptors fall into that large group of pharmacological antagonists that appear to act by occupying "receptive sites" on the effector cell, to the exclusion of agonist molecules, without themselves initiating a response. Typically this antagonism is competitive and reversible.

H_1-RECEPTOR ANTAGONISTS

There are hundreds of compounds of this sort, and discussion will be limited to examples from the main classes (*see* Table 29-1).

Structure-Activity Relationship. The relation between chemical structure and antihistaminic activity is highly complex. Nevertheless, most classical antihistamines can be depicted by the following skeletal structural formula:

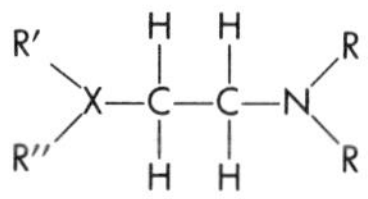

It is at once apparent that the core of this structure is a substituted ethylamine, $-CH_2CH_2N=$, also present in histamine; in most antihistamines, the ethylamine moiety is present as a straight chain, but in others it is part of a ring structure (Table 29-1; *see also* cyproheptadine, below).

Pharmacological Properties. Most of the H_1-receptor antagonists have pharmacological actions and therapeutic applications in common and can be conveniently discussed together. Individual compounds will be mentioned only in those few instances where they depart significantly from the pattern of the group.

Histamine Antagonism. The ability to inhibit effects of histamine on capillary permeability and on vascular, bronchial, and many other types of smooth muscle is the property that characterizes the H_1 antagonists and that provides the basis for their

Table 29-1. REPRESENTATIVE H_1-RECEPTOR ANTAGONISTS AND THEIR STRUCTURAL RELATION TO HISTAMINE

Histamine	imidazole ring—CH_2—CH_2—NH_2
Diphenhydramine* (an ethanolamine)	$(C_6H_5)_2CH$—O—CH_2—CH_2—$N(CH_3)_2$
Pyrilamine† (an ethylenediamine)	H_3CO—C_6H_4—CH_2—$N(\text{pyridyl})$—CH_2—CH_2—$N(CH_3)_2$
Chlorpheniramine‡ (an alkylamine)	Cl—C_6H_4—$CH(\text{pyridyl})$—CH_2—CH_2—$N(CH_3)_2$
Chlorcyclizine§ (a piperazine)	$(C_6H_5)(Cl{-}C_6H_4)CH$—$N\underset{\text{piperazine}}{}N$—$CH_3$
Promethazine (a phenothiazine)	phenothiazine—N—CH_2—$CH(CH_3)$—$N(CH_3)_2$

* Dimenhydrinate is a combination of diphenhydramine and 8-chlorotheophylline in molecular proportions.
† Tripelennamine is the same less H_3CO.
‡ Pheniramine is the same less Cl.
§ Cyclizine is the same less Cl.

prevalent clinical use in hypersensitivity (allergic) states and other conditions where release of endogenous histamine occurs.

Smooth Muscle. H_1-blocking drugs effectively inhibit most smooth muscle responses to histamine. Within the *gastrointestinal tract,* the most numerous studies have been carried out on the guinea pig ileum *in vitro,* a preparation that illustrates the characteristically competitive nature of the antagonism as well as its high degree of specificity. Similar antagonism is also readily demonstrable *in vivo* and in other regions of the gastrointestinal tract.

Antagonism of the *constrictor action of histamine on respiratory smooth muscle* is easily shown *in vivo*, in isolated lungs, or in strips of tracheal, bronchial, or bronchiolar muscle of various species including man. In guinea pigs, death by asphyxia follows quite small doses of histamine, yet the animal may survive a hundred lethal doses of histamine if given an H_1-blocking drug. In the same species, H_1 antagonists offer striking protection against anaphylactic bronchospasm, but this is not so in man, where bronchoconstrictor autacoids beside histamine (*e.g.,* SRS-A) are important.

Within the *vascular tree,* the H_1-blocking drugs inhibit both the vasoconstrictor effects of histamine and, to a degree, the more important vasodilator effects. Apparently, H_2 as well as H_1 receptors are involved, for a combination of H_1- and H_2-blocking drugs is more effective. This is true both of the localized "capillary" dilatation that leads to cutaneous erythema when histamine is injected intradermally and of the more generalized dilatation that results in a fall in blood pressure. The variable, species-dependent, and generally minor stimulant effects of histamine on the heart are little influenced by H_1 blockers.

Capillary Permeability. H_1-blocking drugs strongly antagonize the action of histamine that results in increased capillary permeability and formation of edema. The most striking effect is seen when the antagonist is administered locally, but even following systemic administration a significant reduction in edema formation is usually still obtained.

"Flare" and Itch. The "flare" component of the triple response and the itching caused by intradermal injection of histamine are two different manifestations of a stimulant action of histamine on nerve endings. H_1-blocking drugs suppress both. Although most H_1 antagonists have local anesthetic properties, this cannot entirely account for their effectiveness in countering these effects of histamine. There is little correlation between the anesthetic potency of histamine antagonists and their ability to inhibit neural responses to histamine. Such drugs act apparently in a rather specific manner by blocking histamine receptors, presumably on the nerve endings.

Adrenal Medulla and Autonomic Ganglia. H_1-blocking drugs selectively suppress the stimulant effect of histamine on adrenal chromaffin cells (Staszewska-Barczak and Vane, 1965), as well as the relatively feeble effect of histamine to stimulate autonomic ganglion cells.

Failure to Inhibit Gastric Secretion. The stimulant effect of histamine on *gastric secretion* is among those mediated by H_2 receptors, and it is *not* inhibited by H_1-blocking agents. The failure is illustrated in guinea pigs protected from histamine-induced asphyxial death by H_1-blocking drugs. These animals may subsequently die from perforated ulceration as a result of gastric hypersecretion.

Other Exocrine Glands. There is conflicting evidence on the efficacy of H_1-blocking drugs to suppress histamine-evoked salivary and other exocrine secretions, but some inhibition is generally apparent. The atropine-like properties of many of these antagonists may, however, contribute to lessened secretion in cholinergically innervated glands and reduce ongoing secretion in, for example, the respiratory tree.

Failure to Inhibit Release of Endogenous Histamine. It is essential to note that neither the H_1 nor the H_2 blockers inhibit histamine release. Indeed, the effects of histamine antagonists tend to be in the opposite direction, namely, to facilitate release (*see* below). The beneficial effects of histamine antagonists are thus confined to antagonism of responses to the histamine that is released.

Hypersensitivity Phenomena: Anaphylaxis and Allergy. In the previous discussion of the limitations of the histamine hypothesis of mediation of anaphylaxis and various other allergic responses, it was pointed out that in addition to histamine a number of other potent autacoids are also released, all of which exert effects refractory to inhibition by histamine antagonists. It follows that the efficacy of such antagonists in countering hypersensitivity reactions will vary, depending on the degree to which symptoms are due to histamine. The protection afforded by histamine antagonists thus varies remarkably in different tissues and species. In man, histamine plays an intermediate role. Thus, one finds in man that some phenomena, including edema formation and itch, are fairly well controlled; others, such as hypotension, are less so; and bronchoconstriction is influenced little if at all.

Although laryngeal edema is a prominent feature of fatal anaphylaxis in man and H_1-blocking drugs do antagonize edema formation, the urgency of anaphylactic shock calls for remedies, such as epinephrine, that are more powerful and rapid in their effect and that will additionally counter the relatively refractory bronchoconstrictor and hypotensive effects. The most clinically relevant antagonistic effects of H_1-blocking drugs in experimental human allergic responses are exerted against those of a local nature. Here again the variations in human tissues must be emphasized. Although allergic responses of human skin or mucous membranes are quite well antagonized (presumably histamine is important here), those of human lung are little affected, mainly because of the extraordinary bronchoconstrictor potency of the SRS-A formed and released in the lung. The same general pattern is seen in clinical allergies, and the inefficacy of histamine antagonists in human asthma is especially noteworthy.

Responses to Histamine-Releasing Drugs. These are somewhat better controlled by H_1-blocking drugs in man than are the allergic responses, presumably because the substances involved are fewer and histamine is relatively more important. The limitations of antagonism are, however, essentially those described in connection with allergic responses.

Central Nervous System. The H_1 antagonists can both stimulate and depress the CNS. Stimulation is occasionally encountered in patients given conventional doses, who become restless, nervous, and unable to sleep. Moreover, quite small doses may evoke EEG activation and epileptiform seizures in patients with focal lesions of the cerebral cortex, a property that has been exploited in provocative tests (King and Weeks, 1965). Also, central excitation is a striking feature of poisoning with antihistamines and can result in convulsions, particularly in infants. Central depression, on the other hand, is the usual accompaniment of therapeutic doses. Patients vary in their susceptibility and responses to individual drugs. However, some antihistamines, such as the ethanolamines (Table 29–2, page 609), are particularly active; for example, diphenhydramine causes *somnolence* in about half of those taking it.

Another interesting and useful property of *certain* blockers is the ability to counter *motion sickness.* This effect was first observed with dimenhydrinate and subsequently with diphenhydramine (the active moiety of dimenhydrinate), promethazine, and various piperazine derivatives.

Mechanism of Central Action. How the various histamine-blocking drugs produce their depressant and stimulant effects is not known. Although histaminergic nerves may be present in the brain, there is no obvious correlation between the peripheral histamine-blocking ability of these drugs and their central effects (*see* Faingold and Berry, 1972). Only the antimotion sickness actions have been studied intensively, and even here there is no precise answer. Physiologists debate the causes of motion sickness. All that seems clear is that stimulation of the vestibular apparatus is necessary and sufficient (although the respective roles of semicircular canals and otoliths are uncertain), and that the vestibular cerebellar midbrain "integrative vomiting center" and medullary chemoreceptive trigger zone are somehow involved. It is thus probable that the effective antihistamines exert their action somewhere in these centers (Money, 1970). Electrophysiological recordings in dogs have shown that diphenhydramine diminishes excitability of the vestibular nuclear complex to vestibular afferent activity induced by motion or electrical stimulation of the vestibular nerve (Jaju and Wang, 1971). Similar effects have been obtained with lower doses of scopolamine and atropine, which are more potent antimotion sickness drugs (Jaju et al., 1970). On the whole, the new evidence is in line with the old suggestion (Chinn and Smith, 1955) that the antihistamines effective in motion sickness act by virtue of central antagonism of ACh, as do scopolamine and related atropine-like drugs. All these drugs may act by blocking excitatory labyrinthine impulses at cholinergic synapses in the region of the vestibular nuclei. Promethazine, which is perhaps the antihistamine with the strongest ACh-blocking action, has been found superior to the other antihistamines used to combat motion sickness in a large-scale study that also confirmed the outstanding value of scopolamine as well as the usefulness of centrally active sympathomimetic drugs, especially amphetamine; these findings have prompted speculation on the existence of a noradrenergic mechanism inhibiting motion sickness, and have offered a rationale for concurrent drug therapy (Wood and Graybiel, 1970; *see also* below).

Local Anesthetic Effect. The H_1-blocking drugs possess local anesthetic activity. Some are more potent than procaine. Promethazine and pyrilamine are especially active.

Autonomic Effects. Most antihistamines have some anticholinergic activity, which accounts for the dryness of the mouth experienced by some patients and, more rarely, for other side effects such as difficulty in micturition and impotence. Some intensify responses to norepinephrine or stimulation of adrenergic nerves and inhibit responses to tyramine, apparently by blocking the amine uptake mechanism in the terminals (*see* Johnson and Kahn, 1966).

Cardiovascular System. Rapid intravenous injection of H_1 antagonists causes a transient fall in blood pressure, probably related to local anesthetic activity; but blood pressure is well sustained or may even be elevated when the drug is given slowly, and no significant effects on the cardiovascular system accompany the therapeutic use of antihistamines. In sufficient dosage, some of the drugs have quinidine-like effects on myocardial conduction consistent with their local anesthetic properties.

Absorption, Fate, and Excretion. The H_1 antagonists are readily absorbed from the gastrointestinal tract and parenteral sites of administration. Following oral administration, the effects start within 15 to 30 minutes, are fully developed within 1 hour, and last about 3 to 6 hours, although some of the drugs act much longer (Table 29-2, page 609).

Extensive studies of the metabolic fate of antihistamines have been limited to a few compounds. *Diphenhydramine* rapidly leaves the circulation and reaches a peak concentration in tissues in about 1 hour. The tissues are almost free of the drug in about 6 hours. The highest concentration occurs in the lung, with progressively lower concentrations in the spleen, kidney, brain, muscle, and skin. Little, if any, of the drug is excreted unchanged in the urine; most appears there as degradation products that are almost completely excreted within 24 hours. The main site of metabolic transformation is the liver. Tripelennamine appears to be handled in much the same way. Likewise, chlorcyclizine, chlorpheniramine, and cyclizine are extensively metabolized (*see* Kuntzman *et al.,* 1967; Peets *et al.,* 1972).

Side Effects. In therapeutic doses, all H_1 antagonists elicit side effects. Although these are rarely serious and often disappear with continued therapy, they are sometimes so troublesome that the drug must be withdrawn. Some difference in the incidence and severity of the side effects with different preparations is discernible, but there is such marked variation in the responses of individual subjects that accurate figures of relative incidence of side effects in the population as a whole, even if they were available, would be of doubtful value in assisting the physi-

cian to choose among these drugs. One notable exception is in the tendency to cause somnolence, which is clearly more marked in some of the drugs than in others. About one person in four will experience some bothersome reaction during treatment with a given antihistamine.

The side effect with the highest incidence, and the one common to all drugs in this group, is *sedation.* Although this may be a desirable adjunct in the treatment of some patients in hospital or about to retire for the night, it interferes with the patient's daytime activities and can so dull the mind and slow reflex activity that accidents may occur. Decrease in dosage, the use of a different antihistamine, and combined therapy with stimulants such as caffeine or amphetamine are possible devices for circumventing this undesirable effect. Other untoward reactions referable to *central actions* include dizziness, tinnitus, lassitude, incoordination, fatigue, blurred vision, diplopia, euphoria, nervousness, insomnia, and tremors.

The next most frequent side effects involve the *digestive tract* and include loss of appetite, nausea, vomiting, epigastric distress, and constipation or diarrhea. Their incidence may be reduced by giving the drug with meals. Other side effects include dryness of the mouth, throat, and respiratory passages, sometimes inducing cough; urinary frequency and dysuria; palpitation; hypotension; headache; tightness of the chest; and tingling, heaviness, and weakness of the hands.

Allergy may develop when the antihistamines are given orally, but more commonly it results from topical application. Allergic dermatitis is not uncommon. In addition, histamine-liberating properties have been demonstrated in several of the drugs (Rothschild, 1966) and may contribute to some adverse reactions encountered during therapy. Fortunately, grave complications such as *leukopenia* and *agranulocytosis* are very rare.

The piperazine compounds—cyclizine, chlorcyclizine, and meclizine—have been demonstrated to have *teratogenic effects in laboratory animals,* and their use is contraindicated in women who are pregnant or who may become so (*see* Sadusk and Palmisano, 1965).

Acute Antihistamine Poisoning. Although the H_1-blocking drugs have a relatively high margin of safety, acute poisoning with them is common. Antihistamines are among the drugs most frequently found in medicine cabinets, and all too often they are the cause of accidental poisoning in young children or the instrument of suicide in adults. In children, 20 to 30 tablets or capsules of most commercially available antihistamines represents a lethal or near-lethal dose.

The central effects of the antihistamines constitute their greatest danger and, in a severely poisoned individual, give rise to a constellation of signs and symptoms in which both the depressant and stimulant properties of the drug are in evidence. In the small child, the dominant effect is excitation, and the syndrome of poisoning includes *hallucinations, excitement, ataxia, incoordination, athetosis,* and *convulsions.* The convulsions, sometimes heralded by muscular tremors and athetoid movements, are of the intermittent tonic-clonic type and difficult to control. *Fixed, dilated pupils* with a *flushed face* and *fever* are common, and lend the syndrome a remarkable similarity to that of atropine poisoning. Terminally, there is deepening coma with cardiorespiratory collapse and death, usually within 2 to 18 hours. In the adult, fever and flushing are not usually in evidence, and the phase of excitement leading to convulsions and postictal depression is not uncommonly preceded by drowsiness and coma, so that there is a cycle of depression followed by stimulation and postictal depression. Inasmuch as the treatments of the two types of depression are different, keen judgment is mandatory.

Treatment. There is no specific therapy for antihistamine poisoning, and treatment is along general symptomatic and supportive lines. The direct depressant effect of antihistamines is not as profound as that of the barbiturates. Respiration is usually not seriously embarrassed, and blood pressure is fairly well maintained. Should breathing fail, the mechanical support of ventilation offers a safer and more effective means of maintaining respiration than the use of analeptics, which are prone to initiate or intensify the convulsive phase. When convulsions develop, they are best countered by a short-acting depressant such as thiopental, to provide a rapid, transient, and controllable effect; diazepam is also worthy of a trial.

Preparations. There is a needlessly large number of antihistamines of the H_1-blocking type, and little distinction can be made between them on the basis of efficacy as histamine antagonists. They do vary somewhat, however, with respect to potency, dosage, relative incidence of side effects, and the types of preparations available. Naturally, the physician is desirous of choosing a preparation that will assure him the greatest opportunity for therapeutic success with the minimal chance of side effects. Unfortunately, no antihistamine can be said to be outstanding in this respect. The difficulty lies not only in the quantitative assessment of both therapeutic efficacy and incidence and severity of side effects, but also in the fact that individual variations in response are prominent with these drugs. Such factors tend to undermine the value of generalizations, and the end result is that the physician must often approach the problem in a tentative manner, trying first a thoroughly tested drug known to have the desired pattern of effect in most patients, and employing other drugs only in the event that the first proves unsatisfactory. Since there are many advantages in using the older and well-tried drugs, it would seem wise for the physician to familiarize himself with a few representative compounds from the different classes, and to base his therapy upon these. Few, if any, of the "newer" drugs have any conspicuous therapeutic advantage, and most are more costly. The brief discussion that follows is intended to provide only an indication of the different classes of drugs and their properties. The statements should be interpreted in the light of the foregoing comments. The U.S.P. and N.F. preparations are listed in Table 29-2.

Ethanolamines (Prototype: Diphenhydramine). The drugs in this group are potent and effective H_1 blockers that possess significant anticholinergic activity and have a pronounced tendency to induce sedation. With conventional doses, about half of those who are treated with these drugs experience somnolence, although with carbinoxamine the proportion is rather less. The incidence of gastrointestinal side effects, however, is low in this group.

Ethylenediamines (Prototype: Pyrilamine). These, too, are highly effective H_1 blockers. Although their central effects are relatively feeble and of no therapeutic value, somnolence occurs, nevertheless, in a fair proportion of patients. Gastrointestinal side effects are quite common. This group contains some of the oldest and best-known antihistamines.

Alkylamines (Prototype: Chlorpheniramine). The antihistamines in this group are among the most active H_1 blockers and are generally effective in relatively low doses. The drugs are not so prone to produce drowsiness and are among the more suitable agents for daytime use; but again, a significant proportion of patients do experience this effect. Side effects involving CNS stimulation are more common in this than in other groups.

Piperazines (Prototype: Chlorcyclizine). The oldest member of this group, chlorcyclizine, is an H_1

Table 29-2. PREPARATIONS AND DOSAGE OF REPRESENTATIVE OFFICIAL H₁-BLOCKING ANTIHISTAMINES *

CLASS AND NONPROPRIETARY NAME	STATUS	TRADE NAME	DURATION OF ACTION (HOURS)	USUAL PREPARATION	OTHER PREPARATIONS AVAILABLE	SINGLE DOSE (ADULT)
Ethanolamines						
Diphenhydramine Hydrochloride	U.S.P.	BENADRYL	4–6	Capsules, 25 and 50 mg	Injection (syringes and ampuls); elixir	50 mg
Dimenhydrinate	U.S.P.	DRAMAMINE	4–6	Tablets, 50 mg	Injection; suppositories; syrup	50 mg
Carbinoxamine Maleate	N.F.	CLISTIN	3–4	Tablets, 4 mg; repeat-action tablets, 8 and 12 mg	Elixir	4 mg
Ethylenediamines						
Tripelennamine Hydrochloride	U.S.P.	PYRIBENZAMINE	4–6	Tablets, 25 and 50 mg; delayed-action tablets, 50 and 100 mg	Cream (topical), 2%; ointment (topical), 2%	50 mg
Tripelennamine Citrate	U.S.P.	PYRIBENZAMINE		Elixir, 37.5 mg/5 ml		75 mg
Pyrilamine Maleate	N.F.	HISTALON, NEO-ANTERGAN, NEO-PYRAMINE, NISAVAL	4–6	Tablets, 25 and 50 mg	Various (in combinations)	25–50 mg
Antazoline Phosphate	N.F.	VASOCOR-A	3–4	Ophthalmic solution, 0.5% (less irritating than other antihistamines)		
Methapyrilene Hydrochloride	N.F.	HISTADYL	4–6	Capsules, 25 and 50 mg	Injection; syrup	25–50 mg
Alkylamines						
Chlorpheniramine Maleate	U.S.P.	CHLOR-TRIMETON and many others	4–6	Tablets, 4 mg; repeat-action tablets, 8 and 12 mg	Injection; syrup	2–4 mg
Brompheniramine Maleate	N.F.	DIMETANE, DISOMER	4–6	Tablets, 4 mg	Elixir	4–8 mg
Piperazines						
Cyclizine Hydrochloride	U.S.P.	MAREZINE	4–6	Tablets, 50 mg	Suppositories, 50 and 100 mg; injection	50 mg
Cyclizine Lactate	N.F.	MAREZINE	4–6	Injection, 50 mg/ml in 1-ml ampul		50 mg
Meclizine Hydrochloride	U.S.P.	BONINE	12–24	Tablets (chewing), 25 mg		25–50 mg
Phenothiazines						
Promethazine Hydrochloride	U.S.P.	PHENERGAN	4–6	Tablets, 12.5, 25, and 50 mg	Injection; suppositories; syrup	25–50 mg

* This table contains only those drugs included in U.S.P. and N.F.; for a discussion of phenothiazines, *see* Chapter 12.

antagonist with prolonged action and a comparatively low incidence of drowsiness. The others are used primarily to counter motion sickness. Although the incidence of untoward effects, both CNS depressant and anticholinergic, seems to compare favorably with that of other antihistamines, the side effects may, nevertheless, be disturbing. The possibility of some dulling of mental alertness should be borne in mind when the subject may be called upon to perform exacting and potentially hazardous tasks, such as driving a car. Clearly, in some circumstances the relatively short-acting cyclizine may be preferred to the longer-acting meclizine.

Phenothiazines (Prototype: Promethazine). Most drugs of this class are H_1 antagonists. The prototype, promethazine, was introduced in 1946 for the management of allergic conditions. The prominent sedative effects of this compound and its value in motion sickness were early recognized. Promethazine and its many congeners are now used primarily for their central depressant properties (*see* Chapter 10).

Therapeutic Uses. H_1-Receptor blockers have an established and valued place in the symptomatic treatment of various allergic diseases, in which their usefulness is clearly attributable to their antagonism of histamine. In addition, the central properties of *some* of the series are of considerable therapeutic value, particularly in suppressing motion sickness.

Diseases of Allergy. H_1-Blocking drugs are most useful in acute exudative types of allergy such as *pollinosis* and *urticaria.* Their effect, however, is purely palliative and confined to the suppression in varying degree of symptoms attributable to the pharmacological activity of histamine released by the antigen-antibody reaction. The drugs do not diminish the intensity of this reaction, which is the root cause of the various hypersensitivity diseases. This can be achieved only by other means, such as the removal or avoidance of allergen, specific desensitization, suppression of the reaction by corticosteroids, or, in restricted instances, use of cromolyn (*see* below). This limitation must be clearly recognized because no histamine antagonist is effective against the various other autacoids liberated or formed during allergic responses. Such substances are clearly more important than histamine in *bronchial asthma.* In this disease, histamine antagonists are singularly ineffectual, despite indications that histamine is released and that the asthmatic lung is more sensitive to the bronchoconstrictor actions of administered histamine than is the normal lung. The most important point is that histamine antagonists have no role in the therapy of the severe attack, in which chief reliance must be placed on "physiological antagonists" such as epinephrine, isoproterenol, and theophylline. Equally, in the treatment of *systemic anaphylaxis,* in which autacoids other than histamine are important, the mainstay of therapy is provided by epinephrine, with histamine

antagonists having only a subordinate and adjuvant role. The same is true for severe *angioedema,* in which laryngeal swelling constitutes a threat to life. However, the subordination of histamine antagonists to physiological antagonists in these allergic crises is not based solely on the grounds that autacoids other than histamine are involved. The superiority of physiological antagonists lies in the immediacy of the relief they afford and in the fact that they do not merely reduce the undesirable effects but tend to reverse them.

Other allergies of the respiratory tract are more amenable to therapy with H_1 antagonists. The best results are obtained in *seasonal rhinitis* (hay fever, pollinosis), in which these drugs relieve the sneezing, rhinorrhea, and itching of eyes, nose, and throat. A gratifying response is obtained in most patients, especially at the beginning of the season when pollen counts are low; however, the drugs are rather less effective when the allergens are in abundance, when exposure to them is prolonged, and when nasal congestion has become prominent. Such chronic congestion and the accompanying headache from edema of the paranasal sinus mucosa are rather refractory to antihistamine treatment. In *perennial (vasomotor) rhinitis,* antihistamines are of much less value. Antihistamines have long been employed in elixirs and syrups for controlling *cough,* especially preasthmatic cough in children; but any benefit from their specific antiallergic action or sedation may be offset by the anticholinergic properties of these drugs, which, by excessive drying of the respiratory tree, can render bronchial secretion viscid and make expectoration difficult (Winek, 1969).

Certain of the *allergic dermatoses* respond favorably to antihistamines. Benefit is most striking in acute urticaria, although the itching in this condition is perhaps better controlled than are the edema and the erythema. *Chronic urticaria* is less responsive, but some measure of benefit may be had in a fair proportion of patients. *Angioedema* is also responsive to treatment with antihistamines, but the paramount importance of epinephrine in the severe attack must be reemphasized, especially in the life-threatening involvement of the larynx. Here, however, it may be appropriate to administer *additionally* an antihistamine by the intravenous route. Antihistamines also have a place in the treatment of *itching pruritides.* Some relief may be obtained in many patients suffering from *atopic dermatitis* and *contact dermatitis,* although topical corticosteroids seem to be more valuable, and in such diverse conditions as *insect bites* and *ivy poisoning.* Various other pruritides without allergic basis sometimes respond to antihistamine therapy, usually when the drugs are applied topically but sometimes when they are given orally. However, the considerable danger of producing allergic dermatitis with local application of antihistamines must be recognized. Since antihistamines are effective in blocking allergic dermatoses, it is obvious that the *drugs should be withdrawn prior to skin testing for allergies.*

The value of antihistamines in *systemic allergies* is variable. As described above, they have only an adjuvant role in severe systemic anaphylaxis. The urticarial and edematous lesions of *serum sickness,* however, respond rather well to antihistamine therapy; but often these drugs fail to affect fever or arthralgia. In this condition, the antihistamines should be given in high doses throughout the expected duration of the reaction, in order to avoid relapse. Antihistamines are of some value in controlling *blood transfusion reactions* of the nonhemolytic, nonpyrogenic type, although they are inadequate in controlling the more severe reactions. *Gastrointestinal allergies* are seldom benefited significantly by antihistamines. (*See* Wilhelm, 1961; Hartman, 1969.)

Many *drug reactions* attributable to allergic phenomena respond to therapy with antihistamines, particularly those characterized by itch, urticaria, and angioedema; reactions of the serum-sickness type also respond to intensive treatment. However, explosive histamine release, such as occurs in nitritoid crises or in response to powerful histamine liberators, generally calls for treatment with epinephrine, with antihistamines being accorded a subsidiary role. Nevertheless, prophylactic treatment with an antihistamine may suffice to reduce symptoms to a tolerable level when a drug known to be a powerful histamine liberator is to be given.

Common Cold. Despite early claims and persistent popular belief, antihistamines are of little value in combating the common cold. Their weak anticholinergic effect may, however, lessen rhinorrhea. Persons with chronic allergic rhinitis and superimposed acute colds may benefit directly from the relief of the allergic component and indirectly from the fact that the resistance of the mucosa to infection may be greater when there is no coincidental allergic reaction.

Motion Sickness and Other Conditions. By far the most common application of the central effects of certain antihistamines is in the prophylaxis and treatment of *motion sickness* accompanying air, sea, or land travel. In recent years there has been a tendency to restrict drug therapy to two classes of agents: ACh antagonists of the scopolamine type and H_1 blockers. Early claims that the effective antihistamines were clearly superior have been rebutted by careful studies showing that of all the single agents scopolamine is the most effective in preventing motion sickness (Brand and Perry, 1966). While this has been corroborated in recent very extensive studies, a number of investigators have again demonstrated the usefulness of H_1 blockers—particularly cyclizine, dimenhydrinate, and promethazine in ascending order of effectiveness—and have focused attention on the value of ephedrine and amphetamine alone or in combination with one of the other two classes of drugs. A combination of scopolamine and amphetamine in high dose was outstandingly effective, but side effects were disturbing. Next in effectiveness and better tolerated were combinations of amphetamine in lower dose (10 mg) and scopolamine (0.6 mg) or promethazine (25 mg), with the latter being least prone to induce disturbing side effects (*see* Wood and Graybiel, 1970). At least one antihistamine, promethazine, alone or in combination, is thus one of the best antimotion sickness agents, although its action, like that of scopolamine, is probably due to its potent anticholinergic activity. Such results are a challenge to current therapeutic orthodoxy, which focuses almost exclusively on dimenhydrinate and the piperazine class of antihistamines; these often fail to produce adequate protection. Drugs are best given prophylactically at least 30 minutes before exposure to the disturbing motion.

The antihistamines effective in motion sickness have some beneficial effect in vestibular disturbances such as *Ménière's disease* and other types of *vertigo* (*see* Cohen and deJong, 1972).

The tendency of certain antihistamines, particularly the ethanolamines, to produce somnolence has led to their use as *hypnotics.* They are by no means as powerful or effective as the barbiturates, for example, but they may have some value in selected patients. Antihistamines, particularly methapyrilene, are present in various proprietary remedies for insomnia that are sold "over the counter." While these remedies are generally ineffective in the recommended doses, some singularly sensitive individuals may derive benefit.

The *local anesthetic activity* of antihistamines has often been used to counter itching or painful conditions of skin and mucous membranes. However, as already emphasized, there is danger of drug sensitization following topical application.

H_2-RECEPTOR ANTAGONISTS

As noted above, the histamine antagonists available before 1972 blocked only those effects of histamine mediated by H_1 receptors. Among the histamine-induced responses refractory to inhibition by these antihistamines, the most noteworthy is gastric secretion, a response remarkable for its sensitivity, intensity, clinical importance, and physiological significance. But various other effects of histamine also fall into this category; they include stimulant effects on certain other exocrine secretions and on the force and rate of contraction of various cardiac preparations, and inhibitory effects on the contraction of some smooth muscle preparations, such as the rat uterus. In all these instances, analysis indicates that histamine acts through a common receptor of a different type, termed H_2 receptor, which can be blocked by a new class of histamine antagonists, the H_2-receptor antagonists or H_2-blocking drugs (Black *et al.*, 1972). Some tissues—for example, the smooth muscle of the blood vessels determining total peripheral resistance and hence systemic blood pressure—appear to possess both H_1 and H_2 receptors.

The full extent and importance of H_2 receptors have yet to be defined because it is only recently that the H_2-blocking drugs have become available. What seems most important at this stage is to recognize the existence of H_2 receptors and their susceptibility to block by the newer agents.

Chemistry. The first drug reported to have potent H_2-blocking activity was *burimamide*, N-methyl-N'-(4-[4(5)-imidazolyl]butyl) thiourea (Black *et al.*, 1972). The usefulness of the compound is limited by poor oral absorption. This led to the development of a congener in which a methylene group in the side chain is replaced with an isosteric thioether link to yield *metiamide*, N-methyl-N'-2[(5-methylimidazol-4-yl)methylthio]-ethyl thiourea, a compound with a preferred tautomer of the imidazole ring similar to that of histamine. A pK_a of approximately 7.0 favors ready absorption from the small intestine. The structures of these compounds and their relation to histamine are shown below:

$$\text{HN} \diagdown \text{N:} \quad -CH_2-CH_2-\overset{+}{N}H_3$$

Histamine
(preferred ring tautomer)

$$:N \diagdown NH \quad -CH_2-CH_2-CH_2-CH_2-NH-\underset{\underset{S}{\|}}{C}-NH-CH_3$$

Burimamide

$$H_3C \diagdown \underset{HN \diagdown N:}{} -CH_2-S-CH_2-CH_2-NH-\underset{\underset{S}{\|}}{C}-NH-CH_3$$

Metiamide

Pharmacological Properties.

The two drugs, burimamide and metiamide, are potent H_2 antagonists and produce competitive inhibition of those actions of histamine that are mediated by H_2 receptors, especially gastric acid secretion.

The inhibitory effect of metiamide on gastric acid secretion elicited by infusion of histamine in a *maximally effective dose* in dogs is shown in Figure 29-3. Comparable effects were observed in normal humans in the same study (Black *et al.*, 1973). The inhibitory effects of metiamide and burimamide are all the more remarkable in that they extend to gastric secretion evoked by pentagastrin (lowest curve, Figure 29-3). The latter effect clearly lends fresh weight to the old conjecture that endogenous histamine mediates the effect of gastrin. It also lends a special interest to the use of metiamide and other H_2-blocking drugs in the analysis of gastric function and to the potential value of these drugs in peptic ulceration, the

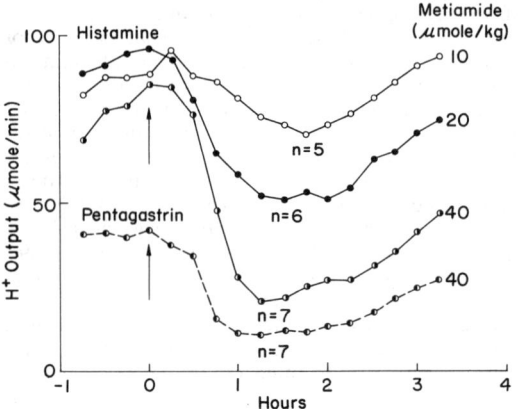

Figure 29-3. *Inhibitory effect of metiamide on gastric acid output in response to histamine or pentagastrin in dogs (Heidenhain pouch technic).*

Histamine (20 μmole/hr) or pentagastrin (10 μmole/kg/hr) was given by continuous intravenous infusion throughout each experiment. Metiamide (10, 20, or 40 μmole/kg) in gelatin capsules was given orally at zero-time (arrows). (After Black, Duncan, Emmett, Ganellin, Hesselbo, Parsons, and Wyllie, 1973. Courtesy of *Agents and Actions*.)

Zollinger-Ellison syndrome, and other gastric hypersecretory states. Patients with duodenal ulcers are known to secrete exceptionally high amounts of gastrin following feeding and also to secrete more acid in response to a given dose of gastrin than do normal individuals; in the Zollinger-Ellison syndrome the huge amounts of circulating gastrin may produce massive gastric ulceration and fatal perforation (Grossman, 1970; McGuigan, 1973). Patients with duodenal ulcers also commonly have an exceptionally high rate of nocturnal acid secretion, which aggravates their condition. In such patients a single oral dose of metiamide brings about a profound reduction in gastric secretion, lasting for hours (Milton-Thompson *et al.*, 1974). This effect, illustrated in Figure 29-4, is unique and unrivaled by any other presently available therapeutic agent or regimen.

In initial reports metiamide unfortunately has been noted to produce agranulocytosis, the incidence of which is sufficiently high to curtail current clinical testing in man. However, active congeners that exhibit a similar pharmacological spectrum may be essentially devoid of this hazard.

The great therapeutic potential and ana-

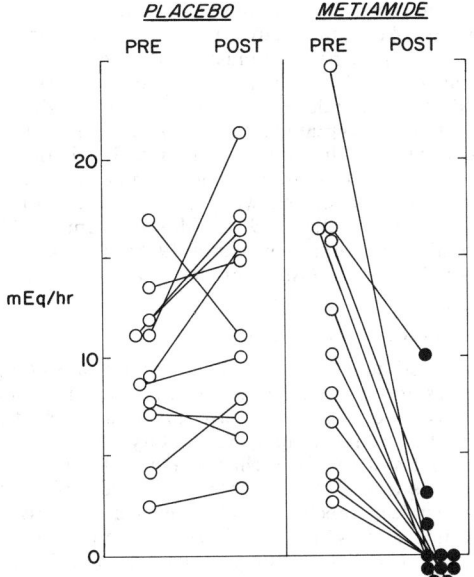

PLACEBO   METIAMIDE

PRE   POST   PRE   POST

mEq/hr

Figure 29-4. *Inhibition of nocturnal gastric acid secretion by a single oral dose of metiamide in patients with duodenal ulcer.*

Gastric juice was collected from 11 males aged 18 to 63 years. Each patient received either metiamide (400 mg) or placebo tablets in predetermined random order. Basal acid output was measured from 10 to 11 P.M. (*pre*); the tablet was then given, and beginning 1 hour later acid output was measured over another 1-hour period (*post*). Note the profound inhibitory effect of metiamide on acid production: 8 of the 11 patients were rendered anacidic. (After Milton-Thompson, Williams, Jenkins, and Misiewicz, 1974. Courtesy of the *Lancet.*)

lytical value of H_2-blocking drugs will certainly generate a flow of pharmacological, physiological, and clinical studies. Reports in a symposium (Wood and Simkins, 1973) provide much useful information.

Histamine, one of the most venerable autacoids, has again been thrust to "front-stage" by pharmacological endeavor.

5-HYDROXYTRYPTAMINE

History. Mammalian physiologists have known for about a century that a vasoconstrictor material appears in serum when blood is allowed to clot. This unidentified vasoconstrictor material, which went by a variety of names, such as *vasotonin,* was a frequent nuisance in perfusion experiments in which defibrinated blood was used, although the older physiologists discovered empirically that it could be eliminated by passing the blood through the lungs, a phenomenon now understood to be due to uptake

and enzymatic destruction. In the late 1940s, the substance appeared in another context during the course of the search for humoral pressor agents such as angiotensin that might play a part in arterial hypertension. In this work the serum vasoconstrictor was a "pest," to be eliminated before the other enquiry could proceed. In 1948, investigators at the Cleveland Clinic succeeded in isolating the serum vasoconstrictor in a crystalline, complex form, to which they gave the name *serotonin* (Rapport *et al.,* 1948). Shortly thereafter, Rapport (1949) made a critical contribution when he deduced that the active moiety of this complex (for which he retained the name *serotonin*) was 5-hydroxytryptamine (5-HT). This compound, when prepared synthetically by Hamlin and Fischer (1951) and others, proved to have all the properties of natural serotonin.

Quite independently of this work on the serum vasoconstrictor, studies had been proceeding in Italy that were destined to establish that 5-HT had a wide distribution in nature and occurred in tissues other than blood. This approach was begun in the 1930s by Erspamer and his colleagues (*see* Erspamer, 1954), whose original purpose was to extract and characterize the substance that imparts peculiar histochemical properties to enterochromaffin cells of the gastrointestinal mucosa. Their work led them to the discovery, first in the gastric mucosa and later in other tissues, of a gut-stimulating factor of basic nature, which they termed *enteramine.* By the late 1940s, Erspamer had accumulated a great deal of information on the pharmacological activity and distribution of enteramine and had suggested that it was an indole alkylamine (Erspamer, 1946). Within a few years of the discovery of 5-HT in the blood, Erspamer and Asero (1952) had established that this too was the chemical structure of enteramine.

Thus, by the time 5-HT had been recognized as such, there already existed a mass of evidence indicating that it was widely distributed in nature and possessed a variety of pharmacological actions. It is therefore not surprising that the introduction of synthetic 5-HT in 1951 touched off an explosion of research. Further interest in 5-HT was provided by the discovery, in 1953, of the presence of the amine in the brain (Twarog and Page, 1953; Amin *et al.,* 1954), and prescient deductions, on this and pharmacological evidence, were made that its function there might be to act as a neurotransmitter substance. An important clue came with the demonstration that the hallucinogen lysergic acid diethylamide (LSD), one of the most potent psychoactive drugs, not only was structurally related to 5-HT but also was a 5-HT antagonist on smooth muscle (Gaddum, 1953; Woolley and Shaw, 1954; Woolley, 1962). Another clue was provided by the discovery that a profound fall in brain 5-HT concentration followed administration of the potent tranquilizer reserpine (*see* Brodie and Shore, 1957). By 1966 a handbook on 5-HT had appeared that cited more than 4000 articles (Erspamer, 1966b) and work has continued apace. There is now compelling evidence that 5-HT is indeed a chemical transmitter released by neurons widely distributed in the brain and probably the target for various centrally active drugs.

Moreover, it is clear that this autacoid has still other functions—some understood well, others little or not at all.

Source and Chemistry. 5-HT is 3-(β-aminoethyl)-5-hydroxyindole. Like histamine, it is widely distributed in the animal and plant kingdoms. It occurs, for example, in vertebrates; in tunicates, mollusks, arthropods, and coelenterates; in fruits such as pineapples, bananas, and plums; and in various nuts. It is also present in numerous stings and venoms, including those of the common stinging nettle, cowhage (the prankster's "itching powder"), wasps, and scorpions (*see* Erspamer, 1966a).

In the mammal, it is synthesized from dietary tryptophan, which is first hydroxylated to 5-hydroxytryptophan (5-HTP) and then decarboxylated to 5-HT, as shown below (Udenfriend, 1959). Normally about 2% of the tryptophan in the diet is converted to 5-HT. Tryptophan-5-hydroxylase is the rate-limiting enzyme in this sequence; however, at least in brain, it is not saturated by its substrate and synthesis *in vivo* depends to some extent on tryptophan concentrations. The enzyme catalyzing conversion of 5-HTP to 5-HT is the relatively nonspecific aromatic L-amino acid decarboxylase, also involved in the synthesis of the catecholamines (*see* Erspamer, 1966b; Symposium, 1968b, 1973, 1974b).

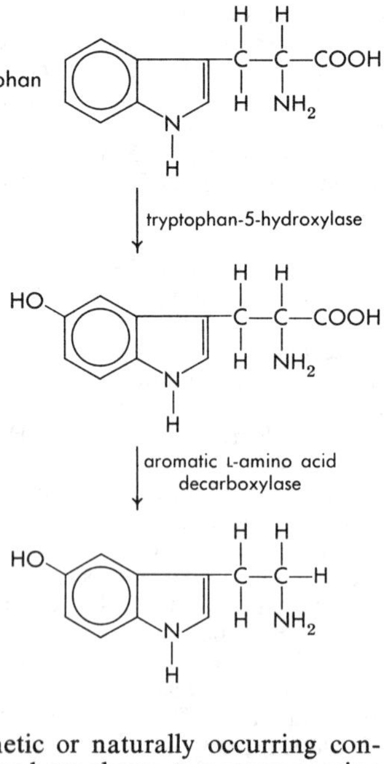

Numerous synthetic or naturally occurring congeners of 5-HT have been shown to possess varying degrees of central and peripheral pharmacological activities, and tryptamine itself, in high doses, is active. It is particularly noteworthy, in view of the possible physiological functions of endogenous 5-HT in the CNS, that several congeneric substances have extraordinarily potent effects on the brain. For example, N,N-dimethyltryptamine and its 5-hydroxy derivative (*bufotenin*) are active principles of the cahobe bean found along the shores of the Carib-

bean and used in aboriginal rites to induce mental changes. Also, the active ingredients of various Mexican hallucinogenic mushrooms (*e.g., Psilocybe mexicana*) used for related purposes are 4-substituted tryptamine derivatives (*psilocine* is 4-hydroxy-N,N-dimethyltryptamine, and *psilocybin* is 4-phosphoryloxy-N,N-dimethyltryptamine). Furthermore, a 4-substituted tryptamine moiety can be recognized in the most potent known psychotomimetic drug, LSD. (*See* Woolley, 1962; Mantegazzini, 1966; Cerletti *et al.,* 1968; Symposium, 1968a, 1968b, 1973, 1974a, 1974b; *see also* Chapters 12 and 16.)

PHARMACOLOGICAL ACTIONS

5-HT stimulates or inhibits a variety of smooth muscles and nerves. These and other actions result in a wide spectrum of responses involving, in particular, the cardiovascular, respiratory, and gastrointestinal systems. It is characteristic of 5-HT that its effects tend to be variable. Responses differ not only between species but also between animals of the same species and even in successive tests in the individual. This variability, which is responsible for many discrepant reports and much controversy, is attributable in large part to two factors: (1) many of the effects of 5-HT are reflexly mediated and hence subject to influences such as pattern of innervation, route and speed of injection, anesthetic state, and spontaneous tone; and (2) tachyphylaxis is common when tests are made at frequent intervals. What follows is a short description of some of the more prominent effects of 5-HT. For further accounts and documentation, the several extensive monographs and reviews should be consulted, particularly the handbook edited by Erspamer (1966b).

Respiratory System. *Stimulation of Afferent Nerves.* Intravenous injection of 5-HT in the dog and man commonly causes a short-lived increase in respiratory minute volume accompanied by variable changes in respiratory rate. With lower doses, the effect is largely attributable to stimulation of carotid and aortic chemoreceptors. With high doses, other ill-defined but possibly central effects contribute. In certain circumstances, particularly in the cat, respiratory movements are strongly inhibited. This again is mainly reflex and due to stimulation of vagal afferent fibers of obscure physiological functions, whose endings are distributed in the region between the great veins and the left atrium.

Bronchoconstriction. 5-HT causes bronchoconstriction in many animals, but this response is uncommon in man, except in asthmatic patients. Its effect is partly reflex but mainly due to direct stimulation of bronchial smooth muscle, a response that can be reproduced *in vitro* (*see* Rodbard and Kira, 1972).

Cardiovascular System. The effects of 5-HT on this system are of unique complexity. By acting directly on the vascular smooth muscle, the drug may evoke vasoconstriction or vasodilatation, depending on the vascular bed, its resting tonus, and the dose given. By its actions on a variety of sensory nerve endings, it sets up pressor and depressor reflexes; in high dose, 5-HT influences ganglionic transmission and adrenal medullary secretion. Finally, by direct and reflex mechanisms, it either stimulates or depresses cardiac output.

Blood Vessels. Direct *vasoconstriction* is the classical effect of 5-HT and the one responsible for its being given names such as *vasotonin* and *serotonin.* Vasoconstriction is prominent in animals when nervous control of the blood vessels has been destroyed. In such circumstances 5-HT given intravenously commonly provokes powerful pressor responses. Renal vessels are very sensitive, and in some laboratory animals the effect may be so intense as to cause necrosis of the renal cortex. Placental, uterine, and umbilical vessels also respond with vasoconstriction, and this effect may interrupt pregnancy in species such as the rat, mouse, and rabbit. The response of the umbilical vessels, which are devoid of innervation, provides a good illustration of the direct action of 5-HT on vascular smooth muscle. Pulmonary vasoconstriction, precapillary and postcapillary, is prominent in dogs and cats but less so in man. Indirect effects mediated by contraction of bronchial muscle complicate interpretation of the effects of low doses. Cerebral blood vessels are constricted powerfully in several species (Lowe and Gilboe, 1973).

Vasodilatation occurs in skeletal muscles, especially with lower doses of 5-HT, and may cause a fall in total peripheral resistance. In the forearm and calf, regions in which muscle is preponderant, this effect tends to increase blood flow. Vasodilatation has also been observed in superficial vessels of the human skin following intradermal or intra-arterial 5-HT. The resulting flush, at first bright red, assumes a dusky hue indicating stagnation, probably as a result of venoconstriction. The effect is direct. However, since arterioles in the skin are constricted by intra-arterial or intravenous 5-HT, the overall effect is a rise in cutaneous vascular resistance. In regions where skin is preponderant, for example, the hand, this reduces blood flow; and even in other regions such as the forearm it may overshadow vasodilatation in skeletal muscle and reduce total blood flow.

Capillary Permeability. 5-HT has no prominent effects on capillary permeability in any species other than rodents, in which it is increased.

Heart. 5-HT has positive inotropic and chronotropic effects of varying intensity on isolated hearts and atria of various species, and increased force of contraction has been observed in experiments on isolated papillary muscles. The autacoid has also been shown, under suitable conditions, to stimulate heart rate, contractile force, and cardiac output in intact animals and man by actions that may include the release of norepinephrine (Fillion *et al.,* 1971). However, the effect may be overwhelmed by autonomic reflexes initiated by concomitant changes in blood pressure or by direct actions of 5-HT on various afferent nerve endings, including baroreceptors, chemoreceptors, and vagal endings in the coronary bed. The last-mentioned reflex effect is particularly noteworthy. It initiates the "coronary chemoreflex" (Bezold-Jarisch reflex), in which there is inhibition of sympathetic outflow and increased activity of the cardiac (efferent) vagus, leading to profound bradycardia and hypotension. Occasionally cardiovascular collapse and fainting occur from such causes when 5-HT is given to man. No significant changes in the electrical properties of the heart have been attributed to 5-HT.

Blood Pressure. The changes in systemic blood pressure that follow an intravenous injection of 5-HT are the result of a mosaic of direct and reflex effects on heart and blood vessels and are notoriously variable. In most species, including man, it is possible to discern three successive phases: a brief depressor phase immediately following the injection; a succeeding pressor phase; and finally, within 1 or 2 minutes of the injection, a prolonged depressor phase. The *early depressor phase* is primarily the result of the coronary chemoreflex; it is abolished by cutting the vagi (which contain both the afferent and the efferent limbs of the reflex) and is suppressed by atropine or by ganglionic blocking drugs. Baroreceptor stimulation may also contribute. The *pressor phase* is due mainly to the direct effects of 5-HT in increasing total peripheral resistance and cardiac output, but chemoreceptor stimulation also plays a part. The *late depressor phase* is attributable to the direct vasodilator effects of 5-HT, principally in skeletal muscle. It persists after ganglionic blocking drugs and other agents that block sympathetic vasoconstrictor outflow. A rise in pulmonary blood pressure is usual in cats and dogs, rarer in man.

Veins are strongly constricted by 5-HT, and intense venospasm commonly accompanies intravenous infusions. The incidence of thrombosis in the injected vein is high.

Kidney and Antidiuresis. In most species, including dog and man, antidiuretic effects are not prominent and are usually encountered only with doses large enough to cause neural and cardiovascular responses. The effect does not depend on the liberation of antidiuretic hormone or on intact renal innervation but seems to be secondary to vascular responses within the kidney or changes in systemic blood pressure that lower glomerular filtration rate. However, modest antidiuresis, accompanied by diminished excretion of electrolytes, has been noted without a fall in glomerular filtration rate in both dog and man. The mechanism is uncertain. Although there is some evidence that 5-HT can stimulate aldosterone output, antidiuresis in response to 5-HT has been observed after adrenalectomy.

Platelets. 5-HT causes platelet aggregation. The effect is small and reversible, and possibly due to adenosine diphosphate formation associated with 5-HT uptake (Mustard and Packham, 1970).

Smooth Muscle. *Alimentary Tract.* Intravenous injections of 5-HT stimulate motility of the small intestine. Man is particularly sensitive, and often responds to doses insufficient to affect the cardiovascular or respiratory system; typically, the response consists in an initial intense spasm followed first by heightened tone with rhythmic propulsive contractions and then by a period of inhibition of spontaneous activity. In experimental animals, injections of 5-HT may also stimulate the large intestine and stomach, but inhibitory effects are not uncommonly encountered. In man, inhibition is the typical response in these regions. Isolated segments of gastrointestinal tract *in vitro* generally exhibit responses qualitatively similar to those obtained *in vivo,* namely, contraction, inhibition, or mixtures of these. The complexity of the pattern is in large measure due to the variety of elements, neural and muscular, responding to 5-HT.

The most thorough analysis of the stimulant effect of 5-HT has been carried out on the isolated guinea pig ileum, where 5-HT contracts the longitudinal muscle partly by acting directly upon it and partly by exciting intramural ganglion cells. The direct action is blocked by various substances antagonizing the smooth muscle effects of 5-HT, including phenoxybenzamine and LSD. The indirect effect mediated through ganglion cells is countered by cocaine, which suppresses the activity of the nerve elements; by atropine, which blocks the action of the ACh that the neurons liberate; and by morphine, which has the dual property of opposing the excitant effect of 5-HT on the ganglion cells and of diminishing the output of ACh from their terminals. In addition, 5-HT can also increase peristaltic activity by stimulating or sensitizing intramural nerve endings.

The inhibitory actions of 5-HT on the gastrointestinal tract have been most intensively studied in the guinea pig stomach (Bülbring and Gershon, 1968). Here the effect is due to a stimulant action of 5-HT on a population of intramural ganglion cells in the myenteric plexus that have an inhibitory effect on the smooth muscle. The action of 5-HT on these ganglion cells is not influenced by substances such as hexamethonium that block stimulant actions of the nicotinic type, but it is blocked by certain "neurotropic" 5-HT antagonists (*see* below). How far inhibitory effects of 5-HT in the colon may also be attributed to stimulation of intrinsic inhibitory neurons is uncertain, but such neurons are certainly present.

Other Smooth Muscle. In addition to the actions on bronchi, blood vessels, and gut, 5-HT stimulates numerous other smooth muscles, including the uterus, urethra, and nictitating membrane. Although the isolated uterus of the estrus rat is exquisitely sensitive, isolated strips of human uterus in various functional states are not, and large doses of 5-HT given intravenously have minor and equivocal actions on the contractile activity of the human pregnant uterus. As in the intestine, the responses of the other viscera are complicated by diverse actions on nervous elements as well as muscle. For example, the contractile response of the bladder shows an initial fast component due to stimulation of pelvic ganglion cells and a second slower component due to a direct action on the muscle, while in the same preparation contractions elicited by preganglionic stimulation are depressed as a result of an action of 5-HT to inhibit pelvic ganglionic transmission (Saum and de Groat, 1973).

Exocrine Glands. Intravenous infusion of 5-HT in the dog reduces the volume, acidity, and pepsin content of *gastric juice* secreted spontaneously or in response to vagal activation, cholinergic drugs, or histamine, but at the same time it increases the production of mucus. Somewhat similar effects have been described in man and various other species and apparently involve reflex as well as direct actions (*see* Thompson, 1971). Variable effects on salivary, pancreatic, and other exocrine secretions have been reported in mammals.

Carbohydrate Metabolism. The intravenous administration of very large doses of 5-HT to dogs raises blood sugar, lowers hepatic glycogen, and increases hepatic phosphorylase activity. The effect seems to be indirect and due to the liberation of epinephrine; it does not occur after adrenalectomy.

Sensory Nerve Endings. 5-HT is capable of stimulating a variety of sensory nerve endings. A few examples will serve to illustrate that this is one of the drug's principal actions. Thus, 5-HT causes intense pain when applied to the base of blisters raised on the skin, sets up electrical activity in a broad spectrum of nerve fibers when given by close intraarterial injection into the skin, and evokes massive centripetal discharges in the abdominal vagus when injected into the aorta. Many of the phenomena accompanying intravenous injections of 5-HT in man are probably due to direct effects on afferent nerves. These include pain at the site of injection, gasping, hyperventilation, substernal "pressure," coughing, "tingling and pricking all over," nausea, and cramps (Hollander *et al.,* 1957).

Autonomic Ganglia. Direct excitation of autonomic ganglion cells has been observed, especially after close arterial injection. Facilitation or inhibition of ganglionic transmission has been noted, the effect depending on experimental conditions (de Groat and Lalley, 1973; Saum and de Groat, 1973).

Adrenal Medulla and Other Endocrine Glands. When injected into the arterial supply to the adrenal glands, 5-HT causes a brisk discharge of catecholamines. A similar response may follow intravenous injection of very large doses of the drug. Intracellular recordings show that 5-HT depolarizes the chromaffin cells (Douglas *et al.,* 1967). 5-HT stimulates or inhibits hormone output from several other endocrine tissues, including the thyroid (Melander and Sundler, 1972), adrenal cortex (Albano *et al.,* 1973), and pancreatic cells (Hellman *et al.,* 1972; Lebovitz and Feldman, 1973). It inhibits release of thyrotropin regulatory hormone from hypothalamic fragments *in vitro* (Grimm and Reichlin, 1973).

Central Nervous System. Although 5-HT is normally present in the CNS and probably has transmitter functions there (*see* below), central effects are not usually encountered when 5-HT is given parenterally, for it is a highly polar substance and poorly penetrates the blood-brain barrier. When injected directly into the lateral cerebral ventricles of cats, 5-HT causes muscular weakness, a swaying gait, a tendency to adopt a sleeping posture, and a catatonic-like state (Feldberg and Sherwood, 1954). Intracisternal administration also results in tremor and changes in body temperature—fever in some animals, hypothermia in others (*see* Feldberg, 1968). Applied by microiontophoresis to randomly encountered neurons throughout the CNS from neo-cortex to spinal cord, 5-HT inhibits some cells and stimulates others (*see* Symposium, 1973, 1974a).

Mode of Action. The actions of 5-HT fall into the pattern described for histamine. *5-HT receptors* are generally believed to reside in the cell membrane and can be selectively blocked by various drugs. *Mechanisms at the Cellular Level.* The chemical nature of 5-HT–receptor interaction is still speculative (*see* Bugg and Thewalt, 1970; Berridge, 1972). It seems that many responses to 5-HT involving such diverse elements as smooth muscle fibers, neurons and their processes, chemoreceptors, and medullary chromaffin cells are attributable, as with other autacoids, to an action exerted on the cell membrane that results in increased permeability to commonly occurring inorganic ions; the ensuing ion movement alters membrane potential and the intracellular ionic environment.

Thus, from intracellular records on individual *neurons* of mollusks, it is evident that excitation in response to 5-HT is attributable to a rise in permeability to sodium, leading to sodium entry and depolarization (*see* Gerschenfeld and Stefani, 1968); a similar effect would explain excitation of mammalian neural elements, including central neurons and ganglion cells and the various sensory terminals associated, for example, with pain, and Bezold-Jarisch or chemosensory reflexes. Intracellular recordings also show that 5-HT depolarizes the chromaffin cells of the adrenal medulla, and this effect, involving influx of calcium, is sufficient to explain catecholamine secretion (*see* Douglas *et al.,* 1967). A membrane action of 5-HT resulting in calcium entry is also generally considered responsible for smooth muscle contraction. As is true of most other drugs, 5-HT fails to evoke secretion or smooth muscle contraction in the absence of calcium. Both in stimulus-secretion coupling (Douglas, 1968, 1974) and in excitation-contraction coupling in smooth muscle (Somlyo and Somlyo, 1970), influx of calcium ions may result from a direct action of 5-HT on the membrane that increases the permeability to calcium, thereby allowing it to run passively down its electrochemical gradient. Depolarization, brought about mainly by a corresponding effect of 5-HT on entry of sodium ions, would also facilitate the entry of calcium, but it appears that calcium movement and functional response can occur independently of sodium influx or fall in membrane potential. Likewise, the inhibitory effects on smooth muscle can also be dissociated from membrane potential; for example, relaxation, like contraction, can be elicited, in fully depolarized muscles. Relaxation is assumed to involve a reduction in the intracellular concentration of free calcium ions, but how 5-HT or any other drug brings this about is unknown. Inhibition in neurons is better understood and involves preferential increases in permeability to potassium ions and, in some cells of mollusks, to chloride ions (Gerschenfeld, 1971). There is much speculation that stimulation of adenylate cyclase activity may explain various effects of 5-HT, including those on nerves (Huang *et al.,* 1971; Skolnick *et al.,* 1973), secretory cells (Prince

and Berridge, 1972; Albano *et al.,* 1973), and muscle (Somlyo and Somlyo, 1970).

ENDOGENOUS 5-HYDROXYTRYPTAMINE

Distribution. In mammals, about 90% of the 5-HT present in the body, which in an adult human probably amounts to 10 mg, is lodged in the gastrointestinal tract, mainly in enterochromaffin cells and enterochromaffin-like cells. A few such 5-HT-containing cells are also present in other tissues (*see* Håkanson, 1970; Thompson, 1971). Of the remaining 5-HT, most is present in platelets and the CNS. Mast cells of rodents and cattle contain 5-HT (*see* Eyre, 1973), but mast cells of other species, including man, do not normally contain 5-HT; however, some has been found in human mast-cell tumors (Morishima, 1970).

Origin, Synthesis, Uptake, Storage, and Release. Enterochromaffin cells, neurons, and rodent mast cells synthesize 5-HT from tryptophan by the enzymatic processes described above, and such synthesis occurs in most tissues where 5-HT is normally stored. However, platelets have little or no capacity to synthesize 5-HT and acquire it by uptake, mainly of 5-HT released into the blood by the intestinal enterochromaffin cells (*see* Sneddon, 1973).

The mechanisms of 5-HT uptake, storage, and release have been most extensively studied in platelets, but there is reason to believe that the results may be applicable, in the main, to neurons and enterochromaffin cells. Uptake of 5-HT into platelets involves two mechanisms: passive diffusion when the extracellular concentration of 5-HT is high and, more noteworthy, an active transport process effective at very low concentrations and transporting 5-HT against a large concentration gradient. The latter mechanism shows striking parallels with the "high-affinity" amine uptake mechanism operating in various monoaminergic neurons and is blocked by the same types of agent—most prominent among them being the tricyclic antidepressant drugs such as imipramine. Inhibition by such drugs is competitive, but the mode of action is uncertain (*see* Todrick and Tait, 1969; Ahtee and Saarnivaara, 1971).

Storage of 5-HT within the platelet is also similar to monoamine storage in other systems, including nerves. It involves membrane-limited vesicles that appear dense cored in electron micrographs. Once within the vesicle, 5-HT is bound as a nondiffusible complex with adenine nucleotides (principally adenosine triphosphate [ATP]) and divalent cations (Pletscher *et al.,* 1971). Again as in nerves, 5-HT in the vesicles may be released by reserpine. Excess 5-HT in the cytoplasm is converted by mitochondrial MAO to 5-hydroxyindoleacetic acid (5-HIAA), in which form it escapes to the extracellular environment. The question whether a sizable cytoplasmic "pool" of 5-HT normally exists outside the vesicles is unsettled (*see* Ahtee and Saarnivaara, 1971; Minter and Crawford, 1971; Sneddon, 1973). During the platelet "release reaction" induced by thrombin, 5-HT is discharged along with ATP and divalent cations apparently as a result of the vesicles fusing with the plasma membrane and emptying by exocytosis (Holmsen *et al.,* 1973). Release of 5-HT from nerves may involve a similar exocytotic mechanism (*see* Douglas, 1968, 1974).

Turnover. An amount of 5-HT roughly equal to that present in the body is synthesized each day (Erspamer, 1966b). Turnover times of 5-HT in brain and gastrointestinal tract have been estimated at about 1 and 17 hours, respectively. However, 5-HT in rodent mast cells turns over very slowly and that bound in platelets appears to be released only on their destruction or during the thrombin-induced "release reaction" (Holmsen *et al.,* 1973).

Role in the Body's Economy. The discovery of a substance that undergoes substantial, unceasing synthesis and destruction in the body and that also possesses intense and varied pharmacological activities has inevitably resulted in a flood of speculation on its physiological function. It is generally agreed that 5-HT has an important role in nervous transmission. In addition, 5-HT is recognized as serving as a precursor metabolite for the pineal hormone, melatonin. Other functions, however, are less evident; no convincing explanations have been advanced, for example, concerning the presence of 5-HT in platelets, enterochromaffin cells, and other cells with established or suspected endocrine function.

Nervous System. There is now compelling evidence that 5-HT serves as the neurotransmitter substance released by a class of neurons commonly referred to as "tryptaminergic." Such neurons are apparently present in the nervous systems of all major animal phyla (Welsh, 1968; Sakharov, 1970; Chase and Murphy, 1973). In suitable invertebrates such as snails and leeches, where neurons are sufficiently large to allow isolation and direct chemical analysis, 5-HT has been shown to be present in some neurons and not in others. Moreover, the stimulant effect of impulses on postsynaptic elements in the 5-HT–containing neurons is mimicked by applied 5-HT (Cottrell, 1971; Lent, 1973; Weinreich *et al.,* 1973).

Central Nervous System. In the mammalian CNS the distribution and projections of the 5-HT–containing neurons have been established by regional analysis of 5-HT content before and after surgical procedures causing tract degeneration (Heller, 1972), and by histochemical fluorescence methods (Dahlström and Fuxe, 1965). The potent inhibitor of tryptophan hydroxylase, *parachlorophenylalanine* (pCPA), has probably provided the most valuable insights into the functions of the tryptaminergic neurons (Koe and Weissman, 1966; Symposium, 1973, 1974a, 1974b). Nevertheless, even with this drug there are some problems of nonspecificity. Other interesting and promising pharmacological tools are the cytotoxic *dihydroxytryptamines* (5,6-dihydroxytryptamine and 5,7-dihydroxytryptamine), which are preferentially taken up into tryptaminergic neurons and thereby cause a preferential degeneration of tryptaminergic fibers (*see* Björklund *et al.,* 1974; Fuxe and Jonsson, 1974).

These technics and others have revealed that the cell bodies of the 5-HT–containing neurons are lodged for the most part in the several raphe nuclei that are scattered through the brain stem from the mescephalon to the lower medulla. Axons from these nuclei are distributed throughout the entire CNS, from forebrain cortex to caudal spinal cord as well as throughout the brain stem itself and the cerebellum. Ascending axons arise mainly from the rostral nuclei and descending (bulbospinal) axons from the caudal nuclei (*see* Symposium, 1973, 1974a).

It is evident that neurons and terminals can take up tryptophan, and that they possess the necessary enzymes to convert it to 5-HT. The neurons and their terminals also have a selective "high-affinity" uptake mechanism for 5-HT; the characteristics of the storage vesicles have already been described. On stimulation of raphe nuclei, turnover of 5-HT increases and its metabolic product, 5-HIAA (or 5-HT itself when MAO is inhibited), can be recovered from the cerebrospinal fluid near the appropriate terminals. From all this, it would seem that 5-HT–containing neurons show all the essential attributes of tryptaminergic function.

Tryptaminergic function implies that the 5-HT released acts as an appropriate transmitter on the postsynaptic "tryptaminoceptive" cells. This has been demonstrated in invertebrates, where a positive visual identification of such cells is relatively simple. Microiontophoretic application of 5-HT mimics the effect of stimulating the presynaptic tryptaminergic neurons (Cottrell, 1971). In the mammalian CNS, cells receiving demonstrable tryptaminergic input are not so easily identified; however, the neurons in certain areas, such as the suprachiasmatic nucleus and the ventrolateral geniculate body, receive a uniform and dense investment of tryptaminergic nerve terminals, and recordings obtained from them can be considered with some confidence to reflect tryptaminergic innervation. Such neurons are almost uniformly inhibited by stimulation of the raphe neurons, and this effect is mimicked by iontophoretic application of 5-HT (Bloom *et al.,* 1972; Haigler and Aghajanian, 1974a). The question of whether tryptaminergic nerves have excitatory as well as inhibitory functions in the mammalian brain is best left open.

Whereas receptor-blocking drugs have contributed outstandingly to analysis of cholinergic and adrenergic nervous function, this is not true of central tryptaminergic transmission. The frustrating fact is that of the many different drugs shown to be 5-HT antagonists on various peripheral structures such as autonomic ganglia or smooth muscle, none has been demonstrated to act as a 5-HT antagonist at any *proven* tryptaminergic synapse within the CNS (Bloom *et al.,* 1973; Haigler and Aghajanian, 1974b). This is all the more remarkable since much early speculation on the existence and function of tryptaminergic transmission in the brain was generated by the discovery of the remarkable hallucinogenic properties of LSD and the demonstration that LSD is a potent antagonist of 5-HT's actions on smooth muscle. Although LSD, in high concentration, does block the action of 5-HT at positively identified *peripheral* tryptaminergic synapses, its effects on positively identified tryptaminoceptive (postsynaptic) neurons in mammalian brain is quite the opposite; here it *mimics* 5-HT and reproduces the effects of stimulating the presynaptic tryptaminergic raphe neurons. Other substances noted for their antagonism toward 5-HT's effects on smooth muscle likewise fail to oppose the effects of 5-HT on these identified tryptaminoceptive cells (Bloom *et al.,* 1973; Haigler and Aghajanian, 1974b). It is true that LSD and some of the other "peripheral 5-HT antagonists" have been noted to inhibit responses to 5-HT applied by microiontophoresis to randomly encountered cells in various regions of the CNS, but none of these cells has been proven to be *physiologically* tryptaminoceptive, that is, to receive tryptaminergic input (*see* Boakes *et al.,* 1970; Bradley and Briggs, 1974a, 1974b). A further complication to be discussed shortly is that LSD proves to have quite unexpected and potent direct actions on the cell bodies of raphe neurons (*see* Haigler and Aghajanian, 1974a).

In the aggregate, the evidence suggests that *one* important general role of the tryptaminergic raphe neurons may be to dampen overreactiveness to various stimuli (external and internal) involving, for example, auditory, visual, olfactory, nociceptive, and other signals affecting social and adaptive behavior (including learning) and involving such parameters as *sleep, sexual behavior, aggressiveness, motor activity, perception* (including *pain*), and *mood*. Since the earliest years of research in the field, the effects of LSD and a host of other psychoactive drugs suspected of interacting with central tryptaminergic systems have focused interest on such complex behavioral functions. Altered tryptaminergic function has been proposed as a cause or factor in various mental illnesses and CNS dysfunctions, including *schizophrenia* (Woolley, 1962), the *affective disorders* (*see* Weil-Malherbe, 1972), *infantile autism,* and *minimal brain dysfunction,* as well as the mental defects accompanying *phenylketonuria* and *Down's syndrome* (*see* Symposium, 1973, 1974b). But this continuing emphasis on some of the most complex physiological and pathophysiological CNS functions should not be allowed to obscure the many indications that tryptaminergic neurons are also involved in other, simpler functions such as *temperature regulation, neuroendocrine control* (*regulation of release of hypophysiotropic hormones*), and *extrapyramidal activity.* (*See* Chase and Murphy, 1973; Symposium, 1973, 1974a, 1974b; de Wied and de Jong, 1974.)

Peripheral Nervous System. Although tryptaminergic nerves innervate effector organs in invertebrates, no such neurons have been unequivocally demonstrated in the peripheral nervous system of mammals. However, it is now evident that mammalian viscera are endowed with neurons that are neither cholinergic nor adrenergic, and there are indications that at least some of these may be tryptaminergic (*see* Robinson and Gershon, 1971; Burks, 1973; Furness and Costa, 1973). There is also some evidence that 5-HT may be the transmitter substance released by certain intrinsic neurons in the gut whose activity contributes to contraction (Burks, 1973; Furness and Costa, 1973). In addition, the untested possibility that tryptaminergic neurons in the intestine may be involved in secretory activity deserves study.

It is worth noting that many different classes of centrally active drugs have been found to affect physiological or biochemical parameters of various tryptaminergic neuronal systems, where they may influence responses to 5-HT or alter uptake, synthesis, storage, release, or catabolism of 5-HT. The list includes hallucinogens such as LSD, N,N-dimethyltryptamine (DMP), and other 5-HT congeners; the psychotogenic phenylethylamines such as mescaline and 2,5-dimethoxy-alpha-4-dimethylphenylethylamine (DOM); reserpine and other drugs that interfere with amine storage; various minor and major tranquilizers; neuroleptic or antipsychotic drugs such as chlorpromazine; thymoleptic or antidepressant drugs, including the tricyclic compounds; MAO inhibitors; amphetamines, particularly the chloroamphetamines; lithium; morphine and other strong analgesics; methylxanthines; and ethyl alcohol. Since almost all of these drugs have been demonstrated to have effects on various types of nervous transmission, it is difficult to discern the functional importance of their effects on tryptaminergic mechanisms. The above list of drugs indicates at least the breadth of current speculation.

Among the most interesting compounds is LSD, the drug responsible more than any other for focusing attention on tryptaminergic mechanisms in the brain. There is abundant evidence that LSD reduces 5-HT turnover in the brain and inhibits the firing of raphe neurons. This effect has been obtained with concentrations of LSD lower than those active at the tryptaminergic synapses formed by the axons of these same raphe cells. Moreover, similar inhibitory effects are seen when 5-HT itself is applied to the raphe cell bodies. These neurons are, in fact, sensitive to the transmitter substance they themselves release at their axon terminals. Whether this sensitivity of the cell bodies reflects the existence of recurrent inhibitory collaterals, or tryptaminergic innervation of the raphe neurons, or has some other explanation, remains to be seen. In any event, the inhibitory effect of LSD on raphe neurons offers a plausible explanation of the drug's hallucinogenic effects, namely, that they result from depression of activity in a system inhibiting visual and other sensory inputs (Haigler and Aghajanian, 1974a).

From the remaining agents listed it seems appropriate to single out morphine, for this is the archetype of the potent analgesics. Profound analgesia can be produced by electrical stimulation of raphe nuclei (*see* Liebeskind *et al.,* 1973). Morphine appears to initiate impulses in bulbospinal fibers descending from raphe neurons, and its analgesic effects are reduced by surgical ablation of raphe nuclei or pharmacological destruction of descending bulbospinal neurons by 5,6-dihydroxytryptamine (*see* Vogt, 1974). Likewise, evidence has been marshaled suggesting the involvement of tryptaminergic neurons in tolerance and other responses to morphine (*see* Way, 1972; Symposium, 1973, 1974b). There is, again, the problem of nonspecificity, for morphine also has actions on cholinergic and adrenergic systems (*see* Kosterlitz *et al.,* 1972); however, the concept that morphine acts by stimulating raphe neurons, thereby inhibiting or occluding sensory input, is an attractive one consistent with the inferences concerning the general role of the raphe system described earlier.

Hypothalamic–Anterior Pituitary Function. The secretory activity of the endocrine cells of the anterior pituitary is controlled by hypophysiotropic hormones (releasing and inhibiting hormones) produced by hypothalamic neuroendocrine cells that are themselves under the control of central neurons of various sorts, including tryptaminergic fibers. The extent of influence of tryptaminergic fibers on hypophysiotropic function, and hence adenohypophyseal activity, is at present only rather vaguely defined. There are indications of involvement of tryptaminergic mechanisms in control of release of corticotropin, thyrotropin, growth hormone, prolactin, and the gonadotropins (*see* Grimm and Reichlin, 1973; Lu and Meites, 1973; de Wied and de Jong, 1974; *see also* Chapter 66). It is thus possible that interference with central tryptaminergic mechanisms may lead to widespread derangement of endocrine function. It is known, for example, that pCPA or precursors of 5-HT such as tryptophan or 5-HTP interfere with the feedback control of pituitary-adrenal function (Berger *et al.,* 1974), and some 5-HT antagonists have been reported to inhibit growth hormone secretion in response to hypoglycemia in man (Bivens *et al.,* 1973).

Endocrine Cells Secreting Polypeptide Hormones. In various species, 5-HT (or another arylethylamine such as dopamine or histamine) occurs in cells known or believed to secrete polypeptide hormones, for example, the parafollicular cells (C cells) of the thyroid, α and β cells of the endocrine pancreas, and various cells secreting gastrointestinal hormones (Owman *et al.,* 1973). In other species, where the endogenous amine is not readily apparent, it can be demonstrated after administering the corresponding amine precursor, 5-HTP, dopa, or histidine. Whereas the amine is stored and released along with the polypeptide hormone in the secretory granules, its function is unknown (*see* Gershon and Nunez, 1973; Lebovitz and Feldman, 1973).

Enterochromaffin System. The 5-HT stored in the gastrointestinal enterochromaffin cells escapes at a basal rate that increases in response to various mechanical and chemical stimuli (Bülbring, 1961; Burks and Long, 1966). The function of the enterochromaffin cells and of this spontaneous and evoked liberation of 5-HT is unknown. The early conjecture (Bülbring, 1961) that 5-HT release is involved in the regulation of peristalsis remains unproven, as does the still older notion that the enterochromaffin cells form a diffuse endocrine system (*see* Thompson, 1971; Owman *et al.,* 1973). A general hormonal role for 5-HT seems unlikely. The 5-HT released to the intestinal blood is avidly taken up by platelets, and what remains is promptly oxidized in the liver and the lungs.

Proliferation of 5-HT–Forming Cells. Tumors of enterochromaffin or related cells (*carcinoid tumors*), in the gastrointestinal or respiratory tract or elsewhere, may synthesize and release large amounts of 5-HT. With massive tumors, so much tryptophan may be diverted to 5-HT synthesis that niacin synthesis suffers and *pellagra* results. More commonly patients show the *carcinoid syndrome* characterized by periodic attacks of flushing, swings in blood pressure, colic and diarrhea, bronchoconstriction, and, when the disease is of long duration, endocardial and other fibroses. Some years ago, when 5-HT was the only substance known to be secreted by these tumors, it was held responsible for this whole spectrum of effects. It has become evident, however, that some features, particularly the flush, are attributable to other autacoids released by the tumors, including kallikrein and prostaglandins (Sandler, 1968). The peculiar patchy "geographical flush" observed in *gastric carcinoid* probably results from histamine release by such tumors. Nevertheless, 5-HT clearly contributes importantly to the carcinoid syndrome. Diarrhea, for example, is sometimes well controlled by 5-HT antagonists such as methysergide and by the inhibitor of 5-HT synthesis, pCPA, although the side effects of the latter may offset its therapeutic value (*see* Sjoerdsma *et al.,* 1970; Hill, 1971; Levine, 1974). Whether 5-HT is the cause of the fibrotic lesions is uncertain. Similar lesions have been found in chronic infections with schistosoma that synthesize large amounts of 5-HT (Bennett *et al.,* 1969); fibrosis is an occasional side effect of methysergide, a chemically related indole (*see* below); and a stimulant effect of 5-HT on fibroblasts in culture has been demonstrated (Boucek and Alvarez, 1971).

Pineal Gland and Melatonin Formation. The pineal gland is one of the richest sources of 5-HT. The amine is synthesized by the pinealocytes and serves as a precursor for the synthesis of the hormone *melatonin* (5-methoxy-N-acetyltryptamine). The initial step is catalyzed by the enzyme 5-hydroxytryptamine-N-acetyltransferase, with the production of 5-hydroxy-N-acetyltryptamine. This is, in turn, converted to melatonin by the enzyme hydroxy-indole-O-methyl transferase. Experiments on rats have shown a remarkable diurnal rhythm. At night the N-acetyltransferase activity is high and the level of the substrate, 5-HT, is low; during the daylight hours this pattern is reversed. Control is by a reflex path involving the retina in the afferent limb and the cervical sympathetic trunk in the efferent limb. Activity in these adrenergic nerves, increasing apparently with darkness, seems to induce N-acetyltransferase activity through receptors in the pinealocytes (*see* Axelrod and Wurtman, 1968; Brownstein *et al.,* 1973), probably involving activation of adenylate cyclase (Klein and Weller, 1973). Whether 5-HT in the pineal gland has a function independent of melatonin synthesis is still conjectural (Owman *et al.,* 1973).

Platelet 5-HT. The function of 5-HT in platelets is obscure. As noted earlier, its potentiating effect on platelet aggregation is small and platelets depleted of 5-HT by reserpine function normally (Mustard and Packham, 1970). One view is that platelets serve simply to sequester the 5-HT escaping from cells, such as those in the enterochromaffin system. There is some evidence that 5-HT liberated from platelets may contribute to the pathophysiology of pulmonary embolism (*see* Spodick, 1972).

Pregnancy, Labor, and Toxemia. There is little evidence that 5-HT is involved in *normal pregnancy, labor,* or *neonatal circulatory adjustments,* despite the responsiveness of the uterus and the uterine, placental, and umbilical vessels. However, the demonstrated ability of 5-HT to induce fetal death and deformity in pregnant rats and mice, probably by constricting uterine vessels and causing ischemia, hints at a possible role in the pathological physiology of gestation, including *toxemia of pregnancy.* Premature labor, with fetuses stillborn or dying shortly after birth, has been observed in pregnancies in women with carcinoid tumors (*see* Robson and Sullivan, 1968; Southgate and Sandler, 1968).

OTHER CONSIDERATIONS

Absorption, Fate, and Excretion. While studies of the actions of 5-HT have generally employed intravenous administration, 5-HT is quite quickly absorbed after parenteral injection. Given orally, it is rapidly degraded and is hence ineffective. The metabolism of 5-HT varies somewhat from one species to another, but in man most of it undergoes oxidative deamination by MAO to form 5-hydroxyindoleacetaldehyde. This aldehyde is promptly degraded, mainly by further oxidation to 5-HIAA by aldehyde dehydrogenase, but also in small part by reduction to the corresponding alcohol, 5-hydroxytryptophol (5-HTOL) (*see* Figure 29–5). The three enzymes are present in liver and various tissues containing 5-HT, including the brain. Uptake and degradation by the lung are important in the metabolism of 5-HT (Vane, 1969); depending on the rate of infusion, 30 to 90% of 5-HT is taken up by pulmonary endothelial cells, there to be metabolized primarily by MAO. This uptake, as in platelets, is dependent on sodium ions and is blocked by drugs such as imipramine (*see* Gillis, 1973).

The principal metabolite, 5-HIAA, is excreted in the urine, along with the very much smaller amounts of 5-HTOL, mainly as the glucuronide or sulfate, and traces of other metabolites. About 2 to 10 mg of 5-HIAA is excreted daily by the normal adult as a result of metabolism of endogenous 5-HT. Larger amounts are excreted by patients with malignant carcinoid, a fact of diagnostic value. It must be remembered, however, that ingestion of 5-HT–containing foods also leads to increased excretion of 5-HT metabolites (*see* Erspamer, 1966a; Levine, 1974).

The pattern of metabolism is strikingly affected by ingestion of ethyl alcohol, which greatly increases 5-HTOL excretion and causes a corresponding reduction in excretion of 5-HIAA. The effect is attributable to diversion of the metabolism of 5-hydroxyindoleacetaldehyde from the normally predominant oxidative route to the reductive pathway. Ethyl alcohol influences catecholamine metabolism similarly (*see* Symposium, 1968a).

Preparations. There is no official preparation, but 5-HT is available as the creatinine sulfate complex for investigational use.

Clinical Use. From a clinical standpoint, the principal interest in 5-HT lies in its role in physio-

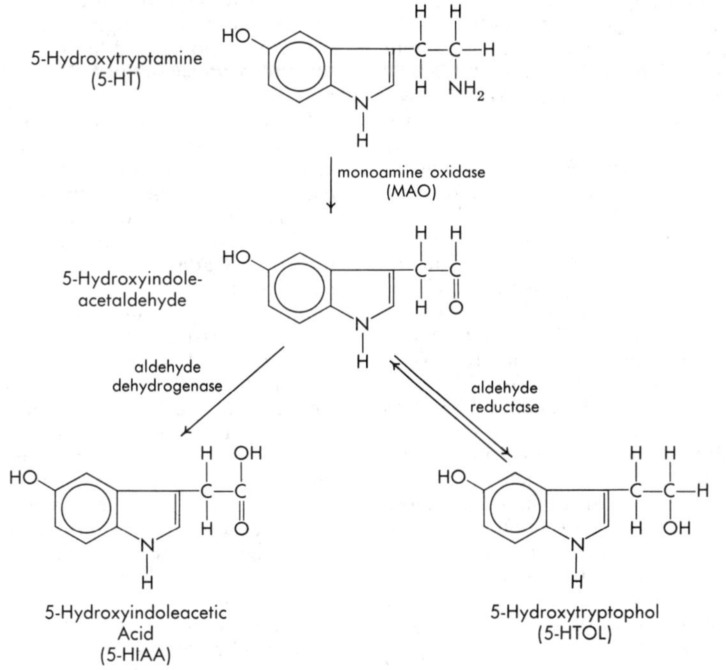

Figure 29–5. *Metabolic degradation of 5-hydroxytryptamine (5-HT).*

logical and pathological processes (*see* Symposium, 1968a, 1968b, 1972, 1973, 1974a, 1974b; Levine, 1974). To date, the drug has not found an accepted therapeutic application. Oral administration of 5-HT followed by measurement of 5-HIAA in the urine provides a simple means of testing the degree of MAO inhibition (Sjoerdsma *et al.*, 1958).

5-HT ANTAGONISTS

There are many drugs that antagonize one or more of the effects of 5-HT. Of these, some are "physiological antagonists" that oppose the effects of 5-HT by exerting counteractions. Other agents act by interrupting transmission in nervous pathways activated, directly or reflexly, by 5-HT. Such drugs are not considered here. There remains a third group of agents that oppose the actions of 5-HT in a more immediate manner by blocking 5-HT receptors; these are more properly considered as 5-HT antagonists. They possess a remarkable diversity of chemical structure. *Ergot alkaloids and related compounds* were early recognized as having anti–5-HT activity, particularly on smooth muscle; in this group the *lysergic acid derivatives* such as the diethylamide (LSD), 2-bromo-LSD, and l-methyl-*d*-lysergic acid butanolamide (methysergide, *see* below) are especially potent. Also, many *indole compounds* are 5-HT antagonists, including derivatives of gramine, harmine, tryptamine (and tryptamine itself), quaternary ammonium salts of N,N-dialkyltryptamines, and indoleacetamidines. These last two indole groups, along with some *arylguanidines and biguanidines*, are principally effective against a variety of 5-HT actions on ganglion cells and peripheral nerve endings, including those in the carotid body. In addition, 5-HT blocking activity, mainly demonstrated on smooth muscle and often of a high order, is present in a host of other drugs, including *antihistamines* of the ethylenediamine type and also, most notably, cyproheptadine (*see* below), *phenothiazines* (particularly chlorpromazine), and *β-haloalkylamines* such as phenoxybenzamine and various other *adrenergic blocking drugs* (*see* Gyermek, 1966).

Several different mechanisms are involved in suppression of responses to 5-HT. Many drugs, such as LSD, methysergide, and cyproheptadine, are classical antagonists of the surmountable competitive type, and their blocking effect on the 5-HT receptors is achieved without evidence of stimulation. With some others, such as tryptamine (or 5-HT itself in high dose), blockade follows activation and involves specific receptor desensitization. Much the same holds for the indoleacetamidines and guanidines. For example, phenylbiguanide, which blocks the actions of 5-HT on nerve endings, including those actions initiating the Bezold-Jarisch reflex, has long been remarkable as a drug precisely because it stimulates the same endings and induces this same reflex. While the effects of most of the 5-HT antagonists are rapidly reversible, those of the β-haloalkylamines are not (*see* Chapter 26).

5-HT antagonists that are active on peripheral structures fall, by and large, into two categories: those that are mainly effective in opposing effects on smooth muscle and those that preferentially block peripheral neural responses. For this reason, Gyermek (1966) has classified them as "musculotropic" and "neurotropic." This indicates at least two types of 5-HT receptors, but in fact there seem to be many types. A substance known to act as a 5-HT antagonist at one site cannot be assumed to act similarly at another, a consideration often ignored in experiments in which these drugs are used as tools without appropriate controls. Particularly, it is fitting to reemphasize the point that it is presently uncertain that any drug known to antagonize an action of 5-HT on a peripheral test object, including neurons, acts as a 5-HT antagonist at any tryptaminergic synapse in the brain (*see* Bloom *et al.*, 1973; Symposium, 1974a, 1974b; Haigler and Aghajanian, 1974b). This is not to say that demonstrated "peripheral" 5-HT antagonists cannot act centrally, but only that several efforts to demonstrate such effects directly have been unsuccessful. The two 5-HT antagonists most used in man, *methysergide* and *cyproheptadine,* are certainly capable of producing effects indicative of central actions; whether these are related to stimulation or block of tryptaminergic mechanisms or to some other action is not known.

Methysergide. This drug (1-methyl-*d*-lysergic acid butanolamide) is a congener of LSD. Its structure is depicted in Table 42–1 (page 873). It inhibits the vasoconstrictor and pressor effects of 5-HT as well as the action of the amine on a variety of extravascular smooth muscles. It is about four times as potent as LSD in blocking edema formation in response to 5-HT in the rat's paw. Unlike LSD, however, it has comparatively little action on the nervous system. Although the drug is an ergot derivative, it possesses only to a slight extent the activity typical of ergot alkaloids, and has only feeble vasoconstrictor and oxytocic activity. Nevertheless, such effects may contraindicate its use during pregnancy.

Clinical interest in methysergide was aroused by a series of publications reporting it to be of value in the prophylactic treatment of *migraine* and other *vascular headaches,* including *Horton's syndrome* (Sicuteri, 1959; Friedman and Elkind, 1963). Prophylactic use of the drug reduces the frequency and intensity of attacks of headache in the majority of patients, and currently constitutes a pharmacological approach to the control of migraine of all types— common, classical, and cluster. The protective effect of methysergide takes 1 to 2 days to develop, and as long to pass off when treatment is terminated. Rebound headaches not uncommonly occur when the drug is withdrawn. Methysergide is without benefit when given during the acute attack and, indeed, may be contraindicated. For comparative evaluation of the prophylactic effects of methysergide and other agents, including cyproheptadine, *see* Speight and Avery (1972) and Nelson (1973).

It is not at all clear why methysergide or any of the other effective agents should be of value in migraine. Numerous attempts to correlate this type of headache with some derangement in 5-HT metabolism have yielded equivocal results, and, therefore, a variety of other autacoids have been incriminated (Symposium, 1968a; Speight and Avery,

1972). The basic etiological mechanism of migraine is unknown, and whether the prophylactic benefit of drugs results from central or peripheral actions is an open question.

Methysergide is of value in combating diarrhea and malabsorption in patients with *carcinoid*. The drug may also be of value in the *postgastrectomy dumping syndrome,* which appears to have a 5-HT–mediated component (Warner, 1967; Levine, 1974).

Side Effects. These are not infrequent but are usually mild and transient; they may, if severe, necessitate withdrawal of the drug. The most common are gastrointestinal and include heartburn, diarrhea, cramps, nausea, and vomiting. Effects attributable to central actions include unsteadiness, drowsiness, weakness, lightheadedness, nervousness, insomnia, confusion, excitement, euphoria, hallucinations, and even frank psychotic episodes. Attention has been drawn to the drug's abuse potential and "street use" (Persyko, 1972). There may be either loss of appetite or weight gain. Reactions suggestive of vascular insufficiency have been observed in a few patients with peripheral vascular disease, and exacerbation of angina pectoris has been noted. One relatively rare, but potentially serious, complication of prolonged treatment is *inflammatory fibrosis.* This gives rise to various syndromes, depending on the site, including retroperitoneal fibrosis, pleuropulmonary fibrosis, and coronary and endocardial fibrosis. Usually the fibrosis retrogresses after withdrawing the drug, but this is not always so and persistent cardiac valvular damage has been reported (Graham, 1967). The phenomenon is of singular theoretical interest because of the structural similarities of methysergide and 5-HT and the suggested causal relationship between endogenous 5-HT concentrations and fibrosis, particularly endothelial, in the carcinoid syndrome (*see* above).

Preparation and Dosage. Methysergide Maleate, U.S.P. (SANSERT), is available in 2-mg tablets. The adult dose is about 2 mg, two or three times per day.

Cyproheptadine. This compound has the following structural formula:

Cyproheptadine

Its structure bears some resemblance to that of the phenothiazine antihistaminic drugs, and, like LSD and other ergot derivatives, it possesses an N-substituted heterocyclic ring.

Although several substances are known that antagonize both histamine and 5-HT, cyproheptadine is unique in that its antagonism toward each of these compounds is of a high order. Its potency against histamine-induced bronchoconstriction in guinea pigs, for example, equals or exceeds that of some of the most active antihistaminic drugs; also, it matches or surpasses LSD in antagonizing the pressor, bronchoconstrictor, uterine stimulant, and edema-forming effects of 5-HT in various laboratory animals. In addition, it has weak anticholinergic activity and possesses mild central depressant properties (Stone *et al.,* 1961).

Preparations, Uses, and Side Effects. Cyproheptadine Hydrochloride, N.F. (PERIACTIN), is available as tablets (4 mg) and as a syrup (2 mg/5 ml). The dose for adults is 4 mg, three or four times per day.

Cyproheptadine has been found to be of use in various allergic diseases. Its antipruritic effect compares favorably with that of other antihistaminic drugs, and it has been used to advantage in the treatment of a variety of pruritic dermatoses (Miller and Fishman, 1961). Its beneficial actions in such conditions are probably attributable to its powerful antihistaminic activity, for there is no evidence that 5-HT is present in significant amounts in the human skin. The 5-HT–antagonizing properties of cyproheptadine, on the other hand, supposedly contribute to its reported beneficial effects in the *postgastrectomy dumping syndrome, intestinal hypermotility of carcinoid,* and some other conditions (*see* Warner, 1967; Levine, 1974). There would seem to be a rationale for preferring cyproheptadine to methysergide in *gastric carcinoid,* in which large amounts of histamine are often secreted along with 5-HT (*see* Levine, 1974).

The most prominent side effect of treatment with cyproheptadine is drowsiness. This sometimes passes off during continued use of the drug. Less frequent effects include dry mouth, anorexia, nausea, dizziness, and, with higher doses, confusion and ataxia. Cyproheptadine also quite commonly causes weight gain accompanied, in children, by an increased rate of growth (*see* Andronic and DiMascio, 1971; Penfold, 1971; Mainguet, 1972). Its therapeutic use for such purposes as an "appetite stimulant" has been questioned (*see* Medical Letter, 1971). The mechanism of action is uncertain, but similar effects have been reported with methysergide and it may be relevant that these drugs can distort the control of secretion of insulin and growth hormone in some individuals (*see* Baldridge *et al.,* 1974).

Ahtee, L., and Saarnivaara, L. The effect of drugs upon the uptake of 5-hydroxytryptamine and metaraminol by human platelets. *J. Pharm. Pharmac.,* **1971,** *23,* 495–501.

Albano, J. D. M.; Brown, B. L.; Ekins, R. P.; Price, I.; Tait, S. A. S.; and Tait, J. F. The effect of increased K+ concentration and serotonin on cyclic AMP and corticosterone output by dispersed adrenal zona glomerulosa cells. *Endocrinology,* **1973,** *58,* xi.

Alonso–De Florida, F.; Del Castillo, J.; García, X.; and Gijón, E. Mechanism of the Schultz-Dale reaction in the denervated diaphragmatic muscle of the guinea pig. *J. gen. Physiol.,* **1968,** *51,* 677–693.

Amin, A. H.; Crawford, T. B. B.; and Gaddum, J. H. The distribution of substance P and 5-hydroxytryptamine in the central nervous system of the dog. *J. Physiol., Lond.,* **1954,** *126,* 596–618.

Andronic, A., and DiMascio, A. Appetite-stimulating and weight-gain properties of cyproheptadine (PERIACTIN) in geriatric subjects. *Curr. ther. Res.,* **1971,** *13,* 40–41.

Ash, A. S. F., and Schild, H. O. Receptors mediating some actions of histamine. *Br. J. Pharmac. Chemother.*, **1966**, *27*, 427–439.

Assem, E. S. K., and Mongar, J. L. Inhibition of allergic reactions in man and other species by cromoglycate. *Int. Archs Allergy appl. Immun.*, **1970**, *38*, 68–77.

Axelrod, J., and Wurtman, R. J. Photic and neural control of indoleamine metabolism in the rat pineal gland. *Adv. Pharmac.*, **1968**, *6A*, 157–166.

Bacq, Z. M. Histamine as protector against ionizing radiation. In, *Histamine and Antihistamines*, Vol. 1. *International Encyclopedia of Pharmacology and Therapeutics*, Sect. 74. (Schacter, M., ed.) Pergamon Press, Ltd., Oxford, **1973**, pp. 109–125.

Baldridge, J. A.; Quickel, K. E.; Feldman, J. M.; and Lebovitz, H. E. Potentiation of tolbutamide-mediated insulin release in adult onset diabetes by methysergide maleate. *Diabetes*, **1974**, *23*, 21–24.

Bartosch, R.; Feldberg, W.; and Nagel, E. Das Freiwerden eines histaminähnlichen Stoffes bei der Anaphylaxie des Meerschweinchens. *Pflügers Arch. ges. Physiol.*, **1932**, *230*, 120–153.

Baylin, S. B.; Beavan, M. A.; Buja, L. M.; and Kreiser, H. R. Histaminase activity: a biochemical marker for medullary carcinoma of the thyroid. *Am. J. Med.*, **1972**, *53*, 723–732.

Bennett, J.; Bueding, E.; Timms, A. R.; and Engstrom, R. G. Occurrence and levels of 5-hydroxytryptamine in *Schistosoma mansoni*. *Molec. Pharmac.*, **1969**, *5*, 542–545.

Berger, P. A.; Barchas, J. D.; and Vernikos-Danellis, J. Serotonin and pituitary-adrenal function. *Nature, Lond.*, **1974**, *248*, 424–426.

Bernstein, I. L.; Siegel, S. C.; Brandon, M. L.; Brown, E. B.; Evans, R. R.; Feinberg, A. R.; Friedlaender, S.; Krumholz, R. A.; Hadley, R. A.; Handelman, N. I.; Thurston, D.; and Yamate, M. A controlled study of cromolyn sodium sponsored by the Drug Committee of the American Academy of Allergy. *J. Allergy clin. Immun.*, **1972**, *50*, 235–245.

Berridge, M. J. The mode of action of 5-hydroxytryptamine. *J. exp. Biol.*, **1972**, *56*, 311–321.

Best, C. H.; Dale, H. H.; Dudley, H. W.; and Thorpe, W. V. The nature of the vasodilator constituents of certain tissue extracts. *J. Physiol., Lond.*, **1927**, *62*, 397–417.

Bivens, C. H.; Lebovitz, H. E.; and Feldman, J. M. Inhibition of hypoglycemia-induced growth hormone secretion by the serotonin antagonists cyproheptadine and methysergide. *New Engl. J. Med.*, **1973**, *289*, 236–239.

Björklund, A.; Baumgarten, H.-G.; and Nobin, A. Chemical lesioning of central monoaminergic axons by means of 5,6-dihydroxytryptamine and 5,7-dihydroxytryptamine. *Adv. biochem. Psychopharmac.*, **1974**, *10*, 13–33.

Black, J. W.; Duncan, W. A. M.; Durant, C. J.; Ganellin, C. R.; and Parsons, E. M. Definition and antagonism of histamine H₂-receptors. *Nature, Lond.*, **1972**, *236*, 385–390.

Black, J. W.; Duncan, W. A. M.; Emmett, J. C.; Ganellin, C. R.; Hesselbo, T.; Parsons, E. M.; and Wyllie, J. H. Metiamide—an orally active histamine H₂-receptor antagonist. *Agents Actions*, **1973**, *3*, 133–137.

Bloom, F. E.; Hoffer, B. J.; Nelson, C.; Sheu, Y.-S.; and Siggins, G. R. The physiology and pharmacology of serotonin mediated synapses. In, *Serotonin and Behavior*. (Barchas, J. D., and Usdin, E., eds.) Academic Press, Inc., New York, **1973**, 249–261.

Bloom, F. E.; Hoffer, B. J.; Siggins, G. R.; Barker, J. L.; and Nicoll, R. A. Effects of serotonin on central neurons: microiontophoretic administration. *Fedn Proc. Fedn Am. Socs exp. Biol.*, **1973**, *31*, 97–106.

Boakes, R. J.; Bradley, P. B.; Briggs, I.; and Dray, A. Antagonism of 5-hydroxytryptamine by LSD 25 in the central nervous system: a possible neuronal basis for the actions of LSD 25. *Br. J. Pharmac.*, **1970**, *40*, 202–218.

Boucek, R. J., and Alvarez, T. R. Increase in survival of

subcultured fibroblasts mediated by serotonin. *Nature, New Biol.*, **1971**, *229*, 61–62.

Bourne, H. R.; Lichtenstein, L. M.; Melmon, K. L.; Henney, C. S.; Weinstein, Y.; and Shearer, G. M. Modulation of inflammation and immunity by cyclic AMP. *Science, Wash.*, **1974**, *184*, 19–27.

Bovet, D.; Horclois, R.; and Walthert, F. Propriétés antihistaminiques de la N-p-méthoxybenzyl-N-diméthylaminoéthyl α amino-pyridine. *C. r. Séanc. Soc. Biol.*, **1944**, *138*, 99–100.

Bovet, D., and Staub, A. Action protectrice des éthers phénoliques au cours de l'intoxication histaminique. *C. r. Séanc. Soc. Biol.*, **1937**, *124*, 547–549.

Bradley, P. B., and Briggs, I. Actions of serotonin and related substances on single neurones in the brain. *Adv. biochem. Psychopharmac.*, **1974a**, *10*, 159–166.

————. Further studies on the mode of action of psychotomimetic drugs: antagonism of the excitatory actions of 5-hydroxytryptamine by methylated derivatives of tryptamine. *Br. J. Pharmac.*, **1974b**, *50*, 345–354.

Breuer, R. I., and Kirsner, J. B. Present status of histalog gastric analysis in man. *Ann. N.Y. Acad. Sci.*, **1967**, *140*, 882–895.

Brezenoff, H. E., and Gertner, S. B. The actions of polymyxin and histamine on ganglionic transmission. *Can. J. Physiol. Pharmac.*, **1972**, *50*, 824–831.

Brodie, B. B., and Shore, P. A. A concept for a role of serotonin and norepinephrine as chemical mediators in the brain. *Ann. N.Y. Acad. Sci.*, **1957**, *66*, 631–642.

Brownstein, M.; Holz, R.; and Axelrod, J. The regulation of pineal serotonin by a *beta* adrenergic receptor. *J. Pharmac. exp. Ther.*, **1973**, *186*, 109–113.

Bugg, C. E., and Thewalt, U. Crystal structure of serotonin picrate, a donor-acceptor complex. *Science, Wash.*, **1970**, *170*, 852–854.

Bülbring, E. The intrinsic nervous system of the intestine and local effects of 5-hydroxytryptamine. In, *Regional Neurochemistry*. (Kety, S. S., and Elkes, J., eds.) Pergamon Press, Ltd., Oxford, **1961**, pp. 437–441.

Bülbring, E., and Gershon, M. D. Serotonin participation in the vagal inhibitory pathway to the stomach. *Adv. Pharmac.*, **1968**, *6A*, 323–333.

Burks, T. F. Mediation by 5-hydroxytryptamine of morphine stimulant actions in dog intestine. *J. Pharmac. exp. Ther.*, **1973**, *185*, 530–539.

Burks, T. F., and Long, J. P. 5-Hydroxytryptamine release into dog intestinal vasculature. *Am. J. Physiol.*, **1966**, *211*, 619–625.

Cerletti, A.; Taeschler, M.; and Weidmann, H. Pharmacologic studies on the structure-activity relationship of hydroxyindole alkylamines. *Adv. Pharmac.*, **1968**, *6B*, 233–246.

Cochrane, D. E., and Douglas, W. W. Calcium-induced extrusion of secretory granules (exocytosis) in mast cells exposed to 48/80 or the ionophores A-23187 and X-537A. *Proc. natn. Acad. Sci. U.S.A.*, **1974**, *71*, 408–412.

Code, C. F.; Hurn, M. M.; and Mitchell, R. G. Histamine in human disease. *Mayo Clin. Proc.*, **1964**, *39*, 715–737.

Code, C. F.; Maslinski, S. M.; Mossini, F.; and Navert, H. Methylhistamines and gastric secretion. *J. Physiol., Lond.*, **1971**, *217*, 557–571.

Cohen, B., and deJong, J. M. B. V. Meclizine and placebo in treating vertigo of vestibular origin. Relative efficacy in a double-blind study. *Archs Neurol., Chicago*, **1972**, *27*, 129–135.

Colebatch, H. J. H. Adrenergic mechanisms in the effects of histamine in the pulmonary circulation. *Circulation Res.*, **1970**, *26*, 379–396.

Cottrell, G. A. Action of imipramine on a serotonergic synapse. *Comp. gen. Pharmac.*, **1971**, *2*, 125–128.

Dahlström, A., and Fuxe, K. Evidence for the existence of monoamine neurons in the central nervous system. II. Experimentally induced changes in the intraneuronal amine levels of bulbospinal neuron systems. *Acta physiol. scand.*, **1965**, *64*, Suppl. 247, 1–36.

Dale, H. H. The anaphylactic reaction of plain muscle in the guinea-pig. *J. Pharmac. exp. Ther.*, **1913**, *4*, 167–223.

———. Some chemical factors in the control of the circulation. *Lancet*, **1929**, *1*, 1179–1183, 1233–1237, 1285–1290.

Dale, H. H., and Laidlaw, P. P. The physiological action of β-imidazolylethylamine. *J. Physiol., Lond.*, **1910**, *41*, 318–344.

———. Further observations on the action of β-imidazolylethylamine. *Ibid.*, **1911**, *43*, 182–195.

———. Histamine shock. *Ibid.*, **1919**, *52*, 355–390.

de Groat, W. C., and Lalley, P. M. Interaction between picrotoxin and 5-hydroxytryptamine in the superior cervical ganglion of the cat. *Br. J. Pharmac.*, **1973**, *48*, 233–244.

Domschke, W.; Domschke, S.; Classen, M.; and Demling, L. Histamine and cyclic 3',5'-AMP in gastric acid secretion. *Nature, Lond.*, **1973**, *241*, 454–455.

Douglas, W. W. Involvement of calcium in exocytosis and the exocytosis-vesiculation sequence. *Biochem. Soc. Symp.*, **1974**, *39*, 1–28.

Douglas, W. W.; Kanno, T.; and Sampson, S. R. Effects of acetylcholine and other medullary secretagogues and antagonists on the membrane potential of adrenal chromaffin cells: an analysis employing techniques of tissue culture. *J. Physiol., Lond.*, **1967**, *188*, 107–120.

Dragstedt, C. A., and Gebauer-Fuelnegg, E. Studies in anaphylaxis. I. The appearance of a physiologically active substance during anaphylactic shock. *Am. J. Physiol.*, **1932**, *102*, 512–519.

Dykes, M. H. M. Evaluation of an antiasthmatic agent cromolyn sodium (AARANE, INTAL). *J. Am. med. Ass.*, **1974**, *227*, 1061–1062.

Emmelin, N. Action of histamine upon salivary glands. In, *Histamine: Its Chemistry, Metabolism and Physiological and Pharmacological Actions.* (Rocha e Silva, M., ed.) *Handb. exp. Pharmak.*, Vol. 18, Part 1. Springer-Verlag, Berlin, **1966**, pp. 294–301.

Erspamer, V. Richerche farmacologiche sull' enteramina. VII. Enteramina e indolalchilamine del veleno di rospo. *Archo Sci. biol.*, **1946**, *31*, 86–95.

———. Occurrence of indolealkylamines in nature. In, *5-Hydroxytryptamine and Related Indolealkylamines.* (Erspamer, V., ed.) *Handb. exp. Pharmak.*, Vol. 19. Springer-Verlag, Berlin, **1966a**, pp. 132–181.

Erspamer, V., and Asero, B. Identification of enteramine, the specific hormone of the enterochromaffin cell system, as 5-hydroxytryptamine. *Nature, Lond.*, **1952**, *169*, 800–801.

Euler, U. S. von. Relationship between histamine and the autonomic nervous system. In, *Histamine: Its Chemistry, Metabolism and Physiological and Pharmacological Actions.* (Rocha e Silva, M., ed.) *Handb. exp. Pharmak.*, Vol. 18, Part 1. Springer-Verlag, Berlin, **1966**, pp. 318–333.

Eyre, P. Histamine H_2-receptors in the sheep bronchus and cat trachea: the action of burimamide. *Br. J. Pharmac.*, **1973**, *48*, 321–323.

Faingold, C. L., and Berry, C. A. A comparison of the EEG effects of the potent antihistaminic (DL-chlorpheniramine) with a less potent isomer (L-chlorpheniramine). *Archs int. Pharmacodyn. Thér.*, **1972**, *199*, 213–218.

Feldberg, W. The monoamines of the hypothalamus as mediators of temperature responses. In, *Recent Advances in Pharmacology*, 4th ed. (Robson, J. M., and Stacey, R. S., eds.) J. & A. Churchill, Ltd., London, **1968**, pp. 349–397.

Feldberg, W., and Sherwood, S. L. Injections of drugs into the lateral ventricle of the cat. *J. Physiol., Lond.*, **1954**, *123*, 148–167.

Fillion, G. M. B.; Lluch, S.; and Uvnas, B. Release of noradrenaline from the dog heart *in situ* after intravenous and intracoronary administration of 5-hydroxytryptamine. *Acta physiol. scand.*, **1971**, *83*, 115–123.

Flacke, W.; Atanackovic, D.; Gillis, R. A.; and Alper, M. H. The action of histamine on the mammalian heart. *J. Pharmac. exp. Ther.*, **1967**, *155*, 271–278.

Foreman, J. C., and Mongar, J. L. Effect of calcium on dextran-induced histamine release from isolated mast cells. *Br. J. Pharmac.*, **1973**, *46*, 767–769.

Friedman, A. P., and Elkind, A. H. Appraisal of methysergide in treatment of vascular headaches of migraine type. *J. Am. med. Ass.*, **1963**, *184*, 125–128.

Furness, J. B., and Costa, M. The nervous release and the action of substances which affect intestinal muscle through neither adrenoceptors nor cholinoceptors. *Phil. Trans. R. Soc. Lond., B*, **1973**, *265*, 123–133.

Fuxe, K., and Jonsson, G. Further mapping of central 5-hydroxytryptamine neurons; studies with the neurotoxic dihydroxytryptamines. *Adv. biochem. Psychopharmac.*, **1974**, *10*, 1–12.

Gaddum, J. H. Antagonism between LSD and 5-hydroxytryptamine. *J. Physiol., Lond.*, **1953**, *121*, 15P.

Garland, L. G., and Mongar, J. L. Inhibition by cromoglycate of histamine release from rat peritoneal mast cells induced by mixtures of dextran, phosphatidyl serine and calcium ions. *Br. J. Pharmac.*, **1974**, *50*, 137–143.

Gerschenfeld, H. M. Serotonin: two different inhibitory actions on snail neurons. *Science, Wash.*, **1971**, *171*, 1252–1254.

Gerschenfeld, H. M., and Stefani, E. Evidence for an excitatory role of serotonin in molluscan synapses. *Adv. Pharmac.*, **1968**, *6A*, 369–392.

Gershon, M. D., and Nunez, E. A. Subcellular storage organelles for 5-hydroxytryptamine in parafollicular cells of the thyroid gland. The effect of drugs which deplete the amine. *J. cell Biol.*, **1973**, *56*, 676–689.

Gillis, C. N. Metabolism of vasoactive hormones by lung. *Anesthesiology*, **1973**, *39*, 626–632.

Graham, J. R. Cardiac and pulmonary fibrosis during methysergide therapy for headache. *Am. J. med. Sci.*, **1967**, *254*, 1–12.

Grimm, Y., and Reichlin, S. Thyrotropin-releasing hormone (TRH): neurotransmitter regulation of secretion by mouse hypothalamic tissue *in vitro*. *Endocrinology*, **1973**, *93*, 626–631.

Grossman, M. I. Gastrin and its activities. *Nature, Lond.*, **1970**, *228*, 1147–1150.

Haigler, H. J., and Aghajanian, G. K. Lysergic acid diethylamide and serotonin: a comparison of effects on serotonergic neurons and neurons receiving a serotonergic input. *J. Pharmac. exp. Ther.*, **1974a**, *188*, 688–699.

———. Peripheral serotonin antagonists: failure to antagonize serotonin in brain areas receiving prominent serotonergic input. *J. neur. Transmiss.*, **1974b**, *35*, 257–273.

Håkanson, R. New aspects of the formation and function of histamine, 5-hydroxytryptamine and dopamine in gastric mucosa. I. Properties of enterochromaffin and enterochromaffin-like cells. II. Properties of mammalian histamine-forming enzymes. *Acta physiol. scand.*, **1970**, *79*, Suppl. 340, 1–134.

Håkanson, R.; Owman, C.; and Sporrong, B. Parakrina celler i mag-tarmkanalen. Upplagringsplats för biogena aminer, gastrointestinola polypeptidhormon och absorptionfaktorer. *Nord. Med.*, **1971**, *85*, 169–174.

Hamlin, K. E., and Fischer, F. E. The synthesis of 5-hydroxytryptamine. *J. Am. chem. Soc.*, **1951**, *73*, 5007–5008.

Hartman, M. M. Capabilities and limitations of major drug groups in allergy: their role within current theories. *Ann. Allergy*, **1969**, *27*, 164.

Heller, A. Neuronal control of brain serotonin. *Fedn Proc. Fedn Am. Socs exp. Biol.*, **1972**, *31*, 81–90.

Hellman, B.; Lernmark, Å.; Sehlin, J.; and Täljedal, I.-B. Transport and storage of 5-hydroxytryptamine in pancreatic β-cells. *Biochem. Pharmac.*, **1972**, *21*, 695–706.

Hill, G. J. Carcinoid tumors: pharmacological therapy. *Oncology*, **1971**, *25*, 329–343.

Hollander, W.; Michelson, A. L.; and Wilkins, R. W. Serotonin and antiserotonins. I. Their circulatory, respiratory and renal effects in man. *Circulation*, **1957**, *16*, 246–255.

Holmsen, H.; Østvold, A.-C.; and Day, J. H. Behaviour of endogenous and newly absorbed serotonin in the platelet release reaction. *Biochem. Pharmac.*, **1973**, *22*, 2599–2608.

Horton, B. T. The use of histamine in the treatment of specific types of headaches. *J. Am. med. Ass.*, **1941**, *116*, 377–383.

Huang, M.; Shimizu, H.; and Daly, J. Regulation of adenosine cyclic 3′,5′-phosphate formation in cerebral cortical slices. Interaction among norepinephrine, histamine, serotonin. *Molec. Pharmac.*, **1971**, *7*, 155–162.

Hughes, M. J., and Coret, I. A. On specificity of histamine receptors in the heart. *Am. J. Physiol.*, **1972**, *223*, 1257–1262.

Impicciatore, M., and Grossman, M. I. Stimulation of gastric acid secretion by 5-methyl histamine in cat. *Am. J. dig. Dis.*, **1973**, *18*, 551–555.

Ivy, A. C., and Bachrach, W. H. Physiological significance of the effect of histamine on gastric secretion. In, *Histamine: Its Chemistry, Metabolism and Physiological and Pharmacological Actions.* (Rocha e Silva, M., ed.) *Handb. exp. Pharmak.*, Vol. 18, Part 1. Springer-Verlag, Berlin, **1966**, pp. 810–891.

Jaju, B. P.; Kirsten, E. B.; and Wang, S. C. Effects of belladonna alkaloids on vestibular nucleus of the cat. *Am. J. Physiol.*, **1970**, *219*, 1248–1255.

Jaju, B. P., and Wang, S. C. Effects of diphenhydramine and dimenhydrinate on vestibular neuronal activity of cat: a search for the locus of their antimotion sickness action. *J. Pharmac. exp. Ther.*, **1971**, *176*, 718–724.

Johnson, A. R., and Erdös, E. G. Release of histamine by vasoactive peptides. *Proc. Soc. exp. Biol. Med.*, **1973**, *142*, 1252–1256.

Johnson, G. L., and Kahn, J. B. Cocaine and antihistaminic compounds: comparison of effects of some cardiovascular actions of norepinephrine, tyramine and bretylium. *J. Pharmac. exp. Ther.*, **1966**, *152*, 458–468.

Johnson, H. L.; Ellis, M.; and Mitoma, C. Non-mast cell histamine kinetics. V. ^{3}H-Histamine formation *in vivo* and effects of precursor pool perturbations. *Eur. J. Pharmac.*, **1973**, *22*, 37–42.

Kagayama, M., and Douglas, W. W. Electron microscopic evidence of calcium-induced exocytosis in mast cells treated with 48/80 or the ionophores A-23187 and X-537A. *J. cell Biol.*, **1974**, *62*, 519–526.

Kakiuchi, S., and Rall, T. W. Studies on adenosine 3′,5′-monophosphate in rabbit cerebral cortex. *Molec. Pharmac.*, **1968**, *4*, 379–388.

Kanno, T.; Cochrane, D. E.; and Douglas, W. W. Exocytosis (secretory granule extrusion) induced by injection of calcium into mast cells. *Can. J. Physiol. Pharmac.*, **1973**, *51*, 1001–1004.

Kay, A. W. Effect of large doses of histamine on gastric secretion of HCl: an augmented histamine test. *Br. med. J.*, **1953**, *2*, 77–80.

Keeton, R. W.; Luckhardt, A. B.; and Koch, F. C. Gastrin studies. IV. The response of the stomach mucosa to food and gastrin bodies as influenced by atropine. *Am. J. Physiol.*, **1920**, *51*, 469–481.

King, G., and Weeks, S. D. Pyribenzamine activation of the electroencephalogram. *Electroenceph. clin. Neurophysiol.*, **1965**, *18*, 503–507.

Klein, D. C., and Weller, J. L. Adrenergic-adenosine 3′,5′-monophosphate regulation of serotonin N-acetyltransferase activity and the temporal relationship of serotonin N-acetyltransferase activity to synthesis of ^{3}H-N-acetylserotonin and ^{3}H-melatonin in the cultured rat pineal gland. *J. Pharmac. exp. Ther.*, **1973**, *186*, 516–527.

Klein, I., and Levey, G. S. Activation of adenyl cyclase by histamine in guinea pig, cat and human heart. *J. clin. Invest.*, **1971**, *50*, 1012–1015.

Koe, B. K., and Weissman, A. Parachlorophenylalanine: a specific depletor of brain serotonin. *J. Pharmac. exp. Ther.*, **1966**, *154*, 499–516.

Koopman, W. J.; Orange, R. P.; and Austen, K. F. Immunochemical and biologic properties of rat IgE. III. Modulation of the IgE-mediated release of slow-reacting substance of anaphylaxis by agents influencing the level of cyclic 3′,5′-adenosine monophosphate. *J. Immun.*, **1970**, *105*, 1096–1102.

Kuntzman, R.; Phillips, A.; Tsai, I.; Klutch, A.; and Burns, J. J. N-oxide formation: a new route for inactivation of the antihistaminic chlorcyclizine. *J. Pharmac. exp. Ther.*, **1967**, *155*, 337–344.

Lebovitz, H. E., and Feldman, J. M. Pancreatic biogenic amines and insulin secretion in health and disease. *Fedn Proc. Fedn Am. Socs exp. Biol.*, **1973**, *32*, 1797–1802.

Lecomte, J. Liberation of endogenous histamine in man. *J. Allergy*, **1957**, *28*, 102–112.

Lent, C. M. Retzius cells: neuroeffectors controlling mucus release by the leech. *Science, Wash.*, **1973**, *179*, 693–696.

Levine, R. J. Serotonin and the carcinoid syndrome; histamine and mastocytosis. In, *Duncan's Diseases of Metabolism: The Genetic and Biochemical Basis of Disease,* 7th ed., Vol. II. (Bondy, P. K., and Rosenberg, L. E., eds.) W. B. Saunders Co., Philadelphia, **1974**, pp. 1651–1684.

Lichtenstein, L. M. The immediate allergic response: *in vitro* separation of antigen activation, decay and histamine release. *J. Immun.*, **1971**, *107*, 1122–1130.

Liebeskind, J. C.; Guilbaud, G.; Besson, J. M.; and Oliveras, J.-L. Analgesia from electrical stimulation of the periaqueductal gray matter in the cat: behavioural observations and inhibitory effects on spinal cord interneurones. *Brain Res.*, **1973**, *50*, 441–446.

Loew, E. R.; MacMillan, R.; and Katser, M. E. The antihistamine properties of BENADRYL, β-dimethylaminoethyl benzhydryl ether hydrochloride. *J. Pharmac. exp. Ther.*, **1946**, *86*, 229–238.

Lowe, R. F., and Gilboe, D. D. Canine cerebrovascular response to nitroglycerine, acetylcholine, 5-hydroxytryptamine, and angiotensin. *Am. J. Physiol.*, **1973**, *225*, 1333–1338.

Lu, K.-H., and Meites, J. Effects of serotonin precursors and melatonin on serum prolactin release in rats. *Endocrinology*, **1973**, *93*, 152–155.

McGuigan, J. E. On the distribution and release of gastrin. *Gastroenterology*, **1973**, *64*, 497–501.

Macmillan, W. H., and Vane, J. R. The effects of histamine on the plasma potassium levels of cats. *J. Pharmac. exp. Ther.*, **1956**, *118*, 182–192.

Mainguet, P. Effect of cyproheptadine on anorexia and loss of weight in adults. *Practitioner*, **1972**, *208*, 797–800.

Majno, G.; Shea, S. M.; and Leventhal, M. Endothelial contraction induced by histamine-type mediators. An electron microscopic study. *J. cell Biol.*, **1969**, *42*, 647–672.

Mannaioni, P. F. Physiology and pharmacology of cardiac histamine. *Archs int. Pharmacodyn. Thér.*, **1972**, *196*, Suppl., 54–67.

Medical Letter. Cyproheptadine (PERIACTIN). **1971**, *13*, 17–18.

Melander, A., and Sundler, F. Interactions between catecholamines, 5-hydroxytryptamine and TSH on the secretion of thyroid hormone. *Endocrinology*, **1972**, *90*, 188–193.

Merchant, F. J.; Bombeck, C. T.; Pissidis, A.; and Nyhus, L. M. Hepatic destruction of synthetic gastrin pentapeptide. *J. natn. med. Ass.*, **1972**, *64*, 246–249.

Miller, J., and Fishman, A. A serotonin antagonist in the treatment of allergic and allied disorders. *Ann. Allergy*, **1961**, *19*, 164–171.

Milton-Thompson, G. J.; Williams, J. G.; Jenkins, D. J. A.; and Misiewicz, J. J. Inhibition of nocturnal acid secretion in duodenal ulcer by one oral dose of metiamide. *Lancet*, **1974**, *1*, 693–694.

Minter, B. F., and Crawford, N. Subcellular distribution of 5-hydroxytryptamine in pig platelets. *Biochem. Pharmac.*, **1971**, *20*, 783–802.

Morishima, T. 5-Hydroxytryptamine (serotonin) and 5-hydroxytryptophan in mast cells of human mastocytosis. *Tohoku J. exp. Med.,* **1970,** *102,* 121–126.

Morley, J. S. Structure-function relationships in gastrin-like peptides. *Proc. R. Soc., B,* **1968,** *170,* 97–111.

Nakajima, S.; Hirschowitz, B. I.; and Sachs, G. Studies on adenyl cyclase in *Necturus* gastric mucosa. *Archs Biochem. Biophys.,* **1971,** *143,* 123–126.

Nelson, R. F. A new prophylactic agent for migraine—four years' experience in seventy-five patients. *Headache,* **1973,** *13,* 96–103.

Orange, R. P., and Austen, K. F. Immunological release of the chemical mediators of anaphylaxis. In, *Identification of Asthma.* Ciba Foundation Study Group No. 38. (Porter, R., and Birch, J., eds.) Churchill-Livingstone, Ltd., London, **1971,** pp. 99–110.

Owman, C.; Håkanson, R.; and Sundler, F. Occurrence and function of amines in endocrine cells producing polypeptide hormones. *Fedn Proc. Fedn Am. Socs exp. Biol.,* **1973,** *32,* 1785–1791.

Paton, W. D. M., and Vane, J. R. An analysis of the responses of the isolated stomach to electrical stimulation and to drugs. *J. Physiol., Lond.,* **1963,** *165,* 10–46.

Payne, R. A., and Kay, A. W. The effect of vagotomy on the maximal acid secretory response to histamine. *Clin. Sci.,* **1962,** *22,* 373–382.

Peets, E. A.; Jackson, M.; and Symchowicz, S. Metabolism of chlorpheniramine maleate in man. *J. Pharmac. exp. Ther.,* **1972,** *180,* 464–474.

Penfold, J. L. Effect of cyproheptadine and a multivitamin preparation on appetite stimulation, weight gain and linear growth. *Med. J. Aust.,* **1971,** *1,* 307–310.

Persyko, I. Psychiatric adverse reactions to methysergide. *J. nerv. ment. Dis.,* **1972,** *4,* 299–301.

Pletscher, A.; Da Prada, M.; Berneis, K. H.; and Tranzer, J. P. New aspects on the storage of 5-hydroxytryptamine in blood platelets. *Experientia,* **1971,** *27,* 993–1002.

Popielski, L. β-Imidazolyläthylamin und die Organextrakte. Erster Teil: β-Imidazolyläthylamin als mächtiger Erreger der Magendrüsen. *Pflügers Arch. ges. Physiol.,* **1920,** *178,* 214–236.

Prince, W. T., and Berridge, M. J. The effects of 5-hydroxytryptamine and cyclic AMP on the potential profile across isolated salivary glands. *J. exp. Biol.,* **1972,** *56,* 323–333.

Rapport, M. M. Serum vasoconstrictor (serotonin). V. The presence of creatinine in the complex: a proposed study of the vasoconstrictor principle. *J. biol. Chem.,* **1949,** *180,* 961–969.

Rapport, M. M.; Green, A. A.; and Page, I. H. Serum vasoconstrictor (serotonin). IV. Isolation and characterization. *J. biol. Chem.,* **1948,** *176,* 1243–1251.

Robinson, R. G., and Gershon, M. D. Synthesis and uptake of 5-hydroxytryptamine by the myenteric plexus of the guinea-pig ileum: a histochemical study. *J. Pharmac. exp. Ther.,* **1971,** *178,* 311–324.

Robson, J. M., and Sullivan, F. M. Effect of 5-hydroxytryptamine on maintenance of pregnancy, congenital abnormalities, and the development of toxemia. *Adv. Pharmac.,* **1968,** *6B,* 187–189.

Rodbard, S., and Kira, S. Lobar, airway, and pulmonary vascular effects of serotonin. *Angiology,* **1972,** *23,* 188–197.

Rosière, C. E., and Grossman, M. I. An analog of histamine that stimulates gastric acid secretion without other actions of histamine. *Science, Wash.,* **1951,** *113,* 651.

Rothschild, A. M. Histamine release by basic compounds. In, *Histamine: Its Chemistry, Metabolism and Physiological and Pharmacological Actions.* (Rocha e Silva, M., ed.) *Handb. exp. Pharmak.,* Vol. 18, Part 1. Springer-Verlag, Berlin, **1966,** pp. 386–430.

Ruoff, H.-J., and Sewing, K.-F. Cyclic 3′,5′-adenosine monophosphate in the rat gastric mucosa after starvation, feeding and pentagastrin. *Scand. J. Gastroent.,* **1973,** *8,* 241–243.

Sadusk, J. F., and Palmisano, P. A. Teratogenic effect of meclizine, cyclizine, and chlorcyclizine. *J. Am. med. Ass.,* **1965,** *194,* 987–989.

Sandler, M. The role of 5-hydroxyindoles in the carcinoid syndrome. *Adv. Pharmac.,* **1968,** *6B,* 127–142.

Saum, W. R., and de Groat, W. C. The actions of 5-hydroxytryptamine on the urinary bladder and on vesical autonomic ganglia in the cat. *J. Pharmac. exp. Ther.,* **1973,** *185,* 70–83.

Schayer, R. W. Histamine and circulatory homeostasis. *Fedn Proc. Fedn Am. Socs exp. Biol.,* **1965,** *24,* 1295–1297.

Schayer, R. W., and Cooper, J. A. D. Metabolism of C^{14} histamine in man. *J. appl. Physiol.,* **1956,** *9,* 481–483.

Schayer, R. W., and Reilly, M. A. Metabolism of ^{14}C-histamine in brain. *J. Pharmac. exp. Ther.,* **1973,** *187,* 34–39.

Sharpey-Schafer, E. P., and Ginsburg, J. Humoral agents and venous tone: effects of catecholamines, 5-hydroxytryptamine, histamine, and nitrites. *Lancet,* **1962,** *2,* 1337–1340.

Shimizu, H.; Creveling, C. R.; and Daly, J. W. The effect of histamines and other compounds on the formation of adenosine 3′,5′-monophosphate in slices from cerebral cortex. *J. Neurochem.,* **1970,** *17,* 441–444.

Sicuteri, F. Prophylactic and therapeutic properties of 1-methyl-lysergic acid butanolamide in migraine (preliminary report). *Int. Archs Allergy appl. Immun.,* **1959,** *15,* 300–307.

Sjoerdsma, A.; Gillespie, L.; and Udenfriend, S. A simple method for the measurement of monoamine-oxidase inhibition in man. *Lancet,* **1958,** *2,* 159–160.

Sjoerdsma, A.; Lovenberg, W.; Engelman, K.; Carpenter, W. T., Jr.; Wyatt, R. J.; and Gessa, G. L. Serotonin now: clinical implications of inhibiting its synthesis with *para*-chlorophenylalanine. *Ann. intern. Med.,* **1970,** *73,* 607–629.

Skolnick, P.; Huang, M.; Daly, J.; and Hoffer, B. Accumulation of adenosine 3′,5′-monophosphate in incubated slices from discrete regions of squirrel monkey cerebral cortex: effect of norepinephrine, serotonin and adenosine. *J. Neurochem.,* **1973,** *21,* 237–240.

Snyder, S. H., and Taylor, K. M. Histamine in the brain: a neurotransmitter? In, *Perspectives in Neuropharmacology: A Tribute to Julius Axelrod.* (Snyder, S. H., ed.) Oxford University Press, New York, **1972,** pp. 43–74.

Southgate, J., and Sandler, M. 5-Hydroxyindole metabolism in pregnancy. *Adv. Pharmac.,* **1968,** *6B,* 179–186.

Spodick, D. H. Electrocardiographic responses to pulmonary embolism. Mechanisms and sources of variability. *Am. J. Cardiol.,* **1972,** *30,* 695–699.

Staszewska-Barczak, J., and Vane, J. R. The release of catecholamines from the adrenal medulla by histamine. *Br. J. Pharmac. Chemother.,* **1965,** *25,* 728–742.

Staub, A.-M., and Bovet, D. Action de la thymoxyéthyldiéthylamine (929F) et des éthers phénoliques sur le choc anaphylactique du cobaye. *C. r. Séanc. Soc. Biol.,* **1937,** *125,* 818–823.

Stone, C. A.; Wenger, H. C.; Ludden, C. T.; Stavorski, I. M.; and Ross, C. A. Antiserotonin-antihistaminic properties of cyproheptadine. *J. Pharmac. exp. Ther.,* **1961,** *131,* 73–84.

Storstein, O.; Calabresi, M.; Nims, R. G.; and Gray, F. D., Jr. The effect of histamine on the pulmonary circulation in man. *Yale J. Biol. Med.,* **1959,** *32,* 197–208.

Taylor, K. M.; Gffeller, E.; and Snyder, S. Regional localization of histamine and histidine in the brain of the rhesus monkey. *Brain Res.,* **1972,** *41,* 171–179.

Todrick, A., and Tait, A. C. The inhibition of human platelet 5-hydroxytryptamine uptake by tricyclic antidepressive drugs. The relation between structure and potency. *J. Pharm. Pharmac.,* **1969,** *21,* 751–762.

Torok, E. E.; Brewer, J. I.; and Dolkart, R. E. Serum diamine oxidase in pregnancy and in trophoblastic diseases. *J. clin. Endocr. Metab.,* **1970,** *30,* 59–65.

Turker, R. K. Presence of histamine H_2-receptors in the

guinea pig pulmonary vascular bed. *Pharmacology,* **1973,** *9,* 306–311.

Twarog, B. M., and Page, I. H. Serotonin content of some mammalian tissues and urine and a method for its determination. *Am. J. Physiol.,* **1953,** *175,* 157–161.

Vogt, M. The effect of lowering the 5-hydroxytryptamine content of the rat spinal cord on analgesia produced by morphine. *J. Physiol., Lond.,* **1974,** *236,* 483–498.

Way, E. L. Role of serotonin in morphine effects. *Fedn Proc. Fedn Am. Socs exp. Biol.,* **1972,** *31,* 113–119.

Weinreich, D.; McCaman, M. W.; McCaman, R. E.; and Vaughn, J. E. Chemical, enzymatic and ultrastructural characterization of 5-hydroxytryptamine-containing neurons from the ganglia of *Aplysia californica* and *Tritonia diomedia. J. Neurochem.,* **1973,** *20,* 969–976.

Welsh, J. H. Distribution of 5-HT in the nervous systems of animals. *Adv. Pharmac.,* **1968,** *6A,* 171–188.

Wilhelm, R. E. The newer anti-allergic agents. *Med. Clins N. Am.,* **1961,** *45,* 887–906.

Winek, C. L. Dangerous cough syrups. *New Engl. J. Med.,* **1969,** *280,* 840.

Wood, C. D., and Graybiel, A. A theory of motion sickness based on pharmacological reactions. *Clin. Pharmac. Ther.,* **1970,** *11,* 621–629.

Woolley, D. W., and Shaw, E. A biochemical and pharmacological suggestion about certain mental disorders. *Science, Wash.,* **1954,** *119,* 587–588.

Yonkman, F. F.; Chess, D.; Mathieson, D.; and Hansen, N. Pharmacodynamic studies of a new antihistamine agent, N'-pyridyl-N'-benzyl-N-dimethylethylene diamine HCl, pyribenzamine HCl. I. Effects on salivation, nictitating membrane, lachrymation, pupil and blood pressure. *J. Pharmac. exp. Ther.,* **1946,** *87,* 256–264.

Monographs and Reviews

Andersson, S. Secretion of gastrointestinal hormones. *A. Rev. Physiol.,* **1973,** *35,* 431–452.

Beraldo, W. T., and Dias da Silva, W. Release of histamine by animal venoms and bacterial toxins. In, *Histamine: Its Chemistry, Metabolism and Physiological and Pharmacological Actions.* (Rocha e Silva, M., ed.) *Handb. exp. Pharmak.,* Vol. 18, Part 1. Springer-Verlag, Berlin, **1966,** pp. 334–366.

Brand, J. J., and Perry, W. L. M. Drugs used in motion sickness. *Pharmac. Rev.,* **1966,** *18,* 895–924.

Chase, T. N., and Murphy, D. L. Serotonin and central nervous function. *A. Rev. Pharmac.,* **1973,** *13,* 181–197.

Chinn, H. I., and Smith, P. K. Motion sickness. *Pharmac. Rev.,* **1955,** *7,* 33–82.

Code, C. F. Histamine and gastric secretion: a later look, 1955–1965. *Fedn Proc. Fedn Am. Socs exp. Biol.,* **1965,** *24,* 1311–1325.

Collier, H. O. J. Endogenous broncho-active substances and their antagonism. *Adv. Drug Res.,* **1970,** *5,* 95–107.

Costa, E., and Meek, J. L. Regulation of biosynthesis of catecholamines and serotonin in the CNS. *A. Rev. Pharmac.,* **1974,** *14,* 491–511.

Cox, J. S. C.; Beach, J. E.; Blair, A. M.; Clarke, A. J.; King, J.; Lee, T. B.; Loveday, D. E. E.; Moss, G. F.; Orr, T. S. C.; Ritchie, J. R.; and Sheard, P. Disodium cromoglycate (INTAL). *Adv. Drug Res.,* **1970,** *5,* 115–196.

de Wied, D., and de Jong, W. Drug effects and hypothalamic-anterior pituitary function. *A. Rev. Pharmac.,* **1974,** *14,* 389–412.

Douglas, W. W. Stimulus-secretion coupling: the concept and clues from chromaffin and other cells. The First Gaddum Memorial Lecture. *Br. J. Pharmac.,* **1968,** *35,* 451–474.

Ebashi, S., and Endo, M. Calcium ion and muscle contraction. *Prog. Biophys. molec. Biol.,* **1968,** *18,* 123–183.

Erspamer, V. Pharmacology of indolealkylamines. *Pharmac. Rev.,* **1954,** *6,* 425–487.

———— (ed.). *5-Hydroxytryptamine and Related Indolealkylamines. Handb. exp. Pharmak.,* Vol. 19. Springer-Verlag, Berlin, **1966b.**

Goth, A. Histamine release by drugs and chemicals. In, *Histamine and Antihistamines,* Vol. 1. *International Encyclopedia of Pharmacology and Therapeutics,* Sect. 74. (Schacter, M., ed.) Pergamon Press, Ltd., Oxford, **1973,** pp. 25–43.

Green, J. P. Histamine. In, *Handbook of Neurochemistry,* Vol. 4. (Lajtha, A., ed.) Plenum Press, New York, **1970,** pp. 221–250.

Gregory, R. A., and Tracy, H. J. A review of recent progress in the chemistry of gastrin. *Am. J. dig. Dis.,* **1966,** *11,* 97–102.

Gyermek, L. Drugs which antagonize 5-hydroxytryptamine and related indolealkylamines. In, *5-Hydroxytryptamine and Related Indolealkylamines.* (Erspamer, V., ed.) *Handb. exp. Pharmak.,* Vol. 19. Springer-Verlag, Berlin, **1966,** pp. 471–528.

Halpern, B. N. Les antihistaminiques de synthèse: essais de chimiothérapie des états allergiques. *Archs int. Pharmacodyn. Thér.,* **1942,** *68,* 339–408.

Kahlson, G., and Rosengren, E. New approaches to the physiology of histamine. *Physiol. Rev.,* **1968,** *48,* 155–196.

————. *Biogenesis and Physiology of Histamine.* Edward Arnold, Ltd., London, **1971.**

Keele, C. A., and Armstrong, D. *Substances Producing Pain and Itch.* The Williams & Wilkins Co., Baltimore, **1964.**

Kosterlitz, H. W.; Collier, H. O. J.; and Villarreal, J. E. (eds.). *Agonist and Antagonist Actions of Narcotic Analgesic Drugs.* University Park Press, Baltimore, **1972.**

Lewis, T. *The Blood Vessels of the Human Skin and Their Responses.* Shaw & Sons, Ltd., London, **1927.**

McIntyre, F. C. Histamine release by antigen-antibody reactions. In, *Histamine and Antihistamines,* Vol. 1. *International Encyclopedia of Pharmacology and Therapeutics,* Sect. 74. (Schacter, M., ed.) Pergamon Press, Ltd., Oxford, **1973,** pp. 45–99.

Mantegazzini, P. Pharmacological actions of indolealkylamines and precursor amino acids on the central nervous system. In, *5-Hydroxytryptamine and Related Indolealkylamines.* (Erspamer, V., ed.) *Handb. exp. Pharmak.,* Vol. 19. Springer-Verlag, Berlin, **1966,** pp. 424–470.

Money, K. E. Motion sickness. *Physiol. Rev.,* **1970,** *50,* 1–39.

Mongar, J. L., and Schild, H. O. Cellular mechanism in anaphylaxis. *Physiol. Rev.,* **1962,** *42,* 226–270.

Mustard, J. F., and Packham, M. A. Factors influencing platelet function: adhesion, release and aggregation. *Pharmac. Rev.,* **1970,** *22,* 97–187.

Page, I. H. *Serotonin.* Year Book Medical Publishers, Inc., Chicago, **1968.**

Paton, W. D. M. Receptors for histamine. In, *Histamine and Antihistamines,* Vol. 1. *International Encyclopedia of Pharmacology and Therapeutics,* Sect. 74. (Schacter, M., ed.) Pergamon Press, Ltd., Oxford, **1973,** pp. 3–24.

Pressman, B. C. Properties of ionophores with broad range cation selectivity. *Fedn Proc. Fedn Am. Socs exp. Biol.,* **1973,** *32,* 1698–1703.

Reite, O. B. Comparative physiology of histamine. *Physiol. Rev.,* **1972,** *52,* 778–819.

Robison, G. A.; Butcher, R. W.; and Sutherland, E. W. *Cyclic AMP.* Academic Press, Inc., New York, **1971.**

Rocha e Silva, M. (ed.). *Histamine: Its Chemistry, Metabolism and Physiological and Pharmacological Actions. Handb. exp. Pharmak.,* Vol. 18, Part 1. Springer-Verlag, Berlin, **1966.**

Sakharov, D. A. Cellular aspects of invertebrate neuropharmacology. *A. Rev. Pharmac.,* **1970,** *10,* 335–352.

Schäfer, E. A. *The Endocrine Organs: An Introduction to the Study of Internal Secretion.* Longmans, Green & Co., New York, **1916.**

Schayer, R. W. Induced synthesis of histamine, microcirculatory regulation and the mechanism of action of the glucocorticoid hormones. *Prog. Allergy,* **1963,** *7,* 187–212.

Sneddon, J. Blood platelets as a model for monoamine-containing neurones. *Prog. Neurobiol.,* **1973,** *1,* 153–198.

Somlyo, A. P., and Somlyo, A. V. Vascular smooth muscle. II. Pharmacology of normal and hypertensive vessels. *Pharmac. Rev.,* **1970,** *22,* 249–353.

Speight, T. M., and Avery, G. S. Pizotifen (B.C-105): a review of pharmacological properties and its therapeutic efficacy in vascular headaches. *Drugs,* **1972,** *3,* 159–203.

Study Group 1971. *Identification of Asthma.* Ciba Foundation Study Group No. 38. (Porter, R., and Birch, J., eds.) Churchill-Livingstone, Ltd., London, **1971.**

Symposium. (Various authors.) Uptake, storage and release of histamine. *Fedn Proc. Fedn Am. Socs exp. Biol.,* **1967,** *26,* 211–240.

Symposium. (Various authors.) Biological role of indolealkylamine derivatives. (Garattini, S., and Shore, P., eds.) *Adv. Pharmac.,* **1968a,** *6A,* 1–440; *6B,* 1–323.

Symposium. (Various authors.) 5-Hydroxytryptamine. (Paasonen, M. K., and Klinge, E., eds.) *Annls Med. exp. Biol. Fenn.,* **1968b,** *46,* 361–519.

Symposium. (Various authors.) Functional significance of serotonin in neuronal systems. *Fedn Proc. Fedn Am. Socs exp. Biol.,* **1972,** *31,* 81–129.

Symposium. (Various authors.) *Serotonin and Behavior.* (Barchas, J. D., and Usdin, E., eds.) Academic Press, Inc., New York, **1973,** pp. 1–642.

Symposium. (Various authors.) Serotonin—new vistas: histochemistry and pharmacology. (Costa, E.; Gessa, G. L.; and Sandler, M.; eds.) *Adv. biochem. Psychopharmac.,* **1974a,** *10,* 1–329.

Symposium. (Various authors.) Serotonin—new vistas: biochemistry and behavioural and clinical studies. (Costa, E.; Gessa, G. L.; and Sandler, M.; eds.) *Adv. biochem. Psychopharmac.,* **1974b,** *11,* 1–428.

Thompson, J. H. Serotonin and the alimentary tract. *Res. Commun. chem. path. Pharmac.,* **1971,** *2,* 687–781.

Udenfriend, S. Biochemistry of serotonin and other indoleamines. *Vitams Horm.,* **1959,** *17,* 133–154.

Vane, J. R. The release and fate of vaso-active hormones in the circulation. *Br. J. Pharmac.,* **1969,** *35,* 209–242.

Warner, R. R. Current status and implications of serotonin in clinical medicine. *Adv. intern. Med.,* **1967,** *13,* 241–282.

Weil-Malherbe, H. The biochemistry of affective disorders. In, *Handbook of Neurochemistry,* Vol. 7. (Lajtha, A., ed.) Plenum Press, New York, **1972,** pp. 371–416.

Wood, C. J., and Simkins, M. A. (eds.). *International Symposium on Histamine H_2-Receptor Antagonists.* Research and Development Division, Smith Kline and French Laboratories, Ltd., Welwyn Garden City, England, **1973.**

Woolley, D. W. *The Biochemical Basis of Psychoses; or, the Serotonin Hypothesis about Mental Illness.* John Wiley & Sons, Inc., New York, **1962.**

Zweifach, B. W. Microcirculation. *A. Rev. Physiol.,* **1973,** *35,* 117–150.

30 POLYPEPTIDES—ANGIOTENSIN, PLASMA KININS, AND OTHER VASOACTIVE AGENTS; PROSTAGLANDINS

William W. Douglas

ANGIOTENSIN

History. In 1898, Tiegerstedt and Bergman found that crude saline extracts of the kidney contained a pressor principle, which they named *renin.* Their discovery had an obvious bearing on the problem of arterial hypertension and its relation to kidney disease that had been posed by Richard Bright's work some 60 years earlier; however, relatively little interest was generated until 1934, when Goldblatt and his colleagues showed convincingly that it was possible to produce persistent hypertension in dogs by constricting the renal arteries. Within a few years, several investigators had detected pressor activity in renal venous blood following renal artery constriction and had attributed the effect to renin. Renin thus came to occupy a central position in the field of experimental hypertension. It was subsequently determined that renin was not itself a pressor substance but was an enzyme that initiated the formation of the pharmacologically active material, a peptide, from a protein substrate present in the plasma (Braun-Menéndez *et al.,* 1940; Page and Helmer, 1940). Two names for the peptide, *angiotonin* and *hypertensin,* persisted until 1958, when it was agreed to rename the pressor substance *angiotensin* and to call the plasma substrate *angiotensinogen* (Braun-Menéndez and Page, 1958). Meanwhile, in the period 1954–1956, Skeggs and his colleagues as well as Elliott and Peart discovered the amino acid composition and sequence of angiotensin, and shortly thereafter it was synthesized by Schwyzer, Bumpus, and their respective coworkers.

A further impetus to research came in 1958, when Gross suggested that the renin-angiotensin system was involved in electrolyte balance and the regulation of aldosterone secretion by the adrenal cortex (*see* Gross, 1968). It was soon shown that the kidneys are important for the increase in aldosterone secretion in response to hemorrhage; that saline extracts of kidney stimulate aldosterone release (Davis *et al.,* 1961; Ganong and Mulrow, 1961); and that synthetic angiotensin, in minute amounts, stimulates aldosterone output in man (Genest *et al.,* 1960; Laragh *et al.,* 1960). Moreover, elevated rates of renin secretion were noted after various maneuvers that lowered plasma sodium concentrations. Thus, the renin-angiotensin system was recognized as a mechanism to stimulate aldosterone secretion and thereby to conserve sodium and maintain blood volume. Such an action, clearly complementary to the usual vasoconstrictor actions, led to a broadening of the concept of the renin-angiotensin system as an important physiological mechanism in the interrelated homeostatic functions concerned with the volume, pressure, and electrolyte composition of body fluids. More recent findings, to be discussed below, have reinforced this interpretation by implicating the system in a variety of other effects, central and peripheral, controlling both electrolyte balance and vasomotor activity.

Chemistry. The formation of pharmacologically active angiotensin *in vivo* is a complex process, described in more detail below, that is initiated when the enzyme renin acts on angiotensinogen ("renin substrate"), an α_2-globulin, to yield the decapeptide angiotensin I (*see* Figure 30–1). This substance has limited pharmacological activity but is acted on by "converting enzyme" (a dipeptidase) to yield the highly active octapeptide angiotensin II. This, in turn, is broken down to less active and inactive peptide fragments by various peptidases, loosely referred to as "angiotensinases." Thus, α-aminopeptidase, by removing the N-terminal amino acid to yield the heptapeptide $Arg^2 \rightarrow Phe^8$, reduces pressor activity twofold to fourfold, and further hydrolysis to remove the next amino acid (arginine) inactivates this heptapeptide almost completely. Hydrolysis in the middle region (by endopeptidases), or the simple removal of the C-terminal phenylalanine by carboxypeptidase, also yields a completely inactive compound. The sequence of reactions is depicted in Figure 30–1. It is customary to refer to angiotensin II simply as angiotensin. Unless there is a possibility of confusion, this convention will be adhered to in the following discussion.

Many analogs of angiotensin have been synthesized, and a considerable body of information on the structure-activity relationship has accumulated. Some analogs have little or no activity. Others are equipotent, for example, $[Val^5]$-angiotensin II, which occurs in cattle. Some appear to be more potent because they are resistant to degradation, for example, $[Sar^1]$-angiotensin II; still others, with various substituents in the place of phenylalanine^8 (which is critical for agonist activity), are inhibitors that constitute an exciting new addition to the field (*see* Khosla *et al.,* 1974; and below).

PHARMACOLOGICAL PROPERTIES

In addition to pressor effects and the ability to stimulate the secretion of aldosterone, angiotensin

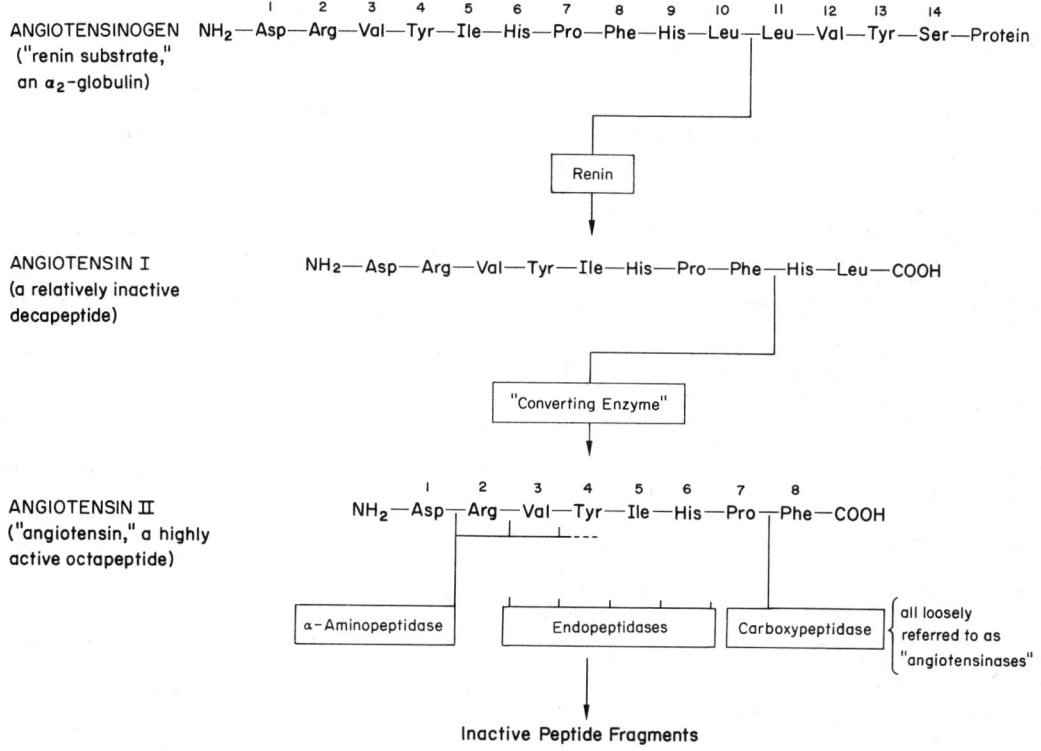

Figure 30-1. *Formation and destruction of angiotensins I and II.*

The structure of angiotensin shown is that found in man, horse, rat, and pig. The bovine form has valine in the 5 position.

possesses several other actions. The physiological and pathophysiological relevance of these are questions of major interest. The reviews by Gross (1971) and Khairallah (1971) and the monograph edited by Page and Bumpus (1974) should be consulted for details and documentation.

Cardiovascular System. *Blood Vessels.* The vasoconstrictor effect of angiotensin intravenously is strongest in the vessels of the skin, splanchnic region, and kidney, and blood flow in these regions falls sharply. The precapillary region is most affected; postcapillary vessels and veins are only feebly constricted. The effect is less in the vessels of skeletal muscle, brain, heart, and adrenal, and blood flow in these tissues is maintained or increased as the relatively weak vasoconstrictor response is opposed by the elevated systemic blood pressure. The pulmonary vessels are constricted very little or not at all.

Vasoconstriction in response to angiotensin has two components, the relative importance of which depends on species, vascular bed, route of injection, and dose: a direct action on the vascular smooth muscle, and an indirect action mediated by the sympathetic nervous system (*see* below). With intravenous infusions in man the direct action accounts for most of the increase in total peripheral resistance

underlying the pressor response; however, in certain vascular beds, such as the hand and the foot, vasoconstriction is mainly due to the sympathetic effect and is suppressed by α-adrenergic blocking drugs. Direct action is demonstrable in these regions when angiotensin is given intra-arterially.

Heart. Experiments on various cardiac preparations have shown that angiotensin has a direct positive inotropic but a weak chronotropic effect (*see* Dempsey *et al.,* 1971). However, *in vivo* such effects are generally complicated by indirect mechanisms. A stimulatory effect of angiotensin on the sympathetic system, within the central nervous system (CNS) or in the periphery, may reinforce or overshadow the direct action (Farr and Grupp, 1971); alternatively, the response of the heart may be dominated by baroreceptor vagal reflexes. In the latter case, the heart rate may slow and end-diastolic pressure rise. Cardiac output may fall but is often maintained. The relatively feeble effect of angiotensin on the veins results in a more modest rise of central venous pressure than is observed with norepinephrine, since venous capacity is not markedly reduced. Although the work of the heart often increases, mainly as the result of the mechanical load, there is usually no coronary insufficiency, presumably because the elevated systemic blood pressure ensures an adequate coronary flow. The coronary constrictor action of angiotensin is comparatively weak. The peptide rarely alters the electrical properties of the heart.

Blood Pressure. Angiotensin is by far the most powerful pressor agent known; on a molecular basis, it is about 40 times more potent than norepinephrine. When a single moderate dose is injected intravenously, systemic blood pressure rises rapidly to a maximum and returns to normal in a few minutes without any secondary fall. When the drug is infused continuously, blood pressure is maintained at an elevated level for hours or days, provided the concentration is not so high as to produce tachyphylaxis. Furthermore, amounts of angiotensin too small to have initial pressor effects will raise blood pressure in various animals and man when exposure to the drug is prolonged (Dickinson and Yu, 1967).

In the lesser circulation, angiotensin commonly causes a moderate rise in pulmonary artery pressure that is due less, perhaps, to its feeble vasoconstrictor action than to an increase of pressure in the pulmonary vein as end-diastolic pressure rises.

Blood Volume, Capillary Permeability, and Lymph Flow. Despite the feeble constrictor effects of angiotensin on *large* veins, some constriction of postcapillary venules seems to take place and there is evidence of increased permeability of the fine vessels (Nickerson and Sutter, 1964), possibly due to contraction of endothelial cells (*see* Robertson and Khairallah, 1974). There is a significant diminution in blood volume and increase in extravascular fluid and lymph flow.

Direct and Indirect Sympathetic Effects. Since pressor effects of angiotensin persist after elimination of possible neural and hormonal components of the response, there is no doubt that the peptide can exert its vasoconstrictor effect by direct action on vascular smooth muscle. Nevertheless, indirect effects mediated by the sympathetic nervous system may contribute to the total cardiovascular response. They include a central stimulatory action to enhance sympathetic outflow, a local action of angiotensin to potentiate adrenergic transmission at peripheral neuroeffector sites, and probably a stimulatory effect on sympathetic ganglia (*see* below).

A number of extravascular smooth muscles are directly stimulated to contract by angiotensin *in vitro;* these effects are often feeble. However, angiotensin can excite or inhibit a variety of such preparations indirectly by stimulating cholinergic or adrenergic ganglion cells or nerve endings.

Central Nervous System. Because the blood-brain barrier is considered generally to be impermeable to peptides, the possibility that angiotensin might have central actions was overlooked for many years. In 1961, however, Bickerton and Buckley demonstrated a centrally mediated hypertensive response in dogs by means of cross-circulation experiments. Since then, many other examples of actions of angiotensin on the CNS have appeared (*see* Severs and Daniels-Severs, 1973).

Central Sympathetic Stimulation. The observation of sympathetic excitation provided by the cross-perfusion experiments was soon complemented by others (Ferrario *et al.,* 1972). Small amounts of angiotensin infused into the vertebral arteries, including those of man, cause a rise in systemic blood pressure that has been maintained for up to a week, and which is demonstrably due to central stimulation. The responsive region appears to lie in the medulla, more specifically in the area postrema where other evidence indicates the blood-brain barrier is deficient.

Drinking and Hydration. Angiotensin, in minute amount, can stimulate drinking by an action within the brain. The effect has been elicited with injections into the third ventricle or anterior hypothalamic areas. The response is striking, and the stimulus seems specific; no such effect has been observed with various other peptides. The response too is specific; it is unaccompanied by eating; indeed, eating is suppressed in favor of drinking. Increased drinking on intravenous injection of angiotensin has been noted in rats and man and may also involve this central effect (Andersson and Eriksson, 1971). In this regard, the peptide increases activity in supraoptic neurons when injected into the brain or third ventricle and appears to stimulate the secretion of antidiuretic hormone (ADH) (Share and Claybaugh, 1972).

Peripheral Autonomic Nervous System. In addition to central enhancement of sympathetic outflow, angiotensin stimulates sympathetic ganglion cells and facilitates ganglionic transmission. The effects are variable, and their contribution to the overall response to circulating angiotensin is controversial. A more consistent response to angiotensin, even in low dose, is stimulation or facilitation at the neuroeffector junctions of sympathetic postganglionic neurons. The mechanism seemingly involves a variety of actions. Increased responsiveness of the innervated organ to norepinephrine has been demonstrated, but the action of angiotensin that leads to an increased concentration of norepinephrine at the synaptic regions is more important. Several mechanisms have been suggested: increased norepinephrine biosynthesis in the adrenergic terminals, depressed re-uptake of the catecholamine, and increased norepinephrine output (*see* Khairallah, 1971; Roth, 1972; Zimmerman *et al.,* 1972).

Adrenal Medulla. Angiotensin releases catecholamines from the adrenal medulla. The effect persists after denervation and seems to be due to a direct depolarizing action on the chromaffin cells (Douglas *et al.,* 1967). Although this is a very sensitive response, it is unlikely that medullary stimulation contributes significantly to the pressor effect of moderate doses of angiotensin given intravenously. (*See also* Peach, 1974.)

Adrenal Cortex and Aldosterone Secretion. Angiotensin has a direct effect on the adrenal cortex, leading to a rather selective stimulation of aldosterone synthesis and secretion with comparatively little effect on the output of other corticosteroids. In man, with intravenous infusion of low doses of the drug that have little or no effect on blood pressure, aldosterone secretion begins within a few minutes and may be maintained for days. This results in retention of sodium and other derangements of electrolyte balance (*see* Davis, 1974).

Kidney and Urine Formation. In addition to its indirect effect on tubular function mediated by aldosterone, angiotensin, given intravenously, influences urine formation directly. The effects are confusing and may be diuretic or antidiuretic, depending on species, dose, sodium balance, and other factors. In man and dog the usual response is a prompt antidiuresis; however, a brisk diuresis commonly occurs in certain hypertensive individuals and in patients with hepatic cirrhosis and ascites. Angiotensin has potent effects within the renal vascular bed that may cause either an increase or a decrease in glomerular filtration rate; this could conceivably explain the diverse patterns observed (Gross and Möhring, 1973). Angiotensin, unlike ADH, has inconsistent and generally weak effects on the transport of water and electrolytes in model epithelial systems, such as toad skin and bladder.

Mechanism of Action. The receptors for angiotensin in smooth muscles, neural tissue, and the adrenal medulla are distinct from those for the biogenic amines and for other peptides.

A membrane-depolarizing action has been demonstrated on chromaffin cells and seemingly accounts for their secretory response; a similar action probably underlies stimulation of ganglion cells and other nervous elements and contributes to smooth muscle contraction. However, smooth muscle depolarized by excess K^+ continues to respond to angiotensin and some other factor must be invoked; this is most likely to be facilitated calcium entry. In essence, then, the mechanism of action of this peptide on these systems appears to be similar to that of the *amine* autacoids such as histamine.

The stimulant action on adrenocortical secretion is attributable to increased synthesis of aldosterone in the zona glomerulosa. In contrast to the adrenal medulla, where secretion can be equated with release of preformed product, the cortex must form new steroid to sustain the response to even a short stimulus. It is uncertain, however, at what stage and by what means angiotensin increases aldosteronogenesis. The effect requires calcium ions, is inhibited by puromycin, and is unaccompanied by a rise in cyclic adenosine 3',5'-monophosphate (cyclic AMP) (Saruta *et al.*, 1972). High-affinity binding sites for angiotensin, possibly related to plasma membrane receptors, have been identified in various tissues, including adrenal cortex (*see* Glossmann *et al.*, 1974).

ENDOGENOUS RENIN-ANGIOTENSIN
SYSTEM

The renin-angiotensin system has been found in each of the vertebrate classes studied. The classical and richest source of renin is the kidney, from which it is secreted by specialized cells, the granular juxtaglomerular cells (JG cells) in the walls of the afferent arterioles as they enter the glomeruli. Secretion of renin is under the control of intrarenal and extrarenal mechanisms that will be discussed later.

Metabolism in Vivo. An understanding of the factors involved in the elaboration and destruction of endogenous angiotensin has become vital to the interpretation of pharmacological and clinical studies of this system.

Renin and the Formation of Angiotensin I. Renin, a protein of about 40,000 molecular weight, is mainly confined to the vascular space after its secretion. It is inactivated by a nonexcretory, catabolic activity within the kidney, and its half-life within the circulation is 15 to 30 minutes. Throughout its sojourn in the blood, renin acts on its substrate, plasma angiotensinogen, which, except in rare instances of severe hepatic disease, is present in such large amounts that it is never rate limiting. The reaction yields the decapeptide angiotensin I, a relatively inactive pressor peptide (*see* Bakhle, 1974; Skeggs *et al.*, 1974).

"Converting Enzyme" and the Formation of Angiotensin II. An enzymatic activity found in blood, "converting enzyme," acts far too slowly to account for the prompt pharmacological responses observed within 20 to 30 seconds of intravenous injection of angiotensin I. Rapid formation of angiotensin II results from the activity of tissue-bound "converting enzyme(s)." Lung is extremely rich in this activity (located on the endothelial surface of the capillaries), so that within the time it takes for blood to traverse the lung over 60% of angiotensin I is converted to angiotensin II; with very low "physiological" concentrations this figure may approach 100%. The fact that the lung processes the whole blood volume indicates the pivotal role of this organ, although "converting enzyme" is present in other tissues and may be very important locally. (*See* Tierney, 1974; Vane, 1974.)

Fate of Angiotensin II. When infused into the vascular beds of various regions or organs in the systemic circulation, most angiotensin II disappears during a single passage and little is recovered in the venous effluent; this is due to its metabolic degradation. The various peptidases ("angiotensinases") that participate in the hydrolysis of angiotensin II and the structures of the inactive degradation products are described above (*see* Figure 30–1). As a result of this degradation by tissue-bound enzymes, the half-life of angiotensin II is only a minute or so, a fact that is reflected in the correspondingly brief course of the pharmacological response to a single intravenous injection. (*See* Ledingham and Leary, 1974; Ryan, 1974; Vane, 1974.)

Functions of the Renin-Angiotensin System. The main events that led to the prevalent view that the renin-angiotensin system is a part of the interrelated homeostatic mechanisms regulating hemodynamics and water and electrolyte balance are described in the historical introduction to this section. Most simply stated, factors that lower blood volume, renal perfusion pressure, or plasma sodium concentration tend to stimulate the secretion of renin, while factors that increase these parameters tend to inhibit its secretion (*see* Figure 30–2). The importance of elevated renin and angiotensin concentrations in certain hypertensive patients and in some experimental hypertensive states has become increasingly evident

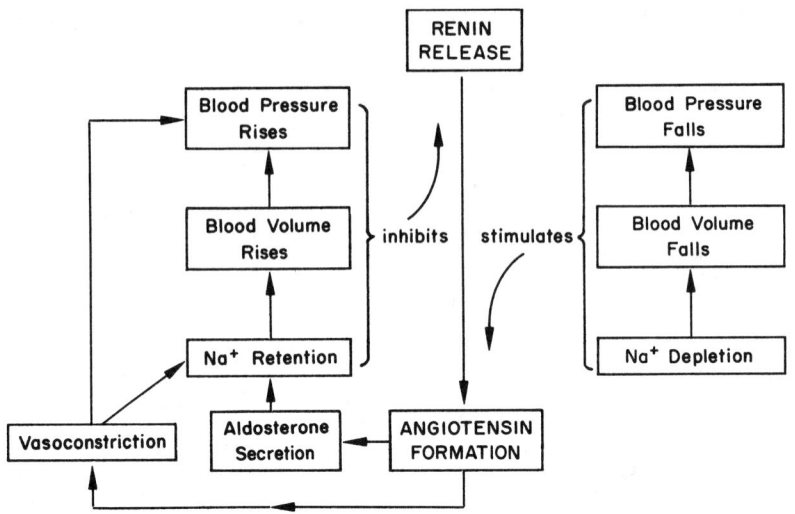

Figure 30-2. *A schematic portrayal of some current speculations on the possible homeostatic role of the renin-angiotensin system.*

from analyses by means of drugs used to block the formation or action of angiotensin II (*see* below). The additional evidence presented above indicating that the renin-angiotensin system can influence cardiovascular function by enhancing central and peripheral sympathetic activity has further heightened interest in the homeostatic functions outlined in Figure 30-2, as have also the other central actions described. While the evidence, taken as a whole, is consonant with the broad homeostatic scheme suggested in Figure 30-2, it cannot be too strongly emphasized that it is difficult to assess the contribution of the renin-angiotensin system in individual patients or experimental models. In no small measure this difficulty springs from the staggering complexity of hemodynamic-water and electrolyte interrelations, a complexity nowhere better illustrated than in the review by Guyton and coworkers (1972).

Control of Renal Renin Secretion. As mentioned, the JG cells in the glomerular afferent arterioles are generally considered the main source of renin secreted in response to the classical stimuli, such as reduced blood volume, reduced renal perfusion pressure, and sodium deprivation. These cells receive input from sympathetic postganglionic efferent fibers, which seemingly exert a secretomotor function that allows the CNS to stimulate renin output in response to appropriate stimuli; this is a β-adrenergic effect. The JG cells also make close contact with the macula densa cells in the wall of the proximal end of the distal tubule and are well placed to act as sensors of sodium and possibly of potassium concentrations of tubular fluid. The macula densa cells are thought to contribute additional local input to the JG cells. Together, JG cells and macula densa form the "juxtaglomerular apparatus." Finally, and possibly most important, JG cells, or some closely related arteriolar receptors, are directly responsive to mechanical stress; renin release is evoked by a variety of manipulations that lower renal perfusion

pressure, such as partial occlusion of the renal artery, reduction of cardiac output, reduction of blood volume by hemorrhage, or chronic sodium depletion. The renal arteriolar receptor involved has been described as a baroreceptor, and either decreased stretch or decreased arteriolar wall tension has been suggested as the essential stimulus. Other factors, of uncertain significance, that are capable of influencing renin release include ADH and angiotensin II, the former stimulating and the latter inhibiting. (*See* Vander, 1967; Assaykeen, 1972; Davis, 1974.)

Role in Aldosterone Secretion. Although it is evident that angiotensin plays a major role in aldosterone secretion, the zona glomerulosa of the adrenal cortex is also stimulated directly by a low sodium and an elevated potassium, by ACTH, and possibly by other factors. Control of aldosterone secretion is not lost in animals and patients from whom both kidneys have been removed. Moreover, humans rendered sodium deficient have circulating plasma concentrations of angiotensin that, when reproduced by infusion, appear to be insufficient to account for the high rate of aldosterone secretion. Interestingly, there may be a role for a metabolite of angiotensin in the control of aldosterone biosynthesis. The angiotensin heptapeptide $Arg^2 \rightarrow Phe^8$ has been shown to exert a potent effect on the zona glomerulosa of the adrenal (Peach and Chiu, 1974). These and other arguments have recently encouraged the view that angiotensin II is but one of several factors required for a completely normal regulation of aldosterone secretion (*see* Page and Bumpus, 1974).

Possible Intrarenal Functions. Since renin is formed and secreted within the kidney, renin and angiotensin could conceivably regulate urine formation locally by actions quite independent of the hormonal loop involving aldosterone secretion. Many different suggestions have been put forward, including autoregulation of the renal circulation, local vasomotor actions tending to alter glomerular filtration or tubular reabsorption, and direct actions of angiotensin on tubular reabsorption (*see* Thurau, 1974).

Involvement in Circulatory Responses and Homeostasis. As indicated in Figure 30–2, factors that *lower* blood pressure or volume tend to *stimulate* renin secretion, while factors that *raise* blood pressure or volume have the opposite effect. The classical vigorous stimuli, severe hemorrhage and "overtransfusion," respectively, and other cardiovascular stimuli involve both the intrarenal "tension-receptive" mechanism and the reflex sympathetic secretomotor control. Milder stimuli of a more common physiological nature may operate mainly through the sympathetic reflex; the increase in renin secretion that occurs in man when changing from the recumbent to the upright position is one well-documented example. Various other reflexes that activate the sympathetic system, such as exercise, hypoglycemia, the cold pressor test, and even emotional stress, increase renin output (*see* Gross, 1971; Assaykeen, 1972; Davis, 1973; Ganong, 1973). In addition to its immediate vasoconstrictor effects and influence on blood volume, the renin-angiotensin system may contribute to circulatory regulation in a variety of indirect ways: by potentiation of central and peripheral sympathetic activity, as already described, and by altering vascular reactivity by inducing chronic changes in the ionic milieu. (*See* Symposium, 1974.)

Involvement in Hypertensive States. The renin-angiotensin system contributes to the constellation of clinical states embraced by the general term *hypertension,* and it is also a factor in experimental renal hypertension induced by partially occluding the renal arteries (Goldblatt hypertension). The main questions at issue are how many, or few, hypertensive conditions, clinical or experimental, involve increased renin-angiotensin activity and what is the magnitude and duration of this involvement. At the outset it must be recognized that hypertension can arise from and be sustained by many factors—it is a symptom rather than a disease. The renin-angiotensin system is but one of the multitude of factors that can contribute, and there is no simple relationship between renin secretion, as reflected by plasma renin activity (PRA), and blood pressure; most patients with hypertension do *not* have high PRA, and high values may occur without hypertension. Elevated PRA is, however, found in most individuals with *malignant hypertension* and, when samples are obtained from the renal vein, is commonly found in *hypertension resulting from stenosis of the renal artery.* Since many cases of stenosis can be corrected by surgery, such measurements may provide a valuable diagnostic aid (*see* Kirkendall and Overturf, 1973). Elevated PRA is constantly present, along with secondary aldosteronism, in renin-secreting tumors, but these are extremely rare. In patients with *essential hypertension,* PRA and plasma angiotensin II concentrations are generally normal but they may be elevated or subnormal. Very low PRA is found in the hypertension accompanying *primary aldosteronism.* Examples of clinical situations in which high PRA and circulating angiotensin II concentrations occur *without* hypertension include various "sodium-wasting" syndromes, such as *Addi-son's disease,* patients with *congestive heart failure of the low-output type,* numerous cases of *secondary hyperaldosteronism* (a condition due to excess renin production), and the very rare condition involving hyperplasia of the juxtaglomerular apparatus known as *Bartter's syndrome.* But perhaps the most remarkable example of elevated PRA unaccompanied by hypertension is normal pregnancy. Extensive discussion of the possible involvement of the renin-angiotensin system in hypertensive states can be found in the monograph edited by Page and Bumpus (1974). (*See also* Peart, 1975.)

Possible Central Nervous System Functions: Thirst, Drinking, and Release of Pituitary Hormones. The central actions of angiotensin that stimulate drinking and release ADH and perhaps other hormones have prompted conjecture that the renin-angiotensin system is physiologically involved in the regulation of these phenomena. Moreover, with the demonstration that renin, angiotensinogen, and "converting enzyme" exist in brain tissue, the argument has been presented that these activities may be endogenous to the brain (*see* Severs and Daniels-Severs, 1973).

Extrarenal Sources of Renin. The persistence of renin in the plasma of nephrectomized animals and patients demonstrates the existence of extrarenal sources of the protein. Renin-like activity is found in *blood vessels* and *nervous tissue,* and some possible functions have been mentioned. Such activity is also found in the *uterus, placenta, amniotic fluid,* and *salivary glands* (*see* Brown *et al.,* 1967; Symposium, 1967; McGiff, 1968; Page and Bumpus, 1974).

CLINICAL CONSIDERATIONS

Preparation. *Angiotensin amide,* the amide of angiotensin II (1-L-asparaginyl-5-L-valyl angiotensin octapeptide; HYPERTENSIN), is available in vials containing 2.5 mg. The drug is diluted and given slowly intravenously at a rate each minute of about 0.01 to 0.2 µg/kg. Blood pressure must be monitored at short intervals until a safe rate of infusion is determined.

Precautions and Untoward Effects. Although considerable elevation of blood pressure may occur without symptoms, angiotensin sometimes causes dizziness and headache. Evidence of coronary insufficiency is occasionally encountered with S-T depression in the ECG and pain in the chest, and has been held responsible for occasional negative inotropic effects. Profound bradycardia and, occasionally, ventricular irregularities may be encountered from overdosage. These are attributable to excessively high blood pressures and intense vagal reflex activity. Angiotensin has no direct arrhythmogenic effects. Mild urticarial reactions have been reported. The greatest danger lies in the powerful pressor activity of the drug; too rapid infusion may easily raise blood pressure to alarming levels.

Clinical Uses. Since angiotensin has become available, interest has centered on its unique pressor properties. It differs from norepinephrine not only in its greater potency but also in a number of qualitative respects that seem to be advantageous in a pressor agent. Thus, its pressor effect is better sustained during prolonged infusion and is less liable to be followed by hypotension. It has little or no tendency to evoke disturbing arrhythmias and, indeed, has been used successfully during anesthesia with cyclopropane and halogenated hydrocarbon agents. Furthermore, it does not cause spasm of the infused vein, nor has it caused tissue necrosis and sloughing when extravasation has occurred at the site of injection. However, angiotensin shares with norepinephrine the disadvantage that it diminishes blood volume by promoting the loss of protein-free fluid from the circulation to tissue spaces. It is inferior to norepinephrine as a constrictor of capacitance vessels, and does not reduce the venous reservoir so effectively. Its lack of prominent stimulant effect on cardiac muscle may also be disadvantageous in certain circumstances.

Angiotensin has been used to restore blood pressure in a variety of hypotensive conditions. It must be emphasized, however, that its value in the treatment of shock is highly controversial, as is that of pressor agents of the sympathomimetic type (*see* Chapter 24). Where hypotension is the consequence of blood loss, treatment, of course, should be aimed at restoring blood volume, and angiotensin must be regarded as only an interim expedient until this can be done.

A relatively high sensitivity to the pressor effects of angiotensin has been suggested as a possible test for identifying women at risk of developing hypertension during pregnancy (Gant *et al.,* 1973).

ANTAGONISTS OF THE
RENIN-ANGIOTENSIN SYSTEM

Any drug that blocks synthesis of angiotensin or blocks tissue receptors for angiotensin may provide a valuable tool for those interested in understanding the involvement of the renin-angiotensin system(s) in physiological and pathological processes, particularly hypertension. One of the earliest approaches was the *immunological,* wherein antibodies to renin were found to lower blood pressure in animals with renal hypertension (Kremen and Wakerlin, 1955). More recently, antibodies directed against angiotensin have also been used in similar experiments, but with less striking results. The difficulties of this approach have been discussed by Bumpus and associates (1973), and Romero and coworkers (1973). A phospholipid fraction of renal extracts has been prepared that possesses renin-inhibiting capacity, and this too has been shown to lower blood pressure in some renal hypertensive animals (*see* Sen *et al.,* 1969). The demonstration of true competitive inhibition of renin by some octapeptide analogs of a segment of angiotensinogen may lead to more useful compounds (Poulsen *et al.,* 1973). Additional, and more immediately applicable, analytical tools and possibly valuable therapeutic agents are provided by two other pharmacological approaches. The first of these is aimed at inhibition of converting enzyme; the second, at blocking angiotensin receptors.

Inhibition of Converting Enzyme. The biochemical characteristics of converting enzyme(s) have

been reviewed in detail by Bakhle (1974), who discussed both peptide and nonpeptide inhibitors. The latter are only useful for *in-vitro* studies. The former, which are quite effective *in vivo,* were originally recognized as bradykinin potentiating factors (BPF), present in viper venom (Ferreira, 1965). It soon became apparent that BPF was a mixture of polypeptides that inhibited bradykininase and, moreover, that these peptides also inhibited converting enzyme. One of these, a nonapeptide, proved particularly potent and long acting. It has been synthesized (Ondetti *et al.,* 1971) and has the following structure: pyroGlu—Trp—Pro—Arg—Pro—Gln—Ile—Pro—Pro. This nonapeptide has little or no depressor activity in normotensive dogs, rats, or man, but inhibits strongly the pressor response to angiotensin I without significantly affecting that to angiotensin II (Bianchi *et al.,* 1973; Collier *et al.,* 1973); it lowers blood pressure significantly in various experimental models of renal hypertension (Engel *et al.,* 1973). It has proven to be of value in the analysis of function of the renin-angiotensin system in normal animals and, along with related inhibitors, has been suggested to be possibly useful in the diagnosis and therapy of hypertension (Collier *et al.,* 1973).

Angiotensin II Antagonists: Peptides Blocking Angiotensin Receptors. There is a group of angiotensin analogs, synthesized in the last few years, that possess the ability to block selectively receptors for angiotensin II in various effector tissues. These antagonists have been developed in several laboratories in a systematic fashion by modifying the parent agonist molecule, angiotensin II, and are thus closely related peptides (*see* Regoli *et al.,* 1973; Khosla *et al.,* 1974). The key modification is in the substitution of the C-terminal phenylalanine, which is essential for the characteristic agonist properties of angiotensin II. Substitution by several different aliphatic amino acids is effective; thus, [Ala[8]]-angiotensin II and [Ile[8]]-angiotensin II are both strong antagonists. Further modification involving replacement of the N-terminal Asp by Sar intensifies and prolongs blocking activity, in part at least by yielding compounds more resistant to degradation by α-aminopeptidase; thus, [Sar[1], Ala[8]]- or [Sar[1], Ile[8]]-angiotensin II are very potent and their effects may last well over an hour.

These various angiotensin antagonists appear to block angiotensin II receptors in a competitive manner and to do so with high specificity (*see* Regoli *et al.,* 1973). Many different responses to angiotensin II have been blocked by these antagonists, including the characteristic circulatory effects, contractions of various smooth muscles, the secretory response of the adrenal cortex, and responses of the CNS and peripheral sympathetic nervous system (*see* Sweet *et al.,* 1973; Zimmerman, 1973). The potential usefulness of such agents in pharmacological analysis and as diagnostic and therapeutic agents is obvious. One illustration of their analytical value has come from experiments showing that angiotensin II antagonists have little effect on resting blood pressure in normal dogs but restore elevated blood pressure to normal levels during the acute but not chronic phases of experimental renal hypertension, thereby illustrating the importance of the renin-angiotensin system in the induction of this phenomenon if not in its maintenance (Pals *et al.,* 1971; Bumpus *et al.,* 1973). In normal individuals the angiotensin II blocking drugs do not lower blood pressure, but a prompt and sustained reduction in systemic blood pressure to near-normal levels has occurred following their administration to patients with hypertensive states of various kinds in which plasma renin activity is elevated (Brunner *et al.,* 1973). Much work remains to be done to determine the full extent of the usefulness of angiotensin II antagonists in the diagnosis and treatment of clinical states involving overactivity of the renin-angiotensin system, but there is clearly great promise in this new class of compounds.

PLASMA KININS (KALLIDIN, BRADYKININ)

History. The discovery of the plasma kinins had its origins in the old observation that urine, injected intravenously, lowers blood pressure. In the 1920s and 1930s, Frey and associates (*see* Frey *et al.,* 1968) characterized the hypotensive substance and showed that similar material could be obtained from saliva, plasma, and a variety of tissues. Since the pancreas was a rich source, they named this material *kallikrein* after the Greek word for that organ (*kallikreas*). By 1937, Werle, Götze, and Keppler had established that kallikreins have an indirect effect and, behaving as enzymes, split off a pharmacologically active substance from some inactive precursor present in plasma. Their discovery preceded by 2 years the analogous finding that renin acts similarly. In 1948, Werle and Berek named the active substance *kallidin* and showed it to be a polypeptide cleaved from a plasma globulin that they termed *kallidinogen* (*see* Frey *et al.,* 1968; Werle, 1970).

Interest in the field intensified with a report by Rocha e Silva and associates (1949) to the effect that the venoms of certain snakes, as well as the enzyme trypsin, acted on plasma globulin to produce a substance, probably a polypeptide, that also lowered blood pressure and caused a slowly developing contraction of the gut. Because of the slow response of the gut, they named this substance *bradykinin,* a term derived from the Greek words *bradys,* meaning "slow," and *kinein,* meaning "to move." Since bradykinin and kallidin were formed under similar conditions and had similar pharmacological actions, it was early suspected that they were closely related. Identification of the pure materials some 10 years later confirmed this suspicion. In 1960, bradykinin, formed by reacting trypsin with globulin, was isolated by Elliott and coworkers and synthesized by Boissonnas and associates (*see* Elliott, 1970). It proved to be a nonapeptide of the structure shown below. Shortly thereafter, this same nonapeptide was found to be a constituent of kallidin, which, however, also contained a pharmacologically similar decapeptide with the same sequence of amino acids but with an additional N-terminal lysine residue (Webster and Pierce, 1963). These substances are now recognized to be but two of a large number of polypeptides that have related pharmacological properties and that are widely distributed in nature. For the whole group the generic term *kinins* has been adopted, and kallidin and bradykinin are referred to as *plasma kinins.*

Chemistry. Because two separate experimental paths led to the identification of the plasma kinins, nomenclature has been confused. The terms adopted here are those recommended by an international committee (*see* Webster, 1970). The term *kallidin* (which formerly embraced both the nonapeptides and decapeptides) is now restricted to the decapeptide, while the term *bradykinin* has been retained for the nonapeptide. Bradykinin has the following amino acid sequence: H—Arg—Pro—Pro—Gly—Phe—Ser—Pro—Phe—Arg—OH. Kallidin has an additional lysine molecule in the N-terminal position and is sometimes referred to as lysylbradykinin. The two peptides are cleaved from common precursor(s), referred to as *kininogen(s),* in the plasma α_2-globulin fraction. This cleavage may be effected by enzymes collectively referred to as *kininogenases.* Among these the greatest interest attaches to the *kallikreins,* a group of proteolytic enzymes of high substrate specificity present in plasma, lymph, various other body fluids (including urine and salivary, pancreatic, and other exocrine secretions), and diverse tissues. Other kininogenases include trypsin, plasmin, and various proteolytic enzymes in certain snake and insect venoms and bacteria. Plasma kallikrein (like trypsin and snake venoms) forms the nonapeptide kinin *bradykinin* directly. Glandular and other kallikreins form the decapeptide kinin *kallidin,* from which bradykinin is rapidly formed by aminopeptidase activity in plasma and tissues (*see* Erdös, 1970).

It is of particular interest that normal blood contains all essential ingredients for kinin formation and is potentially capable of forming pharmacologically massive amounts of kinins. However, kinin formation is normally insignificant because kallikrein is present in an inactive form, prekallikrein. Conversion of prekallikrein to kallikrein, with resulting formation of bradykinin, is readily brought about by various factors disturbing the equilibrium of the plasma. These include changes in pH or temperature, and contact with glass or numerous other water-insoluble materials, particulate matter, crystals, collagen, skin, and damaged tissues. Many of these may be recognized as factors involved in clot formation, and, indeed, endogenous conversion of kininogen to kinin involves a cascade of enzymatic reactions in the plasma reminiscent of the intrinsic clotting mechanism (*see* Chapter 65) and also having origin in activation of Hageman factor (factor XII). Activated Hageman factor (HF_a) can transform prekallikrein to kallikrein directly and can also achieve this same transformation indirectly by activating intermediary factors. The number, sequence of operation, and interaction of the various factors leading to the appearance of kallikrein is still only partially understood, but it is becoming increasingly evident that the process is very complex, and that it interfaces in several areas with the blood clotting mechanism, with fibrinolysis, and with complement and cell lysis; it thus should not be considered as a separate entity. For example, kallikrein seems important for the activation of Hageman factor in fluid phase; the blood clotting factor (Fletcher factor) deficient in patients with Fletcher trait has been identified as plasma prekallikrein (Cochrane *et al.,* 1973; Wuepper, 1973). The plasma kinin-forming system and its relation to clotting, fibrinolysis, and complement are presented in Figure 30-3. (*See also* Erdös, 1970; Movat *et al.,* 1972; Bagdasarian *et al.,* 1973; Cochrane *et al.,* 1973.)

Inactivation of the plasma kinins is very rapid. Their enzymatic destruction in blood results in a half-life of approximately 15 seconds, and further enzymatic inactivation by tissues, particularly the lung, ensures an evanescent effect in the whole animal. Many peptidases and proteases can break down the kinins to inactive fragments and may be referred to as *kininases.* Plasma contains at least two: carboxypeptidase N, which promptly removes the C-terminal arginine to yield virtually inactive peptides, and a dipeptide hydrolase that cleaves the C-terminal dipeptide (*see* Erdös and Yang, 1970). Whether this latter kininase activity or its tissue-bound equivalent in lung is the same enzyme as angiotensin "converting enzyme" is unsettled, but both activities are inhibited by the same agents (*see* above). In a single passage of the kinins through the lesser circulation, the lungs destroy 60 to 90% or

more (*see* Vane, 1969; Alabaster and Bakhle, 1972a, 1972b; Igic *et al.,* 1972; Friedli *et al.,* 1973).

About 200 congeners of the plasma kinins have been synthesized. These have yielded considerable information on the structure-activity relationship, but none has been found to be more intense or significantly longer lasting in its actions, and no useful blocking agent has emerged from this work (*see* Stewart, 1968; Schröder, 1970). Some naturally occurring, related vasodilator peptides of greater potency and duration of action are discussed below.

PHARMACOLOGICAL PROPERTIES

The plasma kinins possess an extraordinarily high degree of pharmacological activity. In extremely low doses they cause vasodilatation, increase capillary permeability and produce edema, evoke pain by some effect on nerve endings, and contract or relax a variety of extravascular smooth muscles (*see* Symposium, 1968; Erdös, 1970; Rocha e Silva and Garcia Leme, 1972).

Cardiovascular System. The kinins are among the most potent vasodilator substances known. On a molar basis, they are about ten times as active as histamine. Intravenously in man they cause flushing in the blush area and conjunctival injection. Blood vessels in muscle, kidney, viscera, and various glands are also dilated, as are coronary and cerebral vessels;

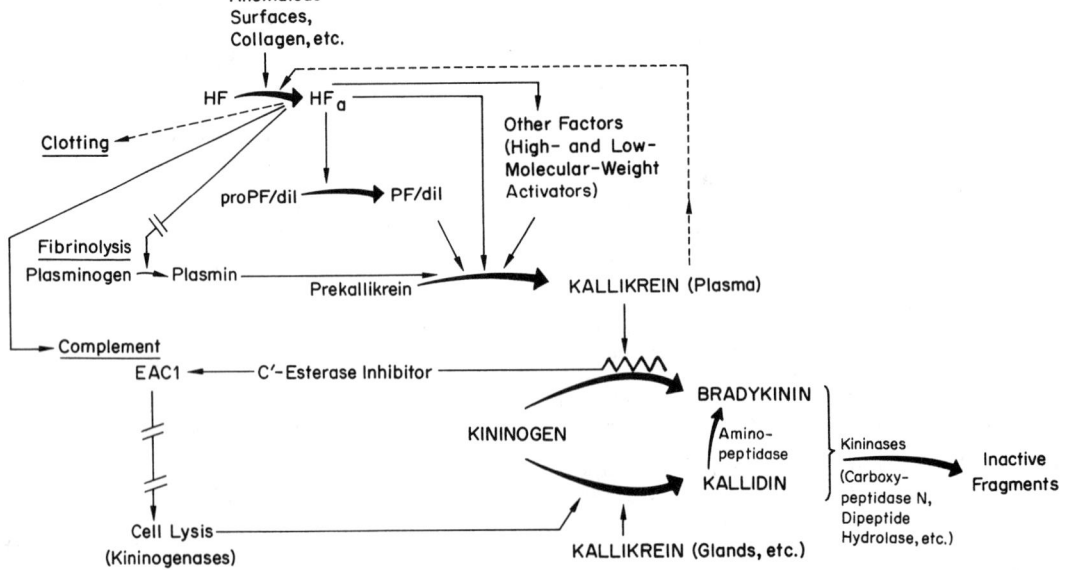

Figure 30-3. *Formation and destruction of the plasma kinins and schematic representation of some suggested interrelations between the kinin-forming system and other functions involving Hageman factor.*

Activated Hageman factor (HF_a) can transform prekallikrein to kallikrein directly or through intermediates by activation of plasmin or PF/dil, a plasma factor so curiously named because its activity was first recognized following dilution of plasma. Activation of the complement cascade leads to cell lysis and the liberation of kininogenases; the kinin and complement systems share a common inhibitor that inactivates both C'1 esterase and kallikrein.

throbbing headache may occur. Effects on pulmonary vessels vary with dose, species, and state of development. These dilator effects, resulting from a direct action of the peptides on arteriolar smooth muscle, cause a sharp fall in systolic and diastolic blood pressures accompanied by an increase in heart rate and cardiac output, mainly, it seems, as a reflex consequence of the fall in the blood pressure and the increased venous return. In contrast to the fine resistance vessels, large arteries and veins tend to contract (*see* Haddy *et al.,* 1970).

Vascular Permeability. The plasma kinins increase permeability in the microcirculation. The effect, like that of histamine and 5-hydroxytryptamine (5-HT), is exerted on the small venules rather than on the true capillaries and involves separation of the junctions between endothelial cells and an increased hydrostatic pressure gradient (Kline *et al.,* 1973). Edema formation, coupled with stimulation of nerve endings (*see* below), results in a "wheal-and-flare" response to intradermal injections in man.

Extravascular Smooth Muscle. Various isolated smooth muscle preparations contract in response to the kinins. The rat uterus is especially sensitive and responds to as little as 0.1 ng/ml. It was the characteristically slow response of the isolated guinea pig ileum that prompted the name *bradykinin.* The kinins act directly on the smooth muscles, and their effect is not blocked by ganglionic blocking agents or atropine. Certain smooth muscles, such as the rabbit aorta or mammary smooth muscle, are little affected; still others, such as the rat duodenum, are relaxed. Tracheobronchial muscle is little affected in many species, but bronchoconstriction is prominent in the guinea pig and in some asthmatic patients, especially when kinins are inhaled (*see* Collier, 1970; Newball and Keiser, 1973).

Stimulation of Nerve Endings and Production of Pain. The plasma kinins are powerful algesic agents. They cause an intense, burning pain when applied to the exposed base of a blister, and a throbbing, burning pain in the hand when injected into the brachial artery. Nociceptive responses or pain occurs when the kinins are injected into animals or man either intraperitoneally or into arteries supplying skin, muscle, or various viscera (*see* Armstrong, 1970). These effects are antagonized by aspirin and other antipyretic analgesics of the anti-inflammatory group, and the important discovery has been made that the antagonism occurs peripherally; these analgesic agents seem to oppose the action of the kinins by some effect on the nerve endings (*see* Lim, 1970).

Stimulation of Autonomic Ganglia and Chromaffin Cells. The kinins, usually in relatively high concentration, stimulate ganglion cells and elicit discharge of catecholamines from the adrenal medulla (*see* Lewis and Reit, 1966); they depolarize chromaffin cells (Douglas *et al.,* 1967). Such actions occasionally contribute significantly to the excitatory and inhibitory responses of the intestine and other organs.

Central Nervous System. The injection of bradykinin into the cerebral ventricles causes a wide spectrum of behavioral, autonomic, and EEG effects (*see* Walaszek, 1970; Ribeiro *et al.,* 1971).

Mechanism of Action. Little is known of the receptors for bradykinin or other kinins, save that they may be distinguished pharmacologically from receptors for various other peptides. Some responses appear to be mediated, at least in part, by generation or liberation of other autacoids, particularly prostaglandins. Release of such substances in response to bradykinin was first demonstrated in guinea pig lung (Piper and Vane, 1969), where they contribute to bronchoconstriction. A similar mechanism may underlie the later phases of vasodilatation, the slowly developing nociceptive responses, and other effects of kinins that are reduced by inhibitors of prostaglandins. (*See* Collier, 1971a, 1971b; Vane, 1971; and discussion of prostaglandins, below.)

Actions of Endogenous Kinins. Since the kinins are such potent pharmacological agents, and since both the substrate and enzymes required to form them are present in abundance in the body, there has been much speculation concerning their possible functions. Their vasodilator activity has provided a principal focus for conjecture. The view that locally formed kinins may mediate atropine-resistant antidromic and functional vasodilatation (especially in exocrine glands) remains controversial (*see* Erdös, 1970). Increased kinin formation has been detected in anaphylaxis and other allergic responses and in shock following burns and mechanical trauma; they may contribute to the accompanying hypotension. Since kinin formation may occur in response to various relatively mild physical and chemical perturbations, such as exposure of plasma or lymph to damaged tissue or even to collagen or heparin, it seems probable that kinins contribute significantly to inflammation (*see* Lepow and Ward, 1972; Movat, 1972). They can certainly produce a reasonable facsimile of the inflammatory response, that is, redness, swelling, pain, and mobilization of leukocytes. A role has also been suggested for kinins in fetal-to-neonatal circulatory adjustments (*see* Campbell *et al.,* 1968; Melmon *et al.,* 1968; Rudolph, 1970).

CLINICAL CONSIDERATIONS

The clinical usefulness of the kinins has yet to be demonstrated. A commercial preparation of pancreatic kallikrein (PADUTIN) has been employed for a number of years with questionable benefit in a variety of vasospastic conditions.

With the kinins, as with histamine and 5-HT, it would seem that from the clinical standpoint the greatest interest attaches to the likelihood that they are involved in a variety of pathological conditions, and that benefit may possibly derive from the use of appropriate antagonists. The possible involvement of kinins in *acute inflammation, shock,* and *anaphylaxis* has been mentioned above. Kinins may also have a role in other acute and chronic allergic and inflammatory states, and in various *arthritides,* including *gout* and *pseudogout* (urate and calcium pyrophosphate crystals are among the many agents activating Hageman factor). Kinin formation by particulate matter such as kaolin and silica may contribute to *foreign-body granulomata* and *pneumoconioses* and to *"blue-velvet disease"* in addicts who inject talc-containing narcotics intravenously. In *hereditary angioneurotic edema*, the plasma lacks a substance (C'1 esterase inhibitor) with kallikrein-inhibiting properties, and evidence of excess kinin formation during an attack has been obtained. Hyperbradykininism has been suggested in explanation of a familial syndrome involving facial erythema with light-headedness or syncope (Streeten *et al.,* 1972). In contrast, failure to produce kinins in response to contact with foreign surfaces is a feature of plasma from patients with *Hageman trait,* namely, the absence of Hageman factor. It is also a feature of plasma from patients with Fletcher trait, mentioned above. Certain *carcinoid tumors* release a kallikrein, and the resulting kinins probably contribute to the carcinoid flush. The occurrence of kinin-forming enzymes in the venoms of snakes may be recalled in the present context. Preformed "kinins" exist in the venoms of wasps and hornets (*see* below).

No specific antagonist of the kinins exists with an effect comparable to that of the antihistamines against histamine, but there are some interesting and possibly clinically relevant instances of drugs that inhibit certain kinin-evoked responses. The effect of aspirin and related analgesics on bradykinin-induced pain has been mentioned and might possibly contribute to the symptomatic relief that such agents afford in inflammatory states and arthritides. Salicylates and glucocorticoids have also been reported to inhibit kallikrein activation. Also, a polyvalent protease and kallikrein inhibitor, a protein extracted from bovine tissues and known commercially as TRASYLOL, has been used with uncertain benefit in various conditions involving excess proteolytic activity, such as *acute pancreatitis,* and in the *carcinoid syndrome.* Current views on the kallikrein-kinin system and its relation to disease and therapy are presented more fully in several reviews (Melmon and Cline, 1967; Kellermeyer and Graham, 1968; Lewis, 1968; Erdös, 1970; Wilhelm, 1971).

OTHER VASOACTIVE POLYPEPTIDES

Kinins. The term *kinins* embraces a number of vasodilator peptides with pharmacological effects resembling those of bradykinin and containing the same nonapeptide fragment (*see* Lewis, 1968; Schachter, 1969). Included are the endecapeptides: *Met—Lys—bradykinin,* which is formed on acidification of plasma; and *phyllokinin* (bradykinin—Ile—Tyr), which is found in an amphibian. Also included are various other kinins of amphibian or mammalian origin such as *colostrokinin* and *urokinin,* and the kinins of wasp and hornet venoms (*see* Schachter, 1969; Pisano, 1970; Erspamer, 1971).

The kinins in the venoms of wasps and hornets doubtless contribute to the reaction to their sting. These insects, however, do not place reliance on a single dolorogen; the wasp cunningly compounds kinins with histamine and 5-HT, and the hornet throws in a fourth substance, acetylcholine (*see* Schachter, 1964).

Others. *Eledoisin* and *physalaemin* are two of a group of polypeptides with powerful depressor and other interesting pharmacological effects that Erspamer and colleagues discovered in various lower vertebrates and invertebrates (*see* Erspamer, 1971). Eledoisin, from octopus salivary glands, and physalaemin, from the skin of an amphibian, are endecapeptides resistant to both carboxypeptidase and aminopeptidase. They are remarkable for the potency and duration of their hypotensive effects. *Caerulein,* a related decapeptide, has more erratic effects on blood pressure but is an extremely potent stimulator of pancreatic and other exocrine secretions. It resembles gastrin and cholecystokinin-pancreozymin both chemically and pharmacologically.

Substance P has now been sequenced (Chang *et al.,* 1971) and synthesized (Tregear *et al.,* 1971). It is an endecapeptide structurally homologous with eledoisin and physalaemin. The gut-stimulating effects and the actions on various nerve preparations have given rise to speculation concerning its normal functions, including the possibility that it may serve as a neurohormone or a neurotransmitter (*see* Sander and Huggins, 1972; Stern *et al.,* 1974).

There also exists a potpourri of pressor peptides formed from plasma by proteolytic activity; *pepsitensin,* a substance closely related to [Val^5]-angiotensin, is discussed by Croxatto (1974). Some amphibian peptides, such as *alytesin* and *bombesin,* also show remarkable pressor activity (*see* reviews by Erspamer, 1971; Sander and Huggins, 1972).

PROSTAGLANDINS

History. There are few substances that currently command more widespread interest in biological circles than do the prostaglandins. Although their history extends back to the early 1930s, it was the isolation, characterization, and synthesis of the representative compounds in the early 1960s that generated such intense interest. The reasons are not hard to find. The prostaglandins are among the most prevalent of autacoids and have been detected in almost every tissue and body fluid; their production increases in response to astonishingly diverse stimuli; they produce, in minute amounts, a remarkably broad spectrum of effects that embraces practically every biological function; they activate or inhibit adenylate cyclase in many types of cells; and, finally, inhibition of their biosynthesis is now recognized as a mechanism of some of the most widely used therapeutic agents, for example, the nonsteroidal anti-inflammatory drugs such as aspirin.

A harbinger of this remarkable development was the observation made by two American gynecologists, Kurzrok and Lieb (1930), that strips of human uterus relax or contract when exposed to human semen. A few years later, Goldblatt in England and Euler in Sweden independently reported smooth-muscle contracting and vasodepressor activity in seminal fluid and accessory reproductive glands, and Euler identified the active material as a lipid-soluble acid, which he named "prostaglandin" (*see* Goldblatt, 1935; Euler, 1936, 1973). More than 20 years were to pass before technical advances allowed the demonstration that prostaglandin was in fact a family of compounds of unique structure, permitted the isolation in crystalline form of two prostaglandins, prostaglandin E_1 (PGE_1) and $PGF_{1\alpha}$, by Bergström and Sjövall in 1957, and led to the elucidation of their structures in 1962 (*see* Bergström and Samuelsson, 1968). Soon, more prostaglandins were characterized and, like the others, proved to be 20-carbon unsaturated carboxylic acids with a cyclopentane ring.

When the general structure of the prostaglandins became apparent, their kinship with essential fatty acids was recognized, and in 1964 Bergström and coworkers and van Dorp and associates independently achieved the biosynthesis of PGE_2 from arachidonic acid using homogenates of sheep vesicular glands (*see* Samuelsson, 1972).

In parallel with these chemical developments, pharmacological studies had shown the presence, in different tissues, of autacoids of acidic lipid nature, which were given names such as *vesiglandin, Darmstoff, irin, menstrual stimulant,* and *medullin,* and these were later recognized to be prostaglandins (*see* Horton, 1972a).

Chemistry. The prostaglandins can be considered as analogs of a hypothetical compound with the trivial name *prostanoic acid,* the structure of which is as follows:

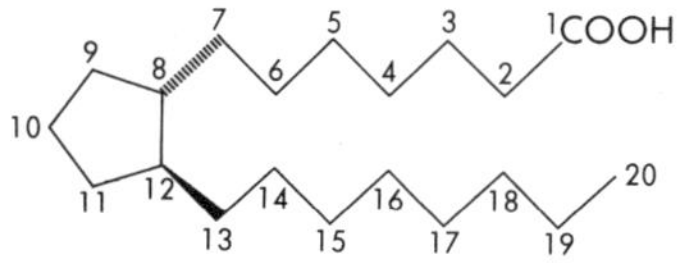

The different prostaglandins fall into several main classes—E, F, A, B, C, and D—distinguished by the constituents of the cyclopentane ring. These structures are shown in Figure 30–4. The main classes are further subdivided in accord with the number of double bonds in the side chains. This is indicated by subscript 1, 2, or 3, and reflects the fatty acid precursor. Thus, prostaglandins derived from 8,11,14-eicosatrienoic acid carry the subscript 1; those derived from 5,8,11,14-eicosatetraenoic acid (arachidonic acid) carry the subscript 2; and the few derived from 5,8,11,14,17-eicosapentaenoic acid carry the subscript 3. These last-mentioned prostaglandins are relatively rare in nature. Prostaglandins of the E and F_α series are sometimes referred to as the "primary prostaglandins." They are the most abundant (especially E_2 and $F_{2\alpha}$) and the most intensively studied. The As, Bs, and Cs are all derivatives of the corresponding Es. Representative formulas are presented in Figures 30–4 and 30–5. (*See* Andersen and Ramwell, 1974.)

Prostaglandin Biosynthesis and Catabolism. *In vivo* most cells seem capable of synthesizing prostaglandins from the essential fatty acid precursors. Concentrations of these acids in free form are generally low, and they cannot be utilized in the esterified form. It is therefore generally believed that endogenous biosynthesis, in the absence of added precursor acid, depends on phospholipase-catalyzed release of precursor acid from cellular phospholipid stores. Indeed, activation of phospholipase A has been suggested as a common rate-limiting step in the enhanced biosynthesis that occurs in response to widely divergent physical, chemical, hormonal, and neurohumoral influences. Synthesis of the primary prostaglandins is accomplished in stepwise manner by a complex of microsomal enzymes referred to as *"prostaglandin synthetase."* The initial events, which involve several steps, result in oxygenation and cyclization of the unesterified precursor acid to form a cyclic peroxide derivative. This *endoperoxide* is then either isomerized (by *endoperoxide isomerase*), thereby yielding a PGE compound, or reduced (by *endoperoxide reductase*), yielding a PGF_α compound (F_β forms do not occur naturally). Thus, with arachidonic acid, the most prevalent precursor, the products are PGE_2 and $PGF_{2\alpha}$ (Figure 30–5), and these are the most abundant mammalian prostaglandins (*see* Samuelsson, 1972; Hamberg and Samuelsson, 1973).

The PGs A, B, and C arise from the corresponding PGE by dehydration and isomerization. Some may be formed chemically only during extraction, but PGA, at least, occurs naturally and is present in abundance in human semen and in smaller amounts in kidney (*see* Lee, 1974). In some species, an isomerase is present that converts PGA to PGC, from which PGB is formed under mildly alkaline conditions (*see* Horton, 1972a). This transformation may explain delayed responses (*e.g.,* delayed hypotension) to injections of PGA.

Apart from the generally slow and species-dependent isomerization, PGs E and F are rather stable in blood, but they are rapidly degraded and inactivated by tissue-bound enzymes; some 80 to 90% or more is destroyed during a single passage through the liver or the lungs (*see* Vane, 1969; Piper, 1973). The initial and major step for both PGEs and PGFs is oxidation of the secondary alcohol group at C 15 by a widely distributed, prostaglandin-specific dehydrogenase (PGDH). This is followed by reduction of the Δ^{13} double bond; the resulting 15-dehydro-13,14-dihydro derivatives have little or no biological activity. These events are followed by β oxidation and ω hydroxylation and oxidation of the side chains (*see* Samuelsson, 1972; Andersen and Ramwell, 1974). PGAs are degraded more slowly; substantial amounts escape degradation in the lung and liver, and their effects are thus more prolonged.

PHARMACOLOGICAL PROPERTIES

No other class of autacoids shows more numerous and diverse effects. Those who have reviewed the field have remarked on this "awesome" and "bewildering" diversity. Not only is the spectrum of actions broad, but also different prostaglandins show different activities, both qualitatively and quantitatively. These differences cannot be discussed in detail here, and the reader is referred to the cited monographs and reviews.

Cardiovascular System. In most species and in most vascular beds PGEs and PGAs are potent vaso-

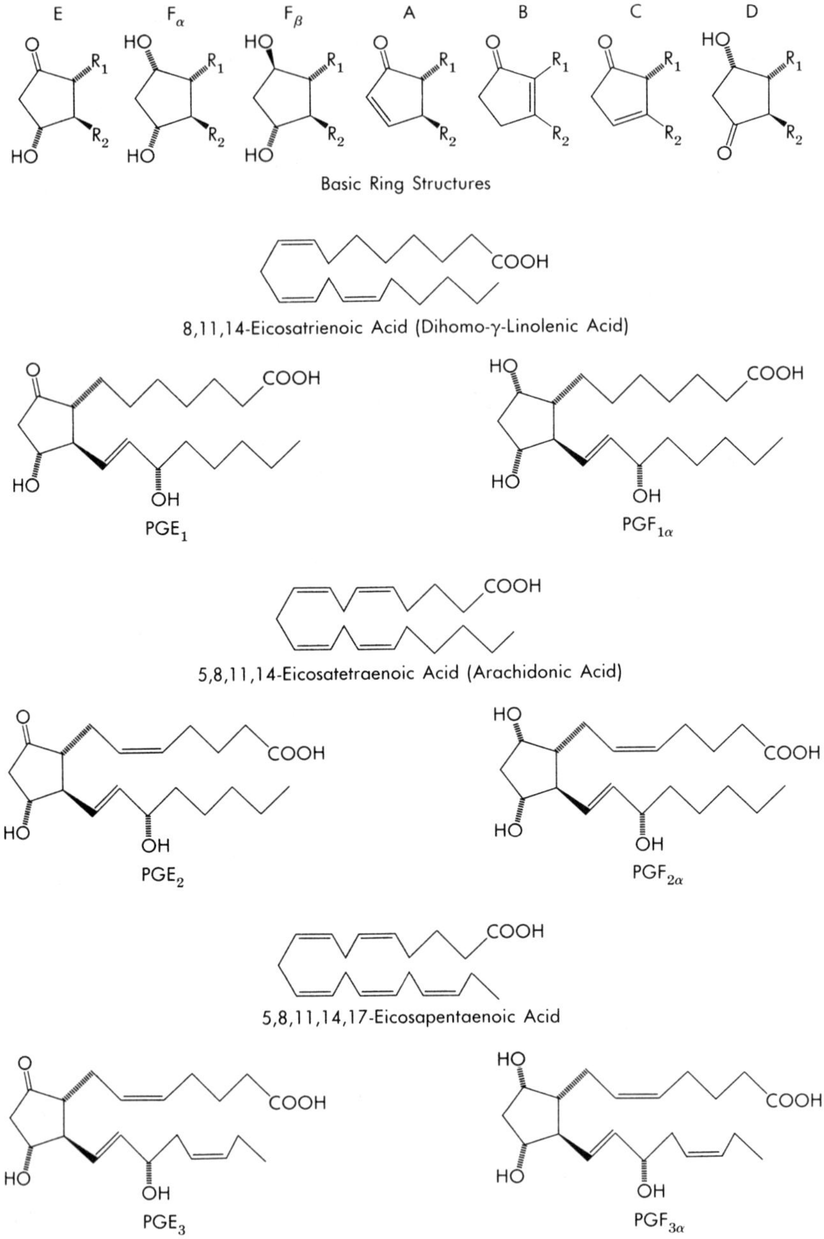

Figure 30-4. *Basic ring structures of the prostaglandins (PGs) and the six "primary" prostaglandins.*

Above each pair of PGs is shown the corresponding fatty acid precursor. In the stereochemical convention followed, the groups indicated by ⁙⁙⁙⁙ lie behind the plane of the cyclopentane ring, while those indicated by ◄—— lie in front of it.

dilators; when injected into the femoral arterial bed in dogs, their potency exceeds that of acetylcholine or histamine, although it is less than that of bradykinin. Responses to $PGF_{2\alpha}$ show species variation, but vasodilatation has been observed following injection into the human brachial artery of $PGF_{2\alpha}$ and PGs A_1, A_2, B_1, E_1, and E_2 (Robinson *et al.*, 1973).

PGA_1 has vasodilatory effects on coronary and other human vascular beds (Barner *et al.*, 1973). Dilatation in response to prostaglandins seemingly involves arterioles, precapillaries, sphincters, and postcapillary venules. PGEs are not universally vasodilatory; constrictor effects have been noted at selected sites. Superficial veins of the hand are contracted by

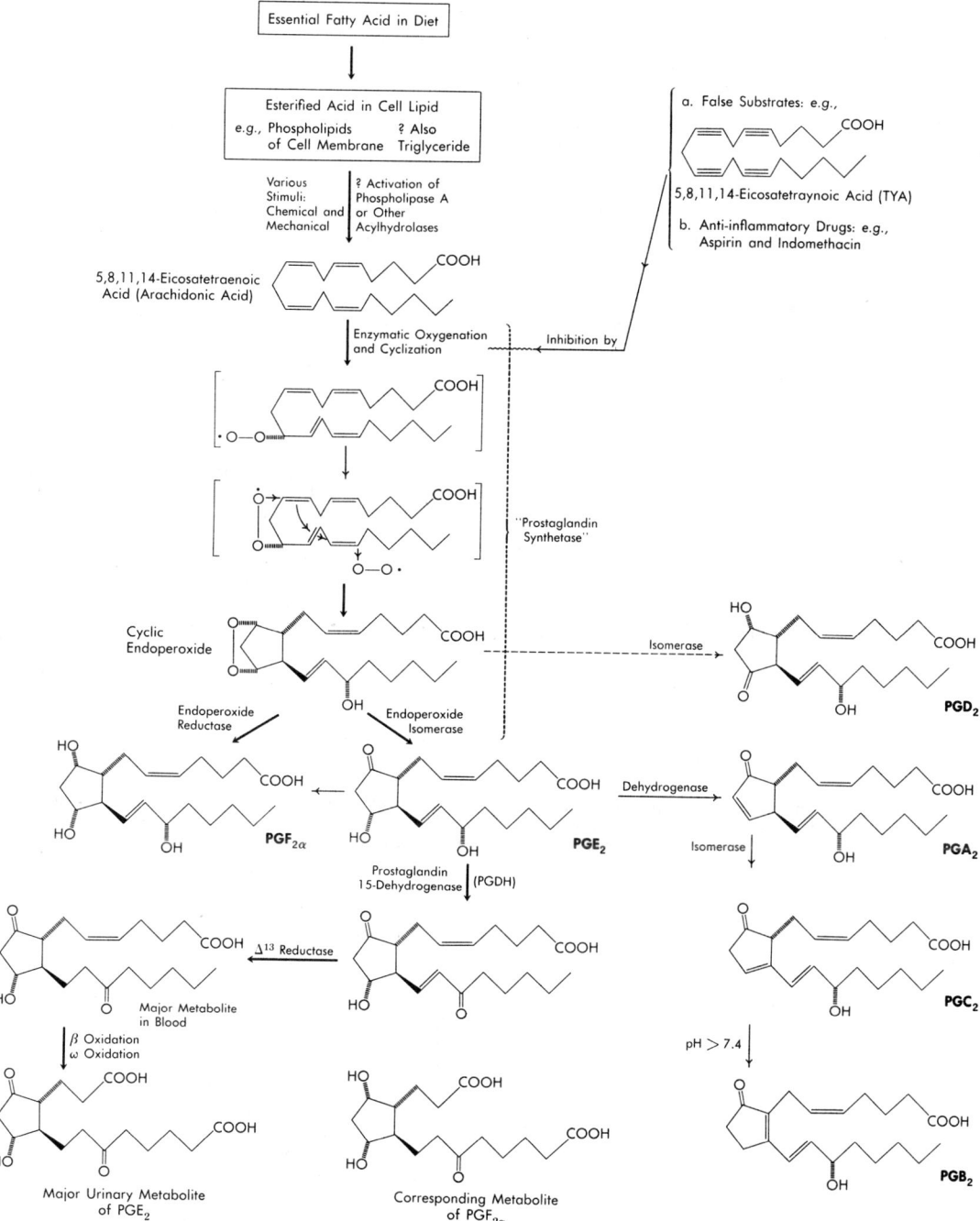

Figure 30–5. *Synthesis and catabolism of the two principal mammalian prostaglandins, PGE$_2$ and PGF$_{2\alpha}$.*

The inhibitors shown act at early stages and prevent formation of the endoperoxide. Enzymatic reduction of PGE to PGF occurs in several tissues. The sequence of breakdown is provided only for PGE$_2$; PGF$_{2\alpha}$ undergoes an analogous series of events. Some additional metabolites are not shown. *See* text for description.

$PGF_{2\alpha}$, but not by PGEs. The behavior of other large-capacitance veins in various animals is similar (*see* Nakano, 1973). In the *pulmonary circulation*, $PGF_{2\alpha}$ constricts both arteries and veins while PGEs and PGAs generally dilate these vessels.

Cardiac output is generally increased by PGs E, F, and A. Direct inotropic effects have been noted in various isolated preparations. In the intact animal, however, increased force of contraction as well as increased heart rate is in large measure a reflex consequence of fall in total peripheral resistance. Systemic blood pressure generally falls in response to PGs E and A, and blood flow to most organs, including the heart and kidney, is increased. These effects are particularly striking in some patients with hypertensive disease (*see* Lee, 1974). To make matters more complex, prostaglandins can influence cardiovascular as well as other systems by indirect means, reminiscent of those of angiotensin, involving actions within the CNS (Lavery *et al.,* 1971) and the peripheral autonomic nervous system, particularly the sympathetic (*see* below).

Capillary permeability is increased by PGs E_1, E_2, $F_{1\alpha}$, and $F_{2\alpha}$. Intradermal injection of these substances in man causes a "wheal and flare." PGE_1 diminishes mean corpuscular volume and increases erythrocyte deformability. This prostaglandin is also the most potent natural inhibitor of platelet aggregation. In contrast, the effects of PGE_2 on both red blood cells and platelets are the opposite of those produced by PGE_1 (*see* Mody, 1972; Allen and Valeri, 1974).

Smooth Muscle. Prostaglandins contract or relax many smooth muscles beside those of the vasculature. Again, responses may vary with species, type of prostaglandin, endocrine status of the tissue, and experimental conditions. However, few smooth muscles are uninfluenced, and many display intense and consistent responses.

Uterus. For historical and practical reasons actions on uterine muscle deserve first consideration. PGEs and PGFs produce strong contraction of isolated guinea pig uteri in estrus or diestrus. Strips of nonpregnant human uterus are contracted by PGFs but relaxed by PGs E, A, and B. The contractile response is most prominent before menstruation, whereas relaxation is greatest at mid-cycle. Uterine strips from pregnant women are uniformly contracted by PGEs and PGFs. In contrast to the *in-vitro* behavior, the human uterus *in vivo,* whether pregnant or not, is always contracted by PGE_1, PGE_2, and $PGF_{2\alpha}$ administered intravenously. The response is prompt and dose dependent, and takes the form of a sharp rise in tonus with superimposed rhythmic contractions, which long outlast the tonic phase. Intravenous infusion results in sustained labor-like contractions with tone falling between each. In contrast to oxytocin (*see* Chapter 42), this effect is observed at all stages of pregnancy, although as with oxytocin sensitivity does increase at term (*see* Karim, 1972; Karim and Hillier, 1973; Behrman and Anderson, 1974).

Bronchial and Tracheal Muscle. In general, PGFs contract and PGEs relax bronchial and tracheal muscle from various species, including man. Asth-

matic individuals are particularly sensitive, and $PGF_{2\alpha}$ has caused intense bronchospasm. In contrast, both PGE_1 and PGE_2 are potent bronchodilators when given to such patients by aerosol; the potency of PGE_1 may exceed that of isoproterenol (*see* Cuthbert, 1973; Parker and Snider, 1973; Zurier, 1974).

Gastrointestinal Muscle. In-vitro responses vary widely with species, segment, type of muscle, and the particular prostaglandin. In the main, longitudinal muscle from stomach to colon is contracted by both PGEs and PGFs, while circular muscle generally relaxes to PGEs and contracts to PGFs. The *in-vivo* effects are also variable in man. Shortened transit times have been observed in the small intestine and colon. Diarrhea, cramps, and reflux of bile have been noted in response to oral PGE; these are common side effects (along with nausea and vomiting) in patients given prostaglandins for abortion (*see* Bennett, 1972; Wilson, 1974).

Gastric, Pancreatic, and Intestinal Secretions. PGs E_1, E_2, and A_1 (but not $F_{2\alpha}$) inhibit gastric secretion, whether basal or stimulated by feeding, histamine, gastrin, or pentagastrin (Robert *et al.,* 1974). Volume, acid, and pepsin are all reduced by some action believed to be exerted directly on secretory cells. On the other hand, an increase in the volume, bicarbonate concentration, and enzyme content of pancreatic secretion has been noted (Rudick *et al.,* 1971). Mucus secretion in the small intestine is also increased, and there is substantial movement of water and electrolytes into the intestinal lumen. Such an effect is probably responsible for the watery diarrhea noted in early experiments in man given PGE_1 orally and subsequently in many individuals given prostaglandins intravenously. Effects of prostaglandins on water and electrolyte transport in other epithelial systems are mentioned below. (*See* Bennett, 1972; Wilson, 1974.)

Kidney and Urine Formation. PGEs and PGAs infused directly into the renal arteries of dogs increase renal blood flow and provoke diuresis, natriuresis, and kaliuresis. The rate of glomerular filtration may change little, and there is debate over whether redistribution of blood from medulla to cortex occurs. In man, the most remarkable effect is seen in certain individuals with hypertension in whom intravenous injection of PGA_1 in amounts below those affecting systemic blood pressure have caused a substantial increase in renal plasma flow, glomerular filtration rate, urine flow, and output of sodium and potassium. When PGA_1 was infused at higher rates in these individuals, parameters of renal function returned toward normal as peripheral resistance fell. This is thus a rather unique situation, where an antihypertensive effect is observed without compromised renal function. (*See* Lee, 1973; Muirhead, 1973; Arendshorst *et al.,* 1974; McGiff *et al.,* 1974.) PGEs inhibit water reabsorption induced by ADH in toad bladder and in rabbit collecting tubules (*see* Nakano and Koss, 1973).

Autonomic Nervous System. Effects of prostaglandins on autonomic ganglia and the adrenal medulla have generally been negligible. On the other hand, prostaglandins often modify sympathetic neuroeffector junctions, sometimes in exceedingly low concentration. PGEs tend to inhibit norepinephrine output from adrenergic nerve endings and to depress the response of the innervated structures. However, such effects are not uniformly observed and vary with species, tissue, and experimental conditions. Moreover, contrary effects leading to increased output of norepinephrine or heightened responsiveness of the effector organ have been noted, particularly with PGFs. Such facilitatory effects contribute to the arteriolar-constricting and venoconstricting actions of $PGF_{2\alpha}$. Evidence on the effects of prostaglandins on cholinergic neuroeffector transmission is fragmentary, but some responses are consistent with increased acetylcholine output. (*See* Hedqvist, 1973; Brody and Kadowitz, 1974.)

Central Nervous System. Many stimulant and depressant effects of prostaglandins on the CNS have been reported (*see* Horton, 1969, 1972a; Coceani, 1974). Among them is sedation in small mammals or young chickens (in which the blood-brain barrier is immature); stupor, catatonia, and other behavioral changes follow injection of PGEs (but not PGFs) into the cerebral ventricles in cats. The firing rates of individual brain cells may be increased or decreased after application of PGE or PGF by microiontophoresis. Especially noteworthy is fever in various species in response to intracerebroventricular PGE, but not PGF or PGA, an effect that involves both increased heat production and reduced heat loss (*see* Feldberg and Saxena, 1971; Milton and Wendlandt, 1971). PGE can also antagonize the inhibitory effect of norepinephrine on cerebellar Purkinje cells (Siggins *et al.*, 1971).

Afferent Nerves and Pain. In man, PGEs cause pain when injected intradermally, and they irritate the mucous membranes of the eyes and respiratory passages. These effects are generally not as immediate or intense as those caused by bradykinin or histamine, but they outlast those caused by the other autacoids and are accompanied by tenderness and potentiation of the pain-producing effects of the other autacoids (*see* Collier and Schneider, 1972; Zurier, 1974).

Endocrine System. A variety of endocrine tissues respond to prostaglandins. These effects include direct and indirect actions on the anterior pituitary (*see* Harms *et al.*, 1974), stimulation of steroid production by the adrenals, stimulation of insulin release (Johnson *et al.*, 1973), thyrotropin-like effects on the thyroid (Mashiter and Field, 1974), and luteinizing hormone–like effects on isolated ovarian tissue, causing increased progesterone secretion from the corpus luteum. This last effect, observed *in vitro*, contrasts with what is perhaps the most remarkable of all the effects of prostaglandins in the endocrine system, namely, luteolysis. This property is possessed especially but not uniquely by $PGF_{2\alpha}$.

Luteolysis. Prompt subsidence of progesterone output and regression of the corpus luteum follows parenteral injection of $PGF_{2\alpha}$ in a wide variety of mammals. This effect interrupts early pregnancy, which is dependent on luteal rather than placental progesterone (*see* Pharriss and Behrman, 1973). The mechanism of luteolysis is uncertain, but it may involve block of the normal ovarian response to circulating gonadotropin. The abortifacient action of prostaglandins in early human pregnancy does not seem to be accompanied by any demonstrable fall in plasma progesterone concentrations, and it is unknown if luteolysis is a significant factor (*see* Behrman and Anderson, 1974; Labhsetwar, 1974).

Metabolic Effects. PGEs, notably PGE_1, inhibit the basal rate of lipolysis from adipose tissue *in vitro* and also lipolysis stimulated by exposure to catecholamines or other lipolytic hormones. Such effects have also been noted *in vivo* in various species, including man, but are more capricious. Indeed, low doses of PGE_1 in man tend to stimulate lipolysis, seemingly by an indirect effect mediated by sympathetic stimulation. PGEs also have some insulin-like effects on carbohydrate metabolism (Nakano, 1973) and exert parathyroid hormone-like effects that result in mobilization of calcium from bone in tissue culture (Klein and Raisz, 1970).

Mechanism of Action. The acidic lipid nature of prostaglandins places them in a unique chemical class of autacoids and raises the question whether their diverse actions can be accommodated within the familiar concept of specific membrane-bound receptors of the sort invoked to explain the actions of autacoids of the classical amine or peptide type. The prevailing view is that such receptors are indeed involved (*see* Weeks, 1972). It is evident, however, that there is no single prostaglandin receptor. The various prostaglandins have quite different patterns of activity; for example, PGEs and PGFs not uncommonly exert opposite effects. The degree of saturation of the side chains commonly affects potency, but may also lead to qualitatively different behavior; examples are provided by the diametrically opposed actions of PGE_1 and PGE_2 on both platelets and erythrocytes. Selective actions of prostaglandin antagonists (*see* below) also testify to the heterogeneity of the receptors. Furthermore, by the use of such antagonists, the receptors for prostaglandins have been distinguished from receptors for all other autacoids.

Conjecture on further details of mechanism revolves around the two factors currently recognized as critically (if somewhat obscurely) involved in the regulation of contraction, secretion, transport, and various metabolic functions, namely, calcium and cyclic AMP—individually or in concert. The evidence buttressing these conjectures follows the familiar pattern. On the one hand, it is possible to demonstrate the calcium dependence of diverse responses to prostaglandins and to observe altered calcium fluxes. On the other, prostaglandins may either stimulate or inhibit the accumulation of cyclic AMP. For example, activation of adenylate cyclase accompanies the stimulatory effects of prostaglandins on the anterior pituitary, ovary, thyroid, and other organs. The responses observed are consistent with those expected from cyclic AMP. In contrast, inhibition of cyclic AMP accumulation is associated with the inhibitory effect of prostaglandins on lipolysis and with the antagonism of the responses of epithelial tissues to ADH. There is good evidence that these are cause-and-effect relationships. (*See* Ramwell and Shaw, 1971; Hittelman and Butcher, 1973; Kahn and Lands, 1973.)

Endogenous Prostaglandins: Possible Functions in Physiological and Pathological Processes. With some autacoids, the scope of permissible conjecture on their possible involvement in normal and abnormal functions is limited by their restricted distribution. This is not so with the prostaglandins. Because these substances can be formed by virtually every tissue and cell type, it is not unreasonable to suspect that each pharmacological effect observed may reflect a physiological or pathophysiological function. And such suspicions have been nurtured and presented in the shape of countless hypotheses bearing on just about every bodily function (*see* appended list of monographs and reviews). Several of these have been supported, or at least encouraged, by the classical gambit of pharmacological analysis by means of blocking agents, of which more will be said later.

Perhaps most interest attaches to the possible involvement of prostaglandins in *reproductive physiology* (*see* Speroff and Ramwell, 1970; Karim and Hillier, 1973; Behrman and Anderson, 1974; Labhsetwar, 1974). Their large number and their very high concentration in human semen, coupled with the substantial absorption of prostaglandins by the vagina, have encouraged speculation that prostaglandins deposited during coitus may facilitate conception by actions on the cervix, uterine body, Fallopian tubes, and transport of semen. However, it should be pointed out that prostaglandins are sparse or absent in the semen of some species. Moreover, antifertility properties can be recognized in some effects of prostaglandins on ovum transport and implantation. Although there does seem to be correlation between the amounts of prostaglandins in the semen and some cases of male infertility, the role of the autacoids in semen remains obscure. In subprimate females a good case can be argued that $PGF_{2\alpha}$ released from the uterine endometrium when conception has not taken place, is the long-sought *luteolytic hormone* (*see* Horton, 1972b; Pharriss and Behrman, 1973), but no clear influence of $PGF_{2\alpha}$ on regression of the human corpus luteum has been demonstrated. On the other hand, prostaglandins rise sharply in the amniotic fluid at term and may participate in parturition. Discharge of endometrial prostaglandins may also contribute to the cramps of dysmenorrhea (and possibly "menstrual" diarrhea). They have also been implicated in habitual abortion and in the constriction of the umbilical artery and vein after delivery of the fetus.

Prostaglandins have been considered as factors regulating tone in many smooth muscles beside the uterus. The interesting notion has been advanced that an abnormal preponderance or imbalance of $PGF_{2\alpha}$ (constrictor) over PGE_2 (dilator) could contribute to high bronchial tone in asthma (*see* Cuthbert, 1973). Many functions in the cardiovascular-

renal system have been proposed. Several signs point to functions within the kidney, including mediation of reactive (ischemic) hyperemia and the autoregulation of renal blood flow (Herbaczynska-Cedro and Vane, 1973, 1974), as well as modulation of the intrarenal effects of the renin-angiotensin system (Aiken and Vane, 1973), and renovascular and tubular effects regulating urine formation. There is, moreover, the possibility that the well-known antihypertensive property of the normally functioning kidney may be related to its capacity to synthesize and release, locally or into the systemic circulation, natriuretic and blood pressure–lowering PGE_2 and PGA_2. Since PGA_2 is only slowly metabolized, a hormonal role is conceivable; but there is some doubt whether the kidney releases it in significant quantities. Escape of PGE_2 from platelets contributes to the second, secretory phase of platelet aggregation and hence to thrombus formation. This prostaglandin, by its actions on erythrocytes, may also be a factor initiating sickle-cell crises (Allen and Valeri, 1974).

Prostaglandins are released by a host of mechanical, thermal, chemical, bacterial, and other insults and are believed to contribute importantly to inflammation, particularly the more slowly developing and persistent aspects (*see* Collier, 1971a, 1971b; Willoughby *et al.*, 1973; Zurier, 1974). They may play a particularly prominent role in inflammatory processes in the eye (*see* Whitelocke *et al.*, 1973). These autacoids are abundant in some arthritic joint fluids. Their release has been detected during allergic reactions, and they may participate in asthmatic attacks, at least in some patients (*see* Tauber *et al.*, 1973; Zurier, 1974). Prostaglandins are known to be released by certain malignant growths, among them medullary carcinoma of the thyroid, and seem to contribute to the accompanying flushing, diarrhea, and occasional hypercalcemia (*see* Sandler *et al.*, 1968; Tashjian *et al.*, 1974). The capacity of prostaglandins to cause bone resorption has been invoked as a cause of alveolar bone loss in periodontal disease.

A modulator (restraining) role for prostaglandins has been suggested to operate in sympathetic nerve transmission, in various transport and secretory functions (including production of gastric juice), and in lipolysis. Finally, prostaglandins may have functions within the CNS; they appear to act as a link in temperature regulation and to be a factor in the fever induced by bacterial pyrogens (*see* Feldberg *et al.*, 1973).

Therapeutic Uses. There has been intense interest in the effects of the prostaglandins on the female reproductive system. The clinical value of the agents, particularly $PGF_{2\alpha}$ and PGE_2, is being assessed in numerous clinics throughout the world. Their actions as *abortifacients* is already clearly established. Given early in pregnancy they are abortifacient, but initial hopes that they might provide a simple, convenient means of postimplantation "contraception," perhaps given as a vaginal suppository, have not been fulfilled. Moreover, the abortifacient action of prostaglandins in the early weeks of pregnancy is inconstant and often incomplete, and may be accompanied by distressing side effects. Nevertheless, prostaglandins appear to be of value in missed abortion and molar gestation, and they have been considered as the agents of choice for inducing midtrimester abortion. They also offer alternatives to oxytocin for induction of labor at term. These actions of prostaglandins are considered more fully in Chapter 42.

The use of prostaglandins for other purposes is currently restricted. PGE_1 has proven valuable for increasing the harvest and storage of blood platelets for therapeutic transfusion (*see* Allen and Valeri, 1974). PGE_2 has been used as an alternative to isoproterenol in bronchial asthma, and it may be of some value in status asthmaticus when sympathomimetic amines fail. However, the value of PGE_2 in such conditions, where it is given by inhalation, is limited by its irritant effect on the respiratory mucosa (*see* Cuthbert, 1973). The possible usefulness of prostaglandins or analogs in treating gastric hyperacidity is attracting interest. Some markedly inhibit gastric secretion when given orally to man and have antiulcer activity (*see* Lippmann and Seethaler, 1973; Robert *et al.*, 1974). There is great promise in the possible usefulness of derivatives that may overcome many of the disadvantages of the natural compounds. The spectrum of uses for such compounds has still to be defined. In addition to the conditions mentioned above, there is the possibility that prostaglandin analogs may yield valuable antihypertensive drugs (*see* Lee, 1973).

The available preparations of the prostaglandins are described in Chapter 42.

INHIBITORS OF THE SYNTHESIS AND ACTIONS OF PROSTAGLANDINS

Therapeutic interest in this area is of course not limited to the possible use of prostaglandins as agonists, but is also very much concerned with the possibility of antagonizing them or interfering with their metabolism, particularly because of their ubiquity, diversity of action, and seeming involvement in so many different physiological and pathological events.

Inhibitors of Synthesis of Prostaglandins. The association between aspirin-like drugs and prostaglandins became clear in 1971, but evidence had accumulated in the late 1960s to suggest that aspirin and related anti-inflammatory agents might owe their actions to interference with autacoids, among them prostaglandins (*see* Collier, 1971a, 1971b; Vane, 1971). In retrospect, several observations can be recognized as providing critical clues. Piper and Vane (1969) discovered that an unknown autacoid, which they named rabbit aorta constrictor substance (RCS), was released along with other compounds from guinea pig lungs during anaphylaxis; aspirin prevented its escape. Aspirin had also been shown to counter responses to arachidonic acid in some preparations, and arachidonic acid was also found to release RCS. In 1971 a series of critical observations was made indicating that aspirin and related anti-inflammatory drugs interfere with the liberation of prostaglandins and, in fact, prevent their synthe-

sis. The anti-inflammatory agents prevented release of prostaglandins from spleen (Ferreira *et al.*, 1971) and platelets (Smith and Willis, 1971) and prevented the synthesis of prostaglandins from arachidonic acid in tissue homogenates (Vane, 1971). It is possible that RCS is related to the cyclic endoperoxide intermediate in the synthetic pathway (*see* Hamberg and Samuelsson, 1973), and that aspirin and related anti-inflammatory drugs prevent production of this critical intermediate (*see also* Flower, 1974). Vane (1971) has argued that inhibition of prostaglandin synthesis may provide an explanation for both the therapeutic effects and several side effects of aspirin and other anti-inflammatory substances of the nonsteroidal type. All these anti-inflammatory compounds inhibit prostaglandin synthesis, and their therapeutic efficacy parallels their ability to inhibit prostaglandin synthetase to a remarkable extent. A clear-cut inhibition of prostaglandin synthesis, as measured by the prostaglandin content of semen or excretion of the principal prostaglandin metabolite in the urine, is evident in man treated with conventional doses of these anti-inflammatory agents.

Beside the aspirin-like inhibitors mentioned (*see also* Chapter 17), it should be noted that analogs of the natural fatty acid precursors serve as competitive inhibitors of prostaglandin production. Among them is the acetylenic analog of arachidonic acid, 5,8,11,14-eicosatetraynoic acid (Figure 30–5) (*see* Lands *et al.*, 1973). The therapeutic potential of agents of this type remains to be assessed. Another exciting possibility lies in the development of drugs with preferential inhibitory actions on the endoperoxide isomerase and reductase that would allow selective depression of E and F_α forms, which so frequently exert different biological effects. Such manipulations are already possible *in vitro* (*see* Hamberg and Samuelsson, 1973; Lands *et al.*, 1973).

Inhibitors of Responses to Prostaglandins. There are presently no universally effective, potent antagonists of responses to the prostaglandins. However, some compounds are effective in selected *in-vitro* tests, and a few of these may be of practical value *in vivo*. Contractions in response to $PGF_{2\alpha}$ in human isolated bronchial muscle are inhibited by *fenamates, phenylbutazone,* and, less potently, *aspirin* (*see* Collier, 1971a, 1971b). Certain prostaglandin analogs, such as 7-oxa-13,14-prostynoic acid, also antagonize some *in-vitro* effects of prostaglandins on muscle and the responses of ovary and thyroid to prostaglandins (*see* Mashiter and Field, 1974). Some *in-vitro* muscle responses to the autacoids are blocked by a dibenzoxazepine hydrazide derivative (SC-19220), and also by a polyester of phloretin and phosphoric acid known as polyphloretin phosphate. References to these substances are in the reviews by Weeks (1972) and Sanner (1974). Polyphloretin phosphate has been found to be of benefit in some inflammatory conditions of the eye (*see* Eakins, 1973; Whitelocke *et al.*, 1973).

Aiken, J. W., and Vane, J. R. Intrarenal prostaglandin release attenuates the renal vasoconstrictor activity of angiotensin. *J. Pharmac. exp. Ther.,* **1973,** *184,* 678.
Alabaster, V. A., and Bakhle, Y. S. The inactivation of

bradykinin in the pulmonary circulation of isolated lungs. *Br. J. Pharmac.*, **1972a**, *45*, 299–310.

————. Converting enzyme and bradykininase in the lung. *Circulation Res.*, **1972b**, *31*, Suppl. II, 72–84.

Andersson, B., and Eriksson, L. Conjoint action of sodium and angiotensin on brain mechanisms controlling water and salt balances. *Acta physiol. scand.*, **1971**, *81*, 18–29.

Arendshorst, W. J.; Johnston, P. A.; and Selkurt, E. E. Effect of prostaglandin E on renal hemodynamics in nondiuretic and volume-expanded dogs. *Am. J. Physiol.*, **1974**, *226*, 218–225.

Bagdasarian, A.; Lahiri, B.; and Colman, R. W. Origin of the high molecular weight activator of prekallikrein. *J. biol. Chem.*, **1973**, *248*, 7742–7747.

Barner, H. B.; Kaiser, G. C.; Jellinek, M.; and Lee, J. B. Effect of prostaglandin A on several vascular beds in man. *Am. Heart J.*, **1973**, *85*, 584–592.

Bianchi, A.; Evans, D. B.; Cobb, M.; Peschka, M. T.; Schaeffer, T. R.; and Laffan, R. J. Inhibition by SQ 20881 of vasopressor response to angiotensin I in conscious animals. *Eur. J. Pharmac.*, **1973**, *23*, 90–96.

Braun-Menéndez, E.; Fasciolo, J. C.; Leloir, L. F.; and Muñoz, J. M. The substance causing renal hypertension. *J. Physiol., Lond.*, **1940**, *98*, 283–298.

Braun-Menéndez, E., and Page, I. H. Suggested revision of nomenclature—angiotensin. *Science, Wash.*, **1958**, *127*, 242.

Brody, M. J., and Kadowitz, P. J. Prostaglandins as modulators of the autonomic nervous system. *Fedn Proc. Fedn Am. Socs exp. Biol.*, **1974**, *33*, 48–60.

Brown, J. J.; Lever, A. F.; and Robertson, J. I. S. Renin and angiotensin in health and disease. *Schweiz. med. Wschr.*, **1967**, *97*, 1635–1639, 1679–1687.

Brunner, H. R.; Gavras, H.; Laragh, J. H.; and Keenan, R. Angiotensin-II blockade in man by sar¹-ala⁸-angiotensin II for understanding and treatment of high blood-pressure. *Lancet*, **1973**, *2*, 1045–1048.

Bumpus, F. M.; Sen, S.; Smeby, R. R.; Sweet, C.; Ferrario, C. M.; and Khosla, M. C. Use of angiotensin II antagonists in experimental hypertension. *Circulation Res.*, **1973**, *32*, Suppl., 150–158.

Campbell, A. G. M.; Dawes, G. S.; Fishman, A. P.; Hyman, A. I.; and Perks, A. M. Release of bradykinin-like pulmonary vasodilator substance in foetal and new-born lambs. *J. Physiol., Lond.*, **1968**, *195*, 83–96.

Chang, M. M.; Leeman, S. E.; and Niall, H. D. Amino-acid sequence of substance P. *Nature, New Biol.*, **1971**, *232*, 86–87.

Cochrane, C. G.; Revak, S. D.; and Wuepper, K. D. Activation of Hageman factor in solid and fluid phases. *J. exp. Med.*, **1973**, *138*, 1564–1583.

Collier, H. O. J. Kinins and prostaglandins. *Proc. R. Soc. Med.*, **1971a**, *64*, 1–16.

————. Prostaglandins and aspirin. *Nature, Lond.*, **1971b**, *232*, 17–19.

Collier, H. O. J., and Schneider, C. Nociceptive response to prostaglandins and analgesic actions of aspirin and morphine. *Nature, New Biol.*, **1972**, *236*, 141–143.

Collier, J. G.; Robinson, B. F.; and Vane, J. R. Reduction of pressor effects of angiotensin I in man by synthetic nonapeptide (B.P.P.₉ₐ or SQ 20,881) which inhibits converting enzyme. *Lancet*, **1973**, *1*, 72–74.

Davis, J. O.; Carpenter, C. C. J.; Ayers, C. R.; Holman, J. E.; and Bahn, R. C. Evidence for secretion of an aldosterone-stimulating hormone by the kidney. *J. clin. Invest.*, **1961**, *40*, 684–696.

Dempsey, P. J.; McCallum, Z. T.; Kent, K. M.; and Cooper, T. Direct myocardial effects of angiotensin II. *Am. J. Physiol.*, **1971**, *220*, 477–481.

Dickinson, C. J., and Yu, R. Mechanisms involved in the progressive pressor response to very small amounts of angiotensin in conscious rabbits. *Circulation Res.*, **1967**, *21*, Suppl. 2, 157–163.

Douglas, W. W.; Kanno, T.; and Sampson, S. R. Effects of acetylcholine and other medullary secretagogues and antagonists on the membrane potential of adrenal chromaffin cells: an analysis employing techniques of tissue culture. *J. Physiol., Lond.*, **1967**, *188*, 107–120.

Engel, S. L.; Schaeffer, T. R.; Waugh, M. H.; and Rubin, B. Effects of the nonapeptide SQ 20881 on blood pressure of rats with experimental renovascular hypertension. *Proc. Soc. exp. Biol. Med.*, **1973**, *143*, 483–487.

Euler, U. S. von. On the specific vasodilating and plain muscle stimulating substance from accessory genital glands in man and certain animals (prostaglandin and vesiglandin). *J. Physiol., Lond.*, **1936**, *88*, 213–234.

Farr, W. C., and Grupp, G. Ganglionic stimulation: mechanism of the positive inotropic and chronotropic effects of angiotensin. *J. Pharmac. exp. Ther.*, **1971**, *177*, 48–55.

Feldberg, W.; Gupta, K. P.; Milton, A. S.; and Wendlandt, S. Effect of pyrogen and antipyretics on prostaglandin activity in cisternal C.S.F. of unanaesthetized cats. *J. Physiol., Lond.*, **1973**, *234*, 279–303.

Feldberg, W., and Saxena, P. N. Fever produced by prostaglandin E₂. *J. Physiol., Lond.*, **1971**, *217*, 547–556.

Ferrario, C. M.; Gildenberg, P. L.; and McCubbin, J. W. Cardiovascular effects of angiotensin mediated by the central nervous system. *Circulation Res.*, **1972**, *30*, 257–262.

Ferreira, S. H. A bradykinin-potentiating factor (BPF) present in the venom of *Bothrops jararaca*. *Br. J. Pharmac. Chemother.*, **1965**, *24*, 163–169.

Ferreira, S. H.; Moncada, S.; and Vane, J. R. Indomethacin and aspirin abolish prostaglandin release from the spleen. *Nature, New Biol.*, **1971**, *231*, 237–239.

Friedli, B.; Kent, G.; and Olley, P. M. Inactivation of bradykinin in the pulmonary vascular bed of newborn and fetal lambs. *Circulation Res.*, **1973**, *33*, 421–427.

Ganong, W. F., and Mulrow, P. J. Evidence of secretion of an aldosterone-stimulating substance by the kidney. *Nature, Lond.*, **1961**, *190*, 1115–1116.

Gant, N. F.; Daley, G. L.; Ghand, S.; Whalley, P. J.; and MacDonald, P. C. A study of angiotensin II pressor response throughout primigravid pregnancy. *J. clin. Invest.*, **1973**, *52*, 2682–2689.

Glossmann, H.; Baukal, A. J.; and Catt, K. J. Properties of angiotensin II receptors in the bovine and rat adrenal cortex. *J. biol. Chem.*, **1974**, *249*, 825–834.

Goldblatt, M. W. Properties of human seminal fluid. *J. Physiol., Lond.*, **1935**, *84*, 208–218.

Hamberg, M., and Samuelsson, B. Detection and isolation of an endoperoxide intermediate in prostaglandin synthesis. *Proc. natn. Acad. Sci. U.S.A.*, **1973**, *70*, 899–903.

Harms, P. G.; Ojeda, S. R.; and McCann, S. M. Prostaglandin-induced release of pituitary gonadotropins: central nervous system and pituitary sites of action. *Endocrinology*, **1974**, *94*, 1459–1464.

Herbaczynska-Cedro, K., and Vane, J. R. Contribution of intrarenal generation of prostaglandin to autoregulation of renal blood flow in the dog. *Circulation Res.*, **1973**, *33*, 428–436.

————. Prostaglandins as mediators of reactive hyperaemia in kidney. *Nature, Lond.*, **1974**, *247*, 492.

Igic, R.; Erdös, E. G.; Yeh, H. S. J.; Sorrells, K.; and Nakajima, T. Angiotensin I converting enzyme of the lung. *Circulation Res.*, **1972**, *31*, Suppl. II, 51–61.

Johnson, D. G.; Fujimoto, W. Y.; and Williams, R. W. Enhanced release of insulin by prostaglandins in isolated pancreatic islets. *Diabetes*, **1973**, *22*, 658–663.

Klein, D. C., and Raisz, L. G. Prostaglandins: stimulation of bone resorption in tissue culture. *Endocrinology*, **1970**, *86*, 1436–1440.

Kline, R. L.; Scott, J. B.; Haddy, F. J.; and Grega, G. J. Mechanism of edema formation in canine forelimbs by locally administered bradykinin. *Am. J. Physiol.*, **1973**, *225*, 1051–1056.

Kremen, S. H., and Wakerlin, G. E. Renin and antirenin

in treatment of long term experimental renal hypertension in the dog. *Proc. Soc. exp. Biol. Med.,* **1955,** *90,* 99–104.

Kurzrok, R., and Lieb, C. C. Biochemical studies of human semen. II. The action of semen on the human uterus. *Proc. Soc. exp. Biol. Med.,* **1930,** *28,* 268–272.

Lands, W. E. M.; Le Tellier, P. R.; Rome, L. H.; and Vanderhoek, J. Y. Inhibition of prostaglandin biosynthesis. In, *International Conference on Prostaglandins. Advances in the Biosciences,* Vol. 9. Pergamon Press, Ltd., Oxford, **1973,** pp. 15–28.

Laragh, J. H.; Angers, M.; Kelly, W. G.; and Lieberman, S. Hypotensive agents and pressor substances: the effect of epinephrine, norepinephrine, angiotensin II and others on the secretory rate of aldosterone in man. *J. Am. med. Ass.,* **1960,** *174,* 234–240.

Lavery, H. A.; Lowe, R. D.; and Scroop, G. C. Central autonomic effects of prostaglandin F_2 on the cardiovascular system of the dog. *Br. J. Pharmac.,* **1971,** *41,* 454–461.

Lewis, G. P., and Reit, E. Further studies on the actions of peptides on the superior cervical ganglia and suprarenal medulla. *Br. J. Pharmac. Chemother.,* **1966,** *26,* 444–460.

Lippmann, W., and Seethaler, K. Oral anti-ulcer activity of a synthetic prostaglandin analogue (9-oxoprostanoic acid: AY-22,469). *Experientia,* **1973,** *29,* 993–995.

Mashiter, K., and Field, J. B. Prostaglandins and the thyroid gland. *Fedn Proc. Fedn Am. Socs exp. Biol.,* **1974,** *33,* 78–80.

Milton, A. S., and Wendlandt, S. Effects on body temperature of prostaglandins of the A, E and F series of injection into the third ventricle of unanaesthetized cats and rabbits. *J. Physiol., Lond.,* **1971,** *218,* 325–336.

Movat, H. Z.; Sottay, M. J.; Fuller, P. J.; and Ozge-Anwar, A. The relationship between the plasma kinin-system and the contact phase of blood-coagulation in man. *Adv. exp. Med. Biol.,* **1972,** *21,* 109–118.

Newball, H. H., and Keiser, H. R. Relative effects of bradykinin and histamine on the respiratory system of man. *J. appl. Physiol.,* **1973,** *35,* 552–556.

Nickerson, M., and Sutter, M. C. Angiotensin in shock. *Can. med. Ass. J.,* **1964,** *90,* 325–327.

Ondetti, M. A.; Williams, N. J.; Sabo, E. F.; Pluščec, J.; Weaver, E. R.; and Kocy, O. Angiotensin-converting enzyme inhibitors from the venom of *Bothrops jararaca.* Isolation, elucidation of structure, and synthesis. *Biochemistry, N.Y.,* **1971,** *10,* 4033–4039.

Page, I. H., and Helmer, O. M. Angiotonin-activator, renin- and angiotonin-inhibitor and the mechanism of angiotonin tachyphylaxis in normal, hypertensive and nephrectomized animals. *J. exp. Med.,* **1940,** *71,* 485–519.

Pals, D. T.; Masucci, F. D.; Denning, G. S.; Sipos, F.; and Fessler, D. C. Role of the pressor action of angiotensin II in experimental hypertension. *Circulation Res.,* **1971,** *29,* 673–681.

Peach, M. J., and Chiu, A. T. Stimulation of aldosterone biosynthesis *in vitro* by angiotensin II and analogs. *Circulation Res.,* **1974,** *34,* Suppl. 1, 7–13.

Peart, W. S. Renin-angiotensin system. *New Engl. J. Med.,* **1975,** *292,* 302–306.

Piper, P. J., and Vane, J. R. Release of additional factors in anaphylaxis and its antagonism by anti-inflammatory drugs. *Nature, Lond.,* **1969,** *223,* 29–35.

Poulsen, K.; Burton, J.; and Haber, E. Competitive inhibitors of renin. *Biochem. J.,* **1973,** *12,* 3877–3882.

Regoli, D.; Park, W. K.; and Rioux, F. II. Pharmacology of angiotensin antagonists. *Can. J. Physiol. Pharmac.,* **1973,** *51,* 114–121.

Ribeiro, S. A.; Corrado, A. P.; and Graeff, F. G. Antinociceptive action of intraventricular bradykinin. *Neuropharmacology,* **1971,** *10,* 725–731.

Robert, A.; Nylander, B.; and Andersson, S. Marked inhibition of gastric secretion by two prostaglandin analogs given orally to man. *Life Sci.,* **1974,** *14,* 533–538.

Robinson, B. F.; Collier, J. G.; Karim, S. M. M.; and Somers, K. Effect of prostaglandins A_1, A_2, B_1, E_2 and F_2 on forearm arterial bed and superficial hand veins in man. *Clin. Sci.,* **1973,** *44,* 367–376.

Romero, J. C.; Hoobler, S. W.; Kozak, T. J.; and Warzynski, R. J. Effect of antirenin on blood pressure of rabbits with experimental renal hypertension. *Am. J. Physiol.,* **1973,** *225,* 810–817.

Rudick, J.; Gonda, M.; Dreiling, D. A.; and Janowitz, H. D. Effects of prostaglandin E_1 on pancreatic endocrine function. *Gastroenterology,* **1971,** *60,* 272–278.

Sandler, M.; Karim, S. M. M.; and Williams, E. D. Prostaglandins in amine-peptide-secreting tumors. *Lancet,* **1968,** *2,* 1053–1055.

Saruta, T.; Cook, R.; and Kaplan, N. M. Adrenocortical steroidogenesis: studies on the mechanism of action of angiotensin and electrolytes. *J. clin. Invest.,* **1972,** *51,* 2239–2245.

Sen, S.; Smeby, R. R.; and Bumpus, F. M. Plasma renin activity in hypertensive rats after treatment with renin preinhibitor. *Am. J. Physiol.,* **1969,** *216,* 499–503.

Siggins, G.; Hoffer, B.; and Bloom, F. Prostaglandin-norepinephrine interactions in brain: microelectrophoretic and histochemical correlates. *Ann. N.Y. Acad. Sci.,* **1971,** *180,* 302–323.

Smith, J. B., and Willis, A. L. Aspirin selectively inhibits prostaglandin production in human platelets. *Nature, New Biol.,* **1971,** *321,* 235–237.

Stern, P.; Catovic, S.; and Stern, M. Mechanism of action of substance P. *Naunyn-Schmiedebergs Arch. Pharmac.,* **1974,** *281,* 233–239.

Stewart, J. M. Structure-activity relationships in bradykinin analogues. *Fedn Proc. Fedn Am. Socs exp. Biol.,* **1968,** *27,* 63–66.

Streeten, D. H. P.; Kerr, L. P.; Kerr, C. B.; Prior, J. C.; and Kalakos, T. G. Hyperbradykininism: a new orthostatic syndrome. *Lancet,* **1972,** *2,* 1048–1053.

Sweet, C. S.; Ferrario, C. M.; Khosla, M. C.; and Bumpus, F. M. Antagonism of peripheral and central effects of angiotensin II by [1-sarcosine, 8-isoleucine]angiotensin II. *J. Pharmac. exp. Ther.,* **1973,** *185,* 35–41.

Tashjian, A. H.; Voelkel, E. F.; Goldhaber, P.; and Levine, L. Prostaglandins, calcium metabolism and cancer. *Fedn Proc. Fedn Am. Socs exp. Biol.,* **1974,** *33,* 81–86.

Tauber, A. I.; Kaliner, M.; Stechschulte, D. J.; and Austen, K. F. Prostaglandins and the immunological release of chemical mediators from human lung. In, *Prostaglandins and Cyclic AMP: Biological Actions and Clinical Applications.* (Kahn, R. H., and Lands, W. E. M., eds.) Academic Press, Inc., New York, **1973,** pp. 29–48.

Tregear, G. W.; Niall, H. D.; Potts, J. T., Jr.; Leeman, S. E.; and Chang, M. M. Synthesis of substance P. *Nature, New Biol.,* **1971,** *232,* 87–89.

Vane, J. R. Inhibition of prostaglandin synthesis as a mechanism of action for aspirin-like drugs. *Nature, New Biol.,* **1971,** *231,* 232–235.

Wuepper, K. D. Prekallikrein deficiency in man. *J. exp. Med.,* **1973,** *138,* 1345–1355.

Zimmerman, B. G. Blockade of adrenergic potentiating effect of angiotensin by 1-sar-8-ala-angiotensin II. *J. Pharmac. exp. Ther.,* **1973,** *185,* 486–492.

Monographs and Reviews

Allen, J. E., and Valeri, C. R. Prostaglandins in hematology. *Archs intern. Med.,* **1974,** *133,* 86–96.

Andersen, N. H., and Ramwell, P. W. Biological aspects of prostaglandins. *Archs intern. Med.,* **1974,** *133,* 30–50.

Armstrong, D. Pain. In, *Bradykinin, Kallidin and Kallikrein.* (Erdös, E. G., ed.) *Handb. exp. Pharmak.,* Vol. 25. Springer-Verlag, Berlin, **1970,** pp. 434–481.

Assaykeen, T. A. (ed.). *Control of Renin Secretion.* Plenum Press, New York, **1972.**

Bakhle, Y. S. Converting enzyme *in vitro* measurement and properties. In, *Angiotensin.* (Page, I. H., and Bumpus,

F. M., eds.) *Handb. exp. Pharmak.*, Vol. 37. Springer-Verlag, Berlin, **1974**, pp. 41–80.

Behrman, H. R., and Anderson, G. G. Prostaglandins in reproduction. *Archs intern. Med.*, **1974**, *133*, 77–84.

Bennett, A. Effects of prostaglandins on the gastrointestinal tract. In, *The Prostaglandins: Progress in Research.* (Karim, S. M. M., ed.) John Wiley & Sons, Inc., New York, **1972**, pp. 205–222.

Bergström, S., and Samuelsson, B. The prostaglandins. *Endeavour*, **1968**, *27*, 109–113.

Coceani, F. Prostaglandins and the central nervous system. *Archs intern. Med.*, **1974**, *133*, 119–129.

Collier, H. O. J. Kinins and ventilation of the lungs. In, *Bradykinin, Kallidin and Kallikrein.* (Erdös, E. G., ed.) *Handb. exp. Pharmak.*, Vol. 25. Springer-Verlag, Berlin, **1970**, pp. 409–420.

Croxatto, H. R. Plasma of serum vasopressor peptides other than angiotensins. In, *Angiotensin.* (Page, I. H., and Bumpus, F. M., eds.) *Handb. exp. Pharmak.*, Vol. 37. Springer-Verlag, Berlin, **1974**, pp. 240–263.

Cuthbert, M. F. Prostaglandins and respiratory smooth muscle. In, *The Prostaglandins: Pharmacological and Therapeutic Advances.* (Cuthbert, M. F., ed.) J. B. Lippincott Co., Philadelphia, **1973**, pp. 253–286.

Davis, J. O. The control of renin release. *Am. J. Med.*, **1973**, *55*, 333–350.

———. The renin-angiotensin system in the control of aldosterone secretion. In, *Angiotensin.* (Page, I. H., and Bumpus, F. M., eds.) *Handb. exp. Pharmak.*, Vol. 37. Springer-Verlag, Berlin, **1974**, pp. 322–336.

Eakins, K. E. Ocular effects. In, *The Prostaglandins*, Vol. 1. (Ramwell, P. W., ed.) Plenum Press, New York, **1973**, pp. 219–238.

Elliott, D. F. The discovery and characterization of bradykinin. In, *Bradykinin, Kallidin and Kallikrein.* (Erdös, E. G., ed.) *Handb. exp. Pharmak.*, Vol. 25. Springer-Verlag, Berlin, **1970**, pp. 7–13.

Erdös, E. G. (ed.). *Bradykinin, Kallidin and Kallikrein. Handb. exp. Pharmak.*, Vol. 25. Springer-Verlag, Berlin, **1970**.

Erdös, E. G., and Yang, H. Y. T. Kininases. In, *Bradykinin, Kallidin and Kallikrein.* (Erdös, E. G., ed.) *Handb. exp. Pharmak.*, Vol. 25. Springer-Verlag, Berlin, **1970**, pp. 289–323.

Erspamer, V. Biogenic amines and active polypeptides of the amphibian skin. *A. Rev. Pharmac.*, **1971**, *11*, 327–350.

Euler, U. S. von. The First Heymans Memorial Lecture. Some aspects of the actions of prostaglandins. *Archs int. Pharmacodyn. Thér.*, **1973**, *202*, Suppl., 295–307.

Ferreira, S. H., and Vane, J. R. New aspects of the mode of action of nonsteroid anti-inflammatory drugs. *A. Rev. Pharmac.*, **1974**, *14*, 57–73.

Fisher, J. W. (ed.). *Kidney Hormones.* Academic Press, Inc., New York, **1971**.

Flower, R. J. Drugs which inhibit prostaglandin biosynthesis. *Pharmac. Rev.*, **1974**, *26*, 33–67.

Frey, E. K.; Kraut, H.; and Werle, E. *Das Kallikrein-Kinin System.* Ferdinand Enke Verlag, Stuttgart, **1968**.

Ganong, W. F. Biogenic amines, sympathetic nerves, and renin secretion. *Fedn Proc. Fedn Am. Socs exp. Biol.*, **1973**, *32*, 1782–1784.

Genest, J.; Nowaczynski, W.; Koiw, E.; Sandor, T.; and Biron, P. Adrenocortical function in essential hypertension. In, *Essential Hypertension: An International Symposium.* (Buchborn, C., and Bock, K. D., eds.) Springer-Verlag, Berlin, **1960**, pp. 126–146.

Gross, F. The regulation of aldosterone secretion by the renin-angiotensin system under various conditions. *Acta endocr., Copenh.*, **1968**, Suppl. 124, 41–64.

———. Angiotensin. In, *Pharmacology of Naturally Occurring Polypeptides and Lipid-Soluble Acids*, Vol. 1. *International Encyclopedia of Pharmacology and Therapeutics*, Sect. 72. (Walker, J. M., ed.) Pergamon Press, Ltd., Oxford, **1971**, pp. 73–286.

Gross, F., and Möhring, J. Renal pharmacology, with special emphasis on aldosterone and angiotensin. *A. Rev. Pharmac.*, **1973**, *13*, 57–90.

Guyton, A. C.; Coleman, T. G.; and Granger, H. J. Circulation: overall regulation. *A. Rev. Physiol.*, **1972**, *34*, 13–46.

Haddy, F. J.; Emerson, T. E., Jr.; Scott, J. B.; and Daugherty, R. M. The effect of the kinins on the cardiovascular system. In, *Bradykinin, Kallidin and Kallikrein.* (Erdös, E. G., ed.) *Handb. exp. Pharmak.*, Vol. 25. Springer-Verlag, Berlin, **1970**, pp. 362–384.

Hedqvist, P. Autonomic neurotransmission. In, *The Prostaglandins*, Vol. 1. (Ramwell, P. W., ed.) Plenum Press, New York, **1973**, pp. 101–132.

Hittelman, K. J., and Butcher, R. W. Cyclic AMP and the mechanism of action of the prostaglandins. In, *The Prostaglandins: Pharmacological and Therapeutic Advances.* (Cuthbert, M. F., ed.) J. B. Lippincott Co., Philadelphia, **1973**, pp. 151–166.

Horton, E. W. Hypotheses on physiological roles of prostaglandins. *Physiol. Rev.*, **1969**, *49*, 122–161.

———. *Prostaglandins. Monographs on Endocrinology*, Vol. 7. Springer-Verlag, Berlin, **1972a**.

———. The prostaglandins. *Proc. R. Soc., B*, **1972b**, *182*, 411–426.

Kahn, R. H., and Lands, W. E. M. (eds.). *Prostaglandins and Cyclic AMP: Biological Actions and Clinical Applications.* Academic Press, Inc., New York, **1973**.

Karim, S. M. M. Prostaglandins and human reproduction: physiological roles and clinical uses of prostaglandins in relation to human reproduction. In, *The Prostaglandins: Progress in Research.* (Karim, S. M. M., ed.) John Wiley & Sons, Inc., New York, **1972**, pp. 71–164.

Karim, S. M. M., and Hillier, K. Pharmacology and therapeutic applications of prostaglandins in the human reproductive system. In, *The Prostaglandins: Pharmacological and Therapeutic Advances.* (Cuthbert, M. F., ed.) J. B. Lippincott Co., Philadelphia, **1973**, pp. 167–200.

Kellermeyer, R. W., and Graham, R. C., Jr. Kinins: possible physiologic and pathologic roles in man. *New Engl. J. Med.*, **1968**, *279*, 754–759, 802–809, 859–866.

Khairallah, P. A. The pharmacology of angiotensin. In, *Kidney Hormones.* (Fisher, J. W., ed.) Academic Press, Inc., New York, **1971**, pp. 130–172.

Khosla, M. C.; Smeby, R. R.; and Bumpus, F. M. Structure-activity relationship in angiotensin II analogs. In, *Angiotensin.* (Page, I. H., and Bumpus, F. M., eds.) *Handb. exp. Pharmak.*, Vol. 37. Springer-Verlag, Berlin, **1974**, pp. 126–161.

Kirkendall, W. M., and Overturf, M. Plasma renin activity and systemic arterial hypertension. In, *Modern Concepts of Cardiovascular Disease.* (Oglesby, P., ed.) American Heart Association, Inc., New York, **1973**, pp. 47–52.

Labhsetwar, A. P. Prostaglandins and the reproductive cycle. *Fedn Proc. Fedn Am. Socs exp. Biol.*, **1974**, *33*, 61–77.

Laragh, J. H.; Baer, L.; Brunner, H. R.; Buhler, F. R.; Sealey, J. E.; and Vaughan, E. D., Jr. Renin, angiotensin and aldosterone system in pathogenesis and management of hypertensive vascular disease. *Am. J. Med.*, **1972**, *52*, 633–652.

Ledingham, J. G., and Leary, W. P. Catabolism of angiotensin II. In, *Angiotensin.* (Page, I. H., and Bumpus, F. M., eds.) *Handb. exp. Pharmak.*, Vol. 37. Springer-Verlag, Berlin, **1974**, pp. 111–125.

Lee, J. Prostaglandins as therapeutic agents. *Archs intern. Med.*, **1973**, *131*, 294–300.

Lee, J. B. Cardiovascular-renal effects of prostaglandins. *Archs intern. Med.*, **1974**, *133*, 56–76.

Lepow, I. H., and Ward, P. A. (eds.). *Inflammation: Mechanisms and Control.* Academic Press, Inc., New York, **1972**.

Lewis, G. P. Pharmacologically active polypeptides. In, *Recent Advances in Pharmacology.* (Robson, J. M., and

Stacey, R. S., eds.) J. & A. Churchill, Ltd., London, 1968, pp. 213–246.

Lim, R. K. S. Pain. *A. Rev. Physiol.,* 1970, *32,* 269–288.

Lowenstein, J. Renin assay in hypertensive disease. *A. Rev. Med.,* 1972, *23,* 333–342.

McGiff, J. C. Tissue hormones: angiotensin, bradykinin and the regulation of regional blood flows. *Med. Clins N. Am.,* 1968, *52,* 263–281.

McGiff, J. C.; Crowshaw, K.; and Itskovitz, H. D. Prostaglandins and renal function. *Fedn Proc. Fedn Am. Socs exp. Biol.,* 1974, *33,* 39–47.

Melmon, K. L., and Cline, M. J. Kinins. *Am. J. Med.,* 1967, *43,* 153–160.

Melmon, K. L.; Cline, M. J.; Hughes, T.; and Nies, A. S. Kinins: possible mediators of neonatal circulatory changes in man. *J. clin. Invest.,* 1968, *47,* 1295–1302.

Mody, N. J. Effects of prostaglandins on platelet function. In, *The Prostaglandins: Progress in Research.* (Karim, S. M. M., ed.) John Wiley & Sons, Inc., New York, 1972, pp. 239–262.

Movat, H. Z. Chemical mediators of the vascular phenomena of the acute inflammatory reaction and of immediate hypersensitivity. *Med. Clins N. Am.,* 1972, *56,* 541–556.

Muirhead, E. E. Vasoactive and anti-hypertensive effects of prostaglandins and other renomedullary lipids. In, *The Prostaglandins: Pharmacological and Therapeutic Advances.* (Cuthbert, M. F., ed.) J. B. Lippincott Co., Philadelphia, 1973, pp. 201–252.

Nakano, J. General pharmacology of prostaglandins. In, *The Prostaglandins: Pharmacological and Therapeutic Advances.* (Cuthbert, M. F., ed.) J. B. Lippincott Co., Philadelphia, 1973, pp. 23–124.

Nakano, J., and Koss, M. C. Pathophysiologic roles of prostaglandins and the action of aspirin-like drugs. *Sth. med. J., Birmingham,* 1973, *66,* 709–721.

Page, I. H., and Bumpus, F. M. (eds.). *Angiotensin. Handb. exp. Pharmak.,* Vol. 37. Springer-Verlag, Berlin, 1974.

Parker, C. W., and Snider, D. E. Prostaglandins and asthma. *Ann. intern. Med.,* 1973, *78,* 963–965.

Peach, M. J. Adrenal medulla. In, *Angiotensin.* (Page, I. H., and Bumpus, F. M., eds.) *Handb. exp. Pharmak.,* Vol. 37. Springer-Verlag, Berlin, 1974, pp. 400–416.

Pharriss, B. B., and Behrman, H. R. Gonadal function. In, *The Prostaglandins,* Vol. 1. (Ramwell, P. W., ed.) Plenum Press, New York, 1973, pp. 347–364.

Piper, P. J. Distribution and metabolism. In, *The Prostaglandins: Pharmacological and Therapeutic Advances.* (Cuthbert, M. F., ed.) J. B. Lippincott Co., Philadelphia, 1973, pp. 125–150.

Pisano, J. J. Kinins of non-mammalian origin. In, *Bradykinin, Kallidin and Kallikrein.* (Erdös, E. G., ed.) *Handb. exp. Pharmak.,* Vol. 25. Springer-Verlag, Berlin, 1970, pp. 589–595.

Ramwell, P. W. (ed.). *The Prostaglandins,* Vol. 1. Plenum Press, New York, 1973.

Ramwell, P. W., and Shaw, J. E. (eds.). Prostaglandins. *Ann. N.Y. Acad. Sci.,* 1971, *180,* 1–568.

Robertson, A. L., and Khairallah, P. A. Effects of angiotensin II on the permeability of the vascular wall. In, *Angiotensin.* (Page, I. H., and Bumpus, F. M., eds.) *Handb. exp. Pharmak.,* Vol. 37. Springer-Verlag, Berlin, 1974, pp. 500–510.

Rocha e Silva, M.; Beraldo, W. T.; and Rosenfeld, G. Bradykinin, a hypotensive and smooth muscle stimulating factor released from plasma globulin by snake venoms and by trypsin. *Am. J. Physiol.,* 1949, *156,* 261–273.

Rocha e Silva, M., and Garcia Leme, J. *Chemical Mediators of the Acute Inflammatory Reaction.* Pergamon Press, Ltd., Oxford, 1972.

Roth, R. H. Action of angiotensin on adrenergic nerve endings: enhancement of norepinephrine biosynthesis. *Fedn Proc. Fedn Am. Socs exp. Biol.,* 1972, *31,* 1358–1364.

Rudolph, A. M. Changes in the circulation after birth. *Circulation,* 1970, *41,* 343–359.

Ryan, J. W. The fate of angiotensin II. In, *Angiotensin.* (Page, I. H., and Bumpus, F. M., eds.) *Handb. exp. Pharmak.,* Vol. 37. Springer-Verlag, Berlin, 1974, pp. 81–110.

Samuelsson, B. Biosynthesis of prostaglandins. *Fedn Proc. Fedn Am. Socs exp. Biol.,* 1972, *31,* 1442–1460.

Sander, G. E., and Huggins, C. G. Vasoactive peptides. *A. Rev. Pharmac.,* 1972, *12,* 227–264.

Sanner, J. H. Substances that inhibit the actions of prostaglandins. *Archs intern. Med.,* 1974, *133,* 133–146.

Schachter, M. Kinins: a group of active peptides. *A. Rev. Pharmac.,* 1964, *4,* 281–292.

———. Kallikreins and kinins. *Physiol. Rev.,* 1969, *49,* 510–547.

Schröder, E. Structure-activity relationships of kinins. In, *Bradykinin, Kallidin and Kallikrein.* (Erdös, E. G., ed.) *Handb. exp. Pharmak.,* Vol. 25. Springer-Verlag, Berlin, 1970, pp. 324–350.

Severs, W. B., and Daniels-Severs, A. E. Effects of angiotensin on the central nervous system. *Pharmac. Rev.,* 1973, *25,* 415–449.

Share, L., and Claybaugh, J. R. Regulation of body fluids. *A. Rev. Physiol.,* 1972, *34,* 235–260.

Skeggs, L. T.; Dorer, F. E.; Kahn, J. R.; Lentz, K. E.; and Levine, M. The biological production of angiotensin. In, *Angiotensin.* (Page, I. H., and Bumpus, F. M., eds.) *Handb. exp. Pharmak.,* Vol. 37. Springer-Verlag, Berlin, 1974, pp. 1–16.

Speroff, L., and Ramwell, P. W. Prostaglandins in reproductive physiology. *Am. J. Obstet. Gynec.,* 1970, *107,* 1111–1130.

Symposium. (Various authors.) Renin mechanisms and hypertension. *Circulation Res.,* 1967, *21,* Suppl. 2, 1–226.

Symposium. (Various authors.) Vasoactive peptides. *Fedn Proc. Fedn Am. Socs exp. Biol.,* 1968, *27,* 49–99.

Symposium. (Various authors.) Prostaglandins. *Fedn Proc. Fedn Am. Socs exp. Biol.,* 1974, *33,* 37–86.

Thurau, K. Intrarenal action of angiotensin. In, *Angiotensin.* (Page, I. H., and Bumpus, F. M., eds.) *Handb. exp. Pharmak.,* Vol. 37. Springer-Verlag, Berlin, 1974, pp. 475–499.

Tierney, D. F. Lung metabolism and biochemistry. *A. Rev. Physiol.,* 1974, *36,* 209–231.

Vander, A. J. Control of renin release. *Physiol. Rev.,* 1967, *47,* 359–382.

Vane, J. R. The release and fate of vaso-active hormones in the circulation. The Second Gaddum Memorial Lecture. *Br. J. Pharmac.,* 1969, *35,* 209–242.

———. The fate of angiotensin I. In, *Angiotensin.* (Page, I. H., and Bumpus, F. M., eds.) *Handb. exp. Pharmak.,* Vol. 37. Springer-Verlag, Berlin, 1974, pp. 17–40.

Walaszek, E. J. The effect of bradykinin and kallidin on smooth muscle. In, *Bradykinin, Kallidin and Kallikrein.* (Erdös, E. G., ed.) *Handb. exp. Pharmak.,* Vol. 25. Springer-Verlag, Berlin, 1970, pp. 430–433.

Webster, M. E. Recommendations for nomenclature and units. In, *Bradykinin, Kallidin and Kallikrein.* (Erdös, E. G., ed.) *Handb. exp. Pharmak.,* Vol. 25. Springer-Verlag, Berlin, 1970, pp. 659–665.

Webster, M. E., and Pierce, J. V. The nature of the kallidins released from human plasma by kallikreins and other enzymes. *Ann. N.Y. Acad. Sci.,* 1963, *104,* 91–107.

Weeks, J. R. Prostaglandins. *A. Rev. Pharmac.,* 1972, *12,* 317–336.

Werle, E. Discovery of the most important kallikreins and kallikrein inhibitors. In, *Bradykinin, Kallidin and Kallikrein.* (Erdös, E. G., ed.) *Handb. exp. Pharmak.,* Vol. 25. Springer-Verlag, Berlin, 1970, pp. 1–6.

Whitelocke, R. A. F.; Eakins, K. E.; and Bennett, A. Prostaglandins and the eye. *Proc. R. Soc. Med.,* 1973, *66,* 429–434.

Wilhelm, D. L. Kinins in human disease. *A. Rev. Med.,* 1971, *22,* 63–84.

Willoughby, D. A.; Giroud, J. P.; Di Rosa, M.; and Velo, G. P.   The control of the inflammatory response with special reference to the prostaglandins. In, *Prostaglandins and Cyclic AMP: Biological Actions and Clinical Applications.* (Kahn, R. H., and Lands, W. E. M., eds.) Academic Press, Inc., New York, 1973, pp. 187–206.

Wilson, D. E.   Prostaglandins. Their actions on the gastro-intestinal tract. *Archs intern. Med.,* **1974,** *133,* 112–118.

Zimmerman, B. G.; Gomer, S. K.; and Liao, J. C.   Action of angiotensin on vascular adrenergic nerve endings: facilitation of norepinephrine release. *Fedn Proc. Fedn Am. Socs exp. Biol.,* **1972,** *31,* 1344–1350.

Zurier, R. B.   Prostaglandins, inflammation and asthma. *Archs intern. Med.,* **1974,** *133,* 101–110.

Cardiovascular Drugs

A large number of drugs have as their major pharmacological action the ability to alter cardiovascular function; these agents will be considered in this section. Many additional drugs, however, also markedly influence the heart and blood vessels; they are described elsewhere in connection with their other important pharmacodynamic properties.

CHAPTER

31 DIGITALIS AND ALLIED CARDIAC GLYCOSIDES

Gordon K. Moe and Alfred E. Farah

Digitalis and certain closely allied drugs have in common a specific and powerful action on the myocardium that is unrivaled in value for the treatment of congestive heart failure. These cardiac drugs are found in a number of plants, but a few are also present in the venom of certain toads. The preparations commonly employed are obtained from digitalis and strophanthus; older preparations also came from squill. In the following discussion, the term *digitalis* is often used to designate the entire group of *cardiac glycosides* rather than those from digitalis alone. The description of the pharmacology and the uses of digitalis applies to all related cardiac glycosides unless otherwise stated.

History. A large number of plant extracts containing cardiac glycosides have been used by natives in various parts of the world as arrow and ordeal poisons. *Squill* was known as a medicine to the ancient Egyptians. The Romans employed it as a diuretic, heart tonic, emetic, and rat poison. *Strophanthus* was introduced into medicine by Sir Thomas Fraser (1890), who discovered its digitalis-like action while studying African arrow poisons. The dried skin of the common toad has been used for centuries as a drug by the Chinese. Powdered toad skins were also commonly employed in the folk medicine of Western countries for dropsy, until replaced by digitalis.

Digitalis, or foxglove, was mentioned in 1250 in the writings of Welsh physicians. It was described botanically 300 years later by Fuchsius (1542), who gave it the name *Digitalis purpurea.* Foxglove was used internally or locally for a number of unrelated diseases ranging from epilepsy to skin ulcers.

In 1785, William Withering published his famous book, entitled *An Account of the Foxglove and Some of Its Medical Uses: with Practical Remarks on Dropsy and Other Diseases.* Withering was aware that digitalis was effective only in certain forms of dropsy but apparently did not associate this with the cardiac actions of the drug. He recognized that the heart was affected, however, for he wrote, "It has a power over the motion of the heart to a degree yet unobserved in any other medicine, and this power may be converted to salutary ends." Apparently, John Ferriar in 1799 was the first to ascribe to digitalis a primary action on the heart and to relegate the diuretic effect to a position of secondary importance. Whereas Withering recorded the benefits to be derived from the proper use of foxglove, his advice was not always heeded. Even during the nineteenth century, digitalis was used indiscriminately for many disorders, often in toxic doses. During the early twentieth century, as a result of the work of Cushny, Mackenzie, Lewis, and others, the drug gradually came to be looked upon as a specific in the treatment of atrial fibrillation. Only within the last 60 years has it become firmly established that the main value of digitalis is in the therapy of congestive heart failure.

Sources and Composition of the Digitalis Principles. Official digitalis is the dried leaf of the foxglove plant, *Digitalis purpurea*. Seeds and leaves of a number of other digitalis species also contain active cardiac principles. *Digitalis lanata* leaves are used in Europe and are the source of certain purified preparations employed in the United States. The formerly official strophanthus is obtained from the seeds of the *Strophanthus Kombé* or *hispidus*. Official ouabain is derived from *Strophanthus gratus*. Squill, the dried, fleshy bulb of the "sea onion," comes from *Urginea (Scilla) maritima*. Another member of this same family, *Convallaria majalis* (lily of the valley), yields a cardiac glycoside, convallatoxin, which is not employed clinically but which possesses potent characteristic digitalis-like activity. Belonging to the same family as the *Strophanthus* plant is a tropical tree, *Thevetia neriifolia* (yellow oleander), the fruit of which contains thevetin, a glycoside that has had desultory clinical trial. Many other plants, including certain members of the Helleborus family, contain cardiac glycosides, none of which has clinical value.

Chemical Nature and Properties of the Cardiac Glycosides. Each glycoside represents the combination of an *aglycone*, or *genin*, with from one to four molecules of sugar (Table 31–1). The pharmacological activity resides in the aglycone, but the particular sugars attached to the aglycone modify the water solubility, cell penetrability, and potency of the resulting glycoside. The major contributions to this field have been reviewed by Chen and Henderson (1954), Fieser and Fieser (1959), and Marshall (1970). The following discussion is only a brief outline of the salient features.

The aglycones can be released from the cardiac glycosides by hydrolysis. They are chemically related to bile acids, sterols, and sex and adrenocortical hormones. The basic structure is a cyclopentanoperhydrophenanthrene nucleus to which is attached an unsaturated lactone ring at C 17. In addition, methyl, hydroxyl, and aldehyde groups are attached in specific positions that vary with the particular aglycone. All the naturally occurring aglycones carry OH groups at position 14 and many have additional OH groups, particularly at position 3, where the sugar moieties are usually attached. The hydroxyl group at C 3 is highly reactive, and semisynthetic derivatives have been made by reaction of aglycones with organic acids, sugars, xanthine, and other

Table 31–1. BOTANICAL SOURCES AND MAJOR CHEMICAL COMPONENTS OF CARDIAC GLYCOSIDES OF CLINICAL IMPORTANCE

PLANT SOURCE	PRECURSOR GLYCOSIDE	SPLIT OFF BY ENZYMATIC AND MILD ALKALINE HYDROLYSIS *	GLYCOSIDE	SPLIT OFF BY ACID HYDROLYSIS *	AGLYCONE, OR GENIN
DIGITALIS — *D. purpurea* (leaf)	Purpurea-glycoside A (deacetyldigilanid A)	Glucose	Digitoxin	Digitoxose (3)	Digitoxigenin
	Purpurea-glycoside B (deacetyldigilanid B)	Glucose	Gitoxin	Digitoxose (3)	Gitoxigenin
		———	Gitalin	Digitoxose (2)	Gitaligenin (gitoxigenin hydrate)
D. lanata (leaf)	Lanatoside A (digilanid A)	Glucose + acetic acid	Digitoxin	Digitoxose (3)	Digitoxigenin
	Lanatoside B (digilanid B)	Glucose + acetic acid	Gitoxin	Digitoxose (3)	Gitoxigenin
	Lanatoside C (digilanid C; cedilanid)	Glucose + acetic acid	Digoxin	Digitoxose (3)	Digoxigenin
STROPHANTHUS — *S. Kombé* (seed)	K-strophanthoside	Glucose	K-strophanthin-β (strophanthin)	Glucose + cymarose	Strophanthidin
	K-strophanthoside	Glucose (2)	Cymarin	Cymarose	Strophanthidin
	K-strophanthin-β	Glucose	Cymarin	Cymarose	Strophanthidin
		———	Cymarol	Cymarose	Strophanthidol
S. gratus (seed)	———	———	Ouabain (G-strophanthin)	Rhamnose	Ouabagenin (G-strophanthidin)
SCILLA (SQUILL) — *Urginea maritima* or *indica* (bulb)	Scillaren A	Glucose	Proscillaridin A	Rhamnose	Scillaridin A

* One mole of sugar or acetic acid is split off, unless the number of moles is otherwise indicated in parentheses.

agents. *Acetylstrophanthidin* is one such semisynthetic derivative. It is not employed clinically but is widely used for experimental purposes because of its rapid onset and short duration of action. The number and the position of other OH groups are important for determining aqueous versus lipid solubility, protein binding, metabolic disposition, and duration of action. Most cardiac aglycones have an angular CH_3 group at C 10, but an aldehyde or alcohol grouping is present in a few. Favorable spatial arrangement in the steroid ring system is also required (Tamm, 1963). A number of naturally occurring cardiac aglycones have been compared with the corresponding glycosides for cardiac activity in animals. In general, the aglycones are more transient and less potent in their myocardial actions but cause similar toxic effects.

The unsaturated lactone ring attached to C 17 possesses the $\Delta^{\alpha,\beta}$ structure, and may be five or six membered. Saturation of the lactone ring reduces activity by tenfold or more, and increases the speed of development of the cardiac actions (Vick *et al.*, 1957); opening of the ring completely abolishes activity.

The structural formulas of *digitoxigenin* and *scillaridin A*, representative cardiac aglycones from the digitalis-strophanthus and the squill–toad venom groups, respectively, are as follows:

Digitoxigenin

Scillaridin A

The essential features of the botanical sources and the component chemical parts of the major cardiac glycosides are summarized in Table 31–1. A special reason for such a tabular summary is the fact that the terminology employed in the literature is confusing and awkward, particularly because the names refer not to chemical structures but to botanical origins. Table 31–1 reveals that the leaves of *D. purpurea* and *D. lanata* yield the same two glycosides—*digitoxin* and *gitoxin*—but that each species, in addition, contains a glycoside not occurring in the other. It has been shown that the cardiac glycosides exist in plants as precursors, called "native," "natural," or "genuine" glycosides. For example, *D. lanata* leaves contain precursors termed *lanatosides* (or digilanids) A, B, and C; upon mild alkaline hydrolysis (loss of acetyl group) and enzymatic hydrolysis (loss of glucose), they yield *digitoxin, gitoxin,* and

digoxin, respectively. Subsequent acid hydrolysis splits off the sugars (digitoxoses) and yields the corresponding aglycones. In *D. purpurea* leaves, however, the precursor glycosides contain no acetyl groups and no analog of lanatoside C; they are known as deacetyldigilanids A and B, and upon enzymatic hydrolysis yield digitoxin and gitoxin, respectively. In addition, this species contains an amorphous mixture of glycosides (*gitalin*) not found in the *D. lanata* leaf.

CARDIOVASCULAR PROPERTIES OF DIGITALIS GLYCOSIDES

The main pharmacodynamic property of digitalis is its ability to increase the force of myocardial contraction. The salutary effects of the drug in congestive heart failure—increased cardiac output; decreased heart size, venous pressure, and blood volume; diuresis and relief of edema—are all explained on the basis of increased contractile force, *a positive inotropic action.*

Because digitalis often dramatically slows the ventricular rate in atrial fibrillation, it was believed for many years that the main effect of the drug was to slow the heart rate. Starting perhaps with Wenckebach in 1910 and continuing with the clinical observations of numerous subsequent investigators, the conviction grew and finally became firmly established that digitalis was effective chiefly in congestive heart failure regardless of cardiac rhythm, and that it brought relief not by virtue of cardiac slowing but by its direct action to increase the force of myocardial contraction.

Cardiac Contractility. The action of digitalis upon the force of systolic contraction has been demonstrated in a variety of preparations of heart muscle and in intact animals and man (*see* Figure 31–1). This effect is clearly independent of extracardiac factors. Cardiac glycosides exert their inotropic stimulation by increasing the rate at which tension or force is developed, not by prolonging the duration of the contractile process (Siegel and Sonnenblick, 1963). The maximal force or tension generated is increased in spite of abbreviation of all phases of systole (Wallace *et al.*, 1963).

The positive inotropic effect of digitalis is not dependent on catecholamine liberation or potentiation, for it can be demonstrated in chronically reserpinized dogs and in the

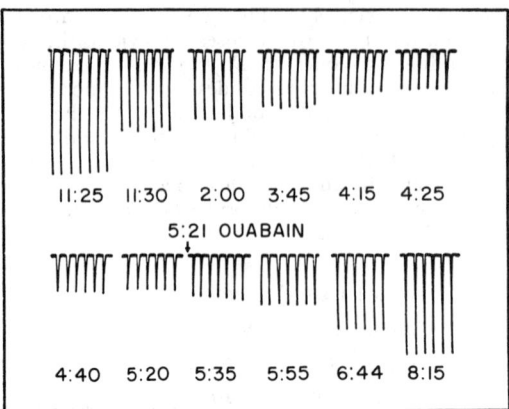

Figure 31-1. *The effect of ouabain on force of contraction of an isolated papillary muscle from the right ventricle of a cat heart.*

The muscle was prepared for isometric recording of contractions induced by rhythmic electrical stimulation. Systolic tension of the muscle, recorded as a downward deflection, decreased spontaneously during 6 hours of perfusion. The addition of ouabain in a concentration of 13 μg per liter (22 nM) restored the force of contraction. (After Gold and Cattell, 1940. Courtesy of the *Archives of Internal Medicine.*)

presence of β-adrenergic blocking agents (Fawaz, 1967).

The force of systolic contraction of the normal heart is under adrenergic neural control. In addition, the heart possesses an intrinsic mechanism for adapting its work output to the load imposed upon it. At any given level of adrenergic influence, the force of contraction of the ventricles increases, within limits, as the initial fiber length or tension just preceding systole increases (Starling's "law of the heart"). In other words, an increase in the end-diastolic volume of the ventricles, or an increased end-diastolic pressure, will be accompanied by an increased work capacity of the muscle. In the failing heart, the work capacity of the ventricle at any given end-diastolic volume or pressure is diminished. The resulting reduction of systolic ejection (stroke volume) leads to an increased residual blood volume within the ventricles at the end of systole. If blood continues to enter the ventricle during diastole at the same rate, the end-diastolic volume and pressure will correspondingly increase; hence, the ventricles must dilate. At the resulting increased fiber tension, an increased

force of systole may be developed (again, within limits). So long as there is any "cardiac reserve" (which may be defined loosely as the degree to which further dilatation can accomplish an increased work output), the heart will compensate for its diminished work capacity by progressive dilatation; this, in turn, will be accompanied (indeed, *caused*) by an increase in the "filling" pressure, reflected as an increased central and peripheral venous pressure. Other compensatory mechanisms are involved, of course, in the chronic adjustment to impaired cardiac function. These include sympathetically mediated reflex increase of heart rate and venomotor tone, and increase in peripheral arteriolar resistance; such responses aid in the maintenance of cardiac output and arterial pressure. Increase in arteriolar resistance in the kidney diverts a large fraction of the renal blood flow to other organs, and the homeostatic functions of the kidney are impaired to the extent that retention of electrolytes and water results.

When digitalis acts to increase the force of systolic contraction, the process described above is reversed. At any given end-diastolic volume or pressure, the increased work capacity permits more nearly complete systolic emptying; the residual systolic blood volume is diminished; the dilatation of the heart is reduced; the venous pressure declines; the reflex cardioacceleration and the arteriolar and venous constriction are diminished; the renal blood flow is increased; and the accumulated salt and water are excreted.

Cardiac Output. In spite of repeated demonstrations of the action of digitalis upon the contractile force of the heart muscle in many varied experimental preparations, it took many years to overcome arguments that the salutary action of the drug in congestive heart failure in man is due to some other action of the drug. After all, Withering himself believed its primary effect was on the kidneys. Mention has already been made of the emphasis long placed upon cardiac slowing as the primary therapeutic action. These arguments have been based in part upon incomplete knowledge of the pathophysiology of heart failure, and in part upon experimental observations made in situations not germane to the problem. Some of the observations may be cited to illustrate the historical development of our present understanding of the importance of the positive inotropic action of the drug.

Action upon "Cardiac Tone." In one of the earliest experimental studies of digitalis, Vulpian observed in 1855 that the drug caused systolic contracture of the frog heart. On the assumption that the failing heart is inefficient *because* it is enlarged, it was taught for many years that digitalis improved cardiac function by reducing cardiac size, a "tonic" effect of the drug. If tone is defined as resistance to stretch, then digitalis does indeed increase the tone of the muscle during *systole;* that is, the force of systolic contraction is increased. But digitalis does not increase the resistance to stretch of the ventricles in *diastole,* not even, except in high concentrations, in the amphibian heart (Kabat and Visscher, 1939). As mentioned above, the failing heart is enlarged *because it is inefficient,* not the reverse; digitalis reduces the size of the failing heart *because it increases the contractile power,* not the reverse.

Action upon Venous Return. Observations that digitalis increases the force of systolic contraction of isolated heart muscle and increases the output of the failing heart in heart-lung preparations cannot be taken as direct evidence that the drug will increase the output of the human heart in failure, for the output of the heart in the intact state is not determined solely by the contractility of the ventricles but is also influenced by total peripheral resistance, blood volume, venomotor "tone," heart rate, and nervous and hormonal agencies. Early studies by Harrison and Leonard (1926) showed that digitalis *decreased* the output of the nonfailing heart in normal dogs. Repeated confirmation of this observation resulted in the conclusion that digitalis reduces venous return, presumably by an action upon the venous capacitance vessels of the circulation (Cohn and Stewart, 1928; Dock and Tainter, 1930; Katz et al., 1938; Cotten and Stopp, 1958). Similar results were obtained in normal human subjects (Stewart and Cohn, 1932; Bing et al., 1950; Williams et al., 1958). In the meantime, many observations showed beyond question that digitalis increases the output of the heart in patients with right, left, or combined ventricular failure. As a result of such observations, the conviction grew that digitalis, although useful in heart failure, had a deleterious effect upon the normal heart, or had an action upon the peripheral veins that obscured or opposed its myocardial effects in the normal subject. For example, it was suggested that digitalis decreased the size of the failing heart toward a more optimal level, but decreased the size of the normal heart below this optimum (Stewart and Cohn, 1932). This would imply a primary action upon cardiac "tone," as described above.

The concept of an extracardiac action upon the peripheral veins received its greatest impetus when it was reported that intravenous administration of digoxin to patients with congestive heart failure caused a reduction of central venous pressure before a measurable increase of cardiac output occurred (McMichael and Sharpey-Schafer, 1944). When the same laboratory reported that venesection also reduced the right atrial pressure and increased the cardiac output in patients in advanced heart failure, it was again suggested that the primary action of digitalis was to diminish venomotor tone, resulting in a "physiological venesection" (Howarth et al., 1946). Explanation of these results was sought in the observations of Patterson and Starling (1914): the output of the isolated heart increases to a maximum and then declines as the venous filling pressure is increased. The failing human heart was assumed to be "over the hump" of the Starling curve, that is, in a state in which reduction of venous pressure could result in an increased cardiac output (*see* Figure 31–3).

If digitalis acted primarily to increase the capacity of the veins, then it could increase cardiac output *only* if the heart were "over the hump," that is, in a state in which cardiac reserve is exhausted. At any level of filling pressure less than that at which maximal output is achieved, a primary reduction of venous pressure would reduce the output.

Within the past few decades, and on the basis of many more studies of digitalis action in the normal state and various stages of cardiac insufficiency, it has become firmly established that digitalis increases the ability of the heart to perform work *at a given filling pressure.* The consequences of this action are illustrated in Figure 31–2; similar results have been obtained repeatedly (*see* Mason, 1973, 1974; Smith and Haber, 1973b).

Digitalis acts not to shift the status of the heart from one point to another on a single curve relating ventricular work to filling pressure, but to shift it to a different member of a continuous family of curves (Figure 31–3). This was demonstrated in the normal dog by Cotten and Stopp (1958). Although digitalis reduced cardiac output and atrial pressures in their experiments, the "function" curve relating left ventricular work to left atrial filling pressure was shifted in the direction of improved contractility. A direct effect of the drug upon contractility of the human heart was subsequently demonstrated (Braunwald et al., 1961; Mason, 1966). In other words, cardiac output may be improved in patients with left ventricular hypertrophy in whom the cardiac reserve at rest has been reduced but not yet exhausted. In support of this concept, Selzer and Malmborg (1962) found that digoxin caused a significant increase of cardiac output in a majority of subjects with "latent" heart failure, that is, in subjects who had heart disease but

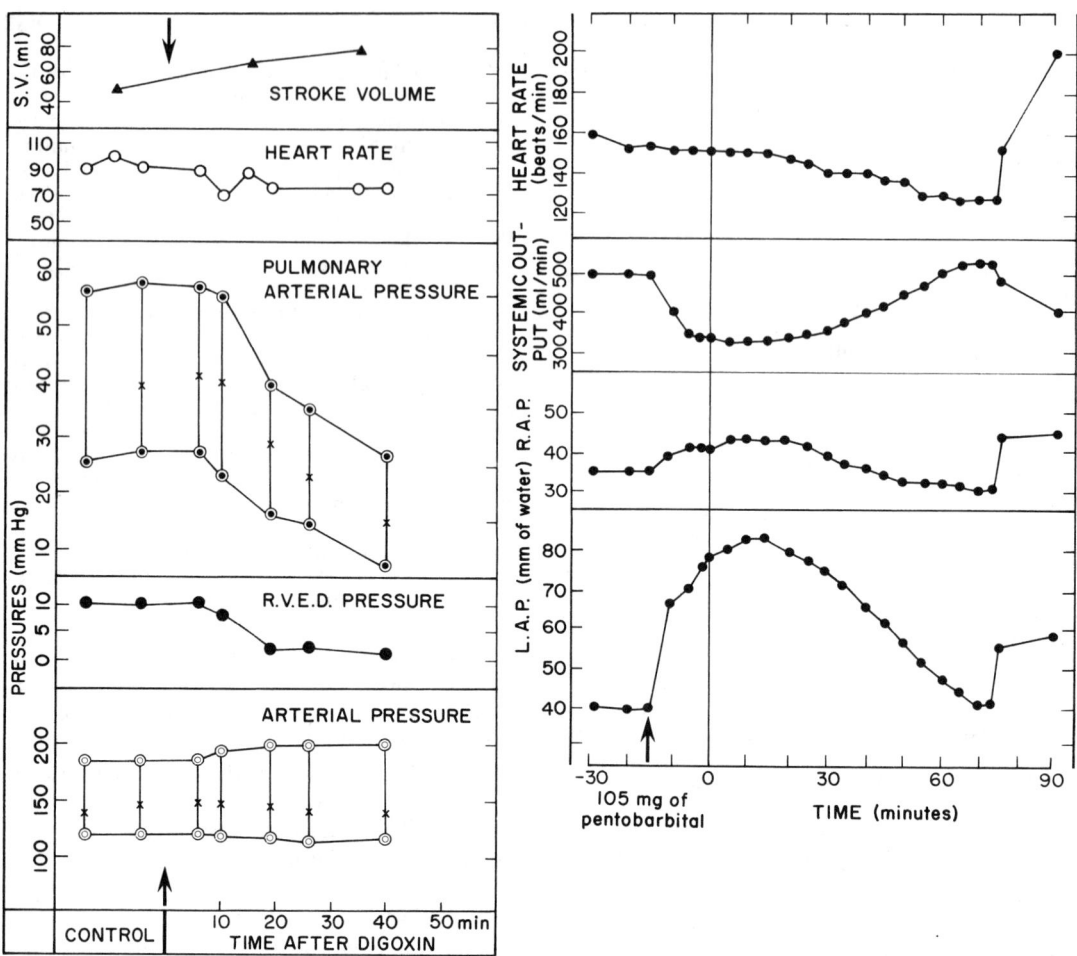

Figure 31-2. *Left.* *Effects of digoxin in a patient with combined right and left ventricular failure and hypertensive cardiovascular disease.*

In addition to systemic hypertension the patient had a reduced cardiac output and pulmonary hypertension. After intravenous digoxin (1.5 mg), cardiac output and stroke volume increased to normal, pulmonary arterial and right ventricular end-diastolic (R.V.E.D.) pressure decreased to normal, and the heart rate decreased to normal. Note the stroke work of the left ventricle was increased as the cardiac output was restored; the work load imposed on the right ventricle was sharply *reduced* by the reduction of pulmonary arterial pressure. (Modified from Harvey, Ferrer, Cathcart, and Alexander, 1951. Courtesy of *Circulation*.)

Right. *Effect of digoxin on experimental heart failure induced by pentobarbital in a dog heart-lung preparation.*

Ordinate scales, top to bottom: heart rate, cardiac output, right atrial pressure, left atrial pressure. At the vertical arrow, sodium pentobarbital was injected to induce heart failure, as evidenced by reduced output and elevated atrial pressures. At time "0" a constant infusion of digoxin was begun at the rate each minute of 0.13 μmole/kg of heart. Within 30 minutes, atrial pressures began to decline and cardiac output to rise. Infusion of the glycoside was continued to the point of toxic manifestations, indicated by the sudden increase of heart rate (ventricular tachycardia), accompanied by a deterioration of cardiac mechanical performance. Note the similarity between the therapeutic response in this preparation and that in the patient depicted in the companion segment of the figure. (After Farah and Maresh, 1948. Courtesy of the *Journal of Pharmacology and Experimental Therapeutics*.)

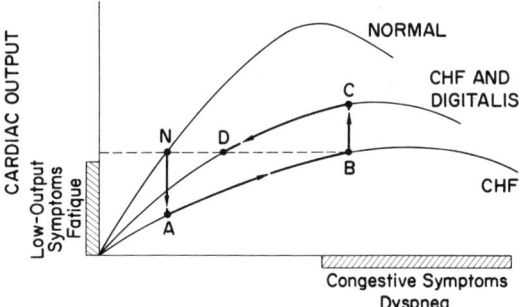

Figure 31-3. *Diagrammatic representation of the use of the Frank-Starling mechanism as a compensation for congestive heart failure.*

The three curves depict ventricular function in normal subjects and in those with congestive heart failure (CHF) and heart failure after treatment with digitalis. The points N through D represent in sequence: initial reduction of contractility due to congestive heart failure (N to A); use of Frank-Starling compensation to maintain cardiac output (A to B); increase in contractility when digitalis is administered (B to C); and reduction in the use of Frank-Starling compensation, which digitalis allows (C to D). Of note is the fact that points N, B, and D all lie on the same line in the vertical axis and thus all represent the same cardiac output, but each is on a different end-diastolic pressure on the horizontal axis. The levels at which symptoms of congestion, such as dyspnea, and symptoms of low cardiac output, such as fatigue, occur are represented by the cross-hatched areas. (After Mason, 1973. Courtesy of *The American Journal of Cardiology*.)

were not in failure and in whom a significant cardiac reserve remained. Finally, attention should be called to careful studies of the hemodynamic effects of cardiac glycosides in normal subjects. Dresdale and associates (1959) and Selzer and coworkers (1959) were unable to confirm the older observations of reduction of cardiac output in normal resting subjects. Both groups concluded that digitalis causes no significant hemodynamic changes in normal individuals.

These observations removed one of the major barriers to the understanding of the effects of digitalis in the human subject. Digitalis does not exert a fundamentally different action upon normal and failing hearts; it increases the contractility in both. The hemodynamic consequences of this action depend upon the status of the cardiovascular system at the time.

Digitalis causes an increase in total peripheral vascular resistance in *normal* subjects by a combination of a moderate direct vasoconstrictor action on both arteriolar and venous smooth muscle and a centrally mediated increase in sympathetic tone (*see* below). This opposes the increased cardiac contractility by increasing impedance to ventricular ejection; the two effects thus counteract each other, and there is essentially no change in cardiac output. In *congestive heart failure,* varying degrees of sympathetically mediated peripheral vasoconstriction already exist as part of the compensatory response; with the increase in myocardial contractility produced by digitalization, the sympathetic hyperactivity is reflexly reduced. This more than compensates for the direct vasoconstrictor action of digitalis, and total peripheral resistance is reduced. Consequently, in congestive heart failure there is no peripheral impedance to increase in cardiac output, such as generally occurs in normal subjects. (*See* Mason, 1966, 1974; Mason *et al.,* 1971.)

In *summary,* while digitalis does not significantly alter cardiac output in human subjects without latent or overt heart failure, the increased cardiac output and work capacity uniformly observed in latent or overt heart failure are the result of a direct action upon cardiac contractility.

Cardiac Rate. In animals, digitalis slows the heart rate by an action mediated in part through the vagus nerve and in part through an extravagal action, which is still present in atropinized animals (McLain *et al.,* 1959). The vagal action is evoked to some extent reflexly by sensitization of the carotid baroreceptors, in part through an action upon receptors in the nodose ganglion, and in part by enhancement of the pacemaker response to acetylcholine (Gaffney *et al.,* 1958; Chai *et al.,* 1967). In relatively high doses digitalis reduces the chronotropic action of epinephrine and of sympathetic nerve stimulation (Méndez *et al.,* 1961a; Nadeau and James, 1963); this may constitute a major component of the extravagal action of the drug. Digitalis in high doses may completely suppress *apparent* pacemaker activity in isolated right atria, but this is probably due to S-A block rather than to actual arrest of the pacemaker cells; continuing activity of S-A nodal cells has been demonstrated in isolated atrial preparations at a time when the atrial muscle can no longer support propagated action potentials.

Cardiac slowing is not a significant feature of digitalis action in normal man (Dresdale *et al.*, 1959; Selzer *et al.*, 1959), but it commonly attends the use of digitalis in congestive heart failure. It is important to recognize that digitalis-induced improvement of the work capacity of the heart in failure may occur before or without a reduction of heart rate. Congestive failure in patients with normal sinus rhythm is often accompanied by tachycardia, along with vasoconstriction, as part of the reflex compensation for a reduction in cardiac output. Digitalis, by improving the cardiac output, will reduce the heart rate. The change in rate, in other words, is *secondary to the improvement of the circulation* and is not the primary therapeutic action of the drug. The point is an important one, for digitalis should not be used with the primary objective of reducing the heart rate when sinus tachycardia is present without evidence of myocardial failure. For example, the heart rate may be reflexly increased as a result of constrictive pericarditis or cardiac tamponade, without any impairment of cardiac contractility. Only toxic doses of digitalis would be likely to reduce the heart rate in such circumstances, and with deleterious results.

Although digitalis in therapeutic doses does not greatly reduce the rate of the heart in normal sinus rhythm, it has a pronounced effect on the ventricular rate in atrial fibrillation by the mechanism discussed below.

Effects on Cardiac Excitability, Conduction Velocity, Refractory Periods, and Automaticity. Because some of the therapeutic and most of the serious toxic effects of digitalis can be related to actions upon the electrophysiological properties of the heart, these actions of the drug have been extensively studied. Understanding of the cellular mechanisms involved has been greatly enhanced in recent years through the application of microelectrode technics to the study of isolated perfused preparations of cardiac tissue. The results obtained have been supplemented by intracardiac records of the electri-

cal behavior of the heart *in situ,* both in experimental animals and in man. The cyclical changes in the transmembrane electrical potential of a spontaneously depolarizing, or pacemaker, fiber of the myocardium (atrial, junctional, or ventricular) are depicted by the solid line of the middle panel of Figure 31-4, as is the concurrent unipolar ECG.

There is general agreement that the *toxic effects* of digitalis on the generation and conduction of cardiac impulses result from inhibition of Na^+,K^+-activated adenosine triphosphatase (Na,K-ATPase), which has been assigned a central role in the active transport of Na^+ and K^+ across the cardiac cell membrane. The possible involvement of this system in the production of increased cardiac contractility is more conjectural (*see* below). Inhibition of the transport mechanism (the "sodium pump") leads to an accumulation of intracellular Na^+, a decrease of intracellular K^+, and a corresponding reduction of the transmembrane potential difference. The direct actions of digitalis on the electrical properties of the heart, like those on the heart rate, are complicated by indirect and reflex actions; these are summarized in Table 31-2.

Cardiac Excitability. The *electrical excitability* of atrium and ventricle in the intact dog heart is slightly increased by lower doses of digitalis, but depressed by higher doses (Méndez and Méndez, 1957). The increased excitability is due largely to the decreased intracellular negativity during diastole (Figure 31-4). The atrium may be rendered electrically inexcitable by doses that do not prevent propagated idioventricular impulses. The specialized conducting pathways of the atria are more resistant than the "ordinary" atrial muscle. Purkinje fibers are gradually depolarized to the stage of inexcitability by high concentrations, but ventricular muscle fibers are more resistant. Thus, resistance to digitalis-induced inexcitability increases progressively from atrium to ventricle. (*See* reviews by Trautwein, 1963; Hoffman and Singer, 1964.)

Conduction Velocity. This property is affected differently in various cardiac tissues. Since the speed of impulse propagation must be a function of the threshold and also of the rate of rise and amplitude of the action potential, it is not surprising that the velocity

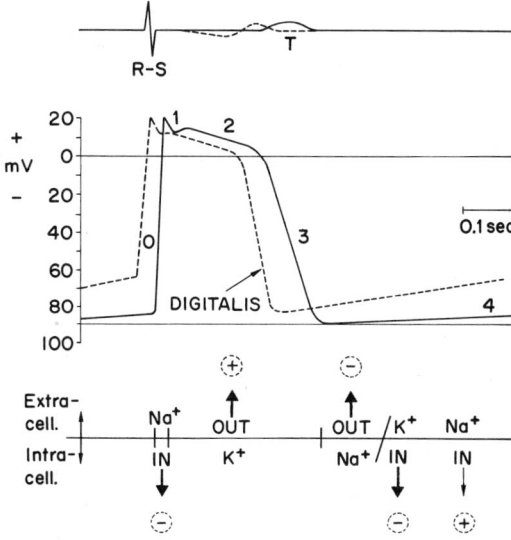

Figure 31-4. *Effects of digitalis on subsidiary pacemaker activity.*

The figure is a diagrammatic representation of the transmembrane electrical potential (middle panel), unipolar ECG (top), and transmembrane monovalent cation movements (bottom) of a spontaneously depolarizing conductive fiber in the atrial, junctional, or ventricular myocardium. In the top and middle panels the effects caused by digitalis are shown by broken lines. In the bottom panel, the sizes of the arrows are related to large or small movements of cations, and the effects of digitalis on the magnitudes of these cation movements are shown by the sign within the broken circles.

During diastole (phase 4), the net effect of the progressive fall in K^+ conductance (not shown) and the concomitant increase in the conductance and slow, passive influx of Na^+ is a gradual depolarization; when the latter reaches the threshold potential, a sudden marked increase in Na^+ permeability causes the rapid depolarization (phase 0), which constitutes the upsweep of the propagated action potential. This is succeeded by the relatively slow phases (1, 2, 3) of repolarization, during which there is a passive egress of K^+. During the plateau of phase 2, there is an inward flux of Ca^{2+}, which is probably an essential step in excitation-contraction coupling (Beeler and Reuter, 1970; New and Trautwein, 1972). The active extrusion of Na^+, coupled with the inward transport of K^+ (shown by the slash line), takes place largely during the early part of phase 4. (Modified from Mason, Zelis, Lee, Hughes, Spann, and Amsterdam, 1971. Courtesy of *The American Journal of Cardiology.*)

is slightly increased in atrium and ventricle by low doses, which increase excitability without reducing membrane-potential or

Table 31-2. SOME MAJOR EFFECTS OF DIGITALIS ON THE ELECTROPHYSIOLOGICAL PROPERTIES OF THE HEART

PROPERTY	EFFECT
Pacemaker Automaticity	
S-A node	→ ↓ (↑, after atropine or toxic doses)
Purkinje fibers	↑
Excitability	
Atrium	→ *
Ventricle	variable *
Purkinje fibers	↑ *
Membrane Responsiveness	
Atrium	variable * (↓, after atropine)
Ventricle	↓ (toxic doses)
Purkinje fibers	↓ (toxic doses)
Conduction Velocity	
Atrium, ventricle	↑ (slight) *
A-V node	↓
Purkinje fibers	↓
Effective Refractory Period	
Atrium	↓ (↑, after atropine)
Ventricle	↓
A-V node	↑
Purkinje fibers	↑ *

Key: The arrows indicate the direction, not the magnitude, of the changes indicated: ↑, increased; ↓, decreased; →, no significant change.
* Decreased with high or toxic doses of digitalis.

action-potential amplitude, and that, correspondingly, conduction is impaired to the point of failure of propagation in the atria when the excitability is depressed by toxic doses. In the ventricles, conduction is depressed in Purkinje fibers before conduction in muscle is seriously impaired (Moe and Méndez, 1951; Swain and Weidner, 1957). Conduction through the A-V node is depressed in isolated preparations and in the intact animal by both vagal and extravagal actions of the drug (Watanabe and Dreifus, 1966, 1970). The slowing of conduction reflects the digitalis-induced decrease in the rate of rise of the action potential (phase 0), which in turn is related to the decreased resting potential (Figure 31-4). In man, these actions are manifested by prolongation of the P-R interval. Intracardiac records of activity in the His (H) bundle localize the effect of moderate doses to the A-H interval, that is, to the node itself. Higher doses may cause prolongation of the H-V interval, reflecting depression of the specialized conduction tissue of the ventricle, and may also cause complete A-V block.

Refractory Periods. Digitalis exerts strikingly different effects upon the refractory periods of the various cardiac tissues. Under conditions that permit reflex vagal activity, digitalis shortens the atrial refractory period and markedly prolongs the functional refractory period of the A-V transmission system. In denervated or atropinized hearts, digitalis *increases* the atrial refractory period; the increase produced at the A-V node with moderate doses is reduced in magnitude by interruption of the vagi (Méndez and Méndez, 1953), and an atropine-insensitive action is prominent with doses bordering on the toxic, both in animals and in man (Gold *et al.,* 1939). The nonvagal effects of digitalis upon atrium and A-V node are due, at least in part, to an antiadrenergic action (Méndez *et al.,* 1961b).

In contrast to its direct effects upon atrial and nodal tissues, digitalis *shortens* the ventricular refractory period (Méndez and Méndez, 1953; Hoffman and Singer, 1964); the effect is accompanied by an abbreviation of the intracellularly recorded action potential, and is apparent in man as a reduced Q-T interval (Figure 31–4). Except for frequency-dependent changes in the refractory period, the ventricular effects of digitalis are not altered by the presence or absence of vagal influences.

Automaticity. Digitalis has profound effects upon automaticity, especially in the ventricles. The increase in automaticity at ectopic pacemaker sites is due to the increased rate of spontaneous diastolic depolarization during phase 4 (Rosen *et al.,* 1973; *see* Figure 31–4). Occasional premature beats may appear at a time when electrical excitability of the ventricle is slightly enhanced, but they increase in frequency as excitability declines with higher doses, until an idioventricular rhythm is manifest. This observation emphasizes the distinction that must be made between *excitability* and *automaticity* (Moe and Méndez, 1951). Ectopic impulse generation may be exposed at an early stage of digitalis intoxication by vagal stimulation, which allows enough time for an accelerated idioventricular focus to "escape" (Vassalle *et al.,* 1963), or by premature stimulation of the

ventricle followed by a compensatory pause, which also permits time for the focus to fire (Lown *et al.,* 1967).

Ectopic impulse generation can be evoked by digitalis in isolated preparations containing specialized conduction fibers of the atria (Hashimoto and Moe, 1973) or Purkinje fibers of the ventricle (Vassalle *et al.,* 1962); the muscle fibers of atria and ventricles depolarize to the stage of inexcitability without exhibiting spontaneous impulse generation. The mechanism of ectopic activity, both in isolated preparations and in the intact heart, has been ascribed to an acceleration of the normal but latent pacemaker activity of the specialized fibers. The accelerated focus is not inhibited by "overdriving"; that is, it does not exhibit the phenomenon of post-pacing depression that is characteristic of the phase-4 depolarization in the S-A node or in spontaneously active Purkinje fibers not exposed to digitalis (Wittenberg *et al.,* 1972; Ferrier *et al.,* 1973).

Digitalis-induced automatic activity in Purkinje fibers is enhanced by increased Ca^{2+} concentration and depressed by increased K^+; circumstantial evidence suggests that the transient depolarizations and the spontaneous responses they generate are due to a transient influx of Ca^{2+} (Ferrier and Moe, 1973).

The activity generated in isolated Purkinje fibers is clearly automatic rather than reentrant. By inference, the first signs of ectopic activity in the intact heart are probably also due to discharge of ectopic pacemakers within the conducting system. As toxicity advances, however, and further depolarization of the cell membrane occurs, conductivity is depressed; the two effects combine to set the stage for reentrant activity and ventricular fibrillation as a terminal event.

The action of digitalis upon automaticity in the intact heart is due, at least in part, to indirect actions mediated by the autonomic nervous system. When adrenergic influences are eliminated by denervation, cardiac arrest rather than fibrillation is often the terminal event (Erlij and Méndez, 1964). There is evidence that ouabain may itself increase preganglionic impulse traffic in cardiac sympathetic nerves as well as in the vagi (Gillis *et al.,* 1972). The β-adrenergic blocking agents offer some protection against digitalis-induced arrhythmias; however, this effect involves "quinidine-like" actions of these agents in addition to β-adrenergic blockade (*see* Chapter 32).

Mechanism of Cardiac Slowing in Atrial Fibrillation. In this arrhythmia the atrial "input" to the A-V transmission system is fractionated, irregular, and rapid, perhaps as high as 500 impulses per minute. Most of the atrial impulses either fail to enter the A-V node or are extinguished by decremental conduction within it. The ventricular rate is rapid and irregular—rapid because the A-V nodal input frequency is so high, and irregular because many impulses that enter the node but fail to emerge will, nevertheless, leave its upper margin refractory to the passage of subsequent impulses ("concealed A-V conduction"). The minimal interval between two ventricular responses will be determined by the effective refractory period of the A-V node; longer ventricular cycles will occur if one or more successive atrial responses enter the node but are extinguished within it. The *average* frequency of the ventricles in this disorder is determined by the conductivity of the A-V node. If vagal tone is high, the functional refractory period of the node is prolonged, the proportion of "concealed" impulses is increased, and the ventricular frequency is reduced; if adrenergic tone is high, the nodal refractory period is reduced and the ventricle accelerates. When fibrillation is accompanied by congestive failure, reflex reduction of vagal tone and increased sympathetic activity combine to increase the frequency with which impulses can traverse the node. The resulting increased frequency of the ventricle may further compromise the cardiac output. The ventricles beat irregularly, and often fire so early in diastole that no systolic ejection occurs (pulse deficit).

The action of digitalis on the ventricular rate in atrial fibrillation has long been attributed to an action upon the refractory period of the A-V node. The action is complex. Digitalis prolongs the apparent or functional refractory period of the A-V transmission system, in part by reflexly increasing vagal and reducing sympathetic activity, in part by a direct action upon the node, and also in part by antagonizing adrenergic influences on the node (Méndez *et al.,* 1961b). The vagal action, in turn, is in large measure the

result of improved contractility and cardiac output.

Increased vagal activity can reduce the ventricular rate in atrial fibrillation without prolonging the A-V functional refractory period. Increased vagal activity, by reducing the duration of the atrial refractory period, will *increase* the average frequency of discharges in the fibrillating atria. When the input frequency to the A-V node is thus increased, the chance of impulses entering the node at a time when they cannot traverse it completely is increased. In other words, the atrial margin of the node will more often be left refractory by "concealed" impulses, and the net ventricular frequency will diminish (Moe and Abildskov, 1964). In *summary,* digitalis reduces the ventricular rate in atrial fibrillation through vagal and extravagal influences that increase the effective refractory period of the A-V transmission system, and through a vagally mediated increase in the atrial frequency.

Action in Atrial Flutter. A circus-movement flutter about an obstacle of crushed atrial tissue in the dog heart will sustain itself at a stable frequency for hours, provided the path length (perimeter of the obstacle) is long enough to permit expiration of the refractory period between circuits (*see* Chapter 32). When such a flutter is established in an animal in which the vagi have been blocked, the administration of digitalis slows the flutter frequency and eventually restores normal sinus rhythm. In similar preparations in which the vagus nerves are intact, digitalis often converts the atrial flutter to atrial fibrillation. Administration of atropine may now restore normal rhythm. The explanation of these results may be found in the direct and indirect effects of digitalis upon the atrial refractory period. When the vagi are blocked, digitalis prolongs the refractory period; however, when the vagus supply is intact, the predominant action is abbreviation (Farah and Loomis, 1950). The vagal effects are not uniformly distributed; the atrial refractory period is greatly reduced at some points and not at all at others. As a result, the flutter wave front becomes fractionated and fibrillation occurs. Conversion of atrial flutter to atrial fibrillation is not uncommon in the clinical use of digitalis; when it occurs it is considered to be a fortunate result, for the ventricular rate is much easier to control during atrial fibrillation than during atrial flutter.

Blood Pressure. In both dogs and man with normal cardiac function, intravenous injection of the cardiac glycosides and particularly of the aglycones causes an elevation of arterial pressure, in part by a direct action on peripheral vessels and in part by central or reflex action (Cotten and Stopp, 1958; Williams *et al.*, 1958). The pressor response is transient as compared with the cardiac actions of the glycosides, probably as the result of reflex adjustments to the elevated pressure.

Mason and Braunwald (1964) found that intravenous injection of ouabain in normal human subjects increases mean arterial pressure, increases systemic vascular resistance, reduces forearm blood flow, and increases venomotor tone. Vasoconstriction occurs in the splanchnic vessels; attention has been called to the possibility of damage to the mesenteric bed when digitalis is used in individuals in whom the splanchnic circulation is already impaired, as in shock (Ulano *et al.*, 1971).

When cardiac output increases in patients with congestive failure, there is a reduction of peripheral resistance, an increase in blood flow, and a reduction of venomotor tone, for the reasons discussed previously, but frequently no increase in arterial pressure. The effects of digitalis upon arterial pressure in patients with congestive failure are variable, and are attributable to the effects upon the heart rather than to a vasoconstrictor action. Elevation of systolic pressure may occur as stroke volume is increased; pulse pressure may increase and diastolic pressure may fall as the circulation improves, tissue oxygenation increases, and reflex vasoconstriction diminishes. Hypertension does not constitute a contraindication to the use of digitalis; patients with hypertension and left ventricular failure may be greatly improved by digitalis therapy. (*See* Figure 31–2.)

Coronary Circulation. Bing and collaborators (1950) found no change in coronary flow or cardiac oxygen consumption in normal human subjects or in patients with heart failure following acute intravenous administration of the strophanthus glycosides. The agents used caused an increase in left ventricular stroke work in the patients in heart failure; the mechanical efficiency of the heart was accordingly increased. The effect on efficiency was undoubtedly related to the reduction in heart size and fiber tension associated with the positive inotropic action (*see* discussion of effects on cardiac energy metabolism, below).

Diuretic Action. Withering employed digitalis in dropsy, and for many years the foxglove was considered to be a diuretic. However, the effects of digitalis on urine flow are primarily the result of its action on the heart and the circulation. In normal persons or in patients with heart failure but without edema or serous effusions, no significant diuresis occurs after digitalis. In cases with anasarca from causes other than congestive heart failure, digitalis does not cause an increase in urine output. Furthermore, when digitalis fails to restore some measure of cardiac compensation in patients with cardiac edema, diuresis fails to develop. Diuresis is often one of the first prominent manifestations of digitalis action in edematous patients with congestive heart failure. Urine output may rise within 24 hours from 200 ml per day to 3 liters or more. The specific gravity of the urine falls, the daily excretion of electrolytes increases, the albuminuria diminishes, and renal clearance tests show improvement in function. The body weight falls even when the edema is occult, provided that there is improvement in the cardiac status. Despite the effect of digitalis therapy, roughly half of all patients require additional and specific measures to promote diuresis. These measures are discussed in Chapter 39.

There are two major causes of edema in heart failure. One cause is the increase in hydrostatic pressure in the capillaries, which retards the net rate of reabsorption of extracellular fluid. When failure is primarily in the left ventricle, pulmonary venous and capillary pressures rise; when the capillary pressure exceeds the osmotic pressure of the plasma proteins, pulmonary edema (accompanied by decreased vital capacity, rales, dyspnea, and cyanosis) occurs. If failure is limited to the right heart, edema occurs in the extrapulmonary tissues. The mechanisms involved are discussed in Chapter 39. As heart failure is relieved and venous pressure is reduced, the edema fluid returns to the blood. The resulting hydremia can often be detected by a fall in specific gravity of the plasma before diuresis is evident. Renal function may also be improved by the relief of vascular congestion in the kidney. The better appetite and the improved gastrointestinal and hepatic functions resulting from a return of cardiac compensation lead to an increase in the concentration of plasma protein, which may be sufficiently low in some patients with chronic congestive heart failure to contribute to edema formation.

A second major cause of cardiac edema results from a presumably compensatory renal mechanism. As the cardiac output diminishes, the renal blood flow and glomerular filtration rate are reduced. Reabsorption of sodium and water from the glomerular filtrate is more complete, and the retained salt and fluid may result in edema, frank or "occult," even without a significant elevation of systemic venous pressure. Increased secretion of aldosterone, together with increased renal sensitivity to mineralocorticoids, is also a major factor in the genesis of cardiac edema (Barger, 1960). The probable sequence of events is: decreased stroke volume → decreased baroreceptor activity → increased adrenergic discharge → decreased renal blood flow → decreased rate of glomerular filtration → increased renin production → increased angiotensin formation → increased aldosterone secretion → inappropriate renal reabsorption of sodium (*see* Davis, 1962). Striking increases in aldosterone secretion have been reported in dogs with experimental heart failure (Carpenter *et al.*, 1962); when cardiac output was improved by administration of digitalis, the aldosterone secretion rate promptly dropped. In some animals with very severe valvular lesions (pulmonary stenosis and complete tricuspid insufficiency), cardiac glycosides failed to increase cardiac output or reduce right atrial pressure; in these animals, digitalis did not reduce aldosterone production. It is thus apparent that the adrenocortical response to digitalis is the result of hemodynamic improvement, and is not due to a direct action of the drug on the kidneys or the adrenals.

Direct Renal Action. A direct action of cardiac glycosides upon the kidneys was suspected for many years. Studies have now shown that a number of aglycones and glycosides (including ouabain, digoxin, and digitoxin) inhibit tubular reabsorption of sodium in the dog kidney (*see* Strickler and Kessler, 1961). This effect is observed when relatively large doses are injected into one renal artery; the opposite kidney serves as the control. The direct effect does not appear to be due to competitive inhibition of corticosteroids, although the structural similarity of the glycosides and the adrenocortical hormones suggested this possibility. It may represent an effect on the Na,K-ATPase in the renal tubular cells. It is doubtful that the action plays a significant role in the diuresis that occurs with the use of digitalis in congestive failure.

Electrocardiographic Effects. Digitalis produces characteristic ECG changes that may assist in determining whether a patient has been receiving digitalis within the previous 2 or 3 weeks. However, these changes cannot in themselves be used for the purpose of quantitatively estimating digitalis dosage or the degree of existing digitalization in a particular patient. Furthermore, the effects of digitalis are often superimposed on changes resulting from the basic cardiac disease. The ECG must be interpreted with these facts in mind.

Within 2 to 4 hours after a large oral dose of digitalis, definite alterations may appear in the ECG. Changes are first noted in the RS-T segment or in the T wave itself. The normally upright T wave becomes diminished in amplitude, isoelectric, or inverted in one or more leads. The RS-T segment may also show depression when the main QRS complex is upward; occasionally the RS-T segment is elevated by digitalis when the main QRS deflection is downward. The changes in the RS-T segment and the T wave may occur alone or may coincide. The alterations caused by digitalis in the T waves and in the RS-T segments of chest leads can simulate those resulting from coronary artery disease or recent coronary occlusion, and can cause confusion in the interpretation of the record if it is not known that a cardiac glycoside has been administered. The RS-T junction of the ECG recorded after exercise in digitalized patients may show depression similar to that of the work ECG in nondigitalized subjects with myocardial ischemia secondary to coronary heart disease. The changes in the RS-T interval and T wave are not affected by atropine.

The P-R interval may be prolonged by digitalis. This effect occurs somewhat later than those changes described above. The interval is rarely greater than 0.25 second. If it is greater than this after digitalis, preexisting disease of the conduction system may be assumed. Atropine can abolish lower degrees of A-V block produced by digitalis, but the direct (or antiadrenergic) actions of the drug causing higher degrees of block are not affected by atropine.

The Q-T portion of the tracing is shortened by digitalis, a reflection of the fact that the drug abbreviates ventricular systole. Large doses occasionally cause changes in the size and the shape of the P wave. Digitalis widens the abnormal QRS complex in the Wolff-Parkinson-White syndrome, probably by slowing A-V nodal propagation without affecting conduction time in the presumed aberrant A-V pathway. This effect is abolished by atropine. Almost every type of ECG tracing associated with cardiac disorders can be simulated by the effects of digitalis on the heart.

Effects on Cardiac Energy Metabolism. The relationship of the effects of digitalis on transmembrane potential, ionic fluxes, and energy metabolism to its production of increased myocardial contractility, as well as toxic effects on the heart, now requires consideration.

A positive inotropic action might result from an increased supply of energy to the contractile mechanism or from an improved efficiency of conversion of chemical to mechanical energy. In the dog heart-lung preparation maintained at constant diastolic volume, Peters and Visscher (1936) recorded increased work output without a corresponding increase in cardiac oxygen consumption. If oxygen consumption is taken as a measure of the total metabolic energy liberated, these results indicate an increased efficiency of conversion of metabolic to mechanical energy. In most subsequent studies of isometric preparations of heart muscle, in all of which digitalis caused an increase in systolic tension, the positive inotropic action was accompanied by an increased oxygen consumption, although the increase in force was often proportionately greater than the increased energy consumption (*see* review by Lee and Klaus, 1971). Because an isometric preparation performs no work, the concept of mechanical efficiency does not, of course, apply. In heart-lung preparations in which the diastolic volume is allowed to diminish in response to enhanced contractility, oxygen consumption may fail to increase, or may even diminish.

An explanation of these apparently contradictory results may be found in the work of Covell and associates (1966). They showed that acetylstrophanthidin increased oxygen

consumption when cardiac volume was small; however, when end-diastolic volume was large, oxygen consumption was not substantially increased in spite of increased contractility. It is now well established that cardiac oxygen consumption is related to the tension within the ventricular wall. According to the Laplace relation, a decrease in fiber length would decrease intramural tension and decrease oxygen consumption, whereas an increase in contractile force at any given fiber length would increase oxygen consumption. The overall effects of cardiac glycosides on cardiac oxygen consumption are thus determined by the relative change in diastolic volume and in the force of contraction; when the work output of the dilated failing heart is increased and its volume is diminished by digitalis, improved mechanical efficiency can result (Bing *et al.*, 1950).

The effect of digitalis on the metabolism of adenosine triphosphate (ATP) and phosphocreatine (PC) has been extensively studied (Wollenberger, 1951; Lee *et al.*, 1960; Lee and Klaus, 1971). Concentrations of ATP and PC in heart muscle are unaffected by doses of ouabain that cause striking inotropic effects, but are reduced by toxic doses that increase oxygen consumption and may thus produce a relative hypoxia (*see* review by Fawaz, 1963). Digitalis has no significant effect on *isolated* enzyme systems of the glycolytic and tricarboxylic acid cycles. The effects on energy metabolism must therefore require an intact cellular organization. Attempts to demonstrate direct physical effects on isolated cardiac muscle proteins (actomyosin, the troponin-tropomyosin system) have been essentially negative (Katz, 1972).

Effects on Na,K-ATPase. In 1957 Skou discovered a membrane adenosine triphosphatase (dependent upon magnesium ions, and activated by sodium and potassium ions; Na,K-ATPase) that is inhibited by digitalis glycosides. Repke (1964) postulated that the Na,K-ATPase is the receptor for cardiac glycosides and that both the positive inotropic effect and the toxic effects result from inhibition of the enzyme (*see* review by Skou, 1965).

There is a striking parallelism between the positive inotropic effect of digitalis in mammalian heart muscle and the degree of inhibition of the ATPase. The enzyme is inhibited by cardioactive glycosides, but not by their inactive congeners. Species differences in sensitivity of the heart to cardiac glycosides are reflected in parallel changes in sensitivity of the ATPase extracted from the hearts of these species.

Thus, rat and toad hearts, as well as the ATPase extracted from them, are resistant; dog, cat, and guinea pig hearts and their corresponding enzymes are sensitive to digitalis glycosides. Changes in ionic composition also influence the cardiac ATPase and the positive inotropic effects of cardiac glycosides in a parallel manner (Caprio and Farah, 1967). Thus, high calcium, high potassium, or low sodium concentrations in the perfusion fluid reduce the positive inotropic effect of ouabain, and also the inhibition of the enzyme. Furthermore, these ionic changes also inhibit the binding of digitalis by cardiac tissue, as well as the binding to a subcellular microsomal fraction known to contain the ATPase (Marks, 1972). The ability of potassium salts to prevent or suppress digitalis toxicity is well known and reinforces the hypothesis that the Na,K-ATPase is the specific receptor for the cardiac glycosides.

Not all studies of the relation between the positive inotropic action of digitalis and the degree of enzyme inhibition have been in agreement. Akera and associates (1970) and Besch and Schwartz (1970) found that the ATPase extracted from mammalian hearts at the height of an inotropic response was inhibited to the extent of 30 to 50%. Okita and coworkers (1973), however, have shown that the positive inotropic effect of a number of digitalis derivatives is terminated by washing, while the inhibition of the ATPase persists. This dissociation of ATPase inhibition and positive inotropic effect is difficult to explain and throws some doubt on the validity of the hypothesis that Na,K-ATPase is the sole cardiac glycoside receptor. However, the array of findings correlating ATPase activity with inotropic effect on heart muscle is very impressive; the hypothesis cannot be rejected.

The membrane ATPase system almost certainly supplies the energy for the active transmembrane transport of *sodium* and *potassium*. Schatzmann (1953) demonstrated that cardiac glycosides can inhibit the transport of sodium and potassium in red blood cells. Similar observations in cardiac muscle explain the decreased intracellular potassium and increased intracellular sodium concentrations that result from digitalis (Calhoun and Harrison, 1931; Wood and Moe, 1942). Many studies have since confirmed these early observations, at least for toxic doses. With therapeutic doses of cardiac glycosides the findings are equivocal; in a number of studies no change or even an increase in intracellular potassium was recorded (for a review, *see* Lee and Klaus, 1971). Some studies in which sensitive radioactive tracer technics were used have demonstrated reduction of intracellular potassium even with subtoxic doses of strophanthidin (Langer and Serena, 1970). If the inotropic action is in fact due to inhibition of the enzyme system that serves the sodium pump, it is difficult to explain a digitalis-induced increase in intracellular potassium concentration; it is possible that the older observations were not sensitive enough to detect such small fractional changes accurately. The role of Na,K-ATPase in the transmembrane transport of cations and the relationship of its inhibition to the mechanism of action of cardiac glycosides are extensively reviewed in the symposium edited by Askari (1974).

The similarities between the actions of *calcium ions* and digitalis on the heart and the demonstration that intracellular calcium ion is necessary for the inotropic response to digitalis have focused attention on the role of calcium (Farah and Witt, 1963). Electrophysiological findings have demonstrated that a slow inward current occurring during the plateau phase of the myocardial action potential is dependent on external calcium concentration (Beeler and Reuter, 1970; New and Trautwein, 1972). It is probable that the inward current is carried by calcium ions and is thus directly related to excitation-contraction coupling; an action of cardiac glycosides on this coupling mechanism has been postulated. This concept is supported by the observation that an increase in an intracellular labile calcium pool follows exposure to digitalis (Bailey and Harvey, 1969; Langer and Serena, 1970). Active transport of calcium into the sarcoplasmic reticulum, a phenomenon thought to be related to relaxation of muscle, is believed not to be directly affected by digitalis (*see* review by Lee and Klaus, 1971). The effect on calcium transport is therefore probably an action at the cell-membrane level.

Langer and Serena (1970) have attempted to relate alterations in intracellular ion concentration and calcium pool changes to inhibition of Na,K-ATPase. In this scheme, inhibition of the ATPase causes an increased intracellular movement of sodium. Transmembrane exchange of sodium for calcium then results in an increase in the intracellular pool of labile calcium ions. This exchange has been demonstrated in squid axon preparations (Baker *et al.,* 1969); if it also occurs in the cardiac cell, the inotropic action could be the result not of the changes in sodium or potassium within the cell but of the indirectly mediated influx of calcium (Langer, 1972).

During diastole, the combination of the movable actin filaments with the stationary filaments of myosin is prevented by the interposed layers of the proteins tropomyosin and troponin (*see* Chapter 37). The Ca^{2+} that flows into the sarcoplasm during the plateau of the action potential combines with troponin, which allows the formation of the actin-myosin complex; the latter is responsible for contraction, utilizing energy supplied by the reaction of myosin ATPase with ATP. The process is reversed with the reduction of intracellular Ca^{2+} by a combination of its uptake into the sarcoplasmic reticulum and extrusion through the transverse tubular system. Digitalis is postulated to increase the ingress of Ca^{2+} as a result of inhibition of the Na,K-ATPase system and thereby to enhance contraction.

Many observations support this scheme, but the present state of our understanding of the highly complex distribution and exchange of ions within the cardiac cell is still too incomplete to permit a final judgment. On the other hand, the excessive loss of intracellular K^+ that results from inhibition of the membrane-bound Na,K-ATPase appears to provide an adequate explanation of many of the toxic effects that are caused by digitalis.

Digitalis Intoxication. Digitalis is said to be the fourth most frequently prescribed drug in the United States. It also has one of the lowest margins of safety. It is therefore not surprising, but it is surely alarming, that estimates of the increase in the incidence of digitalis intoxication since 1950 range from 2 to 14 times (Burch, 1973). The necessity for caution and careful clinical judgment in the use of such potent agents cannot be over-emphasized.

All digitalis preparations cause signs and symptoms of intoxication when given in high doses; there is no "nontoxic" cardiac glyco-side. Accurate determination of the relative "margin of safety" of various glycosides is difficult, for the results depend on the dura-tion of exposure and on the criteria chosen for therapeutic and toxic effects. Farah and Maresh (1948) found no significant differ-ence in the toxic:therapeutic dose ratios of five glycosides tested under identical condi-tions in heart-lung preparations. This is what might be expected if, indeed, the therapeutic and toxic effects are due to a common mech-anism such as inhibition of Na,K-ATPase, as discussed above. The toxic manifestations of glycosides that are more rapidly excreted will be more rapidly dissipated, but the danger of toxicity is present with all preparations.

Manifestations of digitalis toxicity in the heart can be lethal, and it is the obligation of every physician who uses any preparation of the drug to be alert to those signs of tox-icity that call for cessation of therapy. With-ering recognized many of the signs of toxicity of large acute doses: "The foxglove when given in very large and quickly repeated doses, occasions sickness, vomiting, purging, giddiness, confused vision, objects appearing green or yellow; increased secretion of urine, with frequent motions to part with it; slow pulse, even as low as 35 in a minute, cold sweats, convulsions, syncope, death."

Digitalis poisoning, as encountered today, is usually due to the cumulative effect of maintenance doses taken over relatively long periods of time, or to the heroic use of rela-tively large doses administered together with diuretics in the treatment of severe arrhyth-mias, or to "pushing" the drug in situations in which it is ineffectual, or to a failure on the part of the physician to recognize that dosage must be carefully adjusted on an in-dividual basis (*see* Lown *et al.*, 1972).

On the basis of pharmacokinetic data that

have accumulated within the past decade, estimation of digitalis dosage can now be accomplished with more precision than in the past, as discussed below. If patients are followed carefully, and if the plasma glyco-side concentration is determined with the appearance of any indication of overdosage, the incidence of serious digitalis intoxication should decrease.

Gastrointestinal Effects. Anorexia, nausea, and *vomiting* are among the earliest evi-dences of digitalis overdosage. Anorexia usually occurs a day or more before nausea or vomiting. The significance of nausea as an early indication of digitalis poisoning should not be discounted. Salivation often accom-panies the nausea and at times, as Withering noted, it may be copious. Vomiting then occurs, but occasionally it may develop with-out preliminary anorexia or nausea. This is especially likely to happen if a large dose is given rapidly. The episodes of nausea and emesis may start and stop abruptly, only to recur with greater severity. Vomiting requires much physical effort, which the patient with congestive heart failure can ill afford. Nausea and vomiting may be transitory or entirely absent in some patients. The fact that the same symptoms are noted in patients with heart failure is, of course, no deterrent to the use of digitalis. Parallel with the restoration of compensation by digitalis and other meas-ures comes relief from the anorexia, nausea, and vomiting associated with cardiac failure. *Diarrhea* may also be noted, and in rare cases it is the only gastrointestinal manifestation of digitalis toxicity. *Abdominal discomfort* or *pain* often accompanies the gastrointestinal symptoms (65% of patients in a series re-ported by Lely and Enter, 1970). Abdominal pain may be referable to the mesenteric is-chemia described by Ulano and associates (1971). The total dose of glycoside given before nausea and vomiting appear varies greatly in different patients and is inde-pendent of the cardiac status. Once the drug is stopped, gastrointestinal symptoms disap-pear in a few days.

The *mechanism* of nausea and vomiting caused by cardiac glycosides has been extensively investigated (*see* review by Borison and Wang, 1953). Formerly, it was widely believed that gastrointestinal irritation from galenical preparations was the main cause of these symptoms. The type of vomiting that is clinically important and that signifies digitalis intoxication results mainly from the systemic action of the drug. Inasmuch as emesis can be elicited by parenteral administration of digitalis and can be observed (retching movements) after complete removal of the gastrointestinal tract in animals, local irritation is not a factor in its production. The definitive studies of Borison, Wang, and their associates have demonstrated that vomiting induced shortly after intravenous administration of cardiac glycosides results from excitation of a chemoreceptor trigger zone (CTZ), located in the area postrema of the medulla.

Cardiac Effects. The alterations in cardiac rate and rhythm occurring in digitalis poisoning may simulate almost every known type of arrhythmia seen clinically. Indeed, the drug has often been used fraudulently to simulate heart disease. An increasing severity of congestive heart failure may constitute the major evidence of digitalis intoxication; an appropriate decrease in dosage is followed by restoration of cardiac compensation (Batterman and Gutner, 1950). Before deciding whether digitalis or an exacerbation of the patient's disease is the cause of the observed disturbances, one must marshal all the available evidence concerning the cardiac status before the drug was given, the doses used, and the response manifested during the period of digitalization.

Extrasystoles. Probably the most frequent cardiac effect of digitalis overdosage is the occurrence of extrasystoles. They originate most commonly in the ventricle but can arise from the atrium. Extrasystoles and ventricular tachycardia are said to be less common in children. The cause of the ectopic beats is the increased automaticity of the myocardium produced by excessive amounts of digitalis. If the extrasystole recurs after each regular systole, digitalis "coupling" is present (pulsus bigeminus). This is particularly likely to occur in patients with atrial fibrillation and fortunately permits the recognition of overdigitalization, because ventricular ectopic beats may sometimes be difficult to detect in this arrhythmia. Digitalis-induced bigeminy may be the sole indication of intoxication and may precede, follow, or develop simultaneously with other evidence of overdosage of the drug. Pulsus trigeminus may also be observed. The occurrence of ectopic beats does not in itself always signify that digitalis dosage must be curtailed. In some patients relatively small doses can cause this disturbance to appear. Prior existence of extrasystoles does not contraindicate digitalis therapy, which indeed may decrease the number of abnormal beats.

A-V Block. Toxic amounts of digitalis may cause occasional dropped beats or complete A-V dissociation. Partial or complete block must always be viewed as evidence of digitalis intoxication, and should be suspected if the ventricular rate falls below 60 beats per minute. *However, the heart rate may not be slowed at all by digitalis, and an increase in rate—for example, from an accelerated pacemaker in the A-V junctional area—may be the first evidence of digitalis poisoning.*

Other Arrhythmias. *Sinus arrhythmia* may occur as the result of increased vagal activity, especially in the young. *Paroxysmal tachycardia* from digitalis may arise from either the ventricle or the atrium and requires discontinuation of the drug. Nonparoxysmal tachycardias are more common than paroxysmal episodes, but paroxysmal atrial tachycardia with block is considered to be a danger sign (Lown *et al.,* 1960). *Atrial tachycardia* usually arises from an ectopic focus in the atrium rather than from the S-A node. *Ventricular tachycardia* is always serious and calls for immediate cessation of digitalis therapy because ventricular fibrillation may ensue. A particularly ominous type of tachycardia, which is thought to signal the approach of fatal ventricular fibrillation, is characterized by alternation of the QRS complexes. Apparently, this occurs only in badly damaged hearts and is specifically produced by digitalis. Formerly believed to be ventricular in origin, "bidirectional" tachycardia is probably of supraventricular origin with alternating block within the major branches of the ventricular conduction system (Rosenbaum *et al.,* 1969). *Atrial fibrillation* can be caused by large doses of digitalis. That digitalis overdosage can cause fibrillation of the atria is not a deterrent to the use of the drug in this disorder. *Ventricular fibrillation* is undoubtedly the most common cause of death from digitalis poisoning. It is preceded by ventricular extrasystoles. Sudden death in patients receiving large amounts of the drug may well be due to this arrhythmia. It is particularly likely to occur from the injudicious use of large intravenous doses of cardiac glycosides. Other arrhythmias seen after digitalis overdosage include *A-V nodal (junctional) tachycardia, interference dissociation, parasystole, heart block,* and *atrial standstill.*

Neurological Effects. Headache, fatigue, malaise, and *drowsiness* are common symptoms and occur early in the course of digitalis intoxication; generalized muscle weakness and easy fatigability may be particularly prominent. *Neuralgic pain,* usually involving the lower third of the face and simulating trigeminal neuralgia, may be the earliest, most severe, and even the sole manifestation of digitalis intoxication; the extremities and lumbar area may also be involved, and paresthesias often accompany the pain (Batterman and Gutner, 1948). *Mental symptoms* include disorientation, confusion, aphasia, and even delirium and hallucinations ("digitalis delirium"); rarely, *convulsions* have occurred. Neuropsychiatric effects are especially likely to develop in elderly atherosclerotic patients, and the exact role played by digitalis is uncertain. Complicating factors of dehydration, fluid and salt restriction, vomiting, and vigorous diuresis are frequently present, and improvement usually occurs when fluid and electrolyte abnormalities are corrected and therapy with potent diuretics and digitalis is stopped.

Vision. Vision is often blurred. White borders or halos may appear on dark objects ("white vision"), and objects may appear frosted. Color vision can be disturbed; chromatopsia is most common for yellow and green, but less frequently red, brown, and blue vision can occur. Transitory amblyopia, diplopia, and scotomata may also ensue. It has also been reported that digitalis can affect the papillomacular fibers of the optic nerve and cause retrobulbar neuritis. In an epidemic of accidental digitoxin intoxication, 95% of 179 patients complained of visual disturbances; 95% complained of extreme fatigue and weakness. ECG signs considered characteristic of digitalis poisoning were observed in 70% of the subjects (Lely and Enter, 1970).

Skin Rashes, Eosinophilia, and Gynecomastia. These are rare reactions to digitalis. The *skin lesions* may be urticarial or scarlatiniform in character, and are usually not aided by antihistamines. The increase in the number of *eosinophils* is often quite pronounced; atropine has been known to decrease and pilocarpine to increase the number of eosinophils. *Gynecomastia* may be induced in men by digitalis therapy; it has been suggested that the drug, on the basis of its chemical similarity to the sex hormones, may exert estrogenic activity in certain cases (LeWinn, 1953).

Blood Coagulation. Experimental observations in animals appear to indicate that digitalis preparations increase blood coagulability and that heparin reduces the toxicity of digitalis and ouabain. It has been suggested, therefore, that digitalis may exert a thromboplastic effect that contributes to the high incidence of thromboembolic phenomena in patients with cardiovascular disease. The considerable importance of the problem has stimulated fairly extensive animal and clinical research, which has not yet fully settled the issue of whether digitalis shortens

blood coagulation time. Certain clinical data have been presented to suggest that therapeutic doses of digitalis may decrease coagulation time without influencing prothrombin time or clot retraction, and that digitalis exerts a thrombogenic effect, as measured by the increase in tolerance to administered heparin or dicumarol. Nevertheless, most carefully controlled clinical investigations indicate that digitalis has no adverse effect on coagulation time or heparin tolerance. (*See* Cathcart and Blood, 1950; Sutton, 1950; and others.) Very rarely, digitalis may cause thrombocytopenia (Young *et al.,* 1966).

Diagnosis and Treatment of Digitalis Intoxication. Digitalis is often used in situations in which the toxic effects of the drug are difficult to distinguish from the effects of cardiac disease. The diagnostic problem arises most frequently with the hospital admission of a patient with serious arrhythmia and congestive failure from whom a history of recent digitalis therapy cannot be elicited. Full digitalization of such a patient could obviously be lethal if the arrhythmia is induced by digitalis. The use of the extremely short-acting glycoside *acetylstrophanthidin* as a provocative test to detect previous digitalization is hazardous and is no longer employed (Lown *et al.,* 1972).

Sensitive specific methods for the estimation of the concentration of digitalis glycosides in plasma have now been developed to the stage where they are routinely used in a number of general hospitals (*see* below). The laboratory result can indicate whether or not the patient has recently received digitalis, and whether the plasma concentration is within an unquestionably toxic range, but the therapeutic and toxic ranges, not surprisingly, overlap. *Careful and judicious clinical appraisal is still the most important diagnostic tool.*

Probably the most frequent cause of digitalis intoxication in patients who have previously been maintained satisfactorily is hypokalemia; digitalis intoxication can also be precipitated by hypomagnesemia, hypercalcemia, hypoxia, or disturbances in acid-base balance. Cardiac manifestations of toxicity occur when intracellular potassium concentration is reduced, as a result of either excessive doses of the drug itself or too vigorous application of diuretics. Potassium depletion may also result from malnutrition, corticosteroid therapy, hemodialysis, and other causes. The induction of digitalis intoxication by hypoxia or acidosis is probably due, at least in part, to the loss of intracellular potassium.

When digitalis intoxication is diagnosed, therapy with the glycoside and diuretics should be withheld and the patient's progress followed carefully, with frequent monitoring of the ECG. If the condition does not revert spontaneously or if it worsens, appropriate therapy should be instituted. A most useful agent for this purpose is potassium chloride, and antiarrhythmic drugs may occasionally be of value.

Potassium Chloride. Oral administration of potassium chloride to produce a plasma potassium concentration at the upper limit of the normal range may suppress glycoside-induced ectopic arrhythmias. If this measure fails, the salt may be given by slow intravenous infusion with frequent monitoring of the ECG and plasma potassium concentration. Too large or too rapid an increase can induce other arrhythmias, including ventricular fibrillation. Potassium is contraindicated in the presence of A-V block and other disturbances of conduction, since it increases the effective refractory period of the A-V node and enhances the block.

Antiarrhythmic Agents. The most useful drugs of this group for the treatment of digitalis intoxication are phenytoin (diphenylhydantoin), lidocaine, and propranolol. *Phenytoin* can suppress digitalis-induced ventricular tachycardia as well as supraventricular arrhythmias; at the same time, it opposes S-A and A-V nodal block by improving digitalis-prolonged conduction at these sites. In therapeutic concentrations, it has minimal effects on myocardial contractility. The recommended dose is 100 mg infused slowly every 5 minutes until the arrhythmia is reverted or ECG evidence of toxicity is noted; this is followed by a maintenance dose of 400 to 600 mg orally per day for as long as required (Bigger and Strauss, 1972). *Lidocaine* also suppresses ventricular tachycardia, but it is less effective than phenytoin against supraventricular arrhythmias; the dose is 100 mg infused over 3 to 5 minutes, followed by 15 to 50 μg/kg per minute as required to suppress the arrhythmia. *Propranolol* is effective in combating extrasystoles and tachycardia of both ventricular and supraventricular origin; however, it causes a decrease in nodal conduction velocity, which limits its usefulness in the presence of A-V block. Propranolol also depresses myocardial contractility and may produce a marked fall in blood pressure, through a combination of β-adrenergic blockade and a direct action. The dose employed is 1 to 3 mg intravenously, administered at a rate not exceeding 1 mg per minute.

Other Drugs and Procedures. *Atropine* can be employed to control sinus bradycardia, sinoatrial arrest, and second- or third-degree A-V block. *Cholestyramine* (see Chapter 35) has been used experimentally in an attempt to hasten the elimination of cardiac glycosides. By binding glycoside within the intestinal lumen, the exchange resin can interrupt the enterohepatic cycle. Abbreviation of the plasma half-life of digitoxin in man has been demonstrated (Greenberger and Caldwell, 1972). There is little evidence that cholestyramine would be of any use in hastening elimination of digoxin. The use of specific *antiglycoside antibodies* is an additional potential procedure (see Butler *et al.,* 1973). Electrical "countershock" should *not* be employed to convert digitalis-induced arrhythmias; it is hazardous and may cause ventricular fibrillation.

Assay and Unitage of Digitalis Preparations. The U.S.P. requires spectrophotometric assay of digitoxin, digoxin, and ouabain against appropriate reference standards. *Powdered Digitalis,* N.F., requires bioassay, by determination of the lethal dose in pigeons in comparison with that of a reference standard. Tablets or capsules of digitalis powder are prescribed by weight or in units. The official N.F. unit represents the potency of 100 mg of the *N.F. Digitalis Reference Standard Powder* and is roughly equivalent to 0.1 mg of digitoxin.

Product Variability and Bioavailability. Studies of commercial preparations of *digoxin* tablets from several sources have demonstrated that the oral administration of well-known products that have gained wide usage results in predictable plasma concentrations of the glycoside, with understandable intersubject variations. However, other preparations are deficient in that the plasma concentrations achieved are either too low for an adequate therapeutic response or, what is more serious, vary from lot to lot. This is not due to variations in the glycoside content of the tablet but to differences in bioavailability (see Lindenbaum *et al.,* 1971; Lindenbaum, 1973; Wagner *et al.,* 1973). Further studies have revealed that the differences in bioavailability can be correlated with the dissolution rates of the tablets (Lindenbaum *et al.,* 1973). As a result, the U.S.P. describes the official procedure for the determination of the dissolution rate of digoxin tablets and the standards that must be met for each lot that is marketed. The United States Food and Drug Administration has recalled all digoxin preparations that have failed to meet these standards. Future provisions may require bioavailability studies in man before the approval of any new formulation of digoxin in addition to dissolution determinations for lot-to-lot control. Despite these precautions, physicians would be well advised to prescribe the digoxin product with which they are familiar and to indicate the commercial source of the drug to be dispensed if it is prescribed by generic name. Because of complications entailed by the considerably greater degree of metabolism and plasma protein binding of *digitoxin* (see below), comparable data on its bioavailability in various commercial preparations are not yet available. It is predictable that such information will be forthcoming in the near future.

The problems of digoxin bioavailability have been succinctly reviewed in three editorials that appeared in the official publication of the American Heart Association (Harter *et al.,* 1974; Levy and Gibaldi, 1974; New York Heart Association Task Force on Digitalis Preparations, 1974).

No method of assay can eliminate the biological variation of the patient; the response of the patient, not the glycoside content of the pills, is still the primary factor in determining the proper dose schedule.

Preparations Available for Clinical Use. The official and other glycosides in common use listed below provide the physician with appropriate agents for essentially every clinical situation in which a digitalis-type drug is indicated. In former years, the tincture and powdered leaf of digitalis were frequently prescribed. There are few, if any, defensible reasons for their current use.

Digitoxin, U.S.P. (CRYSTODIGIN, PURODIGIN). As officially described, the drug is either pure digitoxin or a mixture of cardioactive glycosides obtained from *Digitalis purpurea, D. lanata,* or other species and consisting chiefly of digitoxin. *Digitoxin Tablets,* U.S.P., are available for oral use, each tablet containing 0.05, 0.1, 0.15, or 0.2 mg of drug. *Digitoxin Injection,* U.S.P., is available for *intravenous* administration and consists of a sterile solution of digitoxin in 40 to 50% alcohol; glycerin may also be present. Each milliliter contains 0.1 to 0.2 mg of the drug. There is evidence that market preparations of crystalline digitoxin may differ somewhat in potency. Studies of bioavailability are in progress.

Digoxin, U.S.P. (LANOXIN). This drug is a glycoside obtained from the leaves of *Digitalis lanata.* It is available for both oral and intravenous administration. *Digoxin Tablets,* U.S.P., contain 0.125, 0.25, 0.375, or 0.5 mg each. *Digoxin Elixir,* U.S.P., contains 0.05 mg/ml. *Digoxin Injection,* U.S.P., is a sterile solution of digoxin in 10% alcohol, each milliliter of solution containing 0.25 mg of drug. Because both the digoxin and the alcohol are tissue irritants, the appropriate dose should be diluted with 10 ml of sterile 0.9% sodium chloride solution before injection. The solution should be administered slowly (5 to 10 minutes), and care taken to avoid extravenous injection.

Lanatoside C (CEDILANID). This drug is no longer official. It is a precursor glycoside obtained from the leaves of *Digitalis lanata.* It is marketed only for oral administration in tablets that contain 0.5 mg of the glycoside. Lanatoside C is assayed in pigeons by the N.F. method for digitalis.

Deslanoside, N.F. (*desacetyl-lanatoside C;* CEDILANID-D). This precursor glycoside is derived from lanatoside C by alkaline hydrolysis, and is more soluble than the parent substance. Deslanoside exhibits the same pharmacological properties as lanatoside C, and for practical purposes merely constitutes the available injectable form of the latter. Deslanoside is assayed spectrophotometrically against a standard preparation. It is marketed as *Deslanoside Injection,* N.F., for intramuscular or intravenous use, in a sterile solution containing 10% ethanol. It is available in 2- and 4-ml ampuls containing 0.2 mg/ml of drug.

Acetyldigitoxin, N.F. (ACYLANID). This is a crystalline glycoside derived from *Digitalis lanata.* It is supplied in tablets of 0.1 or 0.2 mg for oral use only.

Powdered Digitalis, N.F. The source, composition, assay, and unitage of powdered digitalis leaf have been described. The powder can be administered in pill, tablet, or capsule form. *Digitalis Tablets,* N.F., contain 30, 50, 55, 60, 83, or 100 mg of powder. *Digitalis Capsules,* N.F., contain 60 or 100 mg of powder.

Digitalis Tincture. This galenical preparation, formerly in wide use, is no longer official.

Ouabain, U.S.P. (*G-strophanthin*). This glycoside is available as *Ouabain Injection,* U.S.P., a sterile aqueous solution for intravenous injection; it is marketed as 1- and 2-ml ampuls containing 0.25 mg/ml. Various galenical preparations of *strophanthus* and of *squill* are no longer official.

Pharmacokinetics and Metabolism. The doses of the various preparations necessary for digitalization and maintenance are obviously a function not only of their potency but also of the extent of their absorption and the speed of their degradation and excretion. A thorough knowledge of pharmacokinetic principles and of the pharmacokinetics of the commonly used cardiac glycosides is essential for their optimal use and for prevention of the toxic complications that are so prevalent with this class of drugs. This was recognized by Gold and coworkers (1942), who attempted to define the onset and duration of action in quantitative terms by using the response of the ventricular rate in patients with atrial fibrillation as an index of digitalis effect.

Plasma Glycoside Concentrations. In recent years the introduction of sensitive and reliable methods for the determination of particular cardiac glycosides has made it possible to estimate their absorption, distribution, and excretion with great precision (*see* Butler, 1972; Smith and Haber, 1973a). The two procedures that have been employed most extensively are both competitive protein-binding methods: the enzymatic isotopic displacement technic, in which Na,K-ATPase is used as the specific binding protein (Brooker and Jelliffe, 1972), and the radioimmunoassay (Oliver *et al.,* 1971). The latter method, particularly as applied to digoxin, is now employed in many hospital laboratories. However, extremely careful technic and frequent monitoring are necessary in order to minimize inaccuracy and errors.

The radioimmunoassay has been applied to the investigation of many clinical problems, including quantitative estimation of the degree of absorption from the intestine and binding to plasma proteins, correlation of plasma concentrations with therapeutic and toxic responses, duration of action, and metabolic disposition or elimination. The agreement between clinical assessment and estimates based on measurement of plasma glycoside concentrations is surprisingly good. Pertinent data are summarized in Table 31–3, in which the figures represent mean values in subjects with essentially normal renal, thyroid, hepatic, and gastrointestinal function; considerable individual variations may be expected.

**Table 31-3. AVERAGE PHARMACOKINETIC VALUES AND DOSES
FOR CARDIAC GLYCOSIDES**

	DIGITOXIN	DIGOXIN	DESLANOSIDE	OUABAIN
Gastrointestinal absorption	90–100%	60–85%	Unreliable	Unreliable
Onset of action *	½–2 hr	15–30 min	10–30 min	5–10 min
Peak effect *	4–12 hr	1–5 hr	1–2 hr	½–2 hr
Plasma concentration, ng/ml				
Therapeutic	14–26	0.8–1.6		
Toxic	> 34	> 2.4		
Plasma half-life *	5–7 days	36 hr	36 hr	21 hr
Excretory pathway	Hepatic → Renal	Renal	Renal	Renal
Total digitalizing dose (adult) †				
Oral	1.2–1.6 mg ‡	1.0–1.5 mg §		
Intravenous	1.2–1.6 mg ‡	0.75–1.5 mg ¶	1.2–1.6 mg #	0.25–0.5 mg **
Daily oral maintenance dose	0.05–0.2 mg	0.125–0.5 mg		

   * All time values are based on intravenous administration of a single digitalizing dose.

   † The values given represent *average* doses or ranges for complete digitalization; the requirements of *individual* patients may depart considerably from these figures. For the overwhelming majority of patients, only a fraction of the digitalizing dose should be given initially, followed by subsequent fractional doses at appropriate intervals, as indicated for the individual drugs. For complete discussion, *see* text.

   ‡ Digitoxin can be given as a single dose, but is usually administered in divided doses. For rapid digitalization by the oral route, 0.6 mg can be given initially, followed by 0.4 mg 4 to 6 hours later, then 0.2 mg every 6 hours until full digitalization is achieved.

   § Usual initial dose of digoxin is 0.5 to 0.75 mg orally, followed by 0.25 to 0.5 mg at 6-hour intervals until digitalization is achieved. Digitalization can usually be obtained within 1 week by administering 0.5 mg of digoxin daily, without initial loading dose (*see* Mason, 1974).

   ¶ When rapid digitalization is essential, initial intravenous dose of digoxin is 0.5 to 1.0 mg, followed by 0.25 to 0.5 mg at 6-hour intervals until digitalization is achieved. The glycoside can also be given intramuscularly.

   # For emergencies requiring very rapid digitalization, the drug can be given as two doses of 0.6 to 0.8 mg each, intravenously or intramuscularly.

   ** Ouabain is often employed in preference to other glycosides for intravenous use in emergencies.

In practice, determination of the plasma glycoside concentration can be useful in three general situations: when there is a question whether the patient has recently received glycoside medication, when the expected therapeutic response is not obtained, and when there is any indication of digitalis intoxication.

Relationship of Structure to Absorption, Binding, and Disposition. The oral absorption, degree of binding to plasma albumin, and extent of metabolism of cardiac glycosides in general are related directly to their lipid solubility and inversely to their polarity; the latter property is determined primarily by the number of hydroxyl groups attached to the steroid nucleus. Digitoxin, with only one steroidal hydroxyl group, is almost completely absorbed; digoxin, with two, is somewhat less absorbed; ouabain, with five, is absorbed poorly following oral administration (Greenberger and Caldwell, 1972). Digitoxin is nearly completely bound to plasma albumin and is extensively metabolized by the liver to both active and inactive products. Digoxin, in contrast, is bound to only a slight extent and is excreted by the kidney almost completely in unchanged form; consequently, its duration of action is increased in proportion to the degree of any impairment of renal function. Deslanoside and ouabain are likewise not bound extensively to plasma albumin and are excreted largely unchanged.

Relationship of Kinetics to Dosage. The selection of the proper glycoside and the decision whether to employ an initial loading dose or to initiate therapy gradually with the maintenance dose or a multiple thereof should be determined by both the condition of the patient and appreciation of the pharmacokinetic properties of the drugs. The glycosides disappear from the body exponentially (first-order kinetics), with half-lives of approximately a week for digitoxin, 36 hours for digoxin, and less than a day for ouabain. It can be calculated that approximately 10% of the body store of digitoxin, or 37% of that of digoxin, is lost daily; accordingly, the daily administration of these fractions of an initial loading dose should maintain a constant amount of drug within the body. It should also be remembered that in the absence of an initial loading dose, the time required to establish a steady state of drug concentration in the body by administration of fixed doses is four to five half-lives (*see* Chapter 1). If this type of schedule is followed, it would require approximately a month to achieve complete digitalization with digitoxin and approximately a week with digoxin.

The matter of interpatient and intrapatient variation with respect to optimal glycoside dosage requirement cannot be overemphasized. The dosage ranges listed in Table 31-3 are based on *mean* values. A given patient's optimal glycoside requirement may fall outside the ranges indicated on the basis of constitutional factors; residual glycoside from previous medication; acid-base, electrolyte, and fluid balance; renal and hepatic function; endocrine abnormalities; and other determinants. While computer programs and nomograms have been developed to aid in the adjustment of glycoside dosage in accordance with many of these variables, they are not substitutes for clinical acumen. (*See* Jelliffe *et al.,* 1972; Jelliffe and Brooker, 1974.)

Digitoxin. This glycoside is nearly completely absorbed from the gastrointestinal tract. As much as 97% of digitoxin is bound to plasma albumin (Lukas and deMartino, 1969). For this reason the *total* plasma concentration of digitoxin is from 15 to 20 times higher than that of digoxin at comparable therapeutic levels (Smith and Haber, 1973a), and the renal clearance of digitoxin is much lower. The half-life is 5 to 7 days, and, in contrast to digoxin, is relatively uninfluenced by impaired renal function.

Digitoxin is eliminated by hepatic degradation, eventually to inactive genins, which are excreted mainly by the kidneys. Stepwise hydrolysis of the three molecules of digitoxose converts the glycoside to the aglycone digitoxigenin, which is rapidly converted to the inactive epidigitoxigenin (Repke, 1963). Because enterohepatic recirculation occurs, approximately 25% of the metabolic end products appear in the stool. Some conversion to digoxin occurs in the liver, but this is not an important pathway in man. Phenylbutazone and phenobarbital, which are known inducers of hepatic drug-metabolizing enzyme activity, have been shown to accelerate digitoxin metabolism (Bigger and Strauss, 1972).

Digoxin. This glycoside is now the most commonly used digitalis preparation in the United States. While approximately 60 to 85% of oral digoxin is absorbed from the gastrointestinal tract of normal individuals, differences in tablet formulation may lead to wide variation in absorption, as discussed above. Absorption occurs from the small intestine, probably by passive diffusion. Peak plasma concentrations after oral administration of digoxin can be influenced by procedures that modify gastric emptying or intestinal movements, although the total amount absorbed is not greatly affected (Doherty, 1973). The absorption of digoxin is reduced in patients with malabsorption syndrome but is not altered by pancreatic disease.

Digoxin is bound to plasma albumin to the extent of about 25%. The glycoside is also bound to tissue proteins; the concentration in human cardiac tissue may reach 30 times that in the plasma. The average half-life in the plasma is approximately 36 hours. Therapeutic plasma concentrations average 0.8 to 1.6 ng/ml; concentrations of more than 2.4 ng/ml are usually toxic, but considerable overlap occurs in individual cases.

The elimination of digoxin in man is mainly by renal excretion; 60 to 90% of the administered dose appears unchanged in the urine, and only a small fraction is excreted in the stool. Excretion is by glomerular filtration, and the clearance of unbound digoxin is essentially equivalent to that of creatinine in man. Thus, patients with reduced renal function show a longer plasma half-life of digoxin. These considerations are vitally important, since the daily maintenance dose of digoxin is determined by the rate of elimination; ignorance of the status of renal function can result in serious toxic manifestations if renal impairment is present (Doherty, 1973). The increased sensitivity to digoxin observed in geriatric practice is related to the decline of glomerular filtration rate with advancing age, resulting in prolongation of the half-life and elevation of the plasma concentration of the drug. Some enterohepatic recycling of digoxin occurs in man, but only to the extent of 7% of the total dose (Doherty *et al.,* 1970). Hepatic disease does not affect digoxin excretion to any significant extent.

Patients with hyperthyroidism are said to be resistant to digitalis therapy, while hypothyroid patients are more sensitive than normal. In accord with these impressions, plasma digoxin concentrations are low in hyperthyroidism and significantly higher than normal in hypothyroidism.

Routes of Administration. *Oral.* Cardiac glycosides are given orally whenever possible. This is the least expensive and the safest route, and absorption is sufficiently rapid so that early beneficial cardiac effects can be obtained within 2 to 6 hours after adequate doses.

Parenteral. Pain and irritation may result from subcutaneous or intramuscular injection of most preparations; the speed of absorption from intramuscular sites is not significantly faster than from the intestine (Doherty, 1972). The *intravenous* route is preferred when digitalis glycosides must be given parenterally. This route is warranted when minutes may mean the difference between life and death, as in patients with pulmonary edema from acute left ventricular failure. Also, coma, vomiting, or other conditions preventing oral medication may necessitate parenteral therapy. It is preferable to dilute the drug in isotonic sodium chloride solution and to make the injection slowly. The dose must be carefully determined and the facts about previous digitalis medication must be known. The intravenous route for digitalis administration is by far the most dangerous, and its use may be rapidly fatal.

Speed of Onset and Duration of Action. As shown in Table 31–3, the cardiac glycosides differ widely in speed of onset as well as duration of action. It is important to know the time required for a particular digitalis product to develop its full cardiac action, because this determines how far apart one must space subsequent doses in order to avoid excessive medication and toxicity. At one extreme stands digitoxin; even when given intravenously in a single full-digitalizing dose, this glycoside requires 4 or more hours to exhibit its maximal cardiac effect. Two or more weeks are needed for complete regression of its action. Digitalis leaf has the same time constants as digitoxin. At the opposite extreme is ouabain; when administered intravenously, it exerts maximal effects in 30 minutes to 2 hours; the myocardial action disappears completely after 1 to 3 days. The other major glycosides of digitalis, such as deslanoside and digoxin, occupy positions between the two extremes. In general, those that have a rapid onset also have a short duration of action and *vice versa.*

Choice of Glycoside. The physician has the choice of a large variety of digitalis glycosides, as is evident from the listing presented above. The two main criteria in selection are *speed of onset* and *duration* of cardiac action. All digitalis products have the same type of myocardial action, and all have approximately the same therapeutic index; that is, the therapeutic dose is approximately 50 to 60% of the toxic dose. For maintenance therapy, prolonged duration of action is often desirable, such as afforded by digitoxin (Table 31–3); it is somewhat easier to maintain cardiac effects at an optimal level with this glycoside than with those that are rapidly eliminated, such as digoxin or lanatoside C. It must be remembered, however, that a long duration of action carries with it the danger of cumulative development of toxic effects, and their persistence after medication is stopped. For this reason many cardiologists prefer to use a glycoside with a briefer duration of action, such as digoxin. For emergency therapy, rapid onset of action may be imperative and ouabain should then be considered; deslanoside and digoxin may also be used for this purpose. As previously emphasized, care should be exercised when for any reason a patient is shifted from one preparation to another. (*See* Lukas, 1972.)

Dosage for Initial Digitalization and Maintenance. Because of the relatively long half-life of most of the cardiac glycosides, a loading dose ("digitalizing" dose) may be desired to bring body stores rapidly to an effective level, followed by a maintenance dose schedule designed to match the daily rate of elimination (*see* above).

The total *average* dose (by mouth) of *digitoxin* for inducing full therapeutic effects, when given within 36 to 48 hours to an adult who has not received digitalis within 10 days, is 1.2 to 1.6 mg. The total dose should be divided into several equal parts, administered every 6 hours; or one half or one third of the total calculated dose may be given at once, and the remainder in two portions after intervals of 6 hours. If moderately severe cardiac decompensation is present and digitalis has not been taken for the previous 2 weeks, 0.6 mg can be given immediately, followed by 0.4 mg 4 hours later, then 0.2 mg every 4 to 6 hours until optimal benefit is obtained and the maintenance dose can be adjusted (usually 0.05 to 0.2 mg daily). During the initial stages of digitalization the physician must be alert to the signs of toxicity; the *average* doses are certain to be toxic to the susceptible individual.

When *digoxin* is employed for initial and maintenance therapy, the usual initial oral dose is 0.5 to 0.75 mg, followed by 0.25 to 0.5 mg every 6 hours until adequate digitalization is achieved. As discussed above, because of its relatively short half-life, digoxin can usually produce full digitalization within 1 week by daily administration of 0.25 mg, the average maintenance dose, in the absence of an initial loading dose. This is often the procedure of choice when heart failure is not severe and has been developing over a period of months or more.

Children require more digitalis glycoside than do adults, and about 50% more drug than calculated on the basis of body weight must be given in order to obtain similar results (*see* Mathes *et al.,* 1952; Nadas *et al.,* 1953).

If the physician is uncertain of the amount of digitalis taken by the patient within the previous 1 or 2 weeks, the large doses outlined cannot be given safely. It is then best to administer digoxin, 0.25 mg daily, and observe the patient closely for signs of intoxication before *each* subsequent dose is given.

Inasmuch as the major glycoside component of most preparations of powdered digitalis is digitoxin, equivalent to a concentration of 0.1 mg of digitoxin per 100 mg of powdered digitalis or 1 N.F. unit, an equivalent dosage schedule can be employed. Thus, the average digitalizing dose is approximately 1.2 g (12 units) of powdered digitalis, and the average daily maintenance dose is 80 to 160 mg (0.8 to 1.6 units). This preparation is, however, not recommended.

Intravenous Dosage. When beneficial results must be obtained in minutes, rather than hours, intravenous medication may be given. In the United States, the most commonly used intravenous glycosides are deslanoside and digoxin, but these are somewhat slower in onset of action than ouabain. Solutions of digoxin are irritating and may present difficulties in administration. The recommended intravenous dose of deslanoside for full digitalization is 1.2 to 1.6 mg; digoxin, 0.75 to 1.5 mg; and ouabain, 0.25 to 0.5 mg. Once the acute emergency is past, oral administration of a suitable glycoside should be substituted for maintenance therapy. Digitoxin, although available for intravenous injection, is unsuitable for emergency use because of the long latent period of its cardiac action (Table 31–3). Great care and continuous monitoring must be used if cardiac glycosides are given intravenously to patients in whom a careful study of the heart and of the history has not been possible or who have been receiving a digitalis preparation and are still likely to have a significant plasma concentration of glycoside.

Dosage for Maintenance. Most patients receiving a digitalis glycoside must continue therapy for the remainder of their lives. Therefore, in order to maintain the beneficial effects realized by the original digitalization, it is necessary to give the drug daily in an amount sufficient to replace that which is destroyed or eliminated by the body. The general principles that govern estimation of appropriate maintenance dosage have been presented above.

There is no rule of thumb for determining the daily maintenance dose. The amount varies with each case and depends upon the level of digitalis action required. This level should ensure an *optimal digitalis effect.* After the patient has been initially digitalized and has obtained optimal benefit, the dose is adjusted to maintain this level of action. Most patients require approximately 0.1 mg of digitoxin daily or 0.25 mg of digoxin once or twice daily. Others may need as little as one third or as much as four times this amount daily. It is important to understand that in most patients the optimal dose is definitely below that which causes early toxic effects. It is therefore not necessary to increase the dose to the point of producing nausea and vomiting in order to find the maintenance level. In other words, the ideal dose is not necessarily the largest dose tolerated. An amount is sought that will restore the highest degree of cardiac efficiency and relieve all symptoms and signs of heart failure. While the determination of this dose can be assisted materially by various laboratory data and computational aids, as already discussed, it is dependent chiefly upon careful and frequent observation of the patient. It may be large or small and may vary in the same patient according to changes in the status of the myocardium. In some patients, especially those with severe heart failure, the optimal dose occasionally may border for a time on the toxic, and beneficial results will then be obtainable only with amounts of digitalis that produce early symptoms of poisoning.

Average maintenance dosage for cardiac glycosides will vary markedly according to renal function. As an *approximation,* patients with creatinine clearance values of 50 to 80 ml per minute usually require only one half the normal maintenance dose of *digoxin;* the full maintenance dose of *digitoxin* is usually tolerated. When renal failure is severe (creatinine clearance less than 10 ml per minute), one fourth or less of the normal maintenance dose of digoxin may prove toxic; under these circumstances the maintenance dose of digitoxin should also be reduced by one half or more. A loading dose, if administered, need not be adjusted for alterations in renal function (*see* Chapter 1).

THERAPEUTIC INDICATIONS FOR DIGITALIS

Congestive Heart Failure. By far the most important use of digitalis is in congestive heart failure. The devious historical route by which this clear-cut indication for the drug finally became definitely established has already been traced. Digitalis is useful regardless of whether the failure is predominantly of the left or right ventricle, or involves both sides of the heart. The type of rhythm exhibited by the decompensated heart neither indicates nor contraindicates the use of digitalis. Arrhythmias may modify the response to digitalis, but they do not alter the indication for the drug if failure is present.

Digitalis is particularly useful in heart failure resulting from an absolute or relative chronic overload (hypertension, valvular lesions, atherosclerotic heart disease) in which the supply of energy is not impaired. Digitalis does not cause major benefit in situations in which the metabolic energy supply is compromised, as in thyrotoxicosis, hypoxia, and severe thiamine deficiency. Experimentally, it has been shown that failure caused by poisons that reduce high-energy phosphate stores (cyanide, azide, dinitrophenol, etc.) is not relieved by digitalis (Gruhzit and Farah, 1955). Some of the most dramatic responses are seen in patients with congestive heart failure and atrial fibrillation, but excellent and equally significant results are obtained in cases of failure with normal sinus rhythm (Figure 31-2). Exertional and paroxysmal nocturnal dyspnea, cough, cyanosis, ascites, edema, and chronic passive congestion of the lungs and the abdominal viscera are relieved. The diastolic size of the heart is decreased; venous pressure is lowered to normal; cardiac output is increased without a proportional increase in cardiac oxygen consumption; stroke volume and circulatory velocity are enhanced; the diastolic rest period in each cardiac cycle is prolonged; vital capacity is increased, respiratory minute volume is decreased, and arteriovenous oxygen difference is reduced; and the increased blood volume falls toward normal. If tachycardia is present as a compensatory mechanism in failure, the heart rate slows as digitalis returns the functional efficiency of the ventricle toward normal. The mechanisms by which the direct myocardial action of digitalis brings about the above-enumerated changes have been discussed.

Once digitalis has returned the failing heart to a state of compensation, its continued use will do much to prevent the recurrence of heart failure. It is unwise to omit the drug in patients with diminished cardiac reserve who have previously experienced an episode of myocardial insufficiency, even though they have subsequently been free of symptoms. Exceptions, of course, exist. Cardiac failure may be temporary following myocardial infarction; surgical correction of valvular lesions or successful therapy of hypertension may eliminate the need for continuing digitalis medication.

The best results with digitalis are obtained in *hypertensive* or *atherosclerotic* heart disease. In rheumatic, luetic, and congenital heart disease there is no specific defect that either indicates or contraindicates the use of digitalis. In instances of reversible heart disease, such as that associated with infections, anemia, thyrotoxicosis, thiamine deficiency, and arteriovenous fistula, correction of the underlying disease is of greater import than the administration of digitalis. Poor response to digitalis is to be expected in cases of active rheumatic and other forms of toxic or infectious myocarditis. Digitalis is not indicated in shock or in instances of cardiac tamponade. When shock and congestive failure exist together, as they may in myocardial infarction, digitalis may be indicated for therapy of the failure, but little evidence of hemodynamic improvement has been demonstrable (Cohn *et al.*, 1969). In the final analysis, improvement of cardiac function by digitalis depends on the cardiac reserve. In badly damaged hearts digitalis cannot provide much benefit.

Use of Digitalis to Prevent Heart Failure. Numer-

ous studies have shown improved cardiac function in subjects with heart disease without clinical evidence of failure (Selzer and Malmborg, 1962). For example, the oxygen debt after brief episodes of physical exertion is reduced by digitalis in subjects with compensated heart disease (Kahler *et al.*, 1963). Digitalis has also been advocated prophylactically in patients with organic heart disease prior to surgery, particularly thoracic procedures (Wheat and Burford, 1961); whether this is a valid indication is not certain. The major hazard in the prophylactic use is probably that of digitalis intoxication, for the drug is being administered in the absence of the signs and symptoms upon which its beneficial effects are best judged.

Atrial Fibrillation. Even in the absence of congestive heart failure, digitalis is indicated in most cases of atrial fibrillation. The inappropriately rapid ventricular rate in this disorder results in palpitation that may cause great discomfort, and a reduction in cardiac work capacity that may lead to heart failure. The aim of digitalis therapy in patients with atrial fibrillation is to restore myocardial efficiency, reduce the ventricular rate, and eliminate the pulse deficit. The mechanism of ventricular slowing by digitalis in this disorder has been discussed. The fibrillation is rarely halted by digitalis, and the drug should not be employed with this objective. The dosage should be adjusted to maintain the ventricular rate in the range of 60 to 80 per minute at rest, and not to exceed 100 with moderate exercise.

Atrial Flutter. Digitalis is the most useful drug in the management of atrial flutter, whether or not congestive failure is present. There are three possible desirable results of digitalis therapy in this situation. The dysrhythmia may be converted to atrial fibrillation; the degree of A-V block will be increased even if the flutter persists; or normal sinus rhythm may be restored. Conversion to atrial fibrillation is advantageous because management of the ventricular rate is thereby facilitated; when the atria are fibrillating, a graded response of ventricular rate is more likely. In the presence of atrial flutter the degree of block may suddenly shift from 4:1 to 2:1 when, as the result of exercise or excitement, reduced vagal tone and enhanced adrenergic tone combine to increase A-V nodal conductivity; the sudden doubling of ventricular rate may be incapacitating. Not uncommonly normal sinus rhythm occurs, especially when digitalis (with the accompanying increased vagal effects upon the atria) is withdrawn after fibrillation has developed. When the flutter persists in spite of drug therapy, the increased degree of A-V block induced by digitalis will protect against a sudden and excessive increase of ventricular rate.

Paroxysmal Tachycardia. Atrial and A-V nodal paroxysmal tachycardia are the most common tachysystolic dysrhythmias next to atrial fibrillation. The disorders are commonly not associated with cardiac disease, but the attacks may be disabling and hazardous if prolonged. The attacks are often abruptly terminated by measures that enhance vagal activity; these are discussed elsewhere. Digitalis is often successful, probably by virtue of reflex vagal stimulation; intravenous administration of a rapidly acting preparation may be required. Some cases are better controlled by quinidine, particularly when long-term prophylaxis is required in individuals without congestive heart failure (*see* Chapter 32). It should be remembered that *paroxysmal supraventricular tachycardia with partial A-V block may be a result of serious digitalis intoxication.* It is extremely important to be certain of the diagnosis before digitalis is used (Lown *et al.,* 1960).

In *ventricular tachycardia,* digitalis may increase the danger of ventricular fibrillation. If the drug is used at all, great caution is required. Quinidine, procainamide, and electroshock therapy of this disorder is discussed in Chapter 32. If the arrhythmia is caused by digitalis, potassium administration or the use of a suitable antiarrhythmic drug may be indicated.

SPECIAL FACTORS MODIFYING
DIGITALIS THERAPY

Coronary Thrombosis. Coronary occlusion in itself is not an indication for digitalis. Digitalis is contraindicated unless there is congestive heart failure. Following an acute coronary thrombosis, the clinical picture is frequently one of shock rather than of congestive heart failure. Because both myocardial infarction and digitalis toxicity can cause ectopic ventricular rhythms, it has been assumed that digitalis may be particularly dangerous following coronary occlusion. It is true that the diagnosis of digitalis intoxication is difficult in this setting, but it has been stated that no significant increased sensitivity of the heart to digitalis in *therapeutic* concentrations develops in the infarcted myocardium (Lown *et al.,* 1972). Most authorities agree that digitalis is indicated when cardiac decompensation occurs, whether early or late.

Angina Pectoris. Both experimental and clinical data appear to show that digitalis does not decrease coronary blood flow when given to man in therapeutic amounts. In patients with cardiac failure, the restoration of efficient heart action may even improve the coronary circulation. Digitalis is not indicated in angina pectoris without congestive heart failure. In heart failure, however, the coexistence of angina pectoris does not contraindicate digitalis. Cases have been reported in which digitalis was thought to have increased the frequency of attacks of pain. It is possible that digitalis, by restoring cardiac compensation in patients with angina pectoris and heart failure, allows a sufficient increase in physical activity to precipitate anginal attacks. It is well known, for example, that attacks of anginal pain are likely to disappear when congestive failure ensues, probably because the decompensation imposes restricted activity on the patient. There is also evidence that a reduction of heart size, with the attendant decrease of intramural tension and oxygen demand, may reduce the frequency of anginal attacks.

Thyroid Function. Hyperthyroidism in itself is not an indication for digitalis therapy. Tachycardia

due to hyperthyroidism, with or without atrial fibrillation, is poorly controlled by such therapy. If heart failure is present, digitalis is given as in cases without thyrotoxicosis; however, the results obtained are usually not satisfactory until the hyperthyroidism is corrected. If atrial fibrillation occurs and persists despite medical or surgical relief of hyperthyroidism, propranolol may be indicated. The long-standing clinical impression that thyrotoxic patients require more and hypothyroid patients less digitalis than euthyroid subjects is supported by studies of plasma concentrations of digoxin; the plasma half-life is inversely related to the functional status of the thyroid (Doherty and Perkins, 1966).

Acute Myocarditis. If congestive failure occurs in the presence of acute inflammatory processes or myocardial injury induced by toxins (*e.g.*, diphtheria), digitalis may be used, but in smaller-than-usual doses and with close observation.

Arrhythmias. Except for ventricular tachycardia, there is no particular abnormal cardiac rhythm that indicates or contraindicates the use of digitalis in congestive heart failure. In myocardial insufficiency, digitalis should be prescribed regardless of the cardiac rhythm. The use of digitalis in paroxysmal tachycardia and in fibrillation or flutter of the atria has been discussed. In patients with *partial heart block,* the drug may cause complete heart block; nevertheless, it should be used if decompensation exists. Indeed, it has been demonstrated that patients with heart block can be given digitalis safely and that optimal benefit can be obtained with doses that do not increase the grade of block. In *complete heart block* (A-V dissociation), digitalis may be employed safely and is indicated provided failure exists. The idiopathic ventricular rate is usually not accelerated unless toxic amounts are given.

Valvular Defects. There is no specific cardiac valvular defect that indicates or contraindicates the use of digitalis. Severe mechanical obstruction may exist without myocardial failure. Digitalis may cause little improvement in mitral stenosis with normal sinus rhythm, for example, even though the positive inotropic action can be demonstrated in both ventricles (Beiser *et al.,* 1968). Digitalis may also be of little value in hypertrophic subaortic stenosis, probably because the mechanical obstruction to outflow is increased as the heart size diminishes. Poorer results are generally obtained in cases of heart failure associated with aortic than with mitral insufficiency. This may be explainable, in part, by the fact that many cases of mitral disease are rheumatic in origin and have atrial fibrillation associated with failure; these patients respond well to digitalis. On the other hand, cases of aortic insufficiency due to syphilis often respond poorly to digitalis.

Renal and Hepatic Function. As discussed above, lower maintenance doses of *digoxin* will be required in the presence of impaired renal function; patients on hemodialysis or recipients of renal transplants also require appropriate adjustment of dosage schedules. *Digitoxin* dosage is not similarly affected.

In contrast, elimination of *digitoxin,* but not of *digoxin,* is delayed when hepatic function is severely depressed.

Other Drugs. *Catecholamines.* Digitalis and sympathomimetic amines are both capable of causing ectopic pacemaker activity, and their effects may be additive. Accordingly, β-receptor stimulants should be used with caution in digitalized subjects, and *vice versa.* The use of propranolol in the treatment of digitalis intoxication is discussed above.

Antiarrhythmic Drugs. The circumstances under which these agents can be used concurrently with digitalis are described in Chapter 32.

Phenylbutazone, Phenobarbital, and Phenytoin (Diphenylhydantoin). These agents, as discussed above, may accelerate the degradation of digitoxin by induction of the hepatic microsomal drug-metabolizing system. A careful clinical study by Solomon and Abrams (1972) demonstrated that phenobarbital accelerated the conversion of digitoxin to digoxin (otherwise an unimportant metabolic route in man), reduced the plasma concentration of digitoxin by about 50%, and decreased the half-life in plasma by more than 40%. The importance of such observations is clear, since these and related drugs are frequently prescribed concurrently with digitalis glycosides. This requires careful observation of the patient, and readjustment of dosage may be necessary. Patients receiving digitalis should be warned against changing ancillary medications without prior consultation with the physician.

Akera, T.; Larsen, F. S.; and Brody, T. M. Correlation of cardiac sodium- and potassium-activated adenosine triphosphatase activity with ouabain-induced inotropic stimulation. *J. Pharmac. exp. Ther.,* **1970,** *173,* 145–151.

Bailey, L. E., and Harvey, S. C. Effect of ouabain on cardiac ^{45}Ca kinetics measured by indicator dilution. *Am. J. Physiol.,* **1969,** *216,* 123–129.

Baker, P. F.; Blaustein, M. P.; Hodgkin, A. L.; and Steinhardt, R. A. The influence of calcium on sodium efflux in squid axons. *J. Physiol., Lond.,* **1969,** *200,* 431–458.

Barger, A. C. The kidney in congestive heart failure. *Circulation,* **1960,** *21,* 124–128.

Batterman, R. C., and Gutner, L. B. Hitherto undescribed neurological manifestations of digitalis toxicity. *Am. Heart J.,* **1948,** *36,* 582–586.

————. Increasing congestive heart failure: a manifestation of digitalis toxicity. *Circulation,* **1950,** *1,* 1052–1059.

Beeler, G. W., Jr., and Reuter, H. Membrane calcium current in ventricular myocardial fibers. *J. Physiol., Lond.,* **1970,** *207,* 191–209.

Beiser, G. D.; Epstein, S. E.; Stampfer, M.; Robinson, B.; and Braunwald, E. Studies on digitalis. XVII. Effects of ouabain on the hemodynamic response to exercise in patients with mitral stenosis in normal sinus rhythm. *New Engl. J. Med.,* **1968,** *278,* 131–137.

Besch, H. R., and Schwartz, A. On the mechanism of action of digitalis. *J. molec. cell. Cardiol.,* **1970,** *1,* 195–199.

Bigger, J. T., Jr., and Strauss, H. C. Digitalis toxicity: drug interactions promoting toxicity and the management of toxicity. *Semin. Drug Treat.,* **1972,** *2,* 147–177.

Bing, R. J.; Maraist, F. M.; Dammann, J. F.; Draper, A.; Heimbecker, R.; Daley, R.; Gerard, R.; and Calazel, P. Effect of strophanthus on coronary blood flow and cardiac oxygen consumption of normal and failing human hearts. *Circulation,* **1950,** *2,* 513–516.

Braunwald, E.; Bloodwell, R. D.; Goldberg, L. I.; and Morrow, A. G. Studies on digitalis. IV. Observations in man on the effects of digitalis preparations on the contractility of the nonfailing heart and on total vascular resistance. *J. clin. Invest.,* **1961,** *40,* 52–59.

Brooker, G., and Jelliffe, R. W. Serum cardiac glycoside assay based upon displacement of ^{3}H-ouabain from Na-K ATPase. *Circulation,* **1972,** *45,* 20–36.

Burch, G. E. The practice of cardiology today. *Am. Heart J.,* **1973,** *85,* 291–293.

Butler, V. P., Jr. Assay of digitalis in the blood. *Prog. cardiovasc. Dis.,* **1972,** *14,* 571–600.

Calhoun, J. A., and Harrison, T. R. Studies in congestive heart failure. IX. The effect of digitalis on the potassium content of cardiac muscle of dogs. *J. clin. Invest.,* **1931,** *10,* 139–144.

Caprio, A., and Farah, A. The effect of the ionic milieu on the response of rabbit cardiac muscle to ouabain. *J. Pharmac. exp. Ther.,* **1967,** *155,* 403–414.

Carpenter, C. C. J.; Davis, J. O.; Wallace, C. R.; and Hamilton, W. F. Acute effects of cardiac glycosides on aldosterone secretion in dogs with hyperaldosteronism secondary to chronic right heart failure. *Circulation Res.,* **1962,** *10,* 178–187.

Cathcart, R. T., and Blood, D. W. Effect of digitalis on the clotting of the blood in normal subjects and in patients with congestive heart failure. *Circulation,* **1950,** *1,* 1176–1181.

Chai, C. Y.; Wang, H. H.; Hoffman, B. F.; and Wang, S. C. Mechanisms of bradycardia induced by digitalis substances. *Am. J. Physiol.,* **1967,** *212,* 26–34.

Chen, K. K., and Henderson, F. G. Pharmacology of sixty-four cardiac glycosides and aglycones. *J. Pharmac. exp. Ther.,* **1954,** *111,* 365–383.

Cohn, A. E., and Stewart, H. J. Relation between cardiac size and cardiac output per minute following administration of digitalis in normal dogs. *J. clin. Invest.,* **1928,** *6,* 53–77.

Cohn, J. N.; Tristani, F. E.; and Khatri, I. M. Cardiac and peripheral vascular effects of digitalis in clinical cardiogenic shock. *Am. Heart J.,* **1969,** *78,* 318–330.

Cotten, M. de V., and Stopp, P. E. Action of digitalis on the non-failing dog heart. *Am. J. Physiol.,* **1958,** *192,* 114–120.

Covell, J. W.; Braunwald, E.; Ross, J.; and Sonnenblick, E. H. Studies on digitalis. XVI. Effects on myocardial oxygen consumption. *J. clin. Invest.,* **1966,** *45,* 1535–1542.

Davis, J. O. Adrenocortical and renal hormonal function in experimental cardiac failure. *Circulation,* **1962,** *25,* 1002–1014.

Dock, W., and Tainter, M. L. The circulatory changes after full therapeutic doses of digitalis with a critical discussion of views on cardiac output. *J. clin. Invest.,* **1930,** *8,* 467–484.

Doherty, J. E. The metabolism of digitalis glycosides in man. In, *Basic and Clinical Pharmacology of Digitalis.* (Marks, B. H.; and Weissler, A. M., eds.) Charles C Thomas, Pub., Springfield, Ill., **1972,** pp. 230–242.

————. Digitalis glycosides: pharmacokinetics and their clinical implications. *Ann. intern. Med.,* **1973,** *79,* 229–238.

Doherty, J. E.; Flanigan, W. J.; Murphy, M. L.; Bullock, R. T.; Dalrymple, G. L.; Beard, O. W.; and Perkins, W. H. Tritiated digoxin. XIV. Enterohepatic circulation, absorption, and excretion studies in human volunteers. *Circulation,* **1970,** *42,* 867–873.

Doherty, J. E., and Perkins, W. H. Digoxin metabolism in hypo- and hyperthyroidism. *Ann. intern. Med.,* **1966,** *64,* 489–507.

Dresdale, D. T.; Yuceoglu, Y. Z.; Michtom, R. J.; Schultz, M.; and Lunger, M. Effects of lanatoside C on cardiovascular hemodynamics—acute digitalizing doses in subjects with normal hearts and with heart disease without failure. *Am. J. Cardiol.,* **1959,** *4,* 88–99.

Erlij, D., and Méndez, R. The modification of digitalis

intoxication by excluding adrenergic influences on the heart. *J. Pharmac. exp. Ther.*, **1964**, *144*, 97–103.

Farah, A., and Loomis, T. A. The action of cardiac glycosides on experimental auricular flutter. *Circulation*, **1950**, *2*, 742–748.

Farah, A., and Maresh, G. Determination of the therapeutic irregularity, and lethal doses of cardiac glycosides in the heart-lung preparation of the dog. *J. Pharmac. exp. Ther.*, **1948**, *92*, 32–42.

Farah, A., and Witt, P. N. Cardiac glycosides and calcium. In, *Proceedings of the First International Pharmacological Meeting.* Vol. 3, *New Aspects of Cardiac Glycosides.* (Wilbrandt, W., and Lindgren, P., eds.) Pergamon Press, Ltd., Oxford, **1963**.

Fawaz, G. Effect of reserpine and pronethalol on the therapeutic and toxic actions of digitalis in the dog heart-lung preparation. *Br. J. Pharmac. Chemother.*, **1967**, *29*, 302–308.

Ferrier, G. R., and Moe, G. K. Effect of calcium on acetylstrophanthidin-induced transient depolarizations in canine Purkinje tissue. *Circulation Res.*, **1973**, *33*, 508–515.

Gaffney, T. E.; Kahn, J. B., Jr.; Van Maanen, E. F.; and Acheson, G. H. A mechanism of the vagal effect of cardiac glycosides. *J. Pharmac. exp. Ther.*, **1958**, *122*, 423–429.

Gillis, R. A.; Raines, A.; Sohn, Y. J.; Levitt, B.; and Standaert, F. G. Neuroexcitatory effects of digitalis and their role in the development of cardiac arrhythmias. *J. Pharmac. exp. Ther.*, **1972**, *183*, 154–168.

Gold, H., and Cattell, M. Mechanism of digitalis action in abolishing heart failure. *Archs intern. Med.*, **1940**, *65*, 263–278.

Gold, H.; Cattell, M.; Otto, H. L.; Kwit, N. T.; and Kramer, M. L. A method for the bio-assay of digitalis in humans. *J. Pharmac. exp. Ther.*, **1942**, *75*, 196–206.

Gold, H.; Kwit, N. T.; Otto, H.; and Fox, T. On the vagal and extra-vagal factors in cardiac slowing by digitalis in patients with auricular fibrillation. *J. clin. Invest.*, **1939**, *18*, 429–437.

Greenberger, N. J., and Caldwell, J. H. Studies on the intestinal absorption of ^{3}H-digitalis glycosides in experimental animals and man. In, *Basic and Clinical Pharmacology of Digitalis.* (Marks, B. H., and Weissler, A. M., eds.) Charles C Thomas, Pub., Springfield, Ill., **1972**, pp. 15–47.

Gruhzit, C. C., and Farah, A. E. A comparison of the positive inotropic effects of ouabain and epinephrine in heart failure induced in the dog heart-lung preparation by sodium pentobarbital, dinitrophenol, sodium cyanide, and sodium azide. *J. Pharmac. exp. Ther.*, **1955**, *114*, 334–342.

Harrison, T. R., and Leonard, B. W. The effect of digitalis on the cardiac output of dogs and its bearing on the action of the drug in heart disease. *J. clin. Invest.*, **1926**, *3*, 1–36.

Harter, J. G.; Skelly, J. P.; and Steers, A. W. Digoxin—the regulatory viewpoint. *Circulation*, **1974**, *49*, 395–398.

Harvey, R. M.; Ferrer, M. I.; Cathcart, R. T.; and Alexander, J. K. Some effects of digoxin on the heart and circulation in man: digoxin in enlarged hearts not in clinical congestive failure. *Circulation*, **1951**, *4*, 366–377.

Hashimoto, K., and Moe, G. K. Transient depolarizations induced by acetylstrophanthidin in specialized tissue of dog atrium and ventricle. *Circulation Res.*, **1973**, *32*, 618–624.

Howarth, S.; McMichael, J.; and Sharpey-Schafer, E. P. Effects of venesection in low output heart failure. *Clin. Sci.*, **1946**, *6*, 41–50.

Jelliffe, R. W., and Brooker, G. A nomogram for digoxin therapy. *Am. J. Med.*, **1974**, *57*, 63–68.

Jelliffe, R. W.; Buell, J.; and Kalaba, R. Reduction of digitalis toxicity by computer-assisted glycoside dosage regimens. *Ann. intern. Med.*, **1972**, *77*, 891–906.

Kabat, H., and Visscher, M. B. Influence of K-strophanthosid on elasticity of the tortoise ventricle. *Proc. Soc. exp. Biol. Med.*, **1939**, *40*, 8–11.

Kahler, R. L.; Thompson, R. H.; Buskirk, E. R.; Frye, R. L.; and Braunwald, E. Studies on digitalis. VI. Reduction of the oxygen debt after exercise with digoxin in cardiac patients without heart failure. *Circulation*, **1963**, *27*, 397–405.

Katz, A. Effects of digitalis on the cardiac contractile proteins. In, *Basic and Clinical Pharmacology of Digitalis.* (Marks, B. H., and Weissler, A. M., eds.) Charles C Thomas, Pub., Springfield, Ill., **1972**, pp. 128–143.

Katz, L. N.; Rodbard, S.; Friend, M.; and Rottersman, W. The effect of digitalis in the anesthetized dog. 1. Action on the splanchnic bed. *J. Pharmac. exp. Ther.*, **1938**, *62*, 1–15.

Langer, G. A. Effects of digitalis on myocardial ionic exchange. *Circulation*, **1972**, *46*, 180–187.

Langer, G. A., and Serena, S. D. Effects of strophanthidin upon contraction and ionic exchange in rabbit ventricular myocardium: relation to control of active state. *J. molec. cell. Cardiol.*, **1970**, *1*, 65–90.

Lee, K. S.; Yu, D. H.; and Burstein, R. The effect of ouabain on the oxygen consumption, the high energy phosphates and the contractility of the cat papillary muscle. *J. Pharmac. exp. Ther.*, **1960**, *129*, 115–122.

Lely, A. H., and Enter, C. H. J. van. Large-scale digitoxin intoxication. *Br. med. J.*, **1970**, *3*, 737–740.

Levy, G., and Gibaldi, M. Bioavailability of drugs. Focus on digoxin. *Circulation*, **1974**, *49*, 391–394.

LeWinn, E. B. Gynecomastia during digitalis therapy: report of eight additional cases with liver function studies. *New Engl. J. Med.*, **1953**, *248*, 316–320.

Lindenbaum, J.; Butler, V. P.; Murphy, J. E.; and Cresswell, R. M. Correlation of digoxin-tablet dissolution-rate with biological availability. *Lancet*, **1973**, *1*, 1215–1217.

Lindenbaum, J.; Mellow, M. H.; Blackstone, M. O.; and Butler, V. P., Jr. Variation in biological availability of digoxin from four preparations. *New Engl. J. Med.*, **1971**, *285*, 1344–1347.

Lown, B.; Cannon, R. L.; and Rossi, M. A. Electrical stimulation and digitalis drugs: repetitive response in diastole. *Proc. Soc. exp. Biol. Med.*, **1967**, *126*, 698–701.

Lown, B.; Hagemeijer, F.; Barr, I.; and Klein, M. Digitalis intoxication: clinical and experimental assessment of the degree of digitalization. In, *Basic and Clinical Pharmacology of Digitalis.* (Marks, B. H., and Weissler, A. M., eds.) Charles C Thomas, Pub., Springfield, Ill., **1972**, pp. 299–318.

Lown, B.; Wyatt, N. F.; and Levine, H. D. Paroxysmal atrial tachycardia with block. *Circulation*, **1960**, *21*, 129–143.

Lukas, D. S. Of toads and flowers. *Circulation*, **1972**, *46*, 1–4.

Lukas, D. S., and deMartino, A. G. Binding of digitoxin and some related cardenolides to human plasma proteins. *J. clin. Invest.*, **1969**, *48*, 1041–1053.

McLain, P. L.; Kruse, T. K.; and Redick, T. F. The effect of atropine on digitoxin bradycardia in cats. *J. Pharmac. exp. Ther.*, **1959**, *126*, 76–81.

McMichael, J., and Sharpey-Schafer, E. P. The action of intravenous digoxin in man. *Q. Jl Med.*, **1944**, *13*, 123–135.

Marks, B. H. Factors that affect the accumulation of digitalis glycosides by the heart. In, *Basic and Clinical Pharmacology of Digitalis.* (Marks, B. H., and Weissler, A. M., eds.) Charles C Thomas, Pub., Springfield, Ill., **1972**, pp. 69–93.

Mason, D. T. The cardiovascular effects of digitalis in normal man. *Clin. Pharmac. Ther.*, **1966**, *7*, 1–16.

———. Regulation of cardiac performance in clinical heart disease: interactions between contractile state mechanical abnormalities and ventricular compensatory mechanisms. *Am. J. Cardiol.,* 1973, *32,* 437–448.

Mason, D. T., and Braunwald, E. Studies on digitalis. X. Effects of ouabain on forearm vascular resistance and venous tone in normal subjects and in patients in heart failure. *J. clin. Invest.,* 1964, *43,* 532–543.

Mason, D. T.; Zelis, R.; Lee, G.; Hughes, J. L.; Spann, J. F., Jr.; and Amsterdam, E. A. Current concepts and treatment of digitalis toxicity. *Am. J. Cardiol.,* 1971, *27,* 546–559.

Mathes, S.; Gold, H.; Marsh, R.; Greiner, T.; Palumbo, F.; Messeloff, C.; and Pearlmutter, M. Comparison of the tolerance of adults and children to digitoxin. *J. Am. med. Ass.,* 1952, *150,* 191–194.

Méndez, C.; Aceves, J.; and Méndez, R. Inhibition of adrenergic cardiac acceleration by cardiac glycosides. *J. Pharmac. exp. Ther.,* 1961a, *131,* 191–198.

———. The anti-adrenergic action of digitalis on the refractory period of the A-V transmission system. *Ibid.,* 1961b, *131,* 199–204.

Méndez, C., and Méndez, R. The action of cardiac glycosides on the excitability and conduction velocity of the mammalian atrium. *J. Pharmac. exp. Ther.,* 1957, *121,* 402–413.

Méndez, R., and Méndez, C. The action of cardiac glycosides on the refractory period of heart tissues. *J. Pharmac. exp. Ther.,* 1953, *107,* 24–36.

Moe, G. K., and Abildskov, J. A. Observations on the ventricular dysrhythmia associated with atrial fibrillation in the dog heart. *Circulation Res.,* 1964, *14,* 447–460.

Moe, G. K., and Méndez, R. The action of several cardiac glycosides on conduction velocity and ventricular excitability in the dog heart. *Circulation,* 1951, *4,* 729–734.

Nadas, A. S.; Rudolph, A. M.; and Reinhold, J. D. L. The use of digitalis in infants and children: a clinical study of patients in congestive heart failure. *New Engl. J. Med.,* 1953, *248,* 98–105.

Nadeau, R. A., and James, T. N. Antagonistic effects on the sinus node of acetyl strophanthidin and adrenergic stimulation. *Circulation Res.,* 1963, *13,* 388–391.

New, W., and Trautwein, W. The ionic nature of slow inward current and its relation to contraction. *Pflügers Arch. ges. Physiol.,* 1972, *334,* 24–38.

New York Heart Association Task Force on Digitalis Preparations. What should the practicing physician know about digoxin bioavailability and how will FDA action affect him? *Circulation,* 1974, *49,* 399–400.

Okita, G. T.; Richardson, F.; and Roth-Schecter, B. F. Dissociation of the positive inotropic action of digitalis from inhibition of sodium- and potassium-activated adenosine triphosphatase. *J. Pharmac. exp. Ther.,* 1973, *185,* 1–11.

Oliver, G. C.; Parker, B. M.; and Parker, C. W. Radioimmunoassay for digoxin. Technic and clinical application. *Am. J. Med.,* 1971, *51,* 186–192.

Patterson, S. W., and Starling, E. H. On the mechanical factors which determine the output of the ventricles. *J. Physiol., Lond.,* 1914, *48,* 357–379.

Peters, H. C., and Visscher, M. B. Energy metabolism of heart in failure and influence of drugs upon it. *Am. Heart J.,* 1936, *11,* 273–291.

Pickering, G. Starling and the concept of heart failure. *Circulation,* 1960, *21,* 323–331.

Repke, K. Metabolism of cardiac glycosides. In, *Proceedings of the First International Pharmacological Meeting.* Vol. 3, *New Aspects of Cardiac Glycosides.* (Wilbrandt, W., and Lindgren, P., eds.) Pergamon Press, Ltd., Oxford, 1963.

———. Über den biochemischen Wirkungsmodus von Digitalis. *Klin. Wschr.,* 1964, *42,* 157–165.

Rosen, M. R.; Gelband, H.; Merker, C.; and Hoffman, B. F. Mechanisms of digitalis toxicity. Effects of ouabain on phase four of canine Purkinje fiber transmembrane potentials. *Circulation,* 1973, *47,* 681–689.

Rosenbaum, M. B.; Elizari, M. V.; and Lazzari, J. O. The mechanism of bidirectional tachycardia. *Am. Heart J.,* 1969, *78,* 4–12.

Schatzmann, H. J. Herzglykoside als Hemmstoffe für den aktiven Kalium- und Natriumtransport durch die Erythrocytenmembran. *Helv. physiol. pharmac. Acta,* 1953, *11,* 346–354.

Selzer, A.; Hultgren, H. N.; Ebnother, C. L.; Bradley, H. W.; and Stone, A. O. Effect of digoxin on the circulation in normal man. *Br. Heart J.,* 1959, *21,* 335–342.

Selzer, A., and Malmborg, R. O. Hemodynamic effects of digoxin in latent cardiac failure. *Circulation,* 1962, *25,* 695–702.

Siegel, J. H., and Sonnenblick, E. H. Isometric time tension relationships as an index of myocardial contractility. *Circulation Res.,* 1963, *12,* 597–610.

Smith, T. W., and Haber, E. Clinical value of the radioimmunoassay of the digitalis glycosides. *Pharmac. Rev.,* 1973a, *25,* 219–228.

Solomon, H. M., and Abrams, W. B. Interactions between digitoxin and other drugs in man. *Am. Heart J.,* 1972, *83,* 277–280.

Stewart, H. J., and Cohn, A. E. Studies on effect of action of digitalis on output of blood from heart: effect on output in normal human hearts; effect on output of hearts in heart failure with congestion in human beings. *J. clin. Invest.,* 1932, *11,* 917–955.

Strickler, J. C., and Kessler, R. H. Direct renal action of some digitalis steroids. *J. clin. Invest.,* 1961, *40,* 311–316.

Sutton, G. C. Studies on blood coagulation and the effect of digitalis. *Circulation,* 1950, *1,* 271–277.

Swain, H. H., and Weidner, C. L. A study of substances which alter intraventricular conduction in isolated dog heart. *J. Pharmac. exp. Ther.,* 1957, *120,* 137–146.

Tamm, C. The stereochemistry of the glycosides in relation to biological activity. In, *Proceedings of the First International Pharmacological Meeting.* Vol. 3, *New Aspects of Cardiac Glycosides.* (Wilbrandt, W., and Lindgren, P., eds.) Pergamon Press, Ltd., Oxford, 1963.

Ulano, H. B.; Treat, E.; Chang, A. C. K.; and Jacobson, E. D. Splanchnic circulatory responses to ouabain in shock. *Surgery, St. Louis,* 1971, *70,* 678–684.

Vassalle, M.; Greenspan, K.; and Hoffman, B. F. Analysis of arrhythmias induced by ouabain in intact dogs. *Circulation Res.,* 1963, *13,* 132–148.

Vassalle, M.; Karis, J.; and Hoffman, B. F. Toxic effects of ouabain on Purkinje fibers and ventricular muscle fibers. *Am. J. Physiol.,* 1962, *203,* 433–439.

Vick, R. L.; Kahn, J. B., Jr.; and Acheson, G. H. Effects of dihydro-ouabain, dihydrodigoxin and dihydrodigitoxin on the heart-lung preparation of the dog. *J. Pharmac. exp. Ther.,* 1957, *121,* 330–339.

Wagner, J. G.; Christensen, M.; Sakmar, E.; Blair, D.; Yates, J. D.; Willis, P. W., iii; Sedman, A. J.; and Stoll, R. G. Equivalence lack in digoxin plasma levels. *J. Am. med. Ass.,* 1973, *224,* 199–204.

Wallace, A. G.; Mitchell, J. H.; Skinner, N. S.; and Sarnoff, S. J. Duration of the phases of left ventricular systole. *Circulation Res.,* 1963, *12,* 611–619.

Watanabe, Y., and Dreifus, L. S. Electrophysiologic effects of digitalis on A-V transmission. *Am. J. Physiol.,* 1966, *211,* 1461–1466.

———. Interactions of lanatoside C and potassium on atrioventricular conduction in rabbits. *Circulation Res.,* 1970, *27,* 931–940.

Wenckebach, K. F. Discussion on the effects of digitalis on the human heart. *Br. med. J.,* 1910, *2,* 1600–1605.

Wheat, M. W., and Burford, T. H. Digitalis in surgery: extension of classical indications. *J. thorac. cardiovasc. Surg.,* 1961, *41,* 162–168.

Williams, M. H.; Zohman, L. R.; and Ratner, A. C. Hemodynamic effects of cardiac glycosides on normal human subjects during rest and exercise. *J. appl. Physiol.,* 1958, *13,* 417–421.

Wittenberg, S. M.; Gandel, P.; Hogan, P. M.; Kreuger, W.; and Klocke, F. J. Relationship of heart rate to ventricular automaticity in dogs during ouabain administration. *Circulation Res.,* **1972,** *30,* 167–176.

Wollenberger, A. Metabolic action of the cardiac glycosides. II. Effect of ouabain and digoxin on the energy-rich phosphate content of the heart. *J. Pharmac. exp. Ther.,* **1951,** *103,* 123–135.

Wood, E. H., and Moe, G. K. Electrolyte and water content of the ventricular musculature of the heart-lung preparation with special reference to the effects of cardiac glycosides. *Am. J. Physiol.,* **1942,** *136,* 515–522.

Young, R. C.; Nachman, R. L.; and Horowitz, H. I. Thrombocytopenia due to digitoxin. *Am. J. Med.,* **1966,** *41,* 605–614.

Monographs and Reviews

Askari, A. (ed.). Properties and functions of (Na$^+$ + K$^+$)–activated adenosinetriphosphatase. *Ann. N.Y. Acad. Sci.,* **1974,** *242,* 1–741.

Borison, H. L., and Wang, S. C. Physiology and pharmacology of vomiting. *Pharmac. Rev.,* **1953,** *5,* 193–230. (194 references.)

Butler, V. P., Jr.; Watson, J. F.; Schmidt, D. H.; Gardner, J. D.; Mandel, W. J.; and Skelton, C. L. Reversal of the pharmacological and toxic effects of cardiac glycosides by specific antibodies. *Pharmac. Rev.,* **1973,** *25,* 239–248.

Fawaz, G. Cardiovascular pharmacology. *A. Rev. Pharmac.,* **1963,** *3,* 57–90. (199 references.)

Fieser, L. F., and Fieser, M. *Steroids.* Reinhold Publishing Corp., New York, **1959.**

Fisch, C.; Greenspan, K.; Knoebel, S. B.; and Feigenbaum, H. Effect of digitalis on condition of the heart. *Prog. cardiovasc. Dis.,* **1964,** *6,* 343–365. (159 references.)

Fisch, C., and Surawicz, B. (eds.). *Digitalis.* Grune & Stratton, Inc., New York, **1969.**

Glynn, I. M. The action of cardiac glycosides on ion movements. *Pharmac. Rev.,* **1964,** *16,* 381–407. (211 references.)

Hajdu, S., and Leonard, E. The cellular basis of cardiac glycoside action. *Pharmac. Rev.,* **1959,** *11,* 173–209. (196 references.)

Hoffman, B. F., and Singer, D. H. Effects of digitalis on electrical activity of cardiac fibers. *Prog. cardiovasc. Dis.,* **1964,** *7,* 226–260. (107 references.)

Langer, G. A. Ion fluxes in cardiac excitation and contraction and their relation to myocardial contractility. *Physiol. Rev.,* **1968,** *48,* 708–757. (190 references.)

Lee, K. S., and Klaus, W. The subcellular basis for the mechanism of inotropic action of cardiac glycosides. *Pharmac. Rev.,* **1971,** *23,* 193–261. (580 references.)

Lindenbaum, J. Bioavailability of digoxin tablets. *Pharmac. Rev.,* **1973,** *25,* 229–238.

Marks, B. H., and Weissler, A. M. (eds.). *Basic and Clinical Pharmacology of Digitalis.* Charles C Thomas, Pub., Springfield, Ill., **1972.**

Marshall, P. G. Steroids: cardiotonic glycosides and aglycons: toad poisons. In, *Rodd's Chemistry of Carbon Compounds,* 2nd ed., Vol. 2 D. (Coffey, S., ed.) Elsevier Publishing Co., Amsterdam, **1970,** pp. 360–421.

Mason, D. T. Digitalis pharmacology and therapeutics: recent advances. *Ann. intern. Med.,* **1974,** *80,* 520–530.

Skou, J. C. Enzymatic basis for active transport of sodium and potassium across cell membranes. *Physiol. Rev.,* **1965,** *45,* 596–617.

Smith, T. W., and Haber, E. Digitalis. *New Engl. J. Med.,* **1973b,** *289,* 945–952, 1010–1015, 1063–1072, 1125–1129. (336 references.)

Trautwein, W. Generation and conduction of impulses in the heart as affected by drugs. *Pharmac. Rev.,* **1963,** *15,* 277–332. (352 references.)

Withering, W. *An Account of the Foxglove and Some of Its Medicinal Uses: with Practical Remarks on Dropsy and Other Diseases.* C. G. J. & J. Robinson, London, 1785. Reprinted in *Med. Class.,* **1937,** *2,* 305–443.

CHAPTER
32 ANTIARRHYTHMIC DRUGS

Gordon K. Moe and J. A. Abildskov

The principal antiarrhythmic drugs of long-established clinical usefulness are *quinidine* and *procainamide,* in addition to the *digitalis glycosides,* which are discussed in the preceding chapter. More recent additions to the antiarrhythmic group are *lidocaine, phenytoin* (diphenylhydantoin), and *propranolol,* all of which had previously been in clinical use for other purposes. Some agents, such as *bretylium,* are still in the phase of clinical investigation as antiarrhythmic drugs. Before discussing the individual actions and uses of these agents, it will be helpful to consider the physiological abnormalities underlying disorders of cardiac rhythm and the general means of their modification by drugs.

Mechanisms of Antiarrhythmic Drug Action. As discussed in Chapter 31, the cardiac impulse is normally initiated at the automatic, or pacemaker, cells of the S-A node by their spontaneous depolarization (phase 4) during diastole; when the *transmembrane potential* reaches the *threshold potential,* it triggers the rapid depolarization that characterizes phase 0 of the *action potential.* This property of *automaticity* or spontaneous depolarization is shared, although at a lower level, by specialized atrial fibers adjacent to the S-A node and the fibers of the A-V node and Purkinje system. While the bulk of the ordinary atrial and ventricular muscle fibers normally do not exhibit significant spontaneous depolarization, they have the potentiality for such. Under pathological conditions, as discussed below, the automaticity of any cardiac fibers may exceed that of the normal pacemaker cells, which results in the establishment of *ectopic foci,* the basis of certain arrhythmias. Accordingly, one mechanism of antiarrhythmic drug action consists in selective suppression of automaticity at ectopic sites, either by slowing the rate of phase-4 depolarization, or by raising the threshold potential, or by a combination of both actions (Figure 32-1).

The rate of conduction of an impulse is determined primarily by the maximal rate of depolarization (V_{max}) during phase 0, which is characterized as *membrane responsiveness;* this, in turn, is dependent on the level of the transmembrane potential at the moment of excitation. The decrease in membrane responsiveness by quinidine and procainamide results in a decrease in conduction velocity, which actually constitutes a limitation to the efficacy of

these drugs in the treatment of some types of arrhythmias.

The early part of the phases (1–3) of repolarization, when the membrane is inexcitable, constitutes the *absolutely refractory period.* This is succeeded by the *effective refractory period* (ERP) during which the membrane is excitable but an impulse cannot be propagated, followed by the *relatively refractory period* (impulse propagation at reduced velocity) and the *supernormal period.* For practical purposes, the ERP can be considered as the minimal interval required between two propagated impulses. The proportions of the direct and autonomically mediated effects of the various antiarrhythmic agents on the

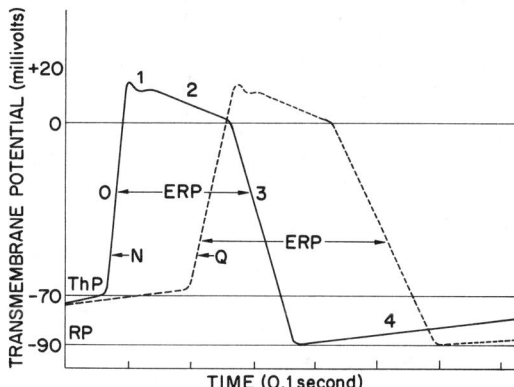

Figure 32-1. *Effects of quinidine on transmembrane potential of isolated Purkinje fiber.*

The solid line (*N*) depicts the transmembrane potential of a hypothetical spontaneously firing, normal Purkinje fiber *in vitro* during the phases (0–4) of the cardiac cycle; the dash line (*Q*) shows its modification by a low concentration of quinidine. Automaticity is suppressed by a decrease in the rate of spontaneous depolarization from the resting potential (RP) during diastole (phase 4) and an increase in the threshold potential (ThP). The rate of depolarization during phase 0 is reduced; the effective refractory period (ERP), action-potential duration (APD), and ERP/APD are increased. At therapeutic concentrations of quinidine *in situ,* automaticity at ectopic sites would be expected to be completely suppressed; the above pattern would be modified further by the vagal blocking action of quinidine, which would result in an increase in heart rate and other changes, as described in the text.

ERP differ. However, with few exceptions, all the drugs of this group prolong the ERP relative to the *action-potential duration* (APD) in Purkinje fibers and ventricular muscle fibers. Also of major importance in determining antiarrhythmic action, particularly in atrial muscle, is the prolongation of the ERP relative to conduction time (or to decrease in conduction velocity), as discussed below. The effects of quinidine on most of these properties are illustrated in Figure 32–1.

Of the major antiarrhythmic agents, *quinidine* and *procainamide* affect nearly all the foregoing parameters in a qualitatively identical manner, and hence they are listed together in Table 32–1; *lidocaine* and *phenytoin* (diphenylhydantoin) also resemble each other in their electrophysiological actions on the heart and are likewise listed together in the table. The other two agents, *propranolol* and *bretylium,* require individual consideration. (*See* Bigger, 1972; Mason *et al.,* 1973a, 1973b; Moss and Patton, 1973.)

Pathological Physiology of Arrhythmias. Disorders of impulse generation include *premature contractions* (*extrasystoles*) originating in abnormal or *ectopic* foci in atria or ventricles, *paroxysmal supraventricular tachycardia, atrial flutter, atrial fibrillation,* and *ventricular tachycardia* and *fibrillation.* Although many attempts have been made on the basis of experimental work to assign to them a common physiological mechanism, there is as yet no agreement on the fundamental processes involved.

Three possible mechanisms for ectopic impulse formation must be considered:

1. *Pacemaker activity,* which is identified electrophysiologically by a slow diastolic depolarization similar to that normally seen in the sinus node, has been observed in isolated preparations of cardiac tissue, particularly in fibers of the specialized conduction system; similar activity occurs in single cells of tissue culture preparations. Under certain conditions true pacemaker activity in an extranodal site may give rise to an ectopic focus. Such a focus may appear as a repetitive ectopic rhythm if its intrinsic frequency exceeds that of the normal pacemaker, or it may be exposed by deceleration of the normal pacemaker or by "entrance block" (*e.g.,* the idioventricular rhythm that occurs after complete A-V block). Isolated extrasystoles of this nature would be expected to occur only late in diastole; however, if local block prevents access of the normal impulse into the ectopic pacemaker site, extrasystoles may occur as a parasystolic rhythm at any time during the nonrefractory phase. Studies indicate that the phase-4 depolarization may of itself provide the entrance block that protects the ectopic focus (Singer *et al.,* 1967). There is also evidence that a "special" type of ectopic impulse generation, differing in important aspects from "normal" phase-4 depolarization, may be produced by digitalis.

2. *"Reentry"* of the *circus-movement* type is commonly invoked to explain flutter and fibrillation of the atria. It is believed to be established when an impulse, blocked temporarily in one direction by refractory tissue, is forced to make a one-way transit about an obstacle. The obstacle may be anatomical (one of the orifices of the atrium), or pathological (an area of damaged or infarcted tissue), or physiological (an area of refractory tissue). Provided the perimeter of the obstacle is long enough, or the ERP of the tissue is brief enough, or the conduction velocity is slow enough, the impulse will, on returning to its source, find the originally refractory tissue recovered and will be able to complete the circuit and establish a repetitive rotation. Reentry is probably responsible also for many cases of paroxysmal

Table 32–1. EFFECTS OF THERAPEUTIC CONCENTRATIONS OF ANTIARRHYTHMIC AGENTS ON ELECTROPHYSIOLOGICAL PROPERTIES OF HEART

	QUINIDINE, PROCAINAMIDE	LIDOCAINE, PHENYTOIN	PROPRANOLOL	BRETYLIUM [1]
Automaticity				
Sinus node	→	→	↓	↑
Ectopic pacemakers	↓	↓	↓	↑
Excitability (Purkinje and myocardial fibers)	↓	→ [2]	↓	→ or ↑
Membrane responsiveness	↓	→, ↑, or ↓	↓	→
Purkinje fibers				
Action-potential duration (APD)	↑	↓	↓	↑
Effective refractory period (ERP)	↑	↓	↓	↑
ERP/APD	↑	↑	↑	→
Conduction velocity (A-V node and Purkinje fibers)	↓ [3]	→ or ↑	↓	→
A-V conduction time	→ or ↑	→ or ↓	→ or ↑	→ or ↑

Key: ↑, increased; ↓, decreased; →, no change.

[1] Increased automaticity and several other effects of bretylium are due to release of catecholamines during early stage of its action.

[2] Lidocaine reduces myocardial excitability; effects at other sites and those of phenytoin are variable.

[3] Effects of quinidine are variable, depending on balance of direct and vagal blocking actions.

(Modified from Bigger, 1972; Mason *et al.,* 1973a; Moss and Patton, 1973; and others.)

supraventricular tachycardia, and may account for ventricular premature beats and tachycardia.

3. A type of *reentry* due to *reciprocal activation between adjacent fibers or groups of fibers* has been postulated as a possible explanation for closely coupled premature beats. It is assumed that if adjacent fibers fail to repolarize simultaneously, the potential difference between them may be sufficient to induce reexcitation of the fiber that recovers first. This mechanism is improbable; the electrotonic interaction between *functionally connected* fibers effectively prevents a gross disparity in their repolarization times and, therefore, limits the potential difference between them (Méndez, C., *et al.,* 1969). Current flow of low magnitude, however, may change the rate of diastolic depolarization in pacemaker fibers and thus alter their firing frequency (Trautwein and Kassebaum, 1961).

Closely coupled extrasystoles probably represent a reentrant phenomenon (Hoffman, 1966). When an impulse is blocked locally (*e.g.,* at a Purkinje-muscle junction), the action potential and ERP of the fibers just proximal to the site of block may be extraordinarily brief (Méndez, C., *et al.,* 1969). Very slow conduction, at rates as low as 5% of normal, may occur in isolated preparations of Purkinje fibers; reentry on this basis has been demonstrated by Wit and associates (1972). The combination of abbreviated ERP and slow conduction permits reentry in a circuit of very limited length (Sasyniuk and Méndez, 1971).

Any of these postulated mechanisms may be responsible for the genesis of occasional or frequent premature contractions, as well as for the initiation of more severe and persistent dysrhythmias, but an understanding of the mechanism by which the latter are maintained, sometimes for very long periods, requires consideration in some detail.

Atrial Fibrillation. Atrial fibrillation is characterized by irregular and asynchronous activation of the atria at high frequency. Because of the fractionated and asynchronous responses, no effective mechanical systole occurs; the atria are distended as in diastole, and only fibrillar twitchings are visible. No P waves are discernible in ECG records, but irregular low-amplitude fluctuations of the "base line" may be recorded at an apparent frequency of 350 to 600 per minute. Only a fraction of the atrial impulses successfully traverse the A-V node; the ventricular rate is in the range of 100 to 200 beats per minute and is usually grossly irregular.

The underlying mechanism of fibrillation is commonly believed to be either an *ectopic focus,* which fires at a frequency that exceeds the capacity of the atria to follow, or a *circus movement,* in which a wave front courses endlessly about an obstacle, again at a frequency too rapid for regular and orderly excitation of the atria. Experimentally, fibrillation can be initiated by rapid, repetitive electrical stimulation, or by the focal injection of small doses of depolarizing drugs into the wall of the atrium. Once established, the arrhythmia may sustain itself indefinitely and independently of the inciting agency. As observed clinically, the arrhythmia may persist for many years; no theory can be considered adequate unless it accounts for the intrinsic stability of the disorder.

Fibrillation can be explained as a self-sustaining arrhythmia in terms of certain normal features of impulse propagation in relatively refractory tissue. The important features are these: (1) the atria are not homogeneous with respect to refractory period (RP) or conduction velocity; (2) the RP is related to the interval between the responses (*i.e.,* inversely related to the frequency); and (3) the conduction velocity is a function of the level of excitability during the relatively refractory period. If the atria were absolutely homogeneous, any impulse, however premature, would be propagated uniformly in all directions from its site of origin; the turbulence characteristic of fibrillation would be impossible. The atria, however, are *not* homogeneous. A premature response will be propagated along an irregular wave front, moving quickly through tissue in an advanced state of recovery, slowly through more refractory tissue, and not at all through tissue still inexcitable. As a result, the interval between the primary and the premature responses will not be constant; consequently, the initial intrinsic variation in RP will be increased. The recovery of excitability following the premature impulse will therefore exhibit a more irregular contour than the excitatory wave front. If still another premature response is generated, the field into which it is propagated will be still more irregularly excitable, and fractionation of the wave front into numerous independent daughter wavelets can occur. When such fractionation and disintegration develop, the process will tend to sustain itself; numerous impulses will course independently, changing in direction and conduction velocity as they encounter tissue in varying stages of refractoriness, dividing into smaller wavelets about islands of completely refractory tissue, or becoming extinguished at refractory barriers (Moe, 1962).

The likelihood of persistence of the arrhythmia will depend upon the number of independent wavelets that can be supported in the tissues. If the number is large, the possibility of chance coalescence or fusion with mutual extinction is small; however, if the number is small, there is a high probability of spontaneous arrest of the process. The number of wavelets, in turn, must depend upon (1) the mass or area of the tissue, (2) the duration of the RP, and (3) the conduction velocity. Large atria can support a larger number of wave fronts; chronic fibrillation is common in the distended and enlarged atria of patients with mitral stenosis. The importance of the RP is also well documented. If the RP were very long, all existing wavelets would encounter refractory tissue and become extinguished. Conversely, vagal stimulation or cholinergic drugs, which abbreviate the atrial RP, are known to facilitate the induction and maintenance of fibrillation. Conduction velocity is less well defined as a factor, for under the conditions of fibrillation it is not an independent variable (the conduction velocity in relatively refractory tissue varies with the stage of refractoriness). Nevertheless, it is clear that, if impulses were propagated rapidly, the whole mass of the tissue would soon be left in the refractory state; that is, the process would be arrested.

Long-standing fibrillation, with accompanying chronic dilatation of the atria, may grossly alter the normal electrophysiological properties of the muscle. These pathological changes may account for the failure of therapeutic attempts at conversion (Singer and TenEick, 1971).

Atrial Flutter. Although a fixed circuit is probably not responsible for sustained fibrillation, it may well account for at least some cases of atrial flutter. A circus movement can be initiated in a ring of excitable tissue if an impulse can be induced to travel in only one direction from a site of stimulation. If the conduction time around the circuit exceeds the duration of the ERP, then the tissue at the site of origin will again be excitable when the wave front reaches it, and the process can sustain itself indefinitely (Rosenblueth, 1953).

The frequency depends upon the path length and the RP of the tissue; if the RP is prolonged, the wave front will engage tissue in a less advanced state of recovery and will decelerate. If the RP is sufficiently prolonged, the wave front will be extinguished and the circus movement will terminate. This has long been the pharmacodynamic explanation of the effect of quinidine. If the wave front is moving at submaximal speed through relatively refractory tissue (*i.e.*, if the path length is a "tight fit"), abbreviation of the RP by vagal stimulation or vagomimetic drugs will increase the frequency. As is often observed in clinical cases, the atria may then be thrown into fibrillation. As is also commonly observed in these cases, withdrawal of the cholinergic agency may then be followed by reversion to sinus rhythm, resumption of the flutter, or persistence of the fibrillation.

The frequency of a circus movement should also be influenced by agents that alter the conduction velocity. An increased speed of propagation should cause the head of the circus wave to engage the refractory tail. However, before extinction of the process occurs, the wave front must enter relatively refractory tissue and slow down. In other words, the effect of increased conduction velocity *per se* cannot be readily assessed as a variable independent of the RP. Primary slowing of conduction, on the other hand, must result in deceleration of the circus movement, and will favor its perpetuation. A circus-movement flutter is likely to be stable if the "excitable gap" is relatively long, that is, if the wave front travels through tissue that has nearly recovered to full excitability.

Initiation of a circus-movement flutter requires at least one premature beat, generated early enough to be propagated in only one direction. One-way propagation can only occur if the tissue is nonhomogeneous. The same considerations apply to the initiation of fibrillation; fibrillation can be easily induced by a single premature stimulus applied to the atrium if the nonuniformity of the tissue with respect to refractory periods is increased, as it is by vagal stimulation. Ventricular fibrillation is also facilitated by agencies that increase the inhomogeneity of the muscle (Han and Moe, 1964).

Paroxysmal Supraventricular Tachycardia. This disorder is characterized by a slower frequency than flutter, in the range of 150 to 200 beats per minute; it is often precisely regular. The dysrhythmia is commonly attributed to a rhythmic ectopic pacemaker, and there is no reason to doubt that this mechanism

occurs; however, certain features of the disorder in many cases suggest that a circus movement may exist, with part of the pathway in the S-A or in the A-V node (Barker *et al.,* 1943). Examples in which reciprocation between atria and ventricles occurs as a result of a longitudinal dissociation of the A-V node have been induced experimentally in animals (Moe and Méndez, 1966) and in man (Schuilenburg and Durrer, 1968; Bigger and Goldreyer, 1970). Episodes of supraventricular paroxysmal tachycardia can often be terminated abruptly by reflexly increased vagal tone (carotid sinus pressure) or cholinomimetic drugs. The use of such agencies is described elsewhere.

QUINIDINE

The main use of quinidine is in the therapy of atrial fibrillation and certain other cardiac arrhythmias. Quinidine is employed much less frequently than digitalis. It must be used with great care, for it is a dangerous as well as an effective drug.

History. Quinidine, an optical isomer of quinine, was first described in 1848 by van Heyningen, and was prepared and given its present name by Pasteur in 1853. In the use of quinine and quinidine for malaria, it was noted many years ago that malarial patients who also had atrial fibrillation would occasionally be cured of arrhythmia by these drugs.

Perhaps the earliest recorded reference to the use of cinchona in atrial fibrillation is that of the French physician Jean-Baptiste de Sénac of Paris, in 1749 (*see* Willius and Keys, 1942). Years later Wenckebach (1914) reported on the effect of quinine alkaloids in certain cardiac arrhythmias. Frey (1918), impressed by the report of Wenckebach, studied quinine, cinchonine, and quinidine in patients with atrial fibrillation and found quinidine to be the most effective. His observations were quickly confirmed by others, and the use of quinidine was extended to additional disorders of cardiac rhythm.

Chemistry. Quinidine is the *d* isomer of quinine and is found with the latter in cinchona bark. The chemistry of the cinchona alkaloids is presented in the discussion of quinine (Chapter 52).

PHARMACOLOGICAL PROPERTIES

Although quinidine shares many of the pharmacological actions of quinine, as employed in therapy the former is more toxic; however, this may be due, in part, to the use of quinidine in clinical conditions that tend to exaggerate its dangers. Both alkaloids are depressant to skeletal and cardiac muscle. The effects of quinine on skeletal muscle are described in Chapter 52. The actions of quinidine on cardiac muscle are more effective than those of quinine.

Cardiac Actions. Quinidine is generally regarded as a myocardial depressant drug, for it depresses excitability, conduction velocity, and contractility. Its direct effects upon the heart are complicated to some extent by indirect effects resulting from an anticholinergic action. Except for differences in potency, the description that follows applies also to procainamide (*see* Table 32–1).

Excitability. The threshold potential for electrical excitation is increased by quinidine, and this is often cited as one of the mechanisms by which it may depress or abolish ectopic impulse generation. In isolated preparations, this has been demonstrated for atria (West and Amory, 1960) and to a lesser extent for Purkinje tissue and papillary muscle (Hoffman, 1958; *see also* Trautwein, 1963). In the intact dog heart, the threshold of excitation of atrial and ventricular muscle is increased and intraventricular conduction is depressed at plasma concentrations within the therapeutic range (Wallace *et al.*, 1966a).

Refractory Period. The ERP is increased by as much as 50% in isolated rabbit atria exposed to quinidine (West and Amory, 1960). Similar effects are observed in isolated ventricular muscle and Purkinje fibers (Hoffman, 1958). In the intact dog, quinidine in doses of 5 to 10 mg/kg causes a significant prolongation of the atrial ERP. The effect is in part direct, but the vagal blocking action of the drug must also play a role. In the ventricles, the ERP is increased by only about 10% by doses of 10 mg/kg, but it may be doubled by doses in the clearly toxic range (20 mg/kg).

The functional RP of the A-V node, defined as the minimal possible interval between two ventricular responses both propagated from the atrium, is slightly prolonged by the direct action of quinidine; however, the vagal blocking action produces the opposite result, an effect that has considerable importance in the clinical use of the drug (*see* below).

The prolongation of the ERP is not accompanied by a comparable increase in the duration of the action potential, as recorded from microelectrodes in single units of atrium, ventricle, or Purkinje tissues. In other words, in the presence of a sufficient concentration of quinidine the tissue *remains refrac-* *tory for an appreciable interval after full restoration of the resting membrane potential.* This is undoubtedly a most important action of the drug; even a slight prolongation of the ERP may prevent the completion of a closely coupled reentrant circuit.

Conduction Velocity. Quinidine decreases the conduction velocity in isolated atria, Purkinje fibers, and ventricular muscle. The slope of the rising phase of the action potential is decreased in these tissues (Hoffman, 1958; Vaughan Williams, 1958), as well as in single units of the A-V node (Sano *et al.*, 1958). Coupled with a reduction of excitability, the decreased speed of depolarization is undoubtedly the reason for the depression of conduction. Delay in the rise time of the action potential is observed with doses that do not alter resting membrane potential or the intracellular Na^+ and K^+ concentrations (Goodford and Vaughan Williams, 1962; Szekeres and Vaughan Williams, 1962); accordingly, it has been suggested that quinidine must reduce the "availability" of the sodium carrier. The hypothesis is attractive, for it would also explain the delay in repolarization and the diminished excitability observed with larger doses (Klein *et al.*, 1960).

Action on Pacemaker Activity. Quinidine in "therapeutic" concentrations causes an increase in the duration of the action potential of cells of the S-A node of isolated rabbit atria; and, by decreasing the slope of slow diastolic depolarization, it reduces spontaneous frequency (West and Amory, 1960). Ectopic pacemaker activity, which often develops spontaneously in the specialized conducting tissue (bundle of His or strands of Purkinje fibers) in isolated preparations of rabbit or dog ventricle, is also inhibited by quinidine. The effect of quinidine on such "ectopic" pacemakers is said to be much more pronounced than on S-A nodal cells (Hoffman, 1958). These results clearly provide an adequate explanation for the efficacy of the drug in reducing the incidence of premature ectopic beats, even when these are not "coupled" to an immediately preceding beat.

Membrane Responsiveness. The maximal rate of depolarization (dv/dt) during phase 0 of the action potential is a sigmoid function of the membrane potential at which excitation occurs (Weidmann, 1955). Accordingly, premature responses initiated before complete repolarization (during phase 3), or after a significant degree of phase-4 depolarization has developed, may be propagated at diminished speed. The curve relating dv/dt to the membrane potential, defined as membrane responsiveness, is shifted to the right by quinidine; that is, the cell membrane must be more completely repolarized before a propagated action potential can occur (*see* review by Singer and TenEick, 1969). In effect, this means that a premature response initiated during the relatively refractory period (*i.e.*, during phase 3) may fail to propagate. Quinidine, therefore, may abolish premature beats whether initiated by ectopic pacemaker activity or by a reentrant circuit.

Vagal Blocking Action. As mentioned above, the direct actions of quinidine are complicated in the intact heart by the vagal blocking action of the drug. Quinidine prevents the cardiac slowing produced by vagal stimulation and by cholinomimetic drugs. Accordingly, in spite of the direct depressant action on pacemaker cells, the drug causes an increased heart rate in unanesthetized animals and in man. The cardioacceleration is partly due to the anticholinergic action, but may also be due to reflex increase of adrenergic influences as a result of the fall of arterial pressure. In fact, it has been found that the frequency of both S-A nodal and idioventricular pacemakers in dogs with complete A-V block is increased by quinidine, even when vagal influences are blocked; after interruption of the cardiac adrenergic nerve supply, quinidine depresses both pacemakers (Roberts *et al.*, 1962).

The ERP of atrial muscle is reduced by vagal stimulation; the anticholinergic action of quinidine here adds to its direct action. It has not been established how much of the clinically useful action of quinidine in the treatment of atrial fibrillation is due to its atropine-like action, but the drug is commonly used in this disorder only after the administration of digitalis, which *increases* vagal activity. Indeed, atropine itself may abolish atrial fibrillation induced by digitalis in experimental animals.

The anticholinergic action of quinidine on the A-V node is an important consideration in the clinical use of the drug. Cholinergic

influences profoundly decrease the A-V conduction velocity and increase apparent ERP; by antagonizing vagal effects, quinidine may *increase* the conductivity of the A-V node—a distinct hazard when the drug is used in the therapy of atrial flutter or fibrillation (*see* Figure 32–2). Because quinidine antagonizes the effects of vagal excitation upon the atrium and A-V node, the administration of parasympathomimetic drugs or the use of any other procedure to enhance vagal activity may fail to terminate paroxysmal supraventricular tachycardia in patients receiving quinidine.

None of the effects of quinidine upon ventricular structures is altered by the vagal

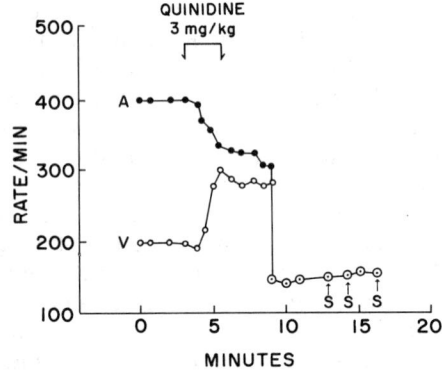

Figure 32–2. *Effect of quinidine on experimental circus-movement flutter.*

A dog was anesthetized with a combination of morphine and chloralose, which preserves a normal level of vagal tone and reflex activity. After creation of a suitable obstacle by crushing the atrial muscle between the superior and inferior venae cavae, flutter was initiated by a brief burst of stimuli applied to the atrium at a frequency of 20 per second. The flutter was stable with an atrial (*A*) frequency of 400 per minute; 2:1 A-V block was present. Quinidine was administered intravenously in a total dose of 3 mg/kg. As the atrial frequency diminished, presumably because of a prolongation of atrial ERP, the ventricular (*V*) frequency increased abruptly to 300. The degree of A-V block was diminished to the range of about 8:7. When the atrial frequency had slowed to 300 per minute, arrest of the flutter occurred abruptly with restoration of sinus rhythm. Repeated attempts to reinitiate flutter (*S*) were unsuccessful. The experimental preparation closely duplicates the response in clinical cases; dangerous acceleration of the ventricles during conversion can be prevented by prior digitalization. (Courtesy of A. E. Farah, Sterling-Winthrop Research Institute.)

blocking actions of the drug, except as indirect consequences of changes in heart rate.

Electrocardiographic Signs of Quinidine Action. The actions of quinidine in moderate and toxic doses may be predicted from the foregoing discussion. Sinus tachycardia results from the anticholinergic action. With higher doses, S-A block may occur as a result of depression of conduction and excitability. The Q-T interval is prolonged, due in part to increased duration of electrical systole, but also in part to diminished intraventricular conduction velocity, reflected also in an increased duration of the QRS complex. Large doses, which increase the temporal dispersion of ventricular refractory periods (Han and Moc, 1964), may *induce* idioventricular impulse generation. Caution is obviously mandatory in the use of the drug for the treatment of ventricular ectopic rhythms; increasing the dose after therapeutic failure may increase the hazard. It is difficult to ascertain how many "intractable" arrhythmias are due to overzealous treatment. In high doses, quinidine is capable of causing ventricular fibrillation. It is generally recognized that this hazard is related to the depressant effect upon intraventricular conduction, and prolongation of QRS complexes is a danger signal in the clinical use of the drug. The introduction of cardiac electroshock therapy for the initial reversion of atrial fibrillation may minimize this iatrogenic hazard, for "prophylactic" doses of the drug are less likely to lead to dangerous concentrations.

Quinidine may cause unpredictable abnormalities of rhythm in digitalized hearts. As its use in atrial fibrillation is not recommended without prior digitalization, very careful surveillance of the patient is necessary.

Myocardial Contractility. Quinidine reduces the tension developed in isolated preparations of atrial and ventricular muscle. The depression of contractility must be regarded as a toxic effect, and may be due in part to depression of conduction leading to a reduction of the synchrony of contraction. In isolated tissues, the negative inotropic action is only slight with concentrations below 5 to 10 μg/ml. Doses in the "safe" therapeutic range probably do not significantly depress contractility in normal hearts, but myocar-

dial depression of even slight degree may be significant in damaged hearts.

Blood Pressure. Large oral doses of quinidine reduce the arterial pressure in human subjects. The depressor action is primarily due to peripheral vasodilatation. Reduction of arterial pressure of serious degree is more likely with parenteral use of the drug.

Action of Quinidine on Cardiac Arrhythmias. In experimental animals, quinidine has been shown to raise the threshold for electrically induced arrhythmias, protect against the idioventricular arrhythmias produced by the combination of epinephrine and myocardial-sensitizing anesthetic agents, prevent or terminate the "late" ventricular tachycardias following coronary artery occlusion, and terminate or prevent circus-movement flutter. These actions of the drug can be explained in terms of the cardiac effects described above.

Ectopic Beats. Premature atrial or ventricular contractions coupled to normal beats are probably suppressed by prolongation of the ERP beyond the termination of the action potential. Premature contractions initiated later in the diastolic phase of either atrium or ventricle are probably not "reentrant." The evidence from isolated preparations suggests that such responses are most likely to originate either in the Purkinje fibers of the ventricle or in electrophysiologically similar cells of the atrium. The action of quinidine to reduce the rate of slow-diastolic depolarization in ectopic pacemakers has been described above. These effects of the drug are of importance not only in its use for the prevention of isolated premature beats but also in its prophylactic use to prevent episodes of tachycardia, flutter, or fibrillation, all of which appear to be initiated by one or more "premature" beats.

Paroxysmal Supraventricular Tachycardia. This dysrhythmia is characterized by sudden onset and sudden termination. If it is due to ectopic atrial or A-V nodal "pacemaker" activity, the effects of quinidine can be understood in terms of the actions described above. If the dysrhythmia is due to a circus movement through a pathway including nodal tissue (*reciprocal rhythm*), the result of various therapeutic maneuvers may be ascribed to actions upon the nodal elements. In general, the frequency of the tachycardias that can clearly be classified in this group is rather narrowly limited to the range of 150 to 200 beats per minute; this implies that the conditions that permit the dysrhythmia are also circumscribed. If this is true, then any major change of the properties of the nodal cells can result in interruption of the circuit. For example, increased vagal activity, which reduces nodal conductivity, can block the intranodal transit of the wave front and abolish the paroxysm; many episodes are readily terminated by this means. On the other hand, an increased velocity of conduction in nodal tissue, which can be expected when anticholinergic drugs are administered, can cause the advancing wave front to extinguish itself in refractory tissue. Precise timing of the events just prior to termination of the paroxysm under the influence of digitalis (*increased vagal* activity) or of quinidine (*antivagal* activity) should provide a clue to the mechanism, but sufficiently careful studies have not been made. Whatever the mechanism, quinidine can be expected to have prophylactic value by suppressing the ectopic impulses that must initiate the tachycardia.

Atrial Flutter. Prolongation of the ERP of the atrium is commonly cited as the one desirable attribute of an "antiflutter" drug. The situation is by no means simple, for the effects of antiarrhythmic drugs upon ERP and upon conduction velocity are inextricably linked. When quinidine is administered to a dog in which a circus-movement flutter has been established, or to a patient with atrial flutter, the frequency invariably declines before reversion abruptly ensues. In the example illustrated in Figure 32–2, the atrial rate diminished by about 25% prior to termination of the circus movement. Quinidine slows conduction velocity in atrial muscle, which could account for the reduction of rate; but it also increases the atrial RP, which could reduce the rate by forcing the circulating impulse to travel in relatively refractory tissue. The two actions are opposed. If the predominant effect of quinidine were a primary reduction of conduction velocity, reversion to sinus rhythm should not be expected to occur until the flutter frequency diminished to less than the prevailing rate of the sinus node. But if the action is primarily upon the ERP, then the conduction velocity will be secondarily depressed until some minimal value is reached below which successful impulse propagation is no longer possible. This may well be the mechanism of action of quinidine in the experimental situation, but the details of the process are still not clearly defined. Méndez (C.) and associates (1969) emphasize the importance of the "wavelength" (*i.e.*, the product of ERP and conduction velocity) in termination of circus-movement flutter. Agents that prolong the ERP without specifically depressing conduction velocity are more effective than those with both actions.

Atrial Fibrillation. If atrial fibrillation were due to a single circus movement about an obstacle so limited in size that activation of the surrounding tissue is irregular and fractionated, then the circuit pathway itself would be unstable. This mechanism seems unlikely, for fibrillation can be, and often is, a very stable arrhythmia. If, however, fibrillation is due to the random wandering of numerous fractionated wavelets, changing in breadth, direction, and number from moment to moment, as suggested by Burn (1961) and by Moe and Abildskov (1959), then the persistence of the arrhythmia is critically related to the degree of inhomogeneity of the tissue and to the mean ERP. Vagal stimulation or cholinomimetic drugs should tend to perpetuate the arrhythmia by reducing the mean ERP and by increasing the range of variation of the ERPs. The action of quinidine here is twofold. By virtue of its direct and antivagal actions, quinidine may be expected to increase the mean ERP and also to reduce the inhomogeneity. The mathematical basis of these actions has been treated in detail by Moe and associates (1964). The action of quinidine, in terms of these concepts, is based not on its ability to snuff out a dominant circus movement but on its ability to reduce the number of wavelets possible in a given mass of tissue.

Toxic Reactions. Quinidine is a dangerous drug, and deaths have occurred from its use. Side effects may require cessation of maintenance therapy in as many as 30% of patients (Lown and Wolf, 1971). In large doses, quinidine can cause the syndrome known as *cinchonism,* which is described in Chapter 52. In the doses generally used, the most common toxic manifestations are gastrointestinal. Diarrhea frequently occurs; nausea and vomiting are also common.

Idiosyncrasy and Hypersensitivity. Idiosyncratic responses to quinidine are not uncommon, and the reaction of the patient to the first dose of the drug should be carefully observed in order to reduce the incidence of dangerous reactions. Occasionally, even small doses cause tinnitus, vertigo, visual disturbances, headache, confusion, skin rashes, angioedema, vomiting, cramps, and diarrhea. Thrombocytopenic purpura occurs as a rare but serious complication. This results from activation of an immune mechanism. In susceptible individuals, antibodies that react *in vitro* with platelets in the presence of quinidine can be demonstrated (Larson, 1953). Hypoprothrombinemic hemorrhage may occur in patients receiving both quinidine and warfarin (Koch-Weser, 1968).

Other serious forms of hypersensitivity are manifested by respiratory embarrassment or vascular collapse. Asthma, depression of breathing, and even respiratory arrest may occur. A precipitous fall in blood pressure associated with restlessness, vertigo, cold sweat, pallor, and syncope characterizes the vascular collapse produced by the drug. Norepinephrine or metaraminol may be useful to combat vascular collapse; artificial respiration and other supportive measures may also be required.

Embolism. The auricular appendages of chronically fibrillating atria often contain mural thrombi. A sudden quinidine-induced reversion to a normal sinus rhythm with resultant complete contractions of the atria may presumably cause the thrombi to be dislodged, whereupon embolic occlusion of the vessels in vital organs may develop. However, it is currently believed that the danger of embolism from quinidine therapy has been exaggerated and that accidents of this type are probably no more frequent after quinidine than when medication is withheld or digitalis employed (Askey, 1962).

"Paradoxical" Tachycardia. When quinidine slows the rate of the fluttering or fibrillating atria, the ventricles may suddenly accelerate as a result of a reduction in the degree of A-V block. The atropine-like effect of the drug on the A-V node, as mentioned above, adds to the hazard. An experimental demonstration of this event is illustrated in Figure 32-2. Tachycardia of this origin can be prevented by prior digitalization. Should arrest of fibrillation or flutter be accompanied by depression of the normal pacemaker, an idioventricular pacemaker may assume control. Occasionally, cardiac asystole may occur.

Ventricular Fibrillation. Selzer and Wray (1964) estimated that paroxysms of ventricular tachycardia or fibrillation may occur in as many as 3 or 4% of patients on quinidine therapy, even at doses not considered to be excessive. The hazard of fibrillation increases with the size of the dose used, and may be heralded by ECG signs of toxicity. The hazard is great when the drug is used in the treatment of ventricular tachycardias, in which the evidence of quinidine toxicity may be impossible to read in the ECG.

Hypotension. A reduction of arterial pressure regularly attends intravenous administration of quinidine; constant observation of pressure as well as of the ECG is mandatory when this route of administration is used.

Contraindications. Most contraindications to quinidine are relative, and each case should be considered individually. One of the few absolute contraindications is that of *complete A-V block* with an A-V nodal or idioventricular pacemaker that may be suppressed by quinidine, thus causing ventricular arrest. Quinidine should also be used with extreme caution in patients with incomplete A-V block since complete block and asystole may be produced. Another absolute contraindication is a history of thrombocytopenic

purpura associated with previous quinidine administration.

The known depressant actions of quinidine on cardiac contractility and arterial blood pressure limit its use in congestive heart failure and hypotensive states. In these situations the risk of quinidine administration must be weighed against the danger of the condition for which it is to be given. Ventricular tachycardia complicating acute myocardial infarction is the prime example of a state in which hypotension and low cardiac output may exist; yet the use of quinidine in this situation may be lifesaving.

Quinidine should *not* be used in the treatment of *digitalis intoxication.* In this situation, phenytoin, lidocaine, or propranolol may be indicated, according to the type of arrhythmia that is present (*see* below, and Chapter 31).

Absorption, Fate, and Excretion. Quinidine is essentially completely absorbed after oral administration; maximal effects occur within 1 to 3 hours, and persist for 6 to 8 or more hours. The biological half-life is about 5 hours; large fluctuations in plasma concentration may be expected if repeated doses are given at this interval. When cumulative effects are sought, repeated doses are given at intervals of 2 to 4 hours. Intramuscular administration of quinidine (usually as the gluconate) yields peak effects in 30 to 90 minutes. Intravenous administration does not produce instantaneous effects; accordingly, the drug should be administered slowly and cautiously by this route to avoid overdosage.

Quinidine is rapidly bound by plasma albumin. When the total plasma concentration of the drug is in the therapeutic range of 3 to 6 μg/ml, approximately 60% of the alkaloid is in the bound form (Conn and Luchi, 1961). The alkaloid and some of its degradation products are also bound to tissue proteins; concentrations 40 times greater than those in plasma have been noted in dog hearts.

Quinidine plasma concentrations have been determined in animals and man to establish the range of values at which therapeutic and toxic effects appear (*see* Table 32-2). The usual analytical method is not specific for quinidine, and the reported values therefore include some inactive as well as some ac-

Table 32–2. PLASMA CONCENTRATIONS OF ANTIARRHYTHMIC AGENTS RECORDED DURING THERAPEUTIC TRIALS IN PATIENTS *

	QUINIDINE ($\mu g/ml$)	PROCAINAMIDE ($\mu g/ml$)	LIDOCAINE ($\mu g/ml$)	PHENYTOIN ($\mu g/ml$)
Partially effective	1.5–2.5	2–4	1–2	4–8
Usually effective	2.5–5.0	4–8	2–5	8–16
Potentially toxic	> 5	> 8	> 5	> 16

* After Koch-Weser, 1972. Courtesy of *Archives of Internal Medicine.*

tive products of quinidine metabolism. In general, it has been reported that therapeutic responses can rarely be expected below 3 μg/ml of plasma, and that toxic reactions are almost certain to occur at levels above 10 μg/ml. The careful studies of Kalmansohn and Sampson (1950a, 1950b), Sokolow and Ball (1956), Conn (1964), and others have provided an excellent understanding of the time course, accumulation, and dosage schedules of oral and parenteral therapy. For example, Sokolow and Ball found that 85% of conversions of atrial fibrillation to normal sinus rhythm occurred with daily doses of 3 g or less, and at plasma concentrations of 8 μg/ml or less.

The metabolic end products of quinidine metabolism have been isolated and identified, and the pharmacological activity of several of these has been assessed (*see* Conn, 1964). Substantially all the administered compound is excreted by the kidney, and about 10 to 50% appears in the urine as unchanged quinidine, within 24 hours.

Preparations and Routes of Administration. *Quinidine Sulfate,* U.S.P., is available for oral administration in the form of 100-, 200-, and 300-mg tablets or capsules. Unofficial preparations for slow absorption are available; these include a 300-mg extended-release tablet of quinidine sulfate, a 330-mg tablet of *quinidine gluconate* (QUINAGLUTE), and a 275-mg tablet of *quinidine polygalacturonate* (CARDIOQUIN). For intravenous use, *Quinidine Gluconate Injection,* U.S.P., is the official form; it is provided in 10-ml vials containing 80 mg/ml. *Quinidine hydrochloride* is also available as an injection in 1-ml ampuls containing 200 mg/ml. Quinidine sulfate is soluble in water to the extent of only 1.0%; the gluconate is soluble to about 10%, but for intravenous injection the necessary dose is further diluted to 800 mg/50 ml in 5% glucose solution and is injected *slowly,* at the rate of 16 mg per minute, with continuous observation of the patient and of the ECG. Intravenous injection should be undertaken only in hospitalized patients. It is important to record the arterial pressure at frequent intervals. Injection should be halted when arterial pressure drops severely, or when the arrhythmia is terminated, or when signs of toxicity (*e.g.,* 25% prolongation of the QRS interval) appear.

THERAPEUTIC USES

The major clinical uses of quinidine are for the prevention or abolition of certain cardiac arrhythmias. These include atrial fibrillation, atrial flutter, paroxysmal supraventricular and ventricular tachycardia, and premature systoles. Quinidine also has a few miscellaneous therapeutic applications, some of which are unrelated to its cardiac actions.

Atrial Fibrillation. *Indications for the Use of Quinidine.* Quinidine is used to convert atrial fibrillation to normal sinus rhythm and to prevent the recurrence of this arrhythmia. Since atrial fibrillation is compatible with a state of well-being for many years, it has been difficult to establish whether and when conversion to normal sinus rhythm is advisable. It is not possible to give a general rule, but certain items should be taken into account in evaluating individual cases. (1) Inadequate cardiac output may be improved by conversion of atrial fibrillation to normal sinus rhythm (Hansen *et al.,* 1952). Conversion thus appears desirable in the patient in whom congestive failure cannot be controlled by other means. (2) When definitive surgical therapy of a cardiac lesion has been accomplished and has not been followed by spontaneous cessation of atrial fibrillation, conversion should be attempted. (3) Conversion is appropriate in the patient with atrial fibrillation in whom palpitation is a major complaint. (4) The likelihood that embolization may occur during chronic atrial fibrillation and at the time of conversion to normal sinus rhythm is a factor to be considered in a decision regarding conversion of atrial fibrillation. It appears that the risk of embolization at the time of conversion is small compared with the continuing danger of thromboembolism when the arrhythmia is allowed to persist (Goldman, 1960; Bloomfield *et al.,* 1973). *Technic of Administration and Dosage.* Attempts to convert atrial fibrillation to normal rhythm should be carried out in the hospital under close observation. In most cases atrial fibrillation is associated with a rapid ventricular rate, and this should be controlled by a digitalis glycoside prior to quinidine administration. If congestive failure is present, its manifestations should be controlled as completely as possible by digitalization, bed rest, diuretics, and other appropriate means prior to administration of quinidine. *In current hospital practice, electrical conversion is far more commonly used than is quinidine* *or procainamide. Drug therapy in prophylactic doses is then used to reduce the chance of recurrence (see below).*

Because of its relatively short half-life, a loading dose of quinidine is unnecessary. Many schedules of quinidine administration have been proposed. A widely used one is the administration of 200 to 300 mg of quinidine orally every 3 or 4 hours for 1 to 3 days. The medication is omitted at night to permit sleep. If such a course of therapy does not result in restoration of sinus rhythm, the individual dose may be increased to 400 mg and a 1- to 3-day course of therapy repeated. Even in the absence of toxic manifestations it is probably wise not to exceed a total daily dose of 4 g, given by any schedule, for the purpose of converting atrial fibrillation to normal rhythm. Therapy may be continued despite mild diarrhea, which is an extremely common side effect. Therapy should be discontinued if frequent ectopic ventricular beats occur. Transient atrial flutter is a frequent occurrence in the course of conversion of atrial fibrillation, but quinidine should be discontinued if *persistent* flutter occurs. When daily doses of 2 g are exceeded, an ECG should be observed, prior to each further dose, for widening of the QRS complex. Unless the need for conversion of atrial fibrillation is compelling and cannot be accomplished by other means, the drug should be discontinued when QRS widening develops.

Maintenance Therapy. When normal rhythm has been reestablished by whatever means, quinidine is usually administered in an attempt to prevent recurrence of atrial fibrillation. The variability of patients and of disease states has made it extremely difficult to evaluate the efficiency of such prophylactic therapy. Probably the most convincing evidence of its effectiveness is the well-known and easily demonstrated effect of the drug to abolish or reduce the frequency of premature beats. Atrial fibrillation is probably initiated by premature excitation; quinidine makes such excitation less likely.

The usual prophylactic dose of quinidine is 200 to 300 mg, three or four times a day. Such doses have been administered for years in situations in which fibrillation is likely to recur. When recurrence of fibrillation is less likely, for example, after surgical therapy of mitral stenosis, prophylactic therapy may be administered for a few weeks and then omitted.

Atrial Flutter. Quinidine has a place in the difficult clinical problem of the management of atrial flutter. It is much less effective in restoring normal rhythm in this disorder than in atrial fibrillation, probably because its actions on the ERP and on conduction velocity in atrial tissue are opposed. It is also less often effective than digitalis. *Digitalis* may result in conversion of atrial flutter to either atrial fibrillation or normal sinus rhythm (*see* Chapter 31).

Quinidine may be used in an attempt to restore normal sinus rhythm when digitalis has failed to convert flutter or has resulted in atrial fibrillation. In either case, quinidine is usually administered along with continued maintenance doses of digitalis. Quinidine alone may slow the atrial rate in flutter to such a level that 1 : 1 A-V transmission becomes possible and an increased ventricular rate results.

Digitalization is effective in preventing this phenomenon. Flutter may sometimes be "captured" and terminated by driving the atrium briefly at a rate in excess of the intrinsic flutter frequency by means of a transvenous intracardiac electrode.

Paroxysmal Supraventricular Tachycardia. Quinidine is sometimes employed for the conversion of paroxysmal A-V nodal or atrial tachycardia to normal sinus rhythm. Other therapeutic measures useful in these disorders include carotid sinus massage, electroshock, and a variety of drugs that activate cholinergic receptors or cause reflex vagal stimulation. Digitalis also has great utility.

Premature Systoles. Quinidine is useful for the suppression of premature systoles. For this purpose oral doses of 200 to 300 mg are given three or four times daily. Premature systoles are extremely common, and it is obviously not appropriate to employ drug therapy in all patients who exhibit such beats. If the premature systoles are frequent or troublesome or if they occur under special circumstances that are likely to lead to more serious arrhythmias, they should be treated. Such circumstances include acute myocardial infarction, in which ventricular premature systoles may presage the occurrence of ventricular tachycardia or fibrillation, or in acute coronary insufficiency without infarction (Bloomfield *et al.*, 1973). Atrial premature beats in patients who have types of heart disease frequently associated with atrial fibrillation, or in patients who have previously had atrial fibrillation, may be treated with quinidine in an attempt to prevent the occurrence of fibrillation.

Ventricular Tachycardia. This arrhythmia is often a complication of acute myocardial infarction and represents a serious hazard to life. Electroshock therapy is used with success to break the fixed, persistent tachycardia; lidocaine is almost universally used in the hospital setting both to treat and to prevent the arrhythmia (*see* below). Quinidine or procainamide is appropriate when the tachycardia occurs in repeated paroxysms. When quinidine is employed, the usual dose is 400 to 600 mg orally every 2 to 3 hours. Much larger doses may be used in resistant cases. As much as 600 mg every hour for 10 hours has been employed. If the patient is vomiting or in shock, intramuscular injections may be given. Intravenous quinidine may also be used, but it should be given slowly while the ECG is being constantly observed (January *et al.*, 1953). It is common practice to dilute 10 ml of the official injection (800 mg of quinidine gluconate) with 40 ml of 5% dextrose injection and administer it by slow intravenous drip during ½ to 1 hour while the blood pressure level and an ECG lead are frequently observed. *It is dangerous to abolish a ventricular tachycardia if A-V block exists, and it should probably not be attempted unless equipment for artificial pacing of the ventricles is at hand.* Unfortunately, it is often difficult to determine whether such block is present, but the prognosis of uncontrolled ventricular tachycardia is so poor that therapy must, nevertheless, be undertaken. When ventricular tachycardia attendant upon myocardial infarction has been broken, whether by electroshock therapy or by drug administration, maintenance therapy should be continued for 3 or 4 weeks until the danger of recurrence has subsided.

Miscellaneous Uses. Quinidine can be used as a diagnostic measure in the *Wolff-Parkinson-White syndrome,* in which it may abolish the ECG abnormality; presumably it depresses the aberrant conduction pathway. The action may be due in part to the atropine-like action of the drug.

Electroshock Therapy of Arrhythmias. Although hardly a pharmacotherapeutic measure, electroshock therapy is a valuable technic for the treatment of cardiac arrhythmias. Originally introduced as a heroic measure in cases of ventricular fibrillation, in which it is essentially the only possible curative procedure, it was successfully applied only after emergency thoracotomy. The introduction of devices generating high-voltage pulses of brief duration has made the method applicable in cases of supraventricular and ventricular tachycardias as well as ventricular fibrillation, by current delivered through electrodes applied to the unopened chest. In the treatment of supraventricular tachycardias, the shock may be triggered by the R wave of the ECG to fall at an instant when the danger of inducing ventricular fibrillation is minimal. The high-current density of the pulse presumably depolarizes all cardiac tissues, thereby arresting all impulse propagation. (Properly timed stimuli of lower intensity may interrupt paroxysms of supraventricular tachycardia or atrial flutter, presumably by occluding a reentrant pathway.) The technic has been applied successfully to arrest atrial flutter and fibrillation, supraventricular and ventricular tachycardias, and ventricular fibrillation, and has become the method of choice for the emergency treatment of these self-sustained arrhythmias (Lown, 1967). Electroshock is dangerous in the presence of digitalis toxicity, probably because the electrical discharge stimulates intrathoracic sympathetic nerves and may lead to serious and intractable ventricular ectopic rhythms (Kleiger and Lown, 1966). Intracardiac stimulation through transvenous probes has been successfully used in the treatment of episodes of paroxysmal supraventricular tachycardia and flutter. This technic is particularly useful in digitalized subjects, for the necessary stimulus strength is only slightly above threshold, and the hazard of massive excitation of intrathoracic nerves does not exist. (For procedures and references, *see* Barold and Linhart, 1970; Ticzon and Whalen, 1973.)

PROCAINAMIDE

History. In 1936, Mautz demonstrated that direct application of procaine to the myocardium elevated the threshold of ventricular muscle to electrical stimulation. Extension of this observation by numerous workers established that the cardiac actions of the local anesthetic resemble those of quinidine. However, the therapeutic value of procaine as an anti-fibrillatory and antiarrhythmic agent is limited by

its short duration of action as a result of the rapid enzymatic hydrolysis of the drug, and by its prominent effects upon the central nervous system (CNS). A systematic study of congeners and metabolites of procaine was undertaken to find a compound with clinically useful quinidine-like actions, and led to the introduction of procainamide as a cardiac drug (Mark *et al.,* 1951). Clinical use of the amide has shown it to be an effective antiarrhythmic agent, particularly in patients with abnormal ventricular rhythms.

Chemistry and Preparations. Procainamide is *p*-amino-N-(2-diethylaminoethyl) benzamide. Its structural formula is as follows:

Procainamide

It differs from procaine merely by replacement of the ester linkage by the amide structure. *Procainamide Hydrochloride,* U.S.P. (PRONESTYL), is a white to tan, odorless, crystalline salt that is readily soluble in water. For oral administration the drug is available as *Procainamide Hydrochloride Capsules,* U.S.P., which contain 250, 375, or 500 mg of the drug. *Procainamide Hydrochloride Injection,* U.S.P., supplied in 10-ml vials containing 100 mg/ml, is suitable for intramuscular and intravenous injection.

Pharmacological Actions. The pharmacological actions of procainamide are qualitatively similar to those of procaine. The advantage of the amide over the parent compound depends upon the more favorable ratio between its cardiac and CNS activities. In addition, the amide is not readily hydrolyzed by plasma esterases, possesses a more satisfactory duration of action, and is effective following oral administration.

The *cardiac actions* of procainamide are essentially identical to those described for quinidine (Wedd *et al.,* 1951; Zapata-Díaz *et al.,* 1952; Woske *et al.,* 1953; and others). The effective concentrations in isolated tissue preparations are approximately ten times as high as equally active concentrations of quinidine (Hoffman, 1958). *Excitability* of both the atrium and the ventricle to electrical stimulation is depressed. *Conduction* in the atrium and ventricle is slowed, but some acceleration of conduction may occur at low doses in specialized conducting fibers as a consequence of an increased membrane potential resulting from suppression of phase-4 depolarization. The ERP of the atrium is prolonged but that of the ventricle is only insignificantly increased. Like quinidine, procainamide usually prolongs the ERP more than the action potential. Cardiac contractility is said to be depressed less by procainamide than by quinidine. In man, *cardiac output* is not markedly decreased unless myocardial damage exists. The occasional accelerating effect of conventional doses of procainamide upon *heart rate* in the absence of arrhythmias indicates that the drug, like quinidine, also produces some degree of vagal block. Larger doses cause A-V block and the appearance of ventricular extrasystoles, which may proceed to ventricular fibrillation. *ECG changes* merely reflect the above-described effects of the drug upon the fundamental properties of the myocardium. Widening of the QRS complex is observed most consistently; prolongation of the P-R and Q-T intervals and alterations of the T waves occur less regularly. Procainamide effectively elevates the threshold of both the atrium and the ventricle to *electrically induced fibrillation*. Ventricular extrasystoles caused by ligation of the coronary arteries are also suppressed, but the drug has only variable protective efficacy against drug-induced arrhythmias.

Intravenous administration of procainamide causes a fall in *blood pressure;* peripheral vasodilatation probably contributes to the hypotensive response, but systolic pressure may be reduced more than diastolic. The hypotension is more pronounced when the control blood pressure is high and when the drug is injected rapidly; it is less marked when the drug is injected intramuscularly, and it is usually absent following oral administration. *CNS actions* of procainamide are not prominent. However, rapid intravenous injection of large doses in animals causes tremors, and death may result from respiratory depression. In man, an occasional patient may experience mental confusion and hallucinations.

Absorption, Fate, and Excretion. Procainamide is rapidly and almost completely absorbed from the gastrointestinal tract. When the drug is given orally, its plasma concentration becomes maximal in about 60 minutes; after intramuscular administration, peak plasma concentrations are reached in 15 to 60 minutes. The drug is relatively slowly hydrolyzed by plasma esterases, and the biological half-life is 3 to 4 hours; therefore, maintenance of effective plasma concentrations requires somewhat more frequent administration than with quinidine. At ordinary plasma concentrations, only 15% of procainamide is bound to macromolecular constituents of plasma. The concentration of drug in most tissues except brain is greater than that in plasma. Approximately 60% of the drug is excreted by the kidney. Two to 10% of an administered dose is recovered in the urine as free and conjugated *p*-aminobenzoic acid. Patients with congestive heart failure and impairment of renal function excrete procainamide more slowly, and cumulative effects during chronic administration are more likely in such individuals. Effective plasma concentrations are in the range of 2 to 8 μg/ml; toxic reactions are common above this range (Table 32–2).

Toxicity and Precautions. In addition to its usual toxic effects, procainamide can cause untoward responses by its actions on an abnormal myocardium or as a result of correction of the arrhythmia for which the drug is employed. As in the case of quinidine therapy of atrial fibrillation or flutter, the ventricular rate may suddenly increase as the atrial rate is slowed (*see* above); adequate digitalization reduces but does not abolish this danger. Ventricular tachysystole is particularly dangerous in the patient with myocardial damage. Procainamide, like quinidine, should not be administered when complete A-V block is present and should be used only cautiously in the presence of partial block because of the danger of asystole. Like quinidine, procainamide must be used with caution and medication must be stopped if the QRS complex is excessively widened.

Procainamide is usually well tolerated. However, it has occasionally caused serious side effects, and deaths have resulted. When the drug is given orally, the most frequently observed untoward effects are anorexia, nausea, and vomiting. Flushing, a bitter taste, diarrhea, weakness, mental depression, giddiness, and psychosis with hallucinations have also been reported. Hypersensitivity to the drug, chills, fever, joint and muscle pain, malaise, itching, angioedema, and urticarial or maculopapular skin rash have also occurred. Cross-sensitivity to procaine and related drugs should be anticipated. Fatal agranulocytosis has been reported, and frequent blood examinations during chronic procainamide therapy are essential. A syndrome similar to systemic lupus erythematosus is a common reaction to chronic administration, and may necessitate termination of therapy (*see* Koch-Weser, 1972, for references). Untoward effects during intravenous administration of procainamide are more frequent and severe than those observed when the drug is given orally. Hypotension commonly occurs and can result in cardiovascular collapse, convulsions, and coronary insufficiency. Serious disturbances of cardiac rhythm, such as ventricular asystole or fibrillation, are also more common when the drug is administered by vein. It should be infused *slowly,* with continuous observation of the ECG and frequent measurement of the blood pressure. Hypotension may occur after intramuscular procainamide, but it is usually not severe. The various dangers of medication must be balanced in each case against the severity of the arrhythmia and the possible benefit to be derived from reversion to a normal sinus mechanism; the drug is then administered or withheld on the basis of such an evaluation.

Dosage and Administration. When oral medication is possible, procainamide should be administered by this route. When parenteral medication is indicated, the drug should be injected intramuscularly. The intravenous route is reserved for cases of severe arrhythmia considered to be life-endangering or failing to respond to oral or intramuscular medication or other therapy. For the treatment of ventricular arrhythmias, the initial *oral* dose for adults is 500 mg to 1.0 g. Larger doses may be required for atrial arrhythmias. If an initial dose of 1.25 g does not produce favorable ECG changes in 1 hour, a second dose of 750 mg may be given, followed by additional doses of 500 mg to 1.0 g at intervals of 2 hours to the limit of tolerance or until the arrhythmia is interrupted. The maintenance dose is usually 500 mg to 1.0 g at intervals of 4 to 6 hours. The *intramuscular* dose is 500 mg to 1.0 g; this may be repeated at 6-hour intervals if oral medication is not feasible. The *intravenous* dose is 200 to 500 mg (occasionally as high as 1.0 g), administered at a rate not exceeding 25 to 50 mg per minute. The commercially available solution (100 mg/ml) should be diluted to permit greater control of the infusion rate. If the blood pressure falls more than 15 mm Hg, the injection should be temporarily discontinued. Solutions of phenylephrine or norepinephrine should be

available to counteract severe hypotensive responses. The infusion is stopped when the arrhythmia is interrupted, or if excessive widening of the QRS complex or other evidence of myocardial toxicity is observed.

Therapeutic Uses and Status. Procainamide has been employed in a wide variety of cardiac arrhythmias. In general, the effectiveness of the drug parallels that of quinidine, and some investigators consider that the two agents are interchangeable. However, procainamide may be effective in patients who have failed to respond to maximally tolerated doses of quinidine and *vice versa.*

Most favorable results have been reported in *ventricular arrhythmias* (except those resulting from digitalis intoxication). Ventricular extrasystoles and paroxysmal ventricular tachycardia are abolished in a large percentage of cases within a few minutes after intravenous injection or within an hour after oral or intramuscular administration. Maintenance therapy may be necessary in some cases. Recurrences usually respond as promptly as the initial episode.

Although ventricular extrasystoles and tachycardia caused by *digitalis intoxication* can be suppressed by procainamide, its effects are unpredictable and fatalities have occurred. If digitalis-induced tachycardia is accompanied by marked conduction disturbances, procainamide readily precipitates ventricular asystole or fibrillation. The complexities and dangers of the combined effects of digitalis and procainamide have been discussed by Zapata-Díaz and coworkers (1952).

In *atrial arrhythmias,* the percentage of failures with procainamide therapy is high (*see* monograph by Moss and Patton, 1973). Procainamide should be used in cases of paroxysmal atrial tachycardia only after reflex vagal stimulation and other measures and drugs of choice have failed. Normal sinus rhythm may be reestablished in cases of atrial fibrillation of short duration, but chronic cases are particularly stubborn. In atrial flutter, in spite of adequate prior digitalization, procainamide often merely slows the atrial rate, whereupon the ventricular rate may be suddenly and dangerously increased if the degree of A-V block is concurrently diminished.

Procainamide has been used in the treatment of *myotonia,* where its effects resemble those of quinine.

LIDOCAINE

Lidocaine is widely used as a local anesthetic (*see* Chapter 20). It has also achieved prominence as an antiarrhythmic agent and is now in common use, particularly in the emergency treatment of ventricular arrhythmias encountered during cardiac surgery or resulting from myocardial infarction. Its mechanism of action differs in some respects from that of quinidine and procainamide, and it possesses certain advantages over the older drugs. Chief among these, especially in the intensive coronary-care unit, is that its antiarrhythmic action develops very rapidly on intravenous administration, and declines quickly when infusion is discontinued. This permits moment-to-moment "titration" of ventricular ectopic activity.

When lidocaine is used in the treatment of ventricular extrasystoles or ventricular tachycardia, the effect of a single intravenous dose, or bolus, of 50 to 100 mg disappears within 10 to 20 minutes in parallel with the fall in its plasma concentration. This is due to *redistribution* to depots that have a more limited blood supply than the heart. When a subsequent continuous infusion, at the rate of 15 to 50 μg/kg per minute, is terminated, the decline of both cardiac effects and plasma concentration reflects the *metabolic* half-life of approximately 2 hours (*see* Harrison *et al.*, 1963; Thompson *et al.*, 1971).

In isolated preparations of canine ventricular tissue exposed to lidocaine concentrations of 0.3 to 30 μg/ml, the drug, like quinidine and procainamide, depresses automaticity of Purkinje fibers. The action may be due to an increased potassium conductance (Arnsdorf and Bigger, 1972). Unlike the older drugs, it abbreviates the APD in both Purkinje and muscle fibers and, to a lesser extent, reduces the ERP of Purkinje fibers. Accordingly, as with quinidine and procainamide, ERP/APD is increased. Membrane responsiveness and conduction velocity of Purkinje fibers are unaffected or increased at concentrations of lidocaine up to 3 μg/ml and depressed only at concentrations above 30 μg/ml (Davis and Temte, 1969; Bigger and Mandel, 1970). However, Singh and Vaughan Williams (1971) attributed these findings in part to the abnormally low concentrations of potassium (3 mEq per liter) present in the standard Tyrode's solution employed by the previous investigators; when the concentration of potassium was raised to 5.6 mEq per liter, they found that lidocaine, as well as phenytoin, caused a decrease in membrane responsiveness at concentrations of 3 μg/ml or higher (*see also* the review by Bassett and Witt, 1973). The electrophysiological properties of atrial mus-

cle are little affected by subtoxic concentrations (Mandel and Bigger, 1971). These observations may account for the lack of efficacy of lidocaine in the treatment of atrial arrhythmias. Doses up to 2 or 3 mg/kg cause little change in A-V conduction time, contractility, intraventricular conduction, or heart rate in anesthetized dogs (Lieberman *et al.*, 1968).

In man, lidocaine appears to cause less depression of arterial pressure and of myocardial contractility than does procainamide in comparable doses (Harrison *et al.*, 1963; Schumacher *et al.*, 1968); this has not been substantiated in experimental animals (Austen and Moran, 1965).

When used in the treatment of ectopic ventricular rhythms, lidocaine usually is administered intravenously, but intramuscular use has also been recommended (Zener *et al.*, 1973). Reports of convulsions are common; intravenous preparations of a suitable barbiturate or diazepam should be readily available. Lidocaine may cause alarming ventricular acceleration during atrial flutter (Marriott and Bieza, 1972), and has been reported to cause S-A nodal arrest when used with quinidine (Jeresaty *et al.*, 1972). *It is not recommended for the treatment of supraventricular arrhythmias.*

Preparations. *Lidocaine Hydrochloride Injection,* U.S.P. (XYLOCAINE), is available for intravenous administration as a 5-ml prefilled syringe or a 50-ml ampul, each containing 20 mg/ml; the injection contains no preservative, sympathomimetic, or other vasoconstrictor, and is the *only preparation of lidocaine that should be given intravenously.* Preparations that are available for use as *local anesthetics* are described in Chapter 20.

PHENYTOIN (DIPHENYLHYDANTOIN)

Phenytoin has long been used in the treatment of seizures (*see* Chapter 13, for complete description). Its interesting effects on the heart prompted clinical investigations to ascertain its potential value in the therapy of cardiac arrhythmias. Harris and Kokernot (1950) observed that large doses abolished ventricular tachycardia in dogs subjected to coronary artery ligation, and suggested that the drug might be useful in the management of cardiac arrhythmias. Subsequent work has demonstrated the efficacy of phenytoin in a variety of experimental and clinical disorders of cardiac rhythm; of particular interest is the demonstration of a unique mechanism of action, quite unlike that of quinidine and procainamide. Also striking is its almost specific antagonism of idioventricular rhythms induced by digitalis.

Cardiac Actions. *Pacemaker Activity.* Phenytoin does not alter the heart rate of dogs under pentobarbital anesthesia (Helfant *et al.*, 1967). In unanesthetized animals, Rosati and coworkers (1967) observed acceleration of the intact heart but deceleration of the chronically denervated heart. They attributed the increased heart rate to an anticholinergic action, but studies in isolated atria indicate that phenytoin has little effect on sinus frequency and does not alter the chronotropic effects of either acetylcholine or isoproterenol. In high concentrations (0.1 mM), a direct depression of phase-4 depolarization in S-A nodal cells was observed (Strauss *et al.*, 1968). Depression of pacemaker activity in Purkinje tissue is apparent with much lower concentrations, and has been demonstrated in the intact heart as well as in isolated preparations (Helfant *et al.*, 1967; Rosati *et al.*, 1967; Bigger *et al.*, 1968a). This action is particularly striking in digitalis-intoxicated hearts, and is undoubtedly responsible for the clinical efficacy of phenytoin in the treatment of ventricular ectopic rhythms.

Excitability and ERP. Like lidocaine, phenytoin neither depresses the excitability nor prolongs the ERP of atrial or ventricular muscle or of the specialized conduction tissue (Strauss *et al.*, 1968). In isolated Purkinje tissue, the APD is abbreviated but the ERP is not diminished in proportion, so that ERP/APD is increased (Bigger *et al.*, 1968a). This is of importance in relation to effects of the drug on intraventricular conduction.

Conduction. Phenytoin produces a striking increase of dv/dt in Purkinje fibers, particularly when this is depressed, as by digitalis. The rate of rise of action potentials initiated early in the relatively refractory period (*i.e.*, before complete repolarization) is increased; membrane responsiveness also is increased. This action, coupled with the effects on APD and ERP, must reduce the chance of impaired conduction and block, and thereby reduce the chance of reentrant rhythms. In rabbit atrial muscle, Katzung and Jensen (1970) observed negative dromotropic and inotropic effects resembling those of quinidine, particularly at K^+ concentrations higher than those used in the studies of Strauss and Bigger and their associates. A-V conduction in man is minimally affected (Caracta *et al.*, 1973).

Effect on Contractility. Most studies indicate that phenytoin causes less depression of contractility than comparable antiarrhythmic concentrations of quinidine and procainamide; it is not certain how much of the negative inotropic action that has been reported (*e.g.*, Mierzwiak *et al.*, 1967) may be due to the diluent. The drug does not reduce the contractile tension of isolated atrial muscle (Strauss *et al.*, 1968), does not prevent the positive inotropic effect of

acetylstrophanthidin in the dog heart (Scherlag *et al.*, 1968), and tends to cause only minor depression of left ventricular function in man (Lieberson *et al.*, 1967).

Blood Pressure. Arterial pressure appears to be reduced less by phenytoin than by quinidine or procainamide, but hypotension does occur on rapid intravenous administration. Here again the diluent may be in part responsible.

Antagonism of Digitalis Arrhythmias. Numerous studies emphasize the almost specific effect of phenytoin in digitalis intoxication. It increases the dose of acetylstrophanthidin necessary to provoke ventricular arrhythmias in the dog and restores normal rhythm when ventricular ectopic rhythms are manifest. Phenytoin is far more effective than procainamide in this regard. It is highly significant that restoration of normal rhythm is accompanied by improvement of A-V and intraventricular conduction, whereas further depression of conductivity is the rule with procainamide (Helfant *et al.*, 1967). When digitalis administration is continued in the presence of phenytoin, the positive inotropic effect of the glycoside continues until a new toxic level is reached. The digitalis-induced depletion of intracellular potassium is also delayed; this presumably is related to the antiarrhythmic action (Scherlag *et al.*, 1968).

Preparations. *Phenytoin Sodium,* U.S.P. (*diphenylhydantoin sodium;* DILANTIN), is available in several oral dosage forms and as an unofficial injectable preparation, as described in Chapter 13.

Therapeutic Uses. Phenytoin has been tried in a wide variety of cardiac arrhythmias (*see* reviews by Mercer and Osborne, 1967; Bigger, 1972). It is of little use in atrial flutter or fibrillation, but has been employed successfully in the treatment of paroxysmal atrial tachycardia, particularly if associated with digitalis intoxication. Phenytoin is much more effective in ventricular ectopic rhythms, whether or not these are the result of digitalis toxicity. Clinical experience bears out the experimental observation that conduction is not further depressed and may even be improved.

Since the plasma half-life of phenytoin is approximately 24 hours, maintenance therapy by oral administration is feasible in addition to its employment intravenously in order to obtain rapid effects. The plasma concentrations of phenytoin at which abolition of ventricular rhythms occurs are in the range of 8 to 16 µg/ml. Appropriate concentrations are reached by intravenous injection of doses of 50 to 100 mg, administered slowly and repeated every 10 to 15 minutes until a therapeutic response occurs or until a maximum of 10 to 15 mg/kg has been administered (Lang *et al.*, 1965; Bigger *et al.*, 1968b). Appropriate blood concentrations may be reached and maintained by an oral medication regimen of 1.0 g on the first day, followed by 0.5 to 0.6 g on each of two subsequent days and 0.4 g thereafter. Drowsiness, vertigo, and nausea develop at plasma concentrations greater than 20 µg/ml, and are a useful guide to therapy (Bigger *et al.*, 1968b).

Toxic Effects. The toxicity of phenytoin is considered fully in Chapter 13. Deaths attending its use in the treatment of arrhythmias have been reported. In two fatal cases the drug was used in an attempt to terminate atrial flutter associated with severe cardiopulmonary disease; cardiac arrest resulted in both (Unger and Sklaroff, 1967). All investigators emphasize the need for caution and close monitoring when intravenous administration is used, particularly when the possibility of S-A nodal depression exists. Caution is also called for in the presence of advanced A-V block. In uremic patients, plasma-protein binding of phenytoin is decreased, the half-life is shortened, and the effective plasma concentration is lower; the defect is not corrected by dialysis.

Status. The use of phenytoin for the treatment of cardiac arrhythmias is still under active clinical investigation, and more experience will be required before its value in comparison with other antiarrhythmic drugs can be properly assessed.

PROPRANOLOL

The pharmacology of the β-adrenergic blocking agents is discussed in detail in Chapter 26. Only those properties related to their use in the treatment of cardiac arrhythmias are considered here. Attention is here focused on propranolol, the drug in this class most commonly used as an antiarrhythmic agent.

Cardiac Actions. In addition to its β-adrenergic blocking action, propranolol has direct quinidine-like actions on the heart.

Actions Due to β-Adrenergic Blockade. In doses of 0.2 mg/kg or less, propranolol effectively blocks the cardiac actions of catecholamines and of sympathetic nerve stimulation in experimental animals. In the presence of significant adrenergic activity, propranolol reduces the heart rate, prolongs A-V conduction time, and reduces contractility. When adrenergic "tone" is minimal, as in trained unanesthetized dogs at rest, propanolol does not alter heart rate, A-V conduction time, intraventricular conduction, or atrial RP. Even under these conditions, however, a significant increase in the ERP of the A-V node has been observed (Wallace *et al.,* 1966b). In dogs with surgically induced heart block, propranolol reduces the idioventricular rate and may even cause asystole (Wallace *et al.,* 1967); this indicates that β-blocking doses suppress the phase-4 depolarization and pacemaker activity of Purkinje tissue. Reduction of idioventricular rate is much more pronounced when this has been enhanced by cardiac glycosides.

Quinidine-like Actions. Shortly after the introduction of selective β-adrenergic blocking agents, it was discovered that they antagonize ventricular ectopic rhythms induced by ouabain (Sekiya and Vaughan Williams, 1963). Many subsequent studies have confirmed this observation, and the β-blocking agents have been used to study the role of adrenergic influences in the genesis of digitalis-induced arrhythmias. It now appears that, whether or not the catecholamines are involved in digitalis toxicity, the effect of propanolol in the experimental situation is largely due to its quinidine-like action. This conclusion is based on the observations that d-propranolol, which has little blocking action, is just as effective in antagonizing digitalis toxicity as the l isomer, that the β-blocking action of l-propranolol is demonstrable at far lower doses than the antiarrhythmic activity, and that newer, "purer" β-blocking agents fail to prevent digitalis toxicity (Somani and Lum, 1965; Lucchesi *et al.,* 1966; Tuttle and Innes, 1966; Koerpel and Davis, 1972). In doses that are capable of terminating digitalis-induced arrhythmias, propranolol, like quinidine, causes a reduction in the velocity of the upstroke of the action potential, and a reduction of the membrane responsiveness. Repolarization of Purkinje fibers is said to be hastened and the ERP diminished, while the APD of ventricular muscle cells remains unchanged (Davis and Temte, 1968). In this respect the drug resembles phenytoin. The maximal frequency to which the isolated tissue can be driven, however, is diminished. Davis and Temte suggested that decremental conduction and block in isolated Purkinje-muscle preparations are prevented by the drug in high concentrations, and that this may have a bearing on the prevention of reentrant rhythms.

Like quinidine, propranolol in high doses (and also its d isomer) has a "direct" negative inotropic action on cardiac muscle, but in equivalent myocardial depressant doses it causes less reduction of blood pressure than does quinidine (Parmley and Braunwald, 1967). Propranolol has been reported also to reduce the extent of myocardial necrosis after transient ischemia in dogs (Sommers and Jennings, 1972).

Dosage and Administration. The official preparations of propranolol are described in Chapter 26. For intravenous administration, an initial dose of 0.5 mg may be given slowly, followed by additional doses to a maximum of 4 mg. Atropine should be available in case excessive cardiac slowing or A-V block occurs. Oral medication is given in divided doses totaling 20 to 80 mg per day. The recommended doses are in the range at which β-adrenergic blockade would be expected; they are lower than the doses resulting in predominantly quinidine-like effects. Therapeutic plasma concentrations for propranolol are in the range of 50 to 100 ng/ml.

Therapeutic Uses. *Supraventricular Tachycardias.* Propranolol has been used principally to control the ventricular rate in cases of supraventricular tachycardia (atrial fibrillation, flutter, and paroxysmal tachycardia). The action, considering the doses used, is undoubtedly due to prolongation of the A-V nodal refractory period, that is, an antiadrenergic action. It is this property of the drug that sets it apart from other antiarrhythmic agents, which commonly increase A-V conduction and accelerate the ventricular rate. Conversion of the atrial arrhythmia to sinus rhythm is uncommon, and probably not related to the drug action *per se*. Propranolol has proven to be effective in numerous cases in which digitalis, with or without quinidine and/or procainamide, failed to reduce the ventricular rate (Wolfson *et al.*, 1966; Frieden *et al.*, 1968) and in cases of paroxysmal atrial tachycardia attributed to digitalis toxicity (Turner, 1966).

Ventricular Arrhythmias. Although propranolol has been used with occasional success in the treatment of ventricular ectopic rhythms, it does not appear to be the drug of choice (Bath, 1966). It has been suggested that propranolol may be especially useful in situations in which electrical conversion of tachysystolic arrhythmias is contraindicated because of the presence of digitalis intoxication (*see* review by Epstein and Braunwald, 1966), and it has been used, in combination with quinidine, to prevent recurrences of a number of supraventricular and ventricular arrhythmias (Fors *et al.*, 1971).

Precautions. Because propranolol antagonizes adrenergic effects on contractility, and because serious arrhythmias are commonly encountered in the presence of overt or incipient heart failure, the use of the drug for its antiarrhythmic actions demands great care. In cases in which cardiac function is severely compromised by the arrhythmia itself, symptoms of heart failure may be relieved as the ventricular rate is controlled. Most investigators, however, recommend the prior and concurrent use of digitalis. Special care is also required, as with other antiarrhythmic agents, in the presence of advanced A-V block. In situations in which the diagnosis of block is uncertain (*e.g.*, when there is a question of supraventricular tachycardia with aberrant conduction or of ventricular tachycardia), propranolol should probably not be used unless emergency pacemaker equipment is available.

BRETYLIUM

Introduced as an antihypertensive agent (*see* Chapter 26), bretylium was suggested for prevention of ventricular fibrillation on the basis of experimental studies by Bacaner (1966). It has since been subjected to clinical and experimental studies. Unlike other antiarrhythmic agents, it causes some enhancement of pacemaker activity in isolated Purkinje fiber preparations, presumably because of liberation of catecholamines. The major effect of bretylium appears to be a prolongation of the ERP

(Wit *et al.*, 1970; Bigger and Jaffe, 1971). How much of its activity in the intact heart is due to catecholamine liberation, how much to its antiadrenergic effect, and how much to a direct action is not yet established. Day and Bacaner (1971) found bretylium effective in controlling postinfarction arrhythmias, and Bernstein and Koch-Weser (1972) suppressed ventricular tachyarrhythmias in more than half of a series of patients in whom other agents had been ineffective. Other studies have failed to demonstrate comparable efficacy (*see* review by Lown *et al.*, 1973). The drug is still under experimental study; it clearly merits further investigation.

GENERAL SUMMARY

Thousands of experimental and clinical studies of antiarrhythmic agents have been published since the original observations on quinine and quinidine. Investigators have believed that, if the mechanism of an arrhythmia were known, it should be possible to select a therapeutic agent with the specific effects necessary to correct the abnormality. Unfortunately, the basic knowledge for precise diagnosis of mechanism (reentry or ectopic pacemaker activity) is still lacking in most cases, with the exception of paroxysmal reciprocal tachycardia and, possibly, atrial flutter. When the cardiologist is faced with an abnormal rhythm, the choice of drugs is still empirical. If quinidine fails, he may try procainamide; if that fails, he may then use lidocaine or phenytoin, or digitalis, or bretylium, or propranolol. If no single agent succeeds, two drugs may be used concurrently. It is distressing that after 60 years no firmer basis for the choice of therapeutic agents has been developed.

A few situations have emerged in which the action of the drugs themselves may contribute to an understanding of mechanisms, and in which something better than coin flipping may dictate the choice. By way of summary, a few of these are listed.

Paroxysmal Supraventricular Tachycardia. The response of this disorder to vagal effects suggested a probable mechanism (Barker *et al.*, 1943), which was confirmed with the advent of transvenous intracardiac stimulation (Bigger and Goldreyer, 1970). The choice of reflex vagal stimulation or digitalis to halt an attack rests on a reasonably sound basis, but the choice of a prophylactic agent to suppress the premature atrial beats that probably initiate the attacks is less certain. The premature beats may be due to an ectopic pacemaker, in which case any of the antiarrhythmic drugs might provide effective prophylaxis, but they also might fail (*see* Fruehan *et al.,* 1974). The premature beats could be reentrant; a case can be made for interruption of a reentrant circuit by the use of those drugs that either prolong or abbreviate the ERP. Prophylaxis, in other words, is still on an empirical basis, and the problem is compounded when the attacks occur in association with the Wolff-Parkinson-White syndrome.

Atrial Flutter. Although much evidence points to a sustained circus movement as the mechanism, atrial flutter is often difficult to halt, perhaps because the pathway is too long to be interrupted by a moderate prolongation of the ERP. It is apparent, however, that quinidine and procainamide, both of which prolong the ERP, may sometimes prove effective, whereas lidocaine, phenytoin, and propranolol rarely are. Méndez (R.) and associates (1969), on the basis of the actions of an antihistamine with profound effects on the atrial ERP, concluded that the drug itself could serve as an aid to defining mechanism. Here, again, prophylaxis is not soundly based. The cardiologist must often resort to digitalis to convert the flutter to fibrillation, or to protect the ventricles by introducing some degree of A-V block with digitalis or propranolol.

Atrial Fibrillation. The high level of success attained with quinidine and procainamide, and the failure of other agents to restore sinus rhythm, suggest that prolongation of the ERP of the atrium is of cardinal importance. The poor success rate of all agents in long-standing fibrillation may suggest a different mechanism (Singer and TenEick, 1971).

Ventricular Premature Responses. It is commonly believed that premature ventricular beats presage more dangerous arrhythmias in patients with coronary artery disease, and that any therapy that would abolish them would reduce the incidence of sudden cardiac death. Idioventricular beats are extremely common, with or without cardiac

disease, and there is no consensus about the value of drug treatment. There is also no agreement about the mechanism. Long-term prophylaxis with antiarrhythmic agents has been recommended, but no effective agent is sufficiently free of troublesome and often serious side effects to merit general use (Koch-Weser, 1972). Even in the postinfarction period in the coronary-care unit, it is being questioned whether drug therapy is useful. Lidocaine, often infused at the first sign of an idioventricular QRS complex, is perhaps used more often to treat the ECG than to benefit the patient. Although there is no doubt that lidocaine will suppress ventricular premature beats, some cardiologists have come to believe that it suppresses responses that occur during the late portion of phase 4, which are benign, and has little effect on the presumably malignant early ("R on T") discharges (*see* Gamble and Cohn, 1972; Bleifeld *et al.,* 1973). The switch from lidocaine to procainamide in some clinics suggests that prolongation of the ERP may be more important than suppression of pacemaker activity, but again the decision is often an empirical one. There is still no clear-cut way of deciding whether premature beats are reentrant or ectopic, no way of being certain whether they are benign or malignant (except that early ones are probably more dangerous), and no way, other than trial and error, of making a logical choice of therapeutic agents.

Nevertheless, empirical observations, based on practical experience, permit the following conclusions:

1. All the drugs considered in this chapter, with the exception of bretylium, are capable of suppressing ectopic pacemaker activity and are therefore potentially useful in preventing those dysrhythmias that are initiated by premature atrial or ventricular contractions.

2. *Quinidine* and *procainamide,* both of which prolong the ERP of atrial and ventricular tissues, are effective in the treatment of atrial flutter and fibrillation, and of ventricular arrhythmias.

3. *Propranolol* is useful in atrial tachyarrhythmias, in which its effect on A-V transmission may control the ventricular rate.

4. *Lidocaine,* which has been almost universally used in the treatment of postinfarc-

tion ventricular arrhythmias, is beginning to be challenged; it has no place in the treatment of supraventricular tachysystolic rhythms.

5. *Phenytoin* is especially useful in the treatment of digitalis-induced arrhythmias, particularly ventricular tachycardia and paroxysmal atrial tachycardia with block, but it is not recommended for the treatment of other atrial arrhythmias. It also has a place, although probably not as the drug of first choice, in the treatment of ventricular ectopic rhythms associated with coronary artery disease.

Arnsdorf, M. F., and Bigger, J. T., Jr. Effect of lidocaine hydrochloride on membrane conductance in mammalian cardiac Purkinje fibers. *J. clin. Invest.*, **1972**, *51*, 2252–2263.

Askey, J. M. Embolism and atrial fibrillation: the effect of restoration of normal rhythm by quinidine. *Am. J. Cardiol.*, **1962**, *9*, 491–495.

Austen, W. G., and Moran, J. M. Cardiac and peripheral vascular effects of lidocaine and procainamide. *Am. J. Cardiol.*, **1965**, *16*, 701–707.

Bacaner, M. Bretylium tosylate for suppression of induced ventricular fibrillation. *Am. J. Cardiol.*, **1966**, *17*, 528–534.

Barker, P. S.; Wilson, F. N.; and Johnston, F. D. The mechanism of paroxysmal atrial tachycardia. *Am. Heart J.*, **1943**, *26*, 435–445.

Barold, S. S., and Linhart, J. W. Recent advances in the treatment of ectopic tachycardias by electrical pacing. *Am. J. Cardiol.*, **1970**, *25*, 698–706.

Bath, J. C. J. L. Treatment of cardiac arrhythmias in unanesthetized patients. *Am. J. Cardiol.*, **1966**, *18*, 415–425.

Bernstein, J. G., and Koch-Weser, J. Effectiveness of bretylium tosylate against refractory ventricular arrhythmias. *Circulation*, **1972**, *45*, 1024–1034.

Bigger, J. T., Jr.; Bassett, A. L.; and Hoffman, B. F. Electrophysiological effects of diphenylhydantoin on canine Purkinje fibers. *Circulation Res.*, **1968a**, *22*, 221–236.

Bigger, J. T., Jr., and Goldreyer, B. N. The mechanism of supraventricular tachycardia. *Circulation*, **1970**, *42*, 673–688.

Bigger, J. T., Jr., and Jaffe, C. C. The effect of bretylium tosylate on the electrophysiologic properties of ventricular muscle and Purkinje fibers. *Am. J. Cardiol.*, **1971**, *27*, 82–92.

Bigger, J. T., Jr., and Mandel, W. J. Effect of lidocaine on the electrophysiological properties of ventricular muscle and Purkinje fibers. *J. clin. Invest.*, **1970**, *49*, 63–77.

Bigger, J. T., Jr.; Schmidt, D. H.; and Kutt, H. Relationship between the plasma level of diphenylhydantoin sodium and its cardiac antiarrhythmic effects. *Circulation*, **1968b**, *38*, 363–374.

Bleifeld, W.; Merx, W.; Heinrich, K. W.; and Effert, S. Controlled trial of prophylactic treatment with lidocaine in acute myocardial infarction. *Eur. J. clin. Pharmac.*, **1973**, *6*, 119–126.

Bloomfield, S. S.; Romhilt, D. W.; Chou, T. C.; and Fowler, N. O. Natural history of cardiac arrhythmias and their prevention with quinidine in patients with acute coronary insufficiency. *Circulation*, **1973**, *47*, 967–973.

Burn, J. H. The cause of fibrillation. *Can. med. Ass. J.*, **1961**, *84*, 625–627.

Caracta, A. R.; Damato, A. N.; Josephson, M. E.; Ricciutti, M. A.; Gallagher, J. J.; and Lau, S. H. Electrophysio-

logic properties of diphenylhydantoin. *Circulation*, **1973**, *47*, 1234–1241.

Conn, H. L., Jr. Quinidine as an antiarrhythmic agent. Basic and clinical considerations. In, *Advances in Cardiopulmonary Diseases*, Vol. II. (Banyai, A. L., and Gordon, B. L., eds.) Year Book Medical Publishers, Inc., Chicago, **1964**, pp. 286–304.

Conn, H. L., Jr., and Luchi, R. J. Ionic influences on quinidine-albumin interaction. *J. Pharmac. exp. Ther.*, **1961**, *133*, 76–83.

Davis, L. D., and Temte, J. V. Effects of propranolol on the transmembrane potentials of ventricular muscle and Purkinje fibers of the dog. *Circulation Res.*, **1968**, *22*, 661–677.

———. Electrophysiological actions of lidocaine on canine ventricular muscle and Purkinje fibers. *Ibid.*, **1969**, *24*, 639–655.

Day, H. W., and Bacaner, M. Use of bretylium tosylate in the management of acute myocardial infarction. *Am. J. Cardiol.*, **1971**, *27*, 177–189.

Fors, W. J.; Vanderark, C. R.; and Reynolds, E. W., Jr. Evaluation of propranolol and quinidine in the treatment of quinidine-resistant arrhythmias. *Am. J. Cardiol.*, **1971**, *27*, 190–194.

Frey, W. Weitere Erfährungen mit Chinidin bei absoluter Herzunregelmässigkeit. *Wien. klin. Wschr.*, **1918**, *55*, 849–853.

Frieden, J.; Rosenblum, R.; Enselberg, C. D.; and Rosenberg, A. Propranolol treatment of chronic intractable supraventricular arrhythmias. *Am. J. Cardiol.*, **1968**, *22*, 711–717.

Fruehan, C. T.; Meyer, J. A.; Klie, J. H.; Johnson, L. W.; Obeid, A. I.; Smulyan, H.; and Eich, R. H. Refractory paroxysmal supraventricular tachycardia. *Am. Heart J.*, **1974**, *87*, 229–237.

Gamble, O. W., and Cohn, K. Effect of propranolol, procainamide, and lidocaine on ventricular automaticity and reentry in experimental myocardial infarction. *Circulation*, **1972**, *46*, 498–506.

Goldman, M. J. Management of chronic atrial fibrillation: indications for and methods of conversion to sinus rhythm. *Prog. cardiovasc. Dis.*, **1960**, *2*, 465–479. (71 references.)

Goodford, P. J., and Vaughan Williams, E. M. Intracellular Na and K concentrations of rabbit atria, in relation to the action of quinidine. *J. Physiol., Lond.*, **1962**, *160*, 483–493.

Han, J., and Moe, G. K. Nonuniform recovery of excitability in ventricular muscle. *Circulation Res.*, **1964**, *14*, 44–60.

Hansen, W. R.; McClendon, R. L.; and Kinsman, J. M. Auricular fibrillation: hemodynamic studies before and after conversion with quinidine. *Am. Heart J.*, **1952**, *44*, 499–516.

Harris, A. S., and Kokernot, R. H. Effects of diphenylhydantoin sodium and phenobarbital sodium upon ectopic ventricular tachycardia in acute myocardial infarction. *Am. J. Physiol.*, **1950**, *163*, 505–516.

Harrison, D. C.; Sprouse, J. H.; and Morrow, A. G. The antiarrhythmic properties of lidocaine and procaineamide. *Circulation*, **1963**, *28*, 486–491.

Helfant, R. H.; Scherlag, B. J.; and Damato, A. N. The electrophysiological properties of diphenylhydantoin sodium as compared to procaineamide in the normal and digitalis-intoxicated heart. *Circulation*, **1967**, *36*, 108–118.

Hoffman, B. F. The action of quinidine and procaineamide on single fibers of dog ventricle and specialized conducting system. *Anais Acad. bras. Cienc.*, **1958**, *29*, 365–368.

———. The electrophysiology of heart muscle and the genesis of arrhythmias. In, *Mechanisms and Therapy of Cardiac Arrhythmias*. (Dreifus, L. S., and Likoff, W., eds.) Grune & Stratton, Inc., New York, **1966**, pp. 29–34.

January, L. E.; Hamilton, H. E.; and Sinton, D. W. Paroxysmal ventricular tachycardia treated with intravenous injections of quinidine. *A.M.A. Archs intern. Med.*, 1953, *91*, 325–332.

Jeresaty, R. M.; Kahn, A. H.; and Landry, A. B., Jr. Sinoatrial arrest due to lidocaine in a patient receiving quinidine. *Chest*, 1972, *61*, 683–685.

Kalmansohn, R. W., and Sampson, J. J. Studies of plasma quinidine content. I. Relation to single dose administration by three routes. *Circulation*, 1950a, *1*, 564–568. II. Relation to toxic manifestations and therapeutic effect. *Ibid.*, 1950b, *1*, 569–575.

Katzung, B. G., and Jensen, R. A. The depressant effect of diphenylhydantoin on electrical and mechanical properties of isolated rabbit and dog atria: dependence on sodium and potassium. *Am. Heart J.*, 1970, *80*, 80–88.

Kleiger, R., and Lown, B. Cardioversion and digitalis. *Circulation*, 1966, *33*, 878–887.

Klein, R. L.; Holland, W. C.; and Tinsley, B. Quinidine and unidirectional cation fluxes in atria. *Circulation Res.*, 1960, *8*, 246–252.

Koch-Weser, J. Quinidine-induced hypoprothrombinemic hemorrhage in patients on chronic warfarin therapy. *Ann. intern. Med.*, 1968, *68*, 511–517.

———. Antiarrhythmic prophylaxis in ambulatory patients with coronary heart disease. *Archs intern. Med.*, 1972, *129*, 763–772.

Koerpel, B. J., and Davis, L. D. Effects of lidocaine, propranolol, and sotalol on ouabain-induced changes in canine Purkinje fibers. *Circulation Res.*, 1972, *30*, 681–689.

Lang, T. W.; Bernstein, H.; Barbieri, F. F.; Gold, H.; and Corday, E. The use of diphenylhydantoin for the treatment of digitalis toxicity. *Archs intern. Med.*, 1965, *116*, 573–580.

Larson, R. K. Mechanism of quinidine purpura. *Blood*, 1953, *8*, 16–25.

Lieberman, N. A.; Harris, R. S.; Katz, R. I.; Lipschutz, H. M.; Dolgin, M.; and Fischer, V. J. The effects of lidocaine on the electrical and mechanical activity of the heart. *Am. J. Cardiol.*, 1968, *22*, 375–380.

Lieberson, A. D.; Schumacher, R. R.; Childress, R. H.; Boyd, D. L.; and Williams, J. F., Jr. The effect of diphenylhydantoin on left ventricular function in patients with heart disease. *Circulation*, 1967, *36*, 692–699.

Lown, B. Electrical reversion of cardiac arrhythmias. *Br. Heart J.*, 1967, *29*, 469–489.

Lown, B., and Wolf, M. Approaches to sudden death from coronary heart disease. *Circulation*, 1971, *44*, 130–142.

Lucchesi, B. R.; Whitsit, L. S.; and Brown, N. L. Propranolol (INDERAL) in experimentally-induced cardiac arrhythmias. *Can. J. Physiol. Pharmac.*, 1966, *44*, 543–547.

Mandel, W. J., and Bigger, J. T., Jr. Electrophysiologic effects of lidocaine on isolated canine and rabbit atrial tissue. *J. Pharmac. exp. Ther.*, 1971, *178*, 81–93.

Mark, L. C.; Kayden, J. J.; Steele, J. M.; Cooper, J. R.; Berlin, I.; Rovenstine, E. A.; and Brodie, B. B. The physiological disposition and cardiac effects of procaineamide. *J. Pharmac. exp. Ther.*, 1951, *102*, 5–15.

Marriott, H. J. L., and Bieza, C. F. Alarming ventricular acceleration after lidocaine administration. *Chest*, 1972, *61*, 682–683.

Mautz, F. R. The reduction of cardiac irritability by the epicardial and systemic administration of drugs as a protection in cardiac surgery. *J. thorac. Surg.*, 1936, *5*, 612–628.

Méndez, C.; Mueller, W. J.; Merideth, J.; and Moe, G. K. Interaction of transmembrane potentials in canine Purkinje fibers and at Purkinje fiber-muscle junctions. *Circulation Res.*, 1969, *24*, 361–372.

Méndez, R.; Kabela, E.; Pastelin, G.; Martínez López, M.; and Sánchez Pérez, S. Antiarrhythmic actions of clemizole as pharmacologic evidence for a circus movement in atrial flutter. *Naunyn-Schmiedebergs Arch. Pharmak.*, 1969, *262*, 325–336.

Mierzwiak, D. S.; Mitchell, J. H.; and Shapiro, W. The effect of diphenylhydantoin and quinidine on left ventricular function in dogs. *Am. Heart J.*, 1967, *74*, 780–791.

Moe, G. K. On the multiple wavelet hypothesis of atrial fibrillation. *Archs int. Pharmacodyn. Thér.*, 1962, *140*, 183–188.

Moe, G. K., and Abildskov, J. A. Atrial fibrillation as a self-sustaining arrhythmia independent of focal discharge. *Am. Heart J.*, 1959, *58*, 59–70.

Moe, G. K., and Méndez, C. The physiological basis of reciprocal rhythm. *Prog. cardiovasc. Dis.*, 1966, *8*, 461–482.

Moe, G. K.; Rheinboldt, W. C.; and Abildskov, J. A. A computer model of atrial fibrillation. *Am. Heart J.*, 1964, *67*, 200–220.

Parmley, W. W., and Braunwald, E. Comparative myocardial depressant and antiarrhythmic properties of *d*-propranolol, *dl*-propranolol, and quinidine. *J. Pharmac. exp. Ther.*, 1967, *158*, 11–21.

Roberts, J.; Stadter, R. P.; Cairoli, V.; and Modell, W. Relationship between adrenergic activity and cardiac actions of quinidine. *Circulation Res.*, 1962, *11*, 758–764.

Rosati, R. A.; Alexander, J. A.; Schaal, S. F.; and Wallace, A. G. Influence of diphenylhydantoin on electrophysiological properties of the canine heart. *Circulation Res.*, 1967, *21*, 757–765.

Rosenblueth, A. The mechanism of auricular flutter and auricular fibrillation. *Circulation*, 1953, *7*, 612–613.

Sano, T.; Tasaki, M.; Ono, M.; Tsuchihashi, T.; Takayama, N.; and Shimamoto, T. Resting and action potentials in the region of the atrio-ventricular node. *Proc. imp. Acad. Japan*, 1958, *34*, 558–563.

Sasyniuk, B., and Méndez, C. A mechanism for reentry in canine ventricular tissue. *Circulation Res.*, 1971, *28*, 3–15.

Scherlag, B. J.; Helfant, R. H.; Ricciutti, M. A.; and Damato, A. N. Dissociation of the effects of digitalis on myocardial potassium flux and contractility. *Am. J. Physiol.*, 1968, *215*, 1288–1291.

Schuilenburg, R. M., and Durrer, D. Atrial echo beats in the human heart elicited by induced atrial premature beats. *Circulation*, 1968, *37*, 680–693.

Schumacher, R. R.; Lieberson, A. D.; Childress, R. H.; and Williams, J. F., Jr. Hemodynamic effects of lidocaine in patients with heart disease. *Circulation*, 1968, *37*, 965–972.

Sekiya, A., and Vaughan Williams, E. M. A comparison of the antifibrillatory actions and effects on intracellular cardiac potentials of pronethalol, disopyramide and quinidine. *Br. J. Pharmac. Chemother.*, 1963, *21*, 473–481.

Selzer, A., and Wray, H. W. Quinidine syncope. *Circulation*, 1964, *30*, 17–26.

Singer, D. H.; Lazzara, R.; and Hoffman, B. F. Interrelationships between automaticity and conduction in Purkinje fibers. *Circulation Res.*, 1967, *21*, 537–558.

Singer, D. H., and TenEick, R. E. Aberrancy: electrophysiologic aspects. *Am. J. Cardiol.*, 1971, *28*, 381–401.

Singh, B. N., and Vaughan Williams, E. M. Effect of altering potassium concentration on the action of lidocaine and diphenylhydantoin on rabbit atrial and ventricular muscle. *Circulation Res.*, 1971, *29*, 286–295.

Sokolow, M., and Ball, R. E. Factors influencing conversion of chronic atrial fibrillation with special reference to serum quinidine concentrations. *Circulation*, 1956, *14*, 568–583.

Somani, P., and Lum, B. K. B. The antiarrhythmic actions of beta adrenergic blocking agents. *J. Pharmac. exp. Ther.*, 1965, *147*, 194–204.

Sommers, H. M., and Jennings, R. B. Ventricular fibrillation and myocardial necrosis after transient ischemia. *Archs intern. Med.*, 1972, *129*, 780–789.

Strauss, H. C.; Bigger, J. T., Jr.; Bassett, A. L.; and Hoffman, B. F. Actions of diphenylhydantoin on the electrical properties of isolated rabbit and canine atria. *Circulation Res.,* **1968,** *23,* 463–477.

Szekeres, L., and Vaughan Williams, E. M. Antifibrillatory action. *J. Physiol., Lond.,* **1962,** *160,* 470–482.

Thompson, P. D.; Rowland, M.; and Melmon, K. L. The influence of heart failure, liver disease, and renal failure on the disposition of lidocaine in man. *Am. Heart J.,* **1971,** *82,* 417–421.

Ticzon, A. R., and Whalen, R. W. Refractory supraventricular tachycardias. *Circulation,* **1973,** *47,* 642–653.

Trautwein, W., and Kassebaum, D. G. On the mechanism of spontaneous impulse generation in the pacemaker of the heart. *J. gen. Physiol.,* **1961,** *45,* 317–330.

Turner, J. R. B. Propranolol in the treatment of digitalis-induced and digitalis-resistant tachycardias. *Am. J. Cardiol.,* **1966,** *18,* 450–455.

Tuttle, R. P., and Innes, I. R. Interaction of pronethalol and ouabain on cardiac rhythm and automaticity. *J. Pharmac. exp. Ther.,* **1966,** *153,* 211–217.

Unger, A. H., and Sklaroff, H. J. Fatalities following use of sodium diphenylhydantoin for cardiac arrhythmias. *J. Am. med. Ass.,* **1967,** *200,* 335–336.

Vaughan Williams, E. M. The mode of action of quinidine on isolated rabbit atria interpreted from intracellular potential records. *Br. J. Pharmac. Chemother.,* **1958,** *13,* 276–287.

Wallace, A. G.; Cline, R. E.; Sealy, W. C.; Young, W. G., Jr.; and Troyer, W. G., Jr. Electrophysiologic effects of quinidine: studies using chronically implanted electrodes in awake dogs with and without cardiac denervation. *Circulation Res.,* **1966a,** *19,* 960–969.

Wallace, A. G.; Schaal, S. F.; Sugimoto, T.; Rozear, M.; and Alexander, J. A. The electrophysiologic effects of beta-adrenergic blockade and cardiac denervation. *Bull. N.Y. Acad. Med.,* **1967,** *43,* 1119–1137.

Wallace, A. G.; Troyer, W. G.; Lesage, M. A.; and Zotti, E. F. Electrophysiologic effects of isoproterenol and beta blocking agents in awake dogs. *Circulation Res.,* **1966b,** *18,* 140–148.

Wedd, A. M.; Blair, H. A.; and Warner, R. S. The action of procaine amide on the heart. *Am. Heart J.,* **1951,** *42,* 399–405.

Weidmann, S. The effect of the cardiac membrane potential on the rapid availability of the sodium carrying system. *J. Physiol., Lond.,* **1955,** *127,* 213–224.

Wenckebach, K. F. *Die unregelmässige Herztätigkeit und ihre klinische Bedeutung.* W. Engelmann, Leipzig, **1914.**

West, T. C., and Amory, D. W. Single fiber recording of the effect of quinidine at atrial pacemaker sites in the isolated right atrium of the rabbit. *J. Pharmac. exp. Ther.,* **1960,** *130,* 183–193.

Willius, F. A., and Keys, T. E. Cardiac clinics. XCIV. A remarkably early reference to the use of cinchona in cardiac arrhythmia. *Proc. Staff Meet. Mayo Clin.,* **1942,** *17,* 294–296.

Wit, A. L.; Hoffman, B. F.; and Cranefield, P. F. Slow conduction and reentry in the ventricular conducting system. *Circulation Res.,* **1972,** *30,* 1–10.

Wit, A. L.; Steiner, C.; and Damato, A. N. Electrophysiologic effects of bretylium tosylate on single fibers of the canine specialized conducting system and ventricle. *J. Pharmac. exp. Ther.,* **1970,** *173,* 344–356.

Wolfson, S.; Robins, S. I.; and Krasnow, N. Treatment of cardiac arrhythmias with beta-adrenergic blocking agents. *Am. Heart J.,* **1966,** *72,* 177–187.

Woske, H.; Belford, J.; Fastier, F. N.; and Brooks, C. McC. The effect of procaine amide on excitability, refractoriness and conduction in the mammalian heart. *J. Pharmac. exp. Ther.,* **1953,** *107,* 134–140.

Zapata-Díaz, J.; Cabrera, C. E.; and Méndez, R. An experimental and clinical study on the effects of procaine amide (PRONESTYL) on the heart. *Am. Heart J.,* **1952,** *43,* 854–870.

Zener, J. C.; Kerber, R. E.; Spivack, A. P.; and Harrison, D. C. Blood lidocaine levels and kinetics following high-dose intramuscular administration. *Circulation,* **1973,** *47,* 984–988.

Monographs and Reviews

Bassett, A. L., and Wit, A. L. Recent advances in electrophysiology of antiarrhythmic drugs. *Prog. Drug Res.,* **1973,** *17,* 33–58. (167 references.)

Bigger, J. T., Jr. Arrhythmias and antiarrhythmic drugs. *Adv. intern. Med.,* **1972,** *18,* 251–281.

DiPalma, J. R., and Schults, J. E. Antifibrillatory drugs. *Medicine, Baltimore,* **1950,** *29,* 123–168. (236 references.)

Epstein, S. E., and Braunwald, E. Beta-adrenergic receptor blocking drugs. *New Engl. J. Med.,* **1966,** *275,* 1175–1183. (140 references.)

Hoffman, B. F., and Cranefield, P. F. *Electrophysiology of the Heart.* McGraw-Hill Book Co., New York, **1960.**

Lown, B.; Temte, J. V.; and Arter, W. J. Ventricular tachyarrhythmias. *Circulation,* **1973,** *47,* 1364–1381.

Mason, D. T.; DeMaria, A. N.; Amsterdam, E. A.; Zelis, R.; and Massumi, R. A. Antiarrhythmic agents. I. Mechanisms of action and clinical pharmacology. *Drugs,* **1973a,** *5,* 261–291.

———. Antiarrhythmic agents. II. Therapeutic considerations. *Ibid.,* **1973b,** *5,* 292–317.

Mercer, E. N., and Osborne, J. A. Current status of diphenylhydantoin in heart disease. *Ann. intern. Med.,* **1967,** *67,* 1084–1107. (121 references.)

Moss, A. J., and Patton, R. D. *Antiarrhythmic Agents.* Charles C Thomas, Pub., Springfield, Ill., **1973.**

Singer, D. H., and TenEick, R. E. Pharmacology of cardiac arrhythmias. *Prog. cardiovasc. Dis.,* **1969,** *11,* 488–514.

Szekeres, L., and Papp, J. G. Antiarrhythmic compounds. *Prog. Drug Res.,* **1968,** *12,* 292–369. (407 references.)

Trautwein, W. Generation and conduction of impulses in the heart as affected by drugs. *Pharmac. Rev.,* **1963,** *15,* 277–332.

33 ANTIHYPERTENSIVE AGENTS AND THE DRUG THERAPY OF HYPERTENSION

Mark Nickerson and John Ruedy

Lack of information regarding the etiology of most cases of hypertension has made the search for effective antihypertensive agents largely empirical. This approach has led to the development of a number of useful drugs with quite diverse mechanisms of action. Several agents that act predominantly on sympathetic nerves or peripheral adrenergic receptors and on autonomic ganglia are described in Chapters 26 and 27. Additional antihypertensive compounds will be discussed in this chapter. The great diversity of proven and postulated mechanisms of antihypertensive drug action makes it obvious that the effectiveness of a given drug cannot be taken as evidence relating its mechanism of action to the etiology of the elevated blood pressure.

I. Antihypertensive Agents

HYDRALAZINE

A considerable number of phthalazine derivatives produce significant hypotension. Several have been used in the treatment of hypertension in Europe, but only *hydralazine* (1-hydrazinophthalazine) is used clinically in North America. It has the following structural formula:

Hydralazine

A number of other compounds, some distant congeners of hydralazine, appear to have very similar hemodynamic effects. *Minoxidil* (6-[1-piperidinyl]-2, 4-pyridiminediamine 3-oxide) (Gottlieb *et al.*, 1972) and also *guancydine* (2-cyano-1-*t*-pentylguanidine) (Hammer *et al.*, 1971) have considerable antihypertensive activity in man, but their advantages and disadvantages relative to hydralazine cannot yet be fully assessed.

Locus and Mechanism of Action. Early studies on hydralazine attributed its antihypertensive effect successively to specific renal vasodilatation and to an action on the central nervous system (CNS). However, present evidence indicates that the major action of hydralazine is direct relaxation of vascular smooth muscle; the effect on arterioles is greater than on veins. In man, intra-arterial is more effective than intravenous administration in raising skin temperature and blood flow of the extremities, and intravenous injection causes a greater vasodilatation in limbs to which vasomotor control has been chronically impaired by sympathectomy or by spinal cord section than in normally innervated limbs. Patients with chronic spinal cord transections as high as T_1 to T_5 and normal blood pressures respond to small doses of hydralazine with a drop in diastolic pressure comparable to that induced in normal subjects. (*See* Åblad, 1963.)

Cardiac stimulation by hydralazine probably involves a reflex response to the fall in blood pressure, but it is somewhat more marked than would be expected on this basis alone and is not well correlated with changes in blood pressure. Tachycardia can be induced by very small doses injected into the cerebral ventricles (Gupta and Bhargava, 1965), and hydralazine tachycardia can be prevented by ganglionic or β-adrenergic blocking agents.

Pharmacological Properties. All major effects of hydralazine are on the *cardiovascular system*. In both laboratory animals and man, adequate doses decrease arterial blood pressure, diastolic often more than systolic, and peripheral vascular resistance, and increase heart rate, stroke volume, and cardiac output. The preferential dilatation of arterioles, as compared to veins, minimizes postural hypotension and promotes the increase in cardiac output. The latter may limit the reduction in mean blood pressure produced by the drug. The effect of hydralazine develops gradually over 15 to 20 minutes even after intravenous administration. The peripheral vasodilatation is widespread but not uniform. Splanchnic, coronary, cerebral, and renal blood flows increase unless the fall in blood pressure is very marked. Glomerular filtration, renal tubular function, and urine volume are not consistently affected; however, in common with many other antihypertensive agents, hydralazine can produce sodium retention and decreased urine volume. Hydralazine usually increases plasma renin activity. Vascular resistance in the cutaneous and muscle beds may decrease, but this is usually in parallel with the fall in blood pressure and blood flow does not increase. (*See* Freis *et al.,* 1953; Åblad, 1963.)

The overall "hyperdynamic" state of the circulation induced by hydralazine may accentuate specific inadequacies; for example, hydralazine can considerably increase the pulmonary artery pressure in patients with mitral valve disease (Aitchison *et al.,* 1955) or cause anginal pain in those with coronary artery insufficiency. Effects of hydralazine on organs other than those of the cardiovascular system are minor and variable. The response to hydralazine administered parenterally usually includes some respiratory stimulation.

Absorption, Fate, and Excretion. Hydralazine is quite well absorbed from the gastrointestinal tract. Blood levels are maximal 3 to 4 hours after oral administration, and small amounts can be detected for as long as 24 hours. Pharmacological effects correlate well with plasma concentrations. Labeled hydralazine has been shown to have a high affinity for, and persistence in, the walls of muscular arteries (Moore-Jones and Perry, 1966). The major metabolic pathways for hydralazine are ring hydroxylation and subsequent conjugation with glucuronic acid, and N-acetylation. The latter is of particular significance because the plasma concentration achieved by a given dose may be almost twice as great in genetic "slow acetylators" as in other patients (Zacest and Koch-Weser, 1972). Only a small fraction is excreted unchanged, but there may be some accumulation of drug in patients with severely impaired renal function. Conversion of a small percentage of administered hydralazine to a hydrazone has been reported; this material could be responsible for some toxic effects of hydralazine, such as peripheral neuropathies, by condensing with and thus depleting pyridoxal.

Preparations, Routes of Administration, and Dosage. *Hydralazine Hydrochloride,* U.S.P. (APRESOLINE), is available in 10-, 25-, 50-, and 100-mg tablets for oral administration, and in 1-ml ampuls containing 20 mg of the drug for intravenous or intramuscular injection. Parenteral administration is usually started with 20 or 40 mg, but the amount and the frequency of administration required to produce a satisfactory lowering of blood pressure are highly variable. The usual oral dose is 100 to 200 mg per day, starting with 10 or 20 mg two to four times daily; this is increased gradually until the desired effect is obtained or unacceptable side effects develop. The dose should not exceed 400 mg per day for any extended period.

Toxicity and Precautions. The incidence of untoward effects of hydralazine therapy is high. Headache, palpitation, anorexia, nausea, dizziness, and sweating are common. Nasal congestion, flushing, lacrimation, conjunctivitis, paresthesias, edema, tremors, and muscle cramps occur less frequently. Side effects are less frequent and less severe when the dose is increased slowly, and tolerance to them may develop with continued administration. In addition, many side effects, particularly palpitation, headache, and dizziness, are less troublesome when hydralazine is given with a β-adrenergic blocking drug. Drug fever, urticaria, skin rash, polyneuritis, gastrointestinal hemorrhage, anemia, and pancytopenia are rare, but require termination of hydralazine therapy. Peripheral neuropathies have been corrected by giving pyridoxine (Raskin and Fishman, 1965). The myocardial stimulation associated with hydralazine administration can produce anginal attacks and ECG changes characteristic of myocardial ischemia. The drug must be used with caution in patients with coronary artery disease.

Chronic administration of hydralazine, particularly in doses of 400 mg or more per day, can produce an *acute rheumatoid state.* This has been reported in approximately 10% of patients receiving high doses, and a syndrome indistinguishable from *disseminated lupus erythematosus* develops in a smaller percentage. A possible immunological basis for these reactions has been reported (Paz and Seifter, 1972). The symptoms regress after hydralazine is discontinued, but relatively long-term treatment with adrenocorticosteroids may be required, and residua have been detected many years later. Lupus erythematosus cells can be found in the blood of some patients receiving hydralazine who are asymptomatic. (*See* Alarcón-Segovia *et al.,* 1967.)

Therapeutic Uses. Hydralazine is used to reduce the blood pressure in a variety of hypertensive conditions, usually in combination with other agents. These uses are discussed as a part of general antihypertensive therapy at the end of this chapter.

METHYLDOPA

Methyldopa (L-α-methyl-3,4-dihydroxyphenylalanine) was shown to be an effective inhibitor of L-aromatic amino acid (dopa) decarboxylase by Sourkes in 1954, but it attracted major attention only after its hypotensive properties were noted during studies of aromatic amino acid metabolism in man (Oates *et al.*, 1960). It has since come to be one of the major agents used in the treatment of essential hypertension. However, the search for its mechanism of action has progressed much less smoothly than has its clinical application. Several blind alleys have held the spotlight, apparently because known biochemical mechanisms that could have been responsible for the antihypertensive effect were accepted without sufficient pharmacological evidence that they were causally involved. Data now available indicate that the major antihypertensive effect of methyldopa is not due to decarboxylase inhibition or to any other effect on peripheral sympathetic nerves or their mediator and, consequently, it should no longer be classified as a peripheral adrenergic neuron blocking agent.

Locus and Mechanism of Action. The mechanism of action of methyldopa as an antihypertensive drug has undergone considerable revision. The earlier views deserve brief mention if only because they appeared at the time to be well documented and plausible.

Methyldopa effectively inhibits the decarboxylation of both dopa and 5-hydroxytryptophan *in vitro* and *in vivo*, and decreases the concentrations of 5-hydroxytryptamine (5-HT), dopamine, and norepinephrine in the CNS and in most peripheral tissues. It was first postulated that methyldopa reduced the blood pressure by inhibiting dopa decarboxylation in sympathetic nerves, which decreased norepinephrine stores and, thus, decreased vasomotor tone. Reductions of tissue dopamine and 5-HT correlated with decarboxylase inhibition, but norepinephrine depletion far outlasted the enzyme inhibition and did not correlate with the hypotensive response. α-Methyldopamine causes a greater reduction in the norepinephrine content of peripheral tissues than does methyldopa, but does not lower blood pressure. Because methyldopa is itself metabolized to α-methylnorepinephrine, which can be stored in sympathetic nerve endings, it was next hypothesized that the latter displaced norepinephrine and acted as an inadequate "false transmitter" (*see* Kopin, 1968). α-Methylnorepinephrine fully meets the definition of a false transmitter, but its pharmacological significance is questionable. The hypotensive effect of methyldopa is not well correlated with the production or tissue content of α-methylnorepinephrine in a variety of circumstances, and the α-methylnorepinephrine formed is readily released by sympathetic nerve activity and effectively constricts peripheral blood vessels in most circumstances. (*See* Sjoerdsma *et al.*, 1963; Muscholl, 1966.) During the period of preoccupation with the norepinephrine-depletion and false-transmitter theories of the action of methyldopa, little attention was paid to the early observation that cardiovascular reflexes and responses to sympathetic nerve stimulation are only slightly inhibited at the time of the maximal hypotensive response (Goldberg *et al.*, 1960). This has been repeatedly confirmed.

The current, generally accepted interpretation is that the major antihypertensive action of methyldopa is on the CNS. Early important evidence for this was that decarboxylase inhibitors that penetrate the CNS abolish the hypotensive response to methyldopa, but those that act only peripherally are ineffective (Henning, 1969; Day *et al.*, 1973). This observation also indicates that the effect is due to a metabolic product of methyldopa rather than to enzyme inhibition by it. α-Methylnorepinephrine is probably the active agent because inhibition of CNS dopamine-β-hydroxylase also antagonizes the hypotension (Day *et al.*, 1973), and it produces more hypotension than do its precursors when administered into the cerebral ventricles (Heise and Kroneberg, 1972). Other observations that point to an important central hypotensive action of methyldopa are that when given intraventricularly it acts in only 1% of the dose required intravenously, it inhibits pressor responses to brain stem but not to peripheral sympathetic nerve stimulation, and the induced hypotension is associated with a decrease in preganglionic sympathetic nerve activity. The acute hypotensive effect of methyldopa has been reported to be abolished by pretreatment with reserpine, imipramine, and intraventricular 6-hydroxydopamine, and to be enhanced by the monoamine oxidase inhibitor tranylcypromine. The hypotension is also blocked by intraventricular administration of a small dose of phentolamine, which suggests that the action, perhaps that of α-methylnorepinephrine, is direct rather than by interference with some adrenergic mechanism. (*See* Kale and Satoskar, 1970; Baum *et al.*, 1972; Day *et al.*, 1973; Finch and Haeusler, 1973.) Many similarities in their effects suggest that methyldopa, through its metabolite, may act on the same central mechanisms as does clonidine (*see* below). Levodopa appears to have a similar antihypertensive action, and it has been reported to augment the antihypertensive effect of methyldopa in man (Gibberd and Small, 1973).

Although present evidence suggests that the major antihypertensive effect of methyldopa is due to an action on the CNS, some contribution of peripheral mechanisms cannot be ruled out. The reduction in renal vascular resistance may be related to the fact that, at least in rats, α-methylnorepinephrine is a much weaker vasoconstrictor in this vascular bed than is norepinephrine (Finch and Haeusler, 1973). In addition, the observation that methyldopa lowers the blood pressure effectively in immunosympathectomized rats suggests some more direct peripheral action (Ayitey-Smith and Varma, 1970).

Pharmacological Properties. Methyldopa causes progressive reductions in blood pressure and heart rate that are maximal at 4 to 6 hours and persist for as long as 24 hours after a single oral dose. Even after intravenous administration the antihypertensive effect is not apparent for 1 to 2 hours. The fall in blood pressure is greater in hypertensive than in normotensive subjects, and has been variously reported to be due to decreases in cardiac output, peripheral resistance, or both. One detailed study of mildly hypertensive patients given methyldopa for a year showed a predominant decrease in cardiac output, and the decrease in mean blood pressure was well correlated with the change in cardiac index (Lund-Johansen, 1972). Bradycardia persisted, and there was little change in stroke volume. The antihypertensive effect was decreased rather than increased during exercise. However, other workers have found dissimilar changes in all these parameters (*see* review by Sannerstedt and Conway, 1970). It is impossible

at this time to assess the reasons for these divergent observations. Methyldopa decreases plasma renin activity, but like most other antihypertensive drugs it tends to cause sodium and water retention. Changes in fluid volumes could contribute to differences in cardiac output. It is also possible that changes observed during chronic administration represent predominantly adaptations to the primary effects of the drug. In general, peripheral resistance and pressor reflexes tend to be more, and heart rate less, decreased after chronic than after acute administration.

Functional competence of sympathetic nerves during acute hypotensive effects of methyldopa is indicated by normal responses to nerve stimulation and to most cardiovascular reflexes in both laboratory animals and man. Responses to the Valsalva maneuver and cold pressor test have been reported inhibited after more prolonged methyldopa administration. However, although blood pressure is lower in the upright than in the supine position, postural hypotension is much less common than with adrenergic neuron blocking drugs such as guanethidine, and exercise hypotension is rare or absent. Consequently, it must be assumed that reflex venoconstriction is relatively intact. Other differences from responses to adrenergic neuron blocking drugs are the absence of most of the signs of sympathetic inadequacy such as miosis, ptosis, and relaxation of the nictitating membrane. The reduction in blood pressure induced by methyldopa has not been shown to involve any major changes in blood flow distribution. Renal blood flow and glomerular filtration are maintained or increased in normotensive subjects and in hypertensive patients with both normal and reduced renal function.

Methyldopa regularly produces *sedation* in laboratory animals and man, and has been shown to have a number of other CNS effects. In contrast to the sedative effect, the drug has been reported to lighten sleep and increase rapid-eye-movement (REM) sleep in man (Baekeland and Lundwall, 1971). It can prevent the rise in body temperature usually induced by bacterial and leukocytic pyrogens, apparently by a central mechanism, and in large doses can cause hypothermia (*see* Miert and Duin, 1972). Methyldopa has also been reported to augment amphetamine-induced hyperactivity in mice, and to increase prolactin release and induce lactation in human patients. These various effects have been consistently attributed to or interpreted as evidence for the involvement of central catecholamine mechanisms of one type or another. However, in most cases the proof of mechanism of action is quite indirect.

Clearly peripheral effects of methyldopa include inhibition of the pressor and other responses to injected dopa, one of the few effects that are due to decarboxylase inhibition, and alteration of responses to indirect-acting sympathomimetics. The latter are augmented by small and inhibited by large doses of methyldopa. The inhibition can occur when responses to adrenergic nerve stimulation are unaffected; in contrast, adrenergic neuron blocking drugs inhibit these two types of responses approximately in parallel (*see* Stone and Porter, 1966).

Absorption, Fate, and Excretion. When methyldopa is administered orally, approximately 50% is absorbed. It appears rapidly in the urine, predominantly as the unaltered compound. Some is excreted as conjugates, and small amounts of decarboxylated derivatives have been identified. Excretion of unchanged methyldopa follows two exponential curves. The first has a half-time of about 1⅔ hours in subjects with normal renal function and accounts for at least 90% of the administered drug. The second phase is much slower. In patients with severely impaired renal function, only about 50% of the drug is excreted during the early phase ($t_{1/2} = 3½$ hours), and some accumulation can occur during chronic administration (Myhre *et al.*, 1972). Both the total quantity absorbed and the distribution of metabolites in the urine can vary considerably in different individuals and in the same patient from day to day. Methyldopa and its metabolites react in the standard chemical tests for catecholamines, and their presence in blood and urine can cause false-positive tests for pheochromocytoma.

Preparations, Routes of Administration, and Dosage. *Methyldopa*, U.S.P. (ALDOMET), is available for oral administration in tablets containing 250 mg. The more soluble preparation, *Methyldopate Hydrochloride*, U.S.P. (ALDOMET ESTER HYDROCHLORIDE), is available in 5-ml vials (50 mg/ml) for parenteral use; it is rapidly hydrolyzed in the body to form methyldopa. The average daily oral dose of methyldopa is 1.0 g. There appears to be little additional effect with doses over 2.0 g. Methyldopa is given in divided doses, usually three times per day. Single parenteral doses are 500 mg to 1.0 g, usually given by intravenous infusion but must be adjusted to the needs of the individual patient.

Toxicity and Precautions. Methyldopa, given either orally or parenterally, regularly causes *sedation*. After a single dose this is of shorter duration than the hypotensive effect and it tends to decrease with continued medication. However, a persistent lassitude and drowsiness, particularly disturbing to individuals doing mental work, represents the overall most important side effect. Other unwanted effects referable to the CNS include vertigo, release of prolactin with resulting lactation, extrapyramidal signs, nightmares, and psychic depression; the last three of these effects are less common with methyldopa than with reserpine. Dry mouth and nasal stuffiness may also be central in origin. Various gastrointestinal upsets occur, but they are only occasionally severe. *Postural hypotension* can develop, but it is considerably less frequent and less severe than during treatment with guanethidine. Exercise hypotension is relatively infrequent. Retention of salt and water with weight gain and *edema* may occur with methyldopa, as with most other antihypertensive drugs. Paradoxical hypertensive reactions to intravenous administration have been reported.

Methyldopa causes a number of reactions that may have an "allergic" basis. Over 20% of patients on chronic methyldopa therapy develop a positive direct-antiglobulin (Coombs') test; the incidence is dose related. In most cases the positive antiglobulin test is of no clinical significance, but a number of cases of *hemolytic anemia* have been reported. The anemia usually regresses when methyldopa is discontinued, but glucocorticoid therapy may be necessary and deaths have been reported. The antiglobulin test commonly remains positive for many months after the last dose of methyldopa. Positive lupus and rheumatoid factor tests have also been reported to result from methyldopa administration. Laboratory evidence of *reversible liver damage* is not uncommon, and several cases of active chronic hepatitis have been identified as due to methyldopa (Goldstein *et al.*, 1973). Other adverse reactions include *drug fever* and, rarely, *granulocytopenia* and *thrombocytopenia*.

Therapeutic Uses. The major clinical use of methyldopa is in the treatment of essential hypertension. It has also been employed in a few cases of *carcinoid disease* with some benefit; in contrast to hypertension, decarboxylase inhibition by methyldopa is probably important in the treatment of this condition.

CLONIDINE

Clonidine hydrochloride (2-[2,6-dichlorophenylamino]-2-imidazoline hydrochloride) is a very active antihypertensive drug closely related chemically to tolazoline (peripheral vasodilator and α-adrenergic blocking agent), naphazoline and tetrahydrozoline (sympathomimetics), and antazoline (an antihistamine). Clonidine has the following structural formula:

Clonidine Hydrochloride

Pharmacological Properties. As expected from the pharmacology of the many 2-imidazoline derivatives previously studied, clonidine has many diverse actions. Although clinical use of the drug is almost entirely on a chronic basis, almost all of the available data on effects in both laboratory animals and man are from acute experiments. After intravenous injection of a few micrograms per kilogram, clonidine produces a brief rise and a subsequent more persistent fall in blood pressure, both of which are prolonged by anesthesia. The initial pressor response to clonidine is due to direct stimulation of α-adrenergic receptors; this action has also been demonstrated on the nictitating membrane and other structures. Clonidine also produces significant α-adrenergic blockade, acting as a *partial agonist*. The pressor response is accentuated and prolonged by drugs and procedures that interfere with reflex blood pressure adjustments (*e.g.*, ganglionic blockade).

In addition to some α-adrenergic blocking activity, clonidine can inhibit the release of norepinephrine and cardiac responses to postganglionic adrenergic nerve stimulation, particularly at low frequencies (*see* Werner *et al.*, 1972). It also appears to produce some

direct peripheral vasodilatation (Shaw *et al.*, 1971). However, these peripheral effects are inadequate to account for the *acute* hypotension and bradycardia produced. This phase of the response is inhibited by spinal cord section and by pretreatment with guanethidine or an α-adrenergic blocking agent, and appears to be due to an action on the CNS. Hypotension results from the injection of small doses of clonidine into the vertebral artery, cisterna magna, or cerebral ventricles, or into the circulation of a vascularly isolated but neurally intact head. The hypotension is associated with a clear reduction in preganglionic splanchnic nerve discharge. Transection experiments indicate that medullary centers are essential for the response (Schmitt and Schmitt, 1969), but the hypothalamus may also be involved. The bradycardia is due to both a decrease in sympathetic and an increase in vagal tone, as would be expected from the known central interactions of these two mechanisms. The increase in vagal tone involves an increased sensitivity of baroreceptor reflexes (Nayler and Stone, 1970).

It has been suggested that the acute central hypotensive and bradycrotic effects are due to stimulation by clonidine of central α-adrenergic receptors that are inhibitory to sympathetic nerve activity. However, such effects are modified inconsistently by various α-adrenergic blocking agents (Schmitt *et al.*, 1973). Pretreatment with intraventricular 6-hydroxydopamine largely abolishes the hypotensive and bradycrotic effects of intraventricular clonidine (Dollery and Reid, 1973), and this observation could indicate a "presynaptic" action on noradrenergic or dopaminergic neurons. However, it could also reflect destruction of some pathway required for the response, but not directly involved in the action of clonidine. Irrespective of the precise mechanism involved, it appears that the major *acute* hypotensive effect of clonidine is due to an action on the CNS.

Clonidine has many effects on the CNS, a number of which are similar to those of chlorpromazine. It produces marked sedation in man and laboratory animals, decreases spontaneous motor activity and conditioned avoidance behavior in animals, increases chloral hydrate sleeping time, and lowers body temperature (Laverty and Taylor, 1969). However, it does not appear to have antipsychotic properties. Centrally but not peripherally induced salivation is inhibited, which probably explains the very frequent occurrence of dry mouth in hypertensive patients receiving clonidine (Putzeys and Hoobler, 1972). The antihypertensive effect in man is largely abolished by concomitant administration of desipramine (Briant *et al.*, 1973).

The effects of *chronic administration* of clonidine

have been reported for several species. In rats it causes irritability and spontaneous aggression rather than sedation, whereas in dogs it fails to block the carotid occlusion reflex or the central bradycrotic effect of angiotensin (Katic *et al.,* 1972). In cats, clonidine in low doses reduces vascular responses to a variety of vasoconstrictors and vasodilators, including norepinephrine, isoproterenol, and angiotensin (Zaimis and Hanington, 1969). In the absence of other data on possible mechanisms of action during prolonged use, it is unclear if this peripheral action is a major factor in the antihypertensive effect of clonidine; it is possible that the acute and chronic effects may involve quite different mechanisms.

Acute antihypertensive responses to intravenous clonidine are maximal within about 20 minutes, and acute effects of either parenteral or oral administration are associated with decreases in cardiac output rather than in peripheral resistance. It has been reported that the further decrease in blood pressure due to tilting does involve a decrease in resistance, and there is probably some reduction in the tone of resistance vessels. Pulmonary artery pressure and cardiopulmonary blood volume are decreased, which indicates a relaxation of capacitance vessels. Glomerular filtration rate is usually decreased, but even when filtration is unaltered sodium excretion is considerably reduced. Clonidine causes an acute increase in cerebral vascular resistance and a decrease in cerebral blood flow in man (James *et al.,* 1970). This was previously noted in laboratory animals (Sherman *et al.,* 1968), and has received surprisingly little attention; changes in cerebral blood flow can have important effects on blood pressure. The acute effects of clonidine on cardiovascular reflexes are variable. It has been reported to block the carotid occlusion reflex but not the response to tilting in laboratory animals, and appears not to alter responses to exercise or to the Valsalva maneuver in man. Reflex control of capacitance vessels is not abolished, and postural hypotension is considerably less than with an adrenergic neuron blocking agent such as guanethidine.

The hemodynamic effects of *chronic clonidine administration* are unclear. Blood pressure is usually reduced less than after a single dose. A relative bradycardia persists, but no marked changes in cardiac output or vascular resistance have been reported. Plasma renin activity is decreased. Sodium retention persists, and the increased extracellular fluid volume could contribute to the maintenance of cardiac output. It probably explains the observation that tolerance to the antihypertensive effect develops more frequently and rapidly when clonidine is given alone than when it is combined with a thiazide diuretic. Postural hypotension does occur, but it is not marked and exercise responses indicate that reflex control of capacitance vessels is not abolished. (*See* Muir *et al.,* 1969; McRaven *et al.,* 1971; Onesti *et al.,* 1971.)

Little is known about the pharmacokinetics of clonidine, at least partly because such small amounts are required to produce an effect. However, it has a short duration of action and three or four doses a day appear to be required to maintain its antihypertensive effect.

Preparations, Routes of Administration, and Dosage. *Clonidine hydrochloride* (CATAPRES) is marketed in 100-µg scored tablets, and as an injection containing 150 µg/ml. The usual total daily dose is from 400 µg to 2.0 mg.

Toxicity and Precautions. The most frequent side effects of clonidine reported in man are dry mouth and sedation, which are very common and not infrequently severe. These tend to decrease with time but do not disappear during chronic therapy. Impotence and constipation are less common, but have been reported to occur in 10 to 20% of cases on chronic therapy. Allergic manifestations, including rashes, pruritus, and angioneurotic edema, have also been observed. Postural hypotension occurs, but is less frequent than with adrenergic neuron blocking agents. Hyperirritability and a marked rebound in blood pressure frequently occur when medication is discontinued. This is associated with a considerable increase in catecholamine excretion and can be controlled by α- and β-adrenergic blocking agents (Hansson *et al.,* 1973). Concomitant administration of a tricyclic antidepressant can largely abolish the antihypertensive effect of clonidine (Briant *et al.,* 1973). Clonidine is still a relatively new drug, and the full range of its adverse effects has probably not yet been determined.

Therapeutic Uses. The use of clonidine in the management of essential hypertension is mentioned at the end of this chapter. The drug has also been shown to be effective in some cases of *migraine* (Shafar *et al.,* 1972).

DIURETIC (SALURETIC) AGENTS

Chlorothiazide was the first of a now-extensive series of benzothiadiazide (thiazide) diuretic agents that are highly effective after oral administration. It greatly simplified long-term management of various conditions requiring the elimination of salt and water, and during such treatment it was noted that chlorothiazide itself had an antihypertensive effect and augmented responses to other antihypertensive drugs. The thiazides and closely related phthalimidine derivatives (*e.g.,* chlorthalidone) have become a mainstay of antihypertensive therapy. They all have equivalent antihypertensive properties and side effects. More recently, other diuretic agents have been shown to have antihypertensive properties. Details of the pharmacology of the diuretics are presented in Chapter 39. Only the antihypertensive effects of these drugs and other properties specifically related to their use in the treatment of hypertension will be considered here.

Benzothiadiazides

The renal actions of the *thiazide* diuretics decrease extracellular fluid and plasma volumes, cardiac output, and total exchangeable sodium in individuals without any evidence of cardiac failure. At this stage, sodium and water depletion appears to provide an adequate basis for the antihypertensive effect and, particularly, for augmentation of the effects of other antihypertensive drugs. It is well known that a reduction in blood volume makes maintenance of the blood pressure highly dependent on vascular tone, particularly that of capacitance vessels. After several months of continuous diuretic administration, plasma volume and total body sodium and water return almost to normal, although in some studies plasma volume has been found to remain significantly reduced (*see* Leth, 1970). Cardiac output may now be slightly above control values. At this time peripheral resistance is clearly decreased, and this appears to be adequate to account

for the persistent antihypertensive effect (Conway and Palmero, 1963). In the early phase, reestablishment of the plasma volume abolishes the antihypertensive effect, but in the later phase expansion of the plasma volume to above normal (as with dextran) does not reverse the reduction in blood pressure. Thus, the persistent antihypertensive effect appears not to be predominantly due to altered fluid volumes, although residual deficits could contribute.

The significance of a very small, persistent deficit in total body sodium is unclear; it does not appear to be reflected in an altered sodium content of arterial walls. The hypotensive effect of diuretics unrelated chemically to the thiazides has led to the suggestion that the ultimate mechanism of the persistent reduction in peripheral resistance may involve altered sodium metabolism or a compensation to it. (*See* Tobian, 1967.) However, sequential studies of body sodium content, plasma volume, and peripheral resistance have not been done with other diuretics and it is not clear whether phases similar to those seen with the thiazides occur.

After cessation of prolonged thiazide diuretic therapy there is a rapid "rebound" of total body sodium, water, and plasma volume to values above normal. This may be a consequence of the considerable elevation in plasma renin activity during treatment (Tarazi *et al.,* 1970). The blood pressure returns toward the pretreatment level much more slowly.

Irrespective of the ultimate mechanism, it appears that the diuretic thiazides relax peripheral arteriolar smooth muscle. Additional support for this conclusion has come from observations on *diazoxide,* a benzothiadiazide that causes marked *salt and water retention,* but produces a much more profound relaxation of arterioles than do its diuretic congeners (*see* below).

The antihypertensive effect of the thiazides appears to have characteristics that are very close to ideal for the management of essential hypertension. The usual pattern involves proportional reductions in systolic and diastolic pressures, maintained or increased cardiac output, little or no postural hypotension, no major changes in regional blood flows, and little or no development of tolerance. Their relatively weak antihypertensive effect does not restrict the range of patients in which they are useful, but it does dictate that other antihypertensive drugs must frequently be used concurrently.

Side effects of the diuretic thiazides are discussed in detail in Chapter 39. Those that most frequently complicate their use in the treatment of hypertension are *hypokalemia, hyperglycemia,* and *hyperuricemia.* The last-named effect may be particularly significant because many hypertensive patients have somewhat elevated blood uric acid concentrations. Some hypokalemia occurs in almost all patients on chronic treatment with a thiazide diuretic, but it is rarely of clinical significance in patients on an adequate diet. Routine potassium supplements are not indicated and may represent a greater hazard than the hypokalemia. Special care is necessary, however, to ensure adequate potassium intake by patients receiving a thiazide and digitalis concurrently.

OTHER DIURETICS

Many diuretics used clinically, including spironolactone, furosemide, ethacrynic acid, and mercurials, have been reported to have antihypertensive properties. However, sufficient reduction of plasma and extracellular volumes by any mechanism will reduce the blood pressure, and in most cases the available data do not allow differentiation between effects on fluid volumes *per se* and effects on vascular resistance.

Spironolactone has been extensively studied, and its pharmacological properties make it suitable for chronic use (*see* Chapter 39). The antihypertensive effects of spironolactone are qualitatively and quantitatively very similar to those of a thiazide. Both drugs increase plasma renin concentration and are most effective in patients with low plasma renin activities. When administered chronically in appropriate doses spironolactone and a thiazide produce similar small reductions in plasma volume and serum sodium (Acchiardo *et al.,* 1972). It has been reported that the antihypertensive effect of spironolactone, but not that of hydrochlorothiazide, is correlated with weight loss (Adlin *et al.,* 1972). Unfortunately, there appear to be no hemodynamic measurements to indicate whether there is an early or late reduction in peripheral resistance during the administration of spironolactone. Some reports suggested that the antihypertensive effects of spironolactone and a thiazide are additive, but with adequate doses of each this does not appear to be the case (Ogilvie and Ruedy, 1969). At the present time the choice between a thiazide and spironolactone in the treatment of hypertension appears to be predominantly on the basis of anticipated side effects in the individual patient. Both produce some gastrointestinal irritation and hypersensitivity reactions, and both can increase the blood urea nitrogen in patients with renal inadequacy. Spironolactone does not cause hypokalemia, hyperglycemia, or hyperuricemia, but amenorrhea, gynecomastia, and hyperkalemia can occur; the last-named effect is particularly hazardous in patients with impaired renal function.

Other diuretics that cause potassium retention, such as *triamterene* and *amiloride,* do not appear to have useful antihypertensive properties.

Furosemide is a powerful diuretic that is used extensively in the treatment of hypertension. Furosemide does have an antihypertensive effect, as is probably true of all drugs that reduce body sodium and fluid volume, but there is no evidence that it significantly reduces arteriolar tone. In comparative chronic trials furosemide tends to have less antihypertensive effect than does a thiazide-type diuretic (Healy *et al.,* 1970; Anderson *et al.,* 1971). In common with the thiazides it causes *hypokalemia, hyperglycemia,* and *hyperuricemia,* and it has a considerably greater potential for producing *serious electrolyte disturbances.* There appears to be no rational role for furosemide in the treatment of the great majority of cases of essential hypertension. It may be useful in special cases, such as those in which renal function is so inadequate that a thiazide or spironolactone cannot prevent sodium accumulation.

Therapeutic Uses. The current role of diuretics in the therapy of essential hypertension and their interactions with other drugs used to lower blood pressure are discussed at the end of this chapter. Other uses of diuretics are covered in Chapter 39.

DIAZOXIDE

Diazoxide is closely related chemically to the thiazide diuretics, as can be seen from their structural formulas.

Chlorothiazide

Diazoxide

Diazoxide appears to have qualitatively the same effects on peripheral blood vessels as do the thiazides. However, it produces much more rapid and profound changes. Consequently, its effects are more amenable to study and have provided information that is probably also applicable to the related diuretics. Rapid intravenous administration of diazoxide to a hypertensive subject causes a prompt fall in both systolic and diastolic pressures associated with a considerable increase in cardiac output and some tachycardia, but the pressure rarely falls below the normal range and postural hypotension does not develop. These characteristics indicate that sympathetic nervous system function is not impaired and that the major action is on resistance rather than capacitance vessels. The differential effect on blood vessels has been confirmed by a variety of more detailed studies that show that diazoxide directly dilates arterioles but has very little effect on large veins (Gaskell and Diosy, 1959; Thirwell and Zsotér, 1972), although it can affect small postcapillary resistance vessels (Ogilvie and Mikulic, 1972).

With single intravenous injections, a marked antihypertensive effect is observed only when the drug is given rapidly (*see* Mroczek *et al.*, 1971). This time dependence has been attributed to the fact that diazoxide is 90% bound to plasma protein and the concentration reaching the vascular smooth muscle is inadequate if time is allowed for equilibration with the binding proteins (Sellers and Koch-Weser, 1969). Once the antihypertensive effect has developed, it usually persists for 4 to 12 hours. Oral diazoxide can produce a slower, sustained fall in blood pressure, but side effects preclude its long-term use.

The major effects of diazoxide on water and electrolyte balance are opposite to those of the diuretic thiazides. It causes marked *retention of sodium and water* in both normotensive and hypertensive individuals, expands plasma volume, and can produce frank edema in patients with myocardial

inadequacy (Thomson *et al.*, 1962). These effects can be readily antagonized by a diuretic thiazide. When diazoxide causes a considerable reduction in blood pressure, glomerular filtration rate and renal plasma flow are also decreased, but sodium retention can occur without any change in blood pressure or renal hemodynamics (Johnson, 1971). In common with its diuretic congeners, diazoxide inhibits tubular excretion of uric acid and can decrease free-water clearance.

Diazoxide is a relatively weak inhibitor of responses of vascular smooth muscle to a variety of stimulants, including norepinephrine and angiotensin. It appears to be a competitive antagonist of barium, and somewhat indirect evidence indicates that it may similarly antagonize the action of calcium (Wohl *et al.*, 1968). The antagonism of calcium may be complex. In a mesenteric vein preparation that contracts spontaneously with the generation of calcium-dependent action potentials, diazoxide blocks the generation of potentials and inhibits responses to agonists that act through these potentials; when the muscle is depolarized, it blocks contractions produced by calcium (Rhodes and Sutter, 1971). As in hemodynamic studies, the weaker effects of diuretic thiazides make it more difficult to study their mechanism of action on vascular smooth muscle, but the evidence available to date is compatible with the assumption that it is similar to that of diazoxide.

Diazoxide inhibits the spontaneous activity and responses of many smooth muscle structures in addition to blood vessels. It is a powerful relaxant of both the gravid and nongravid human uterus, and this has led to the suggestion that it might be used in dysmenorrhea and to arrest premature labor (Landesman *et al.*, 1968).

The major side effects of diazoxide are *salt and water retention*, which can be controlled by a diuretic thiazide; *hyperuricemia;* and *hyperglycemia*. These do not present major problems in short-term therapy, but preclude use of the drug for the long-term management of hypertension. When given chronically for its hyperglycemic effect, diazoxide also causes *hypertrichosis*.

Preparations, Routes of Administration, and Dosage. *Diazoxide*, U.S.P. (HYPERSTAT I.V.), is available for intravenous use, in 20-ml ampuls containing 300 mg of the drug. This is the usual dose. The solution is very alkaline, and care must be taken to avoid extravasation. In Europe, diazoxide is available in 50-mg tablets (EUDEMINE).

Therapeutic Uses. The use of diazoxide in hypertensive emergencies is discussed at the end of this chapter. Although the hyperglycemic effect is a serious obstacle to the use of diazoxide in the management of hypertension, it can be useful in other conditions (*see* Symposium, 1968; *see also* Chapter 71).

NITROPRUSSIDE

Sodium nitroprusside (sodium nitroferricyanide) is a powerful vasodilator that has been used sporadically as a hypotensive agent in man for over 4 decades (*see* Johnson, 1929). The effects of the nitroprusside ion are similar to those of nitrite (*see* Chapter 34), in that it acts directly on the smooth muscle of blood vessels, probably due to the nitroso moiety. Both resistance and capacitance vessels are affected, and the drug would probably cause marked postural hypotension if the patient were ever allowed to assume an upright position. Nitroprusside infused intravenously into a recumbent laboratory animal or man causes a very rapid fall in arterial and central venous pressures, and a moderate increase in heart rate. Cardiac output may increase, considerably so in anesthetized subjects. Vascular resistance is decreased less in the renal than in the femoral and mesenteric vascular beds. The fall in arterial pressure is dose dependent and does not reach a "floor." The effects of nitroprusside are quite transient, due to its rapid conversion in the body to thiocyanate. As soon as infusion of the drug is stopped, the blood pressure begins to rise immediately and reaches the pretreatment level in 1 to 10 minutes. The effect of nitroprusside on smooth muscles other than vascular is not known.

Toxicity, Precautions, and Contraindications. The acute toxicity of nitroprusside is entirely secondary to excessive vasodilatation and hypotension. Symptoms include nausea, vomiting, sweating, restlessness, headache, palpitation, and substernal distress; they disappear promptly when the infusion is stopped or the rate reduced. Patients receiving antihypertensive drug therapy are more sensitive to the anion. Elderly persons should be given lower-than-usual doses. Nitroprusside treatment is a hospital procedure and requires meticulous attention to details of administration (*see* below). The safety of the drug in children and pregnant women has not yet been established. With prolonged therapy (2 to 3 weeks), there is the rare possibility of temporary hypothyroidism from

the effect of the thiocyanate ion to which nitroprusside is converted; cyanide is an intermediate step in this conversion, but it apparently does not accumulate in toxic concentrations. (*See* Page *et al.,* 1955; Ross and Cole, 1973.)

Preparations, Routes of Administration, and Dosage. *Sodium nitroprusside* (NIPRIDE) is a reddish-brown, water-soluble powder, marketed in 5-ml amber-colored, rubber-stoppered vials, each containing 50 mg of the drug. Only fresh solutions should be used, and those more than 4 hours old should be discarded. The solution is made by first adding 2 or 3 ml of 5% dextrose solution in water to the vial and then transferring the contents to an infusion bottle containing 500 ml of the same diluent. Because the compound decomposes in light, the bottle should be covered with an opaque wrapping.

Nitroprusside solution must be administered only by slow intravenous infusion, and a microdrip regulator should be used to ensure a precise flow rate. Other drugs should not be added to the solution. Care should be taken to prevent extravasation. The average adult dose is 3 μg/kg per minute (about 200 μg per minute) for patients not receiving other antihypertensive drugs, but the range of dosage is broad. The maximal dose should not exceed 800 μg per minute. The objective is to reduce the blood pressure by 30 to 40% of the pretreatment diastolic level. *Continuous monitoring of the patient, the blood pressure, and the flow rate is absolutely essential.* With careful supervision, the diastolic blood pressure can be maintained at almost any desired level. Some tolerance to the hypotensive effect of nitroprusside is occasionally observed, but absolute resistance does not occur.

Therapeutic Uses. Nitroprusside is used when short-term, rapid reduction in blood pressure is required. There is no report of any condition in which the blood pressure cannot be lowered by this drug. Its use in *hypertensive emergencies* is mentioned at the end of this chapter, and the drug is also used where hypotension is required to minimize bleeding during surgery (*see* Mani, 1971). In addition, nitroprusside can improve left ventricular function following *acute myocardial infarction* (Franciosa *et al.,* 1972), and it has had preliminary but encouraging trial in patients with *chronic refractory heart failure.* (*See also* Palmer and Lasseter, 1975.)

MINOR ANTIHYPERTENSIVE AGENTS

MONOAMINE OXIDASE (MAO) INHIBITORS

Postural hypotension is a relatively frequent side effect during the use of those antidepressant drugs classified as monoamine oxidase (MAO) inhibitors. One of these, *pargyline* (N-benzyl-N-methyl-2-propynylamine), was introduced specifically as an antihypertensive. However, its effects on the CNS are very similar to those of other members of the group, and it is also an antidepressant. The following discussion will deal predominantly with antihypertensive effects of MAO inhibitors, and, insofar as information is available, major emphasis will be placed on the properties of pargyline. However, the antihypertensive effects of all long-acting members of this group appear to be qualitatively the same and are not well correlated with MAO inhibition (Maxwell, 1963). A more complete discussion of these drugs is presented in Chapter 12.

The mechanism of the antihypertensive effect of MAO inhibitors is a subject on which speculation has far outstripped information. The hypotensive response has a pronounced postural component, which indicates interference with sympathetic venoconstriction. There is little to suggest that this involves the CNS. MAO inhibitors have been reported to reduce transmission through sympathetic but not parasympathetic ganglia, and chronic administration of pargyline has been shown to reduce norepinephrine release in response to preganglionic stimulation (Puig *et al.*, 1972). MAO inhibitors have also been reported to have a "bretylium-like" effect in preventing depletion of tissue norepinephrine by guanethidine and reserpine (Gessa *et al.*, 1963), but they do not markedly or consistently reduce the release of norepinephrine during nerve activity and they augment responses to indirect-acting sympathomimetics (Smith, 1966; Puig *et al.*, 1972). Pargyline has an inconsistent effect on the amount of norepinephrine in tissues, but decreases its rate of synthesis and turnover in both laboratory animals and man. Inhibition of MAO allows the accumulation of dopamine and octopamine, and it has been suggested that these substances could impair adrenergic nerve function by acting as weak "false transmitters" (Kopin *et al.*, 1965); however, their relation to any inadequacy of responses to adrenergic nerve activity has not been established. Whatever the mechanism of action, it should be noted that MAO inhibitors fail to produce many of the signs characteristic of adrenergic nerve failure, including ptosis and relaxation of the nictitating membrane.

The reduction in blood pressure induced by MAO inhibitors develops slowly. Three weeks or more may be required to achieve the maximal effect of daily administration in man, and the effect also disappears very slowly. It is predominantly a postural hypotension without associated tachycardia; reduction of recumbent blood pressure is minimal in most patients. Reports of the hemodynamic changes during treatment with pargyline are inconsistent; the fall in blood pressure has been attributed predominantly to a decrease in peripheral resistance (Onesti *et al.*, 1964) or to a decrease in cardiac output (Sannerstedt, 1967). Reasons for this major discrepancy are not apparent, but a predominant effect on cardiac output is consistent with the considerable tendency to produce postural hypotension that has been reported by many investigators.

Preparations, Routes of Administration, and Dosage. *Pargyline Hydrochloride,* N.F. (EUTONYL), is available in 10-, 25-, and 50-mg tablets for oral use. Administration once daily is as effective as divided doses. The initial dose should not exceed 25 mg, and should be increased only at intervals of a week or more.

Toxicity and Precautions. The MAO inhibitors as a group produce a wide range of toxic reactions (*see also* Chapter 12, and Goldberg, 1964). Pargyline tends to promote fluid retention and nonfluid weight gain. Other untoward effects include CNS stimulation—with insomnia, nightmares, and, occasionally, psychotic reactions—muscle cramps, nausea, diarrhea or constipation, as well as weakness, dizziness, and other symptoms of postural hypotension. Patients may complain less promptly about side effects of pargyline than those of other antihypertensive drugs because of the mood elevation or frank euphoria it can produce. The MAO inhibitors also cause intolerance to a considerable number of other drugs and foods. Severe reactions and death have been reported to result from several combinations (*see* Goldberg, 1964; Blackwell *et al.*, 1967; and Chapter 12), and the full range of incompatibilities is undoubtedly broader than now recognized. Most of these reactions result from altered metabolism of a drug or a food constituent, and emphasize that *many enzymes in addition to MAO are inhibited.* The intolerance may persist for several weeks after the last administration of the inhibitor (Cousins and Maltby, 1971), and involves many drugs that are commonly given without special regard for concurrent antihypertensive therapy or are self-administered, including sedatives, antihistamines, sympathomimetics, antidepressants, narcotics, and hypoglycemic agents. A special precaution is that an MAO inhibitor and methyldopa should never be used together in antihypertensive therapy because this combination can produce severe CNS stimulation and hypertensive reactions.

Therapeutic Uses. Pargyline has been used in the treatment of moderate and severe hypertension, but equally effective and safer drugs are now available.

VERATRUM ALKALOIDS

The veratrum alkaloids are included in this chapter because of the very interesting mechanism by which they reduce blood pressure. Although many alkaloids of at least three pharmacological classes have been isolated from various species of *Veratrum* and members of several other genera, major interest has centered on the hypotensive *ester alkaloids* such as the protoveratrines, and the present discussion will deal only with this group. Major pharmacological properties of the various ester alkaloids are qualitatively the same; thus, to simplify presentation, the general term *veratrum* will be used to refer to them collectively. The relationship of the structure of ester alkaloids to their hypotensive effect has been reviewed by Kupchan (1961), and earlier work on various veratrum alkaloids has been critically and extensively reviewed by Krayer and Acheson (1946).

The veratrum alkaloids act on the membranes of almost all excitable cells to cause repetitive firing after a single stimulus, but usually do not themselves initiate a response. This effect is associated with a delay in repolarization after an evoked discharge, but the relation of negative afterpotential to after-discharge is complex. The actual initiation of subsequent propagated depolarizations is probably dependent on differential repolarization of areas of the cell membrane. The primary action of the alkaloids appears to be to increase the sodium conductivity of the membrane. The effect of veratrum is prevented by local anesthetics or tetrodotoxin, and by increased extracellular calcium or potassium or decreased extracellular sodium. (See reviews by Shanes, 1958; Benforado, 1967.)

The veratrum alkaloids have similar actions on many excitable cells, but sensitivity to them varies considerably. In general, afferent nerve fibers that affect cardiovascular and respiratory function have the lowest thresholds. The increased number of impulses triggered by a given stimulus, often converting phasic to essentially continuous activity, effectively "resets" to a lower level the involved receptors and the reflexes that they initiate. Single small doses of veratrum administered intravenously act predominantly on endings of afferent vagal fibers in the coronary sinus and left ventricle (see Dawes and Comroe, 1954; Juhász-Nagy and Szentiványi, 1961). The response to this increased afferent nerve activity is the Bezold-Jarisch reflex. It is a relatively brief response characterized by hypotension and bradycardia. The bradycardia is prevented and the hypotension attenuated by atropine. Although vagotomy abolishes the Bezold-Jarisch reflex, veratrum can still lower the blood pressure by an action on the baroreceptors of the carotid sinus. Hypotension is a more prominent feature of this response than is bradycardia, and the fall in blood pressure is not markedly reduced by atropine. The response from the carotid sinus develops more slowly than that from the heart, but is more persistent. It appears to be the major factor in the effects induced by veratrum in man under the usual conditions of slow infusion or absorption. Because compensatory mechanisms are "reset" rather than blocked, the fall in blood pressure does not have a major postural component. (See Hoobler et al., 1955.) High concentrations of veratrum have a direct digitalis-like action on the heart.

Doses of veratrum only slightly higher than those required to lower the blood pressure stimulate receptors in the region of the nodose ganglion of the vagus to induce nausea and vomiting; after repeated administration, even this small margin may disappear. The properties of the sensory receptors involved in these two key responses appear to be too similar to allow effective differential sensitization, and this "built-in" adverse effect has prevented effective clinical use of the veratrum alkaloids.

Doses somewhat larger than the minimum necessary to elicit a cardiovascular response cause transient respiratory depression that involves pulmonary stretch receptors and probably other receptors in the thoracic viscera. This reflex rapidly becomes tolerant to repeated injections. Very large doses cause death by central respiratory depression. Both visceral and somatic sensory receptors serving many different modalities are readily activated by veratrum; for example, an intense burning sensation and sneezing can be produced by local application to appropriate areas. Details of the pharmacology of the veratrum alkaloids have been reviewed by Benforado (1967).

Thiocyanate. *Sodium thiocyanate (sodium sulfocyanate or rhodanide)*, one of the first agents to be used in the treatment of hypertension, has had a stormy history, largely because of its toxicity. Antihypertensive activity resides in the thiocyanate anion *per se*. Adequate doses have an undoubted hypotensive effect, but the mechanism of action is obscure. Thiocyanate is distributed in, and handled by, the body in essentially the same manner as are halogen ions. Both its concentration in extracellular fluid and its pharmacological effects are slowly cumulative, and the concentration reached is inversely related to total halogen ion turnover. Toxic reactions include weakness, nausea, vomiting, diarrhea, skin eruptions, arthralgia, palpitation, precordial pain, muscle cramps, facial edema, nephrosis, hepatic necrosis, anemia, depressed thyroid function, irritability, blurred vision, tinnitus, motor aphasia, hallucinations, and delirium. Treatment is largely symptomatic but should include measures to hasten elimination of the offending ion, such as administration of large amounts of chloride (Nickerson and Thomas, 1951; Walser and Rahill, 1965) and, in urgent situations, hemodialysis (Christensen and Williams, 1962).

Mebutamate. *Mebutamate* (2-methyl-2-sec-butyl-1,3-propanediol dicarbamate; CAPLA) differs from *meprobamate* only in the replacement of a propyl group by *sec*-butyl, and it shares the general CNS depressant properties of the latter. There is no convincing evidence that it has any antihypertensive effect in man that cannot be attributed to placebo or sedative effects.

Nitrites. Inorganic nitrite and various organic nitrites and nitrates have a common property of relaxing smooth muscle, including that of blood vessels. In moderate doses, they have little effect on recumbent blood pressure but can produce marked postural hypotension and syncope due to the relaxation of veins. Nitrites do not produce a useful lowering of the blood pressure without the concomitant occurrence of disabling postural hypotension. They are still included in a number of proprietary antihypertensive mixtures, but their effect after oral administration is limited and the amounts are usually too low to produce either a significant decrease in blood pressure or troublesome side effects. The pharmacology of the nitrites and their clinical uses are discussed more fully in Chapter 34.

II. Drug Therapy of Hypertension

It is estimated that the systemic arterial pressures of 20% of the adult population of North America are above the accepted normal range. Several of the causes of these elevations (*e.g.,* pheochromocytoma and primary hyperaldosteronism) are amenable to direct therapeutic intervention. However, these causes are relatively uncommon, and in most cases of systemic hypertension the pathogenesis is obscure and therapy can be directed only to correction of the abnormal pressure. Although such a blind, empirical approach is never ideal, it is now clear that manometric success *per se* can favorably affect prognosis. It has been established that the higher the systolic or diastolic pressure, both within and above the "normal" range, the greater the risk of death from cardiovascular disease. Lowering diastolic pressures of over 105 mm Hg in men reduces the morbidity and mortality due to a variety of cardiovascular complications, including intracerebral hemorrhage, thrombotic cerebrovascular disease, malignant hypertension, dissecting aneurysm, and congestive cardiac failure. To date, there is no evidence that treatment of hypertension reduces the risk of coronary artery disease. There is almost no information on the results of treatment of hypertension in women, and the results of treatment of mild hypertension are still inconclusive. (*See* Veterans Administration Cooperative Study Group on Antihypertensive Agents, 1967, 1970; Page and Sidd, 1972; Aagaard, 1973; Freis, 1973.)

ESSENTIAL HYPERTENSION

Pathophysiology and Classification. Any general discussion of antihypertensive therapy must center on the condition known as essential, or primary, hypertension. This is a somewhat poorly defined condition diagnosed by exclusion, and it is unclear whether it represents a single entity or several, and whether it is distinct from normotension or simply the upper end of a continuous spectrum of blood pressures in the population. Abnormal sympathetic nerve function is probably not responsible for the increases in peripheral vascular resistance and diastolic pressure that characterize essential hypertension. However, in hypertensive as in normotensive individuals, the sympathetic nerves contribute to vascular tone, both arteriolar and venous; even if it is not abnormally high, reduction of this adrenergic vasomotor tone can reduce the blood pressure.

Acute elevation of systemic pressure to a value such as 190/110 mm Hg in a previously normotensive individual acts through the barostatic reflexes to eliminate most of the neurogenic vasomotor tone. However, pressure-sensitive areas such as the carotid sinus can adapt to function in relation to some new "basal" blood pressure far above the normal range in the same way that they operate around a "normal" mean pressure (McCubbin *et al.,* 1956). This "resetting" maintains approximately equivalent sympathetic vasomotor tone in normotensive and hypertensive individuals, and makes it possible for interference with sympathetic nervous system function to lower the pressure in hypertensive states. Conversely, barostatic reflexes will initially tend to oppose a drug-induced reduction in pressure; however, during a sustained antihypertensive effect, these reflexes could reset to maintain the lower pressure. This might explain the finding that, after a period of successful antihypertensive therapy, the pressure may become progressively easier to control. Much more information regarding the time course of baroreceptor changes in human hypertension is required before their role can be reliably interpreted. However, some studies in laboratory animals suggest that adaptation of the receptors may be too rapid to explain the observed changes in responses to antihypertensive drugs (*see* Krieger, 1970).

The selection of agents, the vigor with which antihypertensive therapy is pursued, and the side effects that are acceptable all depend on assessment of the severity and anticipated course of the hypertensive disease. This rests on a weighted consideration of many factors, including the following: (1) The state of peripheral vessels, primarily as determined by examination of the optic fundi. (2) The degree of involvement of organs adversely affected by hypertensive disease, particularly the heart, kidneys, and brain. (3) The blood pressure. Consistent basal diastolic pressures over 110 mm Hg are usually associated with progressive organ damage. It has now been shown that systolic pressure is also a significant determinant of the development of coronary artery disease—indeed, more important than diastolic pressure in women and in men over 45 years of age. However, it is not known whether this risk is reduced by lowering the systolic pressure. Basal blood pressures are usually more reliable than casual blood pressure determinations, but it must be noted that most morbidity and mortality statistics are based on casual pressures. Basal blood pressures are often 10 mm Hg or more below casual readings. Single blood pressure determinations are notoriously unreliable. (4) The duration and rate of progression of the hypertension. The more rapid the development of elevation in diastolic pressure, or of damage to the heart, kidneys, or other organs, the poorer is the prognosis. A prolonged elevation of the pressure with little or no organ damage indicates a relatively good prognosis. (5) The age, sex, race, and family history of the individual. When other findings are equivalent, the prognosis is less favorable in younger than in older individuals, in males than in females, and in Negroes than in Caucasians. (6) The significance of the renin-angiotensin system in hypertensive vascular disease is unclear; at present most evidence suggests that the course of cardiovascular complications of essential hypertension cannot be predicted from the plasma renin activity (Brunner *et al.,* 1972, 1973; Genest *et al.,* 1973; Giese, 1973). However, this system can modify responses to antihypertensive drugs (Crane and Harris, 1970; Spark and Melby, 1971; Bühler *et al.,* 1972; Carey *et al.,* 1972; Beevers *et al.,* 1973), and it now appears necessary to take this factor into consideration, at least in clinical trials. About one fourth of all patients diagnosed as having essential hypertension were found to have low, two thirds to have normal, and the remainder to have elevated plasma renin activity (*see* Lowenstein, 1972).

Although similar factors are involved in all classifications of the severity of hypertensive disease, no single one is generally accepted, and each group working in the field has its own system (*see* Veterans Administration Cooperative Study Group on Antihypertensive Agents, 1967; Ogilvie and Ruedy, 1969; Becker-Christensen *et al.*, 1971; Zacharias *et al.*, 1972). Three very broad categories will be used as a basis for the following discussion of the therapeutic roles of various antihypertensive drugs: (1) *mild hypertension,* with basal diastolic pressure less than 100 mm Hg, no apparent cardiac or cerebral complications, no apparent renal complications, and changes in the optic fundi no more severe than segmental arteriolar narrowing; (2) *moderate hypertension,* which is intermediate in severity between mild and severe; and (3) *severe hypertension,* with basal diastolic pressure more than 130 mm Hg, or cardiac or renal decompensation, or rapid progression of renal damage, or hemorrhages in the optic fundi due to the hypertension. Where there is doubt regarding the severity of the disease process, patients under 50 years of age, males, and Negroes are particularly likely to warrant the more serious classification. Although major consideration in this discussion is given to essential hypertension, "renal" hypertension due to conditions not amenable to surgery can usually be assessed in relation to the same general therapeutic categories.

Therapeutic Regimens. Many hypertension clinics have now demonstrated that in almost all cases of hypertensive cardiovascular disease the blood pressure can be successfully controlled by skillful use of the drugs currently available. However, it has also been estimated that only a small percentage of all hypertensive patients under treatment are even close to optimal control. This disparity emphasizes the fact that *effective use of antihypertensive drugs is not "routine."* Therapy must be tailored to the needs of the individual patient and adjusted as necessary to maintain an optimal balance between therapeutic and side effects; the importance of this principle increases directly with the severity of the disease. Concurrent use of two or more drugs is often desirable, and the reductions in pressure induced by different agents are often approximately additive. Concurrent therapy also allows effective use of smaller doses of the more powerful agents and, therefore, reduces the incidence and the severity of side effects.

However, fixed-dose mixtures of two or more drugs cannot be recommended unless they fit the needs of particular patients. Substantial differences in relative effectiveness have been reported by different groups of investigators, and it is clear that *how drugs are used is at least as important as which are selected for use.* Examples of clinical trials of antihypertensive drugs and of the problems encountered in such studies may be found in many publications, including Aoki and Wilson (1970), Gibb and coworkers (1970), Anderson and associates (1971), Bengtsson (1972), and Putzeys and Hoobler (1972).

A very difficult and important problem in the treatment of hypertension is to determine what constitutes "acceptable" side effects, particularly in the long-term management of relatively mild, asymptomatic cases. All the effective antihypertensive drugs produce quite significant adverse effects, and the reports of several studies have included a comment that, although side effects did not interfere with the management of most cases, the patients very frequently "felt better" while taking a placebo. The physician treating cases of asymptomatic hypertension should remember the difference between prolonging life and making life seem longer.

The drug treatment of hypertension can be obviated in some patients and aided in all by weight control and avoidance of excessive salt (*see* Coleman *et al.,* 1972). In addition, mild elevations of blood pressure can be controlled at least for short periods of time by physical training (Boyer and Kasch, 1970; Choquette and Ferguson, 1973). Oral contraceptive drugs can increase blood pressure, and the use of other contraceptive measures may be desirable in susceptible patients. Since the aim of treatment is primarily to prevent the cardiovascular complications of hypertension, other contributing factors, including obesity, hyperlipidemia, and smoking, should not be neglected.

Mild Hypertension. There appears to be little justification for antihypertensive drug therapy in patients at the lower end of the hypertensive spectrum who are over 45 years of age, especially females. However, the same basic cardiovascular status in a younger individual is often an indication for treatment. Unless there is some specific contraindication, the initial drug to be employed is a *thiazide diuretic,* most commonly hydrochlorothiazide in a dose of 50 mg twice a day. Reduction in blood pressure parallels the saluresis and most of the antihypertensive effect is attained within 3 or 4 days (Wilson and Freis, 1959). Some additional effect may be obtained by increasing the dose to 150 mg per day. The effects of chlorthalidone are indistinguishable from those of hydrochlorothiazide, and its longer duration of action may simplify administration; the maximally effective dose is about 100 mg per day. Spironolactone in adequate doses (100 to 200 mg per day) is probably as effective as a thiazide. Both the thiazide diuretics and spironolactone reduce blood pressure most effectively in patients with low plasma renin activity (Crane and Harris, 1970; Spark and Melby, 1971; Carey *et al.,* 1972).

If diuretic drugs are contraindicated or not tolerated, an alternative initial drug is reserpine, usually 0.5 mg daily. The antihypertensive effect develops slowly over 2 or 3 weeks. This dose of reserpine is usually less effective than a maximal dose of a thiazide diuretic, and side effects increase considerably with higher doses; 1.0 mg per day is probably the absolute maximum for chronic administration. Where a reduction in pressure greater than that produced by the diuretic alone is considered necessary, reserpine can be added with a reasonable expectation that the combination will have a greater effect than that from either agent alone. A few patients may not respond to the above procedures; however, if their hypertension is correctly classified as mild, they may be followed without antihypertensive therapy and more vigorous treatment undertaken if there is evidence of progression.

The association of a much higher-than-normal incidence of *carcinoma of the breast* in women with the long-term use of reserpine in the treatment of hypertension is presented on page 558.

Moderate Hypertension. The initial drug therapy for patients in this category is the same as for mild hypertension, but it will be successful in a smaller percentage of cases. If more vigorous therapy is required to control the blood pressure, the diuretic is continued and some more effective drug is added to the regimen, usually *methyldopa, hydralazine,* or *propranolol.* All antihypertensive drugs except the diuretics frequently cause sodium retention and weight gain, accompanied by a progressive loss of antihypertensive effect that is not easily restored by simply increasing the dose. The addition of a diuretic usually reestablishes the effectiveness of the medication (Finnerty, 1971).

Methyldopa is an antihypertensive drug of intermediate efficacy (*see* Aoki and Wilson, 1970) and a relatively narrow dose range; less than 0.5 g per day is ineffective, and more than 2.0 g per day rarely produces an increased effect. It can be added to basal diuretic therapy in a dose of 0.5 to 1.0 g per day, which is then adjusted according to the response. The most frequent and disturbing side effect is drowsiness and difficulty in performing work that requires concentrated mental effort.

Hydralazine occupies an intermediate position because moderately antihypertensive doses represent a balance between therapeutic and toxic effects. It is generally added to diuretic therapy in a dose as small as 10 mg twice a day and slowly increased to 25 to 50 mg three or four times a day. This procedure appears to reduce side effects. More than 200 mg per day should not be given chronically.

Propranolol is probably as effective as methyldopa or hydralazine when added to diuretic therapy (Prichard, 1970; Bengtsson, 1972; O'Brien and MacKinnon, 1972; Zacharias *et al.,* 1972; Castenfors *et al.,* 1973). When used alone, the antihypertensive response is variable. Patients with high or normal plasma renin activities appear to respond better than do those with low plasma renin (Bühler *et al.,* 1972). Propranolol is usually added to basal diuretic therapy in doses up to 2 to 4 mg/kg per day. Propranolol antagonizes the cardiac stimulation that may limit the effectiveness of hydralazine (Sannerstedt *et al.,* 1971), and the combination has been shown to be more effective than either drug alone. Methyldopa and propranolol reduce plasma renin activity (Bühler *et al.,* 1972; Michelakis and McAllister, 1972), but there is no convincing evidence that this effect is advantageous in the treatment of patients with essential hypertension.

Severe Hypertension. Cases in this prognostic classification must be divided into two distinct groups in determining therapy. One group includes patients in whom chronic changes, particularly in the blood vessels, heart, and kidneys, have produced essentially irreversible damage. In these, therapy must be approached with caution because too rapid or too marked reduction in blood pressure can accentuate angina pectoris or azotemia, impair cerebral function, or predispose to cerebral or coronary thrombosis. It can be dangerous to reduce the blood pressure to the normal range, but full control of the blood pressure is highly beneficial in many patients; aggressive therapy has been shown to be particularly beneficial for many patients with advanced renal damage (Mroczek *et al.,* 1969). Unfortunately, there is no reliable way to predict which patients in this group will benefit from a considerable reduction in blood pressure and which will be adversely affected. Because of this uncertainty, therapy should be started cautiously with the drugs recommended for use in cases of mild hypertension and more powerful agents added only after careful assessment of all aspects of the response.

The approach is entirely different for severe hypertensives who have not yet suffered major irreparable damage to vital organs, or who are in the accelerated phase of the disease. There is convincing evidence that in cases of this type effective antihypertensive therapy will prolong useful life, often markedly. The objective is to reduce the diastolic pressure to the normal range, and the potential benefit, particularly for patients under 50 years of age, justifies whatever discomfort, inconvenience, or expense is required to achieve this end. Many of these patients should be hospitalized for initial evaluation and treatment. As in the other categories, a *diuretic* provides basal therapy, but it is rarely adequate alone. Other drugs used in moderate hypertension may be effective in some cases. Because they increase or sustain renal blood flow, some clinicians have favored hydralazine and methyldopa for use in patients with impaired renal function. However, there is no evidence that their long-range effects on renal function are significantly different from those of other antihypertensive drugs.

Guanethidine and *clonidine* are powerful antihypertensive drugs that are sometimes used in the management of moderate hypertension. However, because of their disturbing side effects they probably should be reserved for cases not adequately controlled by the drugs mentioned above, most commonly in those cases classified as severe. *Guanethidine* can almost completely inhibit sympathetic vasomotor adjustments. Postural and exercise hypotension occur frequently, and standing and post-exercise blood pressures should be considered in determining the optimal dose. The starting dose of guanethidine for ambulatory patients should not be more than 10 mg per day, and it should be increased at intervals of not less than a week until the diastolic pressure is reduced to the normal range or intolerable side effects develop. The initial dose and the

rate of increase can be higher in hospitalized patients under close supervision. The optimal maintenance dose varies widely, from as little as 10 to over 500 mg per day. Since both guanethidine and propranolol can reduce myocardial contractility, they should be used together with caution. Guanethidine and methyldopa have additive effects in some patients. *Bethanidine* (Gibb *et al.,* 1970) and *debrisoquin* (Bauer, 1970) are approximately interchangeable with guanethidine in the treatment of hypertension. Their shorter durations of action and slightly different patterns of adverse effects do not appear to provide a significant advantage.

Clonidine has a much shorter duration of action than does guanethidine and produces much less postural hypotension. However, it has prominent CNS side effects, and its use has not yet been sufficiently extensive to assure full recognition of its toxic potential. (*See* Becker-Christensen *et al.,* 1971; Putzeys and Hoobler, 1972.) Clonidine is usually started at a dose of 0.1 mg four times a day and increased to a maximum of 2.0 mg per day. It has been reported that intravenous clonidine produces predominantly hypertension rather than hypotension in patients with accelerated hypertension (Mroczek *et al.,* 1973).

The impelling objective of therapy in severe hypertension is to reduce the blood pressure. With proper selection of agents and close attention to dosage, it can be reduced to within or near the normal range in most cases. Adjustment of the medications is often facilitated if the patient learns to take his own blood pressure at home. In mild hypertension it is usually undesirable to focus the patient's attention too strongly on his blood pressure. However, the reverse is true of a patient with severe hypertension, and, as in the case of a diabetic, he must realize the danger of having his condition out of control and the importance of his cooperation and assistance in achieving optimal results from drug therapy.

HYPERTENSIVE EMERGENCIES

Situations occasionally arise in which it is essential to reduce the blood pressure very rapidly. Such emergencies include hypertensive encephalopathy, acute heart failure or intracranial hemorrhage associated with hypertension, pressor episodes of pheochromocytoma, acute glomerular nephritis, and toxemia of pregnancy. The infrequency and heterogeneity of hypertensive emergencies make comparative trials of drugs difficult, and therapeutic regimens presently used are largely influenced by the experience of the individual physician.

Patients with severe hypertension but without complications that warrant emergency management will usually respond to bed rest and the treatment described above. The response can be hastened by parenteral therapy. The blood pressure will usually begin to fall within 2 hours after intravenous administration of 0.5 to 1.0 g of methyldopa, and a total of 3.0 g can be given during the first 12 to 18 hours of treatment. Very rarely, an initial rise in pressure is produced (Levine and Strauch, 1966); this can be antagonized by phentolamine. Reserpine has a slower onset and is somewhat less predictable than methyldopa. The recommended dose is 1.0 to 5.0 mg, given intramuscularly. However, because unusual sensitivity is not uncommon, particularly in patients with a recent cerebrovascular accident, administration probably should be started with a test dose of not more than 0.5 mg. The sedation produced by reserpine and methyldopa is desirable in some circumstances, but it can complicate evaluation of the patient's condition. As in other antihypertensive therapy, a diuretic should be included in the regimen.

In real hypertensive emergencies where rapid lowering of the blood pressure is essential, *diazoxide, nitroprusside,* and *trimethaphan* have been found to be particularly useful.

Diazoxide is given as an intravenous bolus of 300 mg within 10 seconds, and produces a prompt, drastic reduction of elevated pressure within 5 minutes. The dose for children is 5 to 10 mg/kg (McLaine and Drummond, 1971). Repeated doses are usually effective. The major disadvantage of diazoxide is that the fall in blood pressure cannot be titrated. Although the pressure rarely falls below the normal range, abrupt reductions can be dangerous in atherosclerotic patients with coronary or cerebrovascular insufficiency.

Sodium nitroprusside is a powerful peripheral vasodilator with which the blood pressure can be rapidly lowered to any desired level, but *its use requires constant and close supervision by trained personnel.* An intravenous infusion of not more than 0.1 mg/ml should be started at a rate of not more than 5 drops per minute and subsequently adjusted to the requirements of the patient (*see* page 715, for details). Drastic hypotension can occur within 2 minutes. Nitroprusside therapy may have to be continued for many hours or several days.

Trimethaphan is second only to nitroprusside as a universally effective hypotensive drug. It is always

given by controlled intravenous infusion, and reliable control of the blood pressure requires constant attention to the rate of administration. Because it acts by both ganglionic blockade and direct peripheral vasodilatation, trimethaphan can reduce the blood pressure to a range below normal. This may occasionally be advantageous, but it is more often dangerous (*see* Magness *et al.,* 1973; Strandgaard *et al.,* 1973).

Hydralazine is less effective than the three drugs mentioned above. It acts quite rapidly when given by infusion or in doses of 20 mg intramuscularly or intravenously, but frequently causes disturbing side effects. Because it stimulates the heart, hydralazine can be dangerous in patients with myocardial or coronary inadequacy. In addition, it can worsen cerebral edema in hypertensive encephalopathy, presumably because of an increased blood flow to the brain (Škinhøj and Strandgaard, 1973). The drug is probably most useful in the treatment of hypertensive crises in acute glomerular nephritis.

Patients with *hypertension complicated by acute cardiac failure* often respond satisfactorily to the standard measures used to reduce cardiac filling pressure rapidly in pulmonary edema. However, some cases require a more direct attack on the elevated arterial pressure, and sodium nitroprusside or trimethaphan is quite suitable for this purpose. Reduction of the arterial pressure reduces myocardial oxygen requirements but it can also reduce coronary blood flow. Consequently, the blood pressure reduction should be controlled and the patient watched carefully for untoward effects.

Although the hypertension of *preeclampsia* and *eclampsia* appears to respond to the drugs described above in much the same manner as do pressure elevations of other etiology, the drug of choice in this situation is probably still *magnesium sulfate* (*see* Pritchard and Stone, 1967). This drug is effective and relatively safe for both reducing the elevated blood pressure and preventing or arresting the convulsions of eclampsia. With the doses used clinically there is little detectable direct effect on the CNS, and the prevention of convulsions is probably secondary to the relief of vasospasm. The dose of magnesium sulfate must be carefully controlled. An effective plasma concentration of magnesium (8 to 10 mEq per liter) can usually be obtained by giving 4.0 g intravenously over 20 minutes and 1.0 g every hour thereafter, or by giving 10 g in divided doses intramuscularly and 5.0 g every 4 to 6 hours. The frequency of administration should be decreased with decreasing renal function. Maternal and fetal hypocalcemia can occur if magnesium sulfate is used over prolonged periods. (*See* Chapter 37.)

Hypertension due to *pheochromocytoma* can be rapidly and completely controlled by *phenoxybenzamine* given intravenously; intravenous or intramuscular *phentolamine* can also be used, but its effect is transient and control of the hypertension is frequently incomplete (*see* Chapter 26).

Aagaard, G. N. The management of hypertension. *J. Am. med. Ass.,* **1973,** *224,* 329–332.

Åblad, B. A study of the mechanism of the hemodynamic

effects of hydralazine in man. *Acta pharmac. tox.*, **1963**, *20*, Suppl. 1, 1–53.

Acchiardo, S.; Dustan, H. P.; and Tarazi, R. C. Similar effects of hydrochlorothiazide and spironolactone on plasma renin activity in essential hypertension. *Cleveland Clin. Q.*, **1972**, *39*, 153–162.

Adlin, V.; Marks, A. D.; and Channick, B. J. Spironolactone and hydrochlorothiazide in essential hypertension. Blood pressure response and plasma renin activity. *Archs intern. Med.*, **1972**, *130*, 855–865.

Aitchison, J. D.; Cranston, W. I.; and Priest, E. A. The effects of 1-hydrazinophthalazine on the pulmonary circulation in mitral disease. *Br. Heart J.*, **1955**, *17*, 425–430.

Alarcón-Segovia, D.; Wakim, K. G.; Worthington, J. W.; and Ward, L. E. Clinical and experimental studies on the hydralazine syndrome and its relationship to systemic lupus erythematosus. *Medicine, Baltimore*, **1967**, *46*, 1–33.

Anderson, J.; Godfrey, B. E.; Hill, D. M.; Munro-Faure, A. D.; and Sheldon, J. A comparison of the effects of hydrochlorothiazide and of furosemide in the treatment of hypertensive patients. *Q. Jl Med.*, **1971**, *40*, 541–560.

Aoki, V. S., and Wilson, W. R. Hydralazine and methyldopa in thiazide-treated hypertensive patients. *Am. Heart J.*, **1970**, *79*, 798–804.

Ayitey-Smith, E., and Varma, D. R. Mechanism of the hypotensive action of methyldopa in normal and immunosympathectomized rats. *Br. J. Pharmac.*, **1970**, *40*, 186–193.

Baekeland, F., and Lundwall, L. Effects of methyldopa on sleep patterns in man. *Electroenceph. clin. Neurophysiol.*, **1971**, *31*, 269–273.

Bauer, G. E. Debrisoquine. A five-year study of a new hypotensive agent. *Med. J. Aust.*, **1970**, *2*, 911–916.

Baum, T.; Shropshire, A. T.; and Varner, L. L. Contribution of the central nervous system to the action of several antihypertensive agents (methyldopa, hydralazine and guanethidine). *J. Pharmac. exp. Ther.*, **1972**, *182*, 135–144.

Becker-Christensen, F.; Bang, H. O.; and Ditzel, J. Treatment of severe hypertension with CATAPRES (St 155). *Acta med. scand.*, **1971**, *190*, 21–26.

Beevers, D. G.; Brown, J. J.; Ferris, J. B.; Fraser, R.; Lever, A. F.; and Robertson, J. I. S. The use of spironolactone in the diagnosis and the treatment of hypertension associated with mineralocorticoid excess. *Am. Heart J.*, **1973**, *86*, 404–414.

Bengtsson, C. Comparison between alprenolol and chlorthalidone as antihypertensive agents. *Acta med. scand.*, **1972**, *191*, 433–499.

Blackwell, B.; Marley, E.; Price, J.; and Taylor, D. Hypertensive interactions between monoamine oxidase inhibitors and foodstuffs. *Br. J. Psychiat.*, **1967**, *113*, 349–365.

Boyer, J. L., and Kasch, F. W. Exercise therapy in hypertensive men. *J. Am. med. Ass.*, **1970**, *211*, 1668–1671.

Briant, R. H.; Reid, J. L.; and Dollery, C. T. Interaction between clonidine and desipramine in man. *Br. med. J.*, **1973**, *1*, 522–523.

Brunner, H. R.; Laragh, J. H.; Baer, L.; Newton, M. A.; Goodwin, F. T.; Krakoff, L. R.; Bard, R. H.; and Bühler, F. R. Essential hypertension: renin and aldosterone, heart attack and stroke. *New Engl. J. Med.*, **1972**, *286*, 441–449.

Brunner, H. R.; Sealey, J. E.; and Laragh, J. H. Renin as a risk factor in essential hypertension: more evidence. *Am. J. Med.*, **1973**, *55*, 295–302.

Bühler, F. R.; Laragh, J. H.; Baer, L.; Vaughan, E. D., Jr.; and Brunner, H. R. Propranolol inhibition of renin secretion. A specific approach to diagnosis and treatment of renin-dependent hypertensive diseases. *New Engl. J. Med.*, **1972**, *287*, 1209–1214.

Carey, R. M.; Douglas, J. G.; Schwelkert, J. R.; and Liddle, G. W. The syndrome of essential hypertension and suppressed plasma renin activity. *Archs intern. Med.*, **1972**, *130*, 849–854.

Castenfors, J.; Johnsson, H.; and Oro, L. Effect of alprenolol on blood pressure and plasma renin activity in hypertensive patients. *Acta med. scand.*, **1973**, *193*, 189–193.

Choquette, G., and Ferguson, R. J. Blood pressure reduction in "borderline" hypertensives following physical training. *Can. med. Ass. J.*, **1973**, *108*, 699–703.

Christensen, J., and Williams, B. J. Thiocyanate psychosis treated by extracorporeal hemodialysis. *J. Am. med. Ass.*, **1962**, *181*, 340–342.

Coleman, T. G.; Manning, R. D., Jr.; Norman, R. A., Jr.; Granger, H. J.; and Guyton, A. C. The role of salt in experimental and human hypertension. *Am. J. med. Sci.*, **1972**, *264*, 103–110.

Conway, J., and Palmero, H. The vascular effect of the thiazide diuretics. *Archs intern. Med.*, **1963**, *111*, 203–207.

Cousins, M. J., and Maltby, J. R. Delayed recovery of sympathetic transmission following ten years of monoamine oxidase inhibition. *Br. J. Anaesth.*, **1971**, *43*, 803–806.

Crane, M. G., and Harris, J. J. Effect of spironolactone in hypertensive patients. *Am. J. med. Sci.*, **1970**, *260*, 311–330.

Day, M. D.; Roach, A. G.; and Whiting, R. L. The mechanism of the antihypertensive action of α-methyldopa in hypertensive rats. *Eur. J. Pharmac.*, **1973**, *21*, 271–280.

Dollery, C. T., and Reid, J. L. Central noradrenergic neurones and the cardiovascular actions of clonidine in the rabbit. *Br. J. Pharmac.*, **1973**, *47*, 206–216.

Finch, L., and Haeusler, G. Further evidence for a central hypotensive action of α-methyldopa in both the rat and cat. *Br. J. Pharmac.*, **1973**, *47*, 217–228.

Finnerty, F. A., Jr. Relationship of extracellular fluid volume to the development of drug resistance in the hypertensive patient. *Am. Heart J.*, **1971**, *81*, 563–565.

Franciosa, J. A.; Guiha, N. H.; Limas, C. J.; Rodriguera, E.; and Cohn, J. N. Improved left ventricular function during nitroprusside infusion in acute myocardial infarction. *Lancet*, **1972**, *1*, 650–654.

Freis, E. D. Changing attitudes to hypertension. *Ann. intern. Med.*, **1973**, *78*, 141–142.

Freis, E. D.; Rose, J. C.; Higgins, T. F.; Finnerty, F. A., Jr.; Kelley, R. T.; and Partenope, E. A. The hemodynamic effects of hypotensive drugs in man. IV. 1-Hydrazinophthalazine. *Circulation*, **1953**, *8*, 199–204.

Gaskell, P., and Diosy, A. Persistence of abnormally high vascular tone in vessels of the finger after digital nerve block in patients with chronic high blood pressure. *Circulation Res.*, **1959**, *7*, 1006–1010.

Genest, J.; Brucher, R.; Kuchel, O.; and Nowaczynski, W. Renin in hypertension: how important a risk factor? *Can. med. Ass. J.*, **1973**, *109*, 475–478.

Gessa, G. L.; Cuenca, E.; and Costa, E. On the mechanism of hypotensive effects of MAO inhibitors. *Ann. N.Y. Acad. Sci.*, **1963**, *107*, 935–941.

Gibb, W. E.; Malpas, J. S.; Turner, P.; and White, R. J. Comparison of bethanidine, α-methyldopa and reserpine in essential hypertension. *Lancet*, **1970**, *2*, 275–277.

Gibberd, F. B., and Small, E. Interaction between levodopa and methyldopa. *Br. med. J.*, **1973**, *2*, 90–91.

Goldberg, L. I. Monoamine oxidase inhibitors: adverse reactions and possible mechanisms. *J. Am. med. Ass.*, **1964**, *190*, 456–462.

Goldberg, L. I.; DaCosta, F. M.; and Ozaki, M. Actions of the decarboxylase inhibitor, α-methyl-3,4-dihydroxyphenylalanine, in the dog. *Nature, Lond.*, **1960**, *188*, 502–504.

Goldstein, G. B.; Lam, K. C.; and Mistilis, S. P. Drug-induced active chronic hepatitis. *Am. J. dig. Dis.*, **1973**, *18*, 177–184.

Gottlieb, T. B.; Katz, F. H.; and Chidsey, C. A., III. Combined therapy with vasodilator drugs and beta-adrenergic blockade in hypertension. A comparative study of minoxidil and hydralazine. *Circulation,* **1972,** *45,* 571–582.

Gupta, K. P., and Bhargava, K. P. Mechanism of tachycardia induced by intracerebroventricular injection of hydralazine (1-hydrazinophthalazine). *Archs int. Pharmacodyn. Thèr.,* **1965,** *155,* 84–89.

Hammer, J.; Ulrych, M.; and Freis, E. D. Hemodynamic and therapeutic effects of guancydine in hypertension. *Clin. Pharmac. Ther.,* **1971,** *12,* 78–90.

Hansson, L.; Hunyor, S. N.; Julius, S.; and Hoobler, S. W. Blood pressure crisis following withdrawal of clonidine (CATAPRES, CATAPRESAN), with special reference to arterial and urinary catecholamine levels, and suggestion for acute management. *Am. Heart J.,* **1973,** *85,* 605–610.

Healy, J. J.; McKenna, T. J.; Canning, B. St. J.; Brien, T. G.; Duffy, G. J.; and Muldowney, F. P. Body composition changes in hypertensive subjects on long-term oral diuretic therapy. *Br. med. J.,* **1970,** *1,* 716–719.

Heise, A., and Kroneberg, G. α-Sympathetic receptor stimulation in the brain and hypotensive activity of α-methyldopa. *Eur. J. Pharmac.,* **1972,** *17,* 315–317.

Henning, M. Studies on the mode of action of α-methyldopa. *Acta physiol. scand.,* **1969,** *76,* Suppl. 322, 1–37.

Hoobler, S. W.; Kabza, T. G.; and Corley, R. W. The effect of protoveratrine on the cardiac output and on some regional circulations in man. *J. clin. Invest.,* **1955,** *34,* 559–564.

James, I. M.; Larbi, E.; and Zaimis, E. The effect of the acute intravenous administration of clonidine (St 155) on cerebral blood flow in man. *Br. J. Pharmac.,* **1970,** *39,* 198P–199P.

Johnson, B. F. Diazoxide and renal function in man. *Clin. Pharmac. Ther.,* **1971,** *12,* 815–824.

Johnson, C. C. The actions and toxicity of sodium nitroprusside. *Archs int. Pharmacodyn. Thèr.,* **1929,** *35,* 480–496.

Juhász-Nagy, A., and Szentiványi, M. Localisation of the receptors of the coronary chemoreflex in the dog. *Archs int. Pharmacodyn. Thèr.,* **1961,** *131,* 39–53.

Kale, A. K., and Satoskar, R. S. Modification of the central hypotensive effect of α-methyldopa by reserpine, imipramine and tranylcypromine. *Eur. J. Pharmac.,* **1970,** *9,* 120–123.

Katic, F.; Lavery, H.; and Lowe, R. D. The central action of clonidine and its antagonism. *Br. J. Pharmac.,* **1972,** *44,* 779–787.

Kopin, I. J.; Fischer, J. E.; Musacchio, J. M.; Horst, W. D.; and Weise, V. K. "False neurochemical transmitter" and the mechanism of sympathetic blockade by monoamine oxidase inhibitors. *J. Pharmac. exp. Ther.,* **1965,** *147,* 186–193.

Krieger, E. M. Time course of baroreceptor resetting in acute hypertension. *Am. J. Physiol.,* **1970,** *218,* 486–490.

Landesman, R.; Coutinho, E. M.; Wilson, K. H.; and Vieira Lopes, A. C. The relaxant effect of diazoxide on nongravid human myometrium *in vivo. Am. J. Obstet. Gynec.,* **1968,** *102,* 1080–1084.

Laverty, R., and Taylor, K. M. Behavioural and biochemical effects of 2-(2,6-dichlorophenylamino)-2-imidazoline hydrochloride (St 155) on the central nervous system. *Br. J. Pharmac.,* **1969,** *35,* 253–264.

Leth, A. Changes in plasma and extracellular fluid volumes in patients with essential hypertension during long-term treatment with hydrochlorothiazide. *Circulation,* **1970,** *42,* 479–485.

Levine, R. J., and Strauch, B. S. Hypertensive responses to methyldopa. *New Engl. J. Med.,* **1966,** *275,* 946–948.

Lund-Johansen, P. Hemodynamic changes in long-term α-methyldopa therapy of essential hypertension. *Acta med. scand.,* **1972,** *192,* 221–226.

McCubbin, J. W.; Green, J. H.; and Page, I. H. Baroceptor function in chronic renal hypertension. *Circulation Res.,* **1956,** *4,* 205–210.

McLaine, P. N., and Drummond, K. N. Intravenous diazoxide for severe hypertension in childhood. *J. Pediat.,* **1971,** *79,* 829–832.

McRaven, D. R.; Kroetz, F. W.; Kioschos, J. M.; and Kirkendall, W. M. The effect of clonidine on hemodynamics in hypertensive patients. *Am. Heart J.,* **1971,** *81,* 482–489.

Magness, A.; Yashon, D.; Locke, G.; Wiederholt, W.; and Hunt, W. E. Cerebral function during trimethaphan-induced hypotension. *Neurology, Minneap.,* **1973,** *23,* 506–509.

Mani, M. K. Nitroprusside revisited. *Br. med. J.,* **1971,** *3,* 407–408.

Maxwell, M. H. Observations pertinent to antihypertensive mechanisms of MAO inhibitors using DL-serine isopropylhydrazine. *Ann. N.Y. Acad. Sci.,* **1963,** *107,* 993–1004.

Michelakis, A. M., and McAllister, R. G. The effect of chronic adrenergic receptor blockade on plasma renin activity in man. *J. clin. Endocr. Metab.,* **1972,** *34,* 386–394.

Miert, A. S. J. P. A. M. van, and Duin, C. T. M. van. The antipyretic effect of α-methyldopa in experimental fever. *J. Pharm. Pharmac.,* **1972,** *24,* 988–990.

Moore-Jones, D., and Perry, H. M., Jr. Radioautographic localization of hydralazine-1-C$_{14}$ in arterial walls. *Proc. Soc. exp. Biol. Med.,* **1966,** *122,* 576–579.

Mroczek, W. J.; Davidov, M.; and Finnerty, F. A., Jr. Intravenous clonidine in hypertensive patients. *Clin. Pharmac. Ther.,* **1973,** *14,* 847–851.

Mroczek, W. J.; Davidov, M.; Gavrilovich, L.; and Finnerty, F. A., Jr. The value of aggressive therapy in hypertensive patients with azotemia. *Circulation,* **1969,** *40,* 893–904.

Mroczek, W. J.; Leibel, B. A.; Davidov, M.; and Finnerty, F. A., Jr. The importance of the rapid administration of diazoxide in accelerated hypertension. *New Engl. J. Med.,* **1971,** *285,* 603–606.

Muir, A. L.; Burton, J. L.; and Lawrie, D. M. Circulatory effects at rest and exercise of clonidine, an imidazoline derivative with hypotensive properties. *Lancet,* **1969,** *2,* 181–185.

Myhre, E.; Brodwall, E. K.; Stenbaek, O.; and Hansen, T. Plasma turnover of methyldopa in advanced renal failure. *Acta med. scand.,* **1972,** *191,* 343–347.

Nayler, W. G., and Stone, J. An effect of ST 155 (clonidine), 2-(2,6-dichlorophenylamino)-2-imidazole hydrochloride, CATAPRES on relationship between blood pressure and heart rate in dogs. *Eur. J. Pharmac.,* **1970,** *10,* 161–167.

Nickerson, M., and Thomas, J. J. Renal excretion of thiocyanate. *J. Lab. clin. Med.,* **1951,** *38,* 194–198.

Oates, J. A.; Gillespie, L.; Udenfriend, S.; and Sjoerdsma, A. Decarboxylase inhibition and blood pressure reduction by α-methyl-3,4-dihydroxy-DL-phenylalanine. *Science, Wash.,* **1960,** *131,* 1890–1891.

O'Brien, E. T., and MacKinnon, J. Propranolol and polythiazide in treatment of hypertension. *Br. Heart J.,* **1972,** *34,* 1042–1044.

Ogilvie, R. I., and Mikulic, E. Effects of diazoxide and ethacrynic acid on sequential vascular segments in the canine gracilis muscle. *J. Pharmac. exp. Ther.,* **1972,** *180,* 368–376.

Ogilvie, R. I., and Ruedy, J. Treatment of hypertension with hydrochlorothiazide and spironolactone. *Can. med. Ass. J.,* **1969,** *101,* 591–594.

Onesti, G.; Novack, P.; Ramirez, O.; Brest, A. N.; and Moyer, J. H. Hemodynamic effects of pargyline in hypertensive patients. *Circulation,* **1964,** *30,* 830–835.

Onesti, G.; Schwartz, A. B.; Kim, K. W.; Paz-Martinez, V.; and Swartz, C. Antihypertensive effect of clonidine. *Circulation Res.,* **1971,** *28,* Suppl. 2, II-53–II-69.

Page, I. H.; Corcoran, A. C.; Dustan, H. P.; and Koppanyi, T. Cardiovascular actions of sodium nitroprusside in animals and hypertensive patients. *Circulation,* **1955,** *11,* 188–198.

Palmer, R. F., and Lasseter, K. C. Sodium nitroprusside. *New Engl. J. Med.,* **1975,** *292,* 294–297.

Paz, M. A., and Seifter, S. Immunological studies of collagens modified by reaction with hydralazine. *Am. J. med. Sci.,* **1972,** *263,* 281–290.

Prichard, B. N. C. Propranolol as an antihypertensive agent. *Am. Heart J.,* **1970,** *79,* 128–133.

Pritchard, J. A., and Stone, S. R. Clinical and laboratory observations on eclampsia. *Am. J. Obstet. Gynec.,* **1967,** *99,* 754–762.

Puig, M.; Wakade, A. R.; and Kirpekar, S. M. Effect on the sympathetic nervous system of chronic treatment with pargyline and L-dopa. *J. Pharmac. exp. Ther.,* **1972,** *182,* 130–134.

Putzeys, M. R., and Hoobler, S. W. Comparison of clonidine and methyldopa on blood pressure and side effects in hypertensive patients. *Am. Heart J.,* **1972,** *83,* 464–468.

Raskin, N. H., and Fishman, R. A. Pyridoxine-deficiency neuropathy due to hydralazine. *New Engl. J. Med.,* **1965,** *273,* 1182–1185.

Rhodes, H. J., and Sutter, M. C. The action of diazoxide on isolated vascular smooth muscle. Electrophysiology and contraction. *Can. J. Physiol. Pharmac.,* **1971,** *49,* 276–287.

Ross, G., and Cole, P. V. Cardiovascular actions of sodium nitroprusside in dogs. *Anaesthesia,* **1973,** *28,* 400–406.

Sannerstedt, R. Hemodynamic effects of pargyline hydrochloride at rest and during exercise in hypertension. *Acta med. scand.,* **1967,** *181,* 699–706.

Sannerstedt, R.; Stenberg, J.; Johnsson, G.; and Werko, L. Hemodynamic interference of alprenolol with dihydralazine in normal and hypertensive man. *Am. J. Cardiol.,* **1971,** *28,* 316–320.

Schmitt, H., and Schmitt, H. Localization of the hypotensive effect of 2-(2-6-dichlorophenylamino)-2-imidazoline hydrochloride (St 155, CATAPRESAN). *Eur. J. Pharmac.,* **1969,** *6,* 8–12.

Schmitt, H.; Schmitt, H.; and Fénard, S. Action of α-adrenergic blocking drugs on the sympathetic centres and their interaction with the central sympatho-inhibitory effect of clonidine. *Arzneimittel-Forsch.,* **1973,** *23,* 40–45.

Sellers, E. M., and Koch-Weser, J. Protein binding and vascular activity of diazoxide. *New Engl. J. Med.,* **1969,** *281,* 1141–1145.

Shafar, J.; Tallett, E. R.; and Knowlson, P. A. Evaluation of clonidine in prophylaxis of migraine. Double-blind trial and follow-up. *Lancet,* **1972,** *1,* 403–407.

Shaw, J.; Hunyor, S. N.; and Korner, P. I. The peripheral circulatory effects of clonidine and their role in the production of arterial hypotension. *Eur. J. Pharmac.,* **1971,** *14,* 101–111.

Sherman, G. P.; Grega, G. J.; Woods, R. J.; and Buckley, J. P. Evidence for a central hypotensive mechanism of 2-(2,6-dichlorophenylamino)-2-imidazoline (CATAPRESAN, ST-155). *Eur. J. Pharmac.,* **1968,** *2,* 326–328.

Sjoerdsma, A.; Vendsalu, A.; and Engelman, K. Studies on the metabolism and mechanism of action of methyldopa. *Circulation,* **1963,** *28,* 492–502.

Skinhøj, E., and Strandgaard, S. Pathogenesis of hypertensive encephalopathy. *Lancet,* **1973,** *1,* 461–462.

Smith, C. B. The role of monoamine oxidase in the intraneuronal metabolism of norepinephrine released by indirectly-acting sympathomimetic amines or by adrenergic nerve stimulation. *J. Pharmac. exp. Ther.,* **1966,** *151,* 207–220.

Sourkes, T. L. Inhibition of dihydroxyphenylalanine decarboxylase by derivatives of phenylalanine. *Archs Biochem. Biophys.,* **1954,** *51,* 444–456.

Spark, R. F., and Melby, J. C. Hypertension and low plasma renin activity: presumptive evidence for mineralo-corticoid excess. *Ann. intern. Med.,* **1971,** *75,* 831–836.

Strandgaard, S.; Olesen, J.; Skinhøj, E.; and Lassen, N. A. Autoregulation of brain circulation in severe arterial hypertension. *Br. med. J.,* **1973,** *1,* 507–510.

Tarazi, R. C.; Dustan, H. P.; and Frohlich, E. D. Long-term thiazide therapy in essential hypertension. Evidence for persistent alteration in plasma volume and renin activity. *Circulation,* **1970,** *41,* 709–717.

Thirwell, M. P., and Zsotér, T. T. The effect of diazoxide on the veins. *Am. Heart J.,* **1972,** *83,* 512–517.

Thomson, A. E.; Nickerson, M.; Gaskell, P.; and Grahame, G. R. Clinical observations on an antihypertensive chlorothiazide analogue devoid of diuretic activity. *Can. med. Ass. J.,* **1962,** *87,* 1306–1310.

U.S. Public Health Service Cooperative Study. Evaluation of antihypertensive therapy. II. Double-blind controlled evaluation of mebutamate. *J. Am. med. Ass.,* **1965,** *193,* 727–729.

Veterans Administration Cooperative Study Group on Antihypertensive Agents. Effects of treatment on morbidity in hypertension: results in patients with diastolic blood pressures averaging 115 through 129 mm Hg. *J. Am. med. Ass.,* **1967,** *202,* 1028–1034.

———. Effects of treatment on morbidity in hypertension. II. Results in patients with diastolic blood pressures averaging 90 through 114 mm Hg. *Ibid.,* **1970,** *213,* 1143–1152.

Walser, M., and Rahill, W. J. Nitrate, thiocyanate, and perchlorate clearance in relation to chloride clearance. *Am. J. Physiol.,* **1965,** *208,* 1158–1164.

Werner, U.; Starke, K.; and Schümann, H. J. Actions of clonidine and 2-(2-methyl-6-ethyl-cyclohexylamino)-2-oxazoline on postganglionic autonomic nerves. *Archs int. Pharmacodyn. Thér.,* **1972,** *195,* 282–290.

Wilson, I. M., and Freis, E. D. Relationship between plasma and extracellular fluid volume depletion and the antihypertensive effect of chlorothiazide. *Circulation,* **1959,** *20,* 1028–1036.

Wohl, A. J.; Hausler, L. M.; and Roth, F. E. Mechanism of the antihypertensive effect of diazoxide: *in vitro* vascular studies in the hypertensive rat. *J. Pharmac. exp. Ther.,* **1968,** *162,* 109–114.

Zacest, R., and Koch-Weser, J. Relation of hydralazine plasma concentration to dosage and hypotensive action. *Clin. Pharmac. Ther.,* **1972,** *13,* 420–425.

Zacharias, F. J.; Cowen, K. J.; Presst, J.; Vickers, J.; and Wall, B. G. Propranolol in hypertension: a study of long-term therapy, 1964–1970. *Am. Heart J.,* **1972,** *83,* 755–761.

Zaimis, E., and Hanington, E. A possible pharmacological approach to migraine. *Lancet,* **1969,** *2,* 298–300.

Monographs and Reviews

Benforado, J. M. The veratrum alkaloids. In, *Physiological Pharmacology.* Vol. 4, *The Nervous System—Part D: Autonomic Nervous System Drugs.* (Root, W. S., and Hofmann, F. G., eds.) Academic Press, Inc., New York, **1967,** pp. 331–398.

Dawes, G. S., and Comroe, J. H., Jr. Chemoreflexes from the heart and lungs. *Physiol. Rev.,* **1954,** *34,* 167–201.

Giese, J. Renin, angiotensin and hypertensive vascular damage: a review. *Am. J. Med.,* **1973,** *55,* 315–322.

Kopin, I. J. False adrenergic transmitters. *A. Rev. Pharmac.,* **1968,** *8,* 377–394.

Krayer, O., and Acheson, G. H. The pharmacology of the veratrum alkaloids. *Physiol. Rev.,* **1946,** *26,* 383–446.

Kupchan, S. M. Hypotensive veratrum ester alkaloids. *J. pharm. Sci.,* **1961,** *50,* 273–287.

Lowenstein, J. Renin assay in hypertensive disease. *A. Rev. Med.,* **1972,** *23,* 333–342.

Muscholl, E. Autonomic nervous system: newer mechanisms of adrenergic blockade. *A. Rev. Pharmac.,* **1966,** *6,* 107–128.

Page, L. B., and Sidd, J. J. Medical management of primary hypertension. *New Engl. J. Med.,* **1972,** *287,* 960–966, 1018–1023, 1074–1081.

Sannerstedt, R., and Conway, J. Hemodynamic and vascular responses to antihypertensive treatment with adrenergic blocking agents: a review. *Am. Heart J.,* **1970,** *79,* 122–127.

Shanes, A. M. Electrochemical aspects of physiological and pharmacological action in excitable cells. *Pharmac. Rev.,* **1958,** *10,* 59–273.

Stone, C. A., and Porter, C. C. Methyldopa and adrenergic nerve function. *Pharmac. Rev.,* **1966,** *18,* 569–575.

Symposium. (Various authors.) Diazoxide and the treatment of hypoglycemia. *Ann. N.Y. Acad. Sci.,* **1968,** *150,* 191–467.

Tobian, L. Why do thiazide diuretics lower blood pressure in essential hypertension? *A. Rev. Pharmac.,* **1967,** *7,* 399–408.

CHAPTER

34 VASODILATOR DRUGS

Mark Nickerson

Differentiation of the drugs discussed in this chapter from those covered in Chapter 33 is primarily on therapeutic rather than pharmacological grounds. From a pharmacodynamic standpoint, "vasodilator" and "antihypertensive" agents are not clearly separable. The two categories are frequently combined at the investigational level, but agents utilized by physicians to lower blood pressure are usually distinct from those that are intended primarily to increase blood flow.

There are a number of clinical conditions in which regional blood flow is inadequate to meet the needs of the tissues (ischemia), and the classical concept was to correct this imbalance by vasodilatation that would presumably increase the delivery of blood. This may be successful in a few situations such as Raynaud's syndrome or shock, where flow is limited by sympathetic overactivity (*see* Chapter 26). However, vasodilators may increase flow to relatively well perfused areas at the expense of ischemic tissues, and therefore clinical benefit may not parallel increased total blood flow to an organ or region. In the most thoroughly studied organ, the heart, it appears that vasodilatation improves the perfusion of ischemic areas if there is redistribution of blood flow. This depends on which sequential segments of the vascular bed are affected, as well as the relation of drug action to the autoregulation of blood flow. Drugs can also improve the balance between blood flow and demand by decreasing the tissue requirements; one mechanism by which this can be accomplished in the heart is by dilatation of capacitance vessels in other, nonischemic areas of the body to decrease venous return and thereby reduce cardiac output and work.

The present chapter deals with the *nitrites* (*organic nitrites and nitrates and nitrite ion*), which are the oldest and still the most important vasodilators, and a small hetero-geneous group of drugs that are discussed together because all are promoted for the treatment of conditions involving regional tissue ischemia. In the discussion of therapeutic uses, consideration will also be given to a number of drugs that, because of their mechanisms of action, have been described in other chapters, but are used in the same clinical situations, particularly in the treatment of *angina pectoris* and of *ischemia of skeletal muscle*.

THE NITRITES

Amyl nitrite and *nitroglycerin (glyceryl trinitrate)* were the first members of this group introduced into medicine, and they have maintained a dominant position among vasodilators for more than 100 years. All their major pharmacological properties are shared qualitatively by the nitrite ion and by a large number of organic nitrate esters. This pharmacological similarity suggested that organic nitrates may act in the body through release of nitrite ion. Many organic nitrates are rapidly metabolized in the liver by glutathione-organic nitrate reductase with the formation of nitrite ion, and only compounds capable of denitration relax smooth muscle. However, the organic nitrates act at least as rapidly as administered nitrite ion and are much more potent; a dose of nitroglycerin could release less than 1% of the nitrite ion required for an equivalent pharmacological effect. These quantitative discrepancies appear to be reconciled by studies that indicate that hepatic denitration is only a model of what occurs in smooth muscle–containing structures during responses to organic nitrates. It appears that the active nitrates react with and are reduced by sulfhydryl groups involved in a "nitrate receptor"; in some ways this interaction or the nitrite ion formed locally causes relaxation. Compounds that are not denitrated by reaction with sulfhydryl groups are inactive, and tolerance to organic nitrates, but not to the nitrite ion, occurs when tissue sulfhydryl is depleted. Responsiveness can be restored by a disulfide-reducing agent such as dithiothreitol. (*See* Needleman and Johnson, 1973.)

PHARMACOLOGICAL PROPERTIES

The basic pharmacological action of nitrites is to relax smooth muscle. The relaxation is nonspecific and affects all smooth muscle irrespective of its innervation or the nature of its responses to adrenergic, cholinergic, or other types of agonists. However, nitrite does not prevent cells from responding to an appropriate stimulus, and its effect can be antagonized by any drug that can activate the smooth muscle under consideration. Thus, nitrite is a *functional antagonist* of norepinephrine, acetylcholine, histamine, and many other agents. The net response can vary from maximal contraction to maximal relaxation, depending on the relative concentrations of the members of any such pair. This antagonism must be kept in mind when assessing overall responses to a nitrite. An increase in vascular resistance does not mean that nitrite does not act on the vessels in question; its effect is simply overcome by compensatory sympathetic activity. Unless another interpretation is specifically indicated, the following discussion will deal with the *net changes* produced by a nitrite under the conditions indicated.

Cardiovascular System. The most prominent and important actions of nitrite are on vascular smooth muscle. The cardiovascular response is dominated by changes in venous return and is very sensitive to gravitational influences. Central venous pressure is decreased, and may fall to negative values with tilting to the upright position. There may be an initial brief increase in cardiac output, during which blood from thoracic reservoirs is shifted to the systemic bed, but subsequently the cardiac output falls. The systemic arterial pressure is usually decreased; the systolic pressure falls more than the diastolic, and the latter may be unchanged or decreased only transiently. A small pulse pressure reflects a decreased cardiac stroke volume. An occasional individual shows marked

sensitivity to the hypotensive effects of nitrite, and severe hypotensive responses can occur even with the usual therapeutic dose, particularly when there is little compensatory tachycardia. They are associated with nausea and vomiting, weakness, restlessness, pallor, cold sweat, and collapse.

Relatively small doses of nitrite can produce syncope in any individual kept in a static upright position. The characteristic response to a change from the horizontal to the vertical position after administration of nitrite is illustrated in Figure 34–1. This is a typical "fainting reaction." The maintained diastolic pressure indicates marked reflex vasoconstriction, which may aggravate the circulatory inadequacy. The tachycardia also reflects attempted reflex compensation. The sharp fall in heart rate just before loss of consciousness is due to enhanced vagal activity resulting from cerebral ischemia; it can be blocked by atropine, but this does not appreciably alter the other cardiovascular parameters or the development of syncope. (*See* Weiss *et al.,* 1937; Wilkins *et al.,* 1937.)

Sequential Vascular Segments. The general features of the cardiovascular response to nitrite have been known for many years, and from them it was possible to deduce the effects on various vascular elements. These deductions have been confirmed and extended by direct measurement. Large arteries are relaxed relatively more than by most other vasodilators. This effect is clearly shown by angiography, and it is reflected in a damped pulse contour and a "bounding" pulse on palpation. The effect on arterioles is relatively less than that of many other agents, and the effect on precapillary sphincters is rather small. The overall response is dominated by the relaxation of relatively large veins, but the ratio of precapillary to postcapillary resistance is not markedly altered, which indicates an equivalent effect on arterioles and venules. (*See* Åblad, 1963; Åblad and Mellander, 1963; Johnsson and Oberg, 1968.) Reflex compensation to the very rapid fall in blood pressure induced by amyl nitrite may explain the observation that it sometimes causes a net increase rather than a decrease in the venous tone of the human forearm. Indeed, most of the reported differences between the effects of amyl nitrite and those of other nitrites are probably due

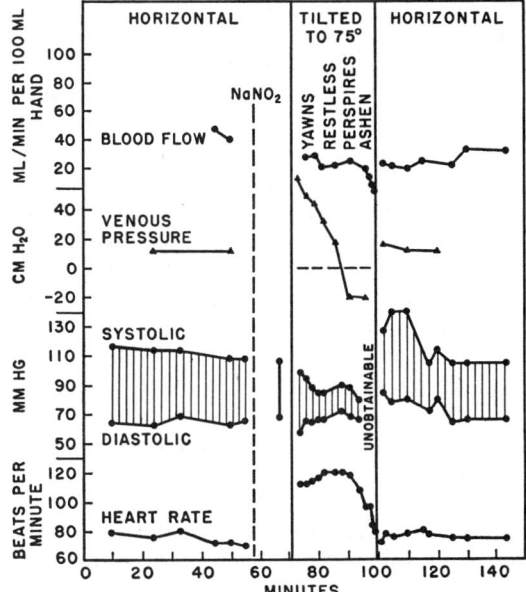

Figure 34–1. *Syncope induced by sodium nitrite.*

Normal adult male given 0.18 g of sodium nitrite by mouth. Only minor changes were recorded while he remained in the horizontal position. When he was tilted to a 75° upright position, his condition began to change rapidly. Yawning appeared and became progressively more prominent; respiration deepened and assumed a sighing character; restlessness, belching, and borborygmus developed; and a cold sweat appeared on the face and extremities and spread over the entire body. Pulse pressure became very narrow due to both a fall in systolic pressure and a significant rise in diastolic pressure. The central venous pressure fell progressively to well below the hydrostatic level of the right atrium. Hand blood flow decreased, and heart rate increased as soon as tilting occurred; both fell precipitously just before loss of consciousness. The subject soon developed the clinical picture of "cardiovascular collapse." He was drowsy, the skin was ashen-gray, and the pupils were dilated. Vision became dim, muscle power was lost, and unconsciousness ensued. The subject was immediately returned to the horizontal position and regained consciousness within 20 seconds. All circulatory abnormalities promptly disappeared. (After Weiss, Wilkins, and Haynes, 1937. Courtesy of the *Journal of Clinical Investigation.*)

to its very rapid action and the consequent reflex adjustments (O'Rourke *et al.,* 1971).

Regional Vascular Beds. Although nitrite can relax all vascular smooth muscle, there are significant differences in the net effects in different beds. The responses mentioned

below are those characteristic of moderate doses of a nitrite in recumbent human subjects or in experimental animals. Relatively small changes in position or in initial blood volume can profoundly modify the response.

Inhalation of amyl nitrite produces a dramatic *cutaneous flush* of the head, neck, and clavicular area (blush zone) in doses that do not alter the blood pressure significantly. Flushing is limited with slower-acting nitrites, and in general they have less effect on cutaneous vessels than on most other vascular beds. The *meningeal vessels* are effectively dilated. This is the basis for the transient pulsating headache experienced by many persons after administration of a nitrite, particularly amyl nitrite. Some increase in intracranial pressure may accompany the dilatation of cerebral vessels, but this is rarely of sufficient magnitude or duration to be clinically significant.

Net *splanchnic* vasoconstriction has been observed to result from nitroglycerin administered to recumbent human subjects (Ferrer *et al.,* 1966). *Renal blood flow* tends to fall with the arterial pressure. Nitrite consistently reduces *pulmonary arterial pressure* in both normal subjects and patients with angina pectoris, probably as a result of both pulmonary vasodilatation and systemic effects of the drug. This is particularly marked in patients with some myocardial inadequacy.

Because of their importance in the treatment of angina pectoris, the effects of nitrites on the *coronary circulation* have been intensively investigated. A clear-cut decrease in coronary resistance and an increase in total blood flow are produced in normal laboratory animals and man, but these effects are usually considerably more transient than the duration of action assessed by peripheral vascular or therapeutic criteria. In most patients with angina pectoris, coronary resistance is only very transiently decreased or is unaltered, and coronary flow in such individuals tends to decrease in parallel with any fall in blood pressure. (*See* Gorlin *et al.,* 1959; Rowe *et al.,* 1961.) However, nitrite produces a more sustained dilatation of the larger coronary vessels, as determined by arteriography in man (Likoff *et al.,* 1964) and by cannulation technics in laboratory animals. A similar, relatively persistent dilatation of collateral vessels has been observed, manifested by an increase in backflow from an adjacent coronary artery beyond a point of chronic narrowing or occlusion and an increase in tissue oxygen tension and myocardial contractility in the area of distribution of the occluded vessel. A greater effect on large than on small coronary vessels is also suggested by the fact that nitrite does not significantly alter the pattern of reactive hyperemia after a short period of acute coronary occlusion. (*See* McGregor and Fam, 1966; Cohen *et al.*, 1973.) The myocardial ischemia associated with coronary artery disease and, particularly, with attacks of angina pectoris results in decreased lactate extraction or actual net lactate production by the myocardium, and there may also be net potassium loss during attacks; nitroglycerin can normalize the lactate and potassium gradients (Chiong *et al.*, 1972). This reflects a decrease in ischemia, but does not indicate the mechanism. A contribution of enhanced perfusion to this improvement is indicated by the observation that sublingual nitroglycerin increases xenon washout from underperfused areas of myocardium in patients with coronary artery disease (Horwitz *et al.*, 1971). It has also been reported that myocardial nutrient blood flow (^{84}Rb extraction) is decreased during anginal attacks induced by pacing and that administration of nitroglycerin then causes a slight increase (Knoebel *et al.*, 1973).

The depressed S-T segment in the ECG and several more direct observations indicate that subendocardial areas of the myocardium are particularly vulnerable to ischemia in coronary artery disease (*see* Moir, 1972), and that the beneficial effect of nitrite can be interpreted as due to an improved blood supply to these areas. The mechanism by which subendocardial perfusion may be increased has not been established, but the two most attractive hypotheses invoke the known effects of nitrite on relatively large collateral (conductance) vessels (*see* McGregor, 1966; McGregor and Fam, 1972) or on systemic capacitance vessels (*see* Becker and Pitt, 1971). The first mechanism has been demonstrated in a variety of animal models; the appropriate redistribution of blood flow and the increase in subendocardial oxygen tension (P_{O_2}) (Weiss and Winbury, 1972) and contractility of ischemic areas (Cohen *et al.*,

1973) have been observed after both intracoronary and systemic administration of nitrite. The second mechanism would involve a decreased venous return, decreased left ventricular diastolic volume and pressure, and, consequently, less mechanical interference with blood flow through perforating arteries to the relatively ischemic subendocardial areas. The involvement of this mechanism is supported by the observations that phlebotomy can relieve and dextran infusion can accentuate the induction of anginal pain by atrial pacing (Parker *et al.*, 1970; Khaja *et al.*, 1971); the major cardiodynamic effects of these volume manipulations are on end-diastolic ventricular pressure and, presumably, volume. It has also been reported that the anginal pain induced by atrial pacing in patients with coronary artery disease is relieved by intravenous but not by intracoronary injection of nitroglycerin (Ganz and Marcus, 1972).

Prolonged administration of nitrite has also been shown to promote the development of interarterial anastomoses in the myocardium and to increase survival rate after experimental narrowing of a coronary artery in pigs, a species that resembles man in normally having little collateral circulation in the myocardium (Lumb and Hardy, 1963).

Heart. No direct action of nitrite on the heart has been proved; changes in rate and in cardiodynamics are secondary to actions on vascular smooth muscle. After a therapeutic dose of nitroglycerin there may be a very transient increase in cardiac output followed by a moderate reduction, which can be considerably accentuated by gravitational stress. Cardiac oxygen consumption increases slightly or does not decrease concomitantly with a decrease in left ventricular work. A great many parameters of cardiac function have been measured and calculated to characterize the effects of nitrite, and they quite consistently show a *decrease in left ventricular energy expenditure.* This is predominantly due to dilatation of systemic capacitance vessels and a decrease in venous return. The only change induced by nitroglycerin that would increase the demand on the myocardium is the reflex increase in heart rate, and this is usually not pronounced. Important changes include decreases in heart size, stroke volume, end-systolic and end-diastolic pressures, and ejection time, leading to a decreased time-tension index. These changes tend to be qualitatively similar in subjects with normal hearts and in those with clinically important occlusive coronary artery disease. However, they are more prominent in the latter and are still more marked when the compromised heart is challenged by exercise, atrial pacing, or an added fluid load. (*See* Gensini, 1972.)

The heart of a patient with severe coronary artery disease appears to be marginally in failure. An increased demand causing anginal pain is associated with a cardiodynamic pattern of acute failure, and the effect of nitrite appears to be to restore compensation. Although there are few measurements of the time course of the primary nitrite effects, many of them appear to be relatively transient, and it is possible that improved left ventricular function may significantly outlast the actions of the drug. Administration of nitrite can decrease the ECG abnormality in patients with a pattern of left ventricular hypertrophy and strain, and can normalize the inadequate ventricular response to exercise in patients with healed myocardial infarcts but without angina (Parker *et al.*, 1967).

Even when blood pressure and coronary blood flow are considerably reduced by a nitrite, normal subjects and most patients with coronary atherosclerosis show no ECG evidence of myocardial hypoxia. However, occasional patients with angina pectoris have a "paradoxical" response in which the nitrite itself causes S-T segment depression and other changes usually induced by exertion. This occurs particularly with a marked and rapid fall in blood pressure, such as that produced by amyl nitrite, and may be largely due to reflex sympathetic effects (Kerber and Harrison, 1972).

Other Effects. The nitrites act on almost all smooth muscle structures. *Bronchial* smooth muscle is relaxed irrespective of the cause of the preexisting tone. The muscles of the *biliary tract,* including those of the gallbladder, biliary ducts, and sphincter of Oddi, are effectively relaxed. In patients with T-tube drainage, a nitrite can rapidly reduce biliary pressure, whether elevated spontaneously or in response to morphine, and can induce rapid emptying of biliary contents into the duodenum. Pain and other symptoms incident to increased pressure are transiently relieved. Smooth muscle of the *gastrointesti-*

nal tract, including that of the esophagus, can be relaxed and its spontaneous motility decreased by nitrite both *in vivo* and *in vitro.* The effect may be transient and incomplete *in vivo,* but abnormal "spasm" is frequently reduced. Similarly, nitrite can relax *ureteral* and *uterine* smooth muscle, but these effects are somewhat unpredictable. Nitrites are singularly devoid of actions on tissues other than smooth muscle.

Absorption, Fate, and Excretion. Most *organic nitrates* are readily absorbed from the sublingual mucosa, and their effects are much more intense and predictable by this route than they are orally. While considerable amounts are absorbed from the gastrointestinal tract, degradation by the liver is so rapid and complete that little of the drug reaches the systemic circulation in active form (Needleman *et al.*, 1972). Some nitrite effect can be demonstrated after large oral or intraportal doses of an organic nitrate, but this is variable, as would be expected when it involves only a very small fraction of the administered drug.

The organic nitrates have traditionally been classified as "short acting" and "long acting," but this distinction is questionable. For example, it has been reported that durations of the pharmacodynamic and therapeutic effects of nitroglycerin and of isosorbide dinitrate are very similar when they are administered sublingually in equieffective doses (Goldstein *et al.*, 1971). Small differences probably can be shown, but the observation that smooth-muscle relaxant potency parallels the rapidity of denitration by the liver makes it unlikely that major alterations in duration of action can be achieved by structural manipulations (Needleman *et al.*, 1969, 1972). Prolongation of action, if it is therapeutically desirable, would probably have to be accomplished by retardation of absorption. The problem of providing effective but delayed absorption has received little attention in relation to modern knowledge of organic nitrate metabolism. Sustained-release oral preparations have had little success and are not promising for compounds that are almost completely cleared by the liver.

Nitroglycerin and other low-molecular-weight organic nitrates are also absorbed through the skin, a route of considerable toxicological importance in the manufacture of explosives, and the venerable 2% nitroglycerin ointment may be the most effective "long-acting" preparation now available (Goldstein and Epstein, 1973).

Many details of the metabolic fates of various organic nitrates have been reported, but most have little bearing on the pharmacology of these compounds. The critical point is that all parent compounds and their pharmacologically active metabolites, if any, are rapidly denitrated by the glutathione–organic nitrate reductase system in the liver. The activity of this system can be augmented by pretreatment with phenobarbital, but it normally is so high that the increase is probably of little practical significance. Unreactive nitrate groups that are only very slowly removed from the carbon skeleton are ineffective in relaxing smooth muscle. For example, pentaerythritol tetranitrate and its very active trinitrate metabolite are very rapidly denitrated; little of either is ever detected in the blood. In contrast, the almost completely inactive mononitrates and dinitrates circulate in the blood for many hours; pentaerythritol and its mononitrate are the major metabolites found in urine. Similarly, glyceryl and isosorbide mononitrates are the major circulating metabolites and excretory products of nitroglycerin and isosorbide dinitrate, respectively. Denitration appears to be limited by the amount of endogenous hepatic glutathione, and the circulation of large amounts of organic nitrate through the liver can deplete glutathione and greatly slow inactivation. (*See* Needleman *et al.,* 1969, 1972; Davidson *et al.,* 1970, 1971; Needleman and Harkey, 1971; Johnson *et al.,* 1972.)

Tolerance. Tolerance, sometimes very great, can develop to various effects of nitrites. Whether or not a preferential tissue tolerance is involved, clinical observations suggest that resistance develops more readily to nitrite-induced headache than to other cardiovascular effects, a fortunate circumstance. A high degree of tolerance of vascular smooth muscle to nitroglycerin can be produced within 2 or 3 days in laboratory animals, and this develops in a few hours when the tissue is incubated *in vitro* with an active nitrate ester in an alkaline medium. The

tolerance developed both *in vivo* and *in vitro* is specific for organic nitrate esters, is associated with a decrease in tissue sulfhydryl content, and can be reversed quickly by a disulfide-reducing agent such as dithiothreitol (Needleman and Johnson, 1973). This sulfhydryl-dependent tolerance does not extend to the nitrite ion. Tolerance to the nitrite ion can occur, but little is known of its specific characteristics or mechanism.

It is clear that extensive tolerance to the effects of organic nitrates can develop in man, but details regarding the conditions required for its induction or its time course have not been established. The scarcity of observations on this matter is probably related to the fact that the available "long-acting" organic nitrate preparations have been generally ineffective in maintaining a continuous effect. However, it has been demonstrated that repeated administration of these preparations can significantly decrease responses, particularly those of veins, to clinical doses of nitroglycerin (Schelling and Lasagna, 1967).

A special aspect of tolerance is observed among individuals exposed to nitroglycerin or nitroglycol in the manufacture of explosives. They frequently suffer from severe headaches, dizziness, and postural weakness during the first several days of employment. Tolerance then develops, but headache and other symptoms may reappear after a few days away from the job, the "Monday disease." It is a common practice for them to rub the responsible agent on their skin or to wear work clothes impregnated with the material during such periods as prophylaxis against unpleasant reactions when they return to work. The most serious effect of chronic exposure is a form of *organic nitrate dependence*. Individuals without demonstrable organic vascular disease have died suddenly or developed myocardial infarctions after a few days' break in chronic exposure, and there are now well-documented cases with typical subjective and objective findings of severe myocardial ischemia, relieved by nitroglycerin, during withdrawal from chronic exposure to an organic nitrate. Coronary and digital arteriospasm during withdrawal and its relaxation by nitroglycerin have also been demonstrated radiographically (*see* Lange *et al.,* 1972). It is probable that the vasospasm and myocardial ischemia are due to the suddenly unopposed effect of some compensatory mechanism, but the nature of this process is unknown. Only a few individuals are now subject to the hazards of chronic exposure to an organic nitrate, and they could probably be protected by adequate industrial safety procedures. However, if present widespread efforts to produce an organic nitrate preparation that would provide an essentially continuous effect are successful, *iatrogenic organic nitrate dependence* could become a very serious and widespread problem.

Toxicity and Untoward Responses. Untoward responses to the therapeutic use of nitrites are almost all secondary to actions on the cardiovascular system. *Headache* is common and can be severe. It usually decreases over a few days if treatment is continued, and often can be controlled by decreasing the dose. Transient episodes of *dizziness, weakness,* and other manifestations of the cerebral ischemia associated with *postural hypotension* may develop occasionally in many patients, particularly if standing immobile, and may occasionally progress to loss of consciousness. This reaction appears to be accentuated by alcohol. Even in the most severe nitrite syncope, positioning and other procedures to facilitate venous return are the only therapeutic measures required. It is widely believed that nitrites can increase intraocular pressure and precipitate glaucoma, but this fear appears to be completely unfounded (Whitworth and Grant, 1964). Drug *rash* is occasionally produced by all the organic nitrates, but it appears to occur most commonly with pentaerythritol tetranitrate.

Methemoglobinemia. Nitrite ion readily oxidizes hemoglobin to methemoglobin both *in vitro* and *in vivo*. Formation of large amounts of methemoglobin can seriously impair the oxygen-carrying capacity of the blood, and anemic hypoxia results. Severe poisoning and even death can result from the ingestion of *nitrate* by infants. The higher pH of their gastrointestinal contents is associated with the presence of certain bacteria, especially *Escherichia coli,* at more proximal enteric loci than in adults. Consequently, nitrite is formed by bacterial reduction of unabsorbed nitrate, and the former is the immediate toxic agent. "Nitrate" poisoning in infants has occurred from the use of bismuth subnitrate as an antidiarrheal agent and from the ingestion of well water with a high nitrate content (*see* Miller, 1971). Whenever a bottle-fed rural infant appears to be cyanotic without obvious cause, the water used in the household should be suspect. The safe limit of nitrate in water for infants under 10 weeks of age may be less than the United States Public Health Service standard of 45 ppm. Ingested nitrate ion has almost no toxicity for older children and adults, but toxic methemoglobinemia can result from the use of high-nitrate water in hemodialysis at home (Carlson and Shapiro, 1970).

Preparations, Routes of Administration, and Dosage. Data for the nitrites and organic nitrates available for clinical use are given in Table 34–1. Sodium nitrite is obsolete except as an intravenous solution for use in the treatment of cyanide poisoning (*see* Chapter 44). Amyl nitrite acts very rapidly after inhalation and is occasionally used for very brief effects. Nitroglycerin is also sufficiently volatile for the tablets to lose activity rapidly unless kept in a tightly sealed glass container; plastic is unsatisfactory (Medical Letter, 1971). Active tablets should produce a distinct burning sensation when placed under the tongue. Only nitroglycerin, erythrityl tetranitrate, and isosorbide dinitrate are available in sublingual tablets. Trolnitrate, which is irritant, and pentaerythritol tetranitrate, which has a very low aqueous solubility, cannot be administered sublingually. The recommended oral doses of the organic nitrates are highly variable because clear-cut therapeutic effects have not been demonstrated by the oral route. *Many sustained-action oral preparations of organic nitrates and combinations with other agents are marketed, but none of these can be recommended.*

THERAPEUTIC USES

The main therapeutic use of nitrites is in the treatment of *angina pectoris,* as discussed at the end of this chapter in relation to other agents employed in this condition. They are used much less frequently for other purposes and, in fact, are often neglected in situations in which they might have a beneficial effect.

Nitroglycerin can provide dramatic relief of *paroxysmal nocturnal dyspnea,* probably as the result of improved left ventricular function and reduced pulmonary arterial pressure. Systemic administration of nitrite is ineffective in peripheral vascular disorders, but *topical application of nitroglycerin ointment* may provide useful cutaneous vasodilatation, particularly in the treatment of *Raynaud's disease* and of slowly healing *trophic ulcers.* Nitrites are sometimes used to dilate peripheral arteries to facilitate differentiation of organic occlusion, functional spasm, and anomalous position of a vessel, by both palpation and angiography. Amyl nitrite produces characteristic changes in pressure gradients and heart murmurs, which can assist in the diagnosis of various congenital and acquired *abnormalities of the heart and great vessels* (*see* Vogelpoel *et al.,* 1959; Marcus *et al.,* 1964).

The nitrites have been used sporadically in almost every condition that involves increased tone or "spasm" of nonvascular smooth muscle, but they have seldom been very successful. The transient action of amyl nitrite or nitroglycerin may occasionally assist in differentiating between morphological defects and functional spasm during *fluoroscopy,* and nitrites have been effective in relieving the pain and dysphagia of diffuse esophageal spasm (Orlando and Bozymski, 1973). Nitroglycerin effectively relaxes the smooth muscle of the gallbladder and bile ducts, and often provides temporary relief of the pain of *biliary colic;* it is less frequently effective in *ureteral colic.* Many other drugs are more useful than the nitrites in *bronchial asthma,* but nitroglycerin

Table 34-1. NITRITES AND ORGANIC NITRATES AVAILABLE FOR CLINICAL USE

NONPROPRIETARY NAME	SOME TRADE NAMES	CHEMICAL STRUCTURE	PREPARATIONS	DOSES AND ROUTES OF ADMINISTRATION
Amyl Nitrite, N.F.	VAPOROLE	H_3C $\quad$CHCH$_2$CH$_2$NO$_2$ H_3C	Pearls: 0.18 and 0.3 ml	0.18 or 0.3 ml, inhalation
Nitroglycerin, U.S.P. (glyceryl trinitrate)	NITRO-BID NITROL NITROSTAT	H_2C—O—NO$_2$ HC—O—NO$_2$ H_2C—O—NO$_2$	Tablets: 0.15, 0.3, 0.4, 0.6, and 2.5 mg Ointment: 2%	0.15 to 0.6 mg, sublingual 2.5 mg, oral, every 12 hr Topical to skin
Sodium Nitrite, U.S.P.		NaNO$_2$	Solution: 3% †	300 to 500 mg (10 to 15 ml), i.v. (to produce methemoglobin)
Erythrityl Tetranitrate, N.F.	CARDILATE	H_2C—O—NO$_2$ HC—O—NO$_2$ HC—O—NO$_2$ H_2C—O—NO$_2$	Tablets: 5, 10, and 15 mg, sublingual and oral	5 to 15 mg, sublingual 15 to 60 mg, oral
Pentaerythritol Tetranitrate, N.F.	DUOTRATE * METRANIL * PENTRITOL PERITRATE VASITOL	O$_2$N—O—H$_2$C$\quad$CH$_2$—O—NO$_2$ $\quad\quad$C O$_2$N—O—H$_2$C$\quad$CH$_2$—O—NO$_2$	Tablets: 10 and 20 mg 30 to 80 mg *	10 to 40 mg, oral 30 to 80 mg, oral, every 12 hr *
Isosorbide Dinitrate, U.S.P.	ISORDIL LASERDIL SORBITRATE	H_2C— HC—O—NO$_2$ CH HC O$_2$N—O—CH CH_2	Tablets: 2.5 and 5 mg, sublingual 5 and 10 mg, oral	2.5 to 10 mg, sublingual 10 to 60 mg, oral
Mannitol Hexanitrate	NITRANITOL	H_2C—O—NO$_2$ O$_2$N—O—CH O$_2$N—O—CH HC—O—NO$_2$ HC—O—NO$_2$ H_2C—O—NO$_2$	Tablets: 30 mg	30 to 60 mg, oral
Trolnitrate Phosphate (triethanolamine trinitrate biphosphate)	METAMINE	$\quad$CH$_2$CH$_2$—O—NO$_2$ N—CH$_2$CH$_2$—O—NO$_2$ $\quad$CH$_2$CH$_2$—O—NO$_2$ $\quad\cdot$ 2H$_3$PO$_4$	Tablets: 10 mg *	20 mg, oral

* Sustained-release preparations.
† Component of cyanide antidote kit (*see* Chapter 44).

occasionally provides relief in an acute attack when other agents fail.

MISCELLANEOUS VASODILATORS

Papaverine. *Papaverine Hydrochloride,* N.F. (6,7-dimethoxy-1-veratrylisoquinoline hydrochloride; CERESPAN, PAVABID), is marketed in tablets (30 to 200 mg) and capsules (150 mg) for oral use, and as a 3% solution for intramuscular or intravenous injection. The usual dose is 100 to 150 mg, two or three times a day. The alkaloid is present to the extent of about 1% in crude opium, but it is unrelated chemically or pharmacologically to the narcotic alkaloids and contributes almost nothing to the overall pharmacology of opium. *Dioxyline phosphate* (PAVERIL) is a synthetic compound that is both structurally and pharmacologically very similar to papaverine. It is available for oral use in 100- and 200-mg tablets. The recommended dose is 100 to 400 mg, three or four times a day.

Pharmacological Properties. Papaverine is the classical example of a nonspecific smooth muscle relaxant (antispasmodic). It is often used as a reference standard in reporting the activity of newly synthesized antispasmodics, possibly because its relatively low potency makes other agents look good by comparison. Papaverine can relax all smooth muscle structures *in vitro,* irrespective of the type of endogenous or exogenous factors inducing tone. However, in the doses tolerated by man, or even in intact laboratory animals, its effects on many structures are limited. Papaverine is a potent inhibitor of a cyclic nucleotide phosphodiesterase found in many tissues and can increase the concentration of cyclic adenosine 3′,5′-monophosphate (cyclic AMP). Since cyclic AMP has been implicated as a possible mediator of β-adrenergic relaxation of smooth muscle, such a mechanism of action of papaverine is plausible.

Papaverine relaxes the smooth muscle of the larger blood vessels and also decreases total peripheral resistance, presumably by an effect on arterioles. It has been shown to produce marked, persistent coronary vasodilatation in experimental animals, but there may be concomitant evidence of myocardial ischemia. Large doses of papaverine can prevent various experimental cardiac arrhythmias, but they can also depress A-V and intraventricular conduction and produce serious arrhythmias. Papaverine decreases cerebrovascular resistance more than do most other vasodilators, and intravenous administration can cause some increase in blood flow in areas of ischemia due to cerebral atherosclerosis. However, the therapeutic value of this small effect is questionable (*see* McHenry *et al.,* 1970).

Therapeutic Uses. Papaverine is mentioned in this chapter because its use to dilate blood vessels has been its last therapeutic application to be discarded. It has not been proved to have therapeutic value in any condition, and its use is now practically obsolete. It is ironic that such a venerable drug has been replaced by agents that, in most therapeutic applications, are not significantly more effective.

Dipyridamole. *Dipyridamole* (2,6-*bis*-[diethanolamino]-4,8-dipiperidinopyrimido-[5,4-*d*]-pyrimidine;

PERSANTINE) is available in 25-mg tablets for oral use. It has many properties qualitatively similar to those of papaverine. Its effects on smooth muscle other than that of the vasculature have received little attention, but it has been reported to antagonize responses such as the contraction of intestinal smooth muscle induced by barium and the bronchospasm induced by either histamine or acetylcholine.

Many different observations have linked the action of dipyridamole to the metabolism of adenosine and adenine nucleotides, which are vasodilators. It increases the persistence of adenosine in the plasma, probably to a large extent by inhibiting its uptake by erythrocytes (an effect similar to that of papaverine), and it blocks such uptake by several other tissues. The presence of an active, saturable uptake process for adenosine has been correlated with the ability of dipyridamole to potentiate responses of a given tissue to the nucleoside; where only passive diffusion is involved, responses are unaffected (Hopkins and Goldie, 1971). Dipyridamole potentiates many diverse responses to adenosine and adenine nucleotides, including coronary dilatation, A-V block in isolated hearts, and contraction of the guinea pig uterus (Stafford, 1966; Afonso and O'Brien, 1967), but it blocks platelet aggregation caused by adenosine diphosphate (Emmons *et al.,* 1965). The marked potentiation of the vasodilatation induced by adenine nucleotides and the fact that responses to most other vasodilatators are unaffected have led to the use of dipyridamole in studies of possible mediators of reactive hyperemia (Parratt and Wadsworth, 1972). Dipyridamole also inhibits phosphodiesterase, and it has been suggested that it causes vasodilatation by allowing the accumulation of cyclic AMP (Hamilton, 1972).

In most situations, dipyridamole decreases blood pressure and increases heart rate and cardiac output, largely as the result of dilatation of systemic resistance vessels. In experiments with controlled cardiac output, 0.3 mg/kg of dipyridamole reduced the blood pressure by 25 to over 50% (Elliot, 1961). Patients with hypertension often respond to intravenous injection of the drug with a marked fall in blood pressure.

Many studies have now demonstrated that dipyridamole greatly decreases coronary vascular resistance, and increases coronary blood flow and coronary sinus oxygen saturation. It clearly does not decrease myocardial work or augment subendocardial oxygen tension. The same general pattern of response has been reported for anesthetized laboratory animals, normal human subjects, and patients with severe coronary artery disease and angina pectoris. Dipyridamole appears to act predominantly on small resistance vessels of the coronary bed. Its full effect abolishes the autoregulatory response to a short period of ischemia, and alters transcapillary exchange in the same way as does severe hypoxemia. Thus, it appears to have little effect on vascular resistance in ischemic areas where small vessels are already dilated. It does not dilate large conducting vessels, as determined either angiographically or by direct-resistance measurements. Prolonged administration to dogs during progressive narrowing of a major coronary artery has been reported to promote the development or enlargement of the arterial anastomoses involved in coronary backflow. No equivalent of this response to chronic administration has been identified in man. (*See* Fam *et al.,* 1964; McGregor, 1966; Winbury *et al.,* 1971.)

In the doses usually employed clinically, dipyridamole is quite nontoxic. Gastrointestinal intolerance with nausea, vomiting, and diarrhea occurs occasionally, as do headache and vertigo. However, the recommended oral dose of 25 to 50 mg, two or three times a day, at least 1 hour before meals, appears to be considerably less than equivalent to the intravenous doses of up to 0.3 mg/kg used in clinical investigation.

Therapeutic Uses. Dipyridamole has been used predominantly in patients with coronary artery disease, particularly when manifested as *angina pectoris.* Although many conflicting observations have been reported, there is no convincing evidence that either acute or chronic administration appreciably decreases the frequency or severity of anginal attacks, and studies involving standardized exercise tolerance tests have quite uniformly failed to show significant improvement (*e.g.,* see Newhouse and McGregor, 1965).

The use of dipyridamole to inhibit *platelet aggregation* and *thrombus formation* is discussed in Chapter 65.

Perhexiline. *Perhexiline maleate* (2-[2,2-dicyclohexylethyl]piperidine maleate; PEXID) is an investigational drug that appears to cause a generalized depression of membrane ionic fluxes. In association with this action, smooth muscle tone, Purkinje fiber automaticity, and A-V and ventricular conduction velocities are decreased, and responses to a variety of agents (*e.g.,* catecholamines, histamine, calcium) are inhibited. The drug does not have a specific β-adrenergic blocking action, and it does not augment responses to adenine nucleotides. Perhexiline has been shown to reduce femoral and coronary vascular resistance, lower heart rate in experimental animals, and cause an overall decrease in left ventricular filling pressure and work. It can also decrease elevated airway resistance and increase pulmonary compliance. In laboratory animals the vascular effect appears to be predominantly on precapillary resistance vessels, but the doses usually administered to man (200 to 400 mg per day) appear to have little antihypertensive effect. Perhexiline also has a moderate thiazide-like diuretic effect that has been observed in both laboratory animals and man.

Perhexiline is well absorbed after oral administration and is excreted in both urine and feces, predominantly as monohydroxylated and dihydroxylated metabolites. The half-life is several days and, consequently, the drug accumulates in the body during chronic administration.

Perhexiline is being tested in patients with *coronary artery disease* for its effects on cardiac arrhythmias, exercise tolerance, and frequency of anginal attacks. It appears to reduce considerably the incidence of ventricular, and perhaps also atrial, ectopic beats in individuals with aberrant pacemaker activity. In patients with *angina pectoris,* perhexiline produces little change in resting heart rate or blood pressure, but tachycardia from exercise is considerably reduced. Cardiac lactate extraction is increased, particularly during exertion, and subjective and ECG evidence of myocardial ischemia is delayed both during standardized exercise and during atrial pacing. It is not clear if the decreased myocardial hypoxia is predominantly due to decreased oxygen requirements or to increased oxygen delivery. Several studies on the chronic administration of perhexiline have reported a decreased incidence of anginal attacks and a reduced consumption of nitroglycerin in a high percentage of patients.

Dizziness is the most prominent side effect of perhexiline reported to date; gastrointestinal upsets and generalized malaise are less frequent. Moderate elevations in plasma SGOT and LDH activities have been reported to occur in almost 20% of patients in some studies. These changes have been reversible in all cases reported to date, sometimes without stopping drug administration, and their significance is still unclear.

It is too early to draw firm conclusions regarding the role that perhexiline may come to play in the treatment of angina pectoris. However, the observations reported to date are very interesting and the drug certainly warrants further study. Many details of the pharmacology of perhexiline are described in a symposium (*see* Symposium, 1973).

Cyclandelate. *Cyclandelate* (3,3,5-trimethylcyclohexyl mandelate; CYCLOSPASMOL) is a general smooth muscle relaxant that differs chemically from the majority of such agents in that it contains no nitrogen. However, most of its pharmacological properties (*see* Bijlsma *et al.,* 1956) are very similar to those of papaverine and of many synthetic antispasmodics promoted primarily for effects on smooth muscle (*see* Chapter 25). Cyclandelate can produce mild vasodilatation in man. This has been noted particularly as increases in digital pulse volume and skin temperature, but increases in cerebral and muscle blood flow have also been reported. The drug is available in 100-mg tablets and 200-mg capsules. Recommended oral doses range up to 1600 mg per day.

Cyclandelate appears to produce little serious toxicity. However, oral doses of 200 mg or more are associated with a significant incidence of unpleasant side effects, including gastrointestinal upsets, flushing, tingling, headache, dizziness, and sweating. Cyclandelate has been used in almost every known type of vascular disease, but its value has not been convincingly demonstrated in any.

Nicotinic Acid and Nicotinyl Alcohol. *Niacin,* N.F. (*nicotinic acid*), and *nicotinyl alcohol* (RONIACOL) have almost identical pharmacological properties. The necessity for oxidation of the latter to the active form, nicotinic acid, does not appear to delay or to increase the duration of its effects. These agents are relatively weak vasodilators with a predominant effect on cutaneous vessels in the blush area; this activity is not shared by nicotinamide. Large doses can lower systemic blood pressure transiently in experimental animals and probably produce some vasodilatation in most vascular beds. However, there is no evidence that the usual clinical doses produce vasodilatation except in the skin. Nicotinic acid and nicotinyl alcohol have very low toxicities. Nausea and vomiting occur occasionally after large oral doses, and syncope, perhaps psychogenic, is even less common. The dose of either drug for cardiovascular effects is selected to produce definite flushing of the face. This is initially about 100 to 150 mg given by mouth, but considerable tolerance can develop. Because the patient is very aware of the flush and associated warmth and tingling, these agents have a strong placebo effect, which may be desirable in some cases. Their vasodilator effect has not been proved to be of therapeutic value. The effects of nicotinic acid on blood lipids and as a vitamin are discussed in Chapters 35 and 73, respectively.

MAJOR THERAPEUTIC USES OF VASODILATORS

Angina Pectoris. The characteristic oppressive pain of angina pectoris appears to arise from ischemia (hypoxia) of some area of the myocardium, precipitated by an imbalance in the demand for and supply of oxygen. Several types of evidence indicate that subendocardial regions are predominantly involved (*see* Moir, 1972). In the past, drug therapy of this condition has centered on attempts to increase coronary blood flow without increasing oxygen consumption, an effect referred to as "benign vasodilatation." However, drugs are now known that greatly increase total coronary blood flow and decrease coronary A-V oxygen difference without increasing exercise tolerance in patients with angina pectoris; dipyridamole is the outstanding example of such pharmacological success and therapeutic failure. In contrast, nitroglycerin effectively decreases ECG evidence of myocardial hypoxia, increases exercise tolerance, and prevents or relieves the characteristic symptoms. Because of this clear therapeutic difference, a comparison of the major cardiovascular effects of nitroglycerin and dipyridamole is instructive. (1) Nitroglycerin increases coronary blood flow and decreases coronary vascular resistance considerably less than does dipyridamole, particularly in patients with a clear-cut anginal syndrome. (2) Nitroglycerin produces a persistent dilatation of large, angiographically visible coronary vessels, but dipyridamole does not. (3) Nitroglycerin dilates collateral vessels in laboratory preparations that involve narrowing or occlusion of a major coronary artery; dipyridamole does not have

a comparable effect. (4) Nitroglycerin does not significantly alter coronary autoregulation, whereas this can be abolished by dipyridamole. (5) Largely because of its action on systemic capacitance vessels, nitroglycerin decreases pulmonary, systemic arterial, and intraventricular diastolic pressures, cardiac output, and heart size; dipyridamole produces much less venous dilatation and clearly does not decrease cardiac work. It appears that the beneficial effect of nitroglycerin is most likely dependent on a reduction of myocardial oxygen requirement or on a specific redistribution of coronary blood flow, or on both.

The possible contribution of decreased cardiac work has received much attention. Indeed, Brunton (1867) first tried amyl nitrite in the treatment of angina pectoris in an attempt to decrease the work of the heart by lowering the blood pressure. Blood pressure, heart rate, and especially ventricular diastolic volume and wall tension quite regularly increase just prior to the onset of an anginal attack. Pain tends to occur at a relatively constant level of myocardial work (heart rate-pressure product or other index) in each individual, and to subside when it drops below this value either spontaneously or as a result of therapy (Robinson, 1968). The major obstacles to acceptance of decreased myocardial work as the dominant or only factor in the relief of anginal pain by nitrite are persistence of the clinical benefit of nitroglycerin beyond the period during which blood pressure, cardiac output, and heart size have been shown to be decreased, particularly in the usual clinical situation of mild exertion (*see* Hoeschen *et al.,* 1966), and the dramatic relief of anginal pain produced by amyl nitrite, which appears not to decrease and may transiently increase cardiac work.

It has been proposed that the beneficial effect of nitroglycerin also involves its predominant action on relatively large coronary arteries, particularly interarterial anastomotic channels, the "conducting vessels." It is reasoned that in the myocardium, as in skeletal muscle, no drug can relax the small resistance vessels more than do the local factors operative in an area of ischemia. Preferential dilatation of conducting vessels could divert more blood to areas of hypoxia where the small resistance vessels are already maximally dilated, while allowing resistance vessels in other areas to maintain their auto-regulatory tone (*see* McGregor and Fam, 1966).

Evaluation of the results of antianginal therapy poses many very difficult problems. The attacks are identified by symptoms rather than by signs and have a large psychosomatic component. Any of the many emotional factors that activate the sympathetic nervous system can increase the oxygen requirement of the myocardium. Thus, fear of an anginal attack can contribute to its production; conversely, confidence in a physician or therapeutic agent *per se* can prevent attacks. Merely the knowledge that they are involved in a test of what may be an effective drug can substantially reduce the incidence of anginal attacks in at least 50% of patient participants. Thus, interpretable observations require a completely double-blind comparison with an appropriate placebo, randomization of patients and medications, and full statistical analysis.

The most appropriate way to prevent the pain of angina pectoris is to prevent myocardial hypoxia. The relationship between pain and hypoxia can often be identified by appropriate exercise tolerance tests. A drug that reduces hypoxia will increase in parallel the amount of exertion required to produce pain and depression of the S-T segment of the ECG. It is generally accepted that drugs that delay the appearance of symptoms without altering the ECG evidence of myocardial ischemia are less desirable and perhaps dangerous.

Aside from the very desirable objective of arresting or reversing pathological changes, which is not pertinent to the present discussion, there are two quite distinct *therapeutic aims of antianginal therapy:* (1) termination of an individual attack, or its prevention by medication taken shortly before a period of stress; and (2) chronic prophylaxis to prevent attacks and increase the patient's exercise capacity.

Individual Anginal Attacks. Nitroglycerin is used much more frequently than any other drug in the treatment or prevention of individual attacks, and it leaves little to be desired. It is always taken sublingually or by chewing the tablet and spreading the material over the buccal mucous membrane; it is ineffective if swallowed. The usual dose is 0.2 to 0.6 mg, which may occasionally need to be repeated once or twice at 5-minute intervals. Many patients learn the dose that gives them the best balance between relief of pain and unpleasant side effects, but there is frequently a tendency to take more than is necessary, particularly when the pain is severe, and this may increase side effects. An effective dose of nitroglycerin administered sublingually usually acts within 2 minutes, and termination of the pain is usually sudden and complete, as in the spontaneous

termination of an attack. However, if the patient immediately stops a precipitating exertion, most anginal attacks last less than 3 minutes, and it is clear that the drug is best taken during the short prodrome experienced by many patients or prior to anticipated exertion. *Amyl nitrite* acts slightly faster than does nitroglycerin, but few patients feel that this difference is enough to justify the considerably greater inconvenience, expense, and side effects associated with its use.

There is general agreement that nitroglycerin given prior to an appropriate exercise tolerance test (Redwood *et al.,* 1971) considerably increases the exertion required for the appearance of subjective and ECG evidence of myocardial hypoxia. Similarly, the use of nitroglycerin shortly before a period of increased activity or other stress can prevent the attack that would otherwise be expected. Nitroglycerin has also been reported to reduce the exertional arrhythmias that occur in patients with coronary artery disease (Gey *et al.,* 1973). Short-term prophylaxis can dramatically improve a patient's outlook by allowing him freely to undertake necessary tasks and to experience pleasures that otherwise are coupled with a threat of excruciating pain.

The acute prophylactic effect of nitroglycerin can persist for more than 30 minutes. Other organic nitrates administered sublingually have a similar effect and duration of action when given in equi-effective doses (Goldstein *et al.,* 1971). Some minor differences in duration may exist, but no real advantages of other organic nitrates over nitroglycerin have been established, and they are considerably more expensive. A more prolonged prophylaxis can be obtained by the use of the slowly absorbed 2% nitroglycerin ointment. Oral administration is ineffective.

Chronic Prophylaxis. Chronic prophylactic therapy attempts to provide a relatively constant drug effect with the objective of decreasing or eliminating anginal attacks and the necessity of intercurrent medication to meet the needs of specific events. Chronic prophylaxis involves factors quite distinct from those encountered in short-term therapy of the acute attack, and proof that a single dose or a few doses of a drug can decrease the incidence of anginal episodes and increase exercise tolerance is not acceptable evidence that its chronic administration will be beneficial.

Studies of long-term therapy in angina pectoris are notoriously difficult to control and evaluate. The criteria most frequently employed to assess the effectiveness of chronic drug therapy are the patients' records of the number of attacks experienced each day and of the number of tablets of nitroglycerin utilized. Standardized exercise tolerance tests are also desirable, but the results are much more difficult to evaluate than in short-term studies. All assessments require careful control of relatively long-term fluctuations in the severity of disease manifestations, climatic conditions, patient activity, and many other factors. (*See* McGregor, 1966; Panels on Cardiovascular Drugs, 1970.)

Propranolol. Increased sympathetic nerve activity can clearly precipitate anginal attacks in susceptible individuals, and block of adrenergic effects can be beneficial by decreasing heart rate, myocardial contractility, cardiac output, and, in some cases, blood pressure. The sympathetic effects are most prominent during exertion, when adrenergic tone is increased. Possible deleterious effects of β-adrenergic blockade are an increase in heart size and in duration of mechanical systole, but in most patients the net effect appears to be a decrease in myocardial oxygen requirements. Coronary blood flow is usually decreased, but the reduction appears to be predominantly in the relatively well perfused subepicardial areas. (*See* Chapter 26 for details of the pharmacology of β-adrenergic blocking drugs.)

Although there are many variations and discrepancies in published observations, as expected in studies on angina pectoris, evidence accumulated over more than 10 years indicates that β-adrenergic blockade has a definite long-term prophylactic value in this condition. Many different β blockers have been studied with similar results, but by far the greatest experience has been with propranolol. Exercise tolerance can be increased by either single-dose or chronic administration of propranolol; both subjective and ECG evidence of myocardial hypoxia are affected, but the two may not be as closely correlated as is the case with nitroglycerin. Most reports indicate that chronic administration of propranolol decreases the frequency of anginal attacks and the consumption of nitroglycerin in a majority of patients. The beneficial effect, in terms of both the percentage of individuals responding and the magnitude of improvement, appears to be roughly related to the dose, up to at least 400 mg per day. An effective dose should decrease the resting heart rate (some experts recommend a reduction of 20 beats or to about 60 per minute), and tachycardia induced by exercise should be greatly attenuated. Some patients do not respond favorably or may be made worse by propranolol, and no clear criteria for patient selection have yet been established. (*See* Amsterdam *et al.,* 1969; Mizgala *et al.,* 1969; Prichard and Gillam, 1971.)

At the present time, many cardiologists consider that propranolol is a suitable "basal" medication for most patients with frequent anginal attacks, unless there is some specific contraindication to its use. The starting dose is 10 mg three or four times a day, and this is gradually increased to the dose giving an optimal balance between benefit and side effects. Patients with evidence of myocardial inadequacy should be digitalized, and patients taking both propranolol and digitalis should be watched carefully for evidence of heart block. The most important complication of propranolol therapy is heart failure, but serious myocardial depression is relatively infrequent when one considers the poor functional state of the heart in many patients with coronary artery disease. It has been reported that sudden withdrawal of propranolol can cause a severe exacerbation of angina or myocardial infarction. This has been noted predominantly in patients with very severe coronary artery disease. Neither the mechanism nor the extent of this problem has been established, but it appears prudent to reduce the dose gradually over 1 to 2 weeks, with careful observation of the patient, if propranolol is to be discontinued.

Complete elimination of anginal attacks by propranolol occurs in only a small percentage of patients, and sublingual nitroglycerin should also be provided to prevent or relieve residual individual attacks. The two types of medication are complementary in that they reduce cardiac work by different mechanisms. In addition, β-adrenergic blockade antagonizes the reflex tachycardia produced by a nitrite, and the nitrite tends to reduce the increase in heart size and the lengthening of mechanical systole caused by the blockade.

"Long-Acting" Organic Nitrates. Attempts at chronic prophylaxis with organic nitrates given orally represent an accumulation of patient-years of "treatment" of angina pectoris second only to that of sublingual nitroglycerin, and the former probably represent the greater dollar expenditure. Reported results have been variable and difficult to evaluate. There have been some reports of increased exercise tolerance; however, in the absence of evidence that a continuous effect had been maintained, even a statistically significant improvement could have represented only the effect of the last dose. Although most of an organic nitrate absorbed from the gastrointestinal tract is inactivated during its first passage through the liver, some effect can be obtained if the dose is sufficiently large.

An analysis of studies reported over a 20-year period on the prophylactic use of organic nitrates clearly shows that the incidence of good results is inversely related to the adequacy of the protocol (placebos, blinding, crossover, etc.) (Stipe and Fink, 1973). The best-controlled studies of chronic oral nitrate administration have shown no greater benefit than was obtained with a placebo (see Cole *et al.,* 1957; Aronow, 1972), but these obviously have not covered all of the many different drugs, schedules, and doses that have been recommended. Although it is still impossible to say categorically that no beneficial effect can be obtained with such agents, studies with propranolol and other β-adrenergic blocking drugs have done much to put oral organic nitrate preparations into perspective. Most of the same problems are involved in evaluating the two types of drugs, and there is now a clear difference in the results; β-adrenergic blockade is the more effective. Since the two are promoted for essentially the same purpose, it appears that the oral organic nitrates now have little to contribute to the management of patients with angina pectoris.

New Drugs and Procedures. Although nitroglycerin is quite satisfactory for the treatment of and short-term prophylaxis against anginal attacks, chronic prophylaxis is still far from optimal. Propranolol and other β-adrenergic blocking drugs should largely displace the older preparations for the latter purpose, but new compounds will continue to appear. It is clear that desirable agents will not be predominantly "coronary vasodilators," and preparations of "long-acting" organic nitrates are not good candidates on the basis of current knowledge of the metabolism of these compounds and of the development of tolerance and dependence. *Perhexiline* may prove to be a useful drug, and more information on its mechanism of action may provide new leads. It has also been suggested that a β-adrenergic blocking agent that specifically inhibits chronotropic responses would be desirable, but no drug with this type of selectivity is known.

It is not appropriate to review here the various surgical procedures being tried to alleviate coronary insufficiency, but pharmacological experience may be pertinent to their assessment.

Other Therapeutic Considerations. Many factors in the daily life of individuals with angina pectoris play a role in determining the frequency and severity of attacks. Patients should be advised to avoid, where possible, situations and activities that are associated with attacks. Smoking is often a contributing factor and should be discouraged. Weight reduction, avoidance of cold, and appropriately graded exercise may also be helpful. An important reduction in the cardiac work of hypertensive patients suffering from angina pectoris can be achieved by lowering the blood pressure. However, this must be done cautiously. The angina may be considerably improved by effective antihypertensive therapy, but it can also be made worse if the decrease in pressure is associated with a considerable reduction in coronary blood flow. Similarly, digitalis can be of value when angina is associated with some degree of myocardial failure, although it is not useful in the absence of this factor. Anxiety and excitement of any type increase sympathetic activity and can precipitate anginal attacks. Where these strong emotions cannot be reasonably avoided within the life style and personality of the individual, the judicious use of a sedative may be helpful. To maintain therapeutic flexibility, sedatives should not be given in fixed-dose combination with more specific antianginal drugs. Alcohol is a good, rapidly acting sedative for many people, and both its pharmacological properties and the convivial atmosphere in which it is often imbibed may help to decrease the tensions that contribute to anginal attacks.

Myocardial Infarction. Angina pectoris and myocardial infarction are two major expressions of coronary atherosclerosis, and an intermediate condition of "accelerated" or "preinfarction" angina has been described. In the past it has been customary to warn against the use of nitroglycerin in angina-like chest pain that is not readily relieved by this drug, because of a postulated danger of decreasing the blood pressure and extending an infarct. However, it is possible that the same reduction in cardiac work that relieves angina could be beneficial in the presence of a coronary occlusion. Studies have indicated that both nitroglycerin (Epstein, 1973) and propranolol (Maroko *et al.*, 1971) can decrease the area of infarction after coronary artery ligation in dogs, and nitroglycerin has been reported to increase cardiac output and decrease pulmonary wedge pressure in patients with heart failure following an infarction (Gold *et al.*, 1972). These data do not allow a recommendation that these antianginal drugs be used in the management of cases of acute myocardial infarction, but they do point to similarities in the responses of patients with these two major complications of coronary artery disease.

Inadequacies of Peripheral Blood Flows. This designation covers a wide variety of conditions in many different parts of the body. Inadequacies of cutaneous, skeletal muscle, and cerebral blood flows are the most commonly treated by drugs, and are largely responsible for the promiscuous, excessive, and generally unsatisfactory use of vasodilators. In many cases the nature of the pathological processes responsible for the ischemia and the characteristics of the physiological regulation of blood flow in the involved area appear to preclude effective therapy with any vasodilator. However, there are few alternatives, and it often appears that a vasodilator drug is prescribed so that the physician will not appear to be completely helpless. If such a "placebo" prescription is used, the doctor should at least recognize what he is doing, and an inexpensive "placebo" should be prescribed.

Cutaneous Circulation. The blood supplies to skin and skeletal muscle in the extremities are commonly affected by the same disease process, but they differ in important ways. Sympathetic nerve activity constricts both cutaneous and muscle vessels; this effect can be readily overcome by local factors in skeletal muscle but not in skin. The difference is well illustrated by a comparison of the therapeutic effects of sympathectomy on conditions involving inadequate blood flow in the two areas (Gillespie, 1967). The most effective cutaneous vasodilators are those that block sympathetic vasoconstriction. These drugs and their use in treating conditions involving inadequate cutaneous circulation are discussed in Chapter 26. Responses to treatment tend to be most favorable when flow is limited more by small than by large vessels. If the major defect is in a large vessel, systemic administration of a blocking agent can actually decrease blood flow in the most seriously ischemic areas by redistributing the limited volume that passes the large-vessel obstruction.

Skeletal Muscle Circulation. Deficient blood flow in skeletal muscle is usually due to morphological changes in large arteries, and is reflected in functional disabilities, of which *intermittent claudication* is the most common. Muscular activity and ischemia *per se* cause massive dilatation of small resistance vessels in this bed, and no vasodilator of any type has been demonstrated to have a greater effect. In contrast to the skin, drugs that stimulate β-adrenergic receptors, such as *nylidrin* and *isoxsuprine*, can cause marked vasodilatation in skeletal muscle (*see* Chapter 24). However, in the presence of arterial disease, the major effect is probably in areas not already dilated by ischemia. In one study of patients with arterial insufficiency, nylidrin was shown to increase total muscle blood flow at rest, but it had no consistent effect on the clearance of a diffusible label and actually decreased the clearance rate during exercise (Zetterquist, 1968). If total blood flow to an extremity is seriously compromised by large-vessel obstruction, cutaneous blood flow can be dangerously reduced when muscle vasodilatation is induced by exercise or reactive hyperemia (Allwood, 1962), and the same hazard probably attends the use of sympathomimetic vasodilators.

In spite of many favorable testimonials, there is no acceptable evidence that any vasodilator drug can improve the exercise capacity of ischemic muscles (*see* Coffman and Mannick, 1972). It also appears doubtful that a drug will be developed that can do more than the autoregulatory mechanisms to get the blood to the areas of skeletal muscle where it is most needed. Many of the problems in assessing and treating peripheral vascular inadequacies in man are discussed in a symposium (*see* Symposium, 1967).

Cerebral Circulation. Reports of decreased functional impairment from the use of vasodilator drugs, sympathetic nerve block, or other procedures assumed to increase cerebral blood flow appear from time to time. However, subsequent work has consistently failed to confirm neurological improvement; this is not unexpected. Resistance in the cerebrovascular bed is very effectively controlled by local autoregulation. Control appears to be most directly related to extracellular pH, which, in turn, is very sensitive to changes in P_{O_2} and P_{CO_2}. This autoregulation functions over a very wide range; indeed, under some circumstances a cerebral blood flow adequate to prevent CNS damage can be maintained when the jugular bulb pressure is only a few millimeters of mercury less than the cerebral arterial pressure (Eckenhoff, 1962). Atherosclerosis reduces the transport of blood to the small vessels involved in autoregulation, and evidence of cerebral ischemia may then result from much smaller reductions in arterial pressure. Conversely, there may be areas of persistent hyperemia adjacent to a recent cerebral infarct in which autoregulation in response to an increase in blood pressure does not occur (Agnoli *et al.*, 1968). As in skeletal muscle, there is a danger that induction of generalized cerebral vasodilatation will redistribute blood flow to the detriment of the most compromised areas. However, deterioration of function or other definite evidence of intracerebral "steal" has not appeared, perhaps because most vasodilators have only a limited effect in this vascular bed. No known drug can decrease cerebral vascular resistance as much as does an increase in arterial P_{CO_2}, and local accumulations of carbon dioxide should have an equivalent effect. Some drugs, such as papaverine given intravenously, can cause a modest increase in cerebral blood flow, including flow in some poorly perfused areas (McHenry *et al.*, 1970), perhaps by dilating relatively large vessels. However, this effect has not been proved to be of clinical value. The effective autoregulation and the dismal history of previous attempts justify a skeptical response to reports of clinical benefit from the action of vasodilator drugs on the cerebral circulation. Many references to studies of the effects of drugs on the cerebral circulation are given in a review by McHenry (1972).

Åblad, B. A study of the mechanism of the hemodynamic effects of hydralazine in man. *Acta pharmac. tox.,* **1963,** *20,* Suppl. 1, 1–53.

Åblad, B., and Mellander, S. Comparative effects of hydralazine, sodium nitrite and acetylcholine on resistance and capacitance blood vessels and capillary filtration in skeletal muscle in the cat. *Acta physiol. scand.,* **1963,** *58,* 319–329.

Afonso, S., and O'Brien, G. S. Enhancement of coronary vasodilator action of adenosine triphosphate by dipyridamole. *Circulation Res.,* **1967,** *20,* 403–408.

Agnoli, A.; Fieschi, C.; Bozzao, L.; Battistini, N.; and Prencipe, M. Autoregulation of cerebral blood flow: studies during drug-induced hypertension in normal subjects and in patients with cerebral vascular diseases. *Circulation,* **1968,** *38,* 800–812.

Allwood, M. J. Redistribution of blood flow in limbs with obstruction of a main artery. *Clin. Sci.,* **1962,** *22,* 279–286.

Amsterdam, E. A.; Gorlin, R.; and Wolfson, S. Evaluation of long-term use of propranolol in angina pectoris. *J. Am. med. Ass.,* **1969,** *210,* 103–106.

Bijlsma, U. G.; Funcke, A. B. H.; Tersteege, H. M.; Rekker, R. F.; Ernsting, M. J. E.; and Nauta, W. T. The pharmacology of CYCLOSPASMOL. *Archs int. Pharmacodyn. Thér.,* **1956,** *105,* 145–174.

Brunton, T. L. On the use of nitrite of amyl in angina pectoris. *Lancet,* **1867,** *2,* 97–98.

Carlson, D. J., and Shapiro, F. L. Methemoglobinemia from well water nitrates: a complication of home dialysis. *Ann. intern. Med.,* **1970,** *73,* 757–759.

Chiong, M. A.; West, R. O.; and Parker, J. O. Influence of nitroglycerin on myocardial metabolism and hemodynamics during angina induced by atrial pacing. *Circulation,* **1972,** *45,* 1044–1056.

Coffman, J. D., and Mannick, J. A. Failure of vasodilator drugs in arteriosclerosis obliterans. *Ann. intern. Med.,* **1972,** *76,* 35–39.

Cohen, M. V.; Downey, J. M.; Sonnenblick, E. H.; and Kirk, E. S. The effects of nitroglycerin on coronary collaterals and myocardial contractility. *J. clin. Invest.,* **1973,** *52,* 2836–2847.

Cole, S. L.; Kaye, H.; and Griffith, G. C. Assay of antianginal agents. I. A curve analysis with multiple control periods. *Circulation,* **1957,** *15,* 405–413.

Davidson, I. W. F.; Miller, H. S.; and DiCarlo, F. J. Absorption, excretion and metabolism of pentaerythritol tetranitrate by humans. *J. Pharmac. exp. Ther.,* **1970,** *175,* 42–50.

Davidson, I. W. F.; Rollins, F. O.; DiCarlo, F. J.; and Miller, H. S. The pharmacodynamics and biotransformation of pentaerythritol trinitrate in man. *Clin. Pharmac. Ther.,* **1971,** *12,* 972–981.

Eckenhoff, J. E. Observations during hypotensive anaesthesia. *Proc. R. Soc. Med.,* **1962,** *55,* 942–944.

Elliot, E. C. The effect of PERSANTIN on coronary flow and cardiac dynamics. *Can. med. Ass. J.,* **1961,** *85,* 469–476.

Emmons, P. R.; Harrison, M. J. G.; Honour, A. J.; and Mitchell, J. R. A. Effect of dipyridamole on human platelet behaviour. *Lancet,* **1965,** *2,* 603–606.

Fam, W. M.; Ragheb, S.; and Hoeschen, R. J. Augmentation of intercoronary anastomosis by long-term administration of a vasodilator drug, dipyridamole (PERSANTIN). *Can. med. Ass. J.,* **1964,** *90,* 970–973.

Ferrer, M. I.; Bradley, S. E.; Wheeler, H. O.; Enson, Y.; Preisig, R.; Brickner, P. W.; Conroy, R. J.; and Harvey, R. M. Some effects of nitroglycerin upon the splanchnic, pulmonary, and systemic circulations. *Circulation,* **1966,** *33,* 357–373.

Ganz, W., and Marcus, H. S. Failure of intracoronary nitroglycerin to alleviate pacing-induced angina. *Circulation,* **1972,** *46,* 880–889.

Gey, G. E.; Fisher, L. D.; Pettet, G. E. M.; and Bruce,

R. A. Exertional arrhythmia and nitroglycerin. *J. Am. med. Ass.,* **1973,** *226,* 287–290.

Gillespie, J. A. The late effects of lumbar sympathectomy on blood flow in the foot in the presence of occlusive arterial disease. *Scand. J. clin. Lab. Invest.,* **1967,** Suppl. 99, 219–221.

Gold, H. K.; Leinbach, R. C.; and Sanders, C. A. Use of sublingual nitroglycerin in congestive failure following acute myocardial infarction. *Circulation,* **1972,** *46,* 839–845.

Goldstein, R. E.; Rosing, D. R.; Redwood, D. R.; Beiser, G. D.; and Epstein, S. E. Clinical and circulatory effects of isosorbide dinitrate. Comparison with nitroglycerin. *Circulation,* **1971,** *43,* 629–640.

Gorlin, R.; Brachfeld, N.; MacLeod, C.; and Bopp, P. Effect of nitroglycerin on the coronary circulation in patients with coronary artery disease or increased left ventricular work. *Circulation,* **1959,** *19,* 705–718.

Hamilton, T. C. The effects of some phosphodiesterase inhibitors on the conductance of the perfused vascular beds of the chloralosed cat. *Br. J. Pharmac.,* **1972,** *46,* 386–394.

Hoeschen, R. J.; Bousvaros, G. A.; Klassen, G. A.; Fam, W. M.; and McGregor, M. Haemodynamic effects of angina pectoris, and of nitroglycerin in normal and anginal subjects. *Br. Heart J.,* **1966,** *28,* 221–230.

Hopkins, S. V., and Goldie, R. G. A species difference in the uptake of adenosine by heart. *Biochem. Pharmac.,* **1971,** *20,* 3359–3365.

Horwitz, L. D.; Gorlin, R.; Taylor, W. J.; and Kemp, H. G. Effects of nitroglycerin on regional myocardial blood flow in coronary artery disease. *J. clin. Invest.,* **1971,** *50,* 1578–1584.

Johnson, E. M., Jr.; Harkey, A. B.; Blehm, D. J.; and Needleman, P. Clearance and metabolism of organic nitrates. *J. Pharmac. exp. Ther.,* **1972,** *182,* 56–62.

Johnsson, G., and Oberg, B. Comparative effects of isoprenaline and nitroglycerin on consecutive vascular sections in the skeletal muscle of the cat. *Angiologica,* **1968,** *5,* 161–171.

Kerber, R. E., and Harrison, D. C. Paradoxical electrocardiographic effects of amyl nitrite in coronary artery disease. *Br. Heart J.,* **1972,** *34,* 851–857.

Khaja, F.; Sanghvi, V.; Mark, A.; and Parker, J. O. Effect of volume expansion on the anginal threshold. *Circulation,* **1971,** *43,* 824–835.

Knoebel, S. B.; McHenry, P. L.; Bonner, A. J.; and Phillips, J. F. Myocardial blood flow in coronary artery disease. Effect of right atrial pacing and nitroglycerin. *Circulation,* **1973,** *47,* 690–696.

Lange, R. L.; Reid, M. S.; Tresch, D. D.; Keelan, M. H.; Bernhard, V. M.; and Coolidge, G. Nonatheromatous ischemic heart disease following withdrawal from chronic industrial nitroglycerin exposure. *Circulation,* **1972,** *46,* 666–678.

Likoff, W.; Kasparian, H.; Lehman, J. S.; and Segal, B. L. Evaluation of "coronary vasodilators" by coronary arteriography. *Am. J. Cardiol.,* **1964,** *13,* 7–9.

Lumb, G. D., and Hardy, L. B. Collateral circulation and survival related to gradual occlusion of the right coronary artery in the pig. *Circulation,* **1963,** *27,* 717–721.

McGregor, M., and Fam, W. M. Regulation of coronary blood flow. *Bull. N.Y. Acad. Med.,* **1966,** *42,* 940–950.

McHenry, L. C., Jr.; Jaffe, M. E.; Kawamura, J.; and Goldberg, H. I. Effect of papaverine on regional blood flow in focal vascular disease of the brain. *New Engl. J. Med.,* **1970,** *282,* 1167–1170.

Marcus, F. I.; Perloff, J. K.; and De Leon, A. C. The use of amyl nitrite in the hemodynamic assessment of aortic valvular and muscular subaortic stenosis. *Am. Heart J.,* **1964,** *68,* 468–475.

Maroko, P. R.; Kjekshus, J. K.; Sobel, B. E.; Watanabe, T.; Covell, J. W.; Ross, J., Jr.; and Braunwald, E. Factors influencing infarct size following experimental coronary artery occlusions. *Circulation,* **1971,** *43,* 67–82.

Medical Letter. Disintegration and storage of nitroglycerin tablets. **1971,** *13,* 13–14.

Miller, L. W. Methemoglobinemia associated with well water. *J. Am. med. Ass.,* **1971,** *216,* 1642–1643.

Mizgala, H. F.; Khan, A. S.; and Davies, R. O. Propranolol in the prophylactic treatment of angina pectoris. *Can. med. Ass. J.,* **1969,** *100,* 756–764.

Needleman, P.; Blehm, D. J.; and Rotskoff, K. S. Relationship between glutathione-dependent denitration and the vasodilator effectiveness of organic nitrates. *J. Pharmac. exp. Ther.,* **1969,** *165,* 286–288.

Needleman, P., and Harkey, A. B. Role of endogenous glutathione in the metabolism of glyceryl trinitrate by isolated perfused rat liver. *Biochem. Pharmac.,* **1971,** *20,* 1867–1876.

Needleman, P., and Johnson, E. M., Jr. Mechanism of tolerance development to organic nitrates. *J. Pharmac. exp. Ther.,* **1973,** *184,* 709–715.

Needleman, P.; Lang, S.; and Johnson, E. M., Jr. Organic nitrates: relationship between biotransformation and rational angina pectoris therapy. *J. Pharmac. exp. Ther.,* **1972,** *181,* 489–497.

Newhouse, M. T., and McGregor, M. Long term dipyridamole therapy of angina pectoris. *Am. J. Cardiol.,* **1965,** *16,* 234–237.

Orlando, R. C., and Bozymski, E. M. Clinical and manometric effects of nitroglycerin in diffuse esophageal spasm. *New Engl. J. Med.,* **1973,** *289,* 23–25.

O'Rourke, R. A.; Bishop, V. S.; Kot, P. A.; and Fernandez, J. P. Hemodynamic effects of nitroglycerin and amyl nitrite in the conscious dog. *J. Pharmac. exp. Ther.,* **1971,** *177,* 426–432.

Panels on Cardiovascular Drugs from the Drug Efficacy Study. Statement on criteria for evaluation of long-acting coronary vasodilators in treatment of angina pectoris. *Circulation,* **1970,** *41,* 149–151.

Parker, J. O.; Case, R. B.; Khaja, F.; Ledwich, J. R.; and Armstrong, P. W. The influence of changes in blood volume on angina pectoris. A study of the effect of phlebotomy. *Circulation,* **1970,** *41,* 593–604.

Parker, J. O.; West, R. O.; and Di Giorgi, S. The hemodynamic response to exercise in patients with healed myocardial infarction without angina; with observations on the effects of nitroglycerin. *Circulation,* **1967,** *36,* 734–751.

Parratt, J. R., and Wadsworth, R. M. The effects of dipyridamole on coronary post-occlusion hyperaemia and on myocardial vasodilatation induced by systemic hypoxia. *Br. J. Pharmac.,* **1972,** *46,* 594–601.

Prichard, B. N. C., and Gillam, P. M. S. Assessment of propranolol in angina pectoris. Clinical dose response curve and effect on electrocardiogram at rest and on exercise. *Br. Heart J.,* **1971,** *33,* 473–480.

Redwood, D. R.; Rosing, D. R.; Goldstein, R. E.; Beiser, G. D.; and Epstein, S. E. Importance of the design of an exercise protocol in the evaluation of patients with angina pectoris. *Circulation,* **1971,** *43,* 618–628.

Robinson, B. F. Mode of action of nitroglycerin in angina pectoris: correlation between haemodynamic effects during exercise and prevention of pain. *Br. Heart J.,* **1968,** *30,* 295–302.

Rowe, G. G.; Chelius, C. J.; Afonso, S.; Gurtner, H. P.; and Crumpton, C. W. Systemic and coronary hemodynamic effects of erythrol tetranitrate. *J. clin. Invest.,* **1961,** *40,* 1217–1222.

Schelling, J.-L., and Lasagna, L. A study of cross-tolerance to circulatory effects of organic nitrates. *Clin. Pharmac. Ther.,* **1967,** *8,* 256–260.

Stafford, A. Potentiation of adenosine and the adenine nucleotides by dipyridamole. *Br. J. Pharmac. Chemother.,* **1966,** *28,* 218–227.

Stipe, A. A., and Fink, G. B. Prophylactic therapy of angina pectoris with organic nitrates: relationship of drug efficacy and clinical experimental design. *J. clin. Pharmac.,* **1973,** *13,* 244–250.

Vogelpoel, L.; Schrire, V.; Nellen, M.; and Swanepoel, A. The use of amyl nitrite in the differentiation of Fallot's tetralogy and pulmonary stenosis with intact ventricular septum. *Am. Heart J.,* **1959,** *57,* 803–819.

Weiss, H. R., and Winbury, M. M. Intracoronary nitroglycerin, pentaerythritol trinitrate and dipyridamole on intramyocardial oxygen tension. *Microvasc. Res.,* **1972,** *4,* 273–284.

Weiss, S.; Wilkins, R. W.; and Haynes, F. W. The nature of circulatory collapse induced by sodium nitrite. *J. clin. Invest.,* **1937,** *16,* 73–84.

Whitworth, C. G., and Grant, W. M. Use of nitrite and nitrate vasodilators by glaucomatous patients. *Archs Ophthal., N.Y.,* **1964,** *71,* 492–496.

Wilkins, R. W.; Haynes, F. W.; and Weiss, S. The role of the venous system in circulatory collapse induced by sodium nitrite. *J. clin. Invest.,* **1937,** *16,* 85–91.

Winbury, M. M.; Howe, B. B.; and Weiss, H. R. Effect of nitroglycerin and dipyridamole on epicardial and endocardial oxygen tension—further evidence for redistribution of myocardial blood flow. *J. Pharmac. exp. Ther.,* **1971,** *176,* 184–199.

Zetterquist, S. Muscle and skin clearance of antipyrine from exercising ischemic legs before and after vasodilating trials. *Acta med. scand.,* **1968,** *183,* 487–496.

Monographs and Reviews

Aronow, W. S. The medical treatment of angina pectoris. V. Long-acting nitrites as antianginal drugs. *Am. Heart J.,* **1972,** *84,* 567–569.

Becker, L., and Pitt, B. Regional myocardial blood flow, ischemia and antianginal drugs. *Ann. clin. Res.,* **1971,** *3,* 353–361.

Epstein, S. E. Hypotension, nitroglycerin, and acute myocardial infarction. *Circulation,* **1973,** *47,* 217–219.

Gensini, G. G. (ed.). *The Study of the Systemic, Coronary and Myocardial Effects of Nitrates.* Charles C Thomas, Pub., Springfield, Ill., **1972.**

Goldstein, R. E., and Epstein, S. E. Nitrates in the prophylactic treatment of angina pectoris. *Circulation,* **1973,** *48,* 917–920.

McGregor, M. Drugs for the treatment of angina pectoris. In, *Clinical Pharmacology,* Vol. 2. *International Encyclopedia of Pharmacology and Therapeutics,* Sect. 6. (Lasagna, L., ed.) Pergamon Press, Ltd., Oxford, **1966,** pp. 377–403.

McGregor, M., and Fam, W. On the site of vasomotion in the coronary vascular bed. In, *The Study of the Systemic, Coronary and Myocardial Effects of Nitrates.* (Gensini, G. G., ed.) Charles C Thomas, Pub., Springfield, Ill., **1972,** pp. 323–333.

McHenry, L. C., Jr. Cerebral vasodilator therapy in stroke. *Stroke,* **1972,** *3,* 686–691.

Moir, T. W. Subendocardial distribution of coronary blood flow and the effect of antianginal drugs. *Circulation Res.,* **1972,** *30,* 621–627.

Symposium. (Various authors.) Clinical studies of peripheral circulation: an international symposium. (Dahn, I., and Lassen, N. A., eds.) *Scand. J. clin. Lab. Invest.,* **1967,** Suppl. 99, 1–248.

Symposium. (Various authors.) Perhexiline. *Postgrad. med. J.,* **1973,** *49,* Suppl. 3, 1–132.

CHAPTER

35 DRUGS USED IN THE PREVENTION AND TREATMENT OF ATHEROSCLEROSIS

Howard A. Eder

Atherosclerosis is manifested anatomically by the occurrence in arteries of atheromatous plaques—pearly gray, elevated lesions that start in the intimal wall of the arteries and contain soft lipid deposits called atheromata. The disease affects large- and medium-sized arteries, including the cerebral, vertebral, coronary, and renal arteries, the aorta, and the principal arteries to the legs. The most important clinical complications of atherosclerosis are coronary heart disease, cerebral vascular disease, and peripheral vascular disease. These complications are, by far, the major cause of death in the United States. Degenerative and arteriosclerotic heart disease is responsible for about one third of deaths from all causes, while cerebral vascular disease is the third most common cause of fatality in the United States, after heart disease and cancer.

Much attention has deservedly been given to the etiology, prevention, and treatment of coronary heart disease, and many prospective studies have demonstrated the presence of certain risk factors that appear to predispose an individual to coronary heart disease. Among these are hyperlipemia, hypertension, cigarette smoking, obesity, sedentary habits, and a positive family history (*see* Cornfield and Mitchell, 1969). In this chapter, attention will be directed toward the use of drugs that are effective in lowering the concentrations of plasma lipids. It must, however, be emphasized that other measures, such as the treatment of hypertension and the cessation of cigarette smoking, are equally important in decreasing the risk of coronary heart disease (*see* Task Force on Arteriosclerosis, 1971).

THE RELATIONSHIP BETWEEN ATHEROSCLEROSIS AND LIPID METABOLISM

The recognition by pathologists in the nineteenth century that lipid deposition is a characteristic fea-

ture of atherosclerosis has emphasized the relationship between atherosclerosis and lipid metabolism. The importance of this relationship has been constantly reaffirmed by further study of the problem. In 1950, Gertler and associates reported that, in patients with coronary heart disease, plasma cholesterol concentrations are higher than in non-affected populations. Subsequently, Albrink and Mann (1959) demonstrated that triglyceride concentrations are also higher in patients with coronary heart disease. In 1950, Gofman and coworkers reported increased concentrations of low-density lipoproteins in patients with coronary heart disease, and this has been confirmed in many other studies by different technics for the measurement of lipoproteins (Barr *et al.,* 1951). In diseases such as familial hypercholesterolemia and diabetes, in which concentrations of low-density lipoproteins are increased, the incidence of atherosclerosis of the coronary arteries is markedly increased. Similarly, in large-scale prospective studies such as those carried out in Framingham, Massachusetts, it was shown that, in a group of middle-aged males followed over a period of 14 years, the incidence of the new occurrence of coronary heart disease was greatest in those individuals with the highest concentrations of plasma lipids and lipoproteins (Kannel *et al.,* 1967). Data obtained earlier in this study showed that the higher the concentration of plasma lipids and lipoproteins the greater was the incidence of coronary heart disease; it also showed that the presence of elevated blood pressure in individuals with elevated concentrations of plasma lipids and lipoproteins increased the risk of coronary heart disease.

It is well known that in those areas of the world, usually the underdeveloped countries, where the mean plasma cholesterol concentration is low, the incidence of coronary heart disease is much lower than in nations such as those in Europe and North America where the plasma lipid concentrations in the population are higher. During World War II, the incidence of coronary heart disease appeared to decrease appreciably in certain countries of Europe at a time when plasma cholesterol concentrations fell, probably in response to changes in diet (Malmros, 1950). In virtually all animals, it has been shown that measures that increase plasma cholesterol concentration produce lesions similar to atherosclerosis in man.

This evidence, while admittedly indirect, strongly suggests that maintenance of plasma lipoprotein concentrations at low levels might well reduce the incidence of coronary heart disease and perhaps other forms of atherosclerosis. Nevertheless, it must be emphasized that definitive clinical studies on the effects of lowering plasma lipid concentrations are only now in progress. Until such data are available, all conclusions regarding the desirability of therapy directed at lowering plasma lipid and lipoprotein concentrations must be considered tentative.

There are two problems that must be considered in relation to therapy. The first is that of the prevention of atherosclerosis in populations at high risk. Since plasma lipoprotein concentrations rise to their adult values during youth, such measures must begin in young individuals. Because of the large number of people involved, and because patients will be treated for a long period of time, any therapy used must have a very large factor of safety. The second problem is that of treatment of individuals with a high risk of developing coronary heart disease. In certain diseases, the risk of acquiring coronary heart disease is greatly increased. Thus, in patients with familial hypercholesterolemia, the occurrence of myocardial infarction in young people is frequent (Epstein et al., 1959). As mentioned previously, the Framingham study showed that hypertension is important as a predisposing cause of coronary heart disease. In Japan, where the incidence of atherosclerosis is low, it is rare to find coronary heart disease in patients with hypertension (Switzer, 1963). Patients with coronary heart disease constitute a special group since the incidence of repeated myocardial infarction is high. The experience during World War II and studies in animals suggest that atherosclerosis may be reversible, and this has encouraged efforts to treat patients with coronary heart disease. In such patients it is perhaps possible to justify the use of agents with a lesser factor of safety. The greater risk, the smaller number of patients involved, and the opportunities for closer observation make this problem different from that of prevention of the disease in the population as a whole.

PLASMA LIPIDS AND LIPOPROTEINS

Many studies of the etiology of atherosclerosis and the effect of therapy thereon depend on measurement of plasma lipids and lipoproteins. The major classes of the plasma lipids are the triglycerides, phospholipids, free cholesterol, cholesterol esters, and free fatty acids. All these lipids, with the exception of the free fatty acids that are bound to albumin,

are present in the plasma as constituents of lipoproteins (see Fredrickson and Levy, 1972; Holmes et al., 1972).

The plasma lipoproteins can be separated into four major classes (Table 35-1). Because of a varying ratio of lipid to protein, their densities differ, and such separation can thus be accomplished by ultracentrifugation; the plasma lipoproteins are also separable by electrophoresis. The patterns of abnormalities observed form the basis for classification of the pathological hyperlipoproteinemias.

The largest lipoprotein particles, the chylomicrons, contain the most lipid and are thus the least dense. They have high molecular weights (10^9 to 10^{10}) and consist of a core of nonpolar lipids (mostly triglycerides) surrounded by a coat of protein, phospholipid, and free cholesterol. Chylomicrons are secreted into the intestinal lymphatics by the intestinal mucosa following the absorption of a lipid-containing meal, and their triglycerides are eventually stored in adipose tissue.

The very-low-density lipoproteins (VLDL), the other triglyceride-rich lipoproteins of plasma, have molecular weights of approximately 5×10^6. These molecules are secreted by the liver, and their triglyceride is in part derived from dietary carbohydrate. Like the chylomicrons, these triglycerides are destined for storage in adipose tissue. On conventional electrophoresis, the VLDL migrate between the β- or low-density lipoproteins (LDL) and the α- or high-density lipoproteins (HDL); the VLDL are thus termed pre-β-lipoproteins in this electrophoretic scheme. Because of the high triglyceride content of the chylomicrons and the VLDL, an increase in their concentration is accompanied by elevation in the concentration of the plasma triglycerides; if this value is sufficiently high, the plasma may be lactescent.

The LDL have molecular weights of 2.3×10^6 and the electrophoretic mobility of β-globulins. These lipoproteins contain the major portion of the total plasma cholesterol. When LDL are present in increased concentration, plasma cholesterol concentration is increased, while the triglyceride concentration is relatively normal.

The HDL are considerably smaller particles of two characterized types: HDL-2, with molecular weights of 186,000; and HDL-3, with molecular weights of 340,000. These lipoproteins have the electrophoretic

Table 35-1. **PROPERTIES OF THE PLASMA LIPOPROTEINS**

LIPOPROTEIN CLASS	DENSITY	ELECTRO-PHORETIC MOBILITY (PAPER)	*Free Cholesterol*	*Cholesterol Esters*	*Phospholipids*	*Triglycerides*	*Protein*
			CHEMICAL COMPOSITION				
			Percent of Class by Weight				
Chylomicrons	<0.95	origin	3.1	6.0	7.1	81.3	2.5
Very low density (VLDL)	<0.95–1.006	pre-β	6.0	16.2	17.9	51.8	7.1
Low density (LDL)	1.006–1.063	β	7.5	39.4	23.1	9.3	20.7
High density (HDL)	1.063–1.21	α	2.0	17.4	26.1	8.1	46.4

mobility of α-globulins and contain about 50% protein; of their lipids, phospholipids predominate.

It is thus possible to classify patients with hyperlipemia on the basis of their plasma lipoprotein pattern (*see* Fredrickson and Levy, 1972). Such classification would be particularly valuable if it could be used as the basis for appropriate treatment of patients with various types of hyperlipoproteinemia. Many workers believe that this is the case. Table 35-2 represents such a classification. It is to be emphasized that the etiology of a given pattern may be genetic, sporadic, or secondary to various other disorders. Possible secondary causes must obviously be investigated. In addition, a given pathophysiological entity may be the cause of more than one abnormal lipoprotein pattern. Discussion of the genetics, enzymatic deficiencies, and secondary causes of these diseases is beyond the scope of this text; the interested reader is referred to the review by Fredrickson and Levy (1972).

Three types of abnormalities occur commonly, and involve the VLDL and the LDL, the two classes of lipoproteins for which there is a positive correlation between plasma concentration and the incidence of atherosclerosis. *Hypercholesterolemia (type IIa)* may be genetic, sporadic, or secondary to various defined causes (*e.g.,* hypothyroidism, nephrotic syndrome, myeloma, excess dietary cholesterol). If genetic, clinical manifestations of the disorder are usually evident before the age of 30; the risk of vascular disease is greatly increased, and about 50% of individuals have myocardial infarction before the age of 50. *Combined hyperlipemia (type IIb)* is also common; both plasma cholesterol and triglyceride concentrations are elevated. In a study of 500 survivors of myocardial infarction, one third had hyperlipemia; familial combined hyperlipemia, often associated with a type-IIb lipoprotein pattern, was the most common genetic cause and accounted for 30% of the hyperlipemic group (*see* Goldstein *et al.,* 1973). *Hypertriglyceridemia (type IV)* is also encountered frequently and is likewise associated with an increased risk of atherosclerosis (Carlson and Böttiger, 1972; Patterson and Slack, 1972). These patients exhibit sensitivity to carbohydrate; that is, a diet high in carbohydrate results in elevated plasma concentrations of VLDL, the triglyceride of which is in part synthesized from carbohydrate by the liver. Glucose tolerance is commonly abnormal, and diabetes mellitus is frequently associated with such an excess of VLDL.

TREATMENT OF HYPERLIPEMIA

Before considering the treatment of hyperlipemia, it is, of course, essential to define the disorder. It is generally agreed that a patient whose plasma cholesterol and triglyceride values lie above those for 95% of the population of the same age group is in the abnormal range and requires treatment. However, since it is also considered that "normal" values in the United States are "high," many workers agree with the suggestion of Levy and coworkers (1972) that any person whose plasma cholesterol concentration is greater than 200 mg/100 ml plus his age in years and whose plasma triglyceride concentration exceeds 150 mg/100 ml has sufficient hyperlipemia to require attention; this, however, does *not necessarily* mean drug therapy. Since the plasma lipid concentrations in patients with hyperlipemia can often be reduced by proper dietary management, all such individuals should have an adequate trial on an appropriately designed diet before institution of drug treatment (*see* Handbook, 1970).

DRUGS AFFECTING PLASMA LIPOPROTEIN CONCENTRATION

With increased interest in the prevention of coronary heart disease and the recognition of the role of hyperlipoproteinemia as a risk factor, a number of drugs have become available for the treatment of hyperlipemia. These agents vary markedly in both their clinical effects and their mechanisms, and there is now evidence indicating that certain drugs are more effective in one type of hyperlipoproteinemia than in others. Only the agents of major importance are discussed

Table 35-2. CLASSIFICATION OF PRIMARY HYPERLIPOPROTEINEMIAS

TYPE	LIPOPROTEIN CLASS AFFECTED	SYNONYMS
I	Chylomicrons	Fat-induced or exogenous hyperlipemia
IIa	β-Lipoproteins (LDL)	Sporadic or familial hypercholesterolemia
IIb	β-Lipoproteins and pre-β-lipoproteins (LDL and VLDL)	Combined hyperlipoproteinemia
III	Abnormal very-low-density (β) lipoproteins	Broad-beta disease
IV	Pre-β-lipoproteins (VLDL)	Carbohydrate-induced or endogenous hyperlipemia
V	Chylomicrons and pre-β-lipoproteins (VLDL)	Mixed hyperlipemia

in this chapter—clofibrate, anion-exchange resins, and nicotinic acid; the status of thyroid hormones and estrogens is also presented.

CLOFIBRATE

In the course of screening tests in rats, Thorp and Waring (1962, 1963) found that a series of aryloxyisobutyric acids were effective in reducing plasma total lipid and cholesterol concentrations. The compound that combined maximal effectiveness with minimal toxicity was clofibrate. Since then, it has been widely used in man and there is now considerable evidence that, in appropriate cases, it is a very effective drug.

Chemistry. Clofibrate, the ethyl ester of *p*-chlorophenoxyisobutyric acid, has the following structural formula:

Clofibrate

Effects on Plasma Lipids. Clofibrate characteristically reduces the plasma triglyceride concentration by lowering the levels of VLDL within 2 to 5 days after initiation of therapy. In most patients, plasma cholesterol and LDL concentrations also fall. However, a large fall in VLDL may be accompanied by a *rise* in LDL, such that the net effect on cholesterol may be slight. The mean value of plasma cholesterol was reduced only 6% in men treated chronically with clofibrate (1.8 g per day) during the Coronary Drug Project (1975); the reduction in plasma triglyceride was 22%. Clofibrate does appear to cause mobilization of cholesterol from tissues, and xanthomatous deposits often regress.

Mechanism of Action. The sites of action of clofibrate are only partially established, and the details of its mechanism of action are largely lacking. It is known to cause inhibition of the hepatic synthesis of cholesterol in the rat (Avoy *et al.,* 1965). In humans, clofibrate also causes inhibition of cholesterol synthesis and increased excretion of neutral sterols (Grundy *et al.,* 1969). Since, as noted, clofibrate is more effective in lowering plasma triglycerides than plasma cholesterol in man (Hunninghake *et al.,* 1969), attention has also been directed to effects of this drug on lipids other than cholesterol. The effect of the drug on VLDL appears to be due primarily to an enhanced rate of their removal from the circulation (Segal *et al.,* 1972; Wolfe *et al.,* 1973). Hepatic synthesis of VLDL is not altered consistently.

Absorption, Fate, and Excretion. In man, clofibrate is completely absorbed from the intestine and appears in the plasma as the deesterified *p*-chlorophenoxyisobutyric acid (CPIB); peak plasma concentrations of the acid occur within 4 hours after the oral administration of clofibrate. The major fraction of CPIB is bound to plasma albumin. The elimination of CPIB proceeds in two kinetic phases, with the slower exponential phase having a mean half-time of 15 hours. Essentially all the acid is excreted in the urine, about 60% as the glucuronide. Concurrent administration of cholestyramine and clofibrate causes only a slight delay in the attainment of peak plasma concentrations of clofibrate. This is an important consideration, since concurrent use of these two drugs may prove to be more effective for certain patients.

Untoward Effects. Clofibrate is well tolerated in man, but occasional patients experience nausea or diarrhea. Drowsiness, weakness, and giddiness have been noted. Langer and Levy (1968) have described an acute syndrome with severe muscle cramps, stiffness, weakness, and muscle tenderness in several patients treated with clofibrate. In these individuals, creatinine phosphokinase was elevated as well as glutamic oxaloacetic transaminase; these enzymes are not infrequently elevated in patients receiving clofibrate. The drug enhances the effect of coumarin anticoagulants, presumably by their displacement from plasma albumin, so that it is necessary in patients receiving both agents to perform frequent determinations of prothrombin time; a reduction in the dose of the anticoagulant drug is usually required (*see* Chapter 65). The drug is contraindicated in patients with impaired renal or hepatic function and in pregnant or nursing women. In males, clofibrate has been reported to cause tenderness of the breasts and to decrease libido.

Preparation, Dosage, and Therapeutic Uses. *Clofibrate,* U.S.P. (ATROMID-S), is available as official capsules containing 500 mg. The drug is administered orally in a dose of 2 g daily, in two or four portions. It is quite effective in reducing the levels of VLDL and, therefore, can be used in hyperlipoproteinemias of types III, IV, and V, and probably in type IIb. Clofibrate is particularly effective in type-III (broad-beta) disease. Opinions differ as to whether clofibrate is effective in type-II hyperlipoproteinemia, and there is probably a great variability of response of the concentration of plasma cholesterol in these patients.

The clinical evidence for the usefulness of clofibrate in preventing deaths from coronary heart disease is incomplete. A number of clinical trials, especially in Great Britain, have suggested that clofibrate therapy reduced the mortality rate in patients with a history of coronary heart disease (*see* Dewar and Oliver, 1971). In these trials, the alleged benefit did not correlate with changes in plasma lipids, and the suggestion has been made that it may be related to removal of cholesterol from slowly metabolized pools, without affecting the concentration of plasma cholesterol, or that it may be unrelated to lipid metabolism and result from other factors, such as inhibition of blood coagulation or thrombosis (Havel and Kane, 1973). To date, the value of clofibrate therapy in the secondary prevention of myocardial infarction in patients with known coronary heart disease remains unproven. Indeed, in the Coronary Drug Project (1975), patients receiving clofibrate for 5 years or more experienced an excess incidence of thromboembolism, angina pectoris, intermittent claudication, and cardiac arrhythmias, and a twofold increase in incidence of gallstones, without any salutary effect on the preexisting coronary heart disease or reduction of total or coronary mortality.

Since clofibrate may increase the LDL concentrations in some patients, the effect of the drug should be monitored by repeated analysis of the plasma lipoprotein pattern. If a shift from VLDL to LDL occurs, it may be necessary to discontinue use of the drug.

BILE ACID–SEQUESTERING RESINS

The first of these agents, *cholestyramine,* was originally used to control pruritus in patients with elevated plasma bile acid concentrations due to cholestasis. While this remains a valid use of the drug, greater interest now centers on the ability of this and similar agents to lower concentrations of plasma cholesterol.

Chemistry. Cholestyramine is the chloride salt of a basic anion-exchange resin. The ion-exchange sites are provided by trimethylbenzylammonium groups in a large copolymer of styrene and divinylbenzene. The average polymeric molecular weight is greater than 10^6. Cholestyramine has the following structural formula:

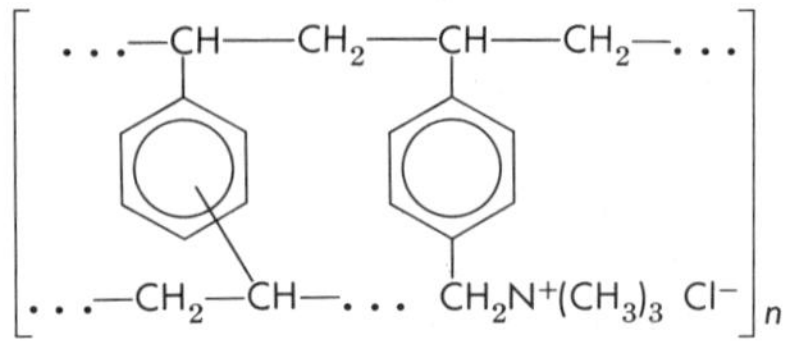

Cholestyramine

A second resin, colestipol hydrochloride, is a copolymer of diethyl pentamine and epichlorohydrin. The tentative structural formula of colestipol is as follows:

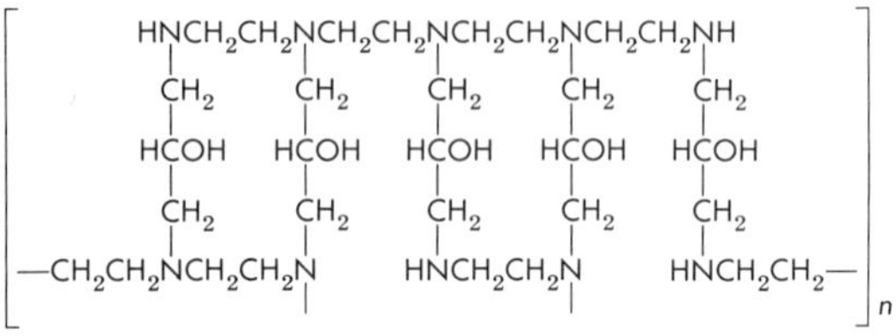

Colestipol

Effects on Plasma Lipids. These resins, administered orally, are not absorbed. They act to bind bile acids in the intestine, and there is thus a large increase in the fecal excretion of the acids. The removal of bile acids increases the hepatic conversion of cholesterol to bile acids, since the acids inhibit the microsomal hydroxylase that catalyzes the rate-limiting step in this reaction sequence (*see* Mosbach, 1969). Furthermore, since bile acids are required for the intestinal absorption (and enterohepatic reabsorption) of cholesterol, there is some additional fecal loss of neutral sterol. Unfortunately, in many patients a compensatory increase in the rate of cholesterol biosynthesis limits the degree of negative cholesterol balance that is obtained (Myant, 1972).

It is logical that the LDL of man are the most altered in response to the administration of a bile acid–sequestering resin. Plasma cholesterol concentrations fall, particularly during the first 2 weeks of therapy. In one study the average reduction of plasma cholesterol in 60 patients with familial hyperbetalipoproteinemia treated with 12 to

24 g of cholestyramine per day was 25%. If treatment with resin is stopped, plasma cholesterol rises rapidly. While there is usually little effect on plasma triglycerides, it is noteworthy that they may increase modestly in some patients.

Untoward Effects and Drug Interactions. These preparations often have an unpleasant sandy or gritty quality, and patients may complain of this. Nausea and constipation are frequent difficulties, and one case of intestinal impaction of cholestyramine has been reported. A large intake of fluid and a diet high in bulk minimize constipation.

With high doses of resins steatorrhea may occur, and preexisting steatorrhea is aggravated by conventional doses. In such cases, the absorption of fat-soluble vitamins is also impaired and vitamin supplementation is recommended. Hypoprothrombinemia has been observed.

The resins obviously may also bind other compounds in the intestine, including drugs administered concurrently. This has been noted particularly with chlorothiazide, phenylbutazone, phenobarbital, anticoagulants, thyroxine, and various digitalis preparations. Cholestyramine has been recommended for the treatment of digitalis intoxication (*see* Chapter 31). As a general rule, it is recommended that other drugs taken orally should be ingested at least 1 hour before or 4 hours after the resin.

Preparations, Dosage, and Therapeutic Uses. *Cholestyramine Resin, U.S.P.* (CUEMID, QUESTRAN), is available in packets of 4 g of resin or in containers of 216 g. *Colestipol hydrochloride* (COLESTID) is not yet generally available. Cholestyramine is administered orally, usually in daily doses of 12 to 32 g, divided into three or four portions to be taken either before meals or before meals and at bedtime. The resin must not be swallowed dry and should be mixed with a pulpy fruit or a liquid.

Cholestyramine and colestipol are most effective in primary hyperbetalipoproteinemia (type IIa) and should be combined with a cholesterol-lowering diet in the treatment of this disorder. In patients with type-IIb lipoprotein patterns, only the LDL are significantly reduced by resin therapy. These agents are of no known benefit in disease of type III, IV, or V. Long-term, prospective studies are now being conducted to evaluate the efficacy of such agents in lowering plasma cholesterol in large populations and in reducing the incidence and consequences of coronary vascular disease.

NICOTINIC ACID

In 1955, Altschul and coworkers showed that large doses of nicotinic acid lower plasma cholesterol concentrations. This property is not shared by nicotinamide and appears to have nothing to do with the role of these compounds as vitamins. The chemistry of nicotinic acid and its function as a vitamin are discussed in Chapter 73.

Effects on Plasma Lipids. When given chronically in large doses, nicotinic acid is effective in lowering the concentrations of both plasma cholesterol and triglycerides in various types of hyperlipoproteinemias. Except for patients with type-III disease, the reduction in cholesterol is usually modest and the reduction in triglyceride is considerably greater (*see* Carlson and Walldius, 1972). In the Coronary Drug Project (1975), cholesterol and triglyceride concentrations were reduced by 10% and 26%, respectively, in men receiving 3 g of nicotinic acid daily.

The *mechanism of action* of nicotinic acid is as yet unclear (*see* Nikkela, 1972). Experiments with isolated fat cells have shown that the drug inhibits the accumulation of cyclic adenosine 3',5'-monophosphate (cyclic AMP) that is stimulated by a variety of lipolytic hormones (Butcher *et al.,* 1968). Lipolysis in adipose tissue is controlled by the concentration of cyclic AMP, which activates a triglyceride lipase. With reduced activity of this enzyme, there is a decreased release of free fatty acid, leading in turn to decreased formation of triglyceride in the liver and hence to diminished release of triglyceride into the plasma.

Other actions of nicotinic acid may also result in reduced triglyceride concentrations in plasma. There is evidence that the drug accelerates the removal of chylomicron triglycerides from the circulation as the result of increased activity of lipoprotein lipase, the enzyme necessary for triglyceride transport into adipose tissue. Furthermore, Langer and associates (1972) have demonstrated that the administration of nicotinic acid reduces the rate of synthesis of LDL in patients with type-II hyperlipoproteinemia. This latter action may explain the effect of the drug on plasma cholesterol.

Untoward Effects. There are several untoward effects of nicotinic acid that limit its usefulness and dictate its relatively minor role in therapy.

The drug produces intense cutaneous flush and pruritus. While these reactions decrease in intensity in most individuals after they have been on therapy for several weeks, they are unpleasant and result in poor patient compliance. There is disagreement as to whether slow upward adjustment of dosage makes this problem better or worse. Gastrointestinal disturbances such as vomiting, diarrhea, and dyspepsia are also common, and peptic ulceration has been reported.

Abnormalities of hepatic function occur in patients taking large doses of nicotinic acid. These include jaundice, a decrease in BSP excretion, and increases of plasma transaminase activities. Hyperglycemia and abnormal glucose tolerance occur in more than half of nondiabetic patients taking nicotinic acid. Plasma uric acid may also be elevated, and the incidence of acute gouty arthritis is increased.

Preparations, Dosage, and Therapeutic Uses. Preparations of *nicotinic acid* (*niacin*) are described in Chapter 73. *Aluminum nicotinate* (NICALEX) is also marketed; it is a complex of aluminum hydroxynicotinate and nicotinic acid. It is hydrolyzed to aluminum hydroxide and nicotinic acid in the gastrointestinal tract. There are no advantages to this preparation, and the aluminum hydroxide may cause decreased absorption of other drugs. The usual dosage of nicotinic acid is 1.5 to 6 g daily; the equivalent for aluminum nicotinate is 1.87 to 7.5 g per day. The daily dose is divided into three or four portions, taken orally with or after meals.

Nicotinic acid is most useful in the treatment of patients with homozygous familial hypercholesterolemia, in whom optimal dietary and resin therapy have not resulted in restoration of plasma lipids to normal. In these patients, as well as others with hypercholesterolemia, the addition of nicotinic acid to such a regimen often produces marked reduction in the concentration of plasma cholesterol. However, the flushing and pruritus are side effects that are difficult to cope with, and the dropout rate of patients on this medication is high.

As with the administration of clofibrate, there is no evidence that treatment with nicotinic acid reduces the mortality rate in men with proven coronary heart disease (Coronary Drug Project, 1975); while the patients receiving nicotinic acid did have significantly fewer myocardial infarctions, the incidence of cardiac arrhythmias was higher.

Because nicotinic acid reduces both LDL and VLDL, it may be effective in all types of hyperlipoproteinemias except type I, and the drug may be used for patients in whom other more agreeable therapy is inadequate. However, in many of these patients the effect of nicotinic acid to impair glucose tolerance and to aggravate or induce hyperuricemia may be particularly disadvantageous.

THYROID HORMONES

Patients with hypothyroidism have elevated concentrations of plasma lipids; when such patients are treated with thyroid hormone, the plasma lipid concentrations decrease, often before there is a significant return of other measurements, such as pulse rate or basal metabolic rate, to normal. Patients with hyperthyroidism often have low concentrations of plasma cholesterol. These findings have led to the attempt to reduce plasma lipid and lipoprotein concentrations in euthyroid individuals by the administration of thyroid hormones. The amounts of hormone required are such as to increase tissue O_2 consumption appreciably, and in patients with coronary heart disease this often produces anginal attacks and can cause myocardial infarction.

The thyroid hormones exert a marked effect on cholesterol metabolism; they cause increased synthesis of cholesterol in the liver, but they also produce increased excretion of sterol in the feces and increased conversion of cholesterol to bile acids. In order to lower plasma cholesterol, the increase in the rate of the latter processes must necessarily be greater than the increase in the rate of cholesterol synthesis (Myant, 1964).

The report that thyroacetic acid analogs of thyroxine can produce a lowering of plasma cholesterol concentration without an increase in basal metabolic rate (Lerman and Pitt-Rivers, 1955) led to the study of a number of analogs of thyroid hormones in an attempt to find agents that affect plasma lipid concentrations without increasing metabolism. D-Thyroxine, the optical isomer of the naturally occurring hormone, was found to lower the plasma cholesterol concentration in rats by 50% at a dose between $\frac{1}{10}$ and $\frac{1}{40}$ of that which produces a 50% increase in O_2 consumption and heart rate. The doses of L-thyroxine required to produce these same effects on cholesterol and O_2 consumption are approximately equal (Boyd and Oliver, 1960).

When D-thyroxine is administered to man in doses of 4 to 8 mg per day, the concentration of LDL is reduced on the average by about 20%. The concentration of VLDL is not changed significantly (Strisower *et al.*, 1968). The most serious adverse effect of this drug is an increase in frequency or severity of anginal attacks in patients with coronary heart disease. The incidence increases with the dose, so that at doses of 10 mg per day the occurrence of angina is frequent whereas at 4 mg per day it is uncommon. Other adverse effects are cardiac arrhythmias and the hypermetabolic effects associated with administration of thyroid hormones, such as nervousness, sweating, tremor, and insomnia. The drug potentiates the effect of concurrently administered oral anticoagulants (*see* Chapter 65).

In the Coronary Drug Project (1972) a large number of patients (survivors of a first myocardial infarction) were treated with D-thyroxine in doses of 6 mg per day. Although the drug did result in reduction in plasma lipid concentrations, there was *increased* mortality from coronary disease in these patients, and hence this portion of the drug study was discontinued. In addition, individuals treated with D-thyroxine developed decreased glucose tolerance, increased plasma bilirubin concentrations, and increased serum glutamic oxaloacetic transaminase and alkaline phosphatase activities.

Preparations, Dosage, and Therapeutic Uses.
Dextrothyroxine Sodium, N.F. (CHOLOXIN), is available as scored tablets containing 1, 2, 4, or 6 mg. The initial oral dose for adults is 1 mg daily for 1 month. This dose is increased by 1 mg at intervals of 1 month until a satisfactory effect is achieved or until a maximal daily dose of 8 mg is reached. For children, the initial daily dose is 0.05 mg/kg and the maximal dose is 4 mg.

Since dextrothyroxine has no consistent effect on VLDL, it is useful only for type-II hyperbetalipoproteinemia. In view of the results of the Coronary Drug Project described above, it is probably undesirable to use this drug in any but young individuals known to be free of coronary artery disease. Its use in hypothyroidism is reserved for patients in whom hypercholesterolemia persists despite adequate therapy with thyroid hormone.

ESTROGENS

The use of estrogens to alter plasma lipoprotein levels was suggested by the observation that young females, who have an appreciably lower incidence of coronary heart disease than do young males, have lower concentrations of LDL (Russ *et al.,* 1951). Following the daily administration of large doses of estrogens (ethinyl estradiol, 1 mg) to males with elevated levels of LDL, the plasma cholesterol decreases by 50% and the concentration of LDL decreases by 30%, while the concentration of HDL almost doubles (Russ *et al.,* 1955). On such large doses of estrogens, male patients experience gynecomastia, loss of libido, and impotence, and often mental depression. With smaller doses of estrogens, the effect on plasma lipoproteins is less, although it is possible to produce some effect with doses of ethinyl estradiol as low as 0.05 mg per day.

It has also been shown that the administration of estrogens results in an increased concentration of VLDL (and elevated plasma triglycerides). This finding, plus the undesirable side effects of estrogen administration in males, makes it highly unlikely that estrogens are useful agents for reducing plasma lipoprotein concentrations. A number of oral contraceptive agents contain estrogens as well as progestins, and the rise in plasma triglycerides observed after ingestion of these preparations is probably due to the estrogens, since progestational agents do not have this effect. Certain women taking oral contraceptives may experience marked hyperlipemia, and pancreatitis has been observed as an apparent result (Davidoff *et al.,* 1973). In the Coronary Drug Project (1973) conjugated estrogens were administered in doses of 2.5 and 5 mg per day. With both dose schedules there occurred an increase in the incidence of new problems related to the preexisting coronary heart disease, and therefore this drug was eliminated from the investigative program. These agents should no longer be considered to be efficacious in the treatment of hyperlipoproteinemia.

It has been reported that the administration of progestins to females with elevated concentrations of VLDL (type V) results in a marked lowering of the levels of these lipoproteins (Glueck *et al.,* 1969).

OTHER DRUGS

Samuel and associates (1967) have noted that the ingestion of *neomycin* in doses as low as 0.5 g per day was effective in lowering the plasma cholesterol concentration. This effect of the antibiotic is described in Chapter 58. Neomycin should be used for this purpose only in patients with type-IIa hyperlipoproteinemia that is not controlled by other measures.

A number of investigations have been conducted with *aminosalicylic acid,* especially in patients with type-II hyperlipoproteinemia. The drug was well tolerated at daily doses of 6 to 8 g and resulted in lowering of both plasma cholesterol and triglycerides. A highly purified preparation of aminosalicylic acid was used in these studies, and there was no evidence of the hepatotoxicity seen with the older preparations (*see* Barter *et al.,* 1974).

Albrink, M. J., and Mann, E. B. Serum triglycerides in coronary artery disease. *Archs intern. Med.,* **1959,** *103,* 4–8.

Altschul, R.; Hoffer, A.; and Stephen, J. D. Influence of nicotinic acid on serum cholesterol in man. *Archs Biochem. Biophys.,* **1955,** *54,* 558–559.

Avoy, D. R.; Swyryd, E. A.; and Gould, R. G. Effects of α-*p*-chlorophenoxyisobutyryl ethyl ester (CPIB) with and without androsterone on cholesterol biosynthesis in rat liver. *J. Lipid Res.,* **1965,** *6,* 369–376.

Barr, D. P.; Russ, E. M.; and Eder, H. A. Protein-lipid relationships in human plasma. II. In atherosclerosis and related conditions. *Am. J. Med.,* **1951,** *11,* 480–493.

Barter, P. J.; Connor, W. E.; Spector, A. A.; Armstrong, M.; Connor, S. L.; and Newman, M. A. Lowering of serum cholesterol and triglyceride by para-aminosalicylic acid in hyperlipoproteinemia. *Ann. intern. Med.,* **1974,** *81,* 619–624.

Butcher, R. W.; Baird, C. E.; and Sutherland, E. W. Effects of lipolytic and antilipolytic substances on adenosine 3′,5′-monophosphate levels in isolated fat cells. *J. biol. Chem.,* **1968,** *243,* 1705–1712.

Carlson, L. A., and Böttiger, L. E. Ischemic heart disease in relation to plasma values of triglycerides and cholesterol. *Lancet,* **1972,** *1,* 865–868.

Cornfield, J., and Mitchell, S. Selected risk factors in coronary disease. *Archs envir. Hlth,* **1969,** *19,* 382–394.

Coronary Drug Project. Findings leading to further modification of its protocol with respect to dextrothyroxine. *J. Am. med. Ass.,* **1972,** *220,* 996–1008.

———. Findings leading to discontinuation of the 2.5 mg/day estrogen group. *Ibid.,* **1973,** *226,* 652–657.

———. Clofibrate and niacin in coronary heart disease. *Ibid.,* **1975,** *231,* 360–381.

Davidoff, F.; Tishler, S.; and Rosoff, C. Marked hyperlipidemia and pancreatitis associated with oral contraceptive therapy. *New Engl. J. Med.,* **1973,** *289,* 552–555.

Dewar, H. A., and Oliver, M. F. Secondary prevention trials using clofibrate. A joint commentary on the Newcastle and Scottish trials. *Br. med. J.,* **1971,** *4,* 784–786.

Epstein, F. H.; Black, W. D.; Hand, E. A.; and Francis, T., Jr. Familial hypercholesterolemia, xanthomatosis and coronary heart disease. *Am. J. Med.,* **1959,** *26,* 39–53.

Gertler, M. M.; Garn, S. M.; and Lerman, J. The interrelationships of serum cholesterol, cholesterol esters and phospholipids in health and in coronary disease. *Circulation,* **1950,** *2,* 205–214.

Glueck, C. J.; Brown, W. V.; Levy, R. I.; Greten, H.; and Fredrickson, D. S. Amelioration of hypertriglyceridemia by progestational drugs in familial type V hyper-lipoproteinemias. *Lancet,* **1969,** *1,* 1290–1291.

Gofman, J. W.; Jones, H. B.; Lindgren, F. T.; Lyon, T. P.; Elliott, H. A.; and Strisower, B. Blood lipids and human atherosclerosis. *Circulation,* **1950,** *2,* 161–178.

Goldstein, J. L.; Schrott, H. G.; Hazzard, W. R.; Bierman, E. L.; and Motulsky, A. G. Hyperlipidemia in coronary heart disease. II. Genetic analysis of lipid levels in 176 families and delineation of a new inherited disorder, combined hyperlipidemia. *J. clin. Invest.,* **1973,** *52,* 1544–1568.

Grundy, S. M.; Ahrens, E. H., Jr.; Salen, G.; and Quintao, E. Mode of action of ATROMID-S on cholesterol metabolism in man. *J. clin. Invest.,* **1969,** *48,* 33a.

Hunninghake, D. B.; Tucker, D. R.; and Azarnoff, D. L. Long-term effects of clofibrate (ATROMID-S) on serum lipids in man. *Circulation,* **1969,** *39,* 675–683.

Kannel, W. B.; Castelli, W. P.; and McNamara, P. M. The coronary profile: 12-year follow-up in the Framingham study. *J. occup. Med.,* **1967,** *9,* 611–619.

Langer, T., and Levy, R. I. Acute muscular syndrome associated with administration of clofibrate. *New Engl. J. Med.,* **1968,** *279,* 856–858.

Langer, T.; Strober, W.; and Levy, R. I. The metabolism of low density lipoprotein in familial type II hyperlipoproteinemia. *J. clin. Invest.,* **1972,** *51,* 1528–1536.

Lerman, J., and Pitt-Rivers, R. Physiological activity of triiodothyroacetic acid. *J. clin. Endocr. Metab.,* **1955,** *15,* 653–655.

Levy, R. I.; Fredrickson, D. S.; Shulman, R.; Bilheimer, D. W.; Breslow, J. L.; Stone, N. J.; Lux, S. E.; Sloan, H. R.; Krauss, R. M.; and Herbert, P. N. Dietary and drug treatment of primary hyperlipoproteinemia. *Ann. intern. Med.,* **1972,** *77,* 267–294.

Malmros, H. Relation of nutrition to health: study of effect of wartime on arteriosclerosis, cardiosclerosis, tuberculosis and diabetes. *Acta med. scand.,* **1950,** *138,* Suppl. 246, 137–153.

Patterson, D., and Slack, J. Lipid abnormalities in male and female survivors of myocardial infarction and their first-degree relatives. *Lancet,* **1972,** *1,* 393–399.

Russ, E. M.; Eder, H. A.; and Barr, D. P. Protein-lipid relationships in human plasma. I. In normal individuals. *Am. J. Med.,* **1951,** *11,* 468–479.

———. Influence of gonadal hormones on protein-lipid relationships in human plasma. *Ibid.,* **1955,** *19,* 4–24.

Samuel, P.; Holtzman, C. M.; and Goldstein, J. Long-term reduction of serum cholesterol levels of patients with atherosclerosis by small doses of neomycin. *Circulation,* **1967,** *35,* 938–945.

Segal, P.; Roheim, P. S.; and Eder, H. A. Effect of clofibrate on lipoprotein metabolism in hyperlipidemic rats. *J. clin. Invest.,* **1972,** *51,* 1632–1638.

Strisower, E. H.; Adamson, G.; and Strisower, B. Treatment of hyperlipidemia. *Am. J. Med.,* **1968,** *45,* 488–501.

Switzer, S. Hypertension and ischemic heart disease in Hiroshima, Japan. *Circulation,* **1963,** *28,* 368–380.

Thorp, J. M., and Waring, W. S. Modification and distribution of lipids by ethyl chlorophenoxyisobutyrate. *Nature, Lond.,* **1962,** *194,* 948–949.

———. An experimental approach to the problem of disordered lipid metabolism. *J. Atheroscler. Res.,* **1963,** *3,* 351.

Wolfe, B. M.; Kane, J. P.; Havel, R. J.; and Brewster, H. P. Mechanism of the hypolipemic effect of clofibrate in postabsorptive man. *J. clin. Invest.,* **1973,** *52,* 2146–2159.

Monographs and Reviews

Boyd, G. S., and Oliver, M. F. Thyroid hormones and plasma lipids. *Br. med. Bull.,* **1960,** *16,* 138–142.

Carlson, L. A., and Walldius, G. Serum and tissue lipid metabolism and effect of nicotinic acid in different types of hyperlipidemia. *Adv. exp. Med. Biol.,* **1972,** *26,* 165–178.

Fredrickson, D. S. A physician's guide to hyperlipidemia. *Mod. Concepts cardiovasc. Dis.,* **1972,** *41,* 31–36.

Fredrickson, D. S., and Levy, R. I. Familial hyperlipoproteinemia. In, *The Metabolic Basis of Inherited Disease,* 3rd ed. (Stanbury, J. B.; Wyngaarden, J. B.; and Fredrickson, D. S.; eds.) McGraw-Hill Book Co., New York, **1972,** pp. 545–614.

Handbook. *The Dietary Management of Hyperlipoproteinemia: A Handbook for Physicians.* National Institutes of Health, NHLI, Bethesda, **1970.**

Havel, R. J., and Kane, J. P. Drugs and lipid metabolism. *A. Rev. Pharmac.,* **1973,** *13,* 287–308.

Holmes, W. L.; Paoletti, R.; and Kritchevsky, D. (eds.). Pharmacological control of lipid metabolism. *Adv. exp. Med. Biol.,* **1972,** *26,* 1–359.

Levy, R. I.; Morganroth, J.; and Rifkind, B. M. Treatment of hyperlipidemia. *New Engl. J. Med.,* **1974,** *290,* 1295–1301.

Mosbach, E. H. Effect of drugs on bile acid metabolism. *Adv. exp. Med. Biol.,* **1969,** *4,* 421–441.

Myant, N. B. The thyroid and lipid metabolism. In, *Lipid Pharmacology.* (Paoletti, R., ed.) Academic Press, Inc., New York, **1964,** pp. 299–323.

———. Effect of drugs on the metabolism of bile acids. *Adv. exp. Med. Biol.,* **1972,** *26,* 137–154.

Nikkela, E. A. Effect of drugs on plasma triglyceride metabolism. *Adv. exp. Med. Biol.,* **1972,** *26,* 113–133.

Task Force on Arteriosclerosis: National Heart and Lung Institute. *Arteriosclerosis,* Vol. 1. Department of Health, Education, and Welfare Publication No. (NIH) 72-137, U.S. Government Printing Office, Washington, D. C., **1971.**

SECTION

VII

Water, Salts, and Ions

CHAPTER

36 AGENTS AFFECTING VOLUME AND COMPOSITION OF BODY FLUIDS

Gilbert H. Mudge and Louis G. Welt

The volume and composition of the body fluids vary tremendously from one compartment to another and from one cell type to another, and are maintained remarkably constant despite the vicissitudes of daily life and the greater stresses imposed by disease. The organization of this remarkable system has developed over millions of years and permits the efficient regulation of homeostasis. The responsible mechanisms reside in a variety of organs and tissues, which include the central nervous system (CNS), the heart and the lungs, the gastrointestinal tract, the kidneys, and, to a remarkable extent, the cell membranes themselves. The failure of the kidney to repair a disordered state to a more nearly normal level is more commonly related to the unavailability of adequate raw material rather than to some primary renal disturbance *per se*. To the extent that this is true, it follows that the wisdom with which the raw materials are supplied may be crucial.

Disturbances in fluid and electrolyte metabolism involve four major properties of the body fluids—volume, osmolality, hydrogen ion concentration (pH), and the concentrations of specific ions. In some disease states an abnormality in one property may dominate the picture. However, severely ill patients often manifest multiple disturbances that coexist and interact. These require particularly thoughtful analysis to determine the separate contribution of each component and its appropriate management.

DISTURBANCES OF VOLUME AND OSMOLALITY

THE DISTRIBUTION AND THE COMPOSITION OF BODY FLUIDS

Distribution of Body Fluids. The total volume of body water in man varies between the approximate limits of 50 and 70% of the body weight. It tends to be closer to 50% in the obese and closer to 70% in the lean. This total volume is divided into two major compartments, the intracellular and the extracellular, and into a much smaller compartment, referred to as the transcellular. This last-named component includes fluids within the tracheobronchial tree, the gastrointestinal tract, the excretory system of the kidneys and glands, the cerebrospinal fluid, and the aqueous humor of the eye. The extracellular compartment is subdivided into two segments, the plasma and the interstitial fluid, with an approximate volume ratio of 1:3 (Maxwell and Kleeman, 1972).

The volumes of these several compartments may be estimated with the use of agents that distribute themselves uniformly throughout a particular compartment (Edelman *et al.,* 1952; Edelman and Leibman, 1959). In this fashion one can estimate the total volume of body water, the extracellular volume, and the plasma volume. The volume of the intracellular compartment cannot be estimated directly, but can be calculated as the difference between total body water and

Table 36-1.   THE MEASUREMENT AND DISTRIBUTION OF BODY WATER

COMPARTMENT	% TOTAL BODY WATER	AGENT USED FOR ESTIMATE *
Total Body Water (TBW)	100	DHO, THO, antipyrine
Intracellular Water (ICW)	55	By difference between TBW and ECW
Extracellular Water (ECW)	35	Inulin, SO_4^{2-}, Cl^-, Br^-
Plasma Volume (PV)	7.5	T1824, ^{131}I-albumin
Interstitial Fluid	27.5	By difference between ECW and PV
Inaccessible Bone Water	7.5	Special technics
Transcellular Water	2.5	Special technics

* DHO = deuterated water; THO = tritiated water; T1824 = plasma-bound dye.

the volume of the extracellular compartment.

A summary of these values and the agents used to estimate their magnitude are presented in Table 36-1.

Composition of Body Fluids.   There are vast differences in the composition of the two major compartments. There is, of course, more information about the extracellular phase, since this is composed of plasma and an ultrafiltrate thereof, and the plasma is accessible for analysis. An average composition for *plasma* is as follows:

CATIONS		ANIONS	
	(mEq/liter)		
Sodium	135–145	Chloride	98–106
Potassium	3.5–5.0	Bicarbonate	24–28
Calcium	4.5–5.3	Phosphate and sulfate	2–5
Magnesium	1.5–2.0	Organic anions	3–6
		Protein	15–20

The concentration of the filterable ions in the *interstitial fluid* can be calculated from the values in serum with a correction for serum water (SW) and the Donnan ratio, which describes the relative concentrations in serum and its ultrafiltrates. This ratio is 0.95 for cations and 1.05 for anions. The calculation is made in the following fashion:

$$Na_{IF} = \frac{Na_S}{SW} \times 0.95$$

$$Cl_{IF} = \frac{Cl_S}{SW} \times 1.05$$

where the subscripts IF and S refer to interstitial fluid and serum, respectively. For precise measurements it should be emphasized that the significant datum is the concentration of an ion in serum water, whereas a clinical laboratory usually reports the con-

centration per liter of serum. Under the vast majority of circumstances, this matters very little since the water content of serum (92%) is reasonably constant within the population and normally varies only to a negligible extent. Since the composition of the interstitial fluid is only slightly but predictably different from that of the plasma, for many purposes the plasma and interstitial fluids may be considered together as *extracellular fluid,* and the electrolyte concentrations in plasma may be used as an estimate of those for the entire compartment.

The composition of *intracellular fluid* is quite different. The major cations are potassium and magnesium with very little sodium, and the major anions are phosphate and protein with less bicarbonate and very little chloride. The composition of intracellular fluid is, of course, estimated with considerable indirection, since the only cells that can be obtained as such are erythrocytes and, to a lesser extent, leukocytes and platelets. Since these are rather specialized tissues, it would seem unlikely that they would necessarily reflect cell composition as a whole. Because muscle tissue represents the largest segment of intracellular fluid, its composition has been studied extensively. Even if one grants the validity of the figures thereby obtained by derived data, simple statements of concentrations per liter of intracellular water tell us little of the physicochemical state of these ions, the characteristics of the phosphate and protein anions, their valence, or other properties. Also, it must be recalled that the intracellular fluids of different tissues differ from each other, and, furthermore, that intracellular fluid is not likely to be homogeneous but probably varies in the several cellular organelles. With all these reservations in mind, it is still useful to examine the data for *muscle-cell fluid* and to compare these with the composition of plasma and interstitial fluid:

CATIONS		ANIONS	
	(mEq/liter)		
Sodium	10	Bicarbonate	10
Potassium	150	Phosphate and	
Magnesium	40	sulfate	150
		Protein	40

The composition of the body can also be studied by the use of radioactive isotopes and by calculation of what is referred to as the *total exchangeable quantity* of a given ion, such as that of sodium or potassium. The method involves the administration of a known quantity of radioactive material, the equilibration of the isotope with all the stable element with which it will readily equilibrate (usually 24 hours is required), the determination of the specific activity in serum, and the calculation of the total quantity of the ion that is exchangeable. This datum is then expressed in terms of some unit, usually a kilogram of body weight. Some of the most extensive data have been collected by Moore and associates (1963), and their values for *total exchangeable sodium, potassium, and chloride* in men and women are as follows:

	MALE	FEMALE
	(mEq/kg of Body Weight)	
Sodium	39.5	38.3
Potassium	48	39.4
Chloride	29.3	28.6

It is known from other analyses that about 75% of total body sodium and 85% of total body potassium are exchangeable.

Another isotopic technic takes advantage of the presence in the body of the naturally occurring isotope of potassium, ^{40}K. With measurement of its specific activity in plasma, the assumption of complete mixing in the entire potassium pool, and a knowledge of the number of counts ascribable to ^{40}K in the body by use of the total-body counter, one can compute the total quantity of potassium in the body. The values average 55 mEq/kg and 49 mEq/kg for male and female, respectively.

Cellular Mechanisms of Electrolyte Control. The manner by which the intracellular and extracellular fluids maintain their major compositional differences has been and continues to be under investigation. These ions are not at equilibrium but exist in a steady state away from equilibrium; this demands an energy-requiring series of operations, referred to in general as "active transport." In the steady-state condition, the concentration of sodium and potassium within the cell is dependent on the rate of pumping of sodium out and potassium in (by the Na^+,K^+-activated adenosine triphosphatase system) and the rates at which these ions move by passive diffusion along the established electrochemical gradients. This steady-state composition will be sustained as long as the extracellular environment does not change and as long as the characteristics of the membrane are stable and the pumping rates are constant.

These ionic transport mechanisms are responsible for the regulation of cell volume. For example, since the cells contain proteins that exert a colloidal osmotic pressure, the cell volume would expand and the cell ultimately disrupt were it not for the mechanisms of active transport that maintain the total quantity (as well as the quality) of the ions fairly constant. In addition, these mechanisms of transport serve to establish and maintain the electrical potential gradients across the cell membrane that are essential for the generation and propagation of action potentials in excitable cells.

Osmotic Pressure. The chief determinant of the passage of fluid from one compartment to another is a change in osmotic pressure (activity of water molecules). The total osmotic pressure of body fluids (300 milliosmoles per liter) is over 7 atmospheres. Those solutes that can freely permeate a cell membrane influence the total osmotic pressure but do not promote a redistribution of water. Those solutes that cannot permeate membranes by free diffusion contribute an *effective osmotic pressure* and one that is responsible for net movement of water.

INTERNAL EXCHANGES OF WATER AND SOLUTE

Intracellular and Extracellular Fluid Volumes. Almost all cell membranes are freely permeable to water. Exceptions include the sweat glands and the distal nephron. However, considering the major tissues of the body, as a consequence of the free diffusion of water, it follows that the extracellular and intracellular fluids are of equal osmolality, and that any transient alteration in the effective osmolality of one fluid must influence a net redistribution of water between the two components until the two fluids are once again of equal osmolality. Primary changes in osmolality occur most often in the extracellular fluid, but there is reason to believe that under some circumstances intracellular osmolality may be directly altered by marked changes in cell metabolism.

The principal determinant of the effective osmolality of the extracellular fluid is the concentration of sodium salts. These ions represent more than 90% of all extracellular solutes that contribute an *effective osmolality.*

Addition of Water. If a subject drinks water faster than he can excrete it, he develops a positive water balance. This water gains access initially to the extracellular phase, where it expands the volume and dilutes the solutes. The decrease in effective osmolality is accompanied by a net movement of water molecules from the extracellular space to the intracellular fluid. Obviously, this will cease when the two fluids are once again of equal osmolality, albeit lower than initially. The result is the distribution of the increment of water through the volume of total body water.

Addition of Salt. If a subject is administered sodium salt in a concentration in excess of that in his extracellular fluid, the concentration of sodium in the extracellular space will increase. Although more sodium tends to diffuse into cells, the rate of extrusion will match the enhanced entry. Thus, one can consider that the increment of salt is confined to the extracellular compartment. The addition of solute diminishes the activity of the molecules of extracellular water, and fewer water molecules enter intracellular fluid than leave it. This promotes a redistribution of water from cells to extracellular space until the two fluids are once again of equal osmolality, albeit higher than initially.

These same net effects on intracellular volume are observed if *hypo*natremia results from a loss of salt in excess of water, or if *hyper*natremia results as a consequence of the loss of water in excess of salt. However, in the last two circumstances, in addition to a redistribution of water between the two major compartments, total body fluid will have been diminished.

The corollary is, of course, that a gain or loss of a saline fluid that is isosmotic with body fluids will cause no shift of water between the cells and the extracellular compartments, but it will expand or contract extracellular volume.

Interstitial and Plasma Fluid Volumes. The same basic principles apply to the steady-state distribution of volume between these two components of the extracellular phase. The determinants are those factors that influence the activity of the molecules of water in the two fluids. The vascular endothelium is permeable to water and to *most* of the solutes. However, it is relatively *im*permeable to the larger molecular species such as proteins and lipids. The segregation of these molecules within the vascular component tends to diminish the activity of the water molecules, and if there were no counteracting force all the extracellular fluid would move into the plasma volume. In the regulation of fluid distribution between the vascular and interstitial fluids, the counteracting force is the hydrostatic pressure within the vascular system. The hydrostatic pressure increases the activity of the molecules of water to such an extent as virtually to nullify the opposite effect on the activity of water exerted by the plasma proteins. In addition, there is a small colloidal osmotic force operating in the interstitial fluid and a minor pressure force referred to as "tissue tension." The *balance* of these forces—the Starling forces—is the determinant of the steady-state distribution of volume between the two compartments.

There is an additional influence that operates owing to the fact that the plasma proteins are charged molecules. Since they are unable to penetrate the endothelial membrane, an equilibrium is set up (the Gibbs-Donnan equilibrium) such that there is a slightly greater concentration of diffusible ions in the fluid associated with the charged impermeant anion. The total influence of the protein on the activity of plasma water is referred to as the "colloidal *oncotic* pressure."

All the above-described Starling forces are usually so adjusted that about one fourth of the extracellular fluid is within the confines of the vascular system and the remainder is in the interstitial space. Furthermore, these forces operate in such a fashion that there is a tendency for water and diffusible solutes to leave the vascular bed at the arteriolar end of the capillaries and return at the same rate at the venous end. In this fashion, there is a large turnover of water and diffusible solutes between the two compartments without a net change in volume. The importance of this turnover is obvious, because this is how the circulation can efficiently bring oxygen and nutrients to the cell and remove carbon dioxide and other end products of metabolism without relying solely on diffusion.

Net shifts can and do occur, however, when there is a dislocation of these Starling forces. Nevertheless, a dislocation of the Starling equilibrium need not necessarily be accompanied by a commensurate change in these two volumes. The overall effect may be mitigated partially by another system of vessels, namely, the lymphatic system. An increase in the hydrostatic pressure transmitted to the capillaries may permit a greater rate of transudation than reabsorption. The same effect may be noted when there is hypoproteinemia and the influence of the colloidal oncotic pressure is thereby diminished. In both circumstances, there is a net movement of volume to the interstitial fluid compartment. An infusion of a concentrated solution of albumin or of some other large molecular species will expand plasma volume at the expense of the interstitial fluid compartment.

One of the important therapeutic implications is that the plasma volume cannot specifically be increased unless the administered fluid contains a colloidal agent. The administration of saline solution to a subject who has lost blood will reexpand the extracellular fluid volume, but virtually all the expansion will be confined to the interstitial compartment.

EXTERNAL EXCHANGES OF WATER AND SOLUTE

The Balance Principle. In the early decades of this century a great deal of research involved measuring the intake and output of various nutrients and their metabolites. While this method has properly become archaic for the study of intermediary metabolism, it nevertheless provides the conceptual basis for our understanding of the pathogenesis and proper therapy of many disturbances of fluid and electrolyte metabolism. With the exceptions that are noted below, one may consider that water and the major solutes do not undergo metabolic alteration. Hence, concentrations within the body fluids represent the balance between intake and output, both for water and the solute in question. By general usage, if a patient gains something, he is in *positive* balance; if he loses something, the balance is *negative;* if there are no significant changes, the balance is *neutral*. The latter is often referred to as "being in balance." As indicated in Table 36–2, the subject who is in a steady state of normal health, and who is neither gaining nor losing weight, is *in balance.*

In general, the greater the change in external balance and the more acutely it occurs, the more accurate is the estimate of the change itself. With large changes, insensible,

Table 36–2. REPRESENTATIVE "NORMAL" VALUES OF FLUID AND ELECTROLYTE INTAKE AND OUTPUT *

	INTAKE		OUTPUT		
	Oral	*Metabolism*	*Urine*	*Feces*	*Insensible*
Water as fluid, ml	1200	0	1500	100	900
Water in food, ml	1000	300			
Nitrogen, g	13	0	12	1.0	0
Sodium, mEq	75	0	74	0.5	0.5
Potassium, mEq	50	0	45	5.0	0
Chloride, mEq	75	0	74	0.5	0.5
Nonvolatile acid, mEq	0	70	70	0	0
Volatile acid, mEq	0	14,000	0	0	14,000

* A single value is selected for each entry to facilitate comparison of intake and output, and all are adjusted to depict a zero net external balance. Nonvolatile acids are largely phosphoric and sulfuric acid residues of metabolism. Volatile acid is exclusively carbon dioxide. All values refer to the amount per 24 hours.

unmeasured or unestimated losses assume relatively less importance. Also, with large external changes, analytical errors become less important. This applies both to the quantitative analysis of either food or excreta and to clinical estimates based on history and physical examination. It is possible to get independent estimates that serve as checks—for example, the change in weight that accompanies a large change in fluid balance. The proper management of many patients includes an accurate record of *intake and output* and daily weights. This is particularly true of severely ill patients with complex disturbances. Intake includes oral intake, infusions, transfusions, and so forth. Output includes urine, vomitus, and fecal and other intestinal losses (*e.g.,* drainage from a common-bile-duct T tube). Except for research purposes, insensible losses through the lungs and skin are not measured, but they should be estimated. Solid food is rarely included in the estimate of intake even though it provides some water of oxidation. In acute renal failure, this assumes importance.

The *initial state* may have two connotations. It may refer to the value presumed to have been present in the state of health (*e.g.,* body water estimated from a patient's normal weight), or it may refer to any state during an illness prior to the initiation of a specific treatment. Balance is the difference between intake and output; for example, balance = infusions + dietary intake − urine − vomitus. The sign of the result obviously indicates if the patient is in positive or negative balance.

From an accurate knowledge of the external balance, or even from a thoughtful guess as to its probable value, it is possible to deduce many pathophysiological mechanisms. Changes in the balance of water and solute may occur simultaneously, but their independent contributions should be evaluated separately. In the case of obligatory extracellular solutes, external balances provide a direct approach to interpreting changes in their concentrations in the plasma. The problem is more complex for intracellular solutes and is discussed in the section on potassium.

It should be emphasized that the effect of a change in external balance on the composition of the body fluids is independent of the discrete physiological mechanisms that may be involved. For example, the loss of 10 liters of water has essentially the same effect on the residual body fluids, whether due to excessive losses through the skin or to the passage of very dilute urine in uncontrolled diabetes insipidus. Because of this, the "black box" mechanisms of fluid and electrolyte balance warrant reemphasis.

Fixed and Labile Ions and Solutes. As indicated above, many solutes do not undergo metabolic alteration. Provided the definitions are not extended too far or applied too rigidly, it is useful to bear in mind the distinction between fixed and labile solutes. This is based on physiological rather than strictly chemical considerations. In the case of charged particles, a *fixed ion* is one that exists in the ionic form under all physiological circumstances. This holds true for strong electrolytes such as sodium, potassium, and chloride. Through metabolic alterations, *labile ions* may either be generated from nonionic precursors or converted to nonionic end products. Thus, labile ions may be added to or removed from the body fluids in a form other than that of the charged ion. For example, the ammonium cation (NH_4^+) can be converted to urea in the liver, and also synthesized from amino acids in the kidney. Bicarbonate ion (HCO_3^-) can be considered labile since at the proper concentration of hydrogen ion (H^+) it can be converted to H_2CO_3, and thence to its volatile form, CO_2. Another example would be the formation of lactic acid from glucose. In addition, the ion of an appropriate weak acid or base may be buffered so as to change its ionic equivalence (*e.g.,* monobasic and dibasic phosphate). Of course, this is not metabolic alteration in the usual sense, but it does denote a degree of partial lability.

The same considerations apply to nonelectrolytes. Mannitol does not undergo metabolic change and may be considered fixed. However, glucose, which has the same osmotic characteristics as mannitol, is highly labile.

These distinctions warrant emphasis to avoid the errors of oversimplification. It is a truism that in electrolyte metabolism the most important attribute of any solute relates to its actual concentration in solution in the body fluids. For many solutes, this is directly related to their external balance. However, this does not apply to those that may be either formed or catabolized within the body. It should be apparent that metabolism may change either ionic or osmotic characteristics.

Consideration of Basal Requirements. A summary of average values for the intake and output of water and the major electrolytes is given in Table 36–2. These values presuppose average diet and physical activity, a normal state of metabolism, and no abnormal losses. There is considerable variation from one individual to another and moderate variation from day to day. The composition of important fluids that may be lost from the body is given in Table 36–3. Abnormal losses will be discussed in a later section.

Insensible Perspiration. Water is continuously lost from the surface of the skin and from the air that is exhaled by the lungs. This is pure water with no solute and is responsible for the dissipation of approximately 25% of the daily heat production.

Sweat. This is a hypotonic solution. The rate of sweating is responsive to internal heat, and, therefore, it is difficult to assign a "daily average." Furthermore, it is exceedingly difficult to estimate, and in some circumstances represents a large and unidentifiable loss.

Gastrointestinal. Although there is a large turnover of ions and water between the gut lumen and the body fluid, the *net* loss from the gastrointestinal tract in the feces is usually trivial.

Urine. A liter of urine per day is adequate to contain the solutes destined for excretion.

Endogenous Water. A certain amount of water is produced by the body each day from the metabolism of nutrients.

Sodium Chloride. The average diet contains 8 to 10 g of salt a day. This value varies widely due to personal tastes. The administration of considerably less will lead to the development of a brief period of negative balance of salt and some loss of fluid volume. To avoid this, unless there is some special indication for the omission of salt, it is probably wise to make 4 to 6 g of salt available daily. If salt is removed from the diet, the normal kidney excretes urine that is virtually free of sodium chloride within 3 to 5 days.

Potassium. In the face of reduced intake this cation is not quite so well conserved by the kidney as is sodium, and with chronic reduction of dietary intake it is important to guard against a deficit.

Magnesium. Renal and gastrointestinal conservation of magnesium is excellent, and about 8 millimoles of this cation is adequate to maintain balance (*see* Chapter 37).

Calcium. Calcium requirements and abnormalities in calcium metabolism are discussed in Chapter 37.

Summary. These approximate daily basal requirements may be summarized as follows:

Water	1500–2000 ml
Potassium chloride	30–60 millimoles
Sodium chloride	75 millimoles
Magnesium salts	8 millimoles

These amounts relate specifically to the adult. Since the requirements for water and

Table 36–3. PRODUCTION RATES AND COMPOSITION OF VARIOUS BODY FLUIDS *

	VOLUME	COMPOSITION			
		Na^+	K^+	Cl^-	HCO_3^-
	ml/24 hr	mEq/liter			
Cutaneous sweat	100–200	50–80	5	40–85	—
Gastrointestinal					
Saliva	1500	10	30	10	10–20
Gastric fluid	2500	10–115	1–35	90–150	0–15
Bile	500	130–160	3–12	90–120	40–50
Pancreatic fluid	700	115–150	3–8	55–95	60–120
Intestinal fluids	3000				
Jejunum	—	85–150	2–10	45–125	—
Ileum	—	85–120	3–10	60–130	—
Ileostomy (old)	—	40–50	3–5	20–30	—
Cecostomy	—	45–135	5–45	20–90	—
Feces					
Normal	100	5	50	5	—
Diarrhea (cholera)	—	130	20	100	50

* Data are summarized from the literature for both average values and their ranges, and refer to an adult in a temperate climate engaging in mild physical activity.

electrolytes are related more closely to the rate of metabolism than to age or body size, the following values may be helpful:

	PER 100 KCAL
Water	100 ml
Sodium	2–3 mEq
Potassium	2–3 mEq
Chloride	4–6 mEq

The probable average caloric expenditure per 24 hours may be estimated from the following:

KG	KCAL
0–10 kg	100/kg
11–20 kg	1000 + 50/kg, for each kg in excess of 10
>20 kg	1500 + 20/kg, for each kg in excess of 20

CLINICAL DISTURBANCES OF VOLUME AND OSMOLALITY

For purposes of classification, several points warrant emphasis. By common clinical usage, the terms *dehydration* and *overhydration* are often inadequate. For an appropriate description, as well as for correct therapy, each condition should be described with two terms—*volume* and *osmolality* (Table 36–4). However, for many purposes the changes in volume and osmolality may be considered independently. (1) The reference point for the classification system is the extracellular fluid. This is justified for two reasons. First, it is the plasma that is available for chemical analysis. Second, it is the extracellular compartment, or its close relative the transcellular compartment, from which abnormal fluid losses occur. (2) The classification is valid for acute changes occurring over hours or days. With more chronic disturbances, compensatory physiological adjustments (*e.g.,* changes in total red-cell volume or total circulating protein) make the classification less accurate. (3) These conditions may or may not be associated with disturbances in acid-base balance. (4) The primary classification refers to changes in *extracellular* volume. If, in response to changes in osmolality, there are secondary changes in *intracellular* volume, these may be in the same or opposite direction to the volume change in the extracellular compartment, but in the direction dictated by extracellular osmolality according to the mechanisms previously described. (5) The classification is based on external changes in water or solute balance, but without any change in red-blood-cell mass or total circulating protein (*i.e.,* without hemorrhage).

It is rare in clinical situations to find pure examples of the categories listed in Table 36–4. This is not surprising since each depends on two factors. Both may be influ-

Table 36-4. TYPES OF ACUTE CHANGES IN VOLUME AND OSMOLALITY *

ACUTE EXTRACELLULAR CHANGE	CLINICAL EXAMPLE	Δ VOLUME		Δ CONC. PLASMA SODIUM	Δ HEMATOCRIT	Δ CONC. PLASMA PROTEIN
		Δ ECW	Δ ICW			
Isotonic contraction	Cholera	↓	0	0	↑	↑
Hypertonic contraction	Excessive sweating	↓	↓	↑	0	↑
Hypotonic contraction	Adrenal insufficiency	↓	↑	↓	↑	↑
Isotonic expansion	Isotonic saline solution	↑	0	0	↓	↓
Hypertonic expansion	Hypertonic saline solution	↑	↓	↑	↓	↓
Hypotonic expansion	Water intoxication	↑	↑	↓	0	↓

* For discussion of hematocrit, *see* text. Direction of change is shown by arrows. 0 = no change; ECW = extracellular water; ICW = intracellular water. Under clinical examples, isotonic and hypertonic saline solutions refer to infusions.

enced by partially independent mechanisms and to slightly variable degrees. For example, excessive water intake is the purest example of hypotonic expansion. It may occur acutely without any significant change in the external balance of sodium. Nevertheless, one of the most common examples within this category is seen in some severely edematous patients, often with prior diuretic therapy. As in the case of pure water intoxication, this is hypotonic expansion, or dilutional hyponatremia. However, in this instance the disorder is preceded by the positive external sodium and water balance that developed during the period of edema formation. Other permutations will be discussed with each subgroup.

Sodium Concentration as an Index of Plasma Osmolality. Since sodium is the major extracellular solute, its concentration may be used as an index of osmolality, directly for the extracellular fluid and indirectly for the intracellular. As a first approximation, osmolality is twice the sodium concentration. There are two conditions in which this estimate is not valid.

Pseudohyponatremia. This is a condition in which the concentration of sodium in the plasma is abnormally low when analyzed by conventional methods (which depend on aliquots measured volumetrically and thus determine molarity and not molality), but in which the concentration would be normal if referred to plasma water. The discrepancy occurs when there is an abnormally high concentration of large molecules and hence an abnormally low percentage of plasma water, most commonly with hyperlipemia or marked hyperproteinemia. A clue to the former is afforded by the lactescence of the serum; the latter occurs particularly in multiple myeloma but also in severe instances of volume depletion.

Sodium as a False Index. This occurs, even with corrections for plasma water, when there is an abnormally high concentration of another solute that is an effective extracellular osmotic particle. It may be seen with severe *hyperglycemia,* either occurring spontaneously in patients with diabetes mellitus or following the infusion of large amounts of glucose. It is also seen after the administration of a nonmetabolizable extracellular solute such as *mannitol.* Glucose slowly gains access to the intracellular space by carrier-mediated transport. Thus, if the plasma level rises abruptly, glucose acts at least transiently as if it were confined to the extracellular space. This may lead to hyperosmolality without hypernatremia and, indeed, due to internal shifts of water, may be associated with hyponatremia. The simplest method of evaluation is to determine the concentrations of sodium and glucose separately, convert these to osmolar terms, and add them together. If hyperglycemia is rapidly corrected under the influence of insulin, a significant amount of extracellular solute

may in effect disappear. This is accompanied by a redistribution of water between the extracellular and intracellular compartments. (*See* Katz, 1973.)

Isotonic Contraction. This occurs when *sodium and water are lost in isotonic proportions.* The most common example is the loss of fluid from the gastrointestinal tract. Cholera is the classical example. Indeed, it was W. B. O'Shaughnessy, in the cholera epidemic of 1831, who pioneered the modern study of fluid and electrolyte disorders by doing chemical analyses that, although crude and difficult, were essentially accurate. This type of disturbance may be complicated by acid-base changes. Loss of strongly acidic fluid from the stomach leads to metabolic alkalosis; loss of alkaline bile and pancreatic fluid, or the less alkaline fluid of severe diarrhea, leads to metabolic acidosis. In addition, varying degrees of potassium and magnesium deficiency may occur concomitantly. The characteristic of this type of dehydration is a normal value for the concentration of sodium in serum. Therefore, regardless of the volume deficit of the extracellular phase, so long as the *concentration* of plasma sodium is normal, there will be no redistribution of water from or into the cellular compartment. The repair of the dehydration simply requires an expansion of the extracellular fluid volume with a solution that approximates the composition of that fluid.

In terms of the extracellular phase one must discriminate between the interstitial fluid component of the extracellular phase and the plasma volume. Although, in general, the interstitial fluid and the plasma volumes are both diminished when the extracellular compartment is reduced, the volume of the plasma is of far greater physiological importance than is that of the interstitial fluid. This is especially true with respect to the microcirculation. The flow of blood is crucial for the delivery of oxygen, substrates, hormones, and vitamins to the tissues, and for the removal of carbon dioxide and other waste products from them. Although in many instances simple restoration of the volume and the tonicity of the extracellular space as a whole will serve to replace the plasma volume proportionately, there are occasions when more prompt and specific attention must be directed to plasma volume in particular, by providing a colloidal solution that will specifically ensure its expansion.

Hypertonic Contraction. This type of dehydration is relatively common and is observed in any circumstance in which there is a *loss of water in excess of sodium.* The classical example involves survival on a life raft under the unremitting impact of the tropical sun (Gamble, 1947). In more common clinical conditions it occurs when the patient is unable to drink water owing to a clouded sensorium and no water (or too little) has been provided parenterally. Other circumstances include diabetes insipidus, excessive sweating (of a hypotonic fluid), and osmotic diuresis. When this occurs in uncontrolled diabetes mellitus, the effect of glucose (a labile solute) in high concentrations is additive to the negative external balance of water in causing extracellular hypertonicity. Less commonly the disturbance may be produced by a high dietary intake of protein if unaccompanied by sufficient water intake to balance the increased urinary losses accompanying the excretion of large amounts of urea.

The effect of hypernatremia on the internal redistribution of water has already been described. In this fashion, the extracellular fluid volume, although diminished, is not as deprived as it would be if the total deficit were derived from this volume alone. In addition, increased concentration of sodium serves as a stimulus to feedback mechanisms that ordinarily promote the acquisition and the conservation of water by provoking thirst and stimulating the secretion of antidiuretic hormone (ADH). On theoretical grounds there should be no change in hematocrit if there is a pure loss of water, since this would occur proportionately from the plasma and the erythrocytes. In most clinical examples, there is also a negative balance of sodium and the hematocrit would therefore rise.

Hypotonic Contraction. This occurs when there is a *loss of sodium in excess of water.* Chief among these conditions are chronic renal insufficiency and adrenocortical insufficiency. It also occurs commonly when isotonic fluid losses are replaced with water (isotonic glucose solution) and too little or

no salt. Essentially the same mechanism is involved when physical exercise in a hot, dry climate is associated with the drinking of water but without the ingestion of salt tablets to replace the loss of salt that occurred through perspiration. The distinguishing features of this type of dehydration is, of course, a reduction in the concentration of sodium in serum. The consequences of this primary reduction in effective osmolality of the extracellular fluid is a passage of water from extracellular fluid into the cells. This type of dehydration greatly reduces the volume of the extracellular phase, for not only has this compartment suffered a loss of volume to the external environment but to the cells as well.

If salt is lost in excess of water, some degree of hyponatremia should develop even if too subtle to be detected by current methods. Salt loss, however, is soon followed by a loss of water in approximately isotonic proportions, so that at an early stage of the disorder there is virtually an isotonic contraction. The reason for this loss of water is not clear. It might be anticipated that it is due to suppression of secretion of ADH, owing to a reduction in the effective osmolality of the body fluids. However, this assumption apparently is untenable, since it has been demonstrated that such a loss of water will occur even if adequate quantities of ADH are ensured (Baker *et al.,* 1961). The deficit of salt appears to influence the urine-concentrating mechanism in such a way as to make it less effective, and as a consequence water is dissipated in the urine. However, as the process develops and more and more salt and then water are lost from the body fluids, there comes a point at which the loss of water consequent to the loss of sodium no longer occurs, and at this point *hyponatremia* is established. The reasons for the ultimate failure to excrete the *relative* excess of water may lie in a reduction in glomerular filtration rate and an increase in tubular reabsorption of sodium in the proximal convolution. These two events would limit the volume of fluid that gains access to the distal segment of the nephron. In this area the slow flow of a small volume of hypotonic fluid may well permit excessive back diffusion of water so that the net effect is a limited volume of urine. Since the contraction of the volume of the extracellular compartment must be substantial before the situation is established, it is implicit that, in most instances of dehydration accompanied by hyponatremia, the intensity of the dehydration is of significant magnitude and warrants prompt and aggressive attention.

Isotonic Expansion. For completeness, the disorders associated with *volume expansion* are briefly discussed with reference to Table 36–4, even though they are more fully presented in Chapter 39.

Of these disorders the most common is isotonic expansion, or the *proportional retention of sodium and water.* This is the basis of edema, most commonly due to cardiac, hepatic, or renal disease. The extracellular compartment may also be expanded by the injudicious use of isotonic saline solution in the overtreatment of dehydration. Even major fluctuations of dietary salt intake rarely give rise to isotonic expansion, at least in the adult. Normal renal function quite rapidly compensates for dietary changes. The changes described in Table 36–4 are most applicable to the rapid and excessive infusion of isotonic saline solution, since with spontaneous disease the slower development of edema is accompanied by changes in red-blood-cell mass and plasma protein. Indeed, the hypoproteinemia of hepatic and renal disease may be an important cause of edema. By definition, in all these examples the concentration of sodium in the plasma is normal. There are no osmotically induced shifts of water between the extracellular and intracellular compartments.

If volume expansion is rapidly induced by infusions of saline solution, this may be accompanied by *dilutional acidosis*—the dilution of extracellular bicarbonate into an abnormally large volume (*see* section on acid-base disturbances).

Hypertonic Expansion. This occurs when *sodium is retained in excess of water.* In its simplest form, it results from the rapid and excessive infusion of hypertonic saline solution. The most common clinical example probably occurs in infants improperly treated for diarrhea and involves the balance between input and output. When treatment consists in oral administration of salt and water, the concentration of salt may be erroneously excessive, or the total quantity administered may be too great to be excreted by the kidneys. Accidental salt poisoning has been reported in infants following the addition of salt instead of sugar to the formula. In these instances, hypertonicity is extreme, but volume expansion is more variable and dependent upon fluid intake and excretion (Finberg *et al.*, 1963). In severe hypernatremia the condition may be fatal, due primarily to damage to the CNS. Osmotically induced water shifts decrease intracellular volume. This contributes to the fall in hematocrit; expansion of plasma volume is obviously also involved.

Hypotonic Expansion. This occurs with *retention of water in excess of sodium.* The simplest example is water intoxication due to the excessive ingestion of water. The concentrations of sodium and protein in the plasma fall by dilution. Since water distributes itself throughout the body fluids in proportion to the compartment size, there is an increase in both the extracellular and the intracellular volumes. It is for this reason that on theoretical grounds the hematocrit does not change since the erythrocytes gain water and enlarge. In a sense, the hematocrit measures imbalances or nonproportional distribution of water between the two compartments. Careful studies provide data that are in close agreement with the theory (Wynn, 1955). Excessive water ingestion is sometimes encountered in emotionally disturbed patients. The dominant symptoms are weakness, presumably of muscular origin, and CNS dysfunction. This may progress from apathy to stupor and coma. In addition, generalized seizures may occur.

Another more complicated example of hypotonic expansion is seen in some patients with edema. In rare instances, during its spontaneous development, edema is associated with a greater retention of water than of salt, often referred to as dilutional hyponatremia. Far more frequently this results from the excessive use of diuretics designed to mobilize edema fluid. Since most of these are in fact saluretic agents, they may produce an imbalance between the losses of salt and water. The syndrome of the inappropriate secretion of ADH also produces hypotonic expansion.

Evaluation of Intensity of Dehydration. For an analysis of a patient's problems in the context of dehydration, one utilizes the same tools employed throughout clinical medicine, namely, a carefully obtained history, a physical examination, and the intelligent, discriminating choice and interpretation of laboratory data. The history should include a careful review of all the events during the course of an illness. To evaluate accurately the state of hydration, it is important to list the nature of the losses of salt and water, as these can be estimated from a knowledge of the basic mandatory losses and the other deficits that have occurred during the course of the illness. In another list, one can estimate the intake of water and ions, and from the two lists come to some *tentative* conclusion as to the qualitative nature of the deficits and the intensity of the dehydration. Information concerning fever, sweating, acute weight change, and thirst (or lack thereof) is all helpful in arriving at the initial evaluation. Also, it must be emphasized that, although the data are crude, they can provide exceedingly useful approximations from which to start. From the history and physical examination one can obtain a reasonable estimate of fluid loss; the probable composition of the lost fluid is readily available (Table 36–3). Except in the rarest of instances, it is not necessary to submit samples of excreta to the laboratory for electrolyte analysis. All physicians should be encouraged to develop some *system of tabulation,* both to make the initial estimate of the degree and the nature of the dehydration and to evaluate the course of therapy. Experience indicates that most complicated problems in fluid-balance therapy are readily understood by arranging the data in tabular form and by the use of simple arithmetic.

The physical examination is helpful in estimating the intensity of the dehydration, and virtually all the useful physical signs reflect the volume of the extracellular phase and of the plasma volume in particular. The blood pressure, the pulse, and the color and temperature of the skin will all provide some insight into the state of the peripheral blood flow. The elasticity of the skin provides additional information concerning the interstitial fluid volume. However, it should be cautioned that patients who have lost subcutaneous fat will have inelasticity of the skin despite a normal state of hydration. The moisture of the mucous membranes can be helpful, but so many ill patients breathe through the mouth that this is frequently of no aid and may actually be quite misleading. The size of the tongue may be the most subtle physical sign that reflects the state of hydration. The state of consciousness is of importance. The characteristics of the respirations may provide some insight to an acid-base disequilibrium, and muscle weakness may suggest potassium depletion.

The useful laboratory data obviously include those determinations of ion concentrations that provide insight into the relationship between solutes and water (*i.e.,* the concentration of sodium in the serum); pH and P_{CO_2}, along with bicarbonate concentrations; creatinine (or blood urea nitrogen values); and potassium and magnesium concentrations, which can be evaluated in terms of deficits or excesses of these ions. The hematocrit and the concentration of total proteins in the serum provide an approximation of the degree of hemoconcentration, but these can be misleading unless one has recent data from the same patient prior to the development of the state of dehydration. The concentration of creatinine in the serum provides a rough estimate of renal function in terms of filtration rate. The urinalysis is helpful in evaluating the state of renal function and in determining whether there is glomerular disease, tubular disturbances, diabetes insipidus, or other disorders.

It would be inappropriate in this textbook to dwell longer on the details of the clinical evaluation of the patient. However, it is exceedingly important to emphasize that a shrewd clinical appraisal of the patient's problem can permit the physician accurately to estimate the state of hydration in both qualitative and quantitative terms (Maxwell and Kleeman, 1972).

Treatment of Fluid and Electrolyte Deficits.

The basic objective of therapy is to restore the volume and composition of the body fluids to normal. However, this requires extensive qualification insofar as priorities are concerned. The present discussion is limited to water and salt balance. The more complex derangements involving blood loss and protein depletion will be considered separately.

Volume Contraction. This is life threatening primarily because of impairment of the circulation. With a decreased circulating blood volume, cardiac output falls and the integrity of the microcirculation is compromised. This occurs whether volume contraction is isotonic, hypertonic, or hypotonic, even though, as outlined above, there are important differences between them. It is urgent, therefore, that in a critical or emergency situation, attention be primarily directed to the deficit of volume. It is probably fair to say that, given volume depletion of sufficient magnitude to threaten life, the prompt infusion of *isotonic sodium chloride solution is indicated;* indeed, it is difficult to contrive a contraindication.

The volume of replacement fluid required for adequate therapy varies enormously. As a general rule, the greater and more acute the depletion, the more urgent the need for replacement. As an extreme example, intravenous therapy at the rate of 100 ml per minute for the first 1000 ml is considered necessary for the successful treatment of cholera (Carpenter, 1966). Most conditions require far less dramatic treatment. As discussed above, the intensity of dehydration must be taken into account. In addition to the factors outlined, attention should also be directed to the speed with which the volume depletion developed. For example, a 4.5-kg (10-lb) weight loss due to the loss of gastrointestinal fluids, from either vomiting or diarrhea, is far more debilitating if it occurs over 2 to 3 hours than over a period of days or weeks.

Disorders of Osmolality. Even with moderately severe hyponatremia or hypernatremia, frequently the disorder may be satisfactorily corrected with isotonic saline solution, provided there is normal renal function. The correction occurs as a result of the physiological adjustments made by the kidney, leading to the excretion of urine at a concentration appropriate to the underlying situation. As emphasized previously, given an adequate supply of raw materials (here best considered in terms of extracellular volume and renal blood flow) the kidney is a remarkably effective regulator of the osmolality of the body.

However, if the disturbance in osmolality is severe, producing symptoms in its own right, or threatening life, it is proper to treat this directly. Clinical judgment should be based on the actual physiological consequences of the disorder, and not on blood chemistry values considered in isolation. As is the case with volume disturbances, a change in osmolality varies in importance depending on the speed of its development. There are examples of virtually asymptomatic extreme hyponatremia that have developed over periods of months, whereas the same degree of hyponatremia, if it appeared over several days, would invariably be accompanied by severe CNS dysfunction. The immediate goal of therapy should be to return osmolality *toward* normal, not necessarily precisely to it, and to judge the urgency of ongoing treatment by the response of the patient. Some of the major effects of abnormal osmolality, either high or low, are on the CNS. For reasons that are incompletely understood, rapid changes in osmolality are poorly tolerated. For example, if the plasma sodium concentration is lowered rapidly in infants with hypernatremia, seizures due to water intoxication may develop even though the plasma is still hypernatremic. When

treating a disturbance in osmolality, it is a conservative goal to return the plasma osmolality halfway to normal within 1 day. Except in extreme instances, this leads to major symptomatic and physiological improvement. In some cases of virtually asymptomatic dilutional hyponatremia it is often debatable whether specific therapy is justified, either because of the absence of any detectable harm or because specific treatment may be of little use (*see* Chapter 39).

Salt or Water Requirements to Correct Disturbances in Osmolality. The principles are best illustrated by considering hyponatremia. As an example, given a plasma sodium concentration of 120 mEq per liter, how much salt (either as dry salt in the diet or as hypertonic saline solution) would be required to elevate this to 130 mEq per liter? For a 70-kg subject without gross volume deficits or excesses, one may assume a total body water of 50 liters. Although the administered sodium will distribute itself in an actual volume equivalent to that of the extracellular compartment, it will exert an osmotic effect to move fluid into that compartment from the intracellular space. This will diminish the induced increment in extracellular osmolality and will also increase intracellular osmolality by the transfer of water. The concentration of sodium in the plasma will not rise by the desired increment of 10 mEq per liter until the osmolality of both the intracellular and extracellular compartments has been raised to a similar extent. Thus, 50 liters × 10 mEq per liter equals 500 mEq of sodium. In this example the volume that is added with the hypertonic saline solution is ignored. A calculation based exclusively on the extracellular volume would be in error. Using TBW for total body water, [Na] for sodium concentration in plasma, and subscripts 1 and 2 for the initial and final states, if TBW is kept constant and one solves for electrolyte balance, then:

$$(TBW_1 \times [Na]_1) + Na\ Balance = TBW_2 \times [Na]_2$$
$$50 \times 120 \quad + 500 \quad = 50 \quad \times 130$$

The same principle applies to the calculation of water requirements for the treatment of hypernatremia. Thus, for the same subject, if the initial concentration of sodium in the plasma were 175 mEq per liter and one desired to dilute this to 160 mEq per liter, this would require a positive water balance of 4.7 liters; with the same equation, now keeping electrolyte content constant, and solving for the change in fluid balance, then:

$$TBW_1 \times [Na]_1 = TBW_2 \times [Na]_2$$
$$50 \times 175 \quad = 54.7 \quad \times 160$$

This equation, or simple modifications for other situations, may be used to estimate requirements involving complex changes in both volume and osmolality.

Technics of Administration of Fluid. Fluids can be administered by mouth, by intermittent gavage, by vein, and by hypodermoclysis. *Oral* intake or administration of fluids by *gavage* is proscribed whenever there is nausea or vomiting or when relatively rapid therapy is necessary; the *parenteral* route is important when the patient is unconscious, since it is wise to eschew gavage feedings in the unconscious patient lest he vomit and aspirate. However, when it is possible, the oral route is desirable since this is truly the only way that adequate calories and other essential nutrients can be made available with ease.

Due consideration must be given to the status of the cardiovascular system in terms of the speed with which fluids are administered. Frequent monitoring of the central venous pressure may be of great help in determining the progress of therapy and the threat of cardiac failure.

Fluids Available for the Repair of Dehydration. There are a variety of *commercially* available solutions that have been designed to repair the average deficits that one might anticipate in most clinical situations. It is suggested that they not be relied upon because their use tends to detract from a careful consideration of the individual problem at hand. In fact, the very premise of this entire discussion is that general principles must be translated to the problems of a specific patient and that individualization of therapy is just as important in this area as it is in the administration of digitalis, antibiotics, and other drugs.

Appropriate fluid regimens can be designed from a small list of simple solutions; these may be designated as raw materials. For the purposes discussed thus far, they include: (1) 5%, 10%, and 50% dextrose in water; (2) solutions of fructose in water; (3) 0.45% NaCl in water (77 mM); (4) 0.45% NaCl and 5% glucose in water; (5) 0.9% NaCl in water (154 mM); (6) 5.0% NaCl in water (855 mM); (7) 5% $NaHCO_3$ in water (595 mM); and (8) 7.5% $NaHCO_3$ in water (900 mM).

With these solutions one can administer water in excess of salt (solutions of dextrose or fructose in water), or 0.45% sodium chloride with or without dextrose; isotonic solutions of sodium chloride adequate, in most instances, for replacement of extracellular fluid *per se;* and solutions of hypertonic saline to correct hyponatremia, in which case about 25% of the sodium may be given as sodium bicarbonate to avoid dilutional acidosis. (The use of alkaline agents is discussed in more detail below, where some of the problems of disorders of acid-base equilibrium are considered.)

The best substitute for the loss of whole blood is obviously suitable and adequately cross-matched whole blood. However, when plasma volume is critically jeopardized, the use of colloid-containing solutions is clearly indicated. These include individual units of plasma, which should have no more serious threat of homologous serum hepatitis (hepatitis virus B) than does a single transfusion of whole blood; a plasma protein solution (5%) prepared from pooled plasma that is heated to 60° C for 10 hours by most manufacturers; 25% solutions of salt-poor human albumin, which may be used as such or diluted with saline; and solutions of dextran. The 25% salt-poor albumin and the plasma protein solutions are safe with respect to hepatitis virus B, but they are expensive. For this reason there has been a widespread effort to find alternative substances that possess the properties desirable for a plasma expander.

Desirable Properties of a Plasma Expander. The major requirement to be sought in an ideal plasma expander is that it should have an oncotic pressure comparable to that of plasma. The substance should remain in the circulation for a period of time adequate to perform its function of immediate expansion of the plasma volume, and yet eventually be disposed of by excretion or metabolic degradation. This period of time is difficult to define and, in fact, would differ with circumstances. The ideal plasma expander should not affect adversely any visceral function, nor should it have an antigenic, allergenic, or pyretic effect. Indeed, except for its physical properties, it should be pharmacologically inert. It should not interfere with typing or cross-agglutination of blood, and it should be able to withstand long periods of storage and wide variations in environmental temperature and still be effective. It should be easily sterilized and have a viscosity suitable for infusion over a reasonable temperature range.

Many substances have been investigated as potential plasma expanders, and at present the only agent, except for plasma and albumin, that is used with any frequency and that appears to meet most of the above requirements is dextran (*see* Fox and Nahas, 1970).

Dextran. Dextran was originally described by the German sugar-chemist Schleibler. The compound was first isolated from solutions of beet sugar, where it is formed by the action of a contaminating bacterium, *Leuconostac mesenteroides.*

Chemistry. In its original form, dextran is a branched polysaccharide of about 200,000 glucose units, with a molecular weight of approximately 40 million. The glucose units in the main chain are bound together through 1:6 glucosidic linkages; those in the shorter branches, through 1:4 linkages. By means of partial hydrolysis and subsequent fractionation, native dextran can be converted to polysaccharides of any desired range of molecular weights.

There are two forms of dextran solution currently available. One has an average molecular weight of 75,000, and the other has an average molecular weight of 40,000. Both agents expand plasma volume specifically. There is evidence to suggest that the lower-molecular-weight dextran may well have advantages (*see* Moore, 1963). Its administration not only corrects hypovolemia but also appears to improve the microcirculation independently of simple volume expansion. It seems to minimize the tendency for sludging of blood that may accompany many forms of shock.

Hemodynamic Action. The hemodynamic action of dextran is that expected of an effective plasma expander. When given to normal individuals, there is a temporary increase in cardiac output, stroke volume, right atrial pressure, and venous pressure. Due to homeostatic adjustments these return to normal within a few hours (Witham *et al.,* 1951). However, the plasma protein concentration remains low for a much longer period. As a result of the hypervolemia produced by dextran, urine flow is increased. There is no reliable evidence that the dextrans influence renal function unfavorably. However, in the presence of hypotension and a reduction in filtration rate, the excessive tubular reabsorption of water may increase the concentration of dextran in the tubular fluid so that viscosity impedes the flow of fluid through the tubule (*see* Fox and Nahas, 1970). In an individual who has sustained a loss of whole blood or plasma, a single infusion of dextran increases the circulating blood volume and improves the hemodynamic status for 24 hours or longer. It has been successfully employed in the treatment of blood and plasma loss in a variety of conditions.

Effects on Blood. Dextran has little effect on the blood. It does not interfere with typing, cross-matching, or Rh determinations. It may produce a hemostatic defect described as an acquired form of von Willebrand's disease (*see* Fox and Nahas, 1970). The properties and uses of dextran 40 for its antiplatelet and antithrombotic effects are described in Chapter 65.

Antigenic Action. Dextran is a potent antigen. This is true of the native polysaccharide and the hydrolysis products used clinically. In man the injection of only 1 mg leads to the development of precipitins and cutaneous erythema and wheal reactions (Kabat and Berg, 1953). Furthermore, dextran occurs in commercial sugar, and dextran-producing organisms can be found in the human gastrointestinal tract. Therefore, a small percentage of individuals who have never received dextran have precipitins to the polysaccharide in the circulation. This accounts for the allergic reactions seen in some patients (*see* below).

The antigenic activity of dextran would seem to preclude its repeated use. However, when given in the massive doses that are employed for infusion, antibody production does not occur, due presumably to the phenomenon of "immunological paralysis." On the other hand, the individual who initially shows a sensitivity reaction to a dextran infusion will also react to subsequent injections.

Distribution, Metabolic Fate, and Excretion. Following the infusion of dextran, the molecules of smaller molecular weight are excreted by the kidney. As much as 50% appears in the urine within 24 hours. However, the remainder traverses the capillary wall very slowly, as judged by its appearance in lymph (Wasserman and Mayerson, 1952; Bollman, 1953). The portion that is not excreted is slowly oxidized over a period of a few weeks. The persistence of dextran and its ultimate metabolic disposal are desirable features of a plasma expander.

Untoward Reactions. Dextran appears to have no significant deleterious effects on renal, hepatic, or other vital functions. Reversible renal tubular lesions have been observed in dogs (Langsjoen, 1965), but they do not appear to have significance for man. However, sensitivity reactions occur for reasons already mentioned. The incidence of such reactions is extremely variable, depending upon the preparation employed. As the technic of manufacture has improved, the number of untoward responses has diminished. These consist in itching, urticaria, joint pains, and other side effects, and are relatively mild in character. Their incidence in normal individuals is less than 10%. They are seldom observed in patients under anesthesia. Dextran may be contraindicated in patients with hypofibrinogenemia or marked thrombocytopenia (Gelin *et al.*, 1961).

Clinical Status. Dextran possesses most of the attributes of an ideal plasma expander, its chief defect being antigenicity. It has been successfully employed in the treatment of the circulatory inadequacies associated with the hypovolemia attending the loss of both whole blood and plasma. It must be realized that the use of a plasma expander is a temporary measure in the treatment of blood loss.

Problems of Carbohydrates, Fats, and Proteins

In the absence of the normal dietary intake of calories and foodstuffs by mouth, intravenous dextrose solution serves to protect against the development of ketosis and to minimize the wasting of protein. For this purpose, on a short-term basis, isotonic or slightly hypertonic dextrose solution is a useful adjuvant, and one should administer approximately 100 g of carbohydrate per day to an adult. For more prolonged treatment, carbohydrate and protein hydrolysates may be given by gavage.

Intravenous Hyperalimentation. This technic has been developed within the last few decades and now represents an important contribution to the management of certain patients, particularly those with intestinal abnormalities or severe dysfunction, trauma, or various surgical complications, both in the pediatric and adult age groups. The success of these procedures justifies their use, but the complications are serious and can be avoided only by meticulous attention to detail involving the pharmacist, nurse, and physician. Such therapy accomplishes a positive nitrogen balance and can be continued for as long as 30 to 60 days. The basic nutrient solution consists of hypertonic dextrose (20 to 25%) and protein hydrolysates or crystalline amino acids (4 to 5%) in water, plus electrolytes and vitamins. The need for hypertonic solutions is dictated by the limits of water intake.

The infusion is given through a percutaneous catheter inserted into a large branch of the superior vena cava. Delivery into a large vein permits prompt adjustment of osmolality by dilution. Rigid sterile surgical technic is essential. A peristaltic pump should be used to drive the infusion through the tubing, which contains a microfilter. Both tubing and filter should be changed frequently. Ancillary medications should be given by another route. Pharmaceutical incompatibilities must be avoided (for other details, *see* Cowan and Sheetz, 1972).

Infrequent mechanical complications are related to the insertion of the catheter. Undoubtedly the most serious complication is that of *infection*. To the extent that this results from the infusion, its incidence is greatly reduced by in-line filters. *Metabolic complications* are common, often mild, and are a direct consequence of the infusions themselves. Since these are acceptable if mild, the regimen should be initiated gradually, then kept constant from day to day and carefully monitored. Mild *glycosuria* is common but may subside after stimulation of endogenous insulin production as a result of the hyperglycemia. However, severe glycosuria may lead to excessive water loss and the undesirable development of hypertonic contraction of body fluids. With the addition of adequate amounts of sodium, potassium, magnesium, chloride, and bicarbonate, electrolyte imbalance may be avoided. Prolonged *hypophosphatemia* may lead to serious neurological and hematological complications, and phosphate is a requirement for prolonged therapy (Lichtman *et al.*, 1971). *Hyperammonemia* may occur, particularly in infants, and can be prevented by reducing the nitrogenous components of the infusion.

The parenteral administration of fat is complicated by pyrogenic reactions. Fat as a source of calories by parenteral administration is the subject of extensive clinical investigation that can be expected to result in the availability of satisfactory preparations in the near future.

Preparations of Fluids Available. Most of the following solutions are now generally available in glass vials, plastic bags, and prefilled syringes with various-size needles. The pH ranges are important with respect to both stability and possible incompatibilities with drugs that may be added. The U.S.P. requires that the concentrations of solutions of dextrose and of dextrose and sodium chloride be labeled in terms of *milliosmoles* of the total solution, that is, the sum of each compound or ion in milligrams per liter divided by its molecular or atomic weight.

Glucose. Dextrose, U.S.P., is commonly referred to as *glucose. Dextrose Injection, U.S.P.*, is a sterile solution, pH 3.5 to 6.5, for parenteral administration. It is marketed in concentrations varying from 2.5 to 50%. *Dextrose and Sodium Chloride Injection, U.S.P.*, pH 3.5 to 6.0, is a sterile solution of glucose and sodium chloride. Available solutions consist of varying concentrations of glucose, 2.5 to 25%, in sodium chloride solution, 0.11 to 0.9%, a complete list of which is given in the U.S.P. Rapid intravenous administration of solutions of glucose may lead to glycosuria. When given at an hourly rate of 800 mg/kg, approximately 95% of the glucose is retained; at half this rate, 100% retention is achieved.

Fructose. Fructose Injection, N.F., is a sterile solution of fructose in water, available as a 10% solution, pH 3.0 to 6.0. One of the advantages of fructose is its rapid removal from the extracellular space, and, therefore, urinary excretion is minimized. Furthermore, it is utilized by the diabetic patient with ketoacidosis, and hence may be useful in the early management of this complication of diabetes mellitus. *Fructose and Sodium Chloride Injection, N.F.*, is a sterile solution of fructose and sodium chloride in water.

Sodium Salts. Sodium Chloride, U.S.P., is the most important single salt for the maintenance of replacement of deficits of extracellular fluid. It is available in a variety of concentrations. Isotonic sodium chloride solution (0.9%) may be administered by different routes. For oral use, tablets or solutions may be used. For subcutaneous injection, an isotonic solution must be employed. *Sodium Chloride Injection, U.S.P.*, is available in various volumes; its pH range is 4.5 to 7.0. Hypertonic solutions (3 and 5%) must be administered intravenously. Hypotonic sodium chloride solution (0.45%) is also available. Sodium chloride may also be incorporated into solutions of glucose and fructose, as described above. *Sodium Bicarbonate, U.S.P.*, is available in the form of *Sodium Bicarbonate Tablets, U.S.P.* A solution of 1.3% is approximately isotonic with body fluids. A sterile solution, *Sodium Bicarbonate Injection, U.S.P.*, is available in ampuls and vials as 1% (20-ml), 1.4% (500-ml), 5% (500-ml), 7.5% (50-ml), and 8.4% (40-ml) solutions; its pH range is up to 8.5.

Human Plasma Protein Fraction, U.S.P. (PLASMANATE, PLASMA-PLEX, PLASMATEIN), is a sterile aqueous solution containing 5% human plasma proteins in sodium chloride solution (0.9%), of which not less than 83% is albumin and the remainder is α- and β-globulins; it is osmotically equivalent to plasma. The risk of transmitting hepatitis B virus is minimized by manufacturers by heating at 60° C for 10 hours. This preparation is available in 250- and 500-ml vials.

Albumin. Normal Human Serum Albumin, U.S.P. (ALBUTEIN, ALBUMINAR, ALBUSPAN), is a sterile preparation of 5 or 25% serum albumin obtained by fractionating blood from healthy human donors. The 5% solution, which is osmotically equivalent to

plasma, is available in 250- and 500-ml vials; the 25% solution is supplied in units of 20, 50, and 100 ml. Risk of hepatitis B virus is minimized by heating in the same manner as described above.

Dextran. Two forms of dextran, which differ in molecular size, are available for use as plasma expanders. *Dextran 70 injection* (GENTRAN, MACRODEX, TRAVERT) contains 6% *dextran* (average molecular weight 70,000) in 0.9% sodium chloride solution or 5% dextrose in water, pH 4.0 to 6.5. *Dextran 40 injection* (GENTRAN 40, LMD 10%, RHEOMACRODEX) contains 10% *dextran 40* (average molecular weight 40,000) in 0.9% sodium chloride solution or 5% dextrose in water. The molecular weight of the former preparation approximates that of human plasma albumin; the smaller molecular size of the latter preparation is said to have the advantage of retarding rouleau formation and sludging of red blood cells. Both preparations are available in units of 500 ml.

Protein Hydrolysates. Mixtures of pure amino acids for parenteral administration are not generally available owing to cost. Preparations of protein hydrolysates are available and are well tolerated. *Protein Hydrolysate Injection, U.S.P.* (AMIGEN, AMINOSOL), is a sterile solution of amino acids and short-chain peptides that represent the approximate nutritive equivalent of the casein, lactalbumin, plasma, fibrin, or other suitable protein from which it is derived by an acidic, enzymatic, or other method of hydrolysis. It may be modified by partial removal and restoration or addition of one or more amino acids. It may contain dextrose or other carbohydrate suitable for intravenous infusion. It is usually available in 5% solution in combination with dextrose, fructose, or alcohol in 500- and 1000-ml volumes.

ACID-BASE DISTURBANCES

It is difficult to review the problem of volume imbalance without some consideration of the acid-base disorder that may be a prominent accompaniment.

Some discussions of this problem in the past have been confusing, in part owing to the various uses of the terms *acid* and *base*. In this discussion an acid will be considered as any substance that can provide a hydrogen ion (a proton donor), and a base as any substance that can accept a proton (a proton acceptor). (For a more complete discussion, *see* Davenport, 1969, and Winters, 1973.) In this context one can view an acid and base in this fashion:

$$\text{Acid} \rightleftarrows \text{Base} + \text{H}^+$$

Some materials can be both an acid or a base, for example, $H_2PO_4^-$, which can either donate or accept a hydrogen ion.

The rate at which an acid dissociates is proportional to its molal concentration. Thus, the acid HA will dissociate at a rate that can be denoted as k_1 [HA]. In contrast, the association of the hydrogen ion and base will be proportional to the product of the two ionic species and can be viewed as equal to:

$$k_2[H^+][A^-]$$

At equilibrium the rates of the two reactions are equal, and one can express this as:

$$k_1[HA] = k_2[H^+][A^-]$$

By rearrangement:

$$[H^+] = \frac{k_1}{k_2}\frac{[HA]}{[A^-]}$$

The ratio of the constants can be expressed as a new constant K, and

$$[H^+] = K\frac{[HA]}{[A^-]}$$

When the convention of Sorenson is used, in which the hydrogen ion concentration is expressed as the negative logarithm, one has the familiar Henderson-Hasselbalch equation:

$$pH = pK + \log\frac{[Base]}{[Acid]}$$

It is clear that the pH is defined by the ratio of the buffer pair. In health, pH of the blood is usually maintained within the limits of 7.35 to 7.45.

The responses that tend to minimize any deviation in pH include buffer reactions, ion-exchange mechanisms, alterations in respiratory activity, and renal mechanisms. Each of the physiological mechanisms that respond to a disturbance in acid-base equilibrium tends to restore pH toward normal. An acid-base disorder can be more or less "compensated." One word of caution should be entered here to emphasize the fact that perfect compensation of a single acid-base disturbance is unlikely; if it occurred and the primary insult remained, the stimulus that induced the mechanisms for compensation would then no longer be operative. In other words, in order for a compensating mechanism to intervene, it must be responding to some stimulus. Hence, if a patient has an acid-base abnormality and has what may be referred to as "perfect compensation," the probability is almost certain that he has more than one disturbance.

Mechanisms of Compensation. *Buffers.* A buffered solution is one that is able to minimize a deviation in pH caused by the addition of acid or base. It contains a *weakly* dissociated acid along with a *highly* dissociated salt of that acid.

Such a buffer pair could be designated as HX and NaX. If a strong acid such as HCl is added to a solution containing this pair, the reaction is as follows:

$$HX + Na^+X^- + H^+Cl^- \rightleftharpoons 2HX + Na^+Cl^-$$

$$\updownarrow (pK_a) \qquad\qquad \updownarrow (pK_a)$$

$$H^+ + X^- \qquad\qquad H^+ + X^-$$

In this fashion 1 mole of the strongly dissociated acid would be converted to approximately 1 mole of an acid that dissociates less, as determined by the pK_a. The concentration of hydrogen ions will increase, but to much less an extent than if the HCl has been added to a system with no buffer.

For significant buffering to occur in biological fluids, the pK_a of the weak acid must be within the pH range of those fluids. Total buffering capacity also depends on the concentration of the buffer itself. The role of true buffer reactions is often inadequately appreciated, particularly in the extent to which the intracellular buffers (principally proteins) are involved in the regulation of bicarbonate concentration in the presence of changing concentrations of carbon dioxide. In the example on the next page, the diffusion reactions between the extracellular and intracellular spaces have been omitted.

Table 36–5. TYPICAL PLASMA VALUES IN THE VARIOUS ACID-BASE DISORDERS *

	pH	HCO_3^-	P_{CO_2}	Cl^-	ANION GAP
Respiratory acidosis	↓	↑	↑	↓	±
Respiratory alkalosis	↑	↓	↓	↑	±
Metabolic acidosis	↓	↓	↓	± or ↑	± or ↑
Metabolic alkalosis	↑	↑	↑	↓	± or ↑

* For calculation of anion gap, *see* text.

$$H^+ + HCO_3^- + B^+Pr^- \rightleftharpoons HPr + B^+ + HCO_3^-$$

$$H_2CO_3$$

B^+Pr^- is the potassium salt of an intracellular protein. It may be seen that the generation of HCO_3^- is reversibly determined by the H_2CO_3 concentration, or the P_{CO_2}. This occurs without any change in the external balance of bicarbonate. This buffer reaction contributes to the changes in bicarbonate that occur in primary respiratory disorders (Table 36–5).

The Bicarbonate–Carbonic Acid System. There are, of course, many buffers in the body fluids, including hemoglobin, phosphates, proteins, and the bicarbonate–carbonic acid pair, which can be expressed as follows:

$$pH = 6.1 + \log \frac{[HCO_3^-]}{[H_2CO_3] + [\text{dissolved } CO_2]}$$

$$CO_2 + H_2O$$

This buffer system has many unique features. Of practical importance is the ease of measurement in serum of the components of the system, the concentrations of which deviate in acid-base disturbances. Such measurements are of great diagnostic value. Of major physiological importance is the manner by which the concentrations of carbonic acid and bicarbonate can be regulated. Since H_2CO_3 is readily converted from or to a gas, CO_2, its concentration is responsive to alveolar P_{CO_2} and can be altered by variations in pulmonary ventilation. Furthermore, the concentration of bicarbonate ion in extracellular fluid can be altered by changes in renal function. Indeed, the *bicarbonate–carbonic acid system is the major buffer system in the body that is subject to compensatory physiological regulation.* Following any alteration in this system, every other buffer pair in body fluids must alter since the ratio of a buffer pair defines and in turn is defined by the pH. Thus, any alteration in the bicarbonate–carbonic acid system achieved by the lungs and the kidneys brings into play the buffer capacity of all other buffer systems in the body fluids. The ratio of the bicarbonate–carbonic acid system at a pH of 7.4 is 20:1. Although a buffer pair is more efficient when the ratio of the pair at body pH is close to

1, the unique qualities of this particular system make it highly effective even at a ratio of 20:1. The mechanisms for the pulmonary and renal control of body pH by alterations in the bicarbonate–carbonic acid ratio will be elaborated below.

Ion Exchange. Cations such as sodium and potassium, and perhaps magnesium and calcium, from muscle and bone may exchange for hydrogen ions in the extracellular fluid, and this may play a significant role in the moderation of alterations in acid-base equilibrium. The exchange of anions probably plays a much less important role except for the shift of chloride and bicarbonate that may occur across the red-cell membrane.

Respiratory Regulation. In terms of quantity alone, the lungs play the major role in the daily excretion of acid as CO_2. The mechanisms in the CNS that are responsible for the rate and the depth of respiratory activity are responsive to the partial pressure of CO_2 and to pH such that a depression in pH or an increase of P_{CO_2} tends to increase ventilatory exchange. This, in turn, serves to eliminate more acid as CO_2 and to minimize the acid-base disturbance.

An interesting and still incompletely evaluated facet of the chemoregulation of respiratory activity relates to an apparent alteration in the sensitivity of the central receptors to an increase of P_{CO_2} after there has been a period of hypercapnia or hypocapnia. A prolonged exposure to increased levels of CO_2 tends to diminish the response to an increment of P_{CO_2} and *vice versa*. This could be due to the magnitude of the pH change induced by the increment of P_{CO_2}. The total *amount* of this buffer system that is available will change during the time that hypercapnia or hypocapnia is present.

Renal Regulation. The renal mechanisms contribute to acid-base regulation by varying the net rate of excretion of hydrogen ions and by selectively reabsorbing and rejecting cations and anions. In terms of combating an acidosis, one can view the major role of the kidney as reabsorbing all the filtered bicarbonate and, in addition, regenerating the bicarbonate that is continually dissipated by the reaction of strong acids with the bicarbonate–carbonic acid buffer system. This can be achieved because more bicarbonate can be returned to the extracellular fluid than is filtered, or, looked at from a different view, more hydrogen ions can be excreted than are filtered. This, of course, implies that hydrogen ions are secreted by the renal tubules. The source of hydrogen ions is $H^+ \cdot HCO_3^-$ formed in the tubular cell by the hydration of CO_2, a reaction catalyzed by the enzyme carbonic anhydrase. The H^+ secreted by the tubular cells exchanges for Na^+ in tubular urine, which, in turn, is returned to the extracellular fluid combined with HCO_3^-. The details of the manner in which the kidney can regenerate the bicarbonate buffer system and regulate the concentration of extracellular bicarbonate are presented elsewhere (*see* introduction to Section VIII).

Laboratory Diagnosis of Acid-Base Disturbances. There are four primary acid-base disturbances of clinical significance: respiratory acidosis and alkalosis, and metabolic acidosis and alkalosis. This classification is based on the original directional change of a single component of the bicarbonate-carbonic acid system. By reference to the Henderson-Hasselbalch equation, the initial change may be either a rise or fall in bicarbonate, or a rise or fall in carbonic acid (or P_{CO_2}). These changes, in turn, may be induced by multiple factors, depending upon the disease entity. There are several technics for the evaluation of these disturbances. The simplest and most common approach is to determine the pH and P_{CO_2} of the blood, and the total CO_2 content of the serum. These data will usually tell one what sort of disturbance or disturbances are present. The history and physical examination should be equally diagnostic as to the general nature of the underlying disorder, but may be less accurate than desired in terms of quantitative evaluation.

Although there are more complex analytical methods for evaluating abnormalities in acid-base metabolism (Singer and Hastings, 1948; Astrup, 1961), they provide little more information than is easily available from the above procedures (Schwartz and Relman, 1963).

The simple calculation of the *anion gap* is also exceedingly helpful. On the basis of the normal cation-anion pattern of the plasma and assuming single normal values in mEq per liter, the difference between the concentration of sodium (140) and the sum of the concentrations of bicarbonate (25) and chloride (105) is 10. A normal range is 8 to 12. Since the anion gap represents the difference between two relatively large numbers, it is subject to accumulative analytical error. Some clinicians add potassium to the calculation, but this contributes little since the observed changes in potassium concentration are, in absolute terms, very small compared to those of the other ions. If the concentration of a normal anion, other than chloride or bicarbonate, is abnormally high, or if an abnormal anion has accumulated, the disorder may be detected by calculation of the anion gap. Major examples of anions that contribute to the anion gap include β-hydroxybutyrate, acetoacetate, lactate, phosphate, and sulfate. The nature of the acid-base disturbance may be assessed with measurements of pH and the bicarbonate-carbonic acid system. The anion gap may provide additional insight into both etiology and compensatory mechanisms.

The four types of acid-base disturbance will now be briefly outlined, and, if the Henderson-Hasselbalch equation is kept in mind, the impact of the primary disturbance will become more clear.

Respiratory Acidosis. In this situation the primary disorder is retention of carbon dioxide because of improper ventilation. The effect is to increase the denominator of the buffer ratio in the Henderson-Hasselbalch equation, and hence to lower the pH. The accession of acid (in this case, CO_2) is buffered, modified by ion-exchange mechanisms, and the kidney responds by increasing the reabsorption of bicarbonate at the expense of chloride. The lungs play no compensatory role, since it is their disability that has induced the disturbance. The chemical characteristics of this disorder are listed in Table 36–5. The diminished response to further increments of P_{CO_2} after a period of hypercapnia presumably makes the degree of hypoxia the major stimulus to breathing. When such patients are exposed to high concentrations of oxygen and the hypoxia is thereby diminished, the major stimulus to breathing may be lessened, further hypoventilation may ensue, and an acute life-threatening increase in P_{CO_2} may result. This is not to be interpreted to mean that such patients should not receive oxygen; rather, it should be administered initially in a concentration less than 100%, and the patient should be watched carefully to ensure that this complication will be recognized readily should it occur. It should also be cautioned that depressant drugs such as the barbiturates or morphine may induce a greater degree of hypoventilation and worsen the problem.

Obviously, the most important aspects of therapy relate to an improvement in the basic cause underlying the hypoventilation. However, conventional therapy may fail or the primary disease process may progress inexorably, and more drastic measures are then indicated. The use of mechanical respiratory devices offers an important therapeutic approach. The improved ventilatory exchange that can be brought about in this fashion may reduce the hypercapnia to such an extent that the patient may once again be more responsive to increments of P_{CO_2}. However, in some instances this may turn out to be self-defeating because the increased work of breathing may result in the production of more CO_2 than the improved ventilatory exchange permits to be excreted.

In severe respiratory acidosis, particularly in asthmatic patients, it may be essential to correct the pH derangement directly. This can be accomplished by the infusion of sodium bicarbonate. At a more normal pH, bronchodilator drugs become more effective and the basic pulmonary disorder may be alleviated. Such therapy expands plasma and extracellular fluid volume, and in the presence of a diminished cardiac reserve should be undertaken with caution (Mithoefer *et al.*, 1965).

The synthetic buffer *tromethamine* (*tris*-[hydroxymethyl] aminomethane) may also be utilized (Manfredi *et al.*, 1960). This base combines with H^+ to raise the pH and to increase the concentration of HCO_3^- at the expense of H_2CO_3.

Respiratory Alkalosis. In this situation the disturbance is caused by an increased excretion of CO_2 by way of the lungs, owing to hyperventilation. It is usually a consequence of an emotional disorder and much less frequently of a lesion of the CNS that presumably stimulates the mechanisms that

drive respiration. It can also be caused by drugs that stimulate respiration, such as the salicylates. The hyperventilation diminishes the P_{CO_2}, which increases the value of the buffer ratio and, therefore, increases the pH. At the same time the plasma concentration of bicarbonate falls as a direct result of the buffer reactions and compensatory mechanisms that come into play. The chemical values are described in Table 36–5. The increased renal excretion of bicarbonate is usually accompanied by some increase in the excretion of potassium as well, so that the disturbance may tend to help initiate an element of potassium depletion. Since the hypocapnia induced in this fashion tends to increase the sensitivity of the central respiratory apparatus to increments of P_{CO_2}, this disorder tends to perpetuate itself.

The therapeutic measures are several. In the patient with hysterical hyperventilation, rebreathing into a paper bag will tend to augment P_{CO_2} and combat the respiratory alkalosis. In the more severe form, in which there is sufficient alkalosis to induce carpopedal spasm, the use of sedation along with breathing a gas mixture with CO_2 (usually about a 5% concentration) may be very helpful. In instances of primary respiratory alkalosis due to a CNS lesion, the therapy must obviously be directed at the specific cause as well. Salicylate poisoning as a cause of respiratory alkalosis is discussed in Chapter 17.

Metabolic Acidosis. The disturbance results either from a loss of proton acceptors (such as bicarbonate in severe diarrhea) or from the accession of an acid load that may result from a metabolic disturbance such as diabetic ketoacidosis, renal insufficiency, lactic acidosis, or that caused by administration of an acidifying salt such as ammonium chloride. Insight into etiology may be obtained from the magnitude of the anion gap. The ketoacids and lactic acid play an obvious role. In renal insufficiency the abnormally large anion gap is attributable to phosphate and sulfate. If acidosis is the result of the ingestion of ammonium chloride, the anion gap is normal since the chloride anion is accounted for in the basic measurement. Whether due to the accession of a potentially acidic load that will be buffered, in part at least, by the bicarbonate system, or to the primary loss of bicarbonate, the impact on the Henderson-Hasselbalch equation is to reduce the value of the numerator and, therefore, to decrease the pH. The buffers, ion-exchange mechanisms, and respiratory and renal responses tend to compensate for the acidosis and are more or less efficient, depending on the intensity of the disturbance on the one hand and the health of the lungs and kidneys on the other.

No effort is made herein to detail the specific therapy of the many types of acidosis, except to mention the fluids that may be useful in combating an overwhelming acidosis. Obviously, the therapy of diabetic acidosis is dependent primarily on improving the utilization of glucose by the administration of insulin as well as correcting the dehydration, the potassium depletion, and the other altered functions; in many instances specific therapy with an alkalinizing agent is unnecessary.

When it is considered advisable to employ an alkalinizing salt, the use of a solution of sodium bicarbonate instead of sodium lactate is recommended. When sodium lactate is employed, the increase in concentration of bicarbonate is dependent on the integrity of cellular oxidative activity. If this is deficient, then the lactate will not be converted to bicarbonate and the therapeutic goal will not have been achieved. This is of particular importance in view of the greater recognition of lactic acidosis itself.

The dose of bicarbonate necessary to correct an acidosis is exceedingly difficult to define antecedently. Formulas have been recommended, but they are so often in error that one should not take such guidelines too rigidly. One suggestion has been to estimate the difference between the normal and the current total HCO_3^- content, expressed in mEq, and multiply this by 50% of the body weight in kilograms. If one elects to use this guideline, appropriate determinations should be made at sufficiently frequent intervals so as to ensure adequate therapy and avoid both undertreatment and overtreatment. Because of the persistent high rate of lactic acid production, undertreatment is more likely in lactic acidosis than in the other forms of metabolic acidosis. Overtreatment is to be avoided since the rapid conversion from acidosis to alkalosis may be harmful.

In more chronic diseases, such as fairly stable chronic renal insufficiency, the metabolic acidosis is correctable with the use of sodium bicarbonate or preparations of sodium citrate. The latter is claimed by many to be more palatable in the form of Shohl's solution (*see* below). In any event, the dose must be found in an empirical fashion. Furthermore, since in the chronic stable situation there is little need for hurry, small doses should be used initially so as not to overtreat. There is a danger of inducing a metabolic alkalosis, especially if the patient has any element of coexistent potassium depletion, and of causing frank carpopedal spasm, if the patient has coincidental hypocalcemia. This danger can be avoided if potassium depletion and hypocalcemia are treated appropriately.

Metabolic Alkalosis. This is characterized by an increase in the concentration of bicarbonate in the extracellular fluid, unattended by a proportionate increase in the P_{CO_2} (*see* Table 36–5), so that the buffer ratio is in excess of 20 and the pH is accordingly increased. This is perhaps the most far-reaching acid-base disturbance, since some of the consequences tend to perpetuate the condition. A metabolic alkalosis can be induced by the loss of hydrogen ions, as in vomiting hydrochloric acid, or by the administration of alkalinizing salts, such as sodium bicarbonate or sodium citrate. The tendency for potassium depletion to produce metabolic alkalosis is associated with complex mechanisms that are discussed in the subsequent section.

The compensatory mechanisms that tend to minimize the deviation in pH may be anticipated from the Henderson-Hasselbalch equation, but in every instance there are serious limits imposed on their efficiency, which is not the case in the acid-base disturbances previously discussed. For example, respiratory compensation may have serious limits imposed upon it, since the increase in pH would tend to suppress ventilation, thus permitting some accumulation of CO_2. However, this might very well be limited owing to hypoxia and hypercapnia, both of which independently tend to increase ventilatory activity by stimulation of peripheral receptors. In addition, although CO_2 penetrates the brain rapidly, equilibration with bicarbonate is slow. Hence, if the cerebrospinal fluid bicarbonate is still relatively normal and the P_{CO_2} is increased, the pH of this fluid is reduced and the central receptors are thereby stimulated to increase ventilatory exchange. The renal response might be expected to promote the excretion of sodium bicarbonate. In fact, this will occur to the point at which a negative balance of sodium develops, in which case all the mechanisms available to promote the retention of sodium are implemented. Stated in different terms, the compensatory renal excretion of bicarbonate requires the obligatory excretion of a fixed cation, principally sodium. When a significant deficit of sodium develops, this ion is no longer excreted in the urine. Hence, bicarbonate excretion also declines despite the persistent alkalosis of the extracellular fluids. *It should be emphasized that sodium depletion (with or without significant potassium depletion) is primarily responsible for the paradoxical aciduria of a metabolic alkalosis.* Little bicarbonate will be excreted without accompanying sodium ions. However, a deficit of potassium augments this phenomenon.

In severe metabolic alkalosis there is another mechanism that may be considered compensatory in nature since it tends to minimize the change in extracellular pH. This involves the accumulation of organic acids in the plasma, and it may be measured indirectly by the anion gap. In the case of metabolic acidosis, the accumulation of such acids is an etiological factor. In the case of metabolic alkalosis, organic acid accumulation may be regarded as compensatory. In its absence, the bicarbonate level would be still higher.

The treatment of the metabolic alkalosis is dependent, in part, on removing the initiating circumstance that induced the concatenation of events leading to this disturbance. When caused by the excessive use of alkalinizing salts, the intensity of the disorder may vary, but even if mild the intake of such salts should be halted. On the basis of early studies of Gamble and Ross (1925) that have been amply supported by subsequent clinical experience, acute metabolic alkalosis may be corrected by the administration of adequate amounts of sodium chloride solution. The ability of a neutral salt to correct an acid-base disturbance is based on physiological rather than simple chemical mechanisms. In the case of alkalosis due to vomiting, the body is depleted of water, hydrogen ion, chloride, and, to a lesser extent, sodium. Once an adequate extracellular volume is reestablished, normal renal mechanisms become effective and sodium, along with bicarbonate, is excreted in the urine. This corrects the compositional abnormality in the plasma. If the situation is more chronic and a significant potassium depletion has developed, supplemental administration of potassium chloride may be required.

Severe metabolic alkalosis may be life threatening. In rare instances, the severity of symptoms requires direct correction of the abnormal pH itself. This can be accomplished with an acidifying salt such as ammonium chloride since, in the presence of normal hepatic function, the alkalosis can be corrected without waiting for renal mechanisms to come into play. Such therapy corrects the acid-base disturbance but not the concomitant volume or solute depletion. Since ammonium is metabolized to urea and H^+, bicarbonate is neutralized, CO_2 is expired, and chloride replaces bicarbonate without any change in total circulating solute. Hepatic failure is considered a contraindication to the administration of ammonium chloride for the correction of a severe alkalosis. However, there are no suitable substitutes. The intravenous injection of dilute hydrochloric acid has been employed on occasion; however, the use of this acid is complicated by hemolysis and thrombophlebitis, and is not recommended if it can possibly be avoided.

Preparations for the Treatment of Acid-Base Disturbances. *Sodium Bicarbonate.* This salt has already been discussed in a previous section. It should be emphasized that it is the preferred alkalinizing salt since it achieves the therapeutic goal promptly.

Sodium Lactate. Sodium Lactate Injection, U.S.P., is a sterile solution of sodium lactate in sterile water. It is usually marketed as an isotonic (⅙ M; 1.9%) solution or as a molar solution that can be appropriately diluted. The reasons for preferring sodium bicarbonate in lieu of sodium lactate have been stated and merit emphasis. If the patient's status demands an increase in the concentration of bicarbonate, the expeditious way to supply it is by administration of sodium bicarbonate rather than a sodium salt of an organic acid that may or may not be converted to bicarbonate.

Shohl's Solution. This is a palatable form in which to prescribe an oral alkalinizing agent. It is prepared as follows: 140 g of citric acid and 90 g of hydrated crystalline salt of sodium citrate are dissolved in water to a final volume of 1 liter. The solution made up in this manner contains sodium in a concentration of 1 mEq/ml of solution.

Tromethamine. Tromethamine, N.F. (THAM), is available as a 0.3 M solution adjusted to pH 8.6 with acetic acid. It is also supplied as a powder (THAM-E) to be dissolved in 1 liter of sterile water. Each liter contains 300 millimoles (36 g) of tromethamine, 30 millimoles of sodium chloride, and 5 millimoles of potassium chloride.

The use of tromethamine is contraindicated in pregnant women or patients with uremia or chronic respiratory acidosis. It should not be given for longer than 1 day.

POTASSIUM

Potassium is important in electrolyte metabolism because of the specific physiological properties of the ion, related primarily to the electrical excitability of cells, the relationship between acid-base disturbances and potassium depletion, and the general effects of imbalance on cellular metabolism.

Potassium Depletion

Etiology of Potassium Depletion. By definition, depletion refers to a significantly negative external balance. This may occur from decreased intake, increased elimination, or both. The former is seen most commonly in patients who are unable to take food by mouth. Increased excretion occurs either from the gastrointestinal tract (vomiting, diarrhea, or surgical drainage of intestinal secretions) or by way of the kidney. Most gastrointestinal fluids have a potassium concentration from two to three times greater than that of the plasma (Table 36–3). The urinary concentration may vary widely. It is increased by adrenal mineralocorticoids, either administered as drugs or secreted endogenously. The mineralocorticoids appear to have no *primary* influence on the tubular secretion of potassium. However, they do increase the rate of sodium reabsorption at a distal site where such reabsorption implements the secretion of potassium. An important consequence of this mechanism is that, when potassium depletion results from primary adrenocortical hyperfunction, it may be lessened by reducing the intake of sodium, and secondarily decreasing the amount of sodium available for distal reabsorption (Seldin *et al.,* 1956). Urinary excretion of potassium is also increased in response to various systemic diseases, in some disorders of renal tubular function, and by the action of certain diuretics (*see* Chapter 39).

Estimation of Deficit. Since the major loss of potassium occurs from the intracellular space, the plasma concentration itself is only a rough index of overall balance. Despite the general correlation between the concentrations of potassium in plasma and in muscle (the major component of the intracellular space), exceptions commonly occur. Some studies show that in the adult an external deficit of 100 to 200 millimoles is necessary before the plasma concentration of potassium falls below normal, and that deficits up to 400 millimoles are required to reduce the plasma concentration below 3 mEq per liter.

The reliability of the plasma level as an index of external balance is further complicated by shifts of potassium between the extracellular and intracellular spaces due to acid-base disorders. In one study, a change of 0.1 unit in plasma pH was accompanied by a reciprocal alteration of about 0.6 mEq per liter in the plasma concentration of potassium. Thus, in diabetic acidosis the plasma potassium concentration may be normal or even elevated despite a significant loss in the urine. Other internal exchanges occur without alterations of pH. The administration of glucose and insulin produces hypokalemia. Hypokalemic periodic paralysis is also the result of potassium movement into the intracellular space. Other methods of evaluating the degree of potassium depletion include examination of alterations that may be seen in the ECG, such as a prolongation of the Q-T interval, a broad and flat T wave, inversion of the T wave, depression of the S-T segment, and defects in conduction.

In arriving at clinical estimates of potassium depletion, perhaps the most important yardstick is the careful assessment of losses of fluids, as obtained from the history, coupled with the knowledge of their probable concentrations of potassium.

A *precise determination* of deficits may be obtained by measuring total exchangeable potassium by the use of ^{42}K, or by the method for estimation of total-body potassium that exploits the presence of the naturally occurring isotope, ^{40}K. The measurement of exchangeable potassium takes at least 24 hours, and determination of total-body potassium demands sophisticated and expensive equipment of limited availability. Analysis of muscle biopsies is another direct approach. These technics are limited to research studies and are unnecessary for routine clinical purposes.

Signs and Symptoms of Potassium Depletion. Potassium depletion may be manifested by impaired neuromuscular function, which may vary from minimal weakness to frank paralysis and the occasional presence of myotonic reflexes; changes in gastric secretions, intestinal dilatation, and ileus; abnormalities of the myocardium with disturbed ECG patterns, conduction defects, and altered sensitivity to digitalis; abnormal functioning of the kidney with impaired tubular secretion of organic acids, alterations in acidification, inability to concentrate the urine appropriately, occasional depression in filtration rate, a possible increased susceptibility to pyelonephritis, and polydipsia independent of the urine-concentrating defect; disturbances in carbohydrate tolerance; and, no doubt, many other functional derangements yet to be documented and explained.

Potassium Depletion and Alkalosis. This syndrome involves the mutual impact of one disorder on the other. Potassium depletion may cause alkalosis, and *vice versa.* The mechanisms involve both external losses and internal shifts. In metabolic alkalosis from vomiting, potassium is lost in the gastric juice and also in the urine. After the excessive administration of sodium bicarbonate, potassium is excreted in the urine to produce a prompt negative balance. However, this tends to stabilize despite the continued intake of the alkalinizing salt (Sanderson, 1954). As emphasized previously, if potassium depletion is mild, the alkalosis may be corrected without specific potassium therapy.

However, if potassium depletion is severe, a state that is often best related to the duration of the disorder, potassium salts may be required to repair the alkalosis. In this instance potassium acts at one or both of two sites, the muscle cell and the renal tubule. When there is an intracellular loss of potassium, it exchanges with extracellular sodium and to a variable extent with hydrogen ion. This produces an *intracellular acidosis.* At the same time the loss of hydrogen ion from the extracellular space produces an *extracellular alkalosis.* This intracellular and extracellular derangement can be corrected by replenishing potassium and presumably is accomplished by the reentry of potassium into the cell in exchange for intracellular sodium and hydrogen ion (Cooke *et al.,* 1952; Orloff *et al.,* 1953). A defect in renal adaptation is of necessity also involved since the extracellular alkalosis would not persist if the kidney were to compensate by increasing the excretion of bicarbonate. In potassium de-

pletion with its accompanying intracellular acidosis, the capacity of the renal tubule to reabsorb bicarbonate is enhanced and the urine may be acidic, the so-called *paradoxical aciduria.* It has already been noted that this is also commonly caused by simple volume depletion. However, with severe potassium depletion the urinary excretion of bicarbonate remains too low to correct the extracellular alkalosis. With potassium therapy this can be corrected and the acid-base balance restored to normal by the reverse of the transcellular exchange of ions described above and by the external loss of bicarbonate.

It must be emphasized that, because of the complexity of the underlying mechanisms involving the discrete balance of both cations and anions and the redistribution of hydrogen ions, there are circumstances in which alkalosis is not an obligatory accompaniment of potassium depletion and, indeed, acidosis may dominate. This is well established for diabetic ketoacidosis, where there is a large anion gap due to the accumulation of organic acids, and for renal tubular acidosis, where the renal deficiency in the secretion of hydrogen ions is associated with an increased excretion of potassium and other cations (Mudge and Vislocky, 1949).

Effects of Potassium Depletion on Certain Tissues. *Skeletal Muscle.* The primary changes in muscle composition, as mentioned, include a diminished concentration of potassium and increased concentration of sodium and hydrogen ion. The pathological lesions visualized in such skeletal muscle are the so-called Zenker's waxy-degeneration type. The lesions are not extensive, and it is unlikely that they are responsible for the neuromuscular abnormality that accompanies potassium depletion. Rather, the latter is due to changes in membrane potential, which are discussed in Chapters 21 and 28.

Heart. There are distinct histological changes in the myocardium that, in the full-blown form, represent necrosis. The earliest changes consist in swelling and loss of striations of the muscle fibers; the fibers, in turn, gradually disappear, leaving the sarcolemma, and provide an appearance best described by the term *myocytolysis.* The lesions may appear anywhere in the myocardium, but there seems to be a striking predilection for the subendocardial area.

There is a most interesting but still poorly understood interrelation between sensitivity to cardiac glycosides and depletion of potassium. It is not uncommon for patients who have been satisfactorily digitalized on a maintenance dose for some period of time to become suddenly intoxicated with digitalis as they develop potassium depletion, usually induced in this circumstance by the administration of potent diuretic agents. Furthermore, the administration of potassium has been of some benefit in digitalis intoxication, even when there is no apparent antecedent potassium deficit. The actions of digitalis as they relate to ion fluxes are discussed in Chapter 31.

Kidney. Potassium depletion has serious effects on the kidney, of both a structural and functional character. Structural alterations in man consist primarily in large, vacuolated cells that appear to be confined to the epithelium of the proximal convolution.

Among the several significant alterations in renal function seen in potassium depletion, the most consistent and profound is the loss of the ability to excrete a concentrated urine. On the basis of micropuncture studies in animals, it is tempting to suggest that in potassium depletion the rate of extrusion of electrolyte from the cells of the ascending limb may be impaired as a consequence of the effects of a diminished level of potassium, either in the luminal fluid or in the contraluminal interstitial fluid. Active transport of chloride and sodium in this segment of the nephron is the initial step in setting up the intrarenal osmotic gradient.

The acute effects of acid-base shifts on potassium secretion by the distal tubule appear to reflect a reciprocal relationship between the concentrations of potassium and hydrogen ions in the secreting cells (Brenner and Berliner, 1973). The resultant effect on external balance has been discussed above. Potassium depletion also appears to promote an increased excretion of ammonia (Tannen *et al.,* 1973).

Treatment of Potassium Deficit. Despite the fact that the consequences of potassium depletion may be serious, and in some respects irreversible, it is wise to proceed cautiously with repair of the deficit, since it is currently impossible to assess the intensity of the depletion with any degree of accuracy. Under such circumstances there are significant hazards that attend overly aggressive therapy. The most serious is the possibility of achieving cardiotoxic concentrations of potassium by administration of potassium salts too rapidly or in too large a quantity. This caution is particularly important in those instances where potassium deficit is coexistent with dehydration and serious contraction of the extracellular fluid volume. The renal excretion of excesses of administered potassium may not be efficient, owing to decompensation of renal function. The route by which potassium should be administered depends on circumstances, but whenever possible the oral route is the safest. However, potassium often must be administered intravenously. If the potassium concentration in plasma is depressed and if renal function is reasonably normal, potassium may be administered at a rate of approximately 20 mEq per hour with considerable safety. There are occasions when the deficit appears more intense and a larger quantity should be administered. In any event, repeated observations should be made at regular intervals, not only of the clinical status of the patient but also of the ECG and the plasma concentration of potassium, to ensure that repletion is proceeding without hazard.

The particular potassium salt that is used has some relevance. If potassium depletion is accompanied by a deficit of chloride, it may be quite difficult to correct that deficit and dissipate the alkalosis unless adequate quantities of chloride are made available. The administration of potassium salts other than the chloride in the context of a regimen free of sodium chloride creates a high concentration of impermeant anions in the tubular fluid, which may in turn facilitate the tubular secretion of potassium and perpetuate a negative external balance for that cation (*see* Gulyassy *et al.,* 1962; Schwartz *et al.,* 1962, 1968).

Miscellaneous Therapeutic Uses. Potassium is sometimes of therapeutic value in conditions not directly associated with a potassium deficiency state. The cation may be of value in the symptomatic control of the cardiac manifestations of digitalis intoxication, especially if there has been some loss of the ion associated with the use of diuretic drugs. A specific therapeutic use of the potassium ion is in the treatment of *familial periodic paralysis*, a rare myopathy characterized by recurrent attacks of flaccid paralysis affecting mainly the muscles of the trunk and limbs. Associated with the periodic attacks, there is a reduction in concentration of potassium in the extracellular fluids. The acute symptoms can be rapidly relieved by the intravenous or oral administration of potassium chloride. The former route should be reserved for emergency use only. If potassium chloride is employed, a solution of 1 g in 50 ml of sterile water is slowly injected. The oral dose is 5 to 10 g. Remission of symptoms occurs within 30 minutes to 2 hours after oral administration. As a prophylactic measure, the administration of 5 g of potassium chloride nightly will help prevent attacks. Rarely, cases of familial periodic paralysis are not associated with hypokalemia and, therefore, do not respond to potassium therapy.

POTASSIUM EXCESS

Hyperkalemia is a common clinical event. The two most common causes of potassium intoxication are the too rapid administration, either by mouth or by vein, of a solution of potassium, and acute or chronic renal insufficiency. In the latter circumstance, hyperkalemia appears, owing to an inability on the part of the kidney to excrete potassium. Hyperkalemia may also occur, even though no potassium is administered, when there has been tissue trauma or when a large postpartum uterus is involuting and cellular potassium thereby gains access to the extracellular fluid. The acute management of this problem includes the intravenous administration of a calcium salt, glucose and insulin, and sodium bicarbonate. Ion-exchange resins (polystyrene sulfonate) that can be given by mouth or instilled by rectum can diminish the hyperkalemia in a day.

Preparations to Repair Potassium Depletion and to Control Hyperkalemia. *Potassium Chloride Oral Solution,* U.S.P., contains 20 mEq of potassium per 15 ml (1 tablespoonful). It is preferable to *Potassium Chloride Tablets,* U.S.P., which are no longer generally available. The tablets may produce considerable gastric irritation; if potassium chloride tablets are enteric coated, they may produce denudation, ulceration, perforation, and stricture of the small bowel. *Potassium Chloride Injection,* U.S.P., is a sterile solution of potassium chloride in water. It is usually marketed as a 15% (2-mEq/ml) or 24% (3.2-mEq/ml) solution in 10-, 20-, or 30-ml ampuls. This solution should never be administered as such but must be suitably diluted to avoid a sudden increase in the concentration of plasma potassium that

could readily be fatal. Various other potassium salts are also available.

Cation-Exchange Resins. Exchange resins have been useful in ridding the body fluids of excess potassium. One of the most efficient is *Sodium Polystyrene Sulfonate,* U.S.P. (KAYEXALATE), which exchanges sodium for potassium. It may be given by mouth, instilled as an enema, or inserted in the rectum in a dialysis bag to facilitate recovery. The resin should be retained in the rectum for 30 to 45 minutes. When administered orally, a laxative should be given concurrently to avoid fecal impaction. The use of resins by mouth is frequently proscribed because there is nausea and vomiting. The usual oral dose is 15 g of the resin one to four times daily. It should be suspended in a palatable vehicle. When used as an enema, 25 g of the resin in 100 ml of a suitable vehicle is inserted through a large Foley catheter with the 30-ml Foley bag inflated. The rectal tube is clamped and the material left in the rectum for the period indicated above. The clamp is then released and the material expelled by the patient. Such enemas are given at 1- to 2-hour intervals until the potassium level is within a safe range.

Calcium Gluconate, U.S.P. Calcium gluconate may be a very useful agent in combating the deleterious effects of hyperkalemia on the heart. It may be administered directly intravenously as a 10% solution while the ECG is monitored. As much as 50 ml of a 10% solution can be administered safely if given slowly. Following this, another 50 ml of the calcium gluconate (10%) can be placed in a larger volume of fluid (glucose in water, etc.) and administered more slowly. Available preparations are described in Chapter 37.

Dialytic Procedures. These technics can be life-saving if the measures described above fail; they are discussed below, in the context of the management of acute renal failure.

ACUTE RENAL INSUFFICIENCY

An acute and significant deterioration in renal function with oliguria or anuria may be transient and due solely to dehydration and diminished blood volume with impaired perfusion of the kidney. Such a disorder may be quickly corrected in the manner described above for the treatment of dehydration and hypovolemia. Return of function eliminates from consideration more serious causes of renal insufficiency.

However, acute tubular necrosis may be provoked by a variety of poisons and drugs, heavy metals, the products of hemolysis, shock, and perhaps other insults. Lesions from these causes are often reversible over a period of weeks, provided the patient can be maintained until resolution occurs and renal function returns.

In the management of acute tubular necrosis the physician is faced with the problem of attempting to maintain the internal environment as nearly normal as is possible. The challenges include the maintenance of a reasonably normal volume of the extracellular fluid, and the combating of the metabolic acidosis, the hyperkalemia, the other ionic disturbances, and the consequences of "uremia."

For the control of the extracellular fluid volume, it seems clear that adult patients need about 400 to 500 ml of water per day to replace the difference between insensible loss and the amount of water that is produced from the metabolism of body tissues. Under such a program a patient should lose 0.2 to 0.4 kg (½ to 1 lb) a day, since without adequate caloric intake this amount of body substance will be consumed. Calories should be provided in the form of carbohydrate, and the usual procedure is to administer the daily allotment of 400 to 500 ml of fluid as a hypertonic solution of glucose. When a catheter is threaded into a rather large vein, this solution can be administered with little discomfort or damage to the wall of the vessel. Nevertheless, the infusion site should be changed every 48 hours to avoid phlebitis and infection. In addition to this fluid regimen, an additional volume of fluid may be added, when necessary, to make up for the volume of urine lost per day and to replace the vomitus and the extra losses of water that may accompany fever and sweating. These additional fluids should contain electrolytes in the approximate concentration in which they are lost, with the exception of potassium.

Hyponatremia is most commonly a consequence of dilution, and the restoration toward normal should be accomplished by the restriction of water intake. This may have some special value, not only from the standpoint of controlling the CNS manifestations of hyponatremia but also of regulating the rate of production of urea nitrogen and perhaps other nitrogenous solutes, as well as of controlling the hyperkalemia (*see* Linhart and Welt, 1963). If the hyponatremia is associated with dehydration, it should be managed with an appropriate hypertonic solution of sodium bicarbonate and sodium chloride. The development of a metabolic acidosis is inevitable, and as long as the patient is not dehydrated the administration of sodium bicarbonate would not appear to be indicated, since one of the complications to avoid is hypervolemia. Hypertension frequently develops during acute tubular necrosis, and in association with hypervolemia it is likely to lead to congestive heart failure and death. Hyperkalemia is usually controllable by ensuring that no potassium is administered, and by the use of exchange resins as outlined above. However, if high concentrations of plasma potassium persist, then more aggressive measures may be indicated in the form of peritoneal or extracorporeal hemodialysis.

The indications for dialysis include uncontrollable hyperkalemia, and the development of signs and symptoms of uremia (*see* Merrill, 1971). Dialysis should be instituted reasonably early rather than delayed until a more critical state is reached.

Peritoneal dialysis is a simple and useful technic, and several commercial preparations of dialytic fluid and tubing for its use are readily available. In general, the solutions are characterized by concentrations that mimic interstitial fluid, with a somewhat higher level of potential bicarbonate and without potassium. The latter can be added when indicated. The commercial preparations of dialytic fluid are made up with 1.5 or 4.25% dextrose. The lower concentration is utilized when the volume of extracellular fluid appears to be normal and it is not desirable to reduce it. The higher concentration of dextrose is used as an osmotic agent to help remove fluid in excess of that which is instilled. Although glucose exchanges across the peritoneal membrane, it does so relatively more slowly than do sodium salts and, therefore, it can act as an effective osmotic agent. In this fashion, one can simultaneously correct the chemical abnormalities, reduce the level of urea and other noxious agents, and correct extracellular fluid volume. Although not as efficient as extracorporeal hemodialysis, peritoneal dialysis obviously is easier to use, and in the course of 24 to 36 hours one can accomplish virtually the same clearance of urea and potassium and the same corrections as with the use of extracorporeal dialytic procedures.

In instances where one wishes to reduce the plasma concentration of potassium and the degree of "uremia" more quickly, extracorporeal hemodialysis (the "artificial kidney") is obviously a more efficient way to accomplish these ends. There are a variety of "artificial kidneys" on the market; an analysis of their relative merits is beyond the scope of this discussion (*see* Bluemle, 1971).

In addition to correctable hyperkalemia, hyponatremia, acid-base disturbances, and the general consequences of the uremic state, the major causes of death aside from the condition in which the complications arose are infection and congestive heart failure. To avoid congestive heart failure, every precaution should be taken to ensure that extracellular fluid volume is not permitted to expand beyond normal and that digitalization is employed as soon as indicated. The control of infection is a serious problem, and most patients are placed on a regimen that is referred to as "reverse isolation," in which every effort is made to prevent their becoming contaminated with microorganisms that the physician may carry with him from other patients or harbors himself.

Solutions for Peritoneal Dialysis. There are several commercial preparations of fluids to be used for peritoneal dialysis; these are marketed with a sterile catheter that is to be introduced into the peritoneal cavity and with tubing for attachment to the bottles of fluid. As stated earlier, these are prepared with 1.5 or 4.25% glucose. In general, the ionic composition per liter is as follows: Na, 140 mEq; Ca, 4 mEq; Mg, 1.5 mEq; Cl, 102 mEq; HCO_3 (by metabolic conversion), 43 mEq.

Throughout this entire chapter, guidelines for therapy have been suggested, and, although exceedingly useful, the reader should be aware that they represent an approach that is an approximation toward an average patient. The physician must examine the details of management as carefully as would be the case in the prescription of a drug or any other therapy in clinical medicine. Individualization of therapy must continuously be practiced.

Astrup, P. New approach to acid-base metabolism. *Clin. Chem.,* **1961,** *7,* 1–15.

Baker, G. P.; Levitin, H.; and Epstein, F. H. Sodium depletion and renal conservation of water. *J. clin. Invest.,* **1961,** *40,* 867–873.

Bluemle, L. W. Dialysis. In, *Diseases of the Kidney,* 2nd ed., Vol. 1. (Strauss, M. B., and Welt, L., eds.) Little, Brown & Co., Boston, **1971,** pp. 343–372.

Bollman, J. L. Extravascular diffusion of dextran from blood. *J. Lab. clin. Med.,* **1953,** *41,* 421–427.

Brenner, B. M., and Berliner, R. W. Transport of potassium. In, *Renal Physiology. Handbook of Physiology,* Sect. 8. (Orloff, J., and Berliner, R. W., eds.) American Physiological Society, Washington, D. C., **1973,** pp. 497–520.

Carpenter, C. C. J. Clinical studies in Asiatic cholera. VI. Overall clinical observations. *Bull. Johns Hopkins Hosp.,* **1966,** *118,* 243–245.

Cooke, R. E.; Segar, W. E.; Cheek, D. B.; Coville, F. E.; and Darrow, D. C. Extrarenal correction of alkalosis associated with potassium deficiency. *J. clin. Invest.,* **1952,** *31,* 798–805.

Edelman, I. S., and Leibman, J. Anatomy of body water and electrolytes. *Am. J. Med.,* **1959,** *27,* 256–277.

Edelman, I. S.; Olney, J. M.; James, A. H.; Brooks, L.; and Moore, F. D. Body composition: studies in the human being by the dilution principle. *Science, Wash.,* **1952,** *115,* 447–454.

Finberg, L.; Kiley, J.; and Luttrell, C. N. Mass accidental salt poisoning in infancy. A study of a hospital disaster. *J. Am. med. Ass.,* **1963.** *184,* 187–190.

Gamble, J. L. Physiological information gained from studies on the life raft ration. *Harvey Lect.,* **1947,** *62,* 247–273.

Gamble, J. L., and Ross, S. G. The factors in the dehydration following pyloric obstruction. *J. clin. Invest.,* **1925,** *1,* 403–423.

Gelin, L.-E.; Korsan-Bengsten, K.; Ygge, J.; and Zederfeldt, B. Influence of low viscous dextran on the hemostatic mechanism. *Acta chir. scand.,* **1961,** *122,* 324–328.

Gulyassy, P. F.; Strihou, C. V. Y. de; and Schwartz, W. B. On the mechanism of nitrate-induced alkalosis: the possible role of selective chloride depletion in acid-base regulation. *J. clin. Invest.,* **1962,** *41,* 1850–1862.

Kabat, E. A., and Berg, D. Dextran, as antigen in man. *J. Immun.,* **1953,** *70,* 514–532.

Katz, M. A. Hyperglycemia-induced hyponatremia —calculation of sodium depression. *New Engl. J. Med.,* **1973,** *289,* 843–844.

Langsjoen, P. H. Observations in the excretion of low molecular dextran. *Angiology,* **1965,** *16,* 148–153.

Lichtman, M. A.; Miller, D. R.; Cohen, J.; and Waterhouse, C. Reduced red cell 2,3-DPG and ATP concentration, and increased hemoglobin-oxygen affinity caused by hypophosphatemia. *Ann. intern. Med.,* **1971,** *74,* 562–568.

Linhart, J. W., and Welt, L. G. The effect of hyponatremia and cellular dilution on tissue catabolism in the rat. *Trans. Ass. Am. Phycns,* **1963,** *76,* 184–198.

Manfredi, F.; Sieker, H. O.; Spoto, A. P.; and Saltzman, H. A. Severe carbon dioxide intoxication: treatment with organic buffer (trihydroxymethylaminomethane). *J. Am. med. Ass.,* **1960,** *173,* 999–1003.

Merrill, J. P. Acute renal failure. In, *Diseases of the Kidney,* 2nd ed., Vol. 1. (Strauss, M. B., and Welt, L. G., eds.) Little, Brown & Co., Boston, **1971,** pp. 637–666.

Mithoefer, J. C.; Runser, R. H.; and Karetsky, M. S. The use of sodium bicarbonate in the treatment of acute bronchial asthma. *New Engl. J. Med.,* **1965,** *272,* 1200–1203.

Moore, F. D. Tris buffer, mannitol, and low viscous dextran. *Surg. Clins N. Am.,* **1963,** *43,* 577–596.

Mudge, G. H., and Vislocky, L. Electrolyte changes in human striated muscle in acidosis and alkalosis. *J. clin. Invest.,* **1949,** *28,* 482–486.

Orloff, J.; Kennedy, T. J., Jr.; and Berliner, R. W. The effect of potassium in nephrectomized rats with hypokalemic alkalosis. *J. clin. Invest.,* **1953,** *32,* 538–542.

Sanderson, P. H. Renal response to massive alkali loading in the human subject. In, *Ciba Foundation Symposium on the Kidney.* (Lewis, A. A. G., and Wolstenholme, G. E. W., eds.) Little, Brown & Co., Boston, **1954,** pp. 165–174.

Schwartz, W. B., and Relman, A. S. A critique of the parameters used in the evaluation of acid-base disorders: "whole blood buffer base" and "standard bicarbonate" compared with blood pH and plasma bicarbonate concentration. *New Engl. J. Med.,* **1963,** *268,* 1382–1388.

Schwartz, W. B.; Strihou, C. V. Y. de; and Gulyassy, P. F. Nitrate alkalosis: the role of anions in acid-base regulation. *Trans. Ass. Am. Physns,* **1962,** *75,* 146–153.

Schwartz, W. B.; Strihou, C. V. Y. de; and Kassirer, J. P. Role of anions in metabolic alkalosis and potassium deficiency. *New Engl. J. Med.,* **1968,** *279,* 630–639.

Seldin, D. W.; Welt, L. G.; and Curt, J. H. The role of sodium salts and adrenal steroids in the production of hypokalemic alkalosis. *Yale J. Biol. Med.,* **1956,** *29,* 229–247.

Singer, R. B., and Hastings, A. B. An improved clinical method for the estimation of disturbances of the acid-base balance of human blood. *Medicine, Baltimore,* **1948,** *27,* 223–242.

Tannen, R. L.; Wedell, E.; and Moore, R. Renal adaptation to a high potassium intake. *J. clin. Invest.,* **1973,** *52,* 2089–2101.

Tosteson, D. C. Active transport, genetics, and cellular evolution. *Fedn Proc. Fedn Am. Socs exp. Biol.,* **1963,** *22,* 19–26.

Wasserman, K., and Mayerson, H. S. Plasma, lymph, and urine studies after dextran infusions. *Am. J. Physiol.,* **1952,** *171,* 218–232.

Witham, A. C.; Fleming, J. W.; and Bloom, W. L. The effect of the intravenous administration of dextran on cardiac output and other circulatory dynamics. *J. clin. Invest.,* **1951,** *30,* 897–902.

Wynn, V. A metabolic study of acute water intoxication in man and dogs. *Clin. Sci.,* **1955,** *14,* 669–680.

Monographs and Reviews

Boen, S. T. Kinetics of peritoneal dialysis: a comparison with the artificial kidney. *Medicine, Baltimore,* **1961,** *40,* 243–287.

Cowan, G., Jr., and Sheetz, W. *Intravenous Hyperalimentation.* Lea & Febiger, Philadelphia, **1972.**

Davenport, H. W. *The ABC of Acid-Base Chemistry,* 5th ed. University of Chicago Press, Chicago, **1969.**

Fox, C. L., Jr., and Nahas, G. G. *Body Fluid Replacement in the Surgical Patient.* Grune & Stratton, Inc., New York, **1970.**

Maxwell, M. H., and Kleeman, C. R. *Clinical Disorders of Fluid and Electrolyte Metabolism.* McGraw-Hill Book Co., New York, **1972.**

Moore, F. D.; Oleson, K. H.; McMurrey, J. D.; Parker, H. V.; Ball, M. R.; and Boyden, C. M. *The Body Cell Mass and Its Supporting Environment.* W. B. Saunders Co., Philadelphia, **1963.**

Nahas, G. G. (ed.). Current concepts of acid-base measurement. *Ann. N.Y. Acad. Sci.,* **1966,** *133,* 1–274.

Pitts, R. F. *Physiology of the Kidney and Body Fluids: An Introductory Text,* 3rd ed. Year Book Medical Publishers, Inc., Chicago, **1974.**

Ussing, H. H.; Kruhøffer, P.; Thaysen, J. H.; and Thorn, N. A. The alkali metal ions in biology. In, *Handb. exp. Pharmak.,* Vol. 13. (Eichler, O., and Farah, A., eds.) Springer-Verlag, Berlin, **1960.**

Winters, R. W. *The Body Fluids in Pediatrics.* Little, Brown & Co., Boston, **1973.**

37 CATIONS: CALCIUM, MAGNESIUM, BARIUM, LITHIUM, AND AMMONIUM

Michael J. Peach

CALCIUM

Calcium is the fifth most abundant element in the body, and the major fraction is in the bony structure. It is present in small quantities in the extracellular fluid and to a minor extent in the structure and cytoplasm of cells of soft tissue. Calcium plays important physiological roles, many of which are only poorly understood. It is essential for the functional integrity of the nervous and muscular systems, where it has a major influence on the excitability of these tissues. It is necessary for normal cardiac function, and is one of the factors involved in the coagulation of the blood.

There are many pathological conditions associated with abnormalities of calcium metabolism. Some of these are accompanied by hypocalcemia or hypercalcemia, and still others are found with normal levels of plasma calcium. Calcium deficiency states may be favorably modified by the use of calcium preparations and vitamin D, and there are drugs that modify *hyper*calcemic states.

Calcium Requirements. The body's needs for calcium are met from food, the prominent source being dairy products. The calcium intake varies from 200 to 1500 mg per day. Calcium requirements are presented in Table XVIII-1.

State of Calcium in the Blood and Its Distribution in the Body. More than 90% of the calcium in the body is in the skeleton as phosphate and carbonate. The steady-state content of skeletal calcium is a consequence of the net effect of bone resorption and new-bone formation (Hancox, 1972). The calcium of bone, therefore, is in a constant exchange with the calcium of the interstitial fluids. The rates of exchange are modifiable by drugs, hormones, vitamins, and other factors that may influence the level of

calcium in the interstitial fluids and also the forms in which the cation is present (*see* Chapters 72 and 76).

The calcium in plasma is maintained at a fairly constant concentration of about 5 mEq per liter. However, this represents the total of three different components: (1) about one third of the plasma calcium is in a nondiffusible complex with proteins; (2) about one tenth is diffusible but complexed with anions (*e.g.,* citrate and phosphate); (3) the remaining fraction represents diffusible ionic calcium. The ionized calcium is the fraction that exerts physiological effects, and symptoms of hypocalcemia occur with its reduction. It is clear that hypocalcemia due to hypoproteinemia and a reduced concentration of protein-bound calcium is not likely to be accompanied by the symptoms and signs of hypocalcemia, unless there is a reduction in the concentration of ionized calcium as well. Hence, the interpretation of the significance of any given value of plasma calcium is impossible without knowledge of the coincident concentration of plasma proteins, and nomograms are available for this purpose.

Absorption and Excretion. In general, the major portion of absorption takes place in the more proximal segments of the small bowel; in man, approximately one third of the ingested calcium is absorbed. Intestinal absorption involves the soluble ionized form of calcium and reflects at least two separate steps: (1) calcium uptake at the mucosal pole and (2) efflux at the serosal pole of the intestinal epithelium. Mucosal uptake of calcium is presumably carrier mediated, and a calcium-binding protein under study is the leading candidate for the transmucosal carrier (Taylor and Wasserman, 1970; Kallfelz and Wasserman, 1972). It has not been established if this transmucosal calcium uptake is active or passive. Calcium efflux at the serosal pole of the intestinal epithelium is generally recognized as an energy-dependent process.

There are factors that clearly augment calcium absorption, and these include vitamin D and parathyroid hormone. Vitamin D_3

(cholecalciferol) is converted in the body to 1,25-dihydroxycholecalciferol by the actions initially of a hepatic and secondly of a renal hydroxylase. This dihydroxy metabolite of the vitamin is required for the active transport of calcium in the small intestine (for additional details, *see* Chapter 76). Parathyroid hormone also causes increased intestinal absorption of calcium. This effect of parathyroid hormone is slow in onset and dependent on dietary calcium and phosphate. The nature of the effects of parathyroid hormone on calcium absorption may be indicative of an indirect action of the hormone—perhaps a modulation of vitamin D metabolism. It is also generally accepted that a low-calcium diet results in increased fractional absorption of calcium.

Glucocorticoids and low concentrations of calcitonin depress calcium transport across the small intestine (Krawitt, 1972; Olson *et al.*, 1972), and there are other factors that also inhibit the absorption of calcium. Some of these are relatively simple, for example, the presence in the bowel of a substance that promotes the formation of a complex or insoluble salt of calcium that is not absorbed through the wall of the gut. Such substances include phytate, oxalate, and probably phosphate. Disease states such as steatorrhea may result in decreased absorption of calcium. This is largely due to decreased absorption of the fat-soluble vitamin D. Other diarrheas with chronic gastrointestinal malabsorption may promote increased fecal losses of calcium as well.

Calcium is secreted into the gastrointestinal tract in saliva, bile, and pancreatic juice. This endogenous calcium and the unabsorbed dietary calcium constitute the sources of the cation excreted in the feces. There is significant calcium loss in milk during lactation, and also daily losses in sweat.

The *urinary excretion* of calcium is the net result of the quantity filtered and the amount reabsorbed. There is no evidence of renal tubular secretion of calcium. The mechanisms for the renal reabsorption of calcium are unknown, and for unexplained reasons there is, in general, a correlation between the urinary excretion of sodium and calcium. This is true when natriuresis is increased by loading with salt, and it also is noted with diuretics that act at the ascending limb of the loop of Henle and the distal tubule (Davis and Murdaugh, 1970).

In animal studies approximately two thirds of the filtered calcium is reabsorbed in the proximal convolution, 20 to 25% in the loop of Henle, and 10% in the distal convolution (Murayama *et al.*, 1972; Massry and Coburn, 1973).

Parathyroid hormone stimulates the reabsorption of calcium by the kidney apparently by means of an effect on the distal tubule, while the active metabolites of vitamin D stimulate proximal tubular reabsorption of calcium (Puschett *et al.*, 1972). Calcitonin inhibits the proximal tubular reabsorption of calcium, thus facilitating excretion of the cation (Paillard *et al.*, 1972).

The influence of renal disease on urinary calcium excretion is varied. In ordinary forms of chronic renal failure, calcium excretion diminishes as filtration rate falls. However, in those instances where filtration is only minimally depressed and the secretion of hydrogen ions is deficient due to an inability to attain a high concentration gradient for hydrogen ions between tubular cell and lumen (renal tubular acidosis), the excretion of calcium may be enhanced. This hypercalciuria may be diminished by the correction of the resulting systemic acidosis.

PHARMACOLOGICAL ACTIONS

Local Actions. Certain salts of calcium, notably the chloride, are intensely irritating to tissue and will cause painful sloughing if injected subcutaneously. Therefore, whenever calcium chloride is administered parenterally, it must be given intravenously and great effort should be made to prevent extravasation. Calcium chloride is also somewhat irritating to the gastrointestinal tract and is usually administered with a demulcent.

Neuromuscular System. Moderate elevations of the level of calcium in the extracellular fluid may have no clinically detectable influences on the neuromuscular apparatus. However, when hypercalcemia becomes extreme, the threshold for excitation of nerve and muscle is increased. In contrast, modest diminution in the level of ionized calcium may decrease the thresholds of excitation in a striking fashion, leading to tetanic seizures and positive Chvostek and Trousseau signs. The role played by calcium in regulating the excitability of tissues is not completely elucidated. Calcium influx across the plasma membrane is thought to be by means of carrier-mediated facilitated diffusion. In excitable tissues a calcium exchange for sodium may be responsible for calcium extrusion from cells (Blaustein and Hodgkin, 1969). However, the concentration of cytoplasmic ionic calcium is not controlled by cellular influx and efflux to nearly the same extent that it is by the mitochondria and sarcoplasmic reticulum, which sequester intracellular calcium. Calcium causes relatively small changes in resting membrane potentials but modifies induced changes of membrane potentials in nerve and muscle. In addition, calcium appears to play an important role in the regulation of cell-membrane permeability to sodium and potassium. Increased concentrations of calcium diminish the permeability of the cell, while decreased calcium concentrations augment permeability.

Calcium plays additional roles both in coupling excitation with muscle contraction and in the release of neurohumoral transmitters. The action potential in muscle stimulates the release of calcium ions from the sarcoplasmic reticulum, and the divalent cation activates contraction. Interaction between actin and myosin, leading to contraction, is inhibited and muscular relaxation occurs when a complex of the proteins troponin and tropomyosin attaches to actin. The binding of calcium to troponin abolishes the inhibitory effect of troponin on the interaction of actin and myosin. Muscle relaxation occurs when ionic sarcoplasmic calcium is pumped back into the sarcoplasmic reticulum, permitting the inhibitory effect of troponin on actin and myosin.

Calcium also plays an important role in stimulus-secretion coupling in certain exocrine and endocrine glands. The release of catecholamines from the adrenal medulla, neurotransmitters at synapses, and autacoids from various sites is dependent on calcium ions. Calcium is necessary for exocytosis. (*See* Douglas, 1968; Rubin, 1970; *see also* Chapters 21 and 29.)

The interrelation between calcium and potassium has been alluded to in Chapter 36.

It was pointed out that a potassium deficiency coincident with hypocalcemia appears to protect against hypocalcemic tetany, and that correction of the potassium deficit without attention to the level of calcium might well provoke tetany without a change in the plasma level of calcium.

Cardiovascular System. It is probable that the above-described processes relating to nerve and skeletal muscle apply to cardiac muscle as well. In the myocardium, a slow inward current has been observed that occurs during the plateau of the action potential and is dependent on ionic calcium (New and Trautwein, 1972). This slow channel probably carries inward calcium current and may be related to excitation-contraction coupling. It has long been recognized that there are certain similarities in the effect of calcium and the cardiac glycosides on the cardiac muscle (Farah and Witt, 1963). Langer (1971) has postulated that the inotropic action of cardiac glycosides is mediated by an influx of calcium ions. However, certain findings are difficult to reconcile with this proposal (*see* Dutta and Marks, 1972; *see also* Chapter 31).

Miscellaneous Effects. Calcium salts may play a role in maintaining the integrity of multicellular mucosal membranes and of individual cell membranes as well. The use of calcium salts to prevent effusions across capillary endothelial membranes is, however, without demonstrated benefit. Calcium is involved in blood coagulation, but the ion is not used to treat disorders of coagulation. Calcium chloride is an acidifying salt and will promote diuresis; however, ammonium salts are much more effective acidifying agents.

ABNORMALITIES OF CALCIUM
METABOLISM

It should be clear from the discussion of some of the factors involved in maintaining calcium homeostasis that there are many ways in which significant alterations in calcium metabolism can occur. Some of these alterations may be accompanied by hypocalcemia and others by hypercalcemia.

Hypocalcemic States. The prominent signs and symptoms of hypocalcemia include tetany and related phenomena such as paresthesias, increased neuromuscular excitability, laryngospasm, muscle cramps, and convulsions (usually grand mal). The hypocalcemic states are as follows:

1. Calcium and vitamin D deprivation may readily promote hypocalcemia. This combination of events is observed in the various malabsorption states, and occurs still too often from inadequate diets owing to poverty. When due to malabsorption, the hypocalcemia is accompanied by a depressed level of phosphorus, the total proteins are usually low, and hypomagnesemia is not uncommon. In adults, low plasma calcium stimulates the release of parathyroid hormone, which causes the release of calcium from bone. This leads to osteomalacia with demineralization principally affecting the spine, rib cage, and long bones. In infants with malabsorption or inadequate calcium intake, the calcium level is usually depressed, there is hypophosphatemia, and the resultant bone disease is *rickets*. Another disorder that is more rare is vitamin D–resistant rickets. It is possible that vitamin D–resistant diseases are due to absent or reduced activity of the hepatic and renal hydroxylases responsible for the synthesis of 1,25-dihydroxycholecalciferol. If hypomagnesemia is also present, its correction may enhance responses to vitamin D and calcium therapy.

2. Hypoparathyroidism may occur spontaneously or result as a consequence of thyroid or other neck surgery. In this disorder, there is distinct hypocalcemia but *hyper*phosphatemia. Although other conditions of hypocalcemia may be associated with opacity of the lens, papilledema, and calcification of the basal ganglia, these occur more commonly with hypoparathyroidism. Other changes include trophic alterations and fungal infections of the skin. Pseudo-hypoparathyroidism is an unusual disorder characterized by multiple structural defects and a failure to respond to exogenous parathyroid hormone. The structural changes are manifested by a round face, short, thick figure, and shortening of some of the metacarpal and metatarsal bones.

3. In the period (1 to 4 days) following removal of a parathyroid adenoma, hypocalcemia is not unusual, especially if there is bone disease.

4. Neonatal tetany may result from a transient hypoparathyroidism that occurs in the newborn of mothers with hyperparathyroidism; indeed, it may be the infant's tetany that provides the clue to the mother's disorder. This is usually transient in the infant and disappears as soon as its own parathyroid glands respond appropriately. Other situations in which neonatal hypocalcemia may supervene include hypernatremia and acute infections.

5. Hypocalcemia is frequently associated with advanced renal insufficiency accompanied by hyperphosphatemia. For reasons that are not clear, many of these patients do not develop tetany unless the severe accompanying acidosis is improved with treatment. The observations of Aviolo and associates (1968) suggest a disturbance in the metabolism of vitamin D in renal insufficiency. High plasma phosphate concentrations appear to facilitate the conversion of 25-hydroxycholecalciferol to a less active metabolite instead of to 1,25-dihydroxycholecalciferol (Tanaka and DeLuca, 1973).

6. Sodium fluoride forms an insoluble salt with calcium and, if ingested in large enough quantities, may induce hypocalcemia and tetany (*see* Chapter 38).

7. Hypocalcemia can also occur following transfusions with citrated blood.

Preparations and Routes of Administration in the Treatment of Hypocalcemia. There are several preparations available if the systemic action of calcium is desired. These differ in calcium content and permissible routes of administration.

Calcium Chloride, U.S.P. ($CaCl_2 \cdot 2H_2O$), contains 27% calcium and consists of white granules freely soluble in water. It is valuable in the treatment of hypocalcemic tetany. The salt can be given either by mouth or intravenously. *It must never be injected into tissues.* It is somewhat irritating to the gastrointestinal tract and should be administered in some demulcent vehicle, such as milk. It should never be given by gavage to infants, as necrosis and ulceration of the gastrointestinal tract may result. *Calcium Chloride Injection,* U.S.P., is irritating to veins. Injections are accompanied by peripheral vasodilatation and a cutaneous burning sensation. The salt is usually given intravenously in a concentration of 5 to 10% (equivalent to 0.68 to 1.36 mEq Ca^{2+}/ml). Injection rate should be slow (not over 1 to 2 ml per minute) to prevent a high concentration of calcium from reaching the heart, because of the danger of cardiac syncope. A moderate fall in blood pressure due to vasodilatation may attend the injection. Since calcium chloride is an acidifying salt, it is usually undesirable in the treatment of the hypocalcemia of renal insufficiency.

Calcium gluceptate injection is a 23% solution (18 mg or 0.9 mEq Ca^{2+}/ml) that is provided in 5-ml ampuls. It is administered intravenously in a dose of 5 to 20 ml (4.5 to 18 mEq Ca^{2+}) for the treatment of severe hypocalcemic tetany; the injection may produce a transient tingling sensation. When the intravenous route is not possible, the injection may be given intramuscularly in a dose up to 5 ml, which may produce a mild local reaction.

Calcium Gluconate, U.S.P. ($[CH_2OH\{CHOH\}_4COO]_2Ca \cdot H_2O$), contains 9% calcium. It is available as *Calcium Gluconate Tablets,* U.S.P., containing 325, 500, 650, or 1000 mg of the salt (equivalent to 1.5, 2.3, 3.0, or 4.6 mEq Ca^{2+}, respectively). It is nonirritating to the gastrointestinal tract. For intramuscular and intravenous injection, *Calcium Gluconate Injection,* U.S.P., is administered as a 10% solution (0.45 mEq Ca^{2+}/ml). It is a readily available source of calcium ions, and the intravenous administration of this salt is the treatment of choice for severe hypocalcemic tetany. The intramuscular route should not be employed in infants, as abscess formation at the site of injection may result.

Calcium Lactate, U.S.P. ($[CH_3CHOHCOO]_2Ca \cdot 5H_2O$), contains 13% calcium. Its physical properties are similar to those of the gluconate. The official tablets are given by the oral route. In the treatment of tetany, its absorption is apparently enhanced by the simultaneous administration of lactose.

Precipitated Calcium Carbonate, U.S.P., is an insoluble, fine, white microcrystalline powder containing 40% calcium. Calcium carbonate is also available as *Calcium Carbonate Tablets,* N.F., containing 600 or 1000 mg. After ingestion, it is converted to soluble calcium salts in the bowel, and calcium is thereby made available for absorption. Patients with achlorhydria may not solubilize calcium from this preparation. It is also used as an antacid.

Dibasic Calcium Phosphate, N.F., and *Tribasic Calcium Phosphate,* N.F., although chiefly used as gastric antacids, are valuable sources of the calcium ion, especially when it is desired to supply both calcium and phosphorus. They are insoluble, tasteless white powders that must be given orally. *Calcium phosphate* is a mixture of normal, basic, and acidic calcium phosphate salts.

Calcium Levulinate, U.S.P., contains 13% calcium. It may be administered orally or parenterally. It is available in powder form or as a 10% solution (0.69 mEq Ca^{2+}/ml), as *Calcium Levulinate Injection,* U.S.P. It has a bitter, saline taste.

Other calcium preparations are described in connection with gastric antacids.

Therapeutic Uses. Calcium salts are specific in the immediate treatment of *low-calcium tetany* regardless of etiology. In severe manifest tetany, the symptoms are best brought under control by intravenous medication. Five to 20 ml of either 10% calcium gluconate or 23% calcium gluceptate solution is injected slowly. For the control of milder symptoms or latent tetany, oral medication suffices. Average doses are *calcium chloride,* 6 to 8 g daily in divided doses, best given in milk; *calcium gluconate,* 15 g daily in divided doses; *calcium lactate,* 4 g, plus lactose, 8 g, with each meal; *calcium carbonate* or *calcium phosphate,* 1 to 2 g with meals, as a watery suspension or sprinkled on food; and *calcium levulinate,* 4 to 5 g with each meal.

Hypercalcemic States. Hypercalcemia occurs in a number of diverse clinical conditions and requires differential diagnosis and appropriate corrective measures.

Ingestion of large quantities of a calcium salt is unlikely by itself to cause hypercalcemia except in patients who have hypothyroidism.

Hyperparathyroidism is also classically associated with significant hypophosphatemia; the latter is due to the diminished ability of the renal tubules to reabsorb phosphorus, owing to the excessive quantities of parathyroid hormone. Some of these patients give a history of renal calculi and peptic ulceration, and a few have mental aberrations with neurotic or even psychotic components. In more advanced stages, characteristic bone lesions are present and the condition can be diagnosed by radiography.

Although very uncommon now, there is the hypercalcemic disorder known as the *milk-alkali syndrome,* caused by the ingestion of large quantities of milk and alkalinizing powders. The pathogenesis of this disorder is still unexplained.

Vitamin D excess is a cause of hypercalcemia. Formerly, large amounts of vitamin D were administered to patients with arthritis, some of whom developed significant hypercalcemia. Vitamin D is increasingly employed in the treatment of the most common form of renal osteodystrophy, which appears to be the result of inadequate calcification of bone matrix (Stanbury, 1968). The treatment is effective; however, unless the chemical values and the clinical course are carefully monitored, the patient may develop hypercalcemia.

Sarcoidosis is associated with about a 20% incidence of hypercalcemia. Increased intestinal absorption of calcium has been attributed to a vitamin D–like substance that these patients may synthesize. Hypercalcemia peaks during summer months with increased exposure to sunlight.

Neoplasms with or without metastases to the bones may be accompanied by hypercalcemia. This is apparently related to the production of vitamin D–like sterols by some mammary tumors. Several other carcinomas have been shown to secrete peptides that resemble parathyroid hormone. The hypercalcemia associated with these peptide-secreting tumors is usually heralded by lethargy, weakness, nausea, and vomiting and not by renal stones or bone disease. Occasionally, patients with *hyperthyroidism* have hypercalcemia. This is presumably due to an increased rate of bone resorption.

Disuse atrophy, as may occur when a patient must lie relatively immobile for a long period of time, may lead to hypercalcemia. This is most common after trauma that has involved large areas of the body and when extensive splinting with casts is necessary.

Idiopathic hypercalcemia of infants is an unusual disease of unknown etiology. There are many similarities to intoxication with vitamin D.

Hypercalcemia is uncommonly noted in *adrenocortical deficiency states,* as in Addison's disease or during the period following operation for a hyperfunctioning tumor of the adrenal cortex or removal of bilateral hyperplastic adrenal glands.

Hypercalcemia occurs occasionally following successful *renal transplantation.* This is due to secondary hyperparathyroidism resulting from the previous chronic renal failure.

The *differential diagnosis* of the various causes of hypercalcemia may be difficult. In contrast to former belief, hypophosphatemia is quite common with hypercalcemia of origins other than hyperparathyroidism. Determination of the percentage of filtered phosphate that is reabsorbed or the maximal ability to reabsorb phosphorus (Tm_P) is of value in discriminating between hyperparathyroidism and other causes for hypercalcemia if renal function is normal. Many other facets of the clinical picture are obviously of help, and the reduction of the calcium concentration in plasma by the use of steroids usually excludes hyperparathyroidism. Immunoassays for parathyroid hormone may be useful in evaluating the role of hyperparathyroidism in abnormalities of calcium metabolism; however, certain carcinomas of nonendocrine tissues secrete peptides that are immunoreactive with antibody to parathyroid hormone.

Hypercalcemia of any etiology can have dire consequences. The predominant and most devastating lesion usually occurs in the kidney with reduction of renal function. Pathological changes are prominent in the collecting ducts and distal tubules.

There are occasions when hypercalcemia is in itself a life-threatening situation. The use of agents that augment the excretion of calcium, such as sodium sulfate, or of compounds that chelate calcium and permit its excretion in a complexed form, such as edetate disodium, is exceedingly helpful. The employment of steroids to reduce hypercalcemia is of benefit in those situations where the hypercalcemia is a consequence of diseases such as sarcoid. The use of sodium phosphate intravenously, as described by Massry and coworkers (1968), is clearly effective in reducing the level of plasma calcium. The mode of action is presumably by promoting the deposition of calcium in bone and decreasing bone resorption. Unfortunately, there is the risk of causing deposition of calcium in soft tissues.

Preparations Used for the Reduction of Hypercalcemia. Sodium Sulfate, U.S.P. (38.9 g of sodium sulfate decahydrate per liter), infused in amounts of 2 to 3 liters over a 9-hour period on 2 successive days, has been reported to promote calcium excretion and a decrease in hypercalcemia (Chakmakjian and Bethune, 1966). A similar solution can be prepared from *Sterile Sodium Sulfate,* U.S.P.

Edetate Disodium, U.S.P., is a chelating agent that forms soluble complexes with calcium. Chelation occurs in the blood and results in a rapid decrease in plasma ionized calcium before excretion of the complex occurs. Among the dangers of such therapy is the possibility that the concentration of calcium may be reduced too quickly and to hypocalcemic levels, thus resulting in tetany, convulsions, severe cardiac arrhythmias, and respiratory arrest. The slow intravenous administration of dilute solutions of the drug minimizes the risk of hypocalcemia. The chelator is usually dissolved in 500 ml of 0.9% saline solution or in 5% dextrose and water and administered intravenously (15 to 50 mg/kg) over a period of 4 hours. This procedure should be undertaken only when the severity of the hypercalcemia justifies the risk. The drug should be used with caution in patients with hypokalemia or congestive heart failure, and it is contraindicated in patients with significant renal disease. (For preparations and further discussion, see Chapter 45.)

Sodium phosphate has been employed intravenously in solutions prepared to contain 0.081 M Na_2HPO_4 and 0.019 M KH_2PO_4 (11.5 and 2.6 g per liter, respectively). Although hypercalcemia may be reduced, the hazards are significant in terms of extraskeletal precipitation of calcium phosphate salts (see Goldsmith and Ingbar, 1966).

Prednisone and other steroids with similar characteristics are capable of reducing hypercalcemic concentrations to normal values, particularly when the hypercalcemia is a consequence of sarcoid. Patients with nonmetastatic carcinomas or hyperparathyroidism are less responsive. Frequently, large doses of 30 to 50 mg of prednisone a day may be necessary initially. The response to glucocorticoid therapy is slow, and 1 to 2 weeks may be required before a fall in serum calcium occurs. A low-calcium intake (virtual elimination of all milk and derivative dairy products) may permit the lowest dose of steroid to accomplish the maintenance of normocalcemia. The complications of the chronic use of steroids must be recalled, and the osteoporosis that results with prolonged administration of glucocorticoid can limit the duration of therapy.

Calcitonin has been used successfully in the treatment of a variety of hypercalcemic states (Sørensen et al., 1970; Bergqvist et al., 1972). The therapeutic potentials of this peptide hormone are still being explored, but it may prove useful in hypercalcemic crisis (see Chapter 72).

Mithramycin, U.S.P. (MITHRACIN), is a cytotoxic antibiotic that has been shown to be very useful in decreasing plasma calcium concentration in hypercalcemia associated with neoplastic disease (Perlia et al., 1970). This agent probably acts directly on bone and blocks calcium resorption. Reduction in plasma calcium concentration occurs within 24 to 48 hours with low doses of this agent (one tenth the antineoplastic dose), and its toxicity is thus less severe (see Chapter 62).

MAGNESIUM

Magnesium is the second most plentiful cation of the intracellular fluids. It is essential for the activity of many enzyme systems and plays an important role with regard to neurochemical transmission and muscular excitability. Deficits are accompanied by a variety of structural and functional disturbances.

The average 70-kg adult has about 2000 mEq of magnesium in his body. About 50% of this magnesium is found in bone, 45% exists as an intracellular cation, and 5% is in the extracellular fluid. Intracellular magnesium concentrations range from 5 to 30 mEq/kg, depending on the tissue. The plasma concentration is 1.5 to 2.2 mEq of magnesium per liter, with about two thirds as free cation in equilibrium with one third bound to plasma proteins. Intracellular and extracellular magnesium concentrations can vary independently, and a deficit in one compartment may not be accompanied by a significant change in the other (Walser, 1967; Wallach and Dimich, 1969). Determination of magnesium concentrations in both plasma and muscle biopsy specimens may thus sometimes be required to diagnose magnesium deficient states. Some form of exchange of magnesium does occur between plasma, the intracellular compartment, and bone; however, very little is known about the mechanisms involved. Estimates of the intracellular ratio of free to bound magnesium are not conclusive at present. About 30% of the magnesium in the skeleton represents an exchangeable pool present either within the hydration shell or on the crystal surface. Mobilization of the cation from this pool in bone is fairly rapid in children but not in adults. The larger fraction of magnesium in bone is apparently an integral part of bone crystal (Alfrey and Miller, 1973).

Absorption and Excretion. The average adult in the United States ingests about 20 to 40 mEq of magnesium a day in an ordinary diet, and of this approximately one third is absorbed from the gastrointestinal tract. The evidence suggests that the bulk of the absorption occurs in the upper small bowel. Absorption is by means of an active process apparently closely related to the transport system for calcium. Ingestion of low amounts of magnesium results in increased absorption of calcium and *vice versa.*

Magnesium is excreted principally by the kidney by glomerular filtration. Under normal conditions 3 to 5% of the filtered ion (4 to 8 mEq per day) is excreted in the urine (Heaton, 1969). Most of the reabsorption of magnesium occurs in the proximal tubule; however, some of the cation is reabsorbed in the distal tubule (Massry and Coburn, 1973). Renal magnesium excretion is increased during diuresis induced by glucose, ammonium chloride, furosemide, ethacrynic acid, and organic mercurials. Hypomagnesemia can occur as a complication of diuretic therapy. Small amounts of magnesium are excreted via the gastrointestinal tract, in milk, and in saliva.

PHYSIOLOGICAL AND PHARMACOLOGICAL ACTIONS

Enzyme Systems. Magnesium is a cofactor of all enzymes involved in phosphate transfer reactions that utilize adenosine triphosphate (ATP) and other nucleotide triphosphates as substrates. Various phosphatases and pyrophosphatases also represent enzymes from an enormous list that are influenced by this metallic ion.

Magnesium plays a vital role in the reversible association of intracellular particles and in the binding of macromolecules to subcellular organelles. For example, the binding of messenger RNA (mRNA) to ribosomes is magnesium dependent, as is the functional integrity of ribosomal subunits.

Central Nervous System. Certain of the effects of magnesium on the nervous system are similar to those of calcium. An increased concentration of magnesium in the extracellular fluid causes depression of the central nervous system (CNS). The effects of extracellular K^+ on seizure threshold and synaptic function are antagonized by magnesium, apparently by a magnesium-mediated decrease in transmitter release. Hypomagnesemia causes increased CNS irritability, disorientation, and convulsions. Significantly elevated concentrations of magnesium in the plasma of manic-depressive and schizophrenic patients or low plasma magnesium values in patients with endogenous and neurotic depressions have been reported in some studies (Brackenridge and McDonald, 1969; Carney et al., 1973). Other studies reveal no correlation between plasma magnesium concentrations and psychosis or neurosis (Brackenridge and Jones, 1971; Naylor et al., 1972).

The flaccid, anesthesia-like state that is produced by the acute intravenous administration of relatively high doses of magnesium sulfate is probably due almost entirely to peripheral neuromuscular blockade by the mechanisms discussed below. In a carefully monitored study of two subjects in whom the plasma concentration of magnesium was raised to approximately 15 mEq per liter, the ensuing profound muscular paralysis was unaccompanied by any significant loss of sensation or consciousness (Somjen et al., 1966).

Neuromuscular System. Magnesium has a direct depressant effect on skeletal muscle. In addition, excess magnesium causes a decrease in acetylcholine release by motor nerve impulses, reduces the sensitivity of the motor end-plate to applied acetylcholine, and decreases the amplitude of the motor end-plate potential. The most critical of these effects is inhibition of acetylcholine release (Hubbard, 1973). The actions of increased magnesium on neuromuscular function are antagonized by calcium. The administration of magnesium sulfate in preeclampsia and eclampsia potentiates neuromuscular blockade produced by *d*-tubocurarine, decamethonium, and succinylcholine (Ghoneim and Long, 1970). Abnormally low concentrations of magnesium in the extracellular fluid result in increased acetylcholine release and increased muscle excitability that can produce tetany.

Cardiovascular System. Certain of the cardiac effects of excess magnesium are similar to those of the potassium ion. High concentrations of magnesium (10 to 15 mEq per liter) cause increased conduction time with lengthened P-R and QRS intervals of the ECG—changes similar to those seen with hyperkalemia (Randall et al., 1964; Seelig,

1969). Magnesium slows the rate of S-A nodal impulse formation. Higher concentrations of magnesium (greater than 15 mEq per liter) produce cardiac arrest in diastole. Magnesium may abolish digitalis-induced premature ventricular contractions (Sodeman, 1965), but the ion is rarely used for this purpose unless hypomagnesemia is also present. States of magnesium deficiency may or may not be associated with decreased potassium in cardiac cells and enhanced toxicity to cardiac glycosides (Seller *et al.*, 1970). The ECG changes seen with magnesium depletion are similar to those seen with hypercalcemia (Seelig, 1969).

Excess magnesium causes vasodilatation by both a direct action on blood vessels and ganglionic blockade.

ABNORMALITIES OF MAGNESIUM METABOLISM

Hypomagnesemia. The *pathology* of magnesium depletion includes changes in skeletal and cardiac muscle and striking nephrocalcinosis. The latter is unique in that it consists in the formation of tiny microliths within the lumen of the nephron, almost entirely confined to the broad ascending limb of Henle's loop. There appears to be no direct initial damage to renal tubular cells, but damage does occur when the microliths grow sufficiently large to cause obstruction and local pressure, leading to necrosis, scar tissue, and dilatation of the more proximal segments of the nephron. In the course of several months on a magnesium-deficient regimen, volunteer subjects have developed hypomagnesemia, with inconsistent occurrence of hypokalemia and hypocalcemia. They may exhibit neuromuscular disorders akin to those seen in hypocalcemia.

Severe acute or chronic diarrhea and steatorrhea may cause loss of magnesium in the stool and lead to magnesium deficiency. Magnesium deficiency can occur in chronic alcoholism; with prolonged intravenous feeding with magnesium-free solutions; during hemodialysis; and in diabetes mellitus, pancreatitis, postdiuretic electrolyte imbalance, renal tubular damage, and other diseases where secondary hypocalcemia and hypokalemia develop (Gitelman and Welt, 1969; Martin, 1969). In primary hyperaldosteronism, the hypokalemia is accompanied by a decrease in plasma magnesium concentration, attributed to a shift of magnesium from the extracellular fluid into cells.

Hypomagnesemia, as well as a decrease in total body magnesium stores, frequently occurs in chronic alcoholic patients (*see* Flink, 1971). The factors responsible probably include increased renal excretion of magnesium (by a combination of direct inhibition of tubular reabsorption of magnesium and the formation of readily excreted complexes of magnesium with lactate and other metabolites that are present in increased amounts in alcoholism), decreased dietary intake of magnesium, vomiting and diarrhea, and hyperaldosteronism in the presence of hepatic cirrhosis. This observation and the similarity between the signs and symptoms of experimental magnesium deficiency in experimental animals and those of delirium tremens have led to the hypothesis that hypomagnesemia is a causative factor in the latter condition. However, convincing evidence of this is lacking (*see* Wacker and Parisi, 1968). As part of the total treatment program for chronic alcoholism, the plasma concentrations of magnesium and of calcium, which is also frequently decreased, should be determined and corrected if found to be low.

Magnesium deficiency is manifested by neuromuscular dysfunction, hyperirritability, and psychotic behavior (Wacker and Parisi, 1968; Shils, 1969). Tetany may occur in the absence of acid-base changes or hypocalcemia and is reversed by magnesium but not calcium administration. A positive Babinski sign, tachycardia, and hypertension may also be associated with hypomagnesemia. Most patients with magnesium deficiency have other electrolyte abnormalities (*i.e.,* hypokalemia and hypocalcemia). Hypomagnesemia may cause these other electrolyte changes (Shils, 1969), and replacement of magnesium may be required to correct hypocalcemia.

During rapid growth periods in newborns and children, hypomagnesemia has been associated with poor intake or excessive losses. A low plasma magnesium concentration in newborns who are fed cow's milk or artificial formulas is apparently related to a high phosphate:magnesium ratio in these diets (Cockburn *et al.,* 1973). In infancy the symptoms reliably associated with hypomagnesemia are seizures, hyperirritability, exaggerated tendon reflexes, and increased muscle tone. There is frequently a concomitant hypocalcemia that is resistant to therapy with calcium and vitamin D. Symptoms may be corrected by the replacement of magnesium (Coussons, 1969; Cockburn *et al.,* 1973). Magnesium therapy also appears to be important in correcting hypocalcemia in infants. Oral administration of calcium for treatment of hypocalcemia without regard to decreased magnesium may only exacerbate a magnesium deficiency by reducing intestinal absorption of the cation. This is consistent with the proposed common transport mechanism for magnesium and calcium in the gastrointestinal tract.

Hypomagnesemia in protein-calorie malnutrition is well documented. Conflicting reports exist on the significance of magnesium therapy in reducing the mortality rate in such patients (Caddell, 1967; Rosen *et al.,* 1970).

There is evidence of parathyroid failure in magnesium deficiency (Rösler and Rabinowitz, 1973). Patients diagnosed as hypoparathyroid have been reported to be resistant to calcium salts and vitamin D and to be hypomagnesemic; they have undetectable plasma concentrations of parathyroid hormone in spite of hypocalcemia (Anast *et al.*, 1972) and show a normal response (increased plasma calcium and phosphaturia) to parathyroid extract (Suh *et al.*, 1973). Treatment with magnesium has resulted in increased plasma parathyroid hormone, increased plasma calcium, and phosphaturia. These reports indicate that hypomagnesemia with hypocalcemia causes either impaired synthesis or impaired release of parathyroid hormone. Acute reduction of plasma magnesium concentration, however, stimulates the secretion of parathyroid hormone.

Parathyroid hormone may cause a fall in magnesium concentration, apparently by provoking a shift of the cation from plasma to bone. Renal tubular reabsorption of magnesium can be stimulated by parathyroid hormone; however, hyperparathyroidism leads to hypomagnesemia. In hyperparathyroidism, the hypercalcemia results in decreased fractional reabsorption of magnesium by the renal tubules and increased renal excretion of filtered magnesium, which eventually leads to magnesium deficiency.

A high proportion of patients who form oxalate and phosphate renal stones have low excretion rates of magnesium. When compared to normal subjects, patients with primary hyperparathyroidism and renal stones have a low urinary magnesium concentration relative to calcium excretion. Hyperparathyroid patients with osteitis fibrosa excrete relatively high concentrations of magnesium, and it has been suggested that magnesium excretion may be a factor in the rarity of urinary calculi in these patients (Sutton and Watson, 1969). These and related observations indicate that magnesium therapy may be of value in preventing the formation of certain types of renal stones (Elliot and Ribeiro, 1973).

Conflicting reports exist regarding changes in magnesium metabolism in women taking oral contraceptive hormones (Goldsmith and Goldsmith, 1966; Simpson and Dale, 1972).

Hypomagnesemia is treated with parenteral fluids containing magnesium sulfate or chloride.

Hypermagnesemia.

An elevated magnesium concentration is usually due to renal insufficiency with decreased ability to excrete absorbed or infused magnesium. The use of magnesium sulfate as a cathartic in patients with impaired renal function can lead to severe toxicity, as can chronic ingestion of magnesium-containing antacids by such individuals. Hypermagnesemia is manifested by muscle weakness, hypotension, ECG changes, sedation, and confusion. As plasma concentrations of magnesium begin to exceed 4 mEq per liter, the deep-tendon reflexes are decreased and may be absent at levels approaching 10 mEq per liter. At 12 to 15 mEq per liter respiratory paralysis is a potential hazard; the respiratory effects can be antagonized to some extent by the intravenous administration of calcium salts. In cases of severe renal impairment, symptomatic hypermagnesemia may be an indication for dialysis. Although man usually tolerates high concentrations of magnesium in plasma, there are occasional instances when cardiac consequences may be seen in the form of complete heart block at concentrations well below 10 mEq per liter.

Elevated plasma magnesium concentration has been shown to influence the function of the parathyroid gland *in vitro*, in experimental animals, and in man (Buckle *et al.*, 1968; Pletka *et al.*, 1971; Targovnik *et al.*, 1971). A twofold to threefold increase of plasma magnesium concentration above the normal range causes decreased release of parathyroid hormone.

Plasma concentrations of magnesium increase in the fetus and approach the maternal blood values after magnesium sulfate administration in eclampsia and preeclampsia. The neonate may be drowsy and exhibit respiratory difficulties and diminished muscle tone (Lipsitz and English, 1967). However, Stone and Pritchard (1970) found no relationship between the plasma magnesium concentration of blood collected from the umbilical cord and the Apgar score. In infants who suffer hypoxia during delivery, hypermagnesemia can result, and the plasma magnesium concentration is inversely correlated with the Apgar score (Engel and Elin, 1970).

Preparations. Magnesium citrate and sulfate are the salts usually employed for their action on the gastrointestinal tract. There are many magnesium preparations used as antacids. For parenteral medication magnesium sulfate is usually employed. The dosage is expressed in terms of the official U.S.P. hydrated salt, $MgSO_4 \cdot 7H_2O$. One gram of this salt is equivalent to 4.06 millimoles (8.12 mEq) of magnesium. *Magnesium Sulfate Injection*, U.S.P., is available in concentrations of 10 and 50%.

Therapeutic Uses. *Gastrointestinal Uses.* The uses of magnesium salts as cathartics and as antacids are discussed elsewhere (*see* Index).

Central Depression. Magnesium sulfate is used in the treatment of seizures associated with acute nephritis and with eclampsia of pregnancy. While it has generally been assumed that the suppression of seizures by magnesium in these conditions is due to a central depressant action, more recent findings, discussed above, indicate that the primary action probably occurs peripherally at the neuromuscular junction. The dose for children is 0.1 to 0.2 ml/kg of body weight (0.16 to 0.32 mEq/kg) of a 20% solution administered intramuscularly. In the treatment of patients with toxemia of pregnancy, Rogers and associates (1969) have developed a system of initial and sustaining dosage, based on body weight. It is possible to attain unduly high plasma concentrations, and the patient must be carefully monitored both clinically and chemically. If magnesium therapy of this sort is to be used, a preparation of a calcium salt should be readily available for intravenous injection to counteract the potential serious hazard of magnesium intoxication. A clinical sign of significance is the presence of deep-tendon reflexes. As long as these are active, it is probable that the patient will not develop respiratory paralysis.

Hypomagnesemia. Intravenous administration of magnesium sulfate is the treatment for severe magnesium deficiency; it should be injected extremely slowly with observance of the same precautions as described above. Two to 4 g (17 to 34 mEq) may be given daily in divided doses.

BARIUM

Barium is extremely toxic when absorbed. The soluble barium salts (chloride, carbonate, hydroxide, and sulfide) should not be used for medicinal purposes. The insoluble barium sulfate is widely employed as an opaque contrast medium for roentgenographic study of the gastrointestinal tract. There is evidence to suggest that radiation-induced gastrointestinal effects may be lessened by the ingestion of barium sulfate (Conard and Scott, 1961).

Systemic Actions and Toxicology. The characteristic systemic action of barium is a very intense stimulation of muscle of all types, regardless of innervation. The major symptoms and signs of poisoning from soluble barium salts are related to this intense muscle stimulation. The action of barium on the gastrointestinal musculature causes vomiting, severe colic and diarrhea, and hemorrhage. The cardiovascular effects consist in marked hypertension due to spasm of the musculature of the arterioles, and cardiac arrhythmias. Ingestion of gram quantities of soluble barium salts may be fatal, with death resulting from cardiac arrest. Muscle tremors are frequent. Respiratory failure and convulsions followed by paralysis of the extremities may also occur. Death usually follows within an hour, but may be delayed.

Poisoning may occur in industry, from the accidental use of a soluble barium salt in x-ray procedures, from the ingestion of certain rodenticides and pesticides that contain barium salts, and from the ingestion of certain depilatories that contain barium sulfide. Certain firework powders also contain soluble barium salts.

The insoluble barium sulfate is not absorbed, and constipation and occasionally impaction may be observed after its oral use. It may rarely produce local granulomatous reactions, for example, granulomas of the rectum and colon, when it is used in roentgenographic procedures (Carney and Stephens, 1973). Perforation of the colon and barium peritonitis have been reported (Gross and Howard, 1972; Gardiner and Miller, 1973). *Barytosis,* a granulomatous disease of the lungs, occurs in workers engaged in mining, sorting, grinding, and bagging of the ore barytes (barium sulfate) (Blum, 1962).

Treatment of barium poisoning consists in the precipitation and removal of the unabsorbed salt remaining in the gastrointestinal tract, by gastric lavage with a 2 to 5% solution of either magnesium sulfate or sodium sulfate. The lavage should be given until the return is clear. In an attempt to counteract the muscular action of barium, 10 ml of a 10% solution of sodium sulfate should be administered intravenously every 30 minutes until symptoms subside. Intravenous potassium has been reported to reverse the effects of barium on skeletal, smooth, and cardiac muscle (Lewi and Bar-Khayim, 1964; Gould et al., 1973). In less severe poisoning, 30 g of sodium sulfate in 250 ml of water may be given by mouth and repeated in 1 hour. Procainamide is useful in treating ventricular arrhythmias, and morphine sulfate and nitroglycerin are effective in relieving cardiac pain. Morphine is also effective for the relief of severe colic. Diuretics appear to be useful in enhancing barium excretion (Gould *et al.,* 1973).

Electrolytes. Barium produces hypokalemia apparently by promoting a shift of potassium from plasma into cells.

Muscle. The use of barium chloride for the symptomatic therapy of Stokes-Adams attacks is obsolete. Barium increases myocardial excitability, as evidenced by premature ventricular contractions, tachycardia, and fibrillation. These cardiac effects are rapidly reversed by potassium (Roza and Berman, 1971).

Barium causes an increase in cell-membrane resistance, a prolongation of action potentials, and depolarization of smooth and skeletal muscle. It has been proposed that these changes are due to barium-induced decreases in potassium conductance (Sperelakis *et al.,* 1967).

Nerve. There is evidence that barium ions may be substituted for sodium ions to produce action potentials in mammalian B and C fibers. In these fibers, the action potentials are remarkably prolonged in an isotonic barium solution. In mammalian A fibers, barium cannot be substituted for sodium, and isotonic barium solution results in conduction block (Greengard and Straub, 1959). Barium has also been shown to release acetylcholine from cholinergic nerves and catecholamines from the adrenal medulla. These actions on neurotransmitter release are due to the ability of barium to substitute for calcium in the neurosecretory process.

Preparations. *Barium Sulfate,* U.S.P., is a fine, white, odorless, tasteless, and bulky powder, free from grittiness. It is practically insoluble in water. In prescribing barium sulfate, the full title should always be written out clearly to avoid confusion with the poisonous barium sulfide or sulfite. There are no official preparations of soluble barium salts.

LITHIUM

Lithium is a member of the same group of elements (Ia) as are sodium and potassium, but it has no known biological role. The ion mimics some of the biological properties of both extracellular sodium and intracellular potassium ions. When introduced into biological systems, lithium acts more like sodium than any other ion. For example, lithium can replace sodium in isolated nerve, muscle, and erythrocyte preparations. However, the counterfeit is not complete, and some differences are observed. Influx of the lithium ion during depolarization is extremely rapid; however, the ion is not effectively removed by the sodium pump, sodium being extruded from cells 10 to 25 times faster than lithium. This makes lithium extremely useful in the study of the ionic basis of membrane potentials. The imperfect substitution of lithium for extracellular and intracellular monovalent cations probably compromises those processes that determine ionic distributions and gradients as well as all physiological functions that depend on these processes (*e.g.*, Na^+,K^+-activated adenosine triphosphatase). The accumulation of lithium in the intracellular environment could be envisioned to perturb any event that is modulated by monovalent cations. These possible interactions signify the enormous magnitude of the task of determining precise mechanisms of action of the lithium ion. Schou (1957), Davis and Fann (1971), and Singer and Rotenberg (1973) have extensively reviewed the subject of the lithium ion.

Absorption, Distribution, and Excretion. Lithium ions are readily and almost completely absorbed from the gastrointestinal tract. Complete absorption occurs in about 8 hours, with peak plasma concentrations occurring 2 to 4 hours after an oral dose. The ion is initially distributed in the extracellular fluid and then gradually accumulated in various tissues to different degrees. The concentration gradients across cellular membranes are much smaller than those for sodium and potassium. The final volume of distribution is equal to that of total body water. Passage through the blood-brain barrier is slow, but when a steady state is achieved the concentration of lithium in the cerebrospinal fluid is about 40% of the plasma concentration (Platman and Fieve, 1968). There is no evidence of the ion binding to plasma proteins.

Approximately 95% of a single dose of lithium is eliminated in the urine. About one third to two thirds of an acute dose is excreted during a 6- to 12-hour initial phase of excretion, followed by a slow excretion over the next 10 to 14 days. With chronic administration, lithium excretion increases during the first 5 to 6 days until equilibrium is reached between ingestion and excretion. When therapy with lithium is stopped, there is a rapid phase of renal excretion followed by a slow 10- to 14-day phase. Since 80% of the filtered lithium is reabsorbed by the renal tubules, renal lithium clearance is about 20% of that for creatinine, ranging between 15 and 30 ml per minute. This is somewhat lower in elderly patients (10 to 15 ml per minute) and higher in young people. Sodium loading enhances the excretion of lithium, and sodium depletion promotes retention of the ion. Determination of clearance is recommended to establish the proper maintenance dose for prolonged lithium therapy. Most of the renal tubular reabsorption of lithium apparently occurs in the proximal tubule and is not altered by diuretics that act in the ascending limb of the loop of Henle and the distal tubule (*e.g.*, ethacrynic acid, organic mercurials, and thiazides). Renal excretion is increased by osmotic diuretics, aminophylline, and acetazolamide. Evidence for distal tubular reabsorption of the ion is based on the lithium diuresis induced by triamterene; however, spironolactone does not increase lithium excretion.

Less than 1% of the lithium ingested leaves the human body in the feces, and 4 to 5% is excreted in the sweat. Lithium is secreted in saliva in concentrations several times greater than that in plasma. Since the ion is excreted in milk, women being treated with lithium should avoid breast feeding to prevent neonatal intoxication.

Therapeutic Uses. In the last 20 years, lithium salts have been used to treat manic-depressive psychosis. Lithium is a useful therapeutic agent in the control of severe mania. Evidence also supports the belief that a certain proportion of patients respond to the ion with a reduced frequency of hypomanic relapse. The use of lithium in obsessional neurosis, childhood psychosis, and excitement in schizophrenia has not been totally convincing. The psychiatric uses of lithium are discussed in detail in Chapter 12.

Lithium has been shown to inhibit the release of iodine from the thyroid and has been utilized in the treatment of thyrotoxicosis. Any advantage of lithium over iodide in the management of Graves' disease remains to be established (*see* Chapter 67). In a limited study, lithium was reported to have a beneficial effect in Huntington's chorea (Dalén, 1973).

Lithium salts have been advocated for the treatment of various illnesses, including gout, diabetes mellitus, and epilepsy, but they have proven of no value in any of these diseases.

Toxicity. Initial lithium therapy is associated with a transient increase in the excretion of 17-hydroxycorticosteroids, sodium, potassium, and water. This effect is usually not sustained beyond 24 hours (Noyes *et al.*, 1971; Platman *et al.*, 1971). After this initial phase, the subsequent 4 to 5 days of lithium therapy is associated with normal potassium excretion, sodium retention, and, in some cases, pretibial edema. Sodium retention has been associated with increased aldosterone excretion and responds to administration of spironolactone (Murphy *et al.*, 1969; Demers and Heninger, 1970). Edema and sodium retention frequently disappear spontaneously after several days.

In 1968, Schou and coworkers reported that a small number of lithium-treated patients developed diffuse, nontender thyroid enlargement, suggestive of compromised thyroid function. In patients treated with lithium, thyroid ^{131}I uptake is increased and plasma protein-bound iodine and free thyroxine tend to be low (*see* Chapter 67). However, patients usually remain euthyroid and obvious hypothyroidism is rare. In rats, the ion has been shown to inhibit thyrotropin activation of thyroid adenylate cyclase (Berens *et al.*, 1970), and inhibitory effects of lithium have been noted on the synthesis of cyclic adenosine 3',5'-monophosphate (cyclic AMP) in several other situations (*see* Dousa and Hechter, 1970; Wang *et al.*, 1974). It is unknown if there is a cause-and-effect relationship between this action of lithium and any of its subsequent effects. In patients who develop goiter, discontinuation of lithium or treatment with thyroid hormone results in shrinkage of the gland.

Polydipsia and polyuria occur in patients treated with lithium, occasionally to a disturbing degree. Several cases of acquired nephrogenic diabetes insipidus have been reported in patients maintained at therapeutic plasma concentrations of the ion (Ramsey *et al.*, 1972; Singer *et al.*, 1972). The polyuria disappears with termination of lithium therapy. The mechanism of this effect may involve inhibition of the action of antidiuretic hormone (ADH) on renal adenylate cyclase, resulting in decreased ADH stimulation of renal reabsorption of water. However, there is also evidence that lithium may exert an action at a step beyond cyclic AMP synthesis to alter both thyroid and renal function. While there is thus uncertainty of the precise site of action of the cation, its effectiveness in blocking the renal response to ADH has aroused interest in its therapeutic usefulness in the treatment of the syndrome of inappropriate secretion of ADH (*see* Forrest, 1975; White and Fetner, 1975).

The lithium ion also has an action on carbohydrate metabolism that resembles somewhat that of insulin (Bhattacharya, 1961). In intact rats, lithium causes an increase in skeletal muscle glycogen accompanied by severe depletion of glycogen from the liver (Plenge *et al.*, 1970). The mechanisms of action of insulin and lithium probably differ inasmuch as maximal amounts of the two agents produce additive effects on glucose metabolism in the isolated rat diaphragm (Haugaard *et al.*, 1974).

The chronic use of lithium causes a benign and reversible depression of the T wave of the ECG, an effect not related to sodium or potassium depletion (Demers and Heninger, 1971).

Lithium causes EEG changes characterized by diffuse slowing, widened frequency spectrum, and potentiation with disorganization of background rhythm. There are conflicting reports with regard to lithium and convulsive disorders. Status epilepticus has been reported in nonepileptic patients with plasma lithium concentrations in the therapeutic range. On the other hand, decreased seizure frequency was reported in severe, poorly controlled epileptics during 6 weeks of treatment with lithium (Erwin *et al.*, 1973).

An increase in circulating leukocytes occurs during the chronic use of lithium and is reversed within 1 week after termination of treatment (Murphy *et al.*, 1971; Shopsin *et al.*, 1971). A case of fatal aplastic anemia possibly related to lithium carbonate therapy has been reported (Hussain *et al.*, 1973).

Allergic reactions such as dermatitis and allergic vasculitis can occur with lithium administration.

Since lithium salts have a low therapeutic index, plasma lithium concentrations must be monitored. A morning plasma lithium concentration between 0.6 and 1.3 mEq per liter is sought. The occurrence of toxicity is related to the plasma lithium concentration and its rate of rise following administration. Acute intoxication is characterized by vomiting, profuse diarrhea, ataxia, coma, and convulsions (Schou *et al.*, 1968). Symptoms of chronic toxicity that are most likely to occur at the plasma lithium absorptive peak include nausea, vomiting, abdominal pain, diarrhea, and sedation. The more serious effects involve the nervous system and consist in mental confusion, hyperreflexia, tremor, dysarthria, seizures, and cranial-nerve and focal neurological signs, progressing to coma and death (Saron and Gaind, 1973). Other toxic effects are cardiac arrhythmias, hypotension, and albuminuria. In pregnancy, concomitant use of natriuretics and low-sodium diets is the most common cause of maternal and neonatal lithium intoxication (Goldfield and Weinstein, 1973). The use of lithium in pregnancy has been associated with neonatal goiter, CNS depression, and cardiac murmur (Amdisen and Skjoldborg, 1969; Woody *et al.*, 1971). All these conditions reverse with time. The safety of lithium in pregnancy has not been established.

Treatment of Lithium Intoxication. Since there is no specific antidote for lithium intoxication, treatment is supportive. If renal function is adequate, excretion can be accelerated with osmotic diuresis and intravenous sodium bicarbonate solution. Aminophylline may also be useful. Dialysis may be the most effective means of removing the ion from the body. When the plasma lithium concentration is lowered by dialysis or other means, recovery is still slow. This suggests that the intracellular lithium concentration may be the prime determinant of the appearance of clinical toxicity.

AMMONIUM

The ammonium ion is of particular interest because it is toxic in high concentrations and because it serves a major role in the maintenance of the acid-base balance of the body.

The ammonium ion is an acid that dissociates to H^+ and NH_3, and the dissociation constant (pK_a 9.3) is such that, in the pH range of body fluids, NH_4^+ constitutes about 99% of the total ammonia ($NH_3 + NH_4^+$) concentration.

The concentration of ammonia in peripheral venous blood ranges between 75 and 200 $\mu g/100$ ml.

Ammonia in the body represents that which is liberated from the deamination of amino acids and the deamidation of amides, and there are several major sources. Portal venous blood contains a high concentration of ammonia. Normally about 20% of the urea produced in the body diffuses into the gut, where it is converted by bacteria to ammonia and carbon dioxide. Intestinal bacteria also produce ammonia from dietary proteins. The ammonia is absorbed and converted back to urea in the liver. In chronic renal failure as much as 75% of the urea produced may enter into this hepatoenteric cycle. Normal renal venous blood contains a high concentration of ammonia that results from the liberation of ammonia from glutamine and certain amino acids in the kidney (see Pitts, 1974). Also, ammonia release has been demonstrated in exercising muscle as well as in brain under certain conditions.

In mammals, the major site of ammonia disposal is the liver, wherein ammonia is converted to urea by way of the ornithine cycle. Another significant fate of ammonia is its participation in the synthesis of glutamine.

Toxicity. Patients with severe hepatic disease or with portacaval shunts often develop derangements of the CNS, which are manifested by disturbance of consciousness, tremor, hyperreflexia, and EEG abnormalities. Since the syndrome is most often associated with elevated blood ammonia concentrations, and since it can be provoked by the feeding of protein as well as by the ingestion of ammonium

salts, it is thought to represent ammonia toxicity to the brain. A direct cause-and-effect relationship between blood ammonia and the clinical status of the patient has not been established; however, a consistent correlation is found between blood ammonia concentration and clinical status. The occurrence of hyperammonemia in children and infants has been associated with defects of enzymes of the urea cycle. Hyperammonemia due to defects of ornithine transcarbamylase or carbamylphosphate synthetase may be related to cyclic vomiting and to at least one form of migraine. The mechanisms by which ammonia induces changes in the CNS are currently unknown. (See Russell, 1973.)

Glutamic acid and *arginine* are of questionable value in the treatment of ammonia intoxication. *Neomycin* has been used to reduce the number of ammonia-producing microorganisms in the intestine, and this therapy is widely accepted as a treatment of hyperammonemia in hepatic disease. However, controlled studies are lacking, and improvement associated with suppression of blood ammonia concentrations has not been established (Zieve, 1966; Chalmers, 1968).

Role in Acid-Base Balance. Ammonia plays a significant role in the maintenance of the hydrogen ion concentration of extracellular fluid within narrow limits. This is accomplished by the participation of ammonia in the renal excretion of hydrogen ions, as discussed in Chapter 36 and in the introduction to Section VIII.

Pharmacological Actions. *Diuresis from Ammonium Salts.* Following the absorption of inorganic salts of ammonium, such as ammonium chloride, the conversion of the ammonium ion to urea frees hydrogen ion (and chloride), and bicarbonate is dissipated. This may result in severe acidosis. Acid-forming salts are diuretic and have been employed for this purpose (see Chapter 39).

Expectorant Action. The ammonium ion supposedly exerts an expectorant action, and its salts are extensively used for this purpose.

Local Actions. Solutions of ammonium hydroxide are local irritants. When applied to the skin in low concentration, they have a rubefacient action, and in high concentrations they are vesicant. Ammonia gas is very irritating, but when inhaled in dilute form it can stimulate reflexly the medullary respiratory and vasomotor centers through irritation of the sensory endings of the trigeminal nerve. High concentrations of ammonia vapor are injurious to the lungs, and death may result from pulmonary edema. Long exposure to low concentrations of ammonia may lead to chronic pulmonary irritation. The maximal concentration of ammonia vapor that can be tolerated without harmful effect is probably less than 250 ppm. High concentrations of neutral ammonium salts are irritating to the gastric mucosa.

Preparations. *Ammonium Chloride,* N.F., is a white crystalline, hygroscopic powder, freely soluble in water. It is available as an official injection, syrup, and tablet. *Ammonium carbonate* consists of a mixture of ammonium bicarbonate and ammonium carbamate. It occurs as white, hard, translucent masses having an ammoniacal odor and taste. The salt is slowly soluble in water to the extent of 25%. *Aromatic Ammonia Spirit*, N.F., is a solution of ammonia, ammonium carbonate, and various essential oils in 70% alcohol.

Therapeutic Uses. The uses of ammonium salts as expectorants, diuretics, and for the correction of metabolic alkalosis are discussed elsewhere (*see* Index). Aromatic ammonia spirit is often employed as a reflex stimulant. It is given by mouth in a dose of 2 ml, well diluted in water.

Alfrey, A. C., and Miller, N. L. Bone magnesium pools in uremia. *J. clin. Invest.*, **1973**, *52*, 3019–3027.

Amdisen, A., and Skjoldborg, H. Haemodialysis for lithium poisoning. *Lancet*, **1969**, *2*, 213.

Anast, C. S.; Mohs, J. M.; Kaplan, S. L.; and Burns, T. W. Evidence for parathyroid failure in magnesium deficiency. *Science, Wash.*, **1972**, *177*, 606–608.

Aviolo, L. V.; Birge, S.; Lee, S. W.; and Slatapolsky, E. The metabolic fate of vitamin D_3-^3H in chronic renal failure. *J. clin. Invest.*, **1968**, *47*, 2239–2252.

Berens, S. C.; Bernstein, R. S.; Robbins, J.; and Wolff, J. Antithyroid effects of lithium. *J. clin. Invest.*, **1970**, *49*, 1357–1367.

Bergqvist, E.; Sjöberg, H. E.; Hjern, B.; Hallberg, D.; and Carlström, A. Calcitonin in the treatment of hypercalcemic crisis. *Acta med. scand.*, **1972**, *192*, 385–389.

Bhattacharya, G. Effects of metal ions on the utilization of glucose and on the influence of insulin on it by the isolated rat diaphragm. *Biochem. J.*, **1961**, *79*, 369–377.

Blaustein, M. P., and Hodgkin, A. L. The effect of cyanide on the efflux of calcium from squid axons. *J. Physiol., Lond.*, **1969**, *200*, 497–528.

Blum, C. K. Radiology of some rarer dust diseases (barytosis, asbestosis and siderosis). *Scot. med. J.*, **1962**, *7*, 478–487.

Brackenridge, C. J., and Jones, I. H. Relation of hyper-magnesemia to activity and neuroleptic drug therapy in schizophrenic states. *J. Neurol. Neurosurg. Psychiat.*, **1971**, *34*, 195–199.

Brackenridge, C. J., and McDonald, C. The concentrations of magnesium and potassium in erythrocytes and plasma of geriatric patients with psychiatric disorders. *Med. J. Aust.*, **1969**, *2*, 390–394.

Buckle, R. M.; Care, A. D.; Cooper, C. W.; and Gitelman, H. J. The influence of plasma magnesium concentration on parathyroid hormone secretion. *J. Endocr.*, **1968**, *42*, 529–534.

Caddell, J. L. Studies in protein-calorie malnutrition. II. A double-blind clinical trial to assess magnesium therapy. *New Engl. J. Med.*, **1967**, *276*, 533–535.

Carney, J. A., and Stephens, D. A. Intramural barium (barium granuloma) of colon and rectum. *Gastroenterology*, **1973**, *65*, 316–320.

Carney, M. W. P.; Sheffield, B. F.; and Sebastian, J. Serum magnesium, diagnosis, ECT and season. *Br. J. Psychiat.*, **1973**, *122*, 427–429.

Chakmakjian, Z. H., and Bethune, J. E. Sodium sulfate treatment of hypercalcemia. *New Engl. J. Med.*, **1966**, *275*, 862–869.

Chalmers, T. C. The management of hepatic coma: a continuing problem. *Med. Clins N. Am.*, **1968**, *52*, 1475–1481.

Cockburn, F.; Brown, J. K.; Belton, N. R.; and Forfar, J. O. Neonatal convulsions associated with primary disturbances of calcium, potassium, and magnesium metabolism. *Archs Dis. Childh.*, **1973**, *48*, 99–108.

Conard, R. A., and Scott, W. A. Modification of radiation-induced gastrointestinal effects by barium meals. *Radiat. Res.*, **1961**, *15*, 527–531.

Coussons, H. Magnesium metabolism in infants and children. *Postgrad. Med.*, **1969**, *46*, 135–139.

Dalén, P. Lithium therapy in Huntington's chorea and tardive dyskinesia (letter to the editor). *Lancet*, **1973**, *1*, 107–108.

Davis, B. B., and Murdaugh, H. V. Evaluation of interrelationship between calcium and sodium excretion by canine kidney. *Metabolism*, **1970**, *19*, 439–444.

Demers, R., and Heninger, G. Pretibial edema and sodium retention during lithium carbonate treatment. *J. Am. med. Ass.*, **1970**, *214*, 1845–1848.

Demers, R. G., and Heninger, G. R. Electrocardiographic T-wave changes during lithium carbonate treatment. *J. Am. med. Ass.*, **1971**, *218*, 381–386.

Dousa, T., and Hechter, O. Lithium and brain adenyl cyclase. *Lancet*, **1970**, *1*, 834–835.

Dutta, S., and Marks, B. H. Species and ionic influences on the accumulation of digitalis glycosides by perfused hearts. *Br. J. Pharmac.*, **1972**, *46*, 401–408.

Elliot, J. S., and Ribeiro, M. E. The effect of varying concentrations of calcium and magnesium upon calcium oxalate solubility. *Invest. Urol.*, **1973**, *10*, 295–297.

Engel, R. R., and Elin, R. J. Hypermagnesemia from birth asphyxia. *J. Pediat.*, **1970**, *77*, 631–637.

Erwin, C. W.; Gerber, C. J.; Morrison, S. D.; and James, J. F. Lithium carbonate and convulsive disorders. *Archs gen. Psychiat.*, **1973**, *28*, 646–648.

Farah, A., and Witt, P. N. Cardiac glycosides and calcium. In, *Proceedings of the First International Pharmacological Meeting.* Vol. 3, *New Aspects of Cardiac Glycosides.* (Wilbrandt, W., and Lindgren, P., eds.) Pergamon Press, Ltd., Oxford, **1963**, pp. 137–171.

Forrest, J. J., Jr. Lithium inhibition of c AMP-mediated hormones: a caution. *New Engl. J. Med.*, **1975**, *292*, 423–424.

Gardiner, H., and Miller, R. E. Barium peritonitis. A new therapeutic approach. *Am. J. Surg.*, **1973**, *125*, 350–352.

Ghoneim, M. M., and Long, J. P. The interaction between magnesium and other neuromuscular blocking agents. *Anesthesiology*, **1970**, *32*, 23–27.

Goldfield, M. D., and Weinstein, M. R. Lithium carbonate in obstetrics: guidelines for clinical use. *Am. J. Obstet. Gynec.*, **1973**, *116*, 15–22.

Goldsmith, N. F., and Goldsmith, J. R. Epidemiological aspects of magnesium and calcium metabolism. Implications of altered magnesium metabolism in women taking drugs for the suppression of ovulation. *Archs envir. Hlth*, **1966**, *12*, 607–619.

Goldsmith, R. S., and Ingbar, S. H. Inorganic phosphate treatment of hypercalcemia of diverse etiologies. *New Engl. J. Med.*, **1966**, *274*, 1–7.

Gould, D. B.; Sorrell, M. R.; and Lupariello, A. D. Barium sulfide poisoning. Some factors contributing to survival. *Archs intern. Med.*, **1973**, *132*, 891–894.

Greengard, P., and Straub, R. W. Restoration by barium of action potentials in sodium-deprived mammalian B and C fibers. *J. Physiol., Lond.*, **1959**, *145*, 562–569.

Gross, G. F., and Howard, M. A. Perforation of the colon from barium enema. *Am. Surg.*, **1972**, *38*, 583–585.

Haugaard, E. S.; Mickel, R.; and Haugaard, N. Actions of lithium ions and insulin on glucose utilization, glycogen synthesis and glycogen synthase in the isolated rat diaphragm. *Biochem. Pharmac.*, **1974**, *23*, 1675–1685.

Heaton, F. W. The kidney and magnesium homeostasis. *Ann. N.Y. Acad. Sci.*, **1969**, *162*, 775–785.

Hussain, M. Z.; Khan, A. G.; and Chandhry, Z. A. Aplastic anemia associated with lithium therapy. *Can. med. Ass. J.*, **1973**, *108*, 724–725.

Kallfelz, F. A., and Wasserman, R. H. Correlation between ^{47}Ca absorption and intestinal calcium-binding activity in the golden hamster. *Proc. Soc. exp. Biol. Med.*, **1972**, *139*, 77–79.

Krawitt, E. L. The role of intestinal transport proteins in cortisone-mediated suppression of calcium absorption. *Biochim. biophys. Acta,* **1972,** *274,* 179–188.

Langer, G. A. Coupling calcium in mammalian ventricle: its source and factors regulating its quantity. *Cardiovasc. Res.,* **1971,** *1,* Suppl. 1, 71–75.

Lewi, Z., and Bar-Khayim, Y. Food poisoning from barium carbonate. *Lancet,* **1964,** *2,* 342–343.

Lipsitz, P. J., and English, I. C. Hypermagnesemia in the newborn infant. *Pediatrics, Springfield,* **1967,** *40,* 856–862.

Massry, S. G., and Coburn, J. W. The hormonal and nonhormonal control of renal excretion of calcium and magnesium. *Nephron,* **1973,** *10,* 66–112.

Massry, S. G.; Muella, E.; Silverman, A. G.; and Kleeman, C. R. Inorganic phosphate treatment of hypercalcemia. *Archs intern. Med.,* **1968,** *12,* 307–312.

Murayama, Y.; Morel, F.; and Le Grimellec, C. Phosphate, calcium and magnesium transfers in proximal tubules and loops of Henle, as measured by single nephron microperfusion experiments in the rat. *Pflügers Arch. ges. Physiol.,* **1972,** *333,* 1–16.

Murphy, D. L.; Goodwin, F. K.; and Bunney, W. E., Jr. Aldosterone and sodium response to lithium administration in man. *Lancet,* **1969,** *2,* 458–461.

———. Leukocytosis during lithium treatment. *Am. J. Psychiat.,* **1971,** *127,* 1559–1561.

Naylor, G. J.; Fleming, L. W.; Stewart, W. K.; McNamee, H. B.; and Le Poidevin, D. Plasma magnesium and calcium levels in depressive psychosis. *Br. J. Psychiat.,* **1972,** *120,* 683–684.

New, W., and Trautwein, W. Inward membrane currents in mammalian myocardium. *Pflügers Arch. ges. Physiol.,* **1972,** *334,* 1–23.

Noyes, R., Jr.; Ringdahl, I. C.; and Andresen, N. J. C. Effect of lithium citrate on adrenocortical activity in manic-depressive illness. *Compreh. Psychiat.,* **1971,** *12,* 337–347.

Olson, E. B., Jr.; DeLuca, H. F.; and Potts, J. T., Jr. The effect of calcitonin and parathyroid hormone on calcium transport of isolated intestine. In, *Calcium, Parathyroid Hormone and the Calcitonins.* (Talmage, R. V., and Munson, P. L., eds.) Excerpta Medica, Amsterdam, **1972,** pp. 240–246.

Paillard, F.; Ardaillou, R.; Malendin, H.; Fillastre, J. P.; and Prier, S. Renal effects on salmon calcitonin in man. *J. Lab. clin. Med.,* **1972,** *80,* 200–216.

Perlia, C. P.; Gubisch, N. J.; Wolter, J.; Edelberg, D.; Dederick, M. M.; and Taylor, S. G., III. Mithramycin treatment of hypercalcemia. *Cancer, N.Y.,* **1970,** *25,* 389–394.

Platman, S. R., and Fieve, R. R. Biochemical aspects of lithium in affective disorders. *Archs gen. Psychiat.,* **1968,** *19,* 659–663.

Platman, S. R.; Hilton, J. G.; Koss, M. C.; and Kelly, W. G. Production of cortisol in patients with manic-depressive psychosis treated with lithium carbonate. *Dis. nerv. Syst.,* **1971,** *32,* 542–544.

Plenge, P.; Mellerup, E. T.; and Rafaelson, O. J. Lithium action on glycogen synthesis in rat brain, liver and diaphragm. *J. psychiat. Res.,* **1970,** *8,* 29–36.

Pletka, P.; Bernstein, D. S.; Hampers, C. L.; Merrill, J. P.; and Sherwood, L. M. Effects of magnesium on parathyroid secretion during chronic haemodialysis. *Lancet,* **1971,** *2,* 462–463.

Puschett, J. B.; Moranz, J.; and Kurnick, W. S. Evidence for a direct action of cholecalciferol and 25-hydroxy-cholecalciferol on the renal transport of phosphate, sodium and calcium. *J. clin. Invest.,* **1972,** *51,* 373–385.

Ramsey, T. A.; Mendels, J.; Stokes, J. W.; and Fitzgerald, R. G. Lithium carbonate and kidney function. *J. Am. med. Ass.,* **1972,** *219,* 1446–1449.

Randall, R. E., Jr.; Cohen, M. D.; Spray, C. C., Jr.; and

Rossmeid, E. C. Hypermagnesemia in renal failure: etiology and toxic manifestations. *Ann. intern. Med.,* **1964,** *61,* 73–88.

Rogers, S. F.; Flowers, C. E., Jr.; and Alexander, J. A. Aggressive toxemia management. *Obstet. Gynec., N.Y.,* **1969,** *33,* 724–728.

Rosen, E. U.; Campbell, P. G.; and Moosa, G. M. Hypomagnesemia and magnesium therapy in protein-calorie malnutrition. *J. Pediat.,* **1970,** *77,* 709–714.

Rösler, A., and Rabinowitz, D. Magnesium-induced reversal of vitamin-D resistance in hypoparathyroidism. *Lancet,* **1973,** *1,* 803–804.

Roza, O., and Berman, L. B. The pathophysiology of barium: hypokalemic and cardiovascular effects. *J. Pharmac. exp. Ther.,* **1971,** *177,* 433–439.

Schou, M.; Amdisen, A.; and Thomsen, K. Clinical and experimental observations concerning the absorption and elimination of lithium and on lithium poisoning. *Acta psychiat. scand.,* **1968,** Suppl. 203, 153–155.

Seelig, M. S. Electrographic patterns of magnesium depletion appearing in alcoholic heart disease. *Ann. N.Y. Acad. Sci.,* **1969,** *162,* 906–917.

Seller, R. H.; Cangiano, J.; Kim, K. E.; Mendelssohn, S.; Brest, A. N.; and Swartz, C. Digitalis toxicity and hypomagnesemia. *Am. Heart J.,* **1970,** *79,* 57–68.

Shils, M. E. Experimental human magnesium depletion. *Medicine, Baltimore,* **1969,** *48,* 61–85.

Shopsin, B.; Friedmann, R.; and Gershon, S. Lithium and leukocytosis. *Clin. Pharmac. Ther.,* **1971,** *12,* 923–928.

Simpson, G. R., and Dale, E. Serum levels of phosphorus, magnesium, and calcium in women utilizing combination oral or long-acting injectable progestational contraceptives. *Fert. Steril.,* **1972,** *23,* 326–330.

Singer, I.; Rotenberg, D.; and Preschett, J. B. Lithium-induced nephrogenic diabetes insipidus: *in vivo* and *in vitro* studies. *J. clin. Invest.,* **1972,** *51,* 1081–1091.

Sodeman, W. A. Diagnosis and treatment of digitalis toxicity. *New Engl. J. Med.,* **1965,** *273,* 35–37, 93–95.

Somjen, G.; Hilmy, M.; and Stephen, C. R. Failure to anesthetize human subjects by intravenous administration of magnesium sulfate. *J. Pharmac. exp. Ther.,* **1966,** *154,* 652–659.

Sørensen, O. H.; Friis, T.; Hindberg, I.; and Nielsen, S. P. The effect of calcitonin injected into hypercalcemic and normocalcemic patients. *Acta med. scand.,* **1970,** *187,* 283–290.

Sperelakis, N.; Schneider, M. F.; and Harris, E. G. Decreased K^+ conductance produced by Ba^{++} in frog sartorius fibers. *J. gen. Physiol.,* **1967,** *50,* 1565–1583.

Stanbury, W. S. Bone disease in uremia. *Am. J. Med.,* **1968,** *44,* 714–724.

Stone, S. R., and Pritchard, J. A. Effect of maternally administered magnesium sulfate on the neonate. *Obstet. Gynec., N.Y.,* **1970,** *35,* 574–577.

Suh, S. M.; Tashjian, A. H., Jr.; Matsuo, N.; Parkinson, D. K.; and Fraser, D. Pathogenesis of hypocalcemia in primary hypomagnesemia: normal end-organ responsiveness to parathyroid hormone, impaired parathyroid gland function. *J. clin. Invest.,* **1973,** *52,* 153–160.

Sutton, R. A., and Watson, L. Urinary excretion of calcium and magnesium in primary hyperparathyroidism. *Lancet,* **1969,** *1,* 1000–1003.

Tanaka, Y., and DeLuca, H. F. The control of 25-hydroxy vitamin D metabolism by inorganic phosphorus. *Archs Biochem. Biophys.,* **1973,** *154,* 566–574.

Targovnik, H. J.; Rodman, J. S.; and Sherwood, L. M. Regulation of parathyroid hormone secretion *in vitro:* quantitative aspects of calcium and magnesium ion control. *Endocrinology,* **1971,** *88,* 1477–1482.

Taylor, A. N., and Wasserman, R. Immunofluorescent localization of vitamin D–dependent calcium-binding protein. *J. Histochem. Cytochem.,* **1970,** *18,* 107–115.

Wallach, S., and Dimich, A. Radiomagnesium turnover studies in hypomagnesemic states. *Ann. N.Y. Acad. Sci.*, **1969**, *162*, 963–972.

Wang, Y.-C.; Pandey, G. N.; Mendels, J.; and Frazer, A. Effect of lithium on prostaglandin E_1-stimulated adenylate cyclase activity of human platelets. *Biochem. Pharmac.*, **1974**, *23*, 845–855.

White, M. G., and Fetner, C. D. Treatment of the syndrome of inappropriate secretion of antidiuretic hormone with lithium carbonate. *New Engl. J. Med.*, **1975**, *292*, 390–392.

Woody, J. N.; London, W. L.; and Wilbanks, G. D., Jr. Lithium toxicity in a newborn. *Pediatrics, Springfield,* **1971**, *47*, 94–96.

Zieve, L. Pathogenesis of hepatic coma. *Archs intern. Med.*, **1966**, *118*, 211–223.

Monographs and Reviews

Davis, J. M., and Fann, W. E. Lithium. *A. Rev. Pharmac.*, **1971**, *11*, 285–298.

Douglas, W. W. Stimulus-secretion coupling: the concept and clues from chromaffin and other cells. (The First Gaddum Memorial Lecture.) *Br. J. Pharmac.*, **1968**, *34*, 451–474.

Flink, E. B. Mineral metabolism in alcoholism. In, *The Biology of Alcoholism*, Vol. 1. (Kissin, B., and Begleiter, H., eds.) Plenum Press, New York, **1971**, pp. 377–395.

Gitelman, H. J., and Welt, L. G. Magnesium deficiency. *A. Rev. Med.*, **1969**, *20*, 233–242.

Hancox, N. M. *Biology of Bone.* Cambridge University Press, London, **1972**.

Hubbard, J. I. Microphysiology of vertebrate neuromuscular transmission. *Physiol. Rev.*, **1973**, *53*, 674–723.

Martin, H. E. Clinical magnesium deficiency. *Ann. N.Y. Acad. Sci.*, **1969**, *162*, 891–900.

Pitts, R. F. *Physiology of the Kidney and Body Fluids: An Introductory Text*, 3rd ed. Year Book Medical Publishers, Inc., Chicago, **1974**.

Rubin, R. P. The role of calcium in the release of neurotransmitter substances and hormones. *Pharmac. Rev.*, **1970**, *22*, 389–428.

Russell, A. The implications of hyperammonemia in rare and common disorders, including migraine. *Mt. Sinai J. Med., N.Y.*, **1973**, *40*, 609–630, 723–735.

Saron, B. M., and Gaind, R. Lithium. *Clin. Toxicol.*, **1973**, *6*, 257–269.

Schou, M. Biology and pharmacology of the lithium ion. *Pharmac. Rev.*, **1957**, *9*, 17–58.

Singer, I., and Rotenberg, D. Mechanisms of lithium action. *New Engl. J. Med.*, **1973**, *289*, 254–260.

Wacker, W. E. C., and Parisi, A. F. Magnesium metabolism. *New Engl. J. Med.*, **1968**, *278*, 658–663, 712–717, 772–776.

Walser, M. Magnesium metabolism. *Ergebn. Physiol.*, **1967**, *59*, 185–296.

CHAPTER

38 ANIONS: PHOSPHATE, IODIDE, FLUORIDE, AND OTHER ANIONS

Michael J. Peach

PHOSPHATE

Phosphorus has important and multifaceted functions in the biochemistry of the body. It is ubiquitous in anatomical terms and is of great significance in a host of reactions throughout virtually all organs and tissues. The bulk of the body's phosphorus is located in the bones, where it plays a key role in osteoblastic and osteoclastic activities. Enzymatically catalyzed phosphate-transfer reactions are numerous and vital in the metabolism of carbohydrate, lipid, and protein, and a proper concentration of the anion is of primary importance in assuring an orderly biochemical sequence. Throughout all the tissues, the storage of energy in biochemical terms is largely as "high-energy phosphate" compounds, and organic phosphate is present in essentially all types of bodily constituents.

In addition, it is well known that phosphorus plays important roles, in terms of modifying the steady state, with respect to tissue concentrations of calcium. Furthermore, the acid-base equilibrium may be modified because phosphate ions are important buffers of the intracellular fluid, and also play a primary role in the renal excretion of hydrogen ion.

Absorption, Distribution, and Excretion. Phosphate is absorbed from, and to a limited extent secreted into, the gastrointestinal tract. The excretion of fecal phosphorus is presumed to be a net consequence of the quantity ingested, absorbed, and secreted. The transport of phosphate from the lumen of the gut is an active, energy-dependent process, and there are factors that appear to modify the degree of its intestinal absorption. The presence of large quantities of calcium or aluminum may lead to the formation of large amounts of insoluble phosphate and may therefore diminish the net absorption of phosphate from the bowel. Vitamin D stimulates phosphate absorption, and this effect is independent of the action of the vitamin on intestinal transport of calcium (Sampson and Matthews, 1972). In general, in adults, about two thirds of the ingested phosphate is absorbed from the bowel, and that which is absorbed from the gut is almost entirely excreted into the urine. In growing children, there is a positive balance of phosphate. Plasma phosphate concentrations are higher in children than in adults. This "hyperphosphatemia" decreases the affinity of hemoglobin for oxygen and is hypothesized to explain the physiological "anemia" of childhood (Card and Brain, 1973).

Phosphorus is present in plasma and extracellular fluid, in cell membranes and intracellular fluid, and in collagen and bone tissue. In the extracellular fluid, phosphate is primarily in inorganic form and only a small component of esterified phosphate is present. Plasma phosphate concentration is inversely related to the action of vitamin D and thus to the rate of renal hydroxylation of 25-hydroxycholecalciferol (*see* Chapter 76). A reduction of the plasma phosphate concentration permits the presence of more calcium in the blood and inhibits deposition of new bone salt. An increased plasma concentration of the phosphate anion facilitates the effect of calcitonin on calcium deposition in bone (Werner *et al.,* 1972). The concentration of plasma inorganic phosphorus may vary with age, and the range has been recorded in great detail by Greenberg and coworkers (1960). The ratio of disodium phosphate and monosodium phosphate in extracellular fluid is 4:1 at a pH of 7.40. The buffer ratio varies, of course, with pH; however, owing to the relatively low concentration, phosphate contributes little to buffering capacity of extracellular fluid. Cell phosphate plays a more important role in intracellular buffering owing to the quantities that are available.

The renal excretion of phosphate has been studied quite extensively (*see* Massry *et al.,* 1973). More than 90% of the phosphate in plasma is filterable, and the bulk is then actively reabsorbed by the initial segment of the proximal tubule. Phosphate reabsorption does not occur in the loop of Henle, and little if any occurs in the distal tubule (Murayama *et al.,* 1972). Plasma volume expansion causes increased urinary phosphate excretion (Steele, 1970). Phosphate excreted in the urine probably represents the net difference between the amount filtered and that reabsorbed. The occurrence of renal tubular secretion of phosphate is still debatable. Parathyroid hormone and calcitonin increase the urinary excretion of phosphate by blocking proximal tubular reabsorption (Agus *et al.,* 1971; Haas *et al.,* 1971). Vitamin D_3 and its metabolites directly stimulate proximal tubular reabsorption of phosphate (Puschett *et al.,* 1972).

Role of Phosphate in the Acidification of the Urine. The interrelations that exist between the rates of excretion of phosphate and titratable acid are referred to in Chapter 36 and in the introduction to Section VIII. Although the concentration of phosphate is low in the extracellular fluid, the anion is progressively concentrated in the renal tubule and represents the most abundant buffer system in the distal tubule. At this site, the secretion of H^+ by the tubular cell in exchange for Na^+ in the tubular urine converts sodium basic phosphate to sodium acid phosphate. In this manner, large amounts of acid can be excreted without lowering the pH of the urine to a degree that would block H^+ transport due to a high concentration gradient between the tubular cell and luminal fluid.

Actions of the Phosphate Ion. Once phosphate gains access to the body fluids and tissues, it exerts little pharmacological effect. If the ion is introduced into the gastrointestinal tract, the absorbed phosphate is rapidly excreted. If large amounts are given by this route, much of it may escape absorption. This leads to a cathartic action, and, therefore, the phosphate salts are employed as mild laxatives. Inorganic phosphate poisoning following ingestion of laxatives that contain phosphate salts has been reported in adults and children (McConnell, 1971; Levitt *et al.,*

1973). The ingestion of large amounts of sodium acid phosphate lowers the pH of the urine. If phosphate salts are introduced intravenously in high concentration, they may prove toxic. Toxicity results from reducing the concentration of Ca^{2+} in the circulation, and the symptoms are those of hypocalcemia. The actions of radioactive phosphate are discussed in Chapter 62.

Phosphate Depletion. There has been a question for some time concerning the possibility of clinical consequences of phosphate depletion (Lotz *et al.,* 1968). Familial hypophosphatemia is an X-linked dominant trait apparently due to defective intestinal absorption and/or renal reabsorption of inorganic phosphate that results in rickets and dwarfism (Glorieux *et al.,* 1972; Short *et al.,* 1973). In a report by Lichtman and coworkers (1969), a patient with striking hypophosphatemia is described who was found to have a significant depression in the steady-state concentration of erythrocyte adenosine triphosphate (ATP). Certain minimal ATP concentrations are required for the viability of red cells in the circulation. In addition to reduced ATP, hypophosphatemia causes a marked decrease in erythrocyte concentrations of 2,3-diphosphoglycerate. Acute hemolytic anemia and impaired tissue oxygenation can occur in severe hypophosphatemia (Jacob and Amsden, 1971). This certainly raises the possibility that other cellular stores of ATP and other critical organic phosphate compounds may be depleted. These biochemical abnormalities, in turn, could well be responsible for certain features of the clinical syndrome.

In general, the phosphorus present in ordinary foods is an adequate source of the ion. The use of expensive preparations of organic phosphates as "tonics" has no validity.

Elemental Phosphorus. Elemental phosphorus exists in two forms. One is a red, granular, nonabsorbable form that is nontoxic. The other is a white or yellow, waxy form that is highly poisonous and will burn on contact with air and, therefore, is preserved under water. Poisoning from this form may occur in industry from breathing volatile fumes or from accidental ingestion.

Phosphorus is used in insecticides, rodent poisons, and fireworks, and in the manufacture of fertilizer. After ingestion, phosphorus exerts a toxic action within the gastrointestinal tract, followed later by injury to the liver, muscles, myocardium, kidney, and central nervous system (CNS). Vomiting may be fairly prompt after ingestion, and the vomitus has a garlic odor and is luminescent. In general, after a short acute episode, there may be a delay of 1 to 3 days before the more profound illness begins.

The *symptoms and signs* of acute phosphorus poisoning are nausea, vomiting, bloody diarrhea, jaundice, pruritus, and abdominal tenderness in the area of an enlarged liver. Hepatic insufficiency may be profound, with hypoglycemia, hypoprothrombinemia, and increase in coagulation time. Ecchymoses and petechiae may be noted in the skin, and one may also find submucosal hemorrhages. Urine flow may become scant, and the urine may be bloody and contain albumin and droplets of free fat. Cardiovascular collapse results from both the metabolic derangements and a direct influence of phosphorus on the myocardium and blood vessels. Death usually follows a period of delirium and coma (Arena, 1973).

Protracted exposure to lesser quantities of phosphorus may produce *chronic poisoning* characterized by necrosis of bone, usually in the lower and upper jaw and the neighboring facial bones. In addition, there may be hepatic cirrhosis and chronic renal damage.

Treatment. If the patient has ingested phosphorus within 5 hours prior to being seen by the physician, it is desirable to employ gastric lavage. This is best accomplished by a solution of 0.1% copper sulfate in water, which tends to form an insoluble coating of copper phosphide. The remaining therapy is addressed primarily to combating the peripheral vascular collapse and the dehydration and acidosis. The mortality rate in acute poisoning cases is close to 50%.

Phosphorus burns should be thoroughly washed with a 1% solution of copper sulfate and then treated like other burns.

Preparations. Only certain of the preparations of *inorganic phosphates* are mentioned here; *calcium phosphates* are described elsewhere, as are organic compounds that contain phosphorus.

Sodium Phosphate, U.S.P., is available as *Sodium Phosphate, Dried,* N.F., as *Sodium Phosphate, Effervescent,* N.F. (a dry, effervescent powder), and as *Sodium Phosphate Solution,* N.F. It is also available in combination with *Sodium Biphosphate,* U.S.P., as *Sodium Phosphate and Biphosphate Oral Solution,* U.S.P., and *Sodium Phosphate and Biphosphate Enema,* U.S.P. *Phosphoric Acid,* N.F., is a colorless, syrupy liquid that is prescribed in the form of *Diluted Phosphoric Acid,* N.F., a solution containing 10% phosphoric acid by weight; it should be further diluted before administration.

Therapeutic Uses. The phosphates are of limited therapeutic usefulness. Sodium phosphate has been employed to diminish hypercalcemia (*see* page 787). The phosphates have a role in the management of the phosphate-depletion syndrome. Phosphate salts are also effective saline cathartics (*see* Chapter 49).

Pathological Conditions Associated with a Disturbance in Phosphate Metabolism. A defect in phosphate metabolism occurs in a variety of diseases, as briefly mentioned below. (*See* Bartter, 1964; *see also* Index.)

Osteoporosis. This condition is considered to be a primary disorder in the formation of bone matrix. There is no primary defect in phosphate metabolism, and plasma concentrations of phosphorus are within usual limits.

Rickets. If the primary defect is a result of inadequate quantities of vitamin D, the consequence is initially a failure adequately to absorb calcium and phosphate from the bowel. This tends to stimulate the secretion of parathyroid hormone, which, in turn, tends to raise the calcium concentration in the plasma toward normal but promotes increased excretion of phosphate. With decreased absorption and increased excretion of phosphate, there is a fall in the plasma concentration. *Familial hypophosphatemia* is due to defective absorption and/or excretion of inorganic phosphate and has been mentioned above. Other forms of rickets are described in Chapter 76.

Osteomalacia. The loss of calcium in stools (due to malabsorption) or the loss from body fluids by way of the kidney (essential hypercalciuria or renal tubular acidosis with augmented calcium excretion) promotes a negative balance of calcium. Such loss deprives the body of calcium stores, and the plasma calcium concentration falls slightly. This, in turn, stimulates the secretion of parathyroid hormone, which restores the calcium concentration to normal but tends to promote some depression of plasma phosphorus.

Osteitis Fibrosa Cystica. In this disorder, there is a primary increase in the secretion of parathyroid hormone that is usually accompanied by an increase in plasma calcium, some reduction of plasma phosphorus, and a decreased renal tubular reabsorption of phosphate.

Secondary Hyperparathyroidism. This condition may be seen in patients with chronic renal insufficiency. The sequence of events probably starts with a high plasma concentration of phosphorus and a low value for calcium; this situation stimulates parathyroid secretion. Since the elevated plasma phosphorus is a consequence of renal insufficiency, it persists. The continuing hyperphosphatemia may be modified by the administration of aluminum hydroxide gel, which tends to inhibit the absorption of phosphate from the bowel, owing to the formation of insoluble aluminum phosphates.

Hypoparathyroidism. In this disorder, characterized by deficient parathyroid secretion, there is a rise in plasma phosphorus and a depressed concentration of calcium. This condition can be readily treated with vitamin D.

IODIDE

There are numerous iodine-containing compounds of pharmacological interest. These include elemental iodine, substances yielding elemental iodine, the inorganic iodides, and iodine-containing organic compounds. Iodine compounds have many unrelated actions and are used in a variety of ways. Consequently, the pharmacology of iodine has been largely subdivided with primary regard to therapeutic applications. The *antiseptic* action of iodine is discussed in Chapter 50, while iodine and the *thyroid* gland are considered in Chapter 67. In this section, discussion will be limited primarily to the general pharmacological aspects of the iodides, their toxicology, and the use of iodine-containing organic compounds in radiography.

Absorption, Distribution, and Excretion. In geographical areas where the iodine supply is adequate, the adult ingests about 150 μg per day. In addition to normal dietary sources of iodine, there are numerous incidental sources such as iodine-containing medicaments, iodine-containing radiographic contrast media, and table salt to which potassium iodide has been added. These nondietary sources may afford confusion in the interpretation of certain laboratory tests employed in the diagnosis of thyroid disorders. Elemental iodine is reduced to iodide in the gastrointestinal lumen, and absorption of iodide has been demonstrated throughout the gastrointestinal tract. Iodide is also absorbed from the enteric tract in the form of iodinated amino acids. Intestinal malabsorption, for example, in protein-calorie malnutrition, has been shown to result in decreased absorption of iodide (Ingenbleek and Beckers, 1973).

Iodide is distributed similarly to the chloride ion, largely extracellularly. However, the volume of distribution is larger than the extracellular space. There are several reasons for a larger distribution. First, the concentration of iodide in the water of red blood cells is almost identical to that in the plasma water. Further, iodide is markedly accumulated by the thyroid gland. Lastly, the concentration of iodide in the gastric and salivary secretions far exceeds its concentration in the extracellular fluid.

The plasma concentration of inorganic iodide is less than 1 μg/100 ml and constitutes only about 10 to 20% of the total plasma iodine concentration. Thus, the thyroid hormones account for the major portion of plasma iodine.

Iodide may be excreted from the body by way of sweat, feces, and milk; however, these routes under ordinary circumstances account for negligible losses from the body. This is illustrated by the fact that 98% of a dose of radioactive iodide administered to an athyreotic individual can be recovered in the urine. Thus, the kidney serves as the chief excretory organ for iodide. The clearance of iodide is always much less than that of inulin under a variety of experimental conditions but is considerably higher than that of other halides. Urinary loss of iodide continues under conditions of serious deficiency, indicating that there is no renal threshold for iodide. Moreover, increasing the filtered load of iodide by inorganic iodide loading does not suggest the existence of a transport maximum for reabsorption of the anion.

Although there are species differences in the rate of renal clearance of iodide and intersubject variations in man, it now seems clear that the major mechanism for the excretion of iodide is similar to that of other halides, namely, glomerular filtration and passive reabsorption due to the electrical gradient produced by the active transport of Na^+; however, Cl^- and Br^- are reabsorbed to a much greater extent than is I^- (see Walser and Rahill, 1965). While the renal excretion of I^- can be increased by procedures that promote Cl^- excretion (e.g., osmotic diuresis, chloruretic diuretics, salt loading), the ratios of their respective clearances remain essentially unchanged. (See also Fregly and McCarthy, 1973.)

Pharmacological Actions. There are few known pharmacological effects of iodide, other than those on the thyroid. After intravenous administration, no specific response has been observed. Neither the CNS nor the circulatory system is affected.

Iodide compounds are employed extensively as expectorants because of the stimulatory effect of iodide on bronchial secretion.

Iodide exerts an effect on granulomatous lesions in that it induces resolution of syphilitic gummata and the granulomatous lesions of tuberculosis, leprosy, and various fungal diseases. This does not depend on the effect of iodide on the responsible microorganism.

Toxicology. *Acute poisoning* from an initial dose of iodide is relatively rare, and even after intravenous injection reactions seldom occur. Ingestion of large amounts of iodide may cause gastrointestinal irritation. An occasional individual, however, shows a marked sensitivity; therefore, before iodide salts or organic iodine preparations are given by the intravenous route, the tolerance of the individual should be determined. The onset of acute iodide poisoning may occur immediately or several hours after the administration of the salt. Angioedema is the outstanding symptom, and swelling of the larynx may lead to suffocation. Multiple cutaneous hemorrhages may be present. Also, manifestations of the serum-sickness type of hypersensitivity, such as fever, arthralgia, lymph node enlargement, and eosinophilia, may appear. Fatal periarteritis nodosa attributed to hypersensitivity to iodide has been described.

The symptoms and therapy of acute *iodine* poisoning are described in Chapter 50.

Chronic iodide poisoning, or *iodism,* is much more common than acute iodide poisoning. There is no way of predicting which patient will react unfavorably, and an individual may vary in his sensitivity to the drug from time to time. Eventually, iodism will occur in all individuals if the dose is sufficiently high.

The symptoms start with an unpleasant brassy taste and burning in the mouth and throat, as well as soreness of the teeth and gums. Increased salivation is noted. Coryza, sneezing, and irritation of the eyes with swelling of the eyelids are commonly observed. Mild iodism simulates a "head cold." The patient often complains of a severe headache that originates in the frontal sinuses. Irritation of the mucous glands of the respiratory tract causes a productive cough. Excess transudation into the bronchial tree may lead to pulmonary edema. In addition, the parotid and submaxillary glands may become enlarged and tender, and the syndrome may be mistaken for mumps parotitis. There also may be inflammation of the pharynx, larynx, and tonsils. Skin lesions are common, and vary in type and intensity. They usually are mildly acneform and distributed in the seborrheic areas. Rarely, severe and sometimes fatal eruptions (ioderma) may occur after the prolonged use of iodides. The lesions are bizarre, resemble those caused by bromide, and, as a rule, involute quickly when iodide is withdrawn. Symptoms of gastric irritation are common; and diarrhea, which is sometimes bloody, may occur. Fever is occasionally observed, and anorexia and depression may be present. The mechanisms involved in the production of these derangements remain unknown.

Treatment of Iodism. Fortunately, the symptoms of iodism disappear spontaneously within a few days after stopping the administration of iodide. Therefore, treatment consists in withdrawing the offending medication and using supportive measures as determined by the particular symptoms. Abundant fluid and sodium chloride intake may be of assistance in hastening iodide elimination. In severe cases, the establishment of an osmotic diuresis by the judicious use of mannitol may be advantageous.

Preparations. The preparations described below may be grouped into three classes, as follows: (1) inorganic iodides, (2) organic compounds that yield the iodide ion, and (3) iodine-containing organic compounds that are used solely as contrast media in roentgenography.

Inorganic Iodides. The important inorganic iodide preparations (*Potassium Iodide,* U.S.P., *Potassium Iodide Solution,* U.S.P., *Sodium Iodide,* U.S.P., and *Strong Iodine Solution,* U.S.P.) used in the treatment of thyroid disorders are described in Chapter 67. *Hydriodic acid syrup* (1.4% hydriodic

acid) is used as a vehicle for many expectorant drugs. Tincture and solution of iodine, and iodophors used as antiseptics, are discussed in Chapter 50.

Organic Compounds Yielding Iodide. These compounds were introduced into therapy because of their sustained action. They are slowly excreted, and during their sojourn in the body iodide is liberated. Most of the preparations consist of iodized proteins, oils, or fatty acids, or simpler iodine-containing compounds. Such compounds are of little therapeutic value in countries where dietary supplements are used. Some, however, are useful to prevent endemic goiter in underdeveloped areas.

Iodine-Containing Organic Compounds for Radiographic Use. Two types of iodinated organic compounds are employed in radiography: the lipid-soluble and the water-soluble agents. The following preparations are among those available.

Iopanoic Acid, U.S.P. (TELEPAQUE), is employed as a contrast medium in cholecystography. After ingestion, it is absorbed promptly, undergoes conjugation with glucuronic acid in the liver, is concentrated and stored in the gallbladder, and is eliminated in the bile. Iopanoic acid seldom causes undesirable reactions and has a low toxicity. However, its use is contraindicated in acute glomerulonephritis, severe chronic renal insufficiency, and acute disorders of the gastrointestinal tract.

Iophendylate Injection, U.S.P. (PANTOPAQUE), is a mixture of isomers of ethyl iodophenylundecylate. It is an absorbable, iodized fatty acid compound of low viscosity designed especially for myelography. This agent should not be used intravascularly. It is equally useful for visualization of all regions of the spinal cord, although this may be technically more difficult in the cervical and thoracic regions. When examination is completed, the compound should be removed by aspiration. When the bulk of the material is removed, the remainder is absorbed within a few months and the incidence of side reactions is low. The agent should not be used when lumbar puncture is contraindicated; and, to avoid subdural and extra-arachnoid extravasation, it should not be employed within 10 days of a previous lumbar puncture.

Iophendylate also is used in emulsified aqueous form as a contrast medium for visualization of the biliary tree, sinus tracts, and certain body cavities.

Diatrizoate Sodium Injection, U.S.P., and *Diatrizoate Sodium Oral Solution,* U.S.P. (HYPAQUE), are perhaps the least toxic of radiopaque media. The oral preparations are used for roentgenographic examination of the gastrointestinal tract. Preparations for intravenous use are available in several formulations with different iodine contents and are used for a wide variety of roentgenographic procedures. After intravenous administration, diatrizoate sodium is excreted unchanged by the kidney.

Diatrizoate Meglumine Injection, U.S.P., and *diatrizoate meglumine oral solution* (CARDIOGRAFIN, GASTROGRAFIN, RENO-M) have the same actions as diatrizoate sodium. They are used for examination of the gastrointestinal tract, angiography, and intravenous urography. The dosages vary depending upon the route of administration as well as the type of examination to be undertaken. Various mixtures of diatrizoate meglumine and diatrizoate sodium are also marketed for intravenous use.

Iodipamide Meglumine Injection, U.S.P. (CHOLO-GRAFIN MEGLUMINE), is one of the best contrast media for intravenous cholangiography and cholecystography. It is also used for angiocardiography and thoracic aortography. This iodinated benzoic acid derivative is also available as the sodium salt, *iodipamide sodium injection* (CHOLOGRAFIN SODIUM).

Iothalamate Meglumine Injection, U.S.P. (CONRAY), is an isomer of diatrizoate meglumine and is freely soluble in water. Following intravenous injection, iothalamate meglumine is rapidly circulated throughout the vascular system and rapidly excreted unchanged in the urine. It is used in intravenous excretory urography, cerebral angiography, peripheral arteriography, and venography. The preparation is also available as the sodium salt, *Iothalamate Sodium Injection,* U.S.P. (ANGIO-CONRAY, CONRAY-400). It is also used in intravenous excretory urography and in intravascular angiocardiography and aortography. It should not be used for cerebral angiography.

A mixture of iothalamate meglumine and sodium salts (VASCORAY) is available and has the same uses as iothalamate sodium.

Ipodate Calcium, U.S.P. (ORGRAFIN CALCIUM), is a water-soluble iodinated organic compound that is administered orally for cholecystography and may be used for cholangiography. This agent should be used with caution in patients with renal or hepatic disease.

The preparation is also available as the sodium salt, *Ipodate Sodium,* U.S.P. (ORGRAFIN SODIUM). The indications for its use are the same as for the calcium salt.

Methiodal Sodium, N.F. (SKIODAN), is a water-soluble compound containing 52% organically bound iodine. It is used for retrograde pyelography. Rarely, oliguria and anuria may follow its use in bilateral procedures.

Acetrizoate sodium (CYSTOKON, PYELOKON-R) is used for retrograde pyelography and cystography.

Tyropanoate sodium (BILOPAQUE) is administered orally, and the compound is absorbed and converted to glucuronic acid conjugates in the liver. The radiopaque conjugates are concentrated in the gallbladder. It is used as a cholecystographic medium.

Sterile propyliodone suspension and *Sterile Propyliodone Oil Suspension,* U.S.P., are suspensions of *Propyliodone,* U.S.P., used for bronchography.

Ethiodized Oil, U.S.P. (ETHIODOL), consists of iodinated, low-viscosity, esterified fatty acids of poppyseed oil. This agent is used as a contrast medium for hysterosalpingography and sialography.

Iodized Oil Injection, N.F. (LIPIODOL), is iodinated poppyseed oil and is used in hysterosalpingography, sialography, and bronchography. This agent is contraindicated in any area where bleeding has occurred and in inflammatory diseases.

Therapeutic Uses. The empirical use of iodide in the treatment of a variety of diseases (*e.g.,* encepha-litis, essential hypertension, portal cirrhosis, and thromboangiitis obliterans) has been of little, if any, value. For many years iodide was used in the treatment of syphilis. Its use was based on the observation that it induced rapid resolution of gummatous lesions. It is no longer employed for this purpose. Similar effects are observed in other granulomatous lesions such as those produced by the fungal diseases sporotrichosis, actinomycosis, and blastomycosis. With the advent of more efficacious drugs for the treatment of these diseases, iodide is rarely employed, with the possible exception of the lymphocutaneous type of sporotrichosis (*see* Seabury and Dascomb, 1964).

Iodide salts are useful *expectorants* when it is desired to liquefy tenacious bronchial secretions, for example, in the later stages of bronchitis, bronchiectasis, and asthma. Sodium or potassium iodide is commonly used in a dose of 0.3 g in aqueous solution every 6 hours. Gastrointestinal irritation, anorexia, and vomiting are frequent side effects (Bernecker, 1969). The drug should not be administered longer than is actually necessary to "loosen" the cough. However, in some patients with chronic bronchitis or asthma, iodide may be prescribed more or less continuously if it appears to afford relief.

Radiographic Uses. Numerous iodine-containing compounds employed as radiographic contrast media are described above. The aim in developing new compounds is to achieve superior contrast material for a given organ system while at the same time eliminating side reactions. In general, iodinated contrast media should be administered with caution in patients with hepatic or renal dysfunction. Media used for gastrointestinal roentgenography and agents administered orally may cause nausea, vomiting, and diarrhea. Acute tubular necrosis has been reported to be the consequence of the ingestion of certain gallbladder dyes (Setter *et al.,* 1963).

The injection of iodized fatty acids is essentially a surgical procedure that involves risk. The following cautions should be especially borne in mind. Preparations that have aged and darkened beyond their original color should not be used. Injection pressure should be carefully controlled to avoid lacerating tissues. Intrauterine injections should be made under fluoroscopic control. The compounds should not be administered to individuals with a history of sensitivity to iodides.

The water-soluble compounds are responsible for two types of severe reactions: (1) Infrequently there may be severe respiratory difficulty with wheezing, bronchial and laryngeal spasm, swelling of the lips and eyelids, and giant urticaria. This is the so-called anaphylactic response and calls for the prompt administration of antiallergic agents together with appropriate supportive measures. (2) Somewhat more frequent is a picture of cardiovascular collapse in which there is a fall in blood pressure, tachycardia, dyspnea, and confusion and cyanosis progressing to unconsciousness. Vasopressor agents as well as antiallergic drugs should be administered. Proper equipment and personnel trained in its use should be available for endotracheal intubation whenever these compounds are being used.

FLUORIDE

The fluoride ion is of interest because of its toxic properties and its effect on dental enamel and bone. Fluoride is widely distributed in nature, and the soils of different regions of the world vary greatly in their fluoride content. Fluoride gains access to plants from the soil as well as from atmospheric sources. The sources of atmospheric fluoride include the burning of soft coal and the manufacturing of superphosphate, aluminum, steel, lead, copper, and nickel. Man obtains fluoride from the ingestion of plants and water. Incidental sources include food additives (*e.g.*, baking powder) that are contaminated with fluoride, and the ingestion of rodenticides and insecticides that contain fluoride compounds.

Absorption, Distribution, and Excretion. Fluorides are absorbed from the gastrointestinal tract, the lungs, and the skin. The gastrointestinal tract is the major site of absorption. The degree of absorption of a fluoride compound is best correlated with its solubility. The relatively soluble compounds, such as sodium fluoride, are almost completely absorbed, whereas relatively insoluble compounds, such as cryolite (Na_3AlF_6) and the fluoride found in bone meal (fluoroapatite), are poorly absorbed. Certain dietary cations (*e.g.*, calcium and iron) retard absorption of fluoride ion by forming low-solubility complexes in the gastrointestinal tract. The second most common route of absorption is by way of the lungs. Pulmonary inhalation of fluoride present in dusts and gases constitutes the major route of industrial exposure. There is evidence that inhalation of fluoride produces the same effects as the ingestion of fluoride (Hodge, 1964). A third, and relatively rare, route of absorption is through the skin (Burke *et al.*, 1973).

Fluoride has been detected in all organs and tissues examined; however, there is no evidence that it is concentrated in any tissues except bone, thyroid, aorta, and perhaps kidney (Armstrong, 1967). Fluoride is preponderantly deposited in the skeleton and teeth, and the degree of skeletal storage is related to intake and age. This is thought to be a function of the turnover rate of skeletal components, with growing bone showing a greater fluoride deposition than bone in mature animals. Prolonged periods of time are required for mobilization of fluoride from bone. Fluoride is accumulated by the aorta, and concentrations increase with age, probably reflecting the calcification that occurs in this artery.

The major route of fluoride excretion is by way of the kidneys; however, fluoride is also excreted in small amounts by the sweat glands, the lactating breast, and the gastrointestinal tract. Under conditions of excessive sweating, the fraction of total fluoride excretion contributed by sweating can reach nearly one half. About 90% of the fluoride ion filtered by the glomerulus is reabsorbed by the renal tubules. Whether tubular secretion of fluoride occurs is unknown.

Pharmacological Actions. The pharmacological actions of fluoride, with the possible exception of its effect on bone and teeth, can be classified as toxic.

Fluoride is an inhibitor of several enzyme systems and diminishes tissue respiration and anaerobic glycolysis. Fluoride is also a useful anticoagulant *in vitro* and is of particular value when it is desired to stop biological activity, such as glycolysis, in erythrocytes.

The chronic administration of sodium fluoride in patients with idiopathic osteoporosis, Paget's disease of bone, and multiple myeloma promotes the retention of calcium (Hodge and Smith, 1968). Fluoride treatment relieves bone pain and tends to strengthen and harden bone. There is an increase in the crystallinity as well as in the fluoride content of bone of patients thus treated, and the microscopic appearance of bone resembles that in patients suffering from chronic fluorosis. (For further detail, *see* Bierman, 1972; Jowsey *et al.*, 1972.) Fluoride has also been used to treat otosclerosis and osteogenesis imperfecta (Castells, 1973; Daniel *et al.*, 1973). Further studies are required to establish the efficacy of the anion in these disorders. The radioactive nuclide ^{18}F has proven useful in bone imaging and the detection of bone metastases (Sharma and Quinn, 1972; Jones *et al.*, 1973).

Acute Poisoning. Acute fluoride poisoning is not rare. It usually results from the accidental ingestion of insecticides or rodenticides containing fluoride salts.

Initial symptoms are secondary to the local action of fluoride on the mucosa of the gastrointestinal tract. Salivation, nausea, abdominal pain, vomiting, and diarrhea are frequent. Systemic symptoms are varied and severe. The patient shows signs of increasing irritability of the nervous system, including paresthesias, a positive Chvostek sign, hyperactive reflexes, and tonic and clonic convulsions. These signs are related to the calcium-binding effect of fluoride. Hypocalcemia and hypoglycemia are frequent laboratory findings. The signs may be delayed for several hours. Pain in various muscle groups may occur. The blood pressure falls, presumably due to central vasomotor depression as well as a direct toxic action on cardiac muscle. The respiratory center is first stimulated and later depressed. Death usually results from either respiratory paralysis or cardiac failure. It is stated that the lethal dose of sodium fluoride for man is about 5 g; however, recovery has been reported in patients ingesting much larger doses, whereas a dose as low as 2 g has been fatal (Arena, 1973). In children, as little as 0.5 g of sodium fluoride may be fatal.

Treatment. The principles of the treatment of fluoride poisoning have been outlined by Peters (1948). (*See also* Waldbott, 1963; Arena, 1973.) They are as follows: (1) Act quickly. (2) Start intravenous therapy with glucose in isotonic saline solution to maintain blood sugar and to have a venous channel available for transfusion in the event of shock. (3) Wash the stomach with limewater (0.15% calcium hydroxide solution) and then give limewater at frequent intervals. (4) Have calcium gluconate available for intravenous administration and watch closely for signs of tetany. (5) Maintain high urine volumes with parenteral fluid. (6) Wash away vomitus, feces, and urine promptly to prevent external burns.

Chronic Poisoning. In man, the major manifestations of the chronic ingestion of excessive amounts of fluoride are osteosclerosis and mottled enamel. Chronic exposure to excess fluoride causes increased osteoblastic activity. Osteosclerosis is a phenomenon wherein the density and calcification of bone are increased; in the case of fluoride intoxication, it is thought to represent the replacement of hydroxyapatite by the denser fluoroapatite. However, the mechanism of its development remains unknown. The degree of skeletal involvement varies from changes that are barely detectable radiologically to marked thickening of the cortex of long bones, numerous exostoses scattered throughout the skeleton, and calcification of ligaments, tendons, and muscle attachments to bone. In its severest form it is a disabling disease and is designated as *crippling fluorosis* (*see* Singh *et al.,* 1963).

Mottled enamel or dental fluorosis is a well-recognized entity that was first described over 50 years ago. The gross changes in very mild mottling consist in small, opaque, paper-white areas scattered irregularly over the tooth surface. In severe cases, discrete or confluent, deep brown- to black-stained pits give the tooth a corroded appearance. Mottled enamel is the result of a partial failure of the enamel-forming cells properly to elaborate and lay down enamel. It is a nonspecific response to a variety of stimuli, one of which is the ingestion of excessive amounts of fluoride.

Since mottled enamel is a developmental injury, the ingestion of fluoride following the eruption of the tooth has no effect. Mottling is one of the first visible signs of an excessive intake of fluoride during childhood. A quantitative relationship between the fluoride concentration of drinking water and mottling has been demonstrated (Muhler and Hine, 1959). Continuous use of water containing about 1.0 ppm of fluoride may result in the very mildest form of mottled enamel in 10% of children. The incidence rises to 40 to 50% at about 1.7 ppm; at 2.5 ppm, it is as high as 80%, with 25% being classified as moderate or severe; between 4.0 and 6.0 ppm, the incidence approaches 100%, with marked increase in severity.

Fluoride and Dental Caries. Experiments in controlling the fluoride content of water took an unexpected and significant turn when it was observed that children born at Bauxite, Arkansas, after a new water supply had been obtained, showed a much higher incidence of caries than those who had been exposed to the former fluoride-containing water (Dean *et al.,* 1941). This led to extensive studies on the part of the United States Public Health Service to ascertain whether the fluoridation of water could be employed as a practical measure to reduce the incidence of tooth decay. It has now been definitely established on the basis of large-scale studies in a number of communities that the fluoridation of water to a concentration of 1.0 ppm is a safe and practical public health measure that results in substantial reduction in the incidence of caries in per-

manent teeth. The Society of Toxicology has studied the question of the safety of water fluoridation and has published the following statement (*see* Statement by the Society of Toxicology, 1969):

> From a critical review of the voluminous and steadily growing literature on the biological effects of inorganic fluoride no evidence has been found of an ill effect of water fluoridation at 1 ppm in temperate climates. In the United States, there are over 10 million people drinking naturally fluoridated water at the near optimal concentration or higher. These waters have been consumed by large numbers of people for many years. Therefore, an extraordinary and exceptional reliability is conferred on the safety of water fluoridation because nature, in a sense, has already made the demonstration in hundreds of communities where the drinking water naturally contains fluoride. Under controlled conditions as recommended by qualified public health authorities, the Society of Toxicology finds water fluoridation to be a safe measure.

There are partial benefits for children who begin drinking fluoridated water at any age; however, optimal benefits are obtained at ages before the permanent teeth erupt. Topical applications of fluoride solutions by dental personnel appear to be particularly effective on newly erupted teeth and can reduce the incidence of caries by 30 to 40%. The prescription of dietary fluoride supplements should be considered for children whose drinking water contains less than 0.7 ppm of fluoride. Conflicting results have been reported from studies of the effectiveness of fluoride-containing toothpastes.

Adequate incorporation of fluoride into teeth causes the outer layers of enamel to be harder and more resistant to demineralization. The deposition of fluoride ion appears to be an anion-exchange process with hydroxyl and/or citrate ions (Gedalia *et al.,* 1969). The fluoride ion occupies the anionic spaces in the enamel apatite crystal surface. The mechanism of prevention of caries exerted by the deposition of minute amounts of fluoride in surface enamel is not completely understood. There is no convincing evidence that fluoride from any source reduces the development of caries after the permanent teeth are completely formed (usually about age 14).

Preparations and Uses. *Sodium Fluoride,* U.S.P., *Sodium Fluoride Solution,* U.S.P., *Sodium Fluoride Tablets,* U.S.P., and *Stannous Fluoride,* U.S.P., are official fluoride preparations. The fluoride salts presently employed in dentifrices are sodium fluoride, stannous fluoride, and *Sodium Fluoride and Orthophosphoric Acid Solution,* N.F. Sodium fluoride, sodium fluosilicate (Na_2SiF_6), and cryolite are the salts commonly used for insecticides.

CHLORIDE

Little need be said about the chloride ion at this point except to refer the reader to Chapter 36 for a complete discussion.

SULFATE

The sulfate ion does not cross cell membranes readily, and its pharmacological properties result from this relative impenetrability. Radioactive sulfate (^{35}S) may be employed to measure the volume of the extracellular space. The parenteral administration of sulfates to augment urinary excretion of calcium is discussed in Chapter 37. When sulfate salts are given by mouth, they tend to be absorbed minimally and, hence, add water to the bowel, thus leading to diarrhea (*see* Chapter 49).

NITRATE

The nitrate ion (NO_3^-) has few clear-cut, specific pharmacological actions. Environmental nitrate and nitrite salts ingested in foods and water have been implicated in cases of methemoglobinemia. (For additional details on toxicological aspects of environmental nitrates, *see* Committee on Nutrition, 1970; Shearer *et al.*, 1972; Chapter 34.) The discussion of the employment of nitrites and nitrates in the management of cardiovascular problems is presented in Chapter 34.

ACETATE

The acetate ion (CH_3COO^-) is used primarily as a vehicle with which to administer a cation. The use of *Potassium Acetate*, U.S.P., is one way by which a potassium deficiency may be repaired. However, it must be remembered, as discussed in Chapter 36, that potassium deficiency may be difficult to repair if chloride is not given. Hence, if other sources of chloride are not available, the potassium is better administered as KCl. Other salts of acetate include sodium acetate and ammonium acetate. Sodium acetate can be used as an alkalinizing agent since acetate is rapidly metabolized.

CITRATE

The citrate ion ($CH_2COO^- \cdot COHCOO^- \cdot CH_2$-$COO^-$) is an intermediary in carbohydrate metabolism. It is of pharmacological interest for the following reasons: (1) it forms a soluble complex with calcium that is poorly dissociable, the property that is the basis of the use of citrate to prevent the coagulation of blood; and (2) its sodium salt is an effective alkalinizing agent used in the management of metabolic acidosis secondary to chronic renal insufficiency or renal tubular acidosis. In certain situations, *Potassium Citrate*, N.F., may be preferable.

Whole blood collected by blood banks is prevented from clotting mainly by the addition of *Anticoagulant Citrate Dextrose Solution*, U.S.P., containing *Citric Acid*, U.S.P., *Sodium Citrate*, U.S.P., and *Dextrose*, U.S.P. Official variants are *Anticoagulant Citrate Phosphate Dextrose Solution*, U.S.P., and *Anticoagulant Sodium Citrate Solution*, N.F. Since the addition of any of these solutions provides an excess of citrate ion over calcium ion in order to be effective, the question arises as to whether massive transfusions can result in citrate intoxication, the manifestations of which are those of hypocalcemia (Cooper *et al.*, 1973). In cardiovascular surgical procedures, the use of citrate-anticoagulated blood has

been shown to decrease plasma concentrations of magnesium as well as calcium ions (Killen *et al.*, 1972).

Citrate is also of therapeutic value in the alleviation of chronic metabolic acidosis such as results from chronic renal insufficiency or the syndrome of renal tubular acidosis (*see* Chapter 36). It is usually prescribed in the form of *Sodium Citrate and Citric Acid Solution*, U.S.P. (*Shohl's solution*). This preparation has a direct irritating effect on oral mucous membranes and can cause necrotic and ulcerative lesions (Newell and Stone, 1974).

OXALATE

The oxalate ion ($COO^- \cdot COO^-$) has no therapeutic uses, and it is of pharmacological interest only because of its toxic properties. It is toxic because it precipitates ionized calcium; furthermore, oxalic acid is a powerful corrosive agent.

Potassium oxalate is the most important of the oxalate salts from a toxicological viewpoint, since it is widely available as a cleaning and bleaching agent.

In general, the symptoms of oxalate poisoning are those of the local irritant effects and hypocalcemia (Arena, 1973). Acute renal failure may develop as a result of precipitation of calcium oxalate crystals in the kidney. In severe cases, the patient develops convulsions and becomes rapidly stuporous and unconscious.

Oxalate is a product of intermediary metabolism. Rarely, due to an inborn error of metabolism, the production and urinary excretion of the anion are excessive (Hagler and Herman, 1973). Persons with such a metabolic error (primary oxalosis) may form renal calculi consisting primarily of calcium oxalate. Calcium oxalate is also deposited in soft tissues throughout the body. Although various therapeutic regimens for the correction of this disorder have been suggested, none has proven efficacious. Secondary oxalosis occurs as a complication of chronic renal failure (Salyer and Keren, 1973). Oxaluria associated with disease or resection of the ileum is apparently due to increased intestinal absorption of oxalate and responds to a low-oxalate diet (Chadwick *et al.*, 1973).

Treatment of oxalate poisoning consists in gastric lavage with limewater (0.15% calcium hydroxide solution) or other calcium salts. Diuresis should be stimulated and maintained by the administration of copious amounts of intravenous fluid to prevent deposition of calcium oxalate crystals in the renal tubules. Sodium bicarbonate should *not* be administered because sodium oxalate is readily absorbed and the systemic effects will become exaggerated.

TARTRATE

The tartrate ion ($COO^- \cdot CHOHCHOHCOO^-$) is absorbed only minimally from the gastrointestinal tract and may, therefore, be employed with safety as a cathartic (*see* Chapter 49). If high concentrations gain access to the circulation, renal damage may result.

CYANATE

The cyanate anion (NCO^-) is of no known importance in normal biological function. However, it has been found to produce irreversible inhibition of red-blood-cell sickling following carbamylation of the amino-terminal valine residue of hemoglobin (Cerami and Manning, 1971). This reaction increases the affinity of hemoglobin for oxygen, which is believed to decrease the aggregation of hemoglobin S that occurs at low oxygen tensions (Cerami et al., 1973b; Jensen et al., 1973).

Preliminary clinical studies have demonstrated that the life-span of the erythrocyte can be increased and that the hemolytic anemia is improved when patients with sickle-cell disease are treated chronically with cyanate, administered orally (Gillette et al., 1974). The toxic effects that have been observed to date have been minor and include occasional gastrointestinal distress and drowsiness. In animal studies, pathological lesions have not been seen. There was an increase in the oxygen affinity of the blood of all species to which cyanate was administered (Cerami et al., 1973a). The value of cyanate in the chronic management of sickle-cell anemia or in the treatment of sickle-cell crisis must obviously await further investigation, but this possibility is of great interest.

Agus, Z. S.; Puschett, J. B.; Senesky, D.; and Goldberg, M. Mode of action of parathyroid hormone and cyclic adenosine 3',5'-monophosphate on renal tubular phosphate reabsorption in the dog. *J. clin. Invest.,* **1971,** *50,* 617–626.

Armstrong, W. D. Body fluid fluoride distribution. *J. dent. Res.,* **1967,** *46,* 60–62.

Bernecker, C. Intermittent therapy with potassium iodide in chronic obstructive disease of the airways. *Acta allerg.,* **1969,** *24,* 216–225.

Bierman, H. R. Fluorides in neoplastic disease. *Postgrad. Med.,* **1972,** *51,* 166–172.

Burke, W. J.; Hoegg, U. R.; and Phillips, R. E. Systemic fluoride poisoning resulting from a fluoride skin burn. *J. occup. Med.,* **1973,** *15,* 39–41.

Card, R. T., and Brain, M. C. The "anemia" of childhood: evidence for a physiologic response to hyperphosphatemia. *New Engl. J. Med.,* **1973,** *288,* 388–392.

Castells, S. New approaches to treatment of osteogenesis imperfecta. *Clin. Orthop.,* **1973,** *93,* 239–249.

Cerami, A.; Allen, T. A.; Graziano, J. H.; DeFuria, F. G.; Manning, J. M.; and Gillette, P. N. Pharmacology of cyanate. I. General effects on experimental animals. *J. Pharmac. exp. Ther.,* **1973a,** *185,* 653–666.

Cerami, A., and Manning, J. M. Potassium cyanate as an inhibitor of the sickling of erythrocytes *in vitro.* *Proc. natn. Acad. Sci. U.S.A.,* **1971,** *68,* 1180–1183.

Cerami, A.; Manning, J. M.; Gillette, P. N.; DeFuria, F.; Miller, D.; Graziano, J. H.; and Peterson, C. M. Effect of cyanate on red blood cell sickling. *Fedn Proc. Fedn Am. Socs exp. Biol.,* **1973b,** *32,* 1668–1672.

Chadwick, V. S.; Modha, K.; and Dowling, R. H. Mechanisms for hyperoxaluria in patients with ileal dysfunction. *New Engl. J. Med.,* **1973,** *289,* 172–176.

Cooper, N.; Brazier, J. R.; Hottenrott, C.; Mulder, D. G.; Maloney, J. V., Jr.; and Buckberg, G. D. Myocardial depression following citrated blood transfusion. *Archs Surg.,* **1973,** *107,* 756–763.

Daniel, H. J.; Shambaugh, G. E.; and Fisch, U. Fluoride and clinical otosclerosis. *Archs Otolar.,* **1973,** *98,* 327–329.

Dean, H. T.; Jay, P.; Arnold, F. A., Jr.; and Elvove, E.

Domestic water and dental caries: study of 2,832 white children, age 12–14 years, of 8 suburban Chicago communities, including *Lactobacillus acidophilus* studies of 1,761 children. *Publ. Hlth Rep., Wash.,* **1941,** *56,* 761–792.

Fregly, M. J., and McCarthy, J. S. Effect of diuretics on renal iodide excretion by humans. *Toxic. appl. Pharmac.,* **1973,** *25,* 289–298.

Gedalia, I.; Azaz, B.; and Schmerling, M. Citrate in the surface enamel of unerupted and erupted teeth. *J. dent. Res.,* **1969,** *48,* 105–108.

Gillette, P. N.; Peterson, C. M.; Lu, Y. S.; and Cerami, A. Sodium cyanate as a potential treatment for sickle-cell disease. *New Engl. J. Med.,* **1974,** *290,* 654–660.

Glorieux, F. H.; Scriver, C. R.; Reade, T. M.; Goldman, H.; and Roseborough, A. Use of phosphate and vitamin D to prevent dwarfism and rickets in X-linked hypophosphatemia. *New Engl. J. Med.,* **1972,** *287,* 481–487.

Greenberg, B. G.; Winters, R. W.; and Graham, J. B. The normal range of serum inorganic phosphorus and its utility as a discriminant in the diagnosis of congenital hypophosphatemia. *J. clin. Endocr. Metab.,* **1960,** *20,* 364–379.

Haas, H. G.; Dambacher, M. G.; Guncaga, J.; and Lauffenburger, T. Renal effects of calcitonin and parathyroid extract in man: studies in hypoparathyroidism. *J. clin. Invest.,* **1971,** *50,* 2689–2702.

Ingenbleek, Y., and Beckers, C. Evidence for intestinal malabsorption of iodine in protein-calorie malnutrition. *J. clin. Nutr.,* **1973,** *26,* 1323–1330.

Jacob, H. S., and Amsden, T. Acute hemolytic anemia with rigid red cells in hypophosphatemia. *New Engl. J. Med.,* **1971,** *285,* 1446–1450.

Jensen, M.; Nathan, D. G.; and Bunn, H. F. The reaction of cyanate with the α and β subunits in hemoglobin. *J. biol. Chem.,* **1973,** *248,* 8057–8063.

Jones, A. E.; Ghaed, N.; Dunson, G. L.; and Hosain, F. Clinical evaluation of orally administered fluorine 18 for bone scanning. *Radiology,* **1973,** *107,* 129–131.

Jowsey, J.; Riggs, B. L.; Kelly, P. J.; and Hoffman, D. L. Effect of combined therapy with sodium fluoride, vitamin D and calcium in osteoporosis. *Am. J. Med.,* **1972,** *53,* 43–49.

Killen, D. A.; Grogan, E. L.; Gower, R. E.; Collins, I. S.; and Collins, H. A. Effect of ACD blood prime on plasma calcium and magnesium. *Ann. thorac. Surg.,* **1972,** *13,* 371–380.

Levitt, M.; Gessert, C.; and Finberg, L. Inorganic phosphate (laxative) poisoning resulting in tetany in an infant. *J. Pediat.,* **1973,** *82,* 479–481.

Lichtman, M. A.; Miller, D. R.; and Freeman, R. B. Erythrocyte adenosine triphosphate depletion during hypophosphatemia. *New Engl. J. Med.,* **1969,** *280,* 240–244.

Lotz, M.; Zisman, E.; and Bartter, F. C. Evidence for a phosphorus-depletion syndrome. *New Engl. J. Med.,* **1968,** *278,* 409–415.

McConnell, T. H. Fatal hypocalcemia from phosphate absorption from laxative preparations. *J. Am. med. Ass.,* **1971,** *216,* 147–148.

Murayama, Y.; Morel, F.; and LeGrimellec, C. Phosphate, calcium and magnesium transfers in proximal tubules and loops of Henle, as measured by single nephron microperfusion experiments in the rat. *Pflügers Arch. ges. Physiol.,* **1972,** *333,* 1–16.

Newell, G. B., and Stone, O. J. Irritant contact stomatitis in chronic renal failure. *Archs Derm.,* **1974,** *109,* 53–55.

Peters, J. H. Therapy of acute fluoride poisoning. *Am. J. med. Sci.,* **1948,** *216,* 278–285.

Puschett, J. B.; Moranz, J.; and Kurnick, W. S. Evidence for a direct action of cholecalciferol and 25-hydroxycholecalciferol on the renal transport of phosphate, sodium and calcium. *J. clin. Invest.,* **1972,** *51,* 373–385.

Salyer, W. R., and Keren, D. Oxalosis as a complication of chronic renal failure. *Kidney Int.,* **1973,** *4,* 61–66.

Sampson, H. W., and Matthews, J. L. Electron microscope autoradiographic investigation of ^{33}P in the intestinal epithelium of rachitic, normal and vitamin-D–treated rats. *Calcif. Tissue Res.,* **1972,** *10,* 58–66.

Seabury, J. H., and Dascomb, H. E. Results of the treatment of systemic mycoses. *J. Am. med. Ass.,* **1964,** *188,* 509–513.

Setter, J. G.; Maher, J. F.; and Schreiner, G. E. Acute renal failure following cholecystography. *J. Am. med. Ass.,* **1963,** *184,* 102–110.

Sharma, S. M., and Quinn, J. L. Sensitivity of ^{18}F bone scans in the search for metastases. *Surgery Gynec. Obstet.,* **1972,** *135,* 536–540.

Shearer, L. A.; Goldsmith, J. R.; Young, C.; Kearns, O. A.; and Tamplin, B. R. Methemoglobin levels in infants in an area with high nitrate water supply. *Am. J. publ. Hlth,* **1972,** *62,* 1174–1180.

Short, E. M.; Binder, J.; and Rosenberg, E. Familial hypophosphatemic rickets: defective transport of inorganic phosphate by intestinal mucosa. *Science, Wash.,* **1973,** *179,* 700–702.

Statement by the Society of Toxicology on the safety of water fluoridation. *Toxic. appl. Pharmac.,* **1969,** *14,* i.

Steele, T. H. Increased urinary phosphate excretion following volume expansion in normal man. *Metabolism,* **1970,** *19,* 29–39.

Walser, M., and Rahill, W. J. Renal tubular reabsorption of iodide as compared with chloride. *J. clin. Invest.,* **1965,** *44,* 1371–1381.

Werner, J. A.; Gorton, S. J.; and Raisz, L. G. Escape from inhibition of resorption in cultures of fetal bone treated with calcitonin and parathyroid hormone. *Endocrinology,* **1972,** *90,* 752–759.

Monographs and Reviews

Arena, J. M. *Poisoning: Toxicology-Symptoms-Treatments,* 3rd ed. Charles C Thomas, Pub., Springfield, Ill., **1973.**

Bartter, F. C. Disturbances of phosphorus metabolism. In, *Mineral Metabolism: An Advanced Treatise.* Vol. 2, *The Elements—Part A.* (Comar, C. L., and Bronner, F., eds.) Academic Press, Inc., New York, **1964,** pp. 315–335.

Committee on Nutrition. Infant methemoglobinemia: the role of dietary nitrate. *Pediatrics, Springfield,* **1970,** *46,* 475–477.

Hagler, L., and Herman, R. H. Oxalate metabolism. *Am. J. clin. Nutr.,* **1973,** *26,* 758–765, 882–889, 1006–1010, 1073–1079.

Hodge, H. C. Fluoride. In, *Mineral Metabolism: An Advanced Treatise.* Vol. 2, *The Elements—Part A.* (Comar, C. L., and Bronner, F., eds.) Academic Press, Inc., New York, **1964,** pp. 573–576.

Hodge, H. C., and Smith, F. A. Fluorides and man. *A. Rev. Pharmac.,* **1968,** *8,* 395–408.

Massry, S. G.; Friedler, R. M.; and Coburn, J. W. Excretion of phosphate and calcium: physiology of their renal handling and relation to clinical medicine. *Archs intern. Med.,* **1973,** *131,* 828–859.

Muhler, J. C., and Hine, M. K. *Fluorine and Dental Health: The Pharmacology and Toxicity of Fluorine.* Indiana University Press, Bloomington, **1959.**

Singh, A.; Jolly, S. S.; Bansal, B. C.; and Mathar, C. C. Endemic fluorosis. *Medicine, Baltimore,* **1963,** *42,* 229–246.

Waldbott, G. L. Acute fluoride intoxication. *Acta med. scand.,* **1963,** *174,* Suppl. 400, 1–44.

SECTION VIII

Drugs Affecting Renal Function and Electrolyte Metabolism

INTRODUCTION

Gilbert H. Mudge

The important homeostatic role of the kidney in maintaining the volume and the composition of the body fluids has already been stressed in preceding chapters. It is not surprising, therefore, to find that drugs that alter renal function comprise a major and indispensable group of therapeutic agents. As knowledge of the fundamental physiological mechanisms of renal function has expanded, the number of drugs that affect specific renal tubular processes has grown in a parallel fashion. Indeed, in many instances the drug has provided the tool to elucidate the finer details of cellular mechanisms. Drugs that alter renal function fall into a variety of classes, depending on both the chemical nature of the drug and the specific renal function upon which it primarily acts. As anticipated, these drugs have wider therapeutic applications than would be included under the designation of diuretics. Therefore, in the following section, drugs with widely different clinical uses will be discussed together because their basic action is on the kidney. It should also be noted that the kidney is the major excretory organ for many therapeutic agents and their metabolites. A knowledge of renal mechanisms is important, therefore, in evaluating the pattern of drug excretion, particularly since, in some instances, alteration of renal function may markedly affect the rate of excretion and hence the duration of drug action or the extent of drug toxicity.

PHYSIOLOGICAL CONSIDERATIONS

The majority of excretory products appear in the glomerular filtrate and are incompletely reabsorbed by the renal tubules. Other substances can also be secreted by the renal tubular cells into the tubular urine and in this manner be eliminated from the body. Certain substances, moreover, undergo both reabsorption and secretion. It should be emphasized that the terms *reabsorption* and *secretion* refer to the direction of net transport without any implication as to underlying cellular mechanisms. Therefore, the factors that are important in the determination of volume and composition of urine are: (1) glomerular filtration, (2) tubular reabsorption, and (3) tubular secretion.

Glomerular Filtration. Functionally and qualitatively, the glomerulus of the kidney is similar to other capillary beds, and filtration is subject to the same physical laws that govern the transport of fluid and permeable solutes across any capillary membrane. Its filtering force is the hydrostatic pressure of the blood derived from the work of the heart. The plasma proteins do not penetrate, to an appreciable extent, the normal glomerular membrane. All the plasma constituents gain access to the glomerular capsule with the exception of the proteins, lipids, and substances bound to proteins.

The glomerular capillary bed has two distinctive features: (1) the efferent vessel is an arteriole rather than a venule, and (2) that portion of the capillary transudate which does not undergo tubular reabsorption is drained to the outside of the body. Glomerular filtration is influenced, therefore, by factors that do not affect other capillary beds.

The hydrostatic pressure within the glomerular capillaries is approximately 60% of the arterial pressure. Thus, systemic blood pressure must be considerably reduced before the rate of glomerular filtration is significantly changed. For example, mean blood pressure must usually fall to a level of 40 mm Hg before filtration ceases. Theoretically, the rate of glomerular filtration may be altered by (1) the hydrostatic pressure within the glomerular capillaries, (2) the osmotic pressure of the nondiffusible constituents of the blood, (3) the number of functioning glomeruli, and (4) back pressure from those structures that drain the glomerular filtrate to the outside.

Urine formation begins in a prodigal way. Included in the glomerular filtrate are not only the waste products but also the essential constituents of the extracellular fluid such as water, electrolytes, and nutrients. These must be largely reabsorbed to maintain the volume and composition of the extracellular fluid. Apparently the excretory function of the kidney demands the filtration of a large volume of extracellular fluid. In turn, the homeostatic function of the organ demands the reabsorption of most of the ingredients of the filtrate.

Although the rate of glomerular filtration is a very important aspect of renal function, drugs that affect the rate of filtration will not be discussed in this section for many reasons. The most common cause of reduction in the filtration rate is organic change in the renal vascular bed. There is no drug available to correct this abnormality. Another common cause of reduction in filtration rate is the reduced renal blood flow secondary to heart failure. For its correction, attention is directed to the heart rather than to the kidney. Many drugs used in the treatment of hypertension reduce renal blood flow and filtration rate, but these represent undesirable side effects. Drugs with marked hemodynamic action, such as epinephrine, alter filtration rate and urine flow by affecting arterial pressure and afferent and efferent renal arteriolar resistance, but no therapeutic application is made of these actions. Finally, there are a few agents, such as dopamine, that significantly increase renal blood flow and filtration rate, but these have only limited therapeutic use. Experience has demonstrated that one can alter the rate of excretion of many substances much more effectively by drugs that alter tubular function than by those that change filtration rate.

Measurement of Glomerular Filtration. The rate of glomerular filtration can be determined very accurately in animals and man by measuring the renal clearance of substances that are freely filtered at the glomerulus and are neither secreted nor reabsorbed by the renal tubule. Thus, the amount of the substance excreted in the urine over a given period of time is a measure of the amount filtered by the glomeruli. It is only necessary to divide this by the concentration of the substance in the filtrate to determine the volume of filtrate from which the urine was derived. Inasmuch as the glomerular filtrate is an ultrafiltrate of plasma, the concentration of such a substance in glomerular fluid can be ascertained by determining the concentration in plasma.

The polysaccharide inulin is accepted as the most valid substance for measuring the filtration rate under almost all circumstances. There is an increasing number of other agents that behave in a similar manner but which, under certain conditions, may or may not undergo tubular transport. Thus, with the introduction of a new compound for measuring filtration rate it is essential that the identity of its clearance with that of inulin be established for each particular experimental condition.

Renal Plasma Flow. Certain substances at low plasma levels are secreted by the renal tubules so efficiently, and undergo so little tubular reabsorption, that essentially all of the substance is removed from the blood in a single passage through the kidney. It therefore follows that the total amount of such a substance appearing in the urine over a given time divided by its plasma concentration is an expression of renal plasma flow. The outstanding example of this type is para-aminohippuric acid.

Tubular Reabsorption. The importance of the reabsorptive function of the renal tubules to the body economy cannot be overemphasized and can best be illustrated by a few numerical considerations. The rate of glomerular filtration in the average adult is approximately 125 ml per minute. In such an individual, the total extracellular fluid volume is approximately 12.5 liters. Thus, a volume equivalent to that of the extracellular fluid is filtered across the glomerular capillary bed within a period of 100 minutes. During this time approximately 100 ml of urine reaches the bladder. Therefore, the tubules normally reabsorb over 99% of the glomerular filtrate. Obviously the composition of the tubular reabsorbate must closely approximate that of the extracellular fluid; otherwise, extreme distortions in the composition of the extracellular fluid would soon result.

The mechanisms of filtration and reabsorption have little in common. The former is a physical process in which the hydrostatic energy is provided by the heart for the transport of water and permeative solute ions and molecules across a permeable membrane. Tubular reabsorption, on the other hand, bears little relationship to the mechanism by which fluid and solutes are returned to the circulation after their egress from other capillary beds. Such reabsorption is largely achieved by active transport of electrolyte and other solutes from tubular fluid to tubular cell and thence to the extracellular fluid. This involves the expenditure of energy derived from metabolic activity. Physical forces involving the oncotic pressure of the peritubular plasma may also contribute to the reabsorption of water. The magnitude of this component is relatively small and uncertain.

Although many of the intimate mechanisms of electrolyte transport are incompletely understood, for operational purposes it is possible to describe them in terms of the scheme summarized in Figure VIII-1. Considered primarily from the point of view of the action of pharmacological agents, the most important tubular mechanisms of electrolyte transport are (1) reabsorption of sodium and chloride, (2) secretion of hydrogen ion, and (3) secretion of potassium. In addition, there are related but separate mechanisms for the reabsorption of calcium, magnesium, phosphate, and sulfate; in the glomerular filtrate these ions are present in low concentrations, and diuretic drugs may influence their transport. It was previously thought that primarily sodium was actively reabsorbed against an electrochemical gradient throughout the nephron, accompanied by the back diffusion of an equivalent amount of fixed anion, mostly chloride. It has now been shown that in the ascending limb of the loop of Henle it is the chloride anion that is transported actively.

The secretion of hydrogen and potassium ions has often been described in terms of a tubular-cell exchange mechanism by which the reabsorption of sodium is visualized as being coupled with the transport of either hydrogen or potassium in the opposite direction. Newer studies, however, cast doubt on the validity of an exchange reaction as an actual cellular mechanism and emphasize that reabsorption occurs by one process and secretion by another. Nevertheless, in terms of the overall events, significant cation secretion (either H^+ or K^+) must be accompanied by Na^+ reabsorption in order to preserve cation-anion balance. From this point of view, therefore, it may still be proper to consider the secretion of either H^+ or K^+ as quantitatively equivalent to a component in the reabsorption of Na^+. It is for this reason that it is at times convenient to refer to exchange reactions involving Na^+-K^+ and Na^+-H^+.

All but a very small fraction of the filtered sodium and water is normally reabsorbed, sodium by active transport and water by diffusion. On the basis of the quantitative relationship between these two processes, it is possible to identify three segments of the nephron on both an anatomical and functional basis. These are intimately related to the processes of concentration and dilution of the urine. As indicated in Figure VIII-1, the reabsorption of sodium and chloride, the major solutes of the glomerular filtrate, can be considered in terms of three different mechanisms: *1-A, 1-B,* and *1-C.* There are at least three criteria by which each of these can be distinguished: anatomical localization, concomitant water permeability, and sensitivity to diuretic drugs. The reabsorptive mechanism labeled *1-A* is in the proximal convolution; *1-B* is in the ascending limb of the loop of Henle; and *1-C*

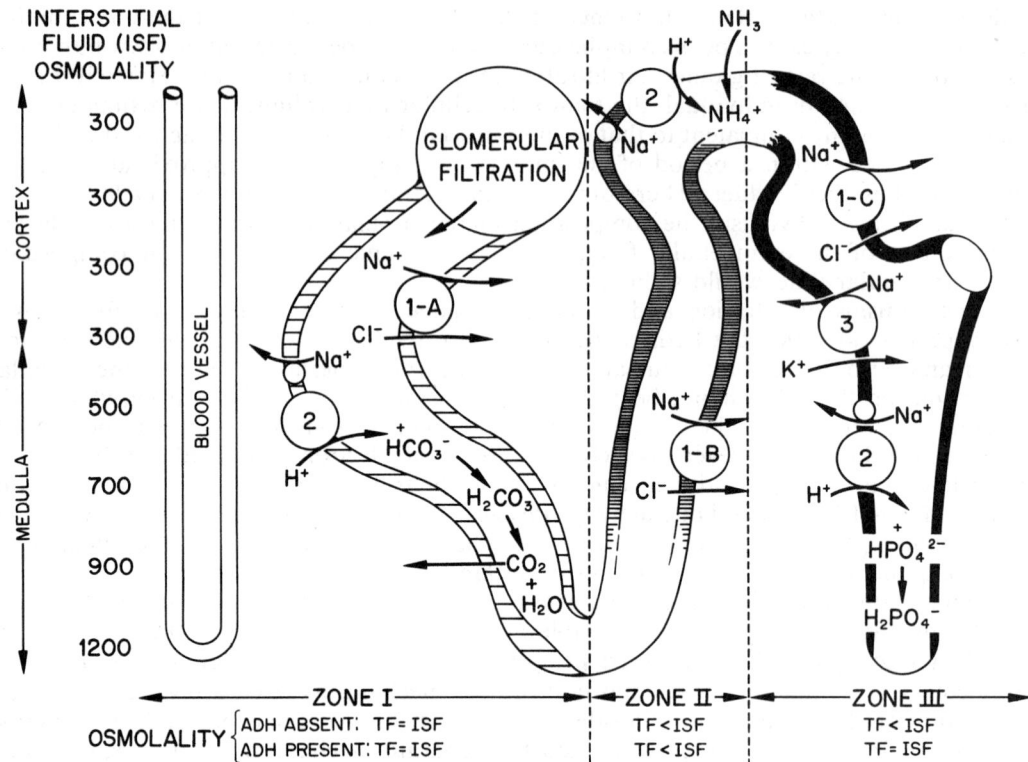

Figure VIII-1. *Schematic representation of the major electrolyte transport systems in the kidney that are susceptible to drug action.* Numbers coincide with the description in the text.

The functional organization of the nephron in relation to the countercurrent system is depicted on the vertical axis to show interstitial osmolality (isosmotic cortex; hypertonic medulla), and also on the horizontal axis to show the water permeability characteristics of the nephron segments. Interstitial osmolality is given in milliosmoles per kilogram of water. In zone I, osmolality of tubular fluid (TF) is approximately equal to that of interstitial fluid (ISF), both being isosmotic to plasma in the cortex but increasingly hypertonic to it in the medulla. The blood vessels are also isosmotic to the adjacent ISF. In zone II, chloride and sodium reabsorptive transport is relatively greater than outward diffusion of water. Hence, osmolality of TF is less than that of adjacent ISF. In zone III, water permeability is under the control of the antidiuretic hormone (ADH). Three types of tubular epithelium are schematically shown to indicate differences in water permeability; the associated mechanisms of sodium reabsorption are indicated by *1–A* and *1–C*, and of chloride reabsorption by *1–B*. The beginning and the end of epithelium in zone II (mostly the ascending limb of the loop of Henle) are left indeterminate because of uncertainty concerning exact functional boundaries.

Mechanisms are also shown for acidification of the urine (*2*) and secretion of potassium (*3*). For a full explanation of these tubular functions, *see* text.

is in the distal nephron, in both the distal convolution and the collecting duct. At *1–A*, there is a high water permeability so that, as solute (Na^+Cl^-) is reabsorbed, water diffuses along the osmotic gradient with such rapidity that the tubular fluid and the adjacent peritubular or interstitial fluid maintain approximately the same osmolality. In the ascending limb (*1–B*) the tubule is relatively impermeable to water despite the active reabsorption of chloride. This has two consequences. First, there is a fall in the concentration of sodium and chloride in the tubular fluid, reaching a minimal value usually in the first portion of the distal convolution; second, the sodium and chloride concentration becomes elevated in the interstitial fluid. A concentration gradient across the tubular epithelium is thus established by active transport at the site of low water permeability. This gradient then becomes multiplied in a longitudinal direction by the countercurrent mechanism, so that within the interstitial fluid a large osmotic gradient becomes established between the isosmotic renal cortex and the hyperosmotic medulla and papilla. The osmotic gradients are partly maintained by the relatively meager blood flow to the medullary region, which acts as a passive countercurrent exchanger. The third sodium transport mechanism ($1-C$) is probably less significant than the others in terms of the total amount of sodium reabsorbed, but is of unique importance in being associated with the area of the nephron susceptible to the antidiuretic hormone (ADH). In the presence of ADH, there is a high permeability to water in this segment. As a result, the tubular fluid, particularly within the collecting ducts, equilibrates with the hyperosmotic interstitium and is then discharged at the end of the collecting duct as a hypertonic or concentrated solution. In the absence of ADH, this portion of the nephron is relatively impermeable to water. Thus, the reabsorption of sodium chloride, as indicated by reactions $1-B$ and $1-C$, progressively lowers the osmolality of the tubular fluid. Under this condition, the tubular fluid does not reach osmotic equilibration with the adjacent interstitium. Thus, in the absence of ADH, the voided urine is characteristically hypoosmotic, or dilute.

There are two other features that characterize distal sodium reabsorption. First, the absolute amount reabsorbed in this area is determined not only by the amount filtered but also by the proportion of the filtrate that has already undergone reabsorption at more proximal sites. This fraction may vary over a wide range, particularly in pathological conditions associated with edema formation or oliguria. Second, the distal mechanisms may have discrete sensitivities to the action of some drugs, including the adrenocortical hormones.

Free-Water Production. By definition, this term refers to the amount of distilled water (*i.e.,* water free of solute) that would have to be added to, or subtracted from, the urine voided over a period of time (usually calculated on a minute basis) in order to render that urine specimen isosmotic with a simultaneous plasma sample. In arithmetical terms, free-water production equals urine volume (V) minus the osmolal clearance (C_{OSM}). The latter term has the usual dimensions of clearance (UV/P) and refers to the sum of the concentrations of all osmotically active solutes in plasma and urine. When the urine is more dilute than plasma, free-water production is positive; when the urine is more concentrated, free-water production is negative. In the first instance, solute-free water is actually excreted as part of the voided urine; in the latter instance, solute-free water can be considered as being returned to the body from the kidney. When the urine has the same osmolality as plasma, free-water production is zero regardless of the rate of urine flow.

Free-water production is an operational concept. At no time, and in no place, does distilled, or solute-free, water exist as such within the kidney. The concept is important in that it takes into account more than just the concentration of osmotically active solute in the urine. By introducing the dimensions of volume per unit time, the net rate at which either the concentrating or diluting mechanism is operating may be accurately described. This has become a useful technic in the analysis of diuretic action.

It should be emphasized that free-water production is *not* synonymous with diuresis. Some of the most potent diuretics may produce a massive diuresis of almost isosmotic urine, and hence with a minimal rate of free-water production. While it is true that free-water production must ultimately influence the solute concentration of the residual body fluids, nevertheless, in the clinical use of diuretics the free-water production has relatively minor therapeutic implications. This is partly due to the fact that urinary excretion is promptly balanced by a variable dietary intake of both solute and water.

The concept of free-water production has played an interesting role in localizing the site of diuretic action within the nephron. It must be strongly emphasized that, in order to infer intrarenal sites of action on the basis of the excretion of solute and water, observations must be made under one or the other of two physiological extremes—either in the absence of ADH or under its maximal influence. The former condition is obtained during unequivocal water diuresis or in patients with diabetes insipidus of posterior pituitary origin; the latter condition

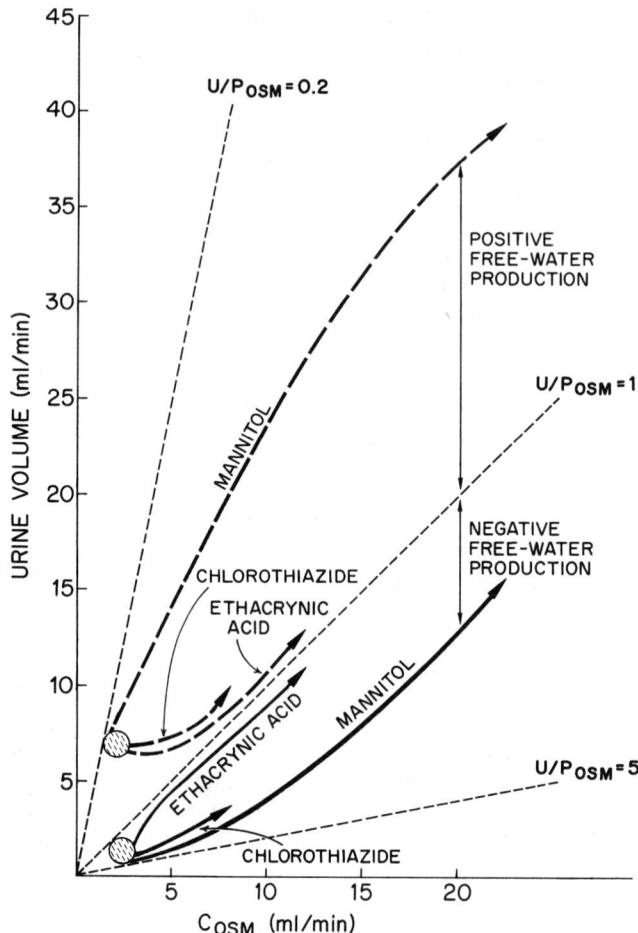

Figure VIII–2. *Relation of urine volume to osmolar clearance* (C_{OSM}).

The diuretic agents were given during a maximal water diuresis, that is, in the absence of ADH (dash lines), or to dehydrated subjects under maximal influence of ADH (solid lines). The magnitude of free-water production is given graphically as the vertical distance between any observed point and the isosmotic line ($U/P_{OSM} = 1$). The shaded circles indicate normal rates of solute excretion (*i.e.*, without diuretics) at extremes of ADH activity. Note that the maximal and minimal urinary osmolalities (as indicated by U/P_{OSM}) are achieved only at normal rates of solute excretion. These data from the literature were obtained in normal man.

may be achieved by water restriction, infusion of hypertonic solute, or administration of exogenous ADH. There is no evidence that the available diuretic drugs directly alter the action of ADH itself.

Figure VIII–2 shows the pattern obtained with three different diuretics. These can be evaluated in terms of the mechanisms and with the nomenclature previously described in Figure VIII–1. The interpretations that have been advanced are essentially as follows. If sodium reabsorption is inhibited in the proximal tubule (*i.e.*, *1–A*), an increased amount of solute will be delivered to the more distal segments, including the ascending limb (*1–B*). With the greater load to this latter site, an increased amount of sodium would be reabsorbed along with chloride, leading to an increase in either the positive or the negative free-water production. This is the result obtained with *mannitol*. In addition, in the case of positive free-water production, some of the increase might also be attributed to augmented sodium reabsorption in the most distal nephron (*1–C*). A second pattern is illustrated by *ethacrynic acid*. If chloride and sodium reabsorption were to be inhibited predominantly in the ascending limb (*1–B*), the urine would tend to remain isosmotic. Despite the resultant diuresis, the production of both positive and negative free water would be impaired. A third possibility is illustrated with *chlorothiazide*. The findings have been interpreted in terms of the inhibition of sodium reabsorption at a distal site, that is, *1–C*. Since the rate of negative free-water production is normal, it is inferred that there is no inhibition of transport in the ascending limb (*1–B*). However, since positive free-water production is partially inhibited, it has been proposed that the drug acts at the most distal site of sodium reabsorption.

Although there is uncertainty about some of the interpretations that have been proposed, there can be no doubt that different diuretics act by distinct and separate mechanisms as judged by free-water production. Of course, the demonstration of an action at one site does not invariably exclude an action elsewhere. By these criteria, osmotic diuretics and acetazolamide act proximally, ethacrynic acid and furosemide act on the ascending limb, and chlorothiazide acts on the distal segment. The site of mercurial action is less conclusive; many studies in the dog appear not to be in agreement with those in man.

In this discussion, the term *free-water production* has been used instead of *free-water clearance*. In the literature, the term *clearance* has been employed, with positive free water being designated as C_{H_2O} and negative free water as $T^c_{H_2O}$. Despite auspicious precedent, the term C_{H_2O} is incorrect if literally translated as "the renal clearance of water," and the term $T^c_{H_2O}$ was initially based on premises that have become obsolete. Despite these semantic difficulties, the concept of free water remains valid, but the term *production* is preferable to that of *clearance*. Fine distinctions between actual generation and net production of free water are beyond the scope of the present discussion.

Hydrogen Ion Secretion. The concept of hydrogen ion secretion has played an important role in the development of modern theories of renal function and of the action of therapeutic agents. Under certain circumstances the amount of titratable acid in the voided urine cannot be accounted for by the selective reabsorption of constituents of the filtrate. This provides proof that hydrogen ion is added to or secreted into the tubular fluid by the tubular cells. The source of the secreted hydrogen ions is carbonic acid derived from the hydration of carbon dioxide. Present evidence strongly suggests that the primary event is the secretion of H^+ itself, rather than the reabsorption of anion (HCO_3^-).

It has long been known that the kidney plays an important role in maintaining acid-base balance. This applies to normal conditions but increases in importance as a homeostatic compensation to metabolic acidosis. The renal response can be described in four separate parameters, as follows: (1) the complete reabsorption of filtered sodium bicarbonate, (2) the acidification of the urinary buffers (*i.e.,* the production of titratable acid), (3) the excretion of fixed anions in combination with NH_4^+ rather than Na^+, and (4) the adjustment of urinary pH or H^+ ion concentration. Each process can be considered in terms of the same underlying mechanism.

In the process of bicarbonate reabsorption, the H^+ derived from $H^+HCO_3^-$ in the tubular cell is exchanged with Na^+ in the tubular urine. The Na^+ combines with the HCO_3^- in the tubular cell and is returned to the extracellular fluid as $Na^+HCO_3^-$. The H^+ in the tubular urine combines with HCO_3^- to form H_2CO_3, which is rapidly broken down to CO_2 and H_2O. This CO_2 then readily back-diffuses across the tubular epithelium to become admixed with the carbonic acid–bicarbonate pool of the body. The overall reaction is the reabsorption of Na^+ and HCO_3^-.

When all the bicarbonate in the tubular urine has been removed, the mechanism of H^+–Na^+ exchange can still continue. Under these circumstances, H^+ will be added to the buffer systems in the urine, primarily phosphate, with the conversion of HPO_4^{2-} to $H_2PO_4^-$. The exchanged Na^+ will be returned to the extracellular fluid as $Na^+HCO_3^-$ and thus contribute to the available fixed cation of the extracellular fluid. If Na^+–H^+ exchange proceeds at a rate insufficient to reabsorb the filtered bicarbonate, an alkaline urine containing large amounts of bicarbonate will be excreted. On the other hand, at maximal rates of H^+ transport, not only will all the bicarbonate disappear from the urine but also the titratable acidity of the urine will rise as a result of acidification of the buffer systems and more $Na^+HCO_3^-$ will be returned to extracellular fluid than was filtered at the glomerulus.

If HCO_3^- and phosphate buffers were not present in the tubular urine, Na^+–H^+ exchange would involve the cation of a neutral salt (*e.g.,* Na^+Cl^-) and would result in formation of a strong acid. This would increase the hydrogen ion concentration of the urine to such an extent that further transport of H^+ would be blocked because of the concentration gradient of H^+ between tubular cell and tubular urine. (The minimal pH that can be achieved in the urine of man is 4.4 to 4.5.) However, in response to the need for conservation of fixed cation, the kidney synthesizes ammonia. When ammonia is formed in the renal tubular cells, it diffuses readily into the tubular urine. If the urine is acidic as a result of Na^+-H^+ exchange, the ammonia that diffuses immediately reacts with H^+ to form NH_4^+. The renal tubule is impermeable to the charged particle (NH_4^+), and hence it does not diffuse back out of the tubular fluid. There are two important consequences of this reaction: first, H^+ is removed, and this permits further Na^+-H^+ exchange to occur; second, NH_3 is removed, and this permits more NH_3 to diffuse from tubular cell to tubular urine. In short, the two processes occur concurrently and can continue only by aiding and abetting each other. By this sequence of events, large amounts of Na^+ can be retrieved from neutral salts and returned to the extracellular fluid as sodium bicarbonate (*2* in Figure VIII–1).

The above discussion is of pharmacological significance because the rate of Na^+-H^+ exchange in the renal tubule can be greatly decreased by drugs that inhibit the enzyme carbonic anhydrase. This catalyzes both the hydration of CO_2 and dehydration of H_2CO_3 and thus determines the relative concentrations of these molecular species. This, in turn, is an important determinant of both the availability of hydrogen ion for secretion and the disposition of the hydrogen ion within the tubular fluid.

Potassium Reabsorption and Secretion. Potassium is an unusual fixed cation in that it undergoes both tubular reabsorption and secretion. Reabsorption occurs largely in the proximal tubule, secretion in the distal tubule (*3* in Figure VIII–1). Since the major fraction of the filtered potassium is reabsorbed, and since this process is relatively immune to physiological stimuli or pharmacological agents, it follows, therefore, that variations in the amount of potassium actually excreted may be attributed to the distal secretory mechanism. As judged by the action of many diuretic agents, the volume of unreabsorbed glomerular filtrate that flows through the distal tubule is one of the determinants of the rate of potassium secretion. Thus, some drugs have the dual effect of increasing the urinary excretion of both sodium and potassium, the former by inhibition of reabsorption and the latter by augmentation of secretion (*3* in Figure VIII–1).

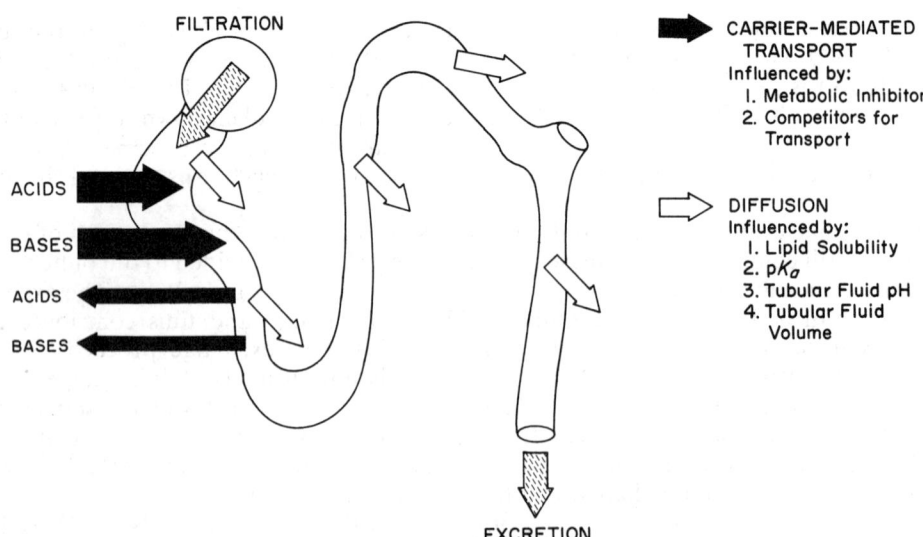

Figure VIII–3.   *Scheme for renal transport of exogenous organic acids and bases.*

Potentially bidirectional transport provides separate mechanisms by which rate of excretion may be altered pharmacologically. Many drugs and drug metabolites are handled by these mechanisms.

Excretion of Organic Acids and Bases. Two major secretory mechanisms for elimination of foreign organic compounds may now be identified in the proximal tubule: one for the transport of organic acids, the other for organic bases (*see* Figure VIII–3). While both mechanisms are dependent on energy derived from cellular metabolism, they are essentially independent systems, particularly to the extent that substances that compete for transport in one system do not influence the other. It has also been shown that some compounds that undergo tubular secretion may not necessarily be excreted in large amounts in the voided urine. This is a consequence of tubular reabsorption. While secretion is an active mechanism, reabsorption of most of these compounds is passive and depends primarily on the permeability of the tubular epithelium to the nonionic moiety of the specific acid or base under consideration. The degree of reabsorption is correlated with the lipid solubility of the nonionic species. Since this appears to be a diffusion process, the magnitude of reabsorption depends on the concentration gradient of the nonionic form from tubular fluid to the peritubular space, and this, in turn, is influenced by the pH and volume of tubular fluid and by the pK_a of the compound in question (*see* Chapter 1). As a consequence, urine flow and urine pH are important factors in determining the rate of excretion for salicylate, probenecid, other benzoates, and many tertiary amines, all of which also undergo active tubular secretion. However, these same physiological variables, urine flow and pH, have relatively little influence on the excretion of hippurates or other lipid-insoluble compounds to which the renal tubular epithelium is impermeable.

This complex system provides two separate means by which therapeutic agents may influence the excretion rate of an organic acid or base. First, carrier-mediated transport mechanisms may be influenced by specific compounds. Second, the extent of ionization of weak acids or bases will be influenced by acidifying or alkalinizing agents; this and the rate of urine flow, which may be directly or indirectly influenced by drugs, will alter the amounts of such compounds that are reabsorbed by diffusion.

CHAPTER

39 DIURETICS AND OTHER AGENTS EMPLOYED IN THE MOBILIZATION OF EDEMA FLUID

Gilbert H. Mudge

Diuretics are agents that increase the rate of urine formation. Despite this simple definition, a large number of physiological and pharmacological factors are involved. It should also be emphasized that by common usage the term *diuresis* has two separate connotations: one refers to the increase in urine volume *per se,* the other to the net loss of solute and water. Under some conditions, the maintenance of an adequate urine volume in itself justifies the use of diuretic agents. However, by far the most important indication is the mobilization of edema fluid, that is, the production of a negative extracellular

fluid balance. The effects of diuretics on solute excretion are of major importance for the understanding both of the underlying mechanisms of drug action and of the consequences of therapy. In general, the different types of diuretics are classified according to the manner by which they alter solute excretion.

Localization of Site of Drug Action. There is uniform agreement that most diuretics act directly on the kidney and, with few exceptions, on tubular rather than glomerular function. Extensive studies have been carried out to localize further the site of action to discrete segments of the nephron. A variety of methods have been employed. These include the clearance technic, stop-flow analysis, micropuncture, histochemistry, enzyme assay, the direct determination of the composition of renal tissue, *in-vitro* studies with kidney slices and isolated tubules, and, by inference, examination of related systems, particularly frog skin and toad bladder preparations.

Despite this intense activity, it is not possible to correlate all observations in a definitive manner. Brief comment on some of the complexities is warranted. First, a drug does not necessarily act at the site at which its concentration is maximal. Second, a drug may act on separate transport mechanisms at different sites—for example, the action of mercurials on the tubular secretion of organic acids proximally and on that of potassium distally. Third, there may be important species differences, most marked in the case of uricosuric agents but also observed with some diuretics. Fourth, although popularly simplified in terms of a single schematic nephron, the operation of the kidney is actually accomplished by millions of individual units that may respond differently both to physiological stress and to the action of diuretics. Fifth, modern concepts of renal function emphasize the architectural integrity of the nephron as an entire unit. This applies to many discrete functions, including solute reabsorption, the operation of the countercurrent system, and the determinants of bidirectional transport, that is, secretion in one segment and reabsorption in another. In the case of the countercurrent mechanism, for example, the magnitude of water reabsorption from the collecting duct is determined primarily by solute reabsorption in the ascending limb. And, sixth, particularly in the case of the quantitative interpretation of sodium and water reabsorption, a drug action on one site may be accompanied by secondary and compensatory changes in transport at another segment. These secondary effects may be mediated by normal mechanisms, rather than by drug action at both sites. Depending on the experimental technic, the compensatory changes may obscure the primary action. It has long been recognized that changes in solute reabsorption in one segment may influence tubular function at more distal sites that are "downstream." However, there is increasing evidence that the reverse may also be true. Distal events may influence more proximal transport. The mechanisms are both intrarenal and extrarenal in nature. Since sodium, the major solute of the tubular fluid, is reabsorbed throughout most portions of the nephron, it is quite possible that many drugs that inhibit its reabsorption act at more than a single site. The apparent localization of drug action to a particular locus may in large part be determined by experimental conditions, as well as by quantitative differences between the actions of the diuretic agent at different sites (*see* Goldberg, 1973; Suki *et al.*, 1973).

Extrarenal Sites of Drug Action. Many of the newer diuretics have proven to be useful in the investigation of electrolyte transport in organs other than the kidney, particularly under *in-vitro* conditions. Not surprisingly, these studies have revealed fundamental mechanisms common to many tissues. However, these are not reviewed systematically in

this chapter unless the action at the extrarenal site occurs with reasonable dosages and is of sufficient magnitude to have clinical relevance. For many drugs, their predominantly renal site of action may be attributed to the high concentration of drug achieved within the kidney.

WATER AND OSMOTIC DIURETICS

Normally the volume of urine is largely determined by the concentrations and types of solutes delivered to the renal tubule. Therefore, water and various electrolytes and nonelectrolytes can act as diuretic agents when given in excess.

WATER

Mechanism of Water Diuresis. Water is a true physiological diuretic. The mechanism of water diuresis is fully discussed in connection with the antidiuretic hormone of the posterior pituitary (*see* Chapter 40).

Therapeutic Uses. Although one seldom regards water as a therapeutic agent, it is often essential to limit or to force fluid intake. The problems of water administration associated with parenteral alimentation are discussed in Chapter 36. There are many other circumstances when one must regulate the volume of fluid intake. For example, it is often desired to attain a given concentration of certain urinary antiseptics in the urine. This can be accomplished by restricting the ingestion of water to a specified amount. On the other hand, when drugs irritating to the urinary tract or of limited solubility are being employed, a higher water intake permits their excretion in sufficiently low concentrations to avoid renal damage. In addition, with many substances, either endogenous such as urea, or exogenous such as drugs or their metabolites, the rate of excretion is partially dependent on the rate of urine flow.

A fundamental problem concerns water intake in edematous individuals. For a long time it was advocated that water should be restricted when edema fluid was present, in the belief that the ingestion of water contributed to edema formation. It is now generally agreed that the intake of extracellular electrolyte rather than of water is of primary importance in this regard and that, if sodium salts are restricted, under most circumstances little is gained by the simultaneous restriction of water.

SODIUM SALTS

Sodium salts occupy a unique position among diuretic salts. Under certain circumstances, the *administration* of sodium salts plays an important and irreplaceable role in assuring and promoting an adequate flow of urine. However, in other situations, the *restriction* of sodium intake is of paramount importance.

Renal Excretion of Sodium Salts. The source of the glomerular filtrate is extracellular fluid. The predominant cation of extracellular fluid is sodium; the predominant anions are chloride and bicarbonate. If the kidneys were to excrete sodium salts excessively with a concomitant loss of water, a rapid reduction in extracellular fluid volume would result. Conversely, an excessive reabsorption of sodium salts and water would soon result in overwhelming edema. The average intake of sodium chloride is approximately 10 g daily, and this amount must be excreted in the urine to maintain electrolyte balance and the constancy of the extracellular environment.

The several processes by which sodium is reabsorbed have been outlined in the introduction to Section VIII. The anionic composition of the tubular fluid may also be of importance. If there is a high concentration of anion to which the tubule is impermeable, the amount of cation reabsorbed necessarily decreases; a large fraction of this cationic component is usually sodium. Current interpretations of the electrochemical gradient indicate that active transport of Na^+ is the primary event in most of the tubule except the ascending limb of the loop of Henle, where Cl^- is actively reabsorbed. Electroneutrality is preserved by the diffusion of the oppositely charged ion, or in certain instances by cationic exchange. Since the mechanisms involve active transport, limitations in tubular capacities are presumed to exist. However, the exact relationship of filtered load to the amount reabsorbed is complex and incompletely understood. The absolute amount reabsorbed in the proximal tubule varies with the amount filtered, the plasma concentration, and the extracellular fluid volume. In the reabsorption of sodium from the more distal portions of the nephron, acid-base balance and adrenocortical steroids also play a role. As a result of normal homeostatic mechanisms the reabsorptive processes adjust themselves so finely that the renal excretion of sodium is normally equivalent to oral intake. In the development of

edema, these renal adjustments fail and urinary sodium excretion decreases. This is true regardless of the nature of the primary disease—most commonly, cardiac, renal, or hepatic.

Therapeutic Uses. *Sodium chloride* is never employed as a diuretic agent in the treatment of edema. Rather, the restriction of sodium intake is of paramount importance. Sodium chloride is used primarily to treat deficits in extracellular fluid volume or concentration. When these are corrected, urinary excretion usually increases to normal rates.

Sodium bicarbonate may be useful in nonedematous states for the purposeful alkalinization of the urine in order to promote the excretion of certain weak organic acids, including such drugs as salicylate, or to enhance the solubility of certain drugs in the urine and thus prevent crystalluria.

Sodium sulfate has very little use as a clinical diuretic for the mobilization of edema fluid. It cannot be taken orally because it is not absorbed and acts as a cathartic. When it is given parenterally, the augmentation of urine volume is primarily the result of the excretion of the administered salt and water. The renal tubule has only a limited capacity to reabsorb the sulfate ion.

Solutions of sodium sulfate undergo complex reactions with calcium and other divalent cations. Sulfate diuresis is associated, therefore, with a marked rise in divalent cation excretion. This has been used as a basis for treating hypercalcemia and possibly radiostrontium poisoning (Walser *et al.,* 1961).

POTASSIUM SALTS

In the past, potassium salts were employed to a limited extent as diuretics. However, they were not very effective for the mobilization of edema fluid and are no longer used for this purpose. Many of the newer diuretics increase the excretion not only of sodium but of potassium as well. As a result, variable degrees of potassium depletion may develop. Under these conditions, the administration of potassium salts is for the purpose of correcting deficits.

OSMOTIC DIURETICS

The term *osmotic diuretic* is generally used for certain nonelectrolytes that have the following attributes in common: (1) they are freely filterable at the glomerulus; (2) they undergo limited reabsorption by the renal tubule; and (3) they are pharmacologically inert by conventional criteria. Taken together, these three characteristics permit the administration of such agents in sufficiently large quantities to contribute significantly to the osmolality of the plasma, the glomerular filtrate, and the tubular fluid. Their action within the kidney depends primarily upon the concentration of osmotically active particles in solution. In addition, most osmotic diuretics are selected because of their resistance to metabolic alteration. However, a sugar such as glucose will act in a similar manner if its concentration becomes excessively high in the plasma and, as a consequence, also in the tubular fluid.

Mechanism of Diuretic Action. When there is a significant increase in the amount of any osmotically active solute in the voided urine, this is usually accompanied by an increase in urine volume. This generalization is subject to quantitative modification by several factors, including the compensatory effects of the rate of release of the antidiuretic hormone (ADH), the magnitude of positive or negative free-water production, and the exact mechanisms by which solute excretion is increased (*see* Figure VIII–2, page 814). In general, there are three separate ways by which the rate of solute excretion may be augmented: the inhibition of electrolyte reabsorption by specific drugs, an increase in the filtered load of electrolytes that are poorly or incompletely reabsorbed, and an increase in the filtered load of the nonelectrolyte osmotic agents.

It is important to appreciate the circumstances under which the osmotic diuretics may play a unique role in either maintaining or increasing urine volume. When the rate of glomerular filtration is acutely reduced, either experimentally in the laboratory or clinically as a result of hypovolemic shock, dehydration, or trauma, the solutes of the glomerular filtrate undergo more complete reabsorption so that there is a disproportionately large fall in the rate of urine flow and solute excretion. As indicated previously, the administration of a normal solute, such as sodium chloride, may restore renal excretory function, but only if there is improvement in renal hemodynamics. If the rate of glomerular filtration remains severely reduced, sodium chloride administration fails to augment urine flow because of the virtually complete tubular reabsorption of this normal electrolyte. Under these same conditions, those diuretics that normally act by inhibiting tubular transport may also be ineffective because the extent to which they reduce tubular reabsorptive capacity is not of sufficient magnitude to compensate for the greatly diminished filtered load.

However, under the same conditions, that is, when the renal circulation is acutely compromised, the osmotic diuretics retain their efficacy. To take mannitol as an example —even though the filtration rate is reduced, mannitol is still filtered at the glomerulus. The tubular impermeability to mannitol is not altered by acute renal ischemia of short duration. Hence, the amount of mannitol that is filtered is also excreted in the voided urine. Unreabsorbed solute limits the back diffusion of water. As a consequence, urine volume can be maintained even in the presence of decreased glomerular function. As a first approximation, urine volume is proportional to the rate of solute excretion, which under these circumstances may be composed largely of the agent administered as the osmotic diuretic. Nephrotoxic agents and prolonged, severe renal ischemia may damage the tubular epithelium and produce acute tubular necrosis with oliguria. The tubule is then no longer selectively impermeable, and osmotic diuretics become ineffective.

An additional action of the osmotic diuretics is to increase the rate of electrolyte excretion, particularly sodium, chloride, and potassium. However, this occurs only with large doses. From a practical point of view, this action should be clearly distinguished from the effect on the rate of urine formation itself. The action on electrolyte reabsorption is related to the isosmotic characteristics of the proximal tubule. Under normal conditions, sodium chloride is the major solute in the proximal fluid and, as it is reabsorbed, water diffuses passively so that the tubular fluid remains isosmotic. Thus, the sodium concentration in the tubular fluid is virtually unaltered, despite the fact that sodium itself is undergoing active reabsorption. However, in the presence of non-reabsorbable solute, the diffusion of water is reduced relative to the movement of sodium in order to maintain an isotonic fluid in the tubule. As a consequence, the concentration of sodium in the tubular fluid decreases, as does the total amount of sodium that is reabsorbed, probably due to the progressively increasing concentration gradient of sodium between the tubular urine and extracellular fluid.

It should be reemphasized that the natriuretic action of osmotic diuretics is largely of experimental interest and is of little importance as a practical means of increasing sodium excretion or mobilizing edema fluid. The same general considerations apply to all osmotic diuretics, even though they may be handled slightly differently by the renal tubule. Mannitol undergoes very little reabsorption, and for many practical purposes the tubule may be considered to be impermeable to it. Sucrose is excreted in a similar manner. In the case of urea, about 50% of the amount filtered at the glomerulus is not reabsorbed. With elevated urea loads, this fraction tends to increase. In the case of glucose, at normal plasma concentrations the amount filtered is virtually completely reabsorbed by an active process in the proximal tubule. As the glucose concentration is increased in both the plasma and the filtrate, the threshold and total reabsorptive capacity of the transport mechanism are exceeded and glucose appears in the voided urine. Hence, with severe hyperglycemia, glucose acts as an osmotic diuretic, even though a portion of the amount filtered continues to be reabsorbed.

The intestinal and renal tubular epithelia have many permeability characteristics in common. Most osmotic diuretics, which, by definition, are poorly reabsorbed by the renal tubules, are also not absorbed from the gastrointestinal tract. Thus, these agents must be administered parenterally in order to achieve effective plasma concentrations. However, urea is absorbed from the intestine.

Therapeutic Uses. Osmotic diuretics may be used for several purposes that are distinct and separate, but all of which depend on the same fundamental characteristics. Their uses include prophylaxis against acute renal failure, differential diagnosis of acute oliguria, and reduction of cerebrospinal and intraocular fluid pressures. Although *urea* and *glucose* have been employed in the past as oral diuretics for the treatment of chronic edema, they have been replaced by superior agents.

Mannitol is extensively employed. Perhaps one of the clearest and most important indications is the *prophylaxis of acute renal failure*. It is used for this purpose in conditions as diverse as cardiovascular operations, severe traumatic injury, operations in the presence of severe jaundice, and management of hemolytic transfusion reactions. In each of these conditions, a precipitous fall in urine flow may be anticipated either as the result of an acutely reduced filtration rate or from acute changes in tubular permeability. The latter may be the consequence of the presence of a noxious agent within the tubular fluid in excessively high concentrations, in some instances sufficient to result in actual precipitation. In these situations, mannitol exerts an osmotic effect within the tubular fluid, inhibits water reabsorption, and maintains the rate of urine flow within reasonably normal limits. As a consequence, the concentration of the noxious agent within the tubular fluid does not reach the excessively high levels that otherwise would have been achieved by the more complete reabsorption of water. Many of the mechanisms responsible for nephrotoxicity are incompletely understood. However, it is clear that under these conditions the use of osmotic diuretics protects the kidney against damage. The maintenance of an adequate flow of relatively dilute urine is probably the single most important factor. Additional factors may also be involved. In the presence of hypotension mannitol is more effective than saline solution in maintaining glomerular filtration (Morris *et al.,* 1972). If given in sufficiently large amounts, mannitol increases extracellular osmolality, which in turn may decrease cellular swelling and improve renal blood flow (Flores *et al.,* 1972). Despite the fact that these mechanisms have been demonstrated experimentally, their clinical significance remains to be evaluated.

A closely related but separate use of mannitol is in the *evaluation of acute oliguria*. With a partial reduction in glomerular function, as might occur from excessive loss of body fluids, urine flow may be increased toward normal by the administration of an osmotic diuretic, and this response may serve as a guide for the additional administration of parenteral fluids. However, if either glomerular or tubular function is too severely compromised, mannitol will not increase urine flow. This may help orient the further management of the patient with acute anuria (Barry and Malloy, 1962).

Mannitol is also used for the *reduction of the pressure and volume of the intraocular and cerebrospinal fluids*. By elevating the osmolality of the plasma, one is able to enhance the diffusion of water from those fluids back into the plasma and the extracellular space.

Mannitol is nearly always given intravenously, and hence it is impractical for the management of chronic edema, regardless of its cause. When administered orally, mannitol produces a catharsis and the fecal fluid has a low sodium concentration. This action has been used rarely in the management of edema and for the correction of hyponatremia in patients refractory to more conventional diuretic measures (James and Evans, 1970).

Toxicity. The major potential toxicity of osmotic diuretics is intrinsically related to the load of solute administered and its effect on the volume and distribution of the body fluids.

In edematous states associated with diminished cardiac reserve, the administration of mannitol introduces a risk that may far outweigh any therapeutic benefit. It should be recalled that mannitol is distributed in the extracellular fluid, and, consequently, the acute administration of hypertonic solutions in amounts sufficient to make a significant contribution to extracellular osmolarity will inevitably be accompanied by an acute expansion of extracellular fluid volume. In the patient with cardiac decompensation, this represents an undesirable hazard. A variety of signs and symptoms suggestive of hypersensitivity reactions has occurred in occasional patients. The repeated administration of large doses of urea and mannitol to experimental animals has not resulted in significant alterations of renal tubular functions.

Preparations and Dosage. *Urea,* U.S.P., is a white crystalline powder, with a slightly bitter taste, freely soluble in water. Sterile preparations (UREAPHIL, UREVERT) are available that may be reconstituted for intravenous use. When administered in this manner, the solution may contain up to 30% urea (w/w) and an isosmotic concentration of dextrose or invert sugar (equal parts of dextrose and levulose), the latter substances being necessary to prevent the hemolysis produced by pure solutions of urea. Intravenous doses of 1 to 1.5 g of urea per kilogram of body weight are optimal in preparation for neurosurgical procedures.

Mannitol, U.S.P. (OSMITROL), is available for intravenous administration as *Mannitol Injection,* U.S.P., and *Mannitol and Sodium Chloride Injection,* U.S.P., in concentrations of 5, 10, 15, 20, or 25% mannitol in volumes ranging from 50 to 1000 ml of water or 0.3 to 0.45% sodium chloride solution. The adult dose for promotion of diuresis ranges from 50 to 200 g over a 24-hour period of infusion; the rate is generally adjusted to maintain a urinary output of at least 30 to 50 ml per hour. It should be preceded by a test dose in patients with marked oliguria or questionable adequacy of renal function. The recommended test dose is 200 mg/kg (approximately 75 ml of a 20% solution for an adult patient), infused over 3 to 5 minutes; if the first or a second test dose fails to promote a urinary flow greater than 30 ml per hour for 2 to 3 hours, the patient's status should be reevaluated prior to continuation of therapy. When used for the prevention of acute renal failure during various types of surgery or for the treatment of oliguria, the total dose is 50 to 100 g of mannitol for an adult patient. The dose for the reduction of intracranial pressure and brain mass prior to neurosurgery, or for the reduction of intraocular tension during an acute attack of congestive glaucoma or for ophthalmic surgery, is 1.5 to 2 g/kg, given as a 15 or 20% solution over a period of 30 to 60 minutes. Contraindications to the administration of mannitol include renal disease of sufficient severity to produce anuria, marked pulmonary congestion or edema, marked dehydration, and intracranial hemorrhage unless craniotomy is to be performed. The infusion of mannitol should be terminated if the patient develops signs of progressive renal dysfunction, heart failure, or pulmonary congestion.

ACID-FORMING SALTS

Salts that tend to produce acidosis have a transient diuretic action. Their effect is greater than would be expected from their "osmotic effect," and one is obliged to consider their acid-forming properties in explaining the mechanism of the diuresis. The most widely used salt is *ammonium chloride.*

Mechanism of Diuretic Action. Before considering the mechanism of diuretic action, the pragmatic definitions of *fixed* and *labile* ions should be reviewed (Chapter 36).

The acidifying salt ($NH_4^+Cl^-$) is the combination of a labile cation and a fixed anion. The conversion, in the liver, of an ammonium ion to urea also results in the net formation of a hydrogen ion. This reacts with the body buffers. The interaction between hydrogen ion and bicarbonate leads to the formation of CO_2, which is excreted by the lungs. The net result is the displacement of bicarbonate by chloride, and the production of a metabolic acidosis. The administration of $NH_4^+Cl^-$, therefore, does not change the *total concentration* of electrolyte in the extracellular fluid, since the addition of a labile cation (NH_4^+) and a fixed anion (Cl^-) leads to the ultimate disappearance of an equivalent amount of labile cation (H^+) and labile anion (HCO_3^-). Thus, while ammonium chloride does not expand extracellular fluid volume, it does alter its *composition.*

As a result of the increase in the chloride concentration of the extracellular fluid, the chloride load to the tubules is acutely augmented and an appreciable amount will escape reabsorption along with an equivalent amount of cation and an isosmotic quantity of water. The cation is obtained from the body fluids and consists predominantly of sodium. Potassium excretion is also increased but to a lesser extent. By enhancing the excretion of both extracellular electrolyte and water, acidifying salts bring about a net loss of extracellular fluid.

As a result of the acidosis produced by acidifying salts, the renal defense of the acid-base pattern of the extracellular fluid comes into play. This calls for the excretion of chloride unaccompanied by fixed cation. The kidney can accomplish this by elaborating ammonia, secreting H^+ in exchange for Na^+, and thereby excreting Cl⁻ in combination with NH_4^+. When full compensation is achieved, the amount of ammonium chloride excreted by the kidney will be equal to that ingested in the usual diuretic dose. Once this balance occurs, ammonium chloride is no longer effective in mobilizing edema fluid (*see* Pitts, 1974).

Therapeutic Uses. The preparations employed in therapy are described elsewhere (*see* Index). The acid-forming diuretics are ordinarily given orally. They may cause gastric irritation and are likely to induce nausea and vomiting. *Ammonium nitrate* produces the least gastrointestinal distress, but occasionally it may cause methemoglobinemia. *Ammonium Chloride*, N.F., is now the most commonly employed agent, and is usually administered in enteric-coated tablets. The dose varies from 8 to 12 g daily, given in divided portions at mealtime. The salt should not be employed when renal function is markedly impaired, as in chronic nephritis, because of the danger of producing uncompensated acidosis. Severe hepatic failure is also a contraindication to the administration of ammonium salts for any purpose.

Acid-forming salts have very limited value as primary diuretics. As discussed above, they are effective only in promoting a net loss of extracellular electrolyte and water for a period of 1 or 2 days. Their chief value is to compensate for the alkalosis induced by the mercurial diuretics, the high-ceiling diuretics, and, less commonly, the thiazides. In the case of the mercurial diuretics, their activity is impaired by alkalosis (*see* below). *Under no circumstances is there justification for the prolonged administration of acidifying salts as the sole diuretic agent.*

MERCURIAL DIURETICS

History. Calomel (mercurous chloride) was used as a diuretic by Paracelsus in the sixteenth century. It was an ingredient of the famous "Guy's Hospital pill" (calomel, squill, and digitalis) and contributed greatly to the diuretic action of this combination of drugs. Despite its efficacy, calomel was displaced by the organic mercurials, because of its cathartic effect and uncertainty of intestinal absorption.

Merbaphen (NOVASUROL), which contains mercury in organic linkage, was originally introduced as an antisyphilitic agent. Its potent diuretic properties were soon discovered by Saxl and Heilig (*see* historical account by Vogl, 1950). For a period of approximately 30 years the organic mercurials were the preeminent diuretics. Following the introduction of potent, less toxic, oral diuretics their use greatly declined. Indeed, only two mercurial diuretics remain as official drugs. Despite their current limited use, they will be discussed in detail since they have made major contributions to our basic understanding of renal tubular function and the therapeutic principles that underlie the mobilization of edema fluid.

PHARMACOLOGICAL PROPERTIES

The pharmacological actions and therapeutic uses of all the organic mercurial diuretics are so similar that they can be discussed as a group.

Mechanism of Diuretic Action. The primary action of the mercurial diuretics is to depress tubular mechanisms responsible for the active reabsorption of sodium and chloride. The advantage of organic mercurials over inorganic compounds lies in the fact that they are rapidly excreted by the kidney. In this way, it is possible to produce reversible functional changes in the renal tubule with minimal danger of producing pathological lesions in the kidney or elsewhere that are characteristic of poisoning by the mercuric ion.

Structure-Activity Relationship. The active form of mercurials has been a controversial subject. Present evidence suggests that the diuretic response is attributable to the intrarenal release of mercuric ions *in vivo* by rupture of the carbon-to-mercury bond, and that, with the drugs commonly employed, this occurs with only a minute fraction of the dose administered (Weiner *et al.*, 1962). This is based on the consideration of a wide variety of factors, as follows: (1) Some organic mercurials are diuretic, others are not; however, there is no specific structural configuration of the organic compound to which diuretic activity can be attributed. (2) All diuretic organic mercurials thus far examined are acid labile in appropriate *in-vitro* systems. This lability involves the rupture of the carbon-to-mercury bond and is catalyzed by thiols. Mercurials that are acid stable in such a system do not have diuretic activity, even though some may be rapidly excreted in the urine and may accumulate within the renal parenchyma. Most diuretic mercurials have the general formula

$$R—\overset{\overset{\textstyle O Y}{|}}{C}H—CH_2—Hg^+,$$ in which Y is usually CH_3 or another alkyl group, and R is a complex organic moiety, frequently with urea groupings or aromatic or heterocyclic rings. The R substituents largely determine the compound's distribution and rate of excretion; they may also be of importance with respect to inducing hypersensitivity reactions. The type formula is acid labile. When the beta carbon is unsubstituted, as in $R—CH_2—CH_2—Hg^+$, the compound is acid stable and nondiuretic. (3) An active diuretic has been shown to release small amounts of mercuric ion in kidney tissue (Clarkson *et al.*, 1965). (4) Under some experimental conditions, inorganic mercuric salts are highly active as diuretics. In contrast to the organic mercurials, their effectiveness is only slightly influenced by changes in acid-base balance. (5) Under a variety of different physiological conditions, there is a high correlation between the action of diuretic organic mercurials and the acidity of the urine. This suggests that urinary acidity may reflect the pH of an intrarenal site at which the organic compounds undergo metabolic alteration.

Mercurials are excreted as the cysteine complex and probably circulate within the body fluids in combination with the thiol groups either of compounds of low molecular weight or of plasma proteins. The capacity of mercurials to complex with thiols is so strong that only vanishingly low, trace amounts of free organic or inorganic mercury can exist within the body. However, mercurial diuresis can be prevented or terminated by the administration of dimercaprol. This agent removes mercury from the kidney; therefore, the renal receptor must have less affinity for mercuric ions than does dimercaprol, a dithiol. Monothiols neither prevent nor terminate diuresis, and some organic mercurials, such as mercaptomerin, are administered complexed with a monothiol and are active in this form. This suggests that the renal receptor has a greater affinity for the mercurial than does a monothiol. Several observations appear to contradict the mercuric ion hypothesis, the most important of which is the finding of inorganic mercury produced *in vivo* after the administration of a nondiuretic organic mercurial compound. The current status of the problem has been evaluated critically by Cafruny and associates (1973) and Clarkson and Vostal (1973).

Effect on Renal Tubular Transport. In therapeutic doses, the important actions of mercurials are limited to the inhibition of the tubular reabsorption of sodium and chloride and to the excretion of potassium. Inhibition of organic acid secretion is seen in man but not in the dog. In the chimpanzee and to a lesser extent in man, certain mercurials have an intense uricosuric action (Fanelli *et al.,* 1973).

During diuresis, the urine contains a high concentration of chloride anion matched by almost equivalent amounts of sodium. (*See* Table 39–1, page 826.) There is also a partial correlation between the plasma chloride concentration and the diuretic response. In metabolic alkalosis induced by sodium bicarbonate, the plasma chloride is low and mercurials are ineffective; in metabolic acidosis induced by ammonium chloride, the plasma chloride is elevated and mercurials are potentiated. However, there are less common conditions in which the correlation fails to hold—the chronic administration of ammonium chloride, the administration of ammonium nitrate, and during hypokalemic alkalosis with paradoxical aciduria. In these situations, mercurials are effective even in the presence of hypochloremia.

The effects of the mercurial diuretics on potassium excretion are complex. The mercurials depress the tubular secretion of potassium. For this reason, diuresis produced by mercurials is accompanied by significantly less potassium loss than occurs with other diuretics that do not inhibit the secretory mechanism. However, mercurials have a paradoxical action in increasing slightly the excretion of potassium when initial excretory rates are low.

The site of mercurial action has been examined extensively. There can be little doubt that inhibition of para-aminohippuric acid (PAH) secretion is proximal and inhibition of potassium secretion is distal. However, as far as the reabsorption of sodium and chloride is concerned, the site of mercurial action is less well established and, indeed, may involve multiple segments of the nephron, each possibly to a variable degree depending upon the precise experimental conditions. Results obtained with different investigative technics have been summarized by Suki and coworkers (1973). From micropuncture studies in the dog, the major site of action has been assigned to the ascending limb (Evanson *et al.,* 1972). At this same site a primary inhibition of chloride transport has been identified (Burg and Green, 1973b). In attempting to define a cellular or biochemical site of action, studies with mercurials have been complicated by the capacity of these agents to react with multiple cell components. Many of the findings appear quantitatively inconsistent, and it is not yet possible to define the mechanisms of mercurial action at the molecular level (*see* Nechay, 1973; Suki *et al.,* 1973).

Effect on Composition of Extracellular Fluid. As a result of the loss of fluid containing sodium and chloride in approximately equal amounts and virtually devoid of bicarbonate, a mercurial diuresis tends to produce a metabolic alkalosis. This has been termed *subtraction alkalosis*. It does not inevitably occur. Most patients receive mercurial diuretics at intervals of several days, and the drug is active only over a period of hours. Therefore, compensation for the distortion in the composition of extracellular fluid produced by the mercurial can be achieved by the kidney after the action of the diuretic has subsided. However, when mercurial diuretics are given in intensive courses or when renal function is inadequate to achieve rapid compensation, and when dietary intake of sodium chloride is excessively low, a persistent systemic alkalosis may develop. When this occurs, the individual may become refractory to the action of the mercurial diuretics.

Refractoriness. Many factors must be involved in the phenomenon of refractoriness. Although pH itself is a determinant of mercurial action at the site of the tubular receptor, other variables play an important role in the overall diuretic response. Individuals in advanced congestive heart failure may have such low filtration rates that they are unresponsive to mercurials. In addition, vigorous diuretic therapy with restriction of dietary sodium chloride intake may result in the renal loss of sodium chloride without a proportional loss of water. This leads to dilutional hyponatremia, which may decrease the diuretic response even without concomitant alkalosis.

Course of Diuresis. Following the parenteral administration of a mercurial diuretic to a responsive edematous patient, an increase in urine flow is evident within 1 to 2 hours and may persist up to 12 hours. A loss of about 2.5% of the body weight represents an average response.

Extrarenal Actions. The organic mercurials normally exert prominent pharmacodynamic actions only on renal tubular function. Should cumulation occur, the signs and symptoms of systemic *mercury poisoning* develop. An action shared by all mercury preparations is the ability in high concentrations to cause *cardiac arrhythmias,* including ventricular fibrillation. The cardiac toxicity of the mercurials is the basis of rare, untoward clinical reactions (*see* below).

Routes of Administration. The organic mercurials were in the past given by many routes, but intramuscular and subcutaneous administration is now almost exclusively used. The intravenous route offers no significant advantage and may precipitate cardiac arrhythmias. Oral administration of a mercurial diuretic is of unpredictable efficacy and is poorly tolerated.

Absorption, Fate, and Excretion. Organic mercurials are rapidly excreted by the kidney. Approximately 50% of injected mercury can be recovered in the urine within 3 hours and up to 95% within 24 hours. Thus, very little appears in the bowel. Excretion is retarded in individuals with impaired renal function. When properly administered even over a span of many years, the mercurials neither accumulate nor show evidence of toxicity.

Untoward Reactions. Untoward reactions to the organic mercurials occur infrequently. There is no evidence that they are in any way influenced by concomitant medication or by the underlying disease.
Immediate Fatal Reactions. These have occurred very rarely and only after intravenous administration. Death in most instances is believed to result from ventricular fibrillation, produced by a transiently high concentration of drug.
Immediate Nonfatal Reactions. These may take a variety of forms, for example, flushing, pruritus, urticaria, dermatitis that may subsequently become exfoliative, fever, and nausea and vomiting. Symptoms are often on an allergic basis. Thrombocytopenia, neutropenia, and agranulocytosis have been reported, and are often the result of sensitization to a specific mercurial.
The classical symptoms of *systemic mercury poisoning* may follow the injudicious use of mercurial diuretics (*see* Chapter 46).

Contraindications. Renal insufficiency or acute nephritis constitutes an absolute contraindication to the use of the mercurial diuretics.

Preparations and Dosage. There are currently only two official preparations of mercurial diuretics. *Mercaptomerin Sodium*, U.S.P. (THIOMERIN), is unique in that it can be administered by either the subcutaneous or intramuscular route. *Mercaptomerin Sodium Injection*, U.S.P., is available in 2-ml cartridge-needle units, and in vials containing 2, 10, and 30 ml; the usual dose is 1 ml (40 mg Hg) but may range from 0.2 to 2 ml daily. *Meralluride*, N.F. (MERCUHYDRIN), is an organic mercurial that is complexed with theophylline to promote absorption. *Meralluride Injection*, N.F., is available in 1- and 2-ml ampuls and is injected intramuscularly; the usual dose is 1 ml (39 mg Hg) and ranges from 0.5 to 2 ml. *Chlormerodrin Hg 197 Injection*, U.S.P., and *Chlormerodrin Hg 203 Injection*, N.F., are organic mercurials employed only as diagnostic agents.

THERAPEUTIC USES

The main use of the mercurial diuretics is in edema of cardiac origin. Good results are sometimes obtained in chronic nephrosis, the nephrotic stage of glomerulonephritis, and ascites due to hepatic cirrhosis or portal obstruction.

Chlormerodrin has also been employed as a *radiopharmaceutical* for diagnostic purposes in the detection of diseases of the kidney and brain. The preferred isotope is [197]Hg. For these purposes the usefulness of chlormerodrin depends on its tissue distribution. The dose of the radiopharmaceutical is itself sufficiently small to be devoid of pharmacological action. However, this may be preceded by the administration of a full diuretic dose of a nonradioactive organic mercurial, in an attempt to reduce radiation to the kidney from renal localization of the radiopharmaceutical.

INHIBITORS OF CARBONIC ANHYDRASE

Acetazolamide is the prototype of a class of agents that have had limited usefulness as diuretics but which have played a major role in the development of fundamental renal physiology and pharmacology.

History. In the early 1930s, Roughton demonstrated the presence in red blood cells of an enzyme, carbonic anhydrase, that catalyzes reaction I:

$$CO_2 + H_2O \overset{I}{\rightleftharpoons} H_2CO_3 \overset{II}{\rightleftharpoons} H^+ + HCO_3^-$$

Both the hydration and the dehydration reactions are under enzymatic control. Reaction II is an ionic dissociation that is virtually instantaneous and not subject to enzymatic acceleration. Carbonic anhydrase has subsequently been found in many sites—including the renal cortex, gastric mucosa, pancreas, eye, and central nervous system (CNS). When sulfanilamide was introduced as a chemotherapeutic agent, metabolic acidosis was recognized as a side effect. The drug was found to inhibit carbonic anhydrase *in vitro* and to inhibit the normal acidification of the urine *in vivo*. Subsequent studies established the role of carbonic anhydrase in renal transport.

Chemistry and Structure-Activity Relationship. An enormous number of sulfonamides have been synthesized and tested for their activity as carbonic anhydrase inhibitors and for their usefulness as diuretics. Acetazolamide has been studied the most extensively. The other three official drugs of this group are dichlorphenamide, ethoxzolamide, and methazolamide. Their structural formulas are as follows:

Acetazolamide

Dichlorphenamide

Ethoxzolamide

Methazolamide

The most important structure-activity relationship is that carbonic anhydrase inhibitory activity is abolished by N-sulfamyl substitutions. Extensive examination has yielded only limited correlations for other structural attributes. The relatively unpredictable relationship between enzyme inhibition *in vitro* and diuretic potency *in vivo* is attributable in some instances to variations in drug distribution, binding, and metabolism (*see* review by Maren, 1967).

PHARMACOLOGICAL PROPERTIES

Mechanism of Action. The major pharmacological action of acetazolamide is the inhibition of the enzyme carbonic anhydrase. Studies with purified enzyme have shown that the inhibition is noncompetitive. The noncatalyzed hydration or dehydration reaction can take place, of course, in the absence of the enzyme. However, the quantitative relationship between the two reaction rates depends on many complex factors. In general, the enzyme is normally present in tissues in huge excess. More than 99% of enzyme activity in the kidney must be inhibited before physiological effects become apparent. The enzyme itself is the dominant tissue component to which the inhibitors become bound.

Action on the Kidney. Following the administration of acetazolamide, the urine volume promptly increases. The normally acidic pH becomes alkaline. The urinary concentration of the bicarbonate anion increases and is matched by sodium and substantial amounts of potassium. (*See* Table 39-1.) The urinary concentration of chloride falls. The increased alka-

linity of the urine is necessarily accompanied by a decrease in the excretion of titratable acid and of ammonia.

The above sequence of events may be attributed to the inhibition of H^+ secretion by the renal tubule. This action was originally attributed exclusively to the distal segment. Current evidence indicates a greater effect on the proximal than on the distal tubule, with little or no effect on the ascending limb. This is supported by measurements of free-water production as well as by micropuncture studies (Goldberg, 1973). Carbonic anhydrase is probably located at the luminal border of the cells of the proximal but not of the distal tubule. Hence, inhibition of the enzyme at the former site may lead to transient changes in pH gradients that limit tubular secretion of H^+ (Rector, 1973).

Within recent years *phosphaturia* has been used as an index of localizing diuretic action since the phosphate anion is thought to be reabsorbed almost exclusively in the proximal tubule. For a given degree of natriuresis, the phosphaturia is greatest for acetazolamide, followed by the thiazides, mercurials, and high-ceiling diuretics in diminishing order. This is consistent with a largely proximal action for acetazolamide (Goldberg, 1973). The phosphaturia may be related to the direct stimulation by acetazolamide of cyclic adenosine $3',5'$-monophosphate (cyclic AMP) production by the kidney. In this sense, the drug acts similarly to the parathyroid hormone in enhancing the urinary excretion of phosphate and cyclic AMP, in contrast to its antagonism of the action of the hormone on bone (Waite, 1972; Rodriguez *et al.*, 1974).

Effect on Plasma Composition. Acetazolamide increases the urinary excretion of bicarbonate and fixed cation, mostly sodium. As a result, the concentration of bicarbonate in the extracellular fluid decreases and metabolic acidosis results. In metabolic acidosis, the renal response to acetazolamide is greatly reduced (Table 39-2). However, with metabolic alkalosis the diuretic response is enhanced. In the edematous patient, the daily administration of acetazolamide leads to a metabolic type of acidosis

Table 39-1. URINARY ELECTROLYTE COMPOSITION DURING DIURESIS *

	VOLUME (*ml/min*)	pH	Na^+	K^+	Cl^-	HCO_3^-
					(*mEq/l*)	
Control	1	6	50	15	60	1
Mannitol	10	6.5	90	15	110	4
Mercurial	7	6	150	8	160	1
Acetazolamide	3	8.2	70	60	15	120
Benzothiadiazides (thiazides)	3	7.4	150	25	150	25
Ethacrynic acid	8	6	140	10	155	1
Furosemide	8	6	140	10	155	1
Triamterene	3	7.2	130	5	120	15
Amiloride	2	7.2	130	5	110	15
Aminophylline	3	6	150	15	160	1

* Data are representative of results that would be observed in man or dog during normal hydration and acid-base balance. Such findings are readily reproducible during the peak of diuresis and following a single maximally effective dose. However, a significant range of urinary values may be anticipated; a single value is given here solely to facilitate comparison of one drug with another. Excretion rates are obtainable as the product of urinary volume and composition.

Table 39–2. EFFECT OF ACID-BASE BALANCE ON ACTION OF DIURETICS *†

PEAK CHANGE IN EXCRETION
($\mu Eq/min$)

	METABOLIC ACIDOSIS			METABOLIC ALKALOSIS		
	Na^+	Cl^-	HCO_3^-	Na^+	Cl^-	HCO_3^-
Mercurial	1000	1100	0	10	10	0
Acetazolamide	5	0	10	300	0	400
Chlorothiazide	200	240	5	380	180	230
Hydrochlorothiazide	300	350	5	430	320	150
Ethacrynic acid	1100	1200	0	1000	1100	0
Furosemide	1240	1280	0	970	880	0
Aminophylline	60	120	0	410	240	170

* Data compiled from references cited in text.
† After Mudge, 1966. Courtesy of the *Annals of The New York Academy of Sciences.*

that is accompanied by the loss of the diuretic response to continued drug therapy. These observations have been interpreted to indicate that renal responsiveness is related to the amount of bicarbonate filtered at the glomerulus. However, factors other than the amount of filtered bicarbonate must be determinants of drug action since the extracellular alkalosis of potassium depletion (with presumed intracellular acidosis) decreases the diuretic response (Maren *et al.,* 1961). In this general phenomenon, the diuretic efficacy of acetazolamide is remotely similar to that of the mercurials in that the diuretic action itself leads to a distortion of extracellular fluid composition, which in turn diminishes the effect of the drug (*see* Mudge, 1966).

Acetazolamide produces a marked increase in potassium excretion, attributable to enhanced secretion in the distal nephron. The effects on potassium are most prominent in acute experiments. With chronic administration, acetazolamide has less effect on potassium balance than do certain other agents.

Eye. The presence of carbonic anhydrase in a number of intraocular structures, including the ciliary processes, and the high concentration of bicarbonate in the aqueous humor have focused attention on the role that the enzyme might play in the secretion of aqueous humor. Acetazolamide reduces the rate of aqueous humor formation; intraocular pressure in patients with glaucoma is correspondingly reduced. This action of the drug appears to be independent of systemic acid-base balance (*see* review by Maren, 1967).

Gastric and Pancreatic Juice. Under appropriate experimental conditions, it is possible to implicate carbonic anhydrase in the formation of gastric and pancreatic juice and to block secretion by enzyme inhibition. These processes are relatively insensitive to ordinary doses of carbonic anhydrase inhibitors, and their pharmacological effect has no therapeutic applications.

Central Nervous System. An action of acetazolamide on the CNS was first suggested by the frequency of paresthesias and somnolence as side effects. Subsequently, the drug has been found to

inhibit epileptic seizures and to decrease the rate of spinal fluid formation. The exact mechanisms by which carbonic anhydrase inhibition is related to these changes in function are not clear, and multiple factors may be involved. Metabolic acidosis from ketogenic diets has long been known to diminish epileptic seizures, and acetazolamide, by virtue of its action on the kidney, leads to the production of a systemic acidosis. However, there is undoubtedly a more direct action on CNS function. An increase in local CO_2 tension may result from inhibition of the enzyme in the brain substance, the choroid plexus, or the erythrocytes of the cerebral blood. The exact role of carbonic anhydrase in brain function remains unknown. The concentration of the enzyme varies from one site to another within the brain (Roth *et al.,* 1959). Acetazolamide may reduce the rate of cerebrospinal fluid formation by the choroid plexus, but it may also transiently elevate cerebrospinal fluid pressure as a result of an increase in intracranial blood flow (Maren, 1967).

Respiration. The dynamic state of CO_2 in the blood and its transport between the blood and both the alveolar air sacs and the peripheral tissues are related to the carbonic anhydrase activity of the circulating erythrocytes. Acetazolamide may create a disequilibrium in the CO_2 transport system, giving rise to increased CO_2 tensions in the tissues and a decreased tension in the pulmonary alveoli. A decrease in the rate of CO_2 elimination may therefore result from acetazolamide administration, but this appears to be transient due to compensatory mechanisms.

At one time it was proposed that patients with respiratory insufficiency might be benefited by acetazolamide. However, the drug has been disappointing as a respiratory stimulant, and is no longer used for this purpose. When employed for other reasons, respiratory insufficiency is not considered a contraindication.

Absorption, Fate, and Excretion. Acetazolamide is readily absorbed from the gastrointestinal tract. Peak plasma concentrations occur within 2 hours. The drug is excreted by the kidney, and both active tubular secretion and passive reabsorption are involved. Excretion is complete within 24 hours. Acetazolamide is tightly bound to carbonic anhydrase and, consequently, is present in greater amounts in those tissues in which the enzyme is present in high concentration, particularly the erythrocytes and the renal cortex. Some carbonic anhydrase inhibitors do not penetrate the erythrocyte. Thus, renal and systemic drug actions may be dissociated on the basis of drug distribution (*see* Maren, 1967). Acetazolamide does not undergo metabolic alteration. Other analogs have been found to be inactive *in vitro* but active *in vivo,* as the result of N-dealkylation to form an active metabolite.

Preparations and Dosage. *Acetazolamide,* U.S.P. (DIAMOX), is available as *Acetazolamide Tablets,* U.S.P., each containing 125 or 250 mg, and as sustained-release capsules containing 500 mg. An effective single oral dose is 250 to 500 mg. Vials of *acetazolamide sodium* are available for parenteral administration. When used as a diuretic, it should be given once daily or every other day. To achieve a sustained metabolic acidosis, the drug should be given at intervals of 8 hours. *Dichlorphenamide,* U.S.P. (DARANIDE), is available as official 50-mg tablets. Optimal effects have been achieved with doses of 200 mg per day. *Methazolamide,* U.S.P. (NEPTAZANE), is available as official 50-mg tablets; the usual dose is 100 to 300 mg per day. *Ethoxzolamide,* U.S.P. (CARDRASE, ETHAMIDE), is available as official 125-mg tablets. An effective dose appears to vary from 125 to 1000 mg per day, given orally in divided doses.

Clinical Toxicity. Serious toxic reactions are infrequent. With large doses, many patients exhibit drowsiness and paresthesias. In hepatic cirrhosis, episodes of disorientation may be induced. The mechanism of this reaction is not clear; it has been postulated that urinary alkalinization diverts ammonia of renal origin from the urine into the systemic circulation. Hypersensitivity reactions are relatively rare. They consist in fever, skin reactions, bone-marrow depression, and sulfonamide-like renal lesions. Calculus formation and ureteral colic have been attributed to the marked reduction in urinary citrate produced by acetazolamide associated with either no change or even a rise in urinary calcium (Gordon and Sheps, 1957). Acetazolamide depresses the uptake of iodine by the thyroid gland. However, drugs of this class are not therapeutically useful as antithyroid agents.

THERAPEUTIC USES

Although undoubtedly effective in evoking a *diuresis,* the carbonic anhydrase inhibitors are relatively ineffective compared to newer and more efficacious agents. Acetazolamide has been given to *reduce intraocular pressure* in the management of glaucoma. It may also be employed for its *anticonvulsant action* for both grand mal and particularly petit mal epilepsy. Neither of these applications has gained wide acceptance.

There are several conditions in which *alkalinization of the urine* may itself be an appropriate thera-peutic goal. For example, chronic alkalinization is useful to prevent precipitation and calculus formation in cystinuria. To maintain electrolyte balance, sodium bicarbonate should be employed, rather than acetazolamide. In acute situations, of which *salicylate poisoning* is the prototype, alkalinization may be used to increase the renal excretion of lipid-soluble weak organic acids. The question of the relative merits of acetazolamide and sodium bicarbonate has been a subject of controversy. Theoretical objections to acetazolamide include its neurological actions and its direct inhibition of the renal tubular secretion of organic acids. The early superimposed respiratory alkalosis seen in some cases is a theoretical objection to the use of sodium bicarbonate, particularly in large doses. The concurrent use of acetazolamide and sodium bicarbonate has provided a satisfactory clinical response (Morgan and Polak, 1969) and has been studied experimentally in detail (Reimold *et al.,* 1973). For reasons that are totally obscure, acetazolamide appears to have a beneficial effect in the management of *periodic paralysis* even when associated with hypokalemia (Griggs *et al.,* 1970). Acetazolamide is also effective in ameliorating the symptoms of *acute mountain sickness* (Gray *et al.,* 1971). A radioactive complex has been proposed for renal scanning (Halpern *et al.,* 1972).

BENZOTHIADIAZIDES

History. This useful and important class of diuretics has an interesting history and provides an instructive example of the manner in which newly synthesized agents may be endowed with unanticipated pharmacological properties. They were first synthesized as an outgrowth of studies on carbonic anhydrase inhibitors. In the examination of certain benzenedisulfonamides, ring closure was found to occur between an acylamino group and the sulfamyl group *ortho* to it. This not only increased diuretic action but also changed fundamental characteristics of the diuresis. The voided urine contained increased amounts of chloride, a response significantly different from that evoked by the parent compounds, which were characteristic carbonic anhydrase inhibitors (*see* Beyer, 1958). Subsequent studies indicated that the benzothiadiazides have a direct effect on the renal tubular transport of sodium and chloride independent of carbonic anhydrase inactivation (Maren and Wiley, 1964).

Chlorothiazide was the first member of this class to be extensively studied. Although many analogs have been subsequently prepared, the basic pharmacological action is the same as for chlorothiazide.

Chemistry and Structure-Activity Relationship. Most compounds of this group are analogs of 1,2,4-benzothiadiazine-1,1-dioxide (*see* Table 39–3 for the parent structural formula and the substituents of the analogs that have received the most intensive study). As a group they can be designated as the "benzothiadiazide," or "thiazide," diuretics. The relationship between structure and activity is complex and depends not only on the chemical configuration of the compound but also on many physiological

Table 39-3. SUMMARY OF CHEMICAL STRUCTURES AND DIURETIC PROPERTIES OF BENZOTHIADIAZIDES *

Agent †	R_2	R_3	R'_3 - R_4	R_6	RANGE OF OPTIMALLY EFFECTIVE ORAL DIURETIC DOSE IN MAN (mg/day)	RELATIVE ORAL NATRIURETIC MAXIMAL RESPONSE IN MAN	EQUIEFFECTIVE CHLORURETIC I.V. DOSE IN THE DOG (mg/kg)	CARBONIC ANHYDRASE 50% INHIBITION IN VITRO (M)	MARKET PREPARATION (TABLETS) (mg)
Chlorothiazide	H	H	‡	Cl	500-2000	0.8	1.25	2×10^{-6}	250,500
Hydrochlorothiazide	H	H	H H	Cl	25-100	1.4	0.05	2×10^{-5}	25,50
Hydroflumethiazide	H	H	H H	CF_3	25-50	1.3	0.25	2×10^{-4}	50
Bendroflumethiazide	H	CH_2—(phenyl)	H H	CF_3	2-5	1.8	0.01	3×10^{-4}	2.5,5,5
Benzthiazide	H	CH_2—S—CH_2—(phenyl)	‡	Cl	25-50	1.3	0.01-0.05	$ca.\ 10^{-7}$	50
Hydrobenzthiazide	H	CH_2—S—CH_2—(phenyl)	H H	Cl	10-100	1.3	0.01-0.05	7×10^{-7}	—
Trichlormethiazide	H	$CHCl_2$	H H	Cl	4-8	1.7	0.01	6×10^{-5}	2,4
Methyclothiazide	CH_3	CH_2Cl	H H	Cl	5-10	1.8			2.5,5
Polythiazide	CH_3	$CH_2SCH_2CF_3$	H H	Cl	4-8	2.0	0.01-0.03	5×10^{-7}	1,2,4
Cyclothiazide	H	(bicyclic CH_2)	H H	Cl	1-6				2
Chlorthalidone	—	—	—	—	25-100	1.8	0.25	3×10^{-7}	50,100
Quinethazone	—	—	—	—	50-200	0.8			50
Metolazone	—	—	—	—	5-10	0.8	0.1	5×10^{-5}	2.5,5,10
Acetazolamide	—	—	—	—	250-375	0.25		7×10^{-8}	125,250

* Note the general agreement between the optimal oral dosage for man relative to the equieffective dosage by intravenous administration in the dog. The relative oral natriuretic response in man is based on the method of Ford (1961), who used careful metabolic regimens and doses in the general range indicated. The numerical values refer to potency ratios, with the natriuretic response to a standard dose of merallide being given the value of 1. Despite the extremely wide range of effective oral dosage, the usual natriuretic response by this assay varies less than threefold.

† The above-listed agents are available under the following nonproprietary and trade names: Chlorothiazide (U.S.P.): DIURIL. Hydrochlorothiazide (U.S.P.): ESIDREX, HYDRODIURIL, ORETIC. Hydroflumethiazide (N.F.): SALURON. Bendroflumethiazide (N.F.): NATURETIN. Benzthiazide (N.F.): EXNA. Trichlormethiazide (N.F.): METAHYDRIN, NAQUA. Methyclothiazide (N.F.): ENDURON. Polythiazide (N.F.): RENESE. Cyclothiazide (N.F.): ANHYDRON. Chlorthalidone (U.S.P.): HYGROTON. Quinethazone (N.F.): HYDROMOX. Metolazone: ZAROXOLYN. Acetazolamide (U.S.P.): DIAMOX.

‡ Unsaturated.

factors such as route of administration, rate of drug excretion, test assay system, and degree of edema or electrolyte imbalance. The problem has been reviewed by Beyer and Baer (1961). A limited number of generalizations can be made: (1) any stable substitution on the 7-sulfonamide group destroys carbonic anhydrase inhibitory activity; (2) substitutions at the same position decrease chloruretic activity but do not abolish it (Maren and Wiley, 1964), although the exact activity of N-7-acetyl derivatives is complicated by *in-vivo* deacetylation (Duggan, 1967); (3) there is no correlation between carbonic anhydrase inactivation *in vitro* and chloruretic response *in vivo;* (4) various halogen substitutions at the 6 position enhance chloruretic potency; (5) saturation of the heterocyclic ring between the 3 and 4 positions also increases potency; (6) a variety of substituents at the 3 position appear to increase diuretic potency; and (7) the addition of various functional groups at the 1, 4, or 5 position decreases diuretic activity. Some compounds have hyperglycemic activity, for which the structural requirements differ from those for diuresis (Wales *et al.,* 1968).

There are some other sulfonamide diuretics that differ chemically from the thiazides by the nature of the heterocyclic ring. However, their pharmacological action is indistinguishable from that of the thiazides. They have the following structures:

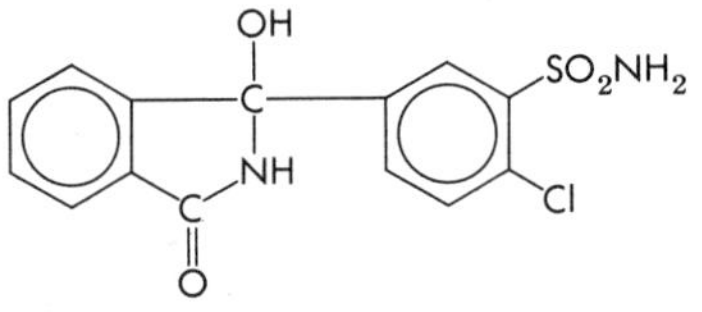

Chlorthalidone

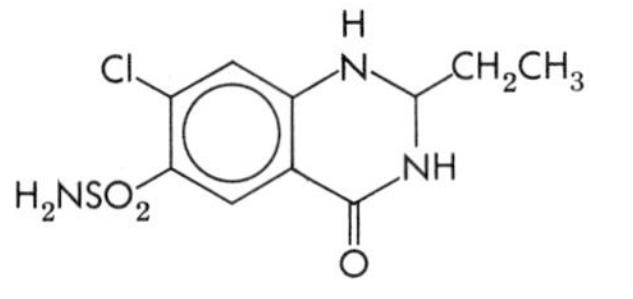

Quinethazone

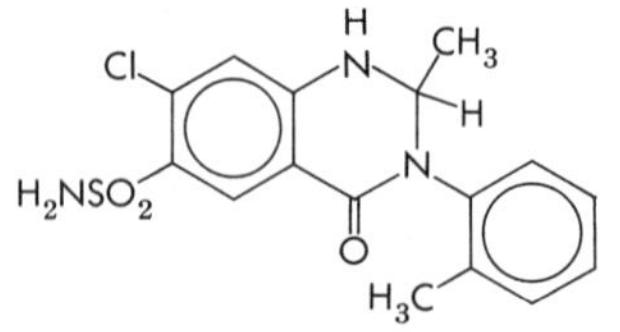

Metolazone

It should be emphasized that all thiazides thus far carefully examined have parallel dose-response curves and comparable maximal chloruretic effects. This implies that they have a similar mechanism of action. The various analogs differ primarily in the dose required to produce a given effect, and do not necessarily differ with respect to their maximal experimental effect or optimal therapeutic response. Comparative potencies vary, depending on the assay system. In general, data obtained in the dog and in clinical trials in man are in reasonable agreement.

In Table 39–3 is given a summary of approximate values from the literature.

PHARMACOLOGICAL PROPERTIES

Mechanism of Diuretic Action. The dominant action of the thiazides is to increase the renal excretion of sodium and chloride and an accompanying volume of water. Unlike both the mercurials and the carbonic anhydrase inhibitors, the action of the thiazides is virtually independent of acid-base balance. The thiazides also evoke a significant augmentation of potassium excretion in amounts sufficient to produce hypokalemia. The thiazides vary widely in their potency as inhibitors of carbonic anhydrase. Those that are active in this respect have the same action on bicarbonate transport by the kidney as does acetazolamide. The pharmacology and the therapeutic use of thiazides as hypotensive agents are considered in Chapter 33. In patients with diabetes insipidus, the thiazides *decrease* urinary volume. These actions are discussed in Chapter 40.

Effect on Renal Function. The unilateral renal intra-arterial injection of thiazides produces a unilateral diuretic response, indicating a direct renal action. Like many other organic acids, the thiazides are themselves secreted into the tubular fluid by an active process located in the proximal segment. The tubular transport of thiazides may be inhibited by probenecid. Depending on the thiazide, its dosage, and the solutes measured, its action on electrolyte transport may or may not be blocked (Beyer and Baer, 1961; Garcia and Yendt, 1970; Belair *et al.,* 1972). The nature of the chemical interaction between the thiazides and specific renal receptors responsible for the chloruretic effect is not known; no critical enzymatic reactions have been identified. It is of interest that nondiuretic thiazide analogs can block the chloruretic action of chlorothiazide without inhibiting urinary alkalinization, a finding interpreted as a competitive reaction for critical renal receptor sites (Ross and Cafruny, 1963).

The thiazides inhibit the reabsorption of sodium and its attendant anion, chloride, in the distal segment. This site of action is documented by different types of experiments, including free-water production, stop-flow analysis, and micropuncture (Goldberg, 1973). Bioelectrical studies suggest a direct action on the movement of sodium itself (Pendleton *et al.,* 1968).

As a class, the thiazides have an important action on *potassium* excretion. In most patients, a satisfactory chloruretic and natriuretic response is also accompanied by significant kaliuresis. (*See* Table 39–1.) Under some experimental conditions, and with selected thiazides, it has been possible partially to separate the effects on sodium and potassium. This can only be observed with minimal saluretic doses. At higher doses, all thiazides appear to share the same action on potassium. The augmented excretion of this cation results from its increased secretion by the distal tubule.

The *glomerular filtration* rate may be reduced by the thiazides, particularly with intravenous administration for experimental purposes. This is presumably the result of a direct action on the renal vasculature (*see* Hook *et al.,* 1966). It has little significance in the interpretation of primary drug action but may be of clinical importance, particularly in patients with diminished renal reserve.

The thiazides may decrease *uric acid* excretion in man, thus increasing its concentration in the plasma. Unlike most other natriuretic agents, the thiazides decrease the renal excretion of *calcium* by failing to block its reabsorption in the distal nephron, where sodium reabsorption is blocked; on the other hand, furosemide reduces the reabsorption of both cations proportionately (Edwards *et al.,* 1973). The excretion of *magnesium* is enhanced by the thiazides, leading to hypomagnesemia.

Iodide and *bromide* are excreted by renal mechanisms qualitatively similar to those for chloride. Diuretic agents that produce chloruresis fail to modify the discriminatory function of the tubule for the different halides (*see* McCarthy *et al.,* 1967). Thus, all chloruretic agents may be useful in the management of bromide intoxication. In addition, increased excretion of iodide, particularly with prolonged diuretic therapy, may produce slight iodine depletion (Mehbod *et al.,* 1967).

Effect on Composition of Extracellular Fluid. The thiazides tend to produce less distortion in the extracellular fluid composition than do other diuretic agents. This results from their multiple action on renal tubular transport, affecting not only the reabsorption of sodium and chloride but also H^+ secretion. For example, in the dog preloaded with sodium bicarbonate, the urine excreted after the administration of a thiazide contains relatively more bicarbonate than chloride. On the other hand, after pretreatment with ammonium chloride, bicarbonate excretion is decreased and chloruresis is enhanced in response to the drug.

Absorption, Fate, and Distribution. The thiazides are absorbed from the gastrointestinal tract and owe their usefulness largely to their effectiveness by the oral route. Absorption is relatively rapid. Most agents show a demonstrable diuretic effect within an hour after oral administration. In general, thiazides with relatively long durations of action show proportionately high degrees of both binding to plasma proteins and reabsorption by the renal tubules (*see* below). Chlorothiazide is distributed throughout the extracellular space and does not accumulate in tissues other than the kidney (Baer *et al.,* 1959). The drug passes readily through the placental barrier to the fetus. All thiazides probably undergo active secretion in the proximal tubule. The extent of this process may vary, as may the degree of subsequent reabsorption. The renal clearances of the drugs are therefore high and may be either above or below the rate of filtration. Most compounds are rapidly excreted within 3 to 6 hours. Bendroflumethiazide and polythiazide have a longer duration of action that is correlated with slower excretion (Piala *et al.,* 1961; Scriabine *et al.,* 1962). The same is true of chlorthalidone and metolazone. In the nephrectomized animal, chlorothiazide may be excreted in the bile; it does not undergo metabolic alteration.

Clinical Toxicity. In animal experiments, the demonstrable toxic dose of all the thiazides is manyfold that required for their pharmacological action. Clinical toxicity is relatively rare and usually results from unexpected hypersensitivity. Cases have been reported with purpura, dermatitis with photosensitivity, depression of the formed elements of the blood, and necrotizing vasculitis (*see* Harber *et al.,* 1959; Björnberg and Gisslén, 1965; Kutti and Weinfeld, 1968).

Plasma *potassium* concentration should be determined periodically in patients who receive thiazide diuretics for extended periods. In order to avoid a negative potassium balance, the thiazides are often prescribed in combination with potassium chloride. The use of *enteric-coated* combinations of potassium chloride and thiazide has been associated with a high incidence of ulceration of the distal jejunum or ileum. It is preferable to prescribe a palatable solution of potassium chloride, several of which are available. Alternatively, thiazide diuretics have been prescribed in combination with an aldosterone antagonist or other potassium-sparing diuretic (*see* below) in order to obtain an additive diuretic effect with maintenance of potassium balance. The plasma *uric acid* is frequently elevated and in susceptible patients may be associated with attacks of gout.

Borderline *renal* and/or *hepatic insufficiency* may be unpredictably aggravated by the thiazides. The mechanisms are not well understood. In patients, particularly those with hypertensive disease and decreased renal reserve, the manifestations of renal insufficiency may be aggravated after intensive or prolonged courses of thiazides that lead to excessive depletion of fluid and electrolyte. In cirrhosis of the liver, deterioration of mental function, including the onset of coma, has been attributed to thiazide therapy. Many observers have noted a correlation with hypokalemia and alkalosis. Increased concentrations of blood ammonia have been reported. The relationship between these findings, the reported signs and symptoms, and the action of the thiazides is not clearly established. Cholestatic hepatitis has also been reported.

The thiazides may induce *hyperglycemia* and aggravate preexisting diabetes mellitus (Dollery, 1973). Several mechanisms have been proposed, including inhibition of pancreatic release of insulin and blockade of peripheral glucose utilization. However, the exact mechanism is in doubt and may involve several factors. The disturbance in carbohydrate metabolism is relatively common and is probably unrelated to the much rarer toxic reaction of acute pancreatitis.

Preparations and Dosage. The thiazides are available as tablets for oral administration. The wide range of dosage is indicated in Table 39-3. In a few instances, preparations of the sodium salt are available for intravenous administration. However, this route offers no advantage for most therapeutic purposes.

Most of the thiazides are given in divided daily doses for the treatment of hypertension, but a single daily dose may be preferable for the mobilization of edema fluid. Trichlormethiazide, chlorthalidone, and polythiazide should be given less frequently, since they have a duration of action longer than 24 hours. The action of quinethazone and metolazone may also persist up to 24 hours. The thiazides are available as the pure preparations and should be administered as such. Combinations in a fixed-dose ratio with other diuretics or with other antihypertensive agents or potassium supplements are usually not recommended. However, fixed-dose combinations of aldosterone antagonists (*see* below) and hydrochlorothiazide are available and can be employed to advantage where the maintenance of potassium balance presents a problem.

THERAPEUTIC USES

The thiazides have their greatest usefulness as diuretics in the management of *edema* of chronic cardiac decompensation. Edema due to chronic hepatic or renal disease also responds favorably. When employed in *hypertensive disease,* with or without overt edema, these agents have a hypotensive action that has proven beneficial (*see* Chapter 33). Although the thiazide diuretics have been reported to produce an elevation of plasma renin activity, the clinical significance of this has not been established (Ganong, 1972). The thiazides have been effective diuretics in some patients with *nephrosis,* but their overall therapeutic usefulness has been unpredictable. When cardiac decompensation or hypertension is accompanied by significant impairment of renal function, the thiazides should be administered with caution because of their capacity to aggravate renal insufficiency.

Less common usages of the thiazides include the treatment of *diabetes insipidus* (*see* Chapter 40) and the management of *hypercalciuria* in patients with recurrent urinary calculi composed of calcium. Probenecid blunts the hypocalciuric action of the thiazides (Garcia and Yendt, 1970).

HIGH-CEILING DIURETICS

The term *high-ceiling* has been used to denote a group of diuretics that have a distinctive action on renal tubular function. These drugs effect a peak diuresis far greater than that observed with other agents. Other features that such drugs share in common are: (1) prompt onset of action, (2) inhibition of sodium and chloride transport in the ascending limb of the loop of Henle, and (3) independence of their action from acid-base balance changes. Ethacrynic acid and furosemide have been studied the most extensively, both clinically and experimentally. Bumetanide has been used in Europe but is not yet available for clinical use in the United States. Indapamide, which also is still unavailable, shares the high potency of bumetanide but has a longer duration of action; unlike the other drugs in this class, it is not a carboxylic acid.

Chemistry and Structure-Activity Relationship. These agents have the following chemical structures:

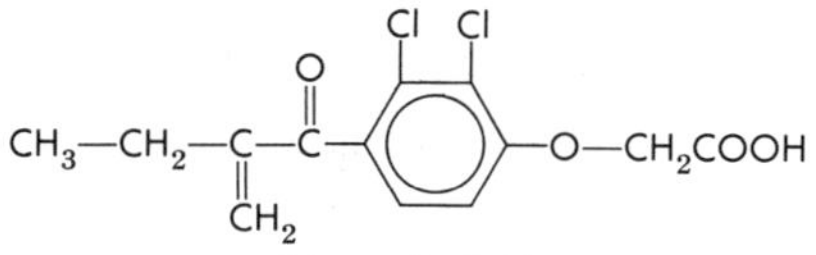

Ethacrynic Acid

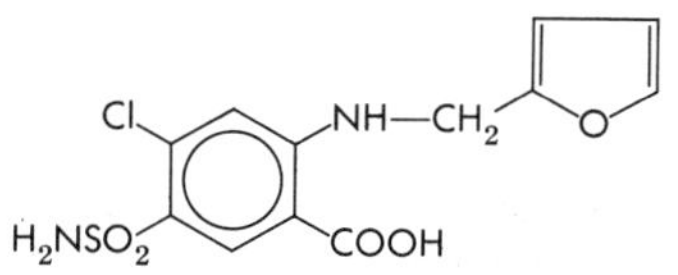

Furosemide

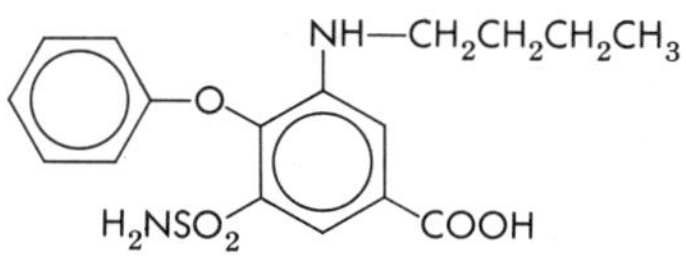

Bumetanide

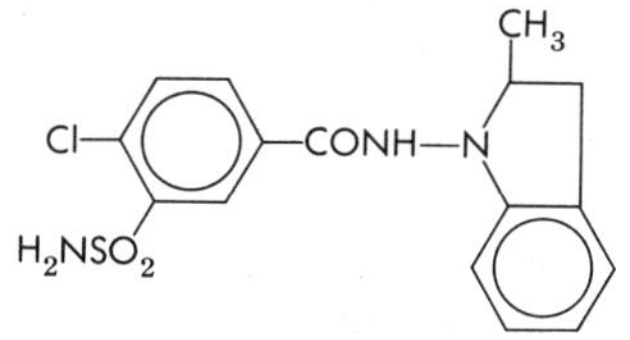

Indapamide

It is apparent that most of these drugs are carboxylic acids of moderately complex compounds having little else in common structurally; thus, they constitute a pharmacological, rather than a chemical, class.

Ethacrynic Acid. Unsaturated ketonic derivatives of aryloxyacetic acid were synthesized in the search for compounds that might react with critical renal sulfhydryl groups in a manner similar to that of the organic mercurials (Schultz *et al.*, 1962). Optimal diuretic activity depends on at least two structural requirements: (1) the methylene and adjacent ketone groups capable of reacting with sulfhydryl radicals of the presumed receptor, and (2) the substituents on the aromatic nucleus.

Furosemide. This drug is one of a series of anthranilic acid derivatives. Congeners differ in milligram potency but exhibit the same pharmacological spectrum.

Bumetanide. This compound is a 3-aminobenzoic acid derivative. Several analogs, which have various substituents, are about equally active in test animals (Feit, 1971). Bumetanide has a higher milligram potency than furosemide, but in other respects the compounds are similar.

Absorption, Distribution, and Excretion. The high-ceiling diuretics are readily absorbed from the gastrointestinal tract, and considerable proportions are bound to plasma proteins. They are rapidly excreted in the urine, by both glomerular filtration and tubular secretion. The rates of excretion are of such a magnitude that cumulation does not occur despite repeated administration. With oral ingestion, a diuretic response may be anticipated within an hour; with intravenous injection, within 2 to 10 minutes. (*See* Beyer *et al.*, 1965; Gayer, 1965; Østergaard *et al.*, 1972.)

Ethacrynic acid is bound to plasma protein. After intravenous injection, about one third of the dose is excreted by the liver and about two thirds by the kidney. The drug recovered from the urine is about equally divided into three fractions: the parent compound, a cysteine adduct, and an unstable metabolite of undetermined nature (Beyer *et al.*, 1965). Ethacrynic acid is secreted by the organic-acid secretory mechanism of the proximal tubule. The net rate of urinary secretion is also dependent on urinary pH. Thus, ethacrynic acid probably normally undergoes substantial back diffusion.

Furosemide is strongly bound to plasma proteins. Although urinary excretion is accomplished both by glomerular filtration and proximal tubular secretion, together this accounts for roughly only two thirds of the ingested dose. The remainder is excreted in the feces. A small fraction is metabolized by cleavage of the side chain (Beyer *et al.*, 1965; Gayer, 1965). An additional product, possibly a glucuronide conjugate, has also been found.

Bumetanide is strongly bound to plasma proteins. While the drug is largely excreted in the urine, in the nephrectomized animal the plasma concentration declines at an appreciable rate. No metabolites have been detected in the dog (Østergaard *et al.*, 1972).

Mechanism of Diuretic Action. In general, the time of onset and duration of diuresis with the agents in this class are shorter than with other classes of diuretics, such as mercurials or thiazides, but this depends to a considerable extent on concomitant changes in fluid balance. The duration of action varies with the particular renal function being measured (Figure 39-1).

The high-ceiling diuretics act primarily to inhibit sodium and chloride reabsorption in the ascending limb of the loop of Henle. This site has been localized as a result of the virtually complete inhibition of both positive and negative free-water production, and by micropuncture technics (*see* Edwards *et al.*, 1973; Goldberg, 1973; Suki *et al.*, 1973). In the isolated tubule, ethacrynic acid acts on the ascending limb to block the active reabsorption of chloride (Burg and Green, 1973c). The magnitude of peak electrolyte excretion is given in Tables 39-1 and 39-2. Unlike that which occurs with the organic mercurials and the inhibitors of carbonic anhydrase, the diuretic response is largely independent of acid-base balance. Inhibition of electrolyte reabsorption has also been observed in the proximal tubule (Morgan *et al.*, 1970). Indeed, the magnitude of the inhibition of tubular reabsorption can be explained only by multiple sites of action. The effect at the proximal site of action has been studied by micropuncture experiments, but it is uncertain to what extent this contributes to the diuresis observed *in vivo*. Actions on the distal tubule and collecting duct are controversial and of a minor degree.

Ethacrynic acid does not inhibit carbonic anhydrase *in vitro* and does not augment bicarbonate excretion (Beyer *et al.*, 1965). Since furosemide and bumetanide have unsubstituted sulfonamide side chains, they might be expected to inhibit carbonic an-

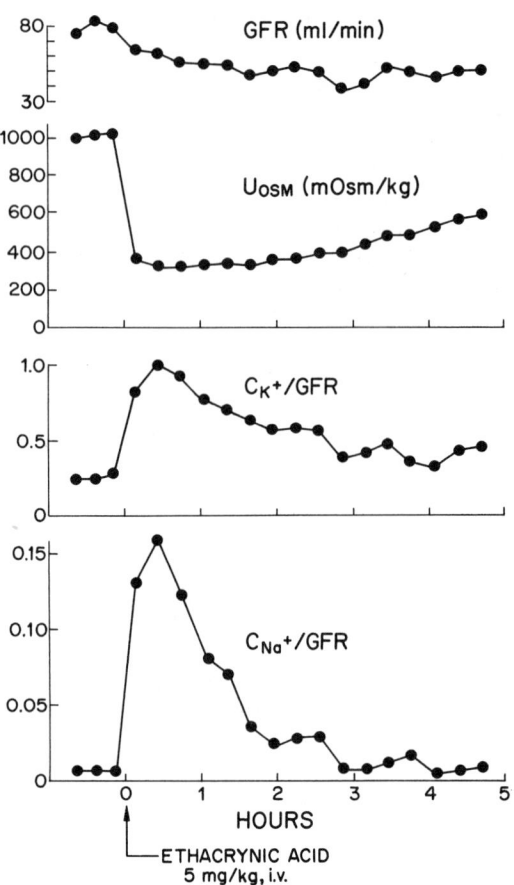

Figure 39-1. *Time course of ethacrynic acid diuresis.*

Observations were made in an anesthetized dog, infused with vasopressin and without volume replacement. Note the gradual reduction in glomerular filtration rate (GFR), which is probably the result of volume depletion. The immediate effect of the drug is a prompt fall in U_{OSM} to a U/P ratio of essentially unity, and an increase in the ratios C_{K^+}/GFR and C_{Na^+}/GFR. Note that the latter ratio returns toward control levels before the urinary concentrating ability is restored, as indicated by U_{OSM}. This discrepancy could be due either to the fact that, with a decrease in GFR, less sodium chloride is available for reabsorption by the ascending limb, or that there is a time lag involving the replenishment of solute to the medullary interstitium.

hydrase; however, as judged by their effect on bicarbonate excretion, such an action, if any, must be extremely weak (Stein *et al.*, 1968; Østergaard *et al.*, 1972).

The increase in *potassium* excretion results from its distal secretion and is approximately proportional to the increased rate of flow in this segment (Duarte *et al.*, 1971). The excretion of *magnesium* and *calcium* is increased by about the same percentage as that of sodium. The phosphaturic response is variable; for unexplained reasons, the natriuresis induced by furosemide may be accompanied by a decrease in the excretion of phosphate (Goldberg, 1973). The high-ceiling diuretics may cause *hyperuricemia* in man. Since these drugs are organic acids that are secreted in the proximal tubule, it is presumed that they act competitively to inhibit urate secretion at this site.

Depending on the experimental conditions, including the dose and speed of administration of the diuretic, either an increase or a decrease in renal blood flow, as well as its redistribution within the kidney, may occur. There is generally an increase in blood flow in the cortex, accompanied by a decrease in the outer medulla. (*See* Hook *et al.*, 1966; Birtch *et al.*, 1967; Dluhy *et al.*, 1970; Kilcoyne *et al.*, 1973; Stowe *et al.*, 1973.) These findings have raised the possibility that changes in intrarenal blood flow might influence electrolyte transport. Conversely, there is good evidence that acute diuresis increases tubular volume and intraluminal pressure; the latter might be transmitted and influence blood flow. Although renal vasodilatation may modify the response to these diuretics, this is a minor effect compared to their direct action on renal tubular transport. With proper clinical usage, renal blood flow is not compromised. These agents, like the thiazide diuretics, also stimulate the release of renin from the kidney (*see* Ganong, 1972). This complicates the analysis of a possible direct vasodilator effect. Furosemide, along with the thiazides and mercurials, greatly augments the urinary excretion of 5-hydroxytryptamine and depletes it from intrarenal stores (Kassab *et al.*, 1973).

Extrarenal Sites of Action. In isolated systems and with high doses, these agents act upon electrolyte transport in a variety of tissues. However, with usual doses the high-ceiling diuretics have no significant pharmacological effects other than on renal function. For example, there may be a slight decrease in bile flow (Erlinger *et al.*, 1970) or changes in the ionic fluxes of isolated erythrocytes (Dunn, 1973). These actions have no known clinical implications. An exception is the action on the inner ear, consisting in a depression of the cochlear microphonic and neural potentials, and a transient increase in the sodium and potassium concentrations in the endolymph (Brusilow and Gordes, 1973). This may result from a direct toxic action on the hair cells (Prazma *et al.*, 1972).

Biochemical Mechanism of Action. Ethacrynic acid was developed as an agent that would combine with thiol groups. There is ample evidence for this type of reaction. For example, the drug irreversibly combines with two thiol groups of glyceraldehyde 3-phosphate dehydrogenase, thus inactivating the enzyme (Birkitt, 1973). However, it is not possible to attribute diuretic action to this type of biochemical reaction, for at least three reasons. First, the other high-ceiling diuretics do not share the same reactivity with thiols. Second, the adduct of ethacrynic acid with cysteine is a more potent inhibitor of electrolyte transport than ethacrynic acid itself (Burg and Green, 1973c). And third, if one considers the thiol-dependent reactions of either aerobic or anaerobic metabolism, it is still unknown to what extent the overall rates of metabolism can be correlated with either electrolyte transport or drug action (Baer and Beyer, 1972; Bowman *et al.*, 1973; Klahr *et al.*, 1973). Some of the high-ceiling diuretics inactivate the Na^+,K^+-dependent adenosine triphosphatase (ATPase) of the kidney, but attempts to implicate this as the mechanism of drug action have encountered quantitative difficulties (Williamson, 1970; Epstein, 1973). Since ATPase is presumably directly related to cation transport, the problem is further compounded by the demonstration that ethacrynic acid acts on the primary transport of the chloride anion, as well as on that of the sodium cation. On an experimental basis, the metabolic actions of furosemide have been used to enhance the preservation of transplanted kidneys (Panijayanond *et al.*, 1973).

Comparative Diuretic Action. From the available data the drugs of this class have remarkably similar actions upon the kidney in most species. Ethacrynic acid and bumetanide are almost inactive in the rat, except at extremely high doses. In the dog and man, bumetanide is effective in a dose about 2% that of furosemide, but its maximal effect is the same. The diuretic action of this group of drugs may be additive to that of less effective agents, but the high-ceiling diuretics themselves are not additive to each other (Hook and Williamson, 1965a). One of the major differences between furosemide and ethacrynic acid is that the former has a broader dose-response curve. Accordingly, the therapeutic regimen may be initiated with rather small doses and adjusted upward to meet the needs of the individual patient.

Effect on Composition of Extracellular Fluid. Metabolic alkalosis may result from the use of the high-ceiling diuretics for essentially the same reason as with the mercurials, namely, the negative balance of extracellular fluid accompanied by a chloride loss relatively greater than that of bicarbonate. In the case of ethacrynic acid, an increase in the rate of hydrogen ion excretion may be a contributing factor (Cannon *et al.,* 1965). For all agents, potassium depletion may contribute to extracellular alkalosis. The *degree* of alkalosis depends on many factors, including the magnitude of diuresis and the intake of chloride salts, either as sodium chloride in the diet or as potassium or ammonium chloride as supplements. The significance of hypokalemia is discussed more fully at the end of the chapter.

Clinical Toxicity. From the extensive experience with ethacrynic acid and furosemide, two generalizations may be made: (1) fluid and electrolyte imbalance is the most common form of clinical toxicity, and (2) side reactions unrelated to primary drug action are quite rare. Hyperuricemia is relatively common, but in most patients it represents little more than a chemical abnormality. In susceptible subjects, attacks of gout may be precipitated. The other reactions include gastrointestinal disturbances (with or without bleeding), depression of formed elements in the blood, skin rashes, paresthesias, and hepatic dysfunction (*see* Kim *et al.,* 1971). Gastrointestinal side effects may be more frequent with ethacrynic acid than with furosemide. Furosemide and thiazides have been implicated as a cause of allergic interstitial nephritis, leading to reversible renal failure (Lyons *et al.,* 1973). A decrease in carbohydrate tolerance may occur, but to a lesser extent than with the thiazides (Dollery, 1973). The development of deafness, either transient or permanent, is a serious and rare complication with ethacrynic acid. Transient deafness has been reported with furosemide. Drug-induced changes in the electrolyte composition of the endolymph represent a possible mechanism. Due to the rarity of this complication, it is not possible to evaluate the contention that it is more common in the presence of renal insufficiency or that it occurs more commonly with one agent than with another. From available data, ototoxity from diuretics is unique to this class of drugs. If a potentially ototoxic antibiotic, such as an aminoglycoside, is being prescribed and concurrent diuretic therapy is indicated, it is advisable to use other diuretic agents such as thiazides or mercurials.

Preparations. *Ethacrynic Acid,* U.S.P. (EDECRIN), is available for oral use as 25- and 50-mg tablets.

The usual dose for adults is from 50 to 200 mg per day. The optimal dose should be determined for each patient, starting with minimal amounts. The sodium salt of ethacrynic acid is available for intravenous use as *Ethacrynate Sodium for Injection,* U.S.P. (EDECRIN SODIUM); the usual dose is 50 mg. *Furosemide,* U.S.P. (LASIX), is available as 20- and 40-mg tablets. In adults, the range of optimal dosage varies from 40 to 200 mg per day. A preparation is also available for parenteral administration, either intravenously or intramuscularly, in ampuls containing 20 mg/2 ml or 100 mg/10 ml of saline solution. The recommended adult dose by this route is 20 or 40 mg, repeated if necessary after not less than 2 hours.

Therapeutic Uses. The high-ceiling diuretics are effective for the treatment of *edema* of cardiac, hepatic, or renal origin. The oral route should be used unless impractical or the clinical situation demands a very prompt diuresis, in which case intravenous or intramuscular administration may be employed. This applies particularly to the management of *acute pulmonary edema.* In this condition the rapid reduction of the volume of extracellular fluid is of sufficient magnitude to reduce venous return and right ventricular output. In the management of refractory edema, the high-ceiling agents may be used in conjunction with other types of diuretics, particularly the potassium-sparing drugs, but there is no rationale for administering two high-ceiling agents concomitantly.

In the presence of *nephrosis* or *chronic renal failure,* doses far higher than usual may be required (Muth, 1973). By conventional measurements, renal function is not compromised by high doses. However, the incidence of undesirable side reactions may be increased (Allison and Kennedy, 1971). Ethacrynic acid and furosemide have been used in *acute renal failure.* Although case reports suggest the possibility that the maintenance of urine flow may prevent further renal damage (Stahl and Stone, 1970), caution is urged in the absence of a better understanding of basic mechanisms. There are increasing instances of renal insufficiency in which the use of multiple drugs, including diuretics, is suspected but not proven as a causative factor. In the case of cephaloridine-induced renal tubular necrosis, high-ceiling diuretics significantly increased renal damage in a controlled experiment (Dodds and Foord, 1970). In symptomatic *hypercalcemia* the high-ceiling diuretics may lower the plasma calcium concentration by increasing the renal excretion of calcium. This requires the replacement of urinary losses of sodium chloride and water (Suki *et al.,* 1970).

ALDOSTERONE ANTAGONISTS

The role of adrenocortical steroids in the regulation of electrolyte and water balance is discussed in Chapter 70. With greater insight into the chemistry of the steroids and with more complete knowledge of their physiological function, it has been possible to synthesize competitive antagonists that are useful as diuretics.

SPIRONOLACTONE

Chemistry. A number of 17-spirolactone steroids have been employed, of which *spironolactone* appears to have the greatest selectivity and efficacy. Its structural formula is as follows:

Spironolactone

Mechanism of Diuretic Action. Compounds of this type are considered as competitive antagonists of aldosterone, the most potent endogenous mineralocorticoid. Presumably they compete for receptor sites because they are homologs of the natural hormone, but they fail to evoke an active response. This concept is based on two general types of indirect evidence obtained from experiments *in vivo:* first, that the antagonist drug is effective only in the presence of either endogenous or exogenous aldosterone; second, that the action of the antagonist may be overcome by increasing the concentration of aldosterone (Kagawa *et al.,* 1959; Liddle, 1961).

The secretion of aldosterone is increased primarily by alterations in electrolyte balance, most importantly by a reduction in effective blood volume, hyponatremia, or hyperkalemia. In addition, angiotensin resulting from the release of renin by the kidney stimulates aldosterone production (*see* Chapter 30). Assay of aldosterone antagonists is usually undertaken experimentally following sodium chloride restriction. In clinical disorders, augmented aldosterone production is commonly associated with cirrhosis and less consistently with cardiac or nephrotic edema. Advanced renal hypertensive disease is accompanied by very high rates of aldosterone secretion.

The mineralocorticoids normally act to augment the renal tubular reabsorption of sodium and chloride, and to increase the excretion of potassium by facilitation of Na^+–K^+ exchange. Excessive mineralocorticoid activity leads to metabolic alkalosis in which potassium depletion plays a major role. Aldosterone has little direct action on the Na^+–H^+ exchange mechanism of the renal tubule; that is, its effect on acid-base balance is secondary to alterations in potassium balance. In the absence of adrenal function, there is an increased excretion of sodium and chloride, or, stated more exactly, sodium and chloride excretion persists even in the presence of depleted body stores, whereas in the normal subject such a condition is associated with extremely low excretory rates. On this basis, one would anticipate that the antagonism of the action of the steroids would result in only a slight increase in electrolyte and water excretion. This is in contrast to the much higher excretion rates evoked by many other diuretics that act on other aspects of the tubular transport mechanisms. In addition, potassium excretion is increased by aldosterone and decreased by the antagonism of its action. Hence, under controlled conditions the urinary Na^+:K^+ ratio serves as an indirect index of aldosterone activity. Spironolactone increases calcium excretion through a direct effect on tubular transport (Wills *et al.,* 1969).

Agents that inhibit the synthesis of aldosterone by the adrenal cortex theoretically have potential diuretic activity, but these are not of practical usefulness.

Preparations. *Spironolactone,* U.S.P. (ALDACTONE), a microcrystalline preparation, is available in official 25-mg oral tablets. It is effective in an average daily dose of 100 mg, given in divided doses.

Clinical Use. The aldosterone antagonists have been used mostly in the management of *refractory edema.* Frequently, they have been employed in conjunction with other diuretic agents rather than as the sole drug. On theoretical grounds, the potassium loss that occurs secondary to the use of other diuretics may be decreased by the coadministration of aldosterone antagonists. In general this has been substantiated by clinical experience. However, the quantitative effects are not exactly predictable, due to the complex interactions of the primary disease, the degree of secondary hyperaldosteronism, and the actions of the diuretics given concomitantly. In edematous patients with advanced renal insufficiency, aldosterone antagonists may induce significant hyperkalemia even if administered concurrently with a thiazide.

Competitive aldosterone antagonists, as well as potassium-retaining agents, are also useful in both the diagnosis and the management of those rare metabolic and renal diseases associated with hypokalemia and potassium depletion (*see* Liddle, 1966).

POTASSIUM-SPARING DIURETICS

During the last several decades, the introduction of new natriuretic agents has been accompanied by parallel studies on the secretion of potassium. These have established (1) that potassium excretion is achieved by distal tubular secretion, (2) that excessive potassium losses may constitute an unfavorable consequence of diuretic action, (3) that the excretion of potassium can be influenced by steroids with mineralocorticoid activity, and (4) that the loss of potassium may also be influenced by drugs that act directly on the distal nephron independently of adrenal steroids. While it is true that triamterene and amiloride possess moderate natriuretic activity, nevertheless their major importance lies in their effect on potassium excretion (Baer and Beyer, 1972).

TRIAMTERENE

Chemistry. Triamterene has the following structural formula:

Triamterene

It is a pteridine compound, related chemically to folic acid. The diuretic activity of closely related homologs of triamterene has been examined, but no specific structural requirements have been established (Maass and Wiebelhaus, 1967). In another series of pteridine compounds, it is possible to demonstrate natriuretic activity with agents that have no potassium-retaining action (Rosenthale and Osdene, 1966). Triamterene is a weak competitive inhibitor of folic acid *in vitro*, but it has no significant antifolic activity *in vivo* (Maass *et al.*, 1967).

Absorption, Distribution, and Excretion. Triamterene is relatively insoluble in water and is administered only by the oral route. It is rapidly absorbed from the gastrointestinal tract and is then excreted in the urine, with a peak in renal excretion within 1 to 2 hours after oral ingestion. From 10 to 88%

of the oral dose can be recovered from the urine within 24 hours. It is probable that this wide range of values is a reflection of variable intestinal absorption. In the plasma, triamterene is about two-thirds bound to protein. Renal excretion is accomplished both by filtration and tubular secretion (Lassen and Nielsen, 1963).

Mechanism of Diuretic Action. Triamterene has no significant pharmacological actions other than those on the kidney. As indicated in Table 39-1, diuresis is characterized by an increase in the excretion of sodium, mostly accompanied by chloride as the anion, and under some circumstances by slight alkalinization of the urine. Compared to acetazolamide, this latter effect is quantitatively of little importance as far as extracellular electrolyte balance is concerned. Triamterene is not an inhibitor of carbonic anhydrase. The exact mechanisms by which it slightly alkalinizes the urine remain unexplained. Under normal circumstances, diuresis is accompanied either by no increase in potassium excretion or by only a slight increase. However, the effect of triamterene on potassium excretion may be greatly modified by pharmacological means, and a sharp reduction in potassium output is then observed. This is particularly noted when other natriuretic agents are given simultaneously, and when there is an excessive amount of mineralocorticoids, either by pretreatment or by spontaneous production (*see* Wiebelhaus *et al.*, 1967). The action of triamterene is not significantly altered by alkalosis or acidosis.

Originally considered a nonsteroidal competitive antagonist of aldosterone, triamterene has subsequently been shown to have a natriuretic effect in the adrenalectomized animal that is not significantly different from that in the normal. It is presumed, therefore, that the action of triamterene is directly on tubular transport and is independent of aldosterone. The reduced rate of potassium excretion results from an inhibition of the secretion of potassium in the distal nephron. This effect is achieved by a primary reduction in sodium reabsorption, which in turn leads to a drop in the transtubular electrical-potential difference. It is the latter that is normally the driving force for potassium secretion (Gatzy, 1971). The slight effect on urinary acidification is also probably distal. Under some circumstances, triamterene may be slightly uricosuric, but the mechanism of this action has not been examined. Unlike other diuretics, triamterene does not appear to cause urate retention.

Clinical Toxicity. Triamterene produces relatively few side effects. The most common are nausea, vomiting, leg cramps, and dizziness. Slight-to-moderate azotemia is relatively common. This does not appear to be directly related to electrolyte and water imbalance and is reversible.

Preparations. *Triamterene,* U.S.P. (DYRENIUM), is administered only by the oral route. It is marketed in capsules containing 100 mg. The usual initial dose is 100 mg, given twice daily. The maximal dose is 300 mg. The maintenance dose should be determined for the individual patient and may be as low as 100 mg every other day.

Therapeutic Uses. Some patients with *edema* have a satisfactory diuretic response to triamterene alone. However, the available clinical data suggest that the greatest usefulness of this drug may be in conjunction with other diuretic agents. In general, the administration of triamterene with another natriuretic compound augments natriuresis and reduces potassium loss. With concurrent drug therapy, it is this latter effect that is more consistently observed. Therefore, the rationale of concomitant drug therapy is primarily in relation to potassium metabolism. Hansen and Bender (1967) summarized the experience obtained from several hundred patients maintained on long-term regimens with triamterene alone, chlorothiazide alone, and both drugs together, and showed that both drugs together provided the highest incidence of normal plasma potassium values. Because of the real possibility of inducing serious hyperkalemia, patients treated with triamterene should *not* receive supplements of potassium.

AMILORIDE

Amiloride is an organic base with the following structural formula:

Amiloride

Absorption, Distribution, and Metabolism. After oral administration, from 15 to 26% of the drug is absorbed from the gastrointestinal tract. When given parenterally, amiloride is almost completely excreted in the urine. The urinary product appears to be identical to the parent compound. However, closely related congeners may become pharmacologically active by conversion to amiloride. After oral administration, the action of amiloride on the kidney reaches a peak within about 6 hours and usually ceases within 24 hours.

Pharmacological Actions. In the usual dosage, amiloride has no important pharmacological actions except those related to the renal tubular transport of electrolytes. Under normal conditions, amiloride slightly increases the renal excretion of sodium and chloride without a significant change in the glomerular filtration rate. At the same time, there may be a moderate increase in urinary pH, indicative of a lesser degree of hydrogen ion secretion. The finding of greatest interest is that, under all conditions tested, natriuresis is associated with either only a slight increase or sometimes an absolute decrease in potassium excretion. This effect of amiloride is undoubtedly most striking when it is given together with more potent saluretic agents. Under these conditions, the effect of amiloride is approximately additive as far as sodium and chloride excretion is concerned, but it is antagonistic with respect to potassium. Many diuretics, such as the thiazides, furosemide, and ethacrynic acid, normally increase potassium output severalfold. This response is greatly ameliorated under the simultaneous influence of amiloride.

By analogy with the more direct studies of the mechanisms of electrolyte transport in the toad bladder, it is postulated that amiloride inhibits the secretion of potassium in essentially the same manner as does triamterene (Gatzy, 1971). The slight action of amiloride on hydrogen ion transport remains unexplained; the drug is not an inhibitor of carbonic anhydrase.

Although amiloride has an overall effect on electrolyte excretion qualitatively similar to that of antagonists of aldosterone, it should be emphasized that it does not act as a competitive antagonist. Since amiloride retains its activity in the absence of adrenal steroids, it is clear that its action at the cellular level of transport is independent of the presence of the steroid hormones (*see* Baer *et al.,* 1967; Bull and Laragh, 1968).

Preparations and Clinical Use. While *amiloride hydrochloride* (MIDAMOR) is employed extensively in Europe, particularly in combination with hydrochlorothiazide, it is not available in the United States.

XANTHINES, PYRIMIDINES, AND TRIAZINES

Historically, the xanthines have long been known for their diuretic action. Their additional pharmacological properties are discussed in Chapter 19. Of the xanthines, theophylline has the greatest action on the kidney. Within recent years, a large number of remotely related heterocyclic nitrogenous compounds have been synthesized and assayed for their diuretic activity. *Amisometradine* and *chlorazanil* are representative aminouracils of this heterogeneous group. Their structural formulas appear on the next page.

Chlorazanil

Amisometradine

Mechanism of Diuretic Action. The stimulatory effect of the xanthines on cardiac function has raised the possibility that diuresis may be the result, in part, of increased renal blood flow and glomerular filtration rate. However, all drugs in this class appear to have a direct action on the renal tubule. The urinary response involves an increase in the rate of sodium and chloride excretion, with no significant effect on urinary acidification. Diuretic action is only slightly affected by changes in acid-base balance, but is potentiated by the coadministration of carbonic anhydrase inhibitors. It has been postulated that intracellular pH directly affects the intrarenal action of these agents (Nechay, 1964). Augmentation of potassium excretion is not remarkable. Unlike the mercurials, the xanthines do not inhibit potassium secretion. Chlorazanil may have a more selective action on potassium transport, as suggested by the blockade of the kaliuretic action of acetazolamide (Williamson et al., 1959); it may possibly act as a weak steroidal antagonist (Skulan and Shideman, 1965). Theophylline has been a useful agent in the study of cellular metabolism and its relation to water and electrolyte permeability (see Handler et al., 1968).

Preparations and Dosage. Preparations of the xanthines are discussed elsewhere. Amisometradine and chlorazinil are not currently available for general use.

Clinical Application. In clinical practice, these agents have received relatively limited application. In general, they do not have the efficacy of other diuretics. Continued use often leads to the loss of their effectiveness for reasons that have not been adequately explained. In addition, gastric irritation becomes a limiting factor with some agents.

THE CLINICAL USE OF DIURETICS

The Pathological Physiology of Edema Formation. The normal volume and composition of the extracellular fluid are regulated by multiple interacting mechanisms. In a healthy adult subject, changes in dietary intake or variations in the extrarenal loss of fluid and electrolytes are accompanied by relatively rapid and sensitive adjustments in the rate of renal excretion. Several factors play an important role in determining the distribution of extracellular fluid within the body and, as a consequence, in defining the nature of the stimuli that directly or indirectly influence the excretory functions of the kidney.

Edema is an increase in extracellular fluid volume. Accordingly, it represents a quantitative change in a normal component of the body. Theoretically, edema could occur in two ways, either from an abnormally high intake of water and electrolyte, or from an abnormally low rate of sodium excretion. Under exceptional experimental circumstances, or as the result of excessively vigorous parenteral fluid therapy, it is possible for edema to result from too great a fluid or electrolyte intake. However, with normal renal function, such a condition is short lived.

In the edematous states usually encountered in clinical medicine, in virtually every instance the underlying abnormality involves a decreased rate of renal excretion. This applies regardless of the underlying pathogenesis of the disease, whether cardiac, hepatic, or renal, or of some other etiology.

The normal relationship between the volumes of interstitial fluid and the circulating plasma depends on dynamic equilibria across the capillary membrane and involves the pressure within the small blood vessels, the osmotic activity of the plasma proteins, the pressure within the tissue spaces, and the flow of lymph (see Chapter 36). Possibly other factors may also be involved, such as the effect of disease or the action of steroids, that may conceivably alter the state of the capillaries themselves. In diseases of hepatic origin, particularly cirrhosis, the pressure relationships are disturbed primarily within the portal circulation, and the formation of edema becomes manifest as ascites. In congestive heart failure, pressure-flow relationships may be disturbed relatively more in either the systemic or the pulmonary circulation, and edema may be localized accordingly. In the nephrotic syndrome or other hypoproteinemic states, the equilibrium across all capillary membranes tends to be altered and edema fluid accumulates in a variety of tissues. However, in each instance the formation of significantly increased amounts of extracellular fluid is either preceded or accompanied by decreased rates of renal excretion.

There is overwhelming evidence to indicate that the primary disturbance in renal function involves the capacity of the kidney to excrete electrolyte. Sodium, chloride, and bicarbonate are quantitatively the most important ions of the extracellular fluid, and, of these, it is primarily the regulation of sodium excretion that is disturbed in the pathogenesis of edema. Retention of extracellular electrolyte is accompanied by the retention of a proportional amount of water and, as a result, the increased volume of extracellular fluid is usually of normal composition and osmolality. However, particularly in severe instances of cardiac or hepatic decompensation, water retention may be relatively greater than that of electrolyte, and hypoosmolality results. Most frequently this is measured in terms of the plasma sodium concentration, that is, as hyponatremia.

The exact mechanisms by which the kidney retains excessive amounts of sodium have been intensively examined. Multiple factors are involved, each of which may vary in importance depending on the underlying etiology. In many edematous states, increased rates of aldosterone secretion have been correlated with increased tubular reabsorption of sodium. In addition, particularly in cardiac decompensation, the glomerular filtration rate may be reduced, thus providing a diminished filtered load on which the tubular reabsorptive mechanism operates. This frequently can be correlated with a decreased concentration of urinary sodium. However, quantitative studies, both in disease and under experimental conditions, have failed to provide a predictable relationship between the rate of sodium excretion and either the amount of sodium filtered or the activity of aldosterone. For this reason, a "third factor" has been postulated that might regulate sodium reabsorption and excretion. However, at the moment, the nature of this factor is obscure and, indeed, several factors may be involved.

Relationship of Drug Action to Pathological Physiology.

When the tubule reabsorbs excessive amounts of electrolyte and edema fluid accumulates, three therapeutic approaches are available to mobilize the fluid and thereafter maintain the constancy of the extracellular fluid volume. The first is to correct the primary disease, if possible. This is, of course, the most desirable goal, but it cannot always be achieved. The second is to suppress renal tubular reabsorptive capacity by the use of drugs. The third is to reduce the amount of sodium salts absorbed from the gastrointestinal tract to a degree commensurate with the diminished renal capacity for their excretion. This is achieved primarily by a low-salt diet. In edema of cardiac origin, the first approach is almost invariably employed. Often all three approaches have to be combined.

Diuretic Drugs in the Treatment of Cardiac Edema.

Our increased understanding of the pathological physiology of cardiac decompensation and of the nature of edema formation makes it clear that the total syndrome cannot be evaluated adequately in terms of a few simple causal relationships, but that multiple interactions are involved, many of a compensatory nature, some representing overcompensations. Granted the primary role of the cardiac dysfunction in the etiology of cardiac decompensation, nevertheless, the additional contributory roles of secondary physiological abnormalities cannot be denied. Yet it is clear that when the extensive electrolyte reabsorption is blocked, either by aldosterone antagonists or other drugs acting directly on the renal tubule, a chain of events is initiated that not only alleviates the symptoms of cardiac failure but also, by objective measurements, leads to an apparent improvement in myocardial

performance. Accordingly, it is reasonable to approach the therapy of cardiac decompensation in the belief that the appropriate correction of edema with diuretic agents may be beneficial to the total cardiac status.

Certain practical distinctions may be made between the therapeutic regimens directed toward the mobilization of edema fluid and toward the maintenance of the edema-free state. In general, these distinctions refer to the choice of the type of diuretic, the route of administration, and the dosage. In all patients with cardiac decompensation, digitalis should be administered in full, adequate dosage and should be considered the primary therapeutic agent. Diuretic drugs acting directly on the kidney, irrespective of their potency or effectiveness, must be considered to have a secondary, albeit important, role. The development of potent new diuretics may have focused excessive attention on diuresis *per se,* and has led to the inadequate digitalization of some patients. With the large number of diuretics now available, the choice of the agent depends primarily on the speed and magnitude of its action.

Ascites. The diuretics are extensively employed in the management of ascites, especially when associated with *cirrhosis* of the liver. Periodic administration either eliminates the necessity for or reduces the interval between paracenteses. Not only does a diuretic regimen contribute to the comfort of the patient, but also his meager protein reserves are spared inasmuch as significant amounts of protein are lost when ascitic fluid is mechanically withdrawn. Many types of diuretics having a direct renal action may be prescribed. If effective, a single drug should be employed. However, since cirrhotic edema may be exceptionally refractory, the concomitant use of different types of agents is often indicated. Secondary hyperaldosteronism is an underlying factor influencing the diuretic response. Electrolyte imbalance is a frequent complication of diuretic therapy in cirrhosis. Because of this, diuretics should be employed in the smallest possible doses. In severely ill patients there is a greater risk of too vigorous therapy, and it may be advisable purposefully to aim for less than the complete mobilization of edema (Sherlock, 1973). With mild, asymptomatic, or residual ascites, no useful purpose is served in attempting to make the patient completely free of edema if this involves the persistent administration of diuretics and the production of hypovolemia or electrolyte imbalances.

Renal Disease. With the introduction of new and more potent diuretics, there has been a gradual change in their use in the management of diseases of the kidney. As a general rule, *chronic renal disease* with edema may be treated in the same manner as other edematous states, with the recognition that these patients are more subject to electrolyte imbalance. In the presence of primary renal disease there is often a lesser effect of the diuretic on tubular function. In the case of the high-ceiling diuretics, particularly furosemide, an increased dose is required. This can be accomplished without any direct deleterious effect on the underlying renal disease

(Muth, 1973). The thiazides are relatively less effective and in high doses may decrease the glomerular filtration rate. The mercurials are effective to a variable degree. However, if the desired diuresis is not obtained, one should discontinue them rather than increase the dose. In *acute glomerular nephritis,* hypervolemia and edema are often self-limited. If diuretics are required, mercurials should be avoided because of their ineffectiveness and their potential nephrotoxicity in this condition.

In the *nephrotic syndrome,* the response to diuretic agents is often disappointing. Although hypoproteinemia is a major etiological factor, the administration of albumin produces a minimal and unpredictable diuretic response. Mercurials are frequently ineffective. Thiazides, ethacrynic acid, furosemide, and aldosterone antagonists are the most successful. The important role of the corticosteroids in the management of the nephrotic syndrome is discussed elsewhere. Their influence on the course of nephrotic edema is related either to an increase in glomerular filtration rate or to an action on the underlying disease process, rather than to a direct effect on the renal handling of electrolyte.

In incipient *acute renal failure,* diuretics have been used to maintain urine flow in the hope that this may diminish further renal damage. The success of this practice is difficult to evaluate. The problem is discussed in the section on osmotic diuretics and in Chapter 36. The theoretical hazards of high-ceiling diuretics have been previously outlined.

Complications of Diuretic Therapy. With the availability of powerful diuretics, there has been an increased incidence of complications in the management of the edematous state that may be directly attributed to the diuresis itself. It should be remembered that the goal of diuretic therapy is the mobilization of edema fluid in such a manner that the extracellular fluid is restored toward normal, in terms of both volume and composition. Electrolyte imbalance occurs when the volume change is excessive or too rapid, or when the diuresis itself results in an alteration in the electrolyte composition of either the extracellular or the intracellular fluid. The deleterious effects of fluid and electrolyte imbalance are seen particularly with the high-ceiling diuretics, not only because of the *magnitude* of the imbalance itself but also, perhaps more importantly, because of the *rapidity* of its development. The *excessively rapid mobilization* of edema may lead to malaise and asthenia. Rapid changes in the pressure-flow relationships in the cardiovascular system may, even in the presence of an expanded extracellular fluid volume, give rise to symptoms usually associated with

hypovolemia. In intensive long-term therapy, the diuretic-induced renal loss of sodium chloride may lead to *extracellular fluid depletion,* with or without hyponatremia. By definition, in both acute and chronic extracellular fluid depletion, there is a reduced amount of sodium in the extracellular space. The condition usually responds to discontinuation of the diuretic agent and the liberalization of sodium chloride intake in the diet. Both these conditions are relatively rare, although undoubtedly more frequent with the introduction of the more efficacious agents.

A far more common condition, particularly in congestive heart failure and hepatic cirrhosis, is *chronic dilutional hyponatremia.* This is associated with persistent edema and expanded extracellular volume. It may occur solely as a result of the underlying disease, but is most often seen as a consequence of diuretic therapy. The physiological defect results from the inability of the patient to excrete an adequately dilute urine. The distal generation of positive free water is defective. This is attributed to an inadequate sodium load to this segment of the nephron. Water restriction is the most direct therapeutic approach, but may be complicated by uncontrollable thirst. Whether the diuretic regimen should be continued or altered is a perplexing problem for which there is no clear answer (*see* Jick, 1966; Walker, 1966).

The *alkalosis* resulting from mercurial or high-ceiling diuretics is largely due to the relatively excessive loss of chloride. Although usually only moderate, the alkalosis may at times be extreme (DeRubertis *et al.,* 1970). It may be corrected by ammonium chloride administration, thus excluding an obligatory role of potassium loss in its pathogenesis. However, supplements of potassium chloride also serve to lessen the alkalosis.

Many diuretics have a variable kaliuretic effect. The resultant *hypokalemia* increases the toxicity of digitalis. In addition, *hyperkalemia* may also result when excessively massive diuresis leads to acute hypovolemia and renal failure, or if potassium-sparing diuretics are used injudiciously. With most diuretics, the magnitude of potassium excretion is often unpredictable. In addition to the type and the dosage of the diuretic itself, the other major determinant of kaliuresis is the activity of the distal secretory mechanism for potassium, which is influenced by aldosterone (Espiner *et al.,* 1967). True *potassium depletion,* with an intracellular deficit, may occur as a result of chronic diuretic therapy. However, there is no simple correlation between the degree of hypokalemia and the total deficit.

Dietary supplements of potassium may be prescribed, but they are contraindicated with triamterene or aldosterone antagonists. The use of *enteric-coated* potassium chloride–diuretic drug preparations should be avoided for reasons stated above. The extent to which supplements prevent or correct potassium depletion in patients on long-term diuretic therapy varies from one patient to another (McKenna *et al.,* 1971; Down *et al.,* 1972; Edmonds and Jasani, 1972). An important variable is the dietary intake of potassium, which is often reduced in chronically ill patients. Inadequate treatment of potassium deficits leads to a sustained catabolic state with progressive nitrogen loss. These derangements are readily prevented or reversed by appropriate supplemental potassium therapy (Walker *et al.,* 1973).

The rationale for the administration of spironolactone and triamterene has been discussed in connection with these agents. The magnitude and the frequency of potassium depletion are undoubtedly greater with the newer oral agents, other than the aldosterone antagonists and triamterene, in comparison to the mercurials. This is usually attributed to an effect of the individual drugs. However, the dosage regimen may be an extremely important factor. The newer agents are often used continually; the mercurials were given intermittently, and, when the kidney was not under their influence, potassium was conserved. *An intermittent dosage schedule for the oral agents would undoubtedly reduce the severity of potassium depletion.*

Both extracellular and intracellular *magnesium depletion* may result from the use of diuretics. Since magnesium and potassium deficits may interact, the problem is complex and warrants more extensive evaluation (*see* Lim and Jacob, 1972).

Refractory Edema. The increasing attention being given to so-called refractory edema is, in fact, partly attributable to the high degree of success in the management of the less severely ill patient. This has enabled many patients with cardiac decompensation to survive longer in an edema-free state. With the progression of the underlying disease, these patients consequently tend to become edematous at a time when their cardiac reserve is significantly more impaired than in the earlier years of their illness. Nevertheless, the patient with persistent and incapacitating edema represents a major therapeutic challenge.

In addition to the factors implicit in the nature of the underlying disease, the pharmacological properties of diuretic drugs must themselves be considered to be important and common causes of diuretic refractoriness. With many drugs, diuretic efficacy is decreased by hyponatremia. With others, specific abnormalities of electrolyte metabolism lead to the refractory state. An additional factor in drug refractoriness is the reduction in glomerular filtration rate. This may be related to the underlying disease state and may also be the result of prior diuretic therapy. It should also be emphasized that diuresis is limited in an overall sense by the extracellular fluid volume. As edema subsides, the response to an individual dose of most drugs diminishes until, as the edema-free state is approached, the magnitude of diuresis is necessarily smaller than at the height of the edema.

When a patient becomes refractory to a diuretic, the entire regimen should be reevaluated. In some instances, minor adjustments of dosage may suffice. Bed rest itself may restore drug responsiveness, due to improvement in the renal circulation. Abnormalities of extracellular fluid composition should be sought for and corrected. The administration of additional diuretics may be appropriate. In some patients, for reasons that are not clear, the use of corticosteroids has appeared to restore responsiveness to a diuretic regimen (Kessler *et al.,* 1962; Jick, 1966).

As a general rule, patients who are refractory to a diuretic of moderate efficacy, such as the thiazides, will show a more satisfactory response to more powerful agents. However, there is great individual variation. In a few patients, for unknown reasons, the less active agents are effective when there is no response to the more powerful drugs.

Use of Multiple Diuretics and Adjuvant Agents. The current availability of many different types of diuretics and many different compounds of the same type has provided the temptation to alter the diuretic regimen at frequent intervals. In the *initial management* of the edematous subject, when *mobilization* of edema fluid is the primary goal of therapy, the changing status of the patient warrants appropriate adjustments in dosage schedules and also in the agents selected for use. However, in the *chronic management* of edema, the best therapeutic results are often correlated with a purposefully constant therapeutic regimen. Minor variations in dosage are warranted on the basis of careful observation.

Despite the widespread use of the high-ceiling diuretics for the treatment of chronic edema, especially of cardiac origin, one may properly raise the question of their overuse in situations in which other diuretics, although less effective by conventional standards, might equally well achieve the desired therapeutic goal with less risk of overtreatment.

In the severely edematous patient, it is becoming apparent that, if a single diuretic agent proves ineffective, it is proper to use more than one type of diuretic agent. Such a program is most easily supervised if one diuretic is given in a relatively constant dose and the second administered intermittently under careful observation. Urine volume or body weight should be accurately measured so that drug effectiveness does not depend on vague impressions. When effective, the results of concomitant therapy are usually supra-additive rather than simply additive. Of course, nothing is to be gained by the administration of two drugs of the same type, such as two different thiazides. Specific examples of rational concurrent therapy with diuretics have been cited in the discussion of individual drugs. It is reemphasized that each agent should be given in an optimally individualized dose and that combinations in a fixed-dose ratio may be less effective unless appropriate for the individual patient.

Allison, M. E. M., and Kennedy, A. C. Diuretics in chronic renal disease: a study of high dosage frusemide. *Clin. Sci.,* **1971,** *41,* 171–187.

Baer, J. E.; Jones, C. B.; Spitzer, S. A.; and Russo, H. F. The potassium-sparing and natriuretic activity of N-amidino-3,5-diamino-6-chloropyrazinecarboxamide hydrochloride dihydrate (amiloride hydrochloride). *J. Pharmac. exp. Ther.,* **1967,** *157,* 472–485.

Baer, J. E.; Leidy, H. L.; Brooks, A. V.; and Beyer, K. H. The physiological disposition of chlorothiazide (DIURIL) in the dog. *J. Pharmac. exp. Ther.,* **1959,** *125,* 295–302.

Barry, K. G., and Malloy, J. P. Oliguric renal failure. Evaluation and therapy by the intravenous infusion of mannitol. *J. Am. med. Ass.,* **1962,** *179,* 510–513.

Belair, E. J.; Cohen, A. I.; and Yelnosky, J. Renal excretion of metolazone, a new diuretic. *Br. J. Pharmac.,* **1972,** *45,* 476–479.

Beyer, K. H. The mechanism of action of chlorothiazide. *Ann. N.Y. Acad. Sci.,* **1958,** *71,* 363–379.

Beyer, K. H.; Baer, J. E.; Michaelson, J. K.; and Russo, H. F. Renotropic characteristics of ethacrynic acid: a phenoxyacetic saluretic diuretic agent. *J. Pharmac. exp. Ther.,* **1965,** *147,* 1–22.

Birkett, D. J. Mechanism of inactivation of rabbit muscle glyceraldehyde 3-phosphate dehydrogenase by ethacrynic acid. *Molec. Pharmac.,* **1973,** *9,* 209–218.

Birtch, A. G.; Zakheim, R. M.; Jones, L. G.; and Barger, A. C. Redistribution of renal blood flow produced by furosemide and ethacrynic acid. *Circulation Res.,* **1967,** *21,* 869–878.

Björnberg, A., and Gisslén, H. Thiazides: a cause of necrotising vasculitis? *Lancet,* **1965,** *2,* 982–983.

Bowman, R. H.; Dolgin, J.; and Coulson, R. Furosemide, ethacrynic acid, and iodoacetate on function and metabolism in perfused rat kidney. *Am. J. Physiol.,* **1973,** *224,* 416–424.

Brusilow, S. W., and Gordes, E. The mutual independence of the endolymphatic potential and the concentrations of sodium and potassium in endolymph. *J. clin. Invest.,* **1973,** *52,* 2517–2521.

Bull, M. B., and Laragh, J. H. Amiloride, a potassium-sparing natriuretic agent. *Circulation,* **1968,** *37,* 45–53.

Burg, M. B., and Green, N. Function of the thick ascending limb of Henle's loop. *Am. J. Physiol.,* **1973a,** *224,* 659–668.

———. Effect of mersalyl on the thick ascending limb of Henle's loop. *Kidney Int.,* **1973b,** *4,* 245–251.

———. Effect of ethacrynic acid on the thick ascending limb of Henle's loop. *Ibid.,* **1973c,** *4,* 301–308.

Cafruny, E. J.; Cho, K. C.; Nigrovic, V.; and Small, A. Organomercurials: why acidosis potentiates effects on renal transport of sodium. In, *Modern Diuretic Therapy in the Treatment of Cardiovascular and Renal Disease.* (Lant, A. F., and Wilson, G. M., eds.) Excerpta Medica, Amsterdam, **1973,** pp. 124–134.

Cannon, P. J.; Heinemann, H. O.; Stason, W. B.; and Laragh, J. H. Ethacrynic acid. Effectiveness and mode of diuretic action in man. *Circulation,* **1965,** *31,* 5–18.

Clarkson, T. W.; Rothstein, A.; and Sutherland, R. The mechanism of action of mercurial diuretics in rats: the metabolism of ^{203}Hg-labelled chlormerodrin. *Br. J. Pharmac. Chemother.,* **1965,** *24,* 1–13.

Clarkson, T. W., and Vostal, J. J. Mercurials, mercuric ion and sodium transport. In, *Modern Diuretic Therapy in the Treatment of Cardiovascular and Renal Disease.* (Lant, A. F., and Wilson, G. M., eds.) Excerpta Medica, Amsterdam, **1973,** pp. 229–240.

DeRubertis, F. R.; Michelis, M. F.; Beck, N.; and Davis, B. B. Complications of diuretic therapy: severe alkalosis and syndrome resembling inappropriate secretion of antidiuretic hormone. *Metabolism,* **1970,** *19,* 709–719.

Dluhy, R. G.; Wolf, G. L.; and Lauler, D. P. Vasodilator properties of ethacrynic acid in the perfused dog kidney. *Clin. Sci.,* **1970,** *38,* 347–357.

Dodds, M. G., and Foord, R. D. Enhancement by potent diuretics of renal tubular necrosis induced by cephaloridine. *Br. J. Pharmac.,* **1970,** *40,* 227–236.

Dollery, C. T. Diabetogenic effect of long-term diuretic therapy. In, *Modern Diuretic Therapy in the Treatment of Cardiovascular and Renal Disease.* (Lant, A. F., and Wilson, G. M., eds.) Excerpta Medica, Amsterdam, **1973,** pp. 320–330.

Down, P. F.; Polak, A.; Rao, R.; and Mead, J. A. Fate of potassium supplements in six outpatients receiving long-term diuretics for oedematous disease. *Lancet,* **1972,** *2,* 721–723.

Duarte, C. C.; Chomety, F.; and Giebisch, G. Effect of amiloride, ouabain, and furosemide on distal tubular function in the rat. *Am. J. Physiol.,* **1971,** *221,* 632–640.

Duggan, D. E. A biochemical basis for the renal activity of N-7-acetylchlorothiazide. *J. Pharmac. exp. Ther.,* **1967,** *156,* 193–199.

Dunn, M. J. Diuretics and red blood cell transport of cations. In, *Modern Diuretic Therapy in the Treatment of Cardiovascular and Renal Disease.* (Lant, A. F., and Wilson, G. M., eds.) Excerpta Medica, Amsterdam, **1973,** pp. 196–208.

Edmonds, C. J., and Jasani, B. Total-body potassium in hypertensive patients during prolonged diuretic therapy. *Lancet,* **1972,** *2,* 8–12.

Edwards, B. R.; Baer, P. G.; Sutton, R. A. L.; and Dirks, J. H. Micropuncture study of diuretic effects on sodium and calcium reabsorption in the dog nephron. *J. clin. Invest.,* **1973,** *52,* 2418–2427.

Epstein, F. H. Role of sodium-potassium-ATPase in sodium reabsorption by the kidney. In, *Modern Diuretic Therapy in the Treatment of Cardiovascular and Renal Disease.* (Lant, A. F., and Wilson, G. M., eds.) Excerpta Medica, Amsterdam, **1973,** pp. 188–195.

Erlinger, S.; Dhumeaux, D.; Berthelot, P.; and Dumont, M. Effect of inhibitors of sodium transport on bile formation in the rabbit. *Am. J. Physiol.,* **1970,** *219,* 416–422.

Espiner, E. A.; Tucci, J. R.; Jagger, P. I.; Pauk, G. L.; and Lauler, D. P. The effect of acute diuretic-induced extracellular volume depletion on aldosterone secretion in normal man. *Clin. Sci.,* **1967,** *33,* 125–134.

Evanson, R. L.; Lockhart, E. A.; and Dirks, J. H. Effect of mercurial diuretics on tubular sodium and potassium transport in the dog. *Am. J. Physiol.,* **1972,** *222,* 282–289.

Fanelli, G. M.; Bohn, D. L.; Reilly, S. S.; and Weiner, I. M. Effects of mercurial diuretics on renal transport of urate in the chimpanzee. *Am. J. Physiol.,* **1973,** *224,* 985–992.

Feit, P. W. Aminobenzoic acid diuretics. 2. 4-Substituted-3-amino-5-sulfamylbenzoic acid derivatives. *J. mednl Chem.,* **1971,** *14,* 432–439.

Flores, J.; DiBona, D. R.; Beck, C. H.; and Leaf, A. The role of cell swelling in ischemic renal damage and the protective effect of hypertonic solute. *J. clin. Invest.,* **1972,** *51,* 118–126.

Ford, R. V. The new diuretics. *Med. Clins N. Am.,* **1961,** *45,* 961–972.

Ganong, W. F. Sympathetic effects on renin secretion; mechanism and physiological role. *Adv. exp. Med. Biol.,* **1972,** *17,* 17–32.

Garcia, D. A., and Yendt, E. R. The effects of probenecid and thiazides and their combination on the urinary excretion of electrolytes and on acid-base equilibrium. *Can. med. Ass. J.,* **1970,** *103,* 473–483.

Gatzy, J. T. The effect of K⁺-sparing diuretics on ion transport across the excised toad bladder. *J. Pharmac. exp. Ther.,* **1971,** *176,* 580–594.

Gayer, J. Die renale Exkretion des neuen Diureticum Furosemide. *Klin. Wschr.,* **1965,** *43,* 898–902.

Gordon, E. E., and Sheps, S. G. Effect of acetazolamide on citrate excretion and formation of renal calculi. *New Engl. J. Med.,* **1957,** *256,* 1215–1219.

Gray, G. W.; Bryan, A. C.; Frayser, R.; Houston, C. S.; and Rennie, I. D. B. Control of acute mountain sickness. *Aerospace Med.,* **1971,** *41,* 81–84.

Griggs, R. C.; Engel, W. K.; and Resnick, J. S. Acetazolamide treatment of hypokalemic periodic paralysis. Prevention of attacks and improvement of persistent weakness. *Ann. intern. Med.,* **1970,** *73,* 39–48.

Hagedorn, C. W.; Kaplan, A. A.; and Hulet, W. H. Prolonged administration of ethacrynic acid in patients with chronic renal disease. *New Engl. J. Med.,* **1965,** *272,* 1152–1155.

Halpern, S.; Tubis, M.; Endon, J.; Walsh, C.; Kunsa, J.; and Zwicker, B. ⁹⁹ᵐTc-penicillamine-acetazolamide complex, a new renal scanning agent. *J. nucl. Med.,* **1972,** *13,* 45–50.

Handler, J. S.; Bensinger, R.; and Orloff, J. Effect of adrenergic agents on toad bladder response to ADH, 3′,5′-AMP, and theophylline. *Am. J. Physiol.,* **1968,** *215,* 1024–1031.

Hansen, K. B., and Bender, A. D. Changes in serum potassium levels occurring in patients treated with triamterene and a triamterene-hydrochlorothiazide combination. *Clin. Pharmac. Ther.,* **1967,** *8,* 392–399.

Harber, L. C.; Lashinsky, A. M.; and Baer, R. L. Photosensitivity due to chlorothiazide and hydrochlorothiazide. *New Engl. J. Med.,* **1959,** *261,* 1378–1381.

Hook, J. B.; Blatt, A. H.; Brody, M. J.; and Williamson, H. E. Effects of several saluretic-diuretic agents on renal hemodynamics. *J. Pharmac. exp. Ther.,* **1966,** *154,* 667–673.

Hook, J. B., and Williamson, H. E. Addition of the saluretic action of furosemide to the saluretic action of certain other agents. *J. Pharmac. exp. Ther.,* **1965a,** *148,* 88–93.

————. Influence of probenecid and alterations in acid-base balance of the saluretic activity of furosemide. *Ibid.,* **1965b,** *149,* 404–408.

James, J. W., and Evans, R. A. Use of oral mannitol in the oedematous patient. *Br. med. J.,* **1970,** *1,* 463–465.

Jick, H. The use of glucocorticoids for diuresis in patients with fluid retention not resulting from renal disease. *Ann. N.Y. Acad. Sci.,* **1966,** *139,* 512–519.

Kagawa, C. M.; Sturtevant, F. M.; and Van Arman, C. G. Pharmacology of a new steroid that blocks salt activity of aldosterone and desoxycorticosterone. *J. Pharmac. exp. Ther.,* **1959,** *126,* 123–130.

Kassab, N.; Zoldy, A.; and Tawab, S. A. Diuretic drugs and serotonin (5-hydroxytryptamine) levels. *Egypt. med. Ass. J.,* **1973,** *78,* 269–282.

Kessler, E.; Hilton, J. G.; and Levy, M. R. Renal and adrenal relationships in refractory edema. *Circulation,* **1962,** *26,* 12–25.

Kilcoyne, M. M.; Schmidt, D. H.; and Cannon, P. J. Intrarenal blood flow in congestive heart failure. *Circulation,* **1973,** *47,* 786–797.

Kim, K. E.; Onesti, G.; Moyer, J. H.; and Swartz, C. Ethacrynic acid and furosemide, diuretic and hemodynamic effects and clinical uses. *Am. J. Cardiol.,* **1971,** *27,* 407–415.

Klahr, S.; Bourgoignie, J.; and Yates, J. Effects of ethacrynic acid and frusemide on renal metabolism. In, *Modern Diuretic Therapy in the Treatment of Cardiovascular and Renal Disease.* (Lant, A. F., and Wilson, G. M., eds.) Excerpta Medica, Amsterdam, **1973,** pp. 241–252.

Kutti, J., and Weinfeld, A. The frequency of thrombocytopenia in patients with heart disease treated with oral diuretics. *Acta med. scand.,* **1968,** *183,* 245–250.

Lassen, J. B., and Nielsen, O. E. Investigations into the diuretic effect and elimination of triamterene. *Acta pharmac. tox.,* **1963,** *20,* 309–316.

Liddle, G. W. Specific and non-specific inhibition of mineralocorticoid activity. *Metabolism,* **1961,** *10,* 1021–1030.

Lim, P., and Jacob, E. Magnesium deficiency in patients on long-term diuretic therapy for heart failure. *Br. med. J.,* **1972,** *3,* 620–622.

Lyons, H.; Pinn, V. W.; Cartell, S.; Cohen, J. J.; and Harrington, J. T. Allergic interstitial nephritis causing reversible renal failure in four patients with idiopathic nephrotic syndrome. *New Engl. J. Med.,* **1973,** *288,* 124–128.

McCarthy, J. S.; Fregly, M. J.; and Nechay, B. R. Effect of diuretics on renal iodide excretion by rats and dogs. *J. Pharmac. exp. Ther.,* **1967,** *158,* 294–304.

McKenna, T. J.; Donohoe, J. F.; Brien, T. G.; Healy, J. J.; Canning, B. St. J.; and Muldowney, F. P. Potassium-sparing agents during diuretic therapy in hypertension. *Br. med. J.,* **1971,** *2,* 739–741.

Maass, A. R., and Wiebelhaus, V. D. Die biologischen und diuretischen Eigenschaften von Triamterene. In, *Therapie mit Triamterene.* (Fellinger, K., ed.) George Thieme Verlag, Stuttgart, **1967,** pp. 2–21.

Maass, A. R.; Wiebelhaus, V. D.; Sosnowski, G.; Jenkins, B.; and Gessner, G. Effect of triamterene on folic reductase activity and reproduction in the rat. *Toxicol. appl. Pharmac.,* **1967,** *10,* 413–423.

Maren, T. H.; Sorsdahl, O. A.; and Dickhaus, A. J. Renal

action of acetazolamide in extracellular alkalosis of K^+ deficiency. *Am. J. Physiol.,* **1961,** *200,* 170–174.

Maren, T. H., and Wiley, C. E. Renal activity and pharmacology of N-acyl and related sulfonamides. *J. Pharmac. exp. Ther.,* **1964,** *143,* 230–242.

Mehbod, H.; Swartz, C. D.; and Brest, A. N. The effect of prolonged thiazide administration on thyroid function. *Archs intern. Med.,* **1967,** *119,* 283–286.

Morgan, A. G., and Polak, A. Acetazolamide and sodium bicarbonate in treatment of salicylate poisoning in adults. *Br. med. J.,* **1969,** *1,* 16–19.

Morgan, T.; Tadokoro, M.; Martin, D.; and Berliner, R. W. Effect of furosemide on Na^+ and K^+ transport studied by microperfusion of the rat nephron. *Am. J. Physiol.,* **1970,** *218,* 292–297.

Morris, C. R.; Alexander, E. A.; Bruns, F. J.; and Levinsky, N. Restoration and maintenance of glomerular filtration by mannitol during hypoperfusion of the kidney. *J. clin. Invest.,* **1972,** *51,* 1555–1564.

Mudge, G. H. Influence of plasma composition on sodium excretion and diuretic action. *Ann. N.Y. Acad. Sci.,* **1966,** *139,* 304–311.

Muth, R. G. Diuretics in chronic renal insufficiency. In, *Modern Diuretic Therapy in the Treatment of Cardiovascular and Renal Disease.* (Lant, A. F., and Wilson, G. M., eds.) Excerpta Medica, Amsterdam, **1973,** pp. 294–305.

Nechay, B. R. Potentiation of diuretic effects of methyl xanthines and pyrimidines by carbonic anhydrase inhibitors. *J. Pharmac. exp. Ther.,* **1964,** *144,* 276–283.

————. Action of mercury on renal sodium transport and adenosine triphosphatase activity. In, *Mercury, Mercurials and Mercaptans.* (Miller, N. W., and Clarkson, J. W., eds.) Charles C Thomas, Pub., Springfield, Ill., **1973,** pp. 111–123.

Østergaard, E. H.; Magnussen, M. P.; Nielsen, C. K.; Eilertsen, E.; and Frey, H.-H. Pharmacological properties of 3-n-butylamino-4-phenoxy-5-sulfamylbenzoic acid (bumetanide), a new potent diuretic. *Arzneimittel-Forsch.,* **1972,** *22,* 66–72.

Panijayanond, P.; Cho, I.; Ulrich, F.; and Nabseth, D. C. Enhancement of renal preservation by furosemide. *Surgery, St. Louis,* **1973,** *73,* 368–373.

Pendleton, R. G.; Sullivan, L. P.; Tucker, J. M.; and Stephenson, R. E., III. The effect of benzothiadiazide on the isolated toad bladder. *J. Pharmac. exp. Ther.,* **1968,** *164,* 348–361.

Piala, J. J.; Poutsiaka, J. W.; Smith, C. I.; Burke, J. C.; and Craver, B. N. Pharmacology of benzydroflumethiazide (NATURETIN). *J. Pharmac. exp. Ther.,* **1961,** *134,* 273–280.

Prazma, J.; Thomas, W. G.; Fischer, N. D.; and Preslar, M. J. Ototoxicity of ethacrynic acid. *Archs Otolar.,* **1972,** *95,* 448–456.

Reimold, E. W.; Warthen, H. G.; and Reilly, T. P., Jr. Salicylate poisoning. Comparison of acetazolamide administration and alkaline diuresis in the treatment of experimental salicylate intoxication in puppies. *Am. J. Dis. Child.,* **1973,** *125,* 668–674.

Rodriguez, H. J.; Walls, J.; Yates, J.; and Klahr, S. Effects of acetazolamide on the urinary excretion of cyclic AMP and on the activity of renal adenyl cyclase. *J. clin. Invest.,* **1974,** *53,* 122–130.

Rosenthale, M. E., and Osdene, T. S. Renal pharmacology of the pteridine diuretic Wy-5356. *Archs int. Pharmacodyn. Thér.,* **1966,** *164,* 11–29.

Ross, C. R., and Cafruny, E. J. Blockade of the diuretic action of benzothiadiazines. *J. Pharmac. exp. Ther.,* **1963,** *140,* 125–132.

Roth, L. J.; Schoolar, J. C.; and Barlow, C. F. Sulfur-35 labelled acetazolamide in cat brain. *J. Pharmac. exp. Ther.,* **1959,** *125,* 128–136.

Schultz, E. M.; Cragoe, E. J., Jr.; Bicking, J. B.; Bolhofer, W. A.; and Sprague, J. A. Alpha,beta-unsaturated ketone derivatives of aryloxyacetic acids, a new class of diuretics. *J. mednl pharm. Chem.,* **1962,** *5,* 660–662.

Scriabine, A.; Schreiber, E. C.; Yu, M.; and Wiseman, E. H. Renal clearance of polythiazide. *Proc. Soc. exp. Biol. Med.,* **1962,** *110,* 872–875.

Sherlock, S. Diuretics in hepatic disease. In, *Modern Diuretic Therapy in the Treatment of Cardiovascular and Renal Disease.* (Lant, A. F., and Wilson, G. M., eds.) Excerpta Medica, Amsterdam, **1973,** pp. 270–280.

Skulan, T. W., and Shideman, F. E. Natriuretic and antiglycogenic activities of a series of symmetrical triazine and pteridine derivatives. *J. Pharmac. exp. Ther.,* **1965,** *148,* 356–362.

Stahl, W. M., and Stone, A. M. Prophylactic diuresis with ethacrynic acid for prevention of postoperative renal failure. *Ann. Surg.,* **1970,** *172,* 361–369.

Stein, J. H.; Wilson, C. B.; and Kirkendall, W. M. Differences in the acute effects of furosemide and ethacrynic acid in man. *J. Lab. clin. Med.,* **1968,** *71,* 654–665.

Storch, T. G., and Layton, W. M., Jr. Teratogenic effects of intrauterine injection of acetazolamide and amiloride in hamsters. *Teratology,* **1973,** *7,* 209–214.

Stowe, N. T.; Wolterink, L. F.; Lewis, A. E.; and Hook, J. B. Diuretic and hemodynamic effects of furosemide in the isolated dog kidney. *Naunyn-Schmiedebergs Archs Pharmac.,* **1973,** *277,* 13–26.

Suki, W. N.; Yium, J. J.; Von Minden, M.; Saller-Hebert, C.; Eknoyan, G.; and Martinez-Maldonado, M. Acute treatment of hypercalcemia with furosemide. *New Engl. J. Med.,* **1970,** *283,* 836–840.

Vogl, A. The discovery of the organic mercurial diuretics. *Am. Heart J.,* **1950,** *39,* 881–883.

Waite, L. C. Carbonic anhydrase inhibitors, parathyroid hormone and calcium metabolism. *Endocrinology,* **1972,** *91,* 1160–1165.

Wales, J. K.; Krees, S. V.; Grant, A. M.; Viktora, J. K.; and Wolff, F. W. Structure-activity relationships of benzothiadiazine compounds as hyperglycemic agents. *J. Pharmac. exp. Ther.,* **1968,** *164,* 82–89.

Walker, W. G. Indications and contraindications for diuretic therapy. *Ann. N.Y. Acad. Sci.,* **1966,** *139,* 481–496.

Walker, W. G.; Sapir, D. G.; Turin, M.; and Cheng, J. T. Potassium homeostasis with diuretic therapy. In, *Modern Diuretic Therapy in the Treatment of Cardiovascular and Renal Disease.* (Lant, A. F., and Wilson, G. M., eds.) Excerpta Medica, Amsterdam, **1973,** pp. 331–342.

Walser, M.; Payne, J. W.; and Browder, A. A. Ion association. IV. Effect of sodium sulfate infusion on renal clearance and body retention of injected radiostrontium in dogs. *J. clin. Invest.,* **1961,** *40,* 234–242.

Weiner, I. M.; Levy, R. I.; and Mudge, G. H. Studies on mercurial diuresis: renal excretion, acid stability and structure-activity relationships of organic mercurials. *J. Pharmac. exp. Ther.,* **1962,** *138,* 96–112.

Wiebelhaus, V. D.; Brennan, F. T.; Sosnowski, G.; Maass, A. R.; Weinstock, J.; and Bender, A. D. The natriuretic and diuretic characteristics of triamterene in the dog. *Archs int. Pharmacodyn. Thér.,* **1967,** *169,* 429–451.

Williamson, H. E. Relationship between ATPase activity and sodium transport and action of diuretics. In, *Proceedings of the Fourth International Congress of Nephrology.* Vol. 2, *Endocrinology: Metabolic Aspects.* (Alwall, N.; Berglund, F.; and Josephson, B.; eds.) S. Karger, Basel, **1970,** pp. 144–152.

Williamson, H. E.; Shideman, F. E.; and LeSher, D. A. Antagonism of the effects of certain steroids on the renal excretion of water and electrolytes by 2-amino-4-(p-chloroanilino)-s-triazine. *J. Pharmac. exp. Ther.,* **1959,** *126,* 82–89.

Wills, M. R.; Gill, J. R., Jr.; and Bartter, F. C. The interrelationships of calcium and sodium excretions. *Clin. Sci.,* **1969,** *37,* 621–630.

Monographs and Reviews

Baer, J. E., and Beyer, K. H.   Subcellular pharmacology of natriuretic and potassium-sparing drugs. *Prog. biochem. Pharmac.,* **1972,** *7,* 59–93.

Beyer, K. H., and Baer, J. E.   Physiological basis for the action of newer diuretic agents. *Pharmac. Rev.,* **1961,** *13,* 517–562.

Goldberg, M.   The renal physiology of diuretics. In, *Renal Physiology. Handbook of Physiology,* Sect. 8. (Orloff, J., and Berliner, R. W., eds.) American Physiological Society, Washington, D.C., **1973,** pp. 1003–1031.

Liddle, G. W.   Aldosterone antagonists and triamterene. *Ann. N.Y. Acad. Sci.,* **1966,** *139,* 466–470.

Maren, T. H.   Carbonic anhydrase: chemistry, physiology, and inhibition. *Physiol. Rev.,* **1967,** *47,* 595–781.

Mudge, G. H.; Berndt, W. O.; and Valtin, H.   Tubular transport of urea, glucose, phosphate, uric acid, sulfate, and thiosulfate. In, *Renal Physiology. Handbook of Physiology,* Sect. 8. (Orloff, J., and Berliner, R. W., eds.) American Physiological Society, Washington, D.C., **1973,** pp. 587–652.

Pitts, R. F.   *Physiology of the Kidney and Body Fluids: An Introductory Text,* 3rd ed. Year Book Medical Publishers, Inc., Chicago, **1974.**

Rector, F. C., Jr.   Acidification of the urine. In, *Renal Physiology. Handbook of Physiology,* Sect. 8. (Orloff, J., and Berliner, R. W., eds.) American Physiological Society, Washington, D.C., **1973,** pp. 431–454.

Suki, W. N.; Eknoyan, G.; and Martinez-Maldonado, M.   Tubular sites and mechanisms of diuretic action. *A. Rev. Pharmac.,* **1973,** *13,* 91–106.

Weiner, I. M.   Transport of weak acids and bases. In, *Renal Physiology. Handbook of Physiology,* Sect. 8. (Orloff J., and Berliner, R. W., eds.) American Physiological Society, Washington, D.C., **1973,** pp. 521–554.

CHAPTER

40 AGENTS AFFECTING THE RENAL CONSERVATION OF WATER

Paul Brazeau

ANTIDIURETIC HORMONE (ADH)

The posterior pituitary antidiuretic hormone (ADH) and closely related polypeptides are substances that evoke a graded increase in the permeability to water of the mammalian nephron and thereby cause free water to be reabsorbed and conserved. Analogous hormones that affect water conservation and the concentration of solutes in body fluids are found in all vertebrates, even the most primitive. Despite the constancy in the chemical structures of the hormones, the target organs and actions have undergone remarkable adaptive changes in fresh- and salt-water fish, amphibians, and terrestrial vertebrates. Thus, in various species the hormones may act by altering blood flow in gill or kidney, sodium transport in skin or bladder, or permeability of these structures to water and solutes. These evolutionary changes have been extensively studied and provide one of the more fascinating chapters in comparative biology (see Sawyer, 1967b, 1972).

In primates, presumably including man, the physiological role of ADH is only to alter the permeability of the terminal portions of the renal tubule to water and urea. However, the property of the hormone first detected in posterior pituitary extracts was a vasoconstrictor action (see below). Unfortunately, the name vasopressin, chosen at that time, persists as the official U.S.P. designation for the hormone. In this chapter, the term vasopressin will be used only in the discussion of natural and synthetic structural analogs and when referring to the preparations of ADH that are available by that name.

The renal excretion of water may also be markedly affected by substances (such as nicotine or alcohol) that are capable of directly altering the rate of release of ADH. In addition, other drugs may modify the volume and osmotic pressure of the urine by inducing alterations in solute excretion or renal hemodynamics (see introduction to Section VIII). However, the latter drugs usually do not seriously interfere with the maintenance of water balance since compensatory readjustments of the rate of ADH release readily occur.

Anatomical and Physiological Considerations. The neurohypophysis is richly innervated with nonmyelinated nerve fibers that originate, for the most part, in the supraoptic and paraventricular nuclei of the hypothalamus. The hypothalamic nuclei are, in turn, linked with subthalamic and thalamic nuclei and through these with the sensory and motor systems and all parts of the cerebral cortex. Thus, the posterior pituitary can be subjected to nerve impulses of diverse origin.

ADH and also oxytocin (see Chapter 42) are formed in cell bodies located principally in the paraventricular and supraoptic nuclei and then migrate along the axons of these cells to perivascular nerve endings in the posterior lobe (see Scharrer and Scharrer, 1954). The hormones accumulate in the nerve endings, largely in "neurosecretory granules," within which they are bound to protein (see below). The neurons originating in the supraoptic nucleus are believed to release ADH almost exclusively, whereas the other hypothalamiconeurohypophyseal tracts contain both hormones in varying ratios (Bisset et al., 1966).

It is generally accepted that the stimuli for the release of hormone are transmitted to or arise in the hypothalamic nuclei and that axonal impulses traversing the hypothalamiconeurohypophyseal tract effect the release of hormone at the nerve endings in the posterior lobe. Electrical stimulation of the supraoptic or paraventricular nuclei results in secretion of hormone, as does the injection into these areas of acetylcholine or physostigmine. Douglas and coworkers have shown that electrical stimulation of the axons leading into the isolated posterior lobe results in ADH release, as does depolarization of these axons and their neurosecretory terminals by high concentrations of potassium ion. They have also shown that calcium ion plays an essential role in linking depolarization to secretion (see Douglas and Poisner, 1964; Mikiten and Douglas, 1965). Less than 20% of the hormone content of the posterior lobe is readily releasable. After this "pool" has been expended, the rate of release falls to very much lower levels, even in the presence of continued intensive stimulation. Little is known of the factors that govern or limit the rates of formation and migration of the hormones. However, severe depletion of the hormone content of the gland has been demonstrated after prolonged physiological stimulation *in vivo.*

There has been intensive investigation of possible mechanisms for the release of ADH and oxytocin into the blood stream. It has been found that a portion of the hormones in the gland is present in protein-bound form in cytoplasm and that calcium ion inhibits this binding. It has been suggested that the influx of calcium associated with the arrival of the nerve impulse thus makes some hormone available for diffusion out of the nerve terminal. It has also been suggested that, although calcium does not cause the release of hormone from isolated neurosecretory granules *in vitro,* the influx of this ion might facilitate the exocytosis of the contents of granules located near the nerve membrane (*see* Ginsberg, 1968). The latter seems likely to constitute the principal mechanism for the release of the hormone.

Together with the mechanisms in the central nervous system (CNS) that govern thirst, the hypothalamiconeurohypophyseal system for the secretion of ADH provides the homeostatic control that maintains the osmotic pressure of body fluids within extremely narrow limits; the rate of secretion of ADH is directly influenced by the degree of body hydration. A large body of evidence indicates that there are osmoreceptors, specifically sensitive to changes in extracellular electrolyte concentration, located in the CNS, probably within the hypothalamic nuclei mentioned above. In well-hydrated subjects the plasma concentration of ADH is generally less than 1 microunit per milliliter (1 μU/ml). Moderate dehydration results in elevation of plasma concentrations to 5 to 10 μU/ml, associated with the excretion of markedly hypertonic urine. Prolonged severe dehydration or the infusion of hypertonic solutions has resulted in the elevation of plasma concentrations to as high as 20 to 100 μU/ml (*see* Lauson, 1967).

There is also evidence for volume receptors that influence the activity of the hypothalamiconeurohypophyseal system (*see* Smith, 1957; Share, 1962; Moore, 1971). It has been suggested that such receptors exist in the left atrium and the pulmonary veins. According to this concept, a decrease or an increase in the circulating blood volume results, respectively, in the stimulation or the suppression of the secretion of ADH. For example, hemorrhage has been shown to be a very powerful stimulus for the release of ADH. The so-called low-salt syndrome is often encountered in patients continuously receiving potent diuretic agents for the control of hypertension, edema, or the ascites of hepatic cirrhosis (White *et al.,* 1953). Although there is usually no impairment of the patient's neurohypophyseal or renal mechanisms for regulation of osmotic pressure, water is retained in spite of the continuing loss of sodium salts so that plasma osmotic pressure falls below normal. It has been suggested that the activation of volume receptors is responsible for the water retention in such patients.

Water retention and hyponatremia also occur in patients suffering from certain tumors, most notably bronchial oat-cell carcinoma (the Schwartz-Bartter syndrome). Such tumors may produce large amounts of an antidiuretic polypeptide, which by all biological and physical criteria is identical to ADH (Sawyer, 1967a).

The above hyponatremic states are examples of what is now referred to as the *syndrome of inappropriate ADH secretion* (SIADH), characterized by hyponatremia secondary to decreased free-water excretion in the presence of otherwise-adequate renal function (Bartter and Schwartz, 1967). It has also been observed in association with certain types of pulmonary disease, in traumatic or disease-related brain injury, and during the use of several drugs other than diuretics, such as the oral hypoglycemic agent chlorpropamide (*see* below). SIADH must be distinguished from pituitary or adrenal insufficiency, hypothyroidism, congestive failure, and so forth, in which hyponatremia may occur due to impairment of the renal capacity for sodium conservation or free-water excretion (Fishman *et al.,* 1971).

Chemistry. In addition to having an antidiuretic action, extracts of the neurohypophysis were found to cause vasoconstriction (pressor principle) and to stimulate the smooth muscle of the uterus (oxytocic principle) and the modified smooth muscle of the mammary glands (milk-ejection factor). Extracts further purified to obtain a high ratio of oxytocic to antidiuretic activity have a vasodilator action that is prominent in some species but weak in man. A protein possessing all these properties in the same proportion as crude gland extracts was isolated from the neurohypophysis of oxen (van Dyke *et al.,* 1942). However, by relatively mild procedures it is possible to separate from this protein, neurophysin, the two polypeptides, ADH and oxytocin, that are responsible for the biological activity of the extracts (*see* Table 40–1). By a modification of the van Dyke procedure, two closely related proteins, neurophysins I and II, have been identified in extracts of the gland. These have molecular weights of approximately 20,000 and selectively bind one to three molecules of ADH or oxytocin. They appear to be identical to the two proteins found in that fraction of the gland obtained by ultracentrifugation, which contains the neurosecretory granules. Neurophysin-like proteins that selectively bind ADH or oxytocin have been found in several target organs (uterus, kidney, mammary gland) but not in other tissues studied.

duVigneaud and coworkers (1953, 1954) determined the structures of ADH and oxytocin and accomplished the complete synthesis of each. The structures are shown in Figure 40–1.

These neurohypophyseal octapeptides are common in all mammals except swine, in which ADH is found to contain lysine in place of arginine. Therefore, the bovine pituitary, when used as the sole source, supplies hormones identical to those of man. However, most available preparations also contain lysine vasopressin due to the use of porcine as well as bovine pituitaries. Pure, synthetic lysine vasopressin, for which the name *lypressin* has been adopted, is now available for therapeutic use. An

Table 40-1.   THE BIOLOGICAL ACTIVITY OF NEUROHYPOPHYSEAL AND
SYNTHETIC OCTAPEPTIDES *

	ACTIVITY (Relative to That of Arginine Vasopressin)		ACTIVITY (Relative to That of Oxytocin)		
	Antidiuretic *(rat)*	*Pressor* *(rat)*	*Milk Ejection* *(rabbit)*	*Oxytocic* *(rat uterus in vitro)*	*Vasode- pressor* *(chicken)*
ADH: Arginine[8] vasopressin	**100**	**100**	15	5	20
Oxytocin	1	1	**100**	**100**	**100**
Lysine[8] vasopressin	80	60	10	2	10
Arginine[8] vasotocin	70	40	40	20	90
Phenylalanine[2]-ly- sine[8] vasopressin	5	15	5	—	2

* Because the activity of the polypeptides has been determined by bioassay procedures that differ somewhat from one laboratory to another, the relative activities shown must be regarded as approximate.

interesting analog, arginine vasotocin, occurs in certain nonmammalian vertebrates. This substance has the ring structure of oxytocin and the side chain of ADH, and has physiological activity in mammals intermediate between that of oxytocin and ADH.

It has been found that optimal or near-optimal antidiuretic and oxytocic activities reside in the structures of the naturally occurring hormones of mammals. The intact pentapeptide ring is essential. Opening the ring, as well as increasing or decreasing its size by even one carbon atom, causes complete or near-complete loss of activity. Removal of the terminal glycine amide, as by trypsin when the hormones are administered orally, also results in inacti-

Antidiuretic Hormone

Oxytocin

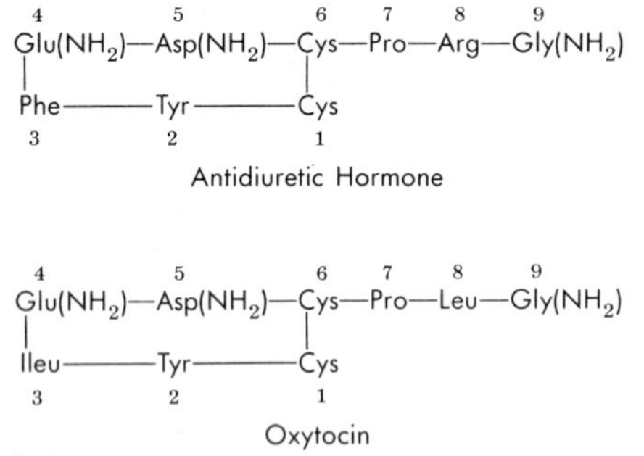

Figure 40-1. *Structures of antidiuretic hormone (ADH) and oxytocin.*

The conventions of symbols and numbering are as follows: Cys—Cys = cystine; Tyr = tyrosine; Phe = phenylalanine; Glu(NH$_2$) = glutamine; Asp(NH$_2$) = asparagine; Pro = proline; Arg = arginine; Gly(NH$_2$) = glycine; Ileu = isoleucine; Leu = leucine. The two cysteine moieties of cystine are numbered separately in these octapeptides. Thus, there are nine, rather than eight, positions in the amino acid sequence. Note that ADH differs from oxytocin only in positions 3 and 8. All the amino acids indicated are the naturally occurring L isomers.

vation. However, congeners in which this glycine is deamidated usually show increased antidiuretic or oxytocic, but not pressor, activity. A basic amino acid, optimally arginine, in position 8 is essential for antidiuretic activity. For appreciable oxytocic activity, isoleucine in position 3 is critical, as is the length but not the composition of the side chain. Modifications of structure other than at positions 3 and 8 alter biological activity to varying degrees. (*See* Walter *et al.,* 1967; Sawyer and Manning, 1973.)

Since ADH and oxytocin exert their primary effects in minute concentrations, an increase in potency would not be of great significance. Therefore, investigation of synthetic congeners has been directed toward increased duration of action, greater selectivity with respect to a single action, or the ability competitively to antagonize an action of the parent hormones. For example, 2-phenylalanine-8-lysine vasopressin, *felypressin,* which shows an increased ratio of pressor-to-antidiuretic activity, is in use in Europe as a vasoconstrictor agent in several applications for which vasopressin has been used (*see* below). Another compound under investigation in man is 1-deamino-8-D-arginine vasopressin (DDAVP). Both of the structural modifications in this congener reduce pressor activity and slow enzymatic inactivation while enhancing antidiuretic activity. Thus, DDAVP is a more potent and significantly longer-acting antidiuretic agent than ADH and has negligible effects, in the doses used, on vascular and other smooth muscle (Vávra *et al.,* 1968; Rudinger *et al.,* 1972).

Secretory Interrelationship between ADH and Oxytocin. It is clear that oxytocin plays a physiological role very different from that of ADH (*see* Chapter 42). Nevertheless, the formation, storage, and release of the two hormones are closely interrelated. Physiological responses (antidiuresis, milk ejection, changes in uterine motility) indicate that their simultaneous release may occur whether the stimulus is appropriate for ADH secretion (hyperosmolarity) or for oxytocin secretion (parturition, suckling, coitus), or is nonspecific (pain, apprehension). However, Holland and coworkers (1958) have observed responses, in lactating rabbits, to the injection of hypertonic saline solution that indicate the release of oxytocin in excess of ADH. Greater depletion of oxytocin than of ADH in the posterior lobe of the dog during lactation was observed by van Dyke and coworkers (1955). The stimulus supplied by hemorrhage appears to be quite specific in that very large amounts of ADH, but little oxytocin, are released. (For details, *see* Sawyer, 1961; Discussion on polypeptide hormones, 1968.)

PHYSIOLOGICAL AND PHARMACOLOGICAL PROPERTIES

As has already been pointed out, the primary action of ADH is to modulate the renal tubular reabsorption of water. In considering the extrarenal responses to ADH, it should be kept in mind that most of these are elicited only by concentrations far higher than those required for antidiuresis and are generally considered to be incidental actions subserving no physiological requirement in mammals.

Renal Action. *The Formation of Hypotonic Urine.* Following the isosmotic reabsorption of the major portion of the glomerular filtrate in the proximal tubule, which is freely permeable to water at all times, electrolyte reabsorption continues in the ascending limb of Henle's loop as well as in the distal convolution and the collecting ducts. However, permeability to water decreases in the ascending thin limb and becomes extremely low in the thick ascending portion. Thus, the fluid entering the distal convolution is always hypotonic and, when circulating concentrations of ADH are low, remains so as electrolyte reabsorption continues along the remainder of the tubule and collecting system. When the secretion of the hormone is completely suppressed by overhydration, 15% or more of the water of the glomerular filtrate may escape into the urine virtually free of electrolyte. The osmotically unobligated water lost during the excretion of hypotonic urine is designated as the *positive free-water clearance*.

The Formation of Isotonic and Hypertonic Urine. Increasing concentrations of circulating ADH result in increasing permeability of the distal segment and the collecting system to water. In some species, this response first appears early in the distal convolution. In primates, it is believed to begin in the cortical collecting tubules or in the terminal

portion of the distal convolution, which is morphologically similar. In either case, since the cortical interstitium is isosmotic with plasma, the graded ADH-induced increases in water permeability permit passive diffusion of water out of the hypotonic luminal fluid toward the point of isosmolarity as this fluid approaches the medullary portion of the collecting system. The final concentration of the urine is then determined in the collecting ducts as they pass through the hypertonic interstitium of the renal papillae. (The mechanism that maintains the hypertonicity of this region is described below.) During dehydration and maximal antidiuresis, water is passively abstracted from the lumen of the collecting duct into the hypertonic peritubular fluid so that the two fluids are in osmotic equilibrium as the urine emerges from the tip of the papilla. Since, under these conditions, papillary osmotic pressure may reach 1400 milliosmoles or more per liter, urine having four to five times the osmotic pressure of plasma may be excreted. The amount of water abstracted and conserved in concentrating the urine to an osmotic pressure greater than that of plasma is known as the *negative free-water clearance*.

The action of ADH in reducing the output of urine to a small volume of fluid having a *markedly elevated osmotic pressure* is striking when the concurrent rate of solute excretion is normal or low, that is, about 2% or less of the filtered load of solutes. For example, 0.6 milliosmole of solute in 2 ml of water (300 milliosmoles per liter) could be concentrated to 0.44 ml of urine (1400 milliosmoles per liter) each minute in the papillary collecting ducts, a conservation or *negative clearance* of 1.56 ml of free water. Thus, at the usual levels of solute excretion, *free* water can be conserved at a far lower rate than it can be excreted. However, when large amounts of solute escape reabsorption, as occurs, for example, during mannitol, glucose, or sodium salt diuresis, the volume of isotonic fluid reaching the concentrating segment is elevated proportionately. The abstraction of a few milliliters of free water from a large volume of isotonic urine then causes a much less striking elevation of osmotic pressure (*see* Orloff *et al.,* 1958).

During extreme osmotic diuresis, the osmotic pressure gradient of the papilla is much reduced (*see* below) and the ability to reabsorb free water is thereby impaired. Under these conditions, the urine approaches isotonicity despite the presence of ADH. In the absence of ADH, however, a large, *positive free-water clearance* may still be superimposed on an osmotic diuresis. During diuresis induced by agents such as the thiazides and furosemide, the renal handling of free water may be impaired by alterations in electrolyte reabsorption in the diluting and concentrating segments of the nephron (*see* Chapter 39).

The Renal Countercurrent Osmotic Multiplier. The net electrolyte reabsorption that occurs as tubular urine traverses the ascending limb of the loop of Henle accounts for only a small portion of the total renal reabsorption of sodium chloride (roughly half of that which escapes proximal reabsorption). However, reabsorption of sodium and chloride in this segment plays an important role in establishing and maintaining the hypertonic milieu in the medulla and papilla that is necessary for the formation of concentrated urine in the collecting ducts. The anatomical arrangement of those loops of Henle that descend deep into the medulla is such that, over a long course, the descending and ascending limbs are in close proximity to each other and to the parallel capillary loops. Movements of solute and water between one and another of these elements can occur readily across the intervening narrow interstitial space. Our present understanding of the events that take place in the loop is as follows. In the descending limb, the low epithelium allows the free passive diffusion of water and, to a lesser extent, urea and other solutes. Thus, at any point along its descent, the luminal fluid approaches osmotic equilibrium with interstitial fluid. Microperfusion studies of isolated segments of the loop indicate that in the ascending thin limb permeability to water decreases and permeability to sodium and chloride increases. Therefore, passive outward movement of these ions could occur as the thin segment returns through areas of progressively decreasing hypertonicity. These studies have confirmed the very low permeability of the thick ascending limb to water and urea and the active reabsorption of chloride accompanied by sodium in this segment (*see* Kokko, 1974). The continuous transfer of sodium and chloride from ascending limbs to interstitial fluid surrounding the parallel permeable structures results in a continous increase in the osmotic pressure within these structures, which reaches its peak at the apex of the papilla. Thus, tubular fluid of very high sodium content and osmotic pressure reaches the bend of the loop of Henle. Then, as sodium reabsorption from the ascending limb proceeds, the tubular fluid again becomes progressively more dilute (*see* Figure 40–2).

At any point along the loop, the osmotic pressures of the fluids in descending limb, interstitium,

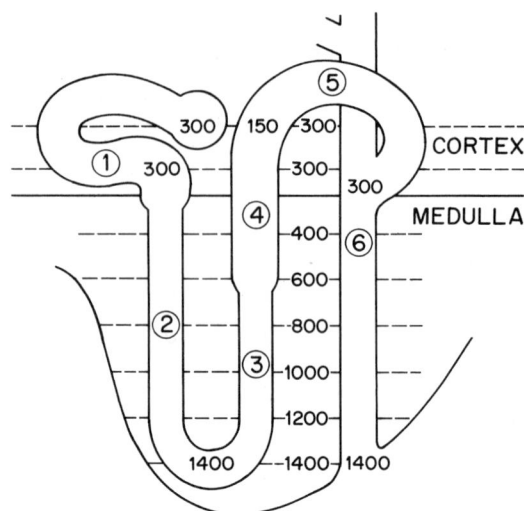

Figure 40–2. *The renal medullary countercurrent multiplier.*

Those nephrons having juxtamedullary glomeruli have long loops of Henle that approach the tip of the papilla and are responsible for the countercurrent multiplication of osmotic pressure in the medulla and papilla. One of these is shown diagrammatically. All numbers refer to the osmotic pressure (milliosmoles per kilogram of H_2O) of tubular or interstitial fluids during maximal ADH-induced antidiuresis in primates. Proximal tubule (*1*)—rapid active reabsorption of Na^+ (with Cl^-), high permeability to H_2O and urea; descending thin limb (*2*)—no active ion transport, permeability to some solutes (including urea); ascending thin limb (*3*)—increasing *passive* permeability to Na^+ and Cl^-, decreasing permeability to H_2O and urea; ascending thick limb (*4*)—active reabsorption of Cl^- (with Na^+), impermeability to H_2O and urea; distal convolution (*5*)—active reabsorption of Na^+ (with Cl^-), very low permeability to H_2O and urea; cortical and medullary collecting system (*6*)—active reabsorption of Na^+ (with Cl^- or by ion exchange), high permeability to H_2O and, in papillary portion, to urea in the presence of ADH (maximal at plasma levels of approximately 4 to 5 $\mu U/ml$).

and capillary are approximately equal; that of the fluid in the chloride-pumping portion of the ascending limb is believed to be about 200 milliosmoles per liter less. In this way a papillary osmotic pressure of 1000 milliosmoles per liter or more *above* that of plasma can be achieved, although the greatest transepithelial concentration gradient required at any one point probably need not exceed 100 mEq of sodium chloride per liter, a gradient consistent with those observed in the distal convolution and collecting ducts. It should be noted that the reabsorption of electrolyte by the collecting ducts also adds solute to the medullary interstitium, as does the passive outward diffusion of urea as the tubular urine is reduced to small volume. The latter has been shown to be facilitated by ADH. Indeed, during maximal antidiuresis, urea accounts for a considerable portion of the osmotically active solute present in tissue near the tip of the papilla. It has been found that the reduction of urea excretion by a protein-free diet results in a sharp reduction of maximal renal concentrating ability, which is reversible by the administration of urea. Thus, urea plays a passive but important role in the concentrating mechanism.

The exchange of solute, water, or heat that occurs between fluids flowing in opposite directions along closely opposed limbs of a folded loop is known as *countercurrent exchange*. When such a loop possesses an intrinsic mechanism for active transfer between the limbs (*e.g.,* chloride transport by the epithelium of the loop of Henle), the system is known as a *countercurrent multiplier*. The existence and characteristics of such systems have long been familiar to the physicist, but they have only recently been recognized in physiological systems. For physical reasons, the achievable gradient increases with increasing length of the loop as well as the rate of active "transfer." In desert rats, for example, the papilla is greatly elongated and the maximal concentrating power of the kidney is thereby greatly increased. A low rate of luminal flow also favors the development of a high gradient between the beginning and the tip of the loop. The low rate of luminal flow prevailing during dehydration therefore favors the establishment of maximal papillary osmotic pressure. Conversely, the high flow rate occurring during osmotic diuresis sharply curtails the efficiency of the countercurrent multiplier. The effectiveness of the system ultimately rests on the rate of sodium and chloride reabsorption in the ascending limb. The effects of aldosterone on this segment await clarification, although it is known that maximal concentrating ability is impaired in the absence of the glucocorticoids.

The microperfusion of isolated nephron segments is now elucidating the pharmacological as well as physiological characteristics of previously inaccessible portions. It has been shown, for example, that active chloride reabsorption in the thick ascending limb is susceptible to inhibition by potent "natriuretic" agents such as furosemide and ethacrynic acid (*see* Symposium, 1974).

The vascular architecture of the medulla and papilla also deserves comment. Were this area perfused by "straight-through" capillaries, randomly associated with the countercurrent mechanism, osmotic gradients would be rapidly dissipated. However, blood perfuses the area by way of elongated capillary loops (vasa recta) that parallel the loops of Henle and constitute a countercurrent exchange system. Plasma in the capillary loops equilibrates passively as it passes through the zone of high interstitial osmotic pressure. It again approaches isotonicity as ascending capillaries emerge from the medulla, carrying away only small amounts of the accumulated solutes. It is believed that elevated rates of medullary blood flow, however, may partially dissipate the osmotic gradient generated by the countercurrent multiplier.

Observation of the high solute content of renal papillary tissue first led to the proposal of the countercurrent mechanism by Wirz and coworkers (1951) as well as by Hargitay and Kuhn (1951). (For details of the evolution of present concepts, *see* Berliner and Bennett, 1967; Symposium, 1974.)

Electrolyte Excretion. An interesting analogy has been drawn between the distal portions of the mammalian nephron and two other epithelial structures involved in fluid conservation, namely, frog skin and toad or frog bladder. In these structures, ADH increases the rate of sodium transport as well as the permeability of the membrane to water and urea. However, there is no experimental evidence that ADH has any direct influence on electrolyte pumps in the mammalian nephron. It has been a common observation in experimental animals that ADH can cause alterations in electrolyte excretion. When these occur, it is usually found that the excretion of sodium, potassium, chloride, and sometimes bicarbonate is at first increased, especially when large amounts of the hormone are administered. The changes in electrolyte excretion in man are absent or not large, and apparently are easily compensated for by normal homeostatic mechanisms. Thus, when water requirements are met, no serious abnormalities of electrolyte metabolism are observed in patients with untreated diabetes insipidus or in patients or normal subjects continuously receiving vasopressin. Therefore, it is generally accepted that the hormone plays no essential role in electrolyte homeostasis and that it can produce no sustained abnormalities other than those secondary to alterations in the volume of body fluid compartments during water retention or depletion.

Although abnormalities of the rate of release or inactivation of ADH have been invoked as contributing factors in the edema formation of a number of disease states, the elevated ADH levels that are sometimes observed tend to be unpredictable and have not been shown to play an etiological role. As mentioned above, ADH in some cases may contribute to the development of hyponatremia. (*See* White *et al.,* 1953; Lauson, 1967.) The interplay of volume- and pressor-receptor systems and ADH, corticosteroids, angiotensin, and so forth, in regulating body fluid volume and electrolyte content is reviewed in a symposium (*see* Symposium, 1971).

Mechanism of Renal Action. Orloff and Handler (1964, 1967), using amphibian bladder, have shown that theophylline and cyclic adenosine 3',5'-monophosphate (cyclic AMP) cause changes in permeability very similar to those caused by ADH. ADH has been shown to increase cyclic AMP production in several tissues, presumably by activation of adenylate cyclase. Theophylline, on the other hand, is believed to inhibit the degradation of cyclic AMP by phosphodiesterase. These investigators therefore proposed that accumulation of cyclic AMP is the common and essential factor that leads to increased permeability of amphibian bladder treated with ADH, theophylline, or cyclic AMP itself. As an extension of this concept, they suggested that cyclic

AMP is an essential intermediate in the antidiuretic action of ADH in the mammalian kidney.

Subsequent studies on the mammalian nephron have shown that cyclic AMP in peritubular fluid mimics the effects of ADH on water permeability. Neither is effective when added to luminal fluid. Thus, it seems clear that the response to ADH is initiated at the peritubular membrane; that cyclic AMP (activation of adenylate cyclase) is involved in the cellular response; and that in mammals the change in permeability is specific for water alone, except in the papillary collecting duct, where permeability to urea is also increased. Experimental studies with a variety of activators of adenylate cyclase or inhibitors of phosphodiesterase support the hypothesis and clarify the mechanism by which a number of drugs and endogenous substances alter the renal response to ADH (Hays and Levine, 1974). The mechanisms responsible for the overall transepithelial change in permeability remain unclear, although the critical permeability barrier or barriers in the ADH response are known to be at the luminal membrane. It has been shown that significant amounts of water pass into lateral interspaces and thence into the peritubular space (*see* Grantham, 1971). For further details, *see* Handler and Orloff (1973) and Hays and Levine (1974).

Cardiovascular System. The pressor effect of posterior pituitary extract on the circulation was first described by Oliver and Schäfer in 1895. In man, ADH, in concentrations many times that required for maximal antidiuresis, can cause contraction of smooth muscle of all parts of the vasculature. The effect is a direct one on contractile elements. It is neither antagonized by adrenergic blocking agents nor prevented by vascular denervation. Circulation in the skin and the gastrointestinal tract is markedly reduced. The coronary vessels are not exempt from the vasoconstrictor effects of vasopressin, and pulmonary arterial pressure also rises.

The effects on *blood pressure* are conditioned by the reactivity of baroreceptor reflexes. Therefore, in normal conscious subjects, very large amounts of vasopressin must be administered to produce a marked and sustained rise in blood pressure. When the efficiency of baroreceptor reflexes is depressed by anesthesia, smaller amounts of the hormone elicit pressor responses. The blockade of autonomic vasomotor and cardioregulatory outflow by ganglionic blocking agents causes a marked increase in sensitivity to the pressor effects. Wagner and Braunwald (1956) have observed that patients with inherent defects in sympathetic outflow are strikingly sensitive to ADH. However, the rate of administration required to produce a rise in blood pressure in such subjects is still larger than that required to produce a maximal renal effect. It seems physiologically unlikely that ADH plays any essential role in the regulation of peripheral resistance.

The effects of vasopressin on the *heart* are indirect and are the result of decreased coronary blood flow and of reflexly induced alterations in vagal and sympathetic tone. Aside from the reflex responses occasioned by the elevation of blood pressure, the effects observed are characteristic of myocardial ischemia.

The effects of ADH on the coronary blood flow can readily be demonstrated in man, provided large doses are employed. In patients with coronary insufficiency, ECG changes similar to those observed after exercise can be observed. The cardiac actions of the hormone are of more than academic interest. Some patients with coronary insufficiency experience anginal pain even in response to the relatively small amounts of ADH required to control diabetes insipidus (*see* below). ADH-induced myocardial ischemia has led to severe reactions and even death (*see* Slotnick and Teigland, 1951).

Other Smooth Muscle. The effects of ADH on smooth muscle also occur in the *enteric tract*. The response is elicited only by large doses (5 to 20 units). Motility of the bowel is markedly increased. Peristaltic activity rather than tone is increased, and, therefore, the propulsive movements are greatly enhanced. The effect is greater on the large than on the small bowel. The smooth muscle of the *uterus* is stimulated by large doses of ADH at all stages of the menstrual cycle and during gestation, when large doses are administered (*see* Chapter 42).

Absorption, Fate, and Excretion. When ADH, lypressin, and their congeners are given orally, they are quickly inactivated by trypsin, which cleaves the 8–9 peptide link. ADH in aqueous solution may be given by the intravenous, intramuscular, or subcutaneous route and by the nasal insufflation of powders or sprays. Due to rapid inactivation, the effects are brief after intravenous administration unless the hormone is given by continuous infusion. After intramuscular or subcutaneous injection, the effects last only a few hours. Repository forms, such as *vasopressin tannate in oil,* are effective for 24 to 48 hours after subcutaneous or intramuscular injection. An inefficient but convenient and inexpensive means of administration has been to apply rather large amounts of the hormone, in the form of posterior pituitary powder, to the nasal mucous membranes. The amounts of ADH absorbed are sufficient for the control of diabetes insipidus for a period of 6 to 12 hours. Lypressin, in the form of a nasal spray, is administered for this purpose.

Upon reaching the circulation, endogenous or injected ADH is rapidly removed. Its half-life in plasma, in concentrations within the physiological range, is approximately 15 minutes in man. ADH is removed from plasma and inactivated largely during passage through the liver and kidneys. A portion of the hormone removed from the plasma by the kidney is enzymatically inactivated. The remainder appears in the urine bound to unidentified large molecules. The urinary clearance of endogenous or exogenous ADH is 5 to 10% of the glomerular filtration rate. Most investigators have found that circulating ADH is largely unbound and is confined to extracellular fluid. The fate of lypressin is similar to that of ADH.

During pregnancy a peptidase appears in plasma that is capable of inactivating a portion of ADH as well as oxytocin (see Chapter 42) by cleavage of the 1-cysteine to 2-tyrosine bond of the ring. For details of the biological fate of ADH, see Sawyer (1961) and Lauson (1967, 1970).

Preparations, Bioassay, and Unitage. ADH is available in two types of preparations. One is an extract in which no separation of the antidiuretic and oxytocic principles has been made. It is assayed for its oxytocic activity, which parallels antidiuretic activity. Activity is compared to that of a U.S.P. bovine pituitary standard and is expressed in terms of U.S.P. *posterior pituitary units. Posterior pituitary* consists of desiccated posterior pituitary powder that contains the equivalent of 1 U.S.P. posterior pituitary unit in each milligram; it is marketed as capsules containing approximately 45 mg, and as an inhalator. *Posterior pituitary injection* (PITUITRIN) is a sterile aqueous extract of the gland that contains the equivalent of 10 U.S.P. posterior pituitary units per milliliter. *Posterior pituitary injection (S)* (PITUITRIN-S), for use as a local hemostatic agent in surgery, contains 20 U.S.P. units per milliliter.

Vasopressin Injection, U.S.P. (PITRESSIN), is prepared from the posterior pituitary glands of domestic animals by separation of ADH from the oxytocic hormone, or by synthesis. It is assayed for pressor activity rather than antidiuretic activity, but these are identical, unit for unit. The test method is the blood pressure of the rat. Activity is designated as *pressor units* and is determined by comparison with a U.S.P. standard. Theoretically, there should be no difference in antidiuretic activity between a U.S.P. posterior pituitary unit and a U.S.P. pressor unit. Vasopressin injection contains 20 pressor units and not more than 1 oxytocic unit per milliliter.

The pure synthetic hormones, when subjected to bioassay, show an activity of approximately 370 U.S.P. pressor units per milligram of arginine vasopressin, and about two thirds of this activity for lysine vasopressin (lypressin). Their ratio of antidiuretic activity is similar. However, for reasons of chemical stability, lysine vasopressin is the more acceptable of the two synthetic hormones for therapeutic use. *Lypressin* (DIAPID) is available as a nasal spray containing 50 U.S.P. posterior pituitary units (pressor) per milliliter. One spray into a nostril provides approximately 2 pressor units.

Vasopressin tannate (PITRESSIN TANNATE) is a water-insoluble tannate of the antidiuretic principle. It is marketed suspended in peanut oil (*vasopressin tannate injection*). Each milliliter contains 5 pressor units.

THERAPEUTIC USES

The actions of ADH on the kidney, the circulation, and the intestinal tract provide the basis for the therapeutic applications of the hormone.

Antidiuretic Action. ADH provides the most effective therapy for *diabetes insipidus* of pituitary origin. If the polyuria is due to a deficiency in secretion of the neurohypophysis, normal urine volume can be restored by administration of the antidiuretic principle in any form. This cannot conveniently be accomplished by injection of aqueous solutions, which must be given either in large dosage or at frequent intervals to provide a continuous action. Sustained absorption can be attained by the nasal insufflation of approximately 40 mg of dry posterior pituitary powder at intervals of 6 to 10 hours. Even more effective control of urine volume is achieved by the intramuscular injection of vasopressin tannate in oil. The dose must be adjusted to the individual and ranges around 0.25 ml (1.25 units) daily. The effects are somewhat cumulative, and the adequacy of a given dose cannot be ascertained for several days. In some patients, adequate control can be obtained by injections at 48-hour intervals. Lypressin nasal spray is usually applied in doses of 4 units by one or two sprays into each nostril four times a day. However, as with the above preparations, the dose required for antidiuresis varies and must be individualized.

The presence of polydipsia and polyuria is not in itself pathognomonic of abnormal function of the pars nervosa. In an occasional individual, a syndrome simulating diabetes insipidus results from a *primary polydipsia*, the secretion of ADH being held in abeyance by continued hydration. Under these circumstances the rate of urine flow is reduced by the injection of hypertonic sodium chloride solution, whereas in diabetes insipidus of pituitary origin urine flow is increased. This procedure provides a rapid means of differential diagnosis. Certain patients with diabetes insipidus are completely refractory to the effects of administered antidiuretic principle. In such individuals, the inability of the kidney to reabsorb water adequately is due to a renal functional anomaly, frequently hereditary, rather than to hypofunction of the pars nervosa, but on rare occasions it may be drug induced (*e.g.,* by lithium). This polyuria, referred to as *nephrogenic diabetes insipidus,* responds, however, to treatment with the thiazide diuretics (*see* below).

The antidiuretic principle is useful in a variety of *diagnostic tests.* The concentrating capacity of the kidney can be rapidly determined by injecting 5 to 10 units of a suitable preparation intramuscularly and measuring the specific gravity of the urine voided 1 and 2 hours later. The increase in concentration obtained is equivalent to that resulting from 18 hours of water deprivation. The test has the advantage that it may be carried out on unprepared patients, is rapidly executed, and is more reliable than water deprivation in edematous individuals. Similarly, posterior pituitary preparations can be administered 15 to 20 minutes prior to the injection of contrast media for *intravenous urography,* to ensure maximal concentration of the contrast material in the urinary tract.

Pressor Action. Despite its unfortunately chosen name, *vasopressin should not be employed as a pressor agent.* If it is desired to produce systemic peripheral vasoconstriction, preference should be given to appropriate sympathomimetic amines that can increase peripheral resistance without reducing coronary blood flow. However, it has been proposed that a justifiable exception may be made for the use of vasopressin as an adjunct in the control of bleeding *esophageal varices* and during abdominal surgery in patients with portal hypertension. When large doses (20 units in 5 minutes) are infused in normal subjects or in patients with cirrhosis and portal hypertension, there is a marked decrease in portal blood flow and pressure lasting approximately 30 minutes (Edmunds and West, 1962). Only a moderate rise in arterial pressure occurs. This effect on portal circulation is attributable to marked splanchnic vasoconstriction. An inactive "hormogen," triglycyl vasopressin, *glypressin,* is under study for such use. After its parenteral administration, continuous conversion to the active octapeptide by the liver results in sustained plasma concentrations that are claimed to provide splanchnic vasoconstriction with minimal effects on other vascular beds.

The use of phenylalanine²-lysine⁸ vasopressin, known as octapressin, *felypressin,* or PLV-II, as a local hemostatic agent has been widely investigated because of its higher ratio of pressor to other activities. It has also been used in place of epinephrine to retard the absorption of local anesthetics. The advantage claimed is that it does not cause cardiac effects in the doses used for these purposes. The preparation is not yet available in the United States.

Intestinal Action. Posterior pituitary extract or vasopressin has been used in the relief of *intestinal paresis* and *distention.* A dose of 5 to 10 units is given by intramuscular injection. However, it should be emphasized that the successful treatment of intestinal distention often calls for varied procedures, including suction decompression and drugs such as neostigmine. Combined therapy may result in addi-

tive effects. The action of vasopressin has also been utilized prior to *cholecystography* in order to remove gas from the bowel.

Untoward Reactions and Contraindications. Following the injection of large doses of posterior pituitary extract or vasopressin, marked facial pallor as a result of cutaneous vasoconstriction is commonly observed. Increased intestinal activity is likely to cause nausea, belching, cramps, and an urge to defecate. Women are apt to experience uterine cramps of a menstrual character. Most serious, however, is the effect on the coronary circulation. Individuals suffering from vascular disease, especially disease of the coronary arteries, should never receive vasopressin, except in the small doses needed for the treatment of diabetes insipidus. Sometimes even these small doses may cause difficulty in a patient who is subject to anginal attacks. The use of chlorothiazide or its congeners is indicated in such patients. When posterior pituitary powder is applied to the nasal mucosa, local irritation is common and hypersensitivity reactions may occur.

BENZOTHIADIAZIDES

Chlorothiazide and other benzothiadiazide (thiazide) diuretics paradoxically cause a reduction in the polyuria of patients with diabetes insipidus (Crawford and Kennedy, 1959). Their clinical use for this purpose is now well established. Other potent natriuretic agents, such as ethacrynic acid, have also been successfully employed (Brown *et al.,* 1966). The chemistry, pharmacology, available preparations, and usual therapeutic applications of these natriuretic agents are discussed in Chapter 39.

The actions of the thiazides in diabetes insipidus differ from those of ADH in two important ways. First, they are effective in diabetes insipidus of nephrogenic as well as pituitary origin. Second, a negative free-water clearance is rarely induced by these agents alone. However, the change from a copious polyuria to the excretion of a smaller volume of urine can reduce or eliminate the handicap of the patient in the pursuit of daily activities. In infants with diabetes insipidus resistant to ADH, the antidiuretic effect may be of more crucial importance since the uncontrolled polyuria may exceed the child's capacity to imbibe and absorb fluids.

The mechanism of the antidiuretic effect is not yet completely understood. Most investigators agree that the natriuretic action of the thiazides plays an important role. When these agents are given continuously to nonedematous subjects, an initial loss of sodium, chloride, and water during the first 2 days is followed by a sustained, moderate state of electrolyte depletion and reduction of extracellular volume. A small reduction in filtration rate may occur, but this is not always observed. It has been proposed that, under these conditions, a significant increase in the fraction of glomerular filtrate reabsorbed in the proximal tubule leads to delivery of reduced amounts of sodium chloride and, most importantly, potential free water to the distal tubule (*see* Earley and Orloff, 1964). Thus, a fluid smaller in volume and less dilute escapes the distal tubule. This explanation is supported by the fact that reduction of filtration rate by dehydration or by drug-induced hypotension has a similar antidiuretic effect in diabetes insipidus. Also, it has been observed that restricted salt intake enhances, and high salt intake antagonizes, the antidiuretic effect of the thiazides. The common denominator among these effects is felt to be the reduction of the amount of filtered water reaching the distal segment (*see* Earley and Orloff, 1962).

It is also believed that the collecting ducts are never completely impermeable to water and that any procedure that reduces the rate of flow of collecting-duct urine allows an increased opportunity for the abstraction of water and the elevation of osmotic pressure of the luminal contents (Berliner and Davidson, 1957). The degree to which the permeability of this segment may be influenced by the thiazides awaits more complete experimental evaluation. However, a number of observations suggest that the thiazides may influence the excretion of free water by actions other than salt depletion (Heineman *et al.*, 1959; Diés *et al.*, 1963).

Therapeutic Use. Chlorothiazide and its congeners are less effective than vasopressin in the treatment of pituitary diabetes insipidus but are invaluable for patients who experience undesirable side effects or allergic reactions after vasopressin and for those who have nephrogenic diabetes insipidus. Since their antidiuretic effects appear to parallel their ability to cause natriuresis, they are given in doses similar to those used for the mobilization of edema fluid. Chlorothiazide, 1.0 to 1.5 g, or hydrochlorothiazide, 50 to 150 mg, in daily divided doses, have been most frequently employed. Reduction of urine volume to 50% or less of pretreatment volumes is considered to be a good response. Moderate restriction of sodium chloride intake has been shown to enhance the antidiuretic effect. Representative clinical studies in adults are described by Havard and Wood (1961) as well as by Earley and Orloff (1962); in infants, by Schotland and associates (1963).

Among the most common of the side effects encountered is potassium depletion. It is essential, therefore, that the patient maintain a high dietary intake of this ion. It is sometimes necessary to administer supplementary oral potassium chloride. Other untoward effects of the thiazides are described in Chapter 39.

OTHER DRUGS

Chlorpropamide, an oral hypoglycemic agent, has been reported to impair free-water excretion, and a number of cases of hyponatremia and water intoxication have resulted from its use (Weissman *et al.*, 1971). It has received clinical trial in diabetes insipidus. Webster and Bain (1970) reported an average reduction in urine volume of 70%, with urine becoming hypertonic during periods of low fluid intake. Inhibition of the antidiuretic effect by ethyl alcohol suggests enhancement of the deficient ADH formation or release, although it has been shown experimentally that the drug may also directly potentiate the renal response to ADH. Hypoglycemia is observed in some patients. The hypolipemic agent *clofibrate* appears to exert a similar effect in pituitary diabetes insipidus without the accompanying risk of hypoglycemia. For details, *see* Hays and Levine (1974).

Two antineoplastic agents, *vincristine* and, in high doses, *cyclophosphamide,* have been reported to have caused hyponatremia with all the clinical features of inappropriate ADH secretion (Cutting, 1971; DeFronzo *et al.*, 1973).

ADH ANTAGONISTS

Although many congeners of ADH have been synthesized, none has the property of blocking the actions of ADH. Such a compound would be useful in the treatment of the syndrome of inappropriate secretion of antidiuretic hormone. The observation that lithium therapy in manic patients is associated with a high incidence of nephrogenic diabetes insipidus has lead to studies on its mechanism of action and possible therapeutic application. Presumably the ion interferes in the sequence of events by which ADH increases the permeability of the collecting tubule to water and urea. (*See* page 793 for further details and references.) Although the ubiquitous actions of lithium make it far from an ideal antagonist of ADH, convincing evidence of its clinical efficacy in this distressing syndrome would certainly stimulate efforts to find a more selective agent to overcome the effects of an inappropriately high concentration of ADH in the circulation.

Bartter, F. C., and Schwartz, W. B. The syndrome of inappropriate secretion of antidiuretic hormone. *Am. J. Med.,* **1967,** *42,* 790–806.

Berliner, R. W., and Bennett, C. M. Concentration of urine in the mammalian kidney. *Am. J. Med.,* **1967,** *42,* 777–789.

Berliner, R. W., and Davidson, D. G. Production of hypertonic urine in the absence of pituitary antidiuretic hormone. *J. clin. Invest.,* **1957,** *36,* 1416–1427.

Bisset, G. W.; Hilton, S. M.; and Poisner, A. M. Hypothalamic pathways for the independent release of vasopressin and oxytocin. *Proc. R. Soc., B,* **1966,** *166,* 422–442.

Brown, D. M.; Reynolds, J. W.; Michael, A. F.; and Ulstrom, R. A. The use and mode of action of ethacrynic acid in nephrogenic diabetes insipidus. *Pediatrics, Springfield,* **1966,** *37,* 447–455.

Crawford, J. D., and Kennedy, G. C. Chlorothiazide in diabetes insipidus. *Nature, Lond.,* **1959,** *183,* 891–892.

Cutting, H. O. Inappropriate secretion of antidiuretic hormone secondary to vincristine therapy. *Am. J. Med.,* **1971,** *51,* 269–271.

DeFronzo, R. A.; Braine, H.; Colvin, O. M.; and Davis, P. J.   Water intoxication in man after cyclophosphamide therapy. *Ann. intern. Med.,* **1973,** *78,* 861–869.

Diés, F.; Suárez, A.; and Rivera, A.   Treatment of diabetes insipidus with orally administered compounds. *Clin. Pharmac. Ther.,* **1963,** *4,* 602–611.

Douglas, W. W., and Poisner, A. M.   Stimulus-secretion coupling in a neurosecretory organ: the role of calcium in the release of vasopressin. *J. Physiol., Lond.,* **1964,** *172,* 1–18.

duVigneaud, V.; Gish, D. T.; and Katsoyannis, P. G.   A synthetic preparation possessing biological properties associated with arginine vasopressin. *J. Am. chem. Soc.,* **1954,** *76,* 4751–4752.

duVigneaud, V.; Ressler, C.; Swan, J. M.; Roberts, C. W.; Katsoyannis, P. G.; and Gordon, S.   The synthesis of an octapeptide amide with the hormonal activity of oxytocin. *J. Am. chem. Soc.,* **1953,** *75,* 4879–4880.

Earley, L. E., and Orloff, J.   The mechanism of antidiuresis associated with the administration of hydrochlorothiazide to patients with vasopressin-resistant diabetes insipidus. *J. clin. Invest.,* **1962,** *41,* 1988–1997.

————.   Thiazide diuretics. *A. Rev. Med.,* **1964,** *15,* 149–166.

Edmunds, R., and West, S. P.   A study of the effect of vasopressin on portal and systemic blood pressure. *Surgery Gynec. Obstet.,* **1962,** *114,* 458–462.

Fishman, M. P.; Vorherr, H.; Kleeman, C. R.; and Telfer, N.   Diuretic-induced hyponatremia. *Ann. intern. Med.,* **1971,** *75,* 853–863.

Ginsberg, M.   Molecular aspects of neurohypophyseal hormone release. *Proc. R. Soc., B,* **1968,** *170,* 27–36.

Grantham, J. J.   Mode of water transport in mammalian renal collecting tubules. *Fedn Proc. Fedn Am. Socs exp. Biol.,* **1971,** *30,* 14–21.

Hargitay, B., and Kuhn, W.   Das Multiplikationprinzip als Grundlage der Harkonzentrierung in der Niere. *Z. Elecktrochem. angew. phys. Chem.,* **1951,** *55,* 539–558.

Havard, C. W. H., and Wood, P. H. N.   The effect of diuretics on renal water excretion in diabetes insipidus. *Clin. Sci.,* **1961,** *21,* 321–332.

Heineman, H. O.; Demartini, F. E.; and Laragh, J. H.   The effect of chlorothiazide on the renal excretion of electrolytes and free water. *Am. J. Med.,* **1959,** *26,* 853–861.

Holland, R.; Cross, B. A.; and Sawyer, C. H.   Milk ejection in the rabbit in response to intracarotid injections of hypertonic saline. *Fedn Proc. Fedn Am. Socs exp. Biol.,* **1958,** *17,* 73.

Kokko, J. P.   Membrane characteristics governing salt and water transport in the loop of Henle. *Fedn Proc. Fedn Am. Socs exp. Biol.,* **1974,** *33,* 25–30.

Lauson, H. D.   Metabolism of antidiuretic hormones. *Am. J. Med.,* **1967,** *42,* 713–744.

Mikiten, T. M., and Douglas, W. W.   Effect of calcium and other ions on vasopressin release from rat neurohypophyses stimulated electrically *in vitro. Nature, Lond.,* **1965,** *207,* 302.

Moore, W. W.   Antidiuretic hormone levels in normal subjects. *Fedn Proc. Fedn Am. Socs exp. Biol.,* **1971,** *30,* 1387–1394.

Oliver, G., and Schäfer, E. A.   On the physiological action of extracts of pituitary body and certain other glandular organs. *J. Physiol., Lond.,* **1895,** *18,* 277–279.

Orloff, J., and Handler, J. S.   The cellular mode of action of antidiuretic hormone. *Am. J. Med.,* **1964,** *36,* 686–697.

————.   The role of adenosine 3',5'-phosphate in the action of the antidiuretic hormone. *Ibid.,* **1967,** *42,* 757–768.

Orloff, J.; Wagner, H. N., Jr.; and Davidson, D. G.   The effect of variations in solute excretion and vasopressin dosage on the excretion of water in the dog. *J. clin. Invest.,* **1958,** *37,* 458–464.

Rudinger, J.; Pliška, V.; and Krejčí, I.   Oxytocin analogues in the analysis of some phases of hormone action. *Recent Prog. Horm. Res.,* **1972,** *28,* 131–172.

Sawyer, W. H.   Pharmacological characteristics of the antidiuretic principle in a bronchogenic carcinoma from a patient with hyponatremia. *J. clin. Endocr. Metab.,* **1967a,** *27,* 1497–1499.

————.   Evolution of the antidiuretic hormones and their functions. *Am. J. Med.,* **1967b,** *42,* 678–686.

————.   Lungfishes and amphibians: endocrine adaptation and the transition from aquatic to terrestrial life. *Fedn Proc. Fedn Am. Socs exp. Biol.,* **1972,** *31,* 1609–1614.

Sawyer, W. H., and Manning, M.   Synthetic analogs of oxytocin and the vasopressins. *A. Rev. Pharmac.,* **1973,** *13,* 5–17.

Scharrer, E., and Scharrer, B.   Hormones produced by neurosecretory cells. *Recent Prog. Horm. Res.,* **1954,** *10,* 183–240.

Schotland, M. G.; Grunbach, M. M.; and Strauss, J.   The effects of chlorothiazides in nephrogenic diabetes insipidus. *Pediatrics, Springfield,* **1963,** *31,* 741–753.

Share, L.   Vascular volume and blood level of antidiuretic hormone. *Am. J. Physiol.,* **1962,** *202,* 791–794.

Slotnick, I. L., and Teigland, J. D.   Cardiac accidents following vasopressin injection (PITRESSIN). *J. Am. med. Ass.,* **1951,** *146,* 1126–1129.

Smith, H. W.   Salt and water volume receptors: an exercise in physiological apologetics. *Am. J. Med.,* **1957,** *23,* 623–652.

van Dyke, H. B.; Adamsons, K.; and Engel, S. L.   Aspects of the biochemistry and physiology of the neurohypophyseal hormones. *Recent Prog. Horm. Res.,* **1955,** *11,* 1–41.

van Dyke, H. B.; Chow, B. F.; Greep, R. O.; and Rothen, A.   The isolation of a protein from the pars neuralis of the ox pituitary with constant oxytocic, pressor and diuresis-inhibiting activities. *J. Pharmac. exp. Ther.,* **1942,** *74,* 190–209.

Vávra, I.; Machová, A.; Holeček, V.; Cort, J. H.; Zaoral, M.; and Sorm, F.   Effect of a synthetic analogue of vasopressin in animals and in patients with diabetes insipidus. *Lancet,* **1968,** *1,* 948–952.

Wagner, H. N., and Braunwald, E.   The pressor effect of the antidiuretic principle of the posterior pituitary in orthostatic hypotension. *J. clin. Invest.,* **1956,** *35,* 1412–1418.

Walter, R.; Rudinger, J.; and Schwartz, I. L.   Chemistry and structure-activity relations of the antidiuretic hormones. *Am. J. Med.,* **1967,** *42,* 653–677.

Webster, B., and Bain, J.   Antidiuretic effect and complications of chlorpropamide therapy in diabetes insipidus. *J. clin. Endocr. Metab.,* **1970,** *30,* 215–227.

Weissman, P. N.; Shenkman, L.; and Gregerman, R. I.   Chlorpropamide hyponatremia. *New Engl. J. Med.,* **1971,** *284,* 65–71.

White, A. G.; Rubin, G.; and Leiter, L.   Studies in edema. IV. Water retention and the antidiuretic hormone in hepatic and cardiac disease. *J. clin. Invest.,* **1953,** *32,* 931–939.

Wirz, H.; Hargitay, B.; and Kuhn, W.   Lokalization des Konzentrierungsprozesses in der Niere durch direkte Kryoskopie. *Helv. physiol. pharmac. Acta,* **1951,** *9,* 196–207.

Monographs and Reviews

Berde, B., and Boisonnas, R. A.   Basic pharmacological properties of synthetic analogues and homologues of the neurohypophysial hormones. In, *Neurohypophysial Hormones and Similar Polypeptides.* (Berde, B., ed.) *Handb. exp. Pharmak.,* Vol. 23. Springer-Verlag, Berlin, **1968,** pp. 802–870.

Discussion on polypeptide hormones.   *Proc. R. Soc., B,* **1968,** *170,* 3–47.

Gottschalk, C. W. Osmotic concentration and dilution of the urine. *Am. J. Med.,* **1964,** *36,* 670–685.

Handler, J. S., and Orloff, J. The mechanism of action of antidiuretic hormone. In, *Renal Physiology. Handbook of Physiology,* Sect. 8. (Orloff, J., and Berliner, R. W., eds.) American Physiological Society, Washington, D.C., **1973,** pp. 791–814.

Harris, G. W. *Neural Control of the Pituitary Gland.* Edward Arnold & Co., London, **1955.**

Hays, R. M., and Levine, S. D. Vasopressin. *Kidney Int.,* **1974,** *6,* 307–322.

Heller, H. (ed.). *The Neurohypophysis.* Butterworth & Co., Ltd., London, **1957.**

Katsoyannis, P. G., and Ginos, J. Z. Chemical synthesis of peptides. *A. Rev. Biochem.,* **1969,** *38,* 891–912.

Lauson, H. D. Fate of the neurohypophysial hormones. In, *Pharmacology of the Endocrine System and Related Drugs,* Vol 1. *International Encyclopedia of Pharmacology and Therapeutics,* Sect. 41. (Heller, H., and Pickering, B. T., eds.) Pergamon Press, Ltd., Oxford, **1970,** pp. 377–397.

Pitts, R. F. *Physiology of the Kidney and Body Fluids: An Introductory Text,* 3rd ed. Year Book Medical Publishers, Inc., Chicago, **1974.**

Rudinger, J. *Oxytocin, Vasopressin and Their Structural Analogues.* Pergamon Press, Ltd., Oxford, **1964.**

———. The design of peptide hormone analogs. In, *Drug Design,* Vol. 2. (Ariëns, E. J., ed.) Academic Press, Inc., New York, **1972,** pp. 319–419.

Sawyer, W. H. Neurohypophysial hormones. *Pharmac. Rev.,* **1961,** *13,* 225–277.

Symposium. (Various authors.) Antidiuretic hormones. (Schwartz, I. L., and Schwartz, W. B., eds.) *Am. J. Med.,* **1967,** *42,* 651–827.

Symposium. (Various authors.) Antidiuretic hormonal secretion. *Fedn Proc. Fedn Am. Socs exp. Biol.,* **1971,** *30,* 1376–1394.

Symposium. (Various authors.) Renal handling of sodium. *Fedn Proc. Fedn Am. Socs exp. Biol.,* **1974,** *33,* 13–36.

Thorn, N. A. Mammalian antidiuretic hormone. *Physiol. Rev.,* **1958,** *38,* 169–195.

Wirz, H., and Dirix, R. Urinary concentration and dilution. In, *Renal Physiology. Handbook of Physiology,* Sect. 8. (Orloff, J., and Berliner, R. W., eds.) American Physiological Society, Washington, D.C., **1973,** pp. 415–430.

CHAPTER

41 INHIBITORS OF TUBULAR TRANSPORT OF ORGANIC COMPOUNDS

Paul Brazeau

The previous chapters have considered those renal tubular functions related to the reabsorption and excretion of electrolytes and water. Of no less importance are the renal tubular transport systems concerned with the reabsorption and secretion of organic compounds. Many substances are now known to influence the function of these systems, usually by inhibition of transport. An inhibitor capable of retarding the active tubular reabsorption of an organic compound augments the renal excretion of that compound. Conversely, an inhibitor capable of depressing the active tubular secretion of a compound retards the urinary excretion of that compound. Such inhibitors, if sufficiently selective in action, can have useful applications as drugs. A number of organic acids and bases have been shown to undergo bidirectional active transport, and many are also subject to passive reabsorption that is influenced principally by the pK_a and lipid solubility of the substance and by urine pH and flow rate (*see* introduction to Section VIII). The effective use of the inhibitors to be described depends on a clear understanding of these complex variables.

Physiological Considerations. In connection with his classical morphological description of the kidney, Bowman speculated that the function of the renal tubular epithelium was the secretion of solutes found in urine. In 1874, 32 years later, Heidenhain carried out experiments that clearly pointed to the tubular secretion of indigo carmine, an organic acid dye. However, the concept that secretion was among the normal functions of the kidney, which was rejected by Ludwig in 1844 and later by Cushny in 1917, remained unpopular. This attitude prevailed when, in 1910, the rate of excretion of phenolsulfonphthalein (PSP) was first used, empirically, for the clinical evaluation of renal function. The great rapidity with which the kidney excreted PSP prompted a critical investigation in the laboratory of E. K. Marshall, Jr., that unequivocally demonstrated the secretion of this dye by the normal kidney. The secretion of other organic acids such as iodopyracet and para-amino-

hippuric acid (PAH) was then confirmed by Marshall and others, notably by A. N. Richards and Homer Smith.

The reabsorption of organic as well as inorganic solutes by the renal tubule, although naively defined and unmeasured, had necessarily been invoked in all the proposed theories of renal function that included the formation of a glomerular filtrate. The development of technics for tubular micropuncture and accurate clearance measurements and the study of isolated renal tissue have now allowed detailed description of the functional characteristics of the transport of organic solutes out of, as well as into, the tubular lumen.

The importance of the renal tubular reabsorption of organic substances is immediately apparent when one considers that most of the nutrients and vitamins in solution in extracellular fluid gain access to the glomerular filtrate. Resources of glucose, amino acids, vitamins, and other essentials would soon be dissipated if these substances were not returned from the tubular urine to body fluids. The efficiency of the kidney in this respect is evident in the absence of body essentials in the urine unless presented to the tubules in unusually large amounts. One of the most familiar examples is the tubular reabsorption of glucose. This process is so efficient that virtually complete removal of the sugar from the tubular urine occurs unless the concentration in the glomerular filtrate, and hence the load delivered to the tubules, is so high that the transport capacity is exceeded.

On the other hand, many organic compounds that reach the kidney are destined to be excreted. These can gain access to the urine either by filtration and incomplete reabsorption or by tubular secretion. The most casual reflection leads to the conclusion that the mechanisms of renal transport must indeed be numerous and complex if substances necessary for the body economy are to be retained and foreign substances plus those end products of metabolism that no longer serve a useful purpose are to be rejected. It is not to be inferred that all excretory functions of the kidney depend upon active tubular transport systems. Many substances gain egress from the body by filtration alone. Their rate of excretion depends upon the extent to which passive back diffusion occurs. At the other extreme are compounds that not only reach the urine by means of glomerular filtration but also are secreted by the renal tubular cells with such efficiency that a single passage through the kidney eliminates them from the renal blood.

Since the secretion of PSP was first proven, little has been learned of the nature of the intracellular mechanisms that accomplish the unidirectional movement of such substances across the renal tubular epithelium. However, a monumental accumulation of experimental and clinical studies has described the active transport of many organic substances. It has been found that reabsorption is accomplished by numerous independent transport systems that tend to be selective for one substance or for a closely related group of substances, such as the amino acids. Secretion has been shown to be attributable largely to two systems. One transports the organic acids already mentioned as well as salicylates, penicillins, many diuretics, sulfonamides, and certain metabolites (such as sulfate esters and glucuronides) of drugs and naturally occurring substances. The other transports bases such as histamine, thiamine, hexamethonium, tolazoline, and many other naturally occurring and synthetic amines. These processes occur throughout the proximal tubule but are believed not to occur in the distal tubule. The clearance data for some substances, for example, uric acid, suggest bidirectional active transport. Organic solute transport proceeds quite independently of the simultaneously occurring reabsorption of inorganic solutes. It is completely dependent on energy from oxidative metabolism. In addition, the *secretion* of organic solutes is specifically dependent on the availability of adenosine triphosphate (ATP). It has been shown that the *rate* of transport of otherwise-independent active transport systems may be affected by changes in the amount of substrate presented for transport by other systems. Weiner and associates (1964) have investigated the structural features of organic acids that favor active transport. Present concepts have been reviewed by Mudge and associates (1973) and Weiner (1973).

Pharmacological Considerations.

It is generally believed that the substance to be transported must be incorporated into some form of carrier complex in or near the cell membrane and subsequently released at the opposite pole. This sequence requires energy for the reactivation of the carrier in order to continue. Thus, the primary component of the carrier mechanism would be located at the luminal membrane in the case of active reabsorption and at the peritubular membrane in the case of secretion. Simple diffusion is often invoked to account for the remainder of the journey into the peritubular or luminal fluid. However, study of the transport of PSP in isolated renal tissue suggests that there may be more than one critical step in the transport of some substances (Forster and Hong, 1958). That this is true of other actively transported substances has been amply confirmed.

There are many conceivable mechanisms by which the intricate process of renal tubular transport of organic compounds could be depressed. The least selective would be to interfere with those reactions that supply energy for transport. A more specific approach is that of competitive inhibition. The capacity of the tubule to transport any one of these organic substances is limited and is termed the "transport maximum" (Tm). It was appreciated early that the aforementioned acids share a common excretory pathway, since the presence of one reduces the Tm of the other. This is believed to be due to competition for an essential intermediary in the transport system.

Let us designate the substance that forms the hypothetical complex with organic acids essential for their transport as "X." The simplest way of depicting the transport of penicillin or PAH would be as follows:

$$
\begin{array}{c}
\text{Penicillin} \\
+ \sim X \rightleftharpoons \\
\text{PAH}
\end{array}
\quad
\begin{array}{c}
\text{Penicillin} \cdot X \\
\rightleftharpoons \\
\text{PAH} \cdot X
\end{array}
\quad
\begin{array}{c}
\text{Penicillin} \\
+ X \\
\text{PAH}
\end{array}
$$

$$\text{Energy Input}$$

Obviously, one limiting factor in this reaction is the supply of activated X ($\sim X$) or the rate at which it can be reformed. If PAH and penicillin had similar association and dissociation rates with the carrier X, they would share the transport system and the Tm of each would be halved if both were present in equally high concentrations. Actually, PAH does reduce the tubular secretion of penicillin and was once employed for this purpose. A commonly encountered effect of this type results from the use of diuretics (ethacrynic acid, furosemide, and the thiazides) that compete with uric acid for secretory transport and thus can cause uric acid retention.

Suppose, however, that an organic acid had a high affinity for the substance X, combined with it, but subsequently did not dissociate readily. The reaction could be depicted as follows:

$$RCOOH + X \rightleftharpoons RCOOH \cdot X$$

Such a compound would exist in the tubular cell primarily as the complex, $RCOOH \cdot X$, and would effectively block the transport of penicillin and yet not be excreted. Probenecid appeared to be an organic acid of this type, since its administration causes prolonged blockade of penicillin secretion and since little probenecid appears in the urine. It has now been shown that probenecid does indeed have a high affinity for the carrier system, and that it is also readily secreted but that subsequently it is reabsorbed by back diffusion (Weiner *et al.,* 1960). The return of the active inhibitor for recirculation accounts for the prolonged action.

PROBENECID

History. Probenecid was developed as a result of a planned pharmacological approach to achieve a specific objective. When penicillin was first introduced into therapy, the antibiotic was expensive and in short supply. The very rapid renal excretion of the antibiotic was of practical significance. For this reason, Beyer and associates began a systematic study to find an organic acid that would depress the renal tubular secretion of penicillin in the manner described above. The first compound to receive clinical trial was CARINAMIDE. It proved to be effective, but the drug was secreted by the renal tubules fairly rapidly so that it was necessary to give large and frequent doses. This problem was overcome with the discovery of probenecid (Beyer *et al.*, 1951).

Chemistry. Probenecid is a benzoic acid derivative with the following structural formula:

Probenecid

Various congeners of probenecid have been studied. Increasing the size of the N-alkyl substitution results in more efficient compounds. Optimal activity appears in probenecid, the N-dipropyl derivative. Gutman (1966) has reviewed the structure-activity relationship of probenecid congeners and that of other uricosuric drugs.

Pharmacological Actions.

The pharmacological actions of probenecid are largely confined to the inhibition of the renal tubular transport of organic acids. It has been widely used in the laboratory and clinical investigation of the excretion of a number of substances. In higher doses than are required for a uricosuric effect, probenecid also inhibits the transport of organic acids at other sites, for example, the transport system that removes organic acids from cerebrospinal fluid (Spector and Lorenzo, 1974). It is a potent inhibitor of certain glycine conjugases. However, its therapeutic applications have been limited principally to the modification of the renal excretion of penicillin and uric acid.

Penicillin. In adequate concentration, probenecid completely blocks the renal tubular secretory transport of penicillin (*see* Chapter 57). This does not mean that the renal excretion of penicillin falls to zero; the antibiotic present in the glomerular filtrate is not reabsorbed by the tubules and continues to be excreted in the urine.

Uric Acid. Normally a high percentage of the uric acid filtered by the glomerulus is reabsorbed by the proximal tubule; this is true even when plasma values are very much elevated. Reabsorption is due to active transport (*see* Berliner *et al.*, 1950). It is now clear that the human proximal tubule also secretes uric acid, as does the proximal tubule of many lower animals (Gutman *et al.*, 1959). Small doses of probenecid and other uricosuric agents, such as phenylbutazone and salicylates, actually depress the excretion of uric acid. This has been attributed to inhibition of secretion (Gutman and Yü, 1958). In support of this, it has been found that pyrazinamide, a tuberculostatic drug that reduces urate excretion in man, also blocks secretion in those species in which secretion is unequivocally demonstrable (Yü *et al.*, 1961). Large doses of probenecid, however, by depressing the more capacious system for reabsorption of uric acid, cause greatly enhanced excretion (Sirota *et al.*, 1952; for further details, *see* Mudge *et al.*, 1973). This uricosuric action of probenecid is of value in the treatment of chronic tophaceous gout.

Miscellaneous Substances. The renal tubular transport of certain diagnostic agents, such as iodopyracet and related iodinated organic acids, and of PAH and PSP is markedly depressed. In fact, the adequacy of the dose level of probenecid can be tested easily by measuring PSP excretion. Following intravenous administration of the dye, the urinary excretion in the first 15 minutes is only 20% of normal because of tubular blockade by probenecid.

The effect of probenecid on the disposition of a number of diagnostic and therapeutic agents in the body is well established. The physician should be alert to the need to modify the dosage of such drugs when they are administered during probenecid therapy.

Among the organic acids normally found in plasma, several have been shown to be transported by the renal tubule. The transport of some of these, for example, pantothenic acid, is known to be inhibited by probenecid. However, no clinical evidence of side effects due to changes in the excretion of essential solutes has been reported.

Absorption, Fate, and Excretion.

Probenecid is completely absorbed after oral administration. Peak plasma concentrations are reached in 2 to 4 hours. The rate of decline of plasma levels is rather variable.

The half-life of the drug in the plasma of most patients is between 6 and 12 hours. Between 85 and 95% of the drug is bound to plasma protein, largely to albumin. The small unbound portion gains access to the glomerular filtrate; a much larger portion is actively secreted by the proximal tubule. In spite of its low pK_a (3.4), the high lipid solubility of the undissociated form results in virtually complete absorption by back diffusion unless the urine is markedly alkaline, in which case amounts well in excess of the filtered load may be excreted. A small amount of probenecid glucuronide appears in the urine. It is also hydroxylated to metabolites that retain their carboxyl function and have uricosuric activity. (For details, *see* Dayton *et al.*, 1963; Israeli *et al.*, 1972.)

Preparations and Dosage. *Probenecid,* U.S.P. (BENEMID), is a white crystalline, odorless powder. The free acid is insoluble in water, but the sodium salt is freely soluble. The compound is marketed as oral tablets (500 mg). The dosage schedule depends upon the objectives of therapy. To block effectively the renal excretion of penicillin, a total daily dose of 2 g is employed in adults. This is administered in four divided doses. The total daily dose for children is from 10 to 25 mg/kg of body weight. In the treatment of chronic gout, a single daily dose of 250 mg is given for 1 week, following which 500 mg is administered twice daily. In some patients it may be necessary to increase the daily dose gradually to a maximum of 2 g, given in four divided portions.

Adjunct in Penicillin Therapy. The oral administration of probenecid in conjunction with penicillin G given by any route results in higher and more prolonged plasma concentrations of the antibiotic than when penicillin is given alone. The elevation in the plasma level is at least twofold and sometimes much greater. Although the reduction of a daily requirement of penicillin G from 1 million to 500,000 units has very little significance, a reduction by 50% or more may be of importance for convenience in the treatment of resistant infections that may require the administration of penicillin G in very large doses.

Probenecid also retards the renal excretion of certain penicillin congeners to a variable degree that is dependent, in part, on the ratio of the amounts secreted and filtered.

Untoward Reactions and Precautions. Probenecid is well tolerated by most patients.

Some degree of gastrointestinal irritation is experienced by at least 2% of patients; the incidence is considerably higher after large doses. Cautious administration is advised in patients with a history of peptic ulcer. Most reports place the incidence of hypersensitivity reactions, usually mild skin rashes, between 2 and 4%. More serious hypersensitivity reactions occur, but they are rare. The appearance of a rash during the concurrent administration of probenecid and penicillin G or a congener presents the physician with an awkward diagnostic dilemma. The hazard of intrarenal precipitation of uric acid during uricosuric therapy is discussed below. The compound also increases to some degree the concentration of sulfonamide in the blood. Huge overdosage of probenecid results in stimulation of the central nervous system, convulsions, and death from respiratory failure (McKinney *et al.*, 1951).

SULFINPYRAZONE

History. Despite its therapeutic efficacy as an anti-inflammatory and uricosuric agent, phenylbutazone (*see* Chapter 17) has undesirable side effects severe enough to preclude its continuous use in the treatment of chronic gout. For this reason, a number of chemical congeners were evaluated for uricosuric and anti-inflammatory activity. One of these, in which a phenyl-thioethyl configuration replaces the butyl side chain of the parent compound, displayed promising activity. Since active metabolites of phenylbutazone were known to be formed, the metabolites of the new compound were also isolated and studied. It was found that side chain oxidation *in vivo* led to the formation of the sulfoxide, *sulfinpyrazone,* a potent uricosuric agent (Burns *et al.*, 1957; Yü *et al.*, 1958).

Chemistry. The chemical structure of sulfinpyrazone is as follows:

Sulfinpyrazone

It is a strong organic acid (pK_a 2.8) that readily forms soluble salts. Burns and coworkers (1958) studied a number of congeners; they found that a low pK_a and polar side chain substitutions favor uricosuric activity (*see also* Gutman, 1966).

Pharmacological Actions. Sulfinpyrazone in sufficient dosage is a potent inhibitor of the renal tubular reabsorption of uric acid. As with other uricosuric agents, small doses may reduce the excretion of uric acid, presumably by inhibiting secretory but not reabsorptive transport. By competitive inhibition, sulfinpyrazone reduces the renal tubular secretion of other organic anions such as PAH and salicylic acid. Its uricosuric action is additive to that of probenecid and phenylbutazone but is mutually antagonistic to that of the salicylates (Yü *et al.*, 1963). Sulfinpyrazone possesses to an unusual degree the ability to displace other organic anions that are bound extensively to plasma proteins (*e.g.*, sulfonamides, salicylates), thus altering their distribution to tissues and their renal excretion (Anton, 1961). The extent to which this property may be a clinical asset or liability depends on concomitant medication.

Sulfinpyrazone lacks the clinically striking anti-inflammatory and analgesic properties of its congener, phenylbutazone.

Platelet Aggregation. The effect of sulfinpyrazone on platelet function is discussed in Chapter 65.

Absorption, Fate, and Excretion. Sulfinpyrazone is well absorbed after oral administration. It is bound to plasma proteins to the extent of 98 to 99%. The half-life of the drug in plasma after its intravenous injection is about 3 hours. After oral administration, however, its uricosuric effect may persist for as long as 10 hours. Although little sulfinpyrazone is available for filtration at the glomerulus, it is secreted by the proximal tubule and undergoes little passive back diffusion because of its low pK_a. Approximately half of the orally administered dose appears in the urine within 24 hours. Most of the drug (90%) in the urine is unchanged; the remainder is eliminated as the N^1-*p*-hydroxyphenyl metabolite, which also is a potent uricosuric substance. (For details, *see* Burns *et al.*, 1957, 1958; Gutman *et al.*, 1960; Dayton *et al.*, 1961.)

Preparations and Dosage. *Sulfinpyrazone,* U.S.P. (ANTURANE), is available as official 100-mg tablets and 200-mg capsules. For the treatment of *chronic gout,* the initial dosage is 100 to 200 mg per day. After the first week, the dose may be gradually increased until a satisfactory lowering of plasma uric acid is achieved and maintained. This may require from 100 to 400 mg per day, divided in two to four doses and preferably given with meals. Occasional resistant patients have been treated successfully with doses as high as 800 mg per day. Larger doses are poorly tolerated and unlikely to produce a further uricosuric effect in the resistant patient. In responsive patients not requiring high dosage, a single daily dose of 100 mg is sometimes satisfactory for maintenance.

Untoward Reactions and Precautions. *Gastrointestinal irritation* occurs in 10 to 15% of all patients receiving sulfinpyrazone, and an occasional patient may require discontinuance of its use. Its frequency and severity increase with dosage. Gastric distress is lessened when the drug is taken in divided doses with meals. Sulfinpyrazone should be given to patients with a history of peptic ulcer only with the greatest caution and careful observation. *Hypersensitivity* reactions, usually a rash with fever, do occur, but less frequently than with probenecid. The severe blood dyscrasias and salt and water retention, hazards of phenylbutazone therapy (*see* Chapter 17), have not been observed during sulfinpyrazone therapy. However, the ability of the drug to depress hematopoiesis has been demonstrated experimentally, and periodic blood-cell counts are therefore advised during prolonged therapy. Adequate precautions must also be taken to prevent intrarenal precipitation of urates (*see* below).

Diagnostic procedures depending on the renal tubular secretion of PAH, PSP, and other organic acids are invalidated by sulfinpyrazone therapy. The effects of sulfinpyrazone on the renal elimination of other drugs are very similar to those of probenecid. The drug also resembles probenecid in that its uricosuric action is antagonized by salicylates.

OTHER DRUGS

A number of drugs having primary pharmacological actions completely unrelated to uric acid metabolism or renal function show moderate-to-marked uricosuric activity. Notable among these are certain anticoagulant coumarins and indandiones and oral hypoglycemic drugs of the sulfonylurea group. However, their use as uricosuric agents is precluded because of the inappropriateness of their primary effects. The degree to which these drugs may complement or antagonize the effects of probenecid and sulfinpyrazone has yet to be established.

Although phenylbutazone and oxyphenbutazone are used during acute attacks of gout primarily for their anti-inflammatory and analgesic effects, it should be remembered that they are also potent uricosuric agents.

THE CLINICAL USE OF URICOSURIC AGENTS

Abnormalities in the rate of formation or renal excretion of uric acid, or both, are the primary etiological factors in gout and other hyperuricemic states. Current knowledge of urate production has been reviewed by Wyngaarden (1974). For details of the role of the kidney in the development of hyperuricemia, *see* Rieselbach and Steele (1974).

In the clinical use of the available uricosuric drugs, it must be kept in mind that they can alter the plasma binding, distribution, and renal excretion of other organic acids (as discussed above), whether these be naturally occurring substances or drugs and drug metabolites.

Gout. The use of probenecid and sulfinpyrazone for the mobilization of uric acid in *chronic gout* is well established. In about two thirds of patients, these agents cause uric acid to be excreted at a rate sufficient to exceed that of formation and thereby promptly lower the plasma uric acid concentration. Although the intravenous administration of large doses of these drugs can cause a fivefold to sevenfold increase in the renal clearance of urate, continuous oral administration to patients with tophaceous gout approximately doubles the daily excretion of urates. In such patients, continued administration prevents the formation of new tophi and causes gradual shrinkage, or even disappearance, of old tophi. In gouty arthritis, there is a reduction in the swelling of chronically enlarged joints and a dramatic degree of rehabilitation may be achieved in patients who suffer severe pain and limitation of joint movement.

The introduction of *allopurinol,* a drug that inhibits the formation of uric acid, constitutes a very important addition to the therapeutic means of controlling hyperuricemia, regardless of its etiology (*see* Chapter 17). In those patients who do not respond well to uricosuric agents because of impaired renal function, allopurinol is especially useful. In patients with gouty nephropathy, it offers the additional advantage over the uricosuric agents that the daily excretion of uric acid is reduced rather than increased. Its administration is compatible with the simultaneous use of the uricosuric agents if necessary (*see* Chapter 17).

Neither the uricosuric agents nor allopurinol alters the course of acute attacks of gout or supplants the use of colchicine and anti-inflammatory agents in their management. Indeed, the acute attacks may increase in frequency or severity during the early months of therapy when urate is being mobilized from affected joints. Therefore, therapy with uricosuric agents should *not be initiated* during an acute attack but may be continued if already begun. Colchicine in small doses (0.5 to 2 mg per day) may be administered at this period (or at any time) to reduce the frequency of attacks. When an acute attack occurs, it is treated with full doses of colchicine or whatever agent has proven most satisfactory in the management of previous attacks (phenylbutazone or oxyphenbutazone, corticosteroids, indomethacin, etc.). The use of salicylates is contraindicated because they antagonize the action of probenecid and sulfinpyrazone. However, for analgesia, acetaminophen may be used. Later in the course of therapy, acute attacks become less frequent or may cease altogether.

In the treatment of gout, the uricosuric drugs are given continually in the lowest dose that will maintain satisfactory plasma uric acid concentrations. Since the pK_a of uric acid is 5.6 and the solubility of the undissociated form is very low, maintaining the output of a large volume of alkaline urine minimizes its intrarenal deposition. This precaution is essential during the early weeks of therapy when uric acid excretion is large, especially in patients with a history of renal disease associated with the passage of urate stones or gravel. It is believed that renal disease of any etiology is a predisposing factor in the development of gouty nephropathy. Eventual improvement in renal function in patients with gouty nephropathy has been reported, but it is uncommon. The use of allopurinol permits a more favorable prognosis in such patients.

There is no universal agreement as to the relative importance of exogenous purines and xanthines, as opposed to those synthesized in the body, as sources of uric acid in gout. However, it is generally agreed that, after a patient has become stabilized on uricosuric therapy, a more liberal diet can be allowed, and only foods of high purine content need be avoided. Since ethyl alcohol in large amounts elevates plasma uric acid concentration, alcoholic beverages must be used in moderation. (For detailed evaluations of uricosuric agents, *see* Gutman, 1966; Yü and Gutman, 1967; Yü, 1974.)

Other Hyperuricemic States. Uricosuric agents, as well as allopurinol, can be useful in those patients who show elevated plasma uric acid concentrations during the administration of chlorothiazide or other diuretics (Beyer and Baer, 1961; Smilo et al., 1962). They are also useful for the control of the hyperuricemia resulting from the use of the cytotoxic antineoplastic agents or from diseases that involve accelerated formation and destruction of blood cells. The use of other drugs, such as levodopa and ethambutol, as well as certain disease states, including toxemia of pregnancy, diabetic ketosis, and uremia, may be accompanied by moderate-to-marked elevation of plasma uric acid. The hyperuricemia may remain asymptomatic, but attacks of gout or renal precipitation of urate may occur. The management of such hyperuricemic states has been outlined by Yü (1974).

Anton, A. H.   A drug-induced change in the distribution and renal excretion of sulfonamides. *J. Pharmac. exp. Ther.,* **1961,** *134,* 291–303.

Berliner, R. W.; Hilton, J. G.; Yü, T.-F.; and Kennedy, T. J., Jr.   The renal mechanism for urate excretion in man. *J. clin. Invest.,* **1950,** *29,* 396–401.

Beyer, K. H., and Baer, J. E. Physiological basis for the action of newer diuretic agents. *Pharmac. Rev.,* **1961,** *13,* 517–561.

Beyer, K. H.; Russo, H. F.; Tillson, E. K.; Miller, A. K.; Verwey, W. F.; and Gass, S. R. "BENEMID," *p*-(di-*n*-propylsulfamyl)-benzoic acid: its renal affinity and its elimination. *Am. J. Physiol.,* **1951,** *166,* 625–640.

Burns, J. J.; Yü, T.-F.; Dayton, P. G.; Berger, L.; Gutman, A. B.; and Brodie, B. B. Relationship between pK_a and uricosuric activity in phenylbutazone analogues. *Nature, Lond.,* **1958,** *182,* 1162–1163.

Burns, J. J.; Yü, T.-F.; Ritterbrand, A.; Perel, J. M.; Gutman, A. B.; and Brodie, B. B. A potent new uricosuric agent, the sulfoxide metabolite of the phenylbutazone analogue G25671. *J. Pharmac. exp. Ther.,* **1957,** *119,* 418–426.

Dayton, P. G.; Secam, L. E.; Landrau, M.; and Burns, J. J. Metabolism of sulfinpyrazone and other thio analogues of phenylbutazone in man. *J. Pharmac. exp. Ther.,* **1961,** *132,* 287–290.

Dayton, P. G.; Yü, T.-F.; Chen, W.; Berger, L.; West, L. A.; and Gutman, A. B. The physiological disposition of probenecid, including renal clearance in man, studied by an improved method for its estimation in biological material. *J. Pharmac. exp. Ther.,* **1963,** *140,* 278–286.

Forster, R. P., and Hong, S. K. *In vitro* transport of dyes by isolated renal tubules of the flounder as disclosed by direct visualization: intracellular accumulation and transcellular movement. *J. cell. comp. Physiol.,* **1958,** *51,* 259–272.

Gutman, A. B.; Dayton, P. G.; Yü, T.-F.; Berger, L.; Chen, W.; Sicam, L. E.; and Burns, J. J. A study of the inverse relationship between pK_a and rate of renal excretion of phenylbutazone analogues in man and dogs. *Am. J. Med.,* **1960,** *29,* 1017–1033.

Gutman, A. B., and Yü, T.-F. Renal regulation of uric acid secretion in normal and gouty man: modification by uricosuric agents. *Bull. N.Y. Acad. Med.,* **1958,** *34,* 387–396.

Gutman, A. B.; Yü, T.-F.; and Berger, L. Tubular secretion of urate in man. *J. clin. Invest.,* **1959,** *38,* 1778–1781.

Israeli, Z. H.; Perel, J. M.; Cunningham, R. F.; Dayton, P. G.; Yü, T.-F.; Gutman, A. B.; Long, K. R.; Long, R. C., Jr.; and Goldstein, J. H. Metabolites of probenecid. Chemical, physical, and pharmacological studies. *J. mednl Chem.,* **1972,** *15,* 709–716.

McKinney, S. E.; Peck, H. M.; Bochey, J. M.; Byham, B. B.; Schuchardt, G. S.; and Beyer, K. H. BENEMID, *p*-(di-*n*-propylsulfamyl)-benzoic acid: toxicologic properties. *J. Pharmac. exp. Ther.,* **1951,** *102,* 208–214.

Sirota, J. H.; Yü, T.-F.; and Gutman, A. B. Effect of BENEMID on urate clearance and discrete renal functions in gouty subjects. *J. clin. Invest.,* **1952,** *31,* 692–701.

Smilo, R. P.; Beisel, W. R.; and Forsham, P. H. Reversal of thiazide-induced transient hyperuricemia by uricosuric agents. *New Engl. J. Med.,* **1962,** *267,* 1225–1227.

Spector, R., and Lorenzo, A. V. The effects of salicylate and probenecid on the cerebrospinal fluid transport of penicillin, aminosalicylic acid and iodide. *J. Pharmac. exp. Ther.,* **1974,** *188,* 55–65.

Weiner, I. M.; Blanchard, K. C.; and Mudge, G. H. Factors influencing renal excretion of foreign organic acids. *Am. J. Physiol.,* **1964,** *207,* 953–963.

Weiner, I. M.; Washington, J. A.; and Mudge, G. H. On the mechanism of action of probenecid on renal tubular secretion. *Bull. Johns Hopkins Hosp.,* **1960,** *106,* 336–346.

Wyngaarden, J. B. Metabolic defects of primary hyperuricemia and gout. *Am. J. Med.,* **1974,** *56,* 651–664.

Yü, T.-F.; Berger, L.; and Gutman, A. B. Suppression of tubular secretion of urate in the dog. *Proc. Soc. exp. Biol. Med.,* **1961,** *107,* 905–908.

Yü, T.-F.; Burns, J. J.; and Gutman, A. B. Results of a clinical trial of G28315, a sulfoxide analogue of phenylbutazone, in gouty subjects. *Arthritis Rheum.,* **1958,** *1,* 532–543.

Yü, T.-F.; Dayton, P. G.; and Gutman, A. B. Mutual suppression of the uricosuric effects of sulfinpyrazone and salicylate: a study in interactions between drugs. *J. clin. Invest.,* **1963,** *42,* 1330–1339.

Monographs and Reviews

Gutman, A. B. Uricosuric drugs, with special reference to probenecid and sulfinpyrazone. *Adv. Pharmac.,* **1966,** *4,* 91–142.

Hitchings, G. H., and Elion, G. B. Drugs and uric acid. *A. Rev. Pharmac.,* **1969,** *9,* 345–362.

Mudge, G. H.; Berndt, W. O.; and Valtin, H. Tubular transport of urea, glucose, phosphate, uric acid, sulfate, and thiosulfate. In, *Renal Physiology. Handbook of Physiology,* Sect. 8. (Orloff, J., and Berliner, R. W., eds.) American Physiological Society, Washington, D.C., **1973,** pp. 587–652.

Pitts, R. F. *Physiology of the Kidney and Body Fluids: An Introductory Text,* 3rd ed. Year Book Medical Publishers, Inc., Chicago, **1974.**

Rieselbach, R. E., and Steele, T. H. Influence of the kidney upon urate homeostasis in health and disease. *Am. J. Med.,* **1974,** *56,* 665–675.

Weiner, I. M. Transport of weak acids and bases. In, *Renal Physiology. Handbook of Physiology,* Sect. 8. (Orloff, J., and Berliner, R. W., eds.) American Physiological Society, Washington, D.C., **1973,** pp. 521–554.

Yü, T.-F. Milestones in the treatment of gout. *Am. J. Med.,* **1974,** *56,* 676–683.

Yü, T.-F., and Gutman, A. B. Principles of current management of primary gout. *Am. J. med. Sci.,* **1967,** *254,* 893–907.

Drugs Affecting Uterine Motility

In this section, only the oxytocics are discussed. The effects of estrogens, androgens, and anterior pituitary hormones on the reproductive system are presented elsewhere.

42 OXYTOCICS

Oxytocin, Prostaglandins, and Ergot Alkaloids

Paul Brazeau

Many drugs possess oxytocic activity, namely, the ability to stimulate the smooth muscle of the uterus. However, only a few have uterine effects sufficiently selective and predictable to justify their use as oxytocic agents in obstetrical practice. These are *oxytocin,* certain of the *prostaglandins,* and the ergot alkaloids *ergonovine* and *methylergonovine.* Each, in appropriate doses during pregnancy, is capable of eliciting graded increases in uterine motility from a moderate increase in the rate and force of spontaneous motor activity to sustained "tetanic" contraction, while causing minimal side effects in healthy subjects. Although these agents have other physiological and pharmacological effects that will be described in some detail, the dangers as well as the value of their use in obstetrics reside largely in this single common action.

The prostaglandins are the latest group of oxytocic agents to be studied. Discussion in this chapter will be limited to the effects of prostaglandins of the E and F types on the uterus and their potential for use as aborti-facients and as oxytocic agents at term. The general discussion of the prostaglandins appears in Chapter 30.

Physiological and Anatomical Considerations. Uterine smooth muscle is characterized by a high degree of spontaneous electrical and contractile activity. Waves of decreased membrane potential with superimposed spike activity are associated with contraction. Cell-to-cell spread of excitation occurs. Increased frequency and duration of spike activity in "pacemaker" areas and more extensive spread of excitation are associated with increases in force of contraction. Widespread depolarization of the myometrium, for example, by high concentrations of potassium ion *in vitro,* results in sustained contracture. As in most excitable tissues, movement of sodium ions appears to play the primary role in depolarization, whereas calcium ions are required for excitation-contraction coupling. The availability of calcium ion strongly influences the response of uterine smooth muscle to physiological and pharmacological stimulation and inhibition.

The uterus has parasympathetic and sympathetic innervation, the former by way of the pelvic nerve and the latter by way of postganglionic fibers from the inferior mesenteric and hypogastric ganglia. Both can elicit increased activity in the mature human uterus, but denervation causes little change in uterine motor activity. Both alpha-(excitatory) and beta-(inhibitory, hyperpolarizing)-adrenergic receptors are clearly demonstrable in the myometrium of mammals. Stimulation of sympathetic nerves supplying the uterus also causes vasoconstriction. Although quite capable of affecting the motility of the uterus, autonomic agonist drugs are not useful for this purpose in clinical practice, largely because they lack the desired selectivity. Since the activity of the uterus is largely independent of its motor innervation, autonomic blocking agents have little effect and do not impair the actions of the clinically used oxytocic agents. Uterine contractile activity is inhibited by local anesthetics and by direct-acting smooth muscle relaxants such as papaverine, nitroglycerin, and caffeine. However, these drugs also lack selectivity.

Uterine smooth muscle is unusually susceptible to endocrine influence, especially that of the estrogens. Thus, spontaneous activity, as well as responsiveness to neurogenic, hormonal, and pharmacological stimulation, increases greatly at puberty and varies thereafter with the ovulatory cycle. In some species, progesterone markedly inhibits uterine activity. Whether progesterone has an important physiological role in regulating the motor activity of the human uterus has yet to be clearly demonstrated.

Experimental Evaluation of Oxytocics. The study of the uterus is complicated by many factors, such as the alterations in its behavior occasioned by physiological variables (maturity, endocrine milieu, period of gestation, etc.). Confusion is compounded by the marked species variations among the experimental animals that have been studied and between these and human beings. *In vitro,* the responses of uterine smooth muscle are strongly influenced by the concentrations not only of calcium but also of magnesium, potassium, and other ions in the bathing medium. The smooth muscle of the cervical region often responds differently than that of the body of the uterus. It is not surprising that there are many conflicting reports of the effects of drugs on this organ. Unless otherwise stated, the effects of the oxytocic drugs to be discussed are those that have been confirmed in human beings.

OXYTOCIN AND POSTERIOR PITUITARY EXTRACTS

The structure, formation, storage, and release of the neurohypophyseal hormones, oxytocin and antidiuretic hormone (ADH), and a comparison of their biological activities have been presented in Chapter 40. The following discussion will deal in more detail with the physiological and pharmacological properties of oxytocin. This hormone has slight, but not insignificant, antidiuretic and vascular activity that may become manifest when large doses are used (*see* below).

Physiological Role of Oxytocin. Oxytocin has stimulant effects on the smooth muscle of the uterus and mammary gland so potent and selective as to suggest that the polypeptide serves a true hormonal function at these sites. Oxytocin is unique in eliciting contractions of the fundus that are indistinguishable in amplitude, duration, and frequency from those seen in late pregnancy and during spontaneous labor. It is well established that the appropriate sensory stimuli, arising in the cervix and vagina or in the mammillae, reflexly cause oxytocin to be released from the posterior pituitary. The initiation of labor occurs without demonstrable dependence on oxytocin. However, dilatation of the birth canal constitutes a well-established reflex stimulus for the release of the hormone. Marked elevation of plasma oxytocin concentrations occurs during delivery and is believed to play an important part in the expulsion of the fetus and placenta. It has not been shown that parturition or lactation fails to occur in the complete absence of oxytocin. However, prolonged labor has been observed and the milk-ejection reflex is absent. It is known that in domestic animals the uterine stimulation, resulting from the release of oxytocin (and ADH), facilitates the ascent of spermatozoa. A corresponding effect in the human reproductive tract has not been established. Oxytocin can thus be considered to play a facilitatory role, at least, in parturition and an essential role in the milk-ejection reflex. Its function, if any, in males is not known. (For detailed discussions, *see* Symposium, 1961; Harris and Donovan, 1966.)

PHARMACOLOGICAL PROPERTIES

Uterus. Oxytocin stimulates both electrical and contractile activity in uterine smooth muscle. With higher concentrations, sustained decreases in resting membrane potential occur. These effects are highly dependent on the presence of estrogen. When estrogen levels are low, the effect of oxytocin is much reduced. The immature uterus is quite resistant (*see* Csapo, 1959). Although progesterone antagonizes the stimulant effect of oxytocin *in vitro,* the corresponding effect in the pregnant human uterus has been difficult to demonstrate. However, progestins have been widely used clinically to attempt to reduce uterine activity in cases of threatened or habitual abortion (*see* Chapter 68).

A very low level of motor activity prevails in the human uterus during the first and second trimesters of pregnancy. During the third trimester, spontaneous motor activity increases progressively until the sharp rise that constitutes the initiation of labor and delivery. The responsiveness of the uterus to oxytocin roughly parallels the increase in spontaneous activity. Oxytocin can initiate or enhance rhythmic contractions at any time, but in early pregnancy only very high doses elicit a response. In a study in which the effect of oxytocin infusions was carefully quantitated in terms of force, duration, and frequency of contractions, Caldeyro-Barcia and Posiero (1959) found an eightfold increase in responsiveness between the twentieth and thirty-ninth week. Most of this increase occurred during the last 9 weeks. Thus, slow intravenous infusion of a few units of oxytocin usually is effective in initiating labor at term. However, there is considerable variability among individuals and labor has been observed to occur after infusion of as little as 25 milliunits (0.05 μg) of oxytocin (*see* below).

Effect of Vasopressin. Paradoxically, the non-pregnant uterus is more responsive to vasopressin than to oxytocin, especially when uterine activity is elevated, as in primary dysmenorrhea (*see* Torpin *et al.*, 1947). However, the effect of vasopressin on uterine smooth muscle shows only a modest increase during pregnancy and is therefore far less than that of oxytocin at term. Vasopressin also differs from oxytocin in that it causes irregular, higher-frequency contractions associated with greater elevation of resting tone.

Mammary Gland. The alveolar ramifications of the mammary gland are surrounded by a network of modified smooth muscle, the myoepithelium. Contraction of these cells forces milk from the alveolar channels into the large sinuses, where it is easily available to the suckling infant. This function is known as milk ejection (milk letdown, in domestic animals). The myoepithelium is highly responsive to oxytocin. Although the catecholamines inhibit milk ejection, the contraction of the myoepithelium is not believed to be dependent on autonomic innervation, but is considered to be under the control of oxytocin and the reflex pathways that initiate the release of the hormone. Oxytocin is occasionally employed to promote milk ejection when this component of lactation appears to be inefficient in nursing mothers. It is also of limited usefulness in the relief of postpartum breast engorgement.

Cardiovascular System. Oxytocin has a marked but transient, direct relaxing effect on vascular smooth muscle when large amounts are administered in man. A decrease in systolic and especially diastolic blood pressure, flushing, and an increase in

limb blood flow are observed (Kitchin *et al.*, 1959). A reflexly induced tachycardia and increase in cardiac output accompany the depressor phase. When high doses are infused continuously, the brief fall in blood pressure is followed by a small but much more sustained rise. With decreased activity of buffer reflexes, for example, during the concomitant use of ganglionic or sympathetic blocking agents, the fall in blood pressure may be more pronounced. The amounts of oxytocin administered for most obstetrical purposes are insufficient to produce marked alterations of blood pressure. However, when very large doses are administered for therapeutic abortion or during uterine surgery, a marked fall in arterial pressure may occur, particularly in deeply anesthetized patients. The smooth muscle of avian blood vessels is highly susceptible to the dilator effect. The hypotensive response of the chicken is the basis of the U.S.P. bioassay for oxytocin.

The vasodilator effect of oxytocin is independent of autonomic receptors. It is readily blocked by small amounts of vasopressin. Infusions of oxytocin within a "physiological" dose range have sometimes been found to cause a marked increase in renal blood flow in dogs (especially in hypophysectomized dogs), an effect that is also blocked by low concentrations of vasopressin. (For further details of the cardiovascular effects of oxytocin, *see* Pickford, 1961; Andersen *et al.*, 1965.)

Other Actions. No predictable changes in electrolyte excretion by the kidney occur in man during the administration of oxytocin, although an increase in sodium excretion is regularly seen when the hormone is given intravenously in experimental animals. When large doses are required for therapeutic purposes, an antidiuretic effect can occur due to the slight intrinsic ADH-like activity of the hormone. Signs of water intoxication have been observed when excessive volumes of intravenous fluids have been administered during such procedures (Saunders and Munsick, 1966). The smooth muscle of tissues other than the uterus, blood vessels, and mammary myoepithelium is not sensitive to oxytocin. In experimental studies, oxytocin, like vasopressin, in high concentrations has effects in numerous tissues that are apparently irrelevant to its primary hormonal actions (for references, *see* Farrell *et al.*, 1968).

Absorption, Fate, and Excretion. If given orally, oxytocin is inactivated by trypsin. However, it is effective after administration by any parenteral route. A less efficient but convenient route is the intranasal application of drops or a spray. The ready absorption of oxytocin from buccal lozenges also permits the use of the oral mucosa as a route of administration.

The distribution and fate of oxytocin in the body are very like those of ADH (*see* Chapter 40). Its half-life in plasma is short. Various investigators have estimated it to be from 1 to several minutes, and even briefer in late pregnancy and during lactation. Its rapid removal from plasma is accomplished largely by the kidney and the liver. The lactating mammary gland also inactivates a significant portion of the circulating hormone. Cell-free extracts of liver and kidney show far higher oxytocin-inactivating activity than do extracts of other tissues. A very small portion of the oxytocin extracted by the kidney reaches the urine in active form, bound, like ADH, to larger nondialyzable molecules. During pregnancy, a glycoprotein aminopeptidase referred to as both "oxytocinase" and "vasopressinase" appears in plasma and is capable of inactivating either hormone by cleavage of the 1-cysteine to 2-tyrosine peptide bond. Plasma enzyme activity increases gradually until, as term approaches, it rises steeply to high levels; these then decline after delivery. High "oxytocinase" activity is also found in the placenta and in uterine tissue during this period. These tissues are thought by most investigators to be the source of the circulating enzyme. (For details, *see* Sawyer, 1954; Berde, 1959; Lauson, 1970.)

Bioassay and Unitage. The oxytocic potency of posterior pituitary extracts is determined by bioassay of their avian vasodepressor activity, which parallels oxytocic activity but is subject to more reproducible assay. Activity is compared to that of a U.S.P. standard preparation, and expressed in terms of *U.S.P. units*. The strength of the preparations of synthetic oxytocin now in use is still expressed in these units, each unit being the equivalent of approximately 2 μg of the pure hormone.

Preparations. *Oxytocin Injection*, U.S.P. (PITOCIN, SYNTOCINON, UTERACON), contains 10 U.S.P. units per milliliter and may be administered intravenously or intramuscularly. Although the U.S.P. allows it to be prepared either from natural sources or by synthesis, all commercial preparations are now synthetic. Oxytocin is also available in the form of a *nasal spray* containing 40 U.S.P. units per milliliter. For sublingual administration of the hormone, *oxytocin citrate buccal tablets* (PITOCIN CITRATE), each containing 200 U.S.P. units, are available.

THERAPEUTIC USES

The uses of oxytocin in *obstetrics* are discussed below.

Use during Lactation. Theoretically oxytocin should be of value for the relief of engorgement of the breasts during lactation and in cases of inadequacy of breast feeding in which insufficient milk ejection is felt to be a contributing factor. The hormone is administered most conveniently by the intranasal route. In cases of inadequacy of breast feeding, it is given by a single burst of the nasal spray in each nostril 2 to 3 minutes before a feeding is to begin. The procedure is seldom successful. However, it is simple and without risk to the patient, and when effective it resolves a frustrating and sometimes painful problem for the patient. Oxytocin does not possess galactopoietic properties and is not useful when inadequate milk production is the underlying problem.

PROSTAGLANDINS

The sources, chemistry, and physiological actions of this ubiquitous group of autacoids are presented in Chapter 30. They have numerous types and sites of direct action and can influence (or be influenced by) the effects of other autacoids, neurotransmitters, hormones, and drugs at these sites. In the female reproductive system, prostaglandins are found in the ovary, myometrium, and menstrual fluid in concentrations that vary with the ovulatory cycle. Following coitus, accessible portions of the female reproductive tract are also exposed to prostaglandins, which occur in high concentrations in human seminal fluid. Seminal prostaglandins can also be absorbed from the vagina in amounts sufficient to produce physiologically active concentrations in plasma. At term and during labor, prostaglandin concentrations rise in amniotic fluid and umbilical cord blood, and prostaglandin may also appear in maternal blood.

In spite of the clearly demonstrable effectiveness of the prostaglandins in stimulating (or, in a few instances, relaxing) smooth muscle in reproductive organs, their physiological role in menstruation, conception, and parturition remains debatable. The semen of a number of mammalian species has been found to be devoid of prostaglandins. Although the widely used drugs aspirin and indomethacin profoundly depress prostaglandin synthesis and release, their use has not yet been reported to influence menstruation or reproduction in patients receiving therapeutic doses. Such facts illustrate the difficulty of assessing the physiological significance of these autacoids.

The prostaglandins have been shown in experimental animals to participate in ovulation and luteolysis and to influence the hormonal events associated with these processes, including the pituitary release of luteinizing hormone. The possible usefulness of prostaglandins or their inhibitors in fertility control is under active investigation. (For reviews, *see* Horton, 1969; Higgins and Braunwald, 1972; Behrman and Anderson, 1974.)

Prostaglandin Inhibitors. In this, as in many other areas of pharmacology, inhibitors or "blocking agents" may have major therapeutic applications. In the case of the prostaglandins, potential uses related to the reproductive system might include dysmenorrhea, premature labor, or fertility control. Aspirin and indomethacin are representative of a number of drugs that inhibit prostaglandin synthetases and thus cause a widespread, nonspecific type of inhibition (*see* Flower, 1974). Substances of diverse structure have been shown to have prostaglandin-receptor blocking activity. However, the more promising agents are synthetic structural analogs that appear to have competitive blocking effects of a more selective nature (*see* Sanner, 1974).

PHARMACOLOGICAL PROPERTIES

The prostaglandins can be considered to be local hormones since, with few exceptions, they exert their effects and are inactivated principally in the tissues or organs in which they are synthesized. Those found in the uterus, and in the menstrual and amniotic fluid, are of the E and F types. Clinical investigation for obstetrical use has been limited almost entirely to prostaglandins E_1, E_2, and $F_{2\alpha}$ (PGE_1, PGE_2, and $PGF_{2\alpha}$).

The members of the PGF series consistently stimulate contractions of both the pregnant or nonpregnant uterus. Although PGE_1 and PGE_2 cause relaxation of nonpregnant uterine tissue *in vitro,* they have a considerably more potent oxytocic action than $PGF_{2\alpha}$ during the last two trimesters of pregnancy. For the induction of labor at term, PGE_1 and PGE_2 have been shown to be as effective as the more widely used $PGF_{2\alpha}$ or oxytocin (Karim *et al.,* 1970). The physiological response of the uterus in late pregnancy to these prostaglandins very closely resembles that to oxytocin. In double-blind studies, experienced obstetricians were unable by objective or subjective criteria to distinguish between the uterine response to, or the effectiveness of, $PGF_{2\alpha}$ and oxytocin (*see* Anderson, 1973). Some investigators have indicated that prostaglandins may show a narrower dose-response range for production of physiological contractions and the occurrence of uterine hypertonus, a potential hazard that may be avoided by very cautious stepwise increments in the rate of infusion.

Although the response of the uterus to prostaglandins also increases as gestation progresses, these agents are much more effective than oxytocin in the earlier months. For abortion in the second trimester, intrauterine instillation by way of a cervical catheter or intra-amniotic injection of PGE_2 or $PGF_{2\alpha}$ results in a high success rate, with frequent but tolerable side effects. However, for very early abortion (menses delayed up to several weeks), the rate of success reported is low and serious side effects have resulted from the doses required.

The *side effects* attending the use of prostaglandins in the second and third trimester and at term are caused by their stimulatory action on the smooth muscle of the alimentary tract, that is, nausea, vomiting, and diarrhea.

Oxytocin and the prostaglandins affect uterine smooth muscle by different mechanisms, and their effects are additive. The possible advantages of their combined use are being explored. The present status of prostaglandins has been reviewed by Behrman and Anderson (1974).

Preparations, Routes of Administration, and Dosage. *Dinoprost tromethamine* (PROSTIN F2 ALPHA) is a solution containing the equivalent of 5 mg of prostaglandin $F_{2\alpha}$ per milliliter; it is available in 4- and 8-ml ampuls for intra-amniotic administration to induce abortion. Dosage is discussed in the final section of this chapter. *Dinoprostone (prostaglandin E_2;* PROSTIN E2) is available currently for investigational use only; it is provided as tablets and as an injection for the induction of labor at term, and as an aerosol for the treatment of asthma.

ERGOT AND THE ERGOT ALKALOIDS

The dramatic effect of ergot ingested during pregnancy has been recognized for over 2000 years, and it was first used by physicians as an oxytocic agent almost 400 years ago. In the early years of this century, the isolation and chemical identification of the active principles of ergot were accomplished and detailed study of their biological activity was begun. The elucidation of the constituents of ergot and their complex actions comprises a most important chapter in the evolution of modern pharmacology. The ergot alkaloids are therefore discussed in detail in this and other chapters, even though the very complexity of their actions limits their therapeutic uses.

Source. *Ergot* is the product of a fungus (*Claviceps purpurea*) that grows upon rye and other grains. Rye is the most susceptible. The parasite can be found in the grainfields of North America and Europe. Rye destined for commercial sale is subject to government inspection and is rejected if it contains more than 0.3% infected grain. In dry years the rejection rate is usually less than 1%, but in other years it has been as high as 36%. Infection of other edible grain by *Claviceps purpurea* or other fungi that produce pharmacologically active alkaloids occurs, but it is less common.

The spores are carried by insects or the wind to the ovaries of young rye, where they germinate into hyphal filaments. As the hyphal filaments penetrate deep into the ovary of the rye, a dense tissue forms. This tissue gradually consumes the entire substance of the grain and hardens into a purple, curved body called the *sclerotium.* This sclerotium is the commercial source of ergot.

Constituents of Ergot. Ergot has been termed a "veritable treasure house of pharmacological constituents." The substances isolated from ergot have been divided by Barger (1931) into two main groups. In the first group are those products peculiar to ergot and not obtainable from any other source. Among these are the ergot alkaloids. The second group consists of a heterogeneous collection of compounds, including several amines of pharmacological importance (*e.g.,* histamine, tyramine, isoamylamine, choline, and acetylcholine). *Claviceps purpurea* and related fungi have also been successfully grown *in vitro* by means of fermentation technics that resemble those used for the antibiotic-producing fungi. Biosynthetic pathways have been established and biosynthetic structural modifications induced.

History. The contamination of an edible grain by a poisonous, parasitic fungus spread death and destruction for centuries. As early as 600 B.C., an Assyrian tablet alluded to a "noxious pustule in the ear of grain"; and in one of the sacred books of the Parsees (400 to 300 B.C.) the following pertinent passage occurs, "Among the evil things created by Angro Maynes are noxious grasses that cause pregnant women to drop the womb and die in childbed." It was fortunate for the ancient Greeks that they objected to the "black malodorous product of Thrace and Macedonia," and therefore did not eat rye. Rye was also comparatively unknown to the early Romans, for it was not introduced into Southwest Europe until after the beginning of the Christian era. Consequently, there is no undisputed reference to ergot poisoning in the early Greek and Roman literature. It was not until the Middle Ages that written descriptions of ergot poisoning first appeared, although it is probable that the disease was prevalent long before this time. Strange epidemics were described in which the characteristic symptom was gangrene of the feet, legs, hands, and arms. In severe cases, the tissue became dry and black and the mummified limbs separated off without loss of blood. Limbs were said to be consumed by the Holy Fire and blackened like charcoal. Mention was also made of agonizing burning sensations in the extremities. The disease was called Holy Fire or St. Anthony's fire, the latter name being in honor of the saint at whose shrine relief was said to be obtained. The relief that followed migration to the shrine of St. Anthony was probably real, for the sufferers received a diet free of contaminated grain during their sojourn at the shrine. The symptoms of ergot poisoning were not restricted to the limbs. Indeed, a frequent complication of ergot poisoning was abortion. A convulsive type of ergotism was also known. There still is no proven explanation as to why, in certain instances, ergotism was associated with symptoms referable to the central nervous system (CNS).

It was not until 1670 that ergot was proved to be the cause of the destructive epidemics that for centuries had raged uncontrolled. At present, our knowledge of the etiology of ergot poisoning makes its prevention quite simple. Yet outbreaks of ergot poisoning have occurred in the present century, epidemics having been reported in Russia in 1926, in Ireland in 1929, and in France in 1953.

Ergot was known as an obstetrical herb before it was identified as the cause of St. Anthony's fire. It was mentioned as early as 1582 by Lonicer as a proven means of producing pains in the womb. It was used by midwives long before it was recognized by the medical profession. The first physician to employ ergot was Desgranges, but he did not publish his observations until 1818. Ten years before, a letter published by John Stearns in the *Medical Repository* of New York, entitled "Account of the Pulvis Parturiens, a Remedy for Quickening Childbirth," marked the official introduction of ergot into medicine (Thoms, 1931). This communication is of sufficient historical interest to quote certain pertinent portions of it:

It [pulvis parturiens] expedites lingering parturition and saves to the accoucheur a considerable portion of time, without producing any bad effects on the patient. . . . Previous to its exhibition it is of the utmost consequence to ascertain the presentation . . . as the violent and almost incessant action which it induces in the uterus precludes the possibility of turning. . . . If the dose is large it will produce nausea and vomiting. In most cases you will be surprised with the suddenness of its operation; it is, therefore, necessary to be completely ready before you give the medicine. . . . Since I have adopted the use of this powder I have seldom found a case that detained me more than three hours. . . .

The use of ergot spread rapidly in the United States, but its adoption in Europe was delayed, per-

haps, as Barger (1931) has suggested, because the Old World had suffered too much from the poisonous properties of ergot. The dangers attending the use of the drug, however, were soon recognized. In 1824, Hosack wrote that the number of stillborn children had increased so greatly since the introduction of ergot that the Medical Society of New York instituted an inquiry. Said Hosack, "The ergot has been called . . . *pulvis ad partum;* as it regards the child, it may, with almost equal truth be denominated the *pulvis ad mortem.*" This astute observer recommended that the drug be used only to control post-partum hemorrhage. Thus, more than a century and a half ago, the indications and contraindications of ergot were accurately defined.

Chemistry. Two series of optically active, isomeric alkaloids can be isolated from ergot. The *l* forms (designated by the suffix "-ine") are pharmacologically active; the *d* forms (designated by the suffix "-inine"), completely inactive. The former are believed to be naturally occurring alkaloids; the latter result from chemical manipulations. The first isolation of a crystalline, pharmacologically active sub-

Table 42-1. ERGOT ALKALOIDS

A. LYSERGIC ACID AND AMINE ALKALOIDS *	B. AMINO ACID ALKALOIDS †

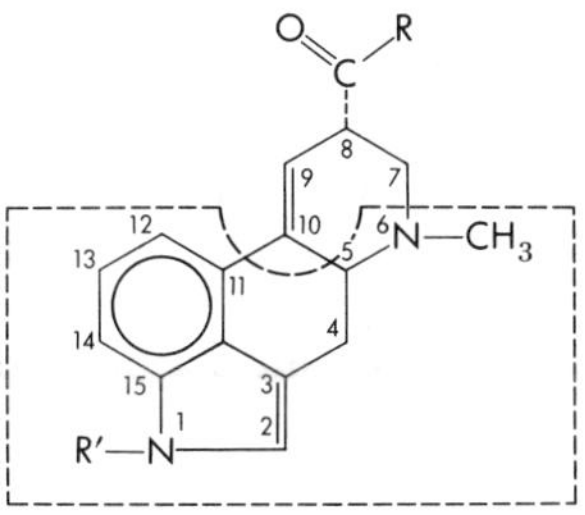

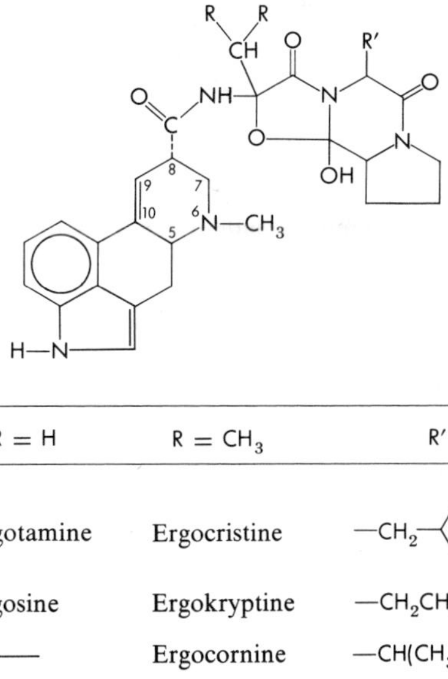

ALKALOID	R	R′		R = H	R = CH$_3$	R′
Lysergic acid	—OH	H		Ergotamine	Ergocristine	—CH$_2$—⟨phenyl⟩ 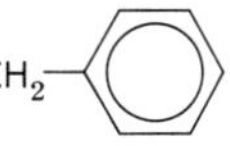
Lysergic acid diethylamide	—N(CH$_2$CH$_3$)$_2$	H		Ergosine	Ergokryptine	—CH$_2$CH(CH$_3$)$_2$
Ergonovine (ergometrine)	—NH—CHCH$_2$OH (CH$_3$)	H		——	Ergocornine	—CH(CH$_3$)$_2$
Methylergonovine	—NH—CHCH$_2$OH (CH$_2$CH$_3$)	H				
Methysergide	—NH—CHCH$_2$OH (CH$_2$CH$_3$)	CH$_3$				

* The dotted enclosure indicates the tryptamine-like portion of the alkaloid.
† The dihydrogenated derivatives differ only in being saturated at C 9 and C 10.

stance from ergot was accomplished in 1906 by Barger, Carr, and Dale as well as by Kraft. This material was called *ergotoxine*. It is now known to be a mixture of three alkaloids, which have been designated *ergocristine, ergocornine,* and *ergokryptine*. What ultimately proved to be the first pure ergot alkaloids were obtained by Stoll in 1920, namely, a pharmacologically active compound, *ergotamine,* and its inactive isomer, ergotaminine. Subsequently, *ergonovine* and then *ergosine* were isolated.

The chemical structure of the alkaloids of ergot has been elucidated largely by the work of Stoll and his associates, following their extensive contribution to the isolation of these substances, and of Jacobs and Craig and their coworkers (*see* Stoll, 1950; Stoll *et al.,* 1951). All are derivatives of lysergic acid, an indole compound. Their structures are shown in Table 42–1. The optical isomerism is due to the presence of two asymmetrical carbon atoms (positions 5 and 8 in the formulas, Table 42–1) in the lysergic acid portion of the molecule. Ergonovine and its derivatives upon hydrolysis yield lysergic acid and an amine; consequently, they are designated as *amine alkaloids.* The alkaloids of higher molecular weight upon hydrolysis yield proline and one other amino acid and are known as *amino acid alkaloids.*

The variety of the ergot alkaloids is further extended by several types of semisynthetic derivatives. One of the double bonds of lysergic acid (C 9 to C 10) can be selectively saturated; in this manner a series of stable *dihydrogenated alkaloids* is obtained. These have been designated *dihydroergotamine, dihydroergocristine,* and so forth, and possess somewhat different pharmacological properties than do the parent alkaloids. In addition, it is possible to combine lysergic acid with different amines than those linked to it in nature. Two products of this series, lysergic acid diethylamide and lysergic acid hydroxybutylamide (methylergonovine), are of pharmacological interest. Methylation of the indole nitrogen of the latter compound yields 1-methyl-methylergonovine (*methysergide*).

Pharmacological Properties

The ergot alkaloids fall into three groups pharmacologically as well as chemically: (1) the amino acid alkaloids, (2) the dihydrogenated amino acid alkaloids, and (3) the amine alkaloids. Inasmuch as the actions of the

individual members of each group differ but little, *ergotamine, dihydroergotamine,* and *ergonovine* can be taken as prototypes.

The pharmacological actions of the ergot alkaloids are varied and complex; some actions are completely unrelated, and some are even mutually antagonistic. The marked effects of ergotamine on the cardiovascular system, for example, are due to simultaneous peripheral vasoconstriction, depression of vasomotor centers, and peripheral adrenergic blockade. The following presentation will be concerned primarily with the responses of the smooth muscle of the uterus and blood vessels. The actions on adrenergic receptors and vasomotor reflexes are discussed in Chapter 26. CNS effects are also discussed in Chapter 26 and in Chapters 12 and 16. A summary of the actions of the ergot alkaloids is presented in Table 42–2.

Uterus. All the natural alkaloids of ergot markedly increase the motor activity of the uterus. The character of the changes elicited is related to the dose administered. After small doses, contractions are increased in force or frequency, or both, but are followed by a normal degree of relaxation. After larger doses, contractions become forceful and prolonged and resting tonus is markedly increased. Although this characteristic precludes their use for induction or facilitation of labor, it is quite compatible with their use post partum or post abortion to control bleeding and maintain uterine contraction. Very high doses can cause sustained contracture. The sensitivity of the uterus to ergot alkaloids varies, especially with the degree of maturity and the stage of gestation, but even an immature uterus is stimulated. The gravid uterus, however, is very sensitive, and small doses of ergot alkaloids can be given at term

Table 42–2. **PHARMACOLOGICAL ACTIONS OF THE ERGOT ALKALOIDS**

CLASS OF COMPOUND	PHARMACOLOGICAL ACTIONS		
	Vasoconstriction and Endothelial Damage	*Oxytocic*	*Adrenergic Blockade*
Natural amino acid alkaloids	Highly active, especially ergotamine	Highly active, delayed onset; ineffective orally	Active
Dihydrogenated alkaloids	Much less active than parent alkaloids	Active on pregnant human uterus	More active than parent alkaloids
Amine alkaloids	Slightly active	Highly active, rapid onset; effective orally	Inactive

or immediately post partum to obtain a marked uterine response unaccompanied by significant side effects. The mechanism of action is one of direct stimulation; the isolated uterus responds equally as well as the uterus *in situ.*

All natural ergot alkaloids have qualitatively the same effect on the uterus, but they exhibit important differences in potency. Ergonovine is the most active. It is superior to ergotamine, the most potent of the amino acid alkaloids, with respect to rapidity of onset of the uterine response following intravenous administration, activity following oral administration, and toxicity (Figure 42–1). For these reasons ergonovine and its semisynthetic derivative, methylergonovine, have replaced other ergot preparations as clinical oxytocics.

Methylergonovine differs little from ergonovine in its uterine actions. The dihydrogenated alkaloids do not have the oxytocic properties of the parent alkaloids when tested in experimental animals. However, they are capable of exerting a marked oxytocic action on the pregnant human uterus at term.

Cardiovascular System. Ergotamine, the other natural amino acid alkaloids, and the dihydrogenated derivatives exert complex actions on the cardiovascular system. These are discussed in detail in Chapter 26.

Ergotamine and related alkaloids that produce *peripheral vasoconstriction* damage the *capillary endothelium.* The mechanism of this toxic action is not clearly understood. Vascular stasis, thrombosis, and gangrene result and are prominent features of ergot poisoning. The susceptibility of different species to gangrene produced by ergot varies greatly. Man unfortunately is particularly sensitive.

The ergot alkaloids vary in vasoconstrictor activity. Ergotamine is the most potent, followed by the other amino acid alkaloids. Dihydroergotamine retains appreciable vasoconstrictor activity, but the dihydrogenated derivatives of the ergotoxine group are far less active. The propensity of the compounds to cause gangrene appears to parallel vasoconstrictor activity. The amine alkaloids cause slight pressor responses and decrease limb blood flow when administered in therapeutic doses.

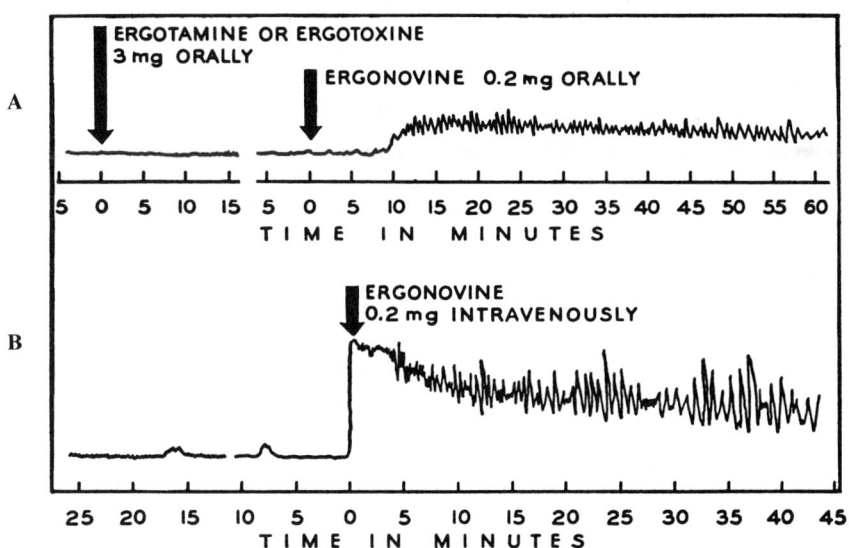

Figure 42–1. *The effect of ergonovine on the human uterus.*

A. The effect on the human uterus of 3 mg of orally administered ergotamine or ergotoxine as compared with 0.2 mg of ergonovine. The record is that of the uterine motility of a woman (para 4) 7 days post partum, obtained by means of a balloon and manometer. Note the inefficacy of ergotoxine and ergotamine when given by mouth and the prompt and sustained response to the small dose of ergonovine. *B.* The effect of 0.2 mg of ergonovine, given intravenously, on the uterine motility of a woman (para 2) 7 days post partum. Note the immediate, marked, and sustained response. Methylergonovine acts in a similar manner. (After Davis, Adair, and Pearl, 1936. Courtesy of the *Journal of the American Medical Association.*)

Vascular Responses in Human Beings and the Relationship to the Therapy of Migraine. Certain ergot alkaloids, notably ergotamine, are effective in relieving migraine headaches. Ergotamine is neither sedative nor analgesic and other forms of pain are not relieved by the drug. Indeed, a study of the action of ergotamine has led to the current concept of the etiology of migraine, which relates the intensity of pain to increased amplitude of pulsations of the cranial arteries, chiefly the branches of the external carotid. This is generally believed to follow a period of vasoconstriction of unknown cause in these vessels, during which many patients experience a subjective "aura," indicating the beginning of an attack. (For details, *see* Wolff, 1972.) Factors that decrease the amplitude of pulsation, for example, digital pressure on the carotid artery, also reduce the intensity of the headache. When ergotamine induces relief of migraine, there is a parallel decline in the amplitude of arterial pulsation.

Other Actions. The ergot alkaloids are antagonists of the actions of 5-hydroxytryptamine and of certain metabolic actions of the catecholamines. These are discussed elsewhere (*see* Index).

Absorption and Fate. The ergot alkaloids of higher molecular weight, such as ergotamine, are poorly and irregularly absorbed from the gastrointestinal tract. The effective oral dose is eight to ten times the intramuscular dose, and the resulting action is delayed and unpredictable (Figure 42–1). There is even a latent period of approximately 20 minutes between the intramuscular injection of the drugs and the onset of uterine response. The action may persist for several hours. Ergonovine, on the other hand, is rapidly and adequately absorbed after oral administration, and its onset of action occurs within 10 minutes. The alkaloids appear to be detoxified by the liver.

Ergot Poisoning. The ergot alkaloids are highly toxic and may cause acute or chronic poisoning. The former is rare and usually results from large amounts of ergot ingested in attempts at abortion. The symptoms consist in vomiting, diarrhea, unquenchable thirst, tingling, itching and coldness of the skin, a rapid and weak pulse, confusion, and unconsciousness. The natural amino acid alkaloids are many times more toxic than their dihydrogenated derivatives. Fatal poisoning has occurred after the oral administration of 26 mg of ergotamine over a period of several days, and also following single injections of only 0.5 to 1.5 mg. Ergonovine is approximately one fourth as toxic as the other natural alkaloids.

At present the epidemic form of chronic ergot poisoning arising from the ingestion of contaminated grain is seldom seen. However, the alkaloids of ergot are extensively employed in therapeutics, and poisoning from their injudicious administration is not rare. Poisoning is usually due to overdosage. There are indications, however, that increased sensitivity to ergot alkaloids may accompany febrile and septic states and disease of the liver. Many cases of ergot poisoning have been reported in patients with puerperal fever. Also, several fatalities from gangrene have occurred in patients with hepatic damage who received ergotamine for relief of the accompanying pruritus. It is assumed that such patients have an unusual vascular sensitivity to ergotamine. Patients having occlusive peripheral vascular disease are extremely susceptible to the vascular complications of ergotamine therapy.

In chronic ergotism, whether due to overdosage or to unusual susceptibility, striking circulatory changes develop. The feet and legs, and somewhat less frequently the hands, become cold, pale, and numb. Muscle pain occurs while walking and later at rest. Arterial pulses in the affected limbs become faint or even disappear. Eventually gangrene develops, beginning usually in the toes but sometimes in the fingers. Two factors are involved in the impairment of the circulation, vasoconstriction and intimal lesions; the latter may result in thrombi that completely occlude the smaller arteries. Additional circulatory disturbances may include anginal pain, tachycardia or bradycardia, and elevation or lowering of the blood pressure.

The most common other symptoms are *headache, nausea, vomiting, diarrhea,* and *dizziness.* Also, there may be noticeable weakness, formication, itching, and coldness of the skin. Symptoms particularly referable to the CNS are confusion, depression, drowsiness, and, rarely, convulsions, hemiplegia, tabetic manifestations, and a fixed miosis.

Methysergide has been implicated in the initiation and exacerbation of fibrotic disease of several types (*see* Chapter 29).

Complications of Ergotamine Therapy. When ergotamine is prescribed in correct dosage in the absence of contraindications, it is a safe and useful drug; few serious complications have been reported from its use in the migraine syndrome.

Nausea and vomiting occur in approximately 10% of patients after oral administration and in about twice that number after parenteral administration, indicating a direct effect of the drug on CNS emetic centers. However, severe nausea is common during attacks of migraine regardless of treatment. Weakness in the legs is common, and muscle pains, which occasionally are quite severe, may occur in the extremities. Numbness and tingling of the fingers and toes are other reminders of the ergotism that this alkaloid may cause. Precordial distress and pain suggestive of angina pectoris, as well as transient tachycardia or bradycardia, have also been noted. Localized edema and itching may occur in an occasional hypersensitive patient. Most of these effects are not alarming and ordinarily do not necessitate interruption of ergotamine therapy.

Treatment. The treatment of ergotism consists in complete withdrawal of the offending drug and symptomatic measures. The latter include attempts to maintain an adequate circulation to the affected parts. Pharmacological agents that have been employed include anticoagulants, low-molecular-weight dextran, and potent vasodilator drugs. Carliner and associates (1974) have reported the successful treatment of a severe case of ergotism by the intravenous infusion of sodium nitroprusside. The initial rate of infusion was 50 μg per minute. Increase in dosage and the duration of infusion were determined by the response of the ischemic limbs and the systemic blood pressure. The patient required two infusions of 20 and 15 hours' duration, respectively. The first infusion was stopped after 20 hours because of a marked fall in systemic blood pressure. The infusion rate at the time was 247 μg per minute. It was resumed 3 hours later (123 μg per minute) because of return of symptoms. Recovery was complete. (*See* Chapter 33 for a further discussion of nitroprusside.)

Nausea and vomiting may be relieved by atropine or by antiemetic compounds of the phenothiazine type.

Preparations. Preparations of the dihydrogenated ergot alkaloids are discussed in Chapter 26. Only a few of the purified ergot alkaloids are available for therapeutic application. *Ergotamine Tartrate,* U.S.P. (GYNERGEN), is usually dispensed in the form of *Ergotamine Tartrate Tablets,* U.S.P., which contain either 1 mg (oral) or 2 mg (sublingual) of the salt, or as an aqueous solution containing 0.5 mg/ml (*Ergotamine Tartrate Injection,* U.S.P.). *Ergotamine Tartrate and Caffeine Tablets,* N.F., and *Ergotamine Tartrate and Caffeine Suppositories,* N.F. (CAFERGOT), are also available; the official tablets contain 1 mg of ergotamine tartrate and 100 mg of caffeine, and the corresponding suppositories 2 mg and 100 mg, respectively. *Ergonovine Maleate,* N.F. (ERGOTRATE), is available in the form of *Ergonovine Maleate Injection,* N.F., which contains 0.2 mg of the salt per milliliter, and in the form of *Ergonovine Maleate Tablets,* N.F., which contain 0.2 mg of the alkaloidal salt. Ergonovine preparations should be kept at temperatures of 0° to 12° C and protected from light.

Methylergonovine Maleate, N.F. (METHERGINE MALEATE), is marketed in solution in 1-ml ampuls containing 0.2 mg and in oral tablets containing 0.2 mg. *Methysergide Maleate,* U.S.P. (SANSERT), is available as oral tablets containing 2 mg.

THERAPEUTIC USES

The major therapeutic uses of the ergot alkaloids fall into two categories: (1) applications in obstetrics (discussed later in this chapter), and (2) treatment of migraine.

Migraine. The etiology of migraine is complex and poorly understood. It is important that the physician should attempt to assess and, if possible, deal with underlying emotional and physical stresses that may markedly influence the incidence and severity of attacks. The nonnarcotic analgesics, caffeine, and other agents may be effective in some patients (*see* Wolff, 1972). Since its first use for the treatment of

migraine in 1926, ergotamine tartrate has remained an important agent for symptomatic relief of this syndrome and is still unique in its effectiveness (Friedman, 1972).

Dosage and Route of Administration. Subcutaneous or intramuscular injection is the usual method of administering ergotamine tartrate. The dose is 0.25 to 0.5 mg, and this may be repeated if the migraine is not relieved or if it recurs. No more than 1.0 mg should be given in 24 hours. Occasionally, ergotamine may be given *intravenously,* but this route should be employed only by those who are thoroughly familiar with the use of the drug. The intravenous dose is usually 0.25 mg and must not be more than 0.5 mg. The latter amount is the maximum allowable in any 24-hour period.

Tablets of ergotamine may be administered *sublingually,* the dose being 3 or 4 mg, given as soon as the headache starts. One or 2 mg may be given hourly thereafter, if necessary, until a total of 10 mg has been taken. The average initial dose for *oral* ingestion is 4 to 5 mg, and 2 mg may be swallowed each hour thereafter until not more than 11 mg has been taken.

The smallest amount effective in relieving the headache should be employed. Overdosage is the chief cause of untoward effects from ergotamine. The therapeutic courses outlined should not be repeated within the same week. After the drug has been given, the patient should lie down in a quiet, dark room for at least 2 hours. The speed and thoroughness of the relief from pain are directly proportional to the promptness with which medication is started after the onset of an attack. The preferred time to administer ergotamine is during the prodromal stage. If the drug is given early, the dose may be decreased considerably. If the seizure has reached its peak, larger amounts of ergotamine are needed. Not only is a longer time then required for effective action but also unpleasant side effects from medication are more pronounced. If a dose of more than 8 mg of ergotamine is necessary by the oral route in order to obtain relief or if the headache is severe, it is better to resort to the subcutaneous injection of 0.5 mg. Oral medication is less effective than parenteral, but it may be satisfactory for mild or incipient attacks of migraine.

Efficacy. It is generally agreed that ergotamine is effective in the vast majority of cases. Approximately 90% of all patients or all attacks are relieved. The specificity of ergotamine for migraine is indicated by the fact that only occasionally are nonmigrainous headaches influenced. Relief is often dramatic. After parenteral injection of ergotamine, the headache may disappear in 15 minutes, but sometimes only after 2 hours or more. Oral medication is much slower in bringing relief, an average of 5 hours being required, and it may fail in severe attacks. Tolerance to ergotamine does not develop. The drug is not a cure and does not decrease the frequency of migraine headaches. Indeed, it has been stated that the frequency may be increased. When this occurs, observance of the specified maximum of weekly doses is particularly important. The drug is not useful in preventing attacks. In fact, it has been claimed that, if the drug is given before the onset of the prodromal stage, an attack may be precipitated, possibly because the migraine attack is preceded by marked constriction of the involved arteries; ergotamine would tend to exaggerate such vasoconstriction.

Ergonovine in Migraine. Ergonovine is only moderately effective in migraine. It has the advantages, however, that it is relatively more effective than ergotamine when given orally and that untoward gastrointestinal symptoms are not so pronounced. Patients in whom ergonovine provides satisfactory relief from attacks of migraine usually prefer the alkaloid to ergotamine.

Dihydroergotamine in Migraine. Dihydroergotamine is also effective in the treatment of migraine (Storch, 1947). It is given parenterally in a dose twice that of ergotamine.

Methysergide in Migraine. Methysergide has only a weak vasoconstrictor action, and it is not useful in the treatment of acute attacks of migraine. However, it is a very potent antagonist of 5-hydroxytryptamine, a substance that has been implicated in the etiology of vascular headaches. Its use as a prophylactic agent in migraine and other forms of vascular headache is discussed in Chapter 29.

Combination with Caffeine. Caffeine enhances the action of the ergot alkaloids in the treatment of migraine, a discovery that must be credited to the sufferers from the disease who observed that strong coffee gave symptomatic relief, especially when combined with the ergot alkaloids. It is now appreciated that the xanthines also constrict cerebral blood vessels and reduce cerebral blood flow.

Contraindications. Because gangrene due to ergotamine has occurred in a number of patients with infection, sepsis is a definite contraindication. It should not be used in patients with vascular disease, such as syphilitic arteritis, marked atherosclerosis, coronary artery disease, thrombophlebitis, and Raynaud's or Buerger's syndrome. Diseases of the liver or kidney are also contraindications. Serious toxicity has been reported from the use of ergotamine in patients with pruritus (Kenney, 1946), especially when the symptom is secondary to hepatic disease. Although very large amounts of ergotamine are required to produce abortion, pregnancy constitutes an objection to use.

THE CLINICAL USE OF OXYTOCICS

There are many indications for, and contraindications to, the clinical use of the oxytocics. In brief, the clearest indications are: (1) to induce labor at term, (2) to control post-partum hemorrhage, (3) to correct postpartum uterine atony, (4) to cause uterine contraction after cesarean section or during other uterine surgery, (5) to induce therapeutic abortion after the first trimester, and (6), in the case of oxytocin, and probably

prostaglandins of the E and F types, to overcome stubborn and prolonged uterine inertia. In general, oxytocics are contraindicated during the first and second stages of labor.

The Induction of Labor at Term. When it is necessary to induce labor at full term, a variety of procedures is available. Often several are used in sequence, starting with the least drastic measure. In many cases, a cathartic or enema is all that is necessary to initiate uterine activity. The cathartic has no direct effect upon the uterus, but apparently the organ is reflexly stimulated.

The drug of choice for the induction of labor in most cases is oxytocin. For all ante-partum indications except abortion, oxytocin should be given by intravenous infusion of a dilute solution, preferably by means of a variable-speed infusion pump. A suitable concentration for use in induction of labor at term is 10 milliunits per milliliter (10 units added to 1 liter of 5% dextrose). The infusion is started at the slow rate of 0.5 ml (5 milliunits) per minute. If no response is obtained within 15 minutes, the rate of administration can be slowly increased to a maximum of 2.0 ml (20 milliunits) per minute. The total dose required to initiate labor ranges from 600 to 12,000 milliunits, with an average of 4000. Oxytocin buccal lozenges may also be used. Although a predictable rate of absorption is claimed, this method of administration lacks the precision and especially the flexibility of intravenous infusion. It shares the advantage that rapid termination of action can be achieved simply by removal of the lozenge from the mouth.

During the entire procedure uterine activity should be carefully monitored. If contractions become too forceful or frequent or resting tone is elevated, the infusion should be immediately discontinued. Changes in fetal heart sounds or rate are useful indicators of fetal distress. Occasionally, even the cautious use of oxytocin will stimulate the uterus to a sustained tetanic contraction, which may so interfere with the placental circulation that it may be necessary to administer a general anesthetic to effect uterine relaxation. When labor is initiated, the infusion of oxytocin is discontinued. The indications for oxytocin during labor are discussed below.

When employed at term, oxytocin induces labor in the majority of cases. If amniotomy is also employed, as it is by many obstetricians, successful induction occurs in 80 to 90% of cases.

Because individual responses to prostaglandins, such as $PGF_{2\alpha}$ and PGE_2, are highly variable and involve a lag period longer than that seen with oxytocin, induction of labor with these agents should be carried out by stepwise increments of the intravenous infusion of dilute solutions. As an example, Behrman and Anderson (1974) reported a schedule in which $PGF_{2\alpha}$ or PGE_2 was infused in appropriate dosage over a period of 10 hours. In comparison with results obtained in patients who received infusions of synthetic oxytocin by a similar schedule, the prostaglandins showed no firm advantages. Efficacy was approximately equal, and an occasional patient who received $PGF_{2\alpha}$ developed uterine hypertonus. The precautions with regard to close monitoring of uterine response and fetal heart sounds are the same for the prostaglandins as for oxytocin. The prostaglandins have the potential advantage of stimulating uterine contractions at any stage of pregnancy; preliminary studies have indicated their usefulness in treating missed abortion, late intrauterine death, molar gestation, and premature rupture of the membranes (*see* Karim, 1970; Barden, 1972).

First and Second Stages of Labor. Oxytocin should not be used during the first and second stages if labor is progressing, albeit slowly. The type of contraction produced often is too forceful and sustained to be compatible with the safety of mother and fetus. In normal labor, events move in an orderly and purposeful manner. Each period of uterine contraction is followed by one of relaxation that not only allows a rest period for the uterine musculature but also assures adequate placental circulation. During the first stage of labor, the cervix gradually dilates. When the uterus, under the stimulus of a drug, contracts too forcibly against an incompletely dilated and rigid cervix, the following accidents may occur: (1) the force of the contraction may drive the presenting part through the incompletely dilated cervical tissues and cause severe laceration of the mother and trauma to the infant; (2) if the soft tissues are unyielding, the uterus may rupture; and (3) the forceful tetanic contraction of the uterus may asphyxiate the fetus.

There are occasions, however, when oxytocin can be used advantageously by the experienced obstetrician to overcome uterine inertia. Cases must be strictly selected and dosage continuously regulated. Even under these circumstances fetal deaths can occur due to the action of oxytocin. Justification for the measure lies in the fact that with proper precautions it entails less risk than operative procedures or indecision. The indication for oxytocics during labor is prolonged, stubborn, uterine inertia in patients who exhibit no disproportion as determined by x-ray. The cautious intravenous infusion of oxytocin is initiated in the manner already described. Multiparous patients (para 4 and over) should not receive oxytocics during the first and second stages of labor because of the greater danger of rupture of the uterus.

Third Stage of Labor and Puerperium. Although there is probably no danger in administering an oxytocic routinely at the beginning of the third stage of labor, and although the stage may thereby be somewhat shortened, the usual procedure is to await the delivery of the placenta before the administration of an oxytocic. At the completion of labor, oxytocic drugs are used routinely. It is at this time and in the puerperium that the oxytocic drugs are especially useful.

After delivery of the fetus, it is desirable to have the uterus firm and active. This reduces greatly the incidence and extent of post-partum hemorrhage. Before the introduction of ergonovine, oxytocin was usually given intramuscularly to control post-partum

bleeding. It was the drug of choice because of the rapid onset of its action. Ergonovine or methylergonovine, due to low toxicity, rapid onset, and sustained duration of action, is usually used for this purpose at present. The intramuscular injection of 0.2 to 0.3 mg produces a rapid and lasting response. Either drug may also be given intravenously in a dose of 0.2 mg if immediate action is desirable (Figure 42–1).

In the normal individual, the period of uterine involution is 8 to 10 weeks, but the process is most rapid during the first 10 days. Although it has not been definitely established whether oxytocic drugs are of material benefit if involution proceeds normally, many obstetricians use small doses of ergonovine orally (0.2 mg, three times daily for 7 days) in order to lessen the possibility of bleeding and infection. However, if involution is delayed, stimulation of the uterus by oxytocics is definitely helpful because delayed involution is usually associated with uterine atony. Under such conditions, ergonovine may be given orally or sublingually in doses of 0.2 to 0.4 mg, three times daily, for as long a period as is necessary to accomplish the desired results. If infection develops in the post-partum uterus, there is evidence that the use of ergonovine may limit its spread. Caution must be observed in the use of ergonovine for an extended period of time.

Therapeutic Abortion and Premature Labor. Abortion during the *first trimester* is most commonly accomplished by means of suction curettage. No satisfactory form of drug-induced abortion during this period is yet available. Beyond the first few weeks of the *second trimester*, intra-amniotic injection of a hypertonic (20%) solution of sodium chloride has been widely employed, but numerous failures occur and the procedure entails serious potential hazards for the patient. Oxytocin is not generally effective, even with infusion of relatively large doses (20 to 30 units). The *prostaglandins* have shown excellent efficacy and safety for second-trimester abortion. For example, of the various modifications tested by Behrman and Anderson (1974), the most satisfactory results were obtained with the intra-amniotic instillation of 40 mg of $PGF_{2\alpha}$, followed by an additional 20 mg 6 hours later. Under these conditions, complete abortion was obtained in over 80% of 70 patients treated, and partial abortion occurred in all the remainder; most patients aborted within 24 and all within 48 hours. Nausea, vomiting, or diarrhea occurred in approximately half the patients, but these side effects were not serious.

After spontaneous or therapeutic abortion or premature delivery, the post-partum indications for ergonovine and oxytocin to control bleeding and maintain uterine tone are similar to those after delivery at term.

Andersen, T. W.; De Padua, C. B.; Stenger, V.; and Prystowsky, H. Cardiovascular effects of rapid intravenous injection of synthetic oxytocin during elective cesarean section. *Clin. Pharmac. Ther.,* **1965,** *6,* 345–349.
Anderson, G. G. Induction of term labor with intravenous PGF_2: a review. *Prostaglandins,* **1973,** *4,* 765–774.
Barden, T. P. Induction of preterm labor with prosta-

glandin F_2 in patients with premature rupture of the membranes. In, *The Prostaglandins.* (Southern, E. M., ed.) Futura Publishing Co., Inc., Mount Kisco, N.Y., **1972**, pp. 193–205.

Barger, G.; Carr, F. H.; and Dale, H. H. An active alkaloid from ergot. *Br. med. J.,* **1906**, *2,* 1792.

Behrman, H. R., and Anderson, G. G. Prostaglandins in reproduction. *Archs intern. Med.,* **1974**, *133,* 77–84.

Caldeyro-Barcia, R., and Posiero, J. J. Oxytocin and the contractility of the human uterus. *Ann. N.Y. Acad. Sci.,* **1959**, *75,* 813–830.

Carliner, N. H.; Denune, D. P.; Finch, C. S., Jr.; and Goldberg, L. I. Sodium nitroprusside treatment of ergotamine-induced peripheral ischemia. *J. Am. med. Ass.,* **1974**, *227,* 308–309.

Csapo, A. Function and regulation of the myometrium. *Ann. N.Y. Acad. Sci.,* **1959**, *75,* 790–808.

Davis, M. E.; Adair, F. L.; and Pearl, S. The present status of oxytocics in obstetrics. *J. Am. med. Ass.,* **1936**, *107,* 261–267.

Friedman, A. P. Reflections on the treatment of headache. *Headache,* **1972**, *11,* 148–155.

Karim, S. M. M. Use of prostaglandin E_2 in the management of missed abortion, missed labor, and hydatidiform mole. *Br. med. J.,* **1970**, *3,* 196–197.

Karim, S. M. M.; Hillier, K.; Trussell, R. R.; Patel, R. C.; and Tamusange, S. Induction of labour with prostaglandin E_2. *J. Obstet. Gynaec. Br. Commonw.,* **1970**, *77,* 200–210.

Kenney, F. R. Gangrene of the hand following treatment for pruritus of hepatotoxic origin. *New Engl. J. Med.,* **1946**, *235,* 35–39.

Kitchin, A. H.; Lloyd, S. M.; and Pickford, M. Some actions of oxytocin on the cardiovascular system in man. *Clin. Sci.,* **1959**, *18,* 399–406.

Kraft, F. Über das Mutterkorn. *Arch. Pharm., Berl.,* **1906**, *244,* 336–359.

Pickford, M. Some extra-uterine actions of oxytocin. In, *Oxytocin.* (Caldeyro-Barcia, R., and Heller, H., eds.) Pergamon Press, Ltd., Oxford, **1961**, pp. 68–83.

Sanner, J. H. Substances that inhibit the actions of prostaglandins. *Archs intern. Med.,* **1974**, *133,* 133–146.

Saunders, W. G., and Munsick, R. A. Antidiuretic potency of oxytocin in women post partum. *Am. J. Obstet. Gynec.,* **1966**, *95,* 5–11.

Sawyer, W. H. Inactivation of oxytocin by homogenates of uteri and other tissues from normal and pregnant rats. *Proc. Soc. exp. Biol. Med.,* **1954**, *87,* 463–465.

Stoll, A. Zur Kenntnis der Mutterkornalkaloide. *Verh. naturf. Ges. Basel,* **1920**, *101,* 190–191.

———. Recent investigations on ergot alkaloids. *Chem. Rev.,* **1950**, *47,* 197–218.

Stoll, A.; Hofmann, A.; and Petrzilka, T. Die Konstitution der Mutterkornalkaloide: Struktur des Peptidteils, III. *Helv. chim. Acta,* **1951**, *34,* 1544–1576.

Thoms, H. John Stearns and pulvis parturiens. *Am. J. Obstet. Gynec.,* **1931**, *22,* 418–423.

Torpin, R.; Woodbury, R. A.; and Child, G. P. The nature of dysmenorrhea. *Am. J. Obstet. Gynec.,* **1947**, *54,* 766–775.

Monographs and Reviews

Barger, G. *Ergot and Ergotism.* Gurney & Jackson, Edinburgh, **1931**.

Berde, B. *Recent Progress in Oxytocin Research.* Charles C Thomas, Pub., Springfield, Ill., **1959**.

Farrell, G.; Fabre, L. F.; and Rauschkolb, E. The neurohypophysis. *A. Rev. Physiol.,* **1968**, *30,* 557–588.

Flower, R. J. Drugs which inhibit prostaglandin biosynthesis. *Pharmac. Rev.,* **1974**, *26,* 33–67.

Friedman, A. P., and Merritt, H. H. *Headache.* F. A. Davis Co., Philadelphia, **1959**.

Harris, G. W., and Donovan, B. T. (eds.). *The Pituitary Gland,* Vol. 3. University of California Press, Berkeley, **1966**.

Higgins, C. B., and Braunwald, E. The prostaglandins. *Am. J. Med.,* **1972**, *53,* 92–112.

Horton, E. W. Hypotheses on physiological roles of prostaglandins. *Physiol. Rev.,* **1969**, *49,* 122–161.

Lauson, H. D. Fate of the neurohypophysial hormones. In, *Pharmacology of the Endocrine System and Related Drugs,* Vol. 1. *International Encyclopedia of Pharmacology and Therapeutics,* Sect. 41. (Heller, H., and Pickering, B. T., eds.) Pergamon Press, Ltd., Oxford, **1970**, pp. 377–397.

Pinkerton, J. M. H. *Advances in Oxytocin Research.* Pergamon Press, Ltd., Oxford, **1965**.

Schacter, M. (ed.). *Polypeptides Which Affect Smooth Muscles and Blood Vessels.* Pergamon Press, Ltd., Oxford, **1960**.

Storch, T. J. C. von. Migraine, 1947: a review. *Am. Practnr, Philad.,* **1947**, *1,* 631–639.

Symposium. (Various authors.) *Oxytocin.* (Caldeyro-Barcia, R., and Heller, H., eds.) Pergamon Press, Ltd., Oxford, **1961**.

Wilson, D. E. (ed.). Symposium on prostaglandins. *Archs intern. Med.,* **1974**, *133,* 29–146.

Wolff, H. G. *Wolff's Headache and Other Pain,* 3rd ed. (Dalessio, D. J., rev.) Oxford University Press, New York, **1972**.

Gases and Vapors

A number of pharmacological agents have in common the property of being gaseous at normal temperatures and pressures. Others are volatile liquids that can yield vapors in sufficiently high concentration to exhibit pharmacological activity. The various gases and vapors have little in common except that they are absorbed chiefly by way of the respiratory tract. In other respects, they are a heterogeneous group of drugs and poisons and are discussed together here only for the purpose of convenience. From a pharmacological standpoint, the gases and vapors may be classified in three large groups—*therapeutic, noxious,* and *inert.* Aside from the anesthetic gases and vapors that are discussed elsewhere, the most important agents of the therapeutic group are *oxygen, carbon dioxide,* and *helium.* Noxious gases and vapors are too numerous for complete discussion, and space is devoted only to the more important members of the group, especially those that produce a high incidence of poisoning. Inert gases assume toxicological importance only when they are present in amounts sufficiently high to reduce the concentration of oxygen below that normally present in the inspired air; this feature does not warrant their discussion as a group. An outstanding example of an inert gas is *nitrogen.* Although helium is commonly viewed as an inert gas, it possesses valuable therapeutic actions due to its unique physical properties and, therefore, is included among the therapeutic gases.

THE THERAPEUTIC GASES

Oxygen, Carbon Dioxide, and Helium

Harry Wollman and Theodore C. Smith

OXYGEN

The importance of oxygen, water, and food to the animal organism is fundamental. Of these three basic essentials for the maintenance of life, the deprivation of oxygen leads to death most rapidly. Oxygen therapy is useful or necessary for life in several diseases and intoxications that interfere with normal oxygenation of the blood or tissues. In addition, pure oxygen administered at ambient pressures greater than 1 atmosphere has both unique applications as a therapeutic agent and multiple toxic effects. Its range of usefulness and toxicity is still being explored and defined.

History. Soon after Priestley's discovery of oxygen in 1772 and Lavoisier's elucidation of its role in respiration, oxygen therapy was introduced in England by Beddoes. His publication in 1794, entitled "Considerations on the Medicinal Use and Production of Factitious Airs," can be considered the beginning of inhalational therapy. Beddoes, overcome with enthusiasm for his project, treated all kinds of diseases with oxygen. They included such diverse conditions as scrofula, leprosy, and paralysis. Such indiscriminate therapeutic applications natu-

881

rally led to many failures, and Beddoes died a disconsolate man. It is interesting to note that Beddoes' collaborator was James Watt, engineer and inventor of the steam engine, and his assistant was Sir Humphry Davy. When Beddoes' experiments proved disappointing, Davy left the laboratory in order to pursue his own investigations on the properties of nitrous oxide. Davy's contribution to the history of anesthesia is mentioned elsewhere.

It was only following such pioneer investigations as those of Haldane, Hill, Barcroft, Krogh, L. J. Henderson, and Y. Henderson that oxygen therapy was placed upon a sound physiological basis.

OXYGEN DEPRIVATION

Etiology of Hypoxia. *Hypoxia* is a broad term used to designate deprivation of oxygen regardless of etiology or site. Since hypoxia can arise from a variety of causes, and because methods of treatment are closely allied to etiology, a classification of the types of hypoxia is useful. One can consider five categories of hypoxia:

1. *Inadequate Oxygen Content of Inspired Gas.* In this situation, pulmonary function is normal but the oxygen tension in the pulmonary alveoli is below normal. This may be due to the low inspired concentration of oxygen at normal ambient pressure, such as occurs when inert gases are present in greater-than-normal concentration. Alternatively, it may be caused by low ambient pressure, such as occurs at high altitude.

2. *Inadequate Delivery of Inspired Gas to the Lungs.* In this category, inspired gas with normal oxygen tension is not delivered to the lungs in adequate amounts. This may be due to respiratory tract obstruction, to muscular weakness induced by disease (*e.g.,* poliomyelitis) or by drugs (*e.g.,* neuromuscular blocking agents), or to lack of respiratory drive because of central nervous system (CNS) disease or the effect of central respiratory depressant drugs (*e.g.,* opioids and barbiturates).

3. *Inadequate Oxygenation of Blood Due to Abnormal Pulmonary Gas Exchange.* In the presence of a normal tension of oxygen in the inspired air and adequate ventilation, a defect in pulmonary function prevents the normal oxygenation of blood. The defect in pulmonary function may be a diffusion block, due to thickening of the alveolar-capillary membrane. It may be caused by venous-arterial (right-to-left) shunts. It may

also reflect a functional inequality of ventilation and perfusion in the lung, such as occurs in most acute and chronic pulmonary diseases.

4. *Inadequate Transport of Oxygen by the Circulation.* The delivery of adequate inspired oxygen to normally ventilated and perfused alveoli results in normal arterial oxygen tension. However, the arterial blood may fail to deliver sufficient oxygen to the tissues. This can be caused by low cardiac output, as in shock, or by maldistribution of the cardiac output, such as occurs following thrombosis or vasospasm. Another cause may be low oxygen-carrying capacity of the blood due to anemia or abnormal hemoglobin function (carboxyhemoglobin; 2,3-diphosphoglyceric acid [2,3-DPG] deficiency).

5. *Inadequate Tissue Utilization.* In this situation, tissues are unable to extract and utilize enough oxygen from the normally oxygenated blood that is delivered. This may be due to abnormally high metabolic demand (*e.g.,* thyrotoxicosis, hyperpyrexia) or to malfunctioning cellular enzyme systems (*e.g.,* cyanide poisoning, uncoupling of oxidative phosphorylation).

Actually, a combination of several kinds of hypoxia may exist and the dangers are then far greater. For instance, an organ with low blood flow due to atherosclerotic changes can sustain serious damage if the oxygen tension of its arterial supply should decrease only slightly.

Effects of Hypoxia. The signs and symptoms of hypoxia are varied and widespread. They are most clearly seen in the individual who is subjected to inadequate oxygenation of the blood acutely or subacutely, as with inhalation of low oxygen mixtures, respiratory depression, or respiratory obstruction. The picture differs in the patient acclimatized to hypoxic conditions; this complex subject cannot be considered here (*see* Van Liere and Stickney, 1963; Tenney and Lamb, 1965). Nor will comment be made on the greater resistance to hypoxia manifested by the newborn of most species (*see* Mott, 1961).

The changes produced by hypoxia include alterations in blood oxygen transport, which sometimes produce cyanosis. In addition, respiratory, cardiovascular, and CNS changes occur, as well as effects on individual organs and tissues and on metabolism. All these effects are discussed below.

Oxygen Saturation and Tension of Blood. The oxygen saturation, or content, of blood is related to its oxygen tension (P_{O_2}), as illustrated by the oxygen-hemoglobin dissociation curve (Figure 43–1). The oxygen tension of the blood *and* the oxygen saturation of the circulating hemoglobin are both reduced when: (1) the partial pressure of oxygen in the inspired air is lowered, (2) the amount of oxygen delivered to the alveoli per minute is below physiological requirements, or (3) the exchange of oxygen from alveoli to blood is inadequate. The resulting reduction of *both* oxygen *tension* and *content* of the blood contrasts with other situations where blood P_{O_2} is normal but oxygen content is low, such as occurs in anemia.

Cyanosis. This is an unreliable guide to the arterial oxygen saturation. Cyanosis appears when about 5 g % of reduced hemoglobin is present in arterial blood. This figure represents an oxygen saturation of 67% when a normal amount of hemoglobin (15 g %) is present. However, when anemia lowers the hemoglobin to 10 g %, then cyanosis does not appear until the arterial blood saturation has decreased to 50%. Furthermore, the ability to recognize cyanosis clinically is extremely variable (Comroe and Botelho, 1947).

Respiration. Hypoxia stimulates both rate and depth of respiration reflexly through the chemoreceptors of the carotid and aortic bodies. Although moderate reductions in oxygen saturation fail to increase the respiratory minute volume markedly, the inhalation of gas mixtures containing 7% or less of oxygen nearly doubles the pulmonary ventilation. Furthermore, the respiratory response to carbon dioxide is considerably enhanced when the P_{O_2} of arterial blood is lowered (*see* Kellogg, 1964). It is important to realize that, as a result of the hyperpnea induced by hypoxia, there is a fall in arterial carbon dioxide tension (P_{CO_2}). Some of the physiological changes observed in hypoxic persons may be partly due to this mild hypocarbia. With decrease in the normal carbon dioxide central respiratory drive, the increase in ventilation due to hypoxia at the peripheral chemoreceptors is somewhat self-limiting.

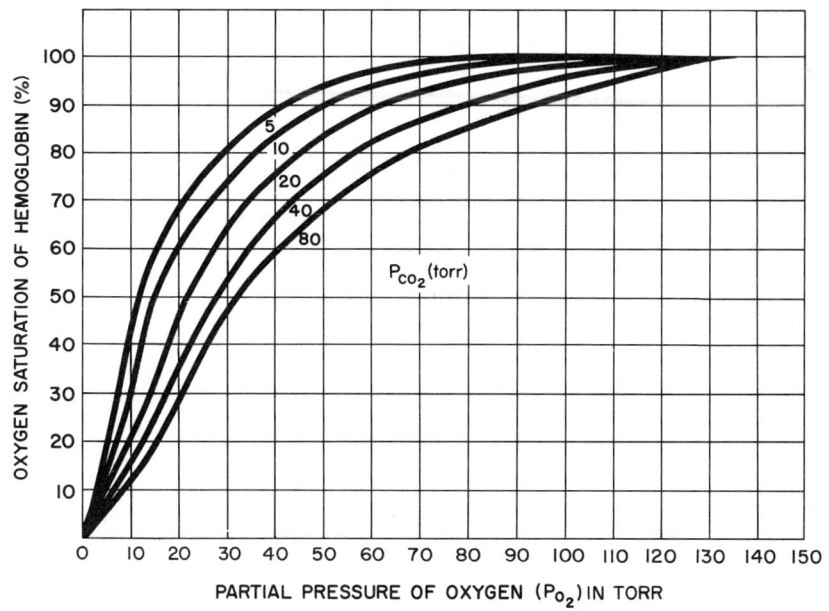

Figure 43–1. *The oxygen-hemoglobin dissociation curve.*

The dissociation of oxygen from hemoglobin is determined by the partial pressure of oxygen (P_{O_2}), and modified by a number of other factors. These include the P_{CO_2} of blood, the influence of which is shown here (Bohr effect). (After Van Liere and Stickney, 1963. Courtesy of the University of Chicago Press.)

Normal individuals breathing low concentrations of oxygen fail to experience dyspnea because hypoxia and dyspnea are not necessarily associated. Dyspnea occurs when the respiratory minute volume approaches the maximal breathing capacity. In the normal individual, with a maximal breathing capacity of 160 liters per minute, an extreme degree of hypoxia does not provide sufficient stimulus for the minute ventilation to reach levels associated with dyspnea. On the other hand, if the maximal breathing capacity is reduced to 15 to 30 liters per minute by pulmonary abnormalities, any slight respiratory stimulation might raise the minute volume sufficiently to cause dyspnea. There are many stimuli to respiration in addition to hypoxia, for example, acidosis, hypercarbia, and activation of stretch receptors originating in the lungs. Thus, the indication for oxygen therapy is not dyspnea but hypoxia. When oxygen is given to a patient who has both hypoxia and dyspnea, therapy should not be stopped if oxygen fails to relieve the dyspnea (see Comroe and Dripps, 1950).

Cardiovascular System. Acute hypoxia results in an increase in *heart rate,* probably mediated through some mechanism other than the carotid and aortic chemoreceptors (Daly and Scott, 1958). In normal individuals exposed to reduced oxygen tensions in the inspired air, the increase in pulse rate varies with the oxygen saturation of arterial blood, reaching about a 30% increase at 70% saturation (Dripps and Comroe, 1947b). Tachycardia is such a consistent response to hypoxia that a reduction in heart rate of 10 beats per minute within a few minutes after the initiation of oxygen therapy has been taken as presumptive evidence that acute hypoxia existed (Comroe and Dripps, 1950). Continuing hypoxia, however, can result in a decrease in heart rate toward normal values, and the prolonged inhalation of 4 to 5% oxygen can produce circulatory failure. The arterial P_{O_2} in this circumstance is below 30 torr (millimeters of mercury) and the saturation is below 50%.

The *blood pressure* increases in normal individuals subjected experimentally to acute hypoxia, but significant increases are not observed unless the inhaled oxygen concentration is below 10%. Both the cardiac output and the coronary blood flow increase during hypoxia. Hypoxia produces cerebral vasodilatation and pulmonary vascular constriction; the latter, in the presence of hypoxia, is an important part of the mechanism that matches pulmonary ventilation and perfusion in the normal lung.

Central Nervous System. Hypoxia affects the CNS both functionally and morphologically. An acute reduction of the arterial oxygen saturation to 85% ($P_{O_2} = 50$ torr) decreases mental effectiveness, visual acuity, emotional stability, and finer muscular coordination. Further reduction to 75% saturation ($P_{O_2} = 40$ torr) leads to faulty judgment, analgesia, and considerable impairment of muscular coordination. If the arterial oxygen saturation is reduced below 65% ($P_{O_2} = 32$ torr), unconsciousness and a progressive, descending depression of the CNS supervene (see Anderson et al., 1946). Finally, circulatory failure occurs. Only mild subjective changes are noted by hypoxic individuals, and a person inhaling a low oxygen mixture may lose consciousness before recognizing that any changes have taken place.

Under certain conditions the inhalation of carbon dioxide may offer some protection to the hypoxic brain, for three reasons. First, it counteracts the hypocarbia produced when hypoxia induces hyperpnea, thus moving the oxygen dissociation curve to the right and making more oxygen available to tissues. Second, it increases the ventilation, resulting in more rapid delivery of oxygen to alveoli and therefore in a higher arterial P_{O_2}. Third, it tends to dilate cerebral vessels and increase blood flow to the brain (see Pierce et al., 1962).

The manifestations of cerebral hypoxia produced by acute arrest of the cerebral circulation are sudden and dramatic. EEG changes, including the appearance of high-voltage slow waves (delta waves), occur within seconds, as does the loss of consciousness. The first histological changes occur in cortical gray matter and some thalamic cells after 3 or 4 minutes of circulatory occlusion; the cerebellum is more resistant to hypoxic damage, and the brain stem and cord are most resistant. Full return of function cannot be expected if circulatory arrest exceeds 3 to 5 minutes, and irreversible damage and death may be expected if the cerebral circulation remains static for longer periods (*see* Plum, 1973).

Individual Organs and Tissues. The brain is usually the first organ to manifest hypoxic damage; the myocardium is also highly susceptible. Hypoxic injury to other organs is slower in onset, but can occur as a result of generalized circulatory insufficiency. Cerebrovascular responses and compensatory vasomotor reflexes combine to deflect an inordinately large proportion of the cardiac output from visceral channels to organs such as the brain and heart. Under these circumstances, hypoxic damage to the liver and kidney as well as other organs can be demonstrated. The effect of oxygen lack on the eye is loss of visual acuity, which is manifested most noticeably by the abrupt development of a sensation of brightening following restoration of the normal supply of oxygen. Muscle tissue is capable of sustaining an oxygen debt for periods of several hours by means of anaerobic metabolism.

Metabolism. Oxygen consumption and carbon dioxide production by the whole body and by various organs do not change measurably until extremes of hypoxia are reached. However, there are changes in carbohydrate metabolism associated with a shift from aerobic to anaerobic metabolic pathways. Those changes most frequently observed are hyperglycemia and increased production of lactic acid, with an increase in the lactate:pyruvate ratio in blood. A summary of the metabolic effects of hypoxia has been provided by Cohen (1972).

OXYGEN ADMINISTRATION

Normally the inspired air contains 20.93% oxygen. At a barometric pressure of 760 torr this represents a partial pressure or tension of oxygen in the inspired air of 159 torr. However, oxygen uptake and dilution with water vapor and carbon dioxide reduce the P_{O_2} in the alveoli to about 100 torr. There is a small tension gradient between alveolar gas and arterial blood, resulting in a normal arterial P_{O_2} of about 90 torr (96% saturation). The inhalation of oxygen at 1 or more atmospheres of ambient pressure raises the arterial P_{O_2} to many times its normal value.

This change is naturally followed by physiological adjustments, and under some circumstances by functional disturbances of the tissues exposed to these high oxygen tensions (*see* Lambertsen, 1965).

Effect on Blood Gases. *Oxygen.* This gas is normally carried by the circulating blood mainly as oxyhemoglobin, with a small amount present in physical solution. However, the relative quantities of oxygen carried in arterial blood by these two mechanisms can vary significantly over the wide range of arterial P_{O_2} observed in different circumstances (*see* Lambertsen *et al.,* 1953, 1955). Table 43-1 illustrates the oxygen content of arterial blood, the amount carried as oxyhemoglobin, the amount carried in solution, and the composition of mixed venous blood under various circumstances. It can be seen that, in most situations, hemoglobin is largely responsible for the transfer of oxygen. However, when oxygen is inhaled at an ambient pressure of 3 atmospheres, sufficient oxygen is carried in physical solution for all the oxygen transfer to be accomplished without desaturating any of the oxyhemoglobin. The consequences of this are discussed below.

Carbon Dioxide. One of the ways in which carbon dioxide is carried by blood is in the form of bicarbonate. This mechanism of carbon dioxide transfer operates more readily when a hydrogen ion acceptor is made available, as occurs in the capillaries when oxyhemoglobin is converted to reduced hemoglobin, a stronger base and therefore a better hydrogen ion acceptor. When large amounts of oxygen are carried in simple solution, the amount of physically dissolved oxygen may be sufficient to satisfy tissue oxygen uptake requirements (*see* Table 43-1). Little or no oxygen is then extracted from oxyhemoglobin, and reduced hemoglobin is not formed. Carbon dioxide is then carried away from tissues less efficiently, and the P_{CO_2} of the tissues rises by several torr (*see* Lambertsen *et al.,* 1953).

Nitrogen. Normally, the blood is in equilibrium with alveolar air, which contains close to 80% nitrogen. As a result, several liters of this inert gas are in solution in body fluids and are present in body cavities. When

Table 43-1. THE CARRIAGE AND TRANSFER OF OXYGEN IN BLOOD *

CONDITIONS	INSPIRED GAS	P_{O_2} OF DRY INSP GAS (torr)	ARTERIAL BLOOD P_{O_2} (torr)	Vol % of Oxygen Carried			MIXED VENOUS BLOOD P_{O_2} (torr)	Vol % of Oxygen Carried		
				as Oxyhgb	in Soln	Total		as Oxyhgb	in Soln	Total
Sea level	Air	159	90	19.3	0.3	19.6	38	14.5	0.1	14.6
	O_2	760	600	20.1	1.9	22.0	50	16.8	0.2	17.0
Altitude of 6.1 km (20,000 ft)	Air	73	35	13.5	0.1	13.6	23	8.5	0.1	8.6
	O_2	350	230	20.1	0.7	20.8	43	15.7	0.1	15.8
Ambient pressure of 3 atmospheres	Air	477	350	20.1	1.1	21.2	45	16.1	0.1	16.2
	O_2	2280	2000	20.1	6.2	26.3	385	20.1	1.2	21.3

* In the first horizontal line, figures for arterial and mixed venous blood are given for normal man breathing air at sea level; in the second, the changes induced by oxygen inhalation are shown. The P_{O_2} is greatly increased in the arterial blood, but oxygen content is increased less than 15%. As hemoglobin is very nearly saturated with oxygen at a P_{O_2} of 90 torr and can carry little more oxygen as P_{O_2} increases, most of the additional oxygen is carried in solution.

In the third horizontal line are figures for acute hypoxia induced by the inhalation of a mixture low in oxygen, equivalent to about 10% oxygen at sea level. Hemoglobin becomes more desaturated as arterial P_{O_2} falls. In the fourth line, one can see complete correction of altitude-induced hypoxia by the breathing of 100% oxygen.

In the final two lines are illustrated the effects of increased ambient pressure. The inhalation of air at 3 atmospheres of pressure produces results intermediate between those of oxygen inhalation at 6.1 km (20,000 ft) and oxygen administration at sea level. When 100% oxygen is inhaled at 3 atmospheres of pressure, arterial P_{O_2} rises to 2000 torr, and the 6.2 vol % of dissolved oxygen in the arterial blood is sufficient to satisfy the oxygen extraction requirements of the body. Thus, no oxygen is extracted from hemoglobin by tissue, and the mixed venous blood contains completely saturated hemoglobin. The consequences of this are discussed in the text.

The figures in this table are approximations based on the assumptions of 15 g % of hemoglobin, 5 vol % of oxygen extraction by the whole body, constant cardiac output, and the ventilatory changes usually observed under the circumstances illustrated. When severe anemia is present, arterial oxygen tensions are little affected, but arterial oxygen content is lower. Oxygen extraction continues, and, therefore, mixed venous blood has considerably lower oxygen content and oxygen tension.

pure oxygen is inhaled, the partial pressure of nitrogen in the alveoli falls rapidly. Nitrogen diffuses from the tissues to be eliminated by the lungs. Most of the nitrogen of the body can be exhaled in this manner within a few hours. The effects of this absence of "inert gas" from the body are discussed under the untoward effects of oxygen inhalation, as well as under therapeutic uses.

Respiration. The immediate effect of the inhalation of 100% oxygen by normal subjects is a mild respiratory depression, presumably due to withdrawal of tonic impulses from the chemoreceptors. After a few minutes the situation becomes far more complex, and there is no general agreement on the steady-state effects of 100% oxygen on respiration (Lambertsen, 1966).

Cardiovascular System. There is a slight decrease in the heart rate of normal subjects inhaling pure oxygen. Cardiac output is reduced by 8 to 20%. There is little change in blood pressure. The inhalation of oxygen also affects blood flow to some important vascular beds. Coronary blood flow in the dog is reduced by the administration of oxygen. Cerebral blood flow is decreased slightly. Some attribute this to the mild hypocarbia attending oxygen inhalation. Whether oxygen itself has any direct effect on cerebral vessels is not yet clear. In the pulmonary vascular bed, high tensions of oxygen cause dilatation and reduced pulmonary arterial pressure. Oxygen inhalation appears to relax the pulmonary vasculature in hypoxic animals and man, and in persons with pulmonary hypertension. (*See* Dripps and Comroe, 1947b; Eckenhoff *et al.,* 1947; Fishman, 1961.)

Metabolism. When 100% oxygen is inhaled by man, changes are not detectable in oxygen consumption, carbon dioxide production, respiratory quotient, or glucose utilization.

UNTOWARD EFFECTS OF OXYGEN INHALATION

The administration of oxygen, particularly at more than 1 atmosphere of pressure, can cause undesirable effects. However, none of these should interdict the use of high partial pressures of oxygen when they are indicated.

Pulmonary Atelectasis. When the alveoli of the lungs are filled predominantly with oxygen, subsequent airway obstruction may result in complete absorption of the gas with consequent alveolar collapse. Similarly, if a body cavity is filled with oxygen and subsequently its access to the atmosphere becomes obstructed, complete absorption of the gas can cause discomforting symptoms. For example, occlusion of the Eustachian tubes may lead to retraction of the eardrums, and obstruction of the paranasal sinuses may produce a "vacuum-type" headache.

Oxygen Apnea. In several situations the response of the respiratory centers to carbon dioxide may be so depressed that respiration is maintained largely by the activity of the carotid and aortic chemoreceptors. This phenomenon may attend cerebral injuries involving the respiratory centers, barbiturate intoxication, or long periods of exposure to hypercarbia or hypoxia (*e.g.,* chronic pulmonary disease). In these instances, the administration of oxygen may cause apnea by the removal of the chemoreceptor drive to respiration. The occurrence of oxygen apnea is not a contraindication to, but rather a convincing indication of the need for, the administration of oxygen. It is better to have the patient well oxygenated with controlled artificial respiration than to have him poorly oxygenated from breathing spontaneously, but inadequately, in response to a hypoxic drive from the chemoreceptor mechanism. Fortunately, in many cases it is possible to administer carefully controlled concentrations of oxygen sufficient to increase arterial oxygenation, but not great enough to cause apnea.

Retrolental Fibroplasia. Retrolental fibroplasia occurs in some premature infants who have been exposed to high concentrations of oxygen at birth. Retinal changes begin to appear between the third and sixth week of life. These may regress entirely or may progress through retinal detachment to blindness. The incidence of this disease has been greatly reduced in recent years by administering oxygen only to those infants who require it and only for as long as it is required, and by limiting the inspired oxygen concentration to 35 to 40% when possible. However, the infant who is cyanotic despite inhalation of 40% oxygen should be exposed to higher concentrations; this can be done without increasing the danger of retrolental fibroplasia, for it is the *arterial* P_{O_2} and not the *inspired* P_{O_2} that is of importance in the causation of this disease. Retinal damage can also occur in adults following inhalation of 100% oxygen at greater-than-atmospheric pressures. This is particularly liable to occur in those patients whose retinal circulation has been previously compromised, for example, by retinal detachment (*see* Nichols and Lambertsen, 1971).

Oxygen Poisoning. *Respiratory Tract Effects.* The inhalation, at atmospheric pressure, of 80% oxygen for more than about 12 hours can cause a symptom complex mainly referable to irritation of the respiratory tract. Normal subjects exposed to these tensions of oxygen in the inspired air manifest a progressive decrease in vital capacity, coughing, nasal stuffiness, sore throat, and substernal distress, followed by tracheobronchitis and later by the development of pulmonary congestion, transudation, exudation, or atelectasis (*see* Clark and Lambertsen, 1971).

This syndrome is not experienced by subjects breathing 50% oxygen, nor by those breathing 100% oxygen at ½ atmosphere for 24 hours or longer. Thus, it is clear that the

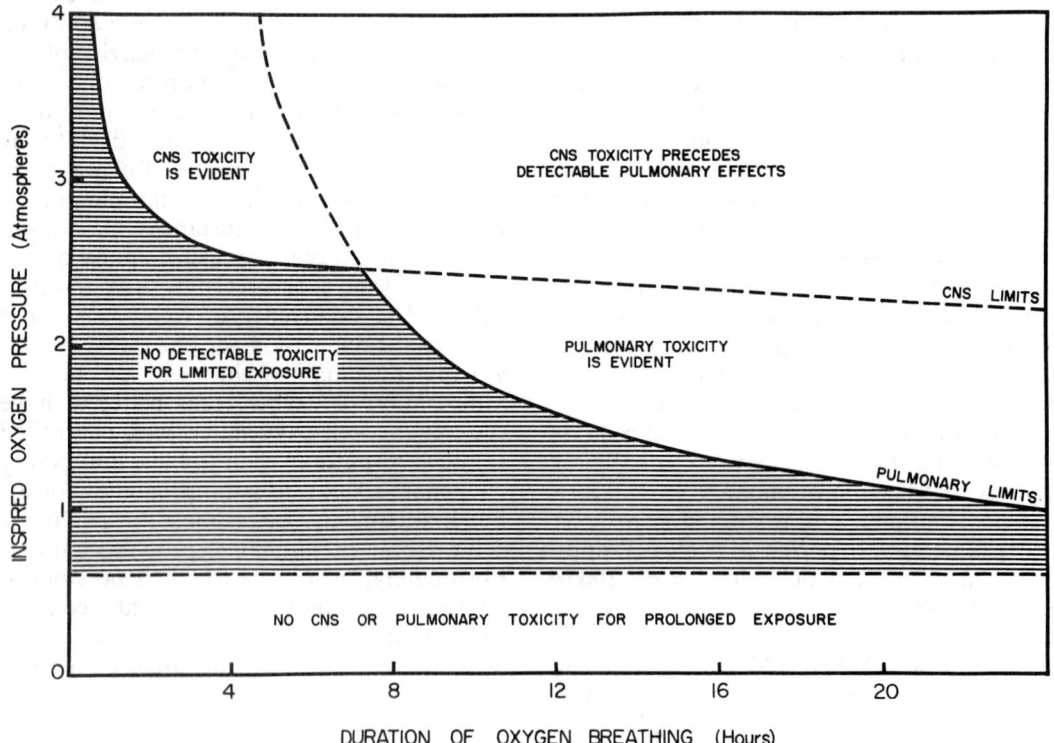

Figure 43-2. *Oxygen-toxicity limits in man.*

   The two areas most affected are the CNS and the lungs. The occurrence of toxicity depends upon both the inspired oxygen pressure (P_{O_2}) and the duration of exposure. The safe duration of exposure becomes shorter as the inspired P_{O_2} increases. Below ½ atmosphere of inspired oxygen, indefinite exposure appears to be safe; between ½ and approximately 2 atmospheres, pulmonary toxicity occurs after prolonged exposures but CNS effects are not detectable; above 2 atmospheres, CNS toxicity appears before pulmonary effects are detectable. (Drawn from suggestions and analysis by C. J. Lambertsen, Institute for Environmental Medicine, University of Pennsylvania.)

important factor in the causation of this symptom complex is the P_{O_2} and *not* the concentration of oxygen in the inhaled gas (*see* Winter and Smith, 1972). The onset and progression of signs and symptoms are more rapid at greater inspired P_{O_2}. When inspired P_{O_2} becomes greater than 2 atmospheres, CNS toxicity is the first symptom to appear (Lambertsen, 1965). Figure 43-2 shows a comparison of the times of onset of pulmonary and CNS symptoms of oxygen toxicity.

Central Nervous System Effects. When pure oxygen is inhaled at pressures greater than 2 atmospheres, a characteristic syndrome is observed. Signs and symptoms include muscular twitching, nausea, vertigo, mood changes, paresthesias, and, finally, loss of consciousness and generalized convulsions. The appearance of this syndrome is related both to the length of exposure and to the ambient P_{O_2}. The symptoms may appear in persons at rest in less than 2 hours at 3 atmospheres, in ½ hour at 4 atmospheres, and in a few minutes at 6 atmospheres of oxygen. However, wide individual variations are observed in the susceptibility to oxygen poisoning. The latent period before oxygen toxicity appears is decreased by physical exertion and by carbon dioxide inhalation. CNS toxicity produced by high pressures of oxygen appears to be reversible with decrease in the inspired P_{O_2}. Following a period of postictal depression, recovery of normal function is complete and relatively rapid.

Although the mechanism of this type of oxygen poisoning is not known, it may be related to the inhibition of certain substances concerned with oxidative metabolism. These include many sulfhydryl-containing enzymes and cofactors, of which coenzyme A is one. Other biochemical changes that may be related to the mechanism of oxygen toxicity include damage to cellular membranes by lipid peroxidation and the oxidation of vital tissue components, including glutathione and ascorbic acid. Some protection against the oxygen toxicity syndrome is offered by the administration of gamma-aminobutyric acid, succinate, chelating agents, certain anesthetics, and tromethamine (*tris*-[hydroxymethyl] aminomethane). The mechanisms by which these agents offer protection are as numerous and conjectural as the possible mechanisms of CNS oxygen toxicity itself. (For detailed discussion, *see* Lambertsen, 1971.)

Preparations. Official U.S.P. preparations of oxygen are of a specified purity. Oxygen is marketed in a compressed form in steel cylinders fitted with reducing valves for delivery of the gas. They are usually color coded (green in the United States), and those for use on anesthetic machines are pin indexed (*see* Chapter 5).

METHODS OF ADMINISTRATION

The various methods for the administration of oxygen will be discussed only briefly. They have been reviewed by Barach (1962) and Egan (1973).

Oxygen Tents and Hoods. These consist of light, portable, tentlike structures usually made of transparent materials. They fit over the patient's head and sometimes over the thorax as well, in a fairly airtight manner. Oxygen is delivered to them at relatively high flow rates, and the exhaled carbon dioxide is usually eliminated with the overflow of gases, just as in many anesthesia circuits. The concentration of oxygen within the tent can be increased by higher flow rates of oxygen, by elimination of leaks, and by the use of smaller tents or hoods. Oxygen tents are desirable for the comfort they offer the patient, and for the cooling and humidification of the atmosphere that some of them offer. However, the oxygen concentration within them is rarely above 50%, and may be as low as 25% when low flow rates are used in large tents that are not carefully closed. Periodic checking of oxygen concentration within tents is easily performed with a paramagnetic or thermal-conductivity oxygen analyzer or with an oxygen electrode, and this should be done whenever possible.

Nasal Cannulas. A simple device for the administration of oxygen is a soft rubber or plastic catheter, which is inserted into a nostril, but not far enough to traverse the nasopharynx and enter the esophagus. Humidified oxygen is then passed through the tube, and the rate of flow largely determines the concentration that enters the alveoli. A double nasal cannula is usually used to increase the inspired oxygen concentration, but it is rare that more than 50% oxygen can be introduced into the lungs by this means. The nasal cannula presents minimal discomfort for the patient, and permits him more freedom of movement than does the tent or the hood, while allowing attending personnel easier access to the patient.

Face Masks. Another, more effective method for the administration of oxygen is a face mask. Such masks may be equipped with a system of valves to permit elimination of carbon dioxide and dilution of the inspired oxygen with ambient air, if this is desired. It is possible to administer nearly 100% oxygen with a tightly fitted face mask. The procedure is economical and efficient, and some of the newer transparent plastic devices enjoy good patient acceptability. Masks are almost essential for use at high altitudes, in aviation, and in pressure chambers. Furthermore, they make possible the use of assisted or controlled ventilation, which can be of value in the treatment of pulmonary edema, asthma, and certain chronic pulmonary diseases. A device similar to the mask is the mouthpiece used in conjunction with a nose clip, but this is less comfortable and is not suitable for the depressed patient, who cannot maintain an airtight seal with this device.

Other Routes. Oxygen administration through an endotracheal tube or a tracheostomy in conjunction with mechanical ventilation is used in the desperately ill. Although oxygen has been given by intravenous and subcutaneous injection and by the gastric and rectal routes as well, it is doubtful whether these methods are of practical value (*see* James *et al.,* 1963). Furthermore, intravenous injection is dangerous in that gas emboli may occur.

In a few cases where patients have been in the final stages of respiratory failure due to pulmonary disease, extracorporeal oxygenation has been used. A heart-lung machine oxygenates part of the patient's blood flow during this procedure. The hope is that several hours or, at the most, several days of such mechanical support may permit sufficient pulmonary improvement to make further extracorporeal support unnecessary (*see* Drinker, 1972).

THERAPEUTIC USES

Haldane stated years ago that *hypoxia not only stops the machine but wrecks the machinery.* The treatment of hypoxia is obviously a medical emergency, and, therefore, all therapeutic measures for its relief should be marshaled. Since the primary objective is the correction of the basic defect responsible for the deficiency, and since the causes of hypoxia are diverse, the therapeutic measures for its relief are numerous and varied. The administration of oxygen frequently does not correct the basic defect. Rather, oxygen is employed as a stopgap until more fundamental measures can be instituted or become effective, or occasionally because specific therapy for the underlying disease is unavailable. In this capacity the administration of oxygen can be lifesaving. The alert therapist does not wait until the signs and symptoms of severe hypoxia are evident but administers the gas in anticipation of its need.

As discussed above, the indication for oxygen therapy is not dyspnea but hypoxia. When oxygen is given to a patient who has both hypoxia and dyspnea, therapy should not be stopped if oxygen fails to relieve the dyspnea.

The therapeutic uses of oxygen are conveniently considered under the same headings that were used above to classify the etiology of hypoxia.

Inadequate Oxygen Content of Inspired Gas. When there is a deficiency of oxygen in the atmosphere, for example, at high altitudes, the administration of supplemental oxygen will assure an adequate oxygen tension in the alveoli. Above an altitude of 3.7 km (12,000 ft), where barometric pressure is below 500 torr, it is necessary to administer supplemental oxygen; above 10.1 km (33,000 ft), even 100% oxygen will not maintain normal alveolar P_{O_2}.

Inadequate Delivery of Inspired Gas to the Lungs. Inadequate oxygenation of the normal lung does not always call for therapy with oxygen. Rather, the basic cause of the hypoxia should be removed. For example, obstruction of the airway can often be corrected by mechanical means; insufficiency of the respiratory muscles or respiratory depression calls for artificial ventilation. However, there are circumstances under which oxygen therapy can be of great value. For instance, when obstruction to breathing is due to bronchoconstriction that proves difficult to overcome, hypoxia can be relieved when oxygen is administered by mask. In instances of respiratory obstruction, the addition of helium to the respiratory mixture may also be of value (*see* below).

Inadequate Oxygenation of Blood Due to Abnormal Pulmonary Gas Exchange. This constitutes the chief indication for oxygen (*see* Bendixen *et al.,* 1965; Pontoppidan *et al.,* 1973). This is especially true when hypoxia is the result of poor diffusion of gases across the alveolar-capillary membrane or of inequality of ventilation and perfusion.

Diffusion Barriers. Oxygen diffuses less readily through the alveolar-capillary membrane than does carbon dioxide. Therefore, in situations where a diffusion barrier exists in the lung, the P_{O_2} of blood may fall considerably while the P_{CO_2} rises little. Oxygen will diffuse poorly across the alveolar-capillary membrane when anatomical changes occur, as in pulmonary fibrosis, or when the membrane is temporarily thickened, as in pulmonary edema. In such situations, oxygen inhalation is of great value in overcoming the diffusion barrier, and adequate arterial oxygenation can usually be obtained with only a small increase in inspired oxygen concentration. Pure diffusion block is rare, and other pulmonary defects in association with it are usually of greater functional importance.

Ventilation-Perfusion Inequalities. When some alveoli are poorly ventilated, the oxygenation of blood flowing past them is decreased. This blood will mix with well-oxygenated blood coming from more normal areas of lung, and the resulting mixed arterial blood will be intermediate in oxygen content. If the ventilation-perfusion defect is serious enough to produce significant desaturation of the arterial blood, therapy with oxygen is indicated. This treatment increases the P_{O_2} of gas in all alveoli, and relief of hypoxia may be expected.

Venous-Arterial Shunts. A small amount of right-to-left shunting of blood is normal from Thebesian and pleural veins. Abnormal degrees of shunting may be due to congenital anatomical defects, or they may be acquired, as with atelectasis or pneumonia. Since the shunted blood is never exposed to respiratory gases, administration of oxygen cannot increase its saturation. The increase in oxygen content of blood draining normal oxygen-containing alveoli is small, as it represents mostly dissolved oxygen (*see* Table 43-1). When this blood mixes with partially unsaturated blood, the resulting arterial pool may still be inadequately oxygenated. Thus, some improvement can be obtained by administering oxygen in the presence of right-to-left shunting, but if the defect is great, as in some patients following operations, arterial blood saturation may not be returned completely to normal. However, compensatory reflexes in the lung will eventually decrease the flow of blood past atelectatic areas, and thus improve overall oxygenation of the blood.

Mixed Defects in Pulmonary Function. In most disease states, more than one factor contributes to the production of hypoxia. For example, in *pneumonia* there is a diffusion defect. Atelectasis is present in some areas of the lung, and there is also a ventilation-perfusion defect. Finally, tachypnea and shallow respiration result in less effective alveolar ventilation. In this disease, as in many others, oxygen administration compensates for some of the abnormalities better than for others. It may overcome the diffusion barrier completely and successfully treat the ventilation-perfusion defect, but may only partially compensate for the shunting of blood past atelectatic alveoli. The inefficient ventilatory pattern usually improves with relief of the hypoxia. However, oxygen does not remove the basic cause of the disease. Improvement is symptomatic until specific chemotherapy proves effective.

In the treatment of *pulmonary edema,* the administration of oxygen by mask with controlled or assisted ventilation can be of value. With this procedure, the increase in airway pressure of 5 to 20 torr at the peak of inspiration has been said to oppose the hydrostatic pressure within the capillaries that contributes to pulmonary edema. More important, the increased intrapulmonary pressure is transmitted to the great veins, thereby retarding the entrance of blood into the right heart. Finally, positive-pressure breathing expands the lung above the closing volume of small airways, opening them for gas flow and reducing the degree of atelectasis.

Another complex pulmonary problem is *pulmonary emphysema and fibrosis.* In this chronic disease, there are diffusion and ventilation-perfusion defects as well as bronchial obstruction. While prolonged oxygen inhalation is impractical, the treatment of such patients with oxygen by mask at intervals is of some use, especially when it is combined with positive-pressure ventilation and other measures such as the use of bronchodilators, anti-infective agents, and postural drainage.

Inadequate Transport of Oxygen by the Circulation. Oxygen is useful in certain types of circulatory disorders, in which it provides a valuable adjunct to more fundamental therapy.

Hemoglobin Deficiency. The administration of oxygen is of importance in the treatment of *carbon monoxide poisoning,* because it accelerates the conversion of carboxyhemoglobin to oxyhemoglobin. In addition, the breathing of pure oxygen leads to increased transport of this gas in physical solution in the plasma, and in this manner tissue hypoxia is partially relieved (*see* Chapter 44). Similarly, oxygen inhalation can also be of value in anemia because the additional oxygen carried in plasma can aid in the relief of tissue hypoxia.

Circulatory Deficiency. Oxygen has been used effectively in certain instances of generalized circulatory deficiency, including cardiac decompensation and shock. In *cardiac decompensation* the oxygen saturation of the blood may be reduced due to pulmonary edema. In addition, there is tissue hypoxia associated with circulatory inadequacy. Oxygen therapy often results in the relief of cyanosis and a slowing of the pulse rate. Although treatment should be directed primarily toward improving cardiac function, oxygen affords temporary relief due to better myocardial oxygenation.

Oxygen administration is of limited value in the therapy of the tissue hypoxia present during *shock.* Nevertheless, oxygen is often administered in peripheral circulatory failure for whatever benefit can be gained from the increase in blood P_{O_2} and the additional oxygen carried in physical solution.

Oxygen may also be of some value in cases of localized circulatory deficiency, such as occurs in *coronary occlusion.* The higher P_{O_2} and oxygen content of the circulating blood may aid in the delivery of oxygen to hypoxic areas of the myocardium. Improvement is frequently noted, with relief of pain and restlessness, improvement of circulation, and relief of cyanosis. Oxygen inhalation may also be of value in some instances of *cerebrovascular accidents,* permitting better oxygenation of marginally hypoxic areas of the brain.

Inadequate Tissue Utilization. Oxygen administration is a temporary therapeutic measure in such situations. It is unlikely to be effective in conditions such as cyanide poisoning. However, it may exert a beneficial effect in those states where the additional oxygen carried in blood can help to satisfy abnormally high tissue demands, as in thyrotoxicosis or hyperthermia.

Miscellaneous Uses of Oxygen. A unique although uncommon use of oxygen, in which advantage is taken of the laws of diffusion of gases, is in the treatment of *abdominal distention.* In such conditions as intestinal obstruction, ileus, or postoperative distention, the gas accumulating in the bowel consists largely of nitrogen. The blood can pick up very little of this nitrogen, for it has already been exposed in the lungs to an atmosphere containing 80% nitrogen. If, however, 100% oxygen is breathed and the partial pressure of nitrogen in the alveoli falls, nitrogen diffuses out of the blood into the exhaled gases. As the nitrogen content of the blood decreases, the gas in the intestine diffuses into the circulation and is eliminated through the lungs.

The symptoms following *pneumoencephalography* with air, consisting in nausea, vomiting, and severe headache, may also be relieved by the inhalation of

100% oxygen. The nitrogen that remains in the subarachnoid space and ventricles following the injection of air can be removed, the mechanism being analogous to that described above. *Subcutaneous emphysema* may be reduced by the same technic. Inhalation of 100% oxygen has also been suggested for treatment of *spontaneous pneumothorax* and *air embolism.*

Oxygen inhalation is also used by workers in *pressurized spaces,* to decrease the inhaled nitrogen concentration and thus to lessen the likelihood of *caisson disease,* or bends, to shorten the required decompression time, and to minimize nitrogen narcosis. Under these conditions one must be careful not to exceed the time and concentration limits for avoidance of oxygen toxicity.

Finally, *in anesthesia,* oxygen is a common diluent for the gaseous and volatile anesthetic agents. The anesthetized patient may inhale up to 98% oxygen when 2% halothane is being administered in a nonrebreathing system, or as little as 20% oxygen when 80% nitrous oxide is given.

Hyperbaric Oxygen Therapy

Although most uses of oxygen do not require more than 1 atmosphere of the gas, there are some conditions where administration of greater tensions may be desirable.

The administration of more than 1 atmosphere of oxygen as a therapeutic measure had its beginnings in the high-pressure experiments of Paul Bert in 1878. In recent decades serious studies of the effects of high-pressure oxygen by investigators such as Behnke, Boerema, and Lambertsen have provided some basis for the use of "hyperbaric oxygen" in clinical medicine.

Hyperbaric oxygenation is accomplished in pressure chambers. These range in size from those designed for a few small experimental animals, through those large enough for a man, up to chambers that accommodate an entire operating suite or an intensive care unit for a number of patients. Since it is neither practical nor economical to fill the larger chambers with oxygen, they may be brought to ambient pressures of more than 1 atmosphere with compressed air. The patients then inhale oxygen at these ambient pressures through a face mask or mouthpiece.

There are many practical difficulties associated with this type of treatment. The facilities and their proper maintenance and operation are expensive; there is a fire hazard in the enclosed space of the chamber; oxygen toxicity and nitrogen narcosis are distinct possibilities; and decompression sickness can occur in patients or attendants (*see* Committee on Hyperbaric Oxygenation, 1966). However, there are some proven and many potential uses for this method of therapy, and they deserve exploration (*see* Trapp *et al.,* 1974).

Anaerobic Infections. Intermittent treatment with hyperbaric oxygen has been of value in the treatment of infections produced by *Clostridium perfrin-*

gens, the anaerobic bacillus causing *gas gangrene.* The increased tissue oxygen pressure achieved may exert an inhibitory effect on the enzyme systems of these bacteria. Antibiotics and other supportive therapy are still necessary. Results can be less satisfactory in the treatment of *tetanus* with hyperbaric oxygen, as the toxin may already be fixed to nerve tissue, and, although the microorganism is killed or prevented from multiplying, irreversible damage may have occurred. However, encouraging results have been reported by some.

Hyperbaric oxygen may prove to be useful in the treatment of other anaerobic infections as well, such as those caused by *Bacteroides* and anaerobic streptococci and cases of actinomycosis that are refractory to other therapy.

Gas Emboli and Bubbles. Hyperbaric oxygenation can be useful in the treatment of decompression sickness. It can also provide immediate relief of symptoms in situations where gas emboli in the vascular tree can be compressed by high pressures, such as diving accidents and postcardiopulmonary-bypass gas emboli. During slow decompression these bubbles, which become filled with oxygen, are gradually absorbed.

Circulatory Disturbances. If the blood flow to a tissue is decreased due to disease such as atherosclerosis, its P_{O_2} might be maintained near normal by increasing the P_{O_2} and oxygen content of its arterial blood. The increase in arterial and venous blood oxygenation produced by inhaling 3 atmospheres of oxygen is shown in Table 43–1. The *diffusion* of significant amounts of oxygen *through the skin* into blood and deeper tissues begins at pressures above 10 atmospheres.

With the hope of improving tissue oxygenation by raising the blood P_{O_2}, hyperbaric oxygen has been used as a therapeutic measure in such *local circulatory disturbances* as acute cerebral edema, various types of peripheral arterial insufficiency, and compromised skin grafts. Additional uses have been suggested in many other localized circulatory problems, but effectiveness has not yet been demonstrated. The possibility of oxygen toxicity makes continuous therapy dangerous, and, therefore, intermittent treatments are used. The efficacy of this method of therapy in these diseases depends on the presence of some circulation to the tissues, that is, with only partial occlusion of vessels or the existence of collateral channels for those that are blocked. One hopes that circulation to the hypoxic areas will develop while hyperbaric oxygenation is supportive through a critical period.

High-pressure oxygen may be of value in some instances of the *generalized circulatory deficiency* occurring in shock and following exceptionally great blood loss. There is not yet general agreement either on the degree of usefulness of hyperbaric oxygen in circulatory disturbances or on the most effective dosage schedules. Clearly, oxygen may provide supplemental therapy, but it will not replace specific and supportive treatment in these cases (*see* McDowall, 1964, 1966).

Acute Respiratory Difficulties. It has been suggested that hyperbaric oxygenation can be of use in the treatment of respiratory abnormalities that result in generalized hypoxia. The use of high-pressure oxygen in the treatment of smoke inhalation or pulmonary embolism may prove to be valuable. It has had little success in treatment of the respiratory distress syndrome of the newborn (*hyaline membrane disease*).

Miscellaneous Uses. *Carbon Monoxide Poisoning.* The use of 2 atmospheres of oxygen will result in faster conversion of carboxyhemoglobin to oxyhemoglobin than will 100% oxygen at sea level. Little practical benefit is gained by increasing pressure much further. One treatment with 2 atmospheres of oxygen for ½ to 1½ hours is usually sufficient even for patients who are comatose on arrival at the hospital. The greatest difficulty encountered in the use of this therapy is the problem of rapidly transporting the patient to a hyperbaric chamber.

Tumor Therapy. Certain rapidly enlarging tumors outgrow their blood supply and develop necrotic areas. Presumably many of the cells in such tumors are hypoxic, and it is known that hypoxic cells exhibit increased resistance to radiation damage. Hyperoxygenation of the blood might increase the P_{O_2} of the more poorly perfused tumor cells, and thereby increase their radiation sensitivity without substantially changing the resistance of normal cells. Therefore, it has seemed reasonable to administer several atmospheres of oxygen to certain patients undergoing radiation therapy, and also cancer chemotherapy. The efficacy of this adjunct to cancer therapy will be difficult to evaluate until considerable numbers of patients have been treated and observed for several years.

Surgical Uses. When cardiovascular operations must be performed on patients with *right-to-left shunts,* additional oxygenation of the nonshunted blood can be of value. It increases the oxygen content of the mixed arterial blood, and may thus increase the patient's tolerance to the stress of surgery. The same type of reasoning has been applied to its intraoperative use in patients with *ventilation-perfusion disturbances.* It has also been suggested that irritability of the hypoxic myocardium during operation is decreased by high-pressure oxygen. In patients with more normal cardiopulmonary status, the additional dissolved oxygen present in tissues under hyperbaric conditions may allow a few additional minutes of *total circulatory occlusion* when this maneuver is necessary for completion of the operation. Surgical uses of hyperbaric oxygenation have been uncommon because of the additional hazards and difficulties entailed, and because other means of safely operating on such patients can be devised.

Cyanide Poisoning. The use of hyperbaric oxygen to overcome the metabolic block in cyanide poisoning deserves further exploration.

Evaluation. The early use of high-pressure oxygen at a few medical centers reflected the first blush of enthusiasm for the clinical exploration of its possible usefulness. Later, the physiological and phar-macological effects of high-pressure oxygen were more fully investigated. Now that its therapeutic indications are beginning to be defined more clearly, it is to be hoped that in the next several years the most effective dosage schedules will be more rigorously defined.

CARBON DIOXIDE

It was not until the end of the eighteenth century that Priestley discovered this gas and Lavoisier described its role in respiration. A century later Miesher demonstrated its effects on the respiration of man. Since then, as the physiological effects of carbon dioxide have been elucidated and quantified, it has become apparent that the gas is of paramount importance in the regulation of many vital functions, and that small changes in P_{CO_2} in the body have marked physiological effects. The potential uses of carbon dioxide as a pharmacological agent and its toxicity lie primarily in its marked effects on respiration, circulation, and the CNS.

TRANSFER AND ELIMINATION OF CARBON DIOXIDE

Several hundred milliliters per minute of carbon dioxide are produced by the body's metabolism at rest, and up to ten times that much during heavy exercise. The gas diffuses readily from the cells that produce it into the blood stream, where it is carried partly as bicarbonate ion, partly in chemical combination with hemoglobin and plasma proteins, and also in physical solution at a partial pressure of about 47 torr in mixed venous blood. It is transported to the lung, where it is normally exhaled at the same rate at which it is produced, leaving a partial pressure of about 40 torr in the alveoli and in the arterial blood.

The P_{CO_2} of air is a fraction of 1 torr. When 4% carbon dioxide is inhaled, the P_{CO_2} of inspired gas rises to about 30 torr. This increases the alveolar P_{CO_2}, decreases the gradient for its transfer from mixed venous blood to alveoli, and temporarily slows its elimination by the lung. However, as carbon dioxide accumulates, the tissue and blood P_{CO_2} rises, and a new steady state is reached in which carbon dioxide tensions are greater than normal. The difference in P_{CO_2} between mixed venous blood and alveoli is reestablished, ventilation is increased, and the volume of carbon dioxide produced each minute by metabolic processes can again be exhaled through the lungs. When 8% carbon dioxide is inhaled, the P_{CO_2} of inspired gas is about 60 torr, which is *higher* than the blood and tissue tensions. Carbon dioxide is thus *taken up* by the body for a period of time. As the gas is both taken up and produced by the body, tissue and blood tensions increase to levels high enough again to provide a gradient from mixed venous blood to the alveoli. With the reestablished gradient and increased ventilation, carbon dioxide elimination can again occur at the same rate as its metabolic production.

Under some circumstances, for example, with certain anesthetic technics (*see* Chapter 5), deliberate hyperventilation is carried out, resulting in a rate of carbon dioxide elimination that exceeds the rate of its production. The body's stores of carbon dioxide become depleted, and the arterial P_{CO_2} may decrease to 25 torr or less. Some of the effects of hypocapnia are discussed below, and also in the chapters on anesthesia.

When carbon dioxide is inhaled, or when alveolar ventilation is decreased, the P_{CO_2} in arterial blood rises and its pH falls. This decrease in pH is referred to as *respiratory acidosis*. When overventilation lowers the P_{CO_2} of blood, the pH rises and *respiratory alkalosis* is present. As carbon dioxide can freely diffuse into and out of cells, the changes in blood P_{CO_2} and pH are soon reflected by intracellular changes of P_{CO_2} and pH (*see* Chapter 36).

EFFECTS OF CARBON DIOXIDE

Alterations of P_{CO_2} and pH have widespread effects in the body. Here a description will be given of the important effects of carbon dioxide on respiration, circulation, and the CNS. (For a more complete discussion of these and other effects, *see* Symposium, 1960.)

Respiration. Carbon dioxide is a potent stimulus to respiration. The inhalation of 2% carbon dioxide produces a measurable increase in both rate and depth of ventilation. Ten percent carbon dioxide can produce respiratory volumes of 75 liters per minute in normal individuals. The inhalation of even higher concentrations produces little additional increase in ventilation. Respiratory stimulation begins in seconds following the inhalation of even low concentrations of carbon dioxide, and maximal stimulation by the inhaled carbon dioxide is usually attained in less than 5 minutes (*see* Lambertsen and Wendel, 1960). The respiratory effects of carbon dioxide inhalation disappear within a few minutes after its withdrawal.

There are at least two *sites* where carbon dioxide acts to stimulate respiration. Respiratory integration areas in the brain stem are acted upon by impulses from medullary chemoreceptors and from peripheral arterial chemoreceptors. *Mechanisms* by which carbon dioxide acts on these receptors probably include changes in carbon dioxide *tension* of blood or sensitive tissues, and decline in blood, cerebrospinal fluid, extracellular fluid, or tissue *pH* produced by carbon dioxide (*see* Mitchell, 1966).

Circulation. The circulatory effects of carbon dioxide are the result of its direct local effects and its centrally mediated effects on the autonomic nervous system. The direct effect of carbon dioxide on the *heart* results from pH changes and produces diminished contractile force and slowing of the rate of contraction (*see* Ng *et al.,* 1967). The cardiac rhythm is usually not affected. The direct effect on *blood vessels* produces vasodilatation.

The autonomic effects of carbon dioxide result in widespread activation of the *sympathetic nervous system* with an increase in plasma concentrations of epinephrine and norepinephrine (*see* Sechzer *et al.,* 1960; Hamilton *et al.,* 1966). The response is mediated by various subcortical centers in the hypothalamus, brain stem reticular formation, and medulla. These areas can be locally excited by carbon dioxide, but they also receive afferents from the carotid and aortic chemoreceptors that are sensitive to changes in carbon dioxide in the blood. The results of sympathetic nervous system activation are, in general, opposite to the local effects of carbon dioxide. The sympathetic effects consist in increase in the force and rate of cardiac contraction and constriction of many vascular beds. The total circulatory response to carbon dioxide, therefore, is determined by the balance of the opposing local and sympathetic nervous system effects. The overall effects of carbon dioxide inhalation in normal man are increase in cardiac output and heart rate, elevation of systolic and diastolic blood pressures, and increase in pulse pressure (*see* Dripps and Comroe, 1947a; Cullen and Eger, 1974). There is a *decrease* in total peripheral resistance when carbon dioxide is breathed. The local vasodilating effects of carbon dioxide, combined with epinephrine-induced dilatation of arterioles of skeletal muscle and the splanchnic circulation, appear to exert more of an influence than do the sympathetically mediated vasoconstrictor effects. In the heart, the marked increase in cardiac output reflects a predominance of the sympathetic over the local effects. When carbon dioxide is breathed by an individual whose vasomotor impulses are blocked, for example, by spinal anesthesia or extensive sympathectomy, the peripheral action of carbon dioxide predominates and the blood pressure falls.

Cardiac arrhythmias due to carbon dioxide inhalation are rare, even when arterial P_{CO_2} reaches 80 torr (Sechzer *et al.*, 1960). However, when the arrhythmia threshold is decreased by factors such as the inhalation of cyclopropane or some of the halogenated anesthetics, carbon dioxide is more likely to produce cardiac arrhythmias.

The cerebral circulation, which does not have functionally important sympathetic innervation, undergoes significant dilatation when carbon dioxide is inhaled (*see* Kety and Schmidt, 1948). To a lesser extent carbon dioxide produces coronary vasodilatation (*see* Berne, 1964).

Following the termination of carbon dioxide inhalation, a mild fall in blood pressure is noted in awake man, along with tachycardia (*see* Dripps and Comroe, 1947a; Sechzer *et al.*, 1960).

The circulatory effects of lower-than-normal tensions of carbon dioxide may be observed during voluntary or mechanical hyperventilation. They consist in vascular dilatation in muscle, and vasoconstriction in skin, intestine, brain, and kidney. Blood pressure is reduced; cardiac output, oxygen consumption, and heart rate are increased (*see* Kety and Schmidt, 1946; McGregor *et*

al., 1962; Rowe *et al.*, 1962). The mechanisms through which these changes are effected are complex. Part of the changes may be attributed to hypocarbia and part to the mechanical effects of hyperventilation or the increased airway pressure caused by mechanical ventilation.

Central Nervous System. The inhalation of low concentrations of carbon dioxide depresses the excitability of the cerebral cortex and increases the threshold for the production of seizures by drugs or electroshock. It also increases the cutaneous pain threshold through a central action. This central depression is of importance in the therapeutic application of the gas, for carbon dioxide can cause further depression of an already depressed brain. However, when high concentrations of carbon dioxide (25 to 30%) are breathed, subcortical areas that have cortical projections are activated. This activation overcomes the depressant effect of carbon dioxide on the cortex. The increased cortical excitability that results can progress to convulsions. The inhalation of even higher concentrations of carbon dioxide (about 50%) produces marked cortical and subcortical depression of a type similar to that produced by anesthetic agents. EEG effects of carbon dioxide inhalation depend on the inhaled concentration. When low concentrations are inhaled and cortical depression is present, EEG waves of increased frequency appear. The inhalation of 30% carbon dioxide produces intermittent high-voltage bursts in the EEG, coinciding with clinical seizure activity. An anesthetic concentration of carbon dioxide (50%) causes flattening of the EEG. A decrease in P_{CO_2} below normal values results in the appearance of high-voltage slow waves (theta and delta), particularly in the frontal leads (*see* Woodbury and Karler, in Symposium, 1960).

Untoward Effects of Carbon Dioxide Inhalation. The normal subject inhaling concentrations of carbon dioxide up to 5 or 6% experiences the sensation of increased respiration, but rarely experiences dyspnea. Some notice an acidic taste, as carbon dioxide forms carbonic acid in the presence of water. The inhalation of higher concentrations, up to about 10%, produces dyspnea, headache, dizziness, sweating, restlessness, paresthesias, and a general feeling of discomfort. Higher concentrations result in pronounced discomfort. The CNS effects of very high concentrations of carbon dioxide are described above. As with oxygen poisoning, the CNS toxicity of carbon dioxide is a reversible phenomenon.

Following the abrupt withdrawal of inhaled concentrations of carbon dioxide above 5%, a few subjects experience headache or dizziness. These symptoms can be avoided by slowly decreasing the inhaled concentration rather than withdrawing it suddenly.

Untoward circulatory effects of carbon dioxide include marked elevation of blood pressure, tachycardia, and possible arrhythmias. The fact that the acidosis resulting from very high concentrations renders effector organs less sensitive to the effect of catecholamines may be beneficial in some circumstances and harmful in others.

Chemistry and Preparations. Carbon dioxide is approximately one and one-half times as dense as air. *Carbon Dioxide,* U.S.P., is of a specified purity. It is marketed in metal cylinders compressed to 58 atmospheres, under which condition it exists as a liquid, vaporizing as it is delivered from the cylinder. For medicinal purposes, carbon dioxide is usually administered in combination with oxygen, and cylinders containing the two gases in varying proportions are available. Since carbon dioxide solidifies at approximately $-78°$ C, it can also be obtained in solid form (dry ice, CO_2 snow).

Methods of Administration. Carbon dioxide is frequently administered by means of a tight-fitting face mask, the gas being supplied from a cylinder containing a mixture of 5 to 10% carbon dioxide in oxygen. It is also possible to deliver 100% carbon dioxide from a cylinder through a tube held a few inches above the patient's face. Carbon dioxide, being heavier than air, falls over the patient's face and is inhaled, diluted with room air. Although this technic requires little equipment, it does not allow one to know the inhaled concentration of carbon dioxide.

Another method of carbon dioxide administration is the rebreathing technic, where the supply of carbon dioxide comes from the patient's exhaled gases, which are rebreathed, for example, from a paper bag. Since the inspired oxygen concentration falls as the inhaled carbon dioxide concentration rises, this should not be continued for longer than a few minutes.

THERAPEUTIC USES

Carbon dioxide inhalation has been suggested as a means of therapy in many commonly encountered situations, but for most of these there are other treatments available that are more effective and offer fewer disadvantages. There remain, however, several interesting and unique uses of the gas in therapy, diagnosis, and research.

Respiratory Depression, Asphyxia, and Coma. The usefulness of carbon dioxide in stimulating depressed respiration is very limited. When respiratory minute volume is reduced, the excretion of carbon dioxide is impaired and the tension of this gas in blood and tissues rises. Thus, there is already an elevated P_{CO_2}. A further elevation of the tension by the administration of carbon dioxide may not increase ventilation and will only worsen the respiratory acidosis. Elevation of P_{CO_2} may even further depress the neurons of the respiratory centers. Therefore, if carbon dioxide is employed as a respiratory stimulant in depression due to drugs, disease, or injury, the effect on respiratory minute volume should be carefully observed and administration of the gas immediately discontinued if the desired response is not obtained. In all types of respiratory depression, asphyxia, and coma, reliance should be placed on mechanical support of the respiration plus the administration of oxygen and, perhaps in some cases, pharmacological respiratory stimulation (*see* Chapter 18).

Intermittent carbon dioxide inhalation has been used postoperatively to increase ventilation, and presumably to aid in the prevention of atelectasis. Intermittent positive-pressure breathing, tracheal suction, coughing, pulmonary physical therapy, and voluntary deep breathing can produce the same results.

Carbon Monoxide Poisoning. The inhalation of 5 to 7% carbon dioxide in oxygen has been used in the treatment of carbon monoxide poisoning, as carbon dioxide increases both the ventilatory exchange and the rate of dissociation of carbon monoxide from carboxyhemoglobin. A possible disadvantage is the production of serious acidosis of brief duration when the respiratory acidosis produced by carbon dioxide is added to the metabolic acidosis already present in cases of severe carbon monoxide poisoning. However, the acidosis further speeds the dissociation of carboxyhemoglobin (*see* Chapter 44).

Uses in Anesthesia. Carbon dioxide inhalation can increase the speed of induction and emergence from anesthesia by increasing minute ventilation (*see* Chapter 5). The disadvantages of respiratory acidosis during anesthesia are presented on page 91. Hyperventilation with its attendant respiratory alkalosis has some uses in anesthesia. It increases the apparent depth of anesthesia. By constricting the cerebral vessels, it decreases brain size slightly and may facilitate the performance of neurosurgical operations.

Uses in Research and Diagnosis. Carbon dioxide inhalation has been of value in the study of the control of respiration and of cerebral blood flow, and carbon dioxide–sensitivity curves have been used to investigate the effects of drugs on respiration and cerebral blood flow. The inhalation of carbon dioxide has been used as a means of testing the depth of respiratory depression. If carbon dioxide stimulates respiration, such responsiveness indicates less intense depression than is present in a patient whose respiration is unaffected or depressed by carbon dioxide. Hyperventilation to lower P_{CO_2} is of use for diagnostic purposes in eliciting the characteristic EEG pattern of absence seizures, but other methods are also available.

Miscellaneous Uses. Carbon dioxide inhalation is one of many suggested treatments for *hiccoughs,* and it has been successful in some cases.

Carbon dioxide inhalation may terminate seizures in patients with *status petit mal.* It has been suggested as a means of increasing cerebral blood flow in cases of *cerebrovascular disease,* but its continuous inhalation for this purpose would obviously be impractical. Furthermore, in patients with vascular disease, the sclerosed cerebral vessels are less able to dilate than are normal vessels; the dilatation of the normal vessels may then produce only undesirable consequences (*see* Meyer *et al.,* 1972). The potential use of carbon dioxide at high altitudes is discussed in the section on central effects of hypoxia. Additional uses include its application in surgery for gas *endarterectomy* and *laparoscopy,* and in *negative contrast roentgenography* where intravenously injected carbon dioxide can permit visualization of the shape and size of the right atrium. Carbon dioxide has also been used to saturate aqueous solutions of the hydrochloride salts of certain *local anesthetics* for the purpose of increasing their rate of penetration into nerve fibers and the extent of their intracellular accumulation, as a consequence of the lowering of intracellular pH. This procedure has been reported to result in increases in the rate of onset and intensity and duration of local anesthetic action (Condouris and Shakalis, 1964; Bromage, 1967). (*See* Chapter 20.)

HELIUM

Helium is an inert gas that owes its pharmacological actions exclusively to its physical properties. Its molecular weight is 4.00, and its specific gravity is 0.14. The low density of helium is the basis for the use of helium-oxygen mixtures when respiration is embarrassed by obstruction. Another physical property of helium, its low aqueous solubility, makes it useful for divers and other workers in high-pressure environments. Its high thermal conductivity increases the rate of heat transfer and heat loss in helium environments; and its high acoustic velocity (1300 m per second) distorts the voice and raises its pitch.

History and Preparations. Helium was identified in 1895 as emanations from radioactive ores (alpha rays). In 1905 it was found in oil and gas wells in Louisiana. Until recently the United States government sponsored the recovery of helium from these wells and its underground storage. There is no other commercial source of the gas, and the present underground supply is limited.

Helium is marketed in compressed form in the usual type of steel cylinder. *Helium,* U.S.P., consists of not less than 95% helium, the remainder being mainly nitrogen. It is available also in various mixtures with oxygen.

Methods of Administration. Helium is usually administered by means of a face mask as a mixture with oxygen and other gases. It can be administered in a non-rebreathing system, but this method is expensive. When it is administered in a closed circuit, the helium is rebreathed; since little helium is dissolved in the body, only oxygen need be added. In closed systems carbon dioxide must be absorbed. In some applications, individuals are placed in closed environments consisting of mixtures of helium and other gases.

Therapeutic Uses. The main uses for helium are in deep-sea diving and prevention of decompression sickness. It is theoretically of use in patients with respiratory obstruction, although beneficial results have rarely been documented.

Deep-Sea Diving and Prevention of Decompression Sickness. Due to its pulmonary and CNS toxicity, the use of oxygen in diving is limited to depths of 9 m (30 ft) of sea water or less. If air is breathed, the limit is increased to 46 m (150 ft). If the oxygen concentration of the inspired mixture is decreased at greater depths, oxygen toxicity can be avoided; however, the addition of nitrogen produces significant nitrogen narcosis at depths of less than 91 m (300 ft) and increases the risk of decompression sickness. When divers or other individuals working under high pressure breathe compressed air, significant amounts of nitrogen dissolve in the blood and tissues. If a person breathing compressed air is too rapidly decompressed, the nitrogen suddenly escapes from the body fluids and causes gas emboli, which produce many untoward phenomena, including excruciating pains and possibly death. Decompression sickness, also known as "divers' bends" or caisson disease, can be avoided only by slow decompression, which permits the dissolved nitrogen to escape from the body fluids gradually and be eliminated by way of the lung without forming gas emboli. Therefore, another diluent of oxygen is needed to permit deeper diving and safer decompression. This function is filled by helium, which has no significant narcotic effects, even at depths of 274 m (900 ft). The very low solubility of helium in body tissues results in shorter decompression times and makes decompression sickness less likely. In addition, the low density of the gas reduces the considerable work of breathing normally required at high pressures.

In some undersea missions an enclosed atmosphere is provided that is filled with a helium-oxygen mixture. Undesirable side effects resulting from helium's physical properties are distortion of speech and increased rate of heat loss.

Respiratory Obstruction. During normal respiration, the flow of gas in the airway is largely laminar. The pressure required to produce laminar flow in the airway is dependent in part on the *viscosity* but not the density of the inhaled gases. On the other hand, when respiratory obstruction exists, there is usually turbulent rather than laminar flow in the area of the obstruction. The energy required to move gases in this situation is inversely related to the *density* of the gases. As helium is so much less dense than nitrogen, a helium-oxygen mixture can be breathed with less effort than can either air or oxygen. When flow is turbulent, the force required for drawing 80% helium with 20% oxygen into the lungs is only one half that necessary for air. Helium, therefore, may be useful in cases of obstruction of the upper tracheobronchial tree or larynx of an acute and self-limiting nature, but it does not replace specific therapy. It is of more use for the increase in ventilation and the resulting carbon dioxide wash-out than for its ability to raise blood P_{O_2}, for which purpose an 80% helium–20% oxygen mixture would be less effective than 100% oxygen. Since flow in distal bronchi is always laminar, even in diseases such as chronic obstructive bronchitis, helium is ineffective for all but upper airway obstruction (*see* Raimondi *et al.*, 1970).

Miscellaneous Uses. As a diluent in anesthetic mixtures containing cyclopropane and oxygen, helium *decreases inflammability;* however, it is not widely used for this purpose. It has also been employed during open-heart surgery; helium-oxygen mixtures are insufflated into the lung during cardio-pulmonary bypass when ventilation of the lung has been discontinued. Helium is not superior to other gases for this purpose, and 100% oxygen or oxygen diluted with nitrous oxide or nitrogen is more commonly used.

Helium's insolubility in body tissues is useful in pulmonary function tests where one does not wish the inspired gas to be taken up from the lung (functional residual capacity, closing volume). Helium has an antiarrhythmic effect in experimental coronary occlusion, which is as yet unexplained (*see* Pifarré *et al.*, 1970).

Anderson, D. P.; Allen, W. J.; Barcroft, H.; Edholm, O. G.; and Manning, G. W. Circulatory changes during fainting and coma caused by oxygen lack. *J. Physiol., Lond.,* **1946,** *104,* 426–434.

Barach, A. L. Historical background. In, Symposium—inhalational therapy. *Anesthesiology,* **1962,** *23,* 407–421.

Barcroft, J. Anoxaemia. *Lancet,* **1920,** *2,* 485–489.

Behnke, A. R., Jr.; Johnson, F. S.; Poppen, J. R.; and Motley, E. P. The effect of oxygen on man at pressures from 1 to 4 atmospheres. *Am. J. Physiol.,* **1935,** *110,* 565–572.

Boerema, I.; Meyne, N. G.; Brummelkamp, W. K.; Bouma, S.; Mensch, M. H.; Kamermans, F.; Stern Hanf, M.; and Van Aalderen, W. Life without blood. *J. cardiovasc. Surg.,* **1960,** *1,* 133–146.

Bromage, P. R. Improved conduction blockade in surgery and obstetrics: carbonated local anesthetics. *Can. med. Ass. J.,* **1967,** *97,* 1377–1384.

Comroe, J. H., Jr., and Botelho, S. The unreliability of cyanosis in the recognition of arterial anoxemia. *Am. J. med. Sci.,* **1947,** *214,* 1–6.

Condouris, G. A., and Shakalis, A. Potentiation of the nerve-depressant effect of local anaesthetics by carbon dioxide. *Nature, Lond.,* **1964,** *204,* 57–59.

Cullen, D. J., and Eger, E. I. Cardiovascular effects of CO_2 in man. *Anesthesiology,* **1974,** *41,* 345–349.

Daly, M. B., and Scott, M. J. The effects of stimulation of the carotid body chemoreceptors on heart rate in the dog. *J. Physiol., Lond.,* **1958,** *144,* 148–166.

Dripps, R. D., and Comroe, J. H., Jr. The respiratory and circulatory response of normal man to inhalation of 7.6 and 10.4 per cent CO_2 with a comparison of the maximal ventilation produced by severe muscular exercise, inhalation of CO_2 and maximal voluntary hyperventilation. *Am. J. Physiol.,* **1947a,** *149,* 43–51.

————. The effect of the inhalation of high and low oxygen concentrations on respiration, pulse rate, ballistocardiogram and arterial oxygen saturation (oximeter) of normal individuals. *Ibid.,* **1947b,** *149,* 277–291.

Eckenhoff, J. E.; Hafkenschiel, J. H.; Landmesser, C. M.; and Harmel, M. Cardiac oxygen metabolism and control of the coronary circulation. *Am. J. Physiol.,* **1947,** *149,* 634–649.

Haldane, J. S.; Meakins, J. C.; and Priestley, J. G. The effects of shallow breathing. *J. Physiol., Lond.,* **1919,** *52,* 433–453.

Haldane, J. S., and Priestley, J. G. The regulation of the lung-ventilation. *J. Physiol., Lond.,* **1905,** *32,* 225–266.

Hamilton, J. T.; Hersey, L. W.; and Twiss, J. L. The role of the adrenal medulla in the blood pressure response to carbon dioxide following hexamethonium. *Archs int. Pharmacodyn. Thér.,* **1966,** *160,* 29–43.

Henderson, Y., and Haggard, H. W. The treatment of carbon monoxide asphyxia by means of oxygen plus carbon dioxide inhalation. *J. Am. med. Ass.,* **1922,** *79,* 1137–1145.

James, L. S.; Apgar, V. A.; Burnard, E. D.; and Moya, F. Intragastric oxygen and resuscitation of the newborn. *Acta paediat., Stockh.,* **1963,** *52,* 245–251.

Kety, S. S., and Schmidt, C. F. The effect of active and passive hyperventilation on cerebral blood flow, cerebral oxygen consumption, cardiac output, and blood pressure of normal young men. *J. clin. Invest.,* **1946,** *25,* 107–119.

————. The effects of altered arterial tension of carbon dioxide and oxygen on cerebral blood flow and cerebral oxygen consumption of normal young men. *Ibid.,* **1948,** *27,* 484–492.

Krogh, M. Diffusion of gases through the lungs of man. *J. Physiol., Lond.,* **1915,** *49,* 271–300.

Lambertsen, C. J.; Ewing, J. H.; Kough, R. H.; Gould, R.; and Stroud, M. W. Oxygen toxicity. Arterial and internal jugular blood gas composition in man during inhalation of air, 100% O_2 and 2% CO_2 in O_2 at 3.5 atmospheres ambient pressure. *J. appl. Physiol.,* **1955,** *8,* 255–263.

Lambertsen, C. J.; Kough, R. H.; Cooper, D. Y.; Emmel, G. L.; Loeschcke, H. H.; and Schmidt, C. F. Oxygen toxicity. Effects in man of oxygen inhalation at 1 and 3.5 atmospheres upon blood gas transport, cerebral circulation and cerebral metabolism. *J. appl. Physiol.,* **1953,** *5,* 471–486.

Lambertsen, C. J., and Wendel, H. An alveolar P_{CO_2} control system: its use to magnify respiratory depression by meperidine. *J. appl. Physiol.,* **1960,** *15,* 43–48.

McDowall, D. G. Hyperbaric oxygen in relation to circulatory and respiratory emergencies. *Br. J. Anaesth.,* **1964,** *36,* 563–571.

————. Hyperbaric oxygen in relation to acute trauma. *Ibid.,* **1966,** *38,* 308–316.

McGregor, M.; Donevan, R. E.; and Anderson, N. M. Influence of carbon dioxide and hyperventilation on cardiac output in man. *J. appl. Physiol.,* **1962,** *17,* 933–937.

Meyer, J. S.; Fukuuchi, Y.; Shimazu, K.; Ohuchi, T.; and Ericsson, A. D. Abnormal hemispheric blood flow and metabolism in cerebrovascular disease. II. Therapeutic trials with 5% CO_2 inhalation, hyperventilation and intravenous infusion of THAM and mannitol. *Stroke,* **1972,** *3,* 157–167.

Mott, J. C. The ability of young mammals to withstand total oxygen lack. *Br. med. Bull.,* **1961,** *17,* 144–147.

Ng, M. L.; Levy, M. N.; and Zieske, H. A. Effects of changes of pH and of carbon dioxide tension on left ventricular performance. *Am. J. Physiol.,* **1967,** *213,* 115–120.

Pierce, E. C., Jr.; Lambertsen, C. J.; Strong, M. J.; Alexander, S. C.; and Steele, D. Blood P_{CO_2} and brain oxygenation at reduced ambient pressure. *J. appl. Physiol.,* **1962,** *17,* 899–908.

Pifarré, R.; Raghunath, T. K.; Vanecko, R. M.; Chua, F. S.; Balis, J. U.; and Neville, W. E. Effect of oxygen and helium mixtures on ventricular fibrillation. *J. thorac. cardiovasc. Surg.,* **1970,** *60,* 648–652.

Plum, F. The clinical problem: how much anoxia-ischemia damages the brain? *Archs Neurol., Chicago,* **1973,** *29,* 359–360.

Raimondi, A. C.; Edwards, R. H. T.; Denison, D. M.; Leaver, D. G.; Spencer, R. G.; and Siddorn, J. A. Exercise tolerance breathing a low density gas mixture, 35% oxygen and air in patients with chronic obstructive bronchitis. *Clin. Sci.,* **1970,** *39,* 675–685.

Rowe, G. C.; Castillo, C. A.; and Crumpton, G. W. Effects of hyperventilation on systemic and coronary hemodynamics. *Am. Heart J.,* **1962,** *63,* 67–77.

Sechzer, P. H.; Egbert, L. D.; Linde, H. W.; Cooper, D. Y.; Dripps, R. D.; and Price, H. L. Effect of CO_2 inhalation on arterial pressure, ECG, and plasma catecholamines and 17-OH corticosteroids in normal man. *J. appl. Physiol.,* **1960,** *15,* 454–458.

Monographs and Reviews

Barcroft, J. *The Respiratory Function of the Blood.* Cambridge University Press, Cambridge, Vol. I, **1925;** Vol. II, **1928.**

Bendixen, H. H.; Egbert, L. D.; Hedley-Whyte, J.; Laver, M. B.; and Pontoppidan, H. *Respiratory Care.* C. V. Mosby Co., St. Louis, **1965.**

Berne, R. M. Regulation of coronary blood flow. *Physiol. Rev.,* **1964,** *44,* 1–29.

Bert, P. *Barometric Pressure: Researches in Experimental Physiology.* (Hitchcock, M. A., and Hitchcock, F. A., transls.) College Book Co., Columbus, Ohio, **1943.**

Clark, J. M., and Lambertsen, C. J. Pulmonary oxygen toxicity: a review. *Pharmac. Rev.,* **1971,** *23,* 37–133.

Cohen, P. J. The metabolic function of oxygen and biochemical lesions of hypoxia. *Anesthesiology,* **1972,** *37,* 148–177.

Committee on Hyperbaric Oxygenation (eds.). *Fundamentals of Hyperbaric Medicine.* National Academy of Sciences–National Research Council, Washington, D.C., **1966.**

Comroe, J. H., Jr., and Dripps, R. D. *The Physiological Basis for Oxygen Therapy.* Charles C Thomas, Pub., Springfield, Ill., **1950.**

Drinker, P. A. Progress in membrane oxygenator design. *Anesthesiology,* **1972,** *37,* 242–260.

Egan, D. F. *Fundamentals of Respiratory Therapy.* C. V. Mosby Co., St. Louis, **1973.**

Fishman, A. P. Respiratory gases in the regulation of the pulmonary circulation. *Physiol. Rev.,* **1961,** *41,* 214–280.

Haldane, J. S., and Priestley, J. G. *Respiration.* The Clarendon Press, Oxford, **1935.**

Henderson, Y. *Adventures in Respiration: Modes of Asphyxiation and Methods of Resuscitation.* The Williams & Wilkins Co., Baltimore, **1938.**

Hill, L. *Caisson Sickness* (an international medical monograph). Edward Arnold & Co., London, **1912.**

Kellogg, R. H. Central chemical regulation of respiration. In, *Respiration,* Vol. 1. *Handbook of Physiology,* Sect. 3. (Fenn, W. O., and Rahn, H., eds.) American Physiological Society, Washington, D. C., **1964,** pp. 507–534.

Lambertsen, C. J. Effects of oxygen at high partial pressure. In, *Respiration,* Vol. 2. *Handbook of Physiology,* Sect. 3. (Fenn, W. O., and Rahn, H., eds.) American Physiological Society, Washington, D. C., **1965,** pp. 1027–1040.

———. Physiological effects of oxygen inhalation at high partial pressures. In, *Fundamentals of Hyperbaric Medicine.* (Committee on Hyperbaric Oxygenation, eds.) National Academy of Sciences–National Research Council, Washington, D. C., **1966,** pp. 12–20.

———(ed.). *Underwater Physiology.* Academic Press, Inc., New York, **1971,** pp. 1–53.

Mitchell, R. A. Cerebrospinal fluid and the regulation of respiration. In, *Advances in Respiratory Physiology.* (Caro, C. G., ed.) The Williams & Wilkins Co., Baltimore, **1966,** pp. 1–47.

Nichols, C. W., and Lambertsen, C. J. Effects of oxygen upon ophthalmic structures. In, *Underwater Physiology.* (Lambertsen, C. J., ed.) Academic Press, Inc., New York, **1971,** pp. 57–66.

Pontoppidan, H.; Geffin, B.; and Lowenstein, E. *Acute Respiratory Failure in the Adult.* Little, Brown & Co., Boston, **1973.**

Symposium. (Various authors.) Carbon dioxide. (Eckenhoff, J. E., ed.) *Anesthesiology,* **1960,** *21,* 585–766.

Tenney, S. M., and Lamb, T. W. Physiological consequences of hypoventilation and hyperventilation. In, *Respiration,* Vol. 2. *Handbook of Physiology,* Sect. 3. (Fenn, W. O., and Rahn, H., eds.) American Physiological Society, Washington, D. C., **1965,** pp. 979–1010.

Trapp, W. G.; Banister, E. W.; Davison, A. J.; and Trapp, P. A. *Proceedings of the Fifth International Hyperbaric Conference,* Vols. I and II. Price Printing, Ltd., Canada, **1974.**

Van Liere, E. J., and Stickney, J. C. *Hypoxia.* University of Chicago Press, Chicago, **1963.**

Winter, P. M., and Smith, G. The toxicity of oxygen. *Anesthesiology,* **1972,** *37,* 210–241.

44 NOXIOUS GASES AND VAPORS

Carbon Monoxide, Hydrocyanic Acid, Benzene, Gasoline, Kerosene, Carbon Tetrachloride, and Miscellaneous Organic Solvents

Ewart A. Swinyard

CARBON MONOXIDE

Carbon monoxide (CO) is a colorless, odorless, tasteless, and nonirritating gas resulting from the incomplete combustion of organic matter. It has no therapeutic value, but its pharmacological properties should be thoroughly understood because CO, except for CO_2, is the most abundant pollutant in the lower atmosphere. Also, a large number of accidental and suicidal deaths occur yearly from its inhalation.

Total CO emissions in the United States are estimated at 102 million tons a year. Approximately 95 million tons per year comes from technological sources; of this, 68% comes from the combustion of various motor fuels, 12% from industrial processes, 8% from solid waste combustion, 2% from fuel (coal, fuel oil, natural gas, and wood) combustion, and 10% from miscellaneous sources (Jaffe, 1970). In volumes % of CO, automobile exhaust contains 4 to 7, coal gas 10, and water gas 30 to 40. The average concentration of CO in the inhaled mixture of cigarette smoke and air is about 0.04 volumes % (Goldsmith and Landaw, 1968).

CO is also produced endogenously in man, during the catabolism of hemoglobin and other heme compounds (Coburn *et al.,* 1963; White, 1970). CO is produced at an average rate of 0.42 ml per hour. The physiological concentration of CO is increased by hemolytic diseases, extensive burns, pregnancy, and surgical anesthesia.

Reaction with Hemoglobin. CO owes its toxic properties to the fact that it combines with hemoglobin to form carboxyhemoglobin (COHb). Hemoglobin in this form is unavailable for the carriage of oxygen. Hemoglobin combines with the same amount

of CO as it does with oxygen, and both gases react with the same group in the hemoglobin molecule. However, CO combines with hemoglobin at a rate about $\frac{1}{10}$ that of oxygen and it dissociates from hemoglobin at a rate about $\frac{1}{2400}$ that of oxygen (Forbes, 1970). Therefore, the affinity of hemoglobin for CO is approximately 240 times greater than for oxygen. Thus, when an individual inhales the gas, there is a rapid removal of CO from the plasma into the red blood cell to combine with hemoglobin. The continual formation of COHb keeps the plasma CO tension at a low level and thereby maintains a steep CO gradient from the pulmonary alveolus to the blood.

COHb, like oxyhemoglobin (O_2Hb), is a dissociable compound; when exposure to the gas is terminated, CO dissociates from its combination with hemoglobin and escapes from the blood. The dissociation of COHb is most rapid in the presence of pure oxygen, which displaces CO in the hemoglobin molecule and converts COHb to O_2Hb. The kinetics of the formation and dissociation of COHb have been reviewed by Roughton (1963) and Holland (1970).

Mechanism of Toxicity. The toxic reactions that follow the inhalation of CO are primarily the result of tissue hypoxia caused by the inability of the blood to carry sufficient oxygen. This point was proved very simply by Haldane in 1895. If mice are subjected to oxygen under a pressure of 2 atmospheres, there is sufficient oxygen in physical solution in the blood for the metabolic requirements of the tissues. Under these conditions, all hemoglobin can be present in the form of COHb without the animals showing any symptoms of poisoning. Thus, under ordinary circumstances of poisoning, CO is not in itself toxic to tissue cells and they are still capable of functioning in a normal manner. The only therapeutic problem is to supply them with adequate amounts of oxygen.

The reduction in the oxygen-carrying *capacity* of blood is proportional to the amount of COHb present. However, the amount of oxygen *available* to the tissues is still further reduced by the inhibitory influence of COHb on the dissociation of any O_2Hb still available. This can be understood best by comparing an anemic individual having a hemoglobin value of 8.0 g % with a person having a hemoglobin value of 16.0 g % but with half of it in the form of COHb (ΔCOHb of 50%). In each instance the oxygen-carrying *capacity* is the same. The anemic individual may show few, if any, symptoms whereas the person suffering from CO poisoning will be near collapse. This is because the presence of COHb interferes with the *release* of oxygen carried by unaltered O_2Hb.

Inspection of the dissociation curve of O_2Hb in the presence of COHb reveals a shift to the left and a flattening of the slope. Therefore, a greater decrease in the oxygen tension (P_{O_2}) of the tissues is necessary before a given amount of oxygen is released. Roughton and Darling (1944) conducted a quantitative study of the effects of CO on the O_2Hb dissociation curve of man. They pointed out that in a normal individual only the upper half of the steep portion of the O_2Hb dissociation curve is operative in oxygen unloading. The lower portion (*i.e.,* 10 to 25 torr P_{O_2}) is kept as reserve (*see* Figure 43–1, page 883). When the ΔCOHb is less than 40%, the dissociation curve is such that oxygen uptake can be kept steady by the use of more or even all of the reserve oxygen available from undissociated O_2Hb at low oxygen tensions. Above this level of ΔCOHb, adequate amounts of oxygen cannot be delivered to the tissues.

A change in total barometric pressure does not affect the relative affinities of hemoglobin for O_2 and CO. However, at high altitudes and other situations where oxygen tensions are low, the effects of a given concentration of CO will be correspondingly more severe (Lilienthal and Pine, 1946; Lilienthal *et al.,* 1946). Thus, the recommended threshold-limit value for workers at 1.5 to 2.4 km (5000 to 8000 ft) is only 25 ppm of inhaled air (*see* American Conference of Governmental Industrial Hygienists, 1966).

Factors Governing Toxicity. Several factors govern the toxicity of CO. The most important are the concentration of the gas in the inspired air, the duration of the exposure, the respiratory minute volume, the cardiac output, the oxygen demand of the tissues, and the hemoglobin concentration of the blood. Therefore, anemic persons are more susceptible to CO than are individuals with normal amounts of hemoglobin. Increased metabolic rate enhances the severity of symptoms in CO poisoning; this is why children succumb earlier than adults, when exposed to a given concentration of the gas. The same principle underlies the use of small animals with high metabolic rates for the detection of toxic quantities of CO, such as the use of canaries in mines. The test animal dies before toxic symptoms are noted in man. Another factor is the contribution made by other sources of CO, especially by smoking cigarettes. Goldsmith and Landaw (1968) have reported that the median COHb level in moderate smokers ($<$ 2 packs per day) who inhale is 5.9%. Chronic exposure to CO under various natural conditions results in mean COHb levels in smokers two to three times those in nonsmokers (Lawther and Commins, 1970; Stewart *et al.,* 1973). Other factors such as ingestion of drugs or alcohol and conditions such as cardiac and respiratory diseases, pregnancy, and anemia are also significant, since they have the effect of lowering the threshold at which CO begins to affect the subject (Rose and Rose, 1971).

Signs and Symptoms of CO Poisoning. The signs and symptoms of CO poisoning are those characteristic of hypoxia. They have been closely correlated with the COHb content of the blood. The relation between symptomatology and COHb concentration is shown in Table 44–1. It is not to be inferred that all of these symptoms are experienced by an individual poisoned with CO. When inhalation of a high concentration causes the blood to become rapidly saturated, transient weakness and dizziness may be the only premonitory warnings before unconsciousness supervenes, and *even these symptoms may be lacking.* Furthermore, the intensity of the symptoms is greatly modified by the oxygen demands of the tissues.

% OF BLOOD SATURATION	SIGNS AND SYMPTOMS
0–10	No symptoms
10–20	Tightness across forehead; possibly slight headache, dilatation of cutaneous blood vessels
20–30	Headache; throbbing in temples
30–40	Severe headache, weakness, dizziness, dimness of vision, nausea and vomiting, collapse
40–50	Same as previous item with greater possibility of collapse or syncope; increased respiration and pulse
50–60	Syncope, increased respiration and pulse; coma with intermittent convulsions; Cheyne-Stokes respiration
60–70	Coma with intermittent convulsions, depressed heart action and respiration, possible death
70–80	Weak pulse and slowed respiration; respiratory failure and death

* Modified from Sayers and Davenport, 1930.

Moderate concentrations of COHb have little effect on vital functions in the human subject at rest. As mentioned previously, the presence of COHb reduces the oxygen-carrying capacity but not the P_{O_2} of arterial blood. As a result, there is no stimulation of the carotid and aortic chemoreceptor mechanism. For example, Apthrop and coworkers (1958) gave four normal men subjected to steady-state exercise sufficient CO to raise their ΔCOHb to between 30 and 50%. No change was observed in *respiratory rate, respiratory minute volume,* or *oxygen consumption,* even when ΔCOHb reached 50%. *Cardiac rate,* on the other hand, was significantly increased in all subjects when ΔCOHb reached 30%.

The clinical findings in patients acutely poisoned by CO are varied. Among those that are not usually thought of as being associated with CO poisoning and yet occur in a fairly large percentage of patients are skin lesions, excessive sweating, hepatic enlargement, bleeding tendency, pyrexia, leukocytosis, albuminuria, and glycosuria (Meigs and Hughes, 1952).

Pathology of Acute CO Poisoning. The severity of pathological changes is directly related to the duration and the degree of hypoxia. The tissues most affected are those most sensitive to oxygen deprivation, such as the brain and the heart. The severe

headache following exposure to CO is believed to be due to cerebral edema and increased intracranial pressure resulting from excessive transudation across hypoxic capillaries.

A study of 351 fatal cases of accidental CO poisoning (Finck, 1966) revealed that there are three major types of gross pathological changes. These changes and their percentage incidence of occurrence in critical tissues are as follows: (1) *congestion* and/or *edema* of lungs (66%), brain (25%), heart (2%), and viscera (7%); (2) *petechiae* of brain (10%) and heart (33%); and (3) *hemorrhage* of lungs (7%), pleura (1%), and brain (2%). Rapidly fatal cases of CO poisoning are characterized by congestion and hemorrhages in all the organs. In less acutely fatal cases, the hypoxic lesions observed are related to the duration of posthypoxic unconsciousness.

Bokonjić (1963) has shown that the maximal period of CO-induced posthypoxic unconsciousness compatible with complete neurological recovery is 21 hours in patients under 48 years of age and 11 hours in patients older than that. Complete recovery of mental function was not observed when the CO-induced unconsciousness exceeded 15 hours in the older group or 64 hours in the younger group. If prolonged posthypoxic unconsciousness occurs, vital organs may be severely damaged. In man, histological studies of the brain have shown extensive demyelination of the white matter, bilateral necrosis of the globus pallidus, and necrotic lesions of Ammon's horn (Brucher, 1967; Lapresle and Fardeau, 1967). The heart is also sensitive to hypoxia and may be permanently damaged by the presence of COHb in the blood. For example, Cosby and Bergeron (1963) reported that nine of ten patients with severe CO poisoning exhibited one or more of the following abnormal ECG changes: sinus tachycardia, T wave abnormalities, S-T segment depression, and atrial fibrillation. Evidences of ischemic changes and subendocardial infarction also have been observed (Anderson *et al.,* 1967). Severe CO poisoning can also produce lesions of the skin, varying from areas of erythema and edema to marked blister and bulla formation (Long, 1968). The pathological lesions that occur in brain, heart, skin, and other organs are primarily vascular, consisting in small hemorrhages and paravascular infiltration with focal necrosis.

Chronic CO Poisoning. The question whether there is a syndrome of chronic CO poisoning remains largely a matter of definition. Some authorities believe that it is quite unlikely that chronic CO poisoning occurs in man. The extensive studies on Holland Tunnel workers (Sievers *et al.,* 1942) and on occupational workers exposed to the gas (Lindgren, 1960) support this view. Nevertheless, illness may develop from tissue injury induced by *repeated acute exposure to toxic concentrations* of CO. Just as in the case of chronic sequelae from an acute severe exposure to the gas, the illness persists and may progress long after the noxious agent has disappeared from the body. In order to minimize the hazard of chronic exposure, the American Conference of Governmental Industrial Hygienists (1966) has reduced the maximal allowable atmospheric concentration for occupational exposure in industry to 0.005 volumes % (50 ppm) for 8 hours of exposure.

Fate and Excretion of CO. The fate of CO in human subjects has been carefully studied by Roughton and Root (1945). Inspired CO first combines with circulating hemoglobin to form COHb. A portion of the CO in dissociable combination with circulating hemoglobin reacts with myoglobin as well as with hemoglobin and possibly with its immediate degradation products outside the confines of the circulation. When air or oxygen containing no CO is breathed, CO dissociates from these combinations and diffuses back into the blood stream and thence into the expired air. CO can be almost completely recovered in the expired air; this fact indicates that there is no significant loss through the skin, sweat, urine, or feces. However, animal experiments indicate that a very small amount is oxidized to CO_2.

There is no excretion of CO unless there is active respiration. Furthermore, COHb is extremely stable and is little affected by putrefaction. Therefore, valid measurements of COHb concentrations in the body can be made long after death. Conversely, little or no CO is absorbed post mortem and analysis of the heart blood provides an accurate measure of the COHb concentration of the blood at death. These facts are of great medicolegal importance.

The quantitative and theoretical aspects of the excretion of CO have been extensively studied by Roughton (1945, 1963). When room air is breathed by a resting subject, the CO content of blood decreases with a half-time of 250 minutes. If oxygen is substituted for air, the equilibrium of the reaction $CO + O_2Hb \rightleftarrows O_2 + COHb$ is shifted toward the left so that the time for halving the concentration of COHb of the blood is reduced to 40 minutes. If 100% oxygen is administered under hyperbaric conditions, the rate of CO elimination is increased even more. These facts provide the basic principles for the treatment of CO poisoning.

Diagnosis of Acute Poisoning. The presumptive diagnosis of acute CO poisoning is usually facilitated by the fact that the victim is commonly found under circumstances that leave little doubt as to the cause of his condition. It is often stated that the unusual combination of pink skin and hypoxia assists with the diagnosis of CO poisoning. Matthew (1971) has emphasized that the "cherry-red cyanosis" is only seen at necropsy; the living patient is commonly cyanotic and pale. Only an occasional living patient will exhibit the unusual combination of hypoxia associated with a bright-red color of the fingernails, mucous membranes, and skin. A final diagnosis depends upon the demonstration of COHb in the blood. Naturally one does not take the time to perform such a test in a severely poisoned individual, but the demonstration of COHb often has medicolegal significance. If a person succumbs in an atmosphere containing CO, a post-mortem blood sample usually contains over 60% of COHb, although death sometimes occurs at lower concentrations. If the patient is removed from such an atmosphere while still breathing, the concentration of COHb rapidly declines, and if respiratory exchange continues to be adequate, the blood is freed of this form of hemoglobin over a course of hours.

Treatment of CO Poisoning. The very first essential is to transfer the patient to fresh air. If respiration has failed, artificial respiration must be immediately instituted. Treatment is then directed toward providing an adequate supply of oxygen to the body cells and hastening the elimination of the CO. The administration of 100% oxygen is the preferred treatment; this not only provides adequate oxygenation for the tissues but also hastens the dissociation of COHb since the half-life of COHb in the blood varies inversely with the partial pressure of oxygen. In severe CO poisoning with loss of consciousness, the treatment of choice is oxygen at 2 to 3 atmospheres pressure (Smith *et al.,* 1962; Norman and Ledingham, 1967; and others). Peterson and Stewart (1970) subjected human volunteers to CO (500 ppm for 2⅓ hours, COHb approximately 25%) and determined the effect of various treatments on the half-life of COHb; the actual half-life under ambient conditions was 320 minutes, whereas with 100% oxygen administered at 1 and 3 atmospheres pressure it was 80 and 23 minutes, respectively. Oxygen administered at high tensions rapidly replaces CO in the hemoglobin molecule, and also dissolves in the plasma in sufficient amounts to provide almost immediate oxygenation of tissue cells. The resultant shortened period of hypoxia limits to the maximal possible extent the tissue damage caused by deprivation of oxygen.

Complete rest and supportive treatment are also essential. The patient should be kept warm. It is especially important that he remains absolutely quiet in order to keep tissue demands for oxygen at a minimum. Clinical or ECG evidence of myocardial damage indicates the need for a period of bed rest (Anderson *et al.,* 1967).

The prognosis should be guarded. The possible aftereffects of severe poisoning have been described. The outcome is especially unfavorable if the patient remains in coma for an extended period. If the patient is not awake in 7 days, his chances of regaining consciousness are remote. This is probably an indication that marked cerebral damage has already resulted.

HYDROCYANIC ACID

Hydrocyanic acid (HCN, prussic acid) is one of the most rapidly acting poisons. Inhalation of vapors of HCN causes severe toxic effects and death within a few minutes to 3 hours, depending upon the concentration breathed. Death has also occurred in young children from eating apricot and other fruit seeds containing cyanogenic glycosides (Sayre and Kaymakcalan, 1964). The action of HCN is due to the cyanide ion; therefore, the toxic properties of the gas are shared by all the soluble inorganic cyanide salts. The following discussion pertains to all compounds that release the cyanide ion.

The cyanides are used extensively in metallurgy, electroplating, metal cleaning, chemical synthesis, and research. In the home, cyanides are present in silver polish, insecticides and rodenticides, and fruit seeds.

Pharmacological Actions. All the pharmacological actions of the cyanide ion result from the cytotoxic hypoxia that it produces.

Mechanism of Action. Cyanide reacts with iron only in the ferric (trivalent) state. It reacts readily with the trivalent iron of *cytochrome oxidase* in mitochondria to form the cytochrome oxidase–CN complex, and with that of methemoglobin to form cyanmethemoglobin. Cytochrome oxidase is particularly reactive with cyanide, and when the two substances combine cellular respiration is inhibited; hence, cyanide produces a cytotoxic hypoxia. The cytochrome oxidase–CN complex is dissociable; the mitochondrial enzyme sulfurtransferase (also called rhodanese) mediates the transfer of sulfur from thiosulfate to the cyanide ion. Thus, thiocyanate is formed, the respiratory enzyme is released, and cell respiration is restored. Tissue sulfurtransferase is adequate to handle relatively large amounts of cyanide, but the reaction is limited by the endogenous supply of thiosulfate. In the presence of high concentrations of methemoglobin, the formation of the cytochrome oxidase–CN complex is minimal. The kinetics of the reactions have been studied by Mintel and Westley (1966), Rodkey (1967), and Schubert and Brill (1968). These facts provide the basis for the therapy of cyanide poisoning.

Central Nervous System. In low concentrations, the cyanide ion stimulates *respiration.* The sites of action are the chemoreceptors of the carotid and aortic bodies. Presumably, the ion acts to block oxidative metabolism in the chemoreceptor cells, and the cells respond as they do to a decreased P_{O_2}. If the medullary respiratory center is unresponsive to

afferent stimulation, for example, in acapnia, cyanide is relatively incapable of increasing respiratory minute volume. Furthermore, the ion is generally toxic. For these reasons, cyanide has no practical value as a respiratory stimulant.

The effect of cyanide on cerebral oxidations is reflected in the electrical activity of the brain. The cortex is first involved, then the basal ganglia, hypothalamus, and midbrain. Moderate or no depression of activity is seen in portions of the pons and the brain stem. The electrical activity of the gray matter of the cord is increased. Recovery proceeds in the reverse direction. The effects of cyanide may therefore be looked upon as a transient functional decerebration, and the behavior of experimental subjects receiving cyanide is consistent with this interpretation (Ward and Wheatley, 1947). It is of interest that repeated daily injections of cyanide, resulting in unconsciousness and convulsions, cause no pathological changes in the central nervous system (CNS) (Wheatley *et al.,* 1947).

Cardiovascular System. The effects of cyanide on the cardiovascular system are similar to those of hypoxia. The effects on the myocardium itself are most prominent. Careful observations have been made of the ECG recorded during the inhalation of lethal amounts of HCN by condemned subjects (Wexler *et al.,* 1947).

Absorption, Fate, and Excretion. The cyanide ion is readily absorbed after oral or parenteral administration. Prolonged local contact with cyanide solutions or with HCN may result in the absorption of toxic amounts through the skin. Part of the absorbed cyanide is excreted unchanged by the lungs. The larger portion, however, is converted by the enzyme sulfurtransferase to the relatively nontoxic thiocyanate ion. Kinetic studies indicate that the cleavage of the thiosulfate sulfur-sulfur bond is the rate-limiting step in this reaction (Mintel and Westley, 1966). Relatively minor metabolic pathways include combination with cystine to form 2-imino-thiazolidine-4-carboxylic acid, oxidation to carbon dioxide and formate, and formation of cyanocobalamin.

Cyanide Poisoning. Most deaths from cyanide have been suicidal or genocidal, but some arise from accidental exposure in industry. The American Conference of Governmental Industrial Hygienists (1973) has established the maximal allowable atmospheric concentration for occupational exposure in industry at 10 ppm (by volume) for 8 hours of exposure. The symptoms of cyanide poisoning appear within a few seconds to minutes after the ingestion of compounds or the breathing of vapors containing the gas. They consist in giddiness, hyperpnea, headache, palpitation, cyanosis, and unconsciousness. Asphyxial convulsions may precede death. Although high doses are fatal within a few minutes, cases have been reported in which death has been delayed for as long as 3 hours. Therefore, prompt treatment can be lifesaving. As long as the heart continues to beat there is a chance for saving the patient, since effective antidotes are available.

Treatment. Treatment for cyanide poisoning is

specific and must be given rapidly if it is to prove effective. It is therefore fortunate that the diagnosis can be made by the characteristic cyanide odor (odor of "oil of bitter almonds") on the breath of the poisoned individual. This sign in association with asphyxia and cyanosis is pathognomonic. The objective in the treatment of cyanide poisoning is to produce a high concentration of methemoglobin (Hb-Fe^{3+}) by the administration of nitrite (Hb-Fe^{2+} + NaNO$_2$ $\rightleftarrows$ Hb-Fe^{3+}). Methemoglobin competes with cytochrome oxidase (Cyt-Fe^{3+}) for the cyanide ion. The concentration gradient favors methemoglobin, cyanmethemoglobin (Hb-FeCN) is formed, and cytochrome oxidase is restored (Hb-Fe^{3+} + Cyt-FeCN $\rightleftarrows$ Hb-FeCN + Cyt-Fe^{3+}). Actual detoxication is then achieved by the administration of thiosulfate, which, under the influence of sulfurtransferase, reacts with cyanide to form thiocyanate (SCN$^-$), a relatively nontoxic substance readily excreted in the urine.

$$Na_2S_2O_3 + CN^- \xrightarrow[\text{SCN}^- \text{ oxidase}]{\text{sulfurtransferase}} SCN^- + Na_2SO_3$$

The final reaction is slowly reversible through the action of thiocyanate oxidase (Williams, 1959). Therefore, if symptoms of poisoning reappear or recovery is slow, the sodium nitrite and sodium thiosulfate treatment should be repeated.

Sodium nitrite is one of the best agents to use for the formation of methemoglobin (Chen et al., 1934). The adult dose is 0.3 to 0.5 g, dissolved in 10 to 15 ml of water. Three to 4 minutes should be taken for the injection. If there is an appreciable delay before the solution can be prepared and injected, the patient may be tided over this period with amyl nitrite inhalations given for 30 seconds of each 2 minutes. Following (but not together with) the sodium nitrite, sodium thiosulfate should be given by slow intravenous injection. The dose is 12.5 g in a total volume of 50 ml. administered over a 10-minute period. If symptoms reappear, the above procedure should be repeated except that in this instance the doses are halved. If the nitrites cause a profound fall in blood pressure, epinephrine or a suitable congener may be administered to control this undesired effect. Also, the severity of the methemoglobinemia may be greater than desired for the purpose of cyanide detoxication; if a severe and prolonged hypoxemia results, it may be necessary to resort to the inhalation of pure oxygen (Cope, 1961; Sheehy and Way, 1968), or even to a blood transfusion. Further treatment is purely symptomatic.

The successful treatment of cyanide poisoning in human beings with sodium nitrite and sodium thiosulfate has been recorded frequently. Chen and Rose (1956) reported that 48 of 49 cases of acute poisoning by HCN were treated successfully with such therapy. Persons who work with and around cyanide preparations should be given specific detailed instructions on the management of cyanide poisoning. A complete cyanide antidote package is marketed by Eli Lilly and Company.

Numerous investigations have been directed toward the discovery of more effective antidotes for the treatment of cyanide poisoning. Several (p-aminopropiophenone, hydroxocobalamin, chlorocobalamin) have been reviewed briefly by Done (1961). Rose and coworkers (1965) have reported that sodium cobaltinitrite is more effective than sodium nitrite in experimental animals. Cittadini and associates (1972) demonstrated that pyruvate significantly decreases the toxicity of cyanide in mice. Pyruvate reacts with cyanide to form the nontoxic pyruvic-cyanhydrin. Whether these approaches will prove of practical value in the treatment of clinical cyanide poisoning remains to be determined.

BENZENE (BENZOL)

Benzene (C$_6$H$_6$, benzol) is a colorless, volatile liquid with a rather pleasant odor. It should be distinguished from *benzine,* a petroleum distillate containing mixed hydrocarbons (such as pentane and hexane) in uncertain proportions. Benzene is present, to some extent, in most gasolines, and it is a common ingredient of paint and varnish removers.

Benzene is toxic when it gains access to the body by any route. Poisoning commonly occurs, however, as a result of the inhalation of the vapors. The inhalation of a concentration of 20,000 ppm is fatal within a period of 5 to 10 minutes; 7500 ppm causes acute symptoms if inhaled for 30 to 60 minutes. The recommended maximal atmospheric concentration (8-hour exposure) is 25 ppm. Notwithstanding its insidious toxicity, benzene continues to be extensively used in the petroleum, explosive, plastics, pesticide, and other industries. It has no therapeutic uses.

Absorption, Fate, and Excretion. Liquid benzene is absorbed from the gastrointestinal tract. Percutaneous absorption is not significant. The vapor gains access to the circulation through the respiratory tract. The compound is mainly deposited in the CNS; its distribution in other organs varies with the time elapsed after exposure. Approximately 50% of absorbed benzene is excreted through the lungs. The remainder is oxidized, for the most part, to phenol, 1,2-benzenediol, 1,4-benzenediol, and 1,2,4-trihydroxybenzene, which are excreted in the urine in the form of ester sulfates and glucuronides (Porteous and Williams, 1949; Laham, 1970). Consequently, the amount of ester sulfates in the urine, expressed as a percentage of the total amount of sulfate, increases with the inhalation of benzene vapors, and the concentration of urinary sulfates has been used as an index of exposure. The concentration of urinary phenols has been used for a similar purpose (Sherwood, 1972). Both methods provide presumptive evidence of exposure to benzene, but they reveal nothing about the health of the individual.

Benzene Poisoning. Benzene poisoning may be acute or chronic. Acute poisoning results when benzene is ingested either by accident or with suicidal intent. It also follows the breathing of concentrated vapors, such as may be encountered when workmen enter storage tanks or large stills for the purpose of cleaning them. Chronic poisoning results from long exposure to vapors in low concentrations.

Acute Poisoning. Symptoms from mild exposure include dizziness, weakness, euphoria, headache, nausea, vomiting, tightness in the chest, and staggering. If exposure is more intense, symptoms progress to blurred vision, tremors, shallow and rapid respiration, ventricular irregularities, paralysis, and unconsciousness; the coma is sometimes preceded by excitement and convulsions. Pathological findings from benzene inhalation include acute granular tracheitis, laryngitis and bronchitis, massive hemorrhage of the lungs, congestive gastritis, infarct of the spleen, acute congestion of the kidneys, and marked cerebral edema (Winek and Collom, 1971). The treatment of this type of poisoning is purely symptomatic.

Chronic Poisoning. In chronic poisoning from inhalation, signs and symptoms referable to the CNS and the gastrointestinal tract are commonly observed, but the major toxic manifestations result from the action of the poison on the bone marrow. Significant chromosomal changes have also been reported after chronic benzene exposure (Vigliani and Forni, 1969; Forni *et al.,* 1971). The toxic effects of chronic poisoning may not become apparent for months or even years after the initial contact with the chemical. Indeed, they may appear after all exposure has ceased.

Symptoms of chronic exposure include headache, loss of appetite, drowsiness, nervousness, and pallor. Anemia, petechiae, and abnormal bleeding have been observed. The anemia may progress to complete aplasia of the bone marrow. Repeated inhalation to the point of euphoria may cause encephalopathy, tremulousness, emotional instability, and apathy.

Benzene may first stimulate leukocyte formation, and the earliest indication of its actions may be leukocytosis (either lymphocytic or polymorphonuclear). Death from myeloid leukemia has been reported (Vigliani and Forni, 1969). This stimulation soon gives way to an inhibition of the precursors of all the formed elements of the peripheral blood. The result is an *aplastic anemia.* In severe cases, the erythrocyte count may be below 1 million per cubic millimeter, with a corresponding decrease in hemoglobin. Usually, however, patients with chronic benzene poisoning have an erythrocyte count approximately 50% of normal. The extensive study of Savilahti (1956) has documented the relative frequency of the various blood abnormalities in chronic benzene poisoning.

Treatment. In acute benzene vapor poisoning, the patient should immediately be removed from the contaminated air. If benzene is ingested, the treatment is the same as that for kerosene (*see* below). If gastric lavage is used, *great care should be exercised to avoid aspiration of the lavage fluid and stomach contents.* Complete bed rest is advisable until respiration is normal. Epinephrine and related substances should be avoided since they may induce fatal ventricular fibrillation. Hematopoietic, respiratory, hepatic, and renal complications should be treated symptomatically. If individuals are known to be exposed to benzene vapors in their working environment, prophylactic measures should be taken. All possible methods should be used to protect such

persons against breathing the fumes. They should have periodic physical examinations, including careful blood studies. In addition, the urine should be examined at intervals to determine the extent of excretion of benzene conjugation products, which serves as a rough index of the degree of exposure. Once poisoning has developed, it is essential to prevent further exposure. Therapy is purely symptomatic. If anemia is very marked, blood transfusion may be advisable and the administration of iron preparations is indicated. If severe neutropenia develops, the therapeutic procedure is the same as that for any other form of agranulocytosis. Thrombocytopenia with purpura may also require blood transfusions.

GASOLINE

Human volunteers exposed for 30 minutes to gasoline vapors in concentrations up to 1000 ppm exhibit irritation of the eyes and dilatation of the conjunctival vessels; exposure for 1 hour to a concentration of 2600 ppm induces dizziness in all subjects. A concentration of 10,000 ppm is rapidly fatal to most animals. Workers, particularly in industries where gasoline is used as a solvent, are often exposed to gasoline vapors and symptoms may ensue. Gasoline consists either of the higher hydrocarbons of the methane series or of unsaturated aromatic hydrocarbons. They differ somewhat in their late central effects (*see* below).

Poisoning. The inhalation of high concentrations of gasoline vapors, such as are encountered by workmen cleaning storage tanks, may cause immediate death. The observation of Chenoweth (1946) that gasoline vapors can sensitize the myocardium so that small amounts of circulating epinephrine may precipitate ventricular fibrillation in a manner analogous to that of cyclopropane may provide the explanation for this type of sudden death. Alternatively, high concentrations of gasoline vapor may lead to rapid central depression and death from respiratory failure.

Milder intoxications are similar to those that follow the ingestion of ethyl alcohol (Machle, 1941). The signs and symptoms include incoordination, restlessness, excitement, confusion, disorientation, ataxia, delirium, and finally coma, which may last for a few hours to several days. The coma following the inhalation of the *aliphatic* hydrocarbons is profound, and deep reflexes are weak or absent. In contrast, the coma attending intoxication with the *aromatic* hydrocarbons is characterized by motor unrest, tremors, and jactitations; reflexes are hyperactive. When low concentrations of gasoline vapor are breathed, prodromal symptoms such as headache, blurred vision, vertigo, ataxia, tinnitus, nausea, anorexia, and weakness are not uncommon.

The signs and symptoms of *chronic exposure* to gasoline vapors are ill defined and may consist in muscular weakness, listlessness, fatigue, nausea, vomiting, abdominal pain, and weight loss. Neurological effects such as confusion, ataxia, tremor, paresthesias, neuritis, and paralysis of peripheral or cranial nerves may also occur.

Habituation to the inhalation of gasoline vapors has been reported in children (Lawton and Malmquist, 1961; Press and Done, 1967). Repeated inhalation induces dizziness, giddiness, a "butterfly feeling," and hallucinations. If the desired end point is exceeded, unconsciousness results.

The *treatment* of acute poisoning from the oral ingestion of gasoline is the same as that for kerosene. Treatment of mild intoxication from the inhalation of gasoline is nonspecific and consists in purely symptomatic and supportive measures.

KEROSENE

Kerosene (kerosine, coal oil) is a mixture of hydrocarbons, chiefly of the methane series, having from 10 to 16 carbon atoms per molecule. It constitutes the fraction distilled from petroleum after the ethers and before the oils. This fraction has a boiling range of 175° to 325° C, and consists mainly of branched paraffins, monocyclic and dicyclic naphthenes, and some aromatic naphthenes. Variable quantities of unsaturated cyclic compounds may also be present. Kerosene is used as aviation fuel, illuminating and heating fuel, and as a vehicle for various insecticides, fungicides, cleaning agents, furniture polishes, and paint thinners. It can often be found around homes, garages, and farms in containers originally designed for milk, carbonated drinks, and other beverages. Hence, it is a *common cause of accidental poisoning in children.* Indeed, petroleum distillate products cause nearly 100 accidental deaths a year in the United States; 90% of these are in children under 5 years of age. It has been estimated that nearly 28,000 nonfatal poisonings due to petroleum distillate products occur annually in children under 5 years of age, and that over 60% of the cases require hospitalization (Subcommittee on Accidental Poisoning, 1962).

Toxicity. Kerosene, unless used as a solvent for more toxic substances, is relatively nontoxic by the oral route. The fatal oral dose for an adult is probably 90 to 120 ml (3 to 4 oz), although at least twice this amount has been tolerated, whereas death has resulted from as little as 15 ml (0.5 oz). The morbidity associated with this agent is attributed to aspiration, which occurs at the time of ingestion or during treatment, and is *not* due to absorption and excretion through the lungs (*see* Arena, 1973). Chemical pneumonitis, complicated by secondary bacterial pneumonia and pulmonary edema, is the most serious sequel to aspiration (Lawton and Malmquist, 1961; Press and Done, 1967). Death in fatal cases is due to hemorrhagic pulmonary edema and usually occurs in the first 16 to 18 hours, but seldom later than 24 hours. Other organs (brain, heart, liver, kidney, and spleen) are frequently involved, but the effects usually clear without residual impairment.

Pathological examination of fatal cases reveals heavy, edematous, and hemorrhagic lungs. The alveoli are filled with proteinaceous exudate, rich in cells and fibrin, and often organized in a pattern resembling that of hyaline membrane disease (Thompson, 1955). Alveolar walls are weakened and may rupture, leading to less frequent sequelae, such as emphysema and pneumothorax. Pulmonary lymph nodes are inflamed, and bronchopneumonia and atelectasis have been noted.

The *symptoms* of kerosene poisoning depend upon the route by which this agent gains access to the body. Poisoning usually results either from *inhalation* of the vapors or from *ingestion* of the liquid. Ingestion of kerosene is more hazardous than inhalation, since vomiting and eructation, as well as the low surface tension of this substance, favor its aspiration into the respiratory tract in toxic amounts.

Inhalation. The inhalation of kerosene vapors induces a transient euphoria that resembles alcoholic intoxication. Other signs and symptoms include a burning sensation in the chest, headache, tinnitus, nausea, weakness, restlessness, muscular incoordination, confusion, disorientation, and, occasionally, convulsions. Drowsiness and eventually coma ensue. Death is usually due to respiratory failure. In rare instances, ventricular fibrillation and sudden death may occur.

Ingestion. The ingestion of kerosene causes local irritation and a burning sensation in the mouth, throat, and esophagus. Vomiting and eructation may result in *aspiration* of the toxic fluid. *Diarrhea* with blood-tinged stools may occur. Drowsiness, cyanosis, low-grade fever, and CNS depression may be present. More serious symptoms include shallow respiration, unconsciousness, and convulsions. The usual clinical course is quite benign unless large quantities have been ingested or the toxic substance has been aspirated. Pulmonary complications, including pneumonia, pneumonitis, and pulmonary edema, result secondarily from unrecognized aspiration of the substance. Death may occur from asphyxia.

The extensive cooperative study of kerosene poisoning, sponsored jointly by the American Academy of Pediatrics and the United States Public Health Service, covers 760 cases in which petroleum distillate products were accidentally ingested; 55% of these and the two reported deaths were due to kerosene (*see* Subcommittee on Accidental Poisoning, 1962). The amount of kerosene ingested was known in 232 of the cases; 35% ingested less than 2 tsp, 35% from 2 tsp to 1 oz, and 30% more than 1 oz. One fatal case, a 1-year-old male infant, ingested 5 to 8 oz of kerosene. Pulmonary complications occurred in 42% of patients. Pulmonary edema was one of the most serious developments and was responsible for one of the two deaths. Spontaneous or induced vomiting resulted in a higher incidence of pulmonary complications (49%) than occurred in those not vomiting (34%). CNS complications (lethargy, stupor, or coma) developed in 31% and appeared to be related to the quantity ingested. For example, such complications were noted in 25% of those ingesting less than 2 tsp and in 41% of those ingesting 1 oz or more.

Treatment. There is no convincing evidence that gastric lavage is superior to emesis or that either is superior to supportive therapy alone in reducing morbidity (Subcommittee on Accidental Poisoning, 1962; Shirkey, 1971; Arena, 1973; and others). It is generally agreed that *gastric lavage or emesis should not be employed* unless the risks involved are justified by the excessive quantity ingested, the presence of more toxic substances in the kerosene, or the condition of the patient. In those few cases in which gastric lavage may be indicated, great care should be taken to pinch the lavage tube firmly in order to forestall the possibility of kerosene leaking and gaining access to the lungs as the opening passes the pharynx. If the patient is conscious, a vegetable oil (olive oil) may be administered to dilute the kerosene and decrease the rate of its absorption. Mineral oil should be avoided because it increases the absorption of petroleum distillates.

The therapy of kerosene poisoning is largely supportive and symptomatic. Oxygen under pressure may be used for pulmonary edema and asphyxia. Antibiotics are sometimes given to prevent secondary bacterial pneumonia, and corticosteroids have been used to prevent pulmonary edema and necrotizing pneumonitis; however, the value of such prophylactic therapy is not supported by experimental studies in dogs (Steele *et al.,* 1972). Caffeine sodium benzoate may be administered parenterally for CNS depression. Epinephrine and related substances should be avoided because of the possibility of inducing cardiac arrhythmias in an already sensitized myocardium. Appropriate therapy is indicated to correct fluid and electrolyte imbalance. All cases of kerosene poisoning, even though asymptomatic, should be hospitalized for at least 24 hours for close observation.

CARBON TETRACHLORIDE

Carbon tetrachloride (CCl_4) is a chlorinated hydrocarbon chemically related to chloroform. The compound, first prepared in 1849, has been used as an anesthetic, a dry shampoo for human hair, and an anthelmintic in the management of hookworm infestation. All these uses have been abandoned because of its extreme toxicity and the development of better and safer substances for these purposes. Today, CCl_4 has no valid clinical application in medicine. Its extensive use in household products has made it an insidious killer around the home. As a result, the United States Food and Drug Administration has banned its sale in any product used in the home, including fire extinguishers. Products containing CCl_4 for industrial, scientific, or other nonhousehold uses are exempt from this regulation.

Pharmacological Actions and Mechanism of Toxicity. Applied locally to the skin, CCl_4 is an irritant and a rubefacient. After its oral ingestion, the irritant action produces a feeling of warmth in the stomach and stimulates intestinal peristalsis. In high concentrations it is toxic to the heart and may cause cardiac arrhythmias and marked hypotension. It is also depressant to the CNS.

The more selective toxicological effects of CCl_4 are upon hepatic and renal tubular cells. Hepatocellular damage in rats, initially manifested by altered lipid metabolism, is apparent within 30 minutes after the intragastric administration of CCl_4. The alteration in lipid metabolism is accompanied and followed by a maze of hepatic pathological disturbances. Histological changes in the endoplasmic reticulum, decreased microsomal enzyme activity, and decreased hepatic protein synthesis are apparent within the first hour of intoxication. This is followed in 2 to 4 hours by a dramatic increase in the concentration of calcium in hepatic mitochondria, a marked alteration in electrolyte distribution, and a swelling of hepatic cells. Depletion of liver glycogen, disruption of lysosomes, and a loss of intracellular enzymes follow. More extensive hepatic damage is apparent within 24 hours; this is characterized by mitochondrial damage and marked centrilobular necrosis of the liver.

Identification of the event that triggers the reaction of the liver to CCl_4 has so far eluded investigators. Damage to the mitochondria and endoplasmic reticulum, sympathoadrenal discharge and subsequent hepatic hypoxia, and peroxidative decomposition of cytoplasmic membrane lipids have all been implicated. The relative importance of these and other factors has been reviewed by Recknagel (1967). Other observations of interest include the destruction of hepatic microsomal cytochrome P-450 in rats by CCl_4 (Sasame *et al.,* 1968), enhancement of CCl_4 hepatotoxicity by phenobarbital (McLean *et al.,* 1969), and the protective effect of proadifen hydrochloride against CCl_4 hepatotoxicity in rats (Marchand *et al.,* 1970, 1971).

Although less is known about the nephrotoxic action of CCl_4, it is, nonetheless, exceedingly important. Experimental studies in rats indicate that CCl_4 produces an early, reversible lesion of the proximal tubule; initial changes occur in the mitochondria, followed by cellular swelling and proliferation of the smooth-surfaced endoplasmic reticulum (Striker *et al.,* 1968). There is a simultaneous increase in the excretion of sodium and water and a decrease in succinic dehydrogenase activity. Mild poisoning in man may be characterized by a reversible oliguria lasting only a few days. In more severe intoxication, the oliguria may be followed in a week or so by almost complete anuria, with red blood cells and albumin in the scanty urine. Hypertension, acidosis, and terminal uremia develop if renal function is not restored. The renal lesion is usually classified as a lower-nephron nephrosis. (For a more detailed account of the toxicity and potential dangers of CCl_4, *see* review by Oettingen, 1955.)

Absorption, Fate, and Excretion. CCl_4 vapor is readily absorbed from the lungs. Orally ingested CCl_4 is readily absorbed from the gastrointestinal tract; this absorption is considerably increased by the concomitant ingestion of fat or alcohol. CCl_4 is also absorbed from the skin, but this is not an important route for systemic toxicity.

CCl_4 is concentrated largely in body fat, liver, and bone marrow (*see* McCollister *et al.*, 1951). Animal experiments indicate that inhaled CCl_4 is excreted over a 2- or 3-month period; about one half is eliminated unchanged in the expired air, and the remainder is exhaled as carbon dioxide and excreted as urea and other metabolites in urine and feces. Because of this slow excretion, chronic intoxication occurs.

Toxicology. CCl_4 poisoning may be acute or chronic. Acute intoxication usually results from inhalation of the vapor while the chemical is being used in a small, unventilated area, or from ingestion of the liquid for suicidal purposes or accidentally. Chronic intoxication is usually due to industrial exposure.

Acute Intoxication Due to Inhalation. Transient exposure to toxic concentrations of CCl_4 vapor results in the following symptoms: irritation of the eyes, nose, and throat; nausea and vomiting; a sense of fullness in the head; dizziness; and headache. If the exposure is soon terminated, these symptoms usually disappear within a few hours. Continued exposure or absorption of larger quantities of the chemical may cause stupor, convulsions, coma, and death from CNS depression. Sudden death may occur from ventricular fibrillation or depression of vital medullary centers.

As indicated above, CCl_4 is a hepatotoxic and nephrotoxic agent. Signs and symptoms of injury to these organs may appear after a delay of from several hours to 2 or 3 days, and may occur in the absence of any severe earlier effect upon the CNS. Other delayed toxic effects include nausea, vomiting, abdominal pain, diarrhea, and hematemesis. Optic neuritis, necrosis of the adrenal cortex, and pancreatitis are infrequent complications. Pulmonary edema, secondary to acute renal failure and myocardial depression, may also occur.

Chronic Intoxication Due to Inhalation. Continued exposure to concentrations of CCl_4 in excess of 100 ppm may result in symptoms of chronic intoxication. Persons exposed to such concentrations complain of nausea, vomiting, loss of appetite, abdominal pain, apathy, mental confusion, and loss of weight. Signs of hepatic or renal damage may also be present if the exposures are of sufficient duration and frequency.

The American Conference of Governmental Industrial Hygienists (1973) has set the maximal safe atmospheric concentration of CCl_4 at 10 ppm for 8 hours of exposure. Since the least concentration detectable by odor is approximately 80 ppm, it is obvious that prolonged exposure to CCl_4 vapor detectable by odor may be hazardous.

Intoxication Due to Ingestion. The ingestion of CCl_4 results in signs and symptoms similar to those of acute intoxication due to inhalation. Gastrointestinal symptoms, including hematemesis and abdominal pain, are more severe and the possibility of hepatic damage is greater when the poison is taken orally. The fatal oral dose has been reported to be

as little as 2 to 4 ml in susceptible persons (Norwood *et al.*, 1950).

Treatment. Emergency treatment should be initiated promptly in any person suspected of having absorbed toxic quantities of CCl_4. The individual exposed to the toxic vapor should be moved to fresh air. If the patient is seen shortly after oral ingestion of CCl_4, the stomach should be emptied immediately, either by inducing vomiting in the conscious patient or by gastric lavage, and a saline laxative should be administered to minimize absorption. If first seen in the stage of advanced CNS depression, every effort should be expended to prevent hypoxia. Oxygen and artificial respiration should be administered if necessary. *Under no circumstances should an attempt be made to elevate the blood pressure by the use of sympathomimetic drugs, because of the danger of producing serious arrhythmias in the sensitized myocardium.*

Treatment of the acute hepatic and renal insufficiency caused by CCl_4 presents one of the most challenging problems in therapy. Although hepatic insufficiency is a very prominent feature of CCl_4 poisoning, renal failure is the most frequent cause of death. Even though the presenting signs and symptoms may be those associated with functional impairment of the liver, renal function should be observed closely and oliguria or anuria anticipated. The therapy of the acute renal failure is that presented in Chapter 36. Fortunately, the basic measures employed in the conservative treatment of acute renal insufficiency, namely, the administration of glucose to provide the major source of calories and careful maintenance of the volume and composition of the body fluids, apply equally well to the management of acute hepatic insufficiency.

The treatment of chronic poisoning differs little from that of acute intoxication. Although renal function may be impaired, the emergency of anuria is usually not a complicating feature. Major attention is therefore directed toward symptomatic therapy and providing an optimal diet.

MISCELLANEOUS ORGANIC SOLVENTS

The deliberate inhalation of the vapors of highly volatile organic solvents is a problem of importance to parents, physicians, and juvenile authorities (*see* Press and Done, 1967). Attention was focused on this problem by the report of Glaser and Massengale (1962) on "glue sniffing" in children. Toxic symptoms reported include pleasant exhilaration, euphoria, excitement, ataxia, slurred speech, diplopia, and tinnitus. Drowsiness, stupor, and unconsciousness may also occur. Repeated exposure may lead to habituation, tolerance, and psychological dependence. The possibility that "glue sniffing" might cause damage to the hematopoietic system, liver, and kidneys has not been excluded.

Many readily available commercial preparations, such as lacquers, enamels, paint thinners, paint and varnish removers, brake and lighter fluids, and plastic cements, provide a source of highly volatile vapors that may be abused by the adolescent looking for the "cheap kick." Socially dangerous acts may be committed by the person under the influence of these vapors. Physicians should be concerned with the underlying factors driving the adolescent to inhale such toxic substances (*see* Chapter 16).

A special class of chemicals subject to abuse by inhalation are the fluorohydrocarbons, such as *dichlorofluoromethane, trichlorofluoromethane, chlorodifluoromethane,* and *1,2-dichlorotetrafluoroethane.* They are widely employed as propellants in various aerosol products. The "sniffing" of such aerosol sprays is a hazardous practice. Bass (1970) identified 110 "sudden sniffing deaths" from inhaling these volatile hydrocarbons. In each case the victim sprayed the aerosol into a plastic bag, inhaled the contents, became excited, ran 90 m or so, collapsed, and died. Necropsy findings were largely negative. Taylor and coworkers (1971) demonstrated that the inhalation of fluoroalkane gases by monkeys induces ventricular premature beats, bigeminy, and tachycardia. Reinhardt and associates (1971) reported that aerosol propellants sensitize the canine heart to epinephrine and cause serious cardiac arrhythmias. These data suggest that "sudden sniffing death" is due to ventricular fibrillation induced by the release of endogenous epinephrine, which then acts on the sensitized myocardium. Although the amount of propellant absorbed into the blood from the use of hairspray, cosmetic, household, and medicated aerosols must vary with circumstances, the physician is advised to counsel his patients on the potential dangers, particularly from their use in poorly ventilated, confined areas. It is possible that patients with cardiac or respiratory disorders may prove especially susceptible.

American Conference of Governmental Industrial Hygienists. *Documentation of Threshold Limit Values,* rev. ed. The Conference, Lansing, Mich., **1966,** pp. 33–36.

————. *Threshold Limit Values for Chemical Substances and Physical Agents in the Workroom Environment with Intended Changes for 1973.* The Conference, Lansing, Mich., **1973,** pp. 10–31.

Anderson, R. F.; Allensworth, D. C.; and de Groot, W. J. Myocardial toxicity from carbon monoxide poisoning. *Ann. intern. Med.,* **1967,** *67,* 1172–1182.

Apthrop, G. H.; Bates, D. V.; Marshall, R.; and Mendel, D. Effect of acute carbon monoxide on work capacity. *Br. med. J.,* **1958,** *2,* 476–478.

Arena, J. M. Emergency treatment of hydrocarbon products ingestion. *J. Am. med. Ass.,* **1973,** *226,* 213.

Bass, M. Sudden sniffing death. *J. Am. med. Ass.,* **1970,** *212,* 2075–2079.

Bokonjić, N. Stagnant anoxia and carbon monoxide poisoning. *Electroenceph. clin. Neurophysiol.,* **1963,** Suppl. 21, 1–102.

Brucher, J. M. Neuropathological problems posed by carbon monoxide poisoning and anoxia. *Prog. Brain Res.,* **1967,** *24,* 75–100.

Chen, K. K., and Rose, C. L. Treatment of acute cyanide poisoning. *J. Am. med. Ass.,* **1952,** *162,* 1154–1155.

Chen, K. K.; Rose, C. L.; and Clowes, G. H. A. Comparative values of several antidotes in cyanide poisoning. *Am. J. med. Sci.,* **1934,** *188,* 767–781.

Chenoweth, M. B. Ventricular fibrillation induced by hydrocarbons and epinephrine. *J. ind. Hyg. Toxicol.,* **1946,** *28,* 151–158.

Cittadini, A.; Caprino, L.; and Terranova, T. Effect of pyruvate on the acute cyanide poisoning in mice. *Experientia,* **1972,** *28,* 943–944.

Coburn, R. F.; Blakemore, W. S.; and Forster, R. E. Endogenous carbon monoxide production in man. *J. clin. Invest.,* **1963,** *42,* 1172–1178.

Cope, C. The importance of oxygen in the treatment of cyanide poisoning. *J. Am. med. Ass.,* **1961,** *175,* 1061–1064.

Cosby, R. S., and Bergeron, M. Electrocardiographic changes in carbon monoxide poisoning. *Am. J. Cardiol.,* **1963,** *11,* 93–96.

Done, A. K. Clinical pharmacology of systemic antidotes. *Clin. Pharmac. Ther.,* **1961,** *2,* 750–793.

Finck, P. A. Exposure to carbon monoxide: review of the literature and 567 autopsies. *Milit. Med.,* **1966,** *131,* 1513–1539.

Forbes, W. H. Carbon monoxide uptake via the lungs. *Ann. N.Y. Acad. Sci.,* **1970,** *174,* 72–75.

Forni, A.; Pacifico, E.; and Limonta, A. Chromosome studies in workers exposed to benzene or toluene or both. *Archs envir. Hlth,* **1971,** *22,* 373–378.

Glaser, H. H., and Massengale, O. N. "Glue-sniffing" in children: deliberate inhalation of vaporized plastic cements. *J. Am. med. Ass.,* **1962,** *181,* 300–303.

Goldsmith, J. R., and Landaw, S. A. Carbon monoxide and human health. *Science, Wash.,* **1968,** *162,* 1352–1359.

Haldane, J. The relation of the action of carbonic oxide to oxygen tension. *J. Physiol., Lond.,* **1895,** *18,* 201–217.

Holland, R. A. B. Reaction rates of carbon monoxide and hemoglobin. *Ann. N.Y. Acad. Sci.,* **1970,** *174,* 154–171.

Jaffe, L. S. Sources, characteristics, and fate of atmospheric carbon monoxide. *Ann. N.Y. Acad. Sci.,* **1970,** *174,* 76–88.

Laham, S. Metabolism of industrial solvents. *Ind. Med. Surg.,* **1970,** *39,* 237–240.

Lapresle, J., and Fardeau, M. The central nervous system and carbon monoxide poisoning. II. Anatomical study of brain lesions following intoxication with carbon monoxide (22 cases). *Prog. Brain Res.,* **1967,** *24,* 31–74.

Lawther, P. J., and Commins, B. T. Cigarette smoking and exposure to carbon monoxide. *Ann. N.Y. Acad. Sci.,* **1970,** *174,* 135–147.

Lawton, J. J., Jr., and Malmquist, C. P. Gasoline addiction in children. *Psychiat. Q.,* **1961,** *35,* 555–561.

Lilienthal, J. L., Jr., and Pine, M. B. The effect of oxygen pressure on the uptake of carbon monoxide at sea level and at altitude. *Am. J. Physiol.,* **1946,** *145,* 345–350.

Lilienthal, J. L., Jr.; Riley, R. L.; Proemmel, D. D.; and Franks, R. E. The relationships between carbon monoxide, oxygen and hemoglobin in the blood of man at altitude. *Am. J. Physiol.,* **1946,** *145,* 351–358.

Lindgren, S. A. A study of the effect of protracted occupational exposure to carbon monoxide. *Acta med. scand.,* **1960,** *167,* Suppl. 356, 5–135.

Long, P. I. Dermal changes associated with carbon monoxide intoxication. *J. Am. med. Ass.,* **1968,** *205,* 51–52.

McCollister, D. D.; Beamer, W. H.; Atchison, G. J.; and Spencer, H. C. The absorption, distribution and elimination of radioactive carbon tetrachloride by monkeys upon exposure to low vapor concentrations. *J. Pharmac. exp. Ther.,* **1951,** *102,* 112–124.

Machle, W. Gasoline intoxication. *J. Am. med. Ass.,* **1941,** *117,* 1965–1971.

McLean, E. K.; McLean, A. E. M.; and Sutton, P. M. Instant cirrhosis. An improved method for producing cirrhosis of the liver in rats by simultaneous administration of carbon tetrachloride and phenobarbitone. *Br. J. exp. Path.,* **1969,** *50,* 502–506.

Marchand, C.; McLean, S.; and Plaa, G. L. The effect of SKF 525A on the distribution of carbon tetrachloride in rats. *J. Pharmac. exp. Ther.,* **1970,** *174,* 232–238.

Marchand, C.; McLean, S.; Plaa, G. L.; and Traiger, G. Protection by 2-diethylaminoethyl-2,2-diphenylvalerate hydrochloride against carbon tetrachloride hepatotoxicity. *Biochem. Pharmac.,* **1971,** *20,* 869–875.

Matthew, H. Acute poisoning: some myths and misconceptions. *Br. med. J.,* **1971,** *1,* 519–522.

Meigs, J. W., and Hughes, J. P. W. Acute carbon monoxide poisoning: an analysis of one hundred five cases. *A.M.A. Archs ind. Hyg.,* **1952,** *6,* 344–356.

Mintel, R., and Westley, J. The rhodanese reaction: mechanism of sulfur-sulfur bond cleavage. *J. biol. Chem.,* **1966,** *241,* 3381–3385.

Norman, J. N., and Ledingham, I. McA. Carbon monoxide poisoning: investigations and treatment. *Prog. Brain Res.,* **1967,** *24,* 101–122.

Norwood, W. D.; Fuqua, P. A.; and Scudder, B. C. Carbon tetrachloride poisoning: more regulation, more education needed. *Archs ind. Hyg.,* **1950,** *1,* 90–100.

Oettingen, W. F. von. *The Halogenated Hydrocarbons: Toxicity and Potential Dangers.* Public Health Service Publication No. 414, U.S. Government Printing Office, Washington, D. C., **1955.**

Peterson, J. E., and Stewart, R. D. Absorption and elimination of carbon monoxide by inactive young men. *Archs envir. Hlth,* **1970,** *21,* 165–171.

Porteous, J. W., and Williams, R. T. Studies in detoxication. 20. The metabolism of benzene. II. The isolation of phenol, catechol, quinol and hydroxyquinol from the ethereal sulphate fraction of the urine of rabbits receiving benzene orally. *Biochem. J.,* **1949,** *44,* 56–61.

Press, E., and Done, A. K. Solvent sniffing. *Pediatrics, Springfield,* **1967,** *39,* 451–461, 611–622.

Recknagel, R. O. Carbon tetrachloride hepatotoxicity. *Pharmac. Rev.,* **1967,** *19,* 145–208.

Reinhardt, C. F.; Azar, A.; Maxfield, M. E.; Smith, P. E., Jr.; and Mullin, L. S. Cardiac arrhythmias and aerosol "sniffing." *Archs envir. Hlth,* **1971,** *22,* 265–279.

Rodkey, F. L. Kinetic aspects of cyanmethemoglobin formation from carboxyhemoglobin. *Clin. Chem.,* **1967,** *13,* 2–5.

Rose, C. L.; Worth, R. M.; Kikuchi, K.; and Chen, K. K. Cobalt salts in acute cyanide poisoning. *Proc. Soc. exp. Biol. Med.,* **1965,** *120,* 780–783.

Rose, E. F., and Rose, M. Carbon monoxide: a challenge to the physician. *Clin. Med.,* **1971,** *78,* 12–18.

Roughton, F. J. W. The average time spent by the blood in the human lung capillary and its relation to the rates of CO uptake and elimination in man. *Am. J. Physiol.,* **1945,** *143,* 621–633.

———. Kinetics of gas transport in the blood. *Br. med. Bull.,* **1963,** *19,* 80–89.

Roughton, F. J. W., and Darling, R. C. The effect of carbon monoxide on the oxyhemoglobin dissociation curve. *Am. J. Physiol.,* **1944,** *141,* 17–31.

Roughton, F. J. W., and Root, W. S. The fate of CO in the body during recovery from mild carbon monoxide poisoning in man. *Am. J. Physiol.,* **1945,** *145,* 239–252.

Sasame, H. A.; Castro, J. A.; and Gillette, J. R. Studies on the destruction of liver microsomal cytochrome P-450 by carbon tetrachloride administration. *Biochem. Pharmac.,* **1968,** *17,* 1759–1768.

Savilahti, M. Mehr als 100 Vergiftungsfälle durch Benzol in einer Schuhfabrik. *Arch. Gewerbepath. Gewerbehyg.,* **1956,** *15,* 147–157.

Sayers, P. R., and Davenport, S. J. Review of carbon monoxide poisoning. *Publ. Hlth Bull., Wash.,* No. 195, U.S. Government Printing Office, Washington, D. C., **1930.**

Sayre, J. W., and Kaymakcalan, S. Cyanide poisoning from apricot seeds among children in Central Turkey. *New Engl. J. Med.,* **1964,** *270,* 1113–1115.

Schubert, J., and Brill, W. A. Antagonism of experimental cyanide toxicity in relation to the *in vivo* activity of cytochrome oxidase. *J. Pharmac. exp. Ther.,* **1968,** *162,* 352–359.

Sheehy, M., and Way, J. L. Effect of oxygen on cyanide intoxication. III. Mithridate. *J. Pharmac. exp. Ther.,* **1968,** *161,* 163–168.

Sherwood, R. J. Evaluation of exposure to benzene vapour during the loading of petrol. *Br. J. ind. Med.,* **1972,** *29,* 65–69.

Shirkey, H. C. Treatment of petroleum distillate ingestion. *Mod. Treat.,* **1971,** *8,* 580–592.

Sievers, R. F.; Edwards, T. I.; and Murray, A. L. A medical study of men exposed to measured amounts of carbon monoxide in the Holland Tunnel for 13 years. *Publ. Hlth Bull., Wash.,* No. 278, U.S. Government Printing Office, Washington, D. C., **1942.**

Smith, G.; Ledingham, I. McA.; Sharp, G. R.; Norman, J. N.; and Bates, E. H. Treatment of coal-gas poisoning with oxygen at 2 atmospheres pressure. *Lancet,* **1962,** *1,* 816–818.

Steele, R. W.; Conklin, R. H.; and Mark, H. M. Corticosteroids and antibiotics for the treatment of fulminant hydrocarbon aspiration. *J. Am. med. Ass.,* **1972,** *219,* 1434–1437.

Stewart, R. D.; Baretta, E. D.; Platte, L. R.; Stewart, E. B.; Kalbfleisch, J. H.; Yserlo, B. V.; and Rimm, A. A. Carboxyhemoglobin concentrations in blood from donors in Chicago, Milwaukee, New York and Los Angeles. *Science, Wash.,* **1973,** *182,* 1362–1364.

Striker, G. E.; Smuckler, E. A.; Kohnen, P. W.; and Nagle, R. B. Structural and functional changes in rat kidney during CCl_4 intoxication. *Am. J. Path.,* **1968,** *53,* 769–789.

Subcommittee on Accidental Poisoning. Co-operative kerosene poisoning study. *Pediatrics, Springfield,* **1962,** *29,* 648–674.

Taylor, G. J., IV; Harris, W. S.; and Bogdonoff, M. B. Ventricular arrhythmias induced in monkeys by the inhalation of aerosol propellants. *J. clin. Invest.,* **1971,** *50,* 1546–1550.

Thompson, P. M. Poisoning due to petroleum products. *Archs Pediat.,* **1955,** *72,* 35–50.

Vigliani, E. C., and Forni, A. Benzene, chromosome change and leukemia. *J. occup. Med.,* **1969,** *11,* 148–149.

Ward, A. A., Jr., and Wheatley, M. D. Sodium cyanide: sequence of changes of activity induced at various levels of the central nervous system. *J. Neuropath. exp. Neurol.,* **1947,** *6,* 292–294.

Wexler, J.; Whittenberger, J. L.; and Dumke, P. R. The effect of cyanide on the electrocardiogram of man. *Am. Heart J.,* **1947,** *34,* 163–173.

Wheatley, M. D.; Lipton, B.; and Ward, A. A., Jr. Repeated cyanide convulsions without central nervous pathology. *J. Neuropath. exp. Neurol.,* **1947,** *6,* 408–411.

White, P. Carbon monoxide production and heme catabolism. *Ann. N.Y. Acad. Sci.,* **1970,** *174,* 23–31.

Williams, R. T. *Detoxification Mechanisms: The Metabolism and Detoxication of Drugs, Toxic Substances and Other Organic Compounds,* 2nd ed. John Wiley & Sons, Inc., New York, **1959.**

Winek, C. L., and Collom, W. D. Benzene and toluene fatalities. *J. occup. Med.,* **1971,** *13,* 259–261.

SECTION
XI

Heavy Metals and Heavy-Metal Antagonists

The heavy metals are conveniently discussed together provided pharmacological organization is not sacrificed in favor of the periodic table of elements. The inorganic salts of the metals can be grouped together because they have many pharmacological and toxicological properties in common. In the case of the organic derivatives of the metals, however, a chemical classification, in some instances, must give way to one based upon therapeutic application. For example, organic mercurial compounds are still used as antiseptics and diuretics and are discussed under each of these classifications. Also, certain metals are excluded from this section because of specific pharmacological actions and therapeutic applications that require their discussion elsewhere. For example, iron is considered in connection with other drugs acting on the blood and the blood-forming organs.

The development of antagonists to the biological actions of certain of the metals is a significant advance of modern pharmacology. The antagonists are both valuable drugs and research tools. They will be discussed before the individual metals because they shed light on the mechanism of action of the metals.

CHAPTER
45   HEAVY-METAL ANTAGONISTS

Walter G. Levine

Heavy metals exert their toxic effects by combining with one or more reactive groups essential for normal physiological functions (*see* Chapter 46). Heavy-metal antagonists are designed specifically to compete with these groups for the metals and thereby to prevent or reverse their toxic effects.

The mechanism of action of these antagonists is best understood in terms of the interaction of metals and various groups known as *ligands*. The heavy metals, particularly those in the transition series, may react with O, S, and N ligands, which, in the body, take the form of $-OH$, $-COO^-$, $-OPO_3H^-$, $>C=O$, $-SH$, $-S-S-$, $-NH_2$, and

$>NH$. The *metal complex* or *coordination compound* that is formed involves a *coordinate* bond, which is similar to a covalent bond except that both electrons are contributed by the ligand.

The drugs discussed in this chapter possess the common property of forming complexes with heavy metals, thereby preventing or reversing the binding of metallic cations to body ligands. The drugs are all *chelating agents*. A chelate is defined as a complex formed between a metal and a compound containing two or more potential ligands (*e.g.*, ethylene*di*amine). The product of such a reaction is a heterocyclic ring. A metal chelate is usually far more stable than is the nonchelate complex of the same metal and one ligand. Five- and six-membered chelate rings are more stable, and a polydentate (multiligand) chelator typically forms a highly stable complex. Chelates are generally less stable at low pH. At a high pH there is a tendency for the metal to hydrolyze and form an insoluble metal hydroxide that is less accessible to the chelating agent. For most therapeutically useful chelating agents, the tendency to form metal hydroxides is probably not an important consideration in physiological systems. Nevertheless, control of the pH of body fluids may be an important consideration during treatment with chelating agents.

The stability of chelates varies with the metal and the ligand atoms. For example, lead and mercury have greater affinities for sulfur and nitrogen than for oxygen ligands, while calcium behaves in the opposite manner. This permits some degree of selectivity of action of a chelating agent in the body. However, absolute specificity of a chelating agent has not yet been demonstrated.

The following requirements have been proposed for an ideal chelating agent: (1) water solubility, (2) resistance to metabolic degradation, (3) ability to penetrate to metal storage sites, (4) ready excretion by the kidney, (5) ability to retain chelating activity at the pH of body fluids, and (6) the property of forming metal complexes that are less toxic than the free metal ion. Another important property is greater affinity for the metal atom than that of the endogenous ligands. The large number of available ligands within the body makes the task of a therapeutic chelating agent a formidable one. In view of the complexity of a biological system, *in-vitro* observations on chelator-metal interactions will serve only as a rough guide to the treatment of heavy-metal poisoning. Only empirical observation can determine the clinical usefulness of these agents. Additionally, a low affinity for calcium is desirable. Since plasma calcium is so readily available for chelation, a drug might serve primarily as a hypocalcemic agent despite its high affinity for heavy metals.

DIMERCAPROL

History. During World War II, an intensive effort was made to develop an antidote to *lewisite,* a vesicant arsenical war gas. Knowing that arsenicals reacted with SH-containing molecules, Stocken and Thompson, at Oxford University, initiated a systematic study of thiol compounds to find one that would successfully compete with the tissue SH groups for the arsenicals. This study represents an excellent but all too rare example of the development of a useful pharmacological agent based on knowledge of biochemical mechanisms (*see* Stocken and Thompson, 1949). Their investigations indicated that the arsenicals would form a very stable and relatively nontoxic chelate ring with the dithiol compound, *dimercaprol* (2,3-dimercaptopropanol). When United States scientists joined their British colleagues in these studies, they designated dimercaprol as British antilewisite (BAL). Pharmacological investigations revealed that this compound would protect against the toxic effects of other heavy metals as well. At the end of the war, when the results of this work were published, it was realized that dimercaprol was effective against poisoning by many heavy metals, a long-sought goal.

Chemistry and Physical Properties. Dimercaprol has the following structure:

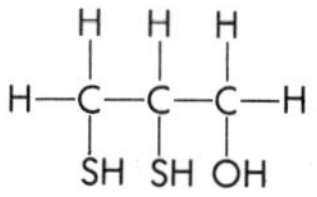

$$
\begin{array}{ccc}
H & H & H \\
| & | & | \\
H-C-C-C-H \\
| & | & | \\
SH & SH & OH
\end{array}
$$

Dimercaprol

It is a clear, colorless, viscous, oily fluid with a pungent, disagreeable odor typical of mercaptans. It will form a 7% aqueous solution and is also soluble in vegetable oils, alcohol, and various other organic solvents. Because of its instability in aqueous solutions, peanut oil is the solvent employed in pharmaceutical preparations.

Dimercaprol and related thiols are readily oxidized *in vitro* in the presence of a number of catalysts. Presumably, oxidation to a cyclic S—S compound can occur *in vivo*. Methemoglobin is reduced instantly to hemoglobin in the presence of dimercaprol, but the drug is too toxic to be used in the treatment of methemoglobinemia.

PHARMACOLOGICAL PROPERTIES

Mechanism of Action. Dimercaprol forms a highly stable chelate with a variety of metals. In the cases of mercury, cadmium, and possibly other metals, a 2:1 complex may form that has even greater stability than does the 1:1 complex. Due to dissociation and oxidation of the complex, the chelated metal can be released to exert again its toxic effects. Thus, Hg^{2+}, Cd^{2+}, and oxophenarsine, injected into experimental animals as their preformed dimercaprol complexes, still retain a considerable degree of toxicity (Gilman *et al.,* 1946a, 1946b; Peters and Stocken, 1947). The dosage regimen is therefore designed to assure the continuous presence of an excess of free dimercaprol in body fluids until excretion of the offending metal has been accomplished to the desired extent.

Dimercaprol prevents inhibition of sulfhydryl enzymes by metals and also reactivates such enzymes. Since the degree of enzyme reactivation diminishes with time, it follows that therapy with dimercaprol is most effective if provided early in the course of poisoning. This therapeutic principle applies to the use of all chelating agents. In the presence of overwhelming amounts of metal, no antagonist is completely effective; this constitutes a limitation to the effectiveness of dimercaprol therapy.

Dimercaprol antagonizes the biological actions of metals that form mercaptides with essential cellular sulfhydryl groups, for example, arsenic, mercury, and cadmium. On the other hand, intoxication by selenites, which inhibit sulfhydryl enzymes by oxidation, is not influenced by dimercaprol. Other metals occupy an intermediate position.

Actions on Enzyme Systems. Dimercaprol is capable of affecting directly a number of enzyme systems that are activated by metals. Among these are catalase, carbonic anhydrase, and peroxidase (Barron *et al.,* 1947; Webb and Van Heyningen, 1947). Potentiation of the hypotensive effect of bradykinin by dimercaprol has been attributed to inhibition of the zinc-containing enzyme carboxypeptidase, which is known to destroy bradykinin (Erdos and Wohler, 1963; Roche e Silva, 1963). In addition, dimercaprol inhibits cytochrome oxidase in tissue slices. The oxidation products of dimercaprol inhibit SH enzymes, while dimercaprol itself reacts with insulin *in vitro* to inactivate the hormone, presumably by reducing essential S—S groups (Barron *et al.,* 1947).

Systemic Actions in Experimental Animals. Dimercaprol exerts rather marked effects on the central nervous system and the cardiovascular system. Toxic doses cause vomiting, tremors, and convulsions, followed by coma and death. Although the convulsions can be controlled with barbiturates, death still occurs because of the severity of the cardiovascular effects. Low doses of dimercaprol constrict peripheral arterioles and thus cause a rise in blood pressure. Larger doses cause capillary damage with a loss of plasma protein and fluid and a marked rise in the hematocrit. The lymph flow increases. Reduction in blood volume results in peripheral circulatory failure, and the animals die in shock (Chenoweth, 1946; Hitchcock, 1946). After toxic doses of dimercaprol, the pH and bicarbonate content of the blood fall due to an increase in plasma lactic acid. The blood sugar rises initially but falls to hypoglycemic levels before death, and the glycogen content of the liver is reduced. The convulsions are not the result of the hypoglycemia.

Human Pharmacology, Side Effects, and Toxicity. The administration of dimercaprol to human subjects results in a variety of side effects that are more alarming than serious; nevertheless, they limit the amount of the dithiol that can be administered. Reactions to dimercaprol occur in approximately 50% of subjects receiving 5 mg/kg intramuscularly. The effects of repeated administration of this dose are not cumulative, provided an interval of at least 4 hours elapses between injections. One of the most consistent responses to dimercaprol is a rise in the systolic and diastolic blood pressures accompanied by tachycardia. The rise in pressure is roughly proportional to the dose administered and may be as great as 50 mm Hg in response to the second of two doses (5 mg/kg) given 2 hours apart. The pressure rises immediately but returns to normal within 2 hours. Other signs and symptoms, many of which tend to parallel the change in blood pressure in time and intensity, are the following, listed in approximate order of frequency: (1) nausea and, in some instances, vomiting; (2) headache; (3) a burning sensation in the lips, mouth, and throat and a feeling of constriction, sometimes even pain, in the throat, chest, or hands; (4) conjunctivitis, lacrimation, rhinorrhea, and salivation; (5) tingling of the hands; (6) a burning sensation in the penis; (7) sweating of the forehead, hands, and other areas; (8) abdominal pain; and (9) occasional appearance of painful sterile abscesses at the injection site. Symptoms are often accompanied by a feeling of anxiety and unrest. Because the dimercaprol-metal complex breaks down easily in an acidic medium, production of an alkaline urine affords protection to the kidney during therapy. The toxicity of the dimercaprol-metal chelate is less than that of dimercaprol itself.

Children react as do adults, although approximately 30% may also experience fever, which disappears upon withdrawal of the drug. A transient reduction of the percentage of polymorphonuclear leukocytes may also be observed. Two children who, through an error in dosage, received inordinately large amounts of dimercaprol (one, 40.5 mg/kg; the other, 25.0 mg/kg, repeated in 4 hours) exhibited vasomotor changes, hypertension, convulsions, and coma. Recovery appeared to be complete within an hour after the onset of convulsions, which were of brief duration.

Dimercaprol may affect thyroid function (Forster *et al.*, 1955; Current *et al.*, 1960). Decreased iodine uptake, increased body weight, and decreased metabolic rate have been observed in experimental animals. Enhanced excretion of some trace metals occurs, but it is considerably less than that observed with edetate or penicillamine. A patient treated with dimercaprol for Wilson's disease was reported to complete two uneventful pregnancies; there were no signs of teratogenicity.

Absorption, Fate, and Excretion. When therapeutic doses of a 10% solution of dimercaprol in oil are administered intramuscularly, peak blood levels are attained in 30 to 60 minutes. Distribution is mainly in the intracellular space. The half-life is short, and metabolic degradation and excretion are essentially complete within 4 hours. Following injection of dimercaprol into experimental animals, there is a sharp rise in the excretion of neutral sulfur in the urine, which accounts for approximately 50% of the sulfur injected as dimercaprol. There is no increase in ethereal sulfur. A rise in urinary glucuronic acid suggests that a portion of dimercaprol may be excreted as glucuronide.

Preparations. *Dimercaprol*, U.S.P. (*2,3-dimercaptopropanol, BAL*), is employed in the form of *Dimercaprol Injection*, U.S.P., a solution of 10% dimercaprol (w/v) and benzyl benzoate in vegetable oil. Each milliliter contains 100 mg of dimercaprol. The preparation is marketed in 3-ml ampuls.

Dosage and Routes of Administration. Dimercaprol is administered by deep intramuscular injection. Rarely, topical application may be employed for the treatment of local lesions of the skin and eyes produced by arsenical vesicants. There may be local pain and tenderness following injection, but severe local reactions are rare.

Dimercaprol must be given in courses to be maximally effective. The duration of a course, the interval between injections, and the dose per injection are best modified to meet the particular situation. All doses should be calculated on a milligram-per-kilogram basis. For the management of toxic reactions accompanying therapy with metals such as arsenic and gold, a prolonged course with relatively low individual doses should be followed. The recommended dose is 2.5 mg/kg, administered at 4-hour intervals during the first 2 days, twice on the third day, and once daily thereafter for 5 to 10 days or until the patient has recovered. For severe acute poisoning, early intensive therapy is indicated. A unit dose of 5 mg/kg should be given at 4-hour intervals for the first 24 hours. Thereafter, both the number of injections and the amount of each injection can be reduced by one half. It should be emphasized, however, that the intensity of any course of dimercaprol therapy should be determined by the severity of the poisoning and the response of the patient. Children tolerate dimercaprol as well as do adults if the drug is given on the basis of body weight; consequently, they should receive full dosages.

THERAPEUTIC USES

The efficacy of dimercaprol in the treatment of poisoning or untoward reactions from arsenicals, mercurials, and gold salts is now well established. The details of treatment and the results that can be anticipated are discussed under the individual metals (*see* Index). Dimercaprol is also of value as an adjunct to calcium disodium edetate (CaNa$_2$EDTA) in the treatment of lead poisoning and to penicillamine in the treatment of Wilson's disease (*see* below). Dimercaprol significantly reduces the toxicity of bismuth, chromium, and nickel, but it is useless in cadmium poisoning and results in intoxication by antimonials are inconclusive.

CALCIUM DISODIUM EDETATE AND DISODIUM EDETATE

Ethylenediaminetetraacetic acid (EDTA, edathamil), its sodium salt (*disodium edetate, Na$_2$EDTA*), and a number of closely related compounds have found application as industrial and analytical reagents for a number of years owing to their property of chelating many divalent and trivalent metals (*see* Chaberek and Martell, 1959; Dwyer and Mellor, 1964). Early investigations into the biological action of EDTA came as a result of a proposal to use it as a food preservative. Although the first animal studies had shown that Na$_2$EDTA caused hypocalcemic tetany, the relatively nontoxic nature of the calcium chelate (calcium disodium edetate, CaNa$_2$EDTA) was soon established (Popovici *et al.,* 1950). It was subsequently observed that CaNa$_2$EDTA was as effective as Na$_2$EDTA as a food preservative by virtue of the ability of metal ions with higher binding constants to displace calcium from the chelate. This raised the possibility that CaNa$_2$EDTA might be used in the treatment of poisoning by metals that displace calcium from the chelate. It was soon found that lead poisoning responded favorably to CaNa$_2$EDTA; this is in fact its principal use today. Poisoning from other metals responds poorly or not at all.

The structure of calcium disodium edetate is as follows:

Calcium Disodium Edetate

PHARMACOLOGICAL PROPERTIES

The rapid intravenous administration of Na$_2$EDTA results in hypocalcemic tetany. However, a slow infusion (less than 15 mg per minute) into a normocalcemic individual elicits no hypocalcemic symptoms, indicating the ready availability of extracirculatory calcium stores (Spencer *et al.,* 1952). In contrast, CaNa$_2$EDTA can be administered intravenously in relatively large quantities with no untoward effects and no change in the plasma or total body calcium concentrations.

Mechanism of Action. All known pharmacological effects of EDTA are due to chelate formation with divalent and trivalent metals. *In vivo,* CaNa$_2$EDTA will bind any metals having greater affinity for EDTA than has calcium, depending, of course, on the availability of such metals. Next to calcium, zinc seems to be most accessible to EDTA in the body. Intravenous administration of CaNa$_2$EDTA increases considerably the urinary excretion of zinc (Perry and Perry, 1959). There is also a slight enhancement of the urinary excretion of cadmium, manganese, lead, iron, and copper.

The successful use of CaNa$_2$EDTA in the treatment of lead poisoning is due, in part, to the ability of lead to displace calcium from the chelate. The fact that EDTA strongly enhances the mobilization and excretion of lead from the body means that lead is to a considerable degree accessible to EDTA. On the contrary, while mercury readily displaces calcium from CaNa$_2$EDTA *in vitro,* mercury poisoning does *not* respond to this drug. The metal is thus unavailable to the chelate. It may be too tightly bound by body ligands (SH) or sequestered in body compartments not penetrated by CaNa$_2$EDTA. Due to its ionic character, it is unlikely that CaNa$_2$EDTA penetrates cells significantly.

Teisinger and associates (1958) and Castellino and Aloj (1965) suggested that CaNa$_2$EDTA chelates only extracellular lead. Due to the consequent increase in concentration gradient the intracellular lead passes out of the cell and is chelated and excreted. Hammond (1971) reported that the primary source of lead that is chelated by CaNa$_2$EDTA is bone, while Castellino and Aloj (1965) found that lead in soft tissues was primarily sequestered and bone lead remained essentially unaffected by CaNa$_2$EDTA. They also showed a biphasic course of elimination that corresponded to rapid excretion of weakly bound extracellular lead followed by the slower excretion of more tightly complexed lead, from intracellular sites.

Absorption, Fate, and Excretion. CaNa$_2$-EDTA is poorly absorbed from the gastrointestinal tract of both man and experimental animals (Foreman *et al.,* 1953; Foreman and Trujillo, 1954), and orally administered drug does not increase urinary calcium excretion (Spencer, 1960). Absorption through the skin is negligible. After intravenous administration, CaNa$_2$EDTA disappears exponentially from the circulation with a half-life of 20 to 60 minutes. About 50% is excreted in the urine in 1 hour and over 95% in 24 hours. For this reason, satisfactory renal function is necessary during therapy. Renal clearance of the compound in dogs equals the inulin clearance, and glomerular filtration accounts for the entire mechanism of urinary excretion (Forland *et al.,* 1966). Altering either the pH or the rate of flow of the urine has no effect on the rate of excretion. Studies with ^{14}C-labeled material indicate that negligible amounts are retained in the body after 24 hours and almost none of the compound is metabolized. It does not enter erythrocytes and is distributed mainly in the extracellular fluids. However, very little gains access to the spinal fluid, and calcium ion levels in the spinal fluid remain unchanged after injection of Na_2EDTA (Soffer and Toribara, 1961).

Toxicity. In general, $CaNa_2EDTA$ is an agent of relatively low toxicity, due in no small part to the fact that it is not metabolized and is rapidly excreted. The principal toxic effect of the drug is on the kidney. Death from lower-nephron nephrosis has occurred during its use in the treatment of metal poisoning. Tubular destruction can be produced by the administration of large doses of either $CaNa_2EDTA$ or Na_2EDTA. Experimentally in rats and also in man, severe hydropic degeneration of proximal tubules has been observed, in some cases with almost total destruction of the proximal tubular epithelium (Dudley *et al.*, 1955; Foreman *et al.*, 1956; Altman *et al.*, 1962). Changes in distal tubules and glomeruli are less conspicuous. The renal effects are usually reversible, and urinary abnormalities disappear rapidly upon cessation of treatment. Hemorrhage and necrosis of intestinal epithelium have been observed in dogs (Ahrens and Aronson, 1971).

The renal toxicity may relate to the fact that large amounts of chelated metals pass through the renal tubule in a relatively short period of time during drug therapy. Some dissociation of chelates may occur, due partly to competition for the metal by physiological ligands or to pH changes within the cell or within the lumen of the tubule (Johnson and Seven, 1960). However, raising the pH of the urine by administration of bicarbonate was found not to diminish the renal toxicity of $CaNa_2EDTA$ in rats (Foreman *et al.*, 1956). Removal of essential metals from the tubular cells may also be a factor in toxicity, although tubular vacuolization during $CaNa_2EDTA$ administration has been observed in the absence of any discernible change in metal content of the kidney (Doolan *et al.*, 1967). Schwartz and coworkers (1970) suggested that vacuolization reflects an induction of pinocytosis by the chelate.

A febrile systemic reaction has been observed in patients 4 to 8 hours after infusion of the drug, characterized by a rapid onset of malaise, fatigue, and excessive thirst, followed by the sudden appearance of fever and chills. This, in turn, is followed by severe myalgia, frontal headache, anorexia, occasional nausea and vomiting, and, rarely, increased urinary frequency and urgency. Other toxic effects include a histamine-like reaction, with sneezing, nasal congestion, and lacrimation; glycosuria; anemia; dermatitis with lesions strikingly similar to those of vitamin B_6 deficiency; transitory lowering of systolic and diastolic blood pressures; prolonged prothrombin time; and inversion of the T wave of the ECG.

Preparations, Routes of Administration, and Dosage. $CaNa_2EDTA$ is available as *Edetate Calcium Disodium*, U.S.P. (CALCIUM DISODIUM VERSENATE). It is marketed as 500-mg tablets, but due to poor oral absorption $CaNa_2EDTA$ is generally not administered by this route. For parenteral use, *Edetate Calcium Disodium Injection*, U.S.P., a 20% solution, is employed. For the diagnosis of lead poisoning, three doses of 25 mg/kg are given intramuscularly in 1.5% procaine hydrochloride solution at intervals of 8 hours.

For therapeutic use, 1.0 g (5 ml) in 250 to 500 ml of 5% glucose in water or isotonic saline solution is administered slowly by intravenous drip over a 1-hour period. A dilute infusion is necessary to avoid thrombophlebitis. Two such courses are administered each day for 3 to 5 days. The drug is then withheld for several days, and further courses of therapy are given if necessary. The total daily dose should not exceed 50 mg/kg of body weight in order to avoid toxic symptoms. For children, maximal dosage is 70 mg/kg of body weight, divided into two doses. In patients with lead encephalopathy and increased intracranial pressure, excess fluids must be avoided. In such cases a 20% solution in 0.5 to 1.5% procaine hydrochloride solution is administered intramuscularly.

Edetate Disodium, U.S.P., is available as *Edetate Disodium Injection*, U.S.P. (ENDRATE DISODIUM). It is marketed in 20-ml ampuls that contain 150 mg/ml of the salt in aqueous solution. The usual dose is 50 mg (0.33 ml)/kg. It is diluted to 500 ml in glucose or isotonic saline solution and administered by intravenous infusion over a period of 2½ to 4 hours. The pH of the final solution may have to be adjusted.

THERAPEUTIC USES

Diagnosis of Lead Poisoning. Because the onset of lead poisoning is usually insidious, it is often desirable to measure the body lead burden of individuals exposed to a high lead environment. The administration of CaNa$_2$EDTA will greatly increase the urinary excretion of lead regardless of previous exposure to the metal. While basal concentrations of urinary lead may not vary with lead exposure, urinary excretion after CaNa$_2$EDTA does reflect the patient's lead burden although wide ranges are seen (Table 45-1). An excretion of over 500 μg in 24 hours is generally indicative of an excess lead burden in the body. After such a test the otherwise symptomless individual can be given courses of treatment until the urinary lead excretion returns to normal.

Treatment of Lead Poisoning. The therapeutic objective in lead poisoning is to mobilize the metal from the tissues and promote its excretion as rapidly as possible. The administration of CaNa$_2$EDTA alleviates symptoms within a short time after treatment is initiated. Colic may disappear within 2 hours, and muscular weakness and tremors disappear after 4 to 5 days. Coproporphyrinuria, stippled red blood cells, and lead lines tend to decrease within 4 to 9 days. The urinary lead excretion is greatest after the first infusion, but decreases with subsequent treatment due to depletion of readily accessible lead. Therefore, a rest period is allowed, during which time redistribution of the lead occurs, thus increasing the amount of available metal. A combination of chelation treatment and peritoneal dialysis has been recommended in acute lead intoxication, where speed of "de-leading" is a crucial factor (Mehbod, 1967).

Childhood Lead Poisoning. Lead poisoning in small children is far more dangerous than in adults. Severe lead encephalopathy has a mortality rate of up to 65% if untreated, and even the survivors have residual effects of brain damage such as ataxia, impaired mental powers, and, in very severe cases, blindness, idiocy, and hemiplegia. Early diagnosis, prompt removal of the child from exposure to lead, and careful supportive management during the first 48 to 72 hours of CaNa$_2$EDTA administration are essential. In view of the unpredictable and fulminating course of lead encephalopathy, it is advisable to view all cases as potentially severe. Unfortunately, CaNa$_2$EDTA alone is not as effective as would be desirable in the treatment of severe lead poisoning in children. Chisolm (1967) recommended that all cases of childhood lead poisoning be treated with both CaNa$_2$EDTA and dimercaprol, with the following dosage schedule: first dose, dimercaprol only,

4 mg/kg intramuscularly; every 4 hours thereafter—in addition to dimercaprol—CaNa$_2$EDTA, 12.5 mg/kg intramuscularly. This regimen is continued for 5 days. In this way toxic effects are minimized, urinary lead excretion is accelerated, and there is a more rapid decrease in blood lead and urinary δ-aminolevulinic acid levels than during therapy with either drug alone. Of great importance is the decreased incidence of residual neurological symptoms so often seen after lead encephalopathy.

Tetraethyl Lead Poisoning. Lead is present in tetraethyl lead in the nonionic form and is thereby inaccessible to CaNa$_2$EDTA. Not unexpectedly the results of administration of CaNa$_2$EDTA intravenously in cases of tetraethyl lead poisoning are rather disappointing. Symptomatic relief is slight, and the excretion of lead in the urine, although somewhat increased, is not as dramatic as for inorganic lead (Boyd, 1957).

Therapeutic Uses of Disodium Edetate. Na$_2$-EDTA has limited usefulness in the diagnosis and treatment of abnormalities in calcium metabolism.

Diagnosis of Hypoparathyroidism. Kaiser and Ponsold (1959) reported that hypoparathyroid patients display an impaired ability to restore calcium levels to normal after they are depressed by Na$_2$EDTA infusion. However, the value of such a diagnostic procedure has been questioned (Stowers et al., 1967).

Cardiac Arrhythmias. The use of Na$_2$EDTA in cases of both atrial and ventricular cardiac arrhythmias, including those associated with digitalis intoxication, has met with some degree of success. The relationship between plasma calcium levels and digitalis toxicity is discussed elsewhere (see Index).

Miscellaneous Uses. Na$_2$EDTA may be useful in the emergency treatment of severe hypercalcemia. Its effectiveness in scleroderma or other diseases involving calcinosis has not been established.

DIETHYLENETRIAMINEPENTAACETIC ACID (DTPA)

DTPA is similar in structure to EDTA but has a somewhat greater affinity for most heavy metals than does EDTA (see Chaberek and Martell, 1959; Dwyer and Mellor, 1964). For this reason, it has been tried in cases of heavy-metal poisoning that do not respond to EDTA. In particular, DTPA has been in-

Table 45-1. EXCRETION OF LEAD IN URINE BEFORE AND AFTER ADMINISTRATION OF CaNa$_2$EDTA *

| PATIENT GROUP | PATIENTS (No.) | URINARY LEAD EXCRETION (μg/LITER) | | | |
| | | *Before Administration* | | *After Administration* | |
		Range	Average	Range	Average
Controls	24	0–160	15	4–405	165
Suspected lead poisoning	11	0–120	24	608–1590	995
Clinical poisoning	8	0–500	146	971–3030	1966

* After Whitaker, Austin, and Nelson, 1962. Courtesy of *Pediatrics.*

vestigated for the treatment of iron-storage disease and poisoning by radioactive metals. The former is now dealt with mainly by the use of deferoxamine (*see* below), and DTPA has had only a limited degree of success in the latter situation.

Like EDTA, DTPA rapidly binds calcium. For this reason, the calcium chelate, $CaNa_2DTPA$, is employed in the treatment of heavy-metal poisoning. Lack of much clinical success with DTPA is probably not surprising, since the affinity of EDTA for many of these metals is very high, and the accessibility of agents of this type to metal storage sites is probably of major importance.

Absorption, Fate, and Excretion. The absorption, fate, and excretion of $CaNa_2DTPA$ are similar to those of $CaNa_2EDTA$. Upon parenteral administration, 90 to 100% of the dose is excreted by the kidneys in 24 hours. DTPA is mainly distributed in the extracellular fluids and does not enter the red blood cell. After administration of ^{14}C-labeled material, very little activity is found in the respiratory CO_2, indicating little or no oxidation. DTPA has fallen into relative disuse, clinically. Its main application, in the mobilization of radioactive metals, is discussed below.

PENICILLAMINE

Penicillamine is β,β-dimethylcysteine. Its structure is as follows:

$$H_3C\underset{\underset{SH}{|}}{\overset{\overset{CH_3}{|}}{C}}-\underset{\underset{NH_2}{|}}{CH}-COOH$$

Penicillamine

It is prepared by the hydrolytic degradation of penicillin. Only the D isomer is recommended for clinical use.

Pharmacological Actions. Penicillamine is an effective chelator of copper, mercury, zinc, and lead and promotes the excretion of these metals in the urine. In addition to its chelating properties, L-penicillamine and, to a lesser extent, its D isomer inhibit enzymes that are pyridoxal dependent (*see* Aposhian, 1961). Experimentally, the toxic effects in rats given high doses of penicillamine resemble those seen in pyridoxine deficiency, and the effects are reversed by feeding pyridoxine (Heddle *et al.,* 1963). In human beings, pyridoxine antagonism is readily demonstrated with the L and the DL forms, but rarely with the D form. There may be no detectable symptoms, but only biochemical evidence of increased urinary excretion of xanthurenic acid and kynurenine. Nevertheless, dietary supplementation of pyridoxine is recommended even when D-penicillamine is used.

Absorption, Fate, and Excretion. Penicillamine is well absorbed from the gastrointestinal tract and, therefore, has a decided advantage over other chelating agents. It is rapidly excreted in the urine. Unlike cysteine, the nonmethylated parent compound, it is somewhat resistant to attack by cysteine desulfhydrase or L-amino acid oxidase (Aposhian, 1961). As a result, penicillamine is relatively stable *in vivo*. This probably explains the effectiveness of penicillamine and the lack of effectiveness of cysteine in promoting the excretion of metals, although *in vitro* both compounds form stable metal chelates. This explanation is further substantiated by the fact that N-acetylpenicillamine is even more effective than penicillamine in protecting against the toxic effects of mercury (Aposhian and Aposhian, 1959). The acetylated derivative is more resistant to metabolic degradation than is the parent compound.

Preparations and Dosage. *Penicillamine,* U.S.P., the D isomer, is a white crystalline, water-soluble powder. In aqueous solution, it is comparatively stable at pH 2 to 4. The drug is dispensed as 250-mg capsules, *Penicillamine Capsules,* U.S.P. (CUPRIMINE). It is administered orally, 1 to 4 g per day, in four divided doses. It is given on an empty stomach to avoid interference by dietary metals. Potassium sulfide, 40 mg, is also given with each meal to minimize absorption of copper. N-Acetylpenicillamine is not yet available as a drug.

Side Effects and Toxicity. D-Penicillamine is relatively nontoxic, and much of the toxicity reported is attributable to use of the L or DL forms. Unfortunately much of the literature on this drug does not indicate the form that was used. Acute sensitivity reactions, manifested by fever, rashes (pruritic, morbilliform, and urticarial), leukopenia, eosinophilia, and thrombocytopenia, have been encountered early in the course of therapy. This requires prompt discontinuation of the drug. Desensitization with small doses of the drug or the administration of corticosteroids may overcome these reactions. Rarely, one or more of these side effects prevent the use of penicillamine. Infrequently, anorexia, nausea, and vomiting occur. Loss of taste for salt and sweet has been observed. Several cases of nephrotoxicity, including patients given only D-penicillamine, have been reported. Presumably they result from hypersensitivity reactions (Adams *et al.,* 1964; Sternlieb and Scheinberg, 1964; Rosenberg and Hayslett, 1967; Elsas *et al.,* 1971). A case of optic neuritis, assumed to be drug related, has also occurred. It responded to treatment with pyridoxine (Tu *et al.,* 1963). After therapy for 1 to 2 years' duration, a systemic lupus erythematosus–like syndrome has been observed. Extravasation of blood into the skin over pressure points (elbows, knees, toes) occurs in some patients after prolonged administration of high doses of penicillamine. Plasma proteins and coagulation tests remain normal. Individuals who are sensitive to penicillin may have a similar reaction to penicillamine.

THERAPEUTIC USES

Wilson's Disease. Penicillamine is an effective drug in the treatment of hepatolenticular degeneration (Wilson's disease) (*see* Sternlieb and Scheinberg, 1964). The disease is due to the deposition of toxic amounts of copper in various tissues and is associated with a deficiency of ceruloplasmin, a copper-containing plasma protein. Therefore, promotion of copper excretion, coupled with a reduction in copper intake, is a rational approach to therapy. Patients treated in this way with penicillamine exhibit marked clinical improvement, particularly in the neurological manifestations. Patients who are originally asymptomatic do not develop clinical symptoms if treated prophylactically. Occasionally it is desirable to use dimercaprol in addition to penicillamine in the treatment of patients with Wilson's disease.

Lead Poisoning. Encouraging reports indicate penicillamine may be of considerable value in lead poisoning (Harris, 1958; Goldberg *et al.,* 1963; Selander, 1967). With doses of 600 to 1500 mg per day, clinical improvement is rapid, with the disappearance of abdominal pain, muscular weakness, vomiting, and diarrhea. Blood concentrations of lead decrease, and urinary excretion of lead is promoted. The amount of coproporphyrin and δ-aminolevulinic acid in the urine diminishes with the increased lead excretion.

Urinary lead concentrations after oral penicillamine may not be as high as those seen after intravenous CaNa$_2$EDTA, and a transient increase in lead within soft tissues has been reported in experimental animals (Hammond, 1973). However, the oral efficacy of penicillamine provides a definite advantage, particularly for the long periods of "deleading" that are often required in lead poisoning. (*See* Chapter 46.)

Cystinuria. Penicillamine has become established in the treatment of cystinuria and the associated nephrolithiasis. In a dose of 30 mg/kg per day, it lowers or eliminates urinary cystine and prevents further stone development (MacDonald and Fellers, 1966). In some cases, reduction in size and finally dissolution of stones are seen after 6 to 12 months of therapy. The mechanism of action is believed to involve the formation of penicillamine-cysteine disulfide, which is 50 times more soluble than the cysteine-cysteine disulfide (cystine).

Rheumatoid Arthritis. There is some promise in the treatment of rheumatoid arthritis with penicillamine (Multicentre Trial Group, 1973). Patients who would be considered suitable for gold therapy also respond well to penicillamine. As with gold therapy, a beneficial effect is seen only after several weeks of treatment, and arthritic symptoms return if the drug is withdrawn prematurely.

DEFEROXAMINE

The structure of this drug is shown below. It is isolated as the iron chelate from *Streptomyces pilosus* and is treated chemically to obtain the metal-free ligand. Deferoxamine has a remarkable affinity for ferric iron ($K_a = 10^{31}$) coupled with a very low affinity for calcium ($K_a = 10^2$), a highly desirable property. It readily competes for the iron of ferritin and hemosiderin, while the iron of transferrin is removed only to a small extent. The iron in cytochromes and hemoglobin is not accessible to deferoxamine. Less than 15% of an oral dose is absorbed, and parenteral administration is required in most cases. Given orally, it binds iron in the lumen of the bowel and thus renders the metal nonabsorbable. This property can be exploited clinically. Deferoxamine is metabolized principally by plasma enzymes, although the pathways have not yet been defined. It is also readily excreted in the urine.

Deferoxamine has been used successfully in the treatment of various *iron-storage dis-*

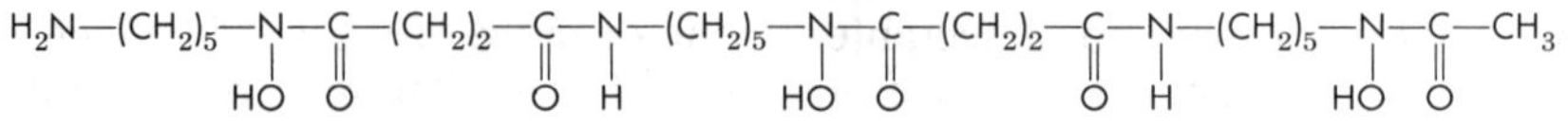

$$H_2N-(CH_2)_5-\underset{\underset{HO}{|}}{N}-\underset{\underset{O}{\|}}{C}-(CH_2)_2-\underset{\underset{O}{\|}}{C}-\underset{\underset{H}{|}}{N}-(CH_2)_5-\underset{\underset{HO}{|}}{N}-\underset{\underset{O}{\|}}{C}-(CH_2)_2-\underset{\underset{O}{\|}}{C}-\underset{\underset{H}{|}}{N}-(CH_2)_5-\underset{\underset{HO}{|}}{N}-\underset{\underset{O}{\|}}{C}-CH_3$$

Deferoxamine

eases as well as *acute iron poisoning.* The latter, a not-uncommon pediatric problem, is the type of iron toxicity most amenable to chelation therapy (Jacobs *et al.,* 1965). Untreated severe iron poisoning has a reported mortality of 50%. Rapid urinary excretion of iron occurs after administration of deferoxamine, and clinical recovery follows. For mild cases, however, deferoxamine therapy has little advantage over supportive measures (Leikin *et al.,* 1967). For optimum results in severe poisoning, both oral and parenteral deferoxamine should be used. Although results in primary hemochromatosis and hemosiderosis secondary to hepatic cirrhosis are disappointing, some cases of *transfusion siderosis* respond well to deferoxamine therapy. *Thalassemia* also responds well to deferoxamine therapy.

Deferoxamine causes a number of toxic and side effects. Among the reactions that have occurred are hypotension, probably due to histamine release (especially during intravenous administration), skin rashes, and gastrointestinal irritation after large oral doses. Occasional cases of cataract formation in man have been reported, and similar effects have been seen experimentally in dogs. In some patients with chronic renal infection, exacerbation may occur, but renal damage in otherwise-normal individuals has not been demonstrated even after 2 years of deferoxamine therapy.

Preparations and Dosage. *Sterile Deferoxamine Mesylate,* U.S.P. (DESFERAL MESYLATE), is available in 5-ml ampuls containing 500 mg. The recommended dose in acute oral iron poisoning is 8 g by nasogastric tube, followed by the parenteral procedures described below. For the mobilization of iron from storage sites the intramuscular route is preferred, unless the patient is in shock. Initially, for *adults and children,* 1 g is given, followed by 500 mg every 4 hours for 2 doses. The injections of 500 mg may be continued at 4- or 12-hour intervals, depending on the clinical response, but the total amount of drug administered should not exceed 6 g in 24 hours. The intravenous route is required in patients in shock. The dosage schedule and limitations are the same as those indicated for the intramuscular route. However, *the infusion rate must never exceed 15 mg/kg per hour.* As soon as the clinical situation permits, intravenous administration should be discontinued and the drug given intramuscularly. For iron-storage diseases, the dosage and the frequency of administration must be tailored to the individual patient, depending on the severity of the disease and the rate of urinary iron excretion.

CHELATING AGENTS AND RADIO-ACTIVE METAL MOBILIZATION

The widespread production and use of radioactive metals have generated a unique medical problem in dealing with cases of accidental poisoning by such metals. Since their toxicity is almost entirely a consequence of ionizing radiation, the therapeutic objective in these cases is not just the chelation of the metals but their removal from the body as rapidly and completely as possible. Two of the most important radioactive metals, radium and strontium, have defied attempts in this direction. This is due primarily to the properties of these elements, which resemble closely those of calcium. Thus, the administration of a calcium chelate results in very little replacement of the calcium within the chelate by the toxic metal, as would occur, for example, with lead.

Plutonium exerts its toxic effects mainly in the bone as soluble ^{239}Pu, or in the lungs and gastrointestinal tract as insoluble ^{239}Pu. DTPA has thus far proven to be the most effective agent for promoting the removal of ^{239}Pu (Rosenthal and Lindenbaum, 1967; Bair and Thompson, 1974). The urinary excretion is enhanced 50- to 100-fold by intravenous DTPA in both animals and man. One gram of DTPA administered by slow intravenous drip on alternate days three times a week for 3 weeks has proven to be an effective dosage schedule. As is seen commonly with heavy-metal poisoning, the effectiveness of treatment diminishes very rapidly with an increased time lag between exposure and beginning of therapy. Oral administration of DTPA is only about 10% as effective as the intravenous route. In mice exposed to ^{239}Pu, prevention of tumor development and ultimate survival are closely related to promotion of ^{239}Pu excretion during treatment with DTPA.

Other homologs, TTHA (triethylenetetraminehexaacetic acid) and TPHA (tetraethylenepentaamineheptaacetic acid), have been tested experimentally in the treatment of poisoning by plutonium, radiocerium, radioyttrium, radioruthenium, and americium. However, none has exhibited substantial advantages over DTPA with regard to promotion of urinary excretion of the metals or to increasing survival after exposure.

The use of ferri-ferrocyanide to promote the excretion of ^{137}Co has shown some promise experimentally, but more clinical experience is required to establish efficacy.

Adams, D. A.; Goodman, R.; Maxwell, M. H.; and Latta, H. Nephrotic syndrome associated with penicillamine therapy of Wilson's disease. *Am. J. Med.,* **1964,** *36,* 330–336.

Ahrens, F. A., and Aronson, A. L. A comparative study of the toxic effects of calcium and chromium chelates of ethylenediaminetetraacetate in the dog. *Toxicol. appl. Pharmac.,* **1971,** *18,* 10–25.

Altman, J.; Wakim, K. G.; and Winkelmann, R. K. Effects of edathamil disodium on the kidney. *J. invest. Derm.,* **1962,** *38,* 215–218.

Aposhian, H. V. Biochemical and pharmacological properties of the metal-binding agent penicillamine. *Fedn Proc. Fedn Am. Socs exp. Biol.,* **1961,** *20,* Suppl. 10, 185–188.

Aposhian, H. V., and Aposhian, M. M. N-acetyl-DL-penicillamine, a new oral protective agent against the lethal effects of mercuric chloride. *J. Pharmac. exp. Ther.,* **1959,** *126,* 131–135.

Barron, E. S. G.; Miller, Z. B.; and Meyer, J. The effect of 2:3-dimercaptopropanol on the activity of enzymes and on the metabolism of tissues. *Biochem. J.,* **1947,** *41,* 78–82.

Boyd, P. R. The treatment of tetraethyl lead poisoning. *Lancet,* **1957,** *1,* 181–185.

Castellino, N., and Aloj, S. Effects of calcium sodium ethylenediaminetetra-acetate on the kinetics of distribution and excretion of lead in the rat. *Br. J. ind. Med.,* **1965,** *22,* 172–180.

Chenoweth, M. B. The cardiovascular actions of 2,3-dimercaptopropanol. *J. Pharmac. exp. Ther.,* **1946,** *87,* 41–54.

Chisolm, J. J., Jr. Treatment of lead poisoning. *Mod. Treat.,* **1967,** *4,* 710–727.

Current, J. V.; Hales, I. B.; and Dobyns, B. M. The effect of 2,3-dimercaptopropanol (BAL) on thyroid function. *J. clin. Endocr. Metab.,* **1960,** *20,* 13–20.

Doolan, P. D.; Schwartz, S. L.; Hayes, J. R.; Mullen, J. C.; and Cummings, N. B. An evaluation of the nephrotoxicity of ethylenediaminetetraacetate and diethylenetriaminepentaacetate in the rat. *Toxicol. appl. Pharmac.,* **1967,** *10,* 481–500.

Dudley, H. R.; Ritchie, A. C.; Schilling, A.; and Baker, W. H. Pathologic changes associated with the use of sodium ethylene diamine tetraacetate in the treatment of hypercalcemia. *New Engl. J. Med.,* **1955,** *252,* 331–337.

Elsas, L. J.; Hayslett, J. P.; Spargo, B. H.; Durant, J. L.; and Rosenberg, L. E. Wilson's disease with reversible renal tubular dysfunction. Correlation with proximal tubular ultrastructure. *Ann. intern. Med.,* **1971,** *75,* 427–433.

Erdos, E. G., and Wohler, J. R. Inhibitors of the *in vivo* enzymatic inactivation of bradykinin and kallidin. *Life Sci.,* **1963,** *4,* 270–274.

Foreman, H. The pharmacology of some useful chelating agents. In, *Metal-Binding in Medicine.* (Seven, M. J., ed.) J. B. Lippincott Co., Philadelphia, **1960.**

Foreman, H.; Finnegan, C.; and Lushbaugh, C. C. Nephrotoxic hazard from uncontrolled edathamil calcium disodium therapy. *J. Am. med. Ass.,* **1956,** *160,* 1042–1046.

Foreman, H., and Trujillo, T. T. The metabolism of C14-labeled ethylenediaminetetraacetic acid in human beings. *J. Lab. clin. Med.,* **1954,** *43,* 566–571.

Foreman, H.; Vier, M.; and Magee, M. The metabolism of C14-labeled ethylenediaminetetraacetic acid in the rat. *J. biol. Chem.,* **1953,** *203,* 1045–1053.

Forland, M.; Pullman, T. N.; Lavender, A. R.; and Aho, I. The renal excretion of ethylenediaminetetraacetate in the dog. *J. Pharmac. exp. Ther.,* **1966,** *153,* 142–147.

Forster, W.; Herrmann, C.; Scharf, J. H.; and Ehrenbrand, F. Korrelation zwischen Stoffwechsel-, Schilddrüsen- und Hypophysenveranderungen bei Ratten nach chronischer Verabreichung von NaJ, BAL und Methionin. *Naunyn-Schmiedebergs Arch. exp. Path. Pharmak.,* **1955,** *225,* 195–209.

Gilman, A.; Allen, R. P.; Philips, F. S.; and St. John, E. The treatment of acute systemic mercury poisoning in experimental animals with BAL, thiosorbitol and BAL glucoside. *J. clin. Invest.,* **1946a,** *25,* 549–556.

Gilman, A.; Philips, F. S.; Allen, R. P.; and Koelle, E. The treatment of acute cadmium intoxication in rabbits with 2,3-dimercaptopropanol (BAL) and other mercaptans. *J. Pharmac. exp. Ther.,* **1946b,** *87,* Suppl., 85–101.

Goldberg, A.; Smith, J. A.; and Lochhead, A. C. Treatment of lead-poisoning with oral penicillamine. *Br. med. J.,* **1963,** *1,* 1270–1275.

Hammond, P. B. The effects of chelating agents on the tissue distribution and excretion of lead. *Toxicol. appl. Pharmac.,* **1971,** *18,* 296–310.

——. The effects of D-penicillamine on the tissue distribution and excretion of lead. *Ibid,* **1973,** *26,* 241–246.

Harris, C. E. C. A comparison of intravenous calcium disodium versenate and oral penicillamine in promoting elimination of lead. *Can. med. Ass. J.,* **1958,** *79,* 664–666.

Heddle, J. G.; McHenry, E. W.; and Beaton, G. H. Penicillamine and vitamin B_6 interrelationships in the rat. *Can. J. Biochem. Physiol.,* **1963,** *41,* 1215–1222.

Hitchcock, P. Effect of dithiols and other enzyme inhibitors on blood vessels. *J. Pharmac. exp. Ther.,* **1946,** *87,* 55–59.

Jacobs, J.; Greene, H.; and Gendel, B. R. Acute iron intoxication. *New Engl. J. Med.,* **1965,** *273,* 1124–1127.

Johnson, L. A., and Seven, M. J. Observations on the *in vivo* stability of metal chelates. In, *Metal-Binding in Medicine.* (Seven, M. J., ed.) J. B. Lippincott Co., Philadelphia, **1960.**

Kaiser, W., and Ponsold, W. Über eine Möglichkeit zur Diagnose der relativen Nebenschilddrüseninsuffizienz durch Infusion von Aethylendiamintetraacetat (ADTA). *Klin. Wschr.,* **1959,** *37,* 1183–1185.

Leikin, S.; Vossough, P.; and Mochir-Fatemi, F. Chelation therapy in acute iron poisoning. *J. Pediat.,* **1967,** *71,* 425–430.

MacDonald, W. B., and Fellers, F. X. Penicillamine in the treatment of patients with cystinuria. *J. Am. med. Ass.,* **1966,** *197,* 396–402.

Mehbod, H. Treatment of lead intoxication: combined use of peritoneal dialysis and edetate calcium disodium. *J. Am. med. Ass.,* **1967,** *201,* 972–976.

Multicentre Trial Group. Controlled trial of D(−) penicillamine in severe rheumatoid arthritis. *Lancet,* **1973,** *1,* 275–280.

Perry, H. M., and Perry, E. F. Normal concentrations of some trace metals in human urine: change produced by ethylenediaminetetraacetate. *J. clin. Invest.,* **1959,** *38,* 1452–1463.

Peters, R. A., and Stocken, L. A. Preparation and pharmacological properties of 4-hydroxymethyl-2-(3′-amino-4′-hydroxyphenyl)-1:3-dithia-2-arsacyclopentane (MAPHARSIDE–BAL compound). *Biochem. J.,* **1947,** *41,* 53–56.

Popovici, A.; Geshickter, C. F.; Reinosky, A.; and Rubin, M. Experimental control of serum calcium levels *in vivo.* *Proc. Soc. exp. Biol. Med.,* **1950,** *74,* 415–417.

Roche e Silva, M. The physiological significance of bradykinin. *Ann. N.Y. Acad. Sci.,* **1963,** *104,* 190–210.

Rosenberg, L. E., and Hayslett, J. P. Nephrotoxic effects of penicillamine in cystinuria. *J. Am. med. Ass.,* **1967,** *201,* 698–699.

Rosenthal, M. W., and Lindenbaum, A. Influence of DTPA therapy on long-term effects of retained monomeric plutonium: comparison with polymeric plutonium. *Radiat. Res.,* **1967,** *31,* 506–521.

Schwartz, S. L.; Johnson, C. B.; and Doolan, P. D. Studies on the mechanism of renal vaculogenesis induced in the rat by ethylenediaminetetraacetate. Comparison of the cellular activities of calcium and chromium chelates. *Molec. Pharmac.,* **1970,** *6,* 54–60.

Selander, S. Treatment of lead poisoning: effects of sodium calcium edetate ($CaNa_2EDTA$) and penicillamine administered orally and intravenously. *Br. J. ind. Med.,* **1967,** *24,* 272–282.

Soffer, A., and Toribara, T. Changes in serum and spinal fluid calcium effected by disodium ethylenediaminetetraacetate. *J. Lab. clin. Med.,* **1961,** *58,* 542–547.

Spencer, H. Studies on the effect of chelating agents in man. *Ann. N.Y. Acad. Sci.,* **1960,** *88,* 435–449.

Spencer, H.; Vankinscott, V.; Lewin, I.; and Laszlo, D. Removal of calcium in man by ethylenediamine tetraacetic acid. A metabolic study. *J. clin. Invest.,* **1952,** *31,* 1023–1027.

Sternlieb, I., and Scheinberg, I. H. Penicillamine therapy for hepatolenticular degeneration. *J. Am. med. Ass.,* **1964,** *189,* 748–754.

Stowers, J. M.; Michie, W.; and Frazer, S. C. A critical evaluation of the trisodium-edetate test for hypothyroidism after thyroidectomy. *Lancet,* **1967,** *1,* 124–127.

Teisinger, J.; Lustinec, K.; and Srbová, J. Effect of edathamil calcium-disodium on retention of lead in the liver. *A.M.A. Archs ind. Hlth,* **1958,** *17,* 302–306.

Tu, J.; Blackwell, R. Q.; and Lee, P. DL-Penicillamine as a cause of optic axial neuritis. *J. Am. med. Ass.,* **1963,** *185,* 83–86.

Webb, E. C., and Van Heyningen, R. The action of British antilewisite on enzyme systems. *Biochem. J.,* **1947,** *41,* 74–78.

Whitaker, J. A.; Austin, W.; and Nelson, J. D. Edathamil calcium disodium (VERSENATE) diagnostic test for lead poisoning. *Pediatrics, Springfield,* **1962,** *29,* 384–388.

Monographs and Reviews

Bair, W. J., and Thompson, R. C. Plutonium: biomedical research. *Science, Wash.,* **1974,** *183,* 715–722.

Chaberek, S., and Martell, A. E. *Organic Sequestering Agents.* John Wiley & Sons, Inc., New York, **1959.**

Chenoweth, M. B. Chelation as a mechanism of pharmacological action. *Pharmac. Rev.,* **1956,** *8,* 57–87.

———. Clinical uses of metal-binding drugs. *Clin. Pharmac. Ther.,* **1968,** *9,* 365–387.

Dwyer, F. P., and Mellor, D. P. (eds.). *Chelating Agents and Metal Chelates.* Academic Press, Inc., New York, **1964.**

Pullman, T. N.; Lavender, A. R.; and Forland, M. Synthetic chelating agents in clinical medicine. *A. Rev. Med.,* **1963,** *14,* 175–194.

Seven, M. J. (ed.). *Metal-Binding in Medicine.* J. B. Lippincott Co., Philadelphia, **1960.**

Soffer, A. *Chelation Therapy.* Charles C Thomas, Pub., Springfield, Ill., **1964.**

Stocken, L. A., and Thompson, R. H. S. Reactions of British antilewisite with arsenic and other metals in living systems. *Physiol. Rev.,* **1949,** *29,* 168–194.

CHAPTER

46 HEAVY METALS

Stewart C. Harvey

At one time the heavy metals occupied a prominent place in the therapeutic armamentarium. They were also formerly of major toxicological importance. However, medical interest in heavy metals has decreased greatly, owing to their replacement by more efficacious and safer synthetic and natural antimicrobial drugs and to public health and hygienic preventive measures against poisoning from their industrial use. Nevertheless, environmental concerns have contributed to the surprisingly active continuing research and literature on the toxicology of certain heavy metals. Except for gold, the valid therapeutic uses of the metals are presented elsewhere (*see* Index).

General Considerations. Although the so-called heavy metals vary widely in their physical, chemical, and biological properties, they share the common property of forming stable coordination complexes with a variety of ligands. They tend to form more stable complexes with sulfur and nitrogen than with oxygen. Although most heavy metals are known to exert biological effects through combination with sulfhydryl groups, they can also combine with other groups, especially in chelate configurations. For example, mercury and silver can combine with amino, imidazole, phosphate, and carboxylate as well as sulfhydryl groups, and lead can combine with phosphate and carboxylate groups. The biological properties of the metals must be sought in the stability, stereochemistry, and magnetic susceptibility of their complexes.

As with other drugs, there often is no correlation between the metal-induced alterations of function of various organs and the concentration of metal therein. Equally important is the metabolic demand of a tissue or the sensitivity of its metabolic systems to disruption. Thus, several heavy metals exert toxic effects on rapidly proliferating tissues such as the gastrointestinal mucosa and bone marrow and on highly specialized cells such as neurons and renal tubular cells. The rapid rate of proliferation of many metal-susceptible pathogenic microorganisms may also explain, in part, the selectivity of heavy-metal agents for the pathogen rather than for the host.

ARSENIC

Arsenic was known as a therapeutic agent to the ancient Greeks and Romans. It has been a classical poison. The history and folklore of arsenic prompted intensive studies by the early pharmacologists. Indeed, the foundations of many of the modern concepts of chemotherapy derive from Ehrlich's early work with the organic arsenicals. The advent of penicillin disposed of antiluetic arsenicals, and other newer drugs have nearly eclipsed the use of other organic arsenicals. In current human therapeutics, arsenicals are of importance only in the treatment of certain tropical diseases. In the United States, the future impact of arsenic on health will be more from industrial and environmental than from medicinal exposure. Interesting reviews of the biological, toxicological, and environmental significance of arsenic have been written by Vallee and associates (1960), Buchanan (1962), Schroeder (1966), Frost (1967), and Lisella and coworkers (1972).

General Considerations. *Chemistry.* The arsenicals may be grouped into inorganic and organic compounds. This classification is partly one of chemical convenience, but the inorganic arsenicals differ from the organic compounds in several important pharmacological respects.

Arsenic trioxide (As_2O_3, often called arsenous acid) is the anhydride of meta-arsenous acid ($HAsO_2$). Nearly all the trivalent inorganic arsenicals can be regarded as salts of meta-arsenous acid. Potassium arsenite was once used promiscuously in medicine. Sodium arsenite, calcium arsenite, copper acetoarsenite (Paris green), and cupric arsenite are employed mainly as insecticides, rodenticides, fungicides, and herbicides. The arsenates ($RAsO_3$) of lead, calcium, and sodium, still used in old formulations of insecticides, are of occasional toxicological interest, as is the parent arsenic pentoxide, used as an herbicide and a defoliant. Arsenic trichloride once enjoyed sporadic use as a substitute for potassium arsenite. Cacodyl, $(CH_3)_2AsAs(CH_3)_2$, and sodium cacodylate, $Na(CH_3)_2AsO_2$, have been classified as inorganic arsenicals because their active form is arsenous acid, to which most of cacodyl is converted in the body. Arsine (AsH_3) is a poisonous gas that is responsible for occasional industrial intoxications. Dimethyl arsine, dimethyl arsinic acid, $(CH_3)_2AsOH$, and methyl arsonic acid, $CH_3AsO(OH)$, as well as their sodium and ammonium salts, occur as biotically formed environmental contaminants and are also used as herbicides.

The major organic arsenicals are derivatives of benzene arsonic acid, $C_6H_5As:O(OH)_2$. Three such pentavalent derivatives are used in medicine: *carbarsone* (4-ureidobenzenearsonic acid), *tryparsamide* (sodium N-carbamylmethyl-*p*-aminobenzenearsonate), and *glycobiarsol* (*see* Index). Benzene arsonic acid and its para-nitro and para-amino derivatives are used in feeds in hog and chicken husbandry. The benzene arsenicals are quite stable with respect to the carbon-arsenic bond and are not converted *in vivo* to inorganic arsenic compounds.

The presence or absence of various substituents on the benzene ring determines not only the solubility of the drug but also its ability to penetrate cell membranes, both of parasitic organisms and of the host. Selectivity is achieved by substituting appropriate groups. Organic arsenicals without highly polar groups are lipid soluble and readily penetrate skin; such compounds usually have a vesicant action.

Trivalent vs. Pentavalent Arsenic. Regardless of whether an arsenical is introduced into the body as trivalent or pentavalent arsenic, all the major toxic and antimicrobial actions can be attributed to the trivalent form. Some pentavalent arsenicals are partly reduced *in vivo* to the active trivalent form, an arsenoxide (R·As:O). However, the redox equilibria *in vivo* favor oxidation, and trivalent arsenic is slowly oxidized in the body to pentavalent arsenic. The low toxicity and high recovery of pentavalent arsenicals in urine and excreta indicate that very little reduction takes place. The pentavalent organic arsenicals, all of which manifest anionic character in body fluids, appear to penetrate the cells of the host less readily than the cells of the susceptible parasite and thus have a higher therapeutic index than do the trivalent forms.

Mechanism of Action. The major toxic action of arsenicals on parasites and the host is one of inhibition of sulfhydryl enzymes. Trivalent organic arsenicals, such as phenylarsenoxide, are more potent inhibitors of representative sulfhydryl enzymes than are inorganic arsenites. The arsenoxide moiety of arsenicals or an active intermediate is not known to combine significantly with any chemical group other than sulfhydryl. Arsenocompounds, such as arsphenamine, and pentavalent arsenicals must be converted to the arsenoxide in the host or parasite before they can act. The general formulation of a complete reaction of an arsenoxide or arsenite with the sulfhydryl of protein is

$$R-As{=}O + 2\,HS-Pr \longrightarrow R-As\Big\langle{}^{S-Pr}_{S-Pr} + H-O-H$$

where R is any group and Pr is protein. The inactivation of essential sulfhydryl enzymes is probably the first step in cell damage. The pyruvate oxidase system and a large number of other enzymes are susceptible to arsenic. The role of arsenical interaction with thioctic (α-lipoic) acid, an essential participant in the pyruvate decarboxylation reaction, is of special interest. Rather than reacting with sulfhydryls of two different molecules, as depicted in the formula above, arsenic can react with both sulfhydryl groups of thioctic acid to form a six-membered ring. Such rings are more stable than noncyclic thioarsenites. Ring formation accounts for the efficacy of dimercaprol in the treatment of arsenic poisoning (*see* Chapter 45).

The selectivity of organic arsenicals for the parasite and not the mammalian host probably derives from several causes. Firstly, arsenoxides may be able to penetrate into the parasite more readily than into mammalian tissue cells. Secondly, the sulfhydryl enzymes of the susceptible parasite may be more sensitive or rate limiting than those of the nonsusceptible parasites or the host. Arsenic-sensitive trypanosomes have very simple metabolic schemes, almost without shunts or convergent pathways, so that inhibition at a single point may prevent nearly all energy production or high-energy phosphorylation. Furthermore, they have a very high metabolic demand, and metabolism probably needs to proceed nearly at capacity. Thirdly, mammalian tissue may oxidize the intracellular arsenical to the inactive arsonic acid more readily than does the parasite. Some species of trypanosomes are virtually devoid of aerobic metabolic systems and thus lack the necessary enzymatic apparatus to oxidize the trivalent form of the arsenical.

Some parasites, especially trypanosomes, become resistant to organic arsenicals. The mechanism of resistance appears to be that of decreased permeability to the arsenical in question. Resistance to one arsenical does not necessarily confer resistance to another, yet it may confer resistance to a nonarsenical. The structure of the organic portion of the molecule appears to be most important.

Arsenate ion is capable of uncoupling phosphorylation through the formation of unstable arsenate esters in lieu of certain phosphate esters that are normally oxidized to high-energy phosphate donors. The importance of this action in animals is unknown. Arsine (AsH_3) combines with hemoglobin and is oxidized to a hemolytic compound that does not appear to act by sulfhydryl inhibition.

PHARMACOLOGICAL AND TOXICOLOGICAL PROPERTIES

Local Effects. Both inorganic and organic arsenicals can penetrate the epithelium and cause necrosis and sloughing. The more water-soluble compounds are the least toxic locally. Tryparsamide, a pentavalent organic arsenical that is generally given intramuscularly, does not cause local irritation; it is soluble and is rapidly absorbed.

Nonallergic contact dermatitis and conjunctivitis are frequent among workers exposed to arsenic-containing dusts. Continued inhalation of arsenical dusts can cause perforation of the nasal septum.

Systemic Effects. *Circulation.* Small doses of *inorganic* arsenic induce mild vasodilatation. Large doses evoke pronounced effects on the circulatory system. Injury may occur in all capillary beds, but is most pronounced in the splanchnic area. It results in the transudation of plasma and a sharp diminution in blood volume. Later, arteriolar and myocardial damage occurs, and the blood pressure falls to shock levels. ECG abnormalities may persist for months after recovery from acute intoxication.

In large doses, the trivalent *organic* arsenicals especially affect the capillaries, resistance vessels, and the heart much as do the inorganic arsenicals. In therapeutic doses, circulatory effects vary with the drug. Rarely, a rapidly developing angioneurotic shocklike reaction follows the intravenous administration of tryparsamide. It occurs too promptly to be attributable to the arsenic moiety. Sympathomimetics effectively elevate the blood pressure during such a crisis, whereas they do not do so during shock from inorganic arsenic. The crisis has been attributed to flocculation of plasma proteins.

Peripheral arteriosclerosis ("blackfoot disease") can result from chronic ingestion of inorganic arsenicals (Heydorn, 1970).

Gastrointestinal Tract. Small doses of *inorganic* arsenicals, especially the trivalent ones, cause mild splanchnic hyperemia. The capillary transudation of plasma resulting from larger doses forms vesicles under the gastrointestinal mucosa. The vesicles eventually rupture, epithelial fragments slough off, and plasma is discharged into the lumen, where it coagulates. Tissue damage and the bulk cathartic action of the increased fluid in the lumen lead to increased peristalsis and the passage of the characteristic "rice-water" stools. The normal proliferation of the epithelium is suppressed, which accentuates the damage. Soon the feces become bloody. Vomiting also frequently occurs, and the vomitus may be bloody. Stomatitis may also occur. The onset of gastrointestinal symptoms may be so gradual that the possibility of arsenic poisoning may be overlooked.

A syndrome of nausea, vomiting, diarrhea, headache, and malaise represents the most frequent type of reaction to the intravenous injection of *organic* arsenicals. The reaction is not immediate, but occurs 4 to 12 hours after injection and lasts from a few hours to several days. It is due to intoxication by the active arsenic moiety of the drug; the incidence is highest after trivalent arsenicals, and lowest after pentavalent arsenicals such as tryparsamide. Large overdoses of organic arsenicals elicit effects similar to those of inorganic arsenicals.

Urinary Tract. The action of arsenic on the renal capillaries, tubules, and glomeruli may cause severe renal damage. The first effect is on the glomeruli. The vessels dilate, allow the escape of protein, and swell to fill the glomerular capsule. Varying degrees of tubular necrosis and degeneration occur. The urine is scant and contains protein, red blood cells, and casts. A few casts, mild albuminuria, and a slight increase in blood urea frequently occur on the day following administration of therapeutic doses of *organic* arsenicals, but the effects are only temporary. Acute renal injury from organic arsenicals is a rare idiosyncrasy.

Skin. Chronic ingestion of low doses of *inorganic* arsenicals causes cutaneous vasodilatation and a "milk and roses" complexion. Prolonged use of arsenic, however, also causes hyperkeratosis and hyperpigmentation. Eventually these actions proceed to atrophy and degeneration, and possibly also to cancer. Skin eruptions are common after inorganic arsenic medication. Systemic trivalent arsenicals interfere with the inflammatory response in skin and favor the occurrence of pyoderma. They also interfere with wound healing in skin and other tissues (Stone, 1969). The incidence of dermatitides from presently used pentavalent *organic* arsenicals is low,

and the reactions are usually mild. The lesions may be localized or generalized in distribution.

Central Nervous System. Chronic use or exposure to inorganic but rarely to organic arsenicals may cause peripheral neuritis. In severe cases, the spinal cord may also be involved. After acute ingestion of toxic doses of inorganic arsenic, approximately 5% of persons will show central depression without gastrointestinal symptoms. Of the arsenicals still used in man, tryparsamide, but not carbarsone or glycobiarsol, causes a high incidence of effects on the central nervous system (CNS) when used in therapeutic doses. These effects are primarily visual. The specific changes and their therapeutic implication are described in Chapter 54.

Encephalopathy is the most common type of toxic response to trivalent organic arsenicals, such as melarsoprol. Of the pentavalent organic arsenicals, glycobiarsol in clinical doses occasionally causes encephalopathy. However, overdoses of carbarsone may also do so. Symptoms include severe headache, high fever, convulsions, and coma. Premonitory signs are increases in the cell count and protein content of the spinal fluid. The cerebral lesions are mainly vascular in origin and occur in both the gray and white matter; characteristic multiple, symmetrical foci of hemorrhagic necrosis occur. In addition to dimercaprol, treatment consists in sedation, anticonvulsant therapy, and measures designed to reduce cerebral edema, such as intravenous injection of hypertonic mannitol or urea solution.

Blood. *Inorganic* arsenicals affect the bone marrow and alter the cellular composition of the blood. The vascularity of the bone marrow is increased. Moderate doses of arsenic lower the erythrocyte count and large amounts cause morphological changes with the appearance of megalocytes and microcytes. Inorganic arsenicals also suppress production of leukocytes. Some of the chronic hematological effects may result from impairment of absorption of folic acid (Van Tongeran *et al.,* 1965). Arsenites also interfere with porphyrin synthesis. Blood and bone-marrow disturbances from *organic* arsenicals are extremely serious, but fortunately they are rare. A few cases of agranulocytosis have been reported to be caused by glycobiarsol.

Liver. Inorganic arsenicals and a number of now-obsolete organic arsenicals are particularly toxic to the liver and produce fatty infiltration, central necrosis, and cirrhosis; tryparsamide may induce hepatic damage in therapeutic doses. The damage may be mild or so severe that acute yellow atrophy and death ensue. The injury is generally to the hepatic parenchyma, but in some cases the clinical picture may closely resemble occlusion of the common bile duct, the principal lesions being pericholangitis and bile thrombi in the finer biliary radicles.

Metabolic Effects. The early toxic actions of inorganic arsenicals give rise to occult edema due to capillary damage and may be mistaken for a gain in weight, which was once misinterpreted as a "tonic" effect. In arsenic poisoning, nitrogen elimination is increased because extensive tissue degeneration occurs in many organs. Attempts to demonstrate a tonic action of arsenic in animals have shown that the element is detrimental to natural growth and development.

Absorption, Distribution, and Elimination. Water-soluble arsenicals are absorbed from all mucous membranes and parenteral sites of administration. The absorption of poorly soluble arsenicals, such as As_2O_3, is greatly dependent upon the fineness of subdivision. In preemergence herbicides, especially, the As_2O_3 is rather coarsely divided. Although pentavalent arsenicals are more highly ionized than the trivalent compounds, the pentavalent inorganic arsenicals are better absorbed than the trivalent, probably because they react less with the intestinal contents and mucosa. The trivalent organic arsenicals, except for melarsoprol, are likewise poorly absorbed from the gastrointestinal tract. They are, however, partially degraded in the intestine, and the resulting inorganic arsenic is readily absorbed. The pentavalent arsenicals are absorbed to varying extents. Carbarsone and melarsoprol are sufficiently absorbed that they have been given by the oral route in the treatment of appropriate systemic infections; in the case of carbarsone there is enough unabsorbed drug to be effective against intraintestinal parasites. Tryparsamide is poorly absorbed from the enteric tract. Absorption through the skin is a function of lipid solubility; in general, trivalent are better absorbed than pentavalent arsenicals. Arsenic compounds can be absorbed through the lungs.

In the United States, the daily intake of arsenic varies widely but averages about 1 mg per day. The body burden in normal adults is usually 14 to 21 mg. The distribution of arsenic depends upon the rate of administration and the particular arsenical involved. Arsenic is stored mainly in liver, kidney, wall of the gastrointestinal tract, spleen, and lung. Much smaller amounts are present in muscle and nervous tissue. Because of the high sulfhydryl content of keratin, high concentrations of arsenic are found in the hair and nails. Deposition in the hair starts within 2 weeks after administration, and arsenic stays fixed at this site for years. It is also deposited in bone and retained there for long periods.

Little is known about the biotransformations of arsenicals in man. From studies in animals it seems probable that trivalent arsenicals are gradually converted to pentavalent forms and that both trivalent and pentavalent forms are partly converted to methylarsenates.

The fraction of a dose of trivalent arsenical that is absorbed is slowly excreted in the urine. After parenteral administration, excretion starts within 2 to 8 hours, but it may take 10 days for complete elimination of arsenic after a single dose and up to 70 days after repeated administration. This slow excretion is the basis for the cumulative toxic action of arsenic. Arsenate and other pentavalent forms are so rapidly excreted in man that very little accumulates unless very large doses are given over a period of time. Lisella and coworkers (1972) have calculated that pentavalent arsenicals taken continually in the maximal allowable concentrations (United States federal regulations) in food and from air and water would require more than 30 years to accumulate a toxic body burden. In spite of the fact that trivalent arsenic is probably oxidized in the tissues and that pentavalent forms are rapidly excreted, arsenate appears to be reabsorbed by the proximal renal tubule and reexcreted as arsenite (Ginsburg, 1965).

Inorganic Arsenic Poisoning. Federal restrictions on the allowable arsenic content in food and in the occupational environment not only have improved safety procedures and decreased the number of intoxications but also have decreased the amount of arsenic in use; only the annual production of arsenic-containing herbicides is increasing.

The incidence of accidental, homicidal, and suicidal arsenic poisoning has greatly diminished in recent decades. From 1949 through 1967 only 140 cases of arsenic poisoning were reported to the National Clearinghouse for Poison Control Centers and the Pesticide Division of the United States Department of Agriculture. Because inorganic arsenical medication is obsolete and organic arsenical use is nearly so, iatrogenic arsenic poisoning is now rare in the United States.

The acute toxic dose of an arsenical varies greatly, depending upon the compound and the physical form. For sodium arsenite in man it ranges from 5 to 50 mg, and the lowest lethal dose is reported to be 128 mg. This is more than ten times as toxic as most As_2O_3 in commercial herbicidal products, but fine pulverization can considerably decrease the toxic dose of the oxide. The toxicity of As_2O_5 in the pellet size marketed in herbicides is about that of commercial As_2O_3; however, the substance is inherently more toxic, owing to a much greater water solubility. The acute toxicity and mortality rates from the lead and calcium arsenates are less than half those of As_2O_3. Commercial methylarsonates are roughly twice as toxic as the As_2O_3 in herbicides (*see* Done and Peart, 1971).

Gastrointestinal discomfort is usually experienced within an hour after an arsenical is taken, although it may be delayed by as much as 12 hours after oral ingestion if food is in the stomach. Burning lips, constriction of the throat, and difficulty in swallowing may be the first symptoms to appear, followed by excruciating gastric pain, projectile vomiting, and diarrhea. The urine is scanty, albuminous, and bloody, and eventually anuria may occur. The patient often complains of marked skeletal muscle cramps and severe thirst. As the loss of fluid proceeds, symptoms of shock appear. Hypoxic convulsions may occur terminally, and coma and death ensue. In severe poisoning, death can occur within an hour, but the usual interval is 24 hours.

In the nervous system form of acute arsenic intoxication, headache, vertigo, restlessness, irritability, loss of memory, stupor, and coma may occur without gastrointestinal symptoms. Muscle contractions and atrophy, incoordination, and blurred and flickering vision are potential sequelae.

Chronic Arsenic Poisoning. The most common early signs of chronic arsenic poisoning are *diarrhea, skin pigmentation* (especially of the neck, eyelids, nipples, and axillae), *hyperkeratosis,* and *circum-*

scribed edema, especially of the lower eyelids, face, and ankles. Other signs and symptoms that should arouse suspicion of arsenic poisoning include garlic odor of the breath and perspiration, excessive salivation and sweating, stomatitis, generalized itching, sore throat, coryza, lacrimation, numbness, burning or tingling of the extremities, dermatitis, vitiligo, and alopecia. Poisoning may begin insidiously with symptoms of weakness, languor, anorexia, occasional nausea and vomiting, and diarrhea or constipation. Subsequent symptoms may simulate an acute coryza. Dermatitis and keratosis of the palms and soles are common features. Desquamation and scaling of the skin may initiate an exfoliative process involving many epithelial structures of the body. The liver may enlarge, and obstruction of the bile ducts may result in jaundice. Eventually cirrhosis may occur from the hepatotoxic action. The renal glomeruli and tubules are damaged.

As intoxication advances, encephalopathy may develop. Peripheral neuritis results in motor and sensory paralysis of the extremities; usually the legs are more severely affected than the arms, in contrast to lead palsy.

The bone marrow is seriously injured by arsenic. All elements of the myeloid tissue may be depressed, and aplastic anemia is the hematopoietic disorder most often encountered.

Arsine gas, generated by electrolytic or metallic reduction of arsenic in metal products, is a cause of rare industrial intoxication. Arsine is bound to erythrocytes, rendering the red blood cells exceedingly fragile, and massive hemolysis occurs if the exposure is sufficient. A few hours after exposure, headache, anorexia, vomiting, paresthesia, abdominal pains, chills, hematemesis, hemoglobinuria, bilirubinemia, and anuria occur. Jaundice appears after 24 hours. Death results from renal failure. Treatment is that for an acute massive hemolysis. Dimercaprol is not effective. The signs, symptoms, and treatment of chronic arsine poisoning are those of anemia.

Treatment of Poisoning. In the event of *acute arsenic poisoning,* dimercaprol in oil should be administered intramuscularly at the earliest possible opportunity. If poisoning is severe, single doses as high as 5 mg/kg should be given at 4-hour intervals during the first 24 hours. Thereafter, the dose may be decreased and the interval between injections prolonged. The duration of the therapeutic regimen should be determined by the status of the patient. Because treatment with dimercaprol is relatively innocuous, a short course (6 doses of 2.5 mg/kg at 4-hour intervals) can be given whenever arsenic poisoning is suspected. In addition to dimercaprol, copious gastric lavage and saline cathartics should be given if the poison was taken orally, particularly if powdered arsenic was ingested, because this material may remain in the stomach for some time. Efforts should be directed as soon as possible toward repair of fluid and electrolyte deficits. Morphine is of great value in controlling pain. Further symptomatic treatment is instituted as indicated but is usually unnecessary if therapy with dimercaprol is prompt and adequate.

Dimercaprol is also generally effective in the treatment of *chronic poisoning* by either inorganic or organic arsenicals. Clinical improvement may occur in 1 to 3 days, and recovery is the rule within 1 to 3 weeks, depending on the organ or system involved. However, if damage has become irreversible, as with aplastic anemia, advanced encephalopathy, and most cases of jaundice, the removal of arsenic from the system is of little help. Chronic intoxication should be treated with prolonged courses of dimercaprol. An exacerbation of symptoms following an initial course of therapy demands the prompt initiation of a second course. Glucocorticoids may be indicated if dermatitis or conjunctivitis exists. (For details of the pharmacology and dosage of dimercaprol, *see* Chapter 45.)

Teratogenesis and Carcinogenesis. Arsenic causes chromosomal breaks in cultured human leukocytes and teratism in hamsters, but whether such effects occur in man is unknown. There is overwhelming epidemiological evidence that, where arsenic appears in certain drinking waters and where arsenic is employed in sheep dip or vineyard sprays, chronic exposure to soluble inorganic arsenicals predisposes to intraepidermal squamous-cell and superficial basal-cell carcinomas of the skin. Evidence is also accumulating that the chronic use of Fowler's solution (potassium arsenite) for psoriasis, asthma, or other disorders also causes skin cancer (*see* Fierz, 1965; Novey and Martel, 1969). Among metal workers, there is a strong correlation between the intensity and duration of exposure and lung cancer (Lee and Fraumeni, 1969). On the basis of present evidence, the therapeutic use of inorganic arsenicals should be condemned. The carcinogenicity of arsenic has been reviewed by Buchanan (1962) and Black (1967).

Therapeutic Use. The present-day use of arsenicals in human medicine is essentially confined to the treatment of *trypanosomiasis* (*see* Chapter 54).

ANTIMONY

Antimony resembles arsenic both chemically and biologically. It was used by the ancients as both a medicine and a cosmetic, and again during the fifteenth and early sixteenth century. In the late sixteenth and early seventeenth century its toxicity and inefficacy caused its abandonment, but it was revived in 1657 because King Louis XIV appeared to respond to an antimonial drug administered by a quack. It was then used for nearly 200 years before it again fell into disrepute. However, in the early twentieth century, organic antimony compounds were introduced as parasiticides, for which purpose they are still useful.

Chemistry. Trivalent antimony readily forms thioantimonites with sulfhydryl groups of cellular constituents; certain trivalent antimonials, such as antimony thioglycollamide and antimony sodium thioglycollate, are thioantimonites. Pentavalent antimony forms thioantimonates, but it is not clear whether it does so *in vivo.* The formulas and preparations of currently employed antimonials are given elsewhere (*see* Index).

Pharmacological and Toxicological Actions.
Upon *local* application, antimony compounds are more caustic than those of arsenic. The salts of antimony, notably the tartrates, are powerful emetics, chiefly by virtue of their irritant action on the gastrointestinal mucosa. However, toxic doses are also emetic by virtue of a central action on the medulla. If a subemetic dose is given, antimony has a nauseant and expectorant action. The salivary and bronchial glands are stimulated reflexly. However, antimony is now considered to be too toxic to be used as an expectorant or an emetic.

Parasiticidal Action. Although it is widely thought that the mechanism of action of antimonials is a reaction with essential sulfhydryl groups, the supposition remains unproven. Trivalent, but not pentavalent, antimonials readily inhibit sulfhydryl enzymes such as pyruvic dehydrogenase. The phosphofructokinase in schistosomes from antimony-treated rats is inhibited (Bueding and Mansour, 1957). However, pentavalent antimonials, used in the treatment of certain protozoal infections, are neither directly parasiticidal nor activated by contact with tissues; consequently, consideration must be given the role of the host in the eradication of the infection.

Absorption, Distribution, and Excretion. Antimony compounds are only slowly absorbed from the gastrointestinal tract. Moreover, they cause marked irritation of the intestinal mucosa. Consequently, they are given only parenterally.

Trivalent and pentavalent antimonials differ greatly in their distribution and excretion. The trivalent compounds have a high affinity for cells. Consequently, they rapidly leave the plasma but remain in the circulation bound in some manner to erythrocytes, where they interfere with the function of hemoglobin (Abdel-Meguid *et al.*, 1967).

Comparatively little is known of the distribution of trivalent antimony in the tissues of man. In animals, abnormally high concentrations are found in the liver and the thyroid. Uptake by the liver is partly by a saturable binding mechanism and partly by diffusion (Smith, 1969). Interestingly, antimony is considerably concentrated in schistosomal ova removed from treated humans (Schulert *et al.*, 1964).

In man, the trivalent antimonials are excreted for the most part by the kidney. Renal excretion is slow, presumably because of the low plasma levels. Therefore, following a single therapeutic dose of a trivalent antimonial, only about 10% is recovered in the urine within 24 hours, and only about 30% within a week (Bartter *et al.*, 1947). As a result, when antimonials are given in courses, the patient is usually in positive antimony balance; plasma and erythrocyte concentrations and urinary excretion increase progressively so that as much as 50% of the preceding dose of antimony may be excreted within 48 hours. When injections are discontinued, plasma and erythrocyte concentrations fall slowly, and antimony can still be detected in the urine after 100 days.

The pentavalent antimonials are not bound by erythrocytes and attain much higher plasma concentrations than do the trivalent compounds. Consequently, they are excreted more rapidly by the kidney. As much as 50% of a pentavalent antimonial may appear in the urine in the 24 hours following a single injection. When the drug is given in courses, the plasma concentration and the urinary excretion both rise, but the patient remains in positive antimony balance. As is true for the trivalent compounds, the pentavalent antimonials are found in large amounts in the liver (hamster); however, significantly high concentrations are also found in the spleen. Gellhorn and van Dyke (1946) have suggested that a high splenic concentration of antimony is essential for the successful treatment of experimental leishmaniasis. Small amounts of pentavalent antimony are reduced to trivalent antimony in the liver.

Toxicity. The symptoms of acute and chronic antimony poisoning are so similar to those caused by arsenic that they need not be repeated here in detail. The shock syndrome is the outstanding feature of acute antimony poisoning. Improper medication with any of the antimony compounds may produce chronic poisoning. Antimony poisoning is rare in the United States, because the element is not widely used in medicine or industry.

Certain untoward reactions of importance are elicited much more frequently by the trivalent than by the pentavalent compounds and appear most often during therapy with tartar emetic. Severe coughing, sometimes associated with vomiting, is likely to develop immediately after intravenous injection. Pneumonia is not an unusual sequel to a therapeutic course of tartar emetic. It is definitely a reaction to the drug and not a complication of the disease being treated. It has not been encountered in the use of pentavalent compounds. Pains in the joints and muscles are common; they do not occur, however, until near the end of a therapeutic course. Acute arthritis is a less common reaction. It generally involves the wrist, knee, and ankle joints. Marked bradycardia occasionally occurs late in a course of antimony therapy. It necessitates the discontinuation of medication. ECG studies in patients receiving medication with trivalent antimonials reveal significant changes during therapy in a high percentage of individuals. These are unassociated with cardiovascular symptoms and disappear within 30 to 60 days after cessation of therapy. Miscellaneous untoward reactions are headache, fainting, dyspnea, apnea, facial edema, abdominal pain, vascular collapse, and mild rashes. Hepatic function may be somewhat depressed during treatment and for several months after its cessation. Hepatitis is a rare but serious reaction and necessitates immediate cessation of medication. An anaphylactoid response, characterized by urticarial rash, husky voice, and, in severe cases, collapse, may be encountered after the sixth or seventh injection in a therapeutic course. Hemolytic anemia, sometimes fatal, may occasionally occur during treatment with stibophen.

The high incidence of urinary bladder tumors seen in patients with schistosomiasis may possibly be caused by antimonials, since tartar emetic has been shown to cause the same defect in tryptophan metabolism that is found in such patients (Kaleda *et al.*, 1972).

Because antimonials are little used in the developed countries, there is only a limited literature on the efficacy of chelating agents in the *treatment of intoxication* by antimony compounds in man. Stevenson and associates (1948) have reported that dimercaprol is effective in ameliorating untoward reactions to stibophen. In experimental animals, dimercaprol is clearly effective against trivalent antimonials, but the efficacy against pentavalent antimony may be species dependent. Adrenocorticosteroids may have some clinical benefit in preventing hepatotoxicity caused by antimonial drugs.

The chief *contraindications* to antimonial therapy are myocarditis, hepatitis, and nephritis.

The trivalent antimonials are locally toxic and, therefore, require intravenous administration for systemic use; the pentavalent compounds may be injected intramuscularly.

Therapeutic Uses. The emetic and expectorant uses of trivalent antimony are obsolete. The pentavalent antimonials occupy an important place in the treatment of the protozoal infection *leishmaniasis,* but trivalent compounds are primarily employed in the management of the helminthic infections *schistosomiasis* and *filariasis* (*see* Chapters 51 and 54). Trivalent antimonials have proven to be effective in the treatment of *granuloma inguinale,* but the antibiotics are more effective and less toxic.

BISMUTH

Bismuth was the last of the group-V metals to be introduced into medicine (1785), but it has the fewest reasons to recommend its continuance in a modern therapeutic armamentarium. While insoluble bismuth compounds are still employed for supposed effects in the gastrointestinal tract, there is no evidence of their efficacy (*see* Chapter 48). Detailed discussions of the absorption, distribution, excretion, toxicity, and former therapeutic applications of bismuth may be found in previous editions of this textbook.

SILVER

Silver was employed medicinally for several thousand years, but it came into prominence only after Paracelsus recommended its use for diseases of the nervous system. The basis for this suggestion was the relationship believed to exist between silver and the moon and the belief that insane individuals ("lunatics") were under the influence of Luna, the moon goddess. Until late in the nineteenth century, silver nitrate (lunar caustic) was still employed for the treatment of epilepsy.

The affinity of silver for sulfur is well known in the tarnishing of silver. Silver salts poison sulfhydryl enzymes, presumably by the formation of hemisilver sulfides with sulfhydryl groups. However, the pharmacological effects of silver salts cannot all be attributed to reactions with sulfhydryl; silver ion also combines with a number of biologically important moieties, including amino, imidazole, carboxyl, and phosphate groups.

Local Actions. The attachment of silver to a reactive group of a protein sharply decreases the solubility of the protein, and denaturation may occur. Precipitation of the protein generally results. When the concentration of silver is low, precipitation is confined to proteins in the interstitial space, and an astringent action is said to have occurred. When the concentration is high, membrane and intracellular structures are damaged, and there is a caustic or corrosive effect. Because they attach so readily to the various active groups on proteins, the silver ions are bound before they diffuse far into the tissues. Precipitation of the silver as silver chloride also limits the extent of movement of the ions. Thus, the local effects of silver are self-limiting, and the spread of damage occurs only when the concentration of silver overwhelms the capacity of the tissues to fix the ion at the site of application. The antiseptic effects of silver probably also derive in part from reactions with bacterial and viral proteins.

Systemic Actions. The systemic actions of silver are not extensive because of its limited absorption, for the reasons mentioned above. However, some silver does gain access to the body from mucous membranes and from burns treated with silver nitrate, and this is in large part retained.

Silver Poisoning. The ingestion of a soluble silver salt in sufficient concentration leads to corrosion of the mucosa of the digestive tract. If this is extensive, death may ensue from local trauma, hemorrhagic gastroenteritis, and shock. Systemic symptoms after parenteral injections of silver compounds have been observed in experimental animals. The fatal oral dose of silver nitrate is approximately 10 g, but recovery has been reported from much larger amounts. Treatment consists in the administration of sodium chloride solution and demulcents, and in the management of shock. Sodium chloride specifically repairs chloride depletion resulting from the precipitation of AgCl. Chloride depletion also occurs in burn patients treated with topical silver nitrate.

Silver gradually accumulates in the body from trace amounts of the metal in the diet, and in the later decades of life reaches an appreciable concentration. High concentrations of silver in the tissues, however, occur only after the careless administration of silver-containing medicinals; systemic effects do not follow absorption. The absorbed silver is widely distributed in the body, and large amounts in the subepithelial portions of the skin can impart a characteristic bluish pigmentation, a condition known as *argyria.* The hue may range from gray to one suggesting marked cyanosis. The pigment may be partly silver sulfide and partly metallic silver, which results from the reduction of silver in tissues. The reduction is photoactivated, so that those portions of the skin exposed to light become discolored. However, the first sign of argyria is often a slate-blue "silver line" in the gingival margins adjacent to the teeth. Argyria can be readily diagnosed and differentiated from other types of pigmentation by direct illumination and dark-field examination of biopsied portions of skin.

The eye is particularly prone to manifest pigmentation from silver, the color ranging from a light bluish-gray to a brownish-black. The discoloration may occur after systemic or local administration and is often the first sign of argyria. Observable pigmentation can occur within 10 days.

Argyria can result either from industrial exposure to silver or from medication with colloidal silver preparations as well as the soluble salts. The current use of silver preparations in the treatment of burns may be expected to cause some cases of argyria.

The only injury sustained in argyria is a cosmetic one, but it remains for life. Successful treatment of argyria is rare and requires the laborious, repetitive intradermal injection of the entire involved area with 6% sodium thiosulfate solution and 1% potassium ferrocyanide solution. Dimercaprol is ineffective, since the pigment is mostly free silver.

The problem of argyria and the pharmacology of silver have been extensively reviewed by Hill and Pillsbury (1939).

Therapeutic Uses. At present silver compounds are used only for their local actions. The nitrate and insoluble silver compounds (*e.g.*, silver sulfadiazine, silver allantoinate, etc.) are employed for their antiseptic and germicidal actions, and the nitrate is also used for its caustic (or corrosive) action (*see* Index).

GOLD

Gold, in elemental form, has been employed for centuries as an antipruritic to relieve the itching palm. In more modern times, the observation by Robert Koch in 1890 that gold inhibited *Mycobacterium tuberculosis in vitro* led to trials in arthritis and lupus erythematosus, thought by some to be tuberculous manifestations. The favorable observations of Forestier (1929) were largely responsible for stimulating interest in gold therapy (chrysotherapy). At present, gold is employed widely in the treatment of rheumatoid arthritis.

Chemistry. The significant preparations of gold are all aurous salts in which the gold is attached to sulfur. The water-soluble compounds employed in therapy all contain hydrophilic groups in addition to the aurothio group. Monovalent gold has a relatively strong affinity for sulfur, weak affinities for carbon and nitrogen, and almost no affinity for oxygen, except in chelates. The strong affinity for sulfur and the inhibitory effect of certain gold salts on pyruvic dehydrogenase suggest that the therapeutic effects of gold salts derive from inhibition of sulfhydryl systems. However, other sulfhydryl inhibitors do not appear to have therapeutic actions in common with gold.

Pharmacological Actions. Although Koch and others found a variable efficacy of gold *in vitro*, little therapeutic effect was observed in experimental infections and none in clinical infections. An exception is experimental syphilis in rabbits and staphylococcal, hemolytic streptococcal, pneumococcal, and leptospiral infections in mice, which respond to high-to-toxic doses of gold compounds. In rats and mice, gold salts prevent polyarthritis caused by *Mycoplasma*-like hemolytic streptococci, but they do not necessarily eradicate the infection. This is of interest because of the widespread belief that microorganisms of the genus *Mycoplasma* are responsible for rheumatoid arthritis in man. Pertinent to this hypothesis is the report that the plasma of arthritic patients receiving gold therapy actually exerts a bacteriostatic action on certain strains of hemolytic streptococci.

Gold compounds can suppress or prevent, but not cure, experimental arthritis and synovitis due to a number of infectious and chemical agents. The generality of the antiarthritic action stands counter to the view that the effects in man are the result of an antibacterial action on *Mycoplasma.*

Gold salts administered *in vivo* alter the properties of collagen in rats, presumably by increasing cross-linkages (*see* Adam and Kühn, 1968). Gold is entrained in lysosomes and phagosomes in the synovial membrane, kidney, mesentery, skin, and probably elsewhere. It does not affect the release of lysosomal hydrolases, but it inhibits these enzymes (Persellin and Ziff, 1966; Ennis *et al.*, 1968; Norton *et al.*, 1968). Gold sodium thiomalate administered subcutaneously to rats inhibits the formation of glucosamine-6-phosphate in connective tissue but not in liver (Bollet and Shuster, 1960).

Gold suppresses the anaphylactic release of histamine more effectively than do glucocorticoids (Norn, 1971). It also prevents prostaglandin synthesis *in vitro* (Deby *et al.*, 1973). In common with other antirheumatic drugs, gold decreases the binding of tryptophan to plasma proteins (McArthur *et al.*, 1971). By several indices, gold moderately suppresses cellular immunity (Strong *et al.*, 1973). Chrysotherapy decreases the elevated plasma concentrations of several trace metals (including copper) in rheumatic patients (Niedermier *et al.*, 1971).

Aurothioglucose, but not other compounds of gold, in toxic doses induces obesity in dogs and certain strains of mice. Gold-induced necrosis of the oligodendroglia in the ventromedial hypothalamus occurs in both rats and mice. Gold is deposited in the scar. The gold of gold thiomalate, which does not induce obesity, is not found in hypothalamic loci.

Absorption, Distribution, and Excretion. The water-soluble gold salts are rapidly absorbed after intramuscular injection, peak blood concentrations being reached in 4 to 6 hours (*see* Freyberg, 1966; Mascarenhas *et al.*, 1972), unless the salt is suspended in oil. Currently marketed gold preparations are erratically absorbed by the oral route. Some chloro (trialkylphosphine) gold compounds appear to be better absorbed orally.

Little is known about the distribution of gold in man, but more is known in animals (*see* Freyberg, 1966). Tissue distribution depends not only on the type of compound administered but also on the time after administration and probably on the duration of treatment. Early in the course of therapy, several percent of the total body content of gold is in the blood. However, the fraction in blood of the normal trace body burden is only about 2×10^{-8} (*see* Schroeder and Nason, 1971). In the blood, soluble gold is first bound (about 95%) to albumin; during the course of the first week, a substantial fraction may be transferred to the erythrocytes in about one third of patients (Smith *et al.*, 1973). During treatment, the concentration in the synovial fluid is about half that in plasma (Gerber *et al.*, 1972); equilibrium occurs in less than 4 hours. Arthritic joints contain more than twice as much gold as do uninvolved ones (*see* Lawrence, 1961). About half of the normal trace body burden of gold is in bone (*see* Schroeder and Nason, 1971), but nothing is known of the bone content during treatment. In animal experiments with the therapeutic gold compounds, the highest concentration in soft tissue is in the kidney, where it tends to deposit in the proximal tubules. Appreciable amounts are also found in the liver and spleen. Throughout the body, gold appears to be concentrated in lysosomes and phagosomes at inflamed sites and in reticuloendothelial cells (*see* Norton *et al.*, 1968).

The pharmacokinetics of gold is complex. With water-soluble preparations, blood concentrations rise sharply after each dose and then decline according to first-order kinetics. There is considerable variation among patients. Furthermore, the kinetics varies with the dose and the duration of treatment. The plasma half-life is about 1 day after an initial dose of 10 mg, but it is 3 to 7 days for a 50-mg dose. However, Rubinstein and Dietz (1973) report a half-life of 27 days after an initial dose of this magnitude. With successive weekly injections the half-life lengthens, and after about the third weekly injection it may be 14 to 40 days, and it is even as long as 168 days after 11 weeks. Therefore, with weekly injections it may take months for the mean blood concentration to reach a plateau. If the interval between injections is increased to 4 weeks, the mean plasma concentration will fall to about one third of that with weekly injections. Lower blood concentrations and longer half-times result with suspensions in oil.

The excretion of gold is 60 to 90% renal and 10 to 40% fecal, the latter probably mostly by biliary secretion. The gold concentration in urine varies among patients. In the first day after injection it ranges from about equal to twice that in plasma; after 7 days it may be slightly above to slightly below the plasma concentration. The half-time for the fall in urine concentration after the first two or three weekly injections appears to be shorter than that of plasma concentration, but it eventually approaches that of the plasma half-life. Fecal excretion is erratic but tends to be low in the first day after injection and to increase during the next several days.

By a double-labeling technic, Gottlieb and co-workers (1972) discovered that during maintenance the total amount excreted during a week is about 40% from the most recent dose and 60% from previ-

ous doses. They reported that, with a biweekly to monthly maintenance dosage schedule, the average weekly excretion is approximately 40%. Although they did not state the mean interval, it is evident that during the 2 weeks or more of excretion most of a dose would have been eliminated; this disagrees sharply with the earlier data of Smith and associates (1958), which indicated that approximately 85% of a dose accumulates. Gottlieb and associates also reported that, after a cumulative dose of 1 g of gold, urinary excretion of gold can be detected for as long as a year. However, blood concentrations fall to the normal trace amounts in about 40 to 80 days (*see* the data of Mascarenhas *et al.*, 1972). Thus, the true cumulative potential of gold is not yet clearly ascertained. Sulfhydryl agents, such as dimercaprol, penicillamine, and N-acetylcysteine, increase the excretion of gold (*see* Lorber *et al.*, 1973b). It is of interest that penicillamine also tends to correct the abnormalities in copper and iron metabolism in rheumatoid arthritis as well as the pathological indices (*see* Jaffe, 1970; Zuckner *et al.*, 1970; Multicentre Trial Group, 1973). Details of the pharmacokinetics of gold can be found in reports by Lorber and associates (1968, 1973a), Gerber and coworkers (1972), Mascarenhas and colleagues (1972), Rubinstein and Dietz (1973), Gottlieb and colleagues (1974), and others.

Preparations and Dosage. *Aurothioglucose,* U.S.P. (SOLGANAL), contains the aurothio group (Au—S—) in lieu of the hydroxyl group at C 1 of the pyranose form of glucose. It contains approximately 50% gold. Although it is water soluble, it is employed mainly as *Aurothioglucose Injection,* U.S.P., a sterile suspension in a suitable fixed oil. Commercial preparations contain 50 or 100 mg/ml in 10-ml vials. *Gold Sodium Thiomalate,* U.S.P. (MYOCHRYSINE), contains the aurothio group in lieu of the hydroxyl group of sodium malate. It contains approximately 50% gold and is very soluble in water. *Gold Sodium Thiomalate Injection,* U.S.P., is a sterile aqueous solution of the drug that is marketed in 1-ml ampuls containing 10, 25, 50, or 100 mg of the salt and in 10-ml multiple-dose vials containing 50 mg/ml. The optimal intramuscular dosage schedule for the treatment of rheumatoid arthritis is still not agreed upon. The U.S.P. dose is 10 mg of gold in the first week, 25 mg in the second and third weeks, and 50 mg a week thereafter, up to a total of 750 mg. If a remission occurs, treatment is continued but reduced to 50 mg biweekly for four doses, then every 3 weeks for four doses, and finally every 4 weeks for a year. If a relapse occurs during this time, the dosage interval should be shortened; if not, therapy may be discontinued. Rheumatologists prefer to base dosage on urine and plasma concentrations of gold. Lorber and associates (1973a) adjust each dose to maintain the plasma concentration at 3 mg per liter. For a variety of other dosage regimens, one may consult the publications of Lockie (1961), Smith (1963), Freyberg (1966), Mathies (1966), and Smyth (1972). Aurothioglucose in oil is absorbed more slowly than gold sodium thiomalate and also appears to yield somewhat lower plasma concentrations (*see* Rubinstein and Dietz, 1973), but the posological and therapeutic implications of these findings are unknown. *Gold Au 198 Injection,* N.F., is employed only for its radiation effects and hence will not be discussed here.

Clinical Toxicity. The incidence of toxicity in the therapeutic use of gold presently ranges from about 25 to 50% of patients, serious toxicity occurring in about 10%. It is commonly believed that clinical remission and toxicity are positively related and that some degree of toxicity is inevitable in any effective treatment with gold (*see* Bayles and Fremont-Smith, 1956; Freyberg, 1966, 1972). However, Gottlieb and coworkers (1972) found the toxicity to be lower among patients undergoing remission than among those refractory to treatment. Smith and associates (1958) marshal strong evidence that toxicity need not be a serious hazard if the maintenance dosage schedule is based upon considerations of the rate of elimination of gold from the body. Lockie and coworkers (1958) state from experience with over 3000 cases that properly supervised therapy can be continued for years without reactions. Note should also be made of the fact that in a double-blind study (Research Sub-committee, 1961b) the incidence of toxic reactions in controls was nearly half that in patients who received gold; hence the real incidence of reactions attributable to gold may be less than past reports would indicate.

The majority of reactions occur relatively early during treatment. Reactions seem to appear more frequently in patients with long-standing rheumatoid disease. There is a positive correlation between age of the patient and toxicity (Ramos *et al.,* 1963). The incidence of toxic reactions has been stated to be unrelated to the *plasma* concentrations of gold (Freyberg *et al.,* 1942; Mascarenhas *et al.,* 1972; Lorber *et al.,* 1973a; Rubinstein and Dietz, 1973). Jessop and Johns (1973) state that hematopoietic toxicity is independent of the plasma concentrations but that the incidence and seriousness of dermatological reactions are correlated with these values when they exceed 3.4 mg per liter. Toxicity may be better correlated with the total body content of gold (Smith *et al.,* 1958).

The most common toxic effects are those involving the skin and the mucous membranes, usually of the mouth. Early transient pruritus is an indication that the tolerance level has been exceeded. A rapid improvement in joint swelling and pain also indicates that the tolerance level is being closely approached. Cutaneous reactions may vary in severity from simple *erythema* to severe *exfoliative dermatitis.* The skin lesions have a characteristic histopathology, and biopsy is important for a differential diagnosis (*see* Gottlieb *et al.,* 1972). Cutaneous reactions have been characterized as manifestations of a type-1 hypersensitivity, in which IgE becomes elevated in reactors (Davis *et al.,* 1973). Lesions of the mucous membranes include *stomatitis, pharyngitis, tracheitis, gastritis, colitis,* and *vaginitis; glossitis* is fairly common. As with silver, a gray-to-blue pigmentation (*chrysiasis*) may occur in the skin and mucous membranes, especially the photoexposed portions (Cox and Marich, 1973).

Severe *blood dyscrasias* may result from aurotherapy. *Thrombocytopenia* occasionally occurs and accounts for many of the fatalities. Thrombocytopenia may develop many months after the gold is administered. *Leukopenia, agranulocytosis,* and *aplastic anemia* may also occur. When panmyelopathy occurs, the urine coproporphyrin and δ-aminolevulinic acid (δ-ALA) levels may increase, as in lead poisoning. Eosinophilia is sometimes observed.

Approximately 50% of patients receiving gold therapy show a trace of proteinuria at some time during therapy. Heavy albuminuria and microscopic hematuria occur in 1 to 3% of cases. The site of damage is usually the proximal tubules. Paradoxically, proteinuria is occasionally cleared by chrysotherapy (Silverberg *et al.,* 1970). Although there are only a few reports in the world literature of gold-induced *nephrosis,* the number reported in some series suggests an incidence of several percent. The nephrosis is usually reversible.

Gold may cause a variety of other severe toxic reactions, including *encephalitis, peripheral neuritis, hepatitis,* and *nitritoid crisis.* Gold can also cause immunological destruction of the synovia. Patients on chrysotherapy may show EEG abnormalities (Dale and Patterson, 1967). Fortunately, the incidence of serious reactions is low, and they generally are the result of failure to discontinue therapy when earlier, less serious symptoms occur.

Avoidance and Treatment. Regular examination of the skin, buccal mucosa, urine, and blood, including cell and platelet counts, should be made. It is the practice in many arthritis clinics to initiate therapy with small doses of gold and to increase the dose gradually. Although untoward effects are not eliminated by this procedure, the severity of those reactions that occur early is somewhat reduced. If an untoward response occurs, therapy should be withheld until it subsides completely. If the reaction is a rash or stomatitis, antihistamines and adrenocorticosteroids may be administered, the latter systemically and/or topically. Glucocorticoids are also indicated in gold-induced nephrosis. Although it has been claimed that glucocorticoids administered during the course of gold therapy increase toxicity (Ramos *et al.,* 1963) and interfere with the therapeutic efficacy of gold (Hill, 1968), not all authorities recognize these claims (*e.g., see* Freyberg, 1972). If gold therapy is initiated in a patient receiving adrenocorticosteroids, the latter should be withdrawn when the accumulated dose of gold is 400 to 600 mg.

If the reaction to gold therapy is not of a serious type and adrenocorticosteroids have been used for its control, injections may be cautiously resumed 2 or 3 weeks after the toxic reaction has subsided and the steroid has been withdrawn. Maintenance dosage should be two thirds to three fourths that previously planned (Smith *et al.,* 1958). However, many experts decline to use the drug again, once toxicity has occurred.

If a severe reaction to gold occurs or if the above-mentioned steps fail to control the toxic effects, treatment with dimercaprol or penicillamine (Bluhm *et al.,* 1962) should be instituted. The administration of dimercaprol may shorten a therapeutic remission induced by gold.

Chrysiasis is treated with strong iodine solution (Lugol's solution) (Silverberg *et al.,* 1970).

Therapeutic Uses. Gold compounds find their chief therapeutic application in *rheumatoid arthritis.* Their exact status continues to be unsettled, in part because of concern over their toxicity and in part because the status of immunosuppressive agents is still uncertain. Furthermore, the only two double-blind trials (*see* Research Sub-committee, 1960, 1961a, 1961b; Cooperating Clinics Committee, 1973) include too few patients to be definitive, and they suffer from other limitations as well. No reliable comparative trials with other drugs have yet been made. At present, gold is used in early, active arthritis that progresses despite an adequate regimen of salicylates, rest, and physical therapy. Gold salts often arrest the progression of the disease in involved joints, at least temporarily; prevent involvement of unaffected joints; improve grip strength; and decrease the erythrocyte sedimentation rate and abnormal plasma glycoprotein and fibrinogen levels. Gold is usually of little benefit when the disease is advanced, with long-standing synovitis or other arthropathies. Chrysotherapy may benefit palindromic rheumatism (Mattingly, 1966).

Despite the dramatic symptomatic improvement in rheumatoid arthritis caused by glucocorticoids, they do not arrest the progress of the disease and are at least equally as toxic as gold. Consequently, gold is usually used in preference to glucocorticoids.

In active rheumatoid arthritis, gold appears rapidly to induce a partial or complete remission in a high percentage of cases. Remissions are usually only moderate, but occasionally they may be dramatic. The most improved patients appear to have a lower fecal and higher renal excretion of gold than do the least improved patients (Gottlieb *et al.,* 1972). The incidence of remissions varies according to the extent to which the therapeutic regimen is individualized and may be as high as 80%.

The duration of the remissions after discontinuation of treatment with gold is extremely variable (from 1 to 18 months). The recurrence is said to be usually not as severe as the original disease, and a high percentage of patients responds favorably to a second course of gold therapy, especially if marked benefits resulted from the first course. In patients who receive gold continuously over many years and who respond favorably, there is little doubt that remissions can be maintained over long periods (*see* Hill, 1968). However, when gold therapy is eventually discontinued and the final status of such patients is compared with those who did not receive chrysotherapy, little difference can be observed (Research Sub-committee, 1961a, 1961b). Even during sustained maintenance therapy, there is roentgenological evidence of progression of the disease.

There is no unanimity of opinion as to the best therapeutic regimen to follow after the completion of a course. Some rheumatologists give no further gold until a relapse occurs; some give a second or even a third course to patients in remission, with rest periods of 6 weeks between courses, and others continue uninterrupted treatment indefinitely, so long as the remission continues (*see* Smyth, 1972). Because of the long period of treatment, requirement for office visits, intramuscular administration, and laboratory tests, patient compliance is poor and there is a high rate of dropout.

Although soluble gold compounds have been administered intra-articularly, the data of Gerber and coworkers (1972) indicate that this route probably offers little advantage. Beneficial effects of intra-articular colloidal ^{198}Au have been reported.

Gold compounds have been successfully employed in the treatment of *nondisseminated lupus erythematosus;* they are given in courses in the same manner as for rheumatoid arthritis. On the other hand, gold compounds should not be used in disseminated lupus. In *pemphigus,* gold compounds have been reported to be of considerable benefit (Pennys *et al.,* 1973).

Contraindications. Gold therapy is contraindicated in patients with *renal disease, hepatic dysfunction* or a *history of infectious hepatitis,* or *hematological disorders.* Patients who have recently had *radiation* should not receive gold because of its depressant action on hematopoietic tissue. Concomitant use of *antimalarials, immunosuppressants, phenylbutazone,* or *oxyphenbutazone* is contraindicated because of the potential of these drugs to cause blood dyscrasias. *Urticaria, eczema,* and *colitis* are also considered to be contraindications to the use of the metal. Finally, gold is poorly tolerated by aged individuals.

MERCURY

The importance of mercury in medicine has steadily diminished since mid-century because of the advent of potent nonmercurial diuretics, the recognized supremacy of nonmercurial antiseptics over mercurials, and the effectiveness of antibiotic and synthetic antibacterial ointments, fields in which the organic or inorganic mercurials were once the agents of choice. Today, the mercurial compounds are mainly of toxicological importance, especially environmental. In this chapter, the general pharmacology and toxicology of mercury will be considered.

Chemistry and Mechanism of Action. Mercury readily forms covalent bonds with sulfur, and it is this property that accounts for most of the biological properties of the metal. When the sulfur is in the form of sulfhydryl groups, divalent mercury replaces the hydrogen atom to form mercaptides, $X—Hg—SR$ and $Hg(SR)_2$, where X is an electronegative radical and R is protein. Organic mercurials form mercaptides of the type $RHg—SR'$. Mercurials even in low concentrations are capable of inactivating sulfhydryl enzymes and thus of interfering with cellular metabolism and function. The affinity of mercury for thiols provides the basis for treatment of mercury poisoning by such agents as dimercaprol and penicillamine. Mercury also combines with other ligands of physiological importance, such as phosphoryl, carboxyl, amide, and amine groups. To what extent combination with such groups contributes to the enzyme-inhibitory, protein-precipitant, and corrosive effects of mercuric ions is unknown.

The various therapeutic and toxic actions of the mercurials are associated with chemical substituents that affect solubility, dissociation, relative affinity for various cellular receptors, distribution, and excretion.

Absorption, Distribution, and Excretion. The absorption, distribution, and excretion of mercury and its compounds vary considerably with the chemical form of the metal. Although *elemental mercury* is below hydrogen in the electromotive series, in the presence of oxygen and chloride in the gastric contents a sufficient amount may dissolve to cause a mild catharsis. The resulting quantities of

the ionic form are small and furthermore are fixed in the chyme and mucosa, so that systemic effects do not usually occur unless the elemental mercury was originally very finely divided. Oxides and sulfides on the surface of mercury that has been well exposed to the atmosphere can contribute to the body burden of the metal and cause diuresis. *Inhaled mercury vapors* rapidly leave the lungs, and the metal is gradually oxidized in erythrocytes and probably other cells; intoxication can result if the exposure is sufficient. Only a small amount of mercury is deposited in the brain, but that which is fixed may be retained for many years. Elemental mercury can be absorbed from the skin, which fact may be attributed to its lipid solubility.

The *soluble inorganic* mercurials (Hg^{2+}) readily gain access to the circulation when taken by mouth, although a considerable portion of the ingested Hg^{2+} may remain fixed to the alimentary mucosa and the intestinal contents. *Insoluble inorganic* mercurous compounds, such as calomel (Hg_2Cl_2), may undergo some oxidation to soluble, absorbable compounds. In suitable vehicles, inorganic mercurials may be absorbed through the intact skin, where some of the mercury may be reduced to elemental mercury and deposited as a gray-to-bluish pigment. In the blood, Hg^{2+} is first fixed to α-globulins and erythrocytes but later shifts to albumin, from which it is redistributed to the tissues with a half-time of about 15 days. Within a few hours the mercury is found in human and animal tissues in the following approximate order of decreasing concentration: pancreas, kidney, liver, spleen, blood, bone marrow, upper respiratory and buccal mucosa, intestinal wall (especially colon), skin, salivary glands, heart, skeletal muscle, brain, and lung. There is some evidence that mercuric salts can be stored in bones. Some tissues have a lower capacity to bind mercury than do others, so that distribution may be dose dependent. Also, the distribution changes over the course of time. In the kidney, mercury is found primarily in the proximal tubules. Excretion of mercury starts immediately after absorption, mainly by way of the kidney and colon, and to a lesser extent via the bile and saliva. Small amounts are also excreted in volatile elemental form, through both the lungs and the skin. Most of the mercury is excreted within 6 days after administration, but traces may be detected for months, even years. Dimercaprol, penicillamine, N-acetyl-D,L-penicillamine, and calcium disodium edetate hasten the urinary excretion of mercury, dimercaprol being superior in this respect. However, dimercaprol effects a redistribution of mercury to the brain (Berlin and Lewander, 1965), the clinical implications of which are not known. Dimercaprol acts similarly on mercury from organomercury compounds.

The absorption, distribution, and excretion of the mercury of *organic* mercurials is determined by physicochemical factors and the extent of *in-vivo* conversion to inorganic mercury. *Methylmercury compounds,* the most important of the environmental mercury contaminants, are lipid soluble and are rapidly and almost completely absorbed from the gastrointestinal tract. In the blood, approximately 90% of a methylmercurial enters the erythrocytes. Initially, liver and kidney have the highest mercury concentrations, about 50% of the total body burden being in the liver in man (Åberg *et al.,* 1969). In the liver, mercury is contained in lysosomes/peroxysomes (Norseth and Brendeford, 1971). The uptake into brain is delayed (Iverson *et al.,* 1973), but the brain concentration ultimately reaches a value one fourth to one half that in the kidney; in man, the amount in the head is 10 to 15% of the body burden. The highest uptake in the nervous system is in the sensory ganglia, where prominent electrophysiological effects occur (Somjen *et al.,* 1973a, 1973b), and this form of mercury is more selective for neurons than for glia and other satellite cells. In rats, about 40% of methylmercury is converted to the inorganic form, but the brain content of inorganic mercury does not exceed 3%. Methylmercury is deposited in hair, the hair: blood ratio being about 300 : 1. Dietary intake can be monitored to predict tissue content and ultimate toxicity; a daily intake of 10 μg/kg at equilibrium will yield a whole-blood concentration of about 570 μg per liter.

In man, urinary excretion is slow at first but accelerates during the first 30 days after exposure (Åberg *et al.,* 1969). However, excretion is primarily fecal; in rats, about 85% is excreted in the feces. Although methylmercury is rapidly excreted into the bile as a complex with cysteine, most of the complex is reabsorbed (Norseth and Clarkson, 1971). Biliary excretion is increased by phenobarbital (Magos and Clarkson, 1973). The fecal mercury comes mainly from mucosal sloughing; it is sloughed mainly as methylmercury, but bacterial flora convert about 50% to inorganic mercury. The total body burden decreases with first a rapid and then a slow phase; the half-time of the slow phase is 70 to 90 days in man. Although hydroxymethyl, methoxyethyl, and ethyl mercurials enter cells in the organic form, they are rapidly converted to inorganic mercury, so that their distribution, excretion, and half-lives are intermediate between those of methylmercury and inorganic mercury. Their toxicity is like that of inorganic mercury. Phenylmercuric compounds are hydroxylated on the ring, conjugated, and then decomposed to inorganic mercury and phenol conjugates. Further details of the metabolism of mercurials may be found in the monographs and reviews by Bidstrup (1964), Brown and Kulkarni (1967), Clarkson (1968, 1972a, 1972b), Hammond (1973), and Miller and Clarkson (1973).

MERCURY POISONING

Principally because mercury is both an environmental and agricultural hazard, not only does mercury intoxication remain a visible medical problem but also there is currently an active literature on various aspects of the environmental effects of mercury and mercury poisoning and its treatment. The interested reader is referred to pertinent reviews and monographs by Bidstrup (1964), Chisolm (1970), Arena (1971), Ciaccio (1971), Fishbein (1971), Grant (1971), Clarkson (1972a, 1972b), Dales (1972), D'Itri (1972), Felton and associates (1972), Friberg and Vostal (1972), Aaronson and Spiro (1973), and Miller and Clarkson (1973).

Acute Mercury Poisoning. *Acute poisoning* usually results from the oral ingestion of highly dissociated inorganic preparations, although it may also result from inhalation of vapors of elemental mercury, from organic mercurials, or even from mercurial ointments applied topically. When mercuric chloride is ingested, the precipitation of the protoplasm of the mucous membranes rapidly causes an ashen-gray appearance of the mouth, pharynx, and gastric mucosa. Intense pain in the affected tissues results, which is aggravated by vomiting. However, vomiting is protective; if the stomach is quickly and effectively emptied, the patient's chance for survival is much greater. A high concentration of the poison may reach the epithelium of the small intestine. The local effect on the bowel soon results in a severe, profuse, bloody diarrhea. Shreds of intestinal mucosa can be identified in the stool; profound shock and death may result. The patient commonly recovers from the local symptoms, especially if vomiting has been extensive or chemical antidotes have been administered. If the poisoning occurs by inhalation of fumes of metallic mercury or organic mercurials, the syndrome is characterized by pneumonitis, lethargy or restlessness, fever, tachypnea, cough, chest pain, cyanosis, diarrhea, and vomiting; atelectasis, emphysema, hemorrhage, and pneumothorax often follow.

The systemic effects of the poison start within a few hours and may last for days; death may ensue. Inorganic mercury and phenylmercuric compounds act diffusely on the capillary walls and specifically at the sites of excretion—the kidney, colon, and mouth. There is first a strong metallic taste; then within 24 to 36 hours, a stomatitis develops, characterized by foul breath, soreness of gums, and excessive salivation. Discoloration of the gingival margins similar to the lead line appears later, and local infection, loosening of the teeth, and necrosis of the alveolar processes may follow. Systemic signs of acute poisoning by elemental mercury and ethylmercuric or methylmercuric compounds include those referable to the CNS, such as lethargy, excitement, hyperreflexia, and tremor.

The renal lesions produced by mercury are confined largely to the tubular epithelium, but the glomeruli are also injured. The kidney may show evidence of disturbed function within a few minutes after the poison reaches the circulation. If the circulation is adequate, the first response of the kidney may be a diuresis due to the suppression of tubular reabsorptive function. Soon, however, the renal damage becomes so extensive that oliguria and finally anuria result. Extrarenal factors may also contribute greatly to the anuria.

Vomiting, diarrhea, and diuresis cause hypovolemia and usually acidosis. In severe cases, widespread capillary damage results in capillary dilatation and shock. Protein and fluid are lost through the vessel walls, and the circulatory volume is markedly diminished. The protein in the plasma may also be reduced as a result of albuminuria and starvation. The excretion of mercury into the colon results in colitis, which intensifies and prolongs the diarrhea.

Treatment. A source of sulfhydryl-rich protein,

such as milk or raw eggs, is introduced into the stomach, and then copious lavage is performed. Sodium formaldehyde sulfoxylate, if available, provides an excellent local antidote. It reduces bivalent mercuric ion to the much less soluble mercurous form. The stomach is lavaged with 250 ml of a 5% solution of the sulfoxylate; an additional 250-ml amount is left in the gastrointestinal tract.

As soon as mercury intoxication is suspected, intramuscular dimercaprol or a penicillamine is given to chelate the mercury and accelerate its excretion. Dimercaprol is maximally effective when given early in the course of poisoning. Prompt therapy with metal-chelating agents affords the kidneys almost complete protection from the toxic effects of mercury. Acutely intoxicated persons have benefited from dimercaprol administered even as late as 5 hours after the ingestion of mercury; patients treated within 4 hours nearly always survive, regardless of the amount of mercury ingested; if such therapy is initiated too late to prevent extensive renal damage and uremia, hemodialysis may be required to relieve uremia and aid in the disposal of the mercury-dimercaprol complex. Fluid, electrolyte, and cardiac abnormalities and shock must be corrected. If the patient survives, a remarkable degree of resolution of the renal lesions occurs in 4 to 5 weeks, and renal function usually returns to normal within several months.

The dosage and the duration of a course of dimercaprol or of penicillamine must be adjusted to the individual case. Dimercaprol is usually given in a dose of 5 to 6 mg/kg intramuscularly, twice a day. Treatment probably should be continued for 10 days, even if recovery is apparently complete at an earlier time.

In the absence of metal-chelating agents, isotonic sodium chloride solution is infused in amounts as great as 10 liters daily to produce a copious diuresis so as to protect the kidney from high concentrations of mercury.

Chronic Mercury Poisoning. Chronic mercury intoxication can result from a wide variety of industrial, agricultural, and domestic exposures, some quite unexpected, such as fumes from mercurial fungicides in latex paints or mercurial catalysts in clandestinely synthesized amphetamines. The use of mercurial preservatives in cosmetics and medicaments has been greatly curtailed, and mercurial ointments are now rarely used, so that poisoning from these sources is almost nonexistent today, except for hypersensitivity. *Methylmercury,* biotically generated from mercurial wastes and incorporated into the aquatic and phytic food chain and also accidentally introduced into foods from fungicide-treated grains, is a source of chronic poisoning, and hundreds of deaths have occurred in a single epidemic.

The signs and symptoms characterizing chronic poisoning from inorganic and hydroxymethyl or phenylmercuric compounds are gingivitis, stomatitis, loosening of the teeth, salivation, metallic taste, colitis, progressive renal damage, loss of appetite, nutritional disturbances, anemia, hypertension, and peripheral neuritis. The CNS is especially involved, as evidenced by behavioral changes, mental depression, irritability, blushing, insomnia, intention tremors and shaking, fatigue and drowsiness, and occasionally hallucinations. The ethylmercuric and methylmercuric compounds mainly cause neurological signs and symptoms, such as motor incoordination, loss of position sense, tremor, constriction of the visual field, hearing loss, spasticity or rigidity with exaggerated reflexes, mental retardation in children, occasionally psychosis, and dysarthria. Polyuria and ECG changes are less common.

Treatment consists in removal from exposure, supportive therapy, and the use of appropriate metal-chelating agents. Chronic mercury poisoning responds slowly to therapy, and the patient may remain in ill health for years. Dimercaprol or penicillamine promotes excretion of mercury in chronically intoxicated patients but often fails to improve the clinical condition. N-Acetyl-D,L-penicillamine appears to be twice as effective as dimercaprol and is less toxic than penicillamine (*see* Kark *et al.,* 1971). In rats, a polythiol resin that sequesters methylmercury in the intestine provides an excellent method of treatment, especially because of the biliary excretion of methylmercury (Norseth and Clarkson, 1971). In *subacute* mercurial poisoning, symptoms are the same as those of chronic poisoning, except that the CNS and the general nutritional condition of the patient are not as seriously affected.

Hypersensitivity. Hypersensitivity to mercury is often unrecognized. Unusual responses to the mercurial diuretics have occurred. Reactions to inorganic preparations of mercury may vary from a slight erythema involving only the area of contact to a severe generalized eruption that may be morbilliform, punctate, or urticarial. Eventually, vesicles and bullae may appear. The skin reactions may be accompanied by fever and prostration. Cases have been reported in which individuals sensitive to mercury have experienced systemic reactions as a result of dental fillings with amalgam. Aaronson and Spiro (1973) speculate that some cases of ulcerative colitis may possibly result from hypersensitivity to mercury. Treatment consists in removal from contact with mercury, appropriate management of the cutaneous lesions, and supportive measures. Metal-chelating agents are often without value.

The syndrome of *acrodynia* (pink disease) in infants and young children is a manifestation of sensitization to mercury. Mercury-induced acrodynia responds to treatment with dimercaprol or N-acetyl-D,L-penicillamine.

Organic mercurials also induce allergic reactions. Contact allergies, even asthma, have been traced to phenylmercuric preservatives in a number of medicaments, suture materials, vaginal contraceptives, and agents employed for laundering hospital linens, as well as in agricultural and household gardening materials.

THERAPEUTIC USES

The specific actions of mercury are considered elsewhere in connection with the several therapeutic uses of the mercury compounds (*see* Index). The inorganic mercuric salts, as well as certain organic compounds of mercury, are employed chiefly as antiseptics and preservatives. Also, certain mercury compounds are effective parasiticides and fungicides when locally applied. Certain complex organic mercurial compounds are employed as diuretics. Mercurous chloride is an obsolete cathartic. The metal is of historical interest in syphilotherapy.

LEAD

Lead is the only early-known heavy metal that does not have some modern therapeutic application. The use of lead compounds as astringents has come and gone within the last 2 centuries. At the present time lead is justifiably *materia non grata* in therapeutics. The modern interest in the metal centers about its toxicological properties.

Like the other heavy metals, lead has an affinity for sulfur, and the metal can combine with sulfhydryl groups in *in-vitro* systems. Although it is usually considered to exert its effects through sulfhydryl inhibition, the fact that the metal is deposited among the bone salts shows that lead has other affinities *in vivo,* and it would be an error to overlook its interactions with carboxyl, phosphoryl, and perhaps other groups in considering possible mechanisms of action.

An overview of the sources, chemical and biological properties, and toxicology of lead may be found in various reviews and monographs. (*See* Symposium, 1964, 1966; Hammond, 1969; Committee on Biologic Effects of Atmospheric Pollutants, 1972; Felton *et al.,* 1972; Guinée, 1972; Hardy *et al.,* 1973; Task Group, 1973.)

Absorption. *Skin.* Inorganic lead does not penetrate normal skin, but it can penetrate abraded skin. *Organic* compounds, such as tetraethyl lead, can rapidly penetrate the intact skin.

Subcutaneous and Intramuscular Sites. Lead projectiles, especially lead shot, embedded in skin or muscle can cause poisoning. Indeed, it has been reported that poisoning occurred less than a month after lead shot had been embedded in tissue.

Gastrointestinal Tract. The majority of cases of household lead poisoning result from the ingestion of the element. Even the normal diet contains appreciable amounts. Many studies on the absorption of lead from the alimentary tract have been conducted (*see* monograph by Cantarow and Trumper, 1944). Such studies are complicated by the variability in intake of dietary lead, the necessity of conducting careful balance studies over long periods of time, the difficulty of distinguishing between intestinal excretion on the one hand and failure of absorption on the other, the technical difficulties of analysis, and other factors.

In a monumental study in the 1930s and 1940s, Kehoe and associates followed continuously the lead metabolism of normal subjects for more than 3 years (for references, *see* Kehoe, 1961, 1964a, 1964b). Their findings showed that only 8 to 12% of orally ingested lead is absorbed, even when the lead is taken in the form of a soluble salt. It was also shown that variations in calcium and phosphorus intake do not affect the absorption of the metal. The only factor found to influence significantly the absorption of lead is the motor activity of the bowel, the absorption varying inversely with motility. Lead is absorbed mainly from the small intestine, to a lesser extent from the colon, and not significantly from the stomach. Absorption is more complete in young than in aged subjects.

Respiratory Tract. Lead can be absorbed from all portions of the respiratory tract, including the nasal passages. Indeed, absorption from the lungs is much more rapid and complete than from the gastrointestinal tract.

Distribution. The distribution of lead in the body is a crucial factor in the development of lead poisoning. In the blood, nearly all the circulating inorganic lead is associated with the erythrocytes. Only when lead is present in relatively large amounts does a significant portion remain in the plasma. The kinetics of distribution and excretion fit a three-compartment model (Rabinowitz *et al.,* 1973).

Following absorption, inorganic lead is distributed in the soft tissues, the highest concentrations being reached in the kidneys. Lead is distributed throughout the tubular epithelial cells (Murakami and Hirosawa, 1973). The concentration in kidneys increases with age (Piscator and Lind, 1972), as probably does the total body burden. The liver usually contains the second highest concentration. Over a period of time the lead is redistributed, becoming deposited especially in bone and also in teeth and hair. Only small quantities of inorganic lead accumulate in the brain; more is found in gray matter and basal ganglia than elsewhere in the CNS (*see* Task Group, 1973). Lead penetrates the placental barrier; although permeative lead can cause congenital abnormalities in animals, teratogenesis in the human has not been reported. However, there are adverse effects on the fetus (*see* Cantarow and Trumper, 1944). Details of the distribution of lead in normal and lead-intoxicated persons have been reviewed by Kehoe (1961, 1964a, 1964b), Schroeder and coworkers (1961), and Committee on Biologic Effects of Atmospheric Pollutants (1972).

The deposition of lead in bone closely resembles that of calcium (*see* Cantarow and Trumper, 1944), but it is deposited as tertiary lead phosphate. After a recent exposure, the concentration of lead is often higher in the flat bones than in the long bones (*see* Kehoe, 1961), although, as a general rule, the long bones contain more lead. In the early period of deposition, the concentration of lead is highest in the epiphyseal portion of the long bones. This is especially true in growing bones, where lead deposits may be detected by x-ray examination as rings of increased density in the ossification centers of the epiphyseal cartilage and as a series of transverse lines in the diaphyses. These may be of diagnostic importance in establishing lead poisoning in children.

Factors that affect the distribution of calcium similarly affect that of lead. Thus, high phosphate intake favors skeletal storage of lead and a lowering of the lead content in soft tissues. Conversely, a low phosphate intake mobilizes lead in bone and elevates its content in soft tissues. High calcium intake in the absence of elevated phosphate intake has a similar effect, owing to competition with lead for available phosphate. Vitamin D tends to promote the deposition of lead in bone, provided a sufficient amount of phosphate is available; otherwise, deposition of calcium preemptively prevents deposition of lead. Lead suppresses enhanced formation of osseous and extraosseus intercellular bone matrix consequent to hypervitaminosis D. Parathyroid hormone and dihydrotachysterol mobilize lead from the skeleton and augment the blood concentration and urinary excretion of the metal. Acidosis promotes the mobilization from bone and the excretion of both lead and calcium. Iodides and bicarbonate also favor movement of lead from bone, but the mechanisms are not known.

Lead in the bone salts does not contribute to toxicity. Consequently, deposition in bone (*see* above) was once promoted to detoxicate lead, and cautious mobilization was undertaken after acute symptoms had subsided. The half-life of lead in bone has been estimated to be 10 years in man (*see* Task Group, 1973). Bone-rarifying diseases may induce episodes of plumbism in persons with a sufficient body burden of lead.

After acute exposure to alkyl lead compounds the initial distribution of lead resembles that after exposure to inorganic lead, in that the highest tissue concentrations are found in the kidney and liver. Tetraethyl lead and trimethyl lead differ in that the latter partitions itself the more evenly among the body tissues, whereas the former never reaches significant concentrations in the skeleton and does not sustain an appreciable concentration in blood. Neither gives rise to high concentrations in the brain, despite the fact that the pharmacological effects are primarily central. The alkyl compounds resist biotransformation; nevertheless, tetraethyl lead is converted to the more toxic triethyl lead, then gradually to inorganic lead, so that chronically it resembles inorganic lead. The disposition of alkyl lead compounds has been reviewed by Hammond (1973).

Excretion. In experimental animals, lead is excreted into the bile, and injected lead may be found in the feces. However, in man, inhaled lead does not reach the feces (*see* Kehoe, 1961). The greatest portion of fecal lead represents unabsorbed lead.

Under normal conditions, during lead balance, the urinary excretion of inorganic lead is approximately 9% of the amount ingested. The concentration of lead in urine is directly proportional to the concentration in plasma (*see* Zielhuis, 1971). Since most of the lead in blood is in the erythrocytes, very little is filtered. However, when blood levels of lead are high, a greater proportion is filtered, so that urinary excretion is at first rapid; gradually it falls to nearly normal rates. Lead also appears to be secreted by the renal tubules. The rate of urinary excretion appears to depend more on the duration of exposure to lead than on the absolute body burden (*see* Kehoe, 1961). The time for complete elimination may exceed the time for accumulation by a factor

of two. In intoxication, the concentration of lead in sweat is about the same as that in urine (Schroeder and Nason, 1971). Lead is also secreted in milk.

The excretion of inorganic lead is enhanced by procedures or conditions that favor mobilization from bone and soft-tissue burdens. Chelating agents, such as dimercaprol, calcium disodium edetate, and penicillamine, increase urinary but not fecal excretion of inorganic lead. The enhanced excretion of lead effected by chelating agents may be helpful in the diagnosis of lead poisoning (*see* Chapter 45).

LEAD POISONING

Despite various regulatory measures, lead poisoning continues to be of significance, especially in children. Even though pediatric cases of lead intoxication are but a fraction of the total number of poisonings, it nevertheless is a major cause of death. Pediatric lead poisoning results commonly from the ingestion of flakes of lead-containing paint or dirt (pica); consequently, it usually occurs in older neighborhoods where painted surfaces are largely undercoated with white lead. Surveys of children in impoverished neighborhoods in several large cities have shown 14 to 20% of children had abnormally high body burdens of lead; in one of these studies (*see* Pueschel *et al.,* 1972), 3.5% had neurological or mental impairment. Children are especially susceptible to lead poisoning (*see* Lin-Fu, 1973), and even the lead in evaporated milk may possibly constitute a hazard to some infants. (For a useful bibliography on childhood lead intoxication, *see* Lin-Fu, 1971.) Among the most common types of nonoccupational exposures among adults are the renovation of old homes and the consumption of "moonshine" whisky that has been distilled through automobile radiators or other lead-soldered apparatus. Frank poisoning from general environmental contamination has not been proven, but the body burdens of some persons working or living close to busy highways or smelters have been found to be considerably elevated (*see* Landrigan *et al.,* 1975).

The rate of excretion of lead is so limited that only a slight excess over the average daily intake may result in a positive lead balance. The normal daily intake of lead is approximately 0.3 mg, although widespread variations occur. Positive lead balance begins at a daily intake of about 0.6 mg. However, at this level of intake, the body burden would not ordinarily reach toxic proportions within a lifetime. As the intake increases, the time for accumulation of toxic amounts shortens disproportionately; whereas a daily intake of 2.5 mg of lead requires nearly 4 years for the accumulation of a toxic burden, a daily intake of 3.5 mg requires but a few months. Furthermore, at levels of intake that require less than a year for accumulation, the toxic amount of lead is a smaller quantity than that accumulated over a longer period of time, because deposition in bone is too slow to buffer the soft tissues during "rapid" accumulation.

Concentrations of lead in blood in excess of 700 μg per liter of whole blood are indicative of lead exposure within some recent period; those in excess of 1 mg per liter indicate that the exposure has been

heavy. Values approximating 5 mg per liter are unusual but may occur when the exposure is quite
severe; higher concentrations are encountered only
in very rare instances of overwhelming accidental
exposure; with such high values contamination of
the specimen should be suspected.

Urine samples also provide a useful source of
evidence of the severity of the preceding exposure.
Cognizance should be taken of urinary volume and
specific gravity. Multiple or 24-hour samples are
preferable to casually voided specimens. The upper
limit of normal urinary lead concentration is 150 μg
per liter. Hazardous lead exposure usually causes
lead excretion at levels above 150 μg per liter, and
most cases of lead poisoning examined during an
episode of intoxication show concentrations between
150 and 300 μg per liter. Concentrations in excess
of 500 μg per liter require verification. However,
urinary and blood levels of lead are only ancillary
to the medical history in establishing the diagnosis
of lead poisoning, since it is the soft-tissue concentration that is important. Shortly after an exposure,
the blood level may be high, but once the lead is
redistributed it may prove to represent a nontoxic
burden. Conversely, toxic symptoms can occur with
blood concentrations in the normal range (Beritić,
1971).

Roentgenographic examination of the metaphyses
of the long bones for the characteristic lines of density, especially in children, examination of the blood
for stippled and fluorescent erythrocytes and anemia,
determination of the coproporphyrin and δ-ALA
concentrations in the urine, and establishment of the
amount of edetate-mobilizable lead in the urine also
aid in the diagnosis of plumbism (see below).

Signs and Symptoms of Lead Poisoning. *Acute
Inorganic Lead Intoxication.* Acute lead poisoning
is quite rare and occurs following the accidental
ingestion of acid-soluble lead compounds. Local
actions in the mouth result in a marked astringent
effect, thirst, and a metallic taste. Nausea, abdominal
pain, and vomiting then ensue, and the vomitus may
be milky in appearance owing to the presence of lead
chloride. The abdominal pain is severe but is unlike
that of chronic poisoning. The stools may be black
from lead sulfide. There may be diarrhea or constipation. If large amounts of lead are rapidly absorbed, the shock syndrome may develop. Acute
CNS symptoms include paresthesias, pain, and muscle weakness. An acute hemolytic crisis sometimes
occurs and results in severe anemia and hemoglobinuria. The kidney is damaged, and oliguria and
urinary changes are evident. Death may result in
1 or 2 days. If the patient survives the acute effects,
characteristic symptoms of chronic lead poisoning
are likely to appear.

Emergency therapy includes copious gastric lavage and magnesium sulfate as a cathartic to rush
the ingested lead through the intestinal tract. Morphine may be needed for pain, but atropine or other
antispasmodics should be given a trial. Shock therapy is instituted if necessary. Large amounts of calcium and phosphate, to assist in the storage of lead
in the bones and thus to prevent late symptoms, as

well as chelating agents are employed, as described
below.

Chronic Inorganic Lead Poisoning. Three fairly
distinct types of chronic lead intoxication are generally described: the gastrointestinal, the neuromuscular, and the CNS syndromes. They may occur separately or in combination. In addition, certain signs,
especially hematological, may be associated with any
of the syndromes. The neuromuscular and CNS
syndromes tend to result more from intense exposure
to lead, whereas the abdominal syndrome tends to
result from a very slowly and insidiously developing
intoxication. In the United States, the CNS syndrome is the most common type among children and
the gastrointestinal syndrome among adults.

The *abdominal syndrome* often begins with vague
symptoms such as *anorexia, muscle discomfort, malaise,* and *headache.* Constipation also is usually an
early sign, especially in adults, but diarrhea occasionally occurs. A *persistent metallic taste* appears
early in the course of the syndrome. As the intoxication advances, anorexia and constipation become
more marked. If obstipation is severe, recurrent *nausea* and *vomiting* usually result. The feces may become tinged with blood. Intestinal spasm, which
gives rise to *abdominal pain,* is often the most distressing feature of the advanced abdominal syndrome. The attacks are paroxysmal and generally
excruciating. The abdominal muscles become rigid,
and tenderness is especially manifested in the region
of the umbilicus, in contrast to that of appendicitis.
In adults, the body temperature may fall, but in
children it usually rises. Pallor, hypertension, and a
slow, hard pulse are common.

The *neuromuscular syndrome,* or *lead palsy,* is rare
in the United States today. It is a manifestation of
advanced subacute poisoning. Muscle weakness and
easy fatigue occur considerably in advance of actual
paralysis, and may be the only signs of the syndrome
to develop. In occult cases, weakness or palsy may
not become evident until after extended muscle activity. The muscle groups involved are usually the
most active ones, generally extensors of the forearm,
wrist, fingers, and extraocular muscles, the palsy
often occurring only on the dominant side. Wrist-
drop and, to a lesser extent, foot-drop have been
considered almost pathognomonic for lead poisoning. There is no sensory involvement, in contrast to
the peripheral neuritis of arsenic poisoning. Degenerative changes in the motoneurons and their axons
as well as impairment of high-energy phosphate
metabolism in the muscle itself have been described.
Long-standing residual paralysis, atrophy, and contractures sometimes result, sequelae that are more
consistent with neural lesions than with interference
with muscle phosphocreatine synthesis. The muscle
and joint pains that are a frequent complaint of
patients with lead poisoning are probably unrelated
to the neuromuscular syndrome; lead impairs the
renal transport of urates and may precipitate an
attack of gout. A detailed summary of lead paralysis
has been presented by Cantarow and Trumper
(1944).

The *CNS syndrome* has been termed *lead encephalopathy.* It is the most serious manifestation of lead

poisoning. It occurs rarely in adults, only as a consequence of rapid, intense absorption of the metal. The first clues to the development of the syndrome may be clumsiness, vertigo, ataxia, falling, headache, insomnia, restlessness, and irritability. As the encephalopathy develops, there may occur excitement and confusion, which may be followed by delirium and repetitive grand mal convulsions or lethargy and coma. Vomiting is a common sign and is usually projectile. Visual disturbances are also present. The signs and symptoms are characteristic of increased intracranial pressure. There may be a proliferative meningitis and intense edema, but punctate hemorrhages, gliosis, and areas of focal necrosis also occur. Demyelination has been seen in nonhuman primates. The fatality rate is about 25%. Approximately 40% of survivors have neurological sequelae, such as mental retardation, EEG abnormalities or frank seizures, cerebral palsy, optic atrophy, or dystonia musculorum deformans.

Although the *renal* effects of lead are not as dramatic as those in the CNS and gastrointestinal tract, nephropathy does occur. In animals, a degenerative tubular necrosis has been observed (Hirsch, 1973). Amino acids, glucose, and phosphate cannot be normally reabsorbed (Fanconi syndrome), and hypophosphatemia may occur. Albumin, erythrocytes, and casts also are frequently found in the urine during poisoning. An increased incidence of chronic nephritis and cerebral hemorrhage occurs later in life among persons who have experienced lead encephalopathy. It is doubtful that the hypertension that frequently attends or follows severe lead poisoning has a renal basis, because renin secretion is actually decreased (Beritić, 1971) and aldosterone levels fail to respond to hypovolemia and hyponatremia.

A widely known *hematological* manifestation of plumbism is the formation of aggregates of ribonucleic acid in erythrocytes to form punctate basophilic stippling, the importance of which was once overemphasized. Among children, stippling is seen in only 60% of cases, and it is frequently absent among adults. Furthermore, stippling occurs in many conditions other than plumbism.

Microcytic hypochromic anemia is more common than stippling and is an almost invariable finding in pediatric cases. The anemia may result in part from the destruction of erythrocytes. The type of hemoglobin (HbA_3) found in the erythrocytes of anemic children with elevated blood lead levels is characteristic of prematurely senescent erythrocytes, but the life-span of the majority of the erythrocytes is normal (Berk et al., 1970); only a small fraction of the erythrocytes is fragile. The erythrocytes from patients with the hemolytic disorder also have a defect in phosphatidic acid synthesis and glucose-6-phosphate dehydrogenase activity during lead poisoning. The permeability to potassium is impaired, probably as the result of inhibition of membrane adenosine triphosphatase (ATPase). The erythrocytes undergo potassium loss and pyknosis and show decreased compliance; the damaged cells are then removed by the reticuloendothelial system. Jaundice often occurs late in lead poisoning. Reticulocytosis, which may result from the stimulant effects of hemolysis on the bone marrow, is common. The anemia is probably also partly dyshematopoietic in nature.

δ-ALA synthetase is inhibited but, because δ-ALA dehydratase is also inhibited, blood and urine levels of δ-ALA increase. δ-ALA dehydratase inhibition occurs even with blood concentrations of lead found in normal urban residents (McIntire et al., 1973). In spite of the substrate-limited decrease in synthesis of coproporphyrinogen III, coproporphyrin blood levels rise, because the conversion to protoporphyrin is also inhibited. Finally, heme synthesis is inhibited. It is the accumulated protoporphyrin that imparts the red fluorescence to fluorocytes. Other hematological disturbances occur, such as alterations in plasma albumin and globulin concentrations. The disturbances of heme synthesis in lead intoxication have been reviewed by de Bruin (1971) and Albahary (1972).

The presence of coproporphyrin and δ-ALA in the urine and fluorocytosis are by no means pathognomonic of lead poisoning, but they are roughly proportional to the blood or urine concentrations of lead. Since they occur as early signs of abnormal lead exposure and their determination is a relatively simple laboratory procedure, these indices can be used routinely in the examination of persons exposed to lead; if positive, more elaborate studies on the lead content of blood and urine can be performed.

Other signs and symptoms of plumbism are an ashen color of the face and a pallor of the lips; retinal stippling; the appearance of "premature aging," with stooped posture, poor muscle tone, and emaciation; and the black or grayish so-called lead line along the gingival margin, which results from the periodontal deposition of lead sulfide. Since it can be removed by good dental hygiene, it is more often absent than present. A similar pigmentation may result from the absorption of mercury, bismuth, silver, thallium, or iron.

Subtle effects may accompany the subclinical toxicity of lead. Mental retardation and hyperactivity have been described in children with only moderate body burdens of lead (Millar et al., 1970; David et al., 1972). By analogy with experimental animals, "subtoxic" doses may possibly decrease the resistance to infections. Chronic exposure causes chromosomal abnormalities in man (Deknudt et al., 1973).

Organic Lead Poisoning. Intoxication by tetramethyl and tetraethyl lead is now rare; owing to vigorous industrial health measures, the hazard resulting from contact with leaded gasoline is minimal. Lead poisoning occurs among "gasoline sniffers." The lead compounds in automobile exhaust are inorganic.

Continued absorption of small amounts of tetraethyl lead can result in the classical syndrome of chronic lead poisoning, inasmuch as the lead is eventually converted in the body to inorganic lead. Since tetraethyl lead can be absorbed much more rapidly than inorganic lead, the onset of poisoning is usually more rapid.

The earliest symptoms of acute tetraethyl lead

poisoning are insomnia and disturbing dreams. Thereafter, anorexia, nausea and vomiting, diarrhea, headache, muscular weakness, and emotional instability may be experienced. Subjective CNS symptoms such as irritability, restlessness, and anxiety are next evident. At this time there is usually hypothermia, bradycardia, and hypotension. With continued exposure, or in the case of intense acute exposure, CNS manifestations progress to delusions, ataxia, exaggerated muscular movements, and, finally, a maniacal state leading to convulsions or coma.

The diagnosis of tetraethyl lead poisoning is established by relating the above signs and symptoms to a history of exposure. The urinary concentration of lead may be elevated, often above 0.15 mg in each liter. The blood concentration of lead may be normal or slightly elevated. Basophilic stippling is uncommon, and coproporphyrinuria is rare. In the case of severe exposure, death may occur within a few hours or may be delayed for several weeks. If death does not occur within this time, recovery is usually complete, but instances of residual CNS damage have been reported. (For further details of tetraethyl lead poisoning, see Cantarow and Trumper, 1944; Sanders, 1964.)

Treatment of Lead Poisoning. Treatment consists in supportive measures and the use of chelating agents. Adequate urine flow is first restored. If necessary, seizures are controlled.

In all symptomatic patients and also asymptomatic ones who have a blood concentration of lead of more than 1 mg per liter, a combination of *intramuscular dimercaprol* and *calcium disodium edetate* is used. The first dose is of dimercaprol only; thereafter, both drugs are given at 4-hour intervals. The dose of dimercaprol is 2.5 mg/kg in adults and 4 mg/kg in children; that of edetate is 8 mg/kg in adults and 12.5 mg/kg in children. In the absence of encephalopathy and if the response to the chelators is prompt, dimercaprol may be discontinued after 2 to 3 days and the daily dose of edetate maintained at 50 mg/kg, in divided doses. In children, a normal course is 5 days, but it is 7 days if marked improvement does not occur by the fourth day. In children with encephalopathy, the course is repeated in 2 to 3 weeks, if necessary. In adults, a course is 3 to 5 days, in the absence of encephalopathy. If an adult patient is intolerant to dimercaprol, *intravenous* edetate is used in lieu of the combination. In asymptomatic patients in whom the blood level is less than 1 mg per liter, edetate alone is used in children and oral penicillamine alone in adults.

A course of dimercaprol-edetate or edetate alone is followed by a course of oral penicillamine. The daily dose is 30 to 40 mg/kg for 3 to 6 months in children who previously manifested encephalopathy or whose blood level of lead exceeds 600 μg per liter and in whom there is prominent radiographic evidence of lead deposition in bone. In adults, the daily dose of penicillamine is 500 to 750 mg for 2 months or until the urinary excretion of lead falls below 500 μg per day. When penicillamine is given for long-term prophylactic chelation, it must not be forgotten that the drug can promote absorption of lead from the gut and thus favor intoxication; every effort must be made to prevent further ingestion of lead, either in the presence or absence of penicillamine. For the pharmacology and adverse effects of the chelating agents, Chapter 45 should be consulted.

In acute lead encephalopathy, quick control of excitement, mania, and convulsions is obtained with diazepam, after which paraldehyde is administered as needed. In the early course of treatment, barbiturates are avoided because of their persistent depressant effects. After an acute episode is over, barbiturates or phenytoin can be used.

In the treatment of acute poisoning by alkyl lead compounds, sedative, anticonvulsant, and fluid and electrolyte therapy may be necessary. Chelating agents are of no avail.

The details of the treatment of lead poisoning have been reviewed by Chisolm (1971).

Abdel-Meguid, M.; Habib, Y. A.; Abdallah, A.; and Sajf, M. The effect of antibilharzial antimonial compounds on the percentage of oxygen saturation of blood. *J. Egypt. med. Ass.,* 1967, *50,* 369–374.

Åberg, B.; Ekman, L.; Falk, R.; Greitz, U.; Persson, G.; and Snihs, J.-O. Metabolism of methyl mercury (^{203}Hg) compounds in man. *Archs envir. Hlth,* 1969, *19,* 478–484.

Adam, M., and Kühn, K. Investigations on the reactions of metals with collagen *in vivo.* I. Comparison of the reaction of gold thiosulfate with collagen *in vivo* and *in vitro. Eur. J. Biochem.,* 1968, *3,* 407–410.

Bartter, F. C.; Cowie, D. B.; Most, H.; Ness, A. T.; and Forbush, S. The fate of radioactive tartar emetic administered to human subjects. *J. trop. Med. Hyg.,* 1947, *27,* 403–416.

Bayles, T. B., and Fremont-Smith, P. Significant clinical remissions in rheumatoid arthritis resulting from "sensitivity" produced by gold salt therapy. *Ann. rheum. Dis.,* 1956, *15,* 394–395.

Beritić, T. Lead concentration found in human blood in association with lead colic. *Archs envir. Hlth,* 1971, *23,* 289–291.

Berk, P. D.; Tschudy, D. P.; Shepley, L. A.; Waggoner, J. G.; and Berlin, N. I. Hematologic and biochemical studies in a case of lead poisoning. *Am. J. Med.,* 1970, *48,* 137–144.

Berlin, M., and Lewander, T. Increased brain uptake of mercury caused by 2,3-dimercaptopropanol (BAL) in mice given mercuric chloride. *Acta pharmac. tox.,* 1965, *22,* 1–7.

Bluhm, G. B.; Sigler, J. W.; and Ensign, D. C. D-Penicillamine therapy of thrombocytopenia secondary to chrysotherapy: a case report. *Arthritis Rheum.,* 1962, *5,* 638.

Bollet, A. J., and Shuster, A. Metabolism of mucopolysaccharides in connective tissue. II. Synthesis of glucosamine-6-phosphate. *J. clin. Invest.,* 1960, *39,* 114–118.

Bueding, E., and Mansour, J. M. The relationship between inhibition of phosphofructokinase activity and the mode of action of trivalent organic antimonials on *Schistosoma mansoni. Br. J. Pharmac. Chemother.,* 1957, *12,* 159–165.

Cooperating Clinics Committee of the American Rheumatism Association. A controlled trial of gold salt therapy in rheumatoid arthritis. *Arthritis Rheum.,* 1973, *16,* 353–358.

Cox, A. J., and Marich, K. W. Gold in the dermis following gold therapy for rheumatoid arthritis. *Archs Derm.,* 1973, *108,* 655–657.

Dale, P. W., and Patterson, M. B. EEG findings in chronic rheumatoid arthritics receiving gold therapy. *Electroenceph. clin. Neurophysiol.,* 1967, *23,* 493.

David, O.; Clark, J.; and Voeller, K. Lead and hyperactivity. *Lancet,* 1972, *2,* 900–903.

Davis, P.; Ezeoke, A.; Munro, J.; Hobbs, J. R.; and Hughes, G. R. V. Immunological studies on the mechanism of gold hypersensitivity reactions. *Br. med. J.,* 1973, *3,* 676–678.

Deby, C.; Bacq, Z.-M.; and Simon, D. *In vitro* inhibition of the biosynthesis of a prostaglandin by gold and silver. *Biochem. Pharmac.,* 1973, *22,* 3141–3143.

Deknudt, G.; Leonard, A.; and Ivanov, B. Chromosome alterations observed in male workers occupationally exposed to lead. *Envir. Physiol. Biochem.,* 1973, *3,* 132–138.

Done, A. K., and Peart, A. J. Acute toxicities of arsenical herbicides. *Clin. Toxicol.,* 1971, *4,* 343–355.

Ennis, R. S.; Granda, J. L.; and Posner, A. S. Effect of gold salts and other drugs on the release and activity of lysosomal hydrolases. *Arthritis Rheum.,* 1968, *11,* 756–764.

Fierz, U. Katamnestische Untersuchungen über die Nebenwirkung der Therapie mit anorganischen Arsen bei Hautkrankheiten. *Dermatologica,* 1965, *131,* 41–58.

Forestier, J. L'aurothérapie dans les rhumatismes chronique. *Bull. Mém. Soc. méd. Hôp. Paris,* 1929, *53,* 323–327.

Gellhorn, A., and van Dyke, H. B. The correlation between distribution of antimony in tissues and chemotherapeutic effect in experimental leishmaniasis. *J. Pharmac. exp. Ther.,* 1946, *88,* 162–172.

Gerber, R. C.; Paulus, H. E.; Bluestone, R.; and Lederer, M. Kinetics of aurothiomalate in serum and synovial fluid. *Arthritis Rheum.,* 1972, *15,* 625–629.

Ginsburg, J. M. Renal mechanism for excretion and transformation of arsenic in the dog. *Am. J. Physiol.,* 1965, *208,* 832–840.

Gottlieb, N. L.; Smith, P. M.; and Smith, E. M. Gold excretion correlated with clinical course during chrysotherapy in rheumatoid arthritis. *Arthritis Rheum.,* 1972, *15,* 582–592.

———. Pharmacodynamics of [197]Au and [195]Au labeled aurothiomalate in blood. Correlation with course of rheumatoid arthritis, gold toxicity and gold excretion. *Ibid.,* 1974, *17,* 171–183.

Heydorn, K. Environmental variation of arsenic levels in human blood determined by neutron activation analysis. *Clinica chim. Acta,* 1970, *28,* 349–357.

Hirsch, G. H. Effect of chronic lead treatment on renal function. *Toxicol. appl. Pharmac.,* 1973, *25,* 84–93.

Iverson, F.; Downie, R. H.; Paul, C.; and Trenholm, H. L. Methyl mercury: acute toxicity, tissue distribution and decay profiles in the guinea pig. *Toxicol. appl. Pharmac.,* 1973, *24,* 545–554.

Jaffe, I. A. The treatment of rheumatoid arthritis and necrotizing vasculitis with penicillamine. *Arthritis Rheum.,* 1970, *13,* 436–443.

Jessop, J. D., and Johns, R. G. S. Serum gold determinations in patients with rheumatoid arthritis receiving sodium aurothiomalate. *Ann. rheum. Dis.,* 1973, *32,* 228–232.

Kaleda, F. S.; Abdel-Taweb, G. A.; Moustafa, M. H.; and Konbar, A. A. Comparative studies on the *in vivo* effects of tartar emetic, vitamin B_6, and the chelating agent 2,3-dimercapropropanol (BAL) on the functional capacity of the tryptophan-niacin pathway in patients with schistosomiasis. *Metabolism,* 1972, *21,* 1105–1112.

Kark, R. A. P.; Poskanzer, D. C.; Bullock, J. D.; and Boylen, G. Mercury poisoning and its treatment with N-acetyl-D,L-penicillamine. *New Engl. J. Med.,* 1971, *285,* 10–16.

Landrigan, P. J.; Gehlbach, S. H.; Rosenblum, B. F.; and coworkers. Epidemic lead absorption near an ore smelter. The role of particulate lead. *New Engl. J. Med.,* 1975, *292,* 123–129.

Lawrence, J. S. Studies with radioactive gold. *Ann. rheum. Dis.,* 1961, *20,* 341–352.

Lee, A. M., and Fraumeni, J. F. Arsenic and respiratory cancer in man: an occupational study. *J. natn. Cancer Inst.,* 1969, *42,* 1045–1052.

Lisella, F.; Long, K. R.; and Scott, H. G. Health aspects of arsenicals in the environment. *J. envir. Hlth,* 1972, *34,* 511–518.

Lockie, L. M.; Norcross, B. M.; and Riordin, D. J. Gold in the treatment of rheumatoid arthritis. *J. Am. med. Ass.,* 1958, *167,* 1204–1206.

Lorber, A.; Atkins, C. J.; Chang, C. C.; Lee, Y. B.; Starrs, J.; and Bovy, R. A. Monitoring serum gold values to improve chrysotherapy in rheumatoid arthritis. *Ann. rheum. Dis.,* 1973a, *32,* 133–139.

Lorber, A.; Baumgartner, W. A.; Bovy, R. A.; Chang, C. C.; and Hollcraft, R. Clinical application for heavy metal-complexing potential of N-acetylcysteine. *J. clin. Pharmac.,* 1973b, *13,* 332–336.

Lorber, A.; Cohen, R. L.; Chang, C. C.; and Anderson, H. E. Gold determination in biological fluids by atomic absorption spectrometry: application to chrysotherapy in rheumatoid arthritis patients. *Arthritis Rheum.,* 1968, *11,* 170–177.

McArthur, J. N.; Dawkins, P. D.; Smith, M. J. H.; and Hamilton, E. B. D. Mode of action of antirheumatic drugs. *Br. med. J.,* 1971, *2,* 677–679.

McIntire, M. S.; Wolf, G. L.; and Angle, C. R. Red cell lead and δ-aminolevulinic acid dehydratase. *Clin. Toxicol.,* 1973, *6,* 183–188.

Magos, L., and Clarkson, T. Effect of phenobarbitone on the biliary excretion of methylmercury in rats and mice. *Nature, New Biol.,* 1973, *246,* 123–124.

Mascarenhas, B. R.; Granda, J. L.; and Freyberg, R. H. Gold metabolism in patients with rheumatoid arthritis treated with gold compounds—reinvestigated. *Arthritis Rheum.,* 1972, *15,* 391–402.

Mattingly, S. Palindromic rheumatism. *Ann. rheum. Dis.,* 1966, *25,* 307–317.

Millar, J. A.; Battistini, V.; Cumming, R. L. C.; Carswell, F.; and Goldberg, A. Lead and δ-aminolevulinic acid dehydratase levels in mentally retarded children and lead-poisoned suckling rats. *Lancet,* 1970, *2,* 695–698.

Multicentre Trial Group. Controlled trial of D(−) penicillamine in severe rheumatoid arthritis. *Lancet,* 1973, *1,* 275–280.

Murakami, M., and Hirosawa, K. Electron microscope autoradiography of kidney after administration of ^{210}Pb in mice. *Nature, Lond.,* 1973, *245,* 153–154.

Niedermier, W.; Prillaman, W. W.; and Griggs, J. H. The effect of chrysotherapy on trace metals in patients with rheumatoid arthritis. *Arthritis Rheum.,* 1971, *14,* 533–538.

Norn, S. Anaphylactic histamine release and influence of antirheumatics. *Acta pharmac. tox.,* 1971, *30,* Suppl. 1, 1–59.

Norseth, T., and Brendeford, M. Intracellular distribution of inorganic and organic mercury in rat liver after exposure to methylmercury salts. *Biochem. Pharmac.,* 1971, *20,* 1101–1107.

Norseth, T., and Clarkson, T. W. Intestinal transport of [203]Hg-labelled methyl mercury chloride. Role of biotransformation in rats. *Archs envir. Hlth,* 1971, *22,* 568–577.

Norton, W. L.; Lewis, D. C.; and Ziff, M. Electron-dense deposits following injection of gold sodium thiomalate and thiomalic acid. *Arthritis Rheum.,* 1968, *11,* 436–443.

Novey, H. S., and Martel, S. H. Asthma, arsenic, and cancer. *J. Allergy,* 1969, *44,* 315–319.

Pennys, N. S.; Eaglestein, W. H.; Indgin, S.; and Frost, P. Gold sodium thiomalate treatment of pemphigus. *Archs Derm.,* 1973, *108,* 56–60.

Persellin, R. H., and Ziff, M. The effect of gold salt on lysosomal enzymes of the peritoneal macrophage. *Arthritis Rheum.,* 1966, *9,* 57–65.

Piscator, M., and Lind, B. Cadmium, zinc, copper, and lead in human renal cortex. *Archs envir. Hlth,* 1972, *24,* 426–431.

Pueschel, S. M.; Kopito, L.; and Schachman, H. Children with an increased lead burden. A screening and follow-up study. *J. Am. med. Ass.,* 1972, *222,* 462–466.

Rabinowitz, M. B.; Wetherill, G. W.; and Kopple, J. D. Lead metabolism in the normal human: stable isotope studies. *Science, Wash.,* **1973,** *182,* 725–727.

Ramos, F. H.; Barrós, B.; Larrosa, R. A.; Dighiero, M.; and Batista, V. Present status of gold in the treatment of rheumatoid arthritis. *A.I.R.,* **1963,** *6,* 105–112.

Research Sub-committee of the Empire Rheumatism Council. Gold therapy in rheumatoid arthritis: report of a multicentre controlled trial. *Ann. rheum. Dis.,* **1960,** *19,* 95–117.

———. Gold therapy in rheumatoid arthritis: final report of a multicentre controlled trial. *Ibid.,* **1961a,** *20,* 315–334.

———. Relation of toxic reactions in gold therapy to improvement in rheumatoid arthritis. *Ibid.,* **1961b,** *20,* 335–340.

Rubinstein, H. M., and Dietz, A. A. Serum gold. II. Levels in rheumatoid arthritis. *Ann. rheum. Dis.,* **1973,** *32,* 128–132.

Schroeder, H. A., and Nason, A. P. Trace-element analysis in clinical chemistry. *Clin. Chem.,* **1971,** *17,* 461–473.

Schulert, A. R.; Browne, H. G.; and Salam, A. H. Human disposition of antimony administered as antimony sodium dimercapto-succinate, with an analysis of antimony concentration in excreted *Schistosoma haematobium* ova. *Trans. R. Soc. trop. Med. Hyg.,* **1964,** *58,* 48–52.

Silverberg, D. S.; Kidd, E. G.; Shnitka, T. S.; and Ulan, R. A. Gold nephropathy. A clinical and pathologic study. *Arthritis Rheum.,* **1970,** *13,* 812–825.

Smith, P. M.; Smith, E. M.; and Gottlieb, N. Gold distribution in whole blood during chrysotherapy. *J. Lab. clin. Med.,* **1973,** *82,* 930–937.

Smith, R. T. Effective antirheumatoid gold therapy. *A.I.R.,* **1963,** *6,* 60–73.

Smith, R. T.; Peak, W. P.; Kron, K. M.; Hermann, I. F.; and Del Toro, R. A. Increasing the effectiveness of gold therapy in rheumatoid arthritis. *J. Am. med. Ass.,* **1958,** *167,* 1197–1204.

Smith, S. E. Uptake of antimony potassium tartrate by mouse liver slices. *Br. J. Pharmac.,* **1969,** *37,* 476–484.

Smyth, C. J. Therapy of rheumatoid arthritis. *Postgrad. Med.,* **1972,** *51,* Suppl., 23–31.

Somjen, G. G.; Herman, S. P.; and Klein, R. Electrophysiology of methyl mercury poisoning. *J. Pharmac. exp. Ther.,* **1973a,** *187,* 579–592.

Somjen, G. G.; Herman, S. P.; Klein, R.; Brubaker, P. E.; Briner, W. H.; Goodrich, J. K.; Krigman, M. R.; and Haseman, J. K. The uptake of methyl mercury (^{203}Hg) in different tissues related to its neurotoxic effects. *J. Pharmac. exp. Ther.,* **1973b,** *187,* 602–611.

Stevenson, D. S.; Suarez, R. M., Jr.; and Marchand, E. J. The use of BAL in heavy metal poisoning with particular reference to antimonial intoxication. *Puerto Rico J. publ. Hlth trop. Med.,* **1948,** *23,* 533–553.

Stone, D. J. The effect of arsenic on inflammation, infection, and carcinogenesis. *Texas Med.,* **1969,** *65,* 40–43.

Strong, J. S.; Bartholomew, B. A.; and Smyth, C. J. Immunoresponsiveness of patients with rheumatoid arthritis receiving cyclophosphamide or gold salts. *Ann. rheum. Dis.,* **1973,** *32,* 233–237.

Van Tongeran, J. H. M.; Kunst, A.; Majoor, C. L. H.; and Schillings, P. H. M. Folic acid deficiency in chronic arsenic poisoning. *Lancet,* **1965,** *1,* 784–786.

Zuckner, J.; Ramsey, R. H.; Dorner, R. W.; and Gantner, G. E., Jr. D-Penicillamine in rheumatoid arthritis. *Arthritis Rheum.,* **1970,** *13,* 131–138.

Monographs and Reviews

Aaronson, R. M., and Spiro, H. M. Mercury and the gut. *Am. J. dig. Dis.,* **1973,** *18,* 583–594.

Albahary, C. Lead and hemopoiesis. The mechanism and consequences of the erythropathy of occupational lead poisoning. *Am. J. Med.,* **1972,** *52,* 367–378.

Arena, J. M. Treatment of mercury poisoning. *Mod. Treat.,* **1971,** *8,* 619–625.

Bidstrup, L. P. *Toxicity of Mercury and Its Compounds.* American Elsevier Publishing Co., New York, **1964.**

Black, M. M. Prolonged ingestion of arsenic. *Pharm. J.,* **1967,** *199,* 593–597.

Brown, J. R., and Kulkarni, M. V. A review of the toxicity and metabolism of mercury and its compounds. *Med. Servs J. Can.,* **1967,** *23,* 786–808.

Buchanan, W. D. *Toxicity of Arsenic Compounds.* Elsevier Publishing Co., Amsterdam, **1962.**

Cantarow, A., and Trumper, A. *Lead Poisoning.* The Williams & Wilkins Co., Baltimore, **1944.**

Chisolm, J. J. Poisoning due to heavy metals. *Pediat. Clins N. Am.,* **1970,** *17,* 591–615.

———. Treatment of lead poisoning. *Mod. Treat.,* **1971,** *8,* 593–611.

Ciaccio, E. I. Mercury: therapeutic and toxic aspects. *Semin. Drug Treat.,* **1971,** *1,* 177–194.

Clarkson, T. W. Biochemical aspects of mercury poisoning. *J. occup. Med.,* **1968,** *10,* 351–355.

———. The pharmacology of mercury compounds. *A. Rev. Pharmac.,* **1972a,** *12,* 375–406. (145 references.)

———. Recent advances in the toxicology of mercury with emphasis on the alkylmercurials. *CRC Crit. Rev. Toxicol.,* **1972b,** *1,* 203–234. (134 references.)

Committee on Biologic Effects of Atmospheric Pollutants. *Lead: Airborne Lead in Perspective.* National Academy of Sciences, Washington, D.C., **1972.**

Dales, L. G. The neurotoxicity of alkyl mercury compounds. *Am. J. Med.,* **1972,** *53,* 219–232.

de Bruin, A. Certain biological effects of lead upon the animal organism. *Archs envir. Hlth,* **1971,** *23,* 249–264. (174 references.)

D'Itri, F. M. *The Environmental Mercury Problem.* CRC Press, Cleveland, **1972.**

Felton, J. S.; Kahn, E.; Salick, B.; Van Natta, F. C.; and Whitehouse, M. W. Heavy metal poisoning. *Ann. intern. Med.,* **1972,** *76,* 779–792.

Fishbein, L. Chromatographic and biologic aspects of inorganic mercury. *Chromat. Rev.,* **1971,** *15,* 195–238. (165 references.)

Freyberg, R. H. Gold therapy for rheumatoid arthritis. In, *Arthritis and Allied Conditions,* 7th ed. (Hollander, J. L., ed.) Lea & Febiger, Philadelphia, **1966,** pp. 302–332.

——— Gold therapy for rheumatoid arthritis. In, *Arthritis and Allied Conditions,* 8th ed. (Hollander, J. L., and McCarty, D. J., Jr., eds.) Lea & Febiger, Philadelphia, **1972,** pp. 455–482.

Freyberg, R. H.; Block, W. D.; and Wells, G. S. Gold therapy for rheumatoid arthritis: considerations based upon studies of the metabolism of gold. *Clinics,* **1942,** *1,* 537–570.

Friberg, L. T., and Vostal, J. J. *Mercury in the Environment.* CRC Press, Cleveland, **1972.**

Frost, D. V. Arsenicals in biology. *Fedn Proc. Fedn Am. Socs exp. Biol.,* **1967,** *26,* 194–208.

Grant, N. Mercury in man. *Environment,* **1971,** *13,* 2–15.

Guinée, V. P. Lead poisoning. *Am. J. Med.,* **1972,** *52,* 283–288.

Hammond, P. B. Lead poisoning. An old problem with a new dimension. In, *Essays in Toxicology,* Vol. 1. (Blood, F. R., ed.) Academic Press, Inc., New York, **1969,** pp. 116–155.

———. Metabolism and metabolic action of lead and other heavy metals. *Clin. Toxicol.,* **1973,** *6,* 353–365.

Hardy, H. L.; Chamberlin, R. I.; Maloof, C. C.; Boylen, G. W., Jr.; and Howell, M. C. Lead as an environmental poison. *Clin. Pharmac. Ther.,* **1973,** *12,* 982–1002.

Hill, D. F. Gold therapy for rheumatoid arthritis. *Med. Clins N. Am.,* **1968,** *52,* 733–738.

Hill, W. R., and Pillsbury, D. M. *Argyria: The Pharmacology of Silver.* The Williams & Wilkins Co., Baltimore, **1939.**

Kehoe, R. A. The Harben Lectures, 1960. The metabolism

of lead in man in health and disease. *Jl R. Inst. publ. Hlth,* **1961,** *24,* 81–97, 101–120, 177–203.

———. Normal metabolism of lead. *Archs envir. Hlth,* **1964a,** *8,* 232–235.

———. Metabolism of lead under abnormal conditions. *Ibid.,* **1964b,** *8,* 235–243.

Lin-Fu, J. S. *Selected Bibliography on Lead Poisoning in Children.* U.S. Government Printing Office, Washington, D.C., **1971.** (201 references.)

———. Vulnerability of children to lead exposure and toxicity. *New Engl. J. Med.,* **1973,** *289,* 1229–1233, 1289–1293.

Lockie, L. M. Current methods of treatment. Adult peripheral rheumatoid arthritis: stages I and II. *Arthritis Rheum.,* **1961,** *4,* 404–407.

Mathies, H. Medikamentöse Therapie der chronischen Polyarthritis. *Medsche Klin.,* **1966,** *61,* 1345–1349.

Miller, M. W., and Clarkson, T. W. (eds.). *Mercury, Mercurials, and Mercaptans.* Charles C Thomas, Pub., Springfield, Ill., **1973.**

Sanders, L. W. Tetraethyl lead intoxication. *Archs envir. Hlth,* **1964,** *8,* 270–277.

Schroeder, H. Abnormal trace metals in man: arsenic. *J. chron. Dis.,* **1966,** *19,* 85–106.

Schroeder, H.; Balassa, J. J.; Gibson, F. S.; and Valanju, S. N. Abnormal trace metals in man: lead. *J. chron. Dis.,* **1961,** *14,* 408–425.

Symposium. (Various authors.) Symposium on lead, University of Cincinnati, February 25–27, 1963. *Archs envir. Hlth,* **1964,** *8,* 202–354.

Symposium. (Various authors.) *Environmental Lead Contamination.* Public Health Service Bulletin No. 1440, U.S. Government Printing Office, Washington, D. C., **1966.**

Task Group on Metal Accumulation. Accumulation of toxic metals with specific reference to their absorption, excretion, and biological half-times. *Envir. Physiol. Biochem.,* **1973,** *3,* 65–107. (210 references.)

Vallee, B. L.; Ulmer, D. D.; and Wacher, W. E. C. Arsenic toxicology and biochemistry. *A.M.A. Archs ind. Hlth,* **1960,** *21,* 132–151.

Zielhuis, R. L. Interrelationship of biochemical responses to the absorption of inorganic lead. *Archs envir. Hlth,* **1971,** *23,* 299–311.

Locally Acting Drugs

Ewart A. Swinyard

A large number of drugs act locally in a purely mechanical or physical manner. Although they possess both therapeutic and pharmaceutical usefulness, their pharmacological properties warrant only brief discussion. Their effects are confined to the site of application when the compounds are employed in reasonable dosage. These effects are described adequately by the names that are applied to the groups into which the drugs can be classified, namely, *demulcents, emollients, protectives, adsorbents,* and *absorbable hemostatics.* Other drugs act primarily at the site of application but have a chemical rather than a physical basis of action; they are *astringents, irritants, sclerosing agents, caustics, keratolytics, antiseborrheics, melanizing and demelanizing agents, mucolytics,* and certain *enzymes.*

DEMULCENTS

The demulcents comprise a group of compounds of high molecular weight that form aqueous solutions having the ability to alleviate irritation, particularly of mucous membranes or abraded surfaces. Chemically, most members of the group are gums, mucilages, or starches. When applied locally to irritated or abraded tissues, the demulcents tend to coat the surface and, by mechanical means, protect the underlying cells from stimuli that result from contact with air or irritants in the environment. The demulcents are applied to the skin in the form of lotions, ointments, or wet dressings; to the gastrointestinal tract in the form of demulcent drinks or enemas; and to the throat in the form of lozenges or gargles. The demulcents also have valuable pharmaceutical properties. They mask the obnoxious taste of certain drugs, and solutions of demulcents are often used

as vehicles for this purpose. They are also employed to provide stable emulsions or suspensions of drugs immiscible with or insoluble in aqueous vehicles. The following preparations are the more important of the demulcents; only their outstanding properties will be described.

Acacia, U.S.P. (*gum arabic*), is the dried gummy exudation from the stems and branches of *Acacia senegal.* When ground, it is a white powder. Acacia is readily soluble in water but insoluble in alcohol. *Acacia Syrup,* N.F., is a vanilla-flavored syrup that contains 10% acacia. Acacia is employed chiefly to suspend or emulsify drugs. It is also incorporated in lozenges.

Tragacanth, U.S.P. (*gum tragacanth*), is the dried gummy exudation from *Astragalus gummifer.* In its powdered form it consists of white, angular fragments. Tragacanth, in contact with sufficient water, swells to form a cloudy gelatinous mass that is 50 times the original volume of gum. It is used as a demulcent base for cutaneous medication, suspending agent for heavy insoluble powders, and emulsifying agent for oils administered orally.

Other natural plant hydrocolloids used to a lesser extent than acacia and tragacanth include *Agar,* U.S.P., *Glycyrrhiza,* U.S.P., and *Sodium Alginate,* N.F.

The synthetic cellulose derivatives also have important demulcent properties. *Methylcellulose,* U.S.P., and *Carboxymethylcellulose Sodium,* U.S.P., two hydrophilic colloid laxatives, have important demulcent properties. These synthetic substitutes for the natural gums are widely used in contact-lens solutions and other ophthalmic preparations, and as suspending agents for nose drops and other drugs that act locally.

Glycerin, U.S.P. (*glycerol*), is a trihydric alcohol, $CH_2OHCHOHCH_2OH$, and consists of a clear, colorless, syrupy liquid that has a sweet taste. Glycerin is miscible with water and alcohol. It is extensively employed as a vehicle for many drugs applied to the skin. Diluted with rose water it is an effective lotion for chapped and roughened hands. In combination with starch it forms a jelly base known as *Starch Glycerite*, N.F., a preparation sometimes employed as an emollient and a vehicle.

Glycerin absorbs water, and, therefore, in high concentration it is somewhat dehydrating and irritating to exposed tissue. Concentrated solutions, for this reason, are slowly bactericidal. The irritant action of glycerin accounts for its efficacy in promoting evacuation of the bowel when used rectally in the form of a suppository (*Glycerin Suppositories*, U.S.P.). It is also available as *glycerin oral solution* (50%). When given orally, glycerin is readily absorbed and serves as a source of calories (4.32 kcal/g). Glycerin by oral and parenteral administration has been used for the management of cerebral edema and to lower ocular tension and cerebrospinal fluid pressure (Tourtellotte *et al.*, 1972). It may be employed as a sweetening agent or vehicle in place of syrups.

Glycerin can exert systemic toxic effects when given orally or parenterally in very large doses. The major toxic effects (hemolysis, hemoglobinuria, and renal failure) are a function of concentration and route of administration. For example, glycerin does not hemolyze red blood cells when it is prepared in concentrations up to 40% in isotonic sodium chloride solution (Tourtellotte *et al.*, 1972). Systemic effects do not follow copious application to the skin.

Various congeners of glycerin are much more toxic than the parent compound. They exert a nephrotoxic effect and also may damage the liver. Indeed, deaths have resulted from the ingestion of drugs dissolved in *diethylene glycol* for oral administration. *Ethylene glycol* is also quite toxic. On the other hand, *propylene glycol* is relatively innocuous. The pharmacology of the glycols has been extensively studied by Hanzlik and associates (Hanzlik *et al.*, 1947; Luduena *et al.*, 1947).

Propylene Glycol, U.S.P., is a clear, colorless, viscous liquid with a slightly acrid taste. It is completely miscible with water and dissolves in many essential oils. It is used as a solvent for oral and injectable drugs, and is also employed in cosmetics, lotions, and ointments, as in *Hydrophilic Ointment*, U.S.P. The topical application of a 40 to 60% aqueous solution of propylene glycol with occlusion has been reported to clear the skin in X-linked ichthyosis and ichthyosis vulgaris (Goldsmith and Baden, 1972).

Polyethylene glycols are high-molecular-weight polymers produced by reacting ethylene oxide with ethylene glycol or water. They have the general formula $H(OCH_2CH_2)_nOH$. The n may range from 1 to a large number; hence, the molecular weights of these substances range from 150 to about 20,000. Substances with molecular weights up to 600 are liquids at room temperature and resemble highly refined petroleum oils in appearance and consistency. Those with molecular weights of 1000 to 9000 are solids at room temperature and resemble petroleum waxes such as paraffin. *Polyethylene glycol 20,000* is a hard, tough solid. The polyethylene glycols are of growing importance to the drug industry, because of their blandness, water solubility, wide compatibility, and low order of toxicity. They are widely employed as water-soluble ointment bases similar to *Polyethylene Glycol Ointment*, U.S.P., as

ingredients of lotions and suppositories, and as tablet coatings. Seven of these substances are listed in the official compendia: *Polyethylene Glycol 300*, N.F., *Polyethylene Glycol 400*, U.S.P., *Polyethylene Glycol 600*, U.S.P., *Polyethylene Glycol 1500*, U.S.P., *Polyethylene Glycol 1540*, N.F., *Polyethylene Glycol 4000*, U.S.P., and *Polyethylene Glycol 6000*, U.S.P.

Several proprietary water-miscible ointment bases, such as AQUAPHOR, POLYSORB, and UNIBASE, are also available. These bases are valuable when large quantities of liquids are to be incorporated into an ointment.

EMOLLIENTS

Emollients are fats or oils used for their local action on the skin and, occasionally, the mucous membranes. They are employed as protectives and as agents for softening the skin and rendering it more pliable, but chiefly as vehicles for more active drugs. These oleaginous substances soften the skin by forming an occlusive oil film on the stratum corneum, thus preventing drying from evaporation of the water that diffuses to the surface from the underlying layers of skin. Only the commonly employed emollients are described below.

Vegetable Oils. Official vegetable oils include *Olive Oil*, U.S.P., *Cottonseed Oil*, U.S.P., *Corn Oil*, U.S.P., *Almond Oil*, N.F., *Peanut Oil*, U.S.P., *Persic Oil*, N.F., and *Cocoa Butter*, U.S.P. (*cacao butter, theobroma oil*). With the exception of the last-named preparation, all are fluids. When taken internally, they act as mild cathartics and as protectives for the gastrointestinal tract in cases of corrosive poisoning. When applied externally, they are emollient to the skin and mucous membranes. They also provide the vehicles for many drugs that are injected in oily solution or suspension. Cocoa butter is a solid that melts at body temperatures. It is widely used as a suppository and an ointment base.

Animal Fats. The outstanding animal fat of pharmacological interest is *Anhydrous Lanolin*, U.S.P. (*wool fat*). This is a yellow, unctuous mass obtained from the wool of sheep. Wool fat is usually employed mixed with 25 to 30% water, in which form it is known as *Lanolin*, U.S.P. (*hydrous wool fat*). These two semisolids are used principally as bases for ointments. Because certain individuals are allergic to wool fat (Masters, 1960), it has been deleted from many official formulations.

Hydrocarbons. The important emollient hydrocarbons are *Paraffin*, N.F., *Petrolatum*, N.F., *White Petrolatum*, U.S.P., *Mineral Oil*, U.S.P., and *Light Mineral Oil*, N.F. *Hydrophilic Petrolatum*, U.S.P., is a widely used ointment base that contains cholesterol, stearyl alcohol, white wax, and white petrolatum. Many official ointments have a base composed of either white wax (5%) and white petrolatum (95%) or yellow wax (5%) and petrolatum (95%). The former combination is official under the name *White Ointment*, U.S.P.; the latter, *Yellow Ointment*, N.F. *Paraffin* is used mainly in ointments to raise their melting points. *White petrolatum* is a common ointment base and also is employed as an emollient and a lubricant. *Light mineral oil* has been used as a vehicle for drugs to be applied to the nasal mucous membranes; however, aqueous vehicles are preferred for this purpose. The more viscous *mineral oil* is an ingredient in various pharmaceutical preparations and is used also as a laxative.

Waxes. *White Wax, U.S.P.* (*bleached beeswax*), and *Yellow Wax, N.F.* (*beeswax*), are employed to harden ointment bases. A base composed of lard hardened with wax is known as a *cerate. Spermaceti,* U.S.P., a waxy substance obtained from the head of the sperm whale, is used to raise the melting point of ointments. A mixture of oil and wax is sometimes used as a vehicle for drugs when slow absorption and sustained effect are desired; the drugs are suspended in the oil-wax vehicle, and the resulting suspension is injected intramuscularly.

A widely employed emollient preparation is *Rose Water Ointment, N.F.* It consists essentially of spermaceti, white wax, almond oil, rose water, and rose oil. Most of the commercial *cold creams* are modifications of this basic preparation. For example, *Cold Cream,* U.S.P., contains mineral oil in place of the almond oil.

PROTECTIVES AND ADSORBENTS

Protectives are designed to cover the skin or mucous membranes in order to prevent contact with possible irritants. Although demulcents and emollients are also protective, common usage restricts the term to certain insoluble and chemically inert substances in a very fine state of subdivision, for example, *dusting powders,* and to the several materials that form an adherent, continuous, flexible or semirigid coat when applied to the skin. Some chemically inert powders also adsorb dissolved or suspended substances, such as gases, toxins, and bacteria; these are known as *adsorbents.* Substances used internally for this purpose are described below, under *gastrointestinal protectives and adsorbents.*

Dusting Powders. These relatively indifferent (inert and insoluble) substances are used to cover and to protect epithelial surfaces, ulcers, and wounds. Those with a smooth surface act mainly by preventing friction; those with a porous structure, by absorbing moisture. The absorption of skin moisture also decreases friction and discourages growth of certain bacteria. The more important dusting powders include *Talc,* U.S.P., *Zinc Oxide,* U.S.P., *Zinc Stearate,* U.S.P., *Magnesium Stearate,* U.S.P., *Starch,* U.S.P., *Boric Acid,* N.F., and *insoluble salts of bismuth.* Water-absorbent powders should not be used on raw surfaces with profuse exudate, as they tend to cake and form adherent crusts. Starch becomes doughy when it absorbs moisture and requires the addition of an antiseptic (2 to 4% boric acid or 1% salicylic acid) to prevent fermentation. Zinc stearate and magnesium stearate are not wetted by moisture, and thus they permit seepage and evaporation and do not crust.

Medicated or perfumed *talc* (mainly magnesium silicate) is widely used as a dusting powder under the name *talcum powder.* Although *talc* is a benign substance when applied to the intact skin, it can induce severe granulomatous reactions when introduced into wounds or an operative field (Antopol, 1933). For this reason, *talc* should never be used as a dusting powder for surgical gloves. A number of substitutes have been proposed, but *Absorbable Dusting Powder,* U.S.P. (BIO-SORB), seems to be the most satisfactory. This is a mixture of amylose and amylopectin, derived from cornstarch, and treated chemically to assure good lubricating properties after sterilization. It has no deleterious effect on rubber gloves, appears to produce no appreciable reaction in tissues, and is absorbed completely in a short time.

Mechanical Protectives. Agents in this category are used to provide occlusive protection from the external environment, to give mechanical support, and as vehicles for various medicaments. *Collodion,* U.S.P., pyroxylon (5%) in an ether-alcohol vehicle, and *Flexible Collodion,* U.S.P., composed of collodion with camphor (2%) and castor oil (3%), are used to seal small wounds and as vehicles for medicated collodions. Their use is diminishing because of the recognition that air helps to maintain a normal cutaneous flora of low pathogenicity. *Zinc Gelatin,* U.S.P., a smooth jelly composed of zinc oxide (10%) and gelatin (15%) in a glycerin-water vehicle, is spread between layers of bandage and used as a protective dressing and support for varicosities and similar lesions. The dressing may be removed by soaking with warm water.

Dimethicone (SILICOTE), a relatively inert silicone oil with skin-adherent and water-repellent properties, is used to protect the skin against exposure to ordinary soap, water, and dermal irritants such as cleansers, decomposition products of urine, and other substances. It is available as an ointment (30%), cream (30%), or spray (33⅓%).

Gastrointestinal Protectives and Adsorbents. A number of chemically inert powders are used internally as protectives and adsorbents. The insoluble salts of bismuth (subcarbonate and subnitrate) and magnesium (trisilicate) are employed as protectives in the management of ulcerations of the stomach and bowel. However, careful clinical studies do not support the popular notion that these substances "coat the crater of the ulcer and provide mechanical protection." Indeed, the bismuth salts are of little value either as protectives or as antacids. The powders that possess adsorptive properties are used to adsorb noxious substances, such as gases, toxins, and bacteria. Unfortunately, adsorption is not a specific action; when substances having significant adsorptive capacity are given by mouth, drugs, nutrients, and enzymes, as well as noxious substances present in the bowel, are adsorbed to their surface. The principal gastrointestinal adsorbents include *magnesium trisilicate, aluminum hydroxide, activated charcoal, kaolin,* and *pectin.*

Magnesium Trisilicate, U.S.P., a relatively weak antacid, is an effective gastrointestinal adsorbent. The gelatinous silicon dioxide, formed by the reaction of magnesium trisilicate with the gastric contents, is said to protect ulcerated mucosal surfaces and favor healing. The salt also interferes with the absorption of tetracyclines, anticholinergics, and other drugs. It is usually given orally suspended in water, in a dose of 1 g four times a day. Chronic use may result in silica kidney stones.

A number of aluminum compounds, such as *Aluminum Hydroxide Gel,* U.S.P., *Dried Aluminum Hydroxide Gel,* U.S.P., and *Aluminum Phosphate Gel,* N.F., are used as adsorbents. These substances also decrease the absorption of tetracyclines, anticholinergics, and other drugs. Since they neutralize hydrochloric acid so efficiently, they are discussed under the gastric antacids (Chapter 48).

Activated Charcoal, U.S.P., an odorless, tasteless, fine black powder, is the residue from the destructive distillation of various organic materials, treated to increase its adsorptive power. The adsorptive capacity of various brands of activated charcoal differs enormously; a finely powdered activated charcoal with a high adsorptive capacity, such as ACTIVATED CHARCOAL-MERCK, NORIT A, and NUCHAR C, has been reported to be satisfactory (Picchioni, 1972). Activated charcoal, because of its broad spectrum of adsorptive activity and its rapidity of action, is considered to be the most valuable single agent for the emergency treatment of certain cases of drug poisoning (Holt and Holz, 1963). According to the *in-vitro* studies of Decker and coworkers (1968), charcoal efficiently adsorbs dextroamphetamine, primaquine, chlorpheniramine, colchicine, phenytoin, aspirin, iodine, phenol, and propoxyphene. Quinacrine, meprobamate, chlorpromazine, quinine, chloroquine, quinidine, glutethimide, 3,4-dichlorophenoxyacetic acid, and methyl salicylate are adsorbed less efficiently; and ferrous sulfate, malathion, DDT, N-methyl carbamate, and boric acid are poorly adsorbed. Mineral acids, alkalis, and compounds insoluble in aqueous acidic solution, such as tolbutamide, are not adsorbed to any appreciable extent. These studies also indicate that the activated charcoal-drug complex is stable for at least 24 hours. The usual dose of activated charcoal is 10 g. In an emergency, this dose can be approximated by stirring sufficient activated charcoal into water to make a thick soup. Although not a substitute for gastric lavage, a suspension of activated charcoal may be used for the lavage fluid.

Kaolin, N.F., is a native, hydrated aluminum silicate, powdered and freed from gritty particles by elutriation. It is used for the treatment of *diarrhea* and *dysentery.* Kaolin has also been used in the treatment of *chronic ulcerative colitis* to adsorb bacteria and toxins in the colon, but it is doubtful whether appreciable activity is retained by the time the material reaches the large bowel. Many proprietary products promoted for the treatment of abnormal intestinal fermentation contain a mixture of kaolin and pectin. It should be noted that kaolin also decreases the absorption of tetracyclines, anticholinergics, and other drugs. Although kaolin is generally considered to be innocuous, granuloma of the stomach has been reported from its use (Cohn *et al.,* 1941).

Pectin, N.F., a purified carbohydrate product ob-tained from the acid extraction of the rind of citrus fruits or from apple pomace, is widely employed in the treatment of *diarrhea.* Chemically, it consists chiefly of polygalacturonic acid, some of the hydroxyl groups of which are methylated. It dissolves in 20 parts of water; the resulting colloidal solution is viscous, opalescent, and acidic in reaction. Pectin is often used in combination with an adsorbent such as kaolin, as indicated above. However, it may be administered simply and conveniently in the form of ground raw apple. The mechanism of action of pectin in diarrheas is unknown. When it is fed to healthy human subjects, only a small amount is recovered in the feces. However, in patients with diarrhea, much larger amounts may be eliminated unchanged. The unchanged material may act in the bowel as an adsorbent and protective. Pectin is decomposed in the colon by bacterial action. The decomposition products have not been identified, but they may consist of acids that provide an unfavorable environment for abnormal bacterial flora causing diarrhea (Werch and Ivy, 1941).

Simethicone, N.F. (MYLICON, SILAIN), a light-gray, translucent liquid of greasy consistency, is a mixture of liquid dimethylpolysiloxanes with antifoaming and water-repellent properties. It is promoted as an adjunct in the treatment of conditions in which gas is a problem, such as flatulence, functional gastric bloating, and postoperative gaseous distention. It has also been used to reduce gas shadows in radiography of the bowel and to improve visualization in gastroscopy. It is believed to be physiologically inert and devoid of toxicity. Simethicone is available as an official oral suspension (40 mg in 0.6 ml) and in official tablets (40, 50, and 80 mg). The usual adult oral dose is 150 to 400 mg daily in divided doses, given after each meal and at bedtime. Simethicone is also used in combination with antacids, antispasmodics, sedatives, and digestants.

ANTIPERSPIRANTS AND DEODORANTS

Antiperspirants and *deodorants,* applied as aerosol sprays, pads, sticks, and roll-on creams, liquids, or semisolids, are vigorously promoted to the public for the control of excessive perspiration and body odor. The average adult produces from 0.5 to 1.5 liters (1 to 3 pt) of perspiration a day. Under normal conditions this secretion is odorless. The unpleasant odor sometimes associated with skin secretions results from chemical and bacterial degradation of the components of perspiration. Consequently, proper skin hygiene is essential to the control of body odors. Many individuals find skin hygiene inadequate and resort to preparations that decrease the flow and/or inhibit the degradation of perspiration. For a more detailed discussion of this subject, the interested reader is referred to the review by Robinson (1973).

Antiperspirants. The agents most commonly used topically as *antiperspirants* include *Aluminum Chloride,* N.F., *aluminum hydroxychloride, aluminum phenolsulfonate, Aluminum Sulfate,* U.S.P., *zinc phenolsulfonate,* and *zirconyl hydroxychloride.*

Aluminum hydroxychloride is the most frequently employed agent. The use of aluminum chloride has declined markedly; it hydrolyzes in aqueous solution to produce aluminum hydroxide and hydrochloric acid. The acidity of such preparations has a deleterious effect on fabrics that come in contact with treated skin. Similar hydrolysis occurs with other aluminum salts of strong inorganic acids such as aluminum sulfate. Aluminum hydroxychloride has a lower acidity than aluminum chloride or sulfate but is still active as an antiperspirant. Aluminum and zinc phenolsulfonate not only are useful astringents with moderate acidity but also are soluble in alcohol, an advantage in liquid aerosol preparations. Aluminum salts are known to cause allergic reactions in susceptible individuals. Zirconium salts, except for the hydroxychloride, have been discarded because of the marked incidence of associated granulomas of the skin.

The mechanism of action of antiperspirants is not completely known. It is generally agreed that these agents are astringent and that this action is largely responsible for their ability to reduce skin secretions.

Deodorants. *Deodorants* reduce the number of resident bacteria on the skin and thus inhibit bacterial decomposition of perspiration. The agents most commonly employed include *Benzalkonium Chloride*, U.S.P., *Methylbenzethonium Chloride*, N.F., *Neomycin Sulfate*, U.S.P., and *Vitamin E*, N.F. (*dl-alpha tocopherol*). These agents are not devoid of untoward side effects. Quaternary ammonium compounds such as benzalkonium are inactivated by soaps and irritate the skin if used in concentrations exceeding 1%, and the use of antibiotics may sensitize the individual and/or result in the production of resistant strains of bacteria. Currently vitamin E is included in some deodorant products; this antioxidant retards degradation of the components of perspiration without specific antibacterial activity.

Available proprietary preparations are either antiperspirant or deodorant or both, depending on the ingredients in the formulation. Consequently, allergic reactions may be induced by any of the above-mentioned agents as well as by the perfume used to scent the preparations. Diagnosis of allergic manifestations is usually not difficult, inasmuch as the allergic response is usually confined to the axilla.

ABSORBABLE HEMOSTATICS

The absorbable hemostatics are not directly concerned in the clotting mechanism; they either arrest bleeding by the formation of an artificial clot or provide a mechanical matrix that facilitates clotting when applied directly to denuded or bleeding surfaces. Since they are absorbed from the site of application after varying periods of time, they are referred to as absorbable hemostatics. It should be emphasized that the agents to be described are used to *control oozing from minute vessels* and will not effectively combat bleeding from arteries or veins when there is appreciable intravascular pressure. The absorbable hemostatics include *absorbable gelatin sponge, oxidized cellulose, human fibrinogen, thrombin,* and *thromboplastin.*

Absorbable Gelatin Sponge, U.S.P. (GELFOAM), is a sterile, absorbable, water-insoluble, gelatin-base sponge. It is used for the control of capillary bleeding. For this purpose it is frequently moistened with sterile isotonic sodium chloride solution or with thrombin solution before use. Since it is completely absorbed in 4 to 6 weeks, it may be left in place after the closure of an operative wound. Contact with tissue does not produce excessive scar formation or untoward cellular reactions. It is usually available as cones, packs, and sponges.

Oxidized Cellulose, U.S.P. (OXYCEL SURGICAL), is a specially treated form of surgical gauze or cotton that promotes clotting by a reaction between hemoglobin and cellulosic acid. Absorption of oxidized cellulose usually occurs within 2 to 7 days after application of the dry material, but complete absorption of large amounts of material may take 6 weeks or longer. It should not be used in combination with thrombin because the low pH interferes with the activity of the thrombin. Oxidized cellulose should not be employed for permanent packing or implantation in fractures because it interferes with bone regeneration and may result in cyst formation. The preparation also inhibits epithelialization and hence should not be used as a surface dressing except for the immediate control of hemorrhage. It is marketed as sterile cotton pledgets, gauze pads, and gauze strips.

Human Fibrinogen, U.S.P., a sterile fraction of normal human plasma, is used for restoring normal plasma fibrinogen levels in hemorrhagic complications caused by acute afibrinogenemia, as discussed elsewhere. Fibrinogen and a solution of thrombin are used locally during certain surgical procedures to create a clot or adhesion *in situ.*

Thrombin, U.S.P., is obtained from bovine plasma and is standardized on the basis of National Institutes of Health (N.I.H.) units. One N.I.H. unit is that amount of thrombin required to clot 1 ml of standard fibrinogen solution in 15 seconds. Thrombin has many applications in surgery. Its use in conjunction with absorbable gelatin sponges has already been mentioned. In addition, the material may be employed alone, either in powder form or in solution, to control capillary bleeding and to promote adhesion of tissue surfaces. For example, it is a valuable agent for the fixation of skin transplants. *Thrombin should be used only for topical application.* It is marketed as a powder in vials containing 1000, 5000, or 10,000 N.I.H. units. Despite its bovine origin, official thrombin appears to be nonantigenic when employed topically.

Thromboplastin (thrombokinase) is a powder prepared from the acetone-extracted brain and/or lung tissue of freshly killed rabbits. It contains thromboplastin, which promotes the conversion of prothrombin to thrombin. It is used for the determination of prothrombin time and activity of the blood, an important guide in anticoagulant therapy. Thromboplastin is also employed in surgery as a local hemostatic.

ASTRINGENTS

Astringents are locally acting drugs that precipitate proteins but have so little penetrability that only the surface of cells is affected. Consequently, the permeability of the cell membrane is greatly reduced but the cell itself remains viable. Many germicidal protein precipitants exert an astringent effect in high dilutions. Certain metallic ions, such as those of zinc and aluminum, are primarily astringent; the astringent effects of the metals are considered in connection with their other pharmacological properties (*see* Index). Of the vegetable astringents, only tannic acid will be mentioned here.

Tannic acid (*tannin, gallotannic acid*) is usually obtained from *nutgalls,* the excrescences on the young twigs of various species of *Quercus* (oak). The term *tannin* is ordinarily used as a synonym for tannic acid. There are many crude plant preparations that possess astringent actions by virtue of their tannin content, but none warrants description here.

Tannic acid was formerly used orally for the symptomatic treatment of diarrhea, topically for the management of extensive burns, and rectally for the relief of various rectal disorders. However, these applications are now practically obsolete because sufficient tannic acid may be absorbed from the gastrointestinal tract, denuded surfaces, and mucous membranes to cause severe centralobular necrosis of the liver (Wells *et al.,* 1942; Barnes and Rossiter, 1943; Krezanoski, 1966). The use of tannic acid as a chemical antidote in poisoning is only of limited value, and some metals and alkaloids are *not* precipitated by it. Furthermore, tannic acid interferes with the highly efficient adsorbent action of activated charcoal (Picchioni *et al.,* 1966). Thus, there are few if any legitimate medical uses for this substance.

IRRITANTS

The irritants are drugs that act locally on cutaneous or mucosal tissue to produce "inflammation." The first response to local irritation is an increased circulation to the injured part. The localized vasodilatation, mediated by way of an axon reflex, is attended by the feeling of comfort, warmth, and sometimes itching. Localized hyperesthesia also occurs. Drugs that evoke only reactive hyperemia are known as *rubefacients.* If the irritant action progresses, the capillaries dilate widely and become more permeable. Plasma escapes into the extracellular spaces, fluid collects under the epidermis, and blisters are formed. Drugs capable of causing this degree of irritation are known as *vesicants.* Irritants of another type readily penetrate into the orifices of the sebaceous glands and cause small multiple abscesses that may become confluent if the irritant action proceeds. Such drugs are called *pustulants.* The pustulants have few if any valid therapeutic applications.

When an irritant agent is used for other than its local effects, it is commonly referred to as a *counterirritant.* The mechanism of action of counterirritation is a dual one. The afferent nerve impulses from the skin are relayed in the cerebrospinal axis to efferent vasomotor fibers supplying internal organs. Thus, the increased circulation to the skin has its counterpart in deeper integumental structures and in viscera innervated from the same segmental level of the central nervous system (CNS). Furthermore, when pain arises from an internal organ, sensory impulses simultaneously coming from the skin, as a result of the action of an irritant, either alter the character of the visceral sensations or, more probably, occupy the final common pathway to the partial or complete exclusion of the impulses arising from the viscera. For example, the use of a rubefacient might relieve pain arising from intestinal spasm either by the salutary effect of an increased circulation to the spastic bowel or by the blocking of visceral afferent impulses. Local irritation can also reflexly stimulate the CNS. Thus, a painful stimulus may reflexly stimulate medullary centers and cause an increase in respiratory rate and blood pressure.

Drugs are the least useful means available for producing hyperemia, irritation, and counterirritation. Physical measures are employed much more frequently than are chemical agents. Heat is often the rubefacient of choice; the hot-water bottle or heating pad, the moist hot pack, and the heat lamp are simple means for applying heat. Short-wave diathermy also is an effective method for producing localized hyperemia.

CAMPHOR

Camphor, formerly used intramuscularly as a reflex respiratory stimulant, is now employed exclusively for its local actions. Natural camphor is obtained from the wood and bark of a tree, *Cinnamomum camphora,* growing especially in Japan and Taiwan. Camphor is also obtained synthetically. Its structural formula is as follows:

Camphor

Pharmacological Actions. *Local.* Camphor is a rubefacient when rubbed on the skin. When not vigorously applied, however, it may produce a feeling of coolness. Camphor also has a mild local anesthetic action, and its application to the skin may be followed by numbness. Camphor has a hot, bitter taste and, when taken in small amounts, produces a feeling of warmth and comfort in the stomach. In large doses it is irritating and causes nausea and vomiting.

Systemic Actions. The systemic effects of camphor are related primarily to stimulation of the CNS. Large doses of the drug, as can occur from ingestion of solid camphor by children, may cause convulsions. Treatment is the same as for poisoning by other central stimulants.

Preparations. *Camphor,* U.S.P., is a transparent, aromatic, crystalline substance that is relatively insoluble in water. It is an ingredient in *paregoric* and a number of proprietary preparations for external application. Official camphor preparations for local application are *Camphor Spirit,* N.F. (10% in alcohol), and *Camphorated Parachlorophenol,* U.S.P. (35% parachlorophenol and 65% camphor).

Therapeutic Uses. Camphor spirit is used as a local irritant. Camphor, applied topically as a 1 to 3% lotion or ointment, is used as an antipruritic and counterirritant. Camphorated parachlorophenol has *antibacterial* properties and is used in dentistry for the treatment of infected root canals.

MISCELLANEOUS AGENTS

Many drugs have an irritant action when applied locally, but this constitutes a minor aspect of their pharmacological properties; included in this category are *Chloroform,* N.F., *Ether,* U.S.P., and *Methyl Salicylate,* U.S.P. Two drugs that are used chiefly as irritants are *mustard* and *cantharides.*

Black mustard is the dried ripe seed of varieties of *Brassica nigra* or *juncea.* On contact with moisture, the preparation yields not less than 0.6% of *allyl isothiocyanate* (C_3H_5NCS), the primary active component. Mustard is usually employed in powder form. It is sometimes used internally as an emetic, but its chief use is as a local irritant in the form of a poultice or plaster. A *mustard plaster* is commonly prepared by adding sufficient tepid water to a mixture of 1 part mustard and 1 to 10 parts flour to make a thin paste. The paste is then spread on a piece of cloth and applied to the affected area. Within 5 minutes after application the area reddens and the skin temperature rises markedly. Since the irritation may proceed to vesication, an undiluted plaster should not remain in contact with the skin longer than 15 to 30 minutes. The local effects persist for 24 to 48 hours.

Cantharides (Spanish fly, Russian flies) consists of the dried insects, *Cantharis vesicatoria.* The active irritant in this crude drug is cantharidin, a white crystalline substance, sparingly soluble in water. It has the following chemical structure:

Cantharidin

Cantharidin exerts a rubefacient and vesicant action on the skin and mucous membranes. When taken orally it causes vomiting, purging, abdominal pain, and shock. The drug is absorbed from the gastrointestinal tract and, to a limited extent, from the skin. It is excreted by the kidney and irritates the entire urinary tract (Presto and Muecke, 1970). Irritation

of the bladder causes urgency of urination, and irritation of the urethra may result in priapism. Cantharides, therefore, is popularly known as an aphrodisiac. However, its use for this purpose is potentially dangerous and deaths have been reported from its promiscuous use by the laity (Craven and Polak, 1954; Nickolls and Teare, 1954). The topical application of a 0.7% solution of cantharidin in equal parts of acetone and flexible collodion is used in the treatment of *digital* and *periungual warts* (Epstein and Kligman, 1958). The blisters induced by this agent heal rapidly, without leaving a scar.

Therapeutic Uses. Irritants were formerly employed topically in the treatment of a variety of systemic diseases, but their use is now almost obsolete. Heat lamps and dry or moist hot packs are usually as effective as medicated plasters or solutions, and are particularly indicated in localized cutaneous infections or cellulitis, myositis, arthritis, bursitis, tenosynovitis, and similar afflictions.

SCLEROSING AGENTS

Sclerosing agents are irritating substances that are used to obliterate varicose veins and fibrose uncomplicated hemorrhoids. For a review of treatment methods for the latter, *see* the symposium (1973) on this subject. They have also been employed for such diverse purposes as the closure of hernial rings, the removal of condylomata acuminata, and in other conditions in which the production of fibrous tissue is the ultimate objective. Numerous irritants have been used as sclerosing agents. Only three, however, warrant even the brief description given below.

Morrhuate Sodium Injection, N.F., is a sterile solution of the sodium salts of the fatty acids of cod liver oil. It is marketed as a 5% aqueous solution, containing 3% benzyl or ethyl alcohol as a preservative. The intravenous dose is 0.5 to 5 ml injected into a localized segment of vein. Hypersensitivity reactions occasionally occur, and appropriate measures should be taken to avoid such effects. *Quinine and urea hydrochloride injection* is a sterile solution of the double salt. Two milliliters of a 5% solution is injected for sclerosing hemorrhoids, especially those that cannot be treated surgically. *Sodium Tetradecyl Sulfate,* N.F. (SOTRADECOL), is an anionic surface-active agent used to sclerose varicose veins. The preparation for this purpose is *Sodium Tetradecyl Sulfate Injection,* N.F., a 1 or 3% aqueous solution with 2% benzyl alcohol and buffered to a pH of 7 to 8. Not more than 0.5 to 2.0 ml should be injected at any one site; total volume should not exceed 10 ml of a 3% solution. A pressure bandage or elastic stocking over the injection site improves the clinical result (Rhodes and Hadfield, 1972). The drug is relatively free from untoward local and systemic reactions, but it may cause pain at the site of the injection and sloughing of the tissue if the solution is allowed to extravasate. Since allergic reactions have been reported, the possibility of an anaphylactic reaction should be kept in mind, and the physician should be prepared to treat it appropriately.

CAUSTICS, ESCHAROTICS, KERATOLYTICS, AND ANTISEBORRHEICS

Caustics and Escharotics. A *caustic* (or *corrosive*) is a topical agent that causes destruction of tissues at the site of application. If the agent also precipitates cell proteins and the inflammatory exudate forms a scab (or eschar) that is later organized into a scar, it is also known as an *escharotic* (or *cauterizant*). Most, but not all, caustics are also escharotics. Certain caustics, especially the alkalis, redissolve precipitated proteins, partly by hydrolysis, so that no scab or only a soft scab forms; such agents penetrate deeply and are generally unsuitable for therapeutic use. Caustics are used to destroy *warts, condylomata, keratoses, certain moles,* and *hyperplastic tissue.* They have also been used in the management of *fungal infections* and *eczematoid dermatitis.* Agents commonly classified in this category include the following: *glacial acetic acid, exsiccated alum, podophyllum, podophyllum resin, phenol,* and *trichloroacetic acid.* The topical uses of certain of these drugs are discussed elsewhere (*see* Index).

Keratolytics (Desquamating Agents). *Benzoic acid, salicylic acid, resorcinol,* various thiols, and certain other agents soften keratin, loosen cornified epithelium, and cause swelling and softening even of viable cells. The epidermis easily *desquamates,* thus ridding the area of invading fungi and making the underlying layers more accessible to medication or surgical debridement. Such agents are used in the treatment of *dermatophytosis, warts, corns,* and *certain acneform* and *eczematous* dermatitides (*see* Index).

Antiseborrheics. A number of drugs, including *benzoic acid, salicylic acid, resorcinol, sulfur,* and some *mercurial compounds,* are sometimes used in the management of disorders of the scalp. These agents are discussed elsewhere (*see* Index). Drugs prepared in pharmaceutical forms especially designed for the treatment of seborrheic dermatitis are considered here.

Selenium Sulfide, U.S.P., is a bright-orange, insoluble powder that is used externally for control of seborrheic dermatitis, dandruff, and nonspecific dermatoses. The toxicity of insoluble selenium sulfide contrasts sharply with the highly toxic soluble selenites, selenates, and organic selenium compounds (Henschler and Kirschner, 1969). Indeed, Cummins and Kimura (1971) have shown in rats that the oral LD50 for the insoluble selenium sulfide is 138 mg/kg (versus 7 mg/kg for the highly soluble sodium selenite) and quite comparable to that for other substances commonly employed in shampoos. Comparatively little absorption occurs after local application of selenium sulfide to normal skin, but the drug is absorbed more readily from inflamed or damaged epithelium. Prolonged contact with skin surfaces may result in burns and dermatitis venenata. Selenium sulfide is employed as *Selenium Sulfide Lotion,* U.S.P. (SELSUN SULFIDE SUSPENSION), a therapeutic shampoo containing 2.5% of the active ingredient in a detergent vehicle. It is also available as a nonprescription drug in a 1% detergent suspension (SEL-

SUN BLUE) in a scented, detergent vehicle. The hair and scalp are washed with a bland soap and rinsed. The shampoo (5 to 10 ml) is worked into the scalp, with warm water to lather. The drug is allowed to remain on the scalp for 2 to 3 minutes and then thoroughly rinsed. Care should be exercised to prevent the shampoo from coming in contact with the conjunctivae; it is irritating and may cause keratitis. The hands should be carefully washed after using this agent. The skin of the neck and external ear may become sensitized to the detergent used in the suspension. Other objectionable features that may result from the use of this preparation include excessive oiliness of the hair and scalp and orange tinting of gray hair. The latter effect may be avoided by thorough rinsing of the hair immediately after each treatment. When prescribing selenium sulfide shampoo, one should caution the patient to keep the preparation out of the reach of children. Weekly or twice-weekly applications successfully control 95% of cases of *seborrhea sicca* (dandruff). It has also been found useful in the treatment of *seborrheic dermatitis* of the scalp and of *tinea versicolor.*

MELANIZING AND DEMELANIZING AGENTS

Many characteristics of skin pigmentation and achromasia are of importance in pharmacology. Skin alterations resulting from untoward effects of drugs are discussed in connection with the agents responsible for such changes. The drugs discussed in this section have clinically useful melanizing (hyperpigmenting) or demelanizing (hypopigmenting) properties. Many details relating to the etiology and management of vitiliginous and lentiginous skin disorders are presented in the review by Fitzpatrick and coworkers (1961) and in the monograph on the pigment cell (*see* Symposium, 1963).

TRIOXSALEN

Trioxsalen, a congener of methoxsalen, is used to facilitate repigmentation in vitiligo, increase tolerance to solar exposure, and enhance pigmentation. Trioxsalen differs from methoxsalen in that the former is 4,5′,8-trimethylpsoralen, whereas the latter is 8-methoxypsoralen. The structural formula is shown below.

Trioxsalen

Pharmacological Actions. The mode of action of trioxsalen in inducing repigmentation of the skin is not yet known. It is believed, however, that its action depends upon the presence of functional melanocytes. Thus, the drug activates the few functional and dopa-positive melanocytes present in the vitiliginous skin area (Jarrett and Szabó, 1956) and evokes a mitotic effect on the melanocytes; the latter mechanism is supported by the autoradiographic studies of Africk and Fulton (1971). The increase in dermal pigment appears gradually over a period of months of repeated exposure.

Side Effects and Contraindications. Side effects are minimal; an occasional patient may experience gastric irritation and nausea. The drug is contraindicated in patients with photosensitizing diseases, such as porphyria, acute lupus erythematosus, or leukoderma of infectious origin. No other photosensitizing drug should be administered with trioxsalen. Children under 12 years of age should not be given the drug.

Preparations. *Trioxsalen,* U.S.P. (TRISORALEN), is a white to off-white, crystalline solid, insoluble in water and slightly soluble in alcohol. It is available as *Trioxsalen Tablets,* U.S.P. (5 mg). The usual oral dose is 10 mg, 2 hours before exposure to sunlight or ultraviolet light. Administration of trioxsalen should not be continued for longer than 14 days. Exposure times should be limited to the manufacturer's recommended schedule, except at high altitudes, where exposure times should be appropriately reduced. If repigmentation is not apparent after 3 months of daily exposure, treatment should be discontinued.

Therapeutic Uses. Trioxsalen is used in *idiopathic vitiligo,* to *increase tolerance to sunlight,* and to enhance *skin pigmentation* (tanning). The drug should be used only under medical supervision.

METHOXSALEN

Methoxsalen is a methoxypsoralen derivative used to increase skin tolerance to sunlight and to facilitate repigmentation in vitiligo. The chemistry of the psoralens has been reviewed by Fowlks (1959). Methoxsalen has the following structural formula:

Methoxsalen

Pharmacological Actions. Methoxsalen is a potent photosensitizer of the skin, particularly to longwave (320 to 400 nm) ultraviolet light (Pathak *et al.,* 1967). Photosensitization selectively inhibits epidermal DNA synthesis without a proportionate inhibition of epidermal-cell function (Cole, 1970). After oral ingestion, increased sensitivity appears in 1 hour, reaches a maximum in 2 hours, and disappears in about 8 hours. Topical application is more effective, and the increased skin sensitivity persists for several days. Exposure of methoxsalen-treated patients to ultraviolet light thickens the stratum corneum, induces an inflammatory reaction in the skin, and increases the amount of melanin in the exposed area (Becker, 1960). Repigmentation persists for 8

to 14 years without further treatment (Kenney, 1971).

Side Effects and Contraindications. Side effects after oral therapy are usually mild and include gastric discomfort, nausea, nervousness, insomnia, and depression. Topical application followed by overexposure to ultraviolet light may result in severe burns. Although Elliott (1959) originally reported abnormal hepatic function in a few patients taking methoxsalen, this observation has not been confirmed (Labby *et al.,* 1959; Tucker, 1959). Indeed, Kligman and Goldstein (1973) were unable to find a single validated case of hepatotoxicity. Nevertheless, methoxsalen is contraindicated in hepatic insufficiency and diseases associated with photosensitivity, such as porphyria, acute lupus erythematosus, hydroa, and polymorphic light eruptions.

Preparations. *Methoxsalen,* U.S.P. (OXSORALEN), is a white crystalline substance, insoluble in water and soluble in alcohol. It is available in 10-mg capsules and as *Methoxsalen Topical Solution,* U.S.P. (1%). For vitiligo the capsules are given orally to adults in a dose of 20 mg once a day, followed in 2 to 4 hours with a 5-minute exposure to sunlight or ultraviolet light; exposure may be gradually increased to 30 minutes. For increased tolerance to sunlight and enhanced pigmentation, the same dosage is employed but should be limited to 14 days of treatment. If the 1% topical solution is used, it is applied at weekly intervals to well-defined vitiliginous lesions followed with a 1-minute exposure to ultraviolet light. Subsequent exposures should be increased with caution. *The topical solution should never be dispensed to the patient for home use.*

Therapeutic Uses. Methoxsalen should be employed only under strict medical supervision. It is possibly effective for the treatment of *idiopathic vitiligo* when employed in conjunction with exposure of affected areas of the skin to ultraviolet light. If the vitiligo is associated with destruction of melanocytes, the drug is ineffective. It may be effective when used to enhance skin tolerance to sunlight. Preliminary clinical studies suggest that oral methoxsalen, followed by exposure to high-intensity, long-wave ultraviolet light, is effective in the management of *psoriasis* (Parrish *et al.,* 1974).

MONOBENZONE

Monobenzone, the monobenzyl ether of hydroquinone, is an amelanotic agent used in severe freckling and other conditions characterized by hyperpigmentation of the skin. Monobenzone (*p*-benzyloxyphenol) has the following structural formula:

Monobenzone

Pharmacological Actions. Monobenzone interferes with the biosynthesis of melanin. It inhibits the enzyme tyrosinase and thereby prevents the conversion of tyrosine to dihydroxyphenylalanine, a precursor of melanin. Since the drug does not destroy melanocytes or facilitate the loss of previously synthesized melanin, response to therapy is usually not apparent until 1 to 4 months. Untoward effects, including mild erythema, dermatitis, and eczematous reactions, have been reported. Unless carefully applied, unsightly depigmented patches may result from its use. Systemic toxicity has not been observed after its local application.

Preparations. *Monobenzone,* N.F. (BENOQUIN), is a white crystalline, odorless powder, freely soluble in alcohol but insoluble in water. It is marketed as *Monobenzone Lotion,* N.F., a 5% solution in isopropyl alcohol and propylene glycol, and *Monobenzone Ointment,* N.F., which contains 20% of the active ingredient in a suitable base. It is applied to hyperpigmented areas two or three times daily for up to 4 months, or until depigmentation has occurred, and then twice weekly to maintain the effect. Treated areas should not be exposed to sunlight; ultraviolet light neutralizes the depigmenting effect. If a satisfactory response is not observed within 4 months, treatment should be discontinued.

Therapeutic Uses. Monobenzone is possibly effective for the treatment of hyperpigmentation caused by the excessive formation of melanin, such as occurs in generalized *lentigo,* severe *freckling, melasma* of pregnancy, and *hyperpigmentation* following inflammation of the skin. Monobenzone is of no value in the treatment of café au lait spots, pigmented nevi, malignant melanoma, or pigmentation resulting from substances other than melanin.

HYDROQUINONE

Hydroquinone (*p*-dihydroxybenzene) is a depigmenting agent used topically in the treatment of hypermelanosis. Although percutaneous application does not, in most instances, completely remove the hyperpigmentation, results are good enough to help the majority of patients become less self-conscious about their pigmentation abnormalities.

Pharmacological Actions. Hydroquinone is thought to inhibit tyrosinase and thus prevent the conversion of tyrosine to melanin. There is a lack of agreement, however, on the specific site of inhibition. Depigmentation is not immediate since hydroquinone interferes only with the formation of new melanin. Likewise, it is only temporary, since melanin production is resumed when the drug is discontinued.

Side Effects and Contraindications. Side effects are usually mild; burning, stinging, rash, and irritation have been reported. Possible allergic reactions have been noted. Therefore, patients should be tested for sensitivity before initiating therapy. The drug should not be used near the eyes, on open cuts, or on children under 12 years of age. It is contraindicated in patients with prickly heat, sunburn, or irritated skin.

Preparations. *Hydroquinone,* U.S.P., is a colorless, crystalline solid, slightly soluble in water and freely soluble in alcohol. It is marketed as *Hydroquinone Ointment,* U.S.P. (ELDOPAQUE), 2% and 4%, in an opaque base to protect treated areas from ultraviolet light; *hydroquinone cream* (ELDOQUIN), 2% and 4%; and *hydroquinone lotion,* 2%, in a stabilized base. These preparations are applied to the area to be lightened once or twice daily and rubbed in well.

Therapeutic Uses. Hydroquinone is used to bleach and lighten localized areas of darkened skin (severe freckling and skin blemishes).

MUCOLYTICS

Although iodides, ammonium chloride, and other drugs have been used orally for many years to loosen viscid sputum and to improve expectoration (*see* Index), the use of nebulized mucolytic agents for this purpose is a comparatively recent development. A number of substances have been reported to be effective mucolytic agents, but more definitive studies have shown them to be either ineffective or undesirable for a variety of clinical reasons (*see* Lieberman, 1970). Therefore, only two such agents will be mentioned here.

Acetylcysteine, N.F. (MUCOMYST), liquefies mucus and DNA (the component of pus responsible for its viscosity) but has no effect on fibrin, blood clots, or living tissue. It exerts its mucolytic activity through its free sulfhydryl group, which acts directly on the mucoproteins to open the disulfide bonds and lower the viscosity of the mucus. The mucolytic activity is greatest at pH 7 to 9. Liquefaction after inhalation is apparent within 1 minute; maximal effect occurs in 5 to 10 minutes; after direct application, the effect is immediate. It is used by inhalation and direct application as adjunct therapy in patients with abnormal, viscid, or inspissated mucous secretions. The agent is marketed as *Acetylcysteine Solution,* N.F. (10 and 20% sterile solution). By inhalation, a nebulized solution, 3 to 5 ml of a 20% solution or 6 to 10 ml of a 10% solution, is used three to four times daily. By direct instillation, 1 or 2 ml of a 10 or 20% solution is used every 1 to 4 hours. Untoward effects include bronchospasm, hemoptysis, and nausea and vomiting. Since acetylcysteine has been reported to inactivate a number of antibiotics, including all of the penicillin-type drugs tested (Lawson and Saggers, 1965), antimicrobial drugs should not be administered in the same solution.

Pancreatic dornase for sterile solution (DORNAVAC) is a purified deoxyribonuclease obtained from beef pancreas. Its use therefore is limited to the liquefaction of purulent secretion, which contains significant amounts of DNA. It is used in reducing the viscosity of pulmonary secretions and as an adjunct in obtaining sputum specimens in suspected bronchogenic carcinoma. Unlike acetylcysteine, pancreatic dornase does not inactivate antibiotics. The usual dose by nebulization is 200,000 units of lyophilized enzyme dissolved in 2 ml of either 10% propylene glycol or

0.9% sodium chloride solution. According to Lieberman (1968), sputum viscosity is reduced almost immediately after aerosol treatment.

ENZYMES

This discussion is limited to enzymes that act at local sites after either topical application or hypodermic injection.

HYALURONIDASE

Hyaluronidase, first studied by Duran-Reynals (1929) and later characterized by Chain and Guthie (1940), is a soluble enzyme product prepared from mammalian testes.

Pharmacological Actions. Hyaluronidase hydrolyzes mucopolysaccharides of the hyaluronic acid class, which are components of intercellular ground substance. It accomplishes this by hydrolyzing the glucosaminidic bonds (Meyer and Rapport, 1952). This temporarily decreases the viscosity of the cellular cement, promotes diffusion of injected fluids or of localized transudates or exudates, and in this way facilitates their absorption. Commercial preparations contain a small amount of bovine serum proteins (Kind and Roffler, 1961), and allergic reactions may sometimes occur; otherwise, systemic effects do not attend its proper use. Sensitivity can be determined by skin testing in the usual manner.

Preparations and Bioassay. *Hyaluronidase for Injection*, N.F. (ALIDASE, HYAZYME, WYDASE), is supplied as a sterile, white, amorphous solid in ampuls containing 150 or 1500 N.F. units and as *Hyaluronidase Injection*, N.F., containing 150 N.F. units per milliliter. Its solutions are colorless, odorless, and unstable. Hyaluronidase activity is assayed on the basis of the ability of the enzyme to decrease the turbidity of colloidal suspensions of hyaluronate and protein *in vitro*.

Therapeutic Uses. Hyaluronidase is effective for enhancing the dispersion and absorption of other injected drugs, for hypodermoclysis, as an adjunct in subcutaneous urography, and for improving resorption of radiopaque agents. It is also employed as an aid in infiltration anesthesia in ocular surgery, for reducing swelling due to trauma, to hasten the onset of action and diffusibility of local anesthetics, to minimize tumefaction during surgery, and for reducing postoperative edema and ecchymosis. The limitations of hyaluronidase as an adjunct in certain types of local anesthesia are discussed on page 394. Hyaluronidase should not be injected into infected or cancerous areas because of the danger of spreading the infection or the malignancy. More detailed information on hyaluronidase is given in the symposium devoted to the enzyme (Symposium, 1950).

STREPTOKINASE AND STREPTODORNASE

Pharmacological Actions. Streptokinase and streptodornase are enzymes produced during the growth of certain strains of hemolytic streptococci.

Streptokinase is a plasminogen activator and dissolves blood clots and the fibrinous portion of exudates. Streptodornase hydrolyzes deoxyribonucleoprotein and hence liquefies the viscous nucleoprotein of dead cells; it has no effect on living cells. These enzymes are used together to aid in the removal of clotted blood and fibrinous or purulent accumulations following trauma or inflammation. The historical development of these agents and more detailed information on their pharmacology and bioassay are presented in the *fourth edition* of this textbook.

Preparations. *Streptokinase-streptodornase* (VARIDASE) is marketed as a *jelly* (100,000 units of streptokinase and 25,000 units of streptodornase in 15 ml), as a *powder for sterile solution for injection* (20,000 units of streptokinase and 5000 units of streptodornase in each vial), as a *powder for solution for topical application* (100,000 units of streptokinase and 25,000 units of streptodornase in each vial), and as *oral tablets* (10,000 units of streptokinase and 2500 units of streptodornase per tablet). Solutions deteriorate at room temperature but remain active for 7 days at 10° C. It should be mentioned that the streptokinase under study for intravenous infusion in the management of patients with myocardial infarction or pulmonary embolism is a highly purified preparation and is available only for investigational use (*see* Chapter 65). The streptokinase described herein is a relatively impure substance and should never be administered intravenously.

Therapeutic Uses and Dosage. Streptokinase-streptodornase is employed to remove clotted blood and fibrinous or purulent exudate resulting from trauma or inflammation. It is also used as an adjunct in the treatment of *hemothorax, hematoma*, and *empyema*, and of chronic suppurations involving draining sinuses, osteomyelitis, and infected wounds or ulcers. Such therapy can be considered only as a supplement to appropriate antibiotic therapy and surgical debridement and drainage.

The enzyme mixture is *contraindicated* in the presence of active hemorrhage because it may interfere with clotting, and in acute cellulitis without suppuration because of the danger of spreading a nonlocalized infection. In cases of active tuberculosis there is danger of reopening previously existing bronchopleural fistulas. When injected into closed cavities or spaces containing clotted blood, thick pus, surface fibrin, or localized effusions, the preparation frequently evokes a local inflammatory reaction and a pyrogenic response. Such reactions have been attributed to pyrogenic substances in the streptokinase-streptodornase mixture and to endogenous pyrogens released from the enzyme-induced inflammatory reaction. Streptokinase and streptodornase are antigenic, and sensitivity reactions have been reported.

Streptokinase-streptodornase is administered by injection into cavities and by topical application in the form of a jelly or wet dressings. It must not be administered intravenously. It is essential that the mixture be placed in intimate contact with the substrate. In enclosed areas, provision must be made for release of increased fluid resulting from the liquefying action of the enzymes. For a *hemothorax* or *thoracic empyema,* the initial dose is 200,000 units of streptokinase and 50,000 units of streptodornase in not less than 10 ml of isotonic sodium chloride solution. A suitable initial dose in *maxillary sinus empyema* is 10,000 to 15,000 units of streptokinase and 2500 to 3750 units of streptodornase in 2 to 3 ml of solution. Similar concentrations may be applied in wet dressings when enzymatic debridement is indicated. The value of oral administration of the enzyme mixture has not been established.

TRYPSIN

Pharmacological Actions. Trypsin is a proteolytic enzyme obtained from bovine pancreas. It acts directly to hydrolyze naturally occurring proteins and is effective within a pH range of 5 to 8; activity is optimal at about pH 7. The specificity of trypsin is quite limited. It hydrolyzes only ester or peptide bonds in which the carboxyl moiety of the amino acid is lysine or arginine (Colman, 1965). Trypsin differs from streptokinase-streptodornase in three ways: it does not require a cofactor, it is effective against a greater number of proteins, and it is capable of hydrolyzing the protein moiety of respiratory tract mucins. Neither oral nor intramuscular administration of the enzyme results in significant blood levels.

Side Effects and Contraindications. Topical application of trypsin may produce a severe burning sensation; this can be prevented by the prior application of a local anesthetic. Local infiltration into closed cavities may cause a slight increase in body temperature and heart rate. This reaction can be prevented by the prior administration of an antihistamine. Aerosol inhalation may cause irritation of the eyes and nose, glossitis, pharyngitis, hoarseness, and systemic reactions. Anaphylactic shock may occur in patients previously treated with trypsin. Trypsin is contraindicated in patients with hepatic dysfunction. It should never be administered intravenously.

Preparations. *Trypsin Crystallized,* N.F. (TRYP-TAR), is a white to yellowish-white, odorless powder standardized in terms of proteolytic activity. Each milligram contains not less than 2500 N.F. trypsin units. It is marketed as a powder and as *Trypsin Crystallized for Aerosol,* N.F., 250,000 N.F. units per milliliter. It is also available in combination with chymotrypsin as a tablet.

Therapeutic Uses. Trypsin is effective when administered as an aerosol for the liquefaction of viscid sputum. It is possibly effective for topical application in the debridement of open wounds and ulcers and for intrapleural use in postoperative or traumatic hemothorax or empyema. It is also useful for the liquefaction of coagulated blood and exudates that have not become organized by fibrous tissue. It should be used with caution in empyema and bronchopleural fistulas of tuberculous origin. Its irritating

effect on respiratory mucosa limits its usefulness as a mucolytic agent. The enzyme is rapidly inactivated when injected into closed cavities.

CHYMOTRYPSIN

Pharmacological Actions. Chymotrypsin, crystallized from an extract of bovine pancreas, is an endopeptidase that hydrolyzes ester and peptide bonds. Although its mechanism of action is thought to be similar to that of trypsin, it differs from the latter in at least three ways: its spectrum of hydrolytic activity is much broader (Colman, 1965), both intramuscular and oral administration of chymotrypsin give measurable blood levels that persist for about 1 hour (Kabacoff *et al.,* 1963), and it is relatively stable for ½ hour in human intestinal juice (Wohlman *et al.,* 1962). Chymotrypsin can be shown to have an anti-inflammatory action in experimental animals, but only when the enzyme is administered parenterally in doses 10 to 20 times those employed clinically and *prior* to the production of the inflammation. Similar effectiveness cannot be demonstrated when the enzyme is administered *after* the inflammation has been established. Therefore, the systemic clinical usefulness of this enzyme remains questionable.

Side Effects and Contraindications. Chymotrypsin is a foreign protein, and sensitivity may develop from repeated injections. Severe anaphylactic reactions with vascular collapse and loss of consciousness have been reported (Colman, 1965). Local irritation at the site of the injection and ulceration after buccal administration have been noted. Although there are no specific contraindications to the oral or buccal administration of chymotrypsin, it is not recommended for use in ophthalmic surgery in patients under 20 years of age because of possible loss of vitreous humor.

Preparations and Dosage. *Chymotrypsin,* U.S.P. (AVAZYME), is a white to yellowish-white, odorless, crystalline or amorphous powder. It is also official as *Chymotrypsin for Ophthalmic Solution,* U.S.P. (CATARASE). Each milligram of chymotrypsin contains not less than 1000 U.S.P. chymotrypsin units. It is marketed as a powder in vials (300 and 750 U.S.P. units) and as tablets (50,000 and 100,000 U.S.P. units). It is also available in combination with trypsin in oral tablets (CHYMORAL, ORENZYME) containing 4000 units of chymotrypsin and 50,000 units of trypsin or 8000 units of chymotrypsin and 100,000 units of trypsin. The usual dosage is 1 to 2 tablets four times a day.

Therapeutic Uses. Chymotrypsin, either alone or in combination with trypsin, is used for the relief of symptoms related to episiotomy. Its usefulness in inflammatory states secondary to surgical or physical trauma remains unproven.

Alpha-chymotrypsin (ALPHA-CHYMAR, QUIMOTRASE, ZOLYSE) is a similar proteolytic enzyme used in cataract operations to loosen the lens after incision of the cornea. After the corneoscleral or corneoscleral-conjunctival incision, the posterior chamber is irrigated with about 2 ml of enzyme solution (150 units per milliliter) to fragment the fibers of the zonule (enzymatic zonulolysis). Untoward effects include temporary glaucoma, moderate uveitis, corneal edema, and striation. Delayed healing has been reported.

OTHER PROTEOLYTIC ENZYMES

A number of other proteolytic enzymes, such as alpha amylase (BUCLAMASE), bromelains (ANANASE), deoxyribonuclease combined with fibrinolysin (ELASE), and papain (PAPASE), were formerly promoted for systemic use in the prevention and treatment of a variety of traumatic inflammatory states. Substantial evidence for such use remains to be established. They are possibly effective for relieving symptoms related to episiotomy. In addition, deoxyribonuclease-fibrinolysin and papain are used topically as debriding agents in a variety of inflammatory and infected open lesions.

Chymopapain (DISCASE) is a proteolytic enzyme isolated from the latex of *Carica papaya*. It is an investigational new drug under study for chemonucleolysis, that is, the removal of the nucleus pulposus of prolapsed intervertebral discs (Smith, 1964; Symposium, 1969). The enzyme attacks the proteoglycan portion of the *nucleus pulposus* but does not affect collagenous components. After conventional discography has confirmed the presence of a defective disc, several milligrams of the enzyme activated in solution with cystine and disodium edetate in water are injected. In some cases, sciatic pain disappears quickly with no other effects. In most cases, however, resolution of pain runs about the same course as that obtained with surgery, but without the associated surgical trauma. Untoward reactions include a 1% incidence of immediate or delayed hypersensitivity and localized but temporary spasmodic back pain. Severe hypersensitivity reactions may be partially ameliorated by prophylactic use of a corticosteroid and an antihistamine. More extensive study is necessary before the advantages and limitations of this interesting technic can be fully evaluated (*see* Wiltse *et al.*, 1975).

Collagenase (COLLAGENASE ABC) is a proteolytic enzyme derived from *Clostridium histolyticum*. It is reported to digest the undenatured collagen fibers involved in the retention of necrotic wound debris (Boxer *et al.*, 1969; Varma *et al.*, 1973). Collagenase is effective against collagen at a pH range of 6 to 8. It is indicated for debridement of severely burned areas and dermal lesions. Its effectiveness in the treatment of other necrotic skin lesions has not been established. Collagenase is available as a 0.5% ointment. It is usually applied to the lesion every day or every other day and covered with a sterile dressing.

Sutilains, N.F., is a proteolytic enzyme elaborated by *Bacillus subtilis*. At body temperature it has optimal activity at a pH range of 6.0 to 6.8. It is available as *Sutilains Ointment*, N.F. (TRAVASE), 1 g of which contains approximately 82,000 casein units of proteolytic activity. It selectively digests necrotic soft tissues. The ointment is used for wound debridement as adjunct therapy to established methods of wound care (Garrett, 1969). It is indicated in second- and third-degree burns, decubitus ulcers, pyogenic wounds, and ulcers secondary to peripheral vascular disease. Patients should be warned to keep the enzyme away from the eyes. Untoward local effects include transient pain, paresthesia, bleeding, and dermatitis. Systemic toxicity has not been observed from the topical application of the ointment.

Africk, J., and Fulton, J. Treatment of vitiligo with topical trimethylpsoralen and sunlight. *Br. J. Derm.*, **1971**, *84*, 151–156.

Antopol, W. Lycopodium granuloma. *Archs Path.*, **1933**, *16*, 326–331.

Barnes, J. M., and Rossiter, R. J. Toxicity of tannic acid. *Lancet*, **1943**, *2*, 218–222.

Becker, S. W., Jr. Use and abuse of psoralens. *J. Am. med. Ass.*, **1960**, *173*, 1483–1485.

Boxer, A. M.; Gottesman, N.; Bernstein, H.; and Mandl, I. Debridement of dermal ulcers and decubiti with collagenase. *Geriatrics*, **1969**, *24*, 75–86.

Chain, E., and Guthie, E. S. Identity of hyaluronidase and spreading factor. *Br. J. exp. Path.*, **1940**, *21*, 324–338.

Cohn, A. L.; White, A. S.; and Weyrauch, H. B. Kaolin granuloma of the stomach. *J. Am. med. Ass.*, **1941**, *117*, 2225–2227.

Cole, R. S. Light-induced cross-linking of DNA in the presence of a furocoumarin (psoralen). *Biochim. biophys. Acta*, **1970**, *217*, 30–39.

Colman, R. W. Proteolytic enzymes in clinical medicine. *Clin. Pharmac. Ther.*, **1965**, *6*, 598–630.

Craven, J. D., and Polak, A. Cantharidin poisoning. *Br. med. J.*, **1954**, *2*, 1386–1388.

Cummins, L. M., and Kimura, E. T. Safety evaluation of selenium sulfide antidandruff shampoos. *Toxicol. appl. Pharmac.*, **1971**, *20*, 89–96.

Decker, W. J.; Combs, H. F.; and Corby, D. G. Adsorption of drugs and poisons by activated charcoal. *Toxicol. appl. Pharmac.*, **1968**, *13*, 454–460.

Duran-Reynals, F. The effect of extracts of certain organs from normal and immunized animals on the infecting power of vaccine virus. *J. exp. Med.*, **1929**, *50*, 327–340.

Elliott, J. A., Jr. Clinical experiences with methoxsalen in the treatment of vitiligo. *J. invest. Derm.*, **1959**, *32*, 311–313.

Epstein, W. L., and Kligman, A. M. Treatment of warts with cantharidin. *A.M.A. Archs Derm.*, **1958**, *77*, 508–511.

Fitzpatrick, T. B.; Seiji, M.; and McGugan, A. D. Melanin pigmentation. *New Engl. J. Med.*, **1961**, *265*, 328–332, 374–378, 430–434.

Fowlks, W. L. The chemistry of the psoralens. *J. invest. Derm.*, **1959**, *32*, 249–254.

Garrett, T. A. *Bacillus subtilis* protease: a new topical agent for debridement. *Clin. Med.*, **1969**, *76*, No. 5, 11–15.

Goldsmith, L. A., and Baden, H. P. Propylene glycol with occlusion for treatment of ichthyosis. *J. Am. med. Ass.*, **1972**, *220*, 579–580.

Hanzlik, P. J.; Lawrence, W. S.; Fellows, J. K.; Luduena, F. P.; and Laqueur, G. L. Epidermal application of diethylene glycol monoethyl ether (CARBITOL) and some other glycols. *J. ind. Hyg. Toxicol.*, **1947**, *29*, 325–341.

Hanzlik, P. J.; Lawrence, W. S.; and Laqueur, G. L. Comparative chronic toxicity of diethylene glycol monoethyl ether (CARBITOL) and some related glycols: results of continued drinking and feeding. *J. ind. Hyg. Toxicol.*, **1947**, *29*, 233–241.

Hanzlik, P. J.; Luduena, F. P.; Lawrence, W. S.; and Hanzlik, H. Acute toxicity and general systemic actions of diethylene glycol monoethyl ether (CARBITOL). *J. ind. Hyg. Toxicol.*, **1947**, *29*, 190–195.

Henschler, D., and Kirschner, U. Zur Resorption und Toxität von Selensulfid. *Arch. Tox.*, **1969**, *24*, 341–344.

Holt, E. L., and Holz, P. H. The black bottle. *J. Pediat.,* **1963,** *63,* 306–314.

Jarrett, A., and Szabó, G. The pathological varieties of vitiligo and their response to treatment with MELADININE. *Br. J. Derm.,* **1956,** *68,* 313–326.

Kabacoff, B. L.; Wohlman, A.; Zombley, M.; and Avakian, S. Absorption of chymotrypsin from the intestinal tract. *Nature, Lond.,* **1963,** *199,* 815–817.

Kenney, J. A., Jr. Vitiligo treated by psoralens. *Archs Derm.,* **1971,** *103,* 475–480.

Kind, L. S., and Roffler, S. Allergic reactions to hyaluronidase. *Proc. Soc. exp. Biol. Med.,* **1961,** *106,* 734–735.

Kligman, A. M., and Goldstein, F. P. Oral dosage in methoxsalen phototoxicity. *Archs Derm.,* **1973,** *107,* 548–550.

Krezanoski, J. Z. Tannic acid: chemistry, analysis, and toxicology. *Radiology,* **1966,** *87,* 655–657.

Labby, D. H.; Imbrie, J. D.; and Fitzpatrick, T. B. Studies of liver function in subjects receiving methoxsalen. *J. invest. Derm.,* **1959,** *32,* 273–275.

Lawson, D., and Saggers, B. A. N.A.C. and antibiotics in cystic fibrosis. *Br. med. J.,* **1965,** *1,* 317.

Lieberman, J. Dornase aerosol effect on sputum viscosity in cases of cystic fibrosis. *J. Am. med. Ass.,* **1968,** *205,* 312–313.

————. The appropriate use of mucolytic agents. *Am. J. Med.,* **1970,** *49,* 1–4.

Luduena, F. P.; Lawrence, W. S.; Fellows, J. K.; Clark, W. H.; and Hanzlik, P. J. Excretion and fate of diethylene glycol monoethyl ether (CARBITOL) after epidermal and other methods of administration. *Archs int. Pharmacodyn. Thér.,* **1947,** *75,* 1–18.

Masters, E. J. Allergies to cosmetic products. *N.Y. St. J. Med.,* **1960,** *60,* 1934–1940.

Meyer, K., and Rapport, M. M. Hyaluronidases. *Adv. Enzymol.,* **1952,** *13,* 199–236.

Nickolls, L. C., and Teare, D. Poisoning by cantharidin. *Br. med. J.,* **1954,** *2,* 1384–1386.

Parrish, J. A.; Fitzpatrick, T. B.; Tanenbaum, L.; and Pathak, M. A. Photochemotherapy of psoriasis with oral methoxsalen and long-wave ultraviolet light. *New Engl. J. Med.,* **1974,** *291,* 1207–1211.

Pathak, M. A.; Worden, L. R.; and Kaufman, K. D. Effect of structural alterations on the photosensitizing potency of furocoumarins (psoralens) and related compounds. *J. invest. Derm.,* **1967,** *48,* 103–118.

Picchioni, A. L. Management of acute poisonings with

activated charcoal. *Am. J. hosp. Pharm.,* **1972,** *28,* 62–64.

Picchioni, A. L.; Chin, L.; Verhulst, H. L.; and Dieterle, B. Activated charcoal vs. "universal antidote" as an antidote for poisons. *Toxicol. appl. Pharmac.,* **1966,** *8,* 447–454.

Presto, A. J., III, and Muecke, E. C. A dose of Spanish fly. *J. Am. med. Ass.,* **1970,** *214,* 591–592.

Rhodes, D. J., and Hadfield, G. J. Treatment of varicose veins by injection and compression. *Practitioner,* **1972,** *208,* 809–817.

Robinson, J. R. Deodorants and antiperspirants. In, *Handbook of Nonprescription Drugs.* (Griffenhagen, G. B., and Hawkins, L. L., eds.) American Pharmaceutical Association, Washington, D. C., **1973,** pp. 209–214.

Smith, L. Enzyme dissolution of the nucleus pulposus in humans. *J. Am. med. Ass.,* **1964,** *187,* 137–140.

Symposium. (Various authors.) Ground substance of mesenchyme and hyaluronidase. *Ann. N.Y. Acad. Sci.,* **1950,** *52,* 945–1195.

Symposium. (Various authors.) The pigment cell: molecular, biological, and clinical aspects. *Ann. N.Y. Acad. Sci.,* **1963,** *100,* 1–1123.

Symposium. (Various authors.) Chemonucleolysis. *Clin. Orthop.,* **1969,** No. 67, 1–104.

Symposium. (Various authors.) Diverse methods of managing hemorrhoids. *Dis. Colon Rectum,* **1973,** *16,* 171–192.

Tourtellotte, W. W.; Reinglass, J. L.; and Newkirk, T. A. Cerebral dehydration action of glycerol. *Clin. Pharmac. Ther.,* **1972,** *13,* 159–171.

Tucker, H. A. Clinical and laboratory tolerance studies in volunteers given oral methoxsalen. *J. invest. Derm.,* **1959,** *32,* 277–280.

Varma, A. D.; Bugatch, E.; and German, F. M. Debridement of dermal ulcers with collagenase. *Surgery Gynec. Obstet.,* **1973,** *136,* 281–282.

Wells, D. B.; Humphrey, H. D.; and Coll, J. J. The relation of tannic acid to the liver necrosis occurring in burns. *New Engl. J. Med.,* **1942,** *226,* 629–636.

Werch, S. C., and Ivy, A. C. A study of the metabolism of ingested pectin. *Am. J. Dis. Child.,* **1941,** *62,* 499–511.

Wiltse, L. L.; Widell, E. H., Jr.; and Yuan, H. A. Chymopapain chemonucleolysis in lumbar disk disease. *J. Am. med. Ass.,* **1975,** *231,* 474–479.

Wohlman, A.; Kabacoff, R. L.; and Avakian, S. Comparative stability of trypsin and chymotrypsin in human intestinal juice. *Proc. Soc. exp. Biol. Med.,* **1962,** *109,* 26–28.

48 GASTRIC ANTACIDS AND DIGESTANTS

Stewart C. Harvey

GASTRIC ANTACIDS

Gastric antacids are agents that neutralize or remove acid from the gastric contents. They are employed by physicians chiefly in the treatment of hyperchlorhydria and peptic ulcer, and by the laity in self-medication for a wide variety of symptoms.

The gastric antacids are a much-abused group of drugs. As a result of irresponsible advertising, the public has come to believe that man is constantly fighting a battle against acidity and that every little belch or upper gastrointestinal upset calls for an antacid. The substantial incidence of placebo responsiveness of individuals with minor gastrointestinal upsets, and even with peptic ulcer, further deludes the laity and often the physician into inappropriate use of antacids. Yet when indicated, they are often used too casually to be of value.

Actions and Effects of Gastric Antacids. The common gastric antacids all contain a weakly basic moiety. The weaker bases, such as the several oxyaluminum compounds, hardly raise the pH of the gastric contents above 4, some not above 3, whereas the mildly strong bases, such as magnesium hydroxide, can raise the pH to about 9 but rarely do so in practice.

All antacids *indirectly* suppress peptic activity when given in sufficient quantity to elevate the pH of human gastric contents above 5 (Piper and Fenton, 1965). Between pH 7 and 8, pepsin is irreversibly inactivated. Although there have been a number of claims that aluminum-, calcium-, and bismuth-containing antacids have *direct* antipeptic activity, such claims have not been supported by studies in which the pH effect was used for control (*see* Kuruvilla, 1971).

The presence of an antacid in the gastric contents increases the volume of gastric juice secreted and the output of HCl. It is not clear whether the effect is purely a function of the pH, and is thus otherwise independent of the antacid employed, or whether some more direct action is involved. Although Clark and Adams (1947) reported differences among antacids in a limited study, theoretical considerations support the view that the effect derives from the elevated pH, which induces the pyloric antrum to release gastrin. In patients with duodenal ulcer the effect is remarkably pronounced. If sodium bicarbonate is continuously administered so that the intragastric pH remains above 4, the 24-hour output of HCl is 6 to 20 times the control continuous-fasting secretion in such patients (Price and Sanderson, 1956). If the pH is kept at 5.5, the gastrin and acid secretory outputs after a meal are approximately doubled (Fordtran and Walsh, 1973). Even though the half-life of gastrin is short, it might be expected that the enhanced rate of secretion would outlast the elevation of pH (*i.e.,* acid rebound would occur). However, Pereira-Lima and Hollander (1959) concluded that rebound does not occur. Nevertheless, evidence for a slight-to-moderate rebound after $Mg(OH)_2$ or $NaHCO_3$ can be found in the data published by Posey and coworkers (1965), Fordtran (1968), and Barreras (1970). Calcium carbonate causes a rebound by a non-pH-related mechanism (Fordtran, 1968).

Gastrin released by neutralization of the gastric contents causes increased gastric motility and elevated lower-esophageal sphincter pressure (Castell and Levine, 1971).

Individual gastric antacids may bring about effects that are unique to the particular compound or to one of its constituent groups. Except for the systemic alkalotic effects of some gastric antacids, other properties and effects are discussed under the individual agents.

Systemic and Nonsystemic Antacids. A *systemic* antacid is one capable of producing metabolic alkalosis, because of appreciable absorption of the cationic moiety. A compound of this type, even if administered in doses that only partially neutralize the gastric contents, may disturb the acid-base balance of the body fluids. A *nonsystemic* antacid is one in which the cationic moiety in the intestine forms insoluble basic compounds that are not subsequently absorbed.

Effects of Systemic Antacids. If a systemic antacid such as sodium bicarbonate is administered, the gastric acid is neutralized by exogenous bicarbonate in lieu of intestinal bicarbonate. The spared equivalent amount of intestinal bicarbonate is then absorbed rather than neutralized. The net effect is the same as though the exogenous sodium bicarbonate had been directly transported into the extracellular fluid. The effect on extracellular bicarbonate is the same whether the antacid is an oxide, carbonate, or any alkaline-reacting compound of an absorbable cation. The kidney must then excrete the excess bicarbonate and cation in order to restore the acid-base balance of the body fluids. Consequently, the urine becomes alkaline. Failure of the renal mechanisms to function adequately would result in a more enduring metabolic alkalosis. Even when the excretory disposal of the bicarbonate is adequate, the repeated alkalinization of the urine during chronic administration of systemic antacids predisposes to phosphatic nephrolithiasis.

For the calcium and magnesium compounds that are partly systemic, the pharmacological and toxicological effects of the cations themselves are of more concern than the alkalosis. The nature of the adverse systemic effects will be discussed under the individual agents.

Effects of Nonsystemic Antacids. A nonsystemic antacid neutralizes the gastric contents but does not tend to cause systemic alkalosis, because not only is the cation very little absorbed but it regains a basic anion in the small intestine. Calcium carbonate may be taken as a good example of a nonsystemic antacid, because it is excreted by the bowel to a considerable degree in the same chemical form as it entered, namely, as $CaCO_3$; thus, the net of the chemical transactions is zero. The equations that describe these events are

$$CaCO_3 + 2H^+ \longrightarrow Ca^{2+} + H_2O + CO_2$$

which takes place in the stomach and

$$Ca^{2+} + CO_3^{2-} \longrightarrow CaCO_3$$

which takes place in the small intestine. At the pH of the jejunum (about 8), there is sufficient CO_3^{2-} in equilibrium with HCO_3^- to precipitate more than 99% of calcium ion present. In the small intestine, calcium ion also combines with fatty acid anions to form insoluble calcium soaps. Were the fatty acid anions not so removed, they would be absorbed and ultimately metabolized to bicarbonate. Thus, it follows that the formation of calcium soaps has the same overall effect to prevent systemic alkalosis as does the intraintestinal precipitation of $CaCO_3$. At the pH of the lower colon (5 to 7.5), some of the $CaCO_3$ will redissolve, but little absorption takes place. Continued formation of insoluble calcium soaps will tend to offset the acid-base effects of the carbonate liberated. Insoluble calcium phosphate also forms in the intestine and contributes to the nonsystemic antacid properties.

Other substances are nonsystemic antacids by virtue of similar mechanisms. The basic aluminum compounds regenerated in the small intestine are probably a mixture of hydrated aluminum oxide, oxyaluminum hydroxide, basic aluminum carbonates of variable composition, and aluminum soaps. Although it is commonly believed that the formation of insoluble $MgCO_3$ accounts for the nonsystemic properies of magnesium-containing antacids, the solubility of magnesium carbonate is 50,000 times higher than that of calcium carbonate, and precipitation at pH 8 cannot occur at clinically achievable concentrations of magnesium ion. The formation of soaps possibly accounts in part for the nonsystemic properties of magnesium compounds.

ALUMINUM HYDROXIDE

So-called aluminum hydroxide is partly aluminum hydroxide and partly aluminum oxide hydrated to a variable extent. As either hydroxide or oxide, it reacts with hydrochloric acid in the stomach to form aluminum chloride. Aluminum hydroxide has a very low equivalent weight and hence a high theoretical neutralizing capacity, but commercial preparations contain a considerable nonreactive bulk, mainly water and some fixed CO_2. Moreover, products differ with respect to antacid efficacy, according to the process of manufacture and to age (*see* Hem *et al.,* 1970). The differences are due in part to the formation of polymers and anhydrous alumina, which dissolve exceedingly slowly in acid. Liquid preparations react faster than do solids. Furthermore, proteins, peptides, amino acids, and certain dietary organic acids greatly impair the neutralizing capacity of aluminum hydroxide (Gibaldi *et al.,* 1964). The insolubility of aluminum hydroxide is a desirable property in that a fraction of sedimented unreacted excess tends to remain in the stomach to yield a sustained effect. There is no acceptable evidence that aluminum hydroxide is superior to other insoluble antacids in this regard.

Although aluminum hydroxide is considered to be nonsystemic, some absorption from the gastrointestinal tract does take place. Seventeen to 31% of dietary aluminum is excreted in the urine (*see* Schroeder and Nason, 1971). A considerable amount of aluminum is distributed to bone and lung (*see* Schroeder and Nason, 1971; Thurston *et al.,* 1972). In renal failure, the administration of aluminum hydroxide can elevate the plasma aluminum concentration to as high as 53 mg per liter (Berlyne *et al.,* 1970).

Among the compounds formed in the intestine from aluminum hydroxide are insoluble aluminum phosphates, which pass through the intestinal tract unabsorbed. Hypophosphatemia, hypophosphaturia, and hypopyrophosphaturia result. Tablets bind more phosphate than do magmas (Krumlovsky and del Greco, 1970). All aluminum-containing antacids except aluminum phosphate have this property. This provides the basis of the therapeutic application of aluminum hydroxide in the occasional treatment of phosphatic nephrolithiasis (*see* below). A phosphate-depletion syndrome is occasionally observed after chronic aluminum hydroxide ingestion. Patients on a therapeutic regimen for peptic ulcer usually have a high phosphate intake, so that binding of phosphate is of no consequence. However, if the phosphate intake is limited, phosphate deprivation can occur. Decreased phosphate absorption is accompanied by increased calcium absorption, which, along with resorption of bone salts, causes hypercalciuria (*see* Lotz *et al.,* 1968; Ansari, 1970). Hypomagnesemia and hypomagnesiuria also occur.

Aluminum ion forms coordinate complexes with a wide variety of substances. Reactions with proteins account for its astringent properties. An astringent action is possibly exerted on gastric and duodenal mucins, but the clinical importance of such an effect is not clear. Mucus secretion is supposedly stimulated by the irritant action of Al^{3+}. Aluminum compounds cause constipation, an effect often attributed to the astringent aluminum ion; inasmuch as the concentration of aluminum in the intestine is extremely low, it is difficult to attribute the effect to an astringent action. Al^{3+} does not affect pepsin (Piper and Fenton, 1961; Anderson and Harthill, 1972; Wenger and Sundy, 1972). Aluminum hydroxide adsorbs pepsin, but the adsorbed enzyme remains active. The compound decreases uropepsin excretion. Aluminum hydroxide is an effective adsorbent and interacts with many drugs in the gastrointestinal tract. Undesirable drug interactions may result. For example, in man the absorption of tetracyclines, chlorpromazine, and aminosalicylic acid is decreased by aluminum hydroxide–containing mixtures. The oral toxicity of atropine and homatropine in mice is reduced by aluminum antacids; such interference with absorption of anticholinergic agents in man could have a considerable bearing on their efficacy in the management of peptic ulcer. In rats, the absorption of aspirin, pentobarbital, and sulfadiazine is decreased, possibly because of effects on pH partition. The absorption of penicillin and pseudoephedrine is increased. Absorption of foodstuffs and nutritional factors, such as amino acids, ascorbic acid, vitamin A, and glucose, is slightly but not importantly depressed. The composition of the feces is unaffected. Aluminum hydroxide has been employed with equivocal results as an adsorbent in intestinal toxemia.

Particles of wet aluminum hydroxide are somewhat adhesive, and the compound is demulcent. The role that the demulcent action plays in the treatment of peptic ulcer is contestable. Dried aluminum hydroxide gel probably does not disperse sufficiently to cover the mucosa. A concentrated suspension has been claimed to provide appreciable coating, but this finding is controversial (Rider *et al.,* 1966; Morrissey *et al.,* 1967). An adherent layer over the crater of an ulcer, if it occurs, can probably be penetrated readily by hydrogen ion but not so by pepsin. Despite the weak effect on intragastric pH after administration of aluminum hydroxide gel, clinical improvement has been reported (Kirsner and Palmer, 1940; Boyd *et al.,* 1942; Smith, 1947), and this has been construed in favor of a demulcent or other non-antacid effect of the drug.

Preparations. *Aluminum Hydroxide Gel,* U.S.P., is an aqueous suspension containing the equivalent of 3.6 to 4.4% Al_2O_3, chiefly in the form of aluminum hydroxide. Flavoring agents may be added. Each milliliter of commercial gel neutralizes from 0.4 to 1.8 mEq of acid in 30 minutes. The average single dose is 15 ml, but this is often insufficient. More than 40 ml (diluted twofold to threefold) per hour is usually given by intragastric drip. *Dried Aluminum Hydroxide Gel,* U.S.P., and *Dried Aluminum Hydroxide Gel Tablets,* U.S.P., contain the equivalent of 50 to 57.5% Al_2O_3. The compound is usually marketed in the form of flavored chewable tablets, each containing 300 to 600 mg of Al_2O_3. The average single dose is 600 mg, which will neutralize approximately 2 to 10 mEq of acid in 30 minutes, depending on the product. Some $Al(OH)_3$-containing products are among the most expensive when the cost is calculated on the basis of the per milliequivalent of acid neutralized.

Therapeutic Uses. The major therapeutic application of aluminum hydroxide is discussed below, under the treatment of peptic ulcer. Mention has already been made of the application of the demulcent and adsorbent properties of aluminum hydroxide. The hypophosphatemic effect has been used in the treatment of *calcinosis universalis* (Nassim and Connolly, 1970) and in hyperparathyroidism secondary to prolonged hemodialysis (Pendras and Erickson, 1966; Goldsmith *et al.,* 1971). Individuals who suffer from recurrent *phosphatic nephrolithiasis* often can be benefited if their urine is kept relatively free of phosphate. A low-phosphate diet and enough aluminum hydroxide (about 40 ml of gel four times a day) to reduce the 24-hour urinary phosphorus excretion to 200 mg or less are prescribed. Although it has been claimed that patients can be maintained on this regimen indefinitely (*see* Shorr and Carter, 1950), some experts are reluctant to continue treatment for long periods of time because of the possibility of mobilizing bone salts. Furthermore, objections to the unpalatable and constipating gel foster noncompliance.

Untoward Reactions. Aluminum hydroxide is a compound of essentially low toxicity. Phosphate depletion and osteomalacia in persons on a low-phosphate diet have been mentioned above. Some individuals are intolerant of the astringent action of the drug and experience nausea and vomiting. Constipation can be circumvented by concurrent therapy with a magnesium-containing antacid. Concretions of fatty acid salts of aluminum may occur in the stools. Several cases of intestinal obstruction by a large mass composed of clotted blood and aluminum hydroxide have been reported. The same complications can result with mixtures containing aluminum hydroxide (Potyk, 1970).

BASIC ALUMINUM CARBONATE

Basic aluminum carbonate is an aluminum oxy-carbonate of indefinite composition. It is marketed in the form of a suspension that contains the equivalent of approximately 5% Al_2O_3 and 2.4% CO_2. Its pharmacological properties are similar to those of aluminum hydroxide gel. One milliliter of the suspension will neutralize at completion 1.2 to 1.5 mEq of acid. However, it is claimed to bind one third more phosphate than does the hydroxide. Since both hydroxide and basic carbonate compounds form the same ions in solution in the gastric contents, the reason for the supposed greater phosphate-retaining power of the carbonate is obscure. It is considered to be the best of the aluminum-containing antacids for the management of phosphatic nephrolithiasis. For antacid use, the dose is 8 ml. To decrease phosphate absorption, the dose is 40 ml 1 hour after each meal and at bedtime (*see* Lavengood and Marshall, 1972).

DIHYDROXYALUMINUM SODIUM CARBONATE

Dihydroxyaluminum sodium carbonate combines in a single chemical entity properties of both sodium bicarbonate and aluminum hydroxide. The drug is a partially systemic antacid. The sodium carbonate moiety reacts rapidly with hydrogen ion, with the evolution of carbon dioxide and aluminum hydroxide. The aluminum hydroxide supposedly exerts a sustained, moderate buffering action that is more reliable than the action of some aluminum hydroxide suspensions. However, present published data on the *in-vivo* properties of dihydroxyaluminum sodium carbonate are unreliable, so that a true comparison is not yet possible. The sole commercial product is expensive when the cost per milliequivalent of available antacid is calculated.

Preparations. *Dihydroxyaluminum Sodium Carbonate,* N.F. (ROLAIDS), is available "over the counter" as tablets containing 300 mg of the drug; the sodium content in 300 mg is 50 mg. The usual dose is 300 to 600 mg.

DIHYDROXYALUMINUM AMINOACETATE

Dihydroxyaluminum aminoacetate is a basic salt of aluminum and glycine. In neutralization four hydrogen ions are used—one for each hydroxyl group, one for the carboxyl group, and one for the amino group. The rate of neutralization equals or exceeds that of the reactive forms of aluminum hydroxide. The aminoacetic acid may possibly delay gastric emptying, but it may also increase gastric secretion. Claims that the substance is less constipating than aluminum hydroxide lack objective clinical support, but there is less aluminum per chemical equivalent.

Preparations. *Dihydroxyaluminum Aminoacetate,* N.F. (ROBALATE), is dispensed as *Dihydroxyaluminum Aminoacetate Magma,* N.F., or *Dihydroxyaluminum Aminoacetate Tablets,* N.F. Most preparations contain 100 mg/ml of the aminoacetate as a magma or 500 mg as a tablet; thus, the aluminum content of the magma is higher but that of the tablet is lower than in the corresponding official aluminum hydroxide preparations. The dose is 500 mg to 2 g. Depending on the product, in 30 minutes 1 g in the tablet form will neutralize approximately 3.8 to 6.3 mEq and in the suspension form (1 g = 10 ml) 5.4 to 8.8 mEq of acid.

ALUMINUM PHOSPHATE

Aluminum phosphate reacts slowly with the hydrochloric acid in gastric juice to yield aluminum chloride and phosphoric acid. In the small intestine aluminum phosphate is largely regenerated from the original antacid constituents, so that endogenous phosphate is spared. The compound is intended for use as an antacid in preference to aluminum hydroxide when interference with phosphate absorption should be avoided, but the data of Fordtran and coworkers (1973) show it to be an ineffective antacid. In patients with impaired renal function, it can cause hyperphosphatemia.

Preparations. *Aluminum phosphate gel* (PHOSPHALJEL) is an aqueous suspension containing 4.0 to 5.0% $AlPO_4$. The dose is 15 to 45 ml. However, no practical dose is sufficient to neutralize the gastric acid in a patient with duodenal ulcer.

CALCIUM CARBONATE

As chalk, calcium carbonate ($CaCO_3$) was the first gastric antacid to be used. It has remained popular for a century and a half. Its antacid effects are rapid in onset and relatively prolonged in duration. $CaCO_3$ has a high neutralizing capacity *in vivo*. Kirsner and Palmer (1940) found it to be the most effective gastric antacid of those they studied, and for nearly 30 years thereafter most authorities considered it to be the antacid of choice in the treatment of peptic ulcer. Today, expert opinion is more cautious, for reasons cited below and elsewhere in this chapter.

$CaCO_3$ has long been considered to be the epitome of a nonsystemic antacid. However, enough is absorbed to cause systemic and renal effects in certain circumstances. A slight-to-moderate metabolic alkalosis occurs during treatment with $CaCO_3$, but it is slow to develop.

The amount of calcium absorbed from $CaCO_3$ probably depends upon the amount of gastric acid; in one study, 0 to 2% of a single 2-g dose was found to be absorbed in achlorhydric persons, 9 to 16% in normal subjects, and 11 to 37% in patients with peptic ulcer (Ivanovich *et al.,* 1967). The fraction absorbed seems to be nearly the same when $CaCO_3$ is given chronically in daily doses of 20 g. A dose-absorption relationship has not been established for $CaCO_3$; however, by analogy with other forms of calcium, the amount absorbed probably reaches a plateau at a dose of about 40 to 50 g.

After a single 4-g dose in normal subjects there is a rise in plasma calcium concentration that lasts less than 3 hours, but after an 8-g dose a longer-lasting hypercalcemia occurs. With a daily dose of 20 g, chronic hypercalcemia is not observed in persons with normal renal function, but it may result from as little as 3.4 g per day when there is azotemia. Calcium excretion varies directly with the creatinine clearance. The amount excreted falls far short of the amount absorbed, less than 1 to 9% of a therapeutic dose usually being excreted, even after weeks of treatment. Some individuals appear to be hyperexcretors of calcium and are among the nephrolithiasis-prone population. Although increased calcium excretion almost always follows the administration of antacid doses of $CaCO_3$, alkaluria does not invariably occur.

Phosphate balance is altered in a positive direction by the administration of $CaCO_3$; plasma phosphate concentrations may or may not be increased, but hyperphosphatemia is the usual finding in patients with the milk-alkali syndrome. Increased calcium intake decreases magnesium absorption. Various details of the absorption, excretion, and systemic effects of $CaCO_3$ can be found in the reports by Wenger and coworkers (1957), McMillan and Freeman (1965), Clarkson and colleagues (1966), Vincent and Radcliff (1966), Ivanovich and associates (1967), Makoff and coworkers (1969), and Malone and Horn (1971).

An acid rebound follows a 4-g but not a 2-g dose of $CaCO_3$ (Fordtran, 1968; Texter et al., 1971). This is not secondary to the neutralization of gastric acid, because equivalent doses of other antacids cause much less effect (Barreras, 1970). Furthermore, gastric hypersecretion is elicited when the stomach is bypassed and appropriately acidified $CaCO_3$ is instilled directly in the small intestine. Although intravenous calcium ion stimulates the release of gastrin and hence increases gastric secretion, the plasma calcium concentration required to do so is much higher than that resulting from oral $CaCO_3$; furthermore, increases in plasma calcium and gastrin concentrations occur dissynchronously (Reeder et al., 1971). Therefore, the effect seems to be attributable to a local action in the intestine.

$CaCO_3$ has been claimed to have antipeptic activity, but this has been shown to be only the result of the increase in gastric pH (Kuruvilla, 1971). Calcium salts have a greater tendency than magnesium salts to precipitate in the intestinal tract. Consequently, they possess no cathartic action but tend to constipate; for this reason magnesium and calcium antacids are often alternated or combined in antacid therapy.

Untoward Effects. The constipating effects and chalky taste of $CaCO_3$ are clinically disadvantageous. Disturbances resulting from the liberation of carbon dioxide have not proven to be a serious problem, although belching occurs in some individuals. Nausea is an occasional complaint. More seriously, infrequent instances of hypercalcemia with alkalosis, calcinosis (including nephro-

calcinosis), and azotemia occur during chronic $CaCO_3$ usage, especially in conjunction with milk and cream (milk-alkali syndrome; see McMillan and Freeman, 1965); renal dysfunction, gastrointestinal hemorrhage, and vomiting or aspiration of the gastric contents through a nasogastric tube seem to predispose to the disorder. When phosphate intake is low, hypophosphatemia may occur. Hypercalciuria and alkaluria predispose to nephrolithiasis. To avoid nephrolithiasis and the milk-alkali syndrome, it has been recommended that no more than 160 mEq (8 g) a day be administered (Fordtran, 1966; see also Edwards, 1973). The gastric hypersecretory action is counterproductive and may possibly account for various reports that $CaCO_3$ is less efficacious than other antacids. However, during continuous neutralization it is doubtful that the secretory rate is any higher than that induced by elevation of the pH alone. $CaCO_3$ has been known to cause fecal concretions.

Preparations. *Precipitated Calcium Carbonate,* U.S.P., is usually dispensed as *Calcium Carbonate Tablets,* N.F., which generally contain either 600 mg or 1.0 g of the salt. In 30 minutes, 1.0 g of $CaCO_3$ neutralizes approximately 13 mEq of acid. Magmas react promptly and completely. The official dose of 1 to 2 g is often inadequate. A 2-g dose of the compound is required every hour to maintain the gastric pH at about 4 in the fasting ulcer patient, yet such dosage greatly exceeds the 8-g daily limit recommended by Fordtran (1966). Since administration 1 hour post cibum appears to prolong the action considerably (Fordtran and Collyns, 1966), the daily dose may be minimized by proper scheduling.

MAGNESIUM CARBONATE

Magnesium carbonate ($MgCO_3$) reacts with acid to generate magnesium cation and carbon dioxide. The rate of reaction is considerably slower than that of $CaCO_3$; when the gastric emptying time is short, the requirement for $MgCO_3$ may be as much as ten times that of $CaCO_3$. Nevertheless, $MgCO_3$ appears to be an excellent antacid under clinical conditions (Kirsner, 1941). The absorption of magnesium and the systemic effects are largely those of $Mg(OH)_2$. The release of CO_2 in the stomach may cause belching.

Preparations. *Magnesium Carbonate,* N.F., is a bulky hydrated powder that contains the equivalent of 40.0 to 43.5% MgO. Although 1 g contains approximately 20 mEq, only a fraction may be available for neutralization *in vivo.* The official dose of 500 mg to 2 g may be inadequate.

MAGNESIUM HYDROXIDE AND OXIDE

Magnesium hydroxide, $Mg(OH)_2$, as milk of magnesia has long been popular among the laity as an antacid and a cathartic, and is also somewhat popular among physicians. The compound is practically insoluble, and solution is not effected until the hydroxide reacts with hydrochloric acid to form magnesium chloride. Unreacted $Mg(OH)_2$ remains in the stomach to react with acid subsequently secreted. Therefore, it has a somewhat prolonged duration of action. However, its neutralizing action is nearly as prompt and complete as that of sodium bicarbonate.

In water, MgO hydrates to $Mg(OH)_2$; consequently, its pharmacology is that of the hydroxide. However, unneutralized MgO may not be completely converted to $Mg(OH)_2$ during its sojourn in the stomach.

Although $Mg(OH)_2$ is claimed not to cause acid rebound, Clark and Adams (1947) reported such an effect; the data of Barreras (1970) also indicate a slight rebound.

In man, a mixture of magnesium and aluminum hydroxide possibly decreases antral motility (Khan et al., 1970); in dogs, the magnesium content of the gastric mucosa and muscularis is increased, and it is possible that the effect to decrease antral motility and uropepsin secretion (Abbott et al., 1967) is from a direct local action. Presumably it is not due to a decrease in gastric secretion since $Mg(OH)_2$ increases lower esophageal sphincter pressure (Castell and Levine, 1971) and acid secretion in Heidenhain pouches (Posey et al., 1965).

A disadvantage of the use of $Mg(OH)_2$ as an antacid in some patients is its cathartic effect (see Chapter 49). In clinical practice, the cathartic effect can be minimized by coadministering calcium carbonate or aluminum hydroxide, which have constipating effects, or alternating such constipating antacids with magnesium hydroxide. Although $Mg(OH)_2$ is classified as a nonsystemic antacid, 5 to 10% of the magnesium can be absorbed; retention of any absorbed magnesium can cause neurological, neuromuscular, and cardiovascular impairment and even death in persons with renal insufficiency (see Randall et al., 1964). Ordinarily the absorbed magnesium ion is rapidly excreted by the kidney. In normal persons, absorption is attended by little or no danger of systemic alkalosis, but the urine may become alkaline. Alkalinization of the urine can decrease the excretion of various weakly basic drugs (e.g., quinidine). $Mg(OH)_2$ increases the absorption of warfarin in man and decreases the absorption of barbiturates in rats. Prolonged use of $Mg(OH)_2$ may rarely cause rectal stones composed of $MgCO_3$ and $Mg(OH)_2$ (Lieber and Alavi, 1970).

Preparations. *Milk of Magnesia*, U.S.P., is an aqueous suspension of magnesium hydroxide containing 7.0 to 8.5% of $Mg(OH)_2$. Each milliliter of milk of magnesia is capable of neutralizing approximately 2.7 mEq of acid. The antacid dose is 5 to 15 ml. Magnesium hydroxide is also available as *magnesium hydroxide tablets;* such tablets generally contain 310 mg each, which can neutralize 10.7 mEq of acid. Magnesium hydroxide is usually marketed in combination with other antacids.

Magnesium Oxide, U.S.P., is usually incorporated into various mixtures. When it is used alone, the official dose is 250 mg, which is inadequate. Although 1 g contains approximately 50 mEq of base, only 8 to 20 mEq may react with the gastric acid in 30 minutes.

MAGALDRATE

Magaldrate is a complex hydroxymagnesium aluminate with the approximate formula $[Mg(OH)^+]_4[Al_2(OH)_{10}^{4-}]\cdot 2H_2O$. It reacts with acid in stages. The hydroxymagnesium is relatively rapidly converted to magnesium ion and the aluminate to hydrated aluminum hydroxide; the aluminum hydroxide then reacts more slowly to give a sustained antacid effect. Magaldrate does not simply simulate physical mixtures of magnesium and aluminum hydroxides, since the aluminum hydroxide freshly generated in the gastric acid does not have time to convert to less reactive forms. Consequently, magaldrate more consistently buffers the gastric contents than do the mixtures. The pH is usually maintained between 3.5 and 4.0. Its systemic effects are those of $Mg(OH)_2$.

Preparations. *Magaldrate*, U.S.P. (RIOPAN), contains the equivalent of 28 to 39% MgO and 17 to 25% Al_2O_3. It is available as official tablets containing 400 mg of antacid or as a suspension containing 80 mg/ml. The dose is 400 to 800 mg.

MAGNESIUM TRISILICATE

There are many silicates of magnesium, but the one employed as an antacid is the magnesium salt of mesotrisilicic acid ($Mg_2Si_3O_8 \cdot nH_2O$). It functions as a nonsystemic antacid. Magnesium trisilicate reacts with acid in the following manner:

$$Mg_2Si_3O_8 \cdot nH_2O + 4H^+ \longrightarrow 2Mg^{2+} + 3SiO_2 + (n + 2)H_2O$$

Magnesium trisilicate has a slow onset of neutralizing action; in 0.1 N HCl less than 30% reacts in 15 minutes and less than 55% in 30 minutes. Two grams per hour is insufficient to raise the gastric pH above 2.5 (Kirsner, 1941).

The gelatinous consistency of the silicon dioxide formed in the stomach is thought to provide an adherent coating that may protect the crater of an ulcer (see Nelson, 1964), but Morrissey and coworkers (1967) did not observe any special adherence. Both silica gel and magnesium trisilicate are good adsorbents. Not only does magnesium trisilicate adsorb pepsin, but it also interferes with the absorption of dietary protein (West and Pennoyer, 1945) and of iron. Its effect on the bioavailability of drugs requires more investigation.

The principal side effect of magnesium trisilicate is the laxation caused by high doses. However, hypermagnesemia and systemic toxicity can occur in patients with renal insufficiency (see Alfrey et al., 1970). Approximately 5% of the magnesium is absorbed. This results in a slight alkaluria. Approximately 7% of the silica may be absorbed (Page et al., 1941). Since 1960, there have been a number of reports of siliceous nephroliths caused by chronic ingestion of magnesium trisilicate (see Joekes et al.,

1973). The stones have a low radiopacity and hence may easily be overlooked. It is probable that the phenomenon occurs moderately often during chronic use. Silica deposits and damage in the renal tubules occur routinely in dogs treated chronically with magnesium trisilicate in doses comparable to *effective* doses in man (Newberne and Wilson, 1970). Similar renal damage is seen in man in geographical regions of high silicate intake. Intestinal impaction from concretions or sediments of magnesium trisilicate occurs, especially if there is gastrointestinal bleeding.

Even if magnesium trisilicate were as reactive as $Mg(OH)_2$, there would nevertheless be no advantage over $Mg(OH)_2$. In the light of its low efficacy and its unique potential toxicity, there seems to be little reason to continue the use of this substance.

Preparations. *Magnesium Trisilicate,* U.S.P. (TRI-SOMIN), contains not less than 20% of magnesium oxide and not less than 45% of silicon dioxide. The powder can be conveniently administered by suspending it in water. One gram of an official preparation theoretically will neutralize 13 to 17 mEq of acid. However, at best only 6 to 7 mEq of dried magnesium trisilicate reacts during the first 30 minutes. The only marketed tablet contains 500 mg of the salt. The tablets should be chewed before they are swallowed, because they do not disintegrate rapidly in the stomach. Although the commonly used dose is 1 g, more than 4 g may be required. Magnesium trisilicate is included in a number of combinations.

SODIUM BICARBONATE

Because of the solubility of sodium bicarbonate ($NaHCO_3$), it exerts an immediate and rapid antacid action in the stomach. Any excess, however, being in solution, rapidly enters the intestine, so that the substance has a shorter duration of action than do other antacids.

The formerly wide use of $NaHCO_3$ has greatly declined, owing not only to the "over-the-counter" promotion of other antacids but also to medical concern about its systemic effects. Chronic use of $NaHCO_3$ alone as an antacid (along with milk) can cause the milk-alkali syndrome (*e.g., see* Ansari, 1970). The systemic toxicity of $NaHCO_3$ in persons with normal renal function has perhaps been overly stressed. Van Goidsenhoven and coworkers (1954) administered daily doses up to 25 mEq/kg to patients for 3 weeks. Although there were changes in the plasma electrolyte concentrations, they were not remarkable; plasma total CO_2 increased by only 5 mEq per liter with the largest dose. Considerable weight gain was the most prominent effect. One of 33 patients developed albuminuria and hematuria with these massive doses. The authors asserted that dehydration with consequent renal ischemia, rather than alkalosis or fluid retention, was the primary cause of complications. Kirsner and Palmer (1942, 1943) reported that even with a combination of 380 mEq of $NaHCO_3$ and 640 mEq of $CaCO_3$ per day only 10% of 1350 patients developed an alkalosis. However, volume expansion can increase the

blood pressure and promote edema, so that the use of even moderate amounts of $NaHCO_3$ may be a hazard to persons with renal insufficiency or incipient or active hypertension or cardiac failure. Alkalinization of the urine favors nephrolithiasis. Consequently, it has been recommended that the daily dose for "over-the-counter" use be limited to 200 mEq in persons under, and 100 mEq in persons over, 60 years of age (*see* Edwards, 1973). Belching and an uncomfortable but rarely dangerous gastric distention occur after ingestion of $NaHCO_3$.

Preparations. The official preparations are *Sodium Bicarbonate,* U.S.P., and *Sodium Bicarbonate Tablets,* U.S.P. One gram of sodium bicarbonate neutralizes 12 mEq of acid. The usual dose is 300 mg to 2 g, but up to 4 g may be needed in some patients. Sodium bicarbonate has a saline taste.

Other Therapeutic Uses. The use of sodium bicarbonate in combating systemic acidosis is discussed elsewhere (*see* Chapter 36). The drug is of great value when it is desired to render the urine alkaline. Sodium bicarbonate is used locally on the skin for various disorders, particularly as an antipruritic, in the form of a moist paste or a solution; there is doubt whether the antipruritic effect derives from anything more than its cooling wetness. Sodium bicarbonate is an ingredient of many solutions employed as douches, mouthwashes, and enemata.

ANTACID MIXTURES

Antacids are presently combined for a variety of reasons: laxative and constipating compounds can correct one another; a fast-acting ingredient can be combined with a slow-acting ingredient to increase the total buffering time; a supposed demulcent or antipeptic ingredient can be included; or promotional claims about a "balanced" product can be made. Often one ingredient has too low a reactivity or is in too small a proportion to contribute significantly to the total activity. Impending regulations that would establish maximal daily doses of individual antacid ingredients and minimal neutralizing capacity for "over-the-counter" antacids will undoubtedly occasion the formulation of new mixtures (*see* Edwards, 1973). In the treatment of peptic ulcer, the use of mixtures has an advantage over the separate administration of the individual components, because patient compliance with antacids is exceptionally poor, even in a hospital setting; the nuisance of separate administration greatly deters compliance.

Beside the several official mixtures, there are many nonofficial mixtures available, among which the patient and physician can search for one that is best suited to the needs of the patient. A mixture that causes laxation in one patient may cause constipation in another. However, mixtures should be selected not only on the basis of the effect on the bowel but also on a knowledge of the antacid efficacy and the potential toxic effects of the separate components in relation to the condition of the patient.

Preparations. *Alumina and Magnesia Oral Suspension,* U.S.P., contains 3.1 to 4.0% Al(OH)$_3$ expressed as Al$_2$O$_3$ and 1.4 to 2.2% Mg(OH)$_2$. One milliliter neutralizes about 1.2 to 2.3 mEq of acid in 30 minutes. The dose is 15 to 30 ml. *Magnesia and Alumina Oral Suspension,* U.S.P., contains 2.9 to 4.2% Mg(OH)$_2$ and 2.0 to 2.4% Al$_2$O$_3$ equivalent of Al(OH)$_3$. One milliliter neutralizes about 1.8 to 2.5 mEq of acid in 30 minutes. The dose is 15 ml. *Alumina and Magnesia Tablets,* U.S.P., and *Magnesia and Alumina Tablets,* U.S.P., may contain different proportions of the two antacid components. *Aluminum hydroxide, magnesium hydroxide, and simethicone tablets* differ from the U.S.P. preparations by the addition of the antifoam agent simethicone. *Magnesia, alumina, and calcium carbonate oral suspension* may contain different proportions of the three antacid ingredients. *Aluminum hydroxide and magnesium trisilicate oral suspension* and *aluminum hydroxide gel and magnesium trisilicate tablets* likewise are available in preparations containing different proportions of the antacid components. In some products the Al(OH)$_3$ is nonreactive.

MISCELLANEOUS GASTRIC ANTACIDS

Dibasic Calcium Phosphate, N.F., *Tribasic Calcium Phosphate,* N.F., and *Magnesium Phosphate,* N.F., are classified as nonsystemic gastric antacids, but their efficacy is low and they are seldom employed. *Sodium Citrate,* U.S.P., partially buffers the gastric contents; however, this salt is absorbed and metabolized to sodium bicarbonate, thus causing systemic alkalosis. Sodium citrate is not marketed as such for antacid use; rather, it is generated from the interaction of NaHCO$_3$ and citric acid. *Sodium tartrate* is similarly generated and is likewise mostly reconverted to NaHCO$_3$ in the bowel and liver. Several *bismuth subsalts* have been promoted as antacids, but none of them is capable of elevating the pH of gastric juice even to 2! Although they are claimed to have demulcent and antipeptic properties, there is sufficient evidence to doubt the claims.

The small amounts of *gastric mucin* or *milk protein* incorporated into some antacid tablets have much too low a neutralizing capacity to be of any conceivable benefit. Even the larger amounts of milk protein contained in some powders add little to the neutralizing capacity. The traditional 90 ml of milk has very little effect on the intragastric pH. After a brief buffer effect, *proteins* induce hypersecretion; although this is somewhat counterproductive, the peptic ulcer patient needs to be kept in nitrogen balance and needs

adequate dietary protein. *Glycine* can delay gastric emptying, but it can also increase gastric secretion.

GASTRIC ANTACIDS IN THE TREATMENT OF PEPTIC ULCER

Pathophysiology of Peptic Ulcer. Since the acid-peptic theory of upper gastrointestinal ulcers was proposed by Abercombie in 1824, only sporadic opposition to it has occurred. Much experimental and clinical evidence has been adduced in favor of the theory. Modern opinion almost uniformly accepts the acid-peptic theory but recognizes that hormonal, circulatory, mechanical, immunological, and other factors contribute to the susceptibility of the duodenal and gastric mucosae to the corrosive effects of gastric juice. The fact that acid secretion in some peptic ulcer patients is normal or even low and that the hypersecretion in most patients remains even after disappearance of the lesion emphasizes the importance of mucosal resistance in peptic ulcer. The etiology and pathophysiology of peptic ulcer will be discussed only briefly here. For further details, the reader is referred to Piper and Heap (1972), Rhodes (1972), Birnbaum (1973), Scratchard (1973), Sleisenger and Fordtran (1973), and Wormsley (1974).

The nocturnal resting secretion of hydrochloric acid in male *duodenal* ulcer patients generally lies between 2 and 6 mEq per hour, which is approximately two to seven times that of the normal male; some patients secrete more than 30 mEq per hour. The output in response to stimuli is also generally much above normal. The mass of parietal cells and the gastrin content of the antrum in persons with duodenal ulcer are approximately twice normal; the gastrin secretion in response to secretagogues or neutralization of the gastric juice is approximately twice that in normal persons, but the fasting gastrin secretion is normal in many patients. Oddly, the resting secretion of acid in *gastric* ulcer patients is below normal, markedly so in women; in these persons, the antral gastrin content may be somewhat below normal, but the fasting and evoked gastric secretion is normal. Probably the reflux of bile causes the gastritis and back diffusion of acid into the mucosa in some of these patients.

Division of the vagus nerves reduces the rate of acid secretion to normal or below in patients with duodenal ulcer and much below normal in patients with gastric ulcer. This has been widely interpreted to mean that the excess secretion in the duodenal ulcer patient is in response to stimuli mediated by the vagus. However, it might just as well be interpreted that resection of the vagus abolishes the normal rather than the hypernormal component of acid secretion; this would be more in keeping with the observation that vagotomy nearly abolishes resting acid secretion in normal dogs and human patients with gastric ulcer. Furthermore, vagotomy also reduces the evoked secretion of gastrin and the parietal secretory response to gastrin and histamine, so that the vagus may simply support the hyperactivity of a humoral system. The predominant medical opinion holds duodenal ulcer to be largely, although not entirely, a psychosomatic disorder, the motor expression of which is mediated through the vagus. If so, the hypernormal component of secretion would of necessity be that which the vagus supports. The psychic and personality factors in peptic ulcer are beyond the scope of this discussion.

Antacid Therapy for Peptic Ulcer.

In spite of the fact that antacids provide only one of several prominent therapeutic measures, they are among the first agents employed and cases are rare, indeed, in which antacids are omitted. Agreement falters over the question whether antacid therapy is more ritualistic than beneficial or whether it does, in fact, aid in the healing of the lesion. Unfortunately, no adequately designed study has been made to answer the question.

Three studies (Doll *et al.*, 1956; Baume and Hunt, 1969; Herrmann and Piper, 1973) are commonly cited in support of the view that antacids do not promote healing. Two of these were conducted in a hospital setting, which in itself accelerates healing and undoubtedly makes it difficult to prove any additional acceleration in the small populations of subjects that were used. In only one study (Doll *et al.*, 1956) were nonmedicated patients used for controls, but the control subjects were spared the continuous intragastric intubation and they were not matched to the test patients for type of ulcer. Since in the other two studies the "placebo" was another antacid in a presumably ineffective regimen, the number of tablets and dose interval could not be matched to simulate the test regimen. Furthermore, no attempt was made to match the small control and test populations for size of the ulcer crater, duration of the attack or the disease, age, or other factors that affect the rate of healing.

In support of the view that antacids do promote healing are the reports by Rossett and coworkers (1952) and Rossett and Kashgarian (1968) that vigorous treatment with alumina and magnesia oral suspension accelerates healing threefold. Although these reports are commendable in that over 1000 patients were included in each study, not only were there no controls (control data were taken from the literature) but antimuscarinic drugs were also employed. The Veterans Administration prospective study (VA Gastric Ulcer Study Group, 1971) is similarly ambiguous, since there were no nonmedicated controls and management included diet and antimuscarinic drugs; the findings were that 76% of 638 treated patients met the criteria for adequate healing. None of these studies was double-blind.

There is no doubt that antacids in appropriate doses relieve the pain of peptic ulcer; such pain is reasonably well established to be the result of the action of acid upon the lesion and subsequent spasm. The disappearance of pain, however, does not necessarily mean that healing is in progress, and numerous instances of "silent," that is, painless, ulcers that progress to the point of perforation are known.

Neutralization and pH. If the aim is simply to relieve pain, the physician need concern himself only with the fact that pain is relieved when the intragastric pH exceeds 2. However, if the physician subscribes to the belief that greater neutralization promotes healing of an ulcer, the following considerations must be addressed.

If the pathogenic role of gastric acid is a *direct* attack on the mucosa to generate a lesion, then any degree of neutralization should be of benefit. Fordtran and coworkers (1973) cite studies in experimental animals that suggest that control of acidity alone, and not peptic activity, is sufficient to confer a therapeutic benefit. The implication that the attack factor is acid and not acid-pepsin is critical to establishing the tenets of effective antacid treatment. For example, to neutralize 80% of gastric acid of pH 1.3, it is necessary only to raise the pH to 2, which most antacids can do. But to inhibit peptic activity of human gastric juice by 80% it is necessary to raise the pH to about 5.5 (*see* Piper and Fenton, 1965). Moreover, the peptic activity is maximal at pH 2, where it is nearly four times what it is at pH 1.3. Therefore, if acid-pepsin is the attack factor, it would be better to leave the gastric acid undisturbed than to neutralize it partially. Not until the pH is elevated to about 5 does the peptic activity drop below that at pH 1.3. Perhaps this explains in part why an effect of antacid treatment on healing eludes conclusive demonstration. At present, it is common to accept an end point of pH 3 or 3.5 as a reasonable goal for antacid treatment. At this pH the acid concentration is only 0.6% that at pH 1.3, but the peptic activity is still three times that at pH 1.3. Piper and Fenton (1965) suggested an alternative, namely, the use of a small but sufficient amount of an antacid such as $Mg(OH)_2$ or $NaHCO_3$ to bring the pH transiently to 8 in order to inactivate pepsin irreversibly, but no therapeutic trial based upon this suggestion has been reported.

Dose. Much has yet to be learned about what constitutes an effective dose and, like the end point, it rests importantly on whether relief of pain or reduction in acidity or peptic activity is the goal. Neutralization of the gastric contents stimulates acid secretion, so that a dose cannot be prescribed on the basis of the basal secretory rate. The maximal augmented rate has been estimated to be 30 to 80 mEq per hour in duodenal ulcer patients (Price and Sanderson, 1956; Fordtran and Walsh, 1973). From the augmented rate and the kinetics of gastric emptying, Myhill and Piper (1964) calculated that 50 mEq per hour of *available* (not theoretical) antacid would be required to neutralize continuously the gastric juice of 90% of patients with duodenal ulcer. This is consistent with the hourly 40- to 80-mEq dose of $CaCO_3$ that Kirsner and Palmer (1940) found necessary to maintain the intragastric pH above 4.0. Translated into weight or volume, 50 mEq requires doses of 4.4 to 63 g among various antacid powders, 12 to 200 g among tablets (10 to 380 tablets!), and 18 to 715 ml among nonconcentrated suspensions (*see* Piper and Fenton, 1964).

On the basis of the peak histamine response, Fordtran and coworkers (1973) were able to distinguish two populations of patients having separate dose requirements for an alumina and magnesia oral suspension; the dose to decrease gastric acidity by 80% was one fifth and by 100% it was one tenth as much in the "hyposecretor" as in the "hypersecretor" group. Further studies are required to establish the general applicability of their findings. Meanwhile, the physician can determine the adequacy of the dose of any given preparation for his patient only by gastric analysis.

Dose Interval. If antacids are prescribed only with the intent to relieve pain, then they may be taken only as needed. However, if the intent is to promote healing, a continuous buffering would be ideal. Except with intragastric drip, continuous buffering is difficult to achieve, and practical considerations force a compromise in which buffering is achieved discontinuously. Gastric emptying limits the duration of action of even the most potent and persistent antacids. The buffering effects of the recommended single dose of a nonconcentrated antacid disappear in an empty stomach in 5 to 40 minutes and those of a concentrated antacid in 45 to 60 minutes (end point, pH 3.5). It has been claimed that if an antacid is ingested 1 hour after a meal, the buffering action may exceed 2 to 3 hours (Fordtran and Collyns, 1966). The data of Powell and coworkers (1971), however, do not show this effect, and the factors that promote the prolonged action need better definition. Based upon the supposition of the universality of the effect, some gastroenterologists give a large dose (80 mEq of $CaCO_3$ or 156 mEq of alumina and magnesia mixture) 1 hour after each meal and at bedtime. Theoretically, it should be possible to achieve buffering for as much as 15 hours a day on this regimen. However, neither the gastric acidity nor the pH during a full day on this regimen has been reported in any study. The daily dose of antacid in this regimen is equal to or less than that required by usual hourly doses of nonconcentrated and bihourly doses of concentrated antacids for approximately the same cumulative time the gastric contents are buffered (*see* Powell *et al.,* 1971). The simplicity of the postcibal schedule should favor a better compliance than do the hourly or bihourly schedules. If continuous buffering is the goal, then hourly doses of about 50 mEq are required.

Choice of Preparation. Drug package information, desk references, and advertisements fail to provide the data critical to a rational choice of antacid products and doses. Only three reports (Brody and Bachrach, 1959; Piper and Fenton, 1964; Fordtran *et al.,* 1973), two partly out-of-date, provide data on neutralization capacity by brand name. The data reveal extreme variations in antacid efficacy among various products. The following guidelines are based on these data and other considerations. (1) Products containing only $Mg(OH)_2$, MgO, $CaCO_3$, or $NaHCO_3$ generally have high neutralization capacities and rapid onsets of action. Dihydroxyaluminum sodium carbonate and magaldrate have intermediate capacities, and $Al(OH)_3$ generally has a low capacity and a slow onset of action. However, an $Al(OH)_3$-hexitol complex (WINGEL) ranks high among nonconcentrated suspensions and among all suspensions for which comparative data are available. Dihydroxyaluminum aminoacetate and

$Mg_2Si_3O_8$ have low neutralizing capacities. (2) Although $NaHCO_3$ and effervescent antacids react very rapidly, they are also easily emptied from the stomach and hence have short durations of action. (3) In adequate doses, MgO, $Mg(OH)_2$, and $NaHCO_3$ can raise the gastric pH above 8 and $CaCO_3$ can raise it above 5. A pH of approximately 4 can sometimes be achieved with magaldrate and dihydroxyaluminum sodium carbonate, but the action is brief and erratic. (4) The antacid capacity, rate of onset, and pH achieved depend upon the proportions of the various constituents in mixtures. When $Al(OH)_3$ is included, the acid reaction of Al^{3+} prevents a high pH from being reached, unless the proportion of $Al(OH)_3$ in the mixture is small. (5) Suspensions generally react faster than tablets. (6) Since claims that certain antacids coat ulcer craters have not been supported, it is unwise to choose on the basis of such claims (*see* Hoon, 1966; Rider *et al.,* 1966; Morrissey *et al.,* 1967). (7) The dosage requirements for antacids that float are no less and possibly may be more than those that sink; whether such antacids protect the esophagus may depend upon the position of the patient. (8) Although simethicone may relieve some gastrointestinal discomfort and decrease gastroesophageal reflux, it does not lessen the antacid requirement. (9) The most effective antacids are also the ones most likely to cause systemic effects; the renal and cardiovascular status should always be weighed in relation to the total daily dose of the various antacid constituents. The sodium contents of antacids are tabulated in the American Pharmaceutical Association's *Handbook of Nonprescription Drugs* (Griffenhagen and Hawkins, 1973). (10) Aspirin-containing antacid mixtures should be avoided, since aspirin is ulcerogenic, unless there is an indication for such analgesic therapy. (11) Proteolytic enzymes in some products must be considered counterproductive. (12) The cost of round-the-clock continuous neutralization may vary from about $2 to $100 per day, depending upon the product; the physician should consider the cost of the regimen to the patient.

For various opinions on the use of antacids, *see* the reviews by Piper and Heap (1972), Piper (1973), Sleisenger and Fordtran (1973), and Morrissey and Barreras (1974).

Other Therapeutic Uses. Antacids have a legitimate place in the treatment of reflex esophagitis. To the extent that heartburn and "sour stomach" are symptoms of such reflux, antacids are indicated. The relationship of other minor gastrointestinal symptoms to gastric acid is usually nil or unproven, and antacids probably exert only a placebo effect in most such conditions.

MISCELLANEOUS ANTIULCER SUBSTANCES

The subject of miscellaneous antiulcer substances has been reviewed by Banks and Marks (1973) and will only be highlighted here. An unequivocally effective, safe antipeptic drug has yet to be perfected; considering the central question of the role of pepsin in ulcerogenesis, the delay is unfortunate.

New and as-yet-experimental H_2-receptor antagonists can dramatically suppress gastrin- and histamine-induced gastric secretion in man. The effect of a single oral dose of *metiamide* on nocturnal acid secretion in patients with peptic ulcer is shown in Figure 29–4 (page 613). These agents may soon assume an important role in the control of pathological gastric acid secretion (*see* Chapter 29).

Certain *esters of prostaglandin E_2* suppress gastric secretion in man for over 4 hours (*see* Karim *et al.*, 1973). *Proglumide* and *gefarnate* (geranyl farnesyl acetate) have been reported to increase mucosal resistance to acid peptic erosion, by uncertain mechanisms.

There have been over 300 reports to date on *carbenoloxone sodium*. Double-blind studies show that it increases the rate of healing of an appreciable proportion of gastric and some duodenal ulcers. The drug increases the secretion of gastric mucoproteins and increases the life-span of the mucosal cells. Although carbenoloxone apparently does not prevent bile-induced gastritis, it does seem to prevent the back diffusion of gastric acid caused by bile acids. (For details of the actions of carbenoloxone, *see* Symposium, 1972.) The use of *cholestyramine* to sequester bile acids and prevent the reflux of bile has not been extensively studied. *Deglycerinized licorice* has a spasmolytic action that decreases ulcer pain, but it does not promote healing. *Metoclopramide* increases the rate of gastric emptying, which may possibly be of benefit in gastric but detrimental in duodenal ulcer patients.

Barbiturates have never been shown to decrease acid secretion, but *diazepam* and *mesoridazine* have been reported to decrease nocturnal secretion by 50% and 70%, respectively (*see* Birnbaum, 1973). *Chlordiazepoxide* has also been alleged to decrease gastric secretion. Several interesting corticothalamic depressants are under investigation.

Antimuscarinic drugs can delay gastric emptying and decrease gastric secretion. Atropine and other belladonna alkaloids are exceptionally poor in this respect, but they continue to be promoted for the adjunctive treatment of duodenal ulcer. There is an unwarranted, pervasive dogma that none of the quaternary antimuscarinic drugs is more selective than atropine for effects on gastric functions, despite an abundance of acceptable evidence to the contrary. The source of the misconception appears to be that secretion-suppressing doses of the quaternary antimuscarinic drugs have been compared for side effects with doses of atropine that have no effect on gastric secretion. Certain quaternary antimuscarinic drugs (*e.g.,* glycopyrrolate, clidinium bromide, and methscopolamine bromide) in tolerated doses can considerably suppress gastric secretion, and some patients have been successfully medicated for several years. Even if this were not true, the relatively short duration of action of some quaternary antimuscarinic agents permits them to be used to suppress nocturnal secretion without causing side effects during the day. (See Chapter 25.) Furthermore, the effect to delay gastric emptying increases the retention of antacids and greatly improves buffering (*see* Marcussen and Vilsvik, 1968). The delay in gastric emptying has been thought to be detrimental in patients with gastric ulcer; however, if the reflux of bile is retarded, the effect may be beneficial.

DIGESTANTS

Digestants are drugs that promote the process of digestion in the gastrointestinal tract. They have occasional usefulness in the treatment of conditions characterized by a lack of one or more of the specific substances that function in the digestion of foodstuffs in the alimentary tract. Thus, they may be classified in a general way as drugs used for replacement therapy in deficiency states. The digestants commonly employed are hydrochloric acid, bile salts, and the enzymes of the stomach and pancreas.

HYDROCHLORIC ACID

The only use of hydrochloric acid is in the treatment of gastric *achlorhydria*. Hypochlorhydria occurs in approximately 10 to 15% of the general population. Achlorhydria may be associated with gastritis, gastric carcinoma, pernicious anemia, and numerous other conditions, but it is also frequently encountered in individuals who are otherwise quite normal. The incidence of idiopathic achlorhydria is greatest among elderly persons. The symptoms of achlorhydria are poorly defined. Indeed, some individuals who repeatedly fail to secrete free hydrochloric acid even in response to a powerful secretagogue such as histamine may experience no gastrointestinal symptoms. The symptoms of other persons with achlorhydria are more definitely related to the attending disorder that gave rise to the achlorhydria. However, certain symptoms may be attributed to achlorhydria itself even though they are not always associated with the complete absence of acid in the stomach. These include vague epigastric distress after meals, belching, abdominal distention, coated tongue, nausea, vomiting, and morning diarrhea (gastrogenous diarrhea). Hydrochloric acid is reported to be effective in relieving this syndrome in a significant percentage of cases, but this may be due to a placebo effect.

Pharmacological Actions. While suitable dilutions of hydrochloric acid do increase somewhat the acidity of the gastric contents, the conventional therapeutic dose of hydrochloric acid, taken during and after a meal, is usually not sufficient to cause the appearance of free hydrochloric acid in the stomach. Rather, most of the acid is bound by the gastric contents.

The absorption of a large amount of hydrochloric acid causes a rise in the chloride and a depletion in the bicarbonate content of the extracellular fluid. The kidney compensates by an increased secretion of H^+ and ammonia formation, and, consequently, fixed cation is not obligatorily excreted. In this manner, metabolic acidosis is prevented; however, if large doses are employed, it is advisable to check the acid-base status of the patient a few days after the start of treatment and occasionally thereafter. Clinically, hydrochloric acid is not usually employed when it is desired to lower the pH of body fluids, because it is much simpler to administer acid-forming salts such as ammonium chloride.

Glutamic acid hydrochloride is sometimes prescribed in lieu of free hydrochloric acid because its solid form allows it to be conveniently administered in capsules. Exposure of the dental enamel to acid is thus avoided. However, it is less effective than free hydrochloric acid in lowering gastric pH.

Preparations and Dosage. *Diluted Hydrochloric Acid,* U.S.P., contains 10% hydrochloric acid. The usual dose of 5 ml contains approximately 15 mEq of acid; before ingestion it must be diluted with 125 to 250 ml of water. Some clinicians recommend that diluted hydrochloric acid be given to the limit of tolerance and claim that optimal results can be obtained only with doses sufficiently large to cause free acid to appear in the stomach. For this purpose, they administer 10 ml (30 mEq) of diluted hydrochloric acid (with water) during and after each meal, usually 2 ml at 15-minute intervals. A dose of this magnitude approaches the amount of acid normally secreted by the stomach in response to a meal.

Hydrochloric acid solutions should be sipped through a glass tube in order to protect the dental enamel from the solvent action of the acid. The subsequent use of a neutralizing alkaline mouthwash is also recommended.

Glutamic acid hydrochloride (ACIDULIN) is administered in the form of capsules that contain 340 mg, only 1.8 mEq of hydrochloric acid. The single dose is 340 mg to 1.0 g.

PEPSINS

Although pepsins normally play an important role in the digestion of dietary protein, the proteolytic enzymes of the intestinal tract function sufficiently to prevent serious digestive disturbances when there is a lack of pepsins. A complete deficiency in the secretion of pepsins does not occur except as an accompaniment of achlorhydria. On the other hand, achlorhydria is not necessarily accompanied by a lack of pepsins. The condition in which the stomach fails to secrete both acid and pepsins in response to an adequate stimulus is known as *gastric achylia.* Gastric achylia is observed most frequently in individuals with pernicious anemia or gastric carcinoma.

The symptoms of gastric achylia cannot be attributed directly to the lack of pepsins. The deficiency in hydrochloric acid appears to be of greater consequence. Therefore, in the treatment of achylia, hydrochloric acid is often used alone, although pepsin is sometimes simultaneously prescribed.

PANCREATIC ENZYMES

The enzymes of the pancreas are obtainable in a preparation known as *pancreatin.* Pancreatin is an amorphous powdered substance obtained from fresh hog pancreas. It contains principally amylase, trypsin, and lipase.

Pancreatin is employed in the treatment of conditions in which the secretion of pancreatic juice is deficient, for example, pancreatitis and mucoviscidosis. The administration of pancreatin provides some benefit; for example, the nitrogen and fat content of the stool can be decreased. Pancreatin should be given in enteric capsules to prevent its destruction by pepsin. The average dose is 0.5 to 1 g.

BILE, BILE SALTS, AND BILE ACIDS

Bile is composed of a variety of substances, inasmuch as its composition is determined both by sec-

retory and excretory activities of the liver. With respect to function and therapeutic application, the most important constituents of bile are the bile acids and their conjugates. The bile acids are derivatives of cholanic acid, which is a steroid. Cholanic acid has the following structural formula:

Cholanic Acid

The important bile acids in human bile are cholic acid (3,7,12-trihydroxycholanic acid) and chenodeoxycholic acid ($3\alpha,7\alpha$-dihydroxycholanic acid), which are present mainly as the sodium salts. However, for the most part, the bile acids are conjugated with glycine or taurine and are secreted as sodium salts of the conjugates (glycocholic acid, taurocholic acid, glycodeoxycholic acid, glycochenodeoxycholic acid, etc.). The conjugates are stable compounds that resist enzymatic hydrolysis in the intestine and are largely reabsorbed as such. The conjugates are sometimes referred to as the *bile salts,* but the term should also include the sodium salts of the unconjugated bile acids. Deoxycholic and lithocholic acids are formed in the intestine by the action of bacteria on the secreted bile acids (*see* Hayakawa, 1973).

It should be emphasized that many bile preparations employed in therapy do not contain natural bile salts; rather, they contain partially synthetic derivatives of the bile acids. The most important of these is *dehydrocholic acid* (triketocholanic acid).

Bile acids are synthesized in the liver, except for deoxycholic acid, which is synthesized by enteric bacteria. The liver normally secretes approximately 24 g of bile salts in 700 to 1000 ml of bile in 24 hours. Most of the bile salts are reabsorbed in the lower small intestine and again become available for secretion. Thus, when the enterohepatic circulation of bile is normal, only about 200 to 800 mg of the daily output of bile salts must be synthesized. The pool of bile salts is approximately 2 to 5 g. Discussions of the chemistry, metabolism, and formation of bile salts may be found in the publications by Nair and Kritchevsky (1971, 1973) and Heaton (1972).

Physiological Functions. Bile has a variety of functions. In solution the conjugated bile salts form micelles in which lipid materials may be entrained. In the absence of bile only about 50% of fat is absorbed and almost none of vitamins A, D, E, and K and carotene. Bile salts also promote the digestion of fats by stimulating pancreatic secretion and by activating pancreatic lipase. The absorption of steroid hormones is only slightly affected. Deoxycholate and dehydrocholate, which do not readily form micelles, only slightly promote the absorption of fat. Bile salts may be involved in the absorption of calcium. Deoxycholic and chenodeoxycholic acids promote a net excretion of sodium, potassium, and water in the colon, and this may be one of the factors regulating colonic absorption.

Exogenous bile salts increase the cholesterol pools, mainly as a result of decreased endogenous production of bile acids with consequent sparing of cholesterol and by a moderate effect upon absorption of cholesterol. Cholesterol absorption is increased by bile salts when there are enough phosphatides, monoglycerides, and fatty acids to enable micelle formation. Bile salts depress cholesterogenesis in the intestinal crypts, but the effect on the systemic cholesterol pool is approximately balanced by increased absorption (see McIntyre and Isselbacher, 1973). Bile salts keep cholesterol in solution in the bile and thus suppress stone formation. They are also involved in the regulation of biliary phospholipid secretion.

Bile salts increase gastrointestinal motility, but the physiological significance is unknown. The large volume of bile that enters the duodenum helps to neutralize the acidic gastric contents but is secondary to pancreatic juice in this respect.

Although bile is of great physiological importance, it is not indispensable, provided fat-soluble vitamins are administered parenterally. Physiological concentrations of the unconjugated bile salts inhibit the growth of anaerobic intestinal bacteria in man.

Pharmacological and Toxic Effects. *Choleretic Actions.* A drug that stimulates the liver to increase the output of bile is called a *choleretic.* A drug that stimulates the liver to increase the output of bile of low specific gravity is called a *hydrocholeretic.* Of all drugs alleged to have choleretic action, the unconjugated bile salts and acids are the most active in this respect. They enhance the flow of bile after intravenous or oral administration. The preparations, however, differ greatly in activity. Dehydrocholic acid is by far the most active. It increases the total volume of bile to a much greater extent than it does the total solids and, therefore, may be designated as a hydrocholeretic. The naturally occurring bile acid conjugates, such as glycocholate and taurocholate, enhance the flow to a much lesser extent, but both volume and total solids are proportionally increased. However, they are not true cholepoietic agents inasmuch as the increment in bile salt excreted does not exceed the amount administered. The hydrocholeretic action of dehydrocholic acid is accompanied by an increase in hepatic arterial blood flow.

The bile salts and acids do not increase the excretion of preformed bile pigment. Any augmentation can be accounted for either by a flushing of bile from the dead space of the duct system or by the hemolytic action of the agents themselves. Dehydrocholate actually decreases bilirubin excretion (Bloomer *et al.,* 1973). Therefore, bile therapy is ineffective in speeding recovery from jaundice following biliary obstruction.

Stone Dissolution. Prolonged treatment with chenodeoxycholic acid gradually dissolves radiolucent gallstones in 50 to 60% of patients (see Thistle and Hoffman, 1973). It was formerly believed that the action was mainly to enhance the solubility of cholesterol in the bile by increasing the bile salt content, but cholic acid does not effect the dissolu-

tion of gallstones. The mechanism is in dispute; chenodeoxycholic acid appears to decrease cholesterol secretion but not to affect the input into, or the size of, the cholesterol pool (for references, see Thistle and Hoffman, 1973). Plasma cholesterol is not affected, but triglyceride concentration is significantly decreased (Bell *et al.,* 1973). There has been concern that lithocholic acid, generated from chenodeoxycholic acid, may cause hepatotoxicity, although lithocholic acid is very little absorbed. A significant number of patients show increases in plasma SGOT activity. In one study, 1 of 11 liver biopsies showed an abnormal cytology, but the cause was undetermined (see Thistle and Hoffman, 1973).

Miscellaneous Choleretics. Various other substances stimulate the flow of bile. The enteric hormone secretin increases both biliary and pancreatic secretion; its brief duration of action limits its clinical usefulness mainly to diagnostic procedures. Gastrin also stimulates biliary secretion. *Tocamphyl* increases the flow of bile severalfold in man and is often superior to other choleretics. Although *florantyrone* is promoted as a hydrocholeretic, the outputs of bile and bile acids are increased proportionately; at best, its action is mild compared to that of bile salts.

Miscellaneous and Toxic Effects. The effect of bile salts to increase the motor and secretory activity of the bowel can cause diarrhea. The administration of dehydrocholic acid has no effect on gastric secretion. Deoxycholate is toxic to the gastrointestinal mucosa if other bile acids are absent. The toxicity of hyocholic and hyodeoxycholic acids is presently unknown, so that it is advisable to avoid using hog bile preparations, in which these foreign bile acids are found.

The toxic actions of bile are of interest both because bile is used as a therapeutic agent and because significantly increased concentrations of the biliary constituents can be found in the blood of patients with biliary obstruction. The outstanding effects of parenterally administered bile are on the circulatory and neuromuscular systems. Following intravenous injection of bile salts there is a marked fall in blood pressure accompanied by bradycardia. The slowing of the heart appears to be the result of stimulation of vagal centers, and it can be blocked by atropine. Bradycardia and hypotension frequently accompany jaundice. The bile salts and acids differ in their depressor activity. Dehydrocholic acid is the least potent and also by far the least toxic of the various compounds. Intravenously, bile salts cause skeletal muscular hyperactivity, twitching, spasm, and a decrease in the threshold for excitation by nerve impulses. Anaphylactoid reactions infrequently follow the intravenous administration of sodium dehydrocholate. In biliary obstruction, pruritus frequently occurs. No direct evidence exists that the pruritus is attributable to bile salts. Nevertheless, the oral administration of *cholestyramine,* which binds bile salts, is followed by relief of the itching.

In dogs, bile salts damage the gastric mucosal barrier, which results in back diffusion of acid. Although the net diffusion into the lumen is diminished, the mucosal concentration is increased and ulceration occurs. It is thought that the reflux of bile into the stomach is a major cause of gastritis and gastric ulcer in man. Dilute solutions of bile acids and bile salts cause lysis of red and white blood cells. In monkeys, lithocholic acid causes the appearance of spur-shaped erythrocytes similar to those seen in persons with hepatocellular damage.

Preparations. *Dehydrocholic Acid,* N.F. (DECHOLIN), is available in tablets containing 250 mg. The usual dose is 250 to 750 mg, three times a day. *Sodium Dehydrocholate Injection,* N.F. (DECHOLIN SODIUM), is marketed as a 20% solution in ampuls containing 3, 5, or 10 ml. The intravenous dose is 3 to 5 ml. *Florantyrone* (ZANCHOL) is marketed as 250-mg tablets; the usual dose is 750 mg to 1.0 g daily. *Tocamphyl* (SYNCUMA) is dispensed as 75-mg tablets. The dose is 75 to 100 mg, three times a day. *Ox bile extract* contains an amount of the sodium salts of ox bile acids equivalent to approximately 45% cholic acid. The composition of ox bile closely resembles that of human bile with respect to bile salts, but hog bile contains acids of undetermined toxicity. Ox bile extract is administered in the form of tablets. The usual dose is 250 to 500 mg. The initial dose of *chenodeoxycholic acid* is 750 mg a day; it is adjusted upward until diarrhea occurs and then diminished by 250 mg for maintenance. Several months to over a year of treatment may be required for the dissolution of gallstones.

Therapeutic Uses. The bile salts or unnatural cholagogues are employed for a limited number of purposes. They are used to replace endogenous bile salts when a deficiency exists. They can be given to promote the flow of bile or to increase intrabiliary pressure; however, much expert medical opinion now holds that the administration of bile salts is often unnecessary or inappropriate and can sometimes cause undue pain or danger to the patient. The special use of chenodeoxycholic acid to dissolve gallstones is discussed above.

When complete or nearly complete biliary obstruction exists, surgery is indicated, not bile salts. Exogenous bile salts further contribute to an already undesirable increase in plasma concentration of bile salts, and they may also initiate an attack of biliary colic. Similarly, bile salts are not indicated in cholestatic jaundice. Proper dietary management can usually reduce the dietary fat to a low level and alter its composition so that a large proportion can be absorbed without bile salts. There has been excessive concern about the absorption of vitamins A and D; deficiency takes months to develop, and surgery for obstruction or recovery from cholestatic jaundice ordinarily will have occurred much earlier. Vitamin K, which is rapidly depleted, may be given as the water-soluble menadione sodium bisulfite. Fats and fat-soluble vitamins can be given parenterally. In partial biliary obstruction the bile output is usually adequate, especially if the diet is properly managed. Bile salts are no better than placebos in nonobstructive, noncholestatic biliary tract disorders or in various malfunctions of the small intestine.

Hydrocholeretics have been administered to increase the flow and reduce the viscosity of bile in postsurgical patients during T-tube drainage. The contention that biliary flush (hydrocholeresis) helps to prevent infections in biliary tract disease or postsurgically remains to be proven. Hydrocholeresis is sometimes used to dislodge small calculi from the biliary tract. According to the location of the calculus, various ancillary postural or manipulative procedures may be required. In choledocholithiasis, in addition to a hydrocholeretic, antispasmodics (antimuscarinic agent or nitroglycerin, and/or oral magnesium sulfate or citrate) may be administered to relax the ductus choledochus and the sphincter of Oddi. If impacted stones fail to dislodge, an attack of biliary colic may result. Controlled studies of this use are lacking. Biliary flush is of assistance to chemolytic procedures for reducing or fragmenting calculi. The filling of the biliary tree during hydrocholeresis may assist the surgeon to visualize the ducts and locate obstructions. Hydrocholeresis also improves the gallbladder shadow for roentgenological examination. Intravenous sodium dehydrocholate is generally used in these diagnostic procedures. There is no acceptable evidence that bile salts hasten the secretion of contrast media into the biliary tract. The rapid intravenous injection of sodium dehydrocholate has been employed to measure circulation time. The end point is the onset of a bitter taste.

Abbott, D. D.; Harrisson, J. W. E.; and Brogle, R. C. Uropepsin excretion and the effect of antacid materials. *J. pharm. Sci.,* **1967,** *56,* 1501–1502.

Alfrey, A. C.; Terman, D. S.; Brettschneider, L.; Simpson, K. M.; and Ogden, D. A. Hypermagnesemia after renal homotransplantation. *Ann. intern. Med.,* **1970,** *73,* 367–371.

Anderson, W., and Harthill, J. E. Aluminum hydroxide and pepsin. *J. Pharm. Pharmac.,* **1972,** *24,* Suppl., 166P.

Ansari, A. Antacid-induced phosphorus depletion and repletion. *Minn. Med.,* **1970,** *53,* 837–838.

Barreras, R. F. Acid secretion after calcium carbonate in patients with duodenal ulcer. *New Engl. J. Med.,* **1970,** *282,* 1402–1405.

Baume, P. E., and Hunt, J. H. Failure of potent antacid therapy to hasten healing in chronic gastric ulcers. *Australas. Ann. Med.,* **1969,** *18,* 113–116.

Bell, G. D.; Lewis, B.; Petrie, A.; and Dowling, R. H. Serum lipids in cholelithiasis: effect of chenodeoxycholic acid therapy. *Br. med. J.,* **1973,** *3,* 520–523.

Berlyne, G. M.; Ben-Ari, J.; Pest, D.; Weinberger, J.; Stern, M.; Gilmore, G. R.; and Levine, R. Hyperaluminaemia from aluminum resins in renal failure. *Lancet,* **1970,** *2,* 494–496.

Bloomer, J. R.; Boyer, J. L.; and Klatskin, G. Inhibition of bilirubin excretion in man during dehydrocholate choleresis. *Gastroenterology,* **1973,** *65,* 929–935.

Boyd, L. J.; Russ, W. R.; and Barowsky, H. Nonreactive alumina in the treatment of peptic ulcer. *Rev. Gastroent.,* **1942,** *9,* 20–25.

Castell, D. O., and Levine, S. M. Lower esophageal sphincter response to gastric neutralization. A new mechanism for treatment of heartburn with antacids. *Ann. intern. Med.,* **1971,** *74,* 223–227.

Clark, B. B., and Adams, W. L. The effect of gastric antacids on gastric secretion as observed in the Cope pouch dog. *Gastroenterology,* **1947,** *9,* 284–292.

Clarkson, E. M.; McDonald, S. J.; and de Wardener, H. E. The effect of a high intake of calcium carbonate in normal subjects and patients with chronic renal failure. *Clin. Sci.,* **1966,** *30,* 425–438.

Doll, R.; Price, A. V.; Pygott, F.; and Sanderson, P. H. Continuous intragastric milk drip in the treatment of uncomplicated gastric ulcer. *Lancet,* **1956,** *1,* 70–73.

Edwards, C. C. Proposal establishing a monograph for OTC antacid products. *Fedl Regis.*, **1973,** *38,* 8714–8724.

Fordtran, J. S. Comparison of antacids for peptic ulcer. *New Engl. J. Med.,* **1966,** *275,* 1316.

Fordtran, J. S., and Collyns, J. A. H. Antacid pharmacology in duodenal ulcer: effect of antacids on postcibal gastric acidity and peptic activity. *New Engl. J. Med.,* **1966,** *274,* 921–927.

Fordtran, J. S.; Morawski, S. G.; and Richardson, C. T. *In vivo* and *in vitro* evaluation of liquid antacids. *New Engl. J. Med.,* **1973,** *288,* 923–928.

Fordtran, J. S., and Walsh, J. H. Gastric acid secretion rate and buffer content of the stomach after eating. Results in normal patients and in patients with duodenal ulcer. *J. clin. Invest.,* **1973,** *52,* 645–657.

Gibaldi, M.; Kanig, J. L.; and Amsel, L. Critical *in vitro* factors in evaluation of gastric antacids. Inhibition of neutralization rate of dried aluminum hydroxide gel. *J. pharm. Sci.,* **1964,** *53,* 1375–1377.

Goldsmith, R. S.; Furzifer, J.; Johnson, W. J.; Fournier, A. E.; and Arnaud, C. D. Control of secondary hyperparathyroidism during long-term hemodialysis. *Am. J. Med.,* **1971,** *50,* 692–699.

Hem, S. L.; Russo, E. J.; Bahal, S. M.; and Levi, R. S. Effect of pH of precipitation on antacid properties of hydrous aluminum oxide. *J. pharm. Sci.,* **1970,** *59,* 317–321.

Herrmann, R. P., and Piper, D. W. Factors influencing the healing rate of chronic gastric ulcer. *Am. J. dig. Dis.,* **1973,** *18,* 1–6.

Hoon, J. R. Observations of antacids by intragastric photography. *Archs Surg.,* **1966,** *93,* 467–474.

Ivanovich, P.; Fellows, H.; and Rich, C. The absorption of calcium carbonate. *Ann. intern. Med.,* **1967,** *66,* 917–923.

Joekes, A. M.; Rose, G. A.; and Sutor, J. Multiple renal silica calculi. *Br. med. J.,* **1973,** *1,* 146–147.

Karim, S. M. M.; Carter, D. C.; Bhana, D.; and Ganesan, P. A. Effect of orally administered prostaglandin E_2 and its 15-methyl analogs on gastric secretion. *Br. med. J.,* **1973,** *1,* 143–146.

Khan, A. A.; Englert, E.; and Moore, J. G. Tissue magnesium and gastric motility after antacids. *Clin. Res.,* **1970,** *18,* 127.

Kirsner, J. B. A further study of the effect of various antacids on the hydrogen ion concentration of the gastric contents. *Am. J. dig. Dis.,* **1941,** *8,* 53–56.

Kirsner, J. B., and Palmer, W. L. The effect of various antacids upon hydrogen ion concentration of the gastric contents. *Am. J. dig. Dis.,* **1940,** *7,* 85–93.

————. Alkalosis complicating the Sippy treatment of peptic ulcer. *Archs intern. Med.,* **1942,** *69,* 789–807.

————. Studies on the effect of massive quantities of sodium bicarbonate on the acid-base equilibrium and renal function. Report of a case with remarkable tolerance. *Ann. intern. Med.,* **1943,** *18,* 100–104.

Krumlovsky, F., and del Greco, F. Use of antacids in patients on chronic dialysis. *Lancet,* **1970,** *2,* 150.

Kuruvilla, J. T. Antipeptic activity of antacids. *Gut,* **1971,** *12,* 897–898.

Lavengood, R. W., Jr., and Marshall, V. F. The prevention of renal phosphatic calculi in the presence of infection by the Shorr regimen. *J. Urol.,* **1972,** *108,* 368–371.

Lieber, A., and Alavi, S. M. Rectal stone. Report of a case. *Am. J. dig. Dis.,* **1970,** *15,* 287–290.

Lotz, M.; Zisman, E.; and Bartter, F. C. Evidence for a phosphorus-depletion syndrome in man. *New Engl. J. Med.,* **1968,** *278,* 409–415.

McMillan, D. E., and Freeman, R. B. The milk-alkali syndrome: a study of the acute disorder with comments on the development of the chronic condition. *Medicine, Baltimore,* **1965,** *44,* 485–501.

Makoff, D. L.; Gordon, A.; Franklin, A. S.; and Gerstein, A. R. Chronic calcium carbonate therapy in uremia. *Archs intern. Med.,* **1969,** *123,* 15–21.

Malone, D. N. S., and Horn, D. B. Acute hypercalcaemia and renal failure after antacid therapy. *Br. med. J.,* **1971,** *1,* 709–710.

Marcussen, J. M., and Vilsvik, J. S. The effect of combined antacid-anticholinergic treatment on the intragastric pH in peptic ulcer disease. *Scand. J. Gastroent.,* **1968,** *3,* 170–176.

Morrissey, J. F.; Honda, T.; and Tanaka, Y. Gastric mucosal coating and gastric emptying time of antacids. *Archs intern. Med.,* **1967,** *119,* 510–517.

Myhill, J., and Piper, D. W. Antacid therapy of peptic ulcer. Part I. A mathematical definition of an adequate dose. *Gut,* **1964,** *5,* 581–584.

Nassim, J. R., and Connolly, C. K. Treatment of calcinosis universalis with aluminum hydroxide. *Archs Dis. Childh.,* **1970,** *45,* 118–121.

Nelson, R. S. Intragastric findings with liquid antacid therapy. *Curr. ther. Res.,* **1964,** *6,* 83–87.

Newberne, P. M., and Wilson, R. B. Renal damage associated with silicon compounds in dogs. *Proc. natn. Acad. Sci. U.S.A.,* **1970,** *65,* 872–875.

Page, R. C.; Heffner, R. R.; and Frey, A. Urinary excretion of silica in humans following oral administration of magnesium trisilicate. *Am. J. dig. Dis.,* **1941,** *8,* 13–15.

Pendras, J. P., and Erickson, R. V. Hemodialysis: a successful therapy for chronic uremia. *Ann. intern. Med.,* **1966,** *64,* 293–311.

Piper, D. W., and Fenton, B. The adsorption of pepsin. *Am. J. dig. Dis.,* **1961,** *6,* 134–141.

————. Antacid therapy of peptic ulcer. Part II. An evaluation of antacids *in vitro. Gut,* **1964,** *5,* 585–589.

————. pH Stability and activity curves of pepsin with special reference to their clinical importance. *Ibid.,* **1965,** *6,* 506–508.

Posey, E. L.; Smith, P.; Turner, C.; and Aldridge, J. Effects of anticholinergics, antacids, and antrectomy on gastrin production and relation of antral motility to gastrin release. *Am. J. dig. Dis.,* **1965,** *10,* 399–410.

Potyk, D. Intestinal obstruction from impacted antacid tablets. *New Engl. J. Med.,* **1970,** *283,* 134–135.

Powell, R. L.; Westlake, W. J.; Longaker, E. D.; and Greene, L. C. A clinical evaluation of a new concentrated antacid. I. Effects on gastric pH. *J. clin. Pharmac.,* **1971,** *11,* 288–295.

Price, A. V., and Sanderson, P. H. Alkali requirement for continuous neutralization of gastric contents in gastric and duodenal ulcer. *Clin. Sci.,* **1956,** *15,* 285–295.

Randall, R. E.; Cohen, M. D.; Spray, C. C.; and Rossmeissl, E. C. Hypermagnesemia in renal failure. Etiology and toxic manifestations. *Ann. intern. Med.,* **1964,** *61,* 73–88.

Reeder, D. D.; Conlee, J. L.; and Thompson, J. C. Calcium carbonate antacid and serum gastrin concentration in duodenal ulcer. *Surg. Forum,* **1971,** *22,* 308–310.

Rider, J. A.; Moeller, H. C.; and Puletti, E. J. Gastroscopic evaluation of the mucosal coating effect of various antacids. *Gastrointest. Endosc.,* **1966,** *12,* 19–22.

Rossett, N. E., and Kashgarian, M. Peptic ulcer: medical cure of ambulatory patients by efficient gastric acid neutralization. *J. Tenn. St. med. Ass.,* **1968,** *61,* 798–801.

Rossett, N. E.; Knox, F. H., Jr.; and Stephenson, S. L., Jr. Peptic ulcer: medical cure by efficient gastric acid neutralization. *Ann. intern. Med.,* **1952,** *36,* 98–109.

Shorr, E., and Carter, A. C. Aluminum gels in the management of renal phosphatic calculi. *J. Am. med. Ass.,* **1950,** *144,* 1549–1556.

Smith, F. H. Nonreactive aluminum hydroxide in the treatment of peptic ulcer. *Gastroenterology,* **1947,** *8,* 494–503.

Texter, E. C., Jr.; Laureta, H. C.; and Martin, G. A.

Absence of acid rebound with two gram doses of calcium carbonate. *Clin. Res.,* **1971,** *19,* 72.

Thistle, J. L., and Hoffman, A. F. Efficacy and specificity of chenodeoxycholic acid therapy for dissolving gallstones. *New Engl. J. Med.,* **1973,** *289,* 655–659.

Thurston, H.; Gilmore, G. R.; and Swales, J. D. Aluminum retention and toxicity in chronic renal failure. *Lancet,* **1972,** *1,* 881–883.

VA Gastric Ulcer Study Group. The Veterans Administration cooperative study on gastric ulcer. *Gastroenterology,* **1971,** *61,* 567–654.

van Goidsenhoven, G. M.-T.; Gray, O. V.; Price, A. V.; and Sanderson, P. H. The effect of prolonged administration of large doses of sodium bicarbonate in man. *Clin. Sci.,* **1954,** *13,* 383–401.

Vincent, P. C., and Radcliff, F. J. Effect of large doses of calcium carbonate on serum and urinary calcium. *Am. J. dig. Dis.,* **1966,** *11,* 286–295.

Wenger, J.; Kirsner, J. B.; and Palmer, W. L. The milk alkali syndrome: hypercalcemia, alkalosis and azotemia following calcium carbonate and milk therapy of peptic ulcer. *Gastroenterology,* **1957,** *33,* 745–769.

Wenger, J., and Sundy, M. Pepsin adsorption by commercial antacid mixtures. *J. clin. Pharmac.,* **1972,** *12,* 136–141.

West, E. S., and Pennoyer, C. Some effects of magnesium trisilicate ingestion upon blood, urine, and feces of human subjects. *Am. J. dig. Dis.,* **1945,** *12,* 199–202.

Monographs and Reviews

Banks, S., and Marks, I. N. Evaluation of new drugs for peptic ulcer. *Clin. Gastroent.,* **1973,** *2,* 379–395.

Birnbaum, D. Peptic ulcer and the central nervous system—etiology and management. *Clin. Gastroent.,* **1973,** *2,* 245–257.

Brody, M., and Bachrach, W. H. Antacids. I. Comparative biochemical and economic considerations. *Am. J. dig. Dis.,* **1959,** *4,* 435–460.

Fordtran, J. S. Acid rebound. *New Engl. J. Med.,* **1968,** *279,* 900–905.

Griffenhagen, G. B., and Hawkins, L. L. (eds.). *Handbook of Nonprescription Drugs.* American Pharmaceutical Association, Washington, D. C., **1973.**

Hayakawa, S. Microbiological transformation of bile acids. *Adv. Lipid Res.,* **1973,** *11,* 143–192. (145 references.)

Heaton, K. W. *Bile Salts in Health and Disease.* The Williams & Wilkins Co., Baltimore, **1972.**

McIntyre, N., and Isselbacher, K. J. Role of the small intestine in cholesterol metabolism. *Am. J. clin. Nutr.,* **1973,** *26,* 647–656.

Morrissey, J. F., and Barreras, R. F. Drug therapy: antacid therapy. *New Engl. J. Med.,* **1974,** *290,* 550–554.

Nair, P. P., and Kritchevsky, D. (eds.). *The Bile Acids.* Vol. 1, *Chemistry.* Plenum Press, New York, **1971.**

——. *The Bile Acids.* Vol. 2, *Physiology and Metabolism.* Plenum Press, New York, **1973.**

Pereira-Lima, J., and Hollander, F. Gastric acid rebound—a review. *Gastroenterology,* **1959,** *37,* 145–153.

Piper, D. W. Antacid and anticholinergic drug therapy. *Clin. Gastroent.,* **1973,** *2,* 361–377.

Piper, D. W., and Heap, T. R. Medical management of peptic ulcer with reference to anti-ulcer agents in other gastro-intestinal diseases. *Drugs,* **1972,** *3,* 366–403.

Rhodes, J. Etiology of gastric ulcer. *Gastroenterology,* **1972,** *63,* 171–181.

Schroeder, H. A., and Nason, A. P. Trace-element analysis in clinical chemistry. *Clin. Chem.,* **1971,** *17,* 461–474.

Scratchard, T. Gastric secretory mechanisms and peptic ulcer. *Clin. Gastroent.,* **1973,** *2,* 259–274.

Sleisenger, M. H., and Fordtran, J. S. *Gastrointestinal Disease: Pathophysiology, Diagnosis, Management.* W. B. Saunders Co., Philadelphia, **1973.**

Symposium. (Various authors.) Symposium on bile salts. *Am. J. Med.,* **1971,** *51,* 565–658.

Symposium. (Various authors.) *Carbenoloxone Sodium.* (Baron, J. H., and Sullivan, F. M., eds.) Appleton-Century-Crofts, New York, **1972.**

Wastell, C. (ed.). *Chronic Duodenal Ulcer.* Appleton-Century-Crofts, New York, **1972.**

Wormsley, K. G. The pathophysiology of duodenal ulceration. *Gut,* **1974,** *15,* 59–81. (284 references.)

CHAPTER
49 LAXATIVES AND CATHARTICS

Edward Fingl

Laxatives and cathartics are drugs that promote defecation. Valid indications for the use of these agents are limited and are clearly less extensive than might be inferred from the frequency with which such drugs are self-prescribed by the laity.

The extensive misuse of self-administered cathartic nostrums by the bowel-conscious public is a result of the many misconceptions concerning bowel function and of the mistaken notions of the value of cathartic medication. Persistence of this misuse reflects the failure of the medical and ancillary health professions to counter the proprietary drug advertising designed to perpetuate these erroneous beliefs.

Classification and Choice of Laxatives and Cathartics. Although often employed interchangeably, the terms *laxative* and *cathartic* correctly imply different intensities of drug effect. Laxative effect suggests the elimination of a soft, formed stool, whereas cathartic effect implies a more fluid evacuation. Thus, the terms *laxative* and *cathartic* are useful for the classification of drugs that pro-

mote defecation, to indicate their maximal efficacy. However, it must be emphasized that an agent designated as a cathartic can, and often should, be administered only in appropriate dosage to produce a laxative rather than a cathartic effect.

The more commonly used agents are classified in Table 49–1, on the basis of general mechanism of action, as emollient or bulk-forming laxatives or as saline or contact cathartics. The emollient laxatives are also often described as fecal softeners. The agents classified as contact cathartics are those formerly designated as stimulant cathartics. The extremely irritant, drastic purgatives are omitted, since these agents are properly considered obsolete.

The individual drugs in each group sometimes have distinguishing pharmacological or clinical characteristics. However, these differences are generally of less practical significance than are the characteristics that the group has in common, and agents in the same category usually have similar clinical usefulness and limitations. The many conflicting claims of clinical superiority of one particular drug over others in the same group can be largely ignored. With rare exception, these claims are based upon inadequately controlled clinical trials or upon comparisons of the drugs at other than equieffective dosage. Consequently, despite the confusingly large number of laxatives and cathartics, the physician need become acquainted with only a few agents to meet the limited valid uses of these drugs.

EMOLLIENT LAXATIVES (FECAL SOFTENERS)

The principal emollient laxatives, the *dioctyl sulfosuccinates* and *mineral oil,* are sufficiently different to require separate description. Nevertheless, their classification together as emollient laxatives serves to em-

Table 49–1. CLASSIFICATION OF LAXATIVES AND CATHARTICS

CLASS	DRUGS
Emollient laxatives (fecal softeners)	Dioctyl sodium sulfosuccinate, dioctyl calcium sulfosuccinate, mineral oil
Bulk-forming laxatives	Methylcellulose, sodium carboxymethylcellulose, psyllium (plantago) preparations, tragacanth and related natural gums, bran
Saline cathartics	Magnesium sulfate, milk of magnesia, magnesium citrate, sodium phosphates, sodium sulfate, potassium sodium tartrate
Contact (stimulant) cathartics	Castor oil, phenolphthalein, bisacodyl, senna, cascara sagrada, danthron

phasize that both types of drugs promote defecation merely by modest softening of the feces. Consequently, their clinical usefulness is limited mainly to situations in which it is desired that the feces be kept soft and that straining at the stool be avoided.

DIOCTYL SULFOSUCCINATES

Dioctyl sodium sulfosuccinate, the prototype for this group of salts, is an anionic surface-active agent widely used in the pharmaceutical industry as an emulsifying agent and as a wetting and dispersing agent in formulations for external application. Its structural formula is shown in Table 49–2. Because of the many potential adverse effects of mineral oil, the surface-active agents are a welcome addition to the group of emollient laxatives. Unfortunately, although the dioctyl sulfosuccinates have been employed as emollient laxatives since 1955, many details of their pharmacology remain uncertain, and controlled clinical comparisons with other laxatives are still limited.

Laxative Effects. In recommended oral dosage, dioctyl sodium sulfosuccinate produces modest softening of the feces within 24 to 48 hours. This effect is attributed to its physical property of lowering surface tension, which is thought to facilitate penetration of the fecal mass by water and fats. In animals, not all surface-active agents are effective laxatives, and more complex effects of dioctyl sodium sulfosuccinate on motor and secretory function of

the digestive tract have been described (Lundholm and Svedmyr, 1959; Lish, 1961). These observations deserve further exploration.

Toxicity. Recommended oral doses of dioctyl sodium sulfosuccinate are well tolerated, and single doses as large as 50 mg/kg in infants have not produced adverse effects. In animals, large doses of the drug produce anorexia, vomiting, and diarrhea.

In ophthalmological formulations, concentrations of dioctyl sodium sulfosuccinate greater than 0.1% may cause conjunctival irritation, and repeated use of the drug may delay healing of corneal lesions. The possible significance of these observations, particularly with regard to use of the drug after hemorrhoidectomy or other anorectal surgery, remains to be determined. Similarly, the reported cytotoxic effect of dioctyl sodium sulfosuccinate on human hepatic cells in tissue culture merits further study, particularly since the drug is absorbed from the gastrointestinal tract and is excreted in significant concentration in the bile (Dujovne and Shoeman, 1972). In animals, dioctyl sodium sulfosuccinate increases the effects of several of the contact cathartics.

Dioctyl Sodium Sulfosuccinate. *Dioctyl Sodium Sulfosuccinate,* U.S.P., is available under a variety of proprietary names, including COLACE and DOXINATE. The drug is supplied as 50-, 60-, and 100-mg capsules and tablets, as 250- and 300-mg capsules, in solution for oral administration (10 and 50 mg/ml), and as a syrup (4 mg/ml).

Although recommended dosage has varied considerably, the usual adult dose is 50 to 480 mg daily, either as a single dose or divided. The higher doses may be required initially. Proportionately smaller doses, as low as 10 to 40 mg daily, are suggested for infants and for children less than 3 years of age. The

Table 49–2. STRUCTURAL FORMULAS OF SELECTED LAXATIVES AND CATHARTICS

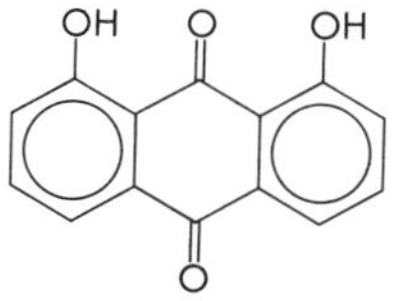

Danthron

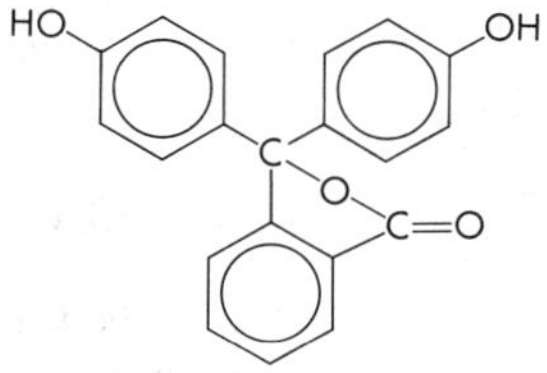

Phenolphthalein

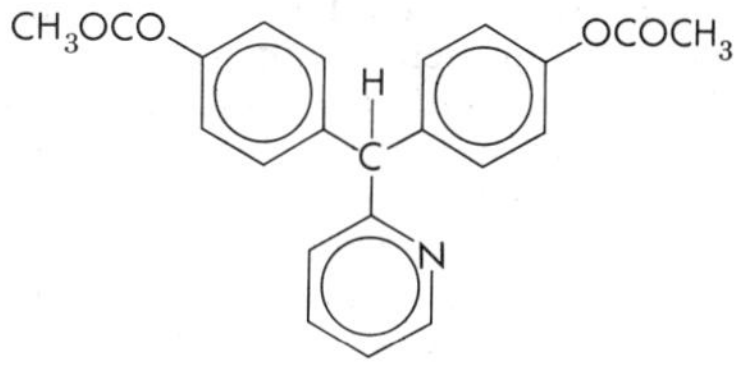

Bisacodyl

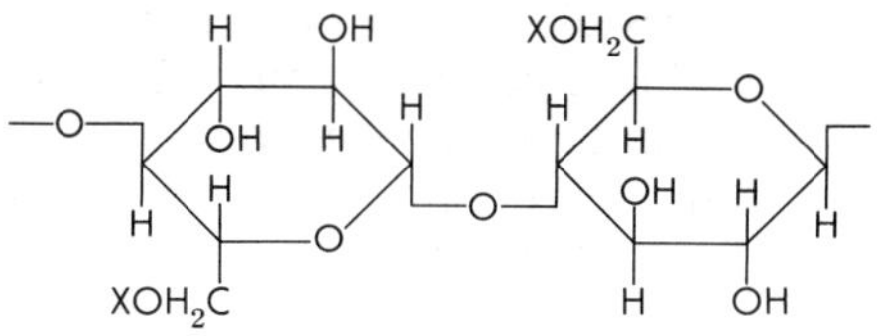

Methylcellulose

X = H or CH₃

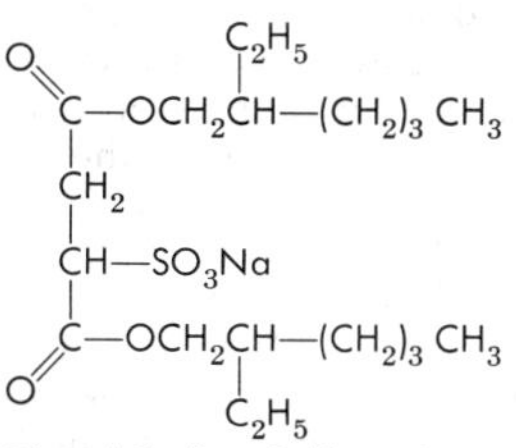

Dioctyl Sodium Sulfosuccinate

solution should be administered in milk or fruit juice to mask its bitter taste. The drug has also been given rectally as a 0.1% solution in doses of 50 to 100 mg.

Mixtures of a surface-active laxative with mineral oil are contraindicated, since the surface-active agent may enhance absorption of the oil. Mixtures with various contact cathartics are also available but cannot be recommended until they have been demonstrated to provide clinical advantages over the contact cathartic given alone.

Dioctyl Calcium Sulfosuccinate. *Dioctyl Calcium Sulfosuccinate,* N.F. (SURFAK), is said to have pharmacological properties and clinical uses and limitations similar to those of the prototype, but the two surface-active agents have not been subjected to careful clinical comparison. Dioctyl calcium sulfosuccinate occasionally causes cramping pains. The drug is available as official 50- and 240-mg capsules. The recommended dosage for adults is 50 to 240 mg daily; proportionately lower doses are suggested for children.

MINERAL OIL

Mineral oil (liquid petrolatum) is a mixture of liquid hydrocarbons obtained from petroleum. The oil is indigestible and absorbed only to a limited extent. In the intestinal tract, it softens the fecal contents, probably by retarding reabsorption of water.

Mineral oil can cause a variety of untoward effects, and its use as an emollient laxative requires adequate appreciation of its potential hazards. Indeed, when the many objections to its use are summed and evaluated, the indictment becomes so grave as to constitute a possible interdiction to its use (Becker, 1952). Clearly, *habitual use of mineral oil must be avoided.*

Toxicity. Mineral oil acts as a lipid solvent and, when administered with meals, may interfere with the *absorption of essential fat-soluble substances.* The absorption of vitamins A and D is affected less than that of provitamin A. The regular ingestion of mineral oil during pregnancy may reduce absorption of vitamin K and produce hypoprothrombinemia.

If it gains access to the lungs, mineral oil is capable of producing *lipid pneumonitis.* This well-known syndrome has been observed most frequently after drugs dissolved in mineral oil are applied to the nasal mucous membranes. However, it should be emphasized that lipid pneumonitis can also occur following the *oral ingestion* of the oil, particularly if it is taken at bedtime. The indiscriminate use of mineral oil by elderly, debilitated, or dysphagic individuals should be discouraged.

Mineral oil is *absorbed* to a limited extent from the intestinal tract. The oil is demonstrable most readily in the mesenteric lymph nodes, but it can also be detected in the intestinal mucosa, liver, and

spleen. At these sites, it elicits a typical foreign-body reaction. Although no physiological disturbances have been related to the presence of the oil at these sites, it must be questioned whether the substance can be used safely over long periods of time.

Leakage of the oil past the anal sphincter is not only an annoying side effect but also an occasional cause of pruritus ani. It is also claimed that the oil interferes with the healing of postoperative wounds in the anorectal region and may induce hemorrhage; therefore, it is recommended by some that it not be employed following hemorrhoidectomy. Furthermore, it is said that continuous presence of the oil in the rectum disturbs normal defecatory reflexes and hence prevents complete evacuation of the bowel.

Preparations and Dosage. *Mineral Oil,* U.S.P. (*liquid petrolatum*), is available in numerous preparations, often under various trade names. They differ greatly in cost but little in efficacy. The dose is 15 to 45 ml, usually taken at night before retiring. It should not be given with meals, since it may interfere with digestion and absorption.

Mineral oil is tasteless, but many individuals object to its consistency. This objection can be overcome if the oil is taken with fruit juice or as *Mineral Oil Emulsion,* N.F. Stable emulsions of the oil penetrate and soften the stool more effectively than does the nonemulsified oil, and they cause less difficulty with leakage of the oil through the anal sphincter. However, emulsification enhances absorption of the oil. Mixtures of mineral oil with other cathartics are also available but are irrational. Mineral oil is also available for rectal administration as *mineral oil enema.*

DIGESTIBLE OILS

Olive Oil, U.S.P., and other digestible oils are also sometimes employed as laxatives. The usual dose is 30 ml or more. A sufficient amount must be given so that enough oil or fatty acid escapes absorption to soften the feces. Digestible oils will, of course, retard gastric secretion and motility and increase the caloric intake; they should not be employed when such effects are undesirable.

BULK-FORMING LAXATIVES

The bulk-forming laxatives include various natural and semisynthetic polysaccharides and cellulose derivatives. These substances dissolve or swell in water to form an emollient gel or viscous solution that serves to maintain the feces soft and hydrated. The resulting bulk promotes peristalsis, and transit time is reduced.

Therapeutic Uses. The *laxative* effect of the bulk-forming agents is usually apparent within 12 to 24 hours, but their full effect may not be achieved until the second or third day of medication. If a constipating, low-residue diet cannot be corrected, as for certain hospitalized or institutionalized patients, the use of the bulk-forming laxatives may be indicated. These agents are also useful in patients in whom it is desired that the feces be maintained soft, to avoid straining at the stool.

Bran and the other bulk-forming agents are also of benefit to reduce intraluminal rectosigmoid pressure and relieve symptoms in patients with *diverticular disease* of the colon (Hodgson, 1972; Painter *et al.,* 1972). The role of lack of dietary bulk as a causal factor in disorders of the large bowel and other diseases remains to be established (*see* Painter and Burkitt, 1971; Goldstein, 1972).

Because of their ability to absorb water and to provide an emollient intestinal mass, the bulk-forming laxatives have some usefulness for the symptomatic relief of *acute diarrhea* and to modify the effluent in patients with an *ileostomy* or *colostomy.* However, sodium, potassium, and water loss may be increased in such patients. The alleged effectiveness of the bulk-forming agents as appetite suppressants in the management of *obesity* has *not* been established.

Adverse Effects. The bulk-forming laxatives are essentially devoid of systemic effects. Flatulence may occur and can sometimes be relieved by increasing the fluid intake. Except for the psyllium preparations, the bulk-forming agents are thought to be excreted more or less quantitatively in the feces.

Intestinal obstruction has been reported after administration of the bulk-forming agents, and *impaction* may result when there is gross intestinal pathology. Occasional cases of *esophageal obstruction* have also occurred when these agents have been swallowed dry or when the tablets are chewed. *Patients who have difficulty swallowing should be warned not to take these preparations dry, and generous amounts of water should be prescribed with all bulk-forming laxatives.*

The distinctive features of the individual bulk-forming laxatives are of limited practical significance. Choice among these preparations often depends upon preference of the individual patient. The bulk-forming laxatives have been reviewed by Gray and Tainter (1941) and Tainter and Buchanan (Symposium, 1954).

Methylcellulose and Carboxymethylcellulose Sodium. *Methylcellulose,* U.S.P., and *Carboxymethylcellulose Sodium,* U.S.P., are hydrophilic semisynthetic cellulose derivatives. They are marketed under many trade names. The two preparations are similar, except that carboxymethylcellulose sodium is insoluble in gastric juice. Both compounds are available as powders, granules, and 500-mg capsules or official tablets. The usual adult dose of methylcellulose or carboxymethylcellulose sodium is 1 to 6 g daily, in divided dosage. During chronic medication, smaller doses may be satisfactory. The dosage of either drug for children is 500 mg, two or three times daily. Both preparations should be taken with 1 or 2 glassfuls of water.

The structural formula of methylcellulose is shown in Table 49–2.

Psyllium (Plantago) Preparations. *Plantago Seed,* N.F., is obtained from various species of plantain. The seeds contain a large amount of natural mucilage and form a gelatinous mass on contact with water. However, the outer seed coat acts as a mechanical irritant that is more harsh than bran. In addition, if the seeds are ground or chewed, a pigment is released, which in animals is deposited as small granules in the renal tubules. For these reasons, the whole seeds have now been largely replaced by powdered preparations of the mucilaginous portion of blond psyllium seeds.

Typical preparations are *plantago ovata coating* (KONSYL) and *psyllium hydrophyllic mucilloid* (META-MUCIL). The latter preparation also contains dextrose as a dispersing agent and provides 14 kcal per 7-g dose. It is claimed that these preparations do not cause renal pigmentation. The usual dose is 4 to 10 g, one to three times daily, stirred in a glassful of water. A similar preparation (L.A. FORMULA) employs equal amounts of lactose and glucose as dispersing agents, readily goes into suspension, and is highly palatable. Chronic administration of the psyllium preparations may produce modest reduction of plasma cholesterol concentration, apparently by interference with reabsorption of bile acids (Forman *et al.,* 1968).

Agar and Tragacanth. *Agar,* U.S.P. (*agar-agar*), is a dried hydrophilic colloidal substance obtained from various species of algae. It is rich in indigestible hemicellulose. It may be eaten as a cereal substitute or added to other foods, or it may be dissolved in hot water and allowed to gel before being taken. However, agar is a relatively ineffective bulk-forming agent in the usual dose of 4 to 16 g. The substance is also employed as an emulsifying agent in a variety of proprietary nostrums combined with mineral oil and other cathartics, but the dose of agar in these preparations is too small to contribute to their laxative effect.

Tragacanth, U.S.P., is the dried gummy exudate from species of *Astragalus.* Closely related products are *karaya (sterculia) gum* and *bassora gum.* These gums are effective bulk-forming laxatives and are available in a variety of proprietary preparations. *Allergic reactions,* characterized by urticaria, rhinitis, atopic dermatitis, and asthma, have been attributed to these agents.

Bran. Bran, a by-product of the milling of wheat, contains almost 20% indigestible cellulose and is an excellent source of intestinal bulk. Crude bran is rather unpalatable, but the processed form makes a pleasant cereal. Bran must be eaten in large doses to be an effective laxative. Several tablespoonfuls a day may be taken as a cereal or in the form of special bran products such as cookies and muffins. Bran and other natural fiber laxatives are not irritating to the normal intestinal mucosa, but these agents should not be employed in individuals with intestinal ulceration, stenosis, or adhesions.

SALINE CATHARTICS

The saline cathartics include several magnesium salts and various sulfates, phosphates, and tartrates. These salts are slowly and incompletely absorbed from the digestive tract and retain water in the intestinal lumen by osmotic forces. Peristalsis is increased indirectly. Latency and intensity of effect vary with the salt and the dosage. Full doses of the saline cathartics (15 g of magnesium sulfate or its equivalent) produce a semifluid or watery evacuation in 3 to 6 hours or less. Since they have many common characteristics and few differences, the saline cathartics are conveniently considered as a group. The distinctive features of the individual drugs are restricted mainly to palatability, cost, maximal efficacy, and risk of untoward systemic effects.

Relative Efficacy. If the saline cathartics were absorbed equally, their relative efficacy could be estimated from their molecular weight and degree of dissociation. However, these salts are not absorbed at equal rates or to the same extent. Consequently, it is not unexpected that such estimates of the relative efficacy of the saline cathartics have been found in error by a factor of 2 or more (Seed and Harris, in Symposium, 1954). Unfortunately, reliable clinical comparison of the saline salts is limited, and these approximate calculations are often the only basis for estimates of relative efficacy. The suggestion that magnesium salts increase motility by causing release of cholecystokinin requires confirmation (Harvey and Read, 1973).

Effect on Water Distribution. Theoretically, if a hypotonic solution of a saline cathartic is ingested, water will be absorbed until the contents of the intestinal tract become isosmotic with body fluids. Conversely, when the cathartic salts are administered in hypertonic solution, water is abstracted from the circulation and is lost in the feces. Indeed, it is possible to dehydrate an individual by the repeated administration of hypertonic solutions of saline cathartics, and these salts were once prescribed for this purpose rather than for evacuation of the bowel. When the objective of medication is the cathartic effect, the saline salts should be administered with

sufficient water by mouth to ensure that no net loss of body water occurs.

Systemic Effects. Some absorption of the component ions of the saline cathartics does occur, and in certain instances they may produce systemic toxicity. This is especially true for magnesium salts, since 20% or more of the administered cation may be absorbed. If renal function is normal, the absorbed magnesium is rapidly excreted. However, if a magnesium cathartic is given to an individual with impaired renal function, the accumulation of magnesium ion in the body fluids may be sufficient to cause magnesium intoxication (see page 790). For this reason, magnesium cathartics must never be administered to patients with impaired renal function. On the other hand, sodium salts may be contraindicated in patients with congestive heart failure, and phosphate salts may reduce the plasma concentration of ionized calcium.

In most instances, the salt that gains access to the systemic circulation is excreted by the kidney, and the absorbed salt acts as a saline diuretic. However, if the saline cathartics are given in strongly hypertonic solution, the consequent loss of body water in the feces may cause noticeable antidiuresis.

Magnesium Salts. *Magnesium Sulfate,* U.S.P. (*Epsom salt*), is one of the more commonly employed saline cathartics. The official dose is 15 g, but significant laxative effect is observed after doses as low as 2 to 5 g, when the salt is administered in dilute solution to a fasting individual. The intensely bitter taste may be partially masked by taking the salt in lemon juice. Strongly hypertonic solutions are likely to be somewhat nauseating.

Milk of Magnesia, U.S.P. (*magnesia magma*), is a 7.0 to 8.5% aqueous suspension of magnesium hydroxide. The usual dose of 15 ml is less effective than 5 g of magnesium sulfate. *Magnesium Hydroxide,* N.F., is also available as tablets. The usual dose is 2 to 4 g. Other magnesium salts, such as magnesium carbonate, magnesium oxide, and magnesium phosphate, have similar laxative properties but are more commonly employed as gastric antacids (see Chapter 48).

Magnesium citrate is a pleasant-tasting, but expensive, saline cathartic. The official preparation, *Magnesium Citrate Solution,* N.F., is a flavored solution containing the equivalent of 1.55 to 1.9 g of magnesium oxide per 100 ml. An excess of citric acid and sodium bicarbonate is added to make the solution effervescent. The official dose is 200 ml.

Sodium and Potassium Salts. *Sodium Phosphate,* U.S.P. (*disodium hydrogen phosphate*), is one of the more pleasant-tasting saline cathartics. The usual dose is 4 to 8 g. It is somewhat less effective than magnesium or sodium sulfate. Still more palatable is *Effervescent Sodium Phosphate,* N.F., a combination of sodium phosphate with sodium bicarbonate and tartaric and citric acids. It is a dry powder that liberates carbon dioxide upon addition of water. The usual dose is 10 to 20 g. Sodium phosphate is also available as a flavored *Sodium Phosphate Solution,*

N.F.; the usual 10-ml dose provides 7.5 g of sodium phosphate. A buffered mixture of sodium phosphates, *Sodium Phosphate and Biphosphate Oral Solution*, U.S.P., and a similar official solution for rectal use are also available.

Sodium Sulfate, U.S.P. (*Glauber's salt*), is one of the cheapest saline cathartics, but it is the most objectionable as far as taste is concerned. The usual dose is 15 g. It is equal in efficacy to magnesium sulfate.

Potassium Sodium Tartrate, N.F. (*Rochelle salt*), is a relatively pleasant-tasting saline cathartic. The official dose is 10 g. The tartrate ion is poorly absorbed from the gastrointestinal tract, and the toxic effect of the ion is not observed when therapeutic doses of this salt are given orally. Potassium sodium tartrate was once a popular laxative in the form of *Seidlitz powder* (*compound effervescent powder*), dispensed as two powders that are dissolved separately in water and mixed just prior to use to provide a pleasant-tasting effervescent solution.

Proprietary Saline Cathartics. A large number of proprietary saline cathartic preparations are available. They range from natural mineral waters, for which extravagant claims are made, to salts that differ little from those described above. The official preparations are less expensive and equally effective.

CONTACT (STIMULANT) CATHARTICS

The three important subgroups of contact cathartics are *castor oil,* the *diphenylmethane* derivatives, and the *anthraquinone* cathartics. These agents are sufficiently different to require separate description. Nevertheless, they have several characteristics in common. All can cause griping, intestinal cramps, increased mucus secretion, and excessively fluid evacuation in some patients. Intensity of effect is proportional to dosage, but individual effective doses of all contact cathartics vary as much as fourfold to eightfold. Consequently, recommended doses that promote the desired effect in the majority of patients can be expected to be relatively ineffective in some and to produce excessive responses in others. Although the contact cathartics are absorbed to different degrees, systemic effects of these agents, other than those secondary to excessive catharsis and water and electrolyte deficits, are relatively unimportant.

The contact cathartics differ with regard to locus of action and latency of response. Since the small intestine is relatively insensitive to the diphenylmethane and anthraquinone cathartics, the effects of these agents are limited primarily to the large intestine and are produced only after a latency of 6 hours or more. In contrast, castor oil acts upon the small intestine and usually produces more thorough catharsis within 3 hours.

The contact cathartics have been reviewed by Travell (Symposium, 1954). Structure-activity relationships among these agents have been summarized by Loewe (1948), Hubacher and Doernberg (1964), and Fairbairn and Moss (1970).

Mechanism of Action. The term *contact cathartic* was originally applied to the diphenylmethane cathartics to indicate that the stimulant effect on the bowel produced by application of these agents to the mucosa could be prevented by prior topical application of a local anesthetic (Göing and Schaumann, 1955; Schmidt, 1955). However, the term is employed here in a more general context for the classification of the diphenylmethane and related agents to indicate that, although the precise mechanism of action is uncertain, it does involve an action on the intestine. In contrast, the other groups of laxatives and cathartics cause hydration of the feces largely or solely by a physical mechanism.

In the past, the contact cathartics were thought to stimulate peristalsis by irritation of the mucosa or by a more selective stimulation of nerves in the mucosa or the intramural neural plexus, or of the intestinal smooth muscle itself. Alternatively, it has been suggested that the primary effect of these drugs may be inhibition of intestinal tone and segmentation activity that provide resistance to normal propulsive activity. In either case, increased hydration of the feces would be attributed to their more rapid transit through the bowel. Still another possible mechanism for the cathartic effect of the contact agents is inhibition of electrolyte and water absorption from the lumen (and possibly enhanced movement of electrolyte and water into the lumen), similar to the effects produced by cholera exotoxin. In this case, motor activity of the intestine would be modified only indirectly by the greater bulk of fluid retained in the bowel.

The relative contribution of each of these mechanisms to the cathartic effect of the individual contact agents *in vivo* remains to be established. However, most have been found to modify electrolyte transport in intestinal segments *in vitro* or *in situ*. An effect on motor activity has been best established for the diphenylmethane derivatives administered rectally or applied directly to the mucosa of the colon. (*See* Forth *et al.*, 1966; Hardcastle and Mann, 1968; Hardcastle and Wilkins, 1970; Christensen, 1971; Phillips, 1972; Ritchie, 1972; Ammon and Phillips, 1973; Nell *et al.*, 1973; Ammon *et al.*, 1974.)

CASTOR OIL

Castor oil, obtained from the seeds of *Ricinus communis,* is composed primarily of the triglyceride of ricinoleic acid, an unsaturated hydroxy fatty acid. Unlike the other contact cathartics, castor oil acts upon the small intestine. For this reason, it is usually administered only when prompt, thorough evacuation of the bowel is desired, as in preparation for certain radiological examinations. Chronic use is not recommended, since absorption of nutrients may be reduced.

Pharmacodynamics. Castor oil itself is a bland oil and is employed locally on the skin for its emollient properties. However, it is hydrolyzed by intestinal lipases to glycerol and ricinoleic acid. This latter substance produces the cathartic effect. The relative importance of effects on electrolyte absorption and secretion and on motor function of the intestine remains to be determined. Ricinoleic acid that is absorbed is metabolized much like other fatty acids (Watson *et al.,* 1963).

Preparations and Dosage. Castor oil is usually administered on an empty stomach, and as little as 4 ml may produce a laxative effect in the fasting adult. However, the usual dose of castor oil for a cathartic effect is 15 to 60 ml for adults and 5 to 15 ml for children. Full doses of castor oil produce one or two copious, semifluid stools within 2 to 6 hours. Because of its prompt action, castor oil should not be administered at bedtime.

Official preparations are *Castor Oil,* U.S.P., and *Aromatic Castor Oil,* N.F. Although the objectionable taste of the oil is partially masked in the latter preparation, flavored *castor oil emulsions* are somewhat more palatable.

DIPHENYLMETHANE CATHARTICS

The primary diphenylmethane cathartics are *phenolphthalein* and *bisacodyl.* These agents have similar pharmacological properties and clinical usefulness and limitations.

Cathartic Effect. The diphenylmethane cathartics exert their greatest effect on the colon. Since they usually do not act in less than 6 hours after oral administration, they are often taken at bedtime, to produce their effect the next morning. The precise mechanism of action of these drugs and the relative importance of an effect upon electrolyte transport and upon motor activity of the bowel remain to be determined.

Phenolphthalein. The cathartic effect of phenolphthalein was discovered in 1902 by Vamossy, during a study undertaken for the Hungarian government to determine its safety as an additive for identification of artificial wines. Since that time, phenol-

phthalein has been widely employed as a cathartic. It is the basic ingredient of numerous proprietary nostrums. The structural formula of phenolphthalein is shown in Table 49–2.

Absorption and Excretion. Up to 15% of a therapeutic dose of phenolphthalein is absorbed; the remainder is excreted in the feces. The absorbed portion is largely eliminated by the kidney, most of it in conjugated form. The urine becomes pink or red if it is sufficiently alkaline. Likewise, the drug excreted in the stool causes a red color if the feces are made alkaline by a soapsuds enema. The patient should be warned of this possible coloring of the urine and feces. Some of the drug absorbed from the intestine may be excreted in the bile, and the resulting enterohepatic cycle may contribute to prolongation of the cathartic effect of the drug.

Toxicity. Phenolphthalein is relatively nontoxic, and large doses of the drug have been ingested by children without untoward systemic effects. Thus, the major danger of phenolphthalein overdosage is fluid and electrolyte deficits resulting from excessive cathartic effect. However, allergic reactions, including fixed-drug eruption, Stevens-Johnson syndrome, and lupus erythematosus, have been reported. The skin lesions may persist for months or years after discontinuation of the drug and leave residual pigmentation. Should the patient take phenolphthalein again, lesions may recur in the same skin areas originally involved. Obviously, such individuals must avoid further exposure to the drug. Deaths have been attributed to allergy to phenolphthalein.

Preparations and Dosage. Phenolphthalein, N.F., is the purified white or faintly yellow preparation. The usual adult dose is 60 to 100 mg (Munch and Calesnick, 1960). Incompletely purified "yellow" phenolphthalein may be somewhat more potent than the purified preparation. Both forms of the drug are odorless and tasteless and, therefore, pleasant to take. Phenolphthalein usually acts in 6 to 8 hours. It is conveniently prescribed in capsules or official tablets. It is also available in many proprietary preparations, often in combination with other cathartics. None of these mixtures affords a distinct advantage over phenolphthalein alone, and many are clearly irrational.

Bisacodyl. Bisacodyl, 4,4′-(2-pyridylmethylene) diphenol diacetate, was introduced as a clinical cathartic in 1953 on the basis of structure-activity studies of compounds related to phenolphthalein. The structural formula of the drug is shown in Table 49–2. Bisacodyl is unique among the contact cathartics only in that it is available for rectal as well as oral administration. Administered rectally, the drug has been compared favorably with glycerin suppositories and with enemas.

Absorption and Excretion. Although it was once thought not to be absorbed from the digestive tract, as much as 5% of an orally administered dose of bisacodyl may be absorbed in man. A portion of the absorbed drug appears in the urine as the glucuronide.

Toxicity. Systemic effects of absorbed bisacodyl have not been noted, and untoward effects of the drug have thus far been limited to excessive cathartic effect. Bisacodyl suppositories may produce a burning sensation in the rectum; mild proctitis has been reported after use of the suppositories for several weeks.

Preparations and Dosage. Bisacodyl, U.S.P. (DULCOLAX), is available as official 5-mg enteric-coated tablets for oral administration and as 10-mg rectal suppositories. The usual *oral dosage* is 10 to 15 mg for adults and 5 to 10 mg for children. To avoid gastric irritation, tablets should be swallowed without chewing or crushing and should not be taken within 1 hour of antacid medication. The drug usually produces one or two soft, formed stools within 6 to 12 hours. Recommended *rectal dosage* is 10 mg for adults and for children over 2 years, and 5 mg for children under 2 years. After rectal administration, the drug usually acts in 15 to 60 minutes.

Oxyphenisatin Acetate. Oxyphenisatin acetate (*acetphenolisatin*) is 3,3-*bis*(*p*-hydroxyphenyl)-2-indolinone diacetate. It has enjoyed sporadic popularity as a cathartic, particularly in Europe. The pharmacological properties of oxyphenisatin acetate closely resemble those of bisacodyl. However, oxyphenisatin acetate has been incriminated as a cause of hepatic injury (Reynolds *et al.,* 1971) and has been withdrawn from the market in many countries. The active desacetyl metabolite, oxyphenisatin, is still available for rectal administration, but it, too, should be abandoned.

The interesting claim that an isatin derivative is the active cathartic constituent of prunes has been challenged (*see* Hubacher and Doernberg, 1964).

ANTHRAQUINONE CATHARTICS

The anthraquinone cathartics are also known as the anthracene or emodin cathartics. The principal agents in this group are *senna, cascara sagrada,* and *danthron.* The major active constituents of the anthraquinone cathartics are anthraquinone or anthrone derivatives related to 1,8-dihydroxyanthraquinone. Individual anthraquinone cathartics vary, depending upon their anthraquinone content and the ease of liberation of the active constituents from their inactive precursor glycosides. In addition, the galenical preparations often employed may contain other active ingredients.

Pharmacodynamics. The cathartic effect of the anthraquinone cathartics is limited mainly to the large intestine. Consequently, they are seldom effective before 6 hours after oral administration, and at times they do not act before 24 hours. The glycosides reach the large intestine both by passage through the digestive tract and by way of the circulation after absorption in the small intestine. The glycosides are hydrolyzed within the lumen of the bowel at least in part by the action of bacterial enzymes. The precise mechanism of the cathartic effect and the relative importance of an effect on electrolyte transport or on intestinal motor function remain to be determined.

Toxicity. Untoward effects of the anthraquinone cathartics are mainly excessive cathartic effects. Although not a consistent observation, the active principles may appear in the milk during lactation in sufficient amount to affect the nursing infant. Certain constituents of the drugs are also excreted by the kidney and may color the urine; patients should be informed of this possibility. A melanotic pigmentation of the colonic mucosa (melanosis coli) has been observed in individuals who have taken anthraquinone cathartics over extended periods of time (Wittoesch *et al.,* 1958). The pigmentation is benign and is usually reversible within 4 to 12 months after medication is discontinued.

Senna. *Senna,* N.F., is obtained from the dried leaflets of *Cassia acutifolia* or *Cassia angustifolia.* It was introduced into Arabian medicine as early as the ninth century A.D. Other preparations official in the N.F. are *Senna Fluidextract* and *Senna Syrup.* The doses of these three compounds for adults are 2 g, 2 ml, and 8 ml, respectively. These preparations usually produce a single, thorough bowel evacuation with considerable griping, within 6 hours. Crystalline senna glycosides, *Sennosides A and B,* N.F. (GLYSENNID), and concentrates of senna pods standardized by chemical or biological assay are also available; they are more stable and more reliable than the preparations of senna leaf (McClure Browne *et al.,* 1957). They are also alleged to cause less cramping and griping than does crude senna. The usual dose of the sennosides is 12 to 36 mg.

Cascara Sagrada. *Cascara Sagrada,* U.S.P. (*sacred bark*), is obtained from the bark of the buckthorn tree, *Rhamnus purshiana.* It was used as a cathartic by the Indians of California. The most commonly employed official preparation is *Aromatic Cascara Fluidextract,* U.S.P. The conventional dose of 5 ml usually causes a single soft or semifluid evacuation of the bowel in approximately 8 hours. The drug is generally taken before retiring. *Cascara Sagrada Fluidextract,* N.F., is used less frequently because it has a very bitter taste; the dose is 1 ml. *Cascara Sagrada Extract,* N.F., a powdered preparation, is available in official tablets but is not as reliable as the fluidextract; the adult dose is 300 mg. Proprietary preparations of the cascara sagrada glycosides (*casanthranol*) are also available.

Danthron. *Danthron,* N.F. (*chrysazin;* DORBANE), is 1,8-dihydroxyanthraquinone. Although danthron is a free anthraquinone rather than a glycoside, its pharmacological properties, uses, and limitations are similar to those of the natural anthraquinone cathartics. The drug is available as official 75-mg scored tablets. The usual adult dose of 75 to 150 mg produces a soft or semifluid stool in 6 to 8 hours.

The structural formula of danthron is shown in Table 49-2.

Aloe. Aloe has not been subjected to controlled clinical comparison with the other anthraquinones but has the reputation of being the most irritating of these cathartics. It produces considerable griping and pelvic congestion, and excessive doses may cause nephritis. It is still described in the U.S.P., but only for pharmaceutical reasons. Both aloe and *aloin,* a mixture of active glycosides, should be abandoned.

Aloin was once a common ingredient of many irrational cathartic mixtures with belladonna and strychnine. Pills of aloin, strychnine, and belladonna (A.S.B. pills) were once a frequent cause of strychnine poisoning in children.

Aloe is alleged to be a cholagogue and is often incorporated in proprietary "liver pills." However, careful studies have revealed that aloe has no detectable effect on the formation of bile by the liver, the evacuation of the gallbladder, or the passage of bile into the duodenum. The drug also has an undeserved reputation as an abortifacient.

USES AND ABUSES OF LAXATIVES AND CATHARTICS

Constipation. Laxatives and cathartics have no role in the management of constipation associated with intestinal pathology, and they are of only secondary importance in the treatment of functional constipation.

Many of the causes of functional constipation are simple to correct, once recognized, and therapy is first attempted without the use of drugs. A diet adequate in indigestible residue, sufficient fluid intake, exercise if necessary, the establishment of a proper "habit time," the reminder that "haste does not make waste," reassurance to overcome emotional factors, and similar measures are often successful. If these efforts alone are not adequate, they may be supplemented by use of the bulk-forming agents or laxative doses of the saline agents. The emollient laxatives are sometimes helpful but are often ineffective. Laxative doses of the contact cathartics may be necessary in the more refractory cases.

When laxatives are employed in the treatment of constipation, they should be administered in the lowest effective dosage, as infrequently as possible, and medication should be discontinued promptly and completely upon termination of the need. In cases of drug-induced constipation, such as that produced by chronic therapy with the opioids, antimuscarinic agents, or certain antihypertensive agents, correction by readjustment of drug dosage or by use of alternative drugs should be considered before resorting to concurrent laxative medication. Antimuscarinic agents are sometimes useful for constipation associated with intestinal hypermotility, and administration of thyroid hormone may produce brilliant results in refractory constipation associated with thyroid deficiency.

The Cornell Conferences on Therapy (1941, 1947) still remain an excellent source of general information about the laxatives and cathartics and the treatment of constipation (*see also* Symposium, 1954).

Other Valid Uses. The use of laxatives is often justified to prevent straining at the stool by patients with *hernia* or *cardiovascular disease.* In addition, they are frequently used, both before and after surgery, to maintain soft feces in patients with *hemorrhoids and other anorectal disorders.* Most laxatives have been recommended for these purposes, but the bulk-forming agents or the emollient laxatives are generally satisfactory and should be preferred. The bulk-forming agents have an established role in the management of *diverticular disease* of the colon.

Cathartics are frequently employed prior to *radiological examination* of the gastrointestinal tract or other abdominal structures and prior to *elective bowel surgery.* Castor oil is the traditional agent for these purposes, but other contact cathartics or full doses of the saline cathartics are also employed. Contact cathartics, either orally or rectally, may also be used instead of enemas for emptying the large bowel prior to *proctological examination.*

In cases of *drug and food poisoning,* full doses of the saline cathartics are sometimes administered to flush the offending substance from the intestinal tract. Magnesium sulfate is often used for this purpose, but sodium sulfate is safer if the toxic substance causes central nervous system depression, and especially if renal function is impaired.

Cathartics are also employed routinely with certain *anthelmintics.* Preliminary cathartic medication facilitates exposure of the parasites to the anthelmintic, and administration of the cathartic after the anthelmintic serves the dual purpose of eliminating the parasites and the toxic vermifuge.

The Cathartic Habit. From earliest times, man has been conscious of his bowel, and purging was long believed a panacea for many ills. Even today, many individuals have unusual notions regarding the frequency, quantity, and consistency of stools necessary for health, and they readily resort to self-prescribed cathartic medication to achieve these goals. The belief that it is of serious consequence to miss a bowel movement is further reinforced by the extensive advertising of proprietary cathartics to the public.

The occasional taking of a laxative, even for an ill-advised reason, can hardly be considered harmful. However, the continued use of these drugs is to be deplored. More important, even the casual use of these drugs can develop into the cathartic habit. After a thorough evacuation of the colon by a cathartic, several days may elapse before a normal bowel movement can again occur. Nevertheless, in the interim, the patient becomes convinced that he is constipated, and he again turns to his favorite remedy. After a time, his bowel habits become so abnormal that he comes to rely entirely on a daily dose of cathartic for a bowel movement.

The patient suffering from the cathartic habit presents a difficult therapeutic problem. Initially, all cathartic medication should be discontinued, and the patient should be informed not to expect a bowel movement for several days. The underlying cause for constipation, if one exists, must be found and corrected; most important, the psychic dependence upon cathartic drugs must be broken. This can sometimes be accomplished by correcting the patient's misconceptions pertaining to bowel function. If necessary, a contact cathartic in minimally effective dosage may be employed during the period in which reestablishment of normal defecatory reflexes is being attempted. Claims that a particular laxative has unique application for this purpose have not been verified, and success is more clearly dependent upon the diligence of the physician and the compliance of the patient. Unfortunately, many individuals suffering from the cathartic habit often promptly return to the use of cathartics, despite the full remedial efforts of the doctor.

Dangers of Cathartic Abuse. In addition to perpetuating dependence upon drugs, the cathartic habit may provide the basis for serious *gastrointestinal disturbances.* Spastic colitis and other functional ills have been traced to the habitual use of the contact cathartics; after prolonged abuse, the appearance of the digestive tract by x-ray examination may resemble that of enterocolitis (Heilbrun and Bernstein, 1955).

Repeated misuse of the stimulant cathartics may also result in excessive *fecal loss of water and electrolyte.* Hypokalemia, sodium depletion, and dehydration have been reported most frequently. Secondary aldosteronism, with loss of potassium in the urine as well as in the feces, may occur if volume depletion is prominent (Fleischer *et al.,* 1969). Steatorrhea and protein-losing gastroenteropathy with hypoalbuminemia have been observed (Heizer *et al.,* 1968), as has excessive excretion of calcium in the stools and osteomalacia of the vertebral column.

Much more dangerous than the cathartic habit is the practice of taking a cathartic for the relief of abdominal pain. An inflamed appendix can be ruptured by the resulting intestinal motor activity, and patients who take purgatives subsequent to the onset of symptoms of acute appendicitis have a mortality rate manyfold higher than the rate for those who do not receive cathartics. *All cathartics are contraindicated in a patient with cramps, colic, nausea, vomiting, or other symptoms of appendicitis or any undiagnosed abdominal pain.*

Ammon, H. V., and Phillips, S. F. Inhibition of colonic water and electrolyte absorption by fatty acids in man. *Gastroenterology,* **1973,** *65,* 744–749.

Ammon, H. V.; Thomas, P. J.; and Phillips, S. F. Effects of oleic and ricinoleic acids on net jejunal water and electrolyte movement: perfusion studies in man. *J. clin. Invest.,* **1974,** *53,* 374–379.

Becker, G. L. The case against mineral oil. *Am. J. dig. Dis.,* **1952,** *19,* 344–348.

Christensen, J. The controls of gastrointestinal movements: some old and new views. *New Engl. J. Med.,* **1971,** *285,* 85–98.

Dujovne, C. A., and Shoeman, L. W. Toxicity of a hepatic laxative preparation in tissue culture and excretion in bile in man. *Clin. Pharmac. Ther.,* **1972,** *13,* 602–608.

Fairbairn, J. W., and Moss, M. J. R. The relative purgative activities of 1,8-dihydroxyanthracene derivatives. *J. Pharm. Pharmac.,* **1970,** *22,* 584–593.

Fleischer, N.; Brown, H.; Graham, D. Y.; and Deleña, S. Chronic laxative-induced hyperaldosteronism and hypokalemia simulating Bartter's syndrome. *Ann. intern. Med.,* **1969,** *70,* 791–798.

Forman, D. T.; Garvin, J. E.; Forestner, J. E.; and Taylor, C. B. Increased excretion of fecal bile acids by an oral hydrophilic colloid. *Proc. Soc. exp. Biol. Med.,* **1968,** *127,* 1060–1063.

Forth, W.; Rummel, W.; and Baldauf, J. Wasser- und Elektrolytbewegung am Dunn- und Dickdarm unter dem Einfluss von Laxantien, ein Beitrag zur Klärung ihres Wirkungsmechanismus. *Naunyn-Schmiedebergs Arch. Pharmak. exp. Path.,* **1966,** *254,* 18–32.

Göing, H., and Schaumann, W. Zum Nachweis reflektorisch von der Darmschleimhaut aus wirksamer Abführmittel. *Arzneimittel-Forsch.,* **1955,** *5,* 282–285.

Goldstein, F. Diet and colonic disease. *J. Am. diet. Ass.,* **1972,** *60,* 499–503.

Gray, H., and Tainter, M. L. Colloid laxatives available for clinical use. *Am. J. dig. Dis.,* **1941,** *8,* 130–139.

Hardcastle, J. D., and Mann, C. V. Study of large bowel peristalsis. *Gut,* **1968,** *9,* 512–520.

Hardcastle, J. D., and Wilkins, J. L. The action of sennosides and related compounds on human colon and rectum. *Gut,* **1970,** *11,* 1038–1042.

Harvey, R. F., and Read, A. E. Effects of oral magnesium sulphate on colonic motility in patients with the irritable bowel syndrome. *Gut,* **1973,** *14,* 983–987.

Heilbrun, N., and Bernstein, C. Roentgen abnormalities of the large and small intestine associated with prolonged cathartic ingestion. *Radiology,* **1955,** *65,* 549–556.

Heizer, W. D.; Warshaw, A. L.; Waldman, T. A.; and Laster, L. Protein-losing gastroenteropathy and malabsorption associated with factitious diarrhea. *Ann. intern. Med.,* **1968,** *68,* 839–852.

Hodgson, J. Effect of methylcellulose on rectal and colonic pressures in treatment of diverticular disease. *Br. med. J.,* **1972,** *3,* 729–731.

Hubacher, M. H., and Doernberg, S. Laxatives. II. Relationship between structure and potency. *J. pharm. Sci.,* **1964,** *53,* 1067–1072.

Lish, P. M. Some pharmacologic effects of dioctyl sodium sulfosuccinate on the gastrointestinal tract of the rat. *Gastroenterology,* **1961,** *41,* 580–584.

Loewe, S. Studies on the laxative activity of triphenyl-methane derivatives. I. Relationship between structure and activity of phenolphthalein congeners. *J. Pharmac. exp. Ther.,* **1948,** *94,* 288–298.

Lundholm, L., and Svedmyr, N. The influence of dioctyl sodium sulfosuccinate on the laxative action of some anthraquinone derivatives. *Acta pharmac. tox.,* **1959,** *15,* 373–383.

McClure Browne, J. C.; Edmunds, V.; Fairbairn, J. W.; and Reid, D. D. Clinical and laboratory assessments of senna preparations. *Br. med. J.,* **1957,** *1,* 436–439.

Munch, J. C., and Calesnick, B. Laxative studies. I. Human threshold doses of white and yellow phenol-phthalein. *Clin. Pharmac. Ther.,* **1960,** *1,* 311–315.

Nell, G.; Overhoff, H.; Forth, W.; Kulenkampff, H.; Specht, W.; and Rummel, W. Influx and efflux of sodium in jejunal and colonic segments of rats under the influence of oxyphenisatin. *Naunyn-Schmiedebergs Archs Pharmac.,* **1973,** *277,* 53–60.

Painter, N. S.; Almeida, A. Z.; and Colebourne, K. W. Unprocessed bran in treatment of diverticular disease of the colon. *Br. med. J.,* **1972,** *1,* 137–140.

Painter, N. S., and Burkitt, D. P. Diverticular disease of the colon: a deficiency disease of Western civilization. *Br. med. J.,* **1971,** *2,* 450–454.

Phillips, S. F. Diarrhea: a current view of the pathophysiology. *Gastroenterology,* **1972,** *63,* 495–518.

Reynolds, T. B.; Peters, R. L.; and Yamada, S. Chronic active and lupoid hepatitis caused by a laxative, oxyphenisatin. *New Engl. J. Med.,* **1971,** *285,* 813–820.

Ritchie, J. Mass peristalsis in the human colon after contact with oxyphenisatin. *Gut,* **1972,** *13,* 211–219.

Schmidt, L. Vergleichende Pharmakologie und Toxikologie der Laxantien. *Naunyn-Schmiedebergs Arch. exp. Path. Pharmak.,* **1955,** *226,* 207–218.

Watson, W. C.; Gordon, R. S., Jr.; Karmen, A.; and Jover, A. The absorption and excretion of castor oil in man. *J. Pharm. Pharmac.,* **1963,** *15,* 183–188.

Wittoesch, J. H.; Jackman, R. J.; and McDonald, J. R. Melanosis coli: general review and a study of 887 cases. *Dis. Colon Rectum,* **1958,** *1,* 172–180.

Monographs and Reviews

Cornell Conferences on Therapy. Management of constipation. *N.Y. St. J. Med.,* **1941,** *41,* 1959–1968.

———. The rational use of cathartic agents. *Ibid.,* **1947,** *47,* 387–393, 504–508.

Symposium. (Various authors.) The colon: its normal and abnormal physiology and therapeutics. *Ann. N.Y. Acad. Sci.,* **1954,** *58,* 293–540.

CHAPTER

50 ANTISEPTICS AND DISINFECTANTS; FUNGICIDES; ECTOPARASITICIDES

Stewart C. Harvey

I. Antiseptics and Disinfectants

Antiseptics and disinfectants are employed very widely and are thus deserving of sober consideration.

Once the germ theory of disease was accepted by the medical profession and antisepsis by chemical agents was demonstrated scientifically, topical antimicrobial drugs were employed with naive enthusiasm by both physicians and laymen. Astute physicians early learned the limitations of antiseptics, but the vast majority of physicians and laymen alike employed such drugs uncritically and often inappropriately, encouraged by promotional propaganda almost from the very beginning. Although several effective and useful antiseptics, such as iodine, were known quite early, in the first half of this century there was a rush to accept a host of lesser and even useless drugs. The euphoria surrounding the discovery of the sulfonamides and antibiotics obscured the need for a thoroughgoing appraisal of the value of antiseptics, collectively and individually. Only a few of the antiseptics have been subjected to controlled clinical comparison with other agents, and clinical standards have yet to be accepted. Both laymen and many physicians still continue to employ the topical antimicrobial drugs in a ritual manner that is often irrational, usually ineffective, and occasionally harmful.

Nevertheless, there are indispensable uses of disinfectants in the household, in hospital sanitation, and in public health measures. Likewise, antiseptics find many legitimate therapeutic applications. Even though systemic antimicrobial drugs have quite properly caused a decline in the use of topical anti-infective agents, antiseptics are sometimes still of value in treating local infections caused by microorganisms refractory to systemic chemotherapy and in the supple-

mentation of such therapy. It is the problem of the physician to choose wisely from the vast number of available drugs and to delineate the beneficial and the harmful uses of germicides.

In this chapter, a drug may receive special attention because of its undoubted efficacy, its toxicity, or the need to deflate an undeserved status.

History. Centuries before the basic researches of Pasteur, Koch, and others established the pathogenicity of bacteria, chemicals were used to control the suppuration of wounds and the spread of contagious diseases. By the time the true significance of microorganisms was appreciated, many drugs were already available as germicides. The earliest written records of man contain references to the use of germicidal agents. Ancient Egyptian embalmers found excellent preservatives among the spices, vegetable oils, and gums, as attested by the fine state of preservation of Egyptian mummies. Ancient Persian laws instructed the populace to store drinking water in bright copper vessels. The practice of salting, smoking, and spicing foods is older than recorded history. The use of wine and vinegar in the dressing of wounds dates back at least to Hippocrates.

During the nineteenth century, the agents used empirically for their germicidal action included several compounds still employed. For example, iodine was used in treating wounds several decades before the bacterial etiology of suppuration was suspected. Because it was then believed that there was an association between putrefaction and the spread of disease, chlorine occupied a prominent place due to the fact that it was a deodorant. Semmelweiss decreased the incidence of puerperal fever in the obstetrical ward of the Allgemeines Krankenhaus of Vienna from 11.4 to 1.3% by ordering the medical students (who were prone to come directly from the autopsy room to the obstetrical ward) to wash their hands in chlorinated lime before examining patients. Following the introduction of the technic of aseptic surgery by Lister, the importance of disinfection of the skin of the patient, the hands of the surgeon, the instruments, and the hospital environment was readily appreciated. Many of the early drugs employed for these purposes are still valuable today. During the early part of this century, the use of germicides in purification of water supplies and in the sanitization of utensils and containers in multiple

987

use by the public became widespread. An interesting review of the ancient and modern uses of germicidal substances is given by Block (1968).

Terminology. The terminology used to describe the actions of drugs on microorganisms is unfortunately somewhat confusing due to the discrepancy between the strict definitions of the terms employed and their usage in loose medical parlance. The origins of these terms, together with their current precise and imprecise connotations, are fully described by Davis (1968) and Lawrence (1968a).

Antiseptics are substances that kill or prevent the growth of microorganisms. This term is used especially for preparations *applied to living tissue*. The definition derives from the original meaning of the term *antiseptic* as a substance that opposes sepsis, putrefaction, or decay. A *disinfectant* is an agent that prevents infection by the destruction of pathogenic microorganisms. It is commonly used in reference to substances *applied to inanimate objects*. A *sanitizer* represents a particular kind of disinfectant; it is an agent that reduces the number of bacterial contaminants to levels judged safe by public health requirements. *Sterilization,* in contrast to *sanitization,* refers to the complete destruction of all forms of life, especially microorganisms, by some chemical or physical process. Under appropriate conditions, a disinfectant may produce complete sterilization. A *germicide,* in the broad and most useful sense, is an agent that destroys microorganisms. Germicides may be further defined by the appropriate use of self-evident terms such as *bactericide, fungicide, virucide,* and *amebicide.*

Properties Desirable in Germicides. The properties of germicides that determine the usefulness and applicability of these agents may appropriately be divided into those desirable for purposes of *disinfection* and those useful in *antiseptics.*

Properties Desirable in Disinfectants. Agents used for disinfection should obviously have high germicidal efficacy. A wide antimicrobial spectrum is also desired, and the most valuable agents are those that are lethal to bacteria, including bacterial spores, as well as fungi, viruses, and protozoa. Rapidly lethal action is a useful property. The ability of the disinfectant to penetrate into crevices and cavities and beneath films of organic matter is desirable. It is also essential that lethal concentrations of the agent can be obtained in the presence of organic matter such as blood, sputum, and fecal material. The agent should be compatible with soaps and with other chemical substances likely to be encountered in the material to be disinfected.

The disinfectant must possess certain physical and chemical properties. A high degree of chemical stability is desired. A universal disinfectant should be noncorrosive to surgical instruments and nondestructive to other materials. Esthetic factors, such as odor, color, or staining quality, are sometimes determinants in the choice of a disinfectant. Cost is often an important consideration.

Properties Desirable in Antiseptics. A high degree of germicidal potency is an important factor in an antiseptic, and a drug that is lethal to microor-

ganisms is obviously superior to one that merely inhibits growth. The clinical usefulness of an antiseptic is related to the breadth of the antimicrobial spectrum; however, agents with narrow spectra find usefulness against infections caused by sensitive microorganisms. Low surface tension is desired in antiseptic solutions for topical application. It is of importance that the drugs retain their activity in the presence of the body fluids, including the exudate present in infection. Rapid germicidal action is desired, but sustained action is likewise of value.

A prime consideration determining the usefulness of an antiseptic is the *therapeutic index.* The therapeutic index is the relationship between the concentration that is effective against microorganisms and one that produces harmful effects, such as local tissue irritation and interference with the mechanisms of healing and tissue repair. Also to be considered are the incidence of hypersensitivity reactions and the degree to which absorption of the drug leads to systemic toxicity. Unfortunately, the chemical properties that give most antiseptics their broad spectrum of activity may make them not only toxic to human tissues but often allergenic as well.

Evaluation of Antimicrobial Activity. The testing of germicides is a complex and controversial field. Many types of tests are presently employed; however, there are many inadequacies in the existing methods, and the procedures are not fully standardized. Detailed aspects of this subject are discussed in the monograph edited by Lawrence and Block (1968).

Soon after the development of technics for growing microorganisms, simple *in-vitro* tests for evaluating *germicidal activity* were proposed. In 1903, Rideal and Walker developed the *phenol coefficient* test, in which the potencies of various germicides are compared to that of phenol against selected bacteria. Although this test introduced some order into the field, certain inadequacies of the technic readily became apparent. Modifications of the phenol coefficient test were therefore made in order to estimate potency of germicides in the presence of organic matter and to distinguish between bacteriostasis and true cell death. Numerous *in-vitro* tests are employed at the present time to evaluate activity of the different chemical classes of germicides against various microorganisms. However, the information obtained from such tests is applicable primarily to the use of the agents in the *disinfection* of inanimate objects.

Methods of testing *antiseptics* are even more varied and less standardized than those employed in testing disinfectants. Two types of information are sought by such tests: evaluation of antimicrobial efficiency under conditions of use and indications of tissue toxicity. A commonly employed test, representative of those designed to estimate antimicrobial efficiency, is that designed by Price for estimating *degermation* of the skin. (*See* Price, 1968, for details and for comparative data on various antiseptics.) Antiseptics are also tested against bacteria on the abraded or incised skin of animals in "infection-prevention" tests. Many other methods have been devised for assessing antiseptics under conditions designed to simulate those of actual use (*see* Miller,

1971). The details of these methods and of the procedures for evaluating tissue toxicity are given by Leary and Stuart (1968) and Ortenzio and Stuart (1968).

Testing of *virucidal agents* requires technics different from those employed in assessing bactericides. Inactivation of bacteriophages and reduction in infectivity of specific virus inocula for chick embryos and for experimental animals are among the procedures employed. The viruses used include the causative agents for poliomyelitis, influenza, and many other communicable diseases. The details concerned with testing antiviral agents are given by Koski and Stuart (1968).

Estimates of *antifungal activity* again require methods different from those used for testing agents against bacteria or viruses. The methods of evaluation of antifungal agents are considered subsequently.

In spite of the many tests for evaluating activity and toxicity of antiseptics, laboratory methods fail to give enough information to determine efficacy of a drug in actual use. It is difficult to ascertain from such tests whether one agent is superior to another. A number of well-controlled clinical trials of surgical and urinary tract antiseptics have been made, but there have been few valid comparisons of antiseptics in the treatment of cutaneous infections. Many commonly used antiseptics are exceedingly weak germicides. Their continued use has the character of folk medicine. It is incumbent upon the physician not only to improve his knowledge about antiseptic use but also to instruct the lay public.

Status of Antiseptics in Relation to Systemic Chemotherapeutic Agents. Most germicides have been employed at one time or another in the local treatment of *wounds* and *infections*. Because of tissue toxicity, inadequate penetration into foci of infection, and reduced activity in the presence of body fluids, dramatic benefit from this use of germicides is the exception rather than the rule. The importance of antiseptics in treating infections is now secondary to that of antibiotics and other systemic chemotherapeutic agents. In experienced hands, selected germicides may be useful in cleansing wounds and in reducing bacterial contamination. However, the common belief that substantial benefit is obtained from the application of antiseptics to wounds, cuts, and abrasions is not supported by the considerable evidence in this field. The various applications of surgical antiseptics have been considered in detail by Price (1968).

In *dermatological infections,* systemic treatment will usually provide more dramatic results than topical therapy. Nevertheless, there are also barriers to the outward movement of systemic drugs, especially into the stratum corneum, so that both systemic and topical treatment may be of value. Also, where resistance or intolerance to systemic antimicrobial drugs exists, topical antiseptics may be indicated. However, topical therapy is not the only recourse; debridement and various cleansing, dressing, and surgical procedures are vital to good management. Germicidal drugs are sometimes useful in prophylaxis against specific infections.

Importance of Germicidal Kinetics. The rate of germicidal action approximates first-order kinetics and is dependent upon the concentration, temperature, pH, and vehicle in which the drug is applied. On the skin of the hands and arms, the time necessary for a 50% reduction in bacterial count is about 0.6 minute for 70% ethanol and 7 minutes for 1:1000 benzalkonium chloride. To effect a 90% reduction in bacterial count, the ethanol would take about 2 minutes whereas the benzalkonium would take about 25 minutes. Obviously, where time is a critical factor, the kinetics are of the utmost importance. The medical and promotional literature frequently grossly neglects this important aspect of the pharmacology of antiseptics.

The kinetics are often much more complex than implied above, because of the superimposed kinetics of diffusion, penetration, binding, redistribution, and other factors. The rate of action is often not directly proportional to the concentration, and for many antiseptics there is an optimal concentration. Furthermore, even though kinetic theory alone predicts 100% kill, many antiseptics fall far short of complete antisepsis; neither of the two agents used in the example above can degerm the skin by much more than 90%. The importance of antibacterial kinetics has been emphasized by Price (1950).

Mechanisms of Antimicrobial Action. The mechanisms by which drugs kill or inhibit the growth of microorganisms are so varied and complex that little can be gained by a general discussion. The monograph edited by Lawrence and Block (1968) and the reviews by Russell (1969) and Drouhet (1970) present general mechanisms of antimicrobial action as well as information on specific germicides. The mechanisms of action of the individual agents will be discussed in the sections that follow.

Antimicrobial Spectra of Germicides. Many germicides exhibit a broad antimicrobial spectrum. Iodine exemplifies a germicide of this type. Some germicides show marked selectivity. For example, hexachlorophene is toxic primarily to gram-positive bacteria. In general, antiseptics are broad-spectrum agents, so that attention will be called only to those drugs that depart significantly from this generalization. For detailed information and references on the antimicrobial spectra of germicides, the reader is referred to the monographs edited by Davis (1950), Reddish (1957), and Lawrence and Block (1968).

It may be stated as a general rule that *bacterial spores* are less readily killed by germicides than are vegetative forms of bacteria. In order to destroy spores it is necessary greatly to increase the time of contact, the concentration of the germicide, or both, above that necessary to kill nonsporulating bacteria. The susceptibility of bacterial spores will be mentioned only in those instances in which the agent is unusually sporicidal or in which it is virtually ineffective against spore forms. The monographs cited above contain detailed data on the effects of germicides on bacterial spores.

Viruses and vegetative forms of *fungi* seem to exhibit approximately the same degrees of sensitivity to chemical agents as do vegetative forms of bacteria (*see* Spaulding, 1968). Improvements in methods of testing for antiviral activity have contributed to the development of a number of agents effective locally or systemically against viral infections. Many germicides have sufficient antifungal activity to warrant their use in the treatment of mycotic diseases. Antifungal agents effective locally are considered subsequently.

Classification. In a discussion of such heterogeneous compounds as the antiseptics and disinfectants, some method of classification is desirable. So varied are the compounds with respect to chemical structure, mechanism of action, and therapeutic use, however, that too strict a classification may be more confusing than elucidating. Thus, by elimination, a chemical classification is the least objectionable and is the one used in the following pages.

PHENOLS, CRESOLS, AND RESORCINOLS

PHENOL

Phenol itself deserves exposition here only because of its historical importance. Certain derivatives are currently of considerably greater importance. The germicidal efficacy of phenol (carbolic acid) was dramatically demonstrated by Lister in 1867, although the compound had been occasionally employed in medicine prior to that time.

Pharmacological Actions. Both the local and the systemic actions of phenol require consideration.

Local Actions. Phenol is bacteriostatic in a concentration of approximately 0.2%, bactericidal above 1%, and fungicidal above 1.3%. The efficacy is greatly reduced at low temperatures and in alkaline media. The drug is much more effective in aqueous solution than in glycerin or lipids. It is relatively inactive when incorporated in soaps.

Phenol presumably exerts its germicidal action by denaturing protein. The protein-phenol complex is a loose one. Therefore, phenol is diffusible and penetrates into tissues. The compound has a markedly toxic action, and because of its penetrability affects even the unabraded skin. When the drug is applied directly to the skin, a white pellicle of precipitated protein is formed. This soon turns red and eventually sloughs, leaving the cutaneous surface stained a light brown. If phenol remains in contact with the skin, it penetrates deeply and may cause extensive necrosis.

When applied locally, phenol exerts a depolarizing local anesthetic action. A 5% solution, even on the unabraded epithelial surface, produces a feeling of warmth and tingling and, eventually, rather complete local anesthesia. Phenol in this concentration is very irritating to exposed tissue and may cause necrosis.

Systemic Actions. Phenol stimulates and then depresses the *central nervous system* (*CNS*). In man, brief stimulation is observed, and the prominent effects are those of CNS depression. The *circulation* is also markedly depressed by phenol. The blood pressure falls, partly as a result of central vasomotor depression but mainly due to a direct toxic action of phenol on the myocardium and the smaller blood vessels. Phenol is a powerful *antipyretic*. The mechanism by which phenol produces a fall in body temperature is not unlike that of the salicylates.

Absorption, Fate, and Excretion. Phenol is absorbed by all routes of administration and can reach the circulation even when applied to the intact skin. A portion of the absorbed drug is oxidized to hydroquinone and pyrocatechol. Another portion is oxidized more completely. Approximately 80% is excreted by the kidney, either unchanged or conjugated with glucuronic and sulfuric acids.

Preparations. *Phenol,* U.S.P. (*carbolic acid*), consists of colorless crystals with a somewhat aromatic odor. It is soluble in water 1:15. *Liquefied Phenol,* U.S.P. (*liquefied carbolic acid*), is phenol maintained in a liquid state by the presence of 10% distilled water. A number of preparations of phenol in water, olive oil, and glycerin, as well as mixtures of phenol and iodine, and phenol and camphor, formerly had official status. *Phenolated Calamine Lotion,* U.S.P. (*compound calamine lotion*), contains 1% phenol.

Phenol Poisoning. When taken orally, phenol produces extensive local corrosion, which causes severe pain and vomiting. Shock and death may rapidly ensue. After absorption, phenol may produce fleeting excitement, but usually the patient rapidly lapses into unconsciousness. The blood pressure is low, cold sweat is prominent, and the body temperature falls markedly. Urine is scanty and contains albumin, casts, and free hemoglobin. Death results from respiratory failure.

Treatment. To remove the agent from the stomach before extensive absorption has occurred, a stomach tube should be passed immediately, and a lavage fluid should be employed that dissolves phenol and yet does not hasten absorption. Olive oil is well suited for this purpose. Alcoholic solutions or mineral oil should be avoided. Alcohol facilitates gastric absorption of phenol; mineral oil is relatively ineffective in dissolving phenol. After copious lavage, fresh oil should be left in the stomach to retard subsequent absorption of phenol and to act as a diluent and demulcent. Treatment of systemic symptoms is purely symptomatic. The fatal dose of phenol for adults has been estimated to be 8 to 15 g. In fatal cases, death usually results within 24 hours or less, but the prognosis should be guarded even after this period of time has elapsed.

If phenol has been applied locally to skin or mucosa, it can be removed effectively with 50% alcohol, glycerin, vegetable oils, sodium bicarbonate solution, or even water.

Therapeutic Uses. Phenol has few legitimate uses as an antiseptic. Most dermatological and anorectal preparations incorporate the phenol in a wax or petrolatum base, which prevents access to the bacteria; others have too low a concentration. In mouth-washes the concentrations used are inadequate for the brief contact time. Crude carbolic acid is sufficiently inexpensive to use for disinfection of excrement. Phenol has been employed as a fungicide but is effective only in concentrations that may cause burns. In full strength, a few drops of liquefied phenol may be employed to cauterize dogbites, snakebites, and other small wounds. It is sometimes used as an antipruritic, either in the form of phenolated calamine lotion or as an ointment or simple aqueous solution. Aqueous solutions stronger than 2%, however, should not be applied to the surface of the body. Solutions containing 4% phenol in glycerin may be employed if necessary. Phenol is no longer used for sclerosing hemorrhoids.

SUBSTITUTED PHENOLS

A number of phenol derivatives are more bactericidal than phenol itself. The most important of these are the *halogenated phenols* and *bis-phenols*, the *alkyl-substituted phenols*, and the *resorcinols*.

Relation of Chemical Structure to Pharmacological Action. Lipid solubility is a prerequisite of most antiseptics, especially those that interact with or pass through the bacterial membrane into the cell. Therefore, chemical modifications of phenol that increase lipid solubility, such as halogenation or alkylation, tend to increase activity, provided that aqueous solubility does not diminish below the level for effective transport. Additional polar groups, as in resorcinol, decrease potency but can be compensated for by alkyl or other nonpolar groups, as in hexylresorcinol. Phenols are less effective in alkaline solution because the phenolate ion is less lipid soluble. The structure-activity relationship of phenol derivatives has been reviewed by Gump and Walter (1968) and Prindle and Wright (1968).

Cresols. Cresol is usually marketed as a mixture of the three isomers of methylphenol. Cresol is no more toxic than phenol and is about three times as active. In spite of this, cresol is incorporated into fewer medicaments than is phenol. Cresol is a fairly efficient bactericide against the common pathogenic organisms, including acid-fast bacilli. The pharmacological properties of cresol are almost identical with those of phenol and do not warrant separate discussion. This is also true for the toxicity and treatment of cresol poisoning. It should be remembered that cresol is just as toxic as phenol; consequently, cresol preparations should not be used with a false sense of security. Many cases of poisoning from cresol have been reported.

Cresol is soluble in water only to the extent of 1:60. Therefore, it is commonly used in the form of *saponated cresol solution (compound cresol solution;*

LYSOL), which is 50% cresol in saponified linseed or other suitable oil. In this form it is miscible with water. Compound cresol solution is used widely for disinfecting inanimate objects. It is superior to and cheaper than phenol. It is probably the preparation of choice for the disinfection of excrement. Also, it may be employed as a handwash in a concentration of 2%. A 1:500 solution of saponated cresol solution is sometimes used as a mildly antiseptic vaginal douche of dubious efficacy. Proprietary preparations are widely advertised for this and other purposes. *Metacresyl acetate,* a derivative, is used in root canal therapy.

Creosote. Creosote is a mixture of phenols obtained from wood tar. It consists mainly of creosol and guaiacol. The bactericidal potency of creosote varies, but in general it is about two to three times that of phenol. *Creosote* is obsolete as an antiseptic and is now used mainly as a household remedy (expectorant), especially in the treatment of croup.

Resorcinol. Resorcinol, *m*-dihydroxybenzene, is both bactericidal and fungicidal but is only about one third as active as phenol. Locally, resorcinol is a protein precipitant. The compound resembles phenol in its systemic actions. Central stimulation is more prominent than with phenol. *Resorcinol,* U.S.P., is a colorless crystalline substance, freely soluble in water and in alcohol and other organic solvents. It is employed in the treatment of *acne, ringworm, eczema, psoriasis, seborrheic dermatitis,* and other cutaneous lesions. Its mild irritant and keratolytic properties may be important to whatever erratic efficacy resorcinol has in these disorders. It is usually applied as an ointment or lotion in strengths varying from 2 to 20%. *Resorcinol lotion* contains 2 to 20% and *Compound Resorcinol Ointment,* N.F., 6% resorcinol. *Resorcinol Monoacetate,* N.F., gradually liberates resorcinol and, therefore, exerts a milder but more lasting action. It is used for the same purposes as resorcinol.

Hexylresorcinol. *Hexylresorcinol,* N.F., is a useful antiseptic that is relatively odorless and does not stain. It is commonly employed in a 1:1000 solution or glycerite in mouthwashes or pharyngeal antiseptic preparations. It is quite irritating to tissue, and an occasional individual exhibits marked sensitivity to its local application.

Hexachlorophene. *Hexachlorophene,* U.S.P., is the most important of the medicinal phenols. It is a polychlorinated *bis*-phenol with the following structure:

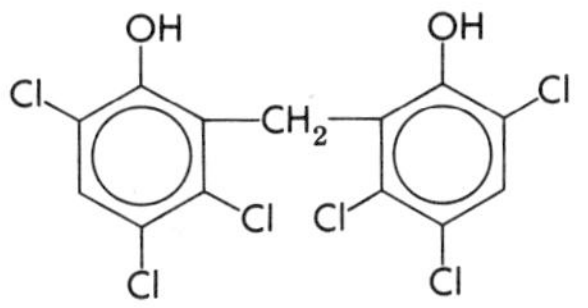

Hexachlorophene

Briefly, hexachlorophene is more effective against gram-positive than gram-negative bacteria. The drug exhibits high bacteriostatic activity, but considerable time is required to kill microorganisms and there is little effect on spores. Growth of many pathogenic fungi is inhibited by the drug. Development of resistance of microorganisms to hexachlorophene has not been reported. The presence of organic matter such as pus or serum reduces the efficiency of hexachlorophene, but activity is retained in the presence of soaps, oils, and vehicles for topical application.

Hexachlorophene accumulates with repeated application to the skin, reaching a maximal concentration in 2 to 4 days. At this time the cutaneous bacterial population may be reduced by 95 to 99% (Price, 1950; Kundsin and Walter, 1973). Removal of the hexachlorophene film and regrowth of the normal flora begin promptly when a soap not containing hexachlorophene is substituted. It should be emphasized that maximal reduction in the flora of the skin is attained only after several days of frequent use of hexachlorophene soap. The reduction in bacterial flora observed immediately after a single scrub with hexachlorophene soap is no greater than that which occurs with nonmedicated soap.

Since most of the potentially pathogenic bacterial residents of the skin are gram positive, hexachlorophene is commonly used by surgeons, physicians, dentists, food handlers, pediatric nurses, and others who routinely are in a position to spread contaminants from their own hands. The drug is also used to degerm the skin of patients scheduled for certain surgical procedures. Because iodophors (see below) are supposedly bactericidal and also initially decrease the skin bacterial population more than does hexachlorophene (King and Zimmerman, 1965; Crowder et al., 1967), the above-named uses of hexachlorophene have been criticized (see Price, 1968). However, although iodophors are initially more effective, before the end of 60 minutes they begin to lose control of the skin flora on the gloved hand, whereas the control by hexachlorophene is at least equal at this time and continues to develop (Kundsin and Walter, 1973). White and Duncan (1972) have shown that the surgical infection rate is the same with either antiseptic in the surgical scrub.

Routine use of hexachlorophene preparations is effective in reducing the incidence and severity of pyogenic skin infections. Bathing of infants with detergents containing hexachlorophene has been shown to reduce markedly the incidence of staphylococcal infections. However, the risk of brain damage to the infant has made this practice controversial (see below).

Hexachlorophene has been used in the treatment of *acne*, but since the associated microorganism is often gram negative and anaerobic, the disorder responds better to certain penetrant oxidizing antiseptics. Hexachlorophene was used effectively for more than 20 years in "over-the-counter" antiseptic and deodorant soaps before they were disapproved by the United States Food and Drug Administration. As a disinfectant, hexachlorophene is inferior to many chemicals and is not used.

Hexachlorophene and the other *bis*-phenols are less irritating to tissue than is phenol. Hexachlorophene is toxic by the oral route. Acute toxic effects include anorexia, nausea, vomiting, abdominal cramps, asthenia, miosis, absence of light reflex, cerebrospinal tract signs, and death. Systemic toxicity can also occur from topical use when the drug is applied daily to the skin of underweight, premature infants or infants with excoriated skin, or several times a day to the skin or vagina of adults. Confusion, diplopia, lethargy, twitching, convulsions, respiratory arrest, and death have occurred. Diffuse status spongiosus of the brain has been demonstrated. In experimental animals this condition appears to be slowly reversible. Details of the toxicity of hexachlorophene may be found in publications by Kimbrough (1971, 1973), Lockhart (1972, 1973), Powell and coworkers (1973), and Plueckhahn (1973), and in Conference (1973); the implications of the continuation or discontinuation of the pediatric use are discussed in the latter two reports.

Hexachlorophene Liquid Soap, U.S.P., contains 0.25% of the antiseptic. A tincture-foam containing 0.23% is reported to be more effective than 3% soap (Gravens *et al.*, 1973).

Parabens. *Methylparaben*, U.S.P., *Ethylparaben*, U.S.P., *Propylparaben*, U.S.P., and *Butylparaben*, U.S.P., aliphatic esters of parahydroxybenzoic acid, are used as preservatives in a great variety of pharmaceutical preparations. Their actions are both those of phenols and an antimetabolite effect of parahydroxybenzoic acid. They have antifungal properties. All are effective in low concentrations (usually 0.1 to 0.3%) that are devoid of systemic toxic effects. However, as constituents of antibacterial ointments, dermatological preparations, and proprietary lotions and skin creams, they are recognized causes of severe and intractable contact dermatitis.

Parabens have been identified as the cause of chronic dermatitis in numerous instances (Epstein, 1968; Schorr, 1968). Patients sensitive to one paraben show cross-sensitivity to the others. The first step in treatment is to eliminate contact with parabens, a difficult task since they are so widely used in proprietary preparations, and their presence is often not indicated on the label.

Miscellaneous Phenols. *Thymol* is both antibacterial and antifungal. It is promoted for the treatment of acne, hemorrhoids, and tinea pedis. It is also present in some mouthwashes; in the concentrations used, it is not effective within any practical contact time. *Chlorothymol* is incorporated in some dental preparations for application to the gingiva and buccal mucosae and in anorectal preparations. *Parachlorometaxylenol* in concentrations of 0.25 to 0.5% is incorporated into preparations for the treatment of superficial burns, acne vulgaris, eczema, seborrheic dermatitis, and diaper rash. *Orthophenylphenol* is contained in several dermatological preparations. Each of the above-named drugs is more potent than phenol; the true efficacy of none is known, because clinical testing has been desultory.

Parachlorophenol, U.S.P., is similar to phenol in its properties and uses. It is a more potent antiseptic than phenol, but the toxicity and caustic actions are also greater. *Camphorated parachlorophenol*, a mixture of approximately 1 part parachlorophenol to 2 parts camphor, is used in root canal therapy; however, it is inferior to sodium hypochlorite and locally instilled antibiotics for this purpose.

TARS

The medicinal tars are obtained from the destructive distillation of various woods and coal and consist mainly of cresols and guaiacols. When suitably diluted, tars act as mild irritants and antiseptics. Preparations include *Coal Tar,* U.S.P., *Pine Tar,* N.F., and *Juniper Tar,* N.F. (*cade oil*). The tars are usually prescribed in ointment form; the only official ointment is *Coal Tar Ointment,* U.S.P. (1% coal tar in paste of zinc oxide). Coal tar is also used as a 1:9 dilution of *Coal Tar Solution,* U.S.P., which contains 20% of the tar. The tars are employed in the treatment of diseases of the skin, such as *psoriasis* and *eczema-dermatitis.*

ALCOHOLS

The aliphatic alcohols are germicidal in varying degree, roughly in logarithmic proportion to their lipid solubility. Thus, potency increases with chain length until solubility limits availability, but branching and additional hydroxyl groups diminish potency.

ETHANOL

Ethanol is an antimicrobial drug of low potency but moderate efficacy in appropriate concentrations. It is bactericidal to all of the common pathogenic bacteria, but some rare species survive and can grow in otherwise-optimal concentrations of the chemical. It is erratic as a fungicide and virucide; it is virtually inactive against dried spores. The optimal concentration depends upon the requirements of use. If a casual wipe of ethanol-wetted cotton is the mode of application, 70% is optimal against *Staphylococcus epidermidis;* however, for disinfection by prolonged contact, 50% is superior. The user deludes himself if he expects more than a 75% reduction in cutaneous bacterial count when 70% ethanol is applied and left to evaporate, except under very humid conditions. Ethanol should not be used for sterilization because it is not sporocidal. *Rubbing Alcohol,* N.F., contains 70% ethanol by weight.

Ethanol precipitates protein. Briefly applied to the skin it does no damage, but it is irritating if left on for long periods of time. Applied to wounds or raw surfaces it not only increases the injury but also forms a coagulum under which bacteria may subsequently thrive. It is thus not used to disinfect open lesions.

ISOPROPANOL

In concentrations above 70%, isopropanol is slightly more germicidal than ethanol, and it is effective in undiluted form. It causes vasodilatation beneath the surface of application, so that needle punctures and incisions at the site bleed more than with ethanol. *Isopropyl Alcohol,* N.F., is undiluted,

but *Isopropyl Rubbing Alcohol,* N.F., contains 70% isopropanol by weight.

ALDEHYDES

Several aldehydes possess bactericidal activity. The aldehyde group condenses with amino groups to form azomethines, and other types of linkages are also formed. In low concentrations, a toxic action is exerted on cells, including microorganisms, even though there is no grossly evident effect on the solubility of proteins; in higher concentrations, proteins are precipitated.

Methenamine is discussed below with the urinary tract antiseptics (page 1006).

FORMALDEHYDE

Formaldehyde is effective against bacteria, fungi, and viruses (*see* McCulloch, 1945; Spaulding, 1968), but the action is slow. In a concentration of 0.5%, 6 to 12 hours is required to kill bacteria and 2 to 4 days to kill spores; even in 8% concentration, 18 hours is required to kill spores. Organic matter is erroneously said not to interfere with the effectiveness of formaldehyde. The aldehyde is bound to organic matter, and a large excess of formaldehyde must be applied to compensate for depletion. In sufficient concentrations, proteins are precipitated.

As a germicide, formaldehyde is mainly used in 2 to 8% concentration to disinfect inanimate objects, such as surgical instruments and gloves. To sterilize tuberculous sputum, it is employed as an 8% solution in 65 to 70% isopropanol. Because formaldehyde cannot be applied safely to the mucous membranes or most of the skin in concentrations high enough to kill microbes rapidly, antiseptic use is mostly an exercise in futility. This is especially true for the presently extant mouthwashes and vaginal douches. Some areas of the skin can tolerate fungicidal concentrations. The astringent properties of 20 to 30% formaldehyde are employed in the treatment of hyperhidrosis; the soles of the feet and palms of the hands can usually tolerate these concentrations. Formaldehyde-containing products for the treatment of ivy poisoning are no longer on the market. The protein-precipitant action is used in the fixation of histological specimens and in the alteration of bacterial toxins to toxoids for vaccines. Preservation of cadavers with formaldehyde rests more on the antimicrobial effects than on hardening of the tissues. It is also used to desensitize teeth.

Alteration of tissue proteins by formaldehyde causes local toxicity and promotes allergic reactions. Repeated contact with solutions of formaldehyde may cause an eczematoid dermatitis. The aldehyde is used to strengthen cellulose fibers in the manufacture of crease-resistant textiles, and dermatitis due to clothing made from such fabrics has occurred (Cronin, 1963). If a solution is ingested, the mucous membranes of the mouth, throat, and intestinal tract are irritated, and severe pain, vomiting, and diarrhea result. After absorption, formaldehyde depresses the CNS and symptoms not unlike those of alcohol intoxication are noted. They consist in vertigo, depression, and coma. Rarely, convulsions are observed. Formaldehyde and its oxidation product, formic acid, are the agents primarily responsible for the systemic toxicity of methanol.

Formaldehyde is official as *Formaldehyde Solution, U.S.P.*, which contains 37% of the aldehyde and 10 to 15% of methanol to retard polymerization.

Glutaraldehyde

Glutaraldehyde is superior to formaldehyde as a sterilizing agent. It is effective against all microorganisms, including viruses and spores. It lacks the disagreeable odor of formaldehyde and is less irritating to the skin and eyes, although it can cause contact dermatitis. It has been marketed as a 2% alkaline solution in 70% isopropanol, which is promoted as rapidly acting. However, a period of 10 hours is necessary to sterilize dried spores. A newly marketed acidic solution kills dried spores in 20 minutes and is also more stable. Neither the alkaline nor the acidic solution is damaging to most surgical instruments. The alkaline solution deposits a polymeric film after a few hours. The two solutions are compared with other sterilants in the review by Boucher (1972). (*See also* Borick, 1968; Smith, 1968.)

ACIDS

Acids have been used in the preservation of foods since antiquity. At present, several acids are employed as antiseptics or cauterizing agents. The germicidal action of some acids is due to hydrogen ions. However, some acidic compounds have a selective type of action that is dependent on a specific chemical group.

The urinary antiseptic acids—nalidixic acid, hippuric acid, and mandelic acid—are discussed in a separate section (page 1006). Fatty acids are included in the discussion of antifungal drugs (page 1010).

Inorganic Acids. The strong inorganic acids are occasionally employed as cauterizing agents for the immediate sterilization of dangerously infected wounds. *Nitric acid* is the one of choice, for it forms a firm eschar and does not penetrate too deeply. It is commonly applied either as concentrated or fuming nitric acid. *Chromic acid* as a 20% solution is sufficiently destructive to tissue to be employed for the removal of *warts.*

Benzoic Acid. This compound has been widely used as a *food preservative.* In a concentration of 0.1% it prevents bacterial and fungal growth if the medium is slightly acidic. It is much less effective at an alkaline pH. Benzoic acid is relatively nontoxic and almost tasteless, and for these reasons it can be added to food. After ingestion, the benzoic acid is conjugated with glycine and excreted in the urine as hippuric acid. A daily intake of 4 to 6 g does not cause toxic symptoms aside from slight gastric irrita-

tion. Larger doses have systemic effects not unlike those of the salicylates.

Benzoic Acid, U.S.P., is a component of *Benzoic and Salicylic Acid Ointment,* U.S.P., which is discussed with the antifungal drugs (page 1012). Benzoic acid can be safely applied to the skin in high concentrations.

Acetic Acid. This acid in 5% concentration is bactericidal to many types of microorganisms and bacteriostatic at lower concentrations. It is occasionally used in 1% solution on the skin for surgical dressings. *Pseudomonas aeruginosa* is particularly susceptible to acetic acid, and the acid may be employed in burn therapy. It is used in vaginal douches to suppress infections with *Trichomonas, Candida,* and *Haemophilus.* It is also a spermatocide.

Boric Acid. Boric acid has an unwarranted reputation as a germicide. It is primarily bacteriostatic, even in saturated aqueous solution. Solutions are nonirritating and, therefore, have been applied to delicate structures such as the cornea.

Toxicity. In the past, boric acid was considered to be a relatively benign and nontoxic substance. Not only was boric acid widely used by the medical profession in the form of ointments and irrigating solutions, but also the compound became a common item in household medicine cabinets and nurseries. The many cases of serious boric acid poisoning have focused attention on the toxic potentialities of the compound. Poisoning has occurred from the accidental substitution of boric acid solution for water or of boric acid powder for glucose in hospital formulations. Consequently, boric acid has been removed from many hospitals and dispensaries. With repeated applications of the powder to the abraded or inflamed skin, sufficient amounts can be absorbed to cause acute poisoning, especially in infants. Lethal amounts can also be absorbed from wound cavities irrigated with boric acid solutions. Approximately half of the persons accidentally intoxicated die. Details of some of the case literature can be found in the reports of Valdes-Dapena and Arey (1962), Wong and coworkers (1964), and Skipworth and associates (1967). The lethal dose has been estimated to be 15 to 20 g in adults and 5 to 6 g in infants. The slow excretion of boric acid contributes to cumulation of the compound and ultimate toxic effects consequent to repeated application.

Acute boric acid poisoning begins with nausea, vomiting, and diarrhea, regardless of the route of administration. The body temperature falls, and an erythematous rash similar to that of scarlet fever develops. This is followed by desquamation, not only in the areas of the rash but also of mucous membranes. At this stage in newborn infants it has been mistaken for staphylococcal toxic epidermal necrolysis. Headache, restlessness, and weakness are also observed. Renal injury often occurs. Death results from circulatory collapse and shock, usually within 5 days. Treatment is purely symptomatic. Plasma volume should be maintained by the infusion of copious amounts of appropriate fluid. *Chronic* intoxication gives rise to anorexia, asthenia, confusion, menstrual disorders, and alopecia. It has occurred from the use of borate-containing mouthwashes.

Absorption, Distribution, and Excretion. Boric acid is readily absorbed from the gastrointestinal tract, serous cavities, and abraded or inflamed skin. It does not penetrate the intact skin. Excretion is primarily by the kidney. Approximately 50% of a given dose is excreted within 24 hours. During chronic administration, a plateau in urinary excretion is reached only after 2 weeks. Relatively large amounts of boric acid are localized in the brain, liver, and kidney. Pathological changes can be detected in the brain and kidney, and Valdes-Dapena and Arey (1962) have called attention to the intracytoplasmic inclusions in the pancreas in fatal cases.

Preparations and Therapeutic Uses. *Boric acid* occurs as colorless, odorless crystals or as a white powder. It is now usually colored to prevent error. Containers of boric acid should bear an autoclavable "poison" label. Boric acid is soluble to the extent of approximately 5% in water and 25% in glycerin. Most modern hospitals limit the use of boric acid to the *ophthalmic ointment.* The use of *boric acid solution* or *powder* on extensive inflamed surfaces or in body cavities fortunately is diminishing and should be considered obsolete. Few commercial dermatological preparations contain the acid today, but sodium borate is sometimes included as a buffer. The inclusion of boric acid in rectal suppositories for hemorrhoids carries the risk of chronic intoxication.

Salicylic Acid. This acid is a weak germicide. Its local actions are discussed under the salicylates (Chapter 17). Uses of this drug in treating fungal infections are given in the discussion of antifungal drugs.

HALOGENS AND HALOGEN-CONTAINING COMPOUNDS

IODINE

Tincture of iodine was first used as an antiseptic by a French surgeon in 1839, and it was employed in treating battle wounds in the U.S. Civil War (*see* Gershenfeld, 1968). Despite the present wide choice of antiseptics, iodine is still among the most valuable agents. The drug has survived on the basis of efficacy, economy, and low tissue toxicity.

Germicidal Action. Elemental iodine is lethal to both microflora and microzoa and to viruses. It is potent and rapidly acting. In the absence of organic matter, most bacteria are killed within 1 minute by exposure to a 1:20,000 solution of iodine; a period of approximately 15 minutes is required to kill wet bacterial spores with this concentration, but certain dry spores may require hours, even at much higher concentrations. A dilution as high as 1:200,000 will destroy all vegetative forms of bacteria in 15 minutes. On the skin, a 1% tincture will kill 90% of the bacteria in 1½ minutes and a 7% tincture in 15

seconds (Price, 1950). The germicidal properties of iodine are reviewed by Gershenfeld (1968).

In the presence of organic matter, some iodine is bound by covalent bonds, but most of it forms loose complexes from which the iodine is slowly released. Thus, the immediate efficacy is somewhat diminished, but over a period of 15 minutes to 1 hour the efficacy is only moderately diminished. All commercial preparations contain iodine in great excess, so that organic matter does not adversely influence immediate efficacy. Even a solution as dilute as 0.1% exerts adequate bactericidal actions in the presence of serum and tissue debris. Although penetration is limited by complex formation with organic matter, the looseness of the complexes allows for the slow progress of diffusion below the surface.

Preparations. *Iodine Tincture,* U.S.P., contains 2% iodine and 2.4% sodium iodide diluted in 50% ethanol. The function of NaI is to increase solubility through formation of I_3^- ions. Official aqueous solutions of iodine are *Strong Iodine Solution,* U.S.P. (*compound iodine solution, Lugol's solution*), and *Iodine Solution,* U.S.P. The former contains 5% iodine and 10% potassium iodide; the latter, 2% iodine and 2.4% sodium iodide.

Toxicity. The local toxicity of iodine is quite low compared to its germicidal potency. Most of the iodine burns that gave iodine a bad reputation were caused by a 7% tincture, which is no longer official. Iodine tinctures sting strongly when applied to raw surfaces, but iodine solution stings only slightly.

In rare instances, an individual may exhibit hypersensitivity to iodine and react markedly to moderate amounts of the element applied to the skin. Symptoms usually take the form of a severe constitutional reaction with fever and a generalized skin eruption of varying type. Seymour (1937) reviewed 15 cases of iodine hypersensitivity and reported a case of his own in which the patient died of exfoliative dermatitis following the application of iodine to the skin.

Iodine has a low toxicity by oral ingestion of therapeutic preparations. Few patients succumb to the effects of the drug. Fatalities have occurred only when large amounts (30 to 250 ml) of iodine tincture have been ingested.

The toxic effects of iodine are largely due to the local actions of the element in the gastrointestinal tract. Iodine is highly corrosive but also readily inactivated. Thus, iodine combines with various foodstuffs in the digestive tract and in this manner is inactivated. Little free iodine is absorbed from the intestinal tract; the element reaches the blood stream mainly in the form of iodide. It is probable that the pathological changes recorded in fatal cases of iodine poisoning and attributed to the systemic effects of iodine are largely the result of shock, tissue hypoxia, and sometimes ethanol intoxication.

Symptoms. The symptoms of iodine poisoning are chiefly gastrointestinal. The diagnosis is facilitated by the fact that the oral mucous membranes are stained brown. Reflex vomiting usually occurs; if starch is present in the stomach, the vomitus is colored blue. The local actions of iodine cause gastro-enteritis, abdominal pain, and diarrhea that may be bloody. Large amounts of fluid are lost by vomiting and diarrhea, and shock may result from dehydration and tissue trauma. In fatal cases, death usually occurs in 1 to 48 hours. The cause of death may be circulatory collapse due to shock, acute corrosive gastritis, asphyxiation from edema of the glottis, or aspiration pneumonia. In rare instances, delayed death from stenosis of the esophagus has been recorded.

Treatment. Gastric lavage with a solution of soluble starch can readily remove all the iodine present in the stomach. Alternative antidotes are sodium thiosulfate (5% solution) or protein. The stomach should be lavaged until all traces of iodine are removed. Further treatment consists in correcting fluid and electrolyte imbalance. Therapy for shock may be necessary.

Therapeutic Uses. The chief use of solutions of elemental iodine is in the *disinfection of the skin.* In this regard iodine is probably superior to any other agent. It is best employed in the form of the tincture, for the alcoholic vehicle facilitates spreading and penetration. Iodine may also be employed in the treatment of *wounds* and *abrasions.* Applied to abraded tissue, aqueous solutions are less irritating than the tincture. Aqueous solutions of 0.5 to 1.0% iodine with iodide are suitable for wounds and abrasions and a 0.1% solution may be used for irrigations. These concentrations can readily be made by proper dilution of the official solutions with water. For application to *mucous membranes,* a 2% solution of iodine in glycerin is the preparation of choice. In the treatment of *cutaneous infections* due to bacteria and fungi, the U.S.P. tincture or solution of iodine may be employed.

Iodine may be used to render contaminated water safe for drinking. The addition of 3 drops of iodine tincture to each quart of water will kill not only amebae but also bacteria within 15 minutes without making the water unpalatable.

IODOPHORS

An iodophor is a combination or complex of iodine with a solubilizing agent or carrier that liberates free iodine in solution. Non-ionic surface-active agents (*see* below) are employed as carriers in many iodophors. Iodophors are widely used at the present time for the purpose of *sanitization* (*see* Gershenfeld, 1968). In addition, *Povidone-Iodine,* U.S.P. (BETADINE, ISODINE), a complex of iodine with polyvinylpyrrolidone, is available as *Povidone-Iodine Solution, U.S.P.,* and *Povidone-Iodine Aerosol,* N.F., for general antiseptic uses. Several other iodophors are found in a variety of proprietary antiseptic preparations. Iodophors produce less pain than do preparations of elemental iodine

when applied to wounds and abrasions. However, superior efficacy of these compounds to iodine solutions has not been demonstrated. Blatt and Maloney (1961) studied three iodophors and found that their germicidal properties were similar to those of iodine solutions with equivalent iodine content. However, King and Price (1963) showed that 1% iodine in 70% alcohol was markedly superior as a skin disinfectant to any of the five iodophors tested. The comparative efficacy of iodophors and hexachlorophene in surgical scrubs and for preoperative preparation is discussed above under hexachlorophene.

CHLORINE AND CHLOROPHORS

The ability of chlorine to arrest putrefaction and prevent associated odors was recognized and utilized long before the concept of microorganisms had originated. Chlorine became widely used in the sterilization of water supplies during the first decade of the twentieth century. It was not until World War I, however, that chlorine-containing compounds were extensively employed in medicine and surgery. As antiseptics, chlorine-containing compounds have largely been replaced by agents that are more efficient and less irritating. However, they are used extensively as sanitizing agents.

CHLORINE

Elemental chlorine is a potent germicidal agent. It exerts its antibacterial action in both the elemental form and as undissociated hypochlorous acid, which is readily formed in aqueous solution from chlorine. In neutral or acidic solution, hypochlorous acid is largely undissociated and exerts a marked bactericidal action. However, in alkaline solution the hypochlorite ion is formed and bactericidal activity is greatly reduced. For example, the bactericidal action of chlorine is ten times greater at pH 6.0 than at pH 9.0. At pH 7.0, the concentration of chlorine necessary to kill most organisms in 15 to 30 seconds varies between 0.10 and 0.25 ppm. However, acid-fast microorganisms are uniquely resistant to chlorine; 500 times the concentrations cited are necessary to destroy *Mycobacterium tuberculosis.* Chlorine is also virucidal and amebicidal.

The bactericidal activity of chlorine can be influenced by a number of factors. Chief of these is the presence of organic matter. Chlorine is a highly reactive element and thus can be bound by organic material. In the presence of excessive organic matter, chlorine is not the disinfectant of choice. In the disinfection of inanimate objects, for example, water, the uptake of chlorine by the organic matter present is known as the *chlorine demand*. It is generally considered that a residual chlorine content of 0.2 to 0.4 ppm of water affords a generous margin of safety. In order to attain this concentration of chlorine in relatively pure water, it is sufficient to add only 0.5 ppm; in grossly polluted waters, 20 ppm is scarcely sufficient.

Elemental chlorine has no medical uses. Its principal relevance to public health is its use in the treatment of community water supplies, although chlorinated lime is often used instead.

CHLOROPHORS

Chlorine itself has limited usefulness as an antiseptic because of difficulties in handling the element in its gaseous state and because chlorine water is very unstable. Many compounds, however, slowly yield hypochlorous acid, and these can be employed for the disinfection of inanimate objects and in surgery. Such compounds may be regarded as chlorophors, even though the ultimate product is hypochlorous acid. The germicidal efficiency of such compounds is related to the ease and extent of the liberation of HOCl.

Hypochlorite Solutions. There are a number of solutions in which chlorine is present in the form of hypochlorites. They are known under various names, such as Dakin's solution, Dakin-Carrel solution, and Labarraque's solution. *Sodium Hypochlorite Solution*, N.F., is the official preparation of this type. It contains 5% NaOCl. This concentration is too high to be employed on tissues, except that it is a valuable agent in root canal therapy. For surgical purposes *Diluted Sodium Hypochlorite Solution*, N.F. (*modified Dakin's solution*), is employed. This preparation contains 0.45 to 0.5% of NaOCl. It may be diluted 1:3.

Solutions of sodium hypochlorite are relatively unstable and should be freshly prepared. They are not only germicidal but also dissolve necrotic tissues. A disadvantage of the hypochlorites is that they dissolve blood clots and delay clotting. Chlorine antiseptics are also somewhat irritating to the skin. *Oxychlorosene* (CLORPACTIN) is a mixture of HOCl and alkylbenzene sulfonates; sodium oxychlorosene contains NaOCl, which is more stable. The surfactant properties of the alkylbenzene sulfonates promote penetration and the antibacterial actions. In addition to its use in topical antisepsis, oxychlorosene, but not the sodium salt, enjoys a special use as a local irrigant during surgery on neoplasms, to destroy detached viable cells in an attempt to prevent metastasis.

Chlorinated Lime. Chlorinated lime consists of a mixture of calcium chloride and calcium hypochlorite and should contain a minimum of 30% available chlorine. It is too irritating to be used on tissues, but it is widely employed for the *disinfection* of inanimate objects and drinking water. Chlorinated lime is relatively unstable and loses much of its activity over a period of a year.

Chloramines. The chloramines are amines, amides, or imides containing an N-chloro substituent. They are unstable in water and slowly release chlorine. Some chloramines also have a direct germicidal action. Chloramines are no longer employed for the irrigation of wounds or as antiseptics but are used in the emergency sterilization of drinking water and for sanitization. In the United States, *Halazone*, N.F., is the only chloramine of importance.

OXIDIZING AGENTS

A number of antiseptic drugs are toxic to microorganisms because they are oxidizing agents. Some compounds release oxygen as an active intermediate, and others probably directly oxidize vulnerable microbial constituents. Their individual properties differ considerably and are influenced by penetration, the rate at which oxygen is liberated, the actions of the cation linked with the oxygen-containing anion, and the effects of the substance remaining after oxygen has been released. For these reasons the drugs require separate discussion.

PEROXIDES

Hydrogen Peroxide. Hydrogen peroxide is a very unstable compound that breaks down readily to form molecular oxygen and water. The official preparation is *Hydrogen Peroxide Solution*, U.S.P., which contains 3% hydrogen peroxide in water. When hydrogen peroxide is applied to tissue, catalase causes rapid decomposition and the germicidal action is brief. Furthermore, solutions of hydrogen peroxide have poor penetrability and are relatively feeble germicides. In view of these defects, the official status of hydrogen peroxide is hard to defend.

The most extensive use of hydrogen peroxide is in the *cleansing of wounds*. The effervescence caused by the release of nascent oxygen affords a weak mechanical means for the removal of tissue debris from inaccessible regions. The drug is somewhat effective in the treatment of *Vincent's infection;* this was an important use before the advent of spirochetcidal antibiotics. The continued use of hydrogen peroxide solution as a mouthwash, even in half strength, may cause the development of hypertrophied filiform papillae of the tongue ("hairy tongue"), but these disappear after the drug is discontinued. Hydrogen peroxide has also been found of value in the treatment of *balanitis* (continuous irrigation with a 2% solution) and of *Trichomonas vaginalis vaginitis*. It is dangerous to inject hydrogen peroxide into closed body cavities from which the released oxygen has no free exit.

Other Peroxides. *Zinc peroxide, magnesium peroxide, calcium peroxide,* and *sodium peroxide* were employed in the past as antiseptics, but only zinc peroxide was received favorably. It was used to treat oropharyngeal and wound infections caused by anaerobes, microaerophils, and even certain aerobes, such as hemolytic streptococci.

Hydrous Benzoyl Peroxide, U.S.P., is used as *Benzoyl Peroxide Lotion,* U.S.P., or as a cream containing 5% of the drug. It slowly releases oxygen, to which its antimicrobial action is attributed. It is also keratolytic, antiseborrheic, and irritant. It is especially indicated for the treatment of acne vulgaris and acne rosacea, which are associated with an anaerobic corynebacterium. After application, there may be transient stinging or burning sensations, which disappear after continued use. It is especially irritating to skin on the neck and circumoral areas. It must be kept away from the eyes. Sudden excess dryness of the skin and desquamation may occur after 1 to 2 weeks of use. The peeling effect is thought to contribute importantly to its efficacy. It can cause contact dermatitis. It also bleaches clothing.

PERMANGANATES

Permanganates are antiseptic and antifungal. Microorganisms vary greatly in their resistance to permanganates. Most bacteria are killed within 1 hour by permanganates in a dilution of 1:10,000, but some microorganisms survive exposure to much higher concentrations. The germicidal efficiency of the permanganate is greatly reduced in the presence of organic matter. Concentrations stronger than 1:5000 are irritating to tissues. *Potassium Permanganate,* U.S.P., forms deep-purple solutions, but it leaves a brown stain of manganese dioxide. Manganous ion resulting from reduction of permanganate is astringent, and this aids in the suppression of inflammation.

Clinical Uses. The permanganates are employed clinically for a variety of purposes, but are used much less than formerly. Their former extensive local application in the treatment of *urethritis* has become obsolete with the advent of effective chemotherapeutic agents. The compound may suppress the vesicular stage of *eczema-dermatitis,* for which purpose a wet dressing of a 1:10,000 solution is employed. Solutions of potassium permanganate are employed in *dermatomycoses,* especially *tinea pedis, tinea cruris,* and *ringworm.* The astringent action probably makes a major contribution, since only the acute or wet stages are much benefited.

The ability of potassium permanganate to oxidize organic substances finds other fields of usefulness aside from the treatment of infections. *Venoms* can be destroyed by oxidation, and application of crystals of potassium permanganate to the site of a *snakebite* is of value provided the wound is opened widely and the circulation is stopped to prevent absorption. However, some believe that the compound does more harm than good in that a crust is formed, which precludes the possibility of suction and drainage from the wound. A wet dressing of permanganate may be employed in the treatment of *ivy poisoning.* Permanganate solution can oxidize many drugs, but it is seldom used as an antidote in poisoning.

HEAVY METALS AND THEIR SALTS

MERCURY COMPOUNDS

The inorganic mercury compounds were among the earliest antiseptics to be used and were highly regarded as potent germicides by Robert Koch. By the end of the last century, discerning bacteriologists had presented evidence that mercury compounds are primarily bacteriostatic, a finding that has been amply confirmed for the inorganic mercurials as well as for the organic mercury compounds introduced in this century. Nevertheless, the belief still persists that these agents are highly effective germicides.

Mechanism of Action. Numerous proposals for the mechanism of antibacterial action of mercury compounds have been advanced (*see* Brewer, 1968). The most plausible explanation at present is that the mercuric ion inhibits sulfhydryl enzymes. However, mercuric ion also combines with amino and other biologically important chemical groups. Bacteria and certain viruses inactivated by mercury can be reactivated by thiols. Bacterial spores exposed to mercurials for many months resume multiplication when the inhibitor is removed. In body fluids, there are many sulfhydryl compounds capable of combining with mercury, for example, glutathione, cysteine, and SH groups of proteins. *Organisms inhibited by mercury can therefore become reactivated when they are introduced into the body.*

The mercury antiseptics inhibit the sulfhydryl enzymes of tissue cells as well as those of bacteria. Such test objects as embryonic tissue and leukocytes are readily injured, and the therapeutic index of mercury compounds is therefore low.

It is obvious that mercury compounds fall far short of being ideal germicides. The claims of high activity for many of the available commercial preparations are based upon testing procedures that fail to take into account the factors outlined. However, some are effective bacteriostatic agents and, as such, find medicinal applications. Finally, it should be noted that in many preparations of organic mercurials the vehicle contains ethyl or benzyl alcohol, which contributes to germicidal activity. Interestingly, with some mercurials it has been shown that the vehicle alone is more active than the mercurial plus the vehicle.

Inorganic Mercurial Antiseptics. Mercuric chloride, the oldest of the mercury antiseptics, was once widely used only for disinfecting inanimate objects or the unabraded skin. It is too irritating and toxic to be applied to an abraded surface. It is now obsolete, and mercuric chloride tablets are no longer available in the United States.

Some insoluble compounds of mercury and metallic mercury itself are incorporated in ointment bases for use as *antiseptics* and as *ectoparasiticides* (*see* below). When compounded in this manner, the mercurial is slowly transferred from the ointment base into the skin, where it exerts its action over long periods of time. *Yellow mercuric oxide ointment* contains 1% HgO. It is employed for application to the eye and in *dermatomycoses, pruritus ani,* and *louse infestation. Ammoniated mercury* is water insoluble and is used in ointment form. *Ammoniated mercury ointment* contains 5% of HgNH$_2$Cl in liquid petrolatum and white ointment. It is used chiefly as a skin antiseptic, especially in *impetigo contagiosa, dermatomycoses,* and certain other dermatoses. It is also employed for scaling in *psoriasis,* in *pruritus ani,* and in *pinworm* and *crab louse infestation.* A 3% ophthalmic ointment has also been used. Sensitization is a common occurrence with these preparations. Furthermore, not only can mercury pass through the skin into the body but also inunction can force the ointments through the skin. Thus, chronic application can cause systemic mercury intoxication. For these reasons and because there are more effective topical antiseptics, the inorganic mercurials are undergoing a much-deserved decline in use.

Organic Mercurial Antiseptics. In the organic mercurial compounds one bond of mercury is directed toward a carbon atom. As a group they are more bacteriostatic, less irritating, and less toxic than the inorganic mercurial salts. Their mechanism of action and limitations have already been discussed. *Merbromin* (MERCUROCHROME) was the first organic mercurial antiseptic to be introduced and for some time had official status. It is only feebly active, even as a bacteriostatic agent. It is the least effective of the commercial mercurial antiseptics. It also has the lowest therapeutic index. The continued inclusion of this drug in first-aid kits is regrettable, and public health would be better served if this drug were removed from the market.

Four organic mercurial antiseptics—*Nitromersol,* N.F. (METAPHEN), *phenylmercuric acetate, phenylmercuric nitrate,* and *Thimerosal,* N.F. (MERTHIOLATE)—have many features in common and thus can be discussed together conveniently. They have the structural formulas shown below.

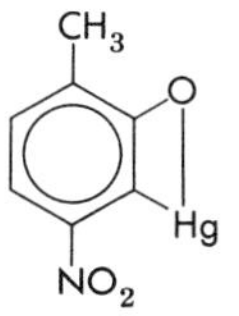

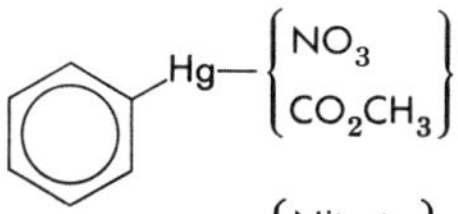

Because organic mercurials are less irritating than soluble inorganic mercurial salts, they can be applied directly to tissue. However, they penetrate poorly, and the tissues fix the mercury so that it is unavailable to the microorganisms. Organic mercurials have been widely used to disinfect instruments and as antiseptics on cutaneous and mucosal surfaces in concentrations from 1 : 100,000 to 1 : 1000. It should be emphasized that these agents are primarily bacteriostatic and are relatively ineffective in killing spores. They are not as efficient for disinfecting instruments as is commonly believed. Sensitization to the organic mercurials occasionally occurs (*see* Mathews, 1968). The organic mercurial antiseptics are marketed in various types of proprietary solutions, tinctures, jellies, ointments, and suppositories.

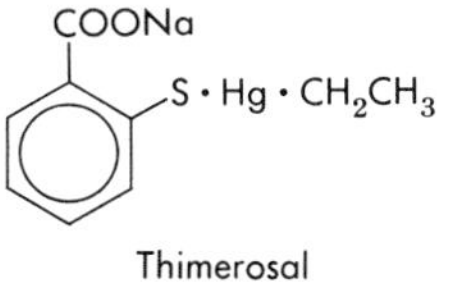

Nitromersol Solution, N.F., contains 0.2% and *Nitromersol Tincture,* N.F., contains 0.5% of the drug. *Thimerosal Aerosol,* N.F., *Thimerosal Solution,* N.F., and *Thimerosal Tincture,* N.F., all contain 0.1% of the compound.

SILVER COMPOUNDS

Many silver compounds have antiseptic properties, but only a few have been used clinically. Soluble, highly ionizable silver salts have astringent and caustic actions as well. Only the local actions of silver are discussed here; the systemic toxicity of silver is discussed in Chapter 46.

Actions. The silver ion combines with sulfhydryl, carboxyl, phosphate, amino, and other biologically important chemical groups. Such interactions involving a protein alter its physical properties and often cause it to precipitate. This is the basis of the astringent and caustic actions of silver ions. This may, in part, explain the antibacterial actions. Yet several poorly ionizable or poorly soluble silver compounds that do not provide enough ion for precipitation of proteins nevertheless are good antiseptics. It must be presumed that silver, like mercury, is capable of interfering with essential metabolic activities in bacterial cells. When solutions of inorganic silver salts are applied to tissue, they exert an immediate germicidal effect. Thereafter, small amounts of ionic silver are liberated from the silver proteinate formed, and this results in a sustained bacteriostatic action.

An interesting bacteriological phenomenon is that distilled water becomes markedly bactericidal after contact with metallic silver. Despite the fact that the concentration of silver ions reaches only 1 part in 20 million, even heavy suspensions of bacteria succumb within a few hours. This action of silver is shared by many heavy metals and is known as *oligodynamic action.* Although diverse theories have been proposed (*see* Romans, 1968), the mechanism of this action is obscure. To the extent that tissue constituents reduce silver ions to metallic silver, the oligodynamic action will contribute to the antibacterial effect.

Inorganic silver salts are highly germicidal in solution. For example, silver nitrate destroys most microorganisms in a concentration of 1 : 1000. Much higher dilutions are bacteriostatic. Silver nitrate is toxic to tissue cells in bactericidal concentrations.

Silver Nitrate. Silver nitrate is the most commonly employed of the inorganic silver salts and is used as a caustic, antiseptic, and astringent agent. The degree of action depends upon the concentration employed and the period of time during which the compound is allowed to act. The silver ion is precipitated by chloride. Thus, the action of the silver salts can be readily stopped by washing with a solution of sodium chloride. This chemical property also accounts for the fact that solutions of simple salts of silver do not readily penetrate into tissues, for the silver ion is precipitated by chloride of tissue fluids. Silver salts stain tissue black due to the deposition of reduced silver. Most of the stain slowly disappears spontaneously, but some may persist indefinitely at some sites.

Therapeutic Uses. Silver Nitrate, U.S.P., is employed either in solid form or in solution. The solid form, *Toughened Silver Nitrate,* U.S.P. (*lunar caustic*), is used for the cauterization of wounds and for removing granulation tissue and warts. It is conveniently dispensed in pencils that should be moistened before use.

Solutions of silver nitrate, in strengths of 0.01 to 10%, are also employed for local application. A 1:10,000 concentration is used as a mildly antiseptic and astringent solution for irrigation of the bladder and urethra. When a strong germicidal action is desired, as for local treatment of infected aphthous ulcers, a 10% solution may be carefully applied. Silver salts are particularly germicidal for gonococci, and *Silver Nitrate Ophthalmic Solution,* U.S.P. (1%), is routinely employed for the *prophylaxis of ophthalmia neonatorum.* A few drops are instilled in the conjunctival sac in newborn infants. If a stronger solution is used, the eyes should be washed immediately with an isotonic sodium chloride solution. At one time, this treatment of the newborn was the established practice in the United States, but the laws were repealed in certain states because some authorities consider penicillin to be superior. However, not only can penicillin cause sensitization but also many gonococci have become resistant to the antibiotic. Hence silver nitrate will continue to be used.

Silver nitrate as a 0.5% solution is used in the treatment of *extensive burns,* usually in conjunction with gentamicin, kanamycin, and/or mafenide. However, since the silver ion combines with chloride to yield insoluble silver chloride, serious hypochloremia can occur. Hyponatremia also results because the cations that accompany the serum chloride are lost into the exudate (Burke *et al.,* 1968). Furthermore, absorbed nitrate can cause methemoglobinemia.

Other Silver Compounds. *Silver sulfadiazine* has been introduced to replace silver nitrate in the topical treatment of *extensive burns* (Fox, 1968). Its solubility is low enough that insufficient silver ion is released to precipitate significant amounts of chloride ion or proteins. Hypochloremia, hyponatremia, and eschars that adhere to dressings are thus avoided. Despite its low solubility, silver sulfadiazine exerts a prominent antibacterial action against *Pseu-*

domonas. The compound is painless upon application. Furthermore, unlike silver nitrate, it does not cause argyrial staining of wounds or bed linens. Insufficient sulfadiazine is absorbed to cause crystalluria.

In the past, a number of colloidal suspensions of insoluble silver compounds or of elemental silver were marketed. Because of the low silver ion concentrations of such preparations, they did not precipitate chloride or protein, and they were usually nonastringent and nonirritating. *Mild silver protein* (19 to 23% silver) and *strong silver protein* (7.5 to 8.5% silver) were the most widely promoted drugs of this class. Although the mild formulation contains more silver than the strong, it is less ionizable and hence is mostly bacteriostatic instead of germicidal. It is nonirritating, even mildly demulcent. The strong form is germicidal and mildly irritating. Claims that colloidal silver preparations are more penetrating than ionizable preparations do not correctly apply to large molecules such as the silver proteins. The silver proteins are usually applied to mucous membranes of the nose and throat, conjunctiva, urethra, bladder, and colon. Colloidal silver preparations have limited value except in the treatment of gonococcal conjunctivitis and gonorrhea, for which use they have largely been displaced by antibiotic therapy. There is no acceptable evidence that the routine use of silver solutions for the prophylaxis of colds or other respiratory tract infections is at all efficacious, and cases of argyria have resulted from this practice. Fortunately, the colloidal silver preparations are now in a deserved oblivion.

ZINC SALTS

The salts of zinc are employed as astringents, antiperspirants, styptics, corrosives, and mild antiseptics. They probably owe their action to the ability of the zinc ion to precipitate protein, but other mechanisms may be involved in the effect on bacteria. The highly ionizable, soluble salts, such as zinc chloride, are quite irritating and can be used as escharotics. When taken internally, the zinc salts irritate the gastric mucosa and cause vomiting; on this basis, zinc sulfate has been employed as an emetic. Otherwise, the main use of zinc salts is for their astringent and antiseptic action on mucous membranes and skin.

Zinc Sulfate, U.S.P., is used in solution as an eyewash (0.1 to 1.0%) in *conjunctivitis* caused by the *Morax-Axenfeld bacillus.* The official preparation for ophthalmological uses is *Zinc Sulfate Ophthalmic Solution,* U.S.P. (OPTHAL-ZIN). For application to the skin, zinc sulfate is used in a concentration of 4%. It is often incorporated with sulfurated potash in equal concentration in a lotion known as *White Lotion,* N.F. Zinc sulfate is useful in such skin diseases and infections as *acne, ivy poisoning, lupus erythematosus,* and *impetigo.* The compound also forms the basis for some deodorant anhidrotics (*see* Chapter 47). A *nasal spray* of zinc sulfate has been used to shrink the mucous membranes so as to allow drainage from infected accessory nasal sinuses. Treatment of this type has a disadvantage in that it inhibits the activity of the cilia of the respiratory mucous membrane. Zinc sulfate accelerates the rate of healing of leg ulcers in patients with sickle-cell abnormalities, in whom the serum zinc concentrations are low (*see* Serjeant *et al.,* 1970). Pressure sores, surgical wounds, and various other lesions have been reported to be benefited. Whether patients who respond well are only those with low serum zinc concentrations is not yet clear. The salt has been applied topically or given orally in a dose of 220 mg three times a day.

Zinc Chloride, U.S.P., is occasionally used as an astringent in solutions of 0.5 to 2%. A 10% solution applied to the teeth is sometimes used to make the teeth less sensitive. *Zinc Acetate,* U.S.P., is used as an astringent and styptic and occasionally as an emetic.

Zinc Oxide, U.S.P., is a fine, white, insoluble salt of zinc that is incorporated in powders, ointments, and pastes. It has a mild astringent and antiseptic action. It is used in skin diseases and infections such as *eczema, impetigo, ringworm, varicose ulcers, pruritus,* and *psoriasis.* Official preparations containing zinc oxide include *Zinc Oxide Ointment,* U.S.P. (20% zinc oxide), *Zinc Oxide Paste,* U.S.P. (25% zinc oxide), and *Zinc Oxide Paste with Salicylic Acid,* N.F. (2% salicylic acid in paste of zinc oxide). *Calamine,* U.S.P., consists of a pink powder containing zinc oxide (not less than 98%) and a small amount of ferric oxide. Official preparations of calamine include *Calamine Lotion,* U.S.P. (8% calamine and 8% zinc oxide), and *Phenolated Calamine Lotion,* U.S.P. (*compound calamine lotion*) (1% phenol in calamine lotion). *Zinc Stearate,* U.S.P., and *zinc oleate* have actions similar to those of zinc oxide. Other antiseptic zinc compounds are *zinc permanganate* and *zinc peroxide.*

SURFACE-ACTIVE AGENTS

Surface-active agents are substances that alter the energy relations at interfaces. They are widely used in industry and in the home as wetting agents, detergents, and emulsifiers. Some compounds possess the ability to precipitate or denature protein and to destroy microorganisms. The major use of surface-active agents in medicine is as bactericides. They have been reviewed by Glassman (1948) and Lawrence (1968b).

Chemistry. Surface-active agents comprise compounds characterized by a structural balance between one or more "water-attracting" (hydrophilic) and "water-repelling" (hydrophobic) groups. Included in this category are cationic, anionic, nonionic, and amphoteric agents. The most important bactericides are the cationic surface-active agents, in which a hydrophobic residue (paraffinic chain, alkyl-substituted benzene or naphthalene ring) is balanced by a positively charged hydrophilic group, most commonly a quaternary ammonium nucleus. The structural formulas of the major cationic agents used in medicine are shown below.

Germicidal Properties. Cationic surface-active agents are bactericidal in low concentrations to a wide variety of gram-positive and gram-negative bacteria. Many fungi and viruses are also susceptible. The anionic agents affect primarily gram-positive microorganisms; the nonionic agents possess little germicidal activity.

The mechanism of action of surface-active agents is unknown, although numerous theories have been proposed (*see* Lawrence, 1968b). The antibacterial action appears to be unrelated to the ability of the compounds to denature protein or to their ability to lower surface tension. Evidence has been presented that the major site of action of these compounds may be the cell membrane, where the agents may cause changes in permeability that permit the escape of enzymes, coenzymes, and metabolic intermediates.

Anionic surface-active agents antagonize the effect of cationic agents. Thus, cationic agents are incompatible with soaps. Within certain time limits, bacteriostatic actions of cationic compounds can be reversed by soaps and other anionic agents. Germicidal activity of the cationic compounds is reduced

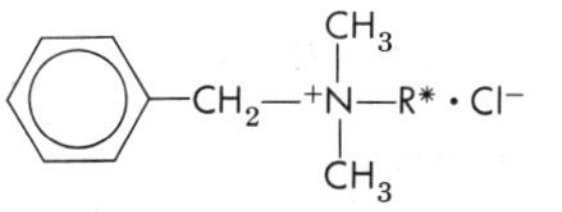

Benzalkonium Chloride

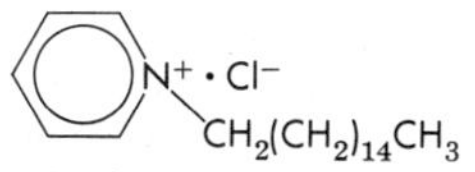

Cetylpyridinum Chloride

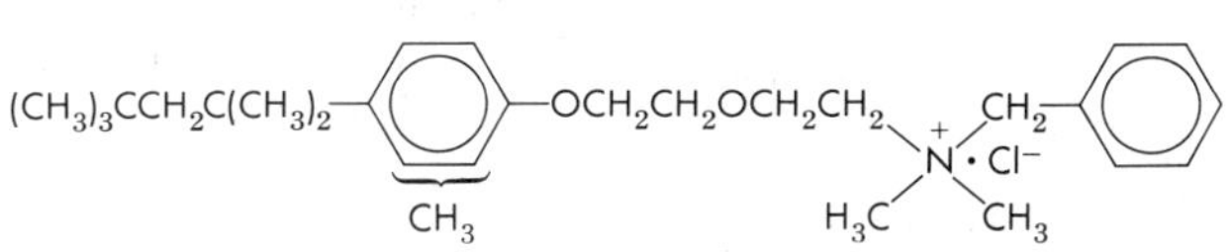

Methylbenzethonium Chloride †

---

* *R* represents any alkyl from C_8H_{17} to $C_{18}H_{37}$; the compound is thus a mixture of molecules in which the alkyls differ.

† Benzethonium differs from methylbenzethonium in lacking the CH_3 in the position indicated by the brace.

by organic matter and by other reactive substances; Lawrence (1968b) lists the more important chemicals that are incompatible with cationic agents. Of special importance is the fact that the surface-active agents are adsorbed to a significant degree by cotton, rubber, and other porous materials. This adsorption reduces the effective concentration of the agent and thereby decreases its germicidal efficiency (*see* below).

Preparations. Only the cationic surface-active agents are employed in medicine. *Benzalkonium Chloride,* U.S.P. (*alkylbenzyldimethylammonium chloride;* ZEPHIRAN), is freely soluble in water, alcohol, or acetone. Aqueous solutions are slightly alkaline. It is available as *Benzalkonium Chloride Solution,* U.S.P. The remaining preparations that have official status are *Benzethonium Chloride,* N.F., *Benzethonium Chloride Solution,* N.F., and *Benzethonium Chloride Tincture,* N.F.; *Cetylpyridinium Chloride,* N.F., *Cetylpyridinium Chloride Lozenges,* N.F., and *Cetylpyridinium Chloride Solution,* N.F.; and *Methylbenzethonium Chloride,* N.F., available as the official lotion, ointment, and powder. Alkylisoquinolinium bromide, cetalkonium chloride, cetyldimethylethylammonium bromide, cetyltrimethylammonium bromide, and laurylisoquinolinium bromide are also contained in a number of topical preparations.

Uses. Surface-active agents are detergents as well as sanitizers and have wide usefulness in the field of sanitation. In medicine they are employed as all-purpose antiseptics for application to skin, tissue, and mucous membranes and as disinfectants for medical and surgical materials.

Antiseptic Uses. Cationic surface-active agents have the following advantages as antiseptics. They are relatively nonirritating to tissue in effective concentrations. They have a rapid onset of action. They wet and penetrate tissue surfaces and possess detergent, keratolytic, and emulsifying actions. They have a relatively low systemic toxicity, but poisoning from oral ingestion has occurred. Nevertheless, certain serious shortcomings must be kept in mind. Their activity is antagonized by soaps, tissue constituents, and pus. Also, when applied to the skin, they tend to form a film under which bacteria may remain viable; the inner surface of the film has low bactericidal power whereas the outer surface is strongly bactericidal. They do not kill spores. Their action is rather slow when compared to that of iodine. A 0.1% solution of benzalkonium chloride applied to the human skin requires about 7 minutes to decrease the bacterial population by a mere 50%; the 0.1% tincture has a slower action than 70% ethanol. Even in the absence of antagonistic tissue constituents, a 0.002% solution requires 9 hours to kill 98% of *Escherichia coli;* this poorly effective concentration is close to that advocated for irrigation and lavage of the urinary tract. The cationic surfactants interact with keratin and cause epidermal damage, although this is minor except during continued use. Lastly, these drugs can cause occasional allergic responses with chronic use, as with certain deodorant preparations and diaper washes. In aggregate, the disadvantages would appear greatly to outweigh the advantages. Since superior agents are available, there seems little reason to use the cationic surfactants as antiseptics.

Benzalkonium chloride is employed in the following concentrations. For preoperative disinfection of unbroken skin or treatment of superficial injuries or fungal infections, the 0.1% tincture is recommended. Aqueous solutions are used for the preoperative disinfection of mucous membranes and denuded skin in 0.01 to 0.05% concentration; for instillation or irrigation of the eye or vagina, 0.02 to 0.05%; for irrigation of widely denuded surfaces, 0.01 to 0.02%; for irrigation of the urinary bladder and urethra, 0.005%; for retention lavage of the bladder, 0.0025%; for disinfection of deep lacerations, 0.1%; for irrigation of infected deep wounds, 0.033%; for treatment of infected denuded areas with wet dressings, 0.02%. The other cationic surface-active agents are employed in essentially the same concentrations. Methylbenzethonium chloride and benzethonium chloride are also used as spermatocides; they can cause vaginal irritation, with burning sensations and itching. Several quaternary surfactants are used in mouthwashes. They are also used as solubilizers in a number of preparations.

Disinfectant Uses. Surface-active agents are widely used for the sterilization of instruments and other materials such as cotton pledgets and rubber gloves. Following sporadic reports that indicated the presence of viable bacteria in solutions of these germicides in which porous materials were stored, Kundsin and Walter (1957) investigated quantitatively the extent of adsorption of benzalkonium chloride by skin, rubber gloves, and surgical sponges of various materials. They demonstrated that these materials adsorb the germicide to such a degree that the concentration of the solution may be materially reduced. Thus, repeated use of the same solution for disinfection of porous materials can reduce the concentration of the agent below the bactericidal limit. The significance of these observations is borne out by the reports of hospital infections traceable to materials stored in ineffective solutions of benzalkonium chloride (*see* Plotkin and Austrian, 1958; Malizia *et al.,* 1960; Lee and Fialkow, 1961). Microorganisms of the *Pseudomonas* and *Enterobacter* genera have been most frequently implicated in such outbreaks.

FURAN DERIVATIVES

Derivatives of furan possess antimicrobial activity. The presence of a nitro group in the 5 position of the furan ring confers antibacterial activity on many 2-substituted furans. The structural formulas of the furan derivatives of principal importance in medicine are as follows:

Nitrofurantoin

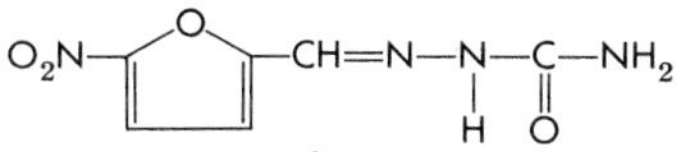

Nitrofurazone

Nitrofurantoin is discussed below with the urinary tract antiseptics (page 1008).

Antibacterial Actions. The furan derivatives affect a variety of gram-positive and gram-negative microorganisms. A bacteriostatic action is exerted upon most bacteria in the concentration range of 1:100,000 to 1:200,000. Bactericidal concentrations are approximately twice as great. Certain strains of bacteria, however, are insensitive to concentrations of the agents far in excess of those mentioned. The mechanism of the antibacterial action of the furan derivatives is unknown, but it is presumed that the compounds interfere with enzymatic processes essential to bacterial growth. Heavy inocula of microorganisms as well as plasma and blood reduce the activity of the drugs. Bacteria develop only a limited resistance to furan derivatives, and cross-resistance between these compounds and sulfonamides or antibiotics does not occur. Some furan derivatives, particularly nifuroxime, possess significant antifungal activity.

Preparations and Therapeutic Uses. *Nitrofurazone*, N.F. (FURACIN), is used as a broad-spectrum *topical* antibacterial agent in the treatment of mixed infections of superficial wounds and diseases of the skin. It is available in the form of the official ointment, cream, and solution; as a powder; as well as in various types of suppositories and dressings. The effects are generally favorable; the bacterial population is greatly reduced, and adverse effects on healing are not observed. However, the compound produces sensitization in approximately 0.5 to 2% of patients, and this sometimes occurs within a few days after the initial application. Although the systemic toxicity of nitrofurazone is relatively low, the drug has been little used in systemic therapy of bacterial infections.

DYES

There is little in common among the clinically used dyes with respect to chemical class or mechanism of action, and their inclusion together expresses a want of a better system of classification. Some of the dyes are not antimicrobial and, therefore, receive only brief mention here.

Gentian Violet. *Gentian Violet*, U.S.P. (*crystal violet, hexamethylrosaniline chloride*), is a triphenylmethane (rosaniline) dye with the following structure:

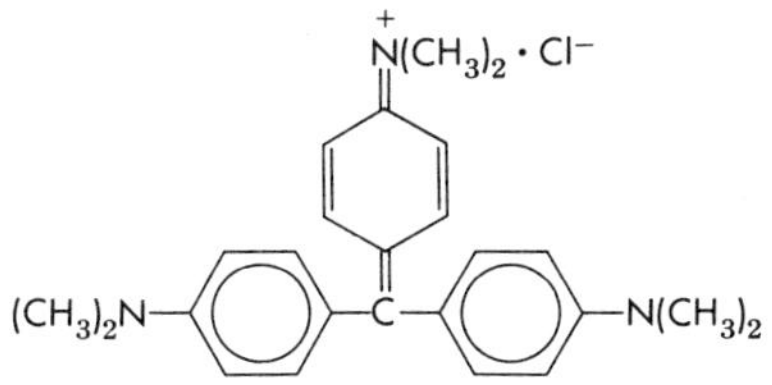

Gentian Violet

Marketed products often contain up to 4% of the tetramethyl and pentamethyl congeners. The pure compound is known as *crystal violet*.

Gentian violet is bacteriostatic and bactericidal to gram-positive bacteria and to many fungi. Gram-negative and acid-fast bacteria are very resistant to the drug. The susceptibility of gram-positive bacteria to the rosaniline dyes is presumably related to the characteristics of the cell that underlie the differential gram stain.

Gentian Violet Solution, U.S.P., contains 1% of the drug in 10% ethanol, and *Gentian Violet Cream*, U.S.P., contains 1.35% in an absorbable base. Gentian violet was once widely employed in the control of many types of infections. It has been used for superficial pyogenic infections, impetigo, Vincent's infection, and chronic and irritative lesions and dermatitides. It is still occasionally employed in treatment of fungal infections. For direct application to tissues, the dye is used in concentrations of 0.02% to 1%. For instillations in closed cavities, the concentration is reduced to 0.01%. It may be used for infected wounds, mucous membranes, and serous surfaces. Tattooing of the skin can result from contact of gentian violet with granulation tissue, and the dye should not be applied to ulcerative lesions of the face. The staining properties are a distinct disadvantage.

Methylene Blue. Methylene blue is tetramethylthionine chloride. It has the following structural formula:

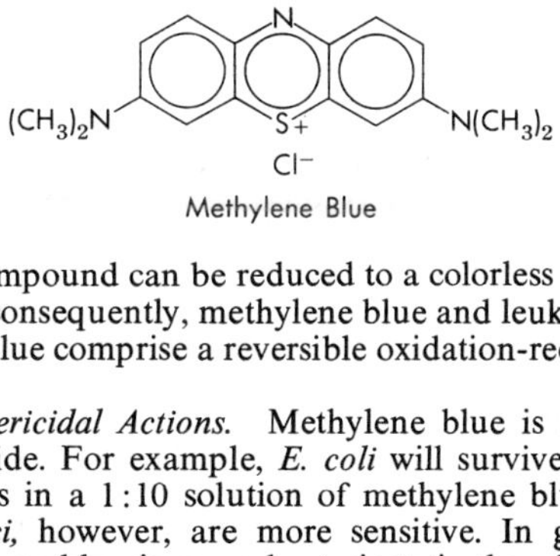

Methylene Blue

The compound can be reduced to a colorless (leuko) form; consequently, methylene blue and leukomethylene blue comprise a reversible oxidation-reduction system.

Bactericidal Actions. Methylene blue is a weak germicide. For example, *E. coli* will survive for 25 minutes in a 1:10 solution of methylene blue. *Micrococci,* however, are more sensitive. In general, methylene blue is more bacteriostatic than bactericidal.

Methemoglobin Formation and Reconversion. Methylene blue has two interesting and opposite actions on hemoglobin. In high concentrations it oxidizes the ferrous iron of reduced hemoglobin to the ferric form, and, as a result, methemoglobin is produced. This action is the basis for the antidotal action of methylene blue in cyanide poisoning. Conversely, *in vivo,* low concentrations of methylene blue or the chemically related thionine are capable of hastening the conversion of methemoglobin to hemoglobin. The reduction of methemoglobin within the intact erythrocyte is accomplished by methemoglobin reductases, which are pyridinenucleotide dependent. Methylene blue can act as an electron acceptor in the transfer of electrons from reduced pyridine nucleotides to methemoglobin. In the reaction, methylene blue is reduced by pyridine nucleotides, and the leukomethylene blue, in turn, reduces methemoglobin to hemoglobin. The dye will not affect methemoglobinemia in persons with glucose-6-phosphate dehydrogenase–deficient erythrocytes. When the formation of reduced pyridine nucleotides is prevented, methylene blue acts purely as an oxidant.

Absorption, Fate, and Excretion. Methylene blue is poorly absorbed from the gastrointestinal tract, and the intravenous toxic dose is much smaller than the oral. In the tissues, methylene blue is rapidly reduced to the leuko form, which is excreted slowly into the urine and the bile. A portion of the leukomethylene blue may be partially demethylated.

Untoward Reactions. Some batches of methylene blue have caused nausea, vomiting, and diarrhea. This may have been the result of their contamination with arsenic and zinc. The intravenous administration of very large doses of methylene blue (500 mg) causes nausea, abdominal and precordial pain, dizziness, headache, profuse sweating, and mental confusion.

Preparations. Methylene Blue, U.S.P. (*methylthionine chloride*), consists of dark-green crystals that are moderately soluble in water and alcohol and form deep-blue solutions. The compound is marketed in the powder form and in aqueous solution in ampuls. For oral administration, the dye is conveniently given in capsules or coated tablets.

Therapeutic Uses. Methylene blue was formerly used as a urinary tract antiseptic but has been replaced by more effective compounds. The uses of methylene blue as an analgesic, antipyretic, and parasiticide have been abandoned. It is of some value as an antidote in cyanide poisoning but is inferior to other drugs. There is no rationale for the use of methylene blue in carbon monoxide poisoning, for which unfortunately it has been recommended and employed. Methylene blue is valuable in the treatment of methemoglobinemia. For *idiopathic methemoglobinemia,* it is given orally in the daily dose of 300 mg in conjunction with large amounts of ascorbic acid. For acute, drug-induced methemoglobinemia, 1 to 2 mg/kg of *Methylene Blue Injection,* U.S.P., can be given intravenously.

Fluorescein. Fluorescein is used medically as the sodium salt, *Fluorescein Sodium,* U.S.P. It has the following structural formula:

Fluorescein Sodium

In aqueous solution it is red but has a green fluorescence that is maximal at the ultraviolet wavelength of 3600Å. *Fluorescein sodium ophthalmic solution* contains 2% of the dye and a suitable antibacterial agent. *Fluorescein Sodium Ophthalmic Strip,* U.S.P.

(FLUOR-I-STRIP), which contains 600 µg of fluorescein sodium, is moistened with sterile water and applied to the conjunctiva.

Fluorescein is devoid of antiseptic properties. Its diagnostic usefulness rests upon its fluorescence. It appears readily in the extracellular fluid and gains access only to viable cells.

The clinical application of fluorescein was originally limited to the field of ophthalmology. When dye in solution or from the strip is applied to the cornea, only portions deprived of epithelium are stained. Ulcerated areas are stained green, foreign bodies are surrounded by a green ring, and loss of substance in the conjunctiva is indicated by a yellow stain.

Fluorescein is now sometimes used for the determination of circulation time, adequacy of blood supply, and viability of tissue. In the determination of circulation time, 500 mg of *Fluorescein Sodium Injection,* U.S.P. (FLUORESCITE), as a 10% solution (for children, 15.4 mg/kg as a 5% solution) is given by rapid intravenous injection. The appearance of fluorescence in the lips, eyes, or intact skin or in wheals (histamine or scratch) raised on any portion of the skin is taken as the end point. Arm-to-lip, arm-to-arm, and arm-to-leg end points may be taken in sequence; the relative circulation times can be of diagnostic importance. The *adequacy of the circulation* to an extremity can also be determined accurately. Acute embolism can be diagnosed immediately, and the role of reflex vasospasm can be assessed by appropriate nerve block. In peripheral vascular disease, the extent and the degree of vascular insufficiency as well as the appropriate level for amputation can be determined by raising a series of wheals and comparing the intensity of fluorescence. In abdominal surgery, the *viability of a strangulated intestine* can be ascertained by the presence of fluorescence, inasmuch as dead cells do not take up the dye. The necessity and extent of resection can thereby be rapidly determined.

Practically no untoward effects accompany the intravenous administration of fluorescein. An occasional patient may experience nausea and vomiting. Fluorescence of the skin persists for several hours, and the dye appears in the urine for as long as 30 hours. Injections may be repeated at intervals of several days without ill effects.

Miscellaneous Dyes. *Aminacrine hydrochloride* exerts germicidal actions against both gram-positive and gram-negative bacteria and against fungi and trichomonads. It is not inactivated by pus, secretions, or body fluids. In the treatment of *vaginal candidiasis, trichomoniasis,* or *Haemophilus infections* it is employed as a 0.1% powder or 0.2% cream, jelly, or suppository. It is also used as a 2% cream for application to the skin.

Sulfobromophthalein Sodium, U.S.P. (*bromsulphalein, BSP*), is available as the disodium salt and used for the determination of hepatic function. *Sulfobromophthalein Sodium Injection,* U.S.P., a 5% solution, is injected intravenously in the dose of 2 to 5 mg/kg of body weight. The dye content of the alkalinized serum is determined 30 minutes later. The normal liver excretes most of the dye within 30 minutes. Anaphylactoid reactions to the dye, occasionally fatal, have been reported (*see* Venger, 1961). Venous induration is frequently associated with the intravenous administration of sulfobromophthalein (Schneider, 1965).

Phenolsulfonphthalein, N.F. (*phenol red, PSP*), is available as the monosodium salt. It is excreted mostly by tubular secretion and is used in the testing of renal function. A 6-mg amount of the dye is given by intramuscular or intravenous injection. The urine is collected at suitable intervals, and the dye content of the voided samples is determined. The normally functioning kidney excretes the dye at approximately the following rate: intravenous administration—35 to 45% in 15 minutes, 50 to 60% in 30 minutes, 65 to 80% in 60 minutes; intramuscular administration—60 to 80% in 120 minutes. Renal insufficiency is evidenced by a failure to excrete the dye at the cited rate. Inasmuch as some of the dye is excreted in the bile, supranormal values are suggestive of hepatic insufficiency.

Evans Blue, U.S.P., is used for diagnostic purposes. After intravenous injection, it is confined to the plasma. From the amount given and the equilibrium plasma concentration, the plasma volume may be calculated.

Scarlet red is used not as an antiseptic but as a wound-healing agent. It probably stimulates tissue proliferation and is used in the treatment of burns, wounds, chronic ulcers, and bedsores. The dye is usually employed in the form of ointments or oily solutions (4 to 8%). There is no unanimity of opinion as to its effectiveness.

MISCELLANEOUS GERMICIDES

Sulfur and Thiosulfates. Sulfur has a long history in medicine. The practice of burning sulfur for the purification of the air is mentioned in the *Odyssey.* Hippocrates considered sulfur an effective antidote against plague. For the layman, sulfur has an undeserved reputation as an intestinal antiseptic, and the practice of an annual "spring cleansing" of the intestinal tract with sulfur and molasses was once prevalent. The legitimate medical uses of sulfur preparations are as fungicides and parasiticides and for the treatment of various cutaneous disorders.

Sulfur must be converted to pentathionic acid ($H_2S_5O_6$) in order to exert germicidal action. Presumably the oxidation of sulfur to pentathionic acid is accomplished by certain microorganisms or by epidermal cells when the element is applied to the skin. Sulfur possesses a keratolytic property, which may be the basis for the therapeutic action of the element in certain cutaneous disorders unassociated with infection.

Sulfur has few outstanding systemic actions. When given orally, it may be partially converted to sulfide, and this is sufficiently stimulating to the intestinal tract to exert a cathartic action. Absorbed sulfide is excreted as sulfate. In certain rare individuals, the absorption of sulfide from the intestine is thought to be associated with the occurrence of episodes of intermittent *enterogenous cyanosis* caused by sulfhemoglobinemia.

Sublimed Sulfur, N.F. (*flowers of sulfur*), is a fine, yellow crystalline, water-insoluble powder. *Precipitated Sulfur,* U.S.P., is a much finer powder and, therefore, has a greater reactive surface than sublimed sulfur. *Colloidal sulfur* has no official status; it is the most active form of sulfur and consists of elemental sulfur in stable aqueous colloidal solutions. The only official ointment of sulfur is *Sulfur Ointment,* U.S.P., which contains 10% precipitated sulfur.

Sulfur is used as a fungicide and parasiticide (*see* below). Sulfur alone, or in combination with other keratolytic agents (often 2% salicylic acid), is widely used in the treatment of cutaneous disorders such as *psoriasis, seborrhea, eczema-dermatitis,* and *lupus erythematosus.* The percentage of sulfur employed may be that of the full-strength ointment, or less if the patient's skin exhibits intolerance. Prolonged local use of sulfur may result in a characteristic dermatitis venenata. Colloidal sulfur has been employed both locally and systemically. Solutions of colloidal sulfur were once administered parenterally in the treatment of a number of diseases, especially arthritis, but were of no proven value in this disease. Furthermore, solutions of colloidal sulfur administered parenterally may cause fever, malaise, severe headache, fatigue, drowsiness, and a temporary increase in joint pain.

Thiosulfates readily generate free sulfur, especially in acidic solution. The pH of the skin is usually low enough to favor a slow release of elemental sulfur, and bacteria also favor the conversion. *White Lotion,* N.F., contains sulfurated potash, which is a complex polysulfide and thiosulfate. *Sodium Thiosulfate,* U.S.P., is intended for parenteral use in the treatment of cyanide poisoning, but it may be applied to the skin in various forms. Cutaneous infections caused by *Staph. aureus* and *Staph. epidermidis* may respond to concentrations as low as 0.5%. Concentrations of 2 to 8% are used to treat acne; they are also antifungal. Wetting of the skin with vinegar increases the activity.

Sulfur Dioxide. Sulfur dioxide has no medical uses, but it is in the U.S.P. as a pharmaceutical necessity. The compound was once popular as a fumigant. It is currently of great environmental interest. Man does not show a respiratory response (bronchoconstriction) until the concentration is close to 5 ppm in air. However, SO_2 is converted to SO_3 and H_2SO_4 in the atmosphere, and it is these products that probably constitute the main threat to the health of man. The report by Alarie and associates (1973) cites several pertinent reviews.

Ichthammol. *Ichthammol,* N.F. (*ammonium ichthosulfonate*), is the product obtained from sulfonating and neutralizing with ammonia, the distillate of certain bituminous schists. The compound contains approximately 10% sulfur in the form of organic sulfonates. It is a brown, viscous fluid with a strong characteristic odor and is soluble in both aqueous and organic solvents. Ichthammol is mildly irritant and somewhat antiseptic. It is used alone, or in combination with other antiseptics, for the treatment of cutaneous disorders such as *psoriasis* and *lupus* *erythematosus* and to promote healing in chronic inflammations. The drug is commonly employed in the form of *Ichthammol Ointment,* N.F. (10% in a petrolatum base). At one time the drug was used widely, but it has deservedly lost much popularity.

Anthralin. *Anthralin,* U.S.P. (1,8,9-anthratriol), is a mild irritant with weak antimicrobial activity. The compound is employed in the treatment of *psoriasis* and *chronic dermatoses.* Anthralin is available as *Anthralin Ointment,* U.S.P., and in proprietary creams or ointments in concentrations of 0.1 to 1.0%. The weakest preparation is first employed, and the strength is then increased according to the tolerance of the patient. Weigand and Everett (1967) found that anthralin was quite effective in cases of psoriasis that had not responded to other treatment. It should be kept away from the eyes and other sensitive surfaces. Anthralin will stain the skin yellow.

Salicylanilides and Carbanilides. *Dibromsalen* and *tribromsalen* are brominated derivatives of salicylanilide. *Chloflucarban* is a polychlorofluoro derivative and *trichlocarban* a trichloro derivative of carbanilide. They are antibacterial and antifungal. Their principal use is in deodorant soaps, for which they appear to be effective. Claims that such soaps reduce the incidence of cutaneous infections require substantiation. All these drugs can cause occasional hypersensitivity; the salicylanilides, especially, may cause photosensitization (*see* Ison and Tucker, 1968).

Ethylene Oxide. Ethylene oxide is a gaseous alkylating germicide with a broad spectrum of activity. It is sporicidal and virucidal. It is used to disinfect and sterilize heat-labile surgical instruments. It alkylates tissue constituents and is thus toxic. Inhalation causes nausea, vomiting, neurological disorders, and even death. Traces of the gas in gloves or clothing may cause burns. Residues in vascular catheters can cause thrombophlebitis; in endotracheal tubes, tracheitis. The gas is explosive in concentrations above 3% and must be mixed with CO_2 or fluorocarbons. The optimal humidity is 30 to 40%. An exposure of 3 hours is used to guarantee killing of desiccated spores. For further information, *see* Boucher (1972).

URINARY TRACT ANTISEPTICS

Several antibacterial drugs cannot be used to treat systemic infections because effective plasma concentrations are not achieved with safe doses. However, because they are concentrated in the renal tubules and can back-diffuse into the renal parenchyma, they can be used to treat urinary tract infections. Furthermore, effective antibacterial concentrations reach the renal pelves and the bladder. Treatment with such drugs can be thought of as local therapy in that only in the kidney and bladder, with the rare exceptions mentioned below, are adequate thera-

peutic levels achieved. The drugs have therefore become known as urinary tract antiseptics.

Methenamine. Methenamine is a urinary tract antiseptic that owes its activity to formaldehyde.

Chemistry. Methenamine is hexamethylenetetramine (hexamethyleneamine). It has the following structure:

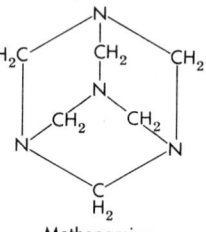

Methenamine

The compound decomposes in water to generate formaldehyde, according to the following reaction:

$$N_4(CH_2)_6 + 6H_2O + 4H^+ \rightleftharpoons 4NH_4^+ + 6HCHO$$

At pH 7.4 almost no decomposition occurs; however, 6% of the theoretical amount of formaldehyde is yielded at pH 6 and 20% at pH 5. Thus, acidification of the urine promotes the formaldehyde-dependent antibacterial action.

Pharmacology and Toxicity. Methenamine is absorbed orally, but 10 to 30% decomposes in the gastric juice unless the drug is protected by an enteric coating. Because of the ammonia produced, methenamine is contraindicated in hepatic insufficiency. So little methenamine decomposes in the blood and tissues that it is virtually nontoxic systemically. Excretion into the urine is nearly quantitative. When the urine pH is 6 and the daily urine volume is 1000 to 1500 ml, a daily dose of 2 g will yield a concentration of 18 to 60 $\mu g/ml$ of formaldehyde; this is more than 20 times the minimal inhibitory concentration for most urinary tract pathogens. Some of the formaldehyde is bound to substances in the urine and in the surrounding tissues, so that daily doses below 0.5 g may not yield much free formaldehyde.

Various poorly metabolized acids can be used to acidify the urine. Low pH alone is bacteriostatic, so that acidification serves a double function. The acids commonly used are mandelic acid, hippuric acid, ascorbic acid, sodium biphosphate, and acid-producing foods such as cranberry juice. Both mandelic and hippuric acids are bacteriostatic *in vitro* beyond their effect on pH, but whether they are superior to acidification alone *in vivo* has not been well established.

Gastrointestinal distress frequently is caused by doses greater than 500 mg four times a day, even with enteric-coated tablets. Bladder irritation, painful and frequent micturition, albuminuria, hematuria, and various rashes may result from doses of 4 to 8 g a day given for longer than 3 to 4 weeks. Once the urine is sterile, a high dose should be reduced. Because systemic methenamine is nontoxic, renal insufficiency is no contraindication to methenamine alone, but the acids may be detrimental. Methenamine mandelate is contraindicated in renal insufficiency. Crystalluria from the mandelate moiety can occur. Methenamine combines with sulfamethizole (Lipton, 1963) and perhaps other sulfonamides in the urine, which results in mutual antagonism.

Preparations and Dosage. Methenamine, N.F., is given as tablets in a dose of 0.5 to 2 (usually 1) g, four times a day. *Methenamine Mandelate,* U.S.P. (MANDELAMINE), is given in an oral suspension or as tablets in the same dose as for methenamine, even though the methenamine equivalence is less. *Methenamine hippurate* (HIPREX) is usually given in a dose of 1 g, twice a day. The recommended dose of *Methenamine and Sodium Biphosphate Tablets,* N.F., 300 mg four times a day, cannot be considered to yield activity equivalent to the usual doses of the other preparations.

Therapeutic Uses and Status. Methenamine is not a primary drug for the treatment of acute urinary tract infections, but it is of value for chronic suppressive treatment. The agent is most useful when the causative organism is *E. coli,* but it can usually suppress the common gram-negative offenders and often *Staph. aureus* and *Staph. epidermidis* as well. *Enterobacter aerogenes* and *Proteus vulgaris* are usually resistant. Urea-splitting bacteria (mostly *Proteus*) make it difficult to control the urine pH. The physician should strive to keep the pH below 5.5. Patient compliance is poor because of the number of pills required with many products. Methenamine is sometimes employed prophylactically in urinary tract instrumentation and catheterization.

Nalidixic Acid. Nalidixic acid has the following chemical structure:

Nalidixic Acid

Pharmacology and Toxicity. Nalidixic acid is bactericidal to most of the common gram-negative bacteria that cause urinary tract infections. It appears to act by inhibiting DNA synthesis. Brumfitt and Pursell (1971) reported that 99% of strains of *E. coli,* 98% of *Proteus mirabilis* and 75 to 97% of other *Proteus* species, 92% of *Klebsiella-Enterobacter,* and 80% of other coliform bacteria are sensitive to the drug. *Pseudomonas* species are resistant. Some strains of *Salmonella* and *Shigella* are also sensitive. Acquired resistance to the drug occurs, but it does not seem to be transferable (*see* Chapter 55).

Approximately 96% of orally administered nalidixic acid is absorbed. Plasma concentrations of 20 to 50 μg/ml may be achieved, but the acid is 93 to 97% bound to plasma proteins. In the body some nalidixic acid is converted to an active hydroxynalidixic acid, and both are excreted into the urine. Most of the drug is conjugated in the liver. The plasma half-life is normally about 8 hours, but it may be as long as 21 hours in the presence of renal failure.

Oral nalidixic acid is usually well tolerated, but nausea, vomiting, and abdominal pain may occur. Allergic reactions such as pruritus, urticaria, various rashes, photosensitivity, eosinophilia, and fever occasionally occur, and cholestasis, thrombocytopenia, leukopenia, and hemolytic anemia rarely occur. Liver function tests and blood-cell counts are advisable if treatment lasts longer than 2 weeks. Effects on the CNS, such as headache, drowsiness, malaise, vertigo, visual disturbances, asthenia, and myalgia, are experienced infrequently. In patients with cerebral vascular insufficiency, parkinsonism, or epilepsy, or in normal children given excessive doses, convulsions occur, perhaps as the result of intracranial hypertension (*see* Boréus and Sundström, 1967). The presence of the drug results in false-positive responses in some urine glucose tests. Nitrofurantoin interferes with the therapeutic action of nalidixic acid.

Therapeutic Uses, Preparations, and Dosage. In the United States, nalidixic acid is approved only for the treatment of urinary tract infections caused by susceptible microorganisms (*see* above). The effectiveness against indole-positive *Proteus* is especially important. Apparent cures are achieved in 30 to 50% of uncomplicated urinary tract infections. Failures in men may be, in part, the result of reinfection from the prostate gland, which is not penetrated. Whether nalidixic acid can effectively penetrate the renal medulla and be of direct value in the treatment of pyelonephritis is uncertain. Rapid development of bacterial resistance has been reported in a widely varying percentage of cases, but 25% is the approximate incidence. Some apparent resistance is an artifact of testing. Oddly, the incidence of nalidixic acid–resistant bacteria in a given community does not seem to rise (*see* Brumfitt and Pursell, 1971).

The use of oral nalidixic acid in the treatment of systemic infections is not usually advised, even when sensitivity testing and blood concentrations seem favorable. However, brucellosis has been successfully managed with oral nalidixic acid. The drug has been given intravenously to treat gram-negative septicemias. Despite the high sensitivity of *E. coli,* Zinsser (1970) found that only half of systemic *E. coli* infections responded to intravenous nalidixic acid. The drug eliminates *Shigella* from the stools less rapidly than does ampicillin and does not significantly affect the course of the disease (*see* Haltalin et al., 1973).

Nalidixic Acid, N.F. (NEGGRAM), is available as *Nalidixic Acid Tablets,* N.F., containing 250 or 500 mg of the drug. The recommended dose for adults is 1 g, four times a day for 1 to 2 weeks; thereafter a daily dose of 2 g is suggested. The recommended daily dose for children is 55 mg/kg of body weight. The drug should not be used in infants under 3 months of age.

Nitrofurantoin. The structure of nitrofurantoin is shown on page 1002. Nitrofurantoin is active against many strains of the common urinary tract pathogens, *E. coli, Proteus* species, *Pseudomonas, Klebsiella, Enterobacter,* and staphylococci, as well as enterococci, streptococci, clostridia, and *Bacillus subtilis.* However, *Proteus, Pseudomonas,* and *Alcaligenes* species are more often resistant than sensitive. Nitrofurantoin is bacteriostatic at concentrations of 5 to 10 μg/ml and bactericidal at 100 μg/ml, but it is not known whether a bactericidal action occurs *in vivo.* The antibacterial activity is higher in an acidic urine.

The compound is rapidly and completely absorbed from the gastrointestinal tract. Antibacterial plasma concentrations are not achieved by recommended doses, because the drug is rapidly eliminated. The plasma half-life is 0.3 to 1 hour. The amount excreted unchanged into the urine is about 40%. The average dose of nitrofurantoin yields a urine concentration of approximately 0.2 mg/ml. This amount is soluble at pH values above 5, but the urine should not be alkalinized; supersaturated solutions of nitrofurantoin do not cause crystalluria. The rate of excretion is linearly related to the creatinine clearance (Sachs et al., 1968), so that in patients with impaired glomerular function the efficacy of the drug may be decreased and the systemic toxicity increased. Nitrofurantoin colors the urine brown.

The most common untoward effects are *nausea, vomiting,* and *diarrhea.* The incidence is less if the drug is administered with milk or other food or is used in a smaller dosage. However, the same effects are sometimes seen after intravenous administration. Various *hypersensitivity reactions* occasionally occur. They may involve the skin, blood, liver, or lungs. They include *chills, fever, leukopenia, granulocytopenia, hemolytic anemia* (when glucose-6-phosphate dehydrogenase deficiency exists in the erythrocyte), *cholestatic jaundice,* and *hepatocellular damage. Allergic pneumonitis* has been observed (*see* DeMasi, 1967; Strauss and Griffin, 1967); it usually resolves within hours after discontinuation of the drug. *Interstitial pulmonary fibrosis* can occur in patients on chronic medication. Elderly patients are especially susceptible to the pulmonary toxicity of nitrofurantoin. Megaloblastic anemia is rare. Various *neurological disorders* are occasionally observed. Headache, vertigo, drowsiness, muscular aches, and nystagmus are readily reversible, but severe *polyneuropathies* with demyelination and degeneration of both sensory and motor nerves have been reported (*see* Roelsen, 1964); signs of denervation and muscle atrophy result. Neuropathies are most likely to occur in patients with impaired renal function and in persons on long-continued treatment. However, Lindholm (1967) has detected electromyographic signs of muscle denervation in 62% of nonuremic patients receiving chronic nitrofurantoin therapy. Nitrofurantoin-induced polyneuropathy has been reviewed by Toole and Parrish (1973).

Nitrofurantoin, U.S.P. (FURADANTIN), is available as *Nitrofurantoin Oral Suspension,* U.S.P., and *Nitrofurantoin Tablets,* U.S.P. The oral adult dose is 50 mg four times a day, with meals and at bedtime, for infections caused by sensitive microorganisms and twice this dose if the microorganisms are relatively resistant. Alternatively, the daily dose is better expressed as 5 to 10 mg/kg in four divided doses.

Bailey and associates (1971) have reported that a single 50- to 100-mg dose at nighttime is sufficient to prevent recurrences. The daily dose for children is 5 to 7 mg/kg, but it may be as low as 2 mg/kg in long-term therapy. A course of therapy should not exceed 14 days, and repeated courses should be separated by rest periods. The incidence of nausea may be lower if the drug is given in the macrocrystalline form (MACRODANTIN). *Nitrofurantoin sodium for injection* is administered intravenously or intramuscularly in daily doses of 360 mg, in two to four divided doses; 720 mg has been successfully given, but the risk of toxicity is considerably increased. Intramuscular injection is painful. For patients who are older than 12 years but who weigh less than 55 kg (120 lb), the daily dose is 6 mg/kg, in two to four divided doses.

Nitrofurantoin is approved only for the treatment of urinary tract infections caused by any of the microorganisms listed above that are sensitive to the drug, but it is not usually as effective as several antibiotics or sulfonamides in the eradication of infections. It is about 50% effective in preventing recurrences. Nitrofurantoin antagonizes the action of nalidixic acid. Injection of nitrofurantoin sodium is indicated only for use in acutely ill patients who cannot tolerate oral nitrofurantoin. Large parenteral doses have been used in treating certain postoperative infections (Rickles, 1965), but such use is only experimental. Pregnancy, impaired renal function (creatinine clearance less than 40 ml per minute), and an age below 3 months are contraindications to the use of nitrofurantoin.

Miscellaneous Urinary Tract Antiseptics. *Mandelic Acid.* This acid is no longer prescribed alone as a urinary tract antiseptic; it is used only in combination with methenamine as *Methenamine Mandelate,* U.S.P. (*see* above). The antibacterial spectrum of the acid is much like that of methenamine. Bacterial resistance does not occur. It is excreted in the urine by glomerular filtration. The mandelic acid is sufficient to acidify the urine, except in the presence of urea-splitting bacteria. Mandelic acid crystalluria occasionally occurs.

Hippuric Acid. Hippuric acid closely resembles mandelic acid in its antibacterial actions and is likewise combined with methenamine to form *methenamine hippurate* (*see* above). Adequately controlled comparisons between the mandelate and the hippurate salts have not been made. However, Gerstein and colleagues (1968) reported that methenamine hippurate caused improvement in the majority of 18 patients with chronic urinary tract infections refractory to other agents, including methenamine mandelate. Hippuric acid is secreted into the urine by the renal tubular transport system and is thus well excreted, even when glomerular filtration is compromised.

Phenazopyridine. Phenazopyridine Hydrochloride, N.F. (PYRIDIUM), has been used in the past as a urinary antiseptic. For this purpose it is of little value, but it is frequently employed to advantage as a urinary tract analgesic. Phenazopyridine is supplied as *Phenazopyridine Hydrochloride Tablets,* N.F., containing 100 or 200 mg of the drug for oral administration. The usual dose is 200 mg, three times daily. The compound is an azo dye, and the urine is colored orange or red; the patient should be so informed. Methemoglobinemia is frequently produced by the drug. Rarer but more serious toxic effects include hemolytic anemia (Gabor *et al.,* 1964; Greenberg and Wong, 1964) and jaundice (Hood and Toth, 1966). It can also precipitate in the urine to cause renal stones. Phenazopyridine is also marketed in combination with sulfisoxazole (AZO GANTRISIN) and sulfamethoxazole (AZO GANTANOL).

II. Antifungal Drugs

In temperate climates, fungal infections comprise a minor fraction of human diseases caused by microorganisms. Nevertheless, their incidence is higher than the ordinary practitioner usually appreciates. Tinea pedis is very common, although the afflicted person rarely consults a physician about it. Drugs for the treatment of the superficial fungal infections are mostly sold "over the counter."

The list of chemicals purported to possess antifungal actions is exceedingly long. The conscientious physician has difficulty discerning the truly efficacious ones, and the layman searching for new remedies for such conditions as dermatophytosis finds many preparations available. Underwood and associates (1946) compiled a catalog of 106 different proprietary preparations available in one locality for the self-treatment of dermatophytosis (*tinea pedis*); contained among them were several-score different chemicals. The investigators tested 400 patients and found 40% sensitive to one or more of the chemicals contained in the remedies; in many instances the sensitization was traceable directly to use of these proprietary preparations. The situation has somewhat improved today; yet, despite the existence at the present time of drugs demonstrably beneficial in dermatophytosis, ineffective preparations are widely advertised and widely purchased.

The majority of antibacterial agents possess fungistatic or fungicidal properties. Therefore, many of the drugs discussed under antiseptics and disinfectants have been employed in the local treatment of fungal infections, and their uses in such mycoses have already been noted in some instances. The present discussion will be restricted to non-antibiotic antifungal drugs. Antifungal antibiotics are discussed in Chapter 61. The antifungal agents have been reviewed by Drube (1972).

Methods of Evaluating Antifungal Agents. Testing of chemicals for antifungal activity is more difficult than evaluation of antibacterial activity. Fungi are maintained less easily in artificial media than are bacteria, their growth requires considerable time, and the phases of growth and morphological forms of fungi are vastly more complex than those of bacteria. For these reasons, the methods for evaluating activity of drugs against fungi are less standard and less adequate than are those for estimating antibacterial potency. The details and shortcomings of the present *in-vitro* methods for measuring antifungal activity are given by Czerkowicz and Stuart (1968).

The *in-vitro* methods for testing drugs against organisms that cause superficial mycoses, such as members of the *Microsporum, Trichophyton,* and *Epidermophyton* genera, estimate either fungistatic or fungicidal activity. Tests of fungistatic activity measure the ability of chemicals to prevent growth of fungi in artificial media. The fungicidal tests determine the ability of agents to kill the mycelial mat or suspensions of spores. Tests of fungicidal activity, like the phenol coefficient test for antibacterial agents, therefore give information that is relevant primarily to the destruction of fungi on inanimate objects. Such tests do not take into account certain factors of great importance in the clinical use of the drugs, particularly the ability of the agent to penetrate into the hair, nails, and horny layers of the skin. For this reason antifungal activity of an agent assessed *in vitro* is an unreliable indicator of its clinical value. Many potent fungicides are inefficacious in treating infections.

Test procedures involving cutaneous fungal infections in experimental animals (*see* Molinas, 1955; Dolan *et al.,* 1957) more nearly approximate the conditions that exist in certain human infections but still do not yield data applicable to human patients.

At the present time, the only reliable evidence for the potential effectiveness of antifungal agents against human infections comes from clinical studies. Unfortunately, controlled clinical studies are all too rare. There is lack of unanimity among experienced practitioners as to the agent of choice in a particular infection caused by a specific microorganism. This disagreement is further compounded by the varied responses of individual patients with similar infections and the different growth characteristics and sensitivities of the various pathogenic fungi. Thus, in many instances it is difficult to state that one agent is clearly superior to others in treating a specific condition.

Antifungal antibiotics and other systemic chemotherapeutic agents (*see* Chapter 61) are frequently employed in treating superficial mycotic infections. In some conditions best results are obtained by the combined use of antibiotics and topical antifungal preparations.

Mechanisms of Antifungal Action. Drugs exert fungistatic and fungicidal actions by a variety of mechanisms. The information on this subject has been reviewed by Stewart (1958), Oster and Woodside (1968), and Drouhet (1970). Many agents used in the treatment of superficial mycoses are virtually devoid of either fungistatic or fungicidal actions in the concentrations employed, and their beneficial effects probably depend upon factors not related to any direct effect on fungi. The keratolytic agents exert their effect mainly by promoting desquamation of the stratum corneum, especially in hyperkeratotic locations. The fungus resides in the stratum corneum, where keratin is its substrate, not in the toxin-induced lesion. Thus, keratolysis removes the offending fungus as well as aids in the penetration of drugs. Drugs that prevent hyperhidrosis indirectly retard proliferation of the fungus by altering the conditions of growth. Astringent drugs exert a palliative effect by allaying the symptoms of acute inflammation and irritation.

FATTY ACIDS AND THEIR SALTS

It has long been known that fatty acids and their salts possess antifungal activity. The antifungal activity of sweat is due to the fatty acids contained therein.

Propionates. Sodium and calcium propionates have long been incorporated in bread dough as nontoxic inhibitors of mold growth. *Sodium propionate* is promoted for the treatment of dermatomycoses. It is relatively weak and possesses only fungistatic activity; both *in vitro* and in human infections, viable fungi can be recovered after exposure to it. Sodium propionate is used in proprietary preparations in concentrations of 5 to 10%. It is also compounded with the more active *undecylenic acid* (*see* below). *Caprylic acid* and its salts are similar in actions to sodium propionate and are used for the same medical purposes.

Undecylenic Acid. The antifungal activity of propionic acid prompted study of the actions of other fatty acids on fungi. Undecylenic acid was found to possess the greatest activity among the agents tested in this large family of compounds. Undecylenic acid is 10-undecenoic acid, an 11-carbon, unsaturated compound.

Undecylenic Acid, U.S.P., is a yellow liquid with a characteristic rancid odor. It is primarily a fungistatic agent, although fungicidal activity may be observed with long exposure to high concentrations of the agent. The drug is active against a variety of fungi, including the common pathogens in superficial mycoses. *Zinc Undecylenate,* U.S.P., is a fine white powder that has antifungal properties similar to those of the acid. The two agents are frequently used together; for example, *Compound Undecylenic Acid Ointment,* U.S.P., contains 5% undecylenic acid and 20% zinc undecylenate in a polyethylene glycol base. The zinc provides an astringent action that aids in the reduction of inflammation. Various other dosage forms include undecylenic acid cream, ointment, powder, lotions, and aerosols. *Calcium undecylenate* is also marketed.

Undecylenic acid preparations are employed in the treatment of various *dermatomycoses,* especially *tinea pedis.* Concentrations of the acid as high as 10%, as well as the compound ointment, may be applied to the skin. For use on mucous membranes the concentration of the acid should not exceed 1%. The preparations are usually not irritating to tissue in the stated concentrations, and sensitization to them is uncommon. It is of undoubted benefit in retarding fungus growth in *tinea pedis,* but the infection frequently persists despite intensive treatment with preparations of the acid and the zinc salt. The value of undecylenic acid in *tinea capitis* is questionable, despite some reports of its efficacy. Kligman and Anderson (1951) failed to demonstrate benefit from the agent in treating this condition; furthermore, they were able to recover viable fungi from hairs infected with *Microsporum audouini* after 33 days exposure *in vitro* to an ointment containing 5% undecylenic acid, 20% zinc undecylenate, and 5% salicylanilide.

MICONAZOLE NITRATE

Miconazole is an imidazolinylmethyl derivative of *bis*-(2,4-dichlorobenzyl) ether. It has the following structure:

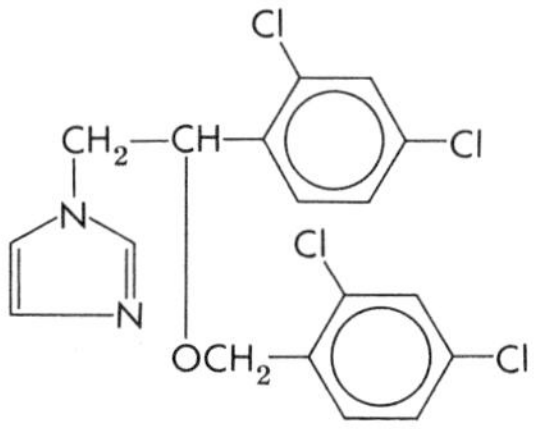

Miconazole

The compound has a broad antifungal spectrum; it is fungicidal to *Trichophyton, Epidermophyton, Microsporum, Candida, Cryptococcus,* and *Aspergillus.*

In the treatment of *tinea pedis,* topical miconazole relieves itching within a few days; vesicles and fissures heal rapidly, but desquamation may continue for several weeks. In one double-blind study in which progress was verified by microscopic examination and cultures (Brugmans *et al.,* 1970), the cure rate was 96%. In the treatment of *tinea cruris,* the drug is comparably effective. *Tinea versicolor, ringworm, onychomycosis,* and *cutaneous candidiasis* have also been reported to respond to topical miconazole. In the treatment of *vulvovaginal candidiasis,* miconazole is considerably superior to nystatin (Proost *et al.,* 1972); pruritus sometimes is relieved after a single application. Some vaginal infections caused by *T. glabratus* also respond.

Miconazole is colorless and odorless. Rarely, burning and maceration follow cutaneous application. Burning, itching, urticaria, headache, and pelvic cramps may occur after intravaginal application, especially during the first week of treatment. However, no such adverse effects were noted among the 194 patients treated by Proost and coworkers (1972). Although the drug penetrates rapidly, only trace amounts can be found in the blood or urine. Miconazole is considered safe for use during pregnancy.

In the United States, *miconazole nitrate* is available as a 2% cream (MICATIN) for use on the skin and nails or as a 2% vaginal cream (MONISTAT). It is applied once or twice daily to the skin for 4 weeks or once daily intravaginally for 14 days. In some countries, it is available in an injectable form for the treatment of systemic mycoses.

TOLNAFTATE

Tolnaftate (TINACTIN) is an excellent topical drug for the treatment of several superficial fungal infections; it is discussed in Chapter 61.

HALOPROGIN

Haloprogin is a halogenated phenolic ether with the following structure:

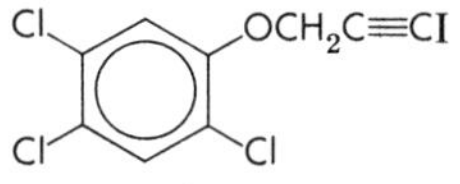

Haloprogin

It is fungicidal to various species of *Epidermophyton, Malassezia, Microsporum,* and *Trichophyton.* During treatment with this drug, irritation, pruritus, burning sensations, vesiculation, increased maceration, and "sensitization" (or exacerbation of the lesion) occasionally occur, especially on the foot if occlusive footgear is worn. It is possible that the sensitization indicates a rapid therapeutic response in which the release of toxins makes the lesion temporarily worse. Photosensitization does not occur. Haloprogin is poorly absorbed through the skin; it is converted to trichlorophenol in the body. The systemic toxicity from topical application appears to be low, but a full evaluation may require years of clinical use. *Haloprogin* (HALOTEX) is available as a 1% cream or solution. It is applied twice a day for 2 to 4 weeks. Its principal use is against *tinea pedis,* for which it appears to be equal in efficacy to tolnaftate; it is also used against *tinea cruris, tinea corporis, tinea manuum,* and *tinea versicolor.* For the results of two double-blind comparative clinical studies, *see* the reports by Hermann (1972) and Katz and Cahn (1972).

BENZOIC ACID AND SALICYLIC ACID

Benzoic and Salicylic Acid Ointment, U.S.P., was long known as *Whitfield's ointment.* It combines the fungistatic action of benzoate with the keratolytic action of salicylate. It contains benzoic acid and salicylic acid in a ratio of 2:1 (usually 6%:3%). It is used mainly in the treatment of *tinea pedis.* Since benzoic acid is only fungistatic, eradication of the infection occurs only after the infected stratum corneum is shed, and continuous medication is required for several weeks to months. The salicylic acid accelerates the desquamation. The ointment is also sometimes used to treat *tinea capitis.* Mild irritation may occur at the site of application.

ACRISORCIN

Acrisorcin, N.F. (AKRINOL), 9-aminoacridinium 4-hexylresorcinolate, is effective against *Malassezia furfur.* Therefore, it is used in the treatment of *tinea versicolor (pityriasis versicolor).* The drug is available as *Acrisorcin Cream,* N.F. (0.2%), and it is applied twice daily to the affected areas; application is continued for 6 weeks after clearing of the lesions. Relapses sometimes occur. Although acrisorcin has mild antibacterial actions, it is not used as an antiseptic. The topical toxicity is low, but it includes production of hives, blisters, and erythematous vesicles. The drug may cause burning sensations when applied to eczematous lesions. Its use may result in photo-induced pruritus. It should be kept away from the eyes.

MISCELLANEOUS ANTIFUNGAL AGENTS

Chlordantoin (SPOROSTACIN) is mainly antifungal against the yeasts, and its use is limited to treatment of *candidiasis* of the skin, nails, buccal mucosa, and vagina. Many such infections fail to respond to the drug. Local irritation and hypersensitivity can occur. It is applied to the vagina as a 1% cream, inserted twice daily for 2 weeks.

Basic fuchsin, a mixture of rosaniline and pararosaniline hydrochlorides, is still marketed in mixtures containing 0.3% basic fuchsin for the treatment of *tinea pedis* and *tinea cruris. Orthochlormercuriphenol* is used as a 0.02% solution, generally in isopropanol, for the treatment of *tinea pedis* and *tinea capitis.* It is also used as a preservative in pharmaceutical and cosmetic products. *Salicylanilide* is used in a 5% ointment for the management of *tinea capitis.* Its efficacy is erratic, and systemic antifungal agents are superior.

Many of the agents discussed in the section on antiseptics and disinfectants are antifungal, and the antimycotic uses of some are mentioned in that section. *Acetic acid* and *aminacrine* require no further discussion. *Gentian violet* (1.35%) is probably used more in the topical treatment of *vaginal candidiasis* than in any other fungal infection. The pure form, *crystal violet,* is used as the *bismuth crystal violet salt* in the treatment of *tinea pedis;* a 1% solution or ointment is applied. The excellent fungicidal properties of *iodine* are usually overlooked. The tincture can be used to treat various dry forms of cutaneous superficial mycoses, and the solution may be applied to wet forms. Various *phenols* (phenol, resorcinol, thymol, chlorothymol, parabens) and the *permanganates* require no further comment. *Sulfur* and the *thiosulfates* still offer useful alternatives to other drugs, and their value in the treatment of the superficial cutaneous mycoses is probably underrated. *Sodium thiosulfate* (2 to 8%) is incorporated into a number of dermatological preparations. Its use in the treatment of *tinea versicolor* is well established, but its value in the treatment of other cutaneous mycoses is largely unexplored. The uses of *selenium sulfide* are described in Chapter 47; its antifungal efficacy is deserving of further study.

Diiodohydroxyquin and *iodochlorhydroxyquin* are incorporated into vaginal preparations to suppress candidal and monilial infections and into dermatological preparations for the treatment of various dermatomycoses and other skin diseases; they are discussed more fully in Chapter 53.

III. Ectoparasiticides

The ectoparasiticides are both ectozoic and ectophytic. In common usage, however, the term *ectoparasiticide* connotes only those drugs that are used against the animal parasites. In the human, these are primarily pediculocides and miticides.

CHLOROPHENOTHANE (DDT)

Chlorophenothane is 1,1,1-trichloro-2,2-*bis*-(*p*-chlorophenyl) ethane. It has the following structure:

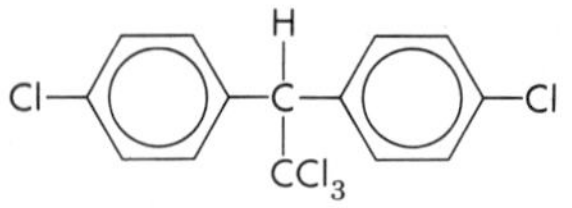

Chlorophenothane (DDT)

It is often improperly called dichlorodiphenyltrichloroethane, from which the term *DDT* is derived. Its insecticidal properties were discovered in Switzerland in 1940, and it was soon used extensively by the armed forces in World War II to control malaria and typhus. Shortly thereafter, it exploded into prominence as an agricultural and household insecticide. Many other polychlorinated hydrocarbons were also introduced as insecticides. For 20 years DDT was used promiscuously in the belief that it was remarkably harmless, but in 1962 it was suddenly realized that DDT was a serious ecological hazard. Subsequently, agricultural and household uses have been severely restricted in the advanced countries. However, medical use is still permitted on a *prescription* basis, and DDT continues to be an important pediculocide.

Insecticidal Action. DDT is toxic to many species of insects and various other arthropods. The LD50 for most insects, when expressed in terms of body weight, differs little from the intravenous LD50 for mammals. However, DDT is as toxic to an insect following topical application as following injection. The high susceptibility of many arthropods to locally applied DDT is due to the ability of the compound to penetrate the chitinous exoskeleton. Nevertheless, certain insects, mites, and ticks are not susceptible to the agent. In addition, acquired resistance to DDT has been observed in most susceptible species, including the human body louse. Resistance results from the selection of naturally occurring resistant mutants.

The primary site of lethal action of DDT in arthropods is on nervous tissue. Studies with arthropod and amphibian axons have shown that the agent acts on the neuronal membrane to render it unstable. DDT combines with lecithin and other phospholipids found in membranes. It also inhibits membrane adenosine triphosphatases. Pertinent references can be found in the report by Bercken (1972).

Pharmacological Effects and Toxicity in Mammals. The approved medical use of DDT is as a pediculocide, so that any effects on the human are classified as side effects or toxicity. Acutely, the only pharmacological effects are toxic ones. Chronically, the effects are subtle and are adverse mainly as they cause drug interactions. However, clinical use has been made of some interactions (*see* below). Accidental acute intoxication with DDT was never frequent; with the present restrictions on the agricultural and household use of DDT, acute intoxication will probably become quite rare. Although the environmental half-life of DDT may possibly measure in decades and body stores of the substance in the population may decline quite slowly, it can be assumed that the importance of the poorly defined problem of chronic toxicity will diminish in the years to come. Consequently, the pharmacological and toxicological effects of DDT will be discussed here only briefly. Various aspects of the pharmacology and toxicology of DDT are reviewed by Hayes (1959, 1969), Symposium (1969), Deichmann and MacDonald (1971), and Deichmann (1972). The most prominent acute actions of DDT in mammals are exerted on the CNS, all portions of which are affected. Signs of stimulation are referable primarily to excitation of supraspinal structures. They include hyperexcitability, tremors, hypothermia, and convulsions. The severity of the convulsions parallels the concentration of DDT in the brain (Dale *et al.,* 1963). The sequence of convulsive manifestations with increasing brain concentrations of DDT consists in tremor, increased reflex excitability, generalized spasms, and tonic-clonic convulsions. After lethal doses, the intervals between convulsions become progressively shorter, and eventually respiration is depressed and death ensues. Sympathetic discharge of central origin accompanies the convulsive episodes. DDT, like other chlorinated hydrocarbons, sensitizes the myocardium to catecholamines so that a sympathoadrenal discharge may cause cardiac arrhythmias, including ventricular fibrillation. Although the central effects of DDT are accompanied by changes in the concentrations of norepinephrine, 5-hydroxytryptamine, and acetylcholine in the brain (*see* Hrdina *et al.,* 1973), such effects are probably secondary to changes in neuronal discharge activity. Significant protection against the central stimulant effects is afforded by central depressants, especially phenobarbital. Animals surviving toxic oral doses of DDT exhibit neuromuscular disturbances for 48 hours or longer. Recovery from toxic intravenous doses is usually complete within 18 hours.

In man, the lethal dose of DDT is sufficiently high that fatal acute poisoning by this agent is not a significant hazard. Nevertheless, deaths have resulted from ingestion of DDT powder, either accidentally or with suicidal intent. The average adult would probably have to ingest 10 to 20 g of DDT in an oily solution to be severely poisoned. This represents several hundred milliliters of the common commercial insecticidal preparations. In such quantities, the vehicle (usually kerosene) would contribute substantially to the toxicity. Deaths have occurred from accidental ingestion of DDT solutions, but the varied symptomatology does not clearly implicate DDT as the major toxic component.

It is generally believed that chronic administration of DDT to experimental animals produces reversible liver damage. Histological changes occur after the daily administration of 10 mg/kg or more over long periods of time. Such doses are much larger than could have occurred through the diet, even at the peak of DDT use, but such chronic exposures conceivably could occur in improperly protected handlers of DDT. The reports on liver damage anteceded knowledge about the cytological changes that accompany the induction of the hepatic microsomal enzyme system. In retrospect, the changes caused by DDT might have been those of hypertrophy of the endoplasmic reticulum, which would explain the ready reversibility and absence of evidences of dysfunction or permanent aftereffects. Induction of microsomal enzymes in animals by DDT has been well documented (for references, *see* Sell and Davison, 1973). In some species of birds it appears that the effect of DDT on shell thickness may be related to increased metabolism of estrogens and thyroid hormones. In other species of birds, DDT appears to inhibit the hepatic metabolism of various substrates, which may possibly relate to changes in breeding habit and population reductions if endogenous hormones are similarly affected. In mammals, DDT and related compounds appear to have estrogenic actions, which may relate to delayed estrous; to decreased libido, fecundity, mammary development, and milk production; and to increased stillbirths and postnatal morbidity, as seen in dogs (Deichmann, 1972). It is generally considered that body burdens of DDT in the general human population are too small to exert such effects, but the potential has not been properly assessed. Hazeltine (1971) adduced evidence that dietary DDT in mothers may reduce plasma bilirubin concentrations in breast-fed infants. DDT has been employed deliberately to accelerate bilirubin metabolism in kernicterus. High does of DDT also accelerate the metabolism of barbiturates, phenylbutazone, antipyrine, and cortisol in man (*see* Conney *et al.,* 1971). The effect of DDT to increase the hepatic metabolism of barbiturates has been used in the treatment of acute barbiturate intoxication (Rappolt, 1973), although there is suspicion that the central stimulant actions of DDT may have been responsible for the rapid recoveries obtained. One can predict confidently that the metabolism of a large number of drugs will ultimately prove to be affected by DDT.

At present, there is little objective evidence that dietary DDT affects human health adversely. In 1956, Hayes and coworkers fed 200 times the then-high average dietary intake of DDT to 35 human volunteers for 18 months; none of the subjects exhibited symptoms that did not have a recognizable cause unrelated to the ingestion of DDT. Clinical and laboratory studies on handlers of DDT, some with 10 to 20 years of exposure, revealed no abnormal incidence of over 50 clinical disorders and no abnormal findings in 33 chemical tests of blood or urine (Laws *et al.,* 1967; Warnick and Carter, 1972). Of interest is the absence of neoplasms in any of these workers; Laws (1971) has reported that DDT suppresses experimental ependymoma in mice. Hypersensitivities, such as dermatitis, anaphylaxis, and fatal periarteritis nodosa and aplastic anemia, have been reported, but they are rare. Whether DDT or other ingredients in commercial mixtures are responsible has never been determined. In a review of the literature, Ercegovich (1973) found no evidence that incidental exposure to DDT adversely affects the immune system in humans.

Absorption, Fate, and Excretion. DDT is slowly and incompletely absorbed from the gastrointestinal tract. As a powder, little is absorbed percutaneously, but in organic solvents appreciable absorption may occur. It can also be absorbed by inhalation, depending upon the particle size.

Absorbed DDT is preferentially distributed to fat. In man, at steady state during chronic administration, the concentration in fat is 10 to 20 times that in liver, over 40 times that in kidney, 70 times that in brain, and 200 times that in plasma. Steady-state concentrations are not reached for 200 to 300 days. Mobilization of fat increases the concentration in plasma and presumably in other tissues. DDT crosses the placenta. It is also excreted into milk.

DDT is dechlorinated by the hepatic microsomal enzyme system to 1,1-dichloro-2,2-*bis*-(*p*-chlorophenyl) ethane (DDD), which is further biotransformed to 2,2-*bis*-(*p*-chlorophenyl) ethane (DDA). A small fraction of the DDD is converted to 1,1-dichloro-2,2-*bis*-(*p*-chlorophenyl) ethene (DDE), which is so avidly retained in the body that tissue concentrations usually exceed those of DDT. Almost no DDT is excreted in the urine. Until steady-state conditions occur, only a tiny fraction of the daily dose of DDT appears in the urine; however, at steady state, 5 to 20% of DDT is excreted as DDA. The fate of the remainder is unknown. DDA excretion has a rapid phase with a half-life of a few days and a slow phase with a half-life that appears to exceed 200 days, which correlates with a biological half-life of DDT of 200 to over 1000 days. The hepatic biotransformation of DDT is accelerated by inducers of the microsomal enzymes, and chronic administration of phenobarbital, phenytoin, and various antianxiety agents and sedatives dramatically lowers the plasma concentrations of both DDT and DDE.

Preparations. *Chlorophenothane* (*DDT*) is used in powder form containing 10% DDT diluted with talc, or as a 0.5 to 2% ointment or emulsion.

Therapeutic Uses. As an ectoparasiticide, DDT is highly effective in the treatment of *pediculosis.* Head lice, body lice, and crab lice are susceptible. For the treatment of head or pubic lice, the powder is rubbed into the hair and allowed to remain for several days. For the treatment of body lice, the underclothes are dusted with the preparation. DDT powder is not irritating to the skin.

DDT is not an effective miticide and therefore should not be employed alone for the treatment of scabies.

GAMMA BENZENE HEXACHLORIDE

Gamma benzene hexachloride is the gamma isomer of hexachlorocyclohexane. It is a white powder that is insoluble in water but soluble in organic solvents.

In insects, gamma benzene hexachloride produces convulsions similar to those caused by DDT, but the onset of action is more rapid. It also produces convulsions in mammals, the toxic dose probably being less than that of DDT. Fatal cases of aplastic anemia have resulted from prolonged exposure to vaporized gamma benzene hexachloride (Loge, 1965). The compound is not readily absorbed through the skin or when taken by mouth.

Gamma benzene hexachloride is an excellent miticide in the treatment of *scabies.* It is employed in 1% concentration in a vanishing cream or lotion. The mixture is applied in a thin layer over the entire cutaneous surface (15 to 25 g for an adult) and is not removed for 24 hours. Pruritus is usually relieved within 24 hours, and the great majority of patients do not require a second treatment. If necessary, however, second and third applications can be made at weekly intervals.

The drug is also a very active pediculocide and is effective in the treatment of *pediculosis pubis, capitis,* and *corporis.* A single application of the 1% ointment or shampoo usually suffices to eradicate the ectoparasite.

Gamma Benzene Hexachloride, U.S.P. (KWELL), is official as a 1% cream or lotion.

MISCELLANEOUS ECTOPARASITICIDES

Benzyl benzoate is a relatively harmless substance that in high concentration is toxic to *Acarus scabiei.* The compound has been widely employed in the treatment of *scabies* and is also useful in the treatment of *pediculosis. Benzyl Benzoate,* U.S.P., is used as a 25% lotion (*Benzyl Benzoate Lotion,* N.F.). In the treatment of *scabies,* the lotion is applied to the entire body, except the face, after thorough cleansing. When the first application is dry, a second coat is applied. After 24 hours, the residue is then washed off.

Pyrethrins are moderately effective as pediculocides. Commercial preparations contain piperonylbutoxide, which enhances the effectiveness by inhibiting enzymatic destruction in the insect. They have been employed as 0.25% aerosols, but the aerosols will probably be discontinued in favor of other dosage forms. Inhaled pyrethrins are detrimental to asthmatics and other persons sensitive to goldenrod pollen; furthermore, the freon vehicle and piperonylbutoxide can cause hepatic neoplasms in mice. Preparations should be kept away from the eyes and mucous membranes. *Malathion* is still employed as a 1% dust, but its use is presently under review and will probably be discontinued. A combination of *tetrahydronaphthalene* and *cupric oleate* is promoted as a pediculocide and niticide, but its true efficacy remains to be determined. *Isobornyl thiocyanoacetate* can eradicate both adult forms and nits of crab, head, and body lice. It is applied as a 5% emulsion, and no more than two applications should be made. The drug is irritant to the eyes and mucous membranes and to the skin of some persons. *Sulfur Ointment,* U.S.P., and other preparations containing sulfur are employed in the treatment of *scabies* and, less frequently, of *pediculosis. Sulfurated lime solution* (16.5% lime, 25% sublimed sulfur) is also used in both types of infestations.

Alarie, Y.; Busey, W. M.; Krumm, A. A.; and Ulrich, C. E. Long-term continuous exposure to sulfuric acid mist in cynomolgus monkeys and guinea pigs. *Archs envir. Hlth,* **1973,** *27,* 16–124.

Bailey, R. R.; Gower, P. E.; Roberts, A. P.; and de Wardener, H. E. Prevention of urinary tract infections with low-dose nitrofurantoin. *Lancet,* **1971,** *3,* 1112–1114.

Bercken, J. van den. The effect of DDT and dieldrin on myelinated nerve fibres. *Eur. J. Pharmac.,* **1972,** *20,* 205–214.

Blatt, R., and Maloney, J. V., Jr. An evaluation of the iodophor compounds as surgical germicides. *Surgery Gynec. Obstet.,* **1961,** *113,* 669–704.

Boréus, L. O., and Sundström, B. Intracranial hypertension in a child during treatment with nalidixic acid. *Br. med. J.,* **1967,** *2,* 744–745.

Brugmans, J. P.; van Cutsem, J. M.; and Thienpont, D. C. Treatment of long-term tinea pedis with miconazole. Double-blind clinical evaluation. *Archs Derm.,* **1970,** *102,* 428–432.

Brumfitt, W., and Pursell, R. Observations on bacterial sensitivities to nalidixic acid and critical comments on the 6-centre survey. *Postgrad. med. J.,* **1971,** *47,* 16–18.

Burke, J. F.; Bondoc, C. C.; and Morris, P. J. Metabolic effects of topical silver nitrate therapy in burns covering more than fifteen percent of the body surface. *Ann. N.Y. Acad. Sci.,* **1968,** *150,* 674–681.

Cronin, E. Formalin textile dermatitis. *Br. J. Derm.,* **1963,** *75,* 267–273.

Crowder, V. H., Jr.; Welsh, J. S.; Bornside, G. H.; and Cohn, I. Bacteriological comparison of hexachlorophene and polyvinylpyrrolidone-iodine surgical scrub soaps. *Am. Surg.,* **1967,** *33,* 906–911.

Dale, W. E.; Gaines, T. B.; Hayes, W. J., Jr.; and Pearce, G. W. Poisoning by DDT: relation between clinical signs and concentration in rat brain. *Science, Wash.,* **1963,** *142,* 1474–1476.

DeMasi, C. J. Allergic pulmonary infiltrates probably due to nitrofurantoin. *Archs intern. Med.,* **1967,** *120,* 631–634.

Dolan, M. M.; Ebelhare, J. S.; Kligman, A. M.; and Bard, R. C. A semi-*in vivo* procedure for testing antifungal agents for topical use. *J. invest. Derm.,* **1957,** *28,* 359–362.

Epstein, S. Paraben sensitivity: subtle trouble. *Ann. Allergy,* **1968,** *26,* 185–189.

Fox, C. L. Silver sulfadiazine—a new topical therapy for *Pseudomonas* in burns. *Archs Surg.,* **1968,** *96,* 184–188.

Gabor, E. P.; Lowenstein, L.; and de Leeuw, N. K. M. Hemolytic anemia induced by phenylazodiaminopyridine (PYRIDIUM). *Can. med. Ass. J.,* **1964,** *91,* 756–759.

Gerstein, A. R.; Okun, R.; Gonick, H. C.; Wilner, H. I.; Kleeman, C. R.; and Maxwell, M. H. The prolonged use of methenamine hippurate in the treatment of urinary tract infection. *J. Urol.,* **1968,** *100,* 767–771.

Gravens, D. L.; Butcher, H. R., Jr.; Ballinger, W. F.; and Dewar, N. F. Septisol antiseptic foam for hands of operating room personnel: an effective antibacterial agent. *Surgery, St. Louis,* **1973,** *73,* 360–367.

Greenberg, M. S., and Wong, H. Methemoglobinemia and Heinz body hemolytic anemia due to phenazopyridine hydrochloride. *New Engl. J. Med.,* **1964,** *271,* 431–435.

Haltalin, K. C.; Nelson, J. D.; and Kusmiesz, H. T. Comparative efficacy of nalidixic acid and ampicillin for severe shigellosis. *Archs Dis. Childh.,* **1973,** *48,* 305–312.

Hayes, W. J., Jr.; Durham, W. F.; and Cueto, C., Jr. The effect of known repeated oral doses of chlorophenothane (DDT) in man. *J. Am. med. Ass.,* **1956,** *162,* 890–897.

Hazeltine, W. DDT and juvenile jaundice. *Clin. Toxicol.,* **1971,** *4,* 55–61.

Hermann, H. W. Clinical efficacy studies of haloprogin, a new topical antimicrobial agent. *Archs Derm.,* **1972,** *106,* 839–842.

Hood, J. W., and Toth, W. N. Jaundice caused by phenazopyridine hydrochloride. *J. Am. med. Ass.,* **1966,** *198,* 116–117.

Hrdina, P. D.; Singhal, R. L.; Peters, D. A. V.; and Ling, G. M. Some neurochemical alterations during acute DDT poisoning. *Toxicol. appl. Pharmac.,* **1973,** *25,* 276–288.

Ison, A. E., and Tucker, J. B. Photosensitive dermatitis from soaps. *New Engl. J. Med.,* **1968,** *278,* 81–84.

Katz, R., and Cahn, B. Haloprogin therapy for dermatophyte infections. *Archs Derm.,* **1972,** *106,* 837–838.

King, T. C., and Price, P. B. An evaluation of iodophors as skin antiseptics. *Surgery Gynec. Obstet.,* **1963,** *116,* 361–365.

King, T. C., and Zimmerman, J. M. Skin degerming practices: chaos and confusion. *Am. J. Surg.,* **1965,** *109,* 695–698.

Kligman, A. M., and Anderson, W. W. Evaluation of current methods for the local treatment of tinea capitis. *J. invest. Derm.,* **1951,** *16,* 155–168.

Kundsin, R. B., and Walter, C. W. Investigations on absorption of Benzalkonium Chloride U.S.P. by skin, gloves, and sponges. *A.M.A. Archs Surg.,* **1957,** *75,* 1036–1042.

————. The surgical scrub—practical consideration. *Archs Surg.,* **1973,** *107,* 75–77.

Lawrence, C. A. Definition of terms. In, *Disinfection, Sterilization, and Preservation.* (Lawrence, C. A., and Block, S. S., eds.) Lea & Febiger, Philadelphia, **1968a,** pp. 9–10.

Laws, E. R., Jr. Evidence of antitumorigenic effects of DDT. *Archs envir. Hlth,* **1971,** *23,* 181–184.

Laws, E. R., Jr.; Curley, A.; and Biros, F. J. Men with intensive exposure to DDT: a clinical and chemical study. *Archs envir. Hlth,* **1967,** *15,* 766–775.

Lee, J. C., and Fialkow, P. J. Benzalkonium chloride—source of hospital infection with gram-negative bacteria. *J. Am. med. Ass.,* **1961,** *177,* 708–710.

Lindholm, T. Electromyographic changes after nitrofurantoin (FURADANTIN) therapy in nonuremic patients. *Neurology, Minneap.,* **1967,** *17,* 1017–1020.

Lipton, J. H. Incompatibility between sulfamethizole and methenamine mandelate. *New Engl. J. Med.,* **1963,** *268,* 92–93.

Lister, J. On a new method of treating compound fractures, abscesses, etc. *Lancet,* **1867a,** *1,* 326–329.

————. On the antiseptic principle in the practice of surgery. *Ibid.,* **1867b,** *2,* 353–356.

Loge, J. P. Aplastic anemia following exposure to benzene hexachloride (lindane). *J. Am. med. Ass.,* **1965,** *193,* 110–114.

Malizia, W. F.; Gangarosa, E. J.; and Goley, A. F. Benzalkonium chloride as a source of infection. *New Engl. J. Med.,* **1960,** *263,* 800–802.

Mathews, K. P. Immediate type hypersensitivity to phenylmercuric compounds. *Am. J. Med.,* **1968,** *44,* 310–318.

Molinas, S. *In vivo* screening of antifungal ointments. *J. invest. Derm.,* **1955,** *25,* 33–42.

Plotkin, S. A., and Austrian, R. Bacteremia caused by *Pseudomonas sp.* following the use of materials stored in solutions of a cationic surface-active agent. *Am. J. med. Sci.,* **1958,** *235,* 621–627.

Powell, M. B.; Swarner, O.; and Lampert, P. Hexachlorophene myelinopathy in premature infants. *J. Pediat.,* **1973,** *82,* 976–981.

Proost, J. M.; Maes-Dockx, F. M.; Nelis, M. O.; and van Cutsem, J. M. Miconazole in the treatment of mycotic vulvovaginitis. *Am. J. Obstet. Gynec.,* **1972,** *112,* 688–692.

Rappolt, R. T., Sr. Use of oral DDT in three human barbiturate intoxications: hepatic enzyme inductions by reciprocal detoxicants. *Clin. Toxicol.,* **1973,** *6,* 147–151.

Rickles, J. A. Nitrofurantoin sodium as a systemic antibacterial in surgical patients. Part I. Therapeutic series. *J. int. Coll. Surg.,* **1965,** *43,* 371–378.

Rideal, S., and Walker, J. T. A. Standardization of disinfectants. *Jl R. sanit. Inst.,* **1903,** *24,* 424–441.

Roelsen, R. Polyneuritis after nitrofurantoin (FURADANTIN) therapy: a survey and report of two new cases. *Acta med. scand.,* **1964,** *175,* 145–154.

Sachs, J.; Geer, T.; Noell, P.; and Kunin, C. M. Effect of renal function on urinary recovery of orally administered nitrofurantoin. *New Engl. J. Med.,* **1968,** *278,* 1032–1035.

Schneider, E. M. Venous abnormalities following intravenous sodium sulfobromophthalein administration. *J. Am. med. Ass.,* **1965,** *194,* 339–342.

Schorr, W. F. Paraben allergy: a cause of intractable dermatitis. *J. Am. med. Ass.,* **1968,** *204,* 107–110.

Serjeant, G. R.; Galloway, R. E.; and Gueri, M. C. Oral zinc sulfate in sickle-cell ulcers. *Lancet,* **1970,** *3,* 891–893.

Seymour, W. B., Jr. Poisoning from cutaneous application of iodine: rare aspect of its toxicologic properties. *Archs intern. Med.,* **1937,** *59,* 952–966.

Skipworth, G. B.; Goldstein, N.; and McBride, W. P. Boric acid intoxication from "medicated talcum powder." *Archs Derm.,* **1967,** *95,* 83–86.

Smith, C. R. Mycobactericidal agents. In, *Disinfection, Sterilization, and Preservation.* (Lawrence, C. A., and Block, S. S., eds.) Lea & Febiger, Philadelphia, **1968,** pp. 504–514.

Stewart, G. T. The mode of action of anti-fungal drugs. In, *Fungous Diseases and Their Treatment.* (Riddell, R. W., and Stewart, G. T., eds.) Butterworth & Co., Ltd., London, **1958,** pp. 183–191.

Strauss, W. G., and Griffin, L. M. Nitrofurantoin pneumonia. *J. Am. med. Ass.,* **1967,** *199,* 765–766.

Toole, J. F., and Parrish, M. L. Nitrofurantoin polyneuropathy. *Neurology, Minneap.,* **1973,** *23,* 554–559.

Underwood, G. B.; Gaul, L. E.; Collins, E.; and Mosby, M. Overtreatment dermatitis of the feet. *J. Am. med. Ass.,* **1946,** *130,* 249–256.

Valdes-Dapena, M. A., and Arey, J. B. Boric acid poisoning: three fatal cases with pancreatic inclusions and a review of the literature. *J. Pediat.,* **1962,** *61,* 531–546.

Venger, N. Fatal reaction to sulfobromophthalein sodium in a patient with bronchial asthma. *J. Am. med. Ass.,* **1961,** *175,* 506–508.

Warnick, S. L., and Carter, J. E. Some findings in a study of workers occupationally exposed to pesticides. *Archs envir. Hlth,* **1972,** *25,* 265–270.

Weigand, D. A., and Everett, M. A. Clearing of resistant psoriasis with ANTHRALIN. *Archs Derm.,* **1967,** *96,* 554–559.

White, J. J., and Duncan, A. The comparative effectiveness of iodophor and hexachlorophene surgical scrub solutions. *Surgery Gynec. Obstet.,* **1972,** *135,* 890–892.

Wong, L. C.; Heimbach, M. D.; Truscott, D. R.; and Duncan, B. D. Boric acid poisoning: report of 11 cases. *Can. med. Ass. J.,* **1964,** *90,* 1018–1023.

Monographs and Reviews

Block, S. S. Historical review. In, *Disinfection, Sterilization, and Preservation.* (Lawrence, C. A., and Block, S. S., eds.) Lea & Febiger, Philadelphia, **1968,** pp. 3–8.

Borick, P. M. Chemical sterilizers (chemosterilizers). *Adv. appl. Microbiol.,* **1968,** *10,* 291–312. (83 references.)

Boucher, R. M. Advances in sterilization techniques: state of the art and recent breakthroughs. *Am. J. hosp. Pharm.,* **1972,** *29,* 661–672.

Brewer, J. H. Mercurials—inorganic and organic. In, *Disinfection, Sterilization, and Preservation.* (Lawrence, C. A., and Block, S. S., eds.) Lea & Febiger, Philadelphia, **1968,** pp. 348–371.

Conference. Hexachlorophene—its usage in the nursery. *Pediatrics, Springfield,* **1973,** *51,* Part II, 329–434.

Conney, A. H.; Welch, R.; Kuntzman, R.; Chang, R.; Jacobson, M.; Munro-Faure, A. D.; Peck, A. W.; Bye, A.; Poland, A.; Poppers, P. J.; Finster, M.; and Wolff, J. A. Effects of environmental chemicals on the metabolism of drugs, carcinogens, and normal body constituents in man. *Ann. N.Y. Acad. Sci.,* **1971,** *179,* 155–172. (98 references.)

Czerkowicz, T. J., and Stuart, L. S. Methods of testing fungicides. In, *Disinfection, Sterilization, and Preservation.* (Lawrence, C. A., and Block, S. S., eds.) Lea & Febiger, Philadelphia, **1968,** pp. 207–220.

Davis, H. L. (ed.). Symposium. Mechanism and evaluation of antiseptics. *Ann. N.Y. Acad. Sci.,* **1950,** *53,* 1–219.

Davis, J. G. Chemical sterilization. *Prog. ind. Microbiol.,* **1968,** *8,* 141–208. (307 references.)

Deichmann, W. B. Toxicology of DDT and related chlorinated hydrocarbon pesticides. *J. occup. Med.,* **1972,** *14,* 285–292.

Deichmann, W. B., and MacDonald, W. E. Organochlorine pesticides and human health. *Fd Cosmet. Toxicol.,* **1971,** *9,* 91–103.

Drouhet, E. Basic mechanisms of antifungal chemotherapy. *Mod. Treat.,* **1970,** *7,* 539–564.

Drube, C. G. Antifungal agents. In, *Annual Reports in Medicinal Chemistry,* Vol. 8. (Heinzelman, R. V., ed.) Academic Press, Inc., New York, **1972,** pp. 116–127.

Ercegovich, C. D. Relationship of pesticides to immune responses. *Fedn Proc. Fedn Am. Socs exp. Biol.,* **1973,** *32,* 2010–2016. (81 references.)

Gershenfeld, L. Iodine. In, *Disinfection, Sterilization, and Preservation.* (Lawrence, C. A., and Block, S. S., eds.) Lea & Febiger, Philadelphia, **1968,** pp. 329–347.

Glassman, H. N. Surface active agents and their application in bacteriology. *Bact. Rev.,* **1948,** *12,* 105–148.

Gump, W. S., and Walter, G. R. The *bis*-phenols. In, *Disinfection, Sterilization, and Preservation.* (Lawrence, C. A., and Block, S. S., eds.) Lea & Febiger, Philadelphia, **1968,** pp. 257–277.

Hayes, W. J., Jr. Pharmacology and toxicology of DDT. In, *The Insecticide Dichlorodiphenyltrichloroethane and Its Significance,* Vol. 2. (Müller, P., ed.) Birkhauser, Basel, **1959,** pp. 11–247. (685 references.)

———. Pesticides and human toxicity. *Ann. N.Y. Acad. Sci.,* **1969,** *160,* 40–54. (81 references.)

Kimbrough, R. D. Review of the toxicity of hexachlorophene. *Archs envir. Hlth,* **1971,** *23,* 119–122.

———. Review of the toxicity of hexachlorophene, including its neurotoxicity. *J. clin. Pharmac.,* **1973,** *13,* 439–444.

Koski, T. A., and Stuart, L. S. Methods of testing virucides. In, *Disinfection, Sterilization, and Preservation.* (Lawrence, C. A., and Block, S. S., eds.) Lea & Febiger, Philadelphia, **1968,** pp. 194–206.

Lawrence, C. A. Quaternary ammonium surface-active disinfectants. In, *Disinfection, Sterilization, and Preservation.* (Lawrence, C. A., and Block, S. S., eds.) Lea & Febiger, Philadelphia, **1968b,** pp. 430–452.

Lawrence, C. A., and Block, S. S. (eds.). *Disinfection, Sterilization, and Preservation.* Lea & Febiger, Philadelphia, **1968.**

Leary, J. S., and Stuart, L. S. Safety evaluations on antimicrobial chemicals. In, *Disinfection, Sterilization, and Preservation.* (Lawrence, C. A., and Block, S. S., eds.) Lea & Febiger, Philadelphia, **1968,** pp. 221–233.

Lockhart, J. D. How toxic is hexachlorophene? *Pediatrics, Springfield,* **1972,** *50,* 229–235.

———. Hexachlorophene and the Food and Drug Administration. *J. clin. Pharmac.,* **1973,** *13,* 445–450.

McCulloch, E. C. *Disinfection and Sterilization.* Lea & Febiger, Philadelphia, **1945.**

Miller, A. K. *In vivo* evaluation of antibacterial chemotherapeutic substances. *Adv. appl. Microbiol.,* **1971,** *14,* 151–183. (149 references.)

Ortenzio, L. F., and Stuart, L. S. Methods of testing antiseptics. In, *Disinfection, Sterilization, and Preservation.* (Lawrence, C. A., and Block, S. S., eds.) Lea & Febiger, Philadelphia, **1968,** pp. 179–198.

Oster, K. A., and Woodside, R. Fungistatic and fungicidal compounds. In, *Disinfection, Sterilization, and Preservation.* (Lawrence, C. A., and Block, S. S., eds.) Lea & Febiger, Philadelphia, **1968,** pp. 305–320.

Plueckhahn, V. D. Hexachlorophene and skin care of newborn infants. *Drugs,* **1973,** *5,* 97–107.

Price, P. B. The meaning of bacteriostasis, bactericidal effect, and rate of disinfection. *Ann. N.Y. Acad. Sci.,* **1950,** *53,* 76–90.

———. Surgical antiseptics. In, *Disinfection, Sterilization, and Preservation.* (Lawrence, C. A., and Block, S. S., eds.) Lea & Febiger, Philadelphia, **1968,** pp. 532–542.

Prindle, R. F., and Wright, E. S. Phenolic compounds. In, *Disinfection, Sterilization, and Preservation.* (Lawrence, C. A., and Block, S. S., eds.) Lea & Febiger, Philadelphia, **1968,** pp. 401–429.

Reddish, G. F. (ed.). *Antiseptics, Disinfectants, Fungicides, and Chemical and Physical Sterilization.* Lea & Febiger, Philadelphia, **1957.**

Romans, I. B. Oligodynamic metals. In, *Disinfection, Sterilization, and Preservation.* (Lawrence, C. A., and Block, S. S., eds.) Lea & Febiger, Philadelphia, **1968,** pp. 372–400.

Russell, A. D. The mechanism of action of some antibacterial agents. *Prog. med. Chem.,* **1969,** *6,* 135–199. (426 references.)

Sell, J. L., and Davison, K. L. Changes in the activities of hepatic microsomal enzymes caused by DDT and dieldrin. *Fedn Proc. Fedn Am. Socs exp. Biol.,* **1973,** *32,* 2003–2009.

Spaulding, E. H. Chemical disinfection of medical and surgical materials. In, *Disinfection, Sterilization, and Preservation.* (Lawrence, C. A., and Block, S. S., eds.) Lea & Febiger, Philadelphia, **1968,** pp. 517–531.

Symposium. (Various authors.) Biological effects of pesticides in mammalian systems. *Ann. N.Y. Acad. Sci.,* **1969,** *160,* 1–946.

Zinsser, H. H. Nalidixic acid in acute and chronic urinary tract infections. *Med. Clins N. Am.,* **1970,** *54,* 1347–1350.

Chemotherapy of Parasitic Diseases

CHAPTER

51 DRUGS USED IN THE CHEMOTHERAPY OF HELMINTHIASIS

Ian M. Rollo

Anthelmintics are drugs used to rid the body of parasitic worms known as helminths. These drugs are of great importance because helminthiasis is the most common disease in the world. Many hundred million, perhaps over a billion, people are hosts to various types of worms. This number is increasing rather than decreasing. For example, with increased agricultural use of land and artificial irrigation, multiplication of aquatic snails has occurred. In endemic areas, this has resulted in a marked increase in the number of people infected with schistosomes. Furthermore, as a result of migration and the ease of air travel to and from regions where such infestations are endemic, worms may appear in countries where previously they had been unknown.

The term *anthelmintic* should not be restricted to drugs acting locally to expel worms from the *gastrointestinal tract.* There are several types of worms that penetrate *tissues,* and drugs used to combat systemic infestations should be included also under the general term *anthelmintic.* Therefore, the anthelmintics may be defined broadly as drugs used to combat any type of helminthiasis. This broad definition would include many drugs that possess anthelmintic activity but have other therapeutic applications of greater importance. For example, oxytetra-cycline is effective in the treatment of enterobiasis. Many tapeworm and fluke infestations respond to certain antimalarial and antimonial drugs. The pharmacological properties of only those agents that are employed primarily as anthelmintics will be discussed in this chapter. However, the applications of all drugs useful in the treatment of helminthiasis will be considered in the section of the chapter in which therapy is discussed.

Worms parasitic for man belong to widely different zoological species and vary with respect to bodily structure, physiology, habitat in the human host, and sensitivity to drugs. There are available now to the physician effective drugs that will bring about a cure in most instances. Considerable advances have been made in the last several years in discovering drugs that surpass the older remedies both in selectivity of action and in relative lack of toxicity, thus relegating the older drugs to a deserved obsolescence. Details of such drugs as aspidium, hexylresorsinol, and gentian violet may be found in earlier editions of this textbook. Increase in selectivity, however, puts greater responsibility on the physician to make an accurate diagnosis and to make proper use of the available agents. It should be remembered also that many of the anthelmintic drugs are toxic; therefore, an unequivocal diagnosis of helminthiasis should precede their use. Physicians and technicians who have few opportunities to deal with specimens in which parasites are presumed to be present should have their findings corroborated by an expert.

In the following presentation, no attempt has been made to group drugs with respect to relative importance or therapeutic application. Rather, individual anthelmintics are presented in *alphabetical order*. A discussion of antimonials then follows. Finally, treatment of specific helminthic infestations is discussed.

BEPHENIUM HYDROXY-NAPHTHOATE

Bephenium was introduced for the treatment of hookworm infestations on the basis of laboratory trials of a series of quaternary ammonium compounds showing activity against a broad range of parasitic nematodes (Copp *et al.*, 1958). The drug is now widely used against infestations due to *Necator americanus* and *Ancylostoma duodenale* (Goodwin *et al.*, 1958; Standen, 1963).

Chemistry. Bephenium is usually employed as the hydroxynaphthoate salt. It has the following structural formula:

Bephenium Hydroxynaphthoate

It is a pale-yellow crystalline substance, sparingly soluble in water and bitter in taste. Standen (1963) has reported the structure-activity relationship of a large series of analogs of bephenium.

Anthelmintic Action. Bephenium hydroxynaphthoate is highly effective, when given in a single dose, against both species of human hookworms and against human infestations with *Ascaris lumbricoides* and *Trichostrongylus orientalis*. It is ineffective against *Strongyloides stercoralis* and has only moderate activity against *Trichuris trichiura*.

Absorption, Fate, and Excretion. After oral administration of a therapeutic dose of bephenium hydroxynaphthoate not more than 0.5% is excreted in the urine within 24 hours.

Preparations, Route of Administration, and Dosage. *Bephenium Hydroxynaphthoate*, U.S.P. (ALCOPARA), is available in official single-dose sachets of 5 g, containing the equivalent of 2.5 g of bephenium base. Bephenium hydroxynaphthoate is given orally on an empty stomach, and food is then withheld for at least 2 hours. The optimal single dose is 5 g. Children under 23 kg of body weight should be given half this dose. In cases of severe diarrhea associated with hookworm disease, daily treatment for 4 to 7 days may be necessary to remove the infestation or to reduce it to negligible proportions. Purging is not required either before or after the administration of bephenium and may even reduce the response obtained. Since residual eggs may be excreted for some days after the adult worms have been eliminated, assessment of the effects of the drug should be deferred until 2 or 3 weeks after treatment.

Toxicity and Side Effects. Bephenium hydroxynaphthoate seems to produce no serious side effects. Because of its bitter taste, the drug may provoke nausea and vomiting; however, most adults and children can take it without difficulty, particularly if the dose is given suspended in a strong sugar solution. Occasionally it may cause mild and temporary looseness of the stool.

Precautions and Contraindications. There are no contraindications to the use of bephenium. However, in view of the possibility of provoking additional vomiting, patients with severe vomiting and suffering from dehydration should have these disturbances corrected before starting treatment with the drug.

Therapeutic Uses. The primary indication for the use of bephenium is in *hookworm disease*. There is little doubt that this drug is an agent of choice against *Ancylostoma duodenale*. Single-dose treatment has resulted in cure rates of from 80 to 98%, with major reduction of worm burden in the remainder. There is less unanimity of opinion concerning the use of bephenium against *Necator americanus*. Fairly high cure rates have been reported following a single dose, but some investigators have found that larger doses and more extended treatment were necessary for a high order of radical cure. In mixed hookworm infestations, all the *A. duodenale* and the majority of *N. americanus* can be removed. In infestations with *Ascaris lumbricoides* or when this roundworm occurs, as it often does, in association with hookworm, bephenium has proven effective in removing or causing a major reduction in the worm burden. Single-dose treatments have resulted in about 80% cures in infestations due to *Trichostrongylus orientalis.*

DICHLOROPHEN

Dichlorophen has been used as a taeniacide in veterinary therapeutics for many years. Because it proved to be a useful drug against the large tapeworms of cats and dogs, trials were carried out to assess its usefulness in *Taenia saginata* and *T. solium* infestations of man. These trials were successful, and later work also showed a considerable measure of success in the treatment of diphyllobothriasis (*see* Standen, 1963).

Chemistry. Dichlorophen is 2,2'-dihydroxy-5,5'-dichlorodiphenylmethane. It has the following structural formula:

Dichlorophen

It occurs as a cream-colored powder with a slightly phenolic odor and taste. The drug is almost insoluble in water.

Anthelmintic Action. Dichlorophen is primarily effective against the large tapeworms of man and domestic animals. The mechanism of action of dichlorophen is not known. Shortly after the administration of an effective dose, the scolex detaches itself from the wall of the intestine, and the worm is killed and digested. For this reason, usually nothing recognizable or only partially disintegrated mature segments can be seen in the stool. This presents difficulty in diagnosing cure, and, therefore, careful follow-up of the patient is required.

Without doubt, dichlorophen produces a high proportion of cures in infestations by *T. saginata.* Good results have also been reported in a few patients with *T. solium* infestation. However, Seaton (1956) considered it might be unwise to use dichlorophen for this purpose because of the risk of cysticercosis from autoinfection by the ova liberated on disintegration of the worm. The drug has some effect also in *Diphyllobothrium latum* and *Hymenolepis nana* infestations of man, but the evidence is meager.

Preparations, Route of Administration, and Dosage. *Dichlorophen* (ANTHIPHEN) is not marketed in the United States. It is supplied as scored tablets containing 500 mg of active material. Dichlorophen is given orally without preliminary fasting or other prior preparation of the patient. Satisfactory results have been obtained by giving 2 to 3 g every 8 hours for three doses (children, 1 to 2 g). Alternatively, a single dose of 6 g (children, 2 to 4 g) may be given on each of 2 successive days. If mass treatment of adults is undertaken, a single dose of 6 to 9 g may

be given. Schneider (1959) extended treatment over 3 days, giving 6 g daily for 2 days and 3 g on the third day, and cured 18 of 30 subjects who had previously failed to respond to other taeniacides. Purgatives are not needed afterward as the drug itself exerts an adequate laxative effect. Purgation may be undesirable, reducing the time of contact of the drug with the scolex.

Toxicity and Side Effects. An appreciable proportion of treated patients experience colic, diarrhea, and nausea lasting from 4 to 6 hours. Vomiting may occur occasionally. Lassitude is another common symptom. Urticaria occurs in a small number of patients, but this disappears without treatment in 24 hours. Late side effects have not been reported.

Precautions and Contraindications. No specific or absolute contraindication has been established, but care should be taken in the presence of hepatic disease. The drug should not be used in circumstances when purgation is undesirable, for example, in febrile disease, late pregnancy, or severe cardiovascular disease.

Therapeutic Uses. Dichlorophen is effective in clearing a large proportion of infestations by *T. saginata. Taenia solium* also appears to be susceptible; however, as already pointed out, there may be a danger of cysticercosis from liberated ova. Available data suggest it may be useful against *D. latum* and *H. nana* infestations. Its lack of serious side effects may recommend its use in patients who are undernourished, weak, or convalescent.

There remains the problem, however, of assessment of cure. Partial digestion of the killed worm results in the passing of grayish-white masses in the feces. The scolex is often unrecognizable. Since *T. saginata* takes no more than 12 weeks to grow from the scolex to the point where the host begins to pass segments, the absence of segments in the stools after this period is taken as the criterion of cure.

DIETHYLCARBAMAZINE

History. During World War II, over 15,000 cases of filariasis occurred in American military personnel quartered on the islands of the Western Pacific. This stimulated the search for effective filaricides. The most promising group of antifilarial compounds to emerge were piperazine derivatives.

Chemistry. *Diethylcarbamazine* is N,N-diethyl-4-methyl-1-piperazinecarboxamide. It has the following structural formula:

Diethylcarbamazine

The drug is marketed as the dicitrate salt, a colorless, crystalline solid with an unpleasant sweetish taste. It is highly soluble in water.

Pharmacological Effects. Diethylcarbamazine causes rapid disappearance of microfilariae of *Wuchereria bancrofti, W. (Brugia) malayi,* and *Loa loa* from the blood of man. The drug is inactive *in vitro;* rather, it appears to sensitize the microfilariae so that they become susceptible to phagocytosis by the fixed macrophages of the reticuloendothelial system. There is no phagocytosis by the circulating phagocytes of the blood (Hawking *et al.,* 1950). The drug causes microfilariae of *Onchocerca volvulus* to disappear from the skin but does not kill microfilariae in the nodules. Nor does it affect the microfilariae of *W. bancrofti* when they are in a hydrocele. There is presumptive evidence that diethylcarbamazine kills adult worms of *W. bancrofti* and definite evidence that it kills adult *W. malayi* and *Loa loa.* However, it has little action against adult *O. volvulus (see* Hawking, 1963).

The pharmacological actions of diethylcarbamazine have been extensively studied by Harned and associates (1948). The compound is relatively nontoxic and possesses a high therapeutic index in experimental animals. The only prominent pharmacological response following intravenous administration in dogs is a rise in blood pressure followed by a fall; both phases are of brief duration. The pressor response is accompanied by tachycardia and peripheral vasoconstriction. The tachycardia is of sinus origin in anesthetized dogs, but frequent ectopic beats are noted in unanesthetized animals. Toxic doses cause vomiting, muscle tremors, and convulsions.

Absorption, Fate, and Excretion. Diethylcarbamazine is readily absorbed from the gastrointestinal tract. After a single oral dose, a peak blood concentration appears in 3 hours; this falls to zero within 48 hours. Excretion is almost entirely urinary, most of the drug appearing as metabolites. The compound is distributed almost equally throughout all body compartments with the exception of fat, and there is little tendency to accumulation when repeated doses are given.

Preparations, Route of Administration, and Dosage. *Diethylcarbamazine Citrate,* U.S.P. (BANOCIDE, HETRAZAN), is available as tablets, each containing 50 mg. The product is stable even under conditions of high temperature and humidity, such as occur in some parts of the tropics. The dosage of diethylcarbamazine used to treat filarial disease has varied considerably. The following are representative of the dosages used most frequently. They may be modified effectively according to individual experience.

Wuchereria bancrofti and *W. malayi.* For mass treatment with the objective of reducing microfilaremia to subinfective levels for mosquitoes, the dose is 2 mg/kg, three times daily after meals, for 7 days. For treatment directed toward possible cure, the dose is 2 mg/kg, three times daily after meals, for at least 3 weeks. Much experience has shown that, if people can be persuaded to take an adequate amount of diethylcarbamazine, the microfilariae and probably some of the adult worms will be destroyed. For practical purposes, an adequate amount seems to be a total dose of about 72 mg of the citrate per kilogram of body weight. The period over which this amount is administered has varied from area to area; spaced doses of 6 mg/kg once a week or once a month give as good an effect as daily doses, and are less likely to cause adverse reaction (World Health Organization, 1967).

Loa loa. Two to 4 mg/kg should be given three times daily after meals for 10 days. If repeated courses are required to produce cure, they should be separated by periods of 3 to 4 weeks.

Onchocerca volvulus. Treatment is effective in removing microfilariae from the skin; however, since the adult worms are not killed, they usually return after some weeks. It may be possible to hold both forms in check by periodic short courses of treatment. When lesions of the eye are present, the initial dose of diethylcarbamazine should not exceed 0.5 mg/kg. This is given once on the first day and twice on the second. The dose is then increased to 1.0 mg/kg, three times daily for the third day, and therapy is continued up to a total of 21 days with a dose of 2 mg/kg three times daily.

In patients infested with *O. volvulus* or *W. malayi,* and to a lesser extent in those infested with *W. bancrofti* and *Loa loa,* the initial systemic reactions provoked by the massive destruction of microfilariae, macrofilariae, or both during treatment may be severe. In such cases the dosage should be lowered or the drug stopped temporarily. Relief of these symptoms is afforded by the use of antihistamines, but, exceptionally, corticosteroids may be required. Once the initial reactions have subsided, continued treatment should not provoke a further series of reactions.

Toxicity and Side Effects. Untoward reactions to diethylcarbamazine, although fairly frequent, are not severe and usually disappear within a few days despite continuation of therapy. Reactions believed to result directly from the drug are headache, general malaise, weakness, joint pains, anorexia, nausea, and vomiting. Other untoward responses result from the filaricidal action. In patients with onchocerciasis, there is usually a violent reaction that is well marked within

16 hours after the first oral dose. This includes swelling and edema of the skin, intense itching, enlargement and tenderness of the inguinal lymph nodes, sometimes a fine papular rash, hyperpyrexia up to 102° F, tachycardia, and headache. These symptoms persist for 3 to 7 days and then subside, after which quite high doses can be tolerated without further reaction. Nodular swellings may occur along the course of the lymphatics, and there is often an accompanying lymphadenitis. The nodules may be the sites of dead worms. The reaction subsides within a few days. Almost all patients receiving therapy exhibit a leukocytosis, first evident on the second day, reaching its peak on the fourth or fifth day, and gradually subsiding over a period of a few weeks. The eosinophilia that frequently occurs in patients with filariasis is intensified for a brief period by diethylcarbamazine therapy.

Precautions and Contraindications. With the exception of the caution that must be exercised in initial treatment with diethylcarbamazine and management of allergic symptoms, particularly in the case of onchocerciasis, there are apparently no contraindications to the use of this drug in recommended doses. In onchocerciasis it is advisable, when treating patients with ocular complications, to have 5% hydrocortisone eyedrops available; when the eye complications are marked, 25 mg of cortisone (or equivalent) may be given with advantage four times a day, 2 days before starting treatment and continued for the first 4 days of treatment. As a precaution in preparing patients for treatment, it may be advisable to give an antimalarial agent if the patient has had a recent history of malaria. This is to prevent relapses that might be provoked by the systemic response to therapy with diethylcarbamazine.

Therapeutic Uses. Diethylcarbamazine can be used effectively to treat infestations with *W. bancrofti*, *W. (Brugia) malayi*, *Loa loa*, and *O. volvulus*. In the first three, radical cure can be achieved by either single or multiple courses of treatment. In onchocerciasis, radical cure is unlikely, but control can be achieved by short periodic courses of treatment. The drug has also been used effectively in the treatment of cutaneous *larva migrans*, although the total number of reported cases is small. Diethylcarbamazine is also effective in clearing *Ascaris* in-

festations, but it has been replaced by other agents for this purpose. In patients with *eosinophilic lung* (*tropical eosinophilia*), treatment with diethylcarbamazine causes a rapid disappearance of symptoms. This, and the finding of microfilariae in lung biopsies, suggest an association between filariasis and the eosinophilic pulmonary syndrome.

HYCANTHONE

The group of xanthones and thioxanthones known as the "MIRACILS" was first synthesized in Germany and studied during World War II as potential chemotherapeutic agents for the treatment of *schistosomiasis* (Kikuth *et al.*, 1946; Mauss, 1948). *Lucanthone* (MIRACIL D) was found to be the most active. This compound was studied extensively in the postwar years in England and the United States and used successfully in the treatment of infestations with *Schistosoma haematobium* and *S. mansoni*. However, intolerance to the drug in a high proportion of patients, particularly in adults, proved to be a considerable disadvantage and led to further investigation of the chemical series. Of the several metabolites of lucanthone appearing in the urine of treated patients, the hydroxymethyl derivative, *hycanthone*, was shown to have very high schistosomicidal activity (Rosi *et al.*, 1965). Early clinical trials provided encouraging results (Katz *et al.*, 1968). Since then the new agent has been used in several programs to control schistosomiasis in the Middle East, Africa, and South America.

Chemistry. Hycanthone is 1-([2-{diethylamino}-ethyl]amino)-4-(hydroxymethyl)-thioxanthen-9-one. It has the following structural formula:

Hycanthone

It is a yellow-orange crystalline powder, highly soluble in water. A solution for injection is stable for at least 24 hours at temperatures of 37° C or lower.

Anthelmintic Action. Hycanthone acts primarily against the adult forms of *S. haematobium* and *S. mansoni*. The drug interferes with the laying of eggs, induces separation of paired worms, produces degenerative changes, and induces a shift of worms to the liver within a period of 3 to 7 days. Death of the adult worm follows. The mechanism of action is unknown but may be associated with stimulation of the worm's low-affinity 5-hydroxytryptamine (5-HT) uptake into nonneuronal tissue. At the same time, there is an impairment of the ability of neuronal structures to store this putative excitatory neurotransmitter (Chou *et al.*, 1973). Clinically, reduced egg excretion becomes most apparent during the second week after treatment.

In some laboratory studies hycanthone-resistant

strains of *S. mansoni* have been produced. There has been a single report of hycanthone resistance in *S. mansoni* from treated patients (Katz *et al.,* 1973); however, in general, the problem of drug resistance has not arisen in the several years the agent has been in use.

Absorption, Fate, and Excretion. Hycanthone is well absorbed after oral administration if the tablet is enteric coated to protect it from degradation by gastric acidity. However, after it was shown that a single intramuscular injection provided the same results as several days of oral treatment, only the parenteral preparation was made available. The drug is well absorbed from the site of intramuscular injection. Peak concentration in the blood is reached in 30 minutes, and in tissues within 1 hour. Only traces remain at the site of injection after 24 hours. The drug appears unchanged in the blood and in all organs with the exception of the liver, where several metabolites of hycanthone have been identified. The main route of excretion is through the bile and feces in the form of conjugated metabolites.

Preparations, Route of Administration, and Dosage. *Hycanthone mesylate* (ETRENOL) is supplied in vials, each containing 200 mg of base to be dissolved in 2 ml of water for injection. The drug is not available in the United States. Hycanthone is given by deep intramuscular injection in a single dose of 2.5 to 3.0 mg of base per kilogram of body weight, up to a maximal adult dose of 200 mg of base. Since there is a high incidence of dose-related side effects, close attention should be paid to the dosage table supplied by the manufacturer. Re-treatment of patients reinfected or harboring a residual infestation may be carried out after 1 to 3 months.

Toxicity and Side Effects. The administration of hycanthone is associated with a high incidence of side effects, varying from 22 to 60% in various trials. These are generally self-limiting and include nausea, vomiting, abdominal discomfort, headache, dizziness, weakness, myalgia, anorexia, diarrhea, and weight loss. Transient, minimal ECG changes have been reported in a few patients, but these appear to have little clinical significance. Vomiting is the most common reaction and usually begins 4 to 8 hours after treatment. In general, side effects rarely persist beyond 24 hours. The onset of severe, persistent vomiting within 2 to 3 hours after injection suggests possible hepatotoxicity, for which treatment should be started promptly. The most serious adverse effect is acute hepatic necrosis, and death may occur in 2 to 5 days. Estimates of the frequency of this complication vary, but in general they are low. The cause is unknown; there may be an association between the administration of the drug and existing pathological changes in the liver brought about by the infestation, other disease process, or the use of other drugs known to affect hepatic function. In several *in-vitro* systems hycanthone has been shown to be mutagenic (*see* Meadows *et al.,* 1973). Results of studies *in vivo* are controversial, but the drug does not appear to be tumorigenic in mice

(Yarinsky *et al.,* 1974). Neither cytogenetic changes nor teratogenic effects have been observed in man. Several analogs of hycanthone have been shown to retain chemotherapeutic activity with much reduced *in-vitro* mutagenic activity (Hulbert *et al.,* 1974). The potential clinical value of these or other derivatives has yet to be determined.

Precautions and Contraindications. Hycanthone should not be administered to pregnant women or to those who have recently given birth until at least 1 month after parturition. The drug is also not recommended for children younger than 3 years of age or weighing less than 15 kg. Patients should be under close medical supervision for at least 2 days after treatment.

Absolute contraindications to treatment with hycanthone are suspected or confirmed jaundice in the present or recent past, hepatic tenderness or nonschistosomal hepatic disease, or recent or concurrent use of drugs known to affect the liver. In particular, phenothiazines should not be administered for the relief of side effects such as nausea or vomiting. Hycanthone should not be given to patients with serious bacterial infection or any acute febrile state. It is also contraindicated when there is a history of previous allergic reaction to the drug, to lucanthone, or to other thioxanthone derivatives.

Therapeutic Uses. Because a single intramuscular injection represents the full course of treatment, hycanthone has great value in mass treatment where schistosomiasis is endemic. Both *S. haematobium* and *S. mansoni* infestations are susceptible; *S. japonicum* is not. The potential for serious, long-term side effects has led to very close examination of the properties of hycanthone by two international consultant groups of the World Health Organization. They found no reason sufficient to justify discontinuation of the use of hycanthone for the treatment of schistosomiasis. Decision to use the drug, especially in mass control programs, should be based on the conditions prevailing in each population to be treated and a realistic assessment of possible benefit against the risks involved.

MEBENDAZOLE

This drug was introduced for the treatment of roundworm infestations as a result of research carried out in Belgium (Brugmans *et al.,* 1971).

Chemistry. Mebendazole is methyl N-(5-benzoyl-2-benzimidazolyl) carbamate. It has the following structural formula:

Mebendazole

It is a yellowish amorphous powder, very slightly soluble in water and most organic solvents, and not unpleasant to taste.

Anthelmintic Action. Mebendazole is highly effective against ascariasis, enterobiasis, trichuriasis, and hookworm infestation in single or in mixed infestation. Variable results have been obtained against *S. stercoralis*. It has shown promise in the treatment of beef and pork tapeworm infestation. The drug is nematocidal by virtue of its ability to inhibit glucose uptake irreversibly (*see* Fierlafijn, 1971). It does not affect blood glucose concentrations in animals, even in high doses (Van den Bossche, 1972). Parasite immobilization and death occur slowly, and clearance from the gastrointestinal tract may not be complete up to 3 days after treatment. The drug inhibits the development of larval hookworms *in vitro* at 50 μg/ml. Much higher concentrations have no effect on fully formed larvae. Shortly after treatment is started, eggs of *Trichuris* and hookworm fail to develop to the larval stage (Wagner and Chavarria, 1974). (*See also* Miller *et al.*, 1974; Wolfe and Wershing, 1974.)

Absorption, Fate, and Excretion. Only a small proportion of an orally administered dose is absorbed, and up to 10% may be recovered in the urine within 24 to 48 hours. Most of the material excreted by the kidney is the decarboxylated derivative of mebendazole.

Preparations, Route of Administration, and Dosage. *Mebendazole* (VERMOX) is available as tablets, each containing 100 mg of the drug. Mebendazole is given orally, and the same dosage schedule applies to adults and children. For control of enterobiasis, a single 100-mg tablet is given. For control of ascariasis, trichuriasis, and hookworm infestation, 100 mg is administered morning and evening on 3 consecutive days. If the patient is not cured 3 weeks after treatment, a second course should be given. Fasting or purging is not required.

Toxicity and Side Effects. Probably as a result of its poor absorption, mebendazole has not caused systemic toxicity in clinical use, even in the presence of anemia and malnutrition. Transient symptoms of abdominal pain and diarrhea have occurred in cases of massive infestation and expulsion of worms.

Precautions and Contraindications. Mebendazole should not be given to pregnant women, nor should it be used in patients who have experienced allergic reactions to the agent.

Therapeutic Uses. Mebendazole is the drug of choice in the treatment of *Trichuris trichiura*. It produces a large proportion of cures and, in those not cured with a first course of treatment, a marked reduction in egg production. It is particularly valuable in the treatment of double or triple infestations, since it also has high activity against *ascariasis, enterobiasis,* and *hookworm* (Chavarria *et al.*, 1973; Sargent *et al.*, 1974).

METRIFONATE

Metrifonate (BILARCIL) is an organophosphorus inhibitor of cholinesterases, used first as an insecticide (DIPTEREX, DYLOX) and later as an anthelmintic. The original trials in man arose from the hope that the anticholinesterase activity of organophosphorus compounds in arthropods would extend to other invertebrates, including the helminths. Metrifonate was selected for trial on the basis of *in-vitro* tests carried out with *Ascaris lumbricoides*. In 1962 it was shown to have high anthelmintic activity in several different human infestations. The substance is O,O-dimethyl-2,2,2-trichloro-hydroxyethyl-phosphonate. It has the following structural formula:

Metrifonate

The drug is, indeed, a potent inhibitor of nematode cholinesterase; 0.1 μM metrifonate inhibits the enzyme from *S. haematobium* by 50%, and lower concentrations inhibit that from *S. mansoni*. In clinical practice, however, the order is reversed, since infestations with *S. haematobium* respond much better to metrifonate. Given in therapeutic doses, metrifonate produces rapid and almost complete inhibition of plasma cholinesterase activity; this recovers to almost normal levels within a few weeks of stopping treatment. Erythrocyte acetylcholinesterase is inhibited to a lesser degree but recovers more slowly. Despite these changes the drug is well tolerated. Treated individuals should, of course, be free from recent exposure to insecticides that might add to the anticholinesterase effect. Metrifonate is recommended only for the treatment of *S. haematobium* infestation. When the recommended dosage scheme is followed, the cure rate is 70 to 80%. In those not freed of parasites, egg output is markedly reduced.

NICLOSAMIDE

Niclosamide was introduced as a taeniacide after laboratory trials in rats with *Hymeno-*

lepis diminuta as a test organism (Gönnert and Schraufstätter, 1960). In the intervening years so much impressive evidence of its high activity and safety has accumulated that, in many places, it has replaced other drugs for the treatment of most cestode infestations (Keeling, 1968).

Chemistry. Niclosamide is N-(2'-chloro-4'-nitrophenyl)-5-chlorosalicylamide. It has the following structural formula:

Niclosamide

It occurs as a yellowish-white powder that is tasteless and odorless. It is insoluble in water.

Anthelmintic Action. Niclosamide acts primarily against cestodes. The drug has been found to be effective against *Echinococcus granulosus* in dogs, as well as against those cestodes infesting man. *Enterobius vermicularis* is also susceptible. In *in-vitro* studies, very little of the drug is absorbed by *H. diminuta* in saline solution. If a homogenate of intestine from normal rats or from rats pretreated with the drug is added, the amount of drug taken up by the worms is greatly increased. Niclosamide has marked effects on metabolism of *H. diminuta* in rats. At low concentrations oxygen uptake is stimulated, but at high concentrations exogenous respiration is inhibited and glucose uptake is blocked. Worms affected by the drug either in the gut or *in vitro* are more susceptible to proteolytic enzymes. After effective doses of the drug, the scolex and segments may be partially digested and unrecognizable.

Preparations, Route of Administration, and Dosage. *Niclosamide* (CESTOCIDE, MANSONIL, YOMESAN) is supplied in vanilla-flavored tablets, each containing 500 mg of the drug. In the United States, this drug is available from the Parasitic Disease Drug Service, Center for Disease Control, Atlanta, Georgia. Niclosamide is given orally. The patient may be prepared by fasting overnight, but there is no conclusive evidence that this is necessary. Those with chronic constipation should be given a laxative before administering the drug. The recommended dose for an adult is 2 g, the tablets to be chewed thoroughly and washed down with water. The dosage for children from 2 to 8 years of age is one half and,

for children under 2 years, one fourth that for adults. For small children it is advisable to grind the tablets as finely as possible and to mix the powder with a little water. A purge may be given 2 hours after the dose in the hope of obtaining less damaged lengths of the worm and an identifiable scolex.

In infestations with *H. nana,* which are usually multiple, it is recommended that the first dose taken after a meal be followed by 1 g daily for an additional 6 days, again each dose after a meal. Discharge of intestinal mucus can be promoted by the administration of sour fruit juices. Worms lodging under accumulations of mucus thus become more readily accessible to the drug.

Toxicity and Side Effects. Niclosamide seems to be singularly free from any undesirable effects, other than very occasional gastrointestinal upset. Very little is absorbed from the gastrointestinal tract, and it has no direct irritant effect. No side effects were observed when niclosamide was given to debilitated or pregnant patients (Gönnert and Schraufstätter, 1960). Follow-up studies showed no alteration in hepatic or renal function or in blood counts of treated patients (Abdallah and Saif, 1961).

Precautions and Contraindications. There are no contraindications to the use of niclosamide as a taeniacide. However, it is important to note that the lethal action of the drug against the adult worm does not extend to the ova contained within the tapeworm segments. This means that the use of niclosamide in *T. solium* infestations may expose the patient to the risk of cysticercosis, since, following digestion of the dead segments, viable ova will be liberated into the lumen of the gut. This makes it mandatory to give an adequate purge within 1 to 2 hours after the drug has been given, to clear the bowel of all dead segments before they can be digested. In *T. saginata* infestations, in which there is no risk of cysticercosis, purging is unnecessary unless immediate proof of cure by finding the scolex is desired.

Therapeutic Uses. Niclosamide can be considered an agent of choice in the treatment of *D. latum, H. nana,* and *T. saginata* infestations (Brown, 1968). It is also effective in the treatment of *T. solium* infestation, but the danger of cysticercosis following its administration detracts from its usefulness. Its ready acceptance by patients, together with the fact that starvation is not necessary, is valuable, particularly in the treatment of children.

NIRIDAZOLE

Niridazole was developed from the synthesis of a large number of nitrothiazole derivatives. The nitrothiazole nucleus was chosen because heterocyclic compounds bearing a nitro group as a characteristic substituent occupy an important position in chemotherapy. Of the many preparations synthesized and tested, derivatives of 5-nitrothiazole substituted by a cyclic urea group in position 2 displayed optimal chemotherapeutic properties. From this category the ethylene-urea derivative, 1-(5-nitro-2-thiazolyl)-2-imidazolidinone (niridazole), was selected for clinical investigation.

Chemistry. Niridazole has the following structural formula:

Niridazole

The substance is a yellow crystalline powder that is odorless and tasteless. It is sparingly soluble in water and most organic solvents.

Pharmacological Effects. Niridazole is both schistosomicidal and amebicidal. Anthelmintic activity is observed first on the vitellogenic gland. The vitelline cells become depleted of egg-shell substance, and there is complete arrest of shell formation in the ootype. Eventually no eggs can be seen in the uterus. Destruction of the vitellogenic gland coincides with a decrease in body length of both male and female worms, and the size of the ovary in the female. The gonads of male worms are less sensitive than those of females. In affected worms, spermatogenesis is stopped; this is followed by complete destruction of the testes. In the liver the female worm is destroyed by leukocytes and the male is immobilized by connective tissue and eventually undergoes autolysis. Niridazole has been shown to decrease the uptake of exogenous glucose by *S. mansoni,* perhaps by inhibiting hexokinase, and to reduce its glycogen stores by inhibiting glycogen phosphorylase phosphatase activity.

In addition to its action on schistosomes, niridazole is an effective amebicide both *in vitro* and in the treatment of intestinal and extraintestinal amebiasis. It is effective in the treatment of guinea worm infestation and has been reported to have some therapeutic effect against the adult worms of *O. volvulus.* It has proven useful in treating a few cases of cutaneous leishmaniasis.

In patients, niridazole produces changes in the ECG after several days of treatment. Flattening or inversion of the T wave occurs. This reverts to normal within 1 to 2 weeks after completion of treatment and has never been associated with clinical evidence of cardiac impairment. The drug may produce EEG changes and may cause agitation, confusional states, visual and auditory hallucinations,

and localized or generalized convulsions. These effects appear to occur largely in patients in whom some degree of impairment of hepatic function exists as a result of the hepatosplenic form of schistosomiasis, concurrent disease, malnutrition, or anemia. As a consequence, the drug is not well metabolized and the concentration of parent substance in the blood is high. Niridazole, in common with some nitrofurazone derivatives, inhibits spermatogenesis in experimental animals by a direct effect on the germinal epithelium of the testes. The effect is reversible on stopping treatment. Human subjects receiving standard doses of niridazole occasionally display a transitory reduction in the number of spermatozoa in ejaculate. Administration of the drug has not been known to impair the fertility of either male or female patients. Treatment with niridazole can provoke hemolysis in individuals with red cells deficient in glucose-6-phosphate dehydrogenase (Doyen *et al.,* 1967).

Further details on the pharmacological effects of niridazole may be found in the proceedings of a symposium (*see* Symposium, 1969a).

Absorption, Fate, and Excretion. Following oral administration, niridazole is absorbed almost entirely over a period of several hours. During its first passage through the liver it is largely metabolized. Owing to slow absorption and rapid metabolism, a low but uniform concentration of parent drug is maintained in the peripheral blood for several hours. The metabolites attain high concentration in the blood and persist there for a long time because they are firmly bound to plasma albumin. The parent compound and its metabolites are uniformly distributed throughout the tissues. The drug is eliminated largely, and almost equally, in the urine and feces, in the latter by way of the bile. The urine becomes dark in color, and there is an unpleasant body odor. The schistosomicidal activity of niridazole is attributable to the parent compound. At least part of its effectiveness must be due to the high concentration in the portal blood and the fact that the various species of *Schistosoma* live mainly or exclusively in the vascular bed supplied by portal blood.

Preparations, Route of Administration, and Dosage. *Niridazole* (AMBILHAR) is supplied in scored tablets, each containing 500 mg. In the United States it is available from the Parasitic Disease Drug Service, Center for Disease Control, Atlanta, Georgia. Niridazole is administered orally. The usual daily dose is 25 mg/kg (maximum of 1.5 g), which may or may not be divided into two portions, depending on the local experience of the physician and practical considerations for ambulatory patients. Treatment is usually continued for 5 days, but this period may be extended to 7 or even 10 days. These longer periods should probably be the rule in *S. mansoni* infestation, which is rather less responsive to therapy than is *S. haematobium,* and also in *S. japonicum* infestation, although the most that can be expected in the latter condition is a reduction in the egg count. The dosage schedule of niridazole in dracontiasis is 25 mg/kg daily for 7 days.

Toxicity and Side Effects. In addition to the side effects alluded to above, the administration of niridazole gives rise to the following less specific effects: abdominal spasm and discomfort, nausea, vomiting, diarrhea, loss of appetite, and headache. Less frequently encountered are insomnia, skin rash, and paresthesias. The incidence and the severity of these side effects are considerably less in children, with the exception of those infested with *S. japonicum.* In this condition, hepatic impairment is seen more frequently than in *S. mansoni* or *haematobium* infestation, with consequent increase in the amount of circulating un-detoxified drug.

Precautions and Contraindications. Since the toxicity of niridazole appears to depend on the amount of parent drug circulating in the blood, any impairment of hepatic function demands the greatest care in its use and contraindicates its employment at least in the ambulatory patient. Evidence of epilepsy or neurotic or psychotic behavior may also be regarded as a contraindication, unless it is deemed necessary to utilize niridazole and the means are at hand to control any symptoms of central nervous system (CNS) excitation. In general, those in poor general condition due to malnutrition, marked anemia, and severe concomitant infections or parasitoses, notably tuberculosis and ancylostomiasis, should not be treated with niridazole. To this group may be added those suffering from the hyperacute exudative form of schistosomiasis. Individuals of races in which genetically determined glucose-6-phosphate dehydrogenase deficiency exists should be treated with care and observed for drug-induced hemolysis. In the United States, the Food and Drug Administration requires that patients receiving niridazole be hospitalized.

Therapeutic Uses. Niridazole is particularly useful in the treatment of schistosomiasis. *Schistosoma haematobium* infestations respond particularly well. *Mansoni* schistosomiasis is not as consistent in its response, but quite good results have followed a slightly more extended course of treatment. Infestations due to *S. japonicum* have given quite varied responses, but reductions in egg count usually follow an adequate course of treatment. Niridazole is effective in the treatment of guinea worm (*D. medinensis*) infestation.

PIPERAZINE

Piperazine was used early in this century for the treatment of gout. It was introduced for this purpose because a solution of piperazine is an excellent solvent for uric acid. Although piperazine proved to be ineffective as a uricosuric agent, extensive clinical experience indicated that the drug was nontoxic. The discovery of the anthelmintic properties of piperazine is usually credited to Fayard (1949), but these were first observed by Boismare, a Rouen pharmacist, whose recipe

is quoted in Fayard's thesis. Clinical studies have shown that the drug is highly effective against both *Ascaris lumbricoides* and *Enterobius* (*Oxyuris*) *vermicularis.* A large number of substituted piperazine derivatives exhibit anthelmintic activity, but apart from diethylcarbamazine none has found a place in human therapeutics (*see* Standen, 1963).

Chemistry. Piperazine has the following structural formula:

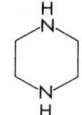

Piperazine

It is available as the hexahydrate, which contains about 44% of base, and, in addition, as various salts such as citrate, adipate, phosphate, calcium edetate, and tartrate. These salts occur as stable, nonhygroscopic, white crystals, freely soluble in water. Aqueous solutions are slightly acidic.

Pharmacological Effects. The effects of piperazine on *Ascaris* have been investigated intensively. The gross effect is a paralysis of muscle that results in expulsion of the worm by peristalsis. Affected worms recover if incubated in a saline medium at 37° C. Further studies have shown that piperazine blocks the response of *Ascaris* muscle to acetylcholine. It has been proposed that piperazine acts on *Ascaris* muscle by altering the permeability of the cell membrane to ions that are responsible for the maintenance of the resting potential. The drug causes hyperpolarization and suppression of spontaneous spike potentials with accompanying paralysis (*see* Saz and Bueding, 1966).

Orally administered piperazine is almost devoid of pharmacological activity. Intravenous administration results in a transient fall in blood pressure. Lethal doses cause convulsions and respiratory depression.

Absorption, Fate, and Excretion. Piperazine is readily absorbed from the gastrointestinal tract. Therefore, it is rather surprising that the compound is effective against a parasite harbored in the large bowel. A portion of the absorbed drug is degraded in the body. The remainder is excreted in the urine. Rogers (1958) observed no significant difference between the rates of urinary excretion of the citrate, phosphate, and adipate. However, there was a wide variation in the rates at which piperazine was excreted by different individuals.

Preparations, Route of Administration, and Dosage. Piperazine salts are available as tablets and wafers, each containing 500 mg, and as syrups and suspensions containing 100 mg/ml, calculated as the hexahydrate. Of the various preparations, one is probably as good as another. The liquid preparations are more acceptable for children. *Piperazine Citrate*, U.S.P., and *Piperazine Phosphate*, N.F., are the official preparations. Trade names include ANTEPAR (citrate and phosphate), MULTIFUGE CITRATE, and PIPIZAN CITRATE.

Piperazine preparations are always given orally. It is unnecessary to supplement treatment with cathartics or enemas. Prior fasting is not necessary. Many different dosage schedules have been investigated, and all have resulted in a considerable measure of success. In *ascariasis,* accepted therapy is to give a single daily dose of 3.5 g for 2 consecutive days; this is the maximal dose. Children should be treated with 75 mg/kg. This dosage schedule will cure almost 100% of patients. A single dose of 4 g has been shown to cure about 50% of patients and to reduce markedly the worm burden in the remainder (Goodwin and Standen, 1958). In *oxyuriasis,* single daily doses of 65 mg/kg, with a maximum of 2.5 g, given for 8 days, will result in 95 to 100% cure. One study in hospital patients showed that a single dose of 4 g of piperazine, with or without senna, cured more than 90% of patients (White and Scopes, 1960). However, because of the possibility of autoinfection shortly after treatment, a second dose would probably have to be given to ambulatory patients less than 3 weeks after the first.

Toxicity and Side Effects. There is a wide range between effective therapeutic and overtly toxic doses of piperazine. Laboratory studies on patients receiving treatment for several days have showed no abnormality. Very occasionally gastrointestinal upset, transient neurological effects, and urticarial reactions have attended its use. Piperazine has been used without ill effect during pregnancy.

Precautions and Contraindications. There are no contraindications to the use of piperazine. Neurotoxic effects have occurred in individuals with renal dysfunction; because urinary excretion is the main route of elimination, care should be exercised in the treatment of such patients.

Therapeutic Uses. Piperazine is the agent of choice in *ascariasis.* It has the advantage of greatly reducing the motility of the worms, thereby reducing the hazard of migration. Since the worms are usually alive when passed, there is little chance of absorption of disintegration products. Where partial intestinal obstruction is a complication of infestation, conservative management together with the administration of piperazine syrup through a drainage tube may obviate the necessity of surgery.

Treatment of *oxyuriasis* is complicated by the readiness with which reinfestation may occur. Many authorities advocate the simultaneous treatment of the entire household with piperazine in lieu of investigation of each member by anal swabs. The palatability of the various preparations, ease of administration to children, and low toxicity make piperazine an agent of choice in pinworm infestations.

PYRANTEL PAMOATE

Pyrantel pamoate was introduced first into veterinary practice as a broad-spectrum anthelmintic effective against pinworm, roundworm, and hookworm (Austin *et al.,* 1966). Its effectiveness and lack of toxicity led to its trial against related helminths that infest the human digestive tract (Bumbalo *et al.,* 1969). Success in these and other trials justifies its addition to the several agents useful in the treatment of nematode infestation. A methyl-thienyl analog of pyrantel, *morantel,* has been introduced as a veterinary nematocide with claims of greater tolerability.

Chemistry. Pyrantel is employed as the pamoate salt. It is *trans*-1,4,5,6-tetrahydro-1-methyl-2-(2-[2-thienyl]-vinyl) pyrimidine. It has the following structural formula:

Pyrantel

The pamoate is a white crystalline salt practically insoluble in either alcohol or water. It is tasteless and stable.

Anthelmintic Action. Pyrantel and its analogs are depolarizing neuromuscular blocking agents. They induce marked, persistent nicotinic activation, which results in spastic paralysis of the worm. Pyrantel also inhibits cholinesterases. It causes a slowly developing contracture of preparations of *Ascaris* at $\frac{1}{100}$ the concentration of acetylcholine required to produce the same effect. In single muscle cells of the helminth, pyrantel causes depolarization and increased spike-discharge frequency, accompanied by increase in tension. In contrast, piperazine causes hyperpolarization with reduction in spike-discharge frequency and relaxation in identical preparations. In the *Ascaris* preparations, pyrantel and piperazine are mutually antagonistic (Aubry *et al.,* 1970; Eyre, 1970). Pyrantel is effective against hookworm, pinworm, and roundworm, but it is ineffective against the whipworm.

Absorption, Fate, and Excretion. Pyrantel pamoate is poorly absorbed from the gastrointestinal tract. Less than 15% is excreted in the urine as parent drug and metabolites. The major proportion of an administered dose may be recovered in the feces.

Preparations, Route of Administration, and Dosage. *Pyrantel Pamoate,* U.S.P. (ANTIMINTH, COMBANTRIN), is supplied as an official oral suspension; each milliliter contains 50 mg of the base. Pyrantel pamoate is given orally at any time without regard to ingestion of food or beverages. A single dose of 11 mg/kg, to a maximum of 1 g, should be given to treat infestations with *Ascaris lumbricoides, Enterobius vermicularis,* or *Ancylostoma duodenale.* In the case of pinworm, it is often wise to repeat the treatment after an interval of 2 weeks. Against *Necator americanus,* the same dose is given once daily for 3 days.

Toxicity and Side Effects. When administered parenterally to rabbits, pyrantel pamoate can produce complete neuromuscular blockade; if given orally, toxic effects are produced only by very large dosage. Gastrointestinal upset is occasionally observed in man, as are headache and dizziness; however, these effects do not persist and are not severe enough to require treatment.

Precautions and Contraindications. Pyrantel pamoate has not been studied in pregnant women, and its use in such patients is thus contraindicated. It is also not recommended for children less than 1 year of age. Since the possibility exists that pyrantel pamoate and piperazine may be mutually antagonistic, it would be unwise to use them together.

Therapeutic Uses. Pyrantel pamoate may be regarded as an agent of choice in the treatment of

ascariasis and *enterobiasis.* High cure rates have been achieved after single-dose treatment. Similarly, high rates of cure have been achieved against both *Ancylostoma* and *Necator hookworm disease,* and the drug appears to be as effective as bephenium in this respect.

PYRVINIUM PAMOATE

Early studies in experimental infestations showed that a series of cyanine dyes possessed marked antifilarial activity (Welch *et al.,* 1947; Peters *et al.,* 1949). One of these, *pyrvinium chloride,* was reported to be active against canine ascarids, trichurids, and hookworms, but to be inactive against tapeworms. The drug was not well tolerated, producing gastrointestinal upset and reversible renal damage (Hales and Welch, 1953). Weston and associates (1953) first observed that the chloride was highly effective against natural pinworm infestations of mice and rats. Its activity against human pinworm infestations was confirmed by Royer (1956) and Sawitz and Karpinski (1956). The chloride, however, produced nausea, abdominal pain, and vomiting, and was later replaced by the pamoate. Both the chloride and the pamoate have shown some degree of effectiveness in strongyloidiasis in man (Brown and Sterman, 1958; Meira *et al.,* 1961; Wagner, 1963).

Chemistry. The structural formula of pyrvinium is as follows:

Pyrvinium

Pyrvinium pamoate is a deep-red crystalline solid, insoluble in water.

Anthelmintic Action. Inhibition of oxygen uptake of adult *Litomosoides* is effected by many compounds containing the amidinium ion system, in which a quaternary nitrogen is separated from a tertiary nitrogen by a resonating carbon chain of alternating double and single bonds. This respiratory inhibition is associated with a compensatory increase in aerobic glycolysis. Concentrations of cyanine dyes a thousand times greater than those exerting an inhibitory effect on the respiration of *Litomosoides* have no effect on the oxygen uptake of mammalian tissues or on the activities of cytochrome c or of cytochrome oxidase. It therefore appears that, in worms, cyanines interfere with respiratory enzyme systems that play only a minor or no role in mammalian tissues. In *Trichuris vulpis,* dog whipworms, cyanine dyes in low concentrations interfere with the anaerobic transport of exogenous glucose; this effect is not seen with *L. carinii.* The dependence of *T. vulpis* on anaerobic metabolism is suggested not only by the low oxygen tension of its habitat, the colon of the dog, but also by the fact that the motility of the parasite is not reduced during incubation for 24 hours in an atmosphere of nitrogen. Hence, the anthelmintic activity of these compounds is associated with inhibition of respiration in aerobes, and interference with the absorption of exogenous glucose in intestinal helminths. Such interference may account for the anthelmintic effects of the cyanines in trichuriasis and in other intestinal helminthiases.

Standen (1963) has reviewed the effects of pyrvinium pamoate on helminth infestations in man and animals. It possesses a marked oxyuricidal action. In trials against *Trichuris* and *Necator* in man, however, repeated treatments gave unimpressive results.

Absorption. When given by the oral route, pyrvinium pamoate is not absorbed from the gastrointestinal tract to any appreciable extent.

Preparations, Route of Administration, and Dosages. *Pyrvinium Pamoate,* U.S.P. (POVAN, VANQUIN), is available as a suspension containing the equivalent of 10 mg of pyrvinium base per milliliter, and as tablets each containing the equivalent of 50 mg of pyrvinium base. For control of *pinworm infestation* in children and adults, pyrvinium pamoate is given orally in a single dose equivalent to 5 mg of pyrvinium base per kilogram of body weight, up to a maximum of 350 mg. A second dose should be administered 2 weeks later, to eliminate worms that have developed from ova ingested after the first dose. As in the case of piperazine, occupants of an entire household may be treated rather than investigating each member by anal swabs. Investigations on the effect of this drug on *strongyloidiasis* have shown promising results. In one series, doses from 2 to 6.4 mg/kg, given daily for 7 days, resulted in a high proportion of cures. Doses of 5 mg/kg, administered for 5 days, cured a smaller proportion but reduced considerably the worm burden in the remainder. Because of the staining quality of the drug, the tablets should be swallowed immediately without chewing. Parents and patients should be informed that the drug will color the stools a bright red, and that the suspension, if spilled, will stain.

Toxicity and Side Effects. Pyrvinium pamoate is well tolerated; the side effects are minimal and should not interfere with therapy. Side effects reported in a small proportion of treated patients included nausea, vomiting, and cramping; the majority of these patients were older children or adults who had received a relatively large dose of either suspension or tablets. Emesis was the most frequent side effect associated with the suspension, but it did not occur in patients who were given tablets.

Therapeutic Uses. Pyrvinium pamoate is an effective alternative drug of choice in treating oxyuriasis. A high cure rate has been achieved following single-dose therapy. However, because of the considerable risk of reinfection, chemotherapy should be combined with vigorous sanitation procedures and a follow-up examination for eggs at the anus

at least 5 weeks after the end of treatment. Its usefulness against strongyloidiasis has been established, but at least 7 days of therapy appears necessary to effect a high proportion of cures. Results obtained in combating infestations by *Trichuris* and *Necator* are unimpressive.

QUINACRINE

Quinacrine is an acridine derivative widely used during World War II as an antimalarial agent. It has almost wholly been superseded for this purpose by other drugs with more desirable properties. It was first used for the treatment of tapeworm infestation in 1939. There have been many reports since then of its efficacy against *Taenia saginata* and *T. solium.* In recent years, however, the availability of equally effective, less toxic agents has resulted in a decrease in its use for this purpose. For a fuller description of its properties, earlier editions of this textbook should be consulted. Quinacrine has the following structural formula:

Quinacrine

It is a bright-yellow crystalline powder with a bitter taste. The hydrochloride is soluble 1:35 in water.

Quinacrine is very readily absorbed from the intestinal tract. Even severe diarrhea does not interfere with absorption. The drug also quickly reaches the circulation from intramuscular sites of injection. It is widely distributed in the tissues and very slowly liberated. Therefore, the drug accumulates progressively in the tissues when it is administered chronically. Significant amounts of quinacrine can still be detected in the urine for at least 2 months after therapy is discontinued. The *metabolic fate* of quinacrine in the body is incompletely understood. Whether quinacrine exerts its antiparasitic actions *per se* or after metabolic transformation remains to be determined. However, its ready intercalation into DNA suggests that the parent drug is the active material, and that its selective toxicity is a function of relative distribution rather than specificity of action (*see* Albert, 1973).

Quinacrine is available as the dihydrochloride, designated *Quinacrine Hydrochloride,* U.S.P. (*mepacrine hydrochloride;* ATABRINE). It contains approximately 80% quinacrine base and is supplied as tablets, containing 100 mg of the dihydrochloride. It is available also as the methanesulfonate for intramuscular administration.

When used as a *taeniacide,* quinacrine is given orally. The patient is placed on a bland, semisolid, nonfat diet for the day before medication. A saline purge or a purge and cleansing enema may be given before treatment. The patient must fast at least from suppertime the evening before, as the gastrointestinal tract should be as empty as possible. Four doses of 200 mg each should be administered 10 minutes apart. Sodium bicarbonate, 600 mg, should be given with each dose to reduce any tendency to nausea and vomiting. A saline purge should be given 1 to 2 hours after the last dose. The expelled worm will be stained yellow, thereby facilitating identification of the scolex. In the treatment of dwarf tapeworm, the treatment is modified as follows: a saline purge is given on the night before medication, followed the next morning by 900 mg in three portions, 20 minutes apart. A saline purge is given 1½ hours later. It has been recommended that this regimen should be followed by 100 mg, three times a day for 3 days. Therapy may be repeated in 1 or 2 weeks if necessary. Children should be given reduced doses according to age. In the treatment of *lambliasis,* 100 mg should be given three times daily for 5 days. A second course of treatment may be given, if necessary, a week later. The dosage for children under 8 years of age should be proportionately reduced.

Because of its widespread use as an antimalarial drug, data on its toxicity are well documented. These have been reviewed extensively by Findlay (1951). The relatively large doses used in the treatment of cestode infestation may cause the transitory *toxic psychosis* that is seen in a small proportion of patients receiving lower doses for conventional treatment of overt malaria. Quinacrine is therefore contraindicated in patients with a history of psychosis. The duration of the drug-induced psychosis is usually 2 to 4 weeks, and the course is relatively benign. Only symptomatic therapy is indicated.

Great caution should be exercised in administering quinacrine (and other antimalarial compounds) to patients with *psoriasis,* since pronounced exacerbation is frequently produced and exfoliative lesions have sometimes developed. Quinacrine is contraindicated in patients receiving antimalarial therapy with primaquine (*see* Chapter 52). Quinacrine should not be given to pregnant women because the drug readily passes the placenta and reaches the fetus.

Quinacrine has proved to be of value in the treatment of the *large tapeworm* infestations of man. Against the *dwarf tapeworm,* however, results have been less conclusive, and more intensive and prolonged treatment, as described above, should be instituted. A number of clinical reports testify to its therapeutic efficacy in *Giardia lamblia* infection. The organisms disappear from the stools, and symptoms referable to the infection rapidly clear.

TETRACHLOROETHYLENE

Although *tetrachloroethylene* replaced carbon tetrachloride as an anthelmintic because of the toxicity of the latter, its physical properties are much like those of carbon tetrachloride. However, the drug is only one fifth as soluble in water and, in the absence of fat in the intestine, it is not absorbed to an appreciable extent. This probably accounts for its relatively low toxicity. Tetrachloroethylene is chiefly of value against hookworm.

Chemistry. Tetrachloroethylene is an unsaturated halogenated hydrocarbon with the following structural formula:

$$Cl_2C=CCl_2$$

Tetrachloroethylene

It is a colorless fluid with an ethereal odor. It is soluble 1:10,000 in water and is miscible with organic solvents. The drug rapidly deteriorates in warm climates and must be stored in a cool, dark place.

Pharmacological Effects. Although it is claimed that little of the administered dose of tetrachloroethylene is absorbed from the gastrointestinal tract, there is not infrequently evidence of central depression. The symptoms are giddiness, inebriation, and, rarely, loss of consciousness. The central actions of tetrachloroethylene are similar to those of chloroform.

Adult hookworms recovered from treated patients after purgation are motile. It has been assumed that affected worms are paralyzed sufficiently to release their attachment to the intestinal wall, and are then expelled by purgation before they can reattach themselves to the intestine. However, purgation is not required for removal of the worms (*see* below). The mechanism of action of tetrachloroethylene may therefore be other than a reversible paralysis. The drug has been shown readily to release lysosomal enzymes from granular fractions prepared from nematodes. Since the gut of nematodes seems to be specialized for lysosomal intracellular digestion of nutrients, an interference with this process may well explain the action of tetrachloroethylene (*see* Allison, 1968).

Preparations, Route of Administration, and Dosage. *Tetrachloroethylene,* U.S.P. (*perchloroethylene*), is available in soft gelatin capsules containing 0.2, 1.0, or 2.5 ml of the drug. It may be difficult to obtain the drug in capsule form for human use. However, the veterinary preparation is perfectly safe and effective to use in the proper dose in man.

Tetrachloroethylene is given orally as a single dose of 0.12 ml/kg, with a maximum of 5 ml. If possible, the diet before the administration of the drug should be low in fat and the patient should eat only a light meal the previous evening. The next morning, the tetrachloroethylene is ingested on an empty stomach; a cathartic is not necessary. A single treatment will generally remove most of the worms, but two or more treatments at 4-day intervals are usually required to clear the infestation. *Necator americanus* is relatively sensitive to tetrachloroethylene, and about 80% of patients harboring this parasite will be cleared after a single treatment. *Ancylostoma duodenale* is more resistant, and the probability of cure is only about 25% after one dose. Tetrachloroethylene has little effect against *Ascaris* and may stimulate this worm to activity and migration within the bowel. This may constitute a danger when massive infestations are present. In these cases the ascariasis may first be removed with a selective agent followed by tetrachloroethylene. The use of bephenium reduces or eliminates both worm burdens simultaneously.

Toxicity and Side Effects. Patients treated with tetrachloroethylene may experience a burning sensation in the stomach, abdominal cramps, nausea, and vomiting. In addition, central effects may be manifested by headache, vertigo, inebriation, and, rarely, loss of consciousness. Hence the patient should be kept at rest for 4 hours after administration of the drug. Severely anemic patients may collapse during therapy.

Precautions and Contraindications. As in the treatment of hookworm infestation with any agent, the first problem is the reestablishment of fluid and electrolyte balance and a reduction of the anemia. Following this treatment, tetrachloroethylene can be tolerated by most patients, but it is probably safer not to give this agent to small, severely ill children and to patients with fatty degeneration of the liver. Because of the central effects of tetrachloroethylene, alcohol should not be taken before or for 24 hours after the drug. (For patients harboring roundworm in addition to hookworm, *see* the comments above.)

Therapeutic Uses. Tetrachloroethylene is useful only against *hookworm* infestations in man. Treatment with this agent is more effective against *Necator americanus* than against *Ancylostoma duodenale* (*see* below).

TETRAMISOLE AND LEVAMISOLE

Tetramisole (ANTHELVET, RIPERCOL) is *racemic* 2,3,5,6-tetrahydro-6-phenylimidazo(2,1-*b*)-thiazole. It was introduced into veterinary practice in 1966 as a nematocidal agent, and it has subsequently been used for the treatment of infestations in man. The *l* isomer is more active than the racemic mixture, and it is now marketed separately as *levamisole* (KETARAX). It has the following structural formula:

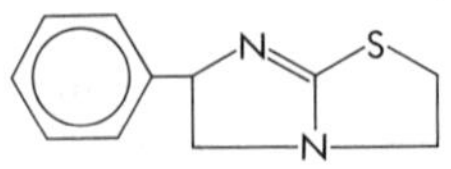

Levamisole

The substance is highly active against a wide range of nematodes. Tetramisole, like pyrantel, is a depolarizing neuromuscular blocking agent and an inhibitor of cholinesterases. The most obvious effect on nematodes is a muscular paralysis, associated with inhibition of fumarate reductase.

There is unanimity about its effectiveness in *ascariasis*. A single, well-tolerated dose produces a very high incidence of cure. Opinions differ, however, regarding its value in other nematode infestations.

THIABENDAZOLE

The development of *thiabendazole* was the result of investigations into anthelmintic activity of several hundred substituted benzimidazole compounds. It is claimed that some of these compounds are among the most potent chemotherapeutic agents known, complete larvicidal activity being manifested *in vitro* at 10 pg/ml. This potency, coupled with the absence of activity toward other microorganisms and negligible mammalian toxicity, suggests a unique interference with a metabolic pathway essential to a variety of helminths (Brown *et al.*, 1961). The drug has been reviewed at length in a symposium (*see* Symposium, 1969b).

Chemistry. Thiabendazole is a 2-(4-thiazolyl)-benzimidazole. It has the following structural formula:

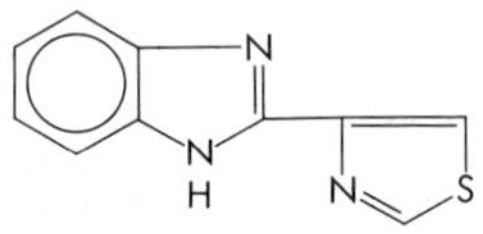

Thiabendazole

The drug occurs as a stable, white crystalline compound. It is almost insoluble in water but readily soluble in dilute acid or alkali.

Pharmacological Effects. Thiabendazole is reported to possess a high degree of activity against a wide range of nematodes infesting the gastrointestinal tract of domestic animals and to be larvicidal *in vitro* at very high dilution (Brown *et al.*, 1961; Standen, 1963). A concentration of 1 ppm has been shown to prevent the embryonic development of *Ascaris* eggs *in vitro* (Egerton, 1961). Its mechanism of action is unknown, although it has been shown to inhibit the helminth-specific enzyme fumarate reductase. Of particular interest are the reports that thiabendazole kills larvae in the muscle of pigs experimentally infected with *Trichinella spiralis*. Several cases of human trichinosis have been treated with thiabendazole and have shown marked clinical improvement. However, in some patients biopsy of deltoid muscle after completion of a course of treatment has revealed actively motile larvae. Generally the drug seems to allay symptoms and reduce eosinophilia, but its effect on larvae that have migrated to muscle is questionable. Anti-inflammatory, antipyretic, and analgesic effects, demonstrated in laboratory animals, may have contributed to the clinical responses. Thiabendazole has no effect on *filariasis*. It is active *in vitro* against a variety of *saprophytic and pathogenic fungi*, particularly against strains of *Trichophyton* and *Microsporum*. Clinically, however, response to treatment of superficial fungal infections has been equivocal.

Absorption, Fate, and Excretion. After oral administration of thiabendazole in man, absorption is rapid. Peak plasma concentrations occur about 1 hour after treatment. Within 48 hours, about 5% of the administered dose is recovered from the feces and about 90% from the urine. Most is excreted in the first 24 hours. Much of the material appearing in the urine is 5-hydroxythiabendazole conjugated either as the glucuronide or as the sulfate.

Preparations, Route of Administration, and Dosage. *Thiabendazole*, U.S.P. (MINTEZOL), is available as an oral suspension containing 500 mg/5 ml, as a topical suspension, and in 500-mg chewable tablets. The drug is preferably given after meals. The maximal daily recommended dose is 3 g. The standard dose for treating all roundworm infestations is 25 mg/kg. This is administered twice daily for 1 day for pinworms, and for 2 successive days for all other infestations. Single-day courses have been utilized quite successfully for all but the treatment of cutaneous larva migrans and trichinosis. A 2-day course is required in treating the former; this may be repeated in 2 days if active lesions are still present. This condition has been treated successfully by the topical application of thiabendazole. In trichinosis, treatment may be continued for 2 additional days, according to the response of the patient. For pinworms, the initial course should be repeated 2 weeks later to decrease the likelihood of reinfection due to the presence of viable ova in the environment. If this is impractical, the 2-successive-day regimen should be followed. Thiabendazole may be tried in the treatment of visceral larva migrans at the usual dosage until either the symptoms subside or toxic effects intervene. Since this is usually a self-limiting disease, however, treatment should be restricted to severe cases.

Toxicity and Side Effects. Side effects frequently encountered are anorexia, nausea, vomiting, and dizziness. Less frequently, diarrhea, epigastric distress, pruritus, weariness, drowsiness, giddiness, and headache occur. Side effects that are experienced rarely include tinnitus, collapse, abnormal sensation in the eyes, numbness, hyperglycemia, xanthopsia, enuresis, decrease in pulse rate and systolic blood pressure, and a transitory rise in cephalin flocculation and SGOT. Fever, facial flush, chills, conjunctival injection, angioneurotic edema, lymphadenopathy, perianal rash, and skin rash occur infrequently, but it is not certain whether these represent hypersensitivity to the drug, hypersensitivity to the parasite, or a manifestation of the disease. Appearance of live *Ascaris* in the mouth and nose has been reported on rare occasions. Some patients may excrete a metabolite that imparts an odor to urine. This is much like that occurring after ingestion of asparagus, and is noted during and for about 24 hours after completion of therapy. Crystalluria without hematuria has been reported on occasion; it promptly subsides with discontinuation of therapy. Transient leukopenia has been noted in a few patients on thiabendazole therapy.

It has been reported that up to one third of patients treated with the recommended dosage have been incapacitated for several hours by one or more symptoms; half were incapacitated for as long as 24 hours by doses of about 50 mg/kg.

Precautions and Contraindications. There are no absolute contraindications to the use of thiabendazole. Because CNS side effects occur quite frequently, activities requiring mental alertness should be prohibited during therapy. Since thiabendazole has hepatotoxic potentialities, it should be used with caution in patients with hepatic disease or decreased hepatic function. No special diet or purgation is needed.

Therapeutic Uses. Thiabendazole is a major advance in the therapy of *S. stercoralis* infestations and of *cutaneous larva migrans*. A 2-day course of treatment produces a better-than-90% cure rate in strongyloidiasis. Pseudo-hookworm infestation (*trichostrongyliasis*) also responds well, although in the United States its use for this purpose and for *dracontiasis* is considered investigational. The majority of patients experience marked relief of symptoms of creeping eruption. Progression of the disease should cease after 2 successive days of treatment. If active lesions persist after a 2-day interval, a second course of treatment is recommended. There is circumstantial evidence that the drug is also beneficial in the treatment of *visceral larva migrans*. Although thiabendazole is effective against *trichinosis* in animals, its value in the human disease is as yet unproven. It seems to allay symptoms and to reduce eosinophilia, but its effect on larvae that have migrated to muscle is open to doubt. Thiabendazole produces a cure rate of more than 90% in *enterobiasis* and a lesser, and more variable, rate in *ascariasis* and *hookworm disease*. The efficacy of the drug against *whipworm* varies greatly, depending on the size of the dose and the duration of treatment. A single 2-day course of treatment produces up to 35% cures. An advantage of thiabendazole is its effectiveness against *Ascaris, Enterobius, Strongyloides,* and *Trichuris* and, consequently, its usefulness in patients with multiple infestations.

ANTIMONY COMPOUNDS

Compounds of antimony are used in the treatment of *trematode* infestations. The general pharmacology and toxicology of these agents are presented in Chapter 46. The following discussion relates only to the uses of antimony compounds in helminthiasis.

Pharmacological Effects. *Anthelmintic Action.* Trivalent antimonials inhibit phosphofructokinase in schistosomes. This inhibition of phosphofructokinase activity can be reversed by increasing the concentration of fructose-6-phosphate and removing the antimony from the supporting medium. This reversibility manifests itself during treatment of the host with subcurative doses of antimonials. Initially the schistosomes migrate from mesenteric veins to the liver, and egg production ceases. After terminating treatment, however, the worms eventually recover and shift back to the mesenteric veins. Mammalian phosphofructokinase is much less sensitive to the action of antimonials, and, therefore, the chemotherapeutic usefulness of antimonials in schistosomiasis is due, in part at least, to differences in the nature of these two enzymes (*see* Saz and Bueding, 1966; Bueding and Schiller, 1968).

ANTIMONY POTASSIUM TARTRATE

Antimony potassium tartrate was introduced in 1918 as the first of the trivalent antimony compounds to be used in the treatment of schistosomiasis.

Chemistry. Antimony potassium tartrate has the following structural formula:

Antimony Potassium Tartrate

The compound occurs as colorless crystals or as a granular powder containing 36.5% trivalent antimony. It is soluble 1:12 in water. Such solutions are stable and may be sterilized by autoclaving or filtration.

Preparations, Routes of Administration, and Dosage. *Antimony Potassium Tartrate,* U.S.P. (*tartar emetic*), is available in crystalline form or in sterile solution in ampuls. The drug is normally administered intravenously, and such treatment is started with 8 ml of a 0.5% solution. If this is well tolerated, subsequent doses are given on alternate days, each dose being increased by 4 ml until the maximal single dose of 28 ml has been reached. A course normally consists of a maximum of 360 ml of the solution.

Precautions and Contraindications. Tartar emetic must be given very slowly by means of a fine needle, and care should be taken to avoid leakage into the perivascular tissue. Too rapid injection may produce a hacking cough, vomiting, and severe or even fatal reactions. The use of antimony potassium tartrate is contraindicated in the presence of severe hepatic, renal, or cardiac insufficiency (*see* Chapter 46).

Therapeutic Uses. Antimony potassium tartrate has been used effectively against all three species of *Schistosoma.* Its use against *S. haematobium* and *S. mansoni* has largely been replaced by more easily employed and less toxic schistosomicides. It remains, however, the drug of choice against *S. japonicum,* which is relatively less susceptible to other agents. For cure of this infestation, a total of 500 ml of 0.5% solution has been used. The drug has also proven valuable in the treatment of *granuloma inguinale.* A small percentage of patients have shown marked improvement after treatment of *mycosis fungoides* with antimony potassium tartrate.

ANTIMONY SODIUM TARTRATE

This compound possesses the same schistosomicidal activity as the potassium salt, but it is claimed to be rather less toxic. Nevertheless, the same precautions must be taken in its use. Antimony sodium tartrate is employed much more widely than the potassium salt in some countries in various parts of the world.

SODIUM ANTIMONYLGLUCONATE

Sodium antimonylgluconate (PENTOSTAM) occurs as an amorphous white powder containing 36% trivalent antimony. The drug is marketed in ampuls containing 190 mg of sterile powder. It is for intravenous use only, and its indications and uses are those of tartar emetic. It is claimed to be less toxic than the tartrates. In the United States the drug is available from the Parasitic Disease Drug Service, Center for Disease Control, Atlanta, Georgia.

Antimony sodium thioglycollate and *antimony thioglycollamide* are both compounds of trivalent antimony, introduced for intramuscular injection in the therapy of schistosomiasis. It is claimed that they are less toxic than antimony potassium tartrate. Both are available in ampuls containing 10 or 20 ml of a 0.4% solution.

ANTIMONY SODIUM-α,α′-DIMER-CAPTOSUCCINATE (STIBOCAPTATE)

Antimony sodium-α,α′-dimercaptosuccinate was reported by Friedheim and coworkers (1954) and Friedheim (1956) to be as effective as stibophen in the treatment of *S. mansoni* and *S. haematobium* infestations and to be less toxic. Subsequent trials have shown high cure rates against both species. It is effective· in a smaller proportion of cases of *S. japonicum.*

Chemistry. Antimony sodium-α,α′-dimercaptosuccinate has the following structural formula:

Antimony Sodium Dimercaptosuccinate

It is a white crystalline substance, readily soluble in water. The aqueous solution is unstable and should be used within 24 hours; if refrigerated, the solution may be used as long as it remains colorless and transparent.

Preparation, Route of Administration, and Dosage. The drug is supplied as a white crystalline powder in ampuls, each containing 0.5 g. The trade name is ASTIBAN. It is prepared for injection by adding 5 ml of water to the ampul, to give a 10% solution. In the United States the compound is available from the Parasitic Disease Drug Service, Center for Disease Control, Atlanta, Georgia.

The drug should be given intramuscularly in a course of five injections, at the rate of one or two per week. Particularly fit hospitalized patients may be given injections on alternate or even on consecutive days with a pause of 1 or 2 days after any injection, if necessary, according to tolerance. The total dose in adults should be between 30 and 50 mg/kg, with a maximum of 2.5 g. In children under 20 kg, total doses of 40 to 60 mg/kg may be given. The higher doses are indicated in *S. mansoni* and *S. japonicum* infestations. There is some evidence that better therapeutic results, greater activity, and less intolerance are obtained if the injection is given once or twice weekly, rather than on 5 consecutive days. Patients with heart disease of various etiologies have been treated successfully and without apparent harm with a total of 50 mg/kg, divided into five weekly intramuscular injections. In areas with highly endemic schistosomiasis, Friedheim and de Jongh (1959) and others have shown that "suppressive management" of *S. haematobium* infestations may be achieved by the monthly injection of the drug. Such treatment, while not providing radical cure, may prove to have considerable value by suppressing the production of eggs by the female para-

sites and thereby interrupting transmission. Ata and Mousa (1961) have used antimony potassium tartrate and stibophen, given weekly, to the same end. Antimony sodium-α,α′-dimercaptosuccinate is ineffective in the "suppressive management" of *S. mansoni* infestations.

Precautions and Contraindications. The appearance of rashes, excessive vomiting, pronounced fatigue, and pyrexia is an indication for temporary suspension of treatment. The drug is contraindicated in the presence of bacterial as well as *herpes simplex* and *zoster* infections; in patients with hepatic, renal, or cardiac insufficiency; and if treatment with antimonials has been carried out within the previous 2 months. It is also contraindicated if there is massive infestation with intestinal helminths.

STIBOPHEN

Since the introduction of antimony potassium tartrate in 1918 as an effective schistosomicide, much effort has gone into a search for less toxic agents. Trivalent antimony compounds are still the most effective in the treatment of schistosomiasis, and stibophen is one of the most widely used.

Chemistry. Stibophen is sodium antimony *bis*-(pyrocatechol-2,4-disulfonate). It has the following structural formula:

Stibophen

The drug occurs as colorless crystals that are freely soluble in water. It is stable in solution after autoclaving but may dissociate and become toxic after prolonged storage. Stibophen oxidizes when the solution is exposed to air for any length of time; hence, unused portions of opened ampuls should be discarded.

Preparation, Route of Administration, and Dosage. *Stibophen,* N.F. (FUADIN), is available in ampuls, each containing 300 mg in 5 ml of a 6.3% aqueous solution with 0.1% sodium bisulfite as preservative. Each milliliter contains the equivalent of 8.5 mg of trivalent antimony. Stibophen is administered intramuscularly. Various dosage schedules are recommended. The best is probably that which best suits local conditions, except in the treatment of *S. japonicum* infestations, for which the most intensive course should be instituted.

Conservative Dosage, Slow Therapy. A total volume of 40 ml is given as follows: 1.5 to 2.0 ml as a sensitivity test dose on the first day, 3.5 ml on the second, and 5 ml on the third; thereafter, six further doses of 5 ml each are given at 2- to 3-day intervals. This course should be repeated after 1 or 2 weeks. Some investigators give adults a total dose of 70 ml in 27 days. In these cases, the final 5-ml doses are given every other day for 12 doses.

Table 51–1. CHOICE OF DRUGS FOR THE CHEMOTHERAPY OF HELMINTHIASIS *

HELMINTH			DRUG ORDER OF CHOICE †	
Class or Subclass	Genus and Species	Synonym	1st	2nd
Nematoda (Roundworms)	Ascaris lumbricoides	Roundworm	Piperazine	Pyrantel pamoate
	Necator americanus	New World hookworm	Bephenium Pyrantel pamoate	Thiabendazole
	Ancylostoma duodenale	Old World hookworm	Bephenium Pyrantel pamoate	Thiabendazole
	Trichuris trichiura	Whipworm	Mebendazole	Thiabendazole
	Strongyloides stercoralis	Threadworm	Thiabendazole	Pyrvinium pamoate
	Enterobius (Oxyuris) vermicularis	Pinworm	Pyrantel pamoate	Piperazine Pyrvinium pamoate
	Trichinella spiralis	Pork roundworm	Corticosteroids ‡	Thiabendazole
	Wuchereria bancrofti Wuchereria (Brugia) malayi Loa loa	Filarial worms	Diethylcarbamazine	———
	Onchocerca volvulus		Diethylcarbamazine + suramin	———
	Dracunculus medinensis	Guinea worm	Thiabendazole	Niridazole
Cestoda (Tapeworms)	Taenia saginata	Beef tapeworm	Niclosamide	Dichlorophen Paromomycin
	Taenia solium	Pork tapeworm		
	Diphyllobothrium latum	Fish tapeworm		
	Hymenolepis nana	Dwarf tapeworm		
Trematoda (Flukes)	Schistosoma haematobium	Blood flukes	Niridazole	Antimony sodium dimercaptosuccinate Hycanthone Metrifonate Stibophen
	Schistosoma mansoni		Antimony sodium dimercaptosuccinate Stibophen	Hycanthone Niridazole
	Schistosoma japonicum		Antimony potassium tartrate	Antimony sodium dimercaptosuccinate Stibophen

Table 51-1. CHOICE OF DRUGS FOR THE CHEMOTHERAPY OF HELMINTHIASIS * (Continued)

	HELMINTH		DRUG ORDER OF CHOICE †	
Class or Subclass	Genus and Species	Synonym	1st	2nd
Trematoda (Flukes)	Paragonimus westermani Paragonimus kellicotti	Lung flukes	Bithionol	Chloroquine
	Clonorchis sinensis	Chinese liver fluke	Chloroquine	Antimony potassium tartrate Bithionol
	Fasciola hepatica	Liver fluke	Emetine	Bithionol Chloroquine
	Fasciolopsis buski	Intestinal fluke	Hexylresorcinol Tetrachloroethylene	——

* For preparations, doses, and administration of the indicated drugs, *see* text.
† When more than one drug is listed, the order is alphabetical.
‡ Used for symptomatic control of severe disease.

Conservative Dosage, Rapid Therapy. A total dosage of 34 ml is given in one course of treatment. On the first day, a 2-ml dose is injected in the morning, followed by 4 ml at midday and 4 ml in the afternoon. On the second and third days, a 4-ml dose is injected three times daily. The course should be repeated after 1 or 2 weeks.

Intensive Therapy. A total dose of 100 ml, given over 14 days, has been used in the treatment of American soldiers infested with *S. japonicum.* On the first, second, and third days, 2, 4, and 6 ml, respectively, were injected, followed by 8 ml daily for 11 days. A cure rate of about 80% was achieved, but nearly all the patients suffered from some toxic reactions. It was considered that the therapeutic benefit outweighed the toxicity.

Precautions and Contraindications. To test the susceptibility of the patient, it is advisable that the first dose be small, only 1.5 to 2.0 ml. Inadvertent intravenous injection should be carefully avoided. Treatment should be stopped in the event of recurrent vomiting, progressive albuminuria, severe and persistent joint pain, or intercurrent febrile infection. Blood dyscrasias, particularly thrombocytopenia with or without purpura, should be watched for and treatment stopped if they occur. The use of stibophen is contraindicated in the presence of severe hepatic, renal, or cardiac insufficiency. This may compromise its use in severe cases of *S. mansoni* and *S. japonicum* infestations because they are often associated with hepatic damage.

Therapeutic Uses. Stibophen is particularly useful in the treatment of *S. haematobium* and *S. mansoni* infestations. It can be successfully employed against *S. japonicum,* but the dosage used is of necessity high and patient cooperation is required because of toxic reactions.

TREATMENT OF WORM INFESTATIONS

A summary of the choice of drugs for the chemotherapy of infestations with specific helminths is provided in Table 51-1. The treatment of these infestations is described in more detail below.

ROUNDWORMS

Ascaris lumbricoides. *Ascaris lumbricoides,* known as the "roundworm," is cosmopolitan. Although cases of ascariasis are not infrequent in temperate climates, the parasite flourishes best in warm localities. In the southern United States, the incidence of ascariasis is very high, especially in the children of families in the poorer economic classes.

Treatment. The older, less efficient, and more toxic ascaricides have largely been discarded in favor of more active, less toxic compounds. One of the several available *piperazine* preparations is, without doubt, the agent of choice. Cure can be achieved in nearly 100% of cases. If ascariasis is a complication of hookworm infestation, great care should be taken in the treatment of the latter to avoid promoting unusual activity of the ascarids. Under such circumstances, the roundworms may block the lumen of the appendix and produce symptoms of appendicitis. They often occlude the common bile duct and occasionally invade the hepatic parenchyma. Perforation of the intestinal wall with subsequent peritonitis may rarely occur. If the worms are stirred to unusual activity, they may form a tangled mass and cause intestinal obstruction. Correct therapy under these circumstances is either the preliminary removal of *Ascaris* with *piperazine* followed by appropriate treatment of the hookworm infestation, or treatment with an agent effective against both roundworms. (For a discussion of this, *see* treatment of hookworm infestation.) *Pyrantel pamoate* is effective in both infestations, but its use against hookworm is considered investigational in the United States. *Bephenium* has been shown to remove or cause a major reduction in the *Ascaris* burden, but its prime indication is in the treatment of hookworm infestation.

Hookworm: Necator americanus, Ancylostoma duodenale.

These related species are commonly known as the *New World,* or *American, hookworm* and the *Old World hookworm,* respectively. The former species was imported into America from Africa. The parasites flourish chiefly between about latitudes 30° south and 40° north. Distribution much further north, into areas where a similar environment prevails, has been brought about by carriers. Such conditions occur in mines and large mountain tunnels, hence the terms *miner's disease* and *tunnel disease.*

Treatment. Treatment of hookworm disease involves two objectives. The first is to restore the blood values to normal, and the second is to expel the intestinal parasites. Often it is necessary to improve the patient's general condition before it is safe to administer an anthelmintic. Proper diet and iron medication are usually quite effective in this regard, but blood transfusion may occasionally be required. However, care must be taken to avoid overloading the circulation, because grave anemia due to hookworm infestation is frequently associated with edema. *Tetrachloroethylene* was the agent of choice in both infestations. Its great disadvantage is that it is dangerous to use alone when, as is frequently the case, the disease is complicated by ascariasis. In such cases, preliminary treatment with piperazine to remove the ascarids should precede treatment with tetrachloroethylene.

Bephenium is now the agent of choice against *Ancylostoma duodenale.* Where there is concurrent infestation with *Ascaris,* the drug will remove or cause a major reduction in the worm burden. There is less agreement about its usefulness against *Necator americanus,* but radical cure can be obtained albeit with larger doses and more extended treatment in most cases. In patients suffering from water and electrolyte imbalance, bephenium should not be used until these are corrected because of the possibility of vomiting induced by its bitter taste. *Pyrantel pamoate* is probably as effective as bephenium against hookworm and is also effective against *Ascaris. Thiabendazole,* while not a drug of first choice in any of the aforementioned infestations, has the advantage of being effective in the treatment of all three. In addition, it is effective in the treatment of trichuriasis, oxyuriasis, and strongyloidiasis, and hence is of special value in patients with multiple infestations.

Larva migrans or "creeping eruption," penetration of the skin of man by larvae of the dog hookworm *Ancylostoma braziliense,* has been successfully treated with *thiabendazole.*

Whipworm: Trichuris trichiura.

Whipworm infestation is encountered throughout the world, especially in warm, humid climates. It is frequently found in areas where ascaris and hookworm are endemic. The worm does not usually cause appreciable trouble except perhaps in heavily infested young children. Rarely, the worms may lodge in the appendix or may penetrate the bowel wall and give rise to peritonitis. Infested children may exhibit mild toxic symptoms and some degree of anemia.

Treatment. Although it is a new drug, *mebendazole* in a dosage of 100 mg twice daily for 3 days is considered the safest and most effective treatment against whipworm. *Thiabendazole* is also effective in an appreciable proportion of cases.

Threadworm: Strongyloides stercoralis.

Strongyloides stercoralis, sometimes called the threadworm or dwarf threadworm, is frequently found in tropical regions, and infestation with this worm is common in the southern United States. Similar environmental conditions are often found underground in the mining industry; hence the worm is occasionally found in mines even in temperate zones.

Treatment. Thiabendazole has been shown to be highly effective and is considered by most to be the drug of choice. Others consider *pyrvinium pamoate* to be equally effective. The relative merits can be assessed only by well-controlled trials, yet to be carried out.

Pinworm: Enterobius (Oxyuris) vermicularis.

Oxyuris is cosmopolitan. It is the most common helminthic infestation in the United States, especially in school children. The systemic symptoms caused by this parasite are mild and often unnoticed. Pruritus in the perianal and perineal regions, however, is especially severe and irritating, and scratching may cause infection. In female patients, the worms may wander into the genital tract and can then penetrate into the peritoneal cavity. Salpingitis or even peritonitis may occur. Because of the ease with which the infestation is distributed throughout the members of a family, a school, or an institution, the physician must decide whether to treat all persons in close contact with an infested person. The possibility of reinfestation demands a rigid standard of personal hygiene, such as keeping nails short, washing hands before meals, and changing cotton undergarments twice a day. Pruritus can be treated symptomatically. It is important also to wash bedroom and bathroom floors at the end of the course of treatment. It is necessary to remember that the time required for development from the egg that is swallowed to the emergence of the sexually mature worm from the anus or to the laying of eggs by the worm is at least 35 days. For this reason it is necessary, in order to prove cure, to show that no eggs can be found at the anus during a period of at least 5 weeks after the end of treatment.

Treatment. The agent of choice is *pyrantel pamoate.* When its use is allied with rigid standards of personal hygiene, a very high proportion of cures can be obtained. Treatment is simple, pleasant, and almost devoid of side effects. Some have used a single dose of *piperazine* combined with a laxative. Satisfactory results have been claimed. However, daily doses for 1 week is a more usual course of treatment. Pyrantel pamoate and piperazine have the added advantage of successfully clearing concurrent ascaris infestation. Also, a single dose of *pyrvinium pamoate* has been shown to produce a high proportion of cures, but its use may be associated with mild-to-severe vomiting. It will also stain clothing or other absorbent material. *Thiabendazole* has also been used as successfully, but associated with its use has been an appreciable incidence of side effects. Until more experience is gained with this drug it should be reserved for patients in whom pyrantel pamoate, piperazine, and pyrvinium pamoate prove ineffective in the treatment of pinworms.

Trichinella spiralis.

The trichina worm does not live at any time outside a host and, being independent of climate, is found all over the earth from the equator to the poles. It is found frequently in Canada, Eastern Europe, and the United States. The only mode of infestation is the eating of raw, or insufficiently cooked, flesh of trichinous animals. All pork, not forgetting pork sausages, should be thoroughly cooked before being eaten. The encysted larvae are killed by exposure to a temperature of 60° C for 5 minutes.

Treatment. *Corticosteroids* are of considerable value in controlling the acute and dangerous systemic manifestations of established infestation. Persons with mild cases may be ill only for a few days. The indefinite symptoms of fever, headache, muscle pain, and weakness seldom lead to a diagnosis of trichinosis. *Thiabendazole,* in well-tolerated doses, has been shown to kill *Trichinella* larvae in the muscle of experimental animals. In human cases, results have been variable. It appears to allay symptoms and to reduce eosinophilia, but its effect on larvae that have migrated to muscle is questionable.

Filariae: Wuchereria bancrofti.

Infestation with this species is especially a risk in Central Africa, South America, India, and southern China. It is found also in the Mediterranean region of southern Spain, Tangier, the Nile Delta, and Turkey; in the Transvaal; and in Brisbane in Australia. The subspecies, *W. bancrofti var. pacifica,* which does not appear periodically in the peripheral blood of man, is found only in New Guinea and the islands of the Central and South Pacific. *Wuchereria (Brugia) malayi* is restricted to Indonesia, the Malay peninsula, Vietnam, southern China, central India, and Ceylon. The migrating filaria, *Loa loa,* is a purely African species. It is found chiefly in western Central Africa, from Sierra Leone to Angola, and chiefly in the region of the large rivers, the Congo, the Niger, the Wellé, and the Ogowé.

Treatment. Although organic antimonials and arsenicals have been shown to have more effect in filariasis, *diethylcarbamazine* is the only agent that should be considered for both suppression and cure. It is advisable to start with a small initial dose to diminish the tendency to allergic reactions resulting from destruction of the microfilariae, particularly those of *Loa loa.* Prophylactic administration of *antihistamines* may diminish the severity of these reactions but will not abolish them altogether. *Corticosteroids* may be required to control acute reactions. In rare instances, serious cerebral allergic reactions have been observed in the treatment of loiasis, probably due to destruction of microfilariae in the brain. If headache is severe or if there is other evidence of an adult *Loa loa* near the orbit, extra care is advisable in initial dosing. The most satisfactory results are achieved in *W. bancrofti* and *W. malayi* infestations if treatment is started early, before obstructive lesions in the lymphatics have occurred. Even in late cases, however, improvement may result. In long-standing *elephantiasis,* surgical measures are required to improve lymph drainage and remove redundant tissue.

The arsenical *melarsonyl* (*Mel W;* TRIMELARSAN) has been employed successfully in the treatment of *W. bancrofti.* However, a number of deaths have occurred following its use, apparently due to encephalopathy. It has been stated that such risks should not be incurred in treating filarial infestations, which are normally nonfatal. Others maintain that with proper attention to the size of dose such accidents need not occur. The physician should, therefore, be fully aware of the risks involved and take all possible precautions in the use of the drug.

Onchocerca volvulus. This filarial worm is very common all over West and Central Africa. It was presumably imported from there into Mexico, northeastern Venezuela, and Guatemala.

Treatment. Migrating microfilariae in the skin in onchocerciasis can readily be eliminated by treatment with *diethylcarbamazine.* Allergic reactions, however, are likely to be even more severe than those occurring in the treatment of *Loa loa.* Great care should be exercised in initial dosing, particularly in cases where lesions of the eye are present (*see* above). The adult worms are relatively insusceptible to the action of the drug. Elimination of adult worms can be achieved by the administration of *suramin* following the schedule recommended by the World Health Organization's Expert Committee on Onchocerciasis (1954). The committee recommended an intravenous dose of 1 g, given weekly for 5 weeks. One fourth of this dose should be given initially to test for intolerance in the patient. Other workers have continued weekly treatment to a total of 10 weeks. Suramin acts principally on the adult female worms; these die or degenerate by the fourth or fifth week of treatment. The male adults are more resistant and remain alive and motile much longer than do the females. In the longer course of treatment, the ova and embryos are destroyed by the sixth to the tenth week. Later, the free microfilariae are also killed. The reaction to suramin is similar to that provoked by diethylcarbamazine, but it is much later in appearing and is more prolonged and less severe. Suramin may therefore be used after a course of diethylcarbamazine or as the initial treatment to destroy the adult worms and to eradicate the infestations. However, since the infestation is not dangerous to life and dangerous side effects may follow the prolonged administration of suramin (*see* Chapter 54), treatment should not be lightly undertaken. *Melarsonyl* also affects adult worms and disrupts intrauterine larval development, thus leading to a gradual decrease in microfilarial densities. However, its use is not without hazard (*see* above under *Wuchereria bancrofti*).

Guinea Worm. *Dracunculus medinensis,* also known as the *dragon* or *Medina* worm, occurs in East and West Africa, India, Pakistan, Bangladesh, Arabia, and Iraq.

Treatment. Traditional treatment is to draw the adult worm out alive. Natives do this by rolling it onto a small piece of wood, drawing out a little of it day by day. If it is ruptured by this procedure, severe secondary infections may appear. It is therefore recommended that the site at which the worm has broken through should be continuously washed with water to cause the worm to discharge all the larvae. After this it may be more easily extracted. Alternatively the worm may be removed by incisions along its course, under a local anesthetic. Satisfactory healing with either extrusion of the worm or, if no worm was extruded, complete symptomatic and functional relief has been obtained by the administration of *niridazole.* No local reactions occur if the worm is ruptured on extrusion (*see* Kothari *et al.,* 1968). *Thiabendazole* has been used with considerable success; such use is considered investigational in the United States.

TAPEWORMS

Taenia saginata. *Taenia saginata,* or the beef tapeworm, is the most common form of tapeworm. It is cosmopolitan.

Treatment. In the United States, the previous drug of choice, *quinacrine,* is becoming obsolete. It is being superseded by *niclosamide* and, in other countries where it is available, also by *dichlorophen.* Both give a high proportion of cures, are simple to administer, and are comparatively free from side effects. Dichlorophen has had more use than niclosamide, but the latter has proved satisfactory to date. Assessment of cure after the use of these drugs is difficult because the worm, segments as well as scolex, is usually passed in a partially digested state. Cure can be assumed only if no further segments have been passed by the end of 3 months. The antibiotic *paromomycin,* given in four doses of 1 g every 4 hours, is also highly effective. Its use for this purpose, however, is considered investigational in the United States.

Taenia solium. *Taenia solium,* or the pork tapeworm, is also cosmopolitan. An attendant danger of *T. solium* infestation, and one that is unique to this type of tapeworm, is that of *cysticercosis,* the harboring of the cysticerci (larvae) in the tissues of the human host. This usually results either from the ingestion of eggs of the parasite, as a result of the contamination of the hands with feces, or from the fact that eggs liberated from a gravid segment may pass upward into the duodenum, where the outer layers are digested. In either case, the free larvae gain access to the circulation and the tissues exactly as in their cycle in the intermediate host, the pig. The seriousness of the symptoms that result depends upon the particular tissue invaded. The usual sites are the brain, orbit, muscles, liver, and lungs.

Treatment. The treatment of infestation with *T. solium* is the same as that with *T. saginata.* It is most important, however, that therapy be successful, for there is a small but real danger that the patient may develop cysticercosis. Because of the action of *dichlorophen, niclosamide,* and *paromomycin,* resulting in partial digestion of the worm, it is obligatory to follow anthelmintic treatment with an adequate purge to clear the bowel before the segments can be digested. Otherwise, autoinfestation by the liberated ova may occur. If the scolex is not identified, courses should be repeated at suitable intervals.

Diphyllobothrium latum. *Diphyllobothrium latum,* the fish tapeworm, is a common parasite in many European countries, the Near East, Siberia, northern Manchuria, Japan, and the lake regions of Canada and the United States. In North America the pike is the most common second intermediate host. The eating of inadequately cooked infested fish introduces the larvae into the human intestine. The tasting of foods containing fish during their preparation is another common cause of infestation. In countries where infestation with fish tapeworm is common, there is a high incidence of megaloblastic anemia, which resembles addisonian pernicious anemia in all respects. This syndrome, which has been termed "bothriocephalus anemia," is especially prevalent in Finland, where until recently 90% of the population of certain provinces harbored worms. The incidence of megaloblastic anemia in infested individuals has been placed as high as 1 case in 136 carriers. The mechanism by which the helminthiasis produces the anemia is discussed in Chapter 64. Expulsion of the worm results in a hematological remission.

Treatment. The previous drug of choice, *quinacrine,* has now been replaced by *dichlorophen, niclosamide,* or *paromomycin;* treatment is the same as that for *T. saginata.* If these newer drugs are used, the presence of eggs in the stool 18 or more days after treatment is indicative of drug failure or reinfestation. The use of paromomycin for the treatment of fish tapeworm is considered investigational in the United States.

Hymenolepis nana. *Hymenolepis nana,* the dwarf tapeworm, with its subspecies *H. nana fraterna,* is the smallest of the tapeworms found in the small intestine of man.

Children are infested more often than adults. It is cosmopolitan, but infestation is more common in warm climates. It is the most frequently occurring tapeworm disease in the southern United States. *Hymenolepis nana* can develop from ovum to mature adult in man without an intermediate host. The cysticerci develop in the villi of the intestine for 3 to 4 days and then regain access to the intestinal lumen. Treatment must therefore be adapted to this form of development.

Treatment. *Dichlorophen, niclosamide,* and *paromomycin* have largely replaced *quinacrine.* Niclosamide has become the agent of choice in North America. Failure of treatment or reinfestation is indicated by the appearance of eggs in the stool about 4 weeks after the last dose. High cure rates have also been obtained with *paromomycin,* an investigational drug in this case, given in a dose of 45 mg/kg daily for 5 to 7 days.

FLUKES

Schistosoma haematobium, S. mansoni. Infestation with these parasites, commonly known as the *blood flukes,* is termed *schistosomiasis* or *bilharziasis.* The disease is widespread throughout Africa and Brazil. Smaller foci also exist in the Near East.

Treatment. The success of therapy depends upon early diagnosis and prompt treatment. If the disease has reached the chronic stage characterized by tissue change, appropriate treatment will be required in addition to chemotherapy if infestation is still present. The drugs of choice differ in the two infestations. *Niridazole* is considered to be the agent of first choice by many experts in the treatment of *S. haematobium* infestation; others prefer *stibophen.* Against *S. haematobium* but not *S. mansoni, metrifonate* has been used with considerable success. The treatment is well tolerated. Other antimonials, such as *antimony sodium dimercaptosuccinate,* also have their proponents. Against *S. mansoni,* the antimonials are to be preferred to niridazole. The response to the latter is not as consistently good as it is in the case of *S. haematobium.* The *antimonial tartrates* have been largely replaced by other trivalent antimony compounds because of a high incidence of side effects. Nevertheless, the employment of any of the drugs is complicated by a high incidence of side effects.

In mass campaigns against both *S. haematobium* and *S. mansoni* in several parts of the world, single-dose intramuscular treatment with *hycanthone* has resulted in a high incidence of cure and reduction in egg output. While the controversy over the possible long-term effects of the drug on the treated population is far from settled, the World Health Organization has found no justification to recommend that its use should cease. Treatment with hycanthone, or any other schistosomicide, in large-scale campaigns should take into account the conditions prevailing in each population to be treated and an assessment of benefit against possible harm. The large-scale control of schistosomiasis has been reviewed by the World Health Organization (1973).

Schistosoma japonicum. This species is restricted to East Asia. Treatment of *S. japonicum* infestation differs from that of infestation by the other species.

Treatment. *Schistosoma japonicum* is apparently insusceptible to *hycanthone* and *metrifonate*. This worm is also less sensitive to the more complex trivalent antimonials; therefore, the tartrates, possessing higher activity albeit greater toxicity for the host, are the agents of choice. *Stibophen* has been used successfully, although a most intensive course of treatment is necessary. Experience with *antimony sodium dimercaptosuccinate* is more limited, but some success has followed its use. There appears to be little consistency in the proportion of patients cured by *niridazole* in various trials. Most investigators are agreed, however, that a course of treatment is followed by a marked reduction in the egg count.

Paragonimus westermani, P. kellicotti.

These two species of *lung fluke* differ morphologically from each other only slightly. *Paragonimus westermani* is prevalent in the Far East, while *P. kellicotti* probably occurs only in the Americas. Infestation with lung fluke, species undetermined, has also been reported in West Africa.

Treatment. *Bithionol* (ACTAMER, BITIN) has been used successfully in the treatment of this infestation. Patients are given 40 to 50 mg/kg orally, in divided doses on alternate days, for a total of 10 to 15 doses. In all cases, stools and sputum become free of eggs after 2 to 5 days of treatment and remain free for at least 12 months. Patients receiving this drug have experienced photosensitivity reactions, urticaria, and gastrointestinal distress. *Chloroquine,* in large doses over an extended period, has also had some success. Treatment with 250 mg three times daily should be continued for 6 weeks.

Clonorchis sinensis. *Clonorchis sinensis,* the Chinese liver fluke, is widely distributed in East Asia.
Treatment. There is no drug that will reliably clear infestation with *C. sinensis.* Prolonged therapy with *chloroquine* offers the best chance of success. However, treatment may have to be discontinued because of the side effects of the large doses required. Treatment with 250 mg, three times daily, should be continued for 6 weeks. Follow-up of treated cases for over 1 year will probably show a disappointing proportion of relapses in those apparently cured. Early cases respond quite well to intravenous *antimony sodium tartrate.* The technic outlined for the treatment of schistosomiasis is followed. *Bithionol,* in the regimen outlined under *P. westermani,* may also be tried. In heavy infestations, therapy can do no more than reduce the number of invading organisms and hence the severity of symptoms. The closely related *Opisthorchis felineus,* the *cat liver fluke,* may develop equally well in man, dogs, and some other fish-eating mammals. No really reliable drug is known for the treatment of this infestation. The therapy outlined for treatment of *C. sinensis* infestation could be tried. Preliminary data indicate that *hexachloroparaxylol* (HETOL) may be used successfully in both parasitoses (*see* Lämmler, 1968).

Fasciola hepatica. *Fasciola hepatica,* the *large liver fluke,* is relatively rare in man but common in sheep, cattle, goats, and other herbivorous animals throughout the world.
Treatment. *Emetine hydrochloride* is the drug of choice. It is given by deep subcutaneous injection in a daily dose of 1 mg/kg (maximum of 60 mg), for up to 10 days. The precautions necessary in treatment with emetine are outlined in Chapter 53. *Bithionol* has been found to be effective when given in the same dosage as in the treatment of lung fluke.

Fasciolopsis buski. *Fasciolopsis buski,* the giant intestinal fluke, occurs chiefly in Southeast Asia.
Treatment. The older drugs used in the treatment of hookworm infestation, *tetrachloroethylene* and *hexylresorcinol,* are very effective against this infestation. The value of *bephenium* is not known.

Heterophyes heterophyes, Metagonimus yokogawai, Watsonius watsoni, Gastrodiscus hominis, Echinostoma ilocanum, Echinostoma lindoënsis. These smaller *intestinal flukes,* occurring in various parts of the world, may cause clinical symptoms only if present as massive infestations.
Treatment. *Tetrachloroethylene,* given in the usual manner, is effective in the treatment of these infestations. *Bephenium* and *niclosamide* are helpful in combating *H. heterophyes.*

Dicrocoelium dendriticum. The small *liver fluke, Dicrocoelium dendriticum,* is primarily a parasite of ruminants, but occasionally it also occurs in man.
Treatment. If massive infestation makes treatment necessary, a course of therapy with *emetine* as outlined above should be tried.

Abdallah, A., and Saif, M. The efficacy of N-2'-chloro-4'-nitrophenyl-5-chlorosalicylamide in the treatment of taeniasis. *J. Egypt. med. Ass.,* **1961,** *44,* 379–381.

Ata, A. H. A., and Mousa, A. H. The evaluation of treating haematobium schistosomiasis in a controlled population with tartar emetic by the slow method. *J. Egypt. med. Ass.,* **1961,** *44,* 695–703.

Aubry, M. L.; Cowell, P.; Davey, M. J.; and Shevde, S. Aspects of the pharmacology of a new anthelmintic: pyrantel. *Br. J. Pharmac.,* **1970,** *38,* 332–344.

Austin, W. C.; Courtney, W.; Danilewicz, J. C.; Morgan, D. H.; Conover, L. H.; Howes, H. L., Jr.; Lynch, J. E.; McFarland, J. W.; Cornwall, R. L.; and Theodorides, V. J. Pyrantel tartrate, a new anthelmintic effective against infections of domestic animals. *Nature, Lond.,* **1966,** *212,* 1273–1274.

Brown, H. D.; Matzuk, A. R.; Ilves, I. R.; Peterson, L. H.; Harris, S. A.; Sarett, L. H.; Egerton, J. R.; Yakstis, J. J.; Campbell, W. C.; and Cuckler, A. C. Antiparasitic drugs. IV. 2-(4'-thiazolyl)-benzimidazole, a new anthelmintic. *J. Am. chem. Soc.*, **1961**, *83*, 1764–1765.

Brown, H. W., and Sterman, M. M. Chemotherapy of strongyloidiasis with pyrrovinylquinium (VANQUIN). *Am. J. trop. Med. Hyg.*, **1958**, *7*, 255–256.

Brugmans, J. P.; Thienpont, D. C.; van Wijngaarden, I.; Vanparijs, O. F.; Schuermans, V. L.; and Lauwers, H. L. Mebendazole in enterobiasis. Radiochemical and pilot clinical study in 1278 subjects. *J. Am. med. Ass.*, **1971**, *217*, 313–316.

Bumbalo, T. S.; Fugazzoto, D. J.; and Wyczalek, J. V. Treatment of enterobiasis with pyrantel pamoate. *Am. J. trop. Med. Hyg.*, **1969**, *18*, 50–52.

Chavarria, A. P.; Swartzwelder, J. C.; Villarejos, V. M.; and Zeledon, R. Mebendazole, an effective broad-spectrum anthelmintic. *Am. J. trop. Med. Hyg.*, **1973**, *22*, 592–595.

Chou, T. T.; Bennett, J. L.; Pert, C.; and Bueding, E. Effect of hycanthone and of two of its structural analogs on levels and uptake of 5-hydroxytryptamine in *Schistosoma mansoni. J. Pharmac. exp. Ther.*, **1973**, *186*, 408–415.

Copp, F. C.; Standen, O. D.; Scarnell, J.; Rawes, D. A.; and Burrows, R. B. A new series of anthelmintics. *Nature, Lond.*, **1958**, *181*, 183.

Doyen, A.; Léonard, J.; Mbendi, S.; and Sonnet, J. Influence des doses thérapeutique du CIBA 32644-Ba sur l'hématopoïèse des patients atteints de bilharziose et d'amibiase. *Acta trop.*, **1967**, *24*, 59–77.

Egerton, J. R. The effect of thiabendazole upon *Ascaris* and *Stephanurus* infections. *J. Parasit.*, **1961**, *47*, Sect. 2, 37.

Eyre, P. Some pharmacodynamic effects of the nematocides: methyridine, tetramisole and pyrantel. *J. Pharm. Pharmac.*, **1970**, *22*, 26–36.

Fayard, C. Ascaridiose et piperazine. Thesis, Paris, **1949**. (Quoted from *Sem. Hôp. Paris*, **1949**, *35*, 1778.)

Fierlafijn, E. Mebendazole in enterobiasis. *J. Am. med. Ass.*, **1971**, *218*. 1051.

Friedheim, E. A. H. Le traitement de la bilharziose urinaire à S. haematobium par le dimercaptosuccinate d'antimoine (TWSb). *Bull. Soc. Path. exot.*, **1956**, *49*, 1247–1252.

Friedheim, E. A. H., and de Jongh, R. T. The effect of a single dose of TWSb in urinary bilharziasis: suggestions for suppressive management of bilharziasis. *Ann. trop. Med. Parasit.*, **1959**, *53*, 316–324.

Friedheim, E. A. H.; Rodrigues da Silva, J.; and Martins, A. V. Treatment of schistosomiasis mansoni with antimony-α,α'-dimercapto-potassium succinate (TWSb). *Am. J. trop. Med. Hyg.*, **1954**, *3*, 714–727.

Gönnert, R., and Schraufstätter, E. Experimentelle Untersuchungen mit N-(2'-chlor-4'-nitrophenyl)-5-Chlorsalicylamid, einen neuen Bandwurmmitel. I. Mitterlung: Chemotherapeutische Versuche. *Arzneimittel-Forsch.*, **1960**, *10*, 881–884.

Goodwin, L. G.; Jayewardene, L. G.; and Standen, O. D. Clinical trials with bephenium hydroxynaphthoate against hookworm in Ceylon. *Br. med. J.*, **1958**, *21*, 1572–1576.

Goodwin, L. G., and Standen, O. D. Treatment of ascariasis with various salts of piperazine. *Br. med. J.*, **1958**, *1*, 131–133.

Hales, D. H., and Welch, A. D. A preliminary study of the anthelmintic activity of cyanine dye No. 715 in dogs. *J. Pharmac. exp. Ther.*, **1953**, *107*, 310–314.

Harned, B. K.; Cunningham, R. W.; Halliday, S.; Vessey, R. E.; Yuda, N. N.; Clark, M. C.; Hine, C. H.; Cosgrove, R.; and SubbaRow, Y. Studies on the chemotherapy of filariasis. VI. Some pharmaco-dynamic properties of 1-diethylcarbamyl-4-methylpiperazine hydrochloride, HETRAZAN. *J. Lab. clin. Med.*, **1948**, *33*, 216–235.

Hawking, F.; Sewell, P.; and Thurston, J. P. The mode of action of HETRAZAN on filarial worms. *Br. J. Pharmac. Chemother.*, **1950**, *5*, 217–238.

Hulbert, P. B.; Bueding, E.; and Hartman, P. R. Hycanthone analogs: dissociation of mutagenic effects from antischistosomal effects. *Science, Wash.*, **1974**, *186*, 647–648.

Katz, N.; Dias, E. P.; Araujo, N.; and Souza, C. P. Estudo de uma cepa humana de *Schistosoma mansoni* resistente a agentes esquistossomicidas. *Revta Soc. bras. Med. trop.*, **1973**, *7*, 381–387.

Katz, N.; Pellegrino, J.; Ferreira, M. T.; Oliveira, C. A.; and Dias, C. B. Preliminary clinical trials with hycanthone, a new antischistosomal agent. *Am. J. trop. Med. Hyg.*, **1968**, *17*, 743–746.

Kikuth, W.; Gönnert, R.; and Mauss, H. MIRACIL, ein neues Chemotherapeuticum gegen die Darmbilharziose. *Naturwissenschaften*, **1946**, *33*, 253.

Kothari, M. L.; Pardnani, D. S.; and Anand, M. P. Niridazole in dracunculiasis. *Am. J. trop. Med. Hyg.*, **1968**, *17*, 864–866.

Mauss, H. Ueber basisch substituierte Xanthon-und Thioxanthon-Abkömmlinge: MIRACIL, ein neues Chemotherapeuticum. *Chemie*, **1948**, *81*, 19.

Meadows, M. G.; Quah, S.; and von Borstel, R. C. Mutagenic action of hycanthone and 1A-4 on yeast. *J. Pharmac. exp. Ther.*, **1973**, *187*, 444–450.

Meira, D. A.; Neto, V. A.; and Campos, R. Tratamento da estrongiloidiase pelo pamoato de pirvinio. *Hospital, Rio de J.*, **1961**, *59*, 1135–1138.

Miller, M. J.; Krupp, I. M.; Little, M. D.; and Santos, C. Mebendazole. An effective anthelmintic for trichuriasis and enterobiasis. *J. Am. med. Ass.*, **1974**, *230*, 1412–1414.

Peters, L.; Bueding, E.; Valk, A. D., Jr.; Higachi, A.; and Welch, A. D. The antifilarial action of cyanine dyes. I. The relative antifilarial activity of a series of cyanine dyes against *Litomosoides carinii, in vitro* and in the cotton rat. *J. Pharmac. exp. Ther.*, **1949**, *95*, 212–239.

Rogers, E. W. Excretion of piperazine salts in urine. *Br. med. J.*, **1958**, *1*, 136–137.

Rosi, D.; Peruzzotti, G.; Dennis, E. W.; Berberian, D. A.; Freele, H.; and Archer, S. A new, active metabolite of 'MIRACIL D.' *Nature, Lond.*, **1965**, *208*, 1005–1006.

Royer, A. Preliminary report on a new antioxyuritic, POQUIL. *Can. med. Ass. J.*, **1956**, *74*, 297.

Sargent, R. G.; Savory, A. M.; Mina, A.; and Lee, P. R. A clinical evaluation of mebendazole in the treatment of trichuriasis. *Am. J. trop. Med. Hyg.*, **1974**, *23*, 375–377.

Sawitz, W. G., and Karpinski, F. E. Treatment of oxyuriasis with pyrrovinylquinium chloride (POQUIL). *Am. J. trop. Med. Hyg.*, **1956**, *5*, 538–543.

Schneider, J. Traitement du taeniases par le 5,5'-dichloro-2,2'-dihydroxydiphenylmethane. *Thérapie*, **1959**, *14*, 63–67.

Wagner, E. D. Pyrvinium pamoate in the treatment of strongyloidiasis. *Am. J. trop. Med. Hyg.*, **1963**, *12*, 60–61.

Wagner, E. D., and Chavarria, A. P. *In vivo* effects of a new anthelmintic, mebendazole (R-17,635) on the eggs of *Trichuris trichiura* and hookworm. *Am. J. trop. Med. Hyg.*, **1974**, *23*, 151–153.

Welch, A. D.; Peters, L.; Bueding, E.; Valk, A. D., Jr.; and Higachi, A. A new class of antifilarial compounds. *Science, Wash.*, **1947**, *105*, 486–488.

Weston, J. K.; Thompson, P. E.; Reinertson, J. W.; Fiskin, R. A.; and Reutner, T. F. Antioxyurid activity, toxicology and pathology in laboratory animals of a cyanine dye, 6-dimethyl-amino-2 (2,5-dimethyl-1-phenyl-3-pyrrol)-vinyl-1-methyl-quinilium chloride. *J. Pharmac. exp. Ther.*, **1953**, *107*, 315–324.

White, R. H. R., and Scopes, J. W. A single-dose treatment of threadworms in children. *Lancet*, **1960**, *1*, 256–258.

Wolfe, M. S., and Wershing, J. M. Mebendazole. Treatment of trichuriasis and ascariasis in Bahamian children. *J. Am. med. Ass.*, **1974**, *230*, 1408–1411.

Yarinsky, A.; Drobeck, H. P.; Freele, H.; Wiland, J.; and Gumaer, K. I. An 18-month study of the parasitologic and tumorigenic effect of hycanthone in *Schistosoma mansoni*-infected and noninfected mice. *Toxicol. appl. Pharmac.*, **1974**, *27,* 169–182.

Monographs and Reviews

Albert, A. *Selective Toxicity: The Physico-Chemical Basis of Therapy,* 5th ed. Chapman & Hall, Ltd., London, **1973.**

Allison, A. The role of lysosomes in the action of drugs and hormones. *Adv. Chemother.,* **1968,** *3,* 253–302.

Brown, H. W. Anthelmintics, new and old. *Clin. Pharmac. Ther.,* **1968,** *10,* 5–21.

Bueding, E., and Schiller, E. Mechanism of action of antischistosomal drugs. In, *Mode of Action of Antiparasitic Drugs,* Vol. 1. (Rodrigues da Silva, J., and Ferreira, M. J., eds.) Pergamon Press, Ltd., Oxford, **1968,** pp. 81–86.

Findlay, G. M. *Recent Advances in Chemotherapy,* Vol. II. J. & A. Churchill, Ltd., London, **1951.**

Hawking, F. Chemotherapy of filariasis. In, *Experimental Chemotherapy,* Vol. I. (Schnitzer, R. J., and Hawking, F., eds.) Academic Press, Inc., New York, **1963,** pp. 893–912.

Keeling, J. E. D. The chemotherapy of cestode infections. *Adv. Chemother.,* **1968,** *3,* 109–152.

Lämmler, G. Chemotherapy of trematode infections. *Adv. Chemother.,* **1968,** *3,* 153–251.

Saz, H. J., and Bueding, E. Relationships between anthelmintic effects and biochemical and physiological mechanisms. *Pharmac. Rev.,* **1966,** *18,* 871–894.

Seaton, D. R. Current therapeutics. CVI. Anthelmintics. *Practitioner,* **1956,** *177,* 507–511.

Standen, O. D. Chemotherapy of helminthic infections. In, *Experimental Chemotherapy,* Vol. I. (Schnitzer, R. J., and Hawking, F., eds.) Academic Press, Inc., New York, **1963,** pp. 701–892.

Symposium. (Various authors.) The pharmacological and chemotherapeutic properties of niridazole and other antischistosomal compounds. *Ann. N.Y. Acad. Sci.,* **1969a,** *160,* 423–946.

Symposium. (Various authors.) Thiabendazole. *Texas Rep. Biol. Med.,* **1969b,** *27,* 533–708.

Van den Bossche, H. Biochemical effects of the anthelmintic drug mebendazole. In, *Comparative Biochemistry of Parasites.* (Van den Bossche, H., ed.) Academic Press, Inc., New York, **1972,** pp. 139–157.

World Health Organization. *Report of the Expert Committee on Onchocerciasis.* Technical Report No. 87, WHO, Geneva, **1954.**

————. *Report of the Expert Committee on Filariasis.* Technical Report No. 359, WHO, Geneva, **1967.**

————. *Report of the Expert Committee on Schistosomiasis Control.* Technical Report No. 515, WHO, Geneva, **1973.**

CHAPTER

52 DRUGS USED IN THE CHEMOTHERAPY OF MALARIA

Ian M. Rollo

In order to understand the actions and uses of antimalarial drugs, it is necessary to appreciate the basic features of the biology of the malarial infection and the major principles and objectives of its treatment, including the problem of multidrug-resistant strains of plasmodia. Accordingly, these aspects will be presented before the pharmacology of the individual drugs is considered.

The chief agents employed in malaria therapy are *chloroquine* and its congeners, *chloroguanide* and related drugs, *pyrimethamine, primaquine,* and *quinine;* they will be described in the order given. Sulfonamides, sulfones, and tetracyclines are also used concurrently with certain of these drugs. *Quinacrine,* a prior mainstay of antimalarial suppression and treatment, is now obsolete for this purpose, but it does have some uses in other infections. It has been replaced almost entirely by chloroquine, which may now be taken to represent the prototype of agents that suppress the malarial infection and control the overt clinical attacks, but neither prevent nor radically cure the disease. Despite its historical importance, *quinine* is discussed last because it is now in most respects the least important of the drugs employed in malaria.

Of considerable importance has been the development of *in-vitro* technics for the assessment of antimalarial activity with, for example, laboratory malarial strains (Richards and Williams, 1973) and strains of falciparum malaria (Rieckmann *et al.,* 1968). The opportunity for experimental chemotherapy of human malarias in a nonhuman, laboratory host has been provided by the successful passage of both falciparum and vivax malarias in the owl monkey (*see* World Health Organization, 1973).

BIOLOGY OF THE MALARIAL INFECTION

Inasmuch as the efficacy of drugs in the prevention and the treatment of malaria is related to the species of infecting parasite and its stage of development, it is essential to review briefly the nature of the malarial infection.

Species of the Genus Plasmodium Infecting Man. (1) *Plasmodium falciparum,* the cause of *malignant tertian* malaria, often produces a fulminating infection in the nonimmune patient; if untreated, the infection may progress rapidly to a fatal termination. Delay in treatment after the demonstration of parasites in the blood may lead to an irreversible state of shock, and death may occur even after the peripheral blood has been cleared of parasites. If treated early, the infection usually responds readily to the administration of effective antimalarial drugs, and relapses will not occur. If treatment is inadequate, however, recrudescence may result from parasites persisting in the blood. (2) *Plasmodium vivax* is the cause of *benign tertian* malaria, which produces milder clinical attacks than those of *P. falciparum* and has a low mortality rate in untreated adults. The infection is characterized by relapses that occur for a period of at least 2 years after primary infection. (3) *Plasmodium malariae* is the cause of *quartan* malaria, an infection that is common in localized areas in the tropics. Relapses do occur but are much rarer than after infection with *P. vivax.* Latent infections of many years' standing may give rise to transfusion-induced malaria. (4) *Plasmodium ovale* is the cause of a rare malarial infection with a periodicity like that of *P. vivax,* but it is milder and more readily cured.

Man is infected by *sporozoites* injected by the bite of infected mosquitoes. The sporozoites disappear rapidly from the circulation and localize in the parenchymal cells of the liver, where they grow, segment, and sporulate. This constitutes the *preerythrocytic stage* of infection, during which the subject remains symptom free. On reaching maturity, *merozoites* are released from the cells of the liver and enter erythrocytes to start the *blood cycle.* In all but falciparum malaria, a proportion of these parasites infects more tissue cells, and this stage of infection, the *exoerythrocytic cycle,* may continue for several years and result in clinical recrudescence or *relapse* in the infected patient. *Schizogony* occurs in the

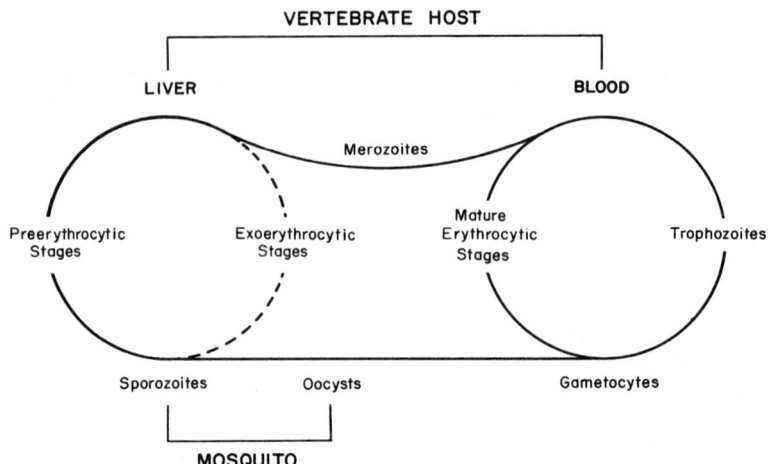

Figure 52-1. *Schematic representation of plasmodial life cycle.* For details, *see* text (——, all malarias; -----, relapsing malarias only). (After Rollo, 1964. Courtesy of Academic Press, Inc.)

infected erythrocytes as a result of growth and segmentation of the merozoites. When the erythrocyte bursts, the liberated *merozoites* are capable of infecting more red blood corpuscles and of starting the cycle anew. It is this periodic breaking of erythrocytes that causes the chill so characteristic of malaria. The fever following the chill is due to the liberated foreign protein and cell products. For reasons not yet understood, some of the merozoites invading erythrocytes fail to follow the asexual pattern of reproduction. They differentiate into male and female parasites known as *gametocytes*. No further development of these forms occurs until blood is ingested by a female mosquito. In the gut of the mosquito, exflagellation of the male gametocyte is followed by fertilization of the female gametocyte; the resulting *zygote,* developing in the gut wall as an *oocyst,* eventually gives rise to the infective *sporozoite.* The various stages are outlined in Figure 52-1.

CHEMOTHERAPY OF MALARIA IN RELATION TO THE BIOLOGY OF THE INFECTION

The chemotherapy of malaria may be conveniently considered under the following six categories: (1) causal prophylaxis, (2) suppressive treatment, (3) clinical cure, (4) radical cure, (5) suppressive cure, and (6) gametocytocidal therapy.

Causal Prophylaxis. A causal prophylactic is an agent that prevents demonstrable infection by exerting a lethal effect on the malarial parasites during their preerythrocytic stages. Inasmuch as man is his own reservoir of infection, causal prophylaxis also

prevents the further transmission of malaria to mosquitoes. To be effective, such therapy must be continued as long as the individual remains in a region where malaria is endemic. The term *true causal prophylaxis* should be reserved for the killing of sporozoites before they can infect the cells of the reticuloendothelium. No agents are known that will affect the viability of sporozoites, in concentrations attainable with therapeutic doses.

Primaquine has causal prophylactic properties, most pronounced against falciparum malaria; unfortunately the possibility of serious side effects makes its use for this purpose unsafe and impracticable. *Chloroguanide* and *pyrimethamine* exert a marked prophylactic effect against falciparum parasites, but they are only partially active against vivax infections.

Suppressive Treatment. Because of the lack of an ideal causal prophylactic agent, attention must be centered on suppressive drug therapy. By suppression is meant the inhibition of the erythrocytic stage of development of the parasites so that the infected individual is kept free of clinical manifestations of the disease. Infection is not prevented by a suppressive drug. The exoerythrocytic stage persists and clinical attacks may supervene at varying intervals after suppressive medication is stopped, particularly in certain types of vivax malaria.

Three particularly effective drugs are available for suppressive purposes, namely, *chloroquine, chloroguanide,* and *pyrimethamine.* Continued suppressive medication is necessary to prevent clinical attacks in *vivax* infections, and relapses occur when therapy is stopped. In contrast, most *falciparum* infections are rather promptly cured by such treatment; the administration of a suppressive drug is continued only if there is the hazard of reinfection. Suppressive treatment is employed during periods of exposure to infected mosquitoes and for some weeks thereafter. It is also used during medical or surgical crises in patients known to have a latent vivax infection. In certain localities, insensitivity or resistance to a particular drug may call for careful selection of the agent to be used.

Clinical Cure. Agents in this category interrupt erythrocytic schizogony of the malarial parasite and in this manner terminate the clinical attack. Such agents are called *schizontocides.* The 4-aminoquinoline derivatives, *chloroquine* and *amodiaquine,* are the drugs of choice. Both vivax and most falciparum malarias respond well. Chloroguanide and pyrimethamine are also highly active schizontocides, but their action is much slower than that of chloroquine. Other differences in therapeutic actions of these drugs are described subsequently. If satisfactory results are not obtained with one of these agents, therapy should be repeated with another. In certain parts of the world, strains of falciparum malaria may be resistant or insensitive to all synthetic antimalarial drugs (*see* above). Under these circumstances recourse must be had to *quinine* or to certain combination therapies to be described later.

Radical Cure. The term *radical cure* refers to eradicating not only the erythrocytic but also the exoerythrocytic parasites of an established infection. The only drugs that accomplish radical cure in *vivax malaria* are the 8-aminoquinoline derivatives, of which only *primaquine* is used now. Usually primaquine is employed concurrently with chloroquine, and a high proportion of cures can be expected (*see* below). Individuals living in endemic areas are not suitable candidates for radically curative therapy because of the

considerable likelihood of reinfection. Such treatment is usually reserved for persons who experience relapsing vivax malaria after leaving malarious regions.

Radical cure of *falciparum malaria* is relatively easy. Proper treatment of the clinical attack is all that is necessary. In persons receiving suppressive medication, mere continuation of such therapy is usually adequate insurance against clinical breakthrough; the suppressive drug should be continued for at least 1 month beyond the time of last exposure to potentially infected mosquitoes. Infection with falciparum sporozoites may recur repeatedly during suppressive medication, but the exoerythrocytic stage does not persist.

Suppressive Cure. The term *suppressive cure* refers to the complete elimination of malarial parasites from the body by continued suppressive treatment, the effect of which is longer than the life-span of the infection. The continued administration of pyrimethamine for 10 weeks after leaving a malarious area has been associated with suppressive cure of certain vivax infections.

Gametocytocidal Therapy. Drugs in this category destroy the sexual forms of malarial parasites in human blood and thereby eliminate the reservoir from which mosquitoes are reinfected. Causal prophylaxis, suppressive therapy, and prompt and adequate treatment of acute clinical attacks all prevent the development or persistence of vivax and falciparum gametocytes. Chloroguanide and pyrimethamine do not destroy gametocytes but prevent their development in mosquitoes. Small doses of primaquine eradicate both vivax and falciparum gametocytes within 3 days. The remaining antimalarial drugs are all effective against *vivax* gametocytes, but *falciparum* gametocytes are quite insensitive.

Mechanisms of Action. Antimalarial agents may be divided rather grossly into two quite distinct groups. The first of these includes the older agents, which may be recognized, even clinically, by the rapidity of their schizontocidal action and the relative difficulty with which resistance to them can be developed by originally sensitive strains. Their fundamental mechanism of action appears to be, at least in part, not specific for the various species. They bind to and alter the properties of both microbial and mammalian DNA. The ability of DNA to serve as a template for replication is thus impaired. This group includes *chloroquine, primaquine,* and *quinine* (*see* Thompson and Werbel, 1972). Their selective toxicity depends upon selective accumulation in the intracellular milieu of the parasite, a process that has not yet been elucidated but may be a function of the partition profile of the drug and plasmodial metabolism (Rollo, 1968), or upon the presence of high-affinity binding sites in sensitive parasites (Fitch, 1970). Primaquine differs from the others in being much less active against the erythrocytic stage of the parasite. The fact that it produces much less change in certain properties of native DNA, when bound to it, than do other potent schizontocidal agents may account for this. Its high activity against the exoerythrocytic stages of the parasite is associated with cytological changes at concentrations that leave the host cells unaffected.

Members of the second group are characterized by a schizontocidal effect that is slow in onset and dependent on the stage of multiplication of the parasite. Resistance to their action can be attained readily in experimental studies, and resistance in the field is not uncommon. Their mechanism of action appears to be much more specific than that of the first group. The biochemical pathway involved is the synthesis of folinic acid from para-aminobenzoic acid (PABA). Agents in this group either interfere with the incorporation of PABA into folic acid, a process that does not occur in mammals, or bind to dihydrofolate reductases; such binding to plasmodial dihydrofolate reductase is very strong in comparison with that to the mammalian heteroenzyme (*see* Table 52-1, page 1057, and Chapter 56). This group includes *chloroguanide, pyrimethamine,* and their derivatives (inhibitors of dihydrofolate reductase), as well as *sulfonamides* and *sulfones* (inhibitors of folic acid synthesis). Mechanisms of action are discussed further under the individual drugs.

ACQUIRED RESISTANCE TO ANTIMALARIAL DRUGS

The foregoing section on mechanisms of action defined the two groups of antimalarial drugs partly in terms of the readiness with which resistance to those agents could be achieved. Strains of plasmodia resistant to the *cinchona alkaloids* or to *4-* or *8-aminoquinolines* can be developed only with difficulty or not at all. In contrast, a high degree of resistance to the *pyrimidines* and *biguanides* has been observed frequently. Acquired drug resistance should not be confused, however, with insensitivity or natural refractoriness, which has nothing to do with previous exposure to a drug. The amount of quinine required to control primary attacks of Roman and Sardinian strains of *P. falciparum,* for example, is eight times more than is required to control infection with other strains. In these cases there is no evidence to suggest that the refractoriness could have been produced by selective pressure exerted by the drug.

The development of resistant strains is often due to the commonly accepted mechanism by which the drug acts simply as a selective agent, allowing the overgrowth of resistant mutants that are likely to occur in any large population. The situation may be complicated, however, by the occurrence, in a large population of parasites, of a small proportion of *less susceptible* plasmodia. Under the circumstances of either no treatment or intensive treatment, these would have little or no opportunity to predominate. During mass prophylaxis, however, a reversal of population pressure, due to the presence of only minimal concentrations of drug in the blood of some individuals of the community, would result in the predominance of the insensitive plasmodia and a change in the characteristic of the strain. Such conditions could occur either as a result of underdosage, malabsorption of the drug, or a combination of both.

Whatever the mechanism, and the foregoing presents the problem in the simplest of terms, the end result is the same. Infections appear, usually in distinct geographical areas, that will no longer respond to previously adequate doses of the antimalarial drug being used. Unfortunately, strains resistant to one drug may exhibit cross-resistance to other agents. For this reason, the utmost care should be exercised in the administration of antimalarial drugs in endemic areas. Schemes of mass prophylaxis either in small localities or over large areas should be designed with the possibility always in mind that improper dosage and methods of drug distribution are very likely to result in the emergence of resistant strains.

A high degree of acquired resistance to *chloroguanide* has been demonstrated conclusively in all species of plasmodia where it has been looked for; the characteristic appears to be stable. Such strains retain their initial sensitivity to quinine and to 4- and 8-aminoquinoline antimalarials. Chloroguanide resistance of a high degree has occurred in *P. falciparum* found in Southeast Asia, West Africa, India, and elsewhere. Also, clinical evidence has accumulated that various strains of *P. vivax* and *P. malariae* may become resistant to the drug.

In several cases where chloroguanide resistance has developed, field observations have pointed to unduly low or too widely spaced doses as an important causal factor. In many areas of the world the development of resistant strains has seriously compromised the value of chloroguanide as a suppressive agent. West African strains of *P. falciparum* are relatively insensitive to the schizontocidal action of chloroguanide, but this is a *natural insensitivity*.

Resistance to *pyrimethamine* can be induced fairly readily in plasmodia of laboratory animals. Cross-resistance to chloroguanide and its derivatives, but not to any other antimalarial drug used clinically, is generally present. Lack of cross-resistance to sulfadiazine in chick malaria, although sulfadiazine-resistant strains are usually cross-resistant to both chloroguanide and pyrimethamine, led to Rollo's hypothesis (1955) on the mode of action of all three substances. Evidence from these experiments, together with data on synergism and antagonism, suggested that all three substances enter the parasite cell by some common mechanism other than passive diffusion. Cross-resistance, or the lack of it, may be explained by changes in the specificity of the uptake mechanism. Subsequently Ferone (1969) found altered dihydrofolate reductase with lesser affinity for the drug in a pyrimethamine-resistant strain of *P. berghei*.

Strains of *P. falciparum* have become resistant to pyrimethamine in several geographical areas, usually as a result of programs of mass suppression. The rapid development of resistance in a strain of *P. malariae* used for malariotherapy in neurosyphilitic patients has been described by Young (1957). The experimental production of resistance in *P. vivax* has also been demonstrated (*see* Rollo, 1964). Combinations of *pyrimethamine* with either dapsone or a long-acting sulfonamide have proven effective in suppression and treatment of pyrimethamine-resistant strains of *P. falciparum* and even of multiresistant strains (*see* below). *Trimethoprim*, either alone or in combination with a sulfonamide, has been found to be particularly effective in similar situations, but only against certain strains.

Resistance to *chloroquine* has become a grave problem in parts of South America and Southeast Asia. Formerly it was considered that chloroquine was one of the available antimalarial drugs to which resistance could not readily be attained. Chloroquine resistance has been associated with a decrease in drug-concentrating capacity of red cells infected with malarial parasites (Macomber *et al.*, 1966).

Despite the widespread use of the drug, chloroquine resistance in the field was not reported until 1961, when Moore and Lanier described falciparum infections in Colombia, relapsing after normally adequate courses of treatment with chloroquine. The strain was normally sensitive to quinine. Further investigation showed that the insensitivity remained after mosquito passage (Young and Moore, 1961). The strain was also insensitive to amodiaquine and hydroxychloroquine but remained sensitive to quinine, quinacrine, and pyrimethamine. Since then, resistance to chloroquine has been reported from several parts of South America and Southeast Asia (*see* Powell and Tigertt, 1968). Currently, active investigation has failed to confirm the presence on the African continent of any strain of *P. falciparum* with a decreased sensitivity to chloroquine.

Many chloroquine-resistant falciparum strains are cross-resistant to other 4-aminoquinolines, quinacrine, chloroguanide, and pyrimethamine, and are termed *multiresistant strains*. Not infrequently, even quinine cannot be relied upon to effect a radical cure, although it can usually control the clinical attack. In response to a standard regimen of chloroquine, there is a spectrum of resistance or insensitivity. An initial response that appears to be adequate may be followed sooner or later by a recrudescence. With other strains, parasitemia may decrease but still remain patent, may show no change, or may even increase. The various categories have been characterized by the World Health Organization (1968). Schedules of treatment vary and obviously depend on the strains involved and local experience. Quinine has been the sheet anchor, given parenterally initially in severely ill patients who cannot tolerate oral medication. Against those strains known to respond inadequately to quinine alone, pyrimethamine in combination with either dapsone, sulfadiazine, or a long-acting sulfonamide such as sulfadoxine should

be administered. The combination itself, without quinine, is also effective, although initial response to treatment is generally slower than when quinine is included. The earlier promise held out by trimethoprim combined with a long-acting sulfonamide in producing a rapid response has not been substantiated; trials with other strains of resistant *P. falciparum* have shown this treatment to be inferior to other established regimens. A tetracycline given in a course of treatment with quinine has also been found effective. Details of the various regimens have been outlined by the World Health Organization (1973).

QUINACRINE

Quinacrine is obsolete as an antimalarial drug; nevertheless, it deserves brief mention because of its historical importance in antimalarial chemotherapy. Full descriptions of its properties can be found in earlier editions of this textbook.

Quinacrine is an acridine derivative introduced for malarial therapy in 1930 mainly as a result of the work of Kikuth. It was first prepared by Mauss and Mietzsch as part of an extensive research program on synthetic antimalarials in Germany, which started when normal supplies of quinine become unavailable during World War I. In World War II, quinine, up to that time the chief antimalarial, was no longer available to the Allies and large-scale production of quinacrine began.

Field experiences gained by the armed forces soon established the superiority of quinacrine over quinine, and quinacrine became the official drug for the treatment of malaria. However, its toxicity and inability to cure benign tertian malaria or to act as a true causal prophylactic provided the incentive for the search for more effective drugs (*see* Wiselogle, 1946).

The concurrent administration of quinacrine greatly enhances the toxicity of the 8-aminoquinoline antimalarials, such as primaquine, by markedly increasing their concentration in the plasma and prolonging their sojourn in the body. This holds particularly with respect to methemoglobinemia and hemolysis. Such combinations should not be used in therapeutics.

Although quinacrine has proven effective in some patients infected with chloroquine-insensitive strains of *P. falciparum*, local experience should determine treatment. The majority of such strains are also insensitive to quinacrine.

CHLOROQUINE

History. Chloroquine is one of a large series of *4-aminoquinolines* investigated in connection with the extensive cooperative program of antimalarial research in the United States during World War II. The objective was to discover more effective and less toxic suppressive agents than quinacrine. Although the 4-aminoquinolines had previously been described as potential antimalarials by Russian investigators, serious attention was not paid to this chemical class until the French reported that

3-methyl-7-chloro-4-(4-diethylamino-1-methylbutyl-amino) quinoline (SN-6911; SONTOCHIN, SONTO-QUIN) was well tolerated and had high activity in human malarias. Beginning in 1943, a large number of these compounds were synthesized and tested for activity in avian malaria and for toxicity in mammals; ten of the series were then examined in humans with experimentally induced malarias. Of these, chloroquine proved most promising and was released for field trial. When hostilities ceased, it was discovered that the chemical had been synthesized and studied under the name of RESOCHIN by the Germans as early as 1934.

Chemistry. Chloroquine has the following structural formula:

Chloroquine

The diphosphate is a white, bitter powder, soluble in water. Its solutions are stable.

Structure-Activity Relationship. Chloroquine contains the same alkyl side chain as quinacrine; it differs from the latter in having a quinoline instead of an acridine nucleus and in lacking the methoxy radical. Chloroquine also bears close resemblance to pamaquine and pentaquine; it differs from them in the position of the alkyl side chain and in having a chlorine instead of a methoxy nuclear substituent. The *d, l,* and *dl* forms of chloroquine are indistinguishable in potency tests in duck malaria, but the *d* isomer is somewhat less toxic than the *l* isomer in mammals. The 4-aminoquinolines showing the most marked antimalarial activity in both avian and human malarias have a chlorine atom in position 7 of the quinoline nucleus. Methyl substitution in position 3 of the nucleus reduces activity, and additional methyl substitution in position 8 completely eliminates activity. The details of the structure-activity relationship of chloroquine and its congeners are discussed by Berliner and coworkers (1948) and Coatney and colleagues (1953).

Pharmacological Effects. Although chloroquine was developed primarily as an *antimalarial agent,* it possesses several other pharmacological properties, all of which are interesting, some of which are useful. Its anti-inflammatory properties are well known, and its usefulness in the treatment of *rheumatoid arthritis* and *discoid lupus erythematosus* is established. Less well established is its efficacy in *systemic lupus erythematosus.* Chloroquine is particularly useful in the treatment of *photoallergic reactions.* Treatment of these conditions requires the administration of much larger doses of the drug than are employed in prophylaxis and treatment of malaria, and involves proper consideration of the toxicity of such large amounts. Chloroquine has been used in the treatment of *cardiac arrhythmias* as an alternative drug to quinidine.

Antimalarial Actions. Chloroquine exerts no significant activity against the exoerythrocytic tissue stages of plasmodia, even when given in massive doses. The drug is thus not a causal prophylactic agent and does not prevent the establishment of infection. However, it is highly effective against the asexual erythrocytic forms of *P. vivax* and *P. falciparum,* and gametocytes of *P. vivax.* It is superior to quinine and quinacrine in suppressing vivax malarias. In the *acute malarial attack,* it rapidly controls parasitemia and clinical symptoms; most patients become completely afebrile within 24 to 48 hours after administration of therapeutic doses, and thick smears of peripheral blood are generally negative by 48 to 72 hours. With the exception of certain South American and Southeast Asian strains, it completely cures falciparum malaria. Chloroquine, like quinine and quinacrine, does not prevent relapses in vivax malaria, but it substantially lengthens the interval between relapses. Chloroquine is well tolerated and is thus easier to administer than quinine or quinacrine. It differs from quinine and quinacrine in that no therapeutic or toxic synergism is manifested when it is administered with primaquine.

Mechanism of Antimalarial Action. The mechanism of plasmodicidal action of chloroquine is not completely certain. While the drug can inhibit certain enzymes, its significant effect is believed to result from its interaction with DNA. Schellenberg and Coatney (1960) have shown that chloroquine inhibits the incorporation of ^{32}P-labeled phosphate into RNA and DNA by *P. gallinaceum in vitro* and *in vivo,* and by *P. berghei in vitro.* Subsequent study has demonstrated that chloroquine combines strongly with DNA, but only if it is double stranded. In addition, it inhibits DNA polymerase markedly and RNA polymerase less so, in both cases by combining with the DNA primer (Allison *et al.,* 1965; Cohen and Yielding, 1965). Changes in several physical parameters are consistent with an intercalation of chloroquine between base pairs of the double helix and, furthermore, with the necessary presence of guanine, more particularly its 2-amino group. Stabilization of the double helix is believed to occur by the formation of additional ionic bonds between the substituted amino side chain of chloroquine and the phosphate anions of complementary strands of DNA across the minor groove (Allison *et al.*, 1966). This appears to be a nonspecific reaction affecting vulnerable DNA regardless of its source. The drug affects both microbial and mammalian cell growth at concentrations of about 10 μM. *In-vitro* erythrocyte-bound parasites are affected by concentrations of the order of 0.1 μM. The apparent anomaly can be explained in part by the accumulation of chloroquine within parasitized erythrocytes to the extent of at least two orders of magnitude greater than the concentration occurring outside (Macomber *et al.*, 1966; Polet and Barr, 1968). The usefulness of chloroquine as a selectively toxic agent is due, at least in part, to this preferential accumulation, since parasitized erythrocytes concentrate more of the drug than do most body organs. The mechanism of this accumulation is unclear but can be explained by passive diffusion of the drug abetted by its partition profile and the metabolic activity of the parasite itself (Rollo, 1968), by sequestration by lysosomes (Homewood *et al.*, 1972), or by the presence of high-affinity receptor sites (Fitch, 1970). However, it should be noted that certain tissues of the host can concentrate chloroquine to an even greater extent (*see* below), and other factors may be involved to cause the selective action of the drug.

Absorption, Fate, and Excretion. Chloroquine is rapidly and almost completely absorbed from the gastrointestinal tract, and only a small proportion of the administered dose is found in the stools. Approximately 55% of the drug in the plasma is bound to nondiffusible plasma constituents. Excretion of chloroquine is quite slow. However, the rate of renal excretion of the drug is increased by acidification of the urine and decreased by alkalinization. Chloroquine is deposited in the tissues in considerable amounts. In animals, from 200 to 700 times the plasma concentration may be found in the liver, spleen, kidney, and lung; leukocytes also concentrate the drug. The brain and spinal cord, in contrast, contain only 10 to 30 times the amount present in plasma.

Chloroquine undergoes appreciable degradation in the body. The main metabolite is desethylchloroquine, which accounts for one fourth of the total material appearing in the urine; bisdesethylchloroquine, a carboxylic acid derivative, and other metabolic products as yet uncharacterized are found in small amounts. Seventy percent can be accounted for as unchanged chloroquine (McChesney *et al.*, 1967). Deethylation to the secondary amine results in a substance that is highly active against avian malaria. Metabolic products of chloroquine may thus be partially responsible for antimalarial activity.

Because of the avidity of tissues for the drug, a loading or priming dose is essential if effective plasma concentrations are to be reached and maintained. When the drug is discontinued, following daily dosage for 2 weeks, plasma concentrations and urinary excretion both decrease with a half-life of 6 to 7 days for the next 4 weeks; subsequently the half-life for urinary excretion increases to 17 days. Small amounts can be found in the urine for long periods of time, some claim for as long as 5 years. Daily oral dosage of 310 mg of chloroquine base results in a plasma plateau of about 125 μg per liter. With a weekly 0.5-g dose, the peak plasma concentration varies between 150 and 250 μg per liter; just prior to the succeeding dose, the range is between 20 and 40 μg per liter. After single or weekly doses, the half-life of the drug in plasma is about 3 days.

Certain antimalarials interfere with the biotransformation of chloroquine. The most effective are amodiaquine, hydroxychloroquine, and pamaquine; and, with their concurrent use, plasma concentrations of chloroquine are elevated for prolonged periods (Gaudette and Coatney, 1961).

Preparations. *Chloroquine Phosphate,* U.S.P. (ARALEN PHOSPHATE, AVLOCLOR, RESOCHIN), is available as tablets containing either 250 or 500 mg of the diphosphate. Approximately 60% of the diphosphate represents the base. Chloroquine is also available as *Chloroquine Hydrochloride Injection,* U.S.P. (ARALEN HYDROCHLORIDE). Chloroquine, coated with cetylsteryl alcohol to protect it from the leaching effect of high humidity, is used in South America to medicate table salt for the purposes of large-scale prophylaxis in remote areas. It is also combined in tablets with pyrimethamine (DARACLOR) or with chloroproguanil (LAPAQUIN) for prophylactic and therapeutic use, and with primaquine for prophylactic use only.

Routes of Administration and Dosage. Chloroquine phosphate is administered in tablet form by the oral route, either before or after meals. The hydrochloride of chloroquine may be employed for parenteral (intramuscular) injection, if necessary.

For the purpose of *suppressive therapy* an oral dose of 500 mg of the phosphate is given on the same day of each week, continuing for at least 1 month after the last exposure in an endemic area. In some parts of the world where malaria transmission is intense, a weekly dose of 1 g is used for nonimmune persons. In certain areas, strains of *P. falciparum* exist that are less sensitive to 4-aminoquinolines than are most commonly encountered strains. In these circumstances, despite apparently adequate suppression, acute attacks may occur on stopping medication, even if maintained for several weeks after leaving the malarious area. With some strains patent infections and acute attacks of falciparum malaria may occur even during suppressive therapy. The management of infections arising from such strains is discussed above.

For the *treatment of the acute attack* of vivax or falciparum malaria, an initial priming or loading dose of 1.0 g is administered; this is followed by an additional 500 mg after 6 or 8 hours and a single dose of 500 mg on each of 2 consecutive days, so that a total of 2.5 g is given in 3 days. This dosage is usually sufficient to cure completely most *P. falciparum* infections and to terminate promptly fever and parasitemia in acute *P. vivax* infections. Freedom from clinical attacks in vivax malaria may then be maintained by suppressive doses of 500 mg weekly.

If parenteral therapy is required for the treatment of coma due to falciparum malaria, the equivalent of 200 mg of chloroquine *base* (250 mg of the hydrochloride) should be administered intramuscularly, half the dose in each buttock. This may be repeated at intervals of 6 hours, but the total dose for the first 24 hours should never exceed the equivalent of 800 mg of the base. Parenteral administration should be terminated as soon as the drug can be taken orally.

Dosages administered to infants or children, orally or intramuscularly, should not exceed 10 mg of chloroquine base per kilogram of body weight per day.

Toxicity and Side Effects. The amounts of chloroquine employed for therapy of the acute malarial attack may cause mild and transient headache, visual disturbances, gastrointestinal upset, and pruritus. Prolonged chronic medication for suppressive purposes causes few significant untoward effects, and only rarely must the drug be discontinued because of intolerance. None of the symptoms is serious, and all readily disappear when the drug is withheld. Chloroquine does not discolor the skin, as does quinacrine. The chief untoward effects are pruritus and gastrointestinal discomfort.

Prolonged treatment with chloroquine causes a lichenoid skin eruption in a small percentage of patients; the condition is mild and subsides promptly when the drug is stopped. Readministration of chloroquine usually does not result in reappearance of the lesion. Large doses given for a year to a group of healthy volunteers occasionally caused some visual symptoms (blurring of vision due to difficulty in accommodation, diplopia), bleaching of the hair, diminution of T waves in some or all leads of the ECG (without evidence of cardiovascular impairment), mild skin eruptions, headache, and slight weight loss; the observed toxic effects caused no incapacity and were reversible upon withdrawal of the drug (Alving *et al.*, 1948). These findings emphasize the relative safety of chloroquine in the recommended dose range.

The administration of chloroquine in the long-term treatment of diseases other than malaria may involve the administration of 250 to 750 mg daily for many months or even years. Such long-term treatment has been shown to result, not infrequently, in a retinopathy. This is characterized by loss of central visual acuity, granular pigmentation of the macula, and retinal artery constriction. The visual loss is not necessarily progressive if the drug is discontinued, but it appears to be irreversible. Bernstein and colleagues (1963) have demonstrated that chloroquine is stored in the iris and choroid of laboratory animals in significantly higher concentrations than in other tissues. Rubin and coworkers (1963) have suggested acidifying the urine of affected patients with ammonium chloride and administering dimercaprol intramuscularly to increase the urinary excretion of chloroquine. Ototoxicity has been reported in a few cases. Hart and Naunton (1964) have implicated chloroquine in the development of fetal abnormalities characterized by severe cochleovestibular paresis.

Precautions and Contraindications. Because of the high concentration that occurs in the liver, chloroquine should be used with caution in the presence of hepatic disease. It should be used cautiously or not at all in the presence of severe gastrointestinal, neurological, or blood disorders. If such disorders occur during the course of therapy, the drug should be discontinued. Concomitant use of gold or phenylbutazone with chloroquine should be avoided because of the tendency of all three agents to produce dermatitis. For patients on long-term, large-dose therapy, ophthalmological examination is recommended before and periodically during treatment (Percival and Meanock, 1968). Chloroquine should not be administered during pregnancy except in the prophylaxis or treatment of malaria when the indications may justify the risk.

Therapeutic Uses. *Malaria.* In human vivax malarias, chloroquine has neither prophylactic nor radically curative value. However, in well-tolerated doses it is highly effective in terminating acute attacks of vivax malaria, and when administered chronically it acts as an effective suppressive agent. When medication is discontinued, relapses occur but the interval for their appearance is prolonged. In falciparum malaria, the drug is markedly effective in controlling acute attacks and as a rule it completely cures the disease. Chloroquine is superior to quinine in that it is more potent and less toxic and it need be given only once weekly as a suppressive agent. It is one of the most generally useful of the antimalarial drugs; however, in some parts of the world, certain strains of *P. falciparum* occur that are much less sensitive or even completely insensitive to the action of the drug.

Other Uses. Apart from the uses mentioned earlier, chloroquine is valuable in the treatment of *extraintestinal amebiasis* (*see* Chapter 53). It has also been reported to be of value in *giardiasis*.

CHLOROQUINE CONGENERS

Of the more than 200 derivatives of 4-aminoquinoline found to be active against avian malarial parasites (Wiselogle, 1946), chloroquine has been the most adequately studied. Other congeners, however, have shown promising therapeutic potentialities. One of these is *Amodiaquine Hydrochloride,* U.S.P. (CAMOQUIN). It is employed for the treatment of overt malarial attacks and for suppression, but it is not used as extensively as chloroquine. Amodiaquine is more active than chloroquine both *in vitro* and *in vivo* against certain strains of *P. falciparum* with decreased sensitivity to chloroquine. *Hydroxychloroquine Sulfate,* U.S.P. (PLAQUENIL), has also been used successfully in place of chloroquine against normally sensitive strains.

CHLOROGUANIDE

History. Chloroguanide represents a distinctly British contribution to antimalarial research during World War II. Its chemical structure is entirely different from that of other antimalarials. The compound was synthesized by Curd and associates (1945), who have reviewed the chemical considerations that resulted in the synthesis of chloroguanide and its congeners. Suffice it to say that early members of the series were synthesized as *pyrimidine* derivatives because of the known importance of pyrimidine-containing compounds in cell metabolism. Later members of the series, of which chloroguanide is one, were simplified by opening the pyrimidine ring to give a biguanide. Curiously enough, metabolism in the body converts this biguanide to a triazine ring, the active form of the drug. Chloroguanide proved to be more potent than quinine in avian malaria and to possess a satisfactory margin of safety in laboratory animals. It was first employed for the treatment of human vivax and falciparum malarias by Adams and coworkers (1945) at the Liverpool School of Tropical Medicine. The compound was then given extensive clinical trial for its prophylactic, curative, and suppressive properties in naturally acquired and experimentally induced falciparum and vivax malarias, particularly by Fairley and associates (1945, 1946). Fairley's investigations delineated the antiplasmodial actions of chloroguanide, and established it as a useful antimalarial. However, the value of the drug is seriously compromised by the development of chloroguanide-resistant strains of plasmodia (*see* below).

Chemistry. Chloroguanide has the structural formula shown at the top of the next column.

Chloroguanide

It is a white powder with a bitter taste. Water solubility at 15° C is approximately 1%.

Structure-Activity Relationship. Chloroguanide is only one of a large series of plasmodicidal biguanides, but it appears to have the widest margin of safety of the homologs examined. The N^5-methyl homolog is also highly active in man but somewhat more toxic. Dihalogen substitution in positions 3 and 4 of the benzene ring yields a compound, *chloroproguanil* (LAPUDRINE), more potent than chloroguanide, whereas the substitution of diethyl for isopropyl in the N^5 position results in lower activity. The bromine analog of chloroproguanil (*bromoguanide*) also possesses high activity and is available commercially in some parts of the world. The details of the structure-activity relationship in the biguanide series may be found in the reports of Curd and associates (1945) and Spinks (1947, 1948).

Pharmacological Effects. *Antimalarial Actions and Efficacy.* Chloroguanide exerts causal prophylactic and suppressive activity in sporozoite-induced falciparum malaria, adequately controls the acute clinical attack, and usually eradicates the infection. The drug exhibits suppressive activity against *P. vivax* infections, and controls the acute clinical attack. It is, however, not fully prophylactic against mosquito-induced vivax malaria because it does not affect the exoerythrocytic tissue stage of this infection. Also, in *P. vivax* infections, erythrocytic forms of the parasite often reappear in the blood shortly after suppressive doses of chloroguanide are withdrawn. Its action on erythrocytic forms of all malarias is slow compared to that of the 4-aminoquinoline antimalarials. Gametocytes are not destroyed, but the development of gametes encysted in the gut wall of the mosquito is prevented.

Chloroguanide and quinine do not act synergistically in the prevention of relapse in vivax malaria as does a combination of an 8-aminoquinoline antimalarial and quinine.

Resistance to chloroguanide, which greatly compromises its general usefulness, is discussed earlier in this chapter.

Mechanism of Antimalarial Action. The elucidation of the mechanism of action of chloroguanide was a rich reward from studies of its metabolic fate (*see* below). The compound is converted in the body to a triazine derivative that is an active inhibitor of the enzyme dihydrofolate reductase. This observation led to a planned program for the synthesis and study of direct inhibitors of the enzyme and the introduction into chemotherapy of the diaminopyrimidines. The mechanism of the chemotherapeutic action of inhibitors of dihydrofolate reductase and the rationale for their concurrent use with sulfonamide compounds that interfere with folate metabolism by other means are discussed in detail under the diaminopyrimidines (page 1056 and *see* Rollo, 1970).

The inhibition of the reduction of folic acid by chloroguanide is consistent with the morphological appearance of affected parasites; nuclear division is prevented and schizogony stops at an early stage. For this reason, chloroguanide acts slowly in the treatment of acute malaria, relief of symptoms occurring only after all the plasmodia have developed to a stage where extensive synthesis of nuclear material is essential for further development. Interest in chloroguanide centers chiefly on the fact that the drug acts not only on the erythrocytic stage of plasmodia but also on the exoerythrocytic tissue stage, especially of *P. falciparum.* This means that some advance has been made toward the goal of discovering causal prophylactic and curative antimalarial agents. Also of considerable interest is the fact that chloroguanide does not destroy gametocytes in the human host but renders them noninfectious for mosquitoes. Development of the fertilized gamete in the gut wall of the mosquito is inhibited, possibly as a result also of increased demand for new nuclear material. However, the gametocytes of different strains of *P. falciparum* are not all adversely affected by the drug.

Absorption, Fate, and Excretion. Chloroguanide is adequately, but rather slowly, absorbed from the gastrointestinal tract. From 70 to 90% of a given dose is absorbed, but only approximately half of it within the first 3 hours after ingestion. After single oral doses, peak plasma concentrations of the drug are attained at 2 to 4 hours; the concentration then declines rather rapidly and is practically zero at 24 hours. During chronic medication the plasma concentration is proportional to the dose, but individuals on the same dosage schedule differ widely in their plasma concentration of drug. Approximately 75% of the plasma chloroguanide is bound to protein, and the concentration of the drug in erythrocytes is six times that in the plasma.

During chronic administration of chloroguanide, the drug accumulates only to a slight extent in the tissues. Thus, chloroguanide differs markedly from chloroquine. Furthermore, chloroguanide is very rapidly eliminated from the tissues after its administration ceases. In man, from 40 to 60% of the chloroguanide absorbed is excreted in the urine, and approximately 10% is secreted directly into the intestinal tract and eliminated in the feces.

As stated above, the drug itself has little effect against plasmodia; activity is dependent upon a substance produced by the action of host tissues on the parent molecule. An active substance, 2,4-diamino-1-*p*-chlorophenyl-1,6-dihydro-6,6-dimethyl-1,3,5-triazine, was isolated from animals treated with chloroguanide and its structure confirmed by synthesis (Carrington *et al.,* 1951; Crowther and Levi, 1953). Smith and colleagues (1961) found that, in man, 60% of the drug excreted in the urine is parent compound, and 30% is the triazine. This latter substance is highly active against avian malarias but has proved to be less active than the parent compound in monkeys infected with *P. cynomolgi* and men infected with *P. falciparum* (Schmidt *et al.,* 1952;

Robertson, 1957). The work of Smith and associates has led to the explanation that, since man and monkey excrete the metabolite rapidly in the urine, such rapid excretion is incompatible with marked therapeutic effect. Hence the active metabolite has little or no usefulness in the therapy of malaria.

Preparations, Route of Administration, and Dosage. *Chloroguanide hydrochloride* (PALUDRINE) is available in tablets containing 100 mg. Chloroguanide is always administered orally.

The *prophylactic* (and *suppressive*) dose for both vivax and falciparum malarias is 100 mg daily for nonimmune subjects. For complete protection of persons in Nigeria, twice this dose is necessary. Semi-immune individuals given 300 mg once weekly are moderately well protected; however, if possible, 200 mg should be given twice weekly. For the treatment of the *acute attack* of vivax malaria in semi-immune or nonimmune subjects, an initial dose of 300 to 600 mg should be followed by 300 mg daily for as long as is required. A single administration of 300 mg usually terminates the clinical attack in semi-immune persons, but many experts prefer to give a 5- or 10-day course. This course of treatment is rarely curative and either suppressive doses must subsequently be employed or radical cure obtained as described below. Chloroguanide should be used in the treatment of overt falciparum malaria only in semi-immune patients and only if the attack is of no more than moderate severity. Daily or twice-daily doses of 300 mg should be continued for 5 days. Chloroguanide is too slow in its action to be useful in the treatment of falciparum malaria in nonimmune patients.

In considering the use of this agent, it is wise to find out how sensitive the local strains are. If resistant strains are encountered, it is a serious error to use higher doses of chloroguanide; one of the 4-aminoquinoline antimalarial agents should be substituted.

Toxicity and Side Effects. Chloroguanide is the most innocuous of the currently employed antimalarials; in therapeutic doses, it causes practically no untoward effects. Large doses (1 g daily) may cause vomiting, abdominal pain, and diarrhea. Excessive amounts may cause hematuria and the transient appearance of epithelial cells and casts in the urine; myelocytes to the extent of 10% may appear in the blood of patients with overt malaria. The drug does not stain the skin, as does quinacrine. As much as 700 mg twice daily for over 2 weeks has been given without the occurrence of serious toxic effects requiring cessation of therapy; this amount is far above that employed in therapy. Gross accidental or deliberate overdosage (as much as 14.5 g) has been followed uniformly by complete recovery. Obviously, the margin of safety of chloroguanide is quite satisfactory.

Precautions and Contraindications. Long-term administration of chloroguanide may result in loss of appetite, perhaps because it has an inhibitory action on gastric secretion. This anorectic effect is more apparent when the drug is taken on an empty stomach; it should therefore be taken after meals or with a glass of milk.

Therapeutic Uses. Chloroguanide is employed only in *malaria;* it has no other established uses. In both falciparum and vivax malarias, the compound adequately controls the overt clinical attack, but it is slower in abolishing fever and parasitemia than are all other antimalarial drugs with the exception of pyrimethamine. For this reason, its use in the treatment of the acute attack of falciparum malaria in nonimmune patients, and in semi-immune patients if the attack is severe, is not recommended. In *falciparum* malaria, chloroguanide is a causal prophylactic, suppressive, and radically curative agent if the plasmodia have not developed resistance to the drug.

In *vivax* malaria, chloroguanide controls the acute clinical attack but has no advantage over more rapidly acting 4-aminoquinoline antimalarial agents. It is also an effective suppressive, but its use does not result in radical cure, particularly of infections caused by highly relapsing strains.

Chloroguanide represents an important chemotherapeutic advance because, in addition to being a potent schizontocide, the drug is lethal to actively developing preerythrocytic tissue forms of certain plasmodia and exerts a sterilizing action on gametocytes. Furthermore, it opened the field for the development of other antifolates.

CYCLOGUANIL EMBONATE

The fact that single doses of antimalarial drugs are effective for only brief periods stimulated Thompson and coworkers (1963) to synthesize compounds that might act for much longer periods of time. Their optimism stemmed from the remarkably high potency of the triazine metabolite of chloroguanide. Their objective was a single-dose, parenteral, repository preparation. Cycloguanil embonate (4,6-diamino-1-[*p*-chlorophenyl]-1,2-dihydro-2,2-dimethyl-*s*-triazine embonate) was prepared and found to possess the desired properties. (It is also known as *chloroguanide triazine embonate* and CAMOLAR.) The results of laboratory tests with *P. berghei*-infected mice and *P. cynomolgi*-infected monkeys showed that well-tolerated doses gave protection for a sufficiently long period of time to encourage trial of the drug in man (Schmidt *et al.*, 1963; Thompson *et al.*, 1963). The prolonged period of protection was found to be due to release of the active moiety from a depot formed at the site of injection and not to a systemic reservoir formed after administration of the drug (Waitz *et al.*, 1963).

Subsequent studies in man showed that a single intramuscular injection of 5 mg/kg protects against *P. falciparum* and *P. vivax* for several months. The results indicated that a single intramuscular injection of the drug provides the equivalent of a prolonged infusion of the soluble dihydrotriazine and appears to prevent the growth or even the survival of both the erythrocytic and the preerythrocytic parasites. Up to 80% of the drug remains at the injection site 2 weeks after administration, and small amounts can be found for as long as 56 weeks later (Thompson *et al.*, 1963).

Field trials confirmed the earlier findings in semi-immune individuals infected with *P. falciparum.* However, a lesser period of protection was afforded to nonimmune subjects with certain *P. vivax* infections. Less protection also occurred when strains of *P. falciparum* with decreased susceptibility to chloroguanide or pyrimethamine were encountered. Indeed, no protection to the multidrug-resistant strains encountered in Southeast Asia was found. Furthermore, use of this compound may lead rapidly to the emergence and spread of drug-resistant strains. In the light of these shortcomings clinical trials have involved the use of two depot preparations in combination. The one is the triazine just described and the other is *acedapsone,* the diacetyl derivative of diaminodiphenylsulfone (N,N'-diacetyl-4,4'-diaminodiphenylsulfone, DADDS; HANSOLAR), which, on slow hydrolysis following intramuscular injection, yields the active antimalarial, diaminodiphenylsulfone (*see* Peters, 1968). There is some evidence that the use of the combination, a 1:1 mixture, may extend the period of protection, delay the emergence of resistant strains, and even provide some protection against strains already less sensitive to either drug alone. However, problems have been encountered with local reactions from its intramuscular administration. The combination is presently termed DAPOLAR. The rationale for the concurrent use of these drugs is discussed below. In the United States, cycloguanil is available only for investigational use.

DIAMINOPYRIMIDINES

History. Of the many 2,4-diaminopyrimidines synthesized and tested for antimicrobial activity, two are outstanding. The first, *pyrimethamine,* was developed and used almost solely as an antimalarial agent; the second, *trimethoprim,* was created as an antibacterial agent and found later to have antimalarial properties. Their development started with a study of substances related to the heterocyclic constituents of the nucleic acids. Several 2,4-diaminopyrimidines were found to antagonize competitively folic and folinic acids in the growth of *Lactobacillus casei.* The prediction was made that *L. casei* would not be unique in its sensitivity to these substances and that eventually, from this group, useful chemotherapeutic agents would be developed. In the consideration of microorganisms that might be sensitive to this new series, a formal analogy between certain of these substances and chloroguanide, as well as certain similarities in microbiological behavior, suggested their trial as antimalarials. The analogy may be carried further by a comparison between the structure of pyrimethamine and that of the triazine metabolite of chloroguanide. The *structure-activity relationship* of these compounds is discussed in previous editions of this textbook.

Experiments with the diaminopyrimidines in the treatment of malaria in experimental animals bore out prediction; a high degree of antimalarial activity was found in several members of the series. The most active, *pyrimethamine*, was later found to be highly effective against the plasmodia infecting man (*see* Falco *et al.,* 1951; Symposium, 1952), and has since been used widely for prophylaxis and suppression. *Trimethoprim* was found not to be outstanding against rodent malaria despite its promise as an antibacterial agent (*see* Bushby and Hitchings, 1968); however, clinical trial showed unexpectedly that it could cure not only normally sensitive *P. falciparum* infections but also infections due to the "Camp" strain, which is resistant to 4-aminoquinolines and to chloroguanide and pyrimethamine (Martin and Arnold, 1967). Unfortunately, later experience with Vietnamese and other strains of *P. falciparum* did not fulfill the promise of the earlier trials. Trimethoprim in combination with sulfalene failed to match the degree of response obtained with the currently accepted treatment regimens.

Chemistry. *Pyrimethamine* has the following structural formula:

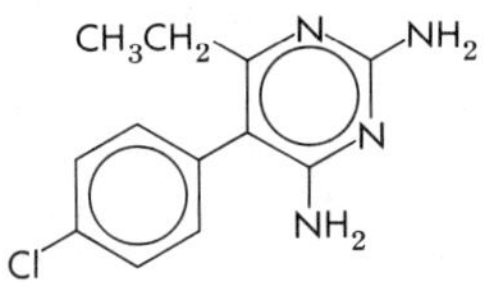

Pyrimethamine

It is a white powder, insoluble in water.

Trimethoprim has the following structural formula:

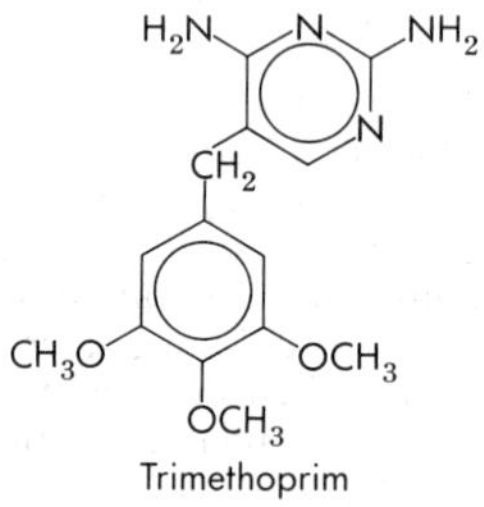

Trimethoprim

It is a pale-yellow crystalline powder.

Pharmacological Effects. *Antimalarial Actions and Efficacy.* The antimalarial effects of pyrimethamine are identical to those of chloroguanide. Its potency, however, is considerably greater, undoubtedly owing to the fact that it acts directly and the half-life is much longer than that of the active metabolite of chloroguanide. *Suppressive cure* of some vivax infections may be achieved by continuing prophylactic medication for 10 weeks after leaving a malarious area. There is a possibility that some causal prophylactic activity may occur in vivax infections. The antimalarial effects of both chloroguanide

and pyrimethamine have been reviewed by Davey (1963) and Hill (1963). The major use of pyrimethamine is in prophylaxis and suppression and in concurrent therapy.

Investigations into the *antimicrobial* actions of 2,4-diaminopyrimidines resulted in novel concepts that may have far-reaching consequences for the development of future chemotherapeutic agents. The enzyme dihydrofolate reductase, catalyzing the reduction of dihydrofolate to tetrahydrofolate, is of vital importance to cells in the biosynthesis of purines, pyrimidines, and certain amino acids. Close structural analogs of the substrate, such as aminopterin and methotrexate, have been used with some success in the treatment of neoplastic disease (*see* Chapter 62). Such agents, however, have little antimicrobial activity, although cell-free preparations of the enzyme from bacterial, protozoal, and mammalian sources are all inhibited by nanomolar concentrations (Ferone *et al.,* 1969). The apparent anomaly can be explained by consideration of the permeability of the cell to folic acid. Mammalian cells, which utilize exogenous folate, must actively transport the vitamin; this uptake mechanism is shared by the folate analogs. Protozoa, like certain bacteria, have in general either lost or never had the ability to utilize preformed folate, and they require a supply of PABA to synthesize their own (Ferone and Hitchings, 1966). The dihydrofolate reductase in intact cells is thus not exposed to these inhibitors. The "small-molecule" antifolates, such as pyrimethamine and trimethoprim, seem to penetrate by nonionic diffusion, and their entrance is unrelated to the ability of the cell to assimilate folic acid (Hitchings and Burchall, 1965). Their selective effect must depend, therefore, on some mechanism other than selective permeability. The answer is to be found in the fact that dihydrofolate reductases from various sources exhibit differences in sensitivity to inhibition by the diaminopyrimidines. Table 52–1 summarizes the pertinent data of Ferone and coworkers. There is an obvious correlation between the inhibitory potency of the agents and their effect on the intact microorganism and the host. For example, pyrimethamine is ineffective as an antibacterial agent although extremely effective as an antimalarial. It has significant tox-

Table 52-1. INHIBITION OF DIHYDROFOLATE REDUCTASES
BY PYRIMETHAMINE AND TRIMETHOPRIM *

| INHIBITOR | CONCENTRATION (nM) FOR 50% INHIBITION OF DIHYDROFOLATE REDUCTASES FROM VARIOUS SOURCES | | |
	Mammalian (rat liver)	Bacterial (E. coli)	Protozoal (P. berghei)
Pyrimethamine	700	2500	~0.5
Trimethoprim	260,000	5	70

* Modified from Ferone, Burchall, and Hitchings, 1969.

icity at doses appreciably higher than the conventional. Trimethoprim, on the other hand, is effective both as an antibacterial and as an antimalarial agent. Its toxicity for the mammalian host seems to be minimal (Kahn et al., 1968).

Drug Combinations. The concept of inhibiting two steps in an essential metabolic pathway with separate drugs was one developed by Hitchings and associates a decade before its practical application was to be realized (*see* Hitchings and Burchall, 1965; Rollo, 1970). Such "sequential blockade" would likely result in a supra-additive effect. In this situation the two steps investigated were the utilization of PABA in the synthesis of dihydropteroic acid, inhibited by sulfonamides, and the reduction of dihydrofolate to the active tetrahydrofolate, inhibited by pyrimethamine. Rollo (1955) showed that about one eighth of the ED50 of pyrimethamine and sulfadiazine administered together was equivalent to the ED50 of either used alone in experimental malarial infections. Later, in a limited trial, Hurly (1959) treated African children infected with *P. falciparum* and *P. malariae* with pyrimethamine and sulfadiazine, alone and in combination. Clinical cure was obtained with the combination of less than one tenth of the curative dose of pyrimethamine plus less than one fourth of the curative dose of sulfadiazine. Subsequently, trials of several combinations of pyrimethamine and either sulfonamides or dapsone have attested to the value of the augmentative effect both in the suppression and in the treatment of acute falciparum infections (*see* Donno et al., 1969; Lucas et al., 1969). Likewise, a combination of trimethoprim with sulfalene (2-sulfanilamido-3-methoxy-pyrazine) has proven valuable in the treatment of some sensitive and multi-

resistant strains of *P. falciparum* (Martin and Arnold, 1968; Donno et al., 1969), but, unfortunately, not others (Canfield et al., 1971).

The value of such combinations is not in reducing the dose of the pyrimidines, since therapeutic doses have a low order of toxicity, but in the possibility of preventing strains of plasmodia from developing resistance to these drugs. Such strains have arisen fairly readily when small doses of pyrimethamine alone were used for long periods of time. Suitable combinations have already shown their value in the treatment of multiresistant strains and in suppression where such strains have been encountered (World Health Organization, 1973). Combinations of trimethoprim with sulfamethoxazole are also of value in the treatment of bacterial infections (*see* Chapter 56).

Absorption, Fate, and Excretion. Smith and Schmidt (1963) found that ^{14}C-labeled *pyrimethamine* was completely and regularly absorbed from the gastrointestinal tract of the monkey. Smith and Ihrig (1959) observed that about 1 mg still remained in the body 30 days after a single dose of 100 mg in volunteers. Pyrimethamine is also excreted in the milk of nursing mothers. Several metabolites of pyrimethamine appear in the urine, but few data are available on either their structure or their antimicrobial activity.

Trimethoprim is rapidly absorbed when given orally. After a single conventional dose, significant plasma levels are detectable in 1 hour, peak levels occur in 2 or 4 hours, and some drug persists in the blood for as long as 24 hours. Tissue concentrations exceed those in the plasma; the lungs and kidney have particularly high concentrations. The level in the cerebrospinal fluid is effectively antibacterial. Four hydroxylated metabolites have been isolated from the urine of man and experimental animals given the drug. About 50% of trimethoprim is excreted in the urine within 24 hours.

Preparations, Route of Administration, and Dosage. *Pyrimethamine,* U.S.P. (DARAPRIM), is marketed in scored tablets, each containing 25 mg of the base. Pyrimethamine is recommended only for prophylaxis and suppression; hence a first dose of 50 mg should be taken just before entering an endemic area. An effective dose is 25 mg once weekly for adults. Dosage is continued weekly as long as residence in endemic areas continues and for 10 weeks after leaving the area, to afford a chance for suppressive cure of vivax infection. The drug is available in combination with dapsone, as MALOPRIM; this preparation is intended for *prophylactic use,* particularly in areas where multiresistant strains are known to occur. It is also available in combination with sulfadoxine, as FANSIDAR, for use in the *treatment* of multiresistant infections. *Trimethoprim* is available in combination with sulfamethoxazole as *trimethoprim-sulfamethoxazole* (BACTRIM, SEPTRA) (*see* Chapter 56).

Toxicity, Precautions, and Contraindications.
With the recommended dosage of 25 mg once weekly, no significant toxic symptoms have been reported for *pyrimethamine*. Excessive doses may be expected to produce a megaloblastic anemia resembling that of folic acid deficiency and readily reversible on discontinuance of treatment or on administration of folinic acid. The dose of pyrimethamine should not be increased over that recommended for suppression, except when used in combination with other agents for the treatment of multiresistant strains. At the same time care should be taken to see that the dose is taken regularly to lessen the possibility of selective emergence of relatively insensitive or resistant strains. In general, the drug should not be used in areas where the plasmodia are predominantly insensitive to the recommended dosage or have become resistant through its misuse. Its use with either dapsone or a sulfonamide has proven beneficial, however, in areas where multiresistant strains are endemic. Used in this way, it is recommended that folinic acid in a daily dose of 10 mg/kg also be given to prevent possible hematological complications.

Available evidence suggests that *trimethoprim* is relatively nontoxic in man. Nausea and vomiting occur after excessively large doses. Skin rashes have been reported. Short-term therapy does not result in hematological abnormalities. The drug should not be given during pregnancy unless treatment is mandatory and alternatives have been excluded. Its use in children under 12 years of age is currently not recommended.

Therapeutic Uses. *Pyrimethamine* administered by itself has little value in the treatment of the acute primary attack of malaria. It is slow in clearing parasitemia, but it prevents development of the fertilized gamete and has some causal prophylactic activity. In combination with sulfadoxine, however, it has shown considerable promise in treating uncomplicated chloroquine-resistant *P. falciparum* infections. Response to treatment has been as adequate as when quinine was included in the regimen (Bartonelli *et al.,* 1967). In a longer course of treatment, a combination of pyrimethamine and either sulfadiazine or dapsone has been used successfully to supplement treatment with quinine in similar situations. Pyrimethamine has had considerable use as a prophylactic and suppressive agent and has proven effective if given once weekly. It is not a radically curative agent in vivax malaria, although continuance of suppressive therapy for 10 weeks after leaving a malarious area will provide "suppressive cure" with certain strains of *P. vivax*.

Pyrimethamine given concurrently with triple sulfonamides has been found useful in the treatment of *toxoplasmosis* (*see* Feldman, 1968). Folinic acid should be given concurrently to obviate the hematological toxicity that may occur with continued daily use of pyrimethamine. Some success has followed the use of pyrimethamine in the treatment of *polycythemia vera* and in the prophylaxis of *meningeal leukemia*.

Trimethoprim, both alone and combined with sulfalene (a long-acting sulfonamide), has received considerable trial in the management of malaria caused by multiresistant strains of *P. falciparum*. Depending on the geographical area and the strain of parasite, results have been highly variable. If therapy with trimethoprim is considered, the fixed-ratio preparation containing sulfamethoxazole should not be used without modification. The dosage of trimethoprim should be increased in order to obtain an adequate antimalarial effect.

PRIMAQUINE

History. In 1891, Ehrlich discovered that methylene blue exhibited weak plasmodicidal activity; the dye was tested because of his observation that it preferentially stained the parasite in the blood stream without staining other tissues. Later it was demonstrated that 8-aminoquinoline had weak schizontocidal activity in infected canaries and also that the slight antimalarial potency of methylene blue could be intensified by substitution of a dialkylaminoalkyl group for one of the N-methyl groups of the dye. Because the methoxy group on the quinoline ring, as in quinine, was believed important for antimalarial activity, a large series of quinoline derivatives was synthesized in which both the methoxy and substituted 8-amino groups were present. *Pamaquine* was the first of the 8-aminoquinoline antimalarials to be introduced into medicine (Mühlens, 1926). Its activity was outstanding, being 60 times that of quinine against canary malaria. During the course of the large-scale cooperative antimalarial research program conducted in the United States during World War II, several hundred derivatives of 8-aminoquinoline were explored in an attempt to discover compounds more potent and less toxic than pamaquine itself (*see* Elderfield *et al.*, 1946; Wiselogle, 1946). From this large number, three agents—*pentaquine, isopentaquine,* and *primaquine*—were selected for further study. Of these three, only primaquine, which received extensive field trials with United Nations forces in Korea, is widely used now. *Quinocide,* a substance very similar in structure to primaquine, is employed in some parts of the world.

Chemistry. Primaquine has the following structural formula:

Primaquine

The diphosphate is the commercially available salt; it is soluble in water, and its solutions are stable, although some decomposition may take place on exposure to light and air.

Structure-Activity Relationship. Since a low chemotherapeutic index was a main drawback to the use of pamaquine, the prime value of the newer 8-aminoquinoline derivatives was a reduction in toxicity without concomitant decrease in antimalarial activity. In a study on toxicity and curative activity against vivax infections, Edgcomb and co-workers (1950) showed that primaquine was the most active, followed by isopentaquine, with pamaquine the least active of the trio. Toxicity decreased as antimalarial activity increased. Hence, primaquine has the highest chemotherapeutic index. The degree of toxicity is related to the degree of substitution of the terminal amino group. Pamaquine, the most toxic, has a tertiary terminal amine, while primaquine, the least toxic, has a primary terminal amine. Intermediate between these two lies isopentaquine, isomeric with pamaquine but with a secondary terminal amine. (For a review, *see* Hill, 1963.)

Pharmacological Effects. Aside from its antimalarial actions, primaquine exerts few pharmacological effects at safe therapeutic doses. Its main actions are of a toxicological nature (*see* below), and are exerted particularly on the blood and the CNS.

Antimalarial Actions and Efficacy. Primaquine is highly active against the primary exoerythrocytic forms of *P. vivax* and *P. falciparum,* especially the latter. Although its causal prophylactic effect is obtained with well-tolerated doses, this activity is of relatively little practical value. The drug is also active against the asexual blood forms of *P. vivax,* but its effect is too erratic to be useful for the treatment of frank clinical attacks of benign tertian malaria. The drug is almost completely ineffective against the asexual blood forms of *P. falciparum.* The 8-aminoquinolines do, however, exert a marked gametocytocidal activity against all four species of plasmodia that infect man, especially against the gametocytes of *P. falciparum.* The great clinical value of primaquine lies in the *radically curative treatment of vivax malaria* and, in certain exceptional circumstances where single-drug administration has proven less than fully effective, in its use as a supplement to chloroquine suppression.

Primaquine is the drug of choice for curative treatment of vivax malaria since it destroys the late tissue forms with greater effectiveness and less danger of toxicity than does any other drug. It is available in combination with chloroquine or with amodiaquine for prophylaxis in endemic areas; however, its routine use for this purpose is not to be encouraged.

Drug Combinations. Neither quinine nor chloroquine, in contrast to quinacrine, exerts a significant effect on the plasma concentration of 8-aminoquinolines. In effecting radical cure of *P. vivax* infection, primaquine is most frequently administered concurrently with a fast-acting schizontocide such as quinine or a 4-aminoquinoline derivative, usually chloroquine. Quinine given concurrently with primaquine appears to reduce the incidence and the intensity of methemoglobinemia; this side effect, however, usually occurs only after the administration of higher doses of the 8-aminoquinoline than are currently recommended. Observations on military personnel in Vietnam suggest that heterozygotes for NADPH methemoglobin reductase are far more common than previously recognized, and that the routine use of primaquine-containing prophylactic combinations in large and continually changing personnel results in a high incidence of methemoglobinemia (Cohen *et al.,* 1968).

Acquired Resistance of Plasmodia to Primaquine. Resistance to 8-aminoquinoline compounds has been developed in avian and monkey malarias (*see* Hill, 1963; Rollo, 1964). Arnold and colleagues (1961) produced primaquine resistance in *P. vivax* by treating partially immune volunteers with subcurative doses of the drug. The asexual erythrocytic forms became resistant to the maximal tolerated dose of the drug after 36 passages. Gametocytes could be transmitted to mosquitoes and developed to the stage of mature and apparently viable sporozoites. These, however, did not infect man. Thus, it appears that the development of primaquine-resistant strains may not become a problem. Nevertheless, it is of the utmost importance that misuse of the drug does not occur, because the 8-aminoquinolines are the only antimalarial agents that can eliminate the late tissue stages of relapsing malaria, and the development of resistant strains would be disastrous.

Mechanism of Antimalarial Action. Little is known of the mode of action of 8-aminoquinolines. Pentaquine, unlike quinine, chloroquine, and quinacrine, does not inhibit the incorporation of ^{32}P-labeled phosphate into DNA or RNA by *P. gallinaceum* or *P. berghei* (Schellenberg and Coatney, 1960). Nevertheless, binding of 8-aminoquinolines to DNA, similar to that observed with chloroquine, has been shown to occur (Whichard *et al.*, 1968). There is considerable evidence that the parent 8-aminoquinoline compounds have only slight antimalarial activity and that *in-vivo* degradation results in more highly active substances (*see* Goodwin and Rollo, 1955).

Absorption, Fate, and Excretion.
After oral administration, the 8-aminoquinoline antimalarial compounds, including primaquine, are readily absorbed. They are, however, rapidly metabolized, and only a small proportion of the administered dose is excreted as the parent drug. The plasma concentration reaches a maximum in about 6 hours, but it falls rapidly thereafter and is barely detectable after 24 hours (Zubrod *et al.*, 1948; Arnold *et al.*, 1955). Considerable variation in peak plasma values is noted among individuals on the same dose schedule. However, neither the hemolytic effect on sensitive erythrocytes (*see* below) nor, probably, the antimalarial effect has much relation to the concentration of the parent drug in the plasma.

Tarlov and coworkers (1962) have outlined a degradation scheme for primaquine modeled after Smith's (1956) proposal for the degradation of pentaquine in monkeys. In this scheme the 6-methoxy group of primaquine is reduced to hydroxy, a second hydroxy group is added in the 5 position, and the resultant compound is converted to a quinonimine by way of the 5,6-quinone derivative of the parent compound. Such a derivative is, or may be, transformed into a resonating compound capable of act-

ing as an oxidation-reduction mediator. Such an agent may accelerate the oxidation of essential substances in sensitive erythrocytes by acting as a hydrogen acceptor and thereby promote hemolysis.

Preparations, Route of Administration, and Dosage. *Primaquine Phosphate,* U.S.P., is supplied in tablets containing 26.3 mg of the salt, equivalent to 15 mg of base. The dosage is usually expressed in terms of the base.

Primaquine is always given orally. Extensive field trials carried out with the United Nations forces in Korea demonstrated the great value of the drug against vivax infections and permitted assessment of the optimal schedule of treatment. Primaquine base (15 mg daily for 14 days) combined with standard chloroquine therapy (1.5 g of base in 3 days) proved to be the regimen of choice for radical cure of Korean vivax malaria treated either during the acute clinical attack or during the late stage of clinical activity. With such a schedule, ambulatory treatment with only minimal medical supervision is possible, clinical toxicity is insignificant, and the relapse rate is less than 3%. Radical cure can be obtained by giving 15 mg of primaquine base alone, daily for 14 days, if administration is carried out during the long-term latent period of the infection.

The above schedule is currently recommended for the treatment and cure of the *temperate zone* variety of vivax malaria. Patients infected with the *Chesson* (*Southwest Pacific*) strain may be treated with two to three times this daily dose of primaquine, that is, 30 to 45 mg of base. Alving and coworkers (1960), however, introduced a schedule involving weekly rather than daily doses of primaquine because of the danger of hemolytic reactions arising from the increased dosage necessary to cure Chesson strain infections. They found that 60 mg of primaquine base together with 300 mg of chloroquine given weekly for 8 weeks resulted in 6% failure compared with about 30% failure following 15 mg of primaquine base alone given daily for 14 days. The use of combinations containing 45 mg of primaquine base resulted in 10% failure; and 30 mg, 55% failure. The highest-dose regimen had negligible hemolytic effect upon the erythrocytes of primaquine-sensitive individuals. The recommended therapy for patients infected with this strain of malaria is, therefore, 600 mg of chloroquine base, followed 6 hours later by 300 mg of chloroquine base combined with 45 mg of primaquine base in one dose. Thereafter 300 mg of chloroquine combined with 45 mg of primaquine should be given as a single dose on the same day of each week for 7 additional weeks. Amodiaquine or hydroxychloroquine may be substituted for chloroquine.

Toxicity and Side Effects.
In the usual therapeutic doses, primaquine has proven quite innocuous when given to Caucasians. Mild-to-moderate abdominal cramps and occasional epigastric distress have occurred in some individuals given the larger doses, and mild anemia, cyanosis (methemoglobi-

nemia), and leukocytosis have been observed. Higher doses (60 to 240 mg of primaquine base daily) accentuate the abdominal symptoms and cause methemoglobinemia and cyanosis in most subjects and leukopenia in some. Hepatic function is unaffected by primaquine, even in patients with infectious hepatitis. Abdominal distress can be alleviated by antacids and by taking the drug at mealtime. Although methemoglobinemia is somewhat greater with primaquine than with pamaquine at all comparable dose levels, in most other respects primaquine has proven less toxic. Granulocytopenia and even agranulocytosis are rare complications of therapy and are usually associated with overdosage. The toxicity of primaquine in most Negroes is as described above; however, there is a fraction of the Negro population (about 10% of males in the United States) who develop anemia due to intravascular hemolysis at daily dose levels of 20 mg (base) and higher. Such primaquine sensitivity of erythrocytes is seen also in some Caucasian ethnic groups, including Sardinians, Sephardic Jews, Greeks, and Iranians, in whom the sensitivity is greater than in the Negro so that the hemolytic reaction from a given dose of drug may well be more severe.

The incidence of hemolysis, in general, follows the same geographical pattern as the distribution of falciparum malaria. A decrease in glucose-6-phosphate dehydrogenase activity has been shown to be characteristic of primaquine-sensitive erythrocytes and appears to represent their major enzymatic deficiency. In normal erythrocytes there are several mechanisms that protect the cells against injury by oxidative drugs such as metabolic derivatives of primaquine. These drugs are capable of accelerating the transfer of hydrogen from reduced nicotinamide adenine dinucleotide phosphate (NADPH), reduced glutathione, hemoglobin, the free sulfhydryl groups of proteins, and other donors. In normal erythrocytes under the stress of oxidant drugs, the rate of NADPH regeneration can be greatly accelerated by increasing the amount of glucose metabolized by means of the pentose phosphate pathway. Sufficient NADPH is therefore readily made available for reduction of oxidized glutathione and methemoglobin through the respective reductase reactions; reduced glutathione also protects the sulfhydryl groups of hemoglobin and the sulfhydryl-containing enzymes against oxidative destruction. Primaquine-sensitive erythrocytes, on the other hand, are incapable of sufficiently rapid regeneration of NADPH because of their deficiency of glucose-6-phosphate dehydrogenase; consequently, all the reductive

processes within the cell that are dependent upon NADPH are impaired. Metabolic processes are diminished so that normal vital functions can no longer be carried out, and alterations in the lipoprotein membrane of the cell result in lysis (*see* Tarlov *et al.,* 1962; Beutler, 1969). Brewer and colleagues (1960) have devised a simple test for detecting such primaquine sensitivity based on the observation that the rate of methemoglobin reduction by erythrocytes from these individuals is markedly slower than normal in the presence of methylene blue. Results from this test correlate very well with the severity of hemolysis. The World Health Organization (1967) and Beutler and Mitchell (1968) have described other simple tests. Since primaquine sensitivity is inherited by a gene carried on the X chromosome, the hemolysis is often of intermediate severity in heterozygous females; because of "variable penetrance," females may be affected less frequently than would be predicted.

At present more than 40 drugs and other substances are known to be capable of inducing hemolysis. These include antimalarials, sulfonamides, nitrofurans, antipyretics, analgesics, sulfones, vitamin K analogs, fava beans (favism), and certain other vegetables.

The severity of the hemolysis is dependent on the dose of drug used. If the initial dose is not too large, the hemolysis is self-limited even when the same dose of drug is continued. This is because older erythrocytes are most susceptible, and, after their destruction, the remaining younger cells and newly produced reticulocytes are relatively resistant to hemolysis. However, the severity of hemolysis can be enhanced or mitigated by many factors and is often unpredictable. For this reason the administration of primaquine or of any other potentially hemolytic drug should be discontinued immediately if marked darkening of the urine or a sudden decrease in hemoglobin concentration occurs (*see* Kellermeyer *et al.,* 1962).

Precautions and Contraindications. Because of the possibility of hemolytic reactions (*see* above), one should watch for suggestive signs. If a daily dose of more than 30 mg of primaquine base (more than 15 mg daily in possibly sensitive patients such as Negroes) is administered, repeated peripheral blood counts and at least gross examination of the urine should be performed during therapy. If the drug is used in schemes for mass administration, some supervision is required.

Primaquine is contraindicated in acutely ill patients suffering from systemic disease characterized by a tendency to granulocytopenia, such as very active forms of rheumatoid arthritis and lupus erythematosus. It should not be given to subjects receiving, at the same time, other potentially hemolytic drugs, agents capable of depressing the myeloid elements of the bone marrow, or quinacrine.

Therapeutic Uses. Primaquine is used mainly for the *radical cure* of vivax and other relapsing malarias. If it is administered during the long-term latent period of the infection, radical cure can be achieved. Its use during an acute clinical attack will prevent subsequent recrudescences. Primaquine should always be given in conjunction with full doses of a 4-aminoquinoline schizontocide, preferably chloroquine, in order to reduce the possibility of developing drug-resistant strains. In appropriate circumstances it may be used in combination with a 4-aminoquinoline for prophylaxis or for the interruption of transmission, especially of *P. falciparum.*

QUININE AND THE CINCHONA ALKALOIDS

History. Quinine is the chief alkaloid of cinchona, the bark of the cinchona tree indigenous to certain regions of South America. The bark is also called Peruvian, Jesuit's, or Cardinal's bark. It is not clear whether the natives were acquainted with the medicinal properties of cinchona. The first written record of the use of cinchona occurs in a religious book written in 1633 and published in Spain in 1639. The author, an Augustinian monk named Calancha, of Lima, Peru, wrote: "A tree grows which they call 'the fever tree' in the country of Loxa, whose bark, the color of cinnamon, is made into powder amounting to the weight of two small silver coins and given as a beverage, cures the fevers and tertians; it has produced miraculous results in Lima." A variety of colorful and fanciful versions of the discovery of the fever bark exist. A popular and persistent version is that the bark was employed in 1638 to treat Countess Anna del Chinchón, wife of the viceroy to Peru, and that her miraculous cure resulted in the introduction of cinchona into Spain in 1639 for the treatment of ague. There is no evidence that the countess ever used the bark; yet for many years the drug was called *los Polvos de la Condesa.* However, the viceroy did bring a large shipment of cinchona to Spain. By 1640, the drug was being employed for fevers in Europe. Its use was first mentioned in European medical literature in 1643 by a Belgian, Herman van der Heyden.

The term *cinchona* was chosen by Linné (who accidentally misspelled it) for the species of plants yielding the drug. Although this term is probably derived from the name of the countess whose alleged cure led to its wide use, some believe that it comes from a word of Incan origin, *kinia,* which means "bark." The Jesuit fathers were the main importers and distributors of cinchona in Europe, and the name *Jesuit bark* soon became attached to the drug. It was sponsored in Rome chiefly by the eminent philosopher Cardinal de Lugo; hence the drug came to be called *Cardinal's bark.* The conservative medical groups viewed the new antipyretic with disdain because its use did not conform to the teachings of Galen. Others looked upon it with suspicion because the Jesuits used it. For these reasons, the drug was dispensed for many years predominantly by charlatans and in the form of secret remedies. The most fabulous of these quacks was the incomparable Robert Talbor. The first official recognition of cinchona came in 1677, when it was included in an edition of the *London Pharmacopoeia* as "Cortex Peruanus."

For almost 2 centuries the bark was employed for medicine as a powder, extract, or infusion. In 1820, Pelletier and Caventou isolated quinine and cinchonine from cinchona, and the use of the alkaloids as such gained favor rapidly.

Chemistry. While quinine has been synthesized, the procedure is too complex and expensive to provide a practical source of the drug. Quinine and the other alkaloids are, therefore, still obtained entirely from natural sources.

Cinchona contains a mixture of more than 20 alkaloids. The most important of these are two pairs of optical isomers, *quinine* and *quinidine,* and *cinchonidine* and *cinchonine.* Quinine and cinchonidine are levorotary. Inasmuch as hundreds of compounds have been derived from quinine and its congeners, each differing in chemical and pharmacological properties, the cinchona alkaloids provide a promising opportunity for the study of the relationship between chemical structure and pharmacological action.

Quinine has the following structural formula:

Quinine

Quinine contains a quinoline group attached through a secondary alcohol linkage to a quinuclidine ring. A methoxy side chain is attached to the quinoline ring and a vinyl to the quinuclidine. *Quinidine* has the same structure as quinine except for the steric configuration of the secondary alcohol grouping. The many natural alkaloids related to quinine and the semisynthetic chemicals derived from quinine differ mainly in the nature of the substitutions on the side chain. Each alteration in the chemical pattern of quinine causes corresponding quantitative but not qualitative changes in the pharmacological actions of the resulting compounds.

Structure-Activity Relationship. The effects of chemical alterations in the quinine molecule on various pharmacological actions have been studied, particularly with regard to antimalarial potency. Since none of the resulting compounds has an antimalarial action superior to that of quinine, the details will not be presented. To summarize, the data indicate that neither the methoxy nor the vinyl radical of the quinine molecule is required for antimalarial activity. In contrast, the secondary alcohol group is absolutely essential, and its reduction increases toxicity and abolishes antiplasmodial potency. Stereoisomerism is a relatively unimportant factor.

Further details of the structure-activity relationship in the cinchona alkaloids may be found elsewhere (*see* Oettingen, 1933; Wiselogle, 1946; and others). Historically, this important field has provided the necessary background for the search for more effective and less toxic antimalarials.

PHARMACOLOGICAL PROPERTIES

The typical actions of cinchona are largely attributable to its quinine content. In the following pages, the pharmacology of quinine will be presented, and the important variations in action of related alkaloids will be pointed out as occasion arises.

Local Actions. Quinine affects such a large variety of biological systems that it has been called a "general protoplasmic poison"; with some reservations this appraisal is probably correct. It is toxic to many bacteria and other unicellular organisms such as trypanosomes, infusoria, yeast, plasmodia, and spermatozoa. Despite this wide range of activity, quinine does exhibit considerable specificity in its action. For example, molds grow freely in quinine solution; only high concentrations of the drug are injurious to sperm cells and bacteria; salt-water, but not fresh-water, amebae are resistant to quinine; and oral spirochetes but not pathogenic spirochetes of relapsing fever are susceptible to the alkaloid.

Local Anesthetic Action. Sensory nerves are briefly stimulated and then paralyzed by quinine. Concentrations only slightly higher than those necessary for anesthesia are likely to cause edema, pain, and reactive fibrosis. The anesthesia may last for many hours or days, and in this respect differs sharply from that produced by the conventional local anesthetics.

Irritant Action. Quinine is a marked local irritant. When taken orally, it may cause gastric pain, nausea, and vomiting. When it is given in solution rectally, the ensuing irritation may result in its rapid expulsion. Subcutaneous or intramuscular injections of the drug are initially painful. Sterile abscesses may result from local tissue damage. Intravenous administration may result in thrombosis of the injected vein from injury to the intima. Vascular damage is the basis for the occasional use of quinine solutions for sclerosing varicose veins. The irritant properties of quinine also appear where the drug is concentrated in the kidney tubule; thus, renal injury may occur.

Antimalarial Actions and Efficacy. Until the third decade of the present century, the cinchona alkaloids represented the sole chemotherapeutic agents for the specific treatment of malaria. Since the advent of synthetic antimalarials, quinine has been relegated to a secondary role.

Quinine is not a true causal prophylactic agent; it is incapable of preventing sporozoite-induced vivax or falciparum malaria in human volunteers.

However, like chloroquine, it is effective both as a suppressive drug and in the control of overt clinical attacks. Its primary action is schizontocidal, and no lethal effect is exerted on sporozoites or preerythrocytic tissue forms. In addition, quinine is gametocytocidal for *P. vivax* and *P. malariae* but not for *P. falciparum.* As both a suppressive and a therapeutic agent, quinine is less well tolerated and less effective than chloroquine. However, a valuable current use of quinine is in the treatment of severe illness due to certain multiresistant strains of *P. falciparum.*

Central Nervous System. Therapeutic doses of quinine have few effects on the central nervous system (CNS) other than to cause *analgesia* and *antipyresis.* The discovery that cinchona lowered the fever of malarial patients quickly led to its use in all forms of febrile illnesses. The rather indifferent results on other fevers indicate that quinine is not a potent antipyretic, and it is rarely used for this purpose. Quinine resembles salicylate and related drugs in its analgesic property. Adequate doses obtund moderate pain, especially muscle and joint pain. The site of action is central.

Cardiovascular System. The actions of quinine on cardiac muscle are qualitatively similar to those of its isomer, quinidine. These are described in full in Chapter 32. Therapeutic doses of quinine have little, if any, effect on the normal heart or blood pressure in man. When given intravenously, quinine causes a definite and sometimes alarming hypotension, particularly when the injection is made rapidly. Epinephrine is a particularly effective resuscitative agent when given after circulatory collapse has developed.

Uterine Muscle. The *oxytocic action* of quinine and related alkaloids is poorly understood. The nongravid human uterus is only slightly influenced by quinine, but as pregnancy proceeds the oxytocic action becomes progressively more noticeable. Although quinine has been used with other drugs to initiate labor, its action is unreliable. Toxic amounts of quinine may cause abortion, but it is questionable whether this is always due to a direct uterine action of the drug. Quinine passes the placental barrier and can produce poisoning in the fetus.

Skeletal Muscle. Quinine and related cinchona alkaloids exert interesting effects on skeletal muscle that have some clinical applicability. Quinine increases the tension response to a single maximal stimulus delivered to the muscle directly or through the nerve, but it increases the refractory period of muscle so that the response to tetanic stimulation is diminished. Quinine also decreases the excitability of the motor end-plate region so that the responses to repetitive nerve stimulation and to acetylcholine are reduced. Thus, it has a curare-like effect on skeletal muscle, and can antagonize the actions of physostigmine on skeletal muscle as effectively as does curare.

The effects of quinine and related alkaloids on skeletal muscle remained purely a matter of academic interest until it was demonstrated that myotonia congenita could be symptomatically relieved by quinine (Wolf, 1936). This disease is the pharmacological antithesis of myasthenia gravis, and investigations soon revealed that drugs effective in one syndrome aggravate the other. Quinine may so aggravate the symptoms of myasthenia that alarming respiratory distress and dysphagia may ensue.

Gastrointestinal Tract. The soluble salts of quinine are extremely bitter, and very small amounts of cinchona preparations are used as *stomachics.* Larger doses may inhibit vagal-mediated gastric secretion. The irritant properties of the cinchona alkaloids cause considerable *gastric distress.* Nausea, vomiting, and diarrhea are prominent when large doses are taken orally. Toxic amounts also produce vomiting by a central action on the medulla. The *musculature* of the intestinal tract is not stimulated by concentrations of the drug reached clinically.

Absorption, Fate, and Excretion. Quinine and its congeners are readily absorbed when given orally. Absorption occurs mainly from the upper small intestine, and is almost complete even in patients with marked diarrhea. Subcutaneous or intramuscular injection of quinine is contraindicated because of local tissue damage.

Peak plasma concentrations of cinchona alkaloids occur within 1 to 3 hours after a single oral dose. After chronic administration of total daily doses of 1 g of drug, the average plasma quinine concentration is approximately 7 μg/ml. After termination of quinine therapy, the plasma level falls rapidly and only a negligible concentration is detectable after 24 hours. A large fraction (approximately 70%) of the plasma quinine is bound to proteins. This explains in part why the concentration of the alkaloid in cerebrospinal fluid is only 2 to 5% of that in the plasma. Quinine readily reaches the tissues of the fetus.

The cinchona alkaloids in large measure are metabolically degraded in the body, especially in the liver, so that less than 5% of an administered dose is excreted *unaltered* in the urine. There is no accumulation of the drugs in the body upon continued administration. The metabolic degradation products are excreted in the urine, where many of them have been identified as hydroxy derivatives (Brodie *et al.,* 1951). The cinchona alkaloids are excreted mainly in the urine, but small amounts also appear in the feces, gastric juice, bile, and saliva. Renal excretion of quinine is twice as rapid when the urine is acidic as when it is alkaline, due to the greater tubular reabsorption of the alkaloidal base. Excretion is also limited by the binding of a large fraction of cinchona alkaloids to plasma proteins.

Toxicity. Poisoning by quinine is usually due to clinical overdosage or to hypersensitivity. The fatal oral dose of quinine for adults is approximately 8 g. When quinine is repeatedly given in full doses, a typical cluster of symptoms occurs to which the term *cinchonism* has been applied. Certain features of the syndrome are seen in salicylate poisoning. In its mildest form it consists in ringing in the ears, headache, nausea, and slightly disturbed vision; however, when medication is continued or after large single doses, symptoms also involve the gastrointestinal tract, the nervous and cardiovascular systems, and the skin.

Hearing and *vision* are particularly disturbed. Functional impairment of the eighth nerve results in tinnitus, decreased auditory acuity, and vertigo. The visual signs are those of blurred vision, disturbed color perception, photophobia, diplopia, night blindness, constricted visual fields, scotomata, and mydriasis. It is not known if the visual and auditory effects are directly neural or secondary to vascular changes. Attention has been directed repeatedly to the marked spastic constriction of the retinal vessels. The retina is ischemic, the discs are pale, and retinal edema may ensue. In severe cases, optic atrophy results. Degenerative changes in the spiral ganglion cells similar to those noted in the ganglion cells of the retina lend support to the belief that the cellular injury from quinine is direct. Perhaps both vascular and neural components of injury are involved.

Gastrointestinal symptoms are also prominent in cinchonism. Nausea, vomiting, abdominal pain, and diarrhea result from the local irritant action of quinine, but the nausea and emesis also have a central basis. The *skin* is often hot and flushed, and sweating is prominent. Rashes frequently appear. Angioedema, especially of the face, is occasionally observed.

CNS symptoms are noted in severer grades of poisoning, particularly headache, fever, vomiting, apprehension, excitement, confusion, delirium, and syncope. *Respiration* is first stimulated and then shallow and depressed. The skin becomes cold and cyanotic as poisoning progresses, the body temperature and the blood pressure fall, weakness is extreme, the pulse is feeble, coma ensues, and death occurs from respiratory arrest. *Death* may result in a few hours or be delayed 1 or 2 days. If the patient recovers, symptoms usually disappear completely except that there may be variable degrees of residual optic and auditory damage in some cases.

At times, *renal damage* may be caused by quinine, and anuria and uremia may ensue. *Acute hemolytic anemia* is a rare complication of quinine therapy; it apparently is caused by the drug only in pregnant women or in patients with malaria. Quinine, like salicylate, is capable of causing *hypoprothrombinemia;* the simultaneous administration of vitamin K counteracts the prolongation of the prothrombin time. Rarely, quinine may cause symptomatic *purpura* in hypersusceptible individuals, by a thrombocytolytic action. In a few instances, the drug appears to have caused *agranulocytosis.* *Abortion* may result from quinine overdosage, but this is not necessarily due to an oxytocic action of the drug. The alkaloid may cause *asthma* in hypersensitive individuals. Transient *ventricular tachycardia* may rarely be observed after massive acute overdosage.

When small doses of cinchona alkaloids cause toxic manifestations, the individual is usually hypersensitive to the drug. Cinchonism may appear after a single dose of quinine, but it is usually mild.

Cutaneous flushing, pruritus, skin rashes, fever, gastric distress, dyspnea, ringing in the ears, and visual impairment are the usual expressions of hypersensitivity; extreme flushing of the skin accompanied by intense, generalized pruritus is the most common form. Hemoglobinuria and asthma from quinine are rare types of idiosyncrasy.

Treatment. Inasmuch as quinine is rapidly destroyed in the body, the longer the patient survives the better the prognosis becomes. Absorption may be slow if fairly insoluble salts have been ingested. Therefore, the stomach should be copiously lavaged or emesis induced with syrup of ipecac. The blood pressure should be supported and symptomatic measures employed to maintain renal function. Artificial respiration may be needed. Hemoglobinuria may necessitate blood transfusion, and the use of alkali to prevent renal blockade may prove helpful. Angioedematous or asthmatic phenomena may require the use of epinephrine, corticosteriods, and antihistamines. Residual visual impairment occasionally yields to vasodilators; in the acute phase of toxic amaurosis caused by quinine, vasodilators administered intravenously may have a salutary effect.

Contraindications. Quinine must be used with considerable caution, if at all, in patients who manifest idiosyncrasy to it, especially when this takes the form of cutaneous, angioedematous, visual, or auditory symptoms. Quinine should be stopped immediately if evidence of hemolysis appears. The drug should not be employed in patients with tinnitus or optic neuritis. In patients with atrial fibrillation, the administration of quinine requires the same precautions as outlined for quinidine (*see* Chapter 32).

Preparations, Routes of Administration, and Dosages. These are numerous preparations of cinchona alkaloids available to the practitioner, particularly in tropical communities where malaria is endemic and where cheap cinchona medication is essential. In the United States, the pure alkaloids are employed rather than the galenical preparations.

The most commonly used salts of quinine are *Quinine Sulfate,* U.S.P., and *quinine dihydrochloride.* Official tablets and capsules of quinine sulfate contain 120, 200, or 300 mg.

The usual oral dose of quinine or its salts is 300 to 600 mg, and the total daily dose is ordinarily not more than 2.0 g. The drug is given after meals, preferably in capsules, to minimize gastric irritation. For young children, quinine may have to be given in solution. The syrup of licorice and the aromatic syrup of eriodictyon are vehicles helpful for this purpose.

Totaquine contains approximately 10% of anhydrous quinine and approximately 75% of the total anhydrous crystallizable cinchona alkaloids. The drug is cheaper than quinine and available in abundance in parts of the world where quinine is expensive or limited in supply. In proper doses, it is as effective as quinine in malaria inasmuch as it contains cinchona alkaloids with approximately the same order of antimalarial potency as quinine. The usual dosage of totaquine for malaria is the same

as that of quinine, namely, 600 mg three times daily after meals, for 7 days.

The *oral route* should be employed for quinine administration whenever possible. Intravenous injection of quinine is to be reserved for certain emergencies such as pernicious or cerebral malaria. The dihydrochloride is employed and the injection should be made very slowly, preferably by the drip method; epinephrine should be available to counteract the untoward effects on the cardiovascular system.

THERAPEUTIC USES

While quinine has been employed in preparations as diverse as douches and hair tonics, it currently has two valid therapeutic applications—for the treatment of malaria and for the relief of nocturnal leg cramps.

Status as an Antimalarial. Except in those parts of the world where the newer antimalarials are unavailable or too expensive, quinine is rarely employed alone as an antimalarial. It is more toxic and less effective than the synthetic antimalarial drugs, and lacks the causal prophylactic and curative properties of chloroguanide and pyrimethamine. A valid antimalarial use of quinine is its administration in combination with primaquine for the radical cure of relapsing vivax malaria and for the treatment of malaria due to strains of *P. falciparum* resistant to chloroquine and cross-resistant to other antimalarial drugs.

Nocturnal Leg Cramps. Recumbency leg muscle cramps (night cramps) are quickly and effectively relieved by quinine in most cases. The dose is 200 to 300 mg before retiring. In some patients, only a brief period of quinine therapy is required to provide long periods of freedom from muscle cramps; in a few individuals, even large doses of the drug may fail to give relief.

ANTIBACTERIAL AGENTS IN ANTIMALARIAL CHEMOTHERAPY

Shortly after their introduction into therapeutics, the sulfonamides were shown to possess antimalarial activity. The sulfones were also shown to be effective; the first trial of dapsone was against *P. falciparum* in 1943. Little attention was paid to the data because of the superiority of other drugs. Current interest stems from their use, usually in combination with pyrimethamine, against resistant strains of falciparum malaria. When antimalarial activity was found in several antibiotics, the tetracyclines and chloramphenicol were tried clinically. Although their action as schizontocides is slow, their activity against drug-resistant malarial parasites is proving useful.

Sulfonamides and Sulfones. Much of the important work on sulfonamides was carried out during the intensive antimalarial program during World War II. This and later work focused attention on sulfadiazine, because of its relatively high activity. It was found, however, to be active only against the asexual blood forms of the human malarial parasites, and to act slowly. Subsequently, two longer-acting sulfonamides, sulfadoxine (FANZIL) and sulfalene (KELFIZINA), have been used for treatment and suppression, mainly in partially immune patients infected with fully sensitive strains of *P. falciparum.* Combinations of sulfadoxine with pyrimethamine are important for the treatment of patients with chloroquine-resistant strains of *P. falciparum.* Sulfadiazine may also be used, depending upon availability.

Parallel studies have demonstrated the value of dapsone used in the same way as sulfonamides, either alone or given concurrently with dihydrofolate reductase inhibitors. Field trials have also shown the value of 4,4'-diacetyldiaminodiphenylsulfone (*acedapsone*), a repository sulfone, given intramuscularly at intervals of several months, either alone or with cycloguanil, for suppression of falciparum infection. Another sulfone, 4,4'-diformamidodiphenylsulfone, is deformylated in the liver after oral administration to provide low sustained plasma concentrations of dapsone. Some success has followed its weekly use for suppression of malaria, in place of dapsone; studies on this substance given concurrently with chloroquine are still experimental. The danger of producing resistant strains not only of malarial parasites but also of pathogenic bacteria by the use of such relatively low dosage has been expressed. Neither sulfonamides nor sulfones are as active against *P. vivax* as they are against *P. falciparum.*

Tetracyclines. The use of tetracyclines in the treatment of the acute attack of multiresistant strains of falciparum malaria reflects sadly the sparsity of primary antimalarial drugs effective in such conditions. Their relative slowness of action makes concurrent treatment with quinine mandatory for rapid control of parasitemia. While several tetracyclines appear equivalent, most data have accumulated for tetracycline itself, and this is recommended. Although tetracycline has shown marked activity against primary tissue schizonts of chloroquine-resistant strains of *P. falciparum,* its long-term use as a prophylactic agent cannot be recommended because of the danger of producing antibiotic-resistant pathogenic bacteria (World Health Organization, 1973).

Miscellaneous Agents. The problems encountered in suppression and treatment of chloroquine-resistant and multiresistant strains of *P. falciparum* have led to intensive reexamination of many series of compounds studied during World War II. Substances have been synthesized that retain the 4-quinolinemethanol nucleus of quinine but in which there is major simplification of the 6-substituent. One of the most active of these, WR 30090 (α-[{dibutylamino} methyl]-6,8-dichloro-2-[3',4'-dichloro]-phenyl-4-quinolinemethanol), has shown rapid blood schizontocidal activity after oral administration to nonimmune patients infected with *P. vivax* and with normally sensitive and chloroquine-resistant strains of *P. falciparum.* Further studies on this compound are underway.

Adams, A. R. D.; Maegraith, B. G.; King, J. D.; Townshend, R. H.; Davey, T. H.; and Havard, R. E. Studies on synthetic antimalarial drugs. XIII. Results of a preliminary investigation of the therapeutic action of 4888 (PALUDRINE) on acute attacks of benign tertian malaria. *Ann. trop. Med. Parasit.,* 1945, 39, 225–231.

Allison, J. L.; O'Brien, R. L.; and Hahn, F. E. DNA: reaction with chloroquine. *Science, Wash.,* 1965, 149, 1111–1113.

———. Nature of the deoxyribonucleic acid—chloroquine complex. In, *Antimicrobial Agents and Chemotherapy—1965.* (Sylvester, J. C., ed.) American Society for Microbiology, Ann Arbor, Mich., 1966, pp. 310–314.

Alving, A. S.; Eichelberger, L.; Craige, B., Jr.; Jones, R., Jr.; Whorton, C. M.; and Pullman, T. N. Studies on the chronic toxicity of chloroquine (SN-7618). *J. clin. Invest.,* 1948, 27, 60–65.

Alving, A. S.; Johnson, C. F.; Tarlov, A. R.; Brewer, G. J.; Kellermeyer, R. W.; and Carson, P. E. Mitigation of the hemolytic effect of primaquine and enhancement of its action against exo-erythrocytic forms of the Chesson strain of *Plasmodium vivax* by intermittent regimens of drug administration. *Bull. Wld Hlth Org.,* 1960, 22, 621–631.

Arnold, J.; Alving, A. S.; and Clayman, C. B. Induced primaquine resistance in vivax malaria. *Trans. R. Soc. trop. Med. Hyg.,* 1961, 55, 345–350.

Arnold, J.; Alving, A. S.; Hockwald, R. S.; Clayman, C. B.; Dern, R. J.; Beutler, E.; Flanagan, C. L.; and Jeffrey, G. M. The antimalarial action of primaquine against the blood and tissue stages of falciparum malaria (Panama, P-F-6 strain). *J. Lab. clin. Med.,* 1955, 46, 391–397.

Bartonelli, P. J.; Sheehy, T. W.; and Tigertt, W. D. Combined therapy for chloroquine-resistant *Plasmodium falciparum* infection. *J. Am. med. Ass.,* 1967, 199, 173–177.

Berliner, R. W.; Earle, D. P., Jr.; Taggart, J. V.; Zubrod, C. G.; Welch, W. J.; Conan, N. J.; Bauman, E.; Scudder, S. T.; and Shannon, J. A. Studies on the chemotherapy of the human malarias. VI. The physiological disposition, antimalarial activity, and toxicity of several derivatives of 4-aminoquinoline. *J. clin. Invest.,* 1948, 27, 98–107.

Bernstein, H. N.; Svaifler, N. J.; Rubin, M.; and Mausour, A. M. The ocular deposition of chloroquine. *Invest. Ophthal.,* 1963, 2, 384–392.

Beutler, E., and Mitchell, M. Special modifications of the fluorescent screening method for glucose-6-phosphate dehydrogenase deficiency. *Blood,* 1968, 32, 816–818.

Brewer, G. J.; Tarlov, A. R.; and Alving, A. S. Methemoglobin reduction test: a new simple, *in vitro* test for identifying primaquine-sensitivity. *Bull. Wld Hlth Org.,* 1960, 22, 633–640.

Brodie, B. B.; Baer, J. E.; and Craig, L. C. Metabolic products of the cinchona alkaloids in human urine. *J. biol. Chem.,* 1951, 188, 567–581.

Bushby, R. S. M., and Hitchings, G. H. Trimethoprim, a sulphonamide potentiator. *Br. J. Pharmac. Chemother.,* 1968, 33, 72–90.

Canfield, C. J.; Whiting, E. G.; Hall, W. H.; and MacDonald, B. S. Treatment of acute falciparum malaria from Vietnam with trimethoprim and sulfalene. *Am. J. trop. Med. Hyg.,* 1971, 20, 524–526.

Carrington, H. C.; Crowther, A. F.; Davey, D. G.; Levi, A. A.; and Rose, F. L. A metabolite of PALUDRINE with high antimalarial activity. *Nature, Lond,* 1951, 168, 1080.

Cohen, R. J.; Sachs, J. R.; Wicker, D. J.; and Conrad, M. E. Methaemoglobinemia provoked by malarial chemoprophylaxis in Vietnam. *New Engl. J. Med.,* 1968, 279, 1127–1131.

Cohen, S. N., and Yielding, K. L. Inhibition of DNA and RNA polymerase reactions by chloroquine. *Proc. natn. Acad. Sci. U.S.A.,* 1965, 54, 521–527.

Crowther, A. F., and Levi, A. A. PROGUANIL: isolation of metabolite with high antimalarial activity. *Br. J. Pharmac. Chemother.,* 1953, 8, 93–97.

Curd, F. H. S.; Davey, D. G.; and Rose, F. L. Studies on synthetic antimalarial drugs. II. General chemical considerations. *Ann. trop. Med. Parasit.,* **1945,** *39,* 157–164. X. Some biguanide derivatives as new types of antimalarial substances with both therapeutic and causal prophylactic activity. *Ibid.,* **1945,** *39,* 208–216.

Donno, L.; Sanguineti, V.; Ricciardi, M. L.; and Soldati, M. Antimalarial activity of kelfizina-trimethoprim and kelfizina-pyrimethamine versus chloroquine in field trials in Nigeria. *Am. J. trop. Med. Hyg.,* **1969,** *18,* 182–187.

Edgcomb, J. H.; Arnold, J.; Yount, E. H., Jr.; Alving, A. S.; and Eichelberger, L. Primaquine, SN 13272, a new curative agent in *vivax* malaria: a preliminary report. *J. natn. Malar. Soc.,* **1950,** *9,* 285–292.

Elderfield, R. C., and others. Alkylaminoalkyl derivatives of 8-aminoquinoline. *J. Am. chem. Soc.,* **1946,** *68,* 1524–1529.

Fairley, N. H. Chemotherapeutic suppression and prophylaxis in malaria: an experimental investigation undertaken by medical research teams in Australia. *Trans. R. Soc. trop. Med. Hyg.,* **1945,** *38,* 311–365.

———. Researches on PALUDRINE (M. 4888) in malaria: an experimental investigation undertaken by the L.H.Q. Medical Research Unit (A.I.F.), Cairns, Australia. *Ibid.,* **1946,** *40,* 105–153.

Falco, E. A.; Goodwin, L. G.; Hitchings, G. H.; Rollo, I. M.; and Russell, P. B. 2:4-Diaminopyrimidines—a new series of antimalarials. *Br. J. Pharmac. Chemother.,* **1951,** *6,* 185–200.

Ferone, R. Altered dihydrofolate reductase in a strain of pyrimethamine-resistant *Plasmodium berghei. Fedn Proc. Fedn Am. Socs exp. Biol.,* **1969,** *28,* 847.

Ferone, R.; Burchall, J. J.; and Hitchings, G. H. *Plasmodium berghei* dihydrofolate reductase: isolation, properties, and inhibition by antifolates. *Molec. Pharmac.,* **1969,** *5,* 49–59.

Ferone, R., and Hitchings, G. H. Folate cofactor biosynthesis by *Plasmodium berghei:* comparison of folate and dihydrofolate as substrates. *J. Protozool.,* **1966,** *13,* 504–506.

Fitch, C. D. *Plasmodium falciparum* in owl monkeys: drug resistance and chloroquine binding capacity. *Science, Wash.,* **1970,** *169,* 289–290.

Gaudette, L. E., and Coatney, G. R. A possible mechanism of prolonged antimalarial activity. *Am. J. trop. Med. Hyg.,* **1961,** *10,* 321–326.

Hart, C. W., and Naunton, R. F. The ototoxicity of chloroquine phosphate. *Archs Otolar.,* **1964,** *80,* 407–412.

Homewood, C. A.; Warhurst, D. C.; Peters, W.; and Baggaley, V. C. Lysosomes, pH and the anti-malarial action of chloroquine. *Nature, Lond.,* **1972,** *235,* 50–52.

Hurly, M. G. D. Potentiation of pyrimethamine by sulphadiazine in human malaria. *Trans. R. Soc. trop. Med. Hyg.,* **1959,** *53,* 412–413.

Kahn, S. B.; Fein, S. A.; and Brodsky, I. Effects of trimethoprim on folate metabolism in man. *Clin. Pharmac. Ther.,* **1968,** *9,* 550–560.

Kellermeyer, R. W.; Tarlov, A. R.; Brewer, G. J.; Carson, P. E.; and Alving, A. S. Hemolytic effect of therapeutic drugs: clinical considerations of the primaquine-type hemolysis. *J. Am. med. Ass.,* **1962,** *180,* 388–394.

Lucas, A. O.; Hendrickse, R. G.; Okubadejo, O. A.; Richards, W. H. G.; Neal, R. A.; and Kofie, B. A. K. The suppression of malarial parasitaemia by pyrimethamine in combination with dapsone or sulphormethoxine. *Trans. R. Soc. trop. Med. Hyg.,* **1969,** *63,* 216–229.

McChesney, E. W.; Fasco, M. J.; and Banks, W. F., Jr. The metabolism of chloroquine in man during and after repeated oral dosage. *J. Pharmac. exp. Ther.,* **1967,** *158,* 323–331.

Macomber, P. B.; O'Brien, R. L.; and Hahn, F. E. Chloroquine: physiological basis of drug resistance in *Plasmodium berghei. Science, Wash.,* **1966,** *152,* 1374–1375.

Martin, D. C., and Arnold, J. D. Trimethoprim in therapy

of acute attacks of malaria. *J. clin. Pharmac.,* **1967,** *7,* 336–341.

———. Treatment of acute falciparum malaria with sulfalene and trimethoprim. *J. Am. med. Ass.,* **1968,** *203,* 476–480.

Moore, D. V., and Lanier, J. E. Observations on two *Plasmodium falciparum* infections with an abnormal response to chloroquine. *Am. J. trop. Med. Hyg.,* **1961,** *10,* 5–9.

Mühlens, P. Die Behandlung der naturlichen menschlichen Malaria-Infektion mit Plasmochin. *Naturwissenschaften,* **1926,** *14,* 1162–1166.

Percival, S. P. B., and Meanock, I. Chloroquine: ophthalmological safety and clinical assessment in rheumatoid arthritis. *Br. med. J.,* **1968,** *3,* 579–584.

Polet, H., and Barr, C. F. Chloroquine and dihydroquinine: in vitro studies of their antimalarial effect upon *Plasmodium knowlesi. J. Pharmac. exp. Ther.,* **1968,** *164,* 380–386.

Richards, W. H. G., and Williams, S. G. Malaria studies in vitro. II. The measurement of drug activities using leucocyte-free blood-dilution cultures of *Plasmodium berghei* and ^{3}H-leucine. *Ann. trop. Med. Parasit.,* **1973,** *67,* 179–190.

Rieckmann, K. H.; McNamara, J. V.; Frischer, H.; Stockert, T. A.; Carson, P. E.; and Powell, R. D. Effects of chloroquine, quinine and cycloguanil upon the maturation of asexual erythrocytic forms of two strains of *Plasmodium falciparum* in vitro. *Am. J. trop. Med. Hyg.,* **1968,** *17,* 661–671.

Robertson, G. I. Experiments with antimalarial drugs in man. V. Experiments with an active metabolite of PROGUANIL and an active metabolite of 5943. *Trans. R. Soc. trop. Med. Hyg.,* **1957,** *51,* 488–492.

Rollo, I. M. The mode of action of sulphonamides, PROGUANIL, and pyrimethamine on *Plasmodium gallinaceum. Br. J. Pharmac. Chemother.,* **1955,** *10,* 208–214.

———. Partition profiles and their possible relation to chloroquine-resistance in plasmodia. *Fedn Proc. Fedn Am. Socs exp. Biol.,* **1968,** *27,* 537.

Rubin, M.; Bernstein, H. N.; and Zvaifler, N. J. Studies on the pharmacology of chloroquine. *Archs Ophthal., N.Y.,* **1963,** *70,* 474–481.

Schellenberg, K. A., and Coatney, G. R. The influence of antimalarial drugs on nucleic acid synthesis in *Plasmodium gallinaceum* and *Plasmodium berghei. Biochem. Pharmac.,* **1960,** *6,* 143–152.

Schmidt, L. H.; Loo, T. L.; Fradkin, R.; and Hughes, H. B. Antimalarial activities of triazine metabolites of chlorguanide and dichlorguanide. *Proc. Soc. exp. Biol. Med.,* **1952,** *80,* 367–370.

Schmidt, L. H.; Rossan, R. N.; and Fisher, K. F. The activity of a repository form of 4,6-diamino-1-(*p*-chlorophenyl)-1,2-dihydro-2,2-dimethyl-s-triazine against infections with *Plasmodium cynomolgi. Am. J. trop. Med. Hyg.,* **1963,** *12,* 494–503.

Smith, C. C. Metabolism of pentaquine in the rhesus monkey. *J. Pharmac. exp. Ther.,* **1956,** *116,* 67–76.

Smith, C. C., and Ihrig, J. Persistent excretion of pyrimethamine following oral administration. *Am. J. trop. Med. Hyg.,* **1959,** *8,* 60–62.

Smith, C. C.; Ihrig, J.; and Menne, R. Antimalarial activity and metabolism of biguanides. I. Metabolism of chloroguanide and chloroguanide triazine in rhesus monkeys and man. *Am. J. trop. Med. Hyg.,* **1961,** *10,* 694–703.

Smith, C. C., and Schmidt, L. H. Observations on the absorption of pyrimethamine from the gastrointestinal tract. *Expl Parasit.,* **1963,** *13,* 178–185.

Spinks, A. Studies on synthetic antimalarial drugs. XVIII. The absorption, distribution and excretion of PALUDRINE in experimental animals. *Ann. trop. Med. Parasit.,* **1947,** *41,* 30–38. XX. The blood concentrations and physiological distribution of some homologues of PALUDRINE in relation to their antimalarial activities. *Ibid.,* **1948,** *42,* 190–197.

Thompson, P. E.; Olszewski, B. J.; Elslager, E. F.; and Worth, D. F. Laboratory studies on 4,6-diamino-1-(*p*-chlorophenyl)-1,2-dihydro-2,2-dimethyl-*s*-triazine pamoate (CI-501) as a repository antimalarial drug. *Am. J. trop. Med. Hyg.,* **1963,** *12,* 481–493.

Waitz, J. A.; Olszewski, B. J.; and Thompson, P. E. Dialysis studies in rats on the long-acting antimalarial CI-501. *Science, Wash.,* **1963,** *141,* 723–725.

Whichard, L. P.; Morris, C. R.; Smith, J. M.; and Holbrook, D. J., Jr. The binding of primaquine, pentaquine, pamaquine, and PLASMOCID to deoxyribonucleic acid. *Molec. Pharmac.,* **1968,** *4,* 630–639.

Wolf, A. Quinine: an effective form of treatment for myotonia. *Archs Neurol. Psychiat., Chicago,* **1936,** *36,* 382–383.

Young, M. D. Resistance of *Plasmodium malariae* to pyrimethamine (DARAPRIM). *Am. J. trop. Med. Hyg.,* **1957,** *6,* 621–624.

Young, M. D., and Moore, D. V. Chloroquine resistance in *Plasmodium falciparum. Am. J. trop. Med. Hyg.,* **1961,** *10,* 317–320.

Zubrod, C. G.; Kennedy, T. J.; and Shannon, J. A. Studies on the chemotherapy of the human malarias. VIII. The physiological disposition of pamaquine. *J. clin. Invest.,* **1948,** *27,* 114–120.

Monographs and Reviews

Albert, A. *Selective Toxicity: The Physico-Chemical Basis of Therapy,* 5th ed. Chapman & Hall, Ltd., London, **1973.**

Beutler, E. Drug-induced hemolytic anemia. *Pharmac. Rev.,* **1969,** *21,* 73–103.

Coatney, G. R.; Cooper, W. C.; Eddy, N. B.; and Greenberg, J. *Survey of Antimalarial Agents: Chemotherapy of Plasmodium gallinaceum Infections; Toxicity; Correlation of Structure and Action.* Public Health Service Monograph No. 9, U.S. Government Printing Office, Washington, D. C., **1953.**

Davey, D. G. Chemotherapy of malaria. Part 1. Biological basis of testing methods. In, *Experimental Chemotherapy,* Vol. 1. (Schnitzer, R. J., and Hawking, F., eds.) Academic Press, Inc., New York, **1963,** pp. 487–511.

Feldman, H. A. Toxoplasmosis. *New Engl. J. Med.,* **1968,** *279,* 1370–1375, 1431–1437.

Goodwin, L. G., and Rollo, I. M. The chemotherapy of malaria, piroplasmosis, trypanosomiasis, and leishmaniasis. In, *Biochemistry and Physiology of Protozoa,* Vol. II.

(Hutner, S. H., and Lwoff, A., eds.) Academic Press, Inc., New York, **1955,** pp. 225–276.

Hill, J. Chemotherapy of malaria. Part 2. The antimalarial drugs. In, *Experimental Chemotherapy,* Vol. 1. (Schnitzer, R. J., and Hawking, F., eds.) Academic Press, Inc., New York, **1963,** pp. 513–601.

Hitchings, G. H., and Burchall, J. J. Inhibition of folate biosynthesis and function as a basis for chemotherapy. *Adv. Enzymol.,* **1965,** *27,* 417–468.

Modell, W. Malaria and victory in Vietnam. *Science, Wash.,* **1968,** *162,* 1346–1352.

Oettingen, W. F. von. *The Therapeutic Agents of the Quinoline Group.* Chemical Catalog Co., New York, **1933.**

Peters, W. Chemotherapeutic agents in tropical diseases. In, *Recent Advances in Pharmacology.* (Robson, J. M., and Stacey, R. S., eds.) J. & A. Churchill, Ltd., London, **1968,** pp. 503–537.

Powell, R. D., and Tigertt, W. D. Drug resistance of parasites causing human malaria. *A. Rev. Med.,* **1968,** *19,* 81–102.

Rollo, I. M. The chemotherapy of malaria. In, *Biochemistry and Physiology of Protozoa,* Vol. III. (Hutner, S. H., ed.) Academic Press, Inc., New York, **1964,** pp. 525–561.

———. Dihydrofolate reductase inhibitors as antimicrobial agents and their potentiation by sulfonamides. *CRC Crit. Rev. clin. lab. Sci.,* **1970,** *1,* 565–583.

Symposium on DARAPRIM. (Various authors.) *Trans. R. Soc. trop. Med. Hyg.,* **1952,** *46,* 467–508.

Symposium. (Various authors.) The synergy of trimethoprim and sulphonamides. *Postgrad. med. J.,* **1969,** *45,* Suppl., 3–104.

Tarlov, A. R.; Brewer, G. J.; Carson, P. E.; and Alving, A. S. Primaquine sensitivity. *Archs intern. Med.,* **1962,** *109,* 209–234.

Thompson, P. E., and Werbel, L. M. *Antimalarial Agents: Chemistry and Pharmacology.* Academic Press, Inc., New York, **1972.**

Wiselogle, F. Y. (ed.). *A Survey of Antimalarial Drugs, 1941–1945.* J. W. Edwards, Pub., Inc., Ann Arbor, Mich., **1946.** (Two volumes.)

World Health Organization. *Standardization of Procedures for the Study of Glucose-6-Phosphate Dehydrogenase.* Technical Report No. 366, WHO, Geneva, **1967.**

———. *Fourteenth Report of the Expert Committee on Malaria.* Technical Report No. 382, WHO, Geneva, **1968.**

———. *Chemotherapy of Malaria and Resistance to Antimalarials.* Technical Report No. 529, WHO, Geneva, **1973.**

CHAPTER

53 DRUGS USED IN THE CHEMOTHERAPY OF AMEBIASIS

Ian M. Rollo

Amebiasis is worldwide in distribution. It can no longer be considered a tropical disease. Indeed, in some districts in the temperate climates where sanitary conditions are poor, the incidence may be almost as high as in warm countries. The disease is widespread in the United States, and surveys have shown an incidence of 20% or more in inhabitants of eleemosynary institutions and rural areas of the southern states. In other areas where standards of hygiene are higher, the incidence is much less but, nevertheless, quite significant. The disease occurs in infants and children as well as in adults.

Dysentery is only one of the protean clinical manifestations of amebiasis. The majority of patients with amebic infections do not have dysentery, but only mild symptoms recognized with difficulty as being caused by pathogenic amebae. Much of the difficulty arises partly from an inability to identify the parasite and partly from a failure to realize the fine interplay of host-parasite relations. The latter may take two forms; either the parasite may remain as a commensal in the lumen of the bowel, producing cysts but with little or no disturbance to the well-being of the host, or it may abuse the hospitality unwittingly offered and invade the tissues (*see* Elsdon-Dew, 1968). Before a definitive diagnosis of amebiasis is made, it is most important that other nonpathogenic amebae found in the human colon—*Dientamoeba fragilis, Endolimax nana, Entamoeba coli, Entamoeba hartmanni,* and *Iodamoeba bütschlii*—are not mistaken for *Entamoeba histolytica.* Differentiation requires the services of a well-trained and experienced microscopist. Evidence of invasive amebiasis can be obtained serologically, and a simple latex agglutination kit is available commercially.

The physician has at his disposal a variety of amebicidal drugs. No one drug can as yet be said to be a cure-all, and treatment must be based on the state of the disease, the condition of the patient, local practice, experience of the practitioner, and, by no means least, the overall cost of a course, or possibly several courses, of treatment.

The most important division of amebicides in the past was into agents effective against *extraintestinal* infections and those effective against *intestinal* amebiasis. Only emetine, the closely related dehydroemetine, and chloroquine were in the first category; all the remaining drugs were in the second. More recently, niridazole and metronidazole have been found to be effective in the treatment of both intestinal and hepatic amebiasis Powell *et al.,* 1966a, 1966b). The former drug has been abandoned as an amebicide because of serious side effects. Successful use of the latter in all states of the disease has, however, revolutionized the treatment of amebiasis (Powell, 1971).

In recent years infection with free-living *Naegleria* species has been recognized as presenting special problems in diagnosis and treatment. In man, the amebae produce a generalized and rapidly progressing, fatal meningoencephalitis. Unfortunately, unless the microorganism is suspected, adequately early diagnosis cannot be made, since the amebae are not readily recognized in the customary gram-stained preparation of cerebrospinal fluid sediment. Evidence from both *in-vitro* and *in-vivo* experiments, and from sparse clinical data, suggests that treatment with amphotericin B may be successful (Duma *et al.,* 1971).

PRINCIPLES OF CHEMOTHERAPY OF AMEBIASIS

The modern therapy of amebiasis includes the treatment not only of patients with acute amebic dysentery but also of those persons who have intestinal amebiasis without acute symptoms. The asymptomatic passer of cysts is, however, a potential source of infection to himself and others and is an extremely serious public health problem, especially if he handles food. Amebic abscesses of the liver, brain, and lung may develop in carriers who have had few or no previous symptoms of intestinal amebiasis. It is important also to remember that hepatic amebiasis has been known to occur during treatment with amebicides acting only at the intestinal site of infection.

In addition to metronidazole, the physician has at his disposal several classes of amebicidal agents, including emetine, chloroquine, antibiotics, halogenated oxyquinolines, organic arsenicals, and synthetic organic compounds of various types. These drugs differ in their usefulness depending upon the character of the amebic infection. *Emetine,* formerly viewed as a specific cure for amebic dysentery, is now known to be the least valuable agent for *curing* the disease but one of the most effective drugs for rapidly controlling the symptoms of severe intestinal infections. Because it does not eradicate cysts, emetine does not cure intestinal amebiasis and is valueless in the treatment of asymptomatic passers of cysts. This shortcoming may be indirect evidence for the part played by the luminal, cyst-producing *minuta* cycle in the etiology of relapse or recrudescence. In sharp contrast to its restricted usefulness in acute amebic dysentery, emetine is of great value in the treatment of amebic hepatitis and amebic involvement of the lung, brain, skin, and other tissues. *Dehydroemetine* is preferred by some physicians. *Chloroquine* is of value only in extraintestinal amebiasis; it resembles emetine in this respect but differs in that it is of no value in acute amebic dysentery. Chloroquine has the advantage of being much less toxic than emetine. *Metronidazole* has become the mainstay of treatment of all forms of the disease, with the exception of asymptomatic intestinal amebiasis and those cases where, because of an idiosyncrasy to the drug or its nonavailability, it cannot be used. Although in the past it seemed unlikely that a drug would ever be discovered that by itself would cure all cases of amebiasis, the successful use of metronidazole indicates that this goal has almost been achieved.

The other amebicides discussed in this chapter are useful in the therapy of intestinal amebiasis, but they are valueless for amebic hepatitis and amebic abscesses. The arsenicals are particularly contraindicated in cases with hepatic involvement. The value of some of the other agents is not necessarily in their greater clinical effectiveness but in the decreased incidence and severity of side effects. The motile forms and hence cysts of pathogenic amebae in the intestinal tract are eradicated by these chemicals. When they are properly employed, especially concurrently or in alternation, approximately 90% of patients can be cured by one or two courses of medication.

The longer the intestinal amebiasis is allowed to continue, the harder it is to cure. Acute cases of amebiasis usually respond very well to adequate therapy, but chronic infections are difficult to eradicate. Chronicity should be prevented by all possible means. Not only are amebicides of importance in therapy but also adjuvant measures can be utilized to advantage. The diet should be low in residue and carbohydrate and high in easily digestible animal proteins. Other antimicrobial agents may be necessary to control associated bacterial invasion, and cure may be impossible without their use. Belladonna or opioids may be required for severe diarrhea.

The criterion of cure of intestinal amebiasis is based on laboratory, not clinical, examination. Disappearance of symptoms does not mean cure of amebiasis. Cure is considered accomplished if no amebae of the *histolytica* species are found in stool specimens properly obtained and examined at weekly intervals for 6 weeks after completion of treatment, at monthly intervals thereafter for 6 months, and at half-yearly intervals for 2 years. Repeated courses of medication are sometimes required to effect a cure. Treatment should be resumed whenever the stools again become positive for pathogenic amebae. It must be emphasized again, however, that many false diagnoses and much unnecessary therapy have resulted from incorrect laboratory reports.

Only the general principles of therapy of amebiasis with specific chemotherapeutic agents can be reviewed here. The details of treatment and of the adjuvant and dietary measures employed should be sought in the specialized literature, references to which are given at the end of this chapter.

Treatment of the Asymptomatic Carrier and Mild Case. Emetine and chloroquine are valueless in the treatment of asymptomatic passers of cysts. Other agents, described below, should be used in such cases; the choice usually depends upon current practice in a particular locale and the personal experience of the physician. These agents, by destroying trophozoites, eradicate amebic cysts. They do not require rest in bed, special routine, or interruption of work. Furthermore, they may be taken orally. If one course of medication does not establish a cure, concurrent drug therapy or alternating courses of two different drugs should be prescribed. Both the asymptomatic cyst passer and the cyst passer who has mild intestinal symptoms may be treated in this manner. The preferred drug is usually an 8-hydroxy-quinoline or diloxanide furoate. Since the presence of cysts in the feces is presumptive evidence of trophozoite activity in the colon, a course of metronidazole or chloroquine is best given to eradicate any unsuspected concurrent hepatic infection, although few authorities actually follow this practice. Metronidazole has proven less effective in the asymptomatic cyst passer than might have been expected from its success in the treatment of other forms of the disease. Although a relatively high rate of cure has resulted from its use, more reliable results can be achieved by the use of purely luminal amebicides. However, the drug has the advantage of dealing effectively with an unsuspected concurrent hepatic infection.

Patients with mild cases of diarrhea or enteritis may remain ambulatory and are best managed by treatment with metronidazole. Severe symptoms may be controlled by injections of emetine in doses of 30 mg twice daily for a few days; otherwise this drug is not employed. If relapse occurs, the course of metronidazole may be repeated or drugs from different chemical classes may be alternated or used concurrently.

Treatment of Acute Amebic Dysentery and Moderately Severe or Chronic Ulcerative Amebic Colitis. With the first successful use of metronidazole in 1966 for the treatment of invasive amebiasis, it became obvious that antiamebic therapy was not only revolutionized but greatly simplified. In place of, for example, emetine and tetracycline followed by a course of an intestinal amebicide, a course of treatment with metronidazole, which is readily acceptable to the patient, provides a high percentage of cures. The drug eliminates not only the intestinal amebae but also any extraintestinal foci of infection.

While such therapy is undeniably effective, there are those who believe that emetine should be used for the rapid relief of symptoms in severely ill patients. In this situation it is injected daily for not more than 10 days, and the total daily dose should not exceed 60 mg. As a rule, symptoms subside within 4 to 6 days and the stools become formed. Emetine is discontinued as soon as the acute symptoms are under control, and either metronidazole or a specific intestinal amebicide is substituted.

As an alternative to metronidazole, concurrent drug therapy may often be employed to advantage in patients with acute amebic dysentery, as well as in those with latent intestinal amebiasis with or without symptoms. Such therapy may hasten cure and reduce the percentage of failures and relapses. For example, emetine and tetracycline have been employed concurrently and then followed with a course of treatment with an intestinal amebicide. Although emetine will most likely have destroyed any amebae reaching the liver, a course of treatment with chloroquine may be advisable to conclude therapy. Dehydroemetine has replaced emetine in some medical centers.

Symptoms and signs suggestive of acute appendicitis may be simulated by acute cecal amebiasis; this complication calls for immediate treatment with emetine, which, as a rule, affords prompt relief. Surgical intervention may cause serious or fatal complications, especially in patients with acute amebic dysentery.

Treatment of Chronic Amebic Dysentery. Patients with acute exacerbations of chronic, long-standing amebic dysentery should be put to bed and managed as outlined for the acute initial attack. If the symptoms are mild or if the disease is in a relatively quiescent stage, the patient may remain ambulatory and should be treated as described for asymptomatic passers of cysts or for those with mild amebic enteritis. Treatment with specific amebicidal agents should not be instituted unless it is established by proper stool examinations that the symptoms are due to infection by *E. histolytica*. Patients who have had amebic dysentery for several years and who eventually have been cured may continue to experience attacks of diarrhea because of altered bowel function and extensive scarring from previous intestinal ulceration. Diarrhea may be noted, especially when the fluid intake is large or after dietary indiscretions. The history of such individuals often reveals that they have received repeated courses of antiamebic therapy, usually with emetine. On the basis of the diarrhea and the history of previous amebic infection, the erroneous diagnosis of recrudescence of infection is made. After repeated stool examinations have failed to reveal pathogenic amebae, the patient should be informed that he is no longer infected but that he may periodically experience episodes of noninfectious diarrhea that do not require amebicidal therapy.

Treatment of Amebic Hepatitis and Abscess. Amebic hepatitis and amebic abscess of the liver and other organs are always secondary to intestinal infection with *E. histolytica*, even though symptoms of intestinal amebiasis may never have been experienced by the patient. Abscesses may occur in asymptomatic passers of cysts. Only motile forms of amebae are found in abscesses.

As in the treatment of acute amebic dysentery, metronidazole has become the agent of first choice. A very high incidence of cure is achieved with a course of treatment readily tolerated by the large majority of patients. Treatment with emetine and chloroquine remains the alternative to metronidazole; despite their limitation in the therapy of intestinal amebiasis, they are extremely effective for treating amebic hepatitis or amebic abscess. Emetine followed by, or used concurrently with, chloroquine has been the usual course of treatment. If myocardial damage is present, emetine and dehydroemetine should be avoided, although the use of chloroquine alone carries a greater chance of relapse (Wilmot *et al.*, 1958). Again, many practitioners prefer to use dehydroemetine rather than emetine, believing it to be as effective and less liable to induce troublesome side effects.

Early recognition of amebic hepatitis and initiation of appropriate treatment may prevent abscess formation. Even if the disease has progressed to the state of frank abscess formation, surgery can often be avoided if chemotherapy is instituted in its early stages. Usually, symptoms and signs of amebic hepatitis are relieved within a week; if not, suppuration has probably occurred. The factors concerned in the choice between medical and surgical measures in the treatment of amebic abscesses cannot be given in detail here. Some authorities claim that intensive medical therapy may completely resolve abscesses of the liver, at times even when these are fluctuating or actually bulging. If striking improvement is not noted after a full course of metronidazole, chloroquine, or emetine with adjuvant agents, surgical intervention is usually indicated. Evidence of perforation ordinarily calls for surgery. Puncture or aspiration of an abscess should not be undertaken unless specific amebicidal agents have been administered for at least 3 days. However, if the size or the location of the abscess suggests imminent rupture, aspiration is done promptly and chemotherapy is started simultaneously. Open drainage is usually avoided. Amebic abscess of the lung or brain is treated in the same manner as hepatic abscess. Surgical measures are usually indicated when an amebic brain abscess is present.

If the patient has been treated with metronidazole and cured of amebic hepatitis or amebic abscess, he will have been cured simultaneously of his intestinal infection. If an alternative course of treatment has been used, attention must be then given to eradicating the infection of the colon with an intestinal amebicide.

METRONIDAZOLE

Probably the most significant advance in the treatment of protozoal infection has been the introduction and successful use of *metronidazole* as an amebicide. Metronidazole was first introduced as a systemic trichomonacidal agent, effective when given orally in both male and female patients. The background of its development, its chemistry and pharmacology, and its place in venereology are described in Chapter 54. The drug is exceedingly active against *E. histolytica.* In culture, the morphology of the microorganisms is altered markedly within 6 to 20 hours by concentrations of 1 to 2 μg/ml of metronidazole. Within 24 hours all microorganisms are

killed. At a concentration of 0.2 μg/ml, the same effect is seen within 72 hours (Gordeeva, 1965). The significance of the advance lies in the usefulness of the drug in the treatment of all forms of amebiasis. The other agents described in this chapter are useful primarily in only one form of the disease, whether it be in the asymptomatic luminal stage, the intestinal invasive stage, or the extraintestinal stage.

The concept of an all-embracing amebicide was first realized in the clinical trial of a somewhat related compound, *niridazole* (Powell *et al.*, 1966b). This drug was found to be effective in the treatment of both amebic liver abscess and amebic dysentery. Unfortunately its side effects were intolerable in the treatment of a disease for which safer drugs already existed. In the same year, Powell and coworkers used metronidazole to treat both forms of invasive amebiasis and found it to be effective. Since then the results of several clinical trials have been published (*see* Powell, 1971). Its acceptance into North American practice as a drug of choice in the treatment of all forms of amebiasis followed confirmation of these initial successes. Since then, various dosage schedules have been investigated, and the trend has been to establish a single schedule of treatment that is adequate for all forms of the disease.

Preparations. Available preparations of metronidazole are described in Chapter 54.

Therapeutic Use. In all geographical areas, regardless of the virulence of the strains, it is recommended that patients with *invasive intestinal infection* be treated with 750 mg of metronidazole, three times daily for 5 to 10 days. The daily dose for children is 35 to 50 mg/kg, given in three equal doses. In areas where the disease is usually less invasive, a smaller daily dose has yielded good results. Nevertheless, for a consistently high rate of parasitological cure, the larger dose is recommended. *Amebic hepatic abscess* also responds to smaller dosage, and any regimen effective in the treatment of amebic dysentery will also cure a concomitant hepatic infection. However, to ensure elimination of the intestinal amebae the above dosage is preferred. Despite the effectiveness of treatment, the need for aspiration in certain cases of hepatic abscess should not be forgotten. There is less unanimity of opinion regarding the treatment of the *asymptomatic* passer of cysts. While metronidazole has proven effective in a large number of cases, it is generally felt that its use incurs more treatment failures than result from the use of purely luminal amebicides; the latter are thus preferred. Despite considerable clinical use over the last several years, resistance of *E. histolytica* to metronidazole has not occurred. Indeed, attempts to produce resistance to the drug *in vitro* have been unsuccessful. *Mass treatment* with a large dose once monthly for a few months and then on alternate months has resulted in a marked decrease in the incidence of amebic dysentery in relatively isolated communities with a high degree of endemicity.

Metronidazole also kills *Giardia lamblia* and, in a dosage of 250 mg three times daily for 10 days, may be considered for treating lambliasis. Such use is considered investigational in North America.

In the relatively large doses used in treating amebiasis, nausea, headache, dry mouth, and metallic taste are frequently encountered but rarely necessitate interruption of treatment. Occasionally, stomatitis, vomiting, diarrhea, dizziness, transient ataxia, confusion, insomnia, paresthesia, and rash are encountered. Patients should be advised to abstain from alcoholic beverages, because metronidazole possesses a disulfiram-like property.

8-HYDROXYQUINOLINES

A number of halogenated 8-hydroxyquinolines have been synthesized and utilized clinically for their amebicidal action. Two such compounds most frequently encountered and official in the United States, *diiodohydroxyquin* and *iodochlorhydroxyquin,* are described here. Other derivatives available in various parts of the world include *broxyquinoline* (5,7-dibromo-8-quinolinol), *chlorquinaldol* (5,7-dichloro-2-methyl-8-quinolinol), and *chiniofon* (8-hydroxy-7-iodo-5-quinolinesulfonic acid).

These agents are directly amebicidal, but the mechanism of this action is unknown. Drugs of this group are ineffective against amebic abscess and hepatitis and apparently act only on microorganisms in the intestinal tract. It is difficult to rank the halogenated 8-hydroxyquinoline amebicides in any order of superiority; authorities differ in their preferences, and each agent has its advocates.

Chemistry. Diiodohydroxyquin and iodochlorhydroxyquin are both dihalogenated derivatives of 8-hydroxyquinoline (8-quinolinol). Their structural formulas are as follows:

Diiodohydroxyquin (X = Y = I)
Iodochlorhydroxyquin (X = I; Y = Cl)

Both compounds are tasteless, brownish-yellow powders that are nearly insoluble in water.

Pharmacological Effects. As mentioned, the 8-hydroxyquinolines are directly amebi-

cidal. They are active against both motile and cystic forms, but their efficacy in eliminating cysts is probably based on their ability to destroy trophozoites. They act only on amebae in the intestinal tract and are ineffective in amebic abscess and hepatitis. While these drugs are effective in the cyst-passing patient, they are much less effective in the treatment of acute amebic dysentery.

Absorption, Fate, and Excretion. After oral administration, a variable but significant portion of the ingested dose is absorbed. In man, up to one fourth of an administered dose of iodochlorhydroxyquin can be recovered in the urine, largely in the form of the glucuronide. The ethereal sulfate is also formed. Berggren and Hansson (1968) compared the gastrointestinal absorption of diiodohydroxyquin with that of iodochlorhydroxyquin and other halogenated 8-hydroxyquinolines. Diiodohydroxyquin was the least well absorbed—only one third as much as iodochlorhydroxyquin. The bulk of these drugs is passed in the feces. However, it is not known if they are effective in intestinal amebiasis solely by virtue of their presence in the lumen of the bowel or also in part by their presence in the circulation.

After a single oral dose of 250 mg, the maximal concentration of iodochlorhydroxyquin in the plasma averages 5 μg/ml within 4 to 8 hours. The half-life of the drug is 11 to 14 hours, and, after repeated, thrice-daily administration in man, a steady-state plasma concentration is reached within a few days (Jack and Riess, 1973).

Preparations. *Diiodohydroxyquin,* U.S.P. (DIODOQUIN, YODOXIN), is available as tablets containing 210 or 650 mg of the drug.

Iodochlorhydroxyquin, N.F. (VIOFORM), is available in several official preparations: as a cream (3% in water-washable base), an ointment (3% in petrolatum base), suppositories (containing 250 mg), a powder, and enteric-coated tablets (containing 250 mg each).

Route of Administration and Dosage. In intestinal amebiasis, the dose of diiodohydroxyquin for adults is 650 mg, three times daily for 20 days. Children should receive a fraction of the adult dosage, depending on age and weight up to 10 years of age; older children should be given the full adult dosage. The initial course should not be repeated without an intervening rest period of 2 to 3 weeks. A daily dose of 650 mg may be adequate in asymptomatic carriers. In the treatment of symptomatic intestinal amebiasis, it is common practice to administer diiodohydroxyquin either concurrently with another effective intestinal amebicide or to give the two drugs in alternating courses.

Iodochlorhydroxyquin is given for amebiasis in the form of oral tablets; a course consists of 500 to 750 mg, three times a day for 10 days. This regimen is repeated after an 8-day rest period. Iodochlorhydroxyquin may be given with another effective intestinal amebicide, or the two drugs may be used in alternating courses. Iodochlorhydroxyquin retention enemas have been employed with considerable success, and rectal irritation does not occur; 2 g of iodochlorhydroxyquin powder in a 1% suspension in water (200 ml) may be instilled on alternate nights for five doses.

Toxicity and Side Effects. While these compounds were thought to have a low order of toxicity and have been widely sold and used for such nonspecific entities as "traveler's diarrhea," such use is apparently associated with significant risk. The most important toxic reaction, ascribed particularly to iodochlorhydroxyquin, is a *subacute myelo-optic neuropathy,* the incidence of which has had a peculiar geographic distribution. The disease is a myelitis-like illness that was first described in Japan, to whose inhabitants it is largely confined; only sporadic cases have been diagnosed elsewhere. As the number of cases increased, a special research council was formed in Japan to investigate the matter. In its findings iodochlorhydroxyquin was implicated as an important etiological factor. This resulted in cessation of sale of the drug in Japan in 1970, and restrictions were imposed on its sale and use in some other countries, including the United States. While there has been considerable controversy over the role of the drug in the etiology of the disease, its discontinuation in Japan led to an immediate and dramatic reduction in the appearance of cases of the syndrome (*see* Oakley, 1973). It seems possible that the epidemic resulted from an interplay between iodochlorhydroxyquin and environmental factors. These may include chemical pollutants, nutritional deficiencies or abnormalities, and infectious agents (Kono, 1971; Cavanaugh, 1973; Zbinden, 1973). The disease is usually preceded by abdominal pain and persistent diarrhea, and it proceeds to bilateral sensory disturbances—paresthesias and dysesthesias, preferentially in the distal parts of the lower limbs. Other frequent symptoms are deep sensory disturbances, muscle weakness in the legs, pyramidal signs, and slight involvement of the upper limbs. Less common are blurred vision and blindness, disturbances of the autonomic nervous system, psychological changes, and greenish discoloration of the tongue.

While subacute myelo-optic neuropathy was epidemic only in Japan and was apparently caused by the administration of iodochlorhydroxyquin, similar toxic effects also have been observed with other 8-hydroxyquinolines in other countries (*see* Oakley, 1973). While the precise relationship is uncertain, administration of diiodohydroxyquin to children for chronic diarrhea has been associated with optic atrophy and permanent loss of vision (*see* Medical Letter, 1974).

Other side effects observed with 8-hydroxyquinolines include severe generalized furunculosis (iodine toxicoderma), chills, fever, mild-to-severe dermatitis, anal irritation and itching, transitory abdominal discomfort, diarrhea, and headache. These drugs are contraindicated in patients with hepatic damage or iodine intolerance. Thyroid enlargement has occasionally been noted, and these agents interfere with certain thyroid function tests for months because of their content of iodine.

Therapeutic Uses. The 8-hydroxyquinolines are effective for *intestinal amebiasis* and are recommended for treatment of asymptomatic passers of cysts. The drugs are useful for ambulatory and mass treatment. They are inexpensive.

The use of these agents to treat "traveler's diarrhea" and chronic nonspecific diarrhea in children cannot be condoned, since such conditions are self-limited and any possible therapeutic benefit does not justify the risk of serious neurotoxicity.

Diiodohydroxyquin has been reported of value in cases of *lambliasis* resistant to quinacrine therapy, in *balantidial dysentery,* and in intestinal infections due to *Dientamoeba fragilis.* Such therapy is regarded as investigational in the United States. Both diiodohydroxyquin and iodochlorhydroxyquin have been used for the treatment of various dermatological disorders, and large doses have been employed orally in the treatment of *acrodermatitis enteropathica,* a rare, potentially fatal pediatric condition (Deffner and Perry, 1973).

IPECAC

Ipecac (ipecacuanha, "Brazil root") was long used by the natives of Brazil in the treatment of diarrheas. It was sold as a secret remedy to the French government in 1658, and its use in dysenteries rapidly spread throughout Europe and India. Its employment was entirely empirical until 1912, when Vedder demonstrated the *in-vitro* efficacy of emetine against *E. histolytica* and suggested that ipecac be used in amebic infections. The source of ipecac is the dried root or rhizome of *Cephaëlis ipecacuanha* or *acuminata,* plants native to Brazil and Central America but also cultivated in India and Malaysia.

Active Principles. The efficacy of ipecac in amebic infections depends upon its content of alkaloids, the principal ones being emetine and cephaëline. Both are amebicidal, but emetine is much more active. Cephaëline is more toxic than emetine, except for the heart, and causes more nausea and vomiting. Emetine constitutes more than one half of the total alkaloidal content of ipecac.

Status and Use. *Ipecac* is official in the U.S.P. in powder form and as a syrup. It is not used in the modern therapy of amebiasis because its administration results in severe gastrointestinal irritation, nausea, and vomiting.

Use as Emetic. Ipecac probably acts both centrally and locally in the enteric tract to cause vomiting. The drug is rather slow in its emetic action, which requires 15 to 30 minutes to become evident. *Ipecac Syrup,* U.S.P., is often used to induce vomiting in cases of poisoning by orally ingested drugs and other chemicals. The dose is 15 to 20 ml, for children and adults alike. This may be repeated after 20 to 30 minutes, if vomiting has not occurred. If the patient still does not vomit, the dosage should be recovered by gastric lavage.

EMETINE

History. The rational use of emetine as an amebicide dates from 1912, when Vedder showed that the drug killed amebae *in vitro;* since then emetine has been one of the most widely used agents in the treatment of both *intestinal* and *extraintestinal* amebiasis. Much of the early work has been reviewed by Craig (1944).

Chemistry and Preparations. *Emetine Hydrochloride,* U.S.P., is a hydrated hydrochloride of an alkaloid obtained from ipecac or prepared synthetically by methylation of cephaëline. Emetine has the following structural formula:

Emetine

Emetine hydrochloride is a white crystalline powder; it is freely soluble in water and alcohol. The drug is very irritating and should not be allowed to come in contact with the cornea or with mucous

membranes, especially of the conjunctiva. It is available in solution in ampuls for parenteral use (20, 30, and 60 mg/ml).

The *structure-activity relationship* in several chemical series allied to emetine has been explored (*see* Woolfe, 1963). However, none of the many congeneric compounds tested by both *in-vitro* and *in-vivo* methods approaches emetine in amebicidal activity.

PHARMACOLOGICAL PROPERTIES

Mechanism of Amebicidal Action. Emetine has a direct lethal action on *E. histolytica.* The drug is much more effective against motile forms than against cysts. *In vitro,* emetine readily kills trophozoites at concentrations that are found in the systemic circulation after therapeutic doses. These values may not be attained in the lumen of the intestine, the site of the *minuta* cycle that is responsible for cyst formation and possibly recrudescence and relapse. Emetine causes degeneration of the nucleus and reticulation of the cytoplasm of amebae; it is thought to eradicate the parasites by interfering with the multiplication of trophozoites.

In experiments elegant in their conception and execution, Grollman (1966) studied the structural basis for the emetine-induced inhibition of protein synthesis in certain mammalian and other cells. He demonstrated the configurational and conformational similarities of (−)-emetine to (−)-cycloheximide and other glutarimide antibiotics, findings that provide the basis for new synthetic approaches to potentially superior chemotherapeutic agents. Later work showed that emetine prevented protein synthesis by inhibiting the translocation of peptidyl-tRNA from the acceptor site to the donor site on the ribosome (Huang and Grollman, 1970).

Local Reactions. A *local reaction* to emetine is very common. It is characterized by aching, tenderness, stiffness, and weakness of the muscles in the area of the injection site, and occurs even after subcutaneous injection. Evidence of local inflammation is lacking, and the reaction is believed to represent a regional myositis. Local eczematous lesions may result from subcutaneous injection of the drug; generalized urticarial and purpuric skin lesions also have been observed. Oral administration results in local irritation of the digestive tract; even when enteric-coated tablets are employed, distressing gastrointestinal symptoms occur. This precludes oral administration.

Systemic Effects. These are essentially *toxic* in nature. *Systemic reactions* involve chiefly the gastrointestinal, skeletal muscular, and cardiovascular systems. Usually more than one system is involved.

Gastrointestinal Effects. These manifestations of emetine toxicity include diarrhea, nausea, and vomiting. Diarrhea may be induced or aggravated in approximately 50% of patients; it is often associated with cramping abdominal pain and, rarely, with blood, mucus, or pus. It may cause marked prostration. The diarrhea is due to increased peristalsis caused by the direct action of emetine on the intestinal musculature. Emetine-induced diarrhea may be mistaken for an exacerbation of the amebic dysentery, from which it can usually be differentiated by the fact that a period of improvement initiated by emetine often precedes the diarrhea. Nausea occurs in approximately one third of patients receiving emetine and may be associated with vomiting; both are probably central in origin when the drug is administered parenterally. Dizziness and faintness often occur, especially in association with the nausea and vomiting. Headache may also be experienced. Gastrointestinal symptoms may disappear despite continued emetine therapy, but occasionally they are so severe that the drug must be discontinued.

Neuromuscular Effects. Neuromuscular manifestations consist in weakness, aching, tenderness, and stiffness of skeletal muscles, especially those of the neck and the extremities. The accompanying fatigability and listlessness are largely subjective. Edema may also occur, perhaps secondary to the muscle injury or inactivity. Mild sensory disturbances and tremor may be observed, but the usual signs of neuritis are absent. Ng (1966) has observed a blocking action of emetine on the neuromuscular junction, which may account for some of the clinical findings. Weakness and muscular pain tend to persist until the drug administration is stopped; they usually appear before more serious symptoms develop and thus serve as a guide for avoiding overdosage.

Cardiovascular System. The most important toxic effects of emetine relate to the cardiovascular system, and include hypotension, precordial pain, tachycardia, dyspnea, and ECG abnormalities; the last two disturbances tend to persist until medication is discontinued, but the others may disappear despite continued emetine therapy. The incidence of cardiovascular involvement varies in different series, and some degree of toxicity may occur in the great majority of patients. Frequently, multiple symptoms are experienced. *Hypotension* is rarely marked. Its cause is unknown, but it is probably unrelated to the direct depressant action of emetine on the myocardium. *Precordial pain* caused by emetine may resemble that of coronary thrombosis, from which it requires differentiation; its cause is unknown, but it is probably not due to any coronary vasoconstrictor action of the drug. *Tachycardia* may occur, especially if the patient is permitted to be ambulatory. It may be due to a direct action of the drug on the S-A node. Tachycardia frequently precedes the appearance of ECG abnormalities, and emetine should be discontinued as soon as it is evident. *Dyspnea* is experienced by some patients, but in most cases it is probably not cardiac in origin. It may be related to the generalized weakness and tends to persist until the drug is stopped.

ECG changes induced by emetine may occur in from 25 to 50% or more of patients. The direct toxic effect of emetine on cardiac muscle has been repeatedly demonstrated in animals and man, and cardiac dilatation, failure, and death have been reported; the ECG affords a sensitive and early index of such toxicity. The major changes from therapeutic doses are flattening and inversion of the T waves in all leads, and prolongation of the Q-T interval (*see* Kent and Kingsland, 1950; Powell, 1967); changes in rhythm are unusual. ECG alterations tend to persist even after emetine is discontinued, in some cases for 2 months or more. In other patients, ECG abnormalities may not appear until the usual course of emetine is completed. Obviously, emetine medication should be stopped as soon as significant ECG changes are evident.

Inasmuch as it is essential to prevent cardiac damage, certain *precautions* must be observed. The patient should be at absolute bed rest during emetine therapy and for several days thereafter. It is probably wise also to recommend that the patient should remain sedentary for several weeks after the drug is given. The patient must be carefully examined each day and questioned concerning his symptoms. The ECG must obviously be monitored. Even in the absence of ECG changes, the drug should be stopped upon the appearance of tachycardia, neuromuscular symptoms, marked gastrointestinal effects, or considerable weakness. From 6 weeks to 2 months should intervene between courses of emetine. In patients with organic heart disease, emetine should not be used unless it is absolutely necessary, as in cases of amebic hepatitis or abscess not controlled by metronidazole or chloroquine. Such forms of amebiasis constitute a greater threat to life than does the potential toxicity of emetine, and with suitable precautions the drug may be employed without undue risk of further cardiac damage.

Absorption, Fate, and Excretion. Emetine is absorbed from parenteral sites of administration and is excreted or detoxicated slowly. The main channel of excretion is the kidney. Although it appears in the urine 20 to 40 minutes after injection, emetine can still be found there 40 to 60 days after treatment has been discontinued. Therefore, cumulative toxic action is an ever-present danger. The highest concentration of the alkaloid is found in the liver, a fact that may account for the greater efficacy of emetine in hepatic than in intestinal amebiasis; appreciable amounts are also found in the lung, kidney, and spleen.

Routes of Administration and Dosages. The preferred routes of emetine administration are by deep subcutaneous or intramuscular injection. The intravenous use of emetine is contraindicated because it is dangerous and offers no therapeutic advantages. The dose of emetine hydrochloride for adults should not exceed 60 mg per day. This amount can be given in a single injection or in 30-mg portions, morning and evening. A course of emetine therapy should not be continued for more than 10 days, and the total dose should not exceed 600 mg. When the patient is underweight or very debilitated, 30 mg should be used instead of the full 60 mg. Children should receive not more than 1.0 mg/kg daily in two divided doses and not over 10 mg/kg in each course. A course of emetine should not be repeated until a rest period of at least 6 weeks has intervened.

Toxicity and Side Effects. Many of the details of emetine toxicity are presented above. Emetine causes a variety of toxic manifestations that may occur with any dose level, depending on individual susceptibility to the drug. In both animals and man, large doses produce acute lesions in the heart, liver, kidney, intestinal tract, and skeletal muscles. Most of the untoward effects observed disappear despite continuation of emetine therapy; this suggests that some degree of tolerance may be acquired. Other toxic effects of the alkaloid, particularly myocardial, are serious and may result in death or prolonged disability. The drug should not be employed unless its potentialities for poisoning are appreciated and unless the patient can be kept under strict medical observation. By paying strict attention to dosage and following the recommendations outlined above, the possibility of cardiac damage can be minimized (*see* Welchman, 1957). Although most deaths from emetine have been in patients given total doses over 1.25 g, several fatalities have occurred from an amount not exceeding the established total dose of 0.6 g (Heilig and Visveswar, 1943). The long persistence of the alkaloid in the body is the basis for cumulative toxicity, and repeated courses of emetine without adequate rest periods frequently result in serious intoxication. The nature, incidence, and mechanisms of the untoward reactions to emetine have been critically reviewed by Klatskin and Friedman (1948).

Precautions and Contraindications. The various precautions to be observed in the use of emetine are presented above. Emetine should not be used if organic disease of the heart or kidneys is present except in patients with amebic abscess or hepatitis, in whom the probable benefits may outweigh the possible hazards. The drug must be employed with considerable caution in aged or debilitated individuals. It is also contraindicated in children unless there is severe dysentery that has failed to respond to other measures. Emetine is best not employed during pregnancy.

Therapeutic Uses. The main use of emetine is for the treatment of *amebiasis;* the alkaloid has also been employed successfully in the treatment of *balantidiasis* (Aréan and Koppisch, 1956), although the preferred drug for this infection is now oxytetracycline. It may also be used successfully in treating infestations with *Fasciola hepatica*. Emetine alone does not result in the *cure* of amebic infection in more than 10 to 15% of patients. Although clinical symptoms are greatly improved and both motile amebae and cysts disappear from the stools during emetine medication in patients with acute amebic dysentery, cysts reappear in approximately 50% of cases at varying periods after therapy has been discontinued. This fact indicates that trophozoites still exist in the bowel. Further emetine therapy usually does not eliminate the cysts. Such patients often become asymptomatic carriers, with all the attendant dangers to themselves and the general public. Treatment of asymptomatic carriers with emetine is notoriously unsuccessful.

The only valid uses of emetine in *intestinal amebiasis* are for severe cases of amebic diarrhea and acute amebic dysentery, or for acute exacerbations of chronic amebic dysentery. The drug should be given only long enough to control the diarrhea or dysenteric symptoms. It should never be administered in doses larger than 60 mg per day or for periods longer than 10 days. Modern practice is to give emetine daily until the acute symptoms subside, usually in 3 to 4 days. Emetine has great value in the treatment of *amebic abscesses* and *amebic hepatitis*. In such conditions, the alkaloid is often lifesaving and is rivaled in efficacy only by metronidazole and chloroquine.

OTHER EMETINE COMPOUNDS

Dehydroemetine. The synthesis of emetine in 1959 led to the ready availability of various analogs (*see* Whittaker, 1969). Of these, dehydroemetine has been studied extensively both in the laboratory and in clinical trial. These studies suggest that dehydroemetine retains the amebicidal property of the parent compound but is less toxic. The substance is identical to emetine except for the lack of hydrogen atoms at positions 2 and 3.

Dehydroemetine is not marketed in North America, but it can be obtained from the Parasitic Disease Drug Service, Center for Disease Control, Atlanta, Georgia. The drug is available in single-dose, 2-ml ampuls, each containing 60 mg of the dihydrochloride in aqueous solution. In adults, a single 10-day course of dehydroemetine, 80 mg daily, is as effective as 60 mg daily of emetine. However, when used alone, neither drug is adequate in the treatment of hepatic amebiasis, and, when metronidazole cannot be used, either course of treatment combined with adequate dosage of chloroquine is favored by many practitioners. A single 10-day course of dehydroemetine, 120 mg daily, is marginally more effective than 65 mg daily of emetine, but with these dosages ECG changes of similar degree are encountered (Powell *et al.*, 1967). The recommended dosage is a single intramuscular or subcutaneous injection of up to 1.5 mg/kg, given daily for 10 days. The total dose should not exceed 1.0 g. The course of treatment should not be repeated in less than 14 days.

Side effects following the use of dehydroemetine are similar to those following emetine; of these, cardiotoxicity has been studied in some detail. While there is no unanimity of opinion, it appears that myocardial changes associated with the administration of dehydroemetine have been less frequent and less severe and have persisted for a shorter period of time than those following the administration of emetine. Nevertheless, the drug should be used cautiously, if at all, in patients with existing cardiac disease, or with primary muscular or neurological disorders. Cardiovascular function should be adequately monitored. Therapy should not be started earlier than 45 days after a previous course of emetine. Concomitant administration of an intestinal amebicide should be employed to eliminate the source of infection and prevent subsequent relapse.

While dehydroemetine has been utilized in the treatment of schistosomiasis and cutaneous leishmaniasis, its usefulness in these conditions has yet to be established. The drug does appear to be useful for fascioliasis. It can definitely be employed with benefit as an alternative to emetine in the treatment of amebic abscess, amebic hepatitis, severe cases of amebic diarrhea, acute amebic dysentery, or acute exacerbations of chronic amebic dysentery. It has no place in the treatment of asymptomatic or mildly symptomatic cyst passers.

CHLOROQUINE

History. The unique therapeutic value of chloroquine in *extraintestinal amebiasis* in man was first reported by Conan (1948, 1949) and Murgatroyd and Kent (1948). *In-vitro* studies with trophozoites of *E. histolytica* had revealed that chloroquine possesses amebicidal activity greater than that of the halogenated 8-hydroxyquinolines and carbarsone but less than that of emetine. This discovery, combined with the knowledge that chloroquine localizes in the liver in a concentration several hundred times greater than that in the plasma, suggested its use in *hepatic amebiasis.* Clinical trial then revealed that the signs and the symptoms of amebic hepatitis disappeared within a few days after the start of chloroquine therapy and that the disease was adequately controlled and often cured. There then followed a large number of studies that delineated the amebicidal properties of the drug in comparison with other agents *in vitro* and in naturally occurring and experimentally induced amebiasis in a variety of animal species. In addition, numerous clinical reports soon fully substantiated the high efficacy of chloroquine in extraintestinal amebiasis, particularly amebic hepatitis and abscess (*see* Lane, 1951; Sodeman *et al.,* 1951; and others). Wilmot and collaborators (1958) and others suggested, however, that chloroquine was somewhat less effective than emetine. It was also determined that the drug is relatively ineffective in intestinal amebiasis, and that an agent effective against amebae in the intestine should be administered concurrently.

Pharmacological Properties. The pharmacology and the toxicology of chloroquine are fully presented in Chapter 52. Only those features of the drug pertinent to its use in amebiasis are described here.

The *clinical response* to chloroquine in patients with hepatic amebiasis is often as prompt and complete as that to emetine, and the drug has proven effective in some individuals failing to respond to emetine. Chloroquine, like emetine, is not always curative, and, therefore, adjuvant medical and surgical measures may be necessary. There is no evidence that amebae develop resistance to chloroquine. The drug is much less effective in amebiasis of the colon, partly because it attains a much lower concentration in the intestinal wall than in the liver and partly because it is almost completely absorbed from the small bowel. Since colonic infection with *E. histolytica* is always the source of extraintestinal amebiasis, it is also necessary routinely to administer a drug effective in intestinal amebiasis to all patients receiving chloroquine for hepatic amebiasis; such therapy reduces the relapse rate. Conversely, because of the clinical impossibility of determining with certainty whether individuals with colonic amebiasis also have hepatic involvement, it is wise to administer chloroquine routinely when a solely intestinal amebicide

is prescribed. Although few cases of *pulmonary amebic abscess* have been treated with chloroquine, the results indicate that this type of infection also responds well to the drug.

The conventional *course* of chloroquine phosphate for extraintestinal amebiasis in adults is 1 g, daily for 2 days, followed by 500 mg, daily for 2 to 3 weeks. Because of the low toxicity of the drug, this dose schedule can be revised upward if necessary. The course of chloroquine may be repeated. Some authorities consider that chloroquine therapy should immediately follow a course of emetine, while others prefer to give the two drugs concurrently.

ARSENICALS

Formerly widely used for the treatment of amebiasis, arsenical compounds are now rarely employed for this purpose in most parts of the world. The pharmacology of the two phenylarsonic acid derivatives in this category, *carbarsone* and *glycobiarsol,* is presented in previous editions of this textbook.

DILOXANIDE FUROATE

History. *Diloxanide* (ENTAMIDE) was introduced by Bristow and associates (1956) as a result of examining a series of substituted acetanilides for amebicidal activity. Clinical trials showed diloxanide to be effective in cyst-passing patients, but to be relatively ineffective in the treatment of acute intestinal amebiasis. This was attributed to the presence of inadequate concentrations of the drug at the sites of infection. Of the many derivatives prepared in attempts to offset this disadvantage, the furoate ester proved to be appreciably more active than the parent compound in experimentally infected rats (Main *et al.,* 1960). The results of early clinical trials showed it to be effective in cases of acute intestinal amebiasis (Shaldon, 1960; Woodruff and Bell, 1960).

Chemistry and Preparations. *Diloxanide furoate* (FURAMIDE) has the following structural formula:

Diloxanide Furoate

It is a white crystalline powder, almost insoluble in water. The ester is hydrolyzed to diloxanide and furoic acid. It is available in oral tablets containing 500 mg of the drug. Its use is currently considered investigational in the United States.

Pharmacological Effects. Diloxanide is directly amebicidal when tested *in vitro*. The furoate ester is active at 0.01 to 0.1 μg/ml, and it is thus considerably more potent than emetine.

Absorption, Fate, and Excretion. In experimental animals, 60 to 90% of an oral dose of diloxanide furoate is excreted in the urine within 48 hours.

More than half of this appears within 6 hours. Excretion in the feces accounts for 4 to 9% of the dose. Peak concentrations appear in the blood within 1 hour but fall to a fraction of this within 6 hours. Hence, a major part of an oral dose is rapidly absorbed from the gastrointestinal tract and is rapidly excreted in the urine. The ester is largely, if not wholly, hydrolyzed in the lumen or mucosa of the intestine, so that only diloxanide appears in the systemic circulation (Wilmshurst and Cliffe, 1964). The drug appears in the urine largely as the glucuronide.

Route of Administration and Dosage. Diloxanide furoate is given only orally. The dosage used in clinical trials in the treatment of both acute and subacute or chronic intestinal amebiasis has varied from 500 mg, three times daily for 5 days (Haddock and Mgaya, 1961), to 3 g, twice daily for 5 days (Schwartz and Geoffroy, 1962). The most generally used dose has been 500 mg, three times daily for 10 days. If necessary, a second course may be given immediately following the first.

Toxicity and Side Effects. Reports of trials to date remark on the lack of serious side effects following the administration of diloxanide furoate; mild gastrointestinal symptoms have been noted, and in some cases there is increased flatulence.

Therapeutic Uses. Diloxanide furoate is regarded by some authorities as an agent of first choice in the treatment of asymptomatic passers of cysts (administered alone) or in the treatment of invasive and extraintestinal amebiasis (administered with other appropriate drugs) (Powell, 1969). It is ineffective when administered alone in the treatment of extraintestinal amebiasis. There is no unanimity of opinion on its efficacy when used alone in the treatment of acute amebiasis with frank dysentery. While good results have been reported from some areas, other trials have been less successful (see Suchak et al., 1962; Wilmot et al., 1962). In trials carried out primarily on asymptomatic subjects passing trophozoites or cysts, or on patients with nondysenteric, symptomatic intestinal amebiasis, treatment with diloxanide furoate resulted in a high percentage of cures (Woodruff and Bell, 1960; Wolfe, 1973). In all cases the drug was well tolerated and suited the cooperative, ambulatory outpatient. Forsyth (1962) compared the value of several forms of treatment and pointed out that the low cost of the drug might be a major factor in underdeveloped countries.

ANTIBIOTIC AMEBICIDES

A number of antibiotics have been found to be of value in the treatment of intestinal amebiasis, especially *erythromycin, paromomycin,* and some of the *tetracyclines.* Inasmuch as paromomycin is the only one that is directly amebicidal, it is the only one discussed in any detail here. Other antibiotics are not amebicidal directly, but act by interfering with the enteric flora essential for the well-being of pathogenic amebae. The older tetracyclines—

tetracycline itself, chlortetracycline, and oxytetracycline—are the most frequently used, their efficacy probably depending on the relatively large proportion of the administered dose that escapes absorption in the bowel. The better-absorbed agents are much less effective (see Chapter 59). If a tetracycline is used, it is recommended that it be administered together with the appropriate drugs for either intestinal or extraintestinal amebic infections.

Paromomycin. This aminoglycoside antibiotic, isolated from cultures of *Streptomyces rimosus,* is amebicidal both *in vitro* and *in vivo.* It acts directly on amebae but is also antibacterial to normal and pathogenic microorganisms in the gastrointestinal tract. Its structural formula is as follows:

Paromomycin

Paromomycin Sulfate, N.F. (HUMATIN), is supplied in capsules, each containing 250 mg of the base, and in a syrup (125 mg/5 ml). The recommended dosage is 25 mg/kg each day, orally in divided doses at mealtimes, for 5 days. Higher doses, up to 66 mg/kg, have been used by some investigators. After oral administration, little of the drug is absorbed into the systemic circulation. Side effects are mainly limited to gastrointestinal upset and diarrhea occurring during the course of therapy. Marked renal damage occurs in animals treated parenterally with the drug. A number of clinical trials have been carried out since the introduction of the drug (see review by Woolfe, 1965). Experience has shown paromomycin to be effective, but by no means infallible, in the treatment of both *acute and chronic intestinal amebiasis;* it is ineffective against extraintestinal forms of the disease. Forsyth (1962), in treating nondysenteric amebiasis in uncooperative patients requiring inpatient treatment, found the drug particularly valuable, because the course of treatment was shorter than that of other amebicides. Paromomycin is also effective in the treatment of *taeniasis.*

Aréan, V. M., and Koppisch, E. Balantidiasis, a review and report of cases. *Am. J. Path.,* **1956,** *32,* 1089–1115.

Berggren, L., and Hansson, O. Absorption of intestinal antiseptics derived from 8-hydroxyquinolines. *Clin. Pharmac. Ther.,* **1968,** *9,* 67–70.

Bristow, N. W.; Oxley, P.; Williams, G. A. H.; and Woolfe, G. ENTAMIDE, a new amoebicide; preliminary note. *Trans. R. Soc. trop. Med. Hyg.,* **1956,** *50,* 182.

Conan, N. J., Jr. Chloroquine in amebiasis. *Am. J. trop. Med.,* **1948,** *28,* 107–110.

———. The treatment of hepatic amebiasis with chloroquine. *Am. J. Med.,* **1949,** *6,* 309–320.

Deffner, N. F., and Perry, H. O. Acrodermatitis enteropathica and failure to thrive. *Archs Derm.,* **1973,** *108,* 658–662.

Duma, R. J.; Rosenblum, W. I.; McGehee, R. F.; Jones, M. M.; and Nelson, E. C.   Primary amoebic meningo-encephalitis caused by *Naegleria. Ann. intern. Med.,* **1971,** *74,* 923–931.

Elsdon-Dew, R.   The epidemiology of amoebiasis. *Adv. Parasit.,* **1968,** *6,* 1–62.

Forsyth, D. M.   The treatment of amoebiasis: a field study of various methods. *Trans. R. Soc. trop. Med. Hyg.,* **1962,** *56,* 400–403.

Gordeeva, L. M.   [A study of the effect of FLAGYL upon *Entamoeba histolytica* in culture.] *Medskaya Parazit.,* **1965,** *34,* 325–329. (In, *Trop. Dis. Bull.,* **1965,** *62,* 1115.)

Grollman, A. P.   Structural basis for inhibition of protein synthesis by emetine and cycloheximide based on an analogy between ipecac alkaloids and glutarimide antibiotics. *Proc. natn. Acad. Sci. U.S.A.,* **1966,** *56,* 1867–1874.

Haddock, D. R. W., and Mgaya, J. K. N.   The treatment of acute amoebic dysentery with ENTAMIDE FUROATE. *E. Afr. med. J.,* **1961,** *38,* 374–378.

Heilig, R., and Visveswar, S. K.   On the cardiac effects of emetine. *Indian med. Gaz.,* **1943,** *78,* 419–424.

Huang, T., and Grollman, A. P.   Novel inhibitors of protein synthesis in animal cells. *Fedn Proc. Fedn Am. Socs exp. Biol.,* **1970,** *29,* 609.

Jack, D. B., and Riess, W.   Pharmacokinetics of iodochlorhydroxyquin in man. *J. pharm. Sci.,* **1973,** *62,* 1929–1932.

Kent, L., and Kingsland, R. C.   Effects of emetine hydrochloride on the electrocardiogram in man. *Am. Heart J.,* **1950,** *39,* 576–587.

Klatskin, G., and Friedman, H.   Emetine toxicity in man: studies on the nature of early toxic manifestations, their relation to the dose level, and their significance in determining safe dosage. *Ann. intern. Med.,* **1948,** *28,* 892–915.

Lane, R.   The treatment of hepatic amoebiasis with chloroquine. *J. trop. Med. Hyg.,* **1951,** *54,* 198–206.

Main, P. T.; Bristow, N. W.; Oxley, P.; Watkins, T. I.; Williams, G. A. H.; Wilmshurst, E. C.; and Woolfe, G. ENTAMIDE. *Ann. Biochem. exp. Med.,* **1960,** *20,* 441–448.

Medical Letter.   Warning on diiodohydroxyquin. **1974,** *16,* 71–72.

Murgatroyd, F., and Kent, R. P.   Refractory amoebic liver abscess treated by chloroquine. *Trans. R. Soc. trop. Med. Hyg.,* **1948,** *42,* 15–16.

Ng, K. K. F.   Blockade of adrenergic and cholinergic transmissions by emetine. *Br. J. Pharmac. Chemother.,* **1966,** *28,* 228–237.

Oakley, G. P., Jr.   The neurotoxicity of the halogenated hydroxyquinolines. *J. Am. med. Ass.,* **1973,** *225,* 395–397.

Powell, S. J.   The cardiotoxicity of systemic amebicides: a comparative electrocardiographic study. *Am. J. trop. Med. Hyg.,* **1967,** *16,* 447–450.

Powell, S. J.; MacLeod, I.; Wilmot, A. J.; and Elsdon-Dew, R.   Metronidazole in amoebic dysentery and amoebic liver abscess. *Lancet,* **1966a,** *2,* 1329–1331.

————.   AMBILHAR in amoebic dysentery and amoebic liver abscess. *Ibid.,* **1966b,** *2,* 20–22.

Powell, S. J.; Wilmot, A. J.; MacLeod, I. N; and Elsdon-Dew, R.   A comparative trial of dehydroemetine hydrochloride in identical dosage in amoebic liver abscess. *Ann. trop. Med. Parasit.,* **1967,** *61,* 26–28.

Schwartz, R., and Geoffroy, H.   [Diloxanides (ENTAMIDE and FURAMIDE).] *Maroc méd.,* **1962,** *41,* 87.

Shaldon, S.   ENTAMIDE FUROATE in the treatment of acute amoebic dysentery. *Trans. R. Soc. trop. Med. Hyg.,* **1960,** *54,* 469–470.

Sodeman, W. A.; Doerner, A. A.; Gordon, E. M.; and Gillikin, C. M.   Chloroquine in hepatic amebiasis. *Ann. intern. Med.,* **1951,** *35,* 331–341.

Suchak, N. G.; Satoskar, R. S.; and Sheth, U. K.   ENTAMIDE FUROATE in the treatment of intestinal amoebiasis. *Am. J. trop. Med. Hyg.,* **1962,** *11,* 330–332.

Vedder, E. B.   An experimental study of the action of ipecacuanha on amoebae. In, *Transactions of the Second Biennial Congress, Far-Eastern Association of Tropical Medicine, 1912, 87.* (Abstracted in, *J. trop. Med. Hyg.,* **1912,** *15,* 313–314.)

Welchman, J. M.   The cardiac toxicity of emetine. *J. trop. Med. Hyg.,* **1957,** *60,* 296–302.

Whittaker, N.   The synthesis of emetine and related compounds. Pt. IX. The use of Wittig-type reagents in the synthesis of 2,3-dehydroemetine. *J. chem. Soc.,* **1969,** *1,* Sect. C, 94–100.

Wilmot, A. J.; Powell, S. J.; and Adams, E. B.   The comparative value of emetine and chloroquine in amebic liver abscess. *Am J. trop. Med. Hyg.,* **1958,** *7,* 197–198.

Wilmot, A. J.; Powell, S. J.; McLeod, I.; and Elsdon-Dew, R.   Some newer amoebicides in acute amoebic dysentery. *Trans. R. Soc. trop. Med. Hyg.,* **1962,** *56,* 85–86.

Wilmshurst, E. C., and Cliffe, E. E.   Absorption and distribution of amoebicides. In, *Absorption and Distribution of Drugs.* (Binns, T. B., ed.) E. & S. Livingstone, Ltd., Edinburgh, **1964,** pp. 191–198.

Wolfe, M. S.   Nondysenteric intestinal amebiasis. Treatment with diloxanide furoate. *J. Am. med. Ass.,* **1973,** *224,* 1601–1604.

Woodruff, A. W., and Bell, S.   Clinical trials with ENTAMIDE FUROATE and related compounds. I. In a non-tropical environment. *Trans. R. Soc. trop. Med. Hyg.,* **1960,** *54,* 389–395.

Monographs and Reviews

Anderson, H. H.   Newer drugs in amebiasis. *Clin. Pharmac. Ther.,* **1960,** *1,* 78–86.

Cavanagh, J. B.   Peripheral neuropathy caused by chemical agents. *CRC Crit. Rev. Toxicol.,* **1973,** *2,* 365–417.

Craig, C. F.   *The Etiology, Diagnosis and Treatment of Amebiasis.* The Williams & Wilkins Co., Baltimore, **1944.**

Kono, R.   Subacute myelo-optico-neuropathy, a new neurological disease prevailing in Japan. *Jap. J. med. Sci. Biol.,* **1971,** *24,* 195–216.

Powell, S. J.   Amebiasis. In, *Current Therapy 1969.* (Conn, H. F., ed.) W. B. Saunders Co., Philadelphia, **1969,** pp. 3–6.

————.   Therapy of amebiasis. *Bull. N.Y. Acad. Med.,* **1971,** *47,* 469–477.

Schneider, J.   Traitement médical de l'amibiase. *Bull. Soc. Path. exot.,* **1961,** *54,* 616–675.

Woolfe, G.   Chemotherapy of amebiasis. In, *Experimental Chemotherapy,* Vol. 1. (Schnitzer, R. J., and Hawking, F., eds.) Academic Press, Inc., New York, **1963,** pp. 355–433.

————.   The chemotherapy of amoebiasis. In, *Progress in Drug Research,* Vol. 8. (Jucker, E., ed.) Birkhäuser Verlag, Basel, **1965,** pp. 11–52.

Zbinden, G.   Geographical toxicology. In, *Progress in Toxicology,* Vol. 1. Springer-Verlag, Berlin, **1973,** pp. 66–71.

54 MISCELLANEOUS DRUGS USED IN THE TREATMENT OF PROTOZOAL INFECTIONS

Ian M. Rollo

SURAMIN

Suramin is one of the few nonmetallic compounds effective in the treatment of *trypanosomiasis.* It was introduced into therapy in 1920 after several years of research in Germany, based on the observed trypanocidal activity of the dyestuffs *trypan red, trypan blue,* and *afridol violet.*

Chemistry and Preparations. *Suramin sodium* (*Bayer 205;* ANTRYPOL, GERMANIN) has the structural formula shown below. It is a white microcrystalline powder, readily soluble in water to yield a neutral solution. Only freshly prepared solutions should be employed. It is marketed in ampuls containing 1.0 g of the drug. Suramin is available in the United States only from the Parasitic Disease Drug Service, Center for Disease Control, Atlanta, Georgia.

Pharmacological Effects. *Trypanocidal Action.* The mechanism of the trypanocidal action of suramin is unknown. The drug inhibits numerous enzyme systems in low concentrations, but trypanocidal activity has not been related to the inhibition of any specific enzyme. Suramin forms firm complexes with protein; this possibly may be related to its chemotherapeutic activity. If trypanosomes are exposed to suramin and then washed, they are no longer infective for animals, although they remain active *in vitro* for over 24 hours. Williamson and Macadam (1965) observed morphological damage in suramin-treated trypanosomes characterized by damage to, or disappearance of, all intracellular membranous structures with the exception of lysosomes. This is remarkable in view of the low concentration of suramin that has been shown to occur in these organelles (*see* Allison, 1968).
Filaricidal Action. Suramin is active against *Onchocerca volvulus.* Its action is primarily against the adult filariae, although the maintenance of high concentrations in the blood is said also to eliminate the microfilariae. It is usually employed following a course of diethylcarbamazine, which is safer and more reliable in its effect on microfilariae (*see* Chapter 51).

Absorption, Fate, and Excretion. Suramin must be administered parenterally. Following its intravenous administration, a high concentration is achieved in the plasma. This falls fairly rapidly for a few hours, then more slowly for a few days, after which a low concentration is maintained for as long as 3 months. The persistence of suramin in the circulation is due to its firm binding to plasma protein. The compound apparently does not enter cells readily since none is present in erythrocytes, and tissue concentrations are uniformly lower than those in the plasma. In experimental animals, however, the kidneys have been found to contain considerably more suramin than other organs. This retention in the kidney may account for the fairly frequent occurrence of albuminuria following injection of the drug in man. Suramin does not penetrate into the cerebrospinal fluid in appreciable amounts. Metabolic destruction of the drug appears to be negligible. The protein-bound suramin dissociates slowly to yield effective concentrations of the drug over long periods of time. Thus, suramin has proven valuable in the *prophylaxis* of trypanosomiasis.

Routes of Administration and Dosage. Suramin is usually given by slow intravenous injection in 10% aqueous solution. Treatment of active *trypanosomiasis* should not be started until 24 hours after diagnostic lumbar puncture, and caution is required if the patient has onchocerciasis. The normal single dose for adults is 1 g. It is advisable to employ a small dose of 200 mg initially to test for sensitivity, after which the normal dose is given on days 1, 3, 7, 14, and 21; weekly doses may be given for an additional 5 weeks. Patients in poor condition should be treated cautiously during the first week. A second

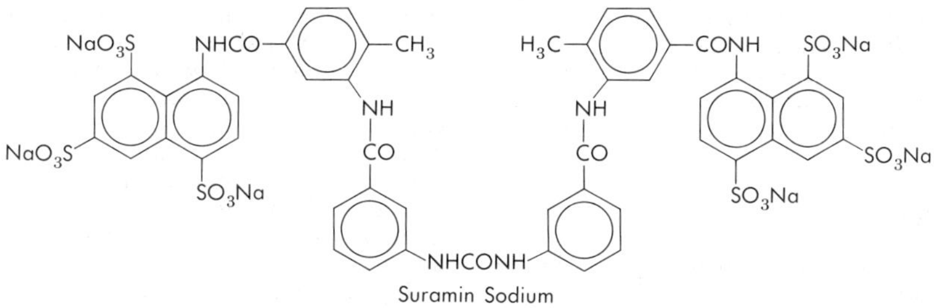

Suramin Sodium

course of treatment should not be given earlier than 3 months after the first. Suramin may be used also as a chemoprophylactic agent. A single dose of 1 g gives protection for about 3 months.

In the treatment of *onchocerciasis,* after initial treatment with diethylcarbamazine, a trial dose of 200 mg should be followed 1 week later by a dose of 1 g; then 1 g is given weekly to a total dose of 4 to 6 g.

Toxicity and Side Effects. Suramin can give rise to a variety of untoward reactions. These vary in intensity and frequency with the nutritional status of the individuals being treated and reach rather serious proportions among the malnourished. The most serious immediate reaction consists in nausea, vomiting, shock, and loss of consciousness. Fortunately, the incidence is low (0.1 to 0.3%). Colic and acute urticaria are other immediate reactions. Later reactions, which occur up to 24 hours after drug administration, are papular eruptions, paresthesia, photophobia, lacrimation, palpebral edema, and hyperesthesia of the palms of the hands and the soles of the feet. Still later reactions consist in albuminuria, hematuria, and cylindruria. Rarely, agranulocytosis or hemolytic anemia may occur.

Precautions and Contraindications. Patients receiving suramin should be followed closely. Therapy should not be continued in patients who show intolerance to initial doses, and the drug should be employed with great caution in individuals with renal insufficiency. A moderate albuminuria is usual during the control of the acute phase, but persisting, heavy albuminuria calls for caution as well as modification of the schedule of treatment. If casts appear, treatment with suramin should be discontinued. The occurrence of palmar-plantar hyperesthesia necessitates caution since it may presage peripheral neuritis.

Therapeutic Uses. Suramin is employed in the treatment of *trypanosomiasis* caused by *T. gambiense* and *T. rhodesiense.* It is of no value in Chagas' disease (*T. cruzi*). When employed alone, the drug is effective only in the early stage of the disease. In the late stage of the disease with central nervous system (CNS) involvement, suramin is commonly used before, or in conjunction with, a course of arsenical therapy because only small amounts of suramin gain access to the cerebrospinal fluid. Suramin is effective in the *prophylaxis* of Rhodesian and Gambian trypanosomiasis. The dose schedule has been outlined. Pentamidine is also useful for this purpose and, indeed, may be a superior agent. Chemoprophylaxis is not recommended for travelers on occasional brief visits to endemic areas since the risk of serious drug toxicity outweighs the risk of acquiring the disease. Suramin is the most effective drug for clearing the adult filariae in *onchocerciasis.* The single dose of 1 g is repeated weekly for 7 to 10 weeks.

PENTAMIDINE

The discovery of chemotherapeutic activity in the diamidine group of drugs, of which pentamidine is a member, was quite fortuitous. It had long been known that cultures of trypanosomes could be maintained only if glucose was present in the medium. Therefore, compounds capable of producing hypoglycemia were tested for trypanocidal activity. One of these, *decamethylenediguanidine* (SYNTHALIN), was highly effective *in vivo.* It was soon learned that the mechanism of trypanocidal action of this drug was entirely unrelated to the production of a hypoglycemic environment, since it was actively trypanocidal *in vitro.* Unfortunately, the compound was much too toxic to be an effective chemotherapeutic agent. (The hypoglycemia produced by decamethylenediguanidine results from a hepatotoxic action.) Therefore, a large number of chemically related compounds were synthesized and screened for protozoicidal action (King *et al.,* 1938). Greatest activity was found among a group of amidines, and it became apparent that the carbon chain served primarily as a carrier for the strongly basic, active amidine groups. Further exploration led to the synthesis of diamidines containing aromatic groups as carriers (Lourie and Yorke, 1939). Of the compounds of this type, three possessed outstanding activity: 4,4'-diamidinostilbene (*stilbamidine*), 4,4'-diamidinophenoxy pentane (*pentamidine*), and 4,4'-diamidinophenoxy propane (*propamidine*). *Pentamidine* is the most valuable because of its stability, low toxicity, and ease of administration. Propamidine is only occasionally used. *Hydroxystilbamidine Isethionate,* U.S.P. (2-hydroxy-4,4'-diamidinostilbene diisethionate), is preferred by some and has proven useful in the treatment of North American blastomycosis (*see* Chapter 61) and visceral leishmaniasis.

Chemistry and Preparations. Pentamidine has the following structural formula:

Pentamidine

Pentamidine isethionate (LOMIDINE), the preparation available commercially, is a white powder, soluble in water to the extent of 10%. It is marketed as a dry powder, in ampuls containing 200 mg of the drug. It is available in the United States only from the Parasitic Disease Drug Service, Center for Disease Control, Atlanta, Georgia.

Pharmacological Effects. *Antiprotozoal Spectrum.* The diamidines are toxic to a number of different protozoa, yet show rather marked selectivity of action. For example, the drugs are curative against *T. rhodesiense* and *T. congolense* infections in experimental animals. However, they are ineffective in curing mice infected with *T. cruzi.* They are also capable of curing *Babesia canis* infections in puppies and *Leishmania donovani* infections in hamsters. These results in animals provide the experimental background for the therapeutic application of diamidines in the treatment of human leishmaniasis and trypanosomiasis.

The diamidines are also fungicidal. This can be

readily demonstrated *in vitro* against *Blastomyces dermatitidis,* and has led to the successful therapeutic trial of the drugs in systemic blastomycosis. The advent of amphotericin B has, however, reduced the value of the diamidines in the treatment of this disease. The antibiotic is to be preferred in initial therapy, but hydroxystilbamidine may prove useful if an inadequate response is obtained. Of particular significance are the excellent results obtained with pentamidine in the treatment of pneumonia caused by *Pneumocystis carinii* (*see* Ivady *et al.,* 1967).

Mechanism of Action. The susceptibility of different species of trypanosomes appears to be related to the relative importance of aerobic and anaerobic glycolysis in their metabolism. However, effects of the drug on mitochondria and on the respiration of intact microorganisms are seen only at very high concentrations of pentamidine (Hill and Hutner, 1968). The basic action of this drug is not known.

Absorption, Fate, and Excretion. Pentamidine isethionate is fairly well absorbed from parenteral sites of administration. Following a single dose, the drug is detectable in the blood for only a very brief period. However, in experimental animals, the liver and the kidney are found to store the drug for months (Launoy *et al.,* 1960). Fixation of pentamidine in tissues seems to be the most important factor in its use as a prophylactic agent in trypanosomiasis.

Routes of Administration and Dosage. Pentamidine is best given by intramuscular injection in individual doses of 4 mg/kg of body weight, daily or on alternate days. The intravenous route may also be used. In the *treatment of early African trypanosomiasis,* a course of ten injections should be given. The drug may be less effective in *T. rhodesiense* infections than in those caused by *T. gambiense.* Because of the rapidity with which *T. rhodesiense* may invade the CNS, treatment with pentamidine is contraindicated unless infection with this species is known with certainty to have occurred within the previous 3 or 4 weeks. Pentamidine has been widely used as a *prophylactic* agent in endemic areas. Single intramuscular injections should be given at intervals of not longer than 6 months; various dosages have been used, but all fall within the range of 3 to 5 mg/kg.

In the treatment of *visceral leishmaniasis (L. donovani* leishmaniasis, or *kala-azar),* pentamidine has been used successfully in courses of 12 to 15 doses. A second course, given after an interval of 1 to 2 weeks, may be necessary in areas where the infection is known to respond less well to treatment. The drug is particularly useful in cases that have failed to respond to antimonials—for example, in the Sudan, where the disease responds only to high doses of antimonials, and in China, where many kala-azar patients are hypersensitive to antimony. Some success has followed the use of pentamidine in the treatment of *cutaneous (L. tropica) leishmaniasis,* or oriental sore (*see* Beveridge, 1963). Hydroxystilbamidine is preferred by some practitioners; the choice probably depends upon the local availability of either compound. Cases of *Pneumocystis carinii pneumonia* should be treated daily with 4 mg/kg intra-muscularly, for 12 to 14 days. In severe cases the drug may be given by slow intravenous injection. If treatment is effective, clinical improvement will occur usually 4 to 6 days after the first injection. A high proportion of cures can be expected, depending on supportive therapy and, if possible, elimination of predisposing conditions. The prognosis is less favorable in debilitated patients with altered immunity or neoplastic disease.

Toxicity and Side Effects. The intravenous injection of pentamidine (and other diamidines) is often followed quickly by alarming reactions, which, fortunately, are not dangerous. They include breathlessness, tachycardia, dizziness or fainting, headache, and vomiting. These reactions are probably connected with the sharp fall in blood pressure that follows too rapid intravenous administration of the drug, and they may be due in part to the release of histamine. Because pentamidine is better tolerated by intramuscular injection and causes little pain, this route is to be preferred. Pentamidine has not been observed to give rise to late neuropathies such as have been reported frequently after courses of stilbamidine. Both hypoglycemia and, paradoxically, hyperglycemia have been reported following administration of pentamidine. Reversible renal dysfunction has been associated with the use of the drug in a small proportion of treated patients (*see* DeVita *et al.,* 1969).

Therapeutic Uses. The diamidines, in particular pentamidine, have three important therapeutic applications. The first is in the treatment of *leishmaniasis.* Although antimonials are generally considered to be the drugs of choice, gratifying results can be obtained with diamidines in cases that fail to respond to antimonial therapy or in patients who cannot tolerate the metal. Pentamidine is given in courses as described above.

Pentamidine is also highly effective in the treatment of *early* cases of Gambian and Rhodesian *trypanosomiasis,* and it has been widely used as a prophylactic against *T. gambiense.* Because the drug does not gain access to the cerebrospinal fluid and cannot be given intrathecally, it should not be employed in the neurological stage of the disease.

Gratifying response may also be obtained in the treatment of *pneumonia* due to *Pneumocystis carinii.* The use of pentamidine in Europe has very markedly reduced mortality in the epidemic form of infection found in debilitated and premature infants. Infected patients suffering from hypogammaglobulinemia or with malignant processes have also been treated successfully.

MELARSOPROL

In 1940, Friedheim described trypanocidal activity in an organic compound of arsenic containing the melamine nucleus. Two compounds made subsequently, the pentavalent melarsen and the trivalent melarsen oxide, were shown to be effective in advanced cases of trypanosomiasis but were considered to be more toxic than tryparsamide. In 1949, Friedheim demonstrated that a dimercaprol derivative of melarsen oxide also could be used effectively and with greater safety in the treatment of such cases; this compound was named *Mel B* and is now known as *melarsoprol*. Of considerable importance was the finding that trypanocidal arsenicals of the melamine type retained their activity against tryparsamide-resistant strains of trypanosomes (VanHoof, 1947; Williamson and Lourie, 1948). On the other hand, Rollo and Williamson (1951) showed that strains made resistant to melarsen were cross-resistant to tryparsamide *and* to the trypanocidal amidines.

Chemistry and Preparations. Melarsoprol has the following structural formula:

Melarsoprol

It is very slightly soluble in water but is readily soluble in propylene glycol. *Melarsoprol (Mel B;* ARSOBAL) is provided as a 3.6% (w/v) sterile solution in propylene glycol. It is available in the United States only from the Parasitic Disease Drug Service, Center for Disease Control, Atlanta, Georgia. The dosage regimens below refer to the 3.6% solution.

Pharmacological Effects. It is surprising perhaps that the combination of arsenic with an antagonist, in this case dimercaprol, should yield an effective drug. Melarsoprol, indeed, retains the high trypanocidal activity of its parent, melarsen oxide, both *in vitro* and *in vivo,* but is less toxic for the host. The mechanism of its trypanocidal action is unknown as yet. The substance either may be dissociated within the microorganism and act as the parent compound, or may act as the intact molecule. Whatever its fate, interaction with SH groups essential for intracellular metabolic processes probably accounts for death of the parasite.

As far as is known, the same mechanism by which melarsoprol is lethal to parasites is concerned in its toxicity to host tissues. However, Flynn and Bowman (1969) have demonstrated that arsenical drugs act differently upon the terminal glycolytic enzyme, pyruvate kinase, depending on whether the source of the enzyme is trypanosomal or mammalian. It is also possible that mammalian tissues oxidize the drug to nontoxic and readily excreted pentavalent compounds more rapidly than does the protozoan. Additionally, melarsoprol may be able to penetrate into the parasite more readily than into mammalian tissue cells. So-called arsenic-resistant parasites may resemble host cells in that they have become less permeable to organic arsenicals (*see* Eagle and Doak, 1951).

The pharmacological effects of melarsoprol in man are regarded as toxic effects, and are discussed below.

Absorption, Fate, and Excretion. Melarsoprol is usually administered intravenously. A small but therapeutically significant amount of the drug penetrates into the cerebrospinal fluid and has a lethal effect on trypanosomes infecting the CNS. The substance is excreted quite quickly, and its prophylactic action lasts no more than a few days (*see* Hawking, 1963).

Route of Administration and Dosages. Melarsoprol is administered by slow intravenous injection of the propylene glycol solution. It should be given through a fine needle, and care must be taken to avoid leakage into surrounding tissues, because it is intensely irritating. Patients with advanced meningoencephalitis, or those who are febrile or wasted, should receive preliminary treatment with suramin (two to four doses of 250 to 500 mg on alternate days). Adults in good condition weighing 50 kg or more and whose cerebrospinal fluid contains less than 40 mg of protein per 100 ml should be given 2 ml on the first day, 2.5 ml on the second, and 3 ml on the third; thereafter, 3.5, 4, and 5 ml on the tenth, eleventh, and twelfth days, respectively, followed by 5 ml on the nineteenth, twentieth, and twenty-first days. For children, underweight patients, and those having excessive amounts of protein in the cerebrospinal fluid, the dosage is based on a similar pattern of increasing doses for 3 days, with weekly intervals between, until a maximal dose of 3.6 mg/kg is attained on the twenty-first day. This dose is repeated on the twenty-eighth, twenty-ninth, and thirtieth days. The initial dose should not be greater than 0.5 ml. Following such regimens, about 80 to 90% of patients are cured. A proportion of those relapsing will be refractory to further treatment with melarsoprol.

Toxicity and Side Effects. Unfortunately, side effects are common during treatment with melarsoprol (*see* Robertson, 1962). Reactive encephalopathy is the most common. The clinical manifestation usually appears after the first 3-day course and then subsides; additional treatment does not produce further deterioration. The administration of dimercaprol produces little benefit, but it is not contraindicated and should perhaps be used if the encephalopathy is severe. The condition may be fatal. Deaths due to this cause, however, have become less frequent with increasing experience in the use of this drug. The reactive encephalopathy occurs more frequently and is more severe in those with pronounced cerebrospinal fluid changes. Hypersensitivity reactions are not common and generally occur during the second or subsequent 3-day course. After recovery, a small dose provokes a lesser reaction, so that desensitization may be carried out by starting with a small dose and increasing this slightly, allowing time for recovery, until it is possible to give a final 3-day course in full dosage. Corticosteroids may be used to control the symptoms during such a procedure. Hemorrhagic encephalopathy is uncommon during treatment, and agranulocytosis is very rare. Occasionally the appearance of numerous casts in the urine or evidence of hepatic disturbance may necessitate modification of treatment. Vomiting and abdominal colic may occur, but their incidence may be reduced by injecting the drug slowly in the supine, fasting patient. The patient should remain in bed and not eat for several hours after the injection is given.

Precautions and Contraindications. Melarsoprol should be given only to patients under hospital supervision so that the dosage regimen may be modified or dimercaprol administered if necessary. It is most important that the initial dosage be based upon clinical assessment of the general condition of the patient, rather than on body weight. It should be recognized that the administration of melarsoprol to leprous patients may precipitate erythema nodosum. The use of the drug is contraindicated during epidemics of influenza.

Therapeutic Uses. Melarsoprol is the drug of choice in the treatment of the meningoencephalitic stage of human trypanosomiasis. It is effective in both Gambian and Rhodesian varieties of the disease. Its great value is in its quick action against both stages of trypanosomiasis, its effectiveness against tryparsamide-resistant strains of trypanosomes, and the absence of ocular toxicity. For these reasons, it has largely superseded tryparsamide. Melarsoprol is extremely effective in the treatment of the hemolymphatic stage of the disease; however, because of its toxicity, it is usually reserved for treatment of the late stage. For this reason also, it has no place in prophylaxis.

Cases of late-stage trypanosomiasis may be encountered that are refractory to treatment with melarsoprol (and hence to treatment with tryparsamide). *Nitrofurazone* may be tried in these difficult cases with some chance of success. A single course of treatment should not exceed 500 mg of the drug at 6-hour intervals for 1 week. Three courses may be given with a week's rest between each. This treatment is unsuitable for febrile or wasted patients. The drug causes severe polyneuropathy and reversible degeneration of the seminiferous tubules. It produces hemolytic anemia in patients with glucose-6-phosphate dehydrogenase deficiency. *Furaltadone* and, presumably, *nifurtimox* may also be used.

MELARSONYL

Melarsonyl (*Mel W;* TRIMELARSAN) is a water-soluble derivative of melarsoprol and may be given intramuscularly. It has been used quite widely in the treatment of human trypanosomiasis, particularly in tropical areas formerly under French influence. Good results have been reported against *T. gambiense* infections. At first the drug seemed to be less toxic than melarsoprol, but this does not seem to have been borne out. Robertson (1963) has reported disappointing results against *T. rhodesiense* infections and has found reactive encephalopathy and relapses to be more common than with melarsoprol. Such relapses were not curable by melarsoprol. Richet (1966) has reviewed the clinical use of melarsonyl.

OTHER ARSENICALS

The introduction of nonarsenical trypanocides and melarsoprol in the treatment of trypanosomiasis has left little place for the use of the older arsenicals. Of these compounds, tryparsamide is still employed in some parts of the world. The many others are described in earlier editions of this textbook.

Tryparsamide. Tryparsamide is a white crystalline powder, containing 25% pentavalent arsenic. It has the following structural formula:

Tryparsamide

Tryparsamide is given *intravenously* in doses of 30 mg/kg in 10 ml of water, at 5- to 7-day intervals for 10 to 12 injections. Children do not tolerate the drug well. A course of treatment may be repeated after an interval of 1 month.

The overall incidence of toxic reactions to tryparsamide is 15% or higher. These also are described in previous editions of this textbook.

Tryparsamide was the mainstay of therapy for *Gambian trypanosomiasis* for several decades. Its trypanocidal activity is only moderate, but its chief value is in its ability to penetrate into the cerebrospinal fluid and hence cure the late stage of the disease. Strains of *T. gambiense* resistant to tryparsamide are not infrequently encountered. Partly for this reason and partly on account of the long duration of treatment and the possibility of causing blindness, it has been largely replaced by melarsoprol. In exceptional cases, such as those with late-stage trypanosomiasis and in very poor general condition, tryparsamide may be given with benefit in a combined course of treatment with either pentamidine or suramin.

SODIUM STIBOGLUCONATE

The history of the development of leishmanicidal antimonial compounds can be divided into three distinct phases. At first, the use of *antimony potassium tartrate (tartar emetic)* in the treatment of trypanosomiasis was followed by its successful use against cutaneous leishmaniasis and, shortly afterward, in cases of kala-azar. Inconvenience in the use of this drug, however, led to the trial of several other trivalent antimonial compounds, notably *antimony sodium tartrate, stibophen,* and *anthiomaline.* These were found to be as effective as and less toxic than tartar emetic. During this period, the successful syntheses of pentavalent antimonial derivatives of phenylstibonic acid were followed by the introduction of a variety of drugs that were as effective as and much less toxic than tartar emetic, thus permitting the use of larger doses and reduction in the period of treatment. Subsequent syntheses reverted to the "tartar-emetic" type of compound in which trivalent antimony was replaced by pentavalent antimony. An early member of this type of compound was *sodium stibogluconate*. This drug is widely used today and, together with *meglumine antimonate* (GLUCANTIME), a compound of the same type that is preferred in territories formerly under French influence, is the mainstay of the treatment of leishmaniasis by antimony. Less widely employed is urea stibamine, one of the phenylstibonic acid derivatives. Because sodium stibogluconate is the most widely used of the antimonial leishmanicides, a brief description of its properties follows. Full details of the investigations on leishmanicides can be found in the reviews of Findlay (1950) and Beveridge (1963).

Chemistry. Sodium stibogluconate probably has the following structural formula:

Sodium Stibogluconate

The precise points of attachment of the antimony, however, are not altogether certain. It is a colorless, amorphous powder, readily soluble in water, and contains 30 to 34% pentavalent antimony.

Pharmacological Effects. Pentavalent antimony compounds such as sodium stibogluconate have little effect on leptomonads growing in tissue culture. Such a marked contrast between *in-vitro* and *in-vivo* activity of these compounds might suggest that reduction of antimony to the trivalent form is necessary for activity. However, the sensitivity of the free, flagellated forms is unlikely to be the same as that of the morphologically different intracellular stage, which cannot be readily cultured. The general pharmacological effects of antimonial compounds are described in Chapter 46.

Preparations. *Sodium stibogluconate (sodium antimony gluconate;* PENTOSTAM, TRIOSTAM) is available in sterile, aqueous solution for parenteral administration. Each milliliter contains 330 mg of the drug, equivalent to 100 mg of pentavalent antimony. It is available in the United States only from the Parasitic Disease Drug Service, Center for Disease Control, Atlanta, Georgia.

Routes of Administration and Dosages. Sodium stibogluconate may be given either intravenously or by the intramuscular route. In cases of *kala-azar,* in which the leishmania are normally sensitive to antimony, the large majority will be cured by a single course of treatment consisting of six daily injections of 6 ml. Against less sensitive strains, three courses, each consisting of ten daily doses of 6 ml intramuscularly and separated by intervals of 10 days, have proven satisfactory. In very debilitated individuals

who appear to react unfavorably to the initial injections, it may be advisable to administer the drug on alternate days or at longer intervals. Reduced dosage is indicated in those who have recently received a course of antimony in another form, and in children. Infants and children, however, tolerate rather larger doses in proportion to body weight than do adults. In the treatment of *Oriental sore,* rapid disappearance of parasites has been reported following an infiltration of the solution around the edges of the lesions. The total volume used should not exceed more than 2 ml at any one time. Otherwise, a single course of treatment as outlined above should prove to be effective in nearly all cases. Less is known of the effectiveness of sodium stibogluconate in the treatment of *mucocutaneous leishmaniasis.* Cautious treatment with *amphotericin B* has proven successful in this condition (Sampaio *et al., 1960). Single injections of *cycloguanil pamoate* have cured a large proportion of patients in Costa Rica, Mexico, and Panama (*see* Johnson, 1968).

The toxicity and side effects of antimonial drugs as well as the precautions and contraindications to be observed in their use are described in Chapter 46.

METRONIDAZOLE

The discovery of *azomycin* (2-nitroimidazole) by Nakamura in 1955 and the demonstration of its trichomonacidal properties by Horie (1956) opened the way for the chemical synthesis and biological testing of many nitroimidazoles. In 1959, Cosar and Julou reported the trichomonacidal activity, both *in vitro* and *in vivo,* of 1-(β-hydroxyethyl)-2-methyl-5-nitroimidazole. Durel and associates (1960) found that oral doses of the drug imparted trichomonacidal activity to semen and urine, and showed that high cure rate could be obtained in both male and female patients suffering from trichomoniasis. Subsequent experience derived from clinical trials in France, the United Kingdom, and North America indicated that the oral administration of the drug, now called *metronidazole,* will cure a high proportion of infected individuals. Its success spurred the synthesis and trial of many similar compounds. Two 5-nitroimidazoles closely related in structure and activity to metronidazole are currently available in some parts of the world. They are *tinidazole* (FASIGYN) and *nimorazole* (NAXOGIN, NULOGYL).

Up to the time of the introduction of metronidazole, topical therapy with many and varied agents effected cure in a large proportion of infected females, but left a hard core of chronic cases for which little could be done other than produce some measure of symptomatic relief. Infection in the male may form a reservoir of parasites for reinfection of the female by sexual contact and cannot be treated topically. By the employment of metronidazole, such cases now stand a very good chance of being cured.

The drug is also very useful in the treatment of intestinal and extraintestinal amebiasis; it is effective in the treatment of lambliasis; and it has a reputation for effectiveness in the treatment of acute ulcerative gingivitis.

Chemistry. Metronidazole has the following structural formula:

Metronidazole

It occurs as pale-yellow crystals that are slightly soluble in water and alcohol.

Pharmacological Effects. Metronidazole is directly trichomonacidal. It destroys 99% of the microorganisms in cultures of *Trichomonas vaginalis* within 24 hours at a concentration of 2.5 μg/ml. It is also directly amebicidal in very low concentrations (*see* Chapter 53). Its mechanism of antiprotozoal action is unknown.

Pharmacologically, metronidazole appears to be practically inert. Large doses in experimental animals affect neither the cardiovascular system nor respiration.

Absorption, Fate, and Excretion. Metronidazole is usually well absorbed after oral administration. Some patients fail to respond to treatment, however, and in such cases a low systemic concentration of the drug may be responsible. Whether this is due to relatively poor absorption from the gastrointestinal tract (Kane *et al.*, 1961) or to a rapid rate of metabolic transformation (Stambaugh *et al.*, 1968) is open to question.

Both unchanged metronidazole and several metabolites are excreted in various proportions in the urine of experimental animals and man after oral administration of the parent compound. The metabolites result from oxidation of side chains and glucuronide formation. The urine of some patients may be reddish-brown in color due to the presence of water-soluble pigments derived from the drug. Low concentrations of metronidazole appear in the saliva and in breast milk during treatment.

Preparations. *Metronidazole*, U.S.P. (FLAGYL), is available as 250-mg tablets. Uncoated vaginal inserts, each containing 500 mg, are also available.

Routes of Administration and Dosages. Many different dosage schedules have been used in the treatment of trichomoniasis in the female. However, the currently accepted regimen is one 250-mg tablet, given orally three times daily for 10 days. When repeated courses of the drug are required for stubborn infections, it is recommended that intervals of 4 to 6 weeks elapse between courses. In such cases, leukocyte counts should be carried out before, during, and after each course of treatment. Vaginal inserts may be used concurrently with oral medication, although there is no evidence that their use yields a higher cure rate than oral medication alone. If their use seems justified because of persistence of infection after normally adequate oral administration, one insert should be used daily for 10 days. At the same time, oral dosage should be reduced to two 250-mg tablets daily. Lack of satisfactory response may indicate the necessity for surgical eradication of foci in the cervical glands or in Skene's and Bartholin's glands.

Reinfection by an infected male partner may also cause apparent lack of satisfactory response. If such is the case, the male may be treated by the oral administration of 250 mg twice daily for 10 days, both partners being treated over the same 10-day period. However, the male should be treated only when trichomonads are demonstrated in the urogenital tract.

While quinacrine is the drug of choice in the treatment of *lambliasis,* its administration is not without unpleasant side effects. Metronidazole has been tried in the same dosage as that used in the treatment of trichomoniasis and found to be effective. Such use is, however, still considered investigational in the United States. The various regimens of treatment for the several forms of amebiasis are discussed in Chapter 53.

Toxicity and Side Effects. Side effects have only rarely been sufficiently severe to cause discontinuance of the drug. The most common have been referable to the gastrointestinal tract. In particular, nausea, anorexia, diarrhea, epigastric distress, and abdominal cramping have occurred; headache and vomiting are occasionally experienced. A metallic, sharp, and unpleasant taste is not unusual. Furry tongue, glossitis, and stomatitis may occur during therapy and be associated with a sudden intensification of moniliasis. Dizziness, vertigo, and, very rarely, incoordination and ataxia have been reported. Numbness or paresthesia of an extremity occurs occasionally. Urticaria, flushing, pruritus, dysuria, cystitis, a sense of pelvic pressure, and dryness of the mouth, vagina, or vulva have been reported. In some individuals the consumption of alcoholic beverages with metronidazole may produce a disulfiram-like effect.

While related chemicals have caused blood dyscrasias, serious difficulties have not been recorded with metronidazole. However, in an appreciable proportion of treated patients, a significant neutropenia has been observed. In all cases the white-cell count returned to normal after the course of medication was completed (*see* Lefebvre and Hesseltine, 1965).

Treatment should be discontinued promptly if ataxia or any other symptom of CNS involvement occurs. Metronidazole is contraindicated in patients with active disease of the CNS or with evidence or a history of blood dyscrasia. The drug has been given in all stages of pregnancy; despite the fact that it passes rapidly into the fetal circulation, there was no evidence that its administration was responsible for fetal abnormality, prematurity, or postnatal incident (*see* Peterson *et al.,* 1966).

Therapeutic Use. The effectiveness of metronidazole in the treatment of *trichomoniasis* in both males and females has been proven without doubt. All investigators have reported very high cure rates. This efficacy and a low incidence of comparatively minor side effects have led to its adoption as the agent of choice. There is also no doubt that persistent re-infection of the female can be prevented if the male partner harboring the parasite is treated concurrently. However, treatment of the male is recommended only if reinfection can be demonstrated to arise from this source.

Metronidazole also kills *Giardia lamblia* and has been shown to be effective in treating *lambliasis* in Europe and South America. It is also an effective amebicide, and has become the agent of choice in the treatment of the several forms of *amebiasis*. There is some evidence of its effectiveness in the treatment of the acute phase of *Vincent's disease* (*see* Emslie, 1967) and in eliminating the guinea worm in *dracontiasis* (Padonu, 1973).

NIFURTIMOX

In Latin America many millions of people are infected with *T. cruzi*, the infective agent of Chagas' disease. Approximately one tenth of those infected die, usually after a chronic and often asymptomatic course. Until recently, there was no drug that, in tolerated doses, could affect the intracellular, leishmanial stage. The nonmultiplying trypanosomes in the blood are more susceptible; primaquine has been found useful in eliminating this initial parasitemia.

Nitrofurans were known to be effective in experimental infections with *T. cruzi*, and numerous congeners have been investigated for their chemotherapeutic usefulness; recent work has proven promising. One drug, 3-methyl-4(5'-nitrofurfurylidene-amino)-tetrahydro-4H-1,4-thiazine-1,1-dioxide, is effective clinically in acute and chronic Chagas' infection (Bock *et al.*, 1972).

Chemistry and Preparations. *Nifurtimox* (*Bayer 2502;* LAMPIT) has the following structural formula:

Nifurtimox

Nifurtimox is marketed in scored tablets that contain 100 mg of the drug; it is available in the United States only from the Parasitic Disease Drug Service, Center for Disease Control, Atlanta, Georgia.

Pharmacological Effects. Nifurtimox is trypanocidal against both the trypamastigote and the amastigote forms of *T. cruzi*. Nothing is known of its mode of action. At a concentration of 1 µg/ml of the drug, vacuolization and mitochondrial swelling occur within a few hours in trypanosomes cultured in HeLa cells. Later changes include a decrease in the number of ribosomes and enlargement of the perinuclear space.

Absorption, Fate, and Excretion. Nifurtimox is well absorbed after oral administration. Despite this, only low concentrations of the drug are found in the blood and tissues, and little is present in the urine. High concentrations of several unidentified metabolites are found, however, and it is obvious that biotransformation occurs rapidly. It is not yet known what effect biotransformation has on trypanocidal activity.

Route of Administration and Dosage. The drug is given orally. *Children* (up to 15 years of age) with *acute* Chagas' disease should receive 25 mg/kg per day in four divided doses for 15 days, followed by 15 mg/kg per day in four divided doses for 75 days. Therapy should be extended to a total of 120 days for *chronic* disease. *Adults* with acute or chronic disease should receive 5 to 7 mg/kg daily for 2 weeks, and this dose is increased by 2 mg/kg at intervals of 2 weeks until 15 to 17 mg/kg is given daily by week 10. Treatment with this dose is continued until the patient has taken the drug for a total of 120 days. Gastric upset resulting from drug administration may be alleviated by simultaneous administration of aluminum hydroxide preparations.

Toxicity and Side Effects. The major toxic effects of nifurtimox in experimental animals given large doses for prolonged periods are referable to the CNS and to the male gonads. Treatment with large doses is associated with stiffness and weakness in the hindlimbs and transitory convulsive episodes. In man, the incidence of undesirable side effects has been high and from 40 to 70% of patients have been affected. Tolerance is generally high, however, and in only a small proportion of patients does treatment have to be interrupted or abandoned. Children appear to tolerate the drug better than do adults. Symptoms are attributable to effects on the CNS and the gastrointestinal tract. All have been reversible on stopping treatment. Phenobarbital affords symptomatic control of effects on the CNS.

Ideally, nifurtimox should be administered only to patients in hospitals, where there is close control of dosage and where appropriate symptomatic treatment of side effects is available. Practical considerations, however, are unlikely to allow this, and hence the disciplining of patients to follow the physician's instructions is particularly important. Because of the nature of the disease and the unique position of the drug, there are no absolute contraindications.

Therapeutic Uses. Nifurtimox is employed in the treatment of *trypanosomiasis* caused by *T. cruzi* (Chagas' disease). It is effective in both the acute and the chronic stages of the infection, although treatment with nifurtimox has no effect on irreversible organ lesions brought about by the disease process. In the acute stage, drug therapy results in disappearance of parasitemia and amelioration of symptoms and cure in over 80% of those treated. In the chronic stage, a cure rate of over 90% has been achieved in trials in Argentina, southern Brazil, Chile, and Venezuela. Much poorer results have been obtained in the middle section of Brazil, where the character of the infection is somewhat different. However, there is no evidence that the intrinsic susceptibility of the parasite differs from that in the other regions.

Bock, M.; Haberkorn, A.; Herlinger, H.; Mayer, K. H.; and Petersen, S. The structure-activity relationship of 4-(5'-nitrofurfurylidine-amino)-tetrahydro-4H-1,4-thiazine-1,1-dioxides active against *Trypanosoma cruzi. Arzneimittel-Forsch.,* **1972,** *22,* 1564–1569. (This issue, 9a of Vol. 22, is devoted to a full discussion of nifurtimox and should be consulted by those interested in obtaining details of the work.)

Cosar, C., and Julou, L. Activité de 1'(hydroxy-2' ethyl)-1 méthyl-2 nitro-5 imidazole (8,823 R.P.) vis-à-vis des infections expérimentales à *Trichomonas vaginalis. Annls Inst. Pasteur, Paris,* **1959,** *96,* 238–241.

DeVita, V. T.; Emmer, M.; Levine, A.; Jacobs, B.; and Berard, C. *Pneumocystis carinii* pneumonia. *New Engl. J. Med.,* **1969,** *280,* 287–291.

Durel, P.; Roiron, V.; Siboulet, A.; and Borel, L. J. Systemic treatment of human trichomoniasis with a derivative of nitroimidazole, 8823 R.P. *Br. J. vener. Dis.,* **1960,** *36,* 21–26.

Emslie, R. D. Treatment of acute ulcerative gingivitis. *Br. dent. J.,* **1967,** *122,* 307–308.

Flynn, I. W., and Bowman, I. B. R. Further studies on the mode of action of arsenicals on trypanosome pyruvate kinase. *Trans. R. Soc. trop. Med. Hyg.,* **1969,** *63,* 121.

Friedheim, E. A. H. L'acide triazine-arsinique dans le traitement de la maladie du sommeil. *Annls Inst. Pasteur, Paris,* **1940,** *65,* 108–118.

——. Mel B in the treatment of human trypanosomiasis. *Am. J. trop. Med.,* **1949,** *29,* 173–180.

Hill, G. C., and Hutner, S. H. Effect of trypanocidal drugs on terminal respiration of *Crithidia fasciculata. Expl Parasit.,* **1968,** *22,* 207–212.

Horie, H. Anti-*Trichomonas* effect of azomycin. *J. Antibiot., Tokyo, A,* **1956,** *9,* 168.

Ivady, G.; Paldy, L.; Koltay, M.; Toth, G.; and Kovaks, Z. *Pneumocystis carinii* pneumonia. *Lancet,* **1967,** *1,* 616–617.

Johnson, C. M. Cycloguanil pamoate in the treatment of cutaneous leishmaniasis: initial trials in Panama. *Am. J. trop. Med. Hyg.,* **1968,** *17,* 819–822.

Kane, P. O.; McFadzean, J. A.; and Squires, S. Absorption and excretion of metronidazole. *Br. J. vener. Dis.,* **1961,** *37,* 276–277.

King, H.; Lourie, E. M.; and Yorke, W. Studies in chemotherapy. XIX. Further report on new trypanocidal substances. *Ann. trop. Med. Parasit.,* **1938,** *32,* 177–192.

Launoy, L.; Guillot, M.; and Jonchère, H. [Storage and elimination of pentamidine in mice and white rats.] *Annls pharm. fr.,* **1960,** *18,* 273–284, 424–439.

Lefebvre, I., and Hesseltine, H. C. The peripheral white blood cells and metronidazole. *J. Am. med. Ass.,* **1965,** *194,* 15–18.

Lourie, E. M., and Yorke, W. Studies in chemotherapy. XXI. The trypanocidal action of certain aromatic diamidines. *Ann. trop. Med. Parasit.,* **1939,** *33,* 289–304.

Padonu, K. O. A controlled trial of metronidazole in the treatment of dracontiasis in Nigeria. *Am. J. trop. Med. Hyg.,* **1973,** *22,* 42–44.

Peterson, W. F.; Stauch, J. E.; and Ryder, C. D. Metronidazole in pregnancy. *Am. J. Obstet. Gynec.,* **1966,** *94,* 343–349.

Richet, P. Le melarsonyl (TRIMELARSAN) en pathologie tropical. *Bull. Séanc. Acad. r. Sci. colon. (outre-Mer),* **1966,** No. 4, 759–785.

Robertson, D. H. H. A trial of Mel W in the treatment of *Trypanosoma rhodesiense* sleeping sickness. *Trans. R. Soc. trop. Med. Hyg.,* **1963,** *57,* 274–289.

Rollo, I. M., and Williamson, J. Acquired resistance to "melarsen," tryparsamide and amidines in pathogenic trypanosomes after treatment with "melarsen" alone. *Nature,* **1951,** *167,* 147–148.

Sampaio, S. A.; Godoy, J. T.; Paiva, L.; Dillon, N. L.; and Lacas, C. da S. The treatment of American (mucocutaneous) leishmaniasis with amphotericin-B. *A.M.A. Archs Derm.,* **1960,** *82,* 627–635.

Stambaugh, J. E.; Feo, L. G.; and Manthei, R. W. The isolation and identification of the urinary oxidative metabolites of metronidazole in man. *J. Pharmac. exp. Ther.,* **1968,** *161,* 373–381.

VanHoof, L. M. J. J. Observations on trypanosomiasis in Belgium Congo. *Trans. R. Soc. trop. Med. Hyg.,* **1947,** *40,* 728–761.

Williamson, J., and Lourie, E. M. "Melarsen" and "melarsen oxide." *Nature, Lond.,* **1948,** *161,* 103–104.

Williamson, J., and Macadam, R. F. Effect of trypanocidal drugs on the fine structure of *Trypanosoma rhodesiense. Trans. R. Soc. trop. Med. Hyg.,* **1965,** *59,* 367–368.

Monographs and Reviews

Allison, A. C. Effects of drugs and toxic agents on lysosomes. In, *The Interaction of Drugs and Subcellular Components in Animal Cells.* (Campbell, P. N., ed.) J. & A. Churchill, Ltd., London, **1968,** pp. 218–235.

Beveridge, E. Chemotherapy of leishmaniasis. In, *Experimental Chemotherapy,* Vol. I. (Schnitzer, R. J., and Hawking, F., eds.) Academic Press, Inc., New York, **1963,** pp. 257–287.

Eagle, H., and Doak, G. O. The biological activity of arsenosobenzenes in relation to their structure. *Pharmac. Rev.,* **1951,** *3,* 107–143.

Findlay, G. M. *Recent Advances in Chemotherapy,* Vol. I. J. & A. Churchill, Ltd., London, **1950.**

Hawking, F. Chemotherapy of trypanosomiasis. In, *Experimental Chemotherapy,* Vol. I. (Schnitzer, R. J., and Hawking, F., eds.) Academic Press, Inc., New York, **1963,** pp. 129–256.

Robertson, D. H. H. Chemotherapy of African trypanosomiasis. *Practitioner,* **1962,** *188,* 80–83.

Williamson, J. Chemotherapy and chemoprophylaxis of African trypanosomiasis. *Expl Parasit.,* **1962,** *12,* 274–322.

Chemotherapy of Microbial Diseases

---

55 ANTIMICROBIAL AGENTS

General Considerations

Louis Weinstein

Historical Aspects. The concept and even the attempt to use substances derived from one living organism to kill another (antibiosis) are almost as old as the science of microbiology. Indeed, the application of antibiotic therapy, without recognition of it as such, is considerably older. The Chinese were aware, over 2500 years ago, of the therapeutic properties of moldy curd of soybean applied to carbuncles, boils, and similar infections and used this material as standard treatment in such disorders. The medical literature has for many centuries contained descriptions of beneficial effects from the application, in certain localized infections, of soil and various plants, most of which probably were sources of antibiotic-forming molds and bacteria.

The first investigators to recognize the clinical potentialities of microorganisms as therapeutic agents were Pasteur and Joubert, who recorded their observations and speculations in 1877. They noted that anthrax bacilli grew rapidly when inoculated into sterile urine but failed to multiply and soon died if one of the "common" bacteria of the air was introduced in the urine at the same time. The same type of experiment in animals produced similar results. They commented on the fact that life destroys life among the lower species even more than among higher animals and plants, and came to the astonishing conclusion that anthrax bacilli could be administered to an animal in large numbers, and it

would not sicken, provided that "ordinary" bacteria were given at the same time. They stated that this observation might hold great promise for therapeutics.

The clinical use of antibiotic agents represents the practical, controlled, and directed application of phenomena that occur naturally and continuously in soil, sewage, water, and other natural habitats of microorganisms. During the latter part of the nineteenth century and the early years of the twentieth century, several antimicrobial substances were demonstrated in bacterial cultures and some were even tested clinically but discarded because they proved to be highly toxic.

The modern era of the chemotherapy of infection started with the clinical use of sulfanilamide in 1936. The "golden age" of antimicrobial therapy began with the production of penicillin in 1941, when this compound, first discovered in 1929, was mass-produced and made available for limited clinical trial for the first time. Although the earliest development of antibiotics involved considerable serendipity, from the discovery of streptomycin by Schatz, Bugie, and Waksman (1944) to the present the search for such agents has been a highly planned, scientifically designed effort.

Definition and Characteristics. Antibiotics are chemical substances produced by various species of microorganisms (bacteria, fungi, actinomycetes) that suppress the growth of other microorganisms and may eventually destroy them. The number of antibiotics now extends into the hundreds, and over 60 have been developed to the stage where they are of value in the therapy of infectious diseases. They differ markedly in physical, chemical, and pharmacological properties, antibacterial spectra, and mechanisms of action. Most have been chemically identified, and some have been synthesized. A few are available only as crude or partially purified extracts. Systemic antibiotic therapy became possible in the early 1940s with the advent of penicillin. The medical, public health, and economic aspects of antibiotics are difficult to overestimate, and the years elapsing since their introduction into therapy have witnessed dramatic reductions in incidence of, and morbidity and mortality due to, a number of infectious diseases.

In addition to antibiotics, the synthetic chemist has added greatly to our therapeutic armamentarium. Thus, drugs such as isoniazid and ethambutol represent important contributions and provide the mainstay for the treatment of tuberculosis. Indeed, little distinction should now be made between compounds of natural and synthetic origin. It is not unlikely that successful chemotherapy of viral diseases and cancer may result from a planned approach directed toward purely synthetic drugs as more is learned about viral replication and malignant cells.

Properties of an Ideal Chemotherapeutic Agent. The *ideal chemotherapeutic agent* should have the following properties. The compound should exhibit selective and effective antimicrobial activity, and it should be bactericidal rather than bacteriostatic. While it might be desirable that an agent kill a broad range of microorganisms, problems of suprainfection often intervene (*see* below). Bacteria should not develop resistance to the drug. Its antimicrobial efficacy must not be materially reduced by body fluids, exudates, plasma proteins, or tissue enzymes. Characteristics of absorption, distribution, fate, and excretion should be such that bactericidal levels in the blood, tissues, and body fluids, including the cerebrospinal fluid, are rapidly reached and maintained for prolonged periods. Excretion of the drug in the urine in bactericidal concentrations is of great value

in urinary tract infections, and renal injury must not result from such excretion. Finally, and obviously, the many general characteristics desirable in any pharmacological agent must also be present.

Classification and Mechanism of Action. The antibacterial agents presently available may be classified into several groups on the basis of their mechanisms of action (Weisblum and Davies, 1968; Pestka, 1971; Symposium, 1974), as follows: (1) *agents inhibiting the synthesis of the bacterial cell wall*—the penicillins, the cephalosporins, cycloserine, vancomycin, ristocetin, and bacitracin; (2) *agents affecting the permeability of the cell membrane*—the polymyxins, colistimethate, and the polyene antifungal agents nystatin and amphotericin; (3) *agents primarily inhibiting protein synthesis by their effects on ribosomes*—chloramphenicol, the tetracyclines, the aminoglycosides, the macrolide antibiotics erythromycin and oleandomycin, and lincomycin and its congener clindamycin; (4) *agents affecting nucleic acid metabolism*—rifampin and nalidixic acid; and (5) *the antimetabolites*—the sulfonamides, trimethoprim, aminosalicylic acid, and the sulfones. Although this classification appears valid at present on the basis of the available evidence, it may require modification as more definitive information is acquired. Furthermore, the general mechanism of action of a few agents remains unknown.

A classification of chemotherapeutic agents based on their clinical effectiveness is related to the "spectrum" of microorganisms that they inhibit. Thus, agents such as penicillin G are considered to have a "narrow spectrum" because, in the doses usually employed, this drug affects primarily gram-positive bacteria and *Neisseria*. The bacitracins fall into the same group since their activity is limited to gram-positive microorganisms. On the other hand, the tetracyclines and chloramphenicol are examples of "broad-spectrum" compounds because they suppress multiplication of both gram-positive and gram-negative bacteria and are also effective in the treatment of rickettsial infections.

To be of practical value in the treatment of infection, an antimicrobial agent must exert its effects upon the invading microorganisms without seriously damaging the cells of the host. It is remarkable that so many compounds with such selective activity have been developed. The principal result of antimicrobial activity is retardation of the rate of bacterial growth. When present in sufficiently high concentration, some drugs kill bacteria *in vivo* as well as *in vitro*. It must be emphasized, however, that the antimicrobial agents, even the most effective ones, do not, except in uncommon instances, cure infection simply by virtue of their activity against the responsible microorganism. Even the bactericidal compounds, in all probability, require the effective intervention of various humoral and cellular defense mechanisms of the host.

Determination of Bacterial Sensitivity to Antimicrobial Agents. The sensitivities of bacteria to various antimicrobial agents are usually determined by a variety of microbiological methods (*see* Ericsson and Sherris, 1971). One accurate technic used in the routine diagnostic laboratory involves inoculation of the microorganism being tested into a liquid culture medium containing serial dilutions of the drug. The lowest concentration of drug inhibiting growth of the bacteria is expressed as the "sensitivity." A more rapid method involves the use of commercially available filter-paper discs impregnated with specific quantities of the drugs. These are placed on the surface of agar plates over which a culture of the microorganism being examined has first been streaked. This is a relatively crude procedure, and its accuracy may be influenced by many factors. It is, however, of practical clinical importance in indicating which antibacterial agent to employ and the general level of dose required to produce a therapeutic effect. Standardized criteria for performance and interpretation of this test have been developed by Bauer and associates (1966).

Resistance of Microorganisms to Antimicrobial Agents. Antibacterial drugs are not effective against all microorganisms. The "spectrum" of activity of each drug is probably the result of several factors, the chief of which relates to the primary mechanism of action. The phenomenon of the development of drug resistance is not universal among either the microorganisms or the drugs. However, it is far more complex than natural resistance. Even after more than 30 years, no significant degree of resistance to penicillin G has developed in *Streptococcus (Diplococcus) pneumoniae* or group-A *Strep. pyogenes.* On the other hand, shortly after this antibiotic came into use, it became apparent that an increasing number of insensitive strains of *Staphylococcus aureus* were being recovered from human infections, for reasons explained below.

The development of resistance to an antibiotic involves a stable genetic change, heritable from generation to generation. Any of the mechanisms that result in alteration of bacterial genetic composition can operate, and bacteria may thus become resistant to antimicrobial agents by *mutation, transduction, transformation,* or *conjugation.* The first three mechanisms are particularly involved in the development of drug insensitivity in gram-positive cocci, while all four may be responsible for the acquisition of resistance by gram-negative bacilli.

Regardless of the genetic mechanism involved in the development of resistance, the basic alterations in susceptibility are related to (1) elaboration of drug-metabolizing enzymes such as penicillinase, cephalosporinase, and adenylylating, phosphorylating, and acetylating enzymes; (2) alteration of the permeability of the bacterial cell to the drug; (3) increased amount of an endogenous antagonist of drug action; or (4) alteration of the amount of drug receptor or the binding characteristics of the compound to its critical target.

Mutation. There is no evidence that mutations resulting in microbial resistance to an antimicrobial agent are caused by exposure to the particular drug. For example, strains of some bacterial species isolated long before certain antibacterial agents were developed have been found to be highly insensitive to them. Such mutations are random events, and the appearance of resistance in a microorganism during therapy merely represents selective multiplication of the resistant mutants that have been present from the beginning of the infection or of a resistant strain introduced from the external environment. Selection also accounts for an increase in the number of resistant strains present in a community or hospital. Widespread and prolonged use of a particular antimicrobial agent, by eliminating the bulk of sensitive microorganisms, selects out the resistant ones, which then become the predominant forms.

The acquisition of resistance to antimicrobial agents by mutation follows different temporal patterns. With some agents, microorganisms become resistant to increasing concentrations of drug in a stepwise manner. Multiple mutations are apparently necessary, each conferring additional degrees of resistance. In other cases, resistance to high concentrations of drug is acquired as a single mutational event. This pattern causes more difficulty for the clinician.

Transduction. The development of resistance by this mechanism involves the intervention of bacteriophage in the transfer of resistance from an insensitive to a sensitive microorganism. A piece of DNA carrying a gene for resistance is enclosed within the coat of the phage and passed from the resistant to the sensitive strain, which then becomes resistant to the drug.

Transformation. This is a process by which a bacterial cell incorporates from its environment one or more genes formed by another bacterium.

Conjugation. An important mechanism for the acquisition of drug resistance is the passage of resistance factors from one microorganism to another during *conjugation.* This involves two factors—the resistance (R) factor and the resistance transfer factor (RTF). The R factor, an extrachromosomal segment of DNA (a plasmid or episome), contains the information for resistance. The RTF unit (also DNA) can exist in combination with the R factor and controls the transfer of the plasmid during conjugation. The presence of the R factor can cause the alteration of components of microorganisms responsible for sensitivity to a drug or the synthesis of enzymes that inactivate antibacterial agents (Davies et al., 1971). Of great importance, the R factor may contain information for resistance to multiple drugs, and all this information may be acquired by a susceptible bacterium as a single event. Primarily gram-negative bacilli have been shown to become drug resistant by this mechanism. Among the microorganisms known to be capable of transferring this type of resistance to susceptible bacteria are *Escherichia coli, Salmonella, Shigella, Klebsiella, Serratia, Vibrio cholerae,* and *Pseudomonas.*

Among the antimicrobial agents to which resistance develops by this method are sulfonamides, aminoglycosides, tetracylines, chloramphenicol, and penicillin. Very important from the clinical standpoint is the frequency with which R factors are passed from nonpathogenic to pathogenic bacterial species. Such passage takes place most often in the intestinal tract. One such contact may result in the sudden acquisition of resistance to two or more of the commonly used antibacterial compounds. The spread of the R factor in the intestinal tract is by successive transfer. While the frequency of transfer of R is low *in vitro* and even lower *in vivo,* antimicrobial drugs exert a powerful selective force. The degree of drug resistance conferred by R factors differs from one host cell to another and from one R factor to another. For example, multiple-drug R factor may cause *E. coli* to be resistant to only 10 μg/ml of streptomycin, but the same R factor may make *Shig. flexneri* insensitive to >1000 μg/ml. There is, accordingly, a wide range of altered drug susceptibility following transfer of one R factor complex, depending on the species of microorganism that is the recipient.

While of special interest to the pharmacologist and microbiologist, this form of drug resistance also has considerable clinical importance. An increasing number of infections due to such microorganisms are being reported from many areas in the world. In some instances, the resistance develops to so many of the commonly used antimicrobial agents that the physician may have to resort to the use of the more dangerous and less-well-known drugs, or there may not be an effective agent for the treatment of a particular infection. (*See* reviews by Watanabe, 1966; Mitsuhashi, 1969.)

The importance of the general problem of bacterial resistance to drugs cannot be overemphasized. Solutions to it, accomplished by the development of new and effective antimicrobial agents, are often only temporary. For example, staphylococci resistant to both the penicillinase-resistant semisynthetic penicillins and the cephalosporin derivatives are presently being recovered from infections. Such strains were present prior to the development of these drugs, the use of which appears to have selected for the resistant mutants. As a rule, microorganisms insensitive to a particular drug tend to be resistant to all other chemically related antimicrobial agents. Bacteria unaffected by tetracycline are usually unresponsive to its congeners. Occasionally, cross-resistance may involve two agents that are chemically dissimilar, for example, erythromycin and lincomycin.

Concurrent therapy with two or more antimicrobial agents may greatly diminish the speed with which bacterial resistance develops, since microorganisms resistant to one drug may still be killed by the other. The classical therapeutic example of this principle is in the drug treatment of tuberculosis. Resistance of the tubercle bacillus to a single tuberculostatic compound such as isoniazid, for example, is appreciably delayed when this drug is given together with another effective agent such as streptomycin or ethambutol. Thus, if a strain of microorganisms can acquire resistance, by independent mutations, to either of two antimicrobial agents at a frequency of once in every 10^5 cell divisions, mutant bacteria simultaneously resistant to both drugs would be expected to arise only once in every 10^{10} divisions.

Treatment Resistance. Not all instances of failure of infections to respond to treatment with antimicrobial agents can be attributed to the activity of drug-resistant microorganisms. A number of other factors related to the host, the antimicrobial agent, and the bacteria exert very important effects on the outcome of therapy, as follows. (1) Delay in therapy. (2) Administration of suboptimal doses of an antimicrobial compound. (3) Alteration in the metabolic state of the microorganisms present in the patient. Dormancy of the bacteria may be responsible for therapeutic failure with some drugs that act only on cells that are actively growing and multiplying. The presence of variant bacterial forms induced by exposure to some antibiotics—for example, forms deficient in cell wall (protoplasts, spheroplasts, L forms)—may make ineffective the antimicrobial agents that act by interfering with cell-wall synthesis. (4) Medication or pathological and physiological processes secondary to infection may antagonize the activity of some of the drugs. For example, chloramphenicol and the tetracyclines antagonize the activity of the penicillins; pus and some metabolites oppose the antibacterial effects of the sulfon-amides; an acidic or alkaline medium may alter the activity of antibacterial substances. (5) In some instances, certain barriers make it difficult or impossible for the drug to reach the site of infection in adequate concentration. Thus, certain sites such as the central nervous system, eye, and prostate are poorly penetrated by relatively hydrophilic antibiotics. (6) The final determinant of cure of infection in many instances is the functional state of host defense mechanisms. Many of these factors are discussed in more detail below.

Selection of an Antimicrobial Agent. The first crucial therapeutic question that the physician must face is *whether or not* to use an antimicrobial agent in a specific situation. Unfortunately, critical thought is often not applied here. If the answer is affirmative, the difficult problem of drug selection obviously arises next. In order to provide maximal benefit for the patient, it is essential for the physician to have a working knowledge of the common pathogenic microorganisms. While the results of bacteriological culture are desirable before therapy is initiated, it is frequently not practical to wait for such data, especially in severe infections in which the outcome may be fatal before the specific etiology is delineated. In many instances, the nature of the responsible microorganism can be determined, within certain limits, by study of stained smears of exudates or body fluids and, when this is not possible, important hints as to the specific cause are often obtained from the study of the clinical features of an infectious disease. It must be stressed, however, that there are many situations in which careful bacteriological studies are absolutely essential to the proper initiation or the modification of treatment, and the conscientious physician must obtain help from those experienced in various bacteriological technics. Even if it is necessary to *begin* antimicrobial therapy without such information, cultures should be obtained if at all possible *prior* to drug administration.

When the etiology of an infectious process has been determined, selection of the most appropriate drug does not follow automatically, because there may be wide variations in susceptibility of different strains of some

species of microorganisms. Essential to the choice of drug is information concerning the *sensitivity pattern* of the infecting agent. In some instances, such tests need not be carried out since long experience has indicated that certain microorganisms have remained highly susceptible to certain antibiotics despite years of exposure (*see* Table 55-1). Thus, when the pneumococcus, group-A beta-hemolytic streptococcus, or *Treponema pallidum* is responsible for disease, the obvious choice is penicillin G. On the other hand, *E. coli, Proteus, Pseud. aeruginosa, Staph. aureus,* and the *viridans* group of *Streptococcus,* among others, have varying sensitivities and must be examined in the laboratory for susceptibility to different drugs.

Although the degree of inhibition of growth of the causative microorganism is an important factor in selecting an antibacterial agent, it must be stressed that it is not the only one. The *nature of the illness* for which therapy is being designed also affects the choice of agent. For example, the physician must know whether a given antimicrobial agent will penetrate to the site of a specific infection; this is particularly true in the treatment of meningitis. An orally administered drug is obviously a poor one for a patient who is vomiting. Injectable preparations must be avoided in individuals who have a bleeding tendency. In critically ill cases, it is sometimes wisest to give more than one drug until culture and sensitivity studies reveal a specific drug requirement. In such instances, cultures must always be taken before therapy is initiated. If a person has previously shown a potentially dangerous type of *hypersensitivity reaction* or a *serious untoward effect* of some other type while receiving an antimicrobial drug, he must not be reexposed to the same agent if this can possibly be avoided. One aspect of the use of anti-infective compounds that is often neglected in the enthusiasm to treat is the *cost of the drug.* Such compounds presently represent one of the most commonly used classes of drugs in private and hospital practice, and the total cost of such agents is a major item in hospital budgets and in the medical care of individuals. The physician must take into consideration, when selecting an antimicrobial compound, whether the same ends might be accomplished, with no more risk, with a drug that is relatively cheap in place of an expensive, but no more effective alternative.

THERAPY WITH COMBINED ANTIMICROBIAL AGENTS

Combination therapy with antimicrobial agents began almost as soon as two such agents became available. Shortly after streptomycin was developed, it was mixed with penicillin and the combination recommended for clinical use, especially in situations in which the definitive etiology was not readily apparent. The advent of other antimicrobial agents, the appearance of increasing numbers of drug-resistant bacterial species, and the reports of enhanced antibacterial activity *in vitro* led to the development of a number of other combinations in which the ratios of the compounds were fixed on the basis of *in-vitro* determinations. These are known as "fixed-dose" combinations. In fact, the results of *in-vitro* tests have correlated very poorly with the clinical results and mixtures of antimicrobial agents have been demonstrated to be superior to a single agent only in a few instances. Most investigators in the field of chemotherapy of infection concur in this view.

A widely accepted basis for predicting the antimicrobial activity of combinations of antibiotics is that suggested by Jawetz and colleagues (1951, 1952). They indicated that mixing one bactericidal drug with another (penicillin and streptomycin) often results in a supra-additive but not an antagonistic effect. On the other hand, the addition of a bacteriostatic compound (tetracycline) to a bactericidal one (penicillin) tends to produce decreased but not additive or supra-additive activity. The penicillins can exert their bactericidal action only against microorganisms that are multiplying. Combinations of two bacteriostatic agents (tetracycline and chloramphenicol) are never inhibitory. While these principles apply *in vitro* and in experimental infections, a number of clinical situations appear to be exceptions. For example, the use of streptomycin together with a tetracycline leads to better results in the therapy of brucellosis. Another approach to the problem of selection of antibacterial agents for concurrent use is based on the known mechanism of action of the individual agents. The combination of sulfamethoxazole and trimethoprim represents such a rational choice, since these two agents inhibit sequential steps in a single, vital biosynthetic pathway (*see* Chapter 56). The studies by Chang and Weinstein (1966) have indicated that the addition of a drug that suppresses protein synthesis to one that inhibits cell-wall synthesis results in abolition of the antibacterial

effects of the latter. On the other hand, the combining of one inhibitor of cell-wall synthesis with another compound that acts in the same manner, or with one that alters cell membranes, results in no loss of activity of either agent. Correlation between laboratory and clinical observations of the action of combinations of antibiotics has been reviewed by Jawetz (1968).

The *simultaneous administration* (but not in the form of "fixed-dose" mixtures) of more than one antimicrobial agent has been suggested for four purposes (Weinstein, 1958): (1) treatment of mixed bacterial infections, (2) delay in rate of emergence of bacterial resistance, (3) enhancement of therapeutic activity, and (4) therapy of severe infectious processes in which the specific etiology has not been established.

1. Treatment of Mixed Bacterial Infections. In some infections, two or more microorganisms are causative. Bronchiectasis, peritonitis, and some instances of acute or chronic otitis media and urinary tract infection are examples. In some cases, the responsible bacteria, although of different species, may be sensitive to a single antimicrobial agent, while in others they have distinctly different drug susceptibilities. This emphasizes the need for determination of the drug sensitivity of each of the components of a mixed flora. If at all possible, such information should be at hand before therapy is initiated. It must be stressed that each microorganism should be studied separately because testing of mixed cultures may produce very misleading information. The anti-infective drugs to be given are selected on the basis of these studies and administered in full doses. In some cases it may be unnecessary and even dangerous to delay initiation of treatment until definitive bacteriological data are available. Peritonitis is an outstanding example; because both gram-positive and gram-negative microorganisms may be involved and because delay in therapy may result in a rapidly fatal outcome, treatment should be started immediately with maximal quantities of the drugs known to be most effective against these types of bacteria. In bronchiectasis, chronic otitis media, and chronic urinary tract infections, therapy need not be initiated before diagnostic bacteriological information becomes available, because these infections have usually been present for such a long time that a delay of 2 or 3 days makes little or no difference in the outcome. This principle does not apply, however, when acute exacerbations of the chronic process develop. Concurrent use of antimicrobial agents does not always lead to cure of an infectious process, even when the responsible microorganisms are sensitive to the individual drugs employed; this is illustrated by chronic urinary tract infections, in which it is known that such therapy may not improve the outlook for recovery.

2. Delay in Rate of Emergence of Bacterial Resistance. *In-vitro* studies have demonstrated that, when

Table 55-1. CURRENT USE OF ANTIMICROBIAL AGENTS IN THE THERAPY OF INFECTIONS

Presentation of choices of specific agents for the treatment of various infections is always provocative of discussion and disagreement because such choices often represent the distillate of personal experiences that may not duplicate those of others. In addition, the current availability of a number of drugs that are approximately equally effective makes an order of choice very difficult, if not impossible. To complicate matters, sensitivity patterns of a number of microorganisms often vary with the hospital or clinic in which they are isolated; in some instances, this reflects a varying degree of exposure to specific agents. The material presented in this table represents not only the practice of the author, based on his experience with the management of these infections, but also that of other experts in the United States. It is important to stress that, as more information accumulates, as recently introduced drugs are used for longer periods, and as entirely new agents are developed, some of the recommendations will require modification not only in the order of choice but even in the specific drugs that are suggested.

Taxonomy is not a static field, and nomenclature of microorganisms changes as further insight into their relationships is obtained. The system used in this table and textbook is that of the eighth edition of *Bergey's Manual of Determinative Bacteriology* (Buchanan and Gibbons, 1974). Older generic and specific names are indicated parenthetically in italic type.

	DISEASES	DRUG ORDER OF CHOICE		
		1st	*2nd* [1]	*3rd* [1]
I. GRAM-POSITIVE COCCI				
Staphylococcus aureus *	Abscesses Bacteremia Endocarditis Pneumonia Meningitis Osteomyelitis	Penicillin G sensitive → Penicillin G	A cephalosporin [2]	Clindamycin [2] Erythromycin Gentamicin Lincomycin Vancomycin [4]
		Penicillin G resistant → A penicillinase-resistant penicillin		
		Methicillin resistant → Vancomycin	A cephalosporin ± kanamycin [3]	
Streptococcus pyogenes (groups A, B, C)	Pharyngitis Scarlet fever Otitis media, sinusitis Cellulitis Erysipelas Pneumonia Bacteremia Other systemic infections	Penicillin G Penicillin V	A cephalosporin [2] Clindamycin [2] Erythromycin Lincomycin	A tetracycline [5]
Streptococcus (viridans group) *	Dental infections Subacute endocarditis Urinary tract infection	Penicillin G ± streptomycin	A cephalosporin [2] Erythromycin	Vancomycin

DISEASES	1st	2nd	3rd [1]
Streptococcus faecalis * (enterococcus) — Urinary tract infection, Bacteremia, Meningitis, Brain abscess	Ampicillin, Penicillin G + an aminoglycoside	Vancomycin	Erythromycin ± an aminoglycoside
Streptococcus bovis — Endocarditis, Urinary tract infection, Bacteremia, Meningitis, Brain abscess	Penicillin G	Erythromycin	Vancomycin
Streptococcus (anaerobic species) * — Bacteremia, Endocarditis, Brain and other abscesses	Penicillin G [6]	Chloramphenicol, Clindamycin, Erythromycin, A tetracycline	—
Streptococcus (Diplococcus) pneumoniae (pneumococcus) — Pneumonia, Meningitis, Endocarditis, Arthritis	Penicillin G	A cephalosporin [2], Chloramphenicol, Clindamycin [2], Erythromycin, Lincomycin	A tetracycline [7]

DRUG ORDER OF CHOICE

II. GRAM-NEGATIVE COCCI / DISEASES	1st	2nd [1]	3rd [1]
Neisseria gonorrhoeae (gonococcus) — Genital infections, Arthritis, Meningitis, Endocarditis	Penicillin G	Ampicillin, Spectinomycin [8]	A cephalosporin [2], Erythromycin, A tetracycline
Neisseria meningitidis (meningococcus) — Meningitis, Bacteremia	Penicillin G	Chloramphenicol	Erythromycin, A sulfonamide [9]
Carrier state	Rifampin, A sulfonamide [9]	—	—

* All strains must be examined *in vitro* for sensitivity to various antimicrobial agents.

[1] Drugs included for second and third choices are (a) indicated in patients hypersensitive to equally or more effective agents, (b) potentially more dangerous than equally active drugs, (c) less likely to produce the desired therapeutic response, or (d) in need, in some cases, of further study in order to allow a valid evaluation of their efficacy.

Lists of drugs within each box are given alphabetically since they are approximately equally effective.

[2] Therapeutic concentrations of this drug are not achieved in the cerebrospinal fluid, and alternative agents should be used to treat infections of the central nervous system.

[3] Not all strains are sensitive to this combination.

[4] As indicated, vancomycin is the drug of first choice for methicillin-resistant staphylococci, since these microorganisms are usually also resistant to all other less toxic antimicrobials.

[5] About 10 to 30% of strains of group-A *Strep. pyogenes* are insensitive to tetracyclines.

[6] Large doses of penicillin G may be required.

[7] Some strains of pneumococci are resistant to tetracyclines.

[8] Spectinomycin is useful for genital infections only.

[9] Although many strains are resistant, sulfonamides are effective for sensitive microorganisms.

Table 55-1. CURRENT USE OF ANTIMICROBIAL AGENTS IN THE THERAPY OF INFECTIONS (Continued)

III. GRAM-POSITIVE BACILLI	DISEASES	DRUG ORDER OF CHOICE		
		1st	2nd [1]	3rd [1]
Bacillus anthracis *	"Malignant pustule" Pneumonia Meningitis	Penicillin G	Erythromycin A tetracycline	A cephalosporin [2] Chloramphenicol Lincomycin
Corynebacterium diphtheriae [10] (Klebs-Loeffler bacillus)	Pharyngitis Laryngotracheitis Pneumonia Other local lesions Carrier state	Penicillin G	Erythromycin	A cephalosporin Lincomycin Rifampin
Corynebacterium species, aerobic and anaerobic * (diphtheroids)	Endocarditis Hepatic disease Wound infections	Penicillin G	Erythromycin	—
Listeria monocytogenes	Meningitis Bacteremia Endocarditis Recurrent abortion	Ampicillin ± streptomycin Penicillin G ± streptomycin	Erythromycin A tetracycline	Chloramphenicol
Erysipelothrix rhusiopathiae	Erysipeloid	Penicillin G	Erythromycin A tetracycline	Chloramphenicol
Clostridium perfringens and other species	Gas gangrene	Penicillin G [11]	Erythromycin A tetracycline	A cephalosporin Chloramphenicol
Clostridium tetani	Tetanus	Penicillin G [12]	A tetracycline	Erythromycin

IV. GRAM-NEGATIVE BACILLI	DISEASES	DRUG ORDER OF CHOICE		
		1st	2nd [1]	3rd [1]
	Urinary tract infection [13]	Ampicillin Nitrofurantoin A sulfonamide Trimethoprim-sulfamethoxazole	Carbenicillin indanyl A cephalosporin Methenamine mandelate Nalidixic acid A tetracycline	Chloramphenicol
Escherichia coli *	Other infections	Ampicillin Gentamicin	A cephalosporin [2] Chloramphenicol	Colistimethate Kanamycin

Strains		Gentamicin Polymyxin B	Kanamycin Neomycin	
Enterobacter (Aerobacter) aerogenes *	Urinary tract and other infections	Gentamicin	Carbenicillin Chloramphenicol Kanamycin A tetracycline	Colistimethate Polymyxin B
Alcaligenes faecalis *	Urinary tract and other infections	Chloramphenicol A tetracycline	Colistimethate Polymyxin B	Gentamicin Kanamycin
Proteus mirabilis	Urinary tract and other infections	Ampicillin Nitrofurantoin [15] A sulfonamide [15]	A cephalosporin [2] Gentamicin Kanamycin	Chloramphenicol A tetracycline
Proteus, other species *	Urinary tract and other infections [16]	Carbenicillin Kanamycin	Gentamicin	Chloramphenicol Streptomycin A tetracycline
Pseudomonas aeruginosa *	Urinary tract and other infections	Carbenicillin [17] Gentamicin ± carbenicillin [17]	Colistimethate Polymyxin B	—
Klebsiella pneumoniae * (Friedlander's bacillus)	Pneumonia Urinary tract infection Biliary tract infection Osteomyelitis	A cephalosporin [18] Kanamycin or gentamicin ± a cephalosporin	Chloramphenicol A tetracycline	Colistimethate Polymyxin B
Salmonella *	Typhoid fever Paratyphoid fever Bacteremia Acute gastroenteritis	Ampicillin [19] Chloramphenicol [19]	Trimethoprim-sulfamethoxazole	—
Shigella *	Acute gastroenteritis [20]	Ampicillin Chloramphenicol	Kanamycin [21] Polymyxin B [21] A tetracycline	A sulfonamide [22] Trimethoprim-sulfamethoxazole

10 Antibiotics alone do not alter the clinical course of diphtheria, but drugs can eradicate the carrier state.

11 Adequate debridement is absolutely essential. Antitoxin therapy is advisable, but newer evidence suggests that this may not play an important role in cure. At least 30 million units of penicillin G should be administered daily.

12 Ten to 20 million units of penicillin G daily, with debridement and adsorbed tetanus toxoid. Human tetanus immune globulin administration may be advisable.

13 Sulfonamides, trimethoprim-sulfamethoxazole, and urinary tract antiseptics are particularly useful for acute urinary tract infections, especially cystitis, in the patient without obstructive uropathy or in whom the disease has not become chronic. These agents also prove useful for chronic suppressive therapy in patients with recurrent urinary tract infection. Some clinicians prefer to reserve the antibiotics for cases in which there are systemic manifestations—particularly in acute pyelonephritis.

14 For toxigenic noninvasive strains of E. coli, poorly absorbed antibiotics (polymyxins, aminoglycosides) are administered orally by some physicians. There is, however, no convincing evidence of the efficacy of antibiotic therapy. For invasive strains, there is debate as to the relative efficacy of systemic antibiotic therapy versus treatment with agents confined to the gastrointestinal tract.

15 Acute lower urinary tract infection can often be controlled by the use of sulfonamide or nitrofurantoin.

16 Some strains are sensitive to chloramphenicol, tetracyclines, or streptomycin. In serious infections, it is best to begin treatment with carbenicillin while the microorganisms are being examined for sensitivity to other drugs. If they prove to be susceptible to other agents, one of these should constitute the therapy of choice.

17 For all serious infections with Pseudomonas, many clinicians prefer gentamicin in combination with carbenicillin, but not in the same solution.

18 An increasing number of strains are becoming resistant to the cephalosporins.

19 Chloramphenicol is the drug of choice for the treatment of typhoid fever. Ampicillin may be used as initial treatment for other types of salmonella infection. However, many strains of this microorganism are presently resistant to a wide variety of drugs; sensitivity testing is mandatory.

20 Many strains of Shigella are now resistant to ampicillin, and some are also resistant to chloramphenicol and tetracyclines.

21 Administered orally; poorly absorbed.

22 May be used if responsible strain is sensitive to sulfonamide.

Table 55-1. CURRENT USE OF ANTIMICROBIAL AGENTS IN THE THERAPY OF INFECTIONS (Continued)

IV. GRAM-NEGATIVE BACILLI	DISEASES	1st	2nd [1]	3rd [1]
		DRUG ORDER OF CHOICE		
Serratia *	Variety of opportunistic infections, primarily in patients receiving immunosuppressive therapy	Gentamicin	Chloramphenicol Kanamycin	Carbenicillin Colistimethate Nalidixic acid Polymyxin B Trimethoprim-sulfamethoxazole
Haemophilus influenzae *	Pharyngitis Otitis media Epiglottitis Laryngotracheobronchitis Pneumonia Meningitis	Ampicillin [23] Chloramphenicol [23]	Streptomycin A sulfonamide A tetracycline [24]	—
Haemophilus ducreyi	Chancroid	A tetracycline	A sulfonamide	Erythromycin Streptomycin
Acinetobacter * (Mima-Herellea group)	Urethritis Bacteremia Endocarditis Meningitis	Gentamicin Kanamycin	Carbenicillin Colistimethate Polymyxin B	—
Brucella	Brucellosis	A tetracycline ± streptomycin [25]	Chloramphenicol ± streptomycin [25]	—
Yersinia (Pasteurella) pestis	Bubonic plague	Streptomycin ± a tetracycline	A tetracycline	Chloramphenicol A sulfonamide
Francisella (Pasteurella) tularensis	Tularemia	Streptomycin	A tetracycline	Chloramphenicol
Pasteurella multocida	Abscesses Bacteremia Meningitis	Penicillin G	A tetracycline	—
Vibrio cholerae (comma)	Cholera [26]	A tetracycline	Chloramphenicol Furazolidone	Erythromycin Trimethoprim-sulfamethoxazole
Flavobacterium meningosepticum	Meningitis	Erythromycin	Rifampin	—
Pseudomonas (Actinobacillus) mallei	Glanders	Streptomycin + a tetracycline	Streptomycin + chloramphenicol	—
Pseudomonas (Actinobacillus)	Melioidosis	A tetracycline ±	Chloramphenicol	Trimethoprim-

(intestinal)	Empyema, Bacteremia	Penicillin G ...	...mycine	Penicillin G

Organism	Diseases	1st	2nd	3rd[1]
Fusobacterium nucleatum (*fusiforme*)	Ulcerative pharyngitis, Lung abscess, empyema, Genital infections, Gingivitis	Penicillin G	Chloramphenicol	Clindamycin, Erythromycin, Lincomycin, A tetracycline
Calymmatobacterium (*Donovania*) *granulomatis*	Granuloma inguinale	A tetracycline	Streptomycin	Ampicillin
Streptobacillus (*Haverhillia*) *moniliformis*	Bacteremia, Arthritis, Endocarditis, Abscesses	Penicillin G	Erythromycin, A tetracycline	A cephalosporin

V. ACID-FAST BACILLI

Organism	Diseases	DRUG ORDER OF CHOICE 1st	2nd[1]	3rd[1]
Mycobacterium tuberculosis (human type)	Pulmonary, miliary, renal, meningeal, and other tuberculous infections	Isoniazid + ethambutol[29], Isoniazid + ethambutol + streptomycin[30]	Rifampin[31]	Aminosalicylic acid[31], Cycloserine[31], Ethionamide[31], Pyrazinamide[31]
Atypical mycobacteria[32]	Lymphadenitis, Pulmonary and other lesions	Isoniazid + ethambutol, Isoniazid + ethambutol + streptomycin	Erythromycin, Rifampin	Aminosalicylic acid, Cycloserine, Ethionamide, Pyrazinamide
Mycobacterium leprae (Hansen's bacillus)	Leprosy	A sulfone	Amithiozone	—

[23] Ampicillin-resistant strains have been reported in many parts of the United States. This requires the concurrent use of penicillin G and chloramphenicol in the *initial* treatment of children with bacterial meningitis. Chloramphenicol can be discontinued if cultures demonstrate *Strep. pneumoniae* or *N. meningitidis*. If *H. influenzae* is causative, sensitivity tests are necessary to determine if ampicillin may be substituted for chloramphenicol.

[24] This agent may be effective when given alone in infections of the pharynx, larynx, trachea, and lungs. In meningitis, it does not produce as good results as when it is combined with streptomycin or as does ampicillin or chloramphenicol.

[25] Such combined therapy is useful in severe infections.

[26] The primary treatment of cholera is prompt replacement of the large loss of water and electrolytes; although this is all that is required, antimicrobial agents will usually shorten the course of the disease. Furazolidone, listed as a second-choice drug for cholera, is no longer generally available in the United States; its pharmacology is discussed in the *fourth edition* of this textbook.

[27] Surgical drainage of abscesses is necessary when they are present.

[28] Many strains of *Bacteroides fragilis* are resistant to conventional doses of penicillin G. Other species of *Bacteroides* (e.g., *B. melaninogenicus*) are sensitive to penicillin G.

[29] For pulmonary tuberculosis. For advanced disease, some experts favor isoniazid plus rifampin.

[30] Recommended by many clinicians for more severe forms of tuberculosis, such as meningitis and the disseminated (miliary) disease. Other physicians use only two of these agents, combining isoniazid with streptomycin, or isoniazid with one of the second- or third-choice drugs.

[31] Always combined with another effective tuberculostatic agent. Capreomycin, viomycin, and kanamycin are additional alternatives.

[32] Atypical mycobacteria are variably sensitive to tuberculostatic drugs. While a number of strains are sensitive to isoniazid and streptomycin, most are resistant to aminosalicylic acid. Scotochromogens may be sensitive to erythromycin. Cycloserine, ethionamide, or pyrazinamide may need to be used and should be given with another drug. All strains must be tested for sensitivity. About 85% of *M. scrofulaceum* and nearly all *M. kansasii* are sensitive to 0.5 to 2 μg/ml of erythromycin. Strains of *M. intracellulare* vary in sensitivity.

Table 55-1.   CURRENT USE OF ANTIMICROBIAL AGENTS IN THE THERAPY OF INFECTIONS (Continued)

		DRUG ORDER OF CHOICE		
VI. SPIROCHETES	DISEASES	1st	2nd [1]	3rd [1]
Treponema pallidum	Syphilis	Penicillin G	A tetracycline	Erythromycin
Treponema pertenue	Yaws	Penicillin G	A tetracycline	Erythromycin
Borrelia recurrentis	Relapsing fever	A tetracycline	Penicillin G	Chloramphenicol
Leptospira	Weil's disease Meningitis	Penicillin G	A tetracycline [33]	—

		DRUG ORDER OF CHOICE		
VII. ACTINOMYCETES	DISEASES	1st	2nd [1]	3rd [1]
Actinomyces israelii	Cervicofacial, abdominal, thoracic, and other lesions	Penicillin G [34]	Erythromycin A tetracycline	A cephalosporin Chloramphenicol Lincomycin
Nocardia *	Pulmonary lesions Brain abscess Lesions of other organs	A sulfonamide + streptomycin	A sulfonamide + ampicillin	A tetracycline + cycloserine Trimethoprim-sulfamethoxazole

		DRUG ORDER OF CHOICE		
VIII. MISCELLANEOUS AGENTS	DISEASES	1st	2nd [1]	3rd [1]
Mycoplasma pneumoniae (Eaton agent)	"Atypical viral pneumonia"	Erythromycin A tetracycline	—	—
Mycoplasma hominis	Nonspecific urethritis Pelvic abscess Septicemia	Clindamycin [35] A tetracycline	Chloramphenicol Erythromycin [36] Gentamicin Streptomycin	Kanamycin
Rickettsia	Typhus fever Murine typhus Brill's disease Rocky Mountain spotted fever Q fever Rickettsialpox	A tetracycline	Chloramphenicol	—
Chlamydia psittaci	Psittacosis (ornithosis)	A tetracycline	Chloramphenicol	Chloramphenicol

| | | DRUG ORDER OF CHOICE | | |
		1st	2nd [1]	3rd [1]
	Inclusion conjunctivitis (blennorrhea)	A tetracycline [38]	Chloramphenicol [39]	—
IX. FUNGI	DISEASES			
Candida albicans	Skin and superficial mucous membrane lesions	Amphotericin B [40] Nystatin [40]	—	—
Candida albicans *Cryptococcus neoformans* *Aspergillus*	Pneumonia Meningitis Skin lesions	Amphotericin B ± flucytosine [41]	Flucytosine	—
Coccidioides immitis *Histoplasma capsulatum* *Mucor*	Isolated lung lesions Bone lesions Disseminated disease	Amphotericin B		
Blastomyces dermatitidis	Blastomycosis (North American) [42]	Amphotericin B	Hydroxystilbamidine	—
Microsporum *Trichophyton* *Epidermophyton*	Skin, hair, and nail infections (tinea)	Griseofulvin		—
Sporothrix (Sporotrichum) schenckii	Sporotrichosis	Iodides	Amphotericin B Griseofulvin	—
X. VIRUSES	DISEASES	1st	2nd [1]	3rd [1]
Herpes simplex virus	Keratoconjunctivitis Encephalitis	Idoxuridine [43]		
Influenza virus	Influenza	Amantadine [44]	—	—

33 Some physicians favor a tetracycline over penicillin G as the drug of first choice.

34 If abscesses are present, they should be drained, regardless of the antibiotic administered.

35 Active against all strains, including T strains.

36 Most active against T strains.

37 A tetracycline may be given orally alone, or it may be applied locally in the conjunctival sac while a sulfonamide is being administered orally.

38 Topical or oral administration.

39 Topical application.

40 Applied locally.

41 Many clinicians give this combination regularly for severe infections due to these microorganisms. There is some evidence that, when a microorganism is resistant to flucytosine, the drug may suppress the activity of amphotericin B.

42 For South American blastomycosis (*Blastomyces brasiliensis*), amphotericin B is the drug of first choice, while a sulfonamide is an alternative.

43 Idoxuridine is of proven value in the therapy of keratoconjunctivitis when applied locally. It is of questionable effectiveness when used in other types of infection due to herpes simplex, including herpetic encephalitis.

44 No evidence of an important therapeutic effect, but apparently effective as prophylaxis for Asian A_2 influenza virus.

a microorganism is exposed to two drugs at the same time, the development of resistance to each agent is appreciably delayed but not completely prevented; this is usually true only when the microorganism is sensitive to both agents. Clinical investigations have indicated that delay of emergence of antibiotic resistance is produced by therapy with two or more antimicrobial drugs in some but not all types of infection. Thus, it is now well established that the concomitant administration of two or more appropriate drugs suppresses strikingly the development of resistance in the tubercle bacillus. Tuberculosis is best treated, therefore, with at least two and in some instances, when the number of infecting microorganisms is great, three tuberculostatic agents simultaneously.

3. Enhancement of Antibacterial Activity in Treatment of Specific Infections.

Increase in antibacterial activity and in clinical effectiveness results from the use of two or more antimicrobial drugs in some but not all infections. In many, a lack of enhancement of, or even a *decrease* in, therapeutic efficiency is observed with such medication.

Infections in Which Concurrent Therapy with Antimicrobial Agents Is Superior to Single Agents. An outstanding example of the superiority of concurrent therapy over the use of a single drug is tuberculosis. Infections produced by *enterococci* respond better, in most instances, in persons treated with penicillin plus streptomycin than with either of these agents alone. Chloramphenicol plus a sulfonamide produces a higher recovery rate in meningitis due to *Haemophilus influenzae* than does the use of the antibiotic alone. *Brucellosis* appears to respond best when treated with a tetracycline together with streptomycin (Killough, 1957). Thus, when chlortetracycline or chloramphenicol is used alone for a period of 12 days, the relapse rate is about 80%; the simultaneous administration of streptomycin and chlortetracycline for 3 weeks reduces this rate to less than 20%. However, duration of therapy is also important, as emphasized by the fact that the number of relapses is only 10% when a tetracycline is given for 6 weeks.

Infections in Which Concurrent Therapy with Certain Antimicrobial Agents Is Inferior to Single Agents. One impressive example of the inferiority of combination therapy in certain infections should serve as sufficient warning. The addition of a broad-spectrum antibiotic to penicillin G in the treatment of pneumococcal meningitis yields a therapeutic result distinctly inferior to that which follows the administration of penicillin alone. In one study, the fatality rate in patients receiving only penicillin was 30%; of those given penicillin plus chlortetracycline, 79% died (Lepper and Dowling, 1951).

It must be stressed that, in many instances, the therapeutic activity of concomitantly administered antimicrobial agents is unpredictable. *Such therapy is often not as good as with the most effective single agent.* Except for cases of severe bacterial infections in which the etiology cannot be delineated and in which delay in treatment may be dangerous, the simultaneous use of two or more anti-infective drugs should be restricted to diseases in which their superiority over single drugs has been proven clinically. When multiple therapy is employed in such situations, the physician should select the agents that he knows are the best and administer each in the same dose as is given when it is administered alone.

4. Therapy of Severe Infections in Which the Specific Etiology Is Unknown.

The most common use of multiple antimicrobial drugs is for the treatment of infections the etiology of which is not immediately apparent. The physician with a patient in whom he suspects an infection often decides that chemotherapy is necessary. Because the exact cause cannot be immediately determined, more than one agent is given in the hope that this will "cover" the situation. In not a small number of cases, the infectious process is due to some virus and the application of *any* currently known antimicrobial agent is not indicated.

In some instances, such multiple therapy results in a broadening of antibacterial activity. This has been demonstrated, for example, with concomitant use of penicillin and streptomycin. It must be emphasized, however, that this phenomenon has followed the use of full therapeutic doses of each drug. If "full-dose" combinations are to be given in the absence of complete bacteriological laboratory reports, the physician must decide, on the basis of the clinical features of the disease, a detailed history, and the initial laboratory investigations, including examination of stained preparations if possible, not only that a patient has a bacterial infection but also the type of organism most likely to be involved. *Under no circumstances must chemotherapy be initiated until all the necessary bacteriological investigations have been started.* Cultures can be taken in only a few minutes and cause no significant delay.

It must be stressed that the initiation of a chemotherapeutic program obviously should not commit the physician to its continuance. If bacteriological studies and sensitivity tests indicate that some drug other than those being used is more effective, this agent should be given promptly, especially if the clinical response has not been optimal. Every effort should be made to treat patients with single antimicrobial agents in maximal therapeutic doses. No one has yet devised a combination of antibiotics, regardless of the number of agents included, that will cure all infections. There probably will never be such a panacea. The use of three or four antibiotics at one time in etiologically obscure infections is a deplorable therapeutic maneuver that must be avoided.

Disadvantages of "Fixed-Dose" Combinations of Antimicrobial Agents. The United States Food and Drug Administration has withdrawn approval of almost all "fixed-dose" combinations for several reasons. These antibiotic combinations encourage inadequate treatment because there is an inevitable tendency to employ the same total dose of the mixture as of a single agent. Such a dose does not necessarily provide an effective amount of any single agent in the combination, particularly of the superior drug. Mixtures provide a false sense of security with regard to a wider coverage or "broad spectrum" of activity. In fact they supply a narrower effective coverage by substituting less effective agents and smaller amounts of individual drugs than if the antimicrobial agents were selected individually, each for its own value, and administered in the proper dose for the purpose intended. They reduce the therapeutic effectiveness that would be anticipated from proper doses of individual drugs or from proper choice of extemporaneous concurrent therapy according to specific requirements, especially when care is taken to choose only agents that may be expected to be most effective against the causative microorganism. Most "fixed-dose" preparations thus have no place in the management of infection. There is, however, one significant exception (trimethoprim-sulfamethoxazole; *see* Chapter 56).

THE PROPHYLAXIS OF INFECTION

Antimicrobial agents have been used in attempts to prevent infection in a variety of situations on the assumption that, if a drug is effective in eradicating microorganisms that have already become established, it should easily discourage their implantation. Because of this view, chemoprophylaxis has been employed, not always wisely, primarily for four purposes, as follows: (1) to protect healthy persons, singly or in groups, against invasion by specific microorganisms to which they have been exposed; (2) to prevent secondary bacterial infection in individuals acutely ill with disease, often due to viruses, for which anti-infective drugs are of no direct help; (3) to reduce the risk of infection in people with various types of chronic illness; and (4) to inhibit the spread of disease from areas of localized infection, or to prevent infection in general, in patients who have been subjected to accidental or surgical trauma. Clinical studies have indicated that there are some areas in which chemoprophylaxis is highly effective and others in which it is totally without value and may, in fact, be associated with either an increased incidence of infection or infection with resistant microorganisms. There are still, however, situations where opinion concerning the efficacy of antimicrobial compounds in preventing bacterial invasion is unsettled.

The following generalizations have been found to apply when antibiotics are administered prophylactically (Weinstein, 1954): (1) *When a single effective drug is used to avoid implantation of a specific microorganism or to eradicate it immediately or shortly after it has become established, but not yet clinically evident, chemoprophylaxis is, with uncommon exception, highly successful.* (2) *If the aim of prophylaxis is to prevent colonization and/or infection by any and all microorganisms that may be present in the internal or external environment of a patient, failure is the rule.* For example, the use of penicillin G to prevent invasion by group-A streptococci or to inhibit the development of gonorrhea after contact is usually highly successful. Contrariwise, administration of any kind of anti-infective drug will not prevent bacterial or mycotic invasion in newborn infants or in patients at increased risk of infection for any of a variety of reasons.

There is no firm evidence that chemoprophylaxis in patients with chronic obstructive pulmonary disease or during catheterization of the urinary tract is effective. Prophylactic drug administration for a week or longer in patients undergoing surgical procedures on the heart, intestinal tract, lungs, and other sites in the attempt to prevent invasion by any or all microorganisms is of questionable efficacy. Furthermore, there is risk of suprainfection, the incidence of which is directly related to the time of exposure to the antibiotic. An approach that may reduce the frequency of suprainfection is to use chemoprophylaxis for only a short period—immediately preoperatively, during certain surgical procedures, and for no more than 24 to 48 hours after the operation is completed. Although sufficient data are not yet available to prove that the incidence of postoperative infections is significantly reduced, this approach merits more study. The specific details of the chemoprophylactic use of anti-infective agents are presented in the discussion of the drugs concerned.

ADVERSE REACTIONS TO
CHEMOTHERAPEUTIC AGENTS

The reactions produced by anti-infective agents are of three general types. There is no difference in concept between *toxic effects* and *hypersensitivity reactions* caused by antimicrobial agents and other classes of drugs. More distinctive, however, are *biological and metabolic alterations in the host,* including alterations in normal microbial flora, suprainfections, and interference with nutrition. These effects may be induced, in varying degree, by the administration of any of the antimicrobials (*see* Weinstein and Weinstein, 1974).

Although practically all individuals who receive therapeutic doses of these agents undergo alterations in the normal microbial population of the intestinal, upper respiratory, and genitourinary tracts, some develop *suprainfection* as a result of such changes. This phenomenon may be defined as the appearance of bacteriological and clinical evidence of a new infection during the chemotherapy of a primary one (*see* Weinstein, 1964). It is relatively common and potentially very dangerous because the microorganisms responsible for the new disease are, in many cases, *Proteus* strains, drug-resistant staphylococci, *Pseudomonas, Candida,* and true fungi; these may be very difficult to eradicate with the presently available anti-infective drugs. Several factors have been found to play a role in the pathogenesis of suprainfection (Weinstein *et al.,* 1954). These are: (1) age under 3 years, (2) the presence of acute or chronic pulmonary disease other than tuberculosis, and (3) the range of antibacterial activity of single or combined drugs. The more "broad" the effect of an antibiotic on microorganisms, the greater is the possibility that a single component of the normal microflora will become predominant, invade, and produce infection. Thus, the incidence of suprainfections is lowest with penicillin G and highest with the tetracyclines and chloramphenicol and with mixtures of broad-spectrum antibiotics.

The proper management of *suprainfections* involves (1) immediate discontinuance of the drug being given, (2) culture of the suspected infected area, and (3) administration of an antimicrobial agent effective against the new offending microorganism. Suprainfections may be prevented, in some cases, by repeated culture of the upper respiratory tract, urine, and feces during chemotherapy. If a potentially pathogenic microorganism becomes highly predominant or is the only constituent of the flora, the administration of a drug to which it is sensitive may be effective.

The fact that harmful effects may follow the therapeutic or the prophylactic use of anti-infective agents must never discourage the physician from their administration in any situation in which they are definitely indicated. It should, however, make him very careful in their use when they are required, and very hesitant to employ them in instances in which indications for their application are either entirely lacking or, at most, only suggestive. To do otherwise is to run the risk, at times, of converting a simple, benign, and self-limited disease into one that may be serious or even fatal.

HOST DETERMINANTS OF RESPONSE
TO ANTIMICROBIAL AGENTS

Although the nature of an infection determines to a great degree the kind of antimicrobial therapy to be employed, innate host factors, completely unrelated to the disorder, are often the prime determinants not only of the type of drug selected but also of its dose, route of administration, risk and nature of untoward effects, and therapeutic effectiveness. Among such factors are age, genetic background, pregnancy, concurrent disease, allergy, nervous system abnormalities, indigenous microbial flora, hepatic function, renal function and electrolyte balance, and host defense mechanisms (*see* Weinstein and Dalton, 1968).

Age. Although the dose schedule of many of the commonly used antimicrobial drugs may be calculated on the basis of body weight or surface area, that of others, especially those excreted in unchanged form by the kidney (*e.g.,* the penicillins), is greatly influenced by the state of renal function, which, in turn, is influenced by age. Age also plays an important role in the risk of some types of reactions, the route of administration, and the therapeutic effectiveness (*see* McCracken, 1974).

Renal function is relatively poor in newborn children, especially those who are premature, and in older persons. Complete renal maturity is probably not reached until the age of 1 year. With advancing age and in old people, glomerular function, effective blood flow, and tubular excretion diminish. Therefore, the dose of a number of antimicrobial agents, especially those excreted in biologically active form by the kidney, must be relatively low in the first month of life, particularly in premature babies, considerably higher in young children, and greatly reduced in individuals over the age of 50, even when blood urea nitrogen and creatinine concentrations are within the normal range.

Because gastric acid secretion is relatively low during the first month of life and in the old (one third of individuals aged 60 to 90 years have achlorhydria), higher-than-expected blood concentrations of penicillin G may follow oral administration of this antibiotic in these age groups.

The type of reaction to an antimicrobial agent is determined by age in some instances. Because the liver of newborn babies contains only small quantities of glucuronyl transferase, the enzyme involved in the inactivation of chloramphenicol by conjugation with uridine diphosphate (UDP) glucuronic acid, death may result from excessively high blood concentrations of unconjugated, biologically active, toxic drug due to improper dosage. The immaturity of the acetylation process in the liver of the newborn may expose babies to high blood concentrations of sulfonamides. Kernicterus may follow the use of sulfisoxazole in newborn infants because the drug competes effectively with bilirubin for binding sites on plasma albumin. The teeth of young children are very susceptible to discoloration and enamel hypoplasia when tetracycline compounds are administered in the period of 2 months to 2 or more years of age. Disturbances in bone growth may also be produced in youngsters receiving this class of antibiotics.

Genetic Factors. The rate at which isoniazid is inactivated in the liver by acetylation is genetically determined. Acute hemolysis may develop in individuals given some antimicrobial compounds in the presence of glucose-6-phosphate dehydrogenase (G-6-PD) deficiency. Although common in Negro males, the defect may result in more severe hemolysis in white people despite a lower incidence. Representative antimicrobial drugs that have provoked episodes of hemolytic anemia in such people are sulfonamides, chloramphenicol, nitrofurantoin, and dapsone. Patients with hemoglobin Zurich and hemoglobin H may also develop hemolysis when given some of these agents.

Pregnancy. Pregnancy imposes an increased risk of reactions to some antimicrobial agents on both the mother and her fetus. Most of these drugs cross the placental barrier (*see* McCracken, 1974). The fetus may suffer some degree of hearing loss when streptomycin is given to its mother. Sulfonamides and isoniazid have produced fetal injury when administered during pregnancy. The tetracyclines pose a special danger to the fetus; the developing teeth may be injured if one of these compounds is given from midpregnancy on, the period when the crowns of the teeth are being formed. The pregnant patient

with pyelonephritis who is treated with a tetracycline may suffer fatal hepatic toxicity; pancreatitis has also been noted in such patients.

Concurrent Disease. Penicillin G and sulfonamides are absorbed from intramuscular and subcutaneous sites to a lesser degree in persons with diabetes mellitus than in those who do not have this metabolic defect. This results in maximal plasma concentrations that are lower and develop more slowly than in normal individuals. If chloramphenicol is given to patients with pernicious anemia or iron-deficiency anemia, the response to therapy with cyanocobalamin or iron, respectively, may be poor.

Atopic Allergy. Persons with a history of atopic allergy are highly susceptible to the development of hypersensitivity to antimicrobial agents, whether or not they have been exposed to them previously.

Nervous System Disorders. Patients with either localized or diffuse nervous system disease are more prone to the development of seizures than are normal individuals when treated with "massive" doses (40 to 80 million units per day) of penicillin G. Penetration of chloramphenicol into cerebrospinal fluid is impaired by the presence of hydrocephalus. The aminoglycosides, polymyxin, and colistin may cause peripheral respiratory arrest in anesthetized patients, especially if they have received a neuromuscular blocking agent. This reaction may particularly occur in patients with myasthenia gravis, and is a problem in the presence of renal failure.

Indigenous Microbial Flora. The microorganisms responsible for suprainfections are, for the most part, members of the normal microbial flora that inhabit various areas of the body such as the intestinal and upper respiratory tracts. In some cases, the microorganisms are derived from the external environment and become part of the indigenous microflora. The normal microflora may condition the response to treatment in special situations. Therapeutic failure or relapse of *Strep. pyogenes* pharyngitis treated with penicillin G may be due to the presence in the throat of penicillinase-producing *Staph. aureus, E. coli, Pseud. aeruginosa,* or *Klebsiella.*

Hepatic Function. Antimicrobial agents that are metabolized, inactivated, or concentrated in the liver may cause abnormal responses when administered to persons with impaired hepatic function. Blood concentrations of chloramphenicol are elevated in such patients, and toxic reactions may supervene. Persons with cirrhosis or chronic or convalescent hepatitis may experience untoward effects when given 2 g of tetracycline orally per day. The half-life of lincomycin is almost doubled in the presence of hepatic dysfunction. Penicillins concentrated in the liver (methicillin, ampicillin, nafcillin) may be absent, or present only in reduced quantities, in the bile in patients with hepatic disease. Erythromycin and rifampin must be used with caution when hepatic dysfunction is present. Those antimicrobial agents that are eliminated in the bile or inactivated in the liver are indicated in Table 55–2.

Table 55–2. ROUTES OF ELIMINATION AND HALF-LIVES OF ANTIMICROBIAL AGENTS AND ADJUSTMENTS OF DOSAGE SCHEDULES ON THE BASIS OF RENAL FUNCTION *

DRUG	ROUTES OF EXCRETION OR INACTIVATION; [1] NORMAL HALF-LIFE (HOURS)	MAINTENANCE DOSE INTERVALS (HOURS) [2]				SIGNIFICANT DIALYSIS OF DRUG [3]
		Creatinine Clearance (ml/min) =				
		>80	*50 to 80*	*10 to 50*	*<10*	
Aminoglycosides						
Gentamicin	Renal; 2	8	12	12–36	48–72	+H; −P
Kanamycin	Renal; 3–4	8	24	24–72	72–96	+H,P
Streptomycin	Renal; 2.5	12	24	24–72	72–96	+H,P
Amphotericin B	Nonrenal; 18–24	24	24	24	24–36	−H
Cephalosporins						
Cefazolin	Renal (hepatic); 1.5	6	12	12 [4]	24 [5]	−H,P
Cephalexin	Renal (nonrenal); 0.6–1	6	6	6–12	18–24	+H,P
Cephaloridine	Renal; 1.5	6	NR [6]	NR	NR	+H,P
Cephalothin	Renal, hepatic; 0.5–0.8	6	6	8	8–12	+H,P
Chloramphenicol	Hepatic (renal); 2.5	6	6	6	6	−H,P
Clindamycin	Hepatic (renal); 2	6	6	6	6	−H,P
Colistimethate	Renal; 2	12	24	36–60	60–90	±H,P
Erythromycin	Hepatic; 1.5	6	6	6	6	−H,P
Flucytosine	Renal; 3–4	6	12	12–24	NR [6]	+H,P
Lincomycin	Hepatic (renal); 5	6	6	6	8–12	−H,P
Penicillins						
Amoxicillin	Renal; 1	8	8	12	16	+H
Ampicillin	Renal, hepatic; 1.5	6	6	9	12	+H; −P
Carbenicillin	Renal, hepatic; 1.5	4	4	6–12	12–16	+H; −P
Cloxacillin Dicloxacillin	Hepatic, renal; 0.5	6	6	6	6	−H
Methicillin	Renal, hepatic; 0.5	4	4	4	8–12	−H,P
Nafcillin	Hepatic (renal); 0.5	6	6	8	12	−H
Oxacillin	Renal, hepatic; 0.5	6	6	6	8–12	−H,P
Penicillin-G	Renal, hepatic; 0.5	8	8	8	12	−H,P
Sulfisoxazole	Renal; 5	6	6	8–12	12–24	+H,P
Tetracyclines						
Chlortetracycline Oxytetracycline Tetracycline	Renal, hepatic; 6–9	6	NR [6]	NR	NR	−H,P
Demeclocycline Methacycline	Renal, hepatic; 15–17	12	NR [6]	NR	NR	−H,P

**Table 55-2. ROUTES OF ELIMINATION AND HALF-LIVES
OF ANTIMICROBIAL AGENTS AND ADJUSTMENTS OF DOSAGE
SCHEDULES ON THE BASIS OF RENAL FUNCTION * (Continued)**

DRUG	ROUTES OF EXCRETION OR INACTIVATION; [1] NORMAL HALF-LIFE (HOURS)	MAINTENANCE DOSE INTERVALS (HOURS) [2] Creatinine Clearance (ml/min) =				SIGNIFICANT DIALYSIS OF DRUG [3]
		>80	50 to 80	10 to 50	<10	
Tetracyclines (Cont.)						
Minocycline	Hepatic, renal; 18	12–24	NR [6]	NR	NR	–H,P
Doxycycline	Hepatic, renal; 20	12–24	12–24	12–24	12–24	–H,P
Tuberculostatic Agents						
Ethambutol	Renal; 6–8	24	24	24–36	48	+H,P
Isoniazid [7]	Renal, hepatic; 2–4	8	8	8	8	+H,P
Rifampin	Hepatic; 3	24	24	24	24	?
Urinary Tract Antiseptics						
Methenamine mandelate	Renal; 4	6	6	NR [6]	NR	?
Nalidixic acid [8]	Renal; 1.5–2	6	6	6	6	?
Nitrofurantoin	Renal; 0.3	8	8	8	NR [6]	+H
Vancomycin	Renal; 6	6	24–72	72–240	240	–H,P

* Most of the data for this table were obtained from Bennett, Singer, and Coggins (1974) and from *Handbook of Antimicrobial Therapy* (1974).

[1] Minor routes of drug disposition are indicated in parentheses.

[2] Maintenance dose intervals (in hours) are based on typical dosage schedules. They should be considered only as representative. Other dosage schedules for an individual agent can be adjusted in proportion to the changes shown. Loading doses are not influenced by alterations of drug disposition.

[3] Significant dialysis indicates a requirement for additional medication following dialysis. H = hemodialysis; P = peritoneal dialysis; + (plus sign) = significant; – (minus sign) = insignificant. A lack of requirement for additional medication following dialysis does not necessarily indicate a lack of utility of dialysis for the treatment of intoxication by the drug.

[4] Reduce dose to 7 mg/kg every 12 hours.

[5] Reduce dose to 5 mg/kg every 24 hours.

[6] NR = not recommended.

[7] There is genetic variation in the hepatic disposition of isoniazid. Slow acetylators of the drug who have reduced renal function may require prolongation of the dose interval.

[8] Inactive, nontoxic metabolite accumulates.

Renal Function. Renal function is one of the most important determinants of the response to antimicrobial agents (Kunin and Finland, 1959; Kunin et al., 1959). It not only is a major consideration in the choice of a drug but also influences the selection of dose and the risk of reactions involving the kidney and other organs. The extent to which elimination of an anti-infective agent is affected by the presence of renal disease and appropriate modifications of dosage schedules are presented in Table 55-2. Drugs that are eliminated almost entirely by the kidney include the penicillins, cephalosporins, aminoglycosides, vancomycin, colistimethate, and polymyxin. The tetracyclines are cleared at varying rates; this determines their degree of toxicity when renal dysfunction is a problem. The amount of erythromycin and lincomycin excreted in the urine is small, whereas that of aminosalicylic acid and isoniazid is large.

The mode of inactivation and excretion of antimicrobial agents should be known by all physicians who use them. It is important that the status of renal function be determined not only before but also during the entire period of treatment, if serious or even lethal effects are to be avoided when potentially toxic agents, especially those that may injure the kidney, are administered. It must be stressed that, even when blood urea nitrogen and creatinine concentrations are normal, older individuals may accumulate a particular drug and experience toxic reactions if the agent is excreted mainly by the kidney, since tubular secretory capacity, not measured by the above indices, may play a predominant role.

Host Defense Mechanisms. Probably the most important determinant of the therapeutic effectiveness of antimicrobial agents is the functional state of the defense mechanisms of the host. Both humoral and cellular phenomena are involved. Inadequacy of type, quantity, and quality of the immunoglobulins, altered or delayed hypersensitivity, and ineffective phagocytosis, acting independently or in varying combination, may result in therapeutic failure despite use of an otherwise effective and appropriate drug. This may occur in Hodgkin's disease, lymphoma, leukemia, cancer of various types, uremia, vasculitis, and granulomatous disease of childhood, disorders in which immunosuppression, abnormal activity of immunoglobulins, or inadequate phagocytosis are problems. In addition, some of the drugs commonly employed to treat these disorders (cytotoxic agents, antimetabolites, corticosteroids), as well as to prevent rejection of transplanted organs, may add to the difficulty because of their immunosuppressive properties.

That the normal activity of defense mechanisms is an absolute requirement for the therapeutic effectiveness of all antimicrobial agents is frequently overlooked. The bacteriostatic drugs should, by definition, never completely eradicate sensitive microorganisms. However, *cure* of some infectious diseases is accomplished by these agents and relapse does not occur when treatment is stopped. This is strong evidence for the intervention of effective host defenses, which, acting on microorganisms after they have been injured by one of these compounds, are responsible for the final eradication of infection. Clinical experience suggests that even bactericidal antibiotics probably require the adjunct activity of cellular and humoral defenses to dispose of bacteria.

MISUSES OF ANTIMICROBIAL DRUGS AND CAUSES OF FAILURE OF THERAPY

Treatment of Untreatable Infections. A common misuse of these agents is in infections that have been proved by experimental and clinical observation to be untreatable. None of the diseases due to the true viruses will respond to any of the presently available anti-infective compounds. Thus, the antimicrobial therapy of measles, chickenpox, mumps, and at least 90% of infections of the upper respiratory tract is totally ineffective and, therefore, worse than useless.

Therapy of Fever of Undetermined Origin. Fever of undetermined etiology may be of two types: one that is present for only a few days to a week and another that persists for an extended period. Both of these are fre-

quently treated with antimicrobial agents when their etiology is unknown. Most instances of pyrexia of short duration, in the absence of localizing signs, are associated with undefined viral infections, often of the upper respiratory tract, and usually do not respond to such drugs; in the bulk of these cases, defervescence takes place spontaneously within a week or less. Studies of prolonged fever have shown that the two most common infectious causes are tuberculosis, often of the disseminated variety, and subacute bacterial endocarditis. Also, the so-called collagen disorders and various neoplasms are frequently responsible for prolonged and significant degrees of fever. A 5-year study in one clinic has shown that the most common cause of persistent fever is lymphoma, often undetectable because it is situated intra-abdominally. Various types of cancer, metabolic disorders, asymptomatic regional enteritis, atypical rheumatoid arthritis, and a number of other noninfectious disorders may present themselves as cases of fever of unknown etiology (Weinstein, 1963).

It has been suggested that fever of longer than 1-week duration merits the use of antimicrobial agents since, if a treatable condition has defied recognition, it will respond, and that failure to improve indicates the presence of nonbacterial disease. Experience has taught, however, that this approach is not only futile but dangerous for three reasons. (1) Untoward reactions to the drugs may occur. (2) The use of antimicrobial agents in an etiologically undefined situation that eventually proves to be noninfectious results in delay in application of more effective therapy, when this is available. Thus, the patient with a malignancy, who in the absence of a diagnosis is given antibacterial drugs, is denied the opportunity of cure or palliation. (3) Difficulty may arise from the nonspecific use of antimicrobial therapy even in instances of fever due to bacterial infection. This is well illustrated by experiences with subacute bacterial endocarditis when the only manifestation is an elevated temperature. Until the diagnosis is made, this situation is frequently treated empirically with one or another anti-infective agent, on and off, sometimes for weeks, before careful studies are finally carried out and blood cultures reveal the true nature of the disease. The dangers of prolonged delay in applying effective therapy in subacute bacterial endocarditis have been thoroughly documented.

It must be stressed that the anti-infective agents are not antipyretics. The most rational approach to the problem of fever of unknown etiology is not one that concentrates on the elevated temperature alone but one that involves a thorough search for its cause, before the patient is exposed to chemotherapy in the hope, often in vain, that, if one agent is not effective, another one or a combination of drugs will be helpful.

Improper Dosage. Erroneous dosage of antimicrobial agents is of two types: administration of excessive amounts and use of suboptimal quantities. There is little doubt that harm may be produced by overdoses of most antimicrobial agents. The difficulties that may arise from drug overdosage in patients with impairment of elimination have already been discussed.

A large area of misuse of antibacterial agents has been created by the administration of doses that are too small or that, although adequate in amount, are given for too short a period of time. As a general rule, the treatment of serious systemic infection requires that patients receive maximal quantities of drug rather than the relatively small amounts usually employed for the therapy of minor illnesses.

Improper Duration of Therapy. One of the most common examples of the problems that may arise from failure to administer antimicrobial drugs for a sufficiently long period is provided by streptococcal pharyngitis. A patient is seen with a sore throat, and, in the absence of a specific diagnosis, a single injection of penicillin G, usually the procaine salt, is administered. Clinical improvement occurs, persists for a few days, and is then followed by recurrence of pharyngeal discomfort. This prompts injection of another dose of the same drug. Again the sore throat disappears, recurs after a short time, and is again treated with a single injection of the antibiotic. This may continue for many days, and a disease that can be eradicated rapidly by continued administration of penicillin for 8 to 10 days is converted into one persisting, with repeated remissions and relapses, until the bacteriological diagnosis is finally established and proper therapy instituted.

There are numerous other examples of difficulty created by abbreviating the duration of therapy. The treatment of staphylococcal pneumonia or endocarditis for less than 4 weeks is accompanied by an unfortunately high incidence of recurrence. In chronic gonococcal diseases such as gonococcal arthritis and salpingitis, cure cannot be expected unless therapy is continued for 10 days to 2 weeks.

Reliance on Chemotherapy with Omission of Surgical Drainage. To rely on anti-infective agents alone to cure some types of infections is to place a demand on them that they cannot always satisfy. The conditions in which this is a problem are usually those with appreciable quantities of purulent exudate or necrotic or avascular infected tissues. A few of many possible examples will be cited. The patient with staphylococcal pneumonia with empyema often fails to be cured by the administration of large doses of an effective drug until constant catheter drainage of the involved area is established. Brain abscess is little affected by antimicrobial therapy alone; for the best results, it must be combined with surgical drainage or extirpation of the lesion. The patient with renal lithiasis will frequently suffer recurrent episodes of acute pyelonephritis, regardless of the number of times he is treated with antimicrobial agents, until the stones are removed. As a generalization, it may be said that, when an appreciable quantity of pus, or necrotic tissue, or a foreign body is a problem, the most effective treatment is a combination of an antimicrobial agent given in adequate dose plus a properly performed surgical procedure; to attempt to treat such conditions with drugs alone represents a misuse of these agents.

Lack of Adequate Bacteriological Information. It has been documented for hospitalized patients that one half of the courses of antimicrobial therapy are administered in the absence of support from the microbiological laboratory. It is clear that the great bulk of the hospital use of these drugs is based on clinical judgment alone. A high proportion of the use is for chemoprophylaxis of questionable value. Bacterial cultures are obtained too infrequently, and the results, when available, are disregarded all too frequently in the selection and application of drug therapy. Frequent use of drug combinations is a cover for diagnostic imprecision. The agents selected are more likely to be those of habit rather than for specific indications, and the dosages employed are routine. Antimicrobial drug therapy must be individualized on the basis of the clinical situation, microbiological information, and the pharmacological considerations presented in this and the subsequent chapters of this section. (For discussions of patterns of antibiotic administration by physicians, *see* Adler *et al.*, 1971; Macaraeg *et al.*, 1971; Resztak and Williams, 1972; Roberts and Visconti, 1972; Jackson, 1973.)

Adler, J. L.; Burke, J. P.; and Finland, M. Infection and antibiotic usage at Boston City Hospital, January, 1970. *Archs intern. Med.,* **1971,** *127,* 460–465.

Bauer, A. W.; Kirby, W. M. M.; Sherris, J. C.; and Turk, M. Antibiotic susceptibility testing by a standardized single disc method. *Am. J. clin. Path.,* **1966,** *45,* 493–496.

Bennett, W. M.; Singer, I.; and Coggins, C. J. A guide to drug therapy in renal failure. *J. Am. med. Ass.,* **1974,** *230,* 1544–1553.

Chang, T. W., and Weinstein, L. Inhibitory effects of other antibiotics on bacterial morphologic changes induced by penicillin G. *Nature, Lond.,* **1966,** *211,* 763–765.

Jawetz, E. Combined antibiotic action: some definitions and correlations between laboratory and clinical results. In, *Antimicrobial Agents and Chemotherapy—1967.* American Society for Microbiology, Ann Arbor, Mich., **1968,** pp. 203–209.

Jawetz, E., and Gunnison, J. B. Studies on antibiotic synergism and antagonism: the scheme of combined antimicrobial activity. *Antibiotics Chemother.,* **1952,** *2,* 243–248.

Jawetz, E.; Gunnison, J. B.; Speck, R. S.; and Coleman, V. B. Studies on antibiotic synergism and antagonism: the interference of chloramphenicol with the action of penicillin. *A.M.A. Archs intern. Med.,* **1951,** *87,* 349–359.

Killough, J. H. Combination antibiotic therapy of brucellosis. *Postgrad. Med.,* **1957,** *22,* 527.

Kunin, C. M., and Finland, M. Persistence of antibiotics in blood of patients with acute renal failure. III. Penicillin, streptomycin, erythromycin and kanamycin. *J. clin. Invest.,* **1959,** *38,* 1509–1519.

Kunin, C. M.; Glazko, A. J.; and Finland, M. Persistence of antibiotics in blood of patients with renal failure. II. Chloramphenicol and its metabolic products in the blood of patients with severe renal diseases and hepatic necrosis. *J. clin. Invest.,* **1959,** *38,* 1498–1508.

Lepper, M. H., and Dowling, H. F. Treatment of pneumococcic meningitis with penicillin compared with penicillin plus AUREOMYCIN. *A.M.A. Archs intern. Med.,* **1951,** *88,* 489–494.

Macaraeg, P. V. J.; Lasagna, L.; and Bianchine, J. R. A study of hospital staff attitudes concerning the comparative merits of antibiotics. *Clin. Pharmac. Ther.,* **1971,** *12,* 1–12.

Pasteur, L., and Joubert, J. Charbonne et septicemie. *C. r. hebd. Séanc. Acad. Sci., Paris,* **1877,** *85,* 101–115.

Resztak, K. E., and Williams, R. B. A review of antibiotic therapy in patients with systemic infections. *Am. J. hosp. Pharm.,* **1972,** *29,* 935–941.

Roberts, A. W., and Visconti, J. A. The rational and irrational use of systemic antimicrobial drugs. *Am. J. hosp. Pharm.,* **1972,** *29,* 828–834.

Schatz, A.; Bugie, E.; and Waksman, S. A. Streptomycin, a substance exhibiting antibiotic activity against gram-positive and gram-negative bacteria. *Proc. Soc. exp. Biol. Med.,* **1944,** *55,* 449–450.

Weinstein, L. Superinfection: a complication of antimicrobial therapy and prophylaxis. *Am. J. Surg.,* **1964,** *107,* 704–709.

Weinstein, L.; Goldfield, M.; and Chang, T. W. Infections occurring during chemotherapy: a study of their frequency, type and predisposing factors. *New Engl. J. Med.,* **1954,** *251,* 247–254.

Monographs and Reviews

Buchanan, R. E., and Gibbons, N. E. (eds.). *Bergey's Manual of Determinative Bacteriology,* 8th ed. The Williams & Wilkins Co., Baltimore, **1974.**

Davies, J.; Brzezinska, M.; and Benveniste, R. R factors: biochemical mechanisms of resistance to aminoglycoside antibiotics. *Ann. N.Y. Acad. Sci.,* **1971,** *182,* 226–233.

Ericsson, H. M., and Sherris, J. C. Antibiotic sensitivity testing. Report of an international collaborative study. *Acta path. microbiol. scand., B,* **1971,** Suppl. 217, 1–90.

Florey, H. W. Historical introduction. *Antibiotics,* Vol. I. (Florey, H. W., *et al.,* authors.) Oxford University Press, New York, **1949.**

Handbook of Antimicrobial Therapy. Medical Letter, Inc., New Rochelle, N.Y., **1974.**

Jackson, G. G. Practice, precision and promise in chemotherapy. *Proceedings, International Congress on Chemotherapy.* Athens, **1973.**

McCracken, G. H., Jr. Pharmacological basis for antimicrobial therapy in newborn infants. *Am. J. Dis. Child.,* **1974,** *128,* 407–419.

Mitsuhashi, S. The R factors. *J. infect. Dis.,* **1969,** *119,* 89–100.

Pestka, S. Inhibitors of ribosome functions. *A. Rev. Microbiol.,* **1971,** *25,* 487–562.

Sabath, L. D. Drug resistance of bacteria. *New Engl. J. Med.,* **1969,** *280,* 91–94.

Sanford, J. P. *Guide to Antimicrobial Therapy.* University of Texas, Southwestern Medical School, Dallas, **1973.**

Symposium. (Various authors.) Mode of action of antibiotics on microbial walls and membranes. (Salton, M. R. J., and Tomasz, A., eds.) *Ann. N.Y. Acad. Sci.,* **1974,** *235,* 1–620.

Watanabe, T. Infectious drug resistance in bacteria. *New Engl. J. Med.,* **1966,** *275,* 888–894.

Weinstein, L. The complications of antibiotic therapy. *Bull. N.Y. Acad. Med.,* **1954,** *31,* 500–518.

———. The use and abuse of antibiotic combinations. *J. Maine med. Ass.,* **1958,** *49,* 176–182.

———. The use and abuse of antimicrobial agents. *Med. Sci.,* **1963,** *14,* 35–40.

Weinstein, L., and Dalton, A. C. Host determinants of response to antimicrobial agents. *New Engl. J. Med.,* **1968,** *279,* 467–473, 524–531, 580–588. (208 references.)

Weinstein, L., and Weinstein, A. J. The pathophysiology and pathoanatomy of reactions to antimicrobial agents. *Adv. intern. Med.,* **1974,** *19,* 109–134.

Weisblum, B., and Davies, J. Antibiotic inhibitors of the bacterial ribosome. *Bact. Rev.,* **1968,** *32,* 493–528. (232 references.)

CHAPTER

56 ANTIMICROBIAL AGENTS

[*Continued*]

Sulfonamides and Trimethoprim-Sulfamethoxazole

Louis Weinstein

SULFONAMIDES

The sulfonamide drugs were the first effective chemotherapeutic agents to be employed systemically for the prevention and cure of bacterial infections in man. The considerable medical and public health importance of their discovery and their subsequent widespread use were quickly reflected in the sharp decline in morbidity and mortality figures for the treatable infectious diseases. Before penicillin became generally available, the sulfonamides were the mainstay of antibacterial chemotherapy. The advent of antibiotics has made large inroads on the popularity and fields of usefulness of the sulfonamides. They continue, however, to occupy an important although relatively small place in the therapeutic armamentarium of the physician and, in some infections, are more effective than other antimicrobial agents. A study of Table 55–1 (page 1096) will indicate the major current uses of sulfonamides.

The term *sulfonamide* is herein employed as a generic name for derivatives of para-aminobenzenesulfonamide (sulfanilamide). More than 5400 congeneric substances were synthesized and studied in the decade that followed the discovery of sulfanilamide. Yet less than a score of them have attained any therapeutic importance.

History. Although sulfanilamide was first prepared in 1908 by Gelmo in the course of investigations of azo dyes, a quarter century was to pass before it was used in human bacterial infections.

Investigations at the I. G. Farbenindustrie resulted, in 1932, in a German patent to Klarer and Mietzsch, covering PRONTOSIL and several other azo dyes containing a sulfonamide group. In the same year, Domagk, a research director of the I. G., working with Klarer and Mietzsch, observed that mice with streptococcal and other infections could be protected by PRONTOSIL (Domagk, 1935a, 1935b). To

Domagk belongs the credit for the discovery of the chemotherapeutic value of PRONTOSIL, for which he was awarded the Nobel Prize in Medicine for 1938. In 1933, the first clinical case study was reported by Foerster, who gave PRONTOSIL to a 10-month-old infant with staphylococcal septicemia and obtained a dramatic cure.

In France, the Tréfouëls, Nitti, and Bovet (1935), working with Fourneau at the Pasteur Institute in Paris, soon communicated the important finding that in the tissues the azo linkage was split so that PRONTOSIL yielded para-aminobenzenesulfonamide, which they thought to be the chemotherapeutic moiety of the molecule. Fourneau then prepared this compound, and he and his associates (1936) demonstrated it to be as effective as PRONTOSIL in curing experimental infections. No great attention was paid elsewhere to these epoch-making advances in chemotherapy until the interest of English investigators was aroused. Colebrook and Kenny (1936) as well as Buttle and coworkers (1936) reported their favorable clinical results with PRONTOSIL and sulfanilamide in puerperal sepsis and meningococcal infections. These two reports awakened the medical profession to the new field of bacterial chemotherapy, and experimental and clinical articles in great profusion soon appeared.

A vast number of derivatives of sulfanilamide were subsequently synthesized; many have been tested for their clinical value in various bacterial, protozoal, and viral diseases. Several achieved important, although temporary, clinical status; relatively few are valuable chemotherapeutic agents today. The major developments have been (1) the introduction of congeners that remain largely unabsorbed in the intestinal tract and hence produce local changes in bacterial flora, (2) the discovery of certain advantages of a combination of sulfonamides (*triple sulfonamides*), (3) the development of sulfonamides with high solubility in urine and hence low renal toxicity, and (4) the establishment of the value of a sulfonamide given concurrently with certain antibiotics or combined with trimethoprim in the therapy of specific infections. One interested in the history of sulfonamides is referred to previous editions of this textbook and the references therein.

Chemistry. The structural formulas of selected sulfonamides are shown in Table 56–1. Most of them are relatively insoluble in water, but their sodium salts are readily soluble. A number of laboratory and

Table 56-1. STRUCTURAL FORMULAS OF SELECTED SULFONAMIDES *

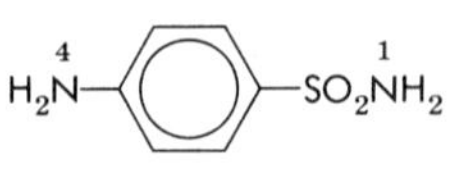

Sulfanilamide

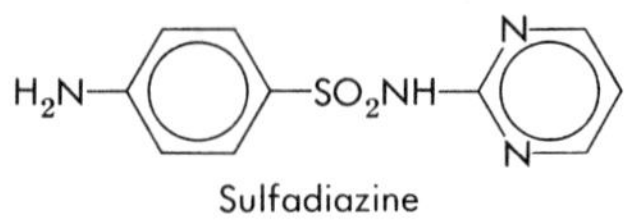

Sulfadiazine

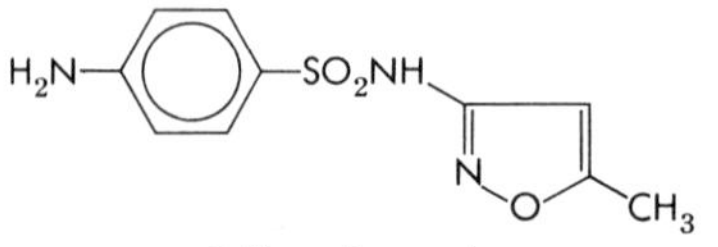

Sulfamethoxazole

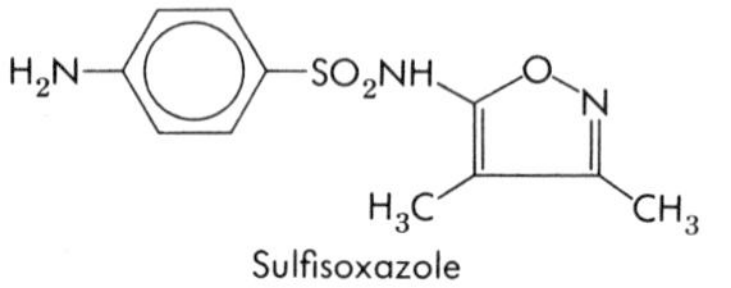

Sulfisoxazole

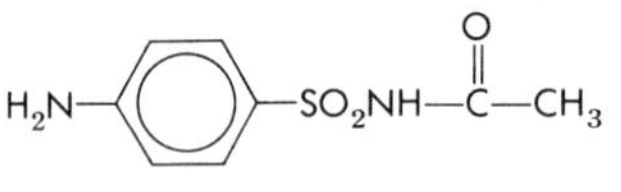

Sulfacetamide

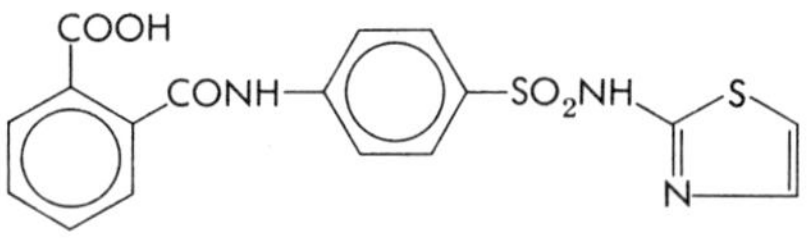

Phthalylsulfathiazole

* The N of the para-NH_2 group is designated as N^4; that of the amide NH_2, as N^1.

bedside methods are available for the *chemical determination* of the sulfonamide concentration in biological fluids.

Structure-Activity Relationship. The number of sulfonamides is so vast and the structure-activity data are so complex that only the major features of this subject will be presented. The minimal structural prerequisites for antibacterial action are all embodied in sulfanilamide itself. The —SO_2NH_2 group is not essential as such, but the important feature is that the sulfur is directly linked to the benzene ring.

The para-NH_2 group (the N of which has been designated as N^4) is essential and can be replaced only by such radicals as can be converted in the tissues to a free amino group. Acylation of the para-NH_2 abolishes *in-vitro* activity; but deacylation may occur *in vivo* with a resulting return of potency, as in the case of the phthalyl derivative of sulfathiazole. Substitutions made in the amide NH_2 group (the N of which has been designated as N^1) have variable effects on antibacterial activity of the molecule. Substitution of heterocyclic aromatic nuclei at N^1 yields highly potent compounds. Bell and Roblin (1942) concluded that the more negative the SO_2 group of an N^1-substituted sulfonamide, the greater is the bacteriostatic activity. They hypothesized that optimal activity had thus been achieved in sulfadiazine. In the main, time has borne out the validity of this prediction. Acetylation at N^1 or its substitution by an amidine group does not interfere with chemotherapeutic activity and may result in compounds with novel properties; for example, the sodium salt of sulfacetamide is nearly neutral in solution, in

contrast to the strong alkalinity of sodium salts of other sulfonamides. Substitution in the benzene ring of sulfonamides usually yields inactive compounds.

EFFECTS ON MICROBIAL AGENTS

Sulfonamides have a wide range of antimicrobial activity against both gram-positive and gram-negative organisms. With a few exceptions, there is a direct correlation between their efficacy *in vitro* and *in vivo*. In general, the sulfonamides exert only a bacteriostatic effect in the body, and cellular and humoral defense mechanisms of the host are essential for the final eradication of the infection.

Antibacterial Spectrum. Among the microorganisms highly susceptible *in vitro* to sulfonamides are group-A *Streptococcus pyogenes* (except types 17 and 19), *Strep. pneumoniae* (pneumococci), some strains of *Bacillus anthracis* and *Corynebacterium diphtheriae, Haemophilus influenzae, H. ducreyi, Brucella, Vibrio cholerae, Yersinia (Pasteurella) pestis, Nocardia, Actinomyces, Calymmatobacterium granulomatis,* and the agents responsible for trachoma, lymphogranuloma venereum, and inclusion conjunctivitis (*Chlamydia trachomatis*).

The widespread use of sulfonamides for the treatment of gonorrhea resulted in the appearance of a large number of cases of this disease in which the responsible microorganisms were resistant to these drugs. Therefore, the sulfonamides were replaced completely by the penicillins and other antimicrobial agents. Consequently, there has been a gradual increase in the number of sulfonamide-sensitive *gonococci*, but this has not reached the point where the use of these compounds is warranted. Although sulfonamides were used successfully for the management of meningococcal infections for many years, a gradual increase in the prevalence of resistant strains became apparent after World War II. By 1963 it was evident that sulfonamide-insensitive strains of *Neisseria meningitidis* were becoming more numerous and producing both the carrier state and disease. While at first this involved group-A strains, resistance also developed in groups B and C. A similar situation prevails with respect to *Shigella.* By 1965, nearly 60% of *Shigella flexneri* and 90% of *Shig. sonnei* were insensitive to this class of drugs (Haltalin and Nelson, 1965).

Some strains of *Escherichia coli* isolated from patients with urinary tract infections are susceptible to sulfonamides. *Nocardia asteroides* is highly sensitive (Black and McNellis, 1971). *Enterobacter (Aerobacter) aerogenes, Pseudomonas aeruginosa,* and *Proteus* species, although occasionally sensitive *in vitro,* seldom respond favorably when they are producing disease. *Francisella (Pasteurella) tularensis, Bordetella pertussis, Leptospira, Borrelia, Treponema, Mycobacterium tuberculosis, M. leprae, Rickettsia, Sarcodina* (amebae), *Plasmodium, Candida, Cryptococcus,* true fungi, and viruses are *not* inhibited by sulfonamides.

Mechanism of Action. The most fruitful theory of the mechanism of action of sulfonamides is known as the Woods-Fildes theory; it is based on the competitive antagonism of para-aminobenzoic acid (PABA) and sulfonamide and proposes that the normal utilization of PABA by bacteria is prevented by these drugs (*see* Fildes, 1940; Woods, 1940). Strong support for this view came with the discovery of pteroylglutamic acid (PGA, folic acid), which contains a PABA moiety. Sulfonamide inhibits bacterial growth by preventing PABA from being incorporated into the PGA molecule. Sensitive microorganisms are those that must synthesize their own PGA. Bacteria that do not require PGA or that can utilize preformed PGA are not affected. Bacteriostasis induced by sulfonamides is counteracted by PABA competitively. Although sulfonamides inhibit PGA synthesis immediately, their effect on bacteria is not manifested until a lag time of several cell divisions has elapsed; presumably in this interval stored PGA is being exhausted. The antagonism described is found *in vivo* as well as *in vitro.* Sulfonamides do not affect animal cells by this mechanism, since they require *preformed* PGA and cannot synthesize it. They are, therefore, comparable to sulfonamide-insensitive bacteria that utilize preformed PGA.

The theory presented above does not explain all the known facts concerning the action of sulfonamide on bacteria. Brown (1962), using cell-free extracts of *E. coli,* found that sulfonamides can also be used as alternative substrates by the enzyme system to form products that are probably analogs of reduced forms of pteroic acid. These analogs could then exert inhibitory effects. The development of knowledge concerning the mode of action of the sulfonamides has been reviewed by Woods (1962).

Synergists and Antagonists of Sulfonamides. One of the most active agents that exerts a supra-additive effect when used with a sulfonamide is *trimethoprim* (*see* Bushby and Hitchings, 1968). This compound is a *powerful* and *selective* inhibitor of microbial dihydrofolate reductase, the enzyme that reduces dihydrofolate to tetrahydrofolate. It is this reduced form of folic acid that is required for one-carbon transfer reactions. The simultaneous administration of a sulfonamide and trimethoprim thus introduces *sequential blocks* in the pathway by which microorganisms synthesize tetrahydrofolate from precursor molecules. The expectation that such a combination would yield supra-additive antimicrobial effects has been realized both *in vitro* and *in vivo* (*see* below; Reisberg *et al.,* 1967).

PABA is the most prominent among the sulfonamide antagonists. Certain local anesthetics that contain PABA antagonize these drugs *in vitro* and *in vivo.* The antagonism between them and PABA finds a practical laboratory use for the improvement of the reliability of bacteriological reports. For example, a culture obtained from a sample of blood or purulent discharge of a patient receiving sulfonamide may be reported falsely sterile because of the concurrent transfer of the drug with the sample. If, on this basis, therapy is prematurely stopped, clinical evidence of the infection soon reappears. To circumvent such errors, PABA is added to culture media; a concentration is employed that is not inhibitory to the common pathogenic organisms but is sufficient to antagonize the antibacterial effect of sulfonamide.

The antibacterial action of sulfonamide is inhibited by blood, pus, and tissue breakdown products.

Effects of Sulfonamide Combined with Other Chemotherapeutic Agents. Investigations of the activity of combinations of sulfonamides and antibiotics *in vitro* and in experimental animals suggest an additive effect when sulfonamide is combined with bacteriostatic agents such as the tetracyclines and either an antagonistic or a supra-additive effect when bacteria are exposed simultaneously to sulfonamides and a bactericidal antibiotic (*see* review by Jawetz and Gunnison, 1953). Experience has validated the effectiveness of sulfadiazine or sulfisoxazole used with chloramphenicol in the treatment of meningitis caused by *H. influenzae.* Other clinical examples are included in Table 55–1 (page 1096) and in the discussion of trimethoprim-sulfamethoxazole.

Acquired Bacterial Resistance to Sulfonamides. Bacteria initially sensitive to sulfonamides can acquire resistance to the drug both *in vitro* and *in vivo.* The clinical importance of sulfonamide resistance was first generally appreciated in the early 1940s, when the cure rate of gonorrhea treated with this class of drugs dropped sharply.

Bacteria resistant to sulfonamide are presumed to originate by random mutation and selection, as discussed in Chapter 55. Transfer of resistance by R factor in gram-negative bacteria has also been demonstrated. Such resistance, once it is maximally developed, is usually persistent and irreversible, particularly when produced *in vivo*. Acquired resistance to sulfonamide usually does not imply *cross-resistance* to chemotherapeutic agents of other classes. The *in-vivo* acquisition of resistance has little or no effect either on virulence or on specific immunological or antigenic characteristics of microorganisms.

Mechanism of Resistance. Resistance to sulfonamide is probably the consequence of an altered enzymatic constitution of the bacterial cell; the alteration may be characterized by (1) an increased capacity to destroy or inactivate the drug, (2) an alternative metabolic pathway for synthesis or degradation of an essential metabolite, or (3) an increased production of an essential metabolite or drug antagonist. The third possibility has received most attention. Woods (1940) was the first to suggest that the resistance of some bacteria to sulfonamide may be based on their ability to synthesize enough PABA to antagonize the drug. Many data support this view. For example, some resistant staphylococci may synthesize 70 times as much PABA as do the susceptible parent strains. Further observations have confirmed this finding and have also substantiated the role of increased production of PGA by sulfonamide-resistant strains of *Staphylococcus aureus* (White and Woods, 1965). Nevertheless, an increased production of PABA is not a constant finding in sulfonamide-resistant bacteria, and resistant mutants may possess enzymes for folate biosynthesis that are less readily inhibited by sulfonamides.

Clinical Aspects and Significance of Resistance to Sulfonamide. Acquired bacterial resistance to sulfonamides plays a significant role in therapeutic failures with this class of drugs, particularly in infections caused by gonococci, staphylococci, meningococci, and streptococci, and to some extent in *Shigella* dysentery and infections caused by *H. influenzae* and *Strep. pneumoniae*.

Much attention centered on the problem created by the emergence of sulfonamide-resistant *Strep. pyogenes* during the mass prophylactic use of sulfadiazine in military personnel during World War II. Indeed, outbreaks of group-A hemolytic streptococcal infections in U.S. military camps, particularly in 1944, were caused by sulfonamide-resistant strains (types 17 and 19) and were a source of considerable concern. Subsequently, the conclusion was reached that such sulfonamide-resistant strains have not constituted any particular problem in civilian medicine. However, large-scale chemoprophylaxis with sulfadiazine favors the development of resistant streptococci and represents a hazard that should be risked only in an emergency. When sulfonamide is given in adequately large doses for relatively short periods of time, drug resistance rarely, if ever, develops in *Strep. pyogenes*. Although one would anticipate that the daily prophylactic use of sulfadiazine in rheumatic fever patients (*see* below) might favor the development of drug-resistant hemolytic streptococci, resistance of clinical importance has not occurred from such medication. The physician should avoid promiscuous use of all antibacterial agents to prevent the occurrence of acquired resistance.

ABSORPTION, FATE, AND EXCRETION

Absorption. Except for sulfonamides especially designed for their local effects in the bowel, this class of drugs is rapidly and adequately absorbed from the *gastrointestinal tract*. Indeed, the agent can often be found in the urine within 30 minutes after its oral ingestion. The small intestine is the major site of absorption, but some of the drug is absorbed from the stomach. Absorption from *other sites,* such as the vagina, respiratory tract, or abraded skin, is variable and unreliable, but a sufficient amount may enter the body to cause toxic reactions in susceptible persons or to produce sensitization. *Subcutaneous* injection of adequate amounts of solutions of sodium salts of sulfonamides results in rapid establishment of antibacterial activity in the blood.

Protein Binding. All sulfonamides are bound in varying degree to plasma proteins, particularly to albumin. The extent to which this occurs is determined by the hydrophobicity of a particular drug and its pK_a; at physiological pH, drugs with a high pK_a exhibit a low degree of protein binding, and vice versa. The extent of binding is decreased in patients with severe renal failure, a phenomenon not totally accounted for by low levels of plasma albumin (Andreasen, 1973). In general, a sulfonamide is bound to a somewhat greater extent in the acetylated than in the free form.

Distribution. Sulfonamides are distributed throughout all tissues of the body. The diffusible fraction of sulfadiazine is uniformly distributed throughout the total body water, while sulfisoxazole is largely confined to the extracellular space. The time (2 to 4 hours) at which equilibrium with plasma is reached varies with the tissue and the compound. The sulfonamides readily enter *pleural, peritoneal, synovial, ocular,* and similar body fluids, and may reach concentrations therein that are 50 to 80% of the simultaneously determined blood concentration.

Since the protein content of such fluids is usually low, the drug is present in the unbound active form.

Cerebrospinal Fluid. After systemic administration of adequate doses, the sulfonamides attain cerebrospinal fluid concentrations that are effective in meningeal infections. At equilibrium, the concentration is usually 50 to 80% of that in the blood. Rate and extent of diffusion vary with each drug and depend on many factors, such as blood concentration, extent of binding by plasma albumin, degree of acetylation, and presence of meningeal inflammation. Inasmuch as the acetylated compounds are more extensively bound by plasma albumin and hence are less available for diffusion, the ratio of free to acetylated drug is higher in the cerebrospinal fluid than in the blood. This also holds true for other body fluids. The cerebrospinal fluid is practically free of protein; consequently, a sulfonamide concentration therein of 5 mg % would be as bacteriostatic as a blood concentration of 10 mg %, half of which is bound to plasma protein.

Fetus. Sulfonamides readily pass through the placenta and reach the fetal circulation. Equilibrium between maternal and fetal blood is usually established within 3 hours after a single oral dose. The concentrations attained in the fetal tissues are sufficient to cause both antibacterial and toxic effects. The blood concentrations of sulfadiazine in the fetus are 50 to 90% of those in the maternal blood. The drug appears more slowly in amniotic fluid than in fetal blood.

Metabolism. The sulfonamides undergo metabolic alterations to a varying extent in the tissues, especially in the liver. Both acetylation and oxidation occur. Some investigators believe that the metabolic products of the sulfonamides, particularly those of oxidation, are responsible for many of the systemic toxic reactions, especially skin lesions and hypersensitivity phenomena. In nearly all species, the major metabolic derivative is the N^4-acetylated sulfonamide. Each sulfonamide is acetylated to a different extent. For example, the percentage of the total plasma sulfonamide that is acetylated ranges between 10 and 40 for sulfadiazine and its methylated derivatives. Acetylation is disadvantageous because the resulting product has no antibacterial activity and yet retains the toxic potentialities of the parent substance. Furthermore, the acetylated forms of some of the older sulfonamides are less soluble and hence contribute to crystalluria and renal complications. Since acetylation is a function of time and hepatic function, the conjugated fraction increases considerably when the sojourn of the drug in the body is prolonged, as in patients with impaired renal function, or decreases when hepatic failure is present. Because of varying degrees of acetylation and other factors, periodic determination of the plasma concentration of free drug is essential when patients with severe bacterial infections are being treated with large doses of sulfonamide.

Excretion. Sulfonamides are eliminated from the body partly as such and partly as metabolic products. The largest fraction is excreted in the urine, and the half-life of sulfonamides in the body is thus dependent on renal function. Small amounts are eliminated in the feces and in bile, milk, and other secretions.

Renal Elimination. Each sulfonamide, free and acetylated, is handled by the kidney in a characteristic manner. In all cases, glomerular filtration is a major factor. Varying degrees of tubular reabsorption occur for most sulfonamides, although sulfacetamide is not appreciably reabsorbed. Tubular secretion also plays a role in some instances. Marked variations in the rate of renal excretion account for the differences in duration of action of the various sulfonamides, as discussed under the individual drugs. As a generalization, the rate of excretion of sulfonamides increases when the value of the acid ionization constant of the drug decreases.

Other Routes. Except for sulfonamides used for intestinal chemotherapy, only small amounts of these drugs are found in the *feces* after oral medication. Various secretions of the body contain low concentrations of these agents. *Prostatic* and *seminal vesicular* fluid contain therapeutic concentrations after adequate oral doses, a matter of importance in the treatment of prostatic and posterior urethral infections. The concentration of sulfonamide in *human milk* is similar to that in plasma. These agents are also secreted in *sweat, tears, saliva, bile,* and *intestinal fluids*. The concentration in bile is similar to that in blood, but the *gastric juice* contains a much lower quantity.

PHARMACOLOGICAL PROPERTIES,
PREPARATIONS, AND DOSAGE OF
INDIVIDUAL SULFONAMIDES

The sulfonamides may be classified into four groups on the basis of the rapidity with which they are absorbed and excreted: (1)

agents absorbed rapidly and excreted rapidly, such as sulfisoxazole and sulfadiazine; (2) *compounds absorbed rapidly but excreted slowly,* such as sulfamethoxypyridazine and sulfadimethoxine; (3) *agents absorbed very poorly when administered orally* and hence active in the bowel lumen, such as succinylsulfathiazole and phthalylsulfathiazole; and (4) *sulfonamides employed mainly for special purposes,* such as sulfacetamide, mafenide, and silver sulfadiazine.

Rapidly Absorbed and Rapidly Eliminated Sulfonamides. *Sulfisoxazole.*

Early studies of sulfisoxazole, reported by Schnitzer and associates (1946), established that it was a rapidly absorbed and rapidly excreted sulfonamide with excellent antibacterial activity (equal to that of sulfadiazine). Since its high solubility eliminates much of the renal toxicity inherent in the use of the older sulfonamides, it has essentially replaced the less soluble agents. Sulfisoxazole should thus be regarded as the prototype of this group.

Sulfisoxazole is distributed only in extracellular body water, and this may explain the fact that the plasma concentration after a given dose is twice that for sulfadiazine. Both the free and acetylated forms of the drug are much more soluble in urine at pH values encountered clinically than are the respective forms of sulfadiazine. After oral ingestion of adequate doses, an effective concentration of free sulfonamide soon appears in the blood. From 28 to 35% of sulfisoxazole in the blood and about 30% in the urine is in the acetylated form. Approximately 95% of a single dose is excreted by the kidney in 24 hours. Concentrations of the drug in urine thus greatly exceed those in blood and may be bactericidal. The cerebrospinal fluid concentration averages about a third of that in the blood.

The recommended daily *oral dose* of sulfisoxazole for children is 150 mg/kg of body weight; one half of this is given initially, followed by one sixth of the daily dose every 4 hours (not to exceed 6 g in 24 hours). The oral dose for adults is 2 to 4 g initially, followed by 1 g every 4 to 6 hours. The *parenteral dose* for adults and children is 100 mg/kg per day, divided into three or four portions. The areas of *clinical usefulness* of sulfisoxazole are discussed below.

Less than 0.1% of patients receiving sulfisoxazole suffer serious *toxic reactions* (Yow, 1953). The untoward effects produced by this agent are similar to those that follow the administration of other sulfonamides, as discussed below. Because of its relatively high solubility in the urine as compared to sulfadiazine, sulfisoxazole only infrequently produces hematuria or crystalluria (0.2 to 0.3%) and the risk of anuria is very small. Despite this, it is advisable that patients taking this drug ingest an adequate quantity of water. Sulfisoxazole and all sulfonamides that are absorbed must be used with caution in patients with impaired renal function. Like all other sulfonamides, sulfisoxazole may produce hypersensitivity reactions,

some of which are potentially lethal. Sulfisoxazole is presently preferred over other sulfonamides by most clinicians, when a rapidly absorbed and rapidly excreted sulfonamide is indicated.

Preparations. *Sulfisoxazole,* U.S.P. (GANTRISIN, SK-SOXAZOLE, and others), is available in 500-mg tablets for *oral* use. It is also marketed as a vaginal cream (10%). *Sulfisoxazole Diolamine,* N.F., is available in 4% solution prepared for *topical* use in the eye, nose, and ear; the same salt is marketed for *parenteral injection,* in 5- and 10-ml ampuls (400 mg/ml). If parenteral therapy is required, *intravenous* or *subcutaneous* administration is employed. Doses are given above. Intravenous administration requires the slow administration of dilute solutions of the drug. *Sulfisoxazole Acetyl,* U.S.P. (GANTRISIN ACETYL), is tasteless and hence preferred for *oral* use in children; it is available as a flavored pediatric syrup and suspension (100 mg/ml). The compound is deacetylated by the enzymes in the small intestine, and this results in a relatively slow absorption of the active form of the drug.

Sulfamethoxazole, N.F. (GANTANOL), is a close congener of sulfisoxazole, but its rates of enteric absorption and urinary excretion are slower. It is employed for both systemic and urinary tract infections. Precautions must be observed to avoid sulfamethoxazole *crystalluria* because of the high percentage of the acetylated, relatively insoluble form of the drug in the urine. Sulfamethoxazole is available for oral use, as 500-mg tablets and as a suspension (100 mg/ml). The *dosage schedules* of sulfamethoxazole for *children* are as follows: 27 kg (60 lb)—1.5 g initially, followed by 750 mg morning and evening; 18 kg (40 lb)—1.0 g initially, followed by 500 mg morning and evening; 9 kg (20 lb)—500 mg for the first dose and then 250 mg morning and evening. The dose for *adults* with mild infections is 2.0 g followed by 1.0 g every 12 hours; for severe disease, the initial dose is 2.0 g and then 1.0 g every 8 hours. The half-life of sulfamethoxazole in babies during the first 10 days of life is considerably longer than in adults. It falls rapidly, being about 9 hours at 3 weeks of age and 4 to 5 hours at 1 year. It then increases toward the half-life characteristic for adults, namely, 10 to 11 hours. The clinical uses of sulfamethoxazole are the same as those for sulfisoxazole. It is presently marketed in fixed-dose combination with phenazopyridine (AZO GANTANOL) as a urinary antiseptic and analgesic, and with trimethoprim (*see* below).

Sulfadiazine. Sulfadiazine given orally is rapidly absorbed from the gastrointestinal tract, and peak blood concentrations are reached within 3 to 4 hours after a single dose. The drug is bound to plasma protein to the extent of about 55% at a concentration of 10 mg% and at normal plasma protein levels. Therapeutic concentrations are attained in cerebrospinal fluid within 4 hours after a single oral dose of 60 mg/kg.

Sulfadiazine is *excreted* quite readily by the kidney in both the free and the acetylated form, rapidly at first and then more slowly over a period of 2 to 3 days. It can be detected in the urine within 30 minutes after oral ingestion. About 15 to 40% of the excreted sulfadiazine is in the *acetylated* form. This form of the drug is excreted more readily than the free fraction, and the administration of alkali accelerates the renal clearance of both forms by further diminishing their tubular reabsorption.

In *adults* who are being treated with sulfadiazine, the initial dose for oral administration is 2 to 4 g, followed by 1 g every 4 to 6 hours. *Children* over 2 months of age should receive one half of a calculated daily dose to initiate therapy and then 65 to 150 mg/kg (to a maximum of 6 g) daily in four to six divided doses. Every precaution must be taken to ensure fluid intake adequate to produce a urine output of at least 1200 ml in adults and a corresponding quantity in children. If this cannot be accomplished, sodium bicarbonate may be given to reduce the risk of crystalluria.

Parenteral therapy with sodium sulfadiazine is not recommended.

Preparations. *Sulfadiazine,* U.S.P., is available as official tablets that usually contain 325 or 500 mg of the drug. *Sulfadiazine Sodium Injection, U.S.P.,* is available for parenteral injection; it is a sterile aqueous solution and usually contains 250 mg/ml. It is rarely used anymore.

Sulfamerazine and Sulfamethazine. Although employed in the past and still official in the U.S.P., these agents are no longer used for the therapy of infections. For a detailed description of their properties, the reader is referred to the *fourth edition* of this textbook.

Sulfonamide Mixtures. A major and frequent toxic reaction to the older sulfonamides was urinary tract injury from precipitation of crystals, usually of acetylated drug, in the renal tubules and ureter. Alkalinization of the urine or intake of adequate fluid is effective in preventing such precipitation; however, these precautions are frequently neglected or undesirable. To offset and circumvent these disadvantages, sulfonamide mixtures were introduced into therapy. The principle that accounts for the value of sulfonamide mixtures is quite simple. Many substances can coexist in solution without interfering with each other's solubility. It is thus possible to saturate a solution with any one sulfonamide and still dissolve in it, almost to the limit of their individual solubilities, a second and a third sulfonamide. Because of the availability of newer agents such as sulfisoxazole that are appreciably more soluble than the older sulfonamides, mixtures of these drugs (*e.g.,* *Trisulfapyrimidines,* U.S.P.) are now little used. For a description of their properties, the interested reader is again referred to the *fourth edition* of this textbook.

Rapidly Absorbed and Slowly Excreted Sulfonamides. *Sulfamethoxypyridazine* and *sulfadimethoxine* offer the advantage of maintenance of effective plasma concentrations when administered only once or twice a day because these agents are rapidly absorbed and slowly excreted. However, they are no longer available in the United States because of the high incidence of severe exudative erythema multiforme (Stevens-Johnson syndrome) resulting from their use.

Poorly Absorbed Sulfonamides. *Succinylsulfathiazole* (SULFASUXIDINE) and *Phthalylsulfathiazole,* N.F.

(SULFATHALIDINE), are very poorly absorbed from the gastrointestinal tract. Both are conjugated at N^4 and are thus inactive until hydrolyzed by intestinal bacteria to sulfathiazole. For this reason, they have been employed in the treatment of some intestinal infections and for reduction of the number of microorganisms in the bowel prior to its surgical manipulation. Such drugs never "sterilize" the intestinal tract, although they may reduce the total number of microorganisms present for varying periods of time. If they are administered long enough, various bacterial species in the intestinal flora become resistant to them and increase in number. Like all such forms of chemoprophylaxis, the use of the poorly absorbed sulfonamides in intestinal surgery probably offers no distinct advantage over meticulous surgical technic and skilled preoperative and postoperative care.

Despite very limited absorption of either of these drugs or of the sulfathiazole derived in the colon, untoward systemic effects do occur. These include fever and allergic reactions. Interference with the normal flora of the intestine can jeopardize bacterial synthesis of vitamin K, and hypoprothrombinemia and hemorrhage may result. It is therefore advisable to administer vitamin K to patients receiving these agents.

If either of these poorly absorbed drugs is to be employed, phthalylsulfathiazole is preferred; its dose is smaller, it is effective even in the presence of watery diarrhea, and it produces soft rather than semiliquid stools. The initial oral *dose* of the drug, prior to intestinal surgery, is 125 mg/kg of body weight each day, divided into equal portions and given at intervals of 6 or 8 hours. The total daily dose should not exceed 8 g unless a watery diarrhea is present, in which case the calculated daily dose may have to be doubled. The diet should be low in residue, and mineral oil is to be avoided. Within 3 to 5 days, the feces become soft and practically odorless, the bowel is found to be empty, and the coliform bacterial count is decreased. Postoperatively, drug treatment is resumed as soon as possible; otherwise, the bacterial count and flora rapidly return to normal. Administration of the drug is continued for 1 to 2 weeks postoperatively.

These agents have also been employed in both the acute and chronic forms of *bacillary dysentery*. However, many strains of *Shigella* are resistant to sulfonamides.

Status. There is no proof of efficacy for the prophylactic use of these drugs prior to bowel surgery. Nevertheless, some surgeons continue to employ them routinely.

Sulfonamides for Special Uses. *Sulfacetamide.* Sulfacetamide is the N^1-acetyl-substituted derivative of sulfanilamide. Its aqueous solubility (1:140) is approximately 90 times that of sulfadiazine. While this agent is no longer used in the therapy of urinary tract infections, solutions of the sodium salt of the drug are used extensively in the management of *ophthalmic infections.* Although topical sulfonamide for most purposes is discouraged because of lack of efficacy and a high risk of sensitization, sulfacetamide has certain advantages. Very high aqueous concentrations are nonirritating to the delicate tissues of the eye and are effectively bactericidal against susceptible microorganisms. A 30% solution of the sodium salt has a pH of 7.4, whereas the solutions of sodium salts of other sulfonamides are highly alkaline. The drug penetrates into ocular fluids and tissues in high concentration. The value of the drug in human cases of acute and chronic conjunctivitis is adequately established. However, a number of antibiotics may be more effective in the treatment and prophylaxis of ophthalmic infections. Sensitivity reactions to sulfacetamide are rare, but the drug should not be used in patients with known hypersensitivity to sulfonamides. Sodium sulfacetamide has no place in the therapy of systemic infections.

The *usual dose* of sodium sulfacetamide solution applied topically to the eye is 1 or 2 drops of a 10 to 30% solution every 2 hours for severe infections and the same amount three or four times a day for chronic conditions. An ophthalmic ointment may be used instead of the solution, provided there is no wound of the cornea; as a rule, the ointment is reserved for application at bedtime.

Preparations. *Sulfacetamide Sodium,* U.S.P. (BLEPH, ISOPTO CETAMIDE, SULAMYD SODIUM), is available only for topical application to the eye, as an *ophthalmic solution* (10, 15, and 30%) and an *ophthalmic ointment* (10 and 30%).

Sulfisoxazole and Phenazopyridine Hydrochloride (AZO GANTRISIN). This preparation is a 10:1 mixture of sulfisoxazole and phenazopyridine hydrochloride. It combines the antibacterial activity of the sulfonamide with the local urinary analgesic activity of phenazopyridine. The preparation is indicated specifically for urinary tract infections associated with pain, burning dysuria, urgency, and frequency. The urine becomes orange-red in color soon after ingestion of this mixture because of the presence of phenazopyridine, an orange-red dye. The dose of the compound for adults is 1 g four times a day. It is supplied as 500-mg tablets.

Salicylazosulfapyridine (AZULFIDINE). This drug is used in the therapy of *ulcerative colitis.* Although improvement in the course of the disease follows the administration of 4 to 8 g of the drug per day, relapses tend to occur in about one third of patients who experience a satisfactory initial response. Salicylazosulfapyridine is preferred to corticosteroids by some gastroenterologists for treatment of patients mildly or moderately ill with ulcerative colitis (Zetzel, 1954; Riis *et al.,* 1973). The drug is also being employed as the first approach to treatment of relatively mild cases of *regional enteritis* and *granulomatous colitis.* Salicylazosulfapyridine is broken down in the gut to sulfapyridine, which is absorbed and eventually excreted in the urine, and 5-aminosalicylate, which reaches high levels in the feces (Peppercorn and Goldman, 1973). Toxic reactions include Heinz-body anemia, acute hemolysis in patients with glucose-6-phosphate dehydrogenase deficiency, and agranulocytosis. Nausea, fever, arthralgias, and rashes occur in up to 20% of patients treated with the drug (Collins, 1968). The use of smaller doses, 2 g per day, is said to reduce the frequency of relapses in patients with ulcerative colitis, as well as the incidence of untoward effects

(Misiewicz *et al.,* 1965). There is no evidence that the compound alters the intestinal microflora of persons with ulcerative colitis (Gorbach *et al.,* 1967). This suggests that any beneficial effect of the drug is probably due to some property other than its antibacterial activity.

Mafenide. This sulfonamide (α-amino-*p*-toluenesulfonamide) is marketed as *Mafenide Acetate Cream,* U.S.P. (SULFAMYLON CREAM). It is effective, when applied topically, for the prevention of invasion of *burns* by a large variety of gram-negative and gram-positive bacteria. It appears to be highly active in inhibiting the implantation of *Pseud. aeruginosa,* but it should not be used in treatment of an established infection. Suprainfection with *Candida* may occasionally be a problem. The drug, in the form of a cream, is applied with aseptic precautions to a thickness of about 1 to 2 mm over the entire burned surface of skin; it is applied twice a day because of its rapid absorption. The wound is left uncovered. Cleansing of the wound and removal of debris should be carried out before each application of the drug. Therapy is continued for up to 60 days; skin grafting is usually possible after 35 to 40 days. The drug appears to be highly effective in patients with burns involving 50% or less of the body surface; the death rate is not appreciably decreased in those in whom 60% or more of the skin has been subjected to thermal injury (Lindberg *et al.,* 1968). The drug is rapidly absorbed systemically and converted to para-carboxybenzenesulfonamide. Studies of absorption from the burn surface indicate that peak plasma concentrations are reached in 2 to 4 hours (*see* Harrison *et al.,* 1972). Adverse effects include intense pain at sites of application, allergic reactions, and loss of fluid by evaporation from the burn surface, since occlusive dressings are not used. The drug and its primary metabolite inhibit carbonic anhydrase. The urine becomes alkaline, and a metabolic acidosis may ensue (White and Asch, 1971). Compensatory tachypnea and hyperventilation with respiratory alkalosis are also observed.

Silver Sulfadiazine (SILVADENE). This drug inhibits the growth *in vitro* of many bacteria and fungi, including some species resistant to sulfonamides (Rosenkranz and Rosenkranz, 1972). The compound is used topically in *burn* therapy, and silver is released slowly from the preparation in concentrations that are selectively toxic to the microorganisms (*see* Chapter 50). While little silver is absorbed, the plasma concentration of sulfadiazine may approach therapeutic levels if a large surface area is involved.

The drug prevents invasion and can eradicate *Pseud. aeruginosa* and other sensitive microorganisms from burns, but it may not be superior to other antimicrobial agents in improving survival from extensive burns. Unlike mafenide, it requires less frequent application, is painless, and does not produce metabolic acidosis (*see* Ballin, 1974).

UNTOWARD REACTIONS TO SULFONAMIDES

All the sulfonamides are potentially dangerous drugs. Awareness by physicians of the incidence and the manner in which reactions occur and of the mechanisms involved can help to circumvent or minimize their occurrence and severity. The untoward effects that develop are numerous and varied. They involve nearly every organ system, often in multiple fashion and in varying degree. An untoward reaction increases the likelihood of a severe response to the subsequent administration of a member of this class of drugs. The overall incidence of reactions is about 5%. Certain untoward effects interdict the subsequent use of these agents; included in this category are drug fever and reactions involving the blood, bone marrow, kidney, liver, skin, and peripheral nerves. (*See* Kutscher *et al.*, 1954; Weinstein *et al.*, 1960.)

Disorders of the Hematopoietic System. Blood dyscrasias are quite uncommon; however, when they do occur, they may be so serious that drug administration must be stopped promptly and appropriate therapy undertaken.

Acute Hemolytic Anemia. The mechanism of the acute hemolytic anemia produced by sulfonamides is not always readily apparent. In some cases, it has been thought to be a sensitization phenomenon. In other instances, the hemolysis is related to an erythrocytic deficiency of glucose-6-phosphate dehydrogenase activity, as discussed in detail on page 1061.

The development of acute hemolytic anemia is unrelated to dosage or blood level of drug. Readministration of sulfonamides to individuals who have had an episode of hemolysis provoked by these compounds is accompanied by a 65% incidence of recurrence. Negroes are more susceptible to this reaction than are white-skinned individuals, and children more so than adults. The hemolytic episode occurs abruptly, usually in the first week of therapy. Nausea, fever, vertigo, jaundice, pallor, hepatosplenomegaly, and shock may develop suddenly. There is a marked decrease in erythrocyte and hemoglobin levels, often by 50 to 70% within a few hours, and leukocytosis, reticulocytosis, bilirubinemia, urobilinuria, and hemoglobin casts are common laboratory findings. Acute renal tubular necrosis may follow the hemoglobinuria.

Hemolytic anemia is rare after sulfadiazine (0.05%); its exact incidence following therapy with sulfisoxazole is unknown.

Agranulocytosis. Agranulocytosis occurs in about 0.1% of patients who receive sulfadiazine; it also can follow the use of other sulfonamides. A sensitization phenomenon is probably the mechanism involved. A direct myelotoxic effect is evident in the bone-marrow maturation arrest at the myeloblast stage. The granulocytopenia is not related to the dose or blood level of drug. Most cases develop only after 10 days of medication. The reaction may appear suddenly and without warning, or only after a period of progressive neutropenia. Although return of granulocytes to normal levels may be delayed for

weeks or months after sulfonamide is withdrawn, most cases recover spontaneously with supportive care.

Aplastic Anemia. Complete suppression of bone-marrow activity with profound anemia, granulocytopenia, and thrombocytopenia is an extremely rare occurrence with sulfonamide therapy. It probably results from a direct myelotoxic effect, and may be fatal.

Thrombocytopenia. Thrombocytopenia of a degree sufficient to permit hemorrhage rarely arises as a result of therapy with the sulfonamides. Transient, mild decreases in platelet counts are a more common occurrence. The mechanism is unknown.

Eosinophilia. Peripheral eosinophilia may occur as an isolated finding and usually disappears promptly after discontinuation of the sulfonamide. It may also accompany other manifestations of sulfonamide hypersensitivity.

Disturbances of the Urinary Tract. The primary factor responsible for the renal damage frequently produced by the older sulfonamides is the formation and deposition of *crystalline aggregates* in the kidneys, calyces, pelvis, ureters, or bladder; this leads to the development of irritation and obstruction. Two other mechanisms, *toxic nephrosis* and *hypersensitivity reaction,* may rarely be involved in the pathogenesis of urinary tract disturbances; thus, anuria and death may occur in patients in whom no evidence of crystalluria or hematuria can be detected and in whom the lesion found at autopsy is tubular necrosis or necrotizing angiitis.

The risk of crystalluria is minimal with more soluble sulfonamides such as sulfisoxazole. Fluid intake should be such as to ensure a daily urine volume of at least 1200 ml (in adults). Alkali therapy may be desirable if urine volume or pH is unusually low, since the solubility of sulfisoxazole increases greatly with slight elevations of pH.

Reactions Due to Sensitization. The incidence of hypersensitivity reactions to sulfonamides is quite variable. Care must be exercised in determining, if possible, whether an observed untoward effect is really related to sensitization or to a direct toxic effect of the drug.

Vascular lesions, involving various organs including the heart and resembling those present in periarteritis nodosa, may appear rarely in the course of sulfonamide administration. The use of sulfisoxazole has been associated with clinical activation of quiescent systemic lupus erythematosus. Eosinophilic migrating pneumonia may occur.

Among the *skin and mucous membrane manifestations* attributed to sensitization to sulfonamide are morbilliform, scarlatinal, urticarial, erysipeloid, pemphigoid, purpuric, and petechial rashes; and erythema nodosum, erythema multiforme of the Stevens-Johnson type, Behçet's syndrome, exfoliative dermatitis, and photosensitivity. Contact dermatitis is very uncommon today, as the result of discontinuation of topical application of these drugs. Although localized sensitization usually leads to a recurrence of the dermatitis when sulfonamide is again administered orally or parenterally, diffuse systemic hypersensitivity states may also develop. Drug eruptions occur most often after the first week of therapy, but may appear earlier in previously sensitized individuals. Fever, malaise, and pruritus are frequently present simultaneously. The incidence of untoward dermal effects is about 1.5% with sulfadiazine therapy and about 2% with sulfisoxazole.

A syndrome similar to *serum sickness* may appear after several days of sulfonamide therapy. Fever, joint pain, urticarial eruptions, conjunctivitis, bronchospasm, and leukopenia are the outstanding features. In persons previously sensitized to these drugs, immediate reactions of the *anaphylactoid type* are sometimes observed.

Drug fever is a common untoward manifestation of sulfonamide treatment and is probably due to sensitization. The incidence approximates 3% with sulfisoxazole. The fever is generally sudden in onset and develops between the seventh and tenth day of sulfonamide administration. It may occur earlier, however, especially if the patient has been previously sensitized to the drug. Headache, chills, malaise, pruritus, and skin rash may or may not accompany the fever. It should be differentiated from the fever that heralds serious toxic reactions to the sulfonamides, such as agranulocytosis and acute hemolytic anemia.

Although *cross-sensitivity* between different sulfonamides does occur, this is not a universal phenomenon; the incidence of sensitivity manifestations following the subsequent administration of a compound other than the one that initially provoked the response is about 20%.

Hepatitis. Focal or diffuse necrosis of the liver due to direct drug toxicity or sensitization occurs in less than 0.1% of patients. Headache, nausea, vomiting, fever, hepatomegaly, jaundice, and laboratory evidence of hepatocellular dysfunction usually appear 3 to 5 days after sulfonamide administration is started, and the syndrome may progress to acute yellow atrophy and death (*see* Dujovne *et al.,* 1967). The development of hepatitis is not influenced by the dose of drug or by the presence of preexisting hepatic disease. Damage to the liver may increase even after drug withdrawal.

Miscellaneous Reactions to the Sulfonamides. Among other untoward effects that may follow the administration of various sulfonamides are *goiter* and *hypothyroidism, arthritis,* and various *neuropsychiatric disturbances.* Coordination and reaction time are not impaired. *Peripheral neuritis* is very rare. *Anorexia, nausea,* and *vomiting* occur in 1 to 2% of persons receiving sulfonamides, and these manifestations are probably central in origin.

The *age* of patients may be an important determinant of the risk of reactions associated with the use of various sulfonamides. Enzymes that acetylate sulfonamides are poorly developed in newborns. In addition, the administration of sulfisoxazole to premature babies may lead to the development of kernicterus due to the displacement of bilirubin from plasma proteins.

SULFONAMIDE THERAPY

The areas in which the sulfonamides are therapeutically useful and constitute drugs of first choice have been sharply reduced by the development of more effective antimicrobial agents and by the gradual but inexorable increase in the resistance of a number of bacterial species to this class of drugs. However, the use of sulfonamides has undergone a revival as a result of the introduction of the combination of trimethoprim and sulfamethoxazole (*see* below).

Urinary Tract Infections. The sulfonamides and the trimethoprim-sulfamethoxazole combination are very useful in the management of infections of the urinary tract. This subject is fully discussed below after the properties of the combination have been considered.

Bacillary Dysentery. Because of the frequency of resistant strains, the sulfonamides are no longer agents of first choice in the management of this disease. An antibiotic such as ampicillin or chloramphenicol should be administered when indicated, depending on the sensitivity of the microorganisms. In instances where the responsible microorganism is sensitive to a sulfonamide, the preferred compound is sulfisoxazole or sulfadiazine and the recommended oral dose is 4 g initially followed by 1 g every 4 hours.

Meningococcal Infections. Resistance to sulfonamides is now common in the various serological groups of *N. meningitidis* (Feldman, 1967; Singer, 1967). All forms of disease produced by meningococci should now be treated with large doses of penicillin G or ampicillin; chloramphenicol has been recommended for patients sensitive to the penicillins. If an epidemic is *proven* to be due to a sulfonamide-sensitive strain of meningococcus, sulfisoxazole or sulfadiazine may be given. In this case, initial sulfonamide therapy is by intravenous administration.

Chemoprophylaxis should be considered for close contacts of patients with meningococcal disease. If the strain of *N. meningitidis* is sensitive to sulfonamides, sulfadiazine (1 g every 12 hours for four doses) should be given. One half of this dose is administered to children 1 to 12 years of age. Penicillin G and several other antibiotics are *not* effective for prophylaxis. Rifampin is a possible alternative when sulfonamide cannot be used; however, there is disagreement as to the utility and advisability of this practice compared to close observation of household contacts, who are usually the only individuals at high risk (*see* Kaiser *et al.,* 1974; Artenstein, 1975). Minocycline should not be used because of the possibility of vestibular toxicity.

Haemophilus Influenzae Meningitis. The present therapy of choice for this disease is ampicillin. Infections with ampicillin-resistant strains are treated with intravenous chloramphenicol. In an unusual circumstance, a combination of streptomycin and sulfonamide may be useful.

Nocardiosis. Sulfonamides are of value in the treatment of infections due to *Nocardia asteroides.* Although the results may be disappointing in some instances, this is often due to erroneous or late diagnosis. A number of instances of complete recovery from the disease, after adequate sulfonamide treatment, have been recorded. If sulfisoxazole is given, the dose must be 6 g per day after a loading dose of 4 g; this schedule is continued for several months after all manifestations have been controlled. The administration of sulfonamide together with an antibiotic has been recommended, especially for advanced cases, and streptomycin or ampicillin has been suggested for this purpose. The clinical response and the results of further sensitivity testing may indicate the necessity of a change in therapy.

Actinomycosis. Penicillin G is currently the drug of choice in the treatment of actinomycosis. Because of occasional failures with this therapy alone, sulfonamide has been used concurrently. Although the effectiveness of such combined medication has been reported, controlled studies in support of its use are not available. Surgical excision of the infected areas is necessary in some cases before the disease can be cured.

Streptococcal Infections. Sulfonamide therapy does not significantly alter the course of *pharyngitis* due to group-A *Strep. pyogenes.* It neither eradicates the microorganisms from the throat nor prevents the development of the late nonsuppurative sequelae such as rheumatic fever and glomerulonephritis. Penicillin therapy, on the other hand, eradicates the microorganisms from practically all patients treated for 10 days.

There is presently no indication for the use of sulfonamides in serious forms of streptococcal diseases, such as erysipelas, cellulitis, bacteremia, and pneumonia. They are readily managed by administration of penicillin or erythromycin.

Trachoma and Inclusion Conjunctivitis. Sulfonamides, in full doses orally and/or applied locally in the conjunctival sac, have been considered the agents of choice for the management of trachoma. In addition, the topical application of one of the tetracyclines has been employed to eradicate common pyogenic organisms in order to shorten the total period of morbidity. Although the therapeutic results are best when therapy is initiated early, even chronic cicatricial cases may respond. The local symptoms may disappear in a few days. Pannus, keratitis, conjunctival granulations, entropion, trichiasis, iritis, and corneal ulcerations improve and may even disappear. Corneal lesions respond more rapidly than do those of the conjunctivae. Blindness may be prevented (*see* Siniscal, 1952). Dawson and associates (1968) reported that some of the reported benefits of chemotherapy in trachoma might be attributable to control of bacterial suprainfection.

Although tetracycline or chloramphenicol is effective, many physicians prefer to treat *inclusion conjunctivitis* (inclusion blenorrhea) with topical application of a 10% sulfacetamide ointment, six times a day for 10 days.

Dermatitis Herpetiformis (Duhring's Disease). Sulfonamides have been used for the management of this skin disorder. The preferred drug appears to be sulfapyridine. Therapy is started with 0.5 g four times a day; this is increased gradually until a total of 4 to 5 g per day is being given, unless intolerance develops. Dermatitis herpetiformis is the only indication for sulfapyridine, an older sulfonamide that is no longer an official drug. In patients in whom this treatment is unsuccessful, the agent of choice is *dapsone;* the initial dose is 25 to 50 mg per day. If this does not produce suppression of the disease and if there is no evidence of toxicity, the dose is increased by 50 mg per day over a period of several days. Rarely, a total daily dose of 500 mg is required.

Toxoplasmosis. Although pyrimethamine is the agent of primary importance in the therapy of infections due to *Toxoplasma gondii,* most clinicians who have had experience with this disease prefer to give full doses of sulfisoxazole simultaneously. In patients with severe chorioretinitis, it is advisable to add a corticosteroid to the therapeutic regimen.

Use of Sulfonamides for Prophylaxis. The effectiveness of penicillin and other antibiotics in preventing certain bacterial infections has decreased but not eliminated the use of sulfonamides for chemoprophylaxis. In a very few situations, sulfonamides serve as satisfactory substitutes for other antimicrobial compounds and may, indeed, be preferable. The sulfonamides exhibit a degree of effectiveness nearly comparable or equal to that of oral penicillin in *preventing streptococcal infections and rheumatic fever recurrences* among susceptible subjects. Despite the efficacy of sulfonamides in the prevention of rheumatic fever recurrence, their toxicity and the possibility of infection by drug-resistant streptococci make them less desirable than penicillin for this purpose. They should be used, however, without hesitation in patients who are hypersensitive to penicillin. Chemoprophylaxis with sulfonamides for even long periods does not lead to important and potentially dangerous alterations in the microflora of the upper respiratory tract. The recommended dose of sulfisoxazole is 1.0 g twice daily; for children under 27 kg (60 lb), the dose is halved. If untoward responses occur, they usually do so during the first 8 weeks of therapy; serious reactions after this time are rare. White-cell counts should be carried out once weekly during the first 8 weeks.

The sulfonamides have been applied prophylactically in a number of situations in which their use is of *doubtful value.* One of the most common of these is the attempt to prevent infection after instrumentation, catheterization, or other manipulation of the *genitourinary tract.* There are no well-controlled observations indicating the value of this measure. Indeed, some studies have demonstrated that such chemoprophylaxis does not produce the desired results; in fact, whereas the number of more readily treatable *E. coli* infections is reduced, those due to *Strep. faecalis, Proteus,* and staphylococci are increased.

TRIMETHOPRIM-SULFA-METHOXAZOLE

The introduction of trimethoprim in combination with sulfamethoxazole constitutes an important advance in the development of clinically effective antimicrobial agents and represents the practical application of a theoretical consideration; that is, if two drugs act on sequential steps in the pathway of an obligate enzymatic reaction in bacteria, the result of their combination will be supra-additive. Extensive biochemical studies of the mode of action of this combination of compounds clearly indicate that this is the case. The details of the mechanisms of action of this preparation were defined well before its range of clinical effectiveness was established. There is little doubt that, in this combination with trimethoprim, sulfonamide will find a broader area of therapeutic usefulness.

Chemistry. Sulfamethoxazole has been discussed on page 1118, and its structural formula is shown in Table 56–1. The history and chemistry of *trimethoprim* are described in Chapter 52.

Antibacterial Spectrum. The antibacterial spectrum of trimethoprim is similar to that of sulfamethoxazole, although the former drug is usually 20 to 100 times more potent than the latter. The data presented here refer to the antimicrobial activity of the *combination* of trimethoprim and sulfamethoxazole.

All strains of *Strep. pneumoniae, C. diphtheriae,* and *N. meningitidis* are sensitive to trimethoprim-sulfamethoxazole. From 50 to 95% of strains of *Staph. aureus, Staph. epidermidis, Strep. pyogenes,* the *viridans* group of streptococci, *Strep. faecalis, E. coli, Pr. mirabilis, Pr. morganii, Pr. rettgeri, Enterobacter (Aerobacter)* species, *Salmonella, Shigella, Pseud. pseudomallei, Serratia,* and *Alcaligenes* species are inhibited. Also sensitive are *Klebsiella* species, *Brucella abortus, Pasteurella haemolytica, Yersinia pseudotuberculosis, Y. enterocolitica,* and *Nocardia asteroides.* Very few strains of *Pseud. aeruginosa* are sensitive. Methicillin-resistant strains of *Staph. aureus,* although also resistant to trimethoprim or sulfamethoxazole alone, are susceptible to the combination. A synergistic interaction between the components of the preparation is apparent *even* when microorganisms are resistant to sulfonamide or resistant to sulfonamide and moderately resistant to trimethoprim. However, a *maximal degree* of synergism occurs when microorganisms are sensitive to both components. The activity of trimethoprim-sulfamethoxazole *in vitro* depends on the medium in which it is determined; for example, traces of thymidine almost completely abolish the antibacterial activity. (*See* Symposium, 1969, 1973.)

Mechanism of Action. The antimicrobial activity of the combination of trimethoprim and sulfamethoxazole results from its actions on two steps of the enzymatic pathway for the synthesis of tetrahydrofolic acid. Sulfonamide inhibits the incorporation of PABA into folic acid, and trimethoprim prevents the reduction of dihydrofolate to tetrahydrofolate. The latter is the form of folate essential for one-carbon transfer reactions, for example, the synthesis of thymidylate from deoxyuridylate. Selective toxicity for microorganisms is achieved in two ways. Mammalian cells utilize preformed folates from the diet and do not synthesize the compound. Furthermore, trimethoprim is a highly *selective* inhibitor of dihydrofolate reductase of lower organisms (*see* Chapter 52). This is vitally important, since this enzymatic function is a crucial one in all species.

The synergistic interaction between sulfonamide and trimethoprim is thus predictable from their respective mechanisms. There is an optimal ratio of the concentrations of the two agents for synergism, and this is equal to the ratio of the minimal inhibitory concentrations of the drugs acting independently. The pharmacokinetic properties of the sulfonamide chosen to be in combination with trimethoprim are thus important, since relative constancy of the concentrations of the two compounds in the body is desired. As mentioned, trimethoprim is usually 20 to 100 times more potent than sulfamethoxazole, and the combination is thus formulated to achieve a sulfamethoxazole concentration *in vivo* 20 times greater than that of trimethoprim. (*See* articles by Hitchings, Burchall, and Bushby in Symposium, 1973.)

Bacterial Resistance. The frequency of development of bacterial resistance to trimethoprim-sulfamethoxazole is lower than it is to either of the agents alone. This is logical, since a microorganism that has acquired resistance to one of the components may still be killed by the other. Resistance in gram-negative bacteria is associated with the presence of R factors, which can be transferred to susceptible microorganisms by conjugation. Resistance to high concentrations of sulfonamides and to moderate concentrations of trimethoprim has been demonstrated to be transferred in this manner. Resistance to trimethoprim in *Staph. aureus* appears to be determined by a chromosomal gene rather than by a plasmid (Nakhla, 1973). The development of resistance to the combination also occurs *in vivo. Escherichia coli* resistant to trimethoprim and *H. influenzae* resistant to trimethoprim-sulfamethoxazole have been isolated from patients treated with the combination (Lacey *et al.,* 1972; May and Davies, 1972).

Absorption, Distribution, and Excretion. The pharmacokinetic profiles of both sulfamethoxazole and trimethoprim follow the general principles discussed in Chapter 1, whether the drugs are administered separately or in combination. After a single oral dose of the combined preparation, trimethoprim is absorbed more rapidly than sulfamethoxazole. The coadministration of the drugs appears to slow the absorption of sulfamethoxazole. Peak blood concentrations of trimethoprim usually occur by 2 hours in most patients, while peak concentrations of sulfamethoxazole are seen by 4 hours after a single oral dose. The half-lives of trimethoprim and sulfamethoxazole are 16 and 10 hours, respectively.

When 400 mg of sulfamethoxazole is given with 80 mg of trimethoprim (the conventional 5:1 ratio), three times daily, the mean minimal steady-state concentrations of the drugs are approximately 20 and 1 $\mu g/ml$, respectively—the optimal ratio that is sought.

Trimethoprim is rapidly distributed and concentrated in tissues, and relatively small quantities are bound to plasma protein in the presence of sulfamethoxazole. The drug enters cerebrospinal fluid and sputum readily. High concentrations of each component of the mixture are also found in bile. About 65% of sulfamethoxazole is bound to plasma protein.

Up to 60% of administered trimethoprim and from 25 to 50% of sulfamethoxazole are excreted in the urine in 24 hours. Two thirds of the sulfonamide is unconjugated. Metabolites of trimethoprim are also excreted. The rates of excretion and the urine concentrations of both compounds are significantly reduced in patients with uremia.

(For details of the pharmacology of trimethoprim-sulfamethoxazole and its components, *see* Bushby and Hitchings, 1968; Sharpstone, 1969; Schwartz and Rieder, 1970; Bergan and Brodwall, 1972; Nolte and Büttner, 1973; Symposium, 1973.)

Preparations, Routes of Administration, and Dosage. *Trimethoprim-sulfamethoxazole* (BACTRIM, SEPTRA) is currently supplied only in oral *tablets* containing 80 mg of trimethoprim and 400 mg of sulfamethoxazole. The usual *adult* dose is 2 tablets every 12 hours for 10 to 14 days for management of most infections. Larger quantities have been given in special circumstances in patients with serious or life-threatening disease. The following dosage should be observed in patients with renal insufficiency: creatinine clearance over 30 ml per minute,

the usual dosage schedule; clearance of 15 to 30 ml per minute, 2 tablets every 24 hours. If the clearance is less than 15 ml per minute, the preparation should not be administered.

Treatment of *children* under 12 years of age is currently not recommended. Since there are as yet insufficient data, the combination must be used with great caution in *pregnant patients.*

Untoward Effects. There is no evidence that trimethoprim-sulfamethoxazole, when given in the recommended doses, induces folate deficiency in normal persons. However, the margin between toxicity for bacteria and that for man may be relatively narrow when the cells of the patient are deficient in folate. In such cases, trimethoprim-sulfamethoxazole may cause or precipitate *megaloblastosis, leukopenia,* or *thrombocytopenia.* In routine use, the combination appears to exert little toxicity. About 75% of the untoward effects involve the *skin.* These are typical of those known to be produced by *sulfonamides,* as already described. *Exfoliative dermatitis, Stevens-Johnson syndrome,* and *toxic epidermal necrolysis* (Lyell's syndrome) are rare, occurring primarily in older individuals. Skin reactions have developed in from 1.6 to 8% of individuals in different series of patients. *Nausea* and *vomiting* constitute the bulk of gastrointestinal reactions; *diarrhea* is rare. *Glossitis* and *stomatitis* are relatively common. Mild and transient *jaundice* has been noted and appears to have the histological features of allergic cholestatic hepatitis. Most patients who have developed icterus have had a history of prior infectious hepatitis. Central nervous system reactions consist in *headache, depression,* and *hallucinations,* manifestations known to be produced by sulfonamides. Hematological reactions, in addition to those mentioned above, are various types of *anemia* (including *aplastic, hemolytic,* and *macrocytic*), *coagulation disorders, granulocytopenia, agranulocytosis, purpura, Henoch-Schönlein purpura,* and *sulfhemoglobinemia.* Previous or simultaneous administration of diuretics with trimethoprim-sulfamethoxazole may carry an increased risk of thrombocytopenia, especially in elderly patients with heart failure; death may occur. (*See* Symposium, 1973.)

Therapeutic Uses. *Urinary Tract Infections.* The sulfonamides remain very useful for the management of most patients with uncomplicated infections of the lower urinary tract. Many physicians still consider sulfisoxazole (2 to 6 g per day for 10 days) the drug of first choice for such urinary tract infections caused by sensitive strains of microorganisms. However, there has been a sharp increase in the incidence of drug resistance among the causative agents, primarily gram-negative bacteria, so that the sulfonamides should not be relied upon for therapy of more serious infections in the upper urinary tract. It is important to distinguish between infections involving the kidney and those that are located in the lower urinary tract. *Acute pyelonephritis* with high-grade fever and other severe constitutional manifestations and the risk of bacteremia and shock is best not treated with a sulfonamide; rather, it requires a bactericidal antimicrobial drug administered parenterally and selected on the basis of the sensitivity of the microorganism cultured from the urine. The sulfonamides should be reserved for the management of *acute and chronic cystitis, chronic infections of the upper urinary tract,* and *asymptomatic bacilluria.* Since acute cystitis is most often caused by *E. coli* or *Pr. mirabilis,* the sulfonamides are highly effective.

Experience with the treatment of uncomplicated lower urinary tract infections with trimethoprim-sulfamethoxazole is now sufficiently extensive to indicate that it is often highly effective, even when the infecting agent is resistant to the sulfonamides alone. A dose of 2 tablets of the combination every 12 hours for 10 days produces cure in the vast majority of cases. The preparation has been shown to produce a better therapeutic effect than does either of its components given separately when the infecting microorganisms are of the family Enterobacteriaceae. It has also been used in the same dose in patients with chronic or recurrent upper and lower urinary tract disease. When *Strep. faecalis* is the causative microorganism, however, resistance often develops within 2 weeks of treatment (Chattopadhyay, 1972). Asymptomatic bacilluria usually responds promptly to treatment with 1 tablet every 6 hours for 2 weeks. Limited experience with use of this combination in 120 pregnant patients with bacilluria revealed no evidence of teratogenicity. It should be remembered that trimethoprim-sulfamethoxazole is a relatively new drug combination with toxic potential equal at least to that of the sulfonamide. Furthermore, the cost of a therapeutic course of this combination is considerably more than that of sulfisoxazole alone. In all such decisions, the results of microbial sensitivity testing must of course be considered.

Recurrent infections of the urinary tract are much more difficult to manage successfully. An integral part of the study of patients with this kind of disease is first to establish whether the chronicity is due to *reinfection* with new microorganisms or whether the same microorganism(s) is persisting, causing *relapse* despite therapy. Reinfection occurs most commonly in sexually active females, is usually a less serious problem, and can often be successfully managed by the initial antimicrobial agent chosen, such as sulfisoxazole. However, relapse with the same microorganism(s) is often more serious, suggesting a persistent focus of infection in the upper urinary tract that is difficult or impossible to eradicate. Reasons for this persistence include: (1) functional or mechanical obstruction preventing complete evacuation of the urinary bladder; (2) resistance of the microorganism(s) to the commonly used antibiotics; (3) impairment of normal host defenses, as in patients with diabetes mellitus; or (4) some combination of the above. These patients must be thoroughly evaluated to rule out remediable obstruction. The microorganisms involved include *Escherichia, Enterobacter (Aerobacter), Alcaligenes, Klebsiella, Proteus,* gram-positive cocci (including the enterococcus), and mixtures of microorganisms. The cure rate for chronic infection of the urinary tract is relatively low, regardless of the type of antimicrobial therapy employed, and *chronic suppressive therapy or intermittent treatment of symptomatic relapses may eventually be the most reasonable goal.* Although many physicians use antibiotics to treat such cases, there is no evidence that such agents produce better results and, because they may have to be administered over long periods, patients are exposed to their untoward effects.

The chemotherapeutic programs that have been employed for this type of disease are variable, and each has its enthusiastic supporters. The writer's program is as follows: As soon as the diagnosis is made, 1 g of sulfisoxazole is given every 6 hours for 10 days. At this time urine bacterial counts are made. If there has been no effect, sulfonamide treatment is stopped and another antibacterial agent (nitrofurantoin, methenamine mandelate) substituted. If, however, the number of microorganisms in the urine is reduced to less than 10,000 per milliliter, the dose of sulfisoxazole is reduced to 1 g every 12 hours and continued for 3 months. Therapy is then omitted, and 1 week later the urine bacterial count is determined. If this is within normal limits, the count is repeated once a month for 3 months. In some but not many instances, this program suffices. In most of the others, relapse follows shortly after the administration of sulfonamide is stopped. Re-treatment is then undertaken with 4 g of sulfonamide per day for the first 10 days and 2 g daily thereafter for 1 year. This results in a small increment of cures. A number of patients require "chronic suppressive therapy." This involves the daily administration of 2 g of sulfisoxazole for a number of years. In older patients, this may have to be carried on for the rest of their lives. Some patients have been treated in this manner for 8 to 10 years because relapse of infection has occurred every time drug has been omitted. It must be stressed that the use of sulfonamides in this fashion for therapy of chronic urinary tract infection fails in a number of cases. With recurrent infection with the same microorganism, a therapeutic course of trimethoprim-sulfamethoxazole may be justified, despite previous failure with sulfonamide alone. Although the initial response to this combination may be satisfactory, relapse is common when obstruction is present, even while therapy is continued. Furthermore, some patients may develop suprainfections with bacteria resistant to this combination. In such cases of relapse, other agents such as nitrofurantoin (100 mg twice a day) or methenamine mandelate (4 g per day and acidification of urine if necessary) may suppress the infection. Patients given "chronic suppressive therapy" have maintained for many years the level of renal function present at the beginning of treatment. (*See* Lindemeyer *et al.,* 1963; McCabe and Jackson, 1965; Turck *et al.,* 1966.)

Genital Infections. Trimethoprim-sulfamethoxazole is effective in the management of *acute gonococcal urethritis* in both men and women. Several regimens have been recommended. Among these are (1) 2 tablets twice a day for 5 days; (2) 4 tablets twice a day for 2 days; (3) 6 tablets once a day for 3 days or 3 tablets twice a day for 3 days. These regimens appear to be as effective as a single dose of 4.8 million units of procaine penicillin G plus 1 g of probenecid. The drug has no effect in preventing incubating *syphilis* or in curing the established disease (Svindland, 1973).

Trimethoprim-sulfamethoxazole appears to produce a beneficial effect in some but not all instances of acute and chronic prostatitis and prostatic abscess. Both short-term therapy (2 tablets twice a day for 2 weeks) and long-term therapy (2 tablets twice a day for 2 months, followed by 1 tablet twice a day for 2 to 9 months) have been recommended.

Respiratory Tract Infections. The response of *Strep. pyogenes acute pharyngitis* to trimethoprim-sulfamethoxazole is not as good as that resulting from treatment with adequate doses of penicillin G.

Pulmonary infections of various types have been treated with the combination. Administration of 2 tablets six times a day or 4 tablets three times a day appears to be very effective in decreasing fever, purulence and volume of sputum, and sputum bacterial count in patients with *acute exacerbations of chronic bronchitis.* The microorganisms involved have been *H. influenzae* and *Strep. pneumoniae.* It has been suggested that trimethoprim-sulfamethoxazole may be an effective prophylactic agent in this kind of disease. A few cases of *lung abscess, pneumonia,* and *bronchiectasis* have been treated successfully. It must be pointed out, however, that experience with therapy of bronchopulmonary infections with this preparation is still too limited to establish the parameters of effectiveness.

Miscellaneous Infections. Several reports have suggested that trimethoprim-sulfamethoxazole may be effective in the therapy of *brucellosis* even when localized lesions such as arthritis, endocarditis, or epididymo-orchitis are present. Doses have ranged from 2 tablets three times a day for 1 week followed by 2 tablets a day for 2 weeks to 4 to 8 tablets per day for 2 months. Most patients recover, particularly when the latter dosage schedule is employed; however, relapse has occurred in 4% of cases even with this regimen. Hassan and associates (1971) have suggested that therapy (2 to 4 tablets per day) be continued for an additional 6 weeks to minimize the risk of relapse.

There is some difference of opinion concerning the therapeutic value of trimethoprim-sulfamethoxazole in *typhoid fever.* The experience of Scragg and Rubidge (1971) suggests that, in children, this drug is not as effective as chloramphenicol. In adults with this disease, trimethoprim-sulfamethoxazole appears to be as effective as chloramphenicol when the dose is 2 tablets every 12 hours for 15 days. The combination has been used in the treatment of *cholera;* it appears to be an effective alternative to tetracycline. Although attempts have been made to treat *subacute bacterial endocarditis* with trimethoprim-sulfamethoxazole, this is not advisable in cases due to the *viridans* group of streptococci, other streptococci, or *Staph. aureus,* since experience is much too limited as yet and highly effective agents for the therapy of this disease are available. However, there is some evidence that valvular infection due to *Pseud. cepacia* may respond favorably, especially when polymyxin is given simultaneously.

Trimethoprim-sulfamethoxazole appears to be effective in the management of *carriers* of *S. typhi* and other species of *Salmonella.* One proposed schedule is 2 tablets twice a day for 3 months; however, relapses have occurred. It has been suggested that the presence of chronic disease of the gallbladder is associated with a high incidence of failure to clear the carrier state (Brodie *et al.,* 1970). (*See* Symposium, 1969, 1973.)

Andreasen, F. Protein binding in plasma from patients with acute renal failure. *Acta pharmac. tox.,* **1973,** *32,* 417–429.

Artenstein, M. S. Prophylaxis for meningococcal disease. *J. Am. med. Ass.,* **1975,** *231,* 1035–1037.

Ballin, J. C. Evaluation of a new topical agent for burn therapy. Silver sulfadiazine (SILVADENE). *J. Am. med. Ass.,* **1974,** *230,* 1184–1185.

Bell, P. H., and Roblin, R. O., Jr. Studies in chemotherapy. VII. A theory of the relation of structure to activity of sulfanilamide type compounds. *J. Am. chem. Soc.,* **1942,** *64,* 2905–2917.

Bergan, T., and Brodwall, E. K. Kidney transport in man of sulfamethoxazole and trimethoprim. *Chemotherapy,* **1972,** *17,* 320–333.

Black, W. A., and McNellis, D. A. Susceptibility of *Nocardia* species to modern antimicrobial agents. In, *Antimicrobial Agents and Chemotherapy—1970.* (Hobby, G. L., ed.) American Society for Microbiology, Bethesda, Md., **1971,** pp. 346–349.

Brodie, J.; MacQueen, I. A.; and Livingstone, D. Effect of trimethoprim-sulfamethoxazole on typhoid and salmonella carriers. *Br. med. J.,* **1970,** *3,* 318–319.

Brown, G. M. The biosynthesis of folic acid. II. Inhibition by sulfonamides. *J. biol. Chem.,* **1962,** *237,* 536–540.

Bushby, S. R. M., and Hitchings, G. H. Trimethoprim, a sulphonamide potentiator. *Br. J. Pharmac. Chemother.,* **1968,** *33,* 72–90.

Buttle, G. A. H.; Gray, W. H.; and Stephenson, D. Protection of mice against streptococcal and other infections by *p*-aminobenzenesulphonamide and related substances. *Lancet,* **1936,** *1,* 1286–1290.

Chattopadhyay, B. Trimethoprim-sulfamethoxazole in urinary tract infection due to *Streptococcus faecalis.* *J. clin. Path.,* **1972,** *25,* 531–533.

Colebrook, L., and Kenny, M. Treatment of human puerperal infections, and of experimental infections in mice, with PRONTOSIL. *Lancet,* **1936,** *1,* 1279–1286.

Collins, J. R. Adverse reactions to salicylazosulfapyridine (AZULFIDINE) in the treatment of ulcerative colitis. *Sth. med. J., Nashville,* **1968,** *61,* 354–358.

Dawson, C. R.; Hanna, L.; Wood, T. R.; and Jawetz, E. Double-blind treatment trials in chronic trachoma of American Indian children. In, *Antimicrobial Agents and Chemotherapy—1967.* American Society for Microbiology, Ann Arbor, Mich., **1968,** pp. 137–142.

Domagk, G. Ein Beitrag zur Chemotherapie der bakteriellen Infektionen. *Dt. med. Wschr.,* **1935a,** *61,* 250–253.

————. Eine neue Klasse von Desinfektionsmitteln. *Ibid.*, **1935b**, *61*, 829–832.

Dujovne, C. A.; Chan, C. H.; and Zimmerman, H. J. Sulfonamide liver injury: review of the literature and report of a case due to sulfamethoxazole. *New Engl. J. Med.*, **1967**, *277*, 785–788.

Feldman, H. A. Sulfonamide-resistant meningococci. *A. Rev. Med.*, **1967**, *18*, 495–506.

Fildes, P. A rational approach to research in chemotherapy. *Lancet*, **1940**, *1*, 955–957.

Fourneau, E.; Tréfouël, J.; Tréfouël, J.; Nitti, F.; and Bovet, D. Chimiothérapie des infections streptococciques par les dérivés du *p*-aminophénylsulfamide. *C. r. Séanc. Soc. Biol.*, **1936**, *122*, 652–654.

Gelmo, P. Sulphamides of *p*-aminobenzenesulphonic acid. *J. Prakt. Chem.*, **1908**, *77*, 369–382.

Gorbach, S. L.; Nahas, L.; Plaut, A.; Weinstein, L.; Patterson, J. F.; and Levitan, R. Studies of intestinal microflora. V. Fecal microbial ecology in ulcerative colitis and regional enteritis: relationship to severity of disease and chemotherapy. *Gastroenterology*, **1967**, *54*, 575–587.

Haltalin, K. C., and Nelson, J. D. *In vitro* susceptibility of shigellae to sodium sulfadiazine and eight antibiotics. *J. Am. med. Ass.*, **1965**, *193*, 705–710.

Harrison, H. N.; Bales, H. W.; and Jacoby, F. J. The absorption into burned skin of SULFAMYLON ACETATE from 5 percent aqueous solution. *J. Trauma*, **1972**, *12*, 994–998.

Hassan, A.; Erian, M. M.; Farid, Z.; Hathout, S. D.; and Sorensen, K. Trimethoprim-sulfamethoxazole in acute brucellosis. *Br. med. J.*, **1971**, *3*, 159–160.

Kaiser, A. B.; Hennekens, C. H.; Saslaw, M. S.; Hayes, P. S.; and Bennett, J. V. Seroepidemiology and chemoprophylaxis of disease due to sulfonamide-resistant *Neisseria meningitidis* in a civilian population. *J. infect. Dis.*, **1974**, *130*, 217–224.

Kutscher, A. H.; Lane, S. L.; and Segall, R. The clinical toxicity of antibiotics and sulfonamides: a comparative review of the literature based on 104,672 cases treated systemically. *J. Allergy*, **1954**, *25*, 135–150.

Lacey, R. W.; Gillespie, W. A.; Bruten, D. M.; and Lewis, E. L. Trimethoprim-resistant coliforms. *Lancet*, **1972**, *1*, 409–410.

Lindberg, R. B.; Moncrief, V. A.; and Mason, A. D., Jr. Control of experimental and clinical burn wound sepsis by topical application of SULFAMYLON compounds. *Ann. N.Y. Acad. Sci.*, **1968**, *150*, 950–960.

Lindemeyer, A. J.; Turck, M.; and Petersdorf, R. G. Factors determining the outcome of chemotherapy in infections of the urinary tract. *Ann. intern. Med.*, **1963**, *58*, 201–216.

McCabe, W. R., and Jackson, G. G. Treatment of pyelonephritis: bacterial, drug and host factors in success or failure among 252 patients. *New Engl. J. Med.*, **1965**, *272*, 1037–1044.

May, J. R., and Davies, J. Resistance of *Haemophilus influenzae* to trimethoprim. *Br. med. J.*, **1972**, *3*, 376–377.

Misiewicz, J. J.; Lennard-Jones, J. E.; Connell, A. M.; Baron, J. H.; and Jones, F. A. Controlled trial of sulphasalazine in maintenance therapy for ulcerative colitis. *Lancet*, **1965**, *1*, 185–188.

Nakhla, L. S. Genetic determinants of trimethoprim resistance in a strain of *Staphylococcus aureus. J. clin. Path.*, **1973**, *26*, 712–715.

Nolte, H., and Büttner, H. Pharmacokinetics of trimethoprim and its combination with sulfamethoxazole in man after single and chronic oral administration. *Chemotherapy*, **1973**, *18*, 274–284.

Peppercorn, M. A., and Goldman, P. Distribution studies of salicylazosulfapyridine and its metabolites. *Gastroenterology*, **1973**, *64*, 240–245.

Reisberg, B.; Herzog, J.; and Weinstein, L. *In vitro* antibacterial activity of trimethoprim alone and in combination with sulfonamides. In, *Antimicrobial Agents and Chemotherapy—1966.* American Society for Microbiology, Ann Arbor, Mich., **1967**, pp. 424–427.

Riis, P.; Anthonisen, P.; Wulff, R.; Folkenborg, O.; Bonnevie, O.; and Binder, V. The prophylactic effect of salicylazosulphapyridine in ulcerative colitis during long-term treatment. *Scand. J. Gastroent.*, **1973**, *8*, 71–74.

Rosenkranz, H. S., and Rosenkranz, S. Silver sulfadiazine: interaction with isolated deoxyribonucleic acid. *Antimicrob. Agents Chemother.*, **1972**, *2*, 373–383.

Schnitzer, R. J.; Foster, R. H. K.; Ercoli, N.; Soo-Hoo, G.; Mangieri, C. N.; and Roe, M. D. Pharmacological and chemotherapeutic properties of 3,4-dimethyl-5-sulfanilamido-isoxazole. *J. Pharmac. exp. Ther.*, **1946**, *88*, 47–57.

Schwartz, D. E., and Rieder, J. Pharmacokinetics of sulfamethoxazole plus trimethoprim in man and their distribution in the rat. *Chemotherapy*, **1970**, *15*, 337–355.

Scragg, J. N., and Rubidge, C. J. Trimethoprim and sulphamethoxazole in typhoid fever in children. *Br. med. J.*, **1971**, *3*, 738–741.

Sharpstone, P. The renal handling of trimethoprim and sulphamethoxazole in man. *Postgrad. med. J.*, **1969**, *45*, Suppl., 38–42.

Singer, R. C. Sulfonamide-resistant meningococcal disease. *Med. Clins N. Am.*, **1967**, *51*, 719–727.

Siniscal, A. A. The sulfonamides and antibiotics in trachoma. *J. Am. med. Ass.*, **1952**, *148*, 637–639.

Svindland, H. B. Treatment of gonorrhoea with sulphamethoxazole-trimethoprim. Lack of effect on concomitant syphilis. *Br. J. vener. Dis.*, **1973**, *49*, 50–53.

Tréfouël, J.; Tréfouël, J.; Nitti, F.; and Bovet, D. Activité du *p*-aminophénylsulfamide sur les infections streptococciques expérimentales de la souris et du lapin. *C. r. Séanc. Soc. Biol.*, **1935**, *120*, 756–758.

Turck, M.; Anderson, K. N.; and Petersdorf, R. G. Relapse and reinfection in chronic bacteriuria. *New Engl. J. Med.*, **1966**, *275*, 70–73.

Weinstein, L., and Samet, C. A. Sulfonamide blood levels and serum antibacterial activity. *Archs intern. Med.*, **1962**, *110*, 794–800.

White, M. G., and Asch, M. J. Acid-base effects of topical mafenide acetate in the burned patient. *New Engl. J. Med.*, **1971**, *284*, 1281–1286.

White, P. J., and Woods, D. D. The synthesis of *p*-aminobenzoic acid and folic acid by staphylococci sensitive and resistant to sulphonamides. *J. gen. Microbiol.*, **1965**, *40*, 243–253.

Woods, D. D. Relation of *p*-aminobenzoic acid to mechanism of action of sulphanilamide. *Br. J. exp. Path.*, **1940**, *21*, 74–90.

————. The biochemical mode of action of the sulphonamide drugs. *J. gen. Microbiol.*, **1962**, *29*, 687–702.

Yow, E. M. Observations on the use of sulfisoxazole (GANTRISIN) in 1000 consecutive patients, with particular reference to the frequency of undesirable side effects. *Am. Practnr Dig. Treat.*, **1953**, *4*, 521–525.

Zetzel, L. Ulcerative colitis. *New Engl. J. Med.*, **1954**, *251*, 610–615, 653–658.

Monographs and Reviews

Hawking, F., and Lawrence, J. S. *The Sulphonamides.* Grune & Stratton, Inc., New York, **1951.**

Henry, R. J. *The Mode of Action of Sulfonamides.* Review series, Vol. 2, No. 1. Josiah Macy, Jr. Foundation, New York, **1944.** (698 references.)

Jawetz, E., and Gunnison, J. B. Antibiotic synergism and antagonism: an assessment of the problem. *Pharmac. Rev.*, **1953**, *5*, 175–192.

Long, P. H., and Bliss, E. A. *The Clinical and Experimental Use of Sulfanilamide, Sulfapyridine and Allied Compounds.* The Macmillan Co., New York, **1939.**

Northey, E. H. *The Sulfonamides and Allied Compounds.* Reinhold Publishing Corp., New York, **1948.** (2668 references.)

Symposium. (Various authors.) The synergy of trimetho-prim and sulphonamides. *Postgrad. med. J.,* **1969,** *45,* Suppl., 3–104.

Symposium. (Various authors.) Trimethoprim-sulfameth-oxazole. *J. infect. Dis.,* **1973,** *128,* Suppl., 425–816.

Weinstein, L.; Madoff, M. A.; and Samet, C. A. The sulfonamides. *New Engl. J. Med.,* **1960,** *263,* 793–800, 842–849, 900–907.

57 ANTIMICROBIAL AGENTS

[Continued]

Penicillins and Cephalosporins

Louis Weinstein

THE PENICILLINS

Penicillin is one of the most important of the antibiotics. Its initial discovery was entirely fortuitous, but its development and therapeutic application represent the results of a well-planned and executed program that brought about one of the major advances in medical science. Although numerous other antimicrobial agents have been produced since penicillin became available, this drug is still probably the most widely used for the treatment of infection. In the years since the first crude product was obtained from fermentation vats, the penicillin molecule has been chemically manipulated, a large number of natural and semisynthetic congeners have been developed, and several new penicillins have become important therapeutic agents.

History. The history of the discovery and the development of penicillin has become common knowledge. It has fortunately been recorded by the chief participants. (*See* Fleming, 1946; Florey, 1946, 1949; Abraham, 1949; Chain, 1954.) Only the highlights are reviewed here. In 1928, while studying staphylococcus variants in the laboratory at St. Mary's Hospital in London, Fleming observed that a mold contaminating one of his cultures caused the bacteria in its vicinity to undergo lysis. Broth in which the fungus was grown was markedly inhibitory and even bactericidal *in vitro* for many microorganisms. Because the mold belonged to the genus *Penicillium*, Fleming named the antibacterial substance *penicillin*.

A decade later penicillin was developed as a systemic therapeutic agent by the concerted and brilliant researches of a group of investigators, headed by H. W. Florey at Oxford University. Starting in 1939, work on the biosynthesis and extraction of penicillin from broth cultures of *Penicillium notatum* was energetically pursued. Within a few months, many of the chemical, physical, and pharmacological properties of the antibiotic were established. By May, 1940, the crude material then available was found to produce dramatic therapeutic effects when administered parenterally to mice with experimentally produced streptococcal infections. Despite great obstacles to its laboratory production, enough penicillin was accumulated by 1941 to conduct therapeutic trials in several patients desperately ill with staphylococcal and streptococcal infections refractory to all other therapy. At this stage, the crude amorphous penicillin was only about 10% pure and it required nearly 100 liters of the broth in which the mold had been grown to obtain enough of the antibiotic to treat one patient for 24 hours. Herrell (1945) records that bedpans were actually used by the Oxford group for growing cultures of *P. notatum*. Case 1 in the 1941 report from Oxford was that of a policeman who was suffering from a severe mixed staphylococcal and streptococcal infection. He was treated with penicillin, some of which had been recovered from the urine of other patients who had been given the drug. It is said that an Oxford professor referred to penicillin as a remarkable substance, grown in bedpans and purified by passage through the Oxford Police Force.

Expansion of the clinical program required the production of larger amounts of penicillin than could be made in the laboratory, and a vast research program was soon initiated in the United States. During 1942, 122 million units of penicillin were made available, and the first clinical trials were conducted at Yale University and the Mayo Clinic with dramatic results (Figure 57–1). By the spring of 1943, 200 cases had been treated with the drug. The results were so impressive that the surgeon general of the United States Army authorized trial of the antibiotic in a military hospital. Soon thereafter, penicillin was adopted throughout the medical services of the United States Armed Forces. By the summer of 1943, the clinical results in 500 cases were reported (National Research Council, 1943).

The deep-fermentation procedure for the biosynthesis of penicillin developed at the Northern Regional Research Laboratories of the Department of Agriculture, Peoria, Illinois, marked a crucial advance in the large-scale production of the antibiotic. From a total production of a few-hundred million units a month in the early days, the quantity manufactured rose to 800 billion units per month by January, 1949. The annual output of the drug per year increased from 222 trillion units (148 tons) in 1950 to 562 trillion units (375 tons) in 1957 (Hirsch and

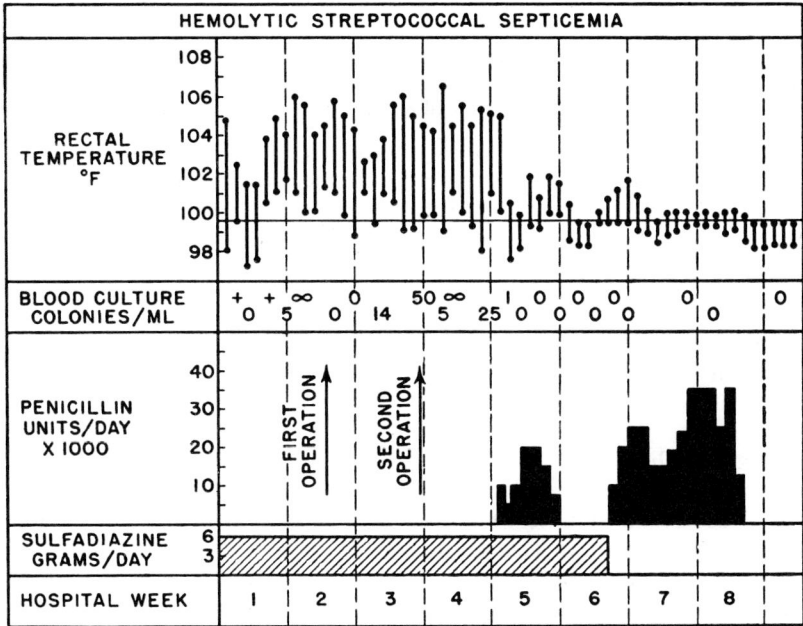

Figure 57-1. *First clinical trial of penicillin in the United States: penicillin therapy of β-hemolytic streptococcal septicemia.*

The patient, a 33-year-old multiparous housewife, entered the New Haven Hospital (Yale University) on February 14, 1942, with the presumptive diagnosis of inevitable abortion of a 4-month-old fetus. Following emptying of the uterus, a chill developed and the temperature rose sharply. (The highest and lowest daily rectal temperature recordings are shown in the figure.) The patient was given sulfadiazine, 6 g daily. High spiking fever persisted despite adequate plasma levels of sulfadiazine, repeated blood transfusions, and supportive therapy. Cultures of the blood and of the fluid aspirated from a septic ankle joint revealed *β-hemolytic streptococcus* type 27. (An "infinite" number of colonies per milliliter of blood is indicated in the figure by the symbol ∞.) The diagnosis of infected abortion, streptococcal septicemia, and thrombophlebitis of the pelvic veins was made. On the eleventh hospital day, surgical exploration of the pelvis was performed (left arrow in figure); the right uterine veins were found to be thrombosed. The right common iliac and left internal iliac veins were ligated. Although blood cultures were negative for several days, the patient's course continued downhill. On the twenty-first hospital day (right arrow), a second operation was undertaken and supravaginal hysterectomy and bilateral salpingo-oophorectomy were performed. The patient's condition remained critical.

On the twenty-ninth hospital day, it was decided to give the patient the carefully husbanded, small supply of penicillin then available. It was injected intravenously every 4 hours day and night for 1 week, in the doses depicted in the figure, until the supply was exhausted. These doses are now known to have been quite small. (The urine was saved for extraction of penicillin for reuse.) The clinical response was dramatic. The temperature fell to normal within a few hours; the blood cultures became sterile and remained so. The persistence of moderate fever was attributable to a pyrogen present in the crude penicillin preparation. The skepticism prevalent at the time resulted in the continuation of sulfadiazine therapy. A new supply of more potent and purer penicillin became available and was given in the depicted doses for 2 weeks, starting on the forty-first hospital day. Convalescence was rapid and uneventful. In its first trial in the United States, penicillin had proved lifesaving. (After Blake, Craige, and Tierney, 1944. Courtesy of the *Transactions of the Association of American Physicians*.)

Putnam, 1958). The first marketable penicillin cost several dollars per 100,000 units; today, the same dose costs only a few cents. Thus did penicillin develop from an insignificant bacteriological tool made in small, impure batches in a university laboratory to an indispensable therapeutic agent industrially manufactured in pure form on an enormous scale.

Source. In the early years of its production, all penicillin came from subcultures of Fleming's original strain. The urgent necessity of producing large amounts of the antibiotic during World War II prompted a vigorous worldwide search for other, more productive strains of *Penicillium*. In addition, mutant strains that arose spontaneously or that were produced by artificial means, such as by exposure to x-rays, were also studied. One of the best was eventually obtained in a culture from the stem of a moldy cantaloupe. After much further selection from this strain, *P. chrysogenum* Thom, NRRL 1951.B 25, was ultimately developed for commercial use. Exposure of this organism to x-rays produced a mutant with a high penicillin yield (X-1612). The production of the antibiotic was enhanced manyfold by growing the mold in corn-steep liquor, a by-product of the maize industry.

Chemistry. The basic structure of the penicillins, as shown in Figure 57–2, consists of a thiazolidine ring (*A*) connected to a beta-lactam ring (*B*), to which is attached a side chain (*R*). The penicillin nucleus itself is the chief structural requirement for biological activity; metabolic transformation or chemical alteration of this portion of the molecule causes loss of all significant antibacterial efficacy. The side chain (*see* Table 57–1, page 1141) determines many of the antibacterial and pharmacological characteristics of a particular type of penicillin. *Penicillin G* is benzylpenicillin.

In the attempt to synthesize penicillin, the greatest obstacle was closure of the beta-lactam ring. Penicilloic acid, the open-chain derivative, was the product of early efforts; attempts to close the ring produced only the isomeric derivative, penicillenic acid. Although closure of the beta-lactam ring has been accomplished, only a token synthesis of penicillin has been achieved, and the process has no commercial application. Biosynthesis of penicillin and synthesis from 6-aminopenicillanic acid, the starting

material for semisynthetic penicillins, remain the current means of obtaining the large amounts of the penicillins used in therapy.

Terminology. The term *penicillin* is generic for the entire group of natural and semisynthetic penicillins. As early as 1943, it became evident that the penicillin prepared in the United States was different from that obtained in Great Britain. It was soon established that the American penicillin had a benzyl side chain whereas the British material had a Δ^2-pentenyl side chain. Still other *natural* penicillins were discovered, and some system of designation became necessary; the American nomenclature was based on capital letters. Several of the early natural penicillins (F, X, K) were studied for clinical efficacy but proved inferior to benzylpenicillin (G).

Semisynthetic Penicillins. The many deficiencies of penicillin G, enumerated below, provided the incentive for the discovery and clinical development of the various semisynthetic penicillins described later in this chapter. In particular, penicillin G is susceptible to inactivation by penicillinases (beta-lactamases); these bacterial enzymes split the beta-lactam ring of penicillin to form the inactive penicilloic acid (Figure 57–2), as a consequence of which the antibiotic is ineffective in the therapy of infections caused by penicillinase-producing microorganisms.

The semisynthetic penicillins can be obtained by the incorporation of specific precursors in mold cultures, by chemical modification of wholly natural penicillins, and by synthesis from 6-aminopenicil-

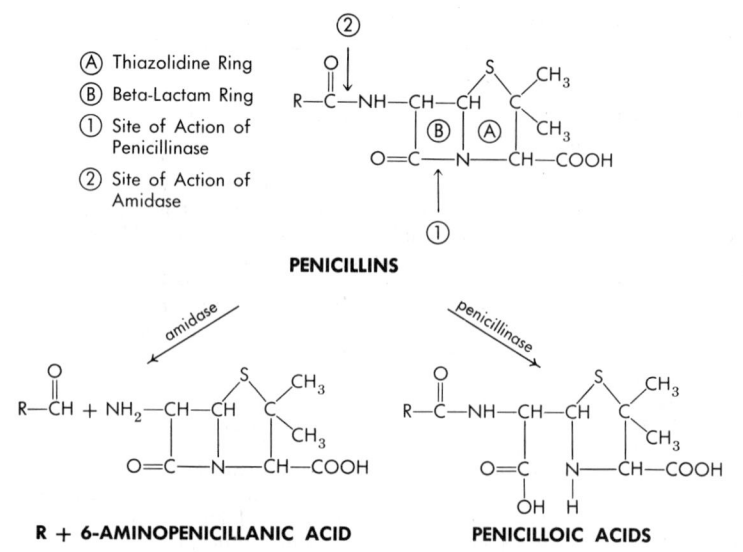

Figure 57–2. *Structure of penicillins and products of their enzymatic hydrolysis.*

lanic acid. The last-named method has been the most fruitful. The important area of research in the development of semisynthetic penicillins had its inception with the commercial production of the penicillin nucleus, *6-aminopenicillanic acid.* The steps leading to this advance have been summarized by Chain (1962) and reviewed by Klein and Finland (1963b). The compound is now produced in large quantities with the aid of an amidase from *P. chrysogenum* (Figure 57–2). This enzyme splits the peptide linkage by which the side chain of penicillin is joined to 6-aminopenicillanic acid (*see* Hamilton-Miller, 1966).

Stability of Penicillin G. The potassium and sodium salts of penicillin G are stable for months in the dry state, even at room temperature; *buffered solutions* may be kept in a refrigerator for several days. Aqueous suspensions of penicillin G procaine are stable for many months at a temperature lower than 25° C, and preparations of penicillin G benzathine are stable at room temperature for at least 2 years. The stability of the *semisynthetic penicillins* is discussed below.

Unitage of Penicillin. A standard system for expressing penicillin potency was adopted by the International Conference on the Standardization of Penicillin, held in London in 1944, which established the *international unit of penicillin* and the *international penicillin master standard.* The latter is a specimen of the crystalline sodium salt of penicillin G; the unit, by definition, is the specific penicillin activity contained in 0.6 μg of the master standard. One milligram of pure penicillin G sodium thus equals 1667 units. Because of the differences in molecular weight, penicillin salts other than the sodium salt have different unitage values; for example, 1.0 mg of pure penicillin G potassium represents 1595 units. The dosage and the antibacterial potency of the semisynthetic penicillins are usually expressed in terms of weight.

Assay. While various methods are available, microbiological assay is the method of choice for clinical purposes. This technic is widely employed for measurement of penicillin concentrations in blood, urine, and spinal and other body fluids, and for studies on the absorption, fate, and excretion of penicillin.

Factors Affecting Antimicrobial Activity. Many factors influence the antimicrobial activity of penicillin and are, therefore, of importance in therapy, bioassay, and determination of bacterial sensitivity. Only the more significant ones will be discussed. The *stability* of the antibiotic obviously affects its potency. Penicillin G is unstable in acidic solutions; fortunately, in the pH range of the body fluids, it displays practically its maximal activity. Variations in the composition of the *culture medium* only slightly influence the potency of the drug as determined *in vitro.* Most *tissue constituents,* blood, and pus do not seriously interfere with the antibacterial action of penicillin. There is no known structural antagonist of penicillin. Although plasma albumin forms an inactive complex with penicillin, the magnitude of the binding is not sufficient to jeopardize its action *in vivo. Penicillinase* rapidly inactivates certain types of the antibiotic, including penicillin G (*see* below).

Density of the bacterial population and *age of the infection* influence penicillin G activity. This drug is a hundred to several thousand times more potent when tested against small than against large inocula of bacteria. Many factors are probably involved in the effect of inoculum size; among these are the greater number of relatively resistant microorganisms in the large populations, the amount of penicillinase produced, and the growth phase of the culture. The intensity and the duration of penicillin therapy needed to abort or cure experimental infections in animals increase with the duration of the infection. The reason is mainly that the bacteria are no longer multiplying as rapidly as in a fresh infection; the antibiotic is most active against bacteria in the logarithmic phase of growth and has no effect on microorganisms in the lag phase (*see* Eagle, 1949, 1952).

EFFECTS OF PENICILLIN G ON MICROORGANISMS

The antimicrobial spectrum of *penicillin G* is presented here, while the antibacterial effects of the various *semisynthetic penicillins,* in comparison with those of penicillin G, are discussed later in this chapter.

Penicillin G is highly effective *in vitro* against many but not all species of gram-positive and gram-negative cocci. Among the *streptococci,* groups A, C, G, H, L, and M are highly sensitive; groups B, E, F, K, and N are less sensitive; *enterococci* are the least susceptible. Whereas most strains of *Staphylococcus aureus* were highly sensitive to penicillin G when this agent was first employed therapeutically, an increasing number of strains resistant to the drug have been recovered over the years. At present, at least 15 to 20% of staphylococci isolated from individuals outside of hospitals are totally resistant to penicillin G; in hospitalized patients, the incidence of such strains is as high as 90 to 95%. *Gonococci* are generally sensitive to penicillin G, although continued exposure of this microorganism to the antibiotic has led to some decrease in sensitivity (Sparling, 1972). A small percentage of strains grow *in vitro* in concentrations of penicillin G as high as 0.1 to 1.0 unit/ml; formerly, all strains were inhibited by 0.06 unit/ml or less. *Meningococci* are quite sensitive to penicillin G. Pneumococci of all serological types are, in general, highly susceptible to penicillin G; however, strains are presently being recovered that are less sensitive but not resistant.

Although the vast majority of strains of *Corynebacterium diphtheriae* are sensitive to penicillin G, some are highly resistant. This is also true for *Bacillus anthracis. Clostridia* are quite susceptible to this antibiotic. *Actinomyces israelii, Streptobacillus (Haverhillia) moniliformis, Pasteurella multocida,* and *Listeria monocytogenes* are inhibited by penicillin G. Most species of *Leptospira* are moderately susceptible to the drug. One of the most exquisitely sensitive microorganisms is *Treponema pallidum.* None of the penicillins is effective against *amebae, plasmodia, rickettsiae, fungi,* or *viruses.*

Although many species of *gram-negative bacilli* are resistant to relatively small quantities of penicillin G, some are affected by moderate-to-high concentrations. The vast majority of strains of *Proteus mirabilis* are inhibited by 10 μg/ml or less of the drug. A study by Weinstein and coworkers (1964a) has indicated that most strains of *Escherichia coli,* all strains of *Salmonella* and *Shigella,* and many strains of *Enterobacter (Aerobacter) aerogenes* and *Alcaligenes faecalis* are susceptible to the high concentrations of penicillin G attained in blood by the parenteral administration of very large doses.

Role of Host Defenses in Penicillin Therapy. As discussed in Chapter 55, host defenses are of importance in the ultimate disposition of certain penicillin-damaged but viable bacteria (group-B hemolytic streptococci) and may at times outweigh the direct bactericidal action of the antibiotic. In man, experiences in the treatment of infections complicating disorders in which specific and nonspecific defense mechanisms are not fully active suggest strongly that penicillin does not cure infection by itself, even when so-called bactericidal levels are present in the blood and tissue fluids. For example, individuals with agranulocytosis who are infected with microorganisms highly sensitive to penicillin often fail to show any response to doses of the drug far in excess of those indicated by the *in-vitro* susceptibility of the offending bacteria (*see* Weinstein and Dalton, 1968).

Effect of Penicillin on Antibody Production. The treatment of human pneumococcal pneumonia with penicillin G does not interfere with the formation of mouse-protective antibodies and agglutinins for the pneumococcus. In streptococcal infections, on the other hand, early penicillin therapy frequently inhibits the development of specific antibodies. Penicillin completely eliminates the appearance of type-specific, M-nucleoprotein (bactericidal) antibody, and sharply reduces the incidence and intensity of development of antistreptolysin and antistreptokinase in cases of scarlet fever. This interferes with the retrospective laboratory diagnosis of *Streptococcus pyogenes* infections.

Effect of Penicillin Coacting with Other Antimicrobial Agents. Penicillin is often given concurrently with other antimicrobial agents for the treatment of infections either in an attempt to increase the total anti-infective effect or to "cover" a situation in which the etiology of a suspected infectious process is not clear. This subject is discussed in more detail in Chapter 55, and examples of clinically beneficial concurrent use of penicillin and other antimicrobial agents are given in the section on therapeutic uses and in Table 55–1 (page 1096).

Mechanism of Action of Penicillin and Related Antimicrobial Agents. Several antimicrobial agents act to inhibit the synthesis of components of the bacterial cell wall, and all will be discussed here.

One layer of the cell wall of both gram-positive and gram-negative microorganisms is formed by *peptidoglycan.* This complex macromolecule provides rigid mechanical stability by virtue of its highly cross-linked latticework structure. In one direction run the glycan strands—alternating molecules of two amino sugars (N-acetylglucosamine and its 3-O-D-lactic acid ether, N-acetylmuramic acid). Peptides of a composition characteristic of individual microbial species form the other dimension and cross-link the glycan strands. In *Staph. aureus,* tetrapeptide units are bonded to the acetylmuramic acid residues, and pentaglycine chains bridge between the tetrapeptide moieties on adjacent strands.

The biosynthesis of the peptidoglycan is usually considered in three stages. The first stage, precursor formation, takes place in the cytoplasm. The product, uridine diphosphate (UDP)–acetylmuramyl-pentapeptide, a "Park nucleotide," accumulates in cells when subsequent synthetic stages are inhibited, and the detection of this accumulation was a major step in the elucidation of the mechanism of action of penicillin (Park and Strominger, 1957). The last reaction in this stage is the addition of a dipeptide, D-alanyl-D-alanine. Synthesis of the dipeptide involves prior racemization of L-alanine and condensation catalyzed by D-alanyl-D-alanine synthetase. D-*Cycloserine* (*see* Chapter 60) is a structural analog of D-alanine and acts as a competitive inhibitor of both the racemase and the synthetase.

During reactions of the second stage, UDP-acetylmuramyl-pentapeptide and UDP-acetylglucosamine are linked (with the release of the uridine nucleotides) to form a long polymer. The sugar pentapeptide is first attached by a pyrophosphate bridge to a phospholipid in the cell membrane. The second sugar is then added, followed by the addition of five glycine residues as a branch of the heteropentapeptide. The first half of the pentaglycine cross-link is thus formed. The completed unit is then cleaved from the membrane-bound phospholipid, a reaction that is inhibited by *vancomycin* and *ristocetin.* For further synthetic reactions to occur the membrane phospholipid, now in a pyrophosphate form, must be dephosphorylated. *Bacitracin* appears to bind to the lipid pyrophosphate and inhibit this reaction.

The third and final stage involves the completion of the cross-link. This is accomplished by a *transpeptidation reaction* that occurs outside the cell membrane. The terminal glycine residue of the pentaglycine bridge is linked to the fourth residue of the pentapeptide (D-alanine), releasing the fifth residue (also D-alanine). This reaction is the one sensitive to the *penicillins* and *cephalosporins.* Perhaps surprisingly, stereomodels reveal that the conformation of penicillin is very similar to that of D-alanyl-D-alanine. The transpeptidase is probably acylated by penicillin; that is, penicilloyl enzyme is apparently formed, with cleavage of the —CO—N— bond of the beta-lactam ring. Strominger (1973) has reviewed this brilliant sequence of investigation (*see also* Blumberg and Strominger, 1974; Symposium, 1974).

The cell walls of gram-negative microorganisms are more complex than those of gram-positive bacteria. However, the peptidoglycan structure is similar, as is the basic action of penicillin. Certain major differences in sensitivity of bacteria are thus not readily explained, nor is the effectiveness of penicillins and cephalosporins with broader antimicrobial spectra. Permeability barriers may offer explanations, as may other as-yet-unidentified sites of drug action.

Deprived of its rigid cell wall, the bacterial cell loses the protection it requires because of its high intracellular osmotic pressure. Lysis of the cell membrane and death follow. In a medium isosmotic with bacterial intracellular fluid, cell-wall–deficient forms (protoplasts or spheroplasts) can survive. It is possible that such cell-wall–deficient forms are responsible for certain failures of therapy with penicillin, despite an initial high level of sensitivity of microorganisms to the antibiotic.

There are other corollaries of these mechanistic studies that have clinical relevance. Since penicillin has no effect on existing cell walls, bacteria must be multiplying for the bactericidal action of penicillin to be manifest. Thus, certain bacteriostatic agents may antagonize the lethal effects of penicillin. Recovery from inhibition of synthesis by penicillin is slow. The continuation of the bactericidal action during "penicillin-free" intervals of therapy that occur with intermittent administration of the drug may be an important factor in the success of such dosage schedules. While penicillin need not be present continuously, the aggregate time during which effective plasma concentrations are maintained is an important determinant of therapeutic success or failure. There is a good correlation between effective concentrations in tissue and *in vitro*.

Bacterial Resistance to Penicillin.
The general phenomenon of resistance to antimicrobial agents is discussed in detail in Chapter 55. With the widespread use of penicillin G, the problem of bacterial resistance has become increasingly prominent and of great clinical importance. Some microorganisms, however, have failed to develop clinically significant degrees of penicillin G resistance despite the fact that infections produced by them have been treated with this agent for more than 30 years; among these are pneumococci and *Strep. pyogenes.*

The percentage of penicillin-resistant staphylococci increased rapidly after the introduction of the antibiotic. For example, Finland and coworkers (*see* Finland and Weinstein, 1953) found that 85% of 120 strains of staphylococci examined for penicillin sensitivity prior to 1946 were inhibited by 0.04 $\mu g/ml$ whereas only 25% of 141 strains studied in the period 1948–1949 were sensitive to this concentration. At the present time almost all staphylococci acquired in the hospital environment are resistant to penicillin G; such strains are less common in the community at large.

Mechanism of Acquired Resistance to Penicillin. The main basis for bacterial resistance to penicillin, occurring naturally or acquired *in vivo,* is the production of the enzyme penicillinase, first described by Abraham and Chain (1940). Penicillin-resistant strains of staphylococci obtained from patients are always capable of elaborating penicillinase; refractory mutants selected by exposure to the drug *in vitro* do not produce this enzyme, and the exact mechanism of their resistance is not known.

Penicillinase is a beta-lactamase that splits the beta-lactam ring of penicillin G and certain congeners between the C and N atoms to form penicilloic acids (*see* Figure 57–2). It is elaborated by a number of different microorganisms, including penicillin-resistant staphylococci, several *Bacillus* species, *E. coli, E. aerogenes, Bacteroides, Proteus* species, *Pseudomonas aeruginosa,* and *Mycobacterium tuberculosis.* Penicillinase-producing gram-positive microorganisms can develop this property by acquisition of a plasmid acquired by transduction; in gram-negative bacteria the ability to produce this enzyme is related to the presence of an R factor acquired by conjugation. Some beta-lactamases are entirely intracellular enzymes, while other bacteria may secrete at least a portion of the enzyme into the environment. The beta-lactamases are both constitutive and inducible. Semisynthetic penicillins such as methicillin, oxacillin, and nafcillin can stimulate the synthesis of penicillinase, despite the fact that they are poor substrates for the enzyme. Penicillinases derived from different microorganisms and from different strains of the same bacterial species have dissimilar kinetic and immunological properties. (*See* Rolinson, 1971; Flynn, 1972.)

The enzyme finds a large area of application in the isolation of microorganisms from blood and exudates from patients receiving penicillin; it should be included in all media in which material obtained from treated individuals is being cultured, in order to eliminate the suppressive effect of any transferred penicillin that may be present. The purified enzyme can be administered intramuscularly to lower plasma concentrations of penicillin when allergic reactions occur. However, this use is *not* recommended, since there is no proof of efficacy and allergic reactions to penicillinase itself may occur. The enzyme is supplied as *penicillinase for injection* (NEUTRAPEN).

ABSORPTION, DISTRIBUTION, EXCRETION, AND METABOLIC ALTERATION OF PENICILLIN G

An enormous literature has accumulated on the absorption, distribution, excretion, and metabolic alteration of the various penicillins available for clinical use. Only the data derived from studies in man and those relevant to the rational therapeutic applications of these compounds will be presented. The following discussion concerns the various forms of *penicillin G*. The properties of the *semisynthetic congeners* are described subsequently.

Absorption. *After Oral Administration.* About one third of an orally administered dose of penicillin G is absorbed from the intestinal tract under favorable conditions. Only a small portion is absorbed from the stomach. Gastric juice at pH 2 rapidly destroys the antibiotic. Because the gastric acidity of full-term newborn babies (after the first 24 to 48 hours) and of premature infants is relatively low, the oral administration of penicillin yields higher plasma concentrations in such patients than in older children or adults. The decrease in gastric acid production with aging, as well as the development of achlorhydria in about 35% of persons over 60 years of age, accounts for better absorption of penicillin G from the gastrointestinal tract of older individuals. Absorption occurs mainly in the duodenum; it is rapid and maximal blood concentrations are attained in 30 to 60 minutes. Two thirds or more of an ingested dose is unabsorbed and passes into the colon, where it is largely inactivated by bacteria; only a small amount is excreted in the feces. The oral dose of penicillin G must be four to five times as large as the intramuscular in order to obtain blood concentrations of comparable height and duration. The two important points to observe in prescribing penicillin G by mouth are to be certain that the dose is adequate, and that it is taken no later than ½ hour before a meal or no earlier than 2 to 3 hours after a meal. Ingestion of food interferes with enteric absorption of penicillin, perhaps by adsorption of the antibiotic on food particles. Although many oral preparations containing buffers are available, these offer no essential advantages over soluble salts of penicillin G taken orally in dry form or (preferably) in aqueous solution.

After Subcutaneous or Intramuscular Injection. The speed of absorption of penicillin G after subcutaneous or intramuscular injection and hence the magnitude and persistence of the blood concentrations attained depend on many factors, including dose, vehicle, concentration, physical form, and solubility of the particular salt or ester of penicillin G. Other factors, especially renal excretion, are also important; for example, so rapid is elimination of penicillin G by the kidney that the plasma concentration falls to half its peak value within 1 hour after injection of aqueous preparations (Figure 57–3). The speed of absorption of soluble penicillin salts is not significantly different after subcutaneous and intramuscular injection; however, the latter is preferred. Peak blood concentrations are reached within 15 to 30 minutes. In most adults with diabetes mellitus, peak plasma concentrations of penicillin G after intramuscular injection are lower than in nondiabetic patients because of poor absorption; the diabetic patient who requires parenteral penicillin G should always be given the drug intravenously.

Many means for prolonging the sojourn of the antibiotic in the body and thereby reducing the frequency of injections have been explored. *Probenecid,* a drug that blocks renal tubular secretion of penicillin, is occasionally used for this purpose; it is discussed in Chapter 41. More commonly, *repository preparations* of penicillin G are employed. Such forms permit injection only once a day or every 2 or 3 days. For special purposes, single-dose administration may suffice. The two repository compounds currently favored are *penicillin G procaine* and *penicillin G benzathine* (*see* section on preparations). Such agents release penicillin G slowly from the area in which they are injected and produce relatively low but persistent concentrations of antibiotic in the blood.

For example, when *penicillin G procaine* is injected intramuscularly (as an aqueous suspension or in oil with aluminum monostearate), a peak plasma concentration is reached within 1 to 3 hours. A conventional dose of 300,000 units of the aqueous suspension results in a maximal plasma concentration of about 1.5 units/ml; this falls gradually so that it averages about 0.2 unit/ml at 24 hours, 0.1 unit/ml at 36 hours, and 0.05 unit/ml at 48 hours. The injection of 300,000 units of penicillin G procaine in oil with aluminum monostearate produces a peak plasma concentration of about 0.25 unit/ml; 0.05 unit/ml or more persists for 96 to 120 hours, and a larger dose (600,000 units) yields somewhat higher values that are maintained more or less uniformly for as long as 4 to 5 days.

Penicillin G benzathine is very slowly absorbed from intramuscular depots and produces the longest

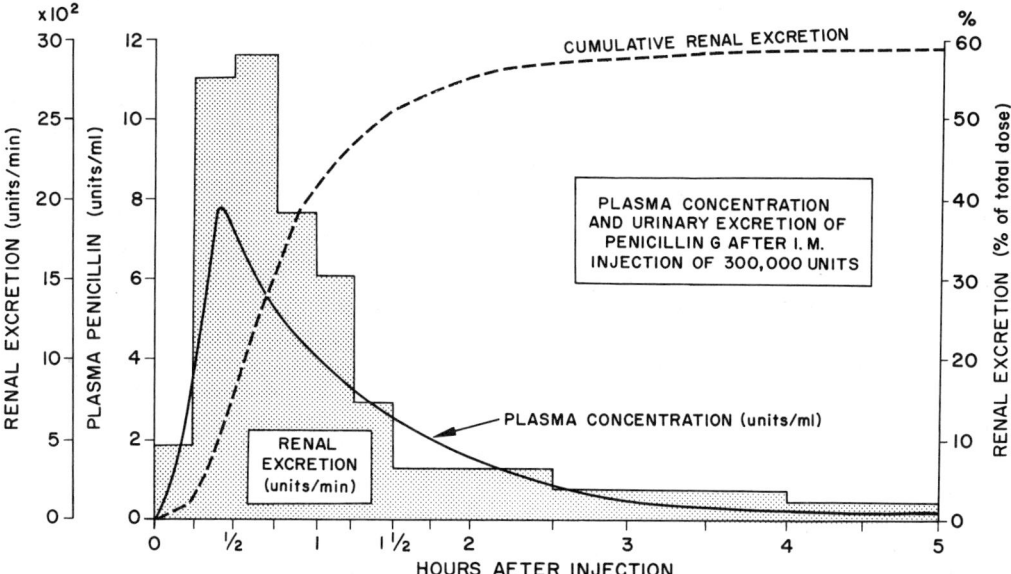

Figure 57–3. *Plasma level and renal excretion of penicillin G.*

This schematic chart is constructed from various reported data on the plasma concentration and the renal elimination of penicillin G in adults with good renal function. In the case shown here, an intramuscular injection of 300,000 units of an aqueous solution of sodium penicillin G was made at zero-time. Observe that the peak plasma level of 8 units/ml was reached between 15 and 30 minutes after the injection and that the concentration then fell quickly to 0.1 unit/ml by the end of 5 hours. This decline is the result of the rapid renal excretion of penicillin G, which is due primarily to tubular secretion. Within the 5-hour period depicted in the chart, nearly 60% (180,000 units) of the administered dose was eliminated in the urine. At the height of the excretory process, nearly 3000 units was being excreted each minute and about 500 ml of plasma was being cleared of penicillin during the same time span.

duration of detectable antibiotic of all the available repository penicillins. For example, in adults, a dose of 1.2 million units given intramuscularly produces an average plasma concentration of 0.15 unit/ml on the first, 0.03 unit/ml on the fourteenth, and 0.003 unit/ml on the thirty-second day after injection. The average duration of demonstrable penicillin in the plasma is about 26 days. Similar pharmacokinetic data are available for newborn infants (Kaplan and McCracken, 1973; Klein *et al.*, 1973).

Absorption from Other Routes. Although suppositories of penicillin G (0.5 to 1.0 million units in cocoa butter) yield therapeutic blood levels when inserted in the *rectum* or *vagina,* such therapy is undependable and not advised. The antibiotic is also absorbed from serous surfaces such as the *pleura, pericardium,* and *peritoneum,* and from *joint cavities* and the *subarachnoid space.* When it is administered as an aerosol by way of the *respiratory tract,* not only are high concentrations produced in the bronchopulmonary tissues despite the presence of mucus but also therapeutic concentrations are attained in the blood and persist for many hours. Penicillin G is not absorbed through the unbroken *skin.*

Distribution. Penicillin G is widely distributed throughout the body, but the con-

centrations in various fluids and tissues differ widely. Its apparent volume of distribution is in about 50% of total body water. More than 90% of the penicillin G in blood is in the plasma and less than 10% is in the erythrocytes; approximately 65% is reversibly bound to plasma albumin. The low concentration of protein in other body fluids and therefore the low degree of binding of penicillin contribute to drug efficacy. Significant amounts appear in liver, bile, kidney, semen, lymph, and intestine.

While probenecid markedly decreases the tubular secretion of the penicillins, this is not the only factor responsible for the elevated plasma concentrations of the antibiotic that follow its administration. Probenecid produces a significant decrease in the volume of distribution of the penicillins (Gibaldi *et al.,* 1970).

Cerebrospinal Fluid. Penicillin does not readily enter the cerebrospinal fluid when the meninges are normal. A plasma concentration of less than 10 units/ml cannot be depended on to establish therapeutically effective concentrations in the cerebrospinal fluid. Even massive intravenous doses of the drug (up to 25 million units in 24 hours) rarely yield spinal fluid concentrations above 0.5 unit/ml, despite the concurrent presence of 50 units/ml of plasma. When the meninges are acutely inflamed, penicillin may penetrate into the spinal fluid more easily; although the concentrations attained vary and are unpredictable, they are often therapeutically effective. Fever appears to increase penetration of the blood-brain barrier by penicillin, probably as a result of vasodilatation and increased cerebral blood flow. Although rarely necessary and fraught with risk if not given properly, the intrathecal route has been used by some clinicians to overcome these difficulties (*see* below); intramuscular penicillin is given at the same time. Direct injection of the antibiotic into the subarachnoid space produces high spinal fluid concentrations immediately; these decline rapidly at first, and then more slowly over a period of 24 hours.

Excretion. Under normal conditions, penicillin G is rapidly eliminated from the body, mainly by the kidney but in small part in the bile and by other channels. The rapid renal excretion of the antibiotic is the reason for the use of measures to prolong its sojourn in the body, such as repository insoluble salts of the drug or the administration of probenecid.

Renal. Approximately 60 to 90% of an intramuscular dose of penicillin G in aqueous solution is eliminated in the urine, largely within the first hour after injection (Figure 57–3). The elimination half-time is about 30 minutes in normal adults. The antibiotic thus reaches high concentrations in the urine; for example, if a dose of 100,000 units of an aqueous solution is injected every 3 hours, the urine will contain from 300 to 1000 units/ml. Approximately 10% of the drug is eliminated by glomerular filtration and 90% by tubular secretion. Renal clearance approximates the total renal plasma flow. The maximal tubular secretory capacity (Tm) for penicillin in the normal male adult is about 3 million units (1.8 g) per hour. Obviously, this maximal transfer capacity is

rarely, if ever, exceeded even when massive doses of the antibiotic are injected intravenously. The rapid renal clearance accounts for the fact that the dose of penicillin G must be increased about fivefold in order to increase the persistence of a plasma concentration of 0.8 unit/ml by only 2 hours.

Clearance values are considerably lower in neonates and infants, because of incomplete development of renal function; as a result, after doses proportionate to surface area, the persistence of penicillin in the blood is several times as long in premature infants as in children and adults. The half-life of the antibiotic in children less than 1 week old is 3 hours; by 14 days of age it is 1⅖ hours (McCracken *et al.*, 1973). After renal function is fully established in young children, the rate of renal excretion of penicillin G is considerably more rapid than in adults. For example, following an intramuscular dose of 300,000 units of penicillin G in aqueous solution in a 3- to 4-year-old child, plasma concentrations of the drug are no longer detectable after 2 to 3 hours. With increasing age and its accompanying decrease in renal tubular excretory function, the rate of elimination of the antibiotic by the kidney is decreased. The renal plasma clearance of penicillin is markedly diminished by other organic acids that are secreted by the renal tubules (Chapter 41).

Approximately 20% of an *oral* dose of penicillin G is excreted in the urine, a reflection of the limited intestinal absorption of the drug; once penicillin has passed the intestinal mucosa, its fate and excretion are the same as for the injected antibiotic.

Anuria increases the half-life of penicillin G from a normal value of ½ hour to about 10 hours. When renal function is impaired, 7 to 10% of the antibiotic may be inactivated per hour by the liver. This probably accounts for its failure to accumulate in excessive concentrations in anuric persons given multiple doses. For this reason, patients with renal shutdown can be treated adequately with penicillin G by the administration of a "loading" dose followed by additional injections every 8 to 12 hours. The dose of the drug must be readjusted during the period of progressive recovery of renal function. If, in addition to renal failure, hepatic insufficiency is also present, the half-life will be prolonged further. It may be necessary to determine the half-life of the drug for the individual patient.

Once penicillin G is released from its repository forms (penicillin G procaine and penicillin G benzathine), it is excreted by the kidney as described above. However, because absorption into the blood from the injection site is continued over a long period, the excretion of active antibiotic in the urine is prolonged. For example, Wright and coworkers (1959) detected penicillin G in the urine of 100% of patients 84 days after an intramuscular injection of 1.2 million units of penicillin G benzathine.

6-Aminopenicillanic acid has been demonstrated in the urine of individuals given oral penicillin (English *et al.*, 1960). It probably is produced by microbial hydrolytic conversion of penicillin in the intestinal tract, and subsequently it is absorbed and then excreted by the kidney.

Bile and Other Channels. Penicillin G is present in human bile, from both the liver and gallbladder, where it is more concentrated and persists longer than in plasma. Indeed, a major site of extrarenal disposition of penicillin is the liver. Biliary excretion of the drug is directly proportional to the adequacy of hepatic function. Because the duodenum is the main site for the enteric absorption of the antibiotic, it is possible that some of the drug excreted in the bile is absorbed by the intestinal mucosa. Some inactivation of the antibiotic takes place in the bile.

A small amount of penicillin G is excreted in human milk and saliva, the concentrations being lower than in plasma. The drug does not appear in detectable quantities in the sweat or tears in man.

Metabolic Alteration. The small fraction of penicillin G that is not excreted in a biologically active form is inactivated in the tissues, but the sites and the mechanisms of inactivation are not well understood. Penicillin G is not readily destroyed in the body.

PREPARATIONS AND ROUTES OF ADMINISTRATION OF PENICILLIN G

Numerous penicillin G preparations are available to the physician, for every route of administration. They are offered under an amazing array of confusing trade names. Many of them are not official. In selecting any penicillin preparation from the large number available, the clinician must keep the following points in mind: (1) the effectiveness of the selected compound for the microorganism responsible for the infection; (2) the route of administration to be em-

ployed; (3) the purpose of drug administration—therapy or prophylaxis; (4) the known risk of untoward effects; and (5) the cost of the preparation.

The presently available, useful preparations of penicillin G can be classified as follows: (1) penicillin G in aqueous solution for parenteral use, (2) repository penicillin G preparations that are slowly absorbed from intramuscular depots, and (3) penicillin G for oral use.

Details of *dosage* of penicillin G preparations are presented subsequently, in the discussion of the treatment of specific infections. The available preparations of *semisynthetic penicillins* are described in connection with their pharmacological and antimicrobial properties.

Although penicillin G preparations for *inhalational therapy* and for *topical application* to skin and mucous membranes are still available, their use is not recommended because proof that they are adequately effective is lacking, and because they produce a high incidence of hypersensitization.

Penicillin G in Aqueous Solution for Parenteral Use. This type of preparation, the first to be marketed, is still widely employed. It is designed for subcutaneous, intramuscular, intravenous, or intrathecal injection. The potassium salts are most frequently used. The two official penicillin salts for injection are *Penicillin G Potassium for Injection,* U.S.P., and *Penicillin G Sodium for Injection,* N.F. The preparations listed are crystalline powders, marketed for parenteral use in sterile dry form in vials or ampuls containing 200,000 to 20 million units each. Solutions are prepared by adding the solvent (sterile distilled water, 0.9% sodium chloride solution, or 5% dextrose solution) directly to the container to yield the desired concentration, usually 100,000 or 200,000 units/ml.

Penicillin G Preparations for Parenteral Use in Repository Form for Prolonged Action. Repository penicillin preparations are designed for deep intramuscular injection, to provide a tissue depot from which the drug is slowly absorbed over a period of 12 hours to several days. The objective is to maintain therapeutic plasma concentrations with as few injections as possible. *Repository penicillin should never be injected intravenously or subcutaneously or into body cavities.*

Sterile Penicillin G Procaine Suspension, U.S.P. (CRYSTICILLIN, DIURNAL-PENICILLIN, DURACILLIN A.S., WYCILLIN SUSPENSION), is an aqueous preparation of the crystalline salt that is soluble in water only to the extent of 0.4%. *Sterile Penicillin G Procaine with Aluminum Stearate Suspension,* U.S.P., contains aluminum monostearate (2% w/v) as a dispersing agent to keep the penicillin G procaine in a homogeneous suspension in oil, to slow absorption of the antibiotic by its hydrophobicity, and to impart *thixotropy* to the preparation, that is, the capability of a gel to become a free-flowing liquid when gently shaken. Penicillin G procaine preparations are marketed for intramuscular injection in 1-, 2-, and 4-ml cartridges and 10-ml vials, each milliliter usually containing 300,000, 500,000, or 600,000 units of the antibiotic.

Procaine combines with penicillin mole for mole; therefore, a dose of 300,000 units contains approximately 120 mg of procaine. This amount is rarely toxic because the procaine is in the form of a poorly soluble salt and hence is only slowly released and absorbed. If the patient is believed to be hypersensitive to procaine, 0.1 ml of 1% solution of the drug should be injected intradermally; individuals exhibiting a positive local response should not be given penicillin G procaine. A slight anesthetic effect of the procaine accounts in part for the fact that injections of penicillin G procaine are virtually painless.

Sterile Penicillin G Benzathine Suspension, U.S.P. (BICILLIN, PERMAPEN), is the aqueous suspension of the salt obtained by the combination of 1 mole of an ammonium base and 2 moles of penicillin G to yield N,N'-dibenzylethylenediamine dipenicillin G. The salt itself is soluble in water only to the extent of 0.02%. The aqueous suspension has advantages in that suspending vehicles containing oily bases and foreign materials are avoided. It is provided for intramuscular injection in 10-ml vials containing 300,000 units/ml and in prefilled syringes (1, 2, and 4 ml) containing 600,000 units/ml. The long persistence of penicillin in the blood after a suitable intramuscular dose reduces cost, need for repeated injections, and local trauma. The local anesthetic effect of penicillin G benzathine is comparable to that of penicillin G procaine.

Certain nonofficial repository preparations for intramuscular use combine an insoluble penicillin G salt (procaine or benzathine) with a soluble salt of penicillin (sodium or potassium). They are designed to provide both the rapid establishment of high plasma concentrations and the prolonged effect of depot penicillin. Some question has been raised concerning the rationale underlying the use of these combinations. Bacteria eradicated by the use of the repository penicillin are not more rapidly killed by the brief exposure to the higher concentration of drug afforded by the rapidly absorbed aqueous penicillin; on the other hand, bacteria that can be eradicated only by the higher concentration are not affected by the low persistent levels afforded by the repository penicillin.

Penicillin G for Oral Use. The oral route for penicillin G administration has the obvious advantages of simplicity and avoidance of trauma of injection. In addition, hypersensitivity reactions are much less frequent after oral than after parenteral administration of penicillin. This mode of administration should be used only in those infections in which clinical experience has proven its efficacy; the dosage to be employed is also determined on this basis. The drug must be given no later than 30 minutes before a meal or earlier than 2 to 3 hours after eating. Oral

therapy should not be employed merely to avoid parenteral injection.

The official oral preparations are *Penicillin G Potassium Tablets,* U.S.P., *Penicillin G Potassium Tablets for Solution,* U.S.P., and *Penicillin G Benzathine Tablets,* U.S.P. They are usually marketed as tablets containing from 50,000 to 1 million units. Various buffer materials are sometimes added; these increase stability of the antibiotic but do not significantly protect against destruction of penicillin G in the acidic gastric contents. Dry salts of penicillin G mixed with flavoring material and various buffers are available for pediatric use. The requisite dose can be mixed with syrup, water, or milk, or added to the milk formula for infants.

SEMISYNTHETIC PENICILLINS: THEIR PHARMACOLOGY AND ANTIMICROBIAL PROPERTIES

As stated previously, the search for penicillin congeners was initiated and continues for the purpose of finding compounds that circumvent, in one or more ways, the shortcomings of penicillin G, particularly its (1) instability in the acidic gastric contents, (2) rapid renal excretion, (3) susceptibility to inactivation by penicillinase and hence inefficacy in infections caused by penicillinase-producing staphylococci, (4) "limited" antibacterial spectrum with particular reference to gram-negative bacteria, (5) rather poor penetrability into the cerebrospinal fluid, and (6) proclivity to induce hypersensitization. Although the last two items listed represent deficiencies of penicillin G not as yet overcome by the semisynthetic congeners to be described, the others have been circumvented in whole or in part. Certainly the "ideal" penicillin has not been discovered as yet, and *penicillin G is still the preferred agent for the vast majority of infections* susceptible to this class of agents, except as otherwise specifically noted throughout this chapter and particularly in the section on therapeutic uses (*see also* Table 55-1, page 1096).

By "semisynthetic" penicillin is here meant *any* congener, whether produced by incorporation of specific precursors in mold cultures (sometimes called semiartificial biosynthetic penicillins) or made by chemical modification of penicillin G (other than salt formation) or of 6-aminopenicillanic acid. By definition, excluded from this category are repository salts of penicillin G, such as those previously described.

Penicillin V. This congener of penicillin is the phenoxymethyl analog of penicillin G. Its sole virtue in comparison with penicillin G is that it is more stable in an acidic medium and, therefore, is better absorbed from the gastrointestinal tract. With respect to its antimicrobial properties, it is similar to penicillin G. It is available only for *oral* administration and hence is not a substitute for parenteral penicillin when such therapy is needed. Its structural formula is shown in Table 57–1. (*See* Klein and Finland, 1963b.)

Table 57–1. CHEMICAL STRUCTURES AND MAJOR PROPERTIES OF VARIOUS PENICILLINS

SIDE CHAIN *	NONPROPRIETARY NAME	MAJOR PROPERTIES		
		Absorption after Oral Administration	*Resistance to Penicillinase*	*Antimicrobial Spectrum*
⬡—CH₂—	Penicillin G	Variable (poor)	No	
⬡—OCH₂—	Penicillin V	Good	No	Narrow
⬡—OCH(CH₃)—	Phenethicillin	Good	No	
Methicillin (OCH₃)	Methicillin	Poor (not given orally)	Yes	
Isoxazolyl	Oxacillin (R₁ = R₂ = H) Cloxacillin (R₁ = Cl; R₂ = H) Dicloxacillin (R₁ = R₂ = Cl) Floxacillin (R₁ = Cl; R₂ = F)	Good	Yes	Narrow
Naphthalene OC₂H₅	Nafcillin	Variable	Yes	
R—⬡—CH(NH₂)—	Ampicillin (R = H) Amoxicillin (R = OH)	Good / Excellent	No	Extended
⬡—CH(COOR)—	Carbenicillin (R = H) Carbenicillin indanyl (R = 5-indanol)	Poor (not given orally) / Good	No	

* Side chain attached to 6-aminopenicillanic acid (*see* Figure 57–2).

Pharmacological Properties. This congener was first produced in 1953 by the addition of suitable precursors to the fermentation medium. It is quite stable on storage, relatively insoluble in the pH range of gastric contents, but more soluble as the pH is increased. Its *antibacterial spectrum* is identical to that of penicillin G. After oral ingestion, the drug escapes destruction in gastric juice, since it is both insoluble and stable at a low pH. It goes into solution in the more alkaline medium of the duodenum and is well but incompletely absorbed from the upper portion of the small intestine. On an equivalent oral-dose basis, the compound yields plasma concentrations two to five times greater than those provided by penicillin G. There is even some evidence that it is better absorbed when ingested after a meal than on an empty stomach. Once absorbed, penicillin V is distributed in the body and excreted by the kidney in the same manner as penicillin G.

The *toxicology* and *therapeutic uses* of penicillin V are presented later in this chapter.

Preparations and Route of Administration. Penicillin V Potassium, U.S.P. (COMPOCILLIN-V K, PEN-VEE K, V-CILLIN K, and others), is supplied for oral use as official tablets (125, 250, or 500 mg each) and granules for solution (125 or 250 mg/5 ml). Suspensions (125 or 250 mg/5 ml) are also available. *Penicillin V,* U.S.P., is marketed under trade names and in official dosage forms and unitages similar to those for the potassium salt. *Penicillin V Benzathine,* N.F., and *Penicillin V Hydrabamine,* N.F., are additional official preparations.

Phenethicillin. This congener of penicillin is a phenoxyethyl analog of penicillin G. Its structural formula is shown in Table 57–1. The drug shares with penicillin V the property of stability in acidic media and better absorption from the gastrointestinal tract. This is its sole advantage in comparison to penicillin G. It is available only for *oral* use and hence is not a substitute for parenteral penicillin, when such therapy is indicated. As a result, its therapeutic applications are limited. (*See* Klein and Finland, 1963b.)

Pharmacological Properties. Phenethicillin is prepared from 6-aminopenicillanic acid. It is available only as the potassium salt, which is freely soluble in water and very resistant to decomposition in acidic solution. Its *antimicrobial spectrum* is almost identical to that of penicillin G. Given orally, the drug is well absorbed and escapes destruction in the acidic gastric contents; despite this fact, intestinal absorption is incomplete. In equal oral doses, it produces higher plasma concentrations than does penicillin G or penicillin V. But this seeming advantage can be overcome by appropriately larger doses of the other two agents. Food retards absorption and thereby prolongs the duration of action of the compound. Peak plasma concentrations occur about 1 hour after oral administration of the drug. Once

phenethicillin is absorbed, its protein binding, distribution, fate, and excretion are similar to those of penicillin G.

The *toxicology* and *therapeutic uses* of phenethicillin are presented later in this chapter.

Preparations and Routes of Administration. The official preparations of this compound are *Phenethicillin Potassium,* N.F. (MAXIPEN, SYNCILLIN), *Phenethicillin Potassium for Oral Solution,* N.F., and *Phenethicillin Potassium Tablets,* N.F. Preparations available for *oral* administration are 250-mg tablets.

Methicillin. This semisynthetic penicillin is prepared from 6-aminopenicillanic acid. Its structural formula is shown in Table 57–1. The drug is highly resistant to cleavage by penicillinase. Its major use is in infections caused by penicillinase-producing strains of *Staph. aureus* not treatable with penicillin G. It is administered only by the *parenteral* route. Methicillin must not be used in preference to penicillin G in infections amenable to treatment with the latter drug. Staphylococci may develop resistance to methicillin by mechanisms not related to penicillinase production. (*See* Klein and Finland, 1963b.)

Pharmacological Properties. Methicillin is bactericidal for nearly all strains of *Staph. aureus;* penicillinase-producing strains are from 15 to 80 times more susceptible to the drug than to penicillin G. It is not as effective as penicillin G against other gram-positive microorganisms. Methicillin is totally without effect on gram-negative bacteria, some of which may even inactivate it.

Resistance of microorganisms to methicillin is an important clinical problem, particularly since staphylococci insensitive to this agent are usually also resistant to all other penicillins, streptomycin, kanamycin, chloramphenicol, and the tetracyclines, and frequently to lincomycin and the cephalosporin derivatives. Although most of the resistant microorganisms belong to phage group III, others are of different phage types; most produce enterotoxin B (Hallander and Laurell, 1971). Such microorganisms have even been isolated in areas where patient exposure to the penicillins has not occurred. While, in general, there is a poor correlation between the incidence of methicillin resistance and the use of this antibiotic, there is a strong association between treatment with orally administered penicillins such as ampicillin and the frequency with which staphylococci resistant to methicillin are recovered (Parker and Hewitt, 1970). The precise mechanism of methicillin resistance has not been completely identified. The difference between staphylococci resistant and sensitive to this antibiotic may be related to chemical differences in their cell wall. An increasing number of human infections due to methicillin-resistant staphylococci are being reported. While many of them have been relatively mild, some have been very severe and have caused death. Vancomycin or ceph- alothin plus kanamycin has been suggested for the management of this kind of disease. (*See* Gill and Hook, 1965; Gravenkemper *et al.,* 1965; Bulger, 1967; Editorial, 1967; Gilbert and Sanford, 1970.)

Methicillin is not employed by the oral route be- cause it is poorly absorbed and readily destroyed by the acidic gastric contents. When the drug is given intramuscularly, peak plasma concentrations are reached in about 30 minutes to 1 hour. After the conventional dose of 1 g in adults, plasma concen- trations in excess of 10 μg/ml are demonstrable; a 2-g dose provides a peak concentration over 20 μg/ml, and approximately 8 μg/ml is still present after 4 hours. About 40% of the methicillin in plasma is bound to protein.

Methicillin does not readily penetrate into cere- brospinal fluid; however, significant concentrations are present in patients with meningitis, but these are not dependable for therapy in such cases. The drug is otherwise well distributed in various body fluids and tissues.

Methicillin is excreted unchanged in the urine, in approximately the same manner as for penicillin G; about two thirds of an intramuscular dose is elimi- nated by this route in 4 hours. Probenecid elevates and prolongs the duration of plasma concentrations of methicillin by blockade of the renal tubular secre- tion, but the total amount of antibiotic eventually excreted in the urine is unaltered. Methicillin persists for a long period and at high concentrations in the plasma in cases of renal failure. Premature babies 4 to 5 days of age have detectable concentrations of methicillin for at least 12 hours after a single dose of 25 mg/kg; however, by the age of 26 to 30 days such infants excrete the drug more rapidly, and its half-life is then about 1½ hours. In normal infants of the same age, the half-life of the antibiotic is about 1 hour (*see* Boe *et al.,* 1967). The portion of injected methicillin that cannot be detected in the urine is excreted into the *bile* and is eliminated by way of the feces. In some cases, the concentration in the bile is higher than in the plasma.

The *toxicology* and *therapeutic uses* of methicillin are discussed later in this chapter.

Preparations and Routes of Administration. The official preparation is *Methicillin Sodium, U.S.P.* (STAPHCILLIN). The salt is stable in dry form and freely soluble in water. It is unstable in acidic media and loses potency when dissolved in 0.85% sodium chloride or in dextrose solution at room temperature. This instability, together with the fact that the drug is excreted rapidly, contraindicates continuous intra- venous infusion unless the solutions are buffered to neutrality. The preparation employed for intra- muscular or intravenous administration is *Methicillin Sodium for Injection, U.S.P.* The drug is marketed in ampuls containing 1, 4, or 6 g of the salt. The solution should be fresh, and other drugs should not be included, since many are incompatible with methicillin in solution. Intramuscular injection of methicillin is more painful than is the case for other penicillins; the need for frequent injections (every 2 to 3 hours) is a definite disadvantage when pro- longed therapy by this route is required.

The Isoxazolyl Penicillins: Oxacillin, Cloxacillin, Dicloxacillin, Floxacillin. These four congeneric semisynthetic penicillins are similar pharmacologically and are thus con- veniently considered together. Their struc- tural formulas are shown in Table 57–1. All are relatively stable in an acidic medium and are adequately absorbed after oral adminis- tration. All are markedly resistant to cleav- age by penicillinase. These drugs are not substitutes for penicillin G in the treatment of diseases amenable to it. Furthermore, be- cause of variability in intestinal absorption, oral administration is not a substitute for the parenteral route in the treatment of serious staphylococcal infections that require a peni- cillin unaffected by penicillinase.

Pharmacological Properties. The isoxazolyl peni- cillins are potent inhibitors of the growth of most penicillinase-producing staphylococci. This is their valid clinical use. Dicloxacillin and floxacillin are more potent than oxacillin and cloxacillin; all are more potent than methicillin. This has little practical significance, however, since dosages are adjusted accordingly. These agents are, in general, less effec- tive against microorganisms susceptible to penicil- lin G, and they are not useful against gram-negative bacteria. Microorganisms can become resistant to these drugs in a stepwise fashion, and cross-resis- tance to all penicillins is usually complete.

These agents are rapidly but incompletely (30 to 50%) absorbed from the gastrointestinal tract. Ab- sorption of the drugs is more efficient when they are taken on an empty stomach. Peak plasma concen- trations are attained by 1 hour and approximate 5 to 10 μg/ml after the ingestion of 1 g of oxacillin, and similar values are obtained with cloxacillin. Somewhat higher concentrations (15 μg/ml) are achieved when 1 g of dicloxacillin or floxacillin is administered. There is little evidence that these differences are of clinical significance. Since absorp- tion is less than complete, higher plasma concen- trations are achieved following intramuscular injec- tion, and larger quantities of the drugs are recoverable in the urine. All these congeners are bound to plasma albumin to a great extent (approxi- mately 90 to 95%); none is removed from the circu- lation to a significant degree by hemodialysis.

The isoxazolyl penicillins are rapidly excreted by the kidney, and the concurrent administration of probenecid results in higher and more persistent plasma concentrations. Normally, 30 to 50% of any of these drugs is excreted in the urine in the first 6 hours after a conventional oral dose. There is also significant hepatic elimination of these agents in the bile. The half-lives for all are between 30 and 60 minutes. Intervals between doses of cloxacillin and dicloxacillin do not have to be altered for patients with renal failure; some adjustment is recommended when oxacillin is so administered (*see* Table 55–2, page 1108). The above-noted differences in plasma concentrations produced by the isoxazolyl penicillins are related mainly to differences in rate of urinary excretion and degree of resistance to degradation in the liver (Rosenblatt *et al.,* 1968).

The *toxicology* and *therapeutic uses* of these agents are presented later in this chapter.

Preparations and Routes of Administration. Oxacillin Sodium, U.S.P. (BACTOCILL, PROSTAPHLIN), is available for oral use in official capsules containing 250 or 500 mg of drug, and as *Oxacillin Sodium for Oral Solution,* U.S.P. (250 mg/5 ml). It is readily soluble in water and stable in the dry state at room temperature. The drug is preferably administered 1 or 2 hours before meals, to ensure better absorption. The daily oral dose of oxacillin for adults is 2 to 4 g, divided into four portions; for children, 50 to 100 mg/kg per day is administered similarly. The injectable form of the drug, *Oxacillin Sodium for Injection,* U.S.P., is available in 250- and 500-mg and 1-g vials. For adults a total of 2 to 12 g per day, and for children 100 to 300 mg/kg per day, may be given intravenously or intramuscularly, injections being given every 4 to 6 hours.

Cloxacillin Sodium, U.S.P. (TEGOPEN), is available in capsules (250 mg) and as an oral solution (125 mg/5 ml). The dose for adults is 250 mg orally every 6 hours for mild-to-moderate infections; for severe infections, it is 500 mg or more every 6 hours. The dose for children is 50 mg/kg per day, divided into equal quantities and given every 6 hours; for those weighing more than 20 kg, adult doses have been recommended.

Dicloxacillin Sodium, U.S.P. (DYNAPEN, PATHOCIL, VERACILLIN), is quite stable at acidic pH, soluble in water, and stable at room temperature. The drug is available only for oral use, in capsules (125 and 250 mg) and as a suspension (62.5 mg/5 ml). The dose for adults and for children weighing more than 40 kg is 250 mg or more every 6 hours; for children weighing less than 40 kg, the recommended daily dose is 25 mg/kg, given in four equal portions at intervals of 6 hours. Because there is incomplete information at present, dicloxacillin should not be given to newborn infants.

Floxacillin sodium (flucloxacillin sodium; FLOXAPEN) is freely soluble in water and is stable in solution at pH 7 for 2 weeks if kept at 5° C. It is not yet available for general clinical use in the United States. Floxacillin has not been used sufficiently long to permit assessment of its therapeutic value.

Nafcillin. This semisynthetic penicillin, derived from 6-aminopenicillanic acid, is highly resistant to penicillinase and has proven effective against infections caused by penicillinase-producing strains of *Staph. aureus.* Its structural formula is shown in Table 57-1.

Pharmacological Properties. Nafcillin is similar to oxacillin in its potency against penicillin G–resistant *Staph. aureus,* but not as active as penicillin G against staphylococci sensitive to the latter agent.

Nafcillin is inactivated to a variable degree in the acidic medium of the gastric contents. Its absorption after oral administration is irregular, regardless of whether the drug is taken with meals or on an empty stomach. After parenteral administration, the plasma concentration of nafcillin is lower than that produced by an equivalent dose of oxacillin. This is associated with a much larger apparent volume of distribution of nafcillin, resulting from a selective sequestration of the antibiotic in the liver and possibly in other tissues (Kind *et al.,* 1970). Nafcillin is bound to plasma protein to the extent of about 90%. Only approximately 10% of an oral dose of nafcillin is recoverable in the urine. Probenecid further reduces its excretion in the urine. The major channel of elimination of nafcillin is the bile, and about 90% of a single intravenous dose can be accounted for by biliary excretion; there is some reabsorption of the drug from the small intestine. Peak concentrations of nafcillin in bile are well above those found in plasma.

The *toxicology* and *therapeutic uses* of nafcillin are presented later in this chapter.

Preparations and Routes of Administration. Nafcillin Sodium, U.S.P. (UNIPEN), is available for oral and parenteral use. Capsules usually contain 250 mg of the drug. A solution is also marketed for oral use. A sterile preparation for injection is supplied in ampuls containing 500 mg, 1 g, or 2 g of the salt. For the therapy of severe *Staph. aureus* infections, nafcillin by the oral route is not reliably effective. Nafcillin is not a substitute for penicillin G in the therapy of infections caused by microorganisms sensitive to the latter agent. The oral and parenteral doses of nafcillin are the same as those described above for oxacillin.

Ampicillin and Congeners: Amoxicillin, Hetacillin. *Ampicillin.* This drug is a semisynthetic compound derived from 6-aminopenicillanic acid, but it differs from the penicillins discussed above by virtue of its extended spectrum of antimicrobial efficacy. Its structural formula is shown in Table 57-1. Ampicillin is degraded by penicillinase and, therefore, is of no value in the management of infections due to staphylococci or other microorganisms that elaborate this enzyme (*see* Klein and Finland, 1963a; Stewart, 1967).

Pharmacological Properties. Ampicillin suppresses the growth of both gram-positive and gram-negative bacteria. It is somewhat less active than penicillin G against gram-positive cocci sensitive to the latter agent. The meningococcus, pneumococcus, gonococcus, and *List. monocytogenes* are sensitive to the drug. *Haemophilus influenzae* and the *viridans* group of streptococci are usually inhibited by very low concentrations of ampicillin. However, several strains of type-b *H. influenzae* highly resistant to ampicillin have been recovered from children with meningitis due to this microorganism (Medical Letter, 1974; Public Health Service, 1974). Enterococci are about twice as sensitive to it, on a weight basis, as to penicillin G. Although most strains of *E. coli, Pr. mirabilis, Salmonella,* and *Shigella* were highly susceptible to this agent when it was first used in the early 1960s, an increasing percentage of these species is now resistant. From 20 to 40% of *E. coli,* a significant number of *Pr. mirabilis,* and practically all species of *Enterobacter (Aerobacter)* are presently insensitive. Resistant strains of *Salmonella* (episome mediated) have been recovered with increasing frequency in various parts of the world, and such strains of *Shigella* are now worldwide. Indole-positive strains of *Proteus, Serratia,* and *Pseudomonas* have always been resistant to the drug.

Ampicillin is stable in acid and is well absorbed after oral administration. An oral dose of 0.5 g produces peak plasma levels of about 3 μg/ml at 2 hours. The drug is detectable in the plasma for about 4 hours after a conventional oral dose. Intake of food prior to ingestion of ampicillin results in less complete absorption. Intramuscular injection of 0.5 or 1.0 g of sodium ampicillin yields peak plasma concentrations of about 7 or 10 μg/ml, respectively, at 1 hour; these decline exponentially with a half-time approximating 90 minutes (*see* Eickhoff *et al.,* 1965).

The administration of probenecid leads to increased concentration and persistence of ampicillin in the plasma. About one fourth of an oral dose is cleared by the kidney in the first 6 hours following ingestion. Approximately 70% of an intramuscular or intravenous dose of 500 mg is eliminated in the urine in this time. Severe renal impairment markedly prolongs the persistence of ampicillin in the plasma. Peritoneal dialysis is ineffective in removing the drug from the blood, but hemodialysis removes about 40% of the body store in about 7 hours. Adjustment of the dose of ampicillin is required in the presence of renal dysfunction, as indicated in Table 55-2 (page 1108).

Ampicillin appears in the bile, undergoes entero-hepatic circulation, and is excreted in appreciable quantities in the feces. Biliary concentration of the drug is markedly dependent on the integrity of the gallbladder and its ducts (Mortimer *et al.,* 1969). When the common bile duct is obstructed, ampicillin is not detectable in the bile.

The *toxicology* and *therapeutic uses* of ampicillin are presented later in this chapter.

Preparations and Routes of Administration. *Ampicillin,* U.S.P. (AMCILL, OMNIPEN, PENBRITIN, POLYCILLIN, and others), is available for oral use in capsules containing 250 or 500 mg; for parenteral use, as the sodium salt in vials containing from 125 mg to 4 g; and as the sodium salt for oral suspension (125 or 250 mg/5 ml). The dose varies with the type and the severity of the infection being treated, with renal function, and with age. For children, doses cannot be prescribed on the basis of body weight or surface area; because the drug is excreted mainly by the kidney, the state of renal function to a great extent determines the dose. Very young babies thus require small doses, while children 3 to 4 years old may receive quantities almost as large as those given to adults. For mild-to-moderately severe disease, the oral dose for adults is 2 to 4 g per day, divided into

equal portions and given every 6 hours. For severe infections, it is best to administer the drug parenterally in doses ranging from 4 to 8 g per day. The treatment of meningitis requires the use of large doses, 300 to 400 mg/kg per day parenterally (in equally divided portions given every 6 hours) for children, and 8 to 12 g or more per day for adults. Solutions should be freshly prepared prior to injection.

Amoxicillin. This drug, a penicillinase-susceptible semisynthetic penicillin, is a close chemical and pharmacological relative of ampicillin (*see* Table 57-1). The drug is stable in acid and is designed for oral use. The antimicrobial spectrum of amoxicillin is essentially identical to that of ampicillin, with the important exception that amoxicillin appears to be less effective than ampicillin for shigellosis. (*See* Sutherland and Rolinson, 1971; Bodey and Nance, 1972; Croydon, 1973; Handsfield *et al.,* 1973; Brusch *et al.,* 1974; International Symposium, 1974; Nelson and Haltalin, 1974.)

Amoxicillin is more rapidly and completely absorbed from the gastrointestinal tract than is ampicillin, which is the major difference between the two. Food does not interfere with absorption. Peak plasma concentrations are reached at 2 hours and average about 4 μg/ml when 250 mg is administered. Perhaps because of more complete absorption of this congener, the incidence of diarrhea with amoxicillin may be less than that following administration of ampicillin. While the half-life of amoxicillin is the same as that of ampicillin, effective concentrations of orally administered amoxicillin are detectable in the plasma for twice as long as with ampicillin, again because of the more complete absorption. About 20% of amoxicillin is protein bound in plasma, a value similar to that for ampicillin. Approximately 60% of a dose of the antibiotic is excreted in an active form in the urine, in contrast to only about 35% of ampicillin. This also correlates with the difference in absorption. Probenecid delays excretion of the drug. (*See* Croydon and Sutherland, 1971; Gordon *et al.,* 1972; Kerrebijn and Michel, 1973; Rolinson, 1973.)

Amoxicillin (AMOXIL, LAROCIN) is available for oral use in capsules (250 or 500 mg), as an oral suspension (125 or 250 mg/5 ml), and as pediatric drops (50 mg/ml). The recommended *dose* of amoxicillin is similar to that of ampicillin (250 to 500 mg in adults), except that it is given three instead of four times a day.

Hetacillin. This drug is also a chemical modification of ampicillin. Indeed, in the body, hetacillin is very rapidly hydrolyzed to ampicillin and acetone. It is acid resistant. The antibacterial spectrum is the same as that of ampicillin, since ampicillin accounts for more than 90% of the biological activity of hetacillin. Peak plasma concentrations are reached 2 hours after an oral dose and are lower than those produced by an equal quantity of ampicillin. The ingestion of food prior to the drug slows absorption further. After intramuscular or oral administration of 450 mg, maximal plasma concentrations are about 6 or 2.5 μg/ml, respectively. Antibacterial activity is still detectable in the blood 8 hours after an oral dose.

While hetacillin has been used successfully in the therapy of a variety of infections, it is doubtful that this congener has any advantages to recommend its use in place of ampicillin. (*See* Bunn *et al.*, 1966; Tuano *et al.*, 1966; Magni *et al.*, 1967.)

Hetacillin (VERSAPEN) is available in capsules, suspension, and pediatric drops for oral use, and also in preparations for intramuscular and intravenous injection. Preparations for intramuscular injection contain lidocaine. Solutions for intravenous use are stable for 6 hours at room temperature. When the drug is prepared for oral use as a suspension or as pediatric drops, it is stable for 7 days at room temperature and 14 days under refrigeration. The doses of hetacillin recommended are often too low; they should be at least as large as those of ampicillin.

Pivampicillin. This drug is yet another congener of ampicillin. It is active only after conversion to ampicillin *in vivo*. Pivampicillin is not currently available in the United States, and there is no indication that its use will offer any advantage.

Carbenicillin and Carbenicillin Indanyl.

Carbenicillin. This drug is a penicillinase-susceptible derivative of 6-aminopenicillanic acid. Its structural formula is shown in Table 57-1. The major advantage of this agent is that it often cures serious infections caused by *Pseudomonas* species, *Proteus* strains resistant to ampicillin, and certain other gram-negative microorganisms. Its major disadvantages are the rapid development of bacterial resistance during treatment in some cases unless large doses are given, the necessity for parenteral injection, and its cost.

Low concentrations of carbenicillin inhibit the growth of *Pr. mirabilis* and many microorganisms sensitive to penicillin G. *Escherichia coli, Enterobacter (Aerobacter)*, and *Salmonella* are less sensitive. The majority of strains of *Pr. vulgaris* and *Pseud. aeruginosa* are sensitive to 25 μg/ml or less of the drug; 85% of *Pseudomonas* are inhibited by 100 μg/ml. Penicillin G–resistant staphylococci, *Klebsiella*, and *Serratia* are, with some exceptions, resistant. Enterococci are suppressed in the range of 50 to 100 μg/ml. Microorganisms rapidly become resistant to carbenicillin *in vitro*. Bacterial resistance also appears *in vivo* during treatment with suboptimal doses of carbenicillin.

Carbenicillin is not absorbed from the gastrointestinal tract and, therefore, must be given parenterally. Large doses are often necessary. Intramuscular injection of 1 g produces peak plasma concentrations of 15 to 20 μg/ml in ½ to 2 hours; activity is practically gone at 6 hours. Maximal plasma concentrations are about four times higher after intravenous than after intramuscular administration of the antibiotic. Intravenous infusion at a rate of 1 g per hour results in average plasma concentrations of approximately 150 μg/ml. About 50% of the antibiotic in plasma is protein bound. The distribution of carbenicillin is similar to that of other penicillins. The half-life of carbenicillin in individuals with normal renal function is about 1 hour; it is prolonged to about 2 hours in the presence of hepatic dysfunction. Hemodialysis reduces the plasma concentration of the antibiotic.

Carbenicillin is excreted primarily by the renal tubules. About 75 to 85% of a dose is recoverable in active form in the urine in 9 hours. Probenecid, by delaying renal excretion of the drug, increases plasma concentrations by about 50%.

The *toxicology* and *therapeutic uses* of carbenicillin are discussed below.

Carbenicillin is available for parenteral injection as the disodium salt (GEOPEN, PYOPEN) in sterile vials containing 1, 2, 5, or 10 g. The daily dose for adults with serious infections is 25 to 30 g; some patients have been given as much as 35 to 40 g. When the drug is administered intravenously, the dosage may be as high as 2 to 2.5 g every 2 hours. Daily doses of 600 to 800 mg/kg have been used to treat very young infants with life-threatening infection. In patients with severe renal failure, the dose should not exceed 2 g every 8 to 12 hours; during hemodialysis, the interval between doses may be reduced to 4 to 6 hours (*see* Table 55-2). Available preparations of carbenicillin contain 4.7 mEq of sodium per gram.

Carbenicillin Indanyl. This congener is the indanyl ester of carbenicillin; it is acid stable and is suitable for oral administration. The ester is rapidly converted to carbenicillin *in vivo* by hydrolysis of the ester linkage. The antimicrobial spectrum of the drug is therefore that of carbenicillin, and bacterial resistance develops as to the parental compound. While relatively low plasma concentrations of carbenicillin are achieved, the active moiety is excreted rapidly in the urine. Thus, the main use of this drug clinically is for the management of urinary tract infections, particularly those caused by *Proteus* species, *Pseud. aeruginosa*, and *E. coli* (Wallace *et al.*, 1971).

Carbenicillin indanyl is rapidly absorbed from the small intestine. The peak plasma concentration, reached about 1 hour after ingestion of 500 mg of the drug, is about 5 μg/ml. About 30% of a dose of 500 mg is excreted in the urine in the first 12 hours; an additional 6% is eliminated in the urine over the next 12 hours. After the administration of 1 g, about 50% is excreted in the first 12 hours and an additional 10% in the next 12 hours. The urine thus contains antimicrobially effective concentrations of carbenicillin after recommended doses of carbenicillin indanyl. Some of the drug is excreted in the bile, and some is detoxified in the liver. (See Butler *et al.*, 1971; English *et al.*, 1972.)

Carbenicillin indanyl sodium (GEOCILLIN) is available in tablets containing 500 mg of the drug (equivalent to 382 mg of carbenicillin). The recommended 6-hour dosage schedules for urinary tract infections due to the various indicated microorganisms are as follows: acute disease due to *E. coli* or *Pr. mirabilis*, 500 mg, and for chronic infection, 1000 mg; for infection caused by *Pseudomonas*, 1000 mg. The drug is expensive.

UNTOWARD AND TOXIC REACTIONS TO PENICILLINS

The penicillins can provoke a variety of untoward effects. The reactions range in severity from very mild and evanescent to severe and fatal. They have followed the use of the drug by any route and have involved most tissues and organs, separately or diffusely (*see* Finland and Weinstein, 1953; Weinstein, 1955).

The *incidence* of untoward effects varies, to some degree, with the type of preparation and the route of administration. Of the injectable penicillins, penicillin G procaine produces the highest incidence of reactions, approximately 5%; aqueous penicillin G, from 2 to 2.5%. The use of penicillin G benzathine causes untoward effects in about 0.3% of patients. Orally administered compounds have a reaction incidence of about 0.3%. In general, the oral route is associated with a lower risk than is the parenteral, but fatalities have occurred when penicillin has been taken by mouth. Suprainfection occurs with varying frequency with the use of all penicillins.

Hypersensitivity Reactions. The mechanism most commonly involved in the pathogenesis of untoward effects from any type of penicillin is *hypersensitization*. Allergic reactions to the penicillins vary from 0.7 to 10% in various reported series (Idsøe *et al.,* 1968). Penicillin is thought to be the most common cause of drug allergy, and the manifestations that develop encompass almost the entire gamut of allergic reactions and immunological mechanisms.

Penicillin can undergo slow conversion *in vivo* to intermediates, such as penicillenic acid, which can react with appropriate constituents of tissues. An important example of this is thought to be the formation of amide derivatives of penicilloic acid by reaction with ε-amino groups of lysine residues in proteins. Such conjugates are frequent major antigenic determinants in penicillin allergy (*see* Levine, 1965; Parker, 1965). Other breakdown products of penicillin appear to act as "minor" antigenic determinants.

Antipenicillin antibodies are detectable in virtually all patients who have received the drug and in many who have never knowingly been exposed to it. Studies on subjects of various ages indicate that 64% of persons have specific IgM antibodies to penicilloyl-polylysine, 13% have specific IgG antibodies for this compound, 5% have both types, and only 16% have neither (Klaus and Fellner, 1973). About 50% of babies in the first year of life have IgM antibodies to this major antigenic determinant, while only 1% have IgG antibody. Recent treatment with the antibiotic induces an increase in major-determinant–specific antibodies that are skin sensitizing. The incidence of positive skin reactors is three to four times higher in atopic than in nonatopic individuals. The synthesis of antibodies to major and minor determinants appears to be linked. Clinical and immunological studies suggest that immediate allergic reactions are mediated by skin-sensitizing antibodies, usually of minor-determinant specificities. Accelerated and late urticarial reactions are usually mediated by major-determinant–specific, skin-sensitizing antibodies. The recurrent-arthralgia syndrome appears to be related to the presence of skin-sensitizing antibodies of minor-determinant specificities. Some maculopapular and erythematous reactions may be due to toxic antigen-antibody complexes of major-determinant–specific IgM antibodies. Accelerated and late urticarial reactions to penicillin appear to terminate spontaneously because of the development of blocking antibodies (*see* Levine *et al.,* 1966).

Hypersensitivity reactions may occur with any dosage form of penicillin; the presence of allergy to one penicillin exposes the patient to a greater risk of reaction if another is given. On the other hand, the occurrence of an untoward effect does not necessarily imply repetition on subsequent exposures. For example, some patients who have had mild-to-moderate skin manifestations may later receive the same penicillin without experiencing a repetition of the allergic response. Hypersensitivity reactions may appear in the absence of previous known exposure to the drug or promptly after the administration of the first dose, especially in individuals who have had prior allergic reactions to other substances. Although elimination of the antibiotic usually results in rapid clearing of the allergic manifestations, they may persist for 1 or 2 weeks or longer after therapy has been stopped. In some cases, the reaction is mild and disappears even while the use of penicillin is continued. In others, it is of serious import and necessitates immediate cessation of penicillin treatment. In a few instances, it is necessary to interdict the future use of penicillin because of the risk of death, and the patient should be so warned. It must again be stressed that fatal episodes of anaphylaxis have followed the ingestion of very small doses of this antibiotic.

Skin rashes of all types have been observed when penicillin sensitization has occurred. Scarlatiniform, morbilliform, urticarial, vesicular, and bullous eruptions may develop. Purpuric lesions are uncommon and are usually the result of a vasculitis; thrombopenic purpura may occur very rarely. Henoch-Schoenlein purpura with renal involvement has been a rare complication. *Contact dermatitis* is observed occasionally in pharmacists, nurses, and physicians who prepare penicillin solutions, even though they may have never received the drug either orally or parenterally; it also results from the ill-advised topical application of penicillin ointments. Fixed-drug reactions have also occurred. More severe reactions involving the skin are exfoliative dermatitis and exudative erythema multiforme of either the erythematopapular or vesiculobullous type; these lesions may be very severe and atypical in distribution and constitute the characteristic Stevens-Johnson syndrome. The incidence of skin rashes appears to be highest following the use of ampicillin, being about 9%; however, it is as high as 50% in patients with infectious mononucleosis due to either the Epstein-Barr (EB) virus or cytomegalovirus (*see* Weary *et al.,* 1970). That the ampicillin-induced skin eruptions in such patients may represent a "toxic" rather than an allergic reaction is suggested by their appearance often within 1 to 2 days after treatment is started in individuals known not to be allergic to penicillin and by the common absence of positive skin reactions to the major and minor determinants of penicillin sensitization.

A variety of *oral lesions* have resulted from sensitization to penicillin. Among these are acute glossitis, severe stomatitis with loss of the buccal mucous membranes, furred tongue, black or brown tongue, and cheilosis. Such manifestations are seen most frequently following the local application of penicillin to the mouth, in the form of lozenges or troches, but they may also be produced by parenteral use of the drug.

Fever may be the only evidence of a hypersensitivity reaction to the penicillins. It may reach high levels and be maintained, remittent, or intermittent; chills occasionally occur. The febrile reaction usually disappears within 24 to 36 hours after administration of the drug is stopped. Fever is often present in association with other manifestations of sensitivity. *Eosinophilia* is an occasional accompaniment of other allergic reactions to penicillin. At times, it may be the sole abnormality and eosinophils may reach levels of 10 to 20% or more of the total number of circulating white blood cells.

Interstitial nephritis may rarely be produced by the penicillins. Hematuria, albuminuria, pyuria, renal-cell and other casts in the urine, elevation of serum creatinine, and even oliguria have been noted in patients receiving methicillin, as reported by Hewitt and associates (1961); eosinophilia and skin rash were present at the same time. In patients with underlying renal disease, penicillin may produce a nephropathy with abnormal urine sediment or acute glomerulonephritis.

The most serious hypersensitivity reactions produced by the penicillins are *angioedema, serum sickness, anaphylaxis,* and the *Arthus phenomenon.* Angioedema with marked swelling of the lips, tongue, face, and periorbital tissues, not infrequently accompanied by asthmatic breathing and "giant hives," has been observed after topical, oral, or systemic administration of penicillins of various types. Serum sickness has followed sensitization, especially to the repository penicillins; the illness varies in severity from mild fever, rash, and leukopenia to severe arthralgia or arthritis, purpura, lymphadenopathy, splenomegaly, mental changes, ECG abnormalities suggestive of myocarditis, generalized edema, albuminuria, and hematuria. This reaction usually appears after penicillin treatment has been continued for 1 week or more; it may be delayed, however, until 1 or 2 weeks after the drug has been stopped. Serum sickness caused by penicillin may persist for a week or longer. In a few instances, patients who have had repeated exposures to penicillin and have experienced various kinds of reactions have been noted later to develop "allergic vasculitis," disseminated lupus erythematosus, or polyarteritis.

Acute *anaphylactic* or *anaphylactoid* reactions induced by various penicillin preparations constitute the most important immediate danger connected with their use. Among all drugs, the penicillins are the most often responsible for this type of untoward effect. Anaphylactoid reactions may occur at any age. Their incidence is thought to be 0.015 to 0.04% in persons treated with penicillins. About 0.002% of patients treated with these agents die from anaphylaxis. It has been estimated that there are at least 300 deaths per year due to this complication of therapy. About 15% of those who succumb have had other types of allergy; 70% have had penicillin previously, and one third of these reacted to it on a prior occasion (Idsøe *et al.*, 1968). Anaphylaxis has most often followed the *injection* of penicillin, although it has also been observed after *oral ingestion* of the drug, and has even resulted from the intradermal instillation of a very small quantity for the purpose of testing for the presence of hypersensitivity. The clinical pictures that develop vary in severity. The most dramatic is sudden, severe hypotension and rapid death. In other instances, bronchoconstriction with severe asthma, or abdominal pain, nausea, and vomiting, or extreme weakness and fall in blood pressure, or diarrhea and purpuric skin eruptions have characterized the anaphylactic episodes.

A history of a previous severe reaction of any type, especially anaphylactic, following the administration of penicillin, or a strong personal or family background of atopic allergy should alert the physician to the possibility of serious difficulty on reexposure to the drug. Such patients should be studied carefully before being exposed to this class of antibiotic. In such cases, a scratch test with penicillin should be carried out. A positive reaction, especially if severe, should interdict the use of the drug. A negative test usually indicates that treatment may be undertaken. However, in some instances, reactions may still occur. For this reason, Levine and Zolov (1969) have suggested that a negative scratch test be followed by intradermal injection of the antibiotic, and have indicated the significance of negative and positive reactions. A *negative response* to injection of the major (benzylpenicilloyl-polylysine) and minor group of determinants suggests that immediate anaphylaxis will not occur, or that the risk of its developing is very small. The incidence of accelerated urticarial, asthmatic, or flush reaction is also very low. A negative intradermal test does not exclude the possibility of exanthematous reactions, the development of Coombs positivity, or the appearance of granulocytopenia. A *positive intradermal reaction* indicates a high probability of an immediate or accelerated allergic response. A positive reaction to benzylpenicilloyl-polylysine is associated with a high risk of an accelerated urticarial reaction. Among the factors important in ascertaining whether a person who has major-determinant–specific reagin

will develop such a response are (1) the dose of penicillin, (2) the presence of major-determinant-specific IgG antibodies (which act as "blocking" antibodies and inhibit or modulate the reaction), and (3) the binding affinity of the reagins. A positive reaction to the minor determinants carries the highest risk of an anaphylactic response when penicillin is administered. Hemagglutination titers are of no value in predicting immediate reactions or accelerated urticaria in individuals with negative skin tests.

Reactions Due to "Toxic" and Irritative Properties of Penicillins. The penicillins are virtually nontoxic to man. Most of the reactions attributed to a toxic mechanism are the result of the irritative effects of excessive concentrations. The actual limit of the dose of penicillin G that can be administered parenterally with safety still remains to be determined. A number of individuals have been treated intravenously with quantities ranging from 40 to 80 million units per day for as long as 4 weeks without untoward effects (Weinstein *et al.*, 1964a). One patient is known to have received 240 million units (144 g) by the intravenous route daily for 6 weeks without any difficulty.

Apparent toxic effects that have been reported include bone-marrow depression, uncommonly observed with conventional doses of methicillin; agranulocytosis with peripheral monocytosis and bone-marrow histiocytosis has been noted following treatment with ampicillin. The administration of carbenicillin has been associated with a potentially significant defect of hemostasis that appears to be due to an impairment of platelet aggregation (Brown *et al.*, 1974).

Most common among the *irritative responses* to penicillin are *pain* and *sterile inflammatory reactions* at the sites of intramuscular injections, reactions that are related to concentration. Serum transaminases and lactic dehydrogenase may be elevated as a result of local damage to muscle. Whereas the administration of 1 million units of penicillin G dissolved in 1 ml of isotonic saline solution may produce severe discomfort for an appreciable period, the injection of the same quantity of drug dissolved in 5 ml is accompanied by only moderate pain that persists only for a short time. Some individuals who receive penicillin intravenously develop *phlebitis* or *thrombophlebitis*. Many persons who take various penicillin preparations by mouth experience nausea, with or without vomiting, and some have mild-to-severe diarrhea. These manifestations are often related to the dose of the drug and, in most instances, represent *irritation of the gastrointestinal tract.*

Another indication of the irritative properties of high concentrations of penicillin is the effect on the *central and peripheral nervous systems.* When penicillin is injected accidentally into the sciatic nerve, severe pain occurs and dysfunction in the area of distribution of this nerve develops and persists for weeks. Intrathecal injection of penicillin G in excessive concentration and dose may produce *arachnoiditis* or severe and fatal *encephalopathy.* The upper limit of safety is about 50,000 units, or approximately 300 units of the drug per milliliter of cerebrospinal fluid, administered intrathecally in the lumbar area. When the antibiotic is given intracisternally, this quantity must be reduced by at least half; when it is administered into a cerebral ventricle, not more than one third of the dose given in the spinal canal should be injected. The concentration of penicillin injected intrathecally is very important. The safest, yet effective, dose in adults is about 30,000 units dissolved in not less than 10 ml of isotonic saline solution or spinal fluid and given over a period of not less than 10 minutes. The parenteral administration of very large doses of penicillin G (40 to 80 million units per day) may produce twitching or localized or generalized epileptiform seizures. These are most apt to occur in the presence of renal insufficiency, localized central nervous system lesions, or hyponatremia. The injection of such quantities of the commonly used preparation, penicillin G potassium, may lead to severe or even fatal hyperkalemia in persons with renal dysfunction.

The accidental injection of penicillin G procaine into a blood vessel may result in a potentially fatal reaction. Since the compound is insoluble, the particles are rapidly deposited in the lungs, where they produce multiple small *pulmonary infarcts* and a clinical syndrome characterized by anxiety, tinnitus, visual difficulty, confusion, disorientation, paresthesias, flushing, chest pain, dyspnea, cyanosis, hypotension, and death in some instances. This picture resembles that produced by fat embolism.

Reactions Due to Biological Alterations in the Host and Unrelated to Hypersensitivity or "Toxicity." The most important biological effect of penicillin, unrelated to hypersensitivity or to a "toxic" reaction, is alteration of the bacterial flora in areas of the body to which it gains access. Regardless of the route by which the drug is administered, but most strikingly when it is given by mouth, penicillin changes the composition of the microflora by eliminating sensitive microorganisms. Thus, profound alterations may be observed in the types and numbers of microorganisms present in the intestinal and upper respiratory tracts; the degree of alteration is related directly to the quantity of penicillin administered. Although this occurs in practically all individuals, it is usually of no clinical significance and the normal microflora is reestablished shortly after therapy is stopped. In some persons, however, *suprainfection* results from the changes in flora (*see* Chapter 55). The incidence of suprainfection with penicillin therapy is about 1%.

Dermatitis involving primarily the scrotal and inguinal skin and resembling that of *pellagra* has been observed in patients receiving penicillin; this may be related to changes in the microbial flora of the intestinal tract with a resultant deficiency in nicotinic acid.

A dramatic effect that may follow the use of penicillin in syphilis is the *Jarisch-Herxheimer reaction;* the mechanism is unknown.

THERAPEUTIC USES OF
THE PENICILLINS

The remarkable influence of penicillin and other antibiotic therapy of infections on the prognosis in infectious diseases is impossible to overestimate and can be appreciated fully only by physicians who dealt with such diseases prior to the advent of the chemotherapeutic era. In this discussion, only the major features of the chief therapeutic uses of penicillin are considered. In Table 55–1 (page 1096), penicillin is compared with other antimicrobial agents with respect to its value in the therapy of various diseases, and alternative drugs are indicated for situations in which penicillin cannot be used.

Pneumococcal Infections. Penicillin G remains the agent of choice for the management of pneumococcal infections of all types. Despite its use for over 3 decades, there is no evidence that pneumococci have developed a clinically significant degree of resistance; all serological types are equally susceptible.

Pneumococcal Pneumonia. A variety of dose schedules and types of penicillin have been employed successfully in the treatment of pneumococcal pneumonia. For parenteral therapy, penicillin G and penicillin G procaine, with or without aluminum monostearate, are the preparations of first choice. Although oral therapy, 250 to 500 mg of penicillin V every 6 hours, has been used with success in this disease, it cannot be recommended for routine use. The semisynthetic penicillins should *not* be used in this situation. The doses of penicillin G currently used are, in all probability, greatly excessive. A dose of 500,000 to 1 million units given intramuscularly every 6 hours is adequate, except in unusual cases. A single daily injection of 600,000 units of penicillin G procaine, with or without the addition of 300,000 units of penicillin G, produces a favorable response in the bulk of cases in which the disease is detected early, the involvement is unilobar, and the patients are otherwise healthy. The generally accepted duration of therapy is 5 days after defervescence, which usually occurs rapidly once therapy is instituted. Although sharply reduced in incidence, complications and death still may supervene in pneumococcal pneumonia treated with penicillin. Bacteremia, infection with type-3 or -8 pneumococci, very young and old age, involvement of more than one lobe, delay in initiating therapy, and the presence of debilitating disorders play very important roles in decreasing the effectiveness of penicillin therapy.

Pneumococcal Empyema. The frequency of this complication of pneumococcal pneumonia has been sharply reduced by penicillin therapy of the primary lung disease. In most cases, it is not necessary to instill the antibiotic intrapleurally when purulent exudate is present in the pleural sac; in such instances, however, the dose of penicillin given intramuscularly should be increased; 1.0 million units every 6 hours has proven effective. As with any collection of pus, drainage is of paramount importance. If the empyema fails to respond, intrapleural injection of 50,000 to 100,000 units of penicillin G in 50 to 100 ml of isotonic saline solution once daily for several days, in addition to the intramuscular drug, may prove helpful in sterilizing the infection and producing cure. If the pleural fluid is very thick, the injection of a mixture of streptococcal deoxyribonuclease with streptokinase-streptodornase intrapleurally results in striking liquefaction of the pus and allows the antibiotic to penetrate the infected area much more efficiently.

Pneumococcal Meningitis. Penicillin has reduced the death rate in this disease from nearly 100% to between 8 and 25%. Several methods of therapy with penicillin have been suggested. Most physicians administer penicillin G intravenously, 2 million units every 2 hours for 2 weeks. An alternative approach involves the cautious intrathecal instillation of the drug. The treatment schedule is as follows: Penicillin G, 30,000 units in 10 ml of isotonic saline solution, is injected into the spinal canal (lumbar sac) over a period of 10 minutes; this is repeated every 12 hours until three doses have been given. In addition, penicillin G, 300,000 to 400,000 units, is given intramuscularly every 3 to 4 hours. Therapy is continued for 2 weeks. The primary objection to intrathecal penicillin therapy is the danger of arachnoiditis and encephalopathy. When very close attention was paid to dose (not greater than 30,000 units for adults and 3000 to 10,000 units for children), dilution of the drug, and speed of injection, untoward effects were not observed in a large group of cases in one clinic in which the fatality rate in patients with good and poor prognoses treated by this method over a period of 20 years was about 8%. In rare instances, especially those in which the spinal fluid contains a very large number of pneumococci but few or no cells, intrathecal injections may have to be given every 12 hours for 3 to 5 days before the bacteria are eradicated. In patients who are sensitized to penicillin, 1 g of erythromycin intravenously every 6 hours for 2 weeks has proven highly successful. Oral or repository penicillins and the semisynthetic congeners have no place in the treatment of this disease. The prognosis is best when the meningitis is "primary" (no obvious focus outside the meninges), next best if it stems from infection in the middle ear or paranasal sinuses, and poorest if it is secondary to pneumococcal pneumonia; infection with type-3 pneumococci has a relatively poor prognosis.

Other Pneumococcal Infections. Penicillin G provides optimal therapy for suppurative *arthritis, osteomyelitis, acute suppurative mastoiditis, endocarditis, peritonitis,* and *pericarditis* due to the pneumococcus. Because of poor penetration of the drug into purulent exudate, in which considerable quantities of fibrin may be present, the plasma and tissue-fluid concentrations must be high; this is best accomplished by the parenteral administration of large doses of a rapidly absorbed preparation. Doses of the order of 10 to 20 million units per day are probably required for cure. Oral and repository penicillins should not be used. The shortest period of treatment for any of these disorders should be 2 weeks; this should be prolonged to at least 4 weeks when endocarditis or poor prognostic factors are present or when complications supervene. *Infections in the middle ear and paranasal sinuses* are treated by some physicians with penicillin G procaine (1.2 million units), given once daily; others prefer oral therapy

because of the convenience. In the writer's opinion, this is not advisable because of the danger of intracranial spread of such infections if they are not rapidly and completely controlled. Ampicillin produces beneficial effects in this type of disease. It is used extensively in children in whom, without rupture of the tympanic membrane, the etiological diagnosis cannot be established; the microorganisms most commonly responsible, *H. influenzae,* the pneumococcus, and group-A *Strep. pyogenes,* are susceptible to ampicillin.

Streptococcal Infections. Group-A *Strep. pyogenes* (beta-hemolytic streptococcus), the microorganism involved in 95% of human streptococcal infections, is highly susceptible to penicillin. The preparation and dose used vary with the nature and the severity of the disease. Alpha-hemolytic and nonhemolytic streptococci show a varying degree of sensitivity to this antibiotic, although a large number of strains, many of which are responsible for subacute bacterial endocarditis, are inhibited by low concentrations of the drug. Anaerobic streptococci are not easily eradicated by penicillin, and many enterococci are resistant to it but are sensitive to concurrent therapy with this antibiotic and an aminoglycoside.

Streptococcal Pharyngitis and Scarlet Fever. These are the two most common diseases produced by group-A *Strep. pyogenes.* The therapy for both these disorders is penicillin, and the oral route is adequate in all but an exceptional case or one in which suppurative complications are present when treatment is started. Penicillin G or penicillin V, 200,000 to 400,000 units given orally at 6- to 8-hour intervals, produces rapid clinical improvement, rids the pharynx of the streptococci in 48 to 96 hours, and completely eliminates the development of suppurative complications such as otitis media and pneumonia. Equally good results are produced by the administration of 600,000 units of penicillin G procaine intramuscularly once daily. Therapy with these preparations must be continued for 10 days. A single injection of 1.2 million units of penicillin G benzathine is also effective. It is widely accepted that penicillin therapy of streptococcal pharyngitis reduces significantly the risk of acute rheumatic fever; however, present evidence suggests that glomerulonephritis is not reduced to a significant degree by treatment with penicillin.

If suppurative complications are present at the time treatment is started, it is best to administer penicillin parenterally; large doses are required. Some patients with streptococcal pharyngitis fail to respond to adequate quantities of penicillin, suffering either a bacteriological or clinical relapse, or both, shortly after therapy is terminated. Some have attributed this to the presence of a penicillinase-producing strain of *Staph. aureus* in the pharynx; its elimination by the use of an antibiotic such as oxacillin, to which both the staphylococcus and the streptococcus are susceptible, is said to produce cure. However, the relation of penicillinase-producing staphylococci to failure to respond to penicillin has been questioned (*see* Quie *et al.,* 1966).

Streptococcal Meningitis. The fatality rate of untreated *Strep. pyogenes* meningitis approaches 100%.

Penicillin G produces dramatic results when used alone in this disease. Although intrathecal therapy may be necessary in an uncommon instance, this type of meningitis responds well to the intramuscular or intravenous administration of large doses of penicillin G; other penicillin preparations are best avoided since they do not produce the high plasma concentrations necessary to provide an inhibitory level of antibiotic in the spinal fluid. The dose for adults is 2 million units every 2 hours; therapy should be continued for no less than 2 weeks.

Streptococcal Pneumonia. Most patients with *Strep. pyogenes* pneumonia are cured by the parenteral administration of penicillin G in doses of 2.5 million units given every 6 hours. Early institution of therapy is essential and helps to reduce the incidence of complications such as empyema. Occasionally, it may be necessary to instill 50,000 to 100,000 units of penicillin G intrapleurally once a day for several days, in addition to the intramuscular or intravenous administration of the drug.

Acute Streptococcal Otitis Media and Mastoiditis. Whereas parenteral penicillin is preferable for the treatment of acute suppurative *otitis media* due to *Strep. pyogenes,* practical considerations often dictate the use of oral therapy. If this route is employed, no less than 400,000 units of penicillin G or 250 mg of penicillin V should be administered orally to adults every 6 hours for 2 weeks. Since this type of disease is most common in children, the dosage has to be adjusted to allow for its more rapid excretion; in this age group, the same dose should be administered at intervals of 3 or 4 hours. Parenteral treatment is mandatory when streptococcal *mastoiditis* has complicated a middle ear infection; children should be hospitalized and given at least 500,000 units of penicillin G intramuscularly every 3 to 4 hours for no less than 2 weeks, if the potentially lethal *intracranial complications* are to be avoided. For adults, the administration of 2 to 4 million units of the same preparation every 6 hours for 2 weeks is effective.

Other Strep. pyogenes Infections. Acute streptococcal endocarditis was almost universally fatal prior to penicillin therapy. Early diagnosis and treatment produce a satisfactory outcome in from 50 to 75% of cases. The drug of choice is penicillin G. It should be given intravenously in a dose of 3 to 5 million units every 6 hours for at least 4 weeks. The need for early therapy cannot be overemphasized; since this type of endocarditis is ulcerative, irreparable damage to the infected valve leaflet with the development of intractable heart failure, despite bacteriological cure, may occur and necessitate immediate valve replacement or lead to death.

Infections of the conjunctiva by this microorganism are not uncommon; they are frequently secondary to streptococcal disease of the upper respiratory tract. Local therapy with penicillin G ointment applied to the eye suffices in most instances; in others, this may have to be supplemented by either oral or parenteral administration of the drug. *Streptococcal impetigo (pemphigus neonatorum)* is a rather common infection of the newborn. It is best treated with parenteral penicillin G; adjustments must be made in the dosage schedule in view of the fact that neo-nates excrete the antibiotic less efficiently than do adults. Topical application of penicillin ointments is inadvisable because this is not only ineffective but also produces a high risk of sensitization.

Streptococcal arthritis and *osteomyelitis* are readily treated with penicillin; the treatment of choice is intramuscular penicillin G. The dosage schedules are the same as those for other systemic streptococcal diseases. Some physicians prefer to instill 50,000 to 100,000 units of penicillin G into the joint cavity when suppurative arthritis is present. This is not necessary in most instances, and should be avoided if possible because of the risk of the introduction of other microorganisms during the injection.

Infections Due to Streptococci Other Than Group-A Strep. pyogenes. The most common infection produced by *alpha-hemolytic streptococci (viridans* group) is subacute bacterial endocarditis. Although the majority of alpha-hemolytic streptococci are sensitive to penicillin, others show varying degrees of resistance to it. Some of the alpha-hemolytic microorganisms that have been recovered from the blood of patients with this disease have proven to be enterococci that are relatively resistant to penicillin. It is essential, therefore, that every strain of streptococcus isolated from cases of subacute bacterial endocarditis be examined quantitatively for sensitivity to penicillin G, since the concurrent administration of penicillin and streptomycin is necessary for the treatment of enterococcal endocarditis. Although unnecessary delay should be avoided, a period of 2 to 3 days of waiting for blood cultures to become positive and for sensitivity testing of the isolated microorganism is not critical in *subacute* endocarditis because this disease has usually been present for 2 weeks to 3 months before the patient presents himself for diagnosis. The fatality rate in subacute bacterial endocarditis prior to the availability of effective chemotherapeutic agents was very close to 100%. The survival rate is presently better than 95% in properly managed cases.

The choice of type and dose of penicillin and the duration of treatment for *subacute bacterial endocarditis* due to penicillin-sensitive microorganisms vary among physicians. Reasonable doses of penicillin G are 2 to 5 million units intravenously every 6 hours for at least 4 weeks.

The treatment of choice for *enterococcal endocarditis* is 3 to 5 million units of penicillin G, administered intravenously every 6 hours, plus 0.5 to 1.0 g of streptomycin, given intramuscularly every 12 hours for 4 weeks. In cases in which penicillin and streptomycin are not synergistic (usually when the microorganism is highly resistant to the aminoglycoside), gentamicin (80 mg every 8 hours in patients with normal renal function) may be substituted for streptomycin. Although some cases will respond to large doses (40 million units or more per day) of penicillin G alone, combined therapy is preferred (Jawetz and Sonne, 1966). Ampicillin and erythromycin are also active against enterococci. However, in patients with hypersensitivity to the penicillins, desensitization to the antibiotic, followed by its concurrent use with an aminoglycoside, has been employed with success. But desensitization is difficult and dangerous. The relative risks posed by the infection and by the drug must be weighed carefully. With the above schedules, the relapse rate, after cessation of treatment, has been less than 1%, and suprainfections have been very rare. The necessity of continuing therapy for at least 4 weeks cannot be overemphasized. However, patients who have been cured of their infections may still die, due to an embolus, heart failure from valvular insufficiency, renal failure in cases not treated sufficiently early, or rupture of a mycotic aneurysm that developed prior to therapy.

Alpha-hemolytic streptococci may be involved in a number of other infections, including brain abscess, urinary tract infection, and purulent meningitis. The therapy for these is based on determination of the sensitivity of the responsible microorganism to penicillin. The agent of choice is penicillin G, and, when serious systemic involvement is present, parenteral administration is preferred.

Nonhemolytic or gamma streptococci may be responsible for subacute bacterial endocarditis and other infections. As with the alpha-hemolytic microorganisms, determination of sensitivity to antibiotics is essential. If penicillin appears to be the drug of choice, it should be used; the details of dose and duration of therapy vary with the location and the severity of the disease.

Anaerobic Streptococcal Infections. Penicillin yields highly inconsistent results when used in infections produced by anaerobic streptococci, because these microorganisms vary markedly in their susceptibility to the drug. In some cases, even huge doses are without effect; in others, relatively small quantities are curative. It is essential, therefore, that all isolates be studied for sensitivity to various antibiotics; if they are susceptible to penicillin G, this drug should be given in large doses (20 to 40 million units per day) intravenously. In severe systemic infections due to anaerobic streptococci, the minimal period of therapy is 4 weeks. Surgical drainage of localized lesions may also be necessary before cure can be accomplished.

Staphylococcal Infections. Staphylococcal resistance to penicillin has been discussed above. It has been estimated that over 90% of staphylococcal infections due to hospital strains and from 15 to 20% of those involving microorganisms present outside a hospital environment are presently resistant to therapy with penicillin G. Therefore, the physician who has a patient with serious disease due to *Staph. aureus* does best to administer one of the penicillinase-resistant penicillins such as oxacillin, nafcillin, or methicillin, but only until the results of sensitivity testing indicate the need for continued use of one of these agents or that penicillin G may be employed. Alternative antimicrobial agents are listed in Table 55–1.

Staphylococcal infections in man are so diverse and have such protean manifestations that discussion of each disease entity will not be attempted. However, several general principles concerning therapy can be formulated, as follows: (1) Staphylococcal infections susceptible to penicillin G should be treated with this agent. (2) Strains that produce penicillinase must be treated with a penicillinase-resistant penicillin. (3) Serious staphylococcal diseases such as pneumonia, bacteremia, and endocarditis must be treated with *maximal doses* of a penicillin or other antibiotic for no less than 4 weeks. (4) Therapy should be administered parenterally in all seriously ill patients. (5) Documented bacteremia indicates the presence of staphylococcal endocarditis in 40 to 50% of cases and requires maximal dose and adequate duration of treatment. (6) Abscesses often interfere with the effectiveness of penicillin therapy and frequently require surgical drainage. (7) Therapy must be instituted early. (8) Topical application of the penicillins for skin infections is not only ineffective but also dangerous because of the high risk of sensitization. (9) There is an increasing incidence of serious infections due to what have come to be known as "methicillin-resistant" staphylococci; physicians must be alert to this possibility early in cases of staphylococcal infection that are responding poorly to treatment with methicillin or other penicillinase-resistant penicillins.

The dose of penicillin G for susceptible staphylococci varies. Quantities of the order of 10 million units, divided into four or six equally spaced doses, are adequate in most instances. The dosages for penicillinase-resistant compounds are discussed above, in the descriptions of each of the drugs.

Meningococcal Infections. Penicillin G is the drug of choice for meningococcal disease. It is very effective in the management not only of meningococcemia and meningitis but also of suppurative arthritis and acute endocarditis due to the meningococcus. The dose for these diseases is 2 million units intravenously every 2 hours. In patients who are hypersensitive to penicillin, chloramphenicol (1 g every 6 hours) is an effective alternative. Therapy should be continued for 12 to 14 days.

Gonococcal Infections. Penicillin G is the agent of choice in all types of gonococcal infection. Although the sensitivity of gonococci to this agent has decreased over the years, most strains can be eliminated if large enough quantities of this antibiotic are administered.

Gonorrhea. The presently recommended treatment of acute uncomplicated gonorrhea in the male or female is the intramuscular injection of 4.8 million units of aqueous penicillin G procaine divided into at least two doses and injected at different sites at one visit; 1 g of probenecid is given orally at least 30 minutes before the injection of penicillin G. If, on the basis of stained smear or culture, or both, there is failure of response, the procedure is repeated. With increasing resistance of *Neisseria gonorrhoeae* to penicillin G, penicillin G benzathine will *not* provide adequate therapeutic concentrations to treat these infections. Treatment of contacts of known cases of gonorrhea is the same as for the active disease. Experiences in the United States Armed Forces in the Far East have indicated, however, a 20 to 30% failure rate with this regimen (Holmes *et al.*, 1967). Treatment of acute gonorrhea with ampicillin is highly effective when a single dose of 3.5 g of the drug is given orally together with probenecid (Kvale *et al.*, 1971). Alternative regimens with spectinomycin or a tetracycline are discussed under the appropriate drugs (*see also* Table 55-1, page 1096). All patients with gonorrhea should have a serological test for syphilis at the time of diagnosis. Repeated tests for such infection are not necessary, for the most part, when penicillin G procaine has been used as described above. Those treated with ampicillin or other agents must have a serological test for syphilis carried out monthly for 4 months.

Gonorrhea complicated by prostatitis, epididymitis, or salpingitis requires the injection of 4.8 million units of aqueous procaine penicillin G once daily for at least 5 days, or until fever has been absent for no less than 48 hours. In some instances of acute "pelvic inflammatory disease," especially when tubo-ovarian abscess is present, hospitalization and the use of large doses of penicillin G (10 to 20 million units per day) for 14 days may be required to cure the disease. The therapy for gonococcal vulvovaginitis in children 2 to 12 years of age is a single dose of 1.2 million units of penicillin G procaine; this is repeated if a response is not produced in 48 hours. In cases of proctitis or pharyngitis due to *N. gonorrhoeae,* a daily injection of 2.4 million units of aqueous pencillin G procaine for 5 days has been recommended.

Extragenital Gonococcal Infections. These require much more intensive therapy than do infections limited to the genitalia. Although the injection of 2.4 million units of aqueous penicillin G procaine once daily for 5 or more days has produced good results in many cases of *gonococcal arthritis,* the writer has had some patients who have required the administration of 10 million units of penicillin G daily for 14 days to produce cure. *Gonococcemia* and *gonococcal endocarditis* are life-threatening infections in which the use of large quantities of penicillin G parenterally over a prolonged period is mandatory. A dose of 2 to 3 million units intravenously or intramuscularly every 6 hours is required; therapy should be continued for 4 weeks. *Ophthalmia neonatorum* is readily cured by penicillin G. It is advisable to give the drug parenterally and also to apply it to the infected conjunctivae. Penicillin G procaine, 300,000 to 600,000 units once daily, plus the local instillation of penicillin G in isotonic saline solution or in an ointment, clears the infection rapidly.

Syphilis. Penicillin G therapy of syphilis is almost ideally safe, inexpensive, and highly effective. However, its availability has hampered education of patients, contact tracing, and serological follow-up. It is so simple and rapid that reinfection is frequent. Despite the availability of such highly effective, relatively cheap (free in some venereal disease clinics), and short-term treatment, the incidence of the infectious forms of syphilis has not decreased and has, in fact, been increasing over the past few years in the United States and other countries.

Several different treatment schedules have been used in the management of syphilis. The one described here has been employed in the clinics of the Massachusetts Department of Public Health (Fiumara, 1964, 1975).

Prophylaxis for contact with syphilis is the same as that for acute gonorrhea, penicillin G procaine being used; a dose of 2.4 million units of penicillin G benzathine has also been found effective (Pirozzi, 1973).

Primary, secondary, latent (asymptomatic), or *late (tertiary) syphilis* is treated with an injection of 600,000 to 900,000 units of penicillin G procaine, either in aqueous suspension or with aluminum monostearate in oil, daily for 10 days. If the patient can return only once a week or is not likely to come back, a dose of 2.4 million units of penicillin G benzathine is administered. If the individual then reappears during the following week, the treatment is repeated. The spinal fluid must be examined in every patient before therapy is undertaken. Cases of *neurosyphilis* (abnormal spinal fluid or suggestive neurological findings, or both) are given 600,000 to 900,000 units of penicillin G procaine (aqueous suspension or aluminum monostearate in oil), once a day for 15 to 20 days. When penicillin G benzathine is used, a dose of 2.4 million units is injected once weekly for 3 weeks. The preferred penicillin preparation in all cases is penicillin G procaine.

Infants with *congenital syphilis* discovered at birth or during the neonatal period are treated daily with 10,000 units/kg of penicillin G procaine, given intramuscularly for 10 days, when there is no evidence of neurological involvement; when there is such involvement, the daily dose is 50,000 units/kg for 10 to 14 days (McCracken and Kaplan, 1974). Children older than 2 years should receive the same dose as for adults.

Positive reagin blood tests may develop during or immediately after treatment in cases of seronegative primary syphilis and a dark-field positive chancre. The serological test usually becomes negative in less than 3 months after therapy has been completed; it remains so unless reinfection or relapse takes place. In patients with seropositive primary syphilis, 6 to 9 months may elapse before seronegativity develops. If the blood test is still positive 9 months after completion of treatment, the patient should again receive penicillin G procaine. About 2% of cases of primary syphilis fail to be cured with one course of therapy; re-treatment more than once is very rarely necessary, except in cases of reinfection.

About 98% of cases of *treated secondary syphilis* are seronegative 1 year after therapy; the other 2% become seronegative in the second year. All patients with a positive blood test after 1 year should have an examination of the spinal fluid and be re-treated in the same manner as those who are seropositive after therapy for primary syphilis. The treatment failure rate in secondary syphilis after one course of penicillin G procaine is 5 to 10%.

Determination of the efficacy of treatment of *latent syphilis* is complicated by the occasional instance in which the patient is "Wassermann-fast." Individuals who have had the disease for 6 months or less react similarly to those with secondary syphilis, except that the number with positive blood tests after 1 year is about 25%. Most of these will be seronegative 2 years after treatment. Patients who have had syphilis for 2 years or less have about a 50% chance of becoming seronegative in 2 years. In general, the blood tests become negative in 75% of patients with early latent disease (less than 4 years' duration) in 5 years or less; the remaining 25% become "Wassermann-fast," some for life. About 25% of cases of *late latent syphilis* (more than 4 years' duration) become seronegative in 5 years or less; the rest become "Wassermann-fast," with very slow reduction of the serological titer. Patients with latent syphilis should have a spinal fluid examination 1 year after therapy has been completed; if this is negative, it should be repeated 1 year later. If the spinal fluid is normal three times (once before treatment and twice after completion of therapy), it need not be examined again. However, all individuals whose blood serological titers remain fixed and fail to show any significant decline 1 year after treatment should be re-treated with the initial dose of penicillin G procaine; if the titer has decreased but still is 1:4 or higher at the end of a year, therapy is repeated.

Patients who have been treated for *neurosyphilis* require spinal fluid analysis every 3 to 6 months, to determine the degree of activity of the disease as gauged by the number of cells, quantity of protein, and the titer of reagin. The most important determinant of active disease is the number of cells; if this is not within normal limits 6 months after therapy has been completed, a full course of penicillin G procaine must be given again. If the protein content is not appreciably reduced after 12 months, re-treatment is indicated. The quantitative spinal fluid serological test may show a decrease in titer after a year but may not revert to negative for many years. Usually, when the titer is fixed at the end of a year or shows only a minimal decline, the patient is re-treated. There is some question whether such repetition of therapy hastens the reversal of the spinal fluid serological reaction.

About 90% or more of patients with secondary syphilis, and to a lesser extent those in any stage of the disease, develop the *Jarisch-Herxheimer reaction.* This occurs several hours after the first injection of penicillin and is characterized by chills, fever, headache, and muscle and joint pains. The syphilitic lesions become more prominent, edematous, and brilliant in color. The manifestations persist for a few hours and are controllable by mild sedation. The rash begins to fade within 48 hours and is usually gone by 14 days. It does not recur after the second or subsequent injections of penicillin. A reduction of the initial dose of antibiotic does not prevent the development of the reaction. *In no case should therapy be withheld or discontinued when the Jarisch-Herxheimer reaction appears.*

Other forms of *late syphilis* respond to the administration of 600,000 units of penicillin G procaine once daily for 10 days. Gummas disappear rapidly. Patients with late syphilis, including those with cardiovascular involvement, may be given full therapeutic doses of penicillin without fear of the *Jarisch-Herxheimer reaction* or therapeutic paradox. In cases in which the risk of local damage is very high, for example, in patients with optic atrophy or nerve deafness, Idsøe and associates (1968) have suggested that therapy might be initiated with small doses of penicillin together with a corticosteroid.

The alternate antibiotic of choice for the treatment of syphilis in individuals who have had reactions to penicillin is one of the tetracyclines, all of which are equally effective. The dose of tetracycline is 0.5 g orally every 6 hours for 10 to 12 days for all stages of disease, except that in neurosyphilis the therapy is continued for 20 days.

Although there is little question that the majority of all types of syphilis are cured by appropriate chemotherapy, the demonstration of *T. pallidum* in the aqueous humor of many patients considered to have been successfully treated has raised questions concerning eradication of the microorganisms from all sites in the body (*see* Smith and Israel, 1971).

Actinomycosis. Penicillin G is the agent of choice for the treatment of all clinical forms of actinomycosis. The dose recommended by various investigators varies from 1 to 20 million units (penicillin G) parenterally per day for 6 weeks; it is probably best to use the larger quantities. Some physicians continue therapy for 2 to 3 months after completion of the parenteral treatment by administering 1 to 2 million units of penicillin G or penicillin V per day orally. Surgical drainage or removal of the local lesion is necessary before cure is accomplished in some cases.

Diphtheria. There is no evidence that penicillin or any other antibiotic alters the incidence of complications or the outcome of diphtheria; specific antitoxin is the only effective treatment. However, penicillin G clears the acute and chronic carrier states. The parenteral administration of 2 to 3 million units per day, in divided doses for 10 to 12 days, eliminates the diphtheria bacilli from the pharynx and other sites in practically 100% of cases. A single daily injection of penicillin G procaine for the same period produces about the same results. Erythromycin appears to be as effective and may be primary treatment or substituted in patients who are sensitized to penicillin (*see* Chapter 61).

Anthrax. Penicillin G is the agent of choice in the treatment of all clinical forms of anthrax. However, strains of *B. anthracis* resistant to this antibiotic have been recovered from human infections. When penicillin G is used, the dose should be 5 to 10 million units per day, given in equally divided and equally spaced doses; therapy should be continued for about 2 weeks.

Clostridial Infections. Although not the only therapy for clostridial infections such as *anaerobic cellulitis, anaerobic myonecrosis (gas gangrene),* and *tetanus,* antimicrobial agents have an important place in the overall management of these diseases. Penicillin G is the agent of choice for *gas gangrene;* the dose is in the range of 5 to 10 million units per day, given parenterally for 2 weeks. Just as important as the use of antitoxin (now questioned) and chemotherapy is adequate debridement of the infected areas; if the blood supply is significantly impaired, amputation of the affected limb may be necessary. Antimicrobial drugs probably have no effect on the ultimate outcome of *tetanus.* Debridement and adsorbed tetanus toxoid (for immunized patients) are proper prophylaxis. The use of human tetanus immune globulin may be indicated. Penicillin is administered, however, to eradicate the vegetative forms of the bacteria that may persist at the site of injury if debridement has been inadequate or if the site at which *Clostridium tetani* has been introduced is no longer apparent; the dose and the duration of penicillin G therapy are the same as for other clostridial infections.

Fusospirochetal Infections. Gingivostomatitis, pulmonary infections, and genital disease produced by the synergistic action of *Fusobacterium nucleatum* (*fusiforme*) and spirochetes present in the respiratory tract are readily treatable with penicillin. The more deep-seated the infection, the larger is the dose of antibiotic required. For simple "trench mouth," 400,000 units of penicillin V every 6 hours usually suffices to clear the disease. When the lung is involved, penicillin G must be given parenterally in a dose ranging from 5 to 10 million units per day and therapy must be initiated early because of the rapidity with which this type of infection produces necrosis of tissue (pulmonary gangrene). Disease of the genitalia produced by these microorganisms is usually severe and requires the same type of therapy as for pulmonary involvement.

Rat-Bite Fever. The two microorganisms responsible for this infection, *Spirillum minor* in the Orient and *Streptobacillus* (*Haverhillia*) *moniliformis* in America and Europe, are sensitive to penicillin G, the therapeutic agent of choice. Since most cases due to the streptobacillus are complicated by bacteremia and, in many instances, by metastatic infections especially of the synovia and endocardium, the dose should be large; a daily dose of 12 to 15 million units given parenterally, for 3 to 4 weeks, has been recommended.

Listeria Infections. Penicillin G is regarded as the drug of choice in the management of infections due to *List. monocytogenes;* ampicillin is also effective in many cases. Neonates and individuals with immunological deficiencies are the most frequent victims of this microorganism and should receive large doses of penicillin G parenterally as early as possible. The most common form of infection in older individuals is meningitis, for which the recommended dose of penicillin G is 15 to 20 million units parenterally per day, for at least 2 weeks. When endocarditis is the problem, the dose is the same, but the duration of treatment should be no less than 4 weeks. Concurrent therapy with streptomycin may be useful.

Pasteurella Infections. The only species of *Pasteurella* highly susceptible to penicillin is *Past. multocida.* Soft-tissue infection, bacteremia, and meningitis are the most common forms of the disease produced by this microorganism in man. Penicillin G, 4 to 6 million units per day parenterally for at least 2 weeks, is effectively curative.

Erysipeloid. The causative agent of this disease, *Erysipelothrix rhusiopathiae,* is sensitive to penicillin. The uncomplicated infection responds well to a single injection of 1.2 million units of penicillin G benzathine. When endocarditis is present, penicillin G, 2 to 20 million units per day in divided parenteral doses, has been found effective; therapy should be continued for 4 to 6 weeks.

Salmonella and Shigella Infections. Infections produced by strains of *Salmonella* and *Shigella* sensitive to ampicillin respond favorably, for the most part, to treatment with this agent. For the less serious diseases that they produce, for example, gastroenteritis, oral therapy with 0.5 to 1.0 g every 6 hours is adequate; for more severe involvement, for example, the enteric fevers or bacteremia (*Salmonella*), parenteral administration is preferred. The primary drawback to the use of ampicillin in such disorders is the increasing incidence of strains of these species that are resistant to the drug. Some investigators have indicated that, even when the microorganism is sensitive to ampicillin, the treatment of choice for typhoid and paratyphoid fever is chloramphenicol. Treatment of acute salmonella gastroenteritis with either ampicillin or chloramphenicol has been reported to prolong the period of postconvalescent excretion of the microorganisms. The acquisition of resistance by the infecting strain *in vivo* was favored by treatment; in most instances, this was due to transfer of resistance factor. It has been suggested that the administration of these antibiotics in this infection may increase the opportunity for person-to-person spread of the disease and for dissemination of resistant bacteria (Aserkoff and Bennett, 1969).

Individuals who have been carriers of *S. typhi* for longer than 1 year can be treated with moderate success with ampicillin, 75 to 100 mg/kg each day for 1 to 3 months (Simon and Miller, 1966; Phillips, 1971). Its efficacy in this situation appears to be related to the presence or absence of gallbladder disease, in the absence of which the drug usually eliminates the bacteria from the stools. Cholecystectomy should probably be reserved for carriers with abnormal gallbladders who relapse after therapy, and ampicillin should be given before, during, and after the operation. The effectiveness of the drug in carriers obviously depends on the sensitivity of the microorganism. Acute gastroenteritis may develop when asymptomatic carriers are treated with ampicillin if the microorganism is resistant to the drug; this syndrome appears to represent an episode of active salmonella infection.

Haemophilus influenzae Infections. Ampicillin is presently a drug of choice for infections caused by sensitive strains of *H. influenzae.* Meningitis in children caused by this microorganism responds rapidly in the vast majority of cases; the daily dose of drug should be no less than 300 to 400 mg/kg, given parenterally for 10 to 14 days. However, ampicillin-resistant strains of *H. influenzae* have appeared and are a source of considerable concern as a cause of therapeutic failures with this antibiotic. In the *initial* treatment of *children* with bacterial meningitis, both penicillin G and chloramphenicol are administered. Chloramphenicol is discontinued if cultures demonstrate *Strep.* (*D.*) *pneumoniae* or *N. meningitidis* as the causative microorganism. If the disease is due to *H. influenzae,* sensitivity tests are necessary to ascertain if ampicillin may be substituted for chloramphenicol. Otitis media, cellulitis, pharyngitis, and osteomyelitis due to *H. influenzae* respond favorably to ampicillin; the oral route is adequate for therapy of the less severe disorders.

Other Gram-Negative Bacillary Infections. Ampicillin is of value in the therapy of infections due to gram-negative bacteria when the microorganisms are sensitive to the drug. Good results have been obtained with this agent in the management of urinary tract infections or other diseases when susceptible bacteria are involved, particularly *E. coli* and *Pr. mirabilis*. This agent is also highly effective in the therapy of infections due to *Haemophilus vaginalis*.

It is common practice to restrict the use of carbenicillin to specific infections with *Pseud. aeruginosa* and indole-positive strains of *Proteus* (*vulgaris, morganii, rettgeri*). Among the serious diseases that have been treated successfully are meningitis (*Pr. vulgaris*), and pneumonia, upper urinary tract infections, and burn infections due to *Pseudomonas*. Children with mucoviscidosis who develop severe pulmonary infections due to *Pseud. aeruginosa* respond favorably when given 350 mg/kg of carbenicillin per day. Although bacteriological cure is not produced, clinical control of the chronic pulmonary infection is achieved. Many clinicians are presently treating serious and life-threatening disease produced by *Pseudomonas* with the concurrent use of carbenicillin and gentamicin, because of the established synergistic activity of the two drugs. These antibiotics should not be mixed in the same solution. The writer prefers to give carbenicillin intravenously and gentamicin intramuscularly when administering these drugs concurrently. (*See* Eastwood and Curtis, 1968; Smith and Finland, 1968; Darrell and Waterworth, 1969; Rodey *et al.*, 1969; Symposium, 1970.)

Carbenicillin indanyl should be reserved for the treatment of urinary tract infections that are caused by the various microorganisms susceptible to carbenicillin.

PROPHYLACTIC USES OF THE PENICILLINS

Demonstration of the effectiveness of penicillin in eradicating microorganisms was quickly, and quite naturally, followed by attempts to prove that it was also effective in preventing the implantation of bacteria in susceptible hosts. As a result, the antibiotic has been administered in almost every situation in which a risk of primary or secondary bacterial invasion has been present. As prophylaxis has been investigated under controlled conditions, it has become clear that penicillin is highly effective in some situations, useless and potentially dangerous in others, and of questionable value in still others.

Penicillin Prophylaxis of Proven Value. *Streptococcal Infections.* The administration of penicillin to individuals exposed to group-A *Strep. pyogenes* affords a predictable and high order of protection. The oral ingestion of 200,000 units of penicillin G or penicillin V, twice a day for 5 days, or a single injection of 600,000 units of either penicillin G procaine in oil with aluminum monostearate or penicillin G benzathine has been found effective. Such therapy administered to all carriers for 10 days may promptly abort an epidemic of streptococcosis and markedly reduce the carrier rate. Some objections have been raised to the routine use of penicillin as prophylaxis in individuals who have had contact with *Strep. pyogenes* on the ground that the risks of reactions to the drug are as great as those associated with the disease. In addition, evidence indicating that the carrier state leads to the development of type-specific immunity has raised serious questions concerning prophylaxis with penicillin, since this tends to suppress or abolish immune responses to *Strep. pyogenes*.

The prevalence and incidence of *streptococcal impetigo* are significantly reduced by two injections of 600,000 units of penicillin G benzathine, given 6 weeks apart, in children 6 years of age or younger, and 1.2 million units in those 7 years of age or older; however, the duration of protection is variable and of lesser degree in younger children (Ferrieri *et al.*, 1974).

Rheumatic Fever Recurrences. Although not all individuals who have had rheumatic fever have residual valvular damage, their susceptibility to recurrent episodes and the risk of cardiac injury in subsequent attacks make it imperative that everyone who has recovered from this disorder be protected against infection by the beta-hemolytic streptococcus. The oral administration of 200,000 units of penicillin G or penicillin V every 12 hours produces a striking decrease in the incidence of rheumatic fever recurrences in susceptible individuals. Because of the difficulties associated with oral treatment, mainly the fact that patients neglect to take the drug, parenteral administration is preferable, especially in children. The intramuscular injection of 1.2 to 2.4 million units of penicillin G benzathine once a month yields excellent results. In cases of hypersensitivity to penicillin, sulfisoxazole or sulfadiazine, 1.0 g twice a day for adults, is also effective; for children weighing under 27 kg (60 lb), the dose is halved. Prophylaxis must be continued throughout the year. The duration of such treatment is an unsettled question. It has been suggested that prophylaxis should be continued for life, because instances of acute rheumatic fever have been observed in the fifth and sixth decades. However, the necessity for such prolonged prophylaxis has not been established. A more common practice is to continue penicillin for 5 years after an episode of rheumatic fever in adults and through the entire period of adolescence when the disease occurs in childhood.

Gonorrhea. The conjunctival instillation of a penicillin G solution in neonates is highly effective in preventing *gonorrheal ophthalmia*. Sex partners of patients with gonorrhea should receive a single intramuscular injection of 4.8 million units of aqueous penicillin G procaine. There is the rare possibility, however, that this may mask the clinical features of syphilis and make the diagnosis of its early stages difficult or impossible.

Syphilis. Prophylaxis for a potential contact with syphilis consists in the intramuscular administration of 4.8 million units of penicillin G procaine (aqueous suspension or in oil with aluminum monostearate) *within 24 hours after exposure.* Persons who have received such prophylaxis should have serological tests for syphilis at monthly intervals for at least 4 months thereafter.

Surgical Procedures in Patients with Valvular Heart Disease. It has been estimated that about 25% of cases of subacute bacterial endocarditis are associated with dental extractions. This observation, together with the fact that 20 to 60% of persons who have teeth removed experience a transient bacteremia, emphasizes the importance of chemoprophylaxis in the presence of congenital or acquired heart disease of any type. Since transient bacterial invasion of the blood stream is known to occur occasionally after other surgical procedures, such as tonsillectomy and operations on the genitourinary and intestinal tracts, prophylaxis is also indicated when these procedures are carried out in individuals with known valvular lesions. Several regimens of penicillin administration have been employed for this purpose. Among them are: (1) intramuscular injection of a single dose of 600,000 to 1.2 million units of penicillin G procaine, 2 to 3 hours before operation; (2) oral administration of 250,000 units of penicillin G or penicillin V every 6 hours for 2 days prior to surgery, on the day of operation, and for 2 days afterward—in addition to the intramuscular injection of 600,000 to 1.2 million units of penicillin G procaine just prior to operation; and (3) injection of 1 million units of penicillin G 1 hour before, immediately after, and 2 hours after surgery. Even such mild manipulations as the scaling of teeth may result in transient bacteremia, and this procedure should be "covered" by penicillin prophylaxis when it is performed in patients with known valvular lesions. Bacteremia is not eliminated by the use of penicillin. Whether the incidence of bacterial endocarditis is actually altered to an appreciable degree by this type of chemoprophylaxis remains to be determined. Should the microorganisms that enter the blood stream from the structures in the mouth or from other sites be resistant to penicillin G, a problem of increasing magnitude, chemoprophylaxis with this agent will obviously be useless. For this reason and in individuals who have been sensitized to penicillin, some physicians prefer to give one of the tetracyclines.

Penicillin Prophylaxis of No Value. A number of disorders in which penicillin has been used prophylactically in the past have been shown by carefully controlled study to be unaffected, as far as secondary bacterial invasion is concerned, by such treatment. Among these are numerous viral infections, coma, shock, burns, heart failure, elective uninfected surgical procedures, "clean" wounds, normal obstetrical delivery, catheterization of the urinary tract, and prematurity.

Penicillin in large doses, often together with streptomycin or gentamicin, has been recommended for "prophylaxis" in patients with pulmonary tuberculosis, bronchiectasis, localized abscesses, urinary tract infections, acute or chronic otitis media, and paranasal sinusitis who are subjected to surgical treatment, inasmuch as these are, in general, "dirty" operations. There is little doubt that such management contributes greatly to a reduction of extension of these infections from the local sites. However, the usual manner in which penicillin and other antimicrobial agents are used in such situations constitutes *therapy* and not *prophylaxis.* Despite such therapy, suprainfection may occur.

Penicillin Prophylaxis of Questionable Value. Penicillin prophylaxis has been used extensively in some situations in which its value has not been completely proven. Among these are cardiac surgery and catheterization, exchange transfusions, transmission of *Staph. aureus* in nurseries and other hospital areas, premature rupture of fetal membranes, and acute diffuse glomerulonephritis. While good results have been noted by some, others have observed no salutary effects.

THE CEPHALOSPORINS

History and Source. *Cephalosporium acremonium,* the first source of the cephalosporins, was isolated in 1948 by Brotzu from the sea near a sewer outlet off the Sardinian coast. Crude filtrates from cultures of this fungus were found to inhibit the *in-vitro* growth of *Staph. aureus* and to cure staphylococcal infections and typhoid fever in man. Culture fluids in which the Sardinian fungus was cultivated were found to contain three distinct antibiotics: (1) *cephalosporin P,* active only against gram-positive microorganisms; (2) *cephalosporin N,* a new type of penicillin with a side chain derived from D-α-aminoadipic acid, effective against both gram-positive and gram-negative bacteria; and (3) *cephalosporin C,* less potent than cephalosporin N but possessing the same range of antimicrobial effectiveness. (For a complete historical review and discussion of the biochemistry of the cephalosporins, *see* Abraham, 1962; Flynn, 1972.)

With the isolation of the active nucleus of cephalosporin C, 7-aminocephalosporanic acid, and with the addition of side chains, it became possible to produce semisynthetic compounds with antibacterial activity very much greater than that of the parent substance.

Chemistry. *Cephalosporin P* is a steroid compound related chemically to helvolic acid and to fusidic acid, an antibiotic elaborated by *Fusidium coccineum. Cephalosporin N* (penicillin N) is an N-acyl derivative of 6-aminopenicillanic acid and is inactivated by penicillinase. It has a polar side chain not previously demonstrated in an antibiotic and yields penicillamine when hydrolyzed. *Cephalosporin C* resembles cephalosporin N in containing a side chain derived from D-α-aminoadipic acid but differs from it because the side chain is condensed with a dihydrothiazine beta-lactam ring system (7-amino-cephalosporanic acid) instead of a thiazolidine beta-lactam ring complex. Compounds containing 7-aminocephalosporanic acid are relatively stable in dilute acid and highly resistant to penicillinase, regardless of the nature of their side chains and their affinity for the enzyme. *Cephalothin* is a semisynthetic derivative of cephalosporin C. Other semisynthetic congeners presently available for clinical use are *cefazolin, cephapirin, cephaloridine, cephalexin, cephradine,* and *cephaloglycin.* Their number can be expected to increase. The structural formulas of these compounds, as well as that of the central nucleus, 7-aminocephalosporanic acid, are shown in Table 57–2.

Antibacterial Activity of Various Cephalosporins. *Cephalothin* is active against both gram-positive and gram-negative microorganisms. Group-A *Strep. pyogenes,* the *viridans* group and nonhemolytic streptococci, *Strep.* (D.) *pneumoniae,* penicillin-resistant and penicillin-sensitive *Staph. aureus, Staph. epidermidis, Cl. perfringens (welchii), List. monocytogenes, B. subtilis, C. diphtheriae, N. gonorrhoeae, N. meningitidis,* and *A. israelii* are highly sensitive to this agent, many being suppressed by concentrations of 0.004 to 1 μg/ml. Gram-negative bacteria are generally less susceptible, but the majority of strains of *Salmonella,* including *S. typhi,* most *Shigella,* all *Pr. mirabilis,* about 75% of *E. coli,* 60% of paracolon strains, and 50% of *H. influenzae* are inhibited by

Table 57–2. STRUCTURAL FORMULAS OF THE CEPHALOSPORINS

COMPOUND	R₁	R₂
7-Aminocephalosporanic acid		
Cephalothin		
Cefazolin		
Cephapirin		
Cephaloridine		
Cephalexin		
Cephradine		
Cephaloglycin		

1 to 6 μg/ml. Almost all strains of *Klebsiella* are sensitive to 4 to 16 μg/ml. Cephalothin is not active against *Enterobacter (Aerobacter)*, other *Proteus* species (*vulgaris, rettgeri, morganii, inconstans*), *Pseud. aeruginosa, Past. multocida, Acinetobacter (Mima-Herellea* group), *Bacteroides, Serratia,* enterococci, viruses, yeasts, and fungi.

Bacteria susceptible to cephalothin are sensitive over approximately the same range of concentrations to cefazolin and cephapirin. However, *cefazolin* is more active than cephalothin against *E. coli, Klebsiella,* and some strains of *Enterobacter (Aerobacter)*. *Cephapirin* is somewhat more inhibitory than cephalothin for group-A *Strep. pyogenes* and the pneumococcus.

The general range of activity and antibacterial spectrum of *cephaloridine* closely approximates that of cephalothin, although some strains of *E. coli* may be somewhat more sensitive to the former. It also appears to be more active than cephalothin against *Cl. perfringens (welchii)*. *Mycobacterium fortuitum* is sensitive to cephaloridine but not to cephalothin.

Cephaloglycin appears to be less potent than cephalothin or cephalexin; this may be related to the difficulty in determining the *in-vitro* activity of the drug because it is inactivated when incubated in broth. Some investigators report that 50% of *E. coli* and *Pr. mirabilis* are inhibited by 1.6 μg/ml of cephaloglycin and that a varying number of members of the *Klebsiella-Enterobacter (Aerobacter)* group are suppressed by a wide range of concentrations, some as low as 12.5 μg/ml. The antimicrobial spectrum of *cephalexin* approximates that of cephalothin. Indole-producing strains of *Proteus, Enterobacter (Aerobacter), Pseudomonas,* and an occasional strain of *Klebsiella* are highly resistant to *cephalexin*. Enterococci and *H. influenzae* are also insensitive to the drug. *Cephradine* is very similar to cephalexin, except that it may be less effective against *E. coli* and *Pr. mirabilis*.

(For details on the antibacterial activity of the cephalosporins, *see* Conference, 1970; Weinstein and Kaplan, 1970; Clinical Symposium, 1973; McGowan *et al.,* 1974.)

Mechanism of Action. Cephalothin and its congeners inhibit bacterial cell-wall synthesis in a manner similar to that of penicillin. This has been described in detail above (*see* page 1134).

Effects of Penicillinase on Cephalosporins.

Cephalosporin C is very resistant to the action of penicillinase, for which it is both a competitive and noncompetitive inhibitor, depending on the substrate tested; however, it does not suppress the breakdown of penicillin G by staphylococcal penicillinase. Cephalosporin C and its semisynthetic congeners induce the synthesis of penicillinase by *B. cereus* and *Staph. aureus*. Cephalothin is highly resistant to this enzyme, but cephaloridine appears to be more susceptible to its effect (Ridley and Phillips, 1965).

Cephalosporinase. Abraham and Newton (1956) first suggested that some bacteria elaborated an enzyme acting specifically on cephalosporin C to destroy its antibacterial activity. This substance, *cephalosporinase,* is also a beta-lactamase (Fleming *et al.,* 1963). Most preparations of the enzyme also exhibit penicillinase activity, and some microorganisms produce one beta-lactamase that acts on both penicillin and the cephalosporins. Others elaborate both penicillinase and cephalosporinase, the activities of the enzymes varying with the strain (*see* Flynn, 1972).

Absorption, Distribution, Fate, and Excretion of the Cephalosporins. *Cephalothin.*

This drug is not well absorbed from the gastrointestinal tract, but it is rapidly absorbed from intramuscular sites of injection. It is fairly widely distributed throughout body tissues and fluids and has a half-life of about 40 minutes, slightly longer than that of the phenoxyalkyl penicillins. It reaches therapeutically active concentrations in the fetus at term. Cephalothin does not normally enter the cerebrospinal fluid despite high plasma concentrations, and in the presence of meningeal inflammation it attains a value only about 1/100 that in the plasma. Approximately 60% of the drug is bound to plasma protein. The administration of 0.5 g of cephalothin intramuscularly to adults produces plasma concentrations of about 10 μg/ml in 30 minutes; administration of 1 g, about 20 μg/ml. From 60 to 80% of a dose of cephalothin is eliminated in unchanged form in the urine, by renal tubular secretion. Probenecid blocks tubular secretion of the antibiotic and thereby prolongs its sojourn in the body and elevates the plasma concentration attained by a given dose. Decreased tubular secretion of the drug also accounts for the higher plasma values observed in premature and newborn infants, because of the incomplete development of their renal function. Twenty to 30% is changed in the body to the weakly antibacterial O-deacetyl metabolite, which is excreted in the urine. The concentrations of cephalothin present in urine after administration of 1 g range from 0.7 to 5 mg/ml. Excretion is delayed in the presence of decreased renal function, and intervals between doses must be lengthened when renal failure is severe (*see* Table 55-2, page 1108). Peritoneal dialysis removes all of cephalothin from the blood in about 48 hours (*see* review by Weinstein and Kaplan, 1970). The drug is also removed from the circulation by hemodialysis; intravenous injections of 1 g at the start and at the conclusion of dialysis produce effective but not excessive concentrations in plasma for 48 to 72 hours (Venuto and Plaut, 1971).

Cefazolin. This cephalosporin is not absorbed from the gastrointestinal tract. The maximal plasma concentration is proportional to dosage and is approximately 17 μg/ml 60 minutes after the intramuscular injection of 250 mg of the drug. This concentration is thus higher than are those obtained following equivalent doses of cephalothin and cephaloridine; however, about 80% of cefazolin is reversibly bound to plasma protein.

Cefazolin is eliminated from the body primarily by renal glomerular filtration with a half-life of 100 minutes, significantly longer than that for cephalothin. Renal tubular and biliary secretion play a secondary role. About 60% of a given dose appears in the urine unaltered within 6 hours, and 80% is recoverable in 24 hours. Peak urine concentrations are thus high (2.5 mg/ml after a 500-mg dose).

The half-life of cefazolin is markedly prolonged in patients with renal insufficiency, and dosage schedules must be altered radically. The drug is removed from the blood to an appreciable extent by hemodialysis. The antibiotic is excreted in the bile even when there is gallbladder disease, and the concentration may normally exceed that in plasma by three times. Concentrations in the bile are higher than those that follow intramuscular injection of equivalent doses of ampicillin. Only very low concentrations of cefazolin are achieved in the cerebrospinal fluid.

(For details of the clinical pharmacology of cefazolin, *see* Bergeron *et al.*, 1973; Clinical Symposium, 1973; Nicholas *et al.*, 1973; Rein *et al.*, 1973.)

Cephapirin. This drug is also not absorbed from the gastrointestinal tract. Intramuscular injection of 0.5 g of cephapirin produces a maximal plasma concentration of about 10 μg/ml at 45 minutes; 1 g, about 16 μg/ml. Plasma concentrations of the drug effective against many sensitive microorganisms are still detectable 6 hours after a single intramuscular dose of 1 g. Close to 50% of cephapirin is bound to plasma protein. The half-life of cephapirin in normal individuals is about 40 minutes and is dependent on renal function. A significant amount of the drug present in the blood is removed by hemodialysis. The antibiotic is excreted mainly by the kidney; only 1% is present in bile. About 30% of an intramuscular dose of cephapirin is excreted in the urine in each of the first two 6-hour periods after injection. The major metabolite of cephapirin is deacetylcephapirin, which has about one half of the antimicrobial activity of the parent compound; 20% of the antibiotic activity in the plasma is due to the deacetylated compound.

Cephaloridine. This congener is also poorly absorbed from the gastrointestinal tract. Peak plasma concentrations are reached about 30 minutes after the drug is injected; 10 to 20% of plasma cephaloridine is bound to protein. While its half-life (60 to 90 minutes) is longer than that of cephalothin, only small amounts are detectable after 8 hours. Intramuscular injections of 0.5 and 1 g yield peak plasma concentrations of 15 and 30 μg/ml, respectively. Approximately 75% of a given dose is excreted in the urine, mainly by glomerular filtration. Cephaloridine accumulates in the blood of patients with decreased renal function, and in azotemic patients plasma concentrations are very high; a single dose of 1 g intramuscularly yields detectable concentrations for as long as 4 days. Peritoneal dialysis or hemodialysis significantly reduces the plasma concentration of the drug. However, cephaloridine should not be given to such patients, since it is nephrotoxic.

Cephalexin. This acid-stable cephalosporin, in contrast to those listed above, is well absorbed from the gastrointestinal tract. Peak plasma concentrations, reached at about 1 hour after ingestion of the drug, are approximately 9 and 18 μg/ml after oral doses of 250 and 500 mg, respectively. The ingestion of food may delay absorption. Less than 10 to 15% of the antibiotic is bound to plasma protein, and plasma drug concentrations fall rapidly, the half-life of cephalexin normally being about 40 minutes. More than 90% of the drug is excreted unaltered in the urine within 6 hours, primarily by renal tubular secretion. The peak concentration of cephalexin in the urine may exceed 1 mg/ml following a 250-mg dose, and therapeutically effective concentrations are still achieved in the urine of patients with decreased renal function. Probenecid is effective in slowing urinary clearance and enhancing the duration of systemic antimicrobial activity. The physician must alter either drug dosage or the interval between doses when renal function is impaired (*see* Table 55-2, page 1108). Cephalexin is efficiently removed from the circulation by hemodialysis or peritoneal dialysis. Cephalexin is also excreted into the bile.

(For details of the clinical pharmacology of cephalexin, *see* Meyers *et al.*, 1969; Conference, 1970; Griffith and Black, 1970; Kunin and Finkelberg, 1970; deMaine and Kirby, 1971; Sales *et al.*, 1972; Boothman *et al.*, 1973.)

Cephradine. The clinical pharmacology of cephradine is very similar to that of cephalexin, and available pharmacokinetic information on the two compounds is essentially identical (*see* Harvengt *et al.*, 1973).

Cephaloglycin. This antibiotic is partially absorbed from the gastrointestinal tract and is administered only by the oral route. Plasma concentrations reach a peak of only 2 to 6 μg/ml at about 2 hours following a single dose of 0.5 g; the drug is no longer detectable in the plasma 8 hours after this dose. The half-life of cephaloglycin is about 4 hours. Most of the cephaloglycin that is absorbed is excreted in the urine as deacetylcephaloglycin, an antimicrobially active metabolite. The urinary concentration of the metabolite averages 350 μg/ml over an 8-hour period following the administration of 500 mg of cephaloglycin; this is sufficient to inhibit most strains of *E. coli, Pr. mirabilis,* and the *Klebsiella-Enterobacter* (*Aerobacter*) group.

Preparations. *Sterile Cephalothin Sodium,* U.S.P. (KEFLIN), is marketed in 10-ml rubber-stoppered vials containing either 1, 2, or 4 g. *Cefazolin sodium* (ANCEF, KEFZOL) is available only for parenteral administration in ampuls containing 250 or 500 mg or 1 g. *Cephapirin sodium* (CEFADYL) is available in vials containing 1 g, for intramuscular and intravenous injection. *Sterile Cephaloridine,* N.F. (LORIDINE), is available in rubber-stoppered ampuls containing 500 mg or 1 g of dry powder. *Cephalexin,* U.S.P. (KEFLEX), is marketed as the monohydrate in several forms, including capsules of 250 and 500 mg, oral suspensions providing, after reconstitution, 125 mg/5 ml or 250 mg/5 ml, and pediatric drops, 100 mg/ml. Preparations of *cephradine* (VELOSEF) include capsules (250 and 500 mg) and an oral suspension (125 mg/5 ml and 250 mg/5 ml). *Cephaloglycin,* N.F. (KAFOCIN), is available as the dihydrate in capsules containing 250 mg.

Dosage and Routes of Administration. *The typical dosage schedules described below for most of the cephalosporins must be modified for patients with impaired renal function.* Suggestions for such changes are presented in Table 55-2 (page 1108).

Cephalothin is administered either intramuscularly or intravenously. The dose varies with the severity of the infection being treated. For mild disease in *adults,* 1 g every 6 hours often suffices; for more serious infection, 1 g every 3 hours; for life-threatening infections, especially when bacteremia is present,

1 g every 2 hours, intravenously. Doses as large as 24 g per day have been administered to adults without apparent ill effects. When the drug is given intravenously, 1 g should be dissolved in 20 to 30 ml of isotonic sodium chloride solution and infused over a period of 20 to 30 minutes; for intramuscular injection, 1 g is dissolved in 4 ml of the saline solution. The daily dose of cephalothin for *infants* and *children* is 40 to 100 mg/kg. The intramuscular injection of this agent is quite painful.

The dose of *cefazolin* for intramuscular or intravenous injection in *adults* with mild infections is 250 to 500 mg every 8 hours; for moderate-to-severe disease, it is 500 mg to 1 g every 6 to 8 hours; daily doses as high as 6 g have been administered. In *children,* the recommended daily dose of cefazolin is 25 to 50 mg/kg; this may be increased to 100 mg/kg if necessary.

The parenteral dose of *cephapirin* for *adults* is 500 mg to 1 g every 4 to 6 hours. For very serious and life-threatening infections, a daily dose of 12 g administered intravenously may be required. *Children* should be given 40 to 80 mg/kg each day, in four equally divided and spaced doses. Patients with serum creatinine levels greater than 5 mg/100 ml should receive 7.5 to 15 mg/kg of the drug every 12 hours. For those undergoing hemodialysis, the same dose is administered just before dialysis is started and every 12 hours thereafter.

Cephaloridine is injected either intramuscularly or intravenously. Because nephrotoxicity has been associated with higher doses, the maximal daily dose must be limited to 4 g. Since other, less toxic cephalosporins are available, there is no reason to recommend this preparation.

Cephalexin and *cephradine* are administered to *adults* in oral doses of 1 to 4 g daily, depending on the nature of the infection. The usual dose is 250 to 500 mg every 6 hours. The daily dose for *children* ranges from 25 to 50 mg/kg, divided into four portions. This may be doubled for more serious infections.

The doses of *cephaloglycin* are very similar to those of cephalexin; however, this preparation is not recommended.

Toxicity and Precautions. About 5% of patients receiving cephalothin or the other semisynthetic cephalosporins develop hypersensitivity reactions, including *fever, eosinophilia, serum sickness, urticarial* or *morbilliform rashes,* or *anaphylaxis. Transient neutropenia* has been observed between the tenth and twentieth days of therapy. A *direct positive Coombs reaction* is frequently (40%) noted when large doses of cephalothin (12 g or more per day) or other cephalosporins are administered or when conventional doses are given in the presence of renal dysfunction. Two mechanisms are responsible for this reaction. (1) Erythrocytes are coated by a cephalothin-globulin (non-antibody) complex; this is rarely associated with hemolysis. (2) Preexisting 7 S cross-reacting antibody to penicillin is bound by cephalothin to red blood cells; this may lead to a significant degree of hemolysis (Lemole *et al.,* 1972).

The incidence of hypersensitivity reactions to cephalosporins is higher in patients who have shown allergic manifestations following the administration of penicillin. This appears to be related to sensitization to the beta-lactam ring common to both these drugs. There is a wide variation in the estimates of the incidence of cross-sensitivity that have been reported. In the writer's experience this is very uncommon. With rare exception, it does not contraindicate the employment of the cephalosporin derivatives in penicillin-sensitive patients in whom the use of these compounds is clearly indicated.

Cephalothin produces renal damage only rarely. Although it has been suggested that this may be a toxic reaction, it is more likely that it is allergic in origin because the lesion is usually an interstitial nephritis. There is suggestive evidence that the coadministration of cephalothin and gentamicin increases the risk of renal tubular necrosis; however, valid data to support this are not yet available. *Cephaloridine is nephrotoxic.* Renal injury due to this drug occurs most often with administration of 6 g or more per day. The clinical picture that develops has all the features of acute tubular necrosis. The mechanism of this reaction is unknown. Large doses of cephaloridine result in a high incidence of granular casts in the urine. The administration of probenecid can ameliorate the nephrotoxicity of cephaloridine.

Other adverse reactions to these agents include *local pain, induration, sterile abscess,* or *tissue slough* after intramuscular injection, particularly with cephalothin. Intravenous infusion of cephalothin is frequently associated with the development of *phlebitis* or *thrombophlebitis;* neutralization of solutions of the drug or its administration together with a small dose of hydrocortisone does little to ameliorate this reaction. The use of intravenous catheters increases the incidence of phlebitis. While cephaloridine produces less irritation, its nephrotoxicity outweighs this advantage. Although it has been suggested that cephapirin is considerably less irritating than cephalothin to blood vessels,

a controlled study has indicated no essential difference between these two agents (Carrizosa *et al.,* 1973). Among other reactions to these drugs that have been observed during treatment are transient elevations of serum transaminases and alkaline phosphatase, hallucinations, nystagmus, and reversible encephalopathy (in a patient with renal failure due to cephaloridine). Cephaloglycin and cephalexin, the orally administered cephalosporins, occasionally produce nausea, vomiting, and diarrhea.

Since cephalothin, cefazolin, and cephapirin are administered as their sodium salts, care should be exercised in the use of large doses in persons with impaired capacity to excrete this cation. Cephaloridine does not have this disadvantage. *Suprainfections,* usually due to gram-negative bacteria, may occur when these antibiotics are employed. (*See* Weinstein and Kaplan, 1970.)

Therapeutic Uses. Cephalothin and the other cephalosporins are highly effective in the therapy of a variety of mild-to-severe infections due to both gram-positive and gram-negative microorganisms.

Diseases produced by *Staph. aureus* (penicillin G-resistant or -sensitive strains), group-A *Strep. pyogenes,* some non-group-A streptococci, *Strep. (D.) pneumoniae, A. israelii,* and *Cl. perfringens* (*welchii*) respond very favorably to proper doses of cephalosporins. Infections due to *enterococci* are usually unaffected by these compounds; unlike concurrent therapy with penicillin and streptomycin or gentamicin, the administration of a cephalosporin with an aminoglycoside may not result in cure of disease produced by these microorganisms. Thus, enterococcal endocarditis cannot be cured with a cephalosporin even when it is given concurrently with gentamicin or streptomycin. However, concomitant therapy with cephalothin and kanamycin appears to be effective in the management of some cases of infection produced by methicillin-resistant staphylococci.

Diseases due to a number of gram-negative bacterial species respond well to the cephalosporins. Among these are infections produced by *E. coli, Klebsiella,* and *Pr. mirabilis,* when the responsible strains are sensitive *in vitro.* Because these bacteria are generally less susceptible to the cephalosporins than are gram-positive microorganisms, the doses required for cure are higher. *Enterobacter (Aerobacter)* infections are, as a rule, resistant to these compounds. Cephaloridine is effective in the therapy of bronchitis due to *H. influenzae,* but other agents often produce better results; this drug has also been found useful when employed as an aerosol in patients with purulent bronchitis. Urinary tract infections due to susceptible microorganisms respond well to oral administration of cephalexin and cephradine. *Cephalosporins should not be used to treat bacterial meningitis.* This is true for all causative microorganisms. Patients receiving high doses of a cephalosporin for treatment of meningitis caused by bacteria that were very sensitive *in vitro* have, nevertheless, succumbed. As noted above, the penetration of cephalosporins into cerebrospinal fluid is poor. Although cephalothin is ineffective in the management of gonorrhea, cephaloridine given in a single intramuscular dose of 2 g has been reported to produce high cure rates in this disease.

The Choice and Status of the Cephalosporins. Inspection of Table 55-1 (page 1096) reveals that a cephalosporin is listed as the drug of first choice just once—for *Klebsiella* infections. The cephalosporins thus seem to be overpromoted and overused. They are, however, valuable secondary agents, and they frequently appear as alternative choices to a penicillin. Some risk is involved in the administration of a cephalosporin to a patient sensitive to penicillin, as discussed above; the physician must be well prepared to deal with hypersensitivity reactions that may arise, particularly in such individuals.

Seven semisynthetic cephalosporins are currently available—four for parenteral and three for oral use. The physician is advised to acquaint himself with only two of these agents, one for parenteral and one for oral use, with the following considerations in mind. There is little difference between cephalothin, cefazolin, and cephapirin; cefazolin is less painful following intramuscular injection. Cephaloridine is nephrotoxic. Of the three compounds available for oral administration, the absorption of cephalexin or cephradine is superior to that of cephaloglycin.

Abraham, E. P., and Chain, E. An enzyme from bacteria able to destroy penicillin. *Nature, Lond.,* **1940,** *146,* 837.

Abraham, E. P., and Newton, G. G. P. A comparison of the action of penicillinase on benzylpenicillin and cephalosporin N and competitive inhibition of penicillinase by cephalosporin C. *Biochem. J.,* **1956,** *63,* 628–634.

Aserkoff, B., and Bennett, J. V. Effect of antibiotic therapy in acute salmonellosis on the fecal excretion of salmonellae. *New Engl. J. Med.,* **1969,** *281,* 636–640.

Bergeron, M. G.; Brusch, J. L.; Barza, M.; and Weinstein, L. Bactericidal activity and pharmacology of cefazolin. *Antimicrob. Agents Chemother.,* **1973,** *4,* 396–401.

Blake, F. G.; Craige, B., Jr.; and Tierney, N. A. Clinical experiences with penicillin. *Trans. Ass. Am. Physns,* **1944,** *58,* 67–74.

Bodey, G. P., and Nance, J. Amoxicillin: *in vitro* and pharmacological studies. *Antimicrob. Agents Chemother.,* **1972,** *1,* 358–362.

Boe, R. W.; Williams, C. P. S.; Bennett, J. V.; and Oliver, T. K., Jr. Serum levels of methicillin and ampicillin in newborn and premature infants in relation to postnatal age. *Pediatrics, Springfield,* **1967,** *39,* 194–201.

Boothman, R.; Kerr, M. M.; Marshall, M. J.; and Burland, W. L. Absorption and excretion of cephalexin by the newborn infant. *Archs Dis. Childh.,* **1973,** *48,* 147–150.

Brown, C. H., III; Natelson, E. A.; Bradshaw, M. W.; Williams, T. W., Jr.; and Alfrey, C. P., Jr. The hemostatic defect produced by carbenicillin. *New Engl. J. Med.,* **1974,** *291,* 265–270.

Brusch, J. L.; Bergeron, M. G.; Barza, M.; and Weinstein, L. An *in vitro* and pharmacological comparison of amoxicillin and ampicillin. *Am. J. med. Sci.,* **1974,** *267,* 41–48.

Bulger, R. J. A methicillin-resistant strain of *Staphylococcus aureus:* clinical and laboratory experiences. *Ann. intern. Med.,* **1967,** *67,* 81–89.

Bunn, P. A.; Milicich, S.; and Lunn, J. S. Pharmacological properties of hetacillin in the human. In, *Antimicrobial Agents and Chemotherapy—1965.* (Hobby, G. L., ed.) American Society for Microbiology, Ann Arbor, Mich., **1966,** pp. 947–950.

Butler, K.; English, A. R.; Knirsch, A. K.; and Korst, J. J. Metabolism and laboratory studies with indanyl carbenicillin. *Delaware med. J.,* **1971,** *43,* 366–375.

Carrizosa, J.; Levison, M. E.; and Kaye, D. Double-blind controlled comparison of phlebitis produced by cephapirin and cephalothin. *Antimicrob. Agents Chemother.,* **1973,** *3,* 306–307.

Chain, E. B. The development of bacterial chemotherapy. *Antibiotics Chemother.,* **1954,** *4,* 215–241.

Croydon, E. A. P. Clinical experience of amoxycillin in the United Kingdom. *Chemotherapy,* **1973,** *18,* 112–118.

Croydon, E. A. P., and Sutherland, R. α-Amino-*p*-hydroxybenzylpenicillin (BRL 2333), a new semisynthetic penicillin: absorption and excretion in man. In, *Antimicrobial Agents and Chemotherapy—1970.* (Hobby, G. L., ed.) American Society for Microbiology, Bethesda, Md., **1971,** pp. 427–430.

Darrell, J. H., and Waterworth, P. M. Carbenicillin resistance in *Pseudomonas aeruginosa* from clinical material. *Br. med. J.,* **1969,** *2,* 141–143.

deMaine, J. B., and Kirby, W. M. M. Clinical pharmacology of cephalexin administered intravenously. In, *Antimicrobial Agents and Chemotherapy—1970.* (Hobby, G. L., ed.) American Society for Microbiology, Bethesda, Md., **1971,** pp. 190–194.

Eagle, H. The recovery of bacteria from the toxic effects of penicillin. *J. clin. Invest.,* **1949,** *28,* 382–386.

————. Experimental approach to the problem of treatment failure with penicillin. I. Group A streptococcal infection in mice. *Am. J. Med.,* **1952,** *13,* 389–399.

Eastwood, J. B., and Curtis, J. R. Carbenicillin administration in patients with severe renal failure. *Br. med. J.,* **1968,** *1,* 486–487.

Eickhoff, T. C.; Kislak, J. W.; and Finland, M. Sodium ampicillin—absorption and excretion of intramuscular and intravenous doses in normal young men. *Am. J. med. Sci.,* **1965,** *249,* 163–171.

English, A. R.; Huang, H. T.; and Sobin, B. A. 6-Aminopenicillanic acid in urine after oral administration of penicillin. *Proc. Soc. exp. Biol. Med.,* **1960,** *104,* 405–406.

English, A. R.; Retsema, J. A.; Ray, V. A.; and Lynch, J. E. Carbenicillin indanyl sodium, an orally active derivative of carbenicillin. *Antimicrob. Agents Chemother.,* **1972,** *1,* 185–191.

Ferrieri, P.; Dajani, A. S.; and Wannamaker, L. W. A controlled study of penicillin prophylaxis against streptococcal impetigo. *J. infect. Dis.,* **1974,** *129,* 429–438.

Fiumara, N. J. The treatment of syphilis. *New Engl. J. Med.,* **1964,** *270,* 1185–1188.

————. Specifics for syphilis. *Drug Ther.,* **1975,** *5,* 191–196.

Fleming, P. C.; Goldner, M.; and Glass, D. G. Observations on the nature, distribution and significance of cephalosporinase. *Lancet*, **1963**, *1*, 1399–1401.

Florey, H. W. The use of micro-organisms for therapeutic purposes. *Yale J. Biol. Med.*, **1946**, *19*, 101–118.

Gibaldi, M.; Davidson, D.; Plaut, M. E.; and Schwartz, M. A. Modification of penicillin distribution and elimination by probenecid. *Int. Z. klin. Pharmak. Ther. Tox.*, **1970**, *3*, 182–189.

Gordon, R. C.; Regamey, C.; and Kirby, W. M. M. Comparative clinical pharmacology of amoxicillin and ampicillin administered orally. *Antimicrob. Agents Chemother.*, **1972**, *1*, 504–507.

Gravenkemper, C. F.; Bennett, J. V.; Brodie, J. L.; and Kirby, W. M. M. Dicloxacillin: *in vitro* and pharmacologic comparisons with oxacillin and cloxacillin. *Archs intern. Med.*, **1965**, *116*, 340–345.

Hallander, H. O., and Laurell, G. Epidemiological and clinical aspects of methicillin resistance and enterotoxin production in *Staphylococcus aureus*. *Ann. N.Y. Acad. Sci.*, **1971**, *182*, 98–105.

Hamilton-Miller, J. M. T. Penicillinacylase. *Bact. Rev.*, **1966**, *30*, 761–771.

Handsfield, H. H.; Clark, H.; Wallace, J. F.; Holmes, K. K.; and Turck, M. Amoxicillin, a new penicillin antibiotic. *Antimicrob. Agents Chemother.*, **1973**, *3*, 262–265.

Harvengt, C.; de Schepper, P.; Lamy, F.; and Hansen, J. Cephradine absorption and excretion in fasting and nonfasting volunteers. *J. clin. Pharmac.*, **1973**, *13*, 36–40.

Hewitt, W. L.; Finegold, S. M.; and Monzon, O. T. Untoward side effects associated with methicillin therapy. In, *Antimicrobial Agents and Chemotherapy*. (Sylvester, J. C., ed.) Braun-Brumfield, Inc., Ann Arbor, Mich., **1961**, pp. 765–769.

Holmes, K. K.; Johnson, D. W.; and Floyd, T. M. Studies of venereal disease. I. Probenecid-procaine penicillin G combination and tetracycline hydrochloride in the treatment of "penicillin-resistant" gonorrhea in men. *J. Am. med. Ass.*, **1967**, *202*, 461–476.

Idsøe, O.; Guthe, T.; Willcox, R. R.; and DeWeck, A. L. Nature and extent of penicillin side-reactions, with particular reference to fatalities from anaphylactic shock. *Bull. Wld Hlth Org.*, **1968**, *38*, 159–188.

Jawetz, E., and Sonne, M. Penicillin-streptomycin treatment of enterococcal endocarditis. *New Engl. J. Med.*, **1966**, *274*, 710–715.

Kaplan, J. M., and McCracken, G. H., Jr. Clinical pharmacology of benzathine penicillin G in neonates with regard to its recommended use in congenital syphilis. *J. Pediat.*, **1973**, *82*, 1069–1072.

Kerrebijn, K. F., and Michel, M. F. Amoxycillin (BRL 2333) in children. *Chemotherapy*, **1973**, *18*, Suppl., 92–96.

Kind, A. C.; Tupasi, T. E.; Standiford, H. C.; and Kirby, W. M. M. Mechanisms responsible for plasma levels of nafcillin lower than those of oxacillin. *Archs intern. Med.*, **1970**, *125*, 685–690.

Klaus, M. V., and Fellner, M. J. Penicilloyl-specific serum antibodies in man. Analysis in 592 individuals from the newborn to old age. *J. Geront.*, **1973**, *28*, 312–316.

Klein, J. O., and Finland, M. Ampicillin: activity *in vitro* and absorption and excretion in normal young men. *Am. J. med. Sci.*, **1963a**, *245*, 544–555.

Klein, J. O.; Schaberg, M. J.; Buntin, M.; and Gezon, H. M. Levels of penicillin in serum of newborn infants after single intramuscular doses of benzathine penicillin G. *J. Pediat.*, **1973**, *82*, 1065–1068.

Kunin, C. M., and Finkelberg, Z. Oral cephalexin and ampicillin: antimicrobial activity, recovery in urine, and persistence of uremic patients. *Ann. intern. Med.*, **1970**, *72*, 349–356.

Kvale, P. A.; Keys, T. F.; Johnson, D. W.; and Holmes, K. K. Single oral dose ampicillin-probenecid treatment of gonorrhea in the male. *J. Am. med. Ass.*, **1971**, *215*, 1449–1453.

Lemole, G. M.; Fadali, A. M. A.; and Molthan, L. Cephalothin-induced tachycardia following aortic valve replacement. *J. Am. med. Ass.*, **1972**, *221*, 593–594.

Levine, B. B. Immunochemical mechanisms involved in penicillin hypersensitivity in experimental animals and in human beings. *Fedn Proc. Fedn Am. Socs exp. Biol.*, **1965**, *24*, 45–50.

Levine, B. B.; Redmond, A. P.; Fellner, M. J.; Voss, H. E.; and Levytska, V. Penicillin allergy and the heterogeneous immune responses of man. *J. clin. Invest.*, **1966**, *45*, 1895–1906.

Levine, B. B., and Zolov, D. M. Prediction of penicillin allergy by immunological tests. *J. Allergy*, **1969**, *43*, 231–244.

McCracken, G. H., Jr.; Ginsberg, C.; Chrane, D. F.; Thomas, M. A.; and Horton, L. J. Clinical pharmacology of penicillin in newborn infants. *J. Pediat.*, **1973**, *82*, 692–698.

McCracken, G. H., Jr., and Kaplan, J. M. Penicillin treatment for congenital syphilis. *J. Am. med. Ass.*, **1974**, *228*, 855–858.

McGowan, J. E.; Garner, C.; Wilcox, C.; and Finland, M. Antibiotic susceptibility of gram-negative bacilli isolated from blood cultures. *Am. J. Med.*, **1974**, *57*, 225–238.

Magni, L.; Örtengren, B.; Sjöberg, B.; and Wahlqvist, S. Stability, absorption and excretion studies with hetacillin. *Scand. J. clin. Lab. Invest.*, **1967**, *20*, 195–201.

Medical Letter. *Haemophilus influenzae* meningitis resistant to ampicillin. **1974**, *16*, 29–30.

Meyers, B. R.; Kaplan, K.; and Weinstein, L. Cephalexin: microbiological effects and pharmacologic parameters in man. *Clin. Pharmac. Ther.*, **1969**, *10*, 810–816.

Mortimer, P. R.; Mackie, D. B.; and Haynes, S. Ampicillin levels in human bile in the presence of biliary tract disease. *Br. med. J.*, **1969**, *3*, 88–89.

National Research Council. Committee on Chemotherapeutic and Other Agents. Division of Medical Sciences. (Keefer, C. S., chrmn.) Penicillin in the treatment of infections; a report of 500 cases. *J. Am. med. Ass.*, **1943**, *122*, 1217–1224.

Nelson, J. D., and Haltalin, K. C. Amoxicillin less effective than ampicillin against *Shigella in vitro* and *in vivo*: relationship of efficacy to activity in serum. *J. infect. Dis.*, **1974**, *129*, Suppl., S222–S227.

Nicholas, P.; Meyers, B. R.; and Hirschman, S. Z. Pharmacology of cefazolin in human volunteers. *J. clin. Pharmac.*, **1973**, *13*, 325–331.

Park, J. T., and Strominger, J. L. Mode of action of penicillin. *Science, Wash.*, **1957**, *125*, 99–101.

Parker, C. W. Immunochemical mechanisms in penicillin allergy. *Fedn Proc. Fedn Am. Socs exp. Biol.*, **1965**, *24*, 51–54.

Parker, M. P., and Hewitt, J. H. Methicillin-resistance in *Staphylococcus aureus*. *Lancet*, **1970**, *1*, 800–804.

Phillips, W. E. Treatment of chronic typhoid carriers with ampicillin. *J. Am. med. Ass.*, **1971**, *217*, 913–915.

Pirozzi, D. J. Syphilis and penicillin. *Ann. intern. Med.*, **1973**, *79*, 447–449.

Public Health Service, U.S. Department of Health, Education, and Welfare. *Morbidity and Mortality*. (Weekly report.) **1974**, *23*, No. 9, 77–78.

Quie, P. G.; Pierce, H. C.; and Wannamaker, L. W. Influence of penicillinase-producing staphylococci on the eradication of group A streptococci from the upper respiratory tract by penicillin treatment. *Pediatrics, Springfield*, **1966**, *37*, 467–476.

Rein, M. F.; Westervelt, F. B.; and Sande, M. A. Pharmacodynamics of cefazolin in the presence of normal and impaired renal function. *Antimicrob. Agents Chemother.*, **1973**, *4*, 366–371.

Ridley, M., and Phillips, I. Relative instability of cephaloridine to staphylococcal penicillinase. *Nature, Lond.*, **1965**, *208*, 1076–1078.

Rodey, G. P.; Rodriguez, V.; and Stewart, D. Clinical

pharmacological studies of carbenicillin. *Am. J. med. Sci.,* **1969,** *257,* 185–190.

Rolinson, G. N. Bacterial resistance to penicillins and cephalosporins. *Proc. R. Soc., B,* **1971,** *179,* 403–410.

———. Laboratory evaluation of amoxycillin. *Chemotherapy,* **1973,** *18,* Suppl., 1–10.

Rosenblatt, J. E.; Kind, A. C.; Brodie, J. L.; and Kirby, W. M. M. Mechanisms responsible for the blood level differences of isoxazolylpenicillins. *Archs intern. Med.,* **1968,** *121,* 345–348.

Sales, J. E. L.; Sutcliffe, M.; and O'Grady, F. Cephalexin levels in human bile in the presence of biliary tract disease. *Br. med. J.,* **1972,** *2,* 441–443.

Simon, H. J., and Miller, R. C. Ampicillin in the treatment of chronic typhoid carriers: report on fifteen treated cases and a review of the literature. *New Engl. J. Med.,* **1966,** *274,* 808–815.

Smith, C. B., and Finland, M. Carbenicillin: activity *in vitro* and absorption and excretion in normal young men. *Appl. Microbiol.,* **1968,** *16,* 1753–1759.

Smith, J. L., and Israel, C. W. Optic atrophy and neurosyphilis. *A. Rev. Med.,* **1971,** *22,* 103–118.

Sparling, P. F. Antibiotic resistance in *Neisseria gonorrheae. Med. Clins N. Am.,* **1972,** *56,* 1133–1144.

Stewart, G. T. Allergenic residues in penicillins. *Lancet,* **1967,** *1,* 1177–1183.

Sutherland, R., and Rolinson, G. N. α-Amino-*p*-hydroxypenicillin (BRL 2333), a new semisynthetic penicillin: *in vitro* evaluation. In, *Antimicrobial Agents and Chemotherapy—1970.* (Hobby, G. L., ed.) American Society for Microbiology, Bethesda, Md., **1971,** pp. 411–415.

Tuano, S. B.; Johnson, L. D.; Brodie, J. L.; and Kirby, W. M. M. Comparative blood levels of hetacillin, ampicillin and penicillin G. *New Engl. J. Med.,* **1966,** *275,* 635–639.

Venuto, R. C., and Plaut, M. E. Cephalothin handling in patients undergoing hemodialysis. In, *Antimicrobial Agents and Chemotherapy—1970.* (Hobby, G. L., ed.) American Society for Microbiology, Bethesda, Md., **1971,** pp. 50–52.

Wallace, J. F.; Atlas, E.; Bear, D. M.; Brown, N. K.; Clark, H.; and Turck, M. Evaluation of an indanyl ester of carbenicillin. In, *Antimicrobial Agents and Chemotherapy—1970.* (Hobby, G. L., ed.) American Society for Microbiology, Bethesda, Md., **1971,** pp. 223–226.

Weary, P. E.; Cole, J. E., III; and Hickam, L. H. Eruptions from ampicillin in patients with infectious mononucleosis. *Archs Derm.,* **1970,** *101,* 86–91.

Weinstein, L.; Lerner, P. I.; and Chew, W. H. Clinical and bacteriologic studies of the effect of "massive" doses of penicillin G on infections caused by gram-negative bacilli. *New Engl. J. Med.,* **1964a,** *271,* 525–533.

Wright, W. W.; Welch, H. W.; Wilner, J.; and Roberts, E. F. Body fluid concentrations of penicillin following intramuscular injection of single doses of benzathine penicillin G and/or procaine penicillin G. *Antibiotic Med. clin. Ther.,* **1959,** *6,* 232–241.

Monographs and Reviews

Abraham, E. P. The action of antibiotics on bacteria. In, *Antibiotics,* Vol. II. (Florey, H. W., *et al.,* authors.) Oxford University Press, New York, **1949,** pp. 1438–1496.

———. The cephalosporins. *Pharmac. Rev.,* **1962,** *14,* 473–500. (110 references.)

Bear, D. M.; Turck, M.; and Petersdorf, R. G. Ampicillin. *Med. Clins N. Am.,* **1970,** *54,* 1145–1159.

Blumberg, P. M., and Strominger, J. L. Interaction of penicillin with the bacterial cell: penicillin-binding proteins and penicillin-sensitive enzymes. *Bact. Rev.,* **1974,** *38,* 291–335.

Chain, E. B. Penicillinase-resistant penicillins and the problem of the penicillin-resistant staphylococci. In, *Resistance of Bacteria to the Penicillins* (Ciba Foundation Study Group No. 13). (De Reuck, A. V. S., and Cameron, M. P., eds.) Little, Brown & Co., Boston, **1962,** pp. 3–19.

Clinical Symposium. (Various authors.) Cefazolin. *J. infect. Dis.,* **1973,** *128,* Suppl., S312–S424.

Conference. (Various authors.) Cephalosporins. *Postgrad. med. J.,* **1970,** *46,* Suppl., 3–159.

Editorial. Methicillin-resistant staphylococci. *New Engl. J. Med.,* **1967,** *277,* 710–711.

Finland, M., and Weinstein, L. Complications induced by antimicrobial agents. *New Engl. J. Med.,* **1953,** *248,* 220–226.

Fleming, A. History and development of penicillin. In, *Penicillin: Its Practical Application.* (Fleming, A., ed.) The Blakiston Co., Philadelphia, **1946,** pp. 1–33.

Florey, H. W. Historical introduction. In, *Antibiotics,* Vol. I. (Florey, H. W., *et al.,* authors.) Oxford University Press, New York, **1949,** pp. 1–73.

Flynn, E. H. (ed.). *Cephalosporins and Penicillins: Chemistry and Biology.* Academic Press, Inc., New York, **1972.**

Gilbert, D. N., and Sanford, J. P. Methicillin: critical appraisal after a decade of experience. *Med. Clins N. Am.,* **1970,** *54,* 1113–1125.

Gill, F. A., and Hook, E. W. Changing patterns of bacterial resistance to antimicrobial drugs. *Am. J. Med.,* **1965,** *39,* 780–795.

Griffith, R. S., and Black, H. R. Cephalexin. *Med. Clins N. Am.,* **1970,** *54,* 1229–1244.

Herrell, W. E. *Penicillin and Other Antibiotic Agents.* W. B. Saunders Co., Philadelphia, **1945.**

Hirsch, H. L., and Putnam, L. E. *Penicillin.* Medical Encyclopedia, Inc., New York, **1958.** (159 references.)

International Symposium. (Various authors.) Amoxicillin: clinical perspectives. *J. infect. Dis.,* **1974,** *129,* Suppl., S121–S274.

Jawetz, E. The use of antimicrobial combinations. *A. Rev. Pharmac.,* **1968,** *8,* 151–170.

Klein, J., and Finland, M. The new penicillins. *New Engl. J. Med.,* **1963b,** *269,* 1019–1025. (214 references.)

Mandell, G. L. Cephaloridine. *Ann. intern. Med.,* **1973,** *79,* 561–565.

Strominger, J. L. The action of penicillin and other antibiotics on bacterial wall synthesis. *Johns Hopkins med. J.,* **1973,** *133,* 63–81.

Strominger, J. L.; Izaki, K.; Matsuhashi, M.; and Tipper, D. J. Peptidoglycan transpeptidase and D-alanine carboxypeptidase: penicillin-sensitive reactions. *Fedn Proc. Fedn Am. Socs exp. Biol.,* **1967,** *26,* 9–22.

Symposium. (Various authors.) Carbenicillin: a clinical profile. *J. infect. Dis.,* **1970,** *122,* Suppl., S1–S117.

Symposium. (Various authors.) Oral indanyl carbenicillin in the treatment of urinary tract infection. *J. infect. Dis.,* **1973,** *127,* Suppl., S93–S165.

Symposium. (Various authors.) Mode of action of antibiotics on microbial walls and membranes. (Salton, M. R. J., and Tomasz, A., eds.) *Ann. N.Y. Acad. Sci.,* **1974,** *235,* 1–160.

Weinstein, L. The complications of antibiotic therapy. *Bull. N.Y. Acad. Med.,* **1955,** *31,* 500–518.

Weinstein, L., and Dalton, A. C. Host determinants of response to antimicrobial therapy. *New Engl. J. Med.,* **1968,** *279,* 467–473, 524–531, 580–588.

Weinstein, L., and Kaplan, K. The cephalosporins. Microbiological, chemical and pharmacological properties and use in chemotherapy of infection. *Ann. intern. Med.,* **1970,** *72,* 729–739.

Weinstein, L.; Kaplan, K.; and Chang, T. W. Treatment of infections in man with cephalothin. *J. Am. med. Ass.,* **1964b,** *189,* 829–834.

58 ANTIMICROBIAL AGENTS

[*Continued*]

Streptomycin, Gentamicin, and Other Aminoglycosides

Louis Weinstein

The aminoglycoside antibiotics—most notably streptomycin, gentamicin, and kanamycin—are discussed in this chapter. As the group name adequately implies, all these drugs contain amino sugars in glycosidic linkage. They are polycations, and their polarity is responsible for pharmacokinetic properties shared by all members of the group. For example, none is adequately absorbed after oral administration, none penetrates into the cerebrospinal fluid with ease, and all are relatively rapidly excreted by the normal kidney.

The aminoglycosides are used almost exclusively to treat infections caused by gram-negative bacteria. They act to inhibit protein synthesis in susceptible microorganisms; the mechanism of this action is best understood for streptomycin and is discussed below. Mutations affecting proteins in the bacterial ribosome, the target for these drugs, can confer marked and rapid resistance to their action. Resistance can also result from the acquisition of a plasmid, and this is associated with the elaboration of drug-metabolizing enzymes. Bacteria that acquire resistance to one aminoglycoside may exhibit resistance to the others.

Serious toxicity is a major limitation to the usefulness of the aminoglycosides, and the same spectrum of toxicity is shared by all members of the group. Most notable is ototoxicity, which can involve both the auditory and vestibular functions of the eighth cranial nerve. Nephrotoxicity is an additional important problem.

STREPTOMYCIN

History and Source. The ineffectiveness of penicillin G in the treatment of infections due to gram-negative microorganisms was the primary stimulus

for the search for antimicrobial agents effective against such bacteria. Unlike the purely accidental discovery of penicillin, the development of streptomycin was the result of a well-planned, scientific search for antibacterial substances. Waksman and coworkers examined a number of soil actinomyces between 1939 and 1943 and demonstrated the elaboration by such fungi of a number of potent antibiotics; however, none of these was clinically useful, being too toxic or not sufficiently active. In 1943, a strain of *Streptomyces griseus* was isolated that elaborated a potent antimicrobial substance. The first public announcement of the discovery of this new antibiotic—*streptomycin*—was made by Schatz, Bugie, and Waksman early in 1944, and it was soon shown to inhibit the growth of the tubercle bacillus and a number of gram-positive and gram-negative microorganisms *in vitro* and *in vivo*. In less than 2 years, extensive bacteriological, chemical, and pharmacological investigations of streptomycin had been carried out, and its clinical usefulness was established. Controlled studies of the therapeutic efficacy of the drug in man were supervised by the National Research Council and supported by large contributions from pharmaceutical and chemical companies; this constituted the first privately financed, nationally coordinated, clinical drug evaluation in history. (*See* Waksman, 1949, 1953.)

Chemistry. Streptomycin is a highly polar organic base with a large number of hydrophilic and functional groups. The drug is made up of three components—streptidine, streptose, and N-methyl-L-glucosamine; its structural formula is on the next page.

Streptomycin base and its inorganic acid salts are soluble in water; streptomycin sulfate is the salt now employed clinically.

Antimicrobial Activity. High concentrations of streptomycin are bactericidal whereas low concentrations are bacteriostatic *in vitro*. Resting cells are less susceptible to the drug than are multiplying bacteria.

Many factors influence the antimicrobial effectiveness of streptomycin. The *pH of the medium* is of particular importance. There is a 20- to 80-fold increase in potency at pH 8.0 as compared to pH 5.8. It is thus considered advantageous to administer an

Streptomycin

alkalinizing agent when streptomycin is used for the therapy of urinary tract infections. Increase in local acidity secondary to tissue damage may be responsible for failure of the drug to eradicate sensitive microorganisms at sites of injury or abscess formation. Streptomycin is considerably less antibacterial under *anaerobic conditions.*

Antimicrobial Activity in Vitro. Bacteria inhibited by less than 10 μg/ml of streptomycin are considered sensitive to it; those suppressed by 10 to 100 μg/ml are classed as moderately sensitive; and those that are affected only by more than 100 μg/ml are classed as resistant.

Among the microorganisms that are sensitive to concentrations of streptomycin readily attainable in man are *Brucella, Erysipelothrix, Haemophilus ducreyi, Listeria monocytogenes, Pseudomonas (Actinobacillus) mallei, Nocardia, Yersinia (Pasteurella) pestis, Francisella (Pasteurella) tularensis,* many but not all strains of *Mycobacterium tuberculosis,* and *Shigella.* The species with strains exhibiting a wide variation in susceptibility include *Streptococcus (Diplococcus) pneumoniae, S. typhi* and other *Salmonella, Escherichia coli, H. influenzae,* the gonococcus and the meningococcus, *Proteus vulgaris, Staphylococcus aureus, Staph. epidermidis, Strep. pyogenes* (group A), *Strep. faecalis,* the *viridans* group of streptococci, and *Vibrio cholerae.* The minimal inhibitory concentrations for some of these vary over more than a thousandfold range. *Bacteroides, Clostridium, Rickettsia, Trypanosoma, Entamoeba histolytica, Trichomonas vaginalis,* fungi, and all viruses are totally resistant to streptomycin.

Mechanism of Action. Streptomycin and other aminoglycosides act directly on the ribosome, where they inhibit protein biosynthesis and decrease the fidelity of translation of the genetic code. The major result of streptomycin action appears to be the prevention of amino acid polymerization after formation of the initiation complex (Weisblum and Davies,

1968). The site of action of streptomycin is the 30 S ribosomal subunit, and mutations in the gene coding for a specific protein of this subunit (P10) control the binding of the antibiotic to the ribosome and the sensitivity of the microorganism to the drug (Nomura *et al.,* 1969). While isolated P10 does not itself bind streptomycin, this protein appears to form a crucial portion of the binding site or to control access of the drug to such a site.

The binding of streptomycin to sensitive ribosomes also causes misreading of the genetic code, perhaps by causing distortion of critical components of the protein synthetic apparatus. Thus, specific aminoacyl tRNA may fail to recognize its proper codon on mRNA and incorrect amino acids are inserted into the peptide chain (Davies and Davis, 1968). Although misreading was originally thought to account for the *lethal* action of aminoglycosides on bacteria, this does not appear to be the case; the fact that the aminoglycosides are bactericidal is still unexplained.

Misreading of the genetic code may, however, account for the phenomenon of bacterial *dependence* on streptomycin, a condition that may be acquired as a single-step mutational event. If there is a mutation at some other site in the bacterial genome that would effectively prevent growth (*e.g.,* an amino acid substitution in a protein essential for normal metabolism), streptomycin-induced misreading of the mutation could result in an acceptable correction of the defect (phenotypic suppression). Bacteria could then resume growth only in the presence of the aminoglycoside. While this is a fascinating phenomenon, it is not of clinical significance.

Resistance to Streptomycin. A major disadvantage and cause of failure of streptomycin therapy is the development of bacterial resistance to the drug. Resistance may be acquired by a single mutational step, and there is selection for such microorganisms in the presence of the antibiotic. The ribosomes from these bacteria are unable to bind streptomycin, and the structure of protein P10 is altered.

Resistant forms may also develop by virtue of their inability to transport streptomycin to an intracellular site or by the induction of enzymes that metabolize the drug (streptomycin phosphotransferase and adenylate synthetase). Such resistance to streptomycin is carried by R factors (plasmids) that may confer resistance to several antibiotics at once (*see* Chapter 55).

As a result of the widespread use of streptomycin over the years, resistant strains of many gram-negative and gram-positive microorganisms have emerged. Insensitivity to the drug may develop with great rapidity, since only a single event followed by selection is required. For example, highly sensitive strains of *H. influenzae* responsible for meningitis have been found to become resistant to concentrations of antibiotic greater than 1000 μg/ml within 48 to 72 hours after initiation of therapy (Weinstein, 1946). The emergence of drug resistance is one of the most important problems in streptomycin therapy and makes it necessary to prove the sensitivity of microorganisms isolated from infected areas if this antibiotic is to be used with the greatest possibility for cure.

Effects of Streptomycin Administered with Other Antimicrobial Agents. Since resistance to streptomycin is a special problem, the concomitant use of streptomycin and other antimicrobial agents offers advantages in specific situations. The outstanding example is the chemotherapy of tuberculosis (*see* Chapter 60). In addition, a number of *in-vitro* studies have suggested that streptomycin combined with penicillin G, ampicillin, a cephalosporin, a sulfonamide, or other anti-infective drugs produces additive or supra-additive antimicrobial effects. Combinations of streptomycin (or other aminoglycosides) with agents that inhibit synthesis of the bacterial cell wall often exert such an effect against enterococci. There may be greater intracellular penetration of streptomycin when combined with such compounds (Moellering *et al.*, 1971; Moellering and Weinberg, 1971).

Absorption, Distribution, and Excretion.
Absorption. Very little streptomycin is absorbed from the intestinal tract, since it is a polycation. The drug is not inactivated in the intestine and is eliminated almost quantitatively in the feces. Absorption from the lung and intrathecal sites is also insignificant. Instillation intrapleurally does result in rapid absorption of streptomycin into the blood, and the drug is also absorbed rapidly from intramuscular and subcutaneous sites of injection.

Distribution. Almost all the streptomycin in blood is present in the *plasma,* and very little enters the erythrocytes. The drug is distributed in all the extracellular fluids. Approximately one third of the antibiotic in the plasma is bound to protein.

The distribution of parenterally administered streptomycin into intracellular and transcellular fluids is more restricted. Little or no streptomycin is detectable in the *cerebrospinal fluid* of individuals with normal meninges; in the presence of meningitis, however, the drug diffuses more readily across the blood–cerebrospinal fluid barrier, but therapeutic concentrations may not necessarily be attained. Intrathecal administration of the drug produces effective concentrations in the cerebrospinal fluid. Diffusion into the *pleural fluid* is relatively slow, but repeated administration of the antibiotic produces pleural fluid concentrations that approximate those in the plasma. *Pericardial* and *synovial fluids* contain appreciable quantities of the antibiotic. Streptomycin penetrates the *fetal plasma* and *amniotic fluid* when it is given late in pregnancy, the concentration in these fluids being about half that in the maternal plasma.

Excretion. Streptomycin is excreted by glomerular filtration. Approximately 50 to 60% of a parenterally administered dose is excreted unchanged in the *urine* in the first 24 hours; most of this appears in the first 12 hours. The rate of renal clearance of streptomycin in man varies from 30 to 70 ml per minute, about 30% lower than the glomerular filtration rate. In the presence of uremia, a single dose of streptomycin may produce reasonably high plasma concentrations for several days, and very little drug is present in the urine. The half-life of the antibiotic, 2 to 3 hours in normal adults, increases to 100 hours when blood urea nitrogen values are in the range of 100 to 150 mg/100 ml. Ototoxicity is strikingly more frequent in the presence of impaired renal function.

A small portion of parenterally administered streptomycin is secreted by the liver into the *bile;* in man, peak concentrations of 10 to 20 μg/ml of bile may be present after large doses. Hepatic dysfunction decreases the quantity of the antibiotic in the bile; in the presence of long-standing obstructive jaundice, streptomycin may not be secreted by the liver.

From 10 to 30% of a parenterally administered dose of streptomycin cannot be accounted for by excretion. However, metabolites of the drug have not been identified.

Plasma and Urinary Concentrations. Peak plasma concentrations are detectable within 1 or 2 hours after intramuscular injection and diminish by about 50% in 5 hours. The antibiotic can be demonstrated in the plasma for at least 8 to 12 hours after a single parenteral dose. Drug accumulation will occur if streptomycin is administered more frequently than this to patients with impaired renal function. In adults, 1 g given intramuscularly produces a peak plasma concentration of 25 to 30 μg/ml.

The intramuscular administration of 0.5 g of streptomycin every 6 hours produces *urinary concentrations* ranging from 200 to 1500 μg/ml, depending on renal function and urine volume.

Preparations. *Streptomycin Sulfate,* U.S.P., is supplied for parenteral injection either as a sterile dry powder or in sterile solution. Each vial contains the equivalent of 1 or 5 g of the base; solutions, which are stable for months, contain 500 mg/ml.

Routes of Administration and Dosage. Streptomycin preparations can be administered by a variety of routes; the choice depends on the type and the location of the infection being treated. *Intermittent, deep intramuscular injection* is the method most often used for parenteral administration. The total daily dose varies from 1 to 2 g (15 to 25 mg/kg); 500 mg to 1.0 g is injected every 12 hours. Children should receive 20 to 30 mg/kg daily, in two divided doses.

Inadequate therapy favors the development of resistant microorganisms. Except in tuberculosis and subacute bacterial endocarditis, it is rarely necessary to give streptomycin for more than 7 to 10 days. Dosage schedules for tuberculosis are described in Chapter 60, and suggestions for adjustment of dosage for patients with impaired renal function are presented in Table 55–2 (page 1108).

Streptomycin may be injected *intravenously;* 500 mg to 1 g is dissolved in 30 to 40 ml of 0.9% sodium chloride solution and injected over a period of 30 to 40 minutes every 12 hours. The *intrathecal* route has been used in conjunction with intramuscular therapy in patients with meningitis. In the rare case in which this is necessary, a number of precautions must be followed.

Only fresh solutions of the drug made from the powder should be used for *intrathecal* injection; commercially prepared solutions contain preservatives that may injure the nervous system. The maximal quantities to be administered in a single dose are as follows: infants less than 1 year of age, 10 to 15 mg; children 1 to 3 years old, 15 to 25 mg; children 4 to 10 years old, up to 50 mg; adults, 75 to 100 mg. The required dose must be given in a volume of no less than 10 ml of 0.9% sodium chloride solution and injected slowly over a period of at least 10 minutes, an approximately equal volume of spinal fluid having previously been withdrawn. The absolute maximal single dose for adults is 100 mg. If intrathecal injections are repeated, the interval between them should be no less than 12 hours. Depending on the microorganism, one to four intrathecal injections may be necessary.

Intrapleural injection of streptomycin has occasionally been used to supplement systemic therapy in some cases of empyema; 500 mg to 1.0 g of streptomycin sulfate dissolved in 0.9% sodium chloride solution can be injected into the pleural cavity; the pus is first aspirated, and the volume of drug solution instilled should equal about two thirds of the volume of exudate removed. The procedure should not be repeated more often than every 24 to 48 hours.

Topical use of streptomycin is not recommended. The drug must never be applied directly to the peritoneal surface because of the possibility of respiratory paralysis (*see* below).

Untoward Effects. Like all other antimicrobial agents, streptomycin produces three types of untoward effects: *hypersensitization reactions,* dose-related *toxic effects,* and those that result from *biological alterations in the host.*

Hypersensitivity Reactions. Skin rashes, *eosinophilia, fever, blood dyscrasias, angioedema, exfoliative dermatitis, stomatitis,* and *anaphylactic shock* are among the hypersensitivity reactions that may follow the administration of streptomycin. *Skin eruptions* develop in about 5% of persons so treated. Morbilliform, maculopapular, erythematous, and urticarial rashes have been observed. Mild cutaneous manifestations do not necessarily require cessation of treatment. *Pruritus, scaling, eosinophilia, lymphadenopathy,* and *fever* may accompany the eruptions, but classical serum sickness does not occur. *Eosinophilia* is common and may develop in 50% of patients receiving streptomycin for an extended period.

Exfoliative dermatitis occurs in less than 1% of individuals given the drug. Most of the allergic cutaneous phenomena subside promptly with cessation of therapy.

Drug fever as an isolated hypersensitivity phenomenon is relatively uncommon; elevations of temperature that occur during therapy more frequently result from sterile inflammatory reactions at the sites of injection of the antibiotic. Although rare, *acute anaphylaxis* may follow the administration of any quantity of streptomycin.

Several types of *blood dyscrasias* have been noted in patients receiving streptomycin. About 0.7% of individuals who receive streptomycin develop *neutropenia.* In a few, the process may progress to *agranulocytosis. Aplastic anemia* and *thrombopenia* with purpura have been described in a few instances.

Toxic and Irritative Reactions. The intramuscular administration of streptomycin commonly produces pain at the site of injection. Hot and tender masses frequently develop in the areas in which the antibiotic is injected. The inflammation is sterile and is frequently accompanied by fever.

Labyrinthine Damage. Nearly 75% of patients given 2 g of streptomycin daily for 60 to 120 days manifest some detectable vestibular disturbance; reduction of the dose to 1 g daily decreases the incidence to approximately 25%. Moderately intense headache lasting 1 or 2 days usually precedes the onset of labyrinthine dysfunction. This is immediately followed by an *acute stage,* in which nausea, vomiting, and equilibratory difficulty develop and persist for 1 to 2 weeks. Vertigo in the upright position, inability to perceive termination of movement ("mental past pointing"), and difficulty in sitting or standing without visual cues are prominent symptoms. Drifting of the eyes at the end of a movement so that focusing and reading are difficult, positive Romberg test, and, rarely, pendular trunk movement and spontaneous nystagmus are outstanding signs. The acute stage ends suddenly and is followed by the appearance of manifestations consistent with *chronic labyrinthitis,* in which, although symptomless while in bed, the patient has difficulty when he attempts to walk or make sudden movements; ataxia is the most prominent feature. The chronic phase persists for approximately 2 months; it is gradually superseded by a *compensatory stage,* in which symptoms are latent and appear only when the eyes are closed. Adaptation to the impairment of labyrinthine function is accomplished by the use of visual cues and deep proprioceptive sensation for determining movement and position; it is more adequate in the young than in the old, but may not be sufficient to permit the high degree of coordination required in many special trades. Full recovery may require 12 to 18 months, and some patients have permanent residual damage. There is no specific treatment for the vestibular deficiency. Although, on the basis of studies in animals, there is controversy concerning the location of the lesions responsible for the vestibular and auditory dysfunction, investigations in man have suggested that streptomycin destroys the ventral cochlear nuclei in the brain stem with extension of pathological changes to the terminals of the nerve fibers in the cochlea.

In a retrospective study of eighth cranial nerve function in children whose mothers, while pregnant, had received streptomycin for the therapy of tuberculosis, Conway and Birt (1965) found that 8 of 17 youngsters, aged 6 to 13 years, had minor defects.

In order to prevent or reduce the incidence and the severity of the toxic effect of streptomycin on vestibular function, several precautions should be observed. As mentioned above, both total daily dose and duration of therapy must be carefully considered. Inflammation of the meninges or the brain appears to predispose to neurotoxic reactions, as do repeated intrathecal injection of the drug and renal insufficiency. When there is evidence of vestibular depression or if headache or ataxia develops, treatment should be discontinued. The patient should be forewarned of the possibility of vestibular impairment before prolonged streptomycin therapy is instituted.

Deafness. Although the toxic effect of streptomycin is greater upon the vestibular than upon the auditory component of the eighth cranial nerve, disturbances in hearing occur, nevertheless, in an appreciable number of patients. Four to 15% of individuals receiving the drug for more than 1 week can be shown to have a measurable decrease in hearing, and complete deafness may ensue in rare cases. A high-pitched tinnitus is often the first symptom of impending difficulty. If the drug is not discontinued, auditory impairment may develop after a few days. The tinnitus may persist for several days to 2 weeks after therapy is stopped. Since perception of sound in the high-frequency range (outside the conversational range) is lost first, the affected individual is not aware of the difficulty, which is not detected unless careful audiometric examination is carried out. If the loss of hearing progresses, the lower sound ranges are affected, and conversation becomes difficult. The results of pathological studies in animals and man are at variance; some workers believe the damage is to the end organ and others believe it is central (see Hawkins and Lurie, 1952; Winston, 1953; Spoendlin, 1966). In any situation in which the possibility of auditory difficulty is suspected, therapy with streptomycin should not be initiated until audiometry has been carried out.

Other Nervous System Effects. The administration of streptomycin may produce dysfunction of the optic nerve. Scotomas, presenting as enlargement of the blind spot, have been induced by the drug.

Among the less common toxic reactions to streptomycin is peripheral neuritis. This may be due either to accidental injection of a nerve during the course of parenteral therapy or to toxicity involving nerves remote from the site of antibiotic administration. Paresthesia, most commonly perioral but also present in other areas of the face or in the hands, occasionally follows the use of the antibiotic and usually appears within ½ to 1 hour after injection of the drug; it may persist for several hours.

The administration of the drug into the lumbar sac, cisterna magna, or cerebral ventricles of man may induce radiculitis, transverse myelitis, arachnoiditis, or paraplegia; root pain may be very severe and intractable. An acute encephalopathy with evidence of brain stem involvement, as indicated by nausea, vomiting, severe occipital headache, nystagmus, cerebellar signs, somnolence, urinary retention, slow and irregular respiration, dyspnea, cyanosis, fever, and delirium, may follow the introduction of excessive quantities of streptomycin into the subarachnoid space or ventricles. A diffuse encephalopathy, characterized by the rapid development of severe and repeated epileptiform seizures and/or coma, may occur if too large a dose of the drug is introduced into the spinal fluid; death may ensue within 6 to 8 hours after the appearance of symptoms in such cases. Pleocytosis and increased protein content of the spinal fluid are present when toxic reactions involve the central nervous system. These untoward effects are associated either with administration of the drug to hypersensitive patients or with the injection of doses in excess of those known to be safe (see above).

A serious and potentially fatal neuromuscular reaction to streptomycin may develop when the drug is instilled into the peritoneal cavity postoperatively, a practice in some surgical clinics. Difficulty in respiration may occur after the instillation of as little as 2 g, but it has been observed most often when larger quantities of the antibiotic have been used. The respiratory difficulty is due to blockade of the neuromuscular junction by streptomycin. The neuromuscular blockade has generally been attributed primarily to suppression of acetylcholine release, with a secondary reduction in sensitivity of the postjunctional membrane (see review by Pittinger and Adamson, 1972), although a more recent study employing neuromuscular preparations from the frog indicates the reverse of this sequence (Dretchen et al., 1973). Death may occur if the respiratory paralysis is not recognized early; therapy consists in administration of a calcium salt, an anticholinesterase agent, or both (see Chapter 28). Patients with myasthenia gravis or those who have received neuromuscular blocking agents are particularly sensitive to this effect.

Renal Effects. Albuminuria, cylindruria, and reduced urine output may develop as a result of streptomycin therapy. Renal irritation is infrequent after daily doses of 1.0 to 1.5 g of the drug, but it is common when doses of 3 to 4 g are administered daily, especially if the urine is acidic. When large doses are to be given for an extended period, agents that alkalinize the urine should also be administered.

Biological Alterations in the Host. The most important "biological" reaction following the administration of streptomycin is suprainfection. Regardless of the route by which it is given, the drug produces significant changes in the normal microflora of the intestinal and respiratory tracts. In a group of 172 patients with a variety of infections treated with streptomycin parenterally, Weinstein and associates (1954) observed suprainfections in about 4%.

Therapeutic Uses. The areas of therapeutic usefulness of streptomycin have become greatly constricted since the development of more effective and less toxic antibacterial drugs (*see* Table 55-1, page 1096). However, this antibiotic still has important applications in the therapy of tuberculosis, as discussed in Chapter 60.

Bacterial Endocarditis. Cases of subacute bacterial endocarditis due to the *viridans* group of streptococci and enterococci, as well as instances of the disease in which the etiology cannot be defined, are treated in many clinics with streptomycin (1 to 2 g per day) and penicillin G (20 to 40 million units per day); therapy is continued for 4 weeks. Endocarditis due to gram-negative bacilli, especially *H. influenzae,* may respond to streptomycin. It is uncommon, however, for this drug to be given alone in this type of disease; it is usually given with full doses of another antibiotic to which the causative microorganism is sensitive.

Tularemia. All forms of tularemia are dramatically benefited by the administration of streptomycin. The course of the disease is shortened, the fatality rate markedly lowered, the incidence of late relapses greatly reduced, and the incidence of complications such as suppuration of buboes and secondary bacterial infection minimized. The best results are obtained when therapy is instituted early; however, chronicity does not exclude the possibility of complete cure. The dose of streptomycin varies with the severity of the infection; most cases respond to the administration of 1 to 2 g per day for 7 to 10 days. The tetracyclines are also highly effective in tularemia and are preferred by some physicians for milder forms of the disease.

Plague. Streptomycin is highly specific and one of the most effective agents for the treatment of all forms of plague. The tetracyclines and chloramphenicol are also beneficial in this disease. When streptomycin is used, a dose of 4 g per day is given for the first 2 days, followed by a 2-g amount each day for an additional 5 to 7 days.

Brucellosis. Mild cases of brucellosis respond well to the administration of a tetracycline. Severe cases, even when complicated, and especially those due to *Br. suis* or *Br. melitensis,* are best treated with a combination of a tetracycline and streptomycin (2 g per day), given for 14 to 21 days. Relapses are managed in the same fashion.

Respiratory Tract Infections. Pneumonitis, pharyngitis, epiglottitis, and tracheobronchitis due to *H. influenzae* respond well to the administration of the usual doses of streptomycin; however, other antimicrobial agents are now preferred in this type of infection.

Peritonitis. Peritonitis resulting from rupture of a viscus presents a problem in mixed infection from spillage of the intestinal flora into the peritoneal cavity. Experience has indicated that concurrent penicillin and streptomycin therapy may be highly effective in favorably influencing the course of this infection. The parenteral administration of 20 to 40 million units of penicillin G plus 2 g of streptomycin per day is recommended. Surgical drainage and repair of the perforation are necessary in some cases before cure can be accomplished; this is especially true when localized collections of pus, such as a subphrenic abscess, are present.

Urinary Tract Infections. The usefulness of streptomycin in the management of urinary tract infections has been greatly reduced by the rapid increase in the number of gram-negative bacilli that are now resistant to this drug. It is now used primarily in severe disease when other drugs have failed to produce benefit, an uncommon event. It may also have a place, in combination with another agent, in the treatment of mixed infections of the urinary tract. Alkalinization of the urine is necessary to produce maximal therapeutic effectiveness.

Bacterial Meningitis. At present, the use of streptomycin for the treatment of meningitis due to gram-negative bacilli such as *H. influenzae, E. coli, Klebsiella pneumoniae,* and *Pseud. aeruginosa* is uncommon because other agents are available that are highly effective and do not require intrathecal administration.

Miscellaneous Infections. Although the tetracyclines and chloramphenicol are the agents of choice at present in the treatment of *granuloma inguinale* and *chancroid,* streptomycin (2 g per day) is indicated in patients who have suffered reactions to the other drugs or in whom the response to these agents is unsatisfactory.

GENTAMICIN

History and Source. *Gentamicin* is a broad-spectrum antibiotic derived from the actinomycete *Micromonospora purpurea.* The drug was first studied and described by Weinstein and coworkers in 1963, and isolated, purified, and characterized by Rosselot and colleagues (1964). It is currently of great value in the therapy of severe infections due to gram-negative bacteria, and it is the most important of the aminoglycosides.

Chemistry. Gentamicin consists of three closely related components, gentamicins C_1, C_2, and C_{1A}, the structures of which follow:

Gentamicin	R	R'
C_1	CH_3	CH_3
C_2	CH_3	H
C_{1A}	H	H

Gentamicin

Antibacterial Activity. The three components of gentamicin have nearly identical antimicrobial activity *in vitro*. It is generally agreed that about 95% of *Pseud. aeruginosa* are inhibited by 10 µg/ml or less of the drug. *Escherichia coli, Klebsiella,* and *Enterobacter* (*Aerobacter*) are also highly sensitive. Practically all penicillin-sensitive and some methicillin-resistant strains of *Staph. aureus* are suppressed by a concentration of 5 µg/ml or less. Group-A streptococci, *Strep.* (*D.*) *pneumoniae, Past. multocida, H. influenzae, Acinetobacter* (*Mima-Herellea* group), and *Bacteroides* are reasonably sensitive to gentamicin. *Serratia* (nonpigmented) are inhibited by concentrations of 1.5 µg/ml or less. Most strains of indole-negative *Proteus* are highly sensitive; the susceptibility of the indole-producing strains is variable. *Mycobacterium tuberculosis* and *Mycoplasma pneumoniae* are highly sensitive. *Citrobacter* (*Paracolobactrum*), *Pr. inconstans, Salmonella, Shigella, Listeria, Brucella,* and some types of streptococci are variably susceptible. *Neisseria gonorrhoeae, N. meningitidis, Pseud. pseudomallei, Clostridium,* and *Corynebacterium* are relatively resistant. The drug is bactericidal in concentrations two to three times those required to produce bacteriostasis. (*See* Klein *et al.,* 1964; Weinstein *et al.,* 1964; Finland, 1969; International Symposium on Gentamicin, 1969.) Gentamicin is more active in alkaline media. The concentration of divalent cations in the medium alters the results of sensitivity tests of *Pseud. aeruginosa* to the drug (Zimelis and Jackson, 1973). Although heparin decreases the antimicrobial activity of gentamicin, the concentration of heparin in the blood of patients given this agent for anticoagulation is too low to produce this effect (Regamey *et al.,* 1972).

The antibacterial activity of gentamicin appears to be additive with ampicillin or kanamycin against *Proteus,* and with colistin against *Pseudomonas.* A supra-additive effect is produced by a combination of gentamicin with cephalothin or penicillin against enterococci, and with carbenicillin against gram-negative bacilli. However, this varies with the bacterial species and even with individual strains. (*See* Rosdahl and Thomsen, 1971; Second International Symposium on Gentamicin, 1971; Watanakunakorn, 1971; Regamey *et al.,* 1973.) The combination of carbenicillin and gentamicin is highly effective for experimental *Pseudomonas* infection in rats. Concurrent use of chloramphenicol or a tetracycline with gentamicin may lead to a reduction in antimicrobial efficacy (Cox, 1970; Sande and Overton, 1973).

Mechanism of Action. The mode of action of gentamicin is qualitatively similar to that of the other aminoglycoside antibiotics. This is discussed above for streptomycin.

Bacterial Resistance. Loss of sensitivity to gentamicin occurs by mechanisms analogous to those discussed for streptomycin. There may be cross-resistance to all members of the aminoglycoside group. Resistant strains of *Pseudomonas* have appeared in clinical settings where gentamicin has been used extensively; this has been especially true in burn units of hospitals. When resistance is transferred by a plasmid, an adenylylating enzyme (gentamicin adenylate synthetase) is responsible for in-

activation of the drug (Benveniste and Davies, 1971). This enzyme can also inactivate kanamycin and tobramycin.

Absorption, Distribution, and Excretion. Gentamicin, a polar aminoglycoside, is poorly absorbed from the gastrointestinal tract. It must be administered parenterally or occasionally topically.

Following *intramuscular* injection of gentamicin, peak concentrations in plasma are reached in 1 to 1½ hours. The values attained are proportional to dosage and are approximately 4 µg/ml when 1 mg/kg of body weight is administered. The antibiotic disappears from the plasma with a half-time of 2 hours, and effective concentrations persist for 6 to 8 hours. Drug disposition is impaired markedly in patients with abnormal renal function.

Gentamicin is very slowly absorbed when applied in an *ointment,* but absorption may be more rapid when a *cream* is used topically. When the antibiotic is applied to large areas of denuded body surface, as may be the case in burned patients, plasma concentrations can reach 1 µg/ml, and 2 to 5% of the drug used may appear in the urine.

Although gentamicin is bound to plasma proteins only to a negligible extent (Gordon *et al.,* 1972), diffusion of the aminoglycoside into certain body fluids is restricted. In the absence of inflammation, little drug penetrates into the cerebrospinal fluid. Even in the presence of meningitis, intrathecal administration of gentamicin appears to be necessary to achieve requisite therapeutic concentrations at this site. Rahal and colleagues (1974) have reported that the simultaneous intramuscular injection of 3.5 mg/kg per day of gentamicin and the instillation of 4 mg into the lumbar sac produce antibiotic concentrations in the cerebrospinal fluid of 20 to 45 µg/ml within 8 hours after the intrathecal injection.

Penetration into secretions of the respiratory tract is also poor. Klastersky and coworkers (1972) have instilled the drug directly into the trachea of patients with tracheostomy, to treat tracheobronchial infections. Therapeutic concentrations of gentamicin are achieved in the aqueous humor following subconjunctival administration; there is little drug in the vitreous or lens. Adequate concentrations of the antibiotic appear in the bile under normal circumstances; however, this is variable when there is biliary obstruction (Mendelson *et al.,* 1973; Pitt *et al.,* 1973).

Gentamicin is excreted in the urine by glomerular filtration. The clearance of the drug roughly parallels that of creatinine. Urinary concentrations range from 50 to 100 times those in the plasma except in cases of very severe renal dysfunction, where they are only about three times the peak concentration in the plasma. During the first few days of intramuscular therapy, about 40% of an administered dose is recoverable in the urine, suggesting accumulation or sequestration of the drug. After this, the amount excreted daily approaches the quantity given. Approximately 80 to 90% of gentamicin is removed from the circulation during 12 hours of hemodialysis; peritoneal dialysis appears to be less effective. In patients undergoing hemodialysis, a replacement dose of 1 mg/kg is recommended at the end of each period of dialysis.

For details of the clinical pharmacology of gentamicin, *see* Finland, 1969; International Symposium on Gentamicin, 1969; Cox, 1970; Second International Symposium on Gentamicin, 1971.

Preparations, Routes of Administration, and Dosage. The official preparation is *Gentamicin Sulfate,* U.S.P. (GARAMYCIN). It is available in various official forms: vials and prefilled syringes containing 40 mg/ml (or 10 mg/ml for pediatric use), an *ointment* and *cream* (0.1%), and an *opthalmic ointment* (0.3%). The preparation available for parenteral administration contains preservatives and is not suitable for intrathecal use. The recommended intramuscular dose for adults is 3 to 5 mg/kg per day, one third being given every 8 hours. Several dosage schedules have been suggested for *infants:* 2 to 2.5 mg/kg every 8 hours has been found to be safe for children up to 2 years of age; 6 mg/kg daily, divided into two equally spaced injections, has been recommended for neonates with severe infections.

Careful studies by a number of investigators have emphasized that the recommended doses of gentamicin do not yield reproducible concentrations in plasma and that there is a considerable degree of individual variation. Gentamicin may be present in the plasma in only subinhibitory or undetectable concentrations for several hours after its injection in some patients given the "standard" dose every 8 hours. Periodic determinations of the plasma concentration of the antibiotic may be necessary.

The presence of any significant degree of renal insufficiency imposes additional difficulty in establishing a regimen of therapy that will yield maximal therapeutic benefit with minimal or no risk of toxic reactions. A number of different approaches to this problem have been suggested. One schedule for treatment with gentamicin, based on endogenous creatinine clearance, is presented in Table 55–2

(page 1108). Nomograms have also been developed (Chan *et al.,* 1972). The writer has often administered a "loading" dose of 2 to 2.3 mg/kg followed by single doses of 0.8 mg/kg at an interval equal in hours to four times the serum creatinine concentration (expressed in milligrams percent). The plasma concentration of gentamicin should be determined at frequent intervals when renal function is impaired. Although it has not yet been established exactly what plasma concentration is toxic, peak concentrations greater than 10 μg/ml and minimal (predose) values in excess of 2 μg/ml for greater than 10 days have been associated with nephrotoxicity.

It is current practice to treat serious infection due to *Pseudomonas* with a combination of gentamicin and carbenicillin. These two drugs must never be mixed in the same bottle because the penicillin inactivates the aminoglycoside to a significant degree; similar *in-vitro* incompatibilities exist between gentamicin and other penicillins, cephalosporins, amphotericin B, and heparin.

Untoward Effects. Untoward effects of gentamicin include *nausea, vomiting, headache, transient proteinuria, elevation of blood urea nitrogen, increase in serum transaminases and alkaline phosphatase,* and *transient macular skin eruptions. Overgrowth of Candida* may follow oral administration of the drug. The most important and serious side effect of the use of gentamicin is *ototoxicity.* This occurs in about 2% of patients receiving the drug and is most common in those with renal failure. The vestibular rather than the auditory portion of the eighth cranial nerve is selectively involved, although hearing loss may occur occasionally. Loss of labyrinthine function may be bilateral, complete, and permanent, or unilateral and partial, and function may be restored either slowly or rapidly after treatment is stopped. Previous therapy with other ototoxic agents, total dose of gentamicin per kilogram of body weight, and possibly age, but not duration of treatment, increase the risk of ototoxicity. In addition, the simultaneous administration of the aminoglycoside with ethacrynic acid and probably other diuretic agents appears to increase the risk. The early signs of ototoxicity are headache, dizziness, and nausea or vomiting with motion. Cessation of therapy when these manifestations appear may reduce the risk of serious damage to the eighth nerve. *Patients receiving gentamicin should have vestibular and auditory function examined at frequent intervals; the drug should be stopped when impairment appears.* Gentamicin may also produce neuromuscular blockade of the type discussed above for streptomycin.

Although very few cases have been studied, it has been reported that combined therapy with gentamicin and cephalothin or cephaloridine produces *acute renal insufficiency* and *acute tubular necrosis* (*see* Opitz *et al.*, 1971; Bobrow *et al.*, 1972). *All persons with any degree of renal failure who are treated with gentamicin should, if possible, have frequent determination of plasma concentrations of the drug, which should not be allowed to exceed 10 to 12 μg/ml, to minimize the risk of toxicity.* Gentamicin should not be administered to pregnant women.

Therapeutic Uses. A large variety of infections have been treated successfully with gentamicin. However, due to the high toxicity of this drug, its use *must* be restricted to the therapy of life-threatening infections and those for which a less toxic antimicrobial agent is ineffective. The antibiotic has its most important field of application in the therapy of serious gram-negative microbial infections, especially those due to *Pseud. aeruginosa, Enterobacter (Aerobacter), Klebsiella, Serratia,* and other species resistant to the more widely used agents. Among these are urinary tract infections, bacteremia, meningitis, ventriculitis, tularemia, infected burns, osteomyelitis, pneumonia, peritonitis, gonorrhea, and infections of the ear, nose, and throat. When the antibiotic is employed in urinary tract infections, the urine pH should be alkaline, since the drug is less active in an acidic medium. Gentamicin has proven effective in the management of pneumonia caused by *Pseudomonas* in patients with mucoviscidosis. Most observers presently agree that severe infections due to *Pseud. aeruginosa* are best treated with gentamicin plus carbenicillin (24 to 30 g per day). Enteritis due to pathogenic strains of *E. coli* may be treated by the daily administration of 4 mg/kg orally, divided into four equal-sized and -spaced doses, plus 2 mg/kg intramuscularly (one half this dose every 12 hours) (Coetzee and Leary, 1971).

Meningitis caused by gram-negative microorganisms presents a grave therapeutic problem. When bacteria are resistant to ampicillin, therapy with gentamicin is necessary; however, adequate concentrations can be obtained only by intrathecal administration. A dose of 4 mg given by this route every 18 hours for 5 to 10 days has been recommended (Rahal *et al.*, 1974). The preparation of gentamicin suitable for intrathecal instillation is not available for general use.

Patients who develop peritonitis as a result of peritoneal dialysis may require therapy with gentamicin. Since suboptimal intraperitoneal concentrations of the antibiotic may follow intramuscular administration, dialysis should be continued with fluids containing 5 to 10 mg of gentamicin per liter of fluid (Smithivas *et al.*, 1971).

Gentamicin has been given parenterally and applied topically at the same time in the treatment of infected burns; some of the bacteria involved have become resistant to the drug during such therapy. It has been suggested that this regimen be restricted to patients with thermal burns that are life endangering, and be used only when 20% or more of the total body surface is involved.

While there are very few indications for the use of gentamicin for gram-positive bacterial infections, it may at times be necessary and lifesaving. Methicillin-resistant staphylococci may be sensitive to gentamicin. In cases of enterococcal endocarditis that fail to respond to concurrent therapy with penicillin and streptomycin, the administration of gentamicin and penicillin may result in control of the disease. Simultaneous treatment with cephalothin and gentamicin is usually ineffective in altering the course of this type of infection.

When a serious infection of unknown etiology is present, many physicians administer gentamicin with a penicillinase-resistant penicillin, until such time as bacteriological diagnosis is obtained and specific therapy can be planned.

TOBRAMYCIN

A complex of antibacterial compounds is produced by the soil microorganism *Streptomyces tenebrarius*. All are basic, water-soluble aminoglycosides. *Tobramycin* is the least toxic of these compounds and is highly active against a variety of bacteria. The structural formula of tobramycin is as follows:

Tobramycin

Tobramycin is active *in vitro* against *Staph. aureus,* most of the family Enterobacteriaceae, and *Pseud. aeruginosa*. Most staphylococci are inhibited by 1 μg/ml or less; most gram-negative bacteria, by 2 μg/ml or less; and *Pseudomonas*, by 5 to 10 μg/ml or less (Dienstag and Neu, 1972; Molavi *et al.*, 1973).

About 70% of *Klebsiella* and *Enterobacter* (*Aerobacter*) are suppressed by 0.75 μg/ml, and over 50% of *E. coli* and indole-positive and -negative *Proteus* are inhibited by at least 3 μg/ml (Meyers and Hirschman, 1972a). Tobramycin is bactericidal for susceptible microbial species. It is less active than gentamicin for most gram-negative bacteria but at least two to four times more active against *Pseudomonas;* its concurrent use with carbenicillin may yield synergistic activity against this microorganism. Strains of bacteria with low-level resistance to gentamicin are apt to be sensitive to tobramycin. However, those that are markedly resistant to gentamicin are also resistant to tobramycin.

Tobramycin is absorbed readily after intramuscular injection; it is not absorbed from the gastrointestinal tract. An injection of 100 mg yields peak plasma concentrations of about 4 μg/ml at ½ hour. The half-life of the antibiotic has been reported to range from 1½ to 3 hours when renal function is normal, and it is over 50 hours in anephric patients. (*See* Black and Griffith, 1971; Meyers and Hirschman, 1972b; Kaplan *et al.,* 1973; Naber *et al.,* 1973; Regamey *et al.,* 1973; Simon *et al.,* 1973.)

Tobramycin is excreted in the urine by glomerular filtration. From 60 to 90% of the drug appears in the urine within 24 hours following injection of a single dose. Seventy percent of tobramycin is removed from the blood by hemodialysis in 12 hours (Lockwood and Bower, 1973); little is removed during peritoneal dialysis (Weinstein *et al.,* 1973).

Tobramycin is as yet not generally available for clinical use. Its optimal dosage has not yet been determined, but it is in the same range as that of gentamicin.

Although there is insufficient experience to indicate the risk of side effects from tobramycin, it must be emphasized that this drug, like other aminoglycosides, should be regarded as potentially ototoxic and nephrotoxic until proven otherwise.

Because its spectrum of antimicrobial activity is similar to that of gentamicin, tobramycin may prove to be an adequate substitute. It will be of obvious value if strains of *Pseud. aeruginosa* resistant to gentamicin remain susceptible to tobramycin.

KANAMYCIN

History and Source. *Kanamycin* is an antibiotic produced by *Streptomyces kanamyceticus*. It was first produced and isolated by Umezawa and coworkers at the Japanese National Institutes of Health in 1957, and was shown to be active against a variety of microorganisms.

Chemistry. *Kanamycin* is a polybasic, water-soluble substance. It contains two amino sugars in glycosidic linkage with 2-deoxystreptamine. Its structural formula is shown at the top of the next column. Commercial preparations of the antibiotic contain two substances, kanamycins A and B; in the United States the latter must represent less than 5% of the total.

Antibacterial Activity. Kanamycin has a broad range of activity against gram-positive and gram-

Kanamycin A
R = NH₂; R′ = OH

Kanamycin B
R = R′ = NH₂

Kanamycin

negative microorganisms. Sensitive bacteria include *E. coli, Enterobacter* (*Aerobacter*) *aerogenes, K. pneumoniae, Proteus* species, *Citrobacter* (*Paracolobactrum*), *Salmonella, Shigella, Vibrio, Neisseria, Brucella, M. tuberculosis,* atypical mycobacteria, and *Staph. aureus.* Most strains of staphylococci are inhibited by 1 μg/ml or less; some are suppressed only by concentrations of 2 to 5 μg/ml. Tubercle bacilli are suppressed by 2.5 to 10 μg/ml. Pneumococci, *Alcaligenes,* and *Strep. pyogenes* are generally insensitive. Resistant microorganisms include *Pseudomonas,* other streptococci, *Bacteroides,* clostridia and other anaerobes, yeasts, and fungi. The concentrations of kanamycin required to produce bacteriostatic and bactericidal effects are not greatly different. (*See* Conference on Kanamycin, 1966.)

Bacterial Resistance. Bacteria may become insensitive to kanamycin by acquisition of a resistance factor during conjugation; this resistance is associated with the presence of enzymes that can phosphorylate, acetylate, or adenylylate the drug. Cross-resistance between kanamycin, neomycin, and paromomycin is complete; it is only of moderate degree between these agents and streptomycin. As kanamycin has been used more extensively, resistant strains of *Staph. aureus* (up to 30% in some hospitals) and many gram-negative bacteria have been isolated from infected patients. Tubercle bacilli rapidly become insensitive *in vitro.*

Absorption, Distribution, and Excretion. Kanamycin is poorly absorbed from the gastrointestinal tract, and most of an ingested dose is eliminated in the feces; very low plasma concentrations are detectable after oral medication in some individuals. Plasma concentrations of the drug after intramuscular injection are adequately described by a one-compartment model characterized by an elimination half-life of 2⅔ hours and a volume of distribution approximating 40% of total body water. Absorption from an intramuscular depot is complete in about 1½ hours (Doluisio *et al.,* 1973). Intramuscular injection of 1 g of kanamycin yields a peak plasma concentration of 20 to 35 μg/ml at about 1 hour; this falls to 1.2 μg/ml or less at 12 hours. The half-life of the drug in premature infants less than 2 days old is 18 hours; in babies 5 to 22 days of age, 6 hours. Excessive concentrations develop in patients with renal insufficiency. The antibiotic is not bound to plasma proteins.

Kanamycin is excreted primarily by the kidney, mostly by glomerular filtration, but some is secreted by the tubules. Only 0.3 to 1.5% of an ingested dose is excreted in the urine because of poor enteric absorption. From 40 to 80% of a parenteral dose is recoverable in the urine in the 24-hour period after injection. Urine concentrations range from 20 to 100 μg/ml in the first 6 hours after single or multiple doses. Very low concentrations of kanamycin are present in feces after parenteral injection; alterations in the intestinal flora do not occur when the drug is given by this route.

Parenteral administration of kanamycin results in the appearance of appreciable concentrations of the drug in pleural, ascitic, synovial, and peritoneal fluids. In the adult, very little antibiotic is detected in the cerebrospinal fluid. The intramuscular injection of kanamycin in normal children produces spinal fluid concentrations, after 3 hours, that average one fifth to one tenth of those simultaneously present in the plasma, and these concentrations are about twice as high in cases of meningitis. However, kanamycin concentrations in the cerebrospinal fluid of newborn infants with bacterial meningitis given 7.5 mg/kg intramuscularly suggest that complete confidence in the use of this agent in such patients may not be justified (McDonald and St. Geme, 1972). The antibiotic diffuses poorly into bile and amniotic and prostatic fluids. (*See* Conference on Kanamycin, 1966.)

Preparations, Routes of Administration, and Dosage. *Kanamycin Sulfate,* U.S.P. (KANTREX), is available as an official injection in vials containing 500 mg in a 2-ml or 1.0 g in a 3-ml volume, in pediatric vials (75 mg/2 ml), and for oral use in official capsules containing 500 mg. The daily oral dose of kanamycin for children is 50 mg/kg, divided equally and given at 6-hour intervals; adults may receive up to 8 g per day by this route. Great care must be exercised when such treatment is carried out in patients with renal insufficiency, and the oral dose must be reduced. The parenteral dose for adults is 15 mg/kg per day (two to three equally divided and spaced doses) with a maximum of 1.5 g per day. The total quantity administered over a period of treatment should not exceed 15 g. For neonates, the intramuscular dose, during the first 3 days of life, is 7.5 mg/kg per day, divided into two to four equal doses; for older infants, it is 5 to 15 mg/kg per day; children may be given up to 15 mg/kg per day. The intravenous dose is the same as the intramuscular; however, intravenous infusion is rarely employed because absorption of kanamycin from intramuscular sites is excellent.

A dosage schedule for parenteral administration of kanamycin to patients with reduced renal function is given in Table 55-2 (page 1108); formulas for dosage have also been derived (*see* Orme and Cutler, 1969). High plasma concentrations of kanamycin are promptly decreased by peritoneal dialysis or hemodialysis, and one of these procedures should be considered when signs of serious kanamycin toxicity appear. Atkins and colleagues (1973) have reported

that during peritoneal dialysis the mean peritoneal clearance of the drug is 8.3 ml per minute; dialysis reduces the half-life of the antibiotic from 84 to 12 hours in anephric patients. Such individuals being treated with kanamycin should receive an additional dose of 3.5 mg/kg for each day of peritoneal dialysis to compensate for removal of the drug in the dialysate. Plasma concentrations can also be maintained by adding twice that desired to the dialyzing fluid; in most cases, the addition of 20 mg of kanamycin to each liter of inflow dialysate is recommended.

Untoward Effects. Among the *hypersensitivity reactions* that have been noted in individuals receiving kanamycin parenterally are *eosinophilia* (in 8 to 10% of cases, without other evidence of allergy), *fever, maculopapular rashes, pruritus,* and *anaphylaxis.* The *irritative properties* of the drug are reflected in the moderately severe *pain* that is produced by its intramuscular injection and the *nodules* and *sterile abscesses* that may develop in muscles into which it has been introduced, as well as by the *diarrhea, stomatitis,* and *proctitis* that sometimes occur when the drug is taken orally.

The most important side effects of kanamycin stem from its *ototoxicity* and *nephrotoxicity.* Both the cochlear and vestibular portions of the auditory nerve may be damaged. Vestibular injury has been noted in 7% of patients. The outstanding symptom is vertigo; this is of short duration and usually disappears shortly after therapy is stopped. When serial audiometric examinations are carried out, impairment of hearing is found to be quite common (up to 30%). Clinically apparent ototoxicity has been observed in about 5% of patients receiving the drug; in about 2%, the damage has been severe (*see* Conference on Kanamycin, 1966). In some persons, only high-tone perception is lost and deafness is unilateral; however, in others, the defect is severe and bilateral and total irreversible hearing loss may supervene. Conversational hearing loss may be prevented by omitting the drug as soon as any evidence of auditory injury is manifest; this requires frequent audiometric study. The factors that may play a role in the pathogenesis of injury to the inner ear are total dose of kanamycin (regardless of the duration of therapy), decreased renal function, and age; older individuals are thought by some to be more susceptible. The administration of ethacrynic acid in patients receiving kanamycin also increases the risk of ototoxicity (West *et al.,* 1973).

Histological studies indicate that the primary toxic effect of kanamycin is on the outer hair cells. These exhibit a severe degree of degeneration; the supporting cells of the organ of Corti are also damaged. Large doses of the drug produce a decrease in the sodium and an increase in the potassium content of the endolymph. Associated with this is a decline in endolymph potential. These phenomena suggest that the antibiotic interferes with active transport processes in the cochlea. The concentration of kanamycin in labyrinthine fluids increases greatly when the dose of the antibiotic is raised slightly, and values that exceed those in plasma are attained. Thus, toxic concentrations may develop in the inner ear even when doses in the low therapeutic range are administered. (*See* Weinstein and Weinstein, 1974.)

Kanamycin, like the other aminoglycosides, exerts a *curare-like effect on the neuromuscular junction.* This is very similar to that described for streptomycin.

Renal injury is usually evidenced by urinary sediment abnormalities such as pyuria, hematuria, proteinuria, and cylindruria; these frequently disappear shortly after therapy is stopped. Elevations in plasma creatinine and blood urea nitrogen are common and mild; they may continue to increase for as long as a week, and values may not return to normal until the drug has been omitted for 3 to 4 weeks. Acute tubular necrosis may occur but is rare. Older individuals and those with renal insufficiency show an increased susceptibility to renal injury by kanamycin.

Among other untoward effects are circumoral and other *paresthesias, restlessness, nervousness, headache, bulging fontanelle, acute brain syndrome, blurring of vision, sensory involvement of the ninth cranial nerve, increased weakness in myasthenia gravis,* and *tachycardia. Prothrombin* and *plasma fibrinogen* may decrease at the beginning of therapy. *Suprainfections* due to *Pseudomonas, Staph. aureus* and other gram-positive and gram-negative bacteria may develop during treatment with kanamycin (*see* Conference on Kanamycin, 1966).

Therapeutic Uses. Kanamycin is used most often for the therapy of infections due to gram-negative microorganisms, especially *Klebsiella, Enterobacter* (*Aerobacter*), *Proteus,* and *E. coli.* It is without effect on disease produced by *Pseudomonas.* Among infections due to gram-positive bacteria, only those caused by *Staph. aureus* benefit significantly from treatment with this drug. With the present availability of other highly effective and less toxic antistaphylococcal agents, there is presently very little need for kanamycin in the management of this kind of disease. However, it may be necessary to treat methicillin-resistant strains of *Staph. aureus* with the conjoint use of a cephalosporin and kanamycin. Kanamycin has been used to treat human tuberculosis in combination with other effective tuberculostatic agents. Since the therapy of this disease is long and involves the administration of large total doses of the drug, with the risk of ototoxicity and nephrotoxicity, the writer does not employ it for this purpose. Concurrent administration of kanamycin and one of the semisynthetic penicillins, penicillin G, or cephalothin has been used to treat serious infections while awaiting microbiological confirmation of the etiology. Each agent is given in full dose.

Oral kanamycin has been used in the treatment of gastroenteritis due to sensitive, enteropathogenic strains of *E. coli.* There is no convincing evidence that kanamycin or any other antibiotic significantly shortens the duration of the disease. Gentamicin is now more often used for this purpose.

The following precautions must be observed when kanamycin is administered: (1) The dose should be reduced in older individuals and in those with any degree of renal insufficiency; (2) audiograms should be made at frequent intervals; (3) the status of renal function should be known at all times; and (4) the daily parenteral dose should not be greater than 15 mg/kg, and the total quantity administered should not exceed 15 g.

Prophylactic Uses. Kanamycin has been administered *orally* to *suppress the intestinal flora prior to surgery* and as adjunct therapy in cases of *hepatic coma.* The first of these uses is discussed in Chapter 55, and the rationale for such therapy in hepatic coma is described under neomycin (*see* below). The dose usually employed for these purposes is 6 to 8 g per day; quantities as large as 12 g per day have been given. The effect on intestinal bacteria may not be sustained even when such large doses of kanamycin are administered.

NEOMYCIN

History and Source. In 1949, Waksman and Lechevalier isolated a soil organism, *Streptomyces fradiae,* which produced a new antibiotic that in crude form contained an antifungal compound (*fradicin*) and a group of antibacterial substances that were labeled "neomycin." *Neomycin* was purified in the same year and found to be a complex of three compounds (neomycins A, B, and C) with different antimicrobial activities; commercial preparations consist almost entirely of neomycin B.

Chemistry. Neomycin is a polybasic, water-soluble substance that readily forms salts with a variety of acids. Neomycin A is *neamine* (deoxystreptamine linked to 2,6-diamino-2,6-dideoxy-D-glucose). Neomycins B and C are isomeric; each contains *neamine* and a *neobiosamine* (D-ribose linked to a diaminohexose). The structural formula of neomycin B is as follows:

Neomycin B

Antibacterial Activity. Neomycin is a broad-spectrum antibiotic. Its antimicrobial activity is presumably exerted by a mechanism analogous to that discussed for streptomycin. Susceptible microorganisms are usually inhibited by concentrations of 5 to 10 µg/ml or less. Gram-negative species that are highly sensitive are *E. coli, Enterobacter (Aerobacter) aerogenes, K. pneumoniae, Pasteurella, Pr. vulgaris, Salmonella, Shigella, H. influenzae, N. meningitidis, V. cholerae,* and *Bordetella pertussis.* Gram-positive microorganisms that are inhibited include *Bacillus anthracis, C. diphtheriae, Staph. aureus, Strep. faecalis, List. monocytogenes,* and *M. tuberculosis. Borrelia* and *Leptospira interrogans (icterohaemorrhagiae)* are also suppressed. The sensitivity of *Pseud. aeruginosa* to neomycin is variable but not very high. Group-A *Strep. pyogenes,* the *viridans* group of streptococci, fungi, and viruses are resistant. (*See* Waksman *et al.,* 1949, 1950.) Neomycin is active against *tubercle bacilli,* regardless of their susceptibility to streptomycin. Neomycin-resistant microorganisms are less susceptible to streptomycin; cross-resistance is induced to a greater degree by neomycin than by streptomycin. The enzyme involved in certain types of resistance is kanamycin phosphotransferase, which can inactivate kanamycin, neomycin, and paromomycin. Neomycin is also a substrate for kanamycin acetyltransferase, but inactivation of neomycin does not occur following this alteration.

Absorption, Distribution, and Excretion. Neomycin is poorly absorbed from the gastrointestinal tract. An *oral* dose of 3 g produces a peak plasma concentration of only 1 to 4 µg/ml; a total daily intake of 10 g for 3 days yields a blood concentration below that associated with systemic toxicity. About 97% of an oral dose of neomycin escapes absorption and is eliminated unchanged in the feces. Although neomycin can be given orally to very young children, in doses as high as 100 mg/kg per day, its use in such patients for longer than 3 weeks should be avoided because of partial absorption from the intestinal tract, especially if it is the site of disease. The drug is well absorbed after *intramuscular* injection and widely distributed in body fluids and tissues. Administration of 1 g parenterally provides plasma concentrations of about 20 µg/ml. However, there is virtually no current indication for the administration of neomycin by this route since safer agents have replaced it.

The antibiotic is rapidly excreted by the kidney; from 30 to 50% of a parenteral dose is detectable in the urine. Neomycin must be given with the greatest care to patients with renal insufficiency because, even when administered orally, it tends to reach toxic concentrations in the circulation. It is probably best not to employ this agent in such individuals. If it must be used, the dose should be sharply reduced or kanamycin, an antibiotic with similar antimicrobial activity but potentially less ototoxic and nephrotoxic, should be substituted. Plasma concentrations approximating those after parenteral injection of the drug may develop when the drug is given orally (4 to 8 g daily) to cirrhotic persons with renal dysfunction (Kunin *et al.,* 1960; Last and Sherlock, 1960).

Preparations, Routes of Administration, and Dosage. *Neomycin Sulfate,* U.S.P. (MYCIFRADIN, NEOBIOTIC), is available for topical, oral, and parenteral administration. Another formulation (MYCIQUENT) is available only for topical use. Neomycin sulfate is marketed as 500-mg oral tablets, in a solution (125 mg/5 ml), in *dermatological* and *ophthalmic ointments,* and as a *sterile powder* in vials containing 500 mg or 5 or 10 g for dilution with isotonic saline solution for topical application or parenteral injection. Ointments or creams should contain 5 mg of neomycin sulfate per gram, and be applied two or three times a day. *Neomycin Sulfate and Polymyxin B Sulfate Solution for Irrigation,* U.S.P. (NEOSPORIN), contains 40 mg of neomycin and 200,000 units of polymyxin B per milliliter. One milliliter of this preparation is added to 1000 ml of 0.9% sodium chloride solution and is used for continuous irrigation of the urinary bladder through appropriate catheter systems. The goal is to prevent bacteriuria and bacteremia associated with the use of indwelling catheters. The bladder is usually irrigated at the rate of 1000 ml every 24 hours. Neomycin is rarely used parenterally; the dose for intramuscular injection is 250 mg every 6 hours, and only in exceptional instances may this be increased to 500 mg every 6 hours. Oral therapy with neomycin sulfate either for "preparation" of the bowel for surgery or for the management of hepatic coma requires the ingestion of 4 to 8 g daily, in divided doses.

Neomycin is presently available in at least 100 different brands of creams, ointments, and sprays, both alone and in combination with polymyxin, bacitracin, other antibiotics, and a variety of corticosteroids. One such preparation, *Neomycin Sulfate, Polymyxin B Sulfate, and Bacitracin Zinc Ointment,* N.F., is official. The drug is also included in deodorants and in MYCOLOG, a preparation often used to treat "diaper rash." There is no evidence that these topical preparations shorten the time required for healing of wounds or that those containing a steroid are more effective (Medical Letter, 1973).

Untoward Effects. *Hypersensitivity reactions,* primarily *skin rashes,* occur in 6 to 8% of patients when neomycin is applied topically. Individuals sensitive to this agent may develop cross-reactions when exposed to other aminoglycosides. The most important toxic effects of neomycin are *renal damage* and *nerve deafness.* Although these tend to be most frequent when relatively large quantities of the antibiotic are used parenterally, they may occur even with conventional doses. Loss of hearing usually develops during the course of treatment; however, it may not become apparent to the patient, unless audiometric studies are carried out, until some time after therapy has been stopped, because of the time required for the defect to progress into the range of sound used in conversation. Loss of hearing has even occurred in patients with normal renal function following topical application or irrigation of wounds with 0.5% neomycin (Kelley *et al.,* 1969). Abnormal urine sediment and azotemia are quite common in patients treated with neomycin. The risk of both ototoxicity and nephrotoxicity is greater in persons with decreased renal function. Another important toxic reaction is a curariform *paralysis of respiration,* described in the section on streptomycin.

The most important *biological effects* resulting from the oral administration of neomycin are *intestinal malabsorption* and *suprainfection.* Individuals treated with 4 to 6 g of the drug by mouth per day sometimes develop a *spruelike syndrome* with diarrhea, steatorrhea, and azotorrhea. The outstanding example of drug-induced *malabsorption* is that caused by neomycin. In man, the drug produces a moderate malabsorption syndrome for a variety of substances, including fat, protein, cholesterol, carotene, glucose, lactose, sodium, calcium, cyanocobalamin, and iron. This effect may be produced by as little as 3 g of the drug per day but is more marked with a dose of 12 g per day. Neomycin produces mild morphological changes of intestinal villi; precipitates bile salts within the lumen of the intestine; inhibits intraluminal hydrolysis of long-chain triglycerides, presumably by inhibition of pancreatic lipase activity; increases the fecal bile acid excretion, presumably by decreasing bile acid absorption; and reduces intestinal lactase activity. The antibiotic causes a marked decrease in plasma cholesterol concentrations. This is out of proportion to the moderate malabsorption produced, and small doses of the drug have been used for long periods of time for this purpose. The drug has been shown to produce intestinal crypt-cell necrosis, and, since cholesterol synthesis may occur at these sites, this may account for the effect. Parenterally administered neomycin in doses of 200 mg per day does not produce malabsorption nor does it lower plasma cholesterol (Dobbins, 1968). *Acute staphylococcal enterocolitis* occasionally follows the ingestion of neomycin; it may not appear until 2 to 3 days after treatment has been stopped. *Overgrowth of yeasts* in the intestine may also occur; this is not associated with diarrhea or other symptoms in most cases. The oral administration of even large doses of neomycin usually has no effect on blood levels of prothrombin.

Therapeutic Uses. Neomycin has been widely used for *topical application* in a variety of infections of the skin and mucous membranes caused by microorganisms susceptible to the drug. These include *burns, wounds, ulcers,* and *infected dermatoses.* However, such treatment does not eradicate bacteria from the lesions.

The *oral administration* of neomycin has been employed primarily for *"preparation" of the bowel for surgery* and as an adjunct to the therapy of *hepatic coma.* As pointed out in Chapter 55, the necessity for preparation of the bowel has not been validated by controlled studies; furthermore, it involves the risk of serious suprainfections. While the significance of reducing the number of bacteria in the intestine in patients with hepatic coma has not been proved, general clinical experience suggests strongly that this may play an important role in producing a satisfactory outcome in this disease. Blood concentrations of ammonia are reduced during therapy. A daily dose of 4 to 8 g by mouth can be given without difficulty to such patients, provided renal function is normal. Because severe renal insufficiency may develop in the late stages of hepatic failure, treatment with neomycin must be followed with the greatest care and stopped if evidence of ototoxicity or further injury to the kidney appears.

Neomycin is occasionally used in the therapy of intestinal infections, primarily in children, due to pathogenic strains of *E. coli.* The dose for this purpose is 100 mg/kg per day, given orally for about 10 days but never longer than for 3 weeks.

There is presently little or no indication for the parenteral administration of neomycin. Other equally effective and safer antibiotics have almost completely replaced it.

PAROMOMYCIN

This aminoglycoside antibiotic shares several properties in common with neomycin. Since the only current indication for its use is in the treatment of intestinal amebiasis, paromomycin is described in Chapter 53. It is also discussed in earlier editions of this textbook.

Atkins, R. C.; Mion, C.; Despaux, E.; Van-Hai, N.; Christian, J.; and Mion, H. Peritoneal transfer of kanamycin and its use in peritoneal dialysis. *Kidney Int.,* **1973,** *3,* 391–396.

Benveniste, R., and Davies, J. R-factor mediated gentamicin resistance: a new enzyme which modifies aminoglycoside antibiotics. *FEBS Lett.,* **1971,** *14,* 293–296.

Black, H. R., and Griffith, R. S. Preliminary studies with NEBRAMYCIN FACTOR 6. In, *Antimicrobial Agents and Chemotherapy—1970.* (Hobby, G. L., ed.) American Society for Microbiology, Bethesda, Md., **1971,** pp. 314–321.

Bobrow, S. N.; Jaffe, E.; and Young, R. C. Anuria and acute tubular necrosis associated with gentamicin and cephalothin. *J. Am. med. Ass.,* **1972,** *222,* 1546–1547.

Chan, R. A.; Benner, E. J.; and Hoeprich, P. D. Gentamicin therapy in renal failure: a nomogram for dosage. *Ann. intern. Med.,* **1972,** *76,* 773–778.

Coetzee, M., and Leary, P. M. Gentamicin in *Esch. coli* gastroenteritis. *Archs Dis. Childh.,* **1971,** *46,* 646–650.

Conway, N., and Birt, B. D. Streptomycin in pregnancy: effect on foetal ear. *Br. med. J.,* **1965,** *2,* 260–263.

Davies, J., and Davis, B. D. Misreading of ribonucleic acid code words induced by aminoglycoside antibiotics: the effect of drug concentration. *J. biol. Chem.,* **1968,** *243,* 3312–3316.

Dienstag, J., and Neu, H. C. *In vitro* studies of tobramycin, an aminoglycoside antibiotic. *Antimicrob. Agents Chemother.,* **1972,** *1,* 41–45.

Dobbins, W. O., III. Drug-induced steatorrhea. *Gastroenterology,* **1968,** *54,* 1193–1195.

Doluisio, J. T.; Dittert, L. W.; and LaPiana, J. C. Pharmacokinetics of kanamycin following intramuscular administration. *J. Pharmacokinet. Biopharm.,* **1973,** *1,* 253–265.

Dretchen, K. L.; Sokoll, M. D.; Gergis, S. D.; and Long, J. P. Relative effects of streptomycin on motor nerve terminals and endplate. *Eur. J. Pharmac.,* **1973,** *22,* 10–16.

Gordon, R. C.; Regamey, C.; and Kirby, W. M. M. Serum protein binding of the aminoglycoside antibiotics. *Antimicrob. Agents Chemother.,* **1972,** *2,* 214–216.

Hawkins, J. E., Jr., and Lurie, M. H. The ototoxicity of streptomycin. *Ann. Otol. Rhinol. Lar.,* **1952,** *61,* 789–809.

Kaplan, J. M.; McCracken, G. H., Jr.; Thomas, M. L.; Horton, L. J.; and Davis, N. Clinical pharmacology of tobramycin in newborns. *Am. J. Dis. Child.,* **1973,** *125,* 656–660.

Kelley, D. R.; Nilo, E. R.; and Berggren, R. B. Deafness after topical neomycin wound irrigation. *New Engl. J. Med.,* **1969,** *280,* 1338–1339.

Klastersky, J.; Geuning, C.; Mouawad, E.; and Daneau,

D. Endotracheal gentamicin in bronchial infections in patients with tracheostomy. *Chest, 1972, 61,* 117–120.

Klein, J. O.; Eickhoff, T. C.; and Finland, M. Gentamicin: activity *in vitro* and observations in 26 patients. *Am. J. med. Sci.,* 1964, *248,* 528–543.

Kunin, C. M.; Chalmers, T. C.; Leevy, C. M.; Sebastyen, S. C.; Lieber, C. S.; and Finland, M. Absorption of orally administered neomycin and kanamycin with special reference to patients with severe hepatic and renal disease. *New Engl. J. Med.,* 1960, *262,* 380–385.

Last, P. M., and Sherlock, S. Systemic absorption of orally administered neomycin in liver disease. *New Engl. J. Med.,* 1960, *262,* 385–389.

Lockwood, W. R., and Bower, J. D. Tobramycin and gentamicin concentrations in the serum of normal and anephric patients. *Antimicrob. Agents Chemother.,* 1973, *3,* 125–129.

McDonald, L. L., and St. Geme, J. W., Jr. Cerebrospinal fluid diffusion of kanamycin in newborn infants. *Antimicrob. Agents Chemother.,* 1972, *2,* 41–44.

Mendelson, J.; Portnoy, J.; and Sigman, H. Pharmacology of gentamicin in the biliary tract of humans. *Antimicrob. Agents Chemother.,* 1973, *4,* 538–541.

Meyers, B. R., and Hirschman, S. Z. Tobramycin: *in vitro* antibacterial spectrum of a new aminoglycoside. *J. clin. Pharmac.,* 1972a, *12,* 313–320.

———. Pharmacologic studies of tobramycin and comparison with gentamicin. *Ibid.,* 1972b, *12,* 321–324.

Moellering, R. C., Jr., and Weinberg, A. N. Studies on antibiotic synergism against enterococci. II. Effect of various antibiotics on the uptake of ^{14}C-labelled streptomycin by enterococci. *J. clin. Invest.,* 1971, *50,* 2580–2584.

Moellering, R. C., Jr.; Wennersten, C.; and Weinberg, A. N. Studies on antibiotic synergism against enterococci. I. Bacteriologic studies. *J. Lab. clin. Med.,* 1971, *77,* 821–828.

Molavi, A.; Barza, M.; Cole, W.; Berman, H.; and Weinstein, L. *In vitro* assessment of tobramycin, a new aminoglycoside with anti-*Pseudomonas* activity. *Chemotherapy,* 1973, *18,* 7–16.

Nomura, M.; Mizushima, S.; Ozaki, M.; Traub, P.; and Lowry, C. V. Structure and function of ribosomes and their molecular components. *Cold Spring Harb. Symp. quant. Biol.,* 1969, *34,* 49–61.

Opitz, A.; Herrmann, I.; Herrath, D.; and Schaefer, K. Acute renal insufficiency after treatment with an association of gentamicin and cephalosporin. *Medsche Welt, Berl.,* 1971, *22,* 434–438.

Orme, B. M., and Cutler, R. E. The relationship between kanamycin pharmacokinetics: distribution and renal function. *Clin. Pharmac. Ther.,* 1969, *10,* 543–550.

Pitt, H. A.; Roberts, R. B.; and Johnson, W. D., Jr. Gentamicin levels in the human biliary tract. *J. infect. Dis.,* 1973, *127,* 299–302.

Rahal, J. J., Jr.; Hyams, P. J.; Simberkoff, M. S.; and Rubinstein, E. Intrathecal and intramuscular gentamicin in meningitis. *New Engl. J. Med.,* 1974, *290,* 1394–1398.

Regamey, C.; Gordon, R. C.; and Kirby, W. M. M. Comparative pharmacokinetics of tobramycin and gentamicin. *Clin. Pharmac. Ther.,* 1973, *14,* 396–403.

Regamey, C.; Schaberg, D.; and Kirby, W. M. M. Inhibitory effect of heparin on gentamicin concentrations in blood. *Antimicrob. Agents Chemother.,* 1972, *1,* 329–332.

Rosdahl, N., and Thomsen, V. F. *In vitro* activity of gentamicin alone and in combination with other antibiotics. *Acta path. microbiol. scand., B,* 1971, *79,* 333–342.

Rosselot, J. P.; Marquez, J.; Meseck, E.; Murawski, A.; Hamdan, A.; Joyner, C.; Schmidt, R.; Migliore, D.; and Herzog, H. L. Isolation, purification, and characterization of gentamicin. In, *Antimicrobial Agents and Chemotherapy—1963.* (Sylvester, J. C., ed.) American Society for Microbiology, Ann Arbor, Mich., 1964, pp. 14–16.

Sande, M. A., and Overton, J. W. *In vivo* antagonism between gentamicin and chloramphenicol in neutropenic mice. *J. infect. Dis.,* 1973, *128,* 247–250.

Schatz, A.; Bugie, S.; and Waksman, S. A. Streptomycin, a substance exhibiting antibiotic activity against gram-positive and gram-negative bacteria. *Proc. Soc. exp. Biol. Med.,* 1944, *57,* 244–248.

Simon, V. K.; Mosinger, E. U.; and Malerczy, V. Pharmacokinetic studies of tobramycin and gentamicin. *Antimicrob. Agents Chemother.,* 1973, *3,* 445–450.

Smithivas, T.; Hyams, P. J.; Matalon, R.; Simberkoff, M. S.; and Rahal, J. J. The use of gentamicin in peritoneal dialysis. I. Pharmacologic results. *J. infect. Dis.,* 1971, *124,* Suppl., S77–S83.

Spoendlin, H. Zur Ototoxizitat des Streptomyzins. *Practica oto-rhino-lar.,* 1966, *28,* 305–322.

Waksman, S. A.; Hutchinson, D.; and Katz, E. Neomycin activity upon *Mycobacterium tuberculosis* and other mycobacteria. *Am. Rev. Tuberc. pulm. Dis.,* 1949, *60,* 78–89.

Waksman, S. A.; Katz, E.; and Lechevalier, H. Antimicrobial properties of neomycin. *J. Lab. clin. Med.,* 1950, *36,* 93–99.

Waksman, S. A., and Lechevalier, H. A. Neomycin, a new antibiotic active against streptomycin-resistant bacteria, including tuberculosis organisms. *Science, Wash.,* 1949, *109,* 305–307.

Watanakunakorn, C. Penicillin combined with gentamicin or streptomycin: synergism against enterococci. *J. infect. Dis.,* 1971, *124,* 581–586.

Weinstein, A. J.; Karchmer, A. W.; and Moellering, R. C. Tobramycin concentrations during peritoneal dialysis. *Antimicrob. Agents Chemother.,* 1973, *4,* 432–434.

Weinstein, L. The treatment of meningitis due to *Hemophilus influenzae* with streptomycin. *New Engl. J. Med.,* 1946, *235,* 101–111.

Weinstein, L.; Golfield, M.; and Chang, T. W. Infections occurring during chemotherapy: a study of their frequency, type, and predisposing factors. *New Engl. J. Med.,* 1954, *251,* 247–255.

Weinstein, M. J.; Luedemann, G. M.; Oden, E. M.; and Wagman, G. H. Gentamicin, a new broad-spectrum antibiotic complex. In, *Antimicrobial Agents and Chemotherapy—1963.* (Sylvester, J. C., ed.) American Society for Microbiology, Ann Arbor, Mich., 1964, pp. 1–7.

Weinstein, M. J.; Luedemann, G. M.; Oden, E. M.; Wagman, G. H.; Rosselot, J. P.; Marquez, J. A.; Conglio, C. T.; Charney, W.; Herzog, H. L.; and Black, J. Gentamicin, a new antibiotic complex from *Micromonospora. J. mednl Chem.,* 1963, *6,* 463–464.

West, B. A.; Brummett, R. E.; and Himes, D. L. Interaction of kanamycin and ethacrynic acid. Severe cochlear damage in guinea pigs. *Archs Otolar.,* 1973, *98,* 32–37.

Winston, J. Clinical problems pertaining to neurotoxicity of streptomycin group of drugs. *A.M.A. Archs Otolar.,* 1953, *58,* 55–61.

Zimelis, V. M., and Jackson, G. G. Activity of aminoglycoside antibiotics against *Pseudomonas aeruginosa:* specificity and site of calcium and magnesium antagonism. *J. infect. Dis.,* 1973, *127,* 663–669.

Monographs and Reviews

Conference on Kanamycin. (Various authors.) Appraisal after eight years of clinical application. *Ann. N.Y. Acad. Sci.,* 1966, *132,* 773–1090.

Cox, C. Gentamicin. *Med. Clins N. Am.,* 1970, *54,* 1305–1315.

Finland, M. Gentamicin: antibacterial activity, clinical pharmacology and clinical applications. *Med. Times, N.Y.,* 1969, *97,* 161–174.

International Symposium on Gentamicin. (Various authors.) A new aminoglycoside antibiotic. *J. infect. Dis.,* 1969, *119,* 341–540.

Medical Letter. Topical neomycin. 1973, *15,* 101–102.

Naber, K. G.; Westenfelder, S. R.; and Madsen, P. O. Pharmacokinetics of the aminoglycoside antibiotic tobramycin in humans. *Antimicrob. Agents Chemother.,* **1973,** *3,* 469–473.

Pittinger, C., and Adamson, R. Antibiotic blockade of neuromuscular function. *A. Rev. Pharmac.,* **1972,** *12,* 169–184.

Second International Symposium on Gentamicin. (Various authors.) An aminoglycoside antibiotic. *J. infect. Dis.,* **1971,** *124,* Suppl., S1-S300.

Waksman, S. A. (ed.). *Streptomycin, Nature and Practical Applications.* The Williams & Wilkins Co., Baltimore, **1949.**

——. *The Literature on Streptomycin, 1944–1952.* Rutgers University Press, New Brunswick, N.J., **1952.** (5550 references.)

——. Streptomycin: background, isolation, properties, and utilization. *Science, Wash.,* **1953,** *118,* 259–266.

Weinstein, L., and Dalton, A. C. Host determinants of response to antimicrobial agents. *New Engl. J. Med.,* **1968,** *279,* 467–473, 525–531, 580–588.

Weinstein, L., and Weinstein, A. J. The pathophysiology and pathoanatomy of reactions to antimicrobial agents. *Adv. intern. Med.,* **1974,** *19,* 109–134.

Weisblum, B., and Davies, J. Antibiotic inhibitors of the bacterial ribosome. *Bact. Rev.,* **1968,** *32,* 493–528. (232 references.)

CHAPTER

59 ANTIMICROBIAL AGENTS

[*Continued*]

Tetracyclines and Chloramphenicol

Louis Weinstein

TETRACYCLINES

History. The development of the tetracycline antibiotics, stimulated by the recognition of the therapeutic significance of penicillin and streptomycin, was the result of a systematic screening, for antibiotic-producing microorganisms, of soil specimens collected from many parts of the world. The first of these compounds, *chlortetracycline,* was introduced in 1948. Two years later, *oxytetracycline* became available. Elucidation of the chemical structure of these agents confirmed their similarity and furnished the basis for the production of a third member of this group, *tetracycline,* in 1952. In 1957, a new family of tetracyclines was developed, characterized chemically by the absence of the ring-attached CH_3 group present in the others. One of these, *demethylchlortetracycline,* subsequently given the official name *demeclocycline,* became available for general use in 1959. The next compound to appear was *rolitetracycline,* a soluble derivative of tetracycline. Other congeners, certain of which have useful properties, have continued to be developed: *methacycline,* a derivative of oxytetracycline, was introduced in 1961; *doxycycline* became available in 1966; and *minocycline,* in 1972.

Soon after their initial development, the tetracyclines were found to be highly effective against rickettsiae, a number of gram-positive and gram-negative bacteria, and the agents responsible for lymphogranuloma venereum, inclusion conjunctivitis, and psittacosis, and hence became known as "broad-spectrum" antibiotics. With establishment of their *in-vitro* antimicrobial activity, effectiveness in experimental infections, and pharmacological properties, the tetracyclines rapidly became widely used in therapy. (*See* Dowling, 1955; Lepper, 1956; Musselman, 1956.)

Although there are specific and useful differences between the seven tetracyclines currently available in the United States, they are in the main very much alike. This permits discussion of this group of drugs as a class. Rolitetracycline is no longer marketed in the United States. It is described in earlier editions of this textbook.

Source. *Chlortetracycline* and *oxytetracycline* are elaborated by *Streptomyces aureofaciens* and *Streptomyces rimosus,* respectively. The antibiotics are produced in broth by deep-tank fermentation.

Tetracycline is produced semisynthetically from chlortetracycline; it has also been obtained from a species of *Streptomyces. Demeclocycline* is the product of a mutant of the strain of *Streptomyces aureofaciens* from which chlortetracycline was first obtained. *Rolitetracycline, methacycline, doxycycline,* and *minocycline* are all semisynthetic derivatives.

Chemistry, Stability, and Assay. The tetracyclines are closely congeneric derivatives of the polycyclic naphthacenecarboxamide. Their structural formulas are shown in Table 59–1.

Table 59-1. STRUCTURAL FORMULAS OF THE TETRACYCLINES

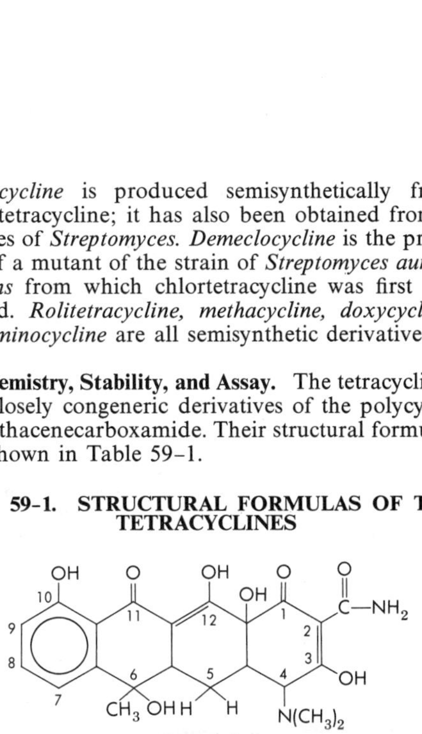

Tetracycline

CONGENER	SUBSTITUENT(S)	POSITION(S)
Chlortetracycline	—Cl	(7)
Oxytetracycline	—OH,—H	(5)
Demeclocycline	—OH,—H; —Cl	(6; 7)
Rolitetracycline	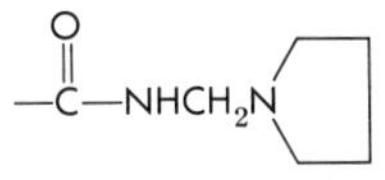 —C(=O)—NHCH₂N⬠	(2)
Methacycline	—OH,—H; =CH₂	(5; 6)
Doxycycline	—OH,—H; —CH₃,—H	(5; 6)
Minocycline	—H,—H; —N(CH₃)₂	(6; 7)

The crystalline bases are faintly yellow, odorless, slightly bitter compounds. They are only slightly soluble in water at pH 7 (0.25 to 0.5 mg/ml), but they form soluble sodium salts and hydrochlorides. While the bases and the hydrochlorides are quite stable as dry powders, most of these agents lose activity relatively rapidly when in solution.

1183

Determination of the concentration of tetracyclines in biological fluids and assay for their degree of antibacterial activity are accomplished by conventional microbiological methods. Because of the instability of solutions of most of these drugs, particularly chlortetracycline, the results of such determinations are only relative and are greatly modified by the assay conditions.

Effects on Microbial Agents. The tetracyclines possess a wide range of antimicrobial activity against gram-positive and gram-negative bacteria, which overlaps that of many other antimicrobial drugs. They are also effective against some microorganisms innately insensitive to many chemotherapeutic agents, such as *rickettsiae, Mycoplasma, Chlamydia* (the agents of *lymphogranuloma venereum, psittacosis, inclusion conjunctivitis,* and *trachoma*), and *amebae.* They are not active against any of the true viruses, yeasts, or fungi.

In vitro, these drugs are primarily bacteriostatic; in high concentrations, they are frequently bactericidal. In general, but not invariably, their *in-vivo* and *in-vitro* efficacies closely parallel each other. Only rapidly multiplying organisms are affected. The sensitivity or resistance of a particular microorganism to each of the congeners is, with some exceptions, quite similar. Although an individual strain of microorganism may be significantly more sensitive to one or another of these antibiotics, *such differences do not follow a general pattern and can only be uncovered by simultaneous sensitivity tests.*

Bacteria. In general, gram-positive microorganisms are affected by lower concentrations of tetracycline than are gram-negative species. However, these agents are less useful for infections caused by gram-positive bacteria because of problems of resistance and the availability of superior antimicrobial agents. For example, in some geographical areas as many as 14% of strains of *Streptococcus (Diplococcus) pneumoniae* may be resistant to the tetracyclines (Gopalakrishna and Lerner, 1973). Forty-three percent of strains of *Strep. pyogenes* isolated in Israel are similarly resistant (Bergner-Rabinowitz and Davies, 1970). It is encouraging that the incidence of tetracycline-resistant staphylococci has been declining, and minocycline appears to be active against strains of *Staphylococcus aureus* that are resistant to other tetracyclines (Finland, 1974). Several gram-positive bacilli are sensitive to these drugs (*see* Table 55–1, page 1096).

While infections with *Neisseria gonorrhoeae* are usually curable with tetracyclines, gonococci may be becoming less sensitive. Many strains of *N. meningitidis* are inhibited.

The order of efficacy of the tetracyclines *in vitro* against most gram-negative bacilli is similar to that of chloramphenicol, although a number of these microorganisms have become less susceptible to the tetracyclines as they have been widely used. Some gram-negative bacilli resistant to other congeners appear to be inhibited by clinically achievable concentrations of minocycline. Tetracyclines are particularly useful for infections caused by *Haemophilus ducreyi, Brucella, Vibrio cholerae, Pseudomonas (Actinobacillus) mallei* and *pseudomallei,* and *Calymmatobacterium (Donovania) granulomatis.* These drugs also inhibit the growth of *Yersinia (Pasteurella) pestis, Francisella (Past.) tularensis,* and *Past. multocida.* More variable success is achieved with infections due to *Escherichia coli, Klebsiella, Enterobacter (Aerobacter), Bacteroides, H. influenzae,* and indole-producing strains of *Proteus.* Nearly all strains of *Pr. vulgaris* and *Pseud. aeruginosa* are resistant.

Rickettsiae. Like chloramphenicol, all the tetracyclines are highly effective against the rickettsiae responsible for *Rocky Mountain spotted fever, murine typhus, epidemic typhus, scrub typhus, rickettsialpox,* and *Q fever,* when they are tested *in vivo.* When given to animals after massive doses of infectious material but before disease appears, these drugs prevent the development of illness, but do not inhibit the formation of specific antibody. The institution of therapy early after the injection of small doses of rickettsiae frequently suppresses the development of both illness and immunity.

Miscellaneous Microbial Agents. The tetracyclines are highly effective in relapsing fever (*Borrelia recurrentis*); they are valuable secondary agents for other diseases caused by the spirochetes *Treponema pallidum, T. pertenue,* and *Leptospira interrogans.* The activity of tetracyclines against *Chlamydia* and *Mycoplasma* has been mentioned. T strains of *Mycoplasma* are not suppressed by these drugs but are susceptible to erythromycin (Harwick and Fekety, 1969; Braun *et al.,* 1970). High concentrations of tetracyclines inhibit the growth of the protozoan *Entamoeba histolytica.*

Effects on Intestinal Flora. Since the tetracyclines are incompletely absorbed from the gastrointestinal tract, high concentrations are reached in the intestinal contents. Within 48 hours after daily administration of conventional doses of these agents, the enteric flora is markedly altered. Coliform microorganisms and gram-positive spore-forming bacteria are particularly sensitive and may be markedly suppressed during chronic medication, before resistant strains reappear. The stools become softer and odorless and acquire a yellow-green color. However, as the fecal coliform count declines, tetracycline-resistant microorganisms, particularly yeasts, fecal streptococci, *Proteus,* and *Pseudomonas* overgrow and the total fecal microbial count may actually increase. Of greater significance is the *frequent overgrowth of antibiotic-resistant strains of staphylococci; suprainfections by coagulase-positive strains of this species have been fatal.* Normal intestinal flora is restored several days after antibiotic medication is withdrawn. Doxycycline, in a daily dose of 100 mg, has been noted to exert a substantially smaller impact on the intestinal flora than does tetracycline (Hinton, 1970).

Effects of Combined Chemotherapeutic Agents. The results of concurrent therapy with tetracyclines and other antimicrobial agents are not predictable in most instances, and deleterious effects have occurred. Striking antagonism between penicillin and the tetracyclines has been observed clinically in pneumococcal meningitis, and the unfortunate therapeutic results emphasize the fact that such antibiotic therapy may be very harmful (*see* Lepper and Dowling, 1951).

Mechanism of Action. The tetracyclines act to inhibit protein synthesis and, like the aminoglycosides, bind specifically to 30 S ribosomes. They appear to prevent access of aminoacyl tRNA to the mRNA-ribosome complex. Only a small portion of the drug is irreversibly bound, and the inhibitory effects of the tetracyclines can be reversed by washing. Therefore, it is probable that the reversibly bound antibiotic is responsible for the antibacterial action. The details of the extensive studies in this field have been reviewed by Weisblum and Davies (1968).

Resistance to the Tetracyclines.
Resistance to the tetracyclines produced *in vitro* appears slowly in a graded, stepwise fashion similar to that observed with penicillin. Microorganisms that have become insensitive to one tetracycline frequently exhibit resistance to the others. Gram-negative bacilli made resistant to tetracycline exhibit moderate-to-great insensitivity to chloramphenicol.

Tetracyclines appear to be accumulated actively by certain bacteria, and resistance to the tetracyclines in *E. coli* strains carrying transferable resistance markers (R factors) has been found to depend on decreased uptake of these antibiotics. Incubation of *E. coli* containing R factor for tetracycline in low concentrations of the drug appears to result in the induction of some factor necessary for its exclusion. (*See* Izaki *et al.,* 1966; Franklin, 1967.)

Absorption, Distribution, and Excretion.
Absorption. All the tetracyclines are adequately but incompletely absorbed from the gastrointestinal tract. Most absorption takes place from the stomach and upper small intestine and is greater in the fasting state; it is much less complete from the lower portions of the intestinal tract. Absorption of these agents is impaired, to a variable degree, by milk and milk products, and particularly by the concomitant administration of aluminum hydroxide gels, sodium bicarbonate, calcium and magnesium salts, and iron preparations (Neuvonen *et al.,* 1970). The mechanisms responsible for the decreased absorption appear to be chelation and an increase in gastric pH (Barr *et al.,* 1971).

The wide range of plasma concentrations present in different individuals following the oral administration of the various tetracyclines is related in large measure to the irregularity of their absorption from the gastrointestinal tract. These drugs can be divided into three groups based on the dosage and frequency of oral administration required to produce effective plasma concentrations.

Chlortetracycline, oxytetracycline, and *tetracycline* are very incompletely absorbed. After a single *oral* dose peak plasma concentrations are attained in 2 to 4 hours. These drugs have half-lives in the range of 6 to 9 hours, and they are frequently administered two to four times daily. The administration of 250 mg every 6 hours produces peak plasma concentrations of approximately 3 μg/ml.

Demeclocycline and *methacycline* are usually administered in lower daily dosage than are the above-mentioned congeners. Their absorption is also incomplete, but their half-lives are about 16 hours and effective plasma concentrations may thus persist for 24 to 48 hours. This is particularly true for demeclocycline. Poor absorption of methacycline may lead to lower plasma concentrations than with recommended doses of tetracycline, despite the difference in half-life.

Doxycycline and *minocycline* should be administered in even lower daily dosage by the oral route, since their half-lives are long (17 to 20 hours) and they are well absorbed. After an oral dose of 200 mg of doxycycline, plasma concentrations of the drug reach a maximum of 3 μg/ml at 2 hours and are well maintained. Plasma concentrations are equivalent when doxycycline is given by the oral or parenteral route (Leibowitz *et al.,* 1972). Food does not interfere with the absorption of doxycycline or minocycline.

Distribution. The volume of distribution of the tetracyclines is relatively larger than that of the body water, indicating sequestration in some tissues. They are bound to plasma proteins in varying degree. The approximate values are as follows: *methacycline,* about 80%; *minocycline,* 70 to 75%; *chlortetracycline,* 50 to 70%; *demeclocycline,* 40 to 50%; *tetracycline,* 25 to 30%; *oxytetracycline,* 20 to 25%; and *doxycycline,* 25 to 30%. However, the values reported in the literature are highly variable (*see* Kunin and Finland, 1959, 1961; Fabre *et al.,* 1966).

All the tetracyclines are removed from the blood by the liver, where they are concentrated and then excreted, by way of the bile, into the intestine, from which they are partially reabsorbed. Biliary concentrations of these agents average at least five to ten times higher than the simultaneous values in plasma (*see* Acocella *et al.,* 1968). Chlortetracycline is more dependent on biliary excretion for its elimination from the body than are the other tetracyclines. Decreased hepatic function or obstruction of the common bile duct results in reduction in the biliary excretion of these agents and their consequent persistence in the blood. Because of their enterohepatic circulation, the tetracyclines may be present in the blood for a long time after cessation of therapy.

Spinal fluid concentrations of *chlortetracycline* average about one fourth those in the plasma; they vary considerably, however, regardless of dose. Inflammation of the meninges is not a prerequisite for the passage of tetracyclines into the cerebrospinal fluid; route and duration of treatment are major determinants. The intravenous injection of a tetracycline results in the gradual appearance of the drug in the spinal fluid over a period of 6 hours. Oral therapy yields very low spinal fluid concentrations.

Penetration of these drugs into most other fluids and tissues is excellent. The tetracyclines are stored in the reticuloendothelial cells of the liver, spleen, and bone marrow, and in bone and the dentine and enamel of unerupted teeth (*see* below). Tetracyclines cross the placenta and enter the fetal circulation and amniotic fluid. Concentrations of tetracycline in umbilical cord plasma reach 60% and in amniotic fluid 20% of those in the circulation of the mother. Relatively high concentrations of these drugs are also found in milk.

Excretion. All the tetracyclines are excreted in the urine and the feces, the primary route for most being the kidney. Since renal clearance of these drugs is by glomerular filtration, their excretion is significantly affected by the state of renal function (*see* below). Twenty to 60% of an intravenous dose of 0.5 g of *tetracycline* is excreted in the urine during the first 24 hours; from 20 to 55% of an oral dose, regardless of size, is excreted by this route. Ten to 35% of a dose of *oxytetracycline* is excreted in active form in the urine, in which it is detectable within ½ hour and reaches a peak concentration in about 5 hours after it is administered. Only 10 to 15% of multiple or single oral doses of *chlortetracycline* is recoverable in the urine; intravenous injection leads to 60% urinary excretion during the first 12 hours. The clearance of chlortetracycline by the kidney is about 35% of the glomerular filtration rate and is less than that of oxytetracycline. The rate of renal clearance of *demeclocycline* is less than half that of tetracycline. About 50% of *methacycline* is excreted in unchanged form in the urine, while about 5% is excreted in the feces over a period of 72 hours.

Minocycline is recoverable both from urine and feces in significantly lower amounts than are the other tetracyclines, and it appears to be metabolized to a considerable extent. Renal clearance of minocycline is slow. The drug persists in the body after its administration is stopped; this may be due to reten-

tion in fatty tissues. The half-life of minocycline is apparently not prolonged in patients with hepatic failure (Devine *et al.,* 1971).

An important distinction should be made in the case of *doxycycline*. It is clear that, with conventional doses, doxycycline is not excreted in the urine to the same extent as are other tetracyclines, and it does not accumulate in the blood of patients with renal failure. It is thus the safest of the tetracyclines for the treatment of extrarenal infections in such individuals. The drug is excreted in the feces (up to 90%) as an inactive conjugate or perhaps as a chelate; for this reason it has relatively less impact on the intestinal microflora. The half-life of doxycycline may be shortened to approximately 7 hours in patients who are receiving chronic treatment with barbiturates or phenytoin (Neuvonen and Penttilä, 1974; Penttilä *et al.,* 1974).

As mentioned, the intestine is an important avenue of elimination of the tetracyclines. Because these agents are incompletely absorbed from the bowel when given orally or when excreted into the intestine in the bile, they are present, in varying concentrations, in the feces. Elimination from the intestinal tract occurs even when the drugs are given parenterally, as a result of excretion in the bile.

Preparations, Routes of Administration, and Dosage. *Chlortetracycline Hydrochloride,* N.F. (Aureomycin), *Oxytetracycline Hydrochloride,* U.S.P. (Terramycin), *Tetracycline Hydrochloride,* U.S.P. (Achromycin, Panmycin, Steclin, Sumycin, Tetrachel, Tetracyn), *Demeclocycline Hydrochloride,* N.F. (Declomycin), *Methacycline Hydrochloride,* N.F. (Rondomycin), *Doxycycline Hyclate,* U.S.P. (Vibramycin), and *Minocycline Hydrochloride,* U.S.P. (Minocin, Vectrin), are available in a wide variety of forms for oral, topical, and parenteral administration.

The tetracyclines are usually prescribed for *oral* use, but they may be administered by intravenous injection. Topical administration is best avoided because of the high risk of sensitization, except for use in the eye. *The tetracyclines should never be injected intrathecally.*

Preparations for Oral Administration. All the tetracyclines listed above are available for oral administration, usually as capsules and occasionally in tablet form, in appropriate dosages ranging from 50 to 500 mg, depending on the preparation. Some of the tetracyclines are also marketed as flavored powders, ophthalmic solutions and ointments, solutions for injection, soluble salts for preparation of oral suspensions and drops, and syrups and elixirs for pediatric use.

The *oral dose* of the tetracyclines varies with the nature and the severity of the disease. For *tetracycline, oxytetracycline,* and *chlortetracycline,* it ranges from 1 to 2 g per day in adults. The recommended dose of *demeclocycline* is somewhat lower, being 150 mg every 6 hours in moderately severe infections and 300 mg every 6 hours when the disease is more serious. The doses for children and infants are calculated on a weight basis. The oral dose of *methacycline* for adults is 150 mg every 6 hours or 300 mg every 12 hours; for children it is 10 mg/kg per day, divided into equal-sized quantities given every 8 hours. The dose of *doxycycline* for adults is 100 mg every 12 hours during the first 24 hours, followed by 100 mg once a day, or twice daily when severe infection is present. Children should receive 4 to 5 mg/kg per day, divided into two equal doses given at a 12-hour interval during the first day, after which a single dose of half this amount is administered; in serious disease, the same quantity is given every 12 hours. The dose of *minocycline* for adults is 200 mg initially, followed by 100 mg every 12 hours; for children it is 4 mg/kg initially, followed by 2 mg/kg every 12 hours.

The *duration* of medication depends upon the character of the disease and the response to therapy. Because the incidence of gastrointestinal distress and particularly of tetracycline-resistant bacterial enteritis rises as the dose of the antibiotic is increased, the minimal dosage compatible with the desired therapeutic response is recommended. Gastrointestinal distress, nausea, and vomiting can be minimized by administration of the tetracyclines with meals. Milk, antacids containing aluminum or magnesium hydroxide or silicate, and iron interfere with the absorption of the drugs and should not be ingested at the same time as is a tetracycline. Mixtures of tetracyclines with nystatin and amphotericin B are available; they have no special value in normal individuals but have been recommended for use in diabetics and patients with other diseases that may increase the risk of suprainfection with fungi; the value of such combinations has not been proven by rigid clinical tests.

Preparations for Parenteral Administration. Chlortetracycline Hydrochloride for Injection, N.F., *Oxytetracycline Hydrochloride for Injection,* U.S.P., *Tetracycline Hydrochloride for Injection,* U.S.P., *doxycycline hyclate for injection,* and *minocycline hydrochloride* are designed for intravenous administration. They are supplied in vials usually containing 100, 250, or 500 mg of the dry, crystalline salt mixed with a suitable buffer. The contents of the vial are dissolved in a convenient volume of sterile distilled water, isotonic sodium chloride solution, or 5% dextrose solution and subsequently diluted to a final concentration of not more than 5 mg/ml of antibiotic. The solution should be injected slowly at a rate not exceeding 2 ml per minute. Oxytetracycline and tetracycline may be given by intermittent intravenous infusion, but chlortetracycline is not sufficiently

stable to be administered in this manner. Infusion of doxycycline must be completed within 12 hours of reconstitution of the powder.

Intravenous administration of the tetracyclines is indicated in severe illness in which the dose may be large and cause nausea and vomiting if given orally, in patients unable to ingest medication, and when the response to oral therapy is inadequate. The total daily intravenous dose of chlortetracycline, oxytetracycline, or tetracycline for most acute infections is 500 mg to 1.0 g, usually administered in two equal portions at 12-hour intervals. Up to 2 g per day may be given in severe infections, but this dose may cause difficulty in some patients (*see* below); quantities larger than 2 g per day must not be given parenterally. The recommended daily intravenous dose for children and infants is 10 to 20 mg/kg of body weight. Because of local irritation and poor absorption, *intramuscular administration* of these tetracyclines is generally unsatisfactory. Preparations containing a local anesthetic are better tolerated on intramuscular injection; the usual adult dose by this route is 100 mg at 8-hour intervals. The usual intravenous dose of doxycycline is 200 mg in one or two infusions on the first day and 100 to 200 mg on subsequent days. The dose for children who weigh less than 45 kg is 4.4 mg/kg on the first day, and this is then reduced correspondingly.

Preparations for Local Application. Except for local use in the eye, topical use of the tetracyclines is not recommended. Official ophthalmic preparations include *Chlortetracycline Hydrochloride Ophthalmic Ointment,* N.F., *Tetracycline Hydrochloride for Ophthalmic Solution,* N.F., and *Tetracycline Hydrochloride Ophthalmic Suspension,* U.S.P. Solutions should be freshly prepared every 7 days and kept refrigerated. One or 2 drops are instilled in the conjunctival sac every 2 hours. The usual concentration of a tetracycline for ophthalmic use is 0.5 to 1%.

UNTOWARD EFFECTS

Hypersensitivity Reactions. Various skin reactions, including *morbilliform rashes, urticaria, fixed drug eruptions,* and generalized *exfoliative dermatitis,* may follow the use of any of the tetracyclines. Among the more severe allergic responses are *angioedema* and *anaphylaxis;* anaphylactoid reactions can occur even after the oral use of these agents. Other effects that may have their origin in hypersensitivity are *burning of the eyes, cheilosis, brown or black coating of the tongue, atrophic or hypertrophic glossitis, pruritus ani or vulvae, and vaginitis;* these effects often persist for weeks or months after cessation of tetracycline therapy. *Fever* of varying degree and *eosinophilia* may occur when these agents are administered. *Serum sickness* has not been observed with the tetracyclines.

It should be emphasized that *cross-sensitization among the various tetracyclines is extremely common* if not universal.

Toxic and Irritative Effects. Irritative effects of the tetracyclines are observed most commonly when they are taken orally. They all produce *gastrointestinal irritation* to a varying degree in some but not all individuals. Epigastric burning and distress, abdominal discomfort, nausea, and vomiting may occur. Oxytetracycline and doxycycline produce these manifestations most frequently; less irritating are chlortetracycline, tetracycline, and demeclocycline, in this order. The larger the dose, the greater is the likelihood of an irritative reaction. If troublesome, gastric distress can be controlled by administration of the tetracyclines with food (not milk or milk products), or antacids that do not contain aluminum, magnesium, or calcium. Nausea and vomiting often subside as medication continues and can frequently be controlled by temporary reduction in dose or by the use of smaller amounts at frequent intervals. *Diarrhea* may also result from the irritative effects of the tetracyclines given orally. In such cases, the stools, while frequent and fluid, do not contain blood or leukocytes. *It is imperative that this type of diarrhea be promptly distinguished from that which results from suprainfection of the bowel by staphylococci,* a life-threatening complication (*see* below).

The intravenous administration of the tetracyclines is frequently followed by *thrombophlebitis,* especially when a single vein is used for repeated infusion. The highly irritative effects of these agents are emphasized by the severe pain that they produce when injected intramuscularly without a local anesthetic.

Long-term therapy with tetracyclines may produce changes in the peripheral blood. *Leukocytosis, atypical lymphocytes, toxic granulation of granulocytes,* and *thrombopenic purpura* have been observed.

Demeclocycline may produce mild-to-severe reactions in the skin of treated individuals exposed to sunlight; this phenomenon is a *phototoxic reaction.* It appears to develop most frequently with a daily dose of 600 mg, but may also occur when smaller quantities are given. High fever, with or without eosinophilia, may be present in some patients. Onycholysis and pigmentation of the nails develop simultaneously in some individuals. The incidence of the "sunburn" reaction was found to be 40 in 2682 patients treated with demeclocycline (Carey, 1960), and doxycycline also is said to produce a high incidence. Phototoxicity is evident only when the skin is exposed to sunlight containing rays in the range of 270 to 320 mμ; these are filtered out by ordinary window glass and are present in the sunlight of temperate zones only in the summer. Oxytetracycline may produce a similar effect; it is less common with tetracycline and has not as yet been observed with minocycline.

That the tetracyclines may *injure the liver* was first observed by Lepper (1951), who reported that patients receiving large doses of tetracycline orally or intravenously developed clinical evidence of hepatic dysfunction; microscopic study of the liver revealed fine vacuoles, cytoplasmic changes, and increase in fat. Oxytetracycline and tetracycline appear to be less hepatotoxic than are the other drugs of this group. Most reactions of this type develop in patients receiving 2 g or more of drug per day parenterally; however, this effect may also occur when large quantities are administered orally. *The tetracyclines pose a special danger in pregnant women,* with respect to possible hepatic injury, particularly if used for the treatment of pyelonephritis, a relatively common occurrence in such patients. Indeed, fatalities have occurred. Jaundice first appears and then progresses to azotemia, acidosis, and terminal shock. The livers are diffusely infiltrated with fat. Although hepatic fat is increased during pregnancy, the quantity appears to be even greater after exposure to a tetracycline. Both renal and hepatic abnormalities may be associated with pregnancy, and this explains the great danger when one of the tetracyclines is administered, especially parenterally or in a daily dose of 2 g or more. Kidney infection appears to be the critical factor because it may lead to decreased renal function and reduced excretion of the drug, resulting in accumulation of toxic concentrations. An instance of disseminated intravascular coagulation has been reported in a pregnant woman who developed hepatorenal failure after being given only two doses of

100 mg each of tetracycline intramuscularly (Pride *et al.*, 1973).

The tetracyclines, with the exception of doxycycline, are not recommended for administration to patients with *renal dysfunction* (*see* Table 55-2, page 1108). The untoward effects are directly related to the particular tetracycline used, the dose, the duration of therapy, and the extent of renal disease. Among the toxic effects are azotemia, hyperphosphatemia, acidosis, weight loss, nausea, and vomiting. Established renal insufficiency may be markedly aggravated by treatment with the tetracyclines. Kuzucu (1970) has called attention to the possibility of the development of severe renal failure in patients who receive tetracycline after being anesthetized with methoxyflurane; in those who died, the kidneys contained numerous calcium oxalate crystals. Transient nephrogenic diabetes insipidus has been observed in some patients receiving demeclocycline.

The tetracyclines exert *profound metabolic effects.* The administration of 2.5 to 3.0 g of chlortetracycline to undernourished adults results in weight loss, increased urinary but not fecal nitrogen excretion, negative nitrogen balance, and elevated serum nonprotein nitrogen concentrations (Gabuzda *et al.*, 1958). Similar changes are observed when a comparable dose of oxytetracycline or 1 g of chlortetracycline is given orally or parenterally; body weight and serum nonprotein nitrogen levels are not altered by the latter agent.

The urinary excretion of riboflavin appears to be increased when doses of 1 to 3 g of chlortetracycline or 2.5 g of oxytetracycline per day are given orally. Increased urinary excretion of folic acid, N'-methylnicotinamide, and certain amino acids also occurs when chlortetracycline is administered. There appears to be no correlation between detectable changes in the fecal bacterial flora and the metabolic abnormalities.

The metabolic abnormalities produced by therapeutic doses of the tetracyclines develop in proportion to the degree of renal dysfunction and to the dosage used and the duration of treatment (Shils, 1963). The basis for the stated changes appears to be an antianabolic effect—inhibition of protein synthesis—of the tetracyclines.

The tetracyclines have been found to *delay blood coagulation.* Although this phenomenon has been attributed to calcium chelation, it has been suggested that it is related to the ability of these drugs to alter plasma lipoproteins. Patients receiving tetracycline intravenously have a slight-to-marked decrease in prothrombin activity and an impairment in the rate of thromboplastin regeneration.

Children receiving long- or short-term therapy with a tetracycline may develop *brown discolorations of the teeth.* The larger the dose of drug relative to body weight, the more severe the deformity, the deeper the color, and the more intense the hypoplasia of enamel. The duration of therapy appears to be less important than the total quantity of antibiotic administered. The risk of this untoward effect is greater when the tetracycline is given to neonates and babies prior to the first dentition. However, pigmentation of the permanent dentition may develop if the drug is given between the ages of 2 months and 5 years, when these teeth are being calcified. An early characteristic of this defect is a yellow fluorescence of the dental pigment, which has an ultraviolet spectrum with an absorption peak at 270 mμ. The *deposition of the drug in the teeth and bones* is probably due to its chelating property and the formation of a tetracycline-calcium orthophosphate complex. As time progresses, the yellow fluorescence is replaced by a nonfluorescent brown color that may represent an oxidation product of the antibiotic, the formation of which is hastened by light. This discoloration is permanent.

Treatment of pregnant patients with tetracyclines may produce discoloration of the teeth in their offspring. The period of greatest danger to the teeth is from midpregnancy to about 4 to 6 months of the postnatal period for the deciduous anterior teeth, and from 6 months to 5 years of age for the permanent anterior teeth (Weyman, 1965), the periods when the crowns of the teeth are being formed. However, children up to 7 years old may be susceptible to this complication of tetracycline therapy.

Tetracyclines are deposited in the *skeleton* of the human fetus and young child. A 40% depression of bone growth, as determined by measurement of fibulas, has been demonstrated in premature infants treated with these agents (Cohlan *et al.*, 1963). This is readily reversible if the period of exposure to the drug is short.

A clinical picture characterized by nausea, vomiting, polyuria, polydipsia, proteinuria, acidosis, glycosuria, and gross aminoaciduria—a form of the *Fanconi syndrome*—has been observed in patients ingesting outdated and degraded tetracycline (Frimpter *et al.*, 1963; Fulop and Drapkin, 1965). All manifestations disappear in about a month after cessation of treatment. A facial lesion typical of systemic lupus erythematosus, as well as sensitivity to sunlight, has also been observed following ingestion of outdated and degraded tetracycline.

The tetracyclines may cause *increased intracranial pressure* and tense bulging of the fontanels (pseudotumor cerebri) in young infants, even when given in the usual therapeutic doses. Except for the elevated pressure, the spinal fluid is normal. Discontinuation of therapy results in prompt return of the pressure to normal.

Recent reports indicate that a substantial percentage of patients receiving the recommended dosage of *minocycline* experience *vestibular toxicity*, manifested by dizziness, ataxia, nausea, and vomiting. The symptoms occur soon after the initial dose and generally disappear within 24 to 48 hours after drug administration is stopped. The vestibular disturbance may pose a hazard for patients engaged in activities requiring unimpaired motor coordination (*see* Williams *et al.*, 1974).

Biological Effects Other Than Allergic or Toxic. Like all antimicrobial agents, the tetracyclines administered orally or parenterally may lead to the development of *suprainfections* that are usually due to strains of bacteria or yeasts resistant to these agents. Oral, pharyngeal, and even systemic infections with yeasts and fungi, particularly *Candida,* are not uncommon; they tend to occur most often in individuals with disorders such as diabetes, leukemia, systemic lupus erythematosus, diffuse vasculitis, and lymphoma, especially if steroids are also being administered. The incidence of suprainfections is much higher with the tetracyclines than with penicillin or streptomycin.

Among the most important suprainfections associated with the administration of the tetracyclines are those that involve the

intestinal tract; they may occur with either oral or parenteral therapy. The possibility that drug-induced diarrhea may be due to active infection of the bowel merits serious consideration in every instance. Three types of infectious enteritis—*staphylococcal enterocolitis, intestinal candidiasis,* and *pseudomembranous colitis*—may follow tetracycline treatment.

Staphylococcal enterocolitis may appear at any time during or shortly after therapy with a tetracycline and is characterized by severe diarrhea with liquid stools that often contain blood and large numbers of polymorphonuclear leukocytes; staining reveals a very marked preponderance of gram-positive cocci, and culture yields almost a pure growth of large numbers of coagulase-positive staphylococci. However, the mere presence of these microorganisms in the stool does not indicate suprainfection, because small numbers of them are normal constituents of the fecal microbial flora. Fever and leukocytosis are common features. *The diagnosis of this disease must be made as rapidly as possible.* Management must be prompt and consists in immediate cessation of tetracycline administration and oral treatment with large doses of another antibiotic to which the staphylococci are sensitive. In many instances, omission of the tetracycline and repair of water and electrolyte disturbances are sufficient to produce rapid cure. When there is any evidence of systemic involvement, *parenteral therapy* with full doses of an appropriate penicillin is indicated.

Although *intestinal candidiasis* has been thought to be a common cause of tetracycline-induced diarrhea, this is probably so only in exceptional instances. Fecal cultures in many individuals with drug-produced diarrhea yield only normal numbers of yeasts. Some patients receiving a tetracycline may harbor large numbers of these microorganisms in the stool and do not have diarrhea. Uncommonly, there appears to be a correlation between the numbers of *Candida* in the stool and the presence of diarrhea. In instances where there is strong evidence for the presence of intestinal candidiasis, the oral administration of nystatin or amphotericin B is indicated.

Pseudomembranous colitis is characterized by severe diarrhea, fever, and stools containing shreds of mucous membrane and a large number of neutrophils; staphylococci are not increased in number. The syndrome develops in some patients who have had intestinal operations but have not been treated with antimicrobial agents. Its causal relation to antibiotic therapy is, therefore, sometimes questionable.

The oral administration of tetracyclines may result in an increase in the quantity of bilirubin and a decrease in the concentration of urobilinogen in the urine. This may cause diagnostic confusion in instances in which differentiation of obstructive from hepatocellular jaundice is important. Plasma prothrombin may be depressed to low levels by the oral administration of tetracyclines given for even moderate periods; this is probably related to the changes in intestinal flora induced by these drugs.

To decrease the incidence of toxic effects, the following precautions should be observed in the use of the tetracyclines. They should not be given to pregnant patients; they should not be employed for the therapy of the common infections in children under the age of 12 years; only doxycycline should be used, if necessary, in patients with overt renal insufficiency; they should be given prophylactically with great care; unused supplies of these antibiotics should be discarded.

THERAPEUTIC USES

The tetracyclines are firmly established as valuable agents in the therapy of a variety of infectious diseases. However, because of increasing bacterial resistance to these drugs and the development of new antimicrobial agents that are more effective for specific infections and less toxic, the indications for the use of tetracyclines have become more restricted (*see* Finland, 1974).

These agents are useful in rickettsial and bacterial diseases, in infections produced by some *Mycoplasma,* and in disorders caused by *Chlamydia;* given concomitantly with other drugs, they are effective in some instances of intestinal amebiasis. Among the infectious diseases for which they are of proven value are *Rocky Mountain spotted fever, murine typhus, recrudescent epidemic typhus, scrub typhus, Q fever, lymphogranuloma venereum, psittacosis, tularemia, brucellosis, gonorrhea, certain urinary tract infections, ocular infections, granuloma inguinale, chancroid, syphilis,* and *disease due to Bacteroides* and *Clostridium.*

The status of the tetacyclines in comparison with other antimicrobial agents for the therapy of various infections is given in Table 55–1 (page 1096). Advantages of these drugs are oral efficacy, relatively low toxicity, and a wide range of antimicrobial activity. Concurrent use of the tetracyclines with other antimicrobial drugs usually has no distinct advantages but has, in a number of instances, resulted in decreased antimicrobial activity.

Rickettsial Infections. The tetracyclines are dramatically effective in rickettsial infections, including Rocky Mountain spotted fever, recrudescent epidemic typhus (Brill's disease), murine typhus, scrub typhus, rickettsialpox, and Q fever. Fever usually subsides in 1 to 3 days, and the rash disappears in 3 to 5 days; striking clinical improvement is evident within 24 hours after initiation of therapy. Con-valescence proceeds uneventfully, and relapses do not occur when medication has been adequate. Clinical recovery in some rickettsial infections, notably Q fever, may be somewhat slower than in others. The tetracyclines are usually merely rickettsiostatic; the development of antibody titers may be delayed or reduced, depending on the severity of infection and the interval between onset of disease and initiation of drug therapy.

Chlamydia (Psittacosis–Lymphogranuloma Venereum Group). *Lymphogranuloma Venereum.* The tetracyclines are currently the treatment of choice in this infection. They exert markedly favorable effects in acute cases and are a valuable adjunct to surgery in management of chronic cases. Decided reduction in the size of buboes is observed within 4 days, and inclusion and elementary bodies entirely disappear from the lymph nodes within 1 week. Lymphogranulomatous proctitis is promptly improved. Benign cicatricial rectal strictures are not significantly ameliorated, although rectal pain, discharge, and bleeding are markedly decreased. The most satisfactory results are obtained with prolonged medication; therapy is continued for 3 to 4 weeks in acute cases and for 1 to 2 months in chronic cases. When relapses occur, treatment is resumed with full doses and is continued for longer periods.

Psittacosis. The tetracyclines are also of value in proven cases of psittacosis. Dramatic and immediate improvement is often observed. Fever and pneumonitis are controlled within 2 to 3 days, and convalescence is rapid and uneventful. Drug therapy for 12 to 14 days is usually adequate. Such treatment may interfere with the development of complement-fixing antibodies.

Inclusion Conjunctivitis. This disease responds rapidly to topical administration of tetracycline, in ointment or liquid form, four times a day for 2 to 3 weeks.

Trachoma. Although the sulfonamides are considered by some to be the most effective agents for the treatment of trachoma, the tetracyclines have proven very effective. These agents are best administered topically in vehicles that cling to the conjunctiva. Some physicians prefer to add oral administration to the therapeutic regimen. In most favorable situations, tetracycline ophthalmic ointment should be applied four times daily for 4 weeks and an oral sulfonamide given for 3 weeks. In endemic areas where ideal therapy is not possible, the application of the ointment to the eyes twice daily for 3 days of each week for 6 months has been suggested. There is evidence that some strains of the agent causing trachoma are becoming insensitive to antibiotics. Doxycycline (0.1 g daily for 28 days) is without effect on the incidence of *Chlamydia* in the conjunctiva and does not significantly influence the bacterial flora of the eye (Dawson *et al.,* 1971).

Mycoplasma Infections. The syndrome known as "primary atypical pneumonia" is caused by *Mycoplasma pneumoniae,* a PPLO that is sensitive to the tetracyclines. Treatment results in a shorter duration of fever, cough, malaise, fatigue, pulmonary rales, and roentgenographic changes in the lungs. Mycoplasma may persist in the sputum following cessation of therapy despite rapid resolution of the active infection (*see* Smith *et al.,* 1967).

Bacillary Infections. *Brucellosis.* Treatment with the tetracyclines produces excellent results in infections caused by *Brucella melitensis, suis,* and *abortus.* Both acute and chronic forms of the disease respond dramatically. The temperature becomes normal within 2 to 5 days, the blood is rapidly cleared of bacilli, palpable liver and spleen recede, and the clinical picture promptly improves. Good results are usually obtained in acute brucellosis with full doses of a tetracycline for 3 weeks. Clinical and bacteriological relapses are not the result of the development of resistant strains of *Brucella* and usually respond to a second course of therapy. The tetracyclines given with streptomycin (1 g daily, intramuscularly) also provide prompt results in patients severely ill with acute brucellosis. Whether such therapy results in a lower incidence of relapse than that observed with a tetracycline alone (for 6 weeks) is unsettled.

Tularemia. Although streptomycin is preferable, therapy with the tetracyclines also produces prompt results in tularemia. Both the ulceroglandular and typhoidal types of the disease respond well. Fever, toxemia, and clinical signs and symptoms are all improved; the bacteria rapidly disappear from blood, sputum, and pleural fluid; and complications are usually prevented.

Cholera. In a controlled trial of the effects of oral antibiotics in the management of cholera in children in Pakistan, Lindebaum and associates (1967) found that tetracycline was the most effective of the agents studied in reducing stool volume, intravenous fluid requirement, and the duration of diarrhea and positive stool culture. Only 1% of the children given tetracycline had diarrhea for more than 4 days. Treatment with tetracycline was significantly more effective than intravenous fluid therapy alone, regardless of the severity of the disease. When oral drug therapy was given for only 48 hours, bacteriological relapse developed in 20% of the cases despite a good clinical response. It must be emphasized that antimicrobial agents are not substitutes for fluid and electrolyte replacement in this disease. The effectiveness of tetracycline as a prophylactic agent in families of cholera patients was demonstrated by McCormack and coworkers (1968). They noted that the administration of the drug for 5 days was effective in preventing infection in contacts.

Other Bacillary Infections. Therapy with the tetracyclines is not uniformly effective in infections caused by *Shigella* and *Salmonella,* because of the increase in incidence of resistant strains. However, these drugs may prove beneficial in some cases. A similar situation holds for infections of various types caused by *E. coli* and *Enterobacter* (*Aerobacter*) *aerogenes.* Although tetracyclines given with a sulfonamide have been used with some success in the therapy of *H. influenzae* meningitis, this is certainly not the therapy of choice. The tetracyclines are without any effect in altering the course of *pertussis;* their use may result in an increased incidence of secondary bacterial infections of the ears and lungs (Weinstein *et al.,* 1954). The tetracyclines are of value in the therapy of most cases of *anthrax* in which the microorganisms are resistant or the patients sensitized to the penicillins. If the disease is severe, it is best to administer the agent intravenously for the first 48 to 72 hours and to follow this with oral therapy. *Yersinia (Past.) pestis,* the causative agent of bubonic plague, is very sensitive to streptomycin, chloramphenicol, and the tetracyclines; however, streptomycin is the agent of choice for the treatment of this disease. When the tetracyclines are used, intravenous therapy for 2 days followed by oral therapy for 1 week is indicated.

Prophylaxis for Bowel Surgery. During chronic oral administration of the tetracyclines, fecal counts of *E. coli* and other susceptible microorganisms may be markedly reduced in some cases, usually within 3 to 4 days. This is particularly true with the poorly absorbed older agents. For this reason, these drugs have been used prophylactically prior to bowel surgery, being given orally in doses of 3 to 4 g per day, for 3 days prior to operation. The intestinal bacteria may become resistant to these agents very rapidly, and overgrowth of *Proteus* and resistant strains of *Staph. aureus* may occur and cause severe and potentially lethal enterocolitis. Because other antibiotics (*e.g.,* neomycin) are more effective in reducing the numbers of intestinal bacteria, and because the evidence is not convincing that "preparation" of the bowel for surgery is of significant value in preventing postoperative complications, the administration of the tetracyclines for this purpose cannot be recommended.

Coccal Infections. Although the tetracyclines were initially effective against a large number of strains of staphylococci, they are presently of limited value in the therapy of disease caused by this microorganism because of the high frequency of resistant strains. Nevertheless, all staphylococci isolated from infected areas should be tested for sensitivity to these agents because their use may be indicated in patients hypersensitive to the penicillins or other antibiotics, and the use of more effective drugs may be accompanied by a higher risk of serious untoward effects. The tetracyclines are distinctly third-order drugs for the management of infection due to group-A *Strep. pyogenes;* a number of strains are resistant to this class of antimicrobial agents. Although streptococcal pharyngitis may appear to respond well during therapy with one of the tetracyclines, the incidence of bacteriological and clinical relapse is high shortly after treatment is stopped. The recovery of tetracycline-resistant strains of *Strep. (D.) pneumoniae* has decreased the applicability of these drugs in the management of pneumonia due to this microorganism. None of the tetracyclines should be used to treat meningococcal infections when other effective drugs are available. Although *minocycline* has been found, when given in a dose of 100 mg every 12 hours for 5 days, to *prevent the development of meningococcal disease* and markedly to *lower the carrier rate* (Guttler and Beatty, 1972), its use for this purpose is not recommended because of the vestibular disturbances that this drug can cause (*see* above). Indeed, such disturbances may be mistaken for early symptoms of meningitis and can cause unnecessary alarm.

Venereal Infections. Although penicillin G is the drug of choice in all clinical forms of *gonorrhea,* it cannot be used in some patients because of the presence of a dangerous degree of hypersensitivity. In such cases, the administration of 0.5 g of a tetracycline (0.3 g of demeclocycline) orally every 6 hours for 1 day is effective in the acute stage of the uncomplicated disease; a single dose of 1.5 g of tetracycline has also been reported to produce a high percentage of cures. In deep-seated infections, it is best to give 2 g of the drug per day for 2 weeks. Studies indicate that a single oral dose of 200 to 300 mg of minocycline (Thatcher *et al.,* 1970) or 300 mg of doxycycline (Moffett *et al.,* 1972) will cure from 92 to 95% of episodes of acute gonorrhea in both females and males. These doses are not sufficient to abort all cases of "incubation" syphilis (Lucas, 1971); hence all patients treated in this manner should have serial examination of the blood for serological evidence of the disease over a period of 2 to 3 months.

The use of the tetracyclines in the therapy of *syphilis* in patients unable to take penicillin is described in Chapter 57. These agents are also effective in *chancroid* and *granuloma inguinale,* but their use in these diseases entails the risk of masking a luetic infection that may have been contracted at the same time. If they are employed, the dose and duration of treatment should be the same as those used to treat syphilis. *Nongonococcal urethritis,* possibly due to *Mycoplasma hominis* or *Chlamydia* species, usually responds to tetracycline therapy.

Urinary Tract Infections. Although the tetracyclines were initially very valuable in the management of urinary tract infection due to gram-negative bacilli, their usefulness has been appreciably reduced by the increase in the number of drug-resistant microorganisms involved in this kind of infection. As a rule, these drugs are not active against *Proteus* and *Pseud. aeruginosa.* Therapy of urinary tract infections with a tetracycline *should never be routine* and should be undertaken only in severe infections, in chronic recurrent disease, and only if the strain isolated from the urine is sensitive. Therapy is usually continued for 7 to 10 days. It is probably best to maintain the urinary pH in the acidic range during treatment because of the lesser antimicrobial activity of the tetracyclines, particularly chlortetracycline but not demeclocycline, in an alkaline medium. For severe acute pyelonephritis, tetracyclines should be used only if no other antimicrobial agent is effective. While doxycycline may be given to patients with high-grade renal dysfunction, the drug concentration in the urine will then not be sufficient for such therapy.

Amebiasis. The tetracyclines that are less well absorbed are effective in *intestinal amebiasis* and eradicate both cysts and trophozoites from the feces, especially if they are administered simultaneously with an amebicidal agent. Tetracycline alone remains the treatment of choice for *Balantidium coli* infestation. Oxytetracycline (0.5 g orally every 6 hours) plus chloroquine (1 g daily for 2 days followed by 0.5 g daily at bedtime for 18 days) produces beneficial results in most instances of *Enta-*

moeba histolytica, and the relapse rate is low. However, the treatment of choice for this disease now appears to be metronidazole (*see* Chapter 53).

Other Infections. *Actinomycosis,* although most responsive to penicillin G, is often beneficially affected by the use of a tetracycline; in severe infections, intravenous therapy for 1 week, followed by oral administration of drug for a month or more, may be required. Minocycline has been suggested for the treatment of *nocardiosis* (Bach *et al.,* 1973). *Yaws* and *relapsing fever* respond favorably to the tetracyclines. *Leptospirosis* (Weil's disease) responds well to penicillin G, but the tetracyclines are also very effective and should be used in the penicillin-sensitive patient; oral therapy for 2 weeks is adequate in most instances. If the kidney is involved and renal function is impaired, doxycycline should be used. Although penicillin G is the drug of choice of many physicians in the therapy of *gas gangrene,* the tetracyclines are also highly effective. They should always be administered intravenously early in the course of therapy. The tetracyclines are effective in the management of some but not all infections due to *Bacteroides.*

Mucoviscidosis. The tetracyclines have been used extensively for the prophylaxis of secondary bacterial infections in patients with mucoviscidosis. In children with this disorder, the daily administration of a tetracycline for months to years has led to a reduction in the incidence of bacterial pneumonia, despite the fact that the microorganisms present in the nasopharyngeal flora become drug resistant during therapy. Doxycycline has been noted to be present in lung and bronchial tissue in concentrations equal to or somewhat higher than those present in plasma (Gartmann, 1972). When used in this manner in young children, the incidence of discoloration of the teeth is high (*see* above).

Chronic Obstructive Pulmonary Disease. A large number of studies have suggested that the oral administration of 0.5 g per day of tetracycline or corresponding doses of the congeneric agents is effective in preventing acute pulmonary infections in individuals with chronic lung disease, especially "bronchitis" or obstructive disorders such as emphysema (Francis *et al.,* 1964). In some instances, such prophylaxis has been used only during the winter months; in others, it has been more prolonged. Although many of the reports are enthusiastic about this procedure, universal agreement as to its effectiveness and safety is lacking. The danger of this kind of prophylaxis is suprainfection with drug-resistant bacteria and with fungi that may be very difficult or impossible to eradicate; death has occurred as a result of such a complication in a number of patients treated in this manner.

Intestinal Disease. Some patients with *Whipple's disease* may respond to antimicrobial agents (penicillin and streptomycin, followed by tetracycline) with a prompt and dramatic cessation of fever, diarrhea, and arthralgia, and with a sustained gain of weight; relapses may disappear promptly on retreatment. The administration of tetracycline to some patients with *tropical sprue* may be associated with folate repletion, a favorable hematological response, decrease in diarrhea, improvement in the enzymatic activity and morphology of the superficial epithelium of the jejunal mucosa, gain in weight, and reversal of the abnormal pattern of lipid distribution. Tetracyclines may also be of value in the *blind-loop syndrome.*

Acne. Tetracyclines have been used for the therapy of acne, and good results have been reported by some workers. Since benefit has been produced by doses too small to exert an antibacterial effect, it has been suggested that these drugs may act by decreasing the fatty acid content of sebum. There is as yet no proof that the tetracyclines or other antibiotics have a beneficial effect in acne, and some placebo crossover studies raise doubt concerning the value of this kind of therapy (Crounse, 1965; Fry and Ramsay, 1966). Use of these drugs may be followed by suprainfection and the development of folliculitis due to gram-negative bacteria (Leyden *et al.,* 1973).

CHLORAMPHENICOL

History and Source. *Chloramphenicol* is an antibiotic produced by *Streptomyces venezuelae,* an organism first isolated by Burkholder in 1947 from a soil sample collected in Venezuela. Filtrates of liquid cultures of the organisms were found to possess marked effectiveness against several gram-negative bacteria and also to exhibit antirickettsial activity (*see* Ehrlich *et al.,* 1948); a crystalline antibiotic substance was then isolated (Bartz, 1948) and named CHLOROMYCETIN because it contained chlorine and was obtained from an actinomycete. When the structural formula of the crystalline material was determined, the antibiotic was prepared synthetically. Pharmacological studies in animals and man were soon undertaken by Smadel and associates (1947 *et seq.*). Late in 1947, the small amount of available chloramphenicol was employed in an outbreak of epidemic typhus in Bolivia, with dramatic results. It was then tried with excellent success in cases of scrub typhus on the Malay peninsula. By 1948, chloramphenicol was produced in amounts sufficient for general clinical use, and was then found to be of value in the therapy of a variety of infections. By 1950, however, it became evident that the drug could cause *serious and fatal blood dyscrasias.*

Chemistry. Chloramphenicol has the following structural formula:

Chloramphenicol

The antibiotic is unique among natural compounds in that it contains a nitrobenzene moiety and is a derivative of dichloroacetic acid. The biologically active form is levorotatory. It is only slightly soluble in water (1:400). The antibiotic is extremely stable. Chloramphenicol is inactivated by enzymes present in filtrates of certain bacteria, which reduce the nitro group and hydrolyze the amide linkage; it is also acetylated (*see* below).

Effects on Microbial Agents. Chloramphenicol possesses a fairly wide spectrum of antimicrobial activity. It is primarily bacteriostatic, although it may be bactericidal to certain species under some conditions. Among the bacteria inhibited by relatively low concentrations of the antibiotic *in vitro* are *Enterobacter* (*Aerobacter*) *aerogenes, E. coli, K. pneumoniae, Bordetella pertussis, H. influenzae, Pasteurella, Pseud. mallei* and *pseudomallei, Bacteroides, Salmonella typhi* and other species, *Proteus* (certain strains), *Neisseria, Shigella, Brucella,* and *V. cholerae.* Some streptococci and staphylococci are suppressed by higher concentrations. *Actinomyces, Bacillus anthracis, Corynebacterium diphtheriae, Clostridium, Listeria, Bartonella,* and *Leptospira* are sensitive to moderate concentrations.

In general, the results of chloramphenicol therapy of *bacterial infections in experimental animals* parallel the *in-vitro* results. Chloramphenicol exerts marked prophylactic and therapeutic effects in experimental infections produced by all rickettsiae. The drug, as a rule, merely suppresses rickettsial growth and thus permits the development of immunity that is responsible for recovery. Chloramphenicol is also effective against *Chlamydia* and *Mycoplasma.*

Resistance to Chloramphenicol. Some species of bacteria, but not rickettsiae, may be made resistant to chloramphenicol *in vitro* by serial culture in increasing concentrations of the drug. Bacterial resistance to chloramphenicol *in vivo* is a problem of increasing *clinical* importance, for both gram-positive and gram-negative microorganisms. Insensitivity of *E. coli, Salmonella,* and other gram-negative bacteria to the drug is due to the presence of a specific resistance (R) factor acquired by conjugation. The resistance of such strains to chloramphenicol appears to be due to the presence of a specific acetyltransferase, which inactivates the drug by using acetyl coenzyme A as the donor of the acetyl group (*see* Shaw, 1971). The enzyme is constitutive in *E. coli.* Resistance of staphylococci to this antibiotic has also increased in incidence; it varies from one hospital to another and is as high as 50% or more in some. Shaw and Brodsky (1968) demonstrated that resistant *Staph. aureus* contains an inducible form of chloramphenicol acetyltransferase.

Mechanism of Action. Chloramphenicol inhibits protein synthesis in bacteria and in cell-free systems. It acts primarily on the 50 S ribosomal subunit and shares this site of action with macrolide antibiotics and lincomycin. The activity of peptidyl transferase, which catalyzes peptide bond formation, is suppressed, although ribosomes may still bind to and move along strands of mRNA. Ribosomal translocation thus appears to be uncoupled from peptide bond synthesis. (*See* Weisberger, 1967; Weisblum and Davies, 1968; Gurgo *et al.*, 1969; Pestka, 1971.)

The effects on mammalian cells, including some of the hematological abnormalities observed in clinical practice, are also thought to be related primarily to inhibition of protein synthesis. However, Godchaux and Herbert (1966) have suggested that the mechanism of action of chloramphenicol on reticulocytes is different from that on bacterial cells. The main effect on reticulocytes is inhibition of the conversion of polysomes to single ribosomes and a decrease in the content of adenosine triphosphate. The synthesis of both RNA and protein is inhibited. It is also clear that chloramphenicol can inhibit mitochondrial protein synthesis in higher cells (Wheeldon and Lehninger, 1966); it is hypothesized that mitochondrial ribosomes resemble bacterial ribosomes (both are 70 S) more than they do the 80 S cytoplasmic ribosomes of mammalian cells.

Absorption, Distribution, Fate, and Excretion. Chloramphenicol is rapidly absorbed from the gastrointestinal tract; significant plasma concentrations are obtained within 30 minutes, and peak values are reached in approximately 2 hours. They range from 20 to 40 μg/ml after 4 g. The half-life of the drug is about 1½ to 3½ hours (Kunin *et al.*, 1959), and it is thus no longer detectable in the blood after 12 to 18 hours. At peak blood concentrations, about 60% of chloramphenicol is bound by plasma albumin.

Chloramphenicol is well distributed in body fluids and readily reaches therapeutic concentrations in cerebrospinal fluid and brain. The drug is present in bile and milk and readily passes the placental barrier. It penetrates into the aqueous humor of the eye after subconjunctival injection. (*See* Brock, 1961.)

The drug is inactivated primarily in the liver by glucuronyl transferase, and chloramphenicol is cleared from the plasma of patients with hepatic cirrhosis more slowly than normally. The half-life of the drug can be correlated directly with the plasma concentration of bilirubin (Azzollini *et al.*, 1972). Chloramphenicol and its metabolites are rapidly excreted in the urine. Over a 24-hour period, 80 to 90% of an orally administered dose is so excreted; about 5 to 10% is in the biologically active form, whereas the remainder is inactive and consists of a hydrolysis product and a glucuronic acid conjugate. The unaltered antibiotic is eliminated mainly by glomerular filtration; the inactive degradation products are eliminated primarily by tubular secretion.

Preparations, Routes of Administration, and Dosage. *Chloramphenicol,* U.S.P. (CHLOROMYCETIN, MYCHEL), is marketed in capsules containing 50, 100, and 250 mg for oral use. *Chloramphenicol Ophthalmic Ointment,* U.S.P., contains 1% of the drug, and *Chloramphenicol Ophthalmic Solution,* U.S.P., is a sterile 0.5% aqueous solution. *Chloramphenicol Palmitate,* U.S.P., is a water-insoluble powder; 1.7 g of this preparation is equivalent to 1 g of chloramphenicol base. *Chloramphenicol Palmitate Oral Suspension,* U.S.P., contains an amount of chloramphenicol palmitate equivalent to 150 mg of chloramphenicol base, mixed with suitable dispersing and flavoring agents, in each 5 ml. This ester is hydrolyzed to free chloramphenicol in the gastrointestinal tract. Lower plasma concentrations may be achieved than those that follow administration of an equivalent dose of chloramphenicol itself. *Chloramphenicol Sodium Succinate for Injection,* U.S.P., is marketed as the dry powder in 1-g quantities; it is intended for solution for *intravenous use,* and it may not be effective when given by the intramuscular route.

Chloramphenicol may be administered orally or intravenously. Dosage schedules for the therapy of specific infections are presented below. Adjustment in dose must be made when chloramphenicol palmitate is used, as indicated above.

Untoward Effects. *Hypersensitivity Reactions.* Although relatively uncommon, *macular* or *vesicular skin rashes* occur as a result of hypersensitization to chloramphenicol. *Fever* may appear simultaneously or be the sole manifestation. Angioedema is a rare complication. Severe *hemorrhage,* involving the skin and mouth as well as the mucosal and serosal surfaces of the intestine and bladder, has been observed to occur shortly after administration of the drug and has been attributed to a hypersensitivity reaction. *Atrophic glossitis,* with or without a black coat on the tongue, is thought to be due to the same mechanism. *Herxheimer reactions* have been observed shortly after institution of chloramphenicol therapy for syphilis, brucellosis, and typhoid fever.

The most important effect of chloramphenicol hypersensitivity is on the *bone marrow;* of all the drugs that may be responsible for *pancytopenia,* chloramphenicol is the most common cause (Erslev and Wintrobe, 1962; Wallerstein *et al.,* 1969). Peripheral blood changes include *leukopenia, thrombopenia,* and *aplasia of the marrow* with *fatal pancytopenia.* This reaction is not related to dose; it occurs almost exclusively in individuals who undergo prolonged therapy and especially in those who are exposed to the drug on more than one occasion. Although the incidence of the reaction is low (one in 40,000 or more courses of therapy), when bone-marrow aplasia is complete the fatality rate is almost 100%.

A compilation of 576 cases of blood dyscrasia due to chloramphenicol indicates that aplastic anemia was the most common type reported, accounting for about 70% of the cases; hypoplastic anemia, agranulocytosis, thrombocytopenia, and bone-marrow inhibition made up the remainder. Among the patients with pancytopenia the outcome was apparently unrelated to the dose of chloramphenicol taken. However, the longer the interval between the last dose of chloramphenicol and the appearance of the first sign of the blood dyscrasia, the greater was the mortality rate; nearly all patients in whom this interval was longer than 2 months died. In most cases the condition for which chloramphenicol had been prescribed did not justify its use (Polak *et al.,* 1972). It has been suggested that, because there are no reported cases in which aplasia of the bone marrow has followed the parenteral administration of chloramphenicol, it is possible that when the drug is taken orally some component of the intestinal flora may degrade it, with the formation and absorption of metabolic products that depress the bone marrow (Holt, 1967).

The risk of aplastic anemia does not contraindicate the use of chloramphenicol in situations in which it is necessary; however, it emphasizes that (1) the drug should never be employed in diseases readily, safely, and effectively treatable with other antimicrobial agents or in undefined situations, (2) repeated courses of the drug must be avoided if at all possible, (3) patients who receive chloramphenicol must be seen frequently by their physicians for blood studies, and therapy must be stopped immediately if bone-marrow effects become apparent, and (4) patients must be instructed to report immediately the occurrence of any bleeding tendency or sore throat or any other symptom that may be indicative of a new infectious process. (See Erslev, 1953; Dameshek, 1960; Best, 1967.)

Toxic and Irritative Effects. Nausea, vomiting, unpleasant taste, diarrhea, and *perineal irritation* may follow the oral administration of chloramphenicol. Differentiation of this type of diarrhea from that due to suprainfection is critical (*see* below); a *low-salt syndrome* may complicate the irritative diarrhea in some instances. Among the rare *toxic effects* produced by this antibiotic are *blurring of vision, digital paresthesias, breaks in chromosomes,* and *inhibition of mitosis in phytohemagglutinin-stimulated lymphocytes. Optic neuritis* may also develop. It occurs in 3 to 5% of children with mucoviscidosis who are given chloramphenicol; there is symmetrical loss of ganglion cells from the retina and atrophy of the fibers in the optic nerve (Cogan *et al.,* 1973). The administration of the vitamin B complex may reverse the neuritis despite continuation of treatment with chloramphenicol (Cocke, 1967).

The development of *anemia* is the most common *toxic* effect of chloramphenicol on the *bone marrow.* This phenomenon is related to dose. It occurs regularly when plasma concentrations are 25 μg/ml or higher, and is observed most often with parenteral therapy and with the use of large doses or prolonged treatment, or both. The drug inhibits the uptake of ^{59}Fe by normoblasts and, to a great extent, the incorporation of this isotope into heme (Ward, 1966). The clinical picture is featured by reticulocytopenia, decrease in hemoglobin, increase in plasma iron, cytoplasmic vacuolation of early erythroid forms and granulocyte precursors, and normoblastosis with a shift to early erythrocyte forms. Complete recovery is the rule after cessation of therapy and occurs in about 12 days (Gussoff and Lee, 1966). The writer has noted this phenomenon frequently in patients given daily doses of 4 g of chloramphenicol.

Fatal chloramphenicol toxicity may develop in *neonates,* especially premature babies, when they are exposed to excessive doses of the drug. Iossifides and coworkers (1963) reported that the antibiotic accumulates in the blood of such children and reaches high concentrations at about the fourth day of treatment. In 1959, Sutherland described three newborn infants who died of "cardiovascular collapse" after receiving daily doses of chloramphenicol of about 200 mg/kg of body weight. Burns and associates (1959) have pointed out that the illness, the *"gray syndrome,"* usually begins 2 to 9 days (average, 4 days) after treatment is started. The manifestations in the first 24 hours are vomiting, refusal to suck, irregular and rapid respiration, abdominal distention, periods of cyanosis, and passage of loose green stools. All the children are severely ill by the end of the first day and, in the next 24 hours, develop flaccidity, an ashen-gray color, and a decrease in temperature. Death occurs in about 40% of the patients, most frequently on the fifth day of life. Those who recover exhibit no sequelae.

Two mechanisms are apparently responsible for this toxic effect in neonates (Weiss *et al.,* 1960): (1) *failure of the drug to be conjugated with glucuronic acid,* due to inadequate activity of glucuronyl transferase in the liver, which is characteristic of the first 3 to 4 weeks of life; and (2) *inadequate renal excretion of unconjugated drug* in the newborn. Excessive plasma concentrations of the glucuronide conjugate are also present, despite low rate of formation, because tubular secretion, the pathway of excretion of this compound, is underdeveloped in the neonate. Children 1 month of age or younger should receive chloramphenicol in a daily dose no larger than 25 mg/kg of body weight; after this age, daily quantities up to 50 mg/kg may be given without difficulty. All babies treated with this antibiotic must be observed very carefully during the entire period of therapy and the drug discontinued at the first sign of toxicity. Toxic effects have not been observed in the newborn when as much as 1 g of the antibiotic has been given every 2 hours to women in labor.

In the *presence of renal insufficiency,* the plasma half-life of biologically active chloramphenicol is not significantly prolonged but that of the conjugated, biologically inactive product is markedly extended (*see* Lindberg *et al.,* 1966). Because of this, the dose of the antibiotic for patients with renal disease is the same as that for normal persons. Although the rate at which chloramphenicol is conjugated with glucuronic acid may be reduced in individuals with hepatic insufficiency, the overall metabolism of the drug is essentially normal. However, the administration of the drug in the *presence of hepatic disease* frequently results in *depression of*

erythropoiesis; this is most intense when ascites and jaundice are present (Suhrland and Weisberger, 1963). About one third of patients with renal insufficiency exhibit the same reaction. Chloramphenicol is removed from the blood to only a very small extent by either peritoneal dialysis or hemodialysis.

Biological Effects Other Than Allergic or Toxic. The administration of chloramphenicol produces changes in the numbers and types of microorganisms that constitute the normal microflora of the alimentary, respiratory, and genital tracts. In some instances, this may lead to *suprainfection* by bacteria (*Staph. aureus, Pseudomonas, Proteus,* and other gram-negative bacteria) and fungi (*Candida* and others). *Oropharyngeal candidiasis* and *acute staphylococcal enterocolitis* may develop. The diagnosis of these suprainfections should be made as early as possible, chloramphenicol therapy must be stopped, and appropriate chemotherapy for the suprainfection must be initiated.

When chloramphenicol is given in large doses by the oral route, the changes in intestinal flora may be responsible, as in the case of the tetracyclines, for a *decrease in plasma prothrombin levels* and a *decrease in urine urobilinogen.* Chloramphenicol can *suppress antibody synthesis* under certain circumstances without altering the normal anamnestic response, and it can prolong homograft survival in animals (Weisberger *et al.,* 1964). However, there is no evidence that the drug inhibits the synthesis of antibody in patients with typhoid or paratyphoid fever.

Therapeutic Uses. *Therapy with chloramphenicol must be limited to those infections in which, on the basis of sensitivity tests, it is the most active agent. When other antimicrobial drugs are available that are equally effective but potentially less toxic than chloramphenicol, they should be used.*

Typhoid Fever. Chloramphenicol is still the drug of choice for the treatment of typhoid fever and other types of systemic salmonella infections. However, epidemics in some parts of the world have been due to strains of *S. typhi* highly resistant to the drug. Although ampicillin is also effective in the management of these infections, studies indicate that, given orally, it is less effective than chloramphenicol in producing a clinical response. However, there are fewer carriers and fewer relapses after ampicillin than after chloramphenicol (*see* Robertson *et al.,*

1968). The occurrence of resistance to the drugs makes it necessary to determine the sensitivity of the microorganisms recovered from patients with these diseases.

Within a few hours after chloramphenicol is administered, *S. typhi* disappears from the blood. Stool cultures frequently become negative in a few days. Clinical improvement is often evident within 48 hours, and fever and other signs of the disease commonly abate within 3 to 5 days. The patient usually becomes afebrile before the intestinal lesions heal; as a result, intestinal hemorrhage and perforation may occur at a time when the clinical condition is rapidly improving. The incidence and the duration of the *carrier state* are not altered. The *dose* of chloramphenicol employed in adults with typhoid fever is 2 g initially, followed by 1 g every 6 hours for 4 weeks. Experience has indicated that intravenous injection of the drug is preferable to the oral route. Relapses usually respond satisfactorily to re-treatment; microorganisms isolated during recurrences are usually still sensitive to the antibiotic *in vitro*.

Bacterial Meningitis. Treatment with chloramphenicol produces excellent results in *H. influenzae meningitis* caused by strains sensitive to the drug. The total daily dose for children should be 50 to 75 mg/kg of body weight, divided into four equal doses given intravenously every 6 hours for 2 weeks. Such therapy is recommended for strains of *H. influenzae* that are resistant to ampicillin; furthermore, dual administration of penicillin G and chloramphenicol is now recommended for *initial* treatment of bacterial meningitis in *children* prior to evaluation of the results of cultures (*see* page 1156).

Anaerobes. Chloramphenicol is quite effective against most anaerobic bacteria; it may be used instead of clindamycin in patients with serious anaerobic infections originating from foci in the bowel or pelvis.

Rickettsial Diseases. The tetracyclines are the preferred agents for the treatment of rickettsial diseases. However, in patients sensitized to these drugs and in those with reduced renal function, as well as in pregnant women, chloramphenicol is the drug of choice. The dramatic effect of chloramphenicol in rickettsial infections has been demonstrated by a number of investigators (*see* Woodward and Wisseman, 1958). *Epidemic, murine, scrub,* and *recrudescent typhus* (Brill's disease) as well as *Rocky Mountain spotted fever* and *Q fever* respond favorably to the antibiotic. The same dose schedule is applicable in all the rickettsial diseases. For adults, the first dose of chloramphenicol is 50 mg/kg of body weight. This is followed by 1 g every 8 hours or 0.5 g every 4 hours. Oral therapy is preferred, whenever possible. The succinate preparation of the drug is used in the same quantities when *intravenous* therapy is necessary. The daily dose of chloramphenicol for children with these diseases is 75 mg/kg of body weight, divided into equal quantities and given every 6 to 8 hours; if chloramphenicol palmitate is used, the daily maintenance dose is 100 mg/kg, given at the same intervals. Therapy should be continued until the general condition has improved and fever has been absent for 24 to 48 hours. The duration of illness and the incidence of relapses and complications are greatly reduced.

Rickettsemia and all manifestations of illness are usually brought under control within a few hours to 2 days.

Brucellosis. Chloramphenicol is not as effective as the tetracyclines in the treatment of brucellosis. In cases in which the use of a tetracycline is contraindicated, 750 mg to 1.0 g of chloramphenicol orally every 6 hours may produce a beneficial effect in both the acute and chronic forms of the disease. Relapses usually respond to re-treatment.

Urinary Tract Infections. Chloramphenicol is very helpful for therapy in some cases of urinary tract infection, although the use of this drug for the management of cystitis is unwarranted except in very unusual circumstances. In patients severely ill with acute pyelonephritis, chloramphenicol may be lifesaving; it can be given intravenously (4 g per day) even in the presence of severe renal failure or anuria. Chloramphenicol should be reserved for cases of acute pyelonephritis in which no other effective and safer agent is available.

Miscellaneous Uses. Chloramphenicol (1 g intravenously every 6 hours) may be useful therapy for infections caused by strains of *K. pneumoniae* resistant to cephalosporins and aminoglycosides. Although chloramphenicol therapy is quite effective in *lymphogranuloma venereum, psittacosis,* and infections caused by *Mycoplasma pneumoniae* and *Yersinia (Past.) pestis*, the tetracyclines or other antimicrobial agents are equally good and are preferred.

Acocella, G.; Mattiussi, R.; Nicolis, F. B.; Pallanza, R.; and Tenconi, L. T. Biliary excretion of antibiotics in man. *J. Br. Soc. Gastroent.,* **1968,** *9,* 536–545.

Azzollini, F.; Gazzaniga, A.; Lodola, E.; and Natangelo, R. Elimination of chloramphenicol and thiamphenicol in subjects with cirrhosis of the liver. *Int. J. clin. Pharmac.,* **1972,** *6,* 130–134.

Bach, M. C.; Monaco, A. P.; and Finland, M. Pulmonary nocardiosis: therapy with minocycline and with erythromycin plus ampicillin. *J. Am. med. Ass.,* **1973,** *224,* 1378–1381.

Barr, W. H.; Adir, J.; and Garnetson, L. Decrease of tetracycline absorption in man by sodium bicarbonate. *Clin. Pharmac. Ther.,* **1971,** *12,* 779–784.

Bartz, Q. R. Isolation and characterization of CHLOROMYCETIN. *J. biol. Chem.,* **1948,** *172,* 445–450.

Bergner-Rabinowitz, S., and Davies, A. M. Sensitivity of *Streptococcus pyogenes* types to tetracycline and other antibiotics. *Israel J. med. Sci.,* **1970,** *6,* 393–398.

Best, W. R. Chloramphenicol-associated blood dyscrasias: a review of cases submitted to the American Medical Association Registry. *J. Am. med. Ass.,* **1967,** *201,* 181–188.

Braun, P.; Klein, J. O.; and Kass, E. Susceptibility of genital mycoplasmas to antimicrobial agents. *Appl. Microbiol.,* **1970,** *19,* 62–70.

Burns, L. E.; Hoggman, J. E.; and Cass, A. B. Fatal circulatory collapse in premature infants receiving chloramphenicol. *New Engl. J. Med.,* **1959,** *261,* 1318–1321.

Carey, B. W. Photodynamic response of a new tetracycline. *J. Am. med. Ass.,* **1960,** *172,* 1196.

Cocke, J. G. Chloramphenicol optic neuritis. *Am. J. Dis. Child.,* **1967,** *114,* 424–426.

Cogan, D. C.; Truman, J. T.; and Smith, T. R. Optic neuropathy, chloramphenicol and infantile genetic agranulocytosis. *Invest. Ophthal.,* **1973,** *12,* 534–537.

Cohlan, S. Q.; Bevelander, G.; and Tiamsic, T. Growth inhibition of prematures receiving tetracycline: clinical and laboratory investigation. *Am. J. Dis. Child.,* **1963,** *105,* 453–461.

Crounse, R. G. The response of acne to placebos and antibiotics. *J. Am. med. Ass.*, **1965**, *193*, 906–910.

Dameshek, W. B. Editorial. Chloramphenicol—a new warning. *J. Am. med. Ass.*, **1960**, *174*, 1853–1854.

Dawson, C. R.; Ostler, H. B.; Hanna, L.; Hoshiwara, I.; and Jawetz, E. Tetracyclines in the treatment of chronic trachoma in American Indians. *J. infect. Dis.*, **1971**, *124*, 255–263.

Devine, L. F.; Johnson, D. P.; Hagerman, C. R.; Pierce, W. E.; Rhode, S. L.; and Peckinpaugh, R. O. The effect of minocycline on meningococcal nasopharyngeal carrier state in naval personnel. *Am. J. Epidem.*, **1971**, *93*, 337–345.

Ehrlich, J.; Gottlieb, D.; Burkholder, P. R.; Anderson, L. E.; and Prindham, T. G. *Streptomyces venezuelae*, N. sp., the source of CHLOROMYCETIN. *J. Bact.*, **1948**, *56*, 467–477.

Erslev, A. Hematopoietic depression induced by CHLOROMYCETIN. *Blood*, **1953**, *8*, 170–174.

Erslev, A. J., and Wintrobe, M. M. Detection and prevention of drug-induced blood dyscrasias. *J. Am. med. Ass.*, **1962**, *181*, 114–119.

Fabre, J.; Pitton, J. S.; and Kunz, J. P. Distribution and excretion of doxycycline in man. *Chemotherapia*, **1966**, *11*, 73–85.

Finland, M. Commentary. Twenty-fifth anniversary of the discovery of AUREOMYCIN: the place of the tetracyclines in antimicrobial therapy. *Clin. Pharmac. Ther.*, **1974**, *15*, 3–8.

Francis, R. S.; May, J. R.; and Spicer, C. C. Influence of daily penicillin, tetracycline, erythromycin, and sulphamethoxypyridazine on acute exacerbations of bronchitis: a report to the research committee of the British Tuberculosis Association. *Br. med. J.*, **1964**, *1*, 728–732.

Franklin, T. J. Resistance of *Escherichia coli* to tetracyclines: changes in permeability to tetracyclines in *Escherichia coli* bearing transferable resistance factors. *Biochem. J.*, **1967**, *105*, 371–378.

Frimpter, G. W.; Timpanelli, A. E.; Eisenmenger, W. J.; Stein, H. S.; and Ehrlich, L. I. Reversible "Fanconi syndrome" caused by degraded tetracycline. *J. Am. med. Ass.*, **1963**, *184*, 111–113.

Fry, L., and Ramsay, C. A. Tetracycline in acne vulgaris: clinical evaluation and the effect on sebum production. *Br. J. Derm.*, **1966**, *78*, 653–660.

Fulop, M., and Drapkin, A. Potassium depletion syndrome secondary to nephropathy apparently caused by "outdated tetracycline." *New Engl. J. Med.*, **1965**, *272*, 986–989.

Gabuzda, G. J.; Gocke, T. M.; Jackson, G. G.; Grigsby, M. E.; Love, B. D., Jr.; and Finland, M. Some effects of antibiotics on nutrition in man including studies of the bacterial flora of the feces. *A.M.A. Archs intern. Med.*, **1958**, *101*, 476–513.

Gartmann, J. Doxycycline concentrations in lung tissue, bronchial wall and bronchial secretions. *Schweiz. med. Wschr.*, **1972**, *102*, 1484–1486.

Godchaux, W., III, and Herbert, E. The effect of chloramphenicol in intact erythroid cells. *J. molec. Biol.*, **1966**, *21*, 537–553.

Gopalakrishna, K. V., and Lerner, P. I. Tetracycline-resistant pneumococci. Increasing incidence and cross resistance to newer tetracyclines. *Am. Rev. resp. Dis.*, **1973**, *108*, 1007–1010.

Gurgo, C.; Aprion, D.; and Schlessinger, D. Polyribosome metabolism in *Escherichia coli* treated with chloramphenicol, neomycin, spectinomycin or tetracycline. *J. molec. Biol.*, **1969**, *45*, 205–220.

Gussoff, B. D., and Lee, S. L. Chloramphenicol-induced hematopoietic depression: a controlled comparison with tetracycline. *Am. J. med. Sci.*, **1966**, *251*, 8–15.

Guttler, R. B., and Beatty, H. N. Minocycline in the chemoprophylaxis of meningococcal disease. *Antimicrob. Agents Chemother.*, **1972**, *1*, 397–402.

Harwick, H. J., and Fekety, F. R., Jr. The antibiotic susceptibility of *Mycoplasma hominis*. *J. clin. Path.*, **1969**, *22*, 483–485.

Hinton, N. A. The effect of oral tetracycline HCl and doxycycline on the intestinal flora. *Curr. ther. Res.*, **1970**, *12*, 341–352.

Holt, R. The bacterial degradation of chloramphenicol. *Lancet*, **1967**, *1*, 1259–1260.

Iossifides, I. A.; Smith, I.; and Keitel, H. G. Chloramphenicol-bilirubin interaction in premature babies. *J. Pediat.*, **1963**, *62*, 735–741.

Izaki, K.; Kiuchi, K.; and Arima, K. Specificity and mechanism of tetracycline resistance in a multiple drug resistant strain of *Escherichia coli*. *J. Bact.*, **1966**, *91*, 628–633.

Kunin, C. M., and Finland, M. Restriction imposed on antibiotic therapy by renal failure. *A.M.A. Archs intern. Med.*, **1959**, *104*, 1030–1050.

Kunin, C. M.; Glazko, A. J.; and Finland, M. Persistence of antibiotics in blood of patients with acute renal failure. II. Chloramphenicol and its metabolic products in the blood of patients with severe renal disease or hepatic cirrhosis. *J. clin. Invest.*, **1959**, *38*, 1498–1508.

Kuzucu, E. Y. Methoxyflurane, tetracycline and renal failure. *J. Am. med. Ass.*, **1970**, *211*, 1162–1164.

Leibowitz, B. J.; Hakes, J. L.; Cohn, M. M.; and Levy, E. J. Doxycycline blood levels in normal subjects after intravenous and oral administration. *Curr. ther. Res.*, **1972**, *14*, 820–831.

Lepper, M. H. Effect of large doses of AUREOMYCIN on human liver. *A.M.A. Archs intern. Med.*, **1951**, *88*, 271–283.

Lepper, M. H., and Dowling, H. F. Treatment of pneumococcic meningitis with penicillin plus AUREOMYCIN: studies including observations on an apparent antagonism between penicillin and AUREOMYCIN. *A.M.A. Archs intern. Med.*, **1951**, *88*, 489–494.

Leyden, J. J.; Marples, R. R.; Mills, O. H., Jr.; and Kligman, A. M. Gram-negative folliculitis—a complication of antibiotic therapy in acne vulgaris. *Br. J. Derm.*, **1973**, *88*, 533–538.

Lindberg, A. A.; Nilsson, L. H.; Bucht, H.; and Kallings, L. O. Concentration of chloramphenicol in the urine and blood in relation to renal function. *Br. med. J.*, **1966**, *2*, 724–728.

Lindebaum, J.; Greenough, W. B.; and Islam, M. R. Antibiotic therapy of cholera in children. *Bull. Wld Hlth Org.*, **1967**, *37*, 529–538.

Lucas, J. B. Gonococcal resistance to antibiotics. *Sth. med. J., Nashville*, **1971**, *59*, 22–28.

McCormack, W. M.; Chowdhury, A. M.; Jahangir, N.; Fariduddin Ahmed, A. B.; and Mosley, W. H. Tetracycline prophylaxis in families of cholera patients. *Bull. Wld Hlth Org.*, **1968**, *38*, 787–792.

Moffett, M.; McGill, M. I.; Masterton, G.; and Schofield, C. B. S. Doxycycline HCl (VIBRAMYCIN) as a single dose oral treatment of gonorrhea in women. *Br. J. vener. Dis.*, **1972**, *48*, 126–128.

Neuvonen, P. J.; Gothoni, G.; Hackman, R.; and Bjorksten, K. Interference of iron with the absorption of tetracyclines in man. *Br. med. J.*, **1970**, *4*, 532–534.

Neuvonen, P. J., and Penttilä, O. Interaction between doxycycline and barbiturates. *Br. med. J.*, **1974**, *1*, 535–536.

Penttilä, O.; Neuvonen, P. J.; Aho, K.; and Lehtovaara, R. Interaction between doxycycline and some antiepileptic drugs. *Br. med. J.*, **1974**, *2*, 470–472.

Polak, B. C. P.; Wesseling, H.; Herxheimer, A.; and Meyler, L. Blood dyscrasias attributed to chloramphenicol. *Acta med. scand.*, **1972**, *192*, 409–414.

Pride, G. L.; Cleary, R. E.; and Hamburger, R. J. Disseminated intravascular coagulation associated with tetracycline-induced hepatorenal failure during pregnancy. *Am. J. Obstet. Gynec.*, **1973**, *115*, 585–586.

Robertson, R. P.; Wahab, M. F. A.; and Raasch, F. O. Evaluation of chloramphenicol and ampicillin in *Sal-*

monella enteric fever. *New Engl. J. Med.,* **1968,** *278,* 171–176.

Shaw, W. V.   Comparative enzymology of chloramphenicol resistance. *Ann. N.Y. Acad. Sci.,* **1971,** *182,* 234–242.

Shaw, W. V., and Brodsky, R. F.   Characterization of chloramphenicol acetyltransferase from chloramphenicol-resistant *Staphylococcus aureus. J. Bact.,* **1968,** *95,* 28–36.

Shils, M. E.   Renal disease and the metabolic effects of tetracycline. *Ann. intern. Med.,* **1963,** *58,* 389–408.

Smadel, J. E., and Jackson, E. B.   CHLOROMYCETIN, an antibiotic with chemotherapeutic activity in experimental rickettsial and viral infections. *Science, Wash.,* **1947,** *106,* 418–419.

Smith, C. B.; Friedewald, W. T.; and Chanock, R. M.   Shedding of *Mycoplasma pneumoniae* after tetracycline and erythromycin therapy. *New Engl. J. Med.,* **1967,** *276,* 1172–1175.

Suhrland, L. F., and Weisberger, A. S.   Chloramphenicol toxicity in liver and renal disease. *Archs intern. Med.,* **1963,** *112,* 747–754.

Sutherland, J. M.   Fatal cardiovascular collapse of infants receiving large amounts of chloramphenicol. *A.M.A. J. Dis. Child.,* **1959,** *97,* 761–767.

Thatcher, R. W.; Pazin, G.; and Domescik, G.   Gonorrheal urethritis in males treated with a single oral dose of minocycline. *Publ. Hlth Rep., Wash.,* **1970,** *85,* 160–162.

Wallerstein, R. O.; Condit, P. K.; Kasper, C. K.; Brown, J. W.; and Morrison, F. R.   Statewide study of chloramphenicol therapy and fatal aplastic anemia. *J. Am. med. Ass.,* **1969,** *208,* 2045–2050.

Ward, H. P.   The effect of chloramphenicol on RNA and heme synthesis in bone marrow cultures. *J. Lab. clin. Med.,* **1966,** *68,* 400–410.

Weinstein, L.; Goldfield, M.; and Chang, T. W.   Infections occurring during chemotherapy: a study of their frequency, type and predisposing factors. *New Engl. J. Med.,* **1954,** *251,* 247–255.

Weisberger, A. S.   Inhibition of protein synthesis by chloramphenicol. *A. Rev. Med.,* **1967,** *18,* 483–494.

Weisberger, A. S.; Daniel, T. M.; and Hoffman, A.   Suppression of antibody synthesis and prolongation of homograft survival by chloramphenicol. *J. exp. Med.,* **1964,** *120,* 183–196.

Weiss, C. F.; Glazko, A. J.; and Weston, J. K.   Chloramphenicol in the newborn infant: a physiologic explanation of its toxicity when given in excessive dose. *New Engl. J. Med.,* **1960,** *262,* 787–794.

Weyman, J.   Tetracyclines and teeth. *Practitioner,* **1965,** *195,* 661–665.

Wheeldon, L. W., and Lehninger, A. L.   Energy-linked synthesis and decay of membrane proteins in isolated rat liver mitochondria. *Biochemistry,* **1966,** *5,* 3533–3545.

Williams, D. N.; Laughlin, L. W.; and Lee, Y.-H.   Minocycline: possible vestibular side-effects. *Lancet,* **1974,** *2,* 744–746.

Monographs and Reviews

Brock, T. D.   Chloramphenicol. *Bact. Rev.,* **1961,** *25,* 32–48. (102 references.)

Dowling, H. F.   *Tetracycline.* Medical Encyclopedia, Inc., New York, **1955.**

Greenberg, P. A., and Sanford, J. P.   Removal and absorption of antibiotics in patients with renal failure undergoing peritoneal dialysis: tetracycline, chloramphenicol, kanamycin, and colistimethate. *Ann. intern. Med.,* **1967,** *66,* 465–479.

Kunin, C. M., and Finland, M.   Clinical pharmacology of the tetracycline antibiotics. *Clin. Pharmac. Ther.,* **1961,** *2,* 51–69. (121 references.)

Lepper, M. H.   AUREOMYCIN (*Chlortetracycline*). Medical Encyclopedia, Inc., New York, **1956.** (769 references.)

Moser, R. H.   Reactions to tetracycline. *Clin. Pharmac. Ther.,* **1966,** *7,* 117–132.

Musselman, M. M.   TERRAMYCIN (*Oxytetracycline*). Medical Encyclopedia, Inc., New York, **1956.** (664 references.)

Pestka, S.   Inhibitors of ribosome functions. *A. Rev. Microbiol.,* **1971,** *25,* 487–562.

Symposium. (Various authors.)   VIBRAMYCIN. *Chemotherapy,* **1968,** *13,* 1–102.

Weisblum, B., and Davies, J.   Antibiotic inhibitors of the bacterial ribosome. *Bact. Rev.,* **1968,** *32,* 493–528. (232 references.)

Woodward, T. E., and Wisseman, C. L., Jr.   CHLOROMYCETIN (*Chloramphenicol*). Medical Encyclopedia, Inc., New York, **1958.** (738 references.)

60 ANTIMICROBIAL AGENTS

[*Continued*]

Drugs Used in the Chemotherapy of Tuberculosis and Leprosy

Louis Weinstein

The pharmacological characteristics and the therapeutic use of each class of compounds employed in the chemotherapy of tuberculosis and leprosy are discussed in this chapter. The treatment of infections in man caused by acid-fast bacteria is still an important and challenging problem. The factors that make the management of mycobacterial diseases difficult in many instances, and even impossible in some, are (1) inadequacy of defense mechanisms in infected human hosts, (2) the metabolic characteristics of mycobacteria, (3) the development of drug resistance in the microorganisms, (4) the lack of bactericidal activity of some of the available drugs, and (5) the capacity of some of the therapeutic agents to produce untoward effects that may preclude their administration or necessitate their use in suboptimal doses.

I. Drugs for Tuberculosis

While all the difficulties mentioned in the first paragraph of this chapter remain, the past decade has witnessed further great improvement in the chemotherapy of tuberculosis, due largely to the availability of two drugs—*ethambutol* and *rifampin*. These have greatly reduced the need for the use of aminosalicylic acid, which now occupies only a minor role, and for streptomycin. *Isoniazid,* however, retains dominant status. These five drugs are discussed in the chronological order of their introduction for tuberculotherapy.

Determination of Drug Sensitivity in Vitro and in Vivo. Microbiological technics, similar to those employed with other microorganisms, have been widely used to determine the *in-vitro* sensitivity of

tubercle bacilli and atypical mycobacteria to various drugs. However, the cultures must be incubated for at least 6 to 8 weeks before the results become significant. Progress in the study of drugs of potential value in the treatment of tuberculosis has also depended greatly on the development of methods for infecting experimental animals with the human strain of *Mycobacterium tuberculosis,* and excellent laboratory technics for the screening of compounds for therapeutic activity are available.

The clinical evaluation of chemotherapy in tuberculosis presents many more and complex problems than does study of the effects of antimicrobial agents in other infections. The chronicity of pulmonary tuberculosis, the unpredictable behavior of untreated lesions, the variability in host resistance, and the emergence of drug-resistant mycobacteria combine to make valid interpretation of the results of treatment difficult; however, in such forms of the disease as miliary dissemination, meningitis, enteritis, and lesions of the bronchi, larynx, and mouth, the changes produced by therapy are usually clear-cut and often dramatic, and evaluation of the effects of drugs is easier and more accurate.

STREPTOMYCIN

A discussion of the pharmacology of streptomycin, including its adverse effects and its uses in infections other than tuberculosis, is presented in Chapter 58. Only those features of the drug related to its antibacterial activity and therapeutic effects in the management of diseases caused by mycobacteria are considered here.

History. Streptomycin was the first clinically effective drug to become available for the treatment of tuberculosis. At first, it was given in large doses, but problems related to toxicity and the development of resistant microorganisms seriously limited its usefulness. This led to administration of the antibiotic in smaller quantities, but streptomycin administered alone still proved to be far from the ideal agent for the management of all forms of this disease. However, after the discovery of other tuberculostatic compounds that, given concurrently with the antibiotic, reduced the rate at which microorganisms became drug resistant despite prolonged exposure, streptomycin reached its full potential in the therapy of tuberculosis.

Antibacterial Activity. Streptomycin is both bacteriostatic and bactericidal for the tubercle bacillus *in vitro*. Concentrations as low as 0.4 μg/ml may inhibit growth. The vast majority of strains of human and bovine *M. tuberculosis* are sensitive to 10 μg/ml. Atypical mycobacteria—photochromogens, scotochromogens, nonchromogens, and rapidly growing species—are not susceptible to streptomycin.

The activity of streptomycin *in vivo* is essentially suppressive. When the antibiotic is administered to experimental animals prior to inoculation with the tubercle bacillus, the development of disease is not prevented. Infection progresses until the animals' immunological mechanisms respond. The presence of viable microorganisms in nonsloughing abscesses at the sites of injection and in the regional lymph nodes, together with the fact that omission of the drug, after many months of therapy, results in rapid spread of infection, adds support to the concept that the only activity of streptomycin *in vivo* is to suppress, not to eradicate, the tubercle bacillus. The antibiotic penetrates tuberculous cavities. Diffusion of streptomycin from extracellular fluid to intracellular fluid is relatively poor.

Bacterial Resistance. Large populations of all strains of tubercle bacilli include a number of cells that are markedly resistant to the antibiotic. These resistant microorganisms arise as a result of random mutations, as discussed in Chapter 55. In a pure culture of *M. tuberculosis,* 1 out of 1 billion is resistant to 1 μg/ml of streptomycin and 1 out of 200 billion is not inhibited by 100 μg/ml; in the presence of the antibiotic, selection for these microorganisms obviously occurs.

There is every reason to believe that selection for resistant tubercle bacilli occurs *in vivo* as it does *in vitro*. In general, the longer therapy is continued, the greater is the incidence of resistance to streptomycin. In some individuals, this develops within 1 month; after 4 months, as many as 80% of patients harbor insensitive tubercle bacilli, half of which are not inhibited by concentrations of drug as high as 1000 μg/ml. If pulmonary cavities fail to close or the sputum is not sterilized within 2 to 3 months, the remaining bacteria are resistant to the antibiotic and treatment is not effective. The concomitant use of streptomycin with another tuberculostatic agent *delays but does not always prevent the emergence of resistance*. If therapy is necessary for a long period, the bacilli may eventually become insensitive to both drugs. The clinical significance of this problem is discussed later in this chapter.

Preparations, Routes of Administration, and Dosage. The preparations and routes of administration of streptomycin are considered in detail in Chapter 58. The dosage schedules used in the treatment of various forms of tuberculosis are discussed below.

Therapeutic Status. Since other effective tuberculostatic agents have become available, the use of streptomycin for the treatment of pulmonary tuberculosis has been very sharply reduced; some schedules for re-treatment still include the drug. Many clinicians prefer to give three drugs, of which streptomycin may be one, for the most serious forms of tuberculosis, such as disseminated disease or meningitis.

The use of streptomycin in the chemotherapy of tuberculosis is described below.

AMINOSALICYLIC ACID

History. The demonstration by Bernheim that benzoic and salicylic acids increase the oxygen consumption of tubercle bacilli, the speculation that similar compounds play a role in the normal metabolism of *M. tuberculosis,* and the theory that related substances might have a reverse effect led to the discovery of the tuberculostatic activity of *aminosalicylic acid* (PAS, para-aminosalicylic acid). The metabolic effect of this acid was found by Lehmann (1946) to be associated with suppression of both growth and multiplication of the microorganisms. When examination of the *in-vivo* effects of the drug in experimental tuberculosis revealed that it altered the course of the disease, aminosalicylic acid was subjected to clinical trial.

Chemistry. The structural formula of aminosalicylic acid is as follows:

Aminosalicylic Acid

Aqueous solutions of the drug are very unstable and undergo decarboxylation. The sodium salt of aminosalicylic acid is much more stable, is highly soluble in water, and forms slightly alkaline solutions that do not decompose at room temperature but are decomposed by heat.

Antibacterial Activity. Aminosalicylic acid is bacteriostatic. *In vitro,* most strains of *M. tuberculosis* are sensitive to a concentration of 1 μg/ml. The antimicrobial activity of aminosalicylic acid is highly specific, and microorganisms other than *M. tuberculosis* are unaffected. Most atypical mycobacteria are not inhibited by the drug.

Studies of the treatment of experimental infections caused by human strains of *M. tuberculosis* indicate that this drug exerts a beneficial effect on the disease. However, the doses of aminosalicylic acid required are relatively large, and the compound must be present continuously. Aminosalicylic acid alone is of little value in the treatment of tuberculosis in man; it is much less effective than either streptomycin or isoniazid.

Bacterial Resistance. Strains of tubercle bacilli insensitive to several hundred times the usual bacteriostatic concentration of aminosalicylic acid can be produced *in vitro*. In general, resistance to aminosalicylic acid is somewhat more difficult to induce *in vitro* than is that to streptomycin.

Resistant strains of tubercle bacilli also emerge in patients treated with aminosalicylic acid, but much more slowly than with streptomycin. Insensitive microorganisms usually are not detectable until the drug has been given for at least 4 months; at the end of about 1 year, over 75% of the strains recovered are no longer highly sensitive.

The tuberculostatic effect of aminosalicylic acid is increased by the addition of either streptomycin or isoniazid, and concurrent exposure of tubercle bacilli to these drugs *in vitro* or *in vivo* delays the emergence of resistant microorganisms to each of the agents. However, appearance of insensitivity is not prevented and will eventually develop to any of the compounds if exposure is sufficiently long.

Mechanism of Action. Aminosalicylic acid is a structural analog of para-aminobenzoic acid, and its mechanism of action appears to be very similar to that of the sulfonamides (*see* Chapter 56). Since the sulfonamides are ineffective against *M. tuberculosis* and aminosalicylic acid is inactive against sulfonamide-susceptible bacteria, it is probable that the enzymes responsible for folate biosynthesis in various microorganisms may be quite exacting in their capacity to distinguish various analogs from the true metabolite (*see* Pratt, 1973).

Pharmacological Actions. Despite the close chemical relationship between aminosalicylic acid and salicylic acid, none of the pharmacodynamic actions of aminosalicylic acid is similar to those of the salicylates. Aminosalicylic acid is neither analgesic nor antipyretic; its administration does not produce the syndrome of salicylism. Indeed, aside from its specific tuberculostatic activity, all pharmacodynamic properties relate to side effects.

Absorption, Distribution, and Excretion. Aminosalicylic acid is readily absorbed from the gastrointestinal tract. A single oral dose of 4 g of the free acid produces maximal plasma concentrations of about 75 μg/ml within 1½ to 2 hours. The sodium salt is absorbed even more rapidly. The drug appears to be distributed throughout the total body water and reaches high concentrations in pleural fluid and caseous tissue. However, values in cerebrospinal fluid are low, perhaps because of active outward transport (Spector and Lorenzo, 1973).

The drug has a half-life of about 1 hour, and plasma concentrations are negligible within 4 to 5 hours after a single conventional dose. Over 80% of the drug is excreted in the urine; more than 50% is in the form of the acetylated compound in man. The largest portion of the remainder is made up of the free acid; small quantities of free and acetylated para-aminosalicyluric and 2,4-dihydroxybenzoic acids are present in the urine (Way *et al.,* 1948). Both aminosalicylic acid and isoniazid are acetylated, and, when both drugs are administered simultaneously, this results in a somewhat higher plasma concentration of free isoniazid than when isoniazid is given alone. The rapid excretion of aminosalicylic acid results in urinary concentrations of 3 to 5 mg/ml when conventional doses are used. The free acid is relatively insoluble; the acetylated form is even less soluble. For this reason, the urine should be neutral or alkaline during treatment in order to prevent crystalluria. The use of the sodium salt of aminosalicylic acid reduces markedly the risk of this complication. Excretion of aminosalicylic acid is greatly retarded in the presence of renal dysfunction, and the use of the drug is not recommended in such patients. Probenecid decreases the renal excretion of this agent.

Preparations, Routes of Administration, and Dosage. *Sodium Aminosalicylate,* U.S.P. (NATRI-PAS, PAMISYL SODIUM, PAS-C, and others), is available in official *tablets* containing 500, 690, and 1000 mg. Capsules, enteric-coated tablets, and granules are also supplied. *Potassium Aminosalicylate,* N.F. (PARASAL POTASSIUM, PASKALIUM), *Calcium Aminosalicylate,* N.F. (PARASAL CALCIUM), and *Aminosalicylic Acid,* N.F. (PAMISYL, PARASAL, REZIPAS), are marketed in a variety of preparations for oral use. Aminosalicylic acid is administered orally in a daily dose of 8 to 12 g; when given simultaneously with isoniazid, the dose may be reduced to 6 to 9 g per day. To obtain an equivalent amount of aminosalicylic acid, the dose of the Na^+ salt must be increased 38%; the corresponding values for the Ca^{2+} and K^+ salts are 30% and 24%, respectively. Because it is a gastric irritant, the drug is best administered after meals, the daily intake being divided into three or four equal-sized doses. If tolerated, the total daily requirement may be administered at one time. Various other clinical problems obviously may dictate the avoidance of a particular salt of the drug.

Untoward Effects. The incidence of untoward effects associated with the use of aminosalicylic acid is 2 to 4%. Irritation of the gastrointestinal tract, as evidenced by *anorexia, nausea, epigastric pain, abdominal distress,* and *increased frequency of bowel evacuation,* is common. Continuation of therapy may result in aggravation of all the symptoms and eventually produces severe *diarrhea.* Drug administration with meals or aluminum hydroxide or a rest period of up to 2 weeks may be beneficial. After such a rest, the starting dose should be small (2 g per day) and gradually increased to the full daily requirement. Patients with peptic ulcer tolerate the drug poorly; indeed, this agent may induce *peptic ulceration* in some individuals. Cessation of treatment is usually followed by rapid healing of such lesions.

A mild degree of malabsorption may be caused by increased peristalsis. Aminosalicylic acid may also cause *renal irritation,* and the drug should not be used in patients with renal disease.

Other untoward effects include inhibition of *prothrombin synthesis* in the liver; however, the prothrombinopenia is usually not sufficiently great to be of clinical significance. Prolonged treatment with 20 g of aminosalicylic acid per day may produce *goiter,* with or without myxedema, in about 20% of patients.

Hypersensitivity reactions to aminosalicylic acid are common. These are most frequent between the second and seventh week of treatment, especially in the fourth and fifth weeks. *High fever* may develop abruptly, with intermittent spiking, or it may appear gradually and be low grade. *Generalized malaise, joint pains,* or *sore throat* may be present at the same time. *Skin eruptions of various types* appear as isolated reactions or accompany the fever. *Neurological manifestations* such as *myeloradiculoneuritis* or *meningitis* have been noted. Continued administration of aminosalicylic acid in the presence of fever or minor complaints such as headache, malaise, and pruritus may lead to *hepatic damage* of varying degree, including acute and fatal *hepatic necrosis; pancreatitis* and *nephritis* may also occur. A clinical picture that resembles *infectious mononucleosis* is an uncommon manifestation of hypersensitivity. The characteristic heterophil agglutinin reaction is negative. If therapy is not stopped when this syndrome develops with high-grade fever, *granulopenia, exfoliative dermatitis,* and *encephalopathy* may supervene. *Death* has occurred from these severe reactions in some cases. Among the hematological abnormalities that have been observed are *leukopenia, agranulocytosis, eosinophilia, lymphocytosis* with abnormal cells, and *thrombopenia. Acute hemolytic anemia* may appear in some instances. The lungs may be the site of two types of allergic reactions to aminosalicylic acid. *Loeffler's syndrome* may develop during the course of therapy. In patients with pulmonary tuberculosis who receive aminosalicylic acid, *perifocal infiltrations* may appear around the tuberculous lesions in the lung; it has been suggested that this may be the counterpart of the Herxheimer reaction and be due to release of tuberculin and the production of a localized tuberculin reaction in the pulmonary tissues.

Because aminosalicylic acid is a relatively strong organic acid, its excretion is accompanied by loss of fixed cation in the urine, and there is the possibility that *acidosis* may develop, especially in children. The administration of the sodium salt of the drug prevents this disturbance. A negative potassium balance of clinical significance may develop in patients receiving aminosalicylic acid. The chief extrarenal cause of the electrolyte disturbance is the loss of fluid and cations during the course of the vomiting and diarrhea induced in some individuals; supplemental potassium therapy may be necessary in such cases.

Therapeutic Status. When first introduced, aminosalicylic acid was employed alone in the treatment of tuberculosis. However, it was distinctly infe-

rior to streptomycin, and this led to concurrent therapy, at first with streptomycin and later with isoniazid. The importance of aminosalicylic acid in the management of pulmonary and other forms of tuberculosis has markedly decreased since more active agents, especially ethambutol, have been developed (*see* discussion of chemotherapy of tuberculosis, below).

ISONIAZID

History. The discovery of isoniazid, a highly effective tuberculostatic drug, was somewhat fortuitous. In 1945, Chorine reported that nicotinamide possesses tuberculostatic action. Examination of the compounds related to nicotinamide revealed that many pyridine derivatives possess tuberculostatic activity; among these are congeners of isonicotinic acid. Because the thiosemicarbazones were known to inhibit *M. tuberculosis,* the thiosemicarbazone of isonicotinaldehyde was synthesized and studied. The starting material for this synthesis was the methyl ester of isonicotinic acid, and the first intermediate was isonicotinylhydrazide (isoniazid), a compound that soon proved to be more effective than any other known synthetic or antibiotic tuberculostatic agent. The interesting history of these chemical studies has been reviewed by Fox (1953).

Chemistry and Structure-Activity Relationship. *Isoniazid* is the hydrazide of isonicotinic acid; the structural formula is as follows:

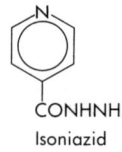

Isoniazid

Only one congener is known that markedly inhibits the multiplication of the tubercle bacillus, the isopropyl derivative *iproniazid* (1-isonicotinyl-2-isopropylhydrazide). This compound, which is a potent inhibitor of monoamine oxidase, is too toxic for use in man, and it is no longer employed, either for tuberculosis or as an antidepressant (Chapter 12).

Antibacterial Activity. Isoniazid is both tuberculostatic and tuberculocidal *in vitro;* the minimal tuberculostatic concentration is 0.025 to 0.05 $\mu g/ml$. The bacteria undergo one or two divisions before multiplication is arrested. The bactericidal effects of isoniazid are exerted only against actively growing tubercle bacilli; "resting" microorganisms resume normal multiplication when removed from contact with the drug.

Among the various atypical mycobacteria, only *M. kansasii* is usually susceptible to isoniazid. However, sensitivity must always be tested *in vitro,* since the inhibitory concentration required may be rather high.

Isoniazid is highly effective for the treatment of experimental tuberculosis in animals and is strikingly superior to streptomycin. Control of induced infection in guinea pigs is achieved with doses as low as 1 mg per day. Unlike streptomycin, isoniazid penetrates cells with ease and is just as effective against intracellularly located bacilli as it is against those growing in culture media.

Bacterial Resistance. Tubercle bacilli grown *in vitro* in increasing concentrations of isoniazid become insensitive to enormous concentrations of the drug. Cross-resistance between isoniazid and other tuberculostatic drugs does not occur. Present evidence suggests that the mechanism of resistance is related to failure of the drug to penetrate or to be taken up by the microorganisms.

As with the other agents described, treatment with isoniazid also leads to the emergence of resistant strains *in vivo*. The shift from primarily sensitive to mainly insensitive microorganisms occasionally occurs within a few weeks after therapy is started; however, there is considerable variation in the time of appearance of this phenomenon from one case to another. The clinical significance of conversion to resistance to isoniazid is considered later in this chapter.

Mechanism of Action. While the mechanism of action of isoniazid is unknown, there are several hypotheses. These include effects on lipids, nucleic acid biosynthesis, and glycolysis. Youatt (1969) has reviewed the available data. Takayama and associates (1972) have suggested a primary action of isoniazid to inhibit the biosynthesis of mycolic acid. Exposure to isoniazid leads to a loss of acid fastness and a decrease in the quantity of methanol-extractable lipid of the microorganisms. Only isoniazid-sensitive tubercle bacilli take up the drug (Wimpenny, 1967). This uptake appears to be an active process, although most of the drug within the bacilli is the isonicotinic acid metabolite (Jenne and Beggs, 1973).

Absorption, Distribution, and Excretion. Isoniazid is readily absorbed when administered either orally or parenterally. Peak plasma concentrations develop 1 to 2 hours after oral ingestion. There is genetic variation in the metabolism of this drug in man, which significantly alters the plasma concentrations achieved and its half-life in the circulation (*see* below). The half-life of the drug may be prolonged in the presence of hepatic insufficiency. The simultaneous administration of aminosalicylic acid produces higher concentrations of free active isoniazid in the blood by reducing the degree of acetylation (*see* Lauener and Favez, 1959).

Isoniazid diffuses readily into all body fluids and cells. The drug is detectable in significant quantities in pleural and ascitic fluids; concentrations in the cerebrospinal fluid are about 20% of those in the plasma. Isoniazid penetrates well into caseous material. The concentration of the agent is initially higher in the plasma and muscle than in the infected tissue, but the latter retains the drug for a long time in quantities well above those required for bacteriostasis (*see* Robson and Sullivan, 1963).

From 75 to 95% of a dose of isoniazid is excreted in the urine in 24 hours; all of this represents drug metabolites (Des Prez and Boone, 1961). The main excretion products in man are acetylisoniazid, formed by acetylation, and isonicotinic acid, a hydrolysis product. Small quantities of an isonicotinic acid conjugate, probably isonicotinyl glycine, one or more isonicotinyl hydrazones, and traces of N-methylisoniazid are also detectable in the urine.

The human population shows genetic heterogeneity with regard to the rate of acetylation of isoniazid (and certain other compounds) (Mandel *et al.,* 1959; Evans *et al.,* 1960; Sunahara *et al.,* 1961). There is bimodal distribution of slow and rapid inactivators of the drug; this variability is due to differences in the activity of an acetyl transferase.

The rate of inactivation is not influenced by sex or age, but the frequency of the "slow" phenotype is dependent on race. The lowest incidence of slow inactivators is found among the Eskimos and Japanese, while the majority of Egyptians, Israelis, and Scandinavians display this phenotype. The incidence of slow inactivators among Americans is approximately 50% (Mattila and Tiitinen, 1967; La Du, 1972). There is a higher percentage of rapid inactivators among diabetics, especially children, than in nondiabetic individuals. The data of Evans and coworkers (1960) indicate that the slow inactivator is an autosomal homozygous recessive. Rapid inactivators are therefore of two genotypes—heterozygotes and homozygous dominants. Heterozygotes have significantly higher plasma isoniazid concentrations than do the homozygous subjects.

Six hours after oral administration of 4 mg/kg of isoniazid to individuals who acetylate the drug slowly, plasma concentrations are higher than 0.8 μg/ml, while in rapid inactivators they are 0.2 μg/ml or less; values in the latter group at 6 hours are about 50% of peak values (Harris, 1963). In general, the concentration of active isoniazid in the circulation of rapid inactivators is about one fifth to one half of that present in persons who acetylate the drug slowly. In the whole population, the half-life of isoniazid varies from 1 to 3 hours; as described, the distribution is bimodal. Patients who inactivate isoniazid at a slow rate tend to develop polyneuritis more often and to experience a higher frequency and more rapid reversal of infectiousness than do those who acetylate the drug rapidly (Evans *et al.*, 1960).

The renal clearance of isoniazid is dependent to only a small degree on the status of renal function, but patients who are slow inactivators of the drug may accumulate toxic concentrations if their renal function is impaired. It has been suggested (Bowersox *et al.*, 1973) that 300 mg per day of the drug can be administered safely to individuals in whom the plasma creatinine concentration is less than 12 mg/100 ml. Patients with more severe renal dysfunction may receive the same daily dose, but the plasma concentrations of the drug should be monitored. In slow inactivators, the dose should be reduced to ensure a concentration of less than 1 μg/ml, 24 hours after the preceding dose; reduction to less than 200 mg per day will rarely be necessary.

Preparations, Routes of Administration, and Dosage. *Isoniazid,* U.S.P. (*isonicotinic acid hydrazide;* HYZYD, NICONYL, NYDRAZID, and others), is available in official tablets containing 100 and 300 mg, as a syrup containing 10 mg/ml, and as an injection in a concentration of 100 mg/ml. The commonly used total daily dose of the drug is 5 mg/kg, with a maximum of 300 mg. This is given orally in two or three equally divided and spaced doses; it has been suggested that the total daily requirement may be administered at one time, but this may lead to an increase in the neurotoxic effects. Young children tolerate up to 20 mg/kg daily without difficulty; in severe disease such as meningitis, doses as high as 25 to 30 mg/kg daily have been given with good results.

The effects on dosage of renal disease and genetic variation in the rate of acetylation of isoniazid have been discussed above.

Untoward Effects. The overall incidence of untoward effects due to isoniazid is dose related; it is only about 1% when the daily intake is 3 mg/kg, but it rises sharply as this is increased.

Hypersensitivity to isoniazid is uncommon, but may result in *fever,* various *skin eruptions, hepatitis,* and *morbilliform, maculopapular, purpuric,* and *urticarial rashes. Hematological reactions* may also occur (agranulocytosis, eosinophilia, thrombopenia, anemia). *Vasculitis* associated with *antinuclear antibodies* may appear during treatment but disappears when it is stopped. *Arthritic*

symptoms (*back pain,* bilateral proximal interphalangeal *joint involvement, arthralgia* of the knees, elbows, and wrists, and the *"shoulder-hand" syndrome*) have been attributed to this agent (Good *et al.*, 1965; Doust and Moatamed, 1968).

The most important side effects of the drug are related to its direct toxicity, especially for the *peripheral* and *central nervous systems. Peripheral neuritis* is the most common reaction and is said to occur in 17% of patients receiving 6 mg/kg of isoniazid daily. The neuropathological changes associated with this untoward effect include disappearance of synaptic vesicles, mitochondrial swelling or condensation, and fragmentation of axon terminals; alterations of the lumbar and sacral spinal ganglia and spinal cord occur occasionally (Schröder, 1970a, 1970b). Because the urinary excretion of pyridoxine is increased and the clinical picture resembles that of pyridoxine deficiency, the prophylactic administration of 100 mg of pyridoxine per day is recommended. The use of this quantity of the vitamin prevents the development not only of peripheral neuritis but also of most other nervous system dysfunction in practically all instances, even when therapy is carried on for as long as 2 years.

Convulsions may occur in patients with no prior history of seizure disorder when they are given conventional doses of isoniazid. Such convulsions are not generally thought to be related to pyridoxine deficiency; however, the writer has studied two patients who, while being treated with the drug but not taking pyridoxine, developed seizures; blood concentrations of the vitamin were undetectable in both cases, and parenteral administration of large doses of pyridoxine rapidly terminated the seizures.

Optic neuritis followed by *atrophy* may occur during therapy with isoniazid. Vision must be monitored, and ophthalmoscopic examination should be carried out at periodic intervals in persons receiving the drug; early cessation of treatment usually results in resolution of the ocular abnormality. *Muscle twitching, dizziness, ataxia, paresthesias, stupor,* and *toxic encephalopathy* that may terminate fatally are among other manifestations of the neurotoxicity of isoniazid. A number of *mental abnormalities* may appear during the use of this drug; among these are euphoria, *transient impairment of memory, separation of ideas and reality, loss of self-control,* and *florid psychoses.*

Signs and symptoms of *excessive sedation* or *incoordination* may develop when isoniazid is given to epileptics who are simultaneously being treated with phenytoin. Isoniazid is known to inhibit the parahydroxylation of this anticonvulsant, but the effect is usually significant only in slow inactivators of isoniazid (Kutt *et al.,* 1966).

Although jaundice has been known for some time to be an untoward effect of exposure to isoniazid, it was not until 1970 that it became apparent that *severe hepatic injury* leading to death may occur in some individuals receiving this drug (Garibaldi *et al.,* 1972). Additional studies in adults and children have confirmed this observation; the characteristic pathology is bridging and multilobular necrosis. Continuation of the drug after symptoms of hepatic dysfunction have appeared tends to increase the severity of damage. Although it has been suggested that allergic mechanisms are responsible, this remains to be proven. This is perhaps not consistent with the observation that slow inactivators of the drug appear more susceptible to the reaction. The contributory role of alcoholic hepatitis has also been questioned. Age appears to be a very important factor in determining the risk of hepatotoxicity due to isoniazid. Hepatic damage is rare in patients less than 20 years of age; the complication is observed in 0.3% of those 20 to 34 years old, and the incidence increases to 1.2% and 2.3% in individuals 35 to 49 and greater than 50 years of age, respectively (Public Health Service, 1974). It is more practical to monitor persons receiving the drug for prodromal symptoms of hepatic injury than it is to measure serum transaminase activities, which may be elevated in asymptomatic patients without heralding hepatitis. Patients being treated with isoniazid should be told of the prodromal manifestations (fatigue, weakness, anorexia, malaise). Isoniazid should be administered only with great care to those with preexisting hepatic disease. (*See* Maddrey and Boitnott, 1973; Stead and Texter, 1973.)

Among miscellaneous reactions associated with isoniazid therapy are *dryness of the mouth, epigastric distress, urinary retention* in the male, *methemoglobinemia,* and *tinnitus.* In those with the predisposition to *pyridoxine-deficiency anemia,* the administration of isoniazid may result in its appearance in full-blown form. Treatment with large doses of the vitamin gradually returns the blood picture to normal in such cases.

Therapeutic Status. Isoniazid is still the most important drug for the treatment of all types of tuberculosis. Toxic effects can be minimized by prophylactic therapy with pyridoxine and careful surveillance of the patient. The drug must be used in combination with another agent for treatment, although it is used alone for prophylaxis.

Details of the use of isoniazid in the chemotherapy of tuberculosis are described below.

ETHAMBUTOL

History. While screening selected compounds, Thomas and coworkers (1961) found that N,N'-di-*iso*propylethylenediamine was effective in the treatment of experimental tuberculous infections in mice. A number of congeners of this compound were examined; the one that eventually proved to be most tuberculostatic was ethylenediimino-di-l-butanol dihydrochloride; in-vitro and in-vivo studies revealed that the *d* form of this substance (ethambutol) exhibited 200 times more activity than did the *l* isomer.

Chemistry. Ethambutol is a water-soluble and heat-stable compound. The structural formula is as follows:

$$H-\underset{\underset{C_2H_5}{|}}{\overset{\overset{CH_2OH}{|}}{C}}-NH-CH_2-CH_2-HN-\underset{\underset{CH_2OH}{|}}{\overset{\overset{C_2H_5}{|}}{C}}-H$$

Ethambutol

Antibacterial Activity. About 75% of strains of the human type of *M. tuberculosis* are sensitive to 1 μg/ml of ethambutol. Bovine tubercle bacilli and photochromogenic microorganisms are inhibited by similar concentrations, but *M. avium* as well as scotochromogenic and nonchromogenic mycobacteria are less predictably affected (Karlson, 1961). Ethambutol has no effect on other bacteria. It suppresses the growth of isoniazid- and streptomycin-resistant tubercle bacilli. Resistance to ethambutol develops very slowly and with difficulty *in vitro.*

Mycobacteria take up ethambutol rapidly when the drug is added to cultures that are in the exponential growth phase. However, growth is not significantly inhibited before about 24 hours. The precise mechanism of action of ethambutol is unknown (*see* Beggs and Ayran, 1972; Jenne and Beggs, 1973).

The therapeutic ratio of ethambutol given orally to animals infected with *M. tuberculosis* is similar to that of isoniazid. When given parenterally, it is superior to streptomycin. Bacterial resistance to the drug develops *in vivo* when it is given alone.

Absorption, Distribution, and Excretion. About 75 to 80% of an orally administered dose of ethambutol is absorbed from the gastrointestinal tract. Plasma concentrations are maximal in man 2 to 4 hours after the drug is taken and are proportional to the dose. A single dose of 25 mg/kg produces a plasma concentration of about 5 μg/ml at 2 hours. The drug has a relatively long half-life; about 50% of the peak concentration is present in the blood at 8 hours and less than 10% at 24 hours. The drug enters erythrocytes with ease; 1 hour after an intravenous dose two to three times as much ethambutol is present in the erythrocytes as in the plasma. Red blood cells thereby serve as a depot from which the drug slowly enters the plasma.

Within 24 hours, 50% of an ingested dose of ethambutol is excreted unchanged in the urine; up to 15% is excreted in the form of two metabolites, an aldehyde and a dicarboxylic acid derivative (Place and Thomas, 1963; Peets *et al.*, 1965). Although it is not certain whether ethambutol is excreted by tubular secretion or solely by glomerular filtration, the latter is thought to play the primary role (Strauss and Erhardt, 1970).

Preparations, Route of Administration, and Dosage. *Ethambutol Hydrochloride*, U.S.P. (MYAMBUTOL), is available in official compressed tablets containing 100 or 400 mg of the *d* isomer. The adult dose is 15 to 25 mg/kg, given once a day. Dosage information is not available for children under 13 years of age.

Ethambutol accumulates in patients with impaired renal function, and adjustment of dosage is necessary. A suggested schedule appears in Table 55–2 (page 1109).

Untoward Effects. Ethambutol produces very few reactions. Daily doses of less than 25 mg/kg are minimally toxic. Among the side effects that have been observed are *dermatitis, pruritus, joint pain, gastrointestinal upset, abdominal pain, fever, malaise, headache, dizziness, mental confusion, disorientation,* and possible *hallucination. Numbness* and *tingling of the fingers* due to *peripheral neuritis* are infrequent. *Anaphylaxis* and *leukopenia* are rare.

The most important side effect is *optic neuritis,* resulting in *decrease of visual acuity* and *loss of ability to perceive the color green.* This is quite uncommon with a dose of 25 mg/kg per day but occurs more often with 50 mg/kg per day. The intensity of the visual difficulty is related to the duration of therapy after decrease in visual acuity first becomes apparent, and it may be unilateral or bilateral. Recovery usually occurs when ethambutol is withdrawn; the time required is a function of the degree of visual impairment (Place and Thomas, 1963).

Ethambutol therapy results in an increased concentration of urate in the blood in about 50% of patients, due to decreased renal excretion of uric acid. The effect may be detectable as early as 24 hours after a single dose or as late as 90 days after treatment is started. This untoward effect is possibly enhanced by isoniazid and pyridoxine (Postlethwaite *et al.*, 1972).

Therapeutic Status. Ethambutol has been used with notable success in the therapy of human tuberculosis of various forms, in combination with isoniazid. Because of greater tuberculostatic activity, lower incidence of toxic side effects, and better patient acceptance, it has essentially replaced aminosalicylic acid.

The use of ethambutol in the chemotherapy of tuberculosis is described below.

RIFAMPIN

The rifamycins are a group of structurally similar, complex macrocyclic antibiotics produced by *Streptomyces mediterranei;* rifampin is a semisynthetic derivative of one of these—rifamycin B.

Chemistry. The drug is a zwitterion and is soluble in organic solvents and in water at acidic pH (Maggi *et al.*, 1966). It has the following structure:

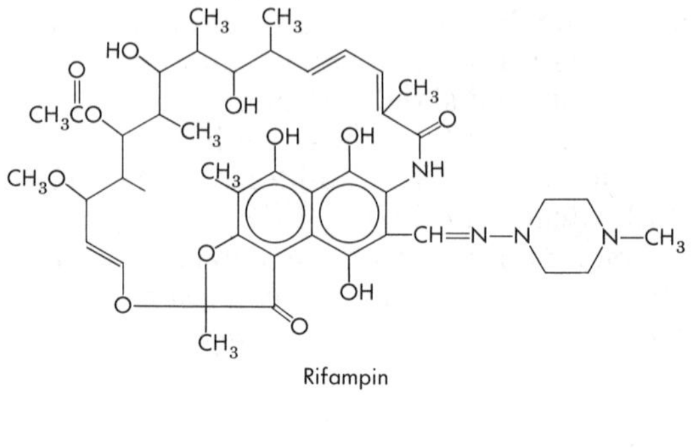

Rifampin

Antibacterial Activity. Rifampin inhibits the growth of most gram-positive bacteria, as well as gram-negative microorganisms such as *Escherichia coli, Pseudomonas,* indole-positive and -negative *Proteus,* and *Klebsiella* (*see* Atlas and Turck, 1968; Kunin *et al.,* 1969). It is less active than penicillin G but slightly more effective than erythromycin, lincomycin, and cephalothin against gram-positive microorganisms; it is distinctly inferior to tetracycline, chloramphenicol, kanamycin, and colistin against gram-negative bacilli (McCabe and Lorian, 1968). The drug is highly active against *Neisseria meningitidis;* minimal inhibitory concentrations range from 0.1 to 0.8 μg/ml (Ivler *et al.,* 1970). There is evidence that the drug may inhibit the growth of certain types of virus (Lester, 1972).

Rifampin in concentrations of 0.005 to 0.2 μg/ml is inhibitory to *M. tuberculosis in vitro* (Verbist and Gyselen, 1968; Lorian and Finland, 1969). Among atypical mycobacteria, *M. kansasii* is inhibited by 0.25 to 1 μg/ml. The majority of strains of *M. scrofulaceum* and *M. intracellulare* are suppressed by concentrations of 4 μg/ml, but certain strains may be resistant to 16 μg/ml. *Mycobacterium fortuitum* is highly resistant to the drug (Molavi and Weinstein, 1971). Rifampin increases the *in-vitro* activity of streptomycin and isoniazid, but not that of ethambutol, against *M. tuberculosis* (Hobby and Lenert, 1972).

Bacterial Resistance. Microorganisms, including mycobacteria, may develop resistance to rifampin rapidly *in vitro* as a one-step process. This also appears to be the case *in vivo,* and the antibiotic must therefore not be used alone in the chemotherapy of tuberculosis. When rifampin has been used for eradication of the meningococcal carrier state, failures have been due to the appearance of drug-resistant bacteria after treatment for as short a period as 2 days (Devine *et al.,* 1971). Microbial resistance to rifampin is due to an alteration of the target of this drug, DNA-dependent RNA polymerase (di Mauro *et al.,* 1969).

Mechanism of Action. Rifampin inhibits DNA-dependent RNA polymerase of mycobacteria and other microorganisms, leading to suppression of initiation of chain formation (but not chain elongation) in RNA synthesis. More specifically, the β subunit of this complex enzyme is the site of action of the drug. RNA polymerase from mammalian cells does not bind rifampin, and RNA synthesis is correspondingly unaffected. (*See* Zillig *et al.,* 1970; Konno *et al.,* 1973.)

Absorption, Distribution, and Excretion. The oral administration of rifampin produces peak plasma concentrations in 2 to 4 hours; after ingestion of 600 mg this value averages 7 μg/ml, but there is considerable variability. Aminosalicylic acid may delay the absorption of rifampin, and adequate plasma concentrations may not be reached. If these agents are used concurrently, they should be given separately at an interval of 8 to 12 hours (*see* Radner, 1973).

Following absorption from the gastrointestinal tract, rifampin is rapidly eliminated in the bile, and an enterohepatic circulation ensues. During this time there is progressive deacetylation of the drug, such that nearly all of the antibiotic in the bile is in the deacetylated form after 6 hours. This metabolite retains essentially full antibacterial activity. Intestinal reabsorption is reduced by deacetylation (as well as by food), and metabolism thus facilitates elimination of the drug. The half-life of rifampin varies from 1½ to 5 hours and is increased in the presence of hepatic dysfunction; it may be *decreased* in patients receiving isoniazid concurrently who are slow inactivators of this drug. There is a progressive shortening of the half-life of rifampin by about 40% during the first 14 days of treatment, due to increased biliary excretion. Up to 30% of a dose of the drug is excreted in the urine; half of this may be unaltered antibiotic. Adjustment of dosage is *not* necessary in patients with impaired renal function.

Rifampin is distributed throughout the body and is present in effective concentrations in many organs and body fluids, including the cerebrospinal fluid. This is perhaps best exemplified by the fact that the drug may impart an orange-red color to the urine, feces, saliva, sputum, tears, and sweat; patients should be so warned. (*See* Furesz *et al.,* 1967; Cohn, 1969; Furesz, 1970; Jenne and Beggs, 1973; Radner, 1973.)

Untoward Effects. Rifampin does not cause untoward effects with great frequency. The most notable problem is the development of *jaundice.* Sixteen deaths associated with this reaction have been recorded in 500,000 treated patients. Alcoholism, preexisting hepatic disease, or the simultaneous administration of other hepatotoxic agents seems to increase the risk of difficulty. Intermittent exposure to rifampin has been reported to be associated with the development of the *hepatorenal syndrome* (Flynn *et al.,* 1974). Elevations of plasma SGOT and alkaline phosphatase activities and bilirubin concentrations have also been reported; these return to normal when therapy is stopped. Biliary excretion of the drug competes with that of contrast media used for study of the gallbladder and may also cause retention of BSP. There is a significant interaction (of unknown mechanism) between rifampin and oral anticoagulants of the coumarin type that leads to a decrease in efficacy of the latter agents. This appears about 5 to 8 days after rifampin administration is started and persists for 5 to 7 days after it is stopped. The drug appears to enhance the catabolism of glucocorticoids and estrogens.

Gastrointestinal disturbances produced by rifampin (*epigastric distress, nausea, vomiting, abdominal cramps, diarrhea*) have occasionally required discontinuation of the drug. Various symptoms related to the nervous system have also been noted, including *fatigue, drowsiness, headache, dizziness, ataxia, confusion, inability to concentrate, generalized numbness, pain in the extremities,* and *muscular weakness.* Among hypersensitivity reactions are *fever, pruritus, urticaria,* various types of *skin eruptions, eosinophilia,* and *soreness of the mouth and tongue. Hemolysis, hemoglobinuria, hematuria, renal insufficiency,* and *acute renal failure* have been observed rarely; these are also thought to be hypersensitivity reactions. *Thrombocytopenia, transient leukopenia,* and *anemia* have occurred during therapy. Since the potential teratogenicity of rifampin is unknown, it is best to avoid the use of this agent during pregnancy; the drug is known to cross the placenta.

Immunoglobulin light-chain proteinurea (either kappa, lambda, or both) has been noted by Graber and associates (1973) in about 85% of patients with tuberculosis treated with rifampin. None of the patients had symptoms or electrophoretic patterns compatible with myeloma. The drug suppresses the transformation of antigen-sensitized lymphocytes by the antigen. The administration of rifampin in conventional doses has been noted to suppress cutaneous hypersensitivity to tuberculin (Mukerjee et al., 1973).

Overdosage with rifampin is characterized by nausea, vomiting, and increasing lethargy. Severe hepatic involvement may follow.

Preparations. *Rifampin,* U.S.P. (RIFADIN, RIMACTANE), is supplied in official capsules containing 300 mg. The dose for adults is 600 mg given once daily, either 1 hour before or 2 hours after a meal.

Children should receive 10 to 20 mg/kg, with a daily maximum of 600 mg, given in the same way.

Therapeutic Status. Despite the long list of untoward effects from rifampin, their incidence is low and treatment seldom has to be interrupted. The drug may find its greatest usefulness in combination with isoniazid in the initial treatment of pulmonary tuberculosis in an outpatient therapeutic regimen (*see* Newman *et al.,* 1974).

The use of rifampin in the chemotherapy of tuberculosis is detailed below.

Rifampin is a drug of choice for chemoprophylaxis of meningococcal disease in household contacts of patients with such infections.

CYCLOSERINE

Cycloserine is a broad-spectrum antibiotic produced by *Streptomyces orchidaceus.* It was first isolated from a fermentation brew in 1955 and was later synthesized.

Chemistry. Cycloserine is D-4-amino-3-isoxazolidone; the structural formula is as follows:

Cycloserine

The drug is stable in alkaline solution but is rapidly destroyed when exposed to neutral or acidic pH.

Antibacterial Activity and Mechanism of Action. Cycloserine is inhibitory for *M. tuberculosis* in concentrations of 5 to 20 µg/ml *in vitro.* There is no cross-resistance between cycloserine and other tuberculostatic agents. While the antibiotic is effective in experimental infections caused by other microorganisms, studies *in vitro* reveal no suppression of growth in cultures made in conventional media. Hoeprich (1963) determined that this is due to the presence of D-alanine in the commonly used culture media and that the amino acid blocks the antibacterial activity of cycloserine. The two compounds are structural analogs, and cycloserine inhibits reactions in which D-alanine is involved in bacterial cell-wall synthesis (*see* Chapter 57, page 1134). The use of media free of D-alanine reveals that the antibiotic inhibits the growth *in vitro* of enterococci, paracolon strains, *E. coli, Staphylococcus aureus,* and *Chlamydia. In vivo,* cycloserine is more effective in man than results in experimental animals would suggest.

Absorption, Distribution, and Excretion. When given orally, cycloserine is rapidly absorbed. Peak plasma concentrations are reached 3 to 4 hours after a single dose and are in the range of 20 to 35 µg/ml in children who receive 20 mg/kg; only small quantities are present after 12 hours. In adults, doses of 750 mg, given at 6-hour intervals, produce plasma concentrations in excess of 50 μg/ml (*see* Storey and McLean, 1957). Multiple doses lead to accumulation of the drug in the circulation after 3 days.

Cycloserine is distributed throughout body fluids and tissues. There is no appreciable blood-brain barrier to the drug, and cerebrospinal fluid concentrations in all patients are approximately the same as those in plasma.

About 50% of a parenteral dose of cycloserine is excreted, in unchanged form, in the urine in the first 12 hours; a total of 65% is recoverable in the active form over a period of 72 hours. Approximately 35% of the antibiotic is metabolized to an as-yet-unidentified substance. The drug may accumulate to toxic concentrations in patients with renal insufficiency; it may be removed from the circulation by dialysis.

Preparations, Routes of Administration, and Dosage. *Cycloserine,* U.S.P. (SEROMYCIN), is available in official capsules containing 250 mg for oral administration. The usual dose for adults is 250 mg twice a day; this is associated with a small risk of toxic reactions. In more severely ill individuals, 500 mg may be given twice a day for short periods. The dose should be adjusted to yield plasma levels no greater than 30 μg/ml in order to minimize toxicity.

Untoward Effects. Reactions to cycloserine most commonly involve the CNS. They tend to appear within the first 2 weeks of therapy and usually disappear when the drug is withdrawn. Among the *central manifestations* are somnolence, headache, tremor, dysarthria, vertigo, confusion, nervousness, irritability, psychotic states with suicidal tendencies, paranoid reactions, catatonic and depressed reactions, twitching, ankle clonus, hyperreflexia, visual disturbances, paresis, and grand mal or absence seizures. In general, seizures can be prevented by the administration of 100 mg of pyridoxine per day. Large doses of cycloserine or the ingestion of ethyl alcohol increases the risk of seizures. Cycloserine is contraindicated in individuals with a history of epilepsy and may be dangerous in persons who are depressed or are experiencing severe anxiety.

Therapeutic Status. Cycloserine should be reserved for those cases in which safer and more effective agents are interdicted either because of a history of clinically significant reactions or because of resistance of the responsible strain of tubercle bacillus. When cycloserine is employed to treat tuberculosis, it must be given together with another effective tuberculostatic agent.

VIOMYCIN

Source and Chemistry. Viomycin is a strongly basic, complex antibiotic produced by an actinomycete. The drug forms essentially neutral sulfate and hydrochloride salts. It is very soluble in water, and aqueous solutions are moderately stable at room temperature.

Antibacterial Activity. Viomycin is most active *in vitro* against *M. tuberculosis.* Practically all strains of this microorganism are inhibited by drug concentrations of 1 to 10 μg/ml. Viomycin is more tuberculostatic than aminosalicylic acid but less so than streptomycin; it is effective in the treatment of experimental tuberculosis produced by streptomycin-resistant microorganisms. Mycobacteria insensitive to kanamycin are also not susceptible to viomycin *in vitro.* On the other hand, viomycin-resistant strains may retain their sensitivity to kanamycin. The drug is not very active against the common gram-negative and gram-positive bacteria. Viomycin inhibits protein synthesis by *M. tuberculosis.*

Absorption, Distribution, and Excretion. The absorption and the excretion of viomycin in man are similar to those of streptomycin. Absorption from the gastrointestinal tract is limited. The intramuscular injection of 25 to 50 mg/kg produces maximal plasma concentrations in 2 hours. A large proportion of a dose of the drug is recoverable in the urine. Penetration into cerebrospinal fluid is poor.

Preparations, Routes of Administration, and Dosage. *Viomycin Sulfate,* U.S.P. (VIOCIN), is available only for parenteral administration. Vials containing 1 or 5 g of powder are marketed. The usual dose of viomycin is two injections of 1 g each, 12 hours apart, not more often than twice weekly. The drug must always be given concurrently with another effective tuberculostatic agent.

Untoward Effects. The incidence of untoward effects produced by viomycin is higher than that which follows the administration of streptomycin. *Allergic reactions* include eosinophilia and urticarial, erythematous, or pruritic skin rashes. The most important toxic manifestations involve the *kidney, labyrinth,* and *electrolyte balance.* Patients receiving the drug over extended periods almost invariably exhibit proteinuria, cylindruria, hematuria, and pyuria; these abnormalities most often appear within 2 weeks of initiation of therapy. Nitrogen retention and serious disturbances in electrolyte balance due to urinary loss of calcium, potassium, and chloride, together with an increase in bicarbonate of the blood, have been observed in a number of instances. Renal function usually recovers quite rapidly when treatment is stopped. *Impairment of vestibular function* is quite common and more frequent than with streptomycin. Partial deafness is also a risk. These usually become manifest within a month or more after the institution of viomycin therapy. *Because both streptomycin and viomycin are ototoxic, these agents must never be given concurrently.* Plasma electrolytes, renal function, and eighth-nerve function must be monitored frequently. Patients with renal insufficiency should not be given this agent unless there are compelling reasons for its use, in which case the dose must be reduced and the patient closely supervised for the appearance of toxic reactions.

Therapeutic Status. Viomycin should not be used to treat primary or minimal tuberculosis. While the drug is highly effective in severe forms of pulmonary and extrapulmonary tuberculous infections, it should not be employed even in these, unless its use is dictated by patient hypersensitization or microbial resistance to safer agents. Viomycin is of relatively little value in cases in which extensive fibrosis or extensive caseous necrosis is present or in infections due to atypical mycobacteria.

PYRAZINAMIDE

Chemistry. Pyrazinamide is the synthetic pyrazine analog of nicotinamide. It has the following structural formula:

Pyrazinamide

Antibacterial Activity. Pyrazinamide exhibits tuberculostatic activity *in vitro* only at a slightly acidic pH. The growth of tubercle bacilli within monocytes *in vitro* is completely inhibited by the drug in a concentration of 12.5 μg/ml. Pyrazinamide is more effective than aminosalicylic acid, cycloserine, or viomycin in experimental infections with the human strain of *M. tuberculosis* in mice and guinea pigs. When the drug is used alone *in vivo*, the disease is initially controlled but soon relapses as resistance develops. When it is administered simultaneously with isoniazid, the bacteria remain sensitive but the infection may not be eradicated.

Absorption, Distribution, and Excretion. Pyrazinamide is well absorbed from the gastrointestinal tract, and it is widely distributed throughout the body. The oral administration of 1 g produces plasma concentrations of about 45 μg/ml at 2 hours and 10 μg/ml at 15 hours. The drug is excreted primarily by renal glomerular filtration; urinary concentrations average 50 to 100 μg/ml over several hours after a single dose (Stottmeier *et al.*, 1968). Pyrazinamide is hydrolyzed to pyrazinoic acid and subsequently hydroxylated to 5-hydroxypyrazinoic acid, the major excretory product (Weiner and Tinker, 1972).

Preparations, Route of Administration, and Dosage. *Pyrazinamide*, U.S.P., is marketed in official tablets containing 500 mg. It is available only in hospitals. The daily dosage is 20 to 35 mg/kg orally, given in three or four equally spaced doses. The maximal quantity to be given is 3 g per day, regardless of weight.

Untoward Effects. Injury to the *liver* is the most common and serious side effect of pyrazinamide. When a dose of 3 g per day is administered orally, signs and symptoms of hepatic disease appear in about 15% of patients, jaundice supervenes in 2 to 3%, and death due to *hepatic necrosis* results in rare instances (McDermott *et al.*, 1954). Elevations of the plasma glutamic-oxaloacetic and glutamic-pyruvate transaminases are the earliest abnormalities produced by the drug. All patients who are being treated with pyrazinamide should have studies of hepatic function carried out before the drug is administered; these should be repeated at frequent intervals during the entire period of treatment. If evidence of significant hepatic damage becomes apparent, therapy must be stopped. Pyrazinamide should not be given to individuals with any degree of hepatic dysfunction, unless this is absolutely unavoidable.

The drug inhibits excretion of urate, and acute episodes of gout have occurred. Among other untoward effects that have been observed with pyrazinamide are *arthralgias, anorexia, nausea and vomiting, dysuria, malaise,* and *fever. Diabetes mellitus* may become difficult to control in patients who are receiving the drug. Fatal *hemoptysis* during the treatment of pulmonary tuberculosis with pyrazinamide has been reported.

Therapeutic Status. Pyrazinamide is a secondary agent. It is less effective and considerably more toxic than several of the other drugs discussed above. *All patients who are being treated with pyrazinamide should be hospitalized.*

ETHIONAMIDE

Chemistry. Synthesis and study of a variety of congeners of thioisonicotinamide revealed that an alpha-ethyl derivative, ethionamide, is considerably more effective than the parent compound. Ethionamide is a yellow substance, practically insoluble in water, with a faint-to-moderate sulfide odor. It has the following structural formula:

Ethionamide

Antibacterial Activity. The multiplication of human strains of *M. tuberculosis* is suppressed by concentrations of ethionamide ranging from 0.6 to 2.5 μg/ml. Resistance can develop rapidly *in vitro.* Bacilli resistant to other tuberculostatic agents are sensitive to ethionamide. Bovine tubercle bacilli and BCG are less susceptible, being suppressed by levels of 5 μg/ml. Approximately 75% of photochromogenic mycobacteria are inhibited by a concentration of 10 μg/ml or less; the scotochromogens are more resistant. Ethionamide is very effective in the treatment of experimental tuberculosis in animals, although its activity varies greatly with the animal model studied (Rist *et al.*, 1959).

Absorption, Distribution, and Excretion. The oral administration of 1 g of ethionamide yields peak plasma concentrations of about 20 μg/ml in 3 hours; the concentration at 9 hours is 3 μg/ml. The drug has a shorter half-life than does isoniazid. Because of gastric irritation, about 50% of patients are unable to tolerate a single dose larger than 500 mg.

Ethionamide is rapidly and widely distributed; the concentrations in the blood and various organs are approximately equal. Significant concentrations are present in cerebrospinal fluid. Ethionamide, like aminosalicylic acid, inhibits the acetylation of isoniazid *in vitro*.

Less than 1% of ethionamide is excreted in active form in the urine. Metabolites detected in the urine include three dihydropyridines: carbamoyl, thiocarbamoyl, and S-oxocarbamoyl (Bieder *et al.*, 1966).

Preparations, Route of Administration, and Dosage. *Ethionamide*, U.S.P. (TRECATOR-SC), is administered only by the oral route. Tablets containing 250 mg of the drug are available. The initial dose for adults is 250 mg, given twice a day. This is increased by 125 mg per day every 5 days until 1 g is being given daily; this dose must not be exceeded. The drug is best taken with meals in order to minimize gastric irritation.

Untoward Effects. The most common reactions to ethionamide involve the stomach; *anorexia, nausea,* and *vomiting* are common problems. A metallic taste may also be noted. *Severe postural hypotension, mental depression, drowsiness,* and *asthenia* are common. *Convulsions* and *peripheral neuropathy* are rare. Other reactions referable to the nervous system include *olfactory disturbances, blurred vision, diplopia, dizziness, paresthesias, headache, restlessness,* and *tremors. Severe allergic skin rashes, purpura, stomatitis, gynecomastia, impotence, menorrhagia, acne,* and *alopecia* have also been observed. *Acute rheumatic symptoms* have been noted. Increased difficulty in the management of *diabetes mellitus* may become a problem in patients with this disease who are taking ethionamide.

Hepatitis has been associated with the use of the drug in about 5% of cases. This has usually appeared in diabetics and is accompanied by elevated plasma transaminase activities (Simon *et al.*, 1969); liver biopsy has revealed periportal round-cell infiltration, a few swollen and destroyed hepatic cells, areas of fibrosis, and hepatic-cell regeneration. The signs and symptoms of hepatotoxicity clear when treatment is stopped (Phillips and Tashman, 1963). Hepatic function should be assessed at regular intervals in patients receiving ethionamide.

Therapeutic Status. Ethionamide is a secondary agent, to be used in combination with other drugs only when therapy with primary agents is ineffective or contraindicated. (*See* Schwartz, 1966; Lees, 1967.)

OTHER DRUGS

Kanamycin, discussed in detail in Chapter 58, inhibits the growth of *M. tuberculosis in vitro* in a concentration of 10 µg/ml or less. Small groups of patients with tuberculosis have been treated with 1 g of kanamycin daily and a slight therapeutic effect has been observed; toxic effects have been common. Kanamycin should not be used alone but must not be given concurrently with other ototoxic agents.

Capreomycin is an antimycobacterial cyclic peptide elaborated by *Streptomyces capreolus.* It consists of four active components—capreomycins IA, IB, IIA, and IIB—the structures of which are being elucidated (Bycroft *et al.*, 1971). Capreomycin and viomycin are members of a closely related family of antibiotics; their chemical and pharmacological properties are similar. The agent used clinically contains primarily IA and IB; the other fractions make up only 20% of the drug. The drug is effective both *in vitro* and in experimental tuberculosis (Wilson, 1967). Bacterial resistance to capreomycin develops when it is given alone; such microorganisms show cross-resistance with kanamycin and viomycin (Tsukamura *et al.*, 1967).

Capreomycin must be given intramuscularly. The recommended daily dose is 20 mg/kg or 1 g for 60 to 120 days, followed by 1 g two to three times a week. Capreomycin should be administered together with another effective tuberculostatic agent. It has proven of value in the therapy of "resistant," or treatment-failure, tuberculosis when given with ethambutol or isoniazid (Wilson, 1967; Donomae, 1968). *Sterile Capreomycin Sulfate,* U.S.P. (CAPASTAT), is supplied in ampuls containing 1 g of the drug for solution in 2 ml of sodium chloride injection or sterile water.

The reactions associated with the use of capreomycin are hearing loss, tinnitus, transient proteinuria, cylindruria, and nitrogen retention. Severe renal failure is rare. These effects are similar to those described for viomycin (*see* above). Eosinophilia is common. Leukocytosis, leukopenia, rashes, and fever have also been observed. Injections of the drug may be painful. Capreomycin should not be used if streptomycin, kanamycin, or viomycin is being administered.

CHEMOTHERAPY OF TUBERCULOSIS

The treatment of tuberculosis is a complex, protracted procedure because of the underlying pathological anatomy and physiology of the disease, persistence of the causative microorganisms, and the variable and often inadequate defense mechanisms of the host. Lung tissue removed from individuals treated intensively for years may contain acid-fast bacilli, some of which grow in special media and produce atypical tuberculosis in guinea pigs (Darzins and Pukite, 1964). This suggests that, in some instances, even prolonged treatment will not eradicate viable microorganisms but may only alter their growth and disease-producing properties.

Chemotherapy is the keystone of the management of all forms of tuberculosis in man. Ancillary treatment such as surgery, corticosteroids, and other measures is of importance only when response to drugs is incomplete, when the initial stage of the disease is so severe as to pose an immediate threat to life, or when unusual complications develop. The availability of effective tuberculostatic agents has so altered the treatment of tuberculosis that the need for sanatorium care has been strikingly reduced. Patients with tuberculosis can and are being admitted to general hospitals. After a period sufficient to establish the diagnosis and to initiate and stabilize therapy, patients may, with uncommon exception, be returned to their homes. Prolonged bed rest has been shown not to be necessary or helpful in speeding recovery. Some clinicians allow such patients to return to work at an early date; others prefer to have them relatively inactive for at least 3 months. Arrangements must be made to minimize the risk of exposure of contacts, especially children, in the home. The patients must be seen at frequent intervals to follow the course of their disease and treatment.

Problems in Chemotherapy. *Bacterial Resistance to Drugs.* One of the more important problems in the chemotherapy of tuberculosis is bacterial resistance. For this reason concurrent administration of two or more tuberculostatic drugs should be invariably employed in the treatment of all active tuberculous infections.

A spate of publications has appeared on the incidence of resistance to tuberculostatic drugs of bacilli isolated from untreated patients. Results are divergent and depend on the population studied (*e.g.,* patients in Veterans Administration hospitals harbor more resistant microorganisms than do those in the United States as a whole), geographical location, and ethnic and socioeconomic factors. As can be said of many microorganisms, the percentage of untreated patients infected with tubercle bacilli resistant to one or more chemotherapeutic agents is slowly rising. However, the choice of agents has broadened and their mechanisms of action differ, so that cross-resistance does not present a problem. Most observers are of the opinion that the frequency of bacterial resistance is presently not rising at a rate so rapid that the effectiveness of programs of concurrent drug therapy is threatened. However, it is incumbent on the physician to obtain sensitivity data at the beginning and during the course of therapy to assure the selection of a proper combination of drugs and its continued effectiveness.

Atypical Mycobacteria. These microorganisms have been recovered from a variety of lesions in man, ranging from a single pulmonary focus to meningeal or disseminated disease; one type is responsible for most instances of tuberculous lymphadenitis (scrofula) in children. Because they are frequently resistant to many of the commonly used tuberculostatic agents, they must be examined for sensitivity *in vitro* and drug therapy selected on this basis. Group-I microorganisms (*M. kansasii*) show

a greater degree of susceptibility to isoniazid than do the other atypical mycobacteria; the majority are also sensitive to ethionamide, cycloserine, streptomycin, rifampin, and viomycin. Group-II strains (*M. scrofulaceum*) are often susceptible to streptomycin, viomycin, kanamycin, ethionamide, and aminosalicylic acid. Groups III (*M. intracellulare*) and IV (*M. fortuitum, M. marinum*) show very little sensitivity to any of the tuberculostatic drugs *in vitro* (Lorian and Finland, 1969). Molavi and Weinstein (1971) have noted that all strains of *M. kansasii* and the majority of *M. scrofulaceum* and *M. intracellulare,* but none of *M. fortuitum,* are sensitive to rifampin; a nearly identical pattern has been seen with clinically attainable concentrations of erythromycin. Because of the variable drug susceptibility of atypical mycobacteria, treatment of infections due to these microorganisms must be individualized. In many instances, surgical removal of the infected tissue followed by long-term treatment with effective tuberculostatic agents is necessary; this is especially so in tuberculous lymphadenitis. In spite of initial partial resistance to most of the antimycobacterial drugs, disease due to these bacteria may respond with 80 to 85% reversal of infectiousness when treated with streptomycin, isoniazid, and aminosalicylic acid in high doses (Mitchell, 1967).

Choice of Tuberculostatic Agents. The primary agents for the treatment of tuberculosis are isoniazid, ethambutol, rifampin, and streptomycin. In some instances (discussed below), administration of a single drug is considered sufficient, and the compound employed is isoniazid. The selection of the specific members for concurrent therapy is determined to a great degree by the nature and the severity of the disease. Some physicians prefer to administer three agents simultaneously in severe forms of the disease. The purposes of concurrent therapy are (1) to delay the emergence of bacterial resistance to drugs and (2) to increase tuberculostatic effects. The degree to which each of these purposes is achieved varies with the drugs employed, but the primary agents mentioned contribute to both goals. Less effective drugs may only delay the emergence of resistance.

The selection of a drug for the treatment of tuberculosis is also determined by (1) bacterial resistance, (2) the risk of development of untoward effects, and (3) the presence of atypical mycobacteria.

Therapy of Specific Types of Tuberculosis. *Pulmonary Tuberculosis.* While some physicians still treat noncavitary disease with 300 mg of isoniazid per day alone, the use of this agent in this manner is distinctly inferior to its administration with another potent tuberculostatic agent, such as ethambutol, for even minimal disease. In cases in which severe cavitary pulmonary tuberculosis is present, concurrent treatment with three drugs—isoniazid, ethambutol, and streptomycin—is recommended. Streptomycin is often given only until the sputum is negative, and therapy is then continued with the two orally effective agents.

Rifampin should not be used alone in the therapy of pulmonary or other clinical forms of tuberculosis because of the risk of the rapid development of resistance to the drug. Many clinicians reserve this valuable drug for treatment failures. It is the drug of choice for isoniazid-resistant microorganisms, and it is an excellent substitute for streptomycin when three drugs are called for. Furthermore, rifampin can be used as a component of a highly effective and simple initial treatment regimen. Combined therapy with rifampin (600 mg per day) and isoniazid (300 mg per day) results in a very rapid conversion of sputum cultures (90% of adult patients with moderately advanced disease within 12 weeks). This program is well tolerated and can have a major impact in hastening the trend toward outpatient treatment. After a period of 20 weeks, the patient can be maintained on the usual regimen of isoniazid and ethambutol for the duration of therapy (Newman *et al.,* 1974).

The writer treats pulmonary tuberculosis with isoniazid (8 to 10 mg/kg daily), ethambutol (25 mg/kg daily), and pyridoxine (100 mg daily), in patients with mild-to-moderate involvement. In the more severe cases, he adds streptomycin (1 g daily for 6 to 12 weeks, followed by 1 g twice a week for 2 to 3 months; in elderly patients, this daily dose is reduced to 0.5 to 0.75 g); in individuals with renal impairment, this agent is not given. *Chemotherapy is continued for a minimum of 1½ years.*

Failure of chemotherapy may be due to (1) irregular or inadequate therapy (resulting in persistent or resistant mycobacteria) due to poor patient compliance during the protracted therapeutic regimen; (2) the use of a single drug, with interruption necessitated by toxicity or hypersensitivity; (3) an inadequate initial regimen; (4) the primary resistance of the microorganism; (5) the presence of other disorders, such as silicosis, diabetes mellitus, or cor pulmonale; (6) a very severe form of tuberculosis; or (7) the failure to remove infected tissue surgically.

In patients in whom the pulmonary infection is due to strains of *M. tuberculosis* or atypical mycobacteria resistant to the most commonly used agents, determination of their sensitivity to all of the available tuberculostatic drugs is mandatory. Therapy is instituted with at least two or sometimes three of the compounds found to be most active *in vitro.* The same considerations apply to re-treatment of recurrent disease.

Clinical improvement is discernible in the majority of instances of progressive pulmonary tuberculosis treated with tuberculostatic agents. It usually becomes obvious within the first 2 to 3 weeks of therapy and is evidenced by a reduction of fever, decrease in cough, gain in weight, and increase in the sense of well-being. In a high percentage of cases, there is progressive roentgenographic improvement. Over 90% of patients who receive optimal treatment will have negative cultures by the sixth month. Residual cavitary lung disease in the presence of consistently negative sputum and gastric cultures is seldom complicated by reactivation if antibacterial therapy is continued for a sufficiently long period. Cultures that remain positive after 6 months of treatment frequently yield resistant microorganisms. The value of using an alternative therapeutic program at this time should be considered. The development of resistance to isoniazid may not require its discontinuation, since under this circumstance the infection often does not become exacerbated as rapidly or as inevitably as it does when treatment is stopped. However, the addition of another drug may be required to produce cure. (*See* Ware *et al.,* 1969; Bobrowitz, 1971; Boman, 1972; Constans *et al.,* 1972; Schonell *et al.,* 1972; Symposium, 1972; Engbaek *et al.,* 1973.)

Surgical treatment is still of value in the management of some cases of pulmonary tuberculosis, particularly in instances in which persistently infected cavities fail to close, or when the disease is due to strains of *M. tuberculosis* or atypical mycobacteria resistant or only slightly sensitive to a variety of tuberculostatic drugs.

Miliary (Disseminated) Tuberculosis. Although some clinicians treat miliary tuberculosis with only two drugs, the use of three agents is recommended. Isoniazid, ethambutol, and streptomycin can be administered in a regimen similar to that described for pulmonary tuberculosis. The writer administers streptomycin in doses of 1 g daily for 1 month, followed by 1 g twice a week for 3 months. Some clinicians continue the administration of streptomycin twice weekly for the entire period of treatment. Isoniazid and ethambutol are prescribed in the doses previously indicated. Rifampin is also quite useful as part of a therapeutic program for extrapulmonary tuberculosis. The addition of 100 mg of pyridoxine daily is helpful in reducing the incidence of toxic reactions to the isoniazid in the regimen. Therapy is continued for at least 2 years; if it is instituted sufficiently early in the course of the disease and sustained for this period, 90% of patients with disseminated tuberculosis recover.

Tuberculous Meningitis. Several regimens of therapy have been advocated for the treatment of tuberculous meningitis and have produced favorable results in the majority of cases. One approach is similar to that described above for miliary disease. The writer treats tuberculous meningitis in adults with 1 g of streptomycin daily for 3 months, followed by the same quantity only twice a week, plus isoniazid, ethambutol, and pyridoxine as described for pulmonary tuberculosis. Treatment with isoniazid plus rifampin, with or without ethambutol, has also proven to be effective. Intrathecal therapy is not necessary in this disease.

Genitourinary Tuberculosis. Chemotherapy has so remarkably altered the management of renal tuberculosis that nephrectomy is now rarely necessary. At present, most clinicians utilize a combination of isoniazid and ethambutol or isoniazid plus rifampin. Cycloserine (250 mg per day) or ethionamide (250 mg three times a day) has also proven beneficial in patients with resistant microorganisms. Tuberculosis of the epididymis, urinary bladder, and prostate responds well to therapy, and a high rate of fertility is preserved. Such regimens are also highly successful in the management of pelvic tuberculosis in women.

Tuberculosis of Bones and Joints. The treatment of infections of the bones and joints due to the tubercle bacillus is the same as for meningitis and other severe forms of the disease. In advanced cases, however, surgical drainage, excision, and debridement of necrotic tissue, with or without subsequent fusion, may be necessary.

Tuberculous Pleurisy with Effusion. Because 25 to 65% of patients with tuberculous pleural effusions develop active pulmonary tuberculosis within 5 years, it is important that the diagnosis of this syndrome be established and that treatment be instituted. The therapeutic program is the same as for pulmonary tuberculosis; drug administration should be continued for at least 18 months; the 5-year cure rate with treatment is at least 95%.

Tuberculosis of Other Organs. Tuberculous infection of the *peritoneum, pericardium, larynx, gastrointestinal tract, adrenal glands,* and other sites responds very satisfactorily to the administration of tuberculostatic drugs in a typical regimen as described above.

Corticosteroids in Tuberculosis. There is no place for corticosteroids in the routine therapy of most cases of pulmonary tuberculosis. The foremost indication for the administration of these agents is in patients in whom there is an immediate threat to life (Committee on Therapy, American Thoracic Society, 1968). In such instances, survival is prolonged for a period sufficiently long to allow the tuberculostatic drugs to exert a beneficial effect. This is particularly true when severe inflammation is present, such as with meningeal or pericardial involvement.

In more routine cases there is evidence that corticosteroids may actually do harm. Johnson and associates (1967) have pointed out that corticosteroids may impair the bacteriological response. Although there may be a moderate radiological improvement associated with the use of corticosteroids, it is suggested that these compounds be avoided in individuals with this kind of infection.

A short course (3 to 5 days) of treatment with corticosteroids may be necessary in the therapy of hypersensitivity reactions produced by tuberculostatic agents.

It has been suggested that patients with inactive tuberculosis or a positive tuberculin reaction who are receiving corticosteroids for nontuberculous disease be given 300 mg of isoniazid per day for the duration of the hormone administration and for an additional 6 months thereafter (Committee on Therapy, American Thoracic Society, 1968). The writer does not agree with this practice and administers tuberculostatic agents (isoniazid alone or together with ethambutol) routinely only to patients with sarcoidosis who require corticosteroids.

The Chemoprophylaxis of Tuberculosis. While there is no question of the efficacy of isoniazid for the chemoprophylaxis of tuberculosis, current appreciation of the hepatotoxicity of the drug has resulted in the modification of former recommendations for its prophylactic use. Prophylaxis is now recommended for the following categories of individuals (Stead and Texter, 1973): (1) tuberculin converters and reactors who have been exposed to tuberculosis and presumably have acquired an inapparent infection; (2) persons with inactive tuberculosis who have never been adequately treated with isoniazid; and (3) tuberculin reactors (10 mm or more to 3 units of PPD) who also have pulmonary scars suggestive of healed postprimary tuberculosis, diabetes mellitus, silicosis, or a need for corticosteroid therapy. It has been suggested that chemoprophylaxis no longer be recommended for healthy adult reactors with none of the above-listed risk factors for developing active disease. Extreme caution in the administration of isoniazid either prophylactically or therapeutically is necessary in older persons, who appear to be at greater risk of developing hepatotoxicity than are younger individuals. Isoniazid prophylaxis is contraindicated for patients who have hepatic disease or who have had reactions to the drug. In pregnant women, prophylaxis should be delayed until after delivery (Public Health Service, 1974). For prophylaxis, isoniazid is generally given to adults in a daily dose of 300 mg. Children should receive 10 mg/kg to a maximal daily dose of 300 mg. Drug administration is continued for 1 year.

II. Drugs for Leprosy

SULFONES

The sulfones, as a class, are derivatives of 4,4'-diaminodiphenylsulfone (dapsone, DDS), all of which have certain pharmacological properties in common. They are discussed here as a class; only the two members that have official status in the United States, *dapsone* and *sulfoxone,* will be mentioned individually.

History. The sulfones first attracted interest because of their chemical relationship to the sulfonamides. Dapsone was found in 1937 to be 30 times more active and only 15 times as toxic as sulfanilamide when used in streptococcal infections in mice. At that time, the drug was considered too toxic for administration to man, and attempts were initiated to find a compound with a better therapeutic index. None of the sulfones that have since been synthesized has proven of value in the therapy of the common acute bacterial infections. However, when Rist and associates (1940) and Feldman and coworkers (1941) noted that dapsone and glucosulfone (PROMIN), a derivative of dapsone, were effective in suppressing experimental tubercle bacillus infections, attention was attracted to the potential value of these agents in the treatment of human tuberculosis. Although dapsone and some of its congeners eventually proved to be of very limited usefulness in this disease, the interest stimulated by the observations that a drug exerted a marked effect on experimental tuberculosis led to the demonstration that glucosulfone exerted a favorable effect in rat leprosy (Cowdry and Ruangsiri, 1941). This was soon followed by successful clinical trials of this agent in human leprosy. The sulfones are presently the most important drugs for the treatment of this disease.

Chemistry. All the sulfones of clinical value are derivatives of dapsone. Despite the study and development of a large variety of sulfones, this drug remains the agent most useful clinically. The structures of dapsone and sulfoxone sodium are as follows:

H_2N—⬡—S(=O)(=O)—⬡—NH_2

Dapsone

NaO_2SCH_2NH—⬡—S(=O)(=O)—⬡—$NHCH_2SO_2Na$

Sulfoxone Sodium

Antibacterial Activity. The sulfones are bacteriostatic, not bactericidal, *in vitro* for the tubercle bacillus. Dapsone suppresses the growth of pathogenic strains of this microorganism in a concentration of about 10 μg/ml. The tubercle bacillus does not develop resistance to the drug *in vitro*. Because *Mycobacterium leprae* does not readily grow on artificial media, conventional methods cannot be applied to determine its susceptibility to potential therapeutic agents *in vitro*.

The *in-vivo* activity of dapsone in patients with leprosy has been studied by Shepard and coworkers (1968). Using the technic of foot-pad inoculation in the mouse as an index, they noted that therapy with this agent for 28 days reduced the degree of infectiousness of leprous material from nasal washings and skin to about 10% of that present before treatment. After 90 days, there were so few *M. leprae* left that they were barely detectable. The drug is bacteriostatic, but not bactericidal, for *M. leprae,* and the estimated sensitivity to dapsone is 0.02 μg/ml in microorganisms recovered from untreated patients (Shepard *et al.,* 1969). *Mycobacterium leprae* may become resistant to the drug during therapy.

The mechanism of action of the sulfones is probably similar to that of the sulfonamides since both possess approximately the same range of antibacterial activity and both are antagonized by para-aminobenzoic acid.

Untoward Effects. The reactions induced by various sulfones are very similar. The most common untoward effect is *hemolysis* of varying degree. This develops in almost every individual treated with 200 to 300 mg of dapsone per day. Doses of 100 mg or less in normal healthy persons and 50 mg or less in healthy individuals with a glucose-6-phosphate dehydrogenase deficiency do not cause hemolysis (DeGowin, 1967). *Methemoglobinemia* is also common, and Heinz-body formation may occur. While diminished red-cell survival usually occurs during the use of sulfones, and is presumed to be a dose-related effect of their oxidizing activity, *hemolytic anemia* is unusual unless there is a disorder either of the erythrocytes or of the bone marrow (Pengelly, 1963). The hemolysis may be so severe that manifestations of hypoxia become striking.

Anorexia, nausea, and *vomiting* may follow the oral administration of sulfones. Isolated instances of

headache, nervousness, insomnia, blurred vision, paresthesia, reversible peripheral neuropathy (thought to be due to axonal degeneration), *drug fever, hematuria, pruritus, psychosis,* and a variety of *skin rashes* have been reported (Rapoport and Guss, 1972). An *infectious mononucleosis–like syndrome,* which may be fatal, occurs occasionally (Leiker, 1956). The sulfones may induce an *exacerbation of lepromatous leprosy;* this is thought to be analogous to the Jarisch-Herxheimer reaction. This "sulfone syndrome" may develop 5 to 6 weeks after initiation of treatment in malnourished people. Its manifestations include fever, malaise, exfoliative dermatitis, jaundice with hepatic necrosis, lymphadenopathy, and methemoglobinemia, and anemia (DeGowin, 1967).

The sulfones may be given safely for many years in doses adequate for the successful therapy of leprosy if proper precautions are observed. Treatment should be initiated with a small dose and the quantity then increased gradually. Patients must be under constant laboratory and clinical supervision. The reactions induced by the sulfones, especially those related to exacerbation of the leprosy, may be very severe and demand the cessation of treatment as well as the institution of specific measures to reduce the threat to life.

Absorption, Distribution, and Excretion. Dapsone is slowly and nearly completely absorbed from the gastrointestinal tract. The disubstituted sulfones, such as sulfoxone, are incompletely absorbed when administered orally, and large amounts are excreted in the feces. Peak plasma concentrations of dapsone are reached in 1 to 3 hours after administration, but the drug is detectable for 8 to 12 days. When repeated doses are given, traces of the compound are detectable for as long as 35 days after therapy has been stopped. A dose of 100 mg of dapsone per day produces an average of 2 μg of "free" dapsone per gram of blood or nonhepatic tissue. About 50% of the drug is bound to plasma protein (Riley and Levy, 1973). Plasma concentrations following conventional doses of sulfoxone sodium are 10 to 15 μg/ml. These values fall relatively rapidly; however, appreciable quantities are still present at 8 hours.

The sulfones are distributed throughout the total body water and are present in all tissues. They tend to be retained in skin and muscle, and especially in liver and kidney; traces of the drug are present in these organs up to 3 weeks after therapy is stopped. The sulfones are retained in the circulation for a long time because of intestinal reabsorption from the bile; periodic interruption of treatment is advisable for this reason. Dapsone is acetylated in the liver, and the degree of acetylation is genetically determined.

The urinary excretion of sulfones varies with the type of drug; about 70 to 80% of a dose of dapsone is so excreted. The drug is present in urine as an acid-labile mono-N-glucuronide and mono-N-sulfamate in addition to an unknown number of unidentified metabolites (Shepard, 1969). Probenecid decreases the urinary excretion of the acid-labile dapsone metabolites significantly and that of free dapsone to a lesser extent (Goodwin and Sparell, 1969).

Preparations, Routes of Administration, and Dosage. *Dapsone,* U.S.P. (*DDS;* AVLOSULFON), is available in tablets containing 25 or 100 mg. It is given primarily by the oral route. One dosage schedule for the treatment of "uncomplicated" lepromatous leprosy with dapsone is as follows: The initial dose is 25 mg. In the first 2-week period, this amount is given once weekly; in the second, twice a week; in the third, three times a week; in the fourth, four times a week; and in the fifth 2-week period, five times a week. The individual dose is then increased to 50 mg, which is administered three times a week for the first month, four times a week for a second month, and five times a week for a third month. Following this, a 100-mg dose is given three times a week for 1 month and then four times a week for an indefinite period (*see* Trautman, 1965). Browne (1967) has suggested that a 100-mg dose of dapsone twice a week for adults and comparably less for children is effective, and that 100 mg once weekly may be adequate.

A long-acting repository sulfone, *acedapsone* (4,4'-diacetyldiaminodiphenyl sulfone; *DADDS*), is presently undergoing clinical trial (Shepard, 1969; Russell *et al.,* 1971; Shepard *et al.,* 1972). The drug releases dapsone or its monoacetylated derivative through the action of tissue enzymes. Patients treated intramuscularly respond as well to it as to dapsone. A single dose of 225 mg is given every 11 weeks. The results of therapy with acedapsone are comparable to those produced by administration of 50 mg of dapsone per day, although loss of infectivity of the microorganisms requires a longer time with acedapsone than with dapsone. Studies of urinary excretion indicate release of an average of 2.4 mg of dapsone per day.

Sulfoxone Sodium, N.F. (DIASONE SODIUM), is the disodium formaldehyde sulfoxylate substitution product of dapsone. It may be substituted for dapsone in patients in whom this drug produces sufficient gastric distress to impede effective therapy. It is a water-soluble, pale-yellow powder, available for oral administration as enteric-coated tablets containing 165 mg. The initial dose for the treatment of leprosy is 330 mg twice weekly for 2 weeks; this dose is then given four times weekly for the next 2 weeks; thereafter 330 mg is given daily 6 days of each week.

The use of sulfones in *malaria* resistant to the usual antimalarial drugs is discussed in Chapter 52.

AMITHIOZONE

The tuberculostatic activity of thiosemicarbazones and related drugs was first observed by Domagk and coworkers (1946). Study of structure-activity relationship suggested that 4-acetylamino benzaldehyde thiosemicarbazone (amithiozone) was the most promising of these compounds. The structural formula of amithiozone is as follows:

Amithiozone

Lowe (1954) was the first to discover the effectiveness of amithiozone in leprosy. It appears to exert a greater effect on the tuberculoid than on the lepromatous form of the disease. *Mycobacterium leprae* tends to become resistant to this agent as treatment is continued, as evidenced by a slower rate of improvement in the second year of therapy and the occurrence of relapse in the third year. It has been suggested that amithiozone can be substituted for the sulfones when the latter, for some reason, cannot be administered.

The most common untoward effects of the thiosemicarbazones and derivatives are *anorexia, nausea,* and *vomiting.* The drugs may *depress bone-marrow function.* Some degree of *anemia* is observed in a large percentage of patients receiving amithiozone. *Leukopenia* and *agranulocytosis* occur; the incidence of serious reactions involving the leukocytes is about 0.5%. *Acute hemolytic anemia* may develop when high doses are administered. *Skin rashes* are not infrequent; they may be of any type, but exfoliative dermatitis has not yet been noted. Although mild *albuminuria* has been observed, the drugs are not regarded as nephrotoxic. The fairly high incidence of *jaundice* in patients receiving amithiozone suggests that it is hepatotoxic; the effect on the liver disappears when treatment is stopped.

Amithiozone (*thiacetazone;* PANRONE, TIBIONE) is well absorbed from the gastrointestinal tract, and large amounts are excreted in the urine (Robson and Sullivan, 1963). The initial dose is 50 mg per day for 1 to 2 weeks, after which the daily quantity is gradually increased to a maximum of 200 mg. The drug appears to be as effective when given in a single dose each day as when the daily dose is divided. Amithiozone is not available in the United States.

CLOFAZIMINE

Many phenazine congeners exhibit antitubercular activity in experimental animals. One of these, *clofazimine,* is now considered by some to be the chief secondary drug for use in patients infected with *M. leprae* that are resistant to the sulfones (Shepard, 1969). It not only is effective in lepromatous leprosy, causing disappearance of morphologically normal *M. leprae* in a few months, but also appears to exert an anti-inflammatory effect when given in the proper dose and prevents the development of erythema nodosum (Browne, 1967). There is growing evidence that persistent and established exacerbations in lepromatous leprosy are improved and cured by *clofazimine.* This compound acts specifically on the chronic skin ulcers (Buruli ulcer) produced by *M. ulcerans.*

The drug is absorbed by the oral route and appears to accumulate in tissues. This makes possible discontinuous therapy with individual doses separated by 2 or more weeks. Human leprosy from which dapsone-resistant bacilli have been recovered has been treated with clofazimine with good results. However, unlike dapsone-sensitive microorganisms in which killing occurs immediately after dapsone is administered, dapsone-resistant strains do not exhibit appreciable effect until 50 days after therapy with clofazimine has been initiated. The dose of clofazimine is 100 to 300 mg; the optimal interval between doses in man remains to be determined. (*See* Convit *et al.,* 1970; Shepard *et al.,* 1971a, 1971b; Levy *et al.,* 1972.) No significant reactions have been observed with a dose of 100 mg per day. Patients treated with *clofazimine* develop red and black pigmentation; this may be very distressing to light-skinned individuals.

Clofazimine (LAMPRENE) is supplied in capsules containing 100 mg.

MISCELLANEOUS AGENTS

The efficacy of a great many agents in the therapy of leprosy has been investigated (*see* International Congress on Leprology, 1963). Browne (1967) has reported considerable enthusiasm for the use of long-acting sulfonamides in this disease in South America and certain areas of Africa. Derivatives of diphenylthiourea such as thiambutosine have also attracted interest. However, exacerbations of the disease have occurred, presumably due to resistance to this agent.

Rifampin (*see* page 1208) also shows promise in this mycobacterial disease. The drug appears to be bactericidal for *M. leprae,* and it may control the disease more rapidly than does dapsone. It is, however, too early to tell if rifampin will have long-term value in the control of leprosy.

CHEMOTHERAPY OF LEPROSY

Few physicians, other than specialists in the field, are called upon to treat leprosy. Therefore, the following discussion will serve mainly to familiarize the reader with the progress that has been made in the treatment of a bacterial disease that has proven very resistant to chemotherapy. The discussion of drug therapy will be limited to dapsone and to the more important agents that are employed to control the lepra reactions that occur during chemotherapy and are apparently part of the therapeutic response.

Four clinical types of leprosy are recognized. (1) *Lepromatous disease* is characterized by diffuse or ill-defined localized infiltration of the skin, which becomes thickened, glossy, and corrugated; areas of decreased sensation may appear. *Mycobacterium leprae* is demonstrable in smears, and granulomas containing bacteria-laden histiocytes (Virchow cells) are present. As the disease progresses, large nerve trunks are invaded and anesthesia, atrophy of skin and muscle, absorption of small bones, ulceration, and spontaneous amputations may supervene. The intradermal injection of a suspension of heat-killed, bacillus-laden tissue (lepromin or Mitsuda-Hayashi test) causes no reaction. (2) *Tuberculoid* leprosy is featured by skin macules with clear centers and well-defined margins; these are invariably anesthetic. *Mycobacterium leprae* is rarely found in smears made from quiescent lesions, but may appear during activity. Virchow cells are not demonstrable. Noncaseating foci with giant cells of the Langhans variety are present. The lepromin reaction is invariably positive. The disease is characterized by prolonged remissions with periodic reactivation. (3) In the *indeterminate* or *mixed* form of leprosy, the skin lesions are flattened and mildly inflamed, and contain small numbers of *M. leprae.* The lepromin test may be positive or negative, and the disease may progress to either the *lepromatous* or *tuberculoid* type. (4) A *borderline form* of leprosy with features of both the lepromatous and tuberculoid types has also been defined; macular skin lesions, atypical granulomas, positive smear for *M. leprae,* and a negative lepromin reaction are the characteristics of this syndrome.

Reactions may occur in the course of the treatment of leprosy, particularly with the sulfones. They must be distinguished from sudden activation with extension of the disease. Reactions in the lepromatous form of the disease (the *erythema nodosum phenomenon*) are characterized by the appearance of raised, tender, intracutaneous nodules, severe constitutional symptoms, and high fever. The feature of the reaction in tuberculoid leprosy is the presence of sharply defined, symmetrical, macular skin lesions that are surrounded by redness and edema, which may ulcerate. The phenomena of activation and reactions in leprosy are complex and involve host tissue responses and many clinical variations that are beyond the scope of this discussion.

The outlook for persons with leprosy has been remarkably altered by successful chemotherapy, surgical procedures that help to restore function and repair disfigurement, and a striking change in the attitude of the public toward patients who have this infection. The social stigma based on ignorance and Biblical castigation of individuals with this affliction is gradually being replaced by the attitude that considers leprosy a disease and not a crime. Patients with leprosy can be classified as "infectious" or "noninfectious" on the basis of the type, duration, and effects of therapy. Thus, even "infectious" patients may be discharged from leprosaria, provided adequate medical supervision and therapy are maintained, the home environment meets specific conditions, and the local health officer concurs in the disposition of the case.

Sulfones. These agents are the drugs of choice for the therapy of all forms of leprosy. Clinical improvement is evident in practically every treated case. Mucosal lesions are the first to respond; oral, nasal, pharyngeal, and laryngeal nodules, infiltrations, and ulcerations regress and disappear, and secondary infections subside. Skin manifestations may require 1 to 3 years to clear; the degree of residual pigmentation or depigmentation, atrophy, and scarring depends upon the extent of the initial involvement. Severe ocular lesions show little response to the sulfones. If treatment is initiated before ocular disease is evident, it may be prevented. Keratoconjunctivitis and corneal ulceration may be secondary to nerve involvement. When only infiltration of the cornea and beading of the circumcorneal nerves are present, improvement is usually produced by the sulfones but relapses may occur. The administration of a corticosteroid is effective in the management of acute exacerbations of iridocyclitis and iritis, but remission is usually only temporary.

Invasion of the peripheral nerves probably occurs in all cases of leprosy, but it is most prominent in the tuberculoid form of the disease. The involved extremity is painful and swollen. Splinting and application of heat to the affected limb produce relief of the discomfort. Nerve stripping is followed by only temporary relief. The intraneural injection of a corticosteroid or a local anesthetic may be helpful in controlling the pain.

Treatment of leprosy with the sulfones produces much more rapid clinical than bacteriological improvement. Patients harbor *M. leprae* in mucous membranes, skin, and nerves long after superficial lesions have disappeared. The mucous membranes are usually the first to become free of the microorganisms; this requires 6 months to 1 year in the tuberculoid and 1 to 2 years in the lepromatous form of the disease. The bacteria in the skin lesions of treated patients may disappear in 1½ to 3 years in tuberculoid and 3 to 5 years in lepromatous leprosy. The delay in eradication of *M. leprae* may be more apparent than real, because microorganisms may remain and be visualized in tissues long after they have been killed by the drugs.

Untoward Reactions to Sulfone Therapy. The reactions directly related to the sulfones have been discussed above. In addition to these, there are a number of untoward changes in the disease that are associated with the use of these drugs. The incidence of some types of acute reactions that occur in the course of leprosy may be increased during therapy. Among these are *erythema nodosum,* acute episodes of *neuritis, erythema multiforme,* and *erythema necroticans;* their appearance is considered to be evidence that the sulfones are exerting a therapeutic effect. Individuals with lepromatous leprosy in the stage of acute reactions or associated with erythema nodosum should be hospitalized and treated with extreme caution. When reactions occur in cases of *tuberculoid* or *dimorphous disease,* the drug being given must be discontinued immediately and prednisone administered promptly in a dose of 40 to 100 mg per day for 3 to 5 days, and then withdrawn gradually. When sulfone therapy is reinstituted, the initial dose must be small (dapsone, 10 mg once a week) and increased slowly. When tuberculoid reactions develop in untreated cases, sulfones should not be given until resolution has taken place.

Progressive lepra reactions are sometimes ameliorated by reduction of the dose of sulfone being administered. The administration of 0.5 g of streptomycin every other day, in addition, has proven of value in some cases. If this or other therapy (*see* below) is ineffective, treatment with prednisone (15 to 20 mg per day) should be undertaken; it is necessary to give relatively high doses for prolonged periods in some patients. However, if improvement is not apparent within 6 months, the steroid should be gradually withdrawn. Individuals who improve during the course of such therapy may need to be given 5 to 10 mg of prednisone per day for indefinite periods because its withdrawal may exacerbate the process.

When *erythema nodosum* develops during treatment, the dose of drug should be reduced if the manifestations are mild; if they are severe, therapy must be stopped. In some instances, the nodose skin lesions may be recurrent and present a serious problem; prednisone (10 to 60 mg per day) may be necessary. If *erythema nodosum* develops prior to the institution of therapy for leprosy, drug administration must not be undertaken until the reaction disappears. Therapy for the infection must then be given with extreme caution (10 mg of dapsone, once a week initially). Potassium antimony tartrate and stibophen are often very useful in the management of drug-induced severe erythema nodosum with appreciable constitutional manifestations.

Corticosteroids are invaluable in the management of severe exacerbations of leprosy that do not respond to rest, sedatives, aspirin, antimalarial compounds (chloroquine), or antimonials. Steroids should be given in doses adequate to control the manifestations and withdrawn as rapidly as possible. A few weeks later, treatment with dapsone may be renewed very cautiously. In protracted and severe cases, it may be necessary to resume treatment for the infection while a corticosteroid is still being given. Acute exacerbation of a tuberculoid leprosy lesion in the area of an important anatomical structure, especially on the face (facial nerve or nasal duct), requires the administration of a corticosteroid, which, by reducing the intensity of the inflammation and shortening the duration of the reactions, may prevent damage to the underlying tissues. *Thalidomide* exerts an immunosuppressive effect in exacerbations of lepromatous leprosy. The use of this agent is dangerous in women of childbearing age because of its teratogenic effects on the fetus. Severe relapse of lepromatous leprosy often follows withdrawal of thalidomide.

Therapeutic Regimen. The doses of the sulfones are discussed above. Treatment must be prolonged until host defense mechanisms can eradicate the microorganisms that have been altered but not killed by the drugs. However, the inability to demonstrate bacilli does not necessarily indicate cure of the disease. There is a significant incidence of relapse after treatment is stopped, even when *M. leprae* has not been detectable in stained smears for as long as a year or more. It is common practice, therefore, to continue sulfone administration indefinitely, at one third the full therapeutic dose, even though all the usual criteria for "cure" have been fulfilled. This is possible, despite the potential toxicity of these agents, if minimally effective quantities are given and treatment is interspersed with rest periods.

Atlas, E., and Turck, M. Laboratory and clinical evaluation of rifampicin. *Am. J. med. Sci.,* **1968,** *256,* 247–254.

Beggs, W. H., and Ayran, N. E. Uptake and binding of ¹⁴C-ethambutol by tubercle bacilli and the relation of binding to growth inhibition. *Antimicrob. Agents Chemother.,* **1972,** *2,* 390–394.

Bieder, A.; Brunel, P.; and Mazeau, L. Identification de trois nouveaux métabolites de l'ethionamide: chromatographie, spectrophotométrie, polarographie. *Annls pharm. fr.,* **1966,** *24,* 493–500.

Bobrowitz, I. D. Ethambutol compared to streptomycin in original treatment of advanced pulmonary tuberculosis. *Chest,* **1971,** *60,* 14–21.

Boman, G. Rifampin-isoniazid compared with PAS-isoniazid-streptomycin in initial treatment of pulmonary tuberculosis. A controlled cooperative trial. *Chest,* **1972,** *61,* 533–538.

Bowersox, D. W.; Winterbauer, R. H.; Stewart, G. L.; Orme, B.; and Barron, E. Isoniazid dosage in patients with renal failure. *New Engl. J. Med.,* **1973,** *289,* 84–87.

Bycroft, B. W.; Cameron, D.; Croft, L. R.; Hassanali-Walji, A.; Johnson, A. W.; and Webb, T. Total structure of capreomycin 1B, a tuberculostatic peptide antibiotic. *Nature, Lond.,* **1971,** *231,* 301–302.

Cohn, H. D. Clinical studies with a new rifamycin derivative. *J. clin. Pharmac.,* **1969,** *9,* 118–125.

Committee on Therapy, American Thoracic Society. Adrenal corticosteroids and tuberculosis. *Am. Rev. resp. Dis.,* **1968,** *97,* 484–485.

Constans, P.; Baron, A.; Parrot, R.; and Coury, C. A study of 200 cases of active, recent pulmonary tuberculosis treated with rifampin-isoniazid. A follow-up history of one and one-half to three years. *Chest,* **1972,** *61,* 539–544.

Convit, J.; Browne, S. G.; Languillon, J.; Pettit, J. H. S.; Ramanujam, K.; Sagher, F.; Sheskin, J.; deSouza Lima, L.; Tarabini, G.; Tolentino, J. G.; Waters, M. F. R.; Bechelli, L. M.; and Martinez Dominguez, V. Therapy of leprosy. *Bull. Wld Hlth Org.,* **1970,** *42,* 667–672.

Cowdry, E. V., and Ruangsiri, C. Influence of promin, starch, and heptaldehyde on experimental leprosy in rats. *Archs Path.,* **1941,** *32,* 632–640.

Darzins, E., and Pukite, A. Cultivation of acid fast organisms from tuberculous patients after prolonged and intensive treatment. *Am. Rev. resp. Dis.,* **1964,** *89,* 271–279.

DeGowin, R. L. A review of the therapeutic and hemolytic effects of dapsone. *Archs intern. Med.,* **1967,** *120,* 242–248.

Des Prez, R., and Boone, I. U. Metabolism of C¹⁴ isoniazid in humans. *Am. Rev. resp. Dis.,* **1961,** *84,* 42–51.

Devine, L. F.; Johnson, D. P.; Rhode, S. L., III; Hagerman, C. R.; Pierce, W. E.; and Peckinpaugh, R. D. Rifampin—effect of two-day treatment on the meningococcal carrier state and the relationship to the levels of the drug in sera and saliva. *Am. J. med. Sci.,* **1971,** *26,* 74–83.

di Mauro, D.; Snyder, L.; Marino, P.; Lamberti, A.; Coppo, A.; and Tocchini-Valentini, G. P. Rifampicin sensitivity of the components of DNA-dependent RNA polymerase. *Nature, Lond.,* **1969,** *222,* 533–537.

Domagk, G.; Behnisch, R.; Mietzsch, F.; and Schmidt, H. Über eine neue, gegen Tuberkelbazillen *in vitro* wirksame Verbindungsklasse. *Naturwissenschaften,* **1946,** *33,* 315.

Donomae, I. The combined use of capreomycin and ethambutol in re-treatment of pulmonary tuberculosis. *Am. Rev. resp. Dis.,* **1968,** *98,* 699–702.

Doust, J. Y., and Moatamed, F. Arthralgia in pulmonary tuberculosis during chemotherapy. *Dis. Chest,* **1968,** *53,* 62–64.

Engbaek, H. C.; Larpen, S. O.; Rasmussen, K. N.; and Vergmann, B. Initial treatment of tuberculosis with streptomycin and isoniazid combined with either aminosalyl or rifampin. *Scand. J. resp. Dis.,* **1973,** *54,* 83–91.

Evans, D. A. P.; Manley, K. A.; and McKusick, V. A. Genetic control of isoniazid metabolism in man. *Br. med. J.,* **1960,** *2,* 485–491.

Feldman, W. H.; Hinshaw, H. C.; and Moses, H. E. Treatment of experimental tuberculosis with promin (sodium salt of *p,p'*-diamino-diphenyl sulfone-N,N'-dextrose sulfonate): preliminary report. *Proc. Staff Meet. Mayo Clin.,* **1941,** *16,* 118–125.

Flynn, C. T.; Rainford, D. J.; and Hope, E. Acute renal failure and rifampicin: danger of unsuspected intermittent dosage. *Br. med. J.,* **1974,** *2,* 482.

Fox, H. H. The chemical attack on tuberculosis. *Trans. N.Y. Acad. Sci.,* **1953,** *15,* 234–242.

Furesz, S.; Scott, R.; Pallanza, R.; and Mapelli, E. Rifampicin: a new rifamycin. III. Absorption, distribution, and elimination in man. *Arzneimittel-Forsch.,* **1967,** *17,* 533–537.

Garibaldi, R. A.; Drusin, R. E.; Ferebee, S. H.; and Gregg, M. B. Isoniazid-associated hepatitis. Report of an outbreak. *Am. Rev. resp. Dis.,* **1972,** *106,* 357–365.

Good, A. E.; Green, R. A.; and Zarafonetis, C. J. D. Rheumatic symptoms during tuberculosis therapy: a

manifestation of isoniazid toxicity. *Ann. intern. Med.,* **1965,** *63,* 800–807.

Goodwin, C. S., and Sparell, G. Inhibition of dapsone excretion by probenecid. *Lancet,* **1969,** *2,* 884–885.

Graber, C. D.; Jebaily, J.; Galphin, R. L.; and Doering, E. Light chain proteinuria and humoral immunocompetence in tuberculous patients treated with rifampin. *Am. Rev. resp. Dis.,* **1973,** *107,* 713–717.

Harris, H. W. Current concepts of the metabolism of antituberculous agents. *Ann. N.Y. Acad. Sci.,* **1963,** *106,* 43–47.

Hobby, G. L., and Lenert, T. F. Observations on the action of rifampin and ethambutol alone and in combination with other antituberculous drugs. *Am. Rev. resp. Dis.,* **1972,** *105,* 292–295.

Hoeprich, P. D. Alanine:cycloserine antagonism. II. Significance of phenomenon to therapy with cycloserine. *Archs intern. Med.,* **1963,** *112,* 405–414. III. Quantitative aspects and relation to heating of culture media. *J. Lab. clin. Med.,* **1963,** *62,* 657–662.

Ivler, D.; Leedom, J. M.; and Mathies, A. W., Jr. *In vitro* susceptibility of *Neisseria meningitidis* to rifampin. In, *Antimicrobial Agents and Chemotherapy—1969.* (Hobby, G. L., ed.) American Society for Microbiology, Bethesda, Md., **1970,** pp. 473–478.

Jenne, J. W., and Beggs, W. H. Correlation of *in vitro* and *in vivo* kinetics with clinical use of isoniazid, ethambutol and rifampin. *Am. Rev. resp. Dis.,* **1973,** *107,* 1013–1021.

Johnson, J. R.; Turk, T. L.; and MacDonald, F. M. Corticosteroids in pulmonary tuberculosis. III. Indications. *Am. Rev. resp. Dis.,* **1967,** *96,* 62–73.

Karlson, A. G. The *in vitro* activity of ethambutol (dextro-2-2'-[ethylenediimino]-di-1-butanol) against tubercle bacilli and other microorganisms. *Am. Rev. resp. Dis.,* **1961,** *84,* 905–906.

Konno, K.; Oizumo, K.; and Oka, S. Mode of action of rifampin on mycobacteria. II. Biosynthetic studies on the inhibition of ribonucleic acid polymerase of *Mycobacterium bovis* BCG by rifampin and uptake of rifampin-¹⁴C by *Mycobacterium phlei. Am. Rev. resp. Dis.,* **1973,** *107,* 1006–1012.

Kunin, C. M.; Brandt, D.; and Wood, H. Bacteriologic studies of rifampin, a new semisynthetic antibiotic. *J. infect. Dis.,* **1969,** *119,* 132–137.

Kutt, H.; Winters, W.; and McDowell, F. H. Depression of parahydroxylation of diphenylhydantoin by antituberculosis chemotherapy. *Neurology, Minneap.,* **1966,** *16,* 594–602.

La Du, B. N. Isoniazid and pseudocholinesterase polymorphisms. *Fedn Proc. Fedn Am. Socs exp. Biol.,* **1972,** *31,* 1276–1285.

Lauener, H., and Favez, G. Inhibition of isoniazid inactivation by means of PAS and benzoyl PAS in man. *Am. Rev. resp. Dis.,* **1959,** *80,* 26–37.

Lees, A. W. Ethionamide, 500 mg daily, plus isoniazid, 500 mg or 300 mg daily, in previously untreated patients with pulmonary tuberculosis. *Am. Rev. resp. Dis.,* **1967,** *95,* 109–111.

Lehmann, J. Para-aminosalicylic acid in treatment of tuberculosis: preliminary communication. *Lancet,* **1946,** *1,* 15–16.

Leiker, D. L. The mononuclear syndrome in leprosy patients treated with sulfones. *Int. J. Lepr.,* **1956,** *24,* 402–405.

Levy, L.; Shepard, C. C.; and Fasal, P. Clofazimine therapy of lepromatous leprosy caused by dapsone-resistant *Mycobacterium leprae. Am. J. trop. Med. Hyg.,* **1972,** *21,* 315–321.

Lorian, V., and Finland, M. *In vitro* effect of rifampin on mycobacteria. *Appl. Microbiol.,* **1969,** *17,* 202–207.

Lowe, J. The chemotherapy of leprosy: late results of treatment with sulfone and with thiosemicarbazone. *Lancet,* **1954,** *2,* 1065–1068.

McCabe, W. R., and Lorian, V. Comparison of the antibacterial activity of rifampicin and other antibiotics. *Am. J. med. Sci.,* **1968,** *256,* 255–265.

McDermott, W.; Ormond, L.; Muschenheim, C.; Deuschle, K.; McCune, R. M.; and Tompsett, R. Pyrazinamide-isoniazid in tuberculosis. *Am. Rev. Tuberc. pulm. Dis.,* **1954,** *69,* 319–333.

Maddrey, W. C., and Boitnott, J. K. Isoniazid hepatitis. *Ann. intern. Med.,* **1973,** *79,* 1–12.

Maggi, N.; Pasqualucci, C. R.; Ballotta, R.; and Sensi, P. Rifampicin: a new orally active rifamycin. *Chemotherapia,* **1966,** *11,* 285–292.

Mandel, W.; Heaton, A. D.; Russell, W. F.; and Middlebrook, G. Combined drug treatment of tuberculosis. II. Studies of antimicrobially active isoniazid and streptomycin serum levels in adult tuberculous patients. *J. clin. Invest.,* **1959,** *38,* 1356–1365.

Mattila, M. J., and Tiitinen, H. The rate of isoniazid inactivation in Finnish diabetic and non-diabetic patients. *Annls Med. exp. Biol. Fenn.,* **1967,** *45,* 423–427.

Molavi, A., and Weinstein, L. *In vitro* susceptibility of atypical mycobacteria to rifampin. *Appl. Microbiol.,* **1971,** *22,* 23–25.

Mukerjee, P.; Schuldt, S.; and Kasik, J. E. Effect of rifampin on cutaneous hypersensitivity to purified protein derivatives in humans. *Antimicrob. Agents Chemother.,* **1973,** *4,* 607–611.

Newman, R.; Doster, B. E.; Murray, F. J.; and Woolpert, S. F. Rifampin in initial treatment of pulmonary tuberculosis. *Am. Rev. resp. Dis.,* **1974,** *109,* 216–232.

Peets, E. A.; Sweeney, W. M.; Place, V. A.; and Buyske, D. A. The absorption, excretion and metabolic fate of ethambutol in man. *Am. Rev. resp. Dis.,* **1965,** *91,* 51–58.

Pengelly, C. D. R. Dapsone-induced hemolysis. *Br. med. J.,* **1963,** *2,* 662–664.

Phillips, S., and Tashman, H. Ethionamide jaundice. *Am. Rev. resp. Dis.,* **1963,** *87,* 896–898.

Place, V. A., and Thomas, J. P. Clinical pharmacology of ethambutol. *Am. Rev. resp. Dis.,* **1963,** *87,* 901–904.

Postlethwaite, A. E.; Bartel, A. G.; and Kelley, W. N. Hyperuricemia due to ethambutol. *New Engl. J. Med.,* **1972,** *286,* 761–762.

Public Health Service, U.S. Department of Health, Education, and Welfare. Isoniazid-associated hepatitis: summary of the report of the Tuberculosis Advisory Committee and special consultants to the Director, Center for Disease Control. *Morbidity and Mortality.* (Weekly report.) **1974,** *23,* No. 11, 97–98.

Radner, D. B. Toxicologic and pharmacologic aspects of rifampin. *Chest,* **1973,** *64,* 213–216.

Rapoport, A. M., and Guss, S. B. Dapsone-induced peripheral neuropathy. *Archs Neurol., Chicago,* **1972,** *27,* 184–186.

Riley, R. W., and Levy, L. Characteristics of the binding of dapsone and monoacetyldapsone by serum albumin. *Proc. Soc. exp. Biol. Med.,* **1973,** *142,* 1168–1170.

Rist, N.; Block, F.; and Hamon, V. Action inhibitrice du sulfamide et d'une sulfone sur la multiplication *in vitro* et *in vivo* du bacilli tuberculeux aviaire. *Annls Inst. Pasteur, Paris,* **1940,** *64,* 203–237.

Rist, N.; Grumbach, F.; and Libermann, D. Experiments on the antituberculous activity of alpha-ethyl thioisonicotinamide. *Am. Rev. Tuberc. pulm. Dis.,* **1959,** *79,* 1–5.

Russell, D. A.; Shepard, C. C.; McRae, D. H.; Scott, G. C.; and Vincin, D. R. Treatment with 4,4-diacetyldiaminodiphenylsulfone (DADDS) of leprosy patients in the Karimui, New Guinea. *Am. J. trop. Med. Hyg.,* **1971,** *20,* 495–501.

Schonell, M.; Dorken, E.; and Grzybowski, S. Rifampin. *Can. med. Ass. J.,* **1972,** *106,* 783–786.

Schröder, J. M. Zur Pathogenese der Isoniazid-Neuropathie. 1. Eine feinstrukturelle Differenzierung gegenüber der Wallerschen Degeneration. *Acta neuropath.,* **1970a,** *16,* 301–323.

——. Zur Pathogenese der Isoniazid-Neuropathie. II. Phasenkontrast- und elektronenmikroskopische Untersuchungen am Rückenmark, an Spinalganglien und Muskelspindeln. *Ibid.,* **1970b,** *16,* 324–341.

Schwartz, W. S. Comparison of ethionamide with isoniazid in original treatment cases of pulmonary tuberculosis. XIV. A report of the Veterans Administration–Armed Forces Cooperative Study. *Am. Rev. resp. Dis.,* **1966,** *93,* 685–692.

Shepard, C. C.; Levy, L.; and Fasal, P. The death of *Mycobacterium leprae* during treatment with 4,4′-diaminodiphenylsulfone (DDS): initial rates in patients. *Am. J. trop. Med. Hyg.,* **1968,** *17,* 769–775.

——. The sensitivity to dapsone (DDS) of *Mycobacterium leprae* from patients with and without previous treatment. *Ibid.,* **1969,** *18,* 258–263.

——. The death rate of *Mycobacterium leprae* during treatment of lepromatous leprosy with acedapsone (DADDS). *Ibid.,* **1972,** *21,* 440–445.

Shepard, C. C.; Walker, L. L.; Van Landingham, R. M.; and Redus, M. A. Discontinuous administration of clofazimine (B663) on *Mycobacterium leprae* infections. *Proc. Soc. exp. Biol. Med.,* **1971a,** *137,* 725–727.

——. Comparison of B1912 and clofazimine (B663) in *Mycobacterium leprae* infections. *Ibid.,* **1971b,** *137,* 728–729.

Simon, E.; Veres, E.; and Banki, G. Changes in SGOT activity during treatment with ethionamide. *Scand. J. resp. Dis.,* **1969,** *50,* 314–322.

Spector, R., and Lorenzo, W. V. The active transport of para-aminosalicylic acid from the cerebrospinal fluid. *J. Pharmac. exp. Ther.,* **1973,** *185,* 642–648.

Stead, W. W., and Texter, E. C., Jr. Isoniazid hepatitis: backlash of progress. *Ann. intern. Med.,* **1973,** *79,* 125–127.

Storey, P. B., and McLean, R. L. A current appraisal of cycloserine. *Antibiotic Med. clin. Ther.,* **1957,** *4,* 223–232.

Stottmeier, K. D.; Beam, R. E.; and Kubica, G. P. The absorption and excretion of pyrazinamide. I. Preliminary study in laboratory animals and man. *Am. Rev. resp. Dis.,* **1968,** *98,* 70–74.

Strauss, I., and Erhardt, F. Ethambutol absorption, excretion and dosage in patients with renal tuberculosis. *Chemotherapy,* **1970,** *15,* 148–157.

Sunahara, S.; Urano, M.; and Ogawa, M. Genetical and geographic studies on isoniazid inactivation. *Science, Wash.,* **1961,** *134,* 1530.

Takayama, K.; Wang, L.; and David, H. L. Effect of isoniazid on the *in vivo* mycolic acid synthesis cell growth, and variability of *Mycobacterium tuberculosis. Antimicrob. Agents Chemother.,* **1972,** *2,* 29–35.

Thomas, J. P.; Baughn, C. O.; Wilkinson, R. G.; and Shepherd, R. G. A new synthetic compound with antituberculous activity in mice: ethambutol (dextro-2-2′-(ethylenediimino)-di-l-butanol). *Am. Rev. resp. Dis.,* **1961,** *83,* 891–893.

Trautman, J. R. The management of leprosy and its complications. *New Engl. J. Med.,* **1965,** *273,* 756–758.

Tsukamura, M.; Toyama, H.; Mizuno, S.; and Tsukamura, S. Cross resistance relationship among capreomycin, kanamycin, viomycin and streptomycin resistances of *Mycobacterium tuberculosis. Kekkaku, Tokyo,* **1967,** *42,* 399–404.

Verbist, L., and Gyselen, A. Antituberculous activity of rifampin *in vitro* and *in vivo* and the concentrations attained in human blood. *Am. Rev. resp. Dis.,* **1968,** *98,* 923–932.

Ware, M.; Heinvaara, O.; Elo, R.; and Tala, E. Clinical experience of the treatment of drug-resistant pulmonary tuberculosis with rifampicin combined with ethambutol and capreomycin. *Scand. J. resp. Dis.,* **1969,** *50,* 59–63.

Way, E. L.; Smith, P. K.; Howie, D. L.; Weiss, R.; and Swanson, R. The absorption, distribution, excretion and fate of para-aminosalicylic acid. *J. Pharmac. exp. Ther.,* **1948,** *93,* 368–382.

Weiner, I. M., and Tinker, J. P. Pharmacology of pyrazinamide: metabolic and renal function studies related to the mechanism of drug-induced urate retention. *J. Pharmac. exp. Ther.*, **1972**, *180*, 411–434.

Wilson, T. M. Current therapeutics. CCXL. Capreomycin and ethambutol. *Practitioner*, **1967**, *199*, 817–824.

Wimpenny, J. W. T. The uptake and fate of isoniazid in *Mycobacterium tuberculosis* var. *bovis* BCG. *J. gen. Microbiol.*, **1967**, *47*, 389–403.

Youatt, J. A review of the action of isoniazid. *Am. Rev. resp. Dis.*, **1969**, *99*, 729–749.

Zillig, W.; Zechel, K.; Rabussay, D.; Schachner, M.; Sethi, U. S.; Palm, P.; Heil, A.; and Seifert, W. On the role of different subunits of DNA-dependent RNA polymerase from *E. coli* in the transcription process. *Cold Spring Harb. Symp. quant. Biol.*, **1970**, *35*, 47–58.

Monographs and Reviews

Browne, S. G. Advances in the treatment of leprosy. *Practitioner*, **1967**, *199*, 525–531.

Carr, D. T. The treatment of renal tuberculosis. *Med. Clins N. Am.*, **1966**, *50*, 1137–1139.

Cochrane, R. G. A critical appraisal of the present position of leprosy. In, *International Review of Tropical Medicine.* (Lincicome, D. P., ed.) Academic Press, Inc., New York, **1961**, pp. 1–42.

Cochrane, R. G., and Davey, T. F. *Leprosy in Theory and Practice.* The Williams & Wilkins Co., Baltimore, **1964**.

Doub, L. *Bis*(4-aminophenyl) sulfone and related compounds in tuberculosis and leprosy. In, *Medical Chemistry*, Vol. V. (Hartung, W. H., ed.) John Wiley & Sons, Inc., New York, **1961**, pp. 350–425.

Doull, J. A.; Wolcott, R. R.; and Brand, P. W. Treatment of leprosy. I. Chemotherapy. *New Engl. J. Med.*, **1956a**, *254*, 20–25. II. The role of surgery. *Ibid.*, **1956b**, *254*, 64–67.

Fox, W. Changing concepts in the chemotherapy of pulmonary tuberculosis. *Am. Rev. resp. Dis.*, **1968**, *97*, 767–790.

Furesz, S. Chemical and biological properties of rifampicin. *Antibiotica Chemother.*, **1970**, *16*, 316–351.

Gould, R. S. Current concepts of renal tuberculosis. *J. Urol.*, **1968**, *100*, 124–127.

International Congress on Leprology. (Various authors.) *Int. J. Lepr.*, **1963**, *31*, 515–610.

Lattimer, J. K. Renal tuberculosis. *New Engl. J. Med.*, **1965**, *273*, 208–210.

Lester, W. Rifampin: a semisynthetic derivative of rifamycin—a prototype for the future. *A. Rev. Microbiol.*, **1972**, *26*, 85–102.

Meade, G. M. Chemoprophylaxis of tuberculosis. *GP*, **1968**, *38*, 113–119.

Mitchell, R. S. Control of tuberculosis. *New Engl. J. Med.*, **1967**, *276*, 842–848, 905–911.

Pratt, W. B. *Fundamentals of Chemotherapy.* Oxford University Press, New York, **1973**.

Robson, J. M., and Sullivan, F. M. Antituberculosis drugs. *Pharmac. Rev.*, **1963**, *15*, 169–223.

Shepard, C. C. Chemotherapy of leprosy. *A. Rev. Pharmac.*, **1969**, *9*, 37–50.

Symposium. (Various authors.) Rifampin in the treatment of tuberculosis. *Chest*, **1972**, *61*, 517–598.

61 ANTIMICROBIAL AGENTS
[*Continued*]

Miscellaneous Antibacterial Agents; Antifungal and Antiviral Agents

Louis Weinstein

I. Miscellaneous Antibacterial Agents

ERYTHROMYCIN

History and Source. *Erythromycin* is an orally effective antibiotic, discovered in 1952 by McGuire and coworkers in the metabolic products of a strain of *Streptomyces erythreus* (Waksman), originally obtained from a soil sample collected in the Philippine Archipelago. These investigators also carried out the initial *in-vitro* observations, determined the range of toxicity, and demonstrated the effectiveness of the drug in experimental and naturally occurring infections due to gram-positive cocci.

Chemistry. Erythromycin is one of the macrolide antibiotics, so named because they contain a many-membered lactone ring to which are attached one or more deoxy sugars. It is a white crystalline compound, soluble in water to the extent of 2 mg/ml. The structural formula of erythromycin is as follows:

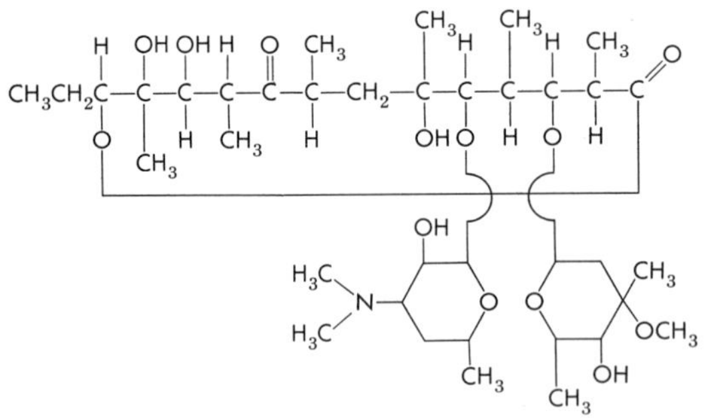

Erythromycin

Antibacterial Activity. Erythromycin may be either bacteriostatic or bactericidal, depending on the nature of the microorganism and the concentration of the drug. It is most effective *in vitro* against gram-positive cocci, such as *Staphylococcus aureus* (penicillin G sensitive or resistant), group-A streptococci, enterococci, and pneumococci; many gram-positive bacilli are also inhibited (*see* Table 55–1,

page 1096). *Neisseria,* some strains of *Haemophilus influenzae, Pasteurella multocida, Brucella, Rickettsia,* and *Treponema* are also inhibited by low concentrations. Erythromycin is effective against *Mycoplasma pneumoniae;* it is without effect on viruses, yeasts, and fungi. Some of the atypical mycobacteria are sensitive to erythromycin *in vitro*. Approximately 85% of strains of *Mycobacterium scrofulaceum* and nearly all of *M. kansasii* are sensitive to 0.5 to 2 µg/ml of the drug; the remainder are inhibited by 4 to 16 µg/ml. Nearly all strains of *M. fortuitum* are resistant, while strains of *M. intracellulare* vary in sensitivity (Molavi and Weinstein, 1971).

While cross-resistance between erythromycin and other antimicrobial agents does not usually occur, it has been noted between lincomycin and erythromycin in strains of the *viridans* group of streptococci isolated from patients treated with either agent (Sprunt *et al.,* 1970). The incidence of erythromycin-resistant strains of *Staph. aureus* has been increasing; in some hospitals 50% of strains are not inhibited by the drug. Occasional strains of *Streptococcus pyogenes* and *Strep. (D.) pneumoniae* resistant to the drug have been recovered from patients.

Mechanism of Action. Erythromycin and other macrolide antibiotics inhibit protein synthesis by binding to 50 S ribosomal subunits of sensitive microorganisms. Erythromycin can interfere with the binding of chloramphenicol, which also acts at this site. Certain resistant microorganisms with mutational changes in components of this subunit of the ribosome fail to bind the drug. The association between erythromycin and the ribosome is reversible but takes place only when the 50 S subunit is free from tRNA molecules bearing nascent peptide chains. The production of small peptides goes on normally in the presence of the antibiotic, but that of highly polymerized homopeptides is suppressed. Gram-positive bacteria accumulate about 100 times more erythromycin than do gram-negative microorganisms. (*See* Mao and Wiegand, 1968; Tanaka *et al.,* 1968; Weisblum and Davies, 1968; Mao and Putterman, 1969; Vogel *et al.,* 1971.)

Absorption, Distribution, and Excretion. *Erythromycin base* is adequately absorbed from the upper part of the small intestine; its activity is destroyed by gastric juice, and food in the stomach delays its ultimate absorption. To overcome these difficulties, the antibiotic can be administered in capsules made with an acid-resistant coating or as the *stearate. Erythromycin estolate* is less susceptible to acid than is the parent compound; it retains its potency at the pH of gastric juice for prolonged periods, and is absorbed to a greater degree than are other forms of the drug. Food does not appreciably alter its absorption. Although erythromycin estolate appears in the blood somewhat more slowly, the peak reached is higher, and high plasma concentrations persist longer when it is administered after a meal (Griffith and Black, 1964). A single, oral 500-mg dose of the estolate produces peak plasma concentrations of approximately 3 μg/ml after 2 hours.

The oral administration of erythromycin base or the stearate produces peak plasma concentrations in 1 to 4 hours, depending on the rapidity of gastric emptying. The values decline strikingly by the fourth to sixth hour. *Erythromycin ethylsuccinate* is another ester that is adequately absorbed following oral administration, particularly when the stomach is empty. However, plasma concentrations of drug are best maintained with administration of the estolate (Griffith and Black, 1969).

Only 2 to 5% of orally administered erythromycin is excreted in active form in the urine; from 12 to 15%, after intravenous infusion. When large doses of erythromycin are given by mouth, the feces may contain as much as 0.5 mg/g. The antibiotic is concentrated in the liver and excreted in active form in the bile, which may contain as much as 250 μg/ml when plasma concentrations are very high.

Erythromycin diffuses readily into intracellular fluids. All tissues except the brain contain higher concentrations than in the blood, and the drug persists for some time in the tissues after it is no longer demonstrable in the circulation. The antibiotic diffuses into pleural and peritoneal fluids. The cerebrospinal fluid concentration in individuals with meningeal inflammation is frequently high enough to eradicate the pneumococcus and the staphylococcus. Erythromycin traverses the placental barrier; fetal plasma concentrations are about 5 to 20% of those in the maternal plasma.

Preparations, Routes of Administration, and Dosage. *Oral Preparations. Erythromycin,* U.S.P. (E-MYCIN, ERYTHROCIN, ILOTYCIN), is available in enteric-coated tablets containing 250 mg of the drug and in suppositories (125 mg). *Erythromycin Stearate Tablets,* U.S.P. (BRISTAMYCIN, ERYTHROCIN STEARATE, ETHRIL), contain 125 or 250 mg each. *Erythromycin Estolate,* N.F. (ILOSONE), is supplied as official capsules (125 and 250 mg), tablets (125, 250, and 500 mg), and as an oral suspension (125 and 250 mg/5 ml). *Erythromycin Ethylsuccinate,* U.S.P. (ERYTHROCIN ETHYL SUCCINATE, PEDIAMYCIN), is available as granules for oral suspension (200 mg/5 ml) and as chewable tablets (200 mg).

Parenteral Preparations. Sterile Erythromycin Gluceptate, U.S.P. (ILOTYCIN GLUCEPTATE), and *Erythromycin Lactobionate for Injection,* U.S.P. (ERYTHROCIN LACTOBIONATE), are available for *intravenous* injection in the form of sterile dry powders (250 or 500 mg or 1 g of antibiotic). *Erythromycin Ethylsuccinate Injection,* N.F. (ERYTHROCIN ETHYL SUCCINATE-I.M.), contains 50 mg/ml in 2- and 10-ml containers for intramuscular injection. This preparation includes butyl aminobenzoate (2%) as a local anesthetic.

The *oral* dose of erythromycin for *adults* ranges from 1 to 4 g per day, in equally divided and spaced amounts, usually given every 6 hours, depending on the nature and severity of the infection. Daily doses of erythromycin as large as 8 g orally, given for 3 months, appear to be well tolerated. Food should not be given immediately before or after oral administration of erythromycin base; this precaution need not be taken when the estolate is administered. The *oral* dose of erythromycin for *children* is 30 to 50 mg/kg per day, divided into four portions. *Intramuscular injection* is limited by the pain it causes. Because of their requirement for larger doses, intramuscular injection usually cannot be carried out in adults; small children do not have the necessary muscle mass. *Intravenous administration* is reserved for the therapy of severe infections. The usual dose used by the writer is 1 g every 6 hours; 1 g of erythromycin gluceptate may be given intravenously every 6 hours for as long as 4 weeks with no difficulty except for thrombophlebitis at the site of injection.

Untoward Effects. The incidence of untoward effects associated with the use of erythromycin preparations is low. Among the *hypersensitivity reactions* are *fever, eosinophilia,* and *skin eruptions,* each of which may occur alone or in combination; they disappear shortly after therapy is stopped. The most striking allergic reaction to this drug is *cholestatic hepatitis.* This apparently occurs only with *erythromycin estolate*. The illness starts after about 10 to 20 days of treatment and is early characterized by nausea, vomiting, and abdominal cramps, often mimicking the pain of acute cholecystitis. These symptoms are shortly followed by jaundice, fever, leukocytosis, eosinophilia, and elevated plasma transaminase and bilirubin concentrations; the cholecystogram is negative. The syndrome resembles acute cholecystitis, extrahepatic biliary obstruction, pancreatitis, or viral hepatitis. The clinical and pathological findings are very similar to those observed with the hepatic disturbance produced by chlorpromazine. All manifestations usually clear entirely within a few days after cessation of drug therapy and rarely are prolonged. Challenge with a small dose of the drug after recovery may reproduce the entire picture. That hypersensitivity is responsible for this syndrome is suggested by its rarity, by the fact that it does not appear with the first exposure to the drug (unless this is continued for at least 10 or more days) and is most frequent in individuals who have been treated more than once, and by the fact that it is not related to dose. False elevation of serum glutamic oxalacetic transaminase may appear in patients taking erythromycin; this seems to be due to an unidentified substance in the blood related to administration of the drug. (*See* Sabath *et al.*, 1968a; Braun, 1969; Tolman *et al.*, 1974.)

Erythromycin may produce *irritative effects*. Oral administration, especially in a dose of 1 g to adults, is very frequently accompanied by epigastric distress, which may be quite severe. Intramuscular injection of quantities larger than 100 mg produces extremely severe pain that persists for hours. Intravenous infusion of 1-g doses, even when dissolved in a large volume, almost regularly is followed by thrombophlebitis.

The writer has studied six patients who developed difficulty in hearing while being treated with 4 g per day of erythromycin intravenously. This effect has appeared as early as the second day of therapy or as late as the third week. Audiometric studies have revealed loss of perception of high-frequency tones at first, progressing to difficulty in the conversational range if therapy is not stopped. Cessation of treatment has led to complete return of normal hearing over a period ranging from several days to 2 or more weeks.

The effects of erythromycin on the intestinal flora are usually insignificant clinically, despite the fact that there may be a sharp reduction in the gram-positive components during its oral administration.

As with all other antimicrobial agents, *suprainfection* may develop during the use of the antibiotic; a variety of gram-negative bacteria as well as yeasts and fungi, especially *Candida*, may be involved.

There are no known contraindications to the use of erythromycin except prior allergic reactions to the drug. Patients with hepatic dysfunction should not receive the estolate. Since very little of the drug is excreted in the urine, full doses may be given safely to patients with renal failure (Kunin and Finland, 1959).

Therapeutic Uses.   Extensive studies of the clinical application of erythromycin have clearly demonstrated its usefulness in a variety of infections due to gram-positive microorganisms.

Staphylococcal Infections.   Erythromycin is very effective in the management of disease produced by both penicillin-sensitive and penicillin-resistant *Staph. aureus.* Excellent results have been obtained in staphylococcal pneumonia, bacteremia, endocarditis, meningitis, osteomyelitis, furuncles, carbuncles, and wound infections. However, the emergence of erythromycin-resistant strains in appreciable numbers in some hospitals is a limiting factor in the use of this drug. The availability of the penicillinase-resistant penicillins and the cephalosporins has reduced the need for erythromycin in this type of disease, but it is still a valuable agent for use in individuals unable to take penicillin because of previous reactions. For staphylococcal skin and wound infections, the oral administration of 0.5 g of erythromycin every 6 hours for 7 to 10 days is usually sufficient. For more serious involvement, for example, bacteremia, endocarditis, pneumonia, meningitis, and osteomyelitis, the drug should be given intravenously in a dose of 1 g every 4 to 6 hours for 4 to 6 weeks.

Other Coccal Infections.   Pharyngitis, scarlet fever, and *erysipelas* produced by group-A *Streptococcus pyogenes* respond dramatically to erythromycin. The oral administration of 250 to 500 mg every 6 hours for 10 days produces rapid cure of these diseases, prevents the appearance of suppurative complications, and suppresses the formation of antistreptolysin. Treatment with 250 mg twice a day appears to produce a rate of cure about equal to that obtained with penicillin G (Shapera *et al.*, 1973). The use of erythromycin should be considered in cases in which the presence of penicillinase-producing staphylococci may be responsible for relapse of streptococcal pharyngitis after adequate treatment with penicillin G. *Pneumococcal pneumonia* responds promptly to oral therapy with 250 to 500 mg of erythromycin every 6 hours; the drug is continued until fever has been absent for 5 days. *Pneumococcal meningitis* in patients sensitive to penicillin has been treated with success by the intravenous injection of 1 g of erythromycin every 4 hours for several days, followed by the same dose every 6 hours for 2 to 3 weeks. Some cases of *subacute bacterial endocarditis* due to streptococci of the *viridans* group have been successfully treated by intravenous infusion of 1 g of erythromycin every 4 to 6 hours for no less than 4 weeks. Endocarditis and other infections due to enterococci may also respond well to the drug.

Miscellaneous Infections. Erythromycin is very effective in eradicating the acute or chronic *diphtheria bacillus carrier state;* an oral dose of 500 mg in adults and 250 mg in children, given every 6 hours for 2 weeks, produces essentially 100% eradication of the microorganisms with no relapse after therapy is stopped. It must be stressed that, in the acute disease, neither this nor any other antibiotic alters the course of the infection or the risk of complications; a proper dose of specific antitoxin must be administered. Erythromycin (500 mg orally every 6 hours for 10 days) has been used with some degree of success in *syphilis* (in penicillin-sensitive persons). *Clostridium tetani* is eradicated by the drug; however, antitoxin must be given simultaneously in cases of tetanus. Erythromycin is very effective in the therapy of *Mycoplasma pneumoniae* pneumonia; however, the microorganisms may persist in the respiratory tract despite adequate plasma concentrations of the antibiotic (Smith *et al.,* 1967). In general, erythromycin is less effective than tetracycline in eliminating the carrier state. The possibility that urinary tract infections due to *Escherichia coli, Klebsiella pneumoniae, Proteus mirabilis, Pseudomonas,* and *Serratia* may be treatable with erythromycin, provided the urine pH is in the alkaline range, has been suggested by Sabath and colleagues (1968b). In the treatment of gonorrhea, an initial dose of 2.5 g of erythromycin stearate followed by the same quantity in divided doses over the following 2 days is said to be a suitable substitute for penicillin therapy (Smith and Osick, 1969); in chronic or deep-seated disease, 500 mg of the drug should be given every 6 hours for about 2 weeks.

Prophylactic Uses. Although penicillin is the drug of choice for the *prophylaxis of rheumatic fever recurrences,* another antistreptococcal agent must be used in individuals sensitized to this antibiotic. The sulfonamides are cheap and effective for this purpose (*see* Chapter 56). In some instances, however, it may be preferable to use erythromycin.

TROLEANDOMYCIN

Troleandomycin is a semisynthetic derivative of *oleandomycin,* a macrolide antibiotic elaborated by *Streptomyces antibioticus.* These agents resemble erythromycin chemically and in their antibacterial activity; they are, however, more toxic and less effective, and it is thus difficult to envision their valid therapeutic application. Troleandomycin is described in earlier editions of this textbook.

LINCOMYCIN

History and Source. *Lincomycin* is an antibiotic elaborated by an actinomycete, *Streptomyces lincolnensis,* so named because it was isolated from soil collected near Lincoln, Nebraska. The drug was first reported in the literature in 1962.

Chemistry and Assay. *Lincomycin* is a derivative of the amino acid trans-L-4-*n*-propylhygrinic acid, attached to a sulfur-containing derivative of an octose. The structural formula of lincomycin is as follows:

Lincomycin

The boldface **C** (position 7) in the structural formula is the site of modification to yield *clindamycin,* the 7-deoxy, 7-chloro derivative. Lincomycin is water soluble and acid stable.

Antibacterial Activity. Concentrations of *lincomycin* less than 0.5 μg/ml inhibit the multiplication *in vitro* of *Strep.* (*D.*) *pneumoniae,* group-A *Strep. pyogenes,* the *viridans* group of streptococci, and *Bacillus anthracis.* However, some strains of pneumococci and group-A streptococci are resistant. The drug is without effect on enterococci. *Corynebacterium diphtheriae, Cl. tetani,* and *Cl. perfringens* are suppressed by concentrations lower than 2 μg/ml. Susceptibility of *Staph. aureus* to the drug is variable; while most strains are sensitive to about 2 μg/ml, about 15% of strains grow in a concentration of 5 μg/ml. A number of strains of staphylococci that are resistant to methicillin or erythromycin are also resistant to lincomycin. The antibiotic is active against some but not all types of *Bacteroides;* in one study, only 7% of strains of *B. fragilis* were found to be susceptible to the drug (Sutter *et al.,* 1973). Lincomycin is bacteriostatic for *Actinomyces* in a concentration of 0.125 to 0.25 μg/ml. *Mycoplasma* are inhibited, but not nearly as effectively as by erythromycin. T strains of *M. hominis* are not susceptible. Lincomycin is not inhibitory for most strains of *Neisseria gonorrhoeae, H. influenzae,* and *enterococci.* Most gram-negative bacilli and all viruses and fungi are resistant. (*See* Meyers *et al.,* 1969; Dixon and Lipinski, 1972.)

Mechanism of Action. Lincomycin binds exclusively to the 50 S subunit of bacterial ribosomes and suppresses protein synthesis. Although lincomycin, erythromycin, and chloramphenicol are not structurally related, they all act at this site, and the binding of one of these antibiotics to the ribosome may inhibit the reaction of the other. There are no clinical indications for the concurrent use of these antibiotics.

Absorption, Distribution, and Excretion. Lincomycin is rapidly but only partially (20 to 35%) absorbed from the gastrointestinal tract. Plasma concentrations are appreciably lower when the drug is taken after a meal. Peak plasma concentrations average about 2 to 5 $\mu g/ml$ after an oral dose of 500 mg; values are maintained above the minimal inhibitory concentration for most gram-positive microorganisms for 6 to 8 hours, and detectable antibacterial activity persists for 12 hours or more. *Intramuscular injection* results in maximal plasma concentrations within 30 minutes. With 600 mg intramuscularly every 12 hours, maximal plasma concentrations are 15 to 20 $\mu g/ml$. *Intravenous infusion* of 600 mg of the drug over a 2-hour period produces concentrations in the therapeutic range for 14 hours. The half-life of lincomycin is about 5 hours. In patients with hepatic insufficiency, the half-life of the drug is almost doubled, even when renal function is normal (Bellamy *et al.,* 1967). Individuals with severe azotemia have plasma concentrations that are three times higher and more sustained than those of normal subjects.

Urinary excretion of lincomycin is limited and quite variable; about 5% of an oral dose and 15% of a parenteral dose appear in the urine. The bile is an important route of excretion of this antibiotic. The drug appears in active form in the feces after oral and parenteral administration, suggesting excretion in the bile, through the intestinal wall, or both.

Lincomycin is distributed in both extracellular and intracellular fluids and is detectable in most human tissues. It reaches insignificant concentrations in cerebrospinal fluid in persons with normal meninges, and attains concentrations that are approximately 40% of those in the plasma in cases of meningitis. The drug appears in adequate concentration in the ocular aqueous humor after parenteral administration; lincomycin penetrates well into bone.

Preparations, Routes of Administration, and Dosage. *Lincomycin Hydrochloride,* U.S.P. (LINCOCIN), is available in capsules containing 250 or 500 mg, as a sterile solution (300 mg/ml) for parenteral use, and in a syrup (50 mg/ml) for use in children.

The recommended *oral dose* of lincomycin for adults is 500 mg every 6 or 8 hours, depending on the severity of the infection; for children it is 30 to 60 mg/kg per day, divided into three or four equal doses. When *intramuscular therapy* is employed, a dose of 600 mg every 6, 8, or 12 hours is recommended, depending on the severity of the infection. *Intravenous therapy* requires the injection of 600 mg dissolved in 250 ml of 5% glucose or isotonic saline solution every 8 to 12 hours; for children, the intravenous dose is 10 to 20 mg/kg daily, divided equally and given as an infusion every 8 to 12 hours. For very severe infections, the quantity administered may be increased.

Untoward Effects. Administration of lincomycin, particularly orally, can cause *diarrhea* in as many as 20% of cases; this diarrhea may be severe, requiring withdrawal of the drug, and some patients develop *pseudomembranous colitis,* which may be fatal. Among the other reactions recorded after oral therapy are *glossitis, stomatitis, nausea, vomiting, pruritus ani, various skin rashes, urticaria, generalized pruritus,* and *vaginitis.* Parenteral administration has been followed rarely by *neutropenia, leukopenia,* and *thrombopenia,* all of which disappear when therapy is stopped. Among other rare untoward effects are *angioedema, serum sickness, anaphylaxis, photosensitivity,* and *cardiopulmonary arrest* (after rapid intravenous infusion). Elevations of serum glutamic oxalacetate transaminase have occasionally been observed after lincomycin, but in some cases this is a false reaction. *Overgrowth of yeasts* may occur in the intestinal tract. *Suprainfections* are uncommon. Renal and neurological abnormalities have not been reported.

Therapeutic Uses. Lincomycin is effective in infections in man due to *pneumococci, Strep. pyogenes* (group A), *Strep. mitis,* and *Staph. aureus;* the *diphtheria carrier state, erysipelas, staphylococcal infections* (strains of proven sensitivity), *streptococcal cellulitis,* and *actinomycosis* have shown very good responses. The drug is not as effective as penicillin in the treatment of otitis media in children. It has been reported to produce good results in acne vulgaris and in suppurative diseases of the skin. Lincomycin appears to have a very high degree of effectiveness in *chronic osteomyelitis.* Concentrations of 1 to 2 $\mu g/g$ are present in bone when those in plasma are 6 to 16 $\mu g/ml$. The antibiotic may have a special affinity for bone or exhibit increased antimicrobial activity when present in osseous structures. The drug is often employed as a substitute for erythromycin because it produces little or no pain on intramuscular injection. However, it is not effective in the management of enterococcal disease and cannot be used in place of erythromycin for this purpose. Furthermore, strains of *Staph. aureus* that are resistant to erythromycin may also be insensitive to lincomycin.

The antibiotic may be of value in the management of some kinds of intestinal disorders (*e.g.,* the blind-loop syndrome), because of its activity against *Bacteroides* and other anaerobes. Oral administration of the drug in man produces a striking decrease or elimination of these bacteria from the intestinal tract, but the number of enterococci may be increased 100,000-fold (Finegold *et al.,* 1966). Lincomycin is of no value in infections due to facultatively anaerobic, gram-negative bacilli.

CLINDAMYCIN

Chemistry. *Clindamycin* is the 7-deoxy, 7-chloro derivative of lincomycin (*see* page 1227).

Antibacterial Activity. While qualitatively similar to lincomycin, clindamycin exhibits, in general, a greater degree of antibacterial activity *in vitro.* It is highly active against most strains of *Staph. aureus* but may not inhibit methicillin-resistant strains. Other sensitive microorganisms include *Strep. (D.) pneumoniae, Strep. pyogenes,* anaerobic streptococci and those of the *viridans* group, other gram-positive species, and *Actinomyces israelii.* The drug is highly active against most strains of *Bacteroides,* especially *B. fragilis,* and *Fusobacterium varium.* An appreciable number of clostridia of clinical importance are resistant. Gram-negative bacilli as well as the gonococcus and the meningococcus are insensitive. (*See* Lerner, 1969; Meyers *et al.,* 1969; Bartlett *et al.,* 1972; Sutter *et al.,* 1973; Wilkins and Thiel, 1973.)

Absorption, Fate, and Excretion. Clindamycin is nearly completely absorbed following oral administration, and peak plasma concentrations of 2 to 3 $\mu g/ml$ are attained within 1 hour after the ingestion of 150 mg. The presence of food in the stomach does not reduce absorption significantly. The half-life of the antibiotic is 2 to 2½ hours, and some drug accumulation is to be expected if it is given at 6-hour intervals.

Clindamycin palmitate, an oral preparation for pediatric use, is itself inactive, but the ester is hydrolyzed rapidly *in vivo.* Its absorption is similar to that of clindamycin. After several oral doses at 6-hour intervals, children attain plasma concentrations of 2 to 4 $\mu g/ml$ with the administration of 8 to 16 mg/kg.

The phosphate ester of clindamycin, which is given parenterally, is also rapidly hydrolyzed *in vivo* to the active parent compound. Following intramuscular injection, peak plasma concentrations are not attained for 3 hours in adults and 1 hour in children. The recommended parenteral dosages provide peak plasma concentrations of 5 to 15 $\mu g/ml$ and effective antimicrobial activity for approximately 8 hours.

While clindamycin is widely distributed in many fluids and tissues, including bone, significant concentrations are apparently not attained in cerebrospinal fluid, even when the meninges are inflamed. The drug readily crosses the placental barrier. Ninety percent or more of clindamycin is bound to plasma proteins. (*See* Panzer *et al.,* 1972; Vacek *et al.,* 1972; Philipson *et al.,* 1973.)

Only about 10% of administered clindamycin is excreted unaltered in the urine, and small quantities are found in the feces. Most of the drug is inactivated by metabolism to N-demethylclindamycin and clindamycin sulfoxide, which are excreted in the urine and bile. The half-life of clindamycin is lengthened only slightly in patients with markedly impaired renal function, and little adjustment of dosage is required for such individuals. Greater accumulation of drug may occur in patients with severe hepatic failure.

The clinical pharmacology of clindamycin is discussed by Lwin and Collipp (1970), DeHaan and associates (1972, 1973), Fass and Saslaw (1972), Kauffman and coworkers (1972), and Balanchandar and colleagues (1973).

Preparations, Routes of Administration, and Dosage. *Clindamycin Hydrochloride,* U.S.P. (CLEOCIN), is supplied for oral administration in capsules containing 75 or 150 mg. *Clindamycin Palmitate Hydrochloride,* N.F. (CLEOCIN PEDIATRIC), is a preparation of flavored granules for suspension to a concentration of 75 mg/5 ml. *Clindamycin Phosphate,* N.F. (CLEOCIN PHOSPHATE), is for intramuscular or intravenous use and is supplied as a solution of 150 mg/ml in 2- and 10-ml containers.

The *oral* dose of clindamycin for *adults* is 150 to 300 mg every 6 hours; for severe infections, 300 to 450 mg every 6 hours. *Children* should receive 8 to 16 mg/kg per day in three or four divided doses; for severe infections, 16 to 20 mg/kg per day. However, children weighing less than 10 kg should receive ½ teaspoonful of clindamycin palmitate hydrochloride (37.5 mg) three times daily as a minimal dose.

When *parenteral* therapy is necessary, *adults* require 600 mg to 3.2 g daily in two, three, or four divided doses, depending on the severity of disease. Daily doses of 4.8 g have been given in unusual circumstances. *Children* should receive 10 to 40 mg/kg per day in three or four divided doses; in severe infections, a minimal daily dose of 300 mg is recommended, regardless of body weight.

Untoward Effects. While the incidence of *diarrhea* caused by clindamycin was originally thought to be low, 5 to 20% of patients may experience this difficulty. More serious, a number of patients have developed *colitis,* with diarrhea, abdominal pain, fever, and blood and mucus in the stools. The cause of this syndrome is uncertain. Some patients have required corticosteroid therapy or colectomy, and deaths have resulted. While the true incidence of this problem is currently unknown, it is clear that serious consideration should be given to the therapeutic indications for this drug. This is particularly true of oral administration for infections that will respond to less toxic agents.

Skin rashes may occur in 10% of patients treated with clindamycin. Other reactions, which are uncommon, include *exudative erythema multiforme* (Stevens-Johnson syndrome), *reversible elevation of SGOT and SGPT, granulocytopenia, thrombopenia,* and *anaphylactoid reactions. Thrombophlebitis* may result from intravenous administration.

Therapeutic Uses. While a number of infections with gram-positive cocci will respond favorably to clindamycin, current uncertainty over the incidence of serious toxicity, especially colitis, requires limitation of its use to infections in which it is clearly superior. The infections studied most intensively to date and for which clindamycin is probably the most effective agent at present are those produced by *Bacteroides*, especially *B. fragilis*. Some species of this genus are, however, variably or poorly sensitive. Abdominal abscesses, bacteremia, pneumonia, lung abscess, empyema, soft-tissue infections, and decubitus ulcers due to *Bacteroides* or *Fusobacterium* respond favorably when parenteral treatment is undertaken and continued for 1 to 2 weeks. In some instances, especially when a mixture of microorganisms is present (*e.g.,* intra-abdominal abscess secondary to rupture of a viscus), adjunct therapy with other antibiotics and particularly surgical drainage are critical in producing cure. (*See* Douglas and Kislak, 1973; Fass *et al.,* 1973; Thadepalli *et al.,* 1973.) Disease due to *Actinomyces israelii* and to anaerobic streptococci has been treated successfully with clindamycin. Chloramphenicol, to which most anaerobes including *Bacteroides* are sensitive, is preferable to clindamycin for the therapy of anaerobic infections of the central nervous system, such as brain abscess, because clindamycin penetrates the blood-brain barrier poorly.

SPECTINOMYCIN

Source and Chemistry. *Spectinomycin* is an antibiotic produced by *Streptomyces spectabilis*. The drug is an aminocyclitol; its structural formula is as follows:

Spectinomycin

Antibacterial Activity and Mechanism. Although spectinomycin is active against a number of gram-negative bacterial species, for which it may be as inhibitory as streptomycin or tetracycline or more suppressive than ampicillin, it is inferior to other drugs to which such microorganisms are susceptible (Schoutens *et al.,* 1972). However, it readily inhibits gonococci at concentrations of 7 to 20 $\mu g/ml$, concentrations produced in plasma by the administration of recommended doses.

Spectinomycin selectively inhibits protein synthesis in gram-negative bacteria. In contrast to the site of action of other such inhibitors described in this chapter, the antibiotic binds to and acts on the 30 S ribosomal subunit. There are similarities in its action to that of the aminoglycosides; however, spectinomycin is not bactericidal and does not cause mis-

reading of polyribonucleotides. High-level bacterial resistance may develop as a result of mutation (Davies *et al.,* 1965).

Absorption, Distribution, and Excretion. Spectinomycin is rapidly absorbed after intramuscular injection. A single dose of 2 g produces peak plasma concentrations averaging 100 $\mu g/ml$ at 1 hour; a 4-g injection, 160 $\mu g/ml$. Eight hours after injection of 2 or 4 g, the plasma concentrations are 15 μg or 30 $\mu g/ml$, respectively. The drug is not significantly bound to plasma protein. Spectinomycin is excreted in biologically active form in the urine; all of an administered dose is recovered within 48 hours after injection.

Preparations. *Spectinomycin hydrochloride* (TROBICIN) is supplied as a sterile powder for reconstitution with water containing 0.9% benzyl alcohol. Vials of 2 and 4 g are available. This solution is for intramuscular injection only.

Untoward Effects. Because of relatively limited clinical experience at present, the full range of toxic reactions to spectinomycin is still uncertain. *Urticaria, chills,* and *fever* have been noted after single doses of the antibiotic, as have *dizziness* and *insomnia.* The injection may be painful. During clinical trials of spectinomycin certain changes in laboratory values were observed after multiple doses. These included a *decrease* in *hemoglobin* and *hematocrit* and *elevations* of serum *alkaline phosphatase* and *glutamate-pyruvate transaminase* activities. Blood urea nitrogen concentrations and creatinine clearance values were altered in some individuals, but no consistent changes indicative of nephrotoxicity have been recorded. A reduction in urine volume has been observed.

Therapeutic Uses. Spectinomycin should be used only for the treatment of *acute genital and rectal gonorrhea.* The recommended dose is a single deep intramuscular injection of 2 g for men with acute gonococcal urethritis; although a dose of 4 g has been recommended for women with this disease, some clinicians have noted that 2 g also produces cure. For patients with gonococcal proctitis the recommended single dose is 4 g. The rate of cure for these forms of gonorrhea is 95 to 100%. Some strains of *N. gonorrhoeae* are resistant to the drug. The antibiotic appears to be a very good choice for the treatment of gonorrhea in individuals sensitized to penicillin and other effective agents, and its use should probably be reserved for such patients for the present. It must be emphasized that spectinomycin is without effect on incubating or established syphilis. (*See* Cornelius and Domescik, 1970; Sinanian *et al.,* 1972; Reyn *et al.,* 1973.)

POLYMYXIN B

History and Source. The *polymyxins,* discovered in 1947, are a group of closely related antibiotic substances (polymyxins A, B, C, D, E) elaborated by various strains of *Bacillus polymyxa,* an aerobic spore-forming rod found in soil. Polymyxin B is available for clinical use and is discussed here. Colistin (polymyxin E) is described below. (*See* Brownlee *et al.,* 1952.)

Chemistry. The polymyxins, which are cationic detergents, are relatively simple, basic peptides with molecular weights of about 1000. They readily form water-soluble salts with mineral acids. The structural formula for polymyxin B, which is itself a mixture of polymyxins B_1 and B_2, is as follows:

$$R - \text{L-DAB} \rightarrow \text{L-Thr} \rightarrow \text{L-DAB} \rightarrow \text{L-DAB} \nearrow \overset{\text{L-DAB} \rightarrow \text{D-Phe} \rightarrow \text{L-Leu}}{\underset{\text{L-Thr} \leftarrow \text{L-DAB} \leftarrow \text{L-DAB}}{\Big\downarrow}}$$

Polymyxin B_1: R = (+)-6-Methyloctanoyl
Polymyxin B_2: R = 6-Methylheptanoyl
DAB = α,γ-Diaminobutyric Acid

Powder forms and aqueous solutions of polymyxin B are quite stable in the physiological ranges of temperature and pH.

Antibacterial Activity. The *in-vitro* and *in-vivo* activity of polymyxin B is sharply restricted to gram-negative bacteria. *Enterobacter, Escherichia, Haemophilus, Klebsiella, Pasteurella, Salmonella, Shigella,* and *Vibrio* are sensitive to concentrations of 0.5 to 2.0 μg/ml. Many strains of *Pseud. aeruginosa* are inhibited *in vitro* by less than 8 μg/ml. *Brucella* is only moderately susceptible. Most strains of *Proteus* are unaffected by the drug. Some *Neisseria* are also resistant, and gram-positive bacteria are singularly unaffected. Orally administered polymyxin B markedly reduces but does not eliminate coliform microorganisms from the feces of man; the drug eradicates *Pseud. aeruginosa* from the intestinal tract.

Polymyxin B is rapidly bactericidal *in vitro*. Substances that antagonize cationic surface-active agents, such as soap, impair the action of the drug.

The development of bacterial resistance to polymyxin B is infrequent in most species. However, insensitive strains are occasionally encountered among susceptible microorganisms. There is complete cross-resistance between polymyxin B and colistin.

Mechanism of Action. Polymyxin B is a surface-active agent, containing lipophilic and lipophobic groups separated within the molecule. The ability of these to become oriented between lipid and protein films is thought to produce a disorientation of the lipoprotein membrane of bacteria, so that it no longer functions as an effective osmotic barrier and thereby allows cell contents to escape. Permeability changes in the membrane begin immediately on contact with the drug. The cell walls of polymyxin B–sensitive bacteria take up more of the antibiotic than do those of resistant bacteria, and sensitivity to polymyxin B may be determined by the composition of the phospholipid fraction. (*See* reviews by Newton, 1956, 1958; Sebek, 1967.)

Absorption, Distribution, and Excretion. Polymyxin B, even in large doses, is not absorbed to a significant degree when given orally. The drug is also poorly absorbed from mucous membranes and the surface of large burns. After daily intramuscular injection of 4.8 mg/kg, plasma concentrations in children range from 3 to 7 μg/ml. The daily administration of 2 to 4 mg/kg parenterally to adults yields values of 1 to 8 μg/ml, the peak occurring about 2 hours after injection. Repeated injections of the antibiotic lead to its accumulation in the circulation. High concentrations develop in patients with renal insufficiency.

Although very little polymyxin B is eliminated by the kidney during the first 12 hours after injection, large amounts are eventually excreted by this route. Concentrations of 20 to 100 μg/ml are found in the urine after continued parenteral therapy with conventional doses. Elimination continues for 1 to 3 days after the drug is stopped. A total of 60% of the administered polymyxin B can be recovered from the urine. The drug apparently does not gain access to the cerebrospinal fluid from the circulation, even when the meninges are inflamed.

Preparations, Routes of Administration, and Dosage. *Polymyxin B Sulfate,* U.S.P. (AEROSPORIN), is available as a *topical powder* (500,000 units in a vial), *otic solution* (10,000 units/ml), and *tablets* (250,000 units). The antibiotic is also marketed in vials containing 500,000 units, for parenteral injection. Pure polymyxin B base contains 10,000 units of polymyxin B activity per milligram. (The official U.S.P. preparation of polymyxin B sulfate contains not less than 6000 units/mg.) Polymyxin B can be given by mouth, by intramuscular injection, by intrathecal instillation, and topically. An official combination of neomycin and polymyxin is used for irrigation of the urinary bladder (*see* page 1179).

The *oral dose* for adults and older children is 750,000 to 1 million units, three times daily; for children 2 to 5 years old, 500,000 to 750,000 units, three times daily; for those under 2 years of age, 250,000 to 500,000 units, three times daily.

The total daily *intramuscular dose* varies from 15,000 to 25,000 units/kg and should not exceed 2 million units; it is ordinarily injected in four equally divided and spaced doses. The intramuscular solution is prepared by dissolving 500,000 units of polymyxin B in 2 ml of 1% sterile procaine hydrochloride solution. The duration of parenteral medication varies with the nature of the illness, the response to therapy, and the severity of toxic reactions but should be at least 3 weeks in most instances. The *intrathecal dose* for children under 2 years of age is 20,000 units daily for 3 or 4 days, then 25,000 units every other day; for older children and adults, 50,000 units daily for 3 or 4 days, then 50,000 units every other day. For adults, each dose may be increased to 100,000 units. The intrathecal solution should contain 50,000 units of the drug in 1 ml of 0.9% sterile sodium chloride solution (not procaine solution); in this concentration, the recommended dose is relatively nonirritating to the meninges and does not cause systemic toxicity. For *topical administration*, polymyxin B can be employed in an ointment, or in solution for use as a spray, irrigation, or wet dressing. A concentration of 0.1 to 0.25% in aqueous solution is nonirritating and effective. Not more than 2 million units should be applied daily to denuded surfaces or open wounds.

Untoward Effects. Polymyxin B applied to intact or denuded skin or mucous membranes produces no systemic reactions because of almost complete lack of absorption of the antibiotic from these sites. *Hypersensitization* is uncommon when the antibiotic is used in this way. Fever and punctate, macular, or urticarial rashes, the primary manifestations of hypersensitivity to the drug, occur infrequently when polymyxin B is administered parenterally. Nausea, vomiting, and diarrhea are produced by large doses (600 mg) taken orally. *Pain* after intramuscular injection is common. A "drawing" or "aching" pain, varying in intensity, may appear about 40 to 60 minutes after an intramuscular injection and radiate along the peripheral nerve distribution; it cannot be prevented by the addition of a local anesthetic to the antibiotic. Intrathecal injection of more than 5 mg of polymyxin B may produce the signs of *meningeal irritation, headache, fever,* and *increase in cells and protein in the spinal fluid* in some individuals.

Other untoward effects of polymyxin B are *facial flushing, dizziness* that may progress to *ataxia, paresthesias* in a circumoral and "glove-and-stocking" distribution, *diplopia* due to peripheral ophthalmoplegia, *ptosis, generalized weakness, slurred speech, generalized areflexia, increase in weakness in myasthenia gravis, blurred vision, difficulty in speaking, dysphagia, dyspnea, acute tubular necrosis,* and *interstitial nephritis.* In some cases, the drug produces noncompetitive *neuromuscular blockade* that results in respiratory paralysis. Respiratory arrest may occur with the first dose of the drug or only after it has been given for as long as 45 days; it is more common when renal failure is present and when plasma concentrations are high, and is very often preceded by dyspnea and restlessness. It is not antagonized by neostigmine or calcium gluconate, as is the case with the aminoglycoside antibiotics (Lindesmith *et al.,* 1968).

The daily injection of 2.5 mg/kg of polymyxin often results in *proteinuria, hematuria,* and *cylindruria.* With doses of 3 mg/kg or more, *azotemia* and *decrease in glomerular filtration rate* are common; these effects tend to increase in severity with continued treatment, but they are reversible if therapy is stopped. Excessively high and sustained plasma concentrations of polymyxin B develop in patients with renal insufficiency; neurotoxicity and nephrotoxicity occur more frequently and with greater intensity in such individuals. If it is absolutely essential that a patient with impaired renal function receive this drug, persons with azotemia should be given only 1.0 to 1.5 mg/kg of polymyxin B each day for not more than 5 to 10 days. Uremic patients can be given two or three injections of the usual dose in order to achieve high blood and tissue concentrations; therapy then must be either stopped or the dosage sharply reduced. *Suprainfection* due to grampositive microorganisms, *Proteus,* yeasts, and fungi may develop during treatment with polymyxin B.

Therapeutic Uses. The primary use of polymyxin B is for treatment of infections caused by gramnegative bacteria, especially *Pseudomonas.* However, the present availability of gentamicin and carbenicillin has reduced markedly the clinical use of this drug. Polymyxin B is effective in the treatment of *urinary tract infections* caused by *Pseudomonas* or other gram-negative bacilli resistant to other antimicrobial agents; it should be reserved for disease involving the kidney and should not be employed in lower urinary tract disease unless this is very severe and accompanied by appreciable systemic manifestations.

Polymyxin B is necessary therapy for the rare *meningeal infections* due to *Pseud. aeruginosa* and other gram-negative bacteria not susceptible to other antibiotics. Since systemically administered polymyxin B does not diffuse into cerebrospinal fluid, treatment of meningitis requires intrathecal injection, as described above, for 3 weeks.

Pulmonary infections due to *Pseud. aeruginosa* may respond to polymyxin B in some instances. *Pseudomonas bacteremia* responds well to this drug; however, metastatic infections in organs are unaffected and, unless these can be drained, the outcome is usually fatal. Polymyxin B is ineffective in most instances of *Pseudomonas endocarditis* since it is not possible to remove the infected vegetations, which are not sterilized by the circulating drug.

Infections of the skin, mucous membranes, eye, and ear due to polymyxin B–sensitive microorganisms respond to local application of the antibiotic in solution or ointment. *External otitis,* frequently due to *Pseudomonas,* may be cured by the topical use of the drug. *Pseudomonas aeruginosa* is a common cause of infection of *corneal ulcers;* local application or subconjunctival injection (up to 10 mg per day) of polymyxin B is often curative.

Patients who require parenteral treatment with polymyxin B should be hospitalized and must be closely monitored for signs of renal toxicity during the entire period of treatment.

COLISTIN

History and Source. *Colistin* is an antibiotic produced by *Bacillus (Aerobacillus) colistinus,* a microorganism isolated from a soil sample obtained from Fukushima Prefecture, Japan (Koyama *et al.,* 1950).

Chemistry. Colistin is polymyxin E, as described above. Polymyxins E_1 and E_2 differ from each other in the same manner as do B_1 and B_2. Colistin is identical to polymyxin B except for the substitution of a residue of D-leucine for that of D-phenylalanine. Solutions of colistin salts are relatively unstable above pH 6.

Colistin is available for clinical use as colistin sulfate, for oral use, and as colistimethate sodium (colistin sodium methanesulfonate), a parenteral preparation.

Antibacterial Activity. The antibacterial spectra of polymyxin B and colistin are very similar (*see* above). Using colistin sulfate, Wright and Welch (1960) demonstrated a greater degree of activity of this compound than of polymyxin B against *Pseudomonas, Salmonella, Shigella,* and members of the *coli-aerogenes* group.

Absorption and Excretion. Colistin is not absorbed from the gastrointestinal tract. Intramuscular injection of 150 mg of colistimethate in adults produces a peak plasma concentration of 6 µg/ml at 2 hours; this declines with a half-time of 2 hours. The same quantity given intravenously yields a maximal plasma concentration of 18 µg/ml; this falls to about 0.4 µg/ml at 12 hours. The drug passes from the maternal to the fetal circulation. Premature infants injected with 1 mg/kg do not develop an effective plasma concentration of the antibiotic; with a dose of 2 mg/kg, a peak value of about 5 µg/ml is reached in 30 minutes. Plasma concentrations are higher in persons with renal insufficiency and are related to the degree of renal dysfunction.

Colistimethate is excreted mainly by glomerular filtration. Urine concentrations exceed 200 µg/ml during the first 2 hours after a usual intramuscular dose. The drug is excreted more rapidly in children than in adults. Colistimethate does not gain access to the cerebrospinal fluid, even when the meninges are inflamed.

Preparations, Routes of Administration, and Dosage. *Colistin Sulfate for Oral Suspension,* U.S.P. (COLY-MYCIN S ORAL SUSPENSION), is marketed as a powder (300 mg) to be suspended in distilled water prior to dispensing (5 mg/ml). *Colistimethate Sodium,* U.S.P. (COLY-MYCIN M PARENTERAL), is marketed for *intravenous* or *intramuscular* injection in vials containing the equivalent of 20 or 150 mg of colistin base to be reconstituted to contain 10 or 75 mg/ml, respectively. The parenteral dose of colistimethate for adults and children is 2.5 to 5 mg/kg per day, in three divided doses. Colistin sulfate is administered *orally* to infants and children with diarrhea caused by bacteria susceptible to the drug; the dose is 3 to 5 mg/kg daily, in three divided portions.

If colistimethate must be used in patients with renal insufficiency, dosage schedules must be altered radically; suggestions are presented in Table 55–2 (page 1108). When patients being treated with the drug are subjected to dialysis, the dose must also be adjusted. Curtis and Eastwood (1968) have recommended the injection of 2 to 3 mg/kg intravenously after each hemodialysis, if this is carried out twice a week. The administration of 2 mg/kg daily during peritoneal dialysis has been suggested by Greenberg and Sanford (1967); this produces effective antibacterial blood levels without excessive accumulation of the drug.

Untoward Effects. Adverse reactions to colistimethate have been noted in 20% of patients given the drug; they are generally reversible (Koch-Weser et al., 1970). Transient *paresthesias, pruritus, dermatoses, visual and speech disturbances, drug fever, diz-*

ziness, and *gastrointestinal disturbances* develop infrequently during the course of therapy with colistimethate. *Suprainfection* may occur during treatment. *Leukopenia* and *granulocytopenia* may possibly be associated with the use of colistimethate. Pain can occur at the site of injection. *Adverse renal effects* appear to be less common than with polymyxin B, but marked azotemia may occasionally develop after large doses in patients with low renal reserve. Acute tubular necrosis has been observed in about 2% of patients given colistimethate; it is usually reversible. *Respiratory paralysis* similar in character to that produced by polymyxin has followed the administration of colistimethate. In general, the incidence and the severity of untoward reactions associated with the use of colistin appear to be less than with polymyxin B.

Therapeutic Uses. The therapeutic indications for colistin are essentially the same as those for polymyxin B. Infections of certain types caused by *Pseud. aeruginosa* are especially susceptible.

NOVOBIOCIN

Novobiocin is a toxic antibiotic with a narrow antibacterial spectrum. A description of the drug is provided in earlier editions of this textbook. There are no current valid indications for its therapeutic use.

VANCOMYCIN

History and Source. *Vancomycin* is an antibiotic produced by *Streptomyces orientalis,* an actinomycete isolated from soil samples obtained in Indonesia and India. Purification of the antibiotic was accomplished and its chemical and antimicrobial properties were described within a short time after its discovery (McCormick et al., 1956).

Chemistry. Vancomycin is a glycopeptide chemically related to *ristocetin,* a defunct antibiotic described in previous editions of this textbook. Vancomycin hydrochloride is a white powder, soluble in water to a concentration of over 100 mg/ml. The structural formula is not yet known.

Antibacterial Activity. The primary activity of vancomycin is against gram-positive bacteria. Many strains of streptococci and staphylococci are sensitive *in vitro* to concentrations of 0.5 to 5 µg/ml. Some strains of *Staph. aureus* have been found to be resistant to clinically achievable concentrations of the antibiotic. Combinations of this drug with streptomycin or gentamicin act synergistically against many but not all strains of enterococci (Watanakunakorn and Bakie, 1973; Westenfelder et al., 1973). The drug is rapidly bactericidal. Cross-resistance with other antimicrobial agents has not been demonstrated.

Mechanism of Action. Bacterial cell-wall synthesis is inhibited by vancomycin. This is discussed in Chapter 57.

Absorption, Distribution, and Excretion. Vancomycin is poorly absorbed after oral administration, and large quantities are excreted in the stool. For parenteral therapy, the drug should be administered intravenously. A single intravenous dose of 500 mg in adults produces plasma concentrations of 6 to 10 μg/ml at the end of 1 to 2 hours; the drug has a half-life in the circulation of about 6 hours. Less than 10% of the antibiotic is bound to plasma protein. Vancomycin appears in various body fluids, including the cerebrospinal fluid when the meninges are inflamed. About 80% of an injected dose is excreted by the kidney; in the presence of renal insufficiency, dangerously high concentrations may accumulate in the blood.

Preparations, Routes of Administration, and Dosage. *Sterile Vancomycin Hydrochloride,* U.S.P. (VANCOCIN), is marketed for *intravenous* use, in 10-ml vials containing powder (500 mg) for solution. The desired dose is preferably diluted and injected intravenously over a 30-minute period, every 6 or 12 hours. The dose of vancomycin for adults is 500 mg every 6 hours or 1 g every 12 hours; in unusually severe infections this may be increased to 1 g every 8 hours. The daily dose for children is 44 mg/kg in equally divided and spaced quantities every 8 to 12 hours. The amount administered daily to premature infants and neonates ranges from 6 to 15 mg/kg. Because of incompletely developed renal function in this age group, the drug must be used with caution. Extreme alteration of dosage is required for patients with impaired renal function (*see* Table 55–2, page 1109). Vancomycin can be given *orally* to patients with staphylococcal enterocolitis. The dose for adults is 500 mg every 6 hours; the total daily dose for children is 44 mg/kg, given in divided doses. *Vancomycin Hydrochloride for Oral Solution,* U.S.P., is available for this purpose. The content of a 10-g container of the antibiotic is mixed with 115 ml of distilled water, so that each 6-ml portion provides approximately 500 mg of the drug.

Untoward Effects. Among the *hypersensitivity reactions* produced by vancomycin are *macular skin rashes* and *anaphylaxis. Phlebitis* and *pain* at the site of intravenous injection are relatively uncommon. *Chills* and *fever* may occur, and a *shocklike state* may develop during the course of intravenous infusion. The most significant untoward reactions are *ototoxicity* and *nephrotoxicity.* Deafness, which is frequently although not always permanent, may follow the use of this drug. In some instances, hearing returns to normal after therapy is stopped; however, in most cases, it progresses despite cessation of treatment. It has been suggested that deafness develops only when excessively high plasma concentrations are produced. A transient rise in blood urea nitrogen may occur. Severe renal damage with death due to uremia has been observed. Since the risk of toxic effects is appreciably increased by high plasma concentrations, vancomycin is best avoided, if possible, in patients with renal insufficiency. If the drug is required in such instances, renal function and level of auditory acuity must be evaluated at frequent intervals. *Suprainfections* due to gram-negative bacteria or fungi may develop during the course of vancomycin therapy.

Therapeutic Uses. There are mercifully few indications for the use of vancomycin; however, the drug assumes great importance when it is required. Vancomycin may be particularly useful in the management of disease produced by methicillin-resistant staphylococci, including *staphylococcal pneumonia, empyema, bacteremia, endocarditis, osteomyelitis, enterocolitis,* and *soft-tissue abscesses.* It may also be needed in the treatment of serious enterococcal infections and those caused by streptococci of the *viridans* group in patients who cannot tolerate penicillin. It may be applied topically in cases of necrotizing ulcerative gingivitis or administered orally to treat staphylococcal enterocolitis. (*See* Griffith and Peck, 1956; Ehrenkranz, 1959; Kirby *et al.,* 1960; Collins and Hood, 1967.) *Vancomycin is interdicted in patients taking or recently exposed to other ototoxic or nephrotoxic agents.*

BACITRACIN

History and Source. *Bacitracin* is an antibiotic produced by the Tracy-I strain of *Bacillus subtilis,* isolated in 1943 from the damaged tissue and street dirt debrided from a compound fracture in a young girl named Tracy; hence the name *bacitracin.* The history, properties, and uses of bacitracin have been reviewed by Meleney and Johnson (1949) and Jawetz (1961).

Chemistry, Assay, and Unitage. The bacitracins are a group of polypeptide antibiotics; multiple components have been demonstrated in the commercial products. The major constituent is *bacitracin A* (*see* Newton and Abraham, 1953); its probable structural formula is as follows:

Bacitracin

A *unit* of the antibiotic is equivalent to 26 μg of the U.S.P. standard.

Antibacterial Activity. A variety of gram-positive cocci and bacilli, *Neisseria, H. influenzae,* and *T. pallidum* are sensitive to 0.1 unit or less of bacitracin per milliliter. *Actinomyces* and *Fusobacterium* are inhibited by concentrations of 0.5 to 5 units/ml. Enterobacteriaceae, *Pseudomonas, Candida, Torula,* and *Nocardia* are resistant to the drug. Bacitracin inhibits bacterial cell-wall synthesis, as described in Chapter 57.

Absorption, Fate, and Excretion. While bacitracin has been employed parenterally in the past, current use is essentially restricted to topical application. The reader is referred to earlier editions of this textbook for descriptions of the pharmacokinetics of this antibiotic.

Preparations, Routes of Administration, and Dosage. Only information pertinent to topical application will be presented. *Bacitracin,* U.S.P. (BACIQUENT), is available in official *ophthalmic* and *dermatological ointments;* these contain 500 units per gram of suitable base. *Bacitracin Zinc,* U.S.P., is marketed for incorporation in ointments. The antibiotic is also available in the form of a *dry powder* (50,000 units per vial) for the preparation of topical solutions. The ointments are applied directly to the involved surface one or more times daily. A number of topical preparations of bacitracin to which neomycin or polymyxin or both have been added are available, and some contain the three antibiotics plus hydrocortisone.

Untoward Effects. Serious *nephrotoxicity* may result from the parenteral use of this antibiotic. *Hypersensitivity reactions* result from topical application, but this is uncommon.

Therapeutic Uses. Although *topical* bacitracin alone or in combination with other antimicrobial agents has been used extensively to treat *furunculosis, pyoderma, carbuncle, impetigo,* and *superficial and deep abscesses,* the value of the drug applied in this fashion is very questionable. For open infections such as *infected eczema, infected dermal ulcers,* and *infected traumatic and surgical wounds,* the local application of the antibiotic may be of some help in eradicating sensitive bacteria. Bacitracin has an advantage over other antibiotics in that topical administration, even in an ointment, rarely produces hypersensitivity. *Suppurative conjunctivitis* and *infected corneal ulcer* respond well to the topical use of bacitracin when they are caused by susceptible bacteria.

TYROTHRICIN

History and Source. *Tyrothricin* is an antibiotic obtained from *Bacillus brevis,* a bacterium isolated from soil by Dubos, who discovered the microorganism and the bactericidal properties of its cultures. Tyrothricin contains two polypeptide components, *gramicidin* (about 20%) and *tyrocidine* (about 80%) (Dubos and Hotchkiss, 1941).

Antibacterial Activity. The antibacterial activity of tyrothricin is the resultant of the sum of the actions of gramicidin and tyrocidine; *gramicidin* is particularly active against *gram-positive bacteria,* while *tyrocidine* shares this activity and also inhibits some *gram-negative bacilli.* Gramicidin is considerably more active than tyrocidine against bacteria sensitive to both agents.

Preparations, Routes of Administration, and Dosage. *Tyrothricin* is employed only *locally* in solution or as an ointment. The concentration of antibiotic usually employed is 0.5 mg/ml or 0.5 mg/g; higher concentrations may be irritating. Gramicidin is also a component of several antibiotic preparations for topical use.

Untoward Effects. Gramicidin and particularly tyrocidine are potent hemolytic agents; therefore, the antibiotic must not be administered by any route that might permit it to enter the blood stream. When properly used by local application, tyrothricin preparations evoke few, if any, untoward effects. *Hemolysis* and even renewed *bleeding* may occur if tyrothricin is employed in fresh surgical or traumatic wounds. Suspensions of the drug should not be used for irrigating paranasal sinuses in close proximity to the subarachnoid spaces, because of the danger of producing potentially fatal chemical meningitis. Other serious complications are *anosmia* and *parosmia,* probably due to injury of the olfactory nerve endings immediately or shortly after topical use of tyrothricin in the nose or paranasal sinuses; recovery is slow and may be incomplete.

Therapeutic Uses. Tyrothricin has been employed to treat infected surface *ulcers* and *wounds, pyodermas,* and infections of the *eye, nose,* and *throat.* The *advantages* of tyrothricin are its absence of sensitizing properties and low tissue toxicity. Its *disadvantages* are its untoward effects and failure to inhibit gram-negative bacteria.

II.   Antifungal Agents

NYSTATIN

History and Source. *Streptomyces noursei* is the source of *nystatin.* The antibiotic inhibits the growth of a variety of pathogenic and nonpathogenic yeasts and fungi but not bacteria. The chemical nature and properties of the drug were reported by Dutcher and colleagues (1954).

Chemistry and Assay. Nystatin is a polyene antibiotic. Its large, conjugated, double-bond ring system is linked to an amino acid sugar, mycosamine. The structural formula is not yet fully elucidated. Nystatin is only slightly soluble in water (10 to 20 units per milliliter). It quickly decomposes in the presence of water or plasma. In the dry form, the drug is stable for at least 3 months at 40° C. The potency of commercial preparations of nystatin is expressed in units; 1.0 mg of the drug contains not less than 2000 units, in order to meet U.S.P. standards. Special assay methods are available for determining sensitivity of microorganisms as well as plasma and body fluid concentrations of the drug.

Antifungal Activity. Nystatin is both fungistatic and fungicidal. *Candida, Cryptococcus, Histoplasma, Blastomyces, Trichophyton, Epidermophyton,* and *Microsporum audouini* are sensitive *in vitro* to concentrations ranging from 1.5 to 6.5 μg/ml. It is generally less susceptible to changes in pH than are other antifungal agents. Nystatin is without effect on bacteria, protozoa, or viruses. Experimental candidiasis, histoplasmosis, coccidioidomycosis, sporotrichosis, and cryptococcosis in animals respond to treatment with nystatin.

Fungal Resistance. Repeated subculture of *Candida albicans* in increasing concentrations of nystatin results in little or no development of resistance, but other species of *Candida* (*C. tropicalis, C. guillermondi, C. krusei,* and *C. stellatoides*) become quite resistant and also insensitive to amphotericin at the same time. Resistance does not, as a rule, develop *in vivo.*

Mechanism of Action. Nystatin is bound by drug-sensitive yeasts and fungi but not by resistant microorganisms. The antifungal activity of the antibiotic is dependent on its binding to a sterol moiety present in the membrane of sensitive fungi. The binding results in a change in permeability of the cell membrane, allowing leakage of a variety of small molecules. (*See* Kinsky, 1962; Weissmann and Sessa, 1967.)

Absorption and Excretion. Absorption of nystatin from the gastrointestinal tract is negligible, and the drug appears in the feces. When doses of 8 million units or more are given, individuals with normal renal function may have plasma concentrations of only 1 to 2.5 μg/ml. Persons with renal insufficiency may occasionally develop significant plasma concentrations of nystatin while taking conventional doses by mouth. Parenteral treatment is not employed. Nystatin is not absorbed from the skin or mucous membranes.

Preparations, Routes of Administration, and Dosage. Official preparations of *Nystatin,* U.S.P. (MYCOSTATIN, NILSTAT, OV-STATIN), are *ointments, oral suspensions,* and *oral tablets. Creams, powders, ointments, suspensions,* and *drops* contain 100,000 units of nystatin per gram or per milliliter; many topical preparations also contain other antibiotics such as neomycin or gramicidin, and hydrocortisone is incorporated in some. Tablets for oral therapy contain 500,000 units; vaginal tablets contain 100,000 units.

The *oral dose for adults* is 500,000 to 1 million units, three times a day; for *children,* 100,000 units, three to four times per day. Topical application is usually made two or three times a day. Vaginal tablets are inserted once or twice daily.

Untoward Effects. Untoward effects of nystatin are uncommon. Mild and transitory nausea, vomiting, and diarrhea may occur after oral administration of the drug. Irritation of the skin and mucous membranes does not result from topical application. Hypersensitivity reactions have not been reported, nor have toxic effects on the blood or blood-forming organs been noted. Since nystatin has no effect on bacteria, suprainfections do not occur even when large doses are used.

Therapeutic Uses. Nystatin is used primarily to treat *Candida* infections of skin, mucous membrane,

and intestinal tract. Paronychia, vaginitis, and stomatitis (thrush) caused by this microorganism are usually benefited by topical therapy. Some instances of *oral candidiasis,* especially those appearing as suprainfections during the use of an antimicrobial agent, may fail to improve when treated with nystatin. *Vaginal candidiasis* usually responds well to topical application of the drug. *Intestinal candidiasis* is a rare disease that is diagnosed and treated more frequently than it is actually present. The recovery of large numbers of *Candida* in the feces does not prove the presence of infection by this microorganism. However, candidiasis of the bowel may occur in individuals predisposed by *diabetes mellitus, leukemia, antibiotic therapy,* or *corticosteroid administration.* The oral ingestion of nystatin appears to produce good results in such cases. It must be stressed that patients receiving antibiotics orally may have overgrowth of yeasts in the intestine without diarrhea, as well as diarrhea without increase of fungi in the stool. This makes the diagnosis of intestinal candidiasis difficult, and the reported beneficial results of therapy are open to considerable question.

Prophylactic Uses. Nystatin has been administered with the tetracyclines for the purpose of preventing the overgrowth of yeasts and fungi in the bowel of patients predisposed to such infections. Although the number of yeasts does not increase when the two drugs are given concurrently, there is no good clinical evidence to indicate that the incidence of mycotic infections is appreciably reduced in such individuals.

AMPHOTERICIN B

History and Source. *Streptomyces nodosus,* a soil actinomycete, is the source of two antifungal agents, amphotericins A and B, which are produced together during the fermentation process. The physical and chemical properties of these agents, methods for separating them, and the preparation of an almost pure *amphotericin B* (containing only 1 to 2% amphotericin A) were elucidated by Vandeputte and coworkers (1956). The antibiotic used clinically is amphotericin B.

Chemistry and Assay. Amphotericin B is another polyene antibiotic; it contains the same nitrogenous moiety present in nystatin, namely, mycosamine, an aminodeoxyhexose. The structural formula is not yet fully elucidated. Amphotericin B is insoluble in water and is quite unstable. The antifungal effects of the antibiotic are maximal between pH 6.0 and 7.5 and decrease at low pH. Microbiological assay is carried out with *C. albicans* as the test microorganism.

Antifungal Activity. *Histoplasma capsulatum, Cryptococcus neoformans, Coccidioides immitis, Candida* species, *Torulopsis glabrata, Rhodotorula, Blastomyces dermatitidis, B. braziliensis,* some strains of *Aspergillus,* and *Sporotrichum schenckii* are sensitive to concentrations of amphotericin B ranging from 0.03 to 1.0 μg/ml *in vitro. Candida tropicalis* is resistant. The antibiotic is either fungistatic or fungicidal, depending on the concentration of the drug and the sensitivity of the fungus. It is without effect on bacteria, rickettsiae, or viruses.

Fungal Resistance. Strains of *C. albicans* and *Coccid. immitis* serially subcultured in increasing concentrations of amphotericin B become resistant to the drug; cross-resistance to nystatin does not develop. There is no evidence at present that resistance develops *in vivo*.

Mechanism of Action. The mechanism of action of amphotericin B is apparently the same as that of other polyene antibiotics, for example, nystatin (*see* above).

Absorption, Distribution, and Excretion. Amphotericin B is poorly absorbed from the gastrointestinal tract. The *oral administration* of about 3 g a day produces plasma concentrations of about 0.1 to 0.5 μg/ml. The *intravenous injection* of 1 to 5 mg of amphotericin B per day initially, followed by the gradual increase of the daily dose to 0.65 mg/kg, yields peak values of approximately 2 to 4 μg/ml. These concentrations are well maintained between doses, since the plasma half-life is about 24 hours. It is probable that most of the antibiotic is bound to sterol-containing membranes in many different tissues. However, details of tissue distribution and possible pathways of drug metabolism are unknown. About 10% of the drug is strongly bound to plasma proteins. Little amphotericin B penetrates into the cerebrospinal fluid or ocular tissues.

The antifungal agent is excreted very slowly in the urine, and only a small fraction of a given dose is excreted in active form; when therapy is stopped, the drug can be detected in the urine for at least 7 to 8 weeks. The concentration of amphotericin B in urine roughly parallels that in plasma. Since this represents only a small fraction of the dose administered, there is no further accumulation of the drug in the plasma of patients with impaired renal function (Feldman *et al.*, 1973).

The clinical pharmacology of amphotericin B is discussed by Bindschalder and Bennett (1969), Diamond and Bennett (1973), Feldman and associates (1973), and Bennett (1974).

Preparations, Routes of Administration, and Dosage. *Amphotericin B*, U.S.P. (FUNGIZONE), is available as an official injection. The sterile, lyophilized *powder* is marketed in vials containing 50 mg of amphotericin B, plus sodium deoxycholate to effect a colloidal dispersion of the insoluble antibiotic, buffers, and diluent. The contents of the vial should be dissolved, with shaking, in 10 ml of sterile water and then added to 5% dextrose in water to make a final concentration of 0.1 mg/ml. *Solutions of electrolytes, acidic solutions, or solutions with preservatives should not be used* because they cause precipitation of the antibiotic. Solutions in which precipitate or foreign material is present must be discarded. Fresh solutions should be prepared for each injection. The addition of 25 to 50 mg of hydrocortisone abolishes or markedly reduces the incidence of severe chills in some but not all patients.

Intravenous infusion by means of a pediatric scalp-vein needle minimizes the risk of thrombophlebitis. A cream, lotion, and ointment containing 3% of amphotericin B are also marketed.

Several schedules have been recommended for intravenous therapy with amphotericin B. One is the administration of 0.25 mg/kg the first day, followed by an increase of 0.25 mg/kg each day until a dose of 1 mg/kg is reached. In very severe infections, the total daily dose may be increased to 1.5 mg/kg; *this must not be exceeded.* The required amount is dissolved in 0.5 to 1 liter of 5% dextrose solution in water and is administered over a 6-hour period. An alternative regimen is the following: 1 mg of amphotericin B dissolved in 250 ml of 5% dextrose solution in water is injected on the first day; this is increased to 5 mg (in 500 ml of 5% dextrose solution) on the second day, and 10 mg (in 1 liter of 5% dextrose solution) on the third day; the dose is then increased by 5 to 10 mg each day until 1 mg/kg is being administered daily. Because of the extended half-life of the drug, the administration of a double dose every other day is also feasible. Still another method is to give an initial dose of 1 mg, followed by a gradual daily increase until the peak plasma concentration achieved is at least twice that required for the *in-vitro* inhibition of the fungus isolated from the patient. (*See* Andrioli and Kravetz, 1962; Drutz *et al.*, 1968; Bindschalder and Bennett, 1969.) Unusually small doses of the drug given intravenously (10 to 355 mg over 4 to 18 days) may be curative in some instances of severe and disabling *Candida* infections (Medoff *et al.*, 1971b). It has been suggested that adjustment of dose on the basis of plasma concentrations and sensitivity testing of the microorganism is of little value, since the technic is difficult and of unproven clinical value (Bennett, 1974).

Intrathecal infusion of amphotericin B may be helpful in cases of fungal meningitis; 0.5 mg of the drug is dissolved in at least 5 ml of spinal fluid and given two to three times a week; a total dose of 15 mg by this route is thought to be adequate. Amphotericin B has also been given intraventricularly to patients with cryptococcal and *Coccid. immitis* meningitis. Intra-articular doses of 5 to 15 mg have been administered.

Untoward Effects. A large number and variety of untoward effects may be associated with the use of amphotericin B. *Hypersensitivity reactions* include *anaphylaxis, thrombopenia, flushing, generalized pain,* and *convulsions.* Among the *irritative and toxic effects* are *chills, fever, phlebitis, headache, anemia, anorexia,* and *decreased renal function.* About 50% of initial intravenous injections of the drug are associated with chills and about 20% with vomiting; the temperature may rise to as high as 40° C. Fever and chills may develop with every injection in the same individual. *Acute hepatic failure* with *jaundice* and *hepatocellular dysfunction* is provoked in some cases by amphotericin B; the hepatic cells exhibit toxic degeneration.

Over 80% of persons given amphotericin B develop *decreased renal function* and *abnormal urine sediment. Mild tubular acidosis* and *hypokalemia* are frequent. *Hypomagnesemia* is also observed, but it is not clear if this problem is of renal origin. The degree of nephrotoxicity is dose related, but there is considerable variation among patients. In general, the extent of impaired function is usually not of lasting clinical importance when a total dose of 4 g or less is administered over at least 6 weeks. With larger doses permanent damage may occur, characterized by thickening and fragmentation of the glomerular basement membrane, hypercellularity, fibrosis as well as hyalination of the glomeruli, nephrocalcinosis, and degeneration and atrophy of the tubules. Alkali therapy during prolonged treatment may be helpful in preventing renal difficulty (McCurdy et al., 1968; Douglas and Healy, 1969). Milder renal manifestations usually disappear when therapy is stopped and do not contraindicate retreatment. *Irreversible renal failure is rarer but obviously may cause death.*

The drug may also produce a normochromic, normocytic *anemia;* the bone marrow reveals a decrease in erythrocyte production; the blood picture usually becomes normal after treatment is stopped. *Leukopenia* and *thrombopenia* may occur rarely.

The *intrathecal injection* of amphotericin B may produce *pain along the distribution of lumbar nerves, headache, paresthesias, nerve palsies* (including *foot-drop*), *chemical meningitis, difficulty in micturition,* and possibly *impairment of vision.*

The subconjunctival injection of amphotericin B may produce permanent yellow discoloration of the conjunctiva. When the dose exceeds 5 mg, salmon-colored, raised nodules develop on the conjunctiva; these resolve gradually after treatment is stopped (Randall and Ritchey, 1973).

For a review of the untoward effects of amphotericin B, *see* Utz and coworkers (1964), Bennett (1974), and Weinstein and Weinstein (1974).

Therapeutic Uses. Amphotericin B is therapeutically effective in a number of *fungal infections* that, prior to the availability of this drug, were almost invariably fatal.

The primary *pulmonary, cutaneous,* and *disseminated* forms of *North American blastomycosis,* with few exceptions, respond very well to amphotericin B therapy. About 50% of cases of severe, *acute pulmonary or progressive disseminated coccidioidomycosis* are cured; pregnancy has an unfavorable effect on this disease, even when it is treated. About 75% of patients with severe *disseminated* or *chronic cavitary pulmonary histoplasmosis* are improved or cured by amphotericin B; resection of the diseased portion of the lung in addition to chemotherapy is recommended. *Histoplasmic uveitis* does not appear to respond to the drug. *Pulmonary, cutaneous,* and *mucous membrane lesions* as well as *meningitis* due to *Cryp. neoformans* are improved or cured by amphotericin B; meningeal infections require both intravenous and intrathecal treatment, and not all are cured.

Pleural, peritoneal, pulmonary, ocular, urinary bladder, cutaneous, mucous membrane, and *disseminated* forms of *candidiasis* are improved or eradicated by the antibiotic, in most instances. Treatment of ocular infection is by subconjunctival or episcleral injection of 5 mg; instillation into the urinary bladder (50 mg per day dissolved in 1 liter of sterile water, via a three-way catheter continuously for 5 days) has produced good results in candidal cystitis (Wise et al., 1973); topical application to lesions of skin or mucous membranes has been effective in some cases. Chronic mucocutaneous candidiasis may respond when treated with amphotericin B orally (Montes, 1971). Although *candidal endocarditis* has been treated with this drug, chemotherapy alone is insufficient to eradicate the infection. Administration of amphotericin B, perhaps in conjunction with flucytosine, followed by surgical removal of the diseased valve and continuation of drug therapy for 4 to 8 weeks after operation, provides the best chance for cure, but even then only in a limited number of cases. Among the other types of mycotic disease that appear to be benefited by amphotericin B are *South American blastomycosis, extracutaneous sporotrichosis, craniofacial mucormycosis, chromoblastomycosis* (local subcutaneous injection of 20 to 35 mg once daily, or intravenous therapy), *aspergillosis,* infection due to *Tor. glabrata,* and *paracoccidiomycosis.*

Healing of the *mucosal, cutaneous,* and *mucocutaneous forms* of American leishmaniasis has been reported to follow administration of amphotericin B in a total dose of 200 to 1450 mg; relapse did not occur after treatment was stopped.

The *duration of amphotericin B therapy* varies with the nature, severity, and course of the infection as well as with the development of untoward effects that may necessitate the temporary cessation of treatment; recurrences require another full course of drug. The minimal period of therapy is usually about 6 weeks; it may need to be extended to as long as 3 to 4 months in some cases. *All patients requiring amphotericin B must be hospitalized,* at least for the initiation of therapy, and they must be under close observation throughout a course of systemic administration of the drug. Hemograms, urinalyses, and hepatic function tests as well as determinations of serum potassium, magnesium, urea nitrogen, and creatinine concentrations should be made two to three times a week, especially during the period when the dose is being increased. If evidence of renal insufficiency appears, treatment should be stopped until renal function returns to normal; it is then reinstituted, as described above.

Amphotericin B has been administered simultaneously with tetracyclines to suppress overgrowth of yeasts and fungi that may be induced by the broad-spectrum antibiotics. There is no clinical evidence that this is either necessary or effective.

FLUCYTOSINE

Chemistry. *Flucytosine* is a fluorinated pyrimidine related to fluorouracil and floxuridine. It is 5-fluorocytosine, the formula of which is as follows:

Flucytosine

Antifungal Activity. Flucytosine inhibits the multiplication of *Cryp. neoformans,* certain strains of *Candida, Tor. glabrata* (more sensitive to amphotericin), *Asp. fumigatus,* and *Spor. schenkii.* Most susceptible strains of *Candida* are suppressed by concentrations of the drug from 0.4 to 8 μg/ml. The minimal fungistatic concentrations for *Aspergillus* and *Sporotrichum* range from 0.14 to 0.6 and 0.6 to 2 μg/ml, respectively. Combination of flucytosine with amphotericin B results in slightly supra-additive activity *in vitro* against *Cryp. neoformans* and sensitive strains of *C. albicans* and *C. tropicalis.* The drug is without effect on *B. dermatitidis, H. capsulatum, Coccid. immitis, Rhizopus oryzae,* and *Absidia corymbifer.* (*See* Marks *et al.,* 1971; Medoff *et al.,* 1971a; Brandsberg and French, 1972; Bennett, 1974.)

Fungal Resistance. Spontaneous mutants of *C. albicans* resistant to flucytosine have been isolated from strains susceptible to the drug. Resistance of this microorganism (not inhibited by 12.5 μg/ml) has developed during therapy; about 40 to 50% of *Candida* species are initially resistant (not inhibited by 100 μg/ml) (Normark and Schönebeck, 1972; Block *et al.,* 1973). Primary resistance is rare in *Cryp. neoformans;* the development of resistance during treatment is a major cause of therapeutic failure (Bennett, 1974).

Mechanism of Action. The precise actions of this new agent are poorly understood at present. Flucytosine is converted in fungal cells to fluorouracil, a known metabolic antagonist. The cytotoxic activity of fluorinated pyrimidines is discussed in detail in Chapter 62.

Absorption, Distribution, and Excretion. Flucytosine is rapidly and well absorbed from the gastrointestinal tract. It is widely distributed in the body, with a volume of distribution closely approximating the total body water. The drug is minimally bound to plasma proteins. Mean peak plasma concentrations are about 30 μg/ml and are reached about 2 hours after administration of a conventional dose; peak values are about 50 μg/ml in anuric patients. Approximately 90% of a given dose is excreted in the urine by glomerular filtration in unchanged form; concentrations in the urine range from 200 to 500 μg/ml. There is no evidence that flucytosine is metabolized to any extent in man. The half-life of the drug is about 3 to 4 hours in normal individuals. In renal failure, the half-life may be as long as 200 hours. There is a linear relation between the elimination rate constant and creatinine clearance; in normal persons, the renal clearance of flucytosine is about 75% of that for creatinine. Because of the obligate renal excretion of the drug, modification of dosage is necessary in *all* patients with renal dysfunction. One possible schedule is presented in Table 55-2 (page 1108); other recommendations have also been made. (*See* Wade and Sudlow, 1972; Dawborn *et al.,* 1973; Schönebeck *et al.,* 1973; Bennett, 1974.)

Flucytosine is present in cerebrospinal fluid at a concentration about 65 to 90% of that simultaneously present in the plasma. The drug also penetrates into the aqueous humor.

Preparations, Routes of Administration, and Dosage. *Flucytosine,* U.S.P. (ANCOBON), is supplied in capsules containing either 250 or 500 mg for oral administration. There are no parenteral preparations. The usual daily dose is 50 to 150 mg/kg, given at 6-hour intervals. This dosage must be altered, as described above, for patients with renal insufficiency.

Untoward Effects. Flucytosine may depress the function of bone marrow and lead to the development of *anemia, leukopenia,* and *thrombocytopenia;* patients are more prone to the appearance of this complication if they have an underlying hematological disorder, are being treated with radiation or drugs that injure the bone marrow, or have a history of treatment with such agents. Other untoward effects include *nausea, vomiting, diarrhea, elevated serum activities of hepatic enzymes* (reversible when therapy is stopped), and, less frequently, *confusion, hallucinations, headache, sedation,* and *vertigo.* All these complications are more frequent in azotemic patients. These effects cannot be explained by deamination of the drug to 5-fluorouracil *in vivo.*

Therapeutic Uses. Although amphotericin B remains the most effective therapeutic agent for the management of infections due to yeasts and fungi, flucytosine is a valuable additional drug in the treatment of certain of these diseases. It is less toxic than amphotericin B, and it can be administered orally.

Some patients with cryptococcal infections of the lungs, joints, and meninges have responded favorably to treatment with flucytosine. Cases of fungemia, urinary tract infection, meningitis, and visceral disease caused by *Candida,* as well as mucocutaneous candidiasis, have improved or have been cured. Experience with disease due to *Tor. glabrata,* although limited, indicates that flucytosine is effective. Some patients with aspergillosis, osteoarticular sporotrichosis, and chromoblastomycosis have also responded favorably. Although mycotic endocarditis has been treated with flucytosine alone, it is best to combine oral administration of this agent with injection of amphotericin B and surgical removal of the infected valve. Such therapy will probably decrease the risk of death to some extent. It has been suggested that flucytosine always be given together with amphotericin B to individuals with serious mycotic infections; this is especially important in cases of cryptococcal meningitis (Bennett, 1974). The duration of therapy with flucytosine for most types of serious mycotic disease should be 4 to 6 weeks. (*See* Utz *et al.,* 1969; Davies and Reeves, 1971; Isacson *et al.,* 1972; Medical Letter, 1972.)

GRISEOFULVIN

History and Source. *Griseofulvin* was first isolated from *Penicillium griseofulvum dierckx* by Oxford and coworkers in 1939. Because it was ineffective against bacteria, no further attention was paid to it for some time. In 1946, Brian and associates found a substance in *Penicillium janczewski* that produced shrinking and stunting of fungal hyphae; they named this the *curling factor;* it was later found to be *griseofulvin.* During the next 10 years, the antibiotic was widely employed in the treatment of a variety of fungal diseases in plants and of ringworm of cattle. In the course of a search for potential therapeutic compounds for the management of fungal infections of the feet of Scottish miners, Gentles (1958) observed that griseofulvin cured experimentally produced mycotic disease of guinea pigs. Soon thereafter, the drug was widely subjected to clinical trial and became available for general use.

Chemistry. The structural formula of griseofulvin is as follows:

Griseofulvin

The drug is practically insoluble in water. It is remarkably thermostable.

Antifungal Activity. Griseofulvin inhibits the growth *in vitro* of various species of the dermatophytes *Microsporum, Epidermophyton,* and *Trichophyton.* The drug has no effect on bacteria or on other fungi, yeasts, *Actinomyces,* or *Nocardia.* Griseofulvin is fungistatic and not fungicidal. Young, actively metabolizing cells are killed by the drug, but the older more dormant elements are not so intensely affected.

Fungal Resistance. *Trichophyton, Epidermophyton,* and *Microsporum* can be made resistant to griseofulvin *in vitro.* Animals infected with resistant strains develop infections similar to those produced by sensitive strains. Isolates from humans receiving the antibiotic appear, with a few exceptions, to retain their sensitivity to the drug when examined *in vitro.* The mycelia of *Microsporum* and *Trichophyton* destroy griseofulvin; the relationship of this phenomenon to fungal resistance to griseofulvin is presently not established.

Mechanism of Action. Actively growing cultures of *M. gypseum* take up very large quantities of griseofulvin, and the drug is bound to cellular lipids. The details of the fungistatic actions of the antibiotic are unfortunately unclear. (*See* El-Nakeeb and Lampen, 1965; Huber and Gottlieb, 1968.)

Absorption, Distribution, and Excretion. The oral administration of griseofulvin produces peak plasma concentrations at about 4 hours, approximately 1 μg/ml when a single dose of 0.5 g is given. These values are quite variable, perhaps due to difficulty in absorption from the intestine (mainly the upper small intestine), because of the insolubility of griseofulvin in aqueous media. Micronized preparations are much better absorbed. The bulk of orally ingested griseofulvin is eliminated in unchanged form in the feces. Less than 1% of an oral dose is excreted in the urine. The drug has a greater affinity for diseased skin than for normal skin. It is deposited in keratin precursor cells. The antibiotic present in such cells when they differentiate is tightly bound to, and persists in, *keratin* and makes this substance resistant to fungal invasion. For this reason, the new growth of hair or nails is the first to become free of disease. As the fungus-containing keratin is shed, it is replaced by normal tissue. Griseofulvin is detectable at the base of the corneum stratum of the skin within 48 to 72 hours and in the midzone about 12 to 19 days after treatment is started; it is probably not present at the intact skin surface. Sweat and transepidermal fluid loss play an important role in the transfer of the drug in the stratum corneum. Only a very small fraction of a dose of the drug is present in body fluids and tissues.

Preparations, Routes of Administration, and Dosage. *Griseofulvin,* U.S.P. (FULVICIN U/F, GRIFULVIN V, GRISACTIN), is marketed in official *capsules* containing 125 or 250 mg and in official *tablets* containing 125, 250, or 500 mg; it is also available as an *oral suspension* (125 mg/5 ml). The daily dose recommended for children is 10 mg/kg; for adults, 500 mg to 1.0 g. Larger doses (1.5 to 2 g per day) may be used for a short time in severe and extensive infections, but the amount should be reduced to 500 mg to 1 g per day when the lesions begin to respond. Best results may be obtained when the calculated dose is divided into four equal parts and given at 6-hour intervals. The length of treatment varies with the location of the infection, as discussed below.

Untoward Effects. The incidence of serious reactions associated with the use of griseofulvin is very low. Among the minor effects, the incidence of which may be as high as 15%, is *headache* that is sometimes severe and usually disappears as therapy is continued. Other *nervous system manifestations* include peripheral neuritis, lethargy, mental confusion, impairment of performance of routine efforts, fatigue, syncope, vertigo, blurred vision, transient macular edema, and augmentation of the effects of alcohol. Among the side effects involving the *alimentary tract* are nausea, vomiting, diarrhea, heartburn, flatulence, dry mouth, thirst, angular stomatitis, glossodynia, and black, furred tongue. *Hepatotoxicity* has also been observed. *Hematological effects* include leukopenia, neutropenia, punctate basophilia, and monocytosis; these often disappear despite continuation of therapy. Blood studies should be carried out at least once a week during the first month of treatment or longer. Common *renal effects* include albuminuria and cylindruria, without evidence of renal insufficiency. Reactions involving the *skin* are cold and warm urticaria, photosensitivity, lichen planus, erythema, erythema multiforme-like rashes, and vesicular and morbilliform eruptions. *Serum-sickness syndromes* and severe *angioedema* develop rarely during treatment with griseofulvin. *Estrogen-like effects* have been observed in children. A moderate but inconsistent increase of *fecal protoporphyrins* has been noted when the drug is used for a long period of time. *Candida intertrigo* may complicate griseofulvin therapy.

Therapeutic Uses. Mycotic disease of the *skin, hair,* and *nails* due to *Microsporum, Trichophyton,* or *Epidermophyton* responds well to griseofulvin therapy. It must be stressed that, since other fungal diseases are not affected by the drug, careful mycological study with identification of the responsible organism is the only basis on which therapy can be selected accurately. Readily treatable with this agent are infections of the *hair* (*tinea capitis*) caused by *M. canis, M. audouini, T. schoenleini,* and *T. verrucosum;* "ringworm" *of the glabrous skin; tinea cruris* and *tinea corporis* caused by *M. canis, T. rubrum, T. verrucosum,* and *Epidermophyton floccosum;* and *tinea of the hands* (*T. rubrum, T. mentagrophytes*) and *beard* (*Trichophyton* species). Griseofulvin is also highly effective in "athlete's foot" or epidermophytosis involving the skin and nails, the vesicular form of which is most commonly due to *T. mentagrophytes* and the hyperkeratotic type to *T. rubrum.*

Symptomatic relief of disease of the skin usually appears after 48 to 96 hours of griseofulvin therapy. The first change is a decrease in erythema and induration of the lesions, followed by involution of scaling and hyperpigmentation over a period of several weeks. Lesions in non-intertriginous areas usually disappear completely in 2 to 4 weeks. Cultures for fungi become negative in 1 to 2 weeks. Treatment should be continued for about 3 weeks, if the palms, soles, and nails are not involved. Infections of the palms and soles respond more slowly and require therapy for 4 to 8 weeks; cultures become negative in 2 to 6 weeks. Since fingernails grow out completely in 4 months and toenails in about 6 months, fungal infections of these tissues require therapy for long periods—4 to 6 months for fingernails and 6 to 12 months for toenails. *Trichophyton rubrum* and *T. mentagrophytes* infections may require higher-than-conventional doses. It has been suggested that the hair be clipped after 2 to 3 weeks of treatment in cases of *tinea capitis;* the advantage of this has not been proved. (For review of griseofulvin therapy, *see* Blank *et al.,* 1959; Goldman *et al.,* 1960; Symposium, 1960; Goldman, 1970.)

MISCELLANEOUS ANTIFUNGAL AGENTS

Tolnaftate. This agent, synthesized in 1960, is the first chemical compound to be effectively fungicidal when applied topically. It has the following structural formula:

Tolnaftate

The drug is a crystalline compound, soluble in most organic solvents but not in water. *In vitro,* it inhibits the growth of *T. mentagrophytes* in a concentration of 7.5 to 75 ng/ml; it is also active against *T. rubrum, T. tonsurans, M. canis, M. gypseum,* and *E. floccosum.* It is without effect on *Candida* species and gram-

positive or gram-negative bacteria. Treatment of human infections with 1% tolnaftate in polyethylene glycol or vanishing-cream base produces a high cure rate in skin disease due to *T. rubrum, T. mentagrophytes, T. tonsurans, E. floccosum, M. canis, M. audouini, M. gypseum,* and *Malassezia furfur.* Tolnaftate solution is effective in *tinea versicolor.* The drug is less effective in the presence of hyperkeratotic lesions, and these should be treated with 10% salicylic acid ointment alternating with tolnaftate. The clinical results produced by the topical application of this agent are thought to be better than those that follow the parenteral administration of griseofulvin in the infections listed above. Lesions on the scalp due to *T. tonsurans* and *M. audouini* do not respond. The drug does not alter the course of onychomycosis. Relapse may occur after cessation of therapy and approximates the rate observed when griseofulvin is employed; it is not due to development of drug resistance in the microorganisms. Retreatment is usually successful. Toxic or allergic reactions have not yet been observed.

Tolnaftate, U.S.P. (TINACTIN), is available as a cream, powder, and solution containing 1% of the drug. The preparations are applied locally twice a day. When pruritus is present, it is usually relieved in 24 to 72 hours. Involution of interdigital lesions due to susceptible fungi is very often complete in 7 to 21 days.

Candicidin. This is a polyene (heptaene) antibiotic obtained from a soil actinomycete. It is both fungistatic and fungicidal and is clinically effective only for treatment of vaginal candidiasis. Adverse reactions to candicidin have been rare. The antibiotic is used topically, twice a day for 2 weeks. *Candicidin,* N.F. (CANDEPTIN, VANOBID), is available as a vaginal ointment (0.06%) with an applicator for insertion; vaginal tablets and capsules containing 3 mg are also supplied.

Hydroxystilbamidine Isethionate. This drug, an aromatic diamidine, is active against fungi and protozoa. Like its congener, *pentamidine* (Chapter 54), it has a suppressive effect on *B. dermatitidis in vitro* and in experimental infections in mice, and has produced favorable results in systemic and pulmonary *human North American blastomycosis;* however, the incidence of relapse has been high. The alarming untoward effects that may be produced by the compound are the same as those caused by pentamidine. *Hydroxystilbamidine Isethionate,* U.S.P., is available in vials containing 225 mg of dry, sterile powder. A freshly prepared solution of 225 mg of the drug in 200 ml of 5% dextrose in water or isotonic sodium chloride solution is infused over a period of 45 to 120 minutes, every 24 hours. The solution must be protected from light. The duration of therapy varies with the location and the severity of the disease; severe blastomycosis may require treatment for as long as 2 to 3 months. Studies of renal and hepatic function should be carried out prior to initiation of therapy and repeated periodically during the course of treatment. In general, pentamidine is preferred to hydroxystilbamidine in the therapy of infections susceptible to both agents.

Other Agents. *Hamycin* (PRIMAMYCIN) is a polyene antifungal antibiotic, related to amphotericin B but fairly well absorbed after oral ingestion. It is highly active *in vitro* against *Candida, Curvularia lunata,* and several species of *Aspergillus.* Hamycin has been used to treat human mycotic infection more extensively in India than in the United States. Several investigations have indicated its usefulness in the therapy of *B. dermatitidis* invasion in man (*see* Emmons *et al.,* 1967). It is thought to be more effective than amphotericin B for blastomycosis. One regimen proposed for the use of this agent is as follows: 10 mg/kg per day during the first week, 20 mg/kg daily during the second week, 10 mg/kg daily during the third week, and 20 mg/kg daily during the fourth week; the daily dose is given in four equal amounts at regularly spaced intervals. A micronized preparation has been found effective in blastomycosis when given in a dose of 10 to 20 mg/kg by mouth daily for 6 weeks (Herrell, 1968). Hamycin has been applied locally with success in *vaginal candidiasis.* It is not generally available in the United States.

Pimaricin (NATAMYCIN) is yet another polyene antifungal agent. The drug has been used primarily as a 5% ophthalmic ointment for topical application in cases of keratitis due to species of *Fusarium* and *Cephalosporium,* in which it has proved to be nontoxic, nonirritating, well tolerated, and therapeutically effective (Newmark *et al.,* 1970, 1971).

Clotrimazole (CANESTEN) (l-[o-chloro-α,α-diphenylbenzyl]imidazole) is structurally unrelated to the other antifungal agents. It has been claimed to be active *in vitro* and in experimental infections against a variety of yeasts and fungi. Despite a few enthusiastic reports from European clinics indicating therapeutic effectiveness in pulmonary candidiasis, a number of studies in the United States have raised doubts about the activity of the drug both *in vitro* and in clinical situations. (*See* Waitz *et al.,* 1971; Bennett, 1974.)

Topical antifungal agents, with the exception of nystatin and tolnaftate, are discussed in Chapter 50.

III. Antiviral Agents

The development of compounds useful for the prophylaxis and therapy of viral disease has presented even more difficult problems than those encountered in the search for drugs effective in disorders produced by other microorganisms. This is so because, in contrast to most other infectious agents, viruses are obligate intracellular parasites that require the active participation of the metabolic processes of the invaded cell. Thus, agents that may inhibit or cause the death of viruses are also very likely to injure the host cells that harbor them. In addition, the clinical manifestations that herald the presence of viral infections represent, in most instances, the final product of the activity of the infectious agent, so that its removal from the scene of action may actually do very little, if anything, to alter appreciably the course of the established disease. Although the search for substances that might be of use in the management of viral infections has been long and intensive, very few agents have been found to have clinical applicability. Indeed, even these have exhibited very narrow activity, limited to one or only a few specific viruses. These drugs are described briefly here. (*See* Weinstein and Chang, 1973.)

Idoxuridine. *Idoxuridine,* U.S.P. (DENDRID, HERPLEX, STOXIL), is 5-iodo-2'-deoxyuridine. It is a white crystalline powder, soluble in water (2 mg/ml) and stable at temperatures up to 65° C but sensitive to light. Official preparations are an ophthalmic ointment (0.5%) and an ophthalmic solution (0.1%).

Idoxuridine may exert several actions on the metabolic pathways involved in pyrimidine synthesis, nucleotide interconversions, and DNA synthesis; for example, thymidine kinase is inhibited. It appears, however, that the greatest effect of the drug results from its conversion to the triphosphate derivative and incorporation into viral DNA. Such DNA is more susceptible to breakage, and altered viral proteins may result from faulty transcription (*see* Pratt, 1973). It is thus logical that the activity of idoxuridine is largely limited to DNA viruses, primarily members of the herpesvirus group. The drug is active *in vitro* against vaccinia, herpesvirus hominis, B virus, varicella, cytomegalovirus, polyoma, SV40, and others. The development of resistance of viruses to the drug both *in vitro* and *in vivo* is common.

Idoxuridine is rapidly inactivated by nucleotidases; this fact precludes its use by other than intravenous or topical administration. After intravenous injection, most of the active form of the drug disappears from the blood in about 30 minutes. A small amount is excreted in the urine.

The primary clinical use of the drug has been in *herpes simplex keratitis.* Maxwell (1963) reported on 1500 cases; he noted a correlation between the type of infection and the response to therapy. Epithelial infections, especially initial attacks in which a dendritic figure is present, respond best. The results are less favorable when the stroma is involved. In recurrent episodes, the acute disease is often controlled, but scarring caused by a previous attack is not altered. It is important to stress that total healing or improvement does not occur in all instances, even in those with the most superficial involvement. *Herpes genitalis* may respond favorably to the topical application of the drug. When applied topically to the conjunctiva, irritation, pain, pruritus, inflammation or edema of the eyelids, and photophobia may develop. Punctate areas may appear in the cornea; it is difficult to ascertain whether these are related to the disease or to therapy.

The *dose* of the official solution is 1 drop in the conjunctival sac every hour during the day and every 2 hours during the night until definite improvement is apparent, after which the same quantity is applied every 2 hours during the day and every 4 hours at night. When the official ointment is used, it is applied every 4 hours during the day and once before bedtime. Therapy is continued for 3 to 5 days after healing is complete, as demonstrated by fluorescein staining. For deep infections, but *not* superficial infections, topical corticosteroids may be employed with *great caution. Boric acid should not be used at the same time.*

Two placebo-controlled double-blind studies of the efficacy of idoxuridine in proven cases of herpes simplex encephalitis have failed to indicate the value of the drug (100 mg/kg per day for 5 days). Myelo-suppression caused by idoxuridine coupled with its failure to prevent death led to the termination of these studies (*see* Boston Interhospital and Cooperative Study, 1975).

The *toxicity* of idoxuridine administered intravenously is related to the dose and duration of treatment. It may be severe, since this cytotoxic drug can inhibit DNA synthesis or function in mammalian cells as well. *Transient bone-marrow depression* is common when the recommended quantity is given. Other untoward effects include *stomatitis, alopecia, hepatic injury,* and *potential carcinogenicity* and *teratogenicity.* Systemic use of the drug is contraindicated in pregnant patients and for diseases that are not potentially lethal.

Amantadine. *Amantadine (1-adamantanamine)* is a synthetic antiviral agent first described by Davies and associates (1964). It is a stable, crystalline, water-soluble amine of unusual structure unrelated to that of any of the other antimicrobial agents. Its structural formula is as follows:

Amantadine

Amantadine is completely absorbed from the gastrointestinal tract. Approximately 90% of an orally administered dose is excreted in the urine (50% within 20 hours) in unchanged form; the drug is not metabolized in the body.

A number of studies have demonstrated the effectiveness of this compound in *preventing* infection of tissue cultures and experimental animals by different strains of Asian (A_2) influenza. This antiviral effect results from the ability of the drug to prevent viral penetration into the host cell. Investigation of the *curative properties* in A_2 influenza in mice has suggested that it may produce a higher survival rate and prolongation of life when given 12 hours after appearance of the first symptom (McGahen and Hoffmann, 1968). An adequate number of studies have been performed to indicate that amantadine is of prophylactic value when administered to humans who have had contact with an active case of A_2 influenza or who have served as experimental subjects for this infection. It is ineffective in influenza due to type-B virus and in measles (Dickinson *et al.*, 1967). In double-blind, placebo-controlled studies of amantadine in patients with naturally occurring and experimentally produced infections due to A_2 influenza virus, the drug has been found to produce a good therapeutic effect even when given as long as 20 hours after onset of illness. Statistically significant increases in the rates of overall clinical improvement, defervescence, and disappearance of signs and symptoms of illness were observed in the patients who received amantadine, compared to those given a placebo. However, virus does persist and the development of specific antibody is not suppressed (Togo *et al.*, 1968; Wingfield *et al.*, 1969; Nafta *et al.*, 1970).

The fact that *its prophylactic activity is limited to a single type of a single virus* cannot be overemphasized. The use of amantadine, with or without vaccine, is recommended in the presence of a documented influenza A_2 epidemic, especially in patients of all ages at high risk. The drug may be of great value in widespread outbreaks of influenza due to antigenic variants of the Asian strain for which effective vaccines may not be available (Council on Drugs, 1967).

The discovery that amantadine is also useful in the treatment of parkinsonism was an act of serendipity. This therapeutic application is discussed in Chapter 14.

Amantadine Hydrochloride, N.F. (SYMMETREL), is available in capsules containing 100 mg and as a syrup (50 mg/5 ml). The dose for children 1 to 9 years of age is 4.4 to 8.8 mg/kg, but it should not exceed a total of 150 mg per day. For older children and adults, the dose is 200 mg once daily or 100 mg twice daily. Therapy should be initiated as soon as possible after contact with a case of active A_2 influenza and continued for at least 10 days. With unknown or repeated exposures, as in an epidemic, drug administration for 30 days has been suggested.

The *adverse reactions* that may be caused by amantadine are discussed in Chapter 14. Persons with cerebral atherosclerosis, psychiatric disorders, or a history of epilepsy must be observed closely when taking this drug. It should not be given to pregnant women.

Methisazone. The structural formula of *methisazone* is as follows:

Methisazone

It is a synthetic antiviral agent. The activity of this type of thiosemicarbazone against the pox group of viruses was first demonstrated by Hamre and associates (1950). The effectiveness of isatin 3-thiosemicarbazone in mice infected with vaccinia virus was reported by Thompson and coworkers (1953); the N-methyl congener, methisazone, was found by Bauer and Sadler (1960) to be markedly active against variola virus in mice.

The mechanism of action of methisazone is unclear. It does not interfere with the production of viral components during the early phases of the infectious cycle, but it appears to prevent proper translation of "late" viral mRNA. Despite the fact that the drug can inhibit the replication of a number of viruses in tissue culture, methisazone is effective *in vivo* mainly against the pox group of viruses.

Methisazone (MARBORAN) is only slightly soluble. For this reason, it is not administered parenterally. It is given as tablets or as a micronized preparation in syrup. The plasma concentrations achieved are variable. The only important reported *side effect* of methisazone is *vomiting;* this is common and may be severe, requiring the use of phenothiazines or other antiemetic agents.

The first clinical studies were carried out by Bauer and associates (1963) in an epidemic of *smallpox* in Madras, India. Most of the contacts had been vaccinated during infancy and again shortly after detection of the index case. Eleven hundred individuals were treated with methisazone (1.5 g twice a day for 4 days, or 3 g twice a day for 4 days, or 3 g initially followed by the same dose 12 hours later). Untreated controls numbered 1126; 78 of these developed smallpox, and 12 died. Among the group given the drug, there were only three instances of the disease (no deaths), a reduction of 96%. This report was hailed "as the most significant advance in smallpox since the days of Jenner" (Editorial, 1963). However, other studies have indicated little or no effect of the drug in variola major; alastrim (mild smallpox) has responded quite favorably.

Although methisazone is without therapeutic effect once smallpox has developed, it has been suggested that it is useful in the treatment of two complications of vaccinia, *vaccinia gangrenosa* and *eczema vaccinatum.* Therapy involves the administration of an initial dose of 200 mg/kg, followed by 50 mg/kg every 6 hours for eight doses. The results of reported studies are difficult to evaluate because controls are lacking and the drug has failed to influence the course of primary immunization with vaccinia virus. The place of methisazone in the therapy of infections produced by the pox group of viruses is unsettled, and the indications for the drug are still under active investigation. Methisazone is currently not generally available in the United States.

Cytarabine. *Cytarabine* (1-β-D-arabinofuranosylcytosine) was originally developed as an antileukemic agent. Its potential effectiveness in viral infections is related to its capacity to inhibit the synthesis of DNA. After the drug is phosphorylated to the corresponding nucleotides *in vivo,* it inhibits both nucleoside reductase and DNA polymerase. It is incorporated into DNA to only a slight extent. The antiviral spectrum is similar to that of idoxuridine. The structural formula of cytarabine and a more detailed description of its actions are presented in Chapter 62.

Cytarabine has several advantages over idoxuridine. In particular, members of the herpesvirus group, especially type 2, are generally more sensitive to cytarabine than to idoxuridine and there have been no reports of the development of resistance to cytarabine. Furthermore, the ready incorporation of idoxuridine into DNA, leading to frequent base-pairing errors, makes this agent a potential mutagen. Cytarabine is rapidly inactivated by deamination

in the liver and kidney. The drug is not detectable in the blood 15 minutes after a single intravenous dose in most patients. The active form of cytarabine persists for much longer after intrathecal injection because it is not deaminated in the central nervous system.

Cytarabine has been applied to the conjunctival sac of patients with herpes keratitis. It has been given systemically in cases of encephalitis and disseminated infection due to herpesvirus hominis, and in infections caused by the varicella-zoster agent; the results have been encouraging. The drug is not effective in the treatment of herpes zoster. Indeed, the course of disseminated herpes zoster may be prolonged and made more severe by treatment with cytarabine (Stevens *et al.,* 1973). Although the drug has been administered to newborn infants infected by cytomegalovirus, the results have been rather poor.

Cytarabine, U.S.P. (CYTOSAR), is variously employed by different investigators. The daily dose has ranged from 10 to 200 mg/sq m for 1 to 7 days. The usual recommended daily dose is 40 mg/sq m for 5 days. Daily intrathecal injections of 10 mg/sq m for 3 to 5 days, in addition to intravenous infusion, have been employed in some cases of encephalitis.

The risk of *adverse reactions* to cytarabine is related to the size of the dose and the duration of treatment. Some degree of *bone-marrow depression* usually occurs when recommended quantities are administered. *Suppression of immunity, hepatic damage,* and *gastrointestinal disturbances* have also accompanied the use of cytarabine.

Andrioli, V. T., and Kravetz, H. M. The use of amphotericin B in man. *J. Am. med. Ass.,* **1962,** *180,* 269–272.

Balanchandar, V.; Collipp, P. J.; and Rising, B. J. Intramuscular clindamycin phosphate in children. *Clin. Med.,* **1973,** *80,* 24–30.

Bartlett, J. G.; Sutter, V. L.; and Finegold, S. M. Treatment of anaerobic infections with lincomycin and clindamycin. *New Engl. J. Med.,* **1972,** *287,* 1006–1010.

Bauer, D. J., and Sadler, P. W. The structure-activity relationships of the antiviral chemotherapeutic activity of isatin β-thiosemicarbasone. *Br. J. Pharmac. Chemother.,* **1960,** *15,* 101–110.

Bauer, D. J.; St. Vincent, L.; Kempe, C. H.; and Downie, A. W. Prophylactic treatment of smallpox contacts with N-methylisatin β-thiosemicarbasone. *Lancet,* **1963,** *2,* 494–496.

Bellamy, H. M., Jr.; Bates, B. B.; and Reinarz, J. A. Lincomycin metabolism in patients with hepatic insufficiency: effect of liver disease on serum concentrations. In, *Antimicrobial Agents and Chemotherapy—1966.* (Hobby, G. L., ed.) American Society for Microbiology, Ann Arbor, Mich., **1967,** pp. 36–41.

Bindschalder, D. D., and Bennett, J. E. A pharmacologic guide to the clinical use of amphotericin B. *J. infect. Dis.,* **1969,** *120,* 427–436.

Blank, H.; Smith, J. G., Jr.; Roth, F. J., Jr.; and Zaias, N. Griseofulvin for the systemic treatment of dermatomycoses. *J. Am. med. Ass.,* **1959,** *171,* 2168–2173.

Block, E. R.; Jennings, A. E.; and Bennett, J. E. 5-Fluorocytosine resistance in *Cryptococcus neoformans. Antimicrob. Agents Chemother.,* **1973,** *3,* 649–656.

Boston Interhospital and Cooperative Study. Boston Interhospital Virus Study Group and the NIAID-Sponsored Cooperative Antiviral Clinical Study. Failure of high dose 5-iodo-2'-deoxyuridine in the therapy of herpes simplex virus encephalitis. Evidence of unacceptable toxicity. *New Engl. J. Med.,* **1975,** *292,* 599–603.

Brandsberg, J. W., and French, M. *In vitro* susceptibility of isolates of *Aspergillus fumigatus* and *Sporothrix schenkii* to amphotericin B. *Antimicrob. Agents Chemother.,* **1972,** *2,* 402–404.

Collins, J. F., and Hood, H. M. Topical antibiotic treatment of acute necrotizing ulcerative gingivitis. *J. oral Med.,* **1967,** *22,* 59–64.

Cornelius, C. E., III, and Domescik, G. Spectinomycin hydrochloride in the treatment of uncomplicated gonorrhoea. *Br. J. vener. Dis.,* **1970,** *46,* 212–213.

Council on Drugs. The amantadine controversy. *J. Am. med. Ass.,* **1967,** *201,* 372–373.

Curtis, J. R., and Eastwood, J. B. Colistin sulphomethate sodium administration with presence of severe renal failure and during haemodialysis and peritoneal dialysis. *Br. med. J.,* **1968,** *1,* 484–485.

Davies, J.; Anderson, P.; and Davis, B. D. Inhibition of protein synthesis by spectinomycin. *Science, Wash.,* **1965,** *149,* 1096–1098.

Davies, R. R., and Reeves, D. S. 5-Fluorocytosine and urinary candidiasis. *Br. med. J.,* **1971,** *1,* 577–579.

Davies, W. L.; Grunert, R. R.; Haff, R. F.; McGahen, J. W.; Neumayer, E. M.; Paulshock, M.; Watts, J. C.; Wood, T. R.; Hermann, E. C.; and Hoffmann, C. E. Antiviral activity of 1-adamantanamine (amantadine). *Science, Wash.,* **1964,** *144,* 862–863.

Dawborn, J. K.; Page, M. D.; and Schiavone, D. J. Use of 5-fluorocytosine in patients with impaired renal function. *Br. med. J.,* **1973,** *3,* 382–384.

DeHaan, R. M.; Metzler, C. M.; Schellenberg, D.; and Vanden Bosch, W. D. Pharmacokinetic studies of clindamycin phosphate. *J. clin. Pharmac.,* **1973,** *13,* 190–209.

DeHaan, R. M.; Metzler, C. M.; Schellenberg, D.; Vanden Bosch, W. D.; and Masson, E. L. Pharmacokinetic studies of clindamycin hydrochloride in humans. *Int. J. clin. Pharmac.,* **1972,** *6,* 105–119.

Diamond, R. D., and Bennett, J. E. A subcutaneous reservoir for intrathecal therapy for fungal meningitis. *New Engl. J. Med.,* **1973,** *288,* 186–188.

Dickinson, P. C. T.; Chang, T.-W.; and Weinstein, L. Effects of amantadines on influenza B and measles virus infection in children. In, *Antimicrobial Agents and Chemotherapy—1966.* (Hobby, G. L., ed.) American Society for Microbiology, Ann Arbor, Mich., **1967,** pp. 521–526.

Dixon, J. M. S., and Lipinski, A. E. Resistance of group A beta-hemolytic streptococci to lincomycin and erythromycin. *Antimicrob. Agents Chemother.,* **1972,** *1,* 333–339.

Douglas, J. B., and Healy, J. K. Nephrotoxic effects of amphotericin B, including renal tubular acidosis. *Am. J. Med.,* **1969,** *46,* 154–162.

Douglas, R. L., and Kislak, J. W. Treatment of *Bacteroides fragilis* bacteremia with clindamycin. *J. infect. Dis.,* **1973,** *128,* 569–571.

Drutz, D. J.; Spickard, A.; Rogers, D. E.; and Koenig, M. G. Treatment of disseminated mycotic infections: a new approach to amphotericin B therapy. *Am. J. Med.,* **1968,** *45,* 405–418.

Dubos, R. J., and Hotchkiss, R. D. The production of bactericidal substances by aerobic sporulating bacilli. *J. exp. Med.,* **1941,** *73,* 629–640.

Dutcher, J. D.; Boyak, G.; and Fox, S. The preparation and properties of crystalline fungicidin (nystatin). In, *Antibiotics Annual, 1953–1954.* Medical Encyclopedia, Inc., New York, **1954,** pp. 191–193.

Editorial. Smallpox prophylaxis. *Lancet,* **1963,** *2,* 501.

Ehrenkranz, N. J. The clinical evaluation of vancomycin in treatment of multiantibiotic refractory staphylococcal infections. In, *Antibiotics Annual, 1958–1959.* Medical Encyclopedia, Inc., New York, **1959,** pp. 587–594.

El-Nakeeb, M. A., and Lampen, J. O. Uptake of griseofulvin by the sensitive dermatophyte, *Microsporum gypseum. J. Bact.,* **1965,** *89,* 564–569.

Emmons, C. W.; Shadomy, H. J.; and Piggott, W. Hamycin: chemotherapeutic studies in systemic mycoses in man. *Am. Rev. resp. Dis.,* **1967,** *95,* 506–509.

Fass, R. J., and Saslaw, S. Clindamycin: clinical and laboratory evaluation of parenteral therapy. *Am. J. med. Sci.,* **1972,** *263,* 369–382.

Fass, R. J.; Scholand, J. F.; Hodges, G. R.; and Saslaw, S. Clindamycin in the treatment of serious anaerobic infections. *Ann. intern. Med.,* **1973,** *78,* 853–859.

Feldman, H. A.; Hamilton, J. D.; and Gutman, R. A. Amphotericin therapy in an anephric patient. *Antimicrob. Agents Chemother.,* **1973,** *4,* 402–405.

Finegold, S. M.; Harada, N. E.; and Miller, L. G. Lincomycin: activity against anaerobes and effect on normal human fecal flora. In, *Antimicrobial Agents and Chemotherapy—1965.* (Hobby, G. L., ed.) American Society for Microbiology, Ann Arbor, Mich., **1966,** pp. 659–667.

Gentles, J. C. Experimental ringworm in guinea pigs: oral treatment with griseofulvin. *Nature, Lond.,* **1958,** *182,* 476–477.

Goldman, L.; Schwarz, J.; Preston, R. H.; Beyer, A.; and Loutzenhiser, J. Current status of griseofulvin: report on one hundred seventy-five cases. *J. Am. med. Ass.,* **1960,** *172,* 532–538.

Griffith, R. S., and Black, H. R. Comparison of the blood levels obtained after single and multiple doses of erythromycin estolate and erythromycin stearate. *Am. J. med. Sci.,* **1964,** *247,* 69–74.

———. Comparison of blood levels following pediatric suspensions of erythromycin estolate and erythromycin ethyl succinate. *Clin. Med.,* **1969,** *76,* 16–18.

Griffith, R. S., and Peck, F. B., Jr. Vancomycin, a new antibiotic. III. Preliminary clinical and laboratory studies. In, *Antibiotics Annual, 1955–1956.* Medical Encyclopedia, Inc., New York, **1956,** pp. 619–622.

Hamre, D.; Bernstein, J.; and Donovick, R. Activity of *p*-aminobenzaldehyde 3-thiosemicarbazone on vaccinia virus in the chick embryo and in the mouse. *Proc. Soc. exp. Biol. Med.,* **1950,** *73,* 275–278.

Herrell, W. E. Hamycin in the treatment of blastomycosis. *Clin. Med.,* **1968,** *75,* 19–20.

Huber, F. M., and Gottlieb, D. The mechanism of action of griseofulvin. *Can. J. Microbiol.,* **1968,** *14,* 111–118.

Isacson, M.; Noah, Z.; Faber, J.; Herishano, Y.; and Gottfried, V. Use of 5-fluorocytosine in systemic candidiasis in infancy. *Archs Dis. Childh.,* **1972,** *47,* 954–959.

Kauffman, R. E.; Shoeman, D. W.; Wan, S. H.; and Azarnoff, D. L. Absorption and excretion of clindamycin-2-phosphate in children after intramuscular injection. *Clin. Pharmac. Ther.,* **1972,** *13,* 704–709.

Kinsky, S. C. Nystatin binding by protoplasts and a particulate fraction of *Neurospora crassa,* and a basis for the selective toxicity of polyene antifungal antibiotics. *Proc. natn. Acad. Sci. U.S.A.,* **1962,** *48,* 1049–1056.

Kirby, W. M. M.; Perry, D. M.; and Bauer, A. W. Treatment of staphylococcal septicemia with vancomycin: report of thirty-three cases. *New Engl. J. Med.,* **1960,** *262,* 49–55.

Koch-Weser, J.; Sidel, V. W.; Federman, E. B.; Kanarek, P.; Finer, D. C.; and Eaton, A. E. Adverse effects of colistimethate. Manifestations and specific reaction rates during 317 courses of therapy. *Ann. intern. Med.,* **1970,** *72,* 857–868.

Koyama, Y.; Kurosawa, A.; Tsuchiya, A.; and Takakuta, K. A new antibiotic, colistin, produced by spore-forming soil bacteria. *J. Antibiot., Tokyo,* **1950,** *3,* 457.

Kunin, C. M., and Finland, M. Restrictions imposed on antibiotic therapy by renal failure. *A.M.A. Archs intern. Med.,* **1959,** *104,* 1030–1050.

Lerner, P. I. Susceptibility of *Actinomyces* species to lincomycin and its 7-halogenated analogues. In, *Antimicrobial*

Agents and Chemotherapy—1968. (Hobby, G. L., ed.) American Society for Microbiology, Bethesda, Md., **1969,** pp. 461–464.

Lindesmith, L. A.; Baines, R. D.; Bigelow, D. B.; and Petty, T. L. Reversible respiratory paralysis associated with polymyxin therapy. *Ann. intern. Med.,* **1968,** *68,* 318–327.

Lwin, H., and Collipp, P. J. Absorption and tolerance of clindamycin-2-palmitate in infants below 6 months of age. *Curr. ther. Res.,* **1970,** *12,* 648–657.

McCormick, M. H.; Stark, W. M.; Pittenger, G. E.; Pittenger, R. C.; and McGuire, J. M. Vancomycin, a new antibiotic. I. Chemical and biologic properties. In, *Antibiotics Annual, 1955–1956.* Medical Encyclopedia, Inc., New York, **1956,** pp. 606–611.

McCurdy, D. K.; Frederic, M.; and Elkinton, J. R. Renal tubular acidosis due to amphotericin B. *New Engl. J. Med.,* **1968,** *278,* 124–131.

McGahen, J. W., and Hoffmann, C. E. Influenza infections of mice. I. Curative activity of amantadine HCl. *Proc. Soc. exp. Biol. Med.,* **1968,** *129,* 678–681.

Mao, J. C.-H., and Putterman, M. The intermolecular complex of erythromycin and ribosome. *J. molec. Biol.,* **1969,** *44,* 347–361.

Mao, J. C.-H., and Wiegand, R. G. Mode of action of macrolides. *Biochim. biophys. Acta,* **1968,** *157,* 404–413.

Marks, M. I.; Steer, P.; and Eickhoff, T. C. *In vitro* sensitivity of *Torulopsis glabrata* to amphotericin B, 5-fluorocytosine, and clotrimazole (Bay 5097). *Appl. Microbiol.,* **1971,** *22,* 93–95.

Maxwell, E. Treatment of herpes keratitis with 5-iodo-2-deoxyuridine (IDU): a clinical evaluation of 1500 cases. *Am. J. Ophthal.,* **1963,** *56,* 571–573.

Medoff, G.; Comfort, M.; and Kobayashi, G. S. Synergistic action of amphotericin B and 5-fluorocytosine against yeast-like organisms. *Proc. Soc. exp. Biol. Med.,* **1971a,** *138,* 571–574.

Medoff, G.; Dismukes, W. E.; Meade, R. H., iii; and Moses, J. Therapeutic program for *Candida* infection. In, *Antimicrobial Agents and Chemotherapy—1970.* (Hobby, G. L., ed.) American Society for Microbiology, Bethesda, Md., **1971b,** pp. 286–290.

Meyers, B. R.; Kaplan, K.; and Weinstein, L. Microbiological and pharmacological behavior of 7-chlorolincomycin. *Appl. Microbiol.,* **1969,** *17,* 653–657.

Molavi, A., and Weinstein, L. *In vitro* activity of erythromycin against atypical mycobacteria. *J. infect. Dis.,* **1971,** *123,* 216–219.

Montes, L. F. Oral amphotericin B on superficial candidiasis. *Clin. Med.,* **1971,** *78,* 14–17.

Nafta, I.; Turcanu, A. G.; Braun, I.; Companetz, W.; Simionescu, A. B. E.; and Florea, V. Administration of amantadine for the prevention of Hong Kong influenza. *Bull. Wld Hlth Org.,* **1970,** *42,* 423–427.

Newmark, E.; Ellison, A. C.; and Kaufman, H. E. Pimaricin therapy of cephalosporium and fusarium keratitis. *Am. J. Ophthal.,* **1970,** *69,* 458–466.

Newmark, E.; Kaufman, H. E.; Polack, F. M.; and Ellison, A. C. Clinical experience with pimaricin therapy in fungal keratitis. *Sth. med. J., Nashville,* **1971,** *64,* 935–941.

Newton, G. G. F., and Abraham, E. P. Observations on the nature of bacitracin A. *Biochem. J.,* **1953,** *53,* 604–613.

Normark, S., and Schönebeck, J. *In vitro* studies of 5-fluorocytosine resistance in *Candida albicans* and *Torulopsis glabrata. Antimicrob. Agents Chemother.,* **1972,** *2,* 114–121.

Panzer, J. D.; Brown, D. C.; Epstein, W. L.; Lipson, R. L.; Mahaffrey, H. W.; and Atkinson, W. H. Clindamycin levels in various body tissues and fluids. *J. clin. Pharmac.,* **1972,** *12,* 259–262.

Philipson, A.; Sabath, L. D.; and Charles, D. Transplacental passage of erythromycin and clindamycin. *New Engl. J. Med.,* **1973,** *288,* 1219–1221.

Randall, R. W., and Ritchey, J. P. Medical therapy for

Aspergillus corneal ulcer. *Archs Ophthal., N.Y.,* **1973,** *90,* 402–404.

Reyn, A.; Schmidt, H.; Trier, M.; and Bentzon, M. W. Spectinomycin hydrochloride (TROBICIN) in the treatment of gonorrhea. Observation of resistant strains of *Neisseria gonorrhoeae. Br. J. vener. Dis.,* **1973,** *49,* 54–59.

Sabath, L. D.; Gerstein, D. A.; and Finland, M. Serum glutamic oxalacetic transaminase: false elevations during administration of erythromycin. *New Engl. J. Med.,* **1968a,** *279,* 1137–1139.

Sabath, L. D.; Gerstein, D. A.; Loder, P. B.; and Finland, M. Excretion of erythromycin and its enhanced activity in urine against gram-negative bacilli with alkalinization. *J. Lab. clin. Med.,* **1968b,** *72,* 916–923.

Schönebeck, J.; Polak, A.; Fernex, M.; and Scholer, H. J. Pharmacokinetic studies on the oral antimycotic agent 5-fluorocytosine in individuals with normal and impaired kidney function. *Chemotherapy,* **1973,** *18,* 321–336.

Schoutens, E.; Peromet, M.; and Yourassowsky, E. Microbiological and clinical study of spectinomycin in urinary tract infections: reevaluation with hospital strains. *Curr. ther. Res.,* **1972,** *14,* 349–357.

Shapera, R. M.; Hable, K. A.; and Matsen, J. M. Erythromycin therapy twice daily for streptococcal pharyngitis. Controlled comparison with erythromycin or penicillin phenoxymethyl four times daily or penicillin G benzathine. *J. Am. med. Ass.,* **1973,** *226,* 531–555.

Sinanian, R.; Panzer, J. D.; and Atkinson, W. H. Time of eradication of gonococcus following spectinomycin therapy. *Clin. Med.,* **1972,** *79,* 15–16.

Smith, C. B.; Friedewald, W. T.; and Chanock, R. B. Shedding of *Mycoplasma pneumoniae* after tetracycline and erythromycin therapy. *New Engl. J. Med.,* **1967,** *276,* 1172–1175.

Smith, D. O., and Osick, P. Erythromycin in the treatment of acute gonococcal urethritis in males. *Curr. ther. Res.,* **1969,** *11,* 1–4.

Sprunt, K.; Leidy, G.; and Redman, W. Cross resistance between lincomycin and erythromycin in *viridans* streptococci. *Pediatrics, Springfield,* **1970,** *46,* 84–88.

Stevens, D. A.; Jordan, G. W.; Waddell, T. F.; and Merigan, T. C. Adverse effect of cytosine arabinoside on disseminated zoster in a controlled trial. *New Engl. J. Med.,* **1973,** *289,* 873–878.

Sutter, V. L.; Kwok, Y.-J.; and Finegold, S. M. Susceptibility of *Bacteroides fragilis* to six antibiotics determined by standardized antimicrobial disc sensitivity testing. *Antimicrob. Agents Chemother.,* **1973,** *3,* 188–193.

Tanaka, K.; Teraoka, H.; Tamaki, M.; Otaka, E.; and Osawa, S. Erythromycin-resistant mutant of *Escherichia coli* with altered ribosomal protein component. *Science, Wash.,* **1968,** *162,* 576–578.

Thadepalli, H.; Gorbach, S. L.; Broido, P. W.; Norsen, J.; and Nyhus, L. Abdominal trauma, anaerobes, and antibiotics. *Surgery Gynec. Obstet.,* **1973,** *137,* 270–276.

Thompson, R. L.; Minton, S. A.; Officer, J. E.; and Hitchings, J. E. The effect of heterocyclic and other thiosemicarbazones on vaccinia infections in the mouse. *J. Immun.,* **1953,** *70,* 229–234.

Togo, Y.; Hornick, R. B.; and Dawkins, A. T. Studies on induced influenza in man. I. Double-blind studies designed to assess prophylactic efficacy of amantadine hydrochloride against A_2/Rockville/1/65 strain. *J. Am. med. Ass.,* **1968,** *203,* 1089–1094.

Tolman, K. G.; Sannella, J. J.; and Freston, J. W. Chemical structure of erythromycin and hepatotoxicity. *Ann. intern. Med.,* **1974,** *81,* 58–60.

Utz, J. P.; Bennett, J. E.; Brandriss, M. W.; Butler, W. T.; and Hill, G. J., ii. Amphotericin B toxicity: combined clinical staff conference at the National Institutes of Health. *Ann. intern. Med.,* **1964,** *61,* 334–354.

Utz, J. P.; Tynes, B. S.; Shadmomy, H. J.; Duma, R. J.; Kannan, M. M.; and Mason, K. N. 5-Fluorocytosine in human cryptococcosis. In, *Antimicrobial Agents and Chemotherapy—1968*. (Hobby, G. L., ed.) American Society for Microbiology, Bethesda, Md., **1969**, pp. 344–346.

Vacek, V.; Heizler, M.; Salvik, M.; and Pavlansky, R. Penetration of clindamycin into bone in man. *Chemotherapy,* **1972**, *17*, 22–25.

Vandeputte, J.; Wachtel, J. L.; and Stiller, E. T. Amphotericins A and B, antifungal antibiotics produced by a streptomyces. II. The isolation and properties of the crystalline amphotericins. In, *Antibiotics Annual, 1955–1956*. Medical Encyclopedia, Inc., New York, **1956**, pp. 587–591.

Vogel, Z.; Vogel, T.; and Elson, D. The effect of erythromycin on peptide bond formation and the termination reaction. *FEBS Lett.,* **1971**, *15*, 249–253.

Wade, D. N., and Sudlow, G. The kinetics of 5-fluorocytosine elimination in man. *Aust. N.Z. J. Med.,* **1972**, *2*, 153–158.

Waitz, J. A.; Moss, E. L.; and Weinstein, M. J. Chemotherapeutic evaluation of clotrimazole [Bay b 5097, 1(*o*-chloro-α-α-diphenylbenzyl) imidazole]. *Appl. Microbiol.,* **1971**, *22*, 891–898.

Watanakunakorn, C., and Bakie, C. Synergism of vancomycin-gentamicin and vancomycin-streptomycin against enterococci. *Antimicrob. Agents Chemother.,* **1973**, *4*, 120–124.

Weissmann, G., and Sessa, G. The action of polyene antibiotics on phospholipid-cholesterol structures. *J. biol. Chem.,* **1967**, *242*, 616–625.

Westenfelder, G. O.; Paterson, R. Y.; Reisberg, B. E.; and Carlson, G. M. Vancomycin-streptomycin synergism in enterococcal endocarditis. *J. Am. med. Ass.,* **1973**, *223*, 37–40.

Wilkins, T. D., and Thiel, T. Resistance of some species of *Clostridium* to clindamycin. *Antimicrob. Agents Chemother.,* **1973**, *3*, 136–137.

Wingfield, W. L.; Pottack, D.; and Grunert, R. R. Therapeutic efficacy of amantadine-HCl and rumantadine-HCl in naturally-occurring influenza A2 respiratory illness in man. *New Engl. J. Med.,* **1969**, *281*, 579–584.

Wise, G. J.; Wainstein, S.; Goldberg, P.; and Kozinn, P. J. Candidal cystitis. Management by continuous bladder irrigation with amphotericin B. *J. Am. med. Ass.,* **1973**, *224*, 1636–1637.

Wright, W. W., and Welch, H. Chemical, biological, and clinical observations on colistin. In, *Antibiotics Annual, 1959–1960*. Antibiotica, Inc., New York, **1960**, pp. 61–74.

Monographs and Reviews

Anderson, D. W. Griseofulvin. Biology and clinical usefulness: a review. *Ann. Allergy,* **1965**, *23*, 103–110.

Bennett, J. E. Chemotherapy of systemic mycoses. *New Engl. J. Med.,* **1974**, *290*, 30–32, 320–323.

Braun, P. Hepatotoxicity of erythromycin. *J. infect. Dis.,* **1969**, *119*, 300–306.

Brownlee, G.; Bushby, S. R. M.; and Short, E. I. The chemotherapy and pharmacology of the polymyxins. *Br. J. Pharmac. Chemother.,* **1952**, *7*, 170–188.

Goldman, L. Griseofulvin. *Med. Clins N. Am.,* **1970**, *54*, 1339–1345.

Greenberg, P. A., and Sanford, J. P. Removal and absorption of antibiotics in patients with renal failure undergoing peritoneal dialysis: tetracycline, chloramphenicol, kanamycin, and colistimethate. *Ann. intern. Med.,* **1967**, *66*, 465–479.

Jawetz, E. Polymyxin, colistin, and bacitracin. *Pediat. Clins N. Am.,* **1961**, *8*, 1057–1071.

Medical Letter. Flucytosine (ANCOBON)—a new antifungal drug. **1972**, *14*, 29–30.

Meleney, F. I., and Johnson, B. A. Bacitracin. *Am. J. Med.,* **1949**, *7*, 794–806.

Newton, B. A. The properties and mode of action of the polymyxins. *Bact. Rev.,* **1956**, *20*, 14–27.

———. Surface active bactericides. In, *Strategy of Chemotherapy,* Vol. 8 (Symposium of the Society for General Microbiology). J. & A. Churchill, Ltd., London, **1958**, pp. 62–93.

Pratt, W. B. *Fundamentals of Chemotherapy.* Oxford University Press, New York, **1973**.

Prusoff, W. H. Recent advances in chemotherapy of viral diseases. *Pharmac. Rev.,* **1967**, *19*, 209–250.

Sebek, O. K. Polymyxins and circulin. In, *Antibiotics.* Vol. 1, *Mechanism of Action.* (Gottlieb, D., and Shaw, P. D., eds.) Springer-Verlag, Berlin, **1967**, pp. 142–152.

Symposium. (Various authors.) Griseofulvin and dermatomycoses. *Archs Derm.,* **1960**, *81*, 650–882.

Weinstein, L., and Chang, T. W. The chemotherapy of viral infections. *New Engl. J. Med.,* **1973**, *289*, 725–730.

Weinstein, L., and Weinstein, A. J. The pathophysiology and pathoanatomy of reactions to antimicrobial agents. *Adv. intern. Med.,* **1974**, *19*, 109–134.

Weisblum, B., and Davies, J. Antibiotic inhibitors of the bacterial ribosome. *Bact. Rev.,* **1968**, *32*, 493–528.

Chemotherapy of Neoplastic Diseases

INTRODUCTION

Paul Calabresi and Robert E. Parks, Jr.

The past decade has witnessed a quiet revolution in the field of cancer chemotherapy. Although there have been no spectacular "breakthroughs," as were seen in the 1940s with the discovery of penicillin and other antibiotics for the treatment of infectious diseases, a wealth of basic knowledge, improved investigative technics, and a substantial number of new antineoplastic agents have emerged. Major developments have occurred in areas such as molecular and cellular biology, which have resulted in a greater understanding of mechanisms of cellular division, tumor immunology, and fundamental factors involved in both viral and chemical carcinogenesis. Although most current antitumor drugs were discovered empirically, considerable insight has been gained into the mechanisms by which many of these compounds affect cellular growth. This has permitted the more rational therapeutic application of these agents, often in synergistic combinations, as well as the evolution of new and more effective drugs. Especially important has been the development of clinical investigative technics, often involving large collaborative studies, that have enabled efficient evaluation and prompt introduction of new drugs or drug combinations into the clinic. Ten years ago significant palliative results were obtained by chemotherapy in a number of human neoplasms, and hope was emerging that choriocarcinoma could be cured by treatment with methotrexate. Today it is possible to list at least ten neoplastic diseases that can be associated with a normal life expectancy after treatment with drugs, alone or in combination with other modalities. These include choriocarcinoma in women; acute leukemia, Wilms' tumor, Ewing's sarcoma, rhabdomyosarcoma, and retinoblastoma in children; and Hodgkin's disease, lymphosarcoma, Burkitt's lymphoma, mycosis fungoides, and testicular carcinoma.

The entire population of neoplastic cells must be eradicated in order to obtain these desired results. The concept of "total cell-kill" applies to chemotherapy as it does to other means of treatment; total excision of tumor is necessary for surgical cure, and complete destruction of all cancer cells is required for a cure with radiation therapy. By investigation of a model tumor system, the L1210 leukemia of mice, Skipper and colleagues have established a number of important principles that have guided and redirected modern cancer chemotherapy. These may be briefly summarized as follows: (1) A single clonogenic malignant cell can give rise to sufficient progeny to kill the host; to achieve cure it is thus necessary to destroy every such cell. Since the doubling-time of most tumors is relatively constant during logarithmic growth, the life-span of the host is inversely related to the number of malignant cells that are inoculated or that survive therapeutic measures. (2) In contrast to antimicrobial chemotherapy where, in most instances, there are major contributions by the immune mechanisms and other host defenses, these play a negligible role in the therapy of neoplastic disease unless only a small number of malignant cells is present. (3) The cell-kill caused by antineoplastic agents follows first-order kinetics; that is, a constant percentage, rather than a constant number, of cells is killed by a given therapeutic maneuver. This finding has had a profound impact on clinical cancer chemotherapy. For example, a patient with advanced acute lymphocytic leukemia might harbor 10^{12} or about 1 kg of malignant cells. A drug capable of killing 99.99% of these cells would reduce the tumor mass to about 100 mg, and this would be apparent as a complete clinical remission. However, 10^8 malignant cells would remain, any of which could cause a relapse in the disease. The logical outgrowth of these concepts has been the attempt to achieve total cell-kill by the use of several chemotherapeutic agents in combination or in rational sequences. The resulting prolonged survival of patients with acute lymphocytic leukemia through the use of such multiple-drug regimens has encouraged the application of these principles to the treatment of other neoplasms.

An understanding of cell-cycle kinetics is essential for the proper use of the current generation of antineoplastic agents. Many of the most potent cytotoxic agents act at specific phases of the cell cycle and, therefore, have activity only against cells that are in the process of division. Accordingly, human malignancies that are currently most susceptible to chemotherapeutic measures are those with a large growth fraction, that is, a high percentage of cells in the process of division. Similarly, normal tissues that proliferate rapidly (bone marrow, hair follicles, and intestinal epithelium) are often subject to damage by some of these potent antineoplastic drugs, and such toxicity often limits drug utility. On the other hand, slow-growing tumors with a small growth fraction, for example, carcinomas of the colon or lung, are often unresponsive to cytotoxic drugs. Although differences in the duration of the cell cycle occur between cells of various types, all cells display a similar pattern during the division process. This may be characterized as follows: (1) there is a presynthetic phase (G_1); (2) the synthesis of DNA occurs (S); (3) an interval follows the termination of DNA synthesis, the postsynthetic phase (G_2); and (4) mitosis (M) ensues—the G_2 cell, containing a double complement of DNA, divides into two daughter G_1 cells. Each of these may immediately reenter the cell cycle or pass into a nonproliferative stage, referred to as G_0. The cells of certain specialized tissues may differentiate into functional cells that are no longer capable of division. On the other hand, many cells, especially those in slow-growing tumors, may remain in the G_0 state for prolonged periods, only to be recruited into the division cycle again at a much later time. Most antineoplastic agents act specifically on processes such as DNA synthesis, transcription, or the function of the mitotic spindle and, therefore, are regarded as cell-cycle specific. It is obvious that further understanding of the cell cycle and of the factors that regulate the recruitment of G_0 cells into the cycle should prove of great value in future attempts to develop chemotherapeutic measures for slow-growing tumors.

A great variety of compounds has been investigated in experimental animals, and a few have proven sufficiently useful in the clinical treatment of human neoplasms, at acceptable levels of toxicity, to deserve the designation of chemotherapeutic agents. It should be emphasized that the compounds selected for discussion represent, for the most part, those that are generally available and have withstood the test of time, although a few have been included either because they illustrate special circumstances or because they are representative of newer developments. Not discussed are several biologically active alkylating agents, hormones, antibiotics, and other compounds that are not commonly used in clinical practice, either because their structural variations offer no particular advantage over existing drugs or because additional investigation is deemed to be necessary. It is also important, in this rapidly changing field, continually to reappraise the current status of available agents, with respect not only to new additions but also to appropriate deletions of compounds the clinical importance of which has declined; information concerning drugs in the latter category may be found in earlier editions of this textbook. Other compounds, particularly certain antimetabolites that were originally developed as antineoplastic agents, have now assumed such important roles in the management of nonneoplastic disorders that they belong more properly in other chapters. Indeed, this spin-off in cancer chemotherapy research represents an area of increasing interest and practical importance to medicine in general. Illustrative examples of such stimulating developments include the use of purine analogs for the suppression of immune responses,

Table XV–1. CHEMOTHERAPEUTIC AGENTS USEFUL IN NEOPLASTIC DISEASE

CLASS	TYPE OF AGENT	NONPROPRIETARY NAMES (OTHER NAMES)	DISEASE *
Alkylating Agents	Nitrogen Mustards	Mechlorethamine (HN₂; MUSTARGEN)	Hodgkin's disease, non-Hodgkin's lymphomas, breast, ovary
		Cyclophosphamide (CYTOXAN, ENDOXAN)	Acute and chronic lymphocytic leukemias, Hodgkin's disease, non-Hodgkin's lymphomas, multiple myeloma, neuroblastoma, breast, ovary, lung, Wilms' tumor, rhabdomyosarcoma
		Melphalan (L-sarcolysin; ALKERAN)	Plasma-cell myeloma, breast, ovary
		Uracil mustard	Chronic lymphocytic leukemia, non-Hodgkin's lymphomas, Hodgkin's disease, ovary, primary thrombocytosis
		Chlorambucil (LEUKERAN)	Chronic lymphocytic leukemia, primary macroglobulinemia, Hodgkin's disease, non-Hodgkin's lymphomas, breast, ovary, testis
	Ethylenimine Derivatives	Triethylenemelamine (TEM)	Hodgkin's disease, non-Hodgkin's lymphomas, retinoblastoma, breast, ovary, chronic leukemias
		Triethylene*thio*-phosphoramide (Thio-TEPA)	Hodgkin's disease, non-Hodgkin's lymphomas, retinoblastoma, breast, ovary
	Alkyl Sulfonates	Busulfan (MYLERAN)	Chronic granulocytic leukemia, polycythemia vera, primary thrombocytosis
	Nitrosoureas	Carmustine (BCNU)	Hodgkin's disease, non-Hodgkin's lymphomas, primary and metastatic brain tumors, melanoma, renal cell
		Lomustine (CCNU)	Hodgkin's disease, non-Hodgkin's lymphomas, primary and metastatic brain tumors, renal cell
		Streptozotocin	Malignant pancreatic insulinoma, malignant carcinoid
	Triazenes	Dacarbazine (DTIC; dimethyltriazeno-imidazolecarboxamide)	Malignant melanoma, Hodgkin's disease, soft-tissue sarcomas
Antimetabolites	Folic Acid Analogs	Methotrexate (amethopterin)	Acute lymphocytic leukemia, choriocarcinoma, mycosis fungoides, breast, testis, oropharyngeal, lung, osteogenic sarcoma
	Pyrimidine Analogs	Fluorouracil (5-fluorouracil; 5-FU)	Breast, colon, stomach, pancreas, ovary, oropharyngeal, urinary bladder, premalignant skin lesions (topical)
		Cytarabine (cytosine arabinoside; CYTOSAR)	Acute granulocytic and acute lymphocytic leukemias
		Azaribine (triacetyl-6-azauridine; TRIAZURE)	Mycosis fungoides, polycythemia vera

* Neoplasms are carcinomas unless otherwise indicated.

CLASS	TYPE OF AGENT	NONPROPRIETARY NAMES (OTHER NAMES)	DISEASE *
Antimetabolites	Purine Analogs	Mercaptopurine (6-mercaptopurine; 6-MP; PURINETHOL)	Acute lymphocytic, acute granulocytic, and chronic granulocytic leukemias
		Thioguanine (6-thioguanine; TG)	Acute granulocytic, acute lymphocytic, and chronic granulocytic leukemias
Natural Products	Vinca Alkaloids	Vinblastine (VLB; VELBAN)	Hodgkin's disease, non-Hodgkin's lymphomas, breast
		Vincristine (VCR; ONCOVIN)	Acute lymphocytic leukemia, neuroblastoma, Wilms' tumor, rhabdomyosarcoma, Hodgkin's disease, non-Hodgkin's lymphomas
	Antibiotics	Dactinomycin (actinomycin D; COSMEGEN)	Choriocarcinoma, Wilms' tumor, rhabdomyosarcoma, testis
		Daunorubicin (daunomycin; rubidomycin; DAUNOBLASTINA)	Acute granulocytic and acute lymphocytic leukemias
		Doxorubicin (adriablastina; ADRIAMYCIN)	Soft-tissue, osteogenic, and other sarcomas; Hodgkin's disease, non-Hodgkin's lymphomas, acute leukemias, breast, genitourinary, thyroid, lung, neuroblastoma
		Bleomycin (BLENOXANE)	Squamous-cell carcinomas of head, neck, skin, esophagus, and genitourinary tract; Hodgkin's disease, non-Hodgkin's lymphomas
		Mithramycin (MITHRACIN)	Testicular tumors, malignant hypercalcemia
	Enzymes	L-Asparaginase	Acute lymphocytic leukemia
Miscellaneous Agents	Substituted Urea	Hydroxyurea (HYDREA)	Chronic granulocytic leukemia, malignant melanoma
	Methyl Hydrazine Derivative	Procarbazine (N-methylhydrazine, MIH; MATULANE, NATULAN)	Hodgkin's disease
	Adrenocortical Suppressant	Mitotane (o,p'-DDD; LYSODREN)	Adrenal cortex
Hormones	Adrenocorticosteroids	Prednisone (METICORTEN; several other equivalent preparations available)	Acute and chronic lymphocytic leukemia, non-Hodgkin's lymphomas, Hodgkin's disease, breast
	Progestins	Hydroxyprogesterone caproate (DELALUTIN) Medroprogesterone acetate (PROVERA) Megestrol acetate (MEGACE)	Endometrium, renal cell, breast, prostate
	Estrogens	Diethylstilbestrol Ethinyl estradiol (ESTINYL) (other preparations available; *see* Chapter 68)	Breast, prostate

Table XV-1. CHEMOTHERAPEUTIC AGENTS USEFUL IN NEOPLASTIC DISEASE (Continued)

CLASS	TYPE OF AGENT	NONPROPRIETARY NAMES (OTHER NAMES)	DISEASE *
Hormones	Androgens	Testosterone propionate Fluoxymesterone (HALOTESTIN) (other preparations available; *see* Chapter 69)	Breast
Radioactive Isotopes	Phosphorus	Sodium phosphate P 32	Polycythemia vera, chronic lymphocytic and granulocytic leukemias
	Iodine	Sodium iodide I 131	Thyroid

* Neoplasms are carcinomas unless otherwise indicated.

the effectiveness of allopurinol in controlling hyperuricemia and gout, the beneficial effects of azaribine and methotrexate in psoriasis, and the inhibitory actions of analogs of pyrimidine and purine nucleosides on the proliferation of certain viruses of the DNA type.

The emphasis in Chapter 62 is placed upon the drugs themselves. Although this is appropriate in a textbook of pharmacology, it is also essential to point out the importance of the role played by the patient. It is generally agreed that patients in good nutritional state and without severe metabolic disturbances, infections, or other complications are better candidates for significant improvement from antineoplastic therapy than are severely debilitated individuals. Ideally, the patient also should have adequate renal, hepatic, and bone-marrow function, uncompromised by tumor invasion, previous chemotherapy, or radiation (particularly of the spine or pelvis). Occasionally, however, even patients with advanced disease have improved dramatically with chemotherapy. Although methods that would enable accurate prediction of the responsiveness of a particular tumor to a given agent are not yet available, efforts are being made to establish better clinical and laboratory criteria for the rational selection of patients prior to therapy. Despite efforts to anticipate the development of complications, anticancer agents, like many other potent drugs with only moderate selectivity, may cause severe toxicity. In such circumstances, the physician must have at his disposal adequate facilities for vigorous supportive therapy; some of these, including platelet transfusions and the administration of allopurinol to prevent the complications of hyperuricemia, have been widely adopted, while others, including better methods to combat or prevent infections, are the subject of intensive investigation.

Among the factors responsible for increased susceptibility of the patient to infections caused by pathogenic bacteria or opportunistic microorganisms is the potential of many antineoplastic agents to produce profound suppression of the immune responses. Some immune responses, particularly cellular immunity mediated by T lymphocytes, are also thought to play an important role in the natural host resistance against malignant tumors; others, including humoral "blocking factors" produced by B lymphocytes, may be deleterious to the patient by actually protecting the neoplastic cells. Since cytotoxic agents can selectively suppress or enhance these immune responses, depending upon dosages or schedules of administration, antineoplastic chemotherapy may cause marked alterations of the delicate balance that exists between the patient and his tumor or microflora. As more effective combinations of potent chemotherapeutic agents approach the desired goal of total cell-kill, the subtle interactions between these drugs and the immunological defenses of the host represent an increasingly important area of investigation, since it is essential that, upon completion of the intensive therapy required, the patient be able to withstand both infection by microorganisms and recurrence of the neoplastic process.

Drugs currently used in chemotherapy of malignant diseases may be divided into several classes, as shown in Table XV-1. This somewhat arbitrary classification is used in Chapter

62 as a convenient framework for describing the various types of agents; the major clinical indications for the drugs are listed in Table XV–1 in order to facilitate rapid reference. Dosage regimens, which are often complex, are discussed under the individual drugs.

Mechanistic classification of these agents is increasingly important, particularly as investigators attempt to utilize this information to design "rational" regimens for chemotherapy. A simplified overview of the sites of action of many of the drugs described in Chapter 62 is shown in Figure XV–1.

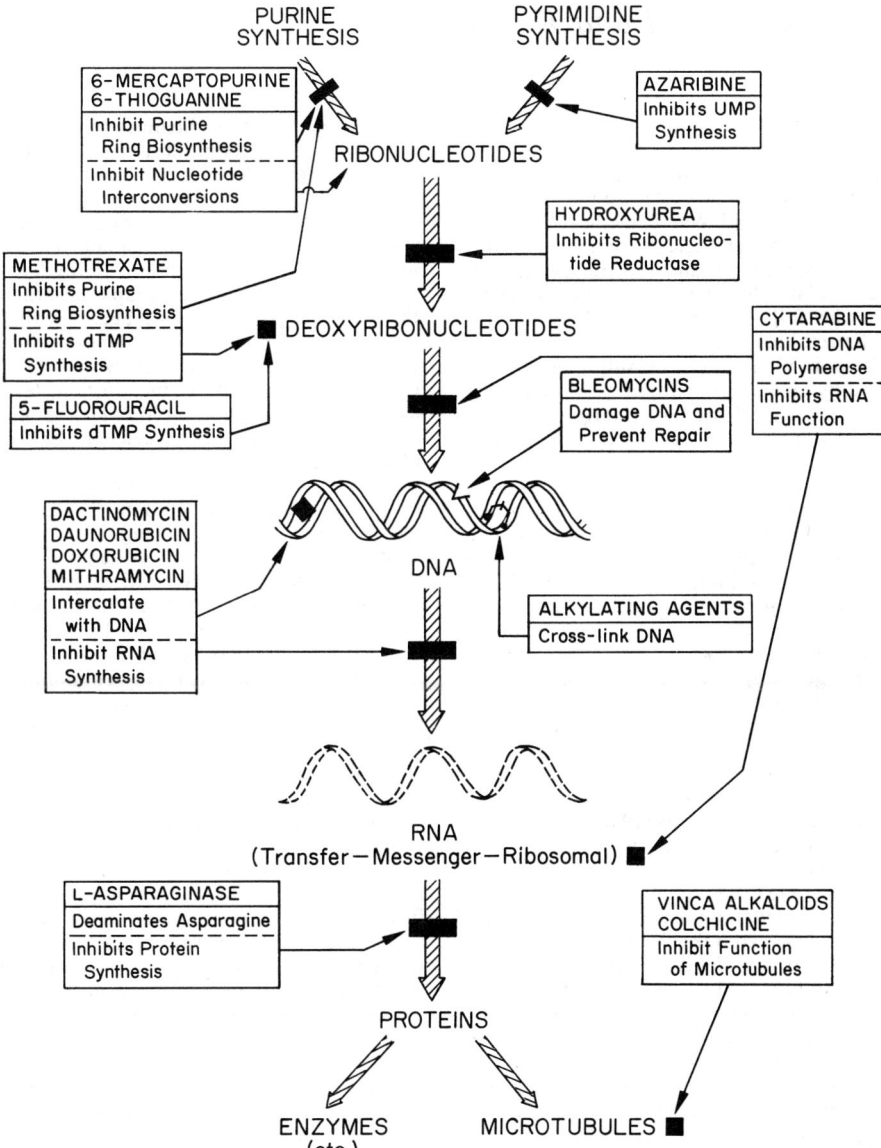

Figure XV–1. *Summary of the mechanisms and sites of action of chemotherapeutic agents useful in neoplastic disease.*

62 ALKYLATING AGENTS, ANTIMETABOLITES, HORMONES, AND OTHER ANTIPROLIFERATIVE AGENTS

Paul Calabresi and Robert E. Parks, Jr.

I. Alkylating Agents

History. Although synthesized in 1854, the vesicant properties of *sulfur mustard* were not described until 1887. During World War I, medical attention was first focused on the vesicant action of sulfur mustard on the skin, eyes, and respiratory tract. It was appreciated later, however, that serious systemic intoxication also follows exposure. In 1919, Krumbhaar and Krumbhaar made the pertinent observation that the poisoning caused by sulfur mustard is characterized by leukopenia and, in cases that came to autopsy, by aplasia of the bone marrow, dissolution of lymphoid tissue, and ulceration of the gastrointestinal tract.

In the interval between World Wars I and II, extensive studies of the biological and chemical actions of the *nitrogen mustards* were conducted. The marked cytotoxic action on lymphoid tissue prompted Gilman, Goodman, and T. F. Dougherty to study the effect of nitrogen mustards on transplanted lymphosarcoma in mice, and in 1942 clinical studies were initiated. This launched the era of modern cancer chemotherapy (Gilman, 1963).

In their early phases, all these investigations were conducted under secrecy restrictions imposed by the use of classified chemical-warfare agents. At the termination of World War II, the nitrogen mustards were declassified and a general review was presented by Gilman and Philips (1946), and shortly thereafter there appeared summaries of clinical research by Goodman and associates (1946), Jacobson and coworkers (1946), and Rhoads (1946). Many reviews have been written on these agents (*see* previous editions of this textbook). More recent discussions include those by Wheeler (1973), Connors (1974, 1975), Ludlum (1975), and Ross (1975).

Thousands of variants of the basic chemical structure of the nitrogen mustards have been prepared. Unfortunately, all attempts at the rational design of "active-site-directed" molecules have failed, and only a few of these agents have proven more useful than the original compound in specific clinical circumstances (*see* below). At the present time five major types of alkylating agents are used in the chemotherapy of neoplastic diseases: (1) the nitrogen mustards, (2) the ethylenimines, (3) the alkyl sulfonates, (4) the nitrosoureas, and (5) the triazenes.

Chemistry. The chemotherapeutic alkylating agents have in common the property of undergoing strongly electrophilic chemical reactions through the formation of carbonium ion intermediates or of transition complexes with the target molecules. These reactions result in the formation of covalent linkages (alkylation) with various nucleophilic substances, including such biologically important moieties as phosphate, amino, sulfhydryl, hydroxyl, carboxyl, and imidazole groups. Several studies on the interaction of alkylating agents with DNA suggest that the key biological compound alkylated is the purine base, guanine, in which the 7 nitrogen is strongly nucleophilic. In addition, less extensive alkylation may occur on the 1 or 3 nitrogens of adenine, the 3 nitrogen of cytosine, or the 6 oxygen of guanine.

The possible consequences of the reaction of nitrogen mustard with guanine residues in DNA chains are illustrated in Figure 62–1. First, one 2-chloroethyl side chain undergoes a first-order (S_N1) intramolecular cyclization, with release of a chloride ion and formation of a highly reactive ethylenimonium intermediate. By this reaction the tertiary amine is converted to a quaternary ammonium compound. The ethylenimonium intermediates can react avidly, through carbonium ion or transition complex intermediate formation, with a large number of inorganic ions and organic radicals by reactions that resemble a second-order (S_N2) nucleophilic substitution reaction (Price, 1975). Alkylation of the 7 nitrogen of guanine residues in DNA, a highly favored reaction, may exert several effects of considerable biological importance, as illustrated in Figure 62–1. Normally, guanine residues in DNA exist predominantly as the keto tautomers and readily make Watson-Crick base pairs by hydrogen bonding with cytosine residues. However, when the 7 nitrogen of guanine is alkylated (to become a quaternary ammonium nitrogen), the guanine residue is more acidic and the enol tautomer is favored. Guanine in this form can make base pairs with thymine residues, thus leading to possible miscoding and the ultimate substitution of an adenine-thymine base pair for a guanine-cytosine base pair. Second, alkylation of the 7 nitrogen labilizes the imidazole ring, making possible the opening of the imidazole ring or depurination by excision of guanine residues, either of which can result in serious damage to the DNA molecule (Shapiro, 1968). Third, with bifunctional alkylators, such as nitrogen mustard, the second 2-chloroethyl side chain can undergo a similar cyclization reaction and alkylate a second guanine residue or another nucleophilic moiety, such as an amino group or a sulfhydryl radical of a protein. This can result in the cross-linking of two nucleic acid chains or the linking of a nucleic acid to a protein by very strong covalent bonds, reactions that would cause a major disruption in nucleic acid function. Any of these effects could adequately explain both the mutagenic and the cytotoxic effects of alkylating agents.

It must be recognized that, in addition to the formation of covalent bonds with guanine residues, a wide variety of other chemical reactions are possible that can result in a number of other important effects on cellular function and viability.

The nitrogen mustards are all regarded as chemically unstable but vary greatly in their degree of instability. Therefore, the specific chemical properties of each member of this class of drugs must be considered individually in therapeutic applications. For example, *mechlorethamine* is so hygroscopic and highly unstable in aqueous form that it is marketed as the dry crystals of the hydrochloride. Solutions are prepared immediately prior to injection and, within a few minutes after administration, mechlorethamine has reacted almost completely within the body. On the other hand, agents such as *chlorambucil* are sufficiently stable to permit oral administration, and *cyclophosphamide,* which is relatively less reactive than mechlorethamine, requires biochemical activation by the cytochrome P-450 system of the liver in order to achieve chemotherapeutic effectiveness.

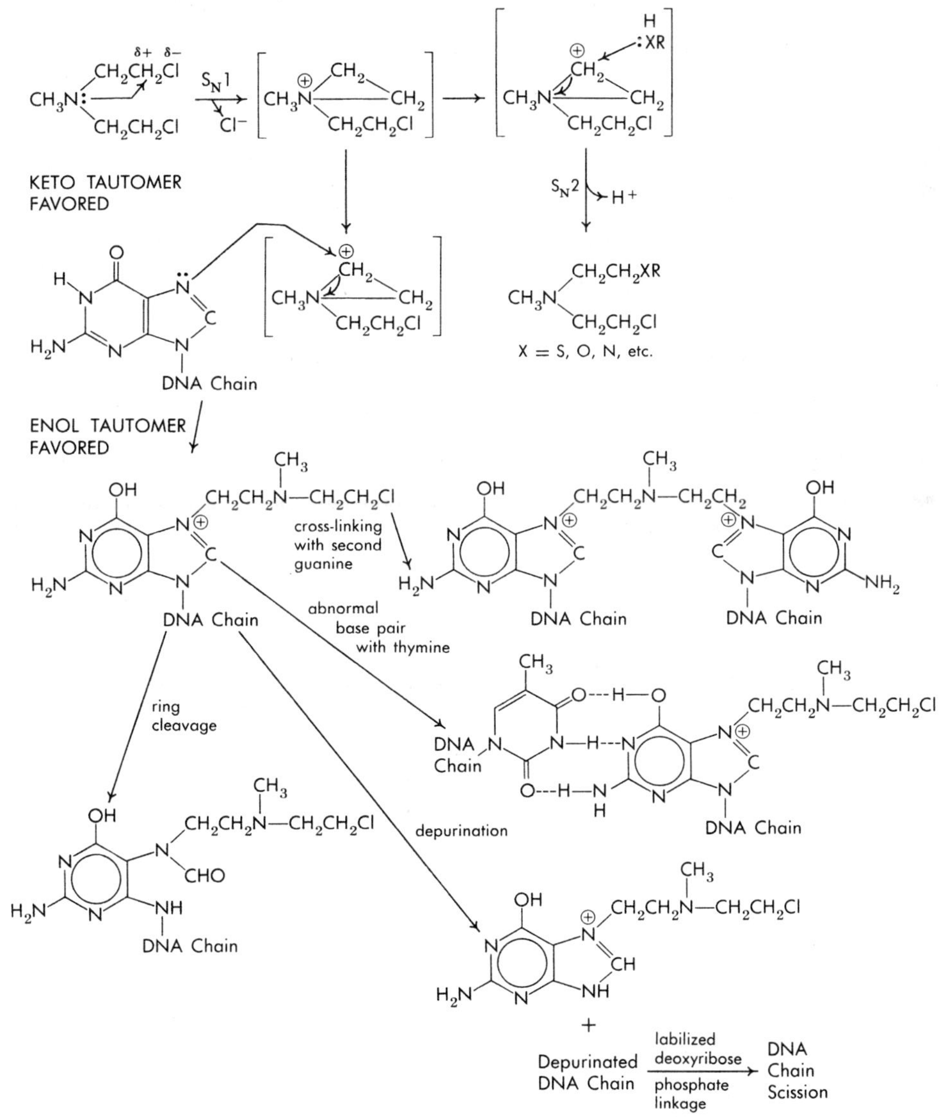

Figure 62-1. *Mechanism of action of alkylating agents.*

The ethylenimine derivatives react by an S_N2 reaction; however, since the opening of the ethylenimine ring is acid catalyzed, they are more reactive at acidic pH. With respect to *busulfan* and certain related compounds used experimentally, "sulfur stripping," a reaction between the compound and sulfhydryl groups, may occur with elimination of the sulfur of the latter (Parham and Wilbur, 1961). Busulfan is an atypical alkylating agent with unusual biological properties that differ significantly from substituted nitrogen mustards and ethylenimines (Fox, 1975).

Structure-Activity Relationship. The alkylating agents used in chemotherapy encompass a diverse group of chemicals that have in common the capacity to contribute, under physiological conditions, alkyl groups to biologically vital macromolecules such as DNA. In most instances, physical and chemical parameters, such as lipophilicity, ability to cross biological membranes, acid dissociation constants, stability in aqueous solution, and so forth, rather than similarity to cellular constituents, have proven crucial to biological activity. With several of the most valuable agents, for example, cyclophosphamide and the nitrosoureas, the active alkylating moieties are generated *in vivo* following complex degradative reactions, some of which are enzymatic. Since many of these physicochemical factors and activation reactions are still poorly understood, most of the agents in use today were discovered by empirical rather than by rational approaches. In most instances where clinically useful agents were uncovered by presumably "rational" methods, it was later learned that the original premises were defective, and the biological usefulness resulted from factors not considered in the original design. Therefore, much more information must become available before the structure-activity relationship of the alkylating agents is fully understood and applied.

The nitrogen mustards may be regarded as nitrogen analogs of sulfur mustard. The biological activity of both types of compounds is based upon the presence of the *bis*-(2-chloroethyl) grouping. In sulfur mustard, the two reactive groups are attached to bivalent sulfur; since nitrogen is trivalent, a third substituent must be present on the nitrogen atom. Although a very large number of alkylating agents have been synthesized and evaluated, the methyl derivative, *mechlorethamine,* has received wide clinical use and has been accepted generally as a standard of reference. Various structural modifications have been made in order to achieve greater selectivity and, therefore, less toxicity. *Bis*-(2-chloroethyl) groups have been linked to (1) amino acids (phenylalanine, glycine, DL-alanine); (2) substituted phenyl groups (aminophenyl butyric acid, as in *chlorambucil*); (3) pyrimidine bases (uracil); (4) benzimidazole; (5) antimalarial agents; (6) sugars (mannitol); and (7) several other substances, including a cyclic phosphamide ester. Although none of these modifications has achieved the goal of producing a highly selective and general cytotoxic action for malignant cells, some of the compounds exhibit notable differences in their secondary pharmacological properties and have attracted much clinical, as well as theoretical, interest. For example, L-phenylalanine mustard (L-PAM) has been reported to be an effective adjuvant to mastectomy in the management of premenopausal patients with primary breast cancer (*see* Fisher *et al.,* 1975).

The structural formulas of some of the more commonly used nitrogen mustards are shown in Table 62-1.

There is no definite evidence that the use of special prosthetic groups, such as phenylalanine, a precursor of melanin, conveys unusual selectivity of action on malignant melanoma. The addition of substituted phenyl groups has produced a series of derivatives that retain the ability to react by an S_N1 mechanism; however, the electron-withdrawing capacity of the aromatic ring greatly reduces the rate of carbonium ion formation, and these compounds can therefore reach distant sites in the body before reacting with components of blood and other tissues. Chlorambucil is the most successful example of such aromatic mustards. It should be emphasized, nevertheless, that

Table 62-1. NITROGEN MUSTARDS EMPLOYED IN THERAPY

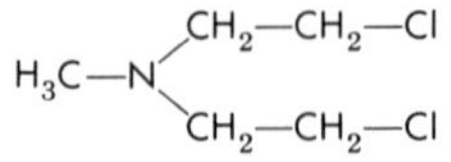

Mechlorethamine

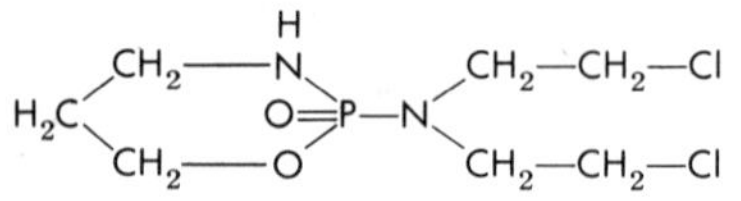

Cyclophosphamide

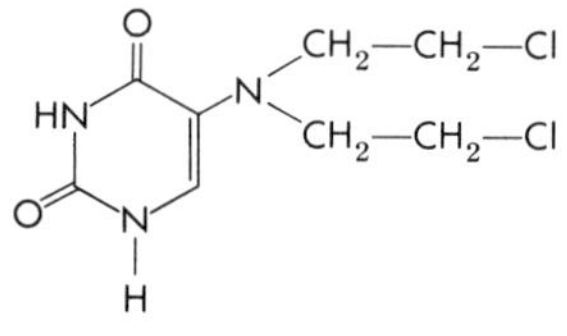

Uracil Mustard

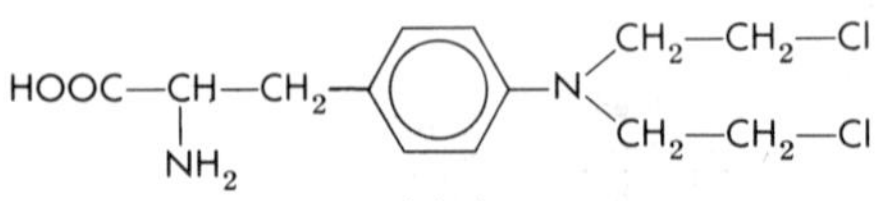

Melphalan

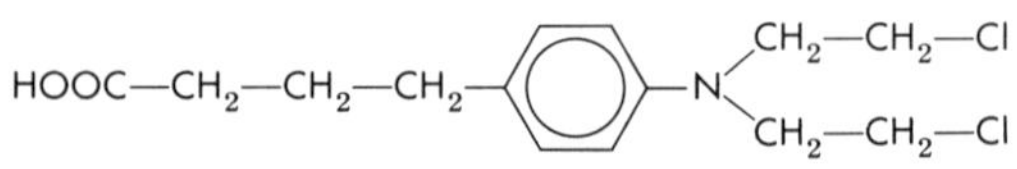

Chlorambucil

these molecular modifications of mechlorethamine have not altered its general spectrum of action; however, by reducing the high reactivity characteristic of the parent compound, the derivatives may be administered orally and are safer and more convenient in the treatment of chronic malignancies of the lymphocytic or plasma-cell series, particularly in the presence of extensive infiltration of the bone marrow.

A classical example of the role of the host metabolism in the activation of an alkylating agent is seen with *cyclophosphamide*—now the most widely used agent of this class. The original rationale that guided design of this molecule was twofold. First, if a cyclic phosphamide group replaced the N-methyl of mechlorethamine, the compound might be relatively inert, presumably because the *bis*-(2-chloroethyl) group of the molecule could not ionize until the cyclic phosphamide was cleaved at the phosphorus-nitrogen linkage. Second, it was hoped that neoplastic tissues might possess high phosphatase or phosphamidase activity capable of accomplishing this cleavage, thus resulting in the selective production of an activated nitrogen mustard in the malignant cells. In accord with these predictions, cyclophosphamide displays only weak cytotoxic, mutagenic, or alkylating activity and is relatively stable in aqueous solution. However, when administered to experimental animals or patients bearing susceptible tumors, marked chemotherapeutic effects, as well as mutagenicity and carcinogenicity, are seen. Although a definite role for phosphatases or phosphamidases in the mechanism of action of cyclophosphamide has not yet been demonstrated, it is clearly established that the drug initially undergoes metabolic activation by the cytochrome P-450 mixed-function oxidase system of the liver, with subsequent transport of the activated intermediate to sites of action, as discussed below. Thus, a crucial factor in the structure-activity relationship of cyclophosphamide concerns its capacity to undergo metabolic activation in the liver, rather than to alkylate malignant cells directly. It also appears that the selectivity of cyclophosphamide against certain malignant tissues may result in part from the capacity of normal tissues, such as liver, to protect themselves against cytotoxicity by further degrading the activated intermediates.

Although initially considered as an antimetabolite, the triazene derivative 5-(3,3-dimethyl-1-triazeno)-imidazole-4-carboxamide, usually referred to as *dacarbazine* or DTIC, is now known to function through alkylation. Its structural formula is as follows:

Dacarbazine

This compound bears a striking resemblance to the known metabolite 5-aminoimidazole-4-carboxamide (AIC), which is capable of conversion to inosinic acid by enzymes of purine synthesis. Thus, it was suspected that dacarbazine acts by inhibiting purine metabolism and nucleic acid synthesis. This resemblance to AIC may be fortuitous, since, for chemotherapeutic effectiveness, dacarbazine requires initial activation by the cytochrome P-450 system of the liver through an N-demethylation reaction. In the target cell, there then occurs a spontaneous cleavage liberating AIC and an alkylating moiety, presumably diazomethane (Oliverio, 1973a).

Although the mechanism of action is not yet fully established, it is generally assumed that the *nitrosoureas,* which include compounds such as 1,3-*bis*-(2-chloroethyl)-1-nitrosourea (carmustine, BCNU), 1-(2-chloroethyl)-3-cyclohexyl-1-nitrosourea (lomustine, CCNU), and its methyl derivative (semustine, methyl-CCNU), as well as the antibiotic *streptozotocin,* exert their cytotoxicity through the liberation of alkylating moieties. Their structural formulas are as follows:

Carmustine (BCNU)

Lomustine (CCNU)

Semustine (Methyl-CCNU)

These compounds have shown unusually high activity against a broad spectrum of experimental tumors. In addition, they are of special interest because, in contrast to many other antineoplastic agents, they are highly lipid soluble and can cross the blood-brain barrier readily. It has been proposed that nitrosoureas are degraded in aqueous media to generate the vinyl carbonium ion, which has high reactivity with nucleophilic centers (Wheeler, 1973). An unusual manifestation of tissue specificity is observed with the glucosamine derivative of nitrosourea, streptozotocin, which is diabetogenic because of its unique cytotoxicity for the beta cells of the pancreatic islets.

Since the formation of the ethylenimonium ion constitutes the initial reaction of the nitrogen mustards, screening programs have been devised to discover useful ethylenimine derivatives. These studies have yielded several active compounds, including triethylenemelamine (TEM), triethylenephosphoramide (TEPA), and triethylene*thio*phosphoramide (thio-TEPA), a more stable sulfur-containing derivative. Their structural formulas are as follows:

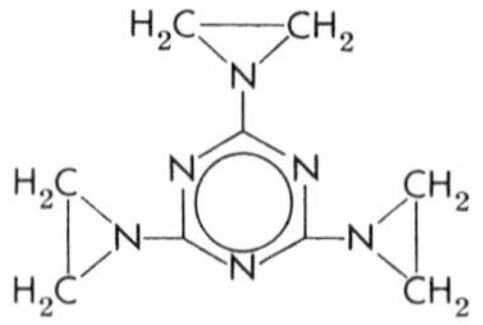

Triethylenemelamine (TEM)

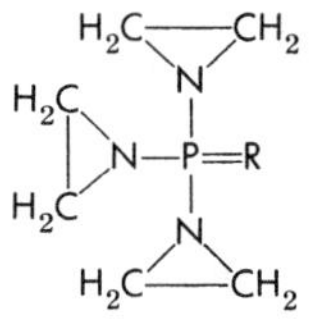

Triethylenephosphoramide (TEPA): R = O
Triethylene*thio*phosphoramide (Thio-TEPA): R = S

While these compounds have cytotoxic activity, they possess no particular advantage. More information on their pharmacological properties may be found in earlier editions of this textbook.

From a large group of esters of alkanesulfonic acids, synthesized as alkylating agents for chemotherapy of neoplastic disease, several interesting compounds have emerged; one of these, busulfan, is of great value in the treatment of chronic granulocytic leukemia; its structural formula is as follows:

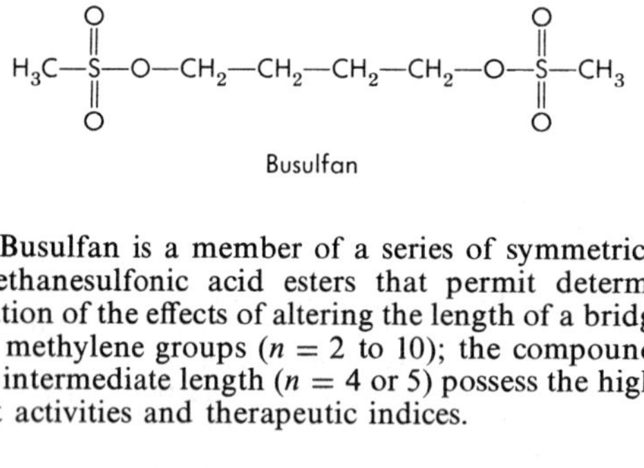

Busulfan

Busulfan is a member of a series of symmetrical methanesulfonic acid esters that permit determination of the effects of altering the length of a bridge of methylene groups ($n = 2$ to 10); the compounds of intermediate length ($n = 4$ or 5) possess the highest activities and therapeutic indices.

PHARMACOLOGICAL ACTIONS

The pharmacological actions of the various groups of alkylating agents are considered together in the following discussion. Although there are many similarities, there are, of course, some notable differences. Primary consideration will be given to the cytotoxic actions that follow the administration of a sublethal dose.

Cytotoxic Actions. The most important pharmacological actions of the alkylating agents are those that disturb the funda-

mental mechanisms concerned with cell growth, mitotic activity, differentiation, and function. The ability of these drugs to interfere with normal mitosis and cell division in all rapidly proliferating tissues provides the basis for their therapeutic applications and for many of their toxic properties. Whereas certain alkylating agents may have damaging effects on tissues with normally low mitotic indices, for example, liver, kidney, and mature lymphocytes, they are most cytotoxic to rapidly proliferating tissues in which a large proportion of the cells are in division. These compounds may readily alkylate nondividing cells, but cytotoxicity is seen only if such cells are stimulated to divide. Thus, the process of alkylation itself may be a relatively nontoxic event, as long as the DNA repair enzymes can correct the lesions in DNA prior to the next cellular division.

In contrast to many other antineoplastic agents, the alkylating drugs, although proliferation dependent, are not cell-cycle specific and may act on cells at any stage of the cycle. However, the toxicity is usually expressed when the cell enters the S phase and progression through the cycle is blocked at the G_2 (premitotic) phase (*see* Wheeler, 1967). While not strictly cell-cycle specific, quantitative differences may be detected when nitrogen mustards are applied to synchronized cells at different phases of the cycle. Cells appear more sensitive in late G_1 or S than in G_2, mitosis, or early G_1. Polynucleotides are more susceptible to alkylation in the unpaired state than in the helical form. During replication of DNA, portions of the molecule are so unpaired.

The cells accumulating behind the block at G_2 may have a double complement of DNA while continuing to synthesize other cellular components, such as protein and RNA. This can result in unbalanced growth, with the formation of enlarged or giant cells that can continue to synthesize DNA, making as much as four or five times the normal complement. Lethal cytotoxic action may occur by so-called interphase death and mitotic death; on the other hand, relatively undifferentiated cells of mammalian germinal tissues may remain nonproliferative during exposure and later undergo nuclear and cytoplasmic hypertrophy, differentiating without further mitosis into more adult cell types. Interphase death is generally regarded as the result of damage to many cellular sites. Nevertheless, this may not be the case; certainly it occurs without any evidence of mitotic activity. For a comprehensive review of the cytotoxic and biochemical effects of alkylating agents, *see* Connors (1975).

Biochemical Actions. An enormous literature deals with the effects of alkylating agents on a wide variety of cellular functions (*see* Ochoa and Hirschberg, 1967). In addition to cytolytic, mutagenic, carcinogenic, and teratogenic effects, they may inhibit glycolysis, respiration, the activity of various enzymes, protein synthesis, and nucleic acid synthesis and function. Thus, one must exert caution in designating any single biochemical event as the cause of all cellular toxicity. However, the great preponderance of evidence now indicates that the primary target of pharmacological doses of alkylating agents is the DNA molecule, as illustrated in Figure 62–1. A crucial distinction that must be emphasized is between the bifunctional agents, in which cytotoxic effects predominate, and the monofunctional agents, which have much greater capacity for mutagenesis and carcinogenesis. This suggests that biochemical events such as the cross-linking of DNA strands, only possible with bifunctional agents, represent a much greater threat to cellular survival than do other effects, such as depurination and chain scission. On the other hand, the latter reactions may cause permanent modifications in DNA structure that are compatible with continued life of the cell and transmissible to subsequent generations; such modifications may result in mutagenesis or carcinogenesis. (*See* Ludlum, 1975.)

The remarkable DNA repair systems found in most cells appear to play a key, if not determining, role in the relative resistance of nonproliferating tissues, the selectivity of action against particular cell types, and acquired resistance to alkylating agents. While alkylation of a single strand of DNA may often be repaired with relative ease, interstrand cross-linkages, such as those produced by the bifunctional alkylating agents, are more difficult to repair and involve more complex mechanisms. Many of the cross-links formed in DNA by these agents at low doses may also be corrected; higher doses cause extensive cross-linkage, and DNA breakdown occurs.

Because of the similarity between the biological effects of alkylation and those of ionizing radiation, alkylating drugs have often been referred to as "radiomimetic" agents. It is generally agreed that this terminology is no longer justified. Since the fundamental biological effects of both ionizing radiation and alkylating agents involve damage to the DNA molecule, with subsequent attempts at correction by the DNA repair enzymes, it is not surprising that a number of similarities in the biological effects are seen.

Mechanisms of Resistance to Alkylating Agents. Acquired resistance to alkylating agents is a common event, and the acquisition of resistance to one alkylating agent usually imparts cross-resistance to other alkylators. While definitive information on the biochemical mechanisms of resistance is lacking, several biochemical mechanisms have been implicated in the development of such resistance by tumor cells. In contrast to the development of resistance to antimetabolites, where single-step mutations can result in almost complete resistance to drug effects, the acquisition of resistance to alkylating agents is usually a slower process, not resulting from single biochemical changes. Resistance of this type may represent the summation of a series of biochemical changes, none of which by itself can confer significant resistance. Among the biochemical changes identified in cells resistant to alkylating agents are

decreased permeability to the drugs and increased production of nucleophilic substances that can compete with the target DNA for alkylation. For example, the administration of cysteine can considerably reduce the antitumor effects of alkylating agents, and there are several examples of animal tumors with acquired resistance that have greater concentrations of free thiol groups than do the sensitive tumor lines from which they were derived. There has been much speculation about the possibility that increased activity of the DNA repair system may permit cells to acquire resistance to alkylating agents. (*See* Connors, 1974.)

Hematological and Immunosuppressive Actions. The hematopoietic system is very susceptible to the effects of alkylating agents. Within 6 to 8 hours after administration of a sublethal dose of a nitrogen mustard, cessation of mitosis and disintegration of formed elements may be evident in the marrow and lymphoid tissues of experimental animals. Lymphocytes appear to be more sensitive to the destructive action of the mustards and relatively resistant to the effects of busulfan, an action that is considered responsible for the immunosuppressive effects observed with the former group, particularly cyclophosphamide. Busulfan seems to be more toxic to granulocytes, and it has been shown that suitable combinations of busulfan and chlorambucil, an aromatic mustard, can simulate closely the hematological effects of whole-body x-radiation. The effects of chlorambucil are followed by rapid recovery, except in lymphoid organs, whereas depression of hematopoiesis after busulfan occurs gradually and is more prolonged. In patients treated with mechlorethamine, lymphocytopenia is usually apparent within 24 hours and becomes progressively more severe for 6 to 8 days; within a few days, granulocytopenia becomes evident and lasts for 10 days to 3 weeks. Variable degrees of depression of platelet and erythrocyte counts may occur during the second or third week after therapy; with ensuing regeneration, hematological recovery is complete at the end of 4 to 6 weeks and rebound hyperplasia may be present from the fifth to the seventh week.

Actions on Reproductive Tissues. In women, amenorrhea of several months' duration sometimes follows a course of therapy with alkylating agents. Impairment of spermatogenesis has been noted both in patients and in experimental animals. Interesting differences and similarities have been found between the effects of these agents and x-rays on the stages of spermatogenesis in rodents. Busulfan mimics most closely the effects of radiation by acting on an early stage of spermatogenesis; this results, after 8 weeks, in a systematic sequential depletion of spermatogonia, spermatocytes, spermatids, and spermatozoa. Triethylenemelamine and the aliphatic mustards affect later stages and produce infertility within 4 weeks. On the other hand, cytotoxic doses of phenylalanine mustard and chlorambucil do not interfere with the fertility of male rats (*see* Jackson, 1959).

Actions on Other Epithelial Tissues. The intestinal mucosa can be damaged by the parenteral administration of minimal lethal doses of a nitrogen mustard in experimental animals; mitotic arrest, cellular hypertrophy, pyknosis, disintegration, and desquamation of the epithelium are evident. Damage to the hair follicles is much more pronounced with cyclophosphamide than with other mustards and frequently results in alopecia; this effect is usually reversible, even with continued therapy. An interesting potential commercial application of this finding involves the administration of this drug to sheep in order to facilitate the harvesting of wool.

Sulfur mustard and the nitrogen mustards are powerful local vesicants. Either direct contact with the compounds or exposure to vapors can lead to serious local reactions. The susceptible tissues are skin, eyes, and respiratory tract. The mustards are not escharotic *per se;* rather, the onset of action is delayed for many hours and the mechanism of tissue injury presumably involves the reaction of their transformation products with essential components of the cell. The vesicant properties of the nitrogen mustards are of concern to the clinician in that local reactions can occur if certain precautions are not observed during the course of administration (*see* below).

Actions on the Nervous System. All nitrogen mustards are powerful stimulants of the central nervous system (CNS). Nausea and vomiting are prominent side effects, particularly of mechlorethamine, and are presumably the result of CNS stimulation. Convulsions, progressive muscular paralysis, and various cholinomimetic effects have been observed. These effects and a poorly understood "delayed-death" syndrome reported in animals indicate that the cytotoxicity of the alkylating agents extends to cellular functions unrelated to proliferative activity. More detailed descriptions and references appear in earlier editions of this textbook.

NITROGEN MUSTARDS

The chemistry and the pharmacological actions of the alkylating agents as a group, and of the nitrogen mustards, have been presented above. Only the unique pharmacological characteristics of the individual agents are considered below.

MECHLORETHAMINE

Mechlorethamine was the first of the nitrogen mustards to be introduced into clinical medicine and is the most rapidly acting of the drugs in this class.

Chemistry. The chemical structure of mechlorethamine has been presented above (*see* Table 62–1).

Absorption, Fate, and Excretion. Mechlorethamine can be absorbed from either the alimentary tract or parenteral sites of administration, but severe local reactions of exposed tissues necessitate intravenous injection for clinical use. In either water or body fluids, at rates affected markedly by pH, mechlorethamine rapidly undergoes chemical transformation and combines with either water or reactive compounds of cells, so that the drug is no longer present in active form after a few minutes. Indeed, it is possible to protect a given tissue from the effects of the agent by the simple expedient of interrupting the blood supply to the area for a few minutes during and immediately after injection of the drug. Conversely, it is possible, but not always feasible, to localize the action of mechlorethamine or related agents to a large extent in a given tissue by injecting the drug into the arterial blood stream supplying that tissue. Less than 0.01% of the drug can be recovered in the urine, since it is altered so rapidly that there is no opportunity for excretion.

Preparations, Dosage, and Routes of Administration. *Mechlorethamine Hydrochloride for Injection,* U.S.P. (MUSTARGEN), is supplied in rubber-stoppered vials containing 10 mg of mechlorethamine hydrochloride triturated with 90 mg of anhydrous sodium chloride. The solution for injection must be freshly prepared before each administration by adding 10 ml of sterile distilled water to the contents of the vial by means of a syringe and needle, with the use of surgical gloves for protection of the hands. The contents of the vial are dissolved while the needle is still in the rubber stopper, and the required volume of solution is then withdrawn and injected immediately. The solution should be injected into the tubing of a rapidly flowing intravenous infusion; this not only reduces the possibility of extravasation of the drug but also lowers the concentration of vesicant that comes in contact with the intima of the vein. The exact rate of injection is relatively unimportant, provided it is completed within a few minutes. In patients who have elevated venous pressure in the antebrachial veins because of compression of the great veins by mediastinal tumors, it is advisable to administer the drug through an indwelling catheter inserted into the femoral vein.

A course of therapy with mechlorethamine consists in the injection of a total dose of 0.4 mg/kg of body weight or 10 mg/sq m. Although this total dose may be given in either two or four daily consecutive injections, a single administration is preferable; the therapeutic response is equal, and the patient is spared an additional 2 or 3 days of anorexia, nausea, and vomiting. The recommended total dosage to be given during a single course should be exceeded only by those who are completely familiar with the use of the drug. Patients without compromised bone-marrow function sometimes can tolerate a total of 0.6 or even 0.8 mg/kg, but dangerous degrees of leukopenia and thrombocytopenia are to be expected if doses of this magnitude are employed. In the presence of extensive infiltration of bone marrow by neoplastic cells, as is often the case in lymphocytic lymphosarcoma, it is wise to reduce the dose to 0.3 or even 0.2 mg/kg, at least for the first course of therapy.

A course of mechlorethamine may be repeated only after bone-marrow function has recovered. This is best ascertained by study of the peripheral blood or by evaluation of bone-marrow granulocyte reserve. Usually at least 6 weeks should elapse between courses of this agent, although other types of mustard therapy may intervene, as discussed below.

Direct intracavitary administration of the drug (0.2 to 0.4 mg/kg) for malignant effusions, particularly of pleural origin, provides valuable palliation.

Therapeutic Uses and Clinical Toxicity. The beneficial results of mechlorethamine in *Hodgkin's disease* and, less predictably, in other *lymphomas* have been extensively confirmed. Although the drug has been effective alone, current practice favors its use in combination with other agents. In generalized Hodgkin's disease (stages III and IV), the so-called MOPP regimen (the combination of mechlorethamine, vincristine (ONCOVIN), procarbazine, and prednisone) is considered the treatment of choice (DeVita *et al.*, 1972). Mechlorethamine-induced remissions in Hodgkin's disease may also be prolonged by the use of chlorambucil, orally in maintenance doses.

In patients with generalized *mycosis fungoides*, very dilute solutions (0.25%) of mechlorethamine may be painted on the involved cutaneous areas with marked beneficial results.

In the treatment of leukemias and related myeloproliferative disorders, mechlorethamine has been superseded by other agents. Although palliative results have been observed in carcinomas of the bronchus, ovary, breast, and other solid tumors, alkylating agents of intermediate or slower reactivity are preferable. (*See* Table XV–1, page 1250, and discussion under individual agents; *see also* Calabresi and Welch, 1962; Brodsky and Kahn, 1972; Holland and Frei, 1973.)

Since the cytotoxic action that is the basis for therapy extends to normal cells, particularly those of the hematopoietic system, mechlorethamine has a low therapeutic index. The safe use of the drug requires an intimate knowledge of its potential toxic effects.

Emesis usually stops within 8 hours after administration of mechlorethamine, but nausea and anorexia may persist for 24 hours. The most effective method of preventing nausea and vomiting is the use of large doses (300 to 400 mg) of a relatively short-acting barbiturate, together with 10 to 20 mg of prochlorperazine, at the time of injection of mechlorethamine. It is customary to administer the mustard at night; thereby the normal sleep pattern is not disturbed.

Of more concern is the *depression of bone-marrow function* and the resulting leukopenia and thrombocytopenia that accompany nitrogen mustard therapy. These have already been described and constitute the major limitation on the amount of drug that can be given in a single course. Rarely, hemorrhagic complications of nitrogen mustard therapy may be due to hyperheparinemia; in such a circumstance, specific therapy with protamine corrects the hemorrhagic diathesis (Chapter 65).

On rare occasions, a maculopapular *skin eruption* may follow therapy with mechlorethamine. The reaction apparently is not one of the hypersensitivity type, does not necessarily recur with subsequent administration of the drug, and does not provide a contraindication to further therapy. *Herpes zoster* is another type of skin lesion frequently associated with nitrogen mustard therapy. Apparently a latent viral infection is not uncommonly present in patients with malignant lymphoma, and therapy with either a nitrogen mustard or radiation may be followed by overt manifestations of the viral disease.

Women should be warned that *menstrual irregularities* may be produced by mechlorethamine, and, since *fetal abnormalities* have been induced in experimental animals, the drug should not be used if pregnancy exists or is suspected. After a course of therapy, catamenia may be delayed or several consecutive menstrual periods may be missed. The effect is presumably the result of arrest of maturation of the Graafian follicles, but there appears to be no permanent damage to ovarian function.

Local Reactions. Local reactions to extravasation of mechlorethamine into the subcutaneous tissue result in a severe, brawny, tender induration that may persist for a long time. If the local reaction is unusually severe, a slough may result. If it is obvious that extravasation has occurred, the involved area should be promptly infiltrated with an isotonic solution of sodium thiosulfate (⅙ M); an ice compress then should be applied intermittently for 6 to 12 hours. The purpose of the thiosulfate is to provide an ion that reacts avidly with the nitrogen mustard and thereby protects tissue constituents. If thiosulfate solution is not available, prompt injections of isotonic sodium chloride solution may have some value by reducing the local concentration of the vesicant agent.

Thrombophlebitis is a potential complication of therapy with mechlorethamine. It rarely occurs if the drug is injected into the tubing during the course of an intravenous infusion.

CYCLOPHOSPHAMIDE

Efforts to modify the chemical structure of mechlorethamine to achieve greater selectivity for neoplastic tissues led to the development of cyclophosphamide. After studies of the pharmacological activity of cyclophosphamide, clinical investigations by European workers demonstrated its effectiveness in selected malignant neoplasms. (For references to the original literature, *see* Calabresi and Welch, 1962; Fairley and Simister, 1965; Symposium, 1967.)

Chemistry. The chemical structure of cyclophosphamide and the interesting rationale that led to its synthesis have been presented above (*see* Table 62-1).

Pharmacological and Cytotoxic Actions. None of the severe acute CNS manifestations reported with the typical nitrogen mustards has been noted with cyclophosphamide. Nausea and vomiting, however, may occur. Although the general cytotoxic action of this drug is similar to that of other alkylating agents, some notable differences have been observed. When compared with mechlorethamine, damage to the megakaryocytes and thrombocytopenia are less common. Another unusual manifestation of selectivity consists in more prominent damage to the hair follicles, resulting frequently in alopecia. The drug is not a vesicant, and local irritation has not been reported.

Absorption, Fate, and Excretion. Cyclophosphamide is well absorbed orally. As mentioned above, the drug is activated by metabolism in the liver by the mixed-function oxidase system of the smooth endo-

plasmic reticulum (Brock, 1967); several toxic metabolites have been identified (Hill *et al.,* 1972a; Sladek, 1973; Connors, 1975). The current view of the metabolism and fate of cyclophosphamide is presented in Figure 62-2. The hepatic cytochrome P-450 mixed-function oxidase system converts cyclophosphamide to 4-hydroxycyclophosphamide, which is in equilibrium with the acyclic tautomer, aldophosphamide. These compounds may be oxidized further by hepatic aldehyde oxidase and perhaps by other enzymes, yielding the metabolites carboxyphosphamide and 4-ketocyclophosphamide, neither of which possesses significant biological activity. It appears that hepatic damage is minimized by these secondary reactions, whereas significant amounts of the activated metabolites, such as aldophosphamide, are transported to the target sites by the circulatory system. It has been proposed that, in cells that are susceptible to cytolysis, the aldophosphamide is cleaved by a β-elimination reaction, generating stoichiometric amounts of phosphoramide mustard and acrolein, both of which are highly cytotoxic (Connors, 1975).

If the cytochrome P-450 system is induced by pretreatment of an animal with phenobarbital or inhibited by administration of proadifen (SKF 525A), however, the antitumor activity and therapeutic index of cyclophosphamide are not significantly modified (Sladek, 1972). The explanation proposed for this unexpected finding illustrates several important pharmacological principles. Cyclophosphamide, which is biologically relatively inactive, is eliminated from the body very slowly. The activated metabolites (*e.g.,* aldophosphamide) alkylate the target sites in susceptible cells in an "all-or-none" type of reaction or are detoxified by formation of inactive metabolites that are rapidly excreted by the kidneys. The cytotoxic effects are related to the total amount rather than to the velocity of generation of the activated metabolites. Thus, it seems likely that the biological actions of cyclophosphamide may be affected more drastically by alterations in the rates of detoxication and elimination than by changes in the rate of generation of the activated metabolites.

Studies with ^{3}H-labeled cyclophosphamide in dogs and humans (Bolt *et al.,* 1961) showed that urinary recovery of unchanged drug was less than 14%, and fecal recovery after intravenous administration was negligible. Maximal plasma concentrations after oral administration were detected at about 1 hour; 31 to 66% of the total radioactivity

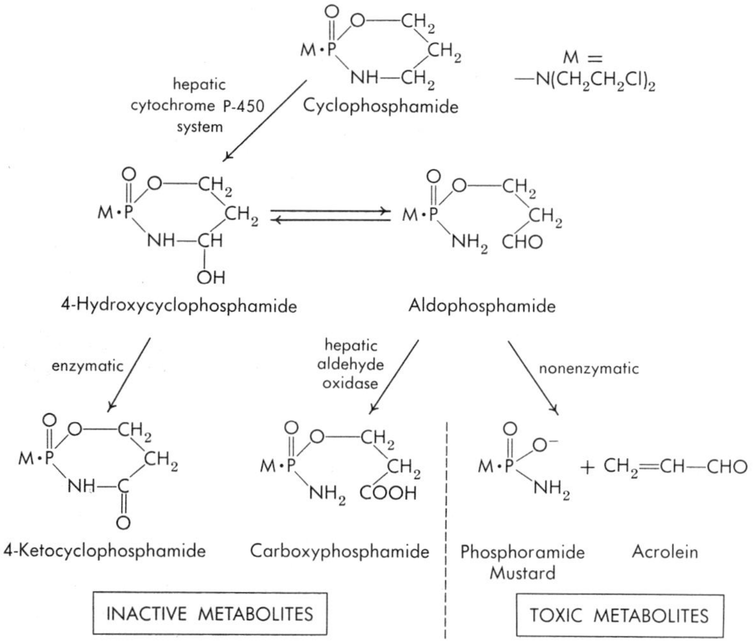

Figure 62–2. *Metabolism of cyclophosphamide.*

administered was recovered in the stools, and 17 to 31% was unchanged drug. After administration of ^{14}C-labeled drug in doses of 6 to 80 mg/kg intravenously, the plasma half-life was 6½ hours, and alkylating metabolites were 56% bound to plasma proteins (Bagley *et al.*, 1973). Prior treatment with allopurinol significantly prolongs the half-life of cyclophosphamide.

Preparations, Dosage, and Routes of Administration. *Cyclophosphamide*, U.S.P. (CYTOXAN, ENDOXAN), is supplied as 25- and 50-mg white tablets and as a powder (100, 200, or 500 mg) in sterile vials. Solutions are prepared by addition of 5 ml of sterile water per 100 mg of drug. Although prompt use is recommended, it is considered satisfactory to administer solutions within 3 hours after preparation.

The drug has been administered orally, intravenously, intramuscularly, intrapleurally, and intraperitoneally. A conservative daily dose of 2 to 3 mg/kg, orally or intravenously, has been recommended for patients with more susceptible neoplasms such as lymphomas and leukemias or with compromised bone-marrow function. A higher daily dosage of 4 to 8 mg/kg intravenously for 6 days, followed by an oral maintenance dose of 50 to 300 mg daily, 5 mg/kg intravenously twice weekly, or 10 to 15 mg/kg intravenously every 7 to 10 days, has been used for the treatment of carcinomas and more resistant neoplasms. Large single doses of 30 mg/kg or 750 to 1000 mg/sq m have been very effective in patients with lymphomas and cause a rapid response approaching that seen with mechlor-

ethamine; in patients without complications or previous therapy, the recommended total initial loading dose is 40 to 50 mg/kg, administered orally or intravenously over a period of 2 to 4 days. Careful evaluation of bone-marrow function is imperative, and prolonged therapy is guided by keeping the total leukocyte count between 2500 and 4000 cells per cubic millimeter of blood or by obtaining the desired response of the tumor.

Therapeutic Uses and Clinical Toxicity. The clinical spectrum of activity for cyclophosphamide is very similar to that of nitrogen mustard, and the initial good results observed in Hodgkin's disease and lymphosarcoma have been confirmed. Complete remissions and even presumed cures have been reported in Burkitt's lymphoma and in acute lymphoblastic leukemia of childhood when the drug is used concurrently with other agents (Zubrod, 1968; Livingston and Carter, 1970; Ziegler, 1972.)

Notable advantages of this drug are the availability of oral as well as parenteral routes of administration and the possibility of giving fractionated doses over prolonged periods of time. For these reasons it possesses a versatility of action that allows an intermediate range of use, between that of the highly reactive intravenous mechlorethamine and that of oral chlorambucil. Beneficial results have been obtained in multiple myeloma, chronic lymphocytic leukemia, and acute leukemia of children.

Complete remissions in lymphoblastic leukemia appear more likely to occur in patients who have responded previously to other agents. Temporary beneficial results also have been obtained in bronchogenic carcinoma, carcinoma of the breast, and ovarian malignancies, as well as in neuroblastoma and other neoplasms of childhood. (*See* Livingston and Carter, 1970; National Conference on Cancer Chemotherapy, 1972; Holland and Frei, 1973.)

Because of its potent *immunosuppressive* properties, cyclophosphamide has received considerable attention in recent years for the control of organ rejection after transplantation and in nonneoplastic disorders associated with altered immune reactivity, including Wegener's granulomatosis, rheumatoid arthritis, the nephrotic syndrome in children, and autoallergic ocular disease. Appropriate caution is advised when the drug is considered for use in these conditions, not only because of its acute toxic effects but also because of its high potential for inducing sterility, teratogenic effects, mutations, and cancer. (*See* Barratt and Soothill, 1970; Starzl *et al.,* 1971; Steinberg *et al.,* 1972; Kaplan and Calabresi, 1973; Gershwin *et al.,* 1974.)

The clinical toxicity of cyclophosphamide differs from that of other nitrogen mustards in that significant degrees of thrombocytopenia are much less common, but there is frequent occurrence of alopecia. Patients should be forewarned of this possible event, which is usually reversible even without interruption of therapy. Nausea and vomiting are common and occur with equal frequency whether the drug is given by the oral or the intravenous route. Mucosal ulcerations, dizziness of short duration, transverse ridging of the nails, increased skin pigmentation, interstitial pulmonary fibrosis, and hepatic toxicity have been reported. Extravasation of the drug into subcutaneous tissues does not produce local reactions, and thrombophlebitis has not complicated intravenous administration. The occurrence of sterile, hemorrhagic cystitis has been reported in 5 to 10% of patients. This has been attributed to chemical irritation produced by reactive derivatives of cyclophosphamide, and its incidence has been reduced in animals by bladder irrigation with a solution of acetylcysteine (Primack, 1971). For routine clinical use, ample fluid intake and frequent voiding are recommended. Administration of the drug should be interrupted at the first indication of dysuria or hematuria. The syndrome of inappropriate antidiuretic hormone (ADH) secretion has been observed in patients receiving cyclophosphamide, usually at doses higher than 50 mg/kg (DeFronzo *et al.,* 1973). It is important to be aware of the possibility of water intoxication, since these patients are usually vigorously hydrated.

MELPHALAN

This phenylalanine derivative of nitrogen mustard is also known as L-sarcolysin. Early clinical studies demonstrated a spectrum of activity similar to that of other alkylating agents.

Chemistry. The chemical structure and the rationale for the synthesis of this amino acid derivative of mechlorethamine have been presented above (*see* Table 62–1; *see also* Livingston and Carter, 1970; Greenwald, 1973; Wheeler, 1975).

Pharmacological and Cytotoxic Actions. The general pharmacological and cytotoxic actions of melphalan are similar to those of other nitrogen mustards. The drug is not a vesicant.

Absorption, Fate, and Excretion. Melphalan is well absorbed when given by the oral route and seems to be equally effective whether given by mouth or intravenously. The drug is said to remain active in the blood for approximately 6 hours.

Preparation, Dosage, and Route of Administration. *Melphalan,* U.S.P. (ALKERAN), is available in scored, 2-mg tablets. Although the general spectrum of action of melphalan seems to resemble that of other nitrogen mustards, the advantages of a gradual but continuous administration by the oral route have made the drug useful in the treatment of *multiple myeloma* (Bergsagel, 1972; George *et al.,* 1972). Beneficial effects have also been reported in malignant melanoma and in carcinoma of the breast and ovary. Its use as adjuvant therapy after surgery for breast cancer is currently under active study, with initial indications of promising results (Fisher, 1972). The usual oral dose is 6 mg daily for a period of 2 to 3 weeks, during which time the blood count should be carefully followed. A rest period of up to 4 weeks should then intervene. When the leukocyte and platelet counts are rising, maintenance therapy, ordinarily 2 to 4 mg daily, is begun. It is usually necessary to maintain a significant degree of bone-marrow depression (total leukocyte count in the range of 3000 to 3500 cells per cubic millimeter) in order to achieve optimal results.

Clinical Toxicity. The clinical toxicity of melphalan is mostly hematological and is similar to that of other alkylating agents. Nausea and vomiting are infrequent. Alopecia does not occur, and changes in renal or hepatic function have not been observed.

URACIL MUSTARD

Uracil mustard was synthesized in an unsuccessful attempt to produce an active-site-directed alkylator by linking the *bis*-(2-chloroethyl) group to the pyrimidine base uracil. Its activity in experimental neoplasms was demonstrated shortly thereafter. No relationship has been demonstrated, however, with the biological functions of uracil.

Chemistry. The structural formula of uracil mustard and its chemical relationship to other alkylating agents are presented above (*see* Table 62–1). It is a crystalline compound that is quite unstable in water.

Pharmacological and Cytotoxic Actions. Uracil mustard may cause nausea and vomiting. The drug is not a vesicant. Cytotoxicity characteristic of the nitrogen mustards has been observed in subacute and chronic toxicity studies of uracil mustard in animals.

Absorption, Fate, and Excretion. Uracil mustard is absorbed quickly but not completely after oral administration in dogs. Plasma concentrations after either oral (2 mg/kg) or intravenous (1 mg/kg) administration decline rapidly, and no evidence of drug is detected at 2 hours. Less than 1% of the administered dose is recovered unchanged in the urine.

Preparation, Dosage, and Route of Administration. *Uracil Mustard,* N.F., is available as a white crystalline powder in capsules containing 1 mg. Two oral dosage schedules are recommended: (1) 1 to 2 mg daily for 3 weeks, repeated after an interruption of 1 week; and (2) 3 to 5 mg daily for 7 days, then 1 mg daily for 3 weeks.

Therapeutic Uses and Clinical Toxicity. The chief advantages of this drug are that it can be administered orally and, in contrast to cyclophosphamide, does not cause frank alopecia. Its clinical spectrum of action is similar to that of other related alkylating agents. Hematopoietic depression is the major manifestation of toxicity, and uracil mustard has been considered useful for controlling thrombocytosis. Nausea, vomiting, diarrhea, and dermatitis have also been noted.

CHLORAMBUCIL

This aromatic derivative of mechlorethamine was synthesized first at the Chester Beatty Research Institute in England. Initial clinical studies demonstrated beneficial results primarily in chronic lymphocytic leukemia, as well as in Hodgkin's disease and related malignant lymphomas. (For references to the early reports, *see* Calabresi and Welch, 1962.)

Chemistry. The chemical formula of chlorambucil and its relation to the nitrogen mustards are presented above (*see* Table 62–1).

Pharmacological and Cytotoxic Actions. Although CNS stimulation can occur, this has been observed only with large doses. Nausea and vomiting may result from single oral doses of 20 mg or more. Cytotoxic effects on the bone marrow, lymphoid organs, and epithelial tissues are similar to those observed with the nitrogen mustards.

Absorption, Fate, and Excretion. Oral absorption is adequate and reliable. There is incomplete information concerning the metabolism, distribution, or elimination of the drug in man.

Preparations, Dosage, and Route of Administration. *Chlorambucil,* U.S.P. (LEUKERAN), is available in 2-mg tablets for oral administration. The standard initial daily dosage is 0.1 to 0.2 mg/kg, continued for at least 3 to 6 weeks. The total daily dose, usually 4 to 10 mg, is given at one time. With fall in the peripheral total leukocyte count or clinical improvement, the dosage is reduced; maintenance therapy (usually 2 mg daily) is feasible and may be required, depending on the nature of the disease.

Therapeutic Uses and Clinical Toxicity. At the recommended dosages, chlorambucil is the slowest-acting and least toxic nitrogen mustard in clinical use. It is the treatment of choice in chronic lymphocytic leukemia and in primary (Waldenström's) macroglobulinemia.

In chronic lymphocytic leukemia, chlorambucil may be given orally over long periods of time, achieving its effects gradually and often without toxicity to a precariously compromised bone marrow. Ease of administration and reliable absorption make it preferable to the ethylenimine derivatives (thio-TEPA and triethylenemelamine) for prolonged palliation. It has largely supplanted these agents in the treatment of carcinoma of the ovary. Its spectrum of action is similar to that of other alkylating agents, and remissions may be expected in Hodgkin's disease and lymphomas, and sometimes in solid tumors. Its use in maintenance therapy to prolong the more immediate beneficial effects of mechlorethamine has been advocated. Clinical improvement comparable to that with melphalan or cyclophosphamide has been observed in some patients with plasma-cell myeloma. In combination with methotrexate and dactinomycin it has been useful in the management of testicular carcinomas. (*See* Livingston and Carter, 1970; Fudenberg, 1972; Gardner, 1972; Knospe *et al.,* 1974.)

Although it is possible to induce marked hypoplasia of the bone marrow with excessive doses of chlorambucil administered over long periods of time, its myelosuppressive action is usually moderate, gradual, and rapidly reversible. Gastrointestinal discomfort, dermatitis, and hepatotoxicity may be encountered occasionally.

ETHYLENIMINES

TRIETHYLENEMELAMINE (TEM) AND TRIETHYLENETHIOPHOSPHORAMIDE (THIO-TEPA)

Triethylenemelamine (TEM) was first synthesized by industrial chemists for use in improving the finish of rayon fabrics. Because of the presence of ethylenimine groups in its structure, the cytotoxic and pharmacological actions were studied by various investigators (*see* Calabresi and Welch, 1962). Triethylene*thio*phosphoramide (thio-TEPA) was introduced clinically in 1953.

Chemistry. The chemical structures of triethylenemelamine and thio-TEPA are discussed above in conjunction with the structure-activity relationship of the alkylating agents.

Status. *Triethylenemelamine,* N.F., is used in the treatment of retinoblastoma. In other neoplasms the ethylenimines are now seldom employed as therapeutic agents, having been replaced by selected nitrogen mustards. Their areas of usefulness are presented in Table XV-1 (page 1250), and their pharmacological properties are described in the *third edition* of this textbook.

ALKYL SULFONATES

BUSULFAN

During the course of an investigation to determine the antineoplastic properties of a series of alkanesulfonic acid esters, the rather selective action of *busulfan* was detected. This finding led to the use of the drug in patients with chronic granulocytic leukemia.

Chemistry. Busulfan is quite stable in dry form. The chemical formula of this compound and the interesting structure-activity relationship of the series have been presented above. Studies on its mechanism of action also have been discussed above.

Pharmacological and Cytotoxic Actions. Busulfan is unique in that it exerts virtually no pharmacological action other than myelosuppression. At low doses, selective depression of granulocytopoiesis is evident. Platelets are also affected by relatively small amounts of drug, and erythroid elements may be suppressed as the dosage is raised; eventually, a pancytopenia results. Cytotoxic action does not appear to extend to either the lymphoid tissues or the gastrointestinal epithelium.

Absorption, Fate, and Excretion. Busulfan is well absorbed after oral administration. Within 3 minutes after its intravenous administration in rats, 90% of the drug disappears from the blood; similar rapid decreases in blood concentrations have been reported in man. In man, as in the rat, almost all administered ^{35}S-busulfan is excreted in the urine as methanesulfonic acid; unchanged drug does not appear in the urine. The metabolism of busulfan with reference to its "sulfur-stripping" action has been discussed above and reviewed in relation to its mechanism of action (Warwick, 1963).

Preparations, Dosage, and Route of Administration. *Busulfan,* U.S.P. (MYLERAN), is available in scored, 2-mg tablets. The initial oral dose varies with the total leukocyte count and the severity of the disease; daily doses from 4 to 12 mg have been given to initiate therapy and are adjusted appropriately to subsequent hematological and clinical responses. It has been reported that reduction of the total leukocyte count to 10,000 or fewer cells per cubic millimeter before discontinuing the drug results in longer remissions. If maintenance doses are required to keep the hematological status under control, 1 to 3 mg may be given daily.

Therapeutic Uses and Clinical Toxicity. The beneficial effects of busulfan in chronic granulocytic leukemia are well established, and remissions may be expected in 85 to 90% of patients after the initial course of therapy. (*See* Galton, 1969; Livingston and Carter, 1970.)

Reduction in morbidity is readily apparent with symptomatic response, characterized by increased appetite and sense of well-being, which may occur within a few days. Reduction of the leukocyte count is noted during the second or third week and regression of splenomegaly follows. Evidence has been advanced (Haut *et al.,* 1961) that median longevity in patients receiving busulfan is increased by 9 months, as compared to a control series. The results obtained are considered to be better than those achieved by treatment with either phosphate-^{32}P, x-radiation, antimetabolites, or other alkylating agents. Beneficial results have been reported in other myeloproliferative disorders, including polycythemia vera and myelofibrosis with myeloid metaplasia. The drug is of no value in acute leukemia or in the "blastic crisis" of chronic granulocytic leukemia.

The major toxic effects of busulfan are related to its myelosuppressive properties, and thrombocytopenia may be a hazard. Occasional instances of nausea, vomiting, diarrhea, impotence, sterility, amenorrhea, and fetal malformation have been reported. Hyperuricemia, resulting from extensive purine catabolism accompanying the rapid cellular destruction, and renal damage from precipitation of urates have been noted. To avoid this complication, the concurrent use of *allopurinol* is recommended. A number of unusual complications have been observed in patients receiving busulfan, but their relation to the drug is poorly understood; these include generalized skin pigmentation, gynecomastia, cheilosis, glossitis, anhidrosis, and pulmonary fibrosis. (For references, *see* Calabresi and Welch, 1962.)

NITROSOUREAS

These highly lipid-soluble, chemically reactive compounds were first synthesized at the Southern Research Institute, Birmingham, Alabama (Johnston *et al.,* 1963; Schabel, 1973). The chemistry, structure-activity relationship, and mechanism of action of the nitrosoureas have been discussed above; their cytotoxic action is exerted at any stage of the cell cycle. Although the nitrosoureas have shown a spectrum of activity similar to that of other alkylating agents in Hodgkin's disease and lymphomas, they are also active against some solid tumors. Because of their unique property of crossing the blood-brain barrier, they have attracted considerable interest in the treatment of meningeal leukemia and brain tumors (Wilson *et al.*, 1970; Walker, 1973).

CARMUSTINE (BCNU)

This compound was the first of the nitrosourea series to receive extensive clinical evaluation. It is effective against a wide range of experimental tumors.

Pharmacological and Cytotoxic Actions. Carmustine is capable of inhibiting the synthesis of DNA, RNA, and protein in a manner similar but not identical to that of other alkylating agents (Livingston and Carter, 1970). Although bone-marrow suppression is observed, there is an unusually delayed onset of leukopenia and thrombocytopenia that is characteristic of this drug. The nadir of the leukocyte and platelet counts may not be reached until 6 weeks after treatment. Cytotoxic effects on the liver, kidneys, and CNS have been reported (Oliverio, 1973b).

Absorption, Fate, and Excretion. Although carmustine is rapidly absorbed by the oral route, it is administered intravenously because tissue uptake and metabolism occur very quickly; disappearance from the plasma takes place within 5 minutes. Approximately 80% of radioactively labeled drug appears in the urine within 24 hours as degradation products of the parent compound. Prolonged plasma concentrations of these degradation products may be the result of binding to plasma protein or active enterohepatic circulation. The active metabolites may be responsible for the delayed bone-marrow toxicity. Entry of these products into the cerebrospinal fluid (CSF) is rapid, and the concentrations in the CSF of man are 15% to 30% of the concurrent plasma values (Oliverio, 1973b).

Preparation, Dosage, and Route of Administration. Carmustine is a light-yellow powder at 4° C; it melts to an oily liquid at room temperature and is stable in the anhydrous state. The half-life of the drug in 0.9% sodium chloride solution at pH 6 is 24 hours at room temperature. Carmustine is usually administered intravenously at doses of 100 to 200 mg/sq m, given as a single injection, and it is not repeated for 6 weeks.

Therapeutic Uses and Clinical Toxicity. The spectrum of activity of carmustine is similar to that of other alkylating agents, with significant responses observed in Hodgkin's disease and to a lesser extent in other lymphomas. Because of its ability to cross the blood-brain barrier, it has been used in meningeal leukemia and in primary and metastatic tumors of the brain, with very encouraging results. Beneficial responses have been reported in melanomas, as well as in gastrointestinal, breast, bronchogenic, and renal-cell carcinomas (Young *et al.*, 1971; Ramirez *et al.*, 1972; Carter, 1973; Moertel, 1973; Walker, 1973).

The most significant clinical toxicity is the characteristically delayed hematopoietic depression described above. The drug is not a vesicant, but local burning pain has been reported after intravenous administration. Nausea and vomiting occur approximately 2 hours after injection, and flushing of the skin, CNS toxicity, esophagitis, diarrhea, dyspnea, and hepatotoxicity have been reported (Young *et al.*, 1971; Ramirez *et al.*, 1972).

LOMUSTINE (CCNU) AND SEMUSTINE (METHYL-CCNU)

Pharmacological and Cytotoxic Actions. Lomustine and its methylated analog, semustine, were selected for clinical studies because of their lipid solubility and superiority to carmustine in the treatment of certain experimental tumors. The cytotoxic effects of these compounds are similar to those of carmustine, as is their clinical toxicity. Delayed bone-marrow depression, reflected by leukopenia and thrombocytopenia, is characteristic and similar to that caused by carmustine (Moertel, 1973).

Absorption, Fate, and Excretion. Lomustine and semustine are rapidly absorbed from the gastrointestinal tract and are administered orally. Although lomustine is rapidly and completely metabolized, prolonged plasma half-life of its metabolites, ranging from 16 to 48 hours, has been reported. Approximately 50% of the administered dose is detectable in the urine within 24 hours and 75% within 4 days. Radioactively labeled semustine is not detectable in either plasma or urine. The chloroethyl moiety has a half-life of 36 hours, while the cyclohexyl portion has a biphasic disappearance curve with an early half-life of 24 hours and a slower secondary phase with a half-life of 72 hours. Although neither drug can be detected intact in the CSF, active metabolites appear in significant concentrations within 30 minutes (Oliverio, 1973b; Carter and Slavik, 1974).

Preparation, Dosage, and Route of Administration. Although parenteral preparations of both lomustine and semustine are available for investigation (Davignon *et al.*, 1973), the drugs are usually administered orally in capsule form. The usual oral dose of lomustine is 130 mg/sq m, while the recommended oral dose of semustine is 200 mg/sq m. Both drugs are administered as a single dose, which is not repeated for 6 weeks.

Therapeutic Uses and Clinical Toxicity. These agents have a wide spectrum of activity. Lomustine appears to be more effective than carmustine in Hodgkin's disease. Beneficial results of therapy with these two nitrosoureas, alone and in combination with other agents, have been reported in patients with malignant gliomas, adenocarcinomas of the gastrointestinal tract, Hodgkin's disease and other lymphomas, carcinoma of the breast, malignant melanoma, hypernephromas, multiple myeloma, and various squamous-cell carcinomas (DeConti *et al.*, 1973; Symposium, 1973; Carter and Slavik, 1974). The clinical toxicity of both drugs is similar, with the characteristically delayed bone-marrow suppression described above being the dose-limiting effect. Nausea and vomiting are frequently encountered.

STREPTOZOTOCIN

This naturally occurring nitrosourea is an antibiotic derived from *Streptomyces acromogenes*. It has been particularly useful in treating functional, malignant pancreatic islet-cell tumors (Livingston and Carter, 1970). The drug is capable of inhibiting synthesis of DNA in microorganisms and mammalian cells (Bhuyan, 1970; Reusser, 1971); it affects all stages of the mammalian cell cycle. Biochemical studies have also revealed potent inhibitory effects on pyridine nucleotides and on key enzymes involved in glyconeogenesis.

Absorption, Fate, and Excretion. Streptozotocin is administered parenterally. After intravenous infusions of 200 to 1600 mg/sq m, peak concentrations in the plasma are 30 to 40 μg/ml; the half-life of the drug is approximately 15 minutes. Only 10 to 20% of a dose is recovered in the urine (Schein *et al.*, 1973).

Preparation, Dosage, and Route of Administration. Although streptozotocin is not commercially available, it can be obtained from the Cancer Therapy Evaluation Branch of the National Cancer Institute, Bethesda, Maryland. The drug is administered intravenously or intraarterially in doses of 1 g/sq m once a week for 4 weeks. It may be continued if a beneficial response is observed.

Therapeutic Uses and Clinical Toxicity. Streptozotocin has been used primarily in patients with metastatic pancreatic islet-cell carcinoma, and beneficial responses are translated into a significant increase in 1-year survival rate and a doubling of median survival time for the responders. It has also been found to be active in malignant carcinoid tumors. Broder and Carter (1973) noted nausea and vomiting in almost all of 52 patients treated for islet-cell carcinoma. Renal or hepatic toxicity occurred in approximately two thirds of cases; although this was usually reversible, renal toxicity was responsible for five deaths. Hematological toxicity, consisting in anemia, leukopenia, or thrombocytopenia, was observed in 20% of patients and was responsible for one fatality.

TRIAZENES

DACARBAZINE (DTIC)

This compound, the chemistry of which is described above, was originally believed to act as an antimetabolite; more recent evidence indicates that it functions as an alkylating agent following metabolic activation in the liver. At present dacarbazine is employed principally for the treatment of malignant melanoma. The overall response rate of malignant melanoma reported for this drug is about 20%, and a similar percentage of responses has been reported for a small series of patients with various sarcomas. The toxicity observed includes nausea and vomiting, usually developing 1 to 3 hours after treatment, and occasional myelosuppression, with both leukopenia and thrombocytopenia. Hepatotoxicity has also been reported. The drug is administered intravenously and has a plasma half-life of about 35 minutes. Almost one half of the compound is excreted intact in the urine in 6 hours. Elevated urinary concentrations of 5-aminoimidazole-4-carboxamide (AIC) have been detected and are derived from the catabolism of dacarbazine, rather than by inhibition of *de-novo* purine biosynthesis.

Since this drug has only recently become available for general use, its status as an antineoplastic agent is still under evaluation. Clinical reports indicate that the agent may have significant activity in some cases of malignant melanoma and Hodgkin's disease. Still to be assessed is the possible use of dacarbazine in combination with other antineoplastic agents. The recommended therapeutic regimen is 3.5 mg/kg per day, administered intravenously for a 10-day period, to be repeated every 28 days.

II. Antimetabolites

FOLIC ACID ANALOGS

METHOTREXATE

Consideration of the analogs of folic (pteroylglutamic) acid is especially important, because this class of antimetabolites not only produced the first striking, although temporary, remissions in leukemia (Farber *et al.,* 1948) but also provided the first drug to cause long-lasting remissions in choriocarcinoma in women, a relatively rare hormone-producing neoplasm (Hertz, 1963). The attainment of a very significant number of apparently permanent remissions in this otherwise-lethal disease has justified the use of the word *cure* and has given great impetus to chemotherapeutic investigation. However, interpretation of these results must be tempered by the knowledge that choriocarcinoma is a transplanted tumor that arises from fetal membranes and, therefore, may be affected by host defense mechanisms. The dramatic clinical results obtained by Farber and coworkers (1948) in the treatment of *acute leukemia in children* with folic acid antagonists constitute a milestone in the history of chemotherapy.

The folate analog methotrexate has also been used with benefit in the therapy of *psoriasis,* a nonneoplastic disease of the skin characterized by abnormally rapid proliferation of epidermal cells (Van Scott *et al.,* 1964; McDonald and Bertino, 1968). Additionally, folate antagonists are potent inhibitors of some types of immune reactions and have been employed as *immunosuppressive agents,* for example, in organ transplantation (Hitchings and Elion, 1963; Schwartz, 1965). (For recent reviews, *see* Johns and Bertino, 1973; Bertino, 1975.)

Structure-Activity Relationship. Folic acid is an essential dietary factor from which is derived a coenzyme, tetrahydrofolic acid, and a group of structurally related derivatives; these are concerned with the metabolic transfer of one-carbon units. A detailed description of the biological functions and therapeutic applications of folic acid appears in Chapter 64.

Although there are many loci where antimetabolites of folate might act, the primary site of action of most of the analogs studied to date is the enzyme *dihydrofolate reductase.* In recent years dihydrofolate reductases from various species and tissues have been subjected to intensive study. The results of

these important investigations have raised the science of chemotherapy to a new level of sophistication, since they demonstrate that, although the various dihydrofolate reductases catalyze identical reactions, they possess subtle differences in structure that are reflected in marked differences in ability to bind various folate antagonists (*see* Chapter 52). The provocative implications of these findings are that other examples of differences in the binding of inhibitors to related enzymes may exist, which, if identified, could be exploited for chemotherapy.

It is probable that other potent dihydrofolate reductase inhibitors can be identified with physical or chemical properties that offer advantages over other antifolates, for example, ability to cross the blood-brain barrier or to penetrate other sites not readily accessible to methotrexate. The partial effectiveness of pyrimethamine, an antimalarial and a relatively weak inhibitor of mammalian dihydrofolate reductase, in the treatment of meningeal infiltration in acute lymphocytic leukemia indicates the potential value of this approach. If such agents can be identified, it seems likely that vital normal tissues may be protected by the simultaneous administration of leucovorin (folinic acid), which, like methotrexate, penetrates the blood-brain barrier with difficulty (*see* below).

An extensive literature exists concerning the relation between structure and action of the folic acid analogs (Handschumacher and Welch, 1960; Hitchings and Burchall, 1965; Johns and Bertino, 1973). In early studies, *aminopterin (i.e.,* 4-amino-4-deoxyfolic acid) was widely used. Currently, however, the folate analog of clinical importance is *methotrexate.* The structures of aminopterin and methotrexate are shown at the bottom of the page.

Mechanism of Action. The major site of action of clinically useful folate antagonists is the enzyme dihydrofolate reductase (Figure 64–1, page 1326). The inhibition caused by methotrexate is so profound and lasts so long, both *in vitro* and *in vivo,* that the kinetics of inhibition often are referred to as "pseudo-irreversible"; indeed, the antagonist cannot be displaced from the enzyme to a significant degree by concentrations of folic acid that are attainable physiologically. Thus, one of the hazards in the use of methotrexate is that its actions cannot be terminated by the administration of folate. A clinically useful derivative of tetrahydrofolate (THF) that can circumvent the inhibition of dihydrofolate reductase is *leucovorin* (folinic acid; N5-formyl-THF; citrovorum factor), available as *Leucovorin Calcium,* U.S.P. Properly timed administration of this normal metabolite following large doses of methotrexate has been employed in order to protect

Aminopterin: R = H
Methotrexate: R = CH₃

normal tissues from the lethal effects of the drug. The procedure has been called leucovorin or folinic "rescue." Although this phenomenon is not yet fully understood, several factors appear to be involved, including the repletion of cellular pools by reduced folate coenzymes, the inhibition by leucovorin of the specific cellular transport mechanism, and the accelerated efflux of intracellular methotrexate (Bertino, 1975). Still unanswered is the fundamental question concerning the achievement of relative selectivity for the salvage of normal cells (*see* below).

An important feature of the binding of active folate antagonists with dihydrofolate reductases is the very low inhibition constants observed (on the order of 1 nM). Covalent bonds are not involved in the enzyme-inhibitor interactions despite the unusually great affinity of the antagonists for dihydrofolate reductase. Huennekens (1968) has pointed out that the negative free-energy change of the binding of aminopterin to chicken liver dihydrofolate reductase is about 3.7 kcal per mole greater than that of dihydrofolate. This is approximately the amount of free energy required for the formation of either a single hydrogen bond or an ionic bond. The substitution of an amino group for a hydroxyl group in the 4 position of the pteridine ring may make possible the formation of a new ionic or hydrogen bond between the analog and the enzyme, which is not feasible with the natural substrate, since the 4-hydroxyl group of natural folates exists largely in the keto form. It is still not established whether a hydrogen or ionic bond is involved, although some evidence favors the latter (Baker, 1967).

As with most inhibitors of cellular reproduction, a selective effect on neoplastic cells is obtainable to only a partial extent with methotrexate. Folate antagonists kill cells during the S phase of the cell cycle, and evidence indicates that methotrexate is much more effective when the cellular population is in the logarithmic phase of growth, rather than in the plateau phase (Hryniuk and Bertino, 1969). Because it is also capable of inhibiting RNA and protein synthesis, however, methotrexate slows the entry of cells into S phase and its cytotoxic action has been referred to as "self-limiting" (Skipper and Schabel, 1973). Since the essential biosynthetic reactions of cellular reproduction appear to be common to all or most types of mammalian cells, opportunities for selective effects on neoplastic cells through ultimate inhibition of dihydrofolate reductase must be sought in such areas as (1) relative rates of cellular reproduction, (2) relative rates and mechanisms of transport of folate antagonists into different types of cells, (3) relative firmness of binding of the analogs within various kinds of cells, (4) relative rates of their metabolic alteration by cells, and (5) possible occurrence of isozymes of dihydrofolate reductase that have different binding properties with folate antagonists.

Mechanism of Resistance to Antifolates. As with other agents now used for treatment of cancer, a major obstacle to clinical success with methotrexate has been the occurrence of resistance to the drug. In experimental microbial and tumor systems, three biochemical mechanisms for acquired resistance to antifolates have been identified: increased levels of dihydrofolate reductase, an alteration in the structure of the enzyme that decreases its affinity for methotrexate, and a decrease in the transport of methotrexate into the cell. Any of these alterations may occur by stable, genetic mutations that give rise to new clones of drug-resistant cells. Although the above-listed resistance mechanisms are clearly demonstrable in experimental systems, little is known of the details of resistance in human malignancies.

It has been shown both in normal man and in other animals, as well as in patients with leukemia, that within a few days after even a single dose of methotrexate there is a temporary appearance in the blood of erythrocytes and leukocytes having greatly augmented levels of dihydrofolate reductase activity (Bertino *et al.*, 1965). In normal blood cells the activity of this enzyme is barely detectable, and the increase, therefore, is striking. These findings may have far-reaching significance with respect to the problems of natural or acquired resistance. The marked increase in dihydrofolate reductase activity may reflect (1) induction of new enzyme synthesis, (2) temporary elimination from the bone marrow of drug-susceptible cells with low enzymatic activity, or (3) protection against catabolic destruction of the enzyme as a result of its complexing with the inhibitor. Dihydrofolate reductase complexed with methotrexate undergoes a conformational change that renders the enzyme remarkably resistant to proteolytic degradation (Hakala and Suolinna, 1966; Burchall, 1968).

General Toxicity and Cytotoxic Action. The actions of 4-amino analogs of folate in animals have been studied extensively. Animals given a minimal lethal dose survive for at least 48 hours and usually die within 3 to 5 days. Anorexia, progressive weight loss, bloody diarrhea, leukopenia, depression, and coma are the outstanding features of fatal intoxication. The major lesions occur in the *intestinal tract* and *bone marrow*. Swelling and cytoplasmic vacuolization of the mucosal cells of the intestinal epithelium are evident within 6 hours. These changes are followed by desquamation of epithelial cells, extrusion of plasma into the lumen of the bowel, and leukocytic infiltration of the submucosa. Terminally, the entire intestinal tract exhibits a severe hemorrhagic desquamating enteritis. Degeneration of bone marrow develops rapidly. Within 24 hours there is evident disturbance in the maturation of erythrocytes. Proliferation of erythroid precursors is inhibited, and significant proportions of primitive erythroid elements have the appearance of megaloblasts. Rapid pathological alteration in myelopoiesis also occurs, and within a few days the bone marrow becomes aplastic. There is diminution in content of lymphoid cells in lymphatic tissue, but there is no evidence of necrosis. The disturbance in hematopoiesis is reflected in the circulating blood by a marked granulocytopenia and reticulocytopenia and a moderate lymphopenia.

Folic acid antagonists seriously interfere with *embryogenesis.* The site of action is on the embryonic mesenchyme. Decidual and placental tissues are unaffected by doses of the drugs that cause fetal death. Young embryos are much more susceptible than are the more developed. The administration of methotrexate during pregnancy obviously is accompanied by great hazards to the fetus.

Absorption, Fate, and Excretion. Methotrexate is readily absorbed from the gastrointestinal tract at doses routinely employed in clinical practice (0.1 mg/kg), but larger doses are incompletely absorbed. The drug is also absorbed from parenteral sites of injection. A direct relationship exists between dose and plasma concentrations. The mean plasma half-life of methotrexate is about 2 hours. Approximately 50% of the drug is bound to plasma proteins. Laboratory studies suggest that it may be displaced from plasma albumin by a number of drugs, including sulfonamides and salicylates, and caution should be used if these are given concomitantly. Of the drug absorbed, from 40 to 50% of a small dose (2.5 to 15 μg/kg) to about 90% of a large dose (150 μg/kg) is excreted unchanged in the urine within 48 hours, mostly within the first 8 hours. A small amount of methotrexate is also excreted in the stool, probably through the biliary tract. Metabolism of methotrexate in man does not seem to occur to a significant degree. The portion of each dose of methotrexate that normally is excreted rapidly gains access to the urine by a combination of glomerular filtration and active tubular secretion. Therefore, the concurrent use of drugs that also undergo tubular secretion, as well as impaired renal function, can influence markedly the response to this drug. Particular caution must be exercised in treating patients with renal insufficiency.

Since methotrexate is a large, polar molecule, it is not surprising that uptake by cells involves a specific transport mechanism. This system is also used for the facilitated uptake of leucovorin and may play a role in the mechanisms of leucovorin "rescue" and acquired drug resistance.

The portion of methotrexate that is retained in human tissues remains for long periods, for example, for weeks in the kidneys and for several months in the liver. The data strongly suggest that methotrexate retained within cells is bound primarily by dihydrofolate reductase, which thereby is prevented from functioning. The affinity of methotrexate for the cytoplasmic enzyme protein is so great that the very gradual release of drug may represent only the minute amounts that are gradually displaced by folate and dihydrofolate, as well as that released by cells that die.

It is important to emphasize that methotrexate is very poorly transported across the blood-brain barrier; hence, neoplastic cells that have entered the CNS probably are not affected by tolerated concentrations of drug in the plasma.

Preparations, Dosage, and Routes of Administration. *Methotrexate,* U.S.P. (*amethopterin*), is provided in scored, 2.5-mg yellow tablets and also as a dry powder (the sodium salt) in vials containing either 2.5 or 25 mg for preparation of sterile injectable solutions.

Although the standard daily oral dosage of methotrexate ordinarily employed in patients with *leukemia* has been 2.5 to 5.0 mg for children and 2.5 to 10.0 mg for adults, newer therapeutic concepts have emerged involving revised dosage schedules and the use of multiple drugs sequentially and concurrently (Zubrod, 1968). Methotrexate *induces* remission slowly, probably because the cells in advanced leukemia are not in the logarithmic phase of growth. For induction of remission it has been superseded by the more rapid and effective therapy with vincristine plus prednisone, with or without daunorubicin. Methotrexate is of great value in the *maintenance* of remissions, particularly when administered intermittently at high doses of 30 mg/sq m, intramuscularly, twice a week (Acute Leukemia Group B, 1965), or by intensive 2-day "pulses" of 175 to 525 mg/sq m at monthly intervals (Djerassi, 1967).

The *intrathecal administration* of methotrexate has been employed, particularly when manifestations of cerebral involvement in either leukemia or choriocarcinoma have appeared, as occurs not infrequently even during systemic remissions. This route of administration achieves high concentrations of methotrexate in the CSF and is effective also in patients whose systemic disease has become resistant to methotrexate, since the leukemic cells in the CNS beyond the blood-brain barrier have survived in a pharmacological sanctuary and retain their original degree of sensitivity to the drug. The recommended intrathecal dose is 0.2 to 0.5 mg/kg, given once or repeated at intervals of 2 to 5 days, depending on the severity of involvement and the response to therapy; another dosage schedule is 12 mg/sq m once weekly for 2 weeks and then monthly. Leucovorin may be administered intramuscularly to counteract the systemic toxicity of methotrexate.

In the treatment of *choriocarcinoma* with methotrexate, intensive treatment is usually employed, for example, 15 mg/sq m (15 to 30 mg) daily for 5 days orally or parenterally. Courses are repeated at 1- to 2-week intervals, toxicity permitting, and urinary gonadotropin titers are used as a guide for persistence of disease.

Methotrexate has been used in the treatment of severe, disabling *psoriasis* in doses of 2.5 to 5.0 mg orally for 5 days or 25 to 50 mg intravenously weekly. An initial parenteral test dose of 5 to 10 mg is recommended to detect any possible idiosyncrasy. Complete awareness of the pharmacology and toxic potential of methotrexate is a prerequisite for its use in this nonneoplastic disorder (Rees *et al.,* 1967; McDonald and Bertino, 1968).

Continuous infusion of relatively large amounts of the drug (up to 50 mg daily for 10 days) has been administered into the arterial blood supply of a *localized neoplasm,* incurable by surgery or irradiation. This procedure has been coupled with intermittent intramuscular injections of leucovorin (6 to 9 mg) every 4 to 6 hours, to reduce the severity of systemic toxicity.

Experimental results in animals (Mead *et al.,* 1963) suggested that the therapeutic index of methotrexate may be improved by administering leucovorin a few hours after the folate antagonist in order to "rescue" preferentially the normal cells of the host after the drug has been bound within the tumor cells. Although the use of methotrexate in high doses and of leucovorin "rescue" has been studied clinically for several years with very encouraging results, the optimal timing, dose of leucovorin required, and proof that the therapeutic index is actually improved remain to be established (*see* Djerassi *et al.,* 1972; Jaffe, 1972; Levitt *et al.,* 1973; Chabner *et al.,* 1975).

Therapeutic Uses and Clinical Toxicity. Methotrexate is a useful drug in the management of *acute lymphoblastic leukemia* in children. It is of established value in *choriocarcinoma* and related trophoblastic tumors of women, with complete and lasting remissions occurring in approximately 75% of women treated sequentially with methotrexate and dactinomycin, and in over 90% when early diagnosis is accompanied by a low urinary gonadotropin titer (Ross *et al.,* 1965). A number of these patients are living without evidence of disease more than 15 years after initiation of therapy. In addition, many women with nonmetastatic trophoblastic disease, *hydatidiform mole,* and *chorioadenoma destruens,* have been treated successfully with methotrexate (Hertz *et al.,* 1963). Beneficial results have also been reported in *mycosis fungoides,* in *carcinomas* of the breast, tongue, pharynx, and testes (in combination with chlorambucil and dactinomycin), as well as in occasional patients with other tumors. Recent reports indicate that high-dose methotrexate, with subsequent leucovorin "rescue," can cause substantial tumor regression in at least two tumors highly refractory to most chemotherapeutic agents: carcinoma of the lung (Djerassi *et al.,* 1972) and osteogenic sarcoma (Jaffe, 1972). (For other references, *see* Calabresi and Welch, 1962; Livingston and Carter, 1970; Bertino and Johns, 1972; Greenwald, 1973.) Striking improvement has been observed with the use of methotrexate in the treatment of severe *psoriasis* (Van Scott *et al.,* 1964; Rees *et al.,* 1967).

Although useful in the management of *acute leukemia* in children, methotrexate is of very limited value in the types of leukemia seen in adult individuals.

Treatment with methotrexate requires constant surveillance of the patient in order to judge dosage properly and to avoid serious toxic reactions. In persons treated with conventional doses or with concomitant leucovorin, it is frequently possible to avoid severe leukopenia or aplasia of the bone marrow. Thrombocytopenia with bleeding can be treated with platelet transfusions, but it may be difficult to control, particularly in the presence of infection. It is imperative that a skilled medical team and sophisticated facilities, particularly abundant platelet transfusions and measures for preventing and combating infections, be available in order to provide the intensive supportive therapy necessary to control the severe toxic manifestations that may result when intensive dosage schedules are used.

Other untoward reactions also may complicate the use of methotrexate. Ulcerative stomatitis and diarrhea are frequent side effects and require interruption of the therapeutic regimen; hemorrhagic enteritis and death from intestinal perforation may occur. Additional toxic manifestations include alopecia, dermatitis, nephrotoxicity, defective oogenesis or spermatogenesis, abortion, teratogenesis, and hepatic dysfunction, usually reversible but sometimes leading to cirrhosis (Coe and Bull, 1968). The long-term complications associated with the use of methotrexate for immunosuppressive therapy are discussed by Schein and Winokur (1975).

PYRIMIDINE ANALOGS

Pyrimidine analogs represent an ingenious development of biochemical pharmacology. The biosynthesis of the pyrimidine base unique to DNA, thymine (5-methyluracil), was selected by Heidelberger and coworkers as a critical point for chemotherapeutic attack. Since it was known that the methyl group of thymine is inserted into 2'-deoxyuridine-5'-phosphate by a sequence of enzymatically catalyzed reactions (the thymidylate synthetase system), it was reasoned that a compound with a stable fluorine substituted for hydrogen in the 5 position of uracil or deoxyuridine conceivably might exert profound effects on the biosynthesis of DNA. This idea was reinforced by the knowledge that fluoroacetate, a fluorine-containing analog of acetate, is an unusually powerful metabolic poison. The analogs, fluorouracil (5-fluorouracil, FU, 5-FU), first synthesized by Duschinsky, Pleven, and Heidelberger in 1957, and floxuridine (fluorodeoxyuridine, FUdR), prepared somewhat later, have proven to be potent antimetabolites that exert some of their effects as predicted, that is, by blocking the synthesis of thymidylic acid. These compounds have been of particular interest because they have significant, although not curative, effects on certain solid tumors in man that do not respond significantly to other antimetabolites. (For references, *see* reviews by Heidelberger, 1973, 1975.)

In addition to fluorouracil and floxuridine, other analogs of the pyrimidine bases and nucleosides have been developed that have proven useful in the treatment of nonneoplastic diseases. Cytarabine (ara-C), idoxuridine (iododeoxyuridine, 5-iododeoxyuridine, IUdR), and trifluoromethyldeoxyuridine display interesting antiviral properties; the clinical value of the first two drugs in viral chemotherapy is discussed in Chapter 61. Fluorocytosine has significant antifungal properties and selectivity (*see* Chapter 61). Azauridine (AzUR) and its triacetyl derivative, azaribine, have proven of considerable value in the treatment of psoriasis. Furthermore, azaribine and cytarabine are effective in the treatment of myeloproliferative and lymphoproliferative disorders. (For references, *see* Chabner *et al.*, 1975; Creasey, 1975a; Ho and Freireich, 1975; Prusoff and Goz, 1975; Skoda, 1975.)

Structure-Activity Relationship. A variety of analogs of natural pyrimidine bases and nucleosides show biological activity. These include compounds altered by substitution on the ring, modifications of the pyrimidine ring structure, and changes in the sugar moiety of the nucleoside. Of particular interest are the halogenated pyrimidines, which include such agents as fluorouracil and idoxuridine. If one compares the van der Waals radii of the various substituents (Table 62–2), the dimension of the fluorine atom resembles that of hydrogen, whereas the bromine and iodine atoms are close in size to the methyl group. Idoxuridine has relatively little effect on the biosynthesis of thymidylic acid; like thymidine, however, it is converted enzymatically within cells to phosphorylated derivatives; it is degraded to the

Table 62–2. STRUCTURAL FORMULAS OF PYRIMIDINE ANALOGS

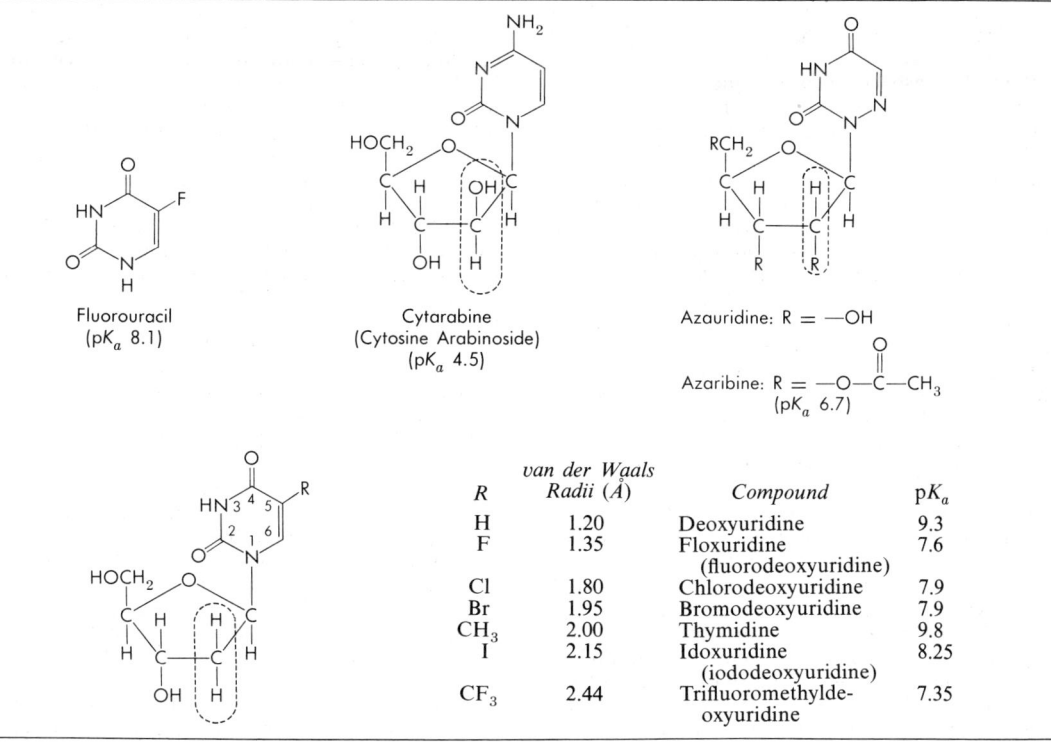

	R	van der Waals Radii (Å)	Compound	pKa
	H	1.20	Deoxyuridine	9.3
	F	1.35	Floxuridine (fluorodeoxyuridine)	7.6
	Cl	1.80	Chlorodeoxyuridine	7.9
	Br	1.95	Bromodeoxyuridine	7.9
	CH₃	2.00	Thymidine	9.8
	I	2.15	Idoxuridine (iododeoxyuridine)	8.25
	CF₃	2.44	Trifluoromethyldeoxyuridine	7.35

corresponding base, iodouracil, which is converted to uracil and iodide. The phosphorylated forms of idoxuridine inhibit competitively the utilization of the analogous derivatives of thymidine and can lead, in appropriate circumstances, to incorporation of the analog, as iododeoxyuridylic acid, into DNA in place of thymidylic acid (Delamore and Prusoff, 1962). These activities can suppress temporarily the growth of both experimental and human neoplasms; in addition, incorporation of the iodo- or bromo-analogs into DNA renders the latter more susceptible to the injurious effects of radiation.

If the hydrogen on position 5 of the pyrimidine ring is replaced with fluorine, the chemical reactivity of the ring is significantly altered, although the molecule, fluorouracil, behaves as does uracil with several enzymes. Fluorine has an inductive (electron-withdrawing) effect, which is reflected in a much lower pK_a with fluorouracil-containing compounds than with the natural compounds. The ionization that occurs is as follows:

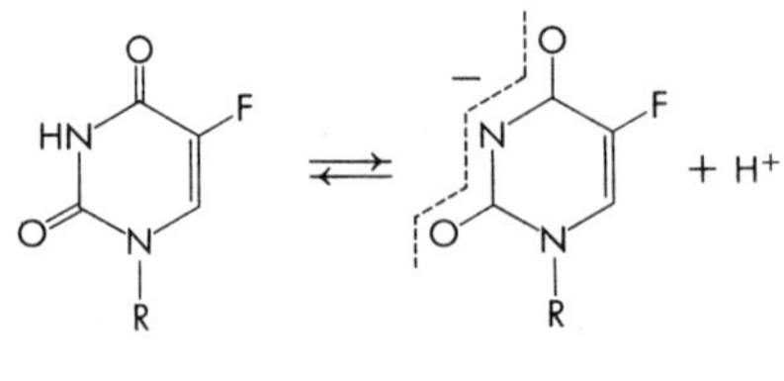

In addition, the carbon-fluorine bond is stronger than the carbon-hydrogen bond and is less susceptible to enzymatic cleavage. Thus, substitution of a halogen atom of the correct dimensions can produce a molecule that sufficiently resembles a natural pyrimidine to interact with enzymes of pyrimidine metabolism and also to interfere drastically with certain other aspects of pyrimidine action.

Similarly, the substitution of a nitrogen for a carbon in position 6 of the pyrimidine ring of uridine yields the analog azauridine (Table 62–2), which is capable of enzymatic conversion to the nucleotide level. However, the fraudulent nucleotide 6-azauradylic acid, because of its increased acidity, binds with and inhibits the enzyme orotidylic acid decarboxylase but cannot react further to form diphosphate and triphosphate nucleotides.

Among the various modifications of the sugar moiety attempted, the replacement of the ribose of cytidine with arabinose has yielded a useful chemotherapeutic agent, cytarabine. As may be seen in Table 62–2, the deviation from normal in this case involves the 2' carbon of the pentose, in which the hydroxyl group is in the opposite configuration from that of natural ribonucleoside, cytidine. This yields a molecule that sufficiently resembles a deoxynucleoside to be capable of conversion to the nucleotide level, but which blocks the synthesis of DNA (*see* reviews by Chabner *et al.*, 1975; Creasey, 1975a). A new agent that appears to behave as a repository form of cytarabine is the anhydro derivative O-2,2-anhydro-1-(β-D-arabinosyl)cytosine (cyclocytidine), in which the 2 carbon of the pyrimidine and the 2' carbon of the ribose are linked by an oxygen bridge. This compound is not susceptible to de-

amination by cytidine deaminase, and the anhydro linkage may be hydrolyzed slowly *in vivo* to liberate cytarabine (Ho, 1974).

FLUOROURACIL AND FLOXURIDINE (FLUORODEOXYURIDINE)

The development, chemistry, and structure-activity relationship of these interesting analogs are discussed above.

Mechanism of Action. Fluorouracil, as such, is without significant inhibitory activity in mammalian systems, and, in order to inhibit cellular growth, it must first be converted enzymatically to the nucleotide level. Several routes of 5'-monophosphate nucleotide (F-UMP) formation are available in animal cells. Fluorouracil may be converted to fluorouridine by uridine phosphorylase and then to F-UMP by uridine kinase (*see* Heidelberger, 1975), or it may react directly with 5-phosphoribosyl-1-pyrophosphate (PRPP), catalyzed by the enzyme orotate phosphoribosyl transferase, to form F-UMP (Reyes, 1969). The latter enzyme is present in higher concentrations in certain tumors than in liver and reacts with orotate as its natural substrate. Many metabolic pathways are available to F-UMP, including incorporation into RNA. However, the reaction sequence crucial for antineoplastic activity involves reduction of the diphosphate nucleotide by the enzyme ribonucleotide diphosphate reductase to the deoxynucleotide level and the eventual formation of 5-fluoro-2'-deoxyuridine-5'-phosphate (F-dUMP). This complex metabolic pathway for the generation of the actual growth inhibitor, F-dUMP, may be bypassed through use of the deoxyribonucleoside of fluorouracil—floxuridine (fluorodeoxyuridine, FUdR)—which is a substrate for intracellular thymidine kinase. Thus, in a single enzymatic step, the inhibitor of thymidylate synthetase, F-dUMP, can be produced in cells by the use of FUdR. Unfortunately, FUdR is a good substrate for both thymidine and deoxyuridine phosphorylases, and it is rapidly degraded to fluorouracil. The formation of FUdR by the reaction of fluorouracil with deoxyribose-1-phosphate has been demonstrated, but the possible significance of this anabolic reaction in chemotherapy is unclear.

The major site of action of F-dUMP derived from fluorouracil is the enzyme thymidylate synthetase, which catalyzes the transfer of a methyl group from N^5,N^{10}-methylenetetrahydrofolic acid to deoxyuridylic acid (dUMP). The fraudulent nucleotide F-dUMP has an unusually great affinity for this enzyme. It behaves as a competitive inhibitor with dUMP. The inhibitory nucleotide is not capable of serving as a substrate but binds to the enzyme from 250 to about 4000 times more tightly than does dUMP. This unusually powerful inhibition of a key enzyme in the synthesis of thymidylate is sufficient to explain most of the cytotoxic effects of fluorouracil and related derivatives (Reyes and Heidelberger, 1965).

Although it has been shown that fluorouracil is much more lethal to logarithmically growing cells than to stationary cells, there is no clearly demonstrated effect at a definite stage of the cell cycle. The phenomenon of "thymineless death" has been invoked to explain the cytotoxic effects of fluorouracil and its derivatives. The blockade of the thymidylate synthetase reaction inhibits DNA synthesis, while cellular production of both RNA and protein continues (Cohen *et al.*, 1958). An imbalance in growth occurs that is not compatible with cell survival. In accord with this proposal, the administration of thymidine can often reverse the toxicity, presumably through bypass of the block at thymidylate synthetase. There has been much speculation that the greater acidity of fluorouracil and its derivatives compared to uracil compounds might lead to incorrect base-pairing and coding errors in transcription or translation of nucleic acids into which fluorouracil has been incorporated. Despite extensive investigations, however, it has not been possible to demonstrate coding errors. Thus, it seems unlikely that such phenomena play a significant role in the biological actions of fluorouracil (*see* Cohen *et al.*, 1958; Heidelberger, 1975).

General Toxicity and Cytotoxic Action. The major sites of action of fluorouracil and floxuridine on normal tissues are the bone marrow and the epithelium of the gastrointestinal and oral mucosa. These are described in detail under clinical toxicity (*see* below).

Absorption, Fate, and Excretion. Fluorouracil and floxuridine are usually administered intravenously, since absorption after ingestion of the drugs is unpredictable and incomplete. Metabolic degradation occurs, particularly in the liver. Floxuridine is converted by thymidine or deoxyuridine phosphorylases into fluorouracil, and the latter is catabolized in much the same way as is uracil. Thus, 5-fluoro-5,6-dihydrouracil is formed, the ring of which is opened to give α-fluoro-β-ureidopropionic acid, which may be degraded further to α-fluoro-β-alanine (Heidelberger, 1975). In man, an important product of the metabolism of fluorouracil is urea.

It is of considerable interest that, given as single daily intravenous doses, the effects of neither fluorouracil nor floxuridine can be prevented by large doses of thymidine (Burchenal *et al.*, 1959); in fact, under these conditions this precursor of DNA *increases* the toxicity of the nucleoside. The apparent paradox is explained by the very rapid metabolic conversion of thymidine to the corresponding base, thymine, which competes

with the enzyme that can attack either fluorouracil, uracil, or thymine. In this manner, an increased concentration of fluorouracil is made available for anabolic utilization. On the other hand, when thymidine is given by intravenous infusion, together with floxuridine, the effects of the latter can be nullified (Sullivan and Miller, 1965), since in this manner enough thymidylate can be provided simultaneously to susceptible cells to circumvent the inhibition of thymidylate synthetase.

Oral absorption of fluorouracil is quite variable and unpredictable (Bruckner and Creasey, 1974). Rapid intravenous administration of fluorouracil produces plasma concentrations of 0.1 to 1.0 mM; plasma clearance is rapid ($t_{1/2} = 10$ to 20 minutes). Urinary excretion of intravenously injected fluorouracil-2-^{14}C, given as a single dose, amounts to only 11% in 24 hours; however, during this period, 63% of the radioactivity is expired as carbon dioxide. Given by continuous intravenous infusion for 24 hours, plasma concentrations in the range of 0.5 to 3.0 μM are obtained and the urinary excretion of fluorouracil is only 4%, while the $^{14}CO_2$ excretion rises to 90% (Mukherjee *et al.*, 1963). These findings probably account for the lower cytotoxicity of fluorouracil administered by infusion, compared to that seen with single doses (Lemon and Mozden, 1964). Fluorouracil readily enters the cerebrospinal fluid, and concentrations of about 7 μM are reached within 30 minutes after intravenous administration; values are sustained for approximately 3 hours and subside slowly during a period of 9 hours (Bourke *et al.*, 1973).

Preparation, Dosage, and Routes of Administration. *Fluorouracil*, U.S.P. (*5-FU*), is available in sterile ampuls containing 500 mg in 10 ml for intravenous administration. The recommended dose for average-risk patients in good nutritional status with adequate hematopoietic, renal, and hepatic function is 12 mg/kg daily for 4 days, by rapid injection, followed by 6 mg/kg on alternate succeeding days for two to four doses if no toxicity is observed. The maximal daily dose has been established arbitrarily at 800 mg. It is prudent to be conservative during the first course of therapy, and treatment should be discontinued at the earliest manifestation of toxicity (usually stomatitis or diarrhea) because the maximal effects of bone-marrow suppression will not be evident until the ninth to fourteenth day. The first course of therapy should be administered either in the hospital or under extremely close supervision in order to establish the tolerance of the individual patient. After a period of 4 weeks from the first injection of the preceding course, a new course of therapy is initiated; the dosage is adjusted on the basis of the previous response and is repeated at monthly intervals. Another type of maintenance schedule is 10 to 15 mg/kg or 600 mg/sq m, administered weekly as a single rapid injection. It is usually necessary to produce mild-to-moderate toxicity in order to achieve significant antineoplastic effects.

In the selection of patients, the roles of nutritional deficiencies and protein depletion have been stressed, particularly in relation to surgery. Reduced tolerance of the hematopoietic system may be present in elderly patients or as a result of invasion of the bone marrow by either neoplastic cells or myelofibrosis. Patients with compromised bone-marrow function as a result of previous therapy either with alkylating agents or x-ray to the pelvis or vertebrae are particularly sensitive to the myelosuppressive action of these compounds. In such circumstances, the granulocyte response after stimulation with a standardized dose of bacterial endotoxin (*pyrexal*) has proven helpful in predicting the functional reserve of the bone marrow (Fink and Calabresi, 1962). In patients with extensive liver metastases, catabolism of the drug may be markedly impaired and therapy may be contraindicated; if treatment is instituted, reduced doses must be administered to prevent the hazards of overdosage. A relatively simple metabolism test, in which the capacity of the subject to convert uracil-2-^{14}C to $^{14}CO_2$ is measured, can be a helpful guide to therapy by assessing the degree of impairment of this hepatic function (Creasey et al., 1967).

Fluorouracil has been administered by infusion into the hepatic artery with favorable results in patients with metastases to the liver (Ansfield et al., 1971; Tandon et al., 1973).

Topical fluorouracil as a 1 or 5% cream or a 1 to 5% solution in propylene glycol (EFUDEX, FLUOROPLEX) has been used successfully in dermatology.

Floxuridine, N.F. (*fluorodeoxyuridine, FUdR*), is available for injection as a powder, 500 mg in 5-ml containers. It may be administered in schedules identical with those of fluorouracil, except that the individual doses, in milligrams, are twice those used with the latter agent. Continuous infusion of floxuridine has produced objective responses with 1/30 to 1/60 the dose necessary with multiple individual doses, but with similar toxicity (Sullivan and Miller, 1965). Continuous infusion of fluorinated pyrimidines into the arterial blood supply of localized tumors, particularly in the liver or in the head and neck region, may provide beneficial clinical effects (Sullivan et al., 1967). Intra-arterial infusions, at doses of 0.1 to 0.6 mg/kg for 24 hours, are administered continuously until local toxicity is encountered.

Therapeutic Uses and Clinical Toxicity. Clinical use of fluorinated pyrimidines has been concerned primarily with *fluorouracil,* and accumulated experience indicates that the drug can be of considerable palliative value in certain types of carcinoma, particularly of the breast and the gastrointestinal tract (*see* Moore et al., 1968); beneficial effects have also been reported in hepatoma, as well as in carcinoma of the ovary, cervix, urinary bladder, prostate, pancreas, and oropharyngeal areas. (For references to the original literature, *see also* Calabresi and Welch, 1962; Livingston and Carter, 1970; Greenwald, 1973; Heidelberger, 1973.) Fluorouracil is widely used with very favorable results for the topical treatment of premalignant keratoses of the skin and multiple superficial basal-cell carcinomas (Klein et al., 1972).

Although fluorouracil and its deoxyribonucleoside are capable of exerting beneficial effects on human tumors, the available evidence indicates that neither agent *per se,* in doses tolerated by the normal tissues, will cause the complete disappearance of any neoplasm. However, remissions for 5 years and even longer have been reported, despite the presence of residual disease. Evidence has been lacking to encourage the expectation that significant overall prolongation of life can be achieved in the majority of patients; however, in patients responding to therapy (Brennan et al., 1964) and in retrospective study of cases with disseminated breast cancer, an increased survival has been reported (Heidelberger, 1965; Ansfield et al., 1969).

The clinical manifestations of toxicity caused by fluorouracil and floxuridine are similar and may be difficult to anticipate because of their delayed appearance. The earliest untoward symptoms during a course of therapy are anorexia and nausea; these are followed shortly after by stomatitis and diarrhea, which constitute reliable warning signs that a sufficient dose has been administered. Stomatitis may be preceded by a sensation of dryness, followed by erythema and formation of a white, patchy membrane that develops into ulceration and necrosis. The occurrence of similar lesions in the stoma of colostomies and at post-mortem examination of the gastrointestinal tract, as well as complaints of dysphagia, retrosternal burning, and proctitis, indicates that enteric injury may occur at any level. The major toxic effects, however, result from the myelosuppressive action of these drugs; clinically, the effects are most frequently manifested as leukopenia, which may begin as early as the second or third day of treatment or as late as the third week. The nadir of the leukopenia is usually between the ninth and fourteenth day after the first injection of drug. Thrombocytopenia and anemia may complicate the picture. Loss of hair, occasionally progressing to total alopecia, nail changes, dermatitis, and increased pigmentation and atrophy of the skin may be encountered. Neurological manifestations have been reported, and myelopathy has been observed after the intrathecal administration of fluorouracil. The low therapeutic indices of these agents emphasize the need for very skillful supervision by physicians familiar with the action of the fluorinated pyrimidines and the possible hazards of chemotherapy.

CYTARABINE (CYTOSINE ARABINOSIDE)

Among the more interesting antimetabolites is cytarabine (cytosine arabinoside, arabinosylcytosine, ara-C), more properly called 1-β-D-arabinofuranosylcytosine. The profound effects of this agent on the growth of certain experimental tumors (Evans *et al.,* 1961) led to its preliminary investigation in man (Talley and Vaitkevicius, 1963). Its clinical usefulness in acute leukemia, alone and in combination with other agents, is well established. (For references, *see* Livingston and Carter, 1970; Greenwald, 1973; Ho and Freireich, 1975.)

Mechanism of Action. This compound may be viewed as an analog of 2'-deoxycytidine in which there is a hydroxyl group on the 2' position that is trans to the hydroxyl group on the 3' position. The structural formula is shown in Table 62–2. The hydroxyl group on the 2' position causes steric hindrance to the rotation of the pyrimidine base around the nucleosidic bond. The bases of polyarabinonucleotide cannot stack normally as do the bases of polydeoxynucleotides. This might lead to nucleic acid dysfunction if arabinosylcytosine residues replace deoxycytidines in a nucleic acid.

As with most purine and pyrimidine antimetabolites, cytarabine must be "activated" by conversion to the 5'-monophosphate nucleotide, in this case catalyzed by deoxycytidine kinase. The nucleotide analog, AraCMP, can react with appropriate nucleotide kinases to form the diphosphate and triphosphate nucleotides (AraCDP and AraCTP).

Despite much investigation and the identification of several potentially important biochemical effects, there is still no agreement on a single site of action to explain the cytotoxicity of cytarabine. Early investigations by Chu and Fischer (1962) suggested a block of ribonucleoside diphosphate reductase by a nucleotide of cytarabine, such as AraCTP, as a crucial effect. Studies with partially purified preparations of the enzyme from Novikoff ascites cells revealed only moderate inhibition by AraCDP and AraCTP (Moore and Cohen, 1967). Since ribonucleoside diphosphate reductase is subject to complex feedback control by deoxynucleotides, it is possible that distortion of the deoxynucleotide pools by cytarabine administration causes secondary inhibition of the enzyme. Several other biochemical effects appear significant. An important observation is that AraCTP, in concentrations achievable in cells, is a potent inhibitor of calf thymus DNA polymerase ($K_i \cong 1\ \mu$M). Recently it has been shown that AraCTP is about 200 times more inhibitory to a virally induced RNA-dependent DNA polymerase (reverse transcriptase) than to the DNA-dependent

enzyme. The inhibition of DNA polymerases can adequately account for the marked inhibition of DNA synthesis and the S-phase–specific action of cytarabine, but it has not yet been definitely correlated with cytotoxicity.

In addition to their ability to block nucleic acid polymerases, nucleotides of cytarabine can become incorporated into both the RNA and DNA of the cell. There is no clear evidence, however, that DNA-chain termination occurs, and little correlation is seen between lethality and the degree of incorporation of cytarabine into DNA. On the other hand, acute cell death, not reversible by deoxycytidine administration, has been correlated with the amount of incorporation of antimetabolites into RNA (Chu and Fischer, 1968; Chu, 1971).

Since most of its actions relate closely to DNA biosynthesis and function, cytarabine is regarded as specific for the S phase of the cell cycle (Skipper and Schabel, 1973).

Mechanism of Resistance to Cytarabine. Both natural and acquired resistance to cytarabine occur. Many normal tissues, as well as some tumors not susceptible to cytarabine, have high concentrations of cytidine deaminase, an enzyme capable of converting cytarabine to the noncytotoxic metabolite, arabinosyl uracil. The ratio of deoxycytidine kinase to cytidine deaminase is a key factor in determining susceptibility of tissues to cytarabine (Chabner *et al.,* 1975). A powerful and apparently irreversible inhibitor of this deaminase, tetrahydrouridine, has been identified (Comiener and Smith, 1968), which causes increases in the plasma half-life and excretion of unchanged drug when administered together with cytarabine. It has not been determined, however, whether inhibition of the deamination of cytarabine effects a favorable change in its therapeutic index. It seems probable that tissues normally protected by cytidine deaminase will suffer adverse effects if cytarabine is administered in combination with tetrahydrouridine.

Several biochemical mutations have been identified that result in acquired resistance to the cytotoxicity of cytarabine. Most frequently seen are deletions or modifications of deoxycytidine kinase, the enzyme required for the "lethal synthesis" of AraCMP (Chu and Fischer, 1965). Less frequent are mutants possessing DNA polymerases with decreased affinity for AraCTP (Creasey, 1975a).

Immunosuppressive Action. In addition to its antineoplastic activity, cytarabine has demonstrated immunosuppressive properties (Calabresi, 1967; Mitchell *et al.,* 1969a, 1969b). It is of interest that variations in dosage or schedule of administration selectively suppress humoral or cellular immunity (Calabresi, 1967; Griswold *et al.,* 1972). These findings have led to the demonstration that plasma blocking factors (humoral antibodies) can be selectively suppressed by cytarabine, with resultant inhibition of tumor growth by cellular immunity (Calabresi *et al.,* 1972; Heppner and Calabresi, 1972).

Although cytarabine is capable of inhibiting DNA

viruses and has been used clinically to treat viral infections (*see* Chapter 61), the use of idoxuridine (iododeoxyuridine, IUdR) is preferred, since this antimetabolite does not demonstrate the potentially deleterious immunosuppressive properties of cytarabine. Adverse effects of cytarabine on disseminated herpes zoster have been reported in a controlled clinical study in which depression of immunological responses was demonstrated (Stevens *et al.,* 1973). Of considerable interest in this respect is the finding that idoxuridine is capable of significantly enhancing antibody production, through mechanisms yet to be explained (Griswold *et al.,* 1975).

Absorption, Fate, and Excretion. Cytarabine is poorly and unpredictably absorbed orally, with less than 20% of the drug reaching the circulation. After intravenous administration of a 5- or 10-mg/kg dose of ^{3}H-labeled drug to patients with neoplastic disease, the blood concentration is no longer measurable after 20 minutes in most patients (Creasey *et al.,* 1966). Other workers describe a biphasic plasma disappearance curve, with an initial rapid phase ($t_{1/2} = 111$ minutes) (Ho and Frei, 1971). Only 4 to 10% of the injected dose is excreted unchanged in the urine within 12 to 24 hours, while 86 to 96% of the radioactivity appears as the inactive, deaminated product, arabinosyl uracil. Higher concentrations of cytarabine are found in CSF after continuous infusion than after rapid intravenous injection. After intrathecal administration of the drug at a dose of 50 mg/sq m, relatively little deamination occurred, even after 7 hours (Ho and Frei, 1971).

Preparation, Route of Administration, and Dosage. *Cytarabine,* U.S.P. (CYTOSAR), is marketed for the treatment of acute leukemias in children and adults. It is supplied as a lyophilized powder in multidose vials containing either 100 or 500 mg of drug, to be reconstituted for injection by adding 5 or 10 ml, respectively, of water. The optimal regimen has not yet been established. From the available data, two dosage schedules are recommended: (1) rapid intravenous injection of 2 mg/kg daily for 10 days—if no toxic or beneficial effects are noted, the dose may be doubled (4 mg/kg daily) and continued until either a therapeutic response or toxicity is encountered; (2) continuous infusion of 0.5 to 1.0 mg/kg (or 30 mg/sq m of body surface) daily, administered by intravenous infusion during a period of 1 to 24 hours—if neither a toxic nor a therapeutic response is obtained in 10 days, the dose may be increased to 2 mg/kg daily, until the desired effect is obtained or toxicity intervenes. In general, children seem to tolerate higher doses than do adults. *Maintenance* therapy with subcutaneous injections of 1.0 mg/kg, weekly or every other week, can be used, although the drug appears more effective for the *induction* of remissions in acute leukemia. Investigations of its efficacy and safety in the treatment of meningeal leukemia, by intrathecal injection, are in progress.

Therapeutic Use and Clinical Toxicity. Cytarabine is indicated for *induction* of remission in acute leukemia in children and adults. Remission rates of 20 to 40% have been reported (Livingston and Carter, 1970; Greenwald, 1973). The drug is particularly useful in acute granulocytic leukemia in adults, since chemotherapy is generally disappointing in this disorder. Clinical studies indicate that cytarabine may be more effective when used with other agents, particularly with thioguanine and daunorubicin (Crowther *et al.,* 1970; Livingston and Carter, 1970; Clarkson, 1972; Heidelberger, 1973). The drug has been studied in patients with a variety of neoplastic diseases. Beneficial effects have been observed in Hodgkin's disease and related lymphomas but very rarely in patients with carcinomas or other tumors. Cytarabine is primarily a potent myelosuppressive agent capable of producing severe leukopenia, thrombocytopenia, and anemia with striking megaloblastic changes. Other toxic manifestations reported include gastrointestinal disturbances and, less frequently, stomatitis, hepatic dysfunction, thrombophlebitis at the site of injection, fever, and dermatitis.

AZARIBINE

The first triazene analog of the series was azauracil, a compound that could not be used clinically because of CNS toxicity. The ribonucleoside, azauridine, exerted antineoplastic activity without neurotoxicity, but only when administered intravenously. The triacetyl derivative, azaribine, was synthesized in order to achieve better absorption by oral administration, since azauridine is metabolized to azauracil by intestinal microorganisms (Handschumacher *et al.,* 1962; Creasey *et al.,* 1963). Azaribine has been extremely effective in the treatment of psoriasis and polycythemia vera (DeConti and Calabresi, 1970; Skoda, 1975).

Chemistry. The structural formulas of azauridine (AzUR) and azaribine (2', 3', 5'-triacetyl-6-azauridine) are shown in Table 62-2, and their chemical relationship to other pyrimidine analogs is discussed above.

Mechanism of Action. Azaribine is deacetylated in the blood to AzUR, and this in turn undergoes intracellular conversion to 6-azauridylic acid (AzUMP). Resistant tumor cells lack uridine kinase, which is required to activate AzUR. AzUMP inhibits the formation of uridylic acid from its carboxylated precursor, orotidylic acid, by blocking the enzyme orotidylate decarboxylase in the *de-novo* pathway of pyrimidine biosynthesis. Significant amounts of orotic acid and orotidine are excreted in the urine. The drug also has demonstrated uricosuric properties.

General Toxicity and Cytotoxic Action. Of particular importance are the evident selectivity of azaribine in man and its remarkable lack of toxicity even when administered at relatively high doses. Normal leukopoiesis and thrombocytopoiesis are not markedly affected by prolonged administration. Moderate anemia, characterized by mild megaloblastic changes, reticulocytopenia, and elevated plasma iron concentrations, occurs after chronic use of high doses of drug and constitutes the basis for its use in polycythemia vera (Calabresi and Turner, 1966). This is readily reversible by discontinuation of drug or by administration of uridine. Hair loss, dermatitis, hepatotoxicity, renal toxicity, and severe gastrointestinal toxicity have not been encountered in several hundred patients treated with this agent.

Absorption, Fate, and Excretion. Azaribine is well absorbed after oral administration. Preparations must be of high quality, because the presence of even small quantities of unacetylated AzUR results in catabolism, by intestinal microorganisms, to azauracil, a neurotoxic metabolite. After absorption, azaribine is almost entirely deacetylated to AzUR in the blood, with some monoacetyl derivative detectable. Peak plasma concentrations of AzUR are reached after 2 to 4 hours, and a plasma disappearance curve with a half-time of approximately 6 to 8 hours is observed. Unlike azauracil, AzUR does not cross the blood-brain barrier and is not detectable in the CSF. When neurotoxic manifestations have been encountered, significant concentrations of azauracil have been measured in the CSF. Approximately 95% of an ingested dose of azaribine is excreted in the urine as AzUR within 16 hours.

Preparation, Dosage, and Route of Administration. *Azaribine* (TRIAZURE) is available for investigational purposes as 500-mg tablets for oral administration. It is indicated for the treatment of severe, recalcitrant, and disabling psoriasis that is not adequately responsive to topical forms of therapy. The recommended dosage is 125 mg/kg daily, administered at 8-hour intervals in three equally divided doses. Occasionally, it may be necessary to use doses up to 200 mg/kg daily. Therapy should be continued until a remission is achieved or moderate anemia intervenes. Clearing of the lesions usually occurs within 8 weeks, after which a remission of several months may ensue. In some patients intermittent maintenance therapy may be required, and reduction of dosage by at least 20% may be necessary if anemia is a significant problem.

At higher dosages in the range of 270 mg/kg daily (administered at 8-hour intervals in three equally divided doses for several weeks), azaribine may result in significant but reversible suppression of erythropoiesis, a finding that prompted its use in polycythemia vera (DeConti and Calabresi, 1970). At these dosages the drug has also been effective in the therapy of mycosis fungoides.

Therapeutic Uses and Clinical Toxicity. Azaribine is extremely effective in the treatment of *generalized psoriasis* (Calabresi and Turner, 1966), and remission rates of 70 to 90% have been reported by several investigators. Although the drug may be of considerable benefit in treating the acute manifestations of psoriatic arthritis, it has caused unexplained exacerbations in patients with rheumatoid arthritis.

When used at higher doses, azaribine has proven more effective and less toxic than other agents in the treatment of *mycosis fungoides* and deserves further study in the management of *polycythemia vera;* clinical toxicity is usually minimal or absent. Hematopoietic suppression appears to be relatively selective

for erythropoiesis, with very little if any effect noted on normal leukocyte or platelet counts. Signs of mild CNS dysfunction, including drowsiness, lethargy, and dizziness, have been reported with lower doses, while hyperreflexia, tremor, diplopia, expressive aphasia, and dysarthria may occur at higher doses. These effects subside promptly upon discontinuation of the medication. Gastrointestinal intolerance may be experienced and can often be circumvented by administering the drug with food. Although thromboembolic manifestations have been encountered in patients with psoriasis treated with azaribine, recent evidence indicates that a previously undetected, increased incidence of this complication occurs in psoriasis and is actually reduced by azaribine therapy (McDonald and Calabresi, 1974).

PURINE ANALOGS

Since the pioneering studies of Hitchings and associates, begun in 1942, a large number of analogs of natural purine bases, nucleosides, and nucleotides have been prepared and studied in a wide variety of biological and biochemical systems. The first of the base analogs found to have marked anticancer activity in experimental tumors were 8-azaguanine and 2,6-diaminopurine; although they did not prove useful in the clinic, they stimulated great interest in the search for more active purine and pyrimidine analogs.

The first clinically effective antipurine, *mercaptopurine* (6-mercaptopurine, 6-MP), was described in Elion and coworkers in 1952 and shortly thereafter was found to have significant activity against human leukemias (Burchenal *et al.*, 1953). Today, mercaptopurine, often used with other drugs, is a valuable purine analog for the treatment of *acute leukemia.* In addition, drugs of this class have been shown to have *immunosuppressive activity,* and a derivative of mercaptopurine, *azathioprine,* is frequently used for the suppression of the immune response, for example, in the prevention of the rejection phenomenon in organ transplantations.

Widespread interest continues in this class of compounds, not only as potential drugs but also as important tools for the dissection of biochemical reactions. As often occurs when a group of chemical agents is subjected to intensive biochemical and pharmacological study, activities are uncovered that lead to uses not originally anticipated. For example, arabinosyl adenine (ara-A) has shown unusual promise against DNA viruses (Ch'ien *et al.*, 1973), and the hypoxanthine analog *allopurinol,* a powerful inhibitor of *xanthine oxidase,* has proven of great value in the treatment of hyperuricemic states (*see* Chapter 17). (For details of the original literature, *see* reviews by Elion and Hitchings, 1965, 1975; Paterson and Tidd, 1975.)

Structure-Activity Relationship. The two purine analogs most useful in the therapy of human leukemia, mercaptopurine and thioguanine, may be viewed as analogs of the natural purines hypoxanthine and guanine, in which the hydroxyl group on the 6 position of the purine ring is replaced by a sulfhydryl group (Table 62–3). Substitution of the hydroxyl group by chloride or selenide also yields compounds with cytotoxic activity. A large number of analogs have been prepared in which the purine ring structure is modified. Of the many other compounds that have been tested, none has yet proved of clinical value. Almost all the purine and purine nucleoside analogs that have cytotoxic activity are capable of cellular enzymatic conversion to nucleotides.

Attempts have been made to modify the structures of mercaptopurine and thioguanine so as to retain biological activity while altering their metabolic degradation. Azathioprine (Table 62–3) was developed with the intent of protecting the sulfhydryl radical of mercaptopurine from rapid methylation or oxidation and to provide a substance from which the active moiety would be released slowly. Azathioprine can react, apparently nonenzymatically, with sulfhydryl groups (most likely with erythrocytic

Table 62–3. STRUCTURAL FORMULAS OF PURINE ANALOGS *

Thioguanine

Mercaptopurine

Azathioprine

* The structures of hypoxanthine and allopurinol are presented in Chapter 17 (Table 17–3, page 353).

glutathione) and thereby cause the slow liberation of free mercaptopurine. Superior immunosuppressive activity is achieved in comparison with the parent compound (Elion, 1967), although this has been questioned (Berenbaum, 1971).

The glutamine antagonists azaserine (O-diazoacetyl-L-serine), 6-diazo-5-oxo-L-norleucine (DON), and duazomycin, although not purine analogs, are potent inhibitors of the *de-novo* pathway of purine nucleotide biosynthesis. These glutamine analogs are diazoketones with chemical reactivities resembling those of diazomethane. They inhibit purine biosynthesis through the formation of covalent bonds with a cysteine residue in the active site of a key enzyme in the pathway, formylglycinamide ribotide amidotransferase. Although these compounds have only weak cytostatic activity when used alone, they can produce significant potentiation when administered with purine analogs such as mercaptopurine or thioguanine (Bennett, 1975).

Mechanism of Action. Although purine analogs and their derivatives have been subjected to intensive study in many laboratories with the disclosure of a number of specific biochemical effects, the mechanisms by which these compounds bring about cell death still are not established, nor is there clear evidence concerning the crucial question why these compounds have greater activity on certain malignant tissues than on most normal tissues. Despite the lack of ultimate answers, one must note that considerable information has been obtained regarding many metabolic effects of these compounds, and such studies have contributed greatly to our understanding of metabolism and its regulation. In the following discussion, it is assumed that the reader understands the biosynthesis of nucleic acids; if this is not the case, he should consult an outline of metabolic pathways.

Most of the antitumor purine analogs examined to date are not active as such, and must undergo a "lethal" synthesis, with formation of *5'-phosphate ribonucleotides*. Many analogs of *hypoxanthine* and *guanine* are substrates for the enzyme hypoxanthine-guanine phosphoribosyl transferase (HGPRT), whereas *adenine* analogs may react with the enzyme adenine phosphoribosyl transferase. These enzymes catalyze the reaction of the base analog with the phosphorylated pentose, 5-phosphoribosyl-1-pyrophosphate (PRPP).

Enzymes capable of catalyzing the direct phosphorylation of *inosine, guanosine,* or their analogs to the nucleotide level have not been unequivocally demonstrated in animal tissues, and analogs of inosine or guanosine must be cleaved by purine nucleoside phosphorylase to liberate the base analog in order to have activity; however, there are enzymes that will convert *adenosine* or its analogs to adenosine-5'-phosphate or its congeners. Adenosine kinase may also convert 6-methylmercaptopurine ribonucleoside (6-MMPR) to the 5'-phosphate ribonucleotide.

The 5'-phosphate ribonucleotide of mercaptopurine, thioinosinate (T-IMP), formed within cells, may inhibit a number of vital metabolic reactions. T-IMP can block the conversion of inosinate (IMP) to adenylosuccinate (AMPS), a key reaction in the formation of adenylate. Also, T-IMP can inhibit, and perhaps react with, inosinic dehydrogenase, the enzyme that catalyzes the conversion of IMP to xanthylate (XMP), a key step in the formation of guanylate (GMP) from IMP. Thus, T-IMP, in concentrations actually demonstrated in tumor cells, can block the synthesis of both AMPS and GMP from the "bridgehead" nucleotide, IMP. In addition, there is evidence that T-IMP is capable of "pseudo-feedback inhibition" of the first committed step in the *de-novo* pathway of purine biosynthesis, the reaction of glutamine and PRPP to form ribosylamine-5-phosphate, catalyzed by PRPP-amidotransferase. The regulation of this enzyme serves as a major control of purine biosynthesis, and it is highly responsive to the intracellular concentrations of 5'-monophosphate ribonucleotides. Analog as well as normal nucleotides can inhibit this enzyme. T-IMP in murine tumor tissue can reach the level of 0.1 mM, or greater, a concentration that is capable of inducing strong inhibition of ribosylamine-5-phosphate synthesis (Paterson, 1959).

The ribonucleotide 6-thioguanosine-5'-phosphate (6-thioGMP) also inhibits several enzymes of purine metabolism. 6-ThioGMP has high affinity but very low reactivity with guanylate kinase, the specific enzyme that converts GMP to GDP, and thus acts as a competitive inhibitor (Miech *et al.*, 1969). Because of the slow rate of removal while synthesis continues, 6-thioGMP may accumulate in tumor tissues to the level of 0.1 mM or higher (Moore and LePage, 1958). The concentrations of 6-thioGMP achieved are sufficient to cause progressive and irreversible inhibition of the enzyme inosinic dehydrogenase, presumably through the formation of disulfide bonds (Hampton, 1963; Anderson and Sartorelli, 1969). In addition, 6-thioGMP is a potent "pseudo-feedback inhibitor" of ribosylamine-5-phosphate synthesis. Despite the accumulation of 6-thioIMP in high concentrations in tissues, the diphosphate and triphosphate nucleotides are not formed. On the other hand, although the diphosphate and triphosphate nucleotides of thioguanine are formed slowly, impressive intracellular concentrations of 6-thioGTP can accumulate with time (Parks *et al.*, 1973).

Although only small amounts of mercaptopurine are incorporated into the nucleic acids, somewhat larger amounts of thioguanine can be incorporated into the DNA of susceptible murine tumors and it has been postulated that this incorporation into DNA is the cause of cell death (LePage, 1968). Arguments both for (Barranco and Humphrey, 1971) and against (Scannell and Hitchings, 1966) this hypothesis have been made.

Of considerable interest is the observation that 6-MMPR is capable of inhibiting the growth of cells that have acquired resistance to purine analogs, such as mercaptopurine, through loss of the enzyme HGPRT. This analog ribonucleoside, although it does not serve as a substrate for purine nucleoside phosphorylase, is mistaken for adenosine by the enzyme adenosine kinase and is converted to the ribonucleotide. Thus, it is possible to form an analog nucleotide by a different enzymatic mechanism than

is employed for the purine base analogs, such as mercaptopurine. Furthermore, the nucleotide formed, 6-methylmercaptopurine ribonucleoside 5'-phosphate (6-MMPR-P), is an unusually potent "pseudo-feedback inhibitor" of the formation of ribosylamine 5-phosphate (Hill and Bennett, 1969). The analog nucleotide 6-MMPR-P can accumulate in unusually high amounts in tumor cells, as well as in human erythrocytes, and can cause a number of unusual biochemical effects (Nelson and Parks, 1972; Warnick and Paterson, 1973). In tumor cells, after a delay of several hours, marked increases occur in the intracellular concentrations of PRPP, in the rate and degree of synthesis of analog nucleotides, such as 6-thioGMP, and in the concentrations of pyrimidine nucleotides, such as uridine triphosphate (UTP) or cytidine triphosphate (CTP). Also, intracellular degradation of 6-thioGMP is impeded. In accord with these biochemical effects, striking synergism occurs in animal tumor systems when 6-MMPR is used in combination with a thiopurine, such as thioguanine or mercaptopurine. These findings suggested the concomitant use of 6-MMPR with purine analogs in the therapy of human malignancy. Clinical reports indicate that a higher incidence of complete remissions can be obtained in acute myelogenous leukemia when mercaptopurine is given with 6-MMPR than when either drug is used alone (Freireich *et al.*, 1967).

Mechanisms of Resistance to Antipurines. As with other tumor-inhibiting antimetabolites, the occurrence of acquired resistance represents perhaps the major obstacle to the successful use of antipurines. Many studies have been performed with experimental systems to determine the mechanisms of resistance to purine analogs, such as mercaptopurine; the most commonly encountered finding is the deficiency or complete lack of the enzyme HGPRT. Since this enzyme is not essential for cell survival but is required for the "lethal" synthesis of fraudulent ribonucleotides of guanine or hypoxanthine analogs, cells deficient in this enzyme would not be damaged by exposure to a drug such as mercaptopurine and would be selected for growth and survival. Cells that are resistant by means of this mechanism usually show cross-resistance between such analogs as mercaptopurine, thioguanine, and azaguanine.

Another mechanism of resistance, identified first with thioguanine-resistant sarcoma 180 tumors, that has recently been found in a number of thiopurine-resistant leukemic patients is an increase in particulate alkaline phosphatase activity (Wolpert *et al.*, 1971). It has been proposed that competitive inhibition of this enzyme by the 5'-mononucleotide of 6-MMPR, by impeding degradation of other analog nucleotides (*e.g.*, 6-thioGMP), may play a role in the synergism seen between 6-MMPR and other thiopurines (Nelson and Parks, 1972).

Other mechanisms of drug resistance to purine antimetabolites have been described (*see* Hutchinson, 1965; Stock, 1966; Brockman, 1974). They include (1) "exclusion" of mercaptopurine from contact with HGPRT in the intact, resistant cell; (2) an increased rate of degradation of the purine base or ribonucleoside analogs; (3) an alteration in the "pseudo-feedback inhibition" of ribosylamine 5-phosphate synthesis (Henderson *et al.*, 1967); and (4) genetic loss of the enzyme adenine phosphoribosyltransferase or adenosine kinase, which makes cells resistant to analogs of adenine or adenosine, for example, 6-MMPR.

The mechanisms whereby human malignancies develop resistance to purine analogs have been difficult to study, and only recently has information become available on this crucial subject. In an early study, the cells of only 1 of 15 leukemic patients resistant to mercaptopurine were found to be deficient in HGPRT (Davidson and Winter, 1964). In another report the HGPRT of leukemic leukocytes from a patient resistant to thioguanine required a much higher concentration of PRPP for maximal velocity than did the enzyme from sensitive cells (Rosman and Williams, 1973). In a study of cells from leukemic patients with acquired resistance to thiopurines, both increased alkaline phosphatase activity and decreased HGPRT activity were detected in 5 of 11 acute nonlymphocytic leukemic patients and 6 of 7 acute lymphocytic leukemic patients. Interestingly, cells from all of the resistant acute lymphocytic leukemics displayed significant increases in particulate alkaline phosphatase activity (Rosman *et al.*, 1974). It is to be hoped that the incidence of acquired resistance to purine analogs in human malignancies can be minimized by the use of appropriate combination chemotherapy. The development of agents that can bypass the enzyme HGPRT or effectively block degradation of thiopurine nucleotides by the particulate alkaline phosphatases is of obvious potential importance.

MERCAPTOPURINE

The introduction of mercaptopurine by Elion and coworkers represents a landmark in the history of antineoplastic and immunosuppressive therapy. Today this antipurine and its derivative, azathioprine, are among the most important and clinically useful drugs of the class. The structure-activity relationship and the mechanism of action and of drug resistance are discussed above. The structural formula of mercaptopurine is presented in Table 62–3.

Absorption, Fate, and Excretion. Mercaptopurine is readily absorbed after oral ingestion. The intestinal epithelium is not damaged in the process. About one half of an oral dose can be accounted for as urinary excretion products in the first 24 hours. After an intravenous dose, the half-life of the drug is relatively short (about 90 minutes) due to uptake by cells, renal excretion, and rapid metabolic degradation. There are two main pathways for the metabolism of mercaptopurine. The first involves methylation of the sulfhydryl group and subsequent oxidation of the methylated derivatives. The formation of nucleotides of 6-methylmercaptopurine has been shown to occur following administration of mercaptopurine or mercaptopurine ribonucleoside (Allan *et al.*, 1966). Substantial amounts of the mono, di, and triphosphate nucleotides of 6-MMPR have been identified in the blood and bone marrow of patients treated with mercaptopurine or azathioprine (Zimmerman *et al.*, 1974). Desulfuration of thiopurines can occur, and relatively large percentages of the administered sulfur are excreted as inorganic sulfate. The second major pathway for mercaptopurine metabolism involves the enzyme xanthine oxidase, which is present in relatively large amounts in the liver. Mercaptopurine is a good substrate for this enzyme, which oxidizes it to 6-thiouric acid, a noncarcinostatic metabolite (Elion, 1967).

An attempt to modify the metabolic inactivation of mercaptopurine by xanthine oxidase led to the development of *allopurinol.* This analog of hypoxanthine is a powerful inhibitor of xanthine oxidase, and not only blocks the conversion of mercaptopurine to 6-thiouric acid but also interferes with the production of uric acid from hypoxanthine and xanthine (*see* Chapter 17). Because of its ability to interfere with the enzymatic oxidation of mercaptopurine and related derivatives, allopurinol increases the exposure of cells to the action of these compounds. Although it greatly potentiates the antineoplastic action of mercaptopurine in tumor-bearing mice, allopurinol increases the toxicity as well, and there is no apparent improvement in the therapeutic index.

Preparation, Dosage, and Route of Administration. *Mercaptopurine,* U.S.P. (*6-mercaptopurine;* PURINETHOL), is marketed as scored, 50-mg tablets. The average daily oral dose is 2.5 mg/kg. The drug is administered as a single dose given at any convenient hour of the day. Starting doses usually range from 100 to 200 mg a day; with hematological and clinical improvement, the dose is diminished to an appropriate multiple of 25 mg and, in general, maintenance therapy of 50 to 100 mg a day is continued. If beneficial effects have not been noted after 4 weeks, the dose may be increased gradually until evidence of toxicity is encountered. The total dose required to produce depression of the bone marrow in patients with nonhematological malignancies is about 45 mg/kg and may range from 18 to 106 mg/kg.

Hyperuricemia with hyperuricosuria may occur during treatment; the accumulation of uric acid presumably reflects the destruction of cells with release of purines that are oxidized by xanthine oxidase, as well as an inhibition of the conversion of inosinic acid to precursors of nucleic acids. This circumstance may be an indication for the use of *allopurinol*. Special caution must be employed if mercaptopurine or its imidazolyl derivative, azathioprine, is used with allopurinol, for reasons presented above. Patients treated simultaneously with both drugs should receive approximately 25% of the usual dose of mercaptopurine.

Therapeutic Uses and Clinical Toxicity. In the early studies with mercaptopurine, bone-marrow remissions were described in over 40% of children with *acute leukemia*, and some benefit was obtained in an additional group (Burchenal, 1954). In the acute leukemias in adults, the results have been much less impressive, but occasional remissions have been obtained with mercaptopurine (Ellison *et al.*, 1972). It is important to emphasize that cross-resistance does not occur between mercaptopurine and other classes of antileukemic agents.

A review of clinical results with mercaptopurine (Burchenal and Ellison, 1961) indicates that in acute leukemia a rapid decrease in the total leukocyte count may begin about 5 or 6 days after the initiation of therapy; on the other hand, a period of 2 to 4 weeks of continuous daily administration may be necessary before a response is observed. The average time necessary for the appearance of bone-marrow remissions in responsive adults is 7 to 8 weeks. The drug has contributed significantly to the treatment of lymphoblastic leukemia, more by maintaining than by inducing remissions (Frei *et al.*, 1965; Zubrod, 1967; Holland and Glidewell, 1972).

In the treatment of chronic granulocytic leukemia, maintenance therapy with mercaptopurine can be useful, but the drug of choice is busulfan, which is less damaging to the proliferation of normal bone-marrow elements. Mercaptopurine, unlike busulfan, may induce a brief remission in the "blastic crisis" that often terminates this disease. Although partial responses have been reported, the drug has not been of value in the therapy of a wide variety of other malignant diseases, including chronic lymphocytic leukemia, Hodgkin's disease, and related lymphomas (*see* Livingston and Carter, 1970; Greenwald, 1973).

The principal toxic effect of this drug is bone-marrow depression, although, in general, this develops more gradually than with folic acid antagonists; accordingly, thrombocytopenia, granulocytopenia, or anemia may not be encountered for several weeks. When depression of normal bone-

marrow elements occurs, cessation of therapy with the drug usually results in prompt recovery. Anorexia, nausea, or vomiting is seen in approximately 25% of adults, but stomatitis and diarrhea are rare; in general, manifestations of gastrointestinal effects are less frequent in children than in adults. The occurrence of jaundice in about one third of adult patients treated with mercaptopurine has been reported (Burchenal and Ellison, 1961); although the pathogenesis of this manifestation is obscure, it usually clears upon discontinuation of therapy. Its appearance has been associated with bile stasis and hepatic necrosis. Dermatological manifestations have been reported. The long-term complications associated with the use of mercaptopurine and its derivative, azathioprine, for immunosuppressive therapy are discussed by Schein and Winokur (1975).

THIOGUANINE

The synthesis of thioguanine was first described by Elion and Hitchings in 1955. It is of particular value in the treatment of acute granulocytic leukemia in combination with cytarabine (Clarkson, 1972). The structural formula of thioguanine is shown in Table 62–3, and its mechanism of action is discussed above.

Absorption, Fate, and Excretion. Peak concentrations in the blood are reached 6 to 8 hours after oral administration of thioguanine, and approximately 40% of the dose is excreted in the urine within 24 hours. When thioguanine is administered to man, the S-methylation product, 2-amino-6-methylthiopurine, rather than free thioguanine appears in the urine. After 8 hours, inorganic sulfate becomes a major urinary metabolite. Lesser amounts of 6-thiouric acid are formed (Elion, 1967), suggesting that deamination catalyzed by the enzyme guanase does not play a major role in the metabolic inactivation of thioguanine. Accordingly, it may be administered in combination with allopurinol without reduction in dosage, unlike mercaptopurine and azathioprine.

Preparation, Dosage, and Route of Administration. *Thioguanine*, U.S.P. (*6-thioguanine, TG*), is available in scored, 40-mg tablets. The average daily dose is 2 mg/kg. If there is no clinical improvement or toxicity after 4 weeks, the dosage may be cautiously increased to 3 mg/kg daily.

Therapeutic Uses and Clinical Toxicity. Clinically, the compound has been used in the treatment of acute leukemia and, in combination with cytarabine, is one of the most effective agents for induction of remissions in acute granulocytic leukemia (Clarkson, 1972); it has not been of value in solid tumors. Thioguanine has been used as an immunosuppressive agent, particularly in patients with nephrosis (Wolff and Goodman, 1962) and with collagen-vascular disorders (Demis et al., 1964). Toxic manifestations include bone-marrow depression and gastrointestinal effects, although the latter may be less pronounced than with mercaptopurine.

III. Natural Products

VINCA ALKALOIDS

History. The beneficial properties of the periwinkle plant (*Vinca rosea* Linn.), a species of myrtle, have been described in medicinal folklore for many years in various parts of the world. An alleged activity as an oral hypoglycemic agent prompted, in 1949, an investigation of crude fractions obtained from this plant. Working with extracts of the periwinkle, Noble and coworkers (1958) were unable to substantiate the claims for hypoglycemic activity in experimental animals; they did, however, observe granulocytopenia and bone-marrow suppression in rats, effects that served to guide the extraction and purification of an active alkaloid, originally termed *vincaleukoblastine*. Other investigations by Johnson and associates demonstrated activity of certain alkaloidal fractions against an acute lymphocytic neoplasm in mice. Fractionation of these extracts yielded four active dimeric alkaloids, now identified by the following nonproprietary names: *vinblastine* (vincaleukoblastine), *vincristine, vinleurosine,* and *vinrosidine.* Only two of these, vinblastine and vincristine, have received extensive clinical investigation. Comprehensive reviews of the vinca alkaloids have been published (Johnson et al., 1963; Symposium, 1968; Johnson, 1973; Creasey, 1975b).

Chemistry. The four vinca alkaloids are very similar chemically. They are asymmetrical dimeric compounds; the structures of vincristine and vinblastine are as follows:

Vincristine

$$R = O{=}\overset{|}{C}{-}H$$

Vinblastine

$$R = \overset{|}{C}H_3$$

No definite information is available regarding metabolic changes that may be necessary for chemical activation or degradative alterations *in vivo.*

Structure-Activity Relationship. The minor differences in structure of these large alkaloidal molecules result in notable differences in toxicity and antitumor spectra of vincristine and vinblastine. Additional minor changes in the structures of the other two active alkaloids apparently are responsible for differences in their experimental antitumor spectra. A number of related dimeric alkaloids are without biological activity; these include neoleurocristine, neoleurosidine, and catharine, which have only one pK_a value, indicating a change, probably to the amide, of the basic nitrogen of the catharanthine portion of the molecule. Removal of the acetyl group at C 4 of one portion of vinblastine destroys its antileukemic activity, as does acetylation of the hydroxyl groups. Either hydrogenation of the double bond or reductive formation of carbinols reduces or destroys activity of these compounds.

Mechanism of Action. The vinca alkaloids are cell-cycle–specific agents and, in common with other drugs such as colchicine and podophyllotoxin, block mitosis with metaphase arrest. The biochemical effects of the vinca alkaloids have been explored extensively, and a number of interesting phenomena have been uncovered. It seems likely, however, that most of the biological activities of these drugs can be explained by their ability to bind specifically with the protein tubulin, a key component of cellular microtubules. When cells are incubated with vinblastine, dissolution of the microtubules occurs, and highly regular crystals are formed that contain 1 mole of bound vinblastine per mole of tubulin. Colchicine and podophyllotoxin also can bind specifically with tubulin, but apparently at a site on the protein different from that bound by vinblastine. Through disruption of the microtubules of the mitotic apparatus, cell division is arrested in metaphase. In the absence of an intact mitotic spindle, the chromosomes may disperse throughout the cytoplasm (exploded mitosis) or may occur in unusual groupings, such as balls or stars. Apparently the inability to segregate chromosomes correctly during mitosis leads ultimately to cellular death.

In addition to their key role in the formation of mitotic spindles, microtubules have been associated with many other cellular functions. Therefore, it is not surprising that vinca alkaloids may affect these functions as well. Some types of cellular movements, phagocytosis, and certain functions of the CNS appear to involve microtubules, which may explain some of the other effects of vinca alkaloids. (See Creasey, 1975b.)

Despite their structural similarity, a remarkable lack of cross-resistance between individual vinca alkaloids has been noted. It has been proposed that their dissimilarities in antitumor spectra, potencies, and toxic effects may be ascribed to variation in their ability to enter specific types of cells, since it is difficult to envision a different mechanism of action for each drug.

Cytotoxic Actions. The growth of a number of experimental tumors in rodents is inhibited by the vinca alkaloids; although the drugs have a similar spectrum of activity, some striking differences are noted. The ability of vinblastine to suppress human choriocarcinoma maintained in the cheek pouch of the hamster is significant in view of subsequent demonstrations of clinical effectiveness in the treatment of this cancer in women. In addition to these and related cytotoxic actions on malignant human cells in culture, the biological spectrum of activity of these compounds extends to certain microorganisms and protozoa.

Clinical as well as experimental studies have demonstrated that bone-marrow depression, chiefly manifested by leukopenia, is the most important cytotoxic effect on normal cells. In this respect, vincristine and vinleurosine are not nearly as potent as vinblastine; with the last, this is the factor that limits the magnitude of dosage. The relatively low toxicity of vincristine for normal cells makes this agent unusual among antineoplastic drugs and one to consider when chemotherapy is required in the presence of impaired bone-marrow function. Loss of hair, presumably secondary to effects on the epithelial cells of the hair follicles, appears to occur more frequently with vincristine than with vinblastine. No definite explanation is available for these and other manifestations of selectivity, such as relative sparing of erythroid elements and megakaryocytes, infrequent cytotoxic effects on the oral and gastrointestinal mucosa, and lack of inhibition of regenerating liver in partially hepatectomized rats (Noble, 1961). Patchy hepatic necrosis has been reported at autopsy in some patients who had received vincristine (Costa *et al.*, 1962).

Neurological Actions. Although neurotoxicity may be occasionally encountered with vinblastine, particularly at high dosage levels, neuromuscular abnormalities are frequently observed with vincristine. Indeed, it is this type of untoward effect that most frequently proves to be the limiting factor during therapy with vincristine. Several types of manifestations have been recognized. In experimental animals, acute toxicity after large doses has been characterized by clonic convulsions, muscular weakness, ataxia, tremors, vomiting, and catalepsy. The development of CNS leukemia in patients receiving vincristine and in hematological remission has been interpreted as evidence that the alkaloid

poorly penetrates the blood-brain barrier. Although torpor, hallucinations, and coma were observed during exploratory clinical studies with very high doses of vincristine (75 µg/kg weekly), peripheral neuropathy is the most common manifestation of neurotoxicity at usual clinical doses. Numbness and tingling of the extremities, followed by weakness, loss of reflexes, foot-drop, ataxia, muscular cramps, and neuritic pains, have been observed frequently. Clinical neurophysiological studies have demonstrated that asymptomatic depression of the Achilles reflex is the earliest and most consistent sign of vincristine-induced neuropathies (Tobin and Sandler, 1968). Muscular weakness involving the larynx and the extrinsic muscles of the eye also has been noted. An effect on the autonomic nervous system may be responsible for severe, and even obstructive, constipation that frequently may develop with prolonged administration of vincristine, but it is seen only rarely with vinblastine. Temporary mental depression, occurring on the second or third day after treatment, especially with vinblastine, may be of clinical significance and is of particular interest because other compounds derived from indole (*e.g.,* lysergic acid diethylamide [LSD], reserpine, and 5-hydroxytryptophan) are known for their effects on mood and behavior.

Absorption, Fate, and Excretion. Unpredictable absorption has been reported after oral administration of vinblastine. The compound is cleared very rapidly from the blood. Within minutes after intravenous injection, radioactively labeled vinblastine is detected mostly in the liver; in less than an hour, significant amounts are no longer present in the circulating blood. Vincristine and vinblastine can be infused into the arterial blood supply of tumors in doses several times larger than those that can be administered intravenously with comparable toxicity; thus, either local uptake or destruction is very rapid. The vinca alkaloids appear to be excreted primarily by the liver into the bile. Radioactively labeled vinblastine has been traced through this route into the intestinal tract, with less than 5% of the label appearing in the urine. Greater toxicity is encountered when vincristine is administered to patients with obstructive jaundice.

Vinblastine

Preparations, Route of Administration, and Dosage. *Vinblastine Sulfate,* U.S.P. (velban), is supplied in ampuls containing 10 mg of dry powder for preparation of fresh solutions (10 ml). Solutions may be stored in the refrigerator for periods of 30 days without significant loss of potency. The drug is given intravenously, either with a needle different from the one employed in filling the syringe or by injection directly into the tubing of an intravenous infusion; special precautions must be taken against subcutaneous extravasation, since this may cause painful irritation and inflammatory changes. The drug should not be injected into an extremity with impaired circulation. After a single dose of 0.1 to 0.15 mg/kg of body weight, hematological responses are observed for 7 to 10 days. If a moderate level of leukopenia (approximately 3000 cells per cubic millimeter) is not attained, the weekly dose may be increased gradually by increments of 0.05 mg/kg of body weight. Beneficial results, however, may occur at lower doses. Once the optimal amount is established, weekly dosage is continued; if the leukocyte count does not return to 4000 cells per cubic millimeter within 10 to 14 days, the treatment schedule is adjusted accordingly. When the disease appears to be under control, cautious prolongation of treatment intervals may be attempted, but in most cases relapse occurs within approximately 3 weeks after the last dose; hence, a maintenance program must be continued indefinitely. Evidence suggests that, particularly in patients with carcinoma, a course of therapy must extend for at least 12 weeks to ensure an adequate trial.

Therapeutic Uses and Clinical Toxicity. Vinblastine can produce beneficial responses in lymphosarcoma, reticulum-cell sarcoma, mycosis fungoides, acute and chronic leukemias, neuroblastoma, and Letterer-Siwe disease (histiocytosis X), as well as in carcinomas of the breast, lung, oral cavity, testis, and bladder (*see* Livingston and Carter, 1970; Greenwald, 1973). The effectiveness of vinblastine in a high proportion of lymphomas is not diminished when the disease process is refractory to alkylating agents. Significant improvement has been reported in 50 to 90% of cases with Hodgkin's disease. The nadir of the leukopenia usually occurs within 4 to 10 days, after which recovery ensues within 7 to 14 days; with higher dosage, the total leukocyte counts may not return to normal until 3 weeks have elapsed. Other toxic effects of vinblastine include neurological manifestations, such as temporary mental depression, paresthesias, loss of deep-tendon reflexes, and, more rarely, headache, convulsions, and psychoses; dysfunction of the autonomic nervous system, with marked constipation, paralytic ileus, urinary retention, bilateral pain and tenderness of the parotid glands associated with dryness of the mouth, and sinus tachycardia, has been reported at higher doses. Gastrointestinal disturbances, including nausea, vomiting, anorexia, and diarrhea, may be encountered. Dermatological manifestations are infrequent, but loss of hair, vesicular mucositis of the mouth, and dermatitis may occur. Extravasation during injection may lead to cellulitis and phlebitis. Local injection of hyaluronidase and application of moderate heat to the area may be of help by dispersing the drug.

Vincristine

Preparations, Route of Administration, and Dosage. *Vincristine Sulfate,* U.S.P. (ONCOVIN), is available as a dry powder in ampuls containing either 1 or 5 mg of drug. Sterile solutions in either water or physiological saline may be stored in a refrigerator for periods up to 2 weeks without significant loss of potency. Vincristine is very useful in acute leukemia in children. The following dosage schedules can be used in this disorder: 0.05 mg/kg for the initial dose, then weekly doses that are increased by increments of 0.025 mg/kg to a maximum of 0.15 mg/kg. Vincristine is often used together with corticosteroids to induce remissions in childhood leukemia; the optimal dosages for these drugs appear to be vincristine, intravenously, 2 mg/sq m of body surface, weekly, and prednisone, orally, 40 mg/sq m, daily. In adults, the usual method of administration is to start therapy with intravenous doses of 0.01 mg/kg of body weight. After observation of the patient for 1 week, the dose is raised by weekly increments of 0.01 mg/kg until either the desired response is obtained or toxicity is encountered. Adult patients with carcinomas or lymphomas often will respond to weekly doses of 0.02 to 0.05 mg/kg. When used in combination with other drugs, for example, in the MOPP regimen (*see* below), the recommended dose of vincristine is 1.0 to 1.5 mg/sq m. High doses of vincristine seem to be tolerated better by children with leukemia than by adults, who would experience severe neurological toxicity. Administration of the drug more frequently than every 7 days or at higher doses seems to increase the toxic manifestations without proportional improvement in the response rate. Maintenance therapy with vincristine is not recommended in children with leukemia (*see* below). The same precautions described for vinblastine should be used to avoid extravasation during intravenous administration.

Therapeutic Uses and Clinical Toxicity. Vincristine has a spectrum of clinical activity that is similar to that of vinblastine, but there are some notable differences. An important feature is the lack of cross-resistance between these agents, a remarkable finding in view of the very close similarity of their chemical structures. Vincristine is effective in Hodgkin's disease and related lymphomas. While it appears to be somewhat less beneficial than vinblastine when used alone in Hodgkin's disease, in combination with mechlorethamine, prednisone, and procarbazine (the so-called MOPP regimen), it is considered the treatment of choice for the advanced stages (III and IV) of this disease (DeVita *et al.,* 1972). Vincristine is more useful than vinblastine in lymphocytic leukemia. Whether this is the result of a more selective action on the lymphocyte or simply a sparing of myelogenous elements in patients whose bone marrows are already compromised by lymphocytic infiltrates is not known. Another area of difference in clinical response to these drugs is acute leukemia, particularly in children; whereas vinblastine is rarely useful in this disease, vincristine is extremely effective.

The rapidity of action of vincristine and its lesser tendency for myelosuppressive action make it a more desirable agent for therapy in the presence of pancytopenia or in combination with other myelotoxic agents. It is particularly useful for the *induction* of remission in acute lymphoblastic leukemia of children when given with prednisone. It is the treatment of choice for this purpose and produces complete remissions in approximately 90% of children on the first course of antileukemic therapy (Symposium, 1968; Holland, 1971; Greenwald, 1973). The approximate rate of second remissions is 70 to 80%. Vincristine and prednisone should be promptly discontinued after remission is induced, since other agents (for example, methotrexate and mercaptopurine) are more effective for *maintenance*. Vincristine has not prevented the occurrence of leukemia in the CNS; for reasons mentioned previously, it should not be given intrathecally. Beneficial responses have been reported in patients with a variety of other neoplasms, particularly Wilms' tumor, neuroblastoma, brain tumors, rhabdomyosarcoma, and carcinomas of the breast, bladder, and the male and female reproductive systems (*see* Symposium, 1968; Livingston and Carter, 1970; Greenwald, 1973; Holland *et al.*, 1973; Creasey, 1975b).

The clinical toxicity of vincristine is mostly neurological, with paresthesias, loss of deep-tendon reflexes, neuritic pain, muscle weakness that may be manifested by foot-drop and inability to walk, hoarseness, headache, ptosis, and double vision. The more severe neurological manifestations may be avoided or reversed by either suspending therapy or reducing the dosage upon occurrence of the earliest symptoms, usually tingling and numbness of the extremities. Severe constipation, sometimes resulting in colicky abdominal pain and obstruction, may be prevented by a prophylactic program of laxatives and hydrophilic agents.

Alopecia occurs in about 20% of patients given vincristine; however, it is always reversible, frequently even without cessation of therapy. Although less common than with vinblastine, leukopenia may occur with vincristine, and thrombocytopenia, anemia, polyuria, dysuria, fever, and gastrointestinal symptoms have been reported occasionally. The syndrome of hyponatremia associated with high urinary sodium and inappropriate ADH secretion has been occasionally observed during vincristine therapy (Fine *et al.*, 1966). In view of the rapid action of the vinca alkaloids, it is advisable to take appropriate precautions to prevent the complication of hyperuricemia. This can be accomplished by the administration of *allopurinol* (*see* above).

ANTIBIOTICS

DACTINOMYCIN (ACTINOMYCIN D)

History. The first crystalline antibiotic agent to be isolated from a culture broth of a species of *Streptomyces* was actinomycin A (Waksman and Woodruff, 1940). Many related antibiotics, including actinomycin D, have subsequently been obtained (Waksman Conference on Actinomycins, 1974). Following the demonstration of marked antineoplastic activity in several experimental tumor systems, clinical investigations were initiated in Europe with actinomycin C (SANAMYCIN) and later with dactinomycin. Beneficial results have been observed in the

therapy of a number of tumors, particularly certain neoplasms that occur in children and choriocarcinoma.

Chemistry and Structure-Activity Relationship. The actinomycins are chromopeptides, and most of them contain the same chromophore, *actinocin,* the fraction that is responsible for the yellow-red color of the molecule. The differences among naturally occurring actinomycins are confined to the peptide side chains, and the variations are in the structure, but not in the number or in the configuration of the α carbon, of the constituent amino acids. By varying the amino acid content of the growth medium it is possible to alter the types of actinomycins produced. It has been demonstrated that changes in the amino acid composition of both polypeptide chains can influence the biological activity of the molecule and that a number of chemical alterations can abolish activity totally (*see* Reich, 1963; Stock, 1966; Waksman Conference on Actinomycins, 1974; Goldberg, 1975). The chemical structure of dactinomycin is as follows:

Dactinomycin

$$\left(\begin{array}{l} \text{Sar} = \text{sarcosine} \\ \text{Meval} = \text{N-methylvaline} \end{array}\right)$$

Mechanism of Action. The ability of actinomycins to bind with double-helical DNA is responsible for their biological activity and cytotoxicity. These complexes require the presence of deoxyguanosine, and apparently intercalation of the antibiotic occurs between a base-paired dG-dC sequence. Similar binding does not occur with RNA. Alterations of the physical properties of DNA, including increases in viscosity and "melting temperature," are induced by the formation of these complexes (Reich, 1963). At the enzymatic level, the synthesis of RNA by DNA-dependent RNA-polymerase is much more sensitive to the effects of dactinomycin than is the synthesis of DNA by DNA-polymerase. The inhibition of RNA synthesis by dactinomycin observed in enzyme preparations and in whole cells is entirely the result of the ability of the antibiotic to form the characteristic complexes with primer DNA. For this reason, the growth of those viruses in which the genome contains predominantly RNA is unaffected by the presence of dactinomycin, while the synthesis of DNA-containing viruses may be significantly inhibited. (For references, *see* Reich, 1963; Stock, 1966; Waksman Conference on Actinomycins, 1974.)

Cytotoxic Action. The drug inhibits rapidly proliferating cells of normal and neoplastic origin and, on a molar basis, is among the most potent antitumor agents known. Atrophy of thymus, spleen, and other lymphatic tissues occurs in experimental animals. Detailed studies of the hematological, gastrointestinal, and other toxic effects of dactinomycin in animals have been described. It may produce damage to the hair roots and is capable of potent local inflammatory action. Erythema sometimes progressing to necrosis has been noted in areas of the skin exposed to x-radiation either before, during, or after administration of the drug.

Absorption, Fate, and Excretion. Dactinomycin is much less potent when given orally than when administered by parenteral injection. Very little active drug can be detected in the circulating blood 2 minutes after its intravenous injection. In rats, approximately 50% of the compound is excreted unchanged in the bile and 10% in the urine. There is no evidence of metabolic modification of the molecule. The drug appears incapable of crossing the blood-brain barrier. Studies on its clinical pharmacology are lacking and information is incomplete.

Preparation, Dosage, and Route of Administration. *Dactinomycin,* U.S.P. (*actinomycin D;* COS-MEGEN), is supplied as a lyophilized powder (0.5 mg in each vial). Solutions should not be exposed to direct sunlight. The usual daily dose is 15 µg/kg; this is given intravenously for 5 days; if no manifestations of toxicity are encountered, additional courses may be given at intervals of 2 to 4 weeks. Daily injections of 100 to 400 µg have been given to children for 10 to 14 days; in other regimens, 3 to 6 µg/kg, for a total of 125 µg/kg, and weekly maintenance doses of 7.5 µg/kg have been used. Although larger amounts have been given in more prolonged courses, in general the total dose necessary to produce antineoplastic effects has been approximately 2.5 to 5.0 mg. Although it is safer to administer the drug into the tubing of an intravenous infusion, direct intravenous injections have been given, with the precaution of discarding the needle used to withdraw the drug from the ampul in order to avoid subcutaneous reaction. Intracavitary use of dactinomycin has been accompanied by considerable toxicity, and there is no evidence that it is more effective or safer than the alkylating agents.

Therapeutic Uses and Clinical Toxicity. Dactinomycin can be lifesaving for women with methotrexate-resistant choriocarcinoma. It is of limited value in other neoplastic disease of adults, except when given with chlorambucil and methotrexate to patients with metastatic testicular carcinomas. Although some response may be observed in Hodgkin's disease and related lymphomas, the beneficial results obtained with rhabdomyosarcoma and Wilms' tumor in children have deserved more attention. In the latter, remissions lasting several years and increased survival have been reported in patients with advanced disease, including pulmonary metastases (Farber, 1966; Livingston and Carter, 1970; Greenwald, 1973; Waksman Conference on Actinomycins, 1974). Antineoplastic activity has been noted in neuroblastoma, Ewing's tumor, melanoma, osteogenic sarcoma, Kaposi's sarcoma, and soft-tissue sarcomas. Its use together with vincristine and cyclophosphamide has been advocated in children with solid tumors (Pratt *et al.,* 1968). Dactinomycin has also been used to inhibit immunological responses, particularly the rejection of renal transplants.

Toxic manifestations include anorexia, nausea, and vomiting, usually beginning a few hours after administration. Hematopoietic suppression with pancytopenia may occur from 1 to 7 days after completion of therapy. A decrease in the platelet count is often the first manifestation of bone-marrow depression, and pancytopenia may develop rapidly. Proctitis, diarrhea, glossitis, cheilitis, and ulcerations of the oral mucosa are common; dermatological manifestations include alopecia, as well as erythema, desquamation, and increased pigmentation in areas subjected to x-radiation. Severe injury may occur as a result of local toxic action.

DAUNORUBICIN AND DOXORUBICIN

These relatively new antineoplastic drugs are glycosidic anthracyclene antibiotics that are fermentation products of the fungus *Streptomyces peucetius* var. *caesius.* Although there are only slight differences in chemical structure, they display markedly different clinical antitumor activity. Daunorubicin, originally isolated in Italy as *daunomycin* (DiMarco *et al.,* 1963) and independently in France as *rubidomycin* (Dubost *et al.,* 1963), has clinical activity only in the acute leukemias. Doxorubicin, also identified and developed in Italy as ADRIAMYCIN (Arcamone *et al.,* 1969), on the other hand, has an impressive record of activity against a wide spectrum of tumors despite a relatively brief period of clinical testing. (*See* Carter *et al.,* 1972; Chabner *et al.,* 1975; DiMarco, 1975.)

Chemistry. The structures of daunorubicin and doxorubicin are shown on the opposite page. Both compounds have tetracycline ring structures with an unusual sugar, daunosamine, attached by glycosidic linkage. The chemical structures of the two anthracyclene antibiotics are identical except for the hydroxyl group on C 14 in doxorubicin.

Mechanism of Action. Although the mechanism of action is not yet fully established, studies of

Daunorubicin: R = H
Doxorubicin: R = OH

daunorubicin involving x-ray diffraction and DNA model building suggest that the anthraclene antibiotics bind tightly with DNA. It has been proposed that intercalation occurs between adjacent base pairs on a DNA strand. The amino sugar daunosamine plays an essential role in this binding. The DNA helix is untwisted to permit intercalation, producing a longer, thinner molecule and causing inhibition of the template activity of the DNA (Pigram *et al.*, 1972).

The evidence on the mechanism of action of doxorubicin is less complete. However, studies performed to date indicate that it binds to DNA and inhibits DNA synthesis in a manner similar to that observed with daunorubicin (DiMarco, 1975). Of special interest is the finding that doxorubicin binds very tightly to myocardial DNA, which is consistent with the unusual cardiomyopathy caused by this drug.

At present there is no satisfactory explanation for the surprisingly and markedly different clinical antitumor activities of daunorubicin and doxorubicin. It is possible, however, that the explanation may lie in differences in their metabolic degradation. Both are subject to rapid and extensive metabolism. In a single passage through the liver about 60% of doxorubicin is extracted, metabolized, and excreted in the bile; at least six metabolites have been identified, the principal one being adriamycinol. This product results from the reduction of the keto group on C 13 by an enzyme found in leukocytes and erythrocytes, and presumably in malignant tissues. An analogous daunomycin metabolite, daunomycinol, has been demonstrated and displays antitumor activity. Responsiveness of patients with acute myelocytic leukemia to daunorubicin has been correlated with the presence of the enzyme, referred to as daunorubicin reductase. In addition to the reduction products, several aglycone metabolites of these antibiotics have been identified. Hopefully, further studies of such metabolites will yield greater insight into the behavior of this important new class of antitumor drugs.

As with other chemotherapeutic agents, resistance is observed to the anthraclenes. As yet, however, there is no clear biochemical explanation of the resistance mechanism. Complete cross-resistance has been reported between daunorubicin and doxorubi-

cin in leukemia L 1210 sublines. Interestingly, cross-resistance has also been described between daunorubicin, dactinomycin, and the vinca alkaloids, which raises the possibility that alteration of cellular permeability may be involved.

As might be expected of the compounds that inhibit the function of DNA, maximal cytotoxic effects are observed during the S phase of the cell cycle, although cytotoxicity is evident during other phases as well.

Absorption, Fate, and Excretion. Daunorubicin and doxorubicin are usually administered intravenously, and data on oral absorption are lacking. The two antibiotics are rapidly cleared from the plasma. Their disappearance curves are biphasic, with an initial half-life of about 1 hour and a long half-life of about 17 hours for both. There is rapid uptake of the drugs in the heart, kidneys, lungs, liver, and spleen. They do not appear to cross the blood-brain barrier. There are notable differences in the metabolism of the two compounds. Two metabolites of daunorubicin appear in human plasma, including daunorubicinol. Doxorubicin appears to have multiple metabolites, with adriamycinol as the primary product. The cumulative 5-day excretion of daunorubicin and its metabolites in the urine has been reported to be 23%, in contrast to 6% for doxorubicin and its metabolites. Both drugs are metabolized primarily in the liver and excreted in the bile. The hepatic clearance of doxorubicin has been estimated to be approximately 60% of hepatic blood flow, and severe clinical toxicity may result if the drug is administered to patients with impaired hepatic function (Alberts *et al.*, 1971; Huffman *et al.*, 1972; Benjamin *et al.*, 1973; Chabner *et al.*, 1975).

Daunorubicin: Preparation, Dosage, and Route of Administration. Daunorubicin (*daunomycin, rubidomycin;* DAUNOBLASTINA) is available as a lyophilized powder in 20-mg vials. The dry, unopened vials are stable at room temperature, but the drug should be used within 6 hours after reconstitution with 5 to 10 ml of sterile water. The recommended dosage is 30 to 60 mg/sq m daily for 3 days or once weekly. The drug has also been given in doses of 0.8 to 1.0 mg/kg daily for 3 to 6 days, and other dosage schedules are being investigated. The agent is administered intravenously with appropriate care to prevent extravasation, since local vesicant action may result.

Daunorubicin: Therapeutic Uses and Clinical Toxicity. Daunorubicin is very useful in the treatment of acute lymphocytic and acute granulocytic leukemias. The drug has some activity against solid tumors in children and in lymphomas; its activity against solid tumors in adults is minimal (Livingston and Carter, 1970; Samuels *et al.*, 1971; Jones *et al.*, 1972; Sutow *et al.*, 1972; Weil *et al.*, 1973). The toxic manifestations of daunorubicin include bone-marrow depression, stomatitis, alopecia, gastrointestinal disturbances, and dermatological manifestations. Cardiac toxicity is a peculiar adverse effect observed with this agent. It is characterized by tachycardia, arrhythmias, dyspnea, hypotension, and congestive failure unresponsive to digitalis (Livingston and Carter, 1970).

Doxorubicin: Preparation, Dosage, and Route of Administration. *Doxorubicin* (ADRIAMYCIN, ADRIBLASTINA) is supplied as a lyophilized powder in 10-mg vials. The dry, unopened vials are stable at room temperature, but the drug should be used within 8 hours after reconstitution with 5 ml of sterile water. The currently recommended dose is 60 to 75 mg/sq m, administered as a single rapid intravenous infusion and repeated after 21 days. The drug has also been given in doses of 0.5 to 1.0 mg/kg daily for 2 to 6 days or in doses of 20 to 30 mg/sq m daily for 3 days or once weekly. Care should be taken to avoid extravasation, since local vesicant action and tissue necrosis may result.

Doxorubicin: Therapeutic Uses and Clinical Toxicity. Doxorubicin is effective in acute leukemias and malignant lymphomas; however, in contrast to daunorubicin, it is also extremely active in a number of solid tumors. The drug is particularly beneficial in a wide range of sarcomas, including osteogenic, Ewing's, and soft-tissue sarcomas. It is one of the most active single agents for the treatment of metastatic adenocarcinoma of the breast, carcinoma of the bladder, bronchogenic carcinoma, and neuroblastoma. In metastatic thyroid carcinoma, doxorubicin is probably the best available agent. Although only preliminary data are available, the drug has demonstrated some activity in carcinomas of the ovary, endometrium, testes, and prostate; squamous-cell carcinomas of the cervix and of the head and neck; and plasma-cell myeloma (Blum and Carter, 1974; Gottlieb and Hill, 1974).

The toxic manifestations of doxorubicin are similar to those of daunorubicin. Myelosuppression is a major dose-limiting complication, with leukopenia usually reaching a nadir during the second week of therapy and recovering by the fourth week; thrombocytopenia and anemia follow a similar pattern but are usually less pronounced. Stomatitis, gastrointestinal disturbances, and alopecia are common but reversible. Cardiomyopathy is a unique characteristic of the anthracyclene antibiotics. Their avid binding to myocardial DNA may be an important pharmacological factor. Tachycardia, arrhythmias, and ST-T wave changes in the ECG may be early manifestations of cardiac toxicity. Severe and rapidly progressive congestive heart failure may follow. Nonspecific alterations, including a decrease in the number of myocardial fibrils, mitochondrial changes, and cellular degeneration, are visible by electron microscopy (LeFrak *et al.*, 1973). Although no predictive tests are available, the frequency of cardiomyopathy is negligible at total doses below 500 mg/sq m. The risk of cardiac toxicity increases markedly (to >20% of patients) at total doses higher than 550 mg/sq m, and this dosage should be exceeded only under exceptional circumstances. Because doxorubicin is primarily metabolized and excreted by the liver, it is important to reduce the dosage in patients with impaired hepatic function (Blum and Carter, 1974; Chabner *et al.*, 1975).

BLEOMYCINS

The bleomycins include a potentially important new group of clinically active antitumor agents discovered by Umezawa and colleagues as fermentation products of *Streptomyces verticillus*. The drug form currently in clinical trial is a complex mixture of glycopeptides; it is to be expected that highly purified and chemically modified bleomycins will become available that perhaps will differ from present preparations in their antineoplastic spectra and toxic manifestations. For recent reviews of the bleomycins, *see* Umezawa (1973a, 1973b) and Chabner and co-workers (1975).

Bleomycins have attracted great interest because of their activity in a variety of human tumors, including squamous carcinomas of skin, head, neck, and lungs, in addition to lymphomas and testicular tumors. In comparison with many other antineoplastic agents, the bleomycins in current use have minimal myelosuppressive and immunosuppressive activities. They do, however, cause unusual cutaneous and pulmonary toxicity. Since the toxic manifestations of the bleomycins do not overlap significantly with those of most other drugs and since their apparent mechanism of action is also unique (*see* below), it seems likely that the bleomycins will find an important place in combination chemotherapy.

Chemistry. The bleomycins are water-soluble, basic glycopeptides that differ from one another in their terminal-amine moieties. Present information indicates that a common chemical structure occurs, as shown on the opposite page, where modification of the **R** radical yields different bleomycins.

It has been possible to prepare bleomycinic acid, where the radical is a hydroxyl group. Nine naturally occurring bleomycins have been isolated in pure form, and chemical addition of various amines to bleomycinic acid has made possible the synthesis of at least 100 artificial bleomycins. The composition of the bleomycins can also be modified by the addition of specific amines to the fermentation mixtures. Of the natural compounds, bleomycin A_2 is the principal component of the bleomycin mixture presently used. It appears that large numbers of natural and semisynthetic bleomycins will become available for experimental and perhaps clinical study.

Mechanism of Action. While the bleomycins have been shown to have a number of interesting biochemical properties, it seems most likely that their cytotoxic action relates to their ability to cause chain scission and fragmentation of DNA molecules. Marked chromosomal abnormalities have also been described that probably are due to the damage to DNA.

Bleomycin B_2 in very low concentrations can bind to DNA and cause nicking. It has been proposed that a chemical reaction occurs between a reactive group on the bleomycin and the DNA, causing the nick (Umezawa, 1973b). Furthermore, an adenosine triphosphate (ATP)–dependent DNA ligase isolated from a rat hepatoma is markedly inhibited by low concentrations of bleomycin. Since DNA ligases play an important role in DNA replication, recombination, and repair, it appears that in the presence of

Bleomycinic Acid: **R** = OH

Bleomycin A$_2$: **R** = NHCH$_2$CH$_2$CH$_2$—S$^+$(CH$_3$)CH$_3$

Bleomycin B$_2$: **R** = NHCH$_2$CH$_2$CH$_2$CH$_2$NHC(=NH)NH$_2$

a bleomycin the repair of chain scission caused by the reaction of the drug or perhaps by an endonuclease cannot be performed, leading to progressive fragmentation of the DNA chain.

Of considerable interest is the apparent mechanism of the selective action of the bleomycins against squamous-cell carcinomas and their toxicity to lung and skin. Evidence indicates that enzymes in most tissues, with the exception of lung and skin, can rapidly inactivate the bleomycins. Furthermore, it has been shown that sarcomas inactivate bleomycin more readily than do carcinomas. The mechanism of the enzymatic inactivation is not yet established, although it appears to involve a deamination or a peptidase reaction.

Studies with synchronized cells have indicated that the bleomycins block the cell cycle, causing accumulation of cells, some severely injured, at G$_2$. Other studies have shown that cells in mitosis are most sensitive to these antibiotics. (*See* Umezawa, 1973a, 1973b.)

Absorption, Fate, and Excretion. Bleomycin is usually administered parenterally, and data on oral absorption are lacking. Microbiological assays have been devised for measuring the distribution of the drug in animals, and relatively high concentrations have been detected in the skin and lungs, the major sites of toxicity. Other tissues contain a soluble enzyme that inactivates the drug by removing 1 mole of ammonia (Umezawa, 1973a, 1973b). In man, bleomycin localizes in various tumors, suggesting a lower level of inactivating enzyme at these sites. Absorption, metabolism, and excretion of the drug

are poorly understood, because of lack of a sensitive method for determining drug concentrations *in vivo* (Chabner *et al.*, 1975).

Preparation, Dosage, and Route of Administration. *Bleomycin* (BLENOXANE) is available as a lyophilized powder in 15-unit ampuls to be reconstituted with 5 ml of sterile water, saline solution, or 5% dextrose solution. The powder is stable at room temperature for 2 years before the drug is dissolved and for 7 days when kept refrigerated after reconstitution. The recommended dose is 10 to 20 units/ sq m, weekly or twice weekly, and the drug is most commonly administered intravenously or intramuscularly. It may also be given by subcutaneous or intra-arterial injection. Total courses exceeding 400 units should be given with great caution.

Therapeutic Uses and Clinical Toxicity. Bleomycin is useful in the palliative treatment of squamous-cell carcinomas of the head, neck, esophagus, skin, and the genitourinary tract, including the cervix, vulva, scrotum, and penis. It has demonstrated effectiveness in testicular carcinomas, with an overall response rate of approximately 30%; this has increased to 90% when the drug is used in combination with vinblastine. Bleomycin is active in Hodgkin's disease and in non-Hodgkin's lymphomas, particularly when administered by slow intravenous infusion. (For details, *see* Ichikawa *et al.*, 1969; Yagoda *et al.*, 1972; Blum *et al.*, 1973.)

In contrast to most other antineoplastic agents, bleomycin causes minimal bone-marrow toxicity. The most commonly encountered adverse effects are mucocutaneous reactions, including stomatitis and alopecia as well as hyperpigmentation, hyperkeratosis, pruritic erythema, ulceration, and vesiculation of the skin. These changes may begin with swelling and hyperesthesia of the hands or erythematous, ulcerating lesions over the pressure areas of the body. Recrudescence of mucocutaneous complications has been reported when other antineoplastic agents are used within 6 weeks after a course of bleomycin. The most serious adverse reaction to this drug is pulmonary toxicity. This poorly characterized manifestation may begin with decreasing pulmonary function, fine rales, cough, and diffuse basilar infiltrates, progressing to severe, and sometimes fatal, pulmonary fibrosis. Approximately 5 to 10% of patients receiving bleomycin develop this severe complication, and about 1% of all individuals treated with the drug have died of pulmonary toxicity. Pulmonary function studies have not been of predictive value. The risk at total doses below 400 units is not dose related. However, a significant increase in the incidence of pulmonary fibrosis has been noted at doses higher than 400 units and in patients over 70 years of age or with underlying pulmonary disease. The use of corticosteroids has been advocated, but their value in reversing or preventing this complication remains to be established. Other toxic manifestations include hyperpyrexia, headache, nausea, and vomiting, as well as a peculiar, acute fulminant reaction observed in patients with lymphomas. This is characterized by profound hyperpyrexia, hypotension, and sustained cardiorespiratory collapse; it does not appear to be a classical anaphylactic reaction and may possibly be related to release of an endogenous pyrogen. Because this reaction has occurred in approximately 6% of patients with lymphomas and has resulted in deaths, it is recommended that patients with lymphomas receive a 1-unit test dose of bleomycin, followed by a 24-hour period of observation, before administration of the drug on standard dosage schedules. Unexplained exacerbations of rheumatoid arthritis have also been reported during bleomycin therapy. (Shastri *et al.*, 1971; Yagoda *et al.*, 1972; Blum *et al.*, 1973; Chabner *et al.*, 1975.)

MITHRAMYCIN

This cytotoxic antibiotic was isolated from cultures of *Streptomyces tanashiensis* by Rao and associates in 1962. Although the drug is highly toxic, it has shown some clinical value in the treatment of advanced embryonal tumors of the testes. Mithramycin appears to have a relatively specific effect on osteoclasts and lowers the plasma calcium concentrations in hypercalcemic patients, including those with various types of cancer and metastatic tumors in bone. The drug has been used experimentally in the treatment of symptomatic Paget's disease, and striking reductions in plasma alkaline phosphatase activity with concomitant relief of bone pain have been observed. For a discussion of the chemistry of mithramycin and related antibiotics, *see* Umezawa (1973a). The structural formula of mithramycin is as shown.

Mechanism of Action. Mithramycin inhibits the synthesis of RNA in a variety of tissues without

Mithramycin

affecting directly the synthesis of protein or DNA (Yarbro *et al.*, 1966; Northrop *et al.*, 1969). It has been postulated that the mechanism of action at the molecular level is similar to that of dactinomycin.

The relatively specific effect of mithramycin on plasma calcium concentrations suggests that the drug may have a direct action on bone (Robins and Jowsey, 1973). Studies with a tissue culture system of embryonic rat bone showed that the release of calcium caused by the addition of parathyroid hormone can be abolished by simultaneous treatment with low concentrations of mithramycin (Cortes *et al.*, 1972). These effects are thought to be the result of a direct action on osteoclasts.

Absorption, Fate, and Excretion. Mithramycin is much less potent when administered orally than when given intravenously. Studies of its clinical pharmacology are lacking, and information on distribution, metabolic fate, and excretion is incomplete.

Preparation, Dosage, and Route of Administration. *Mithramycin,* U.S.P. (MITHRACIN), is available as a freeze-dried powder in vials containing 2.5 mg of drug. The recommended dosage for treatment of testicular tumors is 25 to 30 µg/kg daily or on alternate days for eight to ten doses or until toxicity intervenes. The drug is usually diluted in 1 liter of 5% dextrose in water and administered by slow intravenous infusion over a period of 4 to 6 hours. Extravasation can cause local irritation and cellulitis. For the treatment of hypercalcemia or hypercalciuria, 25 µg/kg has been given daily for one to three doses; this is repeated at intervals of 1 week or more.

Therapeutic Uses and Clinical Toxicity. Mithramycin is of limited value in the treatment of neoplastic disease because of its severe toxicity. It has been beneficial in patients with disseminated testicular carcinomas, especially of the embryonal-cell type (Ream *et al.*, 1968; Kennedy, 1970; Hill *et al.*, 1972b). The drug is useful in treating patients with severe hypercalcemia or hypercalciuria, particularly when associated with advanced or metastatic carcinoma that involves bone or produces parathyroid hormone–like substances (Perlia *et al.*, 1970). Its effectiveness in severe Paget's disease is encouraging but still considered investigational (Ryan *et al.*, 1970; Elias and Evans, 1972). Mithramycin is toxic to the bone marrow, liver, and kidneys. It produces a severe hemorrhagic diathesis, which may be the result of impaired synthesis of various clotting factors in addition to thrombocytopenia. Characteristically, this begins with epistaxis and may proceed to generalized hemorrhagic complications and even death. Adverse gastrointestinal, cutaneous, and neurological manifestations are also frequently observed. At the lower total dose recommended above for the treatment of hypercalcemia, toxicity is less severe. (For additional references, *see* Livingston and Carter, 1970; Greenwald, 1973.)

ENZYMES

L-ASPARAGINASE

History. A unique development in the field of cancer chemotherapy has been the discovery that the enzyme L-asparaginase (L-asparagine amidohydrolase, EC 3.5.1.1.) is an effective chemotherapeutic agent for the treatment of human leukemia. Certain neoplastic tissues, including the lymphoblast in acute lymphoblastic leukemia in children, have as an essential growth requirement the amino acid L-asparagine. In contrast, most normal tissues synthesize their own L-asparagine. The enzyme L-asparaginase, by catalyzing the hydrolysis of asparagine to aspartic acid and ammonia, deprives the malignant cells of an essential amino acid, thus causing cell death without similarly damaging normal tissues.

Discovery of the antitumor action of L-asparaginase derived from an unexpected but highly astute observation by Kidd (1953), who noted that malignancies were suppressed during an immunological experiment that involved leukemic mice injected with guinea pig serum as a source of complement. The effect was specific for guinea pig serum and was not produced by sera from rabbits, horses, or humans. The clue that led to the explanation of this phenomenon was the finding that certain malignant cells grown in culture require L-asparagine, an amino acid not normally needed for the growth of mammalian cells in culture. This led to the discovery by Broome (1963) that the factor in guinea pig serum responsible for suppression of the leukemic cells is the enzyme L-asparaginase.

Preparation and Unitage. A virtually limitless source of L-asparaginase became available when Mashburn and Wriston (1964) identified an L-asparaginase with antileukemic activity in *Escherichia coli*. This microorganism produces two L-asparaginase isozymes, only one of which (EC-2) has anti-

leukemic activity. The *E. coli* enzyme has been purified to homogeneity and is available for therapeutic use as a dry powder in sealed vials containing 10,000 or 50,000 international units (I.U.) per vial. The molecular weight of the enzyme is about 133,000, and it consists of four equivalent subunits (*see* Patterson, 1975). These preparations of *E. coli* L-asparaginase have weak glutaminase activity that may play a role in certain of the biological effects. Also, it is suspected that certain toxic manifestations seen with earlier, less pure preparations may have been due to contamination by bacterial endotoxin.

Mechanism of Action and Clinical Toxicity. When L-asparaginase was first introduced, it was believed that a distinct, qualitative biochemical difference had been detected between normal cells and certain malignant tissues. It is now clear, however, that several functions of some normal tissues are sensitive to L-asparaginase treatment. The synthesis of certain specific proteins, such as plasma albumin, insulin, and clotting factors, may be inhibited. The first wave of mitosis following partial hepatectomy in rats and the transformation of lymphocytes in response to phytohemagglutinin are both inhibited by L-asparaginase.

Of considerable importance in chemotherapy is that, in contrast to most other antitumor drugs, L-asparaginase has minimal effects on the bone marrow, and it does not damage oral or intestinal mucosa or the hair follicles. On the other hand, severe toxicity has been observed that affects the liver, kidneys, pancreas, CNS, and the clotting mechanism (Haskell *et al.*, 1969; Oettgen *et al.*, 1970; Ohnuma *et al.*, 1971). Biochemical evidence of hepatic dysfunction is present in more than 50% of those treated, and most patients display a substantial elevation of blood ammonia (as great as 700 to 900 μg %). Disorders of pancreatic function, including decreased insulin production, are often seen, and approximately 5% of treated adults develop overt pancreatitis; death has resulted from hemorrhagic pancreatitis. CNS dysfunction, ranging from depression to impaired sensorium and coma, has occurred in adults. It is suggested that all or most of these toxic effects result from inhibition of protein synthesis in various tissues of the body. L-Asparaginase has immunosuppressive activity, as seen by inhibition of antibody synthesis, delayed hypersensitivity, lymphocyte transformation, and graft rejection. Thus, both T- and B-lymphocyte functions are affected. Since L-asparaginase is a relatively large, foreign protein, it is antigenic, and hypersensitivity phenomena ranging from mild allergic reactions to anaphylactic shock have been reported in 5 to 20% of treated patients.

Therapeutic Status and Dosage. Unfortunately, L-asparaginase does not appear to be fulfilling its early promise of high tumoricidal activity with minimal toxicity in the treatment of human malignancies. Significant numbers of complete remission have been observed in acute lymphoblastic leukemia, many of which were refractory to other antileukemic agents (Tallal *et al.*, 1970; Sutow *et al.*, 1971); the duration of these remissions, however, has been disappointingly short. Transient remissions have been observed in other forms of leukemia, and occasional beneficial responses have been reported in a few patients with malignant melanoma, lymphosarcoma, and reticulum-cell sarcoma. No objective responses have been seen with most solid tumors (Clarkson *et al.*, 1970). Therefore, unless the antineoplastic spectrum can be broadened by its use in combination with other agents, it appears that the future role of asparaginase in antineoplastic chemotherapy will be limited to the treatment of acute lymphocytic leukemia.

The suggested dosage for the induction of remission in acute lymphoblastic leukemia is 200 I.U./kg daily for 28 days. Higher daily doses (1000 I.U./kg) for periods not exceeding 10 days have also been proposed as a method of avoiding anaphylaxis, which ordinarily appears only after the tenth day.

Currently, L-asparaginase is undergoing clinical trial for its ability to consolidate remissions induced by vincristine and prednisone in acute lymphoblastic leukemia. It is of interest that the toxicity is considerably greater if L-asparaginase is administered before or simultaneously with vincristine, rather than if it is given after the vinca alkaloid. The fact that the toxic effects of L-asparaginase do not coincide with those of most other antineoplastic agents makes reasonable the trial of L-asparaginase in regimens of combination chemotherapy. (For reviews, *see* Adamson and Fabro, 1968; Livingston and Carter, 1970; Capizzi and Handschumacher, 1973; Oettgen, 1975; Patterson, 1975.)

IV. Miscellaneous Agents

HYDROXYUREA

First synthesized in 1869 by Dresler and Stein, hydroxyurea was found to produce leukopenia, anemia, and megaloblastic changes in the bone marrow of rabbits (Rosenthal *et al.*, 1928). It was later shown to have antineoplastic activity against sarcoma 180. Studies of its biological activity and the preliminary assessments of clinical efficacy have been reviewed (*see* Symposium, 1964). The structural formula of hydroxyurea is as follows:

$$H_2N-\overset{\overset{\displaystyle O}{\|}}{C}-NH-OH$$

Hydroxyurea

Cytotoxic Action. Hydroxyurea is representative of a group of compounds that have as their primary site of action the enzyme ribonucleoside diphosphate reductase. Other members of this class that have shown promise in the laboratory are guanazole and the α-N-heterocyclic carboxaldehyde thiosemicarbazones (*see* Agrawal and Sartorelli, 1975). A striking correlation has been observed between the relative growth rate of a series of rat hepatomas and the activity of ribonucleoside diphosphate reductase. This enzyme, which catalyses the reductive conversion of ribonucleotides to deoxyribonucleotides, is a crucial and probably rate-limiting step in the biosynthesis of DNA, and it represents a logical target for the design of chemotherapeutic agents. Nonheme iron is an important component of this enzyme in mammalian tissues, and many of the active inhibitors can chelate or form complexes with iron. These compounds are specific for the S phase of the cell cycle. (For references, *see* Yarbro, 1968; Agrawal and Sartorelli, 1975; Krakoff, 1975.)

Absorption, Fate, and Excretion. In man, hydroxyurea is readily absorbed from the gastrointestinal tract, and peak plasma concentrations are reached in 2 hours; within 24 hours, it is essentially undetectable in the blood. Approximately 80% of the drug is recovered in the urine within 12 hours after either oral or intravenous administration (Beckloff *et al.*, 1965).

Preparation, Dosage, and Route of Administration. *Hydroxyurea*, U.S.P. (HYDREA), is a white powder available for oral use in 500-mg capsules. Two dosage schedules are recommended: (1) intermittent therapy with 80 mg/kg, administered orally as a single dose every third day, and (2) continuous therapy with 20 to 30 mg/kg, administered orally as a single daily dose. Treatment should be continued for a period of 6 weeks in order to determine its effectiveness; if satisfactory antineoplastic results are obtained, therapy can be continued indefinitely, although leukocyte counts at weekly intervals are advisable.

Therapeutic Uses and Clinical Toxicity. At present, the primary role of hydroxyurea in chemotherapy appears to be in the management of chronic granulocytic leukemia, particularly in patients no longer responsive to busulfan (Kennedy and Yarbro, 1966). It has also produced temporary remissions in metastatic malignant melanoma and occasionally in other solid tumors (Ariel, 1970; Livingston and Carter, 1970). Hydroxyurea has been used, in combination with radiotherapy, for carcinomas of the head and neck. Hematopoietic depression, involving leukopenia, megaloblastic anemia, and occasionally thrombocytopenia, is the major toxic effect; recovery of the bone marrow is usually prompt if the drug is discontinued for a few days. Other adverse reactions include gastrointestinal disturbances and mild dermatological reactions; more rarely, stomatitis, alopecia, and neurological manifestations have been encountered.

PROCARBAZINE

A group of antitumor agents, the methylhydrazine derivatives, was discovered among a large number of substituted hydrazines, which had been originally synthesized as potential monoamine oxidase inhibitors. Antineoplastic effects in experimental tumors have been reported with several compounds in this series (Bollag, 1963), including procarbazine, an agent useful clinically in Hodgkin's disease. Comprehensive and detailed descriptions of the biological effects, immunosuppressive activity, physiological disposition, carcinogenicity, and clinical effectiveness of procarbazine have been published (Symposium, 1965; Oliverio, 1973a; Reed, 1975). The structural formula of procarbazine is as follows:

Procarbazine

Cytotoxic Action. The mechanism of action of procarbazine has not been determined. Inhibition of DNA, RNA, and protein synthesis has been observed, although the latter is delayed until after nucleic acid synthesis is inhibited. A progressive decrease in viscosity of DNA solutions is caused by the drug in the presence of oxygen, but not if this is replaced by an inert gas or if peroxidase, catalase, or cysteamine is added. Auto-oxidation occurs in aqueous solutions with production of hydrogen peroxide. The reducing substances also formed are capable of participating in the conversion of hydrogen peroxide to hydroxyl radicals, which may be responsible for the degradation of DNA but not necessarily for the cytotoxic action of the drug. Since only the methyl-substituted hydrazines have been found to be active and only these are capable of forming formaldehyde and its derivatives, it has been suggested that this conversion may play an important role. Cytological studies indicate suppression of mitosis as a result of prolongation of the interphase. A very high percentage of broken chromatids has been observed; these effects may be responsible for disturbances of cell division, as well as for the induction of pulmonary tumors, mammary adenocarcinomas, and leukemia in experimental animals.

Absorption, Fate, and Excretion. Procarbazine is absorbed almost completely from the gastrointestinal tract. After parenteral administration, the drug is readily equilibrated between the plasma and cerebrospinal fluid. It is rapidly metabolized in man, and its half-life in the blood after intravenous injection is approximately 7 minutes. Oxidation of procarbazine produces the corresponding azo compound and hydrogen peroxide. From 25 to 70% of an oral or parenteral dose given to man is recovered from the urine during the first 24 hours after administration; less than 5% is excreted as the unchanged compound and the rest mostly in the form of a metabolite, N-isopropylterephthalanic acid (Oliverio *et al.*, 1964; Bollag, 1965).

Preparation, Dosage, and Route of Administration. *Procarbazine Hydrochloride*, U.S.P. (MATULANE, NATULAN), is marketed in 50-mg capsules. The recommended oral daily dose ranges from 100 to 200 mg for the first week of therapy; then daily doses of 300 mg are given until maximal response is obtained or toxicity intervenes.

Therapeutic Uses and Clinical Toxicity. The greatest therapeutic effectiveness of procarbazine is in Hodgkin's disease, particularly in combination with mechlorethamine, vincristine, and prednisone

(the MOPP regimen) (DeVita *et al.*, 1970). Of major importance is the apparent lack of cross-resistance with other antineoplastic agents. The drug has also demonstrated some activity in oat-cell carcinoma of the lung, non-Hodgkin's lymphomas, myeloma, and melanoma (Livingston and Carter, 1970; Greenwald, 1973; Oliverio, 1973a).

The most common toxic effects include leukopenia, thrombocytopenia, nausea, and vomiting, occurring in 50 to 70% of patients. Other gastrointestinal symptoms as well as neurological and dermatological manifestations have been noted in 5 to 10% of cases; psychic disturbances have also been reported. Because of augmentation of sedative effects, the concomitant use of CNS depressants should be avoided. The ingestion of alcohol by patients receiving procarbazine may cause intense warmth and reddening of the face, as well as other effects resembling the acetaldehyde syndrome produced by disulfiram. Since procarbazine is a weak monoamine oxidase inhibitor, hypertensive reactions may result from its use concurrently with sympathomimetic agents, tricyclic antidepressants, and foods with high tyramine content.

MITOTANE (*o,p'*-DDD)

The principal application of mitotane, a compound chemically similar to the insecticides DDT and DDD, is in the treatment of neoplasms derived from the adrenal cortex. In studies of the toxicology of related insecticides in dogs, it was noted that the adrenal cortex was severely damaged, an effect caused by the presence of the *o,p'* isomer of DDD. Its structural formula is as follows:

Mitotane

Cytotoxic Action. The mechanism of action of mitotane has not been elucidated, but its relatively selective attack upon adrenocortical cells, normal or neoplastic, is well established. Thus, administration of the drug causes a rapid reduction in the levels of adrenocorticosteroids and their metabolites in blood and urine, a response that is useful both in guiding dosage and in following the course of hyperadrenocorticism (Cushing's syndrome) resulting from an adrenal tumor or hyperplasia. Damage to the liver, kidneys, or bone marrow has not been encountered.

Absorption, Fate, and Excretion. Clinical studies indicate that approximately 40% of the drug is absorbed after oral administration. After daily doses of 5 to 15 g, concentrations of 10 to 90 μg/ml of unchanged drug and 30 to 50 μg/ml of a metabolite are present in the blood. After discontinuation of therapy, plasma concentrations of mitotane are still measurable for 6 to 9 weeks. Although the drug is found in all tissues, fat is the primary site of storage. A water-soluble metabolite of mitotane is found in the urine; approximately 25% of an oral or parenteral dose is recovered in this form. About 60% of an oral dose is excreted unchanged in the stool.

Preparation, Dosage, and Route of Administration. *Mitotane*, U.S.P. (*o,p'*-DDD; LYSODREN), is supplied in 500-mg scored tablets. Initial daily oral doses of 8 to 10 g are usually given in three or four divided portions, but the maximal tolerated dose may vary from 2 to 16 g per day. Treatment should be continued for at least 3 months; if beneficial effects are observed, therapy is maintained indefinitely.

Therapeutic Uses and Clinical Toxicity. Mitotane is indicated in the palliative treatment of inoperable adrenocortical carcinoma. In addition to 138 patients reported by Hutter and Kayhoe (1966), 115 have been studied by Lubitz and associates (1973). Clinical effectiveness has been reported in 34 to 54% of these cases. Although the administration of mitotane produces anorexia and nausea in approximately 80% of patients, somnolence and lethargy in about 34%, and dermatitis in 15 to 20%, these effects do not contraindicate the use of the drug at lower doses.

V. Hormones

ADRENOCORTICOSTEROIDS

The pharmacology, major therapeutic uses, and toxic effects of the adrenocorticosteroids are discussed in Chapter 70. Only the applications of the hormones in the treatment of malignant disease will be considered here. Because of their lympholytic effects and their ability to suppress mitosis in lymphocytes, the greatest value of these steroids is in the treatment of acute leukemia in children and of malignant lymphoma. They are especially effective in the management of frank hemolytic anemia and the hemorrhagic complications of thrombocytopenia that frequently accompany malignant lymphomas and chronic lymphocytic leukemia.

In acute lymphoblastic or undifferentiated leukemia of childhood, adrenocorticosteroids may produce prompt clinical improvement and objective hematological remissions in 30 to 50% of children. Although these responses frequently are characterized by complete disappearance of all detectable leukemic cells from the peripheral blood and bone marrow, the duration of remission is extremely variable (2 weeks to 9 months) and relapse of the disease invariably occurs; eventually, drug resistance develops. Remissions occur more rapidly with corticosteroids than with antimetabolites, and there is no evidence of cross-resistance to unrelated agents. For these reasons, therapy is often initiated with a steroid and another type of agent, usually vincristine, conjointly in order to *induce* remissions. This approach followed by continuous *maintenance* treatment with

various agents seems to yield more prolonged remissions (*see* section on methotrexate). Adult leukemia seldom responds to induced hypercorticism, but marked constitutional symptoms of the disease and the hemorrhagic manifestations of thrombocytopenia may be controlled effectively, albeit temporarily, without demonstrable changes in platelet counts.

Corticosteroids have been used in patients with carcinoma, and have been recommended specifically by some for carcinoma of the breast; however, palliative effects are of short duration and complications are frequent. Although the overall results in the treatment of carcinoma with these agents have been disappointing, the judicious short-term use of corticosteroids may be indicated for specific complications such as hypercalcemia and intracranial metastases.

The adrenocorticosteroids are used in conjunction with x-ray therapy to reduce the occurrence of radiation edema in critical areas such as the superior mediastinum, brain, and spinal cord. These drugs are particularly useful in the symptomatic palliation of patients with severe hematopoietic depression secondary to bone-marrow involvement or previous radiation or chemotherapy. They may produce rapid symptomatic improvement in critically ill patients by temporarily suppressing fever, sweats, and pain, and by restoring, to some degree, appetite, lost weight, strength, and sense of well-being. The symptoms tend to recur after the hormone is withdrawn, which indicates that the effects of the disease, but not necessarily the disease process itself, have been affected. Therefore, the value of this type of therapy is to provide the patient with a relatively asymptomatic period during which his general physical condition may improve sufficiently to permit further definitive therapy.

Several preparations are available and at appropriate dosages exert similar effects (*see* Chapter 70). Prednisone, for example, is usually administered orally in doses as high as 60 to 100 mg, or even higher, for the first few days and gradually reduced to levels of 20 to 40 mg per day. A continuous attempt should be made to lower the dosage required to control the manifestations of the disease.

PROGESTINS

Progestational agents (*see* Chapter 68) have been found useful in the management of patients with endometrial carcinoma previously treated by surgery and radiotherapy (Kelley and Baker, 1961). These compounds were tried initially because of the concept that carcinoma of the endometrium results from the prolonged, unopposed overstimulation by estrogen (Hertig and Sommers, 1949). This led to the use of progesterone, which would correct this situation because of its physiological effect in producing maturation and secretory activity of the normal endometrium. Apparently a proportion of neoplastic cells arising from this tissue is still influenced by normal hormonal controls.

There are several preparations available. Hydroxyprogesterone caproate is usually administered intramuscularly in doses of 500 mg twice weekly; medroprogesterone acetate can be administered orally in doses of 100 to 200 mg daily or intramuscularly in doses of 400 mg twice weekly. An alternative oral agent is megestrol acetate, 20 mg twice daily. Beneficial effects, usually characterized by regression of pulmonary metastases, have been observed in approximately one third of patients.

Exceptional but significant responses to progestational agents have been reported in disseminated carcinomas of the breast (Stoll, 1972) and prostate (Fergusson, 1972). Experience with small numbers of patients has led many oncologists to view progestins as the treatment of choice for the palliation of metastatic renal-cell carcinoma (Bloom, 1972).

ESTROGENS AND ANDROGENS

A discussion of the pharmacology of the estrogens and androgens appears in Chapters 68 and 69. Their use in the treatment of certain neoplastic diseases will be discussed here. They are of value in this connection because certain organs that are often the primary site of malignant growth, notably the prostate and the mammary gland, are dependent upon hormones for their growth, function, and morphological integrity. Carcinomas arising from these organs often retain some of the hormonal requirements of their normal counterparts for varying periods of time. By changing the hormonal environment of such tumors it is possible to alter, to some degree, the course of the neoplastic process.

Androgen-Control Therapy of Prostatic Carcinoma. The development of the androgen-control regimen for the treatment of prostatic carcinoma is largely the contribution of Huggins and associates (1941). Their studies are of importance for several reasons: (1) they typify the rational approach to cancer chemotherapy in that the theoretical considerations that led to the trial of the therapeutic regimen were based upon fundamental biochemical concepts; (2) androgen-control therapy represents the first effective chemotherapeutic measure in disseminated carcinomatosis and has provided a great stimulus for research in the field; (3) although no case of prostatic carcinoma has been cured by androgen-control therapy, life expectancy has been increased and thousands of patients have enjoyed the benefit of its ameliorating effects; and (4) approximately 95% of patients with clinical manifestations of carcinoma of the prostate have nonresectable disease and require androgen-control therapy.

History and Rationale. The relationship between the prostate and testicular function was appreciated early in the nineteenth century, when it was noted that regression of the prostate followed orchiectomy. Huggins observed that, in the dog, shrinkage of the gland and cessation of secretion followed castration and that these effects could be reversed by the administration of androgen. Of even greater significance was the observation that the administration of estrogen could block the effects of the androgen. On the basis of these experimental findings, Huggins and associates (1941) postulated that significant clinical improvement should occur after bilateral orchiectomy in patients with advanced prostatic carcinoma, a theory that proved to be correct. It was also demonstrated that similar results could be obtained by the administration of estrogen (Herbst, 1941).

The fundamental mechanism by which the lack of androgen results in regressive changes in normal and malignant prostatic cells is unknown. Relapse eventually occurs in patients on androgen-control therapy, and this constitutes another fundamental problem. The most likely explanation is that in the surviving prostatic cells progressive dedifferentiation occurs, which favors the emergence of cell types that are no longer dependent on androgen.

Therapeutic Regimen. From a statistical analysis of over 1800 cases (Nesbit and Baum, 1950), it appears that 5-year control of prostatic cancer is most effectively obtained by the combined use of orchiectomy and estrogen in patients who, when first treated, are free from metastases. When metastases are already present, orchiectomy seems to be more effective than estrogen therapy, and their combination does not appear to offer any advantage. When either orchiectomy or estrogen alone is employed as a therapeutic measure and the patient relapses, some degree of symptomatic improvement is then obtained by the alternative procedure, but this usually is not outstanding. In view of the fact that orchiectomy is indicated regardless of metastases, and that under certain circumstances further benefit is to be derived from the use of estrogen, it is recommended that both procedures be employed in any case of prostatic carcinoma as soon as the diagnosis is established.

The choice of estrogen is largely determined by cost and convenience. Natural products have no advantage over synthetic preparations, and the oral route of administration causes the least inconvenience to the patient. For these reasons, diethylstilbestrol or a related synthetic compound is the preparation of choice. There is no evidence that survival is improved with excessively large doses. An average dose of diethylstilbestrol is 5 mg three times daily. Indeed, many authorities reduce the daily dose to as little as 1 mg after a few weeks. The dose of other estrogens is in proportion to their potency.

Response to Therapy. Subjective and objective improvements rapidly follow the institution of androgen-control therapy of prostatic carcinoma. From the patient's point of view the most gratifying of these is relief of pain. This is associated with an increase in appetite, weight gain, and a feeling of well-being. Objectively, there are regressions of the primary tumor and soft-tissue metastases. Serial biopsies reveal nuclear and cytoplasmic changes in the malignant tissue; after some months, most of it may be replaced by scar tissue. Malignant cells, however, do not completely disappear. Elevated plasma acid phosphatase activity usually falls to normal. Alkaline phosphatase activity may first rise and then fall. There is often an associated recovery from anemia. Some patients with prostatic carcinoma show no response to androgen-control therapy. Eventually prostatic tumors become insensitive to the lack of androgen or the presence of estrogen; however, it is now well established that effective palliation is afforded by the therapeutic regimen and that the life expectancy of the treated patient is significantly increased.

Untoward Effects. Androgen-control therapy is one of the safest forms of cancer chemotherapy. The psychic trauma of orchiectomy is not inconsequential, but is tempered somewhat by the age of the patient. The same is true of the sexual impotence that usually accompanies either orchiectomy or estrogen therapy. After orchiectomy alone, hot flushes are not uncommon; these can be controlled by the administration of estrogen. Estrogens are capable of producing the untoward responses described in detail in Chapter 68. Mild gastrointestinal disturbances may be noted; occasionally, these may be severe enough to require discontinuation of the drug. There also may be some expansion of extracellular fluid volume in patients with poor cardiac function. In one widely cited study, there was a significant excess mortality from cardiac and cerebrovascular complications when a group of men treated with 5 mg of diethylstilbestrol daily was compared with controls (Veterans Administration Co-Operative Urological Research Group, 1967). Gynecomastia is frequent and may be a disturbing feature in some patients; it is said to be prevented by low-dose radiation of the breasts at the outset of hormonal therapy (Larrson and Sundbom, 1962). In rare instances, carcinoma of the male breast has occurred in patients given estrogen for prolonged periods of time.

Estrogens and Androgens in the Treatment of Mammary Carcinoma. Estrogens and androgens have found application in the treatment of advanced mammary carcinoma. The hormones afford some measure of relief in patients with nonresectable disease in whom the metastatic lesions are too widespread to permit effective radiation.

History and Rationale. Hormonal-control therapy for carcinoma of the breast is by no means a recent development, and late in the nineteenth century castration was recommended. Not long thereafter, radiation of the ovaries was introduced. Both procedures are still practiced. Early experimental work on the relation of ovarian secretions to carcinoma of the breast led to the observation that the incidence of spontaneous breast cancer in female mice could be substantially decreased by castration (Loeb, 1919). Later, Lacassagne (1936) demonstrated that, in a strain of mice in which the females but not the males exhibited a high incidence of spontaneous breast carcinoma, the administration of estrogen to the males resulted in proliferation of the ductal epithelium, from which metastatic adenocarcinoma developed. He was also able, by the injection of estrogen, to increase the incidence of carcinoma of the breast to 100% in a strain of mice that normally had a very low incidence of spontaneous tumors. Among the first reports of the use of testosterone were those of Ulrich in 1939 and Loeser in 1941. In 1944, Haddow and coworkers in Great Britain first reported the results of estrogen therapy. Discussions of results with hormonal-control therapy of carcinoma of the breast may be found in the reports of the Cooperative Breast Cancer Group of the Cancer Chemotherapy National Service Center (*see* Progress Report, 1961, 1962; Kennedy, 1965; Krakoff, 1967).

Therapeutic Regimen. The therapeutic regimen for the use of androgens and estrogens in the treatment of carcinoma of the breast is largely empirical. The first cardinal principle is that hormonal therapy should be reserved for patients for whom surgical treatment or radiotherapy has been fully considered and deemed no longer of value. Once this qualification has been met, androgen therapy may be employed for patients in any age group. Objective remissions are obtained in approximately 20% of patients (Goldenberg, 1964). Estrogen therapy generally is contraindicated in patients who are not at least 5 years past the menopause, regardless of chronological age. Experience has shown that estrogen may accelerate the neoplastic process in women who are still menstruating. In premenopausal women, oophorectomy is the first recommended procedure to institute hormonal control. On the basis of earlier observations, androgen was said to be preferable for the treatment of bone metastases, whereas estrogen was considered to be the preparation of choice for soft-tissue metastases. Subsequent evidence does not entirely substantiate these findings, however, and it is often the practice to change from one type of hormone to the other in unresponsive patients.

Developments in endocrinology have led to extremely important, potentially decisive methods for the selection of patients for ablative or additive hormonal therapy. This may well remove most of the empiricism from this area. Extensive experimental and clinical evidence has shown that estrogen "target" tissues (including approximately 50% of human invasive ductal carcinomas) contain a specific binding protein ("estrogen receptor") (Hilf and Wittliff, 1975). Strong evidence has accumulated that a breast malignancy lacking specific estrogen-binding capacity rarely responds to hormonal manipulation, whereas those tumors containing the receptors usually do so (Jensen *et al.*, 1971; Savlov *et al.*, 1974). The accumulated evidence to date has been derived primarily from patients treated with ablative surgery; further investigation is necessary regarding additive hormonal therapy.

Hormonal therapy utilizes doses much larger than those needed for physiological replacement. Androgen therapy is preferably with oral agents; commonly used regimens include fluoxymesterone, 10 mg orally three times a day, or calusterone, 50 mg orally four times daily. Parenteral androgen therapy may be given as dromostanolone propionate, 100 mg intramuscularly three times weekly. The prototype parenteral androgen preparations, testosterone propionate and testosterone enanthate, while as effective as other androgens, are now rarely employed because of their marked virilizing property.

Compounds with estrogenic activity are numerous. Oral diethylstilbestrol is the most frequently used; it is given initially in doses of 5 mg daily. This dose is gradually increased to a maintenance dose of 5 mg three times daily over a 1- to 2-week period. Ethinyl estradiol is also commonly used, the dosage being gradually increased from 0.5 mg orally once daily to the customary maintenance dose of 3 mg daily, given in three portions. Ethinyl estradiol may be tried if diethylstilbestrol causes intolerable gastrointestinal side effects.

Response to Therapy. The onset of action of the

hormones is slow, and it is necessary to continue therapy for 8 to 12 weeks before a decision can be reached as to effectiveness. If a favorable response is obtained, hormonal treatment should be continued until an exacerbation of symptoms occurs. Withdrawal of the hormone at this time may occasionally be followed by another remission.

In a retrospective study of 944 patients with disseminated mammary carcinoma, objective remissions were noted in approximately 20% of patients receiving androgens and in 30 to 40% of postmenopausal women treated with estrogens. Two major factors appear to temper the rate of response: the menopausal age of the patient and the body system most importantly involved by the disease (local, best; visceral, worst; and osseous, intermediate). It is of interest that, despite regression of the lesions, only rarely is it possible to demonstrate morphological changes in the tumors. The duration of the induced remission averages about 6 months to 1 year; however, some patients may receive benefit for several years. Average survival time in patients who respond to therapy appears to be longer than in untreated controls or in those who do not respond.

Untoward Effects. All the untoward effects that commonly accompany estrogen and androgen therapy have been observed in the use of these agents in the treatment of mammary carcinoma; these effects are described in Chapters 68 and 69. Two toxic manifestations require emphasis. With either hormone, the combined effect of a steroid and osteolytic metastases may result in marked hypercalcemia. The chief dangers are ectopic calcification, particularly in the urinary tract, and the physiological disturbances that may accompany an increase in the concentration of ionized calcium in the extracellular fluid. Patients who show an elevation in plasma calcium should receive a high fluid intake. Severe hypercalcemia, whether spontaneous or drug induced, is a true medical emergency. If an estrogen or androgen is being used, it should be discontinued. Forced hydration, by vein if the patient cannot drink, is mandatory. Further measures may be necessary; these include administration of diuretics, adrenocorticosteroids in large doses, oral or intravenous phosphate supplementation, or the intravenous administration of mithramycin (*see above; see also* Chapter 37). When drug-induced hypercalcemia is corrected, further steroid therapy may be cautiously attempted. The incidence of hypercalcemia in patients receiving androgens is approximately 10%; it occurs less frequently with estrogen therapy. Plasma calcium concentrations should be determined routinely in patients receiving hormonal therapy.

Rarely, either estrogen or androgen therapy may cause exacerbation of the malignant process; this occurs more frequently as a result of estrogen administration.

Androgen-Control Therapy of Carcinoma of the Male Breast. Carcinoma of the male breast is a rare tumor that is seldom diagnosed sufficiently early to permit definitive surgical intervention. The neoplasm regresses in a high proportion of cases in response to androgen-control therapy. Although this may be achieved by either orchiectomy or the administration of estrogen, it is preferable to initiate treatment with orchiectomy; when evidence of exacerbation appears, estrogen therapy is instituted. Remissions of several years can be achieved with this therapeutic regimen (Treves, 1959; Kennedy, 1965).

VI. Radioactive Isotopes

Mechanism of Cytotoxic Action of Ionizing Radiations. It is beyond the scope of this chapter to present a definitive account of present concepts of the mechanism of the cytotoxic actions of ionizing radiations. It is known, however, that radiation interacts with atoms and molecules, and leads to their excitation and ionization (Schwartz, 1966). In irradiated tissue a variety of chemical radicals from water are formed that can further interact with altered irradiated proteins and nucleic acids and lead to cell damage. This damage is often first expressed when cellular division occurs (Kaplan, 1963). In view of the highly technical problems associated with the proper use of radioactive isotopes for either metabolic tracing, diagnostic, or therapeutic purposes, reference should be made to a variety of excellent reviews and books on these subjects (*see* Kaplan, 1963; Schwartz, 1966; Haynie *et al.,* 1973).

SODIUM PHOSPHATE-^{32}P

Preparations, Physical Properties, Distribution, and Excretion. *Sodium Phosphate P 32 Solution,* U.S.P. (*sodium phosphate-^{32}P;* PHOSPHOTOPE), is supplied as a solution for oral use, as well as in sterile form for injection. The half-life is 14.3 days. ^{32}P emits an electron with an average energy of about 0.6 million electron volts (mev) (maximum of about 1.7 mev); the other product of its decomposition is nonradioactive sulfur (^{32}S). The emitted beta particle of ^{32}P penetrates to an average depth of about 2 mm (with a maximum of not more than 8 mm) of tissue. The differential uptake of phosphate by cells is dependent upon at least three factors: (1) the total amount of phosphate in exchangeable form in the tissue; (2) the rate of turnover of the phosphate groups; and (3) the rate at which new cells are formed. The material will enter particularly those tissues in which the metabolic turnover of phosphate groups is high, as in neoplastic cells or in normal cells of the bone marrow, spleen, and lymph nodes, in which cell reproduction also is rapid; in the liver, however, in which cellular reproductive activity is very low, but where the participation of phosphate-containing compounds in metabolism is marked, a large amount of radioactivity also will be assimilated from sodium phosphate-^{32}P.

Ultimately, as phosphate-^{32}P leaves the soft tissues through turnover, the bones become the most radioactive tissue, regardless of the initial distribution of the isotope. The renal elimination of absorbed radioactivity, originally rapid (25 to 50% during the first 4 to 6 days), soon becomes very slow (less than 1% per day). If administered orally, about 25% of the radioactivity of sodium phosphate-^{32}P is unabsorbed and is excreted in the feces. Uptake into osseous tissues, in addition to immediate direct utilization by bone-marrow cells, affords opportunities for both early and long-continued bombardment of both bone-marrow and osseous cells; hence, overdosage can lead to severe depression of bone-marrow function, with resultant leukopenia, thrombocytopenia, and anemia. Indeed, neoplastic changes in these tissues can be produced by large doses of radioactive phosphate.

Therapeutic Uses and Dosage. The high uptake of phosphate-^{32}P by critical normal tissues does not permit a truly selective attack upon malignant tissues. Although the isotope was used at one time for the therapy of chronic leukemias, chemotherapy is now the treatment of choice. Radioactive phosphorus is not effective in the treatment of the acute leukemias, lymphosarcomas, multiple myeloma, or Hodgkin's disease. It has been recommended, by local instillation after surgery, for stage-I and stage-II carcinoma of the ovary (Clark *et al.,* 1970). Occasionally, it has proven helpful for the palliation of bone pain due to metastatic involvement, particularly when used in conjunction with parathyroid hormone (Tong and Rubenfeld, 1967).

Sodium phosphate-^{32}P has been used for palliation in polycythemia vera because of its ability to suppress the overproduction of erythrocytes, as well as the accompanying excessive proliferation of platelets and leukocytes. However, its employment in this disorder has been largely discontinued because of a growing awareness that patients treated with this agent have a higher incidence of leukemia. In the future it will probably be completely replaced by chemotherapy with agents characterized by low or absent mutagenic and carcinogenic potential. When used in severe and refractory polycythemia vera, the initial intravenous dosage of sodium phosphate-^{32}P is usually about 3 mCi, ranging between 2.5 and 5 mCi. Subsequent ^{32}P therapy, with or without phlebotomy, usually is not given for at least 2 or 3 months, and preferably after longer intervals.

GOLD-198

This short-lived isotope of gold (half-life, 2.7 days), which emits both beta particles (principally 0.97 mev; 90 to 94%) and gamma rays (principally 0.41 mev; 6 to 10%), is supplied in the form of colloidal material, 25 to 200 mCi/ml. *Gold Au 198 Injection,* N.F. (AURCOLOID-198, AUREOTOPE), has been used in the treatment of brain tumors in children (D'Angio *et al.,* 1968; Gold *et al.,* 1972). It was also given by injection into closed serous cavities, particularly in the palliative treatment of peritoneal and pleural effusions caused by metastatic neoplasms; the mean effective life of the emissions is about 4 days. It is known that the particles of gold are phagocytized by cells on the walls of serous cavities, where, by mechanisms not clearly understood, their actions lead to diminution in the rate of accumulation of fluid. Since the dosage of ^{198}Au ranges between 35 and 150 mCi, treated patients afford a very significant hazard to nursing and other personnel; in addition, the therapy is costly and offers no therapeutic advantage in the treatment of malignant effusions over the use of alkylating agents, talc, or quinacrine. For these reasons, it has been replaced by these agents.

ISOTOPES OF IODINE

These preparations are discussed in Chapter 67.

Acute Leukemia Group B. New treatment schedule with improved survival in childhood leukemia. *J. Am. med. Ass.,* **1965,** *194,* 187–193.

Alberts, D. S.; Bachur, N. R.; and Holtzman, J. L. The pharmacokinetics of daunomycin in man. *Clin. Pharmac. Ther.,* **1971,** *12,* 96–104.

Allan, P. W.; Schnebli, H. P.; and Bennett, L. L., Jr. Conversion of 6-mercaptopurine and 6-mercaptopurine ribonucleoside to 6-methylmercaptopurine ribonucleotide in human epidermoid carcinoma No. 2 cells in culture. *Biochim. biophys. Acta,* **1966,** *114,* 647–650.

Anderson, J. H., and Sartorelli, A. C. Inhibition of inosinic acid dehydrogenase of sarcoma 180 ascites cells by nucleotides and their analogs. *Biochem. Pharmac.,* **1969,** *18,* 2747–2757.

Ansfield, F. J.; Ramirez, G.; Mackman, S.; Bryan, G. T.; and Curreri, A. R. A ten-year study of 5-fluorouracil in disseminated breast cancer with clinical results and survival times. *Cancer Res.,* **1969,** *29,* 1062–1066.

Ansfield, F. J.; Ramirez, G.; Skibba, J. L.; Bryan, G. T.; Davis, H. L.; and Wirtanen, G. W. Intrahepatic arterial infusion with 5-fluorouracil. *Cancer, N.Y.,* **1971,** *28,* 1147–1151.

Arcamone, F.; Cassinelli, G.; Fantini, G.; Grein, A.; Orezzi, P.; Poli, C.; and Spalla, C. Adriamycin, 14-hydroxy-daunomycin, a new antitumor antibiotic from *S. peucetius* var. *caesius. Biotechnol. Bioeng.,* **1969,** *11,* 1101–1109.

Ariel, I. Therapeutic effects of hydroxyurea. Experience with 118 patients with inoperable solid tumors. *Cancer, N.Y.,* **1970,** *25,* 705–714.

Bagley, C. M.; Bostick, F. W.; and DeVita, V. T., Jr. Clinical pharmacology of cyclophosphamide. *Cancer Res.,* **1973,** *33,* 226–233.

Barranco, S. C., and Humphrey, R. M. The effects of 2′-deoxythioguanosine on survival and progression in mammalian cells. *Proc. Soc. exp. Biol. Med.,* **1971,** *31,* 583–586.

Barratt, T. M., and Soothill, J. F. Controlled trial of cyclophosphamide in steroid-sensitive relapsing nephrotic syndrome of childhood. *Lancet,* **1970,** *2,* 479–482.

Beckloff, G. L.; Lerner, H. J.; Frost, D.; Russo-Alesi, F. M.; and Gitomer, S. Hydroxyurea (NSC-32065) in biological fluids: dose-concentration relationship. *Cancer Chemother. Rep.,* **1965,** *48,* 57–58.

Benjamin, R. S.; Riggs, C. E.; and Bachur, N. R. Pharmacokinetics and metabolism of adriamycin in man. *Clin. Pharmac. Ther.,* **1973,** *14,* 592–599.

Berenbaum, M. C. Is azathioprine a better immunosuppressive than 6-mercaptopurine? *Clin. expl Immun.,* **1971,** *8,* 1–8.

Bertino, J. R.; Cashmore, A.; Fink, N.; Calabresi, P.; and Lefkowitz, E. The induction of leukocyte and erythrocyte dihydrofolate reductase by methotrexate. *Clin. Pharmac. Ther.,* **1965,** *6,* 763–770.

Bhuyan, B. K. The action of streptozotocin on mammalian cells. *Cancer Res.,* **1970,** *30,* 2017–2023.

Bollag, W. The tumor-inhibitory effects of the methyl-hydrazine derivative Ro 4-6467/1 (NSC-77213). *Cancer Chemother. Rep.,* **1963,** *33,* 1–4.

———. Experimental studies with a methylhydrazine derivative, ibenzymethyzin. In, *Natulan (Ibenzymethyzin).* (Jelliffe, A. M., and Marks, J., eds.) John Wright & Sons, Ltd., Bristol, **1965,** pp. 1–8.

Bolt, W. von; Ritzl, F.; Toussaint, R.; and Nahrmann, H. Verteilung und Ausscheidung eines cystostatisch wirkenden mit Tritium markierten N-Lost-Derivatives beim krebskranken Menschen. *Arzneimittel-Forsch.,* **1961,** *11,* 170–175.

Bourke, R. S.; West, C. R.; Chheda, G.; and Tower, D. B. Kinetics of entry and distribution of 5-fluorouracil in cerebrospinal fluid and brain following intravenous injection in a primate. *Cancer Res.,* **1973,** *33,* 1735–1746.

Brennan, M. J.; Talley, R. W.; SanDiego, E. L.; Burrows, J. H.; O'Bryan, R. M.; Vaitkevicius, V. K.; and Horeglad, S. Critical analysis of 594 cancer patients treated with 5-fluorouracil. In, *Proceedings of the International Symposium on Chemotherapy of Cancer, Lugano.* (Plattner, P. A., ed.) Elsevier Publishing Co., Amsterdam, **1964,** pp. 118–150.

Brock, N. Pharmacologic characterization of cyclophosphamide (NSC-26271) and cyclophosphamide metabolites. *Cancer Chemother. Rep.,* **1967,** *51,* 315–325.

Broder, L. E., and Carter, S. K. Pancreatic islet cell carcinoma. II. Results of therapy with streptozotocin in 52 patients. *Ann. intern. Med.,* **1973,** *79,* 108–118.

Broome, J. D. Evidence that the L-asparaginase of guinea pig serum is responsible for its antilymphoma effects. I. Properties of the L-asparaginase of guinea pig serum in relation to those of the antilymphoma substance. *J. exp. Med.,* **1963,** *118,* 99–120.

Bruckner, H. W., and Creasey, W. A. The administration of 5-fluorouracil by mouth. *Cancer, N.Y.,* **1974,** *33,* 14–18.

Burchall, J. T. Protection of microbial dihydrofolate reductase against inactivation by pronase. *Molec. Pharmac.,* **1968,** *4,* 238–246.

Burchenal, J. H.; Holmberg, E. A. D.; Fox, J. J.; Hemphill, S. C.; and Reppert, J. A. The effects of 5-fluorodeoxycytidine, 5-fluorodeoxyuridine, and related compounds on transplanted mouse leukemias. *Cancer Res.,* **1959,** *19,* 494–500.

Burchenal, J. H.; Murphy, M. L.; Ellison, R. R.; Karnofsky, D. A.; Sykes, M. P.; Tan, T. C.; Leone, L. A.; Craver, L. F.; Dargeon, H. W.; and Rhoads, C. P. Clinical evaluation of a new antimetabolite, 6-mercaptopurine, in the treatment of leukemia and allied diseases. *Blood,* **1953,** *8,* 965–999.

Calabresi, P. New techniques for measuring the effects of chemotherapeutic agents upon neoplastic and normal host cells. *Verlag wien. med. Akad.,* **1967,** *7,* 99–111.

Calabresi, P.; Griswold, D.; and Heppner, G. Immunosuppression by drugs in complex immune responses. In, *Proceedings of the Fifth International Congress on Pharmacology,* Vol. 5. (Okita, G. T., and Acheson, G. H., eds.) S. Karger, Basel, **1972,** pp. 421–430.

Calabresi, P., and Turner, R. W. Beneficial effects of triacetyl azauridine in psoriasis and mycosis fungoides. *Ann. intern. Med.,* **1966,** *64,* 352–371.

Chabner, B. A.; Myers, C. E.; Coleman, C. N.; and Johns, D. G. The clinical pharmacology of antineoplastic agents. *New Engl. J. Med.,* **1975,** *292,* 1107–1113, 1159–1168.

Ch'ien, L. T.; Cannon, N. J.; Charamella, L. J.; Dismukes, W. E.; Whitley, R. J.; Buchanan, R. A.; and Alford, C. A., Jr. Adenine arabinoside treatment of severe *Herpesvirus hominis* infections in man. *J. infect. Dis.,* **1973,** *128,* 658–663.

Chu, M. Y. Incorporation of arabinosyl cytosine into 2-7S ribonucleic acid and cell death. *Biochem. Pharmac.,* **1971,** *20,* 2057–2063.

Chu, M. Y., and Fischer, G. A. A proposed mechanism of action of 1-β-D-arabinofuranosylcytosine as an inhibitor of the growth of leukemic cells. *Biochem. Pharmac.,* **1962,** *11,* 423–430.

———. Comparative studies of leukemic cells sensitive and resistant to cytosine arabinoside. *Ibid.,* **1965,** *14,* 333–341.

———. The incorporation of ^{3}H-cytosine arabinoside and its effect on murine leukemic cells (L5178Y). *Ibid.,* **1968,** *17,* 753–767.

Clark, D.; Hilaris, B.; Roussis, C.; and Brunschwig, A. The role of radiation therapy (including isotopes) in the treatment of cancer of the ovary (results of 614 patients treated at Memorial Hospital, New York, N.Y.). *Prog. clin. Cancer,* **1970,** *5,* 227–235.

Clarkson, B. D. Acute myelocytic leukemia in adults. *Cancer, N.Y.,* **1972,** *30,* 1572–1582.

Clarkson, B. D.; Krakoff, I. H.; Burchenal, J. H.; Karnofsky, D. A.; Golbey, R. B.; Dowling, M. D.; Oettgen, H. F.; and Lipton, A. Clinical results of treatment with *E. coli* L-asparaginase in adults with leukemia, lymphosarcoma and solid tumors. *Cancer, N.Y.,* **1970,** *25,* 279–305.

Coe, R. O., and Bull, F. E. Cirrhosis associated with methotrexate treatment of psoriasis. *J. Am. med. Ass.,* **1968,** *206,* 1515–1520.

Cohen, S. S.; Flaks, J. G.; Barner, H. D.; Loeb, M. R.; and Lichtenstein, J. The mode of action of 5-fluorouracil and its derivatives. *Proc. natn. Acad. Sci. U.S.A.,* **1958,** *44,* 1004–1012.

Comiener, G. W., and Smith, C. G. Studies of the enzymatic deamination of ara-cytidine. V. Inhibition *in vitro* and *in vivo* by tetrahydrouridine and other reduced pyrimidine nucleosides. *Biochem. Pharmac.,* **1968,** *17,* 1981–1991.

Cortes, E. P.; Holland, J. F.; Moskowitz, R.; and Depoli, E. Effects of mithramycin on bone resorption *in vitro. Cancer Res.,* **1972,** *32,* 74–76.

Costa, G.; Hreshchyshyn, M. D.; and Holland, J. F. Initial clinical studies with vincristine. *Cancer Chemother. Rep.,* **1962,** *24,* 39–41.

Creasey, W. A.; Fink, M. E.; Handschumacher, R. E.; and Calabresi, P. Clinical and pharmacological studies with 2′,3′,5′-triacetyl-6-azauridine. *Cancer Res.,* **1963,** *23,* 444–453.

Creasey, W. A.; Koutras, G. A.; and Calabresi, P. The metabolism of uracil-2-^{14}C and the granulocyte response to endotoxin as indicators of the toxicity produced in patients receiving 5-fluorouracil. *Clin. Pharmac. Ther.,* **1967,** *8,* 273–282.

Creasey, W. A.; Papac, R. J.; Markiw, M. E.; Calabresi, P.; and Welch, A. D. Biochemical and pharmacological studies with 1-β-D-arabinofuranosylcytosine in man. *Biochem. Pharmac.,* **1966,** *15,* 1417–1428.

Crowther, D.; Bateman, C. J.; Vartan, C. P.; Whitehouse, J. M.; Malpas, J. S.; Hamilton-Fairley, G.; and Scott, R. B. Combination chemotherapy using L-asparaginase, daunorubicin, and cytosine arabinoside in adults with acute myelogenous leukemia. *Br. med. J.,* **1970,** *4,* 513–517.

D'Angio, G.; French, L.; Stadlan, E.; and Keiffer, S. Intrathecal radioisotopes for the treatment of brain tumors. *Clin. Neurol.,* **1968,** *15,* 288–300.

Davidson, J. D., and Winter, T. S. Purine nucleotide pyrophosphorylases in 6-mercaptopurine-sensitive and -resistant human leukemias. *Cancer Res.,* **1964,** *24,* 261–267.

Davignon, J. P.; Yang, K. W.; Wood, H. B., Jr.; and Cradock, J. C. Formulation of three nitrosoureas for intravenous use. *Cancer Chemother. Rep.,* **1973,** *4,* Suppl., 7–11.

DeConti, R. C., and Calabresi, P. Treatment of polycythemia vera with azauridine and azaribine. *Ann. intern. Med.,* **1970,** *73,* 575–579.

DeConti, R. C.; Hubbard, S. P.; Pinch, P.; and Bertino, J. R. Treatment of advanced neoplastic disease with 1-(2-chloroethyl)-3-cyclohexyl-1-nitrosourea (CCNU; NSC-79037). *Cancer Chemother. Rep.,* **1973,** *57,* 201–207.

DeFronzo, R. A.; Braine, H.; and Colvin, O. M. Water intoxication in man after cyclophosphamide therapy. Time course and relation to drug activation. *Ann. intern. Med.,* **1973,** *78,* 861–869.

Delamore, I. W., and Prusoff, W. H. Effect of 5-iodo-2'-deoxyuridine on the biosynthesis of phosphorylated derivatives of thymidine. *Biochem. Pharmac.*, **1962**, *11*, 101–112.

Demis, D. J.; Brown, C. S.; and Crosby, W. H. Thioguanine in the treatment of certain autoimmune, immunologic and related diseases. *Am. J. Med.*, **1964**, *37*, 195–205.

DiMarco, A.; Soldati, M.; Fioretti, A.; and Dasdia, T. Ricerche sull'attivita' della daunomicina su cellule normali e neoplastiche coltivate *in vitro*. *Tumori*, **1963**, *49*, 235–251.

Djerassi, I. Methotrexate infusions and intensive supportive care in the management of children with acute lymphocytic leukemia: follow-up report. *Cancer Res.*, **1967**, *27*, 2561–2564.

Djerassi, I.; Rominger, C. J.; Kim, J. S.; Turchi, J.; Suvansri, U.; and Hughes, D. Phase I study of high doses of methotrexate, with citrovorum factor in patients with lung cancer. *Cancer, N.Y.*, **1972**, *30*, 22–30.

Dubost, M.; Ganter, P.; Maral, R.; Ninet, L.; Pinner, S.; Preud Homme, J.; and Werner, G. H. Un nouvel antibiotique a proprietes antitumorales. *C. r. hebd. Séanc. Acad. Sci., Paris*, **1963**, *257*, 1813–1820.

Elias, E. G., and Evans, J. T. Mithramycin in the treatment of Paget's disease of bone. *J. Bone Jt Surg.*, **1972**, *54-A*, 1730–1736.

Ellison, R. R.; Hoogstraten, B.; Holland, J. F.; Levy, R. N.; Lee, S. L.; Silver, R. T.; ten Pas, A.; Blom, J.; Jacquillat, C.; and Haurani, F. Intermittent therapy with 6-mercaptopurine (NSC-755) and methotrexate (NSC-740) given intravenously to adults with acute leukemia. *Cancer Chemother. Rep.*, **1972**, *56*, 535–542.

Evans, J. S.; Musser, E. A.; Mengel, G. D.; Forsblad, K. R.; and Hunter, J. H. Antitumor activity of 1-β-D-arabinofuranosylcytosine hydrochloride. *Proc. Soc. exp. Biol. Med.*, **1961**, *106*, 350–353.

Farber, S. Chemotherapy in the treatment of leukemia and Wilms' tumor. *J. Am. med. Ass.*, **1966**, *198*, 826–836.

Farber, S.; Diamond, L. K.; Mercer, R. D.; Sylvester, R. F.; and Wolff, V. A. Temporary remissions in acute leukemia in children produced by folic antagonist 4-amethopteroylglutamic acid (aminopterin). *New Engl. J. Med.*, **1948**, *238*, 787–793.

Fine, R. N.; Clarke, R. R.; and Shore, N. A. Hyponatremia and vincristine therapy. Syndrome possibly resulting from inappropriate antidiuretic hormone secretion. *Am. J. Dis. Child.*, **1966**, *112*, 256–259.

Fink, M. E., and Calabresi, P. The granulocyte response to an endotoxin (pyrexal) as a measure of functional marrow reserve in cancer chemotherapy. *Ann. intern. Med.*, **1962**, *57*, 732–742.

Fisher, B. Surgical adjuvant therapy for breast cancer. *Cancer, N.Y.*, **1972**, *30*, 1556–1564.

Fisher, B.; Carbone, P.; Economou, S. G.; and others. L-Phenylalanine mustard (L-PAM) in the management of primary breast cancer. A report of early findings. *New Engl. J. Med.*, **1975**, *292*, 117–122.

Frei, E., III, and others. The effectiveness of combinations of anti-leukemic agents in inducing and maintaining remission in children with acute leukemia. *Blood*, **1965**, *26*, 642–656.

Freireich, E. J.; Bodey, G. P.; Harris, J. E.; and Hart, J. S. Therapy for acute granulocytic leukemia. *Cancer Res.*, **1967**, *27*, 2573–2577.

George, R. P.; Poth, J. L.; Gordon, D.; and Schrier, S. L. Multiple myeloma—intermittent, combination chemotherapy compared to continuous therapy. *Cancer, N.Y.*, **1972**, *29*, 1665–1670.

Gershwin, M. E.; Goetzl, E. J.; and Steinberg, A. D. Cyclophosphamide: use in practice. *Ann. intern. Med.*, **1974**, *80*, 531–540.

Gilman, A. The initial clinical trial of nitrogen mustard. *Am. J. Surg.*, **1963**, *105*, 574–578.

Goldenberg, I. S. Testosterone propionate therapy in breast cancer. *J. Am. med. Ass.*, **1964**, *188*, 1069–1072.

Goodman, L. S.; Wintrobe, M. M.; Dameshek, W.; Goodman, M. J.; Gilman, A.; and McLennan, M. Nitrogen mustard therapy: use of methylbis (β-chlorethyl) amino hydrochloride for Hodgkin's disease, lymphosarcoma, leukemia and certain allied and miscellaneous disorders. *J. Am. med. Ass.*, **1946**, *132*, 126–132.

Gottlieb, J. A., and Hill, C. S., Jr. Treatment of thyroid cancer with adriamycin: experience with 30 patients. *New Engl. J. Med.*, **1974**, *290*, 193–197.

Griswold, D. E.; Heppner, G. H.; and Calabresi, P. Selective suppression of humoral and cellular immunity with cytosine arabinoside. *Cancer Res.*, **1972**, *32*, 298–301.

————. Stimulation of hemolysin plaque-forming cells by idoxuridine. *Ibid.*, **1975**, *35*, 88–92.

Hakala, M. T., and Suolinna, E. M. Specific protection of folate reductase against chemical and proteolytic inactivation. *Molec. Pharmac.*, **1966**, *2*, 465–480.

Hampton, A. Reactions of ribonucleotide derivatives of purine analogues at the catalytic site of inosine 5'-phosphate dehydrogenase. *J. biol. Chem.*, **1963**, *238*, 3068–3074.

Haskell, C. M.; Canellos, G. P.; Leventhal, B. G.; Carbone, P. P.; Serpick, P. P.; and Hansen, H. H. L-Asparaginase toxicity. *Cancer Res.*, **1969**, *29*, 974–975.

Haut, A.; Abbott, W. S.; Wintrobe, M. M.; and Cartwright, G. E. Busulfan in the treatment of chronic myelocytic leukemia: the effect of long-term intermittent therapy. *Blood*, **1961**, *17*, 1–19.

Henderson, J. F.; Caldwell, I. C.; and Paterson, A. R. P. Decreased feedback inhibition in a 6-(methylmercapto) purine ribonucleoside-resistant tumor. *Cancer Res.*, **1967**, *27*, 1773–1778.

Heppner, G. H., and Calabresi, P. Suppression by cytosine arabinoside of serum-blocking factors of cell-mediated immunity to syngeneic transplants of mouse mammary tumors. *J. natn. Cancer Inst.*, **1972**, *48*, 1161–1167.

Herbst, W. P. Effects of estradiol dipropionate and diethyl stilbestrol on malignant prostatic tissue. *Tr. Am. Ass. genito-urin. Surg.*, **1941**, *34*, 195–199.

Hertig, A. T., and Sommers, S. C. Genesis of endometrial carcinoma. I. A study of prior biopsies. *Cancer, N.Y.*, **1949**, *2*, 946–956.

Hertz, R. Folic acid antagonists: effects on the cell and the patient. Clinical staff conference at N.I.H. *Ann. intern. Med.*, **1963**, *59*, 931–956.

Hertz, R.; Ross, G. T.; and Lipsett, M. B. Primary chemotherapy of nonmetastatic trophoblastic disease in women. *Am. J. Obstet. Gynec.*, **1963**, *86*, 808–814.

Hill, D. L., and Bennett, L. L. Purification and properties of 5-phosphoribosyl pyrophosphate amidotransferase from adenocarcinoma 755 cells. *Biochemistry, N.Y.*, **1969**, *8*, 122–130.

Hill, D. L.; Laster, W. R.; and Struck, R. F. Enzymatic metabolism of cyclophosphamide and nicotine and production of a toxic cyclophosphamide metabolite. *Cancer Res.*, **1972a**, *32*, 658–665.

Hill, G. H.; Sedransk, N.; Rochlin, D.; Bisel, H.; Andrews, N. C.; Fletcher, W.; Schroeder, J. M.; and Wilson, W. L. Mithramycin (NSC 24559) therapy of testicular tumors. *Cancer, N.Y.*, **1972b**, *30*, 900–908.

Ho, D. H. W. Biochemical studies of a new antitumor agent, O²2'-cyclocytidine. *Biochem. Pharmac.*, **1974**, *23*, 1235–1244.

Ho, D. H. W., and Frei, E., III. Clinical pharmacology of the 1-β-D-arabinofuranosyl cytosine. *Clin. Pharmac. Ther.*, **1971**, *12*, 944–954.

Holland, J. F., and Glidewell, O. Chemotherapy of acute lymphocytic leukemia of childhood. *Cancer, N.Y.*, **1972**, *30*, 1480–1487.

Holland, J. F., and others. Vincristine treatment of advanced cancer: a cooperative study of 392 cases. *Cancer Res.*, **1973**, *33*, 1258–1264.

Hryniuk, W. M., and Bertino, J. R. The treatment of leukemia with large doses of methotrexate and folinic acid: clinical-biochemical correlates. *J. clin. Invest.,* 1969, *48,* 2140–2155.

Huffman, D. H.; Benjamin, R. S.; and Bachur, N. R. Daunorubicin metabolism in acute nonlymphocytic leukemia. *Clin. Pharmac. Ther.,* 1972, *13,* 895–905.

Huggins, C.; Stevens, R. E., Jr.; and Hodges, C. V. Studies on prostatic cancer: effects of castration on advanced carcinoma of prostate gland. *Archs Surg.,* 1941, *43,* 209–223.

Hutchinson, D. J. Conference on obstacles to the control of acute leukemia: studies on cross-resistance and collateral sensitivity (1962–1964). *Cancer Res.,* 1965, *25,* 1581–1595.

Ichikawa, T.; Nakano, I.; and Hirokawa, I. Bleomycin treatment of the tumors of penis and scrotum. *J. Urol.,* 1969, *102,* 699–707.

Jacobson, L. O.; Spurr, C. L.; Barron, E. S. G.; Smith, T. R.; Lushbaugh, C.; and Dick, G. F. Nitrogen mustard therapy: studies on the effect of methyl-*bis*(beta-chloroethyl) amine hydrochloride on neoplastic diseases and allied disorders of the hemopoietic system. *J. Am. med. Ass.,* 1946, *132,* 263–271.

Jaffe, N. Recent advances in the chemotherapy of metastatic osteogenic sarcoma. *Cancer, N.Y.,* 1972, *30,* 1627–1631.

Johnston, T. P.; McCaleb, G. S.; and Montgomery, J. A. The synthesis of antineoplastic agents. XXXII. N-Nitrosoureas. *J. mednl Chem.,* 1963, *6,* 669–681.

Jones, B., and others. Daunorubicin (NSC-83142) vs. daunorubicin plus prednisone (NSC-10023) vs. daunorubicin plus vincristine (NSC-67574) plus prednisone in advanced childhood acute lymphocytic leukemia. *Cancer Chemother. Rep.,* 1972, *56,* 729–737.

Kaplan, S. R., and Calabresi, P. Drug therapy: immunosuppressive agents. Part I. *New Engl. J. Med.,* 1973, *289,* 952–954.

Kelley, R. M., and Baker, W. H. Progestational agents in the treatment of carcinoma of the endometrium. *New Engl. J. Med.,* 1961, *264,* 216–222.

Kennedy, B. J. Hormone therapy for advanced breast cancer. *Cancer, N.Y.,* 1965, *18,* 1151–1157.

———. Mithramycin therapy in advanced testicular neoplasms. *Ibid.,* 1970, *26,* 755–766.

Kennedy, B. J., and Yarbro, J. W. Metabolic and therapeutic effects of hydroxyurea in chronic myeloid leukemia. *J. Am. med. Ass.,* 1966, *195,* 1038–1043.

Kidd, J. G. Regression of transplanted lymphomas induced *in vivo* by means of normal guinea pig serum. I. Course of transplanted cancers of various kinds in mice and rats given guinea pig serum, horse serum, or rabbit serum. *J. exp. Med.,* 1953, *98,* 565–581.

Klein, E.; Milgrom, H.; Stoll, H. L.; Helm, F.; Walker, H. J.; and Holtermann, O. A. Topical 5-fluorouracil chemotherapy for premalignant and malignant epidermal neoplasms. In, *Cancer Chemotherapy II.* (Brodsky, I., and Kahn, S. B., eds.) Grune & Stratton, Inc., New York, 1972, pp. 147–166.

Knospe, W. H.; Loeb, V.; and Huguley, C. M. Bi-weekly chlorambucil treatment of chronic lymphocytic leukemia. *Cancer, N.Y.,* 1974, *33,* 555–562.

Krakoff, I. H. Chemotherapy and hormonal therapy of carcinoma of the breast. In, *Cancer Chemotherapy.* (Brodsky, I.; Kahn, S. B.; and Moyer, J. H.; eds.) Grune & Stratton, Inc., New York, 1967, pp. 77–83.

Lacassagne, A. Hormonal pathogenesis of adenocarcinoma of the breast. *Am. J. Cancer,* 1936, *27,* 217–228.

Larrson, L. G., and Sundbom, C. M. Roentgen irradiation of the male breast. *Acta radiol.,* 1962, *58,* 253–256.

LeFrak, E. A.; Pitha, J.; Rosenheim, S.; and Gottlieb, J. A. A clinicopathologic analysis of adriamycin cardiotoxicity. *Cancer, N.Y.,* 1973, *32,* 302–314.

Lemon, H. M., and Mozden, P. J. Reduction of toxicity of 5-fluorouracil cancer chemotherapy. *Ann. intern. Med.,* 1964, *60,* 333.

LePage, G. A. The metabolism of α-2′-deoxythioguanosine in murine tumor cells. *Can. J. Biochem.,* 1968, *46,* 655–661.

Levitt, M.; Mosher, M. B.; DeConti, R. C.; Farber, L. R.; Skeel, R. T.; Marsh, J. C.; Mitchell, M. S.; Papac, R. J.; Thomas, E. D.; and Bertino, J. R. Improved therapeutic index of methotrexate with "LEUCOVORIN rescue." *Cancer Res.,* 1973, *33,* 1729–1734.

Loeb, L. Further investigations on the origin of tumors in mice. VI. Internal secretion as a factor in the origin of tumors. *J. med. Res.,* 1919, *40,* 477–496.

Lubitz, J. A.; Freeman, L.; and Okun, R. Mitotane use in inoperable adrenal cortical carcinoma. *J. Am. med. Ass.,* 1973, *223,* 1109–1112.

McDonald, C. J., and Calabresi, P. Psoriasis and occlusive vascular disease. *J. clin. Invest.,* 1974, *53,* 52a.

McDonald, C. J., and Bertino, J. R. Parenteral methotrexate for psoriasis. *Lancet,* 1968, *1,* 864.

Mashburn, L. T., and Wriston, J. C. Tumor inhibitory effect of L-asparaginase from *Escherichia coli. Archs Biochem. Biophys.,* 1964, *105,* 450–452.

Mead, J. A.; Venditti, J. M.; Schrecker, A. W.; Goldin, A.; and Kereszfesgy, J. C. The effect of reduced derivatives of folic acid on toxicity and antileukemic effect of methotrexate in mice. *Biochem. Pharmac.,* 1963, *12,* 371–383.

Miech, R. P.; York, R.; and Parks, R. E., Jr. Adenosine triphosphate-guanosine 5′-phosphate phosphotransferase II. *Molec. Pharmac.,* 1969, *5,* 30–37.

Mitchell, M. S.; Kaplan, S. R.; and Calabresi, P. Alteration of antibody synthesis in the rat by cytosine arabinoside. *Cancer Res.,* 1969a, *29,* 896–904.

Mitchell, M. S.; Wade, M. E.; DeConti, R. C.; Bertino, J. R.; and Calabresi, P. Immunosuppressive effects of cytosine arabinoside and methotrexate in man. *Ann. intern. Med.,* 1969b, *70,* 535–547.

Moertel, C. G. Therapy of advanced gastrointestinal cancer with the nitrosoureas. *Cancer Chemother. Rep.,* 1973, *4,* 27–34.

Moore, E. C., and Cohen, S. S. Effects of arabinonucleotides on ribonucleotide reduction by an enzyme system from rat tumor. *J. biol. Chem.,* 1967, *242,* 2116–2118.

Moore, E. C., and LePage, G. A. The metabolism of 6-thioguanine and neoplastic tissue. *Cancer Res.,* 1958, *18,* 1075–1083.

Moore, G. E.; Bross, D. J.; Ausman, R.; Nadler, S.; Jones, R., Jr.; Slack, N.; and Rimm, A. A. Effects of 5-fluorouracil (NSC-19893) in 389 patients with cancer. *Cancer Chemother. Rep.,* 1968, *52,* 641–653.

Mukherjee, K. L.; Curreri, A. R.; Javid, M.; and Heidelberger, C. Studies on fluorinated pyrimidines. XVII. Tissue distribution of 5-fluorouracil-2-C14 and 5-fluoro-2′-deoxyuridine in cancer patients. *Cancer Res.,* 1963, *23,* 67–77.

Nelson, J. A., and Parks, R. E., Jr. Biochemical mechanisms for the synergism between 6-thioguanine and 6-(methylmercapto) purine ribonucleoside in sarcoma 180 cells. *Cancer Res.,* 1972, *32,* 2034–2041.

Nesbit, R. M., and Baum, W. C. Endocrine control of prostatic carcinoma. *J. Am. med. Ass.,* 1950, *143,* 1317–1320.

Noble, R. L. Symposium on vincaleukoblastine (VLB). In, *Proceedings of the Canadian Cancer Conference,* Vol. 4. (Begg, R. W.; Ham, A.; Leblond, C. P.; and Rossiter, R. J.; eds.) Academic Press, Inc., New York, 1961, pp. 333–338.

Noble, R. L.; Beer, C. T.; and Cutts, J. H. Further biological activities of vincaleukoblastine—an alkaloid isolated from *Vinca rosea* (L.). *Biochem. Pharmac.,* 1958, *1,* 347–348.

Northrop, G.; Taylor, S. G., III; and Northrop, R. L. Biochemical effects of mithramycin on cultured cells. *Cancer Res.,* 1969, *29,* 1916–1919.

Oettgen, H. F., and others. The toxicity of *E. coli* L-asparaginase in man. *Cancer, N.Y.*, **1970**, *25*, 253–278.

Ohnuma, T., and others. Treatment of adult leukemia with L-asparaginase (NSC-109229). *Cancer Chemother. Rep.*, **1971**, *55*, 269–275.

Oliverio, V. T.; Denham, C.; DeVita, V. T.; and Kelly, M. G. Some pharmacologic properties of a new antitumor agent, N-isopropyl-α-(2-methylhydrazino)-*p*-toluamide hydrochloride (NSC-77213). *Cancer Chemother. Rep.*, **1964**, *42*, 1–7.

Parham, W. E., and Wilbur, J. M. The mechanism of action of bisalkylating agents in cancer chemotherapy. II. The reaction of MYLERAN with mercaptans. *J. org. Chem.*, **1961**, *26*, 1569–1577.

Parks, R. E., Jr.; Brown, P. R.; and Kong, C. M. Incorporation of purine analogs into the nucleotide pools of human erythrocytes. *Adv. exp. Med. Biol.*, **1973**, *41A*, 117–127.

Paterson, A. R. P. The formation of 6-mercaptopurine riboside phosphate in ascites tumor cells. *Can. J. Biochem. Physiol.*, **1959**, *37*, 1011–1023.

Perlia, C. P.; Gubisch, N. J.; Wolter, J.; Edelberg, D.; Dederick, M. M.; and Taylor, S. G. Mithramycin treatment of hypercalcemia. *Cancer, N.Y.*, **1970**, *25*, 389–394.

Pigram, W. J.; Fuller, W.; and Hamilton, L. D. Stereochemistry of intercalation: interaction of daunomycin with DNA. *Nature, New Biol.*, **1972**, *235*, 17–19.

Pratt, C. B.; James, D. H., Jr.; Holton, C. P.; and Pinkel, D. Combination therapy including vincristine (NSC-67574) for malignant solid tumors in children. *Cancer Chemother. Rep.*, **1968**, *52*, 489–495.

Primack, A. Amelioration of cyclophosphamide-induced cystitis. *J. natn. Cancer Inst.*, **1971**, *47*, 223–227.

Ramirez, G.; Wilson, W.; Grage, T.; and Hill, G. Phase II evaluation of 1,3-*bis*(2-chloroethyl)-1-nitrosourea (BCNU; NSC-409962) in patients with solid tumors. *Cancer Chemother. Rep.*, **1972**, *56*, 787–790.

Ream, N. W.; Perlia, C. P.; Wolter, J.; and Taylor, S. Mithramycin therapy in disseminated germinal testicular cancer. *J. Am. med. Ass.*, **1968**, *204*, 96–102.

Rees, R. B.; Bennett, J. H.; Maibach, H. I.; and Arnold, H. L. Methotrexate for psoriasis. *Archs Derm.*, **1967**, *95*, 2–11.

Reusser, F. Mode of action of streptozotocin. *J. Bact.*, **1971**, *105*, 580–588.

Reyes, P. The synthesis of 5-fluorouridine 5′-phosphate by a pyrimidine phosphoribosyltransferase of mammalian origin. I. Some properties of the enzyme from P1534J mouse leukemic cells. *Biochemistry, N.Y.*, **1969**, *8*, 2057–2062.

Reyes, P., and Heidelberger, C. Fluorinated pyrimidines. *Molec. Pharmac.*, **1965**, *1*, 14–30.

Rhoads, C. P. Nitrogen mustards in treatment of neoplastic disease: official statement. *J. Am. med. Ass.*, **1946**, *131*, 656–658.

Rosenthal, F.; Wislicki, L.; and Kollek, L. Über die Beziehungen von schwersten Blutgiften zu Abbauprodukten des Eiweisses. *Klin. Wschr.*, **1928**, *7*, 972.

Rosman, M.; Lee, M. H.; Creasey, W. A.; and Sartorelli, A. C. Mechanisms of resistance to 6-thiopurines in human leukemia. *Cancer Res.*, **1974**, *34*, 1952–1956.

Rosman, W., and Williams, H. E. Leukocyte purine phosphoribosyltransferases in human leukemias sensitive and resistant to 6-thiopurines. *Cancer Res.*, **1973**, *33*, 1202–1209.

Ross, G. T.; Goldstein, D. P.; Hertz, R.; Lipsett, M. B.; and Odell, W. D. Sequential use of methotrexate and actinomycin D in the treatment of metastatic choriocarcinoma and related trophoblastic diseases in women. *Am. J. Obstet. Gynec.*, **1965**, *93*, 223–229.

Ryan, W. G.; Schwartz, T. B.; and Northrop, G. Experiences in the treatment of Paget's disease of bone with mithramycin. *J. Am. med. Ass.*, **1970**, *213*, 1153–1157.

Samuels, L. D.; Newton, W. A., Jr.; and Heyn, R. Dauno-

rubicin therapy in advanced neuroblastoma. *Cancer, N.Y.*, **1971**, *27*, 831–834.

Savlov, E. D.; Witliff, J. L.; Hilf, R.; and Hall, T. C. Correlations between certain biochemical properties of breast cancer and response to therapy: a preliminary report. *Cancer, N.Y.*, **1974**, *33*, 303–309.

Scannell, J. P., and Hitchings, G. H. Thioguanine in deoxyribonucleic acid from tumors of 6-mercaptopurine-treated mice. *Proc. Soc. exp. Biol. Med.*, **1966**, *122*, 627–629.

Schein, P.; Kahn, R.; Gorden, P.; Wells, S.; and DeVita, V. T. Streptozotocin for malignant insulinomas and carcinoid tumor. *Archs intern. Med.*, **1973**, *132*, 555–561.

Schein, P. S., and Winokur, S. H. Immunosuppressive and cytotoxic chemotherapy: long-term complications. *Ann. intern. Med.*, **1975**, *82*, 84–95.

Schwartz, R. S. Immunosuppressive drugs. *Prog. Allergy*, **1965**, *9*, 246–303.

Shastri, S.; Slayton, R. E.; Wolter, J.; Perlia, C. P.; and Taylor, S. G., III. Clinical study with bleomycin. *Cancer, N.Y.*, **1971**, *28*, 1142–1146.

Sladek, N. E. Therapeutic efficacy of cyclophosphamide as a function of its metabolism. *Cancer Res.*, **1972**, *32*, 535–542.

———. Evidence for an aldehyde possessing alkylating activity as the primary metabolite of cyclophosphamide. *Ibid.*, **1973**, *33*, 651–658.

Starzl, T. E., and others. Cyclophosphamide and whole organ transplantation in human beings. *Surgery Gynec. Obstet.*, **1971**, *133*, 981–991.

Steinberg, A. D.; Plotz, P. H.; Wolff, S. M.; Wong, V. G.; Agus, S. G.; and Decker, J. L. Cytotoxic drugs in treatment of nonmalignant diseases. *Ann. intern. Med.*, **1972**, *76*, 619–636.

Stevens, D. A.; Jordan, G. W.; Waddell, T. F.; and Merigan, T. C. Adverse effect of cytosine arabinoside on disseminated zoster in a controlled trial. *New Engl. J. Med.*, **1973**, *289*, 873–878.

Sullivan, R. D., and Miller, E. The clinical effects of prolonged intravenous infusion of 5-fluoro-2′-deoxyuridine. *Cancer Res.*, **1965**, *25*, 1025–1033.

Sullivan, R. D.; Watkins, E., Jr.; Oberfield, R. A.; and Khazei, A. M. Current status of protracted arterial infusion chemotherapy for the treatment of solid tumors. *Surg. Clins N. Am.*, **1967**, *47*, 769–784.

Sutow, W. W.; Garcia, F.; Starling, K. A.; Williams, T. E.; Lane, D. M.; and Gehan, E. A. L-Asparaginase therapy in children with advanced leukemia. *Cancer, N.Y.*, **1971**, *28*, 819–824.

Sutow, W. W.; Vietti, T. J.; Lonsdale, D.; and Talley, R. W. Daunomycin in the treatment of metastatic soft tissue sarcoma in children. *Cancer, N.Y.*, **1972**, *29*, 1293–1297.

Tallal, L.; Tan, C.; Oettgen, H.; Wollner, N.; McCarthy, M.; Helson, L.; Burchenal, J.; Karnofsky, D.; and Murphy, M. L. *E. coli* L-asparaginase in the treatment of leukemia and solid tumors in 131 children. *Cancer, N.Y.*, **1970**, *25*, 306–320.

Talley, R. W., and Vaitkevicius, V. K. Megaloblastosis produced by a cytosine antagonist, 1-β-D-arabinofuranosylcytosine. *Blood*, **1963**, *21*, 352–361.

Tandon, R. N.; Bunnell, I. L.; and Cooper, R. G. The treatment of metastatic carcinoma of the liver by the percutaneous selective hepatic artery infusion of 5-fluorouracil. *Surgery, St. Louis*, **1973**, *73*, 118–121.

Tobin, W., and Sandler, G. S. Neurophysiologic alterations induced by vincristine (NSC-67574). *Cancer Chemother. Rep.*, **1968**, *52*, 519–526.

Tong, E. C. K., and Rubenfeld, S. The treatment of bone metastases with parathormone followed by radiophosphorus. *Am. J. Roentg.*, **1967**, *99*, 422–434.

Treves, N. The treatment of cancer of the male breast, especially inoperable by ablative surgery (orchiectomy, adrenalectomy, hypophysectomy) and the hormone therapy with estrogens and corticosteroids: an analysis of 42 patients. *Acta Un. int. Cancr.,* **1959,** *15,* 1169–1178.

Van Scott, E. J.; Auerbach, R.; and Weinstein, G. D. Parenteral methotrexate in psoriasis. *Archs Derm.,* **1964,** *89,* 550–556.

Veterans Administration Co-Operative Urological Research Group. Treatment and survival of patients with cancer of the prostate. *Surgery Gynec. Obstet.,* **1967,** *124,* 1011–1017.

Waksman, S. A., and Woodruff, H. B. Bacteriostatic and bactericidal substances produced by a soil actinomyces. *Proc. Soc. exp. Biol. Med.,* **1940,** *45,* 609–614.

Warnick, C. T., and Paterson, A. R. P. Effect of methylinosine on nucleotide concentrations in L5178Y cells. *Cancer Res.,* **1973,** *33,* 1711–1715.

Weil, M., and others. Daunorubicin in the therapy of acute granulocytic leukemia. *Cancer Res.,* **1973,** *33,* 921–928.

Wilson, C. B.; Boldrey, E. B.; and Enot, K. J. 1,3-*bis*(2-chloroethyl)-1-nitrosourea (NSC-409962) in the treatment of brain tumors. *Cancer Chemother. Rep.,* **1970,** *54,* 273–281.

Wolff, S. M., and Goodman, H. C. Hypogammaglobulinemia produced by administration of 6-thioguanine to patients with nephrosis. *J. clin. Invest.,* **1962,** *41,* 1413–1420.

Wolpert, M. K.; Damle, S. P.; Brown, J. E.; Sznycer, E.; Agrawal, K. C.; and Sartorelli, A. C. The role of phosphohydrolases in the mechanism of resistance of neoplastic cells to 6-thiopurines. *Cancer Res.,* **1971,** *31,* 1620–1626.

Yagoda, A.; Mukherji, B.; Young, C.; Etcubanas, E.; Lamonte, C.; Smith, J. R.; Tan, C. T. C.; and Krakoff, I. H. Bleomycin, an antitumor antibiotic. Clinical experience in 274 patients. *Ann. intern. Med.,* **1972,** *77,* 861–870.

Yarbro, J. W. Further studies on the mechanism of action of hydroxyurea. *Cancer Res.,* **1968,** *28,* 1082–1087.

Yarbro, J. W.; Kennedy, B. J.; and Barnum, C. P. Mithramycin inhibition of ribonucleic acid synthesis. *Cancer Res.,* **1966,** *26,* 36–39.

Young, R. C.; DeVita, V. T., Jr.; Serpick, A. A.; and Canellos, G. P. Treatment of advanced Hodgkin's disease with [1,3 *bis*(2-chloroethyl)-1-nitrosourea] BCNU. *New Engl. J. Med.,* **1971,** *285,* 475–479.

Ziegler, J. L.; Cohen, M. H.; Morrow, R. H.; and Kyalwazi, S. K. Immunologic studies in Burkitt's lymphoma. *Cancer, N.Y.,* **1970,** *25,* 734–738.

Zimmerman, T. P.; Chu, L.-C.; Bugge, J. L.; Nelson, D. J.; Lyon, G. M.; and Elion, G. B. Identification of 6-methylmercaptopurine ribonucleoside 5′-diphosphate and 5′-triphosphate as metabolites of 6-mercaptopurine in man. *Cancer Res.,* **1974,** *34,* 221–224.

Zubrod, C. G. Treatment of the acute leukemias. *Cancer Res.,* **1967,** *27,* 2557–2560.

———. Acute leukemias and Burkitt's lymphoma: present status of therapy. *Cancer, N.Y.,* **1968,** *21,* 553–557.

Monographs and Reviews

Adamson, R. H., and Fabro, S. Antitumor activity and other biological properties of L-asparaginase (NSC-109229): a review. *Cancer Chemother. Rep.,* **1968,** *52,* 617–626.

Agrawal, K. C., and Sartorelli, A. C. α-(N)-heterocyclic carboxaldehyde thiosemicarbazones. In, *Antineoplastic and Immunosuppressive Agents,* Part II. (Sartorelli, A. C., and Johns, D. G., eds.) Springer-Verlag, Berlin, **1975,** pp. 793–807.

Baker, B. R. *Design of Active-Site-Directed Irreversible Enzyme Inhibitors.* John Wiley & Sons, Inc., New York, **1967,** pp. 192–284.

Bennett, L. L. Glutamine antagonists. In, *Antineoplastic and Immunosuppressive Agents,* Part II. (Sartorelli, A. C.,

and Johns, D. G., eds.) Springer-Verlag, Berlin, **1975,** pp. 484–511.

Bergsagel, D. E. Plasma cell myeloma. An interpretive review. *Cancer, N.Y.,* **1972,** *30,* 1588–1594.

Bertino, J. R. Folate antagonists. In, *Antineoplastic and Immunosuppressive Agents,* Part II. (Sartorelli, A. C., and Johns, D. G., eds.) Springer-Verlag, Berlin, **1975,** pp. 468–483.

Bertino, J. R., and Johns, D. G. Folate antagonists. In, *Cancer Chemotherapy II.* (Brodsky, I., and Kahn, S. B., eds.) Grune & Stratton, Inc., New York, **1972,** pp. 9–22.

Bloom, H. J. G. Renal cancer. In, *Endocrine Therapy in Malignant Disease.* (Stoll, B. A., ed.) W. B. Saunders Co., Philadelphia, **1972,** pp. 339–367.

Blum, R. H., and Carter, S. K. Adriamycin. A new anticancer drug with significant clinical activity. *Ann. intern. Med.,* **1974,** *80,* 249–259.

Blum, R. H.; Carter, S. K.; and Agre, K. A clinical review of bleomycin—a new antineoplastic agent. *Cancer, N.Y.,* **1973,** *31,* 903–914.

Brockman, R. W. Resistance to purine analogs. Clinical Pharmacology Symposium. *Biochem. Pharmac.,* **1974,** *23,* Suppl. 2, pp. 107–117.

Brodsky, I., and Kahn, S. B. (eds.). *Cancer Chemotherapy II.* Grune & Stratton, Inc., New York, **1972.**

Burchenal, J. H. The treatment of leukemias. *Bull. N.Y. Acad. Med.,* **1954,** *30,* 429–447.

Burchenal, J. H., and Ellison, R. R. The pyrimidine and purine antagonists. *Clin. Pharmac. Ther.,* **1961,** *2,* 523–541.

Calabresi, P., and Welch, A. D. Chemotherapy of neoplastic diseases. *A. Rev. Med.,* **1962,** *13,* 147–202.

Capizzi, R. L., and Handschumacher, R. E. Asparaginase. In, *Cancer Medicine.* (Holland, J. F., and Frei, E., III, eds.) Lea & Febiger, Philadelphia, **1973,** pp. 850–859.

Carter, S. K. An overview of the status of the nitrosoureas in other tumors. *Cancer Chemother. Rep.,* **1973,** *4,* 35–45.

Carter, S. K.; Schabel, F. M., Jr.; Broder, L. E.; and Johnston, T. P. 1,3-*bis*(2-chloroethyl)-1-nitrosourea (BCNU) and other nitrosoureas in cancer treatment: a review. *Adv. Cancer Res.,* **1972,** *16,* 273–332.

Carter, S. K., and Slavik, M. Chemotherapy of cancer. *A. Rev. Pharmac.,* **1974,** *14,* 157–179.

Connors, T. A. Mechanisms of clinical drug resistance. Clinical Pharmacology Symposium. *Biochem. Pharmac.,* **1974,** *23,* Suppl. 2, 89–100.

———. Mechanism of action of 2-chloroethylamine derivatives, sulfur mustards, epoxides, and aziridines. In, *Antineoplastic and Immunosuppressive Agents,* Part II. (Sartorelli, A. C., and Johns, D. G., eds.) Springer-Verlag, Berlin, **1975,** pp. 18–34.

Creasey, W. A. Arabinosylcytosine. In, *Antineoplastic and Immunosuppressive Agents,* Part II. (Sartorelli, A. C., and Johns, D. G., eds.) Springer-Verlag, Berlin, **1975a,** pp. 232–256.

———. Vinca alkaloids and colchicine. *Ibid.,* **1975b,** pp. 670–694.

DeVita, V. T.; Canellos, G. P.; and Moxley, J. H., III. A decade of combination chemotherapy of advanced Hodgkin's disease. *Cancer, N.Y.,* **1972,** *30,* 1495–1504.

DeVita, V. T., Jr.; Serpick, A. A.; and Carbone, P. P. Combination chemotherapy in the treatment of advanced Hodgkin's disease. *Ann. intern. Med.,* **1970,** *73,* 881–895.

DiMarco, A. Daunomycin and adriamycin. In, *Antineoplastic and Immunosuppressive Agents,* Part II. (Sartorelli, A. C., and Johns, D. G., eds.) Springer-Verlag, Berlin, **1975,** pp. 593–614.

Elion, G. B. Biochemistry and pharmacology of purine analogs. *Fedn Proc. Fedn Am. Socs exp. Biol.,* **1967,** *26,* 898–904.

Elion, G. B., and Hitchings, G. H. Metabolic basis for the actions of analogs of purines and pyrimidines. *Adv. Chemother.,* **1965,** *2,* 91–177.

————. Azathioprene. In, *Antineoplastic and Immunosuppressive Agents,* Part II. (Sartorelli, A. C., and Johns, D. G., eds.) Springer-Verlag, Berlin, **1975,** pp. 404–425.

Fairley, G. H., and Simister, J. M. (eds.). *Cyclophosphamide.* The Williams & Wilkins Co., Baltimore, **1965.**

Fergusson, J. D. Secondary endocrine therapy. In, *Endocrine Therapy in Malignant Disease.* (Stoll, B. A., ed.) W. B. Saunders Co., Philadelphia, **1972,** pp. 263–272.

Fox, B. W. Mechanism of action of methanesulfonates. In, *Antineoplastic and Immunosuppressive Agents,* Part II. (Sartorelli, A. C., and Johns, D. G., eds.) Springer-Verlag, Berlin, **1975,** pp. 35–46.

Fudenberg, H. H. Waldenström's macroglobulinemia. In, *Cancer Chemotherapy II.* (Brodsky, I., and Kahn, S. B., eds.) Grune & Stratton, Inc., New York, **1972,** pp. 393–403.

Galton, D. A. Chemotherapy of chronic myelocytic leukemia. *Semin. Hemat.,* **1969,** *6,* 323–343.

Gardner, F. H. Treatment of lymphoproliferative disease. In, *Cancer Chemotherapy II.* (Brodsky, I., and Kahn, S. B., eds.) Grune & Stratton, Inc., New York, **1972,** pp. 361–373.

Gilman, A., and Philips, F. S. The biological actions and therapeutic applications of the β-chlorethylamines and sulfides. *Science, N.Y.,* **1946,** *103,* 409–415.

Gold, L.; Kieffer, S.; D'Angio, G.; Fallon, V.; and Long, D. Current status of intrathecal radiogold in the treatment of medulloblastoma. *Acta radiol.,* **1972,** *11,* 329–340.

Goldberg, I. H. Actinomycin D. In, *Antineoplastic and Immunosuppressive Agents,* Part II. (Sartorelli, A. C., and Johns, D. G., eds.) Springer-Verlag, Berlin, **1975,** pp. 582–592.

Greenwald, E. S. *Cancer Chemotherapy.* Medical Examination Publishing Co., Inc., Flushing, N.Y., **1973.**

Handschumacher, R. E.; Calabresi, P.; Welch, A. D.; Bono, V.; Fallon, H.; and Frei, E., III. Summary of current information on 6-azauridine. *Cancer Chemother. Rep.,* **1962,** No. 21, 1–18.

Handschumacher, R. E., and Welch, A. D. Agents which influence nucleic acid metabolism. In, *The Nucleic Acids,* Vol. 3. (Chargoff, E., and Davidson, J. N., eds.) Academic Press, Inc., New York, **1960,** pp. 453–526.

Haynie, T. P., III; Johns, M. F.; and Glenn, H. J. Principles of nuclear medicine. In, *Cancer Medicine.* (Holland, J. F., and Frei, E., III, eds.) Lea & Febiger, Philadelphia, **1973,** pp. 567–599.

Heidelberger, C. Fluorinated pyrimidines. *Prog. nucl. acid Res.,* **1965,** *4,* 1–50.

————. Pyrimidine and pyrimidine nucleosides. In, *Cancer Medicine.* (Holland, J. F., and Frei, E., III, eds.) Lea & Febiger, Philadelphia, **1973,** pp. 768–791.

————. Fluorinated pyrimidines and their nucleosides. In, *Antineoplastic and Immunosuppressive Agents,* Part II. (Sartorelli, A. C., and Johns, D. G., eds.) Springer-Verlag, Berlin, **1975,** pp. 193–231.

Hilf, R., and Wittliff, J. L. Mechanisms of actions of hormones: estrogens. In, *Antineoplastic and Immunosuppressive Agents,* Part II. (Sartorelli, A. C., and Johns, D. G., eds.) Springer-Verlag, Berlin, **1975,** pp. 104–138.

Hitchings, G. H., and Burchall, J. J. Inhibition of folate biosynthesis and function as a basis for chemotherapy. *Adv. Enzymol.,* **1965,** *27,* 417–468.

Hitchings, G. H., and Elion, G. B. Chemical suppression of the immune response. *Pharmac. Rev.,* **1963,** *15,* 365–405.

Ho, D. H. W., and Freireich, E. J. Clinical pharmacology of arabinosylcytosine. In, *Antineoplastic and Immunosuppressive Agents,* Part II. (Sartorelli, A. C., and Johns, D. G., eds.) Springer-Verlag, Berlin, **1975,** pp. 257–271.

Holland, J. F. *E pluribus unum:* presidential address. *Cancer Res.,* **1971,** *31,* 1319–1329.

Holland, J. F., and Frei, E., III (eds.). *Cancer Medicine.* Lea & Febiger, Philadelphia, **1973.**

Huennekens, F. M. Folate and B_{12} coenzymes. In, *Biological Oxidations.* (Singer, T. P., ed.) John Wiley & Sons, Inc., New York, **1968,** pp. 439–513.

Hutter, A. M., Jr., and Kayhoe, D. E. Adrenal cortical carcinoma: clinical features of 138 patients. *Am. J. Med.,* **1966,** *41,* 572–592.

Jackson, H. Antifertility substances. *Pharmac. Rev.,* **1959,** *11,* 135–172.

Jensen, E. V.; Black, G. E.; Smith, S.; Kuper, K.; and DeSombre, E. R. Estrogen receptors and breast cancer response to adrenalectomy. *Natn. Cancer Inst. Monogr.,* **1971,** *34,* 55–79.

Johns, D. G., and Bertino, J. R. Folate antagonists. In, *Cancer Medicine.* (Holland, J. F., and Frei, E., III, eds.) Lea & Febiger, Philadelphia, **1973,** pp. 739–754.

Johnson, I. S. Plant alkaloids. In, *Cancer Medicine.* (Holland, J. F., and Frei, E., III, eds.) Lea & Febiger, Philadelphia, **1973,** pp. 840–850.

Johnson, I. S.; Armstrong, J. G.; Gorman, M.; and Burnett, J. P. The vinca alkaloids: a new class of oncolytic agents. *Cancer Res.,* **1963,** *23,* 1390–1427.

Kaplan, H. S. Biochemical basis of reproductive death in irradiated cells. *Am. J. Roentg.,* **1963,** *90,* 907–916.

Krakoff, I. H. Clinical and pharmacologic effects of hydroxyurea. In, *Antineoplastic and Immunosuppressive Agents,* Part II. (Sartorelli, A. C., and Johns, D. G., eds.) Springer-Verlag, Berlin, **1975,** pp. 789–792.

Livingston, R. B., and Carter, S. K. *Single Agents in Cancer Chemotherapy.* Plenum Press, New York, **1970.**

Ludlum, D. B. Molecular biology of alkylation: an overview. In, *Antineoplastic and Immunosuppressive Agents,* Part II. (Sartorelli, A. C., and Johns, D. G., eds.) Springer-Verlag, Berlin, **1975,** pp. 6–17.

National Conference on Cancer Chemotherapy. *Cancer, N.Y.,* **1972,** *30,* 1473–1661.

Ochoa, M., and Hirschberg, E. Alkylating agents. In, *Experimental Chemotherapy,* Vol. 5. (Schnitzer, R. J., and Hawking, F., eds.) Academic Press, Inc., New York, **1967,** pp. 1–132.

Oettgen, H. F. L-Asparaginase: current status of clinical evaluation. In, *Antineoplastic and Immunosuppressive Agents,* Part II. (Sartorelli, A. C., and Johns, D. G., eds.) Springer-Verlag, Berlin, **1975,** pp. 723–746.

Oliverio, V. T. Derivatives of triazenes and hydrazines. In, *Cancer Medicine.* (Holland, J. F., and Frei, E., III, eds.) Lea & Febiger, Philadelphia, **1973a,** pp. 806–817.

————. Toxicology and pharmacology of the nitrosoureas. *Cancer Chemother. Rep.,* **1973b,** *4,* Part 3, No. 3, 13–20.

Paterson, A. R. P., and Tidd, D. M. 6-Thiopurines. In, *Antineoplastic and Immunosuppressive Agents,* Part II. (Sartorelli, A. C., and Johns, D. G., eds.) Springer-Verlag, Berlin, **1975,** pp. 389–403.

Patterson, M. K., Jr. L-Asparaginase: basic aspects. In, *Antineoplastic and Immunosuppressive Agents,* Part II. (Sartorelli, A. C., and Johns, D. G., eds.) Springer-Verlag, Berlin, **1975,** pp. 695–722.

Price, C. C. Chemistry of alkylation. In, *Antineoplastic and Immunosuppressive Agents,* Part II. (Sartorelli, A. C., and Johns, D. G., eds.) Springer-Verlag, Berlin, **1975,** pp. 1–5.

Progress Report. Results of studies by Cooperative Breast Cancer Group, 1956–1960. *Cancer Chemother. Rep.,* **1961,** *11,* 109–141.

Progress Report. Testosterone propionate therapy of breast cancer: Breast Cancer Group. *Cancer Chemother. Rep.,* **1962,** *16,* 273–275.

Prusoff, W. H., and Goz, B. Halogenated pyrimidine deoxyribonucleosides. In, *Antineoplastic and Immunosuppressive Agents,* Part II. (Sartorelli, A. C., and Johns, D. G., eds.) Springer-Verlag, Berlin, **1975,** pp. 272–347.

Reed, D. J. Procarbazine. In, *Antineoplastic and Immunosuppressive Agents,* Part II. (Sartorelli, A. C., and Johns, D. G., eds.) Springer-Verlag, Berlin, **1975,** pp. 747–765.

Reich, E. Biochemistry of actinomycins. *Cancer Res.,* **1963,** *23,* 1428–1441.

Robins, P. R., and Jowsey, J. Effect of mithramycin on normal and abnormal bone turnover. *J. Lab. clin. Med.,* **1973,** *82,* 576–586.

Ross, W. C. J. Rational design of alkylating agents. In, *Antineoplastic and Immunosuppressive Agents,* Part II. (Sartorelli, A. C., and Johns, D. G., eds.) Springer-Verlag, Berlin, **1975,** pp. 33–51.

Schabel, F. M., Jr. Historical development and future promise of the nitrosoureas as anticancer agents. *Cancer Chemother. Rep.,* **1973,** *4,* Part 3, No. 3, 3–6.

Schwartz, E. E. *The Biological Basis of Radiation Therapy.* J. P. Lippincott Co., Philadelphia, **1966.**

Shapiro, R. Chemistry of guanine and its biologically significant derivatives. *Prog. nucl. acid Res. molec. Biol.,* **1968,** *8,* 73–112.

Skipper, H. T., and Schabel, F. M., Jr. Quantitative and cytokinetic studies in experimental tumor models. In, *Cancer Medicine.* (Holland, J. F., and Frei, E., III, eds.) Lea & Febiger, Philadelphia, **1973,** pp. 629–650.

Skoda, J. Azapyrimidine nucleosides. In, *Antineoplastic and Immunosuppressive Agents,* Part II. (Sartorelli, A. C., and Johns, D. G., eds.) Springer-Verlag, Berlin, **1975,** pp. 348–372.

Stock, J. A. Antitumor antibiotics. II. The actinomycins. In, *Experimental Chemotherapy,* Vol. 4. (Schnitzer, R. J., and Hawking, F., eds.) Academic Press, Inc., New York, **1966,** pp. 243–267.

Stoll, B. A. Androgen, corticosteroid and progestin therapy. In, *Endocrine Therapy in Malignant Disease.* (Stoll, B. A., ed.) W. B. Saunders Co., Philadelphia, **1972,** pp. 165–191.

Symposium. (Various authors.) Hydroxyurea. (Thurman, W. G., ed.) *Cancer Chemother. Rep.,* **1964,** *40,* 1–78.

Symposium. (Various authors.) *Natulan.* (Jelliffe, A. M., and Marks, J., eds.) John Wright & Sons, Ltd., Bristol, **1965.**

Symposium. (Various authors.) Cyclophosphamide in pediatric neoplasia. (Oernbach, D. J., ed.) *Cancer Chemother. Rep.,* **1967,** *51,* 315–412.

Symposium. (Various authors.) Vincristine. *Cancer Chemother. Rep.,* **1968,** *52,* 455–535.

Symposium. (Various authors.) The nitrosoureas. *Cancer Chemother. Rep.,* **1973,** *4,* Part 3, 1–82.

Umezawa, H. Studies on bleomycin: chemistry and the biological action. *Biomedicine,* **1973a,** *18,* 459–475.

———. Principles of antitumor antibiotic therapy. In, *Cancer Medicine.* (Holland, J. F., and Frei, E., III, eds.) Lea & Febiger, Philadelphia, **1973b,** pp. 817–826.

Waksman Conference on Actinomycins: their potential for cancer chemotherapy. *Cancer Chemother. Rep.,* **1974,** *58,* 1–123.

Walker, M. D. Nitrosoureas in central nervous system tumors. *Cancer Chemother. Rep.,* **1973,** *4,* 21–26.

Warwick, G. P. The mechanism of action of alkylating agents. *Cancer Res.,* **1963,** *23,* 1315–1333.

Wheeler, G. P. Some biochemical effects of alkylating agents. *Fedn Proc. Fedn Am. Socs exp. Biol.,* **1967,** *26,* 885–892.

———. Alkylating agents. In, *Cancer Medicine.* (Holland, J. F., and Frei, E., III, eds.) Lea & Febiger, Philadelphia, **1973,** pp. 791–806.

———. Mechanism of action of nitrosoureas. In, *Antineoplastic and Immunosuppressive Agents,* Part II. (Sartorelli, A. C., and Johns, D. G., eds.) Springer-Verlag, Berlin, **1975,** pp. 65–84.

Ziegler, J. L. Chemotherapy of Burkitt's lymphoma. *Cancer, N.Y.,* **1972,** *30,* 1534–1539.

Drugs Acting on the Blood and the Blood-Forming Organs

A large number of drugs, including many vitamins and minerals, affect the blood and the blood-forming organs, either directly or indirectly. Agents effective in specific anemias include iron, copper, cobalt, vitamin B_{12}, folic acid, pyridoxine, and riboflavin; these substances are discussed in the following two chapters. In the final chapter of this section, chief attention is devoted to the anticoagulants, heparin and the oral anticoagulants; to thrombolytic agents; and to drugs affecting platelet function.

Many dietary factors are important for normal hematopoiesis, blood coagulation, and the integrity of the vascular wall; some of them are discussed in the section concerning the vitamins. Certain internal secretions can profoundly influence the blood, such as those from the thyroid, the gonads, and the adrenal cortex; these are dealt with in the section devoted to the hormones. A vast array of drugs exert toxic effects on the formed elements of the blood, on hemoglobin, or on the hematopoietic organs. The toxic effects include granulocytopenia, thrombocytopenia, aplastic anemia, hemolytic anemia, and the conversion of hemoglobin into nonfunctional forms. Agents that somewhat selectively depress abnormal proliferation of the cellular elements of the blood are discussed in Chapter 62.

The discovery of liver therapy for pernicious anemia, by Minot and Murphy in 1926, was followed by a marked revival of interest in the field of blood diseases and their therapy. As a result, our knowledge of the mechanisms of blood formation and destruction, the metabolism of iron, the pathological physiology of pernicious and other megaloblastic anemias, and the specificity of hematinic agents is decidedly more complete. The physician now has at his command many reliable procedures for the accurate diagnosis of blood disorders and several drugs for their specific therapy. It is no longer permissible to prescribe these agents without first ascertaining, as nearly as possible, the exact nature of the abnormality. Proper treatment rests upon a clear understanding of the pharmacological properties of the hematopoietic drugs.

The *nutritional anemias* are all treatable by providing the deficient nutrient in appropriate form and dosage. However, the therapeutic goal is not only to restore the body nutrient level to normal, but also to determine and, if possible, eliminate the cause of the deficiency. All nutrient deficiency arises from one or more of the following basic causes: inadequate ingestion, absorption, or utilization, or increased requirement, excretion, or destruction. Knowledge of the food sources and the body metabolism of nutrients is therefore crucial to elimination of the causes of such deficiencies; this information is provided in the following two chapters as it relates to the nutritional anemias.

63 DRUGS EFFECTIVE IN IRON-DEFICIENCY AND OTHER HYPOCHROMIC ANEMIAS

Victor Herbert

IRON AND IRON SALTS

History. The empirical use of iron in the treatment of anemia dates from ancient times. The calcined iron preparation of ancient Hindu medicine, known as *Lauha Bhasma,* was prepared by roasting sheets of iron and then macerating them to a fine white powder in oil, whey, vinegar, cow's urine, and milk. The Greek physicians employed iron for the cure of weakness, a prominent symptom of anemia, in the attempt to impart to the patient the strength of the iron. Indeed, it was believed that Mars, the god of war, had imbued the metal with strength, and the alchemists designated iron as *mars.* Patients with marked pallor were given drinking water in which old swords had been allowed to rust, and Celsus advised that enlarged spleens be treated by using water in blacksmith shops in which white-hot iron had been drenched. He claimed that animals drinking such water had abnormally small spleens.

Sydenham was probably the first physician to employ iron in a manner that would be approved today. In 1681, he wrote the following concerning the treatment of chlorosis:

... I comfort the blood and the spirit belonging to it by giving a chalybeate 30 days running. This is sure to do good. To the worn out or languid blood it gives a spur or fillip whereby the animal spirits which before lay prostrate and sunken under their own weight are raised and excited. Clear proof of this is found in the effect of steel in chlorosis. The pulse gains strength, the face (no longer pale and death-like) a fresh ruddy color.

Sydenham prescribed "steel in substance" or "iron or steel filings steeped in cold Rhenish wine," the dose amounting to 0.5 to 1.0 g of iron daily.

It was not until 1713, however, that Lemery and Goeffy showed that iron is present in blood (ash), and in 1746 Menghini demonstrated that foods rich in iron can elevate the amount of iron in the blood. In 1832, the French physician Pierre Blaud recognized the nature of *chlorosis* when he wrote that the malady "arises from a faulty formation of blood as a result of which the blood is an imperfect fluid or the coloring matter is so defective that it is no longer suitable for stimulating the organism and maintaining the regular exercise of its functions." Blaud recognized that failure in the treatment of chlorosis was due to the use of too small doses of iron, and reported the rapid cure of 30 patients by the use of large doses of the metal. Blaud's original pills consisted of a mixture of equal parts of ferrous sulfate and potassium carbonate, and he gave a sufficient dose to supply 0.4 to 1.6 g of ferrous carbonate daily. This would be considered adequate therapy today. For many years, Blaud's nephew distributed throughout the world the "veritable pills of Doctor Blaud." The Blaud's pills incorporated in the U.S.P. and B.P. differ somewhat from the original pills both in composition and recommended dose. (The history of Blaud's pills has been reviewed by Neuroth and Lee, 1941.)

Also in 1832, Födisch reported that the amount of iron in the blood of chlorotics is greatly diminished, and 10 years later, with the advent of methods for properly examining the blood, Andral and associates noted that iron therapy caused an increase in red blood corpuscles in anemia. Until the last decade of the nineteenth century, iron therapy of anemia followed the principles enunciated by Sydenham and Blaud and was comparable to modern practice. At that time, however, the teachings of Bunge, Quincke, von Noorden, and others caused a radical reduction in the dose of iron in anemia, and it came to be accepted that the metal either was not absorbed in the inorganic form or was necessary only in small doses. The clinical failure of small doses soon brought discredit on iron therapy, and it was not until the end of the second decade of the present century that the lessons taught by the physicians of old were relearned (*see* Haden, 1939). One need only compare the iron dosages in the U.S.P. X with those in the U.S.P. XI (*see* Herbert, 1966) to appreciate the increase that had occurred, due in part to Heath and coworkers (1932) and Reimann and associates (1936), who finally dispelled the ghosts of Bunge, Quincke, and von Noorden by demonstrating that inorganic iron is incorporated into hemoglobin (*see* monograph by Fairbanks *et al.,* 1971).

The only important use of iron in modern medicine is in the treatment of iron-deficiency anemias. The administration of iron to patients with normal blood values serves only to increase the "reserve iron" of the body, and not to increase the red blood cells or hemoglobin above their normal physiological limits.

Distribution and Types of Iron in Nature.
Iron is widely distributed in the animal body, where it exists in both ionic (loosely bound; "inorganic") and nonionic (tightly bound; "organic") forms. Iron is easily oxidized or reduced, and thus is found as a minute but vital part of certain enzymes concerned with electron transfer (the cytochromes, cytochrome oxidase, succinic dehydrogenase, xanthine oxidase). Normally, about 70% of

human body iron is functional or "essential" iron (*i.e.,* in hemoglobin, myoglobin, and intracellular iron-containing enzymes) and 30% is storage or "nonessential" iron (*i.e.,* in hemosiderin and ferritin). In women, the storage reserve tends to be less than half that in men.

Foods high in iron content (greater than 5 mg of iron per 100 g) include organ meats (liver, heart), brewer's yeast, wheat germ, egg yolks, oysters, and certain dried beans and fruits; foods containing 1 to 5 mg of iron per 100 g include most muscle meats, fish and fowl, most green vegetables, and most cereals; foods low in iron (less than 1 mg of iron per 100 g) include milk and milk products and most nongreen vegetables. Iron cooking utensils sharply raise the iron content of foods. Some constituents of foods increase and others decrease the absorption of their content of iron (Symposium, 1968). In general, the mean iron absorption from animal foods is twice that from vegetable foods (Martinez-Torres and Layrisse, in Symposium, 1973).

Since the dietary intake of iron is often marginal, flour has been supplemented with iron (13 to 16.5 mg/lb) in the United States for many years. It is currently proposed to increase the level of this supplementation to 40 mg/lb. However, there has been criticism of this action (*see* Wintrobe, 1973, and references therein), and it is unknown when or if alterations of existing practice will take place.

Iron Metabolism. The past quarter century has witnessed notable advances in our knowledge of iron metabolism, largely because of the use of radioactive isotopes of iron in investigative work (*see* Symposium, 1958, 1964, 1972, 1973; Bothwell and Finch, 1962; Charlton and Bothwell, 1970; Finch *et al.,* 1970; Pollycove and Crosby, in Gordon, 1970; Fairbanks *et al.,* 1971; Jacobs and Worwood, 1974).

Absorption. Control of body iron content rests mainly in the small intestine, which is both the absorptive and an excretory organ for iron (*see* Conrad *et al.,* 1964; Bothwell, 1968b; Jacobs, in Symposium, 1973). This control system is operative primarily in the presence of the amounts of iron found in an ordinary diet, and may be overwhelmed by large quantities of ingested iron. Absorption of iron can occur along the entire length of the alimentary tract, but it is greatest in the duodenum and becomes progressively less distally.

In 1943, Hahn and associates observed that oral administration of a large dose of iron reduced absorption of a second dose given within 6 hours, and proposed a "mucosal block" to absorption of excess iron. Granick (1954) suggested that the protein apoferritin is continuously formed in the mucosal cell and combined with micelles of a colloidal hydrated ferric iron oxide-phosphate complex to yield ferritin; he proposed that the *quantity* of ferritin controls iron absorption by rejecting iron when it is high and accepting iron when it is low. The biochemical mechanisms controlling iron absorption are still not fully understood, but a partial "mucosal block" exists (*see* Conrad *et al.,* 1964; Allgood and Brown, 1967; Crosby, in Gordon, 1970).

Iron absorption is enhanced by iron deficiency, decreased iron stores, or accelerated erythropoiesis (*see* reviews by Bothwell and Finch, 1962; Fairbanks *et al.,* 1971; Moore, in Goodhart and Shils, 1973). The plasma iron level may play a part in controlling iron absorption (*see* Monsen *et al.,* 1967). The role of the pancreas (if any) in control of iron absorption is unclear (*see* review by Crosby, 1968; Bernstein and Herbert, 1973).

There appear to be two mechanisms for iron absorption across the mucosa of the upper small intestine. These mechanisms, operating simultaneously, are: (1) an active transport process with enzymatic or carrier characteristics, perhaps involving attachment of iron to nonferritin protein, and operative primarily at concentrations of iron such as occur in a normal diet; and (2) a first-order passive transport process, perhaps diffusion, that is operative primarily at doses of iron exceeding those in a normal diet (*see* Gitlin and Cruchaud, 1962; Brown and Rother, 1963; Manis and Schachter, 1964).

Iron is absorbed more easily in its ferrous form; ferrous iron passes into and through the mucosal cell directly into the blood stream, where it is immediately bound to transferrin. Small excesses of iron within the villous epithelial cells are oxidized to the ferric state, where they combine with the protein apoferritin to yield ferritin, which is eventually excreted in the feces incorporated in villous absorptive columnar epithelial cells that have been exfoliated at the end of their life-span (*see* Crosby, 1965). This "mucosal block" mechanism for handling excess iron can cope with only small excesses, and it is overwhelmed by large amounts of iron (*see* Smith and Pannacciulli, 1958; Bothwell and Isaacson, 1962). Increasing the size of the oral iron dose increases the *amount* absorbed but decreases the *fraction* of the administered dose that is absorbed.

The absorption of *dietary iron* varies from about 5 to approximately 50% of that of a comparable amount of iron salts. Absorption of food and medicinal iron depends as much on its form as on its absolute amount (*see* Symposium, 1970, 1973; Moore, in Goodhart and Shils, 1973). Of the approximately 6 mg of iron per 1000 kcal in the average daily European or North American diet, about 5 to 10% is absorbed by normal subjects and about 10 to 30% by iron-deficient subjects.

Since it is the ferrous and not the ferric form of iron that is usually absorbed, reducing agents such as ascorbate increase iron absorption, as do also succinate, inosine, and ethionine (*see* monograph by Fairbanks *et al.*, 1971). Phytate may form relatively insoluble and thus unabsorbable complexes with iron; only about 5% of wheat iron is normally absorbed, and this amount increases only to about 7% during iron deficiency (*see* Hussain *et al.*, 1965). Absorption of iron from eggs is also relatively poor, perhaps because the iron is strongly complexed to the phosphate of yolk phosphoproteins. Indeed, a phosphorus-poor diet leads to high iron absorption in animals. Hemoglobin iron (in liver, muscle, blood) is relatively well absorbed as intact heme, which is then split, presumably within the mucosal cell; this mechanism differs from that which handles absorption of inorganic iron (*see* Weintraub *et al.*, 1968); about 10% is absorbed by normal subjects and twice this amount in iron-deficient subjects (*see* Hallberg and Sölvell, 1967; Waxman *et al.*, 1968). Inorganic iron in moderate amounts is absorbed up to twice as well as heme iron by normal subjects; in iron-deficient individuals, absorption of inorganic iron is enhanced far more than the doubled absorption of heme or other food iron. In one study, normal subjects absorbed 7% of iron ascorbate, but iron-deficient subjects absorbed six times as much (*see* Hussain *et al.*, 1965).

Absorption of inorganic iron is decreased by administering it with food; this reduction is related not only to the bulk of the meal but also to its constituents. The relative concentrations of phosphates, phytates, and calcium salts may all play a role in decreasing inorganic iron absorption (*see* review by Crosby, 1968; Conrad, in Symposium, 1970).

The absorption of dietary iron is decreased after partial or complete gastrectomy, but absorption of iron salts is less impaired (*see* review by Bothwell and Finch, 1962). Achlorhydria may decrease iron absorption (*see* Schade *et al.*, 1968). Acid favors the reduction of ferric to ferrous iron and should retard the formation of insoluble complexes of iron with various food constituents, and thus aid absorption of inorganic iron. Antacids such as calcium carbonate, aluminum hydroxide, and magnesium hydroxide decrease iron absorption. Pyridoxine deficiency enhances the absorption of iron, despite an elevated plasma iron level and retardation of hemoglobin synthesis (Gubler *et al.*, 1949).

Transport. Transferrin (siderophilin), a glycoprotein β_1-globulin, transports ferric iron after it has been absorbed to the bone marrow, where the iron is incorporated into hemoglobin (*see* Katz, in Gordon, 1970).

With congenital atransferrinemia, iron absorption continues, and the iron is deposited heavily in all organs except bone marrow. Delivery to the erythron is inadequate, and hypochromic microcytic anemia develops (*see* Heilmeyer, in Symposium, 1964). On the other hand, normal saturated transferrin alone is not sufficient to furnish the erythron with adequate iron, as indicated by another congenital error in iron metabolism, in which there is iron-deficiency anemia with no bone-marrow iron despite adequate transferrin, an elevated plasma iron, and massive hepatic parenchymal iron deposition (Shahidi *et al.*, 1964). Thus, functioning iron-storing reticulum cells in the bone marrow also appear to be essential for iron transfer to the erythron, as suggested by Bessis and Breton-Gorius (1962), and supported by the "experiment of nature" cases of Heilmeyer and of Shahidi and associates.

The plasma iron concentration and the total iron-binding capacity of the plasma vary markedly in different physiological conditions and disease states (Figure 63–1). For example, the plasma iron level is higher in men than in women, and higher in the morning than in the evening; the lower value in women is not caused by menstruation. Hypoferremia characterizes iron-deficiency anemias and a variety of infectious diseases; hyperferremia characterizes hemochromatosis and transfusion hemosiderosis, certain hypochromic and other anemias, and acute hepatitis. Indeed, in hemochromatosis the transferrin is almost completely saturated with iron. The plasma iron concentration is decreased in iron-deficiency anemias because there is insufficient metal for hemoglobin synthesis and the bone marrow is drawing on all available labile stores; it is elevated in pernicious anemia in relapse because little of the metal is being utilized for effective hemoglobin synthesis; it is diminished in anemias of infection because a metabolic defect results in deranged iron metabolism, with low transferrin concentrations. Plasma iron is normally in equilibrium with iron stores, and its level is determined by the balance between iron absorption and deposition, incorporation of the metal into hemoglobin, and its release therefrom; of these multiple factors, hemoglobin synthesis is the primary factor regulating the rate of plasma iron turnover. (*See* reviews by Bothwell and Finch, 1962; Symposium, 1964, 1970, 1973; Finch *et al.*, 1970; Gordon, 1970; Fairbanks *et al.*, 1971.)

Fate. The *distribution* of the approximately 3.5 g of total body iron in the average 70-kg adult male is indicated in Figure 63–2.

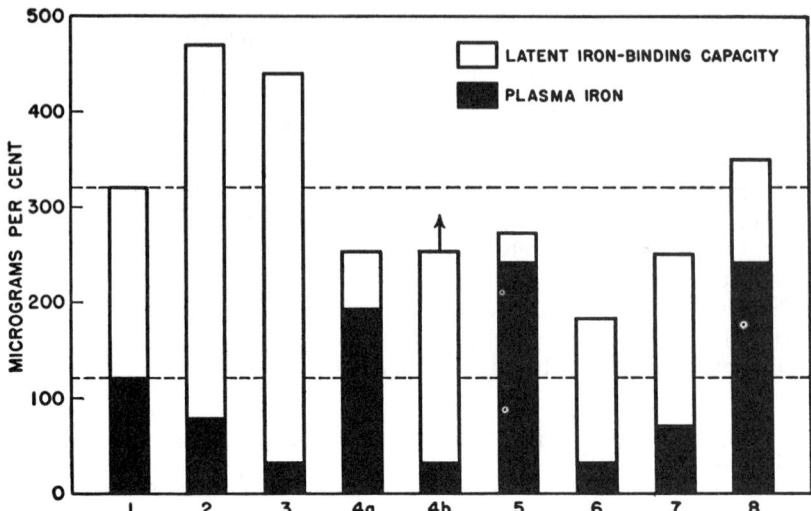

Figure 63-1. *Plasma iron and total iron-binding capacity (total transferrin content) of plasma in various disturbances of iron metabolism.*

(*1*) Healthy adults. (*2*) Late pregnancy. (*3*) Chronic iron deficiency; polycythemia vera. (*4a*) Hemolytic, pernicious, aplastic, and myelophthisic anemias; fetus at parturition. (*4b*) Hemolytic and pernicious anemias during remission. (*5*) Hemochromatosis and transfusion hemosiderosis. (*6*) Acute infections. (*7*) Chronic infections, malignant tumors, myelomatosis, uremia, leukemias, hepatic cirrhosis, acute or subacute liver atrophy. (*8*) Acute hepatitis (second to fifth week).
The lower horizontal dash line represents the normal level of globulin-bound iron in human plasma; the upper line represents the normal level of iron-binding capacity of human plasma. Note that transferrin is normally about one-third saturated with iron. (After Laurell, 1952. Courtesy of *Pharmacological Reviews.*)

Iron exists in man almost exclusively complexed to protein (transferrin, ferritin) or in heme (hemoglobin, myoglobin, heme enzymes). About two thirds is in hemoglobin, about one fourth is in the body's reserve stores as ferritin and hemosiderin, about 3% is in myoglobin, about 0.5% is in heme enzymes, and a minute fraction is in transferrin, which holds about 0.1% of the total body iron (*see* Symposium, 1964).

The *stores* of iron are mainly in reticuloendothelial cells, and thus are found in organs rich in such cells, especially liver, spleen, and bone marrow. Storage iron represents a reserve derived from the diet and from the continuous physiological destruction of red blood cells. The amount of storage iron varies, therefore, with the sources of supply and also with demands made upon it for hemoglobin formation. It amounts to about 1 g in men but only 200 to 400 mg in women (Council on Foods and Nutrition, 1968). The iron reserve in the viscera is *used over and over again,* so that it is almost impossible to produce a severe anemia in an adult male animal by limiting the iron intake. The stored iron, in contrast to enzyme and other parenchymal iron, is available for use by the bone marrow. Approximately 10% of the stores constitutes a "labile pool" of very rapidly

mobilizable iron. The rest of the pool is less rapidly available and is drawn on as the "labile pool" is depleted. A healthy adult in good nutritional condition can compensate, within a relatively short period, for the loss of 30% of his circulating red blood cells without recourse to iron therapy, provided that the iron stores can be adequately mobilized. Under pathological conditions, such as hemochromatosis, more than 50 g of iron may be deposited in the tissues. This abnormal deposition is secondary to excessive absorption of iron; a somewhat similar syndrome can occur in patients given repeated blood transfusions or excessive doses of oral or parenteral iron (*see* Finch *et al.,* 1950; Symposium, 1964, 1973; Charlton and Bothwell, 1966; MacDonald, 1966). Injected iron is quickly linked to the iron stores of the body. When iron is injected intravenously, it is deposited mainly in the liver; approximately half of the injected radioactive metal is present in the liver within 1 to 2 hours. When iron is administered orally, more is taken up by bone marrow and spleen than when it is given intravenously. When iron is liberated from hemolyzed erythrocytes, it is linked to apoferritin in both the liver and the spleen (*see* Hahn *et al.,* 1943; Gabrio *et al.,* 1953; Granick, 1954).

Excretion. Iron is tenaciously conserved. McCance and Widdowson (1943) demonstrated that the body excretes only minimal amounts of iron; normally this amounts to 0.5 to 1 mg daily. This excretion is in nails, hair, feces, and urine, mainly as enzyme iron of exfoliated cells, but there are also trace losses in bile and cell-free sweat. The main excretory pathway is by way of epithelial

cells sloughed from the skin and gastrointestinal tract, which carry out unneeded iron as ferritin (Conrad *et al.,* 1964; Green *et al.,* 1968).

Normally only about 0.1 mg is excreted in sweat, but as much as 2 or 3 mg daily may be lost from large body stores when excessive sweating occurs (*see*

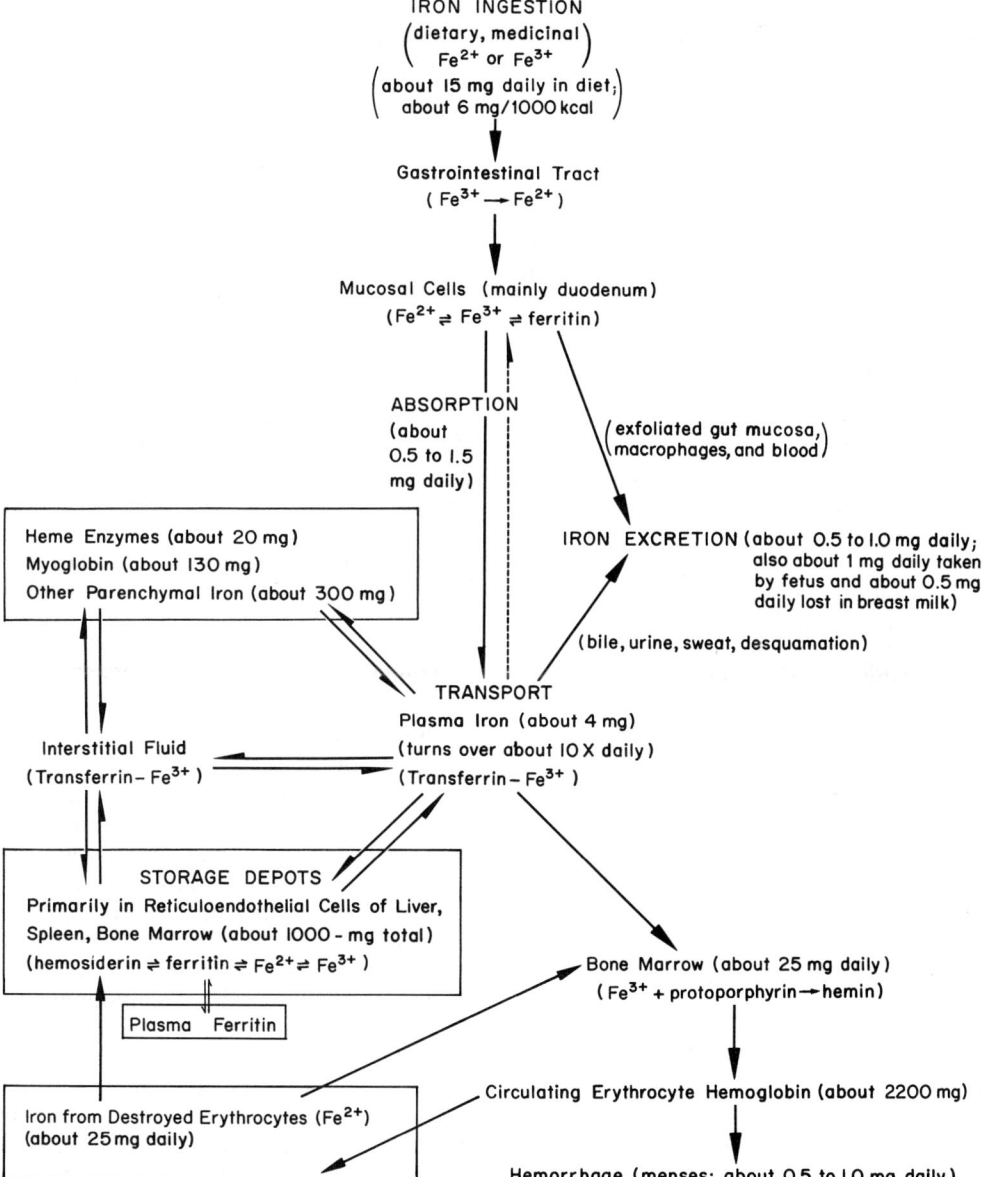

Figure 63-2. *Normal absorption, metabolic pathways, and excretion of iron.*

All amounts are for iron content. The total content of iron in men is about 50 and in women about 35 mg/kg of body weight; this difference is due to the fact that women average only about 300 mg of iron in storage depots. Plasma ferritin is normally about 70 ng/ml in men and 35 ng/ml in women.

Green *et al.,* 1968; Vellar, 1968). Urinary iron excretion averages 0.1 mg daily, but may be raised several-fold in patients with proteinuria or iron overload due to loss in transferrin and exfoliated renal tubular cells (Rifkind *et al.,* 1961). Approximately 1 to 2% of an intravenously administered dose of iron is detectable in the urine, probably derived from non-transferrin-bound iron. Barer and Fowler (1949) have shown that the renal excretion of iron in patients on a normal diet is significantly increased by the ingestion of an acidic salt and markedly decreased by an alkaline salt; the results were ascribed to the effect of intestinal pH on iron absorption. A total of about 4 mg of excess iron may be excreted daily by all routes by a patient compensating for iron overload while continuing to eat a normal diet (Crosby *et al.,* 1963; Green *et al.,* 1968).

The average loss of iron in normal menstruation, spread evenly over the 28 days of the menstrual cycle, is about 0.5 to 1 mg daily. The iron "cost" of a normal pregnancy may vary from 440 to 1050 mg (Table 63–1). To calculate the total added need for iron to support pregnancy, in addition to the "cost" (which is lost iron), one must add iron needed for expansion of the red-cell mass (de Leeuw *et al.,* 1966). The iron lost in lactation is compensated by the iron saved due to the associated amenorrhea.

Iron Requirement. Estimated daily iron requirements are indicated in Table 63–2. The increase in requirement due to pregnancy is indicated in Table 63–1.

Since only about 10% of dietary iron is absorbed, the amount of iron ingested must be tenfold the daily requirement. The average American diet provides about 6 mg of iron per 1000 kcal (Monsen *et al.,* 1967).

Table 63–1.   IRON REQUIREMENTS FOR PREGNANCY

	AVERAGE mg	RANGE mg
External iron loss	170	150–200
Expansion of red-blood-cell mass	450	200–600
Fetal iron	270	200–370
Iron in placenta and cord	90	30–170
Blood loss at delivery	150	90–310
Total requirement *	980	580–1340
Cost of pregnancy †	680	440–1050

* Blood loss at delivery not included.
† Expansion of red-cell mass not included.
(After Council on Foods and Nutrition, 1968. Courtesy of the *Journal of the American Medical Association.*)

Table 63–2.   ESTIMATED DIETARY IRON REQUIREMENTS

	ABSORBED IRON REQUIREMENT mg/day	DIETARY IRON REQUIREMENT * mg/day
Normal men and nonmenstruating women	0.5–1	5–10
Menstruating women	0.7–2	7–20
Pregnant women	2 –4.8	20–48 †
Adolescents	1 –2	10–20
Children	0.4–1	4–10
Infants	0.5–1.5	1.5 mg/kg ‡

* Assuming 10% absorption.
† This amount of iron cannot be derived from diet and should be met by iron supplementation in the latter half of pregnancy.
‡ To a maximum of 15 mg.
(After Council on Foods and Nutrition, 1968. Courtesy of the *Journal of the American Medical Association.*)

Therefore, iron intake from dietary sources is borderline for teenage girls and women, and may be inadequate for infants and pregnant women (Council on Foods and Nutrition, 1968; Food and Nutrition Board, 1974). However, a woman with sufficient iron stores to provide for her increase in hemoglobin mass during pregnancy, who breast-feeds her infant for 6 months, will have her iron needs covered by adequate intake of dietary iron (FAO/WHO Expert Group, 1970).

Hemoglobin contains 0.33% iron; thus, with every 100 ml of blood (containing 15 g of hemoglobin) lost by hemorrhage, a total of 50 mg of iron is lost. Iron in excess of that contained in the diet is necessary for the treatment of iron-deficiency anemia. The average 70-kg adult has about 750 g of circulating hemoglobin containing about 2.5 g of iron; 1% of circulating hemoglobin requires 25 mg of iron for its formation. The patient with an iron-deficiency anemia, even if he absorbs and utilizes completely all the iron in his diet, is still unable to obtain the 25 mg per day necessary to raise his hemoglobin level by 1% per day, not an unreasonable rate. The need for iron is really much greater than that indicated by the hemoglobin rise alone, because of the concomitant increase in blood volume. During the peak of the response to therapy, iron utilization may reach more than 60 mg per day (*see* Hynes, 1949). When it is remembered that *dietary* iron is less well absorbed, and that the anemia may be due to poor absorption of the metal, to chronic blood loss, or to increased physiological demands, it becomes evident why it is so important to administer *medicinal* iron orally in order to attain normal blood values and restore iron balance to normal.

Oral Preparations, Dosage, and Duration of Therapy. (*See* Brown, 1968; Symposium, 1970, 1972; Fairbanks *et al.,* 1971.) Oral *ferrous sulfate,* the least expensive of iron preparations, is the treatment of choice for iron deficiency. Contrary to many advertisements, gastrointestinal tolerance of *all* iron preparations is primarily a function of the total amount of soluble elemental iron per dose and of psychological factors, and is *not* normally a function of the form in which iron is administered. Since absorption of iron is crucially dependent on the dose administered, the largest dose tolerated without side effects should be given. For most persons, that dose is 300 mg of the hydrated salt of ferrous sulfate or 200 mg of the dry salt, thrice daily. The value of spaced daily doses lies in the fact that the absorption rate returns to normal 4 hours after a prior dose (Brown *et al.,* 1958). If gastrointestinal symptoms develop, the dose is reduced by one third or one half. Some patients will tolerate as much as double the usual dose, and may then be given it. When the bone marrow is operating at maximal capacity, in a 70-kg man with iron-deficiency anemia, less than 100 mg of iron daily can be incorporated into hemoglobin. Assuming an average of 25% absorption of iron given as ferrous sulfate, a 2-g dose of the hydrated salt (which is 20% iron) provides 100 mg of absorbed iron. Administration of larger daily doses is without hematopoietic value.

Duration of oral therapy for iron-deficiency anemia should be approximately 6 months, assuming usual therapy (300 mg of $FeSO_4 \cdot 7H_2O$, thrice daily) and severe anemia. Such average therapy will result in absorption of about 45 mg of iron daily during the first month while the iron-deficiency anemia is rapidly improving; about 25 mg daily during the second and third months while the anemia is disappearing but before stores are repleted; and about 5 to 10 mg daily after the third month when the stores

approach repletion. Thus, one can assume absorption of about 1350 mg in the first month, 1500 mg in the next 2 months, and 225 mg in each of the 3 succeeding months, for a total absorption of about 3500 mg (*i.e.,* repletion of body stores) in 6 months. It is important for the physician to remember not only that iron absorption *decreases* as anemia improves but also *that the factors originally producing the iron deficiency may persist.* If these factors are not corrected, oral iron therapy must continue until such correction occurs. Failure to heed this admonition will result in relapse due to persistent negative iron balance.

Iron salts have many incompatibilities and should be prescribed alone, preferably between meals for maximal absorption but just after meals if necessary to minimize gastric symptoms. Gastrointestinal absorption of iron is adequate and essentially equal from the following six *ferrous* salts: *sulfate, fumarate, gluconate, succinate, glutamate,* and *lactate.* Absorption of iron is lower from ferrous *citrate, tartrate, pyrophosphate, cholinisocitrate,* and *carbonate.* Absorption of iron from all *ferric* salts is poor (*see* Brise and Hallberg, 1962). Reducing agents (*e.g.,* ascorbic acid) and some chelating agents (*e.g.,* succinic acid, sulfur-containing amino acids) may increase absorption of iron from ferrous sulfate, but are not worth the extra cost because of the high efficacy of ferrous sulfate when administered alone. Cobalt is especially undesirable because it may produce a rise in hematocrit by an unknown mechanism, and thus obscure the response to iron; additionally it may produce various toxic effects, such as skin rashes, goiter, or angina. (*See* Stevens, in Symposium, 1958; Pollack *et al.,* 1963; *see also* reviews by Bothwell and Finch, 1962; Fairbanks *et al.,* 1971.)

Ferrous Sulfate, U.S.P. (*iron sulfate;* FEOSOL), is the hydrated salt, $FeSO_4 \cdot 7H_2O$, which contains 20% iron; it consists of pale, bluish-green crystals or granules, soluble 1 : 1.5 in water. In moist air, crystals of ferrous sulfate rapidly oxidize and become coated with a brownish-yellow, basic ferric sulfate, and must then not be used for medicinal purposes. The drug is odorless and has a saline, astringent taste. It is usually dispensed as pills or tablets, coated to protect them from moisture. The salt is mixed with glucose or lactose to protect it against oxidation. Official ferrous sulfate tablets usually contain 300 mg of the salt. *Dried Ferrous Sulfate,* U.S.P., is a grayish-white powder that contains not less than 80% of the anhydrous salt. *Ferrous Sulfate Syrup,* N.F., contains 40 mg of the salt (8 mg of iron) in each milliliter. The average adult dose is 2 tsp, thrice daily; for *children* who weigh from 15 to 35 kg, 1 tsp, twice or thrice daily. *Ferrous Sulfate Oral Solution,* U.S.P. (FER-IN-SOL DROPS), contains 125 mg (25 mg of iron) in each milliliter; the average therapeutic dosage is 1 ml, three or four times daily. Palatable *elixirs* of ferrous sulfate are also available.

Ferrous Fumarate, U.S.P., occurs as an anhydrous, reddish-brown granular powder. It contains 33% iron and is moderately soluble in water, stable, and almost tasteless. Unlike ferrous sulfate, it does not require mixing or coating with glucose to protect it against oxidation. Official ferrous fumarate tablets usually contain 200 mg of the salt; the average adult dosage is 600 to 800 mg daily, in divided portions.

Ferrous Gluconate, N.F. (FERGON), and *ferrous lactate* have also been successfully employed in the therapy of iron-deficiency anemia; the gluconate contains 12% metallic iron; the lactate, 19%. Both are tolerated as well as ferrous sulfate. The effective dose of either in terms of iron content is approximately the same as that of the sulfate. The same is true for other compounds of iron occasionally used as hematinics, such as *ferrous carbonate. Ferrous chloride* is a light-brown powder, readily soluble in water. The iron content is 44%, and the formerly recommended dose of 3 or 4 g daily, in divided portions, is too high and may cause marked gastric disturbances.

Reduced iron (*metallic iron, elemental iron*), formerly official, has not been used for many years. However, interest in it is being revived. In the form of carbonyl iron powder, 2- to 6-μm particle size, it has been suggested as a new approach to the treatment of human iron deficiency. It is possibly the best available form of iron for enrichment of bread and cereal because of apparent minimal toxicity even when given in massive oral doses (up to 6 g as a single dose) (Sacks and Crosby, 1974). If further studies support this view, then reduced iron may prove to be an important oral preparation, especially since it would sharply decrease the problem of toxicity to infants who not infrequently find and ingest an oral iron preparation meant for therapy of an adult. In view of the fact that antacids decrease and ascorbic acid enhances absorption of reduced iron, it is possible that both absorbability and toxicity are dependent on solubilization (*i.e.,* ionization) of reduced iron by gastric acid. This solubilization would be limited to subtoxic amounts by the quantity of acid secreted. Should this prove to be the explanation for the low toxicity of large oral doses, reduced iron may be very poorly absorbed in achlorhydric subjects.

There are still other oral preparations, none of which adds anything significantly useful to therapy of iron deficiency. (For a lucid discussion of oral iron therapy, *see* monograph by Fairbanks *et al.,* 1971.) In the words of Bothwell and Finch (1962):

. . . current practice in iron therapy can give the physician little cause for pride. Although a great variety of preparations are being promoted at the present time, their so-called advantages (over ferrous sulfate or related salts) *have no foundation in fact* and, for the most part, depend on some special gimmick to attract the physician's or patient's eye. Such compounds fall into three groups: those advocated on the basis of increased availability, those advocated on the basis of increased tolerance or decreased toxicity, and those in which noniron additives are supposed to assist in the response of the anemic patient.

Sustained-release, delayed-release, and enteric-coated preparations tend to transport iron past the duodenum and proximal jejunum, and thus reduce iron absorption; the claims for sustained action are unjustified (Middleton *et al.,* 1966).

Toxicity and Side Effects of Oral Preparations. (*See* reviews by Aldrich, in Symposium, 1958; Bothwell and Finch, 1962; Moeschlin and Schneider, in Symposium, 1964; Fairbanks *et al.,* 1971.)

Iron Poisoning. All iron preparations are probably equally toxic per unit of soluble iron. Iron poisoning is very rare in adults; it would be very unlikely in adults with ingestion of doses of ferrous sulfate below 50 g. Serious *acute poisoning* in children can result from the ingestion of doses in excess of 1 g (*see* Forbes, 1947). In the United States, there is an average of *at least one death a month* from the ingestion by infants and young children of doses of ferrous sulfate in excess of 2 g. Doses of 1 g may be toxic in children. The colored-sugar coating of many of the commercially available tablets gives them the appearance of candy. All iron preparations should be labeled, "Caution! Keep out of reach of children."

Signs and symptoms may occur within 30 minutes or may be delayed several hours. They are largely those of gastrointestinal irritation and necrosis, often with nausea, vomiting, and shock; they include pallor or cyanosis, lassitude, drowsiness, hematemesis, diarrhea of green and subsequently tarry stools, and cardiovascular collapse. If death does not occur within 6 hours, there may be a transient period of apparent recovery followed by death in 12 to 48 hours. The corrosive injury to the stomach may result in subsequent pyloric stenosis or severe gastric scarring. Hemorrhagic gastroenteritis and hepatic injury are prominent findings at autopsy.

Treatment should begin quickly with the induction of vomiting. Eggs and milk are then fed (to form iron-protein complexes) until it is possible to perform gastric lavage. Within the first hour following ingestion of the iron preparation, the stomach should be lavaged with 1% sodium bicarbonate solution, to convert the iron to a less soluble form. If an iron-chelating drug is available, it is effective for the treatment of both local and systemic effects. The most specific chelating agent for iron is deferoxamine; the regimen for its use in iron poisoning is described in Chapter 45. Dimercaprol should not be used because it may form a toxic complex with iron.

Gastric lavage is dangerous after the first hour because of gastric necrosis, with resultant danger of perforation. Shock, dehydration, and acid-base abnormalities are treated in the conventional manner. Exchange transfusion of blood may be needed in desperate cases not responding to other measures.

Side Effects of Iron Therapy. The patient given iron should be forewarned that conventional oral doses of the iron salts produce constipation in about 10% of cases, diarrhea in about 5%, and nausea and epigastric pain in about 7% (when salts containing the equivalent of 180 mg of ferrous iron per day are given) to 20% (with administration of salts containing 400 mg of ferrous iron per day) (Sölvell, in Symposium, 1970). These side effects are primarily a function of the total amount of absorbable iron per dose, and they can be reduced or eliminated by prescribing iron just after meals instead of between meals (food usually reduces absorbability of medicinal iron) or, more reliably, by reducing the dose by one third to one half. Iron medication colors the feces black, and large amounts may interfere with some tests used for detection of occult blood in the stools; the guaiac test occasionally yields false-positive tests for blood, whereas results with the benzidine test are not as affected by iron medication.

Large chronic doses of iron may so interfere with the assimilation of phosphorus as to cause severe rickets in infants.

When iron balance is restored to normal (usually after about 6 months unless factors favoring negative iron balance persist), therapy with iron should be stopped, to avoid iron-overload hemosiderosis (*see* Symposium, 1964).

Parenteral Preparations and Dosage. (*See* Symposium, 1958, 1970, 1972; Bothwell and Finch, 1962; Figueroa, in Symposium, 1964; Fairbanks *et al.*, 1971.) Parenteral iron is indicated *only* when an iron-deficiency anemia exists *and a trial of oral iron has been ineffective* due to: (1) failure to absorb adequate amounts of oral iron (occasional patients with various malabsorption syndromes); (2) inability to tolerate oral iron (some patients with severe regional enteritis or ulcerative colitis); (3) exhausted iron stores in patients with chronic bleeding, in whom the average daily iron lost equals or exceeds the absorption of iron from oral ferrous sulfate; (4) refusal or inability to take oral iron in necessary dosage (some children, psychiatric and geriatric patients). The last-named problem is sometimes solved

by furtive administration of ferrous sulfate syrup or elixir in fruit juice.

The patient who fails to respond to oral iron should be reevaluated, since he may not have an iron-deficiency anemia (*see* text discussion of Figure 63-3, page 1318). Bone-marrow stores should be demonstrated to be absent (*see* Gale *et al.*, 1963) prior to parenteral iron medication, so that conditions (such as infection) that produce anemia due partly to poor utilization of iron can be excluded. In contrast to the safety, efficacy, and low cost of orally administered iron, the metal given by injection is painful, expensive, and sometimes dangerous.

Intramuscular Preparations. Iron Dextran Injection, U.S.P. (*iron-dextran;* IMFERON), is a sterile, colloidal solution of ferric hydroxide in complex with partially hydrolyzed dextran of low molecular weight, in water for injection; it contains 50 mg of elemental iron per milliliter. The dark-brown solution has a pH of 5.2 to 6.5, and is usually provided in 10-ml vials containing 0.5% phenol as a preservative. It should be injected deeply with a 5- or 7.5-cm (2- or 3-in.), 19- or 20-gauge needle, only into the upper-outer quadrant of the buttock and *not* into the arm or other exposed area. (It is absorbed slowly from subcutaneous tissue, and may stain the skin brown for 1 to 2 years; a Z-track injection technic into muscle should be used to avoid leakage back into subcutaneous tissue.) The iron is absorbed by way of the lymphatic drainage from muscle (*see* Will, 1968). *Total dosage* to restore hemoglobin and replenish stores may be approximated from the formula: $0.3 \times$ body weight in lb $\times$ $\dfrac{(100 - \text{patient's hemoglobin in g \%})}{14.8} \times 100) = $ mg to be injected. Each day's dose should ordinarily not exceed 25 mg for infants under 4 to 5 kg, 50 mg for children under 9 kg, 100 mg for patients under 50 kg, and 100 to 250 mg for others.

Other intramuscular preparations include *Iron Sorbitex Injection,* N.F. (JECTOFER), *green ferric ammonium citrate, ferrous gluconate, iron adenylate,* and *iron polyisomaltose.* They have no clear advantages over iron-dextran, and experience with them is limited.

Intravenous Preparations. Iron Dextran Injection, U.S.P., may also be given intravenously (*see* Marchasin and Wallerstein, 1964); only the preparation without preservatives (2- or 5-ml ampuls) should be used for intravenous administration. To minimize toxic reactions, the initial dose should be limited to 25 mg, followed by daily increments for 2 or 3 days until a 100-mg daily dose is reached. The dose should be given slowly (1 minute per 20 to 50 mg).

Toxicity of Parenteral Preparations. *Local side effects* following intramuscular administration of iron include pain at the injection site, skin discoloration, local inflammation with tender inguinal lymphadenopathy, and lower-quadrant abdominal pain. *Systemic toxicity* occurs in approximately 0.5 to 0.8% of cases, and includes reactions occurring more frequently within 10 minutes of injection, such as headache, muscle and joint pain, hemolysis due to ionized (unbound) iron, faintness, tachycardia, flushing, sweating, nausea, vomiting, bronchospasm with dyspnea, hypotension, dizziness, and circulatory collapse. These reactions are much more common with intravenous than with intramuscular iron preparations. Reactions that occur more frequently from ½ to 24 hours after injection include dizziness, syncope, fever, chills, rash, urticaria, constricting chest pain, backache, generalized body aches, encephalopathy with convulsive seizures, generalized lymphadenopathy, and leukemoid reactions. Approximately one fatal case of anaphylactic shock occurs per 4 million doses administered.

Generally, local inflammatory reactions are much less frequent with intravenous than with intramuscular administration of iron. Conversely, shock or cardiac arrest is more frequent (although rare) with intravenous administration. Other toxic effects of intravenous preparations are the same as with intramuscular preparations.

As should be obvious, *oral iron therapy is preferable to parenteral; the latter should be used as seldom as possible.*

Therapeutic Uses. (*See* Symposium, 1958, 1964, 1970, 1973; *see also* reviews by Bothwell and Finch, 1962; Fairbanks *et al.,* 1971.) The sole established therapeutic use of iron is in the *treatment of iron deficiency.* Use of iron in other conditions does no good and

may do harm by causing iron toxicity or iron-storage disease. Iron-deficiency anemia is very common. As is the case with other nutrients, deficiency of iron may result from inadequate ingestion, absorption, or utilization, or from an increased requirement or increased excretion, or from a combination of these factors. *Blood loss (i.e.,* increased excretion) is almost the sole cause of iron deficiency in adult males and postmenopausal females, and is a major factor in more than half of all instances of iron-deficiency anemia in children and in women in the childbearing period, in North America and Europe. As indicated in Tables 63–1 and 63–2, the daily iron requirement is increased by growth and pregnancy. Thus, iron deficiency is especially common in *infants* and young children on diets low in iron (such as a diet largely of milk), in *pregnant women,* especially multiparas, and in *women with heavy menstrual blood loss* (Rybo, in Symposium, 1973).

The *sequence of events as iron deficiency develops* is depicted in Figure 63–3. The physician must recognize that *not all hypochromic anemias are due to*

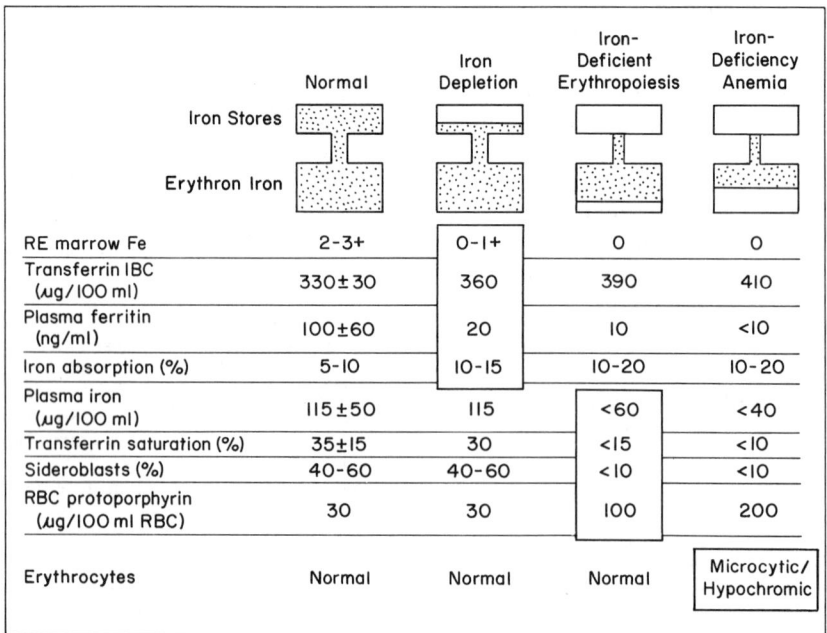

	Normal	Iron Depletion	Iron-Deficient Erythropoiesis	Iron-Deficiency Anemia
Iron Stores				
Erythron Iron				
RE marrow Fe	2-3+	0-1+	0	0
Transferrin IBC (μg/100 ml)	330±30	360	390	410
Plasma ferritin (ng/ml)	100±60	20	10	<10
Iron absorption (%)	5-10	10-15	10-20	10-20
Plasma iron (μg/100 ml)	115±50	115	<60	<40
Transferrin saturation (%)	35±15	30	<15	<10
Sideroblasts (%)	40-60	40-60	<10	<10
RBC protoporphyrin (μg/100 ml RBC)	30	30	100	200
Erythrocytes	Normal	Normal	Normal	Microcytic/ Hypochromic

Figure 63–3. *Sequential changes (from left to right) in the development of iron deficiency.*

Rectangles enclose the first appearance of the indicated abnormal test results. IBC = iron-binding capacity. (After Hillman and Finch, 1974, as modified from Bothwell and Finch, 1962. Courtesy of F. A. Davis Co.)

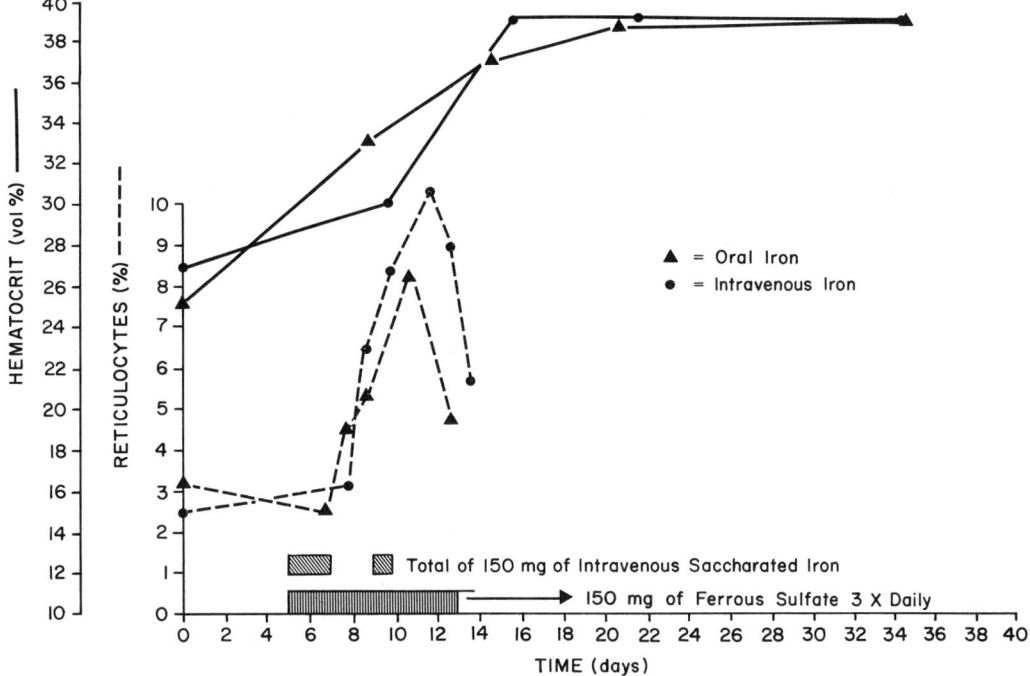

Figure 63–4. *Essentially identical initial response to oral and parenteral iron in identical twins with iron-deficiency anemia.*

After the demonstration that parenteral iron was no more effective than oral iron, both patients were subsequently maintained on oral iron. (After Bothwell and Finch, 1962. Courtesy of Little, Brown & Co.)

iron deficiency, and also that *mild iron-deficiency anemia is often not hypochromic.* Hypochromic anemia may occur with any defect in hemoglobin synthesis: impaired *heme* synthesis (chronic lead poisoning, pyridoxine deficiency), impaired *globin* synthesis (thalassemias), and other unknown or familial causes ("sideroachrestic anemia," etc.) (*see* reviews by Harris and Kellermeyer, 1970; Williams *et al.,* 1972). All these conditions are easily and very quickly separable from iron-deficiency anemia, since the reticuloendothelial cells of the bone-marrow aspirate contain many golden-yellow granules of hemosiderin, easily seen under the microscope without even the necessity of preparing an iron stain; in iron-deficiency anemia, the definitive diagnostic finding is the *absence* of such hemosiderin granules in the bone-marrow aspirate.

The *initial response* to iron therapy (*see* Figure 63–4) will confirm or negate the diagnosis of iron-deficiency anemia. *Ferrous sulfate,* 150 to 300 mg thrice daily, is given for 3 weeks. Beginning about a week after starting therapy, circulating hemoglobin should rise about 0.1 to 0.3 g % daily; the less severe the anemia, the less the daily rise. If oral iron cannot be employed, a total dose of 6 mg/kg of *iron-dextran* intramuscularly or intravenously may be used. *Response* to therapy with equivalent amounts of oral, intramuscular, or intravenous iron preparations is essentially the same (*see* Symposium, 1970). Figure

63–4 illustrates this point. With intravenous iron, initial reticulocytosis and hemoglobin rise may be higher than with oral iron, but this has no practical importance. With oral or parenteral therapy, erythrocytes respond more slowly than does the hemoglobin, but they often reach transiently polycythemic levels about 3 weeks after the start of therapy, since they are pouring into the circulation in the presence of the old, iron-deficient red cells, which have an almost-normal life-span. Reticulocytosis is usually slower and less marked than following specific therapy for megaloblastic anemias. Reticulocytes should rise within 3 to 7 days and reach a peak of about 5 to 15% in 7 to 14 days (mean, 10 days). Reticulocyte responses to iron are more striking in children than in adults; in children with more than 7.5 g % hemoglobin and in adults, the rise in hemoglobin may be the only measure of response to therapy, since there may be no reticulocytosis. Intravenous iron-dextran may frequently produce a reticulocytosis of 3 to 4% in noniron-deficient patients, but the hemoglobin does not rise (*see* Shanbrom and Warner, 1961). Thrombocytosis is said to be present in most patients with iron-deficiency anemias and is corrected by therapy (*see* Schloesser *et al.,* 1965). If hematological response to therapeutic trial with iron is unsatisfactory, the diagnosis of iron deficiency is wrong, or complications that suppress hematopoiesis are present (infection, severe renal or other systemic disease, chloramphenicol administration, etc.), or continued blood loss is exceeding iron intake, or (rarely) there is malabsorption of oral iron.

Not only does iron therapy improve the blood picture, but also it relieves the menorrhagia and other symptoms that often characterize hypochromic anemia, such as soreness of the tongue, dysphagia, dystrophy of the nails and the skin, and fissuring of the angles of the lips. A sense of well-being and increased appetite may occur within 24 to 48 hours; this may relate to tissue iron enzymes in infants (*see* Beutler, 1965) and to placebo effect in adults (*see* Morrow *et al.,* 1968).

Supplementation with 30 to 60 mg of iron daily (*i.e.,* 150 to 300 mg of ferrous sulfate) has been advocated for *pregnant women* (Committee on Maternal Nutrition, 1970) and 0.3 to 0.6 ml of ferrous sulfate pediatric "drops" daily for *low-birth-weight infants* from 1 month until 1 year of age (*see* Burman, in Symposium, 1973). The physician must use his judgment in this regard, based on knowledge of the patient, the dietary habits, and the fact that iron deficiency is frequent in infants and pregnant women both in the United States (Council on Foods and Nutrition, 1968) and around the world (WHO Scientific Group, 1968). To replenish iron stores, *frequent blood donors* should be given 300 mg of ferrous sulfate daily for 1 month after each donation of 500 ml.

COPPER

Deficiency of copper is extremely rare in man (*see* reviews by Cartwright and Wintrobe, 1964; Scheinberg and Sternlieb, 1969; Li and Vallee, in a monograph by Goodhart and Shils, 1973; Food and Nutrition Board, 1974). Although copper is essential in human metabolism, it is so ubiquitous and abundant in food that *there is no evidence that copper need ever be added to a normal diet, either prophylactically or therapeutically.* In "dysproteinemia" in infants, there is edema, hypoproteinemia, anemia, hypoferremia, and hypocupremia. However, the available evidence is that the anemia responds to iron just as quickly without as with added copper (*see* Sturgeon and Brubaker, 1956; Zipursky *et al.,* 1958), and the syndrome was not produced when premature infants were maintained on a copper-deficient homogenized-milk diet (Wilson and Lahey, 1960).

Evidence of clinically significant copper deficiency has not been adduced in various disorders in which hypocupremia occurs (sprue, celiac disease, nephrotic syndrome, Wilson's disease), with the exception of infants depleted of copper by diarrhea superimposed on a copper-deficient milk diet, in whom anemia, neutropenia, and bone disease corrected by copper administration have been recognized (Cordano *et al.,* 1966). However, an inherited defect in copper absorption does not produce anemia (Danks *et al.,* 1972), raising question as to whether copper deficiency *per se* can produce anemia.

Swine and rats deficient in copper develop a severe anemia, morphologically indistinguishable from the anemia of iron deficiency, but it cannot be corrected by iron alone; in this anemia, unlike that of iron deficiency, red-cell survival time is considerably shortened. Severe copper deficiency also produces anemia in rabbits and dogs. Copper and iron metabolism are interrelated in a number of ways. Plasma copper and ceruloplasmin rise in iron deficiency and fall with iron therapy. The enzyme cytochrome oxidase contains both metals. In copper-deficient animals, iron absorption is reduced. Synthesis of heme may be diminished in copper deficiency.

COBALT

Administration of cobalt will induce polycythemia in animals. In man, the substance may improve hematocrit, hemoglobin, and erythrocyte values in some patients with refractory anemia of various types (sickle-cell disease, thalassemia, chronic infection or renal disease, anemia associated with neoplastic disease, various other refractory anemias of unknown cause) (Berk *et al.,* 1949; Symposium, 1955). Rarely, in pure red-cell aplasia, daily doses of 100 to 200 mg of *cobaltous chloride,* given orally in divided amounts, may produce clinical and hematological recovery, obviating the need for blood transfusions; one reported case was maintained in remission *without* and another case only *with* continued cobalt administration (Voyce, 1963). Cobalt deficiency has not been reported in man.

Cobalt stimulates erythropoietin production, but patients with refractory anemia usually already have elevated erythropoietin levels (*see* Stohlman, 1962; Symposium, 1962). Erslev (1962) has shown that erythropoietin enhances uptake of iron by bone-marrow cells. Cobalt blocks certain enzymes involved in iron transport, and *may well stimulate erythrocyte production by causing intracellular hypoxia* (*see* Symposium, 1964). However, large amounts of cobaltous chloride depress erythrocyte production, and accidental intoxication in children may produce cyanosis, coma, and death. Other undesirable effects of cobaltous chloride include cutaneous flushing, retrosternal chest pain, dermatitides, tinnitus, nausea and vomiting, nerve deafness, thyroid hyperplasia with tracheal compression, myxedema, congestive heart failure, malaise, weakness, anorexia, and fatigue. The use of this potentially toxic metal is best left to the expert in clinical hematology; its use as an adjunct to iron therapy for iron deficiency is worthy of the contempt generated by any "shotgun" therapeutic preparation (*see* Crosby, in Symposium, 1955).

PYRIDOXINE

Since the first case of pyridoxine-responsive anemia was described in 1956 by Harris and associates, about 100 such cases have been observed. (*See* reviews by Horrigan and Harris, 1968; Harris and Kellermeyer, 1970). Megaloblastic erythropoiesis has occurred in about 8% of patients, but the great majority had normoblastic, so-called "sideroachrestic" anemia, characterized by abnormally large amounts of nonhemoglobin iron in erythrocyte precursors (with many "ring sideroblasts" and siderocytes), hypochromic microcytic anemia, hyperferremia and almost complete saturation of iron-binding protein, hemosiderosis, increased iron absorption, and minimal evidence of blood regeneration. The anemia is usually of sporadic occurrence in adult males, but familial occurrence has been noted in both sexes and in childhood.

Treatment with oral or intramuscular *pyridoxine hydrochloride*, 20 to 200 mg daily, produces a hemoglobin response *about halfway toward normal* (obviating the necessity for further blood transfusion) in patients whose erythrocytes show extreme variation in size and shape and marked hypochromicity; such therapy produces a hemoglobin rise to *normal levels* in patients whose erythrocytes show only moderate variations in size and shape and moderate hypochromicity.

The anemia is probably never due primarily to nutritional pyridoxine deficiency; it cannot be produced in man by a pyridoxine-deficient diet or by pyridoxine antagonists, and hypochromia and microcytosois persist after pyridoxine therapy. It is probable that pyridoxine acts in its coenzyme role to stimulate heme production, and thereby partially compensates for a deficiency of an unknown enzyme involved in hemoglobin synthesis or for a defect in utilization of pyridoxine (*see* reviews by Horrigan and Harris, 1968; Hines and Grasso, in Seminar, 1970).

Rarely, a patient with pyridoxine-responsive anemia may have a response of still longer duration to an unidentified factor in orally administered crude liver extract or to tryptophan (Horrigan, 1973).

Since pyridoxine is nontoxic in man in the usual doses, a therapeutic trial with this agent should be conducted in all obscure anemias accompanied by iron overload and/or familial involvement. Pyridoxine is further discussed in Chapter 73.

RIBOFLAVIN AND PROTEIN

A pure red-cell aplasia with hypochromic anemia, responding to riboflavin administration, was reported in patients with complicating infections and therapies by Foy and associates (1961). Lane and coworkers (1964) induced riboflavin deficiency in man and demonstrated that an anemia of the pure red-cell aplasia type appeared within a month and was normochromic and normocytic in character. To produce the anemia, it was necessary not only to restrict dietary riboflavin but also to administer galactoflavin, a riboflavin antagonist. The anemia was correctable by oral or intramuscular riboflavin, 10 mg daily. The patients reported by Foy and coworkers (1961) had riboflavin deficiency associated with protein-calorie malnutrition, often complicated by deficiency of iron or anemia of infection (*see* review by Foy and Kondi, 1968). Riboflavin deficiency will probably prove to be a factor in the anemia of patients with protein-calorie malnutrition; in such patients it has not yet been demonstrated that protein deficiency alone is capable of producing anemia, or that feeding of protein alone will correct it (*see* reviews by Finch, 1968; Viteri *et al.*, 1968; Adams, in Seminar, 1970). Other than in patients with gross generalized malnutrition, riboflavin-

deficiency anemia is very unlikely (*see* review by Alfrey and Lane, in Seminar, 1970). Riboflavin has been reported to correct some instances of glutathione reductase deficiency (Beutler, 1969). Riboflavin is discussed further in Chapter 73.

Allgood, J. W., and Brown, E. B. The relationship between duodenal mucosal iron concentration and iron absorption in human subjects. *Scand. J. Haemat.*, **1967**, *4*, 217–229.

Barer, A. P., and Fowler, W. M. Effect of an acid and alkaline salt on the urinary excretion of iron. *J. Lab. clin. Med.*, **1949**, *34*, 932–935.

Berk, L.; Burchenal, J. H.; and Castle, W. B. Erythropoietic effect of cobalt in patients with or without anemia. *New Engl. J. Med.*, **1949**, *240*, 754–761.

Bernstein, L., and Herbert, V. The role of pancreatic exocrine secretions in the absorption of vitamin B_{12} and iron. *Am. J. clin. Nutr.*, **1973**, *25*, 340–346.

Bessis, M. C., and Breton-Gorius, J. Iron metabolism in the bone marrow as seen by electron microscopy: a critical review. *Blood*, **1962**, *19*, 635–663.

Beutler, E. Tissue effects of iron deficiency. *Ser. haemat.*, **1965**, *6*, 41–55.

———. Glutathione reductase: stimulation in normal subjects by riboflavin supplementation. *Science, Wash.*, **1969**, *165*, 613–615.

Blaud, P. Sur les maladies chlorotiques, et sur un mode de traitement spécifique dans ces affections. *Revue méd. fr. étrang.*, **1832a**, *1*, 337.

———. Pilules antichlorotiques. *Bull. gén. thér. méd. chir.*, **1832b**, *2*, 154.

Bothwell, T. H., and Isaacson, C. Siderosis in the Bantu. *Br. med. J.*, **1962**, *1*, 522–524.

Brise, H., and Hallberg, L. Absorbability of different iron compounds. *Acta med. scand.*, **1962**, *171*, Suppl. 376, 23–38.

Brown, E. B., Jr.; Dubach, R.; and Moore, C. V. Studies in iron transportation and metabolism. XI. Critical analysis of mucosal block by large doses of inorganic iron in human subjects. *J. Lab. clin. Med.*, **1958**, *52*, 335–355.

Brown, E. B., Jr., and Rother, M. L. Studies on the mechanism of iron absorption. I. Iron uptake by the normal rat. *J. Lab. clin. Med.*, **1963**, *62*, 357–373.

Charlton, R. W., and Bothwell, T. H. Hemochromatosis: dietary and genetic aspects. *Prog. Hemat.*, **1966**, *5*, 298–323.

Conrad, M. E.; Weintraub, L. R.; and Crosby, W. H. The role of the intestine in iron kinetics. *J. clin. Invest.*, **1964**, *43*, 963–974.

Cordano, A.; Placko, R. P.; and Graham, G. C. Hypocupremia and neutropenia in copper deficiency. *Blood*, **1966**, *28*, 280–283.

Crosby, W. H.; Conrad, M. E., Jr.; and Wheby, M. S. The rate of iron accumulation in iron storage disease. *Blood*, **1963**, *22*, 429–440.

Danks, D. M.; Campbell, P. E.; Stevens, B. J.; Mayne, V.; and Cartwright, E. Menkes's kinky hair syndrome—an inherited defect in copper absorption with widespread effects. *Pediatrics, Springfield*, **1972**, *50*, 188–201.

de Leeuw, N. K. M.; Lowenstein, L.; and Hsieh, Y.-S. Iron deficiency and hydremia in normal pregnancy. *Medicine, Baltimore*, **1966**, *45*, 291–315.

Erslev, A. J. Effect of erythropoietin on uptake and utilization of iron by bone marrow cells *in vitro*. *Proc. Soc. exp. Biol. Med.*, **1962**, *110*, 615–620.

Finch, C. A.; Hegsted, M.; Kinney, T. D.; Thomas, E. D.; Rath, C. E.; Haskins, D.; Finch, S.; and Fluharty, R. G. Iron metabolism: the pathophysiology of iron storage. *Blood*, **1950**, *5*, 983–1008.

Forbes, G. Poisoning with a preparation of iron, copper, and manganese. *Br. med. J.*, **1947**, *1*, 367–370.

Foy, H.; Kondi, A.; and MacDougall, L. Pure red-cell aplasia in marasmus and kwashiorkor treated with riboflavin. *Br. med. J.,* **1961,** *1,* 937–941.

Gabrio, B. W.; Shoden, A.; and Finch, C. A. Relationship between ferritin and hemosiderin in iron storage and iron mobilization. *Fedn Proc. Fedn Am. Socs exp. Biol.,* **1953,** *12,* 47–48.

Gale, E.; Torrance, J.; and Bothwell, T. The quantitative estimation of total iron stores in human bone marrow. *J. clin. Invest.,* **1963,** *42,* 1076–1082.

Gitlin, D., and Cruchaud, A. On the kinetics of iron absorption in mice. *J. clin. Invest.,* **1962,** *41,* 344–350.

Granick, S. Iron metabolism. *Bull. N.Y. Acad. Med.,* **1954,** *30,* 81–105.

Green, R.; Charlton, R.; Seftel, H.; Bothwell, T.; Mayet, F.; Adams, B.; Finch, C.; and Layrisse, M. Body iron excretion in man. *Am. J. Med.,* **1968,** *45,* 336–353.

Gubler, C. J.; Cartwright, G. E.; and Wintrobe, M. M. The effect of pyridoxine deficiency on the absorption of iron by the rat. *J. biol. Chem.,* **1949,** *178,* 989–996.

Haden, R. I. Historical aspects of iron therapy in anemia. *J. Am. med. Ass.,* **1939,** *111,* 1059–1061.

Hahn, P. F.; Bale, W. F.; Ross, J. F.; Balfour, W. M.; and Whipple, G. H. Radioactive iron absorption by gastrointestinal tract. *J. exp. Med.,* **1943,** *78,* 169–188.

Hahn, P. F.; Granick, S.; Bale, W. F.; and Michaelis, L. Ferritin. VI. Conversion of inorganic and hemoglobin iron into ferritin iron in the animal body. Storage function of ferritin iron as shown by radioactive and magnetic measurements. *J. biol. Chem.,* **1943,** *150,* 407–412.

Hallberg, L., and Sölvell, L. Absorption of hemoglobin iron in man. *Acta med. scand.,* **1967,** *181,* 335–354.

Harris, J. W.; Whittington, R. M.; Weisman, R., Jr.; and Horrigan, D. L. Pyridoxin responsive anemia in the human adult. *Proc. Soc. exp. Biol. Med.,* **1956,** *91,* 427–432.

Heath, C. W.; Strauss, M. B.; and Castle, W. B. Quantitative aspects of iron deficiency in hypochromic anemia. *J. clin. Invest.,* **1932,** *11,* 1293–1312.

Herbert, V. Doses and dosing. *New Engl. J. Med.,* **1966,** *274,* 1152.

Horrigan, D. L. Pyridoxine-responsive anemia: influence of tryptophan on pyridoxine responsiveness. *Blood,* **1973,** *42,* 187–193.

Hussain, R.; Walker, R.; Layrisse, M.; Clark, P.; and Finch, C. A. Nutritive value of food iron. *Am. J. clin. Nutr.,* **1965,** *16,* 464–471.

Hynes, M. The iron reserve of a normal man. *J. clin. Path.,* **1949,** *2,* 99–102.

Lane, M.; Alfrey, C. P.; Megel, C. E.; Doherty, M. A.; and Doherty, J. The rapid induction of human riboflavin deficiency with galactoflavin. *J. clin. Invest.,* **1964,** *43,* 357–373.

Laurell, C.-B. Plasma iron and the transport of iron in the organism. *Pharmac. Rev.,* **1952,** *4,* 371–395. (218 references.)

McCance, R. A., and Widdowson, E. M. Iron excretion and metabolism in man. *Nature, Lond.,* **1943,** *152,* 326–327.

MacDonald, R. A. Primary hemochromatosis: inherited or acquired. *Prog. Hemat.,* **1966,** *5,* 324–353. (265 references.)

Manis, J., and Schachter, D. Pathways of iron metabolism in the intestinal mucosa and the regulation of iron absorption. *J. clin. Invest.,* **1964,** *43,* 1240.

Marchasin, S., and Wallerstein, R. O. The treatment of iron-deficiency anemia with intravenous iron dextran. *Blood,* **1964,** *23,* 354–358.

Middleton, E. J.; Nagy, E.; and Morrison, A. B. Studies on the absorption of orally administered iron from sustained-release preparations. *New Engl. J. Med.,* **1966,** *274,* 136–139.

Monsen, E. R.; Kuhn, I. N.; and Finch, C. A. Iron status of menstruating women. *Am. J. clin. Nutr.,* **1967,** *20,* 842–849.

Morrow, J. J.; Dagg, J. H.; and Goldberg, A. A controlled trial of iron therapy in sideropenia. *Scot. med. J.,* **1968,** *13,* 78–83.

Neuroth, M. L., and Lee, C. O. A history of Blaud's pills. *J. Am. pharm. Ass., Sci. Ed.,* **1941,** *30,* 60–63.

Pollack, S.; Kaufman, R.; Crosby, W. H.; and Butkiewicz, J. E. Reducing agents and absorption of iron. *Nature, Lond.,* **1963,** *199,* 384.

Reimann, F.; Fritsch, F.; and Schick, K. Eisenbilanzversuche bei Gesunden und bei Anämischen. II. Untersuchungen über das Wesen der eisenempfindlichen Anämien ("Asiderosen") und der therapeutischen Wirkung des Eisens bei diesen Anämien. *Z. klin. Med.,* **1936,** *131,* 1–50.

Rifkind, D.; Kravetz, H. M.; Knight, V.; and Schade, A. L. Urinary excretion of iron-binding protein in the nephrotic syndrome. *New Engl. J. Med.,* **1961,** *265,* 115–118.

Sacks, P. V., and Crosby, W. H. Bioavailability and toxicity of carbonyl iron. *Clin. Res.,* **1974,** *22,* 562A.

Schade, S. G.; Cohen, R. J.; and Conrad, M. E. Effect of hydrochloric acid on iron absorption. *New Engl. J. Med.,* **1968,** *279,* 672–674.

Schloesser, L. L.; Kipp, M. A.; and Wenzel, F. W. Thrombocytosis in iron deficiency anemia. *J. Lab. clin. Med.,* **1965,** *66,* 107–114.

Shahidi, N. T.; Nathan, D. G.; and Diamond. L. K. Iron deficiency anemia associated with an error of iron metabolism in two siblings. *J. clin. Invest.,* **1964,** *43,* 510–521.

Shanbrom, E., and Warner, G. F. Intravenous iron as a "provocative test" in the diagnosis of iron deficiency. *Clin. Res.,* **1961,** *9,* 68.

Simon, E. R.; Giblett, E. R.; and Finch, C. A. *Red Cell Manual.* University of Washington School of Medicine, Seattle, **1966.**

Smith, M. D., and Pannacciulli, I. M. Absorption of inorganic iron from graded doses: its significance in relation to iron absorption tests and the 'mucosal block' theory. *Br. J. Haemat.,* **1958,** *4,* 428–434.

Sturgeon, P., and Brubaker, C. Copper deficiency in infants: syndrome characterized by hypocupremia, iron deficiency anemia, and hypoproteinemia. *A.M.A. J. Dis. Child.,* **1956,** *92,* 254–265.

Vellar, O. D. Studies on sweat losses of nutrients. 1. Iron content of whole body sweat and its association with other sweat constituents, serum iron levels, hematological indices, body surface area, and sweat rate. *Scand. J. clin. Lab. Invest.,* **1968,** *21,* 157–167.

Voyce, M. A. A case of pure red-cell aplasia successfully treated with cobalt. *Br. J. Haemat.,* **1963,** *9,* 412–418.

Waxman, S.; Pratt, P.; and Herbert, V. Malabsorption of hemoglobin iron in pernicious anemia: correction with intrinsic factor–containing substances. *J. clin. Invest.,* **1968,** *47,* 1819–1825.

Weintraub, L. R.; Weinstein, M. B.; Huser, H.-J.; and Rafal, S. Absorption of hemoglobin iron: the role of a heme-splitting substance in the intestinal mucosa. *J. clin. Invest.,* **1968,** *47,* 531–539.

Will, G. The absorption, distribution and utilization of intramuscularly administered iron-dextran: a radioisotope study. *Br. J. Haemat.,* **1968,** *14,* 395–406.

Wilson, J. F., and Lahey, M. E. Failure to induce dietary deficiency of copper in premature infants. *Pediatrics, Springfield,* **1960,** *25,* 40–49.

Wintrobe, M. M. The proposed increase in the iron fortification of wheat products. *Nutr. Today,* **1973,** *8,* 18–20.

Zipursky, A.; Dempsey, H.; Markowitz, H.; Cartwright, G. E.; and Wintrobe, M. M. Studies on copper metabolism. XXIV. Hypocupremia in infancy. *A.M.A. J. Dis. Child.,* **1958,** *96,* 148–158.

Monographs and Reviews

Bothwell, T. H. Current concepts concerning iron balance. In, *Plenary Session Papers, XII Congress, International Society of Hematology.* (Jaffé, E. R., ed.) The Society, New York, **1968a**, pp. 144–153.

———. The control of iron absorption. *Br. J. Haemat.,* **1968b**, *14,* 453–456.

Bothwell, T. H., and Finch, C. A. *Iron Metabolism.* Little, Brown & Co., Boston, **1962.**

Brown, E. B. Clinical pharmacology of drugs used in the treatment of iron deficiency anemia. *Pharmac. Physns,* **1968,** *2,* 1–7.

Cartwright, G. E., and Wintrobe, M. M. Copper metabolism in normal subjects. *Am. J. clin. Nutr.,* **1964,** *14,* 224–232.

Charlton, R. W., and Bothwell, T. H. Iron deficiency anemia. *Semin. Hemat.,* **1970,** *7,* 67–85.

Committee on Maternal Nutrition, Food and Nutrition Board, National Research Council. *Maternal Nutrition and the Course of Pregnancy.* National Academy of Sciences, Washington, D. C., **1970.**

Council on Foods and Nutrition. Iron deficiency in the United States. *J. Am. med. Ass.,* **1968,** *203,* 119–124.

Crosby, W. H. The control of iron absorption. *Ser. haemat.,* **1965,** *6,* 66–71.

———. Control of iron absorption by intestinal luminal factors. *Am. J. clin. Nutr.,* **1968,** *21,* 1189–1193.

Fairbanks, V. F.; Fahey, J. L.; and Beutler, E. *Clinical Disorders of Iron Metabolism.* Grune & Stratton, Inc., New York, **1971.**

FAO/WHO Expert Group. *Requirements of Ascorbic Acid, Vitamin D, Vitamin B_{12}, Folate, and Iron.* World Health Organization Technical Report, WHO, Geneva, **1970.**

Finch, C. A. Protein deficiency and anemia. In, *Plenary Session Papers, XII Congress, International Society of Hematology.* (Jaffé, E. R., ed.) The Society, New York, **1968,** pp. 154–158.

Finch, C. A.; Deubelbeiss, K.; Cook, J. D.; Eschbach, J. W.; Harker, L. A.; Funk, D. D.; Marsaglia, G.; Hillman, R. S.; Slichter, S.; Adamson, J. W.; Ganzoni, A.; and Giblett, E. R. Ferrokinetics in man. *Medicine, Baltimore,* **1970,** *49,* 17–54.

Food and Nutrition Board, National Research Council. *Recommended Dietary Allowances,* 8th rev. ed. Publication No. 2216, National Academy of Sciences, Washington, D. C., **1974.**

Foy, H., and Kondi, A. Comparison between erythroid aplasia in marasmus and kwashiorkor and the experimentally induced erythroid aplasia in baboons by riboflavin deficiency. *Vitams Horm.,* **1968,** *26,* 653–682.

Goodhart, R. S., and Shils, M. E. (eds.). *Modern Nutrition in Health and Disease,* 5th ed. Lea & Febiger, Philadelphia, **1973.**

Gordon, A. S. (ed.). *Regulation of Hematopoiesis.* Appleton-Century-Crofts, New York, **1970.** (Two volumes.)

Harris, J. W., and Kellermeyer, R. W. *The Red Cell,* rev. ed. Harvard University Press, Cambridge, Mass., **1970.**

Hillman, R. S., and Finch, C. A. *Red Cell Manual.* F. A. Davis Co., Philadelphia, **1974.**

Horrigan, D. L., and Harris, J. W. Pyridoxine-responsive anemias in man. *Vitams Horm.,* **1968,** *26,* 549–568.

Jacobs, A., and Worwood, M. (eds.). *Iron in Biochemistry and Medicine.* Academic Press, Inc., New York, **1974.**

Scheinberg, I. H., and Sternlieb, I. Metabolism of trace metals. In, *Duncan's Diseases of Metabolism,* 6th ed. (Bondy, P. K., ed.) W. B. Saunders Co., Philadelphia, **1969.**

Seminar. (Various authors.) Nutritional anemias. (Herbert, V., ed.) *Semin. Hemat.,* **1970,** *7,* 2–106.

Stohlman, F., Jr. Erythropoiesis. *New Engl. J. Med.,* **1962,** *267,* 342–348, 392–399.

Symposium. (Various authors.) The use of cobalt and cobalt-iron preparations in the therapy of anemia. *Blood,* **1955,** *10,* 852–861.

Symposium. (Various authors.) *Iron in Clinical Medicine.* (Wallerstein, R. O., and Mettier, S. R., eds.) University of California Press, Berkeley, **1958.**

Symposium. (Various authors.) *Erythropoiesis.* (Jacobson, L. O., and Doyle, M., eds.) Grune & Stratton, Inc., New York, **1962.**

Symposium. (Various authors.) *Iron Metabolism.* (Gross, F., ed.) Springer-Verlag, Berlin, **1964.**

Symposium. (Various authors.) Iron deficiency and absorption. (Herbert, V., ed.) *Am. J. clin. Nutr.,* **1968,** *21,* 1138–1193.

Symposium. (Various authors.) *Iron Deficiency.* (Hallberg, L.; Harwerth, H. G.; and Vannotti, A.; eds.) Academic Press, Inc., New York, **1970.**

Symposium. (Various authors.) *Iron.* (Crosby, W. H., ed.) Medcom, Inc., New York, **1972.**

Symposium. (Various authors.) Iron deficiency and iron overload. (Callender, S. T., ed.) *Clins Haemat.,* **1973,** *2,* 241–429.

Viteri, F. E.; Alvarado, J.; Luthringer, D. G.; and Wood, R. P. Hematological changes in protein-calorie malnutrition. *Vitams Horm.,* **1968,** *26,* 573–615.

WHO Scientific Group. *Nutritional Anemias.* World Health Organization Technical Report No. 405, WHO, Geneva, **1968,** pp. 5–37.

Williams, W. J.; Beutler, E.; Erslev, A. J.; and Rundles, R. W. (eds.). *Hematology.* McGraw-Hill Book Co., New York, **1972.**

CHAPTER

64 DRUGS EFFECTIVE IN MEGALOBLASTIC ANEMIAS

Vitamin B_{12} and Folic Acid

Victor Herbert

History. The history of folic acid (pteroylglutamic acid, PGA) and vitamin B_{12} (cyanocobalamin) is a dramatic story of widely divergent investigations in the fields of human deficiency disease, animal nutrition, and microbiology, ultimately converging and resulting in the identification of two vitamins of fundamental importance in cellular metabolism. The story began with Addison's description, in 1849 and 1855, of what his contemporaries evidently recognized as pernicious anemia, or perhaps even earlier with Combe's account in 1822 of a fatal case also said to be one of pernicious anemia, which he correctly ascribed to "some disorder of the digestive and assimilative organs" (*see* review by Castle, 1961).

The Nobel prize-winning discovery of the therapeutic value of liver in pernicious anemia by Minot in 1926 was followed by the demonstration by Castle in 1927 that normal human gastric juice contains an "intrinsic factor" that combines with an "extrinsic factor" contained in animal protein to result in absorption of the "anti–pernicious anemia principle." With the isolation of vitamin B_{12} 2 decades later, Berk and associates (1948) showed that this vitamin was both "extrinsic factor" and "anti–pernicious anemia principle."

In the 1930s, while repeated attempts to isolate and chemically to identify the active "extrinsic factor" were resulting in increased purification of liver extracts, Wills and her associates (1932, 1937) described a macrocytic anemia in Hindu women in Bombay, usually in association with pregnancy, that responded to therapy with MARMITE, a commercial preparation of autolyzed yeast. A similar macrocytic anemia produced by them in monkeys, by feeding the same type of diet that was ingested by their patients, responded to a "Wills factor" present in crude liver extracts but not present in the purer fraction effective in the treatment of pernicious anemia. We now know that the more purified liver extracts used by Wills consisted of a fairly pure solution of vitamin B_{12}, and that the "Wills factor" is folic acid that was removed from the crude liver extracts in the process of purification. However, this knowledge only gradually evolved after the purification of pteroylglutamic acid in 1943 by Stokstad, its crystallization from liver by Pfiffner and associates (1943), its synthesis in 1945 by Angier and coworkers, who also determined its structure (1946), and the isolation in 1948 of *crystalline vitamin B_{12}* from liver concentrates by Rickes and his coworkers in Folkers'

group in the United States and almost simultaneously by Smith and Parker in Great Britain.

Folic acid has proven to be not only the "Wills factor" but also the vitamin M, contained in the dried brewer's yeast, that corrected the deficiency anemia, leukopenia, diarrhea, and gingivitis in monkeys (*see* Day *et al.,* 1945). Folic acid has likewise proven to be the vitamin B_c, contained in yeast, that corrected a deficiency syndrome in chicks characterized by anemia and failure in growth, as described by Stokstad and Manning (1938). In addition, it proved to be the norite eluate factor (*i.e.,* it could be adsorbed on and eluted from charcoal) of liver described by Snell and Peterson (1940), as essential for the growth of *Lactobacillus casei* (also called the "*L. casei* factor" by Stokstad, who purified it in 1943). The term *folic acid* had been coined by Mitchell and coworkers (1941) because they isolated this material, with then-unknown chemical composition, from a leafy vegetable (spinach). In the same year, the paths of the nutritionists and microbiologists crossed when Hutchings and associates recognized that vitamin B_c and the "*L. casei* factor" were interchangeable in supporting bacterial and avian growth.

It now appears that neither vitamin B_{12} (cyanocobalamin) nor folic acid (pteroylglutamic acid) exists as such in either the human body or the various foods from which these agents were isolated. In the body and in foods they are present in various metabolically active coenzyme forms, and frequently also in the form of conjugates with amino acid residues attached to them in peptide linkage. During the extraction procedure these active labile forms are converted to stable pteroylglutamic acid or to cyanocobalamin. The stable forms may not be metabolically active. The delineation of the nature and the action of these coenzyme forms, as well as the unraveling of the independent and interdependent functions of these two vitamins in cellular metabolism in general and in hematopoiesis in particular, is one of the most fascinating stories in biology, many chapters of which remain to be written (*see* Symposium, 1970).

Definition and Nature of Megaloblastic Anemia. This subject has been reviewed by Chanarin (1969), Beck (1972), Stebbins and associates (1973), and Herbert (1975). In most instances, the terms *macrocytic anemia* and *megaloblastic anemia* are interchangeable, because most macrocytic anemias are *macroovalocytic,* and macroovalocytic anemias are nearly always megaloblastic. Nonmegaloblastic (and nonmacroovalocytic) macrocytic anemia may occur with hemolytic anemia (of any type), aplastic anemia, hepatic disease (in which the anemia is usually *macroovalocytic* due to folate deficiency), and hypothyroidism (although this anemia often is *macroovalocytic* due to vitamin B_{12} or folate deficiency). These *macrocytic* anemias are distinguishable from the large body of *macroovalocytic* (megaloblastic) anemias simply by examination of the peripheral blood. Only in megaloblastic anemia does one find in the peripheral blood the combination of *macroovalocytes,* hypersegmentation of the nuclei of the polymorphonuclear leukocytes, and giant platelets.

Megaloblastic anemia is a morphological entity characterized by large germ cells in the bone marrow and by their large progeny in the peripheral blood. Biochemically, it is of diverse etiology, since it may result from blocked DNA synthesis of any cause (Stebbins *et al.,* 1973). Clinically, the cause is almost invariably deficiency of vitamin B_{12} and/or folic acid; the hematological picture produced by folate deficiency is indistinguishable from that produced by vitamin B_{12} deficiency. As with all avitaminoses, deficiency of vitamin B_{12} or folate may occur from *inadequate ingestion, inadequate absorption, inadequate utilization, increased requirement, increased destruction, or increased excretion,* alone or in combination.

The basic abnormality affects all proliferating cells, and, therefore, megaloblasts may be noted not only in the hematopoietic system but also in buccal, bronchial, gastric, jejunal, and vaginal epithelial cells, and probably in other dividing cells as well.

The individual megaloblast is morphologically characterized by the large size of both its nucleus and cytoplasm, with relatively greater increase in the latter. *The basic abnormality appears to be a reduction in the ability to double the nuclear DNA complement in order for the cell to divide,* with cytoplasmic RNA secondarily "building up" behind this bottleneck. Thus, at any given instant in time, the majority of cells in the megaloblastic bone marrow are in the process of slowly doubling their DNA complement (DNA synthesis phase). The hallmark of megaloblastic anemia is this *maturation arrest,* also referred to as *nuclear cytoplasmic dissociation* or *asynchrony,* characterized by a cell with a "young" nucleus and an "old" cytoplasm. The maturation arrest causes the bone marrow to become filled with megaloblastic red-cell precursors, as well as with giant myeloid cells and platelet precursors. These abnormally large progenitors give rise to large offspring, which appear in the peripheral blood as macroovalocytes, polymorphonuclear leukocytes with hypersegmented nuclei ("hypersegmented polys"), and giant platelets. In addition to being an anemia due to ineffective hematopoiesis, megaloblastic anemia is a hemolytic anemia. The macroovalocytes have a shortened life-span, due not only to intrinsic cellular abnormalities but also to extrinsic abnormalities, including a "plasma factor" and moderate splenomegaly.

Not only will deficiency of either vitamin B_{12} or folic acid result in megaloblastic anemia, but also the degree of the anemia caused by the lack of either

agent is conditioned by the quantity of the other agent present. Thus, a patient who has a severe vitamin B_{12} deficiency but who is ingesting and absorbing relatively large quantities of folate may show no anemia and exhibit only moderate hypersegmentation of the nuclei of the polymorphonuclear leukocytes and only moderate macroovalocytosis. Such is often the case with vegetarians. The severity of megaloblastic anemia is almost certainly also conditioned by the relative quantities in the body of many other agents, some indicated in Figure 64-1, such as pyridoxine, serine, histidine, thymine, and methionine.

As might be expected from perusal of Figure 64-1, mass-action effects may transiently lessen the degree of the megaloblastic anemia, as may occur with ingestion of various substrates such as nucleic acid precursors or derivatives, or certain amino acids such as histidine or serine. Other amino acids, such as methionine, may worsen the megaloblastic anemia (Stebbins *et al.,* 1973), despite a reduction in the abnormally elevated excretion of the histidine catabolite formiminoglutamate.

Another factor involved in the severity of overt megaloblastic anemia is *iron.* Iron deficiency tends to produce microcytosis, resulting in partial concealment of the megaloblastosis. The erythroid precursors in the bone marrow are halfway between normoblasts and megaloblasts and, therefore, are called intermediate megaloblasts. In the peripheral blood there may be a *dimorphic anemia* (microcytes and macrocytes present), a *normocytic anemia* (exact balance between the opposing factors), a *microcytic anemia* (when iron deficiency predominates), or a *macroovalocytic anemia* (when iron deficiency does not predominate). Other conditions in which hemoglobin synthesis is blocked, such as Cooley's anemia, may also mask megaloblastosis, as does iron deficiency (*see* reviews by Herbert, 1959, 1975).

Nucleic acid synthesis may be blocked, with resultant megaloblastic anemia, by antimetabolites interfering with any phase of this process. Examples include antifols, antipurines, and antipyrimidines. Megaloblastic anemia will, of course, also develop if nucleic acid synthesis is blocked by congenital absence of a requisite enzyme, an extremely rare occurrence.

Clinical Picture of Megaloblastic Anemia. Megaloblastic anemia, regardless of cause, produces a unitary clinical picture. Symptomatically, as with all anemias, there may be weakness and tiredness, dyspnea, and accentuation of the symptomatology of any associated pulmonary or cardiovascular functional deficit. Peripheral edema may be present, as may a mild icterus due both to hemolysis and to variably disturbed hepatic function. Unlike many other anemias in which only erythrocytes are affected, in megaloblastic anemia all the formed elements are involved. The characteristic morphological changes in the bone marrow and peripheral blood are described above. In association with the leukopenia, the patient may be more susceptible to infection, especially of the genitourinary tract; in association with severe thrombocytopenia, he may have hemorrhagic manifestations.

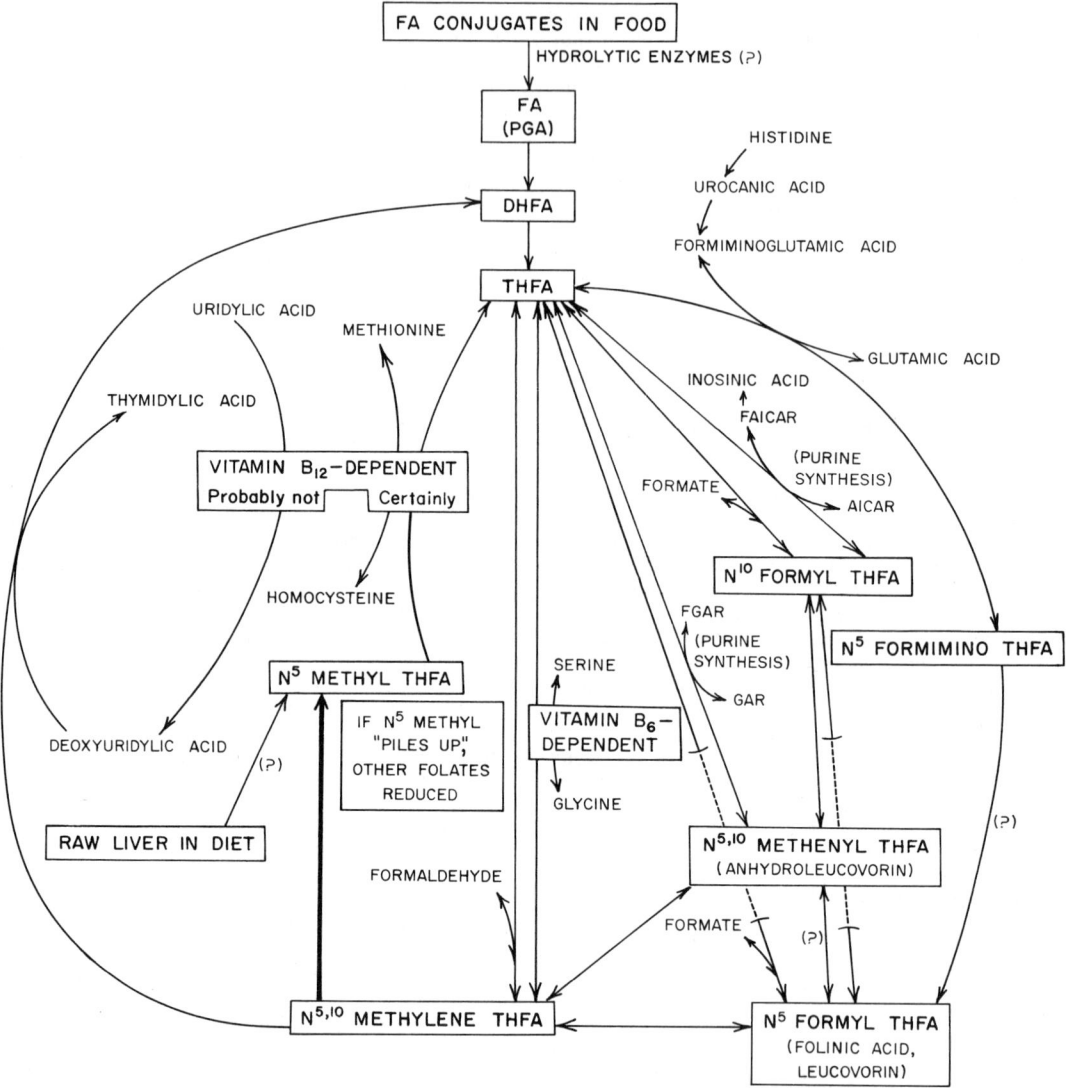

Figure 64–1. *Interrelations of vitamin B_{12} (cyanocobalamin) and folic acid (pteroylglutamic acid) metabolism.*

See text for discussion.

FA = folic acid (pteroylglutamic acid, PGA); *DHFA* = dihydrofolic acid (FH_2); *THFA* = tetrahydrofolic acid (FH_4); *AICAR* = 5-amino-4-imidazolecarboxamide ribonucleotide; *FAICAR* = formyl-AICAR; *GAR* = glycinamide ribonucleotide; *FGAR* = formyl-GAR.

As mentioned above, the megaloblastosis affects all proliferating cells. In association with the gastrointestinal tract involvement there may be diarrhea (especially with folate deficiency) or constipation (especially with vitamin B_{12} deficiency). The tongue may be sore, raw, pale, and smooth (chronic atrophic glossitis), or red and ulcerated (acute glossitis). Anorexia is frequent and, in patients with vitamin B_{12} deficiency, may so reduce food ingestion as to result in secondary folate deficiency.

Addison's clinical description of a patient with megaloblastic anemia, written in 1855, has not been improved upon. He wrote:

The countenance gets pale, the whites of the eyes become pearly, *the general frame flabby rather than wasted;* the pulse perhaps large but remarkably soft and compressible, and occasionally with a slight jerk, especially under the slightest excitement. There is an increasing indisposition to exertion with an uncomfortable feeling of faintness or breathlessness on attempting it; the heart is readily made to palpitate;

the whole surface presents a blanched, smooth and waxy appearance; the lips, gums and tongue seem bloodless; *the flabbiness of the solids increases;* the appetite fails, extreme languor and faintness supervene, breathlessness and palpitation being produced by the most trifling exertion or emotion; some slight edema is probably perceived about the ankles. The debility becomes extreme; the patient can no longer arise from his bed; *the mind occasionally wanders;* he falls into a prostrate and half torpid state, and at length expires. *Nevertheless, to the very last, and after a sickness of perhaps several months' duration, the bulkiness of the general frame and the obesity often present a most striking contrast to the failure and exhaustion observable in every other respect.* [Italics added.]

Addison's classic description perfectly fits patients with megaloblastic anemia due to vitamin B$_{12}$ deficiency; those parts of his description that do not always fit patients with *folate deficiency* have been italicized.

With folate deficiency, the general frame is wasted. Nervous instability is frequent, but damage to myelin does not occur as it does with vitamin B$_{12}$ deficiency and, therefore, there is no peripheral nerve or posterior or lateral column damage.

A low-grade fever is present in 10 to 20% of patients. This may be related to the increased basal metabolic rate that occurs in severe anemia, due to the added work that the heart and respiratory muscles must perform to maintain adequate oxygenation of the tissues. Hyperpigmentation of the skin may occur with deficiency of vitamin B$_{12}$ or folate. Severe deficiency may cause infertility (Jackson *et al.,* 1967).

Interrelations of Vitamin B$_{12}$ and Folic Acid Metabolism. Vitamin B$_{12}$ and folic acid are very closely interrelated metabolically. (*See* Figure 64–1. *See also* Symposium, 1970; Herbert *et al.,* 1973; Tisman and Herbert, 1973.) The pharmacological result is that a large dose of one vitamin will produce a hematological response in a patient whose deficiency is of the other vitamin (*see* review by Herbert, 1963), thus leading the physician erroneously to conclude that the patient suffered from a deficiency of the vitamin administered. *Since folic acid can correct much of the hematological damage due to deficiency of vitamin B$_{12}$ but allows the neurological damage from vitamin B$_{12}$ deficiency to progress, erroneous therapy with folic acid can be disastrous.* For this and other reasons it is imperative that the physician determine the *cause* of megaloblastic anemia in each patient.

Figure 64–1 shows the interrelations of the folate coenzymes and indicates the reactions dependent on vitamin B$_{12}$. The conversion of homocysteine to methionine requires the transfer of a methyl group from 5-methyl tetrahydrofolic acid (THFA) to cobalamin, to form methyl B$_{12}$, and the subsequent transfer of the methyl group from methyl B$_{12}$ to homocysteine, to form methionine (methyl homocysteine). With deficiency of vitamin B$_{12}$, 5-methyl THFA cannot be taken up by cells or converted back to THFA by the vitamin B$_{12}$-dependent pathway and, because of this "methylfolate trap," accumulates in the plasma. This reduces the amounts of folate available to travel along other metabolic pathways, resulting in a functional folate deficiency despite continued ingestion and absorption of folate

by the patient (Metz *et al.,* 1968a; Tisman and Herbert, 1973).

Folate deficiency leads directly to megaloblastic anemia, but it is not yet certain that vitamin B$_{12}$ deficiency leads directly to the disease. It is probable that the megaloblastic anemia that follows vitamin B$_{12}$ deprivation is partly the result of deranged folic acid metabolism caused by deficiency of vitamin B$_{12}$. Vitamin B$_{12}$ is not required for the reduction of uridylic to deoxyuridylic acid or for the reduction of other ribonucleotides to deoxyribonucleotides (*see* Symposium, 1970; Stebbins *et al.,* 1973). It is well established, however, that a folate coenzyme (5,10-methylene THFA) is required to methylate deoxyuridylate to thymidylate (*see* Symposium, 1970).

VITAMIN B$_{12}$ (CYANOCOBALAMIN)

Chemistry. The structural formula of vitamin B$_{12}$, elucidated by Hodgkin and her coworkers, for which work she won the 1964 Nobel prize in chemistry, is shown in Figure 64–2. (*See* Pratt, 1972.)

The two major portions of the molecule are the planar group (the corrin nucleus) and a "nucleotide" lying in a plane nearly at right angles to the corrin nucleus and linked to it by D-1-amino-2-propanol, which is esterified to the "nucleotide" and joined in amide linkage to the corrin nucleus. The "nucleotide" consists of the base 5,6-dimethylbenzimidazole attached to ribose by an α-glycosidic linkage (unlike the β linkage in the nucleic acids). A second bridge between the two major parts of the molecule is the coordinate linkage of the cobalt atom to one of the nitrogen atoms of the benzimidazole. The anionic (—R) group in coordinate linkage with the cobalt atom is cyanide. (The cyanide moiety was present in the originally isolated vitamin B$_{12}$ because it came off the charcoal columns used in the isolation procedure, and replaced the 5'-deoxyadenosyl anionic group naturally present in the liver, from which the vitamin was isolated.) Cyanocobalamin crystallizes as dark-red nodules or prisms; the color is due to the cobalt-containing pigment complex of porphyrin-like nature. The cobalt binding is covalent rather than ionic. It is soluble 1:80 in water and is stable in solution.

Coenzyme B$_{12}$ differs from cyanocobalamin in that, instead of an anionic CN group attached as a ligand of cobalt, the attached moiety is 5'-deoxyadenosine (minus the OH of the 5 carbon of ribose). The vitamin B$_{12}$ coenzymes are very unstable in light. Coenzyme B$_{12}$, in the presence of light and oxygen, undergoes photolysis with formation of aquocobalamin. In the presence of potassium cyanide, coenzyme B$_{12}$ is converted to cyanocobalamin.

Assay. Vitamin B$_{12}$ activity can be assayed in a number of ways, depending on the purity of the material: colorimetrically, spectroscopically, fluorometrically, chemically, by isotope dilution with vitamin B$_{12}$ labeled with radioactive cobalt, microbiologically (by determining ability to promote growth of various vitamin B$_{12}$-dependent microorganisms), by determining ability to promote growth of rats or

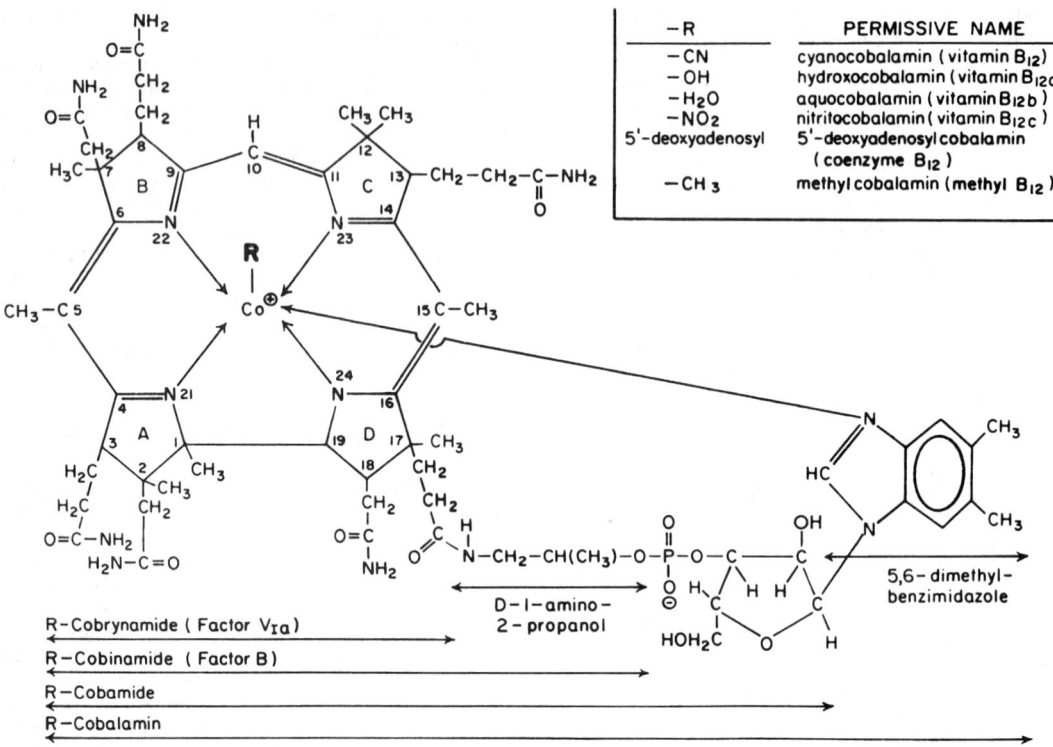

−R	PERMISSIVE NAME
−CN	cyanocobalamin (vitamin B₁₂)
−OH	hydroxocobalamin (vitamin B₁₂a)
−H₂O	aquocobalamin (vitamin B₁₂b)
−NO₂	nitritocobalamin (vitamin B₁₂c)
5′-deoxyadenosyl	5′-deoxyadenosyl cobalamin (coenzyme B₁₂)
−CH₃	methyl cobalamin (methyl B₁₂)

Figure 64-2. *Structural formula of vitamin B₁₂ (cyanocobalamin).*

The numbering system for the corrin nucleus is made to correspond to that of the porphin nucleus by omitting the number 20. The corrin nucleus is in the plane of the page. The **R** group is above it; the rest of the molecule is below it. (Modified from Brown and Reynolds, 1963. Courtesy of the *Annual Review of Biochemistry.*)

chicks, or clinically by administration to humans deficient in the vitamin. (For details, *see* reviews by Smith, 1965; Skeggs, 1967.)

Terminology. The nomenclature in the vitamin B_{12} field is indicated in Figure 64-2. The permissive (semisystematic; trivial) names are less cumbersome and more widely used than the systematic names. For example, the systematic name for vitamin B_{12} is α-(5,6-dimethylbenzimidazolyl) cobamide cyanide. The permissive term *cobalamin* (or B_{12}) is used to describe the vitamin B_{12} molecule minus the cyanide group, and is prefixed by the designation of the anionic R group (*see* Figure 64-2) attached to the cobalt (*i.e.*, 5′-deoxyadenosyl cobalamin or 5′-deoxy-adenosyl B_{12} to describe coenzyme B_{12}). *Cyanocobalamin* is a permissive (semisystematic) name for vitamin B_{12}, and the term *vitamin B_{12}* without qualification means cyanocobalamin exclusively. In practice, however, *the term vitamin B_{12} has two meanings.* To the strict organic chemist it means cyanocobalamin and nothing else. On the other hand, it has become entrenched in the pharmacological literature as a generic term for all the cobamides active in man. All the cobamides so far found to play a role in human metabolism have been cobalamins. The term

vitamin B_{12} is used in this chapter only when the context makes clear which sense is meant. When the context does not make the meaning clear, the proper term will be used (cyanocobalamin for the strict chemical meaning; cobalamin for the loose generic meaning).

There is an entire *family* of natural and semi-synthetic cobalamins, depending on the group that replaces CN (*see* review by Smith, 1965). Vitamin B_{12b} is aquocobalamin, H_2O replacing CN; vitamin B_{12a} (*hydroxocobalamin*) is the anhydrous form of B_{12b}. Both are converted to vitamin B_{12} by treatment with cyanide. Other cobalamins include *dicyanocobalamin, thiocyanatocobalamin, chlorocobalamin,* and *sulfitocobalamin.* These congeners, with the exception of hydroxocobalamin, are not generally available, have no presently known advantage over vitamin B_{12}, and are less stable than cyanocobalamin (Hutchins *et al.,* 1956; Pratt, 1972).

Sources in Nature. On a weight basis, vitamin B_{12} is the most potent of the known vitamins. The original and sole source of the compound in nature appears to be from synthesis by *microorganisms.* It is absent in plant products except as they are contaminated with microorganisms; occurrence in tissues of animals is accounted for by their diet or microbial synthesis in the alimentary tract. In man, synthesis of the vitamin occurs by bacteria in the large bowel, from which site it is not absorbed. The feces of animals and man usually contain large amounts of cyanocobalamin. Both normal persons and pernicious anemia patients in relapse excrete daily about 5 μg of vitamin B$_{12}$ in the feces.

The naturally occurring cobalamins in food are bound to protein and, prior to absorption, this bond must be split by heat or proteolysis.

Rich sources of cobalamin (more than 10 μg/100 g of wet weight) are organ meats, such as lamb and beef liver, kidney, and heart, and bivalves (clams, oysters), which siphon large quantities of vitamin B$_{12}$-synthesizing microorganisms from the sea; moderately high amounts (3 to 10 μg/100 g of wet weight) are present in nonfat dry milk, some seafoods (crabs, striped bass, salmon, sardines), and egg yolk; moderate amounts (1 to 3 μg/100 g of wet weight) are found in muscle meats, some seafoods (lobster, scallops, flounder, haddock, swordfish, tuna), and some cheeses (Camembert, Limburger). There is less than 1 μg/100 g of wet weight in fluid milk products and in cream, Cheddar, and cottage cheeses. One reason for the very slow development of vitamin B$_{12}$ deficiency in strict vegetarians who eat no animal protein of any type is the fact that they ingest legumes, in the nodules of which live microorganisms, such as those of the *Rhizobium* species, that synthesize coenzyme B$_{12}$.

In the United States, the daily cobalamin consumption may be as low as 1 μg or as high as 85 μg. The vitamin resists destruction by cooking.

Metabolic Functions. The cobalamins are involved in many metabolic systems in man (*see* Symposium, 1970, 1971). Cobalamins are essential for normal growth, hematopoiesis, production of all epithelial cells (including those of the gastrointestinal tract), and maintenance of myelin throughout the nervous system. Wherever nucleic acid synthesis occurs, and therefore wherever cells reproduce themselves, cobalamin is required. This requirement is probably proportional to the rapidity of cell proliferation.

Coenzyme B$_{12}$ is required for the hydrogen transfer and isomerization whereby *methylmalonate is converted to succinate,* thus involving cobalamin in both fat and carbohydrate metabolism. Since one pathway of propionic acid utilization in animal tissues involves its conversion by way of methylmalonate to succinate, it is possible that one reason for neurological damage in patients with vitamin B$_{12}$ deficiency is their inability to make the lipid portion of the lipoprotein myelin sheath. This possibility is indirectly supported by the work of Marston and associates (1961), who found that all the biochemical lesions of vitamin B$_{12}$ deficiency in sheep are correctable by folic acid save one, the lesion in propionate metabolism. Inability to form myelin may

relate in part to reduced ability to form the protein part of this lipoprotein. However, so far the only step in protein metabolism in a mammalian system proven to require cobalamin (the conversion of homocysteine to methionine) also requires folate. The concept that neurological damage in patients with cobalamin deficiency is due to blocked RNA synthesis is probably incorrect, since folate has been proven to be required for RNA synthesis and cobalamin has not.

Methylcobalamin is required for the *conversion of homocysteine to methionine* in mammals. In the absence of adequate quantities of cobalamin, folate may be trapped at the 5-methyl level, as indicated in Figure 64–1, resulting in a functional folate deficiency despite otherwise-adequate ingestion and absorption of folate. This "methylfolate trap" hypothesis may explain why all the signs and symptoms of folate deficiency may appear in patients with vitamin B$_{12}$ deficiency (Herbert, in Symposium, 1971). Vitamin B$_{12}$ is thus probably only indirectly involved in DNA synthesis in man (Metz *et al.,* 1968a).

Vitamin B$_{12}$ is concerned in the *maintenance of sulfhydryl groups in the reduced form* necessary for the function of many SH-activated enzyme systems. It may enhance methionine formation in part by diminishing the oxidation of the SH group of homocysteine, which is the methyl acceptor. It has also been suggested that vitamin B$_{12}$ may possibly influence fat metabolism by facilitating the reduction of the S—S form of coenzyme A to the active SH form. Vitamin B$_{12}$ deficiency is characterized by a decrease in reduced SH content (mainly glutathione, which is changed from GSH to GSSG) of erythrocytes and liver. This is correctable by administration of vitamin B$_{12}$. No such reduction is observed in iron or folic acid deficiency. Vitamin B$_{12}$ derivatives have been shown *in vitro* to catalyze the nonenzymatic oxidation of sulfhydryl derivatives. The biochemical "evidence" of ascorbate deficiency in patients with vitamin B$_{12}$ deficiency, despite the absence of clinical scurvy, is probably secondary to the oxidation of SH groups.

Vitamin B$_{12}$ is implicated in *protein synthesis* through its role in the synthesis of the amino acid methionine, and possibly in other ways as well. Since methionine is involved in making available more of the lipotropic substances, choline and betaine, this is another point where cobalamin may play a role in lipid metabolism.

Current Concept of Pathogenesis and Nature of Pernicious Anemia. Classical addisonian pernicious anemia, as understood at present, is a *conditioned vitamin B$_{12}$-deficiency disease* of man caused by idiopathic lack of a specific substance secreted by the normal gastric mucosa. This substance, a glycoprotein, is called the *gastric intrinsic factor of Castle* and is essential for the absorption from the ileum of a dietary (*extrinsic*) factor now known to be vitamin B$_{12}$, a minute amount (less than 1 μg daily) of which is required. (For further details on the mechanism of vitamin B_{12} absorption, *see* below.)

Symptoms of Deficiency. The symptoms of cobalamin deficiency are those of ineffective hematopoiesis, inadequate myelin synthesis, inadequate maintenance of the epithelial cells of the alimentary tract, and generalized debility. As discussed subsequently, these phenomena, except for inadequate myelin synthesis, are common to all megaloblastic anemias regardless of cause. (*See* reviews by Herbert, 1959, 1975.)

Inadequate myelin synthesis is peculiar to vitamin B_{12} deficiency states and results in a wide range of neurological symptoms and signs. Paresthesia, especially numbness and tingling in the hands and feet, is the most frequent neurological symptom. Early frequent signs are diminution of vibration sense and/or position sense (usually occurring first in the ankles and feet), unsteadiness, poor muscular coordination with ataxia, moodiness, mental slowness, poor memory, confusion, agitation, depression, and central scotomata. Delusions, hallucinations, and even overt psychosis may occur. The wide variety of sensory and motor changes tend to be symmetrical, especially if present for a period of weeks or months.

Terms used to describe the nervous system damage due to vitamin B_{12} deficiency included *subacute combined degeneration, combined system disease, posterolateral sclerosis,* and *funicular degeneration.* However, the disease usually starts *insidiously* and not subacutely, combined lesions are often *absent,* and lesions of the peripheral nerves occur much more frequently and much earlier than lesions of the central nervous system. For these reasons, the nervous system changes are more accurately described by direct reference to the actual involvement (*i.e.,* peripheral nerve, or spinal cord, or cerebral damage due to vitamin B_{12} deficiency).

Clinically, there is no relation between the degree of severity of the neurological damage and the degree of severity of the hematological damage, probably because of the highly variable folate intake of different individuals. Patients with high folate intake will have little hematological damage; those with low folate intake will have much hematological damage. This is well illustrated among vegans, who avoid all kinds of animal food and thus get very little vitamin B_{12}, but who have an unusually high folate intake from vegetables and salads.

Human Requirement. In an adult, the minimal daily requirement for crystalline vitamin B_{12} is in the range of 0.1 μg, the quantity of cyanocobalamin or coenzyme B_{12} that will produce a minimal hematological response in a patient with uncomplicated vitamin B_{12} deficiency (Sullivan and Herbert,

1965; Herbert, 1968b). In an individual with normal vitamin B_{12} stores, the daily output of the vitamin, mainly in the bile, is from 3 to 7 μg, of which all but approximately 1 μg is reabsorbed. A 0.6- to 1.2-μg daily quantity orally will sustain modest body stores of vitamin B_{12} in normal adults (Heyssel *et al.,* 1966). (Patients who lack intrinsic factor secretion may require more than normal individuals, since they are unable to reabsorb vitamin B_{12} secreted into the intestinal tract.) To allow for about 60 to 80% absorption from food, the recommended daily dietary intake is 2 μg for adults, 0.3 μg for infants, and 2.5 to 3 μg during pregnancy and lactation (FAO/WHO Expert Group, 1970).

Absorption. Cyanocobalamin is quantitatively and rapidly absorbed from intramuscular and subcutaneous sites of injection; the plasma level of the compound reaches its peak within 1 hour after intramuscular injection. Hydroxocobalamin and coenzyme B_{12} are less rapidly absorbed after parenteral administration, presumably because of their greater affinity for binding to various proteins.

Absorption from the Gastrointestinal Tract. (*See* Symposium, 1962, 1970. *See also* reviews by Herbert, 1968a, 1972; Glass, 1974.) There are two separate and distinct mechanisms for the absorption of cobalamins. The more important of these is *mediated by the gastric intrinsic factor of Castle* and is saturated by 1.5 to 3 μg of B_{12}; interference with this mechanism produces the overwhelming majority of the megaloblastic anemias due to vitamin B_{12} deficiency seen in the United States. The other mechanism of vitamin B_{12} absorption, possibly diffusion, is *independent of intrinsic factor,* and accounts for significant absorption only in the presence of quantities of vitamin B_{12} much greater than those made available from the usual diet. The two mechanisms for vitamin B_{12} absorption overlap to a variable degree in normal man, depending on daily dietary vitamin B_{12} intake and the quantity of the vitamin released from its bound form in the food.

The physiological mechanism for vitamin B_{12} absorption *mediated by intrinsic factor* is unique in that vitamin B_{12} is the only nutrient of man known to require a specific secretion of the gastric mucosa to facilitate its absorption. Vitamin B$_{12}$ in the diet is liberated in the stomach and small intestine from the proteins to which it is bound. The process of splitting vitamin B$_{12}$ from its peptide bonds is facilitated by gastric acid and also by various enzymes secreted into the alimentary tract. The free vitamin B$_{12}$ then attaches to intrinsic factor secreted by gastric parietal cells. The vitamin B$_{12}$–intrinsic factor complex is carried down to the ileum, where it binds to receptors on the ileal surface. The attachment requires calcium (for which magnesium may partially substitute) and a pH above approximately 6 (Carmel *et al.*, 1969). After a delay of several hours at and within the ileal mucosa, the vitamin is transported in the blood stream to the liver and other organs.

Intrinsic factor is a glycoprotein with a molecular weight in the range of 50,000. In man, it is formed in the parietal cells of the stomach. The two most important properties of intrinsic factor are its non-unique ability to bind vitamin B$_{12}$ (a property shared by many proteins, polypeptides, and polysaccharides) and its unique ability to enhance the absorption of vitamin B$_{12}$ from the ileum. (*See* reviews by Gräsbeck, 1969; Allen and Mehlman, 1973; Glass, 1974.)

Intrinsic factor concentrate is a preparation from hog stomach that is active in man in a daily oral dose of 50 mg. It is used in Schilling tests in the differential diagnosis of states of B$_{12}$ malabsorption, as a standard in determining the potency of intrinsic factor concentrates, and as a binder of B$_{12}$ in radioisotopic assay of that vitamin.

The intestinal absorption of cobalamins other than cyanocobalamin is also dependent on intrinsic factor and is equal to or less than that of cyanocobalamin. After intestinal absorption (or parenteral administration), smaller quantities of hydroxocobalamin or coenzyme B$_{12}$ appear in the urine than are found after identical doses of cyanocobalamin because of the greater binding of the former two agents to plasma and tissue protein.

Although the quantity of vitamin B$_{12}$ contained in the daily American diet may vary from as little as 1 μg to as much as 85 μg, the amount of vitamin B$_{12}$ freed from its protein binding in food and made available for absorption will vary with the food, with gastric secretion of acid, and with other factors in the stomach and small intestine. Patients with pernicious anemia, who almost always lack free acid, are probably less able to release vitamin B$_{12}$ from its bound form in food than are normal subjects and, therefore, are less able to make available for absorption by the diffusion mechanism vitamin B$_{12}$ present in diets high in this vitamin.

Patients with pernicious anemia seem to absorb less of a given ingested quantity of cobalamin in food than they do of free cyanocobalamin (Herbert and Sullivan, 1964; Doscherholmen and Swaim, 1973). On the other hand, normal persons given radioactive B$_{12}$ bound in meat or liver absorb almost 100% of quantities up to 3 μg, but absorb very little of the excess over 3 μg. Similar studies indicate that patients with pernicious anemia absorb only about 0.68 μg of vitamin B$_{12}$ from 38 μg ingested as liver, whereas normal *old* people absorb about 1.7 μg (Bozian *et al.*, 1964).

If one measures the intestinal absorption of vitamin B$_{12}$ by the test devised by Schilling (1953), by determining the urinary output of radioactive vitamin B$_{12}$ in patients with pernicious anemia after ingestion of a 2-μg dose, and compares this with the quantity in the urine after ingestion of a 30-μg dose, one finds that the quantity of vitamin excreted after the smaller dose may be markedly enhanced by simultaneous administration of intrinsic factor, whereas the quantity excreted after the larger dose is not significantly affected by intrinsic factor (*see* Herbert *et al.*, 1964). Thus, it is possible that individuals ingesting daily as much as 30 μg of *free* cyanocobalamin (but not cobalamin bound in food) do not need intrinsic factor secretion in order to sustain normality. This statement should not be misinterpreted to mean that daily ingestion of 30 μg of free cyanocobalamin is adequate treatment of patients with pernicious anemia, since such patients frequently have disturbances other than lack of intrinsic factor secretion, such as diarrhea or other intestinal dysfunction, contributing to malabsorption of vitamin B$_{12}$.

Distribution, Storage, Transport, Fate, and Excretion. (*See* Symposium, 1962, 1970, 1971; *see also* review by Gräsbeck, 1969.) Absorbed vitamin B$_{12}$ is transported in the blood stream to the liver and other organs. The liver contains amounts varying from 50 to 90% of the normal adult's total body stores of the vitamin; these stores range from 1 to 10 mg in normal adults. There is no evidence for significant catabolism of vitamin B$_{12}$ in man, and it is probable that loss occurs only by excretion, mainly in the bile. Injected cyanocobalamin or hydroxocobalamin is converted in the liver to coenzyme forms, and thus enters the common storage pool (Rosenblum *et al.*, 1963), mainly coenzyme B$_{12}$ (Stahlberg, 1967). The total body turnover rate of vitamin B$_{12}$ is about 0.05 to 0.2% daily, regardless of pool size; the total daily quantity turned over may be as high as 8 μg in subjects with good body stores and as low as 0.4 μg when body stores are depleted to the point where megaloblastosis is imminent (Heyssel *et al.*, 1966; Reizenstein *et al.*, 1966; Adams and Boddy, 1968).

Since the daily adult requirement of the vitamin is less than 1 μg, and since hematopoietic or neurological evidence of vitamin B$_{12}$ deficiency does not appear until the liver stores are reduced below about 0.1 mg and the plasma level of the vitamin is below about 100 pg/ml, it can be understood why years may pass before a clinical relapse occurs when treatment is stopped, and why it takes 3 to 6 years for vitamin B_{12} deficiency to develop after gastric intrinsic factor secretion ceases.

Not all of the liver stores of vitamin B_{12} are available for blood formation. Patients with pernicious anemia sometimes have a "spontaneous remission" if they develop hepatitis; probably the small amount of residual vitamin B_{12} is released into the blood stream. The liver normally hoards vitamin B_{12} for its own metabolic processes.

Transport. (*See* Herbert, 1968c; Simons, 1968; Gräsbeck, 1969; Hall and Finkler, 1971.) Absorbed vitamin B_{12} binds mainly to a specific B_{12}-binding β-globulin (transcobalamin II) and to a lesser extent to a specific B_{12}-binding α_1-glycoprotein (transcobalamin I) and to an inter-α-glycoprotein (transcobalamin III); both transcobalamins I and III are granulocyte related and together constitute about 10% of the circulating unsaturated vitamin B_{12}-binding capacity (Scott *et al.*, 1974). The B_{12} bound to transcobalamin II is almost instantly delivered to liver, bone marrow, and other tissues. Thus, B_{12} is not normally found associated with transcobalamin II in human serum. The vitamin B_{12} bound to transcobalamin I continues to circulate as a reserve store. Transcobalamin II may be considered as primarily a transport protein, and transcobalamin I as primarily a storage protein for vitamin B_{12} (Retief *et al.*, 1967), which may not be required for normal B_{12} metabolism (Carmel and Herbert, 1969).

The vitamin B_{12} concentration and the vitamin B_{12}-binding capacity of plasma vary markedly in different physiological conditions and disease states (Figure 64–3; compare with Figure 63–1, page 1312). The plasma transcobalamins I and III reflect the size of the body granulocyte pool and are elevated in myeloproliferative disorders and reduced with leukopenia. Peak plasma concentrations of vitamin B_{12} are reached approximately 8 to 12 hours after ingestion of the vitamin in physiological amounts (less than 3 μg of free vitamin), reflecting delay of absorption in the ileum. The mean normal plasma concentration of vitamin B_{12} is 450 pg/ml; the normal range is 200 to 900 pg. Almost all of this vitamin B_{12} is bound to plasma protein; a small fraction (1 to 10%) may be free or very loosely bound.

Excretion in Bile. Approximately 3 to 8 μg of vitamin B_{12} is secreted into the alimentary tract daily, mainly in the bile. Of this, all but approximately 1 μg is reabsorbed by means of the intrinsic factor mechanism. The fact that it takes only about 3 to 6 years for the totally gastrectomized individual to develop vitamin B_{12} deficiency, despite a daily requirement of less than 1 μg and normal body stores of 2 to 5 mg, strongly suggests that a major role in the development of such deficiency is failure adequately to reduce the daily biliary excretion of vitamin B_{12} and thus conserve body stores.

The strict vegetarian, who has both normal intrinsic factor secretion and a normal ileum, maintains an active *enterohepatic circulation of vitamin B_{12}* and thereby economizes his small body store and develops overt deficiency very slowly. On the other hand, the patient who lacks intrinsic factor or has ileal dysfunction cannot reabsorb the vitamin B_{12} excreted in his bile and develops deficiency much more rapidly.

Excretion in Urine. The normal daily urinary excretion of vitamin B_{12} is in the range of 0 to 0.25 μg. Only the small amount of vitamin B_{12} not attached to plasma protein in normal subjects is available for urinary excretion. When the amount of intravenously or intramuscularly administered vitamin B_{12} exceeds the binding capacity of plasma, liver, and other tissues, it is eliminated by glomerular filtration, the clearance approximating that of inulin. Eighty to 95% of an initial injected dose up to 50 μg of vitamin B_{12} is retained, but with doses over this amount the percentage retained falls rapidly at a different rate for each patient.

Vitamin B_{12} crosses the *placenta* from mother to fetus. At birth, the blood level of vitamin in the newborn is three to five times that in the mother.

Preparations, Routes of Administration, and Dosage. A variety of injectable and oral preparations are available for the treatment of pernicious anemia and other vitamin B_{12} deficiency states. *The preparation of choice is vitamin B_{12}, given by intramuscular or deep subcutaneous injection.* Oral preparations are much more expensive and cannot always be depended upon to induce remissions in desperately ill patients, to arrest progression of neurological lesions, or to maintain patients in remission.

Cyanocobalamin Injection, U.S.P. (RUBRAMIN), is a preparation obtained from liver or especially from the growth of suitable microorganisms (bacteria and actinomycetes). The vitamin occurs as a dark-red, crystalline, hygroscopic powder, soluble 1:80 in water. It is very stable at room temperature in sterile physiological saline solution and can be autoclaved for 15 minutes at 121° C. It is marketed in isotonic saline solution in 1-, 5-, 10-, and 30-ml vials, for intramuscular injection; each milliliter contains 30, 50, 60, 100, or 1000 μg of cyanocobalamin. The preparation causes little local discomfort at the site

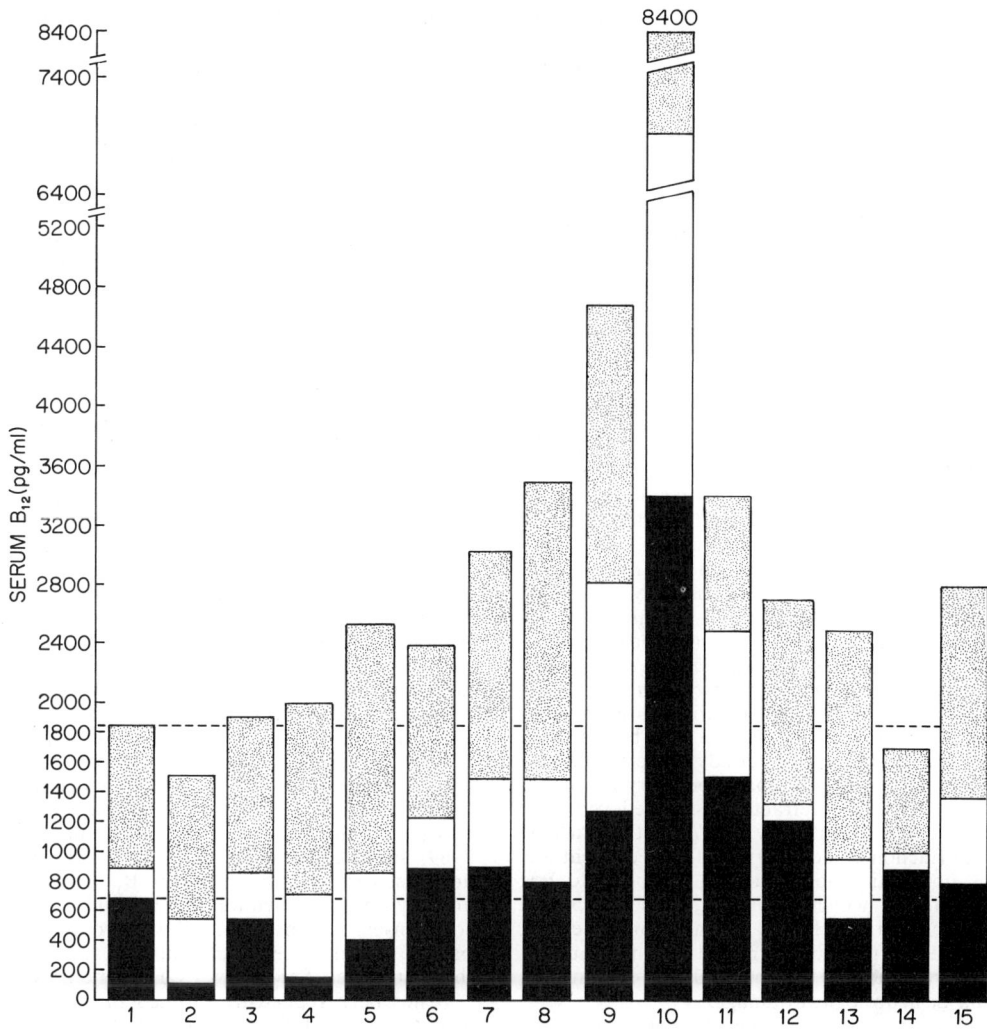

Figure 64-3. *Serum vitamin B$_{12}$ level and total vitamin B$_{12}$-binding capacity in various disturbances of vitamin B$_{12}$ metabolism.*

The lower horizontal dash line represents the mean concentration of vitamin B$_{12}$ in 15 normal human sera; this vitamin B$_{12}$ is nearly all bound to transcobalamin I. The upper horizontal dash line represents the normal level of total vitamin B$_{12}$-binding capacity of the same 15 normal human sera.

The bottom (black) bars represent sera vitamin B$_{12}$ levels. The middle (white) bars represent unsaturated transcobalamin I; the height of the middle bar plus that of the lower bar represents total transcobalamin I (except in hepatic disease, when some B$_{12}$ is bound to the β-globulin). The upper stippled bars represent transcobalamins II and III, which, except in hepatic disease, are generally all but devoid of vitamin B$_{12}$.

The stippled bars would be reduced approximately one third in height if the blood were collected in 47 mM NaF solution, which prevents the *in-vitro* release of granulocyte-related transcobalamin III (Scott *et al.,* 1974).

The values in each column represent averages obtained from the following 15 groups of subjects (parenthetical numbers refer to the numbers below the columns): (*1*) 15 normal healthy adults; (*2*) 20 patients with untreated pernicious anemia; (*3*) 15 patients with treated pernicious anemia; (*4*) 9 untreated patients with B$_{12}$ deficiency not due to pernicious anemia; (*5*) 11 women in the third trimester of pregnancy; (*6*) 24 patients with hepatic cirrhosis; (*7*) 31 patients with polycythemia vera; (*8*) 5 patients with "spent" polycythemia vera; (*9*) 8 patients with myeloid metaplasia; (*10*) 20 patients with chronic myeloid leukemia; (*11*) 8 patients with acute myelogenous leukemia; (*12*) 7 patients with chronic leukopenia for periods in excess of 3 months; (*13*) 4 patients with chronic leukocytosis; (*14*) 3 patients with Di Guglielmo syndrome, all of whom had leukopenia; (*15*) 6 patients with uremia. (After Herbert, 1968c. Courtesy of *Blood.*)

of injection and does not evoke hypersensitivity reactions.

Vitamin B_{12} with Intrinsic Factor Concentrate. This preparation, no longer official, is marketed for oral use, in capsules and tablets. It is a mixture prepared from vitamin B_{12} and dried stomach, pylorus, or duodenum of hogs or other domestic animals used for food by man. The mixture is assayed for hematopoietic activity in pernicious anemia patients, and its potency is expressed in terms of the *oral unit* of activity. Each tablet or capsule usually contains 0.5 oral unit. The amount constituting 1 oral unit contains vitamin B_{12} activity equivalent to not more than 15 μg of cyanocobalamin and not more than 300 mg (dry basis) of the preparation constituting the intrinsic factor concentrate. However, the amount of cyanocobalamin present is not stated on the label, in order to avoid the misleading implication that there is activity in excess of the stated unitage. The preparation is quite expensive, and adequate dosage may cost the patient many times the cost of intramuscular vitamin B_{12} therapy. Stability appears adequate. The possibility of allergic reactions to hog protein should be kept in mind. *The sole valid use of oral vitamin B_{12} with intrinsic factor concentrate is in patients whose primary lesion is lack of secretion of adequate intrinsic factor and who refuse parenteral therapy.* The reason for this is that approximately half the patients who have been treated with such preparations for periods in excess of a year develop refractoriness. Preparations vary in this respect. The reason for refractoriness is believed to be the production of antibody *locally* in the intestine to some fraction of hog intrinsic factor concentrate. It has no relation to circulating antibody to hog intrinsic factor, which, if present, is to *human* and not to hog intrinsic factor (Ramsey and Herbert, 1965). Patients must be examined at a minimum of once every 3 months for any evidence of returning anemia or neurological damage.

Liver injection is a sterile, aqueous parenteral preparation of the soluble thermostable fraction of mammalian livers that contains vitamin B_{12}. Its potency is determined by microbiological assay. *Liver injection* is marketed in 1- and 10-ml vials and contains either 10 or 20 μg/ml of cyanocobalamin activity. *Cyanocobalamin Injection,* U.S.P., is preferred.

Oral liver-extract preparations containing the vitamin B_{12} fraction of mammalian livers are no longer official. They are expensive and difficult for many patients to ingest; their absorption is made uncertain by vomiting or diarrhea, and they cannot be depended upon to supply sufficient vitamin B_{12} to prevent or arrest neurological alteration or rapidly to restore the blood values to normal or to keep them at optimal levels. Such preparations should not be employed.

Oral Cyanocobalamin. Oral treatment with cyanocobalamin alone will allow absorption of approximately 1% of the administered dose by diffusion. Such therapy is expensive and especially uncertain in patients who have vitamin B_{12} deficiency due to sprue or other forms of intestinal malabsorption. The use of large daily doses (100 to 1000 μg) of oral cyanocobalamin should be considered only in patients who refuse parenteral therapy. It may not replenish body stores.

Other Forms of Vitamin B_{12}. Cyanocobalamin is the vitamin B_{12} preparation of choice for oral or intramuscular administration. *Hydroxocobalamin* and *coenzyme B_{12}* have no proven therapeutic advantage over cyanocobalamin when administered orally. Administered parenterally, they produce more sustained elevations of plasma vitamin B_{12} levels than does cyanocobalamin. However, at convenient intervals for parenteral maintenance therapy, such as 1 month, the plasma vitamin B_{12} levels achieved after administration of these agents will have fallen to the same levels as after cyanocobalamin. Furthermore, hydroxocobalamin may give rise to antibody to plasma B_{12}-binding protein in some patients (Skouby *et al.,* 1971). *Hydroxocobalamin,* N.F. (ALPHAREDISOL), is available as a 1-mg/ml injection in 1- and 10-ml vials.

Other Oral Therapies with Vitamin B_{12} and Added Agents. From time to time, it is claimed that vitamin B_{12} combined with another agent is an effective *oral therapy* for pernicious anemia. Such "improved oral therapies" depend for their effect primarily on their content of vitamin B_{12}, and offer no significant advantage over oral treatment with vitamin B_{12} alone. A large number of oral agents may enhance absorption of vitamin B_{12} *by normal individuals,* by stimulating intrinsic factor secretion; however, only intrinsic factor enhances the absorption of vitamin B_{12} in the patient who lacks this factor. ACTH, steroids, vitamin B_{12} itself, folic acid, antibiotics, pancreatic extract, trypsin, and calcium in some cases may improve intestinal absorption of vitamin B_{12} in patients with the malabsorption syndrome (Herbert, 1969; Bernstein and Herbert, 1973). The medical advertisements of oral vitamin B_{12} combinations adroitly omit any mention that the "miraculous absorption-enhancement factor" works only when the patient does not need treatment with vitamin B_{12} in the first place. (*See* review by Herbert, 1959.)

It has been repeatedly claimed that *vitamin B_{12} peptides,* isolated from fermentation of a *Streptomyces* mutant or a propionibacterium, are more readily absorbed from the intestine than is cyanocobalamin. Such claims are not supported by controlled studies, have been refuted by many investigators, and should be regarded as completely invalid.

Depot Preparations of Cyanocobalamin. The usual maintenance treatment of patients with pernicious anemia is with monthly injections of 30 to 1000 μg of cyanocobalamin. However, much of the larger doses is lost in the urine. For these reasons, plus the convenience of injections at intervals greater than a month, several depot preparations have been under study. However, further studies are needed to define whether the relative benefit derived from them warrants their use. Such preparations have also been reported to give rise to antibody to plasma B_{12}-binding protein (Skouby *et al.,* 1971).

"Shotgun" Antianemia Preparations. In spite of the relatively low incidence of pernicious anemia, the number of commercial preparations for the therapy of this disease increases yearly. Many physicians use these agents indiscriminately in any patient with anemia, regardless of the etiology; this practice is not only expensive, but actually may harm the patient, as it often obscures the real nature of the disease. For example, a favorable response to cyanocobalamin in a patient with megaloblastic anemia secondary to gastric carcinoma may obscure and delay the correct diagnosis, and the use of this drug in the treatment of an inadequately diagnosed peripheral neuritis may obscure an underlying pernicious anemia. Employment of mixtures of hematopoietic substances multiplies manyfold the possibility of such errors. Numerous antianemia preparations contain a mixture of liver, stomach, folic acid, iron, copper, cobalt, vitamin B$_{12}$, various other vitamins, and even hormones.

Strauss (1936) has succinctly stated the reasons for not using such mixtures, as follows:

. . . "Shotgun" therapy is to be deplored for a number of reasons. Most mixtures of substances fail to contain enough of any one ingredient to give maximal effects. The patient must pay not only for the material he needs but also for nonessentials. Mixed therapy may so cloud the clinical picture that accurate evaluation of subsequent therapeutic needs becomes impossible. Most patients with addisonian pernicious anemia require life-long treatment whereas the majority of patients with anemia due to iron deficiency, once well, will remain well unless the original cause is re-established. Therefore, if a patient, not definitely known to have pernicious anemia, receives both liver and iron and recovers, no conclusion can be drawn as to which was the effective substance. If both should now be stopped, the patient, should he have pernicious anemia, will sooner or later relapse. In addition *he runs the risk that his relapse may be essentially neurological and may advance to the stage of irreparable spinal cord injury before the nature of the condition is recognized.* On the other hand, if the anemia is of the iron deficiency type and therapy with both liver and iron is continued, the patient is subjected to the expense and inconvenience of taking an unnecessary liver preparation. [Italics added.]

Routes of Administration. As discussed above, the preferred route for administration of cyanocobalamin is the *deep subcutaneous* or the *intramuscular,* with a 25-gauge needle. Such injection of cyanocobalamin is almost devoid of pain. The only recommended use of *oral* maintenance therapy is in the management of strict vegetarians who refuse to eat any animal matter. Such persons respond to 1 μg of cyanocobalamin orally daily.

Dosage. The dose of cyanocobalamin in pernicious anemia depends on the product employed, the route of administration, the severity of the anemia, the presence of complicating factors such as infection and neurological lesions, and the response to therapy. A satisfactory clinical and hematological remission can be obtained in a patient with uncomplicated pernicious anemia or other form of vitamin B$_{12}$-deficiency disease by the daily parenteral administration of 1 μg of cyanocobalamin for 10 days. This is the proper dose to use in *therapeutic trials,* since

it will produce hematological responses only in patients with vitamin B$_{12}$ deficiency, whereas doses in excess of 10 μg daily may produce hematological responses in patients with folate deficiency (*see* review by Herbert, 1963). The purpose of the therapeutic trial is to provide simultaneous *differential diagnosis* and *therapy.* The principles of therapeutic trial were laid down in a classical paper by Minot and Castle (1935). These include a *control period* of a few days to establish the constancy of the reticulocyte level, *elimination of dietary sources of vitamin B$_{12}$ and folic acid,* and a dose of the test material just sufficient to produce a distinct reticulocyte reaction; if a maximally effective amount of active material is given, the bone marrow will not be able to respond further to more potent material.

A therapeutic trial with the proper parenteral dose of cyanocobalamin (1 μg daily) in a patient with pernicious anemia is shown in Figure 64–4. Note especially the following features in the figure: Reticulocytosis occasionally is present in untreated patients with vitamin B$_{12}$ deficiency when they are first seen (but it is not usual); the dyspnea and occasional angina in untreated patients with severe megaloblastic anemia (hematocrit below 15 volumes %) may be immediately relieved by transfusion with 1 unit of packed red cells; 1 μg daily of cyanocobalamin produces an excellent hematological response in the uncomplicated case, accompanied by a gradual rise in the plasma vitamin B$_{12}$ levels, a sharp fall in the plasma iron levels (as iron is utilized in effective hematopoiesis), and a gradual fall in the plasma folate level to normal (if it has been elevated due to vitamin B$_{12}$ deficiency, as often is the case). Not shown in the figure is the leukopenia or thrombocytopenia often seen in patients with untreated megaloblastic anemia; granulocytes and platelets return to normal levels within 1 week after the start of therapy, at approximately the time the reticulocytes reach their peak level.

Initial therapy with doses of cyanocobalamin larger than 1 μg daily is desirable when the vitamin B$_{12}$ deficiency state is complicated by other debilitating illness such as infection, hepatic disease, uremia, coma, severe disorientation, or marked neurological damage. The dose should be 30 μg of vitamin B$_{12}$ daily by *intramuscular* or *deep subcutaneous* injection for 5 to 10 days. Excellent hematopoietic response will follow such therapy, except in cases in which hematopoiesis is suppressed by infection, uremia, chloramphenicol administration, or some other factor. Daily parenteral doses larger than 30 μg have no proven therapeutic advantage. It is possible that the use of such doses may result in slightly more rapid replenishment of body stores, but much of the excess cyanocobalamin is excreted in the urine. *Neural damage* can be completely arrested, and considerable improvement can occur if therapy is instituted early and maintained persistently. Unless the mean corpuscular volume returns to normal, the patient is not fully protected from further damage to the nervous system. The erythrocyte count should be kept above 4.5 million per cubic millimeter and normal hematological morphology should be maintained. Only close and frequent examination of the patient's blood and physical signs can be relied upon to show whether medication is adequate.

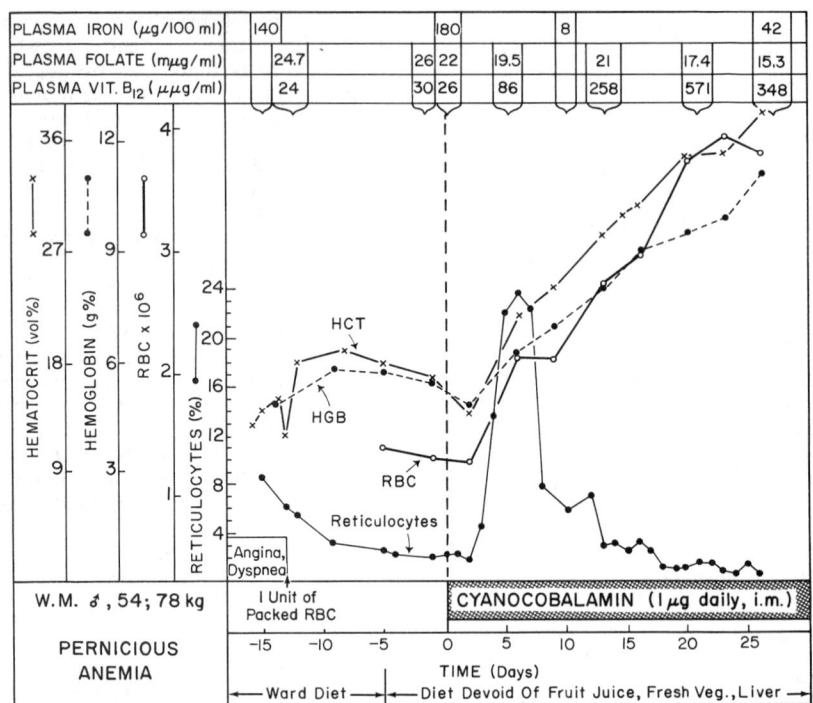

Figure 64-4. *Response of pernicious anemia patient to daily intramuscular injection of 1 μg of cyanocobalamin.*

The parenteral dosage employed constitutes a therapeutic trial of vitamin B$_{12}$ in pernicious anemia. It is not necessarily an optimal dose in complicated cases. (After Herbert, 1963. Courtesy of the *New England Journal of Medicine*.)

There is no evidence that initial therapy with parenteral amounts of cyanocobalamin greater than 30 μg daily for 5 to 10 days followed by maintenance with more than 100 μg monthly is associated with either more rapid arrest of neurological damage or more rapid improvement of such damage. However, the *belief* that larger doses have greater value is entrenched in the literature with almost the force of *fact*, and for this reason larger doses are almost invariably used when patients have neurological complications. A convenient dosage schedule for such patients is 10 to 15 days of 250 μg of cyanocobalamin daily followed by 250 μg once or twice weekly for several months. The dose is kept at 250 μg, but the interval between doses is then gradually increased until, after a period in excess of 1 year, when it appears that no more neurological recovery is likely to occur, the injection is given once monthly. Inasmuch as parenteral cyanocobalamin is relatively inexpensive, and since undertreatment may prolong the time for recovery and undesirable effects have not been reported from overtreatment, one may safely err on the side of overdosage. Persistent treatment with large doses of cyanocobalamin may be required in patients with vitamin B$_{12}$ deficiency who seem refractory to conventional therapy, due to associated infection, myxedema, chronic arthritis, uremia, acromegaly, or some other debilitating illness.

If the patient fails to respond even to parenteral doses as large as 1000 μg daily for 10 days, one is justified in questioning the potency of the material or the correctness of the diagnosis.

To sustain *complete* hematological normality, maintenance therapy should be with a minimum of 100 μg of cyanocobalamin monthly. At this dosage, the plasma vitamin B$_{12}$ level remains normal for a month. Since the patient feels neither malaise prior to each monthly injection nor a perceptible increase in well-being immediately after each injection, it is *imperative that the physician make clear the necessity for continued monthly maintenance therapy,* to avoid the all-too-frequent failure of such patients to continue maintenance therapy, with subsequent insidious development of irreversible neurological damage over a period of several years of vitamin B$_{12}$ deprivation. Maintenance therapy must be given monthly. Because of the limited retention of cyanocobalamin even if one gives as much as 1000 μg in each injection, hematological normality will be sustained for only a little over a month. A single injection of 1000 μg of cyanocobalamin every 12 weeks is inadequate therapy.

Toxic Reactions. Injections of crystalline cyanocobalamin are painless and usually cause no untoward local reactions. Rarely, there may be allergic reactions to impurities in preparations of crystalline cyanocobalamin and hydroxocobalamin. Parenteral injections of *liver extract* can cause mild-to-severe allergic reactions. Local effects resemble a type of Arthus phenomenon without necrosis. General effects include flushing, headache, chill, fever, dyspnea, itching, urticaria, and shock. Patients hypersensitive to liver extract tolerate cyanocobalamin.

THERAPEUTIC USES

The only established clinical use of cyanocobalamin is in the treatment of vitamin B$_{12}$ deficiency. Claims have been made for the value of cyanocobalamin in the therapy of a variety of miscellaneous conditions, including infectious hepatitis, multiple sclerosis, trigeminal neuralgia, poor appetite, miscellaneous neuropathies, poor growth, various psychiatric disorders, aging, thyrotoxicosis, sterility, and various forms of malnutrition. There is no evidence that any of these claims has any validity. The clinical uses of the vitamin are reviewed by Herbert (1959, 1963, 1973a) and Chanarin (1969).

Therapy of the Critically Ill Patient. It is rarely necessary to institute immediate therapy prior to determining the cause of a megaloblastic anemia. The major indications for emergency therapy include severe thrombocytopenia (platelet count less than 50,000 per cubic millimeter) associated with bleeding, severe leukopenia (white-cell count less than 3000 per cubic millimeter) associated with infection, infection itself, coma, severe disorientation, marked neurological damage, severe hepatic disease, uremia, or other debilitating illness complicating the anemia. The anemia itself is not a problem since the dyspnea and occasional angina that may accompany a hematocrit of less than 15 volumes % are relieved by a transfusion of 1 or 2 units of packed red cells. Transfusion is unwarranted in the absence of symptoms of anemia. When venous pressure is elevated, transfusion of packed red cells should be accompanied by withdrawal of an equivalent quantity of whole blood (Duke *et al.,* 1964).

When immediate vitamin therapy is necessary before etiological diagnosis, for one or more of the reasons discussed above, both 100 μg of cyanocobalamin and 15 mg of folic acid are given intramuscularly, followed by 5 mg of folic acid by mouth and 100 μg of vitamin B$_{12}$ intramuscularly daily, for a week.

Pernicious Anemia. Patients with *uncomplicated* addisonian pernicious anemia to whom adequate

doses of cyanocobalamin are given are objectively and subjectively improved within a few days. A sense of well-being often appears within a day. Gastrointestinal disturbances are relieved, and the inflamed, atrophic lingual mucosa returns to normal. Symptoms caused by the anemia are alleviated as the blood values become normal. Strength, mental outlook, and appetite all improve, and within several weeks the patient is symptomatically cured. However, gastric mucosal atrophy and histamine-refractory achlorhydria persist and the ability of the stomach to elaborate intrinsic factor of Castle is not restored. Hence the conditioned deficiency that causes pernicious anemia is not cured, and *therapy must continue for life. This fact must be explained to the patient.*

Individuals with *nervous system involvement* require a longer time for improvement, but progression of the lesions can be immediately arrested. Degree of improvement of neurological defects depends more on their duration than on their severity. The greatest improvement occurs if walking has been impaired for less than 3 months, and little improvement occurs if walking has been affected for more than 2 years. Involvement of the lateral columns of the spinal cord responds more slowly than does that of the posterior columns; consequently, spasticity, exaggerated reflexes, positive Babinski sign, and other reflexes may appear for the first time as posterior-column functions improve; such an event should not be mistaken for a progression of the neural lesions. Cerebral complications may disappear over a period of several months.

The *hematopoietic response* is the earliest and the most dramatic phase of the *recovery from vitamin B$_{12}$ deficiency* and is a good measure of the patient's progress. Serial *bone-marrow* aspirations indicate that, within a few hours after the intramuscular injection of cyanocobalamin, the maturation arrest ceases and the megaloblasts start to develop into reticulated mature cells. Within 48 to 72 hours, normoblastic hematopoiesis is fully restored and the misshapen neutrophilic leukocytes and the abnormal megakaryocytes decrease in number. Thus, as improvement continues, the characteristic macrocytic anemia, leukopenia, and thrombocytopenia disappear. *Reticulocytes* can be observed in the peripheral blood within 2 to 5 days after therapy is started and usually reach their peak about the fifth to twelfth day. The shape and the height of the reticulocyte curve depend on the dose of cyanocobalamin, the route of administration, and, especially, the severity of the anemia. By approximately the time the reticulocytes reach their peak, the *leukocytes* and *platelets* will have returned to normal levels. Frequently, there is a *"platelet overshoot,"* with platelet levels exceeding normal for up to 7 or 10 days before receding to normal. Less frequently, there is a similar *"leukocyte overshoot."* Characteristically, the plasma iron level is elevated in the untreated patient and falls abruptly within 1 to 2 days after the start of therapy.

The reticulocyte peak value is reciprocal to the initial level of erythrocytes; a peak of 50 to 70% is not uncommon after parenteral therapy in patients with initial erythrocyte counts below 1 million per cubic millimeter. Soon after the reticulocyte curve rises, the erythrocytes start to increase rapidly in number and then taper off; values of 4.5 to 5.0 million per cubic millimeter are usually reached in 4 to 8 weeks. In severe cases, the red blood cells increase about 0.5 million per cubic millimeter per week. Because the hemoglobin value is reduced to a lesser extent, it rises more slowly than the erythrocyte count; as a result, the mean corpuscular hemoglobin decreases toward normal. The mean corpuscular volume also decreases, reaching normal in 1 to 3 months. The hypersegmentation of the polymorphonuclear leukocytes gradually disappears over a period of 1 to 2 months. Reticulocyte counts usually recede to preinjection values by the end of the third week, and the blood values are usually normal by the end of the second month. The main features of the hematological response to appropriate therapy in a severe case of pernicious anemia are illustrated in Figure 64–4. If hematological recovery does not follow the initial response pattern outlined above, then either the diagnosis is wrong or complications (such as iron deficiency, renal disease, or neoplasm) suppressing hematopoiesis are present.

In addition to cyanocobalamin therapy, the diet should be adequate in all respects. Iron or folic acid should be prescribed only if overt deficiency appears. If achlorhydria causes gastrointestinal symptoms, 2 to 8 ml of *Diluted Hydrochloric Acid*, U.S.P., may be given in half a glass of water with each meal. Transfusion of blood is required only as an emergency measure in critically anemic patients (*see* Figure 64–4). If the initial hematocrit value is below 15 volumes %, a single transfusion, preferably of packed red cells, is advisable. It is rarely necessary to give more than one such transfusion; in fact, it may be dangerous so to do. The patient with pernicious anemia is usually elderly, has developed the anemia very slowly, and is usually compensated to it. Too rapid a rise in his blood volume may result in circulatory overload (Duke *et al.*, 1964). Potassium supplementation is sometimes given with therapy for megaloblastic anemia, to compensate for the potassium shift accompanying new blood-cell formation.

The most frequent complications of pernicious anemia are infections, especially of the genitourinary tract, and a variable degree of congestive heart failure. The incidence of carcinoma of the stomach in patients with pernicious anemia is approximately threefold higher than occurs in the general population. At yearly intervals, the patient should be examined for this complication.

Vitamin B$_{12}$ Deficiency Other Than Pernicious Anemia. (*See* Herbert, 1959, 1973a, 1975; Sullivan, in Seminar, 1970.) *Dietary deficiency* of vitamin B$_{12}$ occurs in strict vegetarians and in their breast-fed infants (Jadhav *et al.*, 1963). *Malabsorption* of vitamin B$_{12}$ may result from any structural or functional damage to the stomach, where intrinsic factor is secreted, or to the ileum, where intrinsic factor functions to facilitate vitamin B$_{12}$ absorption.

Inadequate secretion of intrinsic factor may occur not only in addisonian pernicious anemia but also as a result of *lesions that destroy the gastric mucosa* (such as the *ingestion of corrosives, linitis plastica of* *nonneoplastic origin,* and *extensive neoplasia* involving the gastric mucosa) and a number of conditions that may be associated with a variable degree of *gastric atrophy* (such as *certain endocrine disorders, iron deficiency, multiple sclerosis,* and *subtotal gastrectomy*) (*see* review by Glass, 1974). *Total gastrectomy* in man always produces vitamin B$_{12}$ deficiency since it completely removes the only source of intrinsic factor.

States of ileal dysfunction include *specific malabsorption of vitamin B$_{12}$*, a rare entity, usually congenital and possibly occasionally acquired. Intrinsic factor secretion is normal, but an unknown defect in the ileum does not allow vitamin B$_{12}$ to be absorbed. A number of conditions that produce *structural* damage to the small intestine *above the ileum* may result in reduced vitamin B$_{12}$ absorption from the ileum, possibly due in part to *functional damage* in the ileum. These conditions include *tropical sprue, nontropical sprue (idiopathic steatorrhea, gluten-induced enteropathy)*, and a variety of structural lesions. Folate deficiency in these patients is usually more severe than vitamin B$_{12}$ deficiency since folate is absorbed from the upper small intestine. These conditions are discussed further, in the section dealing with the uses of folic acid. Lesions leading to vitamin B$_{12}$ deficiency by producing structural derangement in the ileum include *regional ileitis, ileal resection, malignancies, granulomas, strictures,* and *anastomoses involving the ileum.* Since the intrinsic factor mechanism is not operative at low pH, vitamin B$_{12}$ absorption may be low in patients with *pancreatic disease,* which reduces intestinal pH, and may be enhanced by giving sodium bicarbonate; vitamin B$_{12}$ absorption may also be enhanced in such patients by feeding pancreatin (Bernstein and Herbert, 1973; Toskes *et al.*, 1973).

Competition for Vitamin B$_{12}$ by Intestinal Parasites or Bacteria. The *fish tapeworm (Diphyllobothrium latum)* absorbs huge quantities of vitamin B$_{12}$; more than 50% of worm carriers in Finland had low plasma vitamin B$_{12}$ levels, and at least 1 in 50 had overt anemia due to vitamin B$_{12}$ deficiency (Nyberg *et al.*, 1961). *The blind-loop syndrome,* in which an abnormal bacterial flora proliferates in surgically created blind loops, in strictures or anastomoses, or in small-bowel diverticuli, may produce deficiency of vitamin B$_{12}$ or folate, depending in part on the affinity for adsorption and absorption of these two vitamins by the proliferating organism, and in part on the functional or structural derangement in the ileum.

Inadequate utilization of vitamin B$_{12}$ may occur in infants with an inherited *lack of methylmalonyl coenzyme A isomerase* or *defective enzymatic conversion of vitamin B$_{12}$* to one of its coenzyme forms. These infants suffer from vomiting, ketoacidosis, lethargy, failure to grow, and mental retardation. Some respond to large doses of vitamin B$_{12}$ (Barness and Morrow, 1968; Mahoney and Rosenberg, in Symposium, 1970).

Megaloblastic anemia in association with pregnancy or the puerperium, infancy, alcoholism, and *poverty* is usually due primarily to folate deficiency, although associated or even primary vitamin B$_{12}$ deficiency may occur. These conditions are discussed further in the section on the uses of folic acid.

FOLIC ACID
(PTEROYLGLUTAMIC ACID)

Chemistry. Folic acid (pteroylglutamic acid, PGA) has the following structural formula:

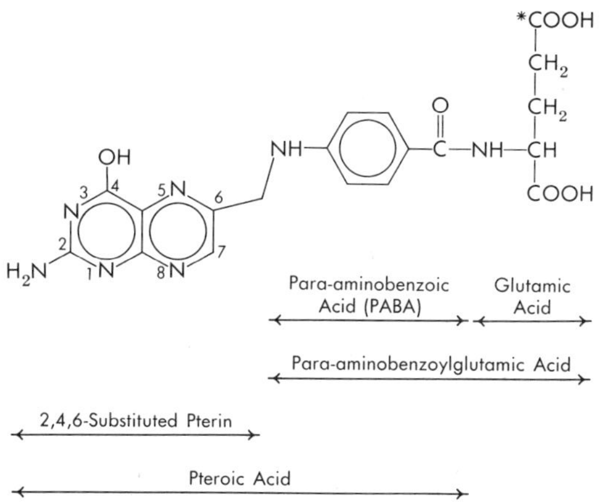

* Site of conjugation of extra glutamate residue(s) of pteroyl di-, tri-, or heptaglutamate.

Folic Acid (Pteroylglutamic Acid)

The major portions of the molecule are a pteridine moiety linked by a methylene bridge to para-aminobenzoic acid, which, in turn, is joined through an amide linkage to glutamic acid.

A variety of synthetic analogs of folic acid act as antivitamins; antagonists to folate (antifols) have found therapeutic application in the treatment of neoplastic disease (*see* Chapter 62).

Terminology. The nomenclature of various folate derivatives is indicated in Figure 64–5. The tentative rules of the International Union of Pure and Applied Chemistry (IUPAC) (1966) state that pteroylglutamic acids may be designated *generically* as *folic acid* and that the pure substance hitherto known as folic acid, folacine, or vitamin B$_c$ shall be named *pteroylglutamic acid.* However, through long usage the term *folic acid* continues to be employed not only generically but also as a synonym for pteroylglutamic acid. This discussion will use the term *folic acid* only when the context makes clear which sense is meant. When the context does not make the meaning clear, the term *folate* will be employed for the generic meaning (as done by WHO Scientific Group, 1968; FAO/WHO Expert Group, 1970). The term *pteroylglutamic acid* will be used when that acid is concerned. *Folinic acid* (*citrovorum factor, leucovorin*) is the term used to designate 5-formyl tetrahydrofolic acid.

Assay. Folate activity can be assayed chemically and microbiologically (*see* Herbert and Bertino, 1967), and also by radioassay (*see* Herbert, in monograph by Surgenor, 1974).

Sources in Nature. Folates are ubiquitous in nature, occurring in nearly all foods. Foodstuffs with the highest folate content per unit of dry weight include yeast, liver, and fresh green vegetables. Some fruits are also relatively high in folate content. From 50 to 95% of the folate content of foods may be destroyed by protracted cooking or by canning. This is a major reason why folate deficiency in man is common (Herbert, 1973b). The quantity of total folate in a "normal" American diet may vary from 50 to 2000 μg daily. The percentage of the total amount of ingested food folate absorbed by man varies, depending on its nature. Folates occur in nature primarily in the form of conjugates, in which more than one molecule of glutamic acid is incorporated in the structure. The product obtained from yeast contains a total of seven glutamic acid molecules and is designated as pteroylheptaglutamic acid. Enzymes present in vegetable and mammalian tissues liberate pteroyldiglutamates and pteroylmonoglutamates from the conjugates to make the folate available for absorption. About 90% of monoglutamate but only about 50% of pure heptaglutamate is absorbed. There is no convincing evidence that pteroylglutamic acid *as such* is found in any natural source; its isolation from natural sources in the past has been due to oxidation and hydrolysis of the naturally occurring reduced conjugated forms (*see* Tamura and Stokstad, 1973).

Metabolic Functions. Pteroylglutamic acid is not active as such in the mammalian organism. Rather, pteroylglutamic acid is enzymatically reduced in the body to tetrahydrofolic acid (THFA), the coenzyme form that acts as an acceptor of various one-carbon units. As indicated in Figure 64–5, THFA is capable of carrying a one-carbon unit as an adduct (designated as R in the figure) on either the 5 or the 10 position, or bridged between the 5 and the 10 positions to form a five-membered ring.

The various other folate coenzymes formed as one-carbon adducts with THFA and the metabolic reactions in which they are involved are indicated in Figures 64–5 and 64–1. The latter also indicates the interrelations of vitamin B$_{12}$ and folate metabolism, and where vitamin B$_6$ is involved. Folate coenzymes participate in a large number of metabolic reactions in which there is a transfer of a one-carbon unit. These reactions include (*see* Figure 64–1): (1) *de-novo* purine synthesis (by the formylation of glycinamide ribonucleotide [GAR] and 5-amino-4-imidazole carboxamide ribonucleotide [AICAR]); (2) pyrimidine nucleotide biosynthesis (by the methylation of deoxyuridylic acid to thymidylic acid); (3) three amino acid conversions—(a) the interconversion of serine and glycine (also requires vitamin B$_6$),

	R	OXIDATION STATE
N^5 formyl THFA	—CHO	formate
N^{10} formyl THFA	—CHO	formate
N^5 formimino THFA	—CH=NH	formate
$N^{5,10}$ methenyl THFA	≫CH	formate
$N^{5,10}$ methylene THFA	>CH$_2$	formaldehyde
N^5 methyl THFA	—CH$_3$	methanol

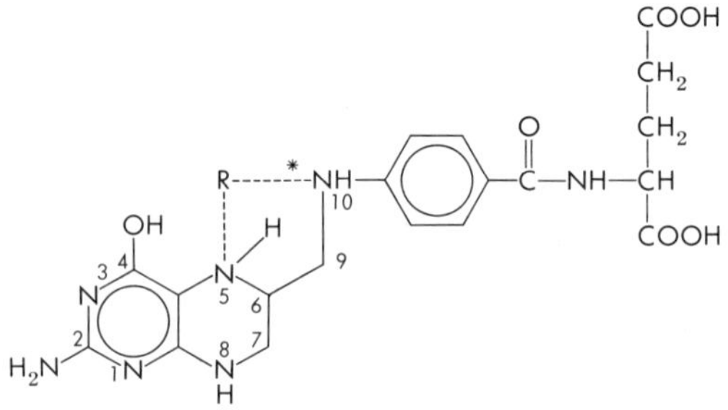

* Broken lines indicate the N^5 and/or N^{10} site of attachment of various
one-carbon units for which THFA acts as a carrier.

5,6,7,8-Tetrahydrofolic Acid (THFA; FH$_4$)(R = —H)

Figure 64–5. *Structures and nomenclature of folate derivatives.*

The table above the formula lists some of the possible one-carbon adducts formed with THFA. It is unknown whether the folates in the human are primarily monoglutamates or polyglutamates.

(b) the catabolism of histidine to glutamic acid, (c) the conversion of homocysteine to methionine (also requires vitamin B_{12}); and (4) the generation of formate into the so-called formate pool, and the utilization of formate therefrom.

The interrelations of folate and vitamin B_{12} are discussed earlier in this chapter.

Symptoms of Deficiency. The most striking feature of folate deficiency is megaloblastic hematopoiesis indistinguishable from that due to vitamin B_{12} deficiency. Glossitis is common, as with vitamin B_{12} deficiency, and diarrhea and weight loss are usually prominent features of the syndrome. In experimental nutritional folate deficiency in man, at the time that megaloblastic anemia has just appeared, there is neither morphological nor functional damage to the gastrointestinal tract; this may suggest that the enteric epithelial cells either retain the tiny amount of food folate in the deficient diet or have a greater avidity for folate (or a lower folate requirement) than do hematopoietic cells.

The pathological state produced by administration of folate antagonists may not be analogous to pure nutritional folate deficiency, since the antagonists produce intracytoplasmic inclusion bodies in the mucosa of the small bowel, observed after various noxious influences but not seen in nutritional folate deficiency (Trier, 1962). However, since folate is required for nucleic acid synthesis, it is evident that sufficiently protracted folate deficiency would produce morphological and functional damage in the small intestine, as well as in every other organ and tissue in which nucleic acid is synthesized.

The most striking clinical difference from vitamin B_{12}–deficiency states is that, with folate deficiency, the neurological signs of damage to myelin do not appear. It is an interesting fact that, unlike vitamin B_{12}, which is selectively *excluded* from spinal fluid, folate is selectively *concentrated* therein (Herbert, 1968d). However, symptoms such as irritability, sleeplessness, and forgetfulness do appear during folate deficiency; such symptoms may be related to disordered cerebral metabolism. It is unlikely that dietary folate deficiency can produce brain damage, except possibly in the newborn (Herbert and Tisman, 1973). Use of antifols during gestation can give rise to deformed offspring.

Human Requirement. The human requirement for folate (*as pteroylglutamic acid*) is approximately 50 μg daily in adults (*see* review by Herbert, 1968b). With allowance for less than 100% absorption, the recommended daily dietary intake is 200 μg of "free" folate (defined as folate available to the microorganism *L. casei* without hydrolysis of conjugates) for adults, 50 μg for infants, 100 μg for children, 400 μg during pregnancy, and 300 μg during lactation (FAO/WHO Expert Group, 1970). The daily folate requirement is hinged to the daily metabolic and cell-division rates. Infection increases metabolic rate and therefore increases folate requirement, and increased cell multiplication (*e.g.,* hyperplastic bone marrow in hemolytic anemias and rapid tissue growth in the fetus and malignant tumors) augments the folate needs. Folate turnover by individual cells is proportional to their rate of one-carbon-unit transfer. The reason why one of the earliest signs of folate deficiency is damage to the hematopoietic system is that the bone marrow normally has one of the most rapid rates of cell division in the body.

Absorption. Folate, in the monoglutamate form, is absorbed rapidly, primarily from the proximal small intestine, although it is capable of being absorbed from the entire length of the small intestine. This absorption may be an active, energy-dependent process for small ("physiological") quantities of the vitamin, but it is probably by diffusion for large quantities.

Pteroylglutamic acid in doses up to 15 mg is almost totally absorbed from the gastrointestinal tract; the percentage absorption of the total folate present in liver and spinach, which contain enzymes that hydrolyze folate conjugates, is high. Absorption of the folate polyglutamates present in most foods is limited by the need for deconjugation prior to absorption, and the presence of inhibitors of deconjugation in some foods, such as yeast. Because of the limited absorption of food folate, only about 5 to 40 μg of free folate activity appears daily in the urine of normal individuals ingesting an average diet. Much of food folate is so poorly absorbed by patients with tropical sprue that up to 1500 μg of it given by mouth will often not produce a hematological response. On the other hand, the absorption of pteroylglutamic acid is so complete, even in the presence of the otherwise-generalized malabsorption of tropical sprue, that some such patients (when they do not also have vitamin B_{12} deficiency) may have hematological responses to only 25 μg orally daily.

Transport, Distribution, Storage, Fate, and Excretion. (*See* Herbert, 1973a, 1973b.) Pteroylglutamic acid appears in the blood plasma within $\frac{1}{2}$ hour after ingestion and is very rapidly converted to various metabolically active folate forms. It is not clear whether there is a discrete transport protein for folate. Approximately two thirds of radioactive folic acid added to normal plasma is bound and unavailable for renal filtration.

When 1 μg of tritium-labeled folic acid per kilogram of body weight is injected intravenously into a normal man, 60% is removed in one circulation time and 90 to 95% is removed in 3 minutes, suggesting that there is a high tissue affinity for "physiological" quantities of folic acid (*i.e.,* quantities such as would be absorbed from an average diet). The folate is distributed to all tissues in the body. There is probably a specific cell-membrane transport process for folic acid (and folinic acid). The very high intracellular concentration of folic acid points to an accumulative process with a high affinity and capacity. Less than 2% of the radioactivity is excreted in the urine in 3 hours, and the later excretion is less than 0.5% an hour (Johns *et al.,* 1961).

When the dose of radioactive folate injected intravenously is 15 μg/kg of body weight, a quantity greater than would be absorbed from an average diet, the fall in plasma concentration is considerably slower. Six hours after injection of such doses, the plasma level finally falls to a level similar to that found after physiological doses. Urinary excretion of radioactivity after injection of the larger dose is also much greater; 20 to 30% of the injected radioactivity is recovered in the urine at the end of 2 hours, but only 5 to 10% more is excreted in the following 24 hours, and less than 2% per day thereafter. After injection of 150 μg/kg of body weight, 60% of the radioactivity appears in the urine within 12 hours (Johns *et al.,* 1961).

Although it is often assumed that folate is enzymatically degraded in man to some extent, there is no convincing evidence for this (*see* review by Jukes and Broquist, 1963). Because the nonenzymatic oxidative deconjugation of reduced folate to pteridine and para-aminobenzoylglutamic acid occurs *in vitro,* the degraded folate found in normal human urine probably results from a reaction *in situ* (*see* below).

In man, at plasma concentrations above 10 μg per liter, urinary folate clearance is independent of the plasma levels and approximates 50 ml per minute. There appears to be renal tubular reabsorption of folic acid by a carrier-mediated mechanism. The maximal tubular reabsorption rate is relatively low, being less than 50 ng per minute.

Only a small amount of folate appears in the urine after ingestion of 0.1 mg of folic acid, but approximately half is excreted when a 5-mg quantity is ingested and up to 90% may be excreted after the ingestion of 15 mg. Most of the folate appears in the urine within 6 hours, and excretion is complete within 24 hours. It is probable that larger quantities may be excreted than stated above, because labile folates in the urine are not protected against oxidative destruction. When such destruction is prevented, it is found that normal subjects eating an average diet may excrete from 1 to 10 μg of folate daily (*see* review by Metz, 1963). The folate activity in the urine may occasionally be as much as tenfold greater if oxidative destruction is prevented by addition of ascorbic acid.

The normal *total body folate stores* are in the range of 5 to 10 mg. The liver contains about half of this total, probably mainly as 5-methyl tetrahydrofolate, which seems also to be the main form of folate normally circulating in human plasma (*see* Chanarin *et al.*, 1966; Herbert, 1968d). As already stated, folate is selectively *concentrated* in the spinal fluid.

Preparations. *Folic Acid,* U.S.P. (FOLVITE), occurs as a yellow or yellowish-orange crystalline powder. It is almost insoluble in water, but with acid and alkali it forms salts that have limited aqueous solubility. Official preparations are *Folic Acid Tablets,* U.S.P., which contain 0.1, 0.4, 5, 10, or 20 mg of the vitamin, and *Folic Acid Injection,* U.S.P., an aqueous solution of the sodium salt of folic acid, marketed in 1-, 2-, and 10-ml ampuls containing 5 mg/ml. There are numerous proprietary preparations in which folic acid is a component of multivitamin mixtures or combined with iron and other substances designed to stimulate hematopoiesis. The danger in the use of such mixtures is described below.

In many patients, much more folic acid is given than is necessary. For therapeutic trials, the physician is advised to add 1 ml (5 mg) of the official *folic acid injection* to 49 ml of *Water for Injection,* U.S.P., to give a solution containing 100 μg/ml of folic acid; 1 ml can be given daily, orally or parenterally.

Folinic acid (*citrovorum factor, leucovorin*) is marketed in 1-ml ampuls containing 3 mg of the vitamin as a racemic mixture. It is used as an antidote to the toxic effect of therapy with antifols (*see* Chapter 62).

Routes of Administration. The oral route of administration of pteroylglutamic acid is preferred unless malabsorption is suspected, in which case the subcutaneous or intramuscular route should be used.

Dosage. The dose of *pteroylglutamic acid* in folate deficiency depends on the severity of the anemia, the presence of complicating factors that may either suppress hematopoiesis or increase the folate requirement, and, in patients with malabsorption, the route of administration. A satisfactory clinical and hematological remission can be obtained in a patient with uncomplicated folate deficiency by the daily oral administration of 0.1 mg for 10 days. This is the proper dose to use in therapeutic trials, since it will produce hematological responses only in patients with folate deficiency, whereas doses in excess of 0.2 mg daily may produce hematological responses in patients with vitamin B_{12} deficiency (*see* review by Herbert, 1963). A therapeutic trial with a parenteral dose of 50 μg of pteroylglutamic acid daily in a patient with folate deficiency and scurvy is shown in Figure 64-6.

Certain features in Figure 64-6 are especially noteworthy. Reticulocytosis is often present in untreated patients with folate deficiency when they are first seen; vitamin C *per se* has no hematopoietic effect in the presence of folate deficiency of severe degree; 50 μg of pteroylglutamic acid daily produces an excellent hematological response in uncomplicated folate deficiency, but the dose is too small to produce a sharp rise in the plasma folate concentration. The expected sharp fall in plasma iron concentration did not occur because ascorbate therapy produced a rise in this value and presumably prevented the early fall that would have been expected in this case. The figure also illustrates that there is often leukopenia in patients with untreated megaloblastic anemia, be it due to deficiency of vitamin B_{12} or folate; frequently there is also thrombocytopenia. These formed elements return to normal levels within 1 week after the start of therapy, at approximately the time of the reticulocyte peak.

Initial therapy with doses of pteroylglutamic acid larger than 0.1 mg daily is desirable when the folate-deficiency state is complicated by conditions that may suppress hematopoiesis (infection, uremia, tumor, chloramphenicol or alcohol administration, and active inflammatory lesions such as rheumatoid arthritis, ulcerative colitis, or hepatitis), or conditions that increase folate requirements (pregnancy, hypermetabolic states, and increased hematopoiesis such as occurs with hemolytic anemia or protracted blood loss). Therapy should then be with doses of 0.5 to 1.0 mg daily, by intramuscular or subcutaneous injection if malabsorption exists. There is no evidence that doses greater than 1 mg daily have any greater efficacy; additionally, loss of folate in the urine becomes roughly logarithmic as the amount administered exceeds 1 mg. *Maintenance therapy* is normally 0.1 mg daily for 1 to 4 months, and then should be stopped only if the diet contains at least one fresh fruit or fresh vegetable daily. If the daily folate requirement is increased due to an increased metabolic or cell-division rate, the maintenance dose should be 0.2 to 0.5 mg daily.

Toxicity. Folic acid is nontoxic in man. Renal toxicity occurs in rats given massive doses, due to precipitation of crystalline folic acid in the tubules and blockade of urine flow. Daily doses of 15 mg in man are without toxic effects; this huge daily dose is well below that which could lead to precipitation of crystalline folic acid in the kidneys. Folic acid has been claimed partially to reverse the antiepileptic effects of phenobarbital, pheny-toin, and primidone, and thereby increase seizure frequency (Reynolds, 1968), but not all workers agree that this can occur (Herbert and Tisman, 1973).

THERAPEUTIC USES

The sole established therapeutic use of pteroylglutamic acid is in the treatment of folate deficiency. Unfortunately, folic acid has been incorporated in "shotgun" anti-anemia mixtures. If preparations containing folic acid are used indiscriminately for the treatment of anemia, without a careful differ-ential diagnosis, the patient with iron-deficiency anemia is being subjected to needless expense whereas the patient with pernicious anemia, despite a hematological

remission, may develop irreparable neuro-logical lesions before the true nature of his disease is recognized. Folic acid is also a component of many multivitamin mixtures. Although folic acid–deficiency syndromes are common, those at risk of developing such syndromes (the pregnant, the poor, alcohol-ics, persons with hemolytic anemia or small-bowel disease) are rarely prophylactically better off by self-medication with multivita-mins than by taking their folate as daily fresh fruit, fruit juice, or vegetables, or by pre-scription of appropriate amounts of folic acid (*see* below), after measurement of serum and red-cell folate concentrations to confirm fo-late status. The use of folic acid in the ther-apy of the *critically ill patient* is discussed on page 1337. The clinical uses of the vitamin

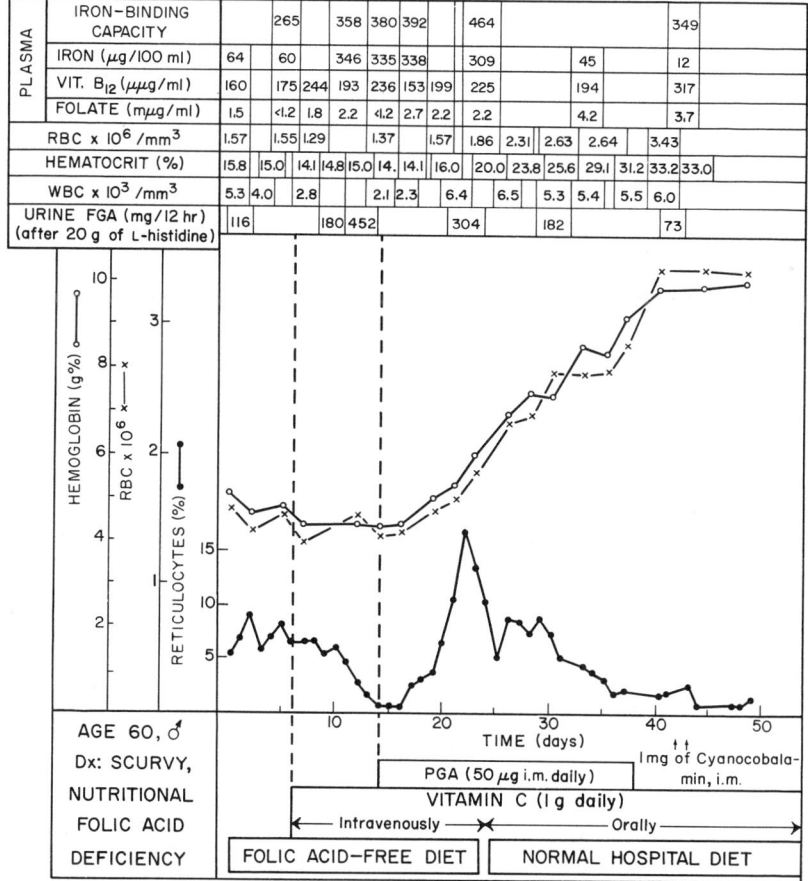

Figure 64–6. *Response to intramuscular injection of 50 µg of folic (pteroylglutamic) acid daily, in a patient with nutritional folate deficiency and scurvy. See* text *for details. (After Herbert, 1963, as modified from Zalusky and Herbert. Courtesy of the* New England Journal of Medicine.)

have been reviewed by Herbert (1959, 1962a, 1962b), Sullivan (1967), Chanarin (1969), and Streiff (in Seminar, 1970).

Nutritional Megaloblastic Anemia (Nutritional Macrocytic Anemia). Nutritional megaloblastic anemia is the hematological manifestation of *inadequate dietary intake* of folate or vitamin B_{12}. The term includes all those megaloblastic anemias resulting from inadequate ingestion with or without superimposed malabsorption of folate and vitamin B_{12}. Frequently, especially in the tropics, the diet is marginal or grossly deficient, and this deficiency is aggravated by the increased demand for folate due to *pregnancy,* the rapid growth in *infancy, malignancy, hemolytic anemia, infection,* or *parasitic infestation.* If the diet is grossly inadequate in both vitamin B_{12} and folate, the patient suffers from a relatively greater deficiency of the latter because body folate stores last only a little over a month whereas body vitamin B_{12} stores last for several years. Nutritional folate deficiency is common, in large measure because food folate is highly susceptible to oxidative destruction by cooking.

Dosage for therapy is described above. Many patients exhibit a multiple deficiency; clinical evidence of associated pellagra, riboflavin deficiency, beriberi, or scurvy is frequent. Not only does folic acid correct the abnormal blood picture, but also improvement in appetite, gain in weight and strength, and disappearance of glossitis and diarrhea are often dramatic. In malnourished young adults, there may be a striking increase in height.

Megaloblastic Anemia in Association with Alcoholism and Liver Disease. (*See* Herbert, 1965; Straus, 1973.) Most alcoholics, with or without overt cirrhosis, have folate deficiency because of their nutritionally inadequate diets. Additionally, alcohol directly suppresses hematopoiesis, in part by blocking folate metabolism. The block may be overcome by doses of folic acid greater than 0.1 mg. Treatment is by withdrawing alcohol and providing a nutritionally balanced diet. Daily oral administration of 0.1 mg may be advisable, especially if the patient returns to alcohol.

Severe hepatic damage, of any cause, may sufficiently reduce the level of enzymes involved in folate metabolism so that therapy with folic acid may have no effect. In such instances, it is possible that therapy with folinic acid may be successful if the deficient enzyme is dihydrofolate reductase. Patients with liver disease, often with alcoholism, occasionally have megaloblastic anemia despite normal or elevated plasma levels of vitamin B_{12} and folate. This anemia may be associated with increased urinary excretion of aminoimidazolecarboxamide, indicating a derangement in purine synthesis similar to that with deficiency of vitamin B_{12} or folate. The cause of this anemia is unknown, but it may be related to temporary inability to utilize vitamin B_{12} or folate. In some of these patients the plasma vitamin B_{12} or folate may be bound to an abnormal protein incapable of delivering the vitamin to sites of utilization.

Treatment consists in an adequate diet and avoidance of alcohol.

Megaloblastic Anemia in Infancy. Megaloblastic anemia in infancy or childhood nearly always is associated with generalized malnutrition, and occurs more readily in infants with infections or diarrhea. The deficiency may be primarily of vitamin B_{12}, especially among the infants of vegetarian parents, but more usually it is of folate, especially when the infant has been on a diet exclusively of boiled milk, goat milk, or gruel (Ford and Scott, 1968). (*Adults* on diets consisting exclusively of milk may also develop folate-deficiency megaloblastic anemia.) Therapy is the same as for nutritional megaloblastic anemia in the adult. Combined deficiency of folate and vitamin B_{12} is common in infants and young children with *protein-calorie malnutrition;* treatment is with a nutritionally adequate diet.

Megaloblastic Anemia in Pregnancy. The requirement of the growing fetus for folate is large, especially in the last trimester of pregnancy and in twin pregnancies. Plasma folate gradually falls during pregnancy. At birth, the plasma folate level of the newborn averages fivefold that of the mother, supporting the concept of parasitization of mother by fetus. Thus, although associated or even occasional primary vitamin B_{12} deficiency may occur, the major cause of megaloblastic anemia in pregnancy is usually deficiency of folate, and therapy with folic acid is usually effective.

Megaloblastic anemia is more frequently seen in multiparous women. Most cases first found during the *puerperium* probably represent cases undiscovered during pregnancy or delivery. In some patients, anemia may have been precipitated by substantial blood loss during or after delivery (resulting in rapid hematopoiesis with an increased folate requirement), by infection, or by the demands of *lactation.* Breast milk has priority over the hematopoietic system for folate (Metz *et al.,* 1968b). *Treatment* should be with 0.5 to 1.0 mg daily, because of the increased folate requirement. An excellent hematopoietic response can be expected. A low plasma vitamin B_{12} level frequently rises without vitamin B_{12} therapy when the patient with megaloblastic anemia of pregnancy is treated with folic acid. Also there is a rapid rise in leukocytes and platelets concomitant with the rise in reticulocytes.

It is not known whether food folate absorption is reduced in pregnancy or if some other factor interferes with folate metabolism. If carefully sought, the incidence of megaloblastic erythropoiesis in pregnant women may be as high as 25% in the third trimester, with a low plasma folate in 50%, and a low erythrocyte folate in 10%, even in temperate zones. For this reason, prophylactic administration of oral folic acid, 0.2 to 0.4 mg daily, throughout pregnancy, is recommended by the Committee on Maternal Nutrition (1970) (*see also* Cooper, 1973).

Megaloblastic Anemia in Association with Anticonvulsant, Antimalarial, and Antibacterial Therapy. Moderate folate deficiency is frequent in association with *anticonvulsant therapy.* It usually is manifested only by a reduced plasma folate level (Herbert and Tisman, 1973), but occasionally overt megaloblastic anemia appears. Certain anticonvulsants probably act as very weak antifols and produce megaloblastic anemia only in patients whose folate stores are already sharply reduced. Whether anticonvulsants block food folate absorption is uncertain. When megaloblastic anemia does occur, it may be corrected either by withdrawing the anticonvulsant or by continuing it and administering 0.1 mg of folic acid orally each day. *Pyrimethamine* will produce megaloblastosis in a high proportion of persons given 25 mg daily for about 2 months (instead of the usual prophylactic dosage of 25 mg weekly). The drug inhibits the enzyme dihydrofolate reductase. Treatment is by cessation of pyrimethamine administration or administration of folinic acid (Stebbins *et al.*, 1973).

Trimethoprim, a weak antifol for man, is used with sulfamethoxazole in antibacterial therapy. It may accentuate a borderline folate or vitamin B_{12} deficiency, producing overt megaloblastosis, and should be used with caution in such subjects (Herbert, 1973b). Folinic acid will restore hematological normality even if trimethoprim therapy is continued.

The diuretic agent *triamterene* is a weak antifol and, therefore, should be used with caution in pregnant woman and alcoholics, who may have borderline folate stores (Corcino *et al.*, 1970).

Megaloblastic Anemia in Association with Rheumatoid Arthritis or Extensive Skin Disease. In Great Britain, patients with rheumatoid arthritis or extensive skin disease may have frank megaloblastic anemia, subnormal plasma folate levels, or excessive excretion of formiminoglutamate in the urine, probably due to a combination of low folate intake and enhanced tissue demand for folate (Gough *et al.*, 1964). The average British diet is lower in folate than is the average American diet, partly because the British often destroy more folate by prolonged cooking. This may be a reason that overt folate deficiency seems to appear more easily in Englishmen than in Americans when stressed by rheumatoid arthritis (or by anticonvulsants, pregnancy, etc.). Factors involved in the possible increased need for folate in patients with rheumatoid arthritis are the use of analgesics or steroids, which may, respectively, increase the metabolic rate or stimulate erythropoiesis; the use of salicylates, which may produce chronic gastrointestinal tract bleeding with consequent increase in need for folate for new blood formation; and the proliferation of the synovial membranes in the diseased joints. *Therapy* is with 0.1 to 0.2 mg of folic acid daily, by mouth. Since there may be an increased incidence of addisonian pernicious anemia in association with rheumatoid arthritis, the possibility of associated vitamin B_{12} deficiency must always be considered.

Malabsorption Syndromes. Varying degrees of reduced absorption of food folate and vitamin B_{12} may occur with any structural or functional disorder of the small intestine. If the disorder is chronic and involves primarily the upper small intestine, folate deficiency is nearly always present, often with an associated vitamin B_{12} deficiency. If the major dysfunction is in the lower small intestine, primary vitamin B_{12} deficiency will occur, sometimes with associated folate deficiency. (*See* review by Herbert, 1968a; Symposium, 1968, 1970; Floch, 1969; Jeffries *et al.*, 1969; Wellcome Trust, 1971.)

Folate deficiency is almost invariably present in *tropical sprue, nontropical sprue (idiopathic steatorrhea),* and *celiac disease;* in these conditions there is usually atrophy of jejunal villi with resulting loss of absorptive surface area. Other vitamin and mineral deficiencies are often present as well as weight loss and osteoporosis from the multiple absorptive defects. Treatment with 0.1 to 1.0 mg of folic acid daily, orally or by injection, is strikingly effective in *tropical sprue,* not only often converting the hematological picture to normal but also often causing subsidence of the anorexia, diarrhea, steatorrhea, soreness of the mouth, atrophy of the lingual papillae, and loss of weight. Impaired intestinal absorption is often dramatically improved. Vitamin B_{12} deficiency is also frequently present, and absorption of vitamin B_{12} may not be improved by folic acid therapy. In such cases, parenteral therapy with vitamin B_{12} in doses identical to those for treatment of pernicious anemia is indicated. For unknown reasons, tetracycline administered over a period of at least 2 months has proven effective in the therapy of tropical sprue, especially the type seen in Puerto Rico. *Steroids* have also improved absorption in some patients with a variety of malabsorption syndromes; the mechanism of this action is unknown.

Celiac disease appears to be a *gluten-induced enteropathy;* a *gluten-free* diet is the single most effective therapy. Folate and vitamin B_{12} deficiency associated with *celiac disease* and *idiopathic steatorrhea* is treated as in *tropical sprue.* In *nontropical sprue,* treatment with folic acid is usually not associated with general improvement of symptoms and signs other than those due to the megaloblastic anemia; not infrequently, some anemia and morphological damage also persist due to untreated associated vitamin B_{12} deficiency.

Extensive organic diseases of the upper small intestine, such as *reticulosis, regional jejunitis,* or *jejunal diverticulosis,* may produce megaloblastic anemia by reducing absorption of food folate, and operative removal of the affected portion of jejunum may restore absorption of folate to normal. Until such restorative surgery is successfully performed, treatment of the folate deficiency is the same as for tropical sprue.

Blind-Loop Syndrome. Any structural defect in the small intestine, either congenital (such as *multiple diverticulosis*) or acquired (such as *stricture* or *anastomosis*) may provide a milieu of intestinal stasis in which there may be an overgrowth of abnormal bacterial flora that may compete with the host for available folate or vitamin B_{12}. Cases have been described in which the resulting megaloblastic anemia was due to folate deficiency, vitamin B_{12} deficiency, or deficiency of both vitamins. Therapy consists in surgical correction of the defect when possible, antibiotic administration to suppress or destroy the abnormal bacterial flora, and vitamin B_{12} or folic acid, depending on the deficiency.

Megaloblastic Anemia in Association with Hemolytic Anemia. Patients in this category usually have been subsisting on a diet marginal in folate content, and the increased demand for folate caused by accelerated hematopoiesis is superimposed. However, some cases have been reported in association with reasonably good diets, and it is possible that the daily folate requirement may be sufficiently increased by constant accelerated hematopoiesis so as to be greater than 0.2 mg of folic acid (Alperin, 1967). Malabsorption syndrome also must be considered in patients who have megaloblastic anemia in association with hemolytic anemia. Therapy is with oral folic acid, 0.5 to 1.0 mg daily, supplemented with a nutritionally adequate diet; this may so reduce the requirement for blood transfusion that some clinicians routinely give folic acid, 0.5 mg daily, to all patients with sickle-cell disease or thalassemia. Treatment is also directed against the hemolytic anemia when possible (antimalarial therapy, splenectomy for hereditary spherocytosis, steroids for "autoimmune" hemolytic anemias, etc.).

Megaloblastic Anemia in Association with Antifols. Antifols bind to dihydrofolate reductase, thereby blocking folate metabolism and producing megaloblastic anemia. Pteroylglutamic acid itself is therapeutically useless (Johns et al., 1964), since there is no dihydrofolate reductase available to convert it to the metabolically active reduced form. Therefore, therapy is with *folinic acid,* which is already reduced and, therefore, is beyond the step blocked by antifols; 3 to 6 mg of the racemic mixture should be given orally or intramuscularly, three times daily (*see* Chapter 62).

Megaloblastic Anemia in Association with Hemochromatosis. When megaloblastic anemia occurs in association with hemochromatosis, especially in alcoholics, there is considerable question as to whether the disease really is hemochromatosis. This is so because vitamin deficiency (vitamin B_{12}, folate, pyridoxine) may result in saturation of the iron-binding capacity and in massive tissue accumulation of iron due to ineffective hematopoiesis. The accumulation may be increased by alcohol ingestion. Treatment should be by cessation of alcohol and administration of cyanocobalamin, folic acid, and pyridoxine for at least 6 months. This will correct the megaloblastic anemia and may "cure" the "hemochromatosis." The megaloblastic anemia sometimes seen with *hemosiderosis* does not respond to vitamin B_{12} but improves on therapy with 150 μg of folic acid intramuscularly daily, indicating that it is due to folate deficiency (Frick and Brunner, 1964).

Megaloblastic Anemia in Association with Malignant Disease. Megaloblastic anemia may occur in various disorders of the hematopoietic system, including erythremic myelosis (Di Guglielmo syndrome), myelofibrosis, polycythemia vera, myeloid metaplasia, acute leukemia, chronic leukemia (especially lymphatic), multiple myeloma, Hodgkin's disease, and lymphomas. Except for erythremic myelosis, the megaloblastosis may result in large part from inadequate ingestion or absorption of folate or (less commonly) of vitamin B_{12} associated with an increased requirement due to the needs of the malignant tissue. A defect in utilization of folate or vitamin B_{12} may exist in some cases that do not respond to administration of either substance. Megaloblastosis due to folate deficiency is sometimes seen with any widespread malignancy; exceptions are malignancies of certain areas of the gastrointestinal tract, which may interfere with vitamin B_{12} absorption (*e.g.,* carcinoma of the stomach, lymphomas involving the ileum). The decision whether patients with lymphoproliferative or myeloproliferative disorders who develop folate deficiency should be treated with folate is difficult; the physician must weigh the benefit to the patient against the possible stimulatory effect of folic acid on growth of malignant tissue. If the decision is to treat, therapy is as for *nutritional megaloblastic anemia.*

Pernicious Anemia. Because folic acid partially (and temporarily) corrects the hematological damage due to vitamin B_{12} deficiency, while allowing the associated neurological damage to proceed uncorrected, it should never be used in the therapy of patients with vitamin B_{12} deficiency of *any* cause, unless there is associated folate deficiency. In the latter situation, 0.1 mg daily should be administered, but not without concomitant cyanocobalamin therapy. Associated nutritional folate deficiency occurs in one third of patients with vitamin B_{12} deficiency, presumably due mainly to the anorexia so frequent in vitamin B_{12}–deficiency states, but probably due also in part to associated diarrhea or other intestinal dysfunction reducing folate absorption. It is possible that gastric acid may help to free folate from its conjugates in food, and the achlorhydria in patients with pernicious anemia may further decrease the amount of folate available for absorption. Additionally, body folate stores may sharply drop for unknown reasons when vitamin B_{12} stores are nearly exhausted. Because the use of multivitamin preparations containing in excess of 0.1 mg of folic acid per daily dose has masked the megaloblastic anemia of persons with vitamin B_{12} deficiency while allowing their neurological damage to progress, the United States Food and Drug Administration prohibits the inclusion of more than 0.1 mg of folic acid per daily dose of any such mixtures sold directly to the public. Nevertheless, these preparations continue to be available by prescription. It is therefore incumbent on the physician *never* to prescribe a multivitamin preparation containing more than 0.1 mg of folic acid per daily dose unless he has evaluated vitamin B_{12} status. The fact that the preparation may also contain cyanocobalamin usually means nothing, since the patient with pernicious anema or with malabsorption for vitamin B_{12} cannot absorb cyanocobalamin, in doses less than 1000 μg daily, in a reliable amount.

Aplastic Anemia and Hypoplastic Anemia. Therapy with folic acid (or cyanocobalamin) is generally useless in these conditions. Rarely, aplastic anemia or erythroid hypoplasia may result from total bone-marrow exhaustion after prolonged deprivation of vitamin B_{12} (or folate). Benefit from folic acid (or cyanocobalamin) in such cases is slow or absent, but large doses of both agents may be tried (1000 μg of cyanocobalamin plus 15 mg of folic acid intramuscularly, daily for a month). A satisfactory response to these agents may occur only following steroid therapy.

Normocytic Anemia. In general, therapy with folic acid or cyanocobalamin has no value in normocytic anemia. For unknown reasons, defective ability to synthesize hemoglobin (*thalassemia, iron deficiency*, etc.) is associated with defective ability to produce megaloblasts despite coexisting deficiency of vitamin B_{12} or folate. Patients with such occult megaloblastic anemia have a peripheral blood picture that is microcytic, normocytic, macrocytic, or dimorphic (both microcytes and macrocytes being present). However, inability normally to synthesize hemoglobin does not prevent the appearance of hypersegmentation of the neutrophil nucleus when deficiency of vitamin B_{12} or folate coexists. Thus, this hallmark of megaloblastic anemia is usually present in the peripheral blood and suggests the presence of associated, treatable deficiency of vitamin B_{12} or folate. Hypersegmentation *without* macroovalocytosis occurs on a congenital basis in approximately 1% of the population; it also occurs with chronic renal disease; therapy with folic acid or cyanocobalamin is usually without value in these two conditions. Hypersegmentation has been claimed to occur as a result of iron deficiency alone, but this is uncommon (Herbert and Tisman, 1971).

MEGALOBLASTIC ANEMIAS RESPONSIVE
TO DRUGS OTHER THAN VITAMIN B_{12}
AND FOLIC ACID

Megaloblastic Anemia in Association with Inhibition of DNA Synthesis. All of the antimetabolites used in chemotherapy of neoplastic disease that are capable of interfering with DNA synthesis are capable of producing megaloblastic anemia. Treatment is by withdrawal of the offending agent or administration of metabolites that function beyond the block.

Hereditary Oroticaciduria. This is a rare autosomal recessive and usually lethal condition in infants due to absence of the enzymes orotidylic pyrophosphorylase and orotidylic decarboxylase. The resultant blockade in pyrimidine synthesis produces megaloblastic anemia. Treatment is with oral steroids and concentrated yeast extract (which contains uridylic and cytidylic acids, and thus bypasses the metabolic block) or with uridine.

Pyridoxine-Responsive Megaloblastic Anemia. Normoblastic erythropoiesis is the rule in patients with anemia responsive to pyridoxine, but occasionally megaloblastic erythropoiesis occurs. The patients are elderly, with hepatomegaly, hepatic damage, excessive sideroblasts, hemosiderosis, hyperferremia, and, eventually, splenomegaly. Dimorphic anemia is usually present. Familial occurrence of hematological abnormalities is significant. Manifestations of overt pyridoxine deficiency (glossitis,

convulsions, peripheral neuropathy, dermatitis) do not occur. Treatment with 100 to 200 mg of pyridoxine, administered orally or intramuscularly daily, produces a hematological response varying from slight to excellent; however, return to hematological normality does not take place, and relapse unresponsive to pyridoxine may occur. Some patients also respond variably to treatment with folic acid, vitamin C, testosterone, and tryptophan. Pyridoxine is involved with folate in amino acid metabolism (*see* Figure 64–1); this may be one metabolic step in which depletion of pyridoxine may lead to megaloblastic anemia. However, the primary lesion in patients with pyridoxine-responsive megaloblastic anemia is unknown. It does not appear to be lack of pyridoxine (*see* Hines and Harris, 1964; Horrigan and Harris, 1968).

Vitamin E-Responsive Megaloblastic Anemias. The hemolytic anemia of some premature infants responds to vitamin E (*see* review by Silber and Goldstein, in Seminar, 1970).

Adams, J. F., and Boddy, K. Metabolic equilibrium of tracer and natural vitamin B_{12}—an experimental study. *J. Lab. clin. Med.,* **1968,** *72,* 392–396.

Addison, T. *On the Constitutional and Local Effects of Disease of the Suprarenal Capsules.* S. Highley, London, **1855.**

Allen, R. H., and Mehlman, C. S. Isolation of gastric vitamin B_{12}-binding proteins using affinity chromatography. I. Purification and properties of human intrinsic factor. *J. biol. Chem.,* **1973,** *248,* 3660–3669.

Alperin, J. B. Folic acid deficiency complicating sickle cell anemia: a study on the response to titrated doses of folic acid. *Archs intern. Med.,* **1967,** *120,* 298–306.

Angier, R. B., and others. The structure and synthesis of *L. casei* factor. *J. Am. chem. Soc.,* **1946,** *103,* 667–669.

Barness, L. A., and Morrow, G., III. Methylmalonic aciduria—a newly discovered inborn error. *Ann. intern. Med.,* **1968,** *69,* 633–635.

Berk, L.; Castle, W. B.; Welch, A. D.; Heinlie, R. W.; Anker, R.; and Epstein, M. Observations on the etiologic relationship of achylia gastrica to pernicious anemia. X. Activity of vitamin B_{12} as food (extrinsic) factor. *New Engl. J. Med.,* **1948,** *239,* 911–913.

Bozian, R. C.; Heyssel, R. M.; and Darby, W. J. Absorption of Co^{60} vitamin B_{12} from natural foodstuff by man. *Am. J. clin. Nutr.,* **1964,** *14,* 239–240.

Carmel, R., and Herbert, V. Deficiency of vitamin B_{12}-binding alpha globulin in two brothers. *Blood,* **1969,** *33,* 1–12.

Carmel, R.; Rosenberg, A. H.; Lau, K.-S.; Streiff, R. R.; and Herbert, V. Vitamin B_{12} uptake by human small bowel homogenate and its enhancement by intrinsic factor. *Gastroenterology,* **1969,** *56,* 548–555.

Chanarin, I.; Hutchinson, M.; MacLean, N.; and Moule, M. Hepatic folate in man. *Br. med. J.,* **1966,** *1,* 396–399.

Corcino, J.; Waxman, S.; and Herbert, V. Mechanism of triamterene-induced megaloblastosis. *Ann. intern. Med.,* **1970,** *73,* 419–424.

Day, P. L.; Mims, V.; Totter, J. R.; Stokstad, E. L. R.; Hutchings, B. L.; and Sloane, N. H. Successful treatment of vitamin M deficiency in monkey with highly purified *Lactobacillus casei* factor. *J. biol. Chem.,* **1945,** *157,* 423–424.

Doscherholmen, A., and Swaim, W. R. Impaired assimilation of egg Co^{57} vitamin B_{12} in patients with hypochlorhydria and achlorhydria and after gastric resection. *Gastroenterology,* **1973,** *64,* 913–920.

Duke, M.; Herbert, V.; and Abelmann, W. H. Hemo-dynamic effects of blood transfusion in chronic anemia. *New Engl. J. Med.,* **1964,** *271,* 975–980.

FAO/WHO Expert Group. *Requirements of Ascorbic Acid, Vitamin D, Vitamin B_{12}, Folate, and Iron.* World Health Organization Technical Report. WHO, Geneva, **1970.**

Ford, J. E., and Scott, K. J. The folic acid activity of some milk foods for babies. *J. Dairy Res.,* **1968,** *35,* 65.

Frick, P. G., and Brunner, H. E. Megaloblastic anemia due to folic acid deficiency in hemochromatosis. *Dt. med. Wschr.,* **1964,** *89,* 161–165.

Gough, K. R.; McCarthy, C.; Read, A. E.; Mollin, D. L.; and Waters, A. H. Folic acid deficiency in rheumatoid arthritis. *Br. med. J.,* **1964,** *1,* 212–217.

Hall, C. A., and Finkler, A. E. Isolation and evaluation of the various B_{12} binding proteins in human plasma. In, *Vitamins and Coenzymes.* (McCormick, D. B., and Wright, L. D., eds.) Academic Press, Inc., New York, **1971,** pp. 108–126.

Herbert, V. Experimental nutritional folate deficiency in man. *Trans. Ass. Am. Physns,* **1962a,** *75,* 307–320.

————. Hematopoietic factors in liver diseases. *Prog. liver Dis.,* **1965,** *2,* 57–68.

————. Transient (reversible) malabsorption of vitamin B_{12}. *Br. J. Haemat.,* **1969,** *17,* 213–219.

Herbert, V.; Streiff, R. R.; and Sullivan, L. W. Notes on vitamin B_{12} absorption: autoimmunity and childhood pernicious anemia; relation of intrinsic factor to blood group substance. *Medicine, Baltimore,* **1964,** *43,* 679–687.

Herbert, V., and Sullivan, L. W. Activity of coenzyme B_{12} in man. *Ann. N.Y. Acad. Sci.,* **1964,** *112,* 855–870.

Herbert, V., and Tisman, G. Iron deficiency and "megalo-blastoid" marrow. *New Engl. J. Med.,* **1971,** *284,* 448.

Herbert, V.; Tisman, G.; Go, L. T.; and Brenner, L. The dU suppression test using ^{125}I-UdR to define biochemical megaloblastosis. *Br. J. Haemat.,* **1973,** *24,* 713–723.

Heyssel, R. M.; Bozian, R. C.; Darby, W. J.; and Bell, M. C. Vitamin B_{12} turnover in man: the assimilation of vitamin B_{12} from natural foodstuff by man and estimates of minimal daily dietary requirements. *Am. J. clin. Nutr.,* **1966,** *18,* 176–184.

Hines, J. D., and Harris, J. W. Pyridoxine-responsive anemia: description of three patients with megaloblastic erythropoiesis. *Am. J. clin. Nutr.,* **1964,** *14,* 137–146.

Horrigan, D. L., and Harris, J. W. Pyridoxine-responsive anemias in man. *Vitams Horm.,* **1968,** *26,* 549–568.

Hutchins, H. H.; Cravioto, P. J.; and Macek, T. J. A comparison of the stability of cyanocobalamin and its analogs in ascorbate solution. *J. Am. pharm. Ass., Sci. Ed.,* **1956,** *45,* 806–808.

International Union of Pure and Applied Chemistry. Ten-tative rules for nomenclature of organic chemistry. *J. biol. Chem.,* **1966,** *241,* 2991–2994.

Jackson, I. M. D.; Doig, W. B.; and McDonald, G. Perni-cious anaemia as a cause of infertility. *Lancet,* **1967,** *2,* 1159–1160.

Jadhav, M.; Webb, J. K. G.; and Baker, S. J. Vitamin-B_{12} deficiency in Indian infants. *Lancet,* **1963,** *1,* 720.

Johns, D. G.; Hollingsworth, J. W.; Cashmore, A. R.; Plenderleith, I. H.; and Bertino, J. R. Methotrexate displacement in man. *J. clin. Invest.,* **1964,** *43,* 621–629.

Johns, D. G.; Sperti, S.; and Burgen, A. S. V. The metab-olism of tritiated folic acid in man. *J. clin. Invest.,* **1961,** *40,* 1684–1695.

Marston, H. R.; Allen, S. H.; and Smith, R. M. Primary metabolic defect supervening on vitamin B_{12} deficiency in the sheep. *Nature, Lond.,* **1961,** *190,* 1085–1091.

Metz, J.; Kelly, A.; Swett, V. C.; Waxman, S.; and Herbert, V. Deranged DNA synthesis by bone marrow from vitamin B_{12}-deficient humans. *Br. J. Haemat.,* **1968a,** *14,* 575–592.

Metz, J.; Zalusky, R.; and Herbert, V. Folic acid binding by serum and milk. *Am. J. clin. Nutr.,* **1968b,** *21,* 289–297.

Minot, G. R., and Castle, W. B. Interpretation of reticulo-cyte reactions: their value in determining potency of

therapeutic materials, especially in pernicious anemia. *Lancet,* **1935,** *2,* 319–320.

Mitchell, H. K.; Snell, E. E.; and Williams, R. J. The concentration of "folic acid." *J. Am. chem. Soc.,* **1941,** *63,* 2284.

Nyberg, W.; Gräsbeck, R.; Saarni, M.; and Bonsdorff, B. von. Serum vitamin B_{12} levels and incidence of tape-worm anemia in a population heavily infested with *Diphyllobothrium latum. Am. J. clin. Nutr.,* **1961,** *9,* 606–612.

Pfiffner, J. J.; Binkley, S. B.; Bloom, E. S.; Brown, R. A.; Bird, O. D.; and Emmett, A. D. Isolation of antianemia factor (vitamin B_{12}) in crystalline form from liver. *Science, N.Y.,* **1943,** *97,* 404–405.

Ramsey, C., and Herbert, V. Dialysis assay for intrinsic factor and its antibody: demonstration of species specifi-city of antibodies to human and hog intrinsic factor. *J. Lab. clin. Med.,* **1965,** *65,* 143–152.

Reizenstein, P.; Ek, G.; and Matthews, C. M. E. Vitamin B_{12} kinetics in man. Implications on total-body-B_{12}-determinations, human requirements and normal and pathological cellular B_{12} uptake. *Physics Med. Biol.,* **1966,** *11,* 295–306.

Retief, F. P.; Gottlieb, C. W.; and Herbert, V. Delivery of $Co^{57}B_{12}$ to erythrocytes from α and β globulin of normal, B_{12}-deficient, and chronic myeloid leukemic serum. *Blood,* **1967,** *29,* 837–851.

Reynolds, E. H. Mental effects of anticonvulsants and folic acid metabolism. *Brain,* **1968,** *91,* 197–214.

Rickes, E. L.; Brink, N. G.; Koniuszy, F. R.; Wood, T. R.; and Folkers, K. Crystalline vitamin B_{12}. *Science, Wash.,* **1948,** *107,* 396–397.

Rosenblum, C.; Reizenstein, P. G.; Cronkite, E. P.; and Meriwether, H. T. Tissue distribution and storage forms of vitamin B_{12} injected and orally administered to the dog. *Proc. Soc. exp. Biol. Med.,* **1963,** *112,* 262–266.

Schilling, R. F. Intrinsic factor studies. II. The effect of gastric juice on the urinary excretion of radioactivity after the oral administration of radioactive vitamin B_{12}. *J. Lab. clin. Med.,* **1953,** *42,* 860–866.

Scott, J. M.; Bloomfield, F. J.; Stebbins, R.; and Herbert, V. Studies on derivation of transcobalamin III from granulocytes. *J. clin. Invest.,* **1974,** *53,* 228–239.

Skouby, A. P.; Hippe, E.; and Olesen, H. Antibody to transcobalamin II and B_{12} binding capacity in patients treated with hydroxycobalamin. *Blood,* **1971,** *38,* 769–774.

Smith, E. L., and Parker, L. F. J. Purification of antiperni-cious anaemia factor. *Biochem. J.,* **1948,** *43,* viii–ix.

Snell, E. E., and Peterson, W. H. Growth factors for bacteria. X. Additional factors required by certain lactic acid bacteria. *J. Bact.,* **1940,** *39,* 273–285.

Stahlberg, K.-G. Studies on methyl-B_{12} in man. *Scand. J. Haemat.,* **1967,** *4,* Suppl. 1, 3–99.

Stebbins, R.; Scott, J.; and Herbert, V. Drug-induced megaloblastic anemias. *Semin. Hemat.,* **1973,** *10,* 235–251.

Stokstad, E. L. R. Some properties of growth factor for *Lactobacillus casei. J. biol. Chem.,* **1943,** *149,* 573–574.

Stokstad, E. L. R., and Manning, P. D. V. Evidence of a new growth factor required by chicks. *J. biol. Chem.,* **1938,** *125,* 687–696.

Strauss, M. B. The pharmacopeia and the physician: use of drugs in treatment of anemias. *J. Am. med. Ass.,* **1936,** *107,* 1633–1636.

Sullivan, L. W., and Herbert, V. Studies on the minimum daily requirement for vitamin B_{12}: hematopoietic re-sponses to 0.1 microgm. of cyanocobalamin or coenzyme B_{12}, and comparison of their relative potency. *New Engl. J. Med.,* **1965,** *272,* 340–346.

Tamura, T., and Stokstad, E. L. R. The availability of food folate in man. *Br. J. Haemat.,* **1973,** *25,* 513–532.

Tisman, G., and Herbert, V. B_{12} dependence of cell uptake of serum folate: an explanation for high serum folate and cell folate depletion in B_{12} deficiency. *Blood,* **1973,** *41,* 465–469.

Toskes, P. P.; Deren, J. J.; and Conrad, M. E. Trypsin-like

nature of the pancreatic factor that corrects vitamin B_{12} malabsorption associated with pancreatic dysfunction. *J. clin. Invest.*, **1973**, *52*, 1660–1664.

Trier, J. S. Morphologic alterations induced by methotrexate in the mucosa of human proximal intestine. I. Serial observations by light microscopy. *Gastroenterology*, **1962**, *42*, 295–305.

Wills, L., and Bilimoria, H. S. Studies in pernicious anaemia of pregnancy: production of macrocytic anaemia in monkeys by deficient feeding. *Indian J. med. Res.*, **1932**, *20*, 391–402.

Wills, L.; Clutterbuck, P. W.; and Evans, P. D. F. A new factor in the production and cure of macrocytic anaemias and its relation to other haemopoietic principles curative in pernicious anaemia. *Biochem. J.*, **1937**, *31*, 2136–2147.

Monographs and Reviews

Beck, W. S. Erythrocyte disorders—anemias related to disturbance of DNA synthesis (megaloblastic anemias). In, *Hematology.* (Williams, W. J.; Beutler, E.; Erslev, A. J.; and Rundles, R. W.; eds.) McGraw-Hill Book Co., New York, **1972**, pp. 249–297.

Bernstein, L., and Herbert, V. The role of pancreatic exocrine secretions in the absorption of vitamin B_{12} and iron. *Am. J. clin. Nutr.*, **1973**, *26*, 340–346.

Blakley, R. L. *The Biochemistry of Folic Acid and Related Pteridines.* North-Holland Publishing Co., Amsterdam; John Wiley & Sons, Inc., New York, **1969**. (Over 2250 references.)

Castle, W. B. A century of curiosity about pernicious anemia. *Trans. Am. clin. climat. Ass.*, **1961**, *73*, 54–80.

Chanarin, I. *The Megaloblastic Anemias.* Blackwell Scientific Publications, Oxford; F. A. Davis Co., Philadelphia, **1969**.

Committee on Maternal Nutrition, Food and Nutrition Board, National Research Council. *Maternal Nutrition and the Course of Pregnancy.* National Academy of Sciences, Washington, D. C., **1970**.

Cooper, B. A. Folate and vitamin B_{12} in pregnancy. *Clins Haemat.*, **1973**, *2*, 461–476.

Floch, M. H. (ed.). Current concepts in intestinal absorption and malabsorption. *Am. J. clin. Nutr.*, **1969**, *22*, 239–351.

Glass, G. B. J. *Gastric Intrinsic Factor and Other Vitamin B_{12} Binders: Biochemistry, Physiology, Pathology and Relation to Vitamin B_{12} Metabolism.* George Thieme Verlag, Stuttgart; Intercontinental Medical Book Co., New York, **1974**.

Gräsbeck, R. Intrinsic factor and the other vitamin B_{12} transport proteins. *Prog. Hemat.*, **1969**, *6*, 233–260.

Herbert, V. *The Megaloblastic Anemias.* Grune & Stratton, Inc., New York, **1959**. (612 references.)

————. The diagnosis and treatment of folic acid deficiency. *Med. Clins N. Am.*, **1962b**, *46*, 1365–1378.

————. Current concepts in therapy: megaloblastic anemia. *New Engl. J. Med.*, **1963**, *268*, 201–203, 368–371.

————. Absorption of vitamin B_{12} and folic acid. *Gastroenterology*, **1968a**, *54*, 110–115.

————. Nutritional requirements for vitamin B_{12} and folic acid. *Am. J. clin. Nutr.*, **1968b**, *21*, 743–752.

————. Diagnostic and prognostic values of measurement of serum vitamin B_{12}–binding proteins. *Blood*, **1968c**, *32*, 305–312.

————. Folic acid deficiency in man. *Vitams Horm.*, **1968d**, *26*, 525–535.

————. Detection of malabsorption of vitamin B_{12} due to gastric or intestinal dysfunction. *Semin. nucl. Med.*, **1972**, *2*, 220–234.

————. Folic acid and vitamin B_{12}. In, *Modern Nutrition*

in Health and Disease, 5th ed. (Goodhart, R. S., and Shils, M. E., eds.) Lea & Febiger, Philadelphia, **1973a**, pp. 221–244.

————. Metabolism of folic acid in man. *J. infect. Dis.*, **1973b**, *128*, Suppl., S601–S606.

————. Megaloblastic anemias. In, *Cecil-Loeb Textbook of Medicine,* 14th ed. (Beeson, P. B., and McDermott, W., eds.) W. B. Saunders Co., Philadelphia, **1975**, pp. 1404–1413.

Herbert, V., and Bertino, J. R. Folic acid. In, *The Vitamins: Chemistry, Physiology, Pathology, Methods,* 2nd ed., Vol. VII. (Gyorgy, P., and Pearson, W. N., eds.) Academic Press, Inc., New York, **1967**, pp. 243–269.

Herbert, V., and Tisman, G. Effects of deficiencies of folic acid and vitamin B_{12} on central nervous system function and development. In, *Biology of Brain Dysfunction,* Vol. 1. (Gaull, G., ed.) Plenum Press, New York, **1973**, pp. 373–392.

Jeffries, G. H.; Weser, E.; and Sleisenger, M. H. Malabsorption. *Gastroenterology*, **1969**, *56*, 777–797.

Jukes, T. H., and Broquist, H. P. Sulfonamides and folic acid antagonists. In, *Metabolic Inhibitors.* (Hochster, R. M., and Quastel, J. H., eds.) Academic Press, Inc., New York, **1963**, pp. 481–534. (182 references.)

Metz, J. Folates in megaloblastic anaemia. *Bull. Wld Hlth Org.*, **1963**, *28*, 517–529.

Pratt, J. M. *Inorganic Chemistry of Vitamin B_{12}.* Academic Press, Inc., New York, **1972**.

Seminar. (Various authors.) Nutritional anemias. (Herbert, V., ed.) *Semin. Hemat.*, **1970**, *7*, 2–106.

Simons, K. Gastric intrinsic factor and other vitamin B_{12} transport proteins: chemical and physiologic properties. *Prog. Gastroent.*, **1968**, *1*, 195–220.

Skeggs, H. R. Vitamin B_{12}. In, *The Vitamins: Chemistry, Physiology, Pathology, Methods,* 2nd ed., Vol. VII. (Gyorgy, P., and Pearson, W. N., eds.) Academic Press, Inc., New York, **1967**, pp. 277–301.

Smith, E. L. *Vitamin B_{12},* 3rd ed. Methuen & Co., London; John Wiley & Sons, Inc., New York, **1965**.

Stokstad, E. L. R., and Koch, J. Folic acid metabolism. *Physiol. Rev.*, **1967**, *47*, 83–116. (223 references.)

Straus, D. J. Hematologic aspects of alcoholism. *Semin. Hemat.*, **1973**, *10*, 183–194.

Sullivan, L. W. Folates in human nutrition. In, *Newer Methods of Nutritional Biochemistry,* Vol. 3. (Albanese, A. A., ed.) Academic Press, Inc., New York, **1967**, pp. 365–406.

Surgenor, D. M. (ed.). *The Red Blood Cell,* 2nd ed. Academic Press, Inc., New York, **1974**.

Symposium (2nd European). (Various authors.) *Vitamin B_{12} and Intrinsic Factor.* (Heinrich, H. C., ed.) Ferdinand Enke Verlag, Stuttgart, **1962**. (82 articles; 61 in English.)

Symposium. (Various authors.) Vitamin B_{12} coenzymes. (Perlman, D., ed.) *Ann. N.Y. Acad. Sci.*, **1964**, *112*, 547–921.

Symposium. (Various authors.) Malabsorption and malnutrition in the tropics. (Klipstein, F. A., ed.) *Am. J. clin. Nutr.*, **1968**, *21*, 933–1127.

Symposium. (Various authors.) Vitamin B_{12} and folate. (Herbert, V., ed.) *Am. J. Med.*, **1970**, *48*, 539–617.

Symposium. (Various authors.) *The Cobalamins.* (Arnstein, H. R. V., and Wrighton, R. J., eds.) Churchill Livingstone, Edinburgh, **1971**.

Wellcome Trust Collaborative Study. *Tropical Sprue and Megaloblastic Anaemia.* Churchill Livingstone, Edinburgh, **1971**.

WHO Scientific Group. *Nutritional Anemias.* World Health Organization Technical Report No. 405, WHO, Geneva, **1968**, pp. 1–37.

CHAPTER

65 ANTICOAGULANT, ANTITHROMBOTIC, AND THROMBOLYTIC DRUGS

Walter G. Levine

MECHANISMS OF BLOOD COAGULATION

In the 4 decades since the introduction of heparin, this drug and others that affect blood coagulation have become widely used in therapy. A complete elucidation of their mode of action is still lacking. However, consideration of some of the reactions involved in the clotting of blood will aid in understanding the mechanisms by which the anticoagulant and antithrombotic effects are exerted.

The factors generally accepted as being involved in blood coagulation are listed in Table 65-1.

Table 65-1. BLOOD CLOTTING FACTORS

FACTOR	COMMON SYNONYMS
I	Fibrinogen
II	Prothrombin
III	Thromboplastin
IV	Calcium
V	Ac globulin, labile factor
VII	Proconvertin, autoprothrombin I
VIII	Antihemophilic globulin
IX	Christmas factor, autoprothrombin II, PTC
X	Stuart factor, autoprothrombin III (C)
XI	PTA
XII	Hageman factor
XIII	Fibrin-stabilizing factor

Certain steps in the coagulation process have been established unequivocally. (1) The final step is the conversion of fibrinogen, a soluble plasma protein, to the insoluble fibrin. (2) This conversion is catalyzed by the enzyme thrombin, which proteolytically splits two small peptides from the fibrinogen molecule, yielding "fibrin monomer"; these monomers then polymerize to form fibrin. (3) Thrombin is derived entirely from prothrombin, a normal constituent of plasma.

The interactions that precede and are required for the activation of prothrombin to thrombin are of great complexity. Two major theories attempt to explain these events.

One theory (Davie and Ratnoff, 1964; Macfarlane, 1964) states that the initiating event in coagulation is the activation of factor XII by contact with a "foreign" surface. Activated factor XII then activates factor XI, which in turn continues the progressive "cascade" of activation that finally yields activated factor V. This substance then directly converts prothrombin to thrombin. The other theory (Seegers, 1969) is based on the premise that factors VII, IX, and X (designated as autoprothrombins by Seegers) are derived from the prothrombin molecule itself. Thus, the concept of autocatalysis is inherent in this theory. Furthermore, the penultimate steps involve the conversion of prothrombin to an intermediary form, "prethrombin," followed by the final activation to thrombin facilitated by activated factor X (autoprothrombin C). Both theories recognize the necessity for platelets during the reactions that culminate in the activation of factor X, and for calcium ions, which are required at a number of stages. Clinicians have been more comfortable in accepting the sequential or cascade theory since apparently it is in accord with many observations made on the clotting defects of patients. Nevertheless, convincing biochemical evidence that the entire cascade of activations occurs as stated is lacking. The autocatalytic theory, in contrast, is founded, for the most part, upon solid biochemical evidence. Despite the obvious conflict over the existence of preformed factors VII, IX, and X, the cascade and autocatalytic theories have come into closer agreement in recent years. It is anticipated that there will be an appropriate blending of the theories into one that will satisfy both chemical and clinical observations.

A useful concept that can be accommodated to either theory is *thromboplastin generation*. Intrinsic thromboplastin is the activity that develops upon mixing platelets with factors V, VIII, IX, X, XI, and XII, while *extrinsic* thromboplastin is formed by mixing tissue extract and factors V, VII, and X. Activated factor X (autoprothrombin C) is probably the "thromboplastin" activity generated in each case. The thromboplastin generation test is often used clinically to evaluate coagulation defects. (For the reader who wishes a more thorough discussion of recent theories of clotting mechanisms, *see* Esnouf and Macfarlane, 1968; Seegers, 1969; Kazal, 1971; Mammen, 1971.)

Additional factors are involved in clot formation and dissolution. The *fibrin-stabilizing factor (factor XIII)* aids in the maintenance of an insoluble fibrin clot. *Profibrinolysin (plasminogen)*, when activated during the final stage of coagulation, can lyse both fibrinogen and fibrin. Another component of plasma, *antithrombin,* inhibits clotting by destroying thrombin. *Antithromboplastin* is an activity attributed to a phospholipid substance or substances that inhibit the activation of prothrombin. A check-and-balance system of anticoagulant and procoagulant factors maintains blood in its proper fluid state, while allowing rapid hemostasis to occur following injury to a blood vessel. The coagulation mechanism thus represents a delicate balance among many factors, the specific functions of which are not clearly defined even today.

The simplified scheme depicted in Figure 65–1 is not intended to present all the complexities of the blood-clotting process discussed above, but it does serve to indicate the major sites of action of anticoagulant drugs.

The anticoagulant drugs in use at the present time inhibit the action or formation of one or more clotting factors. Since the absence of even a single clotting factor is considered a *disease,* one can say that the anticoagulant drugs exert their effects by creating a *clotting defect* resembling that of

certain clinical diseases. In light of this, the physician must exert proper caution in the use of these drugs because the range between insufficient therapy and excessive therapy with undue hemorrhagic risk is narrow and varies considerably from patient to patient. Individualized treatment and frequent laboratory tests are imperative for patients on anticoagulant therapy, who should be considered to be continually on the brink of a bleeding state.

I. Heparin and Oral Anticoagulants

HEPARIN

History. Heparin was discovered in 1916 by a medical student, J. McLean. While preparing thromboplastin extracts of various tissues, he made the surprising observation that some of them con-

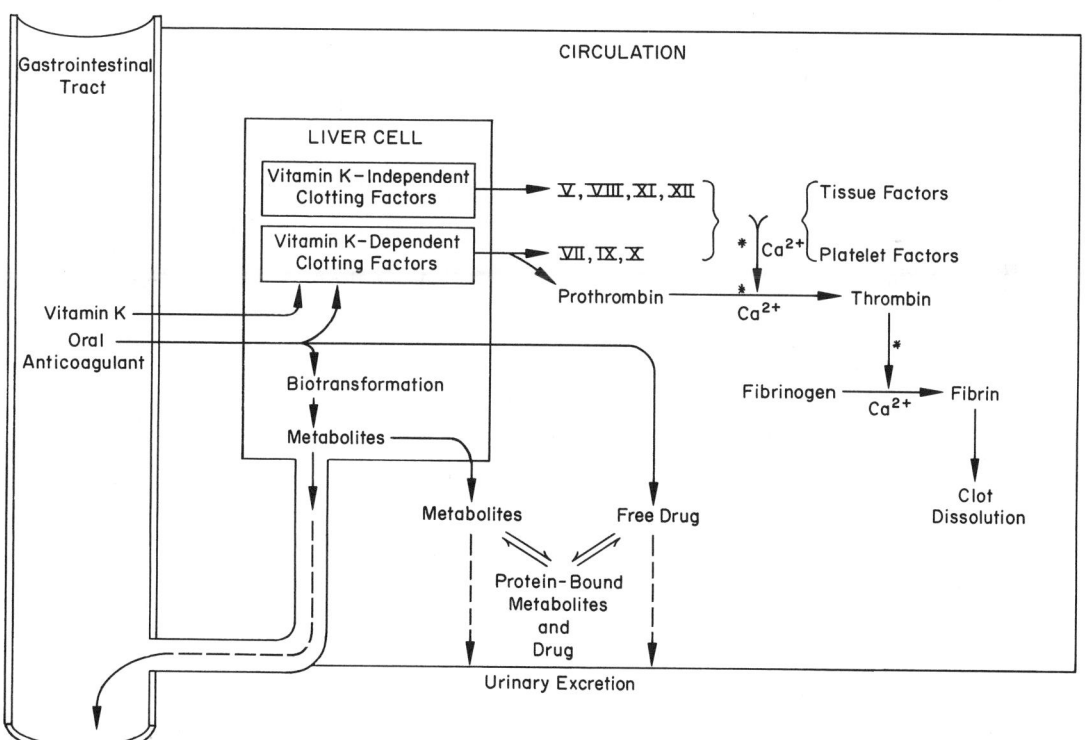

Figure 65–1. *Schematic representation of blood coagulation mechanisms and loci of anticoagulant effects.*

The sites of action of heparin are designated by an asterisk (*). Also shown are the sites of potential interaction between the oral anticoagulants and other drugs (*see* text). Only trace amounts of unaltered dicumarol and warfarin are excreted in the urine. (Modified from Koch-Weser and Sellers, 1971.)

tained a powerful anticoagulant. Howell and Holt (1918) described the characteristics of this anticoagulant and named it *heparin* to indicate its abundant occurrence in the liver. Later, high concentrations were also found in the lung and other tissues. The therapeutic possibilities of such an agent were soon appreciated, but the first relatively crude preparations caused severe reactions upon parenteral administration. Improved methods of extraction and purification (*see* Charles and Scott, 1933; Murray *et al.,* 1937) finally permitted administration of heparin to man (Charles and Scott, 1936). The initial clinical trials of heparin in the prophylaxis of thrombosis were first reported by Crafoord in 1937.

Chemistry. Heparin is a mucopolysaccharide composed of sulfated D-glucosamine and D-glucuronic acid. It has the following unit structure:

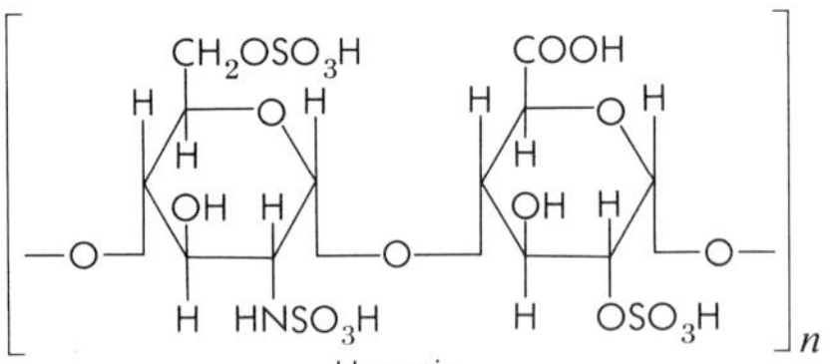

Heparin

Heparin is heterogeneous, and estimates of molecular weight vary from 6000 to 20,000. It contains a large number of O- and N-sulfate linkages and is the strongest organic acid occurring within the body. Anticoagulant activity is related to sulfuric acid content and to molecular shape and size. Hydrolysis of the ester linkage results in an altered molecular shape and a loss of activity. The anticoagulant effect of heparin may be due to reaction of the anionic groups with clotting factors. Sulfated polysaccharides with anticoagulant properties (*heparinoids*) have been synthesized in an attempt to produce a cheap heparin substitute. None of these has met with any clinical success.

Occurrence and Physiological Function. Heparin is found within mast cells and accounts for their characteristic metachromatic staining. Disruption of the cells releases heparin. Heparin can be extracted from many body organs, particularly those with abundant mast cells. The liver and lungs of most species are especially rich in heparin. The circulating blood contains no heparin except after profound disruption of mast cells, such as occurs, for example, during anaphylactic shock.

The physiological function of heparin, if any, is the subject of great speculation. Some evidence suggests that it serves a role in maintaining the blood in a fluid state, as was postulated by Howell many years ago. The discovery of the "heparin clearing factor"

(*see* below) by Hahn (1943) and its identification as a lipoprotein lipase led to speculation that this heparin-activated enzyme may be involved in the "clearing" of postprandial lipemic plasma. Convincing evidence that this is a normal function of heparin is still lacking.

PHARMACOLOGICAL PROPERTIES

The major pharmacological effects of heparin are almost entirely confined to the blood. Even large doses given intravenously have no significant effects except on blood coagulation and blood lipids.

Action on Blood Coagulation. Heparin inhibits the clotting of blood both *in vitro* and *in vivo*. Whole-blood clotting time, thrombin time, and one-stage prothrombin time are prolonged, and thromboplastin generation is abnormal. Clotting time is proportional to the concentration of drug in the blood. However, with therapeutic doses bleeding time is usually unaffected and a patient can carry on normal activities, such as shaving, without danger of bleeding. The anticoagulant action of heparin requires the presence of a plasma α-globulin, referred to as *heparin cofactor,* a substance that appears to be identical with normal plasma antithrombin (antithrombin III). Heparin does not block prothrombin synthesis in the liver as do the oral anticoagulants, but it does inhibit factors involved in the conversion of prothrombin to thrombin. This action is probably exerted by the facilitation of the formation of complexes of the heparin cofactor (antithrombin) with each of the four activated proteases of the coagulation cascade (activated factors IX, X, XI, and XII); a similar heparin-stimulated reaction also occurs between antithrombin and thrombin. The detailed mechanism of this phenomenon may involve a heparin-induced conformational change of the inhibitor (*see* Biggs *et al.,* 1970; Rosenberg, 1974, 1975). It requires 30 to 40 times more heparin to inhibit the action of formed thrombin than it does to prevent thrombin formation. Therefore, the prevention of thrombin formation is probably its primary effect (Jaques, 1967). Heparin also inhibits the aggregation of platelets by thrombin (Eika, 1971; O'Brien *et al.,* 1972).

Heparin and Lipoprotein Lipase. Hahn (1943) was the first to report that the turbidity of post-prandial lipemic plasma could be "cleared" by the injection of heparin, but not by the addition of heparin to lipemic plasma *in vitro*. Anderson and Fawcett (1950) demonstrated that nonheparinized lipemic plasma was cleared *in vitro* by the addition of plasma from a heparinized individual, thus establishing the presence in the circulation of a *clearing factor* produced by heparin. The clearing factor is the enzyme lipoprotein lipase, which catalyzes the hydrolysis of the triglycerides of chylomicra, releasing free fatty acids. The result is a disappearance of chylomicra and a rapid passage of the fatty acids into the tissues. The enzyme has been shown to be distinct from both pancreatic lipase and plasma esterase, and it has been identified in nearly every organ except liver and brain. It appears to be located in or near the vascular wall because, after an intra-arterial injection of heparin, clearing activity can be demonstrated in the venous effluent within a few seconds (Robinson and Harris, 1959). The enzyme also appears in the lymph. Other sulfated polysaccharides likewise produce the clearing reaction.

In man, after an injection of heparin, the circulating lipoprotein lipase rises to peak activity in 9 minutes and the mean half-life is about 25 minutes. A "rebound" hyperlipemia following a period of clearing has been reported to occur after a single injection of heparin (Woldow *et al.,* 1962) despite the fact that the clearing factor could still be demonstrated *in vitro*. The clearing system is highly sensitive to heparin. Detectable levels of lipoprotein lipase appear in the circulation with doses of heparin that do not discernibly prolong clotting times. Protamine and other substances that neutralize the anticoagulant properties of heparin also destroy its clearing function.

A physiological role for lipoprotein lipase has not been established. Its location in, or close to, capillary walls suggests a role in the transport of triglyceride fatty acids through the vessel walls, although direct evidence supporting this view is lacking. Protamine, a heparin antagonist, increases plasma lipid concentrations. However, there is no assurance that protamine acts solely by inactivating heparin. Decreased platelet adhesiveness due to heparin has been associated with activation of the clearing factor (Morris *et al.,* 1971). The relationship, if any, of lipoprotein lipase to certain disease states involving lipid metabolism is unknown.

Miscellaneous Actions. Administration of heparin does not alter the *erythrocyte sedimentation rate,* but use of heparin as an *in-vitro* anticoagulant results in values that differ from those obtained with oxalate or citrate. Routine chemical and morphological studies on blood are unaltered by heparin, although *white-cell counts* should be done within 2 hours due to the tendency of leukocytes to disappear in heparinized blood. Such blood is unsuitable for tests involving *complement* or *isoagglutinins. Fragility* tests should not be performed on heparinized blood because heparin inhibits hemolysis. *Hematocrit* determination may be performed on heparinized blood. Heparin suppression of aldosterone production has

been reported (Ford and Bailey, 1966) as well as an increase in free plasma thyroxine (Saeed-Uz-Zafer *et al.,* 1971). Heparin has also been stated to inhibit fibrinolytic activators as well as antifibrinolysin. Wound healing may be retarded by heparin, but this is controversial. An extensive review of other heparin effects is presented by Jaques (1967).

Absorption, Fate, and Excretion. Heparin is not effective after oral or sublingual administration, but it is well absorbed after intramuscular or subcutaneous injection. In the blood, it is evenly distributed between white cells and plasma. Heparin disappears exponentially from the circulation at a rate dependent upon the dose. The half-lives of 100, 200, and 400 units/kg, injected intravenously, are 56, 96, and 152 minutes, respectively (Olsson *et al.,* 1963). Heparin is metabolized by the liver, and a partially degraded, weakly active form of heparin (uroheparin) is excreted in the urine; after very large intravenous doses in man, up to 50% of nonmetabolized heparin may appear in the urine. The exact mechanism of renal elimination in man is unknown. Heparin does not cross the placenta, and, therefore, is preferred over oral anticoagulants during pregnancy; it also does not pass into the maternal milk.

Unitage and Preparations. The U.S.P. unit of heparin is the quantity that will prevent 1.0 ml of citrated sheep plasma from clotting for 1 hour after the addition of 0.2 ml of a 1:100 $CaCl_2$ solution. *Heparin Sodium,* U.S.P., must contain at least 120 U.S.P. units/mg. The potency of some preparations may far exceed this minimum; therefore, heparin should be prescribed on a unit basis. The drug is available as *Heparin Sodium Injection,* U.S.P. (HEPATHROM, LIPO-HEPIN, LIQUAEMIN, PANHEPRIN), in solutions containing 200, 1000, 5000, 7500, 10,000, 15,000, 20,000, or 40,000 U.S.P. units/ml. A repository form of heparin (DEPO-HEPARIN SODIUM) contains 20,000 U.S.P. units/ml in dextrose-gelatin base to decrease the rate of absorption.

Routes of Administration and Dosage. Heparin must be administered parenterally. The anticoagulant effect is achieved almost immediately after a single intravenous injection but lasts only about 3 to 4 hours. For the *continuous-drip method,* a total of 20,000 to 30,000 units of heparin is added to a liter of 5% glucose or 0.9% sodium chloride solution and administered over a 24-hour period. It may be 2 to 3 hours before the desired anticoagulant effect is established, and it is advisable to give 5000 units directly into the tubing as soon as the infusion is started. In this way the physician is able to maintain a therapeutic blood concentration of a rather evanescent drug. When high doses are required, the large volume of fluid infused may cause hypervolemia and edema. A further disadvantage is the discomfort of a prolonged infusion to a restless or apprehensive patient. For *intermittent intravenous therapy*, usually by means of an indwelling needle, a dose of 10,000 units is administered initially, and 5000 to 10,000 units is then administered every 4 to 6 hours, depending on the weight and the response of the patient. The corresponding dose for pediatric patients is 50 units/kg initially, followed by 100 units/kg every 4 hours. *Deep subcutaneous (intrafat)* injection has been used to offset some of the disadvantages of intravenous administration, but the technic is difficult if local reaction is to be avoided. Absorption is slower, and adequate prolongation of clotting time does not occur for 30 to 60 minutes. Therefore, an initial intravenous dose of 5000 to 10,000 units has been recommended, after which 10,000 to 20,000 units is injected subcutaneously, followed by 8000 to 10,000 units every 8 hours. The repository form of heparin is also administered by this route. Before administration, this gelatin-containing preparation must be liquefied by agitation in hot water. There have been a few reports of tissue slough secondary to hematoma formation at the injection site. The *intramuscular* route is usually avoided due to frequent bleeding and painful hematoma formation at the injection site.

The therapeutic regimens outlined above for the administration of heparin represent average doses. Coagulation time or preferably whole-blood activated partial thromboplastin time must be followed for optimal control.

The use of low-dose, subcutaneous heparin for the prophylaxis of thrombophlebitis in patients undergoing surgery is described later in this chapter.

Side Effects, Toxicity, and Contraindications. Purified commercial preparations of heparin are relatively nontoxic, and the incidence of side effects is low. Acute, reversible thrombocytopenia has been observed after intravenous heparin, but this is uncommon. Heparin blocks the eosinopenic response to corticotropin, adrenocorticosteroids, and insulin. It has an inhibitory effect on antibodies and anaphylaxis. Although hypersensitivity and anaphylactoid reactions are rare, severe asthma, giant urticaria, rhinitis, lacrimation, and fever have been encountered occasionally. Before a full dose is administered to patients with a previous history of allergy, it is advisable to give a trial dose of 1000 units. Some patients develop a transient alopecia several months after heparin administration. The effects of heparin on wound healing are at present controversial (Thompson *et al.*, 1972). Neuropathy is an unusual consequence of heparin therapy (Kubacz, 1971). Osteoporosis and spontaneous fractures have been observed, but only after

prolonged use of heparin. Several cases of priapism have been associated with the use of heparin (Duggan and Morgan, 1970).

The chief danger from heparin is *hemorrhage.* Careful laboratory control reduces the incidence of hemorrhage to a minimum. However, bleeding may be encountered from an unsuspected lesion, such as a peptic ulcer. The hemorrhagic complications recorded include hematuria, hemarthrosis, wound hematoma, and gastrointestinal bleeding. These are more common during prophylactic administration of *conventional doses* after surgery than during treatment of a preexisting thromboembolic condition. The hemorrhage may produce a hematoma in the surgical wound, but this is rarely serious if infection is prevented and larger accumulations of blood are aspirated.

Heparin is contraindicated in patients with active bleeding or bleeding tendencies (*e.g.,* hemophilia, purpura, increased capillary permeability), threatened abortion, subacute bacterial endocarditis, suspected intracranial hemorrhage, inaccessible ulcerative lesions (especially of the gastrointestinal tract), visceral carcinoma, regional or lumbar block anesthesia, severe hypertension, tube drainage of stomach and small intestine, heparin hypersensitivity, and shock. It should also be withheld during and after surgery of the eye, brain, or spinal cord. There may be a higher risk of bleeding in women over 60 years of age, although therapeutic efficacy is unchanged (Jick *et al.*, 1968).

Heparin Antagonists. Mild effects of heparin overdosage usually respond to simple withdrawal of the drug. In the event of major hemorrhage, the use of a specific heparin antagonist is imperative. Protamine sulfate is the only drug presently recommended for this purpose.

Protamine Sulfate. Protamines are simple, low-molecular-weight proteins found in the sperm of certain fish. They are strongly basic and are thus able to combine with the strongly acidic heparin to form a stable complex without anticoagulant activity. No significant dissociation of the complex occurs.

Protamine Sulfate Injection, U.S.P., is available as a solution containing 10 mg/ml. It should be given intravenously very slowly, no more than 50 mg over a 10-minute period. However, doses of 200 mg can be tolerated over a 2-hour period. The usual dose is 1.0 to 1.5 mg to antagonize each 100 units of heparin. After the intravenous administration of heparin, the quantity of protamine required decreases rapidly with the time elapsed after heparin injection. Thirty minutes after a dose of intravenous heparin only about 0.5 mg of protamine is required to antagonize each 100 units injected.

Protamine itself possesses anticoagulant properties. This may be due to an interference with thromboplastin generation (Hougie, 1958). Therefore, it has been recommended not to give more than 100 mg over a short period unless there is certain knowledge of a larger requirement; however, the necessity for this precaution has been disputed (*see* Ellison *et al.,* 1971). Intravenous injection of protamine may cause a sudden fall in blood pressure, bradycardia, dyspnea, transitory flushing, and a feeling of warmth. The untoward cardiovascular effects are believed to be due to direct depression of the myocardium and vascular smooth muscle (Fadali *et al.,* 1974). Slow, careful administration will diminish the incidence and severity of hypotension. Protamine is thought to be nonantigenic.

Therapeutic Uses. The therapeutic uses of heparin are discussed later in this chapter.

ORAL ANTICOAGULANTS

History. The history of the oral anticoagulants dates back to the early 1920s, when Schofield (1922, 1924) described the "sweet clover disease" of cattle, which was characterized by a severe bleeding tendency. This was attributed to feeding the cattle improperly cured sweet clover hay containing a toxic substance that interfered with normal blood-clotting mechanisms. Roderick (1929, 1931) reported a prothrombin deficiency in these animals and suggested that the toxic agent in the hay was probably a decomposition product of coumarin. It was not an irreversible effect, and clotting returned to normal when feeding of the hay was stopped. In 1934, Link and Campbell identified the substance as 3,3'-methylene-*bis*-(4-hydroxycoumarin) (Link, 1943–1944), a chemical synthesized 40 years earlier. This compound, dicumarol, is still widely used in therapy.

Associated with this early progress was the development by Quick of a quantitative method for prothrombin determination, the one-stage prothrombin time, which has evolved into a useful tool for the control of anticoagulant therapy (*see* Quick, 1959). Abnormal prothrombin times occur in obstructive jaundice, in vitamin K deficiency, and during the feeding of spoiled sweet clover. In all three conditions it was assumed that the defect was a lowered prothrombin concentration in the blood. Today, however, it is known that other factors as well are involved both in the Quick one-stage test and in the action of coumarin drugs (*see* below).

In the early 1940s the first promising clinical trials with dicumarol were reported (Bingham *et al.,* 1941; Butt *et al.,* 1941; Meyer *et al.,* 1942; Prandoni and Wright, 1942). There soon followed a profusion of

publications on the clinical use of this compound as an anticoagulant in a variety of medical and surgical conditions. During the past 3 decades, hundreds of chemically related compounds have been studied, but only a few are in use today. These differ mainly in time of onset, duration of action, and side effects (Table 65–4, page 1361). Because the oral route of administration is used almost exclusively, these drugs are often referred to as the *oral anticoagulants.*

Chemistry. The structural formulas of the oral anticoagulants discussed in this chapter appear in Table 65–2. They are either derivatives of 4-hydroxycoumarin or of indan-1,3-dione. Despite the relative simplicity of the chemistry of these drugs, it has proven very difficult to establish the essential chemical characteristics needed to produce anticoagulant activity. For the coumarin derivatives it is known, however, that the minimal structural requirements for activity are an intact 4-hydroxycoumarin residue with the 3 position substituted by a carbon residue or a hydrogen atom. For further discussion of the structure-activity relationship, the reader is referred to the article by Kralt and Claassen (1972).

PHARMACOLOGICAL PROPERTIES

The coumarin and indandione derivatives all have essentially the same action within the body, their differences being mainly quantitative. Because of their widespread use, the pharmacology of dicumarol and warfarin, the two most commonly employed oral anticoagulants, will be considered together in detail. Most of this discussion applies to the other oral anticoagulants as well. The section devoted to the other drugs deals only with features that specifically differ from those of dicumarol and warfarin.

Effect on Blood Coagulation. The oral anticoagulants have only one major pharmacological effect—inhibition of blood-clotting mechanisms by interfering with the hepatic synthesis of the vitamin K–dependent clotting factors. Unlike heparin, they are not active *in vitro* and exert their initial effect *in vivo* only after a latent period of at least 12 to 24 hours. This latent period is accounted for by the natural disappearance of circulating clotting factors. Originally, dicumarol was thought to act solely by diminishing the plasma prothrombin level. It is now appreciated that the oral anticoagulants depress plasma concentrations of factors VII, IX, and X as well. Since it is known that the one-stage prothrombin determination, as originally devised, is more sensitive to factors VII and X than to prothrombin, this test is now

Table 65-2.   STRUCTURAL FORMULAS OF THE ORAL ANTICOAGULANTS *

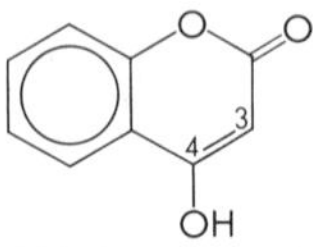

4-Hydroxycoumarin

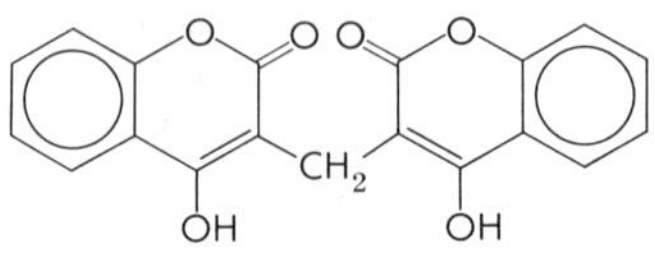

Dicumarol, U.S.P.

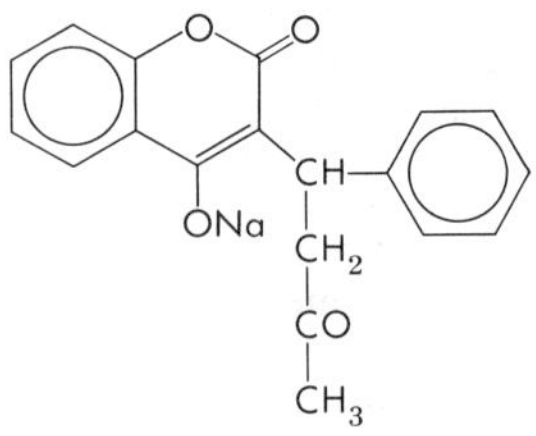

Warfarin Sodium, U.S.P.

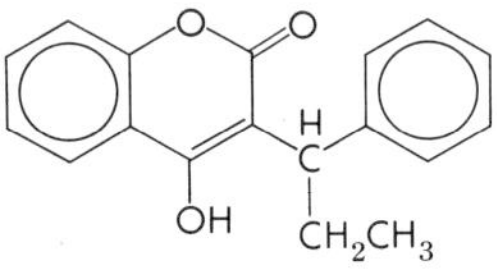

Phenprocoumon, N.F.

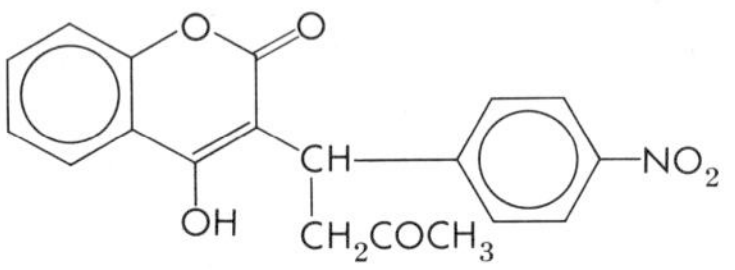

Acenocoumarol, N.F.

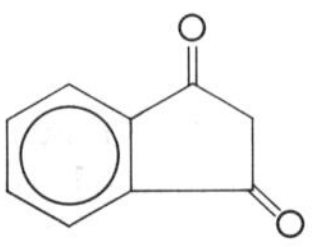

Indan-1,3-dione

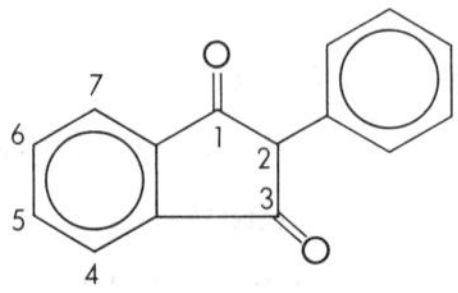

Phenindione, N.F.

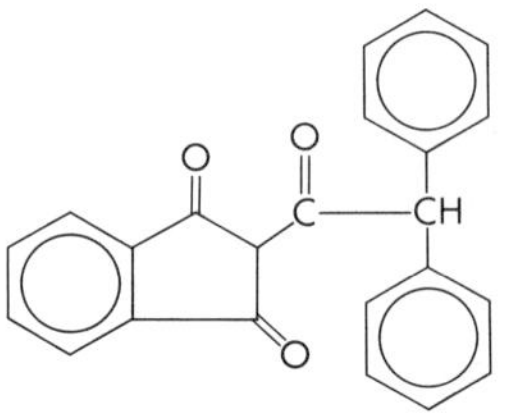

Diphenadione, N.F.

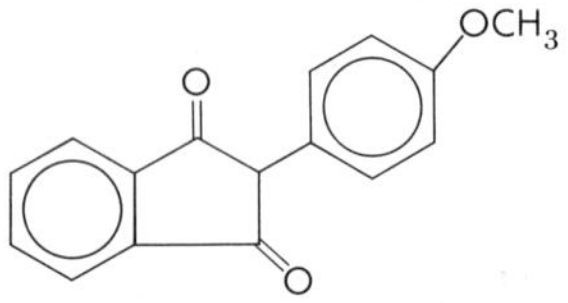

Anisindione

* 4-Hydroxycoumarin and indan-1,3-dione are included to indicate the parent molecules from which the oral anticoagulants are derived.

commonly referred to as the *prothrombin time*. During dicumarol therapy, factor VII decreases more rapidly than do factor IX, factor X, and prothrombin (factor II) (*see* Koch-Weser and Sellers, 1971); this is related to the half-life of these factors in the circulation, estimated to be 6, 20, 40, and 60 hours for factors VII, IX, X, and II, respectively. Whole-blood clotting time in glass tubes is slightly to moderately prolonged during dicumarol therapy; however, in siliconed tubes, a considerable lengthening of clotting time is observed. The recalcification time of citrated plasma is also lengthened. Despite these *in-vitro* observations, bleeding time is unaltered.

Mechanism of Action. The oral anticoagulants have no direct effect on circulating clotting factors. Instead they block the hepatic formation of factors II, VII, IX, and X by competitively inhibiting the action of vitamin K. Synthesis of these factors is dependent upon a sufficient supply of the vitamin. An experimental diet deficient in vitamin K elicits a depression of these factors similar to that seen with the oral anticoagulants. Identity of the site of action of anticoagulants and vitamin K in the liver is indicated by the observation that patients with a genetic resistance to oral anticoagulants also show an increased need for vitamin K (O'Reilly, 1971). Two sites of action for vitamin K have been postulated (Lowenthal and Macfarlane, 1967; Lowenthal and Birnbaum, 1968). The "normal" site is readily blocked by coumarin drugs; the other is responsive only to high concentrations of vitamin K and accounts for the ability of massive doses of vitamin K to overcome oral anticoagulant effects. Coumarin anticoagulants may also affect the transport of vitamin K to its site of action. The major site of action of these drugs and vitamin K may involve a prothrombin precursor subsequent to peptide synthesis (*see* Shah and Suttie, 1972, and Chapter 77). This precursor may also be common to factors VII, IX, and X.

Factors Influencing Activity. Changes in the availability of vitamin K alter the therapeutic response to oral anticoagulants. These include dietary intake of vitamin K and fat, as well as the presence in the large bowel of certain antimicrobial drugs or other agents that alter the normal microflora, an important source of vitamin K. For these reasons, there may be difficulty in stabilizing the therapeutic regimen of ambulatory patients who are undergoing long-term anticoagulant therapy at home, and whose diet cannot be carefully controlled. Apparently age and sex do not modify the effect of the drug, but debilitated and cachectic patients are more sensitive, as are patients with decreased hepatic function. The newborn are particularly sensitive to oral anticoagulants. Corticotropin and adrenocorticosteroids have been reported to cause severe hemorrhage when given with oral anticoagulants (Cauwenberge and Jaques, 1958); this is rather puzzling, since thrombotic episodes are stated to occur more frequently in patients on steroid therapy, and oral anticoagulants have been advised in the prophylaxis of such complications (Rawls, 1955). Renal insufficiency, fever, and scurvy enhance or prolong the oral anticoagulant response. A genetically related resistance to oral anticoagulants has been observed in some patients who require 10 to 20 times the usual dose (*see* O'Reilly and Aggeler, 1970).

Drug Interactions. A large number of drugs, when given concurrently with the oral anticoagulants, alter the magnitude of the observed effect on blood clotting. This subject has received a great deal of attention, since these effects are of notable clinical importance, involving a class of drugs with a narrow margin of safety and complex pharmacokinetic properties. While a similar number of interactions are probable and are being elucidated for other pharmacological agents, the interactions with the oral anticoagulants may be regarded as a model for understanding the intricacies of this subject. The excellent review article by Koch-Weser and Sellers (1971) on drug interactions with coumarin anticoagulants is recommended.

Drugs That Diminish the Response to Oral Anticoagulants. While several mechanisms may be envisioned that would cause this

Table 65–3. DRUG INTERACTIONS OF THE COUMARIN ANTICOAGULANTS *

I. *Drugs That Diminish the Response to Oral Anticoagulants*

A. By Inhibition of Oral Anticoagulant Absorption:
 Griseofulvin †
 (Clofibrate)

B. By Induction of Hepatic Microsomal Enzymes:
 Barbiturates
 Ethchlorvynol
 Glutethimide
 Griseofulvin †
 (Meprobamate)

C. By Stimulation of Synthesis of Clotting Factors:
 Vitamin K
 (Adrenocorticosteroids)
 (Estrogens)

II. *Drugs That Enhance the Response to Oral Anticoagulants*

A. By Displacement of Anticoagulant from Plasma Albumin:
 Chloral hydrate
 Clofibrate †
 Mefenamic acid
 Phenylbutazone
 (Diazoxide)
 (Ethacrynic acid)
 (Nalidixic acid)
 (Sulfinpyrazone)
 (Sulfonamides, long acting)

B. By Increase in Affinity for Receptor:
 D-Thyroxine †

C. By Inhibition of Hepatic Microsomal Enzymes:
 Chloramphenicol
 Clofibrate †
 (Allopurinol)
 (Disulfiram †)
 (Mercaptopurine †)
 (Methylphenidate)
 (Nortriptyline)

D. By Reduction in Availability of Vitamin K:
 Anabolic steroids †
 Clofibrate †
 D-Thyroxine †
 Broad-spectrum antibiotics

E. By Inhibition of Synthesis of Clotting Factors:
 Anabolic steroids †
 Glucagon †
 Quinidine †
 Salicylates †
 (Acetaminophen †)
 (Mercaptopurine †)

F. By Increase in Clotting Factor Catabolism:
 Anabolic steroids †
 D-Thyroxine †

* If the drug name is in parenthesis, the clinical significance of the interaction is minor or has not been firmly established.
† Indicates that the mechanism is still uncertain.

result (*see* Figure 65–1 and Table 65–3), induction of hepatic microsomal enzymes that metabolize the coumarins is the most important. When a drug such as a barbiturate is administered concurrently, the half-life of a coumarin anticoagulant is reduced. After 2 days of such dual therapy, the effect is significant in most patients, although 1 week of administration of the inducing agent may be necessary before a new steady state is established. Under these circumstances, an increased dosage of anticoagulant is required; it must not be forgotten, however, that cessation of administration of an agent that impairs the response to an oral anticoagulant in the manner described requires a decreased dosage of the latter drug. If an enzyme inducer is withdrawn, weeks may be required before the half-life of the anticoagulant returns to normal. Patients must be cautioned *not to alter or to discontinue* any aspect of therapy without consulting their physician.

Drugs That Enhance the Response to Oral Anticoagulants. Similarly, many drugs, acting by the mechanisms listed in Table 65–3, can enhance the action of oral anticoagulants, and adjustments of dosage are required when any of these agents is added to or deleted from a therapeutic regimen. A few of these interactions require additional comment. Large doses of salicylates have often been associated with bleeding problems, especially in patients receiving oral anticoagulants. This may be due to direct gastric irritation, suppression of platelet function, or a true hypoprothrombinemic effect. Only the latter would be antagonized by vitamin K. Since acetaminophen rarely alters the prothrombin time significantly, its substitution for aspirin should be considered in such patients.

Antimicrobials and other agents that alter the intestinal microflora may enhance the anti–vitamin K effect of oral anticoagulants, but this is usually not seen unless there is a dietary deficiency of vitamin K.

Many drugs displace coumarin-type anticoagulants from plasma albumin, and this action can result in a temporary large increase in the plasma concentration of the free anticoagulant, since, for example, 97% of warfarin is so bound at therapeutic concentrations. This results in a prolongation of the prothrombin time. However, it must be appreciated that such displacement also makes more drug available for biotransformation and elimination. The half-life of the anticoagulant is shortened, and a new steady state is eventually established, characterized by the same free anticoagulant concentration and prothrombin time that existed prior to concurrent administration of the displacing drug. Enhancement of anticoagulant effect is thus only temporary, but hemorrhagic catastrophes have resulted when this complication has been overlooked.

The ultimate complexity for this situation (and the others described) is even greater, since the clinical response is dependent on all of the drug concentrations as dictated by the plateau principle (*see* Chapter 1); the half-life of the displacing drug, the half-life of the anticoagulant, and the half-lives of the clotting factors are all involved. It should be obvious that caution, patient cooperation, and close laboratory observation are essential.

Other Concurrent Drug Effects. Dicumarol prolongs the half-lives of *chlorpropamide, phenytoin,* and *tolbutamide,* probably by suppressing their metabolism. Platelet adhesiveness, affected by numerous substances, has been claimed to be decreased during dicumarol therapy, and warfarin may increase the duration of platelet aggregation in response to adenosine diphosphate (ADP).

Absorption, Fate, and Excretion. In man, absorption of dicumarol from the gastrointestinal tract is slow and erratic. Warfarin is more readily and almost completely absorbed. There is considerable variation in absorption rate from one individual to another.

Within the circulation, the two drugs are almost entirely but loosely bound to plasma albumin, and only a small percentage of the total plasma concentration is represented by unbound drug. This accounts in part for the slow rate of degradation of the drugs and for their negligible renal excretion. The half-life of warfarin in man is about 48 (15 to 55) hours; the half-life of dicumarol is dose dependent, ranging from 10 hours at low dosage to 30 hours at high dosage. Appreciable amounts of the drugs are found in erythrocytes, but little or none is present in the cerebrospinal fluid. They accumulate mainly in lung, liver, spleen, and kidney. Studies have demonstrated a correlation between the time the drug remains in the liver and the duration of the hypoprothrombinemic effect. The considerable individual variation in the half-life of dicumarol has been attributed to genetic factors (Vesell and Page, 1968). Vitamin K administration does not alter the half-life of dicumarol in plasma.

There is a considerable lag (24 to 72 hours) between the time of peak plasma concentration and the therapeutic response to oral anticoagulants as measured by the peak effect on prothrombin time (Table 65–4, page 1361). The delay is largely a manifestation of the time required for the depletion of circulating clotting factors and the time required for the establishment of plateau concentrations of drugs with relatively long half-lives. The duration of response is directly proportional to the half-life of the drug in the plasma. The larger the initial dose (loading dose) of the drug, the sooner the desired therapeutic response is attained; however, the size of the dose must be limited so that the maximal response is not excessive.

Dicumarol and warfarin are hydroxylated to inactive compounds by enzymes of the hepatic endoplasmic reticulum. These metabolites and traces of the parent drugs are excreted in the urine. Some unabsorbed dicumarol appears in the feces. The coumarin anticoagulants pass the placental barrier. The normally low prothrombin levels of the newborn may in this way be further reduced. Severe hypoprothrombinemia with cerebral injury has been reported in the newborn infant whose mother received dicumarol *ante partum*. These drugs are also secreted in the milk, although prothrombin times are not known to be significantly altered in nursing infants whose mothers receive full therapeutic doses.

Preparations, Route of Administration, and Dosage. *Dicumarol,* U.S.P. is available in 25-, 50-, and 100-mg tablets and capsules. The recommended dosage schedule is 300 mg the first day, 200 mg the second day, and an average maintenance dose of 75 mg per day (range, 25 to 150 mg), selected on the basis of the therapeutic response. *Warfarin Sodium,* U.S.P. (COUMADIN, PANWARFIN), is available in tablets containing 2, 2.5, 5, 7.5, 10, and 25 mg of the drug as well as an injectable preparation (vials of 50 or 75 mg with ampuls of sterile water). An initial dose of 40 to 60 mg has been commonly used, followed by a daily maintenance dose of 2 to 15 mg. However, O'Reilly and Aggeler (1968) and subsequently others reported a satisfactory response with

a daily dose of 10 to 15 mg for 3 to 5 days *without* a loading dose. It is now accepted practice to avoid a loading dose in order to reduce the danger of hemorrhage, especially in those patients who may prove to be unusually sensitive to the drug. In rare individuals, there is a genetically determined resistance to oral anticoagulants and the dose must be accordingly increased (*see* O'Reilly, 1971). The oral route is used almost exclusively, and only one dose is given daily. The absolute necessity for monitoring the intensity of the anticoagulant effect by means of prothrombin time determination is discussed below.

Toxic Effects. In man, toxic effects other than hemorrhage are seldom seen during dicumarol or warfarin therapy. Occasionally, anorexia, nausea, vomiting, and diarrhea are encountered. A variety of cutaneous lesions has also been reported, including purpura, urticaria, and alopecia. Necrosis of the breast and skin has been observed, and rarely the toes turn purple. Bleeding is the outstanding toxic effect, and may even occur with conventional therapeutic doses and with prothrombin and whole-blood clotting times within the usual expected range. The incidence of hemorrhage is 2 to 4%. *It cannot be emphasized too strongly that treatment of each patient is a highly individualized matter. The patient on anticoagulant therapy must be followed by means of prothrombin time tests and observed carefully for any development of bleeding tendency.*

Bleeding is most common from mucous membranes, skin, and the gastrointestinal and genitourinary tracts. Most frequently encountered is asymptomatic hematuria, which is not fatal and not followed by impairment of renal function. However, intrarenal hematoma and renal colic associated with hematuria may occur. Also seen are ecchymosis, epistaxis, bleeding gums, and hemoptysis. Cerebral hemorrhage is not uncommon in oral anticoagulant–treated patients with subacute bacterial endocarditis, although otherwise rare. Pulmonary interstitial hemorrhage has been reported, and it may be confused clinically with pulmonary embolism. Extensive uterine bleeding has also been observed. It is generally agreed that any hepatic damage occurring in patients without preexisting liver disease is purely secondary to local hemorrhage in the liver or hypoxia from hemorrhagic anemia. Patients have been maintained on therapy for a number of years without hepatic or renal impairment. About 25% of all deaths from therapy with coumarin drugs are due to massive gastrointestinal bleeding, usually from unsuspected peptic ulceration or neoplasm. Indeed, occult carcinoma is often first detected because of bleeding that develops during oral anticoagulant drug therapy.

The *treatment of hemorrhage* caused by therapy with oral anticoagulants first involves immediate withdrawal of the drug. Prothrombin time will usually return to normal, and mild bleeding will cease. For severe hemorrhage, *vitamin K_1* is administered intravenously. Vitamin K_3 (menadione) is of no value under the circumstances. Cessation of bleeding and normal prothrombin times are evident within a few hours after vitamin K_1 is given. This form of treatment should be reserved for severe cases, since the patient then may be refractory for many days to renewed oral anticoagulant therapy. Available preparations and doses of vitamin K are discussed in Chapter 77. Severe hemorrhage may necessitate the transfusion of fresh whole blood or plasma, or banked plasma. If available, a commercial plasma concentrate of factor IX (also rich in factors II, VII, and X) may be administered. The reports of a "rebound" hypercoagulable state resulting from too rapid withdrawal of oral anticoagulant drugs, particularly when coupled with the administration of vitamin K, are controversial. Most authorities are of the opinion that the drug can be withdrawn abruptly with safety; this is in agreement with the fact that it takes several days for the requisite clotting factors to be synthesized in the liver and delivered to the circulation.

Precautions and Contraindications. It is imperative that suitable laboratory facilities be available for accurate control of therapy with coumarin drugs. In addition, a suitable preparation of vitamin K should be available, as well as whole fresh blood or plasma for emergency transfusion. Oral anticoagulants are contraindicated in hemorrhagic tendencies, blood dyscrasias, ulcerative lesions of the gastrointestinal tract, diverticulitis, colitis, subacute bacterial endocarditis, threatened abortion, recent operations on the brain or spinal cord, regional and lumbar-block anesthesia, vitamin K deficiency, and severe hepatic or renal disease. A moderate degree of renal failure is not a contraindica-

tion on a short-term, inpatient basis. It is inadvisable to carry out long-term therapy in a chronic alcoholic, in an individual who may require intensive salicylate therapy, or in cases of malignant hypertension and active tuberculosis. Oral anticoagulant therapy during pregnancy carries a significant hemorrhagic risk for the fetus. Douglas (1962) has expressed the opinion that anticoagulants should not be given to pregnant women. It has been suggested that warfarin therapy during pregnancy may be the cause of an embryopathy, chondroplasia punctata (*see* Becker *et al.*, 1975; Shaul *et al.*, 1975; Warkany, 1975). Patients with congestive heart failure frequently become more sensitive to the drug; an appropriate reduction in dosage may be necessary. As discussed above, interaction between anticoagulants and other drugs must always be considered.

As a precaution, a patient on anticoagulant therapy should carry on his person a notice to this effect (MEDALERT bracelet, wallet card) to alert medical and paramedical personnel should an emergency occur. These drugs should be used only in patients in whom a high degree of compliance can be expected. A written list of directions and warnings should be supplied to the patient, and one should make certain that the instructions are fully understood.

Therapeutic Uses. The clinical uses of dicumarol and warfarin are discussed later in this chapter.

OTHER ORAL ANTICOAGULANTS

As already stated, the pharmacological properties of the oral anticoagulants do not differ greatly from one drug to another. In Table 65-4 can be found their relative durations of action, potency, and side effects. In the following sections, the clinically used coumarin and indandione derivatives are discussed only insofar as they differ from dicumarol and warfarin. More extensive information on these drugs has been presented by Douglas (1962), Poller (1962), and Jaques (1965). Because of the similar nature of all the oral anticoagulants there are few criteria for deciding which one to use clinically. Due to greater degree of control, most clinicians in the United States prefer warfarin.

Phenprocoumon, N.F. This substance, also known as LIQUAMAR, is one of the longest acting of the oral anticoagulants. Peak prolongation of prothrombin time is usually seen in 48 to 72 hours, and the normal value does not return for 1 to 2 weeks. There is a certain amount of danger inherent in the use of such

Table 65–4. DURATION OF ACTION, DOSAGE, AND SIDE EFFECTS OF ORAL ANTICOAGULANTS

DRUG	TRADE NAMES	PEAK PROTHROM-BIN-TIME EFFECT (hr)	DURATION OF EFFECT * (days)	INITIAL DOSE † (mg)	DAILY MAINTENANCE DOSE (mg)	SIDE EFFECTS AND TOXICITY ‡
Dicumarol		36–48	5–6	300, first day; 200, second day	25–150	See text
Warfarin	COUMADIN, PANWARFIN	36–72	4–5	50	2–15	See text
Phenprocoumon	LIQUAMAR	48–72	7–14	21, first day; 9, second day; 3, third day	1–4	Diarrhea, dermatitis
Acenocoumarol	SINTROM	36–48	1½–2	16–28, first day; 8–16, second day	2–10	Mouth ulceration, gastrointestinal disturbances
Phenindione	DANILONE, HEDULIN	24–48	1–4	200, first day; 100, second day	50–100	Leukopenia, agranulocytosis, pyrexia, rashes, jaundice, hepatitis, diarrhea, paralysis of accommodation, oral ulcers, nephropathy, red-orange urine
Diphenadione	DIPAXIN	24–48	15–20	20–30, first day; 10–15, second day	2.5–5	Nausea
Anisindione	MIRADON	24–72	1½–3	300, first day; 200, second day; 100, third day	25–250	Red-orange urine

* After cessation of maintenance medication.
† Loading dose not essential.
‡ In addition to hemorrhagic phenomena.

a long-acting drug, particularly if toxicity occurs; also the return of prothrombin time to normal when vitamin K is given is more difficult to achieve when phenprocoumon has been administered. Side effects are rare; the one usually reported is diarrhea, which disappears upon withdrawal of the drug. Phenprocoumon is available for oral use in 3-mg tablets.

Acenocoumarol, N.F. This substance is also known as SINTROM. Its onset of action is approximately the same as that of dicumarol. Its duration is shorter, however, and recovery is complete 36 to 48 hours after the drug is withdrawn. Acenocoumarol is largely excreted by the kidneys, in unchanged form. The drug is available in 4-mg tablets. The reported toxic effects include ulceration of the mouth and gastrointestinal irritation.

Phenindione, N.F. The hypoprothrombinemic effect of certain indandione derivatives was first recognized over 25 years ago. Since then, phenindione has become a widely used anticoagulant, mainly outside the United States. Both its onset and duration of action are shorter than those of dicumarol and warfarin. A therapeutically effective prothrombin time is attained in 24 to 48 hours. After discontinuation of maintenance therapy, the prothrombin time returns to normal in 1 to 4 days. Although the exact metabolic route of phenindione is unknown, a metabolic product excreted by the kidneys colors the urine red-orange. This coloration is of no clinical importance, but it may be alarming to the patient who is unable to distinguish it from hematuria. Acidification of the urine destroys this color, thus differentiating it from hematuria. There are numerous reports of sensitivity reactions developing during phenindione therapy. The most common of these are rash, pyrexia, and leukopenia; occasionally leukocytosis occurs. These reactions are accompanied by fever, malaise, and headache. The rash is usually erythematous and macular, but occasionally papular, and may become confluent with scaling and itching. Rarely, it progresses to exfoliative dermatitis. Serious renal damage with extensive tubular necrosis has been reported. Albuminuria and massive edema have also been observed. Other recorded toxic effects include diarrhea, paralysis of accommodation, and blurred vision. Most of these effects disappear upon withdrawal of the drug. There have been several reports of hepatitis and agranulocytosis. The incidence of hypersensitivity phenomena is 1.5 to 3.0%. Unfortunately many deaths have occurred from these toxic reactions. It is recommended that use of the drug be limited to patients exhibiting sensitivity to other oral anticoagulants.

Phenindione, also known as DANILONE and HEDULIN, is available for oral use in 20- and 50-mg tablets.

Diphenadione, N.F. Following the advent of phenindione, diphenadione was introduced into medicine. Prothrombin times in the therapeutic range are attained in 24 to 48 hours; however, its duration of action is one of the longest among the oral anticoagulants, 15 to 20 days. The drug is far less toxic than phenindione; occasional nausea is the only

reported side effect. *Diphenadione* (DIPAXIN) is available for oral use in 5-mg tablets.

Anisindione. This compound is also known as MIRADON. It has an action similar to that of phenindione, and the drug produces a red-orange color in alkaline urine. The only reported toxicity is dermatitis; however, the drug has not had such extensive use as phenindione. A therapeutic prothrombin time response is achieved in 24 to 72 hours, and the prothrombin time returns to normal about 36 to 72 hours after the peak effect. Anisindione is available for oral use in 50-mg tablets.

LABORATORY CONTROL OF ANTICOAGULANT MEDICATION

Heparin. *The whole-blood clotting time* (Lee-White time) is an indication of the overall coagulability of the blood and is usually a satisfactory method for measuring the effect of heparin and for adjusting its dosage. The clotting time normally is between 5 and 10 minutes, and should be kept at two to three times normal for a proper therapeutic effect. The test should be performed by the same person for the results to be reliable. It should be done just before the next intravenous dose of heparin is scheduled. The whole-blood activated partial thromboplastin time (known as the PTT time) is more accurate; the PTT should be kept at twice normal, when the test is done 1 hour prior to the next scheduled dose of heparin.

Oral Anticoagulants. The oldest and by far the most widely used method for the control of oral anticoagulant therapy is the *one-stage prothrombin time* (PT), or Quick time. This procedure is sensitive to the levels of factors II, V, VII, and X. *Normal human plasma usually has a PT of about 12.0 (11.0 to 13.0) seconds.* It must be pointed out that, because of variations in technic and reagents, the prothrombin clotting times obtained are relevant only for a particular laboratory and a particular day. The PT for an individual on oral anticoagulants should be two to two and one-half times that of the control. At the onset of oral anticoagulant therapy, daily prothrombin times should be determined. As the response of the patient becomes established, determinations can be made at less frequent intervals. However, even after the regimen is established for long-term treatment, the test should be done at least once a month. Since heparin interferes with the PT determinations, it is advisable to allow a lapse of at least 5 hours after the intravenous administration of heparin and 24 hours after subcutaneous injection before taking the first blood sample.

THERAPEUTIC USES OF HEPARIN AND ORAL ANTICOAGULANTS

Both heparin and the oral anticoagulants are useful in the *prevention* and *treatment* of a variety of *thromboembolic disorders.* Since *heparin* is almost immediately both anticoagulant and antithrombotic, it is of prophylactic and therapeutic value in both venous and arterial thrombosis. Although the *oral anticoagulants* are similarly effective in venous thromboembolic disorders, they are less useful for those occurring in the arterial system. The formation and structure of venous thrombi (red clots, stasis thrombi) resemble those clotting events occurring *in vitro,* whereas arterial clot formation (red thrombus with white head) occurs in a fast-flowing circulation and is critically dependent on initial platelet aggregation, with subsequent adherence of leukocytes to the platelet nidus and development of a fibrin meshwork with entrapped erythrocytes. This process is prevented or arrested by heparin but much less successfully by oral anticoagulants. In any event, clinical experience involving hundreds of thousands of cases over a period of 4 decades has unequivocally established the value of anticoagulant drugs in the management of a variety of thromboembolic conditions.

The complexities of blood coagulation problems are dramatically illustrated by the clinical history of John Hageman, the index patient with Hageman trait—the inherited deficiency of factor XII. He never did show evidence of a bleeding tendency, and in 1968 he died suddenly of a pulmonary embolism after sustaining fractures of the pelvis (Ratnoff *et al.,* 1968).

The following indications for anticoagulants are here considered: (1) myocardial infarction, (2) rheumatic heart disease, (3) cerebrovascular disease, (4) venous thrombosis and pulmonary embolism, and (5) disseminated intravascular coagulation. Detailed discussion is beyond the scope of this textbook. More extensive presentations are those of Sherry and colleagues (1969), Biggs, (1972), and Hume and coworkers (1972).

Heparin vs. Oral Anticoagulants. The question naturally arises whether heparin or an oral anticoagulant is preferable. It is not possible to arrive at a clear-cut answer because each drug has its own distinct advantages and disadvantages, and the value of each varies from one clinical situation to another. Heparin has the important advantage of exerting its effects almost immediately after intravenous injection, while even the most rapidly acting oral anticoagulant requires at least 18 hours to elevate prothrombin time to therapeutic levels. Therefore, therapy is typically instituted by the administration

of heparin, followed in 2 or 3 days, if necessary, by an oral anticoagulant. When both drugs are used, the heparin is continued until the oral anticoagulant takes effect, usually within 2 days. The necessity for parenteral administration places heparin in a disadvantageous position for long-term therapy, for which oral drugs are almost always preferred. The long duration of effect of the oral anticoagulants allows for easier maintenance of a steady anticoagulant effect. Because of its *in-vitro* effects, heparin is employed to prevent clotting in the extracorporeal circulation necessary for hemodialysis and for open-heart surgery. Heparin therapy is quite expensive, and its use almost always requires hospitalization. The oral anticoagulant drugs are inexpensive.

Myocardial Infarction. The acute phase of myocardial infarction was one of the earliest disorders in which therapy with dicumarol was employed (Butt *et al.,* 1941; Lehmann, 1942). It was appreciated that, while anticoagulants obviously could not reduce the immediate mortality due to massive infarction, they should certainly lessen the incidence of secondary thromboembolism. The earlier findings led to a number of large-scale clinical investigations, some of which indicated a marked decrease in mortality (Wright *et al.,* 1948; Tulloch and Gilchrist, 1950), whereas no effect on mortality was seen in others (Honey and Truelove, 1957; Wasserman *et al.,* 1966). However, even when immediate mortality was unaffected, the incidence of subsequent peripheral venous thrombosis and pulmonary embolism was reduced. Griffith and associates (1962) evaluated separately "good-risk" and "bad-risk" patients, those with initially good and poor prognoses, respectively, and found that the mortality rate of "bad-risk" patients was lowered to a greater extent. They recommended, however, that all cases be treated with anticoagulants because a certain percentage of "good-risk" patients suddenly are at grave risk. Gifford and Feinstein (1969) evaluated 32 published studies on anticoagulant therapy in acute myocardial infarction and found that many of the favorable conclusions were not based on sound scientific and medical principles. Drapkin and Merskey (1972) reported that anticoagulants administered to patients after acute myocardial infarction lowered the high mortality rate (31%) among women but had no effect on the lower mortality rate (16%) in men. The current rationale for the use of anticoagulants in this disorder is based mainly on the likelihood of a reduction of the incidence of peripheral venous thrombosis and pulmonary embolism, particularly in patients who are apt to be bedridden for a long period. Ebert (1972) recommends anticoagulants in patients with a large myocardial infarct, a history of previous infarction, congestive heart failure, or complications requiring prolonged bed rest. Currently nearly all patients with acute coronary thrombosis receive heparin for a week to 10 days. If oral anticoagulants are also employed, it is questionable whether they should be continued for more than 2 to 3 months, unless specifically indicated. Careful laboratory control and close observation of the patient will minimize risk of hemorrhage. It is to be remembered that about 50% of all cases of acute myocardial infarction are *not* associated with evidence of coronary thrombosis; indeed, the latter may be secondary to the infarction caused by severe arteriosclerotic coronary narrowing.

Rheumatic Heart Disease. The occurrence of emboli associated with rheumatic heart disease is considered by some to be a major indication for long-term oral anticoagulant treatment. Prophylactic therapy before the first occurrence of an embolic episode has been recommended in severe mitral valve disease. Such a procedure is advisable in patients with atrial fibrillation or an enlarged left atrium. Anticoagulants may be of value in patients who have undergone cardiac surgery for valve replacement, but the newer valves are much less likely to cause embolic episodes and such therapy is now often omitted.

Cerebrovascular Disease. Approximately 20% of cerebrovascular accidents are hemorrhagic, and anticoagulants are of course contraindicated in such cases. For this reason, this therapy should be withheld until the nature of the condition is determined to be cerebral thrombosis. Transient ischemic attacks have been treated with heparin followed by oral anticoagulants, but there is little real proof of efficacy. A stroke in progress is usually an indication for heparin therapy, but a completed stroke is not treated by anticoagulants. These drugs are of value in cerebral embolism from peripheral sites because further emboli may follow; however, it is best to withhold therapy for 3 to 4 days since development of a hemorrhagic infarct is possible. Most stroke clinics do not use oral anticoagulants prophylactically.

Venous Thrombosis and Pulmonary Embolism. Heparin was the first anticoagulant drug to be used in the treatment of *peripheral venous thrombosis* (Murray and Best, 1938), and its value in this condition and in the prevention of pulmonary embolism was recognized immediately. With the introduction of the oral anticoagulants, it was possible to treat a far greater number of cases of venous thrombosis. In a study involving over 1000 cases, Zilliacus (1946) reported a great decrease in the incidence of pulmonary embolism and mortality among patients given heparin or dicumarol. Subsequently, numerous other reports have confirmed the effectiveness of anticoagulants in venous thrombosis, and it is generally agreed that, of all the indications for anticoagulant therapy, this condition is the most readily affected. Of particular importance has been the prevention of postoperative and recumbency thrombosis, the incidence of which has been reduced drastically by the use of anticoagulant drugs. The prophylactic use of *oral* anticoagulants immediately prior to and after surgery waned as surgical technics improved and other measures gained acceptance (early ambulation, bed exercises, elastic stockings, leg elevation, etc.). However, heparin has recently gained prominence for *prophylactic* use, particularly in older patients undergoing surgery and in those prone to thrombosis for other reasons. It is given in "sub-anticoagulant" doses (5000 units subcutaneously) 2 hours before operation and every 12 hours postoperatively for 7 days. Such "low-dose" therapy is based on the theory that a much lower concentration of heparin is necessary to *prevent* activation of factor X than is necessary to *inhibit* factor X already activated. The reduction in incidence of deep-vein thrombosis is most encouraging (from a control incidence of 40% to one as low as 10% in some series). Laboratory control is not necessary since the commonly employed laboratory tests do not reveal effects on the blood clotting mechanisms from the recommended doses; more sensitive procedures are needed. (*See* Kakkar *et al.,* 1972; Gallus *et al.,* 1973; Clagett and Salzman, 1974; Sagar, 1974; Kakkar, 1975.)

So important is immediate and adequate anticoagulation in *pulmonary embolism* that heparin therapy should be started promptly and maintained for a week or more even though oral anticoagulants may also be given (*see* above). Treatment with the oral drugs is continued for at least several weeks, but the exact duration must be determined for each patient, depending on the etiology of the pulmonary embolism.

Miscellaneous Uses. Heparin may be of some value in selected cases of *disseminated intravascular coagulation* (DIC), a syndrome in which the blood is incoagulable and there are extensive small intravascular fibrin thrombi. DIC occurs in patients desperately ill from a variety of serious causes. The widespread development of thrombi consumes the normal clotting factors, and the resultant bleeding then becomes an additional grave problem. Heparin sometimes arrests the intravascular coagulation and thereby allows restoration of normal amounts of coagulation factors, in which case bleeding may cease. However, bleeding may sometimes be aggravated by heparin, or DIC may occur during the course of heparin therapy (*see* Klein and Bell, 1974). The administration of protamine may then be necessary. It is most difficult to select DIC cases for heparin therapy and to forecast the outcome. (*See* Minna *et al.,* 1974.)

The treatment of *severe burns* with heparin has been reported (Saliba *et al.,* 1973); the apparent success of such therapy warrants further investigation.

II. Thrombolytic Agents

Heparin and the oral anticoagulants are inactive against thrombi once they have formed. The blood normally has a lytic system that slowly dissolves fibrin clots; blood plasminogen (profibrinolysin), when activated, releases plasmin, the active fibrinolytic (thrombolytic) substance. However, plasmin normally acts slowly and does not dissolve organized older clots. A most important area of research is the development of substances with direct fibrinolytic activity or that activate or enhance the body's fibrinolytic system. Two such activators currently under intensive study are briefly described here. Unfortunately, neither is totally satisfactory and they are not available for general use. They must be given intravenously, are not devoid of untoward effects, and must be administered within 12 to 14 hours of clot formation or embolization in order to exert any salutary effect.

Urokinase. This substance is found in human urine. It has been concentrated, purified, and tested in the treatment of acute pulmonary embolism. In a nationwide trial, urokinase plus subsequent heparin therapy was shown to accelerate significantly the resolution of pulmonary thromboemboli when compared to heparin alone (Urokinase Pulmonary Embolism Trial, 1973). But the incidence of bleeding was higher with the combined therapy (45%) than with heparin alone (27%). It is recommended that urokinase therapy in pulmonary embolism be reserved for high-risk patients over 50 years of age and for patients with a history of prior cardiopulmonary disease or concurrent severe hemostatic abnormalities. It must be given early, preferably within 12 hours of the onset of the embolic episode. Observations on arterial and venous thromboembolic disorders other than pulmonary embolism suggest a potential role for urokinase therapy. Further clinical investigation is warranted, but at present urokinase must be considered to be strictly an experimental drug. It is very expensive.

Streptokinase. This product of beta-hemolytic streptococci is also an activator of plasminogen. Some success has been reported in its use for thrombolytic therapy in pulmonary embolism (Hirsh et al., 1968). The results of ten large, multicenter, controlled clinical trials of streptokinase in acute myocardial infarction have been critically assessed by Simon and coworkers (1973); the reported results range from a 50% decrease in mortality to no significant effect. The lack of uniformity of experimental conditions among the various investigational groups precludes valid comparisons. Nevertheless, streptokinase deserves further study for its potential value in the treatment of acute myocardial infarction as well as acute pulmonary embolism. The first controlled randomized comparison of urokinase and streptokinase demonstrated some superiority of urokinase to facilitate resolution of pulmonary emboli; however, there was no significant difference in mortality. Both drugs were superior to heparin alone (Urokinase Pulmonary Embolism Trial Study Group, 1974). Streptokinase is an experimental drug and not available commercially. Locally acting preparations of streptokinase plus streptodornase are discussed in Chapter 47.

Aminocaproic Acid, N.F. (AMICAR), is the specific antidote for an overdose of a fibrinolytic agent. It is available as an injection (250 mg/ml), a syrup (250 mg/ml), and tablets (500 mg). The usual dose is 5 g initially (orally or intravenously) followed by 1.25 g per hour until bleeding is under control. The dosage should not exceed 30 g in 24 hours. Rapid intravenous administration should be avoided to prevent hypotension, bradycardia, and other arrhythmias.

III. Drugs Affecting Platelet Function

The drugs discussed thus far in this chapter have little or no discernible effect on platelet function when used in normal therapeutic dosage. However, since platelets play a primary role in the initiation of thrombus formation, particularly in the arterial system, attention has been drawn to several drugs that appear to have effects on platelets that can be utilized clinically.

Aspirin decreases platelet aggregation and thereby prolongs bleeding time (Weiss et al., 1968; Sutor et al., 1971; Mielke et al., 1973). The effect persists for several days. Sodium salicylate and acetaminophen do not elicit this response in normal doses. Insight into the mechanism of this effect of aspirin comes from studies by Zucker and Peterson (1967), who demonstrated a block in ADP-mediated secondary aggregation of platelets, and by Rosenberg and associates (1971), who showed that the inhibition of collagen-induced aggregation was associated with acetylation of platelets by aspirin (*see* page 331). The widespread use of aspirin has led to some concern that this drug in donor blood may be detrimental to the hemostatic mechanisms of blood recipients. However, hemostasis and platelet aggregation in such recipients are unaffected by donor blood containing aspirin (Stuart et al., 1972). Despite the lack of definitive clinical evidence of the value of aspirin in the prevention of coronary and cerebral thrombosis, it is being widely used for this purpose, particularly in patients who are at risk. Large-scale, controlled, long-term prospective studies are required to assess the status of aspirin as a useful drug for prophylaxis of arterial thrombosis.

Sulfinpyrazone, a uricosuric agent, prolongs platelet survival in man. It has been shown to block platelet aggregation in response to collagen and antigen-antibody complexes but not in response to ADP or thrombin (Packham et al., 1967). This appears to be related to a diminished release of ADP and 5-hydroxytryptamine. The drug is being studied for its prophylactive value in thromboembolic disorders. Its pharmacology is presented in Chapter 41.

Dipyridamole, a coronary vasodilator agent, also inhibits ADP-induced platelet aggregation. It has received considerable attention as a prophylactic agent in thromboembolic disorders (*see* Mustard et al., 1972). Alone, it did not alter the course of acute myocardial infarction or deep-vein thrombosis, or prevent thromboembolism occurring after hip surgery, or benefit patients with transient cerebral ischemic attacks. On the other hand, the shortened platelet-survival time occurring in some patients with prosthetic heart valves was returned to normal by use of the drug. Some promise is also apparent when dipyridamole is used in conjunction with an oral anticoagulant; however, bleeding tendencies increase and care must be taken in combined therapy. The use of dipyridamole and aspirin together is also being explored. Clearly, extensive controlled clinical trials are necessary. The pharmacology of dipyridamole is presented in Chapter 34.

Dextran 40, a plasma expander described in Chapter 36, interferes with the function and aggregation of platelets by coating them. It also coats erythrocytes and forms complexes with plasma clotting proteins, and thereby prevents rouleau formation and sludging and inhibits clotting. In addition, dextran 40 affects blood rheology by decreasing blood viscosity. Excessive doses of the polymer can cause hemorrhage by virtue of its antithrombotic effect, and an increase in circulating blood volume may be harmful to patients with congestive heart failure. Dextran 40 has been employed with encouraging results in early thrombophlebitis, pulmonary embolism, and fat embolism. It may be given concurrently with anticoagulant drugs. *Dextran 40* (GENTRAN 40, LMD, RHEOMACRODEX) is given intravenously, 10 ml/kg (10% solution), over a period of several hours; subsequently this dose is repeated every other day, or one half this amount may be given every day. Renal and cardiac functions must be carefully monitored. The drug may cause allergic reactions, occasionally severe. Some clinicians prefer to use *dextran 70* for the prevention of thrombosis. A controlled comparison of dextran 70 with low-dose subcutaneous heparin showed the latter regimen to be superior in the prevention of deep-vein thrombosis in postoperative patients (Multi-unit Controlled Trial, 1974). The status and dangers of dextran 40 therapy of thromboembolic disorders have been reviewed by Data and Nies (1974).

The great potential value of drugs that directly affect platelet function strongly motivates the development and clinical trial of such compounds. Progress in this direction has been slow, however, and the use of these agents must be considered to be on an experimental basis. The dosages of these drugs that have been used for antiplatelet effects are: aspirin, 1 g per day; dipyridamole, 400 mg per day; sulfinpyrazone, 400 to 800 mg per day. They have been used alone as well as in conjunction with heparin and the oral anticoagulants. Since the use of these compounds for this purpose has not yet been established, it is recommended that the doses be adjusted to the requirements of each patient. The status of drugs that inhibit platelets in the management of thrombosis has been reviewed by Didisheim and coworkers (1974).

Other drugs that alter platelet function and thus affect hemostasis are discussed in reviews by Mustard and associates (1972), Weiss (1972), and Zucker (1972), and in the monograph edited by Sherry and Scriabine (1974).

Anderson, N. G., and Fawcett, B. An antichylomicronemic substance produced by heparin injection. *Proc. Soc. exp. Biol. Med.,* **1950,** *74,* 768–771.

Becker, M. H.; Genieser, N. B.; Finegold, M.; Miranda, D.; and Spackman, T. Chondrodysplasia punctata. Is maternal warfarin therapy a factor? *Am. J. Dis. Child.,* **1975,** *129,* 356–359.

Biggs, R.; Denson, K. W. E.; Akman, N.; Borrett, R.; and Hadden, M. Antithrombin III, antifactor Xa and heparin. *Br. J. Haemat.,* **1970,** *19,* 283–305.

Bingham, J. B.; Meyer, O. O.; and Pohle, F. J. Studies on the hemorrhagic agent 3, 3′-methylenebis (4-hydroxycoumarin). I. Its effect on the prothrombin and coagulation time of the blood of dogs and humans. *Am. J. med. Sci.,* **1941,** *202,* 563–578.

Butt, H. R.; Allen, E. V.; and Bollman, J. L. A preparation from spoiled sweet clover [3,3′-methylene-*bis*-(4-hydroxycoumarin)] which prolongs coagulation and prothrombin time of blood. *Proc. Staff Meet. Mayo Clin.,* **1941,** *16,* 388–395.

Cauwenberge, H. van, and Jaques, L. B. Haemorrhagic effect of ACTH with anticoagulant. *Can. med. Ass. J.,* **1958,** *79,* 536–540.

Charles, A. F., and Scott, D. A. Studies on heparin: preparation of heparin. *J. biol. Chem.,* **1933,** *102,* 425–429.
———. Studies on heparin. IV. Observations on the chemistry of heparin. *Biochem. J.,* **1936,** *30,* 1927–1933.

Clagett, G. P., and Salzman, E. W. Prevention of venous thromboembolism in surgical patients. *New Engl. J. Med.,* **1974,** *290,* 93–96.

Crafoord, C. Preliminary report on post-operative treatment with heparin as a preventive of thrombosis. *Acta chir. scand.,* **1937,** *79,* 407–426.

Data, J. L., and Nies, A. S. Dextran 40. *Ann. intern. Med.,* **1974,** *81,* 500–504.

Davie, E. W., and Ratnoff, O. D. Waterfall sequences for intrinsic blood clotting. *Science, Wash.,* **1964,** *145,* 1310–1312.

Drapkin, A., and Merskey, C. Anticoagulant therapy after acute myocardial infarction. *J. Am. med. Ass.,* **1972,** *222,* 541–547.

Duggan, M., and Morgan, C. Heparin: a cause of priapism? *Sth. med. J., Nashville,* **1970,** *63,* 1131–1134.

Ebert, R. V. Use of anticoagulants in acute myocardial infarction. *Circulation,* **1972,** *45,* 903–910.

Eika, C. Inhibition of thrombin-induced aggregation of human platelets by heparin and antithrombin III. *Scand. J. Haemat.,* **1971,** *8,* 250–256.

Ellison, N.; Ominsky, A.; and Wollman, H. Is protamine a clinically important anticoagulant? *Anesthesiology,* **1971,** *35,* 621–629.

Fadali, M. A.; Ledbetter, M.; Papacostas, C. A.; Duke, L. J.; and Lemole, G. M. Mechanism responsible for the cardiovascular depressant effect of protamine sulfate. *Ann. Surg.,* **1974,** *180,* 232–235.

Ford, H. C., and Bailey, R. E. The effect of heparin on aldosterone secretion and metabolism in primary aldosteronism. *Steroids,* **1966,** *7,* 30–40.

Gallus, A. S.; Hirsh, J.; Tuttle, R. J.; Trebilcock, R.; O'Brien, S. E.; Carroll, J. J.; Minden, J. H.; and Hudecki, S. M. Small subcutaneous doses of heparin in prevention of venous thrombosis. *New Engl. J. Med.,* **1973,** *288,* 545–551.

Gifford, R. H., and Feinstein, A. R. A critique of methodology in studies of anticoagulant therapy for acute myocardial infarction. *New Engl. J. Med.,* **1969,** *280,* 351–357.

Griffith, G. C.; Leak, D.; and Hegde, B. Conservative anticoagulant therapy of acute myocardial infarction. *Ann. intern. Med.,* **1962,** *57,* 254–265.

Hahn, P. F. Abolishment of alimentary lipemia following injection of heparin. *Science, N. Y.,* **1943,** *98,* 19–20.

Hirsh, J.; Hale, G. S.; McDonald, I. G.; McCarthy, R. A.; and Pitt, A. Streptokinase therapy in acute major pulmonary embolism: effectiveness and problems. *Br. med. J.,* **1968,** *4,* 729–734.

Honey, G. E., and Truelove, S. C. Prognostic factors in myocardial infarction. *Lancet,* **1957,** *1,* 1155–1161, 1209–1212.

Hougie, C. Anticoagulant action of protamine sulphate. *Proc. Soc. exp. Biol. Med.,* **1958,** *98,* 130–133.

Howell, W. H., and Holt, E. Two new factors in blood coagulation: heparin and antithrombin. *Am. J. Physiol.,* **1918,** *47,* 328–341.

Jick, H.; Slone, D.; Borda, I. T.; and Shapiro, S. Efficacy and toxicity of heparin in relation to age and sex. *New Engl. J. Med.,* **1968,** *279,* 284–286.

Kakkar, V. V. Deep vein thrombosis; detection and prevention. *Circulation,* **1975,** *51,* 8–19.

Kakkar, V. V.; Corrigan, T.; Spindler, J.; Fossard, D. P.; Flute, P. T.; Crellin, R. Q.; Wessler, S.; and Yin, E. T. Efficacy of low doses of heparin in prevention of deep-vein thrombosis after major surgery. A double-blind, randomised trial. *Lancet,* **1972,** *2,* 101–106.

Klein, H. G., and Bell, W. R. Disseminated intravascular coagulation during heparin therapy. *Ann. intern. Med.,* **1974,** *80,* 477–481.

Kubacz, G. J. Femoral and sciatic compression neuropathy. *Br. J. Surg.,* **1971,** *58,* 580–582.

Lehmann, J. Hypoprothrombinemia produced by methylene-*bis*-(hydroxycoumarin): its use in thrombosis. *Lancet,* **1942,** *1,* 318–321.

Lowenthal, J., and Birnbaum, H. Vitamin K and coumarin anticoagulants: dependence of anticoagulant effect on inhibition of vitamin K transport. *Science, Wash.,* **1968,** *164,* 181–183.

Lowenthal, J., and MacFarlane, J. A. Use of a competitive vitamin K antagonist, 2-chloro-3-phytyl-1,4-naptho-quinone, for the study of the mechanism of action of vitamin K and coumarin anticoagulants. *J. Pharmac. exp. Ther.,* **1967,** *157,* 672–680.

Macfarlane, R. G. An enzyme cascade in the blood clotting mechanism, and its function as a biochemical amplifier. *Nature, Lond.,* **1964,** *202,* 498–499.

Meyer, O. O.; Bingham, J. B.; and Axelrod, V. H. Studies on the hemorrhagic agent, 3-3'-methylenebis (4-hydroxy-coumarin). II. The method of administration and dosage. *Am. J. med. Sci.,* **1942,** *204,* 11–21.

Mielke, C. H.; Ramos, J. C.; and Britten, A. F. H. Aspirin as an antiplatelet agent: template bleeding time as a monitor of therapy. *Am. J. clin. Path.,* **1973,** *59,* 236–242.

Morris, C. M.; Kirumba, J.; Furneaux, R. W.; and Ham, J. M. Lipoprotein-lipase responses to heparin. *Br. J. Surg.,* **1971,** *58,* 147–148.

Multi-unit Controlled Trial. Heparin versus dextran in the prevention of deep-vein thrombosis. *Lancet,* **1974,** *2,* 118–120.

Murray, D. W. G., and Best, C. H. The use of heparin in thrombosis. *Ann. Surg.,* **1938,** *108,* 163–177.

Murray, D. W. G.; Jaques, L. B.; Perrett, T. S.; and Best, C. H. Heparin and the thrombosis of veins following injury. *Surgery, St. Louis,* **1937,** *2,* 163–187.

O'Brien, J. R.; Etherington, M.; Jamieson, S.; and Klaber, M. R. Platelet function in venous thrombosis and low-dosage heparin. *Lancet,* **1972,** *1,* 1302–1305.

Olsson, P.; Lagergren, H.; and Ek, S. The elimination from plasma of intravenous heparin: an experimental study on dogs and humans. *Acta med. scand.,* **1963,** *173,* 619–630.

O'Reilly, R. A. Vitamin K in hereditary resistance to oral anticoagulant drugs. *Am. J. Physiol.,* **1971,** *221,* 1327–1330.

O'Reilly, R. A., and Aggeler, P. M. Studies on coumarin anticoagulant drugs: initiation of warfarin therapy without a loading dose. *Circulation,* **1968,** *38,* 169–177.

Packham, M. A.; Warrior, E. S.; Glynn, M. F.; Senyi, A. S.; and Mustard, J. F. Alteration of the response of platelets to surface stimuli by pyrazole compounds. *J. exp. Med.,* **1967,** *126,* 171–188.

Prandoni, A., and Wright, I. The anti-coagulants: heparin and the dicoumarin-3,3'methylene-*bis*-(4-hydroxycoumarin). *Bull. N.Y. Acad. Med.,* **1942,** *18,* 433–458.

Quick, A. J. The development and use of the prothrombin tests. *Circulation,* **1959,** *19,* 92–96.

Ratnoff, O. D.; Busse, R. J., Jr.; and Sheon, R. P. The demise of John Hageman. *New Engl. J. Med.,* **1968,** *279,* 760–761.

Rawls, W. B. A five year study of adrenal steroid compounds. *J. Am. Geriat. Soc.,* **1955,** *3,* 614–622.

Robinson, D. S., and Harris, P. M. The production of lipolytic activity in the circulation of the hind limb in response to heparin. *Q. Jl exp. Physiol.,* **1959,** *44,* 80–90.

Roderick, L. M. The pathology of sweet clover disease in cattle. *J. Am. vet. med. Ass.,* **1929,** *74,* 314–326.

———. A problem in the coagulation of the blood, "sweet clover disease of cattle." *Am. J. Physiol.,* **1931,** *96,* 413–425.

Rosenberg, F. J.; Gimber-Phillips, P. E.; Groblewski, G. E.; Davison, C.; Phillips, D. K.; Goralnick, S. J.; and Cahill, E. D. Acetylsalicylic acid: inhibition of platelet aggregation in the rabbit. *J. Pharmac. exp. Ther.,* **1971,** *179,* 410–418.

Rosenberg, R. D. Heparin action. *Circulation,* **1974,** *49,* 603–605.

———. Actions and interactions of antithrombin and heparin. *New Engl. J. Med.,* **1975,** *292,* 146–151.

Saeed-Uz-Zafar, M.; Miller, J. M.; Breneman, G. M.; and Mansour, J. Observations on the effect of heparin on free and total thyroxine. *J. clin. Endocr. Metab.,* **1971,** *32,* 633–640.

Sagar, S. Heparin prophylaxis against fatal postoperative pulmonary embolism. *Br. med. J.,* **1974,** *2,* 153–155.

Saliba, M. J.; Dempsey, W. C.; and Kruggel, J. L. Large burns in humans. Treatment with heparin. *J. Am. med. Ass.,* **1973,** *225,* 261–269.

Schofield, F. W. A brief account of a disease of cattle simulating hemorrhagic septicaemia due to feeding sweet clover. *Can. vet. Rec.,* **1922,** *3,* 74.

———. Damaged sweet clover: the cause of a new disease in cattle simulating hemorrhagic septicaemia and blackleg. *J. Am. vet. med. Ass.,* **1924,** *64,* 553–575.

Shah, D. V., and Suttie, J. W. The effect of vitamin K and warfarin on rat liver prothrombin concentrations. *Archs Biochem. Biophys.,* **1972,** *150,* 91–95.

Shaul, W. L.; Emery, H.; and Hall, J. G. Chondrodysplasia punctata and maternal warfarin use during pregnancy. *Am. J. Dis. Child.,* **1975,** *129,* 360–362.

Stuart, M. J.; Murphy, S.; Oski, F. A.; Evans, A. E.; Donaldson, M. H.; and Gardner, F. H. Platelet function in recipients of platelets from donors ingesting aspirin. *New Engl. J. Med.,* **1972,** *287,* 1105–1109.

Sutor, A. H.; Bowie, E. J. W.; and Owen, C. A. Effect of aspirin, sodium salicylate and acetaminophen on bleeding. *Mayo Clin. Proc.,* **1971,** *46,* 178–181.

Thompson, R.; Ludewig, R.; Wagensteen, S.; and Rudolf, L. Effect of heparin on wound healing. *Surgery Gynec. Obstet.,* **1972,** *134,* 22–26.

Tulloch, J. A., and Gilchrist, A. R. Anticoagulants in treatment of coronary thrombosis. *Br. med. J.,* **1950,** *2,* 965–971.

Urokinase Pulmonary Embolism Trial Study Group. Urokinase-streptokinase embolism trial. Phase 2 results. *J. Am. med. Ass.,* **1974,** *229,* 1606–1613.

Vesell, E. S., and Page, J. G. Genetic control of dicumarol levels in man. *J. clin. Invest.,* **1968,** *47,* 2657–2663.

Warkany, J. A warfarin embryopathy? *Am. J. Dis. Child.,* **1975,** *129,* 287–288.

Wasserman, A. J.; Gutterman, L. A.; Yoe, K. B.; Kemp, V. E.; and Richardson, D. W. Anticoagulants in acute myocardial infarction: failure of anticoagulants to alter mortality in randomized series. *Am. Heart J.,* **1966,** *71,* 43–49.

Weiss, H. J.; Aledort, L. M.; and Kochwa, S. The effect of salicylates on the hemostatic properties of platelets in man. *J. clin. Invest.,* **1968,** *47,* 2169–2180.

Woldow, A.; Lopez, R. H.; and Goldberg, H. Effect of single injection of heparin on postprandial hyperlipemia. *Am. J. Cardiol.,* **1962,** *10,* 815–818.

Wright, I. S.; Marple, C. D.; and Beck, D. F. Report of

the committee for the evaluation of anticoagulants in the treatment of coronary thrombosis with myocardial infarction. *Am. Heart J.,* **1948,** *36,* 801–815.

Zilliacus, H. On the specific treatment of thrombosis and pulmonary embolism with anticoagulants, with particular reference to post-thrombotic sequelae. *Acta med. scand.,* **1946,** Suppl. 171, 1–221.

Zucker, M. B., and Peterson, J. Inhibition of adenosine diphosphate–induced secondary aggregation and other platelet functions by acetylsalicylic acid. *Proc. Soc. exp. Biol. Med.,* **1967,** *127,* 547–551.

Monographs and Reviews

Biggs, R. (ed.). *Human Blood Coagulation, Haemostasis and Thrombosis.* Blackwell Scientific Publications, Oxford, **1972.**

Didisheim, P.; Kazmier, F. J.; and Fuster, V. Platelet inhibition in the management of thrombosis. *Thromb. Diath. haemorrh.,* **1974,** *32,* 21–34.

Douglas, A. S. *Anticoagulant Therapy.* Blackwell Scientific Publications, Oxford, **1962.**

Ehrlich, J., and Stivala, S. S. Chemistry and pharmacology of heparin. *J. pharm. Sci.,* **1973,** *62,* 517–544.

Engelberg, H. *Heparin: Metabolism, Physiology and Clinical Application.* Charles C Thomas, Pub., Springfield, Ill., **1963.**

Esnouf, M. P., and Macfarlane, R. G. Enzymology and the blood clotting mechanism. *Adv. Enzymol.,* **1968,** *30,* 255–315.

Hume, M.; Levitt, S.; and Thomas, D. P. *Venous Thrombosis and Pulmonary Embolism.* Harvard University Press, Cambridge, Mass., **1972.**

Ingram, G. I. C. Anticoagulant therapy. *Pharmac. Rev.,* **1961,** *13,* 279–328. (252 references.)

Jaques, L. B. *Anticoagulant Therapy: Pharmacological Principles.* Charles C Thomas, Pub., Springfield, Ill., **1965.**

———. The pharmacology of heparin and heparinoids. *Prog. med. Chem.,* **1967,** *5,* 139–198.

Kazal, L. Theories of blood coagulation. Properties and interaction of blood clotting factors. *Ann. clin. lab. Sci.,* **1971,** *1,* 139–154.

Koch-Weser, J., and Sellers, E. M. Drug interactions with coumarin anticoagulants. *New Engl. J. Med.,* **1971,** *285,* 487–498, 547–558.

Kralt, T., and Claassen, V. Anticoagulants structurally related to vitamin K. In, *Drug Design,* Vol. 3. (Ariens, E. J., ed.) Academic Press, Inc., New York, **1972,** pp. 189–203.

Link, K. P. The anticoagulant from spoiled sweet clover. *Harvey Lect.,* **1943–1944,** *39,* 162–216.

Mammen, E. F. Physiology and biochemistry of blood coagulation. In, *Thrombosis and Bleeding Disorders.* (Bang, U. N.; Beller, F. K.; Deutsch, E.; and Mammen, E. F.; eds.) Academic Press, Inc., New York, **1971,** pp. 1–56.

Merskey, C., and Drapkin, A. Anticoagulant therapy. *Blood,* **1965,** *25,* 567–596.

Minna, J. D.; Robboy, S. J.; and Colman, R. W. *Disseminated Intravascular Coagulation in Man.* Charles C Thomas, Pub., Springfield, Ill., **1974.**

Mustard, J. F.; Kinlough-Rathbone, R. L.; Jenkins, C. S. P.; and Packham, M. A. Modification of platelet function. *Ann. N.Y. Acad. Sci.,* **1972,** *201,* 343–359.

O'Reilly, R. A., and Aggeler, P. M. Determinants of the response to oral anticoagulant drugs in man. *Pharmac. Rev.,* **1970,** *22,* 35–96.

Poller, L. *The Theory and Practice of Anticoagulant Treatment.* John Wright & Sons, Ltd., Bristol, **1962.**

Seegers, W. H. Blood clotting mechanisms: three basic reactions. *A. Rev. Physiol.,* **1969,** *31,* 269–288.

Sherry, S.; Brinkhous, K. M.; Genton, E.; and Stengle, J. M. (eds.). *Thrombosis.* National Academy of Sciences, Washington, D.C., **1969.**

Sherry, S., and Scriabine, A. (eds.). *Platelets and Thrombosis.* University Park Press, Baltimore, **1974.**

Simon, T. L.; Ware, J. H.; and Stengle, J. M. Clinical trials of thrombolytic agents in myocardial infarction. *Ann. intern. Med.,* **1973,** *79,* 712–719.

Urokinase Pulmonary Embolism Trial. A national cooperative study. *Circulation,* **1973,** *47,* Suppl. II, II-1–II-108.

Weiss, H. J. The pharmacology of platelet inhibition. *Prog. Hemostasis Thromb.,* **1972,** *1,* 199–231.

Wessler, S. Anticoagulant therapy—1974. *J. Am. med. Ass.,* **1974,** *228,* 757–761.

Zucker, M. B. *In vitro* studies of the platelet aggregation-release reaction. *Curr. Concepts cerebrovasc. Dis. Stroke,* **1972,** *7,* 21–24.

Hormones and Hormone Antagonists

INTRODUCTION

Alfred G. Gilman and Ferid Murad

Preparations containing the active principles of the endocrine glands may be classified from the pharmacological viewpoint as drugs. Whereas most drugs are substances foreign to the body, the hormones are natural secretions of the endocrine glands and exert important functional effects upon other tissues. Consequently, there has been a tendency to place hormones in a different category, although there is really no valid reason for doing so; indeed, some endocrine preparations have unobtrusively broken down this arbitrary distinction. For example, epinephrine is much more frequently viewed as a powerful sympathomimetic drug than as a hormone of the adrenal medulla.

Pharmacological studies on the actions of drugs of endocrine origin have contributed greatly to an understanding of the normal functions of the endocrine glands. Conversely, much can be learned about the effects of a hormonally active drug by observing the consequences of a deficiency or an excess of the hormone in question. The diverse actions of cortisol and its congeners, for instance, are strikingly illustrated by the changes from the normal shown by patients suffering from adrenal deficiency on the one hand and by patients with oversecretion on the other.

It is useful to preserve the distinction between hormones and other active substances of animal origin. By definition, a hormone is a substance secreted by a specific tissue and transported to a distance where it exerts its effect upon other specific tissues. One can quibble with the details of this definition in some instances; for example, growth hormone seems to act upon so many tissues that the term *specific* becomes imprecise, and the distance traveled by the hypothalamic regulatory hormones is rather short. But there are many active substances derived from tissues or body fluids that may not serve any important regulatory function or that may act predominantly at the immediate site of release and thus do not meet the definition of a hormone. The latter compounds are designated as *autacoids* and are discussed in an earlier section (Chapters 29 and 30). Finally, there are some hormones the action of which in man is unknown or poorly understood. Melanocyte-stimulating hormone clearly functions as a hormone in causing darkening of the skin of frogs in response to a black background; although the substance abounds in the mammalian hypophysis, its secretion, transport, and site of action are as obscure as is its function.

To an extent not seen with other drugs, hormones can effect extraordinary changes. The transformation of a tadpole into a frog is hardly more remarkable than the metamorphosis of a myxedematous patient when treated with thyroid. The undeveloped or hypogonadal individual can in some cases be made to resemble the sex to which he should belong and to behave accordingly. Treatment with hydrocortisone can help the arthritic to walk and assist the asthmatic to breathe.

Analogs of the hormones, synthetic compounds resembling the natural products but differing from them in some important respects, have often proven more useful in therapeutics than have the hormones themselves. One aim in endocrinology is the isolation, identification, and synthesis of the active principles of each of the endocrine glands. Sometimes, when these formidable efforts have been crowned with success, the product has been found to be of little use in therapy. It may prove inactive when given by mouth, as are the catecholamines, or it may also be so rapidly degraded that unless injected frequently little effect can be achieved, as in the case of the natural sex hormones. The design of synthetic analogs, compounds altered enough to outwit degradative enzymes but not enough to confuse the receptor sites, is one of the major contributions to endocrine therapy. A striking example was the discovery, 40 years ago, of diethylstilbestrol, a cheap synthetic substance that duplicates the actions of estrogen when given orally. In a number of instances the synthetic analogs, by their more desirable properties, represent striking improvements upon nature.

Other groups of useful drugs can inhibit hormone synthesis or antagonize the cellular actions of hormones. The antithyroid drugs provided the initial example of the first type; they selectively inhibit the synthesis of thyroid hormone, and this action makes them effective in the treatment of hyperthyroidism. More recently, equally specific substances have been developed to block one or another step in the synthesis of the hormones of the adrenal cortex.

Direct inhibition of the action of a hormone upon its receptor sites has been achieved experimentally in several instances and has been put to good use in isolated cases. Inhibition of the action of estrogen seems to account for the remarkable therapeutic effectiveness of clomiphene in reproductive disorders in women. By relieving the inhibitory influence of estrogen upon the pituitary, the substance acts to promote the secretion of gonadotropins.

Usually, when considering the clinical applications of the hormones, one thinks first of their use in replacement therapy—treatment of Addison's disease, myxedema, and so forth, with the appropriate drug. However, if the normal regulatory interactions of an endocrine system are understood, hormones can be exploited for a variety of additional therapeutic and even diagnostic purposes. Regulation of the endocrine systems characteristically takes place on a multitude of levels. Many systems are ultimately responsive to neural or neuroendocrine control of either a stimulatory or inhibitory nature or both. A change in the magnitude of such control results in an appropriate alteration of secretion in a dependent target, and this secretion may serve as the immediate regulator of yet another endocrine organ. The final hormonal secretion in such a chain may "feed back" at any level to regulate the intensity of a controlling signal. Such "feedback" is predominantly negative; thus, a hormone can inhibit its own synthesis and secretion when its critical concentration is exceeded. Positive feedback systems are, however, occasionally utilized. Blood-borne chemicals the concentrations of which are subject to hormonal regulation are also used extensively as feedback regulators in such control systems. This knowledge is useful clinically, and it must be applied in the interpretation of a patient's basal laboratory data and in the performance of a variety of provocative tests of endocrine function. Similarly, therapeutic maneuvers also depend on these regulatory interactions. For example, the activity of the adrenal cortex can be suppressed by an adrenocorticosteroid through inhibition of the secretion of corticotropin; ovulation, if unwanted, can be abolished by ovarian hormones that suppress the secretion of hypophyseal gonadotropins.

The last 15 years have witnessed an explosive increase in knowledge of the mechanisms of hormone action, and this is understood in detail for some endocrine secretions. In a number of cases, hormones interact with specific receptors in cellular plasma membranes that are linked to the enzyme adenylate cyclase, discovered by Sutherland and Rall. This enzyme is stimulated or inhibited in some way by the hormone-receptor complex, and the result is an altered rate of synthesis of cyclic adenosine $3',5'$-monophosphate (cyclic AMP) from adenosine triphosphate (ATP) (Figure XVII-1). Cyclic AMP then acts as the intracellular mediator for the hormone, and the system can thus be viewed as a mechanism for transferring and amplifying the information inherent in the extracellular hormone. Cyclic AMP regulates a variety of intracellular processes, and the ultimate effects are dependent on the cell's capacity to respond—its differentiated repertoire. The mechanism of cyclic AMP action in many cases involves the

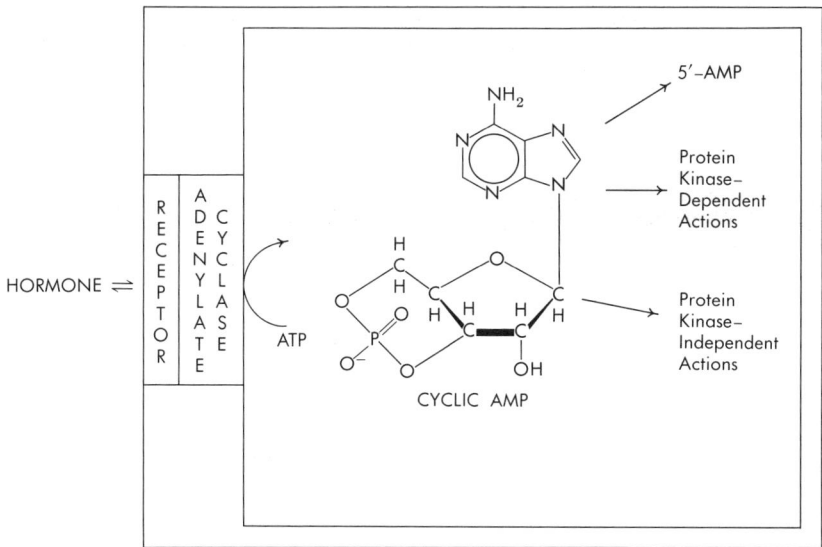

Figure XVII-1. *The role of cyclic AMP in hormonal action.*

activation of protein kinases that phosphorylate cellular constituents and alter the rates at which processes involving these constituents proceed. Cyclic AMP is metabolized to 5'-AMP by specific phosphodiesterases, and inhibitors of these enzymes, such as methylxanthines, can sometimes exert hormone-like effects. The hormones discussed in the following chapters that appear to use this mechanism include the trophic hormones of the adenohypophysis, the melanocyte-stimulating hormones, some of the hypothalamic regulatory hormones, glucagon, parathyroid hormone, and calcitonin.

The steroid hormones and perhaps the thyroid hormones utilize a different mechanism of information transfer. They gain access to the intracellular compartment and bind to cytoplasmic receptor proteins. Following this interaction they are transported to the nucleus and bind there, still accompanied by the initial receptor protein. Changes in various nuclear functions appear to follow. The remaining hormones, which in many ways appear to constitute a group, include growth hormone, somatomedin, prolactin, insulin, and other proteins (not discussed here) such as nerve growth factor. Their mechanisms of action remain more obscure; however, in view of their protein nature, it is appealing to envision interaction with the plasma membrane and the subsequent generation of "second messengers" analogous to cyclic AMP.

Finally, mention should be made of recent methodological advances that have greatly facilitated research and clinical applications in endocrine pharmacology. Foremost, perhaps, is radioimmunoassay, pioneered by Berson and Yalow. Using this sensitive and specific technic, the physician now has rapid access to a wealth of analytical information about his patient. Advances in peptide and protein chemistry are also outstanding. The technics for determination of amino acid sequences developed by Edman and for automated peptide synthesis developed by Merrifield are making the clinical use of various peptides a practical possibility.

CHAPTER

66 ADENOHYPOPHYSEAL HORMONES AND RELATED SUBSTANCES

Alfred G. Gilman and Ferid Murad

The hormones of the adenohypophysis are important more for their potentialities as therapeutic agents of the future than for any established place they may have as remedies for common diseases. By their secretion they regulate many important processes in the body; not only are they the mediators of various disturbances in the endocrine system but they are themselves sensitive to the aberrations of systemic disease. Their secretion is profoundly influenced by many hormones of the peripheral endocrine glands as well as by stimulatory and inhibitory hormones of hypothalamic origin. Similarly striking effects are exerted by many drugs, including natural hormones, hormonal analogs, and inhibitors of hormone synthesis and action.

Three vitally critical endocrine systems are dependent upon the adenohypophysis, not only for the delicate regulation of their secretions but also for the trophic effect necessary for the maintenance of these systems. Without the gonadotropins the entire reproductive system fails and, consequently, the capacity of higher forms of life to perpetuate themselves. Normal growth and development are impossible without growth hormone and thyrotropin; these hormones with those from the adrenal cortex are essential for energy metabolism—the assimilation, storage, and combustion of fuel.

Among the vertebrates, ten adenohypophyseal hormones are recognized: growth hormone, prolactin, two gonadotropins, thyrotropin, corticotropin, two melanocyte-stimulating hormones, and two lipotropins. Of these, the first six are demonstrably important in man. However, it would be premature to deny the possibility that there may be others. With the exception of corticotropin and the melanocyte-stimulating hormones, none has been synthesized, and all the information that has been gained about them has had to be derived from extracts of the pituitary refined to varying degrees. Since the pituitary gland is rich in polypeptides and small proteins, as might be expected of an organ devoted to the synthesis of such a profusion of peptide hormones, the isolation of pure compounds can be a formidable undertaking. Some of these peptides doubtless represent degraded or unfinished precursors of the hormones, and it would be surprising if some of them did not have unusual biological properties.

Interpretation is further complicated by the sharing of an action between two hormones or the expression of an action that may be irrelevant to a hormone's normal function. For example, corticotropin shares with melanocyte-stimulating hormone the property of darkening the skin of melanophore-bearing animals, and several adenohypophyseal hormones are lipolytic. For the want of a better term, these properties have been referred to as overlapping activities or side effects, but many of these relationships can now be understood by study of the chemistry and apparent evolution of the adenohypophyseal hormones.

Recent elucidation of the amino acid sequences of the recognized hormones of the adenohypophysis has shed light on the amazing diversity of the organ (see Li, 1972). Three groups of hormones are apparent (Table 66–1). The members of the first group, growth hormone and prolactin, show considerable sequence homology, a fact that accounts for both the lactogenic activity of growth hormone and the delayed recognition of human prolactin as a distinct entity. Amino acid sequences are said to be homologous if the corresponding amino acid residues are either identical or replaced with similar amino acids. It is hypothesized that both proteins evolved from a single, perhaps prolactin-like molecule. The gonadotropins and thyrotropin (TSH) constitute the second

Table 66-1. PROPERTIES OF THE PROTEIN HORMONES OF THE ADENOHYPOPHYSIS AND PLACENTA

HORMONE—SPECIES	AMINO ACID RESIDUES	MOLECULAR WEIGHT	DISULFIDE BONDS	% CARBOHYDRATE AND SITES OF ATTACHMENT	PEPTIDE CHAINS	COMMENTS
Group 1						
Growth hormone—human	191	22,000	2	0	1	Human growth hormone and human placental lactogen—83% identity of amino acid sequence
Prolactin—ovine	198	23,000	3	0	1	Human growth hormone (1–50) and human prolactin (1–50)—50% homology of amino acid sequence
Placental lactogen—human	191	22,000	2	0	1	
Group 2						
Luteinizing hormone—ovine	α-98 β-119	30,000	α-5 β-6	16% α-56,82 β-13	2	Glycoproteins with nonidentical subunits (α and β); biological specificity in β subunit; Ovine LH-$\alpha \cong$ Bovine TSH-α
Follicle-stimulating hormone—ovine	?	32,000	?	18%	2	Human LH-α: 89 residues / Human LH-β: 115 residues / Human TSH-β: 112 residues
Thyrotropin—bovine	α-96 β-113	28,000	α-5 β-6	13% α-56,82 β-23	2	
Chorionic gonadotropin—human	α-92 β-139	57,000	?	31% α-52,78 β-13,28,118,121,123	2	
Gonadotropin of pregnant mares' serum	?	53,000	?	47%	2	
Group 3						
Corticotropin—human	39	4500	0	0	1	Group shares a common heptapeptide: Met-Glu-His-Phe-Arg-Trp-Gly
α-Melanocyte-stimulating hormone—human	13	1650	0	0	1	Corticotropin (1–13) = α-MSH / β-Lipotropin (1–58) = γ-Lipotropin
β-Melanocyte-stimulating hormone—human	22	2650	0	0	1	
β-Lipotropin—ovine	90	9500	0	0	1	
γ-Lipotropin—ovine	58	5800	0	0	1	

group, closely related glycoprotein hormones. These complex proteins are each composed of two different noncovalently linked subunits (α and β). Remarkably, the α subunits of the group are nearly identical, while specificity resides in unique β subunits. Thus, hybrid hormones can be formed; for example, the α subunit of luteinizing hormone (LH) can be combined with the β subunit of TSH to yield a molecule with thyroid-stimulating activity. Since the β subunits of LH and TSH also show significant homology with the α subunits, it has been proposed that all these peptide chains evolved from a common α subunit-like ancestor. The remaining group comprises corticotropin, the melanocyte-stimulating hormones, and the so-called lipotropins. As part of their sequence, these hormones all share a common heptapeptide (Table 66–1), which itself displays lipolytic and melanocyte-stimulating activity. More extensive structural similarities between members of this group are discussed below and in Chapter 70.

The synthesis of hormones of the first two groups described is not unique to the adenohypophysis, since at least one representative of each group is also produced in quantity by the placenta. The placental lactogen is very similar to growth hormone, and the amino acid sequence of chorionic gonadotropin closely resembles that of LH. A chorionic thyrotropin has also recently been described.

History. As the name *pituitary* implies, it was first thought to be a source of phlegm to moisten the membranes of the nose. But when careful dissection showed it to be closed up in a bony box, it was regarded as a vestigial structure with no function at all. The first tribute of significance was paid in 1887 by Minkowski, who associated the features of acromegaly with a tumor of the gland. Although the cause-and-effect relationship was by no means clear at first, by 1900 Hutchinson was able to conclude that ". . . in the pituitary body we appear to have a sort of growth-regulating centre for the entire body, the disturbance of which in early life will produce the phenomena of gigantism, and in later life those of acromegaly."

The induction of growth by the injection of pituitary extract was first accomplished in rats by Evans and Long in 1921; concurrently they noted for the first time the gonadotropic effect. During most of the 1920s, the pituitary was thought to contain just two hormones.

Hypophysectomy as an experimental approach, introduced by Aschner in 1909 and later used by Dandy, Cushing, and their associates, was first carried out in the dog. This proved to be an unfortunate choice; the operation was difficult, some dogs became obese, and effects on growth were not prominent. The operation did establish that survival was possible and that the gonads atrophied. It was not until 1927 that the true consequences of hypophysectomy in mammals were clarified by Smith's classical experiments in the rat (Smith, 1927, 1930). The obesity was shown to be a consequence of damage to the hypothalamus and could thus be induced whether the pituitary was concurrently extirpated or not. The failure of growth and the atrophy of the gonads, thyroid, and adrenals that followed hypophysectomy were correctable by hypophyseal implants. This work was anticipated 10 years earlier by parallel studies on the hypophysectomized tadpole wherein the several functions of the three parts of the pituitary were correctly assigned (*see* Allen, 1917). Smith's work in the rat was quickly followed by the definition of a thyrotropic hormone by Aron and by Loeb and Bassett in 1929, the preparation of an adrenotropic extract by Collip and coworkers in 1933, and the preparation and naming of prolactin by Riddle and associates in the same year. The year 1933 was further notable for the publication by Fevold and coworkers of the separate identity of a follicle-stimulating and a luteinizing hormone.

This proliferation of proposed adenohypophyseal hormones included several that have not survived as entities. The extent to which the actions of the proposed factors are accounted for by the recognized hormones is, however, a subject of continuing investigation, and the possibility of additional hormones remains.

During the 1950s and 1960s, the development of sophisticated technics of protein purification and analysis (countercurrent distribution, ion-exchange chromatography, gel filtration, electrophoresis) greatly facilitated research in this area. Such purification of the hormones provided better products for biological investigation, and the great importance of species specificity came to be recognized. It was most strikingly shown in the case of growth hormone, only the product from the pituitaries of primates being active in monkeys and man (Knobil and Greep, 1959; Raben, 1959). This reopened the field of clinical investigation to the development of effective and new therapeutic applications. Of immense, recent significance in this regard are technics and instruments for automated amino acid sequence analysis and solid-phase peptide synthesis. These capabilities are now making the clinical use of synthetic peptides feasible.

When it was recognized in the early 1940s that the major vascular supply to the anterior pituitary was made up of blood that had already traversed the capillaries of the median eminence of the hypothalamus, the proper setting for the neurohumoral control of the gland was evident. It has now come to be generally recognized that hypothalamic cells transmit to the anterior lobe individual factors that regulate the secretion of each of its hormones, and this is presently an area of intense research activity (*see* page 1391).

Hypopituitarism. A great deal has been learned about the normal actions of the pituitary hormones by observing the consequences of pituitary deficiency, whether from congenital absence of the gland or secondary to its destruction or removal.

Hypopituitarism in the Adult. The consequences of loss of the adenohypophysis are best shown in nature by the post-partum necrosis described by Sheehan (*see* Sheehan and Summers, 1949). This can amount to complete destruction of the anterior lobe, and the patient may die, presumably from adrenal deficiency. If she survives, recovery of strength and well-being is slow and incomplete. The infant cannot be nursed, as there is no milk; the pubic hair, if shaved, does not grow back, and axillary and other body hair later falls out; the menstrual periods do not resume, and the genital tract atrophies. The skin becomes thin, soft, and finely wrinkled, assuming a waxy pallor from the mild anemia and the loss of dermal pigment. Libido and the sense of sexual identification are lost. There is reduced thyroid function with sensitivity to cold, lack of sweating, low rate of metabolism, low uptake of radioiodine by the thyroid, and increased plasma cholesterol. Various indices of adrenocortical function also show a profound deficit. There is sensitivity to physical stress and to the stress of infection, and there may be frequent episodes of collapse or severe illnesses. Body weight is not grossly altered, but there is a tendency toward plumpness. Survival for 30 years or longer without diagnosis or specific treatment is not unusual. Sometimes one or more of the clinical features are not noted, presumably because pituitary destruction is not complete.

Hypopituitarism from local tumors often seems to affect the secretion of some hormones before others. The menstrual cycle may stop several years before the thyroid or adrenals are affected, or failure of growth may be the first manifestation. There may be features of advanced hypopituitarism at a time when the thyroid seems still to be normal. By contrast, the consequences of hypophysectomy in man resemble the complete picture of Sheehan's syndrome. In recent years, this operation has been carried out extensively for the palliative treatment of cancer and for the amelioration of some of the concomitants of diabetes mellitus.

When hypopituitarism in the adult is treated by replacement with a glucocorticoid, thyroid, and the appropriate sex hormone, complete clinical recovery is apparently achieved. The individual still lacks growth hormone, melanocyte-stimulating hormone, prolactin, and all other factors that have been detected in the adenohypophysis. What deficits are still to be found when only the hormones of the thyroid, adrenal cortex, and gonad are supplied? This question can be answered only by further investigation, because clinically such patients look like normal people, and they feel well and are capable of normal activities. Gametogenesis is lacking, but in isolated cases this has been shown to be correctable with human gonadotropins. Other deficits are by no means obvious. There may be a tendency to excess fat, sparse body and scalp hair, somewhat reduced dermal pigment, and the eyes may seem a bit sunken—little else.

Hypopituitary Dwarfism. Failure of the pituitary to develop during embryogenesis is, surprisingly, compatible with almost normal longevity; the manifestations are ascribable to the lack of the adeno-

hypophyseal hormones, especially growth hormone. Formerly, the condition was recognized only after several years of life, and it was thought that the pituitary might not be necessary for growth until the age of 2 to 4 years. Studies on the growth hormone in the blood of human fetuses and newborns have now shown that the pituitary actively secretes growth hormone early in gestation (Kaplan *et al.,* 1972).

The most striking feature of the condition is, as the name implies, failure to grow normally. At the age of earliest recognition the child is small, with the deviation from the normal becoming more pronounced with advancing years. The dwarfism affects all parts of the body, and the individual comes to resemble a very small version of a normal child. Although growth is very slow, it does not cease; indeed, because it is not arrested by puberty as it is in the normal case, it continues throughout life and almost normal stature may eventually be achieved.

During the years of childhood, the defect in gonadotropic function cannot be recognized clinically and can be detected only by sensitive immunoassays of the blood for *gonadotropic hormones.* In the absence of these hormones there is no sexual development in later years. Although it can be shown that there is no *thyrotropin* or *corticotropin,* there is a small but important amount of activity on the part of the thyroid gland and the adrenal cortex. The dwarfing and retarded osseous development are not as extreme as in cretinism, nor does the hypopituitary dwarf show the mental retardation, the changes in the skin, or the facies of the cretin. However, thyroid function tests indicate hypoactivity, and the thyroid is easily stimulated by thyrotropin. The adrenal cortex is presumed to be usefully functional also, for quite apart from secretion of aldosterone, which does not require corticotropin, some capacity to make a glucocorticoid is presumed because so many bodily functions are not recognizably abnormal. Addisonian crises are not a feature of the condition, and the subjects withstand the stresses of life and of illness rather well. However, it can again be shown that adrenocortical secretions are deficient. The detection of such thyroid and adrenal deficiency helps to differentiate hypopituitarism from the host of other causes of dwarfism.

Hypersecretion of Pituitary Hormones. In acromegaly and in gigantism, the most prominent features are those of excessive action of growth hormone, but it is possible that other hormones are also secreted in excess. Thyrotropin in the blood has been found to be increased, and there is a higher incidence of goiter and enlargement of the adrenal cortex; sometimes lactation is noted. One form of Cushing's syndrome is caused by an oversecretion of corticotropin, and in this condition, as in acromegaly, a tumor of the pituitary is often responsible. Precocious sexual development in association with tumors at the base of the brain appears to be due to isolated hypersecretion of the gonadotropins. Excessive secretion of the several trophic hormones follows impaired function of the individual target glands, owing to the operation of the normal servomechanism; however, except for the above-mentioned conditions associated with tumors, primary overproduction of pituitary hormones is not recognized. Hyperthyroidism is an extremely rare consequence of overproduction of thyrotropin, and no pituitary tumors are known that *individually* oversecrete follicle-stimulating hormone, luteinizing hormone, or melanocyte-stimulating hormone.

GROWTH HORMONE

Chemistry. Of all the active principles of the anterior pituitary, growth hormone is easily the most abundant. In the human gland, up to 10% of the dry weight is growth hormone, and current methods of extraction obtain a high percentage of the hormone from the glands in a form suitable for human use.

Growth hormone is a simple protein of modest size, made up of a single chain of 191 amino acids. There are two intrachain disulfide bonds, and the complete amino acid sequence of the human hormone is known (Li *et al.,* 1966; Niall *et al.,* 1971). While the bovine and ovine hormones are very similar to the human protein in their general features, there are significant differences in primary structure. There is approximately 60% identity of their amino acid sequence with that of human growth hormone; the differences presumably account for their relative inactivity in man.

Recurring regions of amino acid sequence homology within the growth hormone molecule have led to the hypothesis that growth hormone (and the lactogenic hormones) have evolved from smaller ancestors by processes involving the tandem linkage of reduplicated genes (Niall *et al.,* 1971). This concept also suggests the possibility of an "active core" in these hormones. The identification of such an "active core" would be particularly worthwhile, since intact nonprimate growth hormones are poorly active in man. A relatively small active fragment should prove clinically useful, and synthesis might be practical. Promising in this regard are the studies of Sonenberg and coworkers (*see* Yamasaki *et al.,* 1972), who have isolated a 37 amino acid fragment of *bovine* growth hormone that retains growth-promoting activity in rats and has metabolic activity in man. It has also been demonstrated that limited enzymatic digestion of human growth hormone can lead to an increase in biological activity by almost an order of magnitude (Yadley *et al.,* 1973). This raises the possibility that pituitary growth hormone and that found in plasma could be a form of prohormone subject to peripheral alteration and activation. Perhaps consistent with this suggestion are the findings of a "big" growth hormone in the pituitary and plasma (Goodman *et al.,* 1972; Gordon *et al.,* 1973) and four "isohormones," separable by electrophoresis, which are present in nonhomogeneous growth hormone preparations (Yadley *et al.,* 1973). The proportion of these "isohormones" can be altered by treatment with the proteolytic enzyme plasmin.

Physiological Actions. The concept of a growth hormone sprang from clinical observations on gigantism and acromegaly and

was strengthened by the finding that crude extracts of the pituitary gland of the ox, when injected into dogs and rats, elicited increased growth.

Growth. In experiments on the effects of the hormone on growth, the rat has been the favored experimental animal because it is exceptional in several ways. The epiphyses of almost all the long bones remain open throughout life, and growth continues for as long as good nutrition and good health prevail. Maximal sensitivity to growth hormone is brought out when growth in young animals is arrested by hypophysectomy. The rat is also peculiar in responding indiscriminately to the growth hormone of all other mammals thus far explored. However, the response to human growth hormone is limited and seems to decline with continued treatment.

The stimulus to growth provided by growth hormone evidently affects just about every organ and tissue of the body, the possible exceptions in the rat, at least, being the brain and the eye. Thus, hypophysectomy during the early days of life in the rat is eventually fatal, seemingly because the growing brain cannot be accommodated in the dwarfed cranium. The other organs and tissues of the body respond to growth hormone by a proportional increase in size that is in keeping with the total increase in body weight. The growth of bones is reflected in increased body length; the skin and its appendages grow, and the skeletal muscles enlarge. The thoracic and abdominal viscera also grow, sometimes to a greater extent than the rest of the body. Growth of the thymus is a sensitive index of the action of growth hormone; like that of the lymph nodes, it can be countered by a direct action of the corticosteroids. Enlargement of the liver and increased cellular proliferation therein follow brief treatment with growth hormone, and accumulation of fat may augment somewhat the increase in weight. Effects on the size of the spleen are usually obscured by other factors that affect this organ, but the heart, lungs, kidneys, and gastrointestinal tract enlarge in response to growth hormone. There is also slight enlargement of the gonads, adrenals, and thyroid, probably attributable to growth hormone itself rather than to specific trophic hormones that contaminate some preparations.

Studies on the growth effects in other species have not been nearly as detailed as those in the rat; indeed, the animal that has been next best studied is the human being. Such investigation in man represents the first thorough exploration of the effects of growth hormone in the same species from which it was derived. Growth in the human being in response to human growth hormone has been studied largely in dwarfs, and particularly in hypopituitary dwarfs, in whom striking effects, amounting to therapeutic triumphs, have been achieved. The growth is normally proportioned, but there is no sexual maturation, splanchnomegaly, or disproportionate growth of skin or flat bones. No features of gigantism or acromegaly have yet been described, but prolonged treatment with large doses has not yet been attempted.

Effects on the Metabolism of Nitrogen. Growth connotes increased protoplasm and thus protein, the most abundant nitrogen-containing component of the body. It is to be expected that growth is associated with the accumulation of nitrogen in the organism; indeed, a positive nitrogen balance is the classical biochemical expression of growth. In several species, and under a variety of conditions, growth hormone has been shown to cause a retention of nitrogen, and this property has come to be equated with its anabolic effect.

However, it is difficult to measure growth by measuring the retention of nitrogen. Protein contains about 16% nitrogen and most tissue about 10 to 15% protein. The building-up of a kilogram of tissue, then, requires the retention of about 20 g of nitrogen. A rapidly growing boy during the peak of the puberal growth spurt gains, on the average, 15 lb a year. If one third of this is bone and fat, he acquires 10 lb, or 4.5 kg, of tissue containing about 100 g of nitrogen. To accomplish this, he need retain only 0.3 g of nitrogen per day. In careful metabolic studies in man, a positive balance of this magnitude is of borderline significance and would probably be obscured by many inevitable variables. For example, several hundred milligrams of nitrogen are lost each day by desquamation of the skin, sweating, attrition of hair and nails, and possibly exhalation of N_2. These cannot be readily measured and would cause an error in the calculation of balance. When growth hormone is given to human subjects in doses of 5 to 10 mg a day, a total of 3 to 5 g of nitrogen is retained daily—many times the amount needed for a normal rate of growth. Although prolonged balances have not been measured, evidently the effect is evanescent, and the site of storage of this extra nitrogen is unknown. The term *labile protein* has been used in this connection, but it has no enlightening significance.

Along with the retained nitrogen there is accretion of other constituents of tissue—sodium, chloride, potassium, phosphorus, and calcium. In the case of calcium, there is a paradoxical increase in the urinary loss of the element that is balanced by an augmented absorption from the intestinal tract.

Animal experiments have shown that treatment with growth hormone increases the transport of amino acids into tissues and accelerates their incorporation into protein. Thus, in man, one of the early actions of growth hormone is a decrease in the blood concentration of urea, evidently because of diversion of amino acids into anabolic pathways. A variety of anabolic effects can also be observed with isolated tissues incubated *in vitro,* and in this respect the hormone mimics the action of insulin. These anabolic effects likely reflect a hormonal action to increase selectively the rate of information flow from specific regions of DNA to RNA to protein. However, this statement must be made without prejudgment about the number and location of such controlled sites. Their understanding will await far more detailed analysis of the molecular biology of eukaryotic cells.

Effects on Metabolism of Carbohydrate and Lipid. Growth hormone has a number of important and complex effects on carbohydrate and lipid metabolism, most of which are poorly understood. Some of the reasons for this difficulty are obvious. A large number of hormones, notably growth hormone, insulin, glucocorticoids, catecholamines, and glucagon, play important roles in lipid, carbohydrate, and nitrogen homeostasis. As a first important approximation, insulin and growth hormone can be viewed as the major anabolic influences, with the glucocorticoids and catecholamines as their catabolic antagonists. However, the details are not that simple. Each hormone in fact exerts a number of effects at different sites. Their patterns of positive and negative interactions are intimately interwoven, and hormonal alliances shift from site to site. Feedback mechanisms bring direct and indirect secondary forces into play. Temporal separation of phenomena compounds the difficulty, with short-term effects being enforced or overcome by delayed actions that may result from even more complex hormone-cell interactions.

Although an oversimplification of the facts, it might be said that growth hormone seems to switch over the source of fuel for the body from carbohydrate to fat. From another aspect it might be concluded that, if insulin favors the use of sugar and its conversion to fat, growth hormone has just the opposite effect. However, both of these concepts have their limitations.

Houssay's important observation that hypophysectomy relieves the diabetes consequent upon removal of the pancreas did not establish that growth hormone is the responsible agent. Indeed, the work of Long and coworkers later proved that the adrenocorticosteroids are essential to the full expression of pancreatic diabetes. But Houssay showed that crude extracts of the pituitary given to his animals caused the diabetic state to return in full intensity (Houssay, 1942). Later work made it seem highly likely that the responsible agent in his extracts was growth hormone. Thus, from the earliest experiments in this area in the completely depancreatized animal it was clear that the *diabetogenic* action of growth hormone was not *just* an antagonism of insulin. However, in a great many experimental situations, growth hormone can be shown to oppose certain of the actions of insulin. Thus, treatment with growth hormone renders certain species of animals insensitive to insulin, reduces tolerance to glucose, and corrects the hypersensitivity of the hypophysectomized animal to insulin.

In certain species, notably the dog and the cat, growth hormone induces a fully diabetic state and, if injections are continued long enough, permanent diabetes associated with destruction of the beta cells of the pancreatic islets is induced. This drastic end point is far from understood and is evidently peculiar to the species mentioned. It is not known if there is mechanistic relevance to human diabetes.

In patients suffering from diabetes mellitus, growth hormone does exert a clear-cut diabetogenic effect that can be offset by a larger dose of insulin. Some patients with severe diabetes, hypophysectomized for the palliation of ocular or renal lesions and treated with small doses of insulin, have been found to be exquisitely sensitive to growth hormone. A small fraction of the therapeutic dose for promotion of growth can lead to severe intensification of hyperglycemia and ketosis. In the nondiabetic subject, on the other hand, large doses can be given without detectable effects upon tolerance to carbohydrate.

Louis and Conn (1972) have characterized a protein referred to as a *diabetogenic peptide* that causes hyperglycemia and hyperinsulinemia when administered to dogs or man. This material has a molecular weight of approximately 20,000 and can be isolated from the adenohypophysis or from the urine of certain diabetic patients. Interestingly, it is capable of antagonizing the effects of insulin on isolated muscle *in vitro* (Miller and Larner, 1972). It is unknown if there is a direct relationship between this material and growth hormone, although this would offer some appealing explanations.

The antagonism of insulin by growth hormone is, however, not always apparent. Following hypophysectomy there is a tendency toward hypoglycemia that is corrected by the dual administration of glucocorticoids and growth hormone. However, the acute administration of growth hormone does not cause prominent hyperglycemia and may in fact cause a paradoxical and transient insulin-like hypoglycemia. Another insulin-like action of growth hormone involves enhanced uptake of glucose by muscle *in vitro*. Perhaps similarly, hepatic and muscular glycogen stores are depleted after hypophysectomy, and glucocorticoids and growth hormone again suffice to promote glycogen deposition. Thus, growth hormone, glucocorticoids, and insulin all facilitate the storage of carbohydrate in the form of glycogen.

Young (1945) and Russell (1957) have provided extensive evidence in support of the concept that the prominent metabolic actions of growth hormone resemble those brought about by fasting, and they have suggested that increased secretion of the hormone may be of central importance in adaptation to lack of food. With fasting there is increasing intolerance to carbohydrate (hunger diabetes), inhibited lipogenesis, mobilization of fat, and ketosis, responses that can be evoked by growth hormone. In support of this concept, the concentration of circulating growth hormone increases in response to fasting (Roth *et al.*, 1963); it also increases with exercise, and hypoglycemia is a particularly potent stimulus. In teleological terms it is difficult to understand this response. Growth, in the sense of building of protoplasm, cannot take place without food, and one is led to imagine that, without growth hormone, tissue might be broken down during fasting and used indiscriminately for fuel. Growth hormone might hinder this and thereby enforce the use of fat instead.

The first, as well as a most consistent, effect of human growth hormone in man is an increase in free fatty acids in the blood (Raben and Hollenberg, 1959). The response begins about 2 hours after the injection and reflects enhanced mobilization of fatty acids from adipose tissue. On a restricted diet, the hypophysectomized animal loses less fat than does the normal (Lee and Ayres, 1936), but when growth hormone is given there is gain in weight and in length while the fat stores are depleted. Within a few hours of giving growth hormone to normal rats or mice, there is an increase in fat in the liver and it can be shown that this is derived from the depots. Other lipolytic agents, such as epinephrine, corticotropin, and thyrotropin, share this action, but only in the case of epinephrine does the effect seem to have physiological relevance.

Detailed studies have been carried out on the actions of hormones upon adipose tissue and upon isolated fat cells incubated in vitro. Insulin is antilipolytic and strongly stimulates the accumulation of glucose by adipose tissue, the conversion of glucose to fat and glycogen, and its oxidation to CO_2. Epinephrine and several adenohypophyseal hormones promote the hydrolysis of fat and the liberation of free fatty acid, actions that are inhibited in part by insulin and glucose. These lipolytic hormones have a rapid effect that is due to their ability to enhance the synthesis of cyclic adenosine 3',5'-monophosphate (cyclic AMP) (see Chapter 21). Cyclic AMP, in turn, activates a protein kinase that phosphorylates and stimulates a triglyceride lipase—the rate-limiting enzyme in the lipolytic pathway (Huttunen et al., 1970). Growth hormone may also promote lipolysis by influencing the cyclic AMP system, but the nature of its effect is less direct. Fain and coworkers (see Fain, 1973) have shown that exposure of fat cells to growth hormone for 3 hours or more leads to an increased adenylate cyclase activity and ability of the cells to accumulate cyclic AMP. In contrast to the more familiar mechanism of hormonal control of cyclic AMP accumulation, this effect is delayed and appears to require synthesis of both RNA and protein. In addition to these prominent lipolytic effects, growth hormone can also have early transient antilipolytic effects similar to those of insulin. In man, the plasma free fatty acid concentration may be reduced quickly, prior to the delayed characteristic elevation. This is reminiscent, perhaps, of some of the insulin-like effects of growth hormone on carbohydrate metabolism.

Although the effects of fasting mimic some of the actions of growth hormone and may in fact be thus mediated, the analogy by itself cannot be indefinitely extrapolated. On the one hand, growth hormone causes retention of nitrogen, increased assimilation of amino acids by tissue, and growth, whereas starvation has the reverse effects; on the other, growth hormone intensifies those very manifestations of the diabetic state that are ameliorated by fasting. It is difficult to escape the conclusion that the action of growth hormone is closely tied with the action of insulin and that the two hormones work against one another as well as together. When they work together, anabolic effects are dominant; in the fasting state, insulin is inconspicuous but not entirely lacking, and growth hormone then further depresses the use of carbohydrate and promotes the mobilization of fat and mild ketosis; in diabetes, when insulin is lacking or has decreased effectiveness, anabolism is impossible and growth hormone assumes the role of a diabetogenic agent. When growth hormone is lacking, insulin acts unopposed, carbohydrate is burned or converted to fat too quickly, and fasting becomes a major stress because, among other defects, there is difficulty in mobilizing fat for fuel.

The adrenocorticosteroids of the glucocorticoid type are also importantly concerned with the action of growth hormone. They are inhibitory to most anabolic actions but augmentative to the others. In physiological doses, they play a permissive part in numerous processes, such as the mobilization of fat, while in large doses they are strongly catabolic and intensify the diabetic state. Growth ceases when children or young animals are given excessive doses of corticosteroids, and, in hypophysectomized animals, the opposing actions of growth hormone and the corticosteroids can be titrated against one another by the use of some index of growth such as gain in body weight, the size of the thymus, the width of a growing cartilage, or nitrogen balance.

Somatomedin (Sulfation Factor). Serum from normal rats increases the incorporation of sulfate into the constituents of cartilage incubated *in vitro,* while serum from hypophysectomized animals is ineffective (Daughaday *et al.,* 1959). However, if growth hormone is injected into the hypophysectomized animals, their serum becomes endowed with the stimulating property. Added directly to the cartilage or admixed with serum, growth hormone is ineffectual. Normal human serum is also active, that from acromegalic patients more so, and that from patients suffering from hypopituitarism inert. The substance in serum appearing in response to the action of growth hormone is referred to as *sulfation factor* or, more recently, *somatomedin.* It is unknown whether either the restrictions implied by the first name or the all-encompassing implications of the second are valid. However, the factor may also stimulate DNA, RNA, and protein synthesis by chondrocytes *in vitro* (Salmon and DuVall, 1970). It is essential to know how many of the manifold actions of growth hormone are mediated in this way. The operation of such an intermediary substance could explain the lack of effect of growth hormone in many systems *in vitro* unless the hormone is first given *in vivo.* Moreover, this mechanism might clarify the way in which growth is regulated when the secretion of growth hormone itself is subject to minute-to-minute fluctuation dependent on the vicissitudes of the blood sugar and physical exercise.

Growth hormone exhibits a half-life in the circulation of only about 20 minutes, but its effects are much longer lasting. In the treatment of hypopituitary dwarfism, human growth hormone is effective even when injected at weekly intervals. This would be consistent with the operation of an intermediary substance, such as somatomedin, which has a half-life of about 2 days. In the form of familial dwarfism described by Laron, there is an abundance of circulating growth hormone, but somatomedin is lacking and injection of growth hormone fails to stimulate its appearance (Daughaday *et al.,* 1969).

The nature and source of somatomedin are under active investigation. In view of the foregoing discussion of growth hormone as a possible prohormone, it is plausible that somatomedin is an activated fragment or conjugated product derived from growth hormone. Alternatively, it may represent a type of "second messenger," synthesized or released under the influence of growth hormone. Experiments utilizing hypophysectomized and hepatectomized rats suggest that the liver is a major source of somatomedin production (Sledge, 1973). The material is assumed to be a simple peptide, and its molecular weight has been estimated to approximate 8000.

Demonstrations of antilipolytic activity of somatomedin (Underwood *et al.,* 1972) and its apparent ability to inhibit adenylate cyclase (Tell *et al.,* 1973) suggest that this molecule may mediate at least some of the insulin-like effects of growth hormone; they may also indicate the nature of some of the insulin-like material often described in the blood of normal and diabetic subjects.

Regulation of the Secretion of Growth Hormone. Detailed information on the secretion of growth hormone has become available since the development of sensitive radioimmunoassays for the protein (*see* Reichlin, 1973). Such measurements of plasma growth hormone concentration have shown surprisingly large and rapid fluctuations in response to metabolic alterations that are due to changes in the rate of secretion of the hormone from the pituitary. In the resting subject before breakfast, the plasma growth hormone concentration is 1 to 2 ng/ml (range 0 to 3). With continued fasting, the value slowly rises to about 8 ng/ml in 60 hours. After a meal or the drinking of a solution of glucose, the concentration falls rapidly to normal. Hypoglycemia induced by insulin is a particularly potent stimulus, the value rising to 25 to 50 ng/ml in 30 minutes. Hypoglycemia from other causes, as well as interference with the utilization of glucose by 2-deoxyglucose, evokes a similar response. Physical exertion and probably emotional excitement are normal stimuli to enhanced secretion of growth hormone (Roth *et al.,* 1963; Glick *et al.,* 1965). After section of the pituitary stalk, there is no change in the plasma concentration of growth hormone in response to hypoglycemia or to glucose, although the basal concentration of growth hormone is normal. Obesity causes reduction or absence of responses of growth hormone to fasting and other stimuli (Beck *et al.,* 1964). Inhibitory influences on secretion of growth hormone are exerted by free fatty acids (Blackard *et al.,* 1971) and perhaps, by way of a negative-feedback loop, by growth hormone itself (Abrams *et al.,* 1971).

Several provocative tests have been devised to evaluate the capacity of the pituitary to secrete growth hormone. The intravenous infusion of arginine in a dose of 30 g in 30 minutes in adults or 0.5 g/kg in children is safer and just as useful as the induction of hypoglycemia with insulin (Parker *et al.,* 1967). Three to 5 hours after a dose of glucose, as used in the glucose tolerance test, there is normally a rise in the concentration of plasma growth hormone. In this test, excessively obese subjects often do not respond (Theodoridis *et al.,* 1969). The oral administration of levodopa can also be used to evoke secretion of growth hormone (Weldon *et al.,* 1973). In this and other tests there is a relatively high incidence of false-negative responses.

A consistent finding and probably a most important one is the rise in the concentration of growth hormone in the plasma shortly after the onset of deep sleep. This is not just a reflection of a circadian rhythm; if the subject is kept awake all night or fitfully naps often, the rise does not take place until after he falls fast asleep the next day (*see* Parker *et al.*, 1969). In fact, prepubertal children may secrete growth hormone primarily during sleep, while secretion of growth hormone during waking hours becomes more significant in adolescents (Finkelstein *et al.*, 1972). Both prepubertal and pubertal boys have higher concentrations of plasma growth hormone than do adult males (Thompson *et al.*, 1972). Unlike the responses to hypoglycemia and to the other adverse influences mentioned above, this response to sleep makes physiological sense; that is, it fits with one's preconceived notion of how the secretion of growth hormone should be ordered. The old adage to the effect that one grows in his sleep may be right after all.

The increased secretion of growth hormone in response to fasting, hypoglycemia, excitement, and exercise is harder to understand. Under these conditions it seems that it is released when there is a need for fuel. If it caused a rapid release of free fatty acids from adipose tissue, it would accomplish this purpose; however, the time course of these events is such that a more complex explanation seems to be required (*see* Zierler, 1968).

The role of hypothalamic stimulatory and inhibitory hormones in the regulation of the secretion of growth hormone is discussed below.

Assays. The most commonly used bioassays for growth hormone utilize young hypophysectomized rats. *Gain in weight* during 10 days of daily, subcutaneous injection is roughly proportional to the logarithm of the dose. In the *tibia test*, which is more sensitive, the increase in width of the epiphyseal cartilage is measured microscopically. The substances under test are injected subcutaneously daily for 4 days.

Radioimmunoassays for growth hormone are far more sensitive and specific (Utiger *et al.*, 1962). These methods depend upon competition for binding sites on a limited quantity of antibody between pure, radioactive hormone and an unknown quantity of unlabeled hormone. The various methods differ principally in the way in which the bound and the free hormone are separated.

Radioreceptor assays for growth hormone have been described (Lesniak *et al.*, 1973; Tsushima and Friesen, 1973). This technic is conceptually analogous to that of radioimmunoassay. However, a natural binding protein (in these cases, from lymphocytes or liver) is substituted for the antibody. With this method, sensitivity is usually high, and the technic will detect hormonal derivatives with biological activity that may have lost immunoreactivity.

Therapeutic Use. The very limited supply of human growth hormone has restricted its therapeutic use almost exclusively to hypopituitary dwarfism.

The first patient to receive prolonged therapy showed the uninterrupted response depicted in Figure 66–1 (Raben, 1962a, 1962b). At age 17, he was 4 ft 2½ in. tall, weighed 68 lb, and exhibited all the features of hypopituitarism. Treatment with thyroid did not promote growth, and cortisone had little clinical effect. Growth hormone was given subcutaneously in a dose of 2 mg three times weekly for the first 14 months, and over the ensuing years the dose was increased by increments to a maximum of 5 mg three times a week. When he had been treated for 3 years, he had grown to a height of 4 ft 9 in.; although 20 years old, he showed no signs of sexual maturation and, therefore, treatment with androgen was begun. Although he received only 60 mg of testosterone cypionate every 2 weeks, in 4 years there was full development of the penis, growth of axillary and pubic hair, increased body hair, more prominent musculature, and a beginning growth of beard. The bone age, which had advanced slowly with growth hormone, reached 15½ years with androgen therapy. This value is associated with nearly complete closure of the epiphyses of the long bones, implying that growth in height was nearly at an end. As there was an insignificant increase in height during a further 7½ months of treatment, growth hormone was discontinued without stopping the other replacement therapy. He had grown a total of 14 in. in 7 years and had reached the respectable height of 5 ft 4½ in. at the age of 24.

In the majority of cases pituitary dwarfs respond satisfactorily by an increased rate of growth over many years of treatment (*see* Tanner *et al.*, 1971). Usually the gain in height declines with succeeding years, and sometimes this is correctable by increasing the dose. Restoration of responsiveness has also been noted after a 3-month interruption of therapy (Rudman *et al.*, 1973). Antibodies can frequently be detected during treatment, but they do not usually influence the effectiveness of the hormone and a declining response might not correlate with the development of antibodies.

When there is a poor response or none at all, the diagnosis of hypopituitarism or of isolated deficiency of growth hormone may come into question (Rimoin *et al.*, 1968). Normal children and children with short stature from other causes are much less sensitive to growth hormone than are those who are deficient. However, patients with partial deficiency and intermediate concentrations of plasma growth hormone do respond and should be treated (Tanner *et al.*, 1971).

TREATMENT OF A MALE PITUITARY DWARF

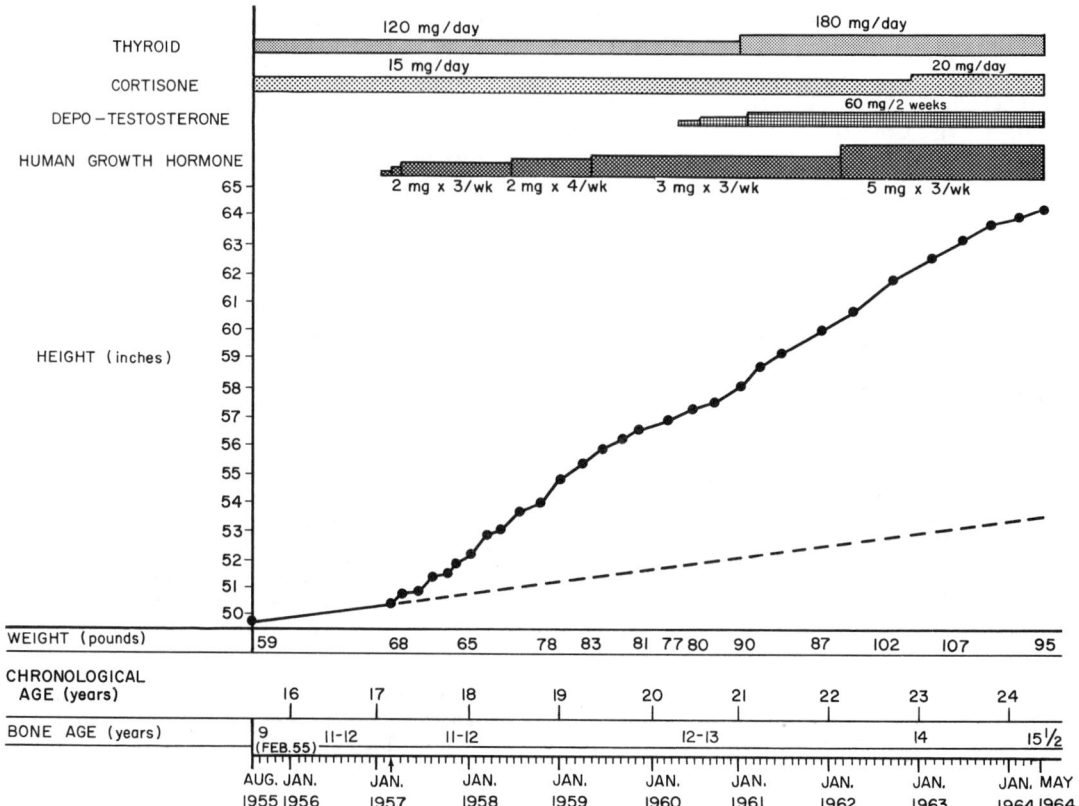

Figure 66–1. *Treatment of a patient with pituitary dwarfism with human growth hormone during replacement therapy with thyroid, cortisone, and testosterone.* (Modified from Raben, 1962b. Courtesy of the *New England Journal of Medicine.*)

To select those cases of short stature that are caused by deficient growth hormone, it is necessary to measure the growth hormone in the serum and to determine whether there is an appropriate response to a provocative stimulus. A requirement for therapy with growth hormone is based on the clinical findings and failure to respond to two or more provocative stimuli for secretion of the hormone. Once initiated, therapy should be evaluated for 8 to 12 months for the expected acceleration of growth. If therapy is successful, it should ideally be continued throughout childhood, and sex hormones, if needed, should be withheld until the possibilities of the response to growth hormone have been fully realized or until deemed necessary.

Undesirable side effects and complications are notably lacking; pain and swelling at sites of injection, allergic reactions, and chronic ill effects do not occur even when serum antibodies can be shown.

Human growth hormone is currently available in the United States only for treatment programs that include research efforts. It is obtained from the National Pituitary Agency of the National Institutes of Health, Bethesda, Maryland, upon approval of its

Medical Advisory Committee. Hormone is supplied for a specific patient, and with yearly reapplication the supply is usually committed until the patient attains a height of 5 ft. It is estimated that the available supply of hormone is sufficient for treatment of only 10% of the hypopituitary children in the United States. All pathologists should cooperate by sending human pituitaries obtained at post-mortem examination to the National Pituitary Agency.

PROLACTIN

Despite a wealth of information about the nature and role of prolactin in a wide variety of species, unequivocal evidence for the existence of the hormone in man was obtained relatively recently (*see* Frantz *et al.,* 1972). It is now appreciated, however, that prolactin plays an important role in normal human function and in certain pathophysiological states.

Prolactin is widely distributed in the pituitaries of vertebrates; it has been found wherever sought in the pituitaries of mammals, birds, reptiles, and amphibia, and has been detected in a few species of fish. Among the amphibia, it has a clear-cut and very striking action in the newt *Triturus*, an action almost as remarkable as the metamorphic one of thyroid hormone on tadpoles. It transforms the terrestrial eft—a small, pink quadruped found under rocks in the woods—into a larger, dark-green, fish-shaped creature with a broad tail designed for swimming. The animal then takes to the water, its normal breeding habitat, which accounts for the term *water-drive factor,* coined before the active principle was equated with prolactin (Bern and Nicoll, 1968).

The term *prolactin* was coined for the hormone responsible for the secretion of milk by the crop glands of the pigeon (Riddle *et al.,* 1933). In this bird there is a bilateral outpouching of the esophagus and, prompted by the psychological concomitants of brooding, a glandular structure grows within each pouch so that by the time of hatching a thick secretion, the crop milk, becomes available to each parent for regurgitating down the throats of the young. The response of the bird is a sensitive one; it is sufficient for one partner to see his mate sitting on the eggs for his pituitary to secrete prolactin and provoke the growth of the crop glands. In so naming the hormone, the tenuous analogy between the mammary gland and the crop sac was correctly drawn because it later was clear that prolactin is also of importance in initiating secretion from the breast.

Chemistry. The difficulty in isolating human prolactin is attributable to the facts that growth hormone is very similar in structure, possesses significant lactogenic activity in conventional bioassays for the hormone, and is present in human pituitaries in quantities far in excess of prolactin. However, refined bioassay technics permitted verification of the existence of human prolactin (Frantz and Kleinberg, 1970), and the technic of affinity chromatography permitted purification of a primate prolactin and subsequent development of a specific radioimmunoassay (Guyda and Friesen, 1971; Hwang *et al.,* 1971). Progress in the purification, chemistry, and physiology of human prolactin has been rapid since these advances.

Amino acid sequence determination of the aminoterminal region of the hormone (residues 1–50) has revealed approximately 25% identity and 50% homology with human growth hormone. There is high conservation of structure between human and ovine prolactin (80% identity), at least in this region, and the structure of the human hormone undoubtedly resembles closely that of sheep (Niall *et al.,* 1973).

Ovine prolactin has been characterized extensively, since the pituitaries of sheep are readily available and constitute a very rich source (Li *et al.,* 1970). The general structural features are very similar to those of the growth hormones (Table 66–1); the proposed evolutionary relationship of these molecules has been discussed above. As with the growth hormones, "isohormones" with presumed minor structural differences can be detected by electrophoresis.

Physiological Actions. *Breast.* The mammary gland is a site of immensely complex interactions among a number of hormones, with the majority of endocrine organs participating vigorously in the initiation and maintenance of lactation. The hormones of the adrenal cortex, thyroid, and ovaries are all necessary, and their presence is dependent on the trophic hormones of the adenohypophysis. Insulin and perhaps growth hormone exert important anabolic influences. The vital participation of prolactin completes the contribution of the anterior pituitary, with all of its major secretions at work. The role of oxytocin is considered in Chapter 42.

The actions of prolactin on the mammary gland have been studied particularly in explanted rodent tissue. However, investigations of normal and aberrant prolactin secretion seem to assure the existence of a comparable function in the human female. In systems *in vitro,* prolactin in the proper hormonal milieu can be shown to promote proliferation and subsequent differentiation of mammary ductal and alveolar epithelium. There is a rapid increase in RNA synthesis and induction of the synthesis of milk proteins and of enzymes necessary for lactose synthesis (Topper, 1970; Turkington *et al.,* 1973). At the subcellular level, activation of the development of rough endoplasmic reticulum, Golgi apparatus, and secretory granules is prominent.

These "mammotrophic" actions of prolactin suggest a possible role of prolactin in mammary tumorigenesis. Prolonged prolactin administration, the grafting of extra pituitaries, or experimental lesions in the median eminence that cause increased prolactin secretion all result in a high percentage of mammary tumors in susceptible rats and mice. Furthermore, estrogen will not produce tumors in the absence of the pituitary; however, in rats treated with carcinogens, prolactin promotes tumorigenesis in the absence of estrogens or progestins. Furthermore, drugs that enhance prolactin secretion (*e.g.,* reserpine, haloperidol—*see* below) facilitate experimental tumor growth, while those that inhibit secretion (*e.g.,* ergot derivatives) impede growth and reduce the incidence of spontaneous tumors in rodent models (*see* Meites *et al.,* 1972; McMahon *et al.,* 1973). Extrapolation between highly susceptible strains of rodents and man is obviously of questionable value, but these observations may provide additional explanations for the effectiveness of hormonal therapy of breast tumors. They may also relate to reports of the increased incidence of breast cancer among women who have been treated with reserpine for hypertension (*see* Armstrong *et al.,*

1974; Boston Collaborative Drug Surveillance Program, 1974; Heinonen *et al.,* 1974).

Ovary. The effects of prolactin on the ovary are species dependent. While the hormone has in the past also been referred to as *luteotropin,* this description was based on observations on rats and mice. In these species prolactin can prolong the life of the functioning corpus luteum, but it probably does not fulfill the role of a true luteotropic hormone. Notably, prolactin will not stimulate progesterone biosynthesis by corpora lutea from a variety of species, including rats (*see* Dorfman, 1972). It may, however, function to promote the luteal synthesis of cholesterol, the steroidal precursor. In contrast, luteinizing hormone is uniformly effective in stimulating progesterone synthesis. Surprisingly, recent evidence suggests that the sharp rise in prolactin secretion seen during proestrus in the rat may be responsible for luteolysis of corpora lutea formed during the previous cycle (Meites *et al.,* 1972).

Significant effects of prolactin on the human ovary are not known, and large variations of plasma prolactin concentrations are not apparent at different stages of the menstrual cycle.

Prolactin Secretion. Refined assay technics not only have been instrumental in the identification and purification of human prolactin but also have allowed exploration of physiological, pathological, and pharmacological influences on prolactin secretion (*see* Frantz *et al.,* 1972; Friesen, 1973).

The normal human plasma concentration of prolactin approximates 5 to 10 ng/ml and is essentially the same in males and females. Prolactin concentrations rise markedly during pregnancy, reaching a maximum at term. In nursing mothers prolactin secretion is critically controlled by the sucking stimulus or breast manipulation. Prolactin concentration can rise 10- to 100-fold within 30 minutes of stimulation. Other stimuli for prolactin secretion include psychic and physical stress, insulin-induced hypoglycemia, and high doses of estrogens. Interestingly, hypertonicity results in large elevations of plasma prolactin (Buckman and Peake, 1973). Future work should reveal whether any physiological significance is attached to this phenomenon or if it represents an undiscarded heritage of the *water-drive factor.*

Secretion of prolactin by the pituitary is under predominantly negative control by the hypothalamus. Thus, a prolactin release–inhibiting hormone (PRIH) is secreted tonically by the hypothalamus and is carried by the hypothalamicoadenohypophyseal portal system to the adenohypophysis, where it inhibits prolactin secretion. There is considerable evidence that the release of PRIH is under adrenergic (dopaminergic) control, or that PRIH might even be dopamine (MacLeod and Lehmeyer, 1974). Thus, the administration of levodopa *in vivo* inhibits prolactin secretion, and dopamine is a highly effective inhibitor when instilled into the third ventricle or when applied to the isolated pituitary *in vitro.* Predictably, the phenothiazine and butyrophenone antipsychotics (*e.g.,* chlorpromazine, haloperidol), which are dopamine antagonists, enhance prolactin secretion, as can reserpine and α-methyldopa. The antipsychotic agents can cause significant galactorrhea associated with elevated plasma prolactin concentrations.

Functional disorders of the hypothalamus (Chiari-Frommel syndrome) and destructive or infiltrative disorders of the hypothalamus or pituitary stalk can also cause prolactin secretion and galactorrhea if there is interference with the tonic inhibitory hypothalamic influence. Pituitary oversecretion of prolactin, often due to functional tumors (Forbes-Albright syndrome), is also known. However, in none of these conditions is there strict correlation between plasma prolactin concentration and the presence or severity of galactorrhea.

Suppression of galactorrhea by administration of levodopa has been attempted with variable success (Turkington, 1972). Some patients who respond initially become refractory to the drug. More promising clinical results have been achieved with ergot derivatives (Floss *et al.,* 1973). Inhibition of lactation in women suffering from ergotism was observed centuries ago. This phenomenon has recently gained scientific credence with the discovery that ergot derivatives profoundly inhibit prolactin secretion *in vivo* and in isolated pituitary preparations *in vitro.* Since the inhibitory effect *in vitro* is antagonized by haloperidol, it is possible to hypothesize that ergot alkaloids activate the dopaminergic receptors that inhibit prolactin release. The experimental compound that has shown significant clinical promise is 2-bromo-α-ergokryptine. An additional finding of potential significance is that this compound can markedly suppress the growth of prolactin-secreting pituitary tumors (Quadri *et al.,* 1972).

Assays. The classical procedure for bioassay of prolactin is based on the original work of Riddle and associates (1933), namely, the increase in weight of the crop sacs of doves and pigeons. Other methods are based on the induction of secretory changes in the suitably prepared mammary glands of guinea pigs and rabbits. As mentioned above, radioimmunoassays have proven invaluable. A radioreceptor assay that utilizes a membrane receptor preparation isolated from rabbit mammary glands should also be useful to assess biological activity (Shiu *et al.,* 1973).

Human Placental Lactogen. Preparations from the human placenta contain growth-promoting and lactogenic activity (*see* Fukushima, 1961); Josimovich and MacLaren (1962) showed that such extracts cross-reacted with antisera to human growth hormone. Purified preparations caused a local response in the crop sac of the pigeon and maintained the function of the corpora lutea of rats but caused little growth in hypophysectomized animals; the active principle was named *placental lactogen.* Friesen (1965, 1966) purified the protein to homogeneity and demonstrated that it was strikingly lactogenic in pseudopregnant rabbits.

The chemical similarity of the substance to human growth hormone was shown by Sherwood (1967), and the complete amino acid sequence has been elucidated by Niall and associates (1971) and Li and coworkers (1973). The resemblance to growth hormone was amply confirmed by these studies, since both hormones contain 191 amino acids that differ in only 32 positions. The greater similarity of amino acid sequence in human placental lactogen and human growth hormone than in human and bovine growth hormones suggests a later evolutionary appearance of the placental lactogen. Its significance is, however, largely unknown. Because of its resemblance to growth hormone, the unwieldy name *chorionic somatomammotropin* is also in use.

GONADOTROPIC HORMONES

The pituitary gland plays an important part in the regulation of gonadal function throughout the vertebrate phylum, but the fullest understanding of the mechanisms involved has been achieved among the mammals. In this class there are striking species differences, with remarkable specialization in some as well as a certain uniformity among others, permitting the formulation of general principles. The adenohypophysis is physiologically and anatomically so situated that it can mediate neural messages that arise from the environment as well as intercept humoral signals from within. It can regulate such diverse phenomena as the annual growth and regression of the gonads of monestrous mammals in response to the changing length of daylight, the release of ova in the rabbit 10 hours after mating, and the reinitiation of follicular growth when a corpus luteum fails for lack of successful impregnation.

For over 40 years it has been known that two gonadotropins are involved, and it seems a general rule among mammals that follicular growth and development on the one hand and ovulation and the formation of a corpus luteum on the other are separately controlled. These same substances stimulate, respectively, the germinal elements of the testis and the androgen-secreting Leydig cells of the interstitial tissue. In the regulation of the function of the corpus luteum, several adaptations have arisen. In some species luteinizing hormone serves as the luteotropin, in others

prolactin plays such a role, while in several species the uterus is somehow involved. During pregnancy the pituitary seems essential in some animals, while in most it is dispensable; luteal function may be autonomous, as in the herbivora, or regulated in part by a placental luteotropin, as in man.

Until very recently the functions of the gonadotropins in man were largely inferred from information derived from other mammals. Direct observations on human beings of the effects of gonadal hormones and their analogs and human gonadotropins have given better understanding and have opened new therapeutic approaches to the disturbances of human reproductive function.

Chemistry. The four gonadotropins considered here (two of pituitary and two of placental origin) are follicle-stimulating hormone (FSH), luteinizing hormone (LH), chorionic gonadotropin (CG), and the gonadotropin of pregnant mares' serum. The gonadotropins, with thyrotropin (TSH), constitute the glycoprotein group of hormones, and their similarities and general chemical features have been mentioned above (*see* Table 66–1).

Follicle-stimulating hormone (FSH) is the least well characterized of the pituitary hormones and the only one for which detailed information on amino acid sequence is not known. However, it is known that the human hormone consists of nonidentical, noncovalently linked subunits (Saxena and Rathnam, 1971). While the α subunit of FSH is significantly different from that of LH or TSH (Papkoff, 1972), there is evidence that the FSH α subunit can combine with the β subunit of chorionic gonadotropin with restoration of chorionic gonadotropin activity (Reichert, 1972).

Luteinizing hormone (LH), also called *interstitial cell–stimulating hormone,* more closely resembles TSH in its physical properties and chemical constitution than it does FSH. Ovine LH-α is identical to bovine TSH-α, and the β subunits show considerable homology. Considerable progress has been made with human LH, and the amino acid sequences of both α and β subunits have been reported (Sairam *et al.,* 1972; Shome and Parlow, 1973). Approximately 70% of the amino acid residues of both subunits are identical to the corresponding portions of the ovine hormone (Liu *et al.,* 1972a, 1972b). Many differences are explicable by a single DNA base change. Human LH-β is even more similar to a major portion of the β subunit of human chorionic gonadotropin, although the latter has a 30 amino acid carboxyl-terminal segment that is not present in human LH-β.

Human chorionic gonadotropin (HCG) is prepared

from the urine of pregnant women. This glyco-protein contains significantly more carbohydrate than do those above, and its high content of sialic acid imparts a very low isoelectric point. The amino acid sequences of both the α and β subunits have been elucidated (Bahl *et al.*, 1972) and, as mentioned, HCG-β and human LH-β resemble each other closely. The α subunits are essentially identical, with the exception of an amino-terminal tripeptide present in HCG and missing from human LH (Papkoff, 1972).

Gonadotropin of pregnant mares' serum, the gonadotropin most in need of a suitable name, is found in maximal concentration in the indicated source between the fiftieth and eightieth days of pregnancy. This gonadotropin has an exceedingly high carbohydrate content (47%) and is rich in sialic acid (14%). Although characterization has been limited, it also appears to have two subunits (Gospodarowicz, 1972).

Physiological Actions. Despite an extraordinarily large number of experimental observations of the actions of gonadotropins, understanding of their functions is far from complete. Most studies have been carried out in species different from that of origin of the hormone, and certain anomalous responses are possibly traceable to this cause. Observations on the responses of the normal human gonads to human gonadotropins are still fragmentary.

Actions on the Ovary. During the follicular phase of the ovarian cycle successive groups of small follicles start to grow, and by the time ovulation is imminent follicles in all stages of development are found. This ovarian response represents the predominant action of FSH, and it is during this phase that estrogen is the main ovarian secretory product (*see* Figure 68–2, page 1427). Since some highly purified preparations of FSH induce follicular growth in hypophysectomized rats without evoking the secretion of estrogen, it is generally believed that small amounts of LH are required (Mills *et al.*, 1971). However, since the hypophysectomized animal suffers multiple deficiencies, further experiments are needed to establish the point.

Shortly before ovulation is to take place, a series of ovarian changes follow in rapid succession, presumably mediated by a burst of LH secretion at this time. The largest follicles expand quickly; those in just the right stage of development to ovulate undergo cytological changes in the granulosa in the direction of luteinization and show intense hyperemia of the theca interna. One area on the surface of the follicle thins and then undergoes dissolution, leaving an aperture through which the viscous follicular fluid oozes, carrying desquamated granulosa cells and the cumulus and its contained ovum with it. Those large follicles not destined to ovulate, perhaps for reasons of improper stage of development, remain avascular and begin to show regressive changes. While ovulation is in progress, widespread atresia involves all the other follicles that shortly before had been flourishing under the influence of FSH, and in certain species the atresic process extends also to the residual corpora lutea of antecedent cycles. It is tempting to attribute the regressive changes in the ovary, which parallel so closely ovulation and luteinization, to an action of LH, but it must be admitted that experimental evidence in support of this concept is not entirely uniform.

With the earliest stages of preovulatory swelling there is evidence of the first secretion of progesterone. This has been shown in species that require the luteotropic action of prolactin as well as in those that do not. The critical influence is exerted by LH.

Measurements of the gonadotropins in plasma throughout the menstrual cycle show that FSH is elevated during the follicular phase and slowly falls before it rises again at midcycle; it is lowest during the luteal phase. LH shows a striking peak at midcycle, usually on the same day that the FSH is highest (*see* Figure 68–2, page 1427). This surge in the secretion of LH is an immediately preovulatory event (*see* Faiman and Ryan, 1967; Midgley and Jaffe, 1968). Further interactions between the gonadotropins and the sex steroids are discussed in Chapters 68 and 69.

Actions on the Testis. Whereas in the ovary both gonadotropins are involved in the secretion of hormones, in the testis LH plays a predominant role. FSH is primarily a gametogenic hormone in males; it is responsible for the anatomical integrity of the seminiferous tubules and only under its influence are the complex stages of gametogenesis carried through to the production of spermatozoa. In the hypophysectomized animal, the major effect of FSH is stimulation of the seminiferous tubules. As the tubules make up the bulk of the testis, tubular growth is accurately reflected by an increase in testicular weight. Possible effects of FSH on testosterone secretion from the Leydig cells are controversial and are discussed in Chapter 69. LH stimulates the interstitial cells to secrete androgen, but the androgen, in turn, exerts a direct effect upon the tubules so that both components of the testis appear to be stimulated.

Mechanism of Action. LH and FSH bind with apparent specificity to various particulate fractions derived from testis and ovary. Furthermore, both gonadotropins are known to stimulate cyclic AMP synthesis in appropriate gonadal preparations (Marsh *et al.,* 1966; Murad *et al.,* 1969). Cyclic AMP then stimulates sex steroid biosynthesis by mechanisms apparently analogous to those operative in the adrenal cortex. The nucleotide has also been shown to induce luteinization of cultured granulosa cells (Channing and Seymour, 1970) and transplanted ovarian follicles (Ellsworth and Armstrong, 1973). It has been suggested that prostaglandins play a role in the stimulation of cyclic AMP synthesis by LH (Kuehl *et al.,* 1970), and similar observations have been made with TSH, a structural cousin (Zor *et al.,* 1969).

Chorionic Gonadotropin (CG). Chorionic gonadotropin is a hormone of human pregnancy; it is secreted by the fetal placenta as early as 7 days after ovulation, and it is absorbed into the blood in sufficient quantity to sustain luteal function and forestall the next menstrual period. The hormone is detectable in the urine by immunoassay several days before the first missed period, and this is the basis of the most commonly used test of pregnancy. The quantity excreted increases rapidly thereafter to a maximum about 6 weeks after ovulation. The urinary content then declines over the next month or so and stabilizes at a lower level for the remainder of pregnancy.

The changes in the corpus luteum in early pregnancy reflect the intense stimulation provided by the LH-like action of chorionic gonadotropin. With the increasing secretion of estrogen and progesterone by the placenta during the third month, the ovaries and the corpus luteum become unessential to the maintenance of gestation, but the corpus luteum does not undergo a pronounced change at this time. Instead, there is a slow regression that, histologically, is not complete even at the time of delivery. In the face of the flood of chorionic gonadotropin during pregnancy, the rest of the ovary remains quiescent; there is no growth or maturation of follicles and no changes suggesting luteinization either of the granulosa or of thecal or stromal elements.

In view of the lack of a clear need for chorionic gonadotropin beyond the first trimester, one is tempted to ask whether chorionic gonadotropin has any other function. Since a mother accepts the immunological insult of the fetus and particularly the fetal trophoblast in intimate contact with the endometrium, Adcock and coworkers (1973) tested the effect of chorionic gonadotropin on the ability of phytohemagglutinin to transform human lymphocytes. Striking and reversible inhibition, presumably due to the carbohydrate portion of the molecule, was noted at concentrations of hormone likely to be achieved or exceeded in the area of contact between endometrium and trophoblast. This suggests a fascinating hypothesis for investigation.

The action on the testis can hardly be regarded as physiological, for the hormone gains access to the male only *in utero,* when it does cause minimal gonadal stimulation; otherwise the hormone is found in the male only in the rare event of a teratomatous tumor containing chorionic elements. Injected into men, however, chorionic gonadotropin stimulates the interstitial cells of the testis to secrete androgen. Activation of the seminiferous epithelium is minimal and may be mediated entirely by the androgen of Leydig-cell origin.

The mechanism of action of chorionic gonadotropin appears to be identical to that of LH.

Absorption, Fate, and Excretion. The gonadotropins of either pituitary or placental origin are effective only if given by injection. The length of survival of the injected and presumably of the endogenously secreted hormones is determined largely by the rate of degradation in the body, because little is excreted in the urine except in the case of chorionic gonadotropin. The period of survival of heterologous gonadotropins is doubtless modified by immune mechanisms. Studies on the rate of disappearance of endogenous human LH, FSH, and chorionic gonadotropin indicate removal from the plasma with at least two distinct half-times. The shorter half-lives for these three hormones approximate 20 minutes, 4 hours, and 11 hours, respectively, while the longer half-lives appear to be 4, 70, and 23 hours (Yen *et al.,* 1968, 1970). Removal of sialic acid from chorionic gonadotropin greatly decreases its half-life, a fact that may provide some insight into the role of the additional carbohydrate of this glycoprotein (Van Hall *et al.*, 1971). While appreciable amounts of chorionic gonadotropin are excreted in the urine, it has been estimated that only 5% of secreted FSH is found in the urine in an active form (Coble *et al.*, 1969). During the latter part of pregnancy, material reacting immunologically like chorionic gonadotropin appears in the urine in quantities several times greater than the quantity of biologically active hormone (Hobson and Wide, 1964), suggesting that there is partial degradation before excretion, and this mechanism may be involved in the rapid clearance of the active hormone from the body after delivery of the placenta.

The gonadotropin of pregnant mares' serum does not appear in the urine of the mare, and it has not been detected in the urine of other animals after injection. In the rat, the duration of action of a single dose is very long; with a moderate dose the maximal ovarian weight is reached about 5 days after the injection, so the substance may enjoy a very long survival in the body.

Assays. Bioassay remains a necessary technic for evaluation of functional activity, which often bears no relationship to immunoreactivity. The gonadotropins pose a special problem because many responses to one hormone are modified by the concurrent action of others, and special conditions must be chosen to minimize this influence. References and descriptions of several technics can be found in the *third* and *fourth editions* of this textbook.

For many purposes, particularly the measurement of gonadotropins in blood and urine, radioimmunoassays are more accurate and far simpler than bioassays. References have been cited by Vande Wiele and Dyrenfurth (1973).

Preparations and Dosages. Currently no purified gonadotropins prepared from human pituitaries are available commercially. For clinical purposes, quite crude preparations are suitable, even though they contain both FSH and LH as well as other active principles. The limiting factor is the scarcity of human pituitary glands and not the preparation of suitable extracts.

Menotropins for injection (PERGONAL) is a preparation of gonadotropins from the urine of postmenopausal women. While FSH and LH activities are present in equal unitage, chorionic gonadotropin is usually required in conjunction with menotropins to induce ovulation. The recommended initial dose is 75 I.U. of each gonadotropin intramuscularly daily for 9 to 12 days. This is followed by 10,000 I.U. of chorionic gonadotropin. If there is no evidence of ovulation, dosage may be increased. In some cases large quantities may be needed. Menotropins for injection is supplied in ampuls containing 75 I.U. of FSH and 75 I.U. of LH. The powder is dissolved in 2 ml of sterile 0.9% sodium chloride solution and is administered intramuscularly, immediately.

Chorionic Gonadotropin for Injection, U.S.P., is a preparation derived from the urine of pregnant women, which is sold under various trade names (ANTUITRIN-S, APL, FOLLUTEIN, LIBIGEN, PREGNYL, RIOGON). It is usually given intramuscularly in doses of 1000 to 4000 I.U. two or three times weekly for several weeks for the treatment of cryptorchism or hypogonadism in men, and in doses of 8000 to 10,000 I.U. one day following treatment with menotropins to evoke ovulation. It is available in packages containing 5000, 10,000, or 20,000 I.U. of powder with an ampul of suitable diluent.

Gonadotropin of pregnant mares' serum is also commercially available under the trade name GESTYL. Although it has been used to a limited extent for 4 decades, no clear-cut indications have emerged and there are few guidelines to dosage.

Purified human LH and FSH are available for investigational use only from the National Pituitary Agency of the National Institutes of Health, Bethesda, Maryland.

Therapeutic Uses. The gonadotropins are used in therapy primarily for the treatment of infertility and cryptorchism.

Infertility. The widest potential usefulness of the gonadotropins is in the induction of ovulation in women who are infertile because of insufficient gonadotropins. An indication of what can be accomplished in this area is provided by the studies of Gemzell (1961, 1965). Following administration of a crude preparation of gonadotropin obtained from human glands, ovulation was successfully induced one or more times in the majority of patients; more than half of the treated women became pregnant. Treatment was uniformly unsuccessful when there was excessive gonadotropin in the urine, indicating intrinsic ovarian failure.

Extensive clinical experience with menotropins and human chorionic gonadotropin, summarized by Thompson and Hansen (1970), indicated the occurrence of ovulation in 75% of patients treated with the drugs. While ovulation was occasionally seen during administration of menotropins before human chorionic gonadotropin was given, it usually took place about 18 hours after administration of the latter hormone. Pregnancy resulted in approximately 25% of the patients; of these, the abortion rate was 25% and fetal abnormalities occurred in 2%. Twenty percent of pregnancies resulted in multiple births (15% twins and 5% with three or more concepti). Interestingly, in another series the male-to-female sex ratio in single births was 0.88, but only 0.43 for births of twins. The growth and development of children born of mothers receiving gonadotropin treatment have been normal (Hack *et al.*, 1970).

The only complications reported for this therapy have been excessive ovarian enlargement and multiple pregnancies. Ovarian hyperstimulation may be seen several days after the administration of chorionic gonadotropin in a few percent of patients. In this condition the enlarged ovaries give rise to pain in the lower abdomen, and, if there is bleeding into the peritoneal cavity, the pain is severe. Under the latter circumstance, hospitalization and observation for ovarian rupture are required, Methods are being devised to avoid these complications (Brown *et al.*, 1969). For example, one can test ovarian responsiveness by measuring the excretion of estrogens in the urine in a preliminary trial and thereby be guided in the dosage appropriate for a therapeutic attempt. If the urinary estrogens exceed 150 μg/24 hours, chorionic gonadotropin should be withheld. Alternatively, several trials may be made with small doses before the larger recommended amounts are used.

It is remarkable how closely the experience with human gonadotropins parallels that following the use of clomiphene (*see* Chapter 68). Further experience will be needed to determine which types of ovarian disorders are best treated with gonadotropin and which with clomiphene; currently clomiphene would seem the better agent in the syndrome of polycystic ovaries whereas gonadotropin would be indicated when the pituitary is primarily at fault.

While the use of human gonadotropin, either from the pituitary gland or from menopausal urine, to promote fertility in the male is a field that has not been extensively explored, men with hypopituitarism have been rendered fertile by this means (Gemzell and Kjessler, 1964; Mancini *et al.*, 1971). As the process of germinal maturation in the tubules requires 10 weeks and the transit of the spermatozoa through the vas deferens several weeks more, investigation of this form of treatment is time consuming. The effectiveness of therapy with gonadotropins when more subtle forms of gametogenic failure are under study is more difficult to evaluate and more extensive experience is required. Often testicular failure appears to be due to an intrinsic fault of the testis itself, and additional gonadotropin would not be expected to be beneficial.

Cryptorchism. Failure of the descent of one testis or both is sometimes noted in childhood; it is most frequent in infancy and is less prevalent with advancing age until it becomes a rare finding in the adult. In the majority of cases, testes undescended in childhood assume their normal position at the time of puberty, a sequence of events that is normal in monkeys. In rare cases, cryptorchism denotes an abnormality of testicular development and in this event descent at puberty does not take place. There is also some indication that testicular development is quite normal if descent is achieved before age seven (Lattimer, 1973). It has been shown that, when normal descent is possible at puberty, the event can be brought on prematurely by the administration of an androgen or chorionic gonadotropin, thus avoiding surgery if early descent is desired. Chorionic gonadotropin is usually used and is customarily given intramuscularly in doses of 1000 to 4000 I.U. two or three times weekly for several weeks, but therapy is stopped as soon as the desired result has been achieved.

THYROTROPIN (TSH)

The regulatory effects of thyrotropin on the thyroid gland are considered in Chapter 67. The essential chemical features of bovine thyrotropin, elucidated by Pierce and coworkers (*see* Pierce, 1971), are summarized in Table 66–1, and the relationship with LH has been discussed.

Recent progress has been made in the amino acid sequence analysis of the human hormone (Sairam and Li, 1973). Again there is evidence that human LH-α and TSH-α are essentially the same. Human TSH-β, the amino acid sequence of which is known, is highly homologous with the bovine TSH-β subunit. Only 11 residues differ, and 9 of these are very conservative replacements.

Assays. A widely used bioassay is that described by McKenzie (1961). Thyroid stimulation is reflected in increased circulating radioactivity in mice with thyroids prelabeled with radioiodine. Radioimmunoassays for human thyrotropin now permit diagnostic studies of the circulating hormone under various clinical circumstances.

Clinical Application. *Thyrotropin* (THYTROPAR) is not used as a therapeutic agent. The single clinical application of this bovine preparation is in the evaluation of thyroid function in conjunction with the use of radioiodine. Hypopituitarism can be differentiated from primary myxedema by the stimulation of thyroid accumulation of radioiodine by thyrotropin in the former condition but not in the latter. In the usual procedure, a dose of 10 units is given as a single intramuscular injection followed by a tracer dose of radioiodine 18 to 24 hours later. Twenty-four hours after the tracer, the uptake in hypopituitarism is usually substantially higher than it was before thyrotropin, whereas it usually remains low in spontaneous myxedema. Plasma thyrotropin concentrations are elevated in primary myxedema, and the increasing availability of radioimmunoassays for thyrotropin should reduce the need for diagnostic thyrotropin administration.

OTHER THYROID STIMULATORS

Three other proteins with varying resemblance to pituitary thyrotropin have been described.

Chorionic Thyrotropin. This protein is the closest apparent relative of the pituitary hormone. Found in the normal placenta, it reacts with antisera to human thyrotropin and appears to have a similar molecular weight. Its significance, if any, is unknown (Hershman, 1972).

Molar Thyrotropin. This material derives its name from its detection in benign and malignant hydatidiform moles, and both *chorionic* and *molar* thyrotropins are thus *trophoblastic* thyrotropins. Molar thyrotropin has also been detected in normal placenta; however, in contrast to chorionic thyrotropin, its activity is not neutralized by antisera to pituitary thyrotropin, and it appears to have approximately twice the molecular weight (Hershman, 1972). This thyroid stimulator has been responsible for thyrotoxicosis in several patients with hydatidiform mole or choriocarcinoma.

Long-Acting Thyroid Stimulator. In the blood of patients suffering from Graves' disease (hyperthyroidism) a substance has been found that exerts a prolonged stimulatory action upon the thyroids of animals used in the assay of thyrotropin. By general agreement, the students of the subject chose to call the substance *long-acting thyroid stimulator* to distinguish it from thyrotropin and to avoid premature inference regarding its etiological role in hyperthyroidism; the term has the unfortunate abbreviation LATS. It was first noted by Adams and Purves (1957), using the guinea pig as the test animal. Later a more satisfactory assay in the mouse was developed by McKenzie (1961). With thyrotropin or with the serum from myxedematous patients, the response in the McKenzie assay is maximal at 2 hours whereas, after giving serum from some patients with hyperthyroidism, the maximal response is not observed until about 10 hours after the injection.

LATS is synthesized by lymphocytes and is an immunoglobulin of the IgG class, a fact that has contributed to the hypothesis that Graves' disease is an autoimmune phenomenon (*see* Kriss, 1970). It is not known if the protein is in fact an antibody. Its actions on the thyroid gland are essentially identical to those of thyrotropin, and this may be logical since both proteins stimulate the synthesis of cyclic AMP (Yamashita and Field, 1972). The protein evidently can traverse the placenta and thereby account for hyperthyroidism of the newborn infants of some hyperthyroid mothers.

The hypothesis that LATS is the cause of hyperthyroidism in Graves' disease has encountered difficulties. The most significant appears to be poor correlation between the amount of circulating LATS activity and the severity of the disease. In fact, some patients with apparent Graves' disease and severe thyrotoxicosis have no demonstrable circulating LATS (*see* Volpe et al., 1972).

EXOPHTHALMOS-PRODUCING SUBSTANCE

Injection of pituitary extract into animals has been noted to cause protrusion of the eyeballs. The phenomenon, first noted in the duck (Shockaert, 1931), has been studied in the guinea pig and several species of fish. It was thought to be caused by thyrotropin, and this seemed logical at a time when thyrotropin was assumed to be an etiological factor in Graves' disease, which is often associated with exophthalmos. However, it is now known that thyrotropin concentrations are very low in Graves' disease. Furthermore, clinical conditions in which thyrotropin secretion is elevated are not characterized by such ocular changes. While apparent dissociation of thyroid-stimulating activity and exophthalmos-producing activity was obtained in the past, it has been shown more recently that homogeneous thyrotropin indeed possesses both activities and that certain proteolytic fragments of the molecule retain exophthalmos-producing activity after loss of most thyroid-stimulating activity (Kohn and Winand, 1971). It is of course possible that there are other substances that can also cause exophthalmos. The etiology of the condition in man remains as obscure as is that of Graves' disease.

CORTICOTROPIN

The discussion of corticotropin (ACTH) appears in Chapter 70 in association with that of the adrenocorticosteroids. The essential features of ACTH chemistry are included in Table 66–1 (page 1373) and Figure 70–1 (page 1474).

MELANOCYTE-STIMULATING HORMONE (MSH)

The intermediate lobe of the pituitary is a part of the adenohypophysis, but in most mammals it is separated from the anterior lobe by the hypophyseal cleft and is composed of a sheet of tissue firmly attached to the contiguous surface of the neurohypophysis.

The term *intermedin* was coined by Zondek for the hormone of the intermediate lobe that mediates various pigmentary responses in the lower vertebrates (*see* Zondek and Krohn, 1932). More recently, Lerner has proposed the term *melanocyte-stimulating hormone* (MSH) (*see* Shizume et al., 1954), a designation that would embrace an action upon the melanocytes of mammalian skin, in keeping with his finding of a darkening of human skin in response to hormone (Lerner and McGuire, 1964). Two compounds have thus far been isolated from pituitary extracts and designated α-MSH and β-MSH. There is evidence for other such proteins that remain uncharacterized (Shapiro et al., 1972).

Chemistry. When strong concentrates of ACTH were first prepared, they were found to be highly active in causing darkening of the skin of frogs. The confusion that arose as a result of this finding was finally resolved when first one component and later two were separated from ACTH. The structures of these substances were elucidated (Dixon, 1964), and they are shown in Figure 70–1 (page 1474) in juxtaposition to ACTH. It is to be noted that the sequence of 13 amino acids making up the molecule of α-MSH is identical with the first 13 residues of ACTH, and that the terminal serine amino group is acetylated. While mammalian α-MSH appears to have a constant amino acid sequence in the species examined, β-MSH does not. Many species synthesize variants of β-MSH with 18 amino acid residues, while in human β-MSH the sequence is extended to 22. Pure ACTH has inherent MSH activity, being about 1/40 as active as α-MSH on a molar basis. The bioassays used are based on hormone-induced darkening of the skin of the frog, chameleon, and related species.

Physiological Actions. Melanocyte-stimulating hormones regulate the pigmentation of fish and amphibian skin by causing dispersal of the pigment granules of the melanophores, thus making the cells appear darker. In keeping with the proposed evolutionary relationship between MSH and ACTH, the members of this group all appear to use cyclic AMP as their intracellular "second messenger" (Abe *et al.,* 1969). While the role of these peptides in regulating normal human pigmentation is unclear, they definitely cause hyperpigmentation when injected in large doses (Lerner and McGuire, 1964). Furthermore, pigmentary changes due to elevated concentrations of MSH and ACTH are noted in human pathological states such as Addison's disease (adrenocortical insufficiency) or rare functional pituitary tumors. It has also been reported that α- and β-MSH are potent natriuretic agents in the rat (Orias and McCann, 1972).

FAT-MOBILIZING FACTORS

It has long been known that the injection of certain pituitary extracts into animals causes ketosis, lowering of the respiratory quotient, and increased fat in the liver. Subsequent studies have shown increased circulating free fatty acids and a direct lipolytic action on isolated adipose tissue *in vitro,* suggesting that mobilization of depot fat is the primary action concerned. As already noted, this is an important part of the action of growth hormone. While TSH, LH, and ACTH have a similar effect, this is not thought to be of physiological consequence, except possibly in the case of TSH. However, the pituitary does contain lipolytic factors that differ from the hormones discussed above. Two such ovine proteins have been purified and analyzed (Li *et al.,* 1965; Chrétien and Li, 1968), and they are included in Table 66–1. Despite their designation as β- and γ-lipotropins, they are potent lipolytic agents in certain species, particularly the rabbit. In view of their structural relationship to ACTH and MSH, it is likely that these materials stimulate lipolysis by a cyclic AMP–dependent mechanism. There is some evidence to favor this hypothesis (Lis *et al.,* 1972). These factors are not active in the rat, and neither they nor their counterparts from human pituitaries are active in man. The possibility of the presence of additional lipolytic substances in human pituitary remains open.

HYPOTHALAMIC CONTROL OF THE ANTERIOR PITUITARY

It is now well established that the influence of the central nervous system upon adenohypophyseal function is mediated by neurohumoral substances transported to the gland

by the hypothalamicoadenohypophyseal-portal system from a capillary network in the region of the median eminence. These substances are referred to as either releasing hormones, releasing factors, or regulatory hormones. Since at least some have been shown to meet the commonly accepted definition of a hormone and also to influence both the synthesis and release of adenohypophyseal hormones, their designation as regulatory hormones (RH) (Schally *et al.,* 1973) seems meritorious. There is great current interest in the identification of hypothalamic regulatory hormones and in their potential use as therapeutic and diagnostic agents. Only a brief summary can be provided here, and several reviews are recommended for detailed discussion and references (Fleischer and Guillemin, 1972; Gual *et al.,* 1972; Kastin *et al.,* 1972; Blackwell and Guillemin, 1973; Schally *et al.,* 1973).

There is evidence to suggest the existence of at least ten regulatory *activities* in the secretions of the hypothalamus. It is not clear at this time whether a lesser or greater number of distinct chemical entities are involved. For at least three adenohypophyseal hormones (prolactin, growth hormone, and MSH), there appears to be dual (stimulatory and inhibitory) regulation. ACTH, TSH, LH, and FSH are perhaps subject only to stimulatory control by this mechanism.

The successful isolation and identification of these hormones have required herculean efforts. In the search for thyrotropin-regulatory hormone, one group utilized 50 tons of hypothalamic starting material. Their ultimate effort involved the purification of 1 mg of the substance from 300,000 ovine hypothalami.

Regulation of Thyrotropin. Thyrotropin-regulatory hormone (TRH) was the first to be identified chemically, in 1970. The porcine and ovine hormone is a tripeptide with both terminal amino and carboxyl groups blocked: L-pyroglutamyl-L-histidyl-L-proline amide. Pyroglutamate is derived from the cyclization of glutamic acid. There is evidence that the hormone from other mammals has the same structure. Synthetic TRH is now available in quantity, and its approval for clinical use is to be expected. Derivatives of TRH have also been synthesized and studied; 3-methyl-His-TRH is eight to ten times more potent than the naturally occurring hormone.

An extremely small quantity of TRH is effective at its site of action; picogram amounts are sufficient to release thyrotropin *in vitro.* Human subjects respond to 50 μg administered intravenously, while a dose of 5 mg or more is required orally. In normal man, intravenous TRH provokes a maximal secretion of thyrotropin within 15 to 30 minutes. Plasma concentrations of thyrotropin remain elevated for 2 to 4 hours, although TRH is inactivated rapidly by human plasma and has a half-life *in vivo* of approximately 5 minutes. There is evidence that TRH stimulates the synthesis as well as the secretion of thyrotropin, although it is not known if this is a primary effect of TRH. In addition, prolactin secretion is also enhanced (*see* below). Specific binding of TRH to pituitary membrane receptors has been demonstrated, as has the associated stimulation of cyclic AMP synthesis. Since cyclic AMP can mimic the actions of TRH *in vitro,* it seems likely that the cyclic nucleotide "second messenger" system is operative here.

The pituitary is the site of negative feedback exerted by the thyroid hormones to inhibit thyrotropin secretion. The action of TRH is antagonized at a molecular site distal to its initial interaction with the plasma membrane. Sites of thyroid hormone feedback may also exist in the central nervous system.

Experimental clinical use is being made of TRH in the diagnosis of thyroid disease; with TRH it can be determined whether secondary hypothyroidism is of pituitary or hypothalamic origin. Hyperthyroid subjects usually fail to respond. Testing involves the intravenous administration of TRH (200 to 500 μg), followed by serial determinations of plasma thyrotropin by immunoassay.

Regulation of Gonadotropins. Predictably, this subject is more complex. Convincing evidence indicates that the secretion of luteinizing hormone is regulated by a hypothalamic hormone, LH-RH, and this material has been purified, identified, and synthesized. Porcine and ovine LH-RH is a decapeptide and has the amino acid sequence pyroGlu-His-Trp-Ser-Tyr-Gly-Leu-Arg-Pro-Gly-NH$_2$. The major current difficulty is that LH-RH definitely stimulates the release of both luteinizing hormone and follicle-stimulating hormone, and it has been proposed that there is but a single gonadotropin-regulatory hormone (LH-RH/FSH-RH).

Synthetic LH-RH is highly active in man. Intravenous administration of 10 to 100 μg causes rapid elevation of plasma gonadotropins. Various temporal patterns of release and sensitivities of gonadotropins to the regulatory hormone have been described. Prolonged or repeated administration results in characteristic and predictable alterations in gonadal function. Ovulation and stimulation of spermatogenesis have been induced in both experimental animals and human subjects. Again, the hormone also stimulates the synthesis of gonadotropin in addition to its release, and cyclic AMP appears to be intimately involved.

While variations in secretion of luteinizing hormone and follicle-stimulating hormone are often simultaneous, normal divergent patterns of secretion

are also well known (*see* Figure 68–2, page 1427). Attempts to explain this invoke, among other observations, the "feedback" effects of sex hormones on responses to the regulatory decapeptide. While important regulatory effects of estrogens and progesterone are thought to occur at neuronal sites in the hypothalamus and elsewhere, direct effects on the pituitary seem probable. Large doses of progesterone can suppress the response of luteinizing hormone to the regulatory hormone, while small amounts of estrogen may enhance the effect. The release of follicle-stimulating hormone may be more susceptible to estrogen inhibition. These interactions are highly complex, and it is impossible at this time to state whether the combined effects of sex hormones and one gonadotropin-regulatory hormone will supply the necessary controls.

The question of paramount importance involves the existence of a separate FSH-RH. Experimental difficulties with follicle-stimulating hormone itself add to the problem. The fact that LH-RH is also a FSH-RH does not exclude the possibility that an additional regulatory hormone is present.

The obvious clinical implications of regulation of gonadotropins have already prompted the synthesis and evaluation of several analogs of LH-RH. Unfortunately, significantly smaller fragments with high activity have not been found. Two analogs with fivefold greater potency have been synthesized by substitution of an amino-terminal ethylamine for glycine amide or by placing D-alanine in the 6 position. A weak antagonist with little stimulatory activity is Des-His²-LH-RH, and better antagonistic activity is observed with Des-His²-D-Ala⁶-LH-RH or Des-His²-Des-Gly¹⁰-LH-RH-ethylamide. These synthetic efforts will certainly continue.

Regulation of Corticotropin. Despite the fact that corticotropin-regulatory hormone (CRH) was the first to be demonstrated by physiological technics, experimental difficulties have delayed its isolation and identification. While antidiuretic hormone and fragments thereof have significant CRH activity, the true hormone is probably an unrelated peptide.

Regulation of Growth Hormone. Growth hormone appears to be subject to regulation by both a GH-RH and a release-inhibiting hormone (GH-RIH). Initial attempts to isolate GH-RH resulted in the characterization of a decapeptide that caused release of growth hormone–like material as detected by bioassay. Unfortunately, corresponding increments in immunoreactive growth hormone could not be observed, and consequently this decapeptide is no longer considered to have physiological significance. Characterization of the true GH-RH awaits further work. Since cyclic nucleotides are effective stimulators of growth hormone secretion *in vitro,* GH-RH may also utilize this mechanism.

Brazeau and associates (1973) have isolated a tetradecapeptide from the ovine hypothalamus that markedly inhibits the secretion of immunoreactive growth hormone *in vivo* and *in vitro.* Its structure is:

Ala—Gly—Cys—Lys—Asn—Phe—Phe—Trp—Lys—Thr—Phe—Thr—Ser—Cys

This peptide is thought to represent a GH-RIH, and for simplicity of nomenclature it has been called *somatostatin.* However, at higher concentrations, somatostatin also inhibits the secretion of TSH, insulin, glucagon, and gastrin (Bloom *et al.,* 1974; Koerker *et al.,* 1974). In addition, the peptide inhibits the action of glucagon on the liver (Oliver and Wagle, 1975) and the effects of pentagastrin and histamine on gastric acid production (Barros D'Sa *et al.,* 1975). While these divergent effects are somewhat perplexing, it should be of interest to explore potential clinical applications of somatostatin in pituitary disease, diabetes mellitus, syndromes associated with hormone-secreting tumors, and acid-pepsin disorders. For example, initial results indicate that infusion of somatostatin can prevent the development of ketoacidosis in patients with juvenile-type diabetes deprived of insulin for 18 hours; this was attributed to inhibition of glucagon secretion (Gerich *et al.,* 1975).

Regulation of Prolactin. Several aspects of hypothalamic regulation of prolactin secretion have been discussed above. The inhibitory influence of a prolactin release–inhibiting hormone appears to predominate. Also as mentioned, TRH has prolactin-releasing activity. It is not known if TRH serves physiologically as the prolactin-regulatory hormone (PRH). However, a rare syndrome characterized by primary hypothyroidism and high circulating prolactin concentration with associated galactorrhea is at least suggestive of pathological function of TRH as a PRH.

Regulation of Melanocyte-Stimulating Hormone. This is a controversial area in which dual control is also suspected. Compounds that inhibit secretion of melanocyte-stimulating hormone have been isolated from the hypothalamus. One such is reported to be Pro-Leu-Gly-NH$_2$, a tripeptide that can be cleaved from oxytocin by enzymes of the hypothalamus. Another is the ring structure of oxytocin, tocinoic acid:

$$\overset{\rule{3cm}{0.4pt}}{Cys—Tyr—Ileu—Gln—Asn—Cys}$$

Regulation of Regulatory Hormones. Although any significant discussion of this important area of neuroendocrinology is beyond the scope of this text, a few points should be made. There is ample evidence to indicate important monoaminergic, particularly adrenergic, control of regulatory hormone release. This has been discussed above in regard to the inhibitor of prolactin secretion. Similar evidence implicates adrenergic mechanisms in the secretion of growth hormone, thyrotropin, and gonadotropins. Drugs that alter central adrenergic mechanisms exert significant influences on the secretion of the adenohypophyseal hormones, and these are discussed under the individual agents involved.

Abe, K.; Robison, G. A.; Liddle, G. W.; Butcher, R. W.; Nicholson, W. E.; and Baird, C. E. Role of cyclic AMP in mediating the effects of MSH, norepinephrine, and melatonin on frog skin color. *Endocrinology,* **1969,** *85,* 674–682.

Abrams, R. L.; Grumbach, M. M.; and Kaplan, S. L. The effect of administration of human growth hormone on the plasma growth hormone, cortisol, glucose, and free fatty acid response to insulin: evidence for growth hormone autoregulation in man. *J. clin. Invest.,* **1971,** *50,* 940–950.

Adams, D. D., and Purves, H. D. The role of thyrotropin in hyperthyroidism and exophthalmos. *Metabolism,* **1957,** *6,* 26–35.

Adcock, E. W., III; Teasdale, F.; August, C. S.; Cox, S.; Meschia, G.; Battaglia, F. C.; and Naughton, M. A. Human chorionic gonadotropin: its possible role in maternal lymphocyte suppression. *Science, Wash.,* **1973,** *181,* 845–847.

Allen, B. M. Effects of extirpation of the anterior lobe of the hypophysis of *Rana pipiens. Biol. Bull. mar. biol. Lab., Woods Hole,* **1917,** *32,* 117–130.

Armstrong, B.; Stevens, N.; and Doll, R. Retrospective study of the association between use of rauwolfia derivatives and breast cancer in English women. *Lancet,* **1974,** *2,* 672–675.

Aron, M. Action de la préhypophyse sur la thyroide chez le cobaye. *C. r. Séanc. Soc. Biol.,* **1929,** *102,* 682–684.

Aschner, B. Demonstration von Hunden nach Extirpation der Hypophyse. *Wien klin. Wschr.,* **1909,** *22,* 1730–1731.

Bahl, O. P.; Carlsen, R. B.; Bellisario, R.; and Swaminathan, N. Human chorionic gonadotropin: amino acid sequence of the α and β subunits. *Biochem. biophys. Res. Commun.,* **1972,** *48,* 416–422.

Barros D'Sa, A. A. J.; Bloom, S. R.; and Baron, J. H. Direct inhibition of gastric acid by growth-hormone releasing-inhibiting hormone in dogs. *Lancet,* **1975,** *1,* 886–887.

Beck, P.; Koumans, J. H. T.; Winterling, C. A.; Stein, M. F.; Daughaday, W. H.; and Kipnis, D. M. Studies of insulin and growth hormone secretion in human obesity. *J. Lab. clin. Med.,* **1964,** *64,* 654–667.

Blackard, W. G.; Hull, E. W.; and Lopez-S, A. Effect of lipids on growth hormone secretion in humans. *J. clin. Invest.,* **1971,** *50,* 1439–1443.

Bloom, S. R.; Mortimer, C. H.; Thorner, M. O.; Besser, G. M.; Hall, R.; Gomez-Pan, A.; Roy, V. M.; Russell, R. C. G.; Coy, D. H.; Kastin, A. J.; and Schally, A. V. Inhibition of gastrin and gastric acid secretion by growth-hormone releasing-inhibiting hormone. *Lancet,* **1974,** *2,* 1106–1109.

Boston Collaborative Drug Surveillance Program. Reserpine and breast cancer. *Lancet,* **1974,** *2,* 669–671.

Brazeau, P.; Vale, W.; Burgus, R.; Ling, N.; Butcher, M.; Rivier, J.; and Guillemin, R. Hypothalamic polypeptide that inhibits the secretion of immunoreactive pituitary growth hormone. *Science, Wash.,* **1973,** *179,* 77–79.

Brown, T. B.; Evans, J. H.; Adey, F. D.; Taft, H. P.; and Townsend, L. Factors involved in the induction of fertile ovulation and human gonadotropins. *J. Obstet. Gynaec. Br. Commonw.,* **1969,** *76,* 289–307.

Buckman, M. T., and Peake, G. T. Osmolar control of prolactin secretion in man. *Science, Wash.,* **1973,** *181,* 755–757.

Channing, C. P., and Seymour, J. F. Effects of dibutyryl cyclic-3′,5′-AMP and other agents upon luteinization of porcine granulosa cells in culture. *Endocrinology,* **1970,** *87,* 165–169.

Chrétien, M., and Li, C. H. Isolation, purification, and characterization of γ-lipotropic hormone from sheep pituitary gland. *Can. J. Biochem.,* **1968,** *45,* 1163–1174.

Coble, Y. D., Jr.; Kohler, P. O.; Cargille, C. M.; and Ross, G. T. Production rates and metabolic clearance rates of human follicle-stimulating hormone in premenopausal and postmenopausal women. *J. clin. Invest.,* **1969,** *48,* 359–363.

Collip, J. B.; Anderson, E. M.; and Thomson, D. L. The

adrenotropic hormone of the anterior pituitary lobe. *Lancet,* **1933,** *2,* 347–348.

Daughaday, W. H.; Laron, Z.; Pertzelan, A.; and Heins, J. N. Defective sulfation factor generation: a possible etiological link in dwarfism. *Trans. Ass. Am. Physns,* **1969,** *82,* 129–140.

Daughaday, W. H.; Salmon, W. D., Jr.; and Alexander, F. Sulfation factor activity of sera from patients with pituitary disorders. *J. clin. Endocr. Metab.,* **1959,** *19,* 743–758.

Dixon, H. B. F. Chemistry of pituitary hormones. In, *The Hormones,* Vol. V. (Pincus, G.; Thimann, K. V.; and Astwood, E. B.; eds.) Academic Press, Inc., New York, **1964,** pp. 1–68.

Ellsworth, L. R., and Armstrong, D. T. Luteinization of transplanted ovarian follicles in the rat induced by dibutyryl cyclic AMP. *Endocrinology,* **1973,** *92,* 840–846.

Evans, H. M., and Long, J. A. The effect of the anterior lobe administered intraperitoneally upon growth, maturity, and oestrous cycles of the rat. *Anat. Rec.,* **1921,** *21,* 62–63.

Faiman, C., and Ryan, R. J. Serum follicle-stimulating hormone and luteinizing hormone concentrations during the menstrual cycle as determined by radioimmunoassays. *J. clin. Endocr. Metab.,* **1967,** *27,* 1711–1716.

Fevold, H. L.; Hisaw, F. L.; Hellbaum, A.; and Hertz, A. Sex hormones of the anterior lobe of the hypophysis: further purification of a follicular stimulating factor and the physiological effects on immature rats and rabbits. *Am. J. Physiol.,* **1933,** *104,* 710–723.

Finkelstein, J. W.; Roffwarg, H. P.; Boyar, R. M.; Kream, J.; and Hellman, L. Age-related change in the twenty-four-hour spontaneous secretion of growth hormone. *J. clin. Endocr. Metab.,* **1972,** *35,* 665–670.

Frantz, A. G., and Kleinberg, D. L. Prolactin: evidence that it is separate from growth hormone in human blood. *Science, Wash.,* **1970,** *170,* 745–747.

Friesen, H. Purification of a placental factor with immunological and chemical similarity to human growth hormone. *Endocrinology,* **1965,** *76,* 369–381.

———. Lactation induced by human placental lactogen and cortisone acetate in rabbits. *Ibid.,* **1966,** *79,* 212–215.

———. Human prolactin in clinical endocrinology: the impact of radioimmunoassays. *Metabolism,* **1973,** *22,* 1039–1045.

Fukushima, M. Studies on somatotropic hormone secretion in gynecology and obstetrics. *Tohoku J. exp. Med.,* **1961,** *74,* 161–174.

Gemzell, C. A. The induction of ovulation in the human by human pituitary gonadotropin. In, *Control of Ovulation.* (Villee, C. A., ed.) Pergamon Press, Ltd., Oxford, **1961.**

Gemzell, C., and Kjessler, B. Treatment of infertility after partial hypophysectomy with human pituitary gonadotropins. *Lancet,* **1964,** *1,* 644.

Gerich, J. E.; Lorenzi, M.; Bier, D. M.; Schneider, V.; Tsalikian, E.; Karam, J. H.; and Forsham, P. H. Prevention of human diabetic ketoacidosis by somatostatin. Evidence for an essential role of glucagon. *New Engl. J. Med.,* **1975,** *292,* 985–989.

Goodman, A. D.; Tanenbaum, R.; and Rabinowitz, D. Existence of two forms of immunoreactive growth hormone in human plasma. *J. clin. Endocr. Metab.,* **1972,** *35,* 868–878.

Gordon, P.; Lesniak, M. A.; Hendricks, C. M.; and Roth, J. "Big" growth hormone components from human plasma: decreased reactivity demonstrated by radioreceptor assay. *Science, Wash.,* **1973,** *182,* 829–831.

Gospodarowicz, D. Purification and physicochemical properties of the pregnant mare serum gonadotropin (PMSG). *Endocrinology,* **1972,** *91,* 101–106.

Guyda, H. J., and Friesen, H. G. The separation of monkey prolactin from monkey growth hormone by affinity chromatography. *Biochem. biophys. Res. Commun.,* **1971,** *42,* 1068–1075.

Hack, M.; Brish, M.; Serr, D. M.; Inster, V.; and Lunenfeld, B. Outcome of pregnancies after induced ovulation. Follow-up of pregnancies and children born after gonadotropin therapy. *J. Am. med. Ass.,* **1970,** *211,* 791–797.

Heinonen, O. P.; Shapiro, S.; Tuominen, L.; and Turunen, M. I. Reserpine use in relation to breast cancer. *Lancet,* **1974,** *2,* 675–677.

Hershman, J. M. Hyperthyroidism induced by trophoblastic thyrotropin. *Mayo Clin. Proc.,* **1972,** *47,* 913–918.

Hobson, B., and Wide, L. The immunological and biological activity of human chorionic gonadotropin in urine. *Acta endocr., Copenh.,* **1964,** *46,* 632–638.

Houssay, B. A. Advancement of knowledge of the role of the hypophysis in carbohydrate metabolism during the last twenty-five years. *Endocrinology,* **1942,** *30,* 884–897.

Huttunen, J. K.; Steinberg, D.; and Mayer, S. E. ATP-dependent and cyclic AMP–dependent activation of rat adipose tissue lipase by protein kinase from rabbit skeletal muscle. *Proc. natn. Acad. Sci. U.S.A.,* **1970,** *67,* 290–295.

Hwang, P.; Guyda, H.; and Friesen, H. A radioimmunoassay for human prolactin. *Proc. natn. Acad. Sci. U.S.A.,* **1971,** *68,* 1902–1906.

Josimovich, J. B., and MacLaren, J. A. Presence in the human placenta and term serum of a highly lactogenic substance immunologically related to pituitary growth hormone. *Endocrinology,* **1962,** *71,* 209–220.

Kaplan, S. L.; Grumbach, M. M.; and Shepard, T. H. The ontogenesis of human fetal hormones. I. Growth hormone and insulin. *J. clin. Invest.,* **1972,** *51,* 3080–3093.

Koerker, D. J.; Ruch, W.; Chideckel, E.; Palmer, J.; Goodner, C.; Ensinck, J.; and Gale, C. C. Somatostatin: hypothalamic inhibitor of the endocrine pancreas. *Science, Wash.,* **1974,** *184,* 482–484.

Kohn, L. D., and Winand, R. J. Relationship of thyrotropin to exophthalmos-producing substance. Formation of an exophthalmos-producing substance by pepsin digestion of pituitary glycoproteins containing both thyrotropic and exophthalmogenic activity. *J. biol. Chem.,* **1971,** *246,* 6570–6575.

Kriss, J. P. The long-acting thyroid stimulator and thyroid disease. *Adv. intern. Med.,* **1970,** *16,* 135–154.

Kuehl, F. A.; Humes, J. L.; Tarnoff, J.; Cirillo, V. J.; and Ham, E. A. Prostaglandin receptor site: evidence for an essential role in the action of luteinizing hormone. *Science, Wash.,* **1970,** *169,* 883–886.

Lattimer, J. K. The optimum treatment for undescended testis. *Med. Coll. Va Q.,* **1973,** *9,* 270–274.

Lee, M., and Ayres, G. B. Composition of weight lost and nitrogen partition of tissues in rats after hypophysectomy. *Endocrinology,* **1936,** *20,* 489–495.

Lerner, A. B., and McGuire, J. S. Melanocyte-stimulating hormone and adrenocorticotrophic hormone: their relation to pigmentation. *New Engl. J. Med.,* **1964,** *270,* 539–546.

Lesniak, M. A.; Roth, J.; Gorden, P.; and Gavin, J. R., iii. Human growth hormone radioreceptor assay using cultured human lymphocytes. *Nature, New Biol.,* **1973,** *241,* 20–22.

Li, C. H.; Barnafi, L.; Chrétien, M.; and Chung, D. Isolation and amino-acid sequence of β-LPH from sheep pituitary glands. *Nature, Lond.,* **1965,** *208,* 1093–1094.

Li, C. H.; Dixon, J. S.; and Chung, D. Amino acid sequence of human chorionic somatomammotropin. *Archs Biochem. Biophys.,* **1973,** *155,* 95–110.

Li, C. H.; Dixon, J. S.; Lo, T.-B.; Schmidt, K. D.; and Pankov, Y. A. Studies on pituitary lactogenic hormone. XXX. The primary structure of the sheep hormone. *Archs Biochem. Biophys.,* **1970,** *141,* 705–737.

Li, C. H.; Liu, W. K.; and Dixon, J. S. Human pituitary growth hormone. XII. The amino acid sequence of the hormone. *J. Am. chem. Soc.,* **1966,** *88,* 2050–2051.

Lis, M.; Gilardeau, C.; and Chrétien, M. Fat cell adenylate cyclase activation by sheep β-lipotropic hormone. *Proc. Soc. exp. Biol. Med.,* **1972,** *139,* 680–683.

Liu, W.-K.; Nahm, H. S.; Sweeney, C. M.; Holcomb, G. N.; and Ward, D. N. The primary structure of ovine luteinizing hormone. II. The amino acid sequence of the reduced, S-carboxymethylated A-subunit (LH-β). *J. biol. Chem.,* **1972a,** *247,* 4365–4381.

Liu, W.-K.; Nahm, H. S.; Sweeney, C. M.; Lamkin, W. M.; Baker, H. N.; and Ward, D. N. The primary structure of ovine luteinizing hormone. I. The amino acid sequence of the reduced and S-aminoethylated S-subunit (LH-α). *J. biol. Chem.,* **1972b,** *247,* 4351–4364.

Loeb, L., and Bassett, R. B. Effect of hormones of anterior pituitary on thyroid gland in the guinea pig. *Proc. Soc. exp. Biol. Med.,* **1929,** *26,* 860–862.

Louis, L. H., and Conn, J. W. Diabetogenic polypeptide from human pituitaries similar to that excreted by proteinuric diabetic patients. *Metabolism,* **1972,** *21,* 1–9.

McKenzie, J. M. Studies on the thyroid activator of hyperthyroidism. *J. clin. Endocr. Metab.,* **1961,** *21,* 635–647.

MacLeod, R. M., and Lehmeyer, J. E. Studies on the mechanism of the dopamine-mediated inhibition of prolactin secretion. *Endocrinology,* **1974,** *94,* 1077–1085.

Mancini, R. E.; Vilar, O.; Donini, P.; and Pérez Lloret, A. Effect of human urinary FSH and LH on the recovery of spermatogenesis in hypophysectomized patients. *J. clin. Endocr. Metab.,* **1971,** *33,* 888–895.

Marsh, J. M.; Butcher, R. W.; Savard, K.; and Sutherland, E. W. The stimulatory effect of luteinizing hormone on adenosine 3′,5′-monophosphate accumulation in corpus luteum slices. *J. biol. Chem.,* **1966,** *241,* 5436–5440.

Midgley, A. R., and Jaffe, R. B. Regulation of human gonadotropins. IV. Correlation of serum concentrations of follicle stimulating and luteinizing hormones during the menstrual cycle. *J. clin. Endocr. Metab.,* **1968,** *28,* 1699–1703.

Miller, T. B., and Larner, J. Anti-insulin actions of a bovine pituitary diabetogenic peptide on glycogen synthesis. *Proc. natn. Acad. Sci. U.S.A.,* **1972,** *69,* 2774–2777.

Mills, T. M.; Davies, P. J. A.; and Savard, K. Stimulation of estrogen synthesis in rabbit follicles by luteinizing hormone. *Endocrinology,* **1971,** *88,* 857–862.

Murad, F.; Strauch, B. S.; and Vaughan, M. The effect of gonadotropins on testicular adenyl cyclase. *Biochim. biophys. Acta,* **1969,** *177,* 591–598.

Niall, H. D.; Hogan, M. L.; Sauer, R.; Rosenblum, I. Y.; and Greenwood, F. C. Sequences of pituitary and placental lactogenic and growth hormones: evolution from a primordial peptide by gene reduplication. *Proc. natn. Acad. Sci. U.S.A.,* **1971,** *68,* 866–869.

Oliver, J. R., and Wagle, S. R. Studies on the inhibition of insulin release, glycogenolysis, and gluconeogenesis by somatostatin in the rat islets of Langerhans and isolated hepatocytes. *Biochem. biophys. Res. Commun.,* **1975,** *62,* 772–777.

Orias, R., and McCann, S. M. Natriuresis induced by alpha and beta melanocyte stimulating hormone (MSH) in rats. *Endocrinology,* **1972,** *90,* 700–706.

Papkoff, H. Subunit interrelationships among the pituitary glycoprotein hormones. *Gen. comp. Endocr.,* **1972,** Suppl. 3, 609–616.

Parker, D. C.; Sassin, J. F.; Mace, J. W.; Gotlin, R. W.; and Rossman, L. G. Human growth hormone release during sleep: electroencephalographic correlation. *J. clin. Endocr. Metab.,* **1969,** *29,* 871–874.

Parker, M. L.; Hammond, J. M.; and Daughaday, W. H. The arginine provocative test: an aid in the diagnosis of hyposomatotropism. *J. clin. Endocr. Metab.,* **1967,** *27,* 1129–1136.

Pierce, J. G. The subunits of pituitary thyrotropin—their relationship to other glycoprotein hormones. *Endocrinology,* **1971,** *89,* 1331–1344.

Quadri, S. K.; Lu, K. H.; and Meites, J. Ergot-induced

inhibition of pituitary tumor growth in rats. *Science, Wash.,* **1972,** *176,* 417–418.

Raben, M. S. Growth hormone. 1. Physiologic aspects. *New Engl. J. Med.,* **1962a,** *266,* 31–35. 2. Clinical use of human growth hormone. *Ibid.,* **1962b,** *266,* 82–86.

Raben, M. S., and Hollenberg, C. H. Effect of growth hormone on plasma fatty acids. *J. clin. Invest.,* **1959,** *38,* 484–488.

Reichert, L. E., Jr. Biological studies on the relatedness of subunits of human follicle stimulating hormone and chorionic gonadotropin. *Endocrinology,* **1972,** *90,* 1119–1132.

Reichlin, S. The physiology of growth hormone regulation: pre- and postimmunoassay eras. *Metabolism,* **1973,** *22,* 987–993.

Riddle, O.; Bates, R. W.; and Dykshorn, S. W. The preparation, identification and assay of prolactin—a hormone of the anterior pituitary. *Am. J. Physiol.,* **1933,** *105,* 191–216.

Roth, J.; Glick, S. M.; Yalow, R. S.; and Berson, S. A. Hypoglycemia: a potent stimulus to secretion of growth hormone. *Science, Wash.,* **1963,** *140,* 987–988.

Rudman, D.; Patterson, J. H.; and Gibbas, D. L. Responsiveness of growth hormone–deficient children to human growth hormone. *J. clin. Invest.,* **1973,** *52,* 1108–1112.

Russell, J. A. Effects of growth hormone on protein and carbohydrate metabolism. *Am. J. clin. Nutr.,* **1957,** *5,* 404–416.

Sairam, M. R., and Li, C. H. Human pituitary thyrotropin: primary structure of the hormone specific β subunit. *Biochem. biophys. Res. Commun.,* **1973,** *54,* 426–431.

Sairam, M. R.; Papkoff, H.; and Li, C. H. Human pituitary interstitial cell stimulating hormone: primary structure of the α subunit. *Biochem. biophys. Res. Commun.,* **1972,** *48,* 530–537.

Salmon, W. D., Jr., and DuVall, M. R. A serum fraction with "sulfation factor activity" stimulates *in vitro* incorporation of leucine and sulfate into protein-polysaccharide complexes, uridine into RNA and thymidine into DNA of costal cartilage from hypophysectomized rats. *Endocrinology,* **1970,** *86,* 721–727.

Saxena, B. B., and Rathnam, P. Dissociation phenomenon and subunit nature of follicle-stimulating hormone from human pituitary glands. *J. biol. Chem.,* **1971,** *246,* 3549–3554.

Shapiro, M.; Nicholson, W. E.; Orth, D. N.; Mitchell, W. M.; Island, D. P.; and Liddle, G. W. Preliminary characterization of the pituitary melanocyte stimulating hormones of several vertebrate species. *Endocrinology,* **1972,** *90,* 249–256.

Sheehan, H. L., and Summers, V. K. The syndrome of hypopituitarism. *Q. Jl Med.,* **1949,** *18,* 319–379.

Sherwood, L. M. Similarities in the chemical structure of human placental lactogen and pituitary growth hormone. *Proc. natn. Acad. Sci. U.S.A.,* **1967,** *58,* 2307–2314.

Shiu, R. P. C.; Kelly, P. A.; and Friesen, H. G. Radioreceptor assay for prolactin and other lactogenic hormones. *Science, Wash.,* **1973,** *180,* 968–971.

Shizume, K.; Lerner, A. B.; and Fitzpatrick, T. B. *In vitro* bioassay for the melanocyte stimulating hormone. *Endocrinology,* **1954,** *54,* 553–560.

Shockaert, J. A. Hyperplasia of thyroid and exophthalmos in treatment with anterior pituitary in young ducks. *Proc. Soc. exp. Biol. Med.,* **1931,** *29,* 306–308.

Shome, B., and Parlow, A. F. The primary structure of the hormone-specific, beta subunit of human pituitary luteinizing hormone (hLH). *J. clin. Endocr. Metab.,* **1973,** *36,* 618–621.

Sledge, C. B. Growth hormone and articular cartilage. *Fedn Proc. Fedn Am. Socs exp. Biol.,* **1973,** *32,* 1503–1505.

Smith, P. E. The disabilities caused by hypophysectomy and their repair. *J. Am. med. Ass.,* **1927,** *88,* 158–161.

———. Hypophysectomy and a replacement therapy. *Am. J. Anat.,* **1930,** *45,* 205–256.

Tanner, J. M.; Whitehouse, R. H.; Hughes, P. C. R.; and Vince, F. P. Effect of human growth hormone treatment for 1 to 7 years on growth of 100 children, with growth hormone deficiency, low birth weight, inherited smallness, Turner's syndrome, and other complaints. *Archs Dis. Childh.,* **1971,** *46,* 745–782.

Tell, G. P. E.; Cuatrecasas, P.; Van Wyk, J. J.; and Hintz, R. L. Somatomedin inhibition of adenylate cyclase activity in subcellular membranes of various tissues. *Science, Wash.,* **1973,** *180,* 312–315.

Theodoridis, C. G.; Brown, G. A.; Chance, G. W.; and Rayner, P. H. W. Growth-hormone response to oral glucose in children with simple obesity. *Lancet,* **1969,** *1,* 1068–1069.

Thompson, C. R., and Hansen, L. M. PERGONAL (menotropins): a summary of clinical experience in the induction of ovulation and pregnancy. *Fert. Steril.,* **1970,** *21,* 844–853.

Thompson, R. G.; Rodriguez, A.; Kowarski, A.; Migeon, C. J.; and Blizzard, R. M. Integrated concentrations of growth hormone correlated with plasma testosterone and bone age in preadolescent and adolescent males. *J. clin. Endocr. Metab.,* **1972,** *35,* 334–337.

Tsushima, T., and Friesen, H. G. Radioreceptor assay for growth hormone. *J. clin. Endocr. Metab.,* **1973,** *37,* 334–337.

Turkington, R. W. Inhibition of prolactin secretion and successful therapy of the Forbes-Albright syndrome with L-dopa. *J. clin. Endocr. Metab.,* **1972,** *34,* 306–311.

Underwood, L. E.; Hintz, R. L.; Voina, S. J.; and Van Wyk, J. J. Human somatomedin, the growth hormone–dependent sulfation factor, is anti-lipolytic. *J. clin. Endocr. Metab.,* **1972,** *35,* 194–198.

Utiger, R. D.; Parker, M. L.; and Daughaday, W. H. Studies on human growth hormone. I. A radioimmunoassay for human growth hormone. *J. clin. Invest.,* **1962,** *41,* 254–261.

Van Hall, E. V.; Vaitukaitis, J. L.; Ross, G. T.; Hickman, J. W.; and Ashwell, G. Effects of progressive desialylation on the rate of disappearance of immunoreactive HCG from plasma in rats. *Endocrinology,* **1971,** *89,* 11–15.

Volpe, R.; Edmonds, M.; Lamki, L.; Clarke, P. V.; and Row, V. V. The pathogenesis of Graves' disease. *Mayo Clin. Proc.,* **1972,** *47,* 824–834.

Weldon, V. V.; Gupta, S. K.; Haymond, M. W.; Pagliara, A. S.; Jacobs, L. S.; and Daughaday, W. H. The use of L-dopa in the diagnosis of hyposomatotropism in children. *J. clin. Endocr. Metab.,* **1973,** *36,* 42–46.

Yadley, R. A.; Rodbard, D.; and Chrambach, A. Isohormones of human growth hormone. III. Isolation by preparative polyacrylamide gel electrophoresis and characterization. *Endocrinology,* **1973,** *93,* 866–873.

Yamasaki, N.; Kangawa, K.; Kobayashi, S.; Kikutani, M.; and Sonenberg, M. Amino acid sequence of a biologically active fragment of bovine growth hormone. *J. biol. Chem.,* **1972,** *247,* 3874–3880.

Yamashita, K., and Field, J. B. Effects of long-acting thyroid stimulator on thyrotropin stimulation of adenyl cyclase activity in thyroid plasma membranes. *J. clin. Invest.,* **1972,** *51,* 463–472.

Yen, S. S. C.; Llerena, O.; Little, B.; and Pearson, O. H. Disappearance rates of endogenous luteinizing hormone and chorionic gonadotropin in man. *J. clin. Endocr. Metab.,* **1968,** *28,* 1763–1767.

Yen, S. S. C.; Llerena, L. A.; Pearson, O. H.; and Littell, A. S. Disappearance rates of endogenous follicle-stimulating hormone in serum following surgical hypophysectomy in man. *J. clin. Endocr. Metab.,* **1970,** *30,* 325–329.

Young, F. G. Growth and diabetes in normal animals treated with pituitary (anterior lobe) diabetogenic extract. *Biochem. J.,* **1945,** *39,* 515–536.

Zierler, K. L. Effects of growth hormone on metabolism of muscle and adipose tissue of the forearm of man. In, *Clinical Endocrinology II.* (Astwood, E. B., and Cassidy, C. E., eds.) Grune & Stratton, Inc., New York, **1968,** pp. 55–68.

Zondek, B., and Krohn, H. Hormon des Zwischenlappens der Hypophyse (Intermedin). *Naturwissenschaften,* **1932,** *8,* 134–136.

Zor, U.; Kaneko, T.; Lowe, I. P.; Bloom, G.; and Field, J. B. Effect of thyroid-stimulating hormone and prostaglandins on thyroid adenyl cyclase activation and cyclic adenosine 3′,5′-monophosphate. *J. biol. Chem.,* **1969,** *244,* 5189–5195.

Monographs and Reviews

Bern, H. A., and Nicoll, C. S. The comparative endocrinology of prolactin. *Recent Prog. Horm. Res.,* **1968,** *24,* 681–713.

Blackwell, R. E., and Guillemin, R. Hypothalamic control of adenohypophysial secretions. *A. Rev. Physiol.,* **1973,** *35,* 357–390.

Dorfman, R. I. Mechanism of action of gonadotropins and prolactin. In, *Biochemical Actions of Hormones,* Vol. II. (Litwack, G., ed.) Academic Press, Inc., New York, **1972,** pp. 295–316.

Fain, J. N. Biochemical aspects of drug and hormone action on adipose tissue. *Pharmac. Rev.,* **1973,** *25,* 67–118.

Fleischer, N., and Guillemin, R. Clinical application of hypothalamic releasing factors. *Adv. intern. Med.,* **1972,** *18,* 303–323.

Floss, H. G.; Cassady, J. M.; and Robbers, J. E. Influence of ergot alkaloids on pituitary prolactin and prolactin-dependent processes. *J. pharm. Sci.,* **1973,** *62,* 699–715.

Frantz, A. G.; Kleinberg, D. L.; and Noel, G. L. Studies on prolactin in man. *Recent Prog. Horm. Res.,* **1972,** *28,* 527–573.

Gemzell, C. Induction of ovulation with human gonadotropins. *Recent Prog. Horm. Res.,* **1965,** *21,* 179–204.

Glick, S.; Roth, J.; Yalow, R. S.; and Berson, S. A. Physiological control of growth hormone. *Recent Prog. Horm. Res.,* **1965,** *21,* 241–283.

Gual, C.; Kastin, A. J.; and Schally, A. V. Clinical experience with hypothalamic releasing hormones. Part 1. Thyrotropin releasing hormone. *Recent Prog. Horm. Res.,* **1972,** *28,* 173–200.

Kastin, A. J.; Gual, C.; and Schally, A. V. Clinical experience with hypothalamic releasing hormones. Part 2. Luteinizing hormone-releasing hormone and other hypophysiotropic releasing hormones. *Recent Prog. Horm. Res.,* **1972,** *28,* 201–217.

Knobil, E., and Greep, R. O. Physiology of growth hormone with particular reference to its action in rhesus monkey and "species specificity" problem. *Recent Prog. Horm. Res.,* **1959,** *15,* 1–69.

Li, C. H. Hormones of the adenohypophysis. *Proc. Am. phil. Soc.,* **1972,** *116,* 365–382.

McMahon, B.; Cole, P.; and Brown, J. Etiology of human breast cancer: a review. *J. natn. Cancer Inst.,* **1973,** *50,* 21–42.

Meites, J.; Lu, K. H.; Wuttke, W.; Welsch, C. W.; Nagasawa, H.; and Quadri, S. K. Recent studies on functions and control of prolactin secretion in rats. *Recent Prog. Horm. Res.,* **1972,** *28,* 471–516.

Niall, H. D.; Hogan, M. L.; Tregear, G. W.; Segre, G. V.; Hwang, P.; and Friesen, H. The chemistry of growth hormones and the lactogenic hormones. *Recent Prog. Horm. Res.,* **1973,** *29,* 387–404.

Papkoff, H.; Sairam, M. R.; Farmer, S. W.; and Li, C. H. Studies on the structure and function of interstitial cell-stimulating hormone. *Recent Prog. Horm. Res.,* **1973,** *29,* 563–588.

Raben, M. S. Human growth hormone. *Recent Prog. Horm. Res.,* **1959,** *15,* 71–114.

Rimoin, D. L.; Merimee, T. J.; Rabinowitz, D.; and McKusick, V. A. Genetic aspects of clinical endocrinology. *Recent Prog. Horm. Res.,* **1968,** *24,* 365–429.

Schally, A. V.; Arimura, A.; and Kastin, A. J. Hypothalamic regulatory hormones. *Science, Wash.,* **1973,** *179,* 341–350.

Topper, Y. J. Multiple hormone interactions in the development of mammary gland *in vitro. Recent Prog. Horm. Res.,* **1970,** *26,* 287–303.

Turkington, R. W.; Majumder, G. C.; Kadohama, N.; MacIndoe, J. H.; and Frantz, W. L. Hormonal regulation of gene expression in mammary cells. *Recent Prog. Horm. Res.,* **1973,** *29,* 417–449.

Vande Wiele, R. L., and Dyrenfurth, I. Gonadotropin-steroid interrelationships. *Pharmac. Rev.,* **1973,** *25,* 189–207.

67 THYROID AND ANTITHYROID DRUGS

Alfred G. Gilman and Ferid Murad

THYROID

The thyroid gland is the source of two fundamentally different types of hormones. *Thyroxine* and *triiodothyronine* are vital for normal growth and development and play an important role in energy metabolism. The other known glandular secretion, *calcitonin,* is considered in Chapter 72.

History. The thyroid gland was first described in 1656 by Wharton, whose investigations were based upon the many older and often amusing opinions concerning the function of this gland (*see* Harington, 1935). He thought, for example, that the viscous fluid within the follicles lubricated the trachea. He also believed that the gland was larger in women to serve a cosmetic function in giving grace to the contour of the neck. Later observers, influenced by the liberal blood supply of the gland, believed that it provided a vascular shunt for the brain. With this function in mind, Rush in 1820 expressed the belief that the larger size of the gland in women was "necessary to guard the female system from the influence of the more numerous causes of irritation and vexation of mind to which they are exposed than the male sex." However, Hofrichter (1820) cleverly opposed this theory by pointing out that, "If it were indeed true that the thyroid contains more blood at some times than at others, this effect would be visible to the naked eye; in this case women would certainly have long ceased to go about with bare necks, for husbands would have learned to recognize the swelling of this gland as a danger signal of threatening trouble from their better halves."

Numerous other theories of thyroid function were advanced, based upon little or no experimental evidence. The belief ultimately became prevalent that the gland served no important physiological role. The thyroid was first recognized as an organ of importance when enlargement was observed to be associated with changes in the eyes and in the heart in the condition we now call hyperthyroidism. It is of interest that this condition, the manifestations of which can on occasion be as striking as any in medicine, escaped description until Parry saw his first case in 1786. Parry's account was not published until 1825 (*see* Parry, 1895) and was followed in 1835 and 1840 by those of Graves and Basedow, whose names became applied to the disorder. It was not until 1874 that Gull first associated atrophy of the gland with the symptoms now known to be characteristic of thyroid deficiency. Hypofunction of the thyroid in adults is still known as *Gull's disease.* The term

myxedema was applied to the clinical syndrome by Ord (1878) in the belief that the characteristic thickening of the subcutaneous tissues was due to excessive formation of mucus.

Extirpation experiments to elucidate the function of the thyroid were at first misinterpreted because of the simultaneous removal of the parathyroids. However, the pioneer research on the latter organs by Gley (1891) allowed the functional differentiation of these two endocrine glands. It was not until after calcitonin was discovered in 1961 that it was realized that the thyroid itself was also concerned with the regulation of calcium. Murray (1891) was the first to treat a case of hypothyroidism by injecting an extract of the thyroid gland; in the following year, Howitz, Mackenzie, and Fox independently discovered that thyroid tissue was fully effective when given by mouth.

Magnus-Levy (1895) discovered the effect of the thyroid on metabolic rate; he found that Gull's disease was characterized by a low rate of metabolism and that the administration of thyroid to hypothyroid or normal individuals increased oxygen consumption.

Chemistry. The active principles of the thyroid gland are the iodine-containing amino acid derivatives of thyronine—*thyroxine* and *triiodothyronine* (Table 67–1). Thyroxine was first isolated in crystalline form from a hydrolysate of thyroid by Kendall (1915), who found that the crystalline product exerted the same physiological effects as the extract from which it was obtained. It was not until 1926, however, that the structural formula of thyroxine was elucidated by Harington, and in the following year Harington and Barger (1927) synthesized the hormone and thus established its chemical constitution.

Following the isolation and the chemical identification of thyroxine, it was generally believed that all the hormonal activity of thyroid tissue could be accounted for by its content of thyroxine. However, careful studies revealed that crude thyroid preparations possessed greater calorigenic activity than could be accounted for by their thyroxine content. The enigma was resolved with the detection, isolation, and synthesis of triiodothyronine (Gross and Pitt-Rivers, 1952; Roche *et al.,* 1952a, 1952b). Further studies revealed that triiodothyronine is qualitatively similar to thyroxine in its biological action but that it is much more potent on a molar basis (Gross and Pitt-Rivers, 1953a, 1953b).

Structure-Activity Relationship. A great many structural analogs of thyroxine have been synthesized in order to define structure-activity relationship, to detect antagonists of thyroid hormones,

Table 67-1. THYRONINE, THYROID HORMONES, AND PRECURSORS

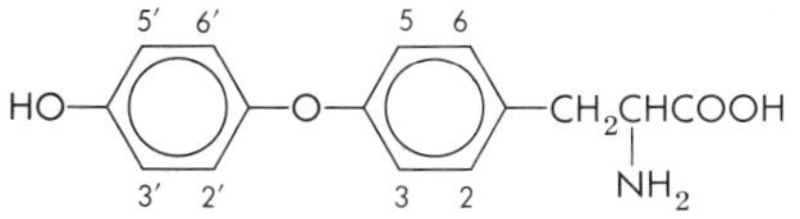

Thyronine

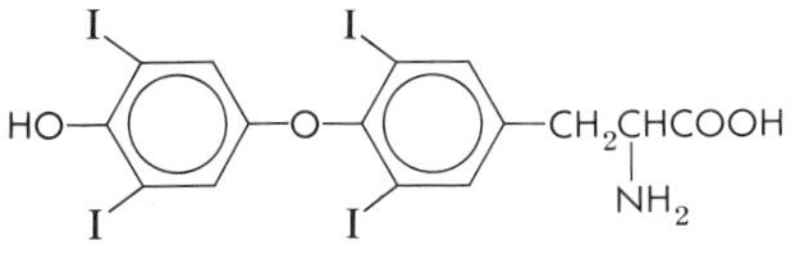

Thyroxine

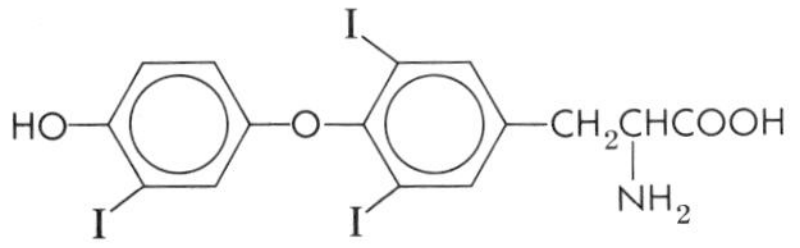

3,5,3'-Triiodothyronine

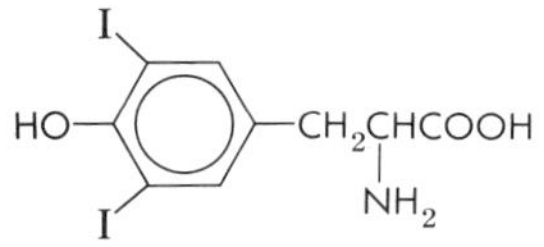

Diiodotyrosine

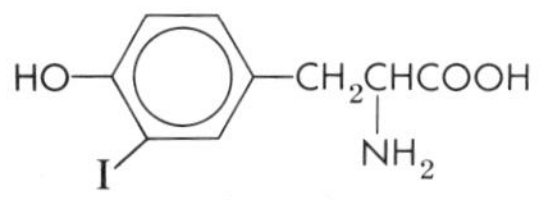

Iodotyrosine

or to find compounds exhibiting one desirable type of activity while not showing unwanted effects. The only significant success has been the partial separation of the cholesterol-lowering action of thyroxine analogs from their calorigenic effect. The *d* isomer of thyroxine is sometimes employed clinically to lower the level of plasma cholesterol (*see* Chapter 35). A complete listing of the compounds tested as of 1955 has been made by Selenkow and Asper.

The structural requirements for a significant degree of thyroid hormone activity have been defined rather precisely (*see* Jorgensen, 1970). The two aromatic rings should be connected by an ether or thioether linkage. However, potent methylene-bridged analogs have been synthesized (Psychoyos *et al.,* 1973). A carboxyl-containing aliphatic side chain in position 1 is important, with L-alanine being the best. Halogen or methyl groups are necessary on positions 3 and 5. Position 4' should be occupied by a hydroxyl group, an amino group, or a group capable of metabolic conversion to a hydroxyl. For maximal activity, halogen atoms, alkyl, or aromatic substituents are necessary at the 3' position or at the 3' and 5' positions. The 3'-monosubstituted compounds are more active than the 3',5'-disubstituted

molecules. Thus, triiodothyronine is four times more potent than thyroxine, while 3'-isopropyl-3,5-diiodo-thyronine has seven times the activity.

While the chemical nature of the 3, 5, 3', and 5' substituents is important, their effects on the conformation of the molecule are apparently even more so. In thyronine, the two rings are angulated at about 120° at the ether oxygen and are free to rotate on their axes. As depicted schematically in Figure 67-1, when the 3,5 iodines are in place there is some restriction to rotation of the two rings, and they tend to take up positions perpendicular to one another; now positions 2' and 3' are no longer equivalent to positions 5' and 6'. Substituents at the 3' position can be either distal (on the convex side, as in Figure 67-1) or proximal to the phenylalanine ring, depending on the rotation. Substitution at the more hindered 2' position probably requires the distal conformation. Much biological evidence indicates that this distal conformation is necessary for activity. Thus, bulky and lipophilic groups in the 3' position enhance activity, and 2' substituents are tolerated. As mentioned, substitutions in the 5' position detract from activity. While not potent, even halogen-free derivatives possess some activity if the proper conformation is possible (Pittman *et al.,* 1973).

According to Jorgensen's formulation, the phenyl-alanine ring with its two iodine atoms is the part of the molecule concerned with its binding to a receptor site. The phenolic ring with its distally oriented group combines with a functional receptor. It is further supposed that the receptor site is of such a shape that substituents on position 5' impair the complementarity of fit.

While analogs that antagonize the actions of the thyroid hormones have been evaluated, none has yet proven clinically useful.

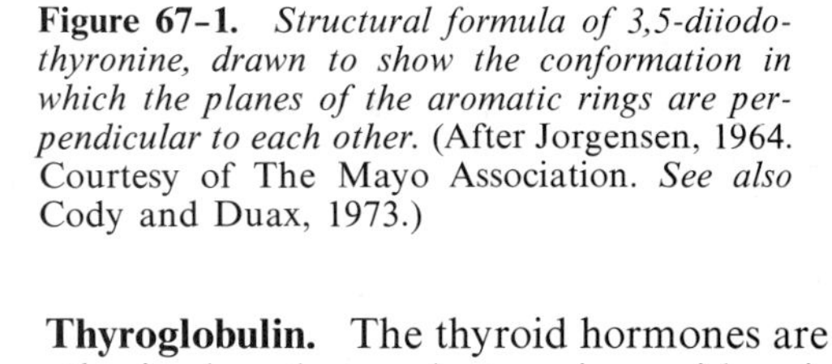

Figure 67-1. *Structural formula of 3,5-diiodo-thyronine, drawn to show the conformation in which the planes of the aromatic rings are perpendicular to each other.* (After Jorgensen, 1964. Courtesy of The Mayo Association. *See also* Cody and Duax, 1973.)

Thyroglobulin. The thyroid hormones are synthesized and stored as amino acid residues of thyroglobulin, a protein constituting the vast majority of the thyroid follicular colloid. The thyroid gland is unique in storing great quantities of potential hormone in this way, and extracellular thyroglobulin can represent a large portion of the mass of the gland. It is a complex and large glycoprotein, made up of several nonidentical subunits. The molecular weight is 660,000 (19 S), and it contains 10% carbohydrate.

Synthesis of Thyroid Hormones. The synthesis of the thyroid hormones is unique, complex, and seemingly grossly inefficient. The major steps involved are the following: (1) the uptake of iodide ion by the gland, (2) the oxidation of iodide and the iodination of tyrosyl groups of thyroglobulin, (3) the conversion of iodotyrosyl radicals to iodothyronyl radicals in this protein, and (4) the proteolysis of thyroglobulin and the release of thyroxine and triiodothyronine into the blood. These processes are summarized in Figure 67–2.

1. *Uptake of Iodide.* Iodine ingested in the diet reaches the circulation in the form of iodide. Under normal circumstances the concentration in the blood is very low, 0.2

to 0.4 µg/100 ml, but the thyroid efficiently and actively transports the ion. As a result, the ratio of thyroid to plasma iodide concentration is usually between 20 and 50 and can far exceed 100 in the stimulated gland. The iodide transport mechanism is inhibited by a number of ions such as thiocyanate and perchlorate (*see* below), appears to require concurrent transport of potassium, and is depressed by cardiac glycosides that inhibit the accumulation of potassium by tissue (*see* Wolff, 1964).

The transport system is subject to regulation by thyrotropin (*see* below) and also apparently by a poorly understood autoregulatory mechanism. Thus, decreased stores of thyroid iodine enhance iodide uptake, and iodide administration can reverse this situation. Some incorporation of iodide into organic form must occur, however, for the inhibitory effect of excess iodide to become apparent (VanderLaan, 1955; Halmi, 1961).

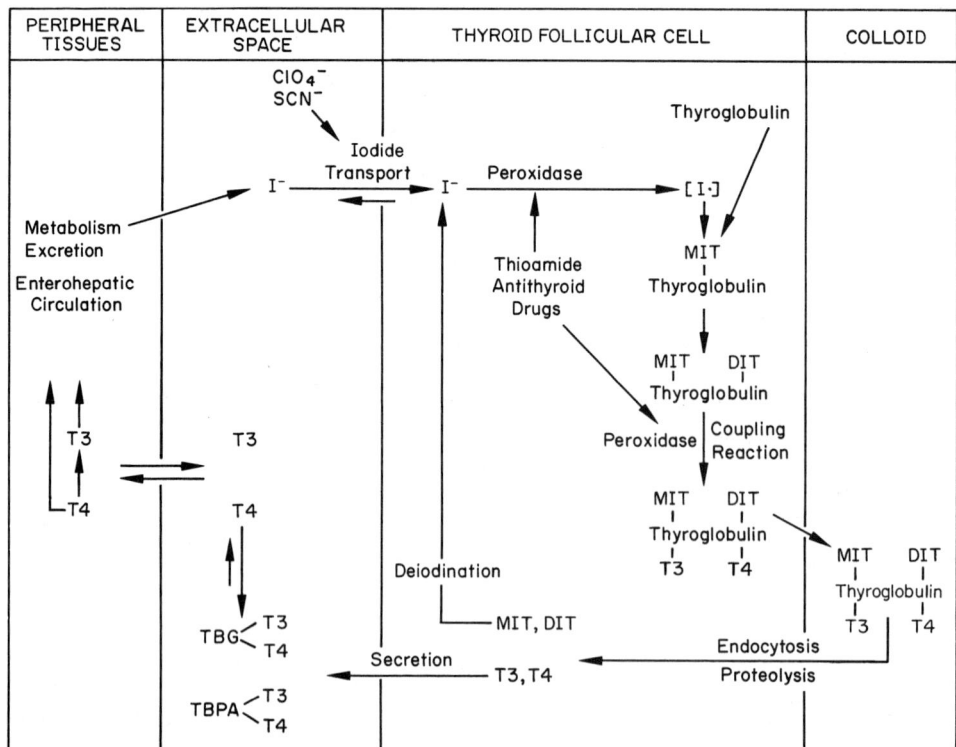

Figure 67-2. *The major pathways of iodine metabolism.*

Abbreviations are as follows: *T3* = triiodothyronine; *T4* = thyroxine; *MIT* = monoiodotyrosine; *DIT* = diiodotyrosine; *TBG* = thyroxine-binding globulin; *TBPA* = thyroxine-binding prealbumin.

If the further metabolism of iodide is blocked by antithyroid drugs, the iodide-concentrating mechanism can more easily be studied. Thus isolated, the mechanism resembles those found in other bodily structures that concentrate iodide, including the salivary glands, gastric mucosa, midportion of the small intestine, skin, mammary gland, and placenta, all of which maintain a concentration gradient of iodide some 10 to 50 times that of the blood. It has been suggested that the accumulation of iodide by the placenta and the mammary gland may be of importance in providing adequate supplies for the young, but no obvious purpose is served by the accumulation of iodide at the other sites. However, the iodide-accumulating system of the thyroid is not unique to the gland and does not account for the specific function of making thyroid hormone.

2. *Oxidation and Iodination.* When iodine and tyrosine are mixed at neutral or slightly alkaline pH, the brown color of iodine rapidly disappears. Two atoms of iodine participate in the reaction at each position on the tyrosine molecule ortho to the phenolic hydroxyl group. One iodine atom combines with hydrogen to form iodide, and the other becomes attached to the ring. Similar reactions take place with tyrosyl residues in protein, and, if excess iodine is added, significant amounts of thyroxine can be made. This helps to define the task the thyroid faces in incorporating iodine into an organic form. Clearly the first hurdle is the oxidation of iodide. Since O_2 and H_2O_2 are the only known biological oxidants with the requisite oxidation-reduction potential, it is believed that generation of H_2O_2 and its utilization in the oxidation of iodide by a peroxidase are the crucial reactions.

The generation of H_2O_2 in the thyroid cell (or any other) is a mysterious process. It is presumed to be formed in close proximity to its site of utilization, and the reactions possibly involve the oxidation of NADPH by NADPH–cytochrome c reductase and the subsequent reduction of O_2 to H_2O_2 (*see* DeGroot *et al.,* 1972).

Taurog and associates (*see* Taurog, 1970) have purified and characterized a heme-containing peroxidase from thyroid particulate fractions that catalyzes the iodination of tyrosyl residues in protein in the presence of H_2O_2. This enzyme appears to be concentrated in membranes at or near the apical surface of the thyroid cell and to catalyze the iodination of thyroglobulin just prior to its storage in the lumen of the thyroid follicle. The precise nature of the "iodinating species" is unknown. There is evidence against oxidation of I^- to I_2 as the crucial step,

even though the enzyme can catalyze this reaction. More probably, the reaction sequence involves the combination of oxidized free radicals of iodine and the tyrosyl acceptor. The initial products of the reaction are monoiodotyrosyl and diiodotyrosyl residues in thyroglobulin.

3. *Formation of Thyroxine and Triiodothyronine from Iodotyrosines.* The remaining synthetic step is the coupling of two diiodotyrosyl residues to form thyroxine or monoiodotyrosyl and diiodotyrosyl residues to form triiodothyronine. These are also oxidative reactions and appear to be catalyzed by the same peroxidase discussed above (Lamas *et al.,* 1972). The mechanism is again largely unknown, but it probably involves the enzymatic transfer of groups, perhaps as radicals, within thyroglobulin. The configuration of the protein is presumed to be important in facilitating this coupling reaction. The possibility of specific amino acid sequences adjacent to thyroxine residues could favor such conformation and enzymatic recognition of appropriate sites (Dunn, 1970). However, unique features of thyroglobulin in this respect are not apparent, since many other proteins can serve as substrates for the peroxidase with the same end result.

The proportions of thyroxine and triiodothyronine formed in the thyroid depend, at least in part, on the relative quantities of monoiodotyrosine and diiodotyrosine available. While a high proportion of monoiodotyrosine seems to favor the formation of triiodothyronine over thyroxine, deficient diiodotyrosine can impair the formation of both thyronines. Thyroxine predominates by a factor of severalfold under most circumstances, and about one fourth of the iodine in the thyroid of most species is in the form of thyroxine. When there is a deficiency of iodine in rat thyroid, however, the ratio of thyroxine to triiodothyronine decreases from 4:1 to 1:3 (Greer *et al.,* 1968). Since triiodothyronine is four times as active as thyroxine and contains only three fourths as much iodine, this change could provide a sixfold increase in hormonal effect from a given quantity of available iodine.

4. *Secretion of Thyroid Hormone.* Since thyroxine and triiodothyronine are synthesized and stored as parts of the molecule of thyroglobulin, proteolysis is an important part of the secretory process. It is generally

believed that thyroglobulin must be completely broken down into its constituent amino acids in order for the hormones to be released. As the molecular weight of thyroglobulin is 660,000 and the protein is made up of about 300 carbohydrate residues and 5500 amino acid residues, only two to five of which are thyroxine (Rall *et al.,* 1964), this is a profligate process indeed. A more frugal arrangement would segregate the iodoamino acids in a small sector of the molecule or near the ends of peptide chains so that some form of selective hydrolysis could take place, but there is little evidence of this type of arrangement. Evidently evolution has not brought economy to the thyroid or perhaps sufficient intelligence to the scientist to understand the rationale of the process utilized. When thyroglobulin is hydrolyzed, monoiodotyrosine and diiodotyrosine are liberated also, but they usually do not leave the thyroid. Instead, they are broken down by an enzyme that attacks them selectively, leaving thyroxine and triiodothyronine untouched, and the iodine, liberated in the form of iodide, is reincorporated into protein (Roche *et al.,* 1952c). Normally, all this iodide is reused; however, when the process is activated intensely by thyrotropin (TSH), some of the iodide reaches the circulation, at times accompanied by trace amounts of the iodotyrosines.

The secretory process is initiated by endocytosis of colloid from the follicular lumen at the apical surface of the cell. This "ingested" thyroglobulin appears as intracellular colloid droplets, which apparently then fuse with lysosomes containing the requisite proteolytic enzymes (Wollman *et al.,* 1964). The liberated hormones presumably exit from the cell at its basal membrane. The daily secretion of thyroxine in normal man is approximately 70 μg and that of triiodothyronine about 25 μg.

Transport of Thyroid Hormone in the Blood. Iodine in the circulation is normally present in several forms, with 95% as organic iodine and approximately 5% as iodide. Most of the organic iodine is thyroxine (90 to 95%), while triiodothyronine represents a relatively minor fraction (about 5%). The thyroid hormones are transported in the blood in strong but noncovalent association with certain plasma proteins.

In 1952, Gordon and coworkers found that, upon electrophoresis of serum, radioactively labeled thyroxine was transported to a site near α-globulin. This binding protein, called *thyroxine-binding globulin,* is the major carrier of thyroid hormones. It is an acidic glycoprotein with a molecular weight of approximately 40,000, and it binds one molecule of thyroxine per molecule of protein with a very high association constant of about 10^{10}. Triiodothyronine is bound less avidly (Sterling *et al.,* 1971). Thyroid hormones are also found associated with *thyroxine-binding prealbumin.* This protein is present in higher concentration than is the thyroxine-binding globulin, but it binds thyroxine and triiodothyronine with association constants near 10^7 and 10^6, respectively (Nilsson and Peterson, 1971). Despite the fact that the prealbumin has four apparently identical subunits, it has a single high-affinity binding site. Albumin can also serve as a carrier for thyroxine when the more avid carriers are overburdened. It is difficult, however, to estimate its quantitative importance.

Protein binding of thyroid hormones protects them from metabolism and excretion, resulting in their long half-life in the circulation. The binding of thyroxine is undoubtedly of importance in the slow onset and prolonged duration of action of the hormone. Of all the congeners of thyroxine studied, none binds as firmly as thyroxine to these proteins. Less than 0.1% of the total thyroxine in plasma is free. While triiodothyronine is much less firmly bound, the quantity that is free is still a small percentage of the total. However, the unbound thyroid hormones constitute the fractions available for action, and their concentrations thus assume particular importance.

Certain drugs and a variety of pathological and physiological conditions can alter the binding of thyroid hormones to proteins or the amounts of these proteins. Thus, the total amounts of thyroid hormones in the plasma and the quantities of *free* hormones can vary somewhat independently. For example, pregnancy or estrogen administration causes elevation of the concentration of thyroxine-binding globulin. This leads to increased thyroxine binding and could lower the concentration of free hormone. Feedback mechanisms compensate, however, and increased thyroid secretion returns the free-hormone concentration to normal. The result is elevated total and bound plasma thyroxine and a normal concentration of free thyroxine. Laboratory tests measuring total thyroxine alone, therefore, would be subject to misinterpretation. Appropriate tests of thyroid function are discussed below.

Conversion of Thyroxine to Triiodothyronine. The hypothesis of conversion of thyroxine to triiodothyronine has returned to favor after years of neglect. This metabolic step has been demonstrated in preparations *in vitro* (Nakagawa and Ruegamer, 1967) and in athyrotic and normal man (Braverman *et al.*, 1970; Sterling *et al.*, 1970). The estimation of the total amount of thyroxine eventually converted to triiodothyronine is a difficult one, but it has been calculated to be in the range of 20% in both rat and man (Pittman, C. S., *et al.*, 1971; Oppenheimer, 1972). This would represent a major source of triiodothyronine production. More importantly, since triiodothyronine is generally estimated to be four times as potent as thyroxine, this would suggest that most of the hormonal activity of thyroxine could be attributed to its conversion to triiodothyronine ($4 \times 20\% = 80\%$). While absolute proof will perhaps await the isolation of a thyroid hormone receptor, the status of triiodothyronine is in ascendance.

Degradation and Excretion. Thyroxine is eliminated slowly from the body and leaves the blood with a half-life of 6 to 7 days. In hyperthyroidism the half-life is shortened to 3 or 4 days, whereas in myxedema it may be 9 to 10 days. These changes are probably due to altered rates of hormonal metabolism. In conditions associated with increased binding to the proteins of plasma, as in pregnancy, elimination is retarded; the reverse is observed when there is reduced protein in plasma, as in nephrosis or hepatic cirrhosis, or when binding to protein is inhibited by certain drugs, such as salicylate or dicumarol. Triiodothyronine, which is less avidly bound to protein, leaves the blood with a half-life of 2 days or less.

Within 3 hours of giving radioiodine-labeled thyroxine intravenously, about one third of the radioactivity can be detected over the liver; indeed, the liver can be out-

lined accurately by scintoscanning at this time (Van Middlesworth *et al.*, 1963). In experimental animals, elimination of thyroxine is greatly slowed after removing the liver (Flock *et al.*, 1956), and preparations made from hepatic tissue are more active in metabolizing thyroxine than are those from other tissues. The liver conjugates thyroxine and triiodothyronine with glucuronic and sulfuric acids through the phenolic hydroxyl group, and excretes these conjugates and a small amount of the free compounds in the bile. There is an enterohepatic circulation of the thyroid hormones, since hydrolysis of the conjugates in the intestine liberates the free compounds, which are then reabsorbed and returned to the liver. A portion of the conjugated material reaches the colon unchanged, is hydrolyzed there, and is eliminated as the free compounds in the feces. In man, approximately 20 to 40% of thyroxine is eliminated in the stool.

As discussed above, a major and important route of thyroxine metabolism is to triiodothyronine. Further deiodination of the molecule can also take place, and these reactions may also be catalyzed by peroxidases. Additional metabolites in which the diphenyl ether linkage is either intact (Pittman *et al.*, 1972) or broken (Wynn and Gibbs, 1962) have been detected both *in vitro* and *in vivo*.

Regulation of Thyroid Function. During the last century, it was appreciated that cellular changes occur in the anterior pituitary in association with endemic goiter or following thyroidectomy. Early in the present century, the classical experimental observations of Cushing (1912) and the clinical observations of Simmonds (1914) established that ablation or disease of the pituitary causes thyroid hypoplasia. It was eventually determined that the anterior pituitary secretes the specific hormone, thyrotropin (TSH) (Chapter 66).

Although there was evidence that thyroid hormone or lack of it causes cellular changes in the pituitary, the control of secretion of thyrotropin by the negative-feedback action of thyroid hormone was not appreciated fully until its central role in the pathogenesis of goiter was elucidated in the early 1940s. It is now recognized that the rate of secretion of thyrotropin is delicately controlled by the quantity of thyroid hormone in the circulation. If extra hormone is given, the secretion of thyrotropin is suppressed and the thyroid becomes inactive and regresses, whereas any decrease in the normal rate of secretion of the thyroid evokes an enhanced secretion of thyrotropin and the thyroid is stimulated to increased growth and function. The mechanism of this effect of thyroid hormone on thyrotropin secretion and the role of the hypothalamic thyrotropin-regulatory hormone (TRH) are discussed in Chapter 66.

Actions of Thyrotropin on the Thyroid. When thyrotropin is given to experimental animals, the first effect on thyroid hormone metabolism that can be measured is an increased secretion. This can be delicately monitored by detecting the radioactivity in the blood leaving the gland that has been prelabeled with radioactive iodine. Under these circumstances, the response can be seen within minutes. Loss of stored radioiodine from the thyroid measured externally in animals or in man also shows the response but less sensitively. All phases of hormone sythesis and release are eventually stimulated: iodide uptake and organification, hormone synthesis, endocytosis, and proteolysis of colloid. There is increased vascularity of the gland and hypertrophy and hyperplasia of thyroid cells.

There is convincing evidence that a primary action of thyrotropin is to activate thyroid adenylate cyclase and to increase the glandular concentration of cyclic adenosine 3′,5′-monophosphate (cyclic AMP) (Gilman and Rall, 1968). Cyclic AMP, acting as the intracellular mediator of thyrotropin, appears to be able to reproduce the important actions of the hormone (*see* Dumont, 1971). Thus, iodide uptake and hormone synthesis are stimulated by the cyclic nucleotide, as are endocytosis and hormone secretion. Protein and nucleic acid synthesis are increased; in fact, cyclic AMP has been shown to be goitrogenic (Pisarev *et al.,* 1970). Several actions of thyrotropin on the intermediary metabolism of thyroid tissue may also be mediated by cyclic AMP, although their immediate importance to hormone metabolism is uncertain.

Prostaglandin E$_1$ is also capable of stimulating accumulation of cyclic AMP in the thyroid (Zor *et al.,* 1969). Predictably, therefore, it too has thyrotropin-like effects on thyroid function. Catecholamines and 5-hydroxytryptamine can also enhance thyroid function, although the mechanisms and significance of their effects are more obscure.

Relation of Iodine to Thyroid Function. Normal thyroid function obviously requires an adequate intake of iodine; without it,

normal amounts of hormone cannot be made, thyrotropin is secreted in excess, and the thyroid hypertrophies. The enlarged and stimulated thyroid becomes remarkably efficient in extracting the residual traces of iodide from the blood. The iodide-concentrating mechanism develops a gradient for the ion that may be ten times the normal, and the vascularity may increase to the point that a bruit is heard. The rush of blood can sometimes be felt by the hand. In this hypertrophied state the thyroid usually succeeds in making sufficient hormone, unless the iodine deficiency is severe.

In some areas of the world *simple* or *nontoxic goiter* is quite prevalent, because iodine is not abundant in most foods. The only rich natural sources commonly eaten are those derived from marine life. Sea fish contain 200 to 1000 µg/kg, shellfish a similar or slightly larger amount, and dried kelp 0.1 to 0.2%, but for those who do not eat marine fish the element can be scarce indeed. To ensure an adequate intake, which is usually taken to be about 100 µg daily, one would have to eat about 5 kg of vegetables or fruit, or 3 kg of meat or fresh-water fish. Milk and eggs are somewhat better sources, but most potable waters contain a negligible amount. However, unnatural sources of iodine in the environment are becoming prevalent and perhaps of concern. A slice of bread may contain 150 µg of iodate, added as a "conditioner" (London *et al.,* 1965). Other sources are as diverse as food colorings and automobile exhaust.

Iodine has been used empirically for the treatment of goiter for 150 years. However, its modern use to prevent goiter was the outgrowth of the extensive studies of Marine, which culminated in the use of iodine to prevent goiter in school children in Akron, Ohio, a region where endemic goiter was prevalent (Marine and Kimball, 1917). The success of these experiments led to the adoption of this form of prophylaxis in many regions of endemic goiter throughout the world.

The most practicable method yet found for providing small supplements of iodine for large segments of the population is the addition of an iodide to table salt, although iodate is now preferred. In some countries, the use of iodine in salt is required by law; in others, including the United States, the use is optional; in newly developing regions, including vast areas of endemic goiter, injection of iodized oil has been used (Thilly *et al.,* 1973); in Japan, supplementation is not needed because kelp is a national delicacy. The quantity of iodide added to table salt varies in different countries; the 100-μg supplement is provided by 1 g of salt in the United States.

Thyroid Hormone Actions. As with other endocrine systems, knowledge of the actions of the hormones has come particularly from observations of the clinical states of both deficient and excess hormone production.

Thyroid Hypofunction. Deficiency of thyroid hormone can be manifested at any age. In the adult, the condition is referred to simply as hypothyroidism or, particularly when severe, as myxedema or Gull's disease. If the gland fails to develop or is congenitally incompetent, the deficiency may be noted soon after birth by the signs of cretinism. Later in childhood, failure of growth and development added to the features of the adult counterpart is recognized as juvenile myxedema.

Myxedema. In its fully developed, classical form, myxedema is associated with degeneration and atrophy of the thyroid gland. The same condition follows surgical removal of the thyroid or its destruction by radioactive iodine. Myxedema is sometimes associated with goiter when there is a severe defect in synthesis of thyroid hormone, when the gland is extensively involved in chronic thyroiditis (Hashimoto's disease), or when antithyroid drugs have been given. In myxedema, the appearance of the patient is pathognomonic. The face is quite expressionless, puffy, and pallid. The skin is cold and dry, the scalp is scaly, and the hair is coarse, brittle, and sparse. The fingernails are thickened and brittle, the subcutaneous tissue appears to be thickened, and there may be true edema. The voice is husky and low pitched, speech is slow, the hearing is often faulty, and mentality is impaired. The appetite is poor, the gastric juice contains little free hydrochloric acid, gastrointestinal activity is diminished, and abdominal distention and constipation are common. Atony of the urinary bladder suggests that the function of other smooth muscles may also be impaired. The voluntary muscles are weak and flabby, and deep-tendon reflexes are slowed. The heart is often dilated, and cardiac output is diminished. There may also be hydropericardium, hydrothorax, and ascites. Refractory anemia, occasionally hyperchromic and macrocytic in character, is often associated with the disease. Menstrual irregularities are prominent. The patient is prone to be drowsy and to sleep a great deal, and he complains of the cold in winter but not of the heat in summer.

Cretinism. Cretinism is usually classified as endemic or sporadic. *Endemic cretinism* is encountered in regions of endemic goiter and is usually due to extreme deficiency of iodine. Goiter may or may not be present. There is a high incidence of nerve deafness in *endemic* but not in *sporadic* cretinism. The latter disease is a consequence of failure of the thyroid to develop normally or the result of a defect in the synthesis of thyroid hormone. Goiter is present if a synthetic defect is at fault.

While detectable at birth, cretinism is often not recognized until 3 to 5 months of age. When untreated, the condition eventually leads to such gross changes as to be unmistakable. The child is dwarfed and the extremities are short, and he is mentally retarded, inactive, uncomplaining, and listless. The face is puffy and expressionless, and the enlarged tongue may protrude through the thickened lips of the half-opened mouth. The skin may have a yellowish hue and a doughy feel, and it is dry and cool to the touch. The heart rate is slow, the body temperature may be low, closure of the fontanels is delayed, and the teeth erupt late. Appetite is poor, feeding is slow and interrupted by choking, constipation is frequent, and there may be an umbilical hernia.

For treatment to be fully effective, the diagnosis must be made long before these obvious changes have come about. Early diagnosis can be made on far more subtle changes noticed by the experienced physician. Small size, reduced length for age, and failure to grow normally, coupled with a hoarse cry, apathy, inertia, and poor muscular tone, may be sufficient to suggest the diagnosis. Once suspected, the diagnosis can easily be confirmed by thyroid function tests.

Thyroid Hyperfunction. Excessive secretion of thyroid hormone may lead to such striking changes that the diagnosis of hyperthyroidism is obvious to the casual observer, or the effects may cause distressing or subtle symptoms that give no clue to their origin. Two major forms of thyroid hyperfunction are recognized. Diffuse toxic goiter (Graves' disease or Basedow's disease) is characterized by thyrotoxicosis and ophthalmopathy. The etiology is obscure, and the disease occurs most commonly in young adults. Toxic nodular goiter (Plummer's disease) occurs primarily in older patients and usually arises from long-standing nontoxic goiter; infiltrative ophthalmopathy is uncommon. At times, however, the distinction between these conditions can be difficult.

Most of the signs and symptoms of hyperthyroidism stem from the excessive production of heat and from increased neuromuscular excitability and increased activity of the sympathetic nervous system. The increased rate of metabolism causes symptoms not unlike those of muscular exercise on a warm day. The skin is flushed, warm, and moist; the muscles are weak and tremulous; the heart rate is rapid, and the heart beat is forceful; and the arterial pulses are prominent and bounding. The increased expenditure of energy gives rise to increased appetite and, if intake is insufficient, to loss of weight. There may also be insomnia, difficulty in remaining still, anxiety and apprehension, intolerance to heat, and increased frequency of bowel movements. Angina and heart failure are more frequently present in older patients. Some individuals may show extensive muscular wasting, suggestive of myopathy. Others have osteoporosis from excessive loss of calcium.

Growth and Development. The most striking and vital effects of thyroid hormone are exemplified by their absence in the cretin, who suffers from deficit in growth and mental retardation. In the absence of thyroxine or triiodothyronine, growth is deficient, particularly at younger ages. The normal response to growth hormone is also dependent on adequate concentrations of thyroid hormone. The restoration of growth in the thyroidectomized animal is one of the most sensitive responses to be seen. In thyroidectomized rats, as little as 0.25 μg of thyroxine injected daily greatly augments growth and 0.5 μg restores it to normal. The basal metabolic rate is little affected by the smallest dose, and more than 1 μg but less than 5 μg daily is required to raise it to normal (Evans *et al.,* 1960).

It is clear that thyroid hormones are important determinants of genetically coded developmental programs. This is seen dramatically in the tadpole, which is almost magically transformed into a frog by thyroxine. Not only does the animal grow limbs, lungs, and other terrestrial accouterments, but also the hormone stimulates the synthesis of a host of enzymes and at the same time so influences the tail that it is digested away and used to build new tissue elsewhere. Does this phenomenon have relevance for man? Perhaps not in its details, but there is little question of a vital role of thyroid hormone in the development of the nervous system. Examination of the brain of hypothyroid animals reveals deficient development, particularly of axonal and dendritic networks. Myelinization is also particularly defective. Several deficits in biochemical development are notable, and it can be hypothesized that thyroid hormone can "push" cells into a differentiative phase and terminate their proliferative phase (Hamburgh, 1969).

The effects of thyroid hormones on protein synthesis and enzymatic activity are certainly not limited to the brain. A large number of enzymatic activities in a variety of tissues are altered in positive and negative directions by the administration of thyroid hormone or by thyroidectomy. However, generalizations about the patterns of results that are seen do not seem possible (*see* Wolff and Wolff, 1964; Pitot and Yatvin, 1973). Detailed understanding of mechanisms of the influence of thyroid hormones on genetic expression is obviously not at hand.

Calorigenic Action. Thyroid hormones increase the metabolic rate of the whole organism, but only certain tissues seem to be affected when their oxygen consumption is measured *in vitro.* Heart, diaphragm, liver, and kidney are markedly stimulated by thyroxine, while, for example, the ovaries and uterus seem unresponsive. This calorigenic action is also dependent upon protein synthesis. Much of it may be secondary to increased cellular work, such as protein synthesis, and increased sodium transport may account for a significant portion of thyroxine-induced energy utilization (Ismail-Beigi and Edelman, 1970). Studies have shown that thyroid hormone administered *in vivo* increases carrier-mediated uptake of adenosine diphosphate (ADP) by mitochondria. The observed increase in mitochondrial oxygen utilization correlates well with the effect on ADP (Babior *et al.,* 1973). The calorigenic response is important in temperature regulation in homeotherms. Thus, thyroid secretion, as regulated by the hypothalamus and pituitary, is stimulated by exposure to cold. While high concentrations of thyroxine can uncouple oxidative phosphorylation in mitochondria, metabolic stimulants such as 2,4-dinitrophenol can also do this without causing other effects characteristic of thyroid hormones. A discussion of the pharmacology of dinitrophenol appears in earlier editions of this textbook.

Cardiovascular System. Hyperactivity of the cardiovascular system is striking in hyperthyroidism, and several factors are probably important (*see* DeGroot, 1972). Cardiac output is undoubtedly augmented secondary to increased peripheral oxygen consumption, but these compensatory mechanisms can explain only a portion of the alterations seen. Chronic treatment with thyroid hormones augments the contractile state of isolated cardiac preparations by mechanisms thought not to involve catecholamines (Buccino *et al.,* 1967). While thyroid hormones have been noted to cause acute changes in myocardial adenylate cyclase activity (Levey and Epstein, 1969), elevated cyclic AMP concentrations have not been observed in preparations of functioning myocardium and cardiac adenylate cyclase activity appears normal in hyperthyroid animals. Thus, there is no clear relationship between the effects of thyroid hormones and cyclic AMP. While it has often been stated that the heart is supersensitive to catecholamines in hyperthyroidism, experimental findings suggest that this is not the case (*see* Levey, 1971). Clinically, however, the stimulatory effects of catecholamines on the stressed hyperthyroid myocardium may be devastating, and there is little doubt of the therapeutic efficacy of drugs that reduce adrenergic function in this condition.

Lipid Metabolism. Hypercholesterolemia is a characteristic feature of hypothyroid states. The predominant effect appears to be impaired disposition of cholesterol. Some separation of actions has been observed between the effects of thyroxine analogs on cholesterol and on calorigenesis, and, as mentioned, D-thyroxine is sometimes used to lower the plasma cholesterol concentration (Chapter 35).

Thyroid hormones appear to enhance the lipolytic responses of fat cells to other hormones, for example, catecholamines, and elevated plasma free fatty acid concentrations are seen in hyperthyroidism. In contrast to the other lipolytic hormones, thyroid hormones do not appear to act by altering cyclic AMP metabolism (*see* Fain, 1973).

Thyroid Function Tests. The laboratory diagnosis of thyroid disease is complicated by the extremely low quantities of thyroid hormones in plasma; by problems of specificity, particularly when analytical technics are directed at iodine; and by variations in the extent of protein binding of the hormones (Fisher, 1973a, 1973b).

The *protein-bound iodine* (PBI) determination measures just that, and it was the first reliable estimate of thyroid status. Variations of this technic (*butanol-extractable iodine* and *thyroxine-iodine by column*) improve its specificity, but these methods are all compromised to varying degrees by other sources of iodine, both endogenous and exogenous.

Particularly troublesome are iodide therapy for hyperthyroidism and certain iodine-containing x-ray contrast media, which can interfere with these determinations for days to years. More satisfactory procedures have become available.

The Murphy-Pattee method for thyroxine is a protein-binding assay, with thyroxine-binding globulin being used in a system analogous to a radioimmunoassay (*see* Murphy, 1969). It is specific, sensitive, and available. While it does require an extraction procedure, this disadvantage is overcome by radioimmunoassays that are specific for thyroxine (Chopra, 1972).

Triiodothyronine presents an even more demanding problem, since its concentration in the plasma is a few percent of that of thyroxine. However, its major contribution to thyroid hormone action and the existence of patients with normal thyroxine and elevated triiodothyronine concentrations ("T3 thyrotoxicosis") demand technics for its routine determination. Progress has been made in specific radioimmunoassays for this hormone, and methods are under evaluation (Gharib *et al.,* 1972).

Accurate determination of total circulating thyroid hormone concentration is, as discussed above, not always sufficient, since the *free* hormone concentration is the determinant of thyroid status. A dialysis technic for free plasma thyroxine has been developed; unfortunately, it is expensive and difficult (Sterling and Brenner, 1966). The acceptable alternative is an estimate of the extent of binding of the hormones or of the total quantity of thyroxine-binding globulin present. The number of unoccupied binding sites can be estimated by determining the competition for radioactive thyroid hormone between the patient's serum (thyroxine-binding globulin) and an ion-exchange resin (*T4 or T3 resin uptake*), or by direct determination of the globulin's binding capacity. Radioimmunoassay of thyroxine-binding globulin is also now feasible. Increased binding capacity (decreased resin uptake) is associated with pregnancy, infectious hepatitis, acute intermittent porphyria, and therapy with perphenazine or estrogens. Decreased binding capacity (increased resin uptake) is noted with the nephrotic syndrome, other major illness, and therapy with androgens, prednisone, phenytoin, phenylbutazone, dicumarol, and salicylates. Other important diagnostic procedures include determination of plasma thyrotropin by radioimmunoassay, provocation of thyroid hormone secretion by injection of thyrotropin or thyrotropin-regulatory hormone, and administration of radioiodine for scanning and estimation of extent of uptake.

Preparations of Thyroid Hormone. Thyroid as well as thyroxine and triiodothyronine are official preparations. *Thyroid,* U.S.P., is a fine powder made from the thyroids of animals slaughtered for food, usually pigs, by defatting and drying with acetone. The U.S.P. specifies that the content of iodine be between 0.17 and 0.23%, and, as most thyroid powders are stronger than this, they are diluted by an inert material. Although neither bioassay nor chemical analyses for thyroxine or triiodothyronine are specified, the product is remarkably uniform. *Thy-*

roid Tablets, U.S.P. (available as THYRAR, THYRO-CRINE, and preparations marketed under the non-proprietary name), are made from the compressed powder in numerous sizes from 15 to 300 mg. *Thyroglobulin,* N.F. (PROLOID), is a purified extract of pig thyroid available in tablets containing from 15 to 300 mg. It conforms to the U.S.P. standard for iodine content and is subjected to bioassay. Its potency is adjusted to be equivalent to *Thyroid,* U.S.P., and it is about twice as expensive. *Levothyroxine Sodium,* U.S.P. (SYNTHROID, LETTER, and nonproprietary preparations), is the sodium salt of the natural isomer of thyroxine and is dispensed in the form of tablets containing 25 to 500 μg and as a powder for reconstitution for injection. *Liothyronine Sodium,* U.S.P. (CYTOMEL), is the somewhat uninformative designation for the salt of L-triiodothyronine. It also is marketed as tablets containing 5, 25, and 50 μg. Kits for preparation of powder for injection are available from the manufacturer. Mixtures of the sodium salts of thyroxine and triiodothyronine in a ratio of 4:1 are also marketed (EUTHROID, THYROLAR). Their only somewhat dubious advantage is replacement therapy with a pure mixture resembling the normal secretion of the gland.

Certain bizarre combinations of thyroid and other drugs (especially amphetamines) are still available and are designed particularly for weight reduction. The use of thyroid or such mixtures for this purpose is dangerous, and sudden deaths from cardiac arrhythmias have occurred. Obesity is not an acceptable indication for thyroid hormone therapy.

Choice of Preparation. The pure compounds carry the attraction of single, reproducible substances of known and constant composition. When thyroxine was first used orally in man, it was considered to be poorly absorbed; the free amino acid is very slightly soluble in water, and it is possible that tablets or large particles escaped solution in the intestinal tract. The sodium salt of thyroxine is better absorbed, probably because a fine suspension is formed in the acid of the stomach. There is still some evidence that absorption of levothyroxine sodium is variable and incomplete, as much as 30 to 40% being recoverable in the stool (Van Middlesworth, 1960). Depending upon the form in which it is given, the proportion of a single oral dose absorbed may vary from 42 to 74% (Hays, 1968); this fraction is rapidly absorbed, while the rest traverses the intestine in a bound unabsorbable form. Nevertheless, levothyroxine sodium has been extensively used with satisfaction and is widely held to be superior to thyroid.

Liothyronine sodium may occasionally be preferred to levothyroxine sodium when a quicker action is desired. It may be useful, therefore, when hypothyroidism has recently supervened from overtreatment with an antithyroid drug or following treatment with radioiodine or thyroidectomy, and in the rare event of coma due to myxedema. It is perhaps less desirable than the other preparations for prolonged therapy because its briefer action might require more frequent doses for steady response. Other disadvantages include altered normal values for thyroid function tests and high cost.

Thyroid, U.S.P., is a highly satisfactory preparation for clinical use. Its continued popularity does not derive merely from a conservative attitude, although at first sight the preparation might seem to be crude, old-fashioned, and poorly standardized. It is well absorbed unless it has an enteric coating or has become hardened because of age or dampness. The potency is sufficiently standard that variation cannot be detected clinically if the official preparation is prescribed.

Comparative Responses to Thyroid Preparations. There is no significant difference in the qualitative response of the patient with myxedema to triiodothyronine, thyroxine, or thyroid. However, there are obvious quantitative differences. Following the subcutaneous administration of a large experimental dose of 1 mg of L-triiodothyronine, a metabolic response can be detected within 4 to 6 hours, at which time the skin becomes detectably warmer and the pulse rate and the temperature increase. With this dose, a metabolic rate of -40% can be raised to normal within 24 hours. The maximal response occurs in 2 days or less, and the effects subside with a half-life of about 8 days. The same single dose of thyroxine exerts much less effect. However, if thyroxine is given in approximately four times the dose of triiodothyronine, a comparable elevation in metabolic rate can be achieved. The peak effect of a single dose is evident in about 9 days, and this declines to half the maximum in 11 to 15 days. In both cases the effects outlast the presence of detectable amounts of hormone; these disappear from the blood with mean half-lives of 2½ and 6 days, respectively. Equivalent clinical responses are obtained from the daily administration of approximately 60 mg of thyroid, 60 mg of thyroglobulin, 100 μg of levothyroxine, or 25 μg of liothyronine.

Therapeutic Uses of Thyroid Hormone.

The two specific indications for the therapeutic use of thyroid hormone are *hypothyroidism* or *myxedema* and *simple goiter.* Inasmuch as they result from thyroid hypofunction, these uses represent true replacement therapy.

Myxedema. According to Means and associates (1963), "Curative treatment of adult myxedema is as perfect a form of therapy as any known to medicine. As long as he takes daily the right amount of thyroid hormone, the patient with Gull's disease can remain normal and may legitimately claim his natural life expectancy." The main objective in the treatment of adult myxedema is to arrive at the proper dose of a suitable thyroid preparation. In most cases, a U.S.P. preparation of thyroid in tablet form is cheapest, most convenient, and most effective. The dose varies somewhat according to complications, especially those involving the heart. The object of therapy is to restore the patient to normal. Often the patient may think he is well when the astute observer can see that he is still hypothyroid. Because long-standing hypothyroidism may have undesirable effects, including a predisposition to atherosclerosis, a full replacement dose should be given if possible. The average daily dose of *Thyroid,* U.S.P., required in myxedema is 120 to 180 mg. Seldom is the requirement greater than this.

While some physicians advocate full and immediate replacement of thyroid hormone in many patients, most argue for more gradual therapy. Since most hypothyroidism has been of long duration at the time of diagnosis, there seems to be little need to be precipitous. In adults, an initial daily dose of 30 mg of thyroid with increments of 30 mg after 2 weeks and of 30 to 60 mg at 2-week intervals thereafter seems reasonable. In older adults or in those with heart disease, more caution is necessary. Initial doses and increments should be halved, and intervals between increments may also be increased. The time of day when medication is taken is unimportant. The patient should be carefully observed during the institution of treatment for untoward reactions such as cardiac pain or palpitations. If angina occurs, care should be exercised but therapy should not be withheld. Cardiac symptoms are the only serious complications of treatment. Arrhythmias have caused death during the initiation of thyroid therapy in myxedema.

In childhood, treatment is the same as in adults, and every attempt should be made to give the largest dose that can be tolerated without causing symptoms or failure to gain weight normally, in order to ensure normal growth and development. Usually a full adult dose is needed, and the schedule above can be used.

Myxedema Coma. A large number of dosage regimens have been advocated for this emergency, and the following serve as examples. Levothyroxine (500 μg, intravenously) or liothyronine (25 μg, intravenously, every 6 to 12 hours, or 100 μg immediately) is preferred initially. Thyroid (120 to 240 mg) may be given by gastric tube if necessary. Further therapy is dictated by the initial clinical response.

Cretinism. Success in the treatment of cretinism depends upon the age at which therapy is started. Unfortunately, many cases do not come to the attention of physicians until the retardation in development has become so obvious as to be alarming to the parents. In such cases, the detrimental effects of the deficiency on mental development will not be completely overcome. If, on the other hand, therapy is started soon after birth, normal physical and mental development may be achieved. Prognosis also depends on the age of onset of the deficiency. If no thyroid develops in the fetus, deficiency probably dates from the fetal age of 3 months, because little hormone is provided from the mother. Perhaps infants with this severe form would not escape mental deficiency no matter how soon treatment was given after birth.

The doses formerly recommended for infants are much too low. Danowski (1962) and associates have shown that doses of 45 mg of thyroid daily at 2 months and 90 mg daily at 1 to 2 years are required. Adult dosages are indicated by 5 years of age. No untoward signs or symptoms accompany these doses. The high requirement and the high tolerance of infants and even premature infants to thyroid have been demonstrated by the fact that doses of 120 to 180 mg do not interfere with gain in weight or produce tachycardia or diarrhea. Although it has not

been shown that these high doses are required in cretinism, the lack of adverse effects from them should allay fears of overtreatment. Intellectual and physical development are the guides for therapy in this condition, and error, if unavoidable, should be made on the side of higher dosage. Excessive dosage will, however, advance the bone age inappropriately.

Mild Hypothyroidism. Hypothyroidism with few of the manifestations of myxedema is a condition that some years ago would have been denied existence by certain physicians. Its reality was firmly established by its similarity to the artificially induced condition in patients in the early stages of their approach to myxedema from overdosage with antithyroid drugs or radioiodine, and by employment of thyroid function tests. In both kinds, the response to treatment provides convincing confirmation. Mild hypothyroidism is frequently encountered among patients with simple goiter. The symptoms may be those of myxedema in mild form, but they may be limited to one or more symptoms such as fatigue, muscle cramps, paresthesias, and intolerance to cold. The treatment for mild hypothyroidism is the same as for myxedema and with the same doses.

Simple Goiter. In simple goiter, or thyroid enlargement without hyperthyroidism, the usual problem is deficient thyroid hormone secretion, causing an excessive output of thyrotropin. The exceptions are unrecognized cases of subacute thyroiditis and autonomous thyroid tumors. As the cause of the condition is frequently some defect in the production of thyroid hormone, treatment with thyroid can properly be regarded as replacement therapy.

Bruns, who was one of the first to report the use of thyroid for the treatment of goiter in 1894, commented when he described 326 treated cases 2 years later ". . . one can theorize that the goiter owes its existence to an increased deficiency of thyroid secretion in the organism which it can take care of by functional hypertrophy."

The aim in treatment is to give full replacement doses of thyroid hormone to suppress the secretion of thyrotropin. Usually this amounts to 120 to 180 mg daily. The effectiveness of treatment can be judged by the uptake of radioiodine by the thyroid, which is greatly reduced to a small percentage of the dose when adequate amounts of thyroid hormone are given. The elevated serum concentration of thyrotropin is also suppressed to normal with therapy, and this serves as an additional index of successful thyroid hormone replacement.

There have been wide differences in the experience of competent observers as to the proportion of goiter cases that respond to treatment with a decrease in the size of the thyroid. Some have observed that only in a minority of the cases is a worthwhile regression achieved. In several large series, however, there has been an appreciable regression in the goiter in about two thirds of the cases and a complete disappearance in half of these. In other series, almost every case showed some response (*see* Doniach *et al.,* 1958; Starr and Goodwin, 1958; Astwood *et al.,* 1960; Higgins *et al.,* 1964). A satisfactory explanation for the discrepant results that have been reported has not been found. Cases of goiter vary widely between individuals as to age, duration, and size, and it is possible that a goitrous population in one area may be quite different from that in another. In areas of endemic goiter where deficiency of iodine is the likely cause, Stanbury and associates have found thyroid medication to be prompt and effective unless the goiter had advanced to the stage of nodular degeneration (*see* Means *et al.*, 1963). However, correction of the iodine deficiency is a more direct approach and is advocated for most cases.

Response to treatment in the kind of goiter commonly seen in the United States may be noticed within a few days; usually, however, it is counted in weeks, and the maximal response may not be seen for many months. Observations on the incidence of relapse when treatment is stopped are insufficient to provide a meaningful figure, but the observation that all do not recur has not been explained.

Nodular Goiter. The transition of diffuse to nodular goiter is much more important than the cosmetic aspect or the infrequent symptoms of compression with difficulty in swallowing. In some instances nodules may secrete hormone and cause hyperthyroidism (*toxic nodular goiter*); however, they are frequently not functional. Herein lies a controversial area of thyroid therapy, since it is necessary to determine if the nonfunctional nodule is malignant. While some advocate excision or biopsy, many prefer to administer replacement doses of thyroid hormone for several months to determine if the nodule will diminish in size—an unlikely occurrence with nonfunctional malignant nodules. Since there is some evidence that nonfunctional nodules are responsive to thyrotropin, there is logic in such efforts; however, it is more difficult to shrink a nodule than to decrease the size of a diffusely enlarged gland.

ANTITHYROID DRUGS AND OTHER THYROID INHIBITORS

A large number of compounds are capable of interfering, directly or indirectly, with the synthesis of thyroid hormones. Several are of great clinical value for the temporary or extended control of hyperthyroid states. These will be discussed in detail. Others are primarily of research or toxicological interest and can only be mentioned. The major inhibitors may be classified into four categories: (1) antithyroid drugs, which interfere directly with the synthesis of thyroid hormones; (2) ionic inhibitors, which block the iodide transport mechanism; (3) iodide itself, which in high concentrations suppresses the thyroid; and (4) radioactive iodine, which damages the gland with ionizing radiations.

ANTITHYROID DRUGS

Regulatory feedback mechanisms are now well appreciated. Thus, a deficient concentration of circulating thyroid hormone evokes increased secretion of thyrotropin, and the result is thyroid hypertrophy—a goiter. It was studies on the mechanism of the development of goiter that first established the central importance of this system of control.

In addition to deficiency of iodine, a great many positive agents were, from time to time, suggested as the cause of simple goiter. Fruitful investigation of this subject dates back to 1928, when Chesney described goiter in laboratory rabbits fed a diet composed largely of cabbage (Chesney *et al.*, 1928). As was learned many years later, this result was probably due to the presence of precursors of the thiocyanate ion in cabbage leaves (*see* below). These experiments led to the work of Hercus and Purves (1936), who showed a clear-cut and reproducible goitrogenic effect from feeding the seeds of the cabbage family of plants. Two pure compounds were soon thereafter shown to produce goiter. Sulfaguanidine, used by the Mackenzies and McCollum (1941) to inhibit intestinal flora for nutritional studies, and phenylthiourea, used by Richter and Clisby (1942) for tests on taste, were found to cause goiter in rats. With such ready means at hand to cause goiter, the mechanism was soon elucidated.

When an effective dose of one of these compounds was fed to young, growing rats, the thyroid glands underwent extraordinary hyperplastic changes characteristic of intense thyrotropic stimulation. However, the animal began to eat less food and eventually to suffer a decreased rate of growth, effects reminiscent of those following thyroidectomy. It was then established that the animals were indeed hypothyroid. Thyroid hormone was then given, with the result that the effects of the goitrogenic agent were altogether abolished. This suggested that the goiter was a compensatory change resulting from the induced state of hypothyroidism. When the hypophysis was removed from the experimental animal, the goitrogen had no visible effect upon the thyroid gland. The conclusion was inescapable that the primary action was an inhibition of the formation of thyroid hormone. The first measurable effect in young rats was a loss of organic iodine from the thyroid; after treatment was begun, no new hormone could be made. Meanwhile the circulating hormone decreased, and compensatory hypertrophy of the thyroid followed (Astwood, 1945).

When it was clear that the primary action of the compounds was to inhibit the formation of thyroid hormone, the therapeutic possibilities in hyperthyroidism were evident and the substances so used became known as *antithyroid drugs.*

Structure-Activity Relationship. The first two compounds found in 1941 proved to be prototypes of two different classes of antithyroid drugs. These two, with one later addition, make up three general categories into which the majority of the agents can be assigned: (1) *thioamides,* of which thiourea is the simplest member, include all the compounds currently used clinically; (2) *aniline derivatives,* of which the sulfonamides make up the largest number, embrace a few substances that have been found to inhibit the human thyroid; and (3) *polyhydric phenols,* such as resorcinol, which have caused goiter in man when applied to the abraded skin. A few other compounds do not fit into any of these categories.

Thioamides. Thiourea and its simpler aliphatic derivatives and heterocyclic compounds containing a thioureylene group make up the majority of the known antithyroid agents that are also effective in man. Although most of them incorporate the entire thioureylene group, in some, one of the nitrogen atoms is replaced by oxygen or another sulfur so that only the thioamide group is common to all (Table 67–2). Among the heterocyclic compounds, the sulfur derivatives that are active are representatives of imidazole, oxazole, hydantoin, thiazole, thiadiazole, uracil, and barbituric acid.

Aniline Derivatives. In this group, optimal antithyroid activity in the rat is associated with a para-substituted aminobenzene grouping with or without aliphatic substitution on the amino nitrogen. While sulfathiazole and sulfadiazine possess significant activity, the sulfonamides are not detectably antithyroid in man in doses used clinically. However, aminosalicylic acid, which is given in doses of many grams daily for months, has caused hypothyroidism and goiter.

Polyhydric Phenols. Hypothyroidism and goiter have followed the use of resorcinol in the form of an ointment for the treatment of leg ulcers. Antithyroid activity seems to be associated with meta substitution on the benzene ring with two polar groups. Thus, phloroglucinol, hexylresorcinol, 2,4-dihydroxybenzoic acid, and *m*-aminophenol are active whereas catechol, hydroquinone, and pyrogallol are not (Arnott and Doniach, 1952; Rosenberg, 1952).

Individual Compounds of Interest. L-5-Vinyl-2-thiooxazolidone (goitrin) has been shown to be responsible for the goiter that results from consuming turnips or the seeds or green parts of cruciferous plants. These plants are eaten by cows, and the compound has been found in cow's milk in areas of endemic goiter in Finland (Arstica *et al.*, 1969); it is about as active as propylthiouracil in man. Van Etten (1969) has reviewed the chemistry of naturally occurring goitrogens.

As the result of industrial exposure, toxicological studies, or clinical trials for various purposes, several other compounds have been noted to possess antithyroid activity. Some of these are aminothiazole, aminotriazole, mercaptoimidazole, tricyanoaminopropene, calcium cyanamide, amphenone B, cobaltous ion, and carbutamide. Among compounds used clinically, phenylbutazone and thiopental are weakly antithyroid in experimental animals. This is not significant at usual doses in man. However, antithyroid effects in man have been observed from dimercaprol.

Mechanism of Action. Antithyroid drugs inhibit the formation of thyroid hormone largely by interfering with the incorporation of iodine into an organic form. This implies that they interfere with the oxidation of iodide ion, but the elucidation of the detailed

Table 67–2. STRUCTURE OF SOME ANTITHYROID COMPOUNDS OF THE THIOAMIDE TYPE FORMERLY AND CURRENTLY USED IN HYPERTHYROIDISM

mechanism involved has been hampered by an incomplete understanding of the iodide-oxidizing system of the thyroid gland. In the consideration of the mechanism of synthesis of thyroid hormone, it was pointed out that oxidation of iodide is probably brought about by a peroxidase. Antithyroid drugs could be inhibitors of this reaction, for example, by binding to the enzyme, by interaction with its substrates or intermediates, or by interfering with the generation of H_2O_2. The iodination reaction catalyzed by purified thyroid peroxidase *in vitro* is very sensitive to inhibition by various antithyroid drugs (Taurog, 1970).

There is considerable evidence that the thyroid peroxidase responsible for iodotyrosine synthesis also functions in the coupling of iodotyrosines to form iodothyronines. The fact that antithyroid drugs also appear to inhibit the coupling reaction *in vivo* is consistent with an action on the peroxidase. Furthermore, the coupling reaction is catalyzed *in vitro* by a purified thyroid peroxidase, and this reaction is inhibited by methimazole (Lamas *et al.*, 1972).

It has also been proposed that the coupling reaction is *more* sensitive to inhibition by antithyroid drugs than is the initial iodination of tyrosyl residues. When, in intact animals, sufficient drug is given to inhibit iodination by about 99%, the small amount of organically bound iodine is found to be largely in the form of monoiodotyrosine. Under these circumstances, formation of diiodotyrosine, triiodothyronine, and thyroxine cannot be detected. With smaller amounts of drug, diiodotyrosine is also formed; when the quantity of inhibitor is reduced still further, the iodothyronines are formed as well. Findings such as these might be interpreted as showing that the coupling reaction is the step most sensitive to inhibition, diiodination the second most sensitive, and the formation of monoiodotyrosine the most resistant of all. However, other interpretations are obviously possible. When the iodine compounds of the thyroid are labeled with radioiodine and then a fully blocking dose of propylthiouracil is given and continued for several days, the thyroid loses triiodothyronine and thyroxine more quickly than it does iodotyrosines. This might also favor the idea that the coupling reaction was blocked, thereby preventing the iodotyrosines from being used to form iodothyronines; again, however, alternative explanations may be more likely. Both types of experiment may merely show that, when the first step in synthesis is impeded, the later steps become progressively more difficult for want of substrate. This might also explain how the coupling reaction can seem to be preferentially inhibited over iodination, even when the two processes are mediated by the same per-

oxidatic enzyme. However, it must be noted that, when hormone synthesis is impaired by inhibiting uptake of iodide ion with perchlorate or thiocyanate, no particular difficulty with the coupling reaction is evident. Furthermore, propylthiouracil inhibition of *thyroxine* synthesis by purified thyroid peroxidase appears to occur at concentrations below those having any effect on the formation of monoiodotyrosyl or diiodotyrosyl residues (Taurog, 1970). The finding that iodination can take place although hormone synthesis is greatly depressed may explain why patients with hyperthyroidism respond well to doses that only partially suppress binding of radioiodine.

There is less agreement on the molecular details of the mechanism of antithyroid drug action. In view of the diversity of goitrogenic chemicals, several mechanisms could be operative. Certain of these compounds can reduce iodine, while some are oxidized by the peroxidase and apparently can form mixed disulfide bonds with protein. There may be reaction with an iodinating intermediate or prevention of its formation.

Several studies have indicated that propylthiouracil can also interfere with the peripheral actions of thyroxine, but not those of triiodothyronine. In view of the evidence of metabolism of thyroxine to triiodothyronine, Oppenheimer and coworkers (1972) have investigated the ability of the antithyroid drugs to influence this conversion in rats. A prominent inhibition was observed. A similar action, accompanied by an elevation of circulating concentrations of thyrotropin, has also been observed in man (Geffner *et al.*, 1975); however, it was not apparent with the administration of methimazole (Saberi *et al.*, 1975). The importance of this action to the overall effect of propylthiouracil or other antithyroid drugs remains to be determined.

Preparations and Dosage. The compounds in current use are *Propylthiouracil*, U.S.P. (6-*n*-propylthiouracil), in the form of 50-mg tablets that can be broken in half, and *Methimazole*, U.S.P. (1-methyl-2-mercaptoimidazole; TAPAZOLE), marketed in 5- and 10-mg tablets. *Methylthiouracil*, N.F. (METHIACIL, THIMECIL), can be obtained in 25- or 50-mg tablets; it is more widely used abroad than in the United States. *Carbimazole* (NEOMERCAZOLE) is a carbethoxy derivative of methimazole, which it closely resembles and into which it is converted in the body; it can be had in 5- and 10-mg tablets, and is widely used in Great Britain.

There are no commercial preparations available for parenteral use in the rare event that treatment cannot be given by mouth. For this eventuality and for experimental purposes, the freely water-soluble compound, methimazole, can be dissolved in saline solution and sterilized by heat.

The usual dose of propylthiouracil for the treatment of hyperthyroidism is 75 to 100 mg every 8 hours. In some cases larger doses, up to 900 mg daily, may be required. Failures of response to treatment with 300 mg daily are sometimes attributable to improper spacing of the doses, since the drug is fully effective for only a few hours. Delayed responses are also sometimes noted when the thyroid is unusually large and when iodine in any form has been given beforehand. When doses larger than 300 mg daily are needed, further subdivision of the time of administration of the daily dose into 4- or 6-hour intervals is perhaps advisable. After the patient is euthyroid, dosage can usually be reduced to one third for maintenance.

The corresponding initial dose of methimazole or carbimazole for the majority of cases is 5 or 10 mg every 8 hours, and seldom are larger quantities needed. Methylthiouracil is usually given in a daily dose of 200 mg, divided into two or four equally spaced doses. When a complete response has been achieved, the dose is reduced but the total daily dose is still subdivided. Only when very small amounts are needed is the frequency of dosage reduced to two or even one dose per day.

Absorption, Metabolism, and Excretion. Measurements of the course of accumulation of radioiodine by the thyroid show that absorption of effective amounts follows within 20 or 30 minutes after an oral dose. They also show that the duration of action of the compounds used clinically is brief. The effect of a dose of 100 mg of propylthiouracil begins to pass off in 2 to 3 hours, and even a 500-mg dose is completely inhibitory for only 6 or 8 hours. By this means it can be shown that as little as 0.5 mg of methimazole stops the accumulation of radioiodine in the thyroid gland, but a single dose of 10 to 25 mg is needed to extend the inhibition to 24 hours.

Studies with radioactive drugs also reveal rapid absorption of the compounds. The half-life of propylthiouracil in plasma approximates 2 hours (Alexander *et al.,* 1969a), while that for methimazole has been estimated to be about 6 hours (Pittman, J. A., *et al.,* 1971). All the useful drugs appear to be concentrated in the thyroid, and methimazole, derived from the metabolism of carbimazole, accumulates after carbimazole is administered (Marchant *et al.,* 1972). Radioactive drugs and metabolites appear largely in the urine.

The antithyroid drugs cross the placenta and can also be found in milk. The use of these drugs in pregnancy is discussed below; women taking these agents should not breast-feed their infants.

Untoward Reactions. When the first drugs of this class (thiouracil, thiobarbital) were used in the treatment of hyperthyroidism, a high incidence of side effects was encountered. Some of these difficulties were,

however, attributable to excessive dosages.

The incidence of side effects from propylthiouracil and methimazole as currently used is very much lower. The overall incidence as compiled by VanderLaan and Storrie (1955) from published cases was 3% for propylthiouracil and 7% for methimazole, with 0.44 and 0.12% of cases, respectively, developing the most serious reaction, agranulocytosis. Further observation suggests that there is little, if any, difference in side effects between these two agents, and that an incidence of agranulocytosis of 1 in 500 is a maximal figure. This reaction usually occurs during the first few months of therapy. Since agranulocytosis can develop rapidly, periodic white-cell counts are of little help. Patients should immediately report the development of sore throat or fever, which usually heralds the onset of this reaction. If the drug is discontinued rapidly, recovery is the rule. Mild granulocytopenia, if noted, may be due to thyrotoxicosis or may be the first sign of this dangerous drug reaction. Caution and frequent leukocyte counts are then required.

The most common reaction is a mild, sometimes purpuric, papular rash. It often subsides spontaneously without interrupting treatment but sometimes calls for changing to another drug, since cross-sensitivity is uncommon. Other less frequent complications are pain and stiffness in the joints, paresthesias, headache, nausea, and loss or depigmentation of the hair. Drug fever, hepatitis, and nephritis are very rare.

Therapeutic Uses. The antithyroid drugs are used in the treatment of *hyperthyroidism* in the following three ways: (1) as definitive treatment, to control the disorder in anticipation of a spontaneous remission; (2) in conjunction with radioiodine, to hasten recovery while awaiting the effects of radiation; and (3) to control the disorder in preparation for surgical treatment. There is no uniformity of opinion as to which form of treatment is the most desirable.

Response to Treatment. Hyperthyroidism may be of two kinds, Graves' disease and hyperthyroidism from one or more overfunctioning thyroid nodules; whichever the cause, the hyperthyroidism seems to respond to antithyroid drugs in the same way. After treatment is instituted, there is usually a latent period of a few days to 2 or more weeks before improvement is clearly manifest; however, in a few cases, and particularly when the hyperthyroidism is severe, definite improvement may be seen in 1 or 2 days. In patients with large goiters and particularly if nodular, the response may be slower. When iodine was commonly used for therapy, it was frequently observed that prior treatment with iodine delayed the response to antithyroid drugs for many weeks. Thus, it would appear that the rate of response is determined by the quantity of stored hormone, the rate of turnover of hormone in the thyroid, and the completeness of the block in synthesis imposed by the dosage given. When large doses are continued, and sometimes with the usual dose, recovery is followed by the development of hypothyroidism. The earliest signs of hypothyroidism call for a reduction in dose; if by chance they have advanced to the point of discomfort, thyroid hormone can be given to hasten recovery. A full dose of 120 to 180 mg daily of thyroid or the equivalent of thyroxine or triiodothyronine for a week will usually suffice. The lower maintenance dose of antithyroid drug discussed above is instituted for continued suppression.

In most cases, treatment with an antithyroid drug requires medical attention only at monthly or bimonthly intervals and adjustment of dosage can be made entirely upon the basis of symptoms and simple clinical signs. If confirmatory tests are desirable, those reflecting the concentration of circulating hormones are the most helpful.

Control of the hyperthyroidism is not associated with further enlargement of the goiter unless hypothyroidism is induced. When this happens, the new enlargement is quickly reversed by giving thyroid hormone. The presumption is, therefore, that thyrotropin is secreted in excessive amounts in response to the hypothyroidism and can be suppressed by thyroid hormone. If this is so, then the overactive thyroid in hyperthyroidism owes its stimulus to something else, perhaps to the long-acting thyroid stimulator that is often found in the blood in this condition (Chapter 66).

Remissions. It has long been said that hyperthyroidism is a condition marked by spontaneous exacerbations and remissions. In modern times, there has been little opportunity to make observations on the course of the disorder undisturbed by treatment and, therefore, a certain degree of skepticism is perhaps understandable. Nonetheless, remissions do take place during treatment. When treatment is continued for about a year, about one half of the patients remain well for long periods, perhaps indefinitely, thereafter. Upon stopping treatment, hyperthyroidism returns promptly within 2 months in about 20% of the patients. Presumably in these patients the disorder is still active and is merely controlled by the medication. Other patients experience remissions lasting several months or many years; after 4 years, relapse is unusual (Solomon et al., 1953).

While there is no good reason to believe that antithyroid drugs have any influence on the basic cause of hyperthyroidism, it is known that treatment causes a loss of iodine from the thyroid and, consequently, a profound depletion of iodine from the body (Harden et al., 1966). The possible importance of this state of iodine deficiency to a favorable outcome is pointed up by the finding that repletion of the stores of iodine after treatment greatly increases the rate of relapse of hyperthyroidism (Alexander et al., 1965). Reduction of iodine intake might be worthwhile when antithyroid drugs are used to treat hyperthyroidism.

Unfortunately, there is no way of predicting before treatment is begun which patients will eventually achieve a lasting remission and which will relapse. It is clear that a favorable outcome is unlikely when the disorder is of long standing and when various forms of treatment have failed. Some observers believe that the prognosis is favorable when the thyroid is not greatly enlarged, and that young women are more apt to recover permanently than are older women or men. Hyperthyroidism in children is particularly obstinate, and drug therapy is often continued for several years.

During treatment, a fairly certain sign that a remission may have taken place is a reduction in the size of the goiter. The persistence of goiter usually indicates failure, unless the patient becomes hypothyroid. Another favorable indication is continued freedom from all signs of hyperthyroidism when the maintenance dose is small. A helpful test to determine whether treatment may safely be discontinued involves measuring the uptake of radioiodine after giving 180 mg of thyroid daily for 3 weeks. Pronounced suppression of uptake implies the reestablishment of the normal feedback mechanism, and a state of remission usually can be correctly inferred (Cassidy and VanderLaan, 1960). Alexander and associates (1969b) have improved upon this test by giving 80 μg of triiodothyronine daily during the whole course of treatment with carbimazole; a 20-minute uptake measurement of radioiodine, which is not influenced by the antithyroid drug, can be made at frequent intervals. If suppression of uptake did not supervene during therapy, relapse always followed when the drug was stopped; similarly it might be concluded that a favorable result would be likely if treatment were discontinued as soon as the thyroid became suppressed.

Disadvantages. The main drawback to therapy with antithyroid drugs is the high incidence of relapse when treatment is stopped. If the 50% of patients relapsing after one course of therapy are retreated once or several times, the number of lasting remissions increases somewhat, but there remain the 20 to 30% of patients who require continuous treatment or treatment with radioiodine or subtotal thyroidectomy. The frequent taking of medication for long periods of time is another disadvantage and, although untoward reactions to the drugs are not frequent and rarely serious, they constitute a further disadvantage. The need for periodic consultation during treatment is probably not a real disadvantage because careful observation at intervals is necessary, whatever the treatment.

Advantages. The obvious advantage of the medical treatment of hyperthyroidism with drugs is the avoidance of a surgical operation and its complications, or of a relatively high incidence of permanent hypothyroidism from radioiodine therapy or surgery. Although it is true that the hyperthyroid patient can be prepared so successfully for an operation that a fatal issue is rare, nevertheless, the attendant dangers of injury to the parathyroids or the recurrent laryngeal nerves are by no means negligible. Another outstanding advantage of the antithyroid drugs is the reversibility of their action. Although the synthesis of thyroid hormone is interrupted, full restoration of function of the gland follows upon their withdrawal. Thus, the remission achieved during treatment is a true remission unattended by loss or destruction of part of the thyroid gland. Finally, the incidence of progressive ophthalmopathy appears to be somewhat less with drug therapy (Aranow and Day, 1965).

The Therapeutic Choice.   Only a brief summary can be presented here. In the "routine" adult patient with Graves' disease, few physicians currently advise subtotal thyroidectomy, and most choose antithyroid drugs or radioiodine. Complications, discomfort, and expense are minimized. Surgery is considered more frequently in children, since most physicians avoid radioiodine in young patients and antithyroid drugs produce fewer permanent remissions. Therapy in young adults is more controversial. It would seem desirable in patients of most ages with Graves' disease to determine whether a remission will be achieved by antithyroid therapy alone, and to use radioiodine or surgical treatment if the disorder shows itself as unremitting.

Radioiodine or surgery is usually chosen for definitive therapy in toxic nodular goiter, since spontaneous remissions are not characteristic of this condition.

There is considerable disagreement about the therapy of thyrotoxicosis during *pregnancy.* The antithyroid drugs cross the placenta and can cause fetal hypothyroidism and goiter. Knowledge of thyroid hormone transport to the fetus is poor. There are three choices of therapy, each with its advocates: minimal doses of antithyroid drugs, full doses of antithyroid drugs with thyroid hormone supplementation, or surgery. The only definitive statement to be made is that radioiodine is contraindicated.

Preoperative Preparation.   An important use of antithyroid drugs is in the preparation of the hyperthyroid patient for subtotal thyroidectomy. It is possible to bring virtually 100% of patients to a euthyroid state; as a consequence, the operative mortality for a single-stage thyroidectomy in expert hands is now very low. The treatment is continued until the patient is judged to be normal or nearly so, and then iodide is added for the 7 to 10 days immediately before the operation. Iodide reduces the vascularity of the gland and makes it less friable, which lessen the difficulties for the surgeon.

Propranolol, Reserpine, and Guanethidine. These antiadrenergic drugs are not thyroid inhibitors, but they have been found useful for the temporary suppression of the signs and symptoms of thyrotoxicosis. As mentioned above, some of the cardiovascular manifestations of hyperthyroidism may be reinforced by the cardiac effects of catecholamines. Reserpine and guanethidine have been found to reduce the heart rate, tremor, and stare in hyperthyroidism and to relieve palpitation, anxiety, and tension. Propranolol appears to be superior to either guanethidine or reserpine; it is far less likely to cause side

effects, and the control of the peripheral manifestations is unmistakable and rapid (*see* Shanks *et al.,* 1969). It is thus valuable in controlling symptoms while awaiting the response to antithyroid drugs or radioiodine, and it may be very useful in a rare but potentially lethal complication, thyroid storm (Das and Krieger, 1969). A usual oral dose is 20 to 40 mg every 6 hours, but the amount should be adjusted according to the response; the heart rate is a reliable indicator. These drugs do not affect the overactivity of the thyroid gland or the rate of secretion of thyroid hormone.

IONIC INHIBITORS

The term *ionic inhibitors* serves to designate the substances that interfere with the concentration of iodide ion by the thyroid gland. The effective agents are themselves anions that in some ways resemble iodide ion; they are all monovalent, hydrated anions of a size similar to that of iodide. The longest known and most studied member, *thiocyanate,* differs from the others qualitatively; it is not concentrated by the thyroid gland, and in large amounts it inhibits the binding of iodine. Wyngaarden and associates (1952) found a number of inorganic ions to be effective in rats; *perchlorate* (ClO_4^-) was ten times as active as thiocyanate and *nitrate* about $\frac{1}{30}$ as active. Other ions, selected on the basis of their size, have also been found to be active; fluoborate (BF_4^-) is as effective as perchlorate, whereas fluosulfonate (SO_3F^-) and difluophosphate ($PO_2F_2^-$) are less so (Anbar *et al.,* 1960). Wolff and Maurey (1963) have related the inhibitory properties of a series of anions to their partial molal ionic volumes. A linear relationship was found in the range of 25 to 46 ml per mole, with bromide (Br^-) the smallest and least effective and pertechnetate (TcO_4^-) the largest and most potent (Wolff and Wolff, 1964).

Thiocyanate.   Chesney's discovery of the goitrogenic action of cabbage leaves in rabbits has been mentioned above. The goitrogenic effect of thiocyanate was discovered in man when, in 1936, Barker described goiter and myxedema in patients being treated for hypertension with potassium thiocyanate. It was soon found that both effects were reversed or prevented by giving thyroid hormone or iodide. The mechanism of thiocyanate action was ultimately determined by the VanderLaans (1947), who demonstrated that thiocyanate abolished the thyroid-to-plasma iodide gradient as accumulated iodide was "discharged" from the gland. Subsequent work has shown that, although thiocyanate does not concentrate in the thyroid, it acts as a competitive inhibitor of the accumulation of iodide. The thyroid gland is in addition capable of metabolizing thiocyanate to sulfate (Maloof and Soodak, 1963).

Thiocyanate ion is produced following the enzymatic hydrolysis of certain plant glycosides. Thus, the eating of some foods (*e.g.,* cabbage) results in an increased concentration of thiocyanate in the blood and urine. Dietary precursors of thiocyanate may be a contributing factor in endemic goiter in certain parts of the world, particularly when the intake of iodine is very low (Delange and Ermans, 1971).

Perchlorate. Unlike thiocyanate, perchlorate is concentrated in the thyroid gland but is not metabolized there and is excreted in the urine unchanged (Anbar *et al.,* 1960; Wolff and Wolff, 1964). Following the finding of Godley and Stanbury (1954) that perchlorate is effective in the control of hyperthyroidism, the ion was used extensively for this purpose. Unfortunately, several cases of aplastic anemia were encountered; consequently, it is very rarely used therapeutically and only when other antithyroid medications cannot be tolerated. Perchlorate can be used to discharge radioiodine from the thyroid gland in a diagnostic test of iodine organification.

IODIDE

Iodide is the oldest remedy for disorders of the thyroid gland. Before the antithyroid drugs were used, it was the only substance available for the medical control of the signs and symptoms of hyperthyroidism. Its use in this way is indeed paradoxical, and the explanation for this paradox is still being sought.

Response to Iodide in Hyperthyroidism. The response of the patient with hyperthyroidism to iodide is often striking and rapid. The effect is usually discernible within 24 hours, and the basal metabolic rate may fall at a rate comparable to that following thyroidectomy. This provides evidence that the release of hormone into the circulation is quickly interrupted. The maximal effect is attained after 10 to 15 days of continuous therapy when the signs and symptoms of hyperthyroidism may have greatly improved.

The changes in the thyroid gland have been studied in detail; vascularity is reduced, the gland becomes much firmer and even hard to the touch, the cells become smaller, colloid reaccumulates in the follicles, and the quantity of bound iodine increases. The changes are those that would be expected if the excessive stimulus to the gland had somehow been removed or antagonized.

Unfortunately, iodide therapy usually does not completely control the manifestations of hyperthyroidism, and after a variable period of time the beneficial effect disappears. With continued treatment, the hyperthyroidism may return in its initial intensity or may become even more severe than it was at first. It is for this reason that, when iodide was the only agent available for the treatment of hyperthyroidism, its use was usually restricted to preoperative preparation of the patient when thyroidectomy was contemplated.

Mechanism of Action. High concentrations of iodide appear to influence all important aspects of iodine metabolism by the thyroid gland (*see* Ingbar, 1972). The autoregulatory effect of iodide to limit iodide transport has been discussed above. Acute effects of iodide to inhibit iodotyrosine and iodothyronine synthesis are also well known (the *Wolff-Chaikoff effect*) (Wolff and Chaikoff, 1948). This inhibition is observed only above critical concentrations of iodide, and the intracellular rather than the extracellular concentration of the anion appears to be the major determinant. With time there is "escape" from this inhibition that is associated with an adaptive decrease in iodide transport and a lowered intracellular iodide concentration. Inhibition of hormone synthesis is also demonstrable *in vitro* with purified thyroid peroxidase. It is hypothesized that iodide could react with the iodinating intermediate of the peroxidase reaction, whether that be I_2, a free radical, or a sulfenyliodide group.

The important clinical effect of high iodide concentration is to inhibit thyroid hormone release. This action is rapid and efficacious in severe thyrotoxicosis. The effect is exerted directly on the thyroid gland, and it can be demonstrated in the euthyroid subject and experimental animals as well as in the hyperthyroid patient. Iodide antagonizes the ability of both thyrotropin and cyclic AMP to stimulate endocytosis of colloid, proteolysis, and hormone secretion (Pisarev *et al.,* 1971). Ingbar (1972) has speculated that the effect may be due to inhibition of glutathione reductase by elemental iodine, with subsequent alteration of the sulfhydryl groups of thyroglobulin. Such changes alter the susceptibility of thyroglobulin to proteolysis.

Other stimulatory effects of thyrotropin also appear to be antagonized. As mentioned above, there is involution of the gland and a reduction of vascularity. Mechanistically, these actions of iodide are particularly obscure.

Iodide-Induced Goiter and Myxedema. In a small proportion of individuals given large doses of iodide for long periods, as in the treatment of asthma or chronic bronchitis, goiter and hypothyroidism supervene. The thyroid gland shows hyperplasia and is depleted of stores of iodine. Thyroid hormone corrects the hypothyroidism and causes the goiter to subside, and the same result follows the withdrawal of the iodide. Before this condition was first recognized, it had been noted by several observers that some patients with hyperthyroidism overreact to iodide by developing hypothyroidism, and evidently this was most often noted in patients who had been unsuccessfully treated by thyroidectomy.

Preparations and Dosage. The dosage or form in which iodide is administered bears little relationship to the response achieved in hyperthyroidism, provided not less than the minimal effective amount is given; this dose is 6 mg per day in most, but not all, patients (Thompson *et al.*, 1930). Lugol's solution (*Strong Iodine Solution,* U.S.P.) is widely used and consists of 5% iodine and 10% potassium iodide. The iodine is reduced to iodide in the intestine before absorption. *Sodium Iodide,* U.S.P., and *Potassium Iodide,* U.S.P., are available in solid form, as is *Potassium Iodide Solution,* U.S.P., for oral administration. While a dosage of 500 mg of iodide per day is often used, 50 to 100 mg per day seems more reasonable.

Therapeutic Uses. The uses of iodide in the treatment of hyperthyroidism are in the immediate preoperative period in preparation for thyroidectomy and, in conjunction with antithyroid drugs and propranolol, in the treatment of thyrotoxic crisis. Prior to surgery, iodide is sometimes employed alone, but more frequently it is used after the hyperthyroidism has been controlled by an antithyroid drug. It is then given during the 10 days that immediately antedate the operation. Optimal control of hyperthyroidism is achieved if antithyroid drugs are first given alone. If iodine is also given from the beginning, variable responses are observed; sometimes the effect of iodide predominates, storage of hormone is promoted, and prolonged antithyroid treatment is required before the hyperthyroidism is controlled.

There are several minor untoward effects of iodide administration, including inflammation of salivary glands (sialadenitis), an unpleasant taste, rhinitis, conjunctivitis, gastritis, and headache. More serious (but infrequent) reactions requiring discontinuation of drug include drug fever, skin rashes, thrombotic thrombocytopenic purpura, and collagen disease-like syndromes.

LITHIUM

Schou and associates (1968) noted goiters in 15 patients during treatment with lithium (*see* Chapter 12). There was apparent hyperstimulation of the thyroid gland accompanied by deficiency of peripheral thyroid hormone. There is now evidence that lithium salts impair thyroid hormone secretion in most patients, although goiter is rare (*see* Temple *et al.*, 1972). Since iodide is the only other compound available that inhibits hormone secretion acutely, these observations have attracted interest. Unfortunately, doses of lithium carbonate that are effective (900 to 1500 mg per day) appear also to interfere with peripheral hormone degradation. There are thus disadvantages, and the clinical use of lithium salts for this purpose is highly experimental.

RADIOACTIVE IODINE

Chemical and Physical Properties. While there are several radioactive isotopes of iodine, greatest use has been made of ^{131}I, ^{125}I, and ^{123}I. ^{131}I has been the most widely employed for biological purposes. It has a half-life of 8 days, and, therefore, over 99% of its radiant energy is expended within 56 days. Its radioactive emissions include both x-rays and β particles. Like that of other radioactive isotopes, its chemical behavior is identical to that of its stable prototype, ^{127}I. ^{125}I is made by bombarding ^{124}Xe with neutrons; its 60-day half-life and its soft radiation made up of x-rays, conversion electrons, and Auger electrons make it highly suitable for many applications (Myers and Vanderleeden, 1960). It has been suggested, on theoretical grounds, that ^{125}I might impair hormone synthesis with less permanent damage to thyroid-cell nuclei (Greig *et al.*, 1970). Of the short-lived radionuclides of iodine, ^{123}I is being used experimentally. ^{123}I is produced from ^{123}Xe, and it emits x-rays with a half-life of only 13 hours, which permits relatively brief radiation exposure during thyroid scans.

Effects on the Thyroid Gland. Like stable iodine, ^{131}I is rapidly and efficiently trapped by the thyroid, incorporated into the iodoamino acids, and deposited in the colloid of the follicles, from which it is slowly liberated. Thus, the destructive beta rays originate within the follicle and act almost exclusively upon the parenchymal cells of the thyroid with little or no damage to surrounding tissue. The x-rays pass through the tissue and can be quantified by external detection. The effects of the radiation depend upon the dosage. When small tracer doses of ^{131}I are administered, thyroid function is not disturbed. However, when large amounts of radioactive iodine gain access to the gland, the characteristic cytotoxic actions of ionizing radiation are observed. Pyknosis and necrosis of the follicular cells are followed by disappearance of colloid and fibrosis of the gland. With properly selected doses of ^{131}I, it is possible completely to destroy the thyroid gland without detectable injury to adjacent tissues. After smaller doses, some of the follicles, usually in the periphery of the gland, retain their function.

Preparations. *Sodium Iodide I 131,* U.S.P. (IODO-TOPE I-131, ORIODIDE-131, THERIODIDE-131, and preparations marketed under the nonproprietary name), is available as a solution or in capsules containing ^{131}I suitable for either oral or intravenous administration. *Sodium iodide I 125* is available in capsules, as a solution for oral administration, and as an injection for intravenous use. The radioactive nuclides are processed in the form of sodium iodide in such a manner that they are essentially carrier free. Other chemical forms of radioactivity are absent. The information on the label includes the activity at a given hour and date, the name and quantity of any added substance (preservative, dye, or stabilizing agent), the intended use, whether oral or intravenous and whether diagnostic or therapeutic, and the recommended dosage. *Sodium iodide I 123* is available only as an investigational drug.

Therapeutic Uses. Radioactive iodine finds its widest use in the treatment of *hyperthyroidism* and in the *diagnosis of disorders of thyroid function.* Discussion will be limited to the uses of ^{131}I.

Hyperthyroidism. Radioactive iodine has proven highly useful in the treatment of hyperthyroidism, and in many circumstances it is regarded as the therapeutic procedure of choice for this condition. ^{130}I was successfully employed in the original studies on the treatment of Graves' disease by endogenous radiation; however, in most subsequent studies, ^{131}I and to a lesser extent ^{125}I have been used.

Dosage and Technic. ^{131}I is administered orally, dissolved in half a glass of water. The amount given is so small that it cannot be detected by taste or odor.

The effective dose of ^{131}I differs for individual patients. It depends primarily upon the size of the thyroid, the iodine uptake of the gland, and the rate of release of radioactive iodine from the gland subsequent to its deposition in the colloid. To determine these variables insofar as possible, many investigators administer a tracer dose of ^{131}I and calculate the iodine uptake by the gland and the rate of loss therefrom. The weight of the gland is estimated. From these data, the dose of isotope necessary to provide from 7000 to 10,000 rads per gram of thyroid tissue is determined. Even when dosage is controlled in this manner, it is difficult to predict the response of an individual to a given amount of the isotope. For these reasons, the optimal dose of ^{131}I, expressed in terms of microcuries taken up per gram of thyroid tissue, varies in different laboratories from 80 to 150 μCi. The usual total dose is 4 to 10 mCi. Lower-dosage ^{131}I therapy (80 μCi/g thyroid) has been advocated to reduce the incidence of subsequent hypothyroidism (Cevallos *et al.,* 1974). While the incidence of hypothyroidism in the early years after such therapy is lower, the ultimate number of patients with this complication may be the same. Since long-term surveillance is difficult, more patients with late hypothyroidism may go undetected (Glennon *et al.,* 1972).

It may prove practical to use ^{131}I safely in the treatment of Graves' disease without resorting to elaborate procedures for the measurement of radioactivity and iodine uptake. For this purpose, a moderate dose of ^{131}I is administered. Again, the dose is determined by the size of the thyroid and the severity of the hyperthyroidism. It averages about 4 mCi. Three months later, the patient is again examined clinically and the need for further treatment determined.

Course of Disease. The course of Graves' disease in a patient who has received an optimal dose of ^{131}I is characterized by progressive recovery. It is very unusual for any tenderness to be noted in the thyroid region, and most observers have failed to detect any exacerbation of hyperthyroidism from loss of hormone from the damaged gland. Beginning after a variable interval of a few days to a few weeks, the symptoms of hyperthyroidism gradually abate over a period of 2 to 3 months. If therapy has been inadequate, the necessity for further treatment is apparent within 3 months.

Depending to some extent upon the dosage schedule adopted, one half to two thirds of patients are cured by a single dose, one third to one fifth require two doses, and in the remainder three or more doses are needed before the disorder is controlled. Although it is usual to allow only about 3 months to elapse before concluding that an incomplete response calls for another dose, late effects of the radiation make it desirable to wait much longer. But, again, this further delays the recovery.

Propranolol or antithyroid drugs or both can be used to hasten the control of hyperthyroidism while awaiting the full effects of the radioiodine. However, the antithyroid drugs should be withheld for a few days or a week after the therapeutic dose of ^{131}I.

Advantages. The advantages of radioactive iodine in the treatment of Graves' disease are many.

No death as a direct result of the use of the isotope has been reported, and only by a gross miscalculation of dose could such an event conceivably occur. In the nonpregnant patient, no tissue other than the thyroid is exposed to sufficient ionizing radiation to be affected. This applies not only to remote organs, such as the kidneys and the gonads, but also to structures adjacent to the thyroid, such as the parathyroid glands and the recurrent laryngeal nerve. The patient is spared the risks, emotional strain, trauma, and cosmetic disfiguration of a surgical procedure. The incidence of progressive exophthalmos appears to be no different than after surgical treatment. Finally, the cost is low, hospitalization is not required, and the patient can indulge in his customary activities during the entire procedure.

Disadvantages. The chief disadvantage of the use of radioactive iodine is the high incidence of hypothyroidism that is induced. Even when elaborate procedures are employed to estimate iodine uptake and gland size, a certain percentage of patients will be overtreated. A distressing feature of this complication is its rising prevalence with the passage of time; the longer the interval after treatment, the higher the incidence. This finding indicates that the earlier estimates of the incidence of hypothyroidism, 5 to 15%, are too low. Several analyses of groups of patients treated 10 or more years previously suggest that after the first 1 or 2 years, when only 5 to 10% of patients may have developed the complication, about 3% more develop hypothyroidism each year so that the eventual rate may exceed 50% (Dunn and Chapman, 1964; Green and Wilson, 1964). However, it now appears that the incidence of hypothyroidism also increases progressively after subtotal thyroidectomy, and such failure of glandular function is suspected to be part of the natural progression of Graves' disease, no matter what the therapy.

Although it is often said that hypothyroidism is not a serious complication because it can so easily be treated with thyroid hormone, it is in fact difficult to ensure that patients who need the hormone actually take it. Treatment is frequently discontinued, and the manifestations of hypothyroidism slowly incapacitate the patient as if he were not aware of what is taking place. Hypothyroidism is obviously a serious complication deserving of painstaking care to make certain that optimal replacement therapy is provided.

Another disadvantage is the long period of time that is sometimes required before the hyperthyroidism is controlled. When a single dose is effective, the response is most satisfactory; however, when multiple doses are needed, it may be many months or a year or more before the patient is well.

Indications. The clearest indication for this form of treatment is hyperthyroidism in older patients and in those with heart disease. Here hyperthyroidism is such a serious disorder that myxedema, as a complication, is of lesser consequence. Radioiodine is also the best form of treatment when hyperthyroidism has relapsed after subtotal thyroidectomy and when prolonged treatment with antithyroid drugs has not led to remission. Other aspects of this problem have been discussed above.

Contraindications. If for no other reason, the risk of hypothyroidism makes radioiodine an unsuitable treatment for hyperthyroidism in childhood. The risk of causing neoplastic changes in the gland has been constantly under consideration since radioiodine was first introduced, and only small numbers of children have been treated in this way. Indeed, many clinics have declined to treat younger patients for fear of causing cancer and have reserved radioiodine for patients over some arbitrary age, such as 25 to 30 years. Since there is now vast experience with ^{131}I, these age limits are lower than they were in the past. While a few reports of thyroid cancer following ^{131}I therapy have appeared, this is hardly surprising in view of the fact that hundreds of thousands of patients with thyroid disease have been treated in this way. There is no evidence that radioiodine therapy has caused thyroid or other forms of cancer in adults. The use of radioiodine during pregnancy is contraindicated; after the first trimester the fetal thyroid would concentrate the isotope and thus suffer damage, but even during the first trimester radioiodine is probably best avoided because there may be adverse effects of radiation on fetal tissues.

Hyperthyroidism with Nodular Goiter. It is often claimed that in patients with nodular goiter the required dose of radioiodine is higher than in those with a diffusely enlarged thyroid gland. Others have been inclined to doubt this and have found that the response is similar if due allowance is made for the somewhat lower uptake in nodular goiter and if the true size of the goiter is not underestimated. It is also thought that the risk of inducing hypothyroidism is less in nodular goiter than in Graves' disease, perhaps because of the natural progression of the latter.

Metastatic Thyroid Cancer. Most thyroid carcinomas accumulate very little iodine. However, follicular carcinomas, which comprise 25% of thyroid malignancies, often do so, although they rarely synthesize sufficient hormone to cause thyrotoxicosis. If metastases accumulate iodine, therapy with large doses of ^{131}I may prolong life, particularly in younger patients (Leeper, 1973). In an attempt to stimulate uptake, thyrotropin has been given or secretion of endogenous thyrotropin has been evoked by inducing hypothyroidism by removal or radiation of the thyroid, or by prolonged treatment with antithyroid drugs. The increased uptake thus achieved is usually not large and may be negligible. Moreover, it has been noted by a number of observers that growth of the metastases may be stimulated by these maneuvers, and they have therefore questioned their advisability (Maloof *et al.*, 1956; Crile, 1957; Thomas, 1958).

Papillary carcinoma is the most common type of thyroid cancer, and some cases may be responsive to thyrotropin. Metastatic lesions occasionally regress when thyrotropin secretion is suppressed by administration of thyroid hormone.

Diagnostic Uses. Tracer studies with radioiodine have found wide application in studies of disorders of the thyroid gland. The uptake of a tracer dose is helpful in the diagnosis of hyperthyroidism, hypothyroidism, and goiter, and the response of the thyroid to thyrotropin or to suppression by thyroid hormone can be evaluated in this way.

Radioiodine is also used to label thyroxine and its congeners to study the absorption, metabolism, and excretion of these substances in various thyroid disorders, and by special methods to measure the quantity of circulating thyroxine and the extent and nature of the binding of thyroxine and triiodothyronine to plasma proteins. Following the administration of a tracer dose, the pattern of localization in the thyroid gland can be depicted by special scanning apparatus, and this technic is sometimes useful in finding ectopic thyroid tissue and occasionally metastatic thyroid tumors.

Various isotopes of iodine have been used successfully in thyroidal scans and to determine percent uptake of the nuclide. Since the pertechnetate anion is trapped in thyroidal tissue in the same manner as iodide, technetium 99m (99m Tc) as pertechnetate has proven useful. The rapidity of the technic with 99m Tc pertechnetate and the greater resolution of thyroid morphology on scanning are advantageous. The radiation dose is less with 99m Tc than with [131]I. [123]I offers additional advantages over the latter isotope due to a greater ratio of thyroidal to non-thyroidal uptake, which results in less radiation exposure and comparable or improved quality of resolution with scanning. [123]I and [132]I can be used with about 1 to 2% of the radiation exposure of ^{125}I or ^{131}I; the very short half-life (2⅓ hours) of [132]I has made it impractical for clinical use. The improvements in thyroid scanning and uptake technics at lower radiation exposure with the more recently available isotopes offer obvious advantages, particularly in the pediatric age group.

Alexander, W. D.; Evans, V.; MacAulay, A.; Gallagher, T. F., Jr.; and Londono, J. Metabolism of ^{35}S-labelled antithyroid drugs in man. Br. med. J., **1969a,** 2, 290–291.

Alexander, W. D.; Harden, R. McG.; Koutras, D. A.; and Wayne, E. Influence of iodine intake after treatment with antithyroid drugs. Lancet, **1965,** 2, 866–868.

Anbar, M.; Guttmann, S.; and Lewitus, Z. The mode of action of perchlorate ions on the iodine uptake of the thyroid gland. Int. J. appl. Radiat. Isotopes, **1960,** 7, 87–96.

Aranow, H., and Day, R. M. Management of thyrotoxicosis in patients with ophthalmopathy: antithyroid regimen determined primarily by ocular manifestations. J. clin. Endocr. Metab., **1965,** 25, 1–10.

Arnott, D. G., and Doniach, J. The effect of compounds allied to resorcinol upon the uptake of radioactive iodine (^{131}I) by the thyroid of the rat. Biochem. J., **1952,** 50, 473–479.

Arstica, A.; Krusius, F.-E.; and Peltola, P. Studies on transfer of thio-oxazolidone-type goitrogens into cow's milk in goiter endemic districts of Finland and in experimental conditions. Acta endocr., Copenh., **1969,** 60, 712–718.

Astwood, E. B. Chemotherapy of hyperthyroidism. Harvey Lect., **1945,** 40, 195–235.

Astwood, E. B.; Cassidy, C. E.; and Aurbach, G. D. Treatment of goiter and thyroid nodules with thyroid. J. Am. med. Ass., **1960,** 174, 459–464.

Babior, B. M.; Creagan, S.; Ingbar, S. H.; and Kipnes, R. S. Stimulation of mitochondrial adenosine diphosphate uptake by thyroid hormones. Proc. natn. Acad. Sci. U.S.A., **1973,** 70, 98–102.

Braverman, L. E.; Ingbar, S. H.; and Sterling, K. Conversion of thyroxine (T4) to triiodothyronine (T3) in

athyreotic human subjects. J. clin. Invest., **1970,** 49, 855–864.

Bruns, P. Beobachtungen und Untersuchungen über die Schilddrüsenbehandlung des Kropfs. Beitr. klin. Chir., **1896,** 16, 521–544.

Buccino, R. A.; Spann, J. F., Jr.; Pool, P. E.; Sonnenblick, E. B.; and Braunwald, E. Influence of thyroid state on the intrinsic contractile properties and energy stores of the myocardium. J. clin. Invest., **1967,** 46, 1669–1682.

Cassidy, C. E., and VanderLaan, W. P. Thyroid-suppression test in the prognosis of hyperthyroidism treated by antithyroid drugs. New Engl. J. Med., **1960,** 262, 1228–1229.

Cevallos, J. L.; Hagen, G. A.; Maloof, F.; and Chapman, E. M. Low-dosage ^{131}I therapy of thyrotoxicosis (diffuse goiters). A five-year follow-up study. New Engl. J. Med., **1974,** 290, 141–143.

Chesney, A. M.; Clawson, T. A.; and Webster, B. Endemic goitre in rabbits. I. Incidence and characteristics. Bull. Johns Hopkins Hosp., **1928,** 43, 261–277.

Chopra, I. J. A radioimmunoassay for measurement of thyroxine in unextracted serum. J. clin. Endocr. Metab., **1972,** 34, 938–947.

Cody, V., and Duax, W. L. Distal conformation of the thyroid hormone 3,5,3′-triiodo-L-thyronine. Science, Wash., **1973,** 181, 757–758.

Crile, G., Jr. The endocrine dependency of certain thyroid cancers and the danger that hypothyroidism may stimulate their growth. Cancer, N.Y., **1957,** 10, 1119–1137.

Cushing, H. The Pituitary Body and Its Disorders. J. B. Lippincott Co., Philadelphia, **1912.**

Das, G., and Krieger, M. Treatment of thyrotoxic storm with intravenous administration of propranolol. Ann. intern. Med., **1969,** 70, 985–988.

DeGroot, L. J. Thyroid and the heart. Mayo Clin. Proc., **1972,** 47, 864–871.

DeGroot, L. J.; Niepomniszcke, H.; Nagasaka, A.; and Hati, R. Mechanism of thyroid hormone formation. Ann. clin. Res., **1972,** 4, 113–120.

Delange, F., and Ermans, A. M. Role of a dietary goitrogen in the etiology of endemic goiter on Idjwi Island. Am. J. clin. Nutr., **1971,** 24, 1354–1360.

Doniach, D.; Hudson, R. V.; Trotter, W. R.; and Waddams, A. Effects of thyroxine, triiodothyronine and TRIAC on metabolic rate, blood lipids and thyroid size and function in subjects with nontoxic goitre. Clin. Sci., **1958,** 17, 519–529.

Dunn, J. T. The amino acid neighbors of thyroxine in thyroglobulin. J. biol. Chem., **1970,** 245, 5954–5961.

Dunn, J. T., and Chapman, E. M. Rising incidence of hypothyroidism after radioactive-iodine therapy in thyrotoxicosis. New Engl. J. Med., **1964,** 271, 1037–1042.

Evans, E. S.; Rosenberg, L. L.; and Simpson, M. E. Relative sensitivity of different biological responses to thyroxine. Endocrinology, **1960,** 66, 433–440.

Flock, E. V.; Bollman, J. L.; Grindlay, J. H.; and Orvis, A. L. Metabolism of L-thyroxine and L-triiodothyronine in the absence of the liver. Am. J. Physiol., **1956,** 187, 407–414.

Geffner, D. L.; Azukizawa, M.; and Hershman, J. M. Propylthiouracil blocks extrathyroidal conversion of thyroxine to triiodothyronine and augments thyrotropin secretion in man. J. clin. Invest., **1975,** 55, 224–229.

Gharib, H.; Ryan, R. J.; and Mayberry, W. E. Triiodothyronine (T3) radioimmunoassay. A critical evaluation. Mayo Clin. Proc., **1972,** 47, 934–937.

Gilman, A. G., and Rall, T. W. Factors influencing adenosine 3′,5′-phosphate accumulation in bovine thyroid slices. J. biol. Chem., **1968,** 243, 5867–5871.

Glennon, J. A.; Gordon, E. S.; and Sawin, C. T. Hypothyroidism after low-dose ^{131}I treatment of hyperthyroidism. Ann. intern. Med., **1972,** 76, 721–723.

Gley, E. Sur les effets de l'extirpation du corps thyroide. C. r. Séanc. Soc. Biol., **1891,** 43, 551–554.

Godley, A. F., and Stanbury, J. B. Preliminary experience in the treatment of hyperthyroidism with potassium perchlorate. *J. clin. Endocr. Metab.,* **1954,** *14,* 70–78.

Gordon, A. H.; Gross, J.; O'Connor, D.; and Pitt-Rivers, R. Nature of the circulating thyroid hormone–plasma protein complex. *Nature, Lond.,* **1952,** *169,* 19–20.

Green, M., and Wilson, G. M. Thyrotoxicosis treated by surgery or iodine-131, with special reference to development of hypothyroidism. *Br. med. J.,* **1964,** *1,* 1005–1010.

Greer, M. A.; Grimm, Y.; and Studer, H. Qualitative changes in the secretion of thyroid hormones induced by iodine deficiency. *Endocrinology,* **1968,** *83,* 1193–1198.

Greig, W. R.; Smith, J. F. B.; and Orr, J. S. Comparative survivals of rat thyroid cells *in vivo* after ^{131}I, ^{125}I, and X irradiations. *Br. J. Radiol.,* **1970,** *43,* 542–548.

Gross, J., and Pitt-Rivers, R. The identification of 3:5:3′-L-triiodothyronine in human plasma. *Lancet,* **1952,** *1,* 439–441.

———. 3:5:3′-Triiodothyronine. 1. Isolation from thyroid gland and synthesis. *Biochem. J.,* **1953a,** *53,* 645–652. 2. Physiological activity. *Ibid.,* **1953b,** *53,* 652–657.

Harden, R. McG.; Alexander, W. D.; Koutras, D. A.; Harrison, M. T.; and Wayne, E. Quantitative studies of iodine metabolism after long-term treatment of thyrotoxicosis with antithyroid drugs. *J. clin. Endocr. Metab.,* **1966,** *26,* 397–401.

Harington, C. R. Chemistry of thyroxine: isolation of thyroxine from thyroid gland. *Biochem. J.,* **1926,** *20,* 293–299.

———. Biochemical basis of thyroid function. *Lancet,* **1935,** *1,* 1199–1204, 1261–1266.

Harington, C. R., and Barger, G. Thyroxine. III. Constitution and synthesis of thyroxine. *Biochem. J.,* **1927,** *21,* 169–183.

Hays, M. Absorption of oral thyroxine in man. *J. clin. Endocr. Metab.,* **1968,** *28,* 749–756.

Hercus, C. E., and Purves, H. D. Studies on endemic and experimental goitre. *J. Hyg., Camb.,* **1936,** *36,* 182–203.

Higgins, H. P.; Elkan, I.; Diosy, A.; Bayley, T. A.; and Buckley, G. C. Prognostic value of high 10-minute ^{131}I uptake in non-toxic goiters. *Can. med. Ass. J.,* **1964,** *91,* 689–693.

Ingbar, S. H. Autoregulation of the thyroid response to iodide excess and depletion. *Mayo Clin. Proc.,* **1972,** *47,* 814–823.

Ismail-Beigi, F., and Edelman, I. S. Mechanism of thyroid calorigenesis: role of active sodium transport. *Proc. natn. Acad. Sci. U.S.A.,* **1970,** *67,* 1071–1078.

Jorgensen, E. C. Stereochemistry of thyroxine and analogues. *Mayo Clin. Proc.,* **1964,** *39,* 560–568.

Kendall, E. C. The isolation in crystalline form of the compound containing iodine which occurs in the thyroid: its chemical nature and physiological activity. *Trans. Ass. Am. Physns,* **1915,** *30,* 420–449.

Lamas, L.; Dorris, M. L.; and Taurog, A. Evidence for a catalytic role for thyroid peroxidase in the conversion of diiodotyrosine to thyroxine. *Endocrinology,* **1972,** *90,* 1417–1426.

Leeper, R. D. The effect of ^{131}I therapy on survival of patients with metastatic papillary or follicular thyroid carcinoma. *J. clin. Endocr. Metab.,* **1973,** *36,* 1143–1152.

Levey, G. S. Catecholamine sensitivity, thyroid hormone and the heart. A reevaluation. *Am. J. Med.,* **1971,** *50,* 413–420.

Levey, G. S., and Epstein, S. E. Myocardial adenyl cyclase: activation by thyroid hormones and evidence for two adenyl cyclase systems. *J. clin. Invest.,* **1969,** *48,* 1663–1669.

London, W. T.; Vought, R. L.; and Brown, F. A. Bread—a dietary source of large quantities of iodine. *New Engl. J. Med.,* **1965,** *273,* 381.

Mackenzie, J. B.; Mackenzie, C. G.; and McCollum, E. V. Effect of sulfanilylguanidine on thyroid of rat. *Science, N.Y.,* **1941,** *94,* 518–519.

Magnus-Levy, A. Über den respiratorischen Gaswechsel unter den Einfluss der Thyroidea sowie unter ver-

schiedenen pathologischen Zustanden. *Berl. klin. Wschr.,* **1895,** *32,* 650–652.

Maloof, F.; Vickery, A. L.; and Rapp, B. An evaluation of various factors influencing the treatment of metastatic thyroid carcinoma with [131]I. *J. clin. Endocr. Metab.,* **1956,** *16,* 1–27.

Marchant, B.; Alexander, W. D.; Lazarus, J. H.; Lees, J.; and Clark, D. H. The accumulation of ^{35}S-antithyroid drugs by the thyroid gland. *J. clin. Endocr. Metab.,* **1972,** *34,* 847–851.

Marine, D., and Kimball, O. P. The prevention of simple goiter in man: a survey of the incidence and types of thyroid enlargements in the schoolgirls of Akron, Ohio, from the 5th to the 12th grades, inclusive; the plan of prevention proposed. *J. Lab. clin. Med.,* **1917,** *3,* 40–48.

Murray, G. R. Note on the treatment of myxedema by hypodermic injection of an extract of the thyroid gland of a sheep. *Br. med. J.,* **1891,** *2,* 796–797.

Myers, W. G., and Vanderleeden, J. C. Radioiodine-125. *J. nucl. Med.,* **1960,** *1,* 149–164.

Nakagawa, S., and Ruegamer, W. R. Properties of a rat tissue iodothyronine deiodinase and its natural inhibitor. *Biochemistry, N.Y.,* **1967,** *6,* 1249–1261.

Nilsson, S. F., and Peterson, P. A. Evidence for multiple thyroxine-binding sites in human prealbumin. *J. biol. Chem.,* **1971,** *246,* 6098–6105.

Oppenheimer, J. H. Thyroid hormones in liver. *Mayo Clin. Proc.,* **1972,** *47,* 854–863.

Oppenheimer, J. H.; Schwartz, H. L.; and Surks, M. I. Propylthiouracil inhibits the conversion of L-thyroxine to L-triiodothyronine. *J. clin. Invest.,* **1972,** *51,* 2493–2497.

Ord, W. M. On myxoedema, a term proposed to be applied to an essential condition in the "cretinoid" affection occasionally observed in middle-aged women. *Med. chir. Trans., Lond.,* **1878,** *61,* 57–78.

Parry, C. H. *Collections from the Unpublished Medical Writings of Dr. C. H. Parry.* Underwood, London, **1895.**

Pisarev, M. A.; DeGroot, L. J.; and Hati, R. KI and imidazole inhibition of TSH and c-AMP induced thyroidal iodine secretion. *Endocrinology,* **1971,** *88,* 1217–1221.

Pisarev, M. A.; DeGroot, L. J.; and Wieber, J. F. Cyclic-AMP production of goiter. *Endocrinology,* **1970,** *87,* 339–342.

Pittman, C. S.; Buck, M. W.; and Chambers, J. B., Jr. Urinary metabolites of ^{14}C-labeled thyroxine in man. *J. clin. Invest.,* **1972,** *51,* 1759–1766.

Pittman, C. S.; Chambers, J. B., Jr.; and Read, V. H. The extrathyroidal conversion rate of thyroxine to triiodothyronine in normal man. *J. clin. Invest.,* **1971,** *50,* 1187–1196.

Pittman, J. A.; Beschi, R. J.; Block, P., Jr.; and Lindsay, R. H. Thyromimetic activity of 3,5,3′,5′-tetramethylthyronine. *Endocrinology,* **1973,** *93,* 201–204.

Pittman, J. A.; Beschi, R. J.; and Smitherman, T. C. Methimazole: its absorption and excretion in man and tissue distribution in rats. *J. clin. Endocr. Metab.,* **1971,** *33,* 182–185.

Psychoyos, S.; Ma, D. S.; Czernik, A. J.; Bowers, H. S.; Atkins, C. D.; Malicki, C. A.; and Cash, W. D. Thyromimetic activity of methylene-bridged thyroid hormone analogs. *Endocrinology,* **1973,** *92,* 243–250.

Richter, C. P., and Clisby, K. H. Toxic effects of bitter-tasting phenylthiocarbamide. *Archs Path.,* **1942,** *33,* 46–57.

Roche, J.; Lissitzky, S.; and Michel, R. Sur la triiodothyronine, produit intermédiare de la transformation de la diiodothyronine en thyroxine. *C. r. hebd. Séanc. Acad. Sci., Paris,* **1952a,** *234,* 997–998.

———. Sur la présence de triiodothyronine dans la thyroglobuline. *Ibid.,* **1952b,** *234,* 1228–1230.

Roche, J.; Michel, R.; Michel, O.; and Lissitzky, S. Sur la déshalogénation enzymatique des iodotyrosine par la corps thyroide et sur son rôle physiologique. *Biochim. biophys. Acta,* **1952c,** *9,* 161–169.

Rosenberg, I. N. The antithyroid activity of some compounds that inhibit peroxidase. *Science, Wash.,* **1952,** *116,* 503–505.

Saberi, M.; Sterling, F. H.; and Utiger, R. D. Reduction in extrathyroidal triiodothyronine production by propylthiouracil in man. *J. clin. Invest.,* **1975,** *55,* 218–223.

Schou, M.; Amdisen, A.; Jensen, S. E.; and Olsen, T. Occurrence of goitre during lithium treatment. *Br. med. J.,* **1968,** *3,* 710–713.

Shanks, R. G.; Hadden, D. R.; Lowe, D. C.; McDevitt, D. G.; and Montgomery, D. A. D. Controlled trial of propranolol in thyrotoxicosis. *Lancet,* **1969,** *1,* 993–994.

Simmonds, M. Ueber Hypophysisschwund mit todlichem Ausang. *Dt. med. Wschr.,* **1914,** *40,* 322–323.

Solomon, D. H.; Beck, J. C.; VanderLaan, W. P.; and Astwood, E. B. Prognosis of hyperthyroidism treated by antithyroid drugs. *J. Am. med. Ass.,* **1953,** *152,* 201–205.

Starr, P., and Goodwin, W. Use of triiodothyronine for reduction of goiter and detection of thyroid cancer. *Metabolism,* **1958,** *7,* 287–292.

Sterling, K., and Brenner, M. A. Free thyroxine in human serum: simplified measurement with the aid of magnesium precipitation. *J. clin. Invest.,* **1966,** *45,* 153–163.

Sterling, K.; Brenner, M. A.; and Newman, E. S. Conversion of thyroxine to triiodothyronine in normal human subjects. *Science, Wash.,* **1970,** *169,* 1099–1100.

Sterling, K.; Hamada, S.; Takemura, Y.; Brenner, M. A.; Newman, E. S.; and Inada, M. Preparation and properties of thyroxine-binding alpha globulin (TBG). *J. clin. Invest.,* **1971,** *50,* 1758–1771.

Temple, R.; Berman, M.; Carlson, H. E.; Robbins, J.; and Wolff, J. The use of lithium in Graves' disease. *Mayo Clin. Proc.,* **1972,** *47,* 872–878.

Thilly, C. H.; Delange, F.; Goldstein-Golaire, J.; and Ermans, A. M. Endemic goiter prevention by iodized oil: a reassessment. *J. clin. Endocr. Metab.,* **1973,** *36,* 1196–1204.

Thomas, C. C., Jr. The use of L-triiodothyronine as a pituitary depressant in the management of thyroid cancer. *Surgery Gynec. Obstet.,* **1958,** *106,* 137–144.

Thompson, W. O.; Thompson, P. K.; Brailey, A. G.; and Cohen, A. C. Prolonged treatment of exophthalmic goiter by iodine alone. *Archs intern. Med.,* **1930,** *45,* 481–502.

VanderLaan, J. E., and VanderLaan, W. P. The iodide concentrating mechanism of the rat thyroid and its inhibition by thiocyanate. *Endocrinology,* **1947,** *40,* 403–416.

VanderLaan, W. P. The biological significance of the iodide-concentrating mechanism of the thyroid gland. *Brookhaven Symp. Biol.,* **1955,** *7,* 30–37.

Van Middlesworth, L. Thyroxine requirement and the excretion of thyroxine metabolites. In, *Clinical Endocrinology I.* (Astwood, E. B., ed.) Grune & Stratton, Inc., New York, **1960,** pp. 103–111.

Van Middlesworth, L.; Turner, J. A.; and Lipscomb, A. Liver function related to thyroxine metabolism. *J. nucl. Med.,* **1963,** *4,* 132–138.

Wolff, J., and Chaikoff, I. L. Plasma inorganic iodide as a homeostatic regulator of thyroid function. *J. biol. Chem.,* **1948,** *174,* 555–564.

Wolff, J., and Maurey, J. R. Thyroidal iodide transport. IV. The role of ion size. *Biochim. biophys. Acta,* **1963,** *69,* 58–67.

Wollman, S. H.; Spicer, S. S.; and Burstone, M. S. Localization of esterase and acid phosphatase in granules and colloid droplets in rat thyroid epithelium. *J. cell Biol.,* **1964,** *21,* 191–201.

Wyngaarden, J. B.; Wright, B. M.; and Ways, P. The effect of certain anions upon the accumulation and retention of iodide by the thyroid gland. *Endocrinology,* **1952,** *50,* 537–549.

Wynn, J., and Gibbs, R. Thyroxine degradation. II. Products of thyroxine degradation by rat liver microsomes. *J. biol. Chem.,* **1962,** *237,* 3499–3505.

Zor, U.; Kaneko, T.; Lowe, I. P.; Bloom, G.; and Field, J. B. Effect of thyroid-stimulating hormone and prostaglandins on thyroid adenyl cyclase activation and cyclic adenosine 3′,5′-monophosphate. *J. biol. Chem.,* **1969,** *244,* 5189–5195.

Monographs and Reviews

Alexander, W. D.; Harden, R. McG.; and Shimmins, J. Studies on the thyroid iodide "trap" in man. *Recent Prog. Horm. Res.,* **1969b,** *25,* 423–439.

Danowski, T. S. *Clinical Endocrinology.* Vol. II, *Thyroid.* The Williams & Wilkins Co., Baltimore, **1962.**

Dumont, J. E. The action of thyrotropin on thyroid metabolism. *Vitams Horm.,* **1971,** *29,* 287–412.

Fain, J. N. Biochemical aspects of drug and hormone action on adipose tissue. *Pharmac. Rev.,* **1973,** *25,* 67–118.

Fisher, D. A. Advances in the laboratory diagnosis of thyroid disease. Part I. *J. Pediat.,* **1973a,** *82,* 1–9. Part II. *Ibid.,* **1973b,** *82,* 187–191.

Halmi, N. S. Thyroidal iodide transport. *Vitams Horm.,* **1961,** *19,* 133–163.

Hamburgh, M. The role of thyroid and growth hormones in neurogenesis. *Curr. Top. devl Biol.,* **1969,** *4,* 109–148.

Jorgensen, E. C. Thyroid hormones and antithyroid drugs. In, *Medicinal Chemistry,* 3rd ed. (Burger, A., ed.) John Wiley & Sons, Inc., New York, **1970,** pp. 838–858.

Liberti, P., and Stanbury, J. B. The pharmacology of substances affecting the thyroid gland. *A. Rev. Pharmac.,* **1971,** *11,* 113–142.

Maloof, F., and Soodak, M. Intermediary metabolism of thyroid tissue and the action of drugs. *Pharmac. Rev.,* **1963,** *15,* 43–95.

Means, J. H.; DeGroot, L. J.; and Stanbury, J. B. *The Thyroid and Its Diseases,* 3rd ed. McGraw-Hill Book Co., New York, **1963.**

Murphy, B. E. P. Protein-binding and the assay of nonantigenic hormones. *Recent Prog. Horm. Res.,* **1969,** *25,* 563–601.

Oppenheimer, J. H.; Surks, M. I.; and Schwartz, H. L. The metabolic significance of exchangeable cellular thyroxine. *Recent Prog. Horm. Res.,* **1969,** *25,* 381–414.

Pitot, H. C., and Yatvin, M. B. Interrelationships of mammalian hormones and enzyme levels *in vivo. Physiol. Rev.,* **1973,** *53,* 228–325.

Rall, J. E.; Robbins, J.; and Lewallen, C. G. The thyroid. In, *The Hormones,* Vol. 5. (Pincus, G.; Thimann, K. V.; and Astwood, E. B.; eds.) Academic Press, Inc., New York, **1964,** pp. 159–439.

Selenkow, H. A., and Asper, S. P., Jr. Biological activity of compounds structurally related to thyroxine. *Physiol. Rev.,* **1955,** *35,* 426–474.

Sterling, K. The significance of circulating triiodothyronine. *Recent Prog. Horm. Res.,* **1970,** *26,* 249–274.

Taurog, A. Thyroid peroxidase and thyroxine biosynthesis. *Recent Prog. Horm. Res.,* **1970,** *26,* 189–241.

VanderLaan, W. P., and Storrie, V. M. A survey of the factors controlling thyroid function, with especial reference to newer views on antithyroid substances. *Pharmac. Rev.,* **1955,** *7,* 301–334.

VanEtten, C. H. Goitrogens. In, *Toxic Constituents of Plant Foodstuffs.* (Liener, I. E., ed.) Academic Press, Inc., New York, **1969,** pp. 103–142.

Werner, S. C., and Ingbar, S. H. (eds.). *The Thyroid.* Harper & Row, Pubs., New York, **1971.**

Wolff, E. C., and Wolff, J. The mechanism of action of the thyroid hormones. In, *The Thyroid Gland,* Vol. 1. (Pitt-Rivers, R., and Trotter, W. R., eds.) Butterworth & Co., Ltd., London, **1964,** pp. 237–282.

Wolff, J. Transport of iodide and other anions in the thyroid gland. *Physiol. Rev.,* **1964,** *44,* 45–90.

CHAPTER

68 ESTROGENS AND PROGESTINS

Ferid Murad and Alfred G. Gilman

The controlled and cyclic formation of estrogens and progesterone is unique to the ovary. These hormones play a vital role in preparing the female reproductive tract for the reception of sperm and implantation of a fertilized ovum. However, it is recognized and appreciated that many attributes of the female habitus are also influenced by these agents. Current knowledge of the synthesis and action of the ovarian hormones has permitted rational therapeutic intervention in certain diseases. Much more clinical use, however, has been made of agents that can mimic the effects of these hormones and that act as contraceptives.

History. It has long been known that removal of the ovaries results in uterine atrophy and a loss of sexual functions. The hormonal nature of the ovarian control of the female reproductive system was established in 1900 by Knauer when he found that ovarian transplants prevented the symptoms of gonadectomy. This observation was extended by Halban (1900), who showed that, if the glands were transplanted even in immature animals, normal sexual development and function were assured. In 1923, Allen and Doisy devised a simple, quantitative bioassay method for ovarian extracts based upon changes produced in the vaginal smear of the rat. Loewe (1925) first reported a female sex hormone in the blood of various species and, shortly thereafter, Frank and associates (1925) detected an active sex principle in the blood of sows in estrus. Of even greater significance was the discovery by Loewe and Lange (1926) of a female sex hormone in the urine of menstruating women and the observation that the concentration of the hormone in the urine varied with the phase of the menstrual cycle. The urinary excretion of large amounts of estrogen in the urine during pregnancy was also reported (Zondek, 1928). This finding was a boon to the chemists, who soon isolated an active substance in crystalline form (Butenandt, 1929; Doisy et al., 1929, 1930). A few years later its chemical structure was elucidated.

The results of early investigations indicated that the ovary secretes two substances. Beard (1897) had postulated that the corpus luteum serves a necessary function during pregnancy, and supporting evidence was offered by Fraenkel (1903), who showed that destruction of the corpora lutea in pregnant rabbits causes abortion. The contributions of Corner and Allen (1929) firmly established the hormonal function of the corpus luteum. These investigators showed that the abortion following extirpation of the corpora lutea in pregnant rabbits can be prevented by the injection of luteal extracts.

ESTROGENS

Synthesis and Chemistry. The ovary is capable of converting acetate to cholesterol and subsequently to other steroids, as summarized in Figure 68-1. The formation of estrogens by ovarian follicles is regulated by follicle-stimulating hormone (FSH). The effects of this gonadotropin are mediated through the formation and subsequent action of cyclic adenosine 3',5'-monophosphate (cyclic AMP) (Fontaine et al., 1971). However, the precise mechanism of the action of cyclic AMP in stimulating the synthesis of estrogen, as well as other steroids, is unknown. In men, the testis can also produce and secrete small amounts of estradiol and estrone (see Chapter 69).

The estrogens are ultimately formed from either androstenedione or testosterone as immediate precursors. The reaction of central importance is the aromatization of ring A. The first step in this reaction involves hydroxylation of C 19, the angular methyl group residing on C 10 of the precursor. Then the newly formed hydroxymethyl group is lost from the nucleus, and ring A is aromatized to yield a phenolic hydroxyl at C 3 (see Heard et al., 1955; Bagget et al., 1956; Ryan, 1959). In certain pathological conditions, this reaction appears to be defective and the androgenic precursor escapes into the circulation. Some cases of hirsutism and some of definite virilism are thought to be caused by this defect, and at least one of the features of the Stein-Leventhal syndrome associated with large polycystic ovaries is attributable to the same biosynthetic difficulty (Mahesh and Greenblatt, 1964).

Of the three main estrogens of human beings, *estradiol-17β* is the most potent and

1423

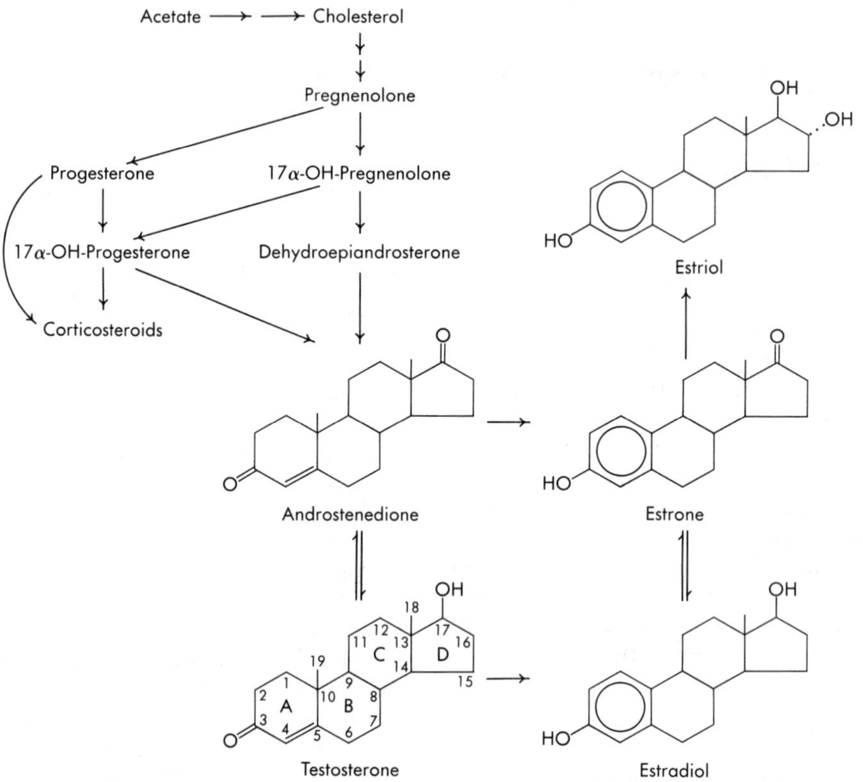

Figure 68-1. *The biosynthetic pathway for the estrogens.* Additional details and structures are shown in Figure 70-3 (page 1479).

the major secretory product of the ovary; it is readily oxidized in the body to *estrone,* which in turn can be hydrated to *estriol.* These transformations take place mainly in the liver, where there is free interconversion between estrone and estradiol (Ryan and Engel, 1953). All three estrogens are excreted in the urine as glucuronides and sulfates, along with a host of related, minor products in water-soluble complexes. During pregnancy, estrogens are synthesized in large quantities by the placenta and apparently by the same enzymatic reactions as used by the ovary. However, there are complex interactions with the fetus, and the fetal adrenal cortex is required for some synthetic steps that are deficient in the placenta (*see* Kellie, 1971). Human urine of pregnancy is thus an abundant source of natural estrogens. Animals of the genus *Equus,* including the horse, are remarkable estrogen factories. The pregnant mare excretes over 100 mg daily, a record exceeded only by the stallion, who,

despite clear manifestations of virility, excretes into his environment more estrogen than any other living creature.

Estrogenic activity is a property shared by a great number of chemical compounds, and in this respect the estrogens are unique among the hormones. The wide distribution of estrogenic activity among natural compounds has sometimes proven to be of economic importance. Sterility in sheep noted in Australia when flocks were allowed to graze on pastures populated by the so-called subterranean clover was eventually traced to the abundant quantity of the weak estrogen *genistein,* an isoflavone contained in this plant (Curnow, 1954).

Among the first nonsteroidal estrogens to be encountered and still the most potent is *diethylstilbestrol* (Dodds *et al.,* 1938), the *trans* configuration of which is as follows:

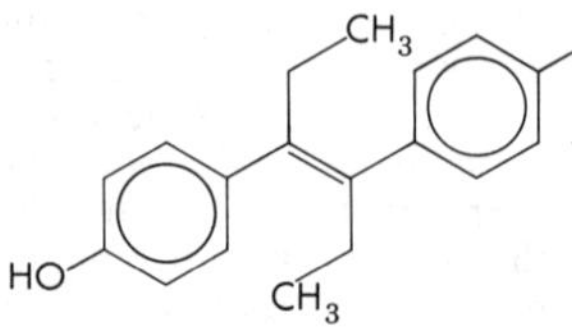

Diethylstilbestrol

In this active *trans* configuration, diethylstilbestrol can be seen to be related structurally to the steroidal compounds. Its estrogenic potency in animals varies somewhat with the assay used, but in most tests it is fully as active as estradiol. In contrast to the natural estrogens, it is highly active when given by mouth and the duration of action of a single dose is longer, properties in keeping with its slower rate of degradation in the body. The introduction of a cheap, plentiful, orally active estrogen at a time when the natural products were scarce and expensive was a milestone in the development of effective endocrine therapy.

A major and controversial use of diethylstilbestrol has been its administration to animals to accelerate weight gain. The past few years have witnessed the ban and the subsequent reapproval of this practice as it is applied to marketable meats in the United States.

Certain chemical alterations of the natural estrogens render them effective by mouth, largely through protection from inactivation by the liver. One of the most highly potent estrogens known, *ethinyl estradiol,* is an example of this type wherein the elements of acetylene are attached at C 17. As little as 20 μg daily serves as replacement therapy in the menopause, and 50 μg may be sufficient to cause withdrawal bleeding. This estrogen and some of its derivatives are widely used and are also incorporated with progesterone-like compounds for regulation of the menstrual cycle and for the control of fertility.

Physiological and Pharmacological Actions. The estrogens are largely responsible for the changes that take place at puberty in girls, and they go a long way toward accounting for the tangible and intangible attributes of femininity. By a direct action, they cause growth and development of the vagina, uterus, and Fallopian tubes. They cause enlargement of the breasts through promotion of ductal growth, stromal development, and the accretion of fat, effects in which pituitary hormones also play a part; they also contribute in a poorly understood manner to molding the body contours, shaping the skeleton, and bringing about changes in the epiphyses of the long bones that condition the puberal spurt in growth and its culmination by fusion of the epiphyses. Growth of axillary and pubic hair and regional pigmentation of the skin of the nipples and areolae and of the genital region are also effects of estrogen.

Psychological and emotional effects, so prominently displayed in lower animals in the form of sexual behavior, estrus, or heat, are partially obscured in human beings by other influences, but presumably estrogen conditions feminine behavior in important ways.

Superimposed upon the feminizing influences of the estrogens is the cyclical component in the intensity of their action, which is responsible for many features of the normal menstrual cycle. During the follicular phase of the cycle, there is proliferation of the vaginal and uterine mucosae, increased secretion of the glands of the uterine cervix, and perhaps noticeable fullness of the breasts. Decline in estrogenic activity at the end of the cycle can bring about menstruation and its attendant phenomena. In the mature cycle with ovulation, progesterone further modifies the genital tract and mammary gland in the direction of pregnancy, and it is the cessation of secretion of progesterone that is the more forceful determinant of menstruation. However, during the first few years of menstruation and again with the approach of the menopause, estrogens dominate the cycle.

Androgens from the Ovary. A question long of interest is whether the androgens secreted by the normal ovary are physiologically important. Measurements of steroid synthesis by ovarian slices *in vitro* and fractionation of steroids contained in venous ovarian blood indicate that both testosterone and androstenedione, precursors of estrogens, are normal ovarian secretions. The daily production rates of testosterone and androstenedione in women are about 0.5 and 1.5 mg, respectively (Sommerville and Collins, 1970; Rosenfield, 1972). Furthermore, studies with rabbit ovary have demonstrated that luteinizing hormone (LH) increases ovarian incorporation of radioactive acetate into testosterone (Mills and Savard, 1972) as well as testosterone secretion (Hilliard *et al.,* 1974).

The remarkably complete sexual development that can be brought about by the administration of estrogen alone and the faithful reproduction of all the features of the menstrual cycle (except the ovarian changes) that can be achieved with estrogen and progesterone seem to leave little place for an androgen in the feminine economy. And yet there may be certain features missing when estrogen-progestin therapy replaces ovarian function. The rapid rate of growth at puberty is hard to explain in view of the limited anabolic and growth-promoting properties of estrogen. The development of axillary and pubic hair under the influence of estrogen alone may not be as complete as it is in the normal girl, and it may be lacking altogether following therapy with estrogen in hypopituitarism. When small doses of androgen are added to the estrogen, growth and distribution of hair on the body are normal even without the pituitary.

Acne, so common during puberty in girls, is closely related to the growth and secretion of the sebaceous glands. The normal development and function of these structures cannot be brought about by estrogen or progesterone, but both can be induced by the administration of small amounts of androgen (*e.g.,* 2.5 mg of methyltestosterone daily; *see* Chapter 69). Furthermore, acne can be effectively treated and the sebaceous glands caused to regress by suppressing gonadotropin secretion and ovarian function with estrogen or with a preparation of an estrogen and a progestin (Briggs *et al.,* 1970).

While estrogen alone is effective replacement therapy in the menopause, some observers believe that a more normal result is achieved when small amounts of androgen are given as well. The small quantities of testosterone and androstenedione secreted by the ovary are probably sufficient to account for the aforementioned observations without being virilizing in the usual sense of that term.

Actions on the Pituitary. The precise actions of estrogens on the secretory activity of the adenohypophysis have been very difficult to define. In the normal sexual cycle of mammals, the structural and the secretory changes in the ovary are brought about by the precisely timed and sequential secretion of gonadotropins from the hypophysis (*see* Yates *et al.,* 1971, and references therein). The improvements in technics available to measure sex steroids and gonadotropins have permitted rapid developments during recent years and have added critical confirmations of certain earlier studies.

One major difficulty has been the demonstration of a single gonadotropin-regulatory hormone (RH), LH-RH/FSH-RH, which increases the pituitary secretion of both LH and FSH (*see* Chapter 66). The varying blood levels of each gonadotropin during the menstrual cycle (Figure 68–2) suggest that another regulatory hormone might exist to explain the apparent independence of their secretion. However, complex feedback effects of sex steroids on the pituitary and hypothalamus influence the secretion and action of LH-RH/FSH-RH, and this could explain the divergent patterns of release of each gonadotropin. This question is still open (*see* Blackwell and Guillemin, 1973; Schally *et al.,* 1973).

While generalization is premature, certain interrelations seem definite. As the ovarian follicle grows under the influence of FSH, the increasing titer of estrogen that is produced decreases the release of LH-RH and thereby suppresses FSH secretion (Minaguchi and Meites, 1967). Estrogen, however, may sensitize the pituitary to the LH-releasing action of LH-RH. The rapid swelling of the follicle, culminating in ovulation, is brought about by the midcycle surge in LH (Figure 68–2), probably due to increased LH-RH release as well as to greater estrogen-induced sensitivity of the pituitary to the regulatory hormone. It is not known why just one of the many follicles that develop under the influence of FSH in primates is selected for rupture and ovulation.

Progesterone begins to be secreted during the formation of the corpus luteum, and secretion continues throughout its functional life. The control of the secretion of the corpus luteum is managed by various species in quite different ways. The mechanism in woman is poorly understood but is probably under the predominant control of LH.

In the rat and mouse, prolactin is essential for the functioning of the corpus luteum. In the rabbit, estrogen can cause the corpus luteum to function; prolactin is probably not involved, and LH may be the normal stimulus. In a number of animals, including the guinea pig and the sheep, the corpus luteum functions autonomously, but in these species the uterus exerts a luteolytic effect to bring an end to the cycle (*see* Anderson *et al.,* 1969). This may be due to prostaglandins, which can be luteolytic and which are found in relatively high concentrations in the menstrual fluid of various species.

Whenever the ovary houses a functional corpus luteum, follicular growth proceeds normally but preovulatory swelling and ovulation do not usually occur. The continued actions of progesterone and estrogen diminish the secretion of LH-RH and perhaps decrease the sensitivity of the pituitary to the releasing hormone. It has also been demonstrated in rats that implantation of LH or FSH in the median eminence or systemic administration of gonadotropins in castrated animals can decrease hypo-

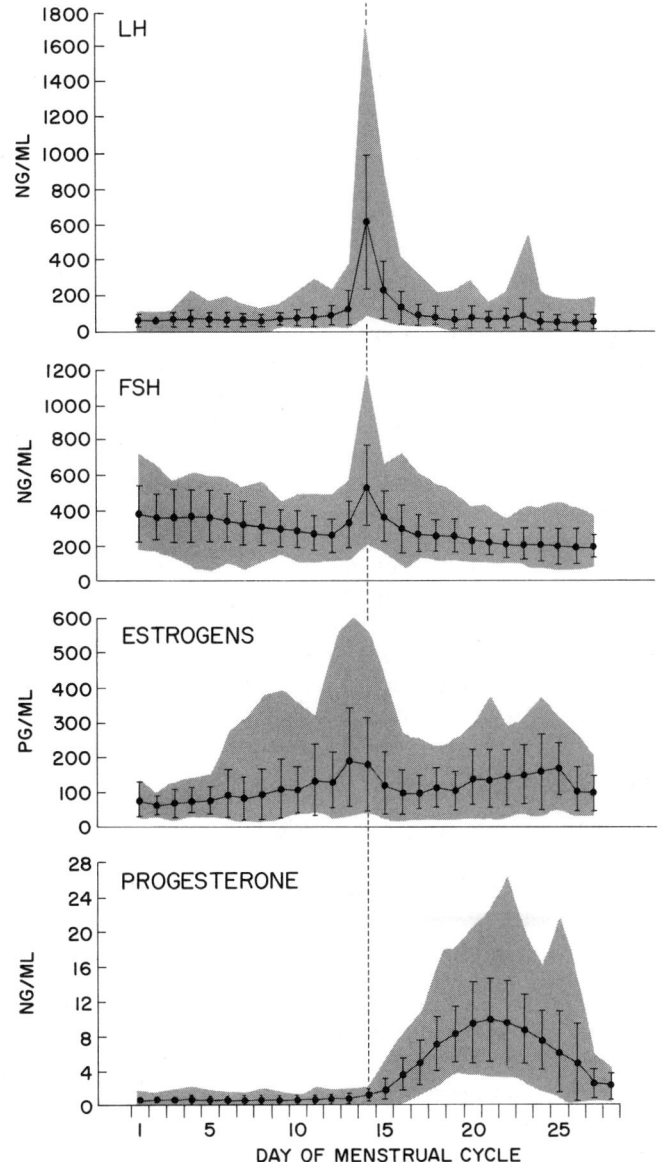

Figure 68-2. *Plasma concentrations of ovarian hormones and gonadotropins in women during normal menstrual cycles.*

Values are the mean ± standard deviation of 40 women. The shaded areas indicate the entire range of observations. Day 1 is the onset of menses. Ovulation on day 14 of the menstrual cycle occurs with the midcycle peak of LH, represented by the dash line. (After Vande Wiele and Dyrenfurth, 1973. Courtesy of *Pharmacological Reviews.* © 1973 The Williams & Wilkins Co., Baltimore.)

thalamic secretion of LH-RH (*see* Schally and Kastin, 1970). However, the physiological significance of this possible feedback mechanism in the regulation of gonadotropin secretion is unknown.

The major mystery in the pituitary secretion of gonadotropins and thus ovarian secretion of estrogens and progesterone is the relatively precise cyclic nature with which this takes place. In addition to the more prolonged and larger oscillations in gonadotropins during the menstrual cycle, smaller

short-term variations in plasma concentrations of gonadotropins have been observed in normal women (Midgley and Jaffe, 1968). The significance of the pulsatile secretion that causes these variations is not known.

In contrast, total daily secretion of gonadotropins in men is quite stable, while secretion during the course of the day is variable (Naftolin *et al.*, 1973). In the male the secretion of both FSH and LH can be inhibited by estrogen; as a result, spermatogenesis is arrested, the testicular tubules become atrophic, and the regressive changes in the genital tract show that the secretion of androgen is reduced (*see* Chapter 69).

When the ovaries or testes are removed or cease to function, there is overproduction of FSH and LH, which are excreted in the urine. Measurements of urinary or plasma gonadotropins are valuable tests in clinical medicine and can be used to show the effectiveness of replacement doses of estrogen or testosterone, which, in amounts that might be considered physiological, specifically inhibit overproduction.

Estrogens and Menstruation. When the ovaries are not functional or have been removed, menstrual flow can be induced by the administration and subsequent withdrawal of estrogen. Both the size of the dose and the duration of treatment are involved in determining whether bleeding will follow, and, within limits, the two determinants can be varied reciprocally with a similar outcome. Bleeding can be induced by a single large dose or by treatment for several weeks with a much smaller amount. When doses within a certain range are given, menstrual flow may ensue even when the treatment is not interrupted. This range lies between the dose that is too small to cause bleeding upon withdrawal and the dose that is large enough to prevent menstrual flow even when continued for a long time. By way of explanation, it is assumed that the longer a certain dose is given, the more sensitive the endometrium becomes to the breakdown that causes bleeding. In the spayed rhesus monkey, Zuckerman (1941) showed that what he termed the "threshold dose" for this kind of bleeding was about 10 μg of estrone injected in oil once daily. With continued treatment for as long as 18 months, periodic bleeding was noted at irregular intervals, averaging 6 weeks in length. It is tempting to relate this type of irregular cycle to the clinical condition called functional uterine bleeding.

The action of progesterone upon the estrogen-treated uterus in causing menstruation is quite unrelated to its action in causing the secretory changes seen microscopically. Hisaw (1942) showed that, when estrogen is given without interruption in amounts well above the threshold dose, brief treatment with progesterone is followed by menstruation a few days later; as little as 1 mg given in a single dose may be enough, whereas the histological changes in the endometrium require many days to develop.

Menstrual bleeding during continuous treatment with threshold doses of estrogen can be prevented by increasing the dose; however, when a brief treatment with progesterone is introduced, estrogen, even in large doses, will not prevent the ensuing menstruation.

Metabolic Actions. The similarity of the estrogens to the androgens in causing retention of salt and water as well as nitrogen and the elements required for the building of protoplasm is discussed in Chapter 69. Estrogens are weaker anabolic agents than the androgens. Retention of salt and water to the point of causing edema is not a common feature of therapy with estrogen. However, edema may be troublesome when estrogen is given in large doses and particularly if an associated condition predisposes to retention of fluid. Thus, the edema of heart failure or renal disease may be accentuated, and excessive fluid retention may complicate therapy with estrogen in older patients and in patients who are bedridden or malnourished. While the edema responds well to diuretics, one should discontinue the estrogen if possible.

Although estrogens have no effect on fasting plasma glucose concentration, alterations in oral and intravenous glucose tolerance tests may be seen when oral contraceptive combinations containing "high" doses of estrogens are given to some patients with preclinical diabetes mellitus or a family history of diabetes mellitus (Briggs *et al.,* 1970; Kalkhoff, 1972). The precise mechanism for the altered glucose tolerance is not known, but it may be due to increased effects of endogenous adrenocorticosteroids, altered gastrointestinal absorption of glucose, or altered plasma concentrations of insulin and growth hormone. The effects are generally reversible when the estrogen is discontinued.

Estrogen, in therapeutic doses or in larger amounts, has been noted to cause alterations in the composition of circulating lipids. These changes are discussed in Chapter 35.

Carcinogenic Action. In a few mammalian species, the administration of estrogens is followed by the development of certain tumors. In extensive investigations, Lacassagne noted the effect of estrogen on male mice of certain strains, the females of which are highly susceptible to spontaneous mammary cancer. These males, after extensive development of the mammary gland, showed epithelial proliferation, dilatation of the ducts, and, after 6 to 18 months, malignant changes. Testicular, lymphoid, and osteogenic tumors have also been induced by estrogen in various animals.

These early experiments disseminated a fear of cancer resulting from estrogen use. Until 1971, however, no evidence of a carcinogenic action of estrogens in man had been reported. Since that time there have been several clinical reports of tumors that may be related to estrogens. In the earliest studies (Greenwald *et al.*, 1971; Herbst *et al.*, 1971, 1972), an increased incidence of vaginal and cervical adenocarcinoma was noted in female offspring of mothers who had taken diethylstilbestrol or other synthetic estrogens during the first trimester of pregnancy. The incidence of this complication is currently unknown, but it is expected to be small. However, pregnant patients should not be given estrogens, particularly during the first trimester—a time when the fetal reproductive tract is developing and may be influenced by exogenous estrogens. In another study, an increased incidence of breast carcinoma was observed in patients who had taken estrogens (Black and Leis, 1972). Those at risk appeared to be nulliparous women and also those who first became pregnant at older ages. The design of this study did not permit determination of the degree of risk. When patients of various ages and parity were grouped, an increased incidence of breast tumors was not apparent, as had been reported in previous studies. In a preliminary report (Baum *et al.*, 1973), benign hepatomas were noted in some young women who had been taking combination preparations of oral contraceptives.

While estrogens have been in use for many years and an increased incidence of tumors was feared on the basis of animal experiments, the demonstrations of such a correlation have been relatively few. If estrogens can, indeed, increase the incidence of various tumors, it seems likely that the number of persons affected will be quite small. However, a long latent period might be required, and this could explain why so few definitive studies are available. If additional observations provide confirmation, the future uses of estrogens will undoubtedly be influenced.

Mechanism of Action. Considerable progress has been made in the elucidation of the mechanism of action of estrogens (*see* Jensen and DeSombre, 1972; Mueller *et al.*, 1972). Putative receptor proteins for the hormone have been detected in quantity only in estrogen-responsive tissues (female reproductive tract, breast, pituitary, and hypothalamus); only the receptor of the uterus has been studied in detail. Estrogens are first bound with very high affinity to a cytoplasmic 8 S receptor protein, which then dissociates into a 4 S form with estrogen attached. Following an additional modification, the estrogen-protein complex is converted to a 5 S species that is transported to the nucleus, where ultimate binding of the estrogen-containing complex occurs. The estrogen-receptor binding reaction is inhibited by antiestrogens such as clomiphene (*see* below). Presumably as a result of this nuclear binding, characteristic metabolic alterations ensue. Specific mRNA and certain specific but unknown proteins are apparently synthesized rapidly, perhaps because of unmasking of restricted regions of DNA. A more general increase in the synthesis of various types of RNA and protein becomes obvious a few hours later, and stimulation of DNA synthesis is an even later event. These effects of estrogens can be blocked by inhibitors of RNA synthesis (dactinomycin) or protein synthesis (cycloheximide). It is not clear whether the prominent general stimulation of RNA synthesis is a result of increased RNA polymerase activity, increased chromatin template activity, altered nuclear transport phenomena, or combinations thereof.

Absorption, Fate, and Excretion. Estrogens used in therapy are, in general, readily absorbed through the skin and mucous membranes. When they are applied for a local action, absorption is often sufficient to cause systemic effects, and in factory workers gynecomastia has followed handling of diethylstilbestrol without gloves.

The urinary excretion rate of estrogens is quite similar whether the agents are given orally or intravenously, which suggests that the absorption of most estrogens from the gastrointestinal tract is prompt and quite complete. The limited oral effectiveness of the natural estrogens and their esters is thus due to metabolic transformation during absorption from the intestine and passage through the liver. Derivatives of the natural estrogens, such as ethinyl estradiol, and the effective nonsteroid estrogens are also readily absorbed when given by mouth and owe their effectiveness to slow inactivation in the body.

The natural estrogens are soluble in water, and, when injected dissolved in oil, are rapidly absorbed and quickly metabolized. The aryl and alkyl esters of estradiol become less and less polar as the size of the substituents increases; correspondingly, the rate of absorption of oily preparations is progressively slowed and the duration of action prolonged. Therapeutic doses of estradiol benzoate are effective for several days; estradiol dipropionate is absorbed over several weeks.

The natural estrogens and their esters, in therapeutic doses, are handled in the body in much the same way as are the endogenous hormones (*see* Fotherby and James, 1972). Inactivation of estrogen in the body is carried out mainly in the liver. A certain proportion of the estrogen reaching that organ is excreted into the bile, only to be reabsorbed from the intestine and carried back again to the liver by the portal vein. During this enterohepatic circulation, degradation of estrogen occurs through conversion to less active products such as estriol and numerous other estrogens, through oxidation to nonestrogenic substances, and through conjugation with sulfuric and glucuronic acids. The natural estrogens circulate in the blood in association with proteins, including sex hormone–binding globulin, and a significant proportion of the estrogen is in the form of conjugates, particularly sulfate. These water-soluble conjugates are strong acids and are thus fully ionized in the body fluids; penetration into cells is therefore limited, and excretion by the kidney is favored because little tubular reabsorption is possible. The course of metabolism of *ethinyl estradiol* is different. Not only is this compound active by mouth but also its inactivation in the liver or other tissues is very slow. This accounts for the high intrinsic potency of the analog. The nonsteroid estrogens are slowly degraded in the body, and little is known of the mechanisms or the excretion products.

As mentioned above, endogenous estrogens appear in the urine as glucuronides and sulfates of estradiol, estrone, and estriol. Small quantities of a great many other derivatives have also been identified. In the normal menstrual cycle the mean daily excretion of estrogens at the midcycle ovulatory maximum is 25 to 100 μg; the second rise during the luteal phase is broader and more prolonged, but the maximal rates of excretion are somewhat smaller (10 to 80 μg). After the menopause the average excretion of estrogens in normal women totals about 5 to 10 μg daily. The values for normal men average 2 to 25 μg per day, quantities about equal to the urinary estrogens of women during the first week of the menstrual cycle. In young children none is detectable. During the first trimester of pregnancy the urinary estrogens derived primarily from the placenta increase and reach levels of about 30 mg per day near term. Their serial determination can be used to assess placental and fetal function.

Assays. Most biological assays for estrogen are based upon the original method of Allen and Doisy, vaginal cornification in the spayed rat or mouse, or upon growth of the uterus in these species. The vaginal response is highly specific, and it is almost by definition that a substance giving rise to a cornified vaginal smear is an estrogen. The test is influenced by other factors, however, and it is inhibited by progesterone and androgen; for this reason, tests on compounds of mixed activity may be difficult to interpret. Most tests based upon the increased weight of the uterus are less specific than the vaginal smear.

Local application of substances to the vagina of spayed animals also provides a very sensitive test for estrogen. With the natural estrogens the test is several hundred times more sensitive than tests based on subcutaneous injection, and the method is especially valuable for the assay of biological materials.

The development of competitive protein-binding and radioimmunoassay methods has accelerated investigation in this and other areas (*see* Niswender and Midgley, 1970; Vande Wiele and Dyrenfurth, 1973). Compared to various bioassay methods, these technics are generally simpler and faster. Since they also usually offer a high degree of sensitivity and specificity, such methods are rapidly becoming routine procedures in many clinical laboratories. However, the immunoassay methods are not useful for studying structure-activity relationship, and it is unlikely that bioassay and sensitive receptor-protein methods will be displaced in research laboratories.

Preparations. Several widely used, orally active nonsteroidal estrogens are available. The most popular have been preparations of *Diethylstilbestrol*, U.S.P., available in tablets containing from 0.1 to 100 mg; injectable preparations containing 5 to 25 mg/ml are also marketed. A number of chemically related compounds for oral use include *Benzestrol*, N.F. (CHEMESTROGEN), *Dienestrol*, N.F. (DIENSTROL, SYNESTROL), *hexestrol*, *methallenestril* (VALLESTRIL), and *promethestrol dipropionate* (MEPRANE).

Estradiol, N.F. (AQUADIOL, PROGYNON, and others), is available in aqueous suspension containing 0.2 to 1 mg/ml for intramuscular injection and as 25-mg pellets for subcutaneous implantation. Various esters of estradiol (benzoate, cypionate, enanthate, propionate, undecylate, and valerate) are prepared in aqueous suspension or oily solution for slow release after intramuscular injection. These preparations contain 0.5 to 40 mg/ml and are sold under various trade names (DELESTROGEN, DEPO-ESTRADIOL, OVOCYLIN, PROGYNON, and many others). *Polyestradiol phosphate* (ESTRADURIN) is also available for intramuscular use in prostatic carcinoma.

Various sulfate esters of *Estrone,* N.F., are available in tablets containing 0.75 to 5 mg (MORESTIN, OGEN, and others). These esters and estrone are also supplied under various trade names in aqueous suspension and oily solution containing 1 to 5 mg/ml for intramuscular injection.

Ethinyl Estradiol, U.S.P. (ESTINYL, FEMINONE, and others), is the most active oral preparation known, and the tablets contain 0.01 to 0.5 mg. It is roughly 25 times as potent as diethylstilbestrol. The 3-methyl ester of ethinyl estradiol, *Mestranol,* U.S.P., is nearly as active and is widely used in the combination oral contraceptives (*see* below).

Conjugated Estrogens, U.S.P. (CONESTRON, PREMARIN, and many others), contains 50 to 65% sodium estrone sulfate and 20 to 35% sodium equilin sulfate; it is available in oral (0.3 to 2.5 mg) and injectable (5 mg/ml) preparations, and as a vaginal cream containing 0.675 mg/g.

Esterified Estrogens, U.S.P. (AMNESTROGEN, EVEX, SK-ESTROGENS, ZESTĒ, and others), contains 75 to 85% sodium estrone sulfate and 6.5 to 15% equilin sodium sulfate in tablets of 0.3 to 2.5 mg. Other mixtures of estrogens available in tablet and injectable forms are also marketed under various trade names.

Chlorotrianisene, N.F. (TACE), is a long-acting oral preparation because of sequestration in adipose tissue and, therefore, is not widely used. It is available in 12-, 25-, and 72-mg capsules and has about one eighth the activity of diethylstilbestrol.

A variety of topical preparations in creams and suppositories are no longer widely used. However, *senile vaginitis* and *kraurosis vulvae* may be effectively treated with such topical preparations. Most of the "over-the-counter" cosmetics and creams that contained estrogens have been removed from the United States market in recent years. However, several are still available that do not require a prescription.

Choice of Preparations.

Since the estrogens used in therapy elicit virtually the same responses, the choice of preparation is largely determined by cost and convenience to the patient. By all odds oral therapy is the best; the action begins promptly and treatment can be terminated at will. With substances such as diethylstilbestrol or ethinyl estradiol, which are not quickly inactivated, a single dose each day is usually sufficient. Conjugated natural estrogens are less effective and if used are given in divided doses. Several doses per day may be needed when high dosage is required. Parenteral therapy has little to recommend it; frequent injections can be avoided by the use of a long-acting preparation, but then the onset and cessation of action are slow, gradual, and uncertain. Conceivably, the long-acting esters given by injection may be useful for long-continued treatment with large doses in the therapy of cancer. The esters are unsuitable in the management of menstrual disorders or as replacement therapy in the menopause when cyclic therapy is desirable; the action slowly declines in a way that is quite unlike the prompt cessation of secretion characteristic of the normal menstrual cycle.

Untoward Responses. The most frequent unpleasant symptom attending the use of estrogen is *nausea*. With large doses there may also be anorexia and even vomiting and mild diarrhea. The nausea is of a peculiar type that seldom interferes with eating and does not cause a loss of weight; it may be noted at various times of the day but, like the "morning sickness" of early pregnancy, it is often troublesome at breakfast time. With continued treatment the symptom usually disappears, and only rarely is it so distressful that treatment must be stopped. Even when very large doses are given, as in the treatment of cancer of the breast, nausea is generally troublesome only for the first 1 or 2 weeks. The symptom can usually be avoided by starting with a small dose and gradually increasing it. One views with skepticism statements that certain preparations are less apt to cause nausea than others. It is likely that the symptom is a part of the estrogenic response and that a lower incidence of nausea implies lower estrogenic potency. Nausea is not avoided by giving estrogens parenterally. Other untoward responses are discussed below, under oral contraceptives.

Therapeutic Uses. *Oral Contraception.* A major use of estrogens is in combination with progestins as oral contraceptives; such use is discussed in a separate section later in this chapter.

Menopause. At a variable age, but usually in the mid or late 40s, the functions of the ovaries decline. Ovulation is lost first, and anovulatory cycles may continue for 1 or 2 years before menstruation ceases altogether. Irregular menstrual cycles are particularly prevalent at this time due to poorly cycling estrogen unaccompanied by sufficient progesterone. Lack of appreciation of the endocrine basis of the menstrual disturbance usually leads to the conclusion that some mechanical factor, such as fibroid tumors, is at fault. Cyclic therapy with a progestin regulates the cycle as the decline in ovarian function progresses to the stage of amenorrhea.

The decline in the secretion of estrogen by the ovary is a slow and gradual process that continues for some years after menstruation has ceased. It is a frequent observation that menopausal symptoms are more severe following oophorectomy than with the natural menopause. Sometimes hot flashes appear for the first time or become more intense if the ovaries are removed after the menopause.

Frequently the decline in ovarian function at the menopause is associated with symptoms that are clearly due to deficiency of estrogen. The characteristic hot flashes may alternate with chilly sensations, inappropriate sweating, and paresthesias, including formication. A variety of other symptoms often occur during the menopause and include muscle cramps, myalgias, arthralgias, anxiety, overbreathing, palpitation, dizziness, faintness, and syncope. These symptoms may or may not be associated with estrogen deficiency. A few women become chronic invalids and experience years of ill health; some feel genuinely miserable and lack vigor and initiative; many, obviously, tolerate the event quite well. About 15 to 25% of menopausal women will seek medical attention and treatment.

Treatment with estrogen is specific and effective. Replacement therapy clearly relieves the hot flashes and other vasomotor symptoms and atrophic vaginitis. The dose needed varies somewhat but can easily be determined by trial. The dose of diethylstilbestrol is about 0.2 to 1 mg once daily by mouth; 0.5 mg is seldom sufficient to cause withdrawal bleeding, 1 mg daily for several weeks sometimes causes bleeding when stopped, and 2 mg often does. Comparable doses of ethinyl estradiol are 0.01 to 0.05 mg; conjugated estrogens may be used in doses of 0.6 to 5 mg daily. Therapy with estrogen is best given in a cyclic manner, 3 or 4 weeks of treatment followed by 1 week without treatment. If withdrawal bleeding is going to occur, it will begin toward the end of the week of no treatment and the estrogen can be resumed before this induced menstrual period ceases. Menopausal symptoms usually do not return in full intensity during the week without treatment. A less popular alternative procedure is to give an effective dose of estrogen without interruption and to evoke a menstrual period every 4 to 6 weeks with a progestin. Occasionally during cyclic therapy with estrogen alone uterine bleeding may continue in an irregular manner after estrogen is resumed. Larger doses of estrogen have been employed to control this bleeding, but the use of a progestin is more uniformly effective. Once a progesterone-withdrawal period has been induced, there may be no further trouble from the use of estrogen alone for many months.

Some students of the menopause have concluded that the use of a small dose of androgen along with estrogen has a decidedly favorable effect. However, many physicians prefer not to administer any androgen. Androgen enhances strength and imparts a sense of well-being. Withdrawal bleeding from estrogen is said to be reduced when androgen is given concurrently. Large doses of androgen in women may increase libido, but in the small doses used in the menopause the effect is seen only in some cases. Excessive dosage leads to undesirable masculinizing effects, but the usual dose of 5 or 10 mg of methyltestosterone daily, interrupted when the estrogen is stopped, does not usually cause detectable virilization. Some observers believe that the estrogen counteracts the masculinizing influence.

Senile or *atrophic vaginitis,* often associated with chronic infection of the atrophic structures, responds well to estrogen. *Kraurosis vulvae,* a distressingly itchy condition due in part to deficiency in estrogen and in part to scratching and other as-yet-unknown factors, is favorably influenced by estrogen supplemented by local treatment, including the application of adrenocorticosteroids.

Some physicians are disinclined to prescribe estrogens in the menopause; they feel that the symptoms are largely emotional in origin and are better managed by reassurance and psychotherapy and with the use of small doses of a sedative. Others prescribe estrogens for periods of months or a few years only. Physicians with these views are undoubtedly concerned about the possible minor and serious side effects of estrogens in light of very little strong evidence to demonstrate their efficacy in preventing the more serious physical disorders accompanying menopause, such as atherosclerosis and osteoporosis. However, indefinite systemic replacement in all menopausal patients, advocated by some, is certainly controversial and may introduce more undesirable effects than the symptomatic improvement warrants (*see* Medical Letter, 1973).

Pregnancy. In the past, large doses of estrogens have been given during pregnancy in attempts to prevent threatened or habitual abortion or because of abnormalities of urinary estrogen excretion in toxemia of pregnancy. There is no evidence that such uses are of any value. Because of this and the possibility of vaginal carcinoma in female offspring (*see* above), the use of estrogens in pregnancy is not recommended. The use of progestins in this condition is discussed subsequently.

Dysmenorrhea. Sturgis and Albright (1940) reported the relief of dysmenorrhea by inhibiting ovulation with estrogen. They injected 1.7 mg of estradiol benzoate intramuscularly every 3 days for six doses, starting within the first week after the onset of menses, and found that the next episode of bleeding was painless. If the estrogen was started later in the cycle, ovulation was not inhibited and the subsequent period was painful. Estrogen treatment proved worthwhile and has since been widely used. Oral dosage can be taken, for example, in the form of diethylstilbestrol in a daily dose of about 2 mg, starting 5 days after the onset of a menstrual period and continuing for 15 to 20 days. Indeed, treatment can be continued for several weeks longer, if desired, so that the artificial periods are less frequent. Also, it has been found that oral therapy in full doses can often be used successfully month after month if too long an interval is not permitted to elapse between courses. The additional use of an orally active progesterone-like steroid facilitates management, as it does when the method is used as a contraceptive measure, and combined oral contraceptive agents are now preferred (*see* below).

The use of estrogens in the treatment of *endometriosis* is discussed in connection with the therapeutic uses of the progestins.

Functional Uterine Bleeding. This disorder usually results from anovulatory cycles with continuous secretion of estrogen unopposed by progesterone. While estrogens can be used with some therapeutic success, progestins are logically preferred (*see* below).

Failure of Ovarian Development. There are several unusual conditions wherein the ovaries do not develop and, in consequence, puberty does not occur. In *ovarian dysgenesis* with dwarfism (Turner's syndrome) diagnosis can often be made before the age of puberty by the associated congenital anomalies and the stature. Therapy with estrogen at the appropriate time brings about a perfect replica of the events of puberty, except for the spurt in growth and, of course, the changes in the ovary. The genital structures grow to normal size. The breasts develop, there is growth of axillary and pubic hair, and the body assumes the normal feminine contour. Also, androgens have been used successfully to promote growth (*see* Chapter 69). It is common practice to start with small doses of estrogen, such as 0.5 mg of diethylstilbestrol or 0.02 mg of ethinyl estradiol, and then increase the dose slowly over a year or so before initiating menstrual periods by cyclic treatment with larger doses. It is felt that there may be some merit in thus imitating the normal sequence of events at puberty.

Failure of ovarian development is also a part of the picture of *hypopituitarism* in childhood. Deficiency of the thyroid and the adrenal cortex is easily corrected with replacement therapy, and the failure of sexual development is treated with estrogen as outlined just above. If human growth hormone is used, these girls can achieve a normal adult stature (*see* Chapter 66). Treatment with estrogen at the normal age of puberty can be expected to cause a small acceleration of growth, but the addition of small doses of androgen has a greater growth-promoting effect, as noted in Chapter 69.

Acne. The common form of acne is a feature of puberty in both sexes, and androgen seems to be the essential factor, operating through stimulation of sebaceous glands (Strauss and Pochi, 1968). Treatment with estrogen is effective in both sexes by suppressing gonadotropins and gonadal androgen secretion, but its usefulness in the male is limited by gynecomastia, suppression of the testis, uncertain effects on skeletal growth, and danger of hastening epiphyseal closure. In young women estrogen is effective therapy in doses designed to suppress the ovary and may be continued with benefit for many months in cyclic fashion. One of the oral contraceptive agents of either the combined or the sequential type is more convenient. It may be given in the same manner as when used to prevent ovulation, and the preparations with larger amounts of estrogen are used. However, tretinoin (all *trans*-retinoic acid) and antibiotics (tetracyclines or erythromycin) are preferred (*see* Chapters 75 and 59).

Hirsutism. In most instances, excessive growth of body hair in women cannot be traced to an endocrine cause, but occasionally a mild androgenic influence of ovarian or adrenal origin is suspected. When suppression of the adrenal cortex by giving a corticosteroid is ineffectual, suppression of the ovary with an estrogen may be worthwhile. If it is to be tried, suppression of the ovary for about a year with continuous therapy may be needed before it can be ascertained whether the maneuver is successful. Doses of about 2 mg daily of diethylstilbestrol or its equivalent are sufficient. Menstrual periods during this time can be evoked at intervals by cyclic use of an oral progestin.

Prevention of Heart Attacks. In view of the favored position of women in the incidence of fatal myocardial infarction, estrogen therapy has been tried as a prophylactic measure in men. A large-scale randomized and double-blind study has been conducted by the Coronary Drug Project Research Group. This study included 8341 male patients aged 30 to 64 years with a previous history of myocardial infarction. The administration of 5 mg of conjugated estrogens daily to a group of these patients led to an increased incidence of nonfatal cardiovascular complications, and this portion of the project was discontinued (Coronary Drug Project Research Group, 1970). Some patients were given 2.5 mg of conjugated estrogens daily for 4 to 5 years, and their mortality rate was no different from that of the placebo group (Coronary Drug Project Research Group, 1973). However, patients in the low-dose group had about a twofold increase in incidence of thromboembolism and about a threefold increase in mortality from cancer, particularly lung cancer. While apparently significant, the number of lung tumors observed was very small.

Osteoporosis. Osteoporosis is a disorder of the skeleton associated with the loss of both hydroxyapatite (calcium phosphate complexes) and protein matrix (colloid). The result is thinning and weakening of the bones and an increased incidence of fractures, particularly compression fractures of the vertebrae. In older patients it is called *senile osteoporosis* and affects both sexes. Coming after menopause it is referred to as *postmenopausal osteoporosis.* Many different methods of treatment have been tried with the aim of increasing bone density and substance, and there is no general agreement that any provides a marked, sustained effect. It has been logical to think that estrogen replacement in postmenopausal patients would be effective. However, postmenopausal patients with osteoporosis have plasma levels of estrogens, testosterone, and gonadotropins that are not significantly different from values in postmenopausal patients without the disorder (Riggs *et al.,* 1973). Nevertheless, several groups (Lafferty *et al.,* 1964; Riggs *et al.,* 1969) have demonstrated that, after several months of estrogen replacement in postmenopausal patients, calcium balance becomes positive and plasma alkaline phosphatase activity and bone resorption decrease to normal. Bone formation is normal before treatment and remains unchanged. The benefits of estrogen replacement, however, last only 9 to 14 months in spite of continued estrogen treatment (Lafferty *et al.,* 1964). Essentially similar conclusions were reached by Riggs and associates (1972), but in their study the use of estrogens for 26 to 42 months led to decreased bone formation that overcame the benefit of decreased resorption. It is not known whether periodic long courses of estrogen therapy would continue to be effective if interrupted by periods of withdrawal. Androgens have effects similar to those of estrogen.

Neoplastic Diseases. Many carcinomas of the breast and prostate are apparently dependent upon the proper hormonal environment for their growth. Estrogens have been used with some success to alter this environment and to decrease the growth of such neoplasms. Their use in these disorders is discussed in Chapter 62.

Suppression of Post-Partum Lactation. Estrogens, progestins, and androgens are used to decrease milk production in the post-partum period. The use of these agents is discussed below and in Chapter 69.

ANTIESTROGENS

The term *antiestrogen* has been rather broadly applied to several different types of compounds that inhibit or modify the action of estrogen. Progestins and androgens have been described as antiestrogenic; some weak estrogens are antiestrogenic by some criteria, and certain compounds are antiestrogenic when applied locally to the responsive tissue. The most striking antiestrogens are the derivatives of chlorotrianisene—*ethamoxytriphetol* and *clomiphene.*

In a physiological sense it is misleading to refer to the action of progesterone as antiestrogenic. Normally progesterone acts upon estrogen-stimulated tissue; indeed, its full effects are displayed only when estrogen is acting at the same time. For example, estrogen characteristically evokes a cornified vaginal smear; when progesterone is given too, the vaginal mucosa is changed to the form typical of pregnancy and cornification disappears. In this instance the two hormones must act together to bring about the pregnancy-like response, and in this sense neither one is the inhibitor of the other. Nonetheless, in the characterization of compounds with mixed activities, tests for their "antiestrogenic" effect may have practical utility.

Certain estrogens are limited in their action in the sense that increasing doses bring about diminishing increments of response. Estriol, in various tests based upon the change in size of the uterus, has this characteristic and, when estriol is given with estradiol, the response to the latter is lessened (Hisaw *et al.,* 1954). Estriol and other compounds of this type have been referred to as *impeded estrogens* and appear to behave as partial agonists. Quite a large number of compounds prove to be antiestrogenic when they are applied directly to the responsive tissue, such as the vaginal mucosa of the mouse, and estrogen is given systemically at the same time. *Dimethylstilbestrol* is a potent antiestrogen of this type, and it is interesting that it is a better inhibitor of estradiol than of diethylstilbestrol (Emmens *et al.,* 1962).

Highly effective inhibitors of estrogen came from an unexpected direction. The weakly estrogenic compound *chlorotrianisene* (Table 68–1), unlike most estrogens, was noted not to cause enlargement of the pituitary when given to rats in large doses.

Table 68–1. STRUCTURAL SIMILARITY OF TWO ANTIESTROGENS TO CHLOROTRIANISENE

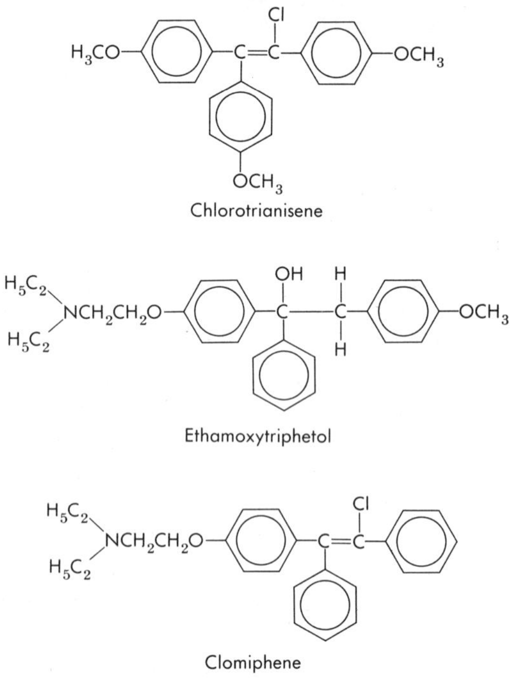

Chlorotrianisene

Ethamoxytriphetol

Clomiphene

Estradiol normally causes pronounced enlargement of the pituitary, but when chlorotrianisene was given concurrently the effect was greatly reduced (Segal and Thompson, 1956). The related, nonestrogenic compound *ethamoxytriphetol* (Table 68–1) was found to be strikingly antiestrogenic. It inhibited endogenous estrogen as well as estrogen given in the form of the natural compounds, diethylstilbestrol, or chlorotrianisene. The inhibition was seen in a variety of effects as well as in several species (Lerner *et al.,* 1958). It did not inhibit estrogen-induced mammary growth or prevent the suppressive effect of estrogen upon the gonadotropic function of the pituitary. Limited studies in man also showed antiestrogenic properties, but more extensive human studies have been carried out with the related compound *clomiphene.*

Clomiphene. Initial animal tests with clomiphene showed very slight estrogenic activity and moderate antiestrogenic activity. The striking effect was inhibition of the pituitary's gonadotropic function. Small doses stopped the estrous cycle of normal rats and reduced the size of the ovary. Somewhat larger doses inhibited spermatogenesis, also by inhibiting the secretion of gonadotropin. Thus, in both sexes the compound was a potent contraceptive. When given to human beings, however, the most prominent effect was impressive enlargement of the ovaries. Properly applied, the compound has proven to be a most remarkable and useful agent for the treatment of infertility. Greenblatt and coworkers (1962) made extensive and careful studies and found that ovulation could be induced in a high proportion of patients with amenorrhea, the Stein-Leventhal syndrome, and functional uterine bleeding with anovulatory cycles. Pregnancy followed in a significant number of cases when infertility had been the problem. Excessive enlargement of the ovaries and the formation of ovarian cysts were common features of the treatment when doses of 100 to 200 mg daily were given for 2 or 3 weeks, but with doses of 50 or 75 mg daily this complication was less frequent and the ovaries returned to normal size after treatment had been completed. The substance gave evidence of antiestrogenic effects. Hot flashes were experienced by some patients, vaginal cornification in precocious puberty in young girls was inhibited, and in one case suppression of ovulation with ethinyl estradiol was prevented by clomiphene. There was no clinical evidence of progestational or androgenic effects.

From these and other earlier studies it was inferred that clomiphene increased pituitary secretion of gonadotropins. Assays of human plasma and urine for FSH and LH have proven this to be the case. Clomiphene prevents the binding of tritiated estradiol in the hypothalamus and anterior pituitary of rats (Kato *et al.,* 1968), and it is presumed to interact with the estrogen "receptor sites" to prevent the normal feedback inhibition of estrogens on the secretion of LH-RH/FSH-RH and gonadotropins. The formation of large and cystic ovaries can be the result of increased gonadotropin concentrations, leading to ovarian stimulation, ovulation, and sustained function of corpora lutea.

Due to the ethylene moiety in the molecule, clomiphene is a mixture of two isomers. The *cis-* form possesses the antiestrogenic activity, while the *trans-* form is estrogenic. Therefore, the mixture possesses less than one half of either activity. The different effects of the isomers undoubtedly added confusion to the interpretation of earlier studies.

Therapeutic Uses. Clomiphene Citrate, U.S.P. (CLOMID), has been used clinically for the treatment of infertility in women in doses varying between 25 and 200 mg daily by mouth, for periods of a few days to a few weeks. It is available in 50-mg tablets. In view of the development of enlarged ovaries with higher doses, a dose of 50 mg daily for 5 days has been recommended. This is started on the fifth day of the menstrual cycle except in patients who have not menstruated recently. In infertility and menstrual disorders, treatment has been repeated at monthly intervals with success (Macgregor *et al.,* 1968). Ovulation is achieved in about 70% and pregnancy in 30% of properly selected patients. The use of clomiphene and gonadotropins in infertility is also discussed in Chapter 66. As with gonadotropins, hyperstimulation of the ovaries with the formation of multiple cysts and a high incidence of multiple births (8%) is seen. The use of clomiphene has not altered the expected incidence of abortions or fetal abnormalities, and infants of mothers treated with clomiphene have developed normally. In addition to the undesirable effects already noted, there have been instances of gastric upset, skin rashes, and visual disturbances. The latter are reversible after withdrawal of the drug.

PROGESTINS

For some years after Corner and Allen had isolated progesterone from the corpora lutea of sows, the small amounts of the hormone available, at first from natural sources and later from synthesis, hampered experimental work and therapeutic application. The hormone had to be given by injection, and the duration of action was brief. With the introduction during the 1950s of new classes of progestational agents with prolonged activity and enhanced oral effectiveness, the structures associated with activity were found to be quite diverse. The number of progestins has proliferated abundantly, and some have had wide clinical use as contraceptive agents.

Chemistry. Some of the progestins have inherent estrogenic or androgenic effects, some show dissociations of effectiveness in various tests, and some have properties that resemble progesterone very closely. The compounds of greatest interest in therapeutics are those that are effective when given by mouth. Some representative progestins are shown in Table 68–2.

The first progestin that was reasonably effective orally was 17α-ethinyltestosterone (*ethisterone*). Derivatives of testosterone lacking the angular methyl group (C 19) attached to C 10, the 19-nortestosterones, were much more effective orally. The parent compound, 19-nortestosterone, is inactive, but a number of 17α-alkyl derivatives are effective. The 17α-methyl derivative is progestational and androgenic. 17α-Ethyl-19-nortestosterone (*norethandrolone*) is also progestational and androgenic and is used clinically as an anabolic agent. Its structural formula is given in Table 69–4 (page 1463). 17α-Ethinyl-19-nortestosterone, or *norethindrone* (*norethisterone*), is a potent oral progestin in man and is only mildly androgenic. Shift of the double bond in norethindrone gives the isomer *norethynodrel*, one of the first compounds to be widely used as a contraceptive. Reduction of the 3-keto group of norethindrone yields a partially reduced derivative of ethinyl estradiol termed *ethynodiol*, the diacetate of which is a particularly potent progestational agent in man. Removal of the oxygen function at position 3 gives rise to an interesting series of compounds, the *estrenols*, the biological activity of which is critically dependent upon the substituent grouping on C 17. Thus, *ethinylestrenol* is a powerful progestational agent free of androgenic and anabolic effects, *allylestrenol* has progestational and other actions, and *ethylestrenol* (Table 69–4, page 1462) is used as an anabolic agent. The 13-ethyl analog of norethindrone, or 18-homonorethisterone (*norgestrel*), was found to be 100 times as progestational as norethindrone in the Clauberg test.

Another series of orally active progestins is typified by the compound *chlormadinone acetate,* which is 6α-chloro-Δ⁶-17α-acetoxy progesterone, a purely progestational agent of high potency (Brennan and Kraay, 1963) previously used in contraceptive formulations. The 6-methyl analog has similar properties and is referred to as *megestrol.*

Additional progestational compounds took origin from a different line of investigation. 17α-Hydroxyprogesterone, first isolated from the adrenal glands in 1940, was virtually inert. On the other hand, the acetic acid ester had appreciable activity and could be taken by mouth, although very large doses were required (Davis and Wied, 1957). When the compound was given by injection in oil, activity was prolonged, a property shared by other esters such as the *valerate* and *caproate*. The caproate has been used extensively as a long-acting progestin, but it is virtually inactive by mouth. Other derivatives of 17α-hydroxyprogesterone were found to be effective orally, and the one most widely studied is the 6-methyl analog, *medroxyprogesterone acetate*. The 16α,17α-dihydroxy derivative of progesterone in the form of the *acetophenone* is moderately active by mouth but has the property of extremely long action when given parenterally (Lerner *et al.*, 1964).

Perhaps the most potent progestin yet encountered is *cyproterone acetate*. It has had only limited use as a progestin, perhaps because of a greater interest in its use as an antiandrogen (Chapter 69).

Synthesis and Secretion. Progesterone is secreted by the ovary mainly from the corpus luteum during the second half of the menstrual cycle. Secretion actually begins just before ovulation from the follicle that is destined to release an ovum. The formation of progesterone from steroid precursors is summarized in Figure 68–1 and occurs in the ovary, testis, adrenal cortex, and placenta. The stimulatory effect of LH on progesterone synthesis and secretion by the corpus luteum is mediated by an increased synthesis of cyclic AMP (Marsh *et al.*, 1966).

If the ovum is fertilized, implantation takes place about 7 days later in the human being and almost at once the developing trophoblast secretes its luteotropic hormone, chorionic gonadotropin, into the maternal circulation, and the functional life of the corpus luteum is sustained. Chorionic gonadotropin, detectable in urine several days before the expected time of the next menstrual period, is excreted in progressively increasing amounts for the next 5 weeks or so, and in much reduced quantities thereafter throughout pregnancy. During the second or third month of pregnancy the developing placenta begins to secrete estrogen and progesterone, and thereafter the corpus luteum

Table 68-2. STRUCTURAL RELATIONSHIP OF VARIOUS PROGESTINS TO PROGESTERONE

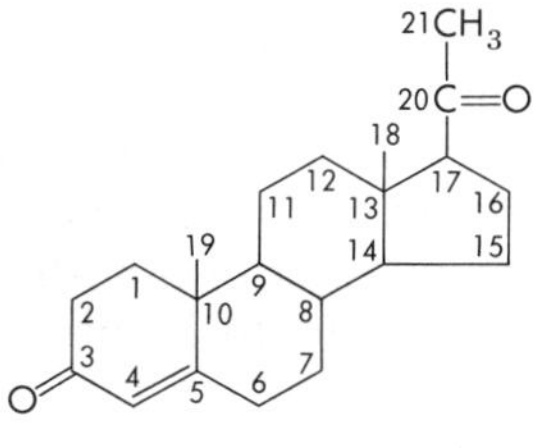

21CH₃
20 C=O
18
12 17 16
11 13
19 14 15
1 9 8
2 10
3 7
4 5 6
O

Progesterone

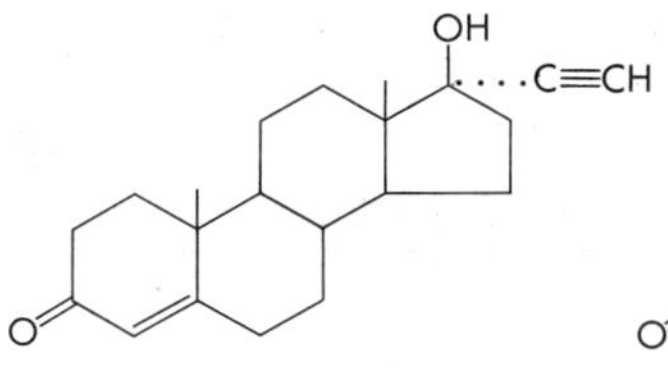

OH
····C≡CH
O

Ethisterone

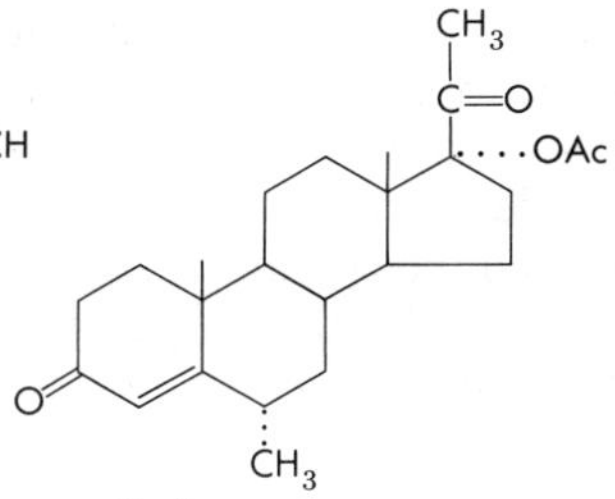

CH₃
C=O
····OAc
O
ĊH₃

Medroxyprogesterone Acetate

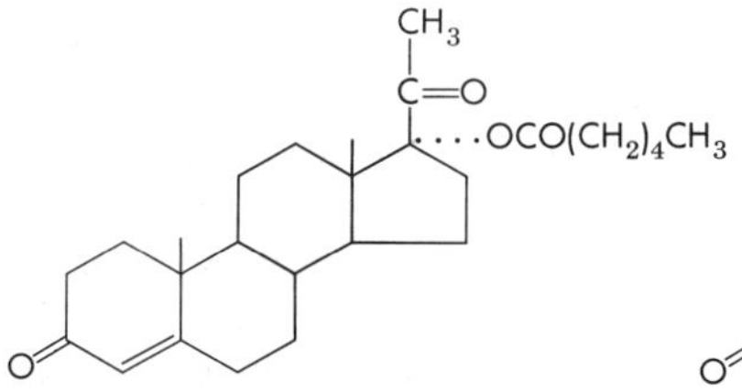

CH₃
C=O
····OCO(CH₂)₄CH₃
O

Hydroxyprogesterone Caproate

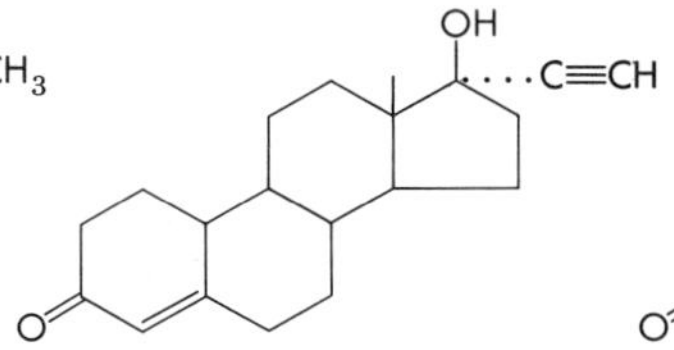

OH
····C≡CH
O

Norethindrone

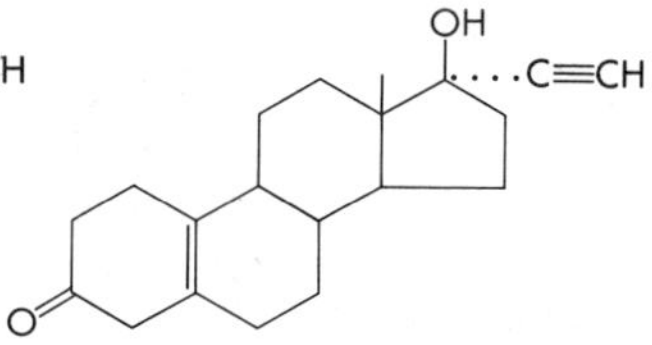

OH
····C≡CH
O

Norethynodrel

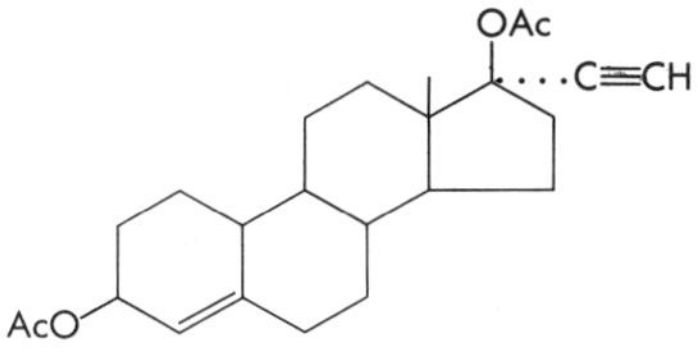

OAc
····C≡CH
AcO

Ethynodiol Diacetate

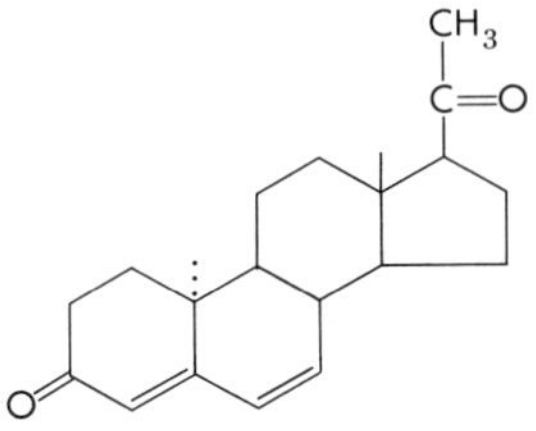

CH₃
C=O
O

Dydrogesterone

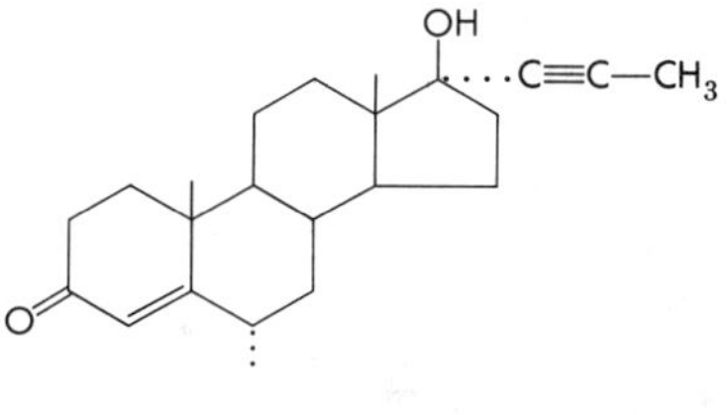

OH
····C≡C—CH₃
O

Dimethisterone

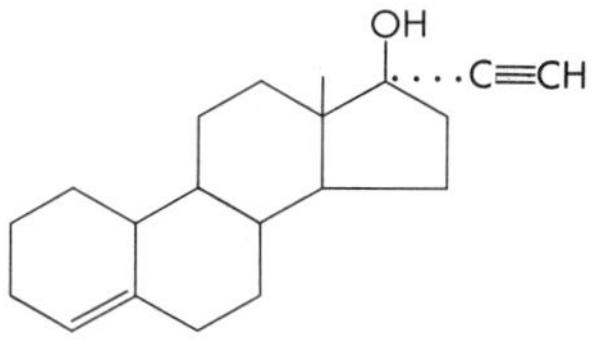

OH
····C≡CH
O

Ethinylestrenol

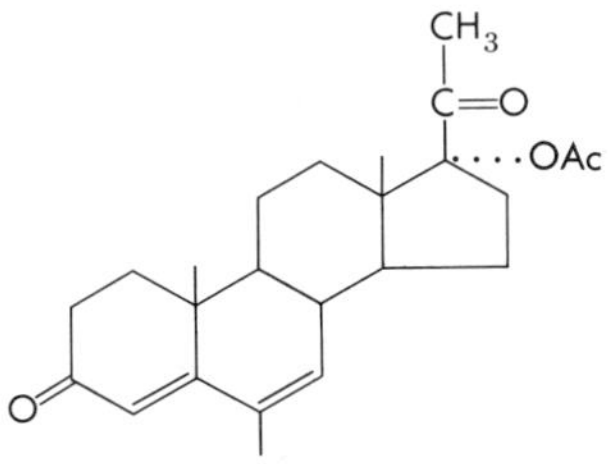

CH₃
C=O
····OAc
O

Megestrol Acetate

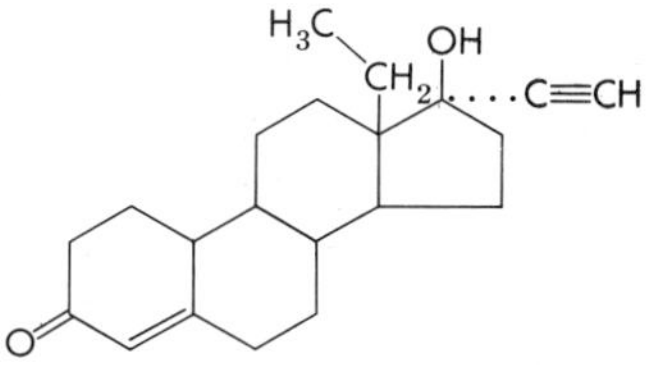

H₃C OH
CH₂ ····C≡CH
O

Norgestrel

is not essential to continued gestation. Estrogen and progesterone continue to be secreted in large amounts by the placenta up to the time of delivery.

Measurements of the rate of secretion of progesterone suggest that, from a few milligrams a day secreted during the follicular phase of the cycle, the rate increases to 10 to 20 mg during the luteal phase and to several hundred milligrams during the latter part of pregnancy (Vande Wiele *et al.,* 1960). Rates of from 1 to 5 mg per day have been measured in men, and are comparable to the values in women during the follicular phase of the cycle.

Physiological and Pharmacological Actions. Progesterone released during the luteal phase of the cycle leads to the development of a secretory endometrium. Abrupt decline in the release of progesterone from the corpus luteum at the end of the cycle is the main determinant of the onset of menstruation. If the duration of the luteal phase is artificially lengthened, either by sustaining luteal function or by treatment with progesterone, decidual changes in the endometrial stroma similar to those seen in early pregnancy can be induced. Estrogen, which under normal circumstances antecedes and accompanies progesterone in its action upon the endometrium, is essential to the development of the normal pattern. When the orally active progestins were first tested and given from day 5 of the cycle for 20 days, the endometrial stroma showed intense luteal action while the glands, stimulated at first, actually became atrophic. It turned out that these patterns were caused by progestins, with little or no intrinsic estrogenic activity; if estrogen was given as well, the response closely resembled the normal.

The endocervical glands are also influenced by progesterone, and the abundant watery secretion of the estrogen-stimulated structures is changed to a scant viscid material. When the estrogen-stimulated secretion dries on a glass slide, sodium chloride crystallizes to form a dendritic pattern called "ferning." Progestins inhibit this pattern.

The estrogen-induced maturation of the human vaginal epithelium is modified toward the condition of pregnancy by the action of progesterone, a change that can be detected in cytological alterations in the vaginal smear. If the quantity of estrogen concurrently acting is known to be adequate, or if it is assured by giving estrogen, the cytological response to a progestin can be used to evaluate its progestational potency.

Mammary Gland. During pregnancy and to a minor degree during the luteal phase of the cycle, progesterone, acting with estrogen, brings about a proliferation of the acini of the mammary gland. Toward the end of pregnancy the acini fill with secretion and the vasculature of the gland is notably increased; however, only after the influences of estrogen and progesterone are withdrawn by the event of parturition does lactation begin. The action of estrogen or estrogen and progesterone, when used post partum for relieving the sensation of engorgement, is probably largely a direct one upon the mammary tissue to inhibit secretion.

Thermogenic Action. If the body temperature is measured each day throughout the normal menstrual cycle, preferably at the same time each morning, an increase of about 1° F may be noted at midcycle, and this correlates with the event of ovulation. The temperature rise persists for the remainder of the cycle until the onset of menstrual flow. The phenomenon is caused by progesterone, as can be shown by giving the hormone to nonovulating women or to men. The minimal detectably effective dose of progesterone is about 5 mg once daily, and a dose of 10 or 20 mg daily is fully effective. These doses also span the range of effectiveness on the changes in the endometrium, cervix, and vagina, as discussed above. The relative effectiveness of other progestins has been evaluated in this way, a single dose usually being sufficient to elicit the response. Thus, 17α-acetoxyprogesterone requires an oral dose of 100 to 125 mg daily, and the slowly absorbed esters of 17α-hydroxyprogesterone are effective upon injection of about 250 mg; certain other progestational compounds, such as ethisterone and dydrogesterone, are not thermogenic.

Mechanism of Action. Progesterone-binding activity is detectable in appropriate target tissues, and the amount of receptor is definitely increased following pretreatment of animals with estrogen (*see* Jensen and DeSombre, 1972; O'Malley and Means, 1974). Following binding to a cytoplasmic receptor protein, the steroid is transported to the nucleus, and the complex is bound there in reactions analogous to those described above for estrogens. However, there is no apparent need for receptor alteration, as with the estrogen receptor. Chromatin template activity is increased, and new species of RNA are synthesized. In the chick oviduct, the synthesis of a specific protein (avidin) is markedly increased, and this is inhibited by dactinomycin and cycloheximide.

Absorption, Fate, and Excretion. Progesterone injected in oily solution is readily absorbed and at a rate that is too rapid for optimal therapeutic efficiency. In animal tests several doses per day are more effective than the same dose once daily, and less frequent dosage is quite inefficient. Inactivation takes place largely in the liver. Many pregnane derivatives and isomers conjugated with glucuronide or sulfate are found in the urine. While most of the metabolites of progesterone are unidentified, one of the major urinary products is the glucuronide of pregnane-3α,20α-diol. The rate of turnover of endogenous progesterone is unusually rapid, the half-life in blood being a few minutes, and doubtless exogenous material is handled in the same way. A small amount of progesterone is stored in body fat, but this is generally regarded as quantitatively unimportant. Although it is quickly disposed of, progesterone given at daily intervals in sufficient dose is thoroughly effective, and one is forced to conclude that its actions upon tissue must continue after it has disappeared from the plasma. When progesterone is given by mouth, it is much less effective, but a similar proportion is eliminated in the urine as pregnanediol. Presumably, absorption from the intestinal tract is prompt, but the compound is rapidly transformed during passage through the liver and possibly also during absorption through the intestinal mucosa.

About 50 to 60% of administered radioactive progesterone appears in the urine and about 10% in feces. Pregnanediol in urine accounts for 12 to 15% of the progesterone metabolized. When progesterone is given for a prolonged period, during the luteal phase of the cycle, or during pregnancy, a larger proportion (25 to 30%) appears in the urine as pregnanediol (see Fotherby and James, 1972). Pregnanediol is a notably specific product, and measurements of urinary pregnanediol provide a valuable index of the secretion and metabolism of progesterone. Approximately 1 mg per day is excreted during the follicular phase of the cycle, after the menopause, and by men. During the luteal phase of the cycle 2- to 4-mg amounts are excreted daily, and during pregnancy the values increase to 50 to 70 mg before term.

Assays. Many of the new steroids are not purely estrogenic, progestational, androgenic, or anabolic but show several types of activity. No one bioassay for progesterone-like action adequately characterizes a compound, and each is modified in one way or another by the estrogenic and androgenic potencies of the material being tested; some bioassays are influenced differently from others. A great deal has been learned about the characteristics and limitations of these tests, but none yields an unequivocal estimate of progestational potency of new compounds. The various bioassay methods available are based on changes in the microscopic appearance or carbonic anhydrase activity of the endometrium of animals. Other methods are based upon the maintenance of pregnancy in oophorectomized animals or inhibition of ovulation. The reader is referred to the *fourth edition* of this textbook for a more complete description of bioassay methods used and for references.

Various chemical assays for progesterone and pregnanediol are also available. As discussed earlier for estrogens, protein-binding assays and immunoassays are also available, specific, and sensitive (see Niswender and Midgley, 1970; Vande Wiele and Dyrenfurth, 1973).

Preparations. Until recent years the only preparations available were progesterone itself and ethisterone. Currently, many orally active substances and combinations of them with estrogen are in wide use (Table 68–2).

Progesterone Injection, U.S.P. (GESTEROL, LIPO-LUTIN, PROLUTON), contains 50 mg of progesterone per milliliter of vegetable oil. Progesterone is peculiar among the commonly used steroids in being locally irritating, and not more than about 50 mg can be given intramuscularly in a single injection; *Sterile Progesterone Suspension,* U.S.P. (GESTEROL AQUE-OUS), is particularly painful and is seldom used.

Medroxyprogesterone Acetate, U.S.P. (DEPO-PROVERA), contains 50, 100, or 400 mg/ml in aqueous medium for intramuscular injection, and *Medroxyprogesterone Acetate Tablets,* U.S.P. (PROVERA), contain 2.5 or 10 mg each.

Hydroxyprogesterone Caproate Injection, U.S.P. (DELALUTIN), is provided as an oily solution of 125 mg/ml (in sesame oil) or 250 mg/ml (in castor oil) for intramuscular injection.

Megestrol acetate (MEGACE) is available in 20-mg tablets.

Dydrogesterone, N.F. (DUPHASTON, GYNOREST), is marketed as 5- and 10-mg tablets.

Norethindrone, U.S.P. (MICRONOR, NOR-Q.D., NOR-LUTIN), and *Norethindrone Acetate,* U.S.P. (NORLU-TATE), are available alone in 0.35- and 5-mg tablets and in combination with estrogens as oral contraceptives (see below).

Ethisterone (DUOSTERONE) is available in 10-, 25-, and 50-mg tablets.

A variety of other oral progestin preparations are also combined with estrogens (ethinyl estradiol or mestranol) as oral contraceptives (see Table 68–3, page 1443).

It is not possible to give accurate values for the relative clinical effectiveness of the several compounds because careful comparisons are limited in number and different responses have been used in the published studies. In various tests in women, as with different bioassays in animals, the relative potencies of the progestins are not the same. Furthermore, some progestins possess more or less estrogenic and androgenic activities than do others.

Therapeutic Uses. Application of physiological principles in the management of ovarian disorders and contraception has made it possible to use these new agents with notable therapeutic success.

Contraception. This undoubtedly represents the major use of these agents and is discussed later in this chapter.

Functional Uterine Bleeding. This is a common disorder, characterized by grossly irregular cycles and episodes of prolonged and sometimes exsanguinating hemorrhage. The condition may arise at any time during the menstrual life, but is more frequent in young girls before regular ovulatory cycles are established and again with the approach of the menopause. The endocrine basis is poorly cycling action of estrogen uninterrupted by the action of progesterone.

The immediate goal is to stop the bleeding, and the long-range aim is to regulate the cycle. Both estrogens and androgens have been used effectively, but a progestin is specific. The condition can be treated with small doses of a progestin for a few days with the aim of inducing progesterone-withdrawal bleeding and counting on the termination of this to stop the bleeding. As little as 5 mg of progesterone, injected once daily for 4 days, or a single dose of 50 mg is effective. It is much better to give an orally active progestin in full doses to stop the bleeding. Five to 10 mg of norethindrone every 4 to 6 hours will usually be effective in 24 hours, and then 5 mg twice daily can be continued for 1 or 2 weeks to give a respite from bleeding. Withdrawal bleeding at the end of treatment will, in effect, be a normal menstrual flow, usually accompanied by cramps; however, it will be self-limited in duration and, if nothing further is done, there will be a free interval of several weeks. Other progestins may also be used, but those without inherent estrogenic activity are more effective if combined with an estrogen such as 2 mg of stilbestrol or 0.1 mg of ethinyl estradiol daily. To prevent a recurrence of functional bleeding, cyclic therapy is called for; an oral progestin, such as norethindrone, in a dose of 5 to 10 mg daily is given for 5 days at monthly intervals, beginning 20 to 25 days after the induced period. Regular menstrual periods can thus be induced for as long as one chooses. This allows time to elapse for the young patient to mature, for the premenopausal patient to age, and for many of the other patients to recover spontaneously from whatever caused the upset. There is some evidence to suggest, moreover, that cyclic therapy may exert a favorable effect upon the establishment of a normal interplay between ovary and pituitary.

Dysmenorrhea. Relief of dysmenorrhea by inhibiting ovulation is discussed under estrogen, where it is pointed out that treatment in successive cycles is sometimes rendered difficult by the delay in onset of withdrawal bleeding. If estrogen is not resumed until this bleeding stops, some 10 days may elapse and ovulation in the next cycle may not be prevented. A progestin can therefore be used to advantage either with the estrogen from days 5 to 25 of the cycle or added to the estrogen during the last 5 days (Greenblatt *et al.,* 1954). In either case menstruation is prompt, the treatment can be resumed 5 days later, and the cycle can be repeated indefinitely. Such cycles are entirely physiological, lacking only the ovarian components and ovulation, and fertility is not usually a consideration when dysmenorrhea is the problem.

Premenstrual Tension. This is an ill-defined condition of uncertain etiology. Changes in hormone concentrations and electrolytes are probably responsible for the irritability, breast tenderness, headache, and weight gain during the luteal phase of the cycle. Progesterone or an oral progestin may be effective when given during the last week or 10 days of the cycle. Sometimes this is not effective, and the symptoms are sufficiently distressing to warrant inhibition of ovulation with combined progestin-estrogen therapy.

Endometriosis. The severe dysmenorrhea of this condition is not completely understood. In many instances, suppression of ovulation with estrogen is followed by a painless, estrogen-withdrawal period; this suggests that the pain in the two conditions is of similar origin. Treatment of this form of endometriosis thus becomes the treatment of dysmenorrhea. In certain severe cases of endometriosis, the major problem is the development of painful extrauterine masses and treatment is aimed at causing regression of the ectopic endometrial growths. Prolonged treatment, designed to prevent menstruation for many months, relieves a major difficulty by preventing bleeding into the endometrial masses or peritoneal cavity. Favorable effects have been achieved even with the continuous use of estrogen alone for this purpose. Better results have been described from the continuous use of oral progestins, and actual regression of the endometrial growths has been observed. In women with normal cycles, Ferin (1962) induced amenorrhea for intervals of as long as 30 months by continual treatment with 5 mg of 17α-methyl-19-nortestosterone and later 2.5 and 1 mg, or with 5 mg daily of ethinylestrenol. There was ovarian and pronounced endometrial regression but no adverse effects upon subsequent cycles and ovulation. Medroxyprogesterone acetate may also be used in doses of 2.5 mg daily for 2 to 3 weeks, after which the dose is increased to 10 to 15 mg daily.

Threatened and Habitual Abortion. In spite of the very considerable experience in the use of progesterone and other progestins to prevent abortion, it is not possible to conclude unequivocally that the treatment is effective in the majority of patients. This is an amazing admission.

Numerous enthusiastic claims have been made for the efficacy of the long-acting parenteral preparations and the orally active 19-nortestosterone derivatives. Skepticism arises from two sources: statistical and embryological. It is common practice to assume that, if several abortions have taken place, the chances of the next pregnancy going to term are greatly reduced. Interpreted in this way, treatment can be shown to be highly successful; an estimated chance of approximately 15% for success may be improved to one of 65%. Others will argue that the chances of a successful pregnancy are no more influenced by former reproductive behavior than are the results of tossing a coin influenced by a run of tails.

There is a good deal of evidence to show that abortion is often caused by abnormalities of the embryo (Hertig and Rock, 1949). An effective treatment might therefore be expected to carry to term a sizable number of monsters, but this is not the usual experience. If progestins are to be used to help prevent abortion, the preparation should be selected with care since those with androgenic properties can cause abnormalities in the genital development of female fetuses (Wilkins *et al.,* 1958; Jacobson, 1962). Ethisterone and some of the 17-nortestosterones are androgenic, and virilizing effects upon the fetus might be expected. However, similar genital deformities have been ascribed to the use of progesterone itself. Nevertheless, there are thought to be a few patients who have an inadequate luteal response with deficient progesterone secretion and who benefit from progestins during the first trimester. To identify these patients, urinary progesterone metabolites must obviously be determined.

Evaluation of Ovarian Function and Diagnosis of Pregnancy. In amenorrhea, some indication of the production of estrogen from the ovary may be derived from administering progesterone or a nonestrogenic progestin to determine whether withdrawal is followed by menstrual bleeding. When bleeding does not take place, it is presumed that secretion of estrogen is minimal. If by rare chance the subject is in the luteal phase of a cycle or is pregnant, bleeding will not immediately follow, and this has been used as a test of pregnancy. However, immunoassay of urinary chorionic gonadotropin, which is increased very early during the first trimester of pregnancy, is a relatively simple technic and is preferred.

Suppression of Post-Partum Lactation. The administration of estrogens and/or progestins is effective in suppressing lactation in the immediate postpartum period. The precise mechanism of action is not known. Significant reduction in milk secretion is seen with concentrations of estrogens and progestins contained in oral contraceptive preparations (Kora, 1969). Doses of 0.1 to 0.15 mg of ethinyl estradiol daily for 5 to 7 days or 5 mg of diethylstilbestrol daily for 5 days followed by tapered doses for several days are more effective. Androgens are also widely used for this purpose (*see* Chapter 69).

Endometrial Carcinoma. Progestins may be used as a palliative measure in recurrent or metastatic endometrial carcinoma. When used in this manner, megestrol acetate may be given in oral doses of 40 mg daily for several months as a trial. Alternative therapy is the weekly intramuscular administration of 400 mg of medroxyprogesterone acetate.

ORAL CONTRACEPTIVES

The incredible growth of the world population stands out as one of the fundamental events of our era. The Old Testament dictum "Be fruitful, and multiply" (Genesis 9:1) has been religiously followed by readers and nonreaders of the Bible alike. In 1798, Thomas Robert Malthus started a great controversy by opposing the prevailing view of unlimited progress for man by making two postulates and a conclusion. He postulated that "food is necessary to the existence of man," and that sexual attraction between woman and man is necessary and likely to persist, since "towards the extinction of the passion between the sexes, no progress whatever has hitherto been made," barring ". . . individual exceptions." Malthus concluded that "the power of population is infinitely greater than the power in the earth to produce subsistence for man," a "natural inequality" that would someday loom "insurmountable in the way to the perfectibility of society." Malthus' essay sparked great controversy and in-

quiry into the principle governing the growth of population. In seeking to discover the causes of population increase, T. R. Edmonds in 1832 suggested that "a deterioration in the condition of the English labourers . . . , the destruction of the feeling of self-respect" was such a great distress that "among the great body of the people . . . , sexual intercourse is the only gratification. . . . When they are better fed they will have other enjoyments at command than sexual intercourse, and their numbers . . . will not increase in the same proportion as at present." Today we realize that our sheer numbers have increased so much that they are straining Earth's capacity to supply food, energy, and raw materials. We also know, perhaps better than T. R. Edmonds, where some of the blame for this growth lies. Advances in medicine and public health have led to a significant decline in mortality and an increased life expectancy. Thus, medical science has begun to assume a portion of the responsibility for overpopulation. To this end, drugs in the form of hormones and their analogs have been developed to control human fertility.

Of drugs requiring a prescription, oral contraceptives are among the most widely used agents, with recent annual sales of about $330 million worldwide and $150 million in the United States. The lives of millions of women are punctuated daily by the taking of a medicine for a condition from which they do not suffer—a prophylactic for a contingency that may not materialize.

A comprehensive investigation of the inhibition of ovulation by the use of progestational agents was initiated by Rock, Pincus, and Garcia in women who seemed normal in every way but who had failed to conceive. There was some basis for the rationale of inducing a kind of pseudopregnant condition in the expectation that, when treatment was stopped, fertility might be enhanced by the operation of compensatory mechanisms. That this aspect of the study met with some success was of passing interest; that the study showed that ovulation could be abolished at will for as long as desired and with great regularity was a fundamental contribution (*see* Rock *et al.,* 1957; Pincus, 1960). The compounds used were derivatives of 19-nortestosterone, given by mouth in an arbitrarily adopted schedule from day 5 to day 25 of the menstrual cycle (the first day of menses is day 1). Withdrawal bleeding occurred within a few days of completing the course, and treatment was begun again 4 days after the first day of flow. Extensive field studies were started in San Juan, Puerto

Rico, in 1955, under the direction of Pincus and associates at the Puerto Rico Family Planning Center. The tablet used was ENOVID, containing 10 mg of the progestin norethynodrel and 0.15 mg of the estrogen mestranol, and it was taken daily on the same schedule. Soon thereafter similar studies were initiated in Humacao, Puerto Rico, and in Port-au-Prince, Haiti. It was soon found that, when the schedule was followed, no pregnancies occurred; when tablets were allegedly missed for 1 to 5 days, some pregnancies followed but the rate was only 4% of that to be expected if no contraception were practiced. When 6 to 19 days of tablet-taking were missed, the pregnancy rate was 25% of expectation. The success of these studies prompted many others, and the results of broad, almost worldwide, experience followed (Pincus, 1965; Kistner, 1969).

Among the first of the orally active steroids to be used in inhibiting ovulation, some had inherent estrogenic activity and some preparations of the progestins were later found to be contaminated with estrogen. In a way this was a happy chance, because it served to show that estrogen enhanced the suppressive effect of the progestin and led to the general use of a mixture of the two. The substance considered to be the most likely estrogenic contaminant of norethynodrel was the 3-methyl ether of ethinyl estradiol, *mestranol,* which was therefore incorporated in ENOVID. As experience was gained, the dose of the progestin was reduced and that of the estrogen was increased without loss of contraceptive efficiency. Experience with the use of the combined estrogen and progestin preparations shows them to be so near to 100% effective that a closer estimate cannot be made. This method of reversible contraception is, then, the most effective yet devised.

Other modifications of the *combination* have also been tried with success. *Sequential* preparations in which an estrogen is taken for 14 to 16 days and a combination of an estrogen and a progestin is then taken for 5 or 6 days have been about 98 to 99% successful as oral contraceptives. The sequential method has the appeal of more closely duplicating the normal cycle, and the menstrual flow is said to resemble the normal in being more abundant, a dubious advantage.

Single-entity preparations are also now available. A progestin alone has come to be called the "minipill," while an estrogen alone is a postcoital or "morning-after pill." The "minipills" were introduced in order to eliminate the estrogen, the agent in *combined* and *sequential* preparations that is thought to be responsible for most if not all of the minor and major side effects of oral contraceptives. The recent availability of "minipills," however, has not yet permitted sufficiently large studies to support the notion of decreased side effects with progestins alone. The contraceptive efficacy of the "minipill" has been about 97 to 98%, which is somewhat less than with the combined preparations, and the menstrual cycles are more irregular. The intramuscular injection of medroxyprogesterone every few months has been more effective but has been associated with an increased incidence of irregular bleeding and particularly of infertility after its discontinuation. Diethylstilbestrol has been approved as a postcoital, "morning-after" contraceptive, but its use is largely restricted to emergency situations such as rape and incest.

Preparations and Dosage. Some of the formulations used as oral contraceptives are listed in Table 68–3. The *combined* preparations contain 0.05 to 0.1 mg of ethinyl estradiol or mestranol and various amounts of a progestin and are taken for 20 or 21 days. The *sequential* tablets provide the estrogen for 20 or 21 days, with the progestin added for the last 5 days. In either case the next course is started 7 days after the last dose or 5 days after the onset of the menstrual flow.

Many contraceptive preparations are dispensed in convenient calendar-like containers that help the user to count the days. Some obviate the need of counting by incorporating seven blank pills in the package to provide 3 weeks of treatment and 1 week off. A pill is taken every day, regardless of when menstruation starts or stops. A suffix "28" in the trade name designates these package forms.

The "minipills" (MICRONOR and NOR-Q.D., containing 0.35 mg of norethindrone, and ORVETTE, containing 75 μg of norgestrel) are taken daily continually. Since they are less effective and pregnancy is possible during their administration, patients should discontinue the "minipill" if they have amenorrhea for more than 60 days, and they should be examined for pregnancy. Likewise, if patients have missed one or more pills and have amenorrhea for more than 45 days, they should be similarly evaluated.

Medroxyprogesterone Acetate, U.S.P. (DEPO-PROVERA), is injected intramuscularly in a dose of 150 mg every 3 months but should be used only if the possibility of permanent infertility is acceptable to the patient. This use is still investigational.

Table 68–3. COMPOSITION AND DOSES OF ORAL CONTRACEPTIVES

TRADE NAME	MG—PROGESTIN	MG—ESTROGEN
Combinations *		
DEMULEN	1 Ethynodiol diacetate	0.05 Ethinyl estradiol
ENOVID 5 MG	5 Norethynodrel	0.075 Mestranol
ENOVID-E	2.5 Norethynodrel	0.10 Mestranol
LOESTRIN 1/20; ZORANE 1/20	1 Norethindrone	0.02 Ethinyl estradiol
LOESTRIN 1.5/30; ZORANE 1.5/30	1.5 Norethindrone	0.03 Ethinyl estradiol
MODICON	0.5 Norethindrone	0.035 Ethinyl estradiol
NORINYL 1 + 50; ORTHO-NOVUM 1/50	1 Norethindrone	0.05 Mestranol
NORINYL 1 + 80; ORTHO-NOVUM 1/80	1 Norethindrone	0.08 Mestranol
NORINYL, 2 MG; ORTHO-NOVUM, 2 MG	2 Norethindrone	0.10 Mestranol
ORTHO-NOVUM, 10 MG	10 Norethindrone	0.06 Mestranol
NORLESTRIN, 1 MG	1 Norethindrone acetate	0.05 Ethinyl estradiol
NORLESTRIN, 2.5 MG	2.5 Norethindrone acetate	0.05 Ethinyl estradiol
OVULEN	1 Ethynodiol diacetate	0.10 Mestranol
OVRAL	0.5 Norgestrel	0.05 Ethinyl estradiol
ZORANE 1/50	1 Norethindrone	0.05 Ethinyl estradiol
Sequentials †		
NORQUEN; ORTHO-NOVUM SQ	2 Norethindrone	0.08 Mestranol
ORACON	25 Dimethisterone	0.10 Ethinyl estradiol
"Minipills" ‡		
MICRONOR; NOR-Q.D.	0.35 Norethindrone	———
ORVETTE	0.075 Norgestrel	———
Postcoital §		
———	———	25 Diethylstilbestrol

* Combination tablets for 20 or 21 days and off for 7 or 8 days.
† Estrogen alone for 14 to 16 days, then combination for 5 or 6 days, and off for 7 or 8 days.
‡ "Minipills" are taken daily continually.
§ 25 mg twice daily for 5 days within 72 hours after sexual intercourse.

The postcoital contraceptive diethylstilbestrol is started within 72 hours after sexual intercourse at a dose of 25 mg twice daily for 5 days. To be effective the tablets must be continued for 5 consecutive days in spite of nausea and vomiting, which commonly occur. Since estrogens are not advised in pregnancy because of the possibility of vaginal carcinoma in female offspring (*see* above), abortion should be performed if diethylstilbestrol is not effective.

Effects on Laboratory Tests. Certain laboratory results may be altered by the use of oral contraceptives. These include the following: hepatic function tests (*e.g.*, increased sulfobromophthalein retention), increase in some clotting factors, tests for thyroid function (due to increased levels of thyroxine-binding globulin), tests of adrenocortical function (due to increased cortisol-binding globulin and altered metyrapone test), and pregnanediol determination.

Mechanism of Action. The administration of estrogen and a progestin, as contained in combination or sequential preparations, could interfere with fertility in any one of several ways. However, it is clear that, as currently used, the mixture inhibits ovulation. The questions then are how is ovulation prevented and what other mechanisms might interfere with impregnation. The effects of ovarian hormones upon the gonadotropic functions of the pituitary are discussed earlier in this chapter; the predominant effect of estrogen is to inhibit the secretion of FSH, while continued action of progesterone serves to inhibit the release of LH. It is clear that ovulation could be prevented either by inhibiting the ovulatory stimulus or by preventing the growth of follicles, and this accords with the experimental facts that ovulation can be prevented by either estrogen or progesterone given singly. The orally active progestins cannot be equated as a group with progesterone because some are inherently estrogenic, some slightly androgenic, and some purely progestational; correspondingly, their ovulation-inhibiting potentialities may be mediated in somewhat different ways.

From the limited number of direct observations on the ovary during treatment with the progestin-estrogen combinations, it appears that follicular growth is largely suppressed, an effect to be attributed to estrogen contained in the mixture. Suppression of ovulation by compounds such as norethindrone, medroxyprogesterone acetate, ethynodiol diacetate, and ethinylestrenol without added estrogen would, presumably, be due largely to inhibition of LH.

Measurements of circulating FSH and LH show that estrogen-progestin combinations suppress both hormones. The plasma levels of FSH and LH are stable; early follicular FSH and midcycle FSH and LH peaks are not seen (Swerdloff and Odell, 1969). With sequential preparations, estrogen alone suppresses FSH but causes an irregular increase in LH; when a progestin is then given, there is a brief rise in LH followed by a sustained decline.

One might reasonably conclude that the most widely used preparations to date owe their effectiveness in inhibiting ovulation to the estrogenic component and that the progestin serves the major purpose of ensuring that withdrawal bleeding will be prompt, brief in duration, and essentially physiological.

Even if ovulation were not prevented, it is easy to imagine that the contraceptive agents could interfere with impregnation by their direct actions upon the genital tract. From animal experiments it is abundantly clear that the endometrium must be just in the right stage of development under estrogen and progesterone for nidation to take place. It seems unlikely that implantation would be possible in the altered endometrium developed under the influence of most of the suppressants. Similarly, the abundant watery secretion of the cervix at the time of ovulation has always been regarded as essential to the well-being of the sperm and the thick tenacious mucus secreted under the influence of progesterone to be a hostile environment. Little is known of the coordinated contractions of the cervix, uterus, and Fallopian tubes that are presumed to be essential for the transport of spermatozoa to the egg and the precisely timed conveyance of the blastocyst to the uterine lumen, but probably the correct hormonal environment is essential for the execution of these important maneuvers. Although it can easily be imagined that estrogen-progestin mixtures could interfere with impregnation in these ways, there has been no opportunity to find out, because ovulation is almost always prevented when the agents are used in the usual way.

The fear that estrogen may have deleterious effects prompted the use of a *progestin alone* in various ways. Continuous administration of a progestin in sufficient dose abolishes the cycle for as long as it is given and leads to ovarian and endometrial atrophy (Ferin, 1962). Very small doses may alter the structure of the endometrium and the consistency of the cervical mucus without disrupting the cycle or inhibiting ovulation. In seeking a dose sufficient to be contraceptive but too small to inhibit the ovary, Martinez-Manautou and coworkers (1967) established that 0.5 mg of chlormadinone acetate, when given without interruption, was fully effective as a contraceptive, with some women showing evidence of ovulation.

The action of the "minipill" with 0.35 mg of norethindrone may be mediated by alteration of the cervical mucus and endometrium without influencing ovulation; however, the precise mechanisms of action are unknown. With continued daily administration, menstruation occurs but the length of the cycle and the duration of bleeding are quite variable, factors that will probably influence their popularity.

Long-acting progestins, given by intramuscular injection, are also effective. For example, 150 mg of medroxyprogesterone acetate, administered every 3 months starting just after parturition, prevented pregnancy in all; irregular bleeding, troublesome at first, gave way to amenorrhea and an atrophic endometrium in most cases (Mishell *et al.*, 1968). This form of contraception also used the highly active, purely progestational compounds by incorporating them in pessaries to provide vaginal absorption, in intrauterine devices, or in plastic capsules for subcutaneous application. Currently in clinical trial is an intrauterine device consisting of a polymer outer membrane over a progesterone-impregnated core, which is claimed to be effective for one year. Since large doses of some progestins may produce virilization of the female fetus if pregnancy is not prevented (Wilkins *et al.,* 1958; Jacobson, 1962), these methods are less acceptable.

The development of *postcoital* contraceptives is an intriguing subject but, unfortunately, a most difficult problem to approach. A vast number of hormones and other agents are effective in this regard in animals, but controlled experiments in women are difficult to design and still more difficult to carry out. It has long been known that the use of large doses of estrogen in women is effective in preventing implantation, but such doses are tolerated only in cases of single or very infrequent exposure. Tests in animals show that there is a rough correlation between the contraceptive potency of these substances and their estrogenic activity (Jacob and Morris, 1969).

Large doses of estrogens used as postcoital contraceptives may act by inhibiting fertilization and nidation in several ways. The motility of the oviduct may be altered, the endometrium is changed, and withdrawal from the large doses of estrogens induces bleeding.

One would think that a large dose of a potent progestin should be effective as a postcoital contraceptive, but no reports have been found that show this to be true. A more exciting possibility would be an effective antiprogestin. Such a substance should precipitate menstruation at any time after ovulation or induce a "physiological" abortion at will.

The use of prostaglandins to produce abortion is discussed in Chapter 42.

Undesirable Effects. The frequent, mild side effects—nausea, occasional vomiting, dizziness, headache, discomfort in the breasts, and gain in weight—are manifestations of early pregnancy and are attributable entirely, or nearly so, to the estrogen in the preparations. These symptoms are more frequent and may be more troublesome than the side effects in menopausal women given estrogen, probably because the contraceptives are not taken for the relief of symptoms. However, most of them are short lived or are noted only in the first cycle or two. Irregular menstrual bleeding, the so-called breakthrough bleeding, is also more frequent at first; it seems to be less troublesome with the preparations containing the larger doses of estrogen.

Many other minor disturbances have been attributed to the oral contraceptives. Some symptoms, including depression of mood, easy fatigue, and lack of initiative, have been attributed to the progestin in the tablets and are less troublesome or even unnoticed with the newer preparations containing smaller amounts.

Various ocular conditions have also been reported, including retinal thrombosis, optic neuritis, diplopia, and others. However, it has not been determined that these are in fact related to oral contraceptives. Skin rashes, alopecia, and hirsutism seldom occur, but chloasma (brownish macules of the face) frequently occurs with prolonged use of most preparations. Cholestatic jaundice due to the 17-alkyl-substituted steroids in all of the preparations is rare; an increased incidence of gallbladder disease with estrogens has been reported by the Boston Collaborative Drug Surveillance Program (1974). Folate absorption may be decreased, but few patients develop anemia or other signs of deficiency. Increases in systolic and diastolic blood pressure may be due to an increased concentration of angiotensin as well as to salt and water retention. The increase in blood pressure is reversible within several months of discontinuation of the preparations (Weir *et al.,* 1974). The impairment in glucose tolerance in some patients was discussed earlier. The resumption of spontaneous menses usually requires about 6 to 10 weeks after oral contraceptives have been discontinued. However, some patients have prolonged periods of anovulation and amenorrhea (sometimes associated with galactorrhea), requiring therapy with clomiphene or gonadotropin. Preliminary studies have indicated that prepregnancy use of oral contraceptives results in a higher incidence of female offspring (Keserü *et al.,* 1974). Continuation of intake of oral contraceptives during pregnancy has been reported to increase congenital limb deformation in the offspring (Janerich *et al.,* 1974). Administration of oral contraceptives soon after delivery will decrease lactation and interfere with breast feeding.

Thromboembolism. Clinical trials in sizable groups of women had been under way for 5 years or so before side effects of any consequence were described. Instances of *thrombophlebitis,* a rare disorder in healthy young women, then began to be noted, and several reports of *thromboembolism* from England were sufficiently alarming to cause the United States Food and Drug Administration to appoint a committee (the Wilson Committee) to study the matter. The conclusion reached was that the incidence of this disorder among the women taking the medication was not greater than the spontaneous incidence of the condition in women of childbearing age (*see* FDA, 1963). The data and conclusions of this report were extended and reaffirmed 2 years later by Winter (1965). However, in 1968 two official documents were published in Great Britain, one from the Committee on Safety of Drugs (Inman and Vessey, 1968) and the other from the Medical Research Council (Vessey and Doll, 1968). The former cited evidence to show that the risk of death from the complications is about six times higher among users than among nonusers of the "pill" (1.3 versus 0.2 deaths per 100,000 per year). In the latter report it was estimated that the incidence of thrombophlebitis in young women was increased tenfold with oral contraceptives.

These retrospective studies, while apparently underestimating the spontaneous incidence of thrombophlebitis, suffer from a statistical dilemma, because what was really studied was the incidence of medication among those with complications versus those without. Retrospective studies are also generally criticized since cause-and-effect relationships cannot be established and because biases are introduced due to the means by which information is obtained.

Because of the British reports, the United States Food and Drug Administration, in 1968, appointed another committee to investigate the matter further. In August, 1969, the FDA released to the press its conclusion that the "pills" are safe. The committee apparently concluded that there might be a small increase in the incidence of thromboembolism but that the reported incidence is erroneously high.

In recent large prospective studies, the incidence of thrombophlebitis (about 1 to 2 cases per 1000 patients per year) was not altered by the use of oral contraceptives (Drill, 1972). Objections to the design of this study have also been raised. Inman and co-workers (1970) reported an increased incidence of deep-vein thrombosis, pulmonary embolism, cerebral thrombosis, and coronary thrombosis in "pill" users. While there were no differences between users of *combined* and *sequential* preparations, the incidence of thromboembolism was greater with preparations containing higher doses of estrogens. In another study no relationship of thromboembolic disease to estrogen content in oral contraceptives was observed (Drill and Calhoun, 1972).

The Collaborative Group for the Study of Stroke in Young Women (1973, 1975) found about a ninefold increase in incidence of thrombotic strokes among oral contraceptive users. The Coronary Drug Project Research Group (1973) also found a twofold increase in the incidence of thrombophlebitis and pulmonary embolism in men who received 2.5 mg of conjugated estrogens daily for 4 to 5 years. Similarly, in men with prostatic carcinoma the administration of 5 mg of diethylstilbestrol daily was associated with an increased incidence of myocardial infarction and strokes (Veterans Administration, 1967).

Therefore, one can find reports supporting either view, and this raging controversy will continue until controlled, large, prospective studies are performed. Obviously, the effect sought with oral contraceptives is prevention of pregnancy, and this precludes an ideal, randomized, double-blind study.

The possible increase in thromboembolism is also supported by studies with various clotting factors. Patients taking estrogens or combined oral contraceptives have been found to have accelerated blood clotting and increased blood concentrations of some clotting factors, as well as increased platelet aggregation. These effects have not been observed with preparations containing only progestin (Poller *et al.,* 1972).

While the amalgamation and interpretation of these numerous studies are somewhat risky, most agree that the morbidity and mortality from thromboembolic diseases are increased about fourfold to tenfold with the use of *combined* or *sequential* oral contraceptives. Experience with the "mini-pill" (only progestin) has been too limited to draw any conclusions.

It is widely believed that thrombophlebitis and its complications occur more frequently during pregnancy and the post-partum period. Furthermore, increased mortality from various causes during pregnancy supports the view that the increased incidence of thromboembolic disorders with oral contraceptives is probably a comparatively minor and acceptable risk, since pregnancy is effectively prevented. Serious complications of pregnancy are perhaps so much more frequent than are those resulting from oral contraceptive use that the incidence of difficulties from unwanted pregnancies might be still higher if all couples switched to other methods of contraception, all of which are less effective.

Cancer. Because of the numerous animal studies that demonstrate an increased incidence of several different types of tumors with estrogen, there has also been much concern that similar problems would occur in oral contraceptive users. Melamed and co-workers (1969) reported an increased incidence of carcinoma of the cervix *in situ* in patients using oral contraceptives compared to those using the diaphragm. However, in view of the many socioeconomic factors that are known to influence the incidence of this disease, the significance of this retrospective study is unclear. Furthermore, extensive earlier studies in Puerto Rico and Haiti showed a lowered incidence of cancer of the uterus and the breast among the users of the contraceptives (Pincus, 1965). Also, cytological changes in cervical smears may be misleading during pregnancy and during medication with the contraceptives (Kyriakos *et al.,* 1968).

As discussed earlier, it is possible that an increased incidence of several types of tumors may be related to the use of estrogens and oral contraceptives. The relatively few incriminating studies, despite the vast use of these agents, may reflect the latent period needed for cellular transformation. Future studies will be particularly important to resolve these questions. (*See* review by Drill, 1975.)

In view of these considerations, it seems highly prudent to continue to evaluate each patient and her need for oral contraceptives. Clearly in some patients pregnancy is either very undesirable or contraindicated due to preexisting disease; the additional risks from oral contraceptives seem minor. However, in most patients the decision is more difficult. There are many alternative means of contraception, but none is as effective as oral contraceptives. For extensive population control, these agents are extremely useful and few complications are to be expected. With the recent United States Supreme Court decision on abortion, the future need for a *totally* effective contraceptive method may be less urgent for some individuals.

If oral contraceptives are prescribed, preparations with lower estrogen content are generally preferred, and patients require periodic evaluation for side effects. The United States Food and Drug Administration exercises strict control over the labeling of estrogens and oral contraceptives. Contraindications to their use are thromboembolic disorders or a past history of these conditions, markedly impaired hepatic function, known or suspected carcinoma of the breast or other estrogen-dependent neoplasia, and undiagnosed genital bleeding. In addition, various warnings and precautions, as well as the possible adverse reactions outlined above, must be listed. The extent to which these possible adverse reactions should be discussed with the patient at first was left to the discretion of the physician, but now a brief description of the hazards of this form of contraception is included in each package dispensed to the patient.

Allen, E., and Doisy, E. A. An ovarian hormone: a preliminary report on its localization, extraction, and partial purification, and action in test animals. *J. Am. med. Ass.,* **1923,** *81,* 819–821.

Bagget, B.; Engel, L. L.; Savard, K.; and Dorfman, R. I. The conversion of testosterone-3-C^{14} to C^{14}-estradiol-17β by human ovarian tissue. *J. biol. Chem.,* **1956,** *221,* 931–941.

Baum, J. K.; Bookstein, J. J.; Holtz, F.; and Klein, E. W. Possible association between benign hepatomas and oral contraceptives. *Lancet,* **1973,** *2,* 926–929.

Beard, J. *The Span of Gestation and the Cause of Birth.* G. Fischer, Jena, **1897.**

Black, M. M., and Leis, H. P. Mammary carcinogenesis. Influence of parity and estrogens. *N.Y. St. J. Med.,* **1972,** *72,* 1601–1605.

Boston Collaborative Drug Surveillance Program. Surgically confirmed gall bladder disease, venous thromboembolism, and breast tumors in relation to postmenopausal estrogen therapy. *New Engl. J. Med.,* **1974,** *290,* 15–18.

Brennan, D. M., and Kraay, R. J. Chlormadinone acetate, a new highly active gestation-supporting agent. *Acta endocr., Copenh.,* **1963,** *44,* 367–379.

Briggs, M. H.; Pitchford, A. G.; Staniford, M.; Barker, H. M.; and Taylor, D. Metabolic effects of steroid contraceptives. *Adv. Steroid Biochem. Pharmac.*, **1970**, *2*, 111–222.

Butenandt, A. Über "PROGYNON," ein crystallisiertes, weibliches Sexualhormon. *Naturwissenschaften*, **1929**, *17*, 879.

Collaborative Group for the Study of Stroke in Young Women. Oral contraception and increased risk of cerebral ischemia or thrombosis. *New Engl. J. Med.*, **1973**, *288*, 871–878.

———. Oral contraceptives and stroke in young women; associated risk factors. *J. Am. med. Ass.*, **1975**, *231*, 718–722.

Corner, G. W., and Allen, W. M. Physiology of the corpus luteum. II. Production of a special uterine reaction (progestational proliferation) by extracts of the corpus luteum. *Am. J. Physiol.*, **1929**, *88*, 326–346.

Coronary Drug Project Research Group. The coronary drug project. Initial findings leading to modifications of its research protocol. *J. Am. med. Ass.*, **1970**, *214*, 1303–1313.

———. The coronary drug project. Findings leading to discontinuation of the 2.5-mg/day estrogen group. *Ibid.*, **1973**, *226*, 652–657.

Curnow, D. H. Oestrogenic activity of subterranean clover. II. Isolation of genistein from subterranean clover and methods of quantitative estimation. *Biochem. J.*, **1954**, *58*, 283–287.

Davis, M. E., and Wied, G. L. 17α-Hydroxyprogesterone acetate: an effective progestational substance on oral administration. *J. clin. Endocr. Metab.*, **1957**, *17*, 1237–1244.

Dodds, E. C.; Goldberg, L.; Lawson, W.; and Robinson, R. Oestrogenic activity of alkylated stilboestrols. *Nature, Lond.*, **1938**, *142*, 34.

Doisy, E. A.; Veler, C. D.; and Thayer, S. A. Folliculin from the urine of pregnant women. *Am. J. Physiol.*, **1929**, *90*, 329–330.

———. The preparation of the crystalline ovarian hormone from the urine of pregnant women. *J. biol. Chem.*, **1930**, *86*, 499–509.

Drill, V. A. Oral contraceptives and thromboembolic disease. I. Prospective and retrospective studies. *J. Am. med. Ass.*, **1972**, *219*, 583–592.

Drill, V. A., and Calhoun, D. W. Oral contraceptives and thromboembolic disease. II. Estrogen content of oral contraceptives. *J. Am. med. Ass.*, **1972**, *219*, 593–596.

FDA. Report on ENOVID. *J. Am. med. Ass.*, **1963**, *185*, 776.

Ferin, J. Artificial induction of hypo-oestrogenic amenorrhea with methylestrenolone or with lynestrenol. *Acta endocr., Copenh.*, **1962**, *39*, 47–67.

Fontaine, Y.-A.; Fontaine-Bertrand, E.; Salmon, C.; and Delerue-Lebelle, N. Stimulation *in vitro* par les deux hormones gonadotropes hypophysaires (LH et FSH) de l'activité adénylcyclasique de l'ovaire chez la ratte prépubère. *C. r. hebd. Séanc. Acad. Sci., Paris*, D, **1971**, *272*, 1137–1140.

Fraenkel, L. Die Funktion des Corpus Luteum. *Arch. Gynaek.*, **1903**, *68*, 483–545.

Frank, R. T.; Frank, M. L.; Gustavson, R. G.; and Weyerts, W. W. Demonstration of the female sex hormone in the circulating blood. I. Preliminary report. *J. Am. med. Ass.*, **1925**, *85*, 510.

Greenblatt, R. B.; Hammond, D. O.; and Clark, S. L. Membranous dysmenorrhea: studies in etiology and treatment. *Am. J. Obstet. Gynec.*, **1954**, *68*, 835–844.

Greenblatt, R. B.; Roy, S.; Mahesh, V. B.; Barfield, W. E.; and Jungck, E. C. Induction of ovulation. *Am. J. Obstet. Gynec.*, **1962**, *84*, 900–909.

Greenwald, P.; Barlow, J. J.; Nasca, P. C.; and Burnett, W. S. Vaginal cancer after maternal treatment with synthetic estrogens. *New Engl. J. Med.*, **1971**, *285*, 390–392.

Halban, J. Ueber den Einfluss der Ovarien auf die Entwicklung des Genitales. *Mschr. Geburtsch. Gynäk.*, **1900**, *12*, 496–503.

Heard, R. D. H.; Jellinck, P. H.; and O'Donnell, V. J. Biogenesis of the estrogens: the conversion of testosterone-4-C^{14} to estrone in the pregnant mare. *Endocrinology*, **1955**, *57*, 200–204.

Herbst, A. L.; Kurman, R. J.; Scully, R. E.; and Poskanzer, D. C. Clear-cell adenocarcinoma of the genital tract in young females. *New Engl. J. Med.*, **1972**, *287*, 1259–1264.

Herbst, A. L.; Ulfelder, H.; and Poskanzer, D. C. Adenocarcinoma of the vagina. Association of maternal stilbestrol therapy with tumor appearance in young women. *New Engl. J. Med.*, **1971**, *284*, 878–881.

Hertig, A. T., and Rock, J. A series of potentially abortive ova recovered from fertile women prior to the first missed menstrual period. *Am. J. Obstet. Gynec.*, **1949**, *58*, 968–988.

Hilliard, J.; Scaramuzzi, R. J.; Pang, C.-N.; Penardi, R.; and Sawyer, C. H. Testosterone secretion by rabbit ovary *in vivo*. *Endocrinology*, **1974**, *94*, 267–271.

Hisaw, F. L. The interaction of the ovarian hormones in experimental menstruation. *Endocrinology*, **1942**, *30*, 301–308.

Hisaw, F. L.; Velardo, J. T.; and Goolsby, C. M. Interaction of estrogens on uterine growth. *J. clin. Endocr. Metab.*, **1954**, *14*, 1134–1143.

Inman, W. H. W., and Vessey, M. P. Investigation of deaths from pulmonary, coronary and cerebral thrombosis and embolism in women of childbearing age. *Br. med. J.*, **1968**, *2*, 193–199.

Inman, W. H. W.; Vessey, M. P.; Westerholm, B.; and Engelund, A. Thromboembolic disease and the steroidal content of oral contraceptives. *Br. med. J.*, **1970**, *2*, 203–209.

Jacob, D., and Morris, J. McL. The estrogenic activity of postcoital antifertility compounds. *Fert. Steril.*, **1969**, *20*, 211–222.

Jacobson, B. D. Hazards of norethindrone therapy during pregnancy. *Am. J. Obstet. Gynec.*, **1962**, *84*, 962–968.

Janerich, D. T.; Piper, J. M.; and Glebatis, D. M. Oral contraceptives and congenital limb-reduction defects. *New Engl. J. Med.*, **1974**, *291*, 697–700.

Kato, J.; Kobayashi, T.; and Villee, C. A. Effect of clomiphene on the uptake of estradiol by the anterior hypothalamus and hypophysis. *Endocrinology*, **1968**, *82*, 1049–1052.

Keserü, T. L.; Maràz, A.; and Szabo, J. Oral contraception and sex ratio at birth. *Lancet*, **1974**, *1*, 369.

Knauer, E. Die Ovarien-Transplantation. *Arch. Gynaek.*, **1900**, *60*, 322–376.

Kora, S. J. Effect of oral contraceptives on lactation. *Fert. Steril.*, **1969**, *20*, 419–423.

Kyriakos, M.; Kempson, R. L.; and Konikov, N. F. A clinical and pathologic study of endocervical lesions associated with oral contraceptives. *Cancer, N.Y.*, **1968**, *22*, 99–110.

Lafferty, F. W.; Spencer, G. E.; and Pearson, O. H. Effects of androgens, estrogens, and high calcium intakes on bone formation and resorption in osteoporosis. *Am. J. Med.*, **1964**, *36*, 514–528.

Lerner, L. J.; Holthaus, F. J., Jr.; and Thompson, C. R. A non-steroidal estrogen antagonist: 1-(*p*-2-diethylaminoethoxyphenyl)-1-phenyl-2-*p*-methoxyphenyl ethanol. *Endocrinology*, **1958**, *63*, 295–318.

Lerner, L. J.; Yiacas, E.; Bianchi, A.; Turkheimer, A. R.; DePhillipo, M.; and Borman, A. Effect of the acetophenone derivative of 16α,17αα-dihydroxyprogesterone on the estrous cycle, mating and fertility in the rat. *Fert. Steril.*, **1964**, *15*, 63–73.

Loewe, S. Nachweis brunsterzeugender Stoffe im weiblichen Blute. *Klin. Wschr.*, **1925**, *4*, 1407–1408.

Loewe, S., and Lange, F. Der Gehalt des Frauenharns an brunsterzeugenden Stoffen in Abhängigkeit von ovariellen Zyklus. *Klin. Wschr.*, **1926**, *5*, 1038–1039.

Macgregor, A. H.; Johnson, J. E.; and Bunde, C. A. Further clinical experience with clomiphene citrate. *Fert. Steril.*, **1968**, *19*, 616–622.

Marsh, J. M.; Butcher, R. W.; Savard, K.; and Sutherland, E. W. The stimulatory effect of luteinizing hormone on adenosine 3′,5′-monophosphate accumulation in corpus luteum slices. *J. biol. Chem.*, **1966**, *241*, 5436–5440.

Martinez-Manautou, J.; Giner-Velasquez, J.; and Rudel, H. Continuous progestogen contraception: a dose relationship study with chlormadinone acetate. *Fert. Steril.*, **1967**, *18*, 57–62.

Medical Letter. Estrogens and the menopausal patient. **1973**, *15*, 6–8.

Melamed, M. R.; Koss, L. G.; Flehinger, B. J.; Kelisky, R. P.; and Dubrow, H. Prevalence rates of uterine cervical carcinoma *in situ* for women using the diaphragm or contraceptive oral steroids. *Br. med. J.*, **1969**, *3*, 195–200.

Midgley, A. R., and Jaffe, R. B. Regulation of human gonadotropins. IV. Correlation of serum concentrations of follicle stimulating and luteinizing hormones during the menstrual cycle. *J. clin. Endocr. Metab.*, **1968**, *28*, 1699–1703.

Mills, T. M., and Savard, K. *In vitro* steroid synthesis by follicles isolated from the rabbit ovary. *Steroids*, **1972**, *20*, 247–262.

Minaguchi, H., and Meites, J. Effects of a norethynodrel-mestranol combination (ENOVID) on hypothalamic and pituitary hormones in rats. *Endocrinology*, **1967**, *81*, 826–834.

Mishell, D. R., Jr.; El-Habashy, M. A.; Good, R. G.; and Moyer, D. L. Contraception with an injectable progestin: a study of its use in postpartum women. *Am. J. Obstet. Gynec.*, **1968**, *101*, 1046–1053.

Naftolin, F.; Judd, H. L.; and Yen, S. C. C. Pulsatile patterns of gonadotropins and testosterone in man: the effects of clomiphene with and without testosterone. *J. clin. Endocr. Metab.*, **1973**, *36*, 285–288.

Pincus, G. Clinical effects of new progestational compounds. In, *Clinical Endocrinology I.* (Astwood, E. B., ed.) Grune & Stratton, Inc., New York, **1960**, pp. 526–531.

Poller, L.; Thomson, J. M.; and Thomas, P. W. Effects of progestogen oral contraceptives with norethisterone on blood clotting and platelets. *Br. med. J.*, **1972**, *4*, 391–393.

Riggs, B. L.; Ryan, R. J.; Wahner, H. W.; Jiang, N.-S.; and Mattox, V. R. Serum concentrations of estrogen, testosterone, and gonadotropins in osteoporotic and non-osteoporotic postmenopausal women. *J. clin. Endocr. Metab.*, **1973**, *36*, 1097–1099.

Riggs, L.; Jowsey, J.; Goldsmith, R. S.; Kelly, P. J.; Hoffman, D. L.; and Arnaud, C. D. Short- and long-term effects of estrogen and synthetic anabolic hormone in postmenopausal osteoporosis. *J. clin. Invest.*, **1972**, *51*, 1659–1663.

Riggs, L.; Jowsey, J.; Kelly, P. J.; Jones, J. D.; and Maher, F. T. Effect of sex hormones on bone in primary osteoporosis. *J. clin. Invest.*, **1969**, *48*, 1065–1072.

Ryan, K. J. Biological aromatization of steroids. *J. biol. Chem.*, **1959**, *234*, 268–272.

Ryan, K. J., and Engel, L. L. The interconversion of estrone and estradiol by human tissue slices. *Endocrinology*, **1953**, *52*, 287–291.

Segal, S. J., and Thompson, C. R. Inhibition of estradiol-induced pituitary hypertrophy in rats. *Proc. Soc. exp. Biol. Med.*, **1956**, *91*, 623–625.

Strauss, S., and Pochi, P. E. The hormonal control of human sebaceous glands: observations in certain endocrine disorders. In, *Clinical Endocrinology II.* (Astwood, E. B., and Cassidy, C. E., eds.) Grune & Stratton, Inc., New York, **1968**, pp. 798–808.

Sturgis, S. H., and Albright, F. The mechanism of estrin therapy in the relief of dysmenorrhea. *Endocrinology*, **1940**, *26*, 68–72.

Swerdloff, R. S., and Odell, W. D. Serum luteinizing and follicle stimulating hormone levels during sequential and nonsequential contraceptive treatment of eugonadal women. *J. clin. Endocr. Metab.*, **1969**, *29*, 157–163.

Vande Wiele, R. L.; Gurpide, E.; Kelly, W. G.; Laragh, J. H.; and Lieberman, S. The secretory rate of progesterone and aldosterone in normal and abnormal late pregnancy. *Acta endocr., Copenh.*, **1960**, *34*, Suppl. 51, 159.

Vessey, M. P., and Doll, R. Investigation of relation between use of oral contraceptives and thromboembolic disease. *Br. med. J.*, **1968**, *2*, 199–205.

Veterans Administration. The Veterans Administration co-operative urological research group: treatment and survival of patients with cancer of the prostate. *Surgery Gynec. Obstet.*, **1967**, *124*, 1011–1017.

Weir, R. J.; Briggs, E.; Mack, A.; Naismith, L.; Taylor, L.; and Wilson, E. Blood pressure in women taking oral contraceptives. *Br. med. J.*, **1974**, *1*, 533–535.

Wilkins, L.; Jones, H. M.; Holman, G. H.; and Stempfel, R. S. Masculinization of the female fetus associated with administration of oral and intramuscular progestins during gestation: non-adrenal female pseudohermaphrodism. *J. clin. Endocr. Metab.*, **1958**, *18*, 559–585.

Winter, I. C. The incidence of thromboembolism in ENOVID users. *Metabolism*, **1965**, *14*, 422–428.

Zondek, B. Darstellung des weiblichen Sexualhormon aus dem Harn, insbesondere dem Harn von Schwageren. *Klin. Wschr.*, **1928**, *7*, 485–486.

Zuckerman, S. Periodic uterine bleeding in spayed rhesus monkeys injected daily with a constant dose of oestrone. *J. Endocr.*, **1941**, *2*, 263–267.

Monographs and Reviews

Anderson, L. L.; Bland, K. P.; and Melampy, R. M. Comparative aspects of uterine-luteal relationships. *Recent Prog. Horm. Res.*, **1969**, *25*, 57–99.

Blackwell, R. E., and Guillemin, R. Hypothalamic control of adenohypophyseal secretions. *A. Rev. Physiol.*, **1973**, *35*, 357–390.

Drill, V. A. Oral contraceptives: relation to mammary cancer, benign breast lesions, and cervical cancer. *A. Rev. Pharmac.*, **1975**, *15*, 367–385.

Emmens, C. W.; Cox, R. I.; and Martin, L. Antiestrogens. *Recent Prog. Horm. Res.*, **1962**, *18*, 415–460.

Fotherby, K., and James, F. Metabolism of synthetic steroids. *Adv. Steroid Biochem. Pharmac.*, **1972**, *3*, 67–165.

Hafez, E. S. E., and Evans, T. N. (eds.). *Human Reproduction: Conception and Contraception.* Harper & Row, Pubs., New York, **1973**.

Jensen, E. V., and DeSombre, E. R. Mechanism of action of the female sex hormones. *A. Rev. Biochem.*, **1972**, *41*, 203–230.

Kalkhoff, R. K. Effects of oral contraceptive agents and sex steroids on carbohydrate metabolism. *A. Rev. Med.*, **1972**, *23*, 429–438.

Kellie, A. E. The pharmacology of the estrogens. *A. Rev. Pharmac.*, **1971**, *11*, 97–112.

Kistner, R. W. *The Pill: Facts and Fallacies about Today's Oral Contraceptives.* Delacorte Press, Dell Publishing Co., Inc., New York, **1969**.

Mahesh, V. B., and Greenblatt, R. B. Steroid secretions of the normal and polycystic ovary. *Recent Prog. Horm. Res.*, **1964**, *20*, 341–394.

Mueller, G. C.; Vanderhaar, B.; Kim, U. H.; and Le Mahieu, M. Estrogen action: an inroad to cell biology. *Recent Prog. Horm. Res.*, **1972**, *28*, 1–45.

Niswender, G. D., and Midgley, A. R. Hapten-radioimmunoassay for steroid hormones. In, *Immunologic Methods in Steroid Determination.* (Peron, F. Q., and Caldwell, B. V., eds.) Appleton-Century-Crofts, New York, **1970**, pp. 149–173.

O'Malley, B. W., and Means, A. R. Female steroid hormones and target cell nuclei. *Science, Wash.*, **1974**, *183*, 610–620.

Pincus, G. *The Control of Fertility.* Academic Press, Inc., New York, **1965**.

Rock, J.; Garcia, C. M.; and Pincus, G. Synthetic progestins in the normal human menstrual cycle. *Recent Prog. Horm. Res.,* **1957,** *13,* 323–339.

Rosenfield, R. L. Role of androgens in growth and development of the fetus, child, and adolescent. *Adv. Pediat.,* **1972,** *19,* 172–213.

Schally, A. V.; Arimura, A.; and Kastin, A. J. Hypothalamic regulatory hormones. At least nine substances from the hypothalamus control the secretion of pituitary hormones. *Science, Wash.,* **1973,** *179,* 341–350.

Schally, A. V., and Kastin, A. J. The role of sex steroids, hypothalamic LH-releasing hormone and FSH-releasing hormone in the regulation of gonadotropin secretion from the anterior pituitary gland. *Adv. Steroid Biochem. Pharmac.,* **1970,** *2,* 41–69.

Sommerville, I. F., and Collins, W. P. Indices of androgen production in women. *Adv. Steroid Biochem. Pharmac.,* **1970,** *2,* 267–314.

Vande Wiele, R. L., and Dyrenfurth, I. Gonadotropin-steroid interrelationships. *Pharmac. Rev.,* **1973,** *25,* 189–207.

Yates, F. E.; Russell, S. M.; and Moran, J. W. Brain-adenohypophyseal communication in mammals. *A. Rev. Physiol.,* **1971,** *33,* 393–444.

CHAPTER

69 ANDROGENS AND ANABOLIC STEROIDS

Ferid Murad and Alfred G. Gilman

ANDROGENS

The testis, ovary, and adrenal cortex are responsible for the normal synthesis of androgens. An understanding of the regulation of the synthesis and secretion of androgens and of the effects of these compounds has led to their clinical use, primarily in hypogonadal conditions in men and to promote anabolism in both sexes. Additional knowledge of gonadotropic and androgenic regulation of spermatogenesis may permit the use of these agents as oral contraceptives in men in the foreseeable future.

History. The observation that castration makes the eunuch, properly credited to primitive man, ushered in the dawn of endocrinology. By the year 1771, John Hunter had induced male characteristics in the hen by transplanting testes from the cock (*see* Forbes, 1947); however, credit for the discovery that the testis is a gland of internal secretion is usually ascribed to Berthold, who in 1849 showed that the transplantation of gonads into castrated roosters prevented the typical signs of castration. This was the first published experimental evidence for the effect of an endocrine gland. However, it was not this observation but the popular belief that failure of testicular function was the cause of the symptoms of old age in men that stimulated many attempts to isolate an active testicular principle. As an example of the wide acceptance of this belief may be cited the experiments of Brown-Séquard (1889), the renowned French physiologist, who prepared a testicular extract and administered it to himself. He was convinced that he had gained in vigor and capacity for work from the treatment, but it is now known that his aqueous extract was devoid of hormone.

Chemistry. The elucidation of the chemistry of the male sex hormones was made possible by the development of methods of assay. The procedure of Koch and coworkers for the determination of androgenic activity utilizing the growth response of the capon's comb was employed in the isolation of active androgenic substances from urine. The isolation of the urinary principle was first accomplished by Butenandt (1931), who by herculean effort obtained 15 mg of crystalline *androsterone* from 15,000 liters of male urine, and in 1932 Butenandt proposed a structural formula that was later shown by synthesis to be correct (Ruzicka *et al.*, 1934).

Further chemical investigations led to the isolation, in 1934, of another androgenic principle from urine, which differed from androsterone by having a double bond in the ring system. At first called *dehydroisoandrosterone*, this compound, *dehydroepiandrosterone*, was later shown to be an excretion product of adrenal origin.

Studies of chemical derivatives of these substances yielded new information. Thus, it was observed that androsterone acetate was as potent as the free alcohol but had a prolonged duration of action. Also, the reduction of androsterone to *androstanediol* increased activity two to three times, in much the same manner as does the reduction of estrone to estradiol.

Attention next focused on the testes as the real source of male sex hormone. It soon became evident that there were physiological and chemical differences between androsterone and the extracts of testicles. For example, active testicular extracts that were equal to androsterone in promoting comb growth in capons had a much greater effect on the seminal vesicles of castrated rats. Active testicular extracts were first prepared as early as 1927 by Loewe, using the mammalian seminal vesicle for assay (*see* Loewe and Voss, 1930). The testicular principle was isolated in crystalline form by Laqueur and associates (*see* David *et al.*, 1935), and soon its chemical structure was elucidated and the hormone synthesized (Ruzicka and Wettstein, 1935); this substance was called *testosterone*.

Testosterone is 10 times as active as androsterone in promoting comb growth in the capon, and about 70 times as potent in its action on the seminal vesicles of castrated rats. Testosterone is the true testicular hormone, and androsterone and its androgenically inert isomer, etiocholanolone or 5β-androsterone, are its major urinary excretion products. *Androstenedione*, an intermediary metabolite, is likewise intermediate in potency between testosterone and androsterone (*see* Table 69–1).

A great many other steroids with androgenic activity soon became known; some were isolated from ovarian and adrenal tissue as well as from the testis, and numerous analogs and derivatives were prepared. The acetic acid ester of testosterone was found to be more potent than testosterone and to have a greatly prolonged action. As the size of the substituent increased, activity by the cock's comb test fell off but duration of action in mammalian tests increased. In short-term tests testosterone propionate was found to be particularly potent and is still widely used in therapeutics; the cypionate (cyclopentylpropionate) and enanthate (heptanoate) esters are current long-acting preparations. 17α-Methyltestosterone was unique among 17α-substituted alkyl

1451

Table 69-1. METABOLISM OF ANDROGENS

Testosterone $\rightleftharpoons$ Androstenedione $\rightarrow$ Androsterone $+$ Etiocholanolone

derivatives in retaining androgenic potency while at the same time being active when given by mouth. The 17α-ethyl and higher derivatives were almost inert and the 17α-ethinyl was androgenically weak but active as a progestin. Efforts to improve upon methyltestosterone as an orally active androgen have been vigorously pursued. Fluoxymesterone, the 9α-fluoro-11β-hydroxy derivative of methyltestosterone, is more active than the parent compound in animal tests, and mesterolone, the 1-methyl derivative of dihydrotestosterone, is a potent, orally active androgen in man. Thus far, no nonsteroid androgen has been discovered.

The adrenal and the ovary also secrete androgenic 17-ketosteroids such as androstenedione that can be metabolized to testosterone in peripheral tissues (Baird *et al.,* 1969a; Sommerville and Collins, 1970). The 17β-hydroxysteroids are more androgenic than their 17-keto analogs (Table 69–2), and the androgenic activities of the latter may be a result of their metabolism to 17β-hydroxysteroids in tissues.

A great many derivatives of testosterone have also been prepared and tested in the search for compounds that might promote general body growth without having masculinizing effects. Such compounds are often called *anabolic steroids,* perhaps somewhat prematurely because a complete dissociation of the two effects has not yet been convincingly achieved. The degree of dissociation of the androgenic and anabolic effects with various compounds is dependent upon the bioassays used and is often

a matter of debate. Testosterone itself is one of the most potent anabolic steroids, and it may be theoretically impossible to separate the two activities totally. However, it would be highly desirable to have anabolic compounds that are not androgenic, for this would permit their use in women without inducing masculinization and in children without causing undesirable effects on sexual and osseous development.

Testosterone Synthesis and Secretion. Through poorly understood mechanisms, the pituitary begins to secrete increased amounts of luteinizing hormone (LH) and follicle-stimulating hormone (FSH) at the time of puberty. At this stage of development (about age 14 in males and age 12 in females), the pituitary becomes less sensitive to sex hormone–feedback inhibition. Prior to puberty, plasma testosterone levels are very low (0 to 13 ng/100 ml), although the immature testes are capable of synthesizing androgens if challenged. In the adult male, plasma testosterone concentrations rise to 0.2 to 1 μg/100 ml, and the production rate is 2.5 to 11 mg per day (Rosenfield, 1972). Pathways of androgen biosynthesis are shown in

Table 69-2. RELATIVE ANDROGENIC ACTIVITY OF SOME STEROIDS *†

	FOWL BIOASSAY	RODENT BIOASSAY	HUMAN VIRILIZATION
17β-Hydroxysteroids			
Dihydrotestosterone	4	4	4
Testosterone	3.5	4	4
Androstanediol-3α	3.5	3	2
Androstenediol	2.5	2	
Androstanediol-3β	0.5		
17-Ketosteroids			
Androstenedione	2.5	3	
Dehydroepiandrosterone	2	1	0

* Semiquantitative scale where 4 = most potent.

† After Rosenfield, 1972. Courtesy of *Advances in Pediatrics.*

Figure 68–1 (page 1424). In plasma, about 98% of testosterone is bound to sex hormone–binding globulin, cortisol–binding protein, and albumin; about 2% is free (*see* Fotherby and James, 1972). The free steroid is active, and its concentration correlates with androgenic effects.

Androgen-Gonadotropin Relationships. LH and FSH together are responsible for increasing testicular growth, spermatogenesis, and steroidogenesis. All of these actions are probably mediated through cyclic adenosine 3′,5′-monophosphate (cyclic AMP) (Murad *et al.*, 1969; *see* Eik-Nes, 1971). LH, also called interstitial cell–stimulating hormone (ICSH), interacts with the interstitial (Leydig) cells of the testes to increase the synthesis of cyclic AMP and subsequently the formation of androgens from acetate and cholesterol. The precise site of stimulation of steroidogenesis by cyclic AMP in this and other tissues is unknown. While the major effects of FSH are thought to be on spermatogenesis in the seminiferous tubules and that of LH on testosterone synthesis by Leydig cells, complex interactions exist in the testis. Some studies in rabbits (Johnson and Ewing, 1971) and men (*see* Sizonenko *et al.*, 1973) have indicated that FSH can also enhance testosterone synthesis and can augment the activity of LH. Furthermore, testosterone is required for spermatogenesis and maturation of sperm. With immunohisto-chemical technics, LH has been localized to Leydig and peritubular cells and FSH to tubular Sertoli cells (Castro *et al.*, 1972). The Sertoli cells of the seminiferous tubules may also produce testosterone (Lacy and Pettit, 1970). It has been speculated that the testosterone from the Sertoli cells is particularly important for spermatogenesis, and that the hormone produced by the Leydig cells is the one released into the circulation. However, both LH and FSH have growth-promoting effects on the testes, and both probably regulate testosterone synthesis. The nonphysiological effects of human chorionic gonadotropin in the male to increase testosterone synthesis appear identical to those of LH (Dufau *et al.*, 1973).

The nature of the mechanism of feedback of the testicular secretions upon the gonadotropic function of the pituitary is a problem of continuing uncertainty. Testosterone sup-presses the secretion of gonadotropins, causes atrophy of both the interstitial tissue and the tubules of the normal testis, and suppresses the excessive secretion of gonadotropins in the urine in eunuchism. The doses needed seem to be larger than one might expect. Implantation of testosterone in the median eminence of rats will inhibit pituitary gonadotropin secretion (*see* Davidson, 1969) by decreasing the level of gonadotropin-regulatory hormone (LH-RH/FSH-RH) (Mittler and Meites, 1966).

Other work has shown that certain testicular extracts devoid of androgenic activity also suppress gonadotropin, suggesting that there might be a second testicular secretion that serves a regulatory function. Excessive excretion of gonadotropin in the urine frequently accompanies pathological conditions that cause atrophy, degeneration, or sclerosis of the seminiferous tubules when the interstitial tissue seems normal or hyperplastic, and when deficient androgen is not clinically evident. This suggests that a tubular secretion, perhaps estrogen, is deficient. Conversely, in the rare association of normal spermatogenesis and deficient androgen, the syndrome of the fertile eunuch, urinary gonadotropin may be only slightly higher than normal, again suggesting that a restraining influence upon the pituitary may arise in the tubule. Because estrogens are produced in the testis and are potent inhibitors of gonadotropin secretion (*see* Chapter 68), an estrogen is thought to be the most likely candidate. In normal men, the concentrations of estradiol and estrone in the spermatic vein exceed those in peripheral plasma (Kelch *et al.*, 1972; Longcope, 1972). Indeed, other studies have indicated that the testis is the major source of estradiol in men (Saez *et al.*, 1972). However, estrogens can also be synthesized from testosterone elsewhere in the body (Lipsett *et al.*, 1966; Baird *et al.*, 1969b), and experimental evidence suggests that estrogens formed from *administered* or *endogenous* androgen may be responsible for the inhibition of gonadotropin secretion that results. Mesterolone (Table 69–3, page 1461) is a potent androgen that is methylated at C 1 on the saturated A ring and thus cannot be aromatized to an estrogen. Experiments in man with mesterolone have shown that pituitary gonadotropin is not suppressed unless very large amounts are given. Oral doses of 30 mg daily are androgenically effective, but doses as high as 150 mg daily influence neither the size nor the microscopic appearance of the testis (Laschet et al., 1967b; Petry et al., 1968). Similarly, oxandrolone (Table 69-4, page 1463), given to normal men in doses as high as 40 mg daily for 6 months, does not reduce the seminal volume or the sperm count; this compound cannot, of course, be aromatized to an estrogen. Findings such as these would suggest that the feedback effect of the testicular secretion on the gonadotropic function of the pituitary is not mediated as much by androgen as by estrogen. This untidy mechanism is unlike most endocrine interrelationships and will be suspect, pending further elucidation.

Gonadotropins are secreted in a pulsatile manner. In adult men, the plasma levels of LH, FSH, and testosterone fluctuate during the course of the day (Naftolin et al., 1973). Similar pulsations in gonadotropins are observed in women, superimposed upon the alterations occurring during the menstrual cycle (Midgley and Jaffe, 1968). At about the sixth or seventh decade of life androgen production in the male slowly declines, and men experience a *pseudoclimacteric,* which is slower in development than is the female menopause (*see* below).

Ovarian and Adrenal Androgens. As mentioned earlier, androgens are also normally secreted by the ovary and the adrenal cortex. Alterations in plasma levels of testosterone and androstenedione have been observed in women during the menstrual cycle. Two peaks of androgen concentration are seen that are qualitatively similar to those of the estrogens at the preovulatory and luteal phases of the cycle (Judd and Yen, 1973). The daily production rate of testosterone in women is about 0.5 mg, and it has been suggested that this is derived from the metabolic conversion of androstenedione to testosterone (*see* Sommerville and Collins, 1970; Rosenfield, 1972, and references therein). However, studies with rabbit ovary *in vivo* and *in vitro* have demonstrated synthesis and secretion of testosterone, which are enhanced by LH administration (Mills and Savard, 1972; Hilliard et al., 1974). In some ovarian disorders, such as the Stein-Leventhal syndrome, ovarian androgen secretion may be markedly increased, resulting in virilization.

In men about 10% of the androgen production is from the adrenal cortex. This amount is not sufficient to maintain spermatogenesis or secondary sexual features of the adult male. However, as discussed in Chapter 68, the androgens secreted by the ovary and adrenal cortex probably have physiological significance in women. In abnormal conditions such as the adrenogenital syndrome, the adrenal cortex can secrete large quantities of steroids and androgenic precursors due to a defect in steroid hydroxylation.

Physiological and Pharmacological Actions. The normal function of androgen in man is familiar to everyone in the remarkable changes of *puberty* that transform the boy into a man. Minimal androgen secretion from the infantile-sized prepuberal testis and adrenal cortex suppresses secretion of gonadotropins until, at a variable age, secretion of gonadotropins breaks out of restraints and the testis starts to enlarge. Shortly thereafter the penis and scrotum begin to grow and pubic hair appears. Almost simultaneously the remarkable growth-promoting property of androgen is revealed in a rapid increase in height and the great development of the skeletal musculature, which, with thickening of the skeleton, contributes to a rapid increase in body weight. The testes reach adult proportions before all the changes of puberty are completed. As a result of androgens, the skin becomes thicker and tends to be oily because of a proliferation of sebaceous glands; the latter are prone to infection, leading in some individuals to acne. Subcutaneous fat is lost, and the veins are prominent under the skin. Axillary hair grows, and hair on the trunk and limbs develops into a pattern typical of the male. Some degree of development of the mammary gland can be detected as a disc of firm tissue in more than half of normal boys at this stage, later to subside or to disappear altogether. Growth of the larynx causes difficulty at first in adjusting the tone of speech and later brings about a permanent deepening of the voice. Early in puberty penile erections become frequent and masturbation becomes a regular phenomenon. As the muscles grow there is increased physical vigor, which probably becomes maximal at the end of puberty or shortly thereafter.

Growth of beard lags well behind the other events of puberty and is the last of the new acquisitions to be completed. Concurrently, those whose inheritance so dictates show the first signs of growing bald, with recession of the hairline at the temples and thinning of the hair at the crown. At about this time the major spurt in growth comes to an end as the epiphyses of the larger long bones begin to unite, and over the next few years only 1 to 2 cm of additional growth is possible.

It is also thought that androgens are responsible for the aggressive and sexual behavior of males (*see* Lunde and Hamburg, 1972). However, this is an area of controversy, and some believe that behavior is predominantly acquired and not biologically determined. While this is a difficult matter to resolve, the differential behavioral patterns of many male and female animals suggest that sex hormones play an important role. Further, the sexual behavior of female rats is changed to that characteristic of males after treatment with testosterone, either as neonates or as adults (Sachs *et al.,* 1973).

When androgen is given before puberty or to a young eunuchoid man, its actions begin almost at once. Within an hour darkening of the skin from increased circulation of blood can be detected by a reflectance photometer, and within a few days dermal areas, which had been untanned by former exposure to the sun, visibly darken (Hamilton, 1948). There is also a dusky reddening of the scrotum and adjoining genital region. Within 1 or 2 days of the start of treatment erections appear, which become embarrassingly inappropriate and frequent even to the point of discomfort; with continued treatment at the same dose this excessive response subsides. Increased muscular strength and physical vigor are noted within a few days, and a general feeling of well-being prevails. Within a few weeks a distinct change in the voice can be noted, and soon thereafter the penis begins to grow and traces of axillary and pubic hair appear. The striking effects on growth are expressed without delay and, if subsequent measurements of height and weight are plotted and extrapolated backward, growth appears to have started at the beginning of treatment. The rapidity of growth is impressive; the height may increase 10 to 12.5 cm during the first year and continue at a somewhat diminished rate for 2 or 3 years. With continued treatment, development follows the course of normal puberty with the growth of a full beard as the final tribute to vigorous and successful therapy.

Eunuchism. The normal actions of androgens are also displayed by the consequences of deficiency. If the testes fail to function or are removed in boyhood, there is no puberty. A boy so afflicted continues to grow and becomes abnormally tall; the hands and feet become especially large and the limbs unduly long. The appearance and demeanor of childhood are in striking contrast to the stature; the larynx does not grow, leaving the voice high pitched and puerile. The skin remains soft and thin and develops a yellowish pallor from deficient melanin and a mild anemia; a characteristic fine wrinkling of the skin is seen about the eyes and mouth. The skeletal musculature is underdeveloped and is made still more inconspicuous by a layer of subcutaneous fat. Accumulation of fat is especially prominent around the shoulders and breasts and over the upper thighs, hips, and abdomen, the whole giving the mistaken impression of femininity. Familial baldness does not appear, the beard is scant or nonexistent, the axillary and pubic hair is very sparse, and the body hair is short and fine. The genitalia are those of a child, and there is no sexual drive.

Hypogonadism after Puberty. Some of the sexual characteristics developed during puberty are self-sustaining, while others must be supported by the continued action of androgen. Hypogonadism in the adult is typified by castration after puberty. The general bodily proportions remain the same, the penis does not shrink, the voice does not change, and the beard and body hair remain unchanged for a long time. Libido and potency are greatly reduced or annihilated, and the oft-quoted exceptions to this generalization are misleading. The prostate and seminal vesicles are atrophic, and the volume of the semen is very small or there is none at all.

Complete failure of the endocrine function of the testis in adult life is not a common event; a partial deficiency is more usual, and it often originates from an incomplete development at puberty. As mentioned earlier, testicular function commonly decreases with age; generally this occurs at a slow rate after the sixth or seventh decade, and alterations in sexual characteristics are minimal or inapparent. The decrease in libido in some men after age 40 or 50 usually cannot be attributed to altered testicular function.

Actions on the Testis and Accessory Structures. As early as fetal life, testicular androgens begin to be secreted and express their important role in the development of the reproductive tract. It has been known for some time that lack of androgens in the genotypic male fetus results in the acquisition of female sex structures (Jost, 1971). However, in the presence of the testes and endogenous androgens the Müllerian ducts of the fetus degenerate and each of the Wolffian ducts differentiates into the epididymis, vas deferens, and seminal vesicle; the penis and scrotum also develop. While differentiation of the external genitalia can be influenced by exogenous androgens, local endogenous testosterone appears to be important for differentiation of the Wolffian ducts. During the latter part of pregnancy fetal androgens begin to decline, and after birth they become undetectable in most assay systems (*see* Rosenfield, 1972).

At puberty and thereafter androgens exert a direct effect upon the testis, at least in certain species. Following hypophysectomy in the rat, shrinkage of the testis is slowed by the injection of androgen and spermatogenesis is maintained for a long time. This peculiar effect is also revealed by the biphasic response of the normal animal to androgen; moderate doses produce atrophy of the testis through suppression of gonadotropins, while with larger doses the atrophy is less because of the direct sustaining effect upon the seminiferous tubules. A great many compounds have been found to exert this effect, and some of them are only very weakly androgenic. Δ^5-Pregnenolone, for example, is highly effective but is almost devoid of androgenic potency (Selye and Albert, 1942); indeed, it has no other known endocrine or pharmacological action.

Androgens are required not only for spermatogenesis in the seminiferous tubules but also for the maturation of sperm in their passage through the epididymis and vas deferens. The nature of the effects of testosterone on sperm formation and maturation is unknown. Such studies are obviously complicated by the 10 weeks required for spermatogenesis in men and the several weeks needed for passage of sperm through the vas deferens and for maturation. In fetal, prepuberal, and puberal life the actions of testosterone result in growth of the clitoris or penis. Androgens are also required for the growth and function of the seminal vesicle and prostate. While these structures act as a reservoir for and sources of secretions that are added to semen, their precise roles are not known.

Anabolic Effects. The nitrogen-retaining effect was first measured in castrated dogs injected with androgen-containing extracts from the urine of normal men (Kochakian and Murlin, 1935). Papanicolaou and Falk (1938) showed that the skeletal muscles of male guinea pigs are much larger than those of the female, and that the difference is abolished by removal of the testes. Injection of testosterone propionate into the female or the castrated male caused pronounced muscular development. The effect of androgen could even be noted by palpation of the head; the temporal and masseter muscles show a large sex difference, but the other skeletal muscles are also involved to a lesser extent. This, at least, is a clear-cut example of a difference between the sexes. The large muscles of the male represent a sexual character dependent upon androgen for its expression, and these agents are sometimes abused by athletes for this purpose. Hypertrophy of the musculature in response to testosterone requires retention of nitrogen and other elements to build protoplasm; protein synthesis is increased.

The anabolic effects of androgen were carefully investigated by Kenyon and associates (*see* Knowlton *et al.,* 1942, and references therein), who showed that the elements required for the building of protoplasm were retained in appropriate proportion. The effects were more pronounced in eunuchoid men, in boys before puberty, and in women than in normal men. A dose of 25 mg of testosterone propionate daily caused an average retention of nitrogen of 63 mg/kg daily in eunuchoid men. There was also retention of potassium, sodium, phosphorus, sulfur, and chloride associated with a gain in weight, which could be accounted for by the water held in association with the retained salts and protein. During recovery, sodium, chloride, and water were quickly lost from the body, and phosphorus and potassium were lost less rapidly and completely, while the stored nitrogen was retained for weeks. The relatively small dose of 5 mg of testosterone propionate daily also was effective. The nitrogen retained was about half that observed after 25 mg daily, and a dose of 50 mg daily was not followed by a greater effect. The daily dose of 5 mg was not accompanied by conspicuous effects on sexual development, suggesting that androgen may normally contribute to adolescent growth at an early stage before sexual development is well advanced.

Estradiol benzoate in the large dose of 5 mg daily exerts metabolic effects similar to those observed after an equal dose of testosterone propionate. Progesterone, on the other hand, is mildly *catabolic;* daily doses of 50 or 100 mg, given intramuscularly, cause a slightly negative balance of nitrogen and a loss of salt in normal men and women (Landau *et al.,* 1955).

While many of the newer steroids used for their anabolic effects have been carefully studied in animals, their anabolic potency compared to testosterone in man is largely unknown. Furthermore, their androgenic activity in man has not been determined with any degree of accuracy. The problem would be simplified if there were some simple indicator of the action of androgen.

Effects on Sebaceous Glands. It has been shown that the prevalence of acne at puberty and during treatment with androgens is related to the growth and secretion of the sebaceous glands. Strauss and Pochi (1963) demonstrated that the effect is specific for androgens. Methyltestosterone is active in doses as small as 5 mg daily, while a dose of 2.5 mg daily of fluoxymesterone has variable effects. However, these effects are not seen in adult males, whose glands are apparently maximally stimulated. When acne results from endogenous androgen stimulation, estrogens will ameliorate this condition, probably by decreasing the secretion of gonadotropins and androgen (*see* Ebling, 1970; Chapter 68, page 1433).

Mechanism of Action. Testosterone is probably not the active form of the hormone. It is converted by a reductase in target tissues to the more active dihydrotestosterone, the

structure of which follows (*see* Liao and Fang, 1969; Wilson and Gloyna, 1970).

Dihydrotestosterone

In the curious inherited condition of male pseudohermaphroditism or in the syndrome of feminizing testes, the genotypic male undergoes normal feminine development associated with secretion from the testes of normal amounts of testosterone. Although the concentration of circulating testosterone is that of a normal man, neither the endogenous hormone nor treatment with large doses of androgen has the slightest masculinizing effect. While some studies have suggested that androstane reductase is reduced or lacking in these subjects, other work indicates that there is altered testosterone binding in plasma and target tissues (Mauvais-Jarvis *et al.,* 1971).

Dihydrotestosterone binds to a cytoplasmic protein receptor and is transferred to the nucleus; increased RNA polymerase activity and increased synthesis of specific RNA and protein result (*see* Liao and Fang, 1969; Bardin *et al.,* 1973). As with other steroid-tissue interactions these events are quite complex, and elucidation of the precise events that result in development and altered function of target tissues will require intensive investigation.

Absorption, Metabolism, and Excretion. Testosterone injected as a solution in oil is so quickly metabolized and excreted that the androgenic effect is small. Testosterone given by mouth is readily absorbed, but such administration is much less effective inasmuch as a considerable proportion of the hormone is altered by passage through the liver before reaching the systemic circulation. Attempts have been made to use absorption through the skin or through the buccal mucosa to bypass the liver and to slow absorption, but with only limited success. The testosterone esters are much less polar and, when injected in oil, greatly favor the lipid phase and are absorbed much more slowly. Testosterone propionate is much more active than testosterone even when each is injected every day, and the ester produces a steady effect when injected at 2- or 3-day intervals. Esters of the larger acids are longer acting; the cypionate and enanthate are fully effective when given at 1- or 2-week intervals in proportionately larger doses. Suspensions of testosterone or its esters in aqueous media are effective and long acting, but they sometimes cause local irritation and the rate of absorption may not always be uniform. Densely compacted pellets of testosterone implanted under the skin are an efficient source from which a steady rate of absorption continues for a long time; the last remnants may not disappear for 6 to 8 months. Some success in clinical trials has also been gained with subcutaneous implantation of silicone-rubber (SILASTIC) capsules containing testosterone to provide prolonged, continuous release of the hormone (*see* Segal, 1973, and references therein).

As mentioned earlier, testosterone in plasma is bound primarily to sex hormone–binding globulin, and about 2% is free. A reciprocal relationship exists between plasma concentrations of testosterone and the sex hormone–binding globulin, and the concentration of the globulin in females is about twice that of males. Thus, the amount of the sex hormone–binding globulin may determine the concentration of *free* testosterone in plasma and thereby its half-life, which is generally 10 to 20 minutes.

Inactivation of testosterone takes place primarily in the liver (Hudson and Coghlan, 1968; Baird *et al.,* 1969b). Metabolism of testosterone and androstenedione involves reduction of ring A to form androstanedione, with markedly reduced activity. The 3-keto group is reduced to form androsterone and its isomer etiocholanolone (Table 69–1); the 17-keto group is further reduced to form androstanediol (*see* Fotherby and James, 1972, and references therein).

After the administration of radioactive testosterone or androstenedione, about 90% of the radioactivity appears in the urine; 6% appears in the feces after undergoing enterohepatic circulation. Urinary products include primarily androsterone and etiocholanolone.

Small amounts of androstanediol and estrogens are also excreted. These steroids are in the form of glucuronide and sulfate conjugates.

Androsterone and etiocholanolone, among many other compounds, are measured as *17-ketosteroids* in the usual clinical tests, but the major fraction of the ketosteroids of urine consists of metabolic products of secretions of the adrenal cortex. About 30% of urinary 17-ketosteroids are derived from metabolism of testicular hormones. Thus, measurement of the excretion of 17-ketosteroids is a poor test for the functional activity of the testis and is a much better index of adrenocortical function. Low values point to adrenal insufficiency rather than to hypogonadism, and high values almost always are indicative of adrenocortical hyperactivity or tumor. Without the testes, the human male is nearly depleted of androgen even though the urinary 17-ketosteroids may be within the normal range. In women, if pronounced virilization is associated with normal or nearly normal excretion of ketosteroids, an ovarian tumor producing testosterone is likely, whereas high values point to an adrenocortical origin of the disorder.

The esters of testosterone are metabolized in much the same way as is testosterone itself, but other changes in the molecule (as in methyltestosterone and fluoxymesterone) alter the course of metabolic degradation. Such synthetic androgens are metabolized to a lesser degree than is testosterone and have longer half-lives. Unaltered compounds, metabolites, and conjugates are excreted in the urine and feces (Fotherby and James, 1972).

Assays. Androgens used in therapeutics are pure substances, and the doses are measured by weight. Bioassay is used in the evaluation of androgenic potency of new compounds and of compounds used primarily as progestins or for their anabolic effect. The classical assay based upon the growth of the comb of the capon is still used.

Better parallelism with clinical effectiveness is given by bioassays in mammals, and the most widely used test depends upon the growth of the seminal vesicles or ventral prostate of the castrated rat.

However, in clinical laboratories quite different assays are widely used; they include the use of sex hormone–binding globulin as well as sensitive and specific radioimmunoassays (*see* Niswender and Midgley, 1970; Vande Wiele and Dyrenfurth, 1973). These methods offer several advantages over bioassay methods; the more notable are simplicity, sensitivity, and lower cost.

Bioassay for Anabolic Potency. An early observation on a dissociation of the effects of androgens was made by Kochakian (1947). In the mouse the kidney is larger in the male than in the female and regresses in size upon castration. The normal male proportions are restored by testosterone and by a variety of other androgens, some of which, such as methylandrostanediol, are androgenically weak. Also, estradiol given with testosterone reduces the response of the seminal vesicles and ventral prostate without impairing the growth of the kidney.

A systematic search for nonandrogenic anabolic steroids has made use of the growth of the levator ani muscle of the castrated rat as an assay, a method developed by Eisenberg and Gordan (1950) and Hershberger and coworkers (1953). The limitations of the method became apparent when the findings were not always borne out by other tests or by actual clinical trials. It is perhaps unfortunate that this particular muscle was chosen as an indicator of "myotropic" activity because it is intimately associated with the genital organs and its response to androgens is not shared by the rest of the skeletal musculature.

Another test for anabolic activity is in the rat given an amount of food just sufficient to maintain a constant body weight. Measurement of the excretion of nitrogen before and after giving the substance to be tested provides an index to nitrogen-retaining potency (Arnold *et al.,* 1959). Stucki and associates (1960) have used the oophorectomized rhesus monkey under strictly controlled environmental conditions and on a constant diet, and measured the nitrogen-retaining effect of steroids. This technic is difficult, expensive, and time consuming, and only a limited number of compounds have been tested in this way.

Preparations and Dosage. Some of the preparations of androgens available for clinical use are summarized in Table 69–3. Additional, little used esters of testosterone (phenylacetate, ketolaurate) are also available.

When full replacement therapy with androgen is required, the intramuscular preparations are the most effective. Dosage should provide at least 10 mg per day; with testosterone propionate this is met by giving 25 mg three times weekly. With the longer-acting esters, which may be somewhat less efficient, the dose is about 200 mg every 2 weeks. Long-term treatment with these doses may not cause full masculine development; there may still be remnants of a eunuchoid habitus, poorly developed muscles, and a sparse beard.

Preparations Used for Their Anabolic Effects. Some of these preparations are summarized in Table 69-4. These compounds have been introduced primarily for use as anabolic agents with the expectation that they would be relatively less androgenic than testosterone and its close relatives. None is free of androgenic activity in man, and in many instances the androgenicity is much greater than the results of animal tests had predicted. Some have come to be used primarily as androgens, and many have

been applied in the palliative treatment of carcinoma of the breast. The very small doses recommended for some of the compounds have detectable anabolic activity without noticeable androgenic effects.

Various mixtures of androgenic and anabolic steroids with estrogens, vitamins, and other agents are also available. However, their use is to be discouraged since there are no clinical indications for such fixed-dose combinations.

Untoward Effects. When used in women, all the androgens carry the risk of causing masculinization. Among the earliest of the undesirable manifestations are acne, the growth of facial hair, and hoarsening or deepening of the voice, and these are the very features that women most dislike. Menstrual irregularities will occur if gonadotropin secretion is suppressed. If treatment is discontinued as soon as these are noticed, they slowly subside. With continued treatment, as in the use of androgen in mammary carcinoma, there may also develop the male pattern of baldness, excessive body hair, prominent musculature and veins, and hypertrophy of the clitoris, all largely irreversible phenomena. With prolonged treatment the deepening of the voice is also irreversible.

The adverse consequences of giving androgens to young children are not fully understood. Serious disturbances of growth and of sexual and osseous development can occur, and the effects of androgens to enhance epiphyseal closure in children may continue for as long as several months after administration. Anabolic agents should be used with great care in children.

Edema. Retention of water in association with sodium chloride appears to be a constant sequel to the administration of androgen and accounts for a portion of the gain in weight, at least in short-term treatment. In the doses used to treat hypogonadism, the retention of water usually does not lead to detectable edema, but edema may become troublesome when large doses are given in the treatment of neoplastic diseases. Water and electrolyte retention is undesirable in patients with heart failure or in patients prone to edema from some other cause, such as cirrhosis of the liver, renal disease, or hypoproteinemia. Edema may limit the use of large doses of androgen for their anabolic effects in states of malnutrition. Salt and water retention from androgens responds to the administration of natriuretics and use can

Table 69-3. SOME ANDROGENIC STEROIDS USED IN THERAPY

NONPROPRIETARY NAME	SOME TRADE NAMES	CHEMICAL STRUCTURE	DOSAGE FORMS	USUAL CLINICAL DOSAGE SCHEDULES FOR ANDROGEN DEFICIENCY *
Testosterone, N.F.	NEO-HOMBREOL F ORETON (many others)		Aqueous suspension: 25 to 50 mg/ml for i.m. use Pellets: 75 mg for s.c. use	I.M.: 50 mg three times weekly S.C.: 4 pellets (300 mg) every 4 to 6 months
Testosterone Propionate, U.S.P.	NEO-HOMBREOL ORETON PROPIONATE (many others)	$O-COCH_2CH_3$	Tablets: 10 mg Aqueous suspension or oily solution: 25, 50, and 100 mg/ml for i.m. use	Buccal: 10 to 20 mg daily I.M.: 25 mg two to four times weekly
Testosterone Enanthate, U.S.P.	DELATESTRYL (many others)	$O-CO(CH_2)_5CH_3$	Oily solution: 100 and 200 mg/ml for i.m. use	I.M.: 100 to 400 mg every 2 to 4 weeks
Testosterone Cypionate, U.S.P.	DEPO-TESTOSTERONE (many others)	$O-COCH_2CH_2$	Oily solution: 50 to 200 mg/ml for i.m. use	I.M.: 100 to 400 mg every 2 to 4 weeks

Methyltestosterone, U.S.P.

METANDREN
NEO-HOMBREOL M
ORETON METHYL
(many others)

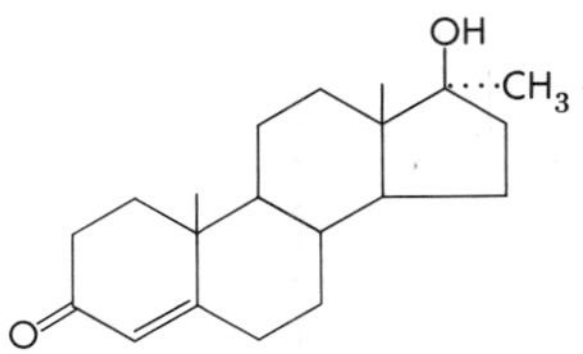

Tablets: 5, 10, and 25 mg

Buccal: 5 to 25 mg daily
Oral: 10 to 50 mg daily

Fluoxymesterone, U.S.P.

HALOTESTIN
ORA-TESTRYL
ULTANDREN

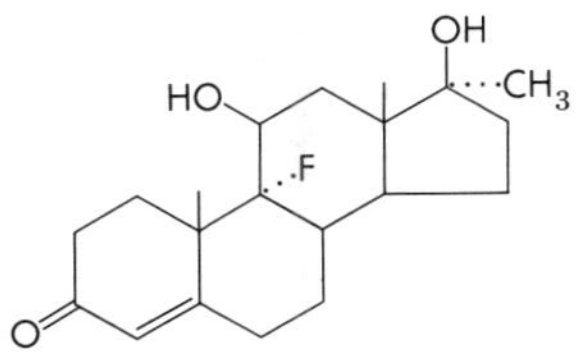

Tablets: 2, 5, and 10 mg

Oral: 2 to 30 mg daily

Mesterolone

ANDROVIRON
PROVIRON

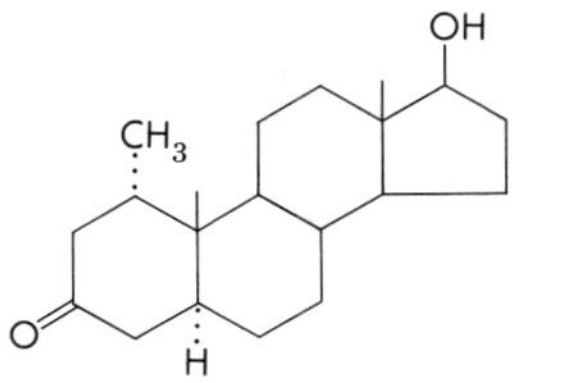

Tablets: 25 mg

Oral: 50 to 100 mg daily

* Dosage schedules for breast carcinoma in females are generally two to three times those for androgen replacement.

1461

Table 69-4. SOME ANABOLIC STEROIDS USED IN THERAPY

NONPROPRIETARY NAME	SOME TRADE NAMES	CHEMICAL STRUCTURE	DOSAGE FORMS	USUAL CLINICAL DOSAGE SCHEDULES FOR ANABOLIC EFFECTS
Dromostanolone Propionate, N.F.	DROLBAN		Oily solution: 50 mg/ml for i.m. use	I.M.: 100 mg three times weekly (for breast carcinoma)
Ethylestrenol *	MAXIBOLIN		Elixir: 2 mg/5 ml Tablets: 2 mg	Oral: 4 to 8 mg daily
Methandriol	STENEDIOL (many others)		Tablets: 50 mg	Oral: 50 to 150 mg daily
Methandrostenolone, N.F.	DIANABOL		Tablets: 2.5 and 5 mg	Oral: 5 mg daily

Nandrolone Decanoate, N.F.

DECA-DURABOLIN

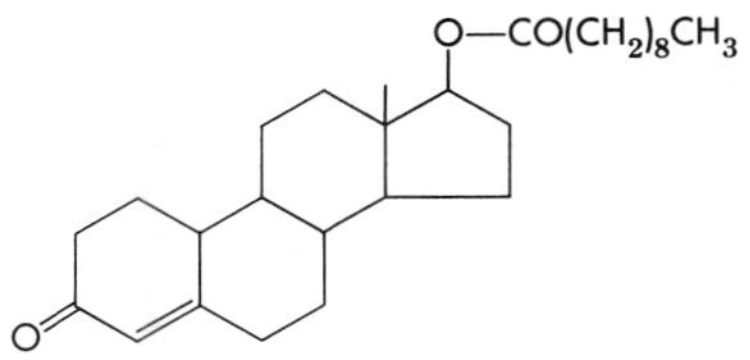

$O-CO(CH_2)_8CH_3$

Oily solution: 50 and
100 mg/ml for i.m. use

I.M.: 50 to 100 mg every
3 to 4 weeks

Nandrolone Phenpropionate, N.F.

DURABOLIN

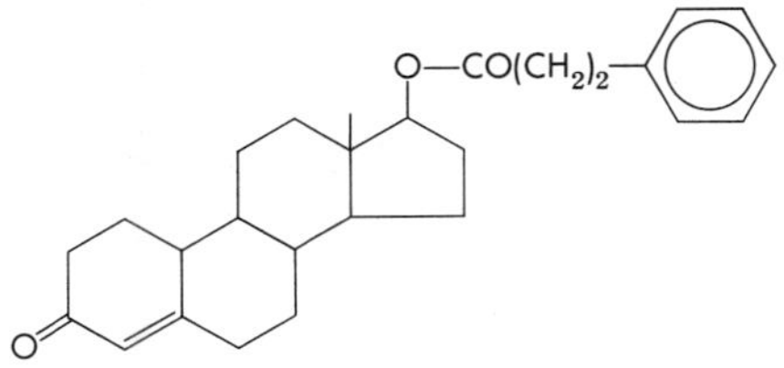

$O-CO(CH_2)_2$

Oily solution: 25 and
50 mg/ml for i.m. use

I.M.: 25 to 50 mg weekly

Norethandrolone *

NILEVAR

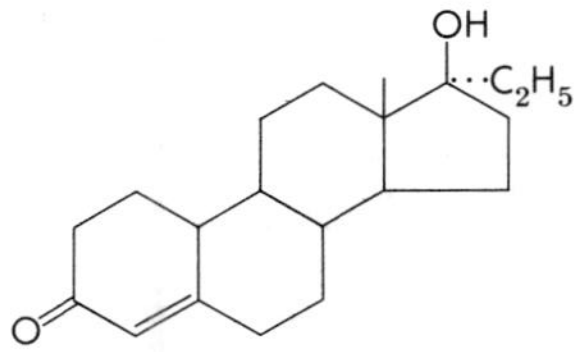

OH
C_2H_5

Liquid: 8.3 mg/ml
Tablets: 10 mg
Oily solution: 25 mg/ml
for i.m. use

Oral: 25 to 50 mg daily
I.M.: 25 to 50 mg daily

Oxandrolone, N.F.

ANAVAR

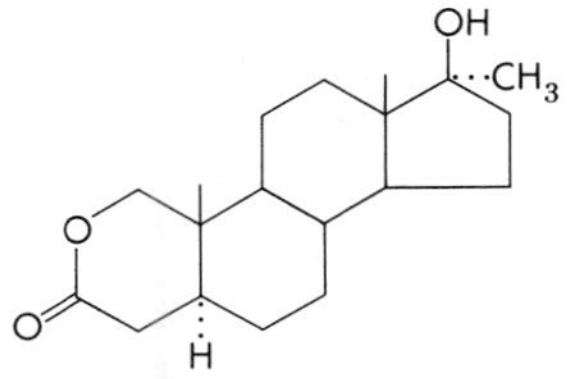

OH
CH_3
H

Tablets: 2.5 mg

Oral: 5 to 10 mg daily

* Not available in the United States.

1463

Table 69–4. SOME ANABOLIC STEROIDS USED IN THERAPY (Continued)

NONPROPRIETARY NAME	SOME TRADE NAMES	CHEMICAL STRUCTURE	DOSAGE FORMS	USUAL CLINICAL DOSAGE SCHEDULES FOR ANABOLIC EFFECTS
Oxymetholone, N.F.	ADROYD ANADROL		Tablets: 2.5, 5, 10, and 50 mg	Oral: 5 to 15 mg daily (as much as 50 to 100 mg daily for anemia)
Stanolone *	ANABOLEX ANDROLONE NEODROL		Tablets: 25 mg Aqueous suspension: 50 mg/ml for i.m. use	Oral: 50 to 100 mg daily I.M.: 100 mg daily
Stanozolol, N.F.	WINSTROL		Tablets: 2 mg	Oral: 6 mg daily
Testolactone, N.F.	TESLAC		Tablets: 50 mg Aqueous suspension: 100 mg/ml for i.m. use	Oral: 150 mg daily I.M.: 100 mg three times weekly (for breast carcinoma)

* Not available in the United States.

1464

be made of this effect to differentiate between growth of protoplasm and gain in weight from expansion of the volume of extracellular fluid.

Jaundice. Methyltestosterone was the first of a number of therapeutic agents discovered to cause a type of liver damage called cholestatic hepatitis. Jaundice is the prominent clinical feature, and the underlying disturbance is stasis and accumulation of bile in the biliary capillaries of the central portion of the lobules, without obstruction in the larger ducts. The contiguous hepatic cells exhibit only minor histological changes and remain viable. This condition is not seen with testosterone or its esters, but steroids with a 17α-methyl substituent are particularly apt to cause it. These include fluoxymesterone, methandrostenolone, 17α-methyl-19-nortestosterone, oxymetholone, and stanozolol. Other steroids substituted in the 17α position also cause the reaction. Norethandrolone (17α-ethyl-19-nortestosterone) has been extensively studied; although frank jaundice is unusual, doses of the order of 25 to 50 mg daily frequently cause some increase in bilirubin and in glutamic-oxaloacetic transaminase and reduced elimination of sulfobromophthalein (Kory *et al.*, 1959; Perez-Mera and Shields, 1962). The response is clearly dependent on dose and becomes a frequent complication when very large amounts are given, as for palliation in neoplastic diseases. With 17α-methyl-19-nortestosterone, for example, given in doses of 30 mg daily, some increase in circulating bilirubin is an almost constant finding (Feldman and Carter, 1960). As even small doses of compounds such as methyltestosterone are metabolized with difficulty by the liver, large doses can be expected to have cumulative effects and to result in the building-up of large amounts of the substance or a metabolite in the body. It has become common practice in the use of the 17α-substituted steroids to give short courses of treatment of 3 or 4 weeks each, interrupted by free intervals of similar length.

Methyltestosterone produces creatinuria, as also do 17α-methylandrostenediol and 17α-methylandrostanediol (*see* Wilkins and Fleischmann, 1945). Again, the esters of testosterone do not have this effect. It seems unlikely that it is merely a coincidence that

the 17α-methyl steroids cause both cholestatic jaundice and creatinuria, but it must be admitted that no causal connection between these two events can be envisioned.

Hepatic Carcinoma. There have been several reports describing relatively small numbers of patients who had received androgens and anabolic steroids for prolonged periods and who developed hepatic adenocarcinoma (Bernstein *et al.*, 1971; Johnson *et al.*, 1972; Henderson *et al.*, 1973). All the patients described received 17-alkyl derivatives for aplastic anemia for 1 to 7 years. These isolated case reports make additional surveillance mandatory in order to evaluate this possible complication.

Steroid Fever. Etiocholanolone, a major excretory metabolite of testosterone that is inactive as an androgen, had always been considered to be pharmacologically inert until Kappas and coworkers (1958) discovered that the administration of the compound intramuscularly to human beings caused an intense local inflammatory response. Subjects developed a prompt rise in body temperature to 103° to 105° F, accompanied by chills and followed by malaise and all the other features of a fever. Other compounds later found to cause fever include 11β-hydroxyetiocholanolone, pregnanediol, pregnanolone, 11-ketopregnanolone, and lithocholic acid. The effect is much less prominent in females because of estrogen antagonism (Wolff *et al.*, 1973) and is not seen in several other species. It is also more pronounced following intramuscular than intravenous injection. The local reaction after intramuscular injection and the frequent induction of thrombophlebitis upon intravenous injection point to the importance of local inflammation in the syndrome. Administration of hydrocortisone at the site of injection of etiocholanolone to diminish the local inflammatory response reduces the fever. Whether the thermogenic response to progesterone, as in the luteal phase of the menstrual cycle, is to be regarded as a similar phenomenon is not clear, and the part played by these steroids in various febrile states in man is still unsettled. It is unlikely that fever will ever be a side effect of therapy with androgens because the compounds known to cause fever are not used therapeutically.

Impotence and Azoospermia. While androgens are required for spermatogenesis and may maintain spermatogenesis for prolonged periods in animals after hypophysectomy, continued use of androgens may result in azoospermia due to inhibition of gonadotropin secretion and conversion to estrogens. After administration of 25 mg of testosterone propionate daily for 6 weeks, spermatogenesis declines. Anabolic steroids may produce the same effect, and since they can also suppress endogenous testosterone production, they can lead to impotence after their withdrawal. Sustained and painful penile erections (*priapism*) are seen with initial androgen-replacement therapy.

Local Irritation. Buccal and sublingual preparations may result in stomatitis, and implantation of androgen-containing pellets may produce localized inflammation.

Therapeutic Uses. The outstanding therapeutic indication for the androgens is deficient endocrine function of the testes. Their use as anabolic agents, although of much wider potential application, is still in the stage of exploration.

Hypogonadism. Failure of the testis to secrete androgen usually cannot be recognized in childhood and is first to be seriously considered when the changes of puberty seem to be delayed. However, there is some evidence that cryptorchism may be associated with primary testicular defects and eventual androgen deficiency.

The age of onset of puberty varies widely among individuals, and, when there is no evidence of maturation at age 15 to 17, there may be great concern on the part of the patient and his parents. There is a good deal of debate about the use of androgen to hasten the changes of puberty in normal boys with delayed sexual maturation. Most physicians would agree that androgens should be withheld if parental pressures can be overcome.

Patients with delayed puberty should be evaluated for pituitary as well as gonadal function. If growth hormone deficiency is also present, androgens should be withheld until acceptable height is achieved with human growth hormone (*see* below). If puberal changes are to be induced with an androgen, it can be given in courses of 4 to 6 months at a time, and stopped for like periods to ascertain whether the testes are enlarging and development is progressing spontaneously. The secretion of gonadotropins must also be reevaluated after discontinuation of androgens.

When there is complete testicular failure and puberty cannot occur, prolonged therapy is required. One of the long-acting esters of testosterone, such as the cypionate or the enanthate, may be given intramuscularly in a dose of about 200 mg every 1 or 2 weeks for a period of 2 to 3 years, and in a similar dose monthly thereafter for maintenance. Testosterone propionate in a dose of 50 mg three times weekly is effective and might be used initially, but for prolonged treatment it is inconvenient.

Methyltestosterone in the recommended dose of 30 to 50 mg daily or fluoxymesterone in a 10- to 20-mg dose daily has been used, but experienced observers find that the androgenic response is limited in patients with gonadotropin deficiency and that even larger doses fail to bring about complete sexual development (*see* McCullagh and Schaffenburg, 1954; Wilkins, 1965; Paulsen, 1974). This does not appear to be the case with patients with primary testicular failure. It is advantageous to initiate treatment of adolescents with small doses and to increase these gradually over the first 6 months or year. Presumably the oral preparations are satisfactory for this purpose, and the gradual changes of early puberty should thereby be duplicated.

When hypogonadism starts in adult life and the maturation of puberty has already come about, it is customary to use somewhat smaller doses as replacement therapy than are used in the undeveloped eunuch. Long-acting esters of testosterone in doses of 200 mg every month may be sufficient, and even methyltestosterone or fluoxymesterone in full doses may be effective.

It is a common clinical observation that individuals with hypogonadism repeatedly discontinue therapy for unstated reasons of their own. They seem to prefer their abnormal state, to which they have adapted through long effort. Perhaps the stresses of an artificial puberty are more uncomfortable than we realize, or perhaps the management of dosage is not as skillful as it might be.

Hypopituitarism. As long as human growth hormone is not readily available, androgen will unfortunately be needed as a growth-promoting agent in the treatment of childhood dwarfism due to hypopituitarism. These children are given replacement doses of thyroid and a suitable corticosteroid. Treatment with androgen is not given until the age of puberty, so that the time of sexual development will be appropriate. Therapy should be deferred even longer if possible in the hope of achieving a maximal increase in height. As an increase of about 30 cm (1 ft) is all that can be expected before growth ceases from closure of the epiphyses, treatment is most satisfactory if a height of 1.2 m (4 ft) or so has been achieved spontaneously. Obviously less growth is achieved in those individuals with advanced radiological bone age. In boys, the same schedule of treatment as that in hypogonadism has been used, and acceleration of growth has been recorded that is just as rapid as in individuals with a normal pituitary. In girls, large doses of androgen cannot be given and treatment with estrogen induces only a slight acceleration of growth. Martin and Wilkins (1958) achieved a substantial spurt in growth by the use of 10 to 20 mg of methyltestosterone with 1 mg of diethylstilbestrol daily. There was no virilization and feminine sexual development was normal, including a normal development of axillary and pubic hair. If the methyltestosterone was stopped and the diethylstilbestrol continued, the body hair was lost only to regrow when the androgen was given again. It would seem reasonable in both sexes to give only small doses during the first year or so of treatment, in the expectation that a greater increment of growth would be achieved before the epiphyses unite. The reason for this conjecture is twofold: the property of androgen to cause closure of the epiphyses was not definitely established until effective preparations of the hormone became plentiful and large doses were used, and small doses of androgen can exert various anabolic effects without pronounced effects upon sexual maturation.

To Accelerate Growth in Childhood. The advisability of using anabolic-androgenic steroids in children is a much-debated question, and no authoritative answer can yet be given. There are many causes of dwarfism, and a few of these can be remedied. Androgens have been used successfully to promote growth in girls with Turner's syndrome (gonadal dysgenesis) (Johanson *et al.,* 1969). In many instances no cause can be found for short stature, and it is here that the question of the advisability of treatment with androgenic-anabolic steroids arises.

Some children with short stature are diagnosed as having *constitutional delay of growth and development* and will eventually attain normal height and sexual development. While treatment should if possible be delayed or withheld, patients and parents may request therapy. Androgens given before puberty reproduce not only the normal puberal spurt in growth but also the inevitable fusion of the epiphyses that puts an end to linear growth. It is possible that doses may be found that promote growth without closing the epiphyses, or perhaps favorable results will be obtained with courses of treatment extending over a few months and alternating with like intervals without treatment. Some compounds, for example, oxandrolone, have been observed to favor growth over epiphyseal maturation (Ray *et al.,* 1965), suggesting that useful effects may be achieved with proper dosage.

The younger the child the greater is the risk of compromising the final mature height. In teen-agers in whom delayed puberty is the reason for short stature, careful treatment with androgen is probably justified. Treatment for a 6-month period might be given with the following drugs, in the indicated daily doses: oxandrolone, 0.1 mg/kg; methandrostenolone, 0.04 mg/kg; ethylestrenol, 0.1 to 0.2 mg/kg; or methyltestosterone, in a total daily dose of 5 mg or less (Sobel, 1968). If positive effects, such as growth or sexual maturation, are seen, treatment might be discontinued for 6 months to observe whether spontaneous puberty has supervened; if it has not, further courses could be given. In younger children, the decision to use this form of treatment is more difficult to make; it is usually undertaken as a last resort and always with awareness of the risk of limiting mature stature.

Use in Aging Men. There is a good deal of continuing debate about the question of a male counterpart to the menopause of women. It is clear that castration in the adult is frequently followed by symptoms typical of the menopause that can be relieved by androgen. It is also well established that the various indices of testicular function show a very gradual decline with advancing years. These include reduced libido, reduced sexual activity, and lessened muscular size and strength. On the average there is a slight rise in urinary gonadotropin with age, with wide individual variation (Albert, 1956) and a similarly variable decline in the volume of the semen and the total number of spermatozoa. Although there is normally no sharp decline in the endocrine function of the testes to justify the term *climacteric,* in analogy with the condition in women, reduction of testicular function seems to be a normal process in older men. Androgen replacement in aging men has not been convincingly shown to be beneficial.

Osteoporosis. As discussed in Chapter 68, androgens and estrogens can improve calcium balance and decrease bone resorption when given to patients with osteoporosis (Lafferty *et al.,* 1964; Riggs *et al.,* 1969). However, these effects of continuous steroid treatment last only for 9 to 14 months. Riggs and co-workers (1972) also demonstrated that after 1 or 2 years of therapy bone formation declines and this counteracts the beneficial effects of androgens. It is not known if this apparent refractoriness to therapy can be overcome with interrupted courses of steroids.

Menstrual Disorders. Heretofore androgens were used in a variety of menstrual disorders, but they have been supplanted by the more effective, orally active progestins and combination contraceptives (*see* Chapter 68).

Anemia. McCullagh and Jones (1942) were the first to show that the mild anemia of eunuchoid individuals can be corrected by replacement therapy with androgen. It was later noted that large doses of androgen sometimes caused excessive erythropoiesis, leading to moderate polycythemia, and advantage was taken of this effect by Gardner and Pringle (1961) in the treatment of hypoplastic anemia and the anemia of neoplastic disease. Doses as high as 1.2 g per week of testosterone enanthate and 200 mg per day of methyltestosterone were used. There was a slight reticulocytosis and an increase in erythrocytes and hemoglobin. There was, of course, intense virilization but no other untoward effect except jaundice from methyltestosterone. The effects of androgens on erythrocyte formation explain the normally higher hematocrit in males.

Androgenic-anabolic steroids are now widely used in the treatment of aplastic anemia, red-cell aplasia, hemolytic anemias, and the anemias associated with renal failure, myeloid metaplasia, lymphoma, leukemia, and various other disorders. Androgens are the most useful nonspecific stimulants of erythropoiesis (*see* Shahidi, 1973, and references therein). Although the response of the bone marrow varies in different conditions, erythropoiesis is stimulated first and most consistently, leukopenia is ameliorated later, and improvement in thrombocytopenia occurs last. Androgens and anabolic steroids are effective in less than half of the patients treated, and up to 3 months may be needed to see an increase in red blood cells and longer for increases in neutrophils and platelets (Li *et al.,* 1972). The consensus is that these agents are beneficial in milder cases and probably of little or no benefit in severe anemia. However, with the poor prognosis of many of these diseases, most agree that a therapeutic trial is appropriate.

The doses of androgenic-anabolic steroids used have been large, and it is not known if smaller doses are effective. Weekly injections of esters of testosterone in doses of 600 mg to 1 g are used. Many other agents, including nandrolone decanoate and oxymetholone, have also been used in variable amounts with success.

The mechanism of action has been sought in the

stimulation of secretion of erythropoietin by the kidney. Although such an action can be shown under some circumstances, androgens have also been found to stimulate directly the synthesis of heme, an action potentiated by erythropoietin. The response of the other elements of the bone marrow suggests a direct effect thereon of the androgenic-anabolic agents.

Promotion of Anabolism. Androgenic-anabolic steroids have been used in a wide assortment of conditions, ranging from postoperative recovery to chronic debilitating diseases. Studies of various designs have shown that the androgens reduce the negative nitrogen balance and may convert a mildly negative balance to a positive one. The effects are intimately related to the intake of protein and the total caloric intake, and, depending upon the conditions, a small increase in either one of these may have a greater effect than the administration of the anabolic agent. While few would disagree that these agents are anabolic and may induce short-term effects, it seems unlikely that their use has altered the outcome of, or shortened the recovery from, the underlying illness. However, they promote a feeling of well-being and improve appetite, and their use in terminal diseases cannot be criticized.

Suppression of Lactation. As discussed in Chapter 68, estrogens and progestins are used when it is advisable to decrease post-partum lactation. Androgens have also proven very effective. Side effects are not seen or are minimal with the administration of 50 to 100 mg of esters of testosterone for 1 to 4 days post partum. Oral preparations are used for 4 to 6 days. These agents should be started at the time of delivery.

Breast Carcinoma. Androgens are used as a palliative measure for recurrent and metastatic carcinoma of the breast in postmenopausal patients and in premenopausal patients after prior oophorectomy (*see* Chapter 62). The use of endocrine organ ablation and hormonal therapy for breast carcinoma was prompted by studies of an altered incidence of mammary tumors in rodents after castration or treatment with estrogens and androgens. The use of these measures in women, however, has been largely empirical. Recent attempts to demonstrate hormonal dependence of an individual patient's tumor *in vitro* may provide a more rational basis for such therapy. Decrease in bone pain and improvement in subjective symptoms occur in about 20 to 30% of patients. Remissions may take 3 months to develop and may last 6 to 12 months. If androgens are used, they are given in large doses such as 50 to 100 mg of testosterone propionate three times a week. In addition to side effects discussed above, some patients with metastases to bone develop hypercalcemia during therapy, an indication to withdraw the androgen. Androgens are contraindicated in men with breast carcinoma.

ANTIANDROGENS

A search for compounds that might inhibit the action of androgen was doubtless prompted by clinical considerations. Treat-

ment of cancer of the prostate was one of the earlier aims; however, the uses of potent antagonists might range from virilization in women to precocious puberty in boys, and from acne to satyriasis. These compounds might also be valuable as male contraceptives. Recent developments suggest that some of these aspirations may be fulfilled in the foreseeable future.

Estrogens, in a restricted sense, may be regarded as antiandrogenic. They may have actions of their own upon genital tissues, which differ from those of androgens and in this way seem to antagonize androgen.

Progesterone comes nearer to being an antiandrogen, albeit a very weak one, and some of the more potent antiandrogens now known are derivatives of progesterone. Two other weak antiandrogens with no known hormonal activity of any other kind are the derivatives dodecahydrophenanthrene (Randall and Selitto, 1958) and A-norprogesterone; the former somewhat resembles progesterone lacking a D ring; the latter is progesterone with one carbon atom missing from ring A (Lerner, 1964). Several other steroids also have weak antiandrogenic activity, although most studies have been confined to animals.

Nonsteroidal antiandrogens have also been examined in animals and in systems *in vitro*. These compounds block the action or synthesis of testosterone and include dimethanesulfonate derivatives, N-(3,5-dimethyl-4-isoxazolylmethyl) phthalimide (DIMP), 4'-nitro-3'-trifluoromethylisobutyranilide, and cyanoketone.

Cyproterone Acetate. In the search for orally active progestins, steroids with a 1,2α-methylene substitution were found to be antiandrogenic. Cyproterone acetate is among the most potent, and its structure is as follows:

Cyproterone Acetate

While it is a potent antiandrogen, it also possesses progestational, androgenic, and antiestrogenic activities. Treatment of the pregnant rat with 1 or 10 mg daily led to the remarkable finding that the male fetuses were "feminized," the penis was underdeveloped and resembled a clitoris, the prostate was missing, and the testes were small and undescended. These changes were permanent (Hamada *et al.*, 1963).

In the mature rat, the compound causes atrophy of the seminal vesicles, prostate, levator ani muscle, and other androgen-responsive organs, as well as cellular changes in the pituitary typical of castration with increased gonadotropin secretion (Neumann, 1966). This latter effect is not observed in men (Jackson and Jones, 1972). The testes are unaffected by small or moderate doses, although larger doses can decrease Leydig cell function and spermatogenesis. In the castrated animal, only about five times as much antagonist as testosterone is needed to reduce the androgenic response by 50%. With large doses of cyproterone acetate the antagonism is almost complete (Neumann *et al.*, 1970).

Laschet and associates (1967a) gave doses of 100 to 200 mg daily to men suffering from severe deviations in sexual behavior and noted that male sexuality virtually disappeared in 10 to 14 days. The effect passed off within 2 weeks after discontinuing treatment; no gynecomastia or other side effects were noted. This loss of libido when the drug is given to males certainly detracts from its possible use as a male contraceptive. The results of trials of the compound in the treatment of hirsutism and virilism in women and for acne have not been consistent, perhaps because quite different dosages have been used. Several studies have been encouraging with regard to its use in prostatic carcinoma (*see* Wein and Murphy, 1973, and references therein). Although cyproterone acetate is the most active antiandrogen so far encountered, closely related analogs are also active. The free alcohol is only about one third as active as the acetate and, surprisingly, is devoid of progestational activity, whereas the acetate is one of the most potent progestins known. Antiandrogen drugs are still in the investigational stage and are not yet generally available.

MALE CONTRACEPTIVES

There are many requirements of the ideal contraceptive drug: simplicity, acceptability, reversibility, lack of toxicity, and, of course, efficacy. Although all these criteria have not even been attained in the oral contraceptives for women, the agents discussed in Chapter 68 seem to come very close. In this respect, women have been liberated long before men. Recent clinical studies of inhibition of spermatogenesis and fertility provide some indication that pharmacological contraception in men will become available, and an optimistic estimate for realization of this aim would be 5 to 10 years.

A variety of compounds, in addition to the antiandrogens discussed above, can inhibit spermatogenesis. These include antineoplastic agents, cadmium, nitrofuranes, α-chlorhydrin, and dinitropyrrole (*see* Jackson and Jones, 1972). However, the irreversible effects of some and the toxicity of many preclude their clinical use. Studies in animals, including primates, have resulted in a rational approach to this problem with androgens, estrogens, progestins, and their combinations.

Perhaps the most promising approach to date is the dual administration of an androgen and progestin. Preliminary clinical trials in which patients received continuous testosterone and a progestin (usually administered in the form of silicone-rubber capsule implants) have resulted in sterility with minimal side effects. The rationale for this combination is to suppress gonadotropin secretion and spermatogenesis with a progestin and to prevent alteration of accessory sexual structures with simultaneous testosterone administration (*see* Segal, 1973, and references therein).

Arnold, A.; Beyler, A. L.; and Potts, C. O. Androstanazole, a new orally active anabolic steroid. *Proc. Soc. exp. Biol. Med.,* **1959,** *102,* 184–187.

Baird, D. T.; Uno, A.; and Melby, J. C. Adrenal secretions of androgens and oestrogens. *J. Endocr.,* **1969a,** *45,* 135–136.

Bernstein, M. S.; Hunter, R. L.; and Yachnin, S. Hepatoma and peliosis hepatitis in Fanconi's anemia. *New Engl. J. Med.,* **1971,** *284,* 1135–1136.

Brown-Séquard, C. E. Des effets produits chez l'homme par des injections souscutanées d'un liquide retiré des testicules frais de cobaye et de chien. *C. r. Séanc. Soc. Biol.,* **1889,** *1,* 420–430.

Butenandt, A. Über die chemische Untersuchung der Sexualhormons. *Z. angew. Chem.,* **1931,** *44,* 905–908.

Castro, A. E.; Alonso, A.; and Mancini, R. E. Localization of follicle stimulating and luteinizing hormones in the rat testis using immunohistological tests. *J. Endocr.,* **1972,** *52,* 129–136.

David, K.; Dingemanse, E.; Freud, J.; and Laquer, E. Über krystallinisches männliches Hormon aus Hoden (Testosteron), wirksamer als aus Harn oder aus Cholesterin bereitetes Androsteron. *Hoppe-Seyler's Z. physiol. Chem.,* **1935,** *233,* 281–282.

Dufau, M. L.; Watanabe, K.; and Catt, K. J. Stimulation of cyclic AMP production by the rat testis during incubation with hCG *in vitro. Endocrinology,* **1973,** *92,* 6–11.

Eisenberg, E., and Gordan, G. S. The levator ani muscle of the rat as an index of myotrophic activity of steroidal hormones. *J. Pharmac. exp. Ther.,* **1950,** *99,* 38–44.

Feldman, E. B., and Carter, A. C. Endocrinologic and

metabolic effects of 17α-methyl-19-nortestosterone in women. *J. clin. Endocr. Metab.,* **1960,** *20,* 842–857.

Forbes, T. R. Crowing hen: early observations on spontaneous sex reversal in birds. *Yale J. Biol. Med.,* **1947,** *19,* 955–970.

Gardner, F. H., and Pringle, J. C. Androgens and erythropoiesis. I. Preliminary clinical observations. *Archs intern. Med.,* **1961,** *107,* 846–862.

Hamada, H.; Neumann, F.; and Junkmann, K. Intrauterine antimaskuline Beinflüssung von Rattenfeten durch ein stark Gestagen wirksames Steroid. *Acta endocr., Copenh.,* **1963,** *44,* 380–388.

Henderson, J. T.; Richmond, J.; and Sumerling, M. D. Androgenic-anabolic steroid therapy and hepatocellular carcinoma. *Lancet,* **1973,** *1,* 934.

Hershberger, L. G.; Shipley, E. G.; and Meyer, R. K. Myotrophic activity of 19-nortestosterone and other steroids determined by modified levator ani muscle method. *Proc. Soc. exp. Biol. Med.,* **1953,** *83,* 175–180.

Hilliard, J.; Scaramuzzi, R. J.; Pang, C.-N.; Penardi, R.; and Sawyer, C. H. Testosterone secretion by rabbit ovary *in vivo. Endocrinology,* **1974,** *94,* 267–271.

Hudson, B., and Coghlan, J. P. Abnormalities of testosterone secretion in the male. In, *Clinical Endocrinology II.* (Astwood, E. B., and Cassidy, C. E., eds.) Grune & Stratton, Inc., New York, **1968.**

Johanson, A. J.; Brasel, J. A.; and Blizzard, R. M. Growth in patients with gonadal dysgenesis receiving fluoxymesterone. *J. Pediat.,* **1969,** *75,* 1015–1021.

Johnson, B. H., and Ewing, L. L. Follicle-stimulating hormone and the regulation of testosterone secretion in rabbit testes. *Science, Wash.,* **1971,** *173,* 635–637.

Johnson, F. L.; Feagler, J. R.; Lerner, K. G.; Majerus, P. W.; Siegel, M.; Hartmann, J. R.; and Thomas, E. D. Association of androgenic-anabolic steroid therapy with development of hepatocellular carcinoma. *Lancet,* **1972,** *2,* 1273–1276.

Judd, H. L., and Yen, S. S. C. Serum androstenedione and testosterone levels during the menstrual cycle. *J. clin. Endocr. Metab.,* **1973,** *36,* 475–481.

Kappas, A.; Hellman, L.; Fukushima, D. K.; and Gallagher, T. F. The thermogenic effect and metabolic fate of etiocholanolone in man. *J. clin. Endocr. Metab.,* **1958,** *18,* 1043–1055.

Kelch, R. P.; Jenner, M. R.; Weinstein, R.; Kaplan, S. L.; and Grumbach, M. M. Estradiol and testosterone secretion by human, simian, and canine testes in males with hypogonadism and in male pseudohermaphrodites with the feminizing testes syndrome. *J. clin. Invest.,* **1972,** *51,* 824–830.

Knowlton, K.; Kenyon, A. T.; Sandiford, I.; Lotwin, G.; and Fricker, R. Comparative study of metabolic effects of estradiol benzoate and testosterone propionate in man. *J. clin. Endocr. Metab.,* **1942,** *2,* 671–684.

Kochakian, C. D., and Murlin, J. R. The effect of male hormone on the protein and energy metabolism of castrate dogs. *J. Nutr.,* **1935,** *10,* 437–459.

Kory, R. C.; Bradley, M. H.; Watson, R. N.; Callahan, R.; and Peters, B. J. A six-month evaluation of an anabolic drug, norethandrolone, in underweight persons. II. Bromsulphalein (BSP) retention and liver function. *Am. J. Med.,* **1959,** *26,* 243–248.

Lacy, D., and Pettit, A. J. Sites of hormone production in the mammalian testis, and their significance in the control of male fertility. *Br. med. Bull.,* **1970,** *26,* 87–91.

Lafferty, F. W.; Spencer, G. E.; and Pearson, O. H. Effects of androgens, estrogens and high calcium intake on bone formation and resorption in osteoporosis. *Am. J. Med.,* **1964,** *36,* 514–528.

Landau, R. L.; Bergenstal, D. M.; Lugibihl, K.; and Kascht, M. E. The metabolic effects of progesterone in man. *J. clin. Endocr. Metab.,* **1955,** *15,* 1194–1215.

Laschet, U.; Laschet, L.; Felzner, H.-R.; Glaesel, H.-U.; Mall, G.; and Naab, M. Results in the treatment of

hyper- and abnormal sexuality of men with antiandrogens. *Acta endocr., Copenh.,* **1967a,** *56,* Suppl. 119, 54.

Laschet, U.; Nierman, H.; Laschet, L.; and Paarmann, H. F. Mesterolone, a potent oral active androgen without gonadotropin inhibition. *Acta endocr., Copenh.,* **1967b,** *56,* Suppl. 119, 55.

Li, F. P.; Alter, B. P.; and Nathan, D. G. The mortality of acquired aplastic anemia in children. *Blood,* **1972,** *40,* 153–162.

Loewe, S., and Voss, H. E. Der Stand der Erfassung des männlichen Sexualhormons (Androkinins). *Klin. Wschr.,* **1930,** *9,* 481–487.

Longcope, C. The metabolism of estrone sulfate in normal males. *J. clin. Endocr. Metab.,* **1972,** *34,* 113–122.

McCullagh, E. P., and Jones, R. Effect of androgens on the blood count of men. *J. clin. Endocr. Metab.,* **1942,** *2,* 243–251.

McCullagh, E. P., and Schaffenburg, C. A. The testes. In, *Glandular Physiology and Therapy,* 5th ed. (Council on Pharmacy and Chemistry, American Medical Association.) J. B. Lippincott Co., Philadelphia, **1954,** pp. 220–257.

Martin, M. M., and Wilkins, L. Pituitary dwarfism: diagnosis and treatment. *J. clin. Endocr. Metab.,* **1958,** *18,* 679–693.

Mauvais-Jarvis, P.; Crepy, O.; and Bercovici, J. P. Further studies on the pathophysiology of testicular feminization syndrome. *J. clin. Endocr. Metab.,* **1971,** *32,* 568–571.

Midgley, A. R., and Jaffe, R. B. Regulation of human gonadotropins. IV. Correlation of serum concentrations of follicle stimulating and luteinizing hormones during the menstrual cycle. *J. clin. Endocr. Metab.,* **1968,** *28,* 1699–1703.

Mills, T. M., and Savard, K. *In vitro* steroid synthesis by follicles isolated from the rabbit ovary. *Steroids,* **1972,** *20,* 247–262.

Mittler, J. C., and Meites, J. Effects of hypothalamic extract and androgen on pituitary FSH release *in vitro. Endocrinology,* **1966,** *78,* 500–504.

Murad, F.; Straugh, B. S.; and Vaughan, M. The effect of gonadotropins on testicular adenyl cyclase. *Biochim. biophys. Acta,* **1969,** *177,* 591–598.

Naftolin, F.; Judd, H. L.; and Yen, S. S. C. Pulsatile patterns of gonadotropins and testosterone in man: the effects of clomiphene with and without testosterone. *J. clin. Endocr. Metab.,* **1973,** *36,* 285–288.

Neumann, H. Auftreton von Kastrationszellen im Hypophysenvorderlappen männlicher Ratten nach Behandlung mit einem Antiandrogen. *Acta endocr., Copenh.,* **1966,** *53,* 53–60.

Papanicolaou, G. N., and Falk, E. A. General muscular hypertrophy induced by androgenic hormones. *Science, N.Y.,* **1938,** *87,* 238–239.

Perez-Mera, R. A., and Shields, C. E. Jaundice associated with norethindrone acetate therapy. *New Engl. J. Med.,* **1962,** *267,* 1137–1138.

Petry, R.; Rausch-Strooman, J.-G.; Heinz, H. A.; Senge, T.; and Mauss, J. Androgen treatment without inhibiting effect on hypophysis and male gonads. *Acta endocr., Copenh.,* **1968,** *59,* 497–507.

Randall, L. O., and Selitto, J. J. Anti-androgenic activity of a synthetic phenanthrene. *Endocrinology,* **1958,** *62,* 693–695.

Ray, C. G.; Kirschvink, J. F.; Waxman, S. H.; and Kelley, V. C. Studies of anabolic steroids. III. The effect of oxandrolone on height and skeletal maturation in mongoloid children. *Am. J. Dis. Child.,* **1965,** *110,* 618–623.

Riggs, L.; Jowsey, J.; Goldsmith, R. S.; Kelly, P. J.; Hoffman, D. L.; and Arnaud, C. D. Short- and long-term effects of estrogen and synthetic anabolic hormone in postmenopausal osteoporosis. *J. clin. Invest.,* **1972,** *51,* 1659–1663.

Riggs, L.; Jowsey, J.; Kelly, P. J.; Jones, J. D.; and Maher,

F. T. Effect of sex hormones on bone in primary osteoporosis. *J. clin. Invest.,* **1969,** *48,* 1065–1072.

Ruzicka, L.; Goldberg, M. W.; Meyer, J.; Brüngger, H.; and Eichenberger, E. Über die Synthese des Testikelhormons (Androsteron) und Stereosomerer desselben durch Abbau hydrierter Sterine. *Helv. chim. Acta,* **1934,** *17,* 1395–1406.

Ruzicka, L., and Wettstein, A. Synthetische Darstellung des Testishormons, Testosteron (Androsten-3-on-17-ol). *Helv. chim. Acta,* **1935,** *18,* 1264–1275.

Sachs, B. D.; Pollak, E. I.; Kreiger, M. S.; and Barfield, R. J. Sexual behavior: normal male patterning in androgenized female rats. *Science, Wash.,* **1973,** *181,* 770–772.

Saez, J. M.; Morera, A. M.; Dazard, A.; and Bertrand, J. Adrenal and testicular contribution to plasma estrogens. *J. Endocr.,* **1972,** *55,* 41–49.

Segal, S. Male fertility control studies: an editorial comment. *Contraception,* **1973,** *8,* 187–188.

Selye, H., and Albert, S. Prevention by certain steroids of testicular atrophy elicited by small doses of testosterone. *Proc. Soc. exp. Biol. Med.,* **1942,** *49,* 227–229.

Shahidi, N. T. Androgens and erythropoiesis. *New Engl. J. Med.,* **1973,** *289,* 72–80.

Sizonenko, P. C.; Cuendet, A.; and Paunier, L. FSH. I. Evidence for its mediating role on testosterone secretion in cryptorchidism. *J. clin. Endocr. Metab.,* **1973,** *37,* 68–73.

Sobel, E. H. Anabolic steroids. In, *Clinical Endocrinology II.* (Astwood, E. B., and Cassidy, C. E., eds.) Grune & Stratton, Inc., New York, **1968.**

Stucki, J. C.; Forbes, A. D.; Northam, J. I.; and Clark, J. J. An assay for anabolic steroids employing metabolic balance in the monkey: the anabolic activity of fluoxymesterone and its 11-keto analogue. *Endocrinology,* **1960,** *66,* 585–598.

Wein, A. J., and Murphy, J. J. Experience in the treatment of prostatic carcinoma with cyproterone acetate. *J. Urol.,* **1973,** *109,* 68–70.

Wilkins, L. *The Diagnosis and Treatment of Endocrine Disorders in Childhood and Adolescence,* 3rd ed. Charles C Thomas, Pub., Springfield, Ill., **1965.**

Wilkins, L., and Fleischmann, W. Studies on the creatinuria due to methylated steroids. *J. clin. Invest.,* **1945,** *24,* 21–32.

Wolff, S. M.; Kimball, H. R.; and Marshall, J. R. The effects of hydrocortisone and estrogen on experimental fever induced by etiocholanolone. *J. infect. Dis.,* **1973,** *128,* 243–247.

Monographs and Reviews

Albert, A. Human urinary gonadotropin. *Recent Prog. Horm. Res.,* **1956,** *12,* 227–296.

Baird, D. T.; Horton, R.; Longcope, C.; and Tait, J. F. Steroid dynamics under steady-state conditions. *Recent Prog. Horm. Res.,* **1969b,** *25,* 611–664.

Bardin, C. W.; Bullock, L. P.; Sherins, R. J.; Mowszowicz, I.; and Blackburn, W. R. Androgen metabolism and mechanism of action in male pseudohermaphroditism: a study of testicular feminization. *Recent Prog. Horm. Res.,* **1973,** *29,* 65–109.

Davidson, J. M. Feedback control of gonadotropin secretion. In, *Frontiers in Neuroendocrinology.* (Ganong, W. F., and Martini, L., eds.) Oxford University Press, New York, **1969,** pp. 343–388.

Ebling, F. J. Steroids, hormones and sebaceous secretion. *Adv. Steroid Biochem. Pharmac.,* **1970,** *2,* 1–39.

Eik-Nes, K. B. Production and secretion of testicular steroids. *Recent Prog. Horm. Res.,* **1971,** *27,* 517–535.

Fotherby, K., and James, F. Metabolism of synthetic steroids. *Adv. Steroid Biochem. Pharmac.,* **1972,** *3,* 67–165.

Hamilton, J. B. Role of testicular secretions as indicated by effects of castration in man and by studies of pathological conditions and short lifespan association with maleness. *Recent Prog. Horm. Res.,* **1948,** *3,* 257–322.

Jackson, H., and Jones, A. R. The effects of steroids and their antagonists on spermatogenesis. *Adv. Steroid Biochem. Pharmac.,* **1972,** *3,* 167–192.

Jost, A. Embryonic sexual differentiation. In, *Hermaphroditism, Genital Anomalies and Related Endocrine Disorders,* 2nd ed. (Jones, H. W., and Scott, W. W., eds.) The Williams & Wilkins Co., Baltimore, **1971,** pp. 16–64.

Kochakian, C. D. The role of hydrolytic enzymes in some of the metabolic activities of steroid hormones. *Recent Prog. Horm. Res.,* **1947,** *1,* 177–214.

Lerner, L. J. Hormone antagonists: inhibitors of specific activities of estrogen and androgen. *Recent Prog. Horm. Res.,* **1964,** *20,* 435–476.

Liao, S., and Fang, S. Receptor-proteins for androgens and the mode of action of androgens on gene transcription in ventral prostate. *Vitams Horm.,* **1969,** *27,* 17–90.

Lipsett, M. B.; Wilson, H.; Kischner, M. A.; Korenman, S. C.; Fishman, L. M.; Sarfaty, G. A.; and Bardin, C. W. Studies on Leydig cell physiology and pathology: secretion and metabolism of testosterone. *Recent Prog. Horm. Res.,* **1966,** *22,* 245–271.

Longson, D. Androgen therapy. *Practitioner,* **1972,** *208,* 338–348.

Lunde, D. T., and Hamburg, D. A. Techniques for assessing the effects of sex steroids on affect, arousal, and aggression in humans. *Recent Prog. Horm. Res.,* **1972,** *28,* 627–663.

Neumann, F.; Berswordt-Wallrabe, R. von; Elger, W.; Steinbeck, H.; Hahn, J.; and Kramer, M. Aspects of androgen-dependent events as studied by antiandrogens. *Recent Prog. Horm. Res.,* **1970,** *26,* 337–405.

Niswender, G. D., and Midgley, A. R. Hapten-radioimmunoassay for steroid hormones. In, *Immunologic Methods in Steroid Determination.* (Péron, F. G., and Caldwell, B. V., eds.) Appleton-Century-Crofts, New York, **1970,** pp. 149–173.

Paulsen, C. A. The testes. In, *Textbook of Endocrinology,* 5th ed. (Williams, R. H., ed.) W. B. Saunders Co., Philadelphia, **1974,** pp. 323–367.

Rosenfield, R. L. Role of androgens in growth and development of the fetus, child, and adolescent. *Adv. Pediat.,* **1972,** *19,* 172–213.

Sommerville, I. F., and Collins, W. P. Indices of androgen production in women. *Adv. Steroid Biochem. Pharmac.,* **1970,** *2,* 267–314.

Strauss, J. S., and Pochi, P. E. The human sebaceous gland: its regulation by steroidal hormones and its use as an end organ for assaying androgenicity *in vivo. Recent Prog. Horm. Res.,* **1963,** *19,* 385–435.

Vande Wiele, R. L., and Dyrenfurth, I. Gonadotropin-steroid interrelationships. *Pharmac. Rev.,* **1973,** *25,* 189–207.

Wilson, J. D., and Gloyna, R. E. The intranuclear metabolism of testosterone in the accessory organs of reproduction. *Recent Prog. Horm. Res.,* **1970,** *26,* 309–336.

70 ADRENOCORTICOTROPIC HORMONE; ADRENOCORTICAL STEROIDS AND THEIR SYNTHETIC ANALOGS; INHIBITORS OF ADRENOCORTICAL STEROID BIOSYNTHESIS

Robert C. Haynes, Jr., and Joseph Larner

The adrenocorticotropic hormone (ACTH, corticotropin) of the adenohypophysis and the steroids of the adrenal cortex are considered together in this chapter because the primary physiological and pharmacological effects of ACTH result from the secretion of adrenocortical steroids. Biologically active synthetic analogs of the adrenocorticosteroids and those nonsteroidal substances that alter the pattern of secretion of the adrenal cortex by inhibiting certain biosynthetic pathways are also included in this chapter. Synthetic steroids and other compounds that inhibit the action of aldosterone on the renal tubule are discussed in Chapter 39.

History. The physiological significance of the adrenals began to be appreciated as a consequence of the description by Addison (1855) of the clinical syndrome resulting from destructive disease of the adrenal glands. His observations interested the physiologist Brown-Séquard (1856), who did the pioneer experiments on the effects of adrenalectomy and concluded that the adrenal glands are essential to life.

By the third decade of this century it was generally recognized that the cortex rather than the medulla is the life-maintaining portion of the gland. Soon the literature was replete with descriptions of the numerous physiological abnormalities exhibited by adrenalectomized animals. The complex nature of adrenocortical deficiency was dramatized in the 1930s by the partisan character of research groups oriented to study either the imbalance of electrolytes or the defects in carbohydrate metabolism present in the deficiency state. Renal loss of sodium was convincingly demonstrated to be a characteristic of adrenocortical insufficiency by Harrop and associates (1933) as well as by Loeb and coworkers (1933). Equally convincing was the demonstration of a depletion of carbohydrate stores (Cori and Cori, 1927). Furthermore, hypoglycemia could be corrected by adrenocortical extracts (Britton and Silvette, 1931). Glucose and glycogen, formed under the influence

of the adrenal cortex during fasting, appeared to be derived from tissue protein (Long *et al.,* 1940). From these studies there emerged the concepts of two types of adrenocortical hormones. The mineralocorticoids primarily regulate electrolyte homeostasis, and the glucocorticoids are hormones concerned with carbohydrate metabolism. This concept of the dichotomy of "salt" and "sugar" hormones has proven useful and survives at the present time in a modified form.

In 1932, the neurosurgeon Cushing described the syndrome of hypercorticism, which bears his name (Cushing, 1932). The cases Cushing described were those of "pituitary basophilism," recognized subsequently as being a condition characterized by hypersecretion of ACTH. The symptom complex is now known to result from excessive plasma concentrations of adrenocortical hormones, regardless of whether they originate endogenously or as the consequence of therapeutic intervention.

The preparation of adrenocortical extracts with a reasonable degree of activity was first accomplished by Swingle and Pfiffner (1930a, 1930b) as well as by Hartman and associates (1930). The existence of biologically active tissue extracts presented a challenge to organic chemists, who by 1942 had isolated, crystallized, and elucidated the structures of 28 steroids from the adrenal cortex (Reichstein and Shoppee, 1943). Five of these compounds—cortisol, cortisone, corticosterone, 11-dehydrocorticosterone, and 11-desoxycorticosterone—were demonstrated to be biologically active. Another decade passed before the principal mineralocorticoid was discovered. Stimulus for the search for this elusive material was provided by the work of Deming and Luetscher (1950), who isolated from the urine of patients with edema a substance that induced sodium retention and potassium excretion in adrenalectomized rats. The definitive evidence for its source was provided by Tait and coworkers (1952), who purified the compound from adrenocortical extracts. The substance was crystallized, the structure was established, and the hormone was eventually named *aldosterone* (Simpson *et al.,* 1954). Shortly thereafter, quantitative estimates of the rates of secretion of the major, biologically active products of the adrenal cortex, namely, cortisol, corticosterone, and aldosterone, were provided (Bush, 1953; Farrell *et al.,* 1955).

Meanwhile, other investigators had turned their attention to the adenohypophysis. The classical studies of Foster and Smith (1926) established the fact that hypophysectomy results in atrophy of the adrenal cortex. Not long thereafter, it was demonstrated that cell-free extracts of the anterior pituitary had a stimulating effect upon the adrenal cortex of the hypophysectomized animal (Collip et al., 1933; Evans, 1933; Houssay et al., 1933). Further chemical fractionation of such extracts led to the isolation of a hormone, ACTH, that acted selectively to cause chemical and morphological changes in the adrenal cortex (Li et al., 1943; Sayers et al., 1943; Astwood et al., 1952). The structure of ACTH was established by Bell and coworkers (1956). Further brilliant chemistry culminated in the synthesis of biologically active peptides (Hofmann et al., 1961) and of an ACTH of 39 amino acid residues (Schwyzer and Sieber, 1963). The rate of release of ACTH from the adenohypophysis was shown to be determined by the balance of inhibitory effects of the secretions of the adrenal cortex (Ingle et al., 1938) and the excitatory effects of the nervous system. The hypothalamus was established as the "final common path" for the variety of stimuli impinging on the adenohypophysis (see Harris, 1955).

A detailed analysis of the morphology of the adrenal cortex had suggested to Swann (1940) and to Deane and Greep (1946) that the glomerulosa zone of the adrenal cortex functions relatively independently of the pituitary. Following hypophysectomy, the glomerulosa zone of the adrenal cortex thickens, whereas the fasciculata shrinks markedly and the reticularis disappears almost entirely. These morphological observations, together with the fact that the hypophysectomized rat, in contrast to the adrenalectomized animal, can survive without salt therapy, prompted Swann as well as Deane and Greep to assign to the glomerulosa zone the specific function of autonomously elaborating a hormone regulating electrolyte balance. This hormone is now known to be aldosterone. Subsequent experimental studies have shown that the rate of secretion of aldosterone is regulated by a complex system, of which the pituitary is a relatively unimportant element.

Throughout the 1940s there was intense interest in the physiological roles of ACTH and adrenocortical steroids, stimulated by the appreciation that many physiological and biochemical responses to noxious stimuli are dependent upon the integrity of the adenohypophyseal-adrenocortical system. The most ardent exponent of the relationship between the adrenal cortex and "stress" was Selye (see Selye, 1946), who developed an elaborate hypothesis that certain "diseases of adaptation" resulted from the complex responses of susceptible tissues to the adrenocortical hormones. Although no such diseases have been demonstrated to occur, Selye's prolific publications were constant reminders of the variegated responses of many tissues to the adrenocortical hormones or to their lack.

It was upon such a background that Hench and coworkers in 1949 announced the dramatic effects of cortisone and ACTH in diseases other than adrenocortical insufficiency. As early as 1929, Hench was impressed by the fact that arthritic patients, when pregnant or jaundiced, experienced a temporary remission; he believed that a metabolite was responsible for the remission. The possibility that the antirheumatic substance might be an adrenocortical hormone was actively entertained, and as soon as cortisone was available in sufficient quantity it was tested in a case of acute rheumatoid arthritis. Fortunately, an adequate dose was employed and the response was dramatic. Thereafter, the salutary effects of ACTH were also demonstrated. The observations (Hench et al., 1949) immediately evoked wide interest. Soon, therapeutic applications were extended to other fields, with results to be presented later in this chapter. The impact upon the medical world can be gained from the fact that, in the year following the first published report of the efficacy of cortisone in the treatment of rheumatoid arthritis, the Nobel Prize in Medicine was jointly awarded to Kendall and Reichstein, who were responsible for much of the basic chemical research that led to the synthesis of the steroid, and to Hench, whose contribution has just been described.

In addition to a surge of clinical investigation, the therapeutic success of cortisone stimulated a wave of basic research in the 1950s related to steroid biogenesis, its control by ACTH, the chemistry and pharmacology of synthetic analogs of adrenocortical hormones, and the physiology of adrenocortical secretion. In that decade knowledge of the biochemistry of adrenal steroid synthesis and metabolism was brought close to its present level. As noted above, aldosterone was discovered; it was established that ACTH controls the reaction of cholesterol side chain scission (Stone and Hechter, 1954) and acts through the intermediacy of cyclic adenosine 3′,5′-monophosphate (cyclic AMP) (Haynes, et al., 1959); most synthetic analogs of cortisol used today were introduced, and practical technics for determination of cortisol became available to the clinician.

Effective clinical use of the corticosteroids has become possible because of their isolation, elucidation of structure, and economical synthesis. In the 1930s and 1940s, the expensive and relatively weak adrenocortical extracts available had to be reserved for the use of patients in crises of Addison's disease. Desoxycorticosterone was the first adrenocortical hormone to be synthesized (Steiger and Reichstein, 1937), and this allowed partial pharmacological control of the addisonian patient. Then followed the synthesis of a number of corticosteroids, including cortisone, cortisol, and aldosterone; large quantities of corticosteroids are now marketed for therapeutic use. Manipulation of structure has yielded a variety of synthetic analogs, a few of which represent significant therapeutic gains in terms of the ratio of anti-inflammatory potency to effects on electrolyte metabolism.

The enthusiasm that followed the announcement of therapeutic activity in the mesenchymal-tissue diseases by Hench and associates in 1949 has been followed by sober evaluation and perspective. The corticosteroids have gained an important and reasonably well-defined place in therapy, but high hopes for elimination of toxicity have not been fulfilled. For this reason, it cannot be overemphasized that the corticosteroids, in pharmacological doses, are powerful drugs with slow cumulative toxic effects on all tissues, which may be inapparent until made manifest by a catastrophe.

ADRENOCORTICOTROPIC HORMONE (ACTH, CORTICOTROPIN)

Chemistry. The structure of human ACTH, a peptide of 39 amino acid residues, is shown in Figure 70–1. Loss of one amino acid from the N-terminal end of the molecule (serine, number 1) by hydrolytic cleavage results in complete loss of biological activity. In contrast, a number of amino acids may be split off the C-terminal end with no effect on potency. A 24–amino acid peptide (sequence 1 through 24, Figure 70–1) retains the activity of the parent hormone, and the eicosopeptide (sequence 1 through 20) likewise is fully active. Potency and duration of action can be enhanced by making substitutions in the amino acid chain, for example, D-serine for L-serine in position 1, norleucine for methionine in position 4, and valine amide for asparagine in position 25; these substitutions increase resistance of the peptide to the action of proteolytic enzymes. However, no advantages have yet been gained in clinical practice by such manipulations (Jubiz *et al.,* 1968; Friedman, 1969).

Actions on Adrenal Cortex. ACTH stimulates the human adrenal cortex to secrete cortisol, corticosterone, aldosterone, and a number of weakly androgenic substances. In the absence of the adenohypophysis, the adrenal cortex undergoes atrophy and the rates of secretion of cortisol and corticosterone are markedly reduced and remain virtually unchanged in response to otherwise-effective stimuli. Although ACTH does stimulate secretion of aldosterone, the rate of this process is relatively independent of the adenohypophysis, and this explains the approximate normality of electrolyte balance in the hypophysectomized animal. The glomerulosa zone is the least involved of the various zones of the adrenal in the atrophic changes that follow hypophysectomy, and it is the glomerulosa that is mainly responsible for the elaboration of aldosterone.

Prolonged administration of large doses of ACTH induces hyperplasia and hypertrophy of the adrenal cortex and continuous high output of cortisol, corticosterone, and weak androgens.

The concentration of ascorbic acid is relatively high in the adrenal cortex, particularly in the rat. ACTH administration selectively induces a prompt reduction in the concentration of the vitamin in the gland. The phenomenon is the basis of a method of bioassay of the hormone (Sayers *et al.,* 1948). There is no convincing evidence to indicate that ascorbic acid is intimately involved in the elaboration of the corticosteroids.

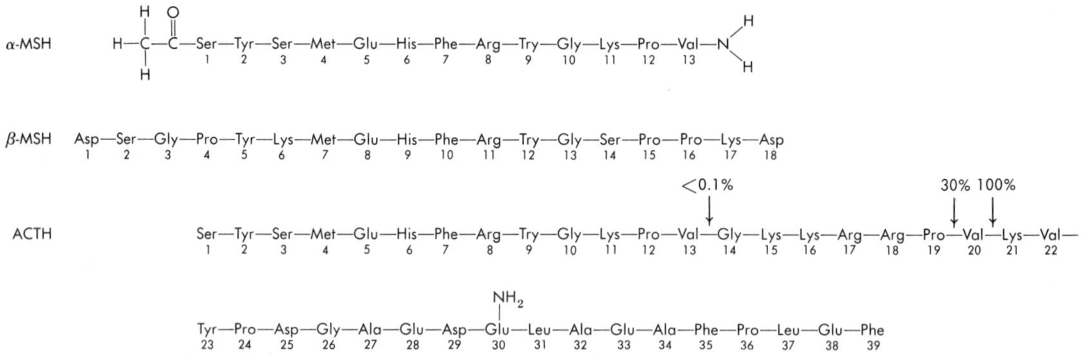

Figure 70–1. *Amino acid sequences for human ACTH and two MSHs.*

Ovine, porcine, and bovine ACTHs differ from human ACTH only at amino acid positions 25, 31, and 33 (Li, 1972). Synthetic peptides with amino acid sequences represented by the structures to the left of the arrows have been prepared and assayed (Hofmann, 1962). Note that full biological activity is retained as the chain is shortened until 19 is reached, at which length a significant reduction in potency develops.

α-Melanocyte-stimulating hormone (α-MSH, α-intermedin) has a sequence of amino acids identical with that of the first 13 residues of ACTH. (Note that an acetyl group is present on the N-terminal serine and there is an amide group on the valine.) It has less than 0.1% of the activity of ACTH on the adrenal cortex.

β-MSH is another potent melanocyte-stimulating hormone found in pituitary tissue. The sequence 4 to 10 of α-MSH and ACTH is identical to the sequence 7 to 13 of β-MSH (*see* Lerner and Lee, 1962; Chapter 66).

Mechanism of Action. ACTH acts to stimulate the *synthesis* of adrenocortical hormones; if it facilitates the release of preformed steroids from the adrenal cortex at all, this effect is overshadowed by the greater effect on synthesis. ACTH, as many other hormones, controls its target tissue through the agency of cyclic AMP. Thus, treatment with ACTH causes an increase in concentration of the cyclic nucleotide within adrenocortical cells (Haynes, 1958); cyclic AMP mimics ACTH in stimulating steroidogenesis (Haynes *et al.*, 1959), in depleting ascorbic acid (Earp *et al.*, 1970), and in maintaining the weight of the adrenal after hypophysectomy (Ney, 1969). ACTH presumably reacts with a specific hormone receptor in the adrenal-cell plasma membrane, and the result is a stimulation of adenylate cyclase activity and the formation of cyclic AMP. The principal metabolic site at which steroidogenesis is regulated by the cyclic nucleotide is the oxidative cleavage of the side chain of cholesterol, the reaction that results in the formation of pregnenolone (*see* Figure 70–3, page 1479). This step is rate limiting in the sequence of reactions that leads to the formation of adrenal steroid hormones (Stone and Hechter, 1954). Exposure of adrenocortical cells to ACTH together with aminoglutethimide (to block side chain cleavage) leads to increased amounts of cholesterol within the adrenal mitochondria, the locus of the side chain–cleaving enzyme (Mahaffee *et al.*, 1974). Furthermore, cholesterol bound to cytochrome P-450 is increased by ACTH (Bell and Harding, 1974). These findings, together with evidence that the availability of cholesterol is the factor that limits the rate of the cleavage reaction in intact mitochondria (Kahnt *et al.*, 1974), suggest that ACTH, via cyclic AMP, stimulates the initial reaction in steroidogenesis from cholesterol by making the substrate, cholesterol, available in increased concentration to the enzyme within the mitochondria.

The trophic effects of ACTH on the adrenal cortex are not understood beyond the fact that they, like stimulation of steroidogenesis, appear to be mediated by cyclic AMP (Ney, 1969).

Extra-adrenal Effects of ACTH, Including Hyperpigmentation. Large doses of ACTH given to adrenalectomized animals cause a number of metabolic changes, including ketosis, lipolysis, hypoglycemia (early after administration), and insulin resistance (late after administration). These extra-adrenal effects are of doubtful physiological significance, particularly since large doses are needed to induce them (Engel, 1961). Intravenous administration of ACTH (synthetic or porcine, but not bovine) leads to a transient elevation of the concentration of growth hormone in the plasma of adults but not children (Lee *et al.*, 1973).

Natural and synthetic corticotropins darken the isolated skin of the frog; this is not surprising since the amino acid sequence, 1 through 13, is identical with that of the melanocyte-stimulating hormone, α-MSH (Figure 70–1). Large doses of highly purified α-MSH and ACTH have been demonstrated to darken the skin of the adrenalectomized human subject. Whether they exert a melanocyte-stimulating effect in man in physiological concentrations remains to be demonstrated. The relative magnitude of influence of ACTH as compared to MSH in hyperpigmentation of the skin in Addison's disease is not known. The plasma concentrations of both are increased (Abe *et al.*, 1967).

Regulation of ACTH Release. The fluctuations in the rates of secretion of cortisol, corticosterone, and, to some extent, aldosterone are determined by the fluctuations in the release of ACTH from the adenohypophysis. The adenohypophysis, in turn, is under the influence of the *nervous system* and a *negative corticosteroid feedback mechanism*.

Nervous System: The Final Common Path. Stimuli that induce release of ACTH are subserved by neural paths converging on the median eminence of the hypothalamus. The functional link between the median eminence and the adenohypophysis, the final common path, is vascular, not neural. In response to an appropriate stimulus, corticotropin-regulatory hormone (CRH) is elaborated at neuronal endings in the median eminence and transported in the hypophyseal-portal vessels to the adenohypophysis, where it releases ACTH. CRH itself remains unsatisfactorily characterized (*see* Chapter 66).

ACTH is synthesized in basophilic cells of the adenohypophysis and, like several other peptide hormones, is probably derived from a larger precursor (Yalow and Berson, 1973). "Big ACTH," a protein of apparent molecular weight greater than 20,000, can be converted to ACTH by a short exposure to trypsin.

MSH appears to be a more primitive hormone in evolution than is ACTH. Scott and associates (1973) have suggested that ACTH is a precursor of MSH, and they have proposed that the immunoreactive ACTH of cyclostomes functions only as a precursor for the older hormone.

Negative Feedback of the Corticosteroids (Cortisol and Corticosterone). Corticosteroid administration, particularly cortisol, suppresses ACTH release, reduces the store of ACTH in the adenohypophysis, and induces morphological changes (hyalinization of the basophilic cells) suggestive of functional impairment of the adenohypophysis. The adrenal cortex itself undergoes atrophy. Contrariwise, adrenalectomized animals and patients with Addison's disease have abnormally high concentrations of ACTH in the blood even under optimal environmental conditions. When a stimulus is applied to an adrenalectomized animal, the titer of ACTH reaches even higher levels. These observations point up the important inhibitory role of the corticosteroids and clearly demonstrate that ACTH release remains under control of the nervous system in the absence of the corticosteroid feedback. ACTH release at any instant is determined in the normal subject by the balance of neural excitatory and corticosteroid inhibitory forces.

Examples of Effective Stimuli of Secretion. A number of conditions have been demonstrated to stimulate adrenocortical secretion in man. These include the agonal state, severe infections, surgery, parturition, cold, exercise, and emotional stress (Hodges *et al.,* 1962). The plasma concentrations of adrenocortical steroids can be elevated within a few minutes of the initiation of an appropriate stimulus.

Diurnal Cycles in Adrenocortical Activity. The rate of secretion of cortisol by the adrenal cortex of a normal human subject under optimal conditions is about 20 mg per day. However, the rate is not steady and exhibits rhythmic fluctuations; plasma concentrations of adrenocortical steroids are relatively high in the early morning hours, decline during the day, and reach a minimum about midnight. Plasma concentrations of ACTH are higher at 6 A.M. than at 6 P.M.

Absorption, Fate, and Excretion. The activity of ACTH is destroyed by the proteolytic enzymes of the gastrointestinal tract; therefore, the hormone is ineffective when given orally. It is readily absorbed from parenteral sites, and is usually administered by intramuscular injection and occasionally by intravenous infusion.

ACTH rapidly disappears from the circulation following its intravenous administration; in man, the plasma half-life is about 15 minutes. No significant biological activity is present in the urine, indicating that ACTH is inactivated in the tissues.

Inasmuch as the maximal effects of a trophic hormone on a target organ are achieved when optimal amounts of the trophic hormone are acting continuously, the quantitative response to ACTH differs markedly with the technic of administration. Renold and associates (1952) continuously infused a fixed dose of 20 units of ACTH for periods varying from 30 seconds to 48 hours. They demonstrated a linear increase in adrenocortical secretion with the duration of infusion. Obviously, when the hormone is given by rapid intravenous injection, much of it fails to act on the adrenal cortex. This also occurs, but to a lesser extent, when ACTH is administered intramuscularly in aqueous solution.

Bioassay. The U.S.P. has adopted the *Third International Standard for Corticotropin* (Bangham *et al.,* 1962) as the reference standard in the United States. Potency is based on an assay in hypophysectomized rats in which depletion of adrenal ascorbic acid is measured after subcutaneous administration of the ACTH. All commercial preparations are now described in these units only.

Preparations, Dosage, and Routes of Administration. *Corticotropin Injection,* U.S.P. (ACTH), is available as a sterile solution or as a lyophilized powder (ACTHAR) for intramuscular or intravenous use. The preparation is derived from the pituitaries of mammals used for food. Maximal adrenocortical secretion is obtained in adults with a total dose of 25 U.S.P. units infused for 8 hours.

Repository Corticotropin Injection, U.S.P. (H.P. ACTHAR GEL, CORTROPHIN GEL), is administered either intramuscularly or subcutaneously. It is a highly purified ACTH in gelatin solution. A typical dose is 40 units, given once daily.

Some gel preparations of ACTH have been approved for intravenous administration. However, it is preferable to utilize the purer *corticotropin for injection* for intravenous therapy and *cosyntropin* (*see* below) for diagnostic use, in order to minimize the possibility of allergic reactions.

Sterile Corticotropin Zinc Hydroxide Suspension, U.S.P. (CORTROPHIN-ZINC), is a preparation of purified corticotropin adsorbed on zinc hydroxide, intended for intramuscular injection. A typical dose is 40 units, given once daily.

Cosyntropin for injection (CORTROSYN) is a synthetic peptide corresponding to amino acid residues 1 to 24 of human ACTH. This preparation, approved for diagnostic purposes, is given intramuscularly or intravenously in a dose of 0.25 mg (equivalent to 25 units).

Therapeutic and Diagnostic Applications of ACTH. At the present time, the most important use of ACTH is as a *diagnostic agent* in adrenal insufficiency. For this purpose, ACTH is administered and the concentration of cortisol in plasma is determined. A normal increase in plasma cortisol rules out primary adrenocortical failure. If there is no acute response, prolonged administration of ACTH is carried out. In cases of pituitary insufficiency, prolonged treatment can be expected to elicit a rise in plasma cortisol concentration.

Therapeutic uses of ACTH have included the treatment of adrenocortical insufficiency and non-endocrine disorders that are responsive to glucocorticoids. However, therapy with ACTH is less predictable and much less convenient than is that with appropriate steroids. In patients who do not have a deficiency of mineralocorticoids, the effect of ACTH to stimulate the secretion of these steroids can cause undesirable effects on electrolyte distribution and excretion. ACTH would obviously be of no value in the treatment of primary adrenocortical failure. Furthermore, there is no substantial evidence that therapeutic goals can be attained with ACTH in secondary adrenocortical insufficiency that cannot be attained with appropriate doses of currently available steroids. It must be kept in mind, however, that ACTH and corticosteroids are not pharmacologically equivalent. Treatment with ACTH exposes the tissues to a rich mixture of glucocorticoids, mineralocorticoids, and androgens, in contrast to the conventional, contemporary practice of administering a single glucocorticoid. It is possible that the steroid mixture resulting from adrenal stimulation by ACTH has effects that differ significantly from those of a single, synthetic glucocorticoid. Thus, Grahame (1969) reported the absence of dermal atrophy in patients treated for prolonged periods of time with ACTH, in contrast to that found with corticosteroid treatment. This has been tentatively attributed to a protective action of androgens against the inhibitory effects of glucocorticoids on fibroblasts (Harvey and Grahame, 1973).

Clinical Toxicity of ACTH.

The toxicity of ACTH, aside from extremely rare hypersensitivity reactions, is entirely attributable to the increased rate of secretion of adrenocorticosteroids (*see* below). Hypersensitivity reactions, ranging from mild fever to anaphylaxis and death, have been reported. The synthetic ACTH peptides are thought to be less antigenic than is the parent molecule. Nevertheless, hypersensitivity to them does occur (Forssman and Mulder, 1973). ACTH may be expected to induce more sodium retention, a greater degree of hypokalemic alkalosis, and more acne than do the synthetic congeners of cortisol.

ACTH Antagonists. When the tryptophan residue (position 9) of ACTH is modified by formation of the *o*-nitrophenyl sulfenyl derivative (Kong *et al.*, 1972) or by substitution with another amino acid (Hofmann *et al.*, 1974), the modified peptides act as weak agonists or as inactive compounds that nevertheless bind to membrane preparations containing adrenocortical adenylate cyclase. They are therefore effective antagonists of ACTH and greatly inhibit the response of adenylate cyclase to the hormone. These, or similar compounds, may prove to be of use in certain clinical situations of excess secretion of ACTH, such as occurs in some pulmonary tumors.

ADRENOCORTICAL STEROIDS (ADRENOCORTICOSTEROIDS, CORTICOSTEROIDS)

From cholesterol, the adrenal cortex synthesizes two classes of steroids: the corticosteroids, with 21 carbons; and the adrenal androgens, with 19 carbons. A typical corticosteroid, *cortisol,* is shown in Figure 70–2; a typical adrenal androgen, *dehydroepiandrosterone,* is shown in Figure 70–3.

Adrenocorticosteroid Biosynthesis. Cholesterol is an obligatory intermediate in the biosynthesis of corticosteroids. Although the adrenal cortex synthesizes cholesterol from acetate by processes similar to those in liver, the greater part of the cholesterol (60 to 80%) utilized for corticosteroidogenesis comes from exogenous sources, both at rest and following ACTH administration (Borkowski *et al.*, 1967). Cholesterol is enzymatically converted to 21-carbon corticosteroids and 19-carbon weak androgens by a series of steps presented in simplified form in Figure 70–3. Oxidation and cleavage of the cholesterol side chain between C 20 and C 22 yield pregnenolone. 17α-Hydroxylation of pregnenolone, yielding 17α-hydroxypregnenolone, followed by oxidative scission of the side chain, results in the formation of dehydroepiandrosterone, the androgen produced by the adrenal cortex in the largest quantity. Androstenedione, another adrenal androgen, is formed either by rearrangement of the ring system of dehydroepiandrosterone from Δ^5-3β-hydroxy configuration to a Δ^4-3-keto configuration or by oxidative removal of the side chain of 17α-hydroxyprogesterone. The adrenal cortex secretes testosterone; however, about half the plasma testosterone of normal women is derived from androstenedione at an extra-adrenal site (Burger *et al.*, 1964; Bardin and Lipsett, 1967). The major pathway from pregnenolone to cortisol comprises the following steps: rearrangement and oxidation of the Δ^5-3β-hydroxy configuration to a Δ^4-3-keto configuration (progesterone); 17α-hydroxylation (17α-hydroxyprogesterone); 21-hydroxylation (11-desoxycortisol); and 11β-hydroxylation (cortisol). Aldosterone is synthesized from pregnenolone by successive rearrangement and oxidation of the Δ^5-3β-hydroxy ring system to the Δ^4-3-keto system, yielding progesterone; 21-hydroxylation, yielding desoxycorticosterone; 11β-hydroxylation, yielding corticosterone; 18-hydroxylation, yielding 18-hydroxycorticosterone (not shown in Figure 70–3); and, finally, oxidation of the 18-hydroxyl to an aldehyde, yielding aldosterone.

Adrenocorticosteroids are not stored in the adrenal. The amounts of corticosteroids found in adrenal tissue are insufficient to maintain normal rates of secretion for more than a few minutes in the absence of continuing biosynthesis. For this reason, the rate of biosynthesis is tantamount to the rate of secretion. Table 70–1 shows typical rates of secretion of the physiologically most important corticosteroids in man—cortisol and aldosterone—and also their ap-

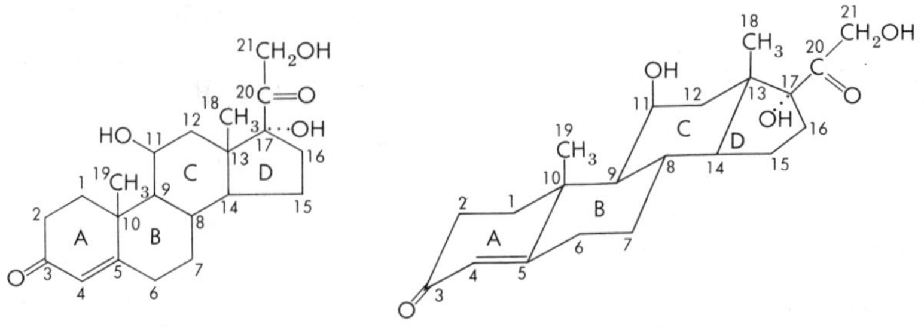

I   II

Figure 70-2. *Structure, stereochemistry, and nomenclature of adrenocorticosteroids, as typified by cortisol (hydrocortisone).*

The four rings—A, B, C, and D—are not in a flat plane, as conventionally represented in *I,* but have the approximate configuration shown in *II.* (The planarity of the valence angles about the double bond between C 4 and C 5 prevents the chair form of ring A, as shown, from being an energetically probable conformational state. As a result, ring A is in a half-chair conformation, not easily represented in two dimensions.) Orientation of the groups attached to the steroid ring system is importantly related to biological activity. The methyl groups at C 18 and C 19, the hydroxyl group at C 11, and the two-carbon ketol side chain at C 17 project above the plane of the steroid and are designated β. Their connection to the ring system is shown by full-line bonds. The hydroxy at C 17 projects below the plane and is designated α, and the connection to the ring is shown by a dotted bond. The ketone at C 3 in association with the double bond between C 4 and C 5 in ring A is an important structural feature of the biologically active corticosteroids. Reduction of the ketone at C 3 leads to the formation of two isomers: one, 3β-hydroxy; the other, 3α-hydroxy. Saturation of the 4,5 double bond leads to the formation of two isomers: 5α and 5β. Reduction of the ketone at C 20 creates an asymmetrical carbon at this site, the two possible isomers being designated α and β.

In formal chemical nomenclature, the adrenocortical hormones are described as derivatives of androstane or of pregnane. Double bonds are indicated by the symbol Δ with superscripts to indicate the position of the double bond. In this convention, cortisol is designated 11β,-17α,21-trihydroxy-Δ^4-pregnene-3,20-dione. Dehydroepiandrosterone is designated 3β-hydroxy-Δ^5-androsten-17-one.

proximate concentrations in peripheral plasma. The mechanism of control of steroidogenesis by ACTH has been discussed above, and the regulation of aldosterone synthesis by renin and angiotensin is described in Chapter 30.

PHYSIOLOGICAL FUNCTIONS AND PHARMACOLOGICAL EFFECTS

The corticosteroids have numerous and diversified physiological functions and pharmacological effects. They influence carbohy-

Table 70-1. RATES OF SECRETION AND TYPICAL PLASMA CONCENTRATIONS OF THE MAJOR BIOLOGICALLY ACTIVE CORTICOSTEROIDS IN MAN

		CORTI-SOL	ALDOSTE-RONE
Rate of secretion under optimal conditions, mg/day		20	0.125
Concentrations in peripheral plasma of man, $\mu g/100$ ml	8 A.M.	16	0.01
	4 P.M.	4	

drate, protein, fat, and purine metabolism; electrolyte and water balance; and the functions of the cardiovascular system, the kidney, skeletal muscle, the nervous system, and other organs and tissues. Furthermore, the corticosteroids endow the organism with the capacity to resist many types of noxious stimuli and environmental change. The adrenal cortex is the organ, *par excellence,* of homeostasis, being importantly responsible for the relative freedom that higher organisms exhibit in a constantly changing environment. In the absence of the adrenal cortex, survival is possible but only under the most rigidly prescribed conditions; for example, food must be available regularly, sodium chloride ingested in relatively large quantities, and environmental temperature maintained within a suitably narrow range.

A given dose of corticosteroid may be *physiological* or *pharmacological,* depending on the environment and the activities of the organism. Under favorable conditions, a small dose of corticosteroid maintains the adrenalectomized animal in a state of well-being. Under adverse conditions a relatively large dose is needed if the animal is to survive. This same large dose given repetitively under optimal conditions induces hyper-

corticism, that is, signs of excess of corticosteroid. The fluctuations in the secretory activity of a normal subject are presumed to reflect the varying needs of the organism for corticosteroids.

Corticosteroids, like other hormones, do

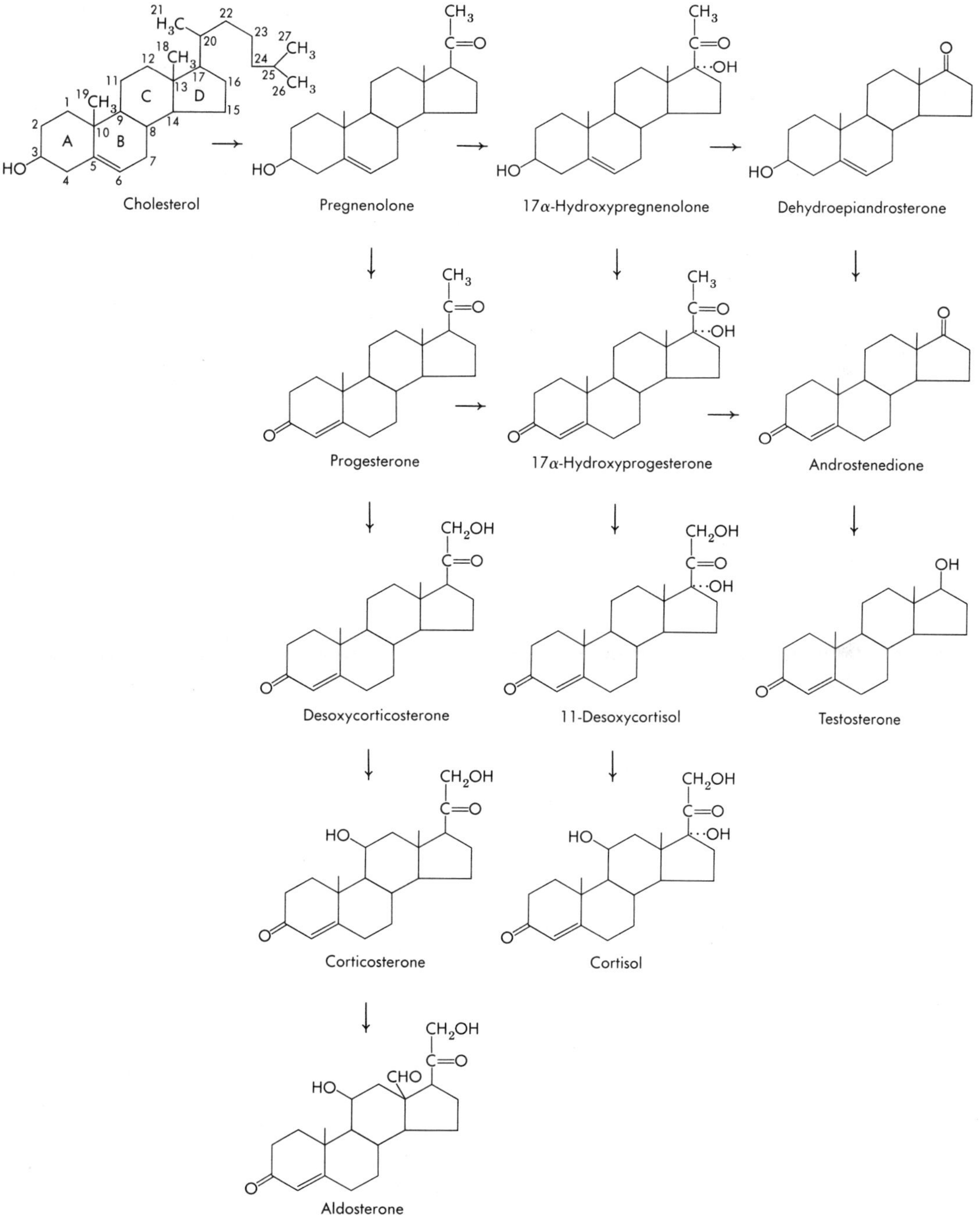

Figure 70-3. *Principal pathways for biosynthesis of adrenocorticosteroids and adrenal androgens.*

not make it possible for cells to perform activities of which they are otherwise incapable, but they do influence the *rates* at which *particular* events occur.

The regulatory actions of corticosteroids are often complexly related to the regulatory actions of other hormones. *In vitro,* in the absence of lipolytic hormones, cortisol even in large concentrations has virtually no effect on the rate of lipolysis in adipose tissue. Likewise, a sympathomimetic amine has only slight effect on the rate of lipolysis if there is a deficiency of glucocorticoids. However, if a necessary minimal amount of cortisol is added together with a range of concentrations of a sympathomimetic amine, the rate of lipolysis will be proportional to the concentration of the sympathomimetic amine. The necessary but not sufficient role of corticosteroids acting in concert with other regulatory forces has been termed "permissive" by Ingle (1954).

Certain of the numerous biological actions of the corticosteroids lend themselves to quantitative measurement. Potency estimates of naturally occurring and synthetic corticosteroids in the categories of *sodium retention* (reduction of sodium excretion by the kidney of the adrenalectomized animal), *liver glycogen deposition,* and *anti-inflammatory effect* (inhibition of the action of an agent that induces inflammation) are presented in Table 70–2. Potencies of steroids as judged by ability to maintain the adrenalectomized animal in a state of well-being closely parallel potencies as judged by ability to induce sodium retention. Potencies based on liver glycogen

deposition, anti-inflammatory effect, work capacity of skeletal muscle, and involution of lymphoid tissue closely parallel one another. Dissociations exist between potencies based on sodium retention and on liver glycogen deposition; traditionally the corticosteroids have thus been classified into *mineralocorticoids* and *glucocorticoids,* according to potencies in the two categories. Desoxycorticosterone, the prototype of the mineralocorticoids, is highly potent in regard to sodium retention but practically without effect on liver glycogen deposition. Cortisol, the prototype of the glucocorticoids, is highly potent in regard to liver glycogen deposition but weak in regard to sodium retention. The naturally occurring corticosteroids cortisol and cortisone as well as the synthetic corticosteroids prednisolone and triamcinolone are glucocorticoids. However, corticosterone is a steriod that has modest but significant activities in both categories. Finally, aldosterone is exceedingly potent with respect to sodium retention, with modest but appreciable potency for liver glycogen deposition. At rates secreted by the adrenal cortex or in doses that exert maximal effects on electrolyte balance, aldosterone has no significant effect on carbohydrate metabolism. Under these conditions, aldosterone may be classified as a mineralocorticoid.

In the descriptions of the physiological functions and the pharmacological effects of the corticosteroids to follow, the terms *mineralocorticoid* and *glucocorticoid* will be employed for convenience. It is to be emphasized that the biological characteristics of the corticosteroids range over a spectrum from that of a strictly mineralocorticoid type at the one end to that of a strictly glucocorticoid type at the other.

Mechanism of Action. Corticosteroids, like other steroid hormones, are thought to act by controlling the rate of synthesis of proteins. As is true with estrogens (Chapter 68), the corticosteroids react with receptor proteins in the cytoplasm of sensitive cells to form a steroid-receptor complex. Such receptors have been identified in many tissues (Ballard *et al.,* 1974). The steroid-receptor complex undergoes a conformational change, as noted by an increase in the sedimentation constant; following this, the complex moves

Table 70–2. RELATIVE POTENCIES OF CORTICOSTEROIDS

	SODIUM RETENTION	LIVER GLYCOGEN DEPOSITION	ANTI-INFLAMMATORY EFFECT
Natural Steroids			
Cortisol	1 *	1	1
Cortisone	0.8 *	0.8	0.8
Corticosterone	15	0.35	0.3
11-Desoxycorticosterone	100	0	0
Aldosterone	3000	0.3	?
Synthetic Steroids			
Prednisolone	<1 *	4	4
Triamcinolone	0	5	5

* Promotes sodium excretion under certain circumstances.

into the nucleus, where it binds to chromatin. Information carried by the steroid or more likely by the receptor protein directs the genetic apparatus to transcribe RNA of all types. Presumably the most important of these RNAs is the giant heterogeneous RNA, which contains nucleotide sequences that act as templates (mRNA) after a complex processing of the polymer has taken place (Scherrer, 1973).

Steroid hormones appear to stimulate transcription and ultimately the synthesis of specific proteins. While this is true for corticosteroids in some tissues, such as the liver, in other tissues, for example, lymphoid cells and fibroblasts, the overall effect of the hormones is a catabolic one. This suggests that the steroid-receptor complex may inhibit rather than stimulate transcription in these instances. However, Makman and coworkers (1971) presented evidence suggesting that steroids act in lymphatic cells to stimulate the synthesis of an inhibitory or toxic protein, which presumably causes the catabolic effects.

Although a broad outline of the action of the corticosteroids is emerging and there are a number of instances in which the synthesis of specific proteins is known to be induced by the hormones, the links between the initial actions of the hormones and the final metabolic effects have not been elucidated for the most part. A comprehensive review of glucocorticoid action is that of Thompson and Lippman (1974).

Carbohydrate and Protein Metabolism. The effects of adrenocortical hormones on carbohydrate and protein metabolism are epitomized in the teleological view that these steroids have evolved to protect glucose-dependent cerebral functions by stimulating the formation of glucose, diminishing its utilization, and promoting its storage as glycogen. Adrenalectomized animals exhibit no marked abnormality in carbohydrate metabolism if food is regularly available. Under such circumstances, normal concentrations of glucose in the plasma are maintained and glycogen is stored in the liver. However, a brief period of starvation rapidly depletes carbohydrate reserves. The concentration of glycogen in the liver, and to a lesser extent that in muscle, decreases and hypoglycemia

develops. In light of these facts, it is not surprising that the adrenalectomized animal is hypersensitive to insulin. Patients with Addison's disease have similar abnormalities in carbohydrate metabolism.

Administration of a glucocorticoid such as cortisol corrects the defect in carbohydrate metabolism of the adrenalectomized animal; glycogen stores, particularly in the liver, are increased; concentrations of plasma glucose remain normal during fasting; sensitivity to insulin returns to normal. Increased excretion of nitrogen accompanies the increased production of glucose, indicating that protein is converted to carbohydrate (Long et al., 1940). Prolonged exposure to large doses of glucocorticoids leads to an exaggeration of these changes in glucose metabolism, so that a diabetic-like state is produced: glucose in the plasma tends to be elevated in the fasting subject, there is increased resistance to insulin, glucose tolerance is decreased, and glucosuria may be present.

The mechanism by which the glucocorticoids inhibit utilization of glucose in peripheral tissues is not understood. Decreased uptake of glucose has been demonstrated in adipose tissue, skin, fibroblasts, and thymocytes as a result of glucocorticoid action.

Glucocorticoids promote gluconeogenesis by both peripheral and hepatic actions. Peripherally these steroids act to mobilize amino acids from a number of tissues. This catabolic action of the glucocorticoids is reflected in the atrophy of lymphatic tissues, reduced mass of muscle, osteoporosis (reduction in protein matrix of bone followed by calcium loss), thinning of the skin, and a negative nitrogen balance. Amino acids funnel into the liver, where they serve as substrates for enzymes involved in the production of glucose and glycogen.

In the liver the glucocorticoids induce de-novo synthesis of a number of enzymes involved in gluconeogenesis and amino acid metabolism. For example, the hepatic enzymes phosphoenolpyruvate carboxykinase, fructose-1,6-diphosphatase, and glucose-6-phosphatase, which catalyze reactions of glucose synthesis, are increased in concentration (Ashmore and Weber, 1968). However, induction of these enzymes requires a matter of hours and cannot account for the earliest effects of the hormones on gluconeogenesis. More rapid effects of glucocorticoids are apparent on hepatic mitochondria, such that they carboxylate pyruvate to form oxaloacetate at an accelerated rate (Adam and Haynes, 1969). This is the first reaction in the synthesis of glucose from pyruvate.

Prolonged, but not acute, treatment with glucocorticoids has been found to elevate the concentration of glucagon in the plasma (Marco et al., 1973; Wise et al., 1973). Inasmuch as glucagon itself stimulates gluconeogenesis, the rise in glucagon should also contribute to the enhanced synthesis of glucose. The deposition of glycogen in the liver found after treatment with glucocorticoids is now thought to be at least in part secondary to the rise in plasma insulin concentration elicited by the elevated plasma glucose (Kreutner and Goldberg, 1967).

Lipid Metabolism. Two effects of corticosteroids on lipid metabolism are firmly established. The first is the dramatic redistribution of body fat that occurs in the hypercorticoid state. The other is the facilitation of the effect of adipokinetic agents in eliciting lipolysis of the triglycerides of adipose tissue. A number of other effects of corticosteroids on lipids have been reported, but in few, if any, instances have they turned out to be clear, direct actions of the corticosteroids themselves.

Administration of large doses of glucocorticoids to human subjects over a long period of time or the hypersecretion of cortisol that occurs in Cushing's syndrome leads to a peculiar alteration in fat distribution. There is a gain of fat in depots in the back of the neck ("buffalo hump"), supraclavicular area, and face ("moon face") and a loss of fat from the extremities. The mode of action of the corticosteroids in bringing about abnormal fat distribution is unknown; the phenomenon illustrates the complexity of the problem of steroids and fat metabolism, for it is apparent that the fat depots are heterogeneous and differ from area to area in their responses to the same hormone.

The mobilization of fat from peripheral fat depots by epinephrine, norepinephrine, or adipokinetic peptides of the adenohypophysis is markedly blunted in the absence of the adrenal cortex or the adenohypophysis. It appears that cortisol acts in adipose tissue to facilitate the lipolytic response to cyclic AMP, rather than to enhance its accumulation. Hypophysectomy in rats has only a slight effect on the accumulation of cyclic AMP after exposure of adipose tissue to graded doses of epinephrine (Birnbaum and Goodman, 1973); however, hypophysectomy greatly decreases the lipolytic response of adipose tissue to the cyclic nucleotide. Treatment with cortisol restores the normal response to lipolytic hormones and to cyclic AMP (Goodman, 1968). Plasma lipids are not changed consistently in either hypocorticism or hypercorticism.

Electrolyte and Water Balance. Mineralocorticoids act on the distal tubules of the kidney to enhance the reabsorption of sodium ions from the tubular fluid into the plasma; they increase the urinary excretion of both potassium and hydrogen ions. The consequences of these three primary effects in concert with similar actions on cation transport in other tissues appear to account for the entire spectrum of physiological and pharmacological activities that are characteristic of the mineralocorticoids. Thus, the primary features of *hypercorticism* are positive sodium balance and expansion of the extracellular fluid volume, normal or slight increase in the concentration of sodium in the plasma, hypokalemia, and alkalosis. In contrast, those of the deficient state, *hypocorticism*, are sodium loss, hyponatremia, hyperkalemia, contraction of the extracellular fluid volume, and cellular hydration. The classical studies of Harrop and Loeb and their associates (*see* Harrop *et al.*, 1933; Loeb, 1933; Loeb *et al.*, 1933) revealed a defect of major consequence in adrenocortical insufficiency, namely, the renal loss of sodium. The renal tubules normally reabsorb practically all the sodium filtered at the glomerulus. For example, on an ordinary diet, 99.5% may be reabsorbed to maintain sodium balance. Typically, in a patient with Addison's disease under the same circumstances of dietary intake, maximal reabsorption attainable is 98.5%. Since approximately 24,000 mEq of sodium is filtered per day, the 1% difference between reabsorption in the normal subject and reabsorption in the patient with Addison's disease amounts to a loss of 240 mEq of sodium per day. The gravity of the situation is obvious when one considers that this amount of sodium is normally present in 1.7 liters of extracellular fluid. Proportionately more sodium than water is lost through the kidney and the concentration of extracellular sodium decreases; extracellular fluid becomes hypoosmotic, and water shifts from the extracellular into the intracellular compartment. This shift, together with the renal loss of water, results in a marked reduction in the volume of the extracellular fluid. Cells are hydrated, and the increase in the hematocrit value is due not only to a shrinkage of the plasma volume but also to the swelling of the erythrocytes. Hyperkalemia and the tendency toward acid-base disturbances are a result of impairments in the excretion of potassium and of hydrogen ions. Without administration of mineralo-corticoids or sodium chloride solution or both, a rapid downhill course ensues in adrenocortical insufficiency. The shrinkage of extracellular fluid volume, the cellular hydration, and the hypodynamic state of the cardiovascular system combine to cause circulatory collapse, renal failure, and death.

In adrenocortical insufficiency, a basic defect in ion transport occurs in a variety of secretory cells. Not only the kidney but also the salivary glands, the sweat glands, the exocrine pancreas, and the mucosa of the gastrointestinal tract elaborate fluids abnormally high in the concentration of sodium and abnormally low in the concentration of potassium. In the patient with Addison's disease, sweating may contribute significantly to the negative balance of sodium. Certain investigators would extend the influence of the corticosteroids on ion transport and water movement to all tissues throughout the organism.

Aldosterone is by far the most potent of the naturally occurring corticosteroids in regard to electrolyte balance. Plasma sodium and potassium concentrations and blood pressure remain normal in adrenalectomized dogs given 10 μg of this potent mineralocorticoid per day. Under the same conditions, the maintenance dose of cortisol is 5000 μg. Aldosterone acts directly on the kidney, as indicated by the fact that a small dose (0.0045 μg per minute) infused into a renal artery of the adrenalectomized dog produces antinatriuresis only on the injected side after a latent period of an hour (Barger *et al.,* 1958).

Aldosterone plays an important role in the regulation of sodium and potassium balance. Evidence of this is the relatively normal electrolyte balance exhibited by the hypophysectomized animal as a result of the secretion of aldosterone by the adrenal cortex. The increased rate of secretion of aldosterone that occurs in man when dietary salt is severely limited would appear to be a compensatory adjustment of physiological importance. However, *changes* in the rate of secretion of aldosterone are not the cause of *rapid* changes that may occur in sodium excretion. The latent period of action of the steroid is too long to account for abrupt changes in ion excretion.

The intravenous administration of aldosterone to a normal subject is followed, after a delay of about an hour, by a decrease in the rate of renal sodium ion excretion and an increase in the rate of potassium ion and hydrogen ion excretion. If the administration of relatively large amounts of aldosterone is continued over a period of more than 2 or 3 days, sodium excretion again equals sodium intake. However, potassium ion and hydrogen ion excretion continues at an accelerated rate, resulting in hypokalemic hypochloremic alkalosis.

This "escape" from acute sodium retention is not understood. Some evidence exists for the presence of a salt-losing hormone that acts to inhibit sodium ion reabsorption in the proximal tubules. The increased sodium ion load delivered to the distal tubule as a consequence overcomes the mineralocorticoid effect, and the resulting excretion of sodium ions creates the "escape" from sodium retention. The tissue effects of the mineralocorticoids have been reviewed by Mulrow and Forman (1972).

The morphological complexity of the mammalian kidney presents a formidable obstacle to an attack on the question as to how aldosterone increases sodium reabsorption. Aldosterone stimulates sodium transport by the toad bladder, and it is only natural that investigators have turned to this structurally simple organ as an experimental system.

Studies with the toad bladder have indicated that aldosterone, like other steroids, probably acts to initiate transcription of RNA that serves as template for the synthesis of a protein or proteins. This hypothetical "aldosterone-induced protein" is thought to facilitate the transport of sodium ions. Two major hypotheses have been developed from experiments with toad bladders to explain the actions of aldosterone in the kidney. Both use the following model of renal sodium ion reabsorption. The sodium ions of the tubular filtrate enter the cells of the distal tubules down a concentration gradient through their surface facing the tubular lumen (apical or mucosal surface). They diffuse through the cell to the serosal surface, which is in contact with extracellular fluid. At this interface the ions are pumped out of the cell against a concentration gradient by an energy-requiring pump that has the operational characteristics of a Na^+,K^+-activated adenosine triphosphatase (Na,K-ATPase). The "permease" hypothesis proposes that mineralocorticoids increase the permeability of the mucosal surface to sodium ions. Sodium ions therefore enter the cells at an accelerated rate and are pumped out into the extracellular space by the sodium ion pump at the serosal surface. The alternative or "pump" hypothesis proposes that the mucosal surface of the tubular cells is freely permeable to sodium ions. Aldosterone increases the sodium-pumping activity at the serosal surface by activating the pump enzyme(s) or by providing additional energy to drive the pump. Thus, in both hypotheses aldosterone accelerates the presumed rate-limiting step in sodium ion reabsorption. In the "permease" hypothesis this is considered to be entrance of sodium ions into the tubular cells; in the variations of the "pump" hypothesis, this step is thought to be the pumping of the sodium ions out of the tubular cells (Feldman *et al.,* 1972).

The mechanisms of the enhanced potassium ion and hydrogen ion excretion are less well understood. For practical purposes one may visualize these ions as being "exchanged" for the additional sodium ions reabsorbed under the influence of the steroids, because the sum of the equivalents of the additional potassium and hydrogen ions excreted is equal to that of the additional sodium ions retained.

The *glucocorticoids* decrease the absorption of calcium from the intestine and increase its renal excretion, thus producing a negative balance of the cation. These effects are considered to be the basis of the favorable therapeutic response to glucocorticoids seen in hypercalcemia (*see* Chapter 37, page 787).

Desoxycorticosterone is a mineralocorticoid of some historical interest for it was the first corticosteroid to be synthesized and made available for the treatment of Addison's disease. Desoxycorticosterone is practically devoid of glucocorticoid effects. Qualitatively, it is identical to aldosterone in its effects on electrolytes; quantitatively, it is about $\frac{1}{30}$ as potent (*see* Table 70–2).

Cortisol induces sodium retention and potassium excretion, but much less effectively than does aldosterone. Acute treatment with cortisol, unlike that with aldosterone, does not increase net acid secretion (Lemann *et al.,* 1970). In striking contrast to aldosterone, cortisol, under certain circumstances, especially sodium loading, enhances sodium excretion. This may be accounted for by the capacity of cortisol to increase the glomerular filtration rate (GFR). Aldosterone and desoxycorticosterone are ineffective in this regard. Furthermore, cortisol has a significant stimulatory influence on tubular secretory activity, as reflected in an increase in Tm_{PAH}.

Impaired water diuresis in response to an administered water load is sufficiently characteristic of adrenal insufficiency to have been used as a diagnostic criterion. In adrenal insufficiency, GFR is reduced and plasma antidiuretic hormone (ADH) concentration is increased; these factors account for failure to excrete a water load (Ahmed *et al.,* 1967). Administration of cortisol, but not of aldosterone, increases GFR and restores water diuresis. The influence of cortisol on plasma concentration of ADH has not been settled. Saline infusion increases GFR, reduces plasma ADH concentration, and restores water diuresis (Gill *et al.,* 1962).

Hypercorticism due to administration of large doses of cortisol (or related glucocorticoids) or to excessive secretion of cortisol by the adrenals is sometimes associated with a hypokalemic hypochloremic alkalosis. However, the changes, particularly the degree of hypokalemia, are moderate in severity and reflect the relatively weak effect of cortisol as compared to aldosterone on electrolyte balance. Muscular weakness associated with glucocorticoid treatment is usually due to a loss of muscle mass rather than of potassium.

Cardiovascular System. The most striking effects of corticosteroids on the cardiovascular system are those that are the consequence of regulation of renal sodium ion excretion. These are seen most vividly in hypocorticism when reduction in blood volume accompanied by increased viscosity can lead to hypotension and cardiovascular collapse. However, the impairment of the cardiovascular system in adrenocortical insufficiency obviously involves complex, poorly understood processes in addition to the defects in water and electrolyte balance that result from excessive loss of salt and water in the urine. The corticosteroids exert important actions on the various elements of the circulatory system, including the capillaries, the arterioles, and the myocardium. In the absence of the corticosteroids, there is increased capillary permeability, inadequate vasomotor response of the small vessels, and reduction in cardiac size and output.

An excess of mineralocorticoids occurs in its purest form in *primary aldosteronism,* the result of excessive secretion of this steroid. In this disease the major clinical findings are hypertension and hypokalemia. The hypokalemia is an obvious consequence of the renal effects of aldosterone, but the genesis of the hypertension has not been clarified. Development of hypertension requires a prolonged excess of mineralocorticoid and increased sodium intake (Mulrow and Forman, 1972). Hypertension occurs in most cases of Cushing's syndrome but rarely, if at all, as the result of administration of synthetic glucocorticoids lacking mineralocorticoid activity. Steroid-induced hypertension may be the result of prolonged, excessive sodium retention; one hypothesis proposes that this leads to edema within the walls of arterioles, thereby reducing their lumina and increasing peripheral vascular resistance (Tobian, 1960).

Glucocorticoids, including those with no demonstrable mineralocorticoid activity, produce a slowly developing vasoconstriction of cutaneous vessels when applied locally (McKenzie and Stoughton,

1962). The mechanism of this vasoconstriction is not known.

It has been suggested that the corticosteroids enhance the response of the cardiovascular system to adrenergic stimuli (Gainesburg, 1958). Yard and Kadowitz (1972) demonstrated that cortisol, in a narrow dose range, augmented the vasoconstrictor response to epinephrine but not to norepinephrine in the extremities of dogs and cats. Aldosterone acted similarly to cortisol, but dexamethasone was inactive. The significance of this effect may be minor considering the fact that the steroids did not influence the response to norepinephrine.

Skeletal Muscle. The maintenance of normal function of skeletal muscle requires adequate concentrations of corticosteroids, but excessive amounts of either mineralocorticoids or glucocorticoids lead to abnormalities.

It is well known that one of the outstanding signs of adrenocortical insufficiency is a diminished work capacity of striated muscle. This is manifested in patients with Addison's disease by weakness and fatigability. Adrenalectomized animals are similarly affected. The most important single factor responsible for this dysfunction appears to be the inadequacy of the circulatory system. Abnormalities in electrolyte balance and carbohydrate metabolism in adrenocortical insufficiency contribute only in small measure to the impairment in skeletal muscle function.

Muscle weakness in primary aldosteronism is in large measure a result of the hypokalemia characteristic of this disease. Glucocorticoids given for prolonged periods in high doses or secreted in abnormal amounts in Cushing's syndrome tend to cause a wasting of skeletal muscle. The mechanism of this is not known. This steroid myopathy is responsible, at least in part, for the weakness and fatigability noted in the syndrome.

Central Nervous System. The corticosteroids affect the central nervous system (CNS) in a number of indirect ways; in particular, they maintain normal concentrations of plasma glucose, an adequate circulation, and the normal balance of electrolytes in the body. The steroids may also have direct effects, but these are as yet poorly defined. An influence of the corticosteroids can be observed on mood, behavior, the EEG, and brain excitability.

Patients with Addison's disease exhibit apathy, depression, and irritability, and some are frankly psychotic. Desoxycorticosterone is ineffective but cortisol is very effective in correcting these abnormalities of psyche and behavior. An array of reactions, varying in degree and kind, is seen in patients to whom glucocorticoids are administered for therapeutic purposes. Most patients respond with elevation in mood, which may be explained in part by the relief of the symptoms of the disease being treated. In some, more definite mood changes occur, characterized by euphoria, insomnia, restlessness, and increased motor activity. A smaller but significant percentage of patients treated with high doses of cortisol become anxious or depressed. This latter type of reaction has been seen particularly in patients who utilize the disease for which they are treated as part of a psychological defense mechanism and, as a result, are threatened by relief of symptoms. A still smaller percentage exhibit psychotic reactions; this is especially true of patients with a previous history of psychiatric illness (*see* Chapter 12, page 196). Among patients with Cushing's syndrome, there is a high incidence of neuroses and psychoses.

The changes induced by excessive quantities of the corticosteroids are reversible. The abnormalities of behavior usually disappear when the corticosteroids are withdrawn or the Cushing's syndrome is effectively treated.

In both hypocorticism and hypercorticism the EEG characteristically shows a significant amount of slow activity, definitely slower than alpha waves. The abnormal EEG pattern exhibited by patients with Addison's disease is corrected by cortisol but not by desoxycorticosterone. The abnormal pattern of the EEG in hypercorticism is also reversible.

Brain excitability may be assessed grossly by incidence of spontaneous seizures or by changes in the threshold to seizure-inducing procedures. Adrenalectomized animals are unusually susceptible to the development of seizures, whether induced electrically, chemically, audiogenically, or by insulin or water intoxication. Seizure thresholds are normal if the animal is maintained on 0.9% sodium chloride solution or on desoxycorticosterone. In normal animals, desoxycorticosterone decreases and cortisol increases brain excitability. Spontaneous seizures in man have been attributed to treatment with large doses of cortisone or ACTH.

The means by which the corticosteroids exert their influence on the CNS are probably numerous, and the discussion will be limited to two possibilities—cerebral blood flow and electrolytes. Blood flow to the brain is less than normal in adrenocortical insufficiency, even when the adrenalectomized animal is maintained on desoxycorticosterone. Cortisol therapy, on the other hand, probably plays an indirect role in the maintenance of normal brain function by exerting a salutary influence on the circulation.

The increase in brain excitability in hypocorticism and the decrease in brain excitability in an animal given large doses of desoxycorticosterone appear to be related to changes in the concentrations of electrolytes in the brain. The ratios of extracellular to intracellular sodium and intracellular to extracellular potassium are decreased in hypocorticism and increased with excess desoxycorticosterone. Furthermore, the administration of sodium chloride in excess to adrenalectomized animals maintains ion concentrations and brain excitability at normal levels. In contrast, chronic administration of cortisol increases brain excitability without influencing the concentrations of sodium and potassium in the brain. It is concluded that the influence of desoxycorticosterone on brain excitability is mediated through its influence on sodium transport, whereas cortisol acts by a different and as-yet-unknown mechanism. That cortisol may act directly on the brain is suggested by the report that there are cortisol-binding proteins possessing the characteristics of steroid receptors in the brain (Ballard *et al.*, 1974).

Thresholds for the perception of taste, smell, and sound stimuli are reduced in adrenocortical insufficiency and elevated in hypercorticism. Glucocorticoids restore thresholds to normal, but desoxycorticosterone is without effect (Henkin, 1970).

A review of adrenal-brain relationships is that edited by De Wied and Weijnen (1970).

Formed Elements of Blood. Glucocorticoids tend to increase the hemoglobin and red-cell content of the blood, as evidenced by the frequent occurrence of polycythemia in Cushing's syndrome and a mild, normochromic, normocytic anemia in Addison's disease.

The corticosteroids also affect circulating white cells. Administration of glucocorticoids leads to an increase in the number of polymorphonuclear leukocytes in the blood, while the numbers of lymphocytes, eosinophils, monocytes, and basophils decrease. The response of platelets is unclear, as both thrombocytosis and thrombocytopenia have been reported to follow glucocorticoid administration.

There is evidence that glucocorticoids retard erythrophagocytosis (Greendyke *et al.*, 1965). A stimulation of erythropoiesis has not been convincingly demonstrated in the healthy individual. However, the steroids do elicit a normoblastic response in the marrow of patients with megaloblastic anemia (Doig *et al.*, 1957).

Steroid-induced granulocytosis is thought to result from the combination of an increased rate of entrance of polymorphonuclear leukocytes into the blood from the marrow and a diminished rate of their removal (Bishop *et al.*, 1968).

The lymphocytopenia that results from the actions of the corticosteroids is presumably related to the widespread effects of the glucocorticoids on lymphoid tissue (*see* following section). A single dose of cortisol in man produces a decline of about 70% in circulating lymphocytes and a decline of over 90% in monocytes in 4 to 6 hours. The thymus-derived lymphocytes are decreased proportionately more than those that are derived from the bone marrow. The profile of cellular responses of the lymphocytes remaining in the blood to various mitogens and antigens is altered when contrasted to that of lymphocytes of untreated subjects. This presumably indicates that subpopulations of lymphocytes are differentially affected by the steroids. It is currently thought that, at least in man, the lymphocytopenia is the result of redistribution rather than of destruction of cells (Fauci and Dale, 1974).

Lymphoid Tissue. The secretion of the adrenal cortex has a striking effect on lymphoid tissue. Addison was the first to observe the increase in mass of lymphoid tissue that accompanies adrenocortical insufficiency; there is also a lymphocytosis. In contrast, Cushing's syndrome is characterized by lymphocytopenia and decreased mass of lymphoid tissue.

In a number of laboratory animals glucocorticoids cause a rapid lysis of lymphatic tissue, especially striking in cells of the thymus (Dougherty and White, 1944, 1947). Man is much more resistant to this lympholytic effect of the steroids, and some investigators doubt that the glucocorticoids have a comparable effect in man (Claman, 1972). This implies that the changes in lymphoid tissue seen in man in chronic hypercorticosteroid or hypocorticosteroid states must result from changes in rates of cellular formation or destruction that become manifest over a prolonged period of time. As noted above, the acute effects of steroids on circulating lymphocytes may be due to sequestration from the blood, rather than to lymphocytolysis.

Within 1 to 3 hours following the administration of glucocorticoids to rats or mice, dissolution of lymphocytes in lymphoid tissue becomes apparent. The nuclei become pyknotic and disintegrate, or the cells may shed their cytoplasm. The cellular debris is phagocytized. Dissolution continues during the period of steroid administration. Thereafter, there is a return to normal lymphoid structure, characterized by differentiation of lymphocytes from reticulum cells and resumption of mitosis (*see* Dougherty and White, 1944, 1947).

The mechanism of the dramatic lympholytic effects of the glucocorticoids in rodents has been the subject of many investigations. The presence of a glucocorticoid "receptor" protein in rat thymus (Munck and Brinck-Johnsen, 1968; Schaumburg and Bojesen, 1968) has increased the probability that these effects are mediated by an interaction between a steroid-receptor complex and the chromatin of the nucleus. Early changes in biochemical functions produced in the thymus by glucocorticoids include decreased transport of amino acids, nucleotides, and ions and decreased glucose utilization, synthesis of RNA, and phosphorylation.

The addition of an inhibitor of protein synthesis, cycloheximide, after the effects of the steroids are established reverses the inhibitions. This strongly suggests that the steroids induce the synthesis of a protein that, in turn, acts to inhibit various cellular functions. In addition, it appears that the synthesis of this protein must continue for the steroids to be effective (Makman *et al.*, 1971).

Immune Responses. Corticosteroids and ACTH modify the clinical course of a variety of diseases in which hypersensitivity is believed to play an important role. However, there is no convincing evidence that the therapeutic use of the corticosteroids has any significant effect on the titer of circulating antibodies, either IgG or IgE, that play a major role in certain allergic and auto-immune states (Grieco and Cushman, 1970). This is true in spite of the fact that the symptoms of the diseases are often alleviated dramatically by the steroids. It is also now believed that in clinical situations in which the glucocorticoids are used to prevent the consequences of cell-mediated (delayed hypersensitivity) immune reactions, for example, graft rejection, the steroids do not interfere with the normal processes in the development of cell-mediated immunity. Rather, they prevent or suppress the inflammatory responses that take place as a consequence of the hypersensitivity reactions (Cohen, 1971; Weston *et al.*, 1972; Balow and Rosenthal, 1973).

The dramatic lympholysis in steroid-treated rodents has possibly proved to be misleading in developing an understanding of the effects of glucocorticoids in suppressing immune reactions. The assumption has been that the steroids act by destroy-ing or damaging lymphoid cells critical to the development of immune reactions. The demonstration that the small number of cells remaining in the thymus of the mouse after treatment with cortisol have an undiminished capacity to establish cell-mediated immune responses has made this concept untenable (Cohen *et al.*, 1970).

One aspect of the glucocorticoid effect in suppressing cell-mediated immune reactions is now beginning to be understood. It is thought that, in delayed sensitivity reactions, lymphocytes previously sensitized to a particular antigen encounter the antigen within a tissue at a site destined to be the location of the inflammatory response. These lymphocytes, activated by the antigen, begin production of a number of soluble factors that control the cellular response. Among the factors produced is the macrophage migration inhibitory factor (MIF), which causes an accumulation of nonsensitized macrophages in the area by inhibiting their mobility (Bloom and Bennett, 1966). Glucocorticoids do not affect the production of MIF by lymphocytes that have been activated by an appropriate antigen, but the steroids do block the effect of MIF on macrophages; that is, the movement of these cells is no longer impeded, and they do not accumulate locally (Balow and Rosenthal, 1973). In contemplating these more recent advances, it is sobering to realize that a stimulatory effect of corticosteroids on the migration of macrophages has been known for over 30 years (Heilman, 1945).

It is reasonable to believe that additional mechanisms responsible for the effects of the steroids in suppressing the immune response will be elucidated. It is possible the glucocorticoids will be found to oppose the actions of other soluble factors released by sensitized lymphocytes following activation by specific antigens.

Anti-inflammatory Properties. ACTH, cortisol, and the synthetic analogs of cortisol have the capacity to prevent or suppress the development of the local heat, redness, swelling, and tenderness by which inflammation is recognized at the gross level of observation. At the microscopic level, they inhibit not only the early phenomena of the inflammatory process (edema, fibrin deposition, capillary dilatation, migration of leukocytes into the inflamed area, and phagocytic activity) but also the later manifestations (capillary proliferation, fibroblast proliferation, deposition of collagen, and, still later, cicatrization).

Although current understanding of these effects is unsatisfactory, many observations have been made that have therapeutic relevance and that must be taken into account in explanatory formulations. Perhaps the most important of these for the physician is that corticosteroids inhibit the inflammatory response whether the inciting agent is radiant, mechanical, chemical, infectious, or immunological. In clinical terms, the administration of corticosteroids for their anti-inflammatory effects is palliative therapy; the underlying cause of the disease remains; the inflammatory manifestations are merely suppressed. It is this suppression of inflammation and its consequences that has made the corticosteroids such valuable therapeutic agents—indeed, at times lifesaving. It is also this property that gives them a nearly unique potential for therapeutic disaster. The signs and symptoms of inflammation are expressions of the disease process that are often used by the physician in diagnosis and in evaluating the effectiveness of treatment. These may be missing in patients treated with glucocorticoids. For example, an infection may continue to progress while the patient superficially appears to improve, and a peptic ulcer may perforate without producing clinical signs. This situation has been epitomized in the grimly facetious remark that the corticosteroids, misused, permit a patient to walk all the way to the autopsy room!

Cortisol and presumably other anti-inflammatory steroids are to be found in inflamed tissues, although they are not selectively concentrated there when account is taken of the edema and increased vascularity of the affected area. Anti-inflammatory effects depend upon the direct local action of the steroid, for some compounds are very effective on topical application to skin or eye without detectable systemic absorption. The hypothesis that glucocorticoids exert their anti-inflammatory actions by inhibiting the rupture of lysosomes (Weissman and Thomas, 1964) has been entertained for a number of years. The evidence supporting this concept is unsatisfactory from a number of points of view, in particular with regard to sensitivity and specificity of the responses of the experimental system. (*See* reviews by Haynes, 1974, and Thompson and Lippman, 1974, for critical discussions of this hypothesis.)

It now appears likely that the effects of glucocorticoids on inflammatory processes will not be found to derive from a single pivotal action, as was proposed in the lysosomal-stabilization hypothesis. Rather, discrete effects on blood vessels, leukocytes, and fibroblasts and other structures will probably be elucidated, and the overall effects on inflammation should prove to be the sum of these separate effects. (In suggesting the unlikelihood of a unitary action on inflammation, it is not the intent to deny the probability of a generalized action of the steroids at the molecular level, such as the formation of steroid-receptor complexes in the cytoplasm of steroid-sensitive cells.)

Several discrete effects of the steroids relevant to their anti-inflammatory properties are beginning to be understood. For example, a considerable amount is known about the inhibitory effects of the glucocorticoids on fibroblasts, phenomena that are of undoubted importance in the suppression of later phases of inflammation (Gray *et al.*, 1971). The mechanism by which glucocorticoids inhibit accumulation of macrophages is discussed in the preceding section. It has been found that cortisol, when added to a mixture of cultured lymphocytes and monocytes, causes the appearance of a factor in the culture medium that stimulates the migration of polymorphonuclear leukocytes (Stevenson, 1973).

Growth and Cell Division. Pharmacological doses of glucocorticoids retard or interrupt the growth of children, indicating an adverse effect on the epiphyseal cartilage. Inhibition of growth is a rather widespread effect of the glucocorticoids. For example, they inhibit cell division or the synthesis of DNA in thymocytes (Dougherty and White, 1945); fibroblasts (Pratt and Aronow, 1966); normal, developing, and regenerating liver (Howard, 1964; Loeb and Sternschein, 1973); gastric mucosa (Loeb and Sternschein, 1973); developing brain (Howard, 1964); developing lung (Carson *et al.*, 1973); and epidermis (Fisher and Maibach, 1971). Nevertheless, this effect is somewhat selective, and corticosteroids do not characteristically produce the bone-marrow depression or the enteritis that follows exposure to nonspecific antimitotic agents. The mechanism of this effect of the steroids is not known. It has been reported that cortisone treatment rapidly decreases the activity of DNA polymerase in rat liver (Henderson and Loeb, 1970).

ABSORPTION, TRANSPORT, METABOLISM, AND EXCRETION

Absorption. Cortisol and numerous congeners, including synthetic analogs, are effective when given by mouth. Desoxycorticosterone acetate is unusual in that it is ineffective by this route.

Water-soluble esters of cortisol and its synthetic congeners are administered intravenously in order to achieve high concentrations in body fluids rapidly. Prolonged effects are obtained by intramuscular injection of suspensions of cortisol, congeners, and esters. Minor changes in chemical structure may result in large changes in the rate of absorption, time of onset of effect, and duration of action.

Glucocorticoids are absorbed from sites of local application such as synovial spaces, the conjunctival sac, and the skin. The absorption may be sufficient, when administration is chronic or large areas of skin are involved, to cause systemic effects, including adrenocortical suppression.

Transport, Metabolism, and Excretion. In the plasma, 90% or more of the cortisol is reversibly bound to protein under normal circumstances (Mills *et al.,* 1960). The binding is accounted for by two protein fractions. One, "corticosteroid-binding globulin," is a glycoprotein; the other is plasma albumin. The globulin has high affinity but low total binding capacity; the albumin has low affinity but relatively large binding capacity. Consequently, at low or normal concentrations of corticosteroids most of the hormone is bound to globulin. When the amount of corticosteroid is increased, concentrations of both free and albumin-bound steroid increase with little change in the concentration of that bound to the globulin. Corticosteroids compete with each other for binding sites on the corticosteroid-binding globulin. Cortisol has high affinity; glucuronide-conjugated steroid metabolites and aldosterone have low affinities (Daughaday, 1960).

During pregnancy and during estrogen treatment in both sexes, corticosteroid-binding globulin, total plasma cortisol, and free cortisol increase several-fold. The physiological significance of these facts is not known. There is some evidence that the unbound and the albumin-bound cortisol, but not the cortisol bound to corticosteroid-binding globulin, are available for hepatic extraction and metabolism.

All the biologically active adrenocortical steroids and their synthetic congeners have a double bond in the 4,5 position and a ketone group at C 3. Reduction of the 4,5 double bond can occur at both hepatic and extrahepatic sites and yields an inactive substance. Subsequent reduction of the 3-ketone substituent to a 3-hydroxyl has been demonstrated only in liver. Most of the ring-A–reduced metabolies are enzymatically coupled through the 3-hydroxyl with sulfate or

with glucuronic acid to form water-soluble sulfate esters or glucuronides, and they are excreted as such. These conjugation reactions occur principally in liver and to some extent in kidney.

Reversible oxidation of the 11-hydroxyl group has been demonstrated to occur slowly in a variety of extrahepatic tissues and rapidly in liver. Corticosteroids with an 11-ketone substituent require reduction to 11-hydroxyl compounds for their biological activity (Sweat and Bryson, 1960). Reduction of the 20-ketone group to a 20-hydroxyl configuration yields a substance having little, if any, biological activity. Corticosteroids with an hydroxyl group at C 17 undergo an oxidation that yields 17-ketosteroids and a two-carbon fragment. These 17-ketosteroids are totally lacking in corticosteroid activity but, in a few instances, have weak androgenic or pyrogenic properties (Kappas *et al.,* 1960).

When radioactive-carbon, ring-labeled steroids are injected intravenously in man, most of the radioisotope is recovered in the urine within 72 hours; no radioactivity can be detected in expired CO_2. Neither biliary nor fecal excretion is of any quantitative importance in man (Hellman *et al.,* 1956). Tait and Burstein (1964) have estimated that the liver metabolizes at least 70% of the cortisol secreted.

The metabolism of cortisol has been studied more extensively than that of all other corticosteroids, and it is generally assumed that the metabolism of its congeners and synthetic derivatives is qualitatively similar. Cortisol has a plasma half-life of about 1½ hours. The metabolism of corticosteroids is greatly slowed by introduction of the 1,2 double bond or a fluorine atom into the molecule, and the half-life is correspondingly prolonged. Corticosteroids are metabolized principally by reduction of ring A, reduction of the ketone at C 20, and cleavage of the side chain. The metabolites are excreted in the urine as glucuronides, sulfates, and unconjugated compounds. By using cortisol labeled with radioactive carbon in ring A, Fukushima and associates (1960) determined the quantitative distribution of its various metabolites in the urine to be: (1) unaltered cortisol—less than 1%; (2) "tetrahydrocortisols," two stereoisomers (5α and 5β), plus "tetrahydrocortisone," one isomer (5β)—about 40% (*see* legend to Figure 70–2); (3) cortols, four stereoisomers (the possible combinations of 5α, 5β, 20α, and 20β), plus cortolones, four stereoisomers (again the possible combinations of stereoisomerism at C 5 and C 20)—about 17%; (4) 11-hydroxyetiocholanolone and 11-

ketoetiocholanolone plus 11-hydroxyandrosterone—about 6%.

Groups (1) and (2) comprise most of the substances measured in clinical laboratories as "17-hydroxy corticosteroids," or "Porter-Silber" steroids (Silber and Porter, 1954). Groups (1), (2), and (3) comprise most of the substances measured in the urine of normal persons by clinical laboratories as "17-ketogenic steroids." Urinary steroids of group (4) make a contribution to the clinically measured 17-ketosteroids (*see* Figure 70–4).

The metabolism of aldosterone follows the general pattern described above for cortisol.

STRUCTURE-ACTIVITY RELATIONSHIP

Cortisone was the first corticosteroid used for its anti-inflammatory effect. The development of sodium retention, reduced carbohydrate tolerance, osteoporosis, and other toxic effects as a consequence of therapy with cortisone led to attempts to synthesize compounds in which anti-inflammatory effect is dissociated from sodium retention and from effects on carbohydrate and protein metabolism. Modifications of structure have led to increases in the ratio of anti-inflammatory to sodium-retaining potency, such that in a number of presently available compounds electrolyte effects are of no serious consequence, even at the highest doses used. However, in all compounds studied to date, effects on inflammation and on carbohydrate and protein metabolism have paralleled one another. It seems likely that effects on inflammation and on organic metabolism are different facets of the same fundamental process.

Changes in molecular structure may bring about changes in biological potency as a result of changes in absorption, protein binding, rate of metabolic transformation, rate of excretion, ability to traverse membranes, and intrinsic effectiveness of the molecule at its site of action. Study of the structure-activity relationship of steroids has provided useful information in the search for new and better drugs. In the following paragraphs, modifications of the pregnane nucleus that have been of value in the commercial production of therapeutic agents are described. The molecular sites of alteration are shown in Figure 70–5 in bold lines and letters. Table 70–3 lists the effects of the modifications discussed relative to cortisol.

Ring A. The 4,5 double bond and the 3-ketone are both necessary for typical adrenocorticosteroid activity. Introduction of a 1,2 double bond, as in prednisone or prednisolone, enhances the ratio of carbohydrate-regulating potency to sodium-retaining potency by selectively increasing the former. Prednisolone is metabolically transformed more slowly than cortisol. However, this cannot fully account for increased carbohydrate-regulating potency, since electrolyte-regulating potency is not increased.

Ring B. 6α-Substitution has unpredictable effects. In the particular instance of cortisol, 6α-methylation increases anti-inflammatory, nitrogen-wasting, and sodium-retaining effects in man (Liddle, 1958). In contrast, 6α-methylprednisolone has slightly greater anti-inflammatory potency and less electrolyte-regulating potency than predniso-

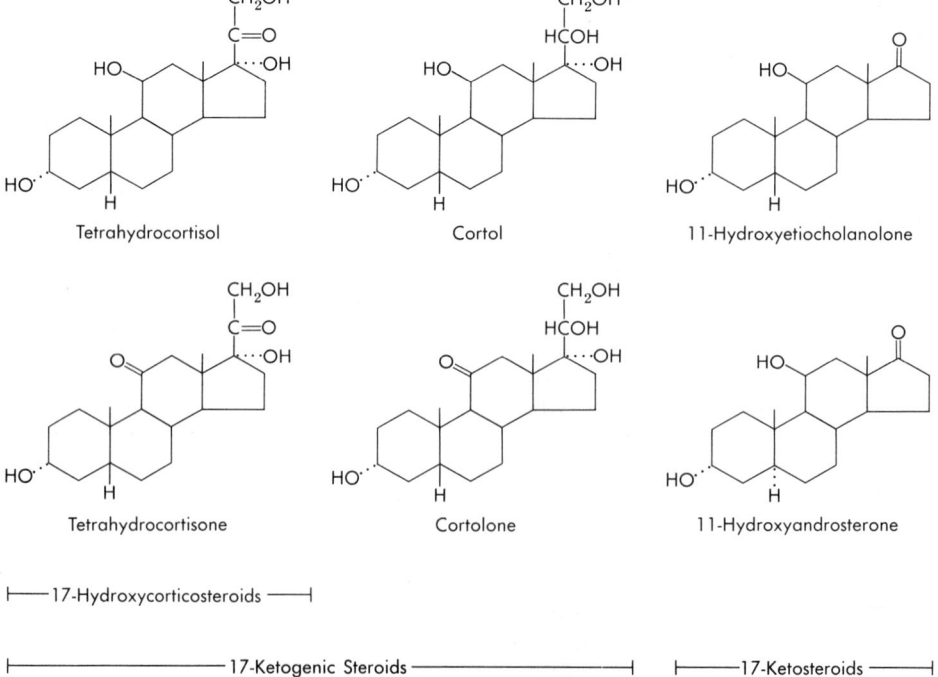

Tetrahydrocortisol   Cortol   11-Hydroxyetiocholanolone

Tetrahydrocortisone   Cortolone   11-Hydroxyandrosterone

|—— 17-Hydroxycorticosteroids ——|

|————————— 17-Ketogenic Steroids —————————| |———— 17-Ketosteroids ————|

Figure 70–4. *Principal products of metabolic transformations of cortisol recovered from urine.*

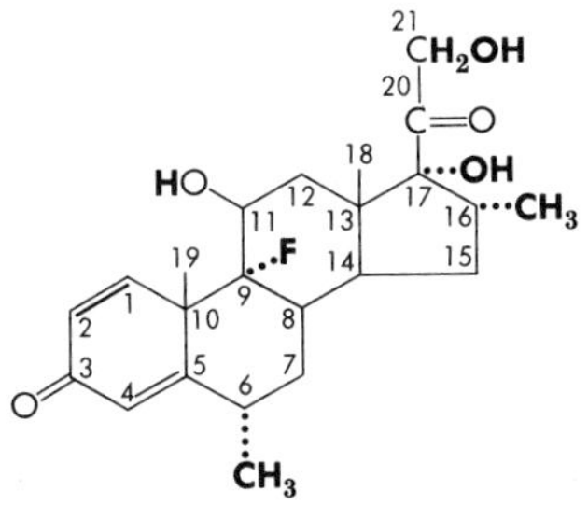

Figure 70-5. *Structure-activity relationship of adrenocorticosteroids.*

Light lines and letters indicate structural features common to compounds having anti-inflammatory action. Bold lines and letters indicate modifications that enhance or suppress characteristic activities. (After Liddle, 1961. Courtesy of *Clinical Pharmacology and Therapeutics.*)

lone. Fluorination in the 9α position enhances all biological activities of the corticosteroids, apparently by its electron-withdrawing effect on the 11β-hydroxy group (Schlagel, 1972).

Ring C. The presence of an oxygen function at C 11 is indispensable for significant anti-inflammatory and carbohydrate-regulating potency (cortisol versus 11-desoxycortisol) but is not necessary for high sodium-retaining potency, as demonstrated by desoxycorticosterone. Oxidation of 11β-hydroxy compounds to 11-keto compounds results in significant losses of activity, and the residual activity depends upon metabolic transformation to the 11β-hydroxy congener (cortisol versus cortisone).

Ring D. 16-Methylation or hydroxylation eliminates the sodium-retaining effect but only slightly modifies potency with respect to effects on organic metabolism and inflammation.

All presently used anti-inflammatory steroids are 17α-hydroxy compounds. Although some carbohydrate-regulating and anti-inflammatory effects may occur in 17-desoxy compounds (cortisol versus corticosterone), the fullest expression of these activities requires the presence of the 17α-hydroxy substituent.

All natural corticosteroids and most of the active synthetic analogs have a 21-hydroxy group. While some glycogenic and anti-inflammatory activities may occur in its absence, its presence is required for significant sodium-retaining activity. 21-Desoxycortisol appears to be without biological activity of any kind.

PREPARATIONS AND ROUTES OF ADMINISTRATION

The organic chemists have synthesized a bewildering number of modified adrenocorticosteroids, many of which share the same properties and differ only with respect to absolute dosage. At the outset it should be reemphasized that, whereas a clear separation has been made between mineralocorticoids and glucocorticoids, there is no member of the latter group that is unique with respect to a separation of therapeutic and toxic effects. A working knowledge of a small number of preparations is sufficient for nearly every clinical purpose.

Corticosteroids are administered orally, parenterally (intravenous, intramuscular, intrasynovial, and intralesional routes), and topically (dermal ointments, creams, and lotions; ophthalmic ointments and solutions; respiratory aerosols; enemas). It is probable that some absorption into the systemic circulation occurs with all forms of topical administration. In the case of most aerosols, absorption is virtually equivalent to that from parenteral or oral administration. Adrenocortical suppression can occur with applications of steroids to the conjunctival sac and to the skin. Absorption from the skin is especially marked when the steroid is applied under plastic film over a large surface area.

Information on available steroid preparations is presented in Table 70-4.

Beclomethasone dipropionate (9α-chloro-16β-methylprednisolone 17,21-dipropionate) is a chlorinated analog of betamethasone that has been used topically in dermatology. A number of clinical reports have indicated that this steroid administered by inhalation in doses of 300 to 600 μg per day will control chronic asthma in a significant proportion of pediatric patients without suppressing the adrenal cortex (Jones, 1973). It appears that beclomethasone is many times more active topically than dexamethasone but equal to or less active than dexamethasone as an adrenocortical suppressing agent. This suggests that it may have an unusually rapid rate of inactivation in the body (Harris *et al.*, 1973). The compound is not yet generally available.

Table 70-3. RELATIVE POTENCIES OF CORTICOSTEROIDS

COMPOUND	RELATIVE ANTI-INFLAMMATORY POTENCY	RELATIVE SODIUM-RETAINING POTENCY
Hydrocortisone (Cortisol)	1	1
Tetrahydrocortisol	0	0
Prednisone (Δ^1-Cortisone)	4	0.8
Prednisolone (Δ^1-Cortisol)	4	0.8
6α-Methylprednisolone	5	0.5
9α-Fluorocortisol	10	125
11-Desoxycortisol	0	0
Cortisone	0.8	0.8
Corticosterone	0.35	15
Triamcinolone (9α-Fluoro-16α-hydroxyprednisolone)	5	0
Paramethasone (6α-Fluoro-16α-methyl-prednisolone)	10	0
Betamethasone (9α-Fluoro-16β-methyl-prednisolone)	25	0
Dexamethasone (9α-Fluoro-16α-methyl-prednisolone)	25	0

Table 70-4. PREPARATIONS OF ADRENOCORTICAL STEROIDS AND THEIR SYNTHETIC ANALOGS *

NONPROPRIETARY NAME	DERIVATIVE	TRADE NAMES	ORAL FORMS		INJECTABLE FORMS	TOPICAL FORMS	TOPICAL OPHTHALMIC PREPARATIONS †
			Tablets	*Liquids*			
Desoxycorticosterone	Acetate, U.S.P.	DOCA ACETATE, PERCORTEN ACETATE	2, 5 mg (buccal)	—	5 mg/ml (oil) ▲; 125 mg (pellets) ‡	—	—
	Pivalate, N.F.	PERCORTEN PIVALATE	—	—	25 mg/ml (susp.) ‡	—	—
Fludrocortisone	Acetate, U.S.P.	FLORINEF ACETATE	0.1 mg ▲	—		—	—
Hydrocortisone, U.S.P.	—	CORTEF, HYDROCORTONE, and others	5, 10, 20 mg ▲	—	25, 50 mg/ml (susp.)	0.125–2% cream ▲; 1% ointment ▲; 0.25% lotion ▲; 100 mg/60 ml enema ▲	0.2% suspension
	Acetate, U.S.P.	CORTEF ACETATE, HYDROCORTONE ACETATE, and others	—	—	25, 50 mg/5 ml (susp.) ▲	1, 2.5% ointment ▲; 15, 25 mg suppositories; 10% rectal foam	2.5% suspension ▲; 1.5% ointment ▲
	Cypionate, N.F.	CORTEF FLUID	—	2 mg/ml (susp.) ‡	—	—	—
	Sodium Phosphate, U.S.P.	HYDROCORTONE PHOSPHATE	—	—	50 mg/ml ▲	—	—
	Sodium Succinate, U.S.P.	SOLU-CORTEF	—	—	100, 250, 500 mg; 1 g (powder) ▲	—	—
—	—	CELESTONE	0.6 mg ‡	0.6 mg/5 ml	—	0.2% cream ‡	—

Drug	Salt/Ester	Trade Name	Tablets	Oral Liquid	Injection	Topical	Ophthalmic/Other
Betamethasone, N.F.	Phosphate and Acetate, N.F.	SOLUSPAN	—	—	(susp.) ‡	—	—
	Valerate, N.F.	VALISONE	—	—	—	0.1% cream ‡ or ointment ‡; 0.01, 0.1% lotion ‡; 0.15% aerosol ‡	—
Cortisone	Benzoate	BENISONE GEL, FLUROBATE GEL	—	—	—	0.025% cream or gel	—
	Acetate, U.S.P.	CORTONE ACETATE	5, 25 mg ▲	—	25, 50 mg/ml (susp.) ▲	—	1.5, 2.5% suspension
Dexamethasone, U.S.P.	—	DECADRON, GAMMACORTEN, and others	0.25–1.5 mg ▲	0.5 mg/5 ml (elixir) ▲	—	0.04% cream; 0.1% gel; 0.011% aerosol (topical) ‡	0.1% suspension
	Sodium Phosphate, U.S.P.	DECADRON PHOSPHATE, HEXADROL PHOSPHATE	—	—	4 mg/ml ▲	0.1% cream ▲; 18 mg/12.6 g aerosol (inhalation)	0.1% solution ▲; 0.05% ointment ▲
	Acetate	DECADRON-L.A.	—	—	8 mg/ml	16.6 mg/50 g aerosol	—
Prednisolone, U.S.P.	—	DELTA-CORTEF and others	1, 2.5, 5 mg ▲	—	—	—	—
	Acetate, U.S.P.	METICORTELONE ACETATE and others	—	—	25, 50, 100 mg/ml (susp.) ▲	—	0.12, 1% suspension

* Preparations above the double line are intended for use as mineralocorticoids.
† Other preparations are available for subconjunctival injection.
▲ U.S.P. preparation.
‡ N.F. preparation.

Table 70-4. PREPARATIONS OF ADRENOCORTICAL STEROIDS AND THEIR SYNTHETIC ANALOGS (Continued)

NONPROPRIETARY NAME	DERIVATIVE	TRADE NAMES	ORAL FORMS		INJECTABLE FORMS	TOPICAL FORMS	TOPICAL OPHTHALMIC PREPARATIONS †
			Tablets	Liquids			
Prednisolone, U.S.P.	Sodium Phosphate, U.S.P.	HYDELTRASOL and others	—	—	20 mg/ml ▲	—	0.125, 0.5, 1% solution ▲; 0.25% ointment
	Sodium Succinate, U.S.P.	METICORTELONE SOLUBLE	—	—	50 mg (powder) ▲	—	—
	Tebutate, U.S.P.	HYDELTA-T.B.A.	—	—	20 mg/ml (susp.)	—	—
Prednisone, U.S.P.	—	DELTA-DOME, PARACORT, and others	1–25 mg ▲	—	—	—	—
Methyl-prednisolone, N.F.	—	MEDROL	2, 4, 16 mg ‡	—	—	—	—
	Acetate, U.S.P.	DEPO-MEDROL, MEDROL ACETATE	—	—	20, 40, 80 mg/ml (susp.) ‡	0.25, 1% cream ‡; 40 mg/unit enema ▲	—
	Sodium Succinate, U.S.P.	SOLU-MEDROL	—	—	40, 125, 500 mg; 1 g (powder) ▲	—	—
Paramethasone	Acetate, N.F.	HALDRONE, STEMEX	1, 2 mg ‡	—	—	—	—
	—	ARISTOCORT, KENACORT	1, 2, 4, 8, 16 mg ‡	—	—	—	—
Triamcinolone, N.F.	Acetonide, U.S.P.	ARISTODERM, KENALOG	—	—	10, 40 mg/ml (susp.) ▲	0.025, 0.1, 0.5% cream ▲; 0.025, 0.1% ointment ▲; 0.1% foam; 0.025, 0.1% lotion; 0.1% spray ‡; 0.1% dental	—

Generic Name	Form	Trade Name					
		KENACORT DIACETATE	—	—	—	—	—
	Hexacetonide, U.S.P.	ARISTOSPAN	—	—	5 mg/ml (susp.) ▲	—	—
Flumethasone	Pivalate, N.F.	LOCORTEN	—	—	—	0.025% cream ‡	—
Fluocinolone	Acetonide, U.S.P.	FLUONID, SYNALAR	—	—	—	0.01, 0.025, 0.2% cream ▲; 0.025% ointment ▲; 0.01% topical solution ▲	—
Fluocinonide, U.S.P.	—	LIDEX, TOPSYN GEL	—	—	—	0.05% cream or gel ▲	—
Fluoromethalone, N.F.	—	OXYLONE	—	—	—	0.025% cream ‡	0.1% suspension
Flurandrenolide, U.S.P.	—	CORDRAN	—	—	—	0.025, 0.05% cream ▲ or ointment ▲; 0.05% lotion; 4 μg/sq cm tape	—
Medrysone	—	HMS LIQUIFILM, MEDROCORT	—	—	—	—	1% suspension

† Other preparations are available for subconjunctival injection.
▲ U.S.P. preparation.
‡ N.F. preparation.

TOXICITY OF ADRENOCORTICAL
STEROIDS

Two categories of toxic effects are observed in the therapeutic use of adrenocorticosteroids: those resulting from *withdrawal* and those resulting from *continued use of large doses.* Acute adrenal insufficiency results from too rapid withdrawal of corticosteroid therapy. Protocols for discontinuing corticosteroid therapy in patients who have been subjected to suppressive therapy for long periods have been described by Harter and associates (1963). There is a characteristic corticosteroid withdrawal syndrome, consisting in fever, myalgia, arthralgia, and malaise, which may be extremely difficult to distinguish from "reactivation" of rheumatoid arthritis or rheumatic fever (Amatruda *et al.,* 1960). Pseudotumor cerebri with papilledema is a rare reaction that follows reduction or withdrawal of corticosteroid therapy (Levine and Leopold, 1973).

Prolonged therapy with corticosteroids may result in suppression of pituitary-adrenal function that can be slow in returning to normal. Graber and coworkers (1965) found that the processes of recovery of normal pituitary and adrenal function required about 9 months in some patients. During this recovery period and for an additional 1 to 2 years, the patient may need to be protected during stressful situations, such as surgery or severe infections, by the administration of corticosteroids.

In addition to pituitary-adrenal suppression, the principal complications resulting from prolonged therapy with corticosteroids are fluid and electrolyte disturbances; hyperglycemia and glycosuria; increased susceptibility to infections, including tuberculosis; peptic ulcers, which may bleed or perforate; osteoporosis; a characteristic myopathy; behavioral disturbances; posterior subcapsular cataracts; and Cushing's habitus, consisting of "moon face," "buffalo hump," supraclavicular fat pads, "central obesity," striae, ecchymoses, acne, and hirsutism.

Hypokalemic alkalosis and *edema* are infrequently encountered in patients being treated with synthetic corticosteroid congeners and almost never in patients taking the 16α-substituted compounds triamcinolone and dexamethasone. *Glycosuria* can

usually be kept within tolerable limits with diet and/or insulin, and its occurrence should not be an important factor in the decision to continue corticosteroid therapy or to initiate it in diabetic patients.

Increased susceptibility to infection in patients treated with corticosteroids is not specific for any particular bacterial or fungal pathogens. If infection develops in a patient treated with corticosteroids, the dose should be maintained or increased and the best available treatment for the infection vigorously administered. Corticosteroid therapy may be initiated in patients having known infections of some consequence if effective, specific chemotherapy can be administered concomitantly with the hormones.

Peptic ulceration is an occasional complication of corticosteroid therapy. The high incidence of hemorrhage and perforation in these ulcers and the insidious nature of their development make them severe therapeutic problems. Some investigators believe that the steroids are not the cause of the ulcers since, of all patients receiving steroids, only those with rheumatoid arthritis have an increased incidence of ulcers. In this disease the nearly universal administration of aspirin makes it difficult to evaluate the evidence. It has been proposed that the glucocorticoids alter the mucosal defense mechanisms. The problem of steroid-associated ulcers is reviewed by Fenster (1973).

Myopathy, characterized by weakness of the proximal musculature of arms and legs and of their associated shoulder and pelvic muscles, is occasionally seen in patients taking large doses of corticosteroids. It may occur soon after treatment is begun and be sufficiently severe to prevent ambulation. It is not specific for synthetic corticosteroid congeners, for it is found in pituitary-dependent Cushing's syndrome. It is a serious complication and an indication for withdrawal of therapy. Recovery may be slow and incomplete.

Behavioral disturbances may take various forms, for example, nervousness, insomnia, changes in mood or psyche, and psychopathies of the manic-depressive or schizophrenic type. Suicidal tendencies are not uncommon. Serious reactions are most likely to occur in individuals who have a previous history of psychosis or other evidence of emotional or mental instability, and usually represent intensification of preexisting personality disorders. However, it should be emphasized that absence of a history of psychotic breakdown or of defective emotional adjustment is no guarantee against the occurrence of psychosis during hormonal therapy.

Posterior subcapsular cataracts have been reported in children receiving corticosteroid therapy (Bihari and Grossman, 1968). Nearly all patients with rheumatoid arthritis who receive 20 mg of prednisone per day for 4 years develop cataracts (Levine and Leopold, 1973); it is possible that patients with this disease are particularly susceptible to this complication.

Osteoporosis and *vertebral compression fractures* are frequent serious complications of corticosteroid therapy in patients of all ages. Osteoporosis is an indication for withdrawal of therapy and should be looked for regularly in radiographs of the spine in patients taking glucocorticoids for longer than a few months. The possibility of development of osteoporosis should be an important consideration in initiating and managing corticosteroid therapy, especially in postmenopausal women.

THERAPEUTIC USES

With the exception of substitution therapy, the use of corticosteroids and their congeners in disease is empirical. From a large experience accumulated since Hench's memorable discovery, at least six therapeutic principles may be abstracted, as follows: (1) for any disease, in any patient, the appropriate dose to achieve a given therapeutic effect must be determined by trial and error and must be reevaluated from time to time as the stage and the activity of the disease alter; (2) a *single* dose of corticosteroid, even a large one, is virtually without harmful effects; (3) a few days of corticosteroid therapy, in the absence of specific contraindications, is unlikely to produce harmful results except at the most extreme dosages; (4) as corticosteroid therapy is prolonged over periods of months, and to the extent that the dose exceeds the equivalent of substitution therapy, the incidence of disabling and potentially lethal effects increases; (5) except in adrenal

insufficiency, the administration of corticosteroids is neither etiological nor curative therapy but only palliative by virtue of the anti-inflammatory effects; and (6) abrupt cessation of prolonged, high-dosage corticosteroid therapy is associated with a significant risk of adrenal insufficiency of sufficient severity to be threatening to life.

Translated into the terms of clinical practice, these general principles are equivalent to the following rules. When corticosteroids are to be administered over long periods, the dose must be the smallest one that will achieve a desired effect. This dose must be found by trial and error. Where the goal of therapy is relief of painful or distressing symptoms not associated with an immediately life-threatening disease, for example, rheumatoid arthritis, the initial dose should be small and gradually increased until pain or distress has been reduced to tolerable levels. Complete relief is not sought. At frequent intervals the dose should be gradually reduced until the development of more severe symptoms signals that the minimal acceptable dose has been found. When therapy is directed at an immediately life-threatening state, for example, pemphigus, the initial dose should be a large one, estimated to achieve, almost with certainty, control of the crisis. If some benefit is not observed in a short time, the dose should be doubled or tripled. When potentially lethal disease is controlled by large amounts of corticosteroid, reduction of the dose should be carried out under conditions that permit frequent, accurate observations. Under these circumstances it is essential to assess constantly the relative dangers of therapy and of the disease being treated.

The apparently innocuous character of a single administration of corticosteroid in amounts within the conventional therapeutic range justifies its use without a definite diagnosis in apparently mortal crises in which there exists some probability that life is threatened by primary adrenal insufficiency, by pituitary insufficiency, or by cerebral edema. If one of these conditions is present, a single intravenous injection of a soluble corticosteroid may prevent immediate death and allow time for diagnostic procedures.

Short courses of systemic corticosteroid therapy in large doses may properly be given for diseases that do not threaten life, in the absence of specific contraindications. The general rule is that long courses of therapy at high dosage should be reserved for life-threatening disease. On occasion, and for definite cause, when the patient is threatened with permanent disability, this rule is justifiably violated.

It is not possible to define the precise dose of glucocorticoids that will produce pituitary and adrenocortical suppression in a given patient, since there is considerable variation in individual responses. In general, the higher the dose and the more prolonged the therapy the greater is the likelihood of suppression.

Harter and associates (1963) have suggested that some dissociation of therapeutic effects from certain undesirable metabolic effects can be achieved by the administration of a single large dose of corticosteroid every other day, in contrast to the usual daily multiple-dose schedule. A single dose every other day or at even longer intervals is acceptable therapy for some, but not all, patients with a variety of diseases modified by corticosteroid therapy. When this therapeutic regimen is possible, the degree of suppression of the pituitary and adrenal cortex can be minimized. Steroids with very prolonged effects, such as those substituted at C 16, are not suitable for use by this dosage schedule.

Substitution Therapy. Insufficiency of secretion of the adrenal cortex results from structural or functional lesions of the adrenal cortex itself or from structural or functional lesions of the anterior pituitary. In either case, the patient may present with acute, catastrophic adrenal insufficiency (adrenal crisis) or chronic adrenal insufficiency. When the adrenal itself is the seat of the lesion, all elements of normal adrenal secretion may be reduced or absent or the deficiency may be selective for one or more components of secretion.

Acute Adrenal Insufficiency. This disease is characterized by gastrointestinal symptoms, dehydration, weakness, lethargy, and hypotension. It is usually associated with disorders of the adrenal, rather than the pituitary, although exceptions occur. It frequently follows abrupt withdrawal of high doses of corticosteroids.

The immediate needs of such patients are water, sodium, chloride, glucose, hydrocortisone, and appropriate therapy for precipitating causes, for example, infection, trauma, or hemorrhage. Inasmuch as these patients have a diminished capacity for a water diuresis and have often undergone some degree of cellular hydration, they are susceptible to water intoxication. The principal intravenous fluid should be isotonic sodium chloride solution. Glucose is required for nutrition and to prevent or treat hypoglycemia, but it should be given intravenously in isotonic sodium chloride solution. The total amount of intravenous fluid administered during the first 24 hours should not, in most instances, exceed 5% of ideal body weight. The patient should be monitored for evidences of rising venous pressure and pulmonary edema, because the functional capacity of the cardiovascular system is reduced by adrenocortical insufficiency. Hydrocortisone hemisuccinate or phosphate must be given in the intravenous fluids at a rate of 100 mg every 8 hours, following an initial rapidly administered intravenous injection of 100 mg. In the period of transition from intravenous fluid therapy to normal diet and activity, intramuscular hydrocortisone hemisuccinate or phosphate may be used in a dose of 25 mg every 6 or 8 hours.

Chronic Adrenal Insufficiency. This disease results from adrenal surgery or destructive lesions of the adrenal cortex. It requires the administration of cortisone acetate, 25 to 37.5 mg per day or equivalent, in single or divided doses. A common dose schedule is 25 mg on arising and 12.5 mg in the late afternoon. Most patients will also require a potent mineralocorticoid. The most convenient drug to use for this purpose is 9α-fluorocortisol acetate. The usual adult dose is 0.1 to 0.3 mg daily. Some patients do not need a mineralocorticoid and are adequately treated with cortisone and generous dietary salt. Therapy is guided by the patient's sense of well-being, alertness, appetite, weight, muscular strength, pigmentation, blood pressure, and freedom from orthostatic hypotension.

Congenital Adrenal Hyperplasia. This is a familial disorder in which activity of one of several enzymes required for biosynthesis of corticosteroids is deficient. With diminished or absent production of cortisol, aldosterone, or both, and consequent lack of inhibitory feedback, the adrenal cortex is stimulated to the overproduction of other hormonally active steroids. The clinical presentation, laboratory findings, and treatment depend on which of the six enzyme deficiencies thus far described is responsible. Only the syndrome of 21-hydroxylase deficiency will be described here.

In about 90% of the patients with congenital adrenal hyperplasia there is a deficiency of 21-hydroxylase activity. When the deficiency is only partial, the usual case, cortisol is secreted at normal rates as a result of continuous hypersecretion of ACTH, with consequent overproduction of adrenal androgens and their precursors. Aldosterone secretion is approximately normal. Female children undergo virilization, female "pseudohermaphroditism," and male children show precocious development of secondary sexual characteristics, "macrogenitosomia." Linear growth is accelerated in childhood, but the height at maturity is reduced by premature closure of the epiphyses.

In about 30% of patients with 21-hydroxylase deficiency, the enzymatic defect is sufficiently severe to compromise increased aldosterone secretion in response to a hypovolemic stimulus. Such patients are unable to conserve sodium normally ("salt wasters"), in addition to manifesting androgenic effects (Bongiovanni *et al.,* 1967).

All patients with congenital adrenal hyperplasia resulting from a 21-hydroxylase deficiency require substitution therapy with cortisol or a suitable congener, and those with a salt-losing tendency require, in addition, a sodium-retaining steroid. The usual oral dose of cortisol is about 0.6 mg/kg daily in four divided doses, the last one being given as late as possible in order to maintain pituitary suppression overnight. When parenteral substitution therapy is desired, cortisone acetate may be given intramuscularly every other day. The mineralocorticoid usually given is 9α-fluorocortisol acetate, 0.05 to 0.1 mg per day. Therapy is guided by gain in weight and height, by excretion of urinary 17-ketosteroids, and by blood pressure. Sudden spurts of linear growth may indicate inadequate pituitary suppression and excessive androgen secretion, whereas growth failure suggests overtreatment.

A number of rare forms of congenital adrenal hyperplasia are known in which enzyme deficiencies of the adrenal cortex, with similar defects of the gonads, result in clinical and laboratory findings very different from those described above for 21-hydroxylase deficiency. The types described thus far are: "desmolase" deficiency (Camacho *et al.,* 1968), 3β-hydroxysteroid dehydrogenase deficiency (Bongiovanni *et al.,* 1967), 17α-hydroxylase deficiency (Goldsmith *et al.,* 1968), 11β-hydroxylase deficiency (Bongiovanni *et al.,* 1967), and 18-hydroxylase deficiency (David *et al.,* 1968). The clinical and laboratory findings and the treatment in these rare forms are quite different from those in 21-hydroxylase deficiency. The publications cited should be consulted for details.

Adrenal Insufficiency Secondary to Anterior Pituitary Insufficiency. This condition is not usually associated with the dramatic signs and symptoms characteristic of adrenal insufficiency resulting from disease of the adrenal cortex unless there are complicating circumstances, for example, unusual fluid losses, trauma, or starvation. Hypoglycemia is the most frequent cause of symptoms. In the absence of unusual demands, fluid and electrolyte balance is normal, apparently as a consequence of the nearly normal regulation of aldosterone secretion in the hypopituitary patient. The administration of 25 mg of cortisone acetate on arising and 12.5 mg in late afternoon is adequate replacement therapy for most patients with anterior pituitary insufficiency. This schedule mimics, to some extent, the normal diurnal cycle of adrenal secretion. When initiating treatment, it is customary to begin cortisol first and to add thyroid replacement therapy after adrenal insufficiency is under some degree of control, on the hypothetical grounds that the administration of thyroid without cortisol to a hypopituitary patient may precipitate acute adrenal insufficiency.

Therapeutic Uses in Nonendocrine Diseases. Brief outlines of important uses of corticosteroids in diseases other than those involving the pituitary-adrenal complex are set forth below.

The dosage of glucocorticoids varies greatly with the condition being treated. In the following discus-sion of therapy of various disease entities, approximate doses of a representative corticosteroid congener, usually prednisone, are suggested. It is not meant to imply that prednisone has peculiar merit in general or for any particular disease over the other corticosteroid congeners. For purpose of comparison, the following is the *equivalent milligram dosage* of the various glucocorticoids: *cortisone,* 25; *hydrocortisone,* 20; *prednisolone,* 5; *prednisone,* 5; *methylprednisolone,* 4; *triamcinolone,* 4; *paramethasone,* 2; *betamethasone,* 0.75; *dexamethasone,* 0.75. These dose relationships apply only to oral or intravenous administration of these compounds. When these substances or their derivatives are injected intramuscularly or into joint spaces, their relative properties may be greatly altered.

Arthritis. In *rheumatoid arthritis,* the criterion for initiating corticosteroid therapy is progressive disease with consequent economic disability, despite intensive treatment with rest, physical therapy, gold, salicylates, and other drugs. The decision to embark upon a program of hormone therapy must be made with due consideration for the fact that corticosteroid therapy, once started, may have to be continued for many years or for life, with the attendant risks of serious complications. The initial dose should be small and increased slowly until the desired degree of control is attained. The symptomatic effect of small reductions should be frequently tested in order to maintain the dose as low as possible. Complete relief is not sought. A regimen of rest, physical therapy, and salicylates is continued. The usual initial dose is about 10 mg of prednisone (or equivalent) per day in divided doses. Optimal therapy for some patients with painful symptoms confined to one or a few joints may be intra-articular injection of the steroid into the affected joints. Typical doses are 5 to 20 mg of triamcinolone acetonide or the equivalent, depending upon the size of the joint cavity.

In *osteoarthritis,* intra-articular injection of corticosteroids is recommended for treatment of episodic manifestations of acute inflammation: local heat, swelling, and pain. Injections for this purpose should be infrequent because, in both rheumatoid arthritis and osteoarthritis, a significant incidence of painless destruction of the joint, reminiscent of Charcot's arthropathy, may be associated with repeated intra-articular injections of corticosteroids (Rheumatism Review Committee, 1963).

Rheumatic Carditis. Corticosteroids are reserved for patients failing to respond to salicylates and as initial therapy for patients severely ill with fever, acute congestive heart failure, arrhythmia, and pericarditis; acute manifestations are more rapidly suppressed by corticosteroids than by salicylates, a possibly lifesaving difference in a moribund patient. A dose of approximately 40 mg of prednisone or equivalent is usually given daily, in divided amounts, although much larger doses may on occasion be required. Reactivation of the disease occurs in a number of instances following withdrawal of steroid therapy. For this reason it has been suggested that salicylates be given concurrently with corticosteroids and be continued through and after the period of withdrawal of hormone therapy (Fischel *et al.,* 1958).

Renal Diseases. Corticosteroids do not modify the course of acute or chronic glomerulonephritis. However, patients with the *nephrotic syndrome* attributable to systemic lupus erythematosus or to primary renal disease, except renal amyloidosis (Maxwell *et al.,* 1964), may be benefited by corticosteroid therapy. A typical therapeutic regimen consists in the daily administration, in divided doses, of 60 mg of prednisone or equivalent (2 mg/kg of edema-free body weight in children) for 3 or 4 weeks. If a remission with a diuresis and decreased proteinuria occurs during this period, maintenance treatment is continued for as long as a year. For this, the daily dose of prednisone is given only for the first 3 days of each week (Bacon and Spencer, 1973).

Collagen Diseases. The manifestations of most of the diseases in this group are controlled by glucocorticoids. An exception is *scleroderma,* which is considered generally refractory to these agents. It is important to distinguish between scleroderma and *mixed connective disease syndrome,* which is responsive to steroids (Yount *et al.,* 1973). *Polymyositis, polyarteritis nodosa,* and the granulomatous-polyarteritis group (*Wegener's granulomatosis, temporal-cranial arteritis,* and *polymyalgia rheumatica*) are treated with daily doses of prednisone, approximately 1 mg/kg or equivalent, to induce a remission. The dose is then tapered down to the minimally effective level. Glucocorticoids decrease morbidity in all these diseases and prolong the survival times of patients with polyarteritis nodosa and Wegener's granulomatosis. *In temporal (giant-cell) arteritis, adequate steroid therapy is necessary to prevent the blindness that occurs in about 20% of untreated cases. Fulminating systemic lupus erythematosus* is a life-threatening condition, the manifestations of which should be suppressed by adrenocorticosteroid therapy with doses large enough to produce a prompt effect. Treatment usually consists in a 1-mg/kg daily dose of prednisone or equivalent. Within 48 hours, reduction of fever and improvement in the signs and symptoms of arthritis, pleuritis, or pericarditis should be observed. If not, the dose should be increased in 20-mg increments daily until a favorable response occurs. After the acute episode has been brought under control, corticosteroid therapy should be reduced by small steps, for example, 5 mg of prednisone per week, until signs or symptoms warn against further reductions. Salicylate or antimalarial drugs are then introduced and may permit a further reduction of corticosteroid dosage (Robinson, 1962). There have been favorable reports on the treatment of systemic lupus erythematosus with a combination of glucocorticoids and antimetabolites, such as azathioprine, or the alkylating agent cyclophosphamide. This combination therapy is still experimental and not recommended for general use (Yount *et al.,* 1973).

Allergic Diseases. The manifestations of allergic disease that are of limited duration such as *hay fever, serum sickness, urticaria, contact dermatitis, drug reactions, bee stings, angioneurotic edema,* and *anaphylaxis* can, if necessary, be suppressed by adequate doses of glucocorticoids given as a supplement to the primary therapy. It must be emphasized, however, that the effects of the steroids require some time to develop, and *severe reactions such as anaphylaxis and angioneurotic edema of the glottis require immediate therapy with epinephrine, 0.5 to 1.0 ml of a 1:1000 solution (0.5 to 1.0 mg) subcutaneously.* In life-threatening situations steroids may be given intravenously; dexamethasone phosphate (8 to 12 mg or equivalent) is appropriate. In less severe diseases, such as serum sickness or hay fever, antihistaminic compounds are the drugs of first choice.

Bronchial Asthma. The corticosteroids should *not* be used in the treatment of any asthmatic condition, acute or chronic, that can be brought under moderate control with other measures. In *status asthmaticus,* cortisol (50 to 100 mg) is administered by intravenous infusion over 8 hours. The procedure is repeated daily until the acute attack is under control, following which the patient is given 10 mg of prednisone twice daily for 4 or 5 days. The dose is then reduced in steps and withdrawal planned for about the tenth day after initiation of the prednisone therapy. Under favorable circumstances, the patient can subsequently be managed once again with his prior medication.

In the treatment of *severe chronic bronchial asthma,* uncontrolled by other measures, corticosteroid therapy may be considered. The decision must be made with great care since the majority of patients, once started on corticosteroid therapy, remain indefinitely on such therapy.

The aim of corticosteroid therapy is the establishment of a dose of steroid effective in reducing the severity but not in eliminating the manifestations of the disease. Such a dose almost invariably induces a mild degree of hypercorticism. The majority of patients are given 5 to 10 mg of prednisone daily by mouth, in divided doses. The patient is encouraged to use his usual medication in combination with corticosteroid therapy in order to keep the dose of steroid at the lowest possible level compatible with amelioration of the disease. When an acute exacerbation occurs, the dose is increased to two or even three times the maintenance dose. (*See* Knowles, 1961; Rees and Williams, 1962.)

Ocular Diseases. Corticosteroids are frequently used to suppress inflammation in the eye, and employed properly they are often responsible for preservation of sight. Levine and Leopold (1973) list 28 disorders of the eye that respond to corticosteroids. They are administered locally for disease of the outer eye and anterior segment. Both natural and synthetic corticosteroids attain therapeutic concentrations in the aqueous humor following instillation into the conjunctival cul-de-sac. For disease of the posterior segment, systemic administration is required.

A typical prescription is 0.1% dexamethasone phosphate solution (ophthalmic), 2 drops in the conjunctival sac every 4 hours while awake, and 0.05% dexamethasone phosphate ointment (ophthalmic) at bedtime. For inflammations of the posterior segment of the eye, usual daily doses are approximately 30 mg of prednisone or equivalent, administered orally in divided doses.

It has been convincingly demonstrated that topical corticosteroid therapy *frequently induces intraocular hypertension* in normal eyes and further increases pressure in eyes with initially elevated pressure. The glaucoma has not always been reversible on cessation of corticosteroid treatment. It has been recommended that, when corticosteroids are applied to the eye for more than 2 weeks, the intraocular pressure be monitored.

The local administration of corticosteroids to patients with bacterial, viral, or fungal conjunctivitis *may mask evidences of progression of the infection until sight is lost.* Corticosteroids are *contraindicated in herpes simplex* (dendritic keratitis) of the eye, because progression of the disease and irreversible clouding of the cornea may occur. Topical steroids should not be used in the treatment of mechanical lacerations and abrasions of the eye. They delay healing and promote the development and spread of infection.

Skin Diseases. The development of corticosteroid preparations suitable for topical administration has revolutionized the therapy of the more common varieties of skin disease. Maibach and Stoughton (1973) have divided 20 dermatological disorders that respond to topical corticosteroids into those that are very responsive and those that require higher concentrations of steroids, occlusion of the drug under a plastic film, or intralesional administration. Attention must be paid to the concentration of steroid used, and there are a large number of preparations of various concentrations available for topical use (Table 70–4). A typical prescription for an eczematous eruption is 1% hydrocortisone ointment applied locally twice daily. Effectiveness is enhanced by application of the cream or ointment under a transparent plastic wrapping. Unfortunately, systemic absorption is also enhanced, occasionally sufficiently to suppress the pituitary-adrenal axis. Adrenocorticosteroids are administered systemically for severe episodes of acute skin disorders and exacerbations of chronic disorders. The dose is usually 40 mg per day of prednisone or equivalent. Systemically administered corticosteroids may be lifesaving in *pemphigus.* Up to 120 mg of prednisone or equivalent per day may be required to control the disease.

Diseases of the Intestinal Tract. Patients severely ill with untreated *celiac sprue* can often benefit from a course of glucocorticoid therapy given at the same time that management with a gluten-free diet is begun. Prednisolone, 30 mg per day or equivalent, is continued for 3 to 4 weeks. Patients who fail to respond to a gluten-free diet are helped by lower doses of prednisolone (7 to 12 mg per day or equivalent) for an indefinite period (Wall, 1973).

Corticosteroid therapy is indicated in selected patients with *chronic ulcerative colitis.* Mildly ill patients with bowel symptoms but without disabling systemic symptoms usually can and should be managed with rest, diet, sedation, anticholinergic agents, and chemotherapy. However, patients who do not improve should have a trial of methylprednisolone acetate, 40 mg or equivalent, in a nightly retention enema, in an attempt to induce remission. Alternate-day therapy may be effective. Severely ill patients with fever, anorexia, anemia, and malnutrition often improve dramatically when given systemic corticosteroid therapy. Large doses, 60 to 120 mg per day of prednisone, or the equivalent, are recommended. Major complications of ulcerative colitis

may occur despite corticosteroid therapy. Signs and symptoms of intestinal perforation and peritonitis may be difficult to detect during corticosteroid treatment (Korelitz and Lindner, 1964).

Cerebral Edema and Increased Intracranial Pressure. Corticosteroids are of value in the reduction or prevention of cerebral edema associated with surgical and other brain trauma, cerebrovascular accidents, and brain malignancies, primary or metastatic. Objective and subjective evidence of improvement may occur within 4 hours following the administration of 50 mg of prednisone or equivalent. Conventional doses are of the order of 100 mg of prednisone or equivalent per day, in divided doses. The clinical benefits are probably derived from suppression of brain inflammation.

Malignancies. The chemotherapy of *acute lymphocytic leukemia* and *lymphomas* has been greatly improved by the introduction of therapy with multiple agents, and glucocorticoids are used because of their antilymphocytic effects. At the present time these diseases are treated in a complex fashion with rigidly scheduled sequences of combined drug therapy. Prednisone is commonly used in conjunction with an alkylating agent such as cyclophosphamide, an antimetabolite, and a vinca alkaloid (*see* Chapter 62). These therapeutic regimens are only suitable for use in medical centers under the supervision of oncologists.

Objective tumor regression in *carcinoma of the breast* can be induced by glucocorticoids in about 15% of patients; prednisolone (30 mg per day) has been the usual treatment. The presumed mechanism by which the corticosteroids act in these patients is through adrenocortical suppression, with an accompanying decrease in production of androgens, which are precursors of tumor-stimulating estrogens (Brennan, 1973). Similar therapy has been suggested to suppress adrenal androgens in the castrated patient with carcinoma of the prostate.

Diseases of the Liver. The use of glucocorticoids in the treatment of hepatic diseases has been the subject of controversy. Careful studies have now indicated several diseases of the liver in which therapy with steroids significantly improves survival rates; these are *subacute hepatic necrosis* and *chronic active hepatitis, alcoholic hepatitis,* and *nonalcoholic cirrhosis in females* (Lesesne and Fallon, 1973; Copenhagen Study Group for Liver Diseases, 1974). Treatment of *subacute hepatic necrosis* and *chronic active hepatitis* includes prednisolone, 60 to 100 mg per day; the dose is tapered as the disease improves. Treatment of *alcoholic hepatitis* with corticosteroids is reserved for patients who are severely ill, with evidence of hepatic encephalopathy. Prednisone (40 mg per day) is given for 1 month, followed by withdrawal over a period of 2 to 4 weeks. *Nonalcoholic cirrhosis in women* should be treated with glucocorticoids if the patient does not have ascites. Daily dosages average 15 to 20 mg of prednisone or equivalent when they are adjusted to the needs of the individual patients. The data indicate that *steroid treatment lowers survival rates when ascites is present.* Treatment of cirrhotic male patients with steroids has not been shown to be beneficial.

Shock. While corticosteroids are often administered to patients in shock, there is little evidence to indicate that such therapy is efficacious. To the contrary, it seems clear that there is no benefit to patients suffering from cardiogenic or hemorrhagic shock. Conflicting reports have appeared regarding septic shock, and this question remains open. Those who have reported favorable results following the administration of glucocorticoids for septic shock have used doses in excess of 300 mg of hydrocortisone or its equivalent as soon as possible. (*See* Reichgott and Melmon, 1973, and references therein.)

Miscellaneous Diseases. *Sarcoidosis* is treated with prednisone, approximately 1 mg/kg per day or equivalent, to induce a remission. Maintenance doses, which are often required for long periods of time, may be 10 mg of prednisone per day or less. In this, as in other diseases treated by prolonged steroid therapy, patients with positive tuberculin reactions or other evidence of tuberculosis should receive prophylactic antituberculosis therapy. In *thrombocytopenia,* prednisone, 0.5 mg/kg or equivalent, is used to decrease the bleeding tendency. In severe cases and for initiation of treatment of *idiopathic thrombocytopenia,* daily doses of prednisolone, 1 to 1.5 mg/kg, are employed. *Hemolytic anemias* with a positive Coombs test are treated with prednisone, 1 mg/kg per day or equivalent. If hemolysis is severe, therapy is initiated with 100 mg of hydrocortisone intravenously; as the disease improves, the dose is decreased. Small maintenance doses may be needed for several months. In *organ transplantation,* high doses of prednisone (50 to 100 mg) are given at the time of the transplant surgery. Smaller maintenance doses (10 to 20 mg per day) are continued indefinitely, and the dosage is increased if rejection is threatened. In *aspiration of gastric contents,* prednisone (50 to 100 mg) is given for 2 to 3 days to suppress the inflammatory reaction in the lung and to prevent development of pulmonary abscess.

DIAGNOSTIC APPLICATIONS OF ADRENOCORTICAL STEROIDS

Potent synthetic congeners of cortisol reduce urinary excretion of cortisol metabolites by inhibition of pituitary ACTH release. The dose required is so small, in gravimetric terms, that it contributes only negligibly to the urinary steroids. Liddle (1960) has reported that the administration of 0.5 mg of dexamethasone or of 9α-fluoroprednisolone every 6 hours for a total of eight doses results in a marked suppression of excretion of cortisol metabolites in normal persons, but has almost no effect on the urinary steroids of persons with pituitary-dependent hypercorticism. This test is useful in distinguishing persons with some nonspecific elevation of steroid excretion, for example, that due to obesity or stress, from patients with Cushing's syndrome. The administration of 2.0 mg of dexamethasone every 6 hours for a total of eight doses causes a definite suppression of excretion of cortisol metabolites in patients with pituitary-dependent hypercorticism, but ordinarily has little if any effect on the urinary steroids of patients with adrenal neoplasms or ACTH-producing tumors (Meador *et al.,* 1962). However, "suppressible" tumors have been reported. The results of these tests are likely to be most definite if the urinary steroids

are measured daily for 2 days before and for at least 2 days during administration of the suppressing agent. Variations of this procedure (shorter test period and measurement of plasma cortisol rather than urinary metabolites) have been described (Sawin *et al.,* 1968).

INHIBITORS OF ADRENOCORTICAL STEROID BIOSYNTHESIS

Three pharmacological agents have proven most useful as inhibitors of adrenocortical secretion. Mitotane (*o,p'*-DDD), an adrenocorticolytic agent, is discussed in Chapter 62. Metyrapone and aminoglutethimide are discussed here. The subject has been reviewed by Temple and Liddle (1970).

Metyrapone. Metyrapone reduces cortisol production by inhibition of the 11β-hydroxylation reaction. The biosynthetic process is terminated at 11-desoxycortisol (Figure 70–3), a compound that has practically no inhibitory influence on ACTH release. In the normal person, a compensatory increase in ACTH release follows, and the secretion of 11-desoxycortisol, a "17-hydroxycorticoid," is markedly accelerated. Consequently, in normal persons, administration of metyrapone induces increased renal excretion of "17-hydroxycorticoids."

Metyrapone is used to test the ability of the pituitary to respond to a decreased concentration of plasma cortisol. Administration of metyrapone to patients with disease of the hypothalamico-pituitary complex who are unable to achieve a compensatory increase in the rate of ACTH release is, of course, not followed by increased renal excretion of "17-hydroxycorticoids."

The ability of the adrenal to respond to ACTH should be demonstrated before metyrapone is employed, for two reasons: (1) administration of metyrapone can be used as a test for normal hypothalamico-pituitary function only if the adrenal glands are capable of responding to ACTH, and (2) the drug may induce acute adrenal insufficiency in patients with reduced adrenal secretory capacity. Metyrapone also inhibits synthesis of aldosterone, which, like cortisol, is an 11β-hydroxylated compound. However, metyrapone does not typically cause a deficiency in mineralocorticoids, with a consequent loss of sodium and retention of potassium, because the inhibition of the 11β-hydroxylation reaction results in an increased production of 11-desoxycorticosterone, a mineralocorticoid.

Metyrapone has been used experimentally to treat the hypercortisolism that results from adrenal neoplasms that function autonomously and from ectopic ACTH production by tumors. It is not suitable for correcting the excessive cortisol secretion of Cushing's syndrome caused by hypersecretion of pituitary ACTH. In this situation, the decline in circulating cortisol produced by metyrapone elicits additional ACTH release. This, in turn, stimulates the incompletely blocked adrenal cortex to secrete cortisol until the concentration in the plasma is the same as before treatment.

Metyrapone, U.S.P. (METOPIRONE), is 2-methyl-1,2-di-3-pyridyl-1-propanone. The drug is marketed as 250-mg oral tablets and as a solution of the ditartrate salt (100 mg/ml equivalent to 43.8 mg/ml of the base) in 10-ml ampuls for intravenous administration. Following two 24-hour control periods, the drug is given orally in the dose of 750 mg every 4 hours for six doses, or intravenously (30 mg/kg), infused over a period of 4 hours. Maximal urinary excretion of 11-desoxycorticosteroids is observed on the next day following oral administration and on the same day following intravenous infusion.

Aminoglutethimide. This compound, α-ethyl-p-aminophenyl-glutarimide, inhibits the conversion of cholesterol to 20α-hydroxycholesterol. This inhibition of the first reaction of steroidogenesis from cholesterol interrupts production of both cortisol and aldosterone.

Aminoglutethimide has been used successfully to decrease the hypersecretion of cortisol in autonomously functioning adrenal tumors and in hypersecretion resulting from ectopic ACTH production. It is not useful in Cushing's syndrome resulting from excessive pituitary ACTH, for the same reason described for metyrapone.

Aminoglutethimide is available only for investigational studies.

Abe, K.; Nicholson, W. E.; Liddle, G. W.; Island, D. P.; and Orth, D. N. Radioimmunoassay of β-MSH in human plasma and tissues. *J. clin. Invest.,* **1967,** *46,* 1609–1616.

Adam, P. A. J., and Haynes, R. C., Jr. Control of hepatic mitochondrial CO_2 fixation by glucagon, epinephrine, and cortisol. *J. biol. Chem.,* **1969,** *244,* 6444–6450.

Addison, T. *On the Constitutional and Local Effects of Disease of the Suprarenal Capsules.* Samuel Highley, London, **1855.**

Ahmed, A. B. J.; George, B. C.; Gonzalez-Auvert, C.; and Dingman, J. F. Increased plasma arginine vasopressin in clinical adrenocortical insufficiency and its inhibition by glucocorticoids. *J. clin. Invest.,* **1967,** *46,* 111–123.

Amatruda, T. T., Jr.; Hollingsworth, D. R.; D'Esopo, N. D.; Upton, G. V.; and Bondy, P. K. A study of the mechanism of the steroid withdrawal syndrome. *J. clin. Endocr. Metab.,* **1960,** *20,* 339–354.

Ashmore, J., and Weber, G. Hormonal control of carbohydrate metabolism in liver. In, *Carbohydrate Metabolism and Its Disorders,* Vol. I. (Dickens, F.; Randle, P. J.; and Whelan, W. J.; eds.) Academic Press, Inc., New York, **1968,** pp. 335–374.

Astwood, E. B.; Raben, M. S.; and Payne, R. W. Chemistry of corticotrophin. *Recent Prog. Horm. Res.,* **1952,** *7,* 1–57.

Bacon, G. E., and Spencer, M. L. Pediatric uses of steroids. *Med. Clins N. Am.,* **1973,** *57,* 1265–1276.

Ballard, P. L.; Baxter, J. D.; Higgins, S. J.; Rousseau, G. C.; and Tomkins, G. M. General presence of glucocorticoid receptors in mammalian tissues. *Endocrinology,* **1974,** *94,* 998–1002.

Balow, J. E., and Rosenthal, A. S. Glucocorticoid suppression of macrophage migration inhibitory factor. *J. exp. Med.,* **1973,** *137,* 1031–1039.

Bangham, D. R.; Mussett, M. V.; and Stack-Dunne, M. P. The third international standard for corticotrophin. *Bull. Wld Hlth Org.,* **1962,** *27,* 395–408.

Bardin, C. W., and Lipsett, M. B. Testosterone and androstenedione blood production rates in normal women and

women with idiopathic hirsutism or polycystic ovaries. *J. clin. Invest.,* **1967,** *46,* 891–902.

Barger, A. C.; Berlin, R. D.; and Tulenko, J. F. Infusion of aldosterone, 9-α-fluorohydrocortisone and antidiuretic hormone into the renal artery of normal and adrenalectomized, unanesthetized dogs: effect on electrolyte and water excretion. *Endocrinology,* **1958,** *62,* 804–815.

Bell, J. J., and Harding, B. W. The acute action of adrenocorticotropic hormone on adrenal steroidogenesis. *Biochim. biophys. Acta,* **1974,** *348,* 285–298.

Bell, P. H.; Howard, K. S.; Shepherd, R. G.; Finn, B. M.; and Meisenhelder, J. H. Studies with corticotropin. II. Pepsin degradation of β-corticotropin. *J. Am. chem. Soc.,* **1956,** *78,* 5059–5066.

Bihari, M., and Grossman, B. J. Posterior subcapsular cataracts related to long term corticosteroid treatment in children. *Am. J. Dis. Child.,* **1968,** *116,* 604–608.

Birnbaum, R. S., and Goodman, H. M. Effects of hypophysectomy on cyclic AMP accumulation and action in adipose tissue. *Fedn Proc. Fedn Am. Socs exp. Biol.,* **1973,** *32,* 535.

Bishop, C. R.; Athens, J. W.; Boggs, D. R.; Warner, H. R.; Cartwright, G. E.; and Wintrobe, M. M. Leukokinetic studies. XIII. A non-steady-state kinetic evaluation of the mechanism of cortisone-induced granulocytosis. *J. clin. Invest.,* **1968,** *47,* 249–260.

Bloom, B. R., and Bennett, B. Mechanism of a reaction *in vitro* associated with delayed hypersensitivity. *Science, Wash.,* **1966,** *153,* 80–82.

Borkowski, A. J.; Levin, S.; Delcroix, C.; Mahler, A.; and Verhas, V. Blood cholesterol and hydrocortisone production in man: quantitative aspects of the utilization of circulating cholesterol by the adrenals at rest and under adrenocorticotropin stimulation. *J. clin. Invest.,* **1967,** *46,* 797–811.

Brennan, M. J. Corticosteroids in the treatment of solid tumors. *Med. Clins N. Am.,* **1973,** *57,* 1225–1239.

Britton, S. W., and Silvette, H. Some effects of corticoadrenal extract and other substances on adrenalectomized animals. *Am. J. Physiol.,* **1931,** *99,* 15–32.

Brown-Séquard, C. E. Recherches expérimentales sur la physiologie et la pathologie des capsules surrenales. *C. r. hebd. Séanc. Acad. Sci., Paris,* **1856,** *43,* 422–425.

Burger, H. G.; Kent, J. R.; and Kellie, A. E. Determination of testosterone in human peripheral and adrenal venous plasma. *J. clin. Endocr. Metab.,* **1964,** *24,* 432–441.

Bush, I. E. Species differences in adrenocortical secretion. *J. Endocr.,* **1953,** *9,* 95–100.

Camacho, A. M.; Kowarski, A.; Migeon, C. J.; and Brough, A. J. Congenital adrenal hyperplasia due to a deficiency of one of the enzymes involved in the biosynthesis of pregnenolone. *J. clin. Endocr. Metab.,* **1968,** *28,* 153–161.

Carson, S. H.; Taeusch, W. H., Jr.; and Avery, M. E. Inhibition of lung cell division after hydrocortisone injection into fetal rabbits. *J. appl. Physiol.,* **1973,** *34,* 660–663.

Claman, H. N. Corticosteroids and lymphoid cells. *New Engl. J. Med.,* **1972,** *287,* 388–397.

Cohen, J. J. The effects of hydrocortisone on the immune response. *Ann. Allergy,* **1971,** *29,* 358–361.

Cohen, J. J.; Fischbach, M.; and Claman, H. N. Hydrocortisone resistance of graft *vs* host activity in mouse thymus, spleen and bone marrow. *J. Immun.,* **1970,** *105,* 1146–1150.

Collip, J. B.; Anderson, E. M.; and Thompson, D. L. The adrenotropic hormone of the anterior pituitary lobe. *Lancet,* **1933,** *2,* 347–348.

Copenhagen Study Group for Liver Diseases. Sex, ascites, and alcoholism in survival of patients with cirrhosis. Effect of prednisone. *New Engl. J. Med.,* **1974,** *293,* 271–273.

Cori, C. F., and Cori, G. T. The fate of sugar in the animal body. VII. The carbohydrate metabolism of adrenalectomized rats and mice. *J. biol. Chem.,* **1927,** *74,* 473–494.

Cushing, H. The basophil adenomas of the pituitary body

and their clinical manifestations. *Bull. Johns Hopkins Hosp.*, **1932**, *50*, 137–195.

Daughaday, W. H. The binding of corticosteroids by serum proteins *in vitro*. In, *Hormones in Human Plasma*. (Antoniades, H. N., ed.) Little, Brown & Co., Boston, **1960**, pp. 495–512.

David, R.; Golon, S.; and Drucker, W. Familial aldosterone deficiency: enzyme defect, diagnosis and clinical course. *Pediatrics, Springfield*, **1968**, *41*, 403–414.

Deane, H., and Greep, R. O. A morphological and histochemical study of the rat's adrenal cortex after hypophysectomy, with comments on the liver. *Am. J. Anat.*, **1946**, *79*, 117–146.

Deming, Q. B., and Luetscher, J. A., Jr. Bioassay of desoxycorticosterone-like material in urine. *Proc. Soc. exp. Biol. Med.*, **1950**, *73*, 171–175.

Doig, A.; Girdwood, R. H.; Duthie, J. J. R.; and Knox, J. D. E. Response of megaloblastic anaemia to prednisolone. *Lancet*, **1957**, *2*, 966–972.

Dougherty, T. F., and White, A. Influence of hormones on lymphoid tissue structure and function: role of pituitary adrenotrophic hormone in regulation of lymphocytes and other cellular elements of the blood. *Endocrinology*, **1944**, *35*, 1–14.

————. Functional alterations in lymphoid tissue induced by adrenal cortical secretion. *Am. J. Anat.*, **1945**, *77*, 81–115.

————. Evaluation of alterations produced in lymphoid tissue by pituitary adrenal cortical secretion. *J. Lab. clin. Med.*, **1947**, *32*, 584–605.

Earp, H. S.; Watson, B. S.; and Ney, R. L. Adenosine 3′,5′-monophosphate as the mediator of ACTH-induced ascorbic acid depletion in the rat adrenal. *Endocrinology*, **1970**, *87*, 118–123.

Engel, F. L. Extra-adrenal actions of adrenocorticotropin. *Vitams Horm.*, **1961**, *19*, 189–227.

Evans, H. M. Present position of our knowledge of anterior pituitary function. *J. Am. med. Ass.*, **1933**, *101*, 425–432.

Farrell, G. L.; Rauschkolb, E. W.; and Royce, P. C. Secretion of aldosterone by the adrenal of the dog: effects of hypophysectomy and ACTH. *Am. J. Physiol.*, **1955**, *182*, 269–272.

Fauci, A. S., and Dale, D. C. The effect of *in vivo* hydrocortisone on subpopulations of human lymphocytes. *J. clin. Invest.*, **1974**, *53*, 240–246.

Feldman, D.; Funder, J. W.; and Edelman, I. S. Subcellular mechanisms in the action of the adrenal steroids. *Am. J. Med.*, **1972**, *53*, 545–560.

Fenster, L. F. The ulcerogenic potential of glucocorticoids and possible prophylactic measures. *Med. Clins N. Am.*, **1973**, *57*, 1289–1294.

Fischel, E. E.; Frank, C. W.; Boltax, A. J.; and Arcasoy, M. Observations on the treatment of rheumatic fever with salicylate, ACTH and cortisone. II. Combined salicylate and corticoid therapy and attempts at rebound suppression. *Arthritis Rheum.*, **1958**, *1*, 351–366.

Fisher, L. B., and Maibach, H. I. The effect of corticosteroids on human epidermal mitotic activity. *Archs Derm.*, **1971**, *103*, 39–44.

Forssman, O., and Mulder, J. Hypersensitivity to different ACTH peptides. *Acta med. scand.*, **1973**, *193*, 557–559.

Foster, G. L., and Smith, P. E. Hypophysectomy and replacement therapy in relation to basal metabolism and specific dynamic action in the rat. *J. Am. med. Ass.*, **1926**, *87*, 2151–2153.

Friedman, M. The duration of action of the synthetic pentacosapeptide D-serine[1]-norleucine[4]-valinamide[25]-β-1-25-corticotrophin (DW-75) in man. *Experientia*, **1969**, *25*, 416–419.

Fukushima, D. K.; Bradlow, H. L.; Hellman, L.; Zumoff, B.; and Gallagher, T. F. Metabolic transformation of hydrocortisone-4-C[14] in normal men. *J. biol. Chem.*, **1960**, *235*, 2246–2252.

Gainesburg, J. Influence of intra-arterial hydrocortisone on adrenergic responses in the hand. *Br. med. J.*, **1958**, *2*, 424–426.

Gill, J. R., Jr.; Gann, D. S.; and Bartter, F. C. Restoration of water diuresis in addisonian patients by expansion of the volume of extracellular fluid. *J. clin. Invest.*, **1962**, *41*, 1078–1085.

Goldsmith, O.; Solomon, D. H.; and Horton, E. Hypogonadism and mineralocorticoid excess: the 17-hydroxylase deficiency syndrome. *New Engl. J. Med.*, **1968**, *277*, 673–677.

Goodman, H. M. Endocrine control of lipolysis. In, *Progress in Endocrinology: Proceedings of the Third International Congress of Endocrinology, Mexico*. (Gual, C., and Ebling, F. J. G., eds.) Excerpta Medica, Amsterdam, **1968**, pp. 115–123.

Graber, A. L.; Ney, R. E.; Nicholson, W. E.; Island, D. P.; and Liddle, G. W. Natural history of pituitary-adrenal recovery following long term suppression with corticosteroids. *J. clin. Endocr. Metab.*, **1965**, *25*, 11–16.

Grahame, R. Elasticity of human skin *in vivo*. A study of the physical properties of the skin in rheumatoid arthritis and the effect of corticosteroids. *Ann. phys. Med.*, **1969**, *10*, 130–136.

Gray, J. G.; Pratt, W. B.; and Aronow, L. Effect of glucocorticoids on hexose uptake by mouse fibroblasts *in vitro*. *Biochemistry, N.Y.*, **1971**, *10*, 277–284.

Greendyke, R. M.; Bradley, E. M.; and Swisher, S. N. Studies on the effects of administration of ACTH and adrenal corticosteroids on erythrophagocytosis. *J. clin. Invest.*, **1965**, *44*, 746–753.

Harris, D. M.; Martin, L. E.; Harrison, C.; and Jack, D. The effect of oral and inhaled beclomethasone dipropionate on adrenal function. *Clin. Allergy*, **1973**, *3*, 243–248.

Harris, G. W. *Neural Control of the Pituitary Gland*. Edward Arnold, London, **1955**.

Harrop, G. A.; Soffer, L. J.; Ellsworth, R.; and Trescher, J. H. Studies on the suprarenal cortex. III. Plasma electrolytes and electrolyte excretion during suprarenal insufficiency in the dog. *J. exp. Med.*, **1933**, *58*, 17–38.

Harter, J. G.; Reddy, W. J.; and Thorn, G. W. Studies on an intermittent corticosteroid dosage regimen. *New Engl. J. Med.*, **1963**, *269*, 591–596.

Hartman, F. A.; Brownell, K. A.; and Hartman, W. E. A further study of the hormone of the adrenal cortex. *Am. J. Physiol.*, **1930**, *95*, 670–680.

Harvey, W., and Grahame, R. Effect of some adrenal steroid hormones on skin fibroblast replication *in vitro*. *Ann. rheum. Dis.*, **1973**, *32*, 272.

Haynes, R. C., Jr. The activation of adrenal phosphorylase by the adrenocorticotropic hormone. *J. biol. Chem.*, **1958**, *233*, 1220–1222.

Haynes, R. C., Jr.; Koritz, S. B.; and Péron, F. G. Influence of adenosine 3′,5′-monophosphate on corticoid production by rat adrenal glands. *J. biol. Chem.*, **1959**, *234*, 1421–1423.

Heilman, D. H. The effect of 11-dehydro-17-hydroxycorticosterone and 11-dehydrocorticosterone on the migration of macrophages in tissue culture. *Proc. Staff Meet. Mayo Clin.*, **1945**, *20*, 318–320.

Hellman, L.; Bradlow, H. L.; Frazell, E. L.; and Gallagher, T. F. Tracer studies of the absorption and fate of steroid hormones in man. *J. clin. Invest.*, **1956**, *35*, 1033–1044.

Hench, P. S.; Kendall, E. C.; Slocumb, C. H.; and Polley, H. F. The effect of a hormone of the adrenal cortex (17-hydroxy-11-dehydrocorticosterone; compound E) and of pituitary adrenocorticotropic hormone on rheumatoid arthritis. *Proc. Staff Meet. Mayo Clin.*, **1949**, *24*, 181–197.

Henderson, I. C., and Loeb, J. N. Fall in liver DNA polymerase activity in cortisone-treated rats. *Nature, Lond.*, **1970**, *228*, 556–557.

Henkin, R. I. The effects of corticosteroids and ACTH on sensory systems. *Prog. Brain Res.*, **1970**, *32*, 270–294.

Hodges, J. R.; Jones, M. T.; and Stockham, M. A. Effect of emotion on blood corticotropin and cortisol concentrations in man. *Nature, Lond.,* **1962,** *193,* 1187–1188.

Hofmann, K. Chemistry and function of polypeptide hormones. *A. Rev. Biochem.,* **1962,** *31,* 213–246.

Hofmann, K.; Montibeller, J. A.; and Finn, F. M. ACTH antagonists. *Proc. natn. Acad. Sci. U.S.A.,* **1974,** *71,* 80–83.

Hofmann, K.; Yajima, H., Yanaihara, N.; Liu, T.; and Lande, S. Studies on polypeptides. XIII. The synthesis of a tricosapeptide possessing essentially the full biological activity of natural ACTH. *J. Am. chem. Soc.,* **1961,** *83,* 487–489.

Houssay, B. A.; Biasotti, A.; Mazzoco, P.; and Sammartino, A. Acción del extracto antero-hipofisario sobre las glandulas adrenales. *Revta Soc. argent. Biol.,* **1933,** *9,* 262–268.

Howard, E. Effects of corticosterone and food restriction on growth and on DNA, RNA, and cholesterol contents of the brain and liver in infant mice. *J. Neurochem.,* **1964,** *12,* 181–191.

Ingle, D. J. Permissive action of hormones. *J. clin. Endocr. Metab.,* **1954,** *14,* 1272–1274.

Ingle, D. J.; Higgins, G. M.; and Kendall, E. C. Atrophy of the adrenal cortex in the rat produced by administration of large amounts of cortin. *Anat. Rec.,* **1938,** *71,* 363–372.

Jones, R. S. Beclomethasone in childhood asthma. *Archs Dis. Childh.,* **1973,** *48,* 663–664.

Jubiz, W.; West, C. D.; and Tyler, F. H. Lack of prolonged activity of a new ACTH preparation (DW-75) in human subjects. *J. clin. Endocr. Metab.,* **1968,** *28,* 1377–1379.

Kahnt, F. W.; Milani, A.; Steffen, H.; and Neher, R. The rate-limiting step of adrenal steroidogenesis and adenosine 3':5'-monophosphate. *Eur. J. Biochem.,* **1974,** *44,* 243–250.

Kappas, A.; Soybel, W.; Glickman, P.; and Fukushima, D. K. Fever-producing steroids of endogenous origin in man. *Archs intern. Med.,* **1960,** *105,* 701–708.

Knowles, J. P. Difficulties in weaning in steroid treatment of asthma. *Br. med. J.,* **1961,** *2,* 1396–1399.

Kong, Y. C.; Moyle, W. R.; and Ramachandran, J. Inhibition of ACTH induced cyclic AMP synthesis in isolated rat adrenal cells by NPS-ACTH. *Proc. Soc. exp. Biol. Med.,* **1972,** *141,* 350–352.

Korelitz, B. I., and Lindner, A. E. The influence of corticotrophin and adrenal steroids on the course of ulcerative colitis: a comparison with the presteroid era. *Gastroenterology,* **1964,** *46,* 671–679.

Kreutner, W., and Goldberg, N. D. Dependence on insulin of the apparent hydrocortisone activation of hepatic glycogen synthetase. *Proc. natn. Acad. Sci. U.S.A.,* **1967,** *58,* 1515–1519.

Lee, P. A.; Keenan, B. S.; Migeon, C. J.; and Blizzard, R. M. Effect of various ACTH preparations on the secretion of growth hormone in normal subjects and in hypopituitary patients. *J. clin. Endocr. Metab.,* **1973,** *37,* 389–396.

Lemann, J., Jr.; Piering, W. F.; and Lennon, E. J. Studies of the acute effects of aldosterone and cortisol on the interrelationship between renal sodium, calcium, and magnesium excretion in normal man. *Nephron,* **1970,** *7,* 117–130.

Lerner, A. B., and Lee, T. H. The melanocyte-stimulating hormones. *Vitams Horm.,* **1962,** *20,* 337–346.

Lesesne, H. R., and Fallon, H. J. Treatment of liver disease with corticosteroids. *Med. Clins N. Am.,* **1973,** *57,* 1191–1201.

Levine, S. B., and Leopold, I. H. Advances in ocular corticosteroid therapy. *Med. Clins N. Am.,* **1973,** *57,* 1167–1177.

Li, C. H. Adrenocorticotropin 45. Revised amino acid sequences for sheep and bovine hormones. *Biochem. biophys. Res. Commun.,* **1972,** *49,* 835–839.

Li, C. H.; Evans, H. M.; and Simpson, M. E. Adrenocorticotropic hormone. *J. biol. Chem.,* **1943,** *149,* 413–424.

Liddle, G. W. Studies of structure-function relationships of steroids. II. The 6α-methylcorticosteroids. *Metabolism,* **1958,** *7,* 405–415.

———. Tests of pituitary-adrenal suppressibility in the diagnosis of Cushing's syndrome. *J. clin. Endocr. Metab.,* **1960,** *20,* 1539–1560.

Loeb, J. N., and Sternschein, M. J. Suppression of thymidine incorporation into the gastric mucosa of cortisone-treated rats: possible relation to glucocorticoid-induced gastric ulceration. *Endocrinology,* **1973,** *92,* 1322–1377.

Loeb, R. F. Effect of sodium chloride in the treatment of a patient with Addison's disease. *Proc. Soc. exp. Biol. Med.,* **1933,** *30,* 808–812.

Loeb, R. F.; Atchley, D. W.; Benedict, E. M.; and Leland, J. Electrolyte balance studies in adrenalectomized dogs with particular reference to the excretion of sodium. *J. exp. Med.,* **1933,** *57,* 775–792.

Long, C. N. H.; Katzin, B.; and Fry, E. G. Adrenal cortex and carbohydrate metabolism. *Endocrinology,* **1940,** *26,* 309–344.

McKenzie, A. W., and Stoughton, R. B. Method for comparing percutaneous absorption of steroids. *Archs Derm.,* **1962,** *86,* 608–610.

Mahaffee, D.; Reitz, R. C.; and Ney, R. L. The mechanism of action of adrenocorticotropic hormone. The role of mitochondrial cholesterol accumulation in the regulation of steroidogenesis. *J. biol. Chem.,* **1974,** *249,* 227–233.

Maibach, H. I., and Stoughton, R. B. Topical corticosteroids. *Med. Clins N. Am.,* **1973,** *57,* 1253–1264.

Makman, M. H.; Dvorkin, B.; and White, A. Evidence for induction by cortisol *in vitro* of a protein inhibitor of transport and phosphorylation in rat thymocytes. *Proc. natn. Acad. Sci. U.S.A.,* **1971,** *68,* 1269–1273.

Marco, J.; Calle, C.; Román, D.; Diaz-Ferros, M.; Villanueva, M. L.; and Valverde, I. Hyperglucagonism induced by glucocorticoid treatment in man. *New Engl. J. Med.,* **1973,** *288,* 128–131.

Maxwell, M. H.; Adams, D. A.; and Golman, R. Corticosteroid therapy of amyloid nephrotic syndrome. *Ann. intern. Med.,* **1964,** *60,* 539–555.

Meador, C. K.; Liddle, G. W.; Island, D. P.; Nicholson, W. E.; Lucas, C. P.; Nuckton, J. G.; and Luetscher, J. A. Cause of Cushing's syndrome in patients with tumors arising from "nonendocrine" tissue. *J. clin. Endocr. Metab.,* **1962,** *22,* 693–703.

Mills, I. H.; Schedl, H. P.; Chen, P. S., Jr.; and Bartter, F. C. The effect of estrogen administration on the metabolism and protein binding of hydrocortisone. *J. clin. Endocr. Metab.,* **1960,** *20,* 515–528.

Munck, A., and Brinck-Johnsen, T. Specific and nonspecific physicochemical interactions of glucocorticoids and related steroids with rat thymus cells *in vitro. J. biol. Chem.,* **1968,** *243,* 5556–5565.

Ney, R. L. Effects of dibutyryl cyclic AMP on adrenal growth and steroidogenic capacity. *Endocrinology,* **1969,** *84,* 168–170.

Pratt, W. B., and Aronow, L. The effect of glucocorticoids on protein and nucleic acid synthesis in mouse fibroblasts growing *in vitro. J. biol. Chem.,* **1966,** *241,* 5244–5250.

Rees, H. A., and Williams, D. A. Long-term steroid therapy in chronic intractable asthma: a study of 317 adult asthmatics on continuous steroid therapy for an average period of 2½ years. *Br. med. J.,* **1962,** *1,* 1575–1579.

Reichgott, M. J., and Melmon, K. L. Should corticosteroids be used in shock? *Med. Clins N. Am.,* **1973,** *57,* 1211–1223.

Renold, A. E.; Jenkins, D.; Forsham, P. H.; and Thorn, G. W. The use of intravenous ACTH: a study in quantitative adrenocortical stimulation. *J. clin. Endocr. Metab.,* **1952,** *12,* 763–797.

Robinson, W. D. Management of systemic lupus erythematosus. *Arthritis Rheum.,* **1962,** *5,* 521–528.

Sawin, C. T.; Bray, G. A.; and Idelson, B. A. Overnight suppression test with dexamethasone in Cushing's syndrome. *J. clin. Endocr. Metab.*, **1968**, *28*, 422–424.

Sayers, G.; White, A.; and Long, C. N. H. Preparation and properties of pituitary adrenotropic hormone. *J. biol. Chem.*, **1943**, *149*, 425–436.

Sayers, M. A.; Sayers, G.; and Woodbury, L. A. The assay of adrenocorticotrophic hormone by the adrenal ascorbic acid–depletion method. *Endocrinology*, **1948**, *42*, 379–393.

Schaumburg, B. P., and Bojesen, E. Specificity and thermodynamic properties of the corticosteroid binding to a receptor of rat thymocytes *in vitro. Biochim. biophys. Acta*, **1968**, *170*, 172–188.

Scherrer, K. Messenger RNA in eukaryotic cells: the life history of duck globin messenger RNA. *Acta endocr., Copenh.*, **1973**, *180*, Suppl., 95–129.

Schlagel, C. A. Penetration and action of glucocorticoids. *Adv. Biol. Skin*, **1972**, *12*, 339–356.

Schwyzer, R., and Sieber, P. Total synthesis of adrenocorticotropic hormone. *Nature, Lond.*, **1963**, *199*, 172–174.

Scott, A. P.; Ratcliffe, J. G.; Rees, L. H.; Landon, J.; Bennett, H. P. J.; Lowry, P. J.; and McMartin, C. Pituitary peptide. *Nature, New Biol.*, **1973**, *244*, 65–67.

Selye, H. General adaptation syndrome and diseases of adaptation. *J. clin. Endocr. Metab.*, **1946**, *6*, 117–230.

Silber, R. H., and Porter, C. C. The determination of 17,21-dihydroxy-20-ketosteroids in urine and plasma. *J. biol. Chem.*, **1954**, *210*, 923–932.

Simpson, S. A.; Tait, J. F.; Wettstein, A.; Neher, R.; Euw, J. V.; Schindler, O.; and Reichstein, T. Konstitution des Aldosterons des neuen Mineralocorticoids. *Experientia*, **1954**, *10*, 132–133.

Steiger, M., and Reichstein, T. Desoxy-cortico-steron (21-Oxy-progesteron) aus Δ⁵-3-Oxy-ätio-cholensäure. *Helv. chim. Acta*, **1937**, *20*, 1164–1179.

Stevenson, R. D. Hydrocortisone and the migration of human leukocytes: an indirect effect mediated by mononuclear cells. *Clin. exp. Immun.*, **1973**, *14*, 417–426.

Stone, D., and Hechter, O. Studies on ACTH action in perfused bovine adrenals: the site of action of ACTH in corticosteroidogenesis. *Archs Biochem. Biophys.*, **1954**, *51*, 457–469.

Swann, H. G. The pituitary-adrenocortical relationship. *Physiol. Rev.*, **1940**, *20*, 493–521.

Sweat, M. L., and Bryson, M. J. The role of phosphopyridinenucleotides in the metabolism of cortisol by peripheral tissue. *Biochim. biophys. Acta*, **1960**, *44*, 217–223.

Swingle, W. W., and Pfiffner, J. J. Experiments with an active extract of the suprarenal cortex. *Anat. Rec.*, **1930a**, *44*, 225–226.

———. An aqueous extract of the suprarenal cortex which maintains the life of bilaterally adrenalectomized cats. *Science, N.Y.*, **1930b**, *71*, 321–322.

Tait, J. F.; Simpson, S. A.; and Grundy, H. M. The effect of adrenal extract on mineral metabolism. *Lancet*, **1952**, *1*, 122–124.

Tobian, L. Interrelationship of electrolytes, juxtaglomerular cells and hypertension. *Physiol. Rev.*, **1960**, *40*, 280–312.

Wall, A. J. The use of glucocorticoids in intestinal disease. *Med. Clins N. Am.*, **1973**, *57*, 1241–1252.

Weissman, G., and Thomas, L. The effect of corticosteroids upon connective tissue and lysosomes. *Recent Prog. Horm. Res.*, **1964**, *20*, 215–245.

Weston, W. L.; Mandel, M. J.; Krueger, G. G.; and Claman, H. N. Differential suppressive effect of hydrocortisone on lymphocytes and mononuclear macrophages in delayed hypersensitivity of guinea pigs. *J. invest. Derm.*, **1972**, *59*, 345–348.

Wise, J. K.; Hendler, R.; and Felig, P. Influence of glucocorticoids on glucagon secretion and plasma amino acid concentrations in man. *J. clin. Invest.*, **1973**, *52*, 2774–2782.

Yalow, R. S., and Berson, S. A. Characteristics of "big ACTH" in human plasma and pituitary extracts. *J. clin. Endocr. Metab.*, **1973**, *36*, 415–423.

Yard, A. C., and Kadowitz, P. J. Studies on the mechanism of hydrocortisone potentiation of vasoconstrictor responses to epinephrine in the anesthetized animal. *Eur. J. Pharmac.*, **1972**, *20*, 1–9.

Yount, W. J.; Utsinger, P. D.; Puritz, E. M.; and Ortbals, D. W. Corticosteroid therapy of the collagen vascular disorders. *Med. Clins N. Am.*, **1973**, *57*, 1343–1355.

Monographs and Reviews

Bongiovanni, A. M.; Eberlein, W. R.; Goldman, A. S.; and New, M. Disorders of adrenal steroid biogenesis. *Recent Prog. Horm. Res.*, **1967**, *23*, 375–449.

De Wied, D., and Weijnen, J. A. W. M. (eds.). Pituitary, adrenal, and the brain. *Prog. Brain Res.*, **1970**, *32*, 1–357.

Grieco, M. H., and Cushman, P., Jr. Adrenal glucocorticoids after twenty years. A review of their clinically relevant consequences. *J. chron. Dis.*, **1970**, *22*, 637–711.

Haynes, R. C., Jr. Hormonal drugs. *Clin. Pharmac. Ther.*, **1974**, *16*, 945–953.

Liddle, G. W. Clinical pharmacology of the anti-inflammatory steroids. *Clin. Pharmac. Ther.*, **1961**, *2*, 615–635.

Mulrow, P. J., and Forman, B. H. The tissue effects of mineralocorticoids. *Am. J. Med.*, **1972**, *53*, 561–572.

Reichstein, T., and Shoppee, C. W. The hormones of the adrenal cortex. *Vitams Horm.*, **1943**, *1*, 346–413.

Rheumatism Review Committee. Rheumatism and arthritis. *Ann. intern. Med.*, **1963**, *59*, 1–125.

Tait, J. F., and Burstein, S. *In vivo* studies of steroid dynamics in man. In, *The Hormones*, Vol. 5. (Pincus, G.; Thimann, K. V.; and Astwood, E. B.; eds.) Academic Press, Inc., New York, **1964**, pp. 441–557.

Temple, T. E., and Liddle, G. W. Inhibitors of adrenal steroid biosynthesis. *A. Rev. Pharmac.*, **1970**, *10*, 199–218.

Thompson, E. B., and Lippman, M. E. Mechanism of action of glucocorticoids. *Metabolism*, **1974**, *23*, 159–202.

Thorn, G. W. (ed.). Symposium on the adrenal cortex. *Am. J. Med.*, **1972**, *53*, 529–700.

CHAPTER

71 INSULIN AND ORAL HYPOGLYCEMIC DRUGS; GLUCAGON

Joseph Larner and Robert C. Haynes, Jr.

INSULIN

History. Credit for the discovery of insulin is given to Banting and Best, who extracted the active principle from the pancreas and demonstrated its therapeutic effects in diabetic dogs and human subjects in the years 1921 and 1922 (*see* Best, 1963). However, many investigators had paved the way for the discovery, and at least one, Paulesco (1921), also demonstrated the presence of a pancreatic material that was capable of producing hypoglycemia in animals. Probably of greatest earlier import was the demonstration by von Mering and Minkowski in 1889 that pancreatectomized dogs exhibit aberrations in carbohydrate metabolism similar to those seen in diabetes mellitus in man. This was a fine example of serendipity, for von Mering and Minkowski were engaged in studies on the digestive, not the islet, functions of the pancreas at the time of their discovery. Banting approached the problem with two working hypotheses: (1) the islet tissue secreted insulin, and (2) previous failures to isolate the active principle had been due in many instances to the proteolytic destruction of insulin by the digestive enzymes of the pancreas during the course of extraction. He devised elegantly simple approaches to circumvent the difficulty. He tied the pancreatic ducts so that the acinar tissue degenerated and left the islet tissue undisturbed, and from the remaining tissue extracted the active principle in relatively high concentration. He also used fetal pancreas as starting material, tissue with functional islets but lacking proteolytic digestive activity. Later on, normal pancreas was used as a commercial source when it was found that acid alcohol not only extracted insulin but also prevented proteolytic destruction.

The first patient to receive the active extracts prepared by Banting and Best was Leonard Thompson, aged 14 (Banting *et al.,* 1922). He appeared at the Toronto General Hospital with a blood glucose of 500 mg %, and he was excreting 3 to 5 liters of urine per day. Despite rigid control of diet (450 kcal per day), he continued to excrete large quantities of glucose, and, without insulin, the most likely course was death after a few months. Extracts were first administered on January 11, 1922, and they induced a reduction in the concentration and excretion of blood glucose. Daily injections were then begun, and there was immediate improvement. The excretion of glucose was reduced from over 100 to as little as 7.5 g per day. Furthermore, ". . . the boy became brighter, looked better and said he felt stronger." Here was as dramatic an interruption of a fatal metabolic disorder as one will find in the annals of the history of medical science.

Immediately after the discovery of insulin there was justifiable excitement and then unfortunate relaxation, an attitude that the problems of treatment and of etiology of diabetes mellitus had been solved. True, the discovery of insulin was a momentous advance, but as time went by it became apparent that treatment was more than simply injection of insulin, that the etiology was more complex in many instances than mere destruction of islet tissue, and that the explanation of the action of the hormone was an exceedingly complex problem involving the elucidation of the intermediary metabolism not only of carbohydrate but also of protein and fat.

The chemistry of insulin has progressed from the preparation of active extracts to the preparation of insulin in crystalline form (Abel, 1926), to the establishment of the amino acid sequence of the polypeptide hormone (Sanger, 1960), and, eventually, to the complete synthesis of the molecule (Katsoyannis, 1966). Of great practical importance in treatment has been the preparation of insulin in a variety of forms that exhibit a wide range in rate of absorption.

The studies on the etiology of diabetes mellitus took an interesting turn when Houssay (1936a, 1936b) reported that hypophysectomy ameliorated diabetes in the dog and that extracts of the anterior pituitary exacerbated the condition. Soon thereafter, Young (1937) induced permanent diabetes in dogs by prolonged administration of anterior pituitary extract. Long and Lukens (1936) provided convincing evidence that the adrenal cortex, as well as the adenohypophysis, exerts effects antagonistic to insulin. A new attitude developed. Diabetes could be caused not only by a deficiency of insulin but also by an excess of certain hormones, for example, growth hormone, glucocorticoids, and glucagon. However, there is little evidence of hypersecretion of any of these hormones in the vast majority of diabetic patients. Possible exceptions are certain products of the adenohypophysis; both growth hormone and an adenohypophyseal "diabetogenic peptide" have been suggested to play etiological roles in the generation of at least certain forms of the disease (Louis *et al.,* 1966; Bornstein *et al.,* 1971; Krahl, 1972; *see also* Chapter 66).

The search for the etiology of diabetes mellitus has recently turned from strictly endocrine to immunological and infectious factors. Reports have appeared of diabetes associated with anti-insulin antibodies in patients never exposed to exogenous hormone (Ohneda *et al.,* 1974). Current research suggests that the disease, particularly the juvenile-onset form, may have an autoimmune etiology (Goldstein *et al.*, 1970), or even that it may result from a viral infection (Craighead and Steinke, 1971). It is clear that questions about the pathogenesis of diabetes have not yielded answers as readily as have those about the chemistry and mechanism of action of insulin.

Chemistry and Biosynthesis. Insulin, with a molecular weight of about 6000, is made up of two chains of amino acids joined together by disulfide linkages (*see* Figure 71-1). The sequence of amino acids in the two chains (termed A for acidic and B for basic) and the arrangement of the three disulfide bridges were worked out in a brilliant series of investigations by Sanger and associates in the period 1945–1955 (*see* Sanger, 1960). The efforts of the chemists culminated in the complete synthesis of both ovine and human insulin (Katsoyannis, 1966).

While it had been assumed that the A and B chains were synthesized separately and then joined together in the β cells of the pancreatic islets, Steiner and colleagues (1967, 1972) and Chance and associates (*see* Chance, 1972) demonstrated that the β cells form insulin from a single-chain precursor termed proinsulin (Figure 71-1). On conversion of human proinsulin to insulin, four basic amino acids (arginine 31, arginine 32, lysine 64, and arginine 65) and the connector or C-peptide, made up of residues 31 through 65, are removed. The resultant insulin molecule has two chains, the A chain with glycine as the amino-terminal residue and the B chain with phenylalanine at the amino terminus. In many commercial preparations of insulin it is possible to detect small amounts of proinsulin and other related molecules resulting from incomplete conversion of the prohormone.

Hodgkin and associates (*see* Hodgkin and Mercola, 1972) have determined the three-dimensional structure of insulin by x-ray analysis of single crystals. Insulin can exist as a monomer, a dimer, or a hexamer composed of three such dimers. Two molecules of Zn^{2+} are coordinated in the hexamer, which is presumably the form stored in the granule of the β cell. The biologically active form of the hormone is thought to be the monomer. X-ray analysis has also shown that the two chains are compactly arranged, with the A chain positioned above the central helical portion of the B chain. From each end of this helical region the terminal portions of the B chain extend as arms, and the A chain is enclosed between them.

Many species variations are known, and some are of clinical significance. For example, the major sites of chemical difference between porcine, ovine, equine, and cetacean insulins are in positions 8, 9, and 10 of the A chain. The porcine hormone is most similar to that of man and differs only by the substitution of an alanine residue at the carboxy terminus of the B chain (Steiner *et al.*, 1972). By the use of porcine insulin as the starting material, human insulin can now be synthesized with relative ease (Ruttenberg, 1972).

The specific activities of various mammalian insulins are very similar (22 to 27 units/mg, *see* below)

(Humbel *et al.*, 1972). Proinsulin has only slight biological activity, while the separated A and B chains are essentially inactive.

The Assay of Insulin in Plasma. In addition to the older *in-vivo* bioassays, which depend on the lowering of blood glucose in rabbits or the production of convulsions in mice (*see* Humbel *et al.*, 1972), several *in-vitro* methods have attained popularity because of their high degree of sensitivity and their relative simplicity of execution. One method is based on the capacity of insulin to increase the glycogen content or the glucose uptake of the rat diaghragm. Adipose tissue assays are based on the capacity of insulin to stimulate glucose metabolism by the epididymal fat pad of the rat or by suspensions of isolated fat cells prepared from the epididymal fat pad. Measured end points are CO_2 production from glucose, incorporation of the ^{14}C of labeled glucose into fat, or glucose uptake from the medium.

The radioimmunoassay of insulin in human plasma is based on the capacity of human insulin to compete with porcine or bovine insulin (labeled with ^{131}I or ^{125}I) for binding sites on an antibody derived from the serum of guinea pigs that have been injected with porcine or bovine insulin. The addition of human insulin to a solution of insulin-^{131}I-antibody complex results in the displacement of insulin-^{131}I from binding sites, the amount displaced being quantitatively related to the amount of human insulin present. Free insulin-^{131}I so displaced is separable from bound insulin by several technics, and quantitated in terms of its radioactivity. This type of method, originally described by Yalow and Berson (1960), has now been applied to many hormones and other molecules. The sensitivity of the radioimmunoassay for insulin is an order of magnitude greater than the *in-vitro* bioassays and two or more orders of magnitude greater than the *in-vivo* bioassays.

Types of Plasma Insulin. Plasma insulin estimated by bioassay is called *insulin-like activity* (ILA), and plasma insulin estimated by immunoassay is called *immunoreactive insulin* (IRI). IRI and ILA differ both quantitatively and qualitatively. The concentration of plasma IRI of normal persons after an overnight fast is under 20 microunits/ml.

When insulin antibody is added to plasma, a decrease in ILA is observed (suppressible ILA); however, a considerable portion (sometimes over 90%) of the ILA may persist, and this is termed nonsuppressible ILA or NSILA. The amount of suppressible ILA corresponds to the amount of IRI (Oelz *et al.*, 1972). Thus, estimates of plasma ILA are invariably higher than are those of IRI. NSILA has been intensively studied. It is not increased in plasma after glucose administration, and it persists in plasma after pancreatectomy. It behaves like insulin in isolated systems in stimulating glucose uptake and glycogenesis in muscle, in stimulating lipogenesis and glucose oxidation in adipose tissue, and in inhibiting lipolysis. It consists of at least two components: NSILA-S (soluble in acid-ethanol), molecular weight 7500; and NSILA-P (precipitated in acid-ethanol), molecular weight 100,000. Neither form is chemi-

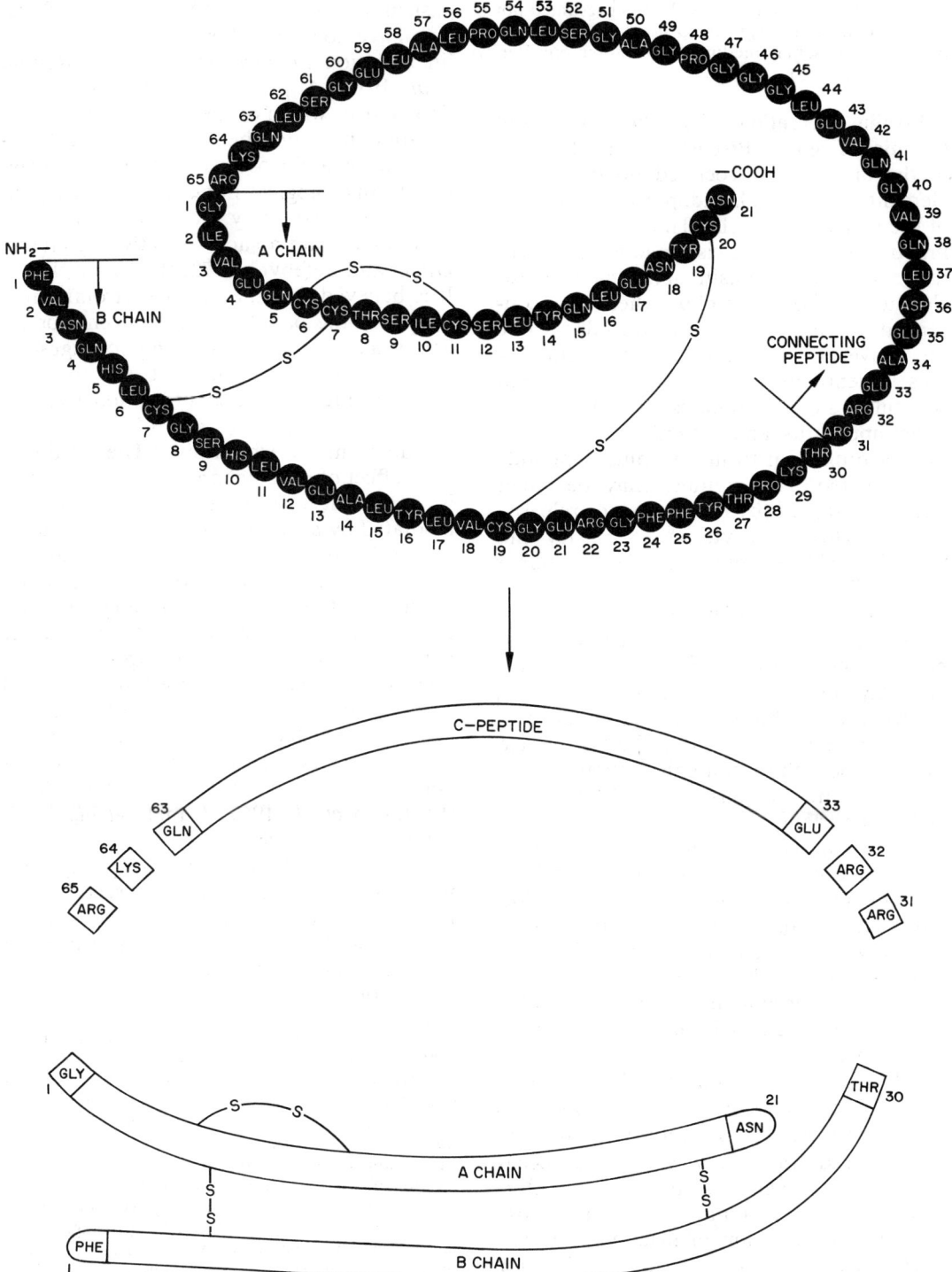

Figure 71-1. *Human proinsulin and its conversion to insulin.*

The amino acid sequence of human proinsulin is shown. By proteolytic removal of four basic amino acids and the C-peptide, proinsulin is converted to insulin. (For details, *see* the text.)

1509

cally related to insulin, and NSILA is presumed not to be of pancreatic origin (Oelz *et al.,* 1972); it may be related to somatomedin (*see* Chapter 66; Van Wyck *et al.,* 1973).

Insulin Secretion: Morphological and Chemical Events. Proinsulin is synthesized in the membrane-associated polyribosomal elements of the rough endoplasmic reticulum of the pancreatic β cells. The prohormone is first transferred to the cisternae of the reticulum and then via transitional elements (vesicles) to the Golgi complex, where it is concentrated within immature granules. Here the conversion of proinsulin to insulin begins. Eventually proinsulin- and insulin-containing storage granules bud off from the Golgi apparatus, and the enzymatic conversion of proinsulin to insulin plus C-peptide is completed. The granules may be either stored, destroyed (by lysosomes), or released by emiocytosis (exocytosis). (*See* Lacy and Greider, 1972; Renold *et al.,* 1972; Steiner *et al.,* 1972.)

Regulation of Insulin Secretion. Gastrointestinal Mechanisms. Insulin release appears to be controlled by the coordinated interplay of the availability of food products, gastrointestinal hormones, and other hormonal and neural stimuli. In the last-named category, both the autonomic nervous system and the central nervous system (CNS) are of major importance.

In keeping with insulin's role to promote the storage of all fuels, it is not surprising that, in addition to glucose, amino acids, fatty acids of all chain lengths, and ketone bodies will call forth its secretion. In man, glucose is most probably the principal stimulus. But in other animals, depending on diet, amino acids or fatty acids may be of primary importance.

It has been known for over 70 years that glucose is more effective in provoking glycosuria when injected intravenously than when administered orally. However, it was recognized only relatively recently that this difference is due to a greater ability of oral glucose to evoke the secretion of insulin (McIntyre *et al.,* 1964); the same may also be true for amino acids (Renold *et al.,* 1972). This strongly suggests the presence of a signal from the gastrointestinal tract to the pancreas, and several of the gastrointestinal hormones, including secretin, pancreozymin,

gastrin, and gastrointestinal or "gut" glucagon, have now been shown to stimulate insulin secretion *in vitro* and *in vivo* (Renold *et al.,* 1972). At present there is considerable debate over which of these, alone or in combination, mediates the response. Secretin appears to be a glucose-sensitive intestinal signal of physiological importance, while pancreozymin may play a similar role as a protein- and amino acid–sensitive signal (*see* Unger and Lefebvre, 1972; Buchanan, 1973). It is believed that the upper gastrointestinal tract and the pancreas form an enteropancreatic axis responsible not only for digestion and absorption of foods but also for their effective and controlled utilization (Kipnis, 1971).

Autonomic Mechanisms. The predominant effect of norepinephrine or epinephrine is to inhibit insulin secretion, a response mediated by α-adrenergic receptors. In addition, *selective* activation of β-adrenergic receptors results in stimulation of the secretion of insulin. Exercise and pathological states associated with activation of the autonomic nervous system, including hypoxia, hypothermia, surgery, and severe burns, all lead to a suppression of insulin secretion via the α-receptor mechanism (Porte and Robertson, 1973). Cholinomimetic drugs and vagalnerve stimulation enhance insulin release (Frohman *et al.,* 1967; Kaneto *et al.,* 1967; Malaisse *et al.,* 1967).

The adrenergic and cholinergic systems may control the basal rate of secretion of insulin as well as the reaction to stress. Thus, α-receptor blockade raises and muscarinic or β-receptor blockade lowers the basal concentration of insulin in plasma.

Control by Other Hormones. It is now recognized that the secretory activity of the pancreatic β cell is affected by a wide variety of hormones. An unexpected finding was the demonstration that glucagon stimulates insulin release (*see* Marks and Samols, 1970). In addition, a variety of peptide hormones and autacoids can either stimulate or inhibit insulin release and modify the secretory response of the β cell to nutrients and drugs (Kipnis, 1971). Among the more interesting are the prostaglandins, certain of which enhance insulin release (Johnson *et al.,* 1973), and somatostatin, a tetradecapeptide of hypothalamic origin that inhibits the secretion of insulin and glucagon in addition to that of growth hormone. (*See* Chapter 66; Gerich *et al.,* 1974; Koerker *et al.,* 1974.)

Biochemical Mechanisms and Kinetics. In man, glucose is the only nutrient that stimulates both insulin *secretion* and *biosynthesis* at physiological concentrations, and this action has been studied extensively. While carbohydrate utilization is an important feature of the glucose-induced release of insulin, convincing evidence indicates that it is the hexose molecule itself that is the secretagogue. Concentrations of glycolytic intermediates and cofactors have been measured in islets within seconds after exposure to glucose; these either do not change or the changes do not explain the secretory phenomenon (Matschinsky *et al.*, 1970). Moreover, certain sugars, such as galactose and 3-O-methylglucose, increase glycolysis without causing insulin secretion. Conversely, a number of agents that block glycolysis do not affect insulin secretion (Matschinsky and Ellerman, 1973). Glucose thus appears to serve a double role; it is hypothesized to act as a secretagogue by means of interaction with a glucoreceptor on the cell membrane, and, of course, it serves as an energy source within the β cell.

The fact that β-adrenergic agonists stimulate insulin secretion suggests that cyclic adenosine 3′,5′-monophosphate (cyclic AMP) mediates the response. Glucagon is also known to increase cyclic AMP concentrations in islets and stimulates insulin secretion (*see* Goldfine *et al.*, 1972). When α receptors are stimulated by norepinephrine, cyclic AMP concentration and insulin secretion are decreased (Turtle and Kipnis, 1967). The exact role of cyclic AMP is not clear, but it may be related to the requirement for Ca^{2+}. Insulinotropic agents act only in the presence of extracellular Ca^{2+} and facilitate its influx. Cyclic AMP and Ca^{2+} may activate the microtubule-microfilament system that is hypothetically involved in the migration and emiocytosis of the insulin-containing granules (*see* Malaisse, 1972).

Of great importance has been the discovery of the biphasic kinetics of the glucose-induced insulin release from the β cell. Both *in vitro* and *in vivo*, there occurs an initial burst of secretion that peaks in minutes and rapidly declines, followed by a second, longer-lasting peak that may duplicate the initial peak value after an hour or longer. The concept of two pools of stored insulin, one more rapidly released than the other, has emerged. The rapidly secreted insulin may be a more important determinant of the rate at which glucose is utilized in the body, and selective impairment of the early phase of secretion is noted in many "prediabetic" and diabetic patients (*see* below). Secretion of insulin during the second phase may depend on protein synthesis (*see,* however, Grodsky, 1971).

Secretion of Insulin by the β Cells: Action of Alloxan and Other Toxins. The insulin content of the pancreas closely parallels the degree of granulation of the β cells (Hartroft and Wrenshall, 1955). If, after 80% of the pancreas is removed, diabetes develops progressively, the progression of the diabetes closely parallels the degenerative changes in the β cells of the remaining fragment of pancreas; the α cells undergo no change. Agents that rather selectively destroy the β cells induce diabetes mellitus. These compounds include alloxan, uric acid, dialuric acid, dehydroascorbic acid, dehydroisoascorbic acid, some quinolones, streptozotocin, and magnesium. Of

these, alloxan (mesoxalylurea) attained great importance in research because its administration is a convenient means for the production of insulin-deficiency diabetes in otherwise-normal experimental animals. Unfortunately, alloxan has not been of value in the treatment of insulin-secreting tumors of the pancreas. When streptozotocin, the N-nitroso derivative of glucosamine produced by *Streptomyces achromogenes,* is injected into rats, degeneration of pancreatic β cells follows. In recent years it has replaced alloxan as the preferred agent to produce a diabetic state in experimental animals (*see* Rerup, 1970), and it is useful clinically to treat insulin-secreting tumors (*see* Chapter 62). *Transient hyperglycemia* may be produced following the administration of certain pharmacological agents capable of inhibiting insulin release (*see* below).

Distribution, Excretion, and Fate. A fraction of the endogenous or exogenous insulin in plasma may be associated with certain proteins, chiefly α- and β-globulins. However, there is doubt that these associations are of importance for the transport of insulin, the bulk of which appears to circulate in blood and lymph as the free hormone. The volume of distribution of insulin approximates the volume of extracellular fluid.

The plasma half-life of insulin injected intravenously is less than 9 minutes in man. While insulin can be detected in urine, the kidney filters and reabsorbs the hormone, and renal excretion is not a major route of elimination (Chamberlain and Stimmler, 1967). The liver and kidney are of primary importance in degrading the hormone, and each is capable of destroying almost 40% of the insulin produced per day (30 to 50 units). Severe impairment of renal function appears to affect the rate of disappearance of circulating insulin to a greater extent than does hepatic disease, since the liver operates closer to its capacity to destroy the hormone and cannot compensate for such loss of renal catabolic function. Although peripheral tissues such as muscle and fat bind and inactivate insulin, this is of minor quantitative significance.

In-vitro experiments suggest that two systems are involved in the degradation of insulin by the liver: (1) an enzyme termed glutathione-insulin transhydrogenase, which utilizes reduced glutathione to reduce the disulfide bridges; and (2) a proteolytic enzyme(s) that cleaves the reduced and separated chains to peptides and amino acids. A highly purified glutathione-insulin transhydrogenase enzyme without proteolytic activity has been isolated from liver by Varandani and Nafz (1972). Presumably because of the reductive separation of the two chains of insulin, free A chains have been demonstrated in the plasma and urine of normal individuals and diabetic patients (Varandani, 1970).

A proteolytic enzyme that degrades both insulin and glucagon has been extensively purified from rat skeletal muscle (Duckworth and Kitabchi, 1974). This enzyme is interesting, because its K_m for insulin is within the physiological range of hormone concentrations.

Insulin and Diabetes Mellitus. Two major syndromes comprise diabetes mellitus—the juvenile-onset (insulin-dependent, ketosis-prone) and the maturity-onset (nonketotic) forms of the disease. The former is clearly characterized by the essential absence of insulin synthesis and secretion. Insulin is present in the latter form of the disease, but impairment of its secretion is suggested by delayed appearance of the hormone in plasma following glucose administration.

Numerous studies have demonstrated the absence of circulating (immunoreactive) insulin in the plasma of patients with juvenile-onset diabetes; analyses of pancreatic insulin have also shown that the hormone is not present (Rastogi *et al.,* 1973). An independent estimate of β-cell function has been devised, based on plasma concentrations of the connector or C-peptide. Its absence from the plasma of patients with juvenile-onset diabetes again indicates failure of β-cell function (Rubenstein *et al.,* 1972). This form of the disease usually begins with marked hyperglycemia or an episode of ketoacidosis associated with extremely low concentrations of immunoreactive insulin and C-peptide in the plasma. A period of clinical remission usually follows, accompanied by improvement in carbohydrate tolerance and a reduction in the requirement for insulin administration. During this time β-cell function returns, as evidenced by restoration of plasma immunoreactive insulin and C-peptide. However, in the fully established disease that follows, the function of the β cell appears to be lost totally.

Individuals with maturity-onset diabetes have functional β cells, as evidenced by the presence of both immunoreactive insulin and C-peptide in plasma. However, there is a delay in the initial secretion of insulin when stimulated by glucose, even in the earliest, so-called latent forms of the disease. Impaired β-cell function is also revealed by the

fact that less insulin is secreted at any given glucose concentration in both diabetic subjects and those with latent disease. The defect may be in the glucoreceptor of the β-cell membrane. (*See* Kipnis, 1971; Cerasi and Luft, 1973a, 1973b; Robertson and Porte, 1973.) However, there is not complete agreement on this point; Reaven and coworkers (1972), for example, described increased plasma insulin concentrations associated with resistance to insulin in patients in early stages of this form of diabetes.

The secretory function of α cells of pancreatic islets is also compromised in diabetes mellitus. Plasma immunoreactive glucagon concentrations are elevated in diabetic patients, particularly during ketoacidosis, and the normal suppression of plasma glucagon by hyperglycemia is impaired (*see* Unger, 1972a). It is not clear whether this is a primary defect in the diabetic state or one that is secondary to β-cell failure and hyperglycemia; it is, however, a characteristic of the disease.

Another vitally important and pathognomonic feature is the capillary basement-membrane thickening that occurs early in the course of diabetes mellitus. This pathological change is probably responsible for the major vascular complications of the disease, including premature atherosclerosis, intercapillary glomerulosclerosis, retinopathy, neuropathy, and ulceration and gangrene of the extremities. While considerable progress has been made in the chemical characterization of normal and "diabetic" basement membrane, it is not known whether the lesion is the result of insulin deficiency or if it is more primary and perhaps of etiological significance (*see* Siperstein, 1972; Spiro, 1973).

Insulin Deficiency: How Insulin Corrects the Metabolic Aberrations of the Diabetic State. Diabetes mellitus due to inadequate insulin secretion by the β cells of the pancreas is characterized by hyperglycemia, hyperlipemia, ketonemia, and azoturia. The purpose of the following discussion is to explain these metabolic aberrations in terms of the effects of insulin on various tissues and organs. The steps described refer to Figure 71-2.

Hyperglycemia. The hyperglycemia of insulin deficiency is a consequence of underutilization and overproduction of glucose.

In the absence of insulin there is a marked reduction in the rate of transport of glucose across certain cell membranes. Lundsgaard (1939) first suggested that insulin acted to enhance glucose transport, and Levine and associates (1949) demonstrated that insulin increased the volume of distribution of ga-

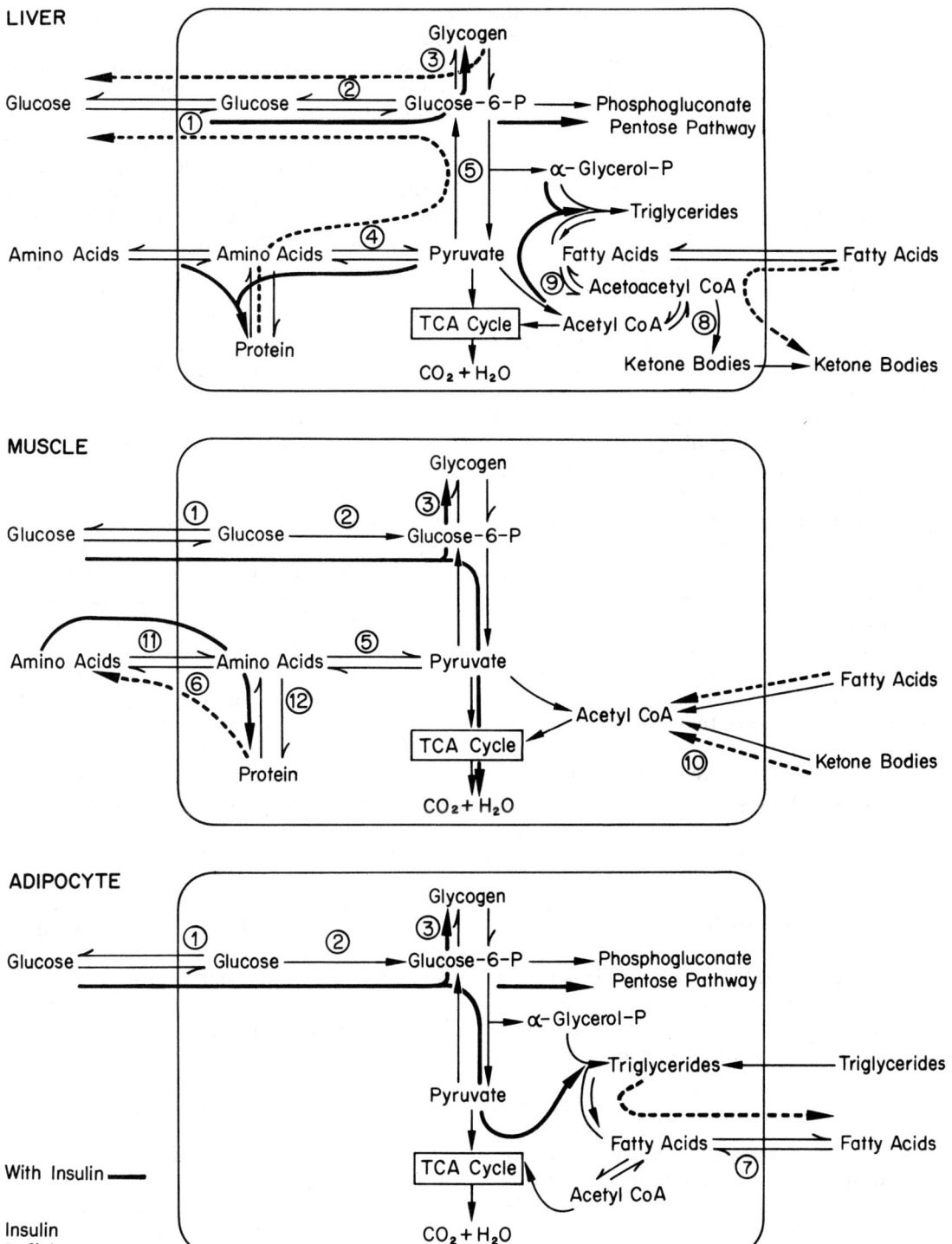

Figure 71-2. *Major metabolic effects of insulin deficiency.*

Thick solid arrows (──►) show the pathways that are favored in the presence of insulin, while thick broken arrows (····►) depict those that predominate when the action of the hormone is insufficient. (For explanation, *see* the text.)

lactose (which is not metabolized) in the nephrectomized, eviscerated dog. They reasoned that the hormone accelerates transport of certain hexoses, including glucose, across cell membranes (steps Muscle-① [M-①] and Adipocyte-① [A-①], Figure 71–2); the exclusion of glucose from the intracellular compartment by a relatively "impermeable" plasma membrane explained the underutilization of glucose in the diabetic state. However, it could also be explained as an effect on the rate of glucose phosphorylation, the obligatory first step in metabolism. That insulin acts to increase transport of glucose independent of rate of phosphorylation was demonstrated in the isolated rat diaphragm preparation by Park and associates (1955). Normally the concentration of glucose is virtually zero within skeletal muscle cells in the presence or the absence of insulin. Once glucose enters the cell, it is quickly phosphorylated to glucose-6-phosphate (steps Liver-② [L-②], M-②, and A-②, Figure 71–2). Park and coworkers showed that at low temperatures, even though the conversion of glucose to glucose-6-phosphate was slowed, insulin clearly increased the transfer of glucose from the medium into the cells. Likewise, it can be shown that insulin accelerates the transfer of glucose into the fat cell, wherein it is transformed to fat or glycogen or oxidized to CO_2.

Obviously, glucose underutilization is to an important degree the consequence of a reduced rate of entrance of the sugar into cells. Because of this inability to gain entrance to the metabolic machinery, the oxidation of glucose to CO_2 and its conversion to glycogen and fat are slowed. It is of practical importance to note that exercise increases the rate of transport of glucose into muscle cells, even in the absence of insulin. Vigorous exercise will induce hypoglycemia in the diabetic subject, and the dose of insulin must be adjusted accordingly. This response may be due to the release of bound insulin or insulin-like material from within the muscle itself or its vasculature (Dieterle et al., 1973).

Insulin does not influence the rate of transfer of glucose across all cell membranes. In insulin deficiency, transport of glucose into the hepatic cell (step L-①) is not significantly reduced; this is not a factor of importance in the development of the metabolic aberrations of the hepatic cell. In diabetes, rate of entry of glucose into the brain is unaffected and function of the nervous system remains normal unless a state of ketoacidosis develops. Erythrocytes, leukocytes, and cells of the renal medulla take up glucose at a rate designed to meet their needs quite independently of insulin. As expected, the rate of glucose oxidation is reduced but by no means to zero in insulin deficiency. This point is illustrated by experiments in which the conversion of labeled glucose to CO_2 is compared in normal and diabetic subjects. A significant reduction characterizes diabetes, but in quantitative terms the reduction may not be dramatic.

In the absence of insulin there is a marked reduction in the activity of the enzyme system that catalyzes the conversion of glucose to glycogen. Insulin added to isolated rat diaphragm or injected into the dog increases the activity of the enzyme (glycogen synthase) that is involved in the conversion of glucose to glycogen in skeletal muscle (step M-③) and in liver (step L-③) (Villar-Palasi and Larner, 1961; Bishop and Larner, 1967). Insulin also activates glycogen synthase in the adipocyte (step A-③).

In the absence of insulin there is an abnormally high rate of conversion of protein to glucose. In insulin deficiency the quantity of glucose excreted in the urine can far exceed the quantity ingested, from which it may be concluded that the metabolic disturbance is characterized by excessive production of glucose as well as by decreased rate of utilization. Estimates of glucose production rates, with the use of ^{14}C-glucose, show excess production in the insulin-deficient state. One can immediately dismiss fat as a source of the excess glucose. Carbohydrates, proteins, and fats share a common pool of intermediates; carbon atoms can shift from fatty acid to glucose and *vice versa,* but *no net* production of glucose from fat has been demonstrated. On the contrary, net production of fat from glucose is easily demonstrated.

Proteins and amino acids are converted to glucose at an abnormally high rate in insulin deficiency. The liver is the site of such conversion (steps L-④ and L-⑤). Protein and amino acids are mobilized from peripheral tissues (*see* the section on azoturia, below). In Figure 71–2, a net loss of amino acid is shown for muscle (step M-⑥); the amino acids so mobilized in insulin deficiency are converted in the liver to glucose and urea (steps L-④ and L-⑤). Among the amino acids, alanine serves a particularly important role.

Hyperlipemia and Ketonemia. The abnormally high concentration of free fatty acids in the plasma of the diabetic subject is due, in large measure, to their increased mobilization from the peripheral fat depots (step A-⑦). Insulin has a direct inhibitory effect on a lipase concerned with the mobilization of fatty acids, while growth hormone, glucocorticoids, thyroid hormones, and catecholamines enhance lipolysis. The marked hyperlipemia that characterizes the diabetic state may be regarded as a consequence of the uninhibited actions of the above hormones on the fat depots.

The source of the ketone bodies in the diabetic subject or the fasting normal subject is the liver (step L-⑧). In the absence of insulin, lipolysis, facilitated by various hormones, proceeds unchecked. The liver takes up large quantities of the free fatty acids thus liberated and oxidizes them to acetyl coenzyme A (CoA) (step L-⑨). The reduced ability of the insulin-deficient liver to synthesize fatty acids from acetyl CoA results in the increased diversion of this substrate to ketone bodies (step L-⑧), which appear in the blood in large quantities. The ketone bodies are utilized as a source of energy by skeletal muscle, heart muscle, and other tissues (step M-⑩).

Azoturia. Insulin deficiency results in conversion of large amounts of protein to glucose with consequent increased production and excretion of urea and ammonia. Increased excretion of ammonia is a renal homeostatic mechanism stimulated by ketoacidosis. In the absence of insulin there is reduced movement of amino acids into muscle and possibly other cells (step M-⑪) and reduced incorporation of amino acids into protein (step M-⑫). Both effects are independent of glucose transport since they can be demonstrated *in vitro* in the absence of glucose in the medium. In insulin deficiency, amino acids do enter the hepatic cell, where they are deaminated and oxidized to yield pyruvate and contribute importantly to the hepatic overproduction of glucose. Hepatic gluconeogenesis from pyruvate and lactate is markedly accelerated by insulin deficiency (Exton *et al.,* 1966; Friedmann *et al.,* 1967). Furthermore, the protein catabolic actions of adrenocorticosteroids and thyroid hormones are unopposed in insulin deficiency, thus tilting the protein anabolic-catabolic balance toward catabolism.

Mechanism of Insulin Action. Major advances have been made in this area, and certain molecular aspects of the action of insulin are rather well understood. Principally through the work of Cuatrecasas (1973) and of Kono (1969), the putative insulin receptor from the cell membrane has been purified and characterized as an insulin-binding protein. The interaction of the hormone with the receptor is highly specific, and the kinetics of the process has been defined. This binding reaction is clearly different from any that results in degradation of insulin. These findings and the fact that the action of insulin is competitively inhibited by a large "diabetogenic peptide" (Miller and Larner, 1972) indicate that the initial action of the hormone is at the cell surface.

The relationship of insulin action to cyclic nucleotide metabolism is of great interest but is unclear. Decreased intracellular concentrations of cyclic AMP (or, perhaps, increased concentrations of cyclic GMP) could explain many of the metabolic effects of insulin. While insulin can cause a lowering of the cyclic AMP concentration in some tissues, this has been observed convincingly only when cyclic AMP synthesis is first stimulated by counterregulatory hormones (Jefferson *et al.,* 1968). Basal concentrations of the cyclic nucleotide are not demonstrably depressed when insulin acts alone (Larner, 1972). This has been the main argument against a direct relationship between the action of insulin and cyclic AMP.

Effects of insulin on the enzymes that catalyze the synthesis and destruction of cyclic AMP have been investigated. While some have observed inhibition of adenylate cyclase, it is more likely that the hormone in some way stimulates cyclic nucleotide phosphodiesterase activity (Manganiello and Vaughan, 1973). The physiological significance is unclear, but the effect may explain the ability of insulin to depress elevated cyclic AMP concentrations.

As described in Chapter 21 (*see* Figure 21–7, page 430), glycogen synthesis and glycogenolysis are controlled by a cascading series of protein phosphorylation reactions. In the presence of cyclic AMP, a protein kinase is activated, and the eventual result is a stimulation of glycogen breakdown and an inhibition of glycogen synthesis. Insulin acts to tip the balance in the other direction—toward glycogen synthesis. The hormone appears to reduce the sensitivity of the protein kinase to cyclic AMP, in effect inhibiting the action of the cyclic nucleotide without the need to lower its concentration (Villar-Palasi and Wenger, 1967; Larner *et al.,* 1974). Glycogen synthase is activated, since a phosphoprotein phosphatase is less opposed and acts to dephosphorylate the enzyme (conversion of the D to the I form; *see*

Chapter 21). By analogous mechanisms, the action of insulin results in dephosphorylation of phosphorylase and of a triglyceride lipase; the metabolic sequelae are inhibition of glycogenolysis and lipolysis, respectively.

Pyruvate dehydrogenase, an important mitochondrial enzyme, is also controlled by insulin (and other hormones) by phosphorylation and dephosphorylation reactions (*see* review by Randle and Denton, 1973). The active form of the enzyme is the dephosphorylated one, and it is increased after insulin treatment by an unknown mechanism. As a result, pyruvate is oxidized or converted to fat and is unavailable for glucose formation.

In addition to the enhanced synthesis of fat, insulin increases the activity of membrane-bound lipoprotein lipase, which makes fatty acids derived from circulating lipoproteins available to the cell (Hollenberg, 1962).

In protein metabolism, insulin promotes amino acid uptake, enhances protein synthesis, and inhibits protein degradation (*see* Manchester, 1972; Morgan *et al.,* 1972). In general, the effects on protein synthesis have been localized to translational events, including polyribosome formation (Wool *et al.,* 1972; Evans *et al.,* 1974) and peptide chain initiation (Morgan *et al.,* 1971). Stabilization of lysosomes has been suggested to explain the inhibition of proteolysis (Mortimore and Mondon, 1970).

The mechanisms of the important actions of insulin to enhance the facilitated diffusion of glucose and the active transport of amino acids are not known. Membrane vesicles that are altered in a stable manner to transport glucose at an enhanced rate can be prepared from fat cells treated with insulin (Carter *et al.,* 1972); this system may facilitate precise biochemical characterization. Of interest in this connection are demonstrations of altered phosphorylation of membrane proteins following exposure to insulin (Benjamin and Singer, 1974).

The action of insulin to promote K^+ uptake into cells, even in the absence of glucose, is classical (*see* Zierler, 1972); a similar effect on Mg^{2+} accumulation has also been demonstrated (Aikawa, 1960). Since K^+ and Mg^{2+} are important in metabolism, for example, in protein biosynthesis, it has been suggested that these cations may play roles as "second messengers" to mediate the actions of insulin (Krahl, 1972).

When one considers the span of membrane and intracellular activities that are modulated by insulin, it is perhaps not surprising that little is known of the hormone's molecular mechanisms of action, except in the case of glycogenesis and antilipolysis, where the role of activated and inactivated catalysts and the mechanisms of their interconversions are defined.

Insulin Unitage. Insulin preparations must be bioassayed as described above in order to ascertain their physiological activity. The assay described in the U.S.P. is based on the ability of samples to lower the blood glucose concentration. The potency is expressed in U.S.P. units, and the standard of comparison is the U.S.P. *Insulin Reference Standard.* The potency of the reference-standard crystals is indicated on the label of each preparation. It is of the order of 22 units/mg. Newer, more pure preparations of the hormone (*see* below) have potencies of 26 to 30 units/mg.

Preparations. Since the previous edition of this textbook, significant advances and changes have been made in the United States in the purity and formulation of insulin preparations. These have been summarized by Rosenbloom (1974).

As a result of a recommendation of the American Diabetes Association's Committee on the Use of Therapeutic Agents, U-40 and U-80 insulins (40 and 80 units/ml) are being eliminated in favor of a single U-100 dosage form for all types of insulin (*see* Committee, 1972). The objective is to reduce the chance of patient error, which is greater with the multiple dosage forms and dually calibrated syringes than with a single dosage form. It is expected that manufacture of the U-80 concentration will cease in the United States in 1975 and that the U-40 formulation will be eliminated within a few years. Concentrated preparations of regular insulin (U-500) are available for patients who are resistant to the hormone (*see* below).

Prior to 1973, insulin preparations available for therapeutic use in the United States contained significant amounts of proinsulin and its incompletely converted products as potentially antigenic components; new procedures have been devised to prepare purer preparations of the hormone. Two such preparations are "single-peak" insulin (essentially one protein peak observed during fractionation by SEPHADEX G50 chromatography) and "single-component" insulin, in which the hormone is subjected to ion-exchange chromatography (Root *et al.,* 1972; Schlichtkrull *et al.,* 1972). The purity of commercial insulin in the United States is now that of "single-peak" insulin (99%). While greatly improved in purity over previous products, "single-peak" insulin appears still to contain antigenic components (Tantillo *et al.,* 1974). However, antibody production is markedly reduced with "single-component" insulin (purity greater than 99%); while this product is not commercially available, it may be obtained from the manufacturer if needed.

Because of the precipitation of impurities formerly contained in insulin preparations, it was necessary to supply regular insulin at an acidic pH. The purer preparations described above have eliminated this difficulty, and most regular insulin preparations (and all regular U-100 preparations) in the United States are now supplied at neutral pH. This has resulted in improved stability of the hormone, and patients need no longer refrigerate the vial of insulin in use. Furthermore, neutral regular insulin can be mixed in any desired proportion with other, modified insulin preparations since all marketed insulin preparations will be at the same pH.

Preparations of insulin are divided into three categories according to promptness, duration, and intensity of action following subcutaneous administration. They are classified as fast-, intermediate-, and long-acting types (*see* Table 71–1). Insulin precipitated from solution in the amorphous (noncrystalline) form and then prepared for subcutaneous injection by solution in water at either neutral or acidic pH

Table 71-1. PROPERTIES OF VARIOUS PREPARATIONS OF INSULIN

TYPE	PREPARATION	APPEARANCE	PROTEIN MODIFIER	APPROXIMATE TIME OF ONSET * (*hours*)	APPROXIMATE DURATION OF ACTION * (*hours*)	COMPATIBLE MIXED WITH
Fast-Acting	*Insulin Injection,* U.S.P. (regular insulin)	Clear solution	None	1	6	All preparations
	Insulin Injection, U.S.P. "Insulin made from zinc-insulin crystals" (regular insulin)	Clear solution	None	1	8	All preparations
	Prompt Insulin Zinc Suspension, U.S.P. (SEMILENTE insulin)	Cloudy suspension	None	1	14	LENTE preparations
Intermediate-Acting	*Isophane Insulin Suspension,* U.S.P. (NPH insulin, isophane insulin)	Cloudy suspension	Protamine	2	24	Insulin injection
	Insulin Zinc Suspension, U.S.P. (LENTE insulin)	Cloudy suspension	None	2	24	Insulin injection, SEMILENTE
	Globin Zinc Insulin Injection, U.S.P.	Clear solution	Globin	2	18	—
Long-Acting	*Protamine Zinc Insulin Suspension,* U.S.P.	Cloudy suspension	Protamine	7	36	Insulin injection
	Extended Insulin Zinc Suspension, U.S.P. (ULTRALENTE insulin)	Cloudy suspension	None	7	36	Insulin injection, SEMILENTE

* These figures are representative. The values may be expected to vary over a relatively wide range, depending on the dose and the individual patient.

(about 3.2) (*Insulin Injection,* U.S.P.) is rapidly absorbed; action is prompt in onset, intense, and short in duration. The term *amorphous* applies to the noncrystalline physical state of the insulin. Crystalline insulin is prepared by the precipitation of the hormone in the presence of zinc (as zinc chloride) in a suitable buffer medium. Crystalline insulin when dissolved in water at neutral or acidic pH is also known as *Insulin Injection,* U.S.P., but may bear the additional label "insulin made from zinc-insulin crystals." Following subcutaneous injection it has a slightly slower onset and a slightly longer duration of action than does amorphous insulin.

By permitting insulin and zinc to react with the basic protein protamine, Hagedorn and associates (1936) prepared a protein complex, *protamine zinc insulin.* When the complex is injected subcutaneously in an aqueous suspension, it dissolves only slowly at the site of deposition, and the insulin is absorbed at a retarded but steady rate. The objective of therapy with protamine zinc insulin suspension is to provide the daily requirement of hormone in a single injection. In the severely diabetic patient,

however, the onset of action of protamine zinc insulin suspension is too slow, and if large doses are employed the duration of action is too prolonged for adequate control. To obviate this difficulty, combination therapy with regular insulin and protamine zinc insulin suspension was introduced. The two insulins can be given either as separate injections or mixed in the proper proportion immediately prior to injection.

Insulin mixtures can be prepared extemporaneously by mixing insulin injection and protamine zinc insulin suspension in the syringe immediately before use. The onset and the duration of action of the resulting mixture differ from those of the two preparations injected separately. This is because the protamine in protamine zinc insulin suspension is capable of reacting with a certain amount of additional regular insulin with the establishment of a new equilibrium. The mixtures commonly employed contain a ratio of 2 to 3 units of regular insulin to 1 unit of protamine zinc insulin. The purpose of such a mixture is to provide a preparation that has a rapid onset as well as a prolonged duration of action. Mixtures in which the ratio of regular to protamine zinc insulin is less than 2:1 possess essentially the properties of protamine zinc insulin suspension. The chief disadvantage in the use of insulin mixtures is that they are unstable and, therefore, must be extemporaneously prepared by the patient. This procedure is too complicated for many patients. The chief advantage is that any mixture can be prescribed to meet the varying needs of different patients.

The search has continued for a stable solution of insulin that possesses the desirable properties of fairly rapid onset and moderately prolonged duration of action. Three preparations of this type are *Globin Zinc Insulin Injection,* U.S.P., developed by Reiner and associates (1939); *Isophane Insulin Suspension,* U.S.P., developed in Hagedorn's laboratory by Krayenbühl and Rosenberg and first reported in the American literature by Peck (1964); and LENTE *insulins.*

Globin Zinc Insulin Injection, U.S.P., is a mixture of insulin and the protein globin (derived from beef hemoglobin) and zinc chloride. The time of onset and the duration of action of this preparation are intermediate between those of regular insulin and protamine zinc insulin suspension. Globin zinc insulin injection is now rarely used.

Isophane Insulin Suspension, U.S.P., is also known as NPH-50 insulin; the *N* denotes a neutral solution (pH 7.2), the *P* refers to the protamine zinc insulin content, the *H* signifies the origin in Hagedorn's laboratory, and the *50* refers to the content of 0.50 mg of protamine per 100 U.S.P. units of insulin. It is a modified protamine zinc insulin suspension. The concentrations of insulin, protamine, and zinc are so arranged that the preparation has an onset and a duration of action intermediate between those of regular insulin and protamine zinc insulin suspension. The advantage of this mixture is its stability in regard to the ratio of "free" to "bound" insulin. Its effects on blood sugar are indistinguishable from those of an extemporaneous mixture of 2 to 3 units of regular insulin and 1 unit of protamine zinc insulin suspension.

The chemical studies of Hallas-Møller and associates (1952a, 1952b) revealed that the solubility of insulin was determined in important measure by its physical state (amorphous, crystalline, size of the crystals) and by the zinc content and the nature of the buffer in which it was suspended. Insulin can thus be prepared in a slowly absorbed, slow-acting form without the use of other proteins, such as protamine or globin, to bind it. Large crystals of insulin with high zinc content, when collected and resuspended in a solution of sodium acetate–sodium chloride (pH 7.1 to 7.5), are slowly absorbed after subcutaneous injection and exert an action of long duration. This preparation is named *Extended Insulin Zinc Suspension,* U.S.P. (ULTRALENTE insulin). Amorphous insulin precipitated at high pH is almost as rapid in onset and as short in duration of action as regular insulin. The preparation is named *Prompt Insulin Zinc Suspension,* U.S.P. (SEMILENTE insulin). The two forms of insulin may be mixed to yield a stable mixture of crystalline (7 parts) and amorphous (3 parts) insulin—*Insulin Zinc Suspension,* U.S.P. (LENTE insulin)—that is intermediate in onset and

duration of action between SEMILENTE and ULTRALENTE preparations.

The properties of the various official insulin preparations are presented in Table 71–1. Most commercial insulin preparations in the United States are mixtures of the bovine and porcine hormones. Pure porcine or pure bovine insulin is also available. The LENTE insulins contain methylparaben as a preservative; the other preparations, either phenol or cresol. All preparations are usually given by subcutaneous injection. *Only insulin injection can be given by the intravenous route.* The insulins are marketed in 10-ml vials.

Hypoglycemia Associated with Hyperinsulinism. Hypoglycemic reactions may occur in any diabetic subject treated with insulin or with an oral hypoglycemic agent. Reactions are seen frequently in the labile form of the disease, a form characterized by unpredictable spontaneous reductions in insulin requirement. In other instances, precipitating causes are usually responsible, for example, failure to eat, unaccustomed exercise, and inadvertent administration of too large a dose of insulin.

The reaction pattern associated with hypoglycemia has been fully described in connection with insulin shock therapy for schizophrenia (long since outmoded) and in carefully controlled clinical studies in normal and diabetic volunteers (Sussman *et al.,* 1963). The pattern and the temporal sequence of signs and symptoms are fairly, but by no means absolutely, constant. When the rate of fall in blood glucose is rapid, the early symptoms are those brought on by the compensating secretion of epinephrine; these include sweating, weakness, hunger, tachycardia, and "inner trembling." When the blood glucose falls slowly, the symptoms and signs are referable to the brain and include headache, blurred vision, diplopia, mental confusion, incoherent speech, coma, and convulsions. If the fall in blood glucose is rapid, profound, and persistent, all such symptoms may be present. In only a few patients, the onset is heralded by hunger or nausea; bradycardia and mild hypotension may occur in association with the gastrointestinal discomfort. These changes are a consequence of excitation of the parasympathetic nervous system.

From a practical point of view, about h˙ of the patients may be expected to c˙ help; nevertheless, another large ˙

presumably as a consequence of the confusion attending hypoglycemia, will not. Fortunately, the patients who have neither signs nor symptoms preceding convulsions and coma are few in number, but they present one of the most difficult problems in the management of diabetes.

The majority of the signs and symptoms of insulin hypoglycemia are the result of functional abnormalities of the CNS, since hypoglycemia deprives the brain of the substrate (glucose) upon which it is almost exclusively dependent for its oxidative metabolism. During insulin coma, oxygen consumption in human brain decreases about 45%. The reduction in glucose consumption is proportionately greater, which indicates that the brain is utilizing either some other substrate or carbohydrate stores in cerebral tissue (Kety *et al.*, 1948). After prolonged fasting in man the brain adapts, and the bulk of the fuel utilized is free fatty acids and ketone bodies (Owen *et al.*, 1967).

Hypoglycemic convulsions appear to be markedly influenced by the degree of cerebral hydration. Yannet (1939) observed in cats that a marked hydration of brain cells accompanies insulin coma, and Drabkin and Ravdin (1937) were able to prevent hypoglycemic convulsions by dehydrating experimental animals prior to the administration of insulin. However, this finding is not unique for hypoglycemic convulsions; the convulsive threshold for other types of stimuli is also reduced by cellular hydration.

A prolonged period of hypoglycemia causes irreversible damage to the brain, as evidenced in experimental animals by histological changes in the cortex, basal ganglia, and rostral parts of the medulla. Animals that recover from prolonged periods of hypoglycemia present the typical signs of functional decortication (Baker, 1939; Yannet, 1939; Ziskind and Tyler, 1940). Brain damage occurs even when hypoglycemic convulsions are prevented by barbiturates (Tyler, 1941). There are isolated reports of neurological or mental changes in man following insulin convulsions and coma, including mental retardation, hemiparesis, ataxia, incontinence, aphasia, choreiform movements, parkinsonism, and epilepsy.

Though the signs and the symptoms of hypoglycemia seem well defined, it is often difficult clinically to distinguish this condition from severe diabetic ketoacidosis (diabetic coma). Unfortunately, many cases of insulin coma have been treated with insulin. The symptoms of hypoglycemia yield almost immediately to the intravenous injection of glucose unless hypoglycemia has been sufficiently prolonged to induce organic changes in the brain. If the patient is not able to take soluble carbohydrate or fruit juice orally and if glucose is not available for intravenous injection, 0.5 to 1 mg of glucagon is given (*see* below).

Every diabetic patient taking insulin should carry an identification card containing pertinent medical information.

Other Adverse Reactions. Local or systemic allergic reactions are often seen in patients receiving insulin for the first time or when insulin treatment is reinstituted. The local reactions that result from skin sensitivity usually subside spontaneously. Allergic urticaria, angioedema, and anaphylactic reactions occur infrequently and usually can be avoided by changing to insulin obtained from a different species. Rarely a hyposensitization procedure may be required.

Patients who experience atrophy of subcutaneous fat at the site of injection (insulin lipoatrophy) should inject the insulin in areas that are usually covered by clothing; the problem may be minimized by changing the site of injection frequently. There have been reports of decreased incidence of lipoatrophy with the newer, more highly purified insulins (Tantillo *et al.*, 1974), and injection of these preparations directly into sites of lipoatrophy may facilitate reversal of the process.

Visual disturbances in uncontrolled diabetes that are due to refractive changes are reversed during the early treatment phase. However, since several weeks may be required to stabilize the osmotic equilibrium in the eye, alterations of prescriptions for corrective lenses should be postponed for 3 to 6 weeks.

ORAL HYPOGLYCEMIC AGENTS

History. An important event in the history of the treatment of diabetes mellitus was the introduction of orally effective hypoglycemic agents. Janbon and coworkers (1942), in the course of clinical studies on the treatment of typhoid fever, discovered that a sulfonamide (*p*-amino-benzene-sulfonamido-isopropylthiadiazole) induced hypoglycemia. Janbon's colleague, Loubatières (1957), made the fundamental discovery that the compound exerted no hypoglycemic effect in the completely pancreatectomized animal and suggested that the action was the result of stimulation of the pancreas to secrete insulin. There was no practical application of these findings until Franke and Fuchs capitalized on the discovery that the antibacterial agent *carbutamide* lowered the blood sugar in patients treated for infectious diseases. These workers demonstrated the apparent usefulness of carbutamide in the treatment of diabetes mellitus. Soon thereafter, the compound *tolbutamide* was introduced. This substance is not antibacterial, is less toxic than carbutamide, and soon became popular for the management of certain diabetic patients. Tolbutamide is a member of the class of oral hypoglycemic agents designated as *sulfonylureas*.

Another group of compounds, the *biguanides,* was developed independently of the sulfonylureas. Historically, the development began with the discovery in 1918 by Watanabe that guanidine is hypoglycemic in rats. Guanidine and its substituted derivatives were found to be too toxic to be therapeutically useful. *Diguanides,* two guanidine molecules joined by a chain of methylene groups, were more effective and less toxic than the substituted guanidines. SYNTHALIN A, a potent diguanide, was given clinical trial in diabetes, but it also was found to be too toxic for therapeutic use. Finally, *phenformin* (Ungar *et al.,* 1957), a member of the biguanide series (derived from two molecules of guanidine with elimination of ammonia), was found to have an apparently acceptable toxicity, and this compound has since had widespread use.

SULFONYLUREAS

Chemistry. A number of sulfonylurea compounds exert hypoglycemic activity. The commercially available preparations are *tolbutamide, acetohexamide, tolazamide,* and *chlorpropamide,* which have the following structural formulas:

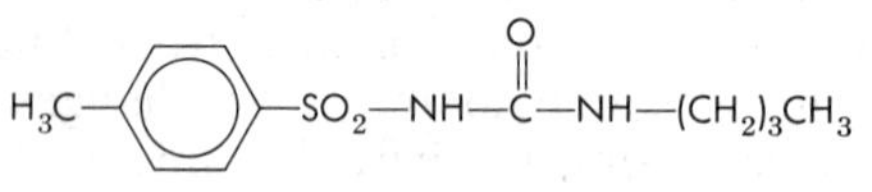

Tolbutamide

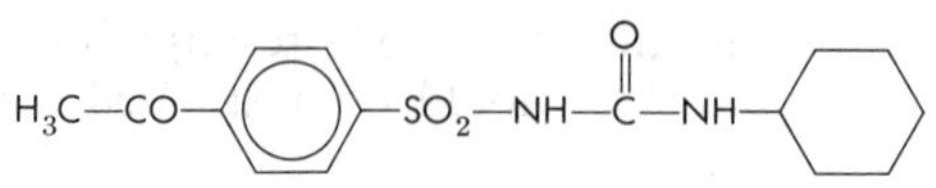

Acetohexamide

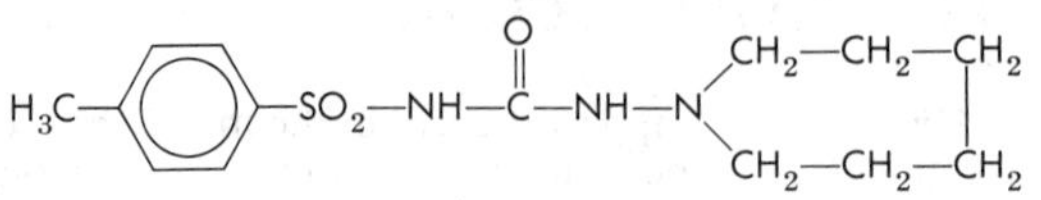

Tolazamide

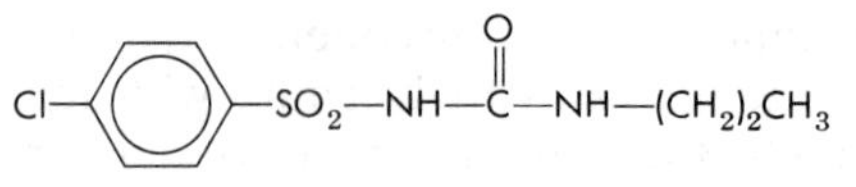

Chlorpropamide

All the effective compounds are arylsulfonylureas with substitutions on the benzene and the urea groups. In the case of tolbutamide, the aryl group is tolyl and the urea substitution is butyl. Tolbutamide differs from the antibacterial compound carbutamide in having methyl instead of amino on the benzene ring. This substitution accounts for the loss of antibacterial properties and for the reduction of toxicity.

Mechanism of Action. The sulfonylureas stimulate the islet tissue to secrete insulin. The evidence, coming as it does from a variety of experimental and clinical studies, unequivocally supports such a conclusion. Administration of sulfonylureas increases the concentration of insulin in the pancreatic vein in cross-circulation experiments. Recipient animals, diabetic or nondiabetic, exhibit hypoglycemia in response to the infusion of pancreatic vein blood from donor animals treated with sulfonylureas but not to the infusion of mesenteric or femoral vein blood from the same animals. Sulfonylureas cause degranulation of the β cells, a phenomenon associated with increased rate of secretion of insulin. Clinical studies demonstrate that the sulfonylureas are ineffective in completely pancreatectomized patients and in juvenile-onset diabetic subjects. On the other hand, they are effective in maturity-onset diabetic patients in whom the pancreas retains the capacity to secrete insulin.

Although the molecular mechanism of action of these agents is not understood, several pertinent observations have been made. Hellman and associates (1971) concluded that labeled tolbutamide is restricted in its action to the extracellular space and does not need to enter the β cell. The invoked release of insulin is immediate and is intimately related to the action of glucose; the drug may sensitize the cell to the normal secretagogue (Widstrom and Cerasi, 1973). Sulfonylureas do not increase the secretion of glucagon.

Extrapancreatic effects of the sulfonylureas have been noted in various organs, and certain of these may potentiate the effects of insulin. A reduction in the hepatic uptake of endogenous insulin has been described (Marshall *et al.,* 1970). Tolbutamide enhances the antilipolytic action of insulin in adipose tissue. This appears to be related to an altered effectiveness of cyclic AMP rather than to any change in metabolism of the cyclic nucleotide (Brown et al., 1972; Fain et al., 1972), and an inhibitory effect of the drug on cyclic AMP–dependent protein kinase has been observed (Wray and Harris, 1973). Other reports indicate a variety of influences on cyclic AMP metabolism in different tissues (Brooker and Fichman, 1971; Kuo et al., 1972; Lasseter et al., 1972); their significance is difficult to assess.

Duration of Action, Fate, and Excretion. The sulfonylureas are absorbed from the gastrointestinal tract and hence are effective when given by mouth. The most important difference among the sulfonylureas, for clinical purposes, is in their duration of action; in increasing order they are tolbutamide, acetohexamide, tolazamide, and chlorpropamide.

Tolbutamide can be detected in the blood within 30 minutes after oral administration; peak concentrations are reached within 3 to 5 hours. The drug is bound to plasma proteins. Tolbutamide is oxidized in the body to butyl-*p*-carboxyphenylsulfonylurea, which is a major excretory product. The half-life of tolbutamide is about 5 hours. Two or occasionally three doses are required daily.

Acetohexamide is rapidly absorbed, and maximal hypoglycemic activity is observed about 3 hours after ingestion. The total duration of action is 12 to 24 hours. Much of the activity is ascribable to a metabolite, *hydroxyhexamide,* which has a plasma half-life of about 6 hours; the parent compound, acetohexamide, has a plasma half-life of 1⅓ hours. In persons with normal renal and hepatic function, more than 80% is excreted, largely as metabolites, in 24 hours. Two doses are usually required daily.

Tolazamide is slowly absorbed; the onset of hypoglycemic action occurs at 4 to 6 hours and persists at a significant level up to 15 hours after a single dose. Tolazamide is metabolized to a number of hypoglycemic substances that are largely excreted by the kidney. For most patients controlled by tolazamide, a single daily dose is sufficient; a few patients require administration of the drug twice daily.

Chlorpropamide is also rapidly absorbed from the gastrointestinal tract and is bound to plasma proteins. In contrast to tolbutamide, chlorpropamide is not metabolically altered to any significant degree and is excreted very slowly in unchanged form. The half-life of a single dose is about 36 hours, or seven times as long as that of tolbutamide. With daily doses of 250 to 500 mg, blood concentrations may not be expected to reach a plateau before 3 or more days. Chlorpropamide is administered in a single daily dose.

Toxicity. O'Donovan (1959) analyzed the incidence of side effects to *tolbutamide* in 9168 cases. The total incidence of side effects was 3.2%; the drug was withdrawn in 1.5% of the patients. The reactions have been classified as hematological (0.24%), cutaneous (1.1%), and gastrointestinal (1.4%). Of the 22 subjects exhibiting hematological abnormalities, 19 had a transient leukopenia; in 9 instances, the leukocyte count returned to normal despite continuation of the drug. Paresthesia, tinnitus, and headache may also occur.

The total incidence of untoward reactions is about 6% for *chlorpropamide* (hematological, 0.6; cutaneous, 3; gastrointestinal, 2; and jaundice, 0.4%). The jaundice is of the cholestatic type and is usually transient. Hyponatremia has been reported in a small number of patients treated with tolbutamide and chlorpropamide.

Experience with *acetohexamide* and *tolazamide* suggests that the frequency and the kinds of toxic reactions are similar to those encountered with tolbutamide and chlorpropamide. Hematological (leukopenia, agranulocytosis, thrombocytopenia, pancytopenia, and hemolytic anemia), cutaneous (rashes, photosensitivity), gastrointestinal (nausea, vomiting, rarely hemorrhage), and hepatic (increased serum alkaline phosphatase, cholestatic jaundice) reactions have been reported.

Hypoglycemic reactions, including coma, may occur (Seltzer, 1972a). While they are usually not severe, several fatalities have been reported. Hypoglycemic episodes may last for several days so that prolonged or repeated glucose administration is required. Reactions have occurred after one dose, after several days of treatment, or after months of drug administration. Most reactions are observed in patients over 50 years of age, and they are more likely to occur in patients with impaired hepatic or renal function. Overdosage or inadequate or irregular food intake may initiate hypoglycemia. Drugs that may increase the risk of hypoglycemia from sulfonylureas include other hypoglycemic agents, sulfonamides, propranolol, salicylates, phenylbutazone, probenecid, dicumarol, chloramphenicol, monoamine oxidase inhibitors, and alcohol.

Sulfonylureas should not be used in a patient with hepatic or renal insufficiency because of the important role of the liver in their metabolism and of the kidney in the excretion of the drugs and their metabolites. Intolerance to alcohol reminiscent of the disulfiram reaction has occurred occasionally in patients taking sulfonylureas.

These agents are also not recommended for use in pregnancy, but only sparse data have been reported on this point. Teratogenesis in animals has been observed to follow the administration of large doses.

A cooperative clinical trial in 12 university-based clinics (University Group Diabetes Program; UGDP) was established in 1961 to determine if the control of blood glucose concentration helps to prevent or delay vascular disease in non-insulin-requiring diabetic patients. About 200 subjects in each of five therapeutic regimens were treated with diet and either placebo, a standard dose of tolbutamide, a standard dose of insulin, a variable dose of insulin, or a standard dose of phenformin.

During a period of over 8 years of observation, there were 120 deaths, including 87 from cardiovascular causes; while 10 to 12 cardiovascular deaths occurred in each of the placebo or insulin groups, 26 such deaths (a significantly higher number) were recorded among the patients in each group taking oral hypoglycemic agents. The overall mortality rate was correspondingly higher in these two groups of diabetic patients. The conclusions of this study were that the combination of diet and either tolbutamide or phenformin was no more effective in prolonging life than diet alone; furthermore, it was felt that diet and either tolbutamide or phenformin may be *less* effective than diet alone or diet together with insulin in preventing cardiovascular mortality. (*See* University Group Diabetes Program, 1970; Knatterud *et al.*, 1971.)

Since the UGDP report, a flood of comments and reports have appeared, both critical (*see* Seltzer, 1972b) and supportive of this massive study. However, no warning has yet been included in the package inserts for these drugs, and there have now appeared a "second generation" of even more potent sulfonylureas (*glimidine* and *glibenclamide*), which are in clinical use in Europe and elsewhere.

Additional studies have continued to indicate an increased incidence of serious difficulties in patients taking oral hypoglycemic drugs. More episodes of ventricular tachycardia and ventricular fibrillation were noted in such diabetic subjects, usually during the early stages of acute myocardial infarction, although there was no difference in the number of deaths (Clayman, 1974; Soler *et al.*, 1974). Patients taking oral hypoglycemic agents in England have been reported to have twice the incidence of myocardial infarctions observed in subjects being treated with diet alone (Boyle *et al.*, 1972; Hadden *et al.*, 1972). Furthermore, at the instigation of the Director of the National Institutes of Health, the Biometric Society appointed a committee to review the UGDP report. The committee concluded that the shortcomings of the study do not invalidate the observations and conclusions, the most pertinent of which are described above, and that other studies do not contradict that of the UGDP. (*See* Chalmers, 1975; Report of the Committee, 1975.)

Preparations and Dosage. *Tolbutamide,* U.S.P. (ORINASE), is marketed in the form of 500-mg tablets. The sodium salt (1 g) is also available for administration intravenously for diagnostic use. *Acetohexamide,* U.S.P. (DYMELOR), is available in 250- and 500-mg tablets. *Tolazamide,* U.S.P. (TOLINASE), is supplied in 100-, 250-, and 500-mg tablets. *Chlorpropamide,* U.S.P. (DIABINESE), is marketed as 100- and 250-mg tablets.

The usual daily dose of tolbutamide is 1000 mg, while 2000 mg is the maximally effective total dose; corresponding dosages are 500 and 1500 mg for acetohexamide. Tolazamide and chlorpropamide are usually administered in a daily dosage of 250 mg, while 750 to 1000 mg is maximal.

Therapeutic Uses. *The sulfonylureas should be used only in subjects with diabetes of the maturity-onset type who cannot be treated with diet alone or who are unwilling or unable to take insulin if weight reduction and dietary control fail.* The physician must realize that he is using these agents only to control symptoms associated with hyperglycemia, and that dietary control with or without insulin is more effective for this purpose. There is no evidence that the oral hypoglycemic agents prevent cardiovascular complications from diabetes, and the best data available suggest that the incidence of such complications is increased in patients taking these drugs. This is obviously too high a price for the convenience of an oral agent, unless *all* other measures have been exhausted.

In general, the likelihood of adequate control with an oral hypoglycemic agent is inversely proportional to the dose of insulin required to maintain the patient. When the insulin requirement is in excess of 40 units per day, the chances of success are relatively low. The sulfonylureas are of no value in the juvenile-onset type of diabetes, in which the pancreas has lost all or nearly all of its capacity to secrete insulin. However, whatever the age of onset, in unstable, ketoacidotic diabetes, sulfonylureas will not provide adequate control. *Such patients require insulin, and attempts to control them with oral therapy are dangerous and doomed to failure.* Deaths from acidosis and dehydration have occurred in patients with unstable ketotic diabetes in whom regulation was attempted with sulfonylureas.

There is no fixed dosage of sulfonylurea to be used in diabetes mellitus. Treatment is guided by the individual patient's response, which must be frequently monitored with chemical determinations, because the requirements change from time to time.

The mildly diabetic patient, whose insulin requirement is fewer than 20 units daily, can be started on the usual dose of the agent chosen, and at the same time all insulin is discontinued. The dose is then adjusted up or down, depending on the patient's response. In the instance of chlorpropamide, about 3 days is required to attain steady-state concentrations in blood. Consequently, upward adjustments of dose should be made at 3-day intervals. Patients of advanced age should begin with about half the usual daily dose, for some are very responsive to sulfonylureas and may develop severe hypoglycemia after usual doses. During the period of initiating treatment, all patients should test their urine four times daily and communicate the results to the physician daily.

The patient who requires more than 20 and fewer than 40 units of insulin daily should be started on the usual dose of the chosen agent and his insulin dosage should simultaneously be reduced by 50%. Thereafter, guided by the patient's response, insulin dosage is progressively reduced and eventually discontinued. Sulfonylurea dosage may need adjustment.

The patient requiring more than 40 units of insulin daily should be given the usual dose of the agent chosen and his insulin dosage should be reduced by 25%. Insulin is then cautiously withdrawn and eventually discontinued, and sulfonylurea is adjusted

according to the observed response. It is to be emphasized that the chance of success is relatively poor. In the patient who requires more than 40 units of insulin daily, it may be desirable to carry out the attempted transfer to the sulfonylurea therapy in the hospital to provide assurance against development of dehydration and acidosis.

Stimulation of the pancreas of the maturity-onset diabetic can often maintain these subjects under ordinary circumstances. However, when insulin requirements are increased, as in fever, surgical interventions, or trauma, the sulfonylureas are inadequate and the patient must be given insulin to carry him through such critical situations.

Weight reduction is of the greatest importance in the treatment of diabetes. A vigorous effort must be made by the patient and the physician to reduce the patient's weight as an integral part of diabetic treatment, irrespective of the drug chosen.

Patients whose diabetes is not controlled by sulfonylureas from the initiation of treatment are said to experience "primary failure." Patients whose diabetes is regulated for a month or more after beginning sulfonylurea treatment, following which inability to maintain control develops, are said to experience "secondary failure." The incidence of this type of failure may be very high, regardless of the agent chosen.

In patients with pancreatic islet-cell tumors, the blood glucose concentration drops rapidly after intravenous injection of tolbutamide and remains low for about 3 hours. A similar effect is not observed in other hypoglycemic states, and tolbutamide administration can thus be used as a diagnostic test. Serum immunoreactive insulin determinations should also be performed. Care is necessary, since fatal hypoglycemia has occurred.

In addition, reports have appeared of the successful treatment of reactive hypoglycemias due to a variety of causes with sulfonylureas (Anderson and Herman, 1971).

BIGUANIDES: PHENFORMIN

Chemistry and Preparations. The only commercially available preparation in the biguanide series of hypoglycemic agents is *phenformin*. Its structural formula is as follows:

Phenformin

Phenformin Hydrochloride, U.S.P. (DBI, MELTROL), is marketed as 25-mg tablets and as 50- and 100-mg timed-disintegration capsules.

Mechanism of Action. The biguanides differ significantly from the sulfonylureas in the mechanism of their hypoglycemic effect. Thus, phenformin does not act by stimulating secretion of insulin by the pancreas, hypoglycemia is not readily induced in normal human subjects, the concentration of insulin in the plasma is not increased, and the morphology of the β cell is uninfluenced. Basically, three actions have been described. *In vitro,* phenformin, in relatively large doses, increases glucose utilization by enhancing anaerobic glycolysis (*see* Williams and Porte, 1974). This is thought to occur as a result of, or coincident with, an inhibition of cellular respiration. As a result, adenosine triphosphate (ATP) concentrations fall and those of lactate increase. A second action of the drug is to decrease gluconeogenesis (*see* Gordon and de Hartog, 1973; Haeckel, 1973). The third and most recently recognized is inhibition of intestinal absorption of glucose and probably certain other substances as well; for example, decreased absorption of vitamin B_{12} has been observed (Berger *et al.,* 1972). Phenformin does not act in the normal subject (at least as readily as it does in the diabetic), presumably because the increase in peripheral glucose utilization is compensated for by an increase in hepatic glucose output.

Phenformin has been used experimentally to correct the hypoglycemia that may follow abnormally rapid intestinal absorption of glucose (Permutt *et al.,* 1973).

Absorption and Duration of Action. Phenformin is adequately absorbed from the gastrointestinal tract. The drug has a short half-life (3 hours) and a correspondingly brief duration of action. The hypoglycemic effect may be prolonged to between 6 and 14 hours with the use of timed-disintegration capsules.

Toxicity. Phenformin may cause a metallic taste, nausea, anorexia, vomiting, diarrhea, or cramps in some patients, particularly if the dose is greater than 200 mg per day. Reduction of the dose or withdrawal of the drug results in prompt disappearance of the untoward reactions. Weight loss and weakness may sometimes occur.

The cause of *ketonuria* during phenformin therapy has been the subject of debate. It is most common in patients with unstable juvenile-onset diabetes treated with a combination of insulin and phenformin. While it may at times reflect an insufficient insulin dosage,

at other times it is associated with normal plasma glucose concentrations. Therefore, in patients taking both insulin and phenformin in whom ketosis develops, plasma glucose concentration should be measured before the insulin dosage is increased, to avoid hypoglycemic reactions. The recommended treatment for ketosis with normal plasma glucose concentrations is a reduction of phenformin dosage or an increase of dietary carbohydrate intake. Increased concentration of lactic acid in the blood without ketosis has been reported to occur in patients with severe renal or cardiovascular impairment under phenformin treatment. However, the drug may not contribute to the lactacidemia, since such severely ill diabetic patients may exhibit lactacidemia even when treated with insulin. Results obtained with phenformin in the UGDP study are discussed above.

Diabetic subjects with severe hepatic or renal insufficiency or congestive heart failure are not suitable candidates for oral hypoglycemic therapy. Almost no data are available concerning the effects of phenformin in pregnancy, and its administration during pregnancy is currently not recommended.

Therapeutic Uses. Phenformin is used in the treatment of maturity-onset diabetes according to the principles presented above for the sulfonylureas.

The patient is started on two tablets, 25 mg each, one before breakfast and the other before supper. The dose is increased until control of the diabetic state is attained or until digestive disturbances limit further increase in dosage. The total daily dose is usually somewhere between 100 and 150 mg. However, doses as high as 400 mg per day are tolerated by some patients. A single 50-mg, timed-disintegration capsule may be substituted as the equivalent of two 25-mg tablets in divided doses.

It is claimed that about 70% of maturity-onset diabetic patients who are imperfectly controlled by either a sulfonylurea or phenformin alone respond favorably to the concurrent use of these agents (Beaser, 1960; Unger *et al.,* 1960). The fact that the sulfonylureas and the biguanides act by different mechanisms to reduce hyperglycemia lends support to this contention (*see* Breidahl *et al.,* 1972). However, since the indications for the use of either phenformin or a sulfonylurea are now severely constricted, such combination therapy should represent the choice of the physician who has exhausted every other alternative.

TREATMENT OF DIABETES MELLITUS

The Ambulatory Patient. The objectives of therapy are maintenance of health and a symptom-free, productively active life. This is attained by attention to diet, body weight, and activity and, if necessary, by the use of insulin. Inability to use insulin in a given patient with maturity-onset diabetes may necessitate the administration of an oral hypoglycemic agent.

Insulin is required for control of diabetes in most persons in whom the disease has its onset before attainment of adult stature (juvenile-onset diabetes), in most underweight persons in whom it appears after cessation of growth, and in pregnant women whose disorder is not controlled by diet. Insulin will be temporarily required in the treatment of keto-acidosis in the obese patient whose diabetes is otherwise controlled by dietary regulation with or without an oral hypoglycemic agent. Insulin is effective in all forms of diabetes. It is the only effective agent for severe manifestations of diabetes and should be used when these are present or threatened, for example, during surgery or infection or following vascular occlusions, irrespective of previous therapy.

Most patients with onset of diabetes in middle or late life are obese. *A serious effort should be made to regulate their diabetes by diet and weight reduction alone.* In doing so, it is important to avoid confusing weight loss resulting from restricted caloric intake with that resulting from uncontrolled diabetes. Weekly determination of weight and 24-hour urine glucose values will prevent this error. Weight, glycosuria, and requirement for insulin or oral hypoglycemic agent should diminish in parallel. Insulin therapy can be satisfactorily initiated on an ambulatory basis in an asymptomatic or mildly symptomatic patient with newly discovered diabetes. However, a short period of hospitalization offers superior opportunities for accurate evaluation of the patient, for the rapid attainment of control, and for education of the patient and his family.

Whether insulin therapy is begun at home or in the hospital, urine should be collected from bedtime to breakfast, from breakfast to lunch, from lunch to supper, and from supper to bedtime. The glucose content of a urine specimen formed during the 2 hours before breakfast is useful in evaluation of patients who require long-acting insulins—protamine zinc insulin suspension or extended zinc insulin suspension. A diet calculated for the patient's needs is begun. Many physicians prefer to use regular insulin in multiple daily doses 20 minutes before meals and at bedtime for the first few days. The usual first dose of regular insulin in the nonketotic patient is 10 units. Subsequent doses are determined by the glycosuria, glycemia, and response to preceding doses. After control is achieved, a single dose of modified insulin given before breakfast is substituted for multiple doses of regular insulin. The total dose of modified insulin is initially equal to 80% of the total daily dose of regular insulin. The basic ingredient of nearly all insulin regimens is an intermediate-acting preparation—isophane insulin suspension or insulin zinc suspension. By adjustment of dose and diet, many patients with maturity-onset diabetes can be satisfactorily regulated with a single prebreakfast injection of intermediate-acting insulin. In other patients, persistence of morning glycosuria, despite afternoon and evening aglycosuria, is an indication for addition of a fast-acting insulin (Table 71–1) to the program. In other patients, persistence of nocturnal glycosuria, despite afternoon and evening aglycosuria, is an indication for the addition of long-acting insulin—extended zinc insulin suspension or protamine zinc insulin suspension. A number of patients with severe, labile diabetes must reconcile themselves to supplementary injections of a fast-acting insulin, before meals or before bedtime. An alternative that is often effective is injection of intermediate-acting insulin in two doses, about three fourths of the total requirement before breakfast and the remainder before supper or before retiring.

Diabetic Ketoacidosis. Diabetic ketoacidosis is a continuum, ranging in severity from slight ketonuria without readily detectable ketonemia (ketosis) to the syndrome of diabetic coma, which is characterized by glycosuria, hypovolemia, ketonuria, ketonemia, metabolic acidosis, and coma, and which may progress to circulatory collapse, anuria, and death. A representative treatment protocol for the more severe form of diabetic ketoacidosis is presented below, but the principles upon which these recommendations are based also govern the treatment of less severe forms of diabetic acidosis.

It is of paramount importance for the patient to be hospitalized and for the physician to remain with the patient until the crisis is past; an accurate running record of all medications, clinical observations, and laboratory tests is essential.

Immediately after the diagnosis of diabetic keto-acidosis is established, insulin injection, 1.0 unit per kilogram of body weight, is administered intravenously and a similar amount is given subcutaneously. In the presence of circulatory collapse, the total amount should be given intravenously.

Insulin is given at approximately 2-hour intervals, the amount adjusted according to plasma glucose concentration and its response to previous injections. Usual doses following the initial dose of 2.0 units per kilogram are of the order of 1.0 unit per kilogram given subcutaneously unless shock is present, in which event it is given intravenously. The plasma glucose concentration should decline progressively. If it does not, insulin is being given at an insufficient rate and there should be no hesitation about increasing the dose twofold. A reasonable goal is to reduce the plasma glucose concentration to approximately 300 mg % in 6 to 8 hours of treatment. It is only by monitoring the plasma glucose response to therapy that the patient with severe insulin resistance can be detected early in the course of treatment and a sufficient amount of insulin given. A few patients will require thousands of units of insulin in a few hours in order to reduce hyperglycemia. Plasma ketone concentrations should also decline progressively in adequately treated patients. However, little change may be observed in ketonemia in the first 4 to 6 hours, even though the plasma glucose declines rapidly. The rate of administration of insulin should be reduced as the plasma glucose concentration approaches 300 mg %. Diminution of plasma ketonemia to grade-1 or trace reactions in undiluted plasma coincides with a reduction in insulin resistance, and the rate of insulin administration should be markedly reduced at that time.

The first fluid administered to a patient with diabetic coma is usually 0.9% sodium chloride solution, approximately 1 liter for an adult. Subsequently, 0.45% sodium chloride solution is administered. Central venous pressure should be monitored in patients with congestive heart failure, renal insufficiency, or shock. If circulatory collapse is present on admission or develops during therapy, plasma should be administered in addition to sodium chloride solutions. In certain patients, hypotension persists in spite of correction of hypovolemia. In such circumstances, appropriate vasopressors may be given when it appears that further administration of plasma will lead to a progressive rise in venous pressure. In order to restore the volume of body fluids, most patients with diabetic coma will need to retain an amount of fluid approximating 5% of body weight. This should be largely achieved in the first 12 hours of treatment. In the presence of a brisk diuresis resulting from glycosuria, it may be necessary to give intravenous fluids at a rate of 20 ml or more per minute in order to achieve a satisfactory rate of rehydration. Observation of the central venous pressure, the hematocrit, and the cumulative hourly difference between fluid intake and urine volume permits avoidance of overhydration. Reduction in plasma glucose and ketone concentrations signals the need for reduction in the rate of insulin administration. At this time 5% glucose solution is substituted for 0.45% sodium chloride solution. Patients who require exceptionally large doses of insulin for control of the critical phase of their acidosis are particularly subject to hypoglycemia for a day or more after the treatment of the critical phase of acidosis, even though insulin may have been completely withdrawn. It is better to tolerate mild glycosuria for 1 or 2 days following treatment of severe acidosis than to risk hypoglycemia.

The administration of alkali is usually not necessary in the treatment of diabetic acidosis and may lead to development of alkalosis. Severe exhausting hyperpnea justifies the administration of 1 liter of isotonic sodium bicarbonate solution.

Patients with diabetic ketoacidosis usually have a normal or moderately elevated plasma concentration of potassium on admission to the hospital, as a consequence of cellular buffering of metabolic acids. At the same time, there exists an intracellular depletion of potassium that may be of the order of hundreds of milliequivalents in patients with severe or prolonged acidosis. During treatment, as the rate of production of ketoacids diminishes and as potassium moves from the extracellular space to the intracellular space under the influence of insulin, hypokalemia may develop, usually beginning after the fourth hour of therapy. When this occurs, there is danger of progressive flaccid paralysis, which may eventually involve muscles of respiration. The administration of small amounts of potassium, considerably less than the estimated deficit, usually prevents paralysis or dramatically increases muscle strength. Symptomatic hypokalemia is not a frequent occurrence during treatment of diabetic ketoacidosis, even when potassium is not given, but occasionally the administration of potassium salts is lifesaving.

Potassium salts should not be administered until it is established that the urinary volume is at least of the order of 1 ml per minute and that hyperkalemia is absent, in order to avoid cardiotoxic concentrations of potassium in the extracellular fluid. If these conditions are met, prophylactic potassium chloride may be given orally, 1.0 g every 4 hours. If the patient is unable to tolerate oral medications, potassium chloride may be given intravenously. The rate of intravenous potassium administration should not exceed 20 mEq per hour. The objective of intravenous potassium therapy is not replacement of the body potassium deficit but the prevention or treatment of symptoms of hypokalemia. For this purpose, a total of 20 to 80 mEq of potassium is often remarkably effective, even in the presence of a total body deficit of hundreds of milliequivalents. Whereas the ECG may provide useful emergency information, it is not a substitute for the measurement of the plasma potassium.

After 6 to 8 hours of treatment, most patients are able to tolerate a liquid diet. In patients treated for uncomplicated ketoacidosis, the usual diet can be resumed in 24 hours. Modified insulin should not be given until the patient is eating regularly.

Nonketotic, hyperosmolar diabetic coma is an important variant of the usual acidotic coma and may occur when β-cell function is sufficient to prevent the development of ketoacidosis. The hyperosmolarity is due to hyperglycemia and hypernatremia. Cerebral dehydration and an increase in brain Na^+ interfere with CNS function, and coma develops. The detailed mechanisms are not known. The treatment is as outlined for ketoacidosis, except that more fluid and less insulin are usually required.

Insulin Resistance. Traditionally, patients requiring more than 200 units of insulin daily are said to be insulin resistant. A physiological definition of insulin resistance is that it is a condition in which the daily insulin requirement is in excess of the amount normally secreted. A useful point of reference is the daily insulin requirement of pancreatectomized man, frequently as low as 30 units. The figure of 200 units per day arbitrarily dividing resistance from nonresistance is undoubtedly too high.

Insulin resistance can be acute or chronic. Acute insulin resistance is associated with surgical or other trauma, emotional disturbances, many infections (especially staphylococcal), and ketoacidosis of any cause. In the latter instance, it seems clear that an increased concentration of glucagon may contribute to the presence of insulin resistance (Unger, 1972a). The high concentrations of free fatty acids and ketoacids in the blood of ketotic patients inhibit glucose uptake by muscle and by insulin-independent tissues such as brain. The anti-insulin factor described by Field and associates (1957) may also contribute.

It is reasonable to postulate that increased blood concentrations of adrenocortical hormones in response to trauma, anxiety, and infection may contribute to insulin resistance; indeed, increased blood concentrations of these hormones have been demonstrated in traumatized, anxious, or infected patients. However, the administration of adrenocorticosteroids to diabetic persons does not cause such abrupt, large increases in insulin requirement as are frequently seen in ketotic diabetic patients, who may require hundreds or thousands of units daily, whereas the increased requirement in hypercorticism is of the order of tens of units. Additional factors must be postulated to account for the insulin requirements of ketotic patients.

Early recognition of exceptionally severe acute insulin resistance may be lifesaving for the patient with diabetic coma (*see* above). The treatment of acute insulin resistance is the treatment of the precipitating cause and the administration of large doses of insulin together with needed water and electrolytes.

Chronic insulin resistance is frequently, but not always, associated with large amounts of plasma insulin-binding antibodies. Insulin resistance often appears after resumption of insulin therapy following a period of discontinuance. Identifiable endocrine disturbances (acromegaly, adrenal hypercorticism, and pheochromocytoma) are rarely the cause of chronic insulin resistance and almost never the cause of extreme insulin resistance (daily insulin requirements in excess of 500 units). A rare and readily recognizable condition associated with chronic insulin resistance is lipoatrophic diabetes, a disorder characterized by absence of normal body fat depots, hyperlipemia and cutaneous xanthomata, hepatomegaly, and cirrhosis, and by insulin-resistant, nonketotic diabetes mellitus (Lawrence, 1955; Craig and Miller, 1960). A type of insulin-resistant diabetes known as "J" disease has been described in patients in the tropics (Alford *et al.*, 1970). Ketosis does not develop even after prolonged insulin withdrawal, but there is marked insulin resistance and a reduced secretion of insulin in response to the administration of glucose. The similarity between this disease and diabetes with hyperosmolar nonketotic coma (described above) has been noted.

In order to supply adequate insulin in chronic insulin resistance, it may be convenient to use the preparation containing 500 units/ml. Some patients may be selectively resistant to bovine insulin while remaining sensitive to porcine insulin. The rationale for using porcine insulin is based on its chemical similarity to human insulin (*see* Figure 71-1).

Chemical alterations have been made to diminish the antigenic properties of porcine insulin. One such modification is dealaninated porcine insulin, where the carboxy-terminal alanine of the B chain is selectively cleaved by enzymatic (carboxypeptidase) action; there is no loss in biological activity. Antibodies to mixed porcine-bovine insulin or to porcine insulin do not react with dealaninated porcine insulin. Reports have appeared of the effectiveness of dealaninated porcine insulin in treating insulin-resistant diabetic patients who failed to respond to the porcine or bovine hormone (Burman *et al.*, 1973). Sulfonylureas reduce the insulin requirement in some insulin-resistant patients, presumably as a consequence of release of endogenous insulin, which has less affinity for circulating antibody than does exogenous bovine or porcine insulin.

GLUCAGON

History. Glucagon was discovered by Murlin and coworkers in 1923—2 years after the discovery of insulin. The contrast between insulin and glucagon, each secreted by adjoining cells in the islets, could hardly be more striking. Because of its immediate therapeutic importance, insulin was well accepted as a hormone and hailed as a major medical advance. Glucagon was of little interest, its discoverers received little recognition, and the hormone was not purified extensively until over 30 years had passed (Staub *et al.*, 1955).

Chemistry. Glucagon is a single-chain polypeptide with a molecular weight of nearly 3500. In contrast to insulin, it contains no cysteine and, consequently, no disulfide linkages; the sequence of its 29 amino acids has been determined by Bromer and associates (1956) (*see* Figure 71-3). Of interest is a striking structural analogy between glucagon and the hormone secretin, suggesting a common genetic origin. The structure of human glucagon has not yet been determined, but it is presumed to be similar to porcine and bovine glucagon, the amino acid compositions of which are identical. The total chemical synthesis of glucagon has been accomplished (*see* Wunsch and Weinges, 1972).

Bioassay and Radioimmunoassay of Glucagon in Plasma. A number of bioassays for glucagon have been developed, based on the ability of the hormone to cause hyperglycemia *in vivo* or to stimulate cyclic AMP production, phosphorylase activity, or glucose production *in vitro*. With the advent of radioimmunoassay, this has become the most widely used method to determine the concentration of glucagon. The chief problem has been cross-reaction of antisera with a related peptide from the gastrointestinal tract—gut glucagon. Since it is becoming increasingly clear that pancreatic and gut glucagons differ chemically and biologically, it is of greatest importance to use specific antisera. The best current methodology yields values for basal plasma pancreatic glucagon concentrations in the range of 0.1 to

NH₂
|
H—His—Ser—Glu—Gly—Thr—Phe—Thr—Ser—Asp—Tyr—Ser—Lys—Tyr—Leu—Asp—

NH₂   NH₂   NH₂
| | |
Ser—Arg—Arg—Ala—Glu—Asp—Phe—Val—Glu—Tyr—Leu—Met—Asp—Thr—OH

Figure 71-3. *The structure of glucagon.*

0.25 ng/ml, very close to those obtained by bioassay (Luyckx, 1972).

Regulation of Glucagon Secretion. Glucagon secretion, like that of insulin, is controlled by the interplay of gastrointestinal food products and other hormones; glucose is again by far the best-understood regulator. A rise in plasma glucose concentration leads to an inhibition of glucagon secretion and *vice versa* (*see* Unger and Lefebvre, 1972). As with insulin secretion, glucose given orally is a more effective signal than glucose administered intravenously. A gastrointestinal signal is thus suggested, and, although the evidence is not complete, secretin may play an important inhibitory role. The suppression of glucagon secretion by glucose is malfunctional in certain diabetic patients (*see* above). It is not clear whether the glucagon-secreting α cell is influenced directly by insulin or if glucose acts alone. It is thus debated whether the α-cell defect in diabetes is a primary lesion (Unger, 1972a; Buchanan and Mawhinney, 1973a, 1973b).

In experimental animals, free fatty acids of various chain lengths and ketones suppress glucagon secretion in a manner analogous to that of glucose; the effects are opposite to those on insulin secretion.

Of the three primary energy sources, amino acids have a unique effect. Their administration leads to an immediate rise in the concentrations of *both* glucagon and insulin in plasma. It has been argued teleologically that the purpose is to promote gluconeogenesis in the liver. This sugar can then replace that which disappears from the plasma as a result of insulin secretion and action, thus preventing hypoglycemia. If sufficient glucose is administered with amino acids to prevent hypoglycemia, enhanced glucagon secretion is not observed. As in the case of glucose, oral amino acids appear to be more potent secretagogues for glucagon than do those given intravenously. Pancreozymin may serve as an additional signal in this case, since it is the only known gastrointestinal hormone that stimulates the secretion of glucagon (*see* Unger and Lefebvre, 1972).

Glucagon secretion is also controlled by autonomic neural mechanisms; both sympathetic nerve stimulation and sympathomimetic amines enhance the secretion of the hormone. Conflicting data have accumulated on the effects of acetylcholine.

Distribution and Inactivation. Pancreatic glucagon circulating in plasma is the same as that extracted from the organ, although 5% of the immunoreactive material in plasma is contained in a biologically inactive fraction of higher molecular weight (7000). Labeled glucagon is more rapidly removed from blood than is insulin. Glucagon is extensively degraded in the liver and kidney, as well as in plasma, and at its tissue receptor sites in plasma membranes.

Enzymatic destruction of glucagon is by proteolysis, and the removal of the amino-terminal histidine leads to loss of biological activity. Cathepsin C inactivates the hormone, as does a proteolytic enzyme purified from rat skeletal muscle that acts on both insulin and glucagon (Duckworth and Kitabchi, 1974).

Physiological and Pharmacological Actions. The hormonal role of glucagon is now well established, and the secretory products of the "organ of Langerhans" are mutual antagonists. Insulin serves as a hormone of fuel storage, while glucagon serves as a hormone of fuel mobilization. Following a meal, β-cell secretion of insulin and suppression of α-cell secretion of glucagon serve to store fuels in liver, muscle, and adipose tissue. Conversely, during starvation, stimulation of glucagon secretion and suppression of insulin secretion direct the breakdown of fuels stored intracellularly to meet the energy needs of the brain and other tissues. A related role for glucagon as the hormone of injury and insult (catabolic illness) has been proposed. For example, impaired glucose tolerance and hyperglycemia noted with infection are associated with increased concentrations of plasma glucagon (Rayfield *et al.,* 1973). Here, glucagon acts to stimulate gluconeogenesis and provide the glucose needed under conditions of insult.

The known actions of glucagon appear to result from stimulation of the synthesis of cyclic AMP. This is particularly true in liver and adipose tissue, and its metabolic effects at these sites are essentially the same as those of epinephrine (*see* Chapter 21). It is worth noting that studies of the mechanism of the hyperglycemic action of glucagon and epinephrine led to the discovery of cyclic AMP (Rall and Sutherland, 1958). In high concentrations, glucagon has a positive cardiac inotropic effect, also presumably related to its ability to stimulate the synthesis of the cyclic nucleotide in the heart.

Therapeutic Use and Preparations. Glucagon hydrochloride is useful in the treatment of insulin-induced hypoglycemia when dextrose solution is not available. It may be given intravenously, intramuscularly, or subcutaneously in a dose of 1.0 mg. When it is given subcutaneously for hypoglycemic coma induced by either insulin or oral hypoglycemic agents, a return to consciousness should be observed within 20 minutes; otherwise, intravenous glucose must be administered as soon as possible. Failure of glucagon to relieve the coma may be due to irreversible brain damage as a consequence of prolonged hypoglycemia or due to marked depletion of glycogen stores in the liver. Nausea and vomiting have been the most frequent adverse effects.

Clinical investigations have been conducted to explore the use of large doses of glucagon in cardiac disorders as an inotropic and chronotropic agent that may be less likely to produce cardiac arrhythmias than are β-adrenergic catecholamines, and for its value as an "antagonist" to β-adrenergic blocking agents. Unfortunately, relatively selective loss of the positive inotropic response to glucagon has been observed in failing hearts that continued to be stimulated by catecholamines (Levey *et al.*, 1970). The hormone has also been used experimentally in the diagnosis and treatment of hypoglycemic disorders and as a stimulus for growth hormone secretion (Galloway, 1972). Although the mechanism is unclear, glucagon has been used to relax the duodenum for x-ray visualization in hypotonic duodenography (Miller *et al.*, 1973).

Glucagon for Injection, U.S.P., the hydrochloride of glucagon, is dispensed as a dry powder in 1- or 10-mg ampuls, packaged with sufficient diluent to make a 1-mg/ml solution.

Miscellaneous Hyperglycemic Agents. *Diazoxide,* a nondiuretic thiazide with antihypertensive activity (*see* Chapter 33), causes hyperglycemia. This effect is usually transitory and is apparently due to both decreased insulin secretion and decreased peripheral utilization of sugar (*see* Speight and Avery, 1971). Diazoxide appears to exert α-adrenergic-like actions on the islet β cell (Culbert *et al.*, 1974), and it also stimulates the release of endogenous catecholamines. The drug has been used experimentally in adults and children to control hypoglycemia, including that caused by insulin-secreting islet-cell tumors (Balsam *et al.*, 1972). *Streptozotocin* has sometimes been employed concurrently (Harell *et al.*, 1972). *Phenytoin* (diphenylhydantoin) can induce hyperglycemia in man and in experimental animals (Levin *et al.*, 1970). The drug inhibits the secretion of insulin, possibly by an effect to decrease intracellular Na$^+$ (Kizer *et al.*, 1970); it has been used to ameliorate hypoglycemia due to insulin-secreting tumors in adults and children (Hofeldt *et al.*, 1974).

Abel, J. J. Crystalline insulin. *Proc. natn. Acad. Sci. U.S.A.,* **1926,** *12,* 132–136.

Aikawa, J. K. Effect of glucose and insulin on magnesium metabolism in rabbits. A study with Mg^{28}. *Proc. Soc. exp. Biol. Med.,* **1960,** *103,* 363–366.

Alford, F. P.; Kiss, Z. S.; Martin, F. I. R.; Pearson, M. J.; Willis, M. F.; and Yeomans, N. D. Type J diabetes in New Guinea—studies of insulin release and insulin sensitivity. *Australas. Ann. Med.,* **1970,** *19,* 111–117.

Anderson, J. W., and Herman, R. H. Treatment of reactive hypoglycemia with sulfonylureas. *Am. J. med. Sci.,* **1971,** *261,* 16–23.

Baker, A. B. Cerebral lesions in hypoglycemia. *Archs Path.,* **1939,** *28,* 298–305.

Balsam, M. J.; Baker, L.; Bishop, H. C.; Hummeler, K.; Yakovac, W. C.; and Kaye, R. Beta cell adenoma in a child with hypoglycemia controlled with diazoxide. *J. Pediat.,* **1972,** *80,* 788–795.

Banting, F. G.; Best, C. H.; Collip, J. B.; Campbell, W. R.; and Fletcher, A. A. Pancreatic extracts in the treatment of diabetes mellitus. *Can. med. Ass. J.,* **1922,** *12,* 141–146.

Beaser, S. B. Orally given combinations of drugs in diabetes mellitus therapy. *J. Am. med. Ass.,* **1960,** *174,* 2137–2141.

Benjamin, W. B., and Singer, I. Effect of insulin on the phosphorylation of adipose tissue protein. *Biochim. biophys. Acta,* **1974,** *351,* 28–41.

Berger, W.; Lauffenburger, T.; and Denes, A. The effect of metformin on the absorption of vitamin B$_{12}$. *Horm. metab. Res.,* **1972,** *4,* 311–312.

Bishop, J. S., and Larner, J. Rapid activation-inactivation of liver uridine diphosphate glucose-glycogen transferase and phosphorylase by insulin and glucagon *in vivo. J. biol. Chem.,* **1967,** *242,* 1354–1356.

Bornstein, J.; Armstrong, J. McD.; Ng, F.; Paddle, B. M.; and Misconi, L. Structure and synthesis of biologically active peptides derived from pituitary growth hormone. *Biochem. biophys. Res. Commun.,* **1971,** *42,* 252–258.

Boyle, D.; Bhatia, S. K.; Hadden, D. R.; Montgomery, D. A. D.; and Weaver, J. A. Ischaemic heart-disease in diabetics. *Lancet,* **1972,** *1,* 338–339.

Breidahl, H. D.; Ennis, G. C.; Martin, F. I. R.; Stawell, J. R.; and Taft, P. Insulin and oral hypoglycaemic agents. II. Clinical and therapeutic aspects. *Drugs,* **1972,** *3,* 204–226.

Bromer, W. W.; Sinn, L. G.; Staub, A.; and Behrens, O. K. The amino acid sequence of glucagon. *J. Am. chem. Soc.,* **1956,** *78,* 3858–3860.

Brooker, G., and Fichman, M. Chlorpropamide and tolbutamide inhibition of adenosine 3′5′ cyclic monophosphate phosphodiesterase. *Biochem. biophys. Res. Commun.,* **1971,** *42,* 824–828.

Brown, J. D.; Steele, A. A.; Stone, D. B.; and Steele, F. A. The effect of tolbutamide on lipolysis and cyclic AMP concentration in white fat cells. *Endocrinology,* **1972,** *90,* 47–59.

Buchanan, K. D. Gut and islet hormones in diabetes. *Postgrad. med. J.,* **1973,** *49,* 117–121.

Buchanan, K. D., and Mawhinney, W. A. A. Glucagon release from isolated pancreas in streptozotocin-treated rats. *Diabetes,* **1973a,** *22,* 797–800.

——. Insulin control of glucagon release from insulin-deficient rat islets. *Ibid.,* **1973b,** *22,* 801–803.

Burman, K. D.; Cunningham, E. J.; Klachko, D. M.; and Burns, T. W. Successful treatment of insulin resistance with dealaninated pork insulin (DPI). *Missouri Med.,* **1973,** *70,* 363–366.

Carter, J., Jr.; Avruch, J.; and Martin, D. B. Glucose transport in plasma membrane vesicles from rat adipose tissue. *J. biol. Chem.,* **1972,** *247,* 2682–2688.

Cerasi, E. S., and Luft, R. Dose-response relationship between plasma-insulin and blood-glucose levels during oral glucose loads in prediabetic and diabetic subjects. *Lancet,* **1973a,** *1,* 794–797.

——. Pathogenesis of genetic diabetes mellitus: further development of a hypothesis. *Mt. Sinai J. Med., N.Y.,* **1973b,** *40,* 334–349.

Chalmers, T. C. Settling the UGDP controversy. *J. Am. med. Ass.,* **1975,** *231,* 624–625.

Chamberlain, M. J., and Stimmler, L. The renal handling of insulin. *J. clin. Invest.,* **1967,** *46,* 911–919.

Chance, R. E. Amino acid sequences of proinsulins and intermediates. *Diabetes,* **1972,** *21,* Suppl. 2, 461–467.

Clayman, C. B. Tolbutamide revisited. *J. Am. med. Ass.,* **1974,** *228,* 1523.

Committee on the Use of Therapeutic Agents of the American Diabetic Association. U100 insulin: a new era in diabetes mellitus therapy. *Diabetes,* **1972,** *21,* 832.

Craighead, J. E., and Steinke, J. Diabetes mellitus–like syndrome in mice infected with encephalomyocarditis virus. *Am. J. Path.,* **1971,** *63,* 119–134.

Cuatrecasas, P. Insulin receptor of liver and fat cell membranes. *Fedn Proc. Fedn Am. Socs exp. Biol.,* **1973,** *32,* 1838–1846.

Culbert, S.; Sharp, R.; Rogers, M.; Felts, P.; and Burr, I. M. Diazoxide modification of streptozotocin-induced diabetes in rats. *Diabetes,* **1974,** *23,* 282–286.

Dieterle, P.; Birkner, B.; Gmeiner, K.-H.; Wagner, P.; Erhardt, F.; Henner, J.; and Dieterle, C. Release of peripherally stored insulin during acute muscular work in man. *Horm. metab. Res.,* **1973,** *5,* 316–322.

Drabkin, D. L., and Ravdin, I. S. The mechanism of convulsions in insulin hypoglycemia: interrelationship of blood concentration, cerebrospinal pressure and convulsions. *Am. J. Physiol.,* **1937,** *118,* 174–183.

Duckworth, W. C., and Kitabchi, A. E. Insulin and glucagon degradation by the same enzyme. *Diabetes,* **1974,** *23,* 536–543.

Evans, R. B.; Morhenn, V.; Jones, A. L.; and Tomkins, G. M. Concomitant effects of insulin on surface membrane conformation and polysome profiles of serum-starved BALB-C 3T3 fibroblasts. *J. cell Biol.,* **1974,** *61,* 95–106.

Exton, J. H.; Jefferson, L. S.; Butcher, R. W.; and Park, C. R. Gluconeogenesis in the perfused liver. *Am. J. Med.,* **1966,** *40,* 709–715.

Fain, J. N.; Rosenthal, J. W.; and Ward, W. F. Antilipolytic action of tolbutamide on brown fat cells. *Endocrinology,* **1972,** *90,* 52–59.

Field, J. B.; Tietze, F.; and Stetten, D., Jr. Further characterization of an insulin antagonist in the serum of patients in diabetic acidosis. *J. clin. Invest.,* **1957,** *36,* 1588–1593.

Friedmann, B.; Goodman, E. H., Jr.; and Weinhouse, S. Effects of insulin and fatty acids on gluconeogenesis in the rat. *J. biol. Chem.,* **1967,** *242,* 3620–3627.

Frohman, L. A.; Ezdinli, E. Z.; and Javid, R. Effect of vagotomy and vagal stimulation on insulin secretion. *Diabetes,* **1967,** *16,* 443–448.

Gerich, J. E.; Lorenzi, M.; Schneider, V.; Karam, J. H.; Rivier, J.; Guillemin, R.; and Forsham, P. H. Effects of somatostatin on plasma glucose and glucagon levels in human diabetes mellitus. *New Engl. J. Med.,* **1974,** *291,* 544–547.

Goldfine, I. D.; Roth, J.; and Birnbaumer, L. Glucagon receptors in β-cells. *J. biol. Chem.,* **1972,** *247,* 1211–1218.

Goldstein, D. E.; Drash, A.; Gibbs, J.; and Blizzard, R. M. Diabetes mellitus: the incidence of circulating antibodies against thyroid, gastric and adrenal tissue. *J. Pediat.,* **1970,** *77,* 304–306.

Hadden, J. W.; Hadden, E. M.; Wilson, E. E.; Good, R. A.; and Coffey, R. G. Direct action of insulin on plasma membrane ATPase activity in human lymphocytes. *Nature, New Biol.,* **1972,** *235,* 174–177.

Haeckel, R. Inhibition of glucose formation from fructose by phenformin in perfused guinea pig livers. *Diabetologia,* **1973,** *9,* 161–164.

Hagedorn, H. C.; Jensen, B. N.; Krarup, N. B.; and Wodstrup, I. Protamine insulinate. *J. Am. med. Ass.,* **1936,** *106,* 177–180.

Hallas-Møller, K.; Jersild, M.; Petersen, K.; and Schlichtkrull, J. Zinc insulin preparations for single daily injection. Clinical studies of new preparations with prolonged action. *J. Am. med. Ass.,* **1952a,** *150,* 1667–1671.

Hallas-Møller, K.; Petersen, K.; and Schlichtkrull, J. Crystalline and amorphous insulin-zinc compounds with prolonged action. *Science, Wash.,* **1952b,** *116,* 394–398.

Harell, A.; Laurian, L.; Ayalon, D.; Kisch, E.; and Cordova, T. Hypoglycemia due to hyperinsulinism treated by streptozotocin and diazoxide. *Israel J. med. Sci.,* **1972,** *8,* 895–896.

Hartroft, W. S., and Wrenshall, G. A. Correlation of beta-cell granulation with extractable insulin of the pancreas. Studies in adult human diabetics and nondiabetics. *Diabetes,* **1955,** *4,* 1–7.

Hellman, B.; Sehlin, J.; and Taljedal, I.-B. The pancreatic β-cell recognition of insulin secretogues. II. Site of

action of tolbutamide. *Biochem. biophys. Res. Commun.,* **1971,** *45,* 1384–1388.

Hofeldt, F. D.; Dippe, S. E.; Levin, S. R.; Karam, J. H.; Blum, M. R.; and Forsham, P. H. Effects of diphenylhydantoin upon glucose-induced insulin secretion in three patients with insulinoma. *Diabetes,* **1974,** *23,* 192–198.

Hollenberg, C. H. The effect of incubation on the characteristics of the lipolytic activity of rat adipose tissue. *Can. J. Biochem. Physiol.,* **1962,** *40,* 703–707.

Houssay, B. A. The hypophysis and metabolism. *New Engl. J. Med.,* **1936a,** *214,* 961–971.

————. Carbohydrate metabolism. *Ibid.,* **1936b,** *214,* 971–982.

Janbon, M.; Chaptal, J.; Vedel, A.; and Schaap, J. Accidents hypoglycemiques graves par un sulfamidothiadiazol (le VK57 ou 2254RP). *Montpell. méd.,* **1942,** *21–22,* 441–444.

Jefferson, L. S.; Exton, J. H.; Butcher, R. W.; Sutherland, E. W.; and Park, C. R. Role of adenosine 3′,5′-monophosphate in the effects of insulin and anti-insulin serum on liver metabolism. *J. biol. Chem.,* **1968,** *243,* 1031–1038.

Johnson, D. G.; Fujimoto, W. Y.; and Williams, R. H. Enhanced release of insulin by prostaglandins in isolated pancreatic islets. *Diabetes,* **1973,** *22,* 658–663.

Kaneto, A.; Kosaka, K.; and Nakao, K. Effects of stimulation of the vagus nerve on insulin secretion. *Endocrinology,* **1967,** *80,* 530–536.

Katsoyannis, P. G. The chemical synthesis of human and sheep insulin. *Am. J. Med.,* **1966,** *40,* 652–661.

Kety, S. S.; Polis, B. D.; Nadler, C. S.; and Schmidt, C. F. The blood flow and oxygen consumption of the human brain in diabetic acidosis and coma. *J. clin. Invest.,* **1948,** *27,* 500–510.

Kipnis, D. M. Nutrient regulation of insulin secretion in human subjects. *Diabetes,* **1971,** *21,* Suppl. 2, 606–616.

Kizer, S.; Vargas-Cordon, M.; Brendel, K.; and Bressler, R. Studies on the mechanism of diphenylhydantoin-induced inhibition of insulin secretion. *J. clin. Invest.,* **1970,** *49,* 52a.

Knatterud, G. L.; Meinert, C. L.; Klimt, C. R.; Osborne, R. K.; and Martin, D. B. Effects of hypoglycemic agents on vascular complications in patients with adult-onset diabetes. *J. Am. med. Ass.,* **1971,** *217,* 777–784.

Koerker, D. J.; Ruch, W.; Chideckel, E.; Palmer, J.; Goodner, C. J.; Ensinck, J.; and Gole, C. C. Somatostatin: hypothalamic inhibitor of the endocrine pancreas. *Science, Wash.,* **1974,** *184,* 482–484.

Kono, T. Destruction of insulin effector systems of adipose tissue cells by proteolytic enzymes. *J. biol. Chem.,* **1969,** *244,* 1772–1778.

Krahl, M. E. Insulin action at the molecular level; facts and speculations. *Diabetes,* **1972,** *21,* Suppl. 2, 695–702.

Kuo, W.-N.; Hodgins, D. S.; and Kuo, J. F. Adenylate cyclase in islets of Langerhans: isolation of islets and regulation of adenylate cyclase activity by various hormones and agents. *J. biol. Chem.,* **1972,** *248,* 2705–2711.

Larner, J. Insulin and glycogen synthase. *Diabetes,* **1972,** *21,* Suppl. 2, 428–438.

Lasseter, K. C.; Levey, G. S.; Palmer, R. F.; and McCarthey, J. S. The effect of sulfonylurea drugs on rabbit myocardial contractility, canine Purkinje fiber automaticity and adenyl cyclase activity from rabbit and human hearts. *J. clin. Invest.,* **1972,** *51,* 2429–2434.

Lawrence, R. D. Three types of human diabetes. *Ann. intern. Med.,* **1955,** *43,* 1199–1208.

Levey, G. S.; Prindle, K. H., Jr.; and Epstein, S. E. Effects of glucagon on adenyl cyclase activity in the left and right ventricles and liver in experimentally-produced isolated right ventricular failure. *J. molec. cell. Cardiol.,* **1970,** *1,* 403–410.

Levin, S. R.; Booker, J., Jr.; Smith, D. F.; and Grodsky, G. M. Inhibition of insulin secretion by diphenylhydantoin in the isolated perfused pancreas. *J. clin. Endocr. Metab.,* **1970,** *30,* 400–401.

Levine, R.; Goldstein, M.; Klein, S.; and Huddlestun, B. The action of insulin on the distribution of galactose in eviscerated nephrectomized dogs. *J. biol. Chem.,* **1949,** *179,* 985–986.

Long, C. N. H., and Lukens, F. D. W. The effects of adrenalectomy and hypophysectomy upon experimental diabetes in the cat. *J. exp. Med.,* **1936,** *63,* 465–490.

Loubatières, A. The hypoglycemic sulfonamides: history and development of the problem from 1942 to 1955. *Ann. N.Y. Acad. Sci.,* **1957,** *71,* 4–11.

Louis, L. H.; Conn, J. W.; and Minick, M. C. A diabetogenic polypeptide from bovine adenohypophysis similar to that excreted in lipoatrophic diabetes. *Metabolism,* **1966,** *15,* 309–324.

Lundsgaard, E. On mode of action of insulin. *Uppsala LäkFör. Förh.,* **1939,** *45,* 143–152.

McIntyre, N.; Holdsworth, C. D.; and Turner, D. S. New interpretation of oral glucose tolerance. *Lancet,* **1964,** *2,* 20–21.

Malaisse, W.; Malaisse-Lagae, F.; Wright, P. H.; and Ashmore, J. Effects of adrenergic and cholinergic agents upon insulin secretion *in vitro. Endocrinology,* **1967,** *80,* 975–978.

Manchester, K. L. Effect of insulin on protein synthesis. *Diabetes,* **1972,** *21,* Suppl. 2, 447–452.

Manganiello, V., and Vaughn, M. An effect of insulin on cyclic adenosine 3′:5′-monophosphate phosphodiesterase activity in fat cells. *J. biol. Chem.,* **1973,** *248,* 7164–7170.

Marks, V., and Samols, E. Intestinal factors in the regulation of insulin secretion. *Adv. metab. Dis.,* **1970,** *4,* 1–38.

Marshall, A.; Gingerich, R. L.; and Wright, P. H. Hepatic effect of sulfonylureas. *Metabolism,* **1970,** *19,* 1046–1052.

Matschinsky, F. M., and Ellerman, J. Dissociation of the insulin releasing and the metabolic functions of hexoses in islets of Langerhans. *Biochem. biophys. Res. Commun.,* **1973,** *50,* 193–199.

Matschinsky, F. M.; Ellerman, J. E.; Krzanowski, J.; Kotler-Brajtburg, J.; Landgraf, R.; and Fertel, R. The dual function of glucose in islets of Langerhans. *J. biol. Chem.,* **1970,** *246,* 1007–1011.

Miller, R. E.; Chernish, S. M.; Rosenak, B. D.; and Rodda, B. E. Hypotonic duodenography with glucagon. *Radiology,* **1973,** *108,* 35–42.

Miller, T. B., and Larner, J. Anti-insulin actions of a bovine pituitary diabetogenic peptide on glycogen synthesis. *Proc. natn. Acad. Sci. U.S.A.,* **1972,** *69,* 2774–2777.

Morgan, H. E.; Jefferson, L. S.; Wolpert, E. B.; and Rannels, D. E. Regulation of protein synthesis in heart muscle. *J. biol. Chem.,* **1971,** *246,* 2163–2170.

Mortimore, G. E., and Mondon, C. E. Inhibition by insulin of valine turnover in liver. Evidence for a general control of proteolysis. *J. biol. Chem.,* **1970,** *245,* 2375–2383.

Murlin, J. R.; Clough, H. D.; Gibbs, C. B. F.; and Stakes, A. M. Aqueous extracts of pancreas. I. Influence on the carbohydrate metabolism of depancreatized animals. *J. biol. Chem.,* **1923,** *56,* 253–296.

O'Donovan, C. J. Analysis of long-term experience with tolbutamide (ORINASE) in the management of diabetes. *Curr. ther. Res.,* **1959,** *1,* 69–87.

Ohneda, A.; Matsuda, K.; Sato, M.; Yamagata, S.; and Sato, T. Hypoglycemia due to apparent autoantibodies to insulin. Characterization of insulin-binding protein. *Diabetes,* **1974,** *23,* 41–50.

Owen, O. E.; Morgan, A. P.; Kemp, H. G.; Sullivan, J. M.; Herrera, M. G.; and Cahill, G. F., Jr. Brain metabolism during fasting. *J. clin. Invest.,* **1967,** *46,* 1589–1595.

Park, C. R.; Bornstein, J.; and Post, R. L. Effect of insulin on free glucose content of rat diaphragm *in vitro. Am. J. Physiol.,* **1955,** *182,* 12–16.

Paulesco, N. C. Action de l'extrait pancréatique injecté dans le sang, chez un animal diabétique. *C. r. Séanc. Soc. Biol.,* **1921,** *85,* 555–557.

Permutt, M. A.; Kelly, J.; Bernstein, R.; Alpers, D. H.; Siegel, B. A.; and Kipnis, D. M. Alimentary hypoglycemia in the absence of gastrointestinal surgery. *New Engl. J. Med.,* **1973,** *288,* 1206–1210.

Porte, D., Jr., and Robertson, R. P. Control of insulin secretion by catecholamines, stress, and the sympathetic nervous system. *Fedn Proc. Fedn Am. Socs exp. Biol.,* **1973,** *32,* 1792–1796.

Rall, T. W., and Sutherland, E. W. Formation of a cyclic adenine ribonucleotide by tissue particles. *J. biol. Chem.,* **1958,** *232,* 1065–1076.

Rastogi, G. K.; Sinha, M. K.; and Dash, R. J. Insulin and proinsulin content of pancreases from diabetic and nondiabetic subjects. *Diabetes,* **1973,** *22,* 804–807.

Rayfield, E. J.; Curnow, R. T.; George, D. T.; and Beisel, W. R. Impaired carbohydrate metabolism during a mild viral illness. *New Engl. J. Med.,* **1973,** *289,* 618–620.

Reaven, G. M.; Olefsky, J.; and Farquhar, J. W. Does hyperglycaemia or hyperinsulinaemia characterize the patient with chemical diabetes? *Lancet,* **1972,** *1,* 1247–1249.

Reiner, L.; Searle, D. S.; and Lang, E. M. On hypoglycemic activity of globin insulin. *J. Pharmac. exp. Ther.,* **1939,** *67,* 330–340.

Report of the Committee for the Assessment of Biometric Aspects of Controlled Trials of Hypoglycemic Agents. *J. Am. med. Ass.,* **1975,** *231,* 583–608.

Rerup, C. C. Drugs producing diabetes through damage of the insulin secreting cells. *Pharmac. Rev.,* **1970,** *22,* 485–518.

Robertson, R. P., and Porte, D., Jr. The glucose receptor. A defective mechanism in diabetes mellitus distinct from the beta adrenergic receptor. *J. clin. Invest.,* **1973,** *52,* 870–876.

Root, M. A.; Chance, R. E.; and Galloway, J. A. Immunogenicity of insulin. *Diabetes,* **1972,** *21,* Suppl. 2, 657–660.

Rosenbloom, A. L. Advances in commercial insulin preparations. *Am. J. Dis. Child.,* **1974,** *128,* 631–633.

Ruttenberg, M. A. Human insulin: facile synthesis by modification of porcine insulin. *Science, Wash.,* **1972,** *177,* 623–626.

Sanger, F. Chemistry of insulin. *Br. med. Bull.,* **1960,** *16,* 183–188.

Schlichtkrull, J.; Brange, J.; Christiansen, A. H.; Hallund, O.; Heding, L. G.; and Jørgensen, K. H. Clinical aspects of insulin-antigenicity. *Diabetes,* **1972,** *21,* Suppl. 2, 649–656.

Seltzer, H. S. Drug-induced hypoglycemia. A review based on 473 cases. *Diabetes,* **1972a,** *21,* 955–966.

———. A summary of criticisms of the findings and conclusions of the University Group Diabetes Program (UGDP). *Ibid.,* **1972b,** *21,* 976–979.

Soler, N. G.; Bennett, M. A.; Lamb, P.; Pentecost, B. L.; FitzGerald, M. G.; and Malins, J. M. Coronary care for myocardial infarction in diabetics. *Lancet,* **1974,** *1,* 475–477.

Speight, T. M., and Avery, G. S. Diazoxide: a review of its pharmacological properties and therapeutic use in hypertensive crises. *Drugs,* **1971,** *2,* 78–137.

Staub, A.; Sinn, L.; and Behrens, O. K. Purification and crystallization of glucagon. *J. biol. Chem.,* **1955,** *214,* 619–632.

Steiner, D. F.; Cunningham, D.; Spigelman, L.; and Aten, B. Insulin biosynthesis: evidence for a precursor. *Science, Wash.,* **1967,** *157,* 697–700.

Sussman, K. E.; Crout, J. R.; and Marble, A. Failure of warning in insulin-induced hypoglycemic reactions. *Diabetes,* **1963,** *12,* 38–45.

Tantillo, J. J.; Karam, J. H.; Burrill, K. C.; Jones, M. A.; Grodsky, G. M.; and Forsham, P. H. Immunogenicity of "single peak" beef-pork insulin in diabetic subjects. *Diabetes,* **1974,** *23,* 276–281.

Turtle, J. R., and Kipnis, D. M. An adrenergic receptor mechanism for the control of cyclic 3′5′ adenosine monophosphate synthesis in tissues. *Biochem. biophys. Res. Commun.,* **1967,** *28,* 797–802.

Tyler, D. B. The mechanism of the production of brain damage during insulin shock. *Am. J. Physiol.,* **1941,** *131,* 554–560.

Ungar, G.; Freedman, L.; and Shapiro, S. L. Pharmacological studies of a new oral hypoglycemic drug. *Proc. Soc. exp. Biol. Med.,* **1957,** *95,* 190–192.

Unger, R. H.; Madison, L. L.; and Carter, N. W. Tolbutamide-phenformin in ketoacidosis-resistant patients. *J. Am. med. Ass.,* **1960,** *174,* 2132–2136.

University Group Diabetes Program. A study of the effects of hypoglycemic agents on vascular complications in patients with adult-onset diabetes. *Diabetes,* **1970,** *19,* Suppl. 2, 747–830.

Varandani, P. T. Urinary excretion of insulin A chain by normal and diabetic subjects. *Diabetes,* **1970,** *19,* 98–101.

Varandani, P. T., and Nafz, M. A. Insulin degradation. I. Purification and properties of glutathione-insulin transhydrogenase of rat liver. *Biochim. biophys. Acta,* **1972,** *286,* 126–135.

Villar-Palasi, C., and Larner, J. Insulin treatment and increased UDPG–glycogen transglucosylase activity in muscle. *Archs Biochem. Biophys.,* **1961,** *94,* 436–442.

Villar-Palasi, C., and Wenger, J. I. *In vivo* effect of insulin on muscle glycogen synthetase: identification of the action pathway. *Fedn Proc. Fedn Am. Socs exp. Biol.,* **1967,** *26,* 563.

Widstrom, A., and Cerasi, E. On the action of tolbutamide in man. I. Role of adrenergic mechanisms in tolbutamide-induced insulin release during normoglycaemia and induced hypoglycaemia. *Acta endocr., Copenh.,* **1973,** *72,* 506–518.

Wray, H. L., and Harris, A. W. Adenosine 3′,5′-monophosphate-dependent protein kinase in adipose tissue: inhibition by tolbutamide. *Biochem. biophys. Res. Commun.,* **1973,** *53,* 291–294.

Yalow, R. S., and Berson, S. A. Immunoassay of endogenous plasma insulin in man. *J. clin. Invest.,* **1960,** *39,* 1157–1175.

Yannet, H. Effect of prolonged insulin hypoglycemia on distribution of water and electrolytes in brain and in muscle. *Archs Neurol. Psychiat., Chicago,* **1939,** *42,* 237–247.

Young, F. G. Permanent experimental diabetes produced by pituitary (anterior lobe) injections. *Lancet,* **1937,** *2,* 372–374.

Ziskind, E., and Tyler, D. B. Decorticate and decerebrate preparations produced by insulin shock. *Proc. Soc. exp. Biol. Med.,* **1940,** *43,* 734–735.

Monographs and Reviews

Avruch, J.; Carter, J. R.; and Martin, D. B. The effect of insulin on the metabolism of adipose tissue. In, *Endocrinology,* Vol. 1. *Handbook of Physiology,* Sect. 7. (Steiner, D. F., and Freinkel, N., eds.) American Physiological Society, Washington, D. C., **1972,** pp. 545–562.

Best, C. H. *Selected Papers of Charles H. Best.* University of Toronto Press, Toronto, **1963.**

Craig, J. W., and Miller, M. Lipoatrophic diabetes. In, *Diabetes.* (Williams, R. H., ed.) Paul B. Hoeber, Inc., New York, **1960,** pp. 700–707.

Galloway, J. A. The pharmacology and clinical use of glucagon. In, *Glucagon: Molecular Physiology, Clinical and Therapeutic Implications.* (Lefebvre, P. J., and Unger, R. H., eds.) Pergamon Press, Ltd., Oxford, **1972,** pp. 299–318.

Gordon, E. E., and de Hartog, M. Gluconeogenesis in renal cortical tubules. Effect of phenformin. *Diabetes,* **1973,** *22,* 50–57.

Grodsky, G. M. A threshold distribution hypothesis for packet storage of insulin. II. Effect of calcium. *Diabetes,* **1971,** *21,* Suppl. 2, 584–593.

Hodgkin, D. C., and Mercola, D. The secondary and tertiary structure of insulin. In, *Endocrinology,* Vol. 1. *Handbook of Physiology,* Sect. 7. (Steiner, D. F., and Freinkel, N., eds.) American Physiological Society, Washington, D. C., **1972,** pp. 139–157.

Humbel, R. E.; Bosshard, H. R.; and Zahn, H. Chemistry of insulin. In, *Endocrinology,* Vol. 1. *Handbook of Physiology,* Sect. 7. (Steiner, D. F., and Freinkel, N., eds.) American Physiological Society, Washington, D. C., **1972,** pp. 111–132.

Lacy, P. E., and Greider, M. H. Ultrastructural organization of mammalian pancreatic islets. In, *Endocrinology,* Vol. 1. *Handbook of Physiology,* Sect. 7. (Steiner, D. F., and Freinkel, N., eds.) American Physiological Society, Washington, D. C., **1972,** pp. 77–89.

Larner, J.; Smith, C. H.; Rosenkrans, A. M.; Miller, T. B., Jr.; Huang, L. C.; Villar-Palasi, C.; and Rebhun, L. Studies on glycogen synthase and its control by hormones. In, *Metabolic Interconversion of Enzymes, 1973: Third International Symposium.* (Fischer, E. H.; Krebs, E. G.; Neurath, H.; and Stadtman, E. R.; eds.) Springer-Verlag, Berlin, **1974,** pp. 63–73.

Lawrence, A. M. Pancreatic alpha-cell function in miscellaneous clinical disorders. In, *Glucagon: Molecular Physiology, Clinical and Therapeutic Implications.* (Lefebvre, P. J., and Unger, R. H., eds.) Pergamon Press, Ltd., Oxford, **1972,** pp. 259–274.

Luyckx, A. S. Immunoassays for glucagon. In, *Glucagon: Molecular Physiology, Clinical and Therapeutic Implications.* (Lefebvre, P. J., and Unger, R. H., eds.) Pergamon Press, Ltd., Oxford, **1972,** pp. 285–298.

Malaisse, W. J. Hormonal and environmental modification of islet activity. In, *Endocrinology,* Vol. 1. *Handbook of Physiology,* Sect. 7. (Steiner, D. F., and Freinkel, N., eds.) American Physiological Society, Washington, D. C., **1972,** pp. 237–260.

Moody, A. J. Gastrointestinal glucagon-like immunoreactivity. In, *Glucagon: Molecular Physiology, Clinical and Therapeutic Implications.* (Lefebvre, P. J., and Unger, R. H., eds.) Pergamon Press, Ltd., Oxford, **1972,** pp. 319–341.

Morgan, H. E.; Rannels, D. E.; Wolpert, E. B.; Giger, K. E.; Robertson, J. W.; and Jefferson, L. S. Effect of insulin on protein turnover in heart and skeletal muscle. In, *Insulin Action.* (Fritz, I. B., ed.) Academic Press, Inc., New York, **1972,** pp. 437–449.

Oelz, O.; Froesch, E. R.; Bunzli, H. F.; Humbel, R. E.; and Ritschard, W. J. Antibody-suppressible and nonsuppressible insulin-like activities. In, *Endocrinology,* Vol. 1. *Handbook of Physiology,* Sect. 7. (Steiner, D. F., and Freinkel, N., eds.) American Physiological Society, Washington, D. C., **1972,** pp. 685–692.

Peck, F. B. Therapy: insulin types. In, *Diabetes Mellitus: Diagnosis and Treatment.* (Danowski, T. S., ed.) American Diabetes Association, Inc., New York, **1964,** pp. 83–86.

Randle, P. J., and Denton, R. M. Rate control by insulin and its mechanism. *Symp. Soc. exp. Biol.,* **1973,** *27,* 401–428.

Renold, A. E.; Stauffacher, W.; and Cahill, G. F., Jr. Diabetes mellitus. In, *Metabolic Basis of Inherited Disease,* 3rd ed. (Stanbury, J. B.; Wyngaarden, J. B.; and Fredrickson, D. S.; eds.) McGraw-Hill Book Co., New York, **1972,** pp. 83–118.

Rubenstein, A. H.; Block, M. B.; Starr, J.; Melani, F.; and Steiner, D. F. Proinsulin and C-peptide in blood. *Diabetes,* **1972,** *21,* Suppl. 2, 661–672.

Siperstein, M. D. Capillary basement membranes and diabetic microangiopathy. *Adv. intern. Med.,* **1972,** *18,* 325–344.

Spiro, R. G. Biochemistry of the glomerular basement

membrane in diabetes. *Adv. metab. Dis.,* **1973,** *2,* Suppl. 2, 179-190.

Steiner, D. F.; Kemmler, W.; Clark, J. L.; Oyer, P. E.; and Rubenstein, A. H. The biosynthesis of insulin. In, *Endocrinology,* Vol. 1. *Handbook of Physiology,* Sect. 7. (Steiner, D. F., and Freinkel, N., eds.) American Physiological Society, Washington, D. C., **1972,** pp. 175-198.

Unger, R. H. Glucagon and diabetes mellitus. *Adv. metab. Dis.,* **1972a,** *6,* 73-98.

———. Glucagon and glucagon immunoreactivity in plasma and pancreatic tissues. In, *Glucagon: Molecular Physiology, Clinical and Therapeutic Implications.* (Lefebvre, P. J., and Unger, R. H., eds.) Pergamon Press, Ltd., Oxford, **1972b,** pp. 205-212.

Unger, R. H., and Lefebvre, P. J. Glucagon physiology. In, *Glucagon: Molecular Physiology, Clinical and Therapeutic Implications.* (Lefebvre, P. J., and Unger, R. H., eds.) Pergamon Press, Ltd., Oxford, **1972,** pp. 213-244.

Van Wyck, J. J.; Underwood, L. E.; Hintz, R. L.; Voina, S. J.; and Weaver, R. P. Chemical properties and some biological effects of human somatomedin. In, *Advances in Human Growth Hormone Research.* (Raiti, S., ed.) Department of Health, Education, and Welfare Publication No. (NIH) 74-612, U.S. Government Printing Office, Washington, D. C., **1973,** pp. 25-45.

Williams, R. H., and Porte, D., Jr. The pancreas. In, *Textbook of Endocrinology,* 5th ed. (Williams, R. H., ed.) W. B. Saunders Co., Philadelphia, **1974,** pp. 502-626.

Wool, I. G.; Castles, J. J.; Leader, D. P.; and Fox, A. Insulin and the function of muscle ribosomes. In, *Endocrinology,* Vol. 1. *Handbook of Physiology,* Sect. 7. (Steiner, D. F., and Freinkel, N., eds.) American Physiological Society, Washington, D. C., **1972,** pp. 385-394.

Wunsch, E., and Weinges, K. F. The synthesis of glucagon. Properties of synthetic glucagon. In, *Glucagon: Molecular Physiology, Clinical and Therapeutic Implications.* (Lefebvre, P. J., and Unger, R. H., eds.) Pergamon Press, Ltd., Oxford, **1972,** pp. 31-46.

Zierler, K. L. Insulin, ions, and membrane potentials. In, *Endocrinology,* Vol. 1. *Handbook of Physiology,* Sect. 7. (Steiner, D. F., and Freinkel, N., eds.) American Physiological Society, Washington, D. C., **1972,** pp. 347-368.

72 PARATHYROID HORMONE AND CALCITONIN

Dixon M. Woodbury

PARATHYROID HORMONE

History. The earliest extirpations of the parathyroid glands were performed unintentionally during thyroidectomies. The resulting symptoms were attributed to the loss of thyroid tissue. Death following experimental thyroidectomy and the unwitting removal of the parathyroids was probably first recorded by Raynard, who in 1834 observed that, whereas older dogs survived thyroidectomy, puppies succumbed within a few days after the operation. Later investigators outlined in detail, without recognizing the cause, the symptoms now associated with parathyroidectomy.

Although there were many earlier references to the yellow glandular bodies attached to the thyroid, credit for the discovery of the parathyroid gland is usually given to Sandstrom, who in 1880 published an anatomical report that attracted little attention among physiologists. The glands were rediscovered by Gley (1891), who determined the effects of their extirpation with the thyroid. Vassale and Generali (1900) successfully removed the parathyroids without interfering with the thyroid and noted that tetany, convulsions, and death quickly followed. They thereby demonstrated that this syndrome was specifically due to parathyroid removal. However, the symptoms following parathyroidectomy varied so greatly in different species that the importance of the organs was not appreciated and controversies continued as to whether they were essential to life. The subsequent discovery of internal and accessory parathyroids accounted for the discrepancies in experimental results and paved the way to the elucidation of the important physiological role played by this endocrine gland.

MacCallum and Voegtlin (1909) first noted the effect of parathyroidectomy on the level of plasma calcium. Since Howell (1899) and Loeb (1901) had previously established the physiological importance of the calcium ion, the relation of low plasma calcium to parathyroprivic symptoms was quickly appreciated and a comprehensive picture of parathyroid function began to form. After various attempts to obtain active extracts of the gland, success was finally attained (Berman, 1924; Collip, 1925; Hanson, 1925). It was readily demonstrated that active extracts could alleviate hypocalcemic tetany in parathyroidectomized animals and raise the plasma calcium concentration in normal animals. For the first time, the relation of certain definite clinical abnormalities to parathyroid hyperfunction was appreciated.

While investigators in the United States, Canada, and England were utilizing the physiological approach to solve the problem of the function of the parathyroid glands, the German and Austrian pathologists were busy associating the skeletal changes of osteitis fibrosa cystica with the presence of parathyroid tumors. In a delightful historical review, Albright (1948) traced the manner in which these two diverse types of investigations finally arrived at the same conclusion. It is hoped that curiosity will lead the reader to this brief classic in medical history. Albright made major contributions to parathyroid physiology, calcium metabolism, and metabolic bone disease, and was largely responsible for stimulating the large advances in knowledge of this field that have occurred in the last 3 decades.

The older literature on the parathyroids and their relation to calcium, phosphate, and bone has been reviewed by Albright and Reifenstein (1948); subsequent developments are presented by Neumann and Neumann (1958), Fourman (1960), Copp (1964), Symposium (1965, 1968, 1971, 1974), and Nichols and Wasserman (1971).

Chemistry. As a result of vigorous efforts in the past decade, the parathyroid hormones (PTH) from various species have been purified to homogeneity and characterized extensively.

Human, bovine, and porcine parathyroid hormones are all single polypeptide chains of 84 amino acid residues; their molecular weights are approximately 9500. The entire amino acid sequence has been established for both bovine and porcine PTH, as has that for the first 34 residues from the amino end of the human hormone. This region includes all the amino acids necessary for biological activity. Bovine and porcine PTH differ by only seven amino acid residues, and the amino-terminal segment of the human hormone differs from the equivalent portion of the bovine and porcine molecules by only four and three amino acid residues, respectively. The three differ little in biological activity, but they are immunologically distinguishable; however, they cross-react with a single antibody and this facilitates an immunoassay for PTH, as discussed below. The sequence comprised of the first 34 amino acids of human and bovine PTH has been synthesized and shown to have characteristic biological activity. (*See* Brewer *et al.,* 1974.)

Synthesis and Immunoassay. PTH is synthesized in the parathyroid glands as a prohormone with a molecular weight of approximately 12,000. The bovine prohormone has six additional amino acid residues on the amino-terminal end; another 15 amino acids are presumably attached to the carboxy terminus, but this has not been established. Proparathyroid hormone (ProPTH) is probably synthesized in the rough endoplasmic reticulum, and it then moves to the Golgi complex, where conversion to PTH commences. There, PTH is stored in granules, and after a period of maturation the hormone is eventually secreted (Cohn *et al.,* 1974). It is not known whether any ProPTH is secreted as such, but the hormone with 84 amino acid residues is the major form secreted from the gland into the circulation. Intact PTH is then cleaved, notably between amino acid residues 33 and 34, into at least two major fragments; this reaction takes place in the blood and/or in the tissues. The larger fragment (molecular weight about 6000) from the carboxy terminus is biologically inactive but is reactive with antibody to the intact hormone. The biologically active fragment(s) shows relatively poor immunoreactivity with such antibody. PTH fragments may also be secreted from the parathyroid glands after proteolysis of the hormone within the cells of the gland. Cleavage into small fragments also takes place, at least in part, in tissues such as liver and kidney, and it is postulated that a small, active hormone moiety is split off at the site of the receptor.

Biological, chemical, and immunological heterogeneity of circulating "PTH" and fragments thereof obviously compounds the difficulties encountered in the immunoassay of plasma PTH, an important procedure in the evaluation of clinical disorders of bone and of calcium metabolism. Present immunoassays measure primarily biologically inactive fragments of PTH, but they are nevertheless useful for the diagnosis of parathyroid disease because the immunoreactive cleavage products are derived predominantly from intact secreted PTH. Antibodies made to smaller biologically active fragments of the human hormone should add considerably to the value of these assay technics, particularly because the half-life of the larger fragment may be considerably longer than that of the biologically active moiety. (*See* Silverman and Yalow, 1973; Arnaud *et al.,* 1974.)

Physiological Function. The primary function of the parathyroid gland is to participate in the cellular mechanisms that maintain the constancy of the concentration of calcium ion in the extracellular fluid. Hormonal control is necessary, because the normal gradient for calcium movement is from plasma to bone. These mechanisms include the absorption of calcium from the gastrointestinal tract, the deposition of calcium in bone and its mobilization therefrom, and the excretion of the ion in urine, feces, sweat, and milk (*see* Figure 72-1 and Chapter 37). There is evidence that PTH accomplishes its functions by an influence on all these mechanisms, but its most prominent effect is to promote the mobilization of calcium from bone.

Regulation of Secretion. The concentration of ionized calcium in the blood (or, more likely, the concentration of ionized calcium in parathyroid cells) is the primary factor that regulates the secretory activity of the parathyroid gland. When the concentration of ionized calcium is low, the secretion of PTH is increased, and hypertrophy and hyperplasia of the gland result if the hypocalcemia is sustained. If the level of ionized calcium is high, the secretion of PTH is decreased, and hypoplasia may result if the hypercalcemia is sustained. *In-vitro* studies show that amino acid uptake, nucleic acid and protein synthesis, cytoplasmic growth, and secretion of PTH are stimulated by exposure to low calcium concentrations and suppressed by exposure to high calcium concentrations. Thus, the calcium ion *per se* appears to regulate growth of the parathyroid gland and its synthesis and secretion of hormone (Roth and Raisz, 1964). It does this by inhibition of one or all of the following steps in the secretory process: amino acid uptake by parathyroid gland cells, synthesis of ProPTH, conversion of ProPTH to PTH, maturation of secretory granules, and secretion of PTH from the cell. In addition, the degradation of newly formed ProPTH or PTH may be enhanced by calcium ion. Inhibition of secretion by calcium ion precedes inhibition of biosynthesis.

There appears to be no direct relation between extracellular phosphate concentrations and the secretion of PTH, except indirectly as changes in phosphate values affect the calcium concentration. Hypermagnesemia also inhibits secretion of PTH, whereas magnesium deficiency increases secretion.

Calcitonin (*see* below) stimulates PTH secretion *in vitro* when there is a high concentration of calcium in the medium, probably by decreasing calcium ion concentration in the parathyroid cell. Also, vitamin D, by its effect to increase ionized calcium concentration in parathyroid-cell cytosol, decreases PTH secretion. Secretory activity of the parathyroid is not regulated by the central nervous system (CNS).

Thus, extracellular ionized calcium concentration is controlled on a minute-to-minute basis by a feedback system, the afferent limb of which is sensitive to the concentration of calcium and the efferent limb of which releases PTH. The hormone acts on various peripheral tissues to mobilize calcium into the extracellular fluid and thereby to restore the normal concentration

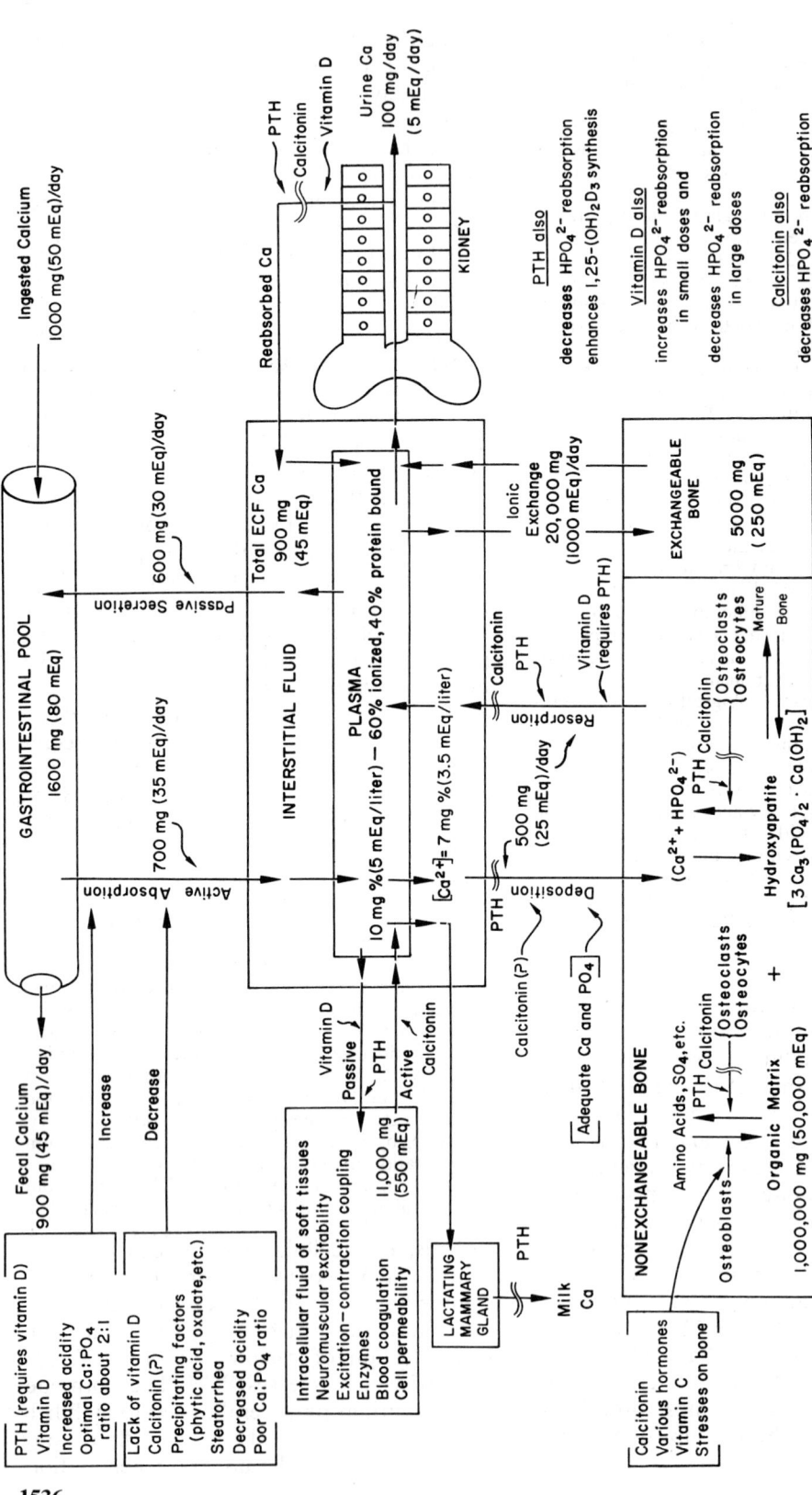

Figure 72-1. *Absorption, distribution, metabolism, and excretion of calcium as affected by parathyroid hormone, vitamin D, calcitonin, and various dietary factors.*

The numerical values inside the blocks representing the various body compartments are the total amounts or concentrations of calcium in that compartment of a 70-kg man. The values on the arrows represent the amount of calcium transferred into or out of the compartment in 1 day. The effects of parathyroid hormone (*PTH*), calcitonin, and vitamin D (1,25-[OH]$_2$D$_3$) are depicted either by *curved arrows*, which indicate an *increased effect or stimula-* *tion* of the process pointed to by the arrow, or *double wavy lines*, which interrupt the arrows going between the various compartments or biochemical processes and indicate a *decreased effect or depression* of the process. Detailed discussion of the effects of PTH and calcitonin is presented in this chapter; of vitamin D, in Chapter 76; and of calcium and phosphate metabolism, in Chapters 37 and 38, respectively.

when it has been lowered. (*See* Symposium, 1965, 1968, 1971, 1974; Sherwood *et al.,* 1968; and others.) (The role of *calcitonin* in regulation of elevated plasma calcium levels is discussed below.) A summary of calcium metabolism and of the effects of PTH and vitamin D thereon is presented in Figure 72–1.

Effects on Gastrointestinal Tract. The main effect of PTH on the gastrointestinal tract is to increase the active absorption of calcium from the small intestine. The effect has been demonstrated both *in vivo* and *in vitro;* it may be a direct effect of PTH that requires the presence of vitamin D, or, more likely, it is an indirect effect that is due to accumulation of the active form of vitamin D as a result of PTH enhancement of the renal conversion of 25-hydroxycholecalciferol (25-OHD$_3$) to 1,25-dihydroxycholecalciferol (1,25-[OH]$_2$D$_3$), as discussed in Chapter 76.

In patients with hyperparathyroidism, there is reduced fecal excretion of calcium as a result of enhanced intestinal absorption; the secretion of calcium into the intestinal tract by way of the bile and the intestinal secretions may also be reduced, but evidence for this is lacking. The enhancement of calcium absorption is of lesser importance for the overall effect of PTH on calcium metabolism than are its effects on other target organs such as bone and kidney. The active uptake of phosphate by the intestine and its flux rate from mucosa to serosa are also increased by PTH, and these effects are blocked by metabolic inhibitors. Thus, the hormone, probably through enhanced formation of 1,25-(OH)$_2$D$_3$, influences both calcium and phosphate absorption.

Effects on Bone. The primary effect of PTH on bone is to increase the rate of resorption of calcium and phosphate. The site of the resorptive effect appears to be on the stable, older portion of bone mineral and not on the labile fraction. PTH, by means of mobilization of calcium from the stable fraction of bone, primarily regulates that portion of the plasma calcium above 7 mg % (3.5 mEq per liter); the portion below this concentration is less dependent on hormonal control and is maintained by the physicochemical equilibrium that exists between the extracellular fluid and the labile (rapidly exchanging) fraction of bone.

Resorption of bone is brought about by osteolytic cells—osteoclasts and osteocytes. PTH stimulates the rate of bone resorption by these cells, increases the rate of conversion (differentiation) of mesenchymal cells to osteoclasts, and lengthens the half-life of these latter cells. With prolonged action of PTH the number of bone-forming osteoblasts is also increased; thus, the rate of bone turnover and remodeling is enhanced. However, individual osteoblasts appear to be less active than normal, and PTH acts to inhibit their synthesis of collagen, a major component of bone matrix.

A direct effect of the hormone on bone is evident from the observations that, in nephrectomized animals, parathyroidectomy promptly decreases plasma calcium concentration and PTH administration increases the concentration. Furthermore, transplantation of parathyroid tissue so as to place it in direct contact with bone *in vivo* causes resorption of bone on the surface in contact with the gland and results in bone deposition on the opposite surface (Barnicot, 1948; Chang, 1951). Gaillard (1961) extended these observations to cultures of bone tissue and limbs and noted, in addition, that PTH produced striking direct effects on bone, cartilage, and connective tissue. He noted disappearance of osteoblasts, formation of many multinuclear osteoclasts in the region of bone resorption, dissolution of bone matrix, complex changes in the growth pattern of the epiphyseal cartilage, and proliferation of the connective tissue filling the shaft. (*See* Symposium, 1965, 1968; Rasmussen and Bordier, 1974.)

Biochemical correlates of PTH action have also been studied extensively. Raisz (*see* Symposium, 1965) demonstrated an increased release of calcium from bone into the culture medium in the presence of PTH. The hormone stimulates production of a collagenase that causes degradation of bone collagen. It also causes depolymerization and solution of the glycoprotein ground substance of bone, inhibits sulfate uptake into the matrix mucopolysaccharides, and inhibits the synthesis of the collagen in bone matrix as measured by ^{14}C-proline incorporation. Thus, the hormone, through its effects on osteoclasts and osteoblasts, simultaneously *enhances resorption* of both the bone mineral and the organic matrix and *inhibits synthesis* of the latter. These conclusions are also supported by observations that RNA, protein, and mucoprotein synthesis is increased in osteoclasts and decreased in osteoblasts by PTH. The resorption of bone is associated with a release of lysosomes from osteoclasts and possibly from osteocytes, by exocytosis into the bone extracellular fluid. The lysosomes contain acid hydrolases but not collagenase.

A further mechanism by which PTH might mobilize calcium and phosphate from the stable portion of bone is by means of stimulating glycolysis and inhibiting citric acid oxidation in osteoclasts and possibly osteocytes. This results in accumulation of lactate, citrate, and other organic acids, thereby producing a decrease in pH at the site of bone resorption. The pH change would cause dissolution of hydroxyapatite.

Insight is also emerging into the subcellular mechanisms by which PTH acts on bone cells to promote the effects just described. The hormone stimulates the membrane-bound adenylate cyclase of bone cells, and cyclic adenosine 3',5'-monophosphate (cyclic AMP) accumulates. Cyclic AMP and/or PTH act to facilitate Ca^{2+} entry into bone cells and to increase Ca^{2+} exit from or decrease Ca^{2+} entry into mitochondria, which contain most of the cellular Ca^{2+}. This action on mitochondria appears to require vitamin D. Calcium transport is also enhanced across the epithelial layer of bone cells that separates bone extracellular space from the general fluid compartment. While further mechanistic details are even more blurred, current hypotheses suggest that cyclic AMP and Ca^{2+} act as intracellular mediators to cause the metabolic changes, such as accumulation of citrate and other organic acids, described above. Cyclic AMP may also play a role in mediating the effects of PTH on bone-cell division and differentiation. (For summaries, *see* Symposium, 1965, 1968, 1971, 1974; Vaes, 1968; Nichols and Wasserman, 1971; Rasmussen and Bordier, 1974.)

Effects on the Kidney. In addition to its prominent effects on bone, PTH also influences the excretion of calcium and phosphate by the kidney. It increases the renal tubular reabsorption of calcium and the excretion of phosphate. Both effects raise the extracellular calcium concentration.

Calcium. Parathyroidectomy, in both animals and man, decreases whereas PTH increases tubular calcium reabsorption at a distal site (*see* Widrow and Levinsky, 1962; Agus *et al.,* 1973). Therefore, when plasma calcium concentration is in the normal range, extirpation of the gland decreases tubular reabsorption of calcium and thereby increases calcium excretion in the urine. When the plasma concentration falls significantly (to less than 7 mg %), there follows a decrease in calcium excretion because the amount of calcium filtered through the glomeruli is lowered to the point that the cation is almost completely reabsorbed despite the reduced tubular reabsorptive capacity. However, when parathyroidectomized animals are kept on a high-calcium diet and plasma calcium remains higher than 7 mg %, the hypercalciuria persists. If PTH is administered to such hypoparathyroid animals or man, tubular reabsorption of calcium is increased and there is initially a decrease in the excretion of calcium. This, along with mobilization of calcium from bone and increased absorption from the gut, results in increased plasma calcium concentration. When the plasma value rises above normal, the hypercalciuria so characteristic of hyperparathyroidism ensues.

Phosphate. It is now well established that PTH increases the renal excretion of inorganic phosphate. The principal site of reabsorption of inorganic phosphate is in the proximal tubule, and this process is inhibited by the hormone. Phosphate reabsorption in the loop of Henle is also inhibited by PTH (Brunette *et al.,* 1973).

Cyclic AMP also appears to mediate these effects of PTH on the kidney. Adenylate cyclase that is stimulated by PTH is located particularly in the renal cortex, and cyclic AMP synthesized in response to the hormone affects tubular transport mechanisms. A portion of the cyclic nucleotide synthesized at this site escapes into the urine, and its assay serves as a measure of parathyroid activity (*see* Chase *et al.,* 1969; *see also* below). Cyclic AMP may inhibit proximal tubular reabsorption of calcium, phosphate, and sodium. The final effect on calcium excretion is, however, inhibitory, since it stimulates distal calcium reabsorption out of proportion to that of sodium. (*See* Symposium, 1968; Agus *et al.,* 1973; Rasmussen and Bordier, 1974.)

Other Ions. PTH also influences the excretion of other ions, most of which are constituents of bone. Renal excretion of magnesium is reduced by the hormone, and the plasma concentration is elevated; in parathyroidectomized animals, magnesium excretion is usually increased and the plasma concentration is reduced. The hormonal effect on magnesium is probably due, as in the case for calcium, to both increased renal tubular reabsorption of magnesium and its mobilization from the exchangeable compartment of bone (MacIntyre *et al.,* 1963). The excretion of water, amino acids, citrate, potassium, bicarbonate, sodium, chloride, and sulfate is increased, whereas the excretion of hydrogen ion is decreased by PTH. The increased excretion of bicarbonate ion appears to be mainly due to inhibition of proximal tubular reabsorption of this anion; it is antagonized by calcium. Although the renal acid-base effects of PTH are similar to those of acetazolamide, they are independent of the carbonic anhydrase system. The effects of PTH on other ions involve actions on both proximal and distal tubules.

Miscellaneous Effects. PTH decreases, whereas parathyroidectomy increases, the calcium concentration of milk and saliva. These effects are the opposite from those that would be expected from the concurrent changes in plasma calcium concentration. It appears likely, therefore, that the hormone can conserve calcium in the extracellular fluid not only by its effects on bone, kidney, and gut but also by reducing the rate of calcium transport from extracellular fluid to milk and saliva.

An association between PTH and the lens of the eye is suggested by the prevalence of cataracts in patients with hypoparathyroidism and the increased content of calcium in the lens in hormone-deficient animals. PTH reduces the calcium concentration of the lens.

Hypoparathyroidism. Extirpation or hypofunction of the parathyroids leads to a characteristic syndrome. Symptoms are the direct result of hypocalcemia and the consequent reduction in the threshold of excitability of polarized membranes. After removal of the parathyroids in dogs, appetite is gradually lost. Fine fibrillary twitchings of skeletal muscles develop and soon become coarser. The animal shows a characteristic awkward gait. Neuromuscular disturbance becomes progressively worse and culminates in convulsions, which may follow in rapid succession or occur at intervals of several days. Death follows respiratory failure, probably resulting from spasm of the muscles of the larynx and diaphragm.

Clinical Hypoparathyroidism. The events leading to abnormalities in calcium metabolism are discussed under the pharmacology of calcium (*see* Chapter 37). Hypoparathyroidism is only one of the many causes of hypocalcemia and occurs relatively rarely. The deficiency syndrome most commonly follows operative procedures on either the thyroid gland or the parathyroids themselves. Less frequently, disease of the parathyroids is the cause (*idiopathic hypoparathyroidism*). Also uncommon is a genetic disorder in which the target organs do not respond to PTH, despite adequate concentrations of the hormone (*pseudohypoparathyroidism*).

In all varieties of hypoparathyroidism, hypocalcemia and its associated symptoms are encountered clinically. The earliest prodromal symptoms of hypocalcemia are paresthesias in the extremities. Mechanical stimulation of peripheral nerves during physical examination usually produces contraction of the appropriate skeletal muscles. These signs and symptoms may be followed by manifest tetany, consisting in muscle spasms, especially carpopedal spasm and laryngospasm. Eventually, generalized convulsions and other CNS manifestations occur. It is highly probable that smooth muscle is also affected. For example, hypocalcemia may be followed by spasm of the ciliary muscle, iris, esophagus, intestine, urinary bladder, and bronchi. ECG changes and a marked tachycardia indicate that the heart is involved. Vascular spasm in the fingers and toes is also commonly observed. In *chronic hypoparathyroidism,* ectodermal changes, consisting in loss of hair, grooved and brittle fingernails, defects of the dental enamel, and cataracts, are frequently encountered; there is also calcification in the basal ganglia. Psychiatric symptoms such as emotional lability, anxiety, depression, and delusions are often present. The EEG may be abnormal. (*See* Albright and Reifenstein, 1948; Fourman, 1960; Rasmussen, 1974.)

Hypoparathyroidism is treated primarily with vitamin D. Dietary supplementation with calcium may also be necessary (*see* Chapters 37 and 76).

Hyperparathyroidism. The administration of a single large dose of PTH to an experimental animal can cause the changes in blood chemistry that are characteristic of hyperparathyroidism. The concentration of ionized calcium in the plasma increases markedly, reaching values as high as 18 to 20 mg % (9 to 10 mEq per liter) in 12 to 18 hours. This is accompanied by a variable decrease in the concentration of plasma phosphate. Chronic administration of the hormone leads to decalcification of bone and the development of bone cysts, deformities, and spontaneous fractures. The calcium mobilized from bone is precipitated in the soft tissues. Metastatic calcification is observed especially in the kidney, the wall of the stomach, the bronchi, the interstitial connective tissue, the heart muscle, and the tunica media of the smaller arteries. The animals exhibit anorexia, vomiting, diarrhea, and muscle atony. They die eventually as a result of renal insufficiency due to diffuse nephrocalcinosis and nephrolithiasis.

Clinical Hyperparathyroidism. Primary hyperparathyroidism results either from hypersecretion of the parathyroid glands (due to hyperplasia, adenoma, or, rarely, carcinoma) or from secretion of "PTH-like" polypeptides from tumors arising at other sites. In some cases such polypeptides may be distinguished from PTH by immunological technics. Plasma calcium concentrations may be normal with primary hyperparathyroidism, but they are usually elevated and plasma phosphate values are usually decreased. Hyperparathyroidism may also be *secondary* to conditions causing negative calcium balance, such as malabsorption and renal disease; in these cases the plasma calcium concentration is low and provides the stimulus for increased secretion of PTH. Hypersecretion of PTH from any cause may lead to a bone disorder known as *osteitis fibrosa generalisata,* or *von Recklinghausen's disease of bone.* However, only one third of cases of hyperparathyroidism exhibit advanced bone changes; another third show minor degrees of decalcification; and the remaining cases present no skeletal abnormalities, although metabolic studies indicate that resorption of bone is actively occurring. In the last-mentioned group, the calcium intake may be sufficient to maintain calcium balance. The symptoms of early decalcification are aching and pain in the bones and joints.

Uncomplicated primary hyperparathyroidism is invariably associated with hypercalciuria and hyperphosphaturia, and is sometimes accompanied by polyuria and polydipsia. The excretion of excessive amounts of calcium and phosphate results in a high incidence of renal calculi, which often cause the presenting symptoms. An equally serious complication is a diffuse nephrocalcinosis, which may progress to a stage of extreme renal insufficiency. It is well to keep in mind that renal insufficiency secondary to nephrocalcinosis or to sequelae of urolithiasis may mask some of the cardinal biochemical features of hyperparathyroidism, namely, hyperphosphaturia, hypercalciuria, and hypophosphatemia, and may also mask the normocalcemic and hypocalcemic varieties of the disease.

Hypercalcemia *per se* can be the cause of some of the signs and symptoms of hyperparathyroidism.

These include hypotonicity of muscle, with general skeletal muscle weakness and smooth muscle dysfunction leading to constipation, flatulence, anorexia, nausea, and vomiting. Occasionally, cardiac irregularities are observed. A higher-than-normal incidence of peptic ulcers and pancreatitis has been reported in patients with the disease. Neuropsychiatric manifestations also occur in many cases (Karpati and Frame, 1964). Advanced cases of osteitis fibrosa generalisata may be associated with anemia and leukopenia.

In addition to laboratory study of calcium and phosphorus, there are certain more specific tests for hyperparathyroidism. The most widely used is the radioimmunoassay of plasma PTH concentration. However, as discussed above, this test is dependent on the antibody preparation used. Another method involves determination of the concentration of cyclic AMP in urine, which is elevated by the action of PTH on the kidney (Murad and Pak, 1972).

Treatment. Surgical resection of the hyperplastic or adenomatous glands is almost always required for the treatment of primary hyperparathyroidism. Surgery can return the patient to a euparathyroid state and prevent continued renal damage and bone dissolution. More commonly, a hypoparathyroid condition ensues. In this case vitamin D therapy and/or supplementation of the diet with calcium is required (*see* Chapter 76). Chronic treatment with oral neutral phosphate, a low-calcium diet, and liberal amounts of fluids is used to lower the plasma calcium concentration in selected patients in whom surgery is contraindicated (Purnell *et al.,* in Symposium, 1974). (For details of clinical hyperparathyroidism and its classification, diagnosis, and treatment, *see* Albright and Reifenstein, 1948; Symposium, 1971, 1974; Rasmussen and Bordier, 1974.)

Preparations, Bioassay, and Unitage. *Parathyroid Injection,* U.S.P., is made from bovine parathyroid glands. Bioassay to determine its activity is performed on healthy mature dogs. One unit of hormone is $\frac{1}{100}$ the amount necessary to raise the concentration of plasma calcium 1 mg % within 16 to 18 hours after subcutaneous injection. Preparations are adjusted to contain approximately 100 units/ml. Bioassay methods for the hormone based on immunochemical procedures have been developed, as described above (*see* Symposium, 1971, 1974). Some batches of commercial parathyroid extract also contain a hypocalcemic factor, probably calcitonin (*see* below; *see also* Copp, 1964). *Synthetic parathyroid hormone* (bovine) is also available for investigational purposes as the (1-34 amino acid) tetratriacontapeptide in 5-ml bottles, 1000 to 1200 units in each.

Absorption, Fate, and Excretion. PTH must be given parenterally, for obvious reasons. The usual route of administration is subcutaneous or intravenous. The maximal effect is obtained approximately 18 hours after a single subcutaneous injection; the response may last for 36 hours. The peak effect of purified preparations or of hormone

given intravenously is seen considerably sooner. Studies in animals with radioiodinated PTH and with the endogenous hormone bioassayed by the immunological method demonstrate that its half-life in the body is about 20 minutes, a value considerably shorter than previously thought. The hormone appears to be carried in the blood, at least in part, in the α-globulin fraction of plasma protein. Excretion in the urine is minimal (less than 1%). The sites of degradation of PTH are still unknown, but they appear to include both the kidney and liver.

Clinical Uses. There are currently no valid therapeutic uses of PTH; while it was formerly employed to elevate the plasma calcium concentration, this can be accomplished with greater safety by the administration of calcium and/or vitamin D.

PTH is used for the *diagnosis* of pseudohypoparathyroidism. Since this disease is characterized by target-organ resistance to the hormone, these patients fail to show an increased concentration of plasma calcium and fail to excrete increased amounts of phosphate and cyclic AMP after the administration of PTH (200 units, intravenously) (*see* Chase *et al.,* 1969).

CALCITONIN

History and Source. The existence of a hypocalcemic hormone, the effects of which are opposite to those of the parathyroid hormone, was discovered and named *calcitonin* by Copp in 1962. It was demonstrated as a result of perfusion of dog's parathyroid and thyroid glands with hypercalcemic blood. This caused an immediate transitory hypocalcemic effect in the systemic blood; it occurred significantly earlier than did hypocalcemia observed after total parathyroidectomy, an indication that suppression of secretion of parathyroid hormone could not account for the rapid effect. The observations led Copp and others to conclude that the parathyroid glands secreted calcitonin in response to hypercalcemia and in this way reduced the elevated plasma calcium concentration to normal. However, Foster and associates (1964), although confirming the presence and hypocalcemic effect of calcitonin in goats, presented evidence that in this species the hormone originates from the *thyroid gland.* Subsequent studies have confirmed the thyroidal origin of calcitonin in other mammals.

The parafollicular "C" cells from the thyroid, which are embryologically derived from the ultimobranchial body, are the site of production and secretion of calcitonin. In nonmammalian vertebrates, calcitonin is found only in ultimobranchial bodies, which are separate organs from the thyroid gland. The hormone from both sources, thyroid and ultimobranchial bodies, is the same. In man, calcitonin is present in the thyroid, parathyroid, and thymus, an indication that the "C" cells are widely distributed.

Chemistry and Immunoreactivity. The calcitonins from the thyroid of the pig and a number of other species, including salmon and man, have been isolated, characterized chemically, and totally synthesized. They are all single-chain polypeptides with a molecular weight of 3600, and contain 32 amino acids. A cystine disulfide bridge exists in the 1-7 position at the amino end of the chain; it is essential for biological activity. The carboxyl-terminal amino acid is prolinamide (*see* Symposium, 1968; Hirsch and Munson, 1969). Calcitonin isolated from human "C"-cell tumors differs from the porcine hormone in 18 of its amino acid residues. Thus, the immunoassay of human tissues and fluids based on antibodies to porcine material has been unreliable because of poor cross-reactivity. However, specific radioimmunoassay for the human hormone has now been developed with calcitonin derived from medullary carcinoma of the human thyroid as the antigen (*see* Tashjian *et al.,* 1974).

Regulation of Secretion. The secretion and biosynthesis of calcitonin in both animals and man are regulated by the concentration of calcium in plasma. When the calcium concentration is high, the amount of the hormone in plasma increases. When the calcium concentration is low, the amount of the hormone decreases markedly and may be undetectable. Normal basal concentrations of calcitonin in plasma as measured by the radioimmunoassay method are <100 pg/ml in more than 75% of subjects. Calcium infusion increases the basal concentration twofold to threefold (Tashjian *et al.,* 1974). The half-life of calcitonin is short (about 10 minutes); hence the hormone most likely is secreted at a fairly continuous rate at normal plasma calcium concentrations. A role of cyclic AMP in the release of calcitonin from "C" cells of the thyroid is indicated by the fact that the dibutyryl derivative of cyclic AMP, epinephrine, and glucagon stimulate its release, as do gastrin and cholecystokinin. The effects of the gastrointestinal hormones could constitute a mechanism for regulation of calcitonin secretion following the ingestion of calcium salts.

While it is clear that calcitonin secretion can be modulated by several different agents under experimental conditions, it is not known to what extent normal physiological variations in secretion occur or if calcitonin plays a significant role in calcium homeostasis. High concentrations of calcitonin have been found in plasma, urine, and tumor tissue (50 to 5000 times normal) in patients with medullary carcinoma of the thyroid gland. The tumor cells originate from the parafollicular cells of the thyroid, and this disease represents a true calcitonin-excess syndrome. The radioimmunoassay of calcitonin appears to be a valuable procedure for detection of thyroid medullary carcinoma, particularly because one form of this disease is inherited as a dominant trait. Relatives of patients must therefore be examined repeatedly (Tashjian *et al.,* 1974).

Mechanism and Actions. There is general agreement from both acute and chronic *in-vivo* experiments and *in-vitro* culture of bones that the hypocalcemic and hypophosphatemic effects of calcitonin are due predominantly to *direct inhibition of bone resorption* by altering osteoclastic and osteocytic activity. This effect on bone resorption is elicited in parathyroidectomized, nephrectomized, and eviscerated animals. Calcitonin enhances bone formation by an effect on osteoblasts. However, the effect is short lived, and osteoclastic as well as osteoblastic activity is decreased with chronic use of the hormone; hence its use is contraindicated in osteoporosis. In addition, calcitonin negates PTH effects on osteolysis mediated by osteocytic and osteoclastic activity.

The intimate biochemical and cellular effects of calcitonin are not yet known, but it does not act as an antiparathyroid hormone. Thus, it does not block the activation of bone-cell adenylate cyclase by PTH and does not inhibit the initial PTH-induced uptake of calcium into bone, the primary effects of PTH on bone cells. It may increase calcium efflux from bone cells by activation of the calcium pump in the cell membrane and may also increase calcium uptake by mitochondria; both these effects are opposite to those produced by PTH and result in a decrease in cytosol calcium ion concentration. Part of the effect of calcitonin appears to be mediated through increasing the cyclic AMP concentration in bone cells, perhaps in cells different from those so activated by PTH (Murad *et al.,* 1970).

Calcitonin also antagonizes the inhibitory effects of PTH on pyrophosphatase activity in isolated Ehrlich ascites tumor cells. Pyrophosphate and pyrophosphatase are intimately involved in the processes of bone formation and resorption. Calcitonin also decreases glucose utilization and lactate production in bone, effects opposite to those of PTH. As a result of depressed bone resorption, the urinary excretion of calcium, magnesium, and hydroxyproline is decreased by calcitonin. Plasma phosphate concentration is also lowered, due mainly to decreased resorption of bone and also to increased urinary phosphate excretion. The direct effects of calcitonin on the kidney are dependent on species. In man, calcitonin increases the excretion of calcium, phosphate, and sodium, effects also mediated in part by cyclic AMP (Murad *et al.,* 1970; Pak, 1971).

Bioassay, Preparations, and Dosage. Bioassay of calcitonin preparations is performed by assessing their ability to lower plasma calcium concentration in the rat. The results are compared with a British Medical Research Council (MRC) Standard and expressed in MRC units. One unit is equivalent to approximately 4 μg of pure porcine calcitonin. (For summaries, *see* Copp, 1964; MacIntyre, 1967; Symposium, 1968, 1974; Tenenhouse *et al.,* 1968; Rasmussen and Bordier, 1974.)

Salmon, porcine, and human calcitonins have been studied experimentally. The hormone from salmon is considerably more potent in man than are the other two, perhaps because it is cleared from the circulation more slowly. Salmon calcitonin is available for clinical use as *calcitonin* (CALCIMAR), a synthetic preparation supplied in vials of 400 MRC units with 4 ml of a diluent containing 16% gelatin. The recommended dosage is 100 units per day, administered subcutaneously or intramuscularly. The drug is expensive.

Therapeutic Uses. Calcitonin is effective in diminishing hypercalcemia and decreasing plasma phosphate concentrations in patients with hyperparathyroidism, idiopathic hypercalcemia of infancy, vitamin D intoxication, and osteolytic bone metastases. The effect of a single dose lasts for 6 to 10 hours. The decrease in plasma calcium and phosphate is the result of their decreased resorption from bone. Although calcitonin is effective in the initial treatment of hypercalcemia from various causes, other measures are recommended and are generally used (*see* Chapter 37).

Calcitonin has proved to be effective in diseases characterized by increased skeletal remodeling (increased bone resorption and bone formation), such as occurs in Paget's disease. In this disease, calcitonin given chronically produces symptomatic relief and reduction in alkaline phosphatase activity, urinary hydroxyproline, and blood flow through the affected area. Calcitonin, alone or with oral phosphate, appears to be the treatment of choice for Paget's disease (*see* Symposium, 1974). Development of antibodies to porcine or salmon calcitonin does occur with long-term therapy in many patients; however, there is no apparent correlation between the development of antibodies and resistance to treatment. While optimal dosage has not been established, favorable results were obtained in one study with 100 MRC units of salmon calcitonin given daily or three times a week by subcutaneous injection. The minimal dose for long-term therapy appeared to be 50 MRC units

injected three times weekly. Side effects included nausea and swelling and tenderness of the hands; urticaria has also been observed (DeRose *et al.,* 1974).

Agus, Z. S.; Gardner, L. B.; Beck, L. H.; and Goldberg, M. Effects of parathyroid hormone on renal tubular reabsorption of calcium, sodium, and phosphate. *Am. J. Physiol.,* **1973,** *224,* 1143–1148.
Albright, F. A page out of the history of hyperparathyroidism. *J. clin. Endocr. Metab.,* **1948,** *8,* 637–657.
Arnaud, C. D.; Goldsmith, R. S.; Bordier, P. J.; and Sizemore, G. W. Influence of immunoheterogeneity of circulating parathyroid hormone on results of radioimmunoassays of serum in man. *Am. J. Med.,* **1974,** *56,* 785–793.
Barnicot, N. A. The local action of the parathyroid and other tissues on the bone in intracerebral grafts. *J. Anat.,* **1948,** *82,* 233–248.
Berman, L. A. Crystalline substance from the parathyroid glands that influences the calcium content of the blood. *Proc. Soc. exp. Biol. Med.,* **1924,** *21,* 465.
Brewer, H. B.; Fairwell, T.; Rittel, W.; Littledike, T.; and Arnaud, C. D. Recent studies on the chemistry of human, bovine and porcine parathyroid hormones. *Am. J. Med.,* **1974,** *56,* 759–766.
Brunette, M. G.; Taleb, L.; and Carriere, S. Effect of parathyroid hormone on phosphate reabsorption along the nephron of the rat. *Am. J. Physiol.,* **1973,** *225,* 1076–1081.
Chang, H. Grafts of parathyroid and other tissues to bone. *Anat. Rec.,* **1951,** *111,* 23–47.
Chase, L. R.; Melson, G. L.; and Aurbach, G. D. Pseudohypoparathyroidism: defective excretion of 3',5'-AMP in response to parathyroid hormone. *J. clin. Invest.,* **1969,** *48,* 1832–1844.
Cohn, D. V.; MacGregor, R. R.; Chu, L. L. H.; Huang, D. W. Y.; Anast, C. S.; and Hamilton, J. W. Biosynthesis of proparathyroid hormone and parathyroid hormone. *Am. J. Med.,* **1974,** *56,* 767–773.
Collip, J. B. The extraction of a parathyroid hormone which will prevent or control parathyroid tetany and which regulates the level of blood calcium. *J. biol. Chem.,* **1925,** *63,* 395–438.
DeRose, J.; Singer, F. R.; Avramides, A.; Flores, A.; Dziadiw, R.; Baker, R. K.; and Wallach, S. Response of Paget's disease to porcine and salmon calcitonins. Effects of long-term treatment. *Am. J. Med.,* **1974,** *56,* 858–866.
Foster, G. B.; Baghdiantz, A.; Kumar, M. A.; Slack, E.; Soliman, H. A.; and MacIntyre, I. Thyroid origin of calcitonin. *Nature, Lond.,* **1964,** *202,* 1303–1305.
Gaillard, P. J. Parathyroid and bone in tissue culture. In, *The Parathyroids.* (Greep, R. O., and Talmage, R. V., eds.) Charles C Thomas, Pub., Springfield, Ill., **1961,** pp. 20–45.
Gley, M. E. Sur les effets de l'extirpation du corps thyroide. *C. r. Séanc. Soc. Biol.,* **1891,** *43,* 551–554.
Hanson, A. M. The hormone of the parathyroid gland. *Proc. Soc. exp. Biol. Med.,* **1925,** *22,* 560–561.
Howell, W. H. On the relation of the blood to the automaticity and sequence of the heartbeat. *Am. J. Physiol.,* **1899,** *2,* 47–81.
Karpati, G., and Frame, B. Neuropsychiatric disorders in primary hyperparathyroidism. *Archs Neurol., Chicago,* **1964,** *10,* 387–397.
Loeb, J. On an apparently new form of muscular irritability (contact irritability?) produced by solutions of salts (preferably sodium salts) whose anions are liable to form insoluble calcium compounds. *Am. J. Physiol.,* **1901,** *5,* 362–373.
MacCallum, S. G., and Voegtlin, C. On the relation of tetany to the parathyroid glands and to calcium metabolism. *J. exp. Med.,* **1909,** *11,* 118–151.

MacIntyre, I.; Boss, S.; and Troughton, V. A. Parathyroid hormone and magnesium homoeostasis. *Nature, Lond.,* **1963,** *198,* 1058–1060.

Murad, F.; Brewer, H. B.; and Vaughan, M. Effect of thyrocalcitonin on adenosine 3′,5′-cyclic phosphate formation by rat kidney and bone. *Proc. natn. Acad. Sci. U.S.A.,* **1970,** *65,* 446–453.

Murad, F., and Pak, C. Y. C. Urinary excretion of adenosine 3′,5′-monophosphate and guanosine 3′,5′-monophosphate. *New Engl. J. Med.,* **1972,** *286,* 1382–1387.

Roth, S. I., and Raisz, L. G. Effect of calcium concentration on the ultrastructure of rat parathyroid in organ culture. *Lab. Invest.,* **1964,** *13,* 331–345.

Sherwood, L. M.; Mayer, G. P.; Ramberg, C. F., Jr.; Kronfeld, D. S.; Aurbach, G. D.; and Potts, J. T., Jr. Regulation of parathyroid hormone secretion: proportional control by calcium, lack of effect of phosphate. *Endocrinology,* **1968,** *83,* 1043–1051.

Silverman, R., and Yalow, R. S. Heterogeneity of parathyroid hormone. Clinical and physiological implications. *J. clin. Invest.,* **1973,** *52,* 1958–1971.

Tashjian, A. H.; Wolfe, H. J.; and Voelkel, E. F. Human calcitonin. Immunologic assay, cytochemical localization and studies on medullary thyroid carcinoma. *Am. J. Med.,* **1974,** *56,* 840–849.

Vaes, G. On the mechanisms of bone resorption: the action of parathyroid hormone on the excretion and synthesis of lysosomal enzymes and on the extracellular release of acid by bone cells. *J. cell Biol.,* **1968,** *39,* 676–697.

Vassale, G., and Generali, F. Fonction parathyroidienne et fonction thyroidienne. *Archs ital. Biol.,* **1900,** *33,* 154–156.

Widrow, S. H., and Levinsky, N. G. The effect of parathyroid extract on renal tubular calcium reabsorption in the dog. *J. clin. Invest.,* **1962,** *41,* 2151–2159.

Monographs and Reviews

Albright, F., and Reifenstein, E. C. *The Parathyroid Gland and Metabolic Bone Disease.* The Williams & Wilkins Co., Baltimore, **1948.**

Aurbach, G. D.; Keutmann, H. T.; Niall, H. D.; Tregear, G. W.; O'Riordan, J. L. H.; Marcus, R.; Marx, S. J.; and Potts, J. T., Jr. Structure, synthesis, and mechanism of action of parathyroid hormone. *Recent Prog. Horm. Res.,* **1972,** *28,* 353–398.

Borle, A. B. Calcium and phosphate metabolism. *A. Rev. Physiol.,* **1974,** *36,* 361–390.

Copp, D. H. Parathyroids, calcitonin, and control of plasma calcium. *Recent Prog. Horm. Res.,* **1964,** *20,* 59–88.

Fourman, P. *Calcium Metabolism and the Bone.* Charles C Thomas, Pub., Springfield, Ill., **1960.**

Hirsch, P. F., and Munson, P. L. Thyrocalcitonin. *Physiol. Rev.,* **1969,** *49,* 548–622.

MacIntyre, I. Calcitonin: a general review. *Calcif. Tissue Res.,* **1967,** *1,* 173–182.

Mallette, L. E.; Bilezikian, J. P.; Heath, D. A.; and Aurbach, G. D. Primary hyperparathyroidism: clinical and biochemical features. *Medicine, Baltimore,* **1974,** *53,* 127–146.

Neumann, W. F., and Neumann, M. *The Chemical Dynamics of Bone Mineral.* University of Chicago Press, Chicago, **1958.**

Nichols, G., and Wasserman, R. H. (eds.). *Cellular Mechanisms for Calcium Transfer and Homeostasis.* Academic Press, Inc., New York, **1971.**

Pak, C. Y. C. Parathyroid hormone and thyrocalcitonin: their mode of action and regulation. *Ann. N.Y. Acad. Sci.,* **1971,** *179,* 450–474.

Rasmussen, H. Parathyroid hormone, calcitonin, and the calciferols. In, *Textbook of Endocrinology,* 5th ed. (Williams, R. H., ed.) W. B. Saunders Co., Philadelphia, **1974,** pp. 660–773.

Rasmussen, H., and Bordier, P. *The Physiological and Cellular Basis of Metabolic Bone Disease.* The Williams & Wilkins Co., Baltimore, **1974.**

Symposium. (Various authors.) *The Parathyroid Glands: Ultrastructure, Secretion, and Function.* (Gaillard, P. J.; Talmage, R. V.; and Budy, A. M.; eds.) University of Chicago Press, Chicago, **1965.**

Symposium. (Various authors.) *Parathyroid Hormone and Thyrocalcitonin (Calcitonin).* (Talmage, R. V., and Bélanger, L. F., eds.) Excerpta Medica, Amsterdam, **1968.**

Symposium. (Various authors.) Hyperparathyroidism. (Forscher, B. K., and Arnaud, C. D., eds.) *Am. J. Med.,* **1971,** *50,* 557–699.

Symposium. (Various authors.) Parathyroid hormone, calcitonin and vitamin D: clinical considerations. (Forscher, B. K., and Arnaud, C. D., eds.) *Am. J. Med.,* **1974,** *56,* 743–870; *57,* 1–62.

Tenenhouse, A.; Rasmussen, H.; Hawker, C. D.; and Arnaud, C. D. Thyrocalcitonin. *A. Rev. Pharmac.,* **1968,** *8,* 319–336.

XVIII

The Vitamins

INTRODUCTION

Paul Greengard

A vitamin may be broadly defined as a substance that is essential for the maintenance of normal metabolic functions but is not synthesized in the body and, therefore, must be furnished from an exogenous source. A healthy individual ingesting a well-balanced diet receives adequate amounts of vitamins from his food. Vitamins obtained in this normal manner can scarcely be regarded as drugs. However, there are many situations in which the concentration of one or more vitamins in the body tissues may be suboptimal. When such exigencies arise or can be anticipated, it is the common practice to administer vitamins in chemically pure form. When employed in this manner, vitamins must be regarded as drugs and a knowledge of their pharmacological properties is desirable. Also, large doses of various vitamins are frequently employed for the treatment of disorders that are not etiologically related to vitamin deficiency. The implication is that such large doses may exert pharmacodynamic actions that are useful in therapy. Although many such claims have been made, few are supported by carefully controlled objective studies. In therapeutic regimens of this type the vitamins often represent nothing more than expensive placebos. Furthermore, excessive administration of certain of the vitamins, notably the lipid-soluble vitamins, can cause toxic manifestations.

Recommended Dietary Allowances. Probably no single class of drugs has been the target of as much quackery, misunderstanding, misrepresentation, and misuse as the vitamins, despite the fact that far more is known about these compounds, including their mechanism of action, than about any other group of substances in the U.S.P. The governments of several countries throughout the world have established scientific committees that have carried out carefully controlled studies to evaluate the vitamin and other nutritional requirements of their citizens. In the United States, a Food and Nutrition Board was established for this purpose under the auspices of the National Academy of Sciences–National Research Council. This Board is composed of a number of scientists of outstanding caliber in the field of human nutrition. Since 1940, the Board has prepared periodically a brochure that contains a set of "Recommended Dietary Allowances" (RDA) for vitamins and other nutrients, based on the existing knowledge of nutritional science. These recommendations are subject to revision as new knowledge becomes available. The 1974 revision of the RDA of the Food and Nutrition Board is reproduced in Table XVIII–1. In large measure, the recommendations of the Board are based on carefully controlled investigations in human volunteers fed diets normal in all respects except the amount of the one nutrient being studied. Through such investigations it has been possible to estimate human requirements for several of the vitamins quite accurately.

The RDA are intended to serve as goals in planning food supplies and as guides for the interpretation of food consumption records. The Board has clearly specified a series of limitations to the usefulness of their data. If, for example, the RDA are used as reference standards for interpreting records of food consumption, it cannot be assumed that food practices are

Table XVIII-1. RECOMMENDED DAILY DIETARY ALLOWANCES [a]

	Age (years)	Weight (kg)	Height (cm)	Energy (kcal)[b]	Protein (g)	FAT-SOLUBLE VITAMINS Vitamin A Activity (RE)[c]	Vitamin A Activity (IU)	Vitamin D (IU)	Vitamin E Activity[e] (IU)	WATER-SOLUBLE VITAMINS Ascorbic Acid (mg)	Folacin[f] (µg)	Niacin[g] (mg)	Riboflavin (mg)	Thiamin (mg)	Vitamin B6 (mg)	Vitamin B12 (µg)	MINERALS Calcium (mg)	Phosphorus (mg)	Iodine (µg)	Iron (mg)	Magnesium (mg)	Zinc (mg)
Infants	0.0–0.5	6	60	kg × 117	kg × 2.2	420[d]	1400	400	4	35	50	5	0.4	0.3	0.3	0.3	360	240	35	10	60	3
	0.5–1.0	9	71	kg × 108	kg × 2.0	400	2000	400	5	35	50	8	0.6	0.5	0.4	0.3	540	400	45	15	70	5
Children	1–3	13	86	1300	23	400	2000	400	7	40	100	9	0.8	0.7	0.6	1.0	800	800	60	15	150	10
	4–6	20	110	1800	30	500	2500	400	9	40	200	12	1.1	0.9	0.9	1.5	800	800	80	10	200	10
	7–10	30	135	2400	36	700	3300	400	10	40	300	16	1.2	1.2	1.2	2.0	800	800	110	10	250	10
Males	11–14	44	158	2800	44	1000	5000	400	12	45	400	18	1.5	1.4	1.6	3.0	1200	1200	130	18	350	15
	15–18	61	172	3000	54	1000	5000	400	15	45	400	20	1.8	1.5	2.0	3.0	1200	1200	150	18	400	15
	19–22	67	172	3000	54	1000	5000	400	15	45	400	20	1.8	1.5	2.0	3.0	800	800	140	10	350	15
	23–50	70	172	2700	56	1000	5000		15	45	400	18	1.6	1.4	2.0	3.0	800	800	130	10	350	15
	51+	70	172	2400	56	1000	5000		15	45	400	16	1.5	1.2	2.0	3.0	800	800	110	10	350	15
Females	11–14	44	155	2400	44	800	4000	400	12	45	400	16	1.3	1.2	1.6	3.0	1200	1200	115	18	300	15
	15–18	54	162	2100	48	800	4000	400	12	45	400	14	1.4	1.1	2.0	3.0	1200	1200	115	18	300	15
	19–22	58	162	2100	46	800	4000	400	12	45	400	14	1.4	1.1	2.0	3.0	800	800	100	18	300	15
	23–50	58	162	2000	46	800	4000		12	45	400	13	1.2	1.0	2.0	3.0	800	800	100	18	300	15
	51+	58	162	1800	46	800	4000		12	45	400	12	1.1	1.0	2.0	3.0	800	800	80	10	300	15
Pregnant				+300	+30	1000	5000	400	15	60	800	+2	+0.3	+0.3	2.5	4.0	1200	1200	125	18+ [h]	450	20
Lactating				+500	+20	1200	6000	400	15	80	600	+4	+0.5	+0.3	2.5	4.0	1200	1200	150	18	450	25

[a] The allowances are intended to provide for individual variations among most normal persons as they live in the United States under usual environmental stresses. Diets should be based on a variety of common foods in order to provide other nutrients for which human requirements have been less well defined.

[b] Kilojoules (kJ) = 4.2 × kcal.

[c] Retinol equivalents.

[d] Assumed to be all as retinol in milk during the first six months of life. All subsequent intakes are assumed to be half as retinol and half as β-carotene when calculated from international units. As retinol equivalents, three fourths are as retinol and one fourth as β-carotene.

[e] Total vitamin E activity, estimated to be 80 percent as α-tocopherol and 20 percent other tocopherols.

[f] The folacin allowances refer to dietary sources as determined by Lactobacillus casei assay. Pure forms of folacin may be effective in doses less than one fourth of the recommended dietary allowance.

[g] Although allowances are expressed as niacin, it is recognized that on the average 1 mg of niacin is derived from each 60 mg of dietary tryptophan.

[h] This increased requirement cannot be met by ordinary diets; therefore, the use of supplemental iron is recommended.

(Modified from Food and Nutrition Board, National Research Council, 1974.)

necessarily poor or that malnutrition exists because the standards are not completely met. The allowances recommended in Table XVIII–1 are those that, in the opinion of the Food and Nutrition Board, will maintain good nutrition in essentially healthy persons in the United States under current conditions of living. The physiological and biochemical bases for the recommended allowances of each specific nutrient are discussed by the Board in great detail in their report (1974), along with the following general comments:

> RDA are recommendations for the amounts of nutrients that should be consumed daily. They are neither estimates of the amounts of nutrients needed per capita in the national or local food supply, nor even in the food purchased. Thus, losses of nutrients that occur during the processing and preparation of food should be taken into consideration in planning diets based on tables of food composition.
>
> RDA *should not be confused with requirements.* Differences in the nutrient requirements of individuals that derive from differences in their genetic makeup are ordinarily unknown. Therefore, as there is no way of predicting whose needs are high and whose are low, RDA (except for energy) are estimated to exceed the requirements of most individuals, and thereby ensure that the needs of nearly all are met.

The Board has also carried out and included in their report an authoritative analysis of the current state of knowledge concerning various other nutrients, including carbohydrate and fat, essential fatty acids, water, sodium, potassium and chloride, copper, fluorine, various trace elements, pantothenic acid, biotin, choline, and vitamin K. A careful perusal of the short, lucid, and authoritative report of the Food and Nutrition Board is highly recommended.

Excessive Intake of Vitamins. The practicing physician is exposed to pressures from two types of extremists in the area of vitaminology. One group of extremists, with representatives both in medical practice and in a few pharmaceutical houses, recommends large intakes of vitamins both for prophylactic purposes and for the treatment of an enormous variety of illnesses for which evidence of therapeutic efficacy of the vitamins is lacking. Many millions of individuals living in the United States regularly ingest quantities of vitamins vastly in excess of the RDA. In the case of the water-soluble vitamins, this would seem to do little harm to the body because of the low toxicity of this class of compounds. However, such practice is economically wasteful and, in some instances, causes financial hardship. The low toxicity of the water-soluble vitamins is probably attributable to the fact that excess quantities of these substances are rapidly excreted in the urine. In the case of the lipid-soluble vitamins, the compounds accumulate in the body fat and can be toxic. The conscientious physician should assure himself that his patients are not victims of the excessive use of vitamins. It is extremely important to distinguish between supplemental and therapeutic vitamin preparations. The latter contain much larger quantities of the individual vitamins than do the supplemental preparations. They should be used only by physicians to cure deficiency diseases or to provide prophylactic treatment of patients with disorders involving greatly increased vitamin requirements. A certain amount of the controversy about the desirability of vitamin supplementation has arisen from a failure to distinguish between the use of vitamins as dietary supplements and their use as therapeutic agents. Unfortunately, a wide variety of therapeutic multivitamin preparations containing many times the daily allowances recommended by the Food and Nutrition Board have been sold as "dietary supplements" without a prescription. A strong argument can be made in favor of placing an upper limit on the potency of vitamin preparations that can be sold without a prescription. Although this has been done for vitamins A and D, the United States Food and Drug Administration, as described below, has proposed regulations concerning the sale of other vitamins and minerals, which, if adopted, should provide the consumer with some protection in this area.

Deficient Intake of Vitamins. The second group of extremists in the area of vitaminology consists of those who, in reaction to the excessive use of vitamins, have campaigned with a certain degree of success against the use of vitamins in any instances except cases of unequivocal vitamin deficiency. In actual fact, the use of vitamins as *dietary supplements* should be considered by the physician in a wide variety of situations. Such situations may result from (1) inadequate intake, (2) disturbance in absorption, and (3) increased tissue requirements. Each of these three categories will be discussed briefly.

Vitamin deficiency due to an *inadequate intake* arises in a variety of circumstances. There are still large parts of the world and even considerable areas in the United States where, owing to poverty, the population eats a diet inadequate in terms of vitamin content. Moreover, there are areas where the prevalence in the diet of one particular type of food results in a relatively high incidence of avitaminosis. Eccentric diets resulting from psychiatric disturbance, individual idiosyncrasies, religious beliefs, or food faddism (such as is observed among vegetarians) are another major cause of vitamin deficiency. A decrease in food consumption because of excess use of alcoholic beverages, poor appetite, dieting to combat obesity, or restricted diets prescribed by physicians for the management of specific diseases represents a further group of situations in which vitamin deficiency can arise.

A *disturbance in absorption* of vitamins is also seen in a variety of conditions. Examples are diseases of the liver and biliary tract, prolonged diarrhea from any cause, hyperthyroidism, pernicious anemia, sprue, and a variety of other disorders of the digestive system. Moreover, since a substantial proportion of certain of the vitamins is provided by the bacteria of the gastrointestinal tract, treatment with antimicrobials that alter the intestinal bacterial flora leads inevitably to a decreased vitamin absorption.

Increased tissue requirements for vitamins also occur under a variety of conditions so that a nutritional deficiency may develop on a diet that had previously been adequate. Such situations can occur in both health and disease. In healthy individuals, for example, there is a greater requirement for various nutrients, including vitamins, during growth, during periods of hard physical work, and during pregnancy, lactation, and menstruation. Diseases associated with an increased metabolism, such as hyperthyroidism, and conditions accompanied by fever or tissue wasting also increase the body's requirements for vitamins. There is also good evidence that vitamin requirements increase during stress.

Multiple-Vitamin Therapy. It is clear from the preceding discussion that supplemental vitamin intake is desirable in a variety of situations. Since deficiency of a single vitamin is rarely encountered clinically, it is customary practice in cases of suspected vitamin deficiency, as well as in prophylactic treatment, to recommend that multiple-vitamin therapy be administered.

The only official multivitamin preparations are decavitamin capsules and tablets. *Decavitamin Capsules,* U.S.P., contain in each capsule not less than the labeled amounts of retinol in the form of vitamin A; vitamin D from natural sources or as ergocalciferol or cholecalciferol or the products obtained by the activation of either ergosterol or 7-dehydrocholesterol; ascorbic acid or its equivalent as sodium ascorbate; calcium pantothenate or its equivalent as racemic calcium pantothenate or as D-panthenol or racemic panthenol; cyanocobalamin; folic acid; nicotinamide; pyridoxine hydrochloride; riboflavin; thiamine hydrochloride or its equivalent as thiamine mononitrate; and a suitable form of alpha-tocopherol. The specifications for *Decavitamin Tablets,* U.S.P., are identical to those for the capsules. There are no longer any official multivitamin-rich concentrates.

New Regulations on Vitamins and Minerals. Based on the study of the Food and Nutrition Board (1974), the United States Food and Drug Administration (FDA) has proposed new regulations on vitamins and minerals (*FDA Drug Bulletin,* December, 1973). The purposes of the regulations are: to distinguish between the three basic uses of nutrients (in food as a part of the ordinary diet, in dietary supplements as insurance against an inadequate diet, and in drugs for therapeutic purposes); to prevent consumer deception by prohibiting unwarranted and false promotional and labeling claims; and to prevent irrational and unjustified combinations of nutrients in dietary supplements. The key factor in the new regulations would be the establishment of a standard for products marketed as dietary supplements. The key change that would result from the regulations is that consumers could be sure that products labeled as dietary supplements contain reasonable and rational amounts and combinations of nutrients to achieve dietary supplementation.

The FDA proposals are based on the United States Recommended Daily Allowances (U.S. RDA), a set of values derived by the FDA from the RDA of the Food and Nutrition Board. FDA has divided all products containing vitamins and minerals into three categories. (1) Products supplemented so they contain up to 50% of the U.S. RDA of vitamins and minerals are *ordinary foods*. (2) With three exceptions, all products supplemented so as to contain 50 to 150% of the U.S. RDA are *dietary supplements*. (The three exceptions are vitamins A and D and folic acid; the upper limits for these are set at 100% of the U.S. RDA.) Dietary supplements in tablets, capsules, or other dosage forms may be composed of any one of the vitamins or minerals listed in Table XVIII–1, as well as of biotin, pantothenic acid, or copper, either alone or in certain specified combinations. Generally, these combinations include vitamins and minerals, vitamins only, minerals only, and vitamins plus iron. (3) Vitamin and mineral preparations that contain more than 150% of the U.S. RDA exceed food requirements and are deemed appropriate only for the treatment of vitamin-mineral deficiencies or for some other medical purpose. It is misleading to represent these high-potency products to the public as dietary supplements. Therefore, they are classified as drugs, and it is proposed that they must be labeled and sold as such.

If these proposals are adopted, existing nonprescription vitamin and mineral drug products will remain on the market unchanged as long as they are prominently designated for drug purposes and are not represented as dietary supplements. Any vitamin or mineral preparation, regardless of potency, that is promoted with claims that it will prevent, treat, or cure a disease is by law not a "food" but a "drug." Therapeutic claims will continue to be permissible for vitamin or mineral drug products if such claims are in fact supported by scientific proof.

Unfortunately, the above-described proposal (3) generated considerable controversy, criticism coming especially from vitamin and health-food manufacturers and other interested parties. The proposals are generally supported by nutrition experts and consumer groups. However, in mid-1975, the FDA reconsidered its position, and the fate of the original proposals is uncertain.

No U.S. RDA have been established for essential nutrients that are not appropriate for addition to general-purpose foods for dietary supplements. These nutrients include choline, vitamin K, chlorine, fluorine, manganese, potassium, sodium, and sulfur. They may be added to special dietary foods, such as infant formulas, and to other foods for use solely under medical supervision to meet nutritional requirements in specific medical conditions.

The FDA singled out vitamins A and D as requiring special attention, and new regulations are now in force. Under current FDA regulations, any preparation of vitamin A with more than 10,000 International Units per dosage unit (twice the U.S. RDA for adults) or any preparation of vitamin D with more than 400 International Units (the U.S. RDA) per dosage unit can be dispensed by prescription only.

CHAPTER

73 WATER-SOLUBLE VITAMINS

The Vitamin B Complex

Paul Greengard

The vitamin B complex comprises a large number of vitamins that differ greatly in chemical structure and biological action. They are grouped together because all are water soluble and can be obtained in relatively high yields from the same sources, notably liver and yeast. However, these are by no means the only natural sources of the various members of the group of vitamins discussed in this chapter.

"Vitamin B" was one of the first of the dietary essentials to be recognized, and the preparation from rice polishings, by Funk in 1911, of a water-soluble concentrate active in the cure of beriberi was an important contribution not only to the chemistry of vitamin B but to the establishment of the concept of deficiency disease. The term *water-soluble vitamin B* was introduced by McCollum and Kennedy in 1916 to describe that dietary substance necessary for growth in rats, and seemingly essential for the prevention of beriberi, which was distinct from fat-soluble vitamin A, the latter having already been described by McCollum and associates. It soon became evident, however, that vitamin B was a complex rather than a single entity. Nine of the compounds generally considered as members of the vitamin B complex, namely, thiamine, riboflavin, nicotinic acid, pyridoxine, pantothenic acid, biotin, choline, inositol, and para-aminobenzoic acid, are discussed in this chapter, although the significance of several of these factors in human nutrition remains to be established. Folic acid (pteroylglutamic acid) and cyanocobalamin (vitamin B_{12}) are considered in Chapter 64 because of their important functions in hematopoiesis. Other possible factors in the B complex have not been characterized sufficiently to warrant discussion of their pharmacological properties or potential uses.

THIAMINE

History. Thiamine was the first member of the vitamin B complex to be identified chemically. Events leading to its isolation actually date back to the late nineteenth century, when Takaki dramatically reduced the incidence of beriberi in the Japanese Navy by instituting certain reforms in the diet. Soon thereafter, Eijkman, a Dutch physician in Java, demonstrated that individuals who developed beriberi while subsisting largely on polished rice could be cured of their disease by the addition of rice polishings to the diet. Moreover, he reproduced these clinical findings experimentally in chickens. Some time later, Funk isolated from rice polishings and yeast a crystalline substance that was effective in the prevention and the cure of experimental beriberi. The compound contained basic nitrogen and was believed to be an amine. It also was essential for life. Therefore, Funk called the substance *vitamine*, a term widely adopted to designate accessory food substances and retained as the word *vitamin* when further research revealed the broad chemical spectrum of the dietary essentials. Following the demonstration of the multiple nature of vitamin B, the anti-beriberi factor was designated *vitamin B_1*.

In 1926, vitamin B_1 was isolated in crystalline form by Jansen and Donath, and in 1936 Williams determined its structure, which he verified by synthesis in the same year. The Council on Pharmacy and Chemistry adopted the name *thiamine* to designate crystalline vitamin B_1, and this is now the official U.S.P. name of the vitamin. Similarly, other members of the vitamin B complex were given official names following their chemical identification.

Chemistry. Thiamine is a complex organic molecule containing a pyrimidine and a thiazole nucleus. The pyrimidine structure is common in nature, but the thiazole nucleus is unique and appears, so far as is known, only in thiamine. Thiamine carries out its function in the body in the form of the coenzyme thiamine pyrophosphate. The structures of thiamine and thiamine pyrophosphate are as follows:

The conversion of thiamine to its coenzyme form is carried out with adenosine triphosphate (ATP) as a pyrophosphate (PP) donor:

$$\text{Thiamine} + \text{ATP} \longrightarrow \text{Thiamine} - \text{PP} + \text{AMP}$$

Antimetabolites to thiamine have been synthesized. The most important of these are neopyrithiamine (pyrithiamine) and oxythiamine.

Pharmacological Actions. Thiamine is practically devoid of pharmacodynamic actions when given in the therapeutic dose range. There may be slight vasodilatation and a fall in blood pressure following rapid intravenous injection, but this is transitory. Even large doses have no effect on the blood sugar concentration despite the fact that the physiological role of the vitamin is concerned with the intermediary metabolism of carbohydrate.

There have been isolated clinical reports of *toxic reactions* to the parenteral administration of thiamine. They probably represent rare instances of hypersensitivity.

Physiological Function. Thiamine pyrophosphate (diphosphothiamine), the physiologically active form of thiamine, functions in carbohydrate metabolism as a coenzyme in the decarboxylation of pyruvic and α-ketoglutaric acids and in the utilization of pentose in the hexose monophosphate shunt. Several facts of clinical importance can be related directly to the cellular action of thiamine. In thiamine deficiency the oxidation of α-keto acids is impaired. An increase in the concentration of pyruvic acid in the blood is one of the diagnostic signs of the deficiency state. A more specific diagnostic test for thiamine deficiency is based upon measurement of transketolase activity in erythrocytes (Brin, 1968). The requirement for thiamine is related to metabolic rate and is greatest when carbohydrate is the source of energy. This is of practical significance in patients being maintained by parenteral alimentation, who receive practically all their calories in the form of dextrose. Such patients should receive a generous allowance of the vitamin.

Symptoms of Deficiency. Severe thiamine deficiency leads to the condition known as beriberi. Beriberi was described as a disease entity long before the concept of vitamins was established. It was one of the first deficiency diseases to be recognized. Beriberi can be diagnosed easily and treated specifically, and its prevalence in the Far East, where it used to be common, is much reduced.

The chief symptoms of thiamine deficiency are related to the nervous and cardiovascular systems. Many of the neurological symptoms and signs are characteristic of peripheral neuritis. A sense of heaviness and weakness in the limbs is followed by marked sensory disturbances in the extremities, such as localized areas of hyperesthesia or anesthesia,

aching, and burning. The nerve trunks are tender to pressure. Muscle strength is gradually lost, and in extreme cases there may be foot-drop or wrist-drop, shuffling gait, and even complete paralysis of a limb. The legs are usually affected more than the arms. The central nervous system (CNS) is also affected by the deficiency. Nervousness, fatigability, personality disturbances, irritability, moodiness, depression, lack of initiative and interest, and poor concentration and memory may result from lack of the vitamin.

Cardiovascular symptoms are also prominent. It is often said that these develop late in the course of the deficiency, but careful observations indicate that severe circulatory disturbances may be evident before the CNS lesions have become sufficiently advanced to cause incapacitation. The following symptoms and signs referable to the cardiovascular system may be the result of thiamine deficiency: dyspnea on exertion, palpitation, tachycardia and embryocardia, gallop rhythm, prominent cardiac and epigastric pulsations, bounding peripheral pulse, enlarged heart, elevated venous pressure, edema, diminished vital capacity, and an abnormal ECG characterized chiefly by flattening or inversion of the T wave and prolongation of the Q-T interval. An interesting finding of considerable diagnostic importance is an abnormally high cardiac output and an increased velocity of blood flow due to arteriolar dilatation associated with the above signs of cardiac insufficiency.

Symptoms referable to the gastrointestinal tract are also observed in severe cases of deficiency. Loss of appetite occurs early and is followed by intestinal atony and constipation, and later by epigastric distress and tenderness. A form of thiamine deficiency known as *wet beriberi* is characterized by extensive edema. The fluid is lost from the plasma largely as a result of hypoproteinemia from an inadequate intake of protein plus the added factor of poor cardiac function.

The more severe grades of the deficiency in infants may run a rapid and fulminating course. Gastrointestinal symptoms may herald the onset. They consist in loss of appetite, vomiting, and greenish stools. This is soon followed by paroxysmal attacks of muscular rigidity, during which the body is held tense and straight. The pulse becomes small and rapid, the face is cyanotic, and the neck veins are engorged. Dysfunction of the vocal cords may result in a characteristic type of plaintive cry or even in aphonia. Death may follow the initial symptoms within 12 to 24 hours unless vigorous treatment is instituted.

The symptoms of *mild thiamine deficiency* are not as characteristic as those of the severe form, and the condition may easily escape diagnosis. It is now appreciated that beriberi is merely the fulminating type of a deficiency disease that is not rare. The symptoms include loss of appetite, muscular weakness, pain and paresthesias in the extremities, a tendency to edema, decreased blood pressure, and low body temperature. The diagnosis may be confirmed by a careful study of the dietary history and by determination of erythrocyte transketolase activity. Thiamine deficiency, however, may occur in association with an apparently adequate diet, for the vitamin is not stored in the body to a great extent. Thus, an increase in metabolic rate or a gastrointestinal disturbance, such as diarrhea of fairly long duration, necessitates an increased thiamine intake. Mild deficiency is also observed in infancy and childhood. The symptoms are pallor, loss of weight, restlessness, slight stiffness of the neck, and spasticity of the extremities.

Human Requirement. Thiamine requirement is a function of metabolic rate. The minimal thiamine requirement in humans approximates 0.33 mg/1000 kcal. However, to provide a margin of safety, the Food and Nutrition Board of the National Research Council recommends a daily thiamine allowance of 0.5 mg/1000 kcal (*see* Table XVIII–1, page 1545).

Absorption, Fate, and Excretion. Absorption of thiamine following intramuscular administration is rapid and complete. In contrast, absorption from the gastrointestinal tract is limited, with a maximal daily absorption of 8 to 15 mg. This can be achieved by the oral administration of 40 mg in divided doses with food. Thiamine is absorbed from the small intestine and the duodenum by two processes, one active and the other passive (Rindi and Ventura, 1972). There is no evidence that the thiamine synthesized by intestinal bacteria represents an available source of vitamin.

Approximately 1 mg of thiamine per day is completely degraded by the tissues. This amount is roughly the minimal daily requirement. When intake is at this low level, little or no thiamine is excreted in the urine. When intake exceeds the minimal requirement, tissue stores are first saturated. Thereafter the excess appears quantitatively in the urine either as pyrimidine or as thiamine. The pyrimidine arises from the degradative splitting of the thiamine molecule. When intake of thiamine exceeds metabolic needs by a few milligrams daily, a large proportion appears in the urine as pyrimidine. As the intake of thiamine is further increased, more of the excess is excreted unchanged, indicating that the capacity of the tissues to split thiamine to pyrimidine is limited.

Preparations. Thiamine can be prescribed as the pure vitamin, in mixtures of pure vitamins, or in the form of vitamin-rich concentrates.

Thiamine Hydrochloride, U.S.P. (*vitamin B$_1$ hydrochloride*), occurs as small, white crystals or as a crystalline powder. *Thiamine Hydrochloride Tablets,* U.S.P., can usually be obtained in sizes ranging from 5 to 250 mg. *Thiamine Hydrochloride Injection,* U.S.P., is a sterile solution of thiamine hydrochloride in water. Preparations available usually contain 50, 100, or 200 mg/ml. Thiamine is also available as *thiamine hydrochloride elixir* (2.25 mg/5 ml). In addition, thiamine is obtainable as the mononitrate salt, *Thiamine Mononitrate,* U.S.P.

Therapeutic Uses. The only established therapeutic value of thiamine is in the treatment or the prophylaxis of thiamine deficiency. When thiamine deficiency has been diagnosed, it is desirable to correct the disorder as rapidly as possible. Therefore, the use of the parenteral route and of doses as large as 30 mg three times daily is justified. Once thiamine deficiency has been corrected, there is no need for parenteral injection or the administration of amounts in excess of daily requirement. The only exception to the above statement is in instances when gastrointestinal disturbances preclude the ingestion or absorption of adequate amounts of the vitamin. A few clinical conditions resulting from dietary deficiency of thiamine will be described briefly.

Alcoholic Neuritis. Jolliffe and coworkers (1936) demonstrated that alcoholic neuritis is basically a nutritional deficiency due to an inadequate intake of thiamine, and alcoholism is the most common cause of thiamine deficiency in the United States. Two factors contribute to bring about an inadequate intake in the chronic alcoholic. Appetite is usually poor, and this leads to a diminished food intake. In addition, a large portion of the caloric intake is in the form of alcohol itself. The symptoms of neurological involvement in alcoholics are those of a polyneuritis with motor and sensory defects. The response to thiamine administration is slow if structural damage has occurred.

Wernicke's syndrome is an additional serious consequence of alcoholism and thiamine deficiency in the Occident. Certain characteristic signs of this disease, notably ophthalmoplegia, nystagmus, and ataxia, respond rapidly to the administration of thiamine but to no other vitamin. However, Wernicke's encephalopathy is usually accompanied by signs of Korsakoff's psychosis, characterized by a striking impairment of retentive memory, inability to acquire new information, and confabulation. Delay in therapy ensures the permanent nature of these changes, and signs of Wernicke's disease are thus considered to constitute a medical emergency. The patient requires *immediate* parenteral therapy with thiamine. It should be recalled that intravenous administration of glucose-containing solutions to the alcoholic may place an additional strain on a limited supply of thiamine, and such treatment may precipitate symptoms if vitamins are not also supplied.

Neuritis of Pregnancy. Pregnancy increases the thiamine requirement slightly. The neuritis of pregnancy takes the form of multiple peripheral nerve involvement, and the signs and symptoms in well-developed cases resemble those described for beriberi. It occurs when the diet is poor or in patients with hyperemesis gravidarum. Proof that the neuritis is due to a thiamine deficiency is gained in those cases in which dramatic clinical improvement is observed after thiamine therapy. The dose employed is from 5 to 10 mg daily, given parenterally if vomiting is severe.

Subacute Necrotizing Encephalomyelopathy (SNE, Leigh's Disease). SNE is a fatal, genetic disease in children, with brain lesions very similar to those in Wernicke's encephalopathy. Extracts of spinal fluid, blood, and urine of patients with SNE inhibit a phosphoryl transferase in brain that catalyzes the synthesis of thiamine triphosphate from thiamine pyrophosphate. Moreover, the brain of SNE patients at autopsy is essentially devoid of thiamine triphosphate, in contrast to normal brains. While the biological role of thiamine triphosphate is unknown, about 10% of the total thiamine in the body is normally in this form. The presence of the inhibitor in urine has been used successfully to diagnose SNE. When patients with SNE are treated daily with large doses of thiamine, most exhibit marked temporary improvement (Pincus *et al.,* 1973).

Cardiovascular Disease. Cardiovascular disease of nutritional origin is observed in chronic alcoholics, pregnant women, persons with gastrointestinal disorders, and those whose diet is deficient for other reasons. When the diagnosis of cardiovascular disease of dietary origin has been correctly made, the response to thiamine therapy is striking. As has already been stated, one of the pathognomonic features of the syndrome is an increased blood flow due to arteriolar dilatation. Within a few hours after the administration of thiamine, the rate of blood flow is reduced and the utilization of oxygen is increased as a result of the improved circulation. If edema is present and due to myocardial insufficiency, diuresis results after proper therapy. The rate of improvement is seemingly inversely proportional to the rate of onset and duration of the disease, and individuals suffering from a chronic deficiency may require protracted treatment. The usual dose of thiamine is 10 to 30 mg three times daily, given parenterally. The dosage can be reduced and the patient maintained on oral medication or by dietary management after signs of the deficiency state have been relieved.

Gastrointestinal Disorders. In experimental and clinical beriberi, certain symptoms are referable to the gastrointestinal tract. On this meager basis, thiamine has been used uncritically as a therapeutic agent for such unrelated conditions as ulcerative colitis, gastrointestinal hypotonia, and chronic diarrhea. Unless the disease being treated is the direct result of a deficiency, there is no reason to expect thiamine to act beneficially. Thiamine may be used, however, as a dietary supplement (along with other vitamins) if it is believed that insufficient amounts are being absorbed. For example, in cases of chronic diarrhea, especially in infants, the prophylactic administration of thiamine may prevent the development of deficiency symptoms. Similar considerations apply for patients with intestinal resections and fistulas.

RIBOFLAVIN

History. Riboflavin was first identified in milk by Blyth in 1879. At that time the substance was called lactochrome because of its source and its intense yellow color. Its physiological significance was not appreciated. At a later date similarly pigmented compounds were isolated from a variety of sources and designated as flavins, prefixed with source names (*e.g.,* lacto-, ovo-, hepato-, etc.) to indicate the material from which they were extracted. It was soon demonstrated that these various flavins are identical in chemical composition.

In the meantime, water-soluble vitamin B had been separated into a heat-labile anti-beriberi factor and a heat-stable growth-promoting factor. The two factors were called vitamins B_1 and B_2 by British and vitamins F and G by American investigators. The British terminology became generally adopted. It was soon appreciated that concentrates of the so-called vitamin B_2 had a yellow color, the intensity of which was related to vitamin activity. It was then demonstrated that crystalline lactoflavin had the same chemical properties and biological activity as the pigmented substance in the vitamin concentrates. All doubt as to the identity of vitamin B_2 and the naturally occurring flavins was removed when lactoflavin was synthesized and the synthetic product was shown to possess full biological activity. The vitamin was designated as *riboflavin* by the Council on Pharmacy and Chemistry because of the presence of ribose in its structure. The term later became official in the U.S.P.

Chemistry. Riboflavin carries out its functions in the body in the form of one or the other of two coenzymes, riboflavin phosphate (flavin mononucleotide, FMN) and flavin adenine dinucleotide (FAD). The structures of riboflavin, FMN, and FAD are shown on the next page. Riboflavin is converted to FMN and FAD by two enzyme-catalyzed reactions (*see* Brown and Reynolds, 1963, for review):

1. Riboflavin + ATP $\longrightarrow$ FMN + ADP

2. FMN + ATP $\longrightarrow$ FAD + PP

Pharmacological Actions. No overt pharmacodynamic actions accompany the oral or parenteral administration of riboflavin.

Physiological Function. FMN and FAD, the physiologically active forms of riboflavin, serve a vital role in metabolism as coenzymes for a wide variety of respiratory proteins.

Symptoms of Deficiency. The symptoms of riboflavin deficiency in man have been thoroughly reviewed by Rivlin (1970). Sore throat and angular stomatitis generally appear first. Later, glossitis, seborrheic dermatitis of the face, and dermatitis over the trunk and extremities occur, followed by anemia and neuropathy. Changes in the epithelium are impressive in experimental riboflavin deficiency, with atrophy, hyperkeratosis, and hyperplasia of the skin. In some subjects, corneal vascularization and cataract formation are prominent.

The anemia that develops in riboflavin deficiency is normochromic and normocytic; this is associated with diminished reticulocytosis, but members of the leukocyte and megakaryocyte series are generally well preserved. Administration of riboflavin to deficient patients restores the reticulocyte count and the hemoglobin concentration to normal, and reticulocytosis is first noted 2 to 5 days after initiation of therapy. Anemia in riboflavin deficiency may be related, at least in part, to disturbances in folic acid metabolism.

The problem in the clinical recognition of riboflavin deficiency is that certain features, such as glossitis and dermatitis, are common signs and may be seen with deficiencies of other vitamins as well. Recognition of riboflavin deficiency is also difficult because it rarely occurs as an isolated finding. In nutritional surveys of children in an urban area and of randomly selected hospitalized patients, deficiency of riboflavin was frequently observed, but almost invariably in conjunction with other vitamin deficiencies.

Human Requirement. The requirements for this vitamin are related fairly closely to energy expenditure (Bro-Rasmussen, 1958). The minimal requirement for riboflavin to prevent clinical signs of deficiency appears to be about 0.3 mg/1000 kcal. Intakes of less than 0.25 mg/1000 kcal have produced, in adult human subjects, clinical signs of deficiency involving ocular, nasal, oral, and genital lesions. Studies of urinary excretion of riboflavin, both endogenous and following a test dose of riboflavin, also suggest the same minimal requirement. However, to provide a margin of safety the Food and Nutrition Board of the National Research Council recommends a somewhat higher riboflavin allowance, which is calculated on the basis of "metabolic body size."

Absorption, Fate, and Excretion. Riboflavin is readily absorbed from the upper gastrointestinal tract (Rivlin, 1970), but the rate of this process is reduced in patients with hepatitis or hepatic cirrhosis and in those receiving probenecid. The vitamin is also readily absorbed following parenteral administration. It is distributed in all tissues, but little is stored and tissue concentrations are uniformly low. The relationship of riboflavin intake to urinary excretion has been studied very thoroughly (Horwitt et al., 1950). When riboflavin is ingested in amounts that approximate the minimal daily requirement, only about 9% appears in the urine. The metabolic fate of the remainder is unknown. As the intake of riboflavin is increased above minimal requirements, larger proportions are excreted unchanged in the urine.

Riboflavin is always present in the feces and probably represents vitamin synthesized by intestinal microorganisms. On low intakes of riboflavin, the amount excreted in the feces is in excess of that ingested. Fecal riboflavin appears to be within the bacterial cells, and there is no evidence that it can be absorbed.

Preparations. *Riboflavin*, U.S.P. (*vitamin B₂*), is a yellow to orange-yellow crystalline powder, having a slight odor, and soluble in water only to the extent of 1 mg in 3 to about 20 ml. The variations in solubility are due to differences in the internal crystalline structure of riboflavin. The vitamin is more soluble in isotonic sodium chloride solution. When dry, riboflavin is not affected appreciably by light; however, when it is in solution, light induces quite rapid deterioration, especially at alkaline pH. *Riboflavin Tablets*, U.S.P., are usually available in sizes ranging from 3 to 100 mg. *Riboflavin Injection*, U.S.P., is a sterile solution of riboflavin in water. For purposes of increasing the solubility of the riboflavin, official preparations may contain suitable, harmless, solubilizing agents. Available preparations for injection usually contain 35 mg/ml.

Therapeutic Uses. The only established therapeutic application of riboflavin is in the treatment or prevention of deficiency disease. Ariboflavinosis seldom occurs as a discrete deficiency but usually accompanies other nutritional diseases, particularly pellagra. Therefore, therapy of ariboflavinosis should include other members of the B complex in addition to riboflavin. Specific therapy with riboflavin consists in the oral administration of 5 to 10 mg daily. The parenteral route may occasionally be necessary to ensure adequate absorption.

NICOTINIC ACID

History. The classical work of Goldberger and coworkers in the United States Public Health Service did much to establish pellagra as a deficiency disease resulting from an inadequate intake of what was then thought to be vitamin B_2. Goldberger fed deficient diets to dogs and produced the condition known as "black tongue," which he believed to be analogous to human pellagra. Indeed, the same diet fed to man produced the classical signs and symptoms of pellagra. In rats, the diet caused a marked dermatitis. The three conditions could be cured by dietary measures.

In 1913, long before Goldberger started his experimental study of pellagra, Funk isolated from rice polishings a compound that he identified as *nicotinic acid*. Funk determined that nicotinic acid was ineffective in the treatment of experimental polyneuritis, and interest in the compound waned. Warburg and associates in 1935 obtained nicotinic acid amide (nicotinamide) from a coenzyme isolated from the red blood corpuscles of the horse. In the same year, Euler and coworkers obtained nicotinic acid from cozymase, and Kuhn and Vetter isolated the compound from heart muscle. These findings stimulated further studies on the nutritional value of nicotinic acid. It was soon found essential for the well-being of many species, but it was not at that time associated with any known dietary deficiency disease.

Meanwhile, riboflavin had been identified as vitamin B_2, and interest centered around the value of this substance in curing black tongue in dogs, dermatitis in rats, and pellagra in man. It soon became evident that a lack of riboflavin was not the cause of this group of nutritional deficiency diseases and that there was another factor to be sought in the vitamin B complex. Liver extracts were known to be highly effective in curing human pellagra and canine black tongue. Elvehjem and associates prepared liver concentrates that were highly effective in the treatment of canine black tongue, and in 1937 they identified the active substance as nicotinic acid. Proof was established by demonstrating that synthetic nicotinic acid derivatives were also effective in alleviating the symptoms of black tongue. On this basis, nicotinic acid was tested for its ability to cure human pellagra and was found to be as effective as liver extract.

Neither nicotinic acid nor riboflavin can cure the dermatitis of rats subsisting on a pellagra-producing diet. Although Goldberger was undoubtedly correct in ascribing to canine black tongue and human pellagra a common etiology, the dermatitis of rats is seemingly unrelated to either of these diseases. Rat dermatitis is relieved by another factor of the vitamin B complex, namely, pyridoxine.

With the recognition of nicotinic acid as the pellagra-preventing vitamin, the compound soon became an official drug. Nicotinic acid is also known as *niacin*, a term introduced in order to avoid any possible confusion between the vitamin and the alkaloid nicotine.

Chemistry. Nicotinic acid is vaguely related chemically to nicotine but possesses none of the latter's pharmacological properties. Nicotinic acid carries out its function in the body by being converted either into nicotinamide adenine dinucleotide (NAD; diphosphopyridine nucleotide, DPN) or nicotinamide adenine dinucleotide phosphate (NADP; triphosphopyridine nucleotide, TPN). It is to be noted that nicotinic acid occurs in the two nucleotides in the form of its amide, nicotinamide. The structures of nicotinic acid, nicotinamide, NAD, and NADP are shown below and on the opposite page, where $R = H$ in NAD and $R = OPO_3H_2$ in NADP.

The metabolic pathway by which nicotinic acid is converted into NAD has been elucidated for a variety of tissues, including human erythrocytes (Preiss and Handler, 1958). The conversion is carried out by three consecutive enzyme-catalyzed reactions (equations 1 to 3 on the next page, where PRPP is 5-phosphoribosyl-1-pyrophosphate). NADP is synthesized from NAD according to equation 4. Nicotinamide and tryptophan can also be converted to NAD (and NADP) in the body, and probable metabolic pathways for these conversions have also been worked out. The biosynthesis from nicotinamide appears to occur in mammalian liver by the deamidation of nicotinamide to nicotinic acid, which is then converted to NAD by way of the Preiss-Handler

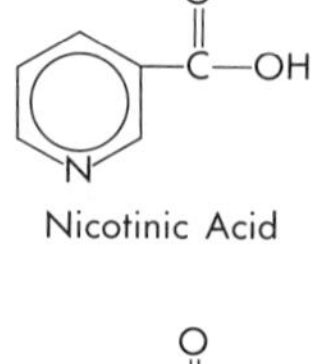

Nicotinic Acid

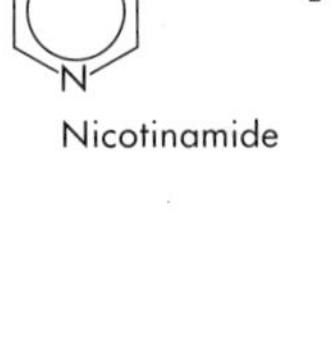

Nicotinamide

NAD and NADP

a vital role in metabolism as coenzymes for a wide variety of proteins involved in tissue respiration. The coenzymes, attached to appropriate protein molecules, function as dehydrogenases, accepting hydrogen from substrates and becoming reduced. The reduced pyridine nucleotides in turn are reoxidized by flavoproteins.

Symptoms of Deficiency. Nicotinic acid is an essential dietary constituent, the lack of which leads to the clinical condition known as pellagra. Pellagra is characterized by signs and symptoms referable especially to the skin, gastrointestinal tract, and CNS. An erythematous cutaneous eruption resembling sunburn first appears on the back of the hands. Other areas exposed to light (forehead, neck, and feet) are later involved, and eventually the lesions may be more widespread. The cutaneous manifestations are characteristically symmetrical and may darken, desquamate, and scar.

The chief symptoms referable to the digestive tract are stomatitis, enteritis, and diarrhea. The tongue becomes very red and swollen and may ulcerate. There is also excessive salivary secretion, and the salivary glands may be enlarged. Diarrhea is recurrent. The stools are watery and may occasionally be bloody. Nausea and vomiting are also common. Gastric achylia is observed in about 50% of cases.

Symptoms referable to the CNS are headache, dizziness, insomnia, depression, and impairment of memory. In severe cases, delusions, hallucinations, and dementia may appear. Motor and sensory disturbances of the peripheral nerves also occur. In addition, certain cases of pellagra manifest a macrocytic anemia. A milder degree of deficiency has been termed "subclinical pellagra." The patients are nervous and irritable and complain of headache and insomnia. They also suffer from indigestion, occasionally nausea and vomiting, and may have diarrhea or constipation. A certain degree of pigmentation of the skin often exists, and there is a burning sensation in the affected cutaneous areas.

pathway (equations 1 to 3) (Petrack *et al.,* 1963). The biosynthesis of NAD from tryptophan is somewhat more complicated. Tryptophan is converted to quinolinic acid by a series of several enzymatic reactions (for review, *see* Brown, 1960); the quinolinic acid is converted to nicotinic acid ribonucleotide (Nishizuka and Hayaishi, 1963), which in turn is converted to NAD by the pathway outlined above.

A variety of compounds that can be converted to nicotinamide in the body possess biological activity. These include derivatives of nicotinic acid substituted on the carboxyl group and derivatives of nicotinamide substituted on the amide nitrogen.

Pharmacological Actions. The pharmacological effects and toxicity of nicotinic acid in man have been carefully reviewed by Mosher (1970), who used data obtained primarily from clinical studies of the compound (tested because of its cholesterol-lowering effect) in the treatment of atherosclerosis. These particularly include flushing, pruritus, gastrointestinal distress, hepatotoxicity, and activation of peptic ulcer disease, in addition to the "therapeutic" effects on lipid metabolism. Nicotinic acid is described in more detail in Chapters 34 and 35.

Physiological Function. NAD and NADP, the physiologically active forms of nicotinic acid, serve

Human Requirement. As indicated above, the dietary requirement for this vitamin can be satisfied not only by nicotinic acid but also by nicotinamide and the amino acid tryptophan. Therefore, the nicotinic acid requirement is influenced by the quantity and the quality of dietary protein. Administration of tryptophan to normal human subjects, as well as to patients with pellagra, and analysis of urinary metabolites indicate that an average of 60 mg of dietary tryptophan is equivalent to 1 mg of nicotinic acid. The minimal requirement of nicotinic acid (including that formed from tryptophan) to prevent pellagra averages 4.4 mg/1000 kcal with an absolute minimal requirement of 1 mg per day if the caloric intake is less than 2000 kcal. The recommended al-

1. Nicotinic Acid + PRPP $\longrightarrow$ Nicotinic Acid Ribonucleotide + PP

2. Nicotinic Acid Ribonucleotide + ATP $\longrightarrow$ Desamido-NAD + PP

3. Desamido-NAD + Glutamine + ATP $\longrightarrow$ NAD + Glutamate + ADP + P

4. NAD + ATP $\longrightarrow$ NADP + ADP

lowance of the Food and Nutrition Board of the National Research Council, expressed in nicotinic acid equivalents, is 6.6 mg/1000 kcal (*see* Table XVIII–1, page 1545).

The relationship between the nicotinic acid requirement and the intake of tryptophan has helped to explain the historical association between the incidence of pellagra and the presence of large amounts of corn in the diet. Corn products are very low in tryptophan content. Therefore, when corn meal provides the major portion of dietary protein, pellagra will develop at levels of intake of nicotinic acid that would be adequate if the dietary protein contained more tryptophan.

Absorption, Fate, and Excretion. Both nicotinic acid and nicotinamide are readily absorbed from all portions of the intestinal tract and from parenteral sites of administration. The vitamin is distributed in all tissues. When therapeutic doses of nicotinic acid or its amide are administered, only small amounts of the unchanged vitamin appear in the urine. When extremely high doses of these vitamins are given, the unchanged vitamin represents the major urinary component. The principal route of metabolism of nicotinic acid and nicotinamide is by the formation of N-methyl nicotinamide, which in turn is further metabolized to N-methyl-2-pyridone-5-carboxamide (for review, *see* Handler, 1960) and N-methyl-4-pyridone-3-carboxamide (Quinn and Greengard, 1966). Nicotinuric acid, the glycine peptide of nicotinic acid, is also a metabolite of nicotinic acid.

Preparations. *Niacin,* N.F. (*nicotinic acid, 3-pyridinecarboxylic acid*), occurs as white crystals or as a crystalline powder. *Niacin Tablets,* N.F., are usually available in 20-, 25-, 50-, 100-, and 500-mg amounts. Several oral preparations containing considerably greater quantities, and intended for use as cholesterol-lowering agents, are also available. *Niacin Injection,* N.F., is a sterile solution of nicotinic acid prepared with the aid of sodium carbonate or sodium hydroxide. Preparations available for injection usually contain 10, 50, or 100 mg/ml. *Niacinamide,* U.S.P. (*nicotinamide, nicotinic acid amide*), occurs as a white crystalline, odorless powder with a bitter taste. *Niacinamide Tablets,* U.S.P., are usually available in 25-, 50-, 100-, and 500-mg amounts. *Niacinamide Injection,* U.S.P., is a sterile solution in water. Preparations available usually contain 100 or 200 mg/ml.

Therapeutic Uses. *Pellagra.* The only established use of nicotinic acid, nicotinamide, and their derivatives is in the prophylaxis and treatment of pellagra. In the acute

exacerbations of the disease, therapy must be intensive. The recommended oral dose is 50 mg, given up to ten times daily. If oral medication is impossible, intravenous injection of 25 mg is given two or more times daily. Pellagra is now quite uncommon in the United States. When observed, it is usually secondary to chronic gastrointestinal disease or to alcoholism. In these cases, multiple nutritional deficiencies often exist.

The response to nicotinic acid or its derivatives is dramatic. Within 24 hours, the fiery redness and swelling of the tongue disappear and sialorrhea diminishes. Associated oral infections heal rapidly. Other infections of mucous membranes frequently seen, notably those involving the pharynx, urethra, vagina, and rectum, also disappear. Nausea, vomiting, and diarrhea may stop within 24 hours, and at the same time the patient is relieved of epigastric distress, abdominal pain, and distention. Appetite also improves. Mental symptoms are quickly relieved, sometimes overnight. Confused patients become mentally clear, and those who are delirious become calm, adjusted to their environment, and remember with insight the events of their psychotic state. So specific are nicotinic acid and its derivatives in this regard that they can be used as diagnostic agents in patients with frank psychoses but with questionable additional evidence of pellagra. Large doses of niacin are recommended, especially when the psychosis is associated with encephalopathy; the syndrome is particularly prone to occur in chronic alcoholics deficient in nicotinic acid. The dermal lesions blanch and heal, but this occurs more slowly. The vitamin has less effect on cutaneous lesions that are moist, ulcerated, or pigmented. The porphyrinuria associated with pellagra also disappears.

Pellagra may be complicated by thiamine deficiency with associated peripheral neuritis. This complication does not respond to nicotinic acid or its congeners and must be treated with thiamine. Many pellagrins are also benefited by additional therapy with riboflavin and pyridoxine.

PYRIDOXINE

History. In the years 1930 to 1935 several groups of workers described a vitamin B factor essential in animal nutrition, which is now believed to have been pyridoxine. However, it was not until 1935 that the complex nature of vitamin B had been sufficiently elucidated to permit Birch and coworkers to conclude that a particular type of dermatitis in rats, which they called acrodynia or florid dermatitis, was due to the lack of a specific vitamin in the diet. In 1936, Birch and György gave the name *vitamin B6* to the substance and presented some of the details of its chemical structure. The compound was later identified chemically by several groups of workers and subsequently synthesized. The nonproprietary name *pyridoxine* was assigned to the vitamin by the Council on Pharmacy and Chemistry on the basis of its chemical structure.

Chemistry. Pyridoxine is one of the three forms in which vitamin B_6 occurs in natural sources. Its structure is as follows:

$$\begin{array}{c} CH_2OH \\ HO-\!\!\!\!\!\!\begin{array}{c}4\\ \end{array}\!\!\!\!\!\!-CH_2OH \\ \underset{5}{\big|} \\ H_3C-\underset{N\ 1}{\big|} \end{array}$$

Pyridoxine

The other two forms of the vitamin are *pyridoxal* and *pyridoxamine*. The three compounds differ in the nature of the substituent on the carbon atom in position 4 of the pyridine molecule: pyridoxal is the corresponding aldehyde, while pyridoxamine contains an aminomethyl group in this position. Each of the three forms of the vitamin can be readily utilized by the mammalian organism. The physiologically active forms of vitamin B_6 are pyridoxal phosphate and pyridoxamine phosphate, where the phosphate is esterified with the alcohol at position 5 of the pyridine ring.

All three forms of vitamin B_6 are converted to pyridoxal phosphate in the body; pyridoxal is converted to pyridoxal phosphate by an enzyme, pyridoxal kinase, according to the reaction:

Pyridoxal + ATP $\longrightarrow$ Pyridoxal Phosphate + ADP

Antimetabolites to pyridoxine have been synthesized and are capable of blocking the action of the vitamin and producing signs and symptoms of deficiency. The most active is 4-deoxypyridoxine, in which the substituent on the carbon atom in position 4 is a methyl group. The anti–vitamin B_6 activity of 4-deoxypyridoxine has been attributed to the formation *in vivo* of 4-deoxypyridoxine-5-phosphate, which is a competitive inhibitor of several pyridoxal phosphate–dependent enzymes.

Isonicotinic acid hydrazide (isoniazid, *see* page 1204) is a potent inhibitor of the reaction catalyzed by pyridoxal kinase. Isoniazid also inhibits enzymatic reactions in which pyridoxal phosphate participates as a coenzyme, but the inhibitory concentrations required in these systems are about 1000 times as great as the concentration required to inhibit the formation of pyridoxal phosphate. Thus, it appears that isoniazid exerts its anti–vitamin B_6 effect primarily by inhibiting the formation of the coenzyme form of the vitamin.

Pharmacological Actions.
Pyridoxine elicits no outstanding pharmacodynamic actions after either oral or intravenous administration. Large doses in the range of 3 to 4 g/kg produce convulsions and death in animals, but lower doses can be given daily without any obvious effects.

Physiological Function. Pyridoxal phosphate serves a vital role in metabolism as a coenzyme for a wide variety of metabolic transformations of amino acids, including decarboxylation, transamination, and racemization, as well as for enzymatic steps in the metabolism of tryptophan, sulfur-containing amino acids, and hydroxy amino acids. In the case of transamination, enzyme-bound pyridoxal phosphate is aminated to pyridoxamine phosphate by the donor amino acid, and the bound pyridoxamine phosphate is then deaminated to pyridoxal phosphate by the acceptor α-keto acid. Determination of alanine transaminase activity of erythrocytes has proven to be a useful method for evaluating the adequacy of pyridoxine concentrations in man (Brin, 1964).

Symptoms of Deficiency. Symptoms referable to pyridoxine deficiency have been produced in all mammalian species that have been studied, including man. The syndrome shows species variation. Important features of the deficiency observed in more than one species relate to the skin, CNS, and erythropoiesis.

Skin. In the rat, *acrodynia* or *florid dermatitis,* which consists in hyperkeratosis and acanthosis of the ears, paws, and snout as well as edema of the corium, is a prominent feature of pyridoxine deficiency. In man, seborrhea-like skin lesions about the eyes, nose, and mouth accompanied by glossitis and stomatitis can be produced within a few weeks by feeding a diet poor in vitamin B complex plus daily doses of the vitamin antagonist 4-deoxypyridoxine. The lesions clear rapidly after the administration of pyridoxine but do not respond to other members of the B complex (Mueller and Vilter, 1950).

Central Nervous System. Rats, pigs, dogs, and man may have convulsive seizures when maintained on a diet deficient in pyridoxine. These seizures can be prevented or cured by low doses of the vitamin. In the pig, degenerative changes in peripheral nerve, dorsal root ganglion cells, and posterior columns of the spinal cord have been described.

The electroshock threshold for producing clonic seizures in rats is substantially lowered by pyridoxine deficiency and can be raised to normal by the administration of pyridoxine. It has been speculated that the induction of convulsive seizures by pyridoxine deficiency is the result of a lowered level of γ-aminobutyric acid, a putative inhibitory CNS neurotransmitter, the synthesis of which is carried out by glutamic acid decarboxylase, a pyridoxal phosphate–requiring enzyme (*see* Roberts, 1963).

Erythropoiesis. In the dog, pig, and monkey, pyridoxine deficiency results in a microcytic, hypochromic anemia. While dietary deficiency of pyridoxine in man may rarely cause anemia, the usual pyridoxine-responsive anemia of man is apparently not due to inadequate supplies of the vitamin as judged by normal standards. This type of anemia is described in Chapter 63.

Human Requirement. The requirement for pyridoxine increases with the amount of protein in the diet. The average adult minimal requirement for pyridoxine is about 1.25 mg per day in individuals ingesting 100 g of protein per day. To provide a reasonable margin of safety, and to allow for daily intakes of more than 100 g of protein, a level of 2.0 mg per day is recommended for adults (*see* Table XVIII–1, page 1545).

Absorption, Fate, and Excretion. Pyridoxine, pyridoxal, and pyridoxamine are readily absorbed from the gastrointestinal tract. The principal excretory product when any of the three forms of the vitamin is fed to man is 4-pyridoxic acid. This product is formed by the action of hepatic aldehyde oxidase on free pyridoxal. Administration of pyridoxine and pyridoxamine also results in an increased excretion of pyridoxal in man, indicating that both compounds are first transformed, directly or indirectly, to pyridoxal, which is then oxidized to 4-pyridoxic acid (for review, *see* Snell, 1960).

Preparations. *Pyridoxine Hydrochloride, U.S.P.,* occurs as colorless or white crystals or as a white crystalline powder. *Pyridoxine Hydrochloride Tablets, U.S.P.,* are usually available in 10-, 25-, 50-, and 100-mg amounts. *Pyridoxine Hydrochloride Injection, U.S.P.,* is a sterile solution of pyridoxine hydrochloride in water, usually containing 50 or 100 mg/ml.

Therapeutic Uses. Although there is no doubt that pyridoxine is essential in human nutrition, the clinical syndrome of pyridoxine deficiency has not been well defined. Nevertheless, it may be presumed that an individual with a deficiency of other members of the B complex may also have a relative pyridoxine deficiency. Therefore, pyridoxine therapy may be advantageous in individuals suffering from a deficiency of other members of the B complex. On the basis that pyridoxine is essential in human nutrition, it is incorporated in many multivitamin preparations for prophylactic use.

Pyridoxine is often given prophylactically to patients receiving isoniazid or hydralazine to prevent the development of peripheral neuritis. This use is well justified. Biochemical evidence of pyridoxine deficiency has been obtained in a fraction of women taking oral contraceptives containing estrogen. This deficiency can be overcome by the administration of pyridoxine (*see* Review, 1973). By contrast, pyridoxine administration should be *avoided* in patients receiving levodopa therapy (*see* Chapter 14).

Pyridoxine-responsive anemia is a well-documented but uncommon condition. The use of the vitamin in this disease is discussed in Chapter 63.

Such anemias in patients without apparent pyridoxine deficiency, as well as a seizure disorder in infants that responds to the administration of pyridoxine, and the abnormalities characterized by xanthurenic aciduria, primary cystathioninuria, or homocystinuria appear to constitute a group of genetically determined clinical states of "pyridoxine dependency," manifested by a requirement for large amounts of the vitamin (*see* Mudd, 1971).

PANTOTHENIC ACID

History. Pantothenic acid was first identified by Williams and associates in 1933 as a substance essential for the growth of yeast. Its name, derived from Greek words signifying "from everywhere," is indicative of the wide distribution of the vitamin in nature. The role of pantothenic acid in animal nutrition was first defined in chicks. A deficiency disease in fowl characterized by skin lesions was known to be cured by filtrate fractions prepared from liver extract. Inasmuch as these same fractions were effective in the treatment of pellagra, it was assumed that the dermatitis in chicks was a form of "chick pellagra." However, following the identification of nicotinic acid it was soon appreciated that, whereas nicotinic acid was effective in pellagra, it failed to correct the nutritional deficiency in fowl. Shortly thereafter, in 1939, Woolley and coworkers and Jukes demonstrated that the chick antidermatitis factor was pantothenic acid.

Chemistry. Pantothenic acid is an optically active organic acid with biological activity residing in the *d* isomer. The vitamin carries out its function in the body by being converted into coenzyme A. Their chemical structures are as follows:

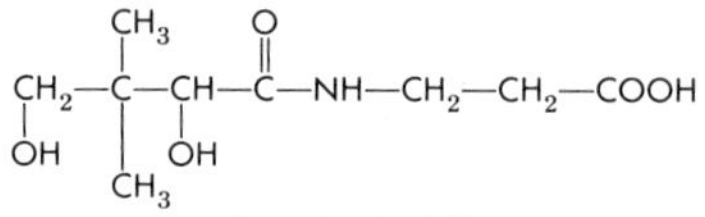

Pantothenic Acid

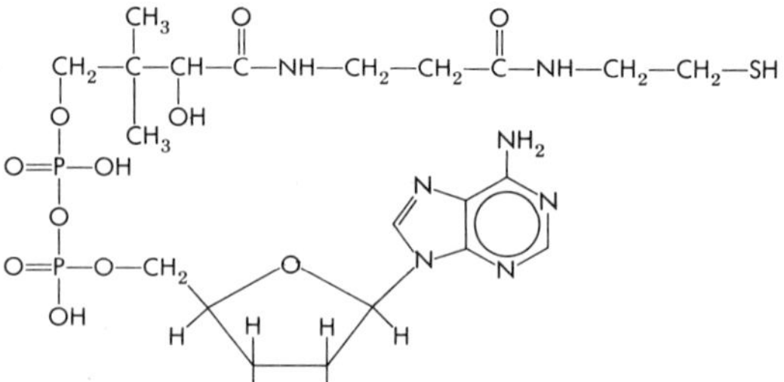

Coenzyme A

The metabolic pathway by which pantothenic acid is converted into coenzyme A involves five consecutive enzyme-catalyzed reactions (*see* Brown and Reynolds, 1963). In this conversion, phosphopantothenic acid, phosphopantothenylcysteine, phosphopantetheine, and dephosphocoenzyme A are successive intermediates.

Many analogs of pantothenic acid have been studied in an attempt to find an antimetabolite. Although active antagonists have been synthesized and are of value as research tools, they are not therapeutic agents.

Pharmacological Actions. Pantothenic acid exhibits no outstanding pharmacodynamic actions following its administration to experimental animals or man. The vitamin is essentially nontoxic.

Physiological Function. Coenzyme A, the physiologically active form of pantothenic acid, serves a vital role in metabolism as a coenzyme for a variety of enzyme-catalyzed reactions involving transfer of acetyl (two-carbon) groups. In these reactions the two-carbon fragment is bound to the sulfhydryl group of coenzyme A.

Symptoms of Deficiency. Pantothenic acid is essential for the growth of various microorganisms, including many strains of pathogenic bacteria. In animals, pantothenic acid deficiency is manifested by symptoms of neuromuscular degeneration, adrenocortical insufficiency, and death. Pantothenic acid deficiency has not been recognized in human beings on a natural diet, presumably because of the ubiquitous occurrence of the vitamin in the ordinary foods. However, by administering a semisynthetic diet low in the vitamin together with a pantothenic acid antagonist, omega-methylpantothenic acid, a syndrome in man is produced that is characterized by fatigue, malaise, headache, sleep disturbances, nausea, abdominal cramps, epigastric distress, occasional vomiting, and flatulence (Hodges *et al.,* 1959; Food and Nutrition Board, 1974). The subjects complain of paresthesias in the extremities, muscle cramps, and impaired coordination. The eosinopenic response to ACTH is lost and increased sensitivity to insulin develops, but there is no change in the concentration of 17-keto steroids in urine or in that of sodium in blood or urine.

Human Requirement. It is reasonable to infer from a review of available literature that pantothenic acid is probably essential for human beings. The Food and Nutrition Board concluded that a daily intake of 5 to 10 mg of pathothenic acid is likely to satisfy human requirements.

Absorption, Fate, and Excretion. Pantothenic acid is readily absorbed from the gastrointestinal tract. It is present in all tissues, in concentrations ranging from 2 to 45 $\mu g/g$. Pantothenic acid apparently is not destroyed in the human body since the intake and the excretion of the vitamin are approximately equal. About 70% of the unchanged pantothenic acid is excreted in the urine and about 30% in the feces.

Preparations. *Calcium Pantothenate,* U.S.P., is available as official tablets containing 10 or 30 mg,

and as an injectable preparation (50 mg/ml). *Racemic Calcium Pantothenate* is also official in the U.S.P.

Therapeutic Uses. There are no generally accepted therapeutic uses for pantothenic acid.

BIOTIN

History. The discovery of biotin resulted from two different experimental approaches: one, the study of a toxic syndrome, which eventually was proven to be due to a substance antagonistic to biotin; the other, a study of the growth requirements of yeast.

In 1916, Batemen observed that a high concentration of egg white in experimental diets was toxic. In 1927, Boas confirmed the fact that rats fed a diet containing raw egg white as the sole source of protein developed a syndrome characterized by neuromuscular disorders, severe dermatitis, and loss of hair. She named the condition *egg-white injury* and demonstrated that it could be prevented by cooking the protein or by the administration of yeast, liver, and other food. Parsons and associates also made notable contributions in this field by producing the toxic syndrome in a variety of species and studying the distribution and the behavior of the protective factor. György also investigated egg-white injury and was convinced that the syndrome induced by the feeding of egg white was a vitamin deficiency. He therefore called the protective substance *vitamin H,* after the German word *Haut* (meaning "skin").

In 1936, Kögl and Tönnis, who were studying yeast growth factors, isolated in crystalline form an essential factor from egg yolk that they called *biotin.* Previously, Allison and coworkers had demonstrated that the growth of certain strains of the genus *Rhizobium* was dependent upon a substance that they called *coenzyme R.* The paths of these various investigations converged when it was demonstrated that biotin, vitamin H, and coenzyme R were the same substance (György, 1940). In 1942, du Vigneaud established the structural formula of biotin, and shortly thereafter the vitamin was synthesized.

In the meantime, the nature of the antagonist to biotin received extensive study. The compound is a protein, first isolated by Eakin and associates in 1940 and called *avidin* ("hungry protein"). Avidin is a glycoprotein of high molecular weight, and it binds biotin with great affinity. The result is inhibition of biotin-dependent enzymatic reactions.

Chemistry. Biotin is a complex, optically active organic acid. Activity resides in the *d* isomer. The vitamin has the following structural formula:

Biotin

The free acid occurs as colorless needles, only slightly soluble in water. The sodium salt is highly soluble. The vitamin in dry state has a high degree of thermostability, and neutral solutions are stable at 100° C.

Three forms of biotin, apart from free biotin itself, have been derived from natural material. These derivatives are biocytin (ϵ-N-biotinyl-1-lysine) and the D and L sulfoxides of biotin. The derived forms of biotin are active in supporting growth of some microorganisms. Their efficacy as substitutes for biotin in human nutrition has not been studied. Biocytin may represent a degradative product of a biotin-protein complex, since, in its coenzyme role, the vitamin is covalently linked to an ϵ-amino group of a lysine residue of the apoenzyme involved.

A number of compounds antagonize the actions of biotin. Among them are biotin sulfone, desthio-biotin, and certain imidazolidone carboxylic acids. The antagonism between avidin and biotin is described above.

Pharmacological Actions. Relatively large amounts of biotin have been administered to both animals and man with impunity (Wright, 1956).

Physiological Function. Biotin is a coenzyme for several enzyme-catalyzed carboxylation reactions and, as such, plays an important role in CO_2 fixation. The CO_2 fixation occurs in a two-step reaction, the first involving binding of CO_2 to the biotin moiety of the biotin enzyme, and the second involving transfer of the biotin-bound CO_2 to an appropriate acceptor. (*See* Review, 1963.)

Symptoms of Deficiency. The ease of producing biotin deficiency varies with the animal. In a few species, a deficiency state can be produced merely by feeding a synthetic diet deficient in this nutrient. In most species, however, presumably owing to synthesis of the vitamin by intestinal bacteria, it is necessary to "sterilize" the intestinal tract, feed raw egg white, or administer biotin antimetabolites in order to produce a biotin deficiency. The symptoms of deficiency vary with the species and include failure of growth, loss of hair, dermatitis, poor lactation, and loss of muscular control. There is no evidence for the spontaneous occurrence of human biotin deficiency. Sydenstricker and associates (1942) produced a deficiency syndrome in man by the feeding of egg white, which responded to the administration of small doses of biotin. Signs and symptoms included dermatitis, hyperesthesia, muscle pain, lassitude, anorexia, slight anemia, and changes in the ECG.

Human Requirement. The human daily requirement for biotin is unknown. Diets providing a daily intake of 150 to 300 μg of biotin are considered adequate by the Food and Nutrition Board. This amount is provided by the average diet in the United States.

Absorption, Fate, and Excretion. Ingested biotin is rapidly absorbed from the gastrointestinal tract and appears in the urine predominantly in the form of free biotin. When synthetic biocytin was administered to man, blood and urine were found to contain biotin rather than biocytin (Wright, 1956). An enzyme present in human blood rapidly hydrolyzes biocytin to yield biotin.

Preparations. There is no official preparation of biotin, and single-entity preparations of the compound are not marketed in the United States.

Therapeutic Uses. There is no established therapeutic application of biotin. Moreover, synthetic biocytin has been administered in various disease states without the disclosure of any valid therapeutic uses (Wright, 1956).

CHOLINE

History. Although choline was identified chemically as a component of lecithin as early as 1862, interest in the compound as a dietary essential stems from the studies of Best and associates on lipotropic substances. Soon after the discovery of insulin, it was observed that depancreatized dogs maintained on insulin therapy developed fatty livers. The fatty infiltration of the liver could be prevented by the inclusion in the diet of crude egg-yolk lecithin or beef pancreas. The substance responsible for this effect was shown to be choline. These studies marked the beginning of an extensive literature on the role of lipotropic substances in animal nutrition, especially that of choline.

Choline has other important functions in addition to those related to fat metabolism. It provides the precursor for the neurochemical mediator acetylcholine. Moreover, the compound is important as a methyl donor in intermediary metabolism.

Despite its essential functions and its presence in the diet, there are several reasons for not classifying choline as a B vitamin. First, choline is present in animal tissues in amounts much greater than those usually associated with the true vitamins. Second, no cofactor essential for an enzymatic reaction has as yet been found that contains choline as a constituent. Finally, choline can be synthesized in the body from serine. In this biosynthesis, serine is first esterified to form phosphatidylserine, then the phosphatidylserine is decarboxylated to phosphatidylethanolamine (cephalin), which in turn is methylated to form phosphatidylcholine (lecithin), and the latter compound is hydrolyzed to liberate free choline. Methionine, in the form of S-adenosyl methionine, serves as the methyl donor in the biosynthesis of choline. This pathway is operative in both mammals and microorganisms. Thus, a choline deficiency can be produced in the mammalian organism only as a result of a combined deficiency of choline and methyl donors. This fact becomes of practical significance in considering the therapeutic value of choline.

Chemistry. Choline (trimethylethanolamine), a cation, has the following structural formula:

$$H_3C-\overset{\overset{\displaystyle CH_3}{|}}{\underset{\underset{\displaystyle CH_3}{|}}{N^+}}-CH_2CH_2OH$$

Choline

Pharmacological Actions. Choline qualitatively has the same pharmacological actions as acetylcholine but is much less active. The acute toxicity of choline, especially by mouth, is relatively low (about 5 g/kg for rats) in comparison with that of some of its esters and many other quaternary ammonium compounds (*see* Best *et al.,* 1956). The oral LD50 for man is estimated to be of the order of 200 to 400 g. Single oral doses of 10 g produce no obvious pharmacodynamic response.

Physiological Function. The important physiological functions of choline have been stated above, but they require amplification.

Lipotropic Action. A full appreciation of the role of choline as a lipotropic substance requires a basic knowledge of fat metabolism, a discussion of which is beyond the scope of this text. It will be recalled that several conditions, including injury to the liver, markedly increase the hepatic fat content. Substances that decrease the fat content of the liver are known as lipotropic agents. Choline may be considered a representative of this class. As a constituent of the phospholipid lecithin, it is essential for normal transport of fat. In its absence, fat accumulates in the liver. In its presence, phospholipid turnover is enhanced and the transport of fat from liver to tissues is promoted. The most dramatic effects of choline as a lipotropic agent are evident when the deposition of fat in the liver is due to a choline deficiency. It should be emphasized, however, that the dramatic lipotropic effects of choline have been demonstrated primarily in experimental animals (chiefly the rat). Data in man are conflicting (*see* below), and choline is no longer considered efficacious in the treatment of hepatic disorders.

Precursor of Acetylcholine. The synthesis of the chemical mediator acetylcholine depends upon the acetylation of choline. This important biological reaction is discussed in Chapter 21.

Transmethylation. Choline can serve as a methyl donor in intermediary metabolism. For example, choline can transfer a labile methyl group to homocysteine to form the essential amino acid methionine. The intricate details of one-carbon metabolism are discussed briefly under cyanocobalamin and folic acid (*see* Chapter 64).

Symptoms of Deficiency. As previously mentioned, choline can be synthesized in the body by the methylation of phosphatidylethanolamine. In this reaction, methionine serves as a methyl donor. Therefore, in mammalian nutrition, methionine can substitute for choline in the diet and a choline deficiency can be achieved only by limiting the intake of both choline and protein or, more specifically, methionine. Under these circumstances, the lipid content of the liver increases, and eventually fibrosis and hepatic cirrhosis occur. This is simple to achieve in experimental animals, but its significance in human nutrition is difficult to assess. No one has performed definitive experiments to indicate the degree and the duration of a choline deficiency that will initiate fatty changes in the human liver. The problem is complicated by the fact that early reversi-

ble pathological changes are not reflected in significant decreases of hepatic function.

The pathological lesions produced by experimental choline deficiency in animals are not limited to the liver. A hemorrhagic degeneration of the kidney has been observed in young rats, young pigs, and calves. Nonhemorrhagic renal lesions have been reported in rabbits. The ocular lesions and hypertension, and possibly the cardiac and vascular lesions, found in choline deficiency are secondary to the renal lesion. Several other effects of choline-deficient diets have been observed in animals. These effects include hemorrhagic lesions in heart muscle and adrenals, involution of the thymus, muscular weakness, muscular dystrophy, skin lesions, pyrosis, and failure of growth (for review, *see* Best *et al.,* 1956). No physiological abnormality relating to the role of choline as a precursor of acetylcholine has been described in choline deficiency.

Human Requirement. The human requirement for choline is not known. The daily intake of adults on average mixed diets is estimated to be 500 to 900 mg. Moreover, as mentioned above, the methionine in the diet promotes the synthesis of choline from serine in the body.

Absorption, Fate, and Excretion. Choline is fairly readily absorbed from the gastrointestinal tract. However, a proportion of choline administered orally to rats or to human patients appears to be converted to trimethylamine and its oxide by intestinal bacteria before absorption takes place. A small amount of choline appears in the urine.

Preparations. Choline is no longer an official drug. It is marketed as choline, choline bitartrate, choline dihydrogen citrate, and choline chloride in various oral dosage forms.

Therapeutic Uses. The necessity for lecithin precursors in the diet in order to prevent fatty infiltration and cirrhosis of the liver in experimental animals has already been discussed. Therefore, it seems obvious that in the treatment of hepatic cirrhosis, a disease associated with deficiencies in diet, an adequate amount of lipotropic substance should be provided. However, there is more to the correction of a grossly inadequate diet than the addition of lipotropic agents; effective resolution of lesions and regeneration in any tissue require optimal amounts of protein and all accessory food factors. Once such a dietary regimen has been established, the intake of preformed choline and of methionine will be more than sufficient to ensure normal fat transport. In addition, many authorities advocate supplemental intake, particularly of thiamine. There have been many studies in which choline in daily doses up to 6 g as well as methionine has been added to the dietary regimen, but evidence is far from convincing that any further degree of benefit can be achieved by such supplementation over long periods of time.

INOSITOL

History. More than a century ago, Scherrer found that patients with diabetes, in contrast to healthy individuals, excreted large quantities of inositol in the urine. Interest in inositol as a possible vitamin was first stimulated by the observation that the compound promoted the growth of certain strains of yeast. Later its importance in animal nutrition was recognized and the compound was assigned to the group of B vitamins (*see* Woolley, 1944). However, the synthesis of inositol in the body, the relatively high concentration in which it occurs in animal tissues, and the failure to find a coenzyme of which inositol is a constituent all argue against its classification as a true vitamin.

Chemistry. Inositol (hexahydroxycyclohexane) is an isomer of glucose. There are seven optically inactive and one pair of optically active stereoisomeric forms of inositol possible, of which only one, the optically inactive *myo*-inositol, is nutritionally active. It has the following structural formula:

Myo-Inositol

Pharmacological Actions. Inositol possesses no outstanding pharmacodynamic actions.

Physiological Function. The physiological function of inositol is unknown, but it is a component of a type of phospholipid, phosphatidylinositol.

Symptoms of Deficiency. These have only been observed in experimental animals and vary with the species. Noteworthy are retarded growth, alopecia, and impaired lactation. Claims by some investigators of lipotropic and antiscorbutic actions of inositol have been disputed by others. Eagle and coworkers (1957) found *myo*-inositol to be an essential growth factor for the *in-vitro* survival and multiplication of all 18 normal and malignant cell lines examined by them.

Human Requirement. A need for inositol in human nutrition has not been established.

Absorption, Fate, and Excretion. The consumption of inositol by man is about 1 g per day. The compound is easily absorbed from the gastrointestinal tract. Inositol is readily converted to glucose, and glucose is readily converted to inositol by the body. Inositol is about one third as effective as glucose in alleviating starvation ketosis. The concentration of inositol in fresh normal human plasma is of the order of 0.5 mg/100 ml of blood. The concentration of inositol is particularly high in heart muscle, brain, and skeletal muscle (1.6, 0.9, and 0.4 g/100 g dry weight, respectively). Only a small amount of ingested inositol is found in the urine.

Preparations. There is no longer an official preparation of inositol.

Therapeutic Uses. Inositol has been used in the management of diseases associated with disturbances in the transport and metabolism of fat, without any convincing evidence of therapeutic benefit.

PARA-AMINOBENZOIC ACID

History. Para-aminobenzoic acid (PABA) has been included as a member of the vitamin B complex although there is no justification for this classification. The compound was first synthesized in 1863, but it remained of little biological interest until Woods and Fildes presented evidence that the sulfonamides exert their antibacterial action by acting as antimetabolites to PABA (*see* Chapter 56). This observation directed attention toward PABA as an essential metabolite in the growth of bacteria and its possible role as a vitamin in mammalian organisms. The requirement of certain microorganisms for PABA results from the necessity for incorporating this molecule into folic acid. However, the mammalian organism is incapable of converting PABA to folic acid and the folic acid requirements of mammals must therefore be met with preformed folic acid. Thus, there is no evidence that PABA is a dietary essential in man. Descriptions of the pharmacological properties of PABA may be found in earlier editions of this textbook.

Best, C. H.; Lucas, C. C.; and Ridout, J. H. Vitamins and the protection of the liver. *Br. med. Bull.,* **1956,** *12,* 9–14.

Brin, M. Use of the erythrocyte in functional evaluation of vitamin adequacy. In, *The Red Blood Cell.* (Bishop, C., and Surgenor, D. M., eds.) Academic Press, Inc., New York, **1964,** pp. 451–476.

———. Blood transketolase determination in the diagnosis of thiamine deficiency. *Heart Bull.,* **1968,** *17,* 86–89.

Bro-Rasmussen, F. The riboflavin requirement of animals and man and associated metabolic relations. Part II. Relation of requirement to the metabolism of protein and energy. *Nutr. Abstr. Rev.,* **1958,** *28,* 369–386.

Brown, G. M. Biosynthesis of water-soluble vitamins and derived coenzymes. *Physiol. Rev.,* **1960,** *40,* 331–368.

Brown, G. M., and Reynolds, J. J. Biogenesis of the water-soluble vitamins. *A. Rev. Biochem.,* **1963,** *32,* 419–462.

Eagle, H.; Oyama, V. I.; Levy, M.; and Freeman, A. E. *myo*-Inositol as an essential growth factor for normal and malignant human cells in tissue culture. *J. biol. Chem.,* **1957,** *226,* 191–205.

György, P. A further note on the identity of vitamin H with biotin. *Science, N.Y.,* **1940,** *92,* 609.

Handler, P. Metabolism of nicotinic acid and the pyridine nucleotides. In, *Proceedings of the Fourth International Congress of Biochemistry.* Vol. 11, *Vitamin Metabolism.* (Umbreit, W., and Molitor, H., eds.) Pergamon Press, Ltd., Oxford, **1960,** pp. 39–49.

Hodges, R. E.; Bean, W. B.; Ohlson, M. A.; and Bleiler, R. Human pantothenic acid deficiency produced by omega-methyl pantothenic acid. *J. clin. Invest.,* **1959,** *38,* 1421–1425.

Horwitt, M. K.; Harvey, C. C.; Hills, O. W.; and Liebert, E. Correlation of urinary excretion of riboflavin with dietary intake and symptoms of ariboflavinosis. *J. Nutr.,* **1950,** *41,* 247–264.

Jolliffe, N.; Colbert, C. N.; and Joffe, P. M. Observations on etiologic relationship of vitamin B (B$_1$) to polyneuritis in alcohol addict. *Am. J. med. Sci.,* **1936,** *191,* 515–526.

Mosher, L. R. Nicotinic acid side effects and toxicity: a review. *Am. J. Psychiat.,* **1970,** *126,* 1290–1296.

Mudd, S. H. Pyridoxine-responsive genetic disease. *Fedn Proc. Fedn Am. Socs exp. Biol.*, **1971**, *30*, 970–976.

Mueller, J. F., and Vilter, R. W. Pyridoxine deficiency in human beings induced with desoxypyridoxine. *J. clin. Invest.*, **1950**, *29*, 193–201.

Nishizuka, Y., and Hayaishi, O. Studies on the biosynthesis of nicotinamide adenine dinucleotide. I. Enzymic synthesis of niacin ribonucleotides from 3-hydroxyanthranilic acid in mammalian tissues. *J. biol. Chem.*, **1963**, *238*, 3369–3377.

Petrack, B.; Greengard, P.; Craston, A.; and Kalinsky, H. J. Nicotinamide deamidase in rat liver and the biosynthesis of NAD. *Biochem. biophys. Res. Commun.*, **1963**, *13*, 472–477.

Pincus, J. H.; Cooper, J. R.; Murphy, J. V.; Rabe, E. F.; Lonsdale, D.; and Dunn, H. G. Thiamine derivatives in subacute necrotizing encephalomyelopathy: a preliminary report. *Pediatrics, Springfield*, **1973**, *51*, 716–721.

Preiss, J., and Handler, P. Biosynthesis of diphosphopyridine nucleotide. II. Enzymatic aspects. *J. biol. Chem.*, **1958**, *233*, 493–500.

Quinn, G. P., and Greengard, P. The pathway for the biosynthesis of N^1-methyl-4-pyridone-3-carboxamide. *Archs Biochem. Biophys.*, **1966**, *115*, 146–152.

Rindi, G., and Ventura, U. Thiamine intestinal transport. *Physiol. Rev.*, **1972**, *52*, 821–827.

Rivlin, R. S. Riboflavin metabolism. *New Engl. J. Med.*, **1970**, *283*, 463–472.

Roberts, E. Some thoughts about the γ-aminobutyric acid system in nervous tissue. *Nutr. Rev.*, **1963**, *21*, 161–165.

Snell, E. E. Some aspects of the metabolism of vitamin B_6. In, *Proceedings of the Fourth International Congress of Biochemistry*. Vol. 11, *Vitamin Metabolism*. (Umbreit, W., and Molitor, H., eds.) Pergamon Press, Ltd., Oxford, **1960**, pp. 250–262.

Sydenstricker, V. P.; Singal, S. A.; Briggs, A. P.; DeVaughn, N. M.; and Isbell, H. Observations on the "egg white injury" in man. *J. Am. med. Ass.*, **1942**, *118*, 1199–1200.

Woolley, D. W. Nutritional significance of inositol. *J. Nutr.*, **1944**, *28*, 305–314.

Wright, L. D. The metabolism of biotin. In, *Symposium on Vitamin Metabolism* (Nutrition Symposium Series, No. 13). National Vitamin Found., New York, **1956**, pp. 104–115.

Monographs and Reviews

Food and Nutrition Board, National Research Council. *Recommended Dietary Allowances*, 8th ed. Publication No. 2216, National Academy of Sciences, Washington, D. C., **1974**.

Goodhart, R. S., and Shils, M. E. (eds.). *Modern Nutrition in Health and Disease*, 5th ed. Lea & Febiger, Philadelphia, **1973**, pp. 186–220.

Review. Mechanism of action of biotin-enzymes. *Nutr. Rev.*, **1963**, *21*, 310–313.

Review. Oral contraceptives and vitamin B_6. *Nutr. Rev.*, **1973**, *31*, 49–50.

Schroeder, H. A. Losses of vitamins and trace minerals resulting from processing and preservation of foods. *Am. J. clin. Nutr.*, **1971**, *24*, 562–573.

Vitamins. *A. Rev. Biochem.* (Reviews on vitamins appear in most volumes.)

CHAPTER
74 WATER-SOLUBLE VITAMINS

[*Continued*]

Ascorbic Acid (Vitamin C)

J. J. Burns

History. Scurvy was the first deficiency disease to be recognized as such. As early as 1720, Kramer observed that medicines gave no relief in this condition, but

. . . if you can get green vegetables, if you can prepare a sufficient quantity of fresh antiscorbutic juices, if you have oranges, lemons, citrons, or their pulp and juice preserved with whey in cask, so that you can make a lemonade, or rather give to the quantity of 3 or 4 ounces of their juice in whey, you will, without other assistance, cure this dreadful evil.

Lind (1757), in his exhaustive treatise on scurvy, showed experimentally in human subjects that oranges and lemons incorporated in the diet could prevent the onset of the disease. In 1804, it became compulsory in Britain to issue a daily ration of lemon or lime juice to all British sailors. This led to the almost complete eradication of scurvy in the British Navy, and to this day the nickname "limies" is applied to British sailors.

Chemistry. The demonstration by Holst and Fröhlich (1907) that experimental scurvy could be produced in guinea pigs provided a bioassay for the antiscorbutic vitamin and greatly aided investigations of its chemical composition. Nevertheless, the combined efforts of many investigators during several decades were required to solve the problem of its chemistry. Zilva (1921) discovered that vitamin C could easily be destroyed by oxidation and could best be protected by reducing agents. He observed that concentrates with high vitamin C content also contained powerful reducing substances but believed the latter merely accompanied the vitamin and protected it. McKinnis and King (1930) were of the opinion, however, that the vitamin itself was responsible for the reducing properties of the concentrates that they obtained from lemon juice.

Meanwhile, Szent-Györgyi had been studying the oxidizing mechanisms of the adrenal cortex, and in 1928 he isolated from the adrenals a powerful reducing agent in crystalline form. He believed it to be a hexuronic acid derivative having the empirical formula $C_6H_8O_6$. Working on the assumption that this same compound might be concerned in the peroxidase system of plants, he succeeded in isolating it from cabbage and orange juice. Szent-Györgyi recognized this crystalline material as probably being identical with the reducing agent reported by Zilva to be present in vitamin C concentrates; but apparently he shared with Zilva the belief that the

compound was merely a protector of the vitamin, for he failed, at that time, to test its antiscorbutic activity.

King and Waugh (1932) finally succeeded in isolating a crystalline compound from lemon juice concentrates, identified it as a hexuronic acid, and demonstrated its potent antiscorbutic properties. A few weeks later, Svirbely and Szent-Györgyi (1932) announced that the hexuronic acid obtained from adrenal glands, cabbages, and oranges also was highly antiscorbutic. Shortly thereafter, the exact chemical constitution of the antiscorbutic hexuronic acid was established independently by workers in several laboratories. It was soon synthesized, and the synthetic product was shown to have the same biological activity as that isolated from natural sources. Because of its physiological role in the prevention of scurvy, the compound was called ascorbic acid. Ascorbic acid is reversibly oxidizable in the body to a form known as dehydroascorbic acid. The latter compound possesses full vitamin activity. Indeed, the physiological functions of the vitamin are probably related to this oxidation-reduction system. The structural formulas of ascorbic acid and dehydroascorbic acid are as follows:

Ascorbic Acid   Dehydroascorbic Acid

Ascorbic acid is optically active. Compounds closely related chemically to L-ascorbic acid possess some antiscorbutic activity, but none compares in potency with the natural vitamin.

Pharmacological Actions. In the strict sense of the word, vitamin C may be said to possess few pharmacological actions. Administration of the compound in amounts greatly in excess of the physiological requirements causes no demonstrable effects. In the

1564

scorbutic individual, however, administration of the vitamin leads to a rapid alleviation of symptoms. Purely secondary symptoms accompanying a deficiency disease are likely to be varied; associated with clinical scurvy may be anemia, infections, metabolic disturbances, and other symptoms. As a result, an extensive literature has accumulated concerning the effect of vitamin C on practically every function of the body. Contributions that may be of great importance have been lost under a deluge of clinical reports, most of them uncritical.

Physiological Function. Although the pathological lesions of vitamin C deficiency have been accurately defined, the biochemical defect that provides the basis for the structural and functional changes in scurvy can be discussed only in very broad terms (*see* King, 1968). Ascorbic acid and dehydroascorbic acid form a readily reversible oxidation-reduction system. Both the oxidized and the reduced form of the vitamin are equally effective as antiscorbutic agents. It is generally believed that this system plays an important role in biological oxidations and reductions and in cellular respiration. Ascorbic acid can be readily oxidized by cytochrome oxidase plus cytochrome c. Dehydroascorbic acid can be reduced by glutathione. Ascorbic acid may subserve an important function in maintaining SH-activated enzyme systems in their reduced form.

A few specific metabolic abnormalities associated with vitamin C deficiency have been described. The metabolism of the aromatic amino acid tyrosine is disturbed, and considerable investigation has been carried out to determine the mechanism involved. It appears that the role of ascorbic acid in tyrosine metabolism is an unusual one for a vitamin. Instead of acting as a cofactor for a particular enzymatic step, as do members of the B family of vitamins, ascorbic acid has the ability to protect an enzyme, *p*-hydroxyphenylpyruvic acid oxidase, from inhibition by its substrate. The protection is necessary only under unusual conditions, when large amounts of tyrosine are being metabolized, since it does not seem to be required under ordinary dietary conditions. The role of ascorbic acid in tyrosine metabolism is nonspecific, since various analogs of ascorbic acid and even a dye, 2,6-dichlorophenolindophenol, which has a similar redox potential, can replace the vitamin (*see* La Du and Zannoni, 1961).

Ascorbic acid is involved in carbohydrate metabolism, as evidenced by the fact that scorbutic animals exhibit hyperglycemia, reduced glucose tolerance, and low hepatic glycogen content and are resistant to insulin. Another metabolic function of ascorbic acid is the role of the vitamin in the conversion of folic acid to folinic acid (leucovorin).

Ascorbic acid occurs in high concentration in both the cortex and the medulla of the adrenals. In the medulla it may function to prevent the oxidation of epinephrine. However, greater interest centers in its possible function in the adrenal cortex. Following

stress or the administration of ACTH, the increased secretion of adrenocorticosteroids is associated with a rapid decrease in the amount of adrenal ascorbic acid and cholesterol. Therefore, it is tempting to assume that ascorbic acid is concerned with the synthesis of adrenocorticosteroids. However, there is no direct evidence in support of such an assumption. Adrenocortical secretion is well maintained in scorbutic animals and man, and the secretion of corticosteroids by the perfused adrenal is uninfluenced by the concentration of ascorbic acid in the perfusion fluid. Therefore, it must be concluded that the increased utilization of ascorbic acid that follows stimulation of the adrenal cortex is a relatively nonspecific response to increased cellular respiratory activity and that other substances can subserve the same functions in the absence of the vitamin.

Symptoms of Deficiency. A deficiency in the intake of vitamin C leads to scurvy. The primary structural changes in vitamin C deficiency result from the fact that ascorbic acid is essential for the formation and the maintenance of intercellular ground substance and collagen. In deficiency states, the collagen bundles in the intercellular ground substance disappear, and the ground substance depolymerizes and becomes thin and watery in appearance. Inasmuch as the ground substance is the essential matrix of connective tissue and the latter constitutes the effective framework of all organs, the reason for the widespread lesions of scurvy becomes apparent. The hemorrhagic manifestations of the disease similarly can be associated with a defect in the so-called cement substance of the capillaries (*see* Sebrell and Harris, 1967).

The chief symptoms of scurvy arise from pathological lesions in the bones and blood vessels. In growing bones, lesions of the epidiaphyseal junction lead to disunion, freedom of movement, and traumatic fragmentation. In the rapidly growing bones of infants, a wide separation of the periosteum from the cortex occurs and massive subperiosteal hemorrhages may result. Subperiosteal hemorrhages also occur in adults. In the teeth, dentin is resorbed and atrophy and degeneration of odontoblasts occur in the pulp. The gums become spongy, bleed easily, and may swell to such an extent that they overlap the teeth. Rarefaction of the alveolar bone results in the loosening of the teeth. Changes in the cells of capillary walls increase their fragility, and hemorrhage occurs in regions subjected to mechanical stress or trauma, such as skin, muscles, bones, and gums (*see* Wolbach, 1937; Sebrell and Harris, 1967). Despite considerable investigation carried out in recent years, there is as yet no mechanism known to explain how ascorbic acid maintains the intercellular ground substance and collagen. The possibility has been suggested that ascorbic acid may exert a direct effect on collagen synthesis by facilitating the hydroxylation of peptide-bound proline and lysine (*see* Barnes and Kodicek, 1972).

Absorption, Distribution, Fate, and Excretion. Ascorbic acid is readily absorbed from the intestinal tract. However, under special circumstances, as in diarrhea, absorption may be limited.

After absorption, increased amounts of vitamin C can be detected in the blood. Ascorbic acid is normally present in both plasma and cells. The concentration in leukocytes and platelets is much higher than in plasma and erythrocytes. Plasma rather than blood concentrations of ascorbic acid are usually determined. Absorbed ascorbic acid is ubiquitously distributed in all body tissues. The highest concentrations are found in glandular tissue, the lowest in muscle and stored fat.

Methods used to estimate the degree of saturation of the tissues with ascorbic acid include determination of urinary excretion, measurement of ascorbic acid in plasma, estimation of ascorbic acid content of the leukocyte-platelet layer of blood, and response to "load" test (*see* Burch, 1961; Goldsmith, 1961). Determination of ascorbic acid in plasma is the usual index of the adequacy of the intake of ascorbic acid, but analysis of ascorbic acid in white blood cells appears to provide the most reliable criterion of the state of tissue saturation. An individual with a plasma concentration of vitamin C of 1 to 2 mg % is completely saturated with the vitamin. Concentrations of approximately 0.5 mg % may be designated as low normal. If the plasma contains less ascorbic acid than 0.5 mg %, the body concentration may be designated as suboptimal. Plasma values below 0.15 mg % are invariably associated with clinical scurvy.

Ascorbic acid is partially destroyed and partially excreted by the body. There is a renal threshold for vitamin C, and the vitamin is excreted by the kidney in large amounts only when the plasma concentration exceeds this threshold, which is approximately 1.4 mg %. The threshold may vary, however, in different individuals. When the body is saturated with ascorbic acid, the plasma concentration will be approximately that of the renal threshold. If further amounts of the vitamin are then administered, most of it escapes into the urine. When the tissues are not saturated and the plasma concentration is low, the ingestion of ascorbic acid results in little or no renal excretion. This forms the basis for the so-called saturation test for determining the vitamin C requirement or the degree of saturation in a particular individual.

Studies with L-ascorbic acid labeled with ^{14}C have shown that the vitamin is oxidized to CO_2 in rats and guinea pigs, but considerably less conversion can be detected in man. A major route of metabolism of L-ascorbic acid in man involves its conversion to urinary oxalate, presumably through the intermediate formation of its oxidized product, dehydroascorbic acid. Ascorbic acid-2-sulfate has recently been identified as a metabolite of the vitamin in human urine. This metabolite may be involved in the action of the vitamin, especially in the sulfation reaction occurring in connective tissue. (*See* Burns, 1959; Atkins *et al.*, 1964; Baker *et al.*, 1966, 1971; Mumma and Verlangieri, 1972.)

Biosynthesis of Ascorbic Acid. Man and other primates as well as the guinea pig are the only mammals known to be unable to synthesize ascorbic acid; consequently, they require dietary vitamin C for the prevention of scurvy. An explanation for this has come from biochemical studies (*see* Burns, 1959). The rat, a typical species that does not require dietary vitamin C, synthesizes ascorbic acid from glucose through the intermediate formation of D-glucuronic acid, L-gulonic acid, and L-gulonolactone (Figure 74-1). Man, monkey, and guinea pig lack the hepatic enzyme required to carry out the last reaction, that is, the conversion of L-gulonolactone to L-ascorbic acid. This reaction is presumably miss-

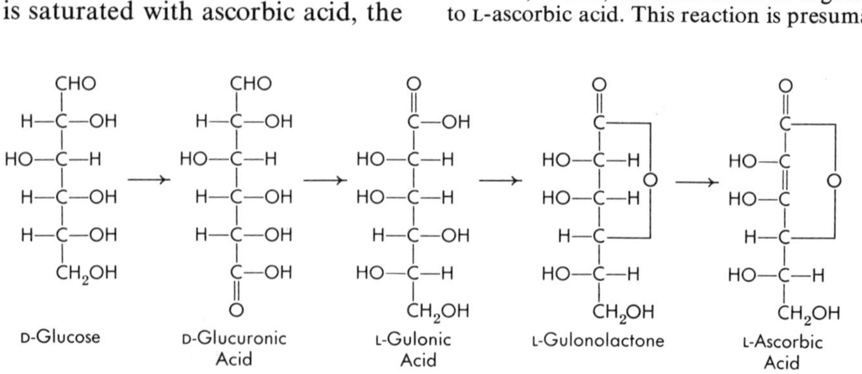

Figure 74-1. *Pathway for the biosynthesis of* L-*ascorbic acid in the rat.* (After Burns, 1959. Courtesy of the *American Journal of Medicine.*)

ing because of a genetically controlled enzyme "deficiency."

Various drugs markedly increase the rate at which ascorbic acid is synthesized from glucose in rats. Included among these are the hypnotics chlorobutanol, meprobamate, and barbital; the analgesics aminopyrine and antipyrine; the muscle relaxant orphenadrine; and the antihistamines diphenhydramine and chlorcyclizine. However, in man and guinea pig drugs stimulate only the formation of increased amounts of D-glucuronic and L-gulonic acids. The mechanism by which drugs stimulate the synthesis of ascorbic acid and its precursors is not known. It is possible that this effect of drugs may represent an adaptive response on the part of the body to foreign compounds. This is suggested from the observation that the drugs that are potent in stimulating the synthesis of ascorbic acid also increase the activity of hepatic microsomal enzymes that metabolize various foreign compounds (*see* Burns and Shore, 1961).

Enhanced pharmacological action of a number of drugs has been observed in vitamin C–deficient guinea pigs. This effect results from decreased activity of drug-metabolizing hepatic microsomal enzymes, which can be restored by administration of ascorbic acid. (*See* Zannoni and Lynch, 1973.) It is not known whether scorbutic man has an impaired ability to metabolize drugs. (*See* Conney *et al.*, 1961.)

Human Requirement. The daily intake of the vitamin must equal the amount oxidized if deficiency is to be avoided. Renal excretion has little influence on the daily requirement because the vitamin is excreted in large amounts only when the body is completely saturated. The human requirement for vitamin C has been studied very extensively, but there is still disagreement on optimal intake. One of the technics that has been widely employed is the saturation test mentioned above. In this test, an individual is first saturated with the vitamin and then placed on a diet free of vitamin C for a given number of days, after which the amount of vitamin required again to produce saturation is determined.

The human daily allowances of vitamin C recommended by the Food and Nutrition Board of the National Research Council are presented in Table XVIII-1 (page 1545). Under certain circumstances, the rate of destruction and, consequently, the requirements for vitamin C are significantly increased. An outstanding example is the increased requirement of patients suffering from certain infectious diseases. An individual with tuberculosis may need 100% more vitamin than does a normal subject in order to remain saturated. Other conditions in which the vitamin C requirements are significantly raised are hyperthyroidism, peptic ulcer, neoplastic disease, pregnancy, lactation, and surgery (Crandon *et al.*, 1961; Goldsmith, 1961). While Pauling has suggested that the human requirement for vitamin C is far higher than that recommended by the Food and Nutrition Board (Pauling, 1970), the validity of his estimate is most questionable (*see* Jukes, 1974).

Preparations and Assay. *Ascorbic Acid,* U.S.P., consists of white or slightly yellow crystals or pow-

der. The vitamin is reasonably stable in the dry state, but solutions deteriorate rapidly if exposed to air. *Ascorbic Acid Tablets,* U.S.P. (CEVALIN, several nonproprietary preparations), usually contain 25, 50, 100, 250, 500, or 1000 mg of the vitamin. Solutions for oral use are also available in various concentrations. *Ascorbic Acid Injection,* U.S.P., is a sterile neutral solution of the vitamin designed for parenteral injection. The currently available preparations contain 50, 100, 250, or 500 mg/ml. Most multivitamin preparations contain ascorbic acid.

There are many foods that have a high vitamin C content. Orange and lemon juices are outstanding in this respect and contain approximately 0.5 mg/ml. This high vitamin content permits the use of fruit juices in therapy in place of pure preparations of the vitamin.

Apart from its role in nutrition, ascorbic acid is commonly used as an antioxidant to protect natural flavor and color of many foods (*e.g.,* processed fruit, vegetables, and dairy products).

Routes of Administration. Vitamin C is usually administered by the oral route; however, in conditions that prevent adequate absorption from the gastrointestinal tract, solutions of the sodium salt may be given by intramuscular or intravenous injection.

Untoward Effects. While serious toxicity from the administration of vitamin C is very uncommon, untoward effects have been reported. The most common is diarrhea. Acidification of the urine by ascorbic acid may cause precipitation of cystine or oxalate stones in the urinary tract and will alter the excretion of certain other drugs administered concurrently. High doses of vitamin C taken during pregnancy have been reported to cause scurvy in infants removed from this environment by birth (Cochrane, 1965).

Therapeutic Uses. The specific therapeutic use for vitamin C is in the prophylaxis and treatment of scurvy. Whether vitamin C deficiency has a causal relationship to clinical syndromes other than scurvy has not been established.

In the prophylaxis of scurvy in infants and children, vitamin C is usually administered in the form of orange juice. The recommended intakes for various age groups are given in Table XVIII-1 (page 1545). An occasional infant is allergic to orange juice, and in such an instance ascorbic acid can be administered in solution. The ascorbic acid should be freshly dissolved.

In conditions in which the demands for ascorbic acid are increased, the vitamin C content of the diet should be fortified either with orange juice or crystalline ascorbic acid. The daily ingestion of 150 mg of ascorbic acid is usually sufficient to meet most requirements.

In the treatment of fully developed scurvy, large doses of ascorbic acid may be given until the symptoms are under control. Toxic effects are very uncommon, and 1 g a day may be administered until the body stores have been replenished.

The reducing properties of vitamin C are of value in the treatment of *idiopathic methemoglobinemia.* Oral doses of 150 mg twice daily are employed. The vitamin is probably less effective than methylene blue in the treatment of methemoglobinemia and should not be relied upon in critical situations.

Marked elevation of plasma tyrosine and modest elevation of plasma phenylalanine can occur in premature infants receiving a high-protein, low–ascorbic acid diet. These high blood amino acid concentrations are restored to normal by administration of a single 100-mg dose of ascorbic acid and are prevented by daily administration of 100 mg of the vitamin, but not by smaller doses. The effect of this aberration of amino acid metabolism in premature infants on subsequent neurological development is, at present, unknown. However, the defect has practical importance, since the abnormal blood values may be confused with those of phenylketonuria (*see* Levine *et al.,* 1941; Light *et al.,* 1966).

Vitamin C has been widely employed for the treatment of such diverse conditions as dental caries, pyorrhea, gum infections, anemia, malnutrition, hemorrhagic states, and miscellaneous infections. While it is true that many of the above conditions may be associated with scurvy, their occurrence is not pathognomonic of scurvy. The final diagnosis of scurvy rests upon roentgenological evidence in the long bones and the chemical evidence of a low ascorbic acid content of the blood. Only then is there assurance that therapy with ascorbic acid will lead to beneficial effects. Despite the vast clinical literature on the various therapeutic indications for vitamin C (the conditions in which the vitamin has been reputed to give specific benefit run the gamut of most known diseases), there is no conclusive evidence that ascorbic acid is of value except in the relief of symptoms causally associated with scurvy.

The possibility that 1- to 3-g or higher daily doses of ascorbic acid can prevent upper respiratory infections has received considerable attention, especially in the lay press. (*See* Pauling, 1970.) While the results of certain double-blind controlled studies have tended to substantiate this suggestion (*see* Anderson *et al.,* 1972; Coulehan *et al.,* 1974), others have not (Walker *et al.,* 1967; Schwartz *et al.,* 1973; Karlowski *et al.,* 1975). Two separate assessments of the status of this controversy have concluded that any potential benefit from ascorbic acid prophylaxis and therapy for upper respiratory infections is slight, if present at all, and does not justify even the small risk (Chalmers, 1975; Dykes and Meier, 1975).

FLAVONOIDS

The flavonoids are discussed in the *fourth edition* of this textbook. No new information has appeared to substantiate their therapeutic use or to indicate that they are dietary essentials.

Anderson, T. W.; Reid, D. B. W.; and Beaton, G. H. Vitamin C and the common cold: a double-blind trial. *Can. med. Ass. J.,* **1972,** *107,* 503–508.

Atkins, G. L.; Dean, B. M.; Griffin, W. J.; and Watts, R.W.E. Quantitative aspects of ascorbic acid metabolism in man. *J. biol. Chem.,* **1964,** *239,* 2975–2980.

Baker, E. M.; Saari, J. C.; and Tolbert, B. M. Ascorbic acid metabolism in man. *Am. J. clin. Nutr.,* **1966,** *19,* 371–378.

Baker, E. M., III; Hammer, D. C.; March, S. C.; Tolbert, B. M.; and Canham, J. E. Ascorbate sulfate: a urinary metabolite of ascorbic acid in man. *Science, Wash.,* **1971,** *173,* 826–827.

Barnes, M. J., and Kodicek, E. Biological hydroxylations and ascorbic acid with special regard to collagen metabolism. *Vitams Horm.,* **1972,** *30,* 1–43.

Burch, H. B. Methods for detecting and evaluating ascorbic acid deficiency in man and animals. *Ann. N.Y. Acad. Sci.,* **1961,** *92,* 268–276.

Burns, J. J. Biosynthesis of L-ascorbic acid: basic defect in scurvy. *Am. J. Med.,* **1959,** *26,* 740–748.

Burns, J. J., and Shore, P. Biochemical effects of drugs. *A. Rev. Pharmac.,* **1961,** *1,* 79–104.

Chalmers, T. C. Effects of ascorbic acid on the common cold. An evaluation of the evidence. *Am. J. Med.,* **1975,** *58,* 532–536.

Cochrane, W. A. Overnutrition in prenatal and neonatal life: a problem? *Can. med. Ass. J.,* **1965,** *93,* 893–899.

Conney, A. H.; Bray, G. A.; Evans, C.; and Burns, J. J. Metabolic interactions between L-ascorbic acid and drugs. *Ann. N.Y. Acad. Sci.,* **1961,** *92,* 115–127.

Coulehan, J. L.; Reisinger, K. S.; Rogers, K. D.; and Bradley, D. W. Vitamin C prophylaxis in a boarding school. *New Engl. J. Med.,* **1974,** *290,* 6–10.

Crandon, J. H.; Lennihan, R., Jr.; Mikal, S.; and Reis, A. E. Ascorbic acid economy in surgical patients. *Ann. N.Y. Acad. Sci.,* **1961,** *92,* 246–267.

Dykes, M. H. M., and Meier, P. Ascorbic acid and the common cold. Evaluation of its efficacy and toxicity. *J. Am. med. Ass.,* **1975,** *231,* 1073–1079.

Goldsmith, G. A. Human requirements for vitamin C and its use in clinical medicine. *Ann. N.Y. Acad. Sci.,* **1961,** *92,* 230–245.

Holst, A., and Fröhlich, T. Experimental studies relating to "ship-beri-beri" and scurvy. II. On the etiology of scurvy. *J. Hyg., Camb.,* **1907,** *7,* 634–671.

Jukes, T. H. Are recommended daily allowances for vitamin C adequate? *Proc. natn. Acad. Sci. U.S.A.,* **1974,** *71,* 1949–1951.

Karlowski, T. R.; Chalmers, T. C.; Frenkel, L. D.; Kapikian, A. Z.; Lewis, T. L.; and Lynch, J. M. Ascorbic acid for the common cold. A prophylactic and therapeutic trial. *J. Am. med. Ass.,* **1975,** *231,* 1038–1042.

King, C. G. Present knowledge of ascorbic acid (vitamin C). *Nutr. Rev.,* **1968,** *26,* 33–36.

King, C. G., and Waugh, W. A. Chemical nature of vitamin C. *Science, N.Y.,* **1932,** *75,* 357–358.

La Du, B. N., and Zannoni, V. G. The role of ascorbic acid in tyrosine metabolism. *Ann. N.Y. Acad. Sci.,* **1961,** *92,* 175–191.

Levine, S. Z.; Gordon, H. H.; and Marples, E. A defect in the metabolism of tyrosine and phenylalanine in premature infants. II. Spontaneous occurrence and eradication by vitamin C. *J. clin. Invest.,* **1941,** *20,* 209–219.

Light, I. J.; Berry, H. K.; and Sutherland, J. M. Aminoacidemia of prematurity, its response to ascorbic acid. *Am. J. Dis. Child.,* **1966,** *112,* 229–236.

McKinnis, R. B., and King, C. G. Nature of vitamin C: study of its electrical transference. *J. biol. Chem.,* **1930,** *87,* 615–623.

Mumma, R. O., and Verlangieri, A. J. Isolation of ascorbic acid-2-sulfate from selected rat organs. *Biochim. biophys. Acta,* **1972,** *273,* 249–253.

Pauling, L. Evolution and the need for ascorbic acid. *Proc. natn. Acad. Sci. U.S.A.,* **1970,** *67,* 1643–1648.

————. *Vitamin C and the Common Cold.* W. H. Freeman & Co., Pubs., San Francisco, **1970**.

Schwartz, A. R.; Togo, Y.; Hornick, R. B.; Tominaga, S.; and Gleckman, R. A. Evaluation of the efficacy of ascorbic acid in prophylaxis of induced rhinovirus 44 infection in man. *J. infect. Dis.,* **1973,** *128,* 500–505.

Sebrell, W. H., and Harris, R. S. (eds.). *The Vitamins: Chemistry, Physiology, Pathology, Methods,* Vol. 1. Academic Press, Inc., New York, **1967,** pp. 306–541.

Svirbely, J. L., and Szent-Györgyi, A. Chemical nature of vitamin C. *Biochem. J.,* **1932,** *26,* 865–870.

Walker, G. H.; Bynoe, M. L.; and Tyrrell, D. A. J. Trial of ascorbic acid in prevention of colds. *Br. med. J.,* **1967,** *1,* 603–606.

Wolbach, S. B. Pathologic changes resulting from vitamin deficiency. *J. Am. med. Ass.,* **1937,** *109,* 7–13.

Zannoni, V. G., and Lynch, M. Role of ascorbic acid in drug metabolism. *Drug Metab. Rev.,* **1973,** *2,* 57–69.

Zilva, S. S. Influence of aeration on stability of antiscorbutic factor. *Lancet,* **1921,** *1,* 478.

CHAPTER

75 FAT-SOLUBLE VITAMINS

Vitamin A

H. George Mandel

History. Certain of the symptoms of vitamin A deficiency were recognized in the middle of the nineteenth century, and their cause was linked to inadequacy of the diet. Thus, the condition known as ophthalmia Brasiliana, a disease of the eyes that primarily afflicted poorly nourished slaves, was first described in 1865. In 1887, endemic night blindness was reported to occur among the orthodox Russian Catholics who fasted during the Lenten period. More pertinent was the observation that the nurslings of mothers who fasted were prone to develop spontaneous sloughing of the cornea. Many other reports of nutritional keratomalacia soon followed from all parts of the world, including the United States.

Experimental rather than clinical observations, however, led to the discovery of vitamin A. In 1913, two groups (Osborne and Mendel; McCollum and Davis) independently reported that animals fed on artificial diets with lard as a sole source of fat developed a nutritional deficiency that could be corrected by the addition of substances such as butter, egg yolk, and cod liver oil to the diet. An outstanding symptom of this experimental nutritional deficiency was xerophthalmia (dryness and thickening of the conjunctiva). Clinical and experimental vitamin A deficiencies were recognized as related during World War I, when it became apparent that xerophthalmia in human beings was a result of a decrease in the content of butterfat in the diet.

Chemistry and Occurrence. The simple observation of Steenbock (1919) that the vitamin A content of vegetables varies with the degree of pigmentation paved the way for the discovery of the chemical nature of the vitamin. Subsequently, Euler and associates (1929) and Moore (1929) demonstrated that the purified plant pigment carotene (provitamin A) is a remarkably potent source of vitamin A. β-Carotene, the most active carotenoid found in plants, has the following structural formula:

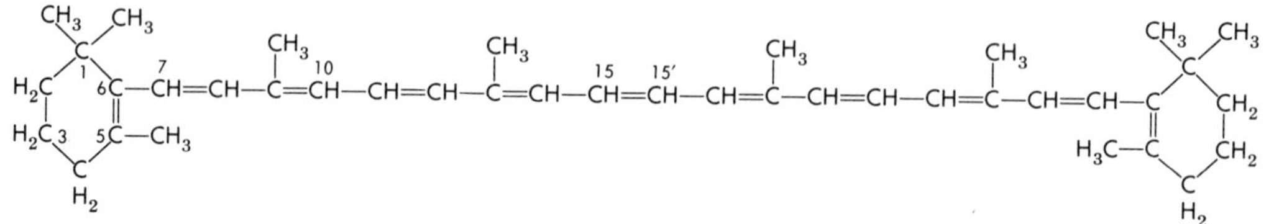

In the United States, the average adult receives about half of his daily intake of vitamin A as carotenoids.

Vitamin A exists in a variety of forms, and the term is frequently used to represent the various compounds. *Retinol* (vitamin A_1), a primary alcohol, is present in esterified form in the tissues of animals and salt-water fishes, mainly in the liver. Its structural formula, established by Karrer and associates (1931), is as follows:

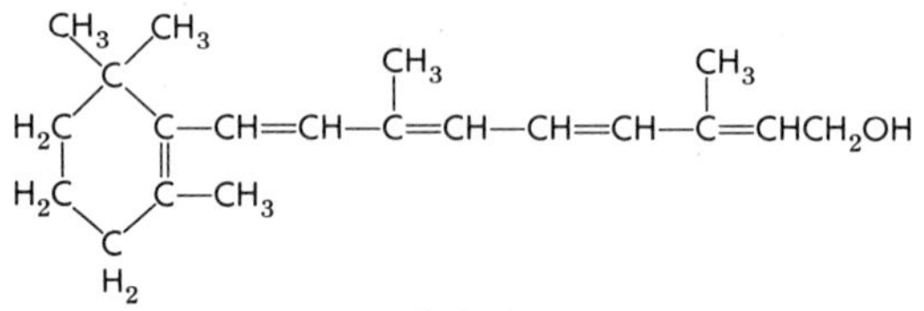

Retinol

A closely related compound, 3-dehydroretinol (vitamin A_2), is obtained from the tissues of fresh-water fishes and usually occurs mixed with retinol. 3-Dehydroretinol contains an additional double bond in the ring, subserves the same functions, follows similar biochemical pathways, but has only 30% of the potency of retinol and is not converted to that form.

A number of geometric isomers of retinol exist because of the possible *cis-trans* configurations of the side chain containing double bonds. Fish liver oils contain mixtures of the stereoisomers; synthetic retinol is exclusively the *trans* isomer. Interconversion between isomers readily takes place in the body. In the visual cycle, the reaction between retinal (vitamin A aldehyde) and opsin to form rhodopsin only occurs with a particular *cis* isomer.

Certain structural modifications of retinol are possible without destroying its activity. Retinoic acid (vitamin A acid), in which the alcohol group has

β-Carotene

1570

been oxidized, shares some but not all of the actions of retinol. Retinoic acid is very potent in promoting growth of vitamin A–deficient animals but is ineffective in visual function and in restoring reproductive function in certain species where retinol is effective.

Ethers and esters derived from the alcohol also show activity. The ring structure of retinol (β-ionone), or the more unsaturated ring in 3-dehydroretinol (dehydro-β-ionone), is essential for activity; hydrogenation destroys biological activity. Of all known derivatives, *trans*-retinol and its aldehyde, retinal, exhibit the greatest biological potency.

Pharmacological Actions. Aside from its essential role in certain biochemical and physiological processes, vitamin A exerts no toxic action in small doses. Significant toxicity is, however, associated with massive administration of the vitamin (*see* below). Comprehensive reviews of the pharmacology of vitamin A are available (Moore, 1957; Dingle and Lucy, 1965; Wolf, 1969).

Physiological Functions. Vitamin A has a number of important functions in the body. It plays an essential role in the function of the retina. It is apparently essential for the integrity of epithelial cells. The vitamin is required for growth, especially of bone, reproduction, and embryonic development. It also has a stabilizing effect on various membranes, acts to regulate membrane permeability, and may be involved in micelle formation (*see* Wasserman and Corradino, 1971).

There are numerous reports that vitamin A acts as a cofactor in various biochemical reactions, such as mucopolysaccharide synthesis, sulfate activation, hydroxysteroid dehydrogenation, cholesterol synthesis, and hepatic microsomal demethylation and hydroxylation of drugs. Although these reactions are diminished in vitamin A deficiency, it now appears more likely that, instead of being produced directly by lack of vitamin A, the effects are caused by the inanition and stress that follow reduced food consumption (Levi *et al.*, 1968; Rogers, 1969). In man, this question is difficult to resolve.

Studies with tissue culture systems suggest that vitamin A deficiency may have an effect on enzyme activities in addition to that resulting from protein deficiency. It is also possible that vitamin A deficiency, by influencing lysosomal activity, alters the turnover of such constituents as sulfated mucopolysaccharides. A possible role in steroid interconversions may be responsible for the observed inhibition of reproduction associated with vitamin A deficiency. Vitamin A also stimulates the synthesis of nuclear RNA, suggesting a role in genetic transcription and cell differentiation (Johnson *et al.*, 1969).

It is likely that retinol is converted to a metabolite that is the true vitamin, but there is no information as to its identity. The major recognized reactions are as follows:

Vitamin A and the Visual Cycle. It has long been known that vitamin A deficiency interferes with vision in dim light, a condition known clinically as nyctalopia (night blindness). The fundamental observations of Hecht (1937), carefully elaborated by Wald and Brown (1965) and Hubbard and colleagues (1965), have contributed greatly to an understanding of this phenomenon (*see* Wald, 1968; Fisher *et al.*, 1970).

Adaptation to dark is a function of both the rods and the cones. Primary adaptation is accomplished by the cones, and the process is completed in a few minutes. Secondary adaptation is a function of the rods, and is not completed for 30 minutes or longer. The process of adaptation is a chemical one, and consists in the formation of photosensitive pigments in the retina that, upon exposure to light of low intensity, are bleached and break down to initiate a nerve impulse. After breakdown, the pigment is resynthesized. The photosensitive pigment of the rods of land vertebrates is known as rhodopsin. Rhodopsin is a combination of a special protein, opsin, and a prosthetic group, 11-*cis*-retinal. The known photosensitive pigment of the cones is iodopsin, and it is probable that many other pigments exist to account for color vision. Iodopsin is a combination of retinal with a protein very similar to opsin, called photopsin. Both photosensitive pigments react similarly but to light of different wavelengths.

In the synthesis of rhodopsin, *cis*-retinol is converted to *cis*-retinal in a reversible reaction that requires nicotinamide adenine dinucleotide (NAD) or nicotinamide adenine dinucleotide phosphate (NADP) and a retinol dehydrogenase (Koen and Shaw, 1966). *Cis*-retinal then combines with the ϵ-amino group of lysine in opsin to form rhodopsin. Photodecomposition of rhodopsin is initiated by light striking the rod. The first step is isomerization of the retinal in rhodopsin to the *trans* configuration.

The *trans* isomer then dissociates from opsin. Energy for the initiation of the nerve impulse may be associated with the exposure of sulfhydryl groups, or conformational changes and charge redistribution of opsin (Hubbard *et al.*, 1965). *Trans*-retinal can be reconverted to *cis*-retinal directly and recombine with opsin again to form rhodopsin. Alternatively, *trans*-retinal can be reduced to *trans*-retinol, which is first converted to *cis*-retinol and then to rhodopsin in the manner described above. The overall sequence of events in the visual cycle is depicted in Figure 75-1.

When human beings are fed diets deficient in vitamin A, their ability for dark adaptation is gradually diminished. Rod vision is affected more than cone vision. Upon depletion of the vitamin from liver and blood (usually at concentrations less than 20 μg of retinol per 100 ml of plasma), the concentration of retinol and of rhodopsin in the retina falls. Unless the deficiency is overcome, opsin, lacking the stabilizing effect of retinal, decays and anatomical deterioration of the rods' outer segments takes place. Irreversible ultrastructural changes in the photoreceptor leading to blindness supervene in rats maintained on a vitamin A–deficient diet for 10 months.

Following short-term vitamin A deprivation, dark adaptation can be restored to normal by the addition of vitamin A to the diet. Some investigators have reported that the effect of vitamin A on nyctalopia of dietary origin can be detected within a few minutes as vitamin A gains access to the retina. Other investigators have shown, however, that normal vision is not regained for months after adequate amounts of the vitamin have been added to the diet. The cause for this delay is unknown.

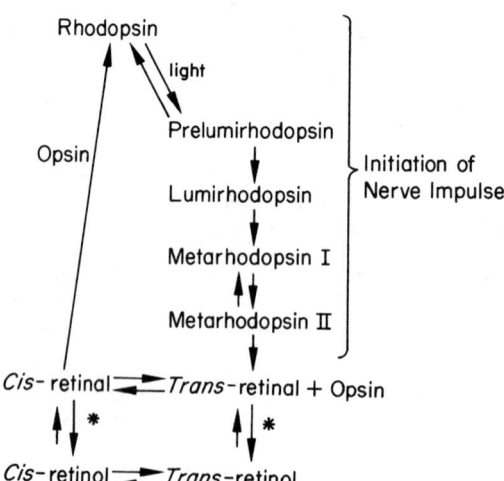

Figure 75-1. *The visual cycle.*

The asterisks(*) refer to the reactions in which retinol dehydrogenase and NAD/NADP are involved. For explanation, *see* the text. (After Hubbard, Bownds, and Yoshizawa, 1965. Courtesy of the Cold Spring Harbor Laboratory of Quantitative Biology.)

Retinol and Epithelial Structures. The functional and structural integrity of epithelial cells throughout the body is dependent upon an adequate supply of vitamin A. The vitamin plays a major role in the induction and control of epithelial differentiation in mucus-secreting or keratinizing tissues. Retinol is required for the formation of a specific fucose-containing glycopeptide, and the vitamin is condensed with mannose to form a glycolipid intermediate (De Luca *et al.*, 1970). In the presence of retinol, basal epithelial cells are stimulated to produce mucus. Excessive retinol leads to the production of a thick layer of mucin, the inhibition of keratinization, and the display of goblet cells.

In the absence of retinol, atrophy of epithelium occurs, followed by a proliferation of basal cells at the expense of mucous cells. The new cells, by their continued growth, undermine and replace the original epithelium with a stratified, keratinizing epithelium.

Tumor Growth. With vitamin A therapy, carcinogen-induced skin tumors of animals may regress. It is possible that the keratinizing squamous metaplasia resulting from carcinogen treatment, which resembles that associated with vitamin A deficiency, is antagonized by vitamin A as a promoter of differentiation (Harris *et al.*, 1972). Alternatively, the increased release of degradative enzymes from lysosomes by vitamin A (or retinoic acid) may produce tumor regression. Vitamin A may also prevent the conversion of the carcinogen to its active metabolites. In other situations, however, vitamin A accelerates tumor development following carcinogen treatment.

Wound Healing. In animals, retinol and retinoic acid antagonize the retardation of wound healing produced by steroids, salicylates, and other anti-inflammatory drugs.

Signs and Symptoms of Deficiency. As is the case with all dietary essentials, a deficiency of retinol retards normal growth and development. Indeed, the bioassay of vitamin A is based upon the ability of the vitamin to restore normal growth in rats fed a diet deficient in vitamin A but complete in all other respects.

Tissue reserves of vitamin A in the normal adult are sufficiently large to require long-term dietary deprivation in order to induce deficiency. Vitamin A deficiency occurs more commonly, therefore, in chronic diseases affecting fat absorption, such as biliary tract or pancreatic disease, sprue, colitis, and portal cirrhosis; following partial gastrectomy; or during extreme, chronic dietary inadequacy.

The deficiency is quite widespread in Southeast Asia, the Middle East, Africa, and South America, particularly in children, and is associated with general malnutrition (*see* McLaren, 1966). Vitamin A deficiency and protein malnutrition are the two most serious nutritional deficiency diseases in the world today. Deficiency of vitamin A may be fatal, especially in infants and young children suffering from kwashiorkor or marasmus. It is estimated that tens of thousands of children in the world go blind every year because of inadequate intake of vitamin A. In the United States, about 15% of the population has plasma or liver vitamin A concentrations below the accepted lower limits of normal (20 μg/100 ml or 40 μg/g, respectively), indicating a risk of deficiency. Most of these individuals are infants or children (*see* Roels, 1970).

Signs and symptoms of mild vitamin A deficiency are easily overlooked. The earliest and most recognizable manifestation is nyctalopia, even though its onset occurs only when vitamin A depletion is severe. Quantitative assessment of retinal function would be useful in the diagnosis of vitamin A deficiency. In addition to effects on growth and development, vitamin A deficiency is associated with keratinization of epithelium, especially of the conjunctiva and cornea. Often there is an impairment of both taste and smell in vitamin A–deficient individuals, which undoubtedly results from a keratinizing effect. Also, hearing may become decreased.

Keratomalacia. This condition, characterized by desiccation, ulceration, and xerosis of the cornea and conjunctiva, is occasionally seen as an acute symptom in the very young who are on severely deficient diets. It is foreshadowed, usually, by xerophthalmia and "Bitot's spots" and ultimately leads to severe visual impairment and even blindness (McLaren, 1966).

Bronchorespiratory Tract. Changes in the bronchorespiratory epithelium from mucus secretion to keratinization lead to increased incidence of respiratory infections in the deficiency state. There is also a decrease in elasticity of the lung and other tissues.

Skin. Keratinization and drying of the epidermis occur and papular eruptions, involving the pilosebaceous follicles, may be found, especially on the extremities.

Genitourinary System. Urinary calculi are frequent concomitants of vitamin A deficiency. Epithelium of the urinary tract shares in the general pathological changes of all epithelial structures. Epithelial debris may thus provide the nidus around which a calculus is formed.

Gastrointestinal Tract. The intestinal mucosa shows a reduction in the number of goblet cells but no keratinization. Alterations in intestinal epithelium and metaplasia of pancreatic ductal epithelium are common. They may be responsible for the diarrhea occasionally seen in vitamin A deficiency.

Sweat Glands. These glands may undergo atrophy and keratinizing squamous-cell metaplasia.

Miscellaneous Signs and Symptoms. In animals, vitamin A deficiency is associated with faulty bone modeling (with production of thick, cancellous bone instead of thinner, more compact bone), nerve lesions, and increased cerebrospinal fluid pressure and hydrocephalus. Abnormalities of reproduction include impairment of spermatogenesis, degeneration of testes, abortion, resorption of fetuses, and production of malformed offspring.

Hypervitaminosis A. An intake of vitamin A greatly in excess of requirement results in a toxic syndrome known as hypervitaminosis A. Several cases in children have been reported (Oliver, 1958); the syndrome has also been detected in a few adults. Excess vitamin E appears to protect against hypervitaminosis A.

All the reported cases in children have been associated with the chronic ingestion of retinol. Usually, high intakes have resulted from overzealous prophylactic vitamin therapy on the part of parents, from extended self-medication, or from confusion between percomorph liver oil and the less potent cod liver oil. Some adults with rare skin diseases, such as ichthyosis and Darier's disease, may receive large doses of vitamin A to ameliorate the skin lesions, and this treatment may result in hypervitaminosis (*see* Bauernfeind *et al.,* 1974).

Early signs and symptoms of chronic vitamin A intoxication include irritability, vomiting, loss of appetite, headache, dry and pruritic skin, and skin desquamation. Fatigue, myalgia, loss of body hair, nystagmus, gingivitis, mouth fissures, hepatosplenomegaly, and lymph node enlargement have been observed. Intracranial pressure may be increased, and neurological symptoms, resembling those of brain tumors, have been reported. The diagnosis is usually made following the appearance of tender, deep, hard swellings on the extremities and the occipital region of the head. Hyperostoses in the underlying bone are easily demonstrated roentgenographically. The only consistent abnormality of the blood is a striking and diagnostic elevation of the plasma vitamin A concentration; values ranging from 300 to 2000 μg (1000 to 6600 units) per 100 ml have been reported.

Treatment consists merely in withdrawal of the vitamin. Most signs and symptoms disappear within a week, but the hyperostoses remain evident for several months after clinical recovery has occurred.

Acute poisoning in man is known to follow the ingestion of polar bear liver. Signs and symptoms include drowsiness, sluggishness, irritability or irresistible desire to sleep, severe headache, vomiting, papilledema, and, after 24 hours, generalized peeling of the skin. The high content of vitamin A in polar bear liver, up to 12,000 μg of retinol per gram (Russell, 1967), is responsible for the syndrome. The acute consumption of more than 500,000 μg or a daily intake exceeding 50,000 μg of retinol frequently results in toxic effects in adults.

Acute poisoning has been noted in infants following ingestion of lesser amounts. The signs are those of increased intracranial pressure; the bulging fontanel and vomiting usually disappear within 36 hours after cessation of ingestion of the vitamin. Ingestion of as little as 7500 to 15,000 μg (25,000 to 50,000 units) of retinol daily for 30 days can also induce signs of increased intracranial pressure in infants (Yaffe and Filer, 1971). The toxicity of the vitamin depends on age, dose, and duration of administration.

Hypervitaminosis A has been studied extensively in experimental animals. The most characteristic lesions occur in the bones and result from accelerated bone and cartilage resorption and new-bone formation. Bones continue to grow in length but not in thickness, with increased susceptibility to fractures. These changes are unassociated with any detectable abnormalities in calcium, phosphorus, or phosphatase levels of the blood. In young animals, premature closure of epiphyses inhibits growth of bones. In general, changes in bone depend on the species, the age of the animal, and the degree of hypervitaminosis. Other manifestations of hypervitaminosis A are anorexia, cutaneous lesions, temporary thickening of skin, deposition of lipid in Kupffer cells, exophthalmos, hypoprothrombinemia, and eventually death in animals. There is considerable interspecies variation in toxic effects. Certain congenital abnormalities have been reported in the offspring of hypervitaminotic mothers (e.g., hydrocephalus and encephalocele). The hypoprothrombinemia observed may be successfully treated with vitamin K.

Large amounts of vitamin A activate the lysosomes to release a protease, cathepsin D, that degrades the structural protein component of bone and cartilage matrix and results in a loss of mucopolysaccharide (Fell and Dingle, 1963; see review by Dingle and Lucy, 1965). Lipoprotein membranes exhibit increased permeability and decreased stability in the presence of excessive concentrations of vitamin A, leading to mitochondrial swelling, lysosomal rupture, and probably the decreased cohesiveness of keratin. Such effects may stimulate mitosis and the proliferation of lower epidermis, but this area is still controversial (Logan, 1972). There is evidence to suggest that these results of vitamin A administration may be pharmacological rather than physiological since α-retinol, an isomer of retinol, apparently has the same effects as retinol on membranes but lacks the growth-promoting activity of vitamin A. Furthermore, it has only limited ability to transform keratinizing to mucus-secreting epithelium. The effects of vitamins A and E on membrane stability appear to be mutually antagonistic (Anderson et al., 1967).

Table 75-1 compares the effects of hypervitaminosis A and hypovitaminosis A.

Human Requirement. Human requirements for vitamin A have been approximated from studies that have attempted to correct experimentally produced deficiency states. The present recommendations of the Food and Nutrition Board of the National Research Council are based upon the amount of vitamin necessary to maintain normal dark adaptation plus an additional factor of safety to cover variations in absorption and utilization of the vitamin. The recommended daily allowances for the normal male and female adult are 1000 and 800 retinol equivalents (5000 and 4000 units) per day, respectively. It is assumed that 50% of dietary vitamin A is derived from retinol and 50% from β-carotene in the United States. For the requirements of infants and children, see Table XVIII-1 (page 1545) and below.

Absorption, Fate, and Excretion. In this discussion the absorption and the fate of both vitamin A and carotene will be con-

Table 75-1. GENERAL CONSEQUENCES OF VITAMIN A DEFICIENCY AND EXCESS *

SITE	HYPOVITAMINOSIS A	HYPERVITAMINOSIS A
General	Growth retardation; susceptibility to infection; death	Malaise; lethargy; deposition of carotenoids; death
Skin and mucous membranes	Xerosis; keratinizing metaplasia; xerophthalmia; keratomalacia	Mucous cell formation, desquamation
Skeletal tissues and bone	Cancellous structure; defective remodeling	Decalcification, fractures, early epiphyseal closure; cortical thickening
Reproductive system	Degeneration of testes; gonadal resorption; congenital malformation	Resorption; congenital malformation
Nervous system	Compression by bone, increased intracranial pressure, atrophy and ataxia	Elevated intracranial pressure
Retina	Night blindness	

* After Fisher, Carr, Huff, and Huber, 1970, as modified from McLaren, 1966. Courtesy of *Federation Proceedings*.

sidered, since both represent important sources of the vitamin. Most of this information has been derived from animal experiments, but it is likely that similar considerations are true for man. More than 90% of the intake of preformed vitamin A is in the form of retinol esters, usually as retinyl palmitate.

Vitamin A is readily absorbed from the normal gastrointestinal tract. If the amount ingested is not much greater than the requirement, absorption is complete; however, when a large excess is taken, some of the vitamin escapes in the feces. Inasmuch as vitamin A is fat soluble, it is not unexpected to find that the absorption of the vitamin is related to that of lipid and is enhanced by bile; nevertheless, aqueous dispersions of retinol or its ester are absorbed more rapidly than are oily solutions.

In the presence of disordered fat absorption, the absorption of vitamin A is materially reduced. In such patients water-miscible preparations should be used. Intestinal absorption of vitamin A is reduced when diets are low in protein. The absorption of vitamin A is also disturbed in hepatic disease. In hepatitis, cirrhosis, or biliary obstruction, the absorption of the vitamin is reduced to an extent that is roughly related to the degree of hepatic insufficiency. In certain infections, absorption may also be reduced.

Intestinal absorption apparently occurs by active transport and is sensitive to metabolic inhibitors (Loran et al., 1961). Retinol esters are hydrolyzed in the lumen of the intestine by pancreatic enzymes and within the brush border of the intestinal cell before absorption, followed by reesterification, mainly to the palmitate (Ganguly, 1969). There may be several cycles of hydrolysis and reesterification (Lawrence et al., 1966). Significant quantities of vitamin A are also absorbed directly into the circulation.

The long-chain fatty acid ester enters the circulation by transport in the chylomicron fraction of lymph (Goodman et al., 1966). Plasma concentrations of esterified retinol reach a peak about 4 hours after the administration of the vitamin. Most of the vitamin is stored in the liver, mainly in parenchymal hepatocytes as the palmitate ester, and a small amount of retinol is present in the Kupffer cells (Linder et al., 1971).

The population median concentration of vitamin A in man is about 100 μg/g of liver. Other tissues, such as kidney, lung, adrenal, and intraperitoneal fat, contain about 1 μg of vitamin A per gram. There is also selective localization of the vitamin in the retina of the eye. Administration of low doses of vitamin E markedly increases the tissue storage of vitamin A. Until hepatic saturation takes place, the administration of vitamin A leads mainly to its accumulation in the liver rather than to increased blood concentrations.

Prior to entering the circulation, the hepatic retinol ester is hydrolyzed and bound to an α_1-globulin (Raz et al., 1970). This retinol-binding protein (RBP) circulates in the blood in man complexed with a prealbumin protein, similar to but apparently not identical with a prealbumin carrier for thyroxine (White et al., 1972). This prevents the circulating RBP (and retinol) from glomerular filtration in the kidney. Also, the protein-carrier transport system limits the quantity of vitamin that reaches a particular organ after the administration of excessive retinol. A small amount of retinol ester is also present in the blood, associated with lipoproteins.

The normal plasma concentration of vitamin A is about 30 to 70 μg (100 to 230 units) per 100 ml, but much higher levels have been reported when vitamin A supplements are taken. The concentration varies with age, geographical location, seasonal food availability, and socioeconomic factors.

If an individual ingests a diet free of vitamin A or its precursors, plasma concentrations are maintained over many months at the expense of hepatic reserves. Blood concentrations, therefore, are not an accurate guide to an individual's vitamin A status, but low plasma values of vitamin A imply that hepatic storage of the vitamin may be exhausted. Signs and symptoms of vitamin A deficiency appear when the plasma concentration falls below 10 to 20 μg/100 ml.

In kwashiorkor, although hepatic stores of vitamin A may be normal, low vitamin A concentrations in the plasma reflect an impairment of the hepatic release of the retinol-RBP complex, which can be overcome by the administration of protein and calories. Nevertheless, when signs of vitamin A deficiency exist, vitamin A supplementation is indicated since feeding results in the release of the RBP-retinol complex by the liver and also in an increase in vitamin A requirements (Smith *et al.,* 1973). Plasma concentrations of vitamin A may also be reduced in hepatic disease, probably because of a defect in the mechanism whereby the vitamin is released from the liver into the circulation. Thus, the RBP concentration and function may be an important determinant of a person's vitamin A status. In infections with fever, such as pneumonia, the vitamin A concentration in the blood may be reduced drastically, partially because of increased urinary excretion.

Pregnancy also alters the vitamin A blood concentrations. Shortly after the onset of pregnancy there is a fall in the mean plasma content of vitamin A, followed by a slow rise, and another sharp fall at parturition. Blood values then rapidly return to normal. It is likely that the increased demands for vitamin A lead to the withdrawal of the vitamin from the blood at a rate exceeding that of mobilization from the hepatic reserve. The placental barrier prevents the extensive transfer of vitamin A or carotenoids. The vitamin concentration in fetal blood is thus less than in maternal blood. Both colostrum and milk offer the newborn an adequate supply of vitamin A (Lübke and Finkbeiner, 1958). The concentration of vitamin A in the milk is maintained at a fixed maximal level if the dietary intake of the vitamin is adequate to permit storage in the liver. With reduced intake, the liver stores are utilized before this characteristic level is diminished.

Retinol is in part conjugated to form a β-glucuronide, which undergoes enterohepatic circulation and is oxidized to retinal and retinoic acid. Several other water-soluble metabolites are also excreted in urine and feces (Dunagin *et al.,* 1966; Roberts and De Luca, 1967). Retinoic acid is decarboxylated and further degraded, and also forms a glucuronide that is rapidly secreted into the bile and excreted in the feces.

Normally no vitamin A can be recovered unchanged from human urine, but in disease states in which urinary excretion of the vitamin A is increased, such as pneumonia or chronic nephritis, the unaltered vitamin is excreted by this route.

Carotene is less well absorbed than vitamin A in man. Absorption depends upon the presence of bile and absorbable fat in the intestinal tract and is greatly decreased by steatorrhea and chronic diarrhea. The ingestion of mineral oil decreases the absorption of carotene, whereas water-soluble dispersing agents enhance absorption. The conversion of carotene to vitamin A occurs in the wall of the small intestine. Two molecules of retinal are produced by cleavage of the 15,15′ double bond (Goodman *et al.,* 1967). This reaction is mediated by the dioxygenase system, requires molecular oxygen, and is influenced by the amount of dietary protein. Some of the retinal is further oxidized to retinoic acid; however, most of it is reduced to retinol, which is then esterified and transported in the lymph, as described above. Carotene is biologically active only following conversion to retinol. Some carotene gains access to the circulation. If very large amounts of carotene are ingested, very high blood concentrations may be achieved, and the hypercarotenemia results in a yellow discoloration of the skin, which is reversible; this can be distinguished from jaundice by the absence of scleral pigmentation. Hypervitaminosis does not develop, however.

Bioassay and Unitage. Most commercial preparations are synthetic retinol esters, which have largely replaced natural vitamin A obtained from fish liver oils. Animal-source preparations must be biologically assayed to establish their activity. This assay depends upon the ability of the vitamin to support growth in vitamin-depleted rats of specified age and weight and fed a standard vitamin A–deficient diet over a given period of time. The activity of suitably purified preparations can be determined by spectrophotometric analysis. The U.S.P. reference standard consists of a solution of *trans*-vitamin A acetate in vegetable oil, each gram of which contains 100,000 units. One U.S.P. vitamin A unit is the specific biological activity of 0.3 μg of retinol, 0.34 μg of retinyl acetate, or 0.6 μg of β-carotene. Because of the relatively inefficient dietary utilization of β-carotene compared to retinol, the new nomenclature is in terms of the retinol equivalent, which represents 1 μg of retinol, 6 μg of dietary β-carotene, or 12 μg of other provitamin A carotenoids. Thus, 1 retinol equivalent equals 3.3 U.S.P. units of vitamin A activity as supplied by retinol or 10 units of vitamin A activity as supplied by β-carotene. Some of the difficulties and inconsistencies attending the spectrophotometric analysis and bioassay of vitamin A as well as the errors that may be encountered have been summarized by Kofler and Rubin (1960) and Harris (1960).

Preparations. There are many types of preparations that contain vitamin A. These range from solutions of pure synthetic vitamin A in oil to numerous fish liver oils and concentrates that contain both vitamin A and vitamin D in various proportions. In the United States, commercial production of synthetic vitamin A is about 1000 tons per year. Absorption is greatest for aqueous preparations, intermediate for emulsions, and slowest for oil solutions. Whereas oil-soluble preparations may lead to greater hepatic storage of the vitamin, water-miscible preparations usually provide higher plasma concentrations (Srikantia and Reddy, 1970).

Vitamin A, U.S.P., is either fish liver oil or a solution of natural or synthetic vitamin A or its fatty acid esters. *Vitamin A Capsules,* U.S.P., contain 1.5 to 15 mg of retinol (5000 to 50,000 U.S.P. vitamin A units) per capsule.

Water-miscible vitamin A (AQUASOL A) is a concentrate of vitamin A dispersed in water by means of a suitable agent.

There are also many multivitamin preparations that include vitamin A, such as *Decavitamin Capsules,* U.S.P., and *Decavitamin Tablets,* U.S.P., each of which contains 1200 μg of retinol per capsule or tablet.

Tretinoin, U.S.P. (*all* trans-*retinoic acid;* RETIN-A), is available for topical use as a 0.1% cream and a 0.05% lotion. It is an irritant, causes skin peeling, and is used for the treatment of acne vulgaris (*see* below).

Therapeutic Uses. The normal adult requirement for vitamin A is supplied by an adequate food intake. The rational uses of vitamin A are in the treatment of vitamin A deficiency and in its prophylactic administration during periods of increased requirement, such as infancy, pregnancy, and lactation. However, limitation in diet due to economic stress or food fads can give rise to the symptoms of deficiency outlined above. In addition, the ingestion of large doses of vitamin E or C may alter the vitamin A status of an individual, judging from animal experiments. Once a vitamin A deficiency has been diagnosed, intensive therapy should be instituted. The patient should then be maintained on a proper diet.

During infancy, pregnancy, or lactation, it is best to supply supplemental vitamin A rather than to rely solely on the diet. Infants usually receive vitamin A in conjunction with vitamin D. A daily intake of 400 to 700 retinol equivalents of vitamin A should be provided for infants and growing children. During pregnancy (especially the second and third trimesters) and lactation, the intake of vitamin A should be maintained at approximately 1000 retinol equivalents per day.

Rarely, the absorption, mobilization, or the storage of vitamin A may be adversely affected, and under such circumstances long-continued therapy with the vitamin may be indicated, as, for example, in an individual with steatorrhea, severe biliary obstruction, cirrhosis of the liver, or following a total gastrectomy. In other disease states where considerable vitamin A is lost from the body, replacement therapy may be necessary. In various infections in which mucous cell turnover is accelerated and urinary excretion of the vitamin is increased, the need for retinol is further enhanced. Individuals already suffering from vitamin A deficiency who develop infections, especially of the respiratory tract, will benefit from the inclusion of adequate amounts of vitamin A in the diet. There is no evidence, however, that an excessive intake of vitamin A will influence the incidence of infections in an individual whose intake of vitamin A is adequate. However, moderate amounts of vitamin A apparently do no harm. If vitamin A is prescribed as a dietary supplement, intake of 1500 μg of retinol represents one and one-half times the recommended daily allowance. Long-term ingestion of much larger amounts may lead to hypervitaminosis.

In kwashiorkor and other severe vitamin A deficiencies in children, a single intramuscular injection of 30,000 μg of retinol as the water-miscible palmitate has been advocated, followed by intermittent oral treatment with vitamin A in oil (*see* Bauernfeind *et al.,* 1974). In areas of the world where protein malnutrition and vitamin A deficiencies abound, 60,000 to 120,000 μg of retinol in oil should be administered to children, under supervision, every 3 to 6 months, depending on the age. Vitamin E should be coadministered since it apparently increases the efficacy of vitamin A therapy and also protects against vitamin A hypervitaminosis.

Vitamin A has been prescribed in many systemic conditions and for the local treatment of infections, burns, and wounds. Carefully controlled observations fail to substantiate the claims advanced for such uses. It may be helpful in certain skin diseases, such as psoriasis and ichthyosis. The use of tretinoin (retinoic acid) in these conditions has also been suggested. The compound is quite irritating when applied directly to the skin (*see* Logan, 1972). The efficacy of such therapy has not been validated by properly controlled clinical trials. However, the topical use of tretinoin for acne vulgaris now has many advocates (*see* Kligman *et al.,* 1974). It is applied topically each day in an amount that initially causes flushing. A moderate amount of redness and peeling is said to favor the therapeutic response. After a few weeks of application, local reaction becomes less severe. The topical application of tretinoin and the oral administration of an antibiotic (a tetracycline or erythromycin) may be required for more severe cases.

Anderson, O. R.; Roels, O. A.; and Pfister, R. M. Dietary retinol and alpha-tocopherol and erythrocyte structure in rats. *Nature, Lond.,* **1967,** *213,* 47–49.

Bauernfeind, J. C.; Newmark, H.; and Brin, M. Vitamin A and E nutrition via intramuscular or oral route. *Am. J. clin. Nutr.,* **1974,** *27,* 234–253.

De Luca, L.; Schumacher, M.; and Wolf, G. Biosynthesis of a fucose-containing glycopeptide from rat small intestine in normal and vitamin A–deficient conditions. *J. biol. Chem.,* **1970,** *245,* 4551–4558.

Dunagin, P. E., Jr.; Zachman, R. D.; and Olson, J. A. The identification of metabolites of retinal and retinoic acid in rat bile. *Biochim. biophys. Acta,* **1966,** *124,* 71–85.

Euler, B. von; Euler, H. von; and Karrer, P. Zur Biochemie der Carotinoide. *Helv. chim. Acta,* **1929,** *12,* 278–285.

Fell, H. B., and Dingle, J. T. Studies on the mode of action of excess vitamin A. 6. Lysosomal protease and the degradation of cartilage matrix. *Biochem. J.,* **1963,** *87,* 403–408.

Fisher, K. D.; Carr, C. J.; Huff, J. E.; and Huber, T. E. Dark adaptation and night vision. *Fedn Proc. Fedn Am. Socs exp. Biol.,* **1970,** *29,* 1605–1638.

Ganguly, J. Absorption of vitamin A. *Am. J. clin. Nutr.,* **1969,** *22,* 923–933.

Goodman, DeW. S.; Blomstrand, R.; Werner, B.; Huang, H. S.; and Shiratori, T. The intestinal absorption and metabolism of vitamin A and β-carotene in man. *J. clin. Invest.,* **1966,** *45,* 1615–1623.

Goodman, DeW. S.; Huang, H. S.; Kanai, M.; and Shiratori, T. The enzymatic conversion of all-*trans* β-carotene into retinal. *J. biol. Chem.,* **1967,** *242,* 3543–3554.

Harris, C. C.; Sporn, M. B.; Kaufman, D. G.; Smith, J. M.; Jackson, F. E.; and Saffiotti, U. Histogenesis of squamous metaplasia in the hamster tracheal epithelium caused by vitamin A deficiency or benzo[α]pyrene–ferric oxide. *J. natn. Cancer Inst.,* **1972,** *48,* 743–761.

Harris, P. L. Bioassay of vitamin A compounds. *Vitams Horm.,* **1960,** *18,* 341–370.

Hecht, S. Rods, cones, and chemical basis of vision. *Physiol. Rev.,* **1937,** *17,* 239–290.

Hubbard, R.; Bownds, D.; and Yoshizawa, T. The chemistry of visual photoreception. *Cold Spring Harb. Symp. quant. Biol.,* **1965,** *30,* 301–315.

Johnson, B. C.; Kennedy, M.; and Chiba, N. Vitamin A and nuclear RNA synthesis. *Am. J. clin. Nutr.,* **1969,** *22,* 1048–1058.

Karrer, P.; Morf, R.; and Schöpp, K. Zur Kenntnis des Vitamins A aus Fischtranen. *Helv. chim. Acta,* **1931,** *14,* 1431–1436.

Kligman, A. M.; Mills, O. H., Jr.; and Leyden, J. J. Acne vulgaris. A treatable disease. *Postgrad. Med.,* **1974,** *55,* 99–105.

Koen, A. L., and Shaw, C. R. Retinol and alcohol dehydrogenases in retina and liver. *Biochim. biophys. Acta,* **1966,** *128,* 48–54.

Kofler, M., and Rubin, S. H. Physicochemical assay of vitamin A and related compounds. *Vitams Horm.,* **1960,** *18,* 315–339.

Lawrence, C. W.; Crain, F. D.; Lotspeich, F. J.; and Krause, R. F. Absorption, transport and storage of retinyl-15-^{14}C palmitate-9,10-^{3}H in the rat. *J. Lipid Res.,* **1966,** *7,* 226–229.

Levi, A. S.; Geller, S.; Rood, D. M.; and Wolf, G. The effect of vitamin A and other dietary constituents on the activity of adenosine triphosphate sulphurylase. *Biochem. J.,* **1968,** *109,* 69–74.

Linder, M. C.; Anderson, G. H.; and Ascarelli, I. Quantitative distribution of vitamin A in Kupffer cells and hepatocyte populations of rat liver. *J. biol. Chem.,* **1971,** *246,* 5538–5540.

Logan, W. S. Vitamin A and keratinization. *Archs Derm.,* **1972,** *105,* 748–753.

Loran, M. R.; Althausen, T. L.; Spicer, F. W.; and Goldstein, W. I. Transport of vitamin A across human intestine *in vitro. J. Lab. clin. Med.,* **1961,** *58,* 622–626.

Lübke, F., and Finkbeiner, H. Beitrag zum Verhalten des Vitamin-A- und β-Carotinspiegels in der Gravidität, unter der Geburt und im Wochenbett. *Int. Z. Vitam-Forsch.,* **1958,** *29,* 45–68.

McCollum, E. V., and Davis, M. The necessity of certain lipins in the diet during growth. *J. biol. Chem.,* **1913,** *15,* 167–175.

McLaren, D. S. Present knowledge of the role of vitamin A in health and disease. *Trans. R. Soc. trop. Med. Hyg.,* **1966,** *60,* 436–462.

Moore, T. Relation of carotin to vitamin A. *Lancet,* **1929,** *2,* 380–381.

Oliver, T. K., Jr. Chronic vitamin A intoxication: report of a case in an older child and review of the literature. *A.M.A. J. Dis. Child.,* **1958,** *95,* 57–68.

Osborne, T. B., and Mendel, L. B. The relation of growth to the chemical constituents of the diet. *J. biol. Chem.,* **1913,** *15,* 311–326.

Raz, A.; Shiratori, T.; and Goodman, DeW. S. Studies on the protein-protein and protein-ligand interactions involved in retinol transport in plasma. *J. biol. Chem.,* **1970,** *245,* 1903–1912.

Roberts, A. B., and De Luca, H. F. Pathways of retinol and retinoic acid metabolism in the rat. *Biochem. J.,* **1967,** *102,* 600–605.

Roels, O. A. Vitamin A physiology. *J. Am. med. Ass.,* **1970,** *214,* 1097–1102.

Rogers, W. E., Jr. Reexamination of enzyme activities thought to show evidence of a coenzyme role for vitamin A. *Am. J. clin. Nutr.,* **1969,** *22,* 1003–1013.

Russell, F. E. Vitamin A content of polar bear liver. *Toxicon,* **1967,** *5,* 61–62.

Smith, F. R.; Goodman, DeW. S.; Arroyave, G.; and Viteri, F. Serum vitamin A, retinol-binding protein, and prealbumin concentrations in protein-calorie malnutrition. II. Treatment including supplemental vitamin A. *Am. J. clin. Nutr.,* **1973,** *26,* 982–987.

Srikantia, S. G., and Reddy, V. Effect of a single massive dose of vitamin A on serum and liver levels of the vitamin. *Am. J. clin. Nutr.,* **1970,** *23,* 114–118.

Steenbock, H. White corn vs. yellow corn, and a probable relation between the fat-soluble vitamin and yellow plant pigments. *Science, N.Y.,* **1919,** *50,* 352–353.

Wald, G. The molecular basis of visual excitation. *Nature, Lond.,* **1968,** *219,* 800–807.

Wald, G., and Brown, P. K. Human color vision and color blindness. *Cold Spring Harb. Symp. quant. Biol.,* **1965,** *30,* 345–361.

White, G. A.; Weston, S.; Kirby, W.; and Glover, J. The form of retinol-binding in human serum. *Biochem. J.,* **1972,** *126,* 10P.

Yaffe, S. J., and Filer, L. J. The use and abuse of vitamin A. American Academy of Pediatrics, Joint Committee Statement, Committee on Drugs and Nutrition. *Pediatrics, Springfield,* **1971,** *48,* 655–656.

Monographs and Reviews

Dingle, J. T., and Lucy, J. A. Vitamin A, carotenoids, and cell function. *Biol. Rev.,* **1965,** *40,* 422–461.

Moore, T. *Vitamin A,* 2nd ed. American Elsevier Publishing Co., New York, **1957.**

Olson, J. A. Metabolism and function of vitamin A. *Fedn Proc. Fedn Am. Socs exp. Biol.,* **1969,** *28,* 1670–1677.

Wasserman, R. H., and Corradino, R. A. Metabolic role of vitamins A and D. *A. Rev. Biochem.,* **1971,** *40,* 501–532.

Wolf, G. International symposium on the metabolic function of vitamin A. *Am. J. clin. Nutr.,* **1969,** *22,* 897–1138.

CHAPTER

76 FAT-SOLUBLE VITAMINS

[Continued]

Vitamin D

James A. Straw

History. Vitamin D is the name applied to two related fat-soluble substances that have in common the ability to prevent rickets or cure the rachitic state once it is established.

Prior to the discovery of vitamin D a high percentage of urban children, especially in the temperate zones, developed rickets. Some thought that the disease was due to lack of fresh air and sunshine; others claimed a dietary factor caused the disease. By 1920 the work of Mellanby and Huldschinsky had shown both of these notions to be correct: the addition of cod liver oil to the diet or exposure to sunlight would either prevent or cure the disease. In 1924 it was found that irradiation of animal rations was as efficacious in curing rickets as was irradiation of the animal itself (Hess and Weinstock, 1924; Steenbock and Black, 1924). The detailed elucidation of the metabolism of the vitamin, its distribution, and its mechanisms of action awaited more sophisticated radiochemical technics.

Chemistry and Occurrence. Ultraviolet irradiation of a variety of animal and plant sterols results in the conversion of these provitamins to compounds with vitamin D (antirachitic) activity. Cleavage of the carbon-to-carbon bond between C 9 and C 10 is the essential alteration produced by the photochemical process. Not all sterols that undergo this cleavage possess antirachitic activity. The principal provitamin found in animal tissues is 7-dehydrocholesterol, and its physiologically significant irradiation product is vitamin D_3 (cholecalciferol, activated dehydrocholesterol). The provitamin 7-dehydrocholesterol is synthesized in the skin, where under the influence of sunlight it is converted to vitamin D_3 (see Figure 76-1).

Ergosterol, which is present in yeasts and fungi, is the provitamin for vitamin D_2 (calciferol). Vitamin D_2 is the active constituent in a number of commercial vitamin preparations as well as in irradiated bread and irradiated milk. The material historically designated as vitamin D_1 was later shown to be a mixture of antirachitic substances.

In some species the antirachitic potencies of vitamin D_2 and vitamin D_3 differ greatly from each other. In man there is no practical difference between the two. In the following discussion vitamin D will be used as the collective term for vitamins D_2 and D_3.

CALCIUM METABOLISM AND THE ROLE OF VITAMIN D

Calcium is essential for many physiological and biochemical processes in the body (see Chapter 37). It is convenient to classify the functions of calcium in these processes as structural (mineralization of bone) and metabolic (participation in neuromuscular and neuronal activity, maintenance of membrane integrity, blood coagulation, and enzyme activity). Under conditions of normal calcium homeostasis, the concentration of ionized calcium in plasma is maintained within the narrow range that is suitable for the metabolic functions. Calcium is present in bone as the relatively insoluble bone salt (hydroxyapatite). Bone, however, is a dynamic tissue that undergoes constant remodeling. Indeed, the simultaneous transfer of calcium, in both directions, between bone and plasma is an essential feature of the homeostatic regulation of the calcium concentration in plasma (see Chapter 72). Since the metabolic functions of calcium are essential to life, it is not surprising that bone salts may be sacrificed to maintain appropriate concentrations of plasma calcium. It also follows that, on a chronic basis, normal mineralization of bone is contingent upon maintenance of adequate amounts of total body calcium.

Regulation of plasma calcium within narrow limits is accomplished by parathyroid hormone, calcitonin, and vitamin D (or its metabolites). A detailed description of the role of parathyroid hormone and calcitonin is presented in Chapter 72. For purposes of the present discussion, the action of these hormones may be summarized as follows. Parathyroid hormone is secreted in response

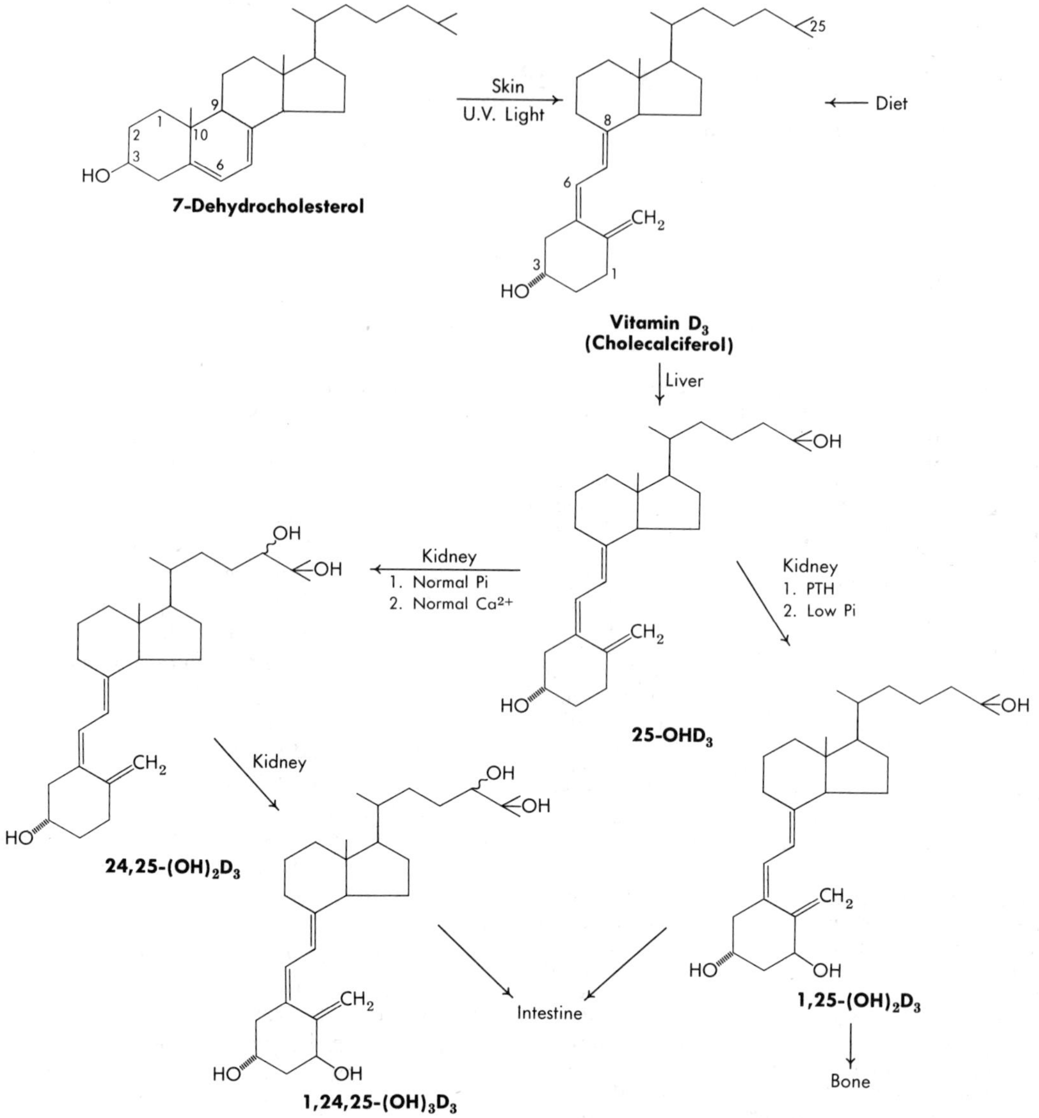

Figure 76–1. *Current concepts of the functional metabolism of vitamin D_3. See* text for discussion and abbreviations. (After DeLuca, 1974. Courtesy of the *American Journal of Medicine*.)

to a fall in plasma calcium ion concentration, and the hormone acts to increase this concentration by accelerating transfer of calcium from the bone compartment, enhancing intestinal absorption of calcium, and increasing reabsorption of calcium by the kidney. In addition, parathyroid hormone promotes phosphate excretion in the urine. While calcitonin secretion can be stimulated by a rise in plasma calcium ion concentration and acts to lower this concentration, presumably by decreasing calcium resorption from bone,

the precise role of this hormone in calcium homeostasis is unknown.

Traditionally, vitamin D was assigned a passive role in calcium metabolism in that its presence in adequate concentrations was thought to permit proper absorption of dietary calcium and to allow full expression of the actions of parathyroid hormone. Recent findings indicate a much more active role of vitamin D in the homeostatic mechanisms that control calcium metabolism. It now appears that vitamin D (or its active metabolite) deserves the status of a hormone that regulates the movement of calcium from both intestine and bone and that plays a major role in the precise control of the concentration of calcium ion in plasma. The following characteristics of vitamin D are consistent with hormonal activity rather than with dietary vitamin activity: vitamin D is synthesized in the skin and under ideal conditions probably is not required in the diet; it is transported by the blood to distant sites in the body, where it is activated; its active form then affects target tissues, resulting in increased plasma calcium concentration; and the conversion of vitamin D to its active form is a reaction that is regulated in a negative-feedback system by plasma calcium.

METABOLIC ACTIVATION

Until recently it was generally believed that vitamin D was directly responsible for its physiological effects. In the late 1960s, the availability of tritium-labeled vitamin D_3 and its analogs made possible a series of studies demonstrating that vitamin D requires further metabolic activation in order to exert its characteristic actions on target tissues. Appreciation of the importance of the biological activation of vitamin D is primarily attributable to studies conducted in the laboratories of DeLuca in the United States and Kodicek in England. The probable events involved in the activation of vitamin D are also shown in Figure 76–1.

25-Hydroxylation of Vitamin D. The initial step in the activation of vitamin D_3 occurs in the liver, and the product is 25-hydroxycholecalciferol (25-OHD$_3$) (Ponchon and DeLuca, 1969). The hepatic enzyme system responsible for 25-hydroxylation of vitamin D has not been fully characterized, but it is associated with the microsomal fraction of liver homogenates and requires the presence of an unidentified cytoplasmic factor (Bhattacharyya and DeLuca, 1974). The fact that the reaction is not inhibited by carbon monoxide indicates that the 25-hydroxylase system differs from the cytochrome P-450–containing drug-metabolizing enzyme system of the liver.

Experiments with rats have shown that the level of 25-hydroxylase activity in the liver

is regulated by the amount of vitamin D_3 administered to the animal. Within 15 minutes after the intravenous injection of vitamin D_3, the activity of the enzyme is depressed and the plasma concentration of 25-OHD$_3$ plateaus after about an hour (Bhattacharyya and DeLuca, 1973). These findings indicate that a mechanism operates to maintain a constant concentration of 25-OHD$_3$ in the blood. Although the exact details of the regulation of vitamin D metabolism at this step are unclear, it is an important control mechanism that serves not only to protect against an overdose of vitamin D but also to conserve vitamin D stores in the body.

1-Hydroxylation of 25-OHD$_3$. After being produced in the liver, 25-OHD$_3$ enters the blood stream, where it circulates in association with vitamin D–binding globulin. Final activation to 1,25-dihydroxycholecalciferol (1,25-[OH]$_2$D$_3$) occurs in the kidney. The enzyme system responsible for 1-hydroxylation of 25-OHD$_3$ is associated with the heavy mitochondrial fraction from renal homogenates; it requires molecular oxygen, Mg^{2+}, and malate and is inhibited by carbon monoxide (Fraser and Kodicek, 1970). The mechanisms by which plasma calcium exerts feedback control over the production of 1,25-(OH)$_2$D$_3$ in the kidney are discussed below.

The Active Form of Vitamin D. Several lines of evidence show conclusively that 1,25-(OH)$_2$D$_3$ is the physiologically active form of the vitamin. When renal production of 1,25-(OH)$_2$D$_3$ is impaired or absent (uremic man or nephrectomized rats), the response to small (physiological) doses of 1,25-(OH)$_2$D$_3$ is normal, whereas even large doses of vitamin D_3 or 25-OHD$_3$ have little or no effect on calcium absorption. Furthermore, in isolated perfused rat intestine, 1,25-(OH)$_2$D$_3$ is at least 200 times as effective as 25-OHD$_3$ in promoting calcium transport (see review by Omdahl and DeLuca, 1973).

The effects of vitamin D_3 and its metabolites on bone resorption have been studied *in vitro*. The dihydroxy metabolite was 100 times more potent than 25-OHD$_3$, while vitamin D_3 itself had no effect on the resorption of bone (Renolds, 1973).

Regulation of Metabolic Activation. The rate of synthesis of 1,25-$(OH)_2D_3$ in the kidneys is closely linked to variations in plasma calcium concentration. Renal mitochondria are capable of converting 25-OHD_3 to either 1,25-$(OH)_2D_3$ or to 24,25-dihydroxycholecalciferol (24,25-$[OH]_2D_3$; Figure 76-1). Under conditions of hypocalcemia produced by dietary calcium deprivation, the kidney produces primarily 1,25-$(OH)_2D_3$, whereas normal plasma calcium concentration or hypercalcemia is associated with synthesis of the less active metabolite, 24,25-$(OH)_2D_3$ (Boyle *et al.,* 1971). It is generally accepted that production of 1,25-$(OH)_2D_3$ is regulated in response to variations in calcium intake, but considerable controversy exists concerning the exact mechanism of the feedback regulation.

One scheme proposes that parathyroid hormone plays a central role in the regulation of renal synthesis of 1,25-$(OH)_2D_3$, as described by Omdahl and DeLuca (1973). These workers proposed that a fall in plasma calcium concentration is detected by the parathyroid gland, which then secretes parathyroid hormone. It, in turn, stimulates 1,25-$(OH)_2D_3$ synthesis in the kidney. The actions of 1,25-$(OH)_2D_3$ to promote calcium absorption in the gastrointestinal tract and mobilization from bone raise the plasma calcium concentration, which ultimately inhibits parathyroid hormone secretion to complete the feedback loop. The above hypothesis is supported by considerable evidence from animal experiments and is consistent with the clinical observation that hypoparathyroid patients require large doses of vitamin D to maintain normal calcium balance.

In a further elaboration of the above scheme, it was proposed that the concentration of inorganic phosphate in the renal cortex functions as the final common pathway for regulation of production of 1,25-$(OH)_2D_3$. Tanaka and DeLuca (1973) found that synthesis of 1,25-$(OH)_2D_3$ occurred when plasma phosphate concentrations were low and that high concentrations of plasma phosphate promoted synthesis of the less active metabolite, 24,25-$(OH)_2D_3$. Parathyroid hormone was proposed to stimulate synthesis of 1,25-$(OH)_2D_3$ by its action to promote renal excretion of inorganic phosphate and thus to decrease plasma phosphate concentrations.

Although the above scheme is attractive, not all observations are consistent with the hypothesis that parathyroid hormone is essential for regulation of vitamin D metabolism. Larkins and coworkers (1973) were able to demonstrate enhanced synthesis of 1,25-$(OH)_2D_3$ in thyroparathyroidectomized rats fed a low-calcium diet, and the effect could not be explained by a fall in plasma phosphate. They suggested that the intracellular concentration of calcium in some critical compartment of the renal cell determines the rate of synthesis of 1,25-$(OH)_2D_3$.

Despite the controversy concerning the details of the control mechanism, there is little doubt that under normal conditions a decrease in plasma calcium results in increased synthesis of the active metabolite of vitamin D.

1,24,25-Trihydroxyvitamin D_3. While 1,25-$(OH)_2D_3$ can carry out all the known functions of vitamin D, other molecular species may also be of importance. It has been demonstrated that 24,25-$(OH)_2D_3$ can support growth, calcium absorption by the intestine, and the mineralization of bone; however, this appears to require its conversion to 1,24,25-trihydroxyvitamin D_3 (1,24,25-$[OH]_3D_3$) by the kidney (Figure 76-1). While this derivative has little ability to promote mobilization of calcium from bone, it is particularly effective in enhancing intestinal calcium transport. The physiological significance of this compound is unknown. (*See* Holick *et al.,* 1973; DeLuca, 1974.)

The Special Case of Dihydrotachysterol. Dihydrotachysterol (DHT) is an analog of vitamin D that may be regarded as the reduction product of either vitamin D_2 (DHT$_2$) or vitamin D_3 (DHT$_3$). DHT is about $\frac{1}{450}$ as active as vitamin D in the usual antirachitic assay, but at high doses it is much more effective than high doses of vitamin D in mobilizing calcium from bone (Suda *et al.,* 1970). The latter effect is the basis for the use of DHT to increase plasma calcium in the treatment of hypoparathyroidism.

Studies describing the metabolic activation of DHT$_3$ provide an explanation for the above findings. DHT$_3$ undergoes 25-hydroxylation to yield 25-hydroxydihydrotachysterol$_3$ (25-$OHDHT_3$), which appears to be the active form of DHT in both intestine and bone (Hallick and DeLuca, 1972). The structure of 25-$OHDHT_3$ follows:

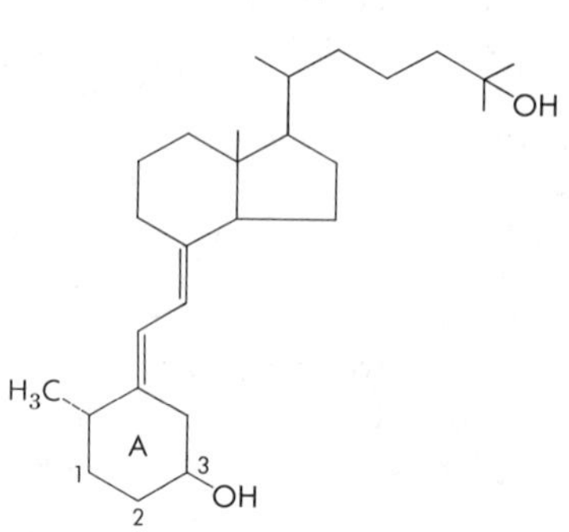

25-Hydroxydihydrotachysterol$_3$ (25-$OHDHT_3$)

Of even greater significance are the observations that 25-hydroxylation of DHT_3 in the liver is not subject to feedback regulation, as is 25-hydroxylation of vitamin D, and that both DHT_3 and $25\text{-}OHDHT_3$ are active in nephrectomized rats (*see* review by Omdahl and DeLuca, 1973). The latter observation implies that DHT_3 does not require 1-hydroxylation in the kidney. A comparison of the structures of $25\text{-}OHDHT_3$ and $1,25\text{-}(OH)_2D_3$ shows that ring A of $25\text{-}OHDHT_3$ is rotated so as to place the 3-hydroxyl group of $25\text{-}OHDHT_3$ in approximately the same geometrical position as the 1-hydroxyl group of $1,25\text{-}(OH)_2D_3$. It seems reasonable that $25\text{-}OHDHT_3$ could interact with receptor sites for $1,25\text{-}(OH)_2D_3$ without undergoing 1-hydroxylation in the kidney. Thus, DHT_3 bypasses both the hepatic and renal mechanisms of metabolic control, allowing the physiologically active form ($25\text{-}OHDHT_3$) of the vitamin D analog to appear in the plasma in proportion to the dose of DHT_3. Presumably DHT_2 behaves in a manner analogous to that described for DHT_3.

PHYSIOLOGICAL FUNCTIONS, MECHANISM OF ACTION, AND PHARMACOLOGICAL PROPERTIES OF VITAMIN D

Vitamin D has two important physiological functions. It is required for normal mineralization of bone, and it plays an essential role in the homeostatic regulation of plasma calcium concentration.

The primary way in which vitamin D promotes normal mineralization of bone is by providing an adequate supply of calcium and phosphate to bone by means of its action to stimulate intestinal absorption of calcium and phosphate. The participation of vitamin D in the homeostatic regulation of plasma calcium is by its action to promote mobilization of calcium from bone. This effect serves to maintain plasma calcium at concentrations required for normal neuromuscular and other functions. Furthermore, since mobilization of calcium occurs from old bone, the calcium and phosphate contributed to the plasma pool may simultaneously participate in mineralization at sites of new-bone formation.

The role of vitamin D in the physiological regulation of calcium and phosphate excretion by the kidneys is not clear, but some findings suggest that the direct effect of physiological doses is to promote reabsorption of both calcium and phosphate. In contrast, large amounts of vitamin D have been shown to promote phosphate excretion.

The mechanisms by which vitamin D exerts its effects on intestinal absorption of calcium, mobilization of bone salts, and reabsorption of calcium and phosphate in the kidney are discussed below.

Intestinal Absorption of Calcium. A defect in intestinal absorption of calcium in vitamin D–deficient rats was demonstrated in the late 1930s (Nicolaysen, 1937). Since that time, numerous methods have been used to study the effects of vitamin D on calcium absorption by the intestine. Movement of calcium from the mucosal to the serosal surface of the intestine has been shown to be a process involving a carrier and active transport against an electrochemical gradient (Adams and Norman, 1970). The active-transport mechanism is present in the microvilli of the brush border (luminal side) of the intestinal epithelial cells.

Three components of the brush border have been implicated in the vitamin D–responsive translocation of calcium from the lumen of the intestine into the epithelial cells. One component, calcium-binding protein, is thought to concentrate calcium in the brush-border membrane. The other two components are calcium-dependent adenosine triphosphatase (ATPase) and alkaline phosphatase, which are probably part of a single enzyme complex and are thought to mediate active transport of calcium into the cytosol of the cell.

Calcium-binding protein has been shown to be localized in the brush-border membrane (Taylor and Wasserman, 1970), and a high correlation exists between the capacity for intestinal absorption of calcium and the content of calcium-binding protein (Taylor and Wasserman, 1969). Both calcium-dependent ATPase and alkaline phosphatase activity in the brush border are induced by vitamin D, and the increased activity is temporally correlated with increased calcium absorption (Haussler et al., 1970). Known inhibitors of alkaline phosphatase also inhibit calcium-dependent ATPase in brush-border preparations, which suggests that these two enzymes may be part of a coupled enzyme system involved in vitamin D–dependent calcium transport.

Movement of calcium through the epithelial cell to the serosal surface has not been extensively investigated, but mitochondria are thought to play a role in this process (Matthews et al., 1971). The final step in absorption is translocation of calcium across the serosal surface membrane into the extracellular fluid; it appears to be linked to Na^+,K^+-activated adenosine triphosphatase (Na,K-ATPase) (Martin and DeLuca, 1969). Neither of these steps has been shown to be involved in the acute response to vitamin D.

Mobilization of Bone Salts. It has been known for many years that large doses of vitamin D cause decalcification of bone. In 1952, Carlsson demonstrated that physiological doses of vitamin D promote mobilization of calcium from bone. In 1963, Rasmussen and coworkers showed that small doses of vitamin D are required for parathyroid hormone to promote such mobilization. More recently,

1,25-$(OH)_2D_3$ has been shown to be active *in vitro* to promote calcium resorption from bone explants (Renolds, 1973).

The molecular mechanisms responsible for mobilization of bone salts are unclear, and the mechanisms by which vitamin D, parathyroid hormone, and calcitonin modify this process are even less well understood. Active translocation of calcium across osteocytes (Talmage, 1972) or across a hypothetical bone membrane (Neuman and Ramp, 1971) has been proposed as the mechanism by which plasma calcium is maintained as a supersaturated solution that is not in chemical equilibrium with calcium in bone fluid. In such a scheme, mobilization of calcium from the bone compartment occurs when active transport of calcium from bone fluid to extracellular fluid is enhanced. Thus, vitamin D could promote mobilization of calcium from bone by stimulating active transport of calcium in osteocytes, perhaps by the same mechanisms that stimulate intestinal absorption of calcium. Proof of such a mechanism requires further investigation.

Renal Effects of Vitamin D. In any attempt to describe the effects of vitamin D on renal excretion of calcium and phosphate, it is essential to separate the direct effects on the kidney from indirect effects that occur when the plasma calcium concentration is altered by the actions of vitamin D on absorption and mobilization of calcium. Administration of vitamin D to a deficient animal will increase plasma calcium concentration and inhibit secretion of parathyroid hormone. The resultant decrease in both phosphate excretion and calcium reabsorption by the kidney may be explained by the removal of these effects of parathyroid hormone. In contrast, hypoparathyroid patients respond to vitamin D or DHT with an enhanced renal reabsorption of calcium (Nordin *et al.*, 1972). Furthermore, physiological doses of vitamin D, 25-OHD_3, or 1,25-$(OH)_2D_3$ have been shown to increase calcium and phosphate reabsorption in thyroparathyroidectomized dogs (Puschett *et al.*, 1972).

It thus seems likely that the direct effects of vitamin D on the kidney are to promote calcium and perhaps phosphate reabsorption. The contribution of such an effect to overall calcium metabolism in the intact animal is unknown, but quantitatively it is probably much less important than the effects of vitamin D on intestine and bone (Omdahl and DeLuca, 1973).

The Role of RNA and Protein Synthesis. Zull and associates (1966) reported that inhibition of RNA synthesis with dactinomycin prevented the *in-vivo* actions of vitamin D in both bone and intestine. This and similar studies were interpreted to indicate that the actions of vitamin D in target tissues were mediated at the molecular level by way of DNA-directed RNA synthesis and ultimately protein synthesis. Recent studies have cast doubt on this interpretation. Gray and DeLuca (1971) showed that administration of dactinomycin or cycloheximide to rats 2 to 5 hours before the administration of 25-OHD_3 prevented its conversion to 1,25-$(OH)_2D_3$. It was also shown that the action of 1,25-$(OH)_2D_3$ to stimulate the intestinal transport of calcium was not blocked by doses of dactinomycin that effectively inhibited the actions of 25-OHD_3 (Tanaka *et al.*, 1971). It now appears that inhibition of RNA and protein synthesis blocks the actions of vitamin D because the 1-hydroxylase system of the kidney has a rapid rate of turnover.

Signs and Symptoms of Deficiency. A deficiency of vitamin D results in inadequate absorption of calcium and phosphate. The consequent decrease in plasma calcium stimulates parathyroid hormone secretion, which acts to restore plasma calcium at the expense of bone calcium. In infants and children, this results in a failure to mineralize newly formed osteoid tissue and cartilage matrix, causing the defect in bone growth known as *rickets*. Due to the lack of calcification, the bone of individuals suffering from rickets is unusually soft and the stress and strain of weight bearing gives rise to the characteristic deformities of the disease.

In adults, vitamin D deficiency results in *osteomalacia* or adult rickets, which is most likely to occur during times of increased calcium need, such as pregnancy or lactation. The disease is characterized by a generalized decrease in bone density. Unlike osteoporosis, the remaining bone is abnormal in that it contains excessive amounts of uncalcified matrix. Gross bone deformities occur only in advanced stages of the disease.

Hypervitaminosis. The acute or chronic administration of excessive amounts of vitamin D or enhanced responsiveness to normal amounts of the vitamin leads to a number of clinical syndromes that are probably the result of deranged calcium metabolism. The physiological or pathological responses to vitamin D are a function of endogenous vitamin D production, tissue reactivity to the vitamin, and particularly vitamin D intake.

Infantile hypercalcemia reached epidemic proportions in England following World War II, at a time when food supplementation with vitamins resulted in intakes far in excess of those required for normal bone growth and development. Although high vitamin D intake was not the sole causative factor of the syndrome, it vanished after dietary vitamin D supplementation was reduced. Some infants seem to be hyperreactive to relatively small doses of vitamin D.

Clinically, most cases of hypervitaminosis D seen in adults are the result of large doses of the vitamin used for the treatment of conditions that are unassociated with vitamin D deficiency but that have been wrongly purported to be benefited by vitamin D therapy, notably rheumatoid arthritis.

There is wide individual variation in the amount of vitamin D that causes hypervitaminosis. As a rough approximation, it may be stated that the continued ingestion of 50,000 units or more daily by a person with normal vitamin D sensitivity may result in poisoning.

Signs and Symptoms. The initial signs and symptoms of vitamin D toxicity are those associated with hypercalcemia and consist in weakness, fatigue, lassitude, headache, nausea, vomiting, and diarrhea. Early impairment of renal function from hypercalcemia is manifest by polyuria, polydipsia, nocturia, decreased urinary concentrating ability, and proteinuria. With prolonged hypercalcemia there may be deposition of calcium salts in soft tissues, most significantly within the kidney; this results in nephrolithiasis and/or diffuse nephrocalcinosis. Other sites of calcification may include blood vessels, heart, lungs, and skin. Some individuals exhibit hypertension. The characteristic changes in blood chemistry are elevated concentrations of plasma calcium and nonprotein nitrogen; phosphate concentrations are variable. Mobilization of calcium from bone contributes to the hypercalcemia and is also responsible for the roentgenographic finding of localized or generalized osteoporosis in a significant percentage of cases of hypervitaminosis D (Holman, 1952).

Vitamin D toxicity may be manifested in the fetus. There is a clinically and experimentally demonstrated relationship between excess maternal vitamin D intake or extreme sensitivity to the vitamin and nonfamilial congenital supravalvular aortic stenosis. In infants, this anomaly is often found in association with other stigmata of hypercalcemia. Many of the offspring of pregnant rabbits that have been treated with large doses of vitamin D have lesions anatomically similar to those of supravalvular aortic stenosis. In addition, other offspring with no aortic narrowing show vascular injury similar to that seen in adults following acute vitamin D

toxicity (Friedman and Roberts, 1966; Taussig, 1966). Maternal hypercalcemia may also result in suppression of parathyroid function in the newborn, with resultant hypocalcemia, tetany, and seizures.

Another potentially toxic action of vitamin D is its effect on fat metabolism. In animals, not only does the vitamin stimulate $^{32}P_i$ incorporation into phospholipid but also it causes increases in hepatic cholesterol, total fat, and fatty acid content (Dalderup, 1968). In man, there is some evidence that 700 to 2500 units daily in adults may raise the plasma cholesterol level (*see* Dalderup *et al.,* 1965). An occasional and interesting sequela resulting from an acute episode of hypercalcemia in patients treated for hypoparathyroidism is a marked increase in response to vitamin D after the disappearance of the hypercalcemia (Leeson and Fourman, 1966).

Treatment of hypervitaminosis D consists in immediate withdrawal of the vitamin, a low-calcium diet, administration of glucocorticoids, and a generous intake of fluid. With this regimen the plasma calcium falls to normal and the calcium in the soft tissue tends to be mobilized. Hydrocortisone has been shown experimentally to decrease calcium absorption, and in man it does cause a more rapid reversion of the elevated plasma calcium concentrations to normal (Verner *et al.,* 1958). Similar symptoms may be associated with toxicity from dihydrotachysterol; treatment is the same as for hypervitaminosis D, that is, treatment of the hypercalcemia. Other aspects of the treatment of hypercalcemia are discussed in Chapter 37.

A conspicuous improvement in renal function is often noted with return of the plasma calcium to normal, but this may not occur if renal damage has been severe.

In children, a single episode of moderately severe hypercalcemia may arrest growth completely for 6 months or more, and the deficit in height may never be fully corrected (Parfitt, 1972).

Absorption, Fate, and Excretion. Vitamin D is usually given by mouth, and gastrointestinal absorption is adequate under most conditions. Both vitamin D_2 and vitamin D_3 are absorbed without esterification from the small intestine, although vitamin D_3 may be absorbed more completely and more rapidly. The exact portion of the gut that is most effective in vitamin D absorption may be a function of the vehicle in which the vitamin is suspended or dissolved. Most of the vitamin appears first in lymph and primarily in the chylomicron fraction as a lipoprotein complex (Schachter *et al.,* 1964).

In animals and man, bile is essential for adequate intestinal absorption and deoxycholic acid is the most important constituent of bile in this regard (Greaves and Schmidt, 1933). Thus, hepatic or biliary dysfunction may seriously impair absorption of vitamin D. Likewise, other abnormalities of gastrointestinal function, especially those associated with steatorrhea, may interfere with proper absorption of orally administered vitamin D.

Absorbed vitamin D circulates in the blood in association with vitamin D–binding protein, which has been shown to be a specific α-globulin (Smith and Goodman, 1971). Vitamin D disappears from plasma with a half-life of 19 to 25 hours, but it is stored in the body for prolonged periods (6 months or longer in the rat), apparently in fat deposits throughout the body (Rosenstreich *et al.,* 1971).

As discussed above, the liver is the site of conversion of vitamin D to its 25-hydroxy derivative, which also circulates in association with vitamin D–binding protein. In fact, 25-OHD$_3$ has been shown to have a higher affinity for the binding protein than does the parent compound (Belsey *et al.,* 1971). The 25-hydroxy derivative has been reported to have a biological half-life of 19 days and constitutes the major circulating form of vitamin D (Smith and Goodman, 1971).

The primary route of excretion of vitamin D is in the bile, and only a small percentage of an administered dose is found in the urine. The metabolites of vitamin D have not been identified in either bile or urine; however, there is evidence to suggest that the hepatic microsomal drug-metabolizing system is involved in the inactivation of vitamin D.

The implication of hepatic drug-metabolizing enzymes in the inactivation of vitamin D resulted from the clinical observations that prolonged use of anticonvulsant drugs known to induce hepatic drug-metabolizing enzymes was associated with a high incidence of rickets and osteomalacia (Dent *et al.,* 1970; Hunter *et al.,* 1971). It was shown that plasma concentrations of 25-OHD$_3$ are decreased in patients receiving anticonvulsant drugs (Hahn *et al.,* 1972b) and that phenobarbital administration could induce increased rates of metabolism of vitamin D to inactive products in animals and patients (Hahn *et al.,* 1972a). Additional studies are needed to define clearly the role of the microsomal drug-metabolizing system in the overall metabolic disposition of vitamin D. However, the clinical implications are clear. Christiansen and coworkers (1973) showed that administration of 2000 units daily of vitamin D, but not calcium lactate alone, restored bone mineral mass to normal values in epileptic patients on anticonvulsant drugs, and Hahn and coworkers (1975) have recommended that most children treated chronically with anticonvulsant drugs should receive supplemental vitamin D. This is particularly true for children on multiple-drug regimens, for whom a weekly intake of at least 10,000 units was recommended. Since a wide variety of commonly used drugs are known to be nonspecific inducers of hepatic drug-metabolizing enzymes, it is apparent that chronic administration of such drugs has the potential for causing drug-induced vitamin D deficiency.

Human Requirements. An exhaustive and critical summary of the prophylactic requirements for vitamin D has been compiled by the Committee on Nutrition of the American Academy of Pediatrics (*see* Committee on Nutrition, 1963). In the more than 50 years that have elapsed since Mellanby (1921) demonstrated the efficacy of cod liver oil in the prevention of rickets, the disease has become a clinical rarity in the United States. Although sunlight provides adequate antirachitic prophylaxis in the equatorial belt, in the temperate climates insufficient cutaneous solar radiation may necessitate dietary vitamin D supplementation.

Previously the recommended allowance of vitamin D could be achieved only by the addition of oral vitamin D supplements to a normal diet. Since the advent of the addition of the vitamin to foodstuffs (especially milk, milk products, cereals, and candy), individuals of all ages receive variable and even excessive vitamin D without its special addition to the diet. Thus, the supplemental requirements vary not only with age, pregnancy, and lactation but also with the quality of the diet. According to the Committee on Nutrition (1963), hypothetical average and high vitamin D diets at various ages would lead to the intake of the following amounts of the vitamin per day without any special vitamin supplements:

6 months, average 400 units; 3 years, average 600 units, high 1600 units; 8 years, average 800 units, high 1900 units. Serious toxicity may result from excessive ingestion of the vitamin, and even as little as 1800 U.S.P. units per day in infants may lead to possible growth inhibition (Jeans and Stearns, 1938). It is clear, therefore, that any recommendation for vitamin D supplementation must be made only after careful scrutiny of the diet.

In both the premature and the normal infant, a total of 400 units per day of vitamin D ensures full antirachitic prophylaxis and optimal growth. Whether this is obtained by way of the diet, by vitamin D supplementation, or by a combination of both is of no consequence. During adolescence and adulthood this amount is probably also sufficient. There is some evidence that vitamin D requirements are greater than normal during pregnancy and lactation, although a daily intake of 400 units is sufficient in these conditions as well (*see* Table XVIII-1, page 1545).

Assay and Unitage. Material to be tested is saponified, purified by column chromatography, and compared spectrophotometrically with the U.S.P. Calciferol Reference Standard. The U.S.P. unit is identical with the international unit and is equivalent to the specific biological activity of 0.025 μg of vitamin D_3 (*i.e.,* 1 mg equals 40,000 units). Bioassay procedures have been used in the past and depend upon evidence of alleviation of the rachitic state. Experimentally they are still in use.

Preparations. There are four main types of vitamin D preparations: (1) fish liver oils or their concentrates, with or without vitamin A and/or vitamin D supplementation; (2) multivitamin preparations containing vitamin D; (3) preparations containing vitamin D and calcium salts, with or without other vitamins; and (4) preparations containing vitamin D activity alone. Although many preparations containing vitamin D are marketed, only official U.S.P. preparations are listed below.

Ergocalciferol, U.S.P. (*calciferol;* DRISDOL, VIOS-TEROL), is pure vitamin D_2. *Ergocalciferol Capsules,* U.S.P., consists of ergocalciferol in edible vegetable oil solution, encapsulated with gelatin. The capsules must contain not less than 100% of the labeled amount of ergocalciferol. Capsules usually contain 625 μg (25,000 U.S.P. units) or 1.25 mg (50,000 U.S.P. units) each. *Ergocalciferol Solution,* U.S.P., is a solution of the vitamin in an edible vegetable oil, polysorbate 80, or propylene glycol. Each gram of solution must contain at least 250 μg (10,000 U.S.P. units) of ergocalciferol.

Cholecalciferol, U.S.P., is pure vitamin D_3.

Decavitamin Capsules, U.S.P., and *Decavitamin Tablets,* U.S.P., contain at least 400 U.S.P. vitamin D units (10 μg of vitamin D as ergocalciferol or cholecalciferol) per capsule or tablet. The vitamin can be from natural sources, or as vitamin D_2 or vitamin D_3, or as the irradiation products of ergosterol or 7-dehydrocholesterol.

Dihydrotachysterol, U.S.P. (HYTAKEROL), is the pure crystalline compound obtained by reduction of

vitamin D_2 and is available as tablets (0.2 mg), capsules (0.125 mg), and solution in oil (0.25 mg/ml). These preparations are all for oral administration.

It is anticipated that functional metabolites of vitamin D will soon be available to treat patients with specific deficiencies of vitamin D activation. 25-$(OH)D_3$ has been shown to be useful in patients receiving anticonvulsant drugs concurrently (*see* above) or with hepatic disease. While 1,25-$(OH)_2D_3$ would be valuable for patients with chronic renal disease or vitamin D–dependent disease (*see* below), this compound is very expensive. Another derivative, 1-$(OH)D_3$, may meet this need. (For discussion and references, *see* DeLuca, 1974, 1975.)

THERAPEUTIC USES

The major therapeutic uses of vitamin D may be divided into three categories: (1) prophylaxis and cure of nutritional rickets, (2) treatment of metabolic rickets and osteomalacia, and (3) treatment of hypoparathyroidism.

Nutritional Rickets. Nutritional rickets is due to inadequate exposure to sunlight or a deficiency of vitamin D in the diet. The condition is extremely rare in the United States and other countries where milk and other foods contain added vitamin D. Infants and children receiving adequate amounts of vitamin D–fortified food do not require additional vitamin D; however, breast-fed infants or those fed unfortified formula should receive 400 units of vitamin D daily as a supplement. The usual pediatric practice is to administer vitamin A in combination with vitamin D. A number of well-balanced vitamin A and D preparations are available for this purpose. Premature infants are more susceptible to rickets and may require supplemental vitamin D, since the fetus acquires more than 85% of its calcium stores during the third trimester.

The curative dose of vitamin D for the treatment of *fully developed rickets* is larger than the prophylactic dose. One thousand units daily will produce normal plasma calcium and phosphate values in approximately 10 days and roentgenographic evidence of healing within about 3 weeks. However, a daily dose of 3000 to 4000 units is often prescribed for more rapid healing; this is of particular importance in severe cases of thoracic rickets when respiration is embarrassed.

There are certain conditions that are known to lead to *poor absorption of vitamin D.* If untreated with vitamin, a frank deficiency may develop. Therefore, vitamin D may be of definite prophylactic value in such disorders as diarrhea, steatorrhea, biliary obstruction, and any other abnormality in gastrointestinal function in which absorption is appreciably diminished. Parenteral administration may be used in such cases.

Metabolic Rickets and Osteomalacia. This group of diseases, which presents as rickets in infants and children and osteomalacia in adults, is characterized by a failure to respond to physiological doses of vitamin D. Three types of metabolic rickets are discussed below, and the reader is referred to articles by Parfitt (1972) and Smith (1972) for more complete discussions of other forms of the disease.

Hypophosphatemic vitamin D–resistant rickets is an X-linked inherited disorder of calcium and phosphate metabolism. It is *not* characterized by a defect in vitamin D metabolism, but treatment with large doses of vitamin D in combination with phosphate salts has been reported to lead to clinical improvement (Brickman *et al.*, 1973).

Vitamin D–dependent rickets (pseudo–vitamin D deficiency rickets) is an inherited, autosomal recessive disease that appears to be due to an inborn error of vitamin D metabolism involving defective conversion of 25-OHD$_3$ to 1,25-(OH)$_2$D$_3$ (Fraser *et al.*, 1973). The condition responds to physiological doses of 1,25-(OH)$_2$D$_3$. However, at the present time this active metabolite of vitamin D is not available for clinical use, and the disease is treated with large doses of vitamin D. Daily doses of from 20,000 to 60,000 units of vitamin D are required for management of the disease (Parfitt and Frame, 1972).

Renal osteodystrophy (renal rickets) is associated with chronic renal failure, and it also is characterized by a decreased ability of the kidney to convert 25-OHD$_3$ to 1,25-(OH)$_2$D$_3$ (Brickman *et al.*, 1972). The initial management of renal osteodystrophy may be achieved with the use of 20,000 to 200,000 units of vitamin D daily; however, as renal failure becomes more severe, DHT may be more desirable (Parfitt and Frame, 1972).

Hypoparathyroidism. Hypoparathyroidism is characterized by hypocalcemia and hyperphosphatemia (*see* Chapter 72). Vitamin D in large doses corrects these abnormalities by its action to promote calcium absorption, calcium mobilization from bone, and perhaps increased renal phosphate excretion. The dose of vitamin D required for maintenance varies from 50,000 to 250,000 units daily. Some patients may require additional calcium in their diet. Overdosage with vitamin D in the treatment of this condition may result in hypercalcemia, which persists for weeks and can cause renal damage.

Dihydrotachysterol is also capable of correcting the abnormalities of hypoparathyroidism and may offer certain advantages over vitamin D. Dihydrotachysterol has a more rapid onset of action; more importantly, it has a shorter duration of action than does vitamin D, and it is thus possible to make more rapid correction for overdosage. At the present time the cost of dihydrotachysterol is not sufficiently higher than vitamin D to make this a consideration in the choice of therapy for hypoparathyroidism. Whichever preparation is used, dosage should be carefully adjusted by frequent measurement of serum calcium.

Miscellaneous Uses of Vitamin D. Miscellaneous uses of vitamin D include treatment of the hypophosphatemia seen in the *Fanconi syndrome* and the osteomalacia of children or adults with *malabsorption syndromes.*

The use of large doses of vitamin D in patients with osteoporosis is of doubtful value and can be dangerous. Furthermore, the indiscriminate use of "over-the-counter" vitamin D preparations for conditions other than the aforementioned is irrational, can be dangerous, and should not be condoned.

Adams, T. H., and Norman, A. W. Studies on the mechanism of action of calciferol. I. Basic parameters of vitamin D–mediated calcium transport. *J. biol. Chem.,* 1970, *245,* 4421–4431.

Belsey, R.; DeLuca, H. F.; and Potts, J. T., Jr. Competitive binding assay for vitamin D and 25-OH vitamin D. *J. clin. Endocr. Metab.,* 1971, *33,* 554–557.

Bhattacharyya, M. H., and DeLuca, H. F. The regulation of rat liver calciferol-25-hydroxylase. *J. biol. Chem.,* 1973, *248,* 2969–2973.

———. Subcellular location of rat liver calciferol-25-hydroxylase. *Archs Biochem. Biophys.,* 1974, *160,* 58–62.

Boyle, I. T.; Gray, R. W.; and DeLuca, H. F. Regulation by calcium of *in vivo* synthesis of 1,25-dihydroxycholecalciferol and 21,25-dihydroxycholecalciferol. *Proc. natn. Acad. Sci. U.S.A.,* 1971, *68,* 2131–2134.

Brickman, A. S.; Coburn, J. W.; Kurokawa, K.; Bethune, J. E.; Harrison, H. E.; and Norman, A. W. Actions of 1,25-dihydroxycholecalciferol in patients with hypophosphatemic, vitamin-D-resistant rickets. *New Engl. J. Med.,* 1973, *289,* 495–498.

Brickman, A. S.; Coburn, J. W.; and Norman, A. W. Action of 1,25-dihydroxycholecalciferol, a potent, kidney-produced metabolite of vitamin D, in uremic man. *New Engl. J. Med.,* 1972, *287,* 891–895.

Carlsson, A. Tracer experiments on the effect of vitamin D on skeletal metabolism of calcium and phosphorus. *Acta physiol. scand.,* 1952, *26,* 212–222.

Christiansen, C.; Rodbro, P.; and Lund, M. Effects of vitamin D on bone mineral mass in normal subjects and in epileptic patients on anticonvulsants: a controlled therapeutic trial. *Br. med. J.,* 1973, *2,* 208–209.

Committee on Nutrition. The prophylactic requirement and toxicity of vitamin D. *Pediatrics, Springfield,* 1963, *31,* 512–523.

Dalderup, L. M. Vitamin D, cholesterol, and calcium. *Lancet,* 1968, *1,* 645.

Dalderup, L. M.; Stockmann, V. A.; Rechsteiner, H. de Vos; and Slikke, G. J. van der. Survey on coronary heart disease in relation to diet in physically active farmers. *Voeding,* 1965, *26,* 245–275.

Dent, C. E.; Richens, A.; Rowle, D. J. F.; and Stamp, T. C. B. Osteomalacia with long-term anticonvulsant therapy in epilepsy. *Br. med. J.,* 1970, *4,* 69–72.

Fraser, D.; Kooh, S. W.; Kind, H. P.; Holick, M. F.; Tanaka, Y.; and DeLuca, H. F. Pathogenesis of hereditary vitamin-D-dependent rickets: an inborn error of vitamin D metabolism involving defective conversion of 25-hydroxyvitamin D to 1α,25-dihydroxyvitamin D. *New Engl. J. Med.,* 1973, *289,* 817–822.

Fraser, D. R., and Kodicek, E. Unique biosynthesis by kidney of a biologically active vitamin D metabolite. *Nature, Lond.,* 1970, *228,* 764–766.

Friedman, W. R., and Roberts, W. C. Vitamin D and the supravalvular aortic stenosis syndrome. *Circulation,* 1966, *34,* 77–86.

Gray, R. W., and DeLuca, H. F. Metabolism of 25-hydroxycholecalciferol and its inhibition by actinomycin D and cycloheximide. *Archs Biochem. Biophys.,* 1971, *145,* 276–282.

Greaves, J. D., and Schmidt, C. L. A. Role played by bile in absorption of vitamin D in rat. *J. biol. Chem.,* 1933, *102,* 101–112.

Hahn, T. J.; Birge, S. J.; Scharp, C. R.; and Avioli, L. V.

Phenobarbital-induced alterations in vitamin D metabolism. *J. clin. Invest.*, *1972a*, *51*, 741–748.

Hahn, T. J.; Hendin, B. A.; Scharp, C. R.; Boisseau, V. C.; and Haddad, J. G., Jr. Serum 25-hydroxycalciferol levels and bone mass in children on chronic anticonvulsant therapy. *New Engl. J. Med.*, *1975*, *292*, 550–554.

Hahn, T. J.; Hendin, B. A.; Scharp, C. R.; and Haddad, J. G., Jr. Effect of chronic anticonvulsant therapy on serum 25-hydroxycalciferol levels in adults. *New Engl. J. Med.*, *1972b*, *287*, 900–904.

Hallick, R. B., and DeLuca, H. F. Metabolites of dihydrotachysterol$_3$ in target tissues. *J. biol. Chem.*, *1972*, *247*, 91–97.

Haussler, M. R.; Nagode, L. A.; and Rasmussen, H. Induction of intestinal brush border alkaline phosphatase by vitamin D and identity with Ca-ATPase. *Nature, Lond.*, *1970*, *228*, 1199–1201.

Hess, A. F., and Weinstock, M. Antirachitic properties imparted to inert fluids and to green vegetables by ultraviolet irradiation. *J. biol. Chem.*, *1924*, *62*, 301–313.

Holick, M. F.; Kleiner-Bossaller, A.; Schnoes, H. K.; Kasten, P. M.; Boyle, I. T.; and DeLuca, H. F. 1,24,25-Trihydroxyvitamin D$_3$. A metabolite of vitamin D$_3$ effective on intestine. *J. biol. Chem.*, *1973*, *248*, 6691–6696.

Holman, C. B. Roentgenologic manifestations of vitamin D intoxication. *Radiology*, *1952*, *59*, 805–816.

Hunter, J.; Maxwell, J. D.; Stewart, D. A.; Parsons, V.; and Williams, R. Altered calcium metabolism in epileptic children on anticonvulsants. *Br. med. J.*, *1971*, *4*, 202–204.

Jeans, P. C., and Stearns, G. Effect of vitamin D on linear growth in infancy: effect of intakes above 1,800 U.S.P. units daily. *J. Pediat.*, *1938*, *13*, 730–740.

Larkins, R. G.; Colston, K. W.; Galante, L. S.; MacAuley, S. J.; Evans, I. M. A.; and MacIntyre, I. Regulation of vitamin D metabolism without parathyroid hormone. *Lancet*, *1973*, *2*, 289–291.

Leeson, P. M., and Fourman, P. Increased sensitivity to vitamin D after vitamin D poisoning. *Lancet*, *1966*, *1*, 1182–1185.

Martin, D. L., and DeLuca, H. F. Influence of sodium on calcium transport by the rat small intestine. *Am. J. Physiol.*, *1969*, *216*, 1351–1359.

Matthews, J. L.; Martin, J. H.; Arsenis, C.; Eisenstein, R.; and Kuettner, K. The role of mitochondria in intracellular calcium regulation. In, *Cellular Mechanisms for Calcium Transfer and Homeostasis.* (Nichols, G., Jr., and Wasserman, R. H., eds.) Academic Press, Inc., New York, *1971*, pp. 239–255.

Mellanby, E. Experimental rickets. *Spec. Rep. Ser. med. Res. Coun.*, *1921*, Series 61, 1–78.

Neuman, W. F., and Ramp, W. K. The concept of a bone membrane: some implications. In, *Cellular Mechanisms for Calcium Transfer and Homeostasis.* (Nichols, G., Jr., and Wasserman, R. H., eds.) Academic Press, Inc., New York, *1971*, pp. 197–206.

Nicolaysen, R. Studies upon the mode of action of vitamin D. III. The influence of vitamin D on the absorption of calcium and phosphorus in the rat. *Biochem. J.*, *1937*, *31*, 122–129.

Nordin, B. E. C.; Peacock, M.; and Wilkinson, R. The relative importance of gut, bone, and kidney in the regulation of serum calcium. In, *Calcium, Parathyroid Hormone, and the Calcitonins.* (Talmage, R. V., and Munson, P. L., eds.) International Congress Series No. 243, Excerpta Medica, Amsterdam, *1972*, pp. 263–272.

Parfitt, A. M. Hypophosphatemic vitamin D refractory rickets and osteomalacia. *Orthop. Clins N. Am.*, *1972*, *3*, 653–680.

Parfitt, A. M., and Frame, B. Treatment of rickets and osteomalacia. *Semin. Drug Treat.*, *1972*, *2*, 83–115.

Ponchon, G., and DeLuca, H. F. Metabolites of vitamin D$_3$ and their biologic activity. *J. Nutr.*, *1969*, *99*, 157–167.

Puschett, J. B.; Moranz, J.; and Kurnick, W. S. Evidence for a direct action of cholecalciferol and 25-hydroxycholecalciferol on the renal transport of phosphate, sodium, and calcium. *J. clin. Invest.*, *1972*, *51*, 373–385.

Rasmussen, H.; DeLuca, H.; Arnaud, C.; Hawker, C.; and Stedingk, M. von. The relationship between vitamin D and parathyroid hormone. *J. clin. Invest.*, *1963*, *42*, 1940–1946.

Renolds, J. J. Bone remodeling: *in vitro* studies on vitamin D metabolites. In, *Symposium on Hard Tissue Growth, Repair, and Remineralization.* (Elliott, K., and Fitzsimons, D. W., eds.) Ciba Foundation Symposium 11, Mouton Pubs., The Hague, Netherlands, *1973*, pp. 315–330.

Rosenstreich, S. J.; Rich, C.; and Volwiler, W. Deposition in and release of vitamin D$_3$ from body fat; evidence for a storage site in the rat. *J. clin. Invest.*, *1971*, *50*, 679–687.

Schachter, D.; Finkelstein, J. D.; and Kowarski, S. Metabolism of vitamin D. I. Preparation of radioactive vitamin D and its intestinal absorption in the rat. *J. clin. Invest.*, *1964*, *43*, 787–796.

Smith, J. E., and Goodman, DeW. S. The turnover and transport of vitamin D and of a polar metabolite with the properties of 25-hydroxycholecalciferol in human plasma. *J. clin. Invest.*, *1971*, *50*, 2159–2167.

Smith, R. The pathophysiology and management of rickets. *Orthop. Clins N. Am.*, *1972*, *3*, 601–621.

Steenbock, H., and Black, A. Fat-soluble vitamins. XVII. The induction of growth-promoting and calcifying properties in a ration by exposure to ultraviolet light. *J. biol. Chem.*, *1924*, *61*, 405–422.

Suda, T.; Hallick, R. B.; DeLuca, H. F.; and Schnoes, H. K. 25-Hydroxydihydrotachysterol$_3$. Synthesis and biological activity. *Biochemistry, N.Y.*, *1970*, *9*, 1651–1657.

Talmage, R. V. Further studies on the control of calcium homeostasis by parathyroid hormone. In, *Calcium, Parathyroid Hormone, and the Calcitonins.* (Talmage, R. V., and Munson, P. L., eds.) International Congress Series No. 243, Excerpta Medica, Amsterdam, *1972*, pp. 422–429.

Tanaka, Y., and DeLuca, H. F. The control of 25-hydroxyvitamin D metabolism by inorganic phosphorous. *Archs Biochem. Biophys.*, *1973*, *154*, 566–574.

Tanaka, Y.; DeLuca, H. F.; Omdahl, J.; and Holick, M. F. Mechanism of action of 1,25-dihydroxycholecalciferol on intestinal calcium transport. *Proc. natn. Acad. Sci. U.S.A.*, *1971*, *68*, 1286–1288.

Taussig, H. B. Possible injury to the cardiovascular system from vitamin D. *Ann. intern. Med.*, *1966*, *65*, 1195–1200.

Taylor, A. N., and Wasserman, R. H. Correlations between the vitamin D–induced calcium binding protein and intestinal absorption of calcium. *Fedn Proc. Fedn Am. Socs exp. Biol.*, *1969*, *28*, 1834–1838.

————. Immunofluorescent localization of vitamin D-dependent calcium-binding protein. *J. Histochem. Cytochem.*, *1970*, *18*, 107–115.

Verner, J. V., Jr.; Engel, F. L.; and McPherson, H. T. Vitamin D intoxication: report of two cases treated with cortisone. *Ann. intern. Med.*, *1958*, *48*, 765–773.

Zull, J. E.; Czarnowska-Misztal, E.; and DeLuca, H. F. On the relationship between vitamin D action and actinomycin-sensitive processes. *Proc. natn. Acad. Sci. U.S.A.*, *1966*, *55*, 177–184.

Monographs and Reviews

DeLuca, H. F. Vitamin D—1973. *Am. J. Med.*, *1974*, *57*, 1–12.

————. The kidney as an endocrine organ involved in the function of vitamin D. *Ibid.*, *1975*, *58*, 39–47.

Nichols, G., Jr., and Wasserman, R. H. (eds.). *Cellular Mechanisms for Calcium Transfer and Homeostasis.* Academic Press, Inc., New York, **1971.**

Omdahl, J. L., and DeLuca, H. F. Regulation of vitamin D metabolism and function. *Physiol. Rev.,* **1973,** *53,* 327–372. (231 references.)

Sebrell, W. H., Jr., and Harris, R. S. (eds.). *The Vitamins: Chemistry, Physiology, Pathology, Methods,* 2nd ed., Vol. 3. Academic Press, Inc., New York, **1971,** pp. 156–301.

Talmage, R. V., and Munson, P. L. (eds.). *Calcium, Parathyroid Hormone, and the Calcitonins.* International Congress Series No. 243, Excerpta Medica, Amsterdam, **1972.**

CHAPTER
77 FAT-SOLUBLE VITAMINS
[*Continued*]
Vitamin K and Vitamin E

Victor H. Cohn

VITAMIN K

History. Vitamin K is a dietary principle essential for the normal biosynthesis of several factors required for clotting of blood. In 1929, Dam observed that chickens fed on inadequate diets developed a deficiency disease in which the outstanding symptom was spontaneous bleeding, apparently due to a low content of prothrombin in the blood. In subsequent publications, Dam and coworkers (1935, 1936) reported that, although the condition was not cured by any of the known vitamins, it could be rapidly alleviated by feeding an unidentified fat-soluble substance. To this substance Dam gave the name *vitamin K* (*Koagulation* vitamin). Independently, Almquist and Stokstad (1935) described the same hemorrhagic disease in chickens and the method for its prevention.

The investigations of Dam and Almquist and their respective associates were reported at a time when the attention of several groups of workers was centered on the cause of the hemorrhagic tendency in patients with obstructive jaundice and diseases of the liver. For example, Quick and coworkers (1935) made the pertinent observation that the coagulation defect in jaundiced individuals was due to a decrease in the concentration of prothrombin in the blood. In the same year, Hawkins and Whipple reported that animals with biliary fistulas were likely to develop excessive bleeding. Hawkins and Brinkhous (1936) subsequently showed that this was due to a deficiency in prothrombin and that the condition could be relieved by the feeding of bile salts.

The culmination of these experimental studies came with the demonstration of Butt and coworkers (1938) as well as Warner and associates (1938) that combination therapy with vitamin K and bile salts was effective in the treatment of the hemorrhagic diathesis in cases of jaundice. Thus, the relationship between vitamin K, adequate hepatic function, and the physiological mechanisms operating in the normal clotting of blood was established.

Occurrence and Chemistry. The early investigations described above showed that vitamin K is a fat-soluble substance present in hog liver fat and in alfalfa. Subsequently, it has been demonstrated that the vitamin is concentrated in the chloroplasts of plant leaves and in many vegetable oils. The feces of most species of animals contain large amounts of the vitamin, which is synthesized by the bacteria in the intestinal tract (*see* Pennock, 1966).

The isolation and the elucidation of the chemical structure of vitamin K were carried out concurrently and independently by several groups of investigators. It was soon appreciated that vitamin K activity was associated with at least two distinct substances, designated as vitamin K_1 and vitamin K_2. Vitamin K_1, or phylloquinone, is 2-methyl-3-phytyl-1,4-naphthoquinone; vitamin K_2 represents a series of compounds (the menaquinones) in which the phytyl side chain of phylloquinone has been replaced by a side chain built up of 2 to 13 prenyl units (*see* Isler and Wiss, 1959). Phylloquinone is found in plants; it is the only natural vitamin K available for therapeutic use. The menaquinones are synthesized, in particular, by gram-positive bacteria.

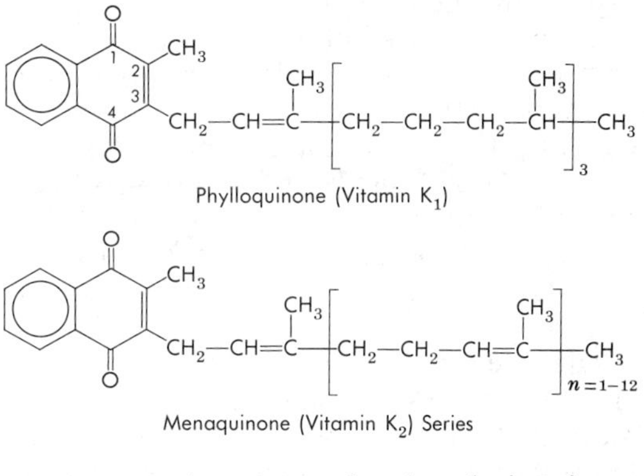

Phylloquinone (Vitamin K_1)

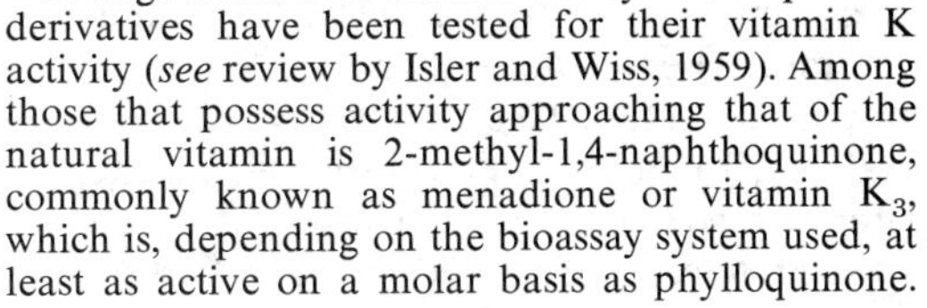

Menaquinone (Vitamin K_2) Series

A large number of natural and synthetic quinone derivatives have been tested for their vitamin K activity (*see* review by Isler and Wiss, 1959). Among those that possess activity approaching that of the natural vitamin is 2-methyl-1,4-naphthoquinone, commonly known as menadione or vitamin K_3, which is, depending on the bioassay system used, at least as active on a molar basis as phylloquinone.

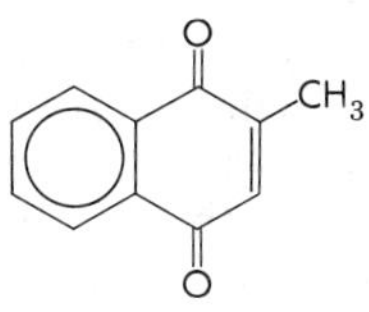

Menadione

The natural vitamins K and menadione are lipid-soluble substances. It is possible to make active water-soluble derivatives of menadione by forming the sodium bisulfite salt or the tetrasodium salt of the diphosphoric acid ester. These compounds are converted in the body to menadione.

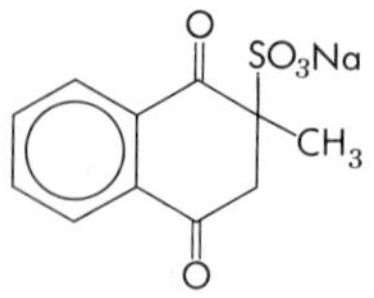

Menadione Sodium Bisulfite

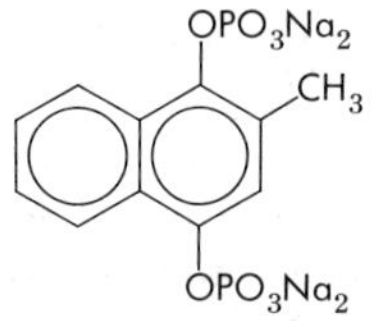

Menadiol Sodium Diphosphate

Pharmacological Actions and Physiological Function.

In normal animals and man, phylloquinone and the menaquinones are virtually devoid of pharmacodynamic activity. In animals and man deficient in vitamin K, the pharmacological action of vitamin K is related to its normal physiological function, that is, to promote the hepatic biosynthesis of prothrombin, proconvertin (factor VII), plasma thromboplastin component (PTC, Christmas factor, factor IX), and the Stuart factor (factor X). (No other body proteins have been shown to be similarly dependent on the presence of vitamin K for their biosynthesis.) The role of these factors in blood clotting is discussed in Chapter 65.

The precise mechanism by which vitamin K enhances formation of these clotting proteins is still not known. While there seems to be general agreement that vitamin K acts at a step in protein synthesis beyond transcription, there is little agreement concerning its precise action (see review by Wasserman and Taylor, 1972). Possibilities include an effect on translation or beyond, at a site involving release of stored clotting factors, or the transformation of a precursor protein to the final product. Some evidence suggests that there is a precursor protein in the liver, and that the vitamin participates in its conversion to active prothrombin, which is then released (Suttie, 1970, 1973). There is considerable other evidence that vitamin K does not function in the synthesis of the polypeptide portion of prothrombin but, rather, in the incorporation of the carbohydrate moiety into its glycoprotein structure (see Martius et al., 1971).

Human Requirement. There is no generally accepted figure for the human requirement of vitamin K; it appears to be extremely small. Frick and associates (1967) estimated the minimal daily requirement, in patients made vitamin K deficient by a starvation diet and antibiotic therapy for 3 to 4 weeks, to be approximately 0.03 μg/kg of body weight. In the infant, 10 μg/kg of body weight of phylloquinone is sufficient to prevent hypoprothrombinemia. Needs are satisfied by the average diet, and, in addition, the vitamin synthesized by intestinal bacteria is also available to the host.

Symptoms of Deficiency. The chief clinical manifestation of vitamin K deficiency is increased bleeding tendency. Ecchymoses, epistaxis, hematuria, gastrointestinal bleeding, and postoperative hemorrhage are common; intracranial hemorrhage may occur. Hemoptysis is uncommon. A further discussion of hypoprothrombinemia is presented in the section on oral anticoagulants (Chapter 65).

Toxicity. Phylloquinone and the menaquinones are nontoxic to animals, even when given in huge amounts. In man, rapid intravenous administration of phylloquinone has produced flushing, dyspnea, chest pains, and rarely death. Whether these reactions were due to the vitamin itself or to the agents used to disperse and emulsify the preparation is not clear.

The administration of large doses of menadione and its derivatives to animals has resulted in the production of anemia, polycythemia, splenomegaly, renal and hepatic damage, and death (see Finkel, 1961). In man, menadione is irritating to the skin and the respiratory tract. Its solutions have vesicant properties. Menadione and its derivatives have been implicated in producing hemolytic anemia, hyperbilirubinemia, and kernicterus in the newborn, especially premature infants (see below). Menadione also can induce hemolysis in individuals who have a glucose-6-phosphate dehydrogenase deficiency in their erythrocytes (Zinkham and Childs, 1957). In patients who have severe hepatic disease, the administration of large doses of menadione or phylloquinone may further depress function of the liver (see below).

Absorption, Fate, and Excretion. The mechanism of intestinal absorption of compounds with vitamin K activity varies with their solubility. Phylloquinone and the menaquinones are adequately absorbed from the gastrointestinal tract only if bile salts are present. Menadione and its water-soluble derivatives, however, are absorbed even in the absence of bile. Phylloquinone and the menaquinones are absorbed almost entirely by way of the lymph; menadione and its water-soluble derivatives enter directly into the blood stream (*see* Woolf and Babior, 1972). Following intramuscular injection, both natural and synthetic vitamin K preparations are readily absorbed. After absorption, phylloquinone is initially concentrated in the liver, but the concentration declines rapidly. Very little vitamin K accumulates in tissues.

Little is known about the metabolic fate of vitamin K. Almost no free unmetabolized vitamin K appears in bile or urine. One metabolite common to both phylloquinone and the menaquinones has been identified in which the side chain has been shortened to seven carbon atoms, to yield a terminal carboxylic acid that forms a γ-lactone excreted as a glucuronide. The considerable amount of fecal vitamin K, which is primarily of bacterial origin, can be greatly reduced by the administration of drugs that exert a bacteriostatic effect in the bowel. In animals treated with warfarin, a major fraction of phylloquinone is metabolized to phylloquinone oxide (Matschiner *et al.*, 1970). Menadione is apparently reduced to the diol (hydroquinone) form and excreted as glucuronide and sulfate conjugates.

Martius and associates (*see* Martius, 1967) have shown in experimental animals that both phylloquinone and menadione can be converted to the more potent menaquinone series. Whether this can occur in man and of what significance these transformations are to the action of phylloquinone and menadione are still unknown.

Apparently there is little storage of vitamin K in the body. The limited stores of the vitamin present in tissue are slowly destroyed. Under circumstances where lack of bile interferes with vitamin K absorption, for example, hypoprothrombinemia develops slowly over a period of several weeks.

Assay and Unitage. Drugs with vitamin K activity may be chemically assayed and do not require bioassay. For the determination of the vitamin K content of foods, an assay based upon the ability of the preparation to increase the prothrombin level of deficient chicks is employed.

Preparations. *Phytonadione,* U.S.P. (*vitamin K_1,* AQUAMEPHYTON, KONAKION, MEPHYTON), is a viscous liquid that is insoluble in water. It is marketed in 5-mg tablets, and in ampuls containing an emulsion of 2 or 10 mg/ml of phytonadione dispersed in a solution of buffered polysorbate and propylene glycol (KONAKION) or polyethylated fatty acid derivatives and dextrose (AQUAMEPHYTON). KONAKION is administered only intramuscularly; AQUAMEPHYTON may be given by any parenteral route.

Menadione, N.F. (*vitamin K_3*), is a bright-yellow crystalline powder that is practically insoluble in water. Menadione is available for oral administration in tablets containing 2, 5, or 10 mg, and as a sterile solution of menadione in oil (usually 2, 10, or 25 mg/ml) designed for intramuscular administration. *Menadione Sodium Bisulfite,* N.F. (HYKINONE), occurs as a white crystalline, hygroscopic powder. It is highly soluble in water and is marketed in 5-mg tablets and in ampuls containing 5 to 10 mg/ml. *Menadiol Sodium Diphosphate Injection,* N.F. (KAPPADIONE, SYNKAVITE), is marketed in ampuls containing 5, 10, or 37.5 mg/ml. *Menadiol Sodium Diphosphate Tablets,* N.F., contain 5 mg of the salt for oral use.

THERAPEUTIC USES

The rational therapeutic use of vitamin K is based on its ability to correct the bleeding tendency or hemorrhage associated with its deficiency. A deficiency of vitamin K and its attendant deficiency of prothrombin and related clotting factors can result from inadequate intake, absorption, or utilization of the vitamin, or as a consequence of the action of a vitamin K antagonist.

Inadequate Intake. After infancy, hypoprothrombinemia arising from a dietary deficiency of vitamin K is extremely rare, because not only is the vitamin present in many foods but also it is synthesized by intestinal bacteria. The combination of an inadequate diet and the prolonged use of drugs that inhibit intestinal bacterial growth may lead, however, to vitamin K deficiency (*see* Frick *et al.*, 1967). Occasionally, the use of a poorly absorbed sulfonamide or a broad-spectrum antibiotic may of itself produce a hypoprothrombinemia that responds readily to small doses of vitamin K and reestablishment of normal bowel flora. Hypoprothrombinemia can occur in patients receiving prolonged intravenous alimentation (Ham, 1971).

Hypoprothrombinemia of the Newborn. Newborn infants have a hypoprothrombinemia due to vitamin K deficiency for the few days after birth, the time required to obtain an adequate dietary intake of the vitamin and to establish a normal intestinal bacterial flora. At birth, the normal infant has only 20 to 40% of the adult plasma concentrations of prothrombin, proconvertin, plasma thromboplastin component, and the Stuart factor. These concentrations decline even further during the first 2 or 3 days after birth, before they begin to rise toward the adult values. In premature infants and in infants with hemorrhagic disease of the newborn, these concentrations are depressed even further (*see* Aballi and deLamerens, 1962). Hemorrhagic disease of the newborn has been associated with breast feeding; human milk has low concentrations of vitamin K (*see* Sutherland *et al.,* 1967), and, in addition, the intestinal flora of breast-fed infants apparently lacks microorganisms that synthesize the vitamin (Keenen *et al.,* 1971).

Administration of vitamin K to the normal newborn infant prevents the decline in concentration of the clotting factors on the days following birth; it does not, however, raise these concentrations to the adult level. Premature infants usually display less of a response to vitamin K administration. In the infant with hemorrhagic disease of the newborn, the administration of vitamin K raises the concentration of these clotting factors to the level normal for the newborn infant and controls the bleeding tendency within about 6 hours (Wefring, 1962).

Although small doses of menadione and its derivatives are considered safe, moderate doses have produced hemolytic anemia, hyperbilirubinemia, and kernicterus in newborn, especially premature, infants, even when administered to the mother prior to delivery. Menadione is excreted in part as a glucuronide and competes with bilirubin for a detoxication mechanism of limited capacity in the newborn. Moreover, menadione may induce some hemolysis, especially in the newborn infant with a congenital defect in erythrocyte glucose-6-phosphate dehydrogenase or with a low alpha-tocopherol blood concentration; this causes a further increase in bilirubin concentration (*see* Finkel, 1961; Wynn, 1963).

The routine prophylactic administration of a small dose of phylloquinone to the newborn infant is now recommended (*see* below). Phylloquinone is the drug of choice since it appears to be nontoxic. A single dose of 0.5 to 1 mg should be administered parenterally to the infant immediately after delivery. This dose may have to be increased or repeated if the mother has received anticoagulant or anticonvulsant drug therapy, or if the infant develops bleeding tendencies.

Infants 1 to 5 months old seem to be quite vulnerable to vitamin K deficiency, especially if they have not received prophylactic administration of the vitamin at birth. Infant formulas that do not contain cows' milk are frequently inadequate in vitamin K. Inadequate intake may be exacerbated by diarrhea, antibiotics that reduce intestinal flora, or any of the malabsorption syndromes (*see* below). The Committee on Nutrition (1971) recommends 50 to 100 μg daily or 1 mg monthly of phylloquinone for this age group (*see* Lukens, 1972).

Inadequate Absorption. Hypoprothrombinemia may be associated with either intrahepatic or extrahepatic biliary obstruction, because the lipid-soluble vitamin is poorly absorbed in the absence of bile. A severe defect in the intestinal absorption of fat from other causes can also interfere with absorption of the vitamin.

Biliary Obstruction or Fistula. Bleeding that accompanies obstructive jaundice or biliary fistula responds promptly to the administration of vitamin K. Oral phylloquinone administered with bile salts is both safe and effective and should be used in the care of the jaundiced patient, both preoperatively and postoperatively. In the absence of significant hepatocellular disease, the prothrombin activity of the blood rapidly returns to normal. If for some reason oral administration is not feasible, a parenteral preparation should be employed. The usual dose is 10 mg of vitamin K or menadione per day.

The treatment of a patient during hemorrhage is more difficult. Significant hemorrhage will obviously require blood replacement therapy. In such cases transfusion of fresh blood or reconstituted fresh plasma accomplishes the dual purposes of combating shock and furnishing an immediate supply of prothrombin. Vitamin K should also be given. If biliary obstruction has caused injury to hepatic cells, the response to vitamin K therapy may be poor. Under these circumstances, bleeding associated with hypoprothrombinemia may require continuing administration of fresh blood or reconstituted plasma.

Malabsorption Syndromes. Various disorders that result in inadequate absorption from the intestinal tract may lead to a vitamin K deficiency and hypoprothrombinemia. These include mucoviscidosis, sprue, regional enteritis and enterocolitis, ulcerative colitis, dysentery, and extensive bowel resection. Since drugs that greatly reduce the bacterial population of the bowel are frequently used in many of these disorders, the availability of the vitamin may be further reduced. Moreover, dietary restrictions may also limit the availability of the vitamin. For immediate correction of the deficiency, parenteral therapy should be given.

Inadequate Utilization. *Hepatocellular Disease.* Hypoprothrombinemia may accompany or follow hepatocellular disease, for example, toxic or infectious hepatitis, or advanced cirrhosis. Hepatocellular damage may also be secondary to long-lasting bile duct obstruction. In these conditions the damaged parenchymal cells may not be able to produce the vitamin K–dependent clotting factors, even if excess vitamin is available. Thus, hypoprothrombinemia under these circumstances is usually not favorably influenced by the administration of vitamin K. However, in some instances an inadequate secretion of bile salts may contribute to the syndrome and some benefit may be obtained from the parenteral administration of 10 mg of phylloquinone daily. Paradoxically, the administration of large doses of vitamin K or its analogs in an attempt to correct the hypoprothrombinemia associated with severe hepatitis or cirrhosis may actually result in a further depression of the prothrombin concentration. The mechanism for this is unknown. The vitamin does not, apparently, further depress hepatic function.

The response of hypoprothrombinemia to parenteral vitamin K administration has been used as a test to distinguish between jaundice due to obstruction and that due to hepatocellular disease (Deutsch, 1966).

Drug-Induced Hypoprothrombinemia. Anticoagulant drugs such as dicumarol and its congeners act as competitive antagonists of vitamin K and interfere with the hepatic biosynthesis of prothrombin and factors VII, IX, and X (*see* Chapter 65). These proteins then disappear from the blood at rates dependent on their individual turnover rates: factor VII declines first, followed by factor IX, factor X, and prothrombin.

Excessive hypoprothrombinemia or bleeding produced by the administration of coumarin or indanedione anticoagulants can be corrected in a period of a few hours by the administration of vitamin K. Phylloquinone is much more effective than menadione or its derivatives (*see* Griminger, 1966) and should be used to counteract the effects of overdosage or overresponse to these anticoagulants. Mild overdosage may be treated simply by drug withdrawal or dose reduction, or by the administration of a single dose of 1 to 5 mg of phylloquinone. Larger doses of phylloquinone may interfere with subsequent oral anticoagulant therapy for several days. If bleeding is severe, the immediate administration of 20 to 40 mg of phylloquinone is indicated. Additional doses at 4-hour intervals may be necessary to return the prothrombin time to normal. Transfusion of fresh whole blood may also be needed.

If severe hypoprothrombinemia should occur as a result of the administration of large amounts of salicylate, the treatment is the same as that outlined for dicumarol-induced hypoprothrombinemia, after withdrawal of the salicylate.

Vitamin K may be of help in combating the bleeding and hypoprothrombinemia following the bite of the tropical American pit viper or other species whose venom destroys or inactivates prothrombin.

Hypoprothrombinemia is also associated with excessive intake of vitamin A. Two mechanisms appear to be involved: an inhibition of intestinal bacterial biosynthesis of menaquinone and a direct antagonism of the hepatic actions of vitamin K (*see* Green, 1966).

VITAMIN E

Few vitamins have been more extensively investigated in recent years than has vitamin E. In animals, the signs of deficiency include structural and functional abnormalities of many organs and organ systems. Attending these morphological alterations are biochemical defects that appear to involve fatty acid metabolism and numerous other enzyme systems. Notable is the fact that many signs and symptoms of vitamin E deficiency in animals superficially resemble disease states in humans; however, there is little unequivocal evidence that vitamin E is of nutritional significance in man or is of any value in therapy.

History. The existence of vitamin E was first demonstrated in 1922 by Evans and Bishop, who found that female rats required a then-unrecognized dietary principle in order to sustain a normal pregnancy. Deficient animals were found to ovulate and conceive normally, but at some time during the period of gestation death and resorption of the fetuses occurred. Lesions in the testes were also described, and for a while vitamin E was referred to as the "antisterility vitamin." Further studies, however, revealed the more widespread effects of deficiency of the vitamin (*see* below). Some experiments seem to indicate that vitamin E is not an essential dietary constituent in animals; at present, the significance of these reports must still be evaluated, but they add further complexities to an already complex and sometimes confusing picture (*see* Wagner and Folkers, 1963).

Chemistry. The vitamin was isolated by Evans and coworkers (1936) from wheat germ oil. Eight naturally occurring tocopherols with vitamin E activity are now known. Alpha-tocopherol (5,7,8-trimethyl tocol) is considered to be the most important tocopherol since it comprises about 90% of the tocopherols in animal tissues and displays the greatest biological activity in most bioassay systems. It was identified chemically by Fernholtz (1938) and synthesized by Karrer and associates (1938). Optical isomerism affects activity; *d* forms are more active than *l* forms.

Alpha-tocopherol

Alpha-tocopherol bears a striking structural similarity to the 6-chromanol form of coenzyme Q_4, with which it shares biological activity in several systems (*see* Smith *et al.*, 1963).

One of the important chemical features of the tocopherols is that they are antioxidants. Furthermore, the compounds form reversible oxidation-reduction systems (*see* Dam, 1957). The tocopherols deteriorate slowly on exposure to air or ultraviolet light.

Pharmacological Actions and Physiological Function. Aside from relieving symptoms of its deficiency in animals, vitamin E displays no notable pharmacological effects or toxicity. There is, as yet, no unifying concept to explain its mode of action. Numerous contradictory findings and claims for the actions and mechanisms of action characterize the literature on vitamin E. A major part of the nutritive or therapeutic value of vitamin E in animals appears to be related to its properties as an antioxidant (*see* Dam, 1957; Horwitt, 1965; Molenaar *et al.,* 1972). In acting as an antioxidant, vitamin E presumably prevents oxidation of essential cellular constituents, or prevents the formation of toxic oxidation products such as the peroxidation products formed from unsaturated fatty acids that have been detected in its absence. Diets high in polyunsaturated fatty acids increase an animal's vitamin E requirement (*see* Witting, 1972). However, other chemically unrelated substances, such as synthetic antioxidants, selenium, some sulfur-containing amino acids, and the coenzyme Q group, are able to prevent or reverse certain symptoms of vitamin E deficiency in animal species (*see* Wasserman and Taylor, 1972).

Some symptoms of vitamin E deficiency in animals are not relieved by other antioxidants, and it is presumed in these cases that the vitamin is acting in a more specific manner (*see* Schwarz, 1965; Diplock *et al.,* 1968; Green, 1972). Olsen and Carpenter (1967) suggested that vitamin E functions as a repressor and thereby regulates the synthesis of specific proteins and enzymes required in differentiation or adaptation of tissues.

Wagner and Folkers (1963) have cited experiments that question the essential nature of vitamin E. By dietary manipulations, animals have been raised that are capable of producing normal offspring in the absence of vitamin E or other antioxidants in their diet. Tissues of these animals appear to be devoid of the vitamin. Wagner and Folkers have further questioned whether vitamin E may not merely be mimicking the actions of a member of the coenzyme Q group, which is almost identical in structure to alpha-tocopherol, possesses similar biological activities, and is present normally in tissues. (*See also* Symposium, 1965.)

There is an apparent relationship between vitamins A and E. Vitamin E may facilitate the absorption, hepatic storage, and utilization of vitamin A. In addition, it seems to protect against various effects of hypervitaminosis A (*see* Bauernfeind *et al.,* 1974).

Symptoms of Deficiency. Although manifestations of vitamin E deficiency in experimental animals are protean in nature, various effects on the reproductive, muscular, cardiovascular, and hematopoietic systems are most important because they bear the closest resemblance to the clinical syndromes alleged to be benefited by vitamin E therapy.

Reproductive System. With the exception of the work cited by Wagner and Folkers (1963), evidence indicates that vitamin E is essential for normal reproduction in several mammalian species below the primate level. The most complete observations have been made on rats. In the male rat, prolonged deficiency produces irreversible sterility due to degeneration of the germinal epithelium. In the vitamin E–deficient female, pregnancy terminates in about 10 days with fetal death and resorption of the uterine contents. The fundamental mechanism by which vitamin E deficiency interferes with reproduction is obscure. Fat metabolism and the antioxidant properties of the vitamin appear to be involved and

probably are interrelated, at least in the rat. As mentioned above, the amounts of vitamin E and unsaturated fatty acids in the diet affect reproduction, and antioxidants incorporated into the diet can completely obviate the need for vitamin E for normal growth and reproduction in the rat (Crider *et al.,* 1961). Thus, the essential nature of vitamin E in pregnancy is unclear.

On the basis of such animal studies, vitamin E has been used in man for the treatment of habitual abortion and sterility in the male and female. It has also been used in toxemia of pregnancy, disorders of menstruation, vaginitis, and menopausal symptoms. In spite of early enthusiastic usage of vitamin E, there is no conclusive evidence that the vitamin is of any beneficial effect in any of these conditions.

Muscular System. In many species a vitamin E–deficient diet leads to the development of muscular dystrophy. In addition to well-defined anatomical lesions, metabolic abnormalities, including creatinuria, increased oxygen uptake of affected muscles, and changes in the activity of numerous enzyme systems, are also seen (*see* Mason, 1973). The anatomical and biochemical changes can be prevented, reversed, or ameliorated with alpha-tocopherol or other lipid-soluble antioxidants, including coenzyme Q. The pathogenesis of the dystrophy is unknown. Tappel and associates (1963) attributed tissue damage to the release of cathepsin, ribonuclease, β-galactosidase, and sulfatase from lysosomes damaged by the action of fatty acid peroxidation products. Even though muscular dystrophy accompanies vitamin E deficiency in the monkey (Dinning and Day, 1957), there is no evidence of a vitamin E deficiency or a therapeutic response to the administration of the vitamin in muscular dystrophy in man (*see* Pappenheimer, 1943; Berneske *et al.,* 1960). Similarly, patients with mucoviscidosis or chronic steatorrhea frequently have flabby and atrophic muscles with focal lesions similar to those seen in experimental animals with muscular dystrophy induced by vitamin E depletion, but treatment of these patients with vitamin E likewise has failed to produce a significant improvement in muscle strength (Levin *et al.,* 1961).

Cardiovascular System. The lesions produced in skeletal muscle by a deficiency of vitamin E apparently are also found in cardiac muscle of several species, although involvement of the heart is generally less common and less severe. The cardiac lesions are sometimes associated with ECG alteration, pathological changes, and even heart failure. On this basis, vitamin E has been used in many types of cardiac disorder and in peripheral vascular disease in man. Carefully controlled clinical studies have failed to demonstrate any benefit from the vitamin that could not be matched by the use of a placebo (*see* Report of the Council, 1950). There is thus no rationale for the use of vitamin E in any cardiovascular disease (Olsen, 1973).

Hematopoietic System. In several animal species a deficiency of vitamin E is associated with an anemia that has features of both abnormal hematopoiesis and decreased erythrocyte lifetime. Erythrocytes from such animals have increased susceptibility to hemolysis by oxidizing agents. Indeed, in man this *in-vitro* laboratory test is the only consistent finding associated with low plasma tocopherol levels (*see* Leonard and Losowsky, 1967). Presumably, tocopherol protects the lipids in the erythrocyte membrane from peroxidation, which results in membrane destruction and hemolysis.

Four clinical situations have now been reported to include alpha-tocopherol–responsive anemia (*see* Darby, 1968; Symposium, 1968). (1) A macrocytic, megaloblastic anemia observed in children with severe protein-calorie malnutrition, while unresponsive to treatment with iron, cyanocobalamin, folic acid, or ascorbic acid, was successfully reversed with large doses of alpha-tocopherol acetate (Majaj *et al.*, 1963; Whitaker *et al.*, 1967). This anemia resembles that produced by vitamin E depletion in the monkey (*see* Fitch, 1968) and, like it, also responds to coenzyme Q (Dinning *et al.*, 1962, 1963). (2) Premature infants may develop a hemolytic anemia that is sometimes associated with increased erythrocyte susceptibility to peroxide hemolysis and low plasma tocopherol concentrations. This anemia, while not responsive to iron, cyanocobalamin, or folic acid, does respond to 200 to 800 mg of alpha-tocopherol acetate (Oski and Barness, 1967). In addition to the hematological response, alpha-tocopherol was also reported to relieve the edema and skin lesions accompanying vitamin E deficiency and a diet high in polyunsaturated fatty acids (Hassan *et al.*, 1966). (3) Erythrocytes that hemolyze spontaneously *in vitro* constitute one characteristic of the acanthocytosis syndrome. Patients with this rare genetic disease lack plasma β-lipoprotein and, therefore, have little or no circulating alpha-tocopherol. Further, they have impaired intestinal absorption of the vitamin. Parenteral administration of 100 mg of alpha-tocopherol acetate raised the plasma alpha-tocopherol concentrations and apparently corrected the autohemolytic feature of the disease for several weeks (Kayden *et al.*, 1965). (4) In malabsorption syndromes characterized by steatorrhea (*e.g.*, sprue, mucoviscidosis, chronic pancreatitis), alpha-tocopherol is not absorbed. Here, too, decreased erythrocyte lifetime and increased erythrocyte sensitivity to hydrogen peroxide are coincident with low plasma alpha-tocopherol concentrations. These patients after long-term deprivation may develop other abnormalities associated with vitamin E deficiency in animals, such as muscle weakness and necrosis, creatinuria, and deposition of ceroid pigment in intestinal smooth muscle. Only the creatinuria and hematological abnormalities are responsive to alpha-tocopherol administration. Adult man, intentionally deprived of vitamin E over an extended period of time, has similar hematological lesions and responds to alpha-tocopherol administration (Horwitt *et al.*, 1963).

While the evidence outlined above seems to implicate vitamin E in normal hematopoiesis, other factors must also be considered. Patients with each of the above syndromes have multiple deficiencies. Furthermore, the ability of the coenzymes Q, selenium, and the sulfur-amino acids to relieve "tocopherol-deficient" syndromes to varying degrees provides further complications for a definitive interpretation. (*See* Symposium, 1965, 1968; Whitaker *et al.*, 1967.)

Human Requirement. In a long-term controlled study of vitamin E depletion in man, Horwitt and coworkers (*see* Horwitt, 1962) found that plasma vitamin E concentration declined significantly only after months on a deficient diet. There were no clinical manifestations of the depletion. From these studies, Horwitt estimated that a daily intake of 10 to 30 mg of vitamin E is sufficient to maintain vitamin E blood concentrations within the normal range. Diets containing large amounts of unsaturated fatty acids increase the daily requirement (Harris and Embree, 1963; Witting, 1972); diets containing selenium, sulfur-amino acids, chromenols, or antioxidants decrease the requirement.

The 1974 recommendations of the Food and Nutrition Board of the National Research Council include 15 I.U. of vitamin E per day for adult men and 12 I.U. per day for adult women. (*See* Table XVIII-1, page 1545.) Human milk (in contrast to cows' milk) has sufficient alpha-tocopherol to meet normal infant requirements. Tocopherols are present in adequate amounts in the normal adult diet. Indeed, vitamin E deficiency has not been detected as a primary deficiency disease in otherwise-healthy children or adults.

Absorption, Fate, and Excretion. Vitamin E is absorbed from the gastrointestinal tract by a mechanism probably similar to that for the other fat-soluble vitamins. Vitamin E enters the blood stream by way of the lymph. It appears first in chylomicrons and then primarily associated with plasma β-lipoproteins (McCormick *et al.*, 1960). Vitamin E is distributed to all tissues. However, newborn infants have plasma tocopherol concentrations only about one fifth those of their mothers, suggesting poor placental transfer. Tissue stores can provide a source of the vitamin for long periods of time, as evidenced by the long time animals must be kept on a vitamin E–deficient diet before signs of deficiency appear.

Seventy to 80% of an intravenously administered dose of radioactive vitamin E is excreted by the liver over a period of a week; the balance appears as metabolites in the urine. The urinary metabolites are glucuronides of tocopheronic acid and its γ-lactone (Simon *et al.*, 1956). Several other metabolites with quinone structures have been found in tissues: one of these is very similar in structure to ubiquinone and may be related to an active form of the vitamin (*see* Green and McHale, 1965); dimer and trimer forms of the vitamin are believed to result from reaction with lipid peroxides (*see* Draper and Csallany, 1970).

Plasma concentrations vary widely among normal individuals. Many attempts have been made to correlate the plasma tocopherol values with disease states. In general, tocopherol concentrations in plasma appear to be related more closely to dietary intake and defects in intestinal absorption of fat than to the presence or absence of disease (*see* Darby *et al.,* 1949; Dju *et al.,* 1958). Low tocopherol values are generally associated, however, with an increased susceptibility of erythrocytes to hemolysis by oxidizing agents (Leonard and Losowsky, 1967).

Assay and Unitage. The vitamin E activity of foods may be determined chemically, or bioassayed for the protection afforded pregnant female rats against death of the fetus. One international unit (I.U.) is equivalent to the activity of 1 mg of *dl*-alpha-tocopheryl acetate. *d*-Alpha-tocopheryl acetate has a potency of 1.36 I.U./mg; *d*-alpha-tocopherol, 1.49 I.U./mg; *d*-alpha-tocopheryl succinate, 1.21 I.U./mg.

Preparations. *Vitamin E,* N.F. (ᴀǫᴜᴀsᴏʟ ᴇ, ᴇ-ꜰᴇʀᴏʟ, and others), is a form of alpha-tocopherol that includes the *d* or the *d* and *l* isomers of alpha-tocopherol, alpha-tocopheryl acetate, or alpha-tocopheryl succinate. Official capsules contain 30 to 1000 I.U. of the vitamin. Tablets of many sizes and injectable forms (100 or 200 I.U./ml) are also available. Several multivitamin tablets, capsules, and drops contain small amounts of vitamin E, including *Decavitamin Capsules,* U.S.P.

Therapeutic Uses. The lack of efficacy of vitamin E in the treatment of those diseases in man that bear some resemblance to vitamin E deficiency in animals, namely, habitual abortion, progressive muscular dystrophy, and cardiovascular disease, has been discussed. These are by no means the only disorders in which vitamin E therapy has been studied. The list extends from minor skin ailments to schizophrenia. With the possible exception of its potential value in treating the anemias associated with extreme protein-calorie malnutrition, prematurity, or acanthocytosis (*see* above), results with alpha-tocopherol have in general been so disappointing that the conclusion seems justified that, at present, there is no persuasive evidence that vitamin E has any therapeutic use.

Aballi, A. J., and deLamerens, S. Coagulation changes in the neonatal period and in early infancy. *Pediat. Clins N. Am.,* **1962,** *9,* 785–815.

Almquist, H. J., and Stokstad, C. L. R. Hemorrhagic chick disease of dietary origin. *J. biol. Chem.,* **1935,** *111,* 105–113.

Bauernfeind, J. C.; Newmark, H.; and Brin, M. Vitamin A and E nutrition via intramuscular or oral route. *Am. J. clin. Nutr.,* **1974,** *27,* 234–253.

Berneske, G. M.; Butson, A. R. C.; Gauld, E. N.; and Levy, D. Clinical trial of high dosage vitamin E in human muscular dystrophy. *Can. med. Ass. J.,* **1960,** *82,* 418–421.

Butt, H. R.; Snell, A. M.; and Osterberg, A. E. The use of vitamin K and bile in treatment of hemorrhagic diathesis in cases of jaundice. *Proc. Staff Meet. Mayo Clin.,* **1938,** *13,* 74–80.

Committee on Nutrition, American Academy of Pediatrics. Vitamin K supplementation for infants receiving milk substitute infant formulas and for those with fat malabsorption. *Pediatrics, Springfield,* **1971,** *48,* 483–487.

Crider, Q.; Alaupovic, P.; and Johnson, B. C. Function and metabolism of vitamin E. III. Vitamin E and antioxidants in the nutrition of the rat. *J. Nutr.,* **1961,** *73,* 64–70.

Dam, H. Cholesterinstoffwechsel in Hühnereiern und Hühnchen. *Biochem. Z.,* **1929,** *215,* 475–492.

Dam, H., and Schønheyder, F. The antihaemorrhagic vitamin of the chick. *Nature, Lond.,* **1935,** *135,* 652–653.

Dam, H.; Schønheyder, F.; and Tage-Hansen, E. Studies on the mode of action of vitamin K. *Biochem. J.,* **1936,** *30,* 1075–1079.

Darby, W. J.; Ferguson, M. E.; Furman, R. H.; Lemley, J. M.; Ball, C. T.; and Meneely, G. R. Plasma tocopherols in health and disease. *Ann. N.Y. Acad. Sci.,* **1949,** *52,* 328–333.

Dinning, J. S., and Day, P. L. Vitamin E deficiency in the monkey. *J. exp. Med.,* **1957,** *105,* 395–402.

Dinning, J. S.; Fitch, C. D.; Shunk, C. H.; and Folkers, K. The response of the anemic and dystrophic monkey to treatment with coenzyme Q. *Jl Am. chem. Soc.,* **1962,** *84,* 2007–2008.

Dinning, J. S.; Majaj, A. S.; Azzam, S. A.; Darby, W. J.; Shunk, C. H.; and Folkers, K. Response of macrocytic anemia in children to the coenzyme Q_4-chromanol. *Am. J. clin. Nutr.,* **1963,** *13,* 169–172.

Diplock, A. T.; Cawthorne, M. A.; Murrell, E. A.; Green, J.; and Bunyan, J. Measurement of lipid peroxidation and α-tocopherol destruction *in vitro* and *in vivo* and their significance in connection with the biological function of vitamin E. *Br. J. Nutr.,* **1968,** *22,* 465–472.

Dju, M. Y.; Mason, K. E.; and Filer, L. J. Vitamin E (tocopherol) in human tissues from birth to old age. *Am. J. clin. Nutr.,* **1958,** *6,* 50–60.

Draper, H. H., and Csallany, A. S. Metabolism of vitamin E. In, *The Fat Soluble Vitamins.* (DeLuca, H. F., and Suttie, J. W., eds.) University of Wisconsin Press, Madison, **1970,** pp. 347–353.

Evans, H. M., and Bishop, K. S. On the relationship between fertility and nutrition. II. The ovulation rhythm in the rat on inadequate nutritional regimes. *J. metab. Res.,* **1922,** *1,* 319–356.

Evans, H. M.; Emerson, O. H.; and Emerson, G. A. The isolation from wheat germ oil of an alcohol, α-tocopherol, having properties of vitamin E. *J. biol. Chem.,* **1936,** *113,* 319–332.

Fernholtz, E. On the constitution of α-tocopherol. *J. Am. chem. Soc.,* **1938,** *60,* 700–705.

Frick, P. G.; Riedler, G.; and Brögli, H. Dose response and minimal daily requirement for vitamin K in man. *J. appl. Physiol.,* **1967,** *23,* 387–389.

Green, J. Vitamin E and the biological antioxidant theory. *Ann. N.Y. Acad. Sci.,* **1972,** *203,* 29–44.

Griminger, P. Biological activity of the various vitamin K forms. *Vitams Horm.,* **1966,** *24,* 605–618.

Ham, J. M. Hypoprothrombinemia in patients undergoing prolonged intensive care. *Med. J. Aust.,* **1971,** *2,* 716–718.

Harris, P. L., and Embree, N. D. Quantitative consideration of the effect of polyunsaturated fatty acid content of the diet upon the requirement for vitamin E. *Am. J. clin. Nutr.,* **1963,** *13,* 385–392.

Hassan, H.; Hashim, S. A.; Van Itallie, T. B.; and Sebrell, W. H. Syndrome in premature infants associated with low plasma vitamin E levels and high polyunsaturated fatty acid diet. *Am. J. clin. Nutr.,* **1966,** *19,* 147–157.

Hawkins, W. B., and Brinkhous, K. M. Prothrombin deficiency the cause of bleeding in bile fistula dogs. *J. exp. Med.,* **1936,** *63,* 795–801.

Horwitt, M. K. Interrelations between vitamin E and polyunsaturated fatty acids in adult men. *Vitams Horm.,* **1962,** *20,* 541–558.

———. Role of vitamin E, selenium, and polyunsaturated fatty acids in clinical and experimental muscle disease. *Fedn Proc. Fedn Am. Socs exp. Biol.,* **1965,** *24,* 68–72.

Horwitt, M. K.; Century, B.; and Zeman, A. A. Erythrocyte survival time and reticulocyte level after tocopherol depletion in man. *Am. J. clin. Nutr.,* **1963,** *12,* 99–106.

Karrer, P.; Fritzsche, H.; Ringier, B. H.; and Salomon, H. α-Tocopherol. *Helv. chim. Acta,* **1938,** *21,* 520–525.

Kayden, H. J.; Silber, R.; and Kossman, C. E. The role of vitamin E deficiency in the abnormal autohemolysis of acanthocytosis. *Trans. Ass. Am. Physns,* **1965,** *78,* 334–342.

Keenan, W. J.; Jewett, T.; and Glueck, H. I. Role of feeding and vitamin K in hypoprothrombinemia of the newborn. *Am. J. Dis. Child.,* **1971,** *121,* 271–277.

Leonard, P. J., and Losowsky, M. S. Relationship between plasma vitamin E level and peroxide hemolysis test in human subjects. *Am. J. clin. Nutr.,* **1967,** *20,* 795–798.

Levin, S.; Gordon, M. H.; Nitowsky, H. M.; Goldman, C.; di Sant'Agnese, P.; and Gordon, H. H. Studies of tocopherol deficiency in infants and children. VI. Evaluation of muscle strength and effect of tocopherol administration in children with cystic fibrosis. *Pediatrics, Springfield,* **1961,** *27,* 578–588.

Lukens, J. H. Vitamin K and the older infant. *Am. J. Dis. Child.,* **1972,** *124,* 639–640.

McCormick, E. C.; Cornwell, D. G.; and Brown, J. B. Studies on the distribution of tocopherol in human serum. *J. Lipid Res.,* **1960,** *1,* 221–228.

Majaj, A. S.; Dinning, J. S.; Azzam, S. A.; and Darby, W. J. Vitamin E responsive megaloblastic anemia in infants with protein-calorie malnutrition. *Am. J. clin. Nutr.,* **1963,** *12,* 374–379.

Martius, C.; Burkart, W.; and Stalder, R. Mechanism of action of vitamin K in vertebrates and bacteria. *FEBS Lett.,* **1971,** *18,* 257–260.

Matschiner, J. T.; Bell, R. G.; Amelotti, J. M.; and Knauer, T. E. Isolation and characterization of a new metabolite of phylloquinone in the rat. *Biochim. biophys. Acta,* **1970,** *201,* 309–315.

Olsen, R. E. Vitamin E and its relation to heart disease. *Circulation,* **1973,** *48,* 179–184.

Olsen, R. E., and Carpenter, P. C. The regulatory function of vitamin E. *Adv. Enzyme Regul.,* **1967,** *5,* 325–334.

Oski, F. A., and Barness, L. A. Vitamin E deficiency: a previously unrecognized cause of hemolytic anemia in the premature infant. *J. Pediat.,* **1967,** *70,* 211–220.

Quick, A. J.; Stanley-Brown, M.; and Bancroft, F. W. A study of the coagulation defect in hemophilia and in jaundice. *Am. J. med. Sci.,* **1935,** *190,* 501–511.

Report of the Council on Foods and Nutrition. Deficiencies of the fat-soluble vitamins. *J. Am. med. Ass.,* **1950,** *144,* 34–45.

Schwarz, K. Role of vitamin E, selenium, and related factors in experimental nutritional liver disease. *Fedn Proc. Fedn Am. Socs exp. Biol.,* **1965,** *24,* 58–67.

Simon, E. J.; Gross, C. S.; and Milhorat, A. T. The metabolism of vitamin E. *J. biol. Chem.,* **1956,** *221,* 797–817.

Smith, J. L.; Bhagavan, H. N.; Hill, R. B.; Gaetani, S.; RamaRao, P. B.; Crider, Q. E.; Johnson, B. C.; Shunk, C. H.; Wagner, A. F.; and Folkers, K. Biological activities of compounds in the vitamin E, vitamin K and coenzyme Q groups in chicks, rabbits and rats. *Archs Biochem. Biophys.,* **1963,** *101,* 388–395.

Sutherland, J. M.; Glueck, H. I.; and Glaser, G. Hemorrhagic disease of the newborn. Breast feeding as a necessary factor in the pathogenesis. *Am. J. Dis. Child.,* **1967,** *113,* 524–533.

Suttie, J. W. Mechanism of action of vitamin K. In, *The Fat Soluble Vitamins.* (DeLuca, H. F., and Suttie, J. W., eds.) University of Wisconsin Press, Madison, **1970,** pp. 447–462.

————. Mechanism of action of vitamin K. Demonstration of a liver precursor of prothrombin. *Science, Wash.,* **1973,** *179,* 192–194.

Tappel, A. L.; Savant, P. L.; and Shibko, S. Lysosomes: distribution in animals, hydrolytic capacity and other properties. In, *Lysosomes* (a Ciba Foundation symposium). (de Reuck, A. V. S., and Cameron, M. P., eds.) Little, Brown & Co., Boston; J. & A. Churchill, Ltd., London, **1963.**

Wagner, A. F., and Folkers, K. Considerations of veristic and quasi-biological activities for coenzyme Q and vitamins E and K. *Perspect. Biol. Med.,* **1963,** *6,* 347–356.

Warner, E. D.; Brinkhous, K. M.; and Smith, H. P. Bleeding tendency of obstructive jaundice: prothrombin deficiency and dietary factors. *Proc. Soc. exp. Biol. Med.,* **1938,** *37,* 628–630.

Wefring, K. W. Hemorrhage in the newborn and vitamin K prophylaxis. *J. Pediat.,* **1962,** *61,* 686–692.

Whitaker, J.; Fort, E. G.; Vimokesant, S.; and Dinning, J. S. Hematologic response to vitamin E in the anemia associated with protein-calorie malnutrition. *Am. J. clin. Nutr.,* **1967,** *20,* 783–789.

Witting, L. A. The role of polyunsaturated fatty acids in determining vitamin E requirements. *Ann. N.Y. Acad. Sci.,* **1972,** *203,* 192–198.

Woolf, I. L., and Babior, B. M. Vitamin K and warfarin. Metabolism, function, and interaction. *Am. J. Med.,* **1972,** *53,* 261–267.

Wynn, R. M. The obstetrical significance of factors affecting the metabolism of bilirubin, with particular reference to the role of vitamin K. *Obstet gynec. Surv.,* **1963,** *18,* 333–354.

Zinkham, W. H., and Childs, B. Effect of vitamin K and naphthalene metabolites on glutathione metabolism of erythrocytes from normal newborns and patients with naphthalene hemolytic anemia. *A.M.A. J. Dis. Child.,* **1957,** *94,* 420–423.

Monographs and Reviews

Dam, H. Influence of antioxidants and redox substances on signs of vitamin E deficiency. *Pharmac. Rev.,* **1957,** *9,* 1–16.

Dam, H., and Søndergaard, E. Vitamin K. In, *The Enzymes,* 2nd ed., Vol. 3. (Boyer, P. D.; Lardy, H.; and Myrbäck, K.; eds.) Academic Press, Inc., New York, **1960,** pp. 329–352.

Darby, W. J. Tocopherol-responsive anemias in man. *Vitams Horm.,* **1968,** *26,* 685–699.

DeLuca, H. F., and Suttie, J. W. (eds.). *The Fat Soluble Vitamins.* University of Wisconsin Press, Madison, **1970.**

Deutsch, E. Vitamin K in medical practice: adults. *Vitams Horm.,* **1966,** *24,* 665–680.

Finkel, M. J. Vitamin K_1 and vitamin K analogues. *Clin. Pharmac. Ther.,* **1961,** *2,* 794–814.

Fitch, C. D. Experimental anemias in primates due to vitamin E deficiency. *Vitams Horm.,* **1968,** *26,* 501–514.

Green, J. Antagonists of vitamin K. *Vitams Horm.,* **1966,** *24,* 619–631.

Green, J., and McHale, D. Quinones related to vitamin E. In, *Biochemistry of Quinones.* (Morton, R. A., ed.) Academic Press, Inc., New York, **1965,** pp. 261–285.

Isler, O., and Wiss, O. Chemistry and biochemistry of the K vitamins. *Vitams Horm.,* **1959,** *17,* 54–92.

Martius, C. Chemistry and function of vitamin K. In, *Blood Clotting Enzymology.* (Seeger, W. H., ed.) Academic Press, Inc., New York, **1967,** pp. 557–575.

Mason, K. E. Effects of nutritional deficiencies on muscle. In, *The Structure and Function of Muscle,* 2nd ed., Vol. 4. (Bourne, G. H., ed.) Academic Press, Inc., New York, **1973,** pp. 155–206.

Molenaar, I.; Vos, J.; and Hommes, F. A. Effect of vitamin E deficiency on cellular membranes. *Vitams Horm.,* **1972,** *30,* 45–82.

Oski, F. A., and Naiman, J. L. *Hematological Problems in the Newborn.* W. B. Saunders Co., Philadelphia, **1966.**

Pappenheimer, A. M. Muscular disorders associated with deficiency of vitamin E. *Physiol. Rev.,* **1943,** *23,* 37–50.

Pennock, J. F.   Occurrence of vitamins K and related quinones. *Vitams Horm.,* **1966,** *24,* 307–329.

Symposium. (Various authors.)   Interrelationships among vitamin E, coenzyme Q, and selenium. *Fedn Proc. Fedn Am. Socs exp. Biol.,* **1965,** *24,* 55–92.

Symposium. (Various authors.)   Recent advances in research on vitamins K and related quinones (vitamins K, ubiquinones or coenzyme Q, plastoquinones). *Vitams Horm.,* **1966,** *24,* 293–689.

Symposium. (Various authors.)   Hematological aspects of vitamin E. *Am. J. clin. Nutr.,* **1968,** *21,* 1–56.

Symposium. (Various authors.)   Vitamin E. Biochemistry, nutritional requirements, and clinical studies. *Am. J. clin. Nutr.,* **1974,** *27,* 937–1037.

Wasserman, R. H., and Taylor, A. N.   Metabolic roles of fat-soluble vitamins D, E, and K. *A. Rev. Biochem.,* **1972,** *41,* 179–201.

PRINCIPLES OF PRESCRIPTION ORDER WRITING AND PATIENT COMPLIANCE INSTRUCTION

Ewart A. Swinyard

The prescription order is the most important therapeutic transaction between the physician and his patient. It represents a summary of the physician's diagnosis, prognosis, and treatment of the patient's illness. It brings to focus on one slip of paper the diagnostic acumen and therapeutic proficiency of the physician with instructions for palliation or restoration of the patient's health. The most carefully conceived prescription order may become therapeutically useless, however, unless it communicates clearly with the pharmacist and adequately instructs the patient on how to take the prescribed medication.

The importance of clarity in the physician's communication with the pharmacist cannot be overemphasized. Some drugs look alike when they are written or sound alike when spoken. Over 500 pairs of such drugs have been identified by Teplitsky (1972). When these like-appearing names are written unclearly, or when like-sounding names are garbled over the telephone, the burden of avoiding misinterpretation falls mainly on the pharmacist who fills the prescription order. This problem can be avoided by indicating clearly the complete English name of the drug.

Numerous studies suggest that too many physicians fail adequately to instruct patients on how to take their prescription medication. A review of such studies by Stewart and Cluff (1972) indicates that from 20 to 82% of patients in a variety of clinical situations failed to take their prescription medication as directed. Most errors were related to the prescription order directions; the patient took the medication either in the wrong dose, for the wrong purpose, or at the wrong time. Also, some patients either missed doses or failed to complete the treatment regimen. Data of this kind emphasize the physician's need for training in the basic principles of prescription order writing and in patient compliance instruction.

PRESCRIPTION ORDER WRITING

Prescription order writing is a neglected art both in the medical school curriculum and in medical practice. This is largely because the practice of writing long, complicated prescription orders containing many active ingredients, adjuvants, correctives, and elegant vehicles has been abandoned in favor of single drugs and drug mixtures compounded by pharmaceutical companies. Even when two or more active ingredients are desired for oral administration, they are preferably prescribed separately so that the physician may adjust the dose of each to the individual requirements of the patient.

The National Prescription Audit (1972) reveals that virtually all (98.7%) prescription orders are for precompounded drug items and that only a few (1.3%) require compounding. This is desirable in most instances, but such simplicity does present an unfortunate aspect. Many physicians have lost the art of prescription order writing and no longer take pride in their ability to prescribe drugs. Furthermore, too many physicians rely upon fixed-dose combinations rather than adjust the doses of the agents to the particular needs of the patient. For example, the prescription audit referred to above shows that 40 of the 200 most frequently prescribed drugs are combination products. Other forms of irrational prescribing (Task Force on Prescription Drugs, 1969) include "the use of drugs without demonstrated efficacy; the use of drugs with an inherent hazard not justified by the seriousness of the illness; the use of drugs in excessive amounts, or for excessive periods of time, or inadequate amounts for inadequate periods; the simultaneous use of two or more drugs without appropriate consideration of their possible interaction; [and] the multiple prescribing, by one or several physicians for the same patient, of drugs which may be unnecessary, cumulative, interacting, or needlessly expensive." Certainly such conditions are to be deplored and can be corrected only by concerted cooperative teaching efforts on the part of pharmacologists and of instructors in the clinical and postgraduate divisions.

To be able accurately and speedily to write prescription orders requires considerable practice. The prescription order should be written legibly. If one has a poor handwriting, the prescription order should be printed or typewritten. It is convenient and the accepted form to have one's name, address, telephone number, office hours, and Drug Enforcement Administration (DEA) registry number (formerly known as the Bureau of Narcotics and Dangerous Drugs [BNDD] number) printed on the prescription order blank. However, prescription order blanks bearing the name of a particular pharmacy or other advertising material should be avoided. Because prescription orders are medicolegal documents, they should be written in ink, although this is compulsory only for controlled substances in schedule II. It is also an excellent custom, too infrequently followed, for the doctor to keep an exact or carbon copy for his files. This copy protects him and serves to complete the record of treatment.

The actual writing of a prescription order, if possible, should be done in the presence of the patient. This tends to impress upon the patient that the order is being written for his particular illness and increases his confidence in the physician. One should write without hesitation and with a degree of determination, concentration, and celerity indicative of the fact that the writer is perfectly acquainted with what he is doing. Erasing, crossing out, and tearing up a prescription order in the presence of the patient are poor procedures psychologically and should be avoided. The prescription order should be laid aside for a few minutes and then proofread before affixing one's signature. This is important because errors do occur, especially if the physician has been distracted by talkative patients or relatives. For other general suggestions on prescription order writing, the interested reader is referred to the excellent articles by Friend (1965) and Mazzullo and Lasagna (1972).

Choice of Language. Years ago prescription orders were written exclusively in Latin. Today prescription orders are written *entirely* in English; abbreviations and empirical jargon, whether in Latin or English, should *not* be employed. The reasons for this are so well known they need not be repeated here.

Choice of Drug Name. Most drugs can be prescribed by their official names (U.S.P. or N.F.), by their nonproprietary names (United States Adopted Names; USAN), or by the manufacturers' proprietary (trade) names. The nonproprietary name is often referred to incorrectly as the generic name; the latter term, based on strict definition, is properly used to designate a chemical relationship among drugs, such as sulfonamides, barbiturates, and so forth, and is not synonymous with nonproprietary name. When the proprietary name is used, the pharmacist filling the prescription order must dispense only the drug of the specified manufacturer. In the other cases he may select any of the available preparations.

There is much discussion concerning the relative advantages of prescribing by nonproprietary versus proprietary name. Arguments in favor of the use of nonproprietary names are based, for the most part, on the elimination of duplication of drug products and the possibility of an economic benefit to the patient. Arguments against such practice usually include the lack of quality control, variability in the formulation and, consequently, in the biological availability of the drug (*see* Chapter 1), and the fact that many nonproprietary names are difficult to remember and to spell. For more detailed discussions of the problems associated with drug nomenclature, the interested reader is referred to the informative articles by Lowenthal (1967) and Teplitsky (1972).

Nonproprietary names are now selected by the United States Adopted Name (USAN) Council, formed in 1964 to succeed the A.M.A.–U.S.P. Nomenclature Committee established in 1961. The USAN Council is sponsored jointly by the American Medical Association, the United States Pharmacopeial Convention, Inc., and the American Pharmaceutical Association. Provision was made in 1967 for a liaison representative of the United States Food and Drug Administration also to serve on the Council. The USAN Council follows carefully established principles in coining nonproprietary names for use in the United States and designates nonproprietary names of compounds of demonstrated or potential therapeutic interest. The program of the Council is indispensable, since the number of nonproprietary names increases steadily and, once assigned, the name remains on record even though the agent it designates has been abandoned. (*See* Jerome and Sagan, 1975.)

In writing prescription orders it is *best to use the nonproprietary name followed by the name of the manufacturer in parentheses*. This not only eliminates the necessity for memorizing multiple drug names but also assures the physician that the product of a particular manufacturer will be dispensed. Furthermore, the nonproprietary name is commonly used in teaching pharmacology to medical students. For these reasons, nonproprietary names will be used exclusively in this Appendix. For purposes of identification, proprietary names, designated by SMALL-CAP TYPE, appear throughout the text in chapter sections dealing with preparations as well as in the Index. This does not imply a complete listing of proprietary names, since the number for a single drug may

Table A-1. WEIGHTS AND MEASURES

METRIC SYSTEM

Mass

1000	grams	=	kilogram	(kg)ʳ *
1.0	gram *	=		(g)
0.001	gram	=	milligram	(mg) *
10^{-6}	gram	=	microgram	(μg) *
10^{-9}	gram	=	nanogram	(ng)
10^{-12}	gram	=	picogram	(pg)

Capacity

1000	cubic centimeters	=	liter	(l) *
100	cubic centimeters	=	deciliter	(dl)
10	cubic centimeters	=	centiliter	(cl)
1.0	cubic centimeter *	=	milliliter	(ml, cc)
0.001	cubic centimeter	=	{ microliter	(μl)
			{ cubic millimeter	(cmm)

* Commonly employed units.

be large and since proprietary names differ from country to country.

Choice of a System of Weights and Measures. Prescription orders should always be written in the metric system. It is a self-explanatory decimal system, employed throughout the scientific world and official in the U.S.P. and the N.F. Most medical publications give quantities and doses exclusively in the metric system. The metric system simplifies the calculation of dosage because the terms for both weight and measure—the gram (g) and the milliliter (ml)—are based on a common unit, the meter. The apothecaries' system employs roman numerals and archaic symbols; it is not a decimal system and does not allow for simplicity of calculation. Hence, it should be abandoned.

Metrology. *The Metric System.* The *milliliter (ml)* is the unit of measure, and is equal to ¹⁄₁₀₀₀ part of a liter, the content of a cube measuring 10 cm on each edge. The *gram (g)* is the unit of weight and is equal to the weight of 1 ml of distilled water at 4° C *in vacuo*. The weights and measures of the metric system are given in Table A–1.

In the metric system, only Arabic numbers are used. In the United States, fluids are measured and solids are weighed, and ordinarily no attention is paid to differences in specific gravity of fluids. It is necessary, therefore, only to designate amounts of drug by numbers without writing "g" to indicate that the metric system was employed.

In the prescription order itself, the Arabic number is placed after the official name of the drug and, if several ingredients are prescribed, the decimal points are placed in the same vertical line. Many physicians substitute a vertical line for decimal points, and this "decimal line" may be printed on the prescription order pad. Above this line one may place "g or ml," although this is not necessary inasmuch as the decimal line pre-

supposes the metric system. It should be emphasized, however, that when the decimal line is used all ingredient quantities must be expressed in the basic units of the metric system (g or ml) and this line cannot be used to express decimal fractions of *milligrams*.

Apothecaries' System. Although the apothecaries' system should never be used in writing prescription orders, physicians should be familiar with its basic units. The basic unit of mass is the grain (20 grains = 1 scruple; 60 grains = 1 dram; 480 grains = 1 ounce; 5760 grains = 1 pound or 12 ounces). The basic unit of capacity is the minim (60 minims = 1 fluid dram; 480 minims = 1 fluid ounce; 7680 minims = 16 fluid ounces or 1 pint). Effective communication with older practitioners and patients may require conversion from the apothecaries' system to the metric system. The more commonly employed equivalents are listed in Table A–2.

Table A-2. METRIC AND APOTHECARIES' EQUIVALENTS *

1 milligram	=	¹⁄₆₅	grain	(¹⁄₆₀)
1 gram	=	15.43	grains	(15)
1 kilogram	=	2.20	pounds	[avoirdupois]
1 milliliter	=	16.23	minims	(15)
1 grain	=	0.065	gram	(60 mg)
1 ounce	=	31.1	grams	(30)
1 minim	=	0.062	ml	(0.06)
1 fluid ounce	=	29.57	ml	(30)
1 pint	=	473.2	ml	(500)
1 quart	=	946.4	ml	(1000)

* Figures in parentheses are approximate values and are *not* used in compounding prescription orders.

Household Measures. Unfortunately, the drugs prescribed so carefully by the physician in milligrams and milliliters are usually measured by the patient with convenient kitchen utensils. Therefore, the physician must know the approximate contents of the various household measures that his patient is likely to employ. These are given in Table A–3.

The "drop," which varies in size, presents a special problem. Its size depends on the particular fluid being dropped—its specific gravity, temperature, and viscosity—as well as on the orifice of the dropper and the angle at which the dropper is held (Hirschorn and Silverman, 1968). The U.S.P. does not sanction the prescribing of doses in drops but provides an official standardized dropper for those who wish to use it. This official dropper, when held vertically, delivers drops of water, each of which weighs between 45 and 55 mg. Most commercial products provide a calibrated dropper for this type of preparation. Physicians who find it necessary to prescribe medicines for oral administration in "drop dosage" should request the pharmacist to mark the medicine dropper to deliver the desired amount of drug or to supply a calibrated dropper. The volume error incurred in measuring any liquid by means of a calibrated dropper should not exceed 10%.

The size of the household teaspoon varies con-

Table A–3. HOUSEHOLD MEASURES

MEASURE	APPROXIMATE METRIC EQUIVALENTS
1 drop *	½₀ ml
1 teaspoon *	5 ml
1 dessertspoon	8 ml
1 tablespoon	15 ml
1 wineglass	60 ml
1 glass	250 ml

* *See* text.

siderably, and a given teaspoon will yield different volumes of medicine depending on the technic of measuring the powder or liquid. For household purposes, an American Standard Teaspoon has been established by the American National Standards Institute, containing 4.93 ± 0.24 ml. The U.S.P. specifies that this teaspoon may be regarded as containing 5 ml. Therefore, a prescription order calling for 120 ml should be considered as containing 24, not 30, teaspoonful doses.

Construction of the Prescription Order. Traditionally, a prescription order follows a definite pattern that facilitates its interpretation. The major elements of a model order are illustrated in example No. 1. This pediatric formulation is used in the symptomatic therapy of asthma. The numbers at the left call attention to the several parts of a prescription order, which are explained below. (These numbers do not appear on the prescription order itself.)

1. *Date.* The date when the prescription order is written is important. Federal law requires that prescription orders for drugs listed in schedules II, III, and IV of the Controlled Substances Act of 1970 be dated; orders for schedule-II substances cannot be filled more than 10 days from date of issuance, whereas those for substances in schedules III and IV cannot be filled or refilled more than 6 months from date of issuance.

2. *Name and Address of the Patient.* These are necessary in order to expedite the handling of the prescription order and to avoid possible confusion with medications intended for someone else. The age should also be included if the patient is a minor; otherwise it may be sufficient to indi-

(No. 1)

1.	May 28, 1975
2.	John Jones, Age 6 596 South Main Street Salt Lake City, Utah 84101
3.	℞
4.	Ephedrine Sulfate 0|3 Secobarbital Sodium 0|6 Syrup, to make 180|0
5.	M.
6.	Label: Take 1 teaspoonful at first sign of asthma. Repeat every 4 hours as necessary. Ephedrine Sulfate and Secobarbital Sodium.
7.	Refill *three* times.
8.	Thomas A. Brown, M.D. DEA No. AB1234321 508 South Main Street Salt Lake City, Utah 84101

cate *adult.* The pharmacist should place the name of the patient on the bottle or container exactly as the doctor has written it. Therefore, it is important that the physician write the full name of the patient on the prescription order and that it be spelled correctly. Prescription orders for schedule-II drugs are required to contain the full name and address of the patient, and the pharmacist must transfer this information to the label that is placed on the container of the completed prescription.

3. *Superscription.* The superscription consists of the symbol ℞ (not "Rx"), an abbreviation for *recipe,* the Latin for "take thou." This was formerly of considerable importance in prescription order writing, since the expression "take thou" determined the Latin ending to be used for the names and amounts of the ingredients.

4. *Inscription.* The inscription is the body of the prescription order and contains the name and the amount of each ingredient. Drugs are prescribed by official English names. Abbreviations should be avoided since their use frequently results in error. For example, "sulf." may be mistaken for sulfide or sulfonate, and "chlor." may be mistaken for chlorate or chloral. The name of each drug is placed on a separate line directly under the preceding one. The names of the drugs are capitalized. Traditionally, the order of ingredients, should there be more than one, is as follows:

Basis. The basis is the principal drug and gives the prescription its chief action.

Adjuvant. As the name suggests, the adjuvant is a drug that aids or increases the action of the principal ingredient.

Corrective. The corrective modifies or corrects undesirable effects of the basis or adjuvant.

Vehicle. The vehicle is the agent used as the solvent in the solution, to increase the bulk, or to dilute the mixture.

Practically, prescription orders seldom contain more than one drug name. However, when three agents are prescribed, the most potent or principal drug is listed first, the other ingredient second, and the vehicle last, as shown in the example.

5. *Subscription.* The subscription contains the directions to the pharmacist, which usually consist in a short sentence such as, "Make a solution," "Mix and place into 10 capsules," or "Dispense 10 tablets"; or it is only a word such as "Mix." The latter is commonly written as the letter "M," from the Latin *misce* ("mix"), which the pharmacist proceeds to do according to his art. English is also the preferred language for writing the subscription.

6. *Signature.* The signature of the prescription order consists in the directions to the patient. The term *signature* does not refer to the physician's name; rather, it is derived from the Latin *signa,* meaning "write," "mark," or "label." Since English is the preferred language, the directions are preceded by the word *Label.* Many older physicians still use the Latin *Signa* or the abbreviation "Sig." or "S." Occasionally, this part of the prescription order is called the *transcription* and the term *signature* is then reserved for the physician's name.

The directions to the patient should always be written in English. Nevertheless, some physicians continue to insert Latin abbreviations into the directions. Some may, for example, write 1 cap. t.i.d.p.c., which the pharmacist translates into English as "Take one capsule three times daily after meals." Since the pharmacist *always* writes the label in English, the use of such abbreviations or symbols should be discouraged.

The directions to the patient contain instructions as to the amount of drug to be taken, the time and frequency of the dose, and other factors such as dilution and route of administration. If the drug is to be used externally only, or to be shaken well before using, or if it is a poison, such facts are included. The pharmacist has printed labels, covering many of these points, which he attaches to the container, and often he affixes them at his own discretion, except for a poison label. Directions should be clear but brief, and should occupy no more space than is available on the label to be placed on the container.

The expression "take as directed" is *never* satisfactory and should be avoided. An ill patient or a distracted and worried parent or relative cannot always be relied upon to remember clearly the verbal directions given by the physician, or he may remember them incorrectly. If the directions are too lengthy or too complicated to be placed in the prescription order, they should be written on a separate instruction sheet and left with the patient. To avoid possible error, the first word of the directions to the patient should be employed as a reminder of the correct route of administration. Thus, the directions for a preparation for internal use should start with the word *take;* for an ointment or lotion, the word *apply;* for suppositories, the word *insert;* and for drops to be placed in the conjunctival sac, external auditory canal, or nostril, the word *place.* The directions to the patient should also be employed as a reminder of the intended purpose of the prescription, by including such phrases as "for relief of pain," "for relief of headache," or "to relieve itching." However, directions that would be embarrassing to the patient if placed on the prescription order or label should be given in private.

There are many cogent reasons why prescription medication should be identified on the label. For example, the rapid identification of a drug may be the difference between life and death in the case of adverse drug reactions, or accidental or deliberate overdosage. Therefore, many states require that the name, strength, and quantity of drug dispensed be indicated on the label.

The pharmacist is always on the alert to detect overdoses of potent drugs in the prescriptions he dispenses. This serves as an added check for the safety of the patient. If it is desirable to administer a drug in a larger amount than is customarily employed, it is best for the prescriber to underline the dose, and to write "correct amount" or "correct dose" and his initials at the side. This notation informs the pharmacist that a mistake has not been made, and saves time otherwise lost in verifying the physician's dosage. It is regrettable that some uniform system of indicating unusual doses has not been adopted by physicians.

7. *Refill Information.* Under the Durham-Humphrey Amendment to the Federal Food, Drug, and Cosmetic Act (*see* page 1614), prescription orders for drugs that bear the caution legend, "Federal law prohibits dispensing without prescription," may not be refilled without the consent of the prescriber. Under the Drug Abuse Control Amendments to the above act (*see* page 1615) prescription orders for schedule-III and schedule-IV drugs cannot be refilled *more than five times* and the prescription order is invalid 6 months from date of issue. For these reasons, the physician should indicate his wishes with respect to refills on each original prescription order. This may be indicated by instruction to refill a certain number of times or not to refill. Such restriction may prevent a well-meaning but none-too-wise patient from passing on the prescription to a friend who may be suffering from superficially similar symptoms. Such information need not be written on narcotic prescription orders for schedule-II substances, since by law these cannot be refilled.

8. *Prescriber's Signature.* The prescription order is completed by the physician writing his signature at the bottom of the blank, with the traditional "M.D." following it. Federal law requires that the physician's address and DEA registry number also appear on every prescription order for schedule-II drugs and that such an order be signed (last name in full) with ink or indelible pencil.

Classes of Prescription Orders. On the basis of the availability of the prescribed medication, prescription orders may be divided into two large classes, *extemporaneous* and *precompounded.* An *extemporaneous* prescription order, also called *magistral* or *compounded,* is the type in which the physician selects the drugs, doses, and pharmaceutical form that he desires and the pharmacist prepares the medication according to his art. The *precompounded* prescription order, on the other hand, is one that calls for a drug or mixture of drugs supplied by a pharmaceutical company by its official or proprietary name and in a form that the pharmacist dispenses without pharmaceutical alteration. The extemporaneous prescription order is considerably more difficult to construct and to write; hence, many physicians avoid this type of order by writing for a precompounded official or proprietary preparation. Examples of prescription orders for extemporaneous and precompounded preparations are given below and will serve to illustrate the principles of prescription order writing.

Examples of Prescription Orders for Extemporaneous Preparations. In writing prescription orders for an extemporaneous preparation for oral administration, it is necessary to know the single dose of each ingredient, the number of doses to be taken each day, and the number of days of medication. This knowledge allows the calculation of the total dosage of each ingredient in the prescription. Suppose that it is desired to prescribe an antitussive-expectorant mixture to be taken orally every 4 hours for a nonproductive, exhausting cough. This means that at least four doses will be taken daily. If teaspoonful doses (5 ml) are used and enough medicine is dispensed to last 6 days, approximately 24 doses or a 120-ml total volume will be needed. If the mixture is to contain codeine phosphate (antitussive), ammonium chloride (expectorant), and terpin hydrate elixir (vehicle), the calculation and the construction of the prescription are as shown in example No. 2. (*Obviously, the calculations should not appear on the completed prescription order.*) Extemporaneous prescription orders for other liquid preparations for oral administration, such as syrups, suspensions, and drop medication, are constructed similarly.

The principles of calculation of dosage illustrated above apply also to prescription orders for dry forms of medication to be taken internally. Since pharmacists are ordinarily not adequately equipped to compound compressed tablets, dry forms of medication are commonly prescribed in capsule form. Whereas it is fairly easy to ingest liquid medicines, it may be difficult to swallow capsules that are too large. Therefore, these are limited to approximately 0.5 g in bulk (for adults) for most medicines. If a larger amount is required for the single dose, then the drug must be divided into 2 or more capsules for each dose. If the

(No. 2)

March 5, 1975

Tom Brown, adult
43 Englewood Drive
White Plains, N.Y. 11703

℞

Codeine Phosphate	0	24
Ammonium Chloride	7	2
Terpin Hydrate Elixir,		
to make	120	0

M.

Single dose × No. of doses
⟷ 10 mg × 24
⟷ 0.3 g × 24

⟷ 5.0 ml × 24

Label: Take 1 teaspoonful in a tumbler of water every
4 hours, if necessary for cough. Codeine Phosphate
and Ammonium Chloride.

Jane Morris, M.D.
DEA No. AD1234567
608 East South Street
White Plains, N.Y. 11705

---

ingredients make too small a bulk to be dispensed conveniently in solid form, an inert powder may be added. There are many such powders and excipients (talc, licorice, lactose, etc.), and the pharmacist often selects and adds them at his own discretion.

Suppose that it is desired to prescribe in capsule form an analgesic mixture containing aspirin, phenacetin, and amobarbital for a patient with painful myositis. The medicine is to be taken every 4 hours during waking hours (*i.e.,* four doses per day) and enough is to be prescribed to last 5 days. The construction of the prescription order is as follows:

(No. 3)

July 29, 1975

Mary Thomas, adult
606 Constitution Avenue, N.W.
Washington, D. C. 20001

℞

		Single dose × No. of doses
Aspirin	6 0	⟷ 0.3 g × 20
Phenacetin	6 0	⟷ 0.3 g × 20
Amobarbital	1 0	⟷ 0.05 g × 20

Mix and divide into 40 capsules.

Label: Take 2 capsules every 4 hours for muscle pain,
if necessary. Aspirin, Phenacetin, and Amobarbital.

Do not refill.

Prescription orders for medicines to be taken internally may also be written by the *single-dose method.* The pharmacist is then instructed to prepare a given number of doses, and he must carry out the calculations illustrated above. For example, prescription order No. 3, if written by the single-dose method, would appear as follows:

(No. 4)

℞

Aspirin	0	3
Phenacetin	0	3
Amobarbital	0	05

Make 20 such doses and place in 40 capsules.

Label: Take 2 capsules every 4 hours for muscle pain, if necessary. Aspirin, Phenacetin, and Amobarbital.

Do not refill.

Prescription orders for ointments are usually fairly simple to construct because the ingredients may be calculated on a *percentage basis* rather than by absolute doses. Suppose that it is desired to prescribe an ointment for a fungal infection of the feet, and that benzoic acid (6%) and salicylic acid (3%) are to be incorporated in a base of hydrophilic petrolatum and white petrolatum. If a 60-g amount of ointment is to be dispensed, the order appears as follows:

(No. 5)

℞

Benzoic Acid	3	6
Salicylic Acid	1	8
Hydrophilic Petrolatum		
White Petrolatum, of each an equal		
amount to make	60	0

Make an ointment.

Label: Apply a thin film to the affected parts night and morning. Benzoic Acid and Salicylic Acid.

When prescribing locally acting drugs, the *percentage form may be used as such* rather than as a basis for calculating absolute amounts of ingredients. Prescription order No. 5 thus may be written as follows:

(No. 6)

℞

Benzoic Acid	6%	
Salicylic Acid	3%	
Hydrophilic Petrolatum		
White Petrolatum, of each an equal amount to make		60|0

Make an ointment.

Label: etc.

One may desire to prescribe an ointment containing 5% sulfur. The U.S.P. includes an official *Sulfur Ointment*, which contains 10% precipitated sulfur in mineral oil (10%) and white ointment (80%). This prescription order may be written as follows:

(No. 7)

℞

Sulfur Ointment	5%	60|0

Label: Apply twice daily to affected skin. Sulfur Ointment.

Although this order does not call for the U.S.P. percentage of sulfur, the use of the official title indicates to the pharmacist that the physician wishes the U.S.P. preparation diluted to a 5% sulfur content by addition of the proper ointment base.

A prescription order for a lotion for external use on the skin is similar in construction to that for an ointment in that only the approximate percentages of the ingredients and not absolute doses need be ordered. An order for a simple lotion incorporating 8% calamine (essentially a pink insoluble powder of zinc oxide), 8% zinc oxide, and 2% glycerin in bentonite magma (native, colloidal, hydrated aluminum silicate) and limewater is written as follows:

(No. 8)

℞

Calamine	19	2
Zinc Oxide	19	2
Glycerin	4	8
Bentonite Magma	60	0
Calcium Hydroxide Solution, to make	240	0

M.

Label: Shake well and apply to sunburned areas as needed. Calamine Lotion.

This lotion is identical with *Calamine Lotion,* U.S.P. It is often modified to suit the specific needs of the patient. A pleasant odor can be obtained by the substitution of rose water for the limewater. If the skin lesion itches, phenol may be added to the lotion in 1 or 2% concentration. Olive oil to the extent of 30% may be substituted for bentonite magma.

Prescription orders for many liquid preparations for local administration, such as ophthalmic solutions, nasal sprays, inhalants, gargles, and douches, are constructed similarly to those cited above. For example, a sterile ophthalmic solution of zinc sulfate and phenylephrine hydrochloride for use in mild conjunctivitis may be prescribed as follows:

(No. 9)

℞

Zinc Sulfate	0	08
Phenylephrine Hydrochloride	0	04
Purified Water, to make	30	00

Make a sterile solution.

Label: Place 2 or 3 drops in affected eye every 3 hours. Zinc Sulfate and Phenylephrine Hydrochloride.

Aqueous solutions prepared for use in the eye are less irritating if they are adjusted to isotonicity with the lacrimal fluid. If it is desired to prescribe an isotonic ophthalmic solution, this fact can be indicated by inserting the phrase, "Sodium Chloride, to make isotonic." The pharmacist will then add sufficient sodium chloride to make the solution isotonic with the fluids of the eye. The above order should then be written as follows:

℞

Zinc Sulfate	0	08
Phenylephrine Hydrochloride	0	04
Sodium Chloride, to make isotonic		
Purified Water, to make	30	00

Make a sterile solution.

Label: etc.

Nasal and otic prescription orders follow the same general form, it being necessary to know only the approximate concentration of each ingredient. Solutions to be used in the nose can also be employed with much greater comfort if made approximately isotonic. The physician can instruct the pharmacist to make nasal solutions isotonic with the body fluids by inserting the phrase, "Dextrose, to make isotonic" or "Sodium Chloride, to make isotonic." The pharmacist will then add the requisite quantity of dextrose or sodium chloride to adjust the tonicity of the preparation to that of the nasal fluid.

Summary. The steps taken in the construction of the average *extemporaneous* prescription order may now be summarized.

1. The date, name, address, and age of the patient, and the superscription (symbol ℞) are written first.

2. The best remedy for the patient's illness is then ordered by its official name, followed by any additional drugs necessary to aid, modify, or correct the effect of the main ingredient.

3. Depending on the form in which the medicine is to be given (solution, powder, capsule, etc.), the proper vehicles, flavors, or excipients are then recorded.

4. The directions to the patient are now written. This determines the size of the dose, the number of doses per day, and, occasionally, the duration of medication. The total number of doses and the total bulk of the prescription can then be readily calculated.

5. The correct total amounts for each drug may now be filled in because the single dose of each is known and need only be multiplied by the total number of doses.

6. The directions to the pharmacist, including instructions with respect to refilling the prescription order, are now written. The order should be examined for incompatibilities, reread, and signed.

Examples of Prescription Orders for Precompounded Preparations. Prescription orders for precompounded preparations direct the pharmacist to dispense remedies that have been compounded in advance by pharmaceutical companies and that require no further manipulation on his part. Practically all the official preparations in the United States, that is, those formulations included in the U.S.P. and N.F., are available in precompounded form. Thus, such remedies are prescribed by their official names and, if they contain more than one substance, the specific ingredients need not be listed. A survey of the U.S.P. and N.F. will acquaint the physician with the wide scope and value of the official preparations. Innumerable precompounded nonofficial preparations are also available under various proprietary names. Some of these represent valuable therapeutic agents that ultimately may be included in an official compendium. Others are merely chemical or pharmaceutical variants of well-established drugs.

In writing a prescription order for a precompounded remedy, it is necessary to know the name of the preparation desired, the pharmaceutical form in which it is available (*i.e.,* ointment, tablet, etc.), the single dose, the route and the frequency of administration, and the approximate number of days of therapy. Suppose one wishes to renew a prescription order for a 3-month supply of digoxin for continued maintenance digitalization of an adult patient with congestive heart failure, who is well stabilized and has been thoroughly instructed regarding compliance.

Since digoxin is available under eight different trade names and is marketed by over 50 different companies, it is good practice to prescribe the drug by its USAN, but to indicate a manufacturer's product that will ensure adequate, dependable bioavailability, as shown below.

(No. 10)

℞

Digoxin Tablets
(Burroughs Wellcome Co.)   0|0005
Dispense 100 such tablets.

Label: Take 1 tablet each morning. Digoxin, 0.5 mg.

It should be noted that when the decimal line is used the unit dose *must* be expressed in grams. When the decimal line is not used, the unit dose *must be clearly stated.* For example, the above prescription could also be written as follows:

℞

Digoxin Tablets
(Burroughs Wellcome Co.)   0.5 mg

or

℞

Digoxin Tablets
(Burroughs Wellcome Co.)   500 μg

Precompounded prescription orders for orally administered liquid preparations are constructed in the same manner as are those for extemporaneous liquid medications, except that the preparation is ordered by name. It is necessary, however, to know the concentration of the active ingredient(s) in the preparation. Suppose that it is desired to prescribe the official U.S.P. phenobarbital elixir (4 mg/ml) as a sedative for a 6-month-old infant with acute pruritic eczema. A prescription order providing 6 days of medication may be written as follows:

(No. 11)

℞

Phenobarbital Elixir, U.S.P.   90|0

Label: Give ½ teaspoonful every 4 hours, as necessary for restlessness. Phenobarbital Elixir.

Do not refill.

Prescription orders for other orally administered precompounded remedies, such as solutions, syrups, suspensions, and tinctures, are written as illustrated in the previous example. However, for some of these the physician is required to provide additional information, whereas others may necessitate special instructions to the pharmacist. Assume that it is desired to prescribe *Paregoric,* U.S.P., for an adult patient for the control of diarrhea.

(No. 12)

July 24, 1975

Mrs. Mary Smith, adult
185 11th Street
Charlottesville, Virginia 22903

℞

    Paregoric, U.S.P.   90|0

Label: Take 1 teaspoonful three times a day, as needed for diarrhea. Paregoric.

        John Doe, M.D.
        DEA No. AD1234567
        608 Temple Street
        Charlottesville, Virginia 22903

Since paregoric is a schedule-III substance according to federal law, the physician must write the name and address of the patient, and his own address and DEA registry number on the prescription order.

Dermatological preparations may also be ordered in precompounded form. For example, assume it is desired to prescribe *Compound Undecylenic Acid Ointment,* U.S.P., for the management of a fungal infection of the feet. The prescription order may be written as follows:

(No. 13)

℞

    Compound Undecylenic Acid
        Ointment, U.S.P.   30|0

Label: Apply to affected area each evening after bathing feet. Compound Undecylenic Acid Ointment.

Other precompounded preparations for external application, such as those for the eye and nose, are prescribed similarly. However, preparations for application to the nasal mucous membrane can be dispensed in either a dropper bottle or atomizer bottle. The physician may wish to indicate the type of container desired. For example, assume that it is desired to prescribe *Phenylephrine Hydrochloride Nasal Solution,* U.S.P., for the treatment of acute rhinitis. This preparation usually is available in 0.125, 0.167, 0.25, 0.5, and 1% solutions. The prescription order may be written as follows:

(No. 14)

℞

    Phenylephrine Hydrochloride Nasal
        Solution, U.S.P.   0.25%   15|0
    Dispense in atomizer bottle.

Label: Spray in each nostril every 3 hours. Phenylephrine Hydrochloride Nasal Solution.

As a final example, suppose it is desired to prescribe an antiemetic in suppository form to control nausea and vomiting in a 4-year-old child, and to provide sufficient medication for 3 days. The prescription order may be written as follows:

(No. 15)

℞

    Prochlorperazine Suppository   2.5 mg
    Dispense 6 such suppositories.

Label: Insert 1 suppository in rectum once or twice daily, for vomiting. Prochlorperazine Suppository, 2.5 mg.

Many precompounded suppositories have protective coverings of tin or aluminum foil, and the physician should instruct his patients on the removal of the coverings and the insertion of the suppositories. Insertion may be facilitated if the suppository is first moistened with tepid water.

Summary. The steps taken in the construction of a *precompounded* prescription order may now be summarized.

1. The date, name, address, and age of the patient, and the superscription (symbol ℞) are written first.

2. The best remedy for the patient's illness is then ordered by name, indicating the desired dosage form and concentration (if available in more than one strength) or the single dose.

3. The directions to the patient are written next. This determines the number of doses per day and, occasionally, suggests the duration of medication. The total bulk of the prescription or the total number of unit doses can then be readily calculated.

4. The directions to the pharmacist, including instructions with respect to renewing the prescription order and identification of the medication, are then written. The prescription order should be carefully reread and signed.

Dosage. Dosage is extremely important in prescription order writing. One must know the method of calculating doses (*see* prescription orders Nos. 2 and 3) and the factors influencing the amount of drug to be prescribed (*see* Chapter 1).

Factors Influencing the Total Bulk of the Prescription. The number of days for which medication is contemplated, the number of doses per day, and the size of each dose determine the bulk of the prescription. There is *no minimal limit* to the total quantity of prescribed medication, and as little as a single dose may be ordered, if this is all that is required. On the other hand, a *maximal limit* is indicated for most prescriptions, even when medication is to continue for an indefinite period; this limit is influenced by the stability and cost of the drug and the possible necessity for alteration of the treatment. The size of standard bottles and ointment containers is also a factor. Most pharmacies stock only containers that are multiples of the apothecaries' ounce (30 ml or

30 g). Consequently, the total quantity of a bulk prescription should be 15, 30, 60, 90, 120, 240, 360, or 480 ml (or grams), corresponding to ½, 1, 2, 3, 4, 8, 12, or 16 oz, respectively. When all factors are considered, a convenient rule of thumb is to prescribe only enough medication for 7 to 14 days. Only under special circumstances should more than this quantity of medication be prescribed. An example of such an exception would be an intelligent, cooperative epileptic patient under good control and exhibiting no drug toxicity.

Size and Form of Unit-Dose Medication. The upper limit of the bulk of unit-dose medication (capsules, tablets, etc.) is usually *0.5 g total,* for adults. However, this arbitrary limit based on what the patient can comfortably swallow may be exceeded in the case of dense materials, such as bismuth subcarbonate. Conversely, even a smaller unit dosage may be indicated for light, bulky medication or for certain patients, especially the very young or old.

Many drugs are commercially available only in a limited variety of dose forms (*e.g.,* only capsules of a single weight). For obvious reasons of convenience and economy, these "standard" forms of medication should be preferred, except under unusual circumstances. Until knowledge of the unit-dose forms available for the various drugs is acquired through experience, the physician is well advised to rely upon his pharmacist for this information. Other useful sources of information include *AMA Drug Evaluations* (*AMA–DE*), a publication of the American Medical Association; *Remington's Pharmaceutical Sciences; Hospital Formulary,* published by the American Society of Hospital Pharmacists; and the *Physicians' Desk Reference* (*PDR*).

Accuracy of Dosage. Extreme accuracy of dosage is unnecessary except for very potent drugs that are given in amounts of a few milligrams or less, and it is absurd when prescribing relatively nontoxic drugs that can be given in a single dose of 0.5 g or more. Therefore, in calculating the total amount of a drug to be ordered in a prescription, a "rounding-off" process is employed. For example, 0.52 g may be taken as 0.5 g; 0.68 g, as 0.7 g; and so forth. In general, a variation of not more than 10% in dosage is permissible. Accuracy in dispensing small amounts of toxic drugs is not obtained with the pharmacist's balance but by the use of ready-made dose forms supplied by reliable pharmaceutical companies.

Official Doses. Official doses in the United States are those listed in the U.S.P. and N.F. These represent the *Usual Doses* that should produce the recognized therapeutic effects in adults, following oral administration unless otherwise specified. The *Usual Dose* is intended to serve only as a guide to the physician, who may vary it in the best interests of the patient's welfare. The official compendia also give the *Usual Dose Range,* intended primarily to guide the pharmacist with respect to confirmation of prescription orders calling for unusually large dosages. Dose information on nonofficial drugs can be obtained from package inserts or the references listed above. Doses of drugs given in this textbook are taken from the above sources and ordinarily represent the *Usual Dose.*

Latin Phrases and Abbreviations. Although the use of Latin in writing prescription orders has largely been abandoned, there are a number of phrases and abbreviations that stubbornly persist despite the fact that their use is not recommended. The more common phrases and abbreviations are as follows:

ad libitum (ad lib.)	at pleasure; freely; as much as wanted
ana (aa. or a̅a̅)	of each
ante (ā)	before
ante cibum (a.c.)	before meals
bis in die (b.i.d.)	twice daily
cum (c̄)	with
gutta; guttae (gtt.)	a drop; drops
hora (h.)	hour
hora somni (h.s.)	hour of sleep; at bedtime
misce (M.)	mix
non repetatur (non rep.)	do not repeat
numerus (No.)	number
post (p̄)	after
post cibum (p.c.)	after meals
pro re nata (p.r.n.)	according to circumstances; occasionally
quantum satis, sufficit, or sufficiat (q.s.)	a sufficient amount; as much as is necessary
(q.s.ad)	a sufficient amount to make
quaque die (qq.d.)	every day
quaque hora (qq.h.)	every hour
(qq.4 h.)	every 4 hours
quarter in die (q.i.d.)	four times a day
semis (ss. or s̅s̅)	one-half
signa (sig.)	write on label
sine (s̄)	without
statim (stat.)	immediately
ter in die (t.i.d.)	three times a day

Vehicles, Flavors, and Coloring Agents. The oral route of administration of drugs is more widely accepted by patients than is any other route. Oral medication should be in the form of tablets and capsules, if at all possible. Children and geriatric patients, however, usually find the liquid forms of oral medication more acceptable; indeed, if bitter, salty, or other objectionable-tasting drugs could be disguised in a liquid preparation, this would be one of the most useful forms of drug administration for such patients. In addition, there are instances when orally administered liquid preparations are essential. It is therefore necessary for the physician to know how to prescribe medicines in a form sufficiently palatable so that they will be taken by the patient.

The effective flavoring and coloring of a drug formulation often present formidable problems. Pharmaceutical manufacturers spend considerable sums of money and devote much time and effort to assure that an otherwise distasteful drug is marketed in an acceptable, elegant form. In such cases, it is probably best to prescribe the drug in a proprietary formulation. Nevertheless, acceptable extemporaneous liquid medications can be obtained by the careful selection of coloring, flavoring, and diluting agents. The physician is well advised to enlist a pharmacist's aid in demonstrating the use of available agents.

A. *Vehicles.* The many vehicles available to the physician for flavoring and diluting drugs may conveniently be divided into three groups: watery (aqueous), hydroalcoholic, and alcoholic vehicles. Their use is largely governed by the solubility characteristics of the active medicinal agent. Listed below are the more commonly employed official vehicles.

1. Watery Vehicles. Watery vehicles include the aromatic waters, the syrups, and the mucilages.

a. AROMATIC WATERS. Aromatic waters, saturated aqueous solutions of volatile oils, are used as vehicles for water-soluble substances and salts. They cannot mask the taste of very disagreeable drugs. The two official aromatic waters are:

> *Orange Flower Water,* N.F.
> *Peppermint Water,* N.F.

b. SYRUPS. Syrups, concentrated aqueous solutions of sugar, are useful as vehicles for water-soluble drugs and act as both solvents and flavoring agents. Some of the more common syrups are as follows:

> *Syrup,* U.S.P.
> *Acacia Syrup,* N.F.
> *Aromatic Eriodictyon Syrup,* N.F.
> *Cherry Syrup, N.F.*
> *Cocoa Syrup,* U.S.P.
> *Orange Syrup,* N.F.
> *Tolu Balsam Syrup,* N.F.

c. MUCILAGES. Mucilages are thick, viscid, adhesive liquids, produced by dispersing gum in water. They are also suitable as vehicles for water-soluble substances, and are especially useful for suspensions and emulsions.

Acacia, U.S.P., the dried gummy exudation from *Acacia senegal,* is used in a 10 to 15% concentration. It is precipitated by strong alcohol.

Tragacanth, U.S.P., the dried gummy exudation from *Astragalus gummifer,* is used in 3 to 6% concentration. Tragacanth, in contrast to acacia, is not precipitated by weak alcoholic solutions.

Methylcellulose, U.S.P., a synthetic substitute for the natural gums, is used in 0.5 to 2.0% concentration. It is also used to prolong the duration of contact of ophthalmic drops.

Carboxymethylcellulose Sodium, U.S.P., a synthetic hydrophilic colloid, is used in a 2% concentration.

2. Hydroalcoholic Vehicles. The most important hydroalcoholic vehicles are the *elixirs.* The elixirs are sweetened hydroalcoholic solutions that contain approximately 25% alcohol. They are suitable vehicles for drugs soluble in either water or dilute alcohol. There are many official *medicated elixirs* containing specific drugs, such as *Diphenhydramine Hydrochloride Elixir,* U.S.P., *Phenobarbital Elixir,* U.S.P., *Acetaminophen Elixir,* U.S.P., and others. The common *nonmedicated* elixirs used exclusively as vehicles and diluents are as follows:

Aromatic Elixir, U.S.P., is a useful vehicle for flavoring or diluting preparations containing approximately 25% alcohol. It may precipitate strongly alcoholic solutions such as tinctures and fluidextracts.

Compound Benzaldehyde Elixir, N.F., has an odor of bitter almonds and contains 3 to 5% alcohol. This is a useful vehicle when a low alcoholic content is desired.

Iso-Alcoholic Elixir, N.F., is a hydroalcoholic vehicle with the flavor and the taste of aromatic elixir. It consists of two formulas, designated as low-alcoholic elixir (8 to 10% alcohol) and high-alcoholic elixir (73 to 78% alcohol). Iso-alcoholic elixir represents a mixture of the two formulas adjusted by the pharmacist to meet the alcoholic requirements of the drugs for which it serves as a vehicle or diluent.

3. Alcoholic Vehicles. Alcoholic vehicles are useful for substances soluble in strong alcohols, or as flavors to be added in small quantities to syrups or elixirs. The alcohol content of these vehicles is approximately 50%, two or more times the alcohol content of the elixirs. There are two types of alcoholic vehicles, the *tinctures* and the *spirits.*

a. TINCTURES. Tinctures are alcoholic or hydroalcoholic solutions of the active principles of drugs. They are *medicated* or *nonmedicated. Medi-*

cated tinctures include such well-known preparations as *Belladonna Tincture,* U.S.P., and *Paregoric,* U.S.P. The nonmedicated tinctures listed below are used as flavoring agents.

> *Sweet Orange Peel Tincture,* N.F.
> *Vanilla Tincture,* N.F.

b. SPIRITS. Spirits are alcoholic solutions of volatile drugs, usually oils. Spirits are also medicated or nonmedicated. Medicated spirits include *Aromatic Ammonia Spirit,* N.F., and *Camphor Spirit,* N.F. Nonmedicated spirits are used in low concentration to impart a pleasing flavor to an otherwise-tasteless or -distasteful liquid. *Peppermint Spirit,* N.F., and *Compound Orange Spirit,* N.F., are most commonly used for this purpose.

The following illustrations will suffice to show how these vehicles and flavoring agents may be used in extemporaneous prescription orders. Suppose that it is desired to prescribe an antibiotic in liquid form for oral administration. The prescription order may be written as follows:

(No. 16)

℞

Tetracycline Hydrochloride	3	0
Cherry Syrup, to make	60	0

Label: Shake well and take 1 teaspoonful orally 1 hour before each meal and at bedtime. Tetracycline Hydrochloride.

Because of its flexibility, iso-alcoholic elixir can be used to advantage in numerous extemporaneous prescription orders. For example, if the physician wishes to prescribe an elixir, tincture, or fluidextract in a vehicle in order to increase the volume and thus make the dose more convenient to measure, it is important that the alcoholic strength of the vehicle be approximately the same as that of the preparation to be diluted; otherwise, the active principles may be precipitated. The physician need not remember the particular alcohol concentration required but should merely prescribe the iso-alcoholic elixir. The pharmacist then ascertains how much of the elixirs of low and high alcohol content to mix in order to obtain the same alcohol concentration as the solution of drug that is being prescribed. Thus, if phenobarbital elixir is ordered in iso-alcoholic elixir, the alcohol content is adjusted to 15%, which is the alcoholic concentration of the phenobarbital elixir, and the barbiturate will not be precipitated out of solution.

(No. 17)

℞

Phenobarbital Elixir	45	0
Iso-Alcoholic Elixir, to make	90	0
M.		

Label: Take 1 teaspoonful in water every 4 hours, as necessary for restlessness. Phenobarbital Elixir.

By diluting the phenobarbital elixir with the iso-alcoholic elixir, fractional teaspoonful doses or "drop dosages" are avoided, since a teaspoonful dose can be adjusted to contain the desired quantity of the barbiturate.

Paregoric, U.S.P., is an example of a medicated tincture that is frequently used as both a vehicle and a therapeutic agent. Suppose it is desired to prescribe paregoric and bismuth subcarbonate for the treatment of diarrhea. The prescription order may be written as follows:

(No. 18)

℞

Bismuth Subcarbonate	8	0
Paregoric, to make	60	0
M.		

Label: Shake well and take ½ teaspoonful every 2 hours, for diarrhea. Bismuth Subcarbonate and Paregoric.

B. *Coloring Agents.* The addition of a color to an otherwise-colorless preparation is of little importance from a therapeutic standpoint, but it is of considerable importance from a psychological standpoint. Many vehicles have their own distinct color. When color is to be added, however, it is best to use the color that is conventionally associated with the taste. Three commonly used coloring agents are as follows:

Amaranth Solution, U.S.P., is a 1.0% solution of F.D.&C. Red No. 2. It has good color stability in both acidic and alkaline solutions. It is used primarily to impart a red color to aqueous pharmaceutical preparations.

Compound Amaranth Solution, N.F., contains 0.9% amaranth, 10% caramel, and 25% alcohol. This solution is used to impart a red color to hydroalcoholic solutions.

Caramel, U.S.P., is a concentrated aqueous solution of burnt sugar. It is used to produce a brown color in elixirs, syrups, and other preparations.

Some physicians prefer to leave the coloring to the pharmacist. In this case, the words *color red* or *color appropriately* are written on the prescription order.

C. *Flavoring Agents.* Wesley (1957) studied the flavors employed in 200 popular pharmaceuticals. His study revealed that several pharmacological classes of agents present common taste problems that may be solved with a relatively few flavoring agents. *Cherry Syrup,* N.F., was the flavor of choice for antibiotics, cough preparations, and sulfonamide-antibiotic mixtures; *Cocoa Syrup,* U.S.P., for sulfonamides; and *Orange Syrup,* N.F., for vitamins. *Raspberry syrup* was also very acceptable for antibiotics, cough preparations, and antihistamines. Wesley suggested that problems presented by most extemporaneous prescription orders for liquids can be solved by the use of the four above-mentioned preparations.

Incompatibility. An incompatibility exists when two or more ingredients in a prescription order interfere with each other in a manner not intended by the physician. Three types of incompatibilities are generally recognized. A *therapeutic* incompatibility occurs when two drugs that either increase or decrease the expected physiological response are unwittingly prescribed concurrently (*see* Chapter 1, pages 36–37). A *physical* incompatibility occurs when liquefaction, deliquescence, precipitation, incomplete solution, or other change in physical state takes place. A *chemical* incompatibility occurs when two ingredients in a prescription react chemically to give new compounds. Most physical and chemical incompatibilities can be avoided, provided the physician keeps a few broad concepts in mind when writing prescription orders.

The physical and chemical incompatibilities most likely to be encountered in prescription order writing may be divided into three groups: solubility phenomena, cationic-anionic incompatibilities, and acid-base or pH effects. The summary that follows covers only those concepts considered helpful to the physician.

Solubility Phenomena. Most organic drugs have both polar (hydrophilic) and nonpolar (hydrophobic) groups in the molecule. Usually a drug of low molecular weight will be soluble in water ($\geq 3\%$) if there is at least one polar group ($-OH$, $-NH_2$, $-SO_3H$, $-CHO$, $-COOH$, etc.) and not more than four carbons in a straight-chain compound or five carbons in a branched chain. This rule of thumb applies to alcohols, aldehydes, ketones, acids, ethers, esters, and other low-molecular-weight compounds. In compounds with higher molecular weights, spatial arrangements profoundly influence solubility. Thus, nonpolar solutes or drugs (*e.g.,* testosterone) are most soluble in nonpolar solvents (vegetable and mineral oils) and polar solutes or drugs (*e.g.,* ascorbic acid) are most soluble in polar solvents (glycerin and water). Many drugs are intermediate in polarity (*e.g.,* acetaminophen) and are soluble in alcohol or hydroalcoholic vehicles.

Cationic-Anionic Incompatibilities. Combination reactions of ionized organic species with each other can be predicted by the method suggested by Miller (1952). Most organic drugs of *high* molecular weight that ionize or dissociate in solution can be divided into three classes, as follows:

Cationic. Organic bases (amines) and their salts, such as acetate, citrate, hydrochloride, phosphate, sulfate, and tartrate; for example, mepazine acetate, chlorothen citrate, erythro-

mycin hydrochloride, phenacaine hydrochloride, phenylephrine hydrochloride, codeine phosphate, amphetamine sulfate, atropine sulfate, ergotamine tartrate, and methscopolamine bromide.

Anionic. Organic acids and their salts, such as ammonium, calcium, potassium, and sodium; for example, cyclobarbital calcium, novobiocin calcium, phenobarbital sodium, penicillin G potassium, phenytoin sodium, fluorescein sodium and some other dyes, and soaps.

Nonionic. Nonionizing esters, ethers, alcohols, and so forth; for example, benzocaine, benzyl benzoate, most glycosides, methylcellulose, sorbitan fatty acid esters (arlacels), polysorbates (tweens), and sugars.

Cationic substances and anionic substances are usually compatible with compounds of their own type and with nonionic substances but are often incompatible with each other, for example, soap and benzalkonium chloride.

Acid-Base or pH Effects. The *addition of acids* to prescriptions containing salts of weak organic acids (anionic drugs such as phenobarbital sodium) will cause the less soluble, free organic acid (phenobarbital) to form. Acids also produce color changes in certain compounds (phenolphthalein), produce effervescence with carbonates and bicarbonates, catalyze hydrolysis of certain esters (aspirin), or cause degradation of some antibiotics (penicillin G). The *addition of bases* to prescriptions containing salts of weak organic bases (cationic drugs such as atropine sulfate) will cause the less soluble, free base (atropine) to form. Whether the free acids and bases liberated in these reactions will form precipitates depends on their solubility in the total mixture at the final pH value. Bases can also facilitate other chemical reactions, such as the oxidation of compounds like catecholamines and ascorbic acid.

Knowledge of these basic principles should enable the physician to select drugs that can be combined in a prescription order without danger of interaction or precipitation.

Prescription Refills. Prescription drugs were formerly controlled by several federal laws, including the Federal Food, Drug, and Cosmetic Act, the Federal Narcotic–Internal Revenue Regulations (historically known as the Harrison Narcotic Act), and the Federal Marihuana Regulations. On May 1, 1971, the *Comprehensive Drug Abuse Prevention and Control Act* of 1970 became fully effective and, except for the Durham-Humphrey Amendment (Section 503B), repealed all the aforementioned laws controlling prescription drugs.

The Durham-Humphrey Amendment defines certain types of drugs that may be sold by the pharmacist only on the prescription order of a practitioner licensed by law to administer such drugs. These drugs are required to bear the label, *"Caution: Federal law prohibits dispensing without prescription."* Under the Durham-Humphrey Amendment, a prescription order cannot be refilled unless authorized by the prescriber. The prescriber may indicate the number of times a prescription order may be refilled, in the blank space in the statement, "Refill _____ times"; this statement may be printed on the prescription order blank.

The Comprehensive Drug Abuse Prevention and Control Act, commonly referred to as the Controlled Substances Act, is designed to control the distribution of all depressant and stimulant drugs (*e.g.,* narcotics, barbiturates, and amphetamines) and other drugs with abuse potential as designated by the Drug Enforcement Administration, Department of Justice. This act requires the pharmacist to keep a record of the receipt and the disposition of all Controlled Substances; such drugs are identified on the label of the *original* container by a symbol, consisting of either the Roman numeral of the schedule within a large letter "C" or the letter "C" followed by the schedule (*e.g.,* C-II). The records must be maintained for a period of at least 2 years and be available for inspection by authorized persons. Prescription orders for Controlled Substances in schedule II must be typewritten, or written in ink or indelible pencil, and signed by the practitioner; such prescription orders must be *limited to a 34-day supply and cannot be refilled.* Prescription orders for drugs covered by schedule III or IV may be issued either orally or in writing by a practitioner and may be refilled, *if so authorized, not more than five times* and may *not* be filled or refilled *more than 6 months* after date of issue. After five refills or after 6 months, the prescribing practitioner may write or authorize a new prescription order. Drugs in schedule V may be prescribed the same as drugs in schedules III and IV, and, under certain conditions, may be dispensed without a prescription.

Physicians should do all they can to prevent refill abuses of prescription orders. It is a good practice to write out the number of refills desired on every prescription order; Arabic numerals may easily be altered and, if not indicated, instructions may easily be forged. Furthermore, when a refill authorization is not given on the prescription order, it cannot be refilled without *personal* authorization by the prescriber.

Controlled Substances Act. Various federal, state, and city laws exist to control the standard of purity of drugs and their manufacture, sale, and dispensing. These laws must be known and

observed by the practitioner. It should be noted that the most stringent law takes precedence, whether it be federal, state, or local. The most important laws are embodied in the *Comprehensive Drug Abuse Prevention and Control Act of 1970 (see* Federal Regulations, April 24, 1971). This act divides narcotic and other drugs into five schedules.

Schedule I. Drugs in this schedule have a high abuse potential and *no* currently accepted medical use in treatment in the United States. Examples of such drugs include heroin, marihuana, LSD, peyote, mescaline, psilocybin, tetrahydrocannabinols, ketobemidone, levomoramide, racemoramide, benzylmorphine, dihydromorphine, morphine methylsulfonate, nicocodeine, nicomorphine, and others. Substances listed in this schedule are not for prescription use but may be obtained for research and instructional use or for chemical analysis by application to the Drug Enforcement Administration, Department of Justice (Form 225), supported by a protocol of the proposed use.

Schedule II. Drugs in this schedule have a high abuse potential with severe psychic or physical dependence liability. Schedule-II controlled substances consist of the former class-A narcotic drugs and drugs containing amphetamines or methamphetamines as the single active ingredient or in combination with each other. Examples of substances included in this schedule are opium, morphine, codeine, hydromorphone (DILAUDID), methadone (DOLOPHINE), PANTOPON, meperidine (DEMEROL), cocaine, oxycodone (PERCODAN), anileridine (LERITINE), oxymorphone (NUMORPHAN), straight amphetamines, and methamphetamines. Also included in schedule II are phenmetrazine (PRELUDIN), methylphenidate (RITALIN), methaqualone (PAREST, QUAALUDE, SOMNAFAC, and SOPOR) and its salts, and amobarbital (AMYTAL), pentobarbital (NEMBUTAL), and secobarbital (SECONAL) and their salts alone, in combination with each other, or in combination with controlled substances.

Schedule III. The drugs in this schedule have an abuse potential less than those in schedules I and II; their abuse may lead to moderate or low physical dependence or high psychological dependence. This schedule includes those drugs formerly known as class-B narcotics (any compound, mixture, or preparation containing limited quantities of codeine, hydrocodone, dihydrocodeine, ethylmorphine, opium, or morphine [*e.g.,* 1.8 g of codeine per 100 ml and not more than 90 mg per dosage unit with an equal or greater quantity of an isoquinoline alkaloid of opium]) and some nonnarcotic drugs such as chlorhexadol, glutethimide (DORIDEN), methyprylon (NOLUDAR), phencyclidine, sulfondiethylmethane, sulfonmethane, nalorphine, benzphet-amine, chlorphentermine, clortermine, mazindol, phendimetrazine, and barbiturates (except those listed in another schedule). Paregoric is in this schedule.

Schedule IV. The drugs in this schedule have a low abuse potential, lead to only limited physical dependence or psychological dependence relative to drugs in schedule III, and include barbital, phenobarbital, methylphenobarbital, chloral betaine (BETA-CHLOR), chloral hydrate, ethchlorvynol (PLACIDYL), ethinamate (VALMID), meprobamate (EQUANIL, MILTOWN), paraldehyde, pentaerythritol chloral (PETRICHLORAL), methohexital, fenfluramine, diethylpropion, phentermine, chlordiazepoxide (LIBRIUM), diazepam (VALIUM), and clorazepate dipotassium (TRANXENE). Flurazepam (DALMANE) and oxazepam (SERAX) are under review for possible inclusion in this schedule.

Schedule V. The drugs in this schedule have an abuse potential less than those listed in schedule IV and, with the exception of paregoric, consist of those preparations formerly known as "exempt" narcotics (narcotic preparations containing nonnarcotic active medicinal ingredients, *e.g.*, not more than 2.5 mg of diphenoxylate and not less than 2.5 μg of atropine sulfate per dosage unit). Substances in this schedule may be prescribed the same as those in schedules III and IV. In addition, drugs in schedule V may be dispensed without a prescription order provided (1) such distribution is made only by a pharmacist; (2) not more than 240 ml of any schedule-V substance containing opium, nor more than 120 ml of any other schedule-V substance, is distributed at retail in a 48-hour period without a prescription order; (3) the purchaser at retail is at least 18 years of age; (4) the pharmacist obtains suitable identification; (5) a record book is maintained that contains the name and address of the purchaser, name and quantity of Controlled Substance purchased, date of sale, and initials of the pharmacist; and (6) other federal, state, or local law does not require a prescription order.

The label of any Controlled Substance in schedule II, III, or IV, when dispensed to or for a patient pursuant to a prescription order, must contain the following warning: *"Caution: Federal law prohibits the transfer of this drug to any person other than the patient for whom it was prescribed."*

In order to prescribe Controlled Substances, a physician must register with the Drug Enforcement Administration, Department of Justice. The registration must be renewed annually, and the certificate of registration kept posted in the same manner as the former Narcotic Tax Stamp. The number on the certificate of registration must then be indicated on all prescription orders for Controlled Substances. He must also file an inventory of the Controlled Substances on hand every 2 years; file a revised form if his location is changed; keep a record of controlled substances listed in schedules II through V that he dispenses, if he regularly charges patients either separately or together with professional services for such medication; and order his supplies of narcotic drugs, listed in schedule II for dispensing or administration, on special order forms obtainable from the Registration Branch, Drug Enforcement Administration, Department of Justice, P.O. Box 28083, Central Station, Washington, D. C. 20005.

Both the physician and the pharmacist are legally responsible for the proper prescribing and dispensing of drugs covered by the Controlled Substances Act. There are many technical details in the regulations and, as a result, the physician may innocently violate the law in his professional use of Controlled Substances, especially as related to the use of narcotics for patients with incurable diseases or in the management of drug addiction (*see* 1971 Regulations, Section 306.07; *see also* the *fourth edition* of this textbook, pages 1718–1719).

PATIENT COMPLIANCE INSTRUCTION

Most physicians assume that once the diagnosis is made and the prescription order is written the patient will benefit from his diagnostic and therapeutic acumen. While this assumption seems reasonable, reviews of compliance reveal an alarming incidence of patient medication errors and noncompliance with regard to taking the prescribed drugs (Marston, 1970; Stewart and Cluff, 1972). A review of over 50 studies indicates that between one fourth and over one half of all outpatients failed to take the medication as prescribed (Blackwell, 1972a). The most common types of noncompliance are errors in the interpretation of the directions, so that the medicine is taken for the wrong reason, in the wrong dose, or at the wrong time (Mazzullo and Lasagna, 1972). Observations of this kind suggest that attention should be directed to some of the basic principles of patient compliance instruction.

Factors Associated with Noncompliance. The drug defaulter, like the placebo reactor, is not a consistent, readily identifiable individual. Patients who are unreliable under one treatment regimen may not be under another. Porter (1969), after a detailed study of this problem, concluded that ". . . it has not proved possible to identify an uncooperative type. Every patient is a potential defaulter; compliance can never be assumed." Nevertheless, it is possible to identify a constellation of factors that may be associated with noncompliance, some of which have been mentioned in the previous discussion on prescription order writing. Several of these factors are briefly reviewed here, in order to emphasize the things the physician can do to improve patient compliance. For a more detailed analysis, the interested reader is referred to the excellent articles by Blackwell (1972b) and Hulka and associates (1975).

The Patient's Illness. After the prescription order has been written, the physician should make sure the patient understands the nature and prognosis of his illness, what he may expect from his medication, and how the medication alters the disease process. Patients frequently discontinue taking a medication such as penicillin for streptococcal pharyngitis because they have not been told the necessity for continuing the drug after the acute symptoms have subsided. Similarly, patients on antidepressant medication frequently discontinue treatment because the physician failed to mention the untoward effects that might appear or to advise the patient that 10 days or more may elapse before he notices any improvement. Patients with chronic illnesses are prone to lapse in compliance, especially if the treatment is prophylactic or suppressive, the condition is mild or asymptomatic, or the consequences of missing a dose or two are not immediate. In contrast, when relapse is immediate or severe, the patient is much less likely to deviate from the prescribed regimen.

The Patient. Errors and noncompliance occur more frequently at the extremes of age. Geriatric patients present problems because of lapses in memory or self-neglect. Poor compliance among children is related to problems of taste and swallowing, although the mother's impression of the severity of the illness has a marked influence on compliance in pediatric patients (Becker *et al.,* 1972). The physician must explore in some detail the patient's eating, sleeping, and working habits. Otherwise, he might prescribe a drug to be taken three times a day with meals for a patient who either eats only twice a day or sleeps all day and works at night. Educational, economic, ethnic, and personality factors have also been shown to influence patient compliance. In general, the less educated, poor patient with a risk-prone personality is more likely to be a drug defaulter (Blackwell, 1972b).

The Physician. The physician's relationship with the patient and how clearly he explains the treatment regimen have a powerful impact on compliance. All too frequently the prescription order is used as a symbol to terminate the visit, rather than as an opportunity to educate the patient. Since most patient errors result from inability to interpret directions, the physician should write the prescription order legibly and in English. He should avoid the use of abbreviations, particularly those that are not well accepted or may be misunderstood. Prescription order directions should include all the details necessary for a patient to know how, with what, when, and how long to take the medication. For example, patient directions for a prescription order for tetracycline capsules might read as follows: "Take orally one capsule with a half glass of water 1 hour before each meal and at bedtime for 10 days." The prescription order should be proofread aloud and the patient cautioned not to take the medication with milk and to avoid antacids while on the drug. Finally, the patient should be asked if he understands the directions and what the treatment is expected to accomplish.

The Medication Prescribed. Multiple medications, frequent-dose regimens, and the physical features of the medication itself often foster poor compliance. Patients taking three or more medications are less likely to use them as directed. Likewise, the more frequently a medication is directed to be taken, the less likely it will be taken as prescribed. One general practitioner reported that the number of drug defaulters doubled when the number of tablets was increased from one to four (Gatley, 1968). Considerable confusion may also develop when multiple drugs of similar appearance are prescribed for the same patient, as has been emphasized by Mazzullo (1972) and Mazzullo and Lasagna (1972). They have also stressed the desirability of providing the patient with an identifying name for each medication prescribed, for example, "heart pill" or "water pill," assuming he has been told what each medication is designed to accomplish. The color plates in the *Physicians' Desk Reference* can be used to show patients what their medication will look like.

Patients frequently discontinue medication upon the appearance of minor untoward effects because they have not been told that such reactions are common and indicate that the drug is working. Special instruction should be given the patient relative to symptoms that indicate overdosage, such as dizziness from antihypertensive agents.

The Treatment Environment. The setting in which the prescribed medication is to be taken has a marked influence on compliance. A series of studies in the same psychiatric hospital revealed that noncompliance increased progressively from 19% in inpatients to 37% in day patients and 48% in outpatients (Hare and Wilcox, 1967). This emphasizes the need to teach the principles of self-medication before the patient leaves the hospital and the added responsibility the physician must assume if he is to achieve satisfactory patient compliance with clinic and private office patients.

The Pharmacist and Patient Compliance. The pharmacist is usually the last professional to contact the ambulatory private patient (or his kin) before the medication regimen is started. Pharmacists can effectively cooperate with the physician in patient compliance education and can counsel the patient on how to take his prescription medication. The physician may be well advised carefully to select a pharmacist to assist him with this problem; such a coordinated effort should have a favorable influence on patient compliance behavior.

Becker, M. H.; Drachman, R. H.; and Kirscht, J. P. Predicting mother's compliance with pediatric medical regimens. *J. Pediat.*, **1972,** *81,* 843–854.

Blackwell, B. The drug defaulter. *Clin. Pharmac. Ther.,* **1972a,** *13,* 841–848.

———. Patient compliance. *New Engl. J. Med.,* **1972b,** *289,* 249–252.

Friend, D. G. Principles and practices of prescription writing. *Clin. Pharmac. Ther.,* **1965,** *6,* 411–416.

Gatley, M. S. To be taken as directed. *Jl R. Coll. gen. Pract.,* **1968,** *16,* 39–44.

Hare, E. H., and Wilcox, D. R. C. Do psychiatric inpatients take their pills? *Br. J. Psychiat.,* **1967,** *113,* 1435–1439.

Hirschorn, J. O., and Silverman, H. I. The ubiquitous medicine dropper. *Am. J. Pharm.,* **1968,** *140,* 1–6.

Hulka, B. S.; Kupper, L. L.; Cassell, J. C.; Efird, R. L.; and Burdette, J. A. Medication use and misuse: physician-patient discrepancies. *J. chron. Dis.,* **1975,** *28,* 7–21.

Jerome, J. B., and Sagan, P. The USAN nomenclature system. *J. Am. med. Ass.,* **1975,** *232,* 294–299.

Lowenthal, W. The controversy over generic equivalency of drugs. *Med. Coll. Va Q.,* **1967,** *3,* 113–118.

Marston, M. V. Compliance with medical regimens: a review of the literature. *Nurs. Res.,* **1970,** *19,* 312–323.

Mazzullo, J. The nonpharmacologic basis of therapeutics. *Clin. Pharmac. Ther.,* **1972,** *13,* 157–158.

Mazzullo, J. M., and Lasagna, L. Take thou . . . but is your patient really taking what you prescribed? *Drug Ther.,* **1972,** *2,* 11–15.

Miller, O. H. Predicting incompatibilities of new drugs. *J. Am. pharm. Ass., Pract. Pharm. Ed.,* **1952,** *13,* 657–659.

The National Formulary, 14th ed. (American Pharmaceutical Association.) Mack Printing Co., Easton, Pa., published **1974,** became official **1975.**

National Prescription Audit and National Hospital Audit, 11th ed. Lea, Inc., Ambler, Pa., **1972.**

The Pharmacopeia of the United States of America, 19th rev. (The United States Pharmacopeial Convention, Inc.) Mack Printing Co., Easton, Pa., published **1974,** became official **1975.**

Porter, A. M. W. Drug defaulting in general practice. *Br. med. J.,* **1969,** *1,* 218–222.

Stewart, R. B., and Cluff, L. E. A review of medication errors and compliance in ambulant patients. *Clin. Pharmac. Ther.,* **1972,** *13,* 463–468.

Task Force on Prescription Drugs. *Final Report.* U.S. Department of Health, Education, and Welfare, Washington, D. C., **1969.**

Teplitsky, B. Caution! 1,000 drugs whose names look-alike or sound-alike. *Pharm. Times,* **1972,** *38,* 29–31.

Wesley, F. Flavor and the modern pharmaceutical. *J. Am. pharm. Ass., Pract. Pharm. Ed.,* **1957,** *18,* 674–677.

INDEX

1619

Trolnitrate phosphate, preparations and dosage, 734
  structural formula, 734
TROLONE (sulthiane), 218
Tromethamine, 775
TRONOTHANE (pramoxine hydrochloride), 391
Tropicamide, ocular effects and uses, 528
  preparations, 527
  structural formula, 527
Trypanosomiasis, melarsonyl in, 1085
  melarsoprol in, 1085
  nifurtimox in, 1088
  nitroflurazone in, 1085
  pentamidine in, 1083
  suramin in, 1082
  tryparsamide in, 1085
Tryparsamide, 924, 1085
  use in trypanosomiasis, 1085
Trypsin, actions and toxicity, 957
  preparations and uses, 957
TRYPTAR (trypsin crystallized), 957
TUAMINE (tuaminoheptane sulfate), 505
Tuaminoheptane, dosage and preparations, 505
  receptor-type activity, 481
  structural formula, 481
  use in nasal congestion, 481, 505
TUBARINE (tubocurarine chloride), 585
Tuberculosis, adrenocorticosteroids in, 1216
  aminosalicylic acid in, 1204
  capreomycin in, 1213
  chemoprophylaxis, 1216
  chemotherapy, 1101, 1213–1216
    atypical mycobacteria, 1214
    bacterial resistance, 1214
    bones and joints, 1215
    choice of tuberculostatic agents, 1214
    general considerations, 1213
    genitourinary, 1215
    meningitis, 1215
    miliary, 1215
    pleurisy with effusion, 1216
    pulmonary, 1214
  cycloserine in, 1211
  determination of drug sensitivity, 1201
  ethambutol in, 1208
  ethionamide in, 1213
  isoniazid in, 1207
  kanamycin in, 1213
  pyrazinamide in, 1212
  rifampin in, 1210
  streptomycin in, 1201–1202
  viomycin in, 1211
Tubocurarine. See also Curare
  pharmacological actions, 579
  preparations and dosage, 585
  structural formula, 576
Tularemia, choice of drugs in, 1100
  gentamicin in, 1175
  streptomycin in, 1172
  tetracyclines in, 1192
Tybamate, preparations and dosage, 192
TYBATRAN (tybamate), 192
TYLENOL (acetaminophen), 346

Typhoid carriers, ampicillin in, 1156
  trimethoprim-sulfamethoxazole in, 1127
Typhoid fever, ampicillin in, 1156
  chloramphenicol in, 1197
  choice of drugs in, 1099
  trimethoprim-sulfamethoxazole in, 1127
Typhus, choice of drugs in, 1102
  epidemic, tetracycline in, 1191
  murine, chloramphenicol in, 1198
    tetracyclines in, 1191
  scrub, chloramphenicol in, 1198
    tetracyclines in, 1191
Tyramine, mechanism of adrenergic action, 434
  receptor-type activity, 481
  structural formula, 481
  uses, 481
Tyrocidine, 1235
Tyropanoate sodium, 803
Tyrosine, structural formula, 423
Tyrothricin, antibacterial activity, 1235
  history and source, 1235
  preparations, administration, and dosage, 1235
  toxicity, 1235
  uses, 1235
TYZINE (tetrahydrozoline hydrochloride), 505

Ulcer. See Peptic ulcer
Ulcerative colitis. See Colitis
ULTANDREN (fluoxymesterone), 1461
ULTRALENTE insulin (extended insulin zinc suspension), 1517
Undecylenic acid, 1010
UNIBASE, 947
UNIPEN (nafcillin sodium), 1144
United States Adopted Name, 43, 1602
United States Pharmacopeia, 42
Upper motoneuron disorders, diazepam in, 192
Upper respiratory infections. See Common cold
Uracil mustard, 1264. See also Alkylating agents
  chemistry, 1254
  use in neoplastic diseases, 1250
Urea, 822
  use as osmotic diuretic, 821
UREAPHIL, 822
URECHOLINE (bethanechol chloride), 470
Urethanes, 126
Urethritis, choice of drugs in, 1096
UREVERT (sterile urea powder), 822
Urinary retention, bethanechol in, 471
  neostigmine in, 460
Urinary tract antiseptics, 1006. See also individual agents
Urinary tract infections, ampicillin in, 1157
  carbenicillin indanyl in, 1157
  cephalosporins in, 1163
  chloramphenicol in, 1198
  choice of drugs in, 1096
  erythromycin in, 1227
  gentamicin in, 1175
  methanamine in, 1007
  nalidixic acid in, 1008